BNF
for Children

2017
2018

September 2017 – 18

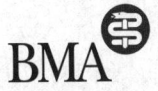
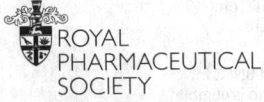

ROYAL
PHARMACEUTICAL
SOCIETY

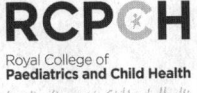

Royal College of
Paediatrics and Child Health
Leading the way in Children's Health

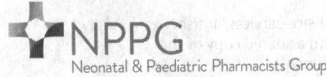

Neonatal & Paediatric Pharmacists Group

Published jointly by
BMJ Group
Tavistock Square, London, WC1H 9JP, UK

and

Pharmaceutical Press
Pharmaceutical Press is the publishing division of the Royal Pharmaceutical Society.
66-68 East Smithfield, London E1W 1AW, UK

ISBN: 978 0 85711 248 4

ISBN: 978 0 85711 321 4 (NHS edition)

ISBN: 978 0 85711 322 1 (ePDF)

Printed by GGP Media GmbH, Pößneck, Germany

Typeset by Data Standards Ltd, UK

Text design by Peter Burgess

A catalogue record for this book is available from the British Library.

Requesting copies of BNF publications
Paper copies may be obtained through any bookseller or direct from:

Pharmaceutical Press
c/o Macmillan Distribution (MDL)
Hampshire International Business Park
Lime Tree Way
Basingstoke
Hampshire
RG24 8YJ
Tel: +44 (0) 1256 302 699
Fax: +44 (0) 1256 812 521
direct@macmillan.co.uk
or via our website www.pharmpress.com

For all bulk orders of more than 20 copies:
Tel: +44 (0) 207 572 2266
pharmpress-support@rpharms.com

The BNFC is available as a mobile app, online (https://bnfc.nice.org.uk/) and also through MedicinesComplete; a PDA version is also available. In addition, BNFC content can be integrated into a local formulary by using BNFC on FormularyComplete; see www.bnf.org for details.

Distribution of printed BNFCs
In **England**, NICE purchases print editions of BNFC for distribution within the NHS. For details of who is eligible to receive a copy and further contact details, please refer to the NICE website:
www.nice.org.uk/about/what-we-do/evidence-services/british-national-formulary. If you are entitled to a shared copy of the BNFC, please call (0) 1268 495 609 or email:
bnf@wilmingtonhealthcare.com.

In **Scotland**, email:
nss.psd-bnf@nhs.net

In **Wales**, contact NHS Wales Shared Services Partnership—Contractor Services:
Tel: 01792 607420

In **Northern Ireland**, email:
ni.bnf@hscni.net

About BNFC content
The BNF *for Children* is for rapid reference by UK health professionals engaged in prescribing, dispensing, and administering medicines to children.

BNF *for Children* has been constructed using robust procedures for gathering, assessing and assimilating information on paediatric drug treatment, but may not always include all the information necessary for prescribing and dispensing. It is expected that the reader will be relying on appropriate professional knowledge and expertise to interpret the contents in the context of the circumstances of the individual child. BNF *for Children* should be used in conjunction with other appropriate and up-to-date literature and, where necessary, supplemented by expert advice. Information is also available from Medicines Information Services.

Special care is required in managing childhood conditions with unlicensed medicines or with licensed medicines for unlicensed uses. Responsibility for the appropriate use of medicines lies solely with the individual health professional.

Please refer to digital versions of *BNF for Children* for the most up-to-date content. *BNF for Children* is published in print but interim updates are issued and published in the digital versions of *BNF for Children*. The publishers work to ensure that the information is as accurate and up-to-date as possible at the date of publication, but knowledge and best practice in this field change regularly. *BNF for Children's* accuracy and currency cannot be guaranteed and neither the publishers nor the authors accept any responsibility for errors or omissions. While considerable efforts have been made to check the material in this publication, it should be treated as a guide only. Prescribers, pharmacists and other healthcare professionals are advised to check www.bnf.org for information about key updates and corrections.

Pharmaid
Numerous requests have been received from developing countries for BNFCs. The Pharmaid scheme of the Commonwealth Pharmacists Association will dispatch old BNFCs to certain Commonwealth countries. For more information on this scheme see commonwealthpharmacy.org/what-we-do/pharmaid/. If you would like to donate your copy email:
admin@commonwealthpharmacy.org

Access the BNF *your* way

The *British National Formulary* (BNF) and *BNF for Children* are updated monthly online via MedicinesComplete, ensuring healthcare professionals always have the latest prescribing advice.

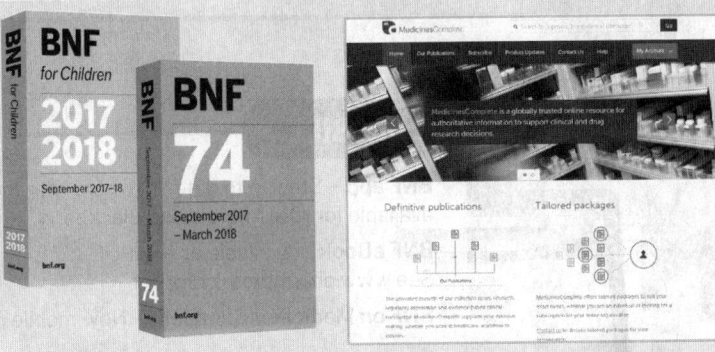

ONLINE

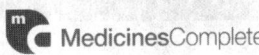

BNF on MedicinesComplete

Access BNF and *BNF for Children* on MedicinesComplete and receive the very latest drug information through monthly online updates.

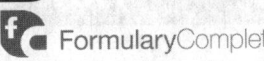

FormularyComplete Create, edit and manage your own local formulary content built upon the trusted prescribing advice of the BNF and *BNF for Children*.

BNF on Evidence Search

Search the BNF and *BNF for Children* alongside other authoritative clinical and non-clinical evidence and best practice at www.evidence.nhs.uk from NICE.

PRINT

Eligible health professionals will now receive one print copy a year – the September issue – to supplement online access. If you are entitled to an NHS copy please refer to page ii for full details on distribution, call 01268 495 609 or email **bnf@binleys.com**.

Turn the page for more details...

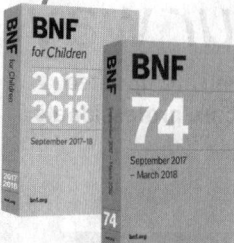
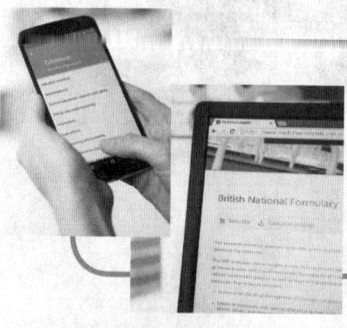

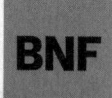
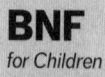

Preface

BNF for Children aims to provide prescribers, pharmacists, and other healthcare professionals with sound up-to-date information on the use of medicines for treating children.

A joint publication of the British Medical Association, the Royal Pharmaceutical Society, the Royal College of Paediatrics and Child Health, and the Neonatal and Paediatric Pharmacists Group, BNF for Children ('BNFC') is published under the authority of a Paediatric Formulary Committee which comprises representatives of these bodies, the Department of Health for England, and the Medicines and Healthcare products Regulatory Agency.

Many areas of paediatric practice have suffered from inadequate information on effective medicines. BNFC addresses this significant knowledge gap by providing practical information on the use of medicines in children of all ages from birth to adolescence. Information in BNFC has been validated against emerging evidence, best-practice guidelines, and crucially, advice from a network of clinical experts.

Drawing information from manufacturers' literature where appropriate, BNFC also includes a great deal of advice that goes beyond marketing authorisations (product licences). This is necessary because licensed indications frequently do not cover the clinical needs of children; in some cases, products for use in children need to be specially manufactured or imported. Careful consideration has been given to establishing the clinical need for unlicensed interventions with respect to the evidence and experience of their safety and efficacy; local paediatric formularies, clinical literature and national information resources have been invaluable in this process.

BNFC has been designed for rapid reference and the information presented has been carefully selected to aid decisions on prescribing, dispensing and administration of medicines. Less detail is given on areas such as malignant disease and the very specialist use of medicines generally undertaken in tertiary centres. BNFC should be interpreted in the light of professional knowledge and it should be supplemented as necessary by specialised publications. Information is also available from Medicines Information Services (see inside front cover).

It is **important** to use the most recent BNFC information for making clinical decisions. The print edition of *BNF for Children* is updated in September each year. Monthly updates are provided online via the BNF Publications website www.bnf.org, MedicinesComplete and the NHS Evidence portal. The more important changes listed under Changes p. xix are cumulative (from one print edition to the next), and can be printed off each month to show the main changes since the last print edition as an aide memoire for those using print copies.

The website (www.bnf.org) includes additional information of relevance to healthcare professionals. Other digital formats of BNFC—including versions for mobile devices and integration into local formularies—are also available.

BNF Publications welcomes comments from healthcare professionals. Comments and constructive criticism should be sent to:

British National Formulary,
Royal Pharmaceutical Society,
66–68 East Smithfield
London
E1W 1AW
editor@bnf.org

The contact email for manufacturers or pharmaceutical companies wishing to contact BNF Publications is manufacturerinfo@bnf.org

Contents

Acknowledgements

The Paediatric Formulary Committee is grateful to individuals and organisations that have provided advice and information to the *BNF for Children* (BNFC).

The principal contributors for this update were:

M.N. Badminton, S. Bailey, G.D.L. Bates, H. Bedford, M.W. Beresford, R.M. Bingham, L. Brook, K.G. Brownlee, I.F. Burgess, A. Cant, R. Carr, T.D. Cheetham, A.G. Cleary, A.J. Cotgrove, J.B.S. Coulter, B.G. Craig, J.H. Cross, A. Dhawan, P.N. Durrington, A.B. Edgar, J.A. Edge, D.A.C. Elliman, N.D. Embleton, A. Freyer, P.J. Goadsby, J. Gray, J.W. Gregory, P. Gringras, J.P. Harcourt, C. Hendriksz, R.F. Howard, R.G. Hull, H.R. Jenkins, S. Jones, B.A. Judd, E. Junaid, P.T. Khaw, J.M.W. Kirk, E.G.H. Lyall, P.S. Malone, S.D. Marks, D.F. Marsh, P. McHenry, P.J. McKiernan, L.M. Melvin, E. Miller, S. Moledina, R.E. Morton, P. Mulholland, C. Nelson-Piercy, J.M. Neuberger, K.K. Nischal, C.Y. Ng, L.P. Omerod, J.Y. Paton, G.A. Pearson, J. Puntis, J. Rogers, K.E. Rogstad, J.W. Sander, N.J. Scolding, M.R. Sharland, N.J. Shaw, O.F.W Stumper, A.G. Sutcliffe, E.A. Taylor, S. Thomas, M.A. Thomson, J.A. Vale, S. Vijay, J.O. Warner, N.J.A. Webb, A.D. Weeks, R. Welbury, W.P. Whitehouse, A. Wright, M.M. Yaqoob, Z. Zaiwalla, and S.M. Zuberi.

Members of the British Association of Dermatologists' Therapy & Guidelines Subcommittee, D.A. Buckley, N. Chiang, M. Cork, K. Gibbon, R.Y.P. Hunasehally, G.A. Johnston, T.A. Leslie, E.C. Mallon, P.M McHenry, J. Natkunarajah, C. Saunders, S. Ungureanu, S. Wakelin, F.S. Worsnop, A.G. Brain (Secretariat), and M.F. Mohd Mustapa (Secretariat) have provided valuable advice.

Members of the Advisory Committee on Malaria Prevention, R.H. Behrens, D. Bell, P.L. Chiodini, V. Field, F. Genasi, L. Goodyer, A. Green, J. Jones, G. Kassianos, D.G. Lalloo, D. Patel, H. Patel, M. Powell, D.V. Shingadia, N.O. Subair, C.J.M. Whitty, M. Blaze (Secretariat), and V. Smith (Secretariat) have provided valuable advice.

Members of the UK Ophthalmic Pharmacy Group have also provided valuable advice.

The MHRA have provided valuable assistance.

Correspondents in the pharmaceutical industry have provided information on new products and commented on products in BNFC.

Numerous doctors, pharmacists, nurses, and others have sent comments and suggestions.

BNFC interactions are provided by C.L. Preston, S.L. Jones, H.K. Sandhu, and S. Sutton.

The BNFC has valuable access to the *Martindale* data banks by courtesy of A. Brayfield and staff.

Valuable technical assistance provided by J. Macdonald, N. Judd, J. Stott, K. Parsons, R. Calle, J. Marsden-Hockham, H. Rowland, M. Kingsbury, O. Griffiths.

C. Cadart, S. Frau, D. Jones, A. Kalaparan, M. Leon-Alonso, M. Lynn, J. MacKershan, J. Martin, J. McCall, S. Powell, A. Raju, M. Sills, J. Smith, and A. Sparshatt provided considerable assistance during the production of this update of the BNFC.

BNF Staff

BNF DIRECTOR
Karen Baxter
BSc, MSc, MRPharmS

HEAD OF CONTENT
Kate Towers
BPharm (AU), GCClinPharm

CONTENT MANAGERS
Thomas F. Corbett
BScPharm (IRL), MPharm (IRL)

Kristina Fowlie
MPharm, CertPharmPract, MRPharmS

Claire McSherry
BPharm (NZ), PGCertClinPharm (NZ)

Heenaben Patel
MPharm, DipClinPharm, MRPharmS

QUALITY AND PROCESS MANAGER
Angela M.G. McFarlane
BSc, DipClinPharm

CLINICAL WRITERS
Abby Calder
BPharm (NZ), PGCertClinPharm (NZ)

Naimah Callachand
MPharm

Holly Hayne
BSc (Pharmacology) (NZ), BPharm (NZ)

Angela L. Kam
BPharm (NZ), PGDipPharmPrac (NZ), PGCertPharmPres (NZ)

Philip D. Lee
BSc, PhD

Kirsty Luck
BPharm (AU)

Nafeesa Mussa
BPharm (NZ), PGCertClinPharm (NZ)

Kere Odumah
MPharm

Paridhi K. Prashar
MPharm, MRPharmS

Jacob M. Warner
BPharm (AU)

Sharyn Young
BPharm (NZ), PGDipClinPharm (NZ)

CLINICAL ASSISTANTS
Elizabeth King

EDITORIAL ASSISTANTS
Hima Bhatt
BSc, MA

Jaya Venkitachalam
BSc, MRes

SENIOR BNF ADMINISTRATOR
Heidi Homar
BA

MANAGING DIRECTOR, PHARMACEUTICAL PRESS
Alina Lourie
B.Ed, MSc

SENIOR MEDICAL ADVISER
Derek G. Waller
BSc, MB, BS, DM, FRCP

Paediatric Formulary Committee 2017-2018

CHAIR
David Tuthill
MB, BCh, FRCPCH

DEPUTY CHAIR
Neil A. Caldwell
BSc, MSc, MRPharmS, FFRPS

COMMITTEE MEMBERS
Indraneel Banerjee
MB BS, MD, FRCPCH

Martin G. Duerden
BMedSci, MB BS, DRCOG, MRCGP, DipTher, DPH

Jessica Higson
BN, MSc, DipHE, RN (Adult), RN (Child), IP

James H. Larcombe
MB, ChB, PhD, FRCGP, DipAdvGP

John Marriott
BSc, PhD, MRPharmS, FHEA

E. David G. McIntosh
MB BS, MPH, LLM, PhD, FAFPHM, FRACP, FRCPCH, FFPM, DRCOG, DCH, DipPharmMed

Angeliki Siapkara
MSc, MD, CCST (Ortho)

Adam Sutherland
MPharm, MSc, FFRPS, MRPharmS

LAY MEMBER
Emily Lam

EXECUTIVE SECRETARY
Heidi Homar
BA

Dental Advisory Group 2017-2018

CHAIR
Sarah Manton
BDS, FDSRCS Ed, FHEA, PhD

COMMITTEE MEMBERS
Karen Baxter
BSc, MSc, MRPharmS

Andrew K. Brewer
BSc, BchD

Alexander Crighton

Kristina Fowlie
MPharm, CertPharmPract, MRPharmS

Michelle Moffat
BDS, MFDS RCS Ed, M Paed Dent RPCS, FDS (Paed Dent) RSC Ed

Kate Towers
BPharm (AU), GCClinPharm

SECRETARY
Arianne J. Matlin
MA, MSc, PhD

EXECUTIVE SECRETARY
Heidi Homar
BA

ADVICE ON DENTAL PRACTICE
The **British Dental Association** has contributed to the advice on medicines for dental practice through its representatives on the Dental Advisory Group.

Nurse Prescribers' Advisory Group 2017–2018

CHAIR
Molly Courtenay
PhD, MSc, Cert Ed, BSc, RGN

COMMITTEE MEMBERS
Karen Baxter
BSc, MSc, MRPharmS

Kristina Fowlie
MPharm, CertPharmPract, MRPharmS

Penny M. Franklin
RN, RCN, RSCPHN(HV), MA, PGCE

Matt Griffiths
BA (Hons), FAETC, RGN, Cert A&E, NISP, PHECC

Tracy Hall
BSc, MSc, RGN, DN, Dip N, Cert N

Penny Harrison
BSc (Hons)

Julie MacAngus
BSc (Hons), RGN, RM, PGCE

Joan Myers
MSc, BSc, RGN, RSCN, Dip DN

Fiona Peniston-Bird
BSc (Hons), NIP, RHV, RGN

Kathy Radley
BSc, RGN

Kate Towers
BPharm (AU), GCClinPharm

EXECUTIVE SECRETARY
Heidi Homar
BA

How BNF Publications are constructed

Overview

The BNF *for Children* (BNFC) is an independent professional publication that addresses the day-to-day prescribing information needs of healthcare professionals involved in the care of children. Use of this resource throughout the health service helps to ensure that medicines are used safely, effectively, and appropriately.

Hundreds of changes are made between print editions, and are published monthly in some digital formats. The most clinically significant updates are listed under Changes p. xix.

BNFC is unique in bringing together authoritative, independent guidance on best practice with clinically validated drug information.

Information in BNFC has been validated against emerging evidence, best-practice guidelines, and advice from a network of clinical experts. BNFC includes a great deal of advice that goes beyond marketing authorisations (product licences or summaries of product characteristics). This is necessary because licensed indications frequently do not cover the clinical needs of children; in some cases, products for use in children need to be specially manufactured or imported. Careful consideration has been given to establishing the clinical need for unlicensed interventions with respect to the evidence and experience of their safety and efficacy.

Validation of information follows a standardised process. Where the evidence base is weak, further validation is undertaken through a process of peer review. The process and its governance are outlined in greater detail in the sections that follow.

Paediatric Formulary Committee

The Paediatric Formulary Committee (PFC) is responsible for the content of BNFC. The PFC comprises pharmacy, medical and nursing representatives with a paediatric background, and lay representatives who have worked with children or acted as a carer of a paediatric patient; there are also representatives from the Medicines and Healthcare products Regulatory Agency (MHRA) and the Department of Health for England. The PFC decides on matters of policy and reviews amendments to BNFC in the light of new evidence and expert advice.

Dental Advisory Group

The Dental Advisory Group oversees the preparation of advice on the drug management of dental and oral conditions; the group includes representatives from the British Dental Association and a representative from the UK Health Departments.

Nurse Prescribers' Advisory Group

The Nurse Prescribers' Advisory Group oversees the list of drugs approved for inclusion in the Nurse Prescribers' Formulary; the group includes representatives from a range of nursing disciplines and stakeholder organisations.

Expert advisers

BNFC uses about 80 expert clinical advisers (including doctors, pharmacists, nurses, and dentists) throughout the UK to help with the clinical content. The role of these expert advisers is to review existing text and to comment on amendments drafted by the clinical writers. These clinical experts help to ensure that BNFC remains reliable by:

- commenting on the relevance of the text in the context of best clinical practice in the UK;
- checking draft amendments for appropriate interpretation of any new evidence;
- providing expert opinion in areas of controversy or when reliable evidence is lacking;
- advising on the use of unlicensed medicines or of licensed medicines for unlicensed uses ('off-label' use);
- providing independent advice on drug interactions, prescribing in hepatic impairment, renal impairment, pregnancy, breast-feeding, neonatal care, palliative care, and the emergency treatment of poisoning.

In addition to consulting with regular advisers, BNFC calls on other clinical specialists for specific developments when particular expertise is required.

BNFC also works closely with a number of expert bodies that produce clinical guidelines. Drafts or pre-publication copies of guidelines are often received for comment and for assimilation into BNFC.

Editorial team

BNFC clinical writers have all worked as pharmacists or possess a pharmacy degree and further, relevant post-graduate qualification, and have a sound understanding of how drugs are used in clinical practice. A number of the clinical writers have specific experience of paediatric practice. As a team, the clinical writers are responsible for editing, maintaining, and updating BNFC content. They follow a systematic prioritisation process in response to updates to the evidence base in order to ensure the most clinically important topics are reviewed as quickly as possible. In parallel the team of clinical writers undertakes a process of rolling revalidation, aiming to review all of the content in the BNF over a 3- to 4-year period.

Amendments to the text are drafted when the clinical writers are satisfied that any new information is reliable and relevant. A set of standard criteria define when content is referred to expert advisers, the Joint Formulary Committee or other advisory groups, or submitted for peer review.

Clinical writers prepare the text for publication and undertake a number of validation checks on the knowledge at various stages of the production.

Sources of BNFC information

BNFC uses a variety of sources for its information; the main ones are shown below.

Summaries of product characteristics

BNFC reviews the summaries of product characteristics (SPCs) of all new products as well as revised SPCs for existing products. The SPCs are a key source of product information and are carefully processed. Such processing involves:

- verifying the approved names of all relevant ingredients including 'non-active' ingredients (BNFC is committed to using approved names and descriptions as laid down by the Human Medicines Regulations 2012);
- comparing the indications, cautions, contra-indications, and side-effects with similar existing drugs. Where these are different from the expected pattern, justification is sought for their inclusion or exclusion;
- seeking independent data on the use of drugs in pregnancy and breast-feeding;
- incorporating the information into BNFC using established criteria for the presentation and inclusion of the data;
- checking interpretation of the information by a second clinical writer before submitting to a content manager; changes relating to doses receive a further check;
- identifying potential clinical problems or omissions and seeking further information from manufacturers or from expert advisers;
- constructing, with the help of expert advisers, a comment on the role of the drug in the context of similar drugs.

Much of this processing is applicable to the following sources as well.

Literature

Clinical writers monitor core medical, paediatric, and pharmaceutical journals. Research papers and reviews relating to drug therapy are carefully processed. When a difference between the advice in BNFC and the paper is noted, the new information is assessed for reliability (using tools based on SIGN methodology) and relevance to UK clinical practice.

If necessary, new text is drafted and discussed with expert advisers and the Paediatric Formulary Committee. BNFC enjoys a close working relationship with a number of national information providers.

In addition to the routine process, which is used to identify 'triggers' for changing the content, systematic literature searches are used to identify the best quality evidence available to inform an update. Clinical writers receive training in critical appraisal, literature evaluation, and search strategies.

Consensus guidelines

The advice in BNFC is checked against consensus guidelines produced by expert bodies. The quality of the guidelines is assessed using adapted versions of the AGREE II tool. A number of bodies make drafts or pre-publication copies of the guidelines available to BNFC; it is therefore possible to ensure that a consistent message is disseminated. BNFC routinely processes guidelines from the National Institute for Health and Care Excellence (NICE), the All Wales Medicines Strategy Group (AWMSG), the Scottish Medicines Consortium (SMC), and the Scottish Intercollegiate Guidelines Network (SIGN).

Reference sources

Paediatric formularies and reference sources are used to provide background information for the review of existing text or for the construction of new text. The BNFC team works closely with the editorial team that produces *Martindale: The Complete Drug Reference*. BNFC has access to *Martindale* information resources and each team keeps the other informed of significant developments and shifts in the trends of drug usage.

Peer review

Although every effort is made to identify the most robust data available, inevitably there are areas where the evidence base is weak or contradictory. While the BNF has the valuable support of expert advisers and the Paediatric Formulary Committee, the recommendations made may be subject to a further level of scrutiny through peer review to ensure they reflect best practice.

Content for peer review is posted on bnf.org and interested parties are notified via a number of channels, including the BNF e-newsletter.

Statutory information

BNFC routinely processes relevant information from various Government bodies including Statutory Instruments and regulations affecting the Prescription only Medicines Order. Official compendia such as the British Pharmacopoeia and its addenda are processed routinely to ensure that BNFC complies with the relevant sections of the Human Medicines Regulations 2012.

BNFC maintains close links with the Home Office (in relation to controlled drug regulations) and the Medicines and Healthcare products Regulatory Agency (including the British Pharmacopoeia Commission). Safety warnings issued by the Commission on Human Medicines (CHM) and guidelines on drug use issued by the UK health departments are processed as a matter of routine.

Relevant professional statements issued by the Royal Pharmaceutical Society are included in BNFC as are guidelines from bodies such as the Royal College of Paediatrics and Child Health.

Medicines and devices

NHS Prescription Services (from the NHS Business Services Authority) provides non-clinical, categorical information (including prices) on the medicines and devices included in BNFC.

Comments from readers

Readers of BNFC are invited to send in comments. Numerous letters and emails are received by the BNF team. Such feedback helps to ensure that BNFC provides practical and clinically relevant information. Many changes in the presentation and scope of BNFC have resulted from comments sent in by users.

Comments from industry

Close scrutiny of BNFC by the manufacturers provides an additional check and allows them an opportunity to raise issues about BNFC's presentation of the role of various drugs; this is yet another check on the balance of BNFC advice. All comments are looked at with care and, where necessary, additional information and expert advice are sought.

Market research

Market research is conducted at regular intervals to gather feedback on specific areas of development.

Assessing the evidence

From January 2016, recommendations made in BNFC have been evidence graded to reflect the strength of the recommendation. The addition of evidence grading is to support clinical decision making based on the best available evidence.

The BNFC aims to revalidate all content over a rolling 3- to 4-year period and evidence grading will be applied to recommendations as content goes through the revalidation process. Therefore, initially, only a small number of recommendations will have been graded.

Grading system

The BNFC has adopted a five level grading system from A to E, based on the former SIGN grading system. This grade is displayed next to the recommendation within the text.

Evidence used to make a recommendation is assessed for validity using standardised methodology tools based on AGREE II and assigned a level of evidence. The recommendation is then given a grade that is extrapolated from the level of evidence, and an assessment of the body of evidence and its applicability.

Evidence assigned a level 1- or 2- score has an unacceptable level of bias or confounding and is not used to form recommendations.

Levels of evidence

- **Level 1++**
  High quality meta-analyses, systematic reviews of randomised controlled trials (RCTs), or RCTs with a very low risk of bias.
- **Level 1+**
  Well-conducted meta-analyses, systematic reviews, or RCTs with a low risk of bias.
- **Level 1-**
  Meta-analyses, systematic reviews, or RCTs with a high risk of bias.
- **Level 2++**
  High quality systematic reviews of case control or cohort studies; or high quality case control or cohort studies with a very low risk of confounding or bias and a high probability that the relationship is causal.
- **Level 2+**
  Well-conducted case control or cohort studies with a low risk of confounding or bias and a moderate probability that the relationship is causal.
- **Level 2-**
  Case control or cohort studies with a high risk of confounding or bias and a significant risk that the relationship is not causal.
- **Level 3**
  Non-analytic studies, e.g. case reports, case series.

- **Level 4**
  Expert advice or clinical experience from respected authorities.

Grades of recommendation

- **Grade A: High strength**
  NICE-accredited guidelines; or guidelines that pass AGREE II assessment; or at least one meta-analysis, systematic review, or RCT rated as 1++, and directly applicable to the target population; or a body of evidence consisting principally of studies rated as 1+, directly applicable to the target population, and demonstrating overall consistency of results.

- **Grade B: Moderate strength**
  A body of evidence including studies rated as 2++, directly applicable to the target population, and demonstrating overall consistency of results; or extrapolated evidence from studies rated as 1++ or 1+.

- **Grade C: Low strength**
  A body of evidence including studies rated as 2+, directly applicable to the target population and demonstrating overall consistency of results; or extrapolated evidence from studies rated as 2++.

- **Grade D: Very low strength**
  Evidence level 3; or extrapolated evidence from studies rated as 2+; or tertiary reference source created by a transparent, defined methodology, where the basis for recommendation is clear.

- **Grade E: Practice point**
  Evidence level 4.

How to use BNF Publications in print

How to use the BNF *for Children* in print

This edition of the BNF *for Children* (BNFC) continues to display the fundamental change to the structure of the content that was first shown in BNFC 2015-2016. The changes were made to bring consistency and clarity to BNFC content, and to the way that the content is arranged within print and digital products, increasing the ease with which information can be found.

For reference, the most notable changes to the structure of the content include:

— Drug monographs – where possible, all information that relates to a single drug is contained within its drug monograph, moving information previously contained in the prescribing notes. Drug monographs have also changed structurally: additional sections have been added, ensuring greater regularity around where information is located within the publication.
— Drug class monographs – where substantial amounts of information are common to all drugs within a drug class (e.g. macrolides p. 314), a drug class monograph has been created to contain the common information.
— Medicinal forms – categorical information about marketed medicines, such as price and pack size, continues to be sourced directly from the Dictionary of Medicines and Devices provided by the NHS Business Services Authority. However, clinical information curated by the BNF team has been clearly separated from the categorical pricing and pack size information and is included in the relevant section of the drug monograph.
— Section numbering – the BNF and BNFC section numbering has been removed. This section numbering tied the content to a rigid structure and enforced the retention of defunct classifications, such as mercurial diuretics, and hindered the relocation of drugs where therapeutic use had altered. It also caused constraints between the BNF and BNFC, where drugs had different therapeutic uses in children.
— Appendix 4 – the content has been moved to individual drug monographs. The introductory notes have been replaced with a new guidance section, Guidance on intravenous infusions p. 15.

Introduction

In order to achieve the safe, effective, and appropriate use of medicines, healthcare professionals must be able to use the BNFC effectively, and keep up to date with significant changes in the BNFC that are relevant to their clinical practice. This *How to Use the BNF for Children* is key in reinforcing the details of the new structure of the BNFC to all healthcare professionals involved with prescribing, monitoring, supplying, and administering medicines, as well as supporting the learning of students training to join these professions.

As with previous editions, the BNFC provides information on the use of medicines in children ranging from neonates (including preterm neonates) to adolescents. The terms infant, child, and adolescent are not used consistently in the literature; to avoid ambiguity actual ages are used in the dose statements in BNFC. The term neonate is used to describe a newborn infant aged 0–28 days. The terms child or children are used generically to describe the entire range from infant to adolescent in BNFC.

Structure of the BNFC

This BNFC edition continues to broadly follow the high level structure of earlier editions of the BNFC (i.e. those published before BNFC 2015-2016):

Front matter, comprising information on how to use the BNFC, the significant content changes in each edition, and guidance on various prescribing matters (e.g. prescription writing, the use of intravenous drugs, particular considerations for special patient populations).

Chapters, containing drug monographs describing the uses, doses, safety issues and other considerations involved in the use of drugs; drug class monographs; and treatment summaries, covering guidance on the selection of drugs. Monographs and treatment summaries are divided into chapters based on specific aspects of medical care, such as Chapter 5, Infections, or Chapter 16, Emergency treatment of poisoning; or drug use related to a particular system of the body, such as Chapter 2, Cardiovascular.

Within each chapter, content is organised alphabetically by therapeutic use (e.g. Airways disease, obstructive), with the treatment summaries first, (e.g. Asthma p. 142), followed by the monographs of the drugs used to manage the conditions discussed in the treatment summary. Within each therapeutic use, the drugs are organised alphabetically by classification (e.g. Antimuscarinics, Beta$_2$-agonist bronchodilators) and then alphabetically within each classification (e.g. Formoterol fumarate, Salbutamol, Salmeterol, Terbutaline sulfate).

Appendices, covering interactions, borderline substances, and cautionary and advisory labels.

Back matter, covering the lists of medicines approved by the NHS for Dental and Nurse Practitioner prescribing, proprietary and specials manufacturers' contact details, and the index. Yellow cards are also included, to facilitate the reporting of adverse events, as well as quick reference guides for life support and key drug doses in medical emergencies, for ease of access.

Navigating the *BNF for Children*

The contents page provides the high-level layout of information within the BNFC; and in addition, each chapter begins with a small contents section, describing the therapeutic uses covered within that chapter. Once in a chapter, location is guided by the side of the page showing the chapter number (the *thumbnail*), alongside the chapter title. The top of the page includes the therapeutic use (the *running head*) alongside the page number.

Once on a page, visual cues aid navigation: treatment summary information is in black type, with therapeutic use titles similarly styled in black, whereas the use of colour indicates drug-related information, including drug classification titles, drug class monographs, and drug monographs.

Although navigation is possible by browsing, primarily access to the information is via the index, which covers the titles of drug class monographs, drug monographs and treatment summaries. The index also includes the names of branded medicines and other topics of relevance, such as abbreviations, guidance sections, tables, and images.

Content types

Treatment summaries

Treatment summaries are of three main types;

- an overview of delivering a drug to a particular body system (e.g. Skin conditions, management p. 682),
- a comparison between a group or groups of drugs (e.g. beta-adrenoceptor blockers (systemic) p. 100),
- an overview of the drug management or prophylaxis of common conditions intended to facilitate rapid appraisal of options (e.g. Hypertension p. 95, or Malaria, prophylaxis p. 370).

In order to select safe and effective medicines for individual children, information in the treatment summaries must be used in conjunction with other prescribing details about the drugs and knowledge of the child's medical and drug history.

Monographs

Overview

In earlier editions (i.e. before BNFC 2015-2016), a systemically administered drug with indications for use in different body systems was split across the chapters relating to those body systems. So, for example, codeine phosphate was found in chapter 1, for its antimotility effects and chapter 4 for its analgesic effects. However, the monograph in chapter 1 contained only the dose and some selected safety precautions.

Now, all of the information for the systemic use of a drug is contained within one monograph, so codeine phosphate p. 265 is now included in chapter 4. This carries the advantage of providing all of the information in one place, so the user does not need to flick back and forth across several pages to find all of the relevant information for that drug. Cross references are included in chapter 1, where the management of diarrhoea is discussed, to the drug monograph to assist navigation.

Where drugs have systemic and local uses, for example, chloramphenicol, and the considerations around drug use are markedly different according to the route of administration, the monograph is split, as with earlier editions, into the relevant chapters.

This means that the majority of drugs are still placed in the same chapters and sections as earlier editions, and although there may be some variation in order, all of the relevant information will be easier to locate.

One of the most significant changes to the monograph structure is the increased granularity, with a move from around 9 sections to over 20 sections; sections are only included when relevant information has been identified. The following information describes these sections and their uses in more detail.

Nomenclature

Monograph titles follow the convention of recommended international non-proprietary names (rINNs), or, in the absence of a rINN, British Approved Names. Relevant synonyms are included below the title and, in some instances a brief description of the drug action is included. Over future editions these drug action statements will be rolled out for all drugs.

In some monographs, immediately below the nomenclature or drug action, there are a number of cross references used to signpost the user to any additional information they need to consider about a drug. This is most common for drugs formulated in combinations, where users will be signposted to the monographs for the individual ingredients (e.g. senna with ispaghula husk p. 46) or for drugs that are related to a drug class monograph (see Drug class monographs, p. xviii).

Indication and dose

User feedback has highlighted that one of the main uses of the BNFC is identifying indications and doses of drugs. Therefore, indication and dose information has been promoted to the top of the monograph and highlighted by a coloured panel to aid quick reference.

The indication and dose section is more highly structured than in earlier editions, giving greater clarity around which doses should be used for which indications and by which route. In addition, if the dose varies with a specific preparation or formulation that dosing information has been moved out of the preparations section and in to the indication and dose panel, under a heading of the preparation name.

Doses are either expressed in terms of a definite frequency (e.g. 1 g 4 times daily) or in the total daily dose format (e.g.

6 g daily in 3 divided doses); the total daily dose should be divided into individual doses (in the second example, the child should receive 2 g 3 times daily).

Doses for specific patient groups (e.g. neonates) may be included if they are different to the standard dose. Doses for children can be identified by the relevant age range and may vary according to their age or body-weight.

Selecting the dose

The dose of a drug may vary according to different indications, routes of administration, age, body-weight, and body surface area. The right dose should be selected for the right age and body-weight (or body surface area) of the child, as well as for the right indication, route of administration, and preparation.

In earlier editions of the BNFC, age ranges and weight ranges overlapped. For clarity and to aid selection of the correct dose, wherever possible these age and weight ranges now do not overlap. When interpreting age ranges it is important to understand that a child is considered to be 11 up until the point of their 12th birthday, meaning that an age range of child 12 to 17 years is applicable to a child from the day of their 12th birthday until the day before their 18th birthday. All age ranges should be interpreted in this way. Similarly, when interpreting weight ranges, it should be understood that a weight of up to 30 kg is applicable to a child up to, but not including, the point that they tip the scales at 30 kg and a weight range of 35 to 59 kg is applicable to a child as soon as they tip the scales at 35 kg right up until, but not including, the point that they tip the scales at 60 kg. All weight ranges should be interpreted in this way.

A pragmatic approach should be applied to these cut-off points depending on the child's physiological development, condition, and if weight is appropriate for the child's age.

For some drugs (e.g. vancomycin p. 312) the neonatal dose varies according to the *corrected gestational* age of the neonate. Corrected gestational age is the neonate's total age expressed in weeks from the start of the mother's last menstrual period. For example, a 3 week old baby born at 27 weeks gestation is treated as having a corrected gestational age of 30 weeks. A term baby has a corrected gestational age of 37–42 weeks when born. For most other drugs, the dose can be based on the child's actual date of birth irrespective of corrected gestational age. However, the degree of prematurity, the maturity of renal and hepatic function, and the clinical properties of the drug need to be considered on an individual basis.

Many children's doses in BNFC are standardised by *body-weight*. To calculate the dose for a given child the weight-standardised dose is multiplied by the child's weight (or occasionally by the child's ideal weight for height). The calculated dose should not normally exceed the maximum recommended dose for an adult. For example, if the dose is 8 mg/kg (max. 300 mg), a child of 10 kg body-weight should receive 80 mg, but a child of 40 kg body-weight should receive 300 mg (rather than 320 mg). Calculation by body-weight in the overweight child may result in much higher doses being administered than necessary; in such cases, the dose should be calculated from an ideal weight for height.

Occasionally, some doses in BNFC are standardised by *body surface area* because many physiological phenomena correlate better with body surface area. In these cases, to calculate the dose for a given child, the body surface area-standardised dose is multiplied by the child's body surface area. The child's body surface area can be estimated from his or her weight using the tables for Body surface area in children, see inside back cover.

Wherever possible, doses are expressed in terms of a definite frequency (e.g. if the dose is 1 mg/kg twice daily, a child of body-weight 9 kg would receive 9 mg twice daily).

Occasionally, it is necessary to include doses in the total daily dose format (e.g. 10 mg/kg daily in 3 divided doses); in these cases the total daily dose should be divided into individual doses (in this example a child of body-weight 9 kg would receive 30 mg 3 times daily).

Most drugs can be administered at slightly irregular intervals during the day. Some drugs, e.g. antimicrobials, are best given at regular intervals. Some flexibility should be allowed in children to avoid waking them during the night. For example, the night-time dose may be given at the child's bedtime.

Special care should be taken when converting doses from one metric unit to another, and when calculating infusion rates or the volume of a preparation to administer. Where possible, doses should be rounded to facilitate administration of suitable volumes of liquid preparations, or an appropriate strength or tablet or capsule.

Other information relevant to Indication and dose

The dose panel also contains, where known, an indication of **pharmacokinetic considerations** that may affect the choice of dose, and **dose equivalence** information, which may aid the selection of dose when switching between drugs or preparations.

The BNFC includes **unlicensed use** of medicines when the clinical need cannot be met by licensed medicines; such use should be supported by appropriate evidence and experience. When the BNFC recommends an unlicensed medicine or the 'off-label' use of a licensed medicine, this is shown below the indication and dose panel in the unlicensed use section.

Minimising harm and drug safety

The drug chosen to treat a particular condition should minimise the patient's susceptibility to adverse effects and, where co-morbidities exist, have minimal detrimental effects on the patient's other diseases. To achieve this, the *Contra-indications*, *Cautions* and *Side-effects* of the relevant drug should be reviewed.

The information under Cautions can be used to assess the risks of using a drug in a patient who has co-morbidities that are also included in the Cautions for that drug—if a safer alternative cannot be found, the drug may be prescribed while monitoring the patient for adverse-effects or deterioration in the co-morbidity. Contra-indications are far more restrictive than Cautions and mean that the drug should be avoided in a patient with a condition that is contra-indicated.

The impact that potential side-effects may have on a patient's quality of life should also be assessed. For instance, in a child who has constipation, it may be preferable to avoid a drug that frequently causes constipation.

Clinically relevant *Side-effects* for drugs are included in the monographs or drug class monographs. Side-effects are listed in order of frequency, where known, and arranged alphabetically. The frequency of side-effects follows the regulatory standard:

- Very common — occurs more frequently than 1 in 10 administrations of a drug
- Common — occurs between 1 in 10 and 1 in 100 administrations of a drug
- Uncommon — between 1 in 100 and 1 in 1,000 administrations of a drug
- Rare — between 1 in 1,000 and 1 in 10,000 administrations of a drug
- Very rare — occurs less than 1 in 10,000 administrations of a drug
- Frequency not known

An exhaustive list of side-effects is not included, particularly for drugs that are used by specialists (e.g. cytotoxic drugs and drugs used in anaesthesia). The BNFC also omits effects

that are likely to have little clinical consequence (e.g. transient increase in liver enzymes).

Recognising that hypersensitivity reactions can occur with virtually all medicines, this effect is generally not listed, unless the drug carries an increased risk of such reactions, when the information is included under *Allergy and cross sensitivity*.

The *Important safety advice* section in the BNFC, delineated by a coloured outline box, highlights important safety concerns, often those raised by regulatory authorities or guideline producers. Safety warnings issued by the Commission on Human Medicines (CHM) or Medicines and Healthcare products Regulatory Agency (MHRA) are found here.

Drug selection should aim to minimise drug interactions. If it is necessary to prescribe a potentially serious combination of drugs, patients should be monitored appropriately. The mechanisms underlying drug interactions are explained in Appendix 1, followed by details of drug interactions.

Use of drugs in specific patient populations

Drug selection should aim to minimise the potential for drug accumulation, adverse drug reactions, and exacerbation of pre-existing hepatic or renal disease. If it is necessary to prescribe drugs whose effect is altered by hepatic or renal disease, appropriate drug dose adjustments should be made, and patients should be monitored adequately. The general principles for prescribing are outlined under *Prescribing in hepatic impairment p. 16*, and *Prescribing in renal impairment p. 16*. Information about drugs that should be avoided or used with caution in hepatic disease or renal impairment can be found in drug monographs under *Hepatic impairment* and *Renal impairment* (e.g. fluconazole p. 358).

Similarly, drug selection should aim to minimise harm to the fetus, nursing infant, and mother. The infant should be monitored for potential side-effects of drugs used by the *mother during pregnancy or breast-feeding*. The general principles for prescribing are outlined under Prescribing in pregnancy p. 18 and Prescribing in breast-feeding p. 18. The Treatment Summaries provide guidance on the drug treatment of common conditions that can occur during pregnancy and breast-feeding (e.g. Asthma p. 142). Information about the use of specific drugs during pregnancy and breast-feeding can be found in their drug monographs under *Pregnancy*, and *Breast-feeding* (e.g. fluconazole p. 358).

A new section, *Conception and contraception*, containing information around considerations for females of childbearing potential or men who might father a child (e.g. isotretinoin p. 727) has been included.

Administration and monitoring

When selecting the most appropriate drug, it may be necessary to screen the patient for certain genetic markers or metabolic states. This information is included within a section called *Pre-treatment screening* (e.g. abacavir p. 397). This section covers one-off tests required to assess the suitability of a patient for a particular drug.

Once the drug has been selected, it needs to be given in the most appropriate manner. A *Directions for administration* section contains the information about intravenous administration previously located in Appendix 4. This provides practical information on the preparation of intravenous drug infusions, including compatibility of drugs with standard intravenous infusion fluids, method of dilution or reconstitution, and administration rates. In addition, general advice relevant to other routes of administration is provided within this section (e.g. fentanyl p. 268) and further details, such as masking the bitter taste of some medicines.

Whenever possible, intramuscular injections should be **avoided** in children because they are painful.

After selecting and administering the most appropriate drug by the most appropriate route, patients should be monitored to ensure they are achieving the expected benefits from drug treatment without any unwanted side-effects. The *Monitoring* section specifies any special monitoring requirements, including information on monitoring the plasma concentration of drugs with a narrow therapeutic index (e.g. theophylline p. 162). Monitoring may, in certain cases, be affected by the impact of a drug on laboratory tests (e.g. hydroxocobalamin p. 547), and this information is included in *Effects on laboratory tests*.

In some cases, when a drug is withdrawn, further monitoring or precautions may be advised (e.g. clonidine hydrochloride p. 99); these are covered under *Treatment cessation*.

Choice and supply

The prescriber, the child's carer, and the child (if appropriate) should agree on the health outcomes desired and on the strategy for achieving them (see *Taking Medicines to Best Effect*). Taking the time to explain to the child (and the child's carer if appropriate) the rationale and the potential adverse effects of treatment may improve adherence. For some medicines there is a special need for counselling (e.g. appropriate posture during administration of doxycycline p. 338, or recognising signs of blood, liver, or skin disorders with carbamazepine p. 189); this is shown in *Patient and carer advice*.

Other information contained in the latter half of the monograph also helps prescribers and those dispensing medicines choose medicinal forms (by indicating information such as flavour or when branded products are not interchangeable e.g. modified-release theophylline p. 162), assess the suitability of a drug for prescribing, understand the NHS funding status for a drug (e.g. sildenafil p. 117), or assess when a patient may be able to purchase a drug without prescription (e.g. loperamide hydrochloride p. 47).

Medicinal forms

In the BNFC, preparations follow immediately after the monograph for the drug that is their main ingredient.

In earlier editions, when a particular preparation had safety information, dose advice or other clinical information specific to the product, it was contained within the preparations section. This information has been moved to the relevant section in the main body of the monograph under a heading of the name of the specific medicinal form (e.g. peppermint oil p. 34).

The medicinal forms (formerly preparations) section provides information on the type of formulation (e.g. tablet), the amount of active drug in a solid dosage form, and the concentration of active drug in a liquid dosage form. The legal status is shown for prescription-only medicines and controlled drugs, as well as pharmacy medicines and medicines on the general sales list. Practitioners are reminded, by a statement under the heading of "Medicinal Form" that not all products containing a specific drug ingredient may be similarly licensed. To be clear on the precise licensing status of specific medicinal forms, practitioners should check the product literature for the particular product being prescribed or dispensed.

Details of all medicinal forms available on the dm+d for each drug in BNF Publications appears online on MedicinesComplete. In print editions, due to space constraints, only certain branded products are included in detail. Where medicinal forms are listed they should not be inferred as equivalent to the other brands listed under the same form heading. For example, all the products listed under a heading of "Modified release capsule" will be available as modified release capsules, however, the brands listed under that form heading may have different release profiles, the available strengths may vary and/or the

products may have different licensing information. As with earlier editions of the BNFC, practitioners must ensure that the particular product being prescribed or dispensed is appropriate.

As medicinal forms are derived from dm+d data, some drugs may appear under names derived from that data; this may vary slightly from those in earlier BNFC versions, e.g. sodium acid phosphate, is now sodium dihydrogen phosphate anhydrous.

Children should be prescribed a preparation that complements their daily routine, and that provides the right dose of drug for the right indication and route of administration. When dispensing liquid preparations, a sugar-free preparation should always be used in preference to one containing sugar. Patients receiving medicines containing cariogenic sugars should be advised of appropriate dental hygiene measures to prevent caries.

Earlier editions of the BNFC only included excipients and electrolyte information for proprietary medicines. This information is now covered at the level of the dose form (e.g. tablet). It is not possible to keep abreast of all of the generic products available on the UK market, and so this information serves as a reminder to the healthcare professional that, if the presence of a particular excipient is of concern, they should check the product literature for the particular product being prescribed or dispensed.

Cautionary and advisory labels that pharmacists are recommended to add when dispensing are included in the medicinal forms section. Details of these labels can be found in Appendix 3, Guidance for cautionary and advisory labels p. 1016. These labels have now been applied at the level of the dose form.

In the case of compound preparations, the prescribing information for all constituents should be taken into account.

Prices in the BNFC

Basic NHS **net prices** are given in the BNFC to provide an indication of relative cost. Where there is a choice of suitable preparations for a particular disease or condition the relative cost may be used in making a selection. Cost-effective prescribing must, however, take into account other factors (such as dose frequency and duration of treatment) that affect the total cost. The use of more expensive drugs is justified if it will result in better treatment of the patient, or a reduction of the length of an illness, or the time spent in hospital.

Prices are regularly updated using the Drug Tariff and proprietary price information published by the NHS dictionary of medicines and devices (dm+d, www.dmd.nhs.uk). The weekly updated dm+d data (including prices) can be accessed using the dm+d browser of the NHS Business Services Authority (apps.nhsbsa.nhs.uk/DMDBrowser/DMDBrowser.do). Prices have been calculated from the net cost used in pricing NHS prescriptions and generally reflect whole dispensing packs. Prices for extemporaneously prepared preparations are not provided in the BNFC as prices vary between different manufacturers.

BNFC prices are not suitable for quoting to patients seeking private prescriptions or contemplating over-the-counter purchases because they do not take into account VAT, professional fees, and other overheads.

A fuller explanation of costs to the NHS may be obtained from the Drug Tariff. Separate drug tariffs are applicable to England and Wales (www.ppa.org.uk/ppa/edt_intro.htm), Scotland (www.isdscotland.org/Health-Topics/Prescribing-and-Medicines/Scottish-Drug-Tariff/), and Northern Ireland (www.hscbusiness.hscni.net/services/2034.htm); prices in the different tariffs may vary.

Typical layout of a monograph and associated medicinal forms

❶ Class Monographs and drug monographs

In most cases, all information that relates to an individual drug is contained in its drug monograph and there is no symbol. Class monographs have been created where substantial amounts of information are common to all drugs within a drug class, these are indicated by a flag symbol in a circle: ▣

Drug monographs with a corresponding class monograph are indicated by a tab with a flag symbol: ⚑1234

The page number of the corresponding class monograph is indicated within the tab. For further information, see How to use BNF Publications

❷ Drug classifications

Used to inform users of the class of a drug and to assist in finding other drugs of the same class. May be based on pharmacological class (e.g. opioids) but can also be associated with the use of the drug (e.g. cough suppressants)

❸ Review date

The date of last review of the content

❹ Specific preparation name

If the dose varies with a specific preparation or formulation it appears under a heading of the preparation name

❺ Evidence grading

Evidence grading to reflect the strengths of recommendations will be applied as content goes through the revalidation process. A five level evidence grading system based on the former SIGN grading system has been adopted. The grades Ⓐ Ⓑ Ⓒ Ⓓ Ⓔ are displayed next to the recommendations within the text, and are preceded by the symbol: EvGr

For further information, see How BNF Publications are constructed

---

Class monograph ❶

CLASSIFICATION ❷

 ⚑1234

Drug monograph ❶   ❸ 01-Jun-2017

(Synonym) another name by which a drug may be known

● **DRUG ACTION** how a drug exerts its effect in the body

● **INDICATIONS AND DOSE**

Indications are the clinical reasons a drug is used. The dose of a drug will often depend on the indications

Indication

▸ ROUTE

▸ Age groups: [Neonate/Child]
   Dose and frequency of administration (max. dose)

SPECIFIC PREPARATION NAME ❹

Indication

▸ ROUTE

▸ Age groups: [Neonate/Child]
   Dose and frequency of administration (max. dose)

DOSE EQUIVALENCE AND CONVERSION information around the bioequivalence between formulations of the same drug, or equivalent doses of drugs that are members of the same class

PHARMACOKINETICS how the body affects a drug (absorption, distribution, metabolism, and excretion)

POTENCY a measure of drug activity expressed in terms of the concentration required to produce an effect of given intensity

DOSES AT EXTREMES OF BODY-WEIGHT dosing information for patients who are overweight or underweight

● **UNLICENSED USE** describes the use of medicines outside the terms of their UK licence (off-label use), or use of medicines that have no licence for use in the UK

> **IMPORTANT SAFETY INFORMATION**
> Information produced and disseminated by drug regulators often highlights serious risks associated with the use of a drug, and may include advice that is mandatory

● **CONTRA-INDICATIONS** circumstances when a drug should be avoided

● **CAUTIONS** details of precautions required

● **INTERACTIONS** when one drug changes the effects of another drug; the mechanisms underlying drug interactions are explained in Appendix 1

● **SIDE-EFFECTS** listed in order of frequency, where known, and arranged alphabetically

● **ALLERGY AND CROSS-SENSITIVITY** for drugs that carry an increased risk of hypersensitivity reactions

● **CONCEPTION AND CONTRACEPTION** potential for a drug to have harmful effects on an unborn child when prescribing for a woman of childbearing age or for a man trying to father a child; information on the effect of drugs on the efficacy of latex condoms or diaphragms

● **PREGNANCY** advice on the use of a drug during pregnancy

● **BREAST FEEDING** EvGr advice on the use of a drug during breast feeding Ⓐ ❺

- **HEPATIC IMPAIRMENT** advice on the use of a drug in hepatic impairment
- **RENAL IMPAIRMENT** advice on the use of a drug in renal impairment
- **PRE-TREATMENT SCREENING** covers one off tests required to assess the suitability of a patient for a particular drug
- **MONITORING REQUIREMENTS** specifies any special monitoring requirements, including information on monitoring the plasma concentration of drugs with a narrow therapeutic index
- **EFFECTS ON LABORATORY TESTS** for drugs that can interfere with the accuracy of seemingly unrelated laboratory tests
- **TREATMENT CESSATION** specifies whether further monitoring or precautions are advised when the drug is withdrawn
- **DIRECTIONS FOR ADMINISTRATION** practical information on the preparation of intravenous drug infusions; general advice relevant to other routes of administration
- **PRESCRIBING AND DISPENSING INFORMATION** practical information around how a drug can be prescribed and dispensed including details of when brand prescribing is necessary
- **HANDLING AND STORAGE** includes information on drugs that can cause adverse effects to those who handle them before they are taken by, or administered to, a patient; advice on storage conditions
- **PARENT AND CARER ADVICE** for drugs with a special need for counselling
- **PROFESSION SPECIFIC INFORMATION** provides details of the restrictions certain professions such as dental practitioners or nurse prescribers need to be aware of when prescribing on the NHS
- **NATIONAL FUNDING/ACCESS DECISIONS** details of NICE Technology Appraisals and SMC advice
- **LESS SUITABLE FOR PRESCRIBING** preparations that are considered by the Paediatric Formulary Committee to be less suitable for prescribing
- **EXCEPTION TO LEGAL CATEGORY** advice and information on drugs which may be sold without a prescription under specific conditions

- **MEDICINAL FORMS**
  Form
  CAUTIONARY AND ADVISORY LABELS if applicable
  EXCIPIENTS clinically important but not comprehensive [consult manufacturer information for full details]
  ELECTROLYTES if clinically significant quantities occur
  ▸ **Preparation name** (Manufacturer/Non-proprietary)
    Drug name and strength pack sizes PoM ⑤ Prices

  Combinations available this indicates a combination preparation is available and a cross reference page number is provided to locate this preparation

⑤ Legal categories

PoM This symbol has been placed against those preparations that are available only on a prescription issued by an appropriate practitioner. For more detailed information see *Medicines, Ethics and Practice*, London, Pharmaceutical Press (always consult latest edition)

CD1 CD2 CD3 CD4-1 CD4-2 CD5 These symbols indicate that the preparations are subject to the prescription requirements of the Misuse of Drugs Act

For regulations governing prescriptions for such preparations, see Controlled Drugs and Drug Dependence

Not all monographs include all possible sections; sections are only included when relevant information has been identified

Drug class monographs

In earlier editions of the BNFC, information relating to a class of drug sharing the same properties (e.g. tetracyclines p. 337), was contained within the prescribing notes. In the updated structure, drug class monographs have been created to contain the common information; this ensures such information is easier to find, and has a more regularised structure.

For consistency and ease of use, the class monograph follows the same structure as a drug monograph. Class monographs are indicated by the presence of a flag ● (e.g. beta-adrenoceptor blockers (systemic) p. 100). If a drug monograph has a corresponding class monograph, that needs to be considered in tandem, in order to understand the full information about a drug, the monograph is also indicated by a flag ◢ 1234 (e.g. metoprolol tartrate p. 103). Within this flag, the page number of the drug class monograph is provided (e.g. 1234), to help navigate the user to this information. This is particularly useful where occasionally, due to differences in therapeutic use, the drug monograph may not directly follow the drug class monograph (e.g. sotalol hydrochloride p. 78).

Evidence grading

The BNF has adopted a five level evidence grading system (see How BNF Publications are constructed p. ix). Recommendations that are evidence graded can be identified by a symbol appearing immediately before the recommendation. The evidence grade is displayed at the end of the recommendation.

Other content

Nutrition

Appendix 2 includes tables of ACBS-approved enteral feeds and nutritional supplements based on their energy and protein content. There are separate tables for specialised formulae for specific clinical conditions. Classified sections on foods for special diets and nutritional supplements for metabolic diseases are also included.

Other useful information

Finding significant changes in the BNFC

- *Changes*, provides a list of significant changes, dose changes, classification changes, new names, and new preparations that have been incorporated into the BNFC, as well as a list of preparations that have been discontinued and removed from the BNFC. Changes listed online are cumulative (from one print edition to the next), and can be printed off each month to show the main changes since the last print edition as an aide memoire for those using print copies. So many changes are made for each update of the BNFC, that not all of them can be accommodated in the *Changes* section. We encourage healthcare professionals to review regularly the prescribing information on drugs that they encounter frequently;

- *Changes to the Dental Practitioners' Formulary*, are located at the end of the Dental List;

- *E-newsletter*, the BNF & BNFC e-newsletter service is available free of charge. It alerts healthcare professionals to details of significant changes in the clinical content of these publications and to the way that this information is delivered. Newsletters also review clinical case studies, provide tips on using these publications effectively, and highlight forthcoming changes to the publications. To sign up for e-newsletters go to www.bnf.org.

- An e-learning programme developed in collaboration with the Centre for Pharmacy Postgraduate Education (CPPE), enables pharmacists to identify and assess how significant changes in the BNF affect their clinical practice. The module can be found at www.cppe.ac.uk.

Using other sources for medicines information

The BNFC is designed as a digest for rapid reference. Less detail is given on areas such as malignant disease and anaesthesia since it is expected that those undertaking treatment will have specialist knowledge and access to specialist literature. The BNFC should be interpreted in the light of professional knowledge and supplemented as necessary by specialised publications and by reference to the product literature. Information is also available from medicines information services.

Changes

Monthly updates are provided online via MedicinesComplete and the NHS Evidence portal. The changes listed below are cumulative (from one print edition to the next).

Significant changes

Significant changes that appear in the print edition of *BNF for Children* 2017–2018:

- Acetylcysteine p. 814 for paracetamol overdose [MHRA advice]
- Anal fissure p. 67: new guidance on management.
- Antibacterials, principles of therapy p. 287: new guidance on early management of sepsis.
- Biological medicines: new guidance, see Guidance on prescribing p. 1.
- Biosimilar medicines: new guidance, see Guidance on prescribing p. 1.
- Cholestasis p. 62: updated guidance on management.
- Coeliac disease p. 33: new guidance on management.
- Constipation p. 38: updated guidance on management.
- Contraceptive, interactions p. 474: updated guidance.
- Crohn's disease p. 24: updated guidance on management.
- Diabetes p. 424: updated guidance on management.
- Epilepsy p. 184: updated guidance on epilepsy and driving.
- Etonogestrel p. 489 (*Nexplanon*®) contraceptive implants: reports of device in vasculature and lung [MHRA/CHM advice].
- Exocrine pancreatic insufficiency p. 69: updated guidance on management.
- Food allergy p. 59: updated guidance on management.
- Haemorrhoids p. 67: new guidance on management.
- Hyoscine butylbromide (*Buscopan*®) injection p. 61: risk of serious adverse effects in patients with underlying cardiac disease [MHRA/CHM advice].
- Hypoglycaemia p. 443: updated guidance on sources of oral glucose.
- Imatinib p. 532: risk of hepatitis B reactivation [MHRA/CHM advice].
- Inborn errors of primary bile acid synthesis p. 63: updated guidance on management.
- Irritable bowel syndrome p. 33: updated guidance on management.
- Lumacaftor with ivacaftor p. 179 for treating cystic fibrosis homozygous for F508del mutation [NICE guidance].
- National funding advice: update to inclusion in BNF Publications, see Guidance on prescribing p. 1.
- Nocturnal enuresis in children p. 467: updated guidance on management.
- Paraffin-based skin emollients on dressings or clothing p. 683: fire risk [MHRA/CHM advice].
- Pegaspargase p. 526 for treating acute lymphoblastic leukaemia [NICE guidance].
- Primary biliary cholangitis p. 63: updated guidance on management.
- Risk of severe harm and death due to withdrawing insulin from pen devices [NHS Improvement Patient Safety Alert], see Insulins p. 432.
- Risk of death and severe harm from error with injectable phenytoin [NHS Improvement Patient Safety Alert], see phenytoin p. 198.
- Short bowel syndrome p. 34: new guidance on management.
- Smith-Lemli-Opitz syndrome p. 63: updated guidance on management.
- Sodium valproate p. 200: resources to support the safety of girls and women who are being treated with valproate [NHS improvement patient safety alert].
- Tuberculosis p. 345 updated guidance on management.
- Ulcerative colitis p. 25: updated guidance on management.
- Urinary retention p. 469: updated guidance on management.
- Vaccines p. 747: updated guidance on influenza vaccination for winter 2017–2018.
- Valproic acid p. 205: resources to support the safety of girls and women who are being treated with valproate [NHS improvement patient safety alert].
- Warfarin sodium p. 94: reports of calciphylaxis [MHRA/CHM advice].

Dose changes

Changes in dose statements that appear in the print edition of *BNF for Children* 2017–2018:

- Etoricoxib p. 624 [rheumatoid arthritis and ankylosing spondylitis].
- Fenofibrate p. 127 [dose in renal impairment].
- Nystatin p. 680

Classification changes

Classification changes that appear in the print edition of *BNF for Children* 2017–2018:

New names

Name changes that appear in the print edition of *BNF for Children* 2017–2018:

Deleted preparations

Preparations discontinued in the print edition of *BNF for Children* 2017–2018:

- *Ketek*®.

New preparations

New preparations that appear in the print edition of *BNF for Children* 2017–2018:

- *Benepali*® [etanercept p. 616].
- *Briviact*® [brivaracetam p. 188].
- *Cilodex*® [dexamethasone with ciprofloxacin p. 663].
- *Delmosart*® [methylphenidate hydrochloride p. 218].
- *Descovy*® [emtricitabine with tenofovir alafenamide p. 400].
- *Edurant*® [rilpivirine p. 396].
- *Exjade*® [deferasirox p. 548].
- *Genvoya*® [elvitegravir with cobicistat, emtricitabine and tenofovir alafenamide p. 399].
- *Odefsey*® [emtricitabine with rilpivirine and tenofovir alafenamide p. 400].
- *Oncaspar*® [pegaspargase p. 526].
- *Orkambi*® [lumacaftor with ivacaftor p. 179].
- *Monuril*® [fosfomycin p. 340].
- *Repatha*® [evolocumab p. 131].
- *Revestive*® [teduglutide p. 35].
- *Revolade*® [eltrombopag p. 554].
- *Raxone*® [idebenone p. 659].
- *Spectrila*® [asparaginase p. 523].
- *Sialanar*® [glycopyrronium bromide p. 780].
- *Translarna*® [ataluren p. 618].
- *Vantobra*® nebuliser solution [tobramycin p. 300].
- *Vimizim*® [elosulfase alfa p. 582].
- *Votubia*® dispersible tablets [everolimus p. 531].

Guidance on prescribing

General guidance

Medicines should be given to children only when they are necessary, and in all cases the potential benefit of administering the medicine should be considered in relation to the risk involved. This is particularly important during pregnancy, when the risk to both mother and fetus must be considered.

It is important to discuss treatment options carefully with the child and the child's carer. In particular, the child and the child's carer should be helped to distinguish the adverse effects of prescribed drugs from the effects of the medical disorder. When the beneficial effects of the medicine are likely to be delayed, this should be highlighted.

Prescribing competency framework The Royal Pharmaceutical Society has published a Prescribing Competency Framework that includes a common set of competencies that form the basis for prescribing, regardless of professional background. The competencies have been developed to help healthcare professionals be safe and effective prescribers with the aim of supporting patients to get the best outcomes from their medicines. It is available at www.rpharms.com/resources/frameworks/ prescribers-competency-framework.

Taking medicines to best effect

Difficulties in adherence to drug treatment occur regardless of age. Factors that contribute to poor compliance with prescribed medicines include:

- difficulty in taking the medicine (e.g. inability to swallow the medicine);
- unattractive formulation (e.g. unpleasant taste);
- prescription not collected or not dispensed;
- purpose of medicine not clear;
- perceived lack of efficacy;
- real or perceived adverse effects;
- carers' or child's perception of the risk and severity of side-effects may differ from that of the prescriber;
- instructions for administration not clear.

The prescriber, the child's carer, and the child (if appropriate) should agree on the health outcomes desired and on the strategy for achieving them ('concordance'). The prescriber should be sensitive to religious, cultural, and personal beliefs of the child's family that can affect acceptance of medicines.

Taking the time to explain to the child (and carers) the rationale and the potential adverse effects of treatment may improve adherence. Reinforcement and elaboration of the physician's instructions by the pharmacist and other members of the healthcare team can be important. Giving advice on the management of adverse effects and the possibility of alternative treatments may encourage carers and children to seek advice rather than merely abandon unacceptable treatment.

Simplifying the drug regimen may help; the need for frequent administration may reduce adherence, although there appears to be little difference in adherence between once-daily and twice-daily administration. Combination products reduce the number of drugs taken but at the expense of the ability to titrate individual doses.

Drug treatment in children

Children, and particularly neonates, differ from adults in their response to drugs. Special care is needed in the neonatal period (first 28 days of life) and doses should always be calculated with care; the risk of toxicity is increased by a reduced rate of drug clearance and differing target organ sensitivity. The terms infant, child and adolescent are used inconsistently in the literature. However, **for reference purposes only**, the terms generally used to describe the paediatric stages of development are:

Preterm neonate	Born at < 37 weeks gestation
Term neonate	Born at 37 to 42 weeks gestation
Post-term neonate	Born at ≥42 weeks gestation
Neonate	From 0 up to 28 days of age (or first 4 weeks of life)
Infant	From 28 days up to 24 months of age
Child	From 2 years up to 12 years of age
Adolescent	From 12 years up to 18 years of age

In BNF for *Children*, the term neonate is used to describe a newborn infant aged 0–28 days. The terms child or children are used generically to describe the entire range from infant to adolescent (1 month–17 years). An age range is specified when the dose information applies to a narrower age range than a child from 1 month–17 years.

Administration of medicines to children

Children should be involved in decisions about taking medicines and encouraged to take responsibility for using them correctly. The degree of such involvement will depend on the child's age, understanding, and personal circumstances.

Occasionally a medicine or its taste has to be disguised or masked with small quantities of food. However, unless specifically permitted (e.g. some formulations of pancreatin p. 70), a medicine should **not** be mixed with large quantities of food because the full dose might not be taken and the child might develop an aversion to food if the medicine imparts an unpleasant taste. Medicines should not be mixed or administered in a baby's feeding bottle.

Children under 5 years (and some older children) find a liquid formulation more acceptable than tablets or capsules. However, for long-term treatment it may be possible for a child to be taught to take tablets or capsules.

An oral syringe should be used for accurate measurement and controlled administration of an oral liquid medicine. The unpleasant taste of an oral liquid can be disguised by flavouring it or by giving a favourite food or drink immediately afterwards, but the potential for food-drug interactions should be considered.

Advice should be given on dental hygiene to those receiving medicines containing cariogenic sugars for long-term treatment; sugar-free medicines should be provided whenever possible.

Children with nasal feeding tubes in place for prolonged periods should be encouraged to take medicines by mouth if possible; enteric feeding should generally be interrupted before the medicine is given (particularly if enteral feeds reduce the absorption of a particular drug). Oral liquids can be given through the tube provided that precautions are taken to guard against blockage; the dose should be washed down with warm water. When a medicine is given through a nasogastric tube to a neonate, **sterile water** must be used to accompany the medicine or to wash it down.

The intravenous route is generally chosen when a medicine cannot be given by mouth; reliable access, often a central vein, should be used for children whose treatment involves irritant or inotropic drugs or who need to receive the medicine over a long period or for home therapy. The subcutaneous route is used most commonly for insulin administration. Intramuscular injections should preferably be **avoided** in children, particularly neonates, infants, and young children. However, the intramuscular route may be advantageous for administration of single doses of medicines when intravenous cannulation would be more problematic or painful to the child. Certain drugs, e.g. some vaccines, are only administered intramuscularly.

The intrathecal, epidural and intraosseous routes should be used **only** by staff specially trained to administer medicines by these routes. Local protocols for the management of intrathecal injections must be in place.

Managing medicines in school

Administration of a medicine during schooltime should be avoided if possible; medicines should be prescribed for once or twice-daily administration whenever practicable. If the medicine is to be taken in school, this should be discussed with parents or carers and the necessary arrangements made in advance; where appropriate, involvement of a school nurse should be sought. *Managing Medicines in Schools and Early Years Settings* produced by the Department of Health provides guidance on using medicines in schools (www.dh.gov.uk).

Patient information leaflets

Manufacturers' patient information leaflets that accompany a medicine, cover only the licensed use of the medicine. Therefore, when a medicine is used outside its licence, it may be appropriate to advise the child and the child's parent or carer that some of the information in the leaflet might not apply to the child's treatment. Where necessary, inappropriate advice in the patient information leaflet should be identified and reassurance provided about the correct use in the context of the child's condition.

Biological medicines

Biological medicines are medicines that are made by or derived from a biological source using biotechnology processes, such as recombinant DNA technology. The size and complexity of biological medicines, as well as the way they are produced, may result in a degree of natural variability in molecules of the same active substance, particularly in different batches of the medicine. This variation is maintained within strict acceptable limits. Examples of biological medicines include insulins and monoclonal antibodies. EvGr Biological medicines must be prescribed by brand name and the brand name specified on the prescription should be dispensed in order to avoid inadvertent switching. Automatic substitution of brands at the point of dispensing is not appropriate for biological medicines. ⟨A⟩

Biosimilar medicines

A **biosimilar medicine** is a biological medicine that is highly similar and clinically equivalent (in terms of quality, safety, and efficacy) to an existing biological medicine that has already been authorised in the European Union (known as the reference biological medicine or originator medicine). The active substance of a biosimilar medicine is similar, but not identical, to the originator biological medicine. Once the patent for a biological medicine has expired, a biosimilar medicine may be authorised by the European Medicines Agency (EMA). A biosimilar medicine is not the same as a generic medicine, which contains a simpler molecular structure that is identical to the originator medicine.

Therapeutic equivalence EvGr Biosimilar medicines should be considered to be therapeutically equivalent to the originator biological medicine within their authorised indications. ⟨A⟩ Biosimilar medicines are usually licensed for all the indications of the originator biological medicine, but this depends on the evidence submitted to the EMA for

authorisation and must be scientifically justified on the basis of demonstrated or extrapolated equivalence.

Prescribing and dispensing The choice of whether to prescribe a biosimilar medicine or the originator biological medicine rests with the clinician in consultation with the patient. EvGr Biological medicines (including biosimilar medicines) must be prescribed by brand name and the brand name specified on the prescription should be dispensed in order to avoid inadvertent switching. Automatic substitution of brands at the point of dispensing is not appropriate for biological medicines. ⟨A⟩

Safety monitoring Biosimilar medicines are subject to a black triangle status (▼) at the time of initial authorisation. EvGr It is important to report suspected adverse reactions using the Yellow Card Scheme (see Adverse reactions to drugs p. 12). For all biological medicines, adverse reaction reports should clearly state the brand name and the batch number of the suspected medicine. ⟨A⟩

UK Medicines Information centres have developed a validated tool to determine potential safety issues associated with all new medicines. These 'in-use product safety assessment reports' will be published for new biosimilar medicines as they become available, see www.ukmi.nhs.uk/activities/patientSafety/default.asp?pageRef=20.

National funding/access decisions The Department of Health has confirmed that, in England, NICE can decide to apply the same remit, and the resulting technology appraisal guidance, to relevant biosimilar medicines which appear on the market subsequent to their originator biological medicine. In other circumstances, where a review of the evidence for a particular biosimilar medicine is necessary, NICE will consider producing an evidence summary (see *Evidence summary: new medicines*, www.nice.org.uk/about/what-we-do/our-programmes/nice-advice/evidence-summaries-new-medicines).

National information In England, see www.nice.org.uk/Media/Default/About/what-we-do/NICE-guidance/NICE-technology-appraisals/biosimilars-statement.pdf. In Northern Ireland, see niformulary.hscni.net/ManagedEntry/bios/Pages/default.aspx. In Scotland, see www.scottishmedicines.org.uk/About_SMC/Policy_statements/Biosimilar_Medicines. In Wales, see www.wales.nhs.uk/sites3/Documents/814/BIOSIMILARS-ABUHBpositionStatement%5BNov2015%5D.pdf.

Availability The following drugs are available as a biosimilar medicine:

- Epoetin alfa p. 537
- Epoetin zeta p. 539
- Etanercept p. 616
- Filgrastim p. 551
- Infliximab p. 31
- Insulin glargine p. 435
- Somatropin p. 454

Complementary and alternative medicine

An increasing amount of information on complementary and alternative medicine is becoming available. Where appropriate, the child and the child's carers should be asked about the use of their medicines, including dietary supplements and topical products. The scope of *BNF for Children* is restricted to the discussion of conventional medicines but reference is made to complementary treatments if they affect conventional therapy (e.g. interactions with St John's wort). Further information on herbal medicines is available at www.mhra.gov.uk.

BNF for Children and marketing authorisation

Where appropriate the *doses, indications, cautions, contra-indications,* and *side-effects* in *BNF for Children* reflect those in the manufacturers' Summaries of Product Characteristics

(SPCs) which, in turn, reflect those in the corresponding marketing authorisations (formerly known as Product Licences). *BNF for Children* does not generally include proprietary medicines that are not supported by a valid Summary of Product Characteristics or when the marketing authorisation holder has not been able to supply essential information. When a preparation is available from more than one manufacturer, *BNF for Children* reflects advice that is the most clinically relevant regardless of any variation in the marketing authorisation. Unlicensed products can be obtained from 'special-order' manufacturers or specialist importing companies.

As far as possible, medicines should be prescribed within the terms of the marketing authorisation. However, many children require medicines not specifically licensed for paediatric use. Although medicines cannot be promoted outside the limits of the licence, the Human Medicines Regulations 2012 do not prohibit the use of unlicensed medicines.

BNF for Children includes advice involving the use of unlicensed medicines or of licensed medicines for unlicensed uses ('off-label' use). Such advice reflects careful consideration of the options available to manage a given condition and the weight of evidence and experience of the unlicensed intervention. Where the advice falls outside a drug's marketing authorisation, *BNF for Children* shows the licensing status in the drug monograph. However, limitations of the marketing authorisation should not preclude unlicensed use where clinically appropriate.

Prescribing unlicensed medicines Prescribing unlicensed medicines or medicines outside the recommendations of their marketing authorisation alters (and probably increases) the prescriber's professional responsibility and potential liability. The prescriber should be able to justify and feel competent in using such medicines, and also inform the patient or the patient's carer that the prescribed medicine is unlicensed.

Drugs and skilled tasks

Prescribers and other healthcare professionals should advise children and their carers if treatment is likely to affect their ability to perform skilled tasks (e.g. driving). This applies especially to drugs with sedative effects; patients should be warned that these effects are increased by alcohol. General information about a patient's fitness to drive is available from the Driver and Vehicle Licensing Agency at www.dvla. gov.uk.

A new offence of driving, attempting to drive, or being in charge of a vehicle, with certain specified controlled drugs in excess of specified limits, came into force on 2nd March 2015. This offence is an addition to the existing rules on drug impaired driving and fitness to drive, and applies to two groups of drugs—commonly abused drugs, including amfetamines, cannabis, cocaine, and ketamine p. 790, and drugs used mainly for medical reasons, such as opioids and benzodiazepines. Anyone found to have any of the drugs (including related drugs, for example, apomorphine hydrochloride) above specified limits in their blood will be guilty of an offence, whether their driving was impaired or not. This also includes prescribed drugs which metabolise to those included in the offence, for example, selegiline hydrochloride. However, the legislation provides a statutory "medical defence" for patients taking drugs for medical reasons in accordance with instructions, *if their driving was not impaired*—it continues to be an offence to drive if actually impaired. Patients should therefore be advised to continue taking their medicines as prescribed, and when driving, to carry suitable evidence that the drug was prescribed, or sold, to treat a medical or dental problem, and that it was taken according to the instructions given by the prescriber, or information provided with the medicine (e.g. a repeat prescription form or the medicine's patient

information leaflet). Further information is available from the Department for Transport at www.gov.uk/government/collections/drug-driving.

Oral syringes

An **oral syringe** is supplied when oral liquid medicines are prescribed in doses other than multiples of 5 mL. The oral syringe is marked in 0.5-mL divisions from 1 to 5 mL to measure doses of less than 5 mL (other sizes of oral syringe may also be available). It is provided with an adaptor and an instruction leaflet. The 5-*mL spoon* is used for doses of 5 mL (or multiples thereof).

Excipients

Branded oral liquid preparations that do not contain *fructose, glucose,* or *sucrose* are described as 'sugar-free' in *BNF for Children*. Preparations containing hydrogenated glucose syrup, mannitol, maltitol, sorbitol, or xylitol are also marked 'sugar-free' since they do not cause dental caries. Children receiving medicines containing cariogenic sugars, or their carers, should be advised of dental hygiene measures to prevent caries. Sugar-free preparations should be used whenever possible, particularly if treatment is required for a long period.

Where information on the presence of *alcohol, aspartame, gluten, sulfites, tartrazine, arachis (peanut) oil* or *sesame oil* is available, this is indicated in *BNF for Children* against the relevant preparation.

Information is provided on *selected excipients* in skin preparations, in vaccines, and on *selected preservatives* and *excipients* in eye drops and injections.

The presence of *benzyl alcohol* and *polyoxyl castor oil* (polyethoxylated castor oil) in injections is indicated in *BNF for Children*. Benzyl alcohol has been associated with a fatal toxic syndrome in preterm neonates, and therefore, parenteral preparations containing the preservative should not be used in neonates. Polyoxyl castor oils, used as vehicles in intravenous injections, have been associated with severe anaphylactoid reactions.

The presence of *propylene glycol* in oral or parenteral medicines is indicated in *BNF for Children*; it can cause adverse effects if its elimination is impaired, e.g. in renal failure, in neonates and young children, and in slow metabolisers of the substance. It may interact with metronidazole p. 319.

The *lactose* content in most medicines is too small to cause problems in most lactose-intolerant children. However in severe lactose intolerance, the lactose content should be determined before prescribing. The amount of lactose varies according to manufacturer, product, formulation, and strength.

Important In the absence of information on excipients in *BNF for Children* and in the product literature (available at www.medicines.org.uk/emc/), contact the manufacturer if it is essential to check details.

Health and safety

When handling chemical or biological materials particular attention should be given to the possibility of allergy, fire, explosion, radiation, or poisoning. Care is required to avoid sources of heat (including hair dryers) when flammable substances are used on the skin or hair. Substances, such as corticosteroids, some antimicrobials, phenothiazines, and many cytotoxics, are irritant or very potent and should be handled with caution; contact with the skin and inhalation of dust should be avoided. Healthcare professionals and carers should guard against exposure to sensitising, toxic or irritant substances if it is necessary to crush tablets or open capsules.

EEA and Swiss prescriptions

Pharmacists can dispense prescriptions issued by doctors and dentists from the European Economic Area (EEA) or Switzerland (except prescriptions for controlled drugs in Schedules 1, 2, or 3, or for drugs without a UK marketing authorisation). Prescriptions should be written in ink or otherwise so as to be indelible, should be dated, should state the name of the patient, should state the address of the prescriber, should contain particulars indicating whether the prescriber is a doctor or dentist, and should be signed by the prescriber.

Security and validity of prescriptions

The Councils of the British Medical Association and the Royal Pharmaceutical Society have issued a joint statement on the security and validity of prescriptions.

In particular, prescription forms should:
- not be left unattended at reception desks;
- not be left in a car where they may be visible;
- when not in use, be kept in a locked drawer within the surgery and at home.

Where there is any doubt about the authenticity of a prescription, the pharmacist should contact the prescriber. If this is done by telephone, the number should be obtained from the directory rather than relying on the information on the prescription form, which may be false.

Patient group direction (PGD)

In most cases, the most appropriate clinical care will be provided on an individual basis by a prescriber to a specific child. However, a Patient Group Direction for supply and administration of medicines by other healthcare professionals can be used where it would benefit the child's care without compromising safety.

A Patient Group Direction is a written direction relating to the supply and administration (or administration only) of a licensed prescription-only medicine (including some Controlled Drugs in specific circumstances) by certain classes of healthcare professionals; the Direction is signed by a doctor (or dentist) and by a pharmacist. Further information on Patient Group Directions is available in Health Service Circular HSC 2000/026 (England), HDL (2001) 7 (Scotland), and WHC (2000) 116 (Wales); see also the Human Medicines Regulations 2012.

NICE, Scottish Medicines Consortium and All Wales Medicines Strategy Group

Advice issued by the National Institute for Health and Care Excellence (NICE), the Scottish Medicines Consortium (SMC) and the All Wales Medicines Strategy Group (AWMSG) is included in *BNF for Children* when relevant. Details of the advice together with updates can be obtained from: www.nice.org.uk, www.scottishmedicines.org.uk and www.awmsg.org.

Prescription writing

Shared care

In its guidelines on responsibility for prescribing (circular EL (91) 127) between hospitals and general practitioners, the Department of Health has advised that legal responsibility for prescribing lies with the doctor who signs the prescription.

Requirements

Prescriptions should be written legibly in ink or otherwise so as to be indelible (it is permissible to issue carbon copies of NHS prescriptions as long as they are signed in ink), should be dated, should state the name and address of the patient, the address of the prescriber, an indication of the type of prescriber, and should be signed in ink by the prescriber (computer-generated facsimile signatures do not meet the legal requirement). The age and the date of birth of the patient should preferably be stated, and it is a legal requirement in the case of prescription-only medicines to state the age for children under 12 years. These recommendations are acceptable for **prescription-only medicines**. Prescriptions for controlled drugs have additional legal requirements.

Wherever appropriate the prescriber should state the current weight of the child to enable the dose prescribed to be checked. Consideration should also be given to including the dose per unit mass e.g. mg/kg or the dose per m² body-surface area e.g. mg/m² where this would reduce error. The following should be noted:

- The strength or quantity to be contained in capsules, lozenges, tablets etc. should be stated by the prescriber. In particular, strength of liquid preparations should be clearly stated (e.g. 125 mg/5 mL).
- The unnecessary use of decimal points should be avoided, e.g. 3 mg, not 3.0 mg. Quantities of 1 gram or more should be written as 1 g etc. Quantities less than 1 gram should be written in milligrams, e.g. 500 mg, not 0.5 g. Quantities less than 1 mg should be written in micrograms, e.g. 100 micrograms, not 0.1 mg. When decimals are unavoidable a zero should be written in front of the decimal point where there is no other figure, e.g. 0.5 mL, not .5 mL. Use of the decimal point is acceptable to express a range, e.g. 0.5 to 1 g.
- 'Micrograms' and 'nanograms' should **not** be abbreviated. Similarly 'units' should **not** be abbreviated.
- The term 'millilitre' (ml or mL) is used in medicine and pharmacy, and cubic centimetre, c.c., or cm³ should not be used. (The use of capital 'L' in mL is a printing convention throughout the BNF; both 'mL' and 'ml' are recognised SI abbreviations).
- Dose and dose frequency should be stated; in the case of preparations to be taken 'as required' a **minimum dose interval** should be specified. Care should be taken to ensure children receive the correct dose of the active drug. Therefore, the dose should normally be stated in terms of the mass of the active drug (e.g. '125 mg 3 times daily'); terms such as '5 mL' or '1 tablet' should be avoided except for compound preparations. When doses other than multiples of 5 mL are prescribed for *oral liquid preparations* the dose-volume will be provided by means of an **oral syringe**, (except for preparations intended to be measured with a pipette). Suitable quantities:

  - Elixirs, Linctuses, and Paediatric Mixtures (5-mL dose), 50, 100, or 150 mL
  - Adult Mixtures (10 mL dose), 200 or 300 mL
  - Ear Drops, Eye drops, and Nasal Drops, 10 mL (or the manufacturer's pack)
  - Eye Lotions, Gargles, and Mouthwashes, 200 mL

- The names of drugs and preparations should be written clearly and **not** abbreviated, using approved titles **only**;

avoid creating generic titles for modified-release preparations).

- The quantity to be supplied may be stated by indicating the number of days of treatment required in the box provided on NHS forms. In most cases the exact amount will be supplied. This does not apply to items directed to be used as required—if the dose and frequency are not given then the quantity to be supplied needs to be stated. When several items are ordered on one form the box can be marked with the number of days of treatment provided the quantity is added for any item for which the amount cannot be calculated.
- Although directions should preferably be in **English without abbreviation**, it is recognised that some Latin abbreviations are used.

Sample prescription

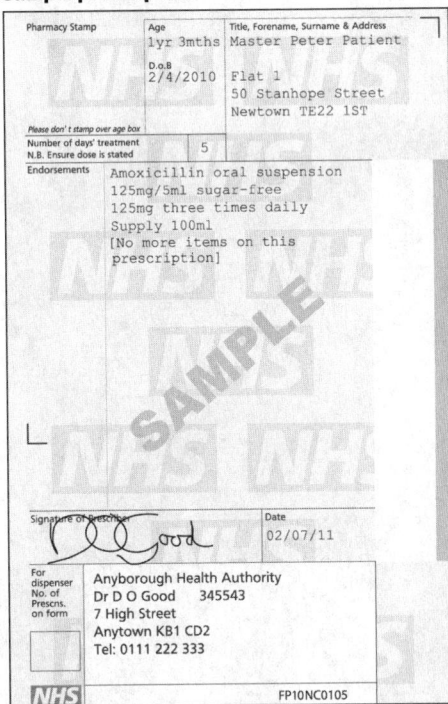

Pharmacy Stamp	Age	Title, Forename, Surname & Address
	1yr 3mths	Master Peter Patient
	D.o.B 2/4/2010	Flat 1
		50 Stanhope Street
		Newtown TE22 1ST

Please don't stamp over age box

Number of days' treatment N.B. Ensure dose is stated   **5**

Endorsements

Amoxicillin oral suspension
125mg/5ml sugar-free
125mg three times daily
Supply 100ml
[No more items on this
prescription]

Signature of Prescriber   *D O Good*

Date   02/07/11

For dispenser No. of Prescns. on form

Anyborough Health Authority
Dr D O Good   345543
7 High Street
Anytown KB1 CD2
Tel: 0111 222 333

NHS   FP10NC0105

Abbreviation of titles In general, titles of drugs and preparations should be written *in full*. Unofficial abbreviations should **not** be used as they may be misinterpreted.

Non-proprietary titles Where non-proprietary ('generic') titles are given, they should be used for prescribing. This will enable any suitable product to be dispensed, thereby saving delay to the patient and sometimes expense to the health service. The only exception is where there is a demonstrable difference in clinical effect between each manufacturer's version of the formulation, making it important that the child should always receive the same brand; in such cases, the brand name or the manufacturer should be stated.

Non-proprietary names of compound preparations Non-proprietary names of **compound preparations** which appear in *BNF for Children* are those that have been compiled by the British Pharmacopoeia Commission or another recognised body; whenever possible they reflect the names of the active ingredients. Prescribers should avoid creating their own compound names for the purposes of generic prescribing; such names do not have an approved definition and can be misinterpreted.

Special care should be taken to avoid errors when prescribing compound preparations; in particular the hyphen in the prefix 'co-' should be retained. Special care should also be taken to avoid creating generic names for **modified-release** preparations where the use of these names could lead to confusion between formulations with different duration of action.

BNFC 2017–2018
Supply of medicines 7
Supply of medicines

Supply of medicines

Overview

When supplying a medicine for a child, the pharmacist should ensure that the child and the child's carer understand the nature and identity of the medicine and how it should be used. The child and the carer should be provided with appropriate information (e.g. how long the medicine should be taken for and what to do if a dose is missed or the child vomits soon after the dose is given).

Safety in the home

Carers and relatives of children must be warned to keep all medicines out of the reach and sight of children. Tablets, capsules and oral and external liquid preparations must be dispensed in a reclosable *child-resistant container* unless:

- the medicine is in an original pack or patient pack such as to make this inadvisable;
- the child's carer will have difficulty in opening a child-resistant container;
- a specific request is made that the product shall not be dispensed in a child-resistant container;
- no suitable child-resistant container exists for a particular liquid preparation.

All patients should be advised to dispose of *unwanted medicines* by returning them to a pharmacy for destruction.

Labelling of prescribed medicines

There is a legal requirement for the following to appear on the label of any prescribed medicine:

- name of the patient;
- name and address of the supplying pharmacy;
- date of dispensing;
- name of the medicine;
- directions for use of the medicine;
- precautions relating to the use of the medicine.

The Royal Pharmaceutical Society recommends that the following also appears on the label:

- the words 'Keep out of the sight and reach of children';
- where applicable, the words 'Use this medicine only on your skin'.

A pharmacist can exercise professional skill and judgement to amend or include more appropriate wording for the name of the medicine, the directions for use, or the precautions relating to the use of the medicine.

Unlicensed medicines

A drug or formulation that is not covered by a marketing authorisation may be obtained from a pharmaceutical company, imported by a specialist importer, manufactured by a commercial or hospital licensed manufacturing unit, or prepared extemporaneously against a prescription.

The safeguards that apply to products with marketing authorisation should be extended, as far as possible, to the use of unlicensed medicines. The safety, efficacy, and quality (including labelling) of unlicensed medicines should be assured by means of clear policies on their prescribing, purchase, supply, and administration. Extra care is required with unlicensed medicines because less information may be available on the drug and any formulation of the drug.

The following should be agreed with the supplier when ordering an unlicensed or extemporaneously prepared medicine:

- the specification of the formulation;
- documentation confirming the specification and quality of the product supplied (e.g. a certificate of conformity or of analysis);
- for imported preparations product and licensing information should be supplied in English.

Extemporaneous preparations

A product should be dispensed extemporaneously only when no product with a marketing authorisation is available. Every effort should be made to ensure that an extemporaneously prepared product is stable and that it delivers the requisite dose reliably; the child should be provided with a consistent formulation regardless of where the medicine is supplied to minimise variations in quality. Where there is doubt about the formulation, advice should be sought from a medicines information centre, the pharmacy at a children's hospital, a hospital production unit, a hospital quality control department, or the manufacturer.

In many cases it is preferable to give a licensed product by an unlicensed route (e.g. an injection solution given by mouth) than to prepare a special formulation. When tablets or capsules are cut, dispersed, or used for preparing liquids immediately before administration, it is important to confirm uniform dispersal of the active ingredient, especially if only a portion of the solid content (e.g. a tablet segment) is used or if only an aliquot of the liquid is to be administered. In some cases the child's clinical condition may require a dose to be administered in the absence of full information on the method of administration. It is important to ensure that the appropriate supporting information is available at the earliest opportunity.

Preparation of products that produce harmful dust (e.g. cytotoxic drugs, hormones, or potentially sensitising drugs such as neomycin sulfate p. 692) should be **avoided** or undertaken with appropriate precautions to protect staff and carers.

The BP direction that a preparation must be *freshly prepared* indicates that it must be made not more than 24 hours before it is issued for use. The direction that a preparation should be *recently prepared* indicates that deterioration is likely if the preparation is stored for longer than about 4 weeks at 15–25°C.

The term **water** used without qualification means either potable water freshly drawn direct from the public supply and suitable for drinking or freshly boiled and cooled purified water. The latter should be used if the public supply is from a local storage tank or if the potable water is unsuitable for a particular preparation.

Emergency supply of medicines

Emergency supply requested by member of the public

Pharmacists are sometimes called upon by members of the public to make an emergency supply of medicines. The Human Medicines Regulations 2012 allows exemptions from the Prescription Only requirements for emergency supply to be made by a person lawfully conducting a retail pharmacy business provided:

a) that the pharmacist has interviewed the person requesting the prescription-only medicine and is satisfied:

   i) that there is immediate need for the prescription-only medicine and that it is impracticable in the circumstances to obtain a prescription without undue delay;

   ii) that treatment with the prescription-only medicine has on a previous occasion been prescribed for the person requesting it;

   iii) as to the dose that it would be appropriate for the person to take;

b) that no greater quantity shall be supplied than will provide 5 days' treatment of phenobarbital p. 208, *phenobarbital sodium*, or Controlled Drugs in Schedules 4 or 5 (doctors or dentists from the European Economic Area and Switzerland, or their patients, cannot request an emergency supply of Controlled Drugs in Schedules 1, 2, or 3, or drugs that do not have a UK marketing authorisation) or 30 days' treatment for other prescription-only medicines, except when the prescription-only medicine is:

   i) insulin, an ointment or cream, or a preparation for the relief of asthma in an aerosol dispenser when the smallest pack can be supplied;

   ii) an oral contraceptive when a full cycle may be supplied;

   iii) an antibiotic in liquid form for oral administration when the smallest quantity that will provide a full course of treatment can be supplied;

c) that an entry shall be made by the pharmacist in the prescription book stating:

   i) the date of supply;

   ii) the name, quantity and, where appropriate, the pharmaceutical form and strength;

   iii) the name and address of the patient;

   iv) the nature of the emergency;

d) that the container or package must be labelled to show:

   i) the date of supply;

   ii) the name, quantity and, where appropriate, the pharmaceutical form and strength;

   iii) the name of the patient;

   iv) the name and address of the pharmacy;

   v) the words 'Emergency supply';

   vi) the words 'Keep out of the reach of children' (or similar warning);

e) that the prescription-only medicine is not a substance specifically excluded from the emergency supply provision, and does not contain a Controlled Drug specified in Schedules 1, 2, or 3 to the Misuse of Drugs Regulations 2001 except for phenobarbital p. 208 or *phenobarbital sodium* for the treatment of epilepsy: for details see *Medicines, Ethics and Practice,* London, Pharmaceutical Press (always consult latest edition). Doctors or dentists from the European Economic Area and Switzerland, or their patients, cannot request an emergency supply of Controlled Drugs in Schedules 1, 2, or 3, or drugs that do not have a UK marketing authorisation.

Emergency supply requested by prescriber

Emergency supply of a prescription-only medicine may also be made at the request of a doctor, a dentist, a supplementary prescriber, a community practitioner nurse prescriber, a nurse, pharmacist, or optometrist independent prescriber, or a doctor or dentist from the European Economic Area or Switzerland, provided:

a) that the pharmacist is satisfied that the prescriber by reason of some emergency is unable to furnish a prescription immediately;

b) that the prescriber has undertaken to furnish a prescription within 72 hours;

c) that the medicine is supplied in accordance with the directions of the prescriber requesting it;

d) that the medicine is not a Controlled Drug specified in Schedules 1, 2, or 3 to the Misuse of Drugs Regulations 2001 except for phenobarbital p. 208 or *phenobarbital sodium* for the treatment of epilepsy: for details see *Medicines, Ethics and Practice,* London, Pharmaceutical Press (always consult latest edition); (Doctors or dentists from the European Economic Area and Switzerland, or their patients, cannot request an emergency supply of Controlled Drugs in Schedules 1, 2, or 3, or drugs that do not have a UK marketing authorisation).

e) that an entry shall be made in the prescription book stating:

   i) the date of supply;

   ii) the name, quantity and, where appropriate, the pharmaceutical form and strength;

   iii) the name and address of the practitioner requesting the emergency supply;

   iv) the name and address of the patient;

   v) the date on the prescription;

   vi) when the prescription is received the entry should be amended to include the date on which it is received.

Royal Pharmaceutical Society's guidelines

1. The pharmacist should consider the medical consequences of not supplying a medicine in an emergency.

2. If the pharmacist is unable to make an emergency supply of a medicine the pharmacist should advise the patient how to obtain essential medical care.

For conditions that apply to supplies made at the request of a patient see Medicines, Ethics and Practice, London Pharmaceutical Press, (always consult latest edition).

Controlled drugs and drug dependence

Regulations and classification

The Misuse of Drugs Act, 1971 prohibits certain activities in relation to 'Controlled Drugs', in particular their manufacture, supply, and possession. The penalties applicable to offences involving the different drugs are graded broadly according to the *harmfulness attributable to a drug when it is misused* and for this purpose the drugs are defined in the following three classes:

- **Class A** includes: alfentanil p. 788, cocaine, diamorphine hydrochloride (heroin) p. 267, dipipanone hydrochloride, lysergide (LSD), methadone hydrochloride p. 286, methylenedioxymethamfetamine (MDMA, 'ecstasy'), morphine, opium, pethidine hydrochloride p. 276, phencyclidine, remifentanil p. 789, and class B substances when prepared for injection.
- **Class B** includes: oral amfetamines, barbiturates, cannabis, cannabis resin, codeine phosphate p. 265, ethylmorphine, glutethimide, ketamine p. 790, nabilone p. 251, pentazocine, phenmetrazine, and pholcodine p. 181.
- **Class C** includes: certain drugs related to the amfetamines such as benzfetamine and chlorphentermine, buprenorphine p. 263, mazindol, meprobamate, pemoline, pipradrol, most benzodiazepines, tramadol hydrochloride p. 276, zaleplon, zolpidem tartrate, zopiclone, androgenic and anabolic steroids, clenbuterol, chorionic gonadotrophin (HCG), non-human chorionic gonadotrophin, somatotropin, somatrem, and somatropin p. 454.

The Misuse of Drugs Regulations 2001 (and subsequent amendments) define the classes of person who are authorised to supply and possess controlled drugs while acting in their professional capacities and lay down the conditions under which these activities may be carried out. In the regulations drugs are divided into five schedules each specifying the requirements governing such activities as import, export, production, supply, possession, prescribing, and record keeping which apply to them.

- **Schedule 1** includes drugs such as lysergide which is not used medicinally. Possession and supply are prohibited except in accordance with Home Office authority.
- **Schedule 2** includes drugs such as diamorphine hydrochloride (heroin) p. 267, morphine p. 271, nabilone p. 251, remifentanil p. 789, pethidine hydrochloride p. 276, secobarbital, glutethimide, the amfetamines, sodium oxybate and cocaine and are subject to the full controlled drug requirements relating to prescriptions, safe custody (except for secobarbital), the need to keep registers, etc. (unless exempted in Schedule 5).
- **Schedule 3** includes the barbiturates (except secobarbital, now Schedule 2), buprenorphine p. 263, mazindol, meprobamate, midazolam p. 215, pentazocine, phentermine, temazepam p. 790, and tramadol hydrochloride p. 276. They are subject to the special prescription requirements. Safe custody requirements do apply, except for any 5,5 disubstituted barbituric acid (e.g. phenobarbital), mazindol, meprobamate, midazolam, pentazocine, phentermine, tramadol hydrochloride, or any stereoisomeric form or salts of the above. Records in registers do not need to be kept (although there are requirements for the retention of invoices for 2 years).
- **Schedule 4** includes in Part I benzodiazepines (except temazepam p. 790 and midazolam p. 215, which are in Schedule 3), zaleplon, zolpidem tartrate, and zopiclone which are subject to minimal control. Part II includes androgenic and anabolic steroids, clenbuterol, chorionic gonadotrophin (HCG), non-human chorionic gonadotrophin, somatotropin, somatrem, and

somatropin p. 454. Controlled drug prescription requirements do not apply and Schedule 4 Controlled Drugs are not subject to safe custody requirements.
- **Schedule 5** includes those preparations which, because of their strength, are exempt from virtually all Controlled Drug requirements other than retention of invoices for two years.

Prescriptions

Preparations in Schedules 2, 3, and 4 of the Misuse of Drugs Regulations 2001 (and subsequent amendments) are identified throughout *BNF for children* using the following symbols:

CD2	for preparations in Schedule 2
CD3	for preparations in Schedule 3
CD4-1	for preparations in Schedule 4 (Part I)
CD4-2	for preparations in Schedule 4 (Part II)
CD5	for preparations in Schedule 5

The principal legal requirements relating to medical prescriptions are listed below (see also Department of Health Guidance).

Prescription requirements Prescriptions for Controlled Drugs that are subject to prescription requirements (all preparations in Schedules 2 and 3) must be indelible and must be *signed* by the prescriber, be *dated*, and specify the prescriber's *address*. A machine-written prescription is acceptable, but the prescriber's signature must be handwritten. Advanced electronic signatures can be accepted for Schedule 2 and 3 Controlled Drugs where the Electronic Prescribing Service (EPS) is used. All prescriptions for Controlled Drugs that are subject to prescription requirements must always state:

- the name and address of the patient;
- in the case of a preparation, the form (The dosage form e.g. tablets must be included on a Controlled Drugs prescription irrespective of whether it is implicit in the proprietary name e.g. *MST Continus* or whether only one form is available) and where appropriate the strength (when more than one strength of a preparation exists the strength required must be specified) of the preparation;
- for liquids, the total volume in millilitres (in both words and figures) of the preparation to be supplied; for dosage units, the number (in both words and figures) of dosage units to be supplied; in any other case, the total quantity (in both words and figures) of the Controlled Drug to be supplied;
- the dose (the instruction 'one as directed' constitutes a dose but 'as directed' does not);
- the words 'for dental treatment only' if issued by a dentist.

A pharmacist is **not** allowed to dispense a Controlled Drug unless all the information required by law is given on the prescription. In the case of a prescription for a Controlled Drug in Schedule 2 or 3, a pharmacist can amend the prescription if it specifies the total quantity only in words or in figures or if it contains minor typographical errors, provided that such amendments are indelible and clearly attributable to the pharmacist (implementation date for *N. Ireland* not confirmed). Failure to comply with the regulations concerning the writing of prescriptions will result in inconvenience to patients and delay in supplying the necessary medicine. A prescription for a Controlled Drug in Schedules 2, 3, or 4 is valid for 28 days from the date stated thereon (the prescriber may forward-date the prescription; the start date may also be specified in the body of the prescription).

Instalments and 'repeats'

A prescription may order a Controlled Drug to be dispensed by instalments; the amount of instalments and the intervals to be observed must be specified (A total of 14 days' treatment by instalment of any drug listed in Schedule 2 of the Misuse of Drugs Regulations, buprenorphine p. 263, and diazepam p. 212 may be prescribed in England. In *England*, forms FP10(MDA) (blue) and FP10H (MDA) (blue) should be used. In *Scotland*, forms GP10 (peach), HBP (blue), or HBPA (pink) should be used. In *Wales* a total of 14 days' treatment by instalment of any drug listed in Schedules 2–5 of the Misuse of Drugs Regulations may be prescribed. In *Wales*, form WP10(MDA) or form WP10HP(AD) should be used. Instalment prescriptions must be dispensed in accordance with the directions in the prescription. However, the Home Office has approved specific wording which may be included in an instalment prescription to cover certain situations; for example, if a pharmacy is closed on the day when an instalment is due. For details, see *Medicines, Ethics and Practice*, London, Pharmaceutical Press (always consult latest edition) or see *Home Office approved wording for instalment prescribing* (Circular 027/2015), available at www.gov.uk/.

Prescriptions ordering 'repeats' on the same form are **not** permitted for Controlled Drugs in Schedules 2 or 3.

Private prescriptions

Private prescriptions for Controlled Drugs in Schedules 2 and 3 must be written on specially designated forms provided by Primary Care Trusts in England, Health Boards in Scotland, Local Health Boards in Wales, or the Northern Ireland Central Services Agency; in addition, prescriptions must specify the *prescriber's identification number*. Prescriptions to be supplied by a pharmacist in hospital are exempt from the requirements for private prescriptions.

Department of Health guidance

Guidance (June 2006) issued by the Department of Health in England on prescribing and dispensing of Controlled Drugs requires:

- in general, prescriptions for Controlled Drugs in Schedules 2, 3, and 4 to be limited to a supply of up to 30 days' treatment; exceptionally, to cover a justifiable clinical need and after consideration of any risk, a prescription can be issued for a longer period, but the reasons for the decision should be recorded on the patient's notes;
- the patient's identifier to be shown on NHS and private prescriptions for Controlled Drugs in Schedules 2 and 3.

Further information is available at www.gov.uk/dh.

See sample prescription:

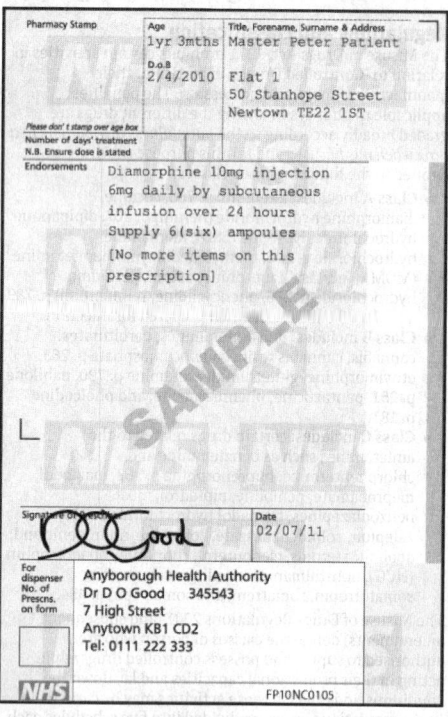

Dependence and misuse

The most serious drugs of addiction are **cocaine**, diamorphine hydrochloride (heroin) p. 267, morphine p. 271, and the **synthetic opioids.**

Despite marked reduction in the prescribing of **amfetamines**, there is concern that abuse of illicit amfetamine and related compounds is widespread. **Benzodiazepines** are commonly misused. However, the misuse of **barbiturates** is now uncommon, in line with declining medicinal use and consequent availability. **Cannabis** (Indian hemp) has no approved medicinal use and cannot be prescribed by doctors. Its use is illegal but widespread. Cannabis is a mild hallucinogen seldom accompanied by a desire to increase the dose; withdrawal symptoms are unusual. However, cannabis extract is licensed as a medicinal product. **Lysergide** (lysergic acid diethylamide, LSD) is a much more potent hallucinogen; its use can lead to severe psychotic states which can be life-threatening.

There are concerns over increases in the availability and misuse of other drugs with variously combined hallucinogenic, anaesthetic, or sedative properties. These include ketamine p. 790 and gamma-hydroxybutyrate (sodium oxybate, GHB).

Prescribing drugs likely to cause dependence or misuse

The prescriber has three main responsibilities:

- To avoid creating dependence by introducing drugs to patients without sufficient reason. In this context, the proper use of the morphine-like drugs is well understood. The dangers of other Controlled Drugs are less clear because recognition of dependence is not easy and its effects, and those of withdrawal, are less obvious.

- To see that the patient does not gradually increase the dose of a drug, given for good medical reasons, to the point where dependence becomes more likely. This tendency is seen especially with hypnotics and anxiolytics. The prescriber should keep a close eye on the amount prescribed to prevent patients from accumulating stocks. A minimal amount should be prescribed in the first instance, or when seeing a new patient for the first time.
- To avoid being used as an unwitting source of supply for addicts and being vigilant to methods for obtaining medicines. Methods include visiting more than one doctor, fabricating stories, and forging prescriptions.

Patients under temporary care should be given only small supplies of drugs unless they present an unequivocal letter from their own doctor. It is sensible to reduce dosages steadily or to issue weekly or even daily prescriptions for small amounts if dependence is suspected.

The stealing and misuse of prescription forms could be minimised by the following precautions:

- do not leave unattended if called away from the consulting room or at reception desks; do not leave in a car where they may be visible; when not in use, keep in a locked drawer within the surgery and at home;
- draw a diagonal line across the blank part of the form under the prescription;
- the quantity should be shown in words and figures when prescribing drugs prone to abuse; this is obligatory for controlled drugs;
- alterations are best avoided but if any are made they should be clear and unambiguous; add initials against altered items;
- if prescriptions are left for collection they should be left in a safe place in a sealed envelope.

Travelling abroad

Prescribed drugs listed in Schedule 4 Part II (CD Anab) and Schedule 5 of the Misuse of Drugs Regulations 2001 are not subject to export or import licensing. However, patients intending to travel abroad for more than 3 months carrying any amount of drugs listed in Schedules 2, 3, or 4 Part I (CD Benz) will require a personal export/import licence. Further details can be obtained at www.gov.uk/guidance/controlled-drugs-licences-fees-and-returns or from the Home Office by contacting DFLU.ie@homeoffice.gsi.gov.uk (in cases of emergency, telephone (020) 7035 6330).

Applications must be supported by a covering letter from the prescriber and should give details of:

- the patient's name and address;
- the quantities of drugs to be carried;
- the strength and form in which the drugs will be dispensed;
- the country or countries of destination;
- the dates of travel to and from the United Kingdom.

Applications for licences should be sent to the Home Office, Drugs Licensing & Compliance Unit, Fry Building, 2 Marsham Street, London. SW1P 4DF.

Alternatively, completed application forms can be emailed to dlcucommsofficer@homeoffice.gsi.gov.uk with a copy of the covering letter from the prescriber as a pdf. A minimum of two weeks should be allowed for processing the application. Patients travelling for less than 3 months do not require a personal export/import licence for carrying Controlled Drugs, but are advised to carry a letter from the prescribing doctor. Those travelling for more than 3 months are advised to make arrangements to have their medication prescribed by a practitioner in the country they are visiting.

Doctors who want to take Controlled Drugs abroad while accompanying patients may similarly be issued with licences. Licences are not normally issued to doctors who want to take Controlled Drugs abroad solely in case a family emergency should arise.

Personal export/import licences do not have any legal status outside the UK and are issued only to comply with the Misuse of Drugs Act and to facilitate passage through UK Customs and Excise control. For clearance in the country to be visited it is necessary to approach that country's consulate in the UK.

Notification of drug misusers

Doctors should report cases of drug misuse to their regional or national drug misuse database or centre.

In **England**, doctors should report cases where they are providing structured drug treatment for substance dependence to their local National Drug Treatment Monitoring System (NDTMS) Team. General information about NDTMS can be found at www.nta.nhs.uk/ndtms.aspx. Enquiries about NDTMS, and how to submit data, should initially be directed to:
EvidenceApplicationTeam@phe.gov.uk

In **Scotland**, doctors should report cases to the Substance Misuse Programme (SMP).

Tel: (0131) 275 6348

In **Northern Ireland**, the Misuse of Drugs (Notification of and Supply to Addicts) (Northern Ireland) Regulations 1973 require doctors to send particulars of persons whom they consider to be addicted to certain controlled drugs to the Chief Medical Officer of the Department of Health and Social Services. The Northern Ireland contacts are:
Medical contact:

Dr Ian McMaster, C3 Castle Buildings, Belfast, BT4 3FQ
Tel: (028) 9052 2421, Fax: (028) 9052 0718
ian.mcmaster@dhsspsni.gov.uk

Administrative contact:
Public Health Information & Research Branch
Department of Health
Annexe 2, Castle Buildings, Stormont, Belfast, BT4 3SQ
Tel: 028 9052 2504

Public Health Information & Research Branch also maintains the Northern Ireland Drug Misuse Database (NIDMD) which collects detailed information on those presenting for treatment, on drugs misused and injecting behaviour; participation is not a statutory requirement.

In **Wales**, doctors should report cases where they are providing structured drug treatment for substance dependence on the Welsh National Database for Substance Misuse; enquiries should be directed to:
substance.misuse-queries@wales.nhs.uk.

Adverse reactions to drugs

Yellow card scheme

Any drug may produce unwanted or unexpected adverse reactions. Rapid detection and recording of adverse drug reactions is of vital importance so that unrecognised hazards are identified promptly and appropriate regulatory action is taken to ensure that medicines are used safely. Healthcare professionals and coroners are urged to report suspected adverse drug reactions directly to the Medicines and Healthcare products Regulatory Agency (MHRA) through the Yellow Card Scheme using the electronic form at www.mhra.gov.uk/yellowcard. Alternatively, prepaid Yellow Cards for reporting are available from the address below and are also bound in the inside back cover of *BNF for Children*.

Send Yellow Cards to:

FREEPOST YELLOW CARD
(No other address details required).
Tel: 0800 731 6789

Suspected adverse drug reactions to any therapeutic agent should be reported, including drugs (*self-medication* as well as those *prescribed*), blood products, vaccines, radiographic contrast media, complementary and herbal products. For biosimilar medicines and vaccines, adverse reaction reports should clearly state the brand name and the batch number of the suspected medicine or vaccine.

Suspected adverse drug reactions should be reported through the Yellow Card Scheme at www.mhra.gov.uk/yellowcard. Yellow Cards can be used for reporting suspected adverse drug reactions to medicines, vaccines, herbal or complementary products, whether self-medicated or prescribed. This includes suspected adverse drug reactions associated with misuse, overdose, medication errors or from use of unlicensed and off-label medicines. Yellow Cards can also be used to report medical device incidents, defective medicines, and suspected fake medicines.

Report all suspected adverse drug reactions that are:

- **serious, medically significant or result in harm**. Serious events are fatal, life-threatening, a congenital abnormality, disabling or incapacitating, or resulting in hospitalisation;
- associated with **newer drugs and vaccines**; the most up to date list of black triangle medicines is available at: www.mhra.gov.uk/blacktriangle

If in doubt whether to report a suspected adverse drug reaction, please complete a Yellow Card.

The identification and reporting of adverse reactions to drugs in children and neonates is particularly important because:

- the action of the drug and its pharmacokinetics in children (especially in the very young) may be different from that in adults;
- drugs may not have been extensively tested in children;
- many drugs are not specifically licensed for use in children and are used either 'off-label' or as unlicensed products;
- drugs may affect the way a child grows and develops or may cause delayed adverse reactions which do not occur in adults;
- suitable formulations may not be available to allow precise dosing in children or they may contain excipients that should be used with caution in children;
- the nature and course of illnesses and adverse drug reactions may differ between adults and children.

Even if reported through the British Paediatric Surveillance Unit's Orange Card Scheme, any identified suspected adverse drug reactions should also be submitted to the Yellow Card Scheme.

Spontaneous reporting is particularly valuable for recognising possible new hazards rapidly. An adverse reaction should be reported even if it is not certain that the drug has caused it, or if the reaction is well recognised, or if other drugs have been given at the same time. Reports of overdoses (deliberate or accidental) can complicate the assessment of adverse drug reactions, but provide important information on the potential toxicity of drugs.

A freephone service is available to all parts of the UK for advice and information on suspected adverse drug reactions; contact the National Yellow Card Information Service at the MHRA on 0800 731 6789. Outside office hours a telephone-answering machine will take messages.

The following Yellow Card Centres can be contacted for further information:

Yellow Card Centre Northwest
2nd Floor, 70 Pembroke Place, Liverpool, L69 3GF
Tel: (0151) 794 8122

Yellow Card Centre Wales
Cardiff University, Department of Pharmacology, Therapeutics and Toxicology, Heath Park, Cardiff, CF14 4XN
Tel: (029) 2074 4181

Yellow Card Centre Northern & Yorkshire
Regional Drug and Therapeutics Centre, 16/17 Framlington Place, Newcastle upon Tyne, NE2 4AB
Tel: (0191) 213 7855

Yellow Card Centre West Midlands
City Hospital, Dudley Road, Birmingham, B18 7QH
Tel: (0121) 507 5672

Yellow Card Centre Scotland
CARDS, Royal Infirmary of Edinburgh, 51 Little France Crescent, Old Dalkeith Road, Edinburgh, EH16 4SA
Tel: (0131) 242 2919
YCCScotland@luht.scot.nhs.uk

The MHRA's database facilitates the monitoring of adverse drug reactions. More detailed information on reporting and a list of products currently under additional monitoring can be found on the MHRA website: www.mhra.gov.uk.

MHRA Drug Safety Update

Drug Safety Update is a monthly newsletter from the MHRA and the Commission on Human Medicines (CHM); it is available at www.gov.uk/drug-safety-update.

Self-reporting

Patients and their carers can also report suspected adverse drug reactions to the MHRA. Reports can be submitted directly to the MHRA through the Yellow Card Scheme using the electronic form at www.mhra.gov.uk/yellowcard, by telephone on 0808 100 3352, or by downloading the Yellow Card form from www.mhra.gov.uk. Alternatively, patient Yellow Cards are available from pharmacies and GP surgeries. Information for patients about the Yellow Card Scheme is available in other languages at www.mhra.gov.uk/yellowcard.

Prescription-event monitoring

In addition to the MHRA's Yellow Card Scheme, an independent scheme monitors the safety of new medicines using a different approach. The Drug Safety Research Unit identifies patients who have been prescribed selected new medicines and collects data on clinical events in these patients. The data are submitted on a voluntary basis by general practitioners on green forms. More information about the scheme and the Unit's educational material is available from www.dsru.org.

Newer drugs and vaccines

Only limited information is available from clinical trials on the safety of new medicines. Further understanding about the safety of medicines depends on the availability of information from routine clinical practice.

The black triangle symbol identifies newly licensed medicines that require additional monitoring by the European Medicines Agency. Such medicines include new active substances, biosimilar medicines, and medicines that the European Medicines Agency consider require additional monitoring. The black triangle symbol also appears in the Patient Information Leaflets for relevant medicines, with a brief explanation of what it means. Products usually retain a black triangle for 5 years, but this can be extended if required.

Medication errors

Adverse drug reactions where harm occurs as a result of a medication error are reportable as a Yellow Card or through the local risk management systems into the National Reporting and Learning System (NRLS). If reported to the NRLS, these will be shared with the MHRA. If the NRLS is not available and harm occurs, report using a Yellow Card.

Adverse reactions to medical devices

Suspected adverse reactions to medical devices including dental or surgical materials, intra-uterine devices, and contact lens fluids should be reported. Information on reporting these can be found at: www.mhra.gov.uk.

Side-effects in the *BNF for Children*

The *BNF for Children* includes clinically relevant side-effects for most drugs; an exhaustive list is not included for drugs that are used by specialists (e.g. cytotoxic drugs and drugs used in anaesthesia). Where causality has not been established, side-effects in the manufacturers' literature may be omitted from the *BNF for Children*.

Description of the frequency of side-effects	
Very common	greater than 1 in 10
Common	1 in 100 to 1 in 10
Uncommon [formerly 'less commonly' in BNF publications]	1 in 1000 to 1 in 100
Rare	1 in 10 000 to 1 in 1000
Very rare	less than 1 in 10 000

Special problems

Symptoms

Children may be poor at expressing the symptoms of an adverse drug reaction and parental opinion may be required.

Delayed drug effects

Some reactions (e.g. cancers and effects on development) may become manifest months or years after exposure. Any suspicion of such an association should be reported directly to the MHRA through the Yellow Card Scheme.

Congenital abnormalities

When an infant is born with a congenital abnormality or there is a malformed aborted fetus doctors are asked to consider whether this might be an adverse reaction to a drug and to report all drugs (including self-medication) taken during pregnancy.

Prevention of adverse reactions

Adverse reactions may be prevented as follows:
- never use any drug unless there is a good indication. If the patient is pregnant do not use a drug unless the need for it is imperative;
- allergy and idiosyncrasy are important causes of adverse drug reactions. Ask if the child has had previous reactions to the drug or formulation;

- prescribe as few drugs as possible and give very clear instructions to the child, parent, or carer;
- whenever possible use a familiar drug; with a new drug be particularly alert for adverse reactions or unexpected events;
- consider if excipients (e.g. colouring agents) may be contributing to the adverse reaction. If the reaction is minor, a trial of an alternative formulation of the same drug may be considered before abandoning the drug;
- obtain a full drug history including asking if the child is already taking other drugs *including over-the-counter medicines*; interactions may occur;
- age and hepatic or renal disease may alter the metabolism or excretion of drugs, particularly in neonates, which can affect the potential for adverse effects. Genetic factors may also be responsible for variations in metabolism, and therefore for the adverse effects of the drug;
- warn the child, parent, or carer if serious adverse reactions are liable to occur.

Drug allergy (suspected or confirmed)

Suspected drug allergy is any reaction caused by a drug with clinical features compatible with an immunological mechanism. All drugs have the potential to cause adverse drug reactions, but not all of these are allergic in nature. A reaction is more likely to be caused by drug allergy if:

- The reaction occurred while the child was being treated with the drug, or
- The drug is known to cause this pattern of reaction, or
- The child has had a similar reaction to the same drug or drug-class previously.

A suspected reaction is less likely to be caused by a drug allergy if there is a possible non-drug cause or if there are only gastro-intestinal symptoms present.

The following signs, allergic patterns and timing of onset can be used to help decide whether to suspect drug allergy:

Immediate, rapidly-evolving reactions (onset usually less than 1 hour after drug exposure)

- Anaphylaxis, with erythema, urticaria or angioedema, and hypotension and/or bronchospasm. See also Antihistamines, allergen immunotherapy and allergic emergencies p. 165
- Urticaria or angioedema without systemic features
- Exacerbation of asthma e.g. with non-steroidal anti-inflammatory drugs (NSAIDs)

*Non-immediate reactions, **without** systemic involvement* (onset usually 6–10 days after first drug exposure or 3 days after second exposure)

- Cutaneous reactions, e.g. widespread red macules and/or papules, or, fixed drug eruption (localised inflamed skin)

*Non-immediate reactions, **with** systemic involvement* (onset may be variable, usually 3 days to 6 weeks after first drug exposure, depending on features, or 3 days after second exposure)

- Cutaneous reactions with systemic features, e.g. drug reaction with eosinophilia and systemic signs (DRESS) or drug hypersensitivity syndrome (DHS), characterised by widespread red macules, papules or erythroderma, fever, lymphadenopathy, liver dysfunction or eosinophilia
- Toxic epidermal necrolysis or Stevens–Johnson syndrome
- Acute generalised exanthematous pustulosis (AGEP)

EvGr Suspected drug allergy information should be clearly and accurately documented in clinical notes and prescriptions, and shared among all healthcare professionals. Children and parents or carers should be given information about which drugs and drug-classes to avoid and encouraged to share the drug allergy status. Ⓐ

EvGr If a drug allergy is suspected, consider stopping the

suspected drug and advising the child and parent or carer to avoid this drug in future. Symptoms of the acute reaction should be treated, in hospital if severe. Children presenting with a suspected anaphylactic reaction, or a severe or non-immediate cutaneous reaction, should be referred to a specialist drug allergy service. Children presenting with a suspected drug allergic reaction or anaphylaxis to NSAIDs, and local and general anaesthetics may also need to be referred to a specialist drug allergy service, e.g. in cases of anaphylactoid reactions or to determine future treatment options. Children presenting with a suspected drug allergic reaction or anaphylaxis associated with beta-lactam antibiotics should be referred to a specialist drug allergy service if their disease or condition can only be treated by a beta-lactam antibiotic or they are likely to need beta-lactam antibiotics frequently in the future (e.g. immunodeficient children). For further information see Drug allergy: diagnosis and management. NICE Clinical Guideline 183 (September 2014) www.nice.org.uk/guidance/cg183.

Defective medicines

During the manufacture or distribution of a medicine an error or accident may occur whereby the finished product does not conform to its specification. While such a defect may impair the therapeutic effect of the product and could adversely affect the health of a patient, it should **not** be confused with an Adverse Drug Reaction where the product conforms to its specification.

The Defective Medicines Report Centre assists with the investigation of problems arising from licensed medicinal products thought to be defective and co-ordinates any necessary protective action. Reports on suspect defective medicinal products should include the brand or the non-proprietary name, the name of the manufacturer or supplier, the strength and dosage form of the product, the product licence number, the batch number or numbers of the product, the nature of the defect, and an account of any action already taken in consequence. The Centre can be contacted at:

The Defective Medicines Report Centre
Medicines and Healthcare products Regulatory Agency,
151 Buckingham Palace Road, London, SW1W 9SZ
Tel: (020) 3080 6574
dmrc@mhra.gsi.gov.uk

Guidance on intravenous infusions

Intravenous infusions for neonatal intensive care

Intravenous policy A local policy on the dilution of drugs with intravenous fluids should be drawn up by a multi-disciplinary team and issued as a document to the members of staff concerned.

Centralised additive services are provided in a number of hospital pharmacy departments and should be used in preference to making additions on wards.

The information that follows should be read in conjunction with local policy documents.

Guidelines

- Drugs should only be diluted with infusion fluid when constant plasma concentrations are needed or when the administration of a more concentrated solution would be harmful.
- In general, only one drug should be mixed with an infusion fluid in a syringe and the components should be compatible. Ready-prepared solutions should be used whenever possible. Drugs should not normally be added to blood products, mannitol, or sodium bicarbonate. Only specially formulated additives should be used with fat emulsions or amino-acid solutions.
- Solutions should be thoroughly mixed by shaking and checked for absence of particulate matter before use.
- Strict asepsis should be maintained throughout and in general the giving set should not be used for more than 24 hours (for drug admixtures).
- The infusion syringe should be labelled with the neonate's name and hospital number, the name and quantity of drug, the infusion fluid, and the expiry date and time. If a problem occurs during administration, containers should be retained for a period after use in case they are needed for investigation.
- Administration using a suitable motorised syringe driver is advocated for preparations where strict control over administration is required.
- It is good practice to examine intravenous infusions from time to time while they are running. If cloudiness, crystallisation, change of colour, or any other sign of interaction or contamination is observed the infusion should be discontinued.

Problems

Microbial contamination The accidental entry and subsequent growth of micro-organisms converts the infusion fluid pathway into a potential vehicle for infection with micro-organisms, particularly species of Candida, Enterobacter, and Klebsiella. Ready-prepared infusions containing the additional drugs, or infusions prepared by an additive service (when available) should therefore be used in preference to making extemporaneous additions to infusion containers on wards etc. However, when this is necessary strict aseptic procedure should be followed.

Incompatibility Physical and chemical incompatibilities may occur with loss of potency, increase in toxicity, or other adverse effect. The solutions may become opalescent or precipitation may occur, but in many instances there is no visual indication of incompatibility. Interaction may take place at any point in the infusion fluid pathway, and the potential for incompatibility is increased when more than one substance is added to the infusion fluid.

Common incompatibilities Precipitation reactions are numerous and varied and may occur as a result of pH, concentration changes, 'salting-out' effects, complexation or other chemical changes. Precipitation or other particle formation must be avoided since, apart from lack of control of dosage on administration, it may initiate or exacerbate adverse effects. This is particularly important in the case of drugs which have been implicated in either thrombophlebitis (e.g. diazepam) or in skin sloughing or necrosis caused by extravasation (e.g. sodium bicarbonate and parenteral nutrition). It is also especially important to effect solution of colloidal drugs and to prevent their subsequent precipitation in order to avoid a pyrogenic reaction (e.g. amphotericin).

It is considered undesirable to mix beta-lactam antibiotics, such as semi-synthetic penicillins and cephalosporins, with proteinaceous materials on the grounds that immunogenic and allergenic conjugates could be formed.

A number of preparations undergo significant loss of potency when added singly or in combination to large volume infusions. Examples include ampicillin in infusions that contain glucose or lactates.

Blood Because of the large number of incompatibilities, drugs should not be added to blood and blood products for infusion purposes. Examples of incompatibility with blood include hypertonic mannitol solutions (irreversible crenation of red cells), dextrans (rouleaux formation and interference with cross-matching), glucose (clumping of red cells), and oxytocin (inactivated).

If the giving set is not changed after the administration of blood, but used for other infusion fluids, a fibrin clot may form which, apart from blocking the set, increases the likelihood of microbial growth.

Intravenous fat emulsion These may break down with coalescence of fat globules and separation of phases when additions such as antibacterials or electrolytes are made, thus increasing the possibility of embolism. Only specially formulated products such as *Vitlipid N®* may be added to appropriate intravenous fat emulsions.

Other infusions Infusions that frequently give rise to incompatibility include amino acids, mannitol, and sodium bicarbonate.

Method

Ready-prepared infusions should be used whenever available. When dilution of drugs is required to be made extemporaneously, any product reconstitution instructions such as those relating to concentration, vehicle, mixing, and handling precautions should be strictly followed using an aseptic technique throughout. Once the product has been reconstituted, further dilution with the infusion fluid should be made immediately in order to minimise microbial contamination and, with certain products, to prevent degradation or other formulation change which may occur; e.g. reconstituted ampicillin injection degrades rapidly on standing, and also may form polymers which could cause sensitivity reactions.

It is also important in certain instances that an infusion fluid of specific pH be used (e.g. **furosemide** injection requires dilution in infusions of pH greater than 5.5).

When drug dilutions are made it is important to mix thoroughly; additions should not be made to an infusion container that has been connected to a giving set, as mixing is hampered. If the solutions are not thoroughly mixed, a concentrated layer of the drug may form owing to differences in density. **Potassium chloride** is particularly prone to this 'layering' effect when added without adequate mixing to infusions; if such a mixture is administered it may have a serious effect on the heart.

A time limit between dilution and completion of administration must be imposed for certain admixtures to guarantee satisfactory drug potency and compatibility. For admixtures in which degradation occurs without the formation of toxic substances, an acceptable limit is the time taken for 10% decomposition of the drug. When toxic substances are produced stricter limits may be imposed. Because of the risk of microbial contamination a maximum time limit of 24 hours may be appropriate for additions made elsewhere than in hospital pharmacies offering central additive service.

Certain injections must be protected from light during continuous infusion to minimise oxidation, e.g. sodium nitroprusside.

Drugs given by continuous intravenous infusion to neonates

The information provided in *BNF for Children* covers dilution with *Glucose intravenous infusion* 5% and 10% and *Sodium chloride intravenous infusion* 0.9%. Compatibility with glucose 5% and with sodium chloride 0.9% indicates compatibility with *Sodium chloride and glucose intravenous infusion*.

Infusion of a large volume of hypotonic solution should be avoided, therefore care should be taken if water for injections is used.

Prescribing in hepatic impairment

Overview

Children have a large reserve of hepatic metabolic capacity and modification of the choice and dosage of drugs is usually unnecessary even in apparently severe liver disease. However, special consideration is required in the following situations:

- liver failure characterised by severe derangement of liver enzymes and profound jaundice; the use of sedative drugs, opioids, and drugs such as diuretics and amphotericin p. 357 which produce hypokalaemia may precipitate hepatic encephalopathy;
- impaired coagulation, which can affect response to oral anticoagulants;
- in cholestatic jaundice elimination may be impaired of drugs such as fusidic acid p. 342 and rifampicin p. 349 which are excreted in the bile;

- in hypoproteinaemia, the effect of highly protein-bound drugs such as phenytoin p. 198, prednisolone p. 421, warfarin sodium p. 94, and benzodiazepines may be increased;
- use of hepatotoxic drugs is more likely to cause toxicity in children with liver disease; such drugs should be avoided if possible;
- in neonates, particularly preterm neonates, and also in infants metabolic pathways may differ from older children and adults because liver enzyme pathways may be immature.

Where care is needed when prescribing in hepatic impairment, this is indicated under the relevant drug in *BNF for Children*.

Prescribing in renal impairment

Issues encountered in renal impairment

The use of drugs in children with reduced renal function can give rise to problems for several reasons:

- reduced renal excretion of a drug or its metabolites may produce toxicity;
- sensitivity to some drugs is increased even if elimination is unimpaired;
- many side-effects are tolerated poorly by children with renal impairment;
- some drugs are not effective when renal function is reduced;
- neonates, particularly preterm, may have immature renal function.

Many of these problems can be avoided by reducing the dose or by using alternative drugs.

Principles of dose adjustment in renal impairment

The level of renal function below which the dose of a drug must be reduced depends on the proportion of the drug eliminated by renal excretion and its toxicity.

For many drugs with only minor or no dose-related side-effects, very precise modification of the dose regimen is unnecessary and a simple scheme for dose reduction is sufficient.

For more toxic drugs with a small safety margin dose regimens based on glomerular filtration rate should be used.

When both efficacy and toxicity are closely related to plasma-drug concentration, recommended regimens should be regarded only as a guide to initial treatment; subsequent doses must be adjusted according to clinical response and plasma-drug concentration.

The total daily maintenance dose of a drug can be reduced either by reducing the size of the individual doses or by increasing the interval between doses. For some drugs, although the size of the maintenance dose is reduced it is important to give a loading dose if an immediate effect is required. This is because it takes about five times the half-life of the drug to achieve steady-state plasma concentration. Because the plasma half-life of drugs excreted by the kidney is prolonged in renal impairment, it can take many doses at the reduced dosage to achieve a therapeutic plasma concentration. The loading dose should usually be the same as the initial dose for a child with normal renal function.

Nephrotoxic drugs should, if possible, be avoided in children with renal disease because the consequences of nephrotoxicity are likely to be more serious when the renal reserve is already reduced.

Glomerular filtration rate is low at birth and increases rapidly during the first 6 months. Thereafter, glomerular filtration rate increases gradually to reach adult levels by 1–2 years of age, when standardised to a typical adult body surface area ($1.73\,m^2$). In the first weeks after birth, serum creatinine falls; a single measure of serum creatinine provides only a crude estimate of renal function and observing the change over days is of more use. In the neonate, a sustained rise in serum creatinine or a lack of the expected postnatal decline, is indicative of a reduced glomerular filtration rate.

Dose recommendations are based on the severity of renal impairment. This is expressed in terms of **glomerular filtration rate** (mL/minute/1.73 m^2).

The following equations provide a guide to glomerular filtration rate.

Child over 1 year:
Estimated glomerular filtration rate (mL/minute/1.73 m^2)= 40 × height (cm)/serum creatinine (micromol/litre)

Neonate:
Estimated glomerular filtration rate (mL/minute/1.73 m^2)= 30 × height (cm)/serum creatinine (micromol/litre)

The values used in these formulas may differ according to locality or laboratory.

The serum-creatinine concentration is sometimes used as a measure of renal function but is only a **rough guide** even when corrected for age, weight, and sex.

Important The information on dose adjustment in *BNF for Children* is expressed in terms of estimated glomerular filtration rate. Renal function in adults is increasingly being reported as estimated glomerular filtration rate (eGFR) normalised to a body surface area of 1.73 m^2; however, eGFR is derived from the MDRD (Modification of Diet in Renal Disease) formula which is not validated for use in children. eGFR derived from the MDRD formula should **not** be used to adjust drug doses in children with renal impairment.

In *BNF for Children*, values for measures of renal function are included where possible. However, where such values are not available, the *BNF for Children* reflects the terms used in the published information.

Degrees of renal impairment defined using estimated glomerular filtration rate (eGFR)

Chronic kidney disease in adults: UK guidelines for identification, management and referral (March 2006) defines renal function as follows:	
Degree of impairment	eGFR[1] mL/minute/1.73 m^2
Normal: Stage 1	More than 90 (with other evidence of kidney damage)
Mild: Stage 2	60–89 (with other evidence of kidney damage)
Moderate[2]: Stage 3	30–59
Severe: Stage 4	15–29
Established renal failure: Stage 5	Less than 15

1. Estimated glomerular filtration rate (eGFR) derived from the Modification of Diet in Renal Disease (MDRD) formula for use in patients over 18 years
2. NICE clinical guideline 73 (September 2008)–Chronic kidney disease: Stage 3A eGFR = 45–59, Stage 3B eGFR = 30–44

Drug prescribing should be kept to the minimum in all children with severe renal disease.

If even mild renal impairment is considered likely on clinical grounds, renal function should be checked before prescribing **any** drug which requires dose modification. Where care is needed when prescribing in renal impairment, this is indicated under the relevant drug in *BNF for Children*.

Dialysis

For prescribing in children on renal replacement therapy consult specialist literature.

Prescribing in pregnancy

Overview

Drugs can have harmful effects on the embryo or fetus at any time during pregnancy. It is important to bear this in mind when prescribing for a woman of *childbearing age* or for men *trying* to *father* a child.

During the *first trimester* drugs can produce congenital malformations (teratogenesis), and the period of greatest risk is from the third to the eleventh week of pregnancy.

During the *second* and *third trimesters* drugs can affect the growth or functional development of the fetus, or they can have toxic effects on fetal tissues.

Drugs given shortly before term or during labour can have adverse effects on labour or on the neonate after delivery.

Not all the damaging effects of intra-uterine exposure to drugs are obvious at birth, some may only manifest later in life. Such late-onset effects include malignancy, e.g. adenocarcinoma of the vagina after puberty in females exposed to diethylstilbestrol in the womb, and adverse effects on intellectual, social, and functional development. The BNF and *BNF for Children* identifies drugs which:

- may have harmful effects in pregnancy and indicates the trimester of risk
- are not known to be harmful in pregnancy

The information is based on human data, but information from *animal* studies has been included for some drugs when its omission might be misleading. Maternal drug doses may require adjustment during pregnancy due to changes in maternal physiology but this is beyond the scope of the *BNF* and *BNF for Children*.

Where care is needed when prescribing in pregnancy, this is indicated under the relevant drug in the BNF and *BNF for Children*.

Important

Drugs should be prescribed in pregnancy only if the expected benefit to the mother is thought to be greater than the risk to the fetus, and all drugs should be avoided if possible during the first trimester. Drugs which have been extensively used in pregnancy and appear to be usually safe should be prescribed in preference to new or untried drugs; and the smallest effective dose should be used. Few drugs have been shown conclusively to be teratogenic in humans, but no drug is safe beyond all doubt in early pregnancy. Screening procedures are available when there is a known risk of certain defects.

Absence of information does not imply safety. It should be noted that the BNF and *BNF for Children* provide independent advice and may not always agree with the product literature.

Information on drugs and pregnancy is also available from the UK Teratology Information Service.www.uktis.org. Tel: 0344 892 0909 (09.00–17:00 Monday to Friday; urgent enquiries only outside these hours).

Prescribing in breast-feeding

Overview

Breast-feeding is beneficial; the immunological and nutritional value of breast milk to the infant is greater than that of formula feeds.

Although there is concern that drugs taken by the mother might affect the infant, there is very little information on this. In the absence of evidence of an effect, the potential for harm to the infant can be inferred from:

- the amount of drug or active metabolite of the drug delivered to the infant (dependent on the pharmacokinetic characteristics of the drug in the mother);
- the efficiency of absorption, distribution, and elimination of the drug by the infant (infant pharmacokinetics);
- the nature of the effect of the drug on the infant (pharmacodynamic properties of the drug in the infant).

Most medicines given to a mother cause no harm to breast-fed infants and there are few contra-indications to breast-feeding when maternal medicines are necessary. However, administration of some drugs to nursing mothers can harm the infant. In the first week of life, some such as preterm or jaundiced infants are at a slightly higher risk of toxicity. Toxicity to the infant can occur if the drug enters the milk in pharmacologically significant quantities. The concentration in milk of some drugs (e.g. fluvastatin p. 129) may exceed the concentration in maternal plasma so that therapeutic doses in the mother can cause toxicity to the infant. Some drugs inhibit the infant's sucking reflex (e.g. phenobarbital p. 208) while others can affect lactation (e.g. bromocriptine). Drugs in breast milk may, at least theoretically, cause hypersensitivity in the infant even when concentration is too low for a pharmacological effect. *BNF for Children* identifies drugs:

- which should be used with caution or which are contra-indicated in breast-feeding for the reasons given above;
- which, on present evidence, may be given to the mother during breast-feeding, because they appear in milk in amounts which are too small to be harmful to the infant;
- which are not known to be harmful to the infant although they are present in milk in significant amounts.

Where care is needed when prescribing in breast-feeding, this is indicated under the relevant drug in the *BNF for Children*.

Important

For many drugs insufficient evidence is available to provide guidance and it is advisable to administer only essential drugs to a mother during breast-feeding. Because of the inadequacy of information on drugs in breast-feeding, absence of information does not imply safety.

Prescribing in palliative care

Overview

Palliative care is the active and total approach to the care of children and young adults with life-limiting and life-threatening conditions, embracing physical, emotional, social, and spiritual elements of their care. It focuses on enhancing the quality of life for the child and support for their family, and includes the management of distressing symptoms, provision of respite, and care following death and bereavement.

Effective palliative care requires a broad multidisciplinary approach that includes the whole family, and ideally should start as soon as possible after diagnosis or recognition of a life-threatening condition.

Drug treatment The number of drugs should be as few as possible. Oral medication is usually appropriate unless there is severe nausea and vomiting, dysphagia, weakness, or coma, when parenteral medication may be necessary. For further information on the use of medicines in paediatric palliative care, see the Association for Paediatric Palliative Medicine (APPM) Master Formulary available at www.appm.org.uk/10.html.

Pain

Pain management in palliative care is focused on achieving control of pain by administering the right drug in the right dose at the right time. Analgesics can be divided into three broad classes: non-opioid (paracetamol p. 260, NSAID), opioid (e.g. codeine phosphate p. 265 'weak', morphine p. 271 'strong') and adjuvant (e.g. antidepressants, antiepileptics). Drugs from the different classes are used alone or in combination according to the type of pain and response to treatment. Analgesics are more effective in preventing pain than in the relief of established pain; it is important that they are given regularly.

Paracetamol or a NSAID given regularly will often be sufficient to manage mild pain. If non-opioid analgesics alone are not sufficient, then an opioid analgesic alone or in combination with a non-opioid analgesic at an adequate dosage, may be helpful in the control of moderate pain. Codeine phosphate or tramadol hydrochloride p. 276 can be considered for moderate pain. If these preparations do not control the pain then morphine is the most useful opioid analgesic. Alternatives to morphine, including transdermal buprenorphine, transdermal fentanyl p. 268, hydromorphone hydrochloride p. 271, methadone hydrochloride p. 286, or oxycodone hydrochloride p. 273, should be initiated by those with experience in palliative care. Initiation of an opioid analgesic should not be delayed by concern over a theoretical likelihood of psychological dependence (addiction).

Bone metastases In addition to the above approach, radiotherapy and bisphosphonates may be useful for pain due to bone metastases.

Neuropathic pain Patients with neuropathic pain may benefit from a trial of a tricyclic antidepressant, most commonly amitriptyline hydrochloride p. 229, for several weeks. An antiepileptic such as carbamazepine p. 189, may be added or substituted if pain persists. Ketamine p. 790 is sometimes used under specialist supervision for neuropathic pain that responds poorly to opioid analgesics. Pain due to nerve compression may be reduced by a corticosteroid such as dexamethasone p. 419, which reduces oedema around the tumour, thus reducing compression. Nerve blocks can be considered when pain is localised to a specific area. Transcutaneous electrical nerve stimulation (TENS) may also help.

Pain management with opioids

Oral route Treatment with morphine p. 271 is given by mouth as immediate-release or modified-release preparations. During the titration phase the initial dose is based on the previous medication used, the severity of the pain, and other factors such as presence of renal impairment or frailty. The dose is given either as an immediate-release preparation 4-hourly (for starting doses, see Morphine), or as a 12-hourly modified-release preparation, in addition to rescue doses. If replacing a weaker opioid analgesic (such as codeine phosphate p. 265), starting doses are usually higher. If pain occurs between regular doses of morphine ('breakthrough pain'), an additional dose ('rescue dose') of immediate-release morphine should be given. An additional dose should also be given 30 minutes before an activity that causes pain, such as wound dressing. The standard dose of a strong opioid for breakthrough pain is usually one-tenth to one-sixth of the regular 24-hour dose, repeated every 2–4 hours as required (up to hourly may be needed if pain is severe or in the last days of life). Review pain management if rescue analgesic is required frequently (twice daily or more). Each child should be assessed on an individual basis. Formulations of fentanyl p. 268 that are administered nasally, buccally or sublingually are not licensed for use in children; their usefulness in children is also limited by dose availability.

Children often require a higher dose of morphine in proportion to their body-weight compared to adults. Children are more susceptible to certain adverse effects of opioids such as urinary retention (which can be eased by bethanechol chloride), and opioid-induced pruritus. When adjusting the dose of morphine, the number of rescue doses required and the response to them should be taken into account; increments of morphine should not exceed one-third to one-half of the total daily dose every 24 hours. Thereafter, the dose should be adjusted with careful assessment of the pain, and the use of adjuvant analgesics should also be considered. Upward titration of the dose of morphine stops when either the pain is relieved or unacceptable adverse effects occur, after which it is necessary to consider alternative measures.

Once their pain is controlled, children started on 4-hourly immediate-release morphine can be transferred to the same total 24-hour dose of morphine given as the modified-release preparation for 12-hourly or 24-hourly administration. The first dose of the modified-release preparation is given with, or within 4 hours of the last dose of the immediate-release preparation. For preparations suitable for 12-hourly or 24-hourly administration see modified-release preparations under morphine. Increments should be made to the dose, not to the frequency of administration. The patient must be monitored closely for efficacy and side-effects, particularly constipation, and nausea and vomiting. A suitable laxative should be prescribed routinely.

Oxycodone hydrochloride p. 273 can be used in children who require an opioid but cannot tolerate morphine. If the child is already receiving an opioid, oxycodone hydrochloride should be started at a dose equivalent to the current analgesic. Oxycodone hydrochloride immediate-release preparations can be given for breakthrough pain.

Prescribing in palliative care

Equivalent doses of opioid analgesics.

This table is only an **approximate** guide (doses may not correspond with those given in clinical practice); children should be carefully monitored after any change in medication and dose titration may be required.

Analgesic/Route	Dose
Codeine: PO	100 mg
Diamorphine: IM, IV, SC	3 mg
Dihydrocodeine: PO	100 mg
Hydromorphone: PO	2 mg
Morphine: PO	10 mg
Morphine: IM, IV, SC	5 mg
Oxycodone: PO	6.6 mg
Tramadol: PO	100 mg

PO = by mouth; IM = intramuscular; IV = intravenous; SC = subcutaneous

Parenteral route Diamorphine hydrochloride p. 267 is preferred for injection because, being more soluble, it can be given in a smaller volume. The equivalent subcutaneous dose is approximately a third of the oral dose of morphine p. 271. Subcutaneous infusion of diamorphine hydrochloride via a continuous infusion device can be useful (for details, see Continuous Subcutaneous Infusions).

If the child can resume taking medicines by mouth, then oral morphine may be substituted for subcutaneous infusion of diamorphine hydrochloride. See the table *Equivalent doses of Morphine and Diamorphine* p. 23.

Rectal route Morphine p. 271 is also available for rectal administration as suppositories.

Transdermal route Transdermal preparations of fentanyl p. 268 and buprenorphine p. 263 [not licensed for use in children] are available; they are not suitable for acute pain or in those children whose analgesic requirements are changing rapidly because the long time to steady state prevents rapid titration of the dose. Prescribers should ensure that they are familiar with the correct use of transdermal preparations (see under fentanyl p. 268) because inappropriate use has caused fatalities.

The following 24-hour oral doses of morphine are considered to be *approximately* equivalent to the buprenorphine and fentanyl patches shown, however when switching due to possible opioid-induced hyperalgesia, reduce the calculated equivalent dose of the new opioid by one-quarter to one-half.

Buprenorphine patches are *approximately* equivalent to the following 24-hour doses of oral morphine

morphine salt 12 mg daily	≡ buprenorphine '5' patch
morphine salt 24 mg daily	≡ buprenorphine '10' patch
morphine salt 36 mg daily	≡ buprenorphine '15' patch
morphine salt 48 mg daily	≡ buprenorphine '20' patch
morphine salt 84 mg daily	≡ buprenorphine '35' patch
morphine salt 126 mg daily	≡ buprenorphine '52.5' patch
morphine salt 168 mg daily	≡ buprenorphine '70' patch

Formulations of transdermal patches are available as 72-hourly, 96-hourly and 7-day patches, for further information see buprenorphine in BNF. Conversion ratios vary and these figures are a guide only. Morphine equivalences for transdermal opioid preparations have been approximated to allow comparison with available preparations of oral morphine.

72-hour Fentanyl patches are *approximately* equivalent to the following 24-hour doses of oral morphine

morphine salt 30 mg daily	≡ fentanyl '12' patch
morphine salt 60 mg daily	≡ fentanyl '25' patch
morphine salt 120 mg daily	≡ fentanyl '50' patch
morphine salt 180 mg daily	≡ fentanyl '75' patch
morphine salt 240 mg daily	≡ fentanyl '100' patch

Fentanyl equivalences in this table are for children on well-tolerated opioid therapy for long periods; fentanyl patches should not be used in opioid naive children. Conversion ratios vary and these figures are a guide only. Morphine equivalences for transdermal opioid preparations have been approximated to allow comparison with available preparations of oral morphine.

Symptom control

Unlicensed indications or routes Several recommendations in this section involve unlicensed indications or routes.

Anorexia Anorexia may be helped by prednisolone p. 421 or dexamethasone p. 419.

Anxiety Anxiety can be treated with a long-acting benzodiazepine such as diazepam p. 212, or by continuous infusion of the short-acting benzodiazepine midazolam p. 215. Interventions for more acute episodes of anxiety (such as panic attacks) include short-acting benzodiazepines such as lorazepam p. 214 given sublingually or midazolam given subcutaneously. Temazepam p. 790 provides useful night-time sedation in some children.

Capillary bleeding Capillary bleeding can be treated with tranexamic acid p. 80 by mouth; treatment is usually continued for one week after the bleeding has stopped but it can be continued at a reduced dose if bleeding persists. Alternatively, gauze soaked in tranexamic acid 100 mg/mL p. 80 or adrenaline/epinephrine solution 1 mg/mL (1 in 1000) p. 132 can be applied to the affected area.
Vitamin K may be useful for the treatment and prevention of bleeding associated with prolonged clotting in liver disease. In severe chronic cholestasis, absorption of vitamin K may be impaired; either parenteral or water-soluble oral vitamin K should be considered.

Constipation Constipation is a common cause of distress and is almost invariable after administration of an opioid analgesic. It should be prevented if possible by the regular administration of laxatives. Suitable laxatives include osmotic laxatives (such as lactulose p. 40 or macrogols), stimulant laxatives (such as co-danthramer p. 44 and senna p. 45) or the combination of lactulose and a senna preparation. Naloxone hydrochloride p. 813 given by mouth may help relieve opioid-induced constipation; it is poorly absorbed but opioid withdrawal reactions have been reported.

Convulsions Intractable seizures are relatively common in children dying from non-malignant conditions. Phenobarbital p. 208 by mouth or as a continuous subcutaneous infusion may be beneficial; continuous infusion of midazolam p. 215 is an alternative. Both cause drowsiness, but this is rarely a concern in the context of intractable seizures. For breakthrough convulsions diazepam p. 212 given rectally (as a solution), buccal midazolam, or paraldehyde p. 215 as an enema may be appropriate.
See *Continuous subcutaneous infusions*, below, for the use of midazolam by subcutaneous infusion using a continuous infusion device.

Dry mouth Dry mouth may be caused by certain medications including opioid analgesics, antimuscarinic drugs (e.g. hyoscine), antidepressants and some antiemetics;

if possible, an alternative preparation should be considered. Dry mouth may be relieved by good mouth care and measures such as chewing sugar-free gum, sucking ice or pineapple chunks, or the use of artificial saliva, dry mouth associated with candidiasis can be treated by oral preparations of nystatin p. 680 or miconazole p. 680, alternatively, fluconazole p. 358 can be given by mouth.

Dysphagia A corticosteroid such as dexamethasone p. 419 may help, temporarily, if there is an obstruction due to tumour. See also *Dry mouth*, above.

Dyspnoea Breathlessness at rest may be relieved by regular oral morphine p. 271 in carefully titrated doses. Diazepam p. 212 may be helpful for dyspnoea associated with anxiety. Sublingual lorazepam p. 214 or subcutaneous or buccal midazolam p. 215 are alternatives. A nebulised short-acting beta₂ agonist or a corticosteroid, such as dexamethasone p. 419 or prednisolone p. 421, may also be helpful for bronchospasm or partial obstruction.

Excessive respiratory secretion Excessive respiratory secretion (death rattle) may be reduced by hyoscine hydrobromide patches or by subcutaneous or intravenous injection of hyoscine hydrobromide p. 256, however, care must be taken to avoid the discomfort of dry mouth. Alternatively, glycopyrronium bromide p 780 may be given. Hyoscine hydrobromide can be administered by subcutaneous or intravenous infusion using a continuous infusion device.

Fungating tumours Fungating tumours can be treated by regular dressing and antibacterial drugs; systemic treatment with metronidazole p. 319 is often required to reduce malodour, but topical metronidazole p. 692 is also used.

Gastro-intestinal pain The pain of bowel colic may be reduced by loperamide hydrochloride p. 47. Hyoscine hydrobromide p. 256 may also be helpful in reducing the frequency of spasms; it is given sublingually as *Kwells* ® tablets and also by subcutaneous infusion.
Gastric distension pain due to pressure on the stomach may be helped by a preparation incorporating an antacid with an antiflatulent and a prokinetic such as domperidone before meals.

Hiccup Hiccup due to gastric distension may be helped by a preparation incorporating an antacid with an antiflatulent.

Insomnia Children with advanced cancer may not sleep because of discomfort, cramps, night sweats, joint stiffness, or fear. There should be appropriate treatment of these problems before hypnotics are used. Benzodiazepines, such as temazepam p. 790, may be useful.

Intractable cough Intractable cough may be relieved by moist inhalations or by regular administration of oral morphine p. 271 every 4 hours. Methadone hydrochloride linctus p. 286 should be avoided because it has a long duration of action and tends to accumulate.

Mucosal bleeding Mucosal bleeding from the mouth and nose occurs commonly in the terminal phase, particularly in a child suffering from haemopoeitic malignancy. Bleeding from the nose caused by a single bleeding point can be arrested by cauterisation or by dressing it. Tranexamic acid p. 80 may be effective applied topically or given systemically.

Muscle spasm The pain of muscle spasm can be helped by a muscle relaxant such as diazepam p. 212 or baclofen p. 620.

Nausea and vomiting Nausea and vomiting are common in children with advanced cancer. Ideally, the cause should be determined before treatment with an antiemetic is started. Nausea and vomiting with opioid therapy are less common in children than in adults but may occur particularly in the initial stages and can be prevented by giving an antiemetic. An antiemetic is usually necessary only for the first 4 or 5 days and therefore combined preparations containing an opioid with an antiemetic are not recommended because they lead to unnecessary antiemetic therapy (and associated side-effects when used long-term).
Metoclopramide hydrochloride p. 252 has a prokinetic action and is used by mouth for nausea and vomiting associated with gastritis, gastric stasis, and functional bowel obstruction. Drugs with antimuscarinic effects antagonise prokinetic drugs and, if possible, should not therefore be used concurrently.
Haloperidol p. 237 is used by mouth or by continuous intravenous or subcutaneous infusion for most metabolic causes of vomiting (e.g. hypercalcaemia, renal failure).
Cyclizine p. 250 is used for nausea and vomiting due to mechanical bowel obstruction, raised intracranial pressure, and motion sickness.
Ondansetron p. 253 is most effective when the vomiting is due to damaged or irritated gut mucosa (e.g. after chemotherapy or radiotherapy).
Antiemetic therapy should be reviewed every 24 hours; it may be necessary to substitute the antiemetic or to add another one.
Levomepromazine p. 257 can be used if first-line antiemetics are inadequate. Dexamethasone p. 419 by mouth can be used as an adjunct.
See *Continuous subcutaneous infusions*, below, for the administration of antiemetics by subcutaneous infusion using a continuous infusion device.

Pruritus Pruritus, even when associated with obstructive jaundice, often responds to simple measures such as application of emollients. Ondansetron p. 253 may be effective in some children. Where opioid analgesics cause pruritus it may be appropriate to review the dose or to switch to an alternative opioid analgesic. In the case of obstructive jaundice, further measures include administration of colestyramine p. 125.

Raised intracranial pressure Headache due to raised intracranial pressure often responds to a high dose of a corticosteroid, such as dexamethasone p. 419, for 4 to 5 days, subsequently reduced if possible; dexamethasone should be given before 6 p.m. to reduce the risk of insomnia. Treatment of headache and of associated nausea and vomiting should also be considered.

Restlessness and confusion Restlessness and confusion may require treatment with haloperidol p. 237. Levomepromazine p. 257 is also used occasionally for restlessness.

Continuous subcutaneous infusions

Although drugs can usually be administered *by mouth* to control symptoms in palliative care, the parenteral route may sometimes be necessary. Repeated administration of *intramuscular injections* should be avoided in children, particularly if cachectic. This has led to the use of portable continuous infusion devices such as syringe drivers to give a *continuous subcutaneous infusion*, which can provide good control of symptoms with little discomfort or inconvenience to the patient.
Indications for the **parenteral route** are:

- inability to take medicines by mouth owing to *nausea and vomiting, dysphagia, severe weakness*, or *coma*;
- *malignant bowel obstruction* for which surgery is inappropriate (avoiding the need for an intravenous infusion or for insertion of a nasogastric tube);
- refusal by the child to take regular medication by mouth.

Syringe driver rate settings Staff using syringe drivers should be **adequately trained** and different rate settings should be **clearly identified** and **differentiated**; incorrect use of syringe drivers is a common cause of medication errors.

Bowel colic and excessive respiratory secretions Hyoscine hydrobromide p. 256 effectively reduces respiratory secretions and is sedative (but occasionally causes paradoxical agitation); it is given in a *subcutaneous* or *intravenous infusion*. Glycopyrronium bromide p. 780 may also be used.

Hyoscine butylbromide p. 61 is effective in bowel colic, is less sedative than hyoscine hydrobromide, but is not always adequate for the control of respiratory secretions; it is given by *subcutaneous infusion* (**important**: *hyoscine butylbromide* must not be confused with *hyoscine hydrobromide*, above).

Confusion and restlessness Haloperidol p. 237 has little sedative effect. Levomepromazine p. 257 has a sedative effect. Midazolam p. 215 is a sedative and an antiepileptic that may be suitable for a very restless patient.

Convulsions If a child has previously been receiving an antiepileptic drug or has a primary or secondary cerebral tumour or is at risk of convulsion (e.g. owing to uraemia) antiepileptic medication should not be stopped. Midazolam p. 215 is the benzodiazepine antiepileptic of choice for *continuous subcutaneous infusion*.

Nausea and vomiting Levomepromazine p. 257 causes sedation in about 50% of patients. Haloperidol p. 237 has little sedative effect.

Cyclizine p. 250 is particularly likely to precipitate if mixed with diamorphine hydrochloride p. 267 or other drugs (see under *Mixing and compatibility*); it is given by *subcutaneous infusion*.

Pain control Diamorphine hydrochloride p. 267 is the preferred opioid since its high solubility permits a large dose to be given in a small volume (see under *Mixing and compatibility*). The table shows approximate equivalent doses of morphine and diamorphine hydrochloride.

Mixing and compatibility The general principle that injections should be given into separate sites (and should not be mixed) does not apply to the use of syringe drivers in palliative care. Provided that there is evidence of compatibility, selected injections can be mixed in syringe drivers. Not all types of medication can be used in a subcutaneous infusion. In particular, chlorpromazine hydrochloride p. 236, prochlorperazine p. 258, and diazepam p. 212 are **contra-indicated** as they cause skin reactions at the injection site; to a lesser extent cyclizine p. 250 and levomepromazine p. 257 also sometimes cause local irritation.

In theory injections dissolved in water for injections are more likely to be associated with pain (possibly owing to their hypotonicity). The use of physiological saline (sodium chloride 0.9% p. 561) however increases the likelihood of precipitation when more than one drug is used; moreover subcutaneous infusion rates are so slow (0.1– 0.3 mL/hour) that pain is not usually a problem when water is used as a diluent.

Compatibility with diamorphine Diamorphine can be given by *subcutaneous infusion* in a strength of up to 250 mg/mL; up to a strength of 40 mg/mL either *water for injections* or *physiological saline* (sodium chloride 0.9%) is a suitable diluent—above that strength only *water for injections* is used (to avoid precipitation).

The following can be mixed with *diamorphine*:

- **Cyclizine**, may precipitate at concentrations above 10 mg/mL or in the presence of sodium chloride 0.9% or as the concentration of diamorphine relative to cyclizine increases; mixtures of diamorphine and cyclizine are also likely to precipitate after 24 hours.
- **Dexamethasone**, special care is needed to avoid precipitation of dexamethasone when preparing it.
- **Haloperidol**, mixtures of haloperidol and diamorphine are likely to precipitate after 24 hours if haloperidol concentration is above 2 mg/mL.

- **Hyoscine butylbromide**
- **Hyoscine hydrobromide**
- **Levomepromazine**
- **Metoclopramide**, under some conditions infusions containing metoclopramide become discoloured; such solutions should be discarded.
- **Midazolam**

Subcutaneous infusion solution should be monitored regularly both to check for precipitation (and discolouration) and to ensure that the infusion is running at the correct rate.

Problems encountered with syringe drivers The following are problems that may be encountered with syringe drivers and the action that should be taken:

- if the subcutaneous infusion runs *too quickly* check the rate setting and the calculation;
- if the subcutaneous infusion runs *too slowly* check the start button, the battery, the syringe driver, the cannula, and make sure that the injection site is not inflamed;
- if there is an *injection site reaction* make sure that the site does not need to be changed—firmness or swelling at the site of injection is not in itself an indication for change, but pain or obvious inflammation is.

Equivalent doses of morphine sulfate and diamorphine hydrochloride given over 24 hours

These equivalences are *approximate only* and should be adjusted according to response

ORAL MORPHINE	PARENTERAL MORPHINE	PARENTERAL DIAMORPHINE
Oral morphine sulfate **over 24 hours**	Subcutaneous infusion of morphine sulfate **over 24 hours**	Subcutaneous infusion of diamorphine hydrochloride **over 24 hours**
30 mg	15 mg	10 mg
60 mg	30 mg	20 mg
90 mg	45 mg	30 mg
120 mg	60 mg	40 mg
180 mg	90 mg	60 mg
240 mg	120 mg	80 mg
360 mg	180 mg	120 mg
480 mg	240 mg	160 mg
600 mg	300 mg	200 mg
780 mg	390 mg	260 mg
960 mg	480 mg	320 mg
1200 mg	600 mg	400 mg

If breakthrough pain occurs give a subcutaneous injection equivalent to one-tenth to one-sixth of the total 24-hour subcutaneous infusion dose. With an intermittent subcutaneous injection absorption is smoother so that the risk of adverse effects at peak absorption is avoided (an even better method is to use a subcutaneous butterfly needle). To minimise the risk of infection no individual subcutaneous infusion solution should be used for longer than 24 hours.

Drugs and sport

Anti-doping

UK Anti-Doping, the national body responsible for the UK's anti-doping policy, advises that athletes are personally responsible should a prohibited substance be detected in their body. Information regarding the use of medicines in sport is available from:

UK Anti-doping
Fleetbank House
2-6 Salisbury Square
London
EC4Y 8AE
Tel: (020) 7842 3450
ukad@ukad.org.uk
www.ukad.org.uk

Information about the prohibited status of specific medications based on the current World Anti-Doping Agency Prohibited List is available from Global Drug Reference Online: www.globaldro.com/UK/search

General Medical Council's advice

Doctors who prescribe or collude in the provision of drugs or treatment with the intention of improperly enhancing an individual's performance in sport contravene the GMC's guidance, and such actions would usually raise a question of a doctor's continued registration. This does not preclude the provision of any care or treatment where the doctor's intention is to protect or improve the patient's health.

Prescribing in dental practice

General guidance

Advice on the drug management of dental and oral conditions has been integrated into the main text. For ease of access, guidance on such conditions is usually identified by means of a relevant heading (e.g. Dental and Orofacial Pain) in the appropriate sections.

The following is a list of topics of particular relevance to dentists.

Prescribing by dentists, see Prescription writing p. 5
Oral side-effects of drugs, see Adverse reactions to drugs p. 12
Medical emergencies in dental practice, see BNF
Medical problems in dental practice, see BNF

Drug management of dental and oral conditions

Dental and orofacial pain, see Analgesics p. 258

Neuropathic pain p. 281
Non-opioid analgesics and compound analgesic preparations, see Analgesics p. 258
Opioid analgesics, see Analgesics p. 258
Non-steroidal anti-inflammatory drugs p. 621

Oral infections

Bacterial infections, see Antibacterials, principles of therapy p. 287

Phenoxymethylpenicillin p. 324
Broad-spectrum penicillins (amoxicillin p. 325 and ampicillin p. 326)
Cephalosporins (cefalexin p. 304 and cefradine p. 305)
Tetracyclines p. 337
Macrolides (clarithromycin p. 315, erythromycin p. 316 and azithromycin p. 314)
Clindamycin p. 313
Metronidazole p. 319
Fusidic acid p. 342

Fungal infections

Local treatment, see Oropharyngeal fungal infections p. 679
Systemic treatment, see Antifungals, systemic use p. 355

Viral infections

Herpetic gingivostomatitis, local treatment, see Oropharyngeal viral infections p. 681
Herpetic gingivostomatitis, systemic treatment, see Oropharyngeal viral infections p. 681 and Herpesvirus infections p. 386
Herpes labialis p. 691

Anaesthetics, anxiolytics and hypnotics

Sedation, anaesthesia, and resuscitation in dental practice p. 774
Hypnotics, see Hypnotics and anxiolytics p. 281
Sedation for dental procedures, see Hypnotics and anxiolytics p. 281
Local anaesthesia p. 792

Minerals

Fluoride p. 675

Oral ulceration and inflammation p. 676
Mouthwashes and gargles, see Mouthwashes and other preparations for oropharyngeal use p. 673
Dry mouth, see Treatment of dry mouth p. 671
Aromatic inhalations, see Aromatic inhalations, cough preparations and systemic nasal decongestants p. 180
Nasal decongestants, see Aromatic inhalations, cough preparations and systemic nasal decongestants p. 180

Dental Practitioners' Formulary p. 1019

Drugs and sport

Chapter 1
Gastro-intestinal system

CONTENTS

1 Chronic bowel disorders

Chronic bowel disorders

Overview

Individual symptoms of chronic bowel disorders need specific treatment including dietary manipulation as well as drug treatment and the maintenance of a liberal fluid intake.

Clostridium difficile infection

Clostridium difficile infection is caused by colonisation of the colon with *Clostridium difficile* and production of toxin. It often follows antibiotic therapy and is usually of acute onset, but may become chronic. It is a particular hazard of ampicillin p. 326, amoxicillin p. 325, co-amoxiclav p. 328, second- and third-generation cephalosporins, clindamycin p. 313, and quinolones, but few antibacterials are free of this side-effect. Oral metronidazole p. 319 or oral vancomycin p. 312 are used as specific treatment; vancomycin may be preferred for very sick patients. Metronidazole can be given by intravenous infusion if oral treatment is inappropriate.

1.1 Inflammatory bowel disease

Crohn's disease

20-Dec-2016

Description of condition

Crohn's disease is a chronic, inflammatory bowel disease that mainly affects the gastro-intestinal tract. It is characterised by thickened areas of the gastro-intestinal wall with inflammation extending through all layers, deep ulceration and fissuring of the mucosa, and the presence of granulomas; affected areas may occur in any part of the gastro-intestinal tract, interspersed with areas of relatively normal tissue. Crohn's disease may present as recurrent attacks, with acute exacerbations combined with periods of remission or less active disease. Symptoms depend on the site of disease but may include abdominal pain, diarrhoea, fever, weight loss, and rectal bleeding.

Complications of Crohn's disease include intestinal strictures, abscesses in the wall of the intestine or adjacent structures, fistulae, anaemia, malnutrition, colorectal and small bowel cancers, and growth failure and delayed puberty in children. Crohn's disease may also be associated with extra-intestinal manifestation: the most common are arthritis and abnormalities of the joints, eyes, liver and skin. Crohn's disease is also a cause of secondary osteoporosis and those at greatest risk should be monitored for osteopenia and assessed for the risk of fractures.

Up to a third of patients with Crohn's disease are diagnosed before the age of 21 years but there is a lack of evidence regarding treatment for children. Paediatric practice is often based on extrapolation from adult studies.

Fistulating Crohn's disease

Fistulating Crohn's disease is a complication that involves the formation of a fistula between the intestine and adjacent structures, such as perianal skin, bladder, and vagina. It occurs in about one quarter of patients, mostly when the disease involves the ileocolonic area.

Aims of treatment

Treatment is largely directed at the induction and maintenance of remission and the relief of symptoms. Active treatment of acute Crohn's disease should be distinguished from preventing relapse. The aims of drug treatment are to reduce symptoms and maintain or improve quality of life, while minimising toxicity related to drugs over both the short and long term. Drug treatment should always be initiated by a paediatric gastroenterologist.

In fistulating Crohn's disease, surgery and medical treatment aim to close and maintain closure of the fistula.

Non-drug treatment

EvGr In addition to drug treatment, management options for Crohn's disease include smoking cessation and attention to nutrition, which plays an important role in supportive care. Surgery may be considered in certain children with early disease limited to the distal ileum and in severe or chronic active disease. Ⓐ

Drug treatment

Treatment of acute disease

Monotherapy

EvGr A corticosteroid (either prednisolone p. 421 or methylprednisolone p. 421 or intravenous hydrocortisone p. 420), is used to induce remission in children with a first presentation or a single inflammatory exacerbation of Crohn's disease in a 12-month period.

Enteral nutrition is an alternative to a corticosteroid when there is concern about growth or side effects.

In children with distal ileal, ileocaecal or right-sided colonic disease, in whom a conventional corticosteroid is unsuitable or contra-indicated, budesonide p. 31 [unlicensed] may be considered. Budesonide is less effective but may cause fewer side-effects than other corticosteroids, as systemic exposure is limited. Aminosalicylates (such as sulfasalazine p. 30 and mesalazine p. 27) are an alternative option in these children. They are less effective than a corticosteroid or budesonide [unlicensed], but may be preferred because they have fewer side-effects. Aminosalicylates and budesonide are not appropriate for severe presentations or exacerbations. Ⓐ

Add-on treatment

EvGr Add on treatment is prescribed if there are two or more inflammatory exacerbations in a 12-month period, or the corticosteroid dose cannot be reduced.

Azathioprine p. 495 or mercaptopurine p. 516 [unlicensed indications] can be added to a corticosteroid or budesonide to induce remission. In children who cannot tolerate azathioprine or mercaptopurine or in whom thiopurine methyltransferase (TPMT) activity is deficient, methotrexate p. 517 can be added to a corticosteroid.

Under specialist supervision, monoclonal antibody therapies, adalimumab p. 614 and infliximab p. 31, are options for the treatment of severe, active Crohn's disease, following inadequate response to conventional therapies or in those who are intolerant of or have contra-indications to conventional therapy. Ⓐ See also *National funding/access decisions* for adalimumab and infliximab.

EvGr Adalimumab and infliximab can be used as monotherapy or combined with an immunosuppressant, although there is uncertainty about the comparative effectiveness. Ⓐ There are concerns about the long-term safety of adalimumab and infliximab in children; malignancies, including hepatosplenic T- cell lymphoma, have been reported.

Maintenance of remission

EvGr Children, and their parents or carers, should be made aware of the risk of relapse with and without drug treatment, and symptoms that may suggest a relapse (most frequently unintended weight loss, abdominal pain, diarrhoea and general ill-health). For those who choose not to receive maintenance treatment during remission, a suitable follow up plan should be agreed upon and information provided on how to access healthcare if a relapse should occur.

Azathioprine or mercaptopurine [unlicensed indications] as monotherapy can be used to maintain remission when previously used with a corticosteroid to induce remission. They may also be used in children who have not previously received these drugs (particularly those with adverse prognostic factors such as early age of onset, perianal disease, corticosteroid use at presentation, and severe presentations). Methotrexate [unlicensed] can be used to maintain remission only in children who required methotrexate to induce remission, or who are intolerant of or are not suitable for azathioprine or mercaptopurine for maintenance. Corticosteroids or budesonide should not be used. Ⓐ

Maintaining remission following surgery

EvGr Azathioprine or mercaptopurine can be considered to maintain remission after surgery in children with adverse prognostic factors such as more than one resection, or previously complicated or debilitating disease (for example, abscess, involvement of adjacent structures, fistulating or penetrating disease). Aminosalicylates can also be considered as an option, however budesonide or enteral nutrition should not be used. Ⓐ

Other treatments

EvGr Loperamide hydrochloride p. 47 can be used to manage diarrhoea associated with Crohn's disease in children who do not have colitis. Ⓐ Colestyramine p. 125 is licensed for the relief of diarrhoea associated with Crohn's disease. See also Acute diarrhoea p. 46.

Fistulating Crohn's disease

Perianal fistulae are the most common occurrence in children with fistulating Crohn's disease. EvGr Treatment may not be necessary for simple, asymptomatic perianal fistulae. When fistulae are symptomatic, local drainage and surgery may be required in conjunction with medical therapy.

Metronidazole p. 319 or ciprofloxacin p. 333 [unlicensed indications], alone or in combination, can improve symptoms of fistulating Crohn's disease but complete healing occurs rarely. Metronidazole should be given for at least 6 weeks but no longer than 3 months because of concerns about peripheral neuropathy. Other antibacterials should be given if specifically indicated (e.g. in sepsis associated with fistulae and perianal disease) and for managing bacterial overgrowth in the small bowel.

Either azathioprine p. 495 or mercaptopurine p. 516 [unlicensed indications] is used to control the inflammation in perianal and enterocutaneous fistulating Crohn's disease and they are continued for maintenance.

Infliximab p. 31 is recommended for children with perianal and enterocutaneous active fistulating Crohn's disease who have not responded to conventional therapy (including antibacterials, drainage and immunosuppressive treatments), or who are intolerant of or have contra-indications to conventional therapy. Infliximab should be used after ensuring that all sepsis is actively draining.

Abscess drainage, fistulotomy, and seton insertion may be appropriate, particularly before infliximab treatment.

Azathioprine, mercaptopurine or infliximab should be continued as maintenance treatment for at least one year.

For the management of non-perianal fistulating Crohn's disease (including entero-gynaecological and enterovesical fistulae) surgery is the only recommended approach. Ⓐ

Useful Resources

Crohn's disease: management in adults, children and young people. Clinical guideline 152. October 2012 (updated May 2016).
www.nice.org.uk/guidance/cg152

Ulcerative colitis
20-Feb-2017

Description of condition

Ulcerative colitis is a chronic inflammatory condition, characterised by diffuse mucosal inflammation—it has a relapsing-remitting pattern. It is a life-long disease that is associated with significant morbidity. Ulcerative colitis is more common in adults; however in children it predominately presents between the ages of 5 and 16 years.

The pattern of inflammation is continuous, extending from the rectum upwards to a varying degree. Inflammation of the rectum is referred to as **proctitis**, and inflammation of the rectum and sigmoid colon as **proctosigmoiditis**. **Left-sided colitis** refers to disease involving the colon distal to the splenic flexure. **Extensive colitis** affects the colon proximal to the splenic flexure, and includes pan-colitis, where the whole colon is involved. Child-onset ulcerative colitis is classified as extensive in 60–80 % of all cases. Common symptoms of active disease or relapse include bloody diarrhoea, an urgent need to defaecate, and abdominal pain.

Ulcerative colitis is classified as **subacute** if it is moderate-to-severely active disease which can be managed in an outpatient setting, and does not require hospitalisation or consideration of urgent surgical intervention.

Complications associated with ulcerative colitis include an increased risk of colorectal cancer, secondary osteoporosis, venous thromboembolism and toxic megacolon. Growth and pubertal development can be affected in children.

Aims of treatment

Treatment is focussed on treating active disease to manage symptoms and to induce and maintain remission.

Drug treatment

Overview

[EvGr] Management of ulcerative colitis is dependent on factors such as clinical severity, extent of disease, and the child's preference. As limited distal disease is uncommon in children, paediatric treatment strategy depends mainly on disease severity rather than the extent of disease. Clinical and laboratory investigations are used to determine the extent and severity of disease and to guide treatment. Severity is classified as mild, moderate or severe (or in remission) by using the Paediatric Ulcerative Colitis Activity Index to assess bowel movement, limitations on daily activity and the presence of abdominal pain or melaena—see the NICE guideline for Ulcerative Colitis for further information (*Useful resources* below).

The extent of disease should be considered when choosing the route of administration for aminosalicylates and corticosteroids; whether oral treatment, topical treatment or both are to be used. ⟨A⟩

If the inflammation is distal, a rectal preparation is adequate, but if the inflammation is extended, systemic medication is required. Either suppositories or enemas can be offered, taking into account the child's preferences. [EvGr] Rectal foam preparations and suppositories can be used when children have difficulty retaining liquid enemas.

Diarrhoea that is associated with active ulcerative colitis is sometimes treated with anti-diarrhoeal drugs (such as loperamide hydrochloride p. 47 [unlicensed under 4 years]) on the advice of a specialist; however their use is contra-indicated in acute ulcerative colitis as they can increase the risk of toxic megacolon.

A macrogol-containing osmotic laxative (such as macrogol 3350 with potassium chloride, sodium bicarbonate and sodium chloride p. 41) may be useful for proximal faecal loading in proctitis. ⟨E⟩

Oral aminosalicylates for the treatment of ulcerative colitis are available in different preparations and release forms. [EvGr] The preparation and dosing schedule should be chosen taking into account the delivery characteristics and suitability for the patient. When used to maintain remission, single daily doses of oral aminosalicylates can be more effective than multiple daily dosing, but may result in more side-effects. ⟨A⟩

Treatment of acute mild-to-moderate ulcerative colitis

[EvGr] Acute treatment to induce remission generally consists of an aminosalicylate with or without a corticosteroid.

Aminosalicylates are recommended as first-line treatment for children at first presentation or with an exacerbation. Oral aminosalicylates (balsalazide sodium p. 27 [unlicensed], mesalazine p. 27 [unlicensed under 6 years], olsalazine sodium p. 30 [unlicensed under 12 years] or sulfasalazine p. 30 [unlicensed under 2 years]) are recommended as first line **except** in children with **proctitis** or **proctosigmoiditis** where a rectal aminosalicylate (mesalazine or sulfasalazine [both unlicensed under 6 years])

is more effective. A rectal corticosteroid (budesonide p. 31 [unlicensed], hydrocortisone p. 420 [unlicensed under 2 years] or prednisolone p. 421) or oral prednisolone [unlicensed under 2 years] alone can be considered in children with proctitis or proctosigmoiditis who are intolerant to or decline treatment with aminosalicylates, or in whom aminosalicylates are contra-indicated.

Addition of oral beclometasone dipropionate p. 154 [unlicensed] or a rectal aminosalicylate to oral aminosalicylate treatment may also be considered in children with **left-sided** or **extensive disease**. Oral prednisolone [unlicensed under 2 years] alone is recommended for children who cannot tolerate or who decline aminosalicylates, or in whom aminosalicylates are contra-indicated.

Oral prednisolone [unlicensed under 2 years] should be considered for the treatment of children with subacute proctitis or proctosigmoiditis.

In all extents of disease, if there are no improvements within four weeks of initial treatment or if symptoms worsen, addition of oral prednisolone to aminosalicylate therapy can be considered (discontinue beclometasone dipropionate if adding oral prednisolone). If there is still no response after 2–4 weeks of treatment with prednisolone, consider adding oral tacrolimus p. 499 [unlicensed indication] to prednisolone to induce remission. ⟨A⟩

[EvGr] Alternatively, on specialist advice, infliximab p. 31 [unlicensed indication; can be used in children over 6 years] or intravenous tacrolimus [unlicensed indication] can be added, if there is no response after 2–4 weeks of treatment with prednisolone. ⟨E⟩

[EvGr] Evaluation of response should be done early to allow tapering of corticosteroids and ongoing treatment. Unnecessary corticosteroid exposure is to be avoided to minimise growth retardation and other corticosteroid-related side effects. ⟨A⟩

Treatment of acute severe ulcerative colitis

Acute severe ulcerative colitis of any extent can be life-threatening and is regarded as a medical emergency. [EvGr] Immediate hospital admission is required for treatment.

Intravenous corticosteroids (such as hydrocortisone or methylprednisolone p. 421) should be given to induce remission in children with acute severe ulcerative colitis (whether it is a first presentation or an inflammatory exacerbation) while assessing the need for surgery. If intravenous corticosteroids are contra-indicated, declined or cannot be tolerated, then intravenous ciclosporin p. 496 [unlicensed indication], or surgery should be considered. A combination of intravenous ciclosporin with intravenous corticosteroids, or surgery is second line therapy for children who have little or no improvement within 72 hours of starting intravenous corticosteroids or in children whose symptoms worsen despite treatment with a corticosteroid. ⟨A⟩

[EvGr] Alternatively, infliximab can be used on specialist advice in children over 6 years, if there is little or no improvement within 72 hours of starting intravenous corticosteroids or in children whose symptoms worsen despite treatment with a corticosteroid.

In patients who experience an initial response to steroids followed by deterioration, stool cultures should be taken to exclude pathogens; cytomegalovirus activation should be considered. ⟨E⟩

Infliximab for ulcerative colitis

[EvGr] Infliximab p. 31 can be used to treat acute severe active ulcerative colitis in children over 6 years who have had an inadequate response to conventional treatment (including corticosteroids and azathioprine p. 495 or mercaptopurine p. 516) or if conventional treatment is not tolerated or contra-indicated. Treatment with these agents is continued into the maintenance phase if effective and tolerated. ⟨A⟩ See also *National funding/access decisions* for infliximab.

EvGr Infliximab can also be used to treat acute exacerbations of severely active ulcerative colitis in children over 6 years, if ciclosporin p. 496 is contra-indicated or clinically inappropriate. ⟨A⟩

Maintaining remission in mild, moderate or severe ulcerative colitis

EvGr To reduce the chances of relapse occurring, maintenance therapy with an aminosalicylate is recommended in most children. Corticosteroids are **not** suitable for maintenance treatment because of their side-effects.

After a mild-to-moderate inflammatory exacerbation of *proctitis* or *proctosigmoiditis*, a rectal aminosalicylate can be started alone or in combination with an oral aminosalicylate, administered daily or as part of an intermittent regimen (such as twice to three times weekly or the first seven days of each month). An oral aminosalicylate can be used alone in children who prefer not to use enemas or suppositories, although, this may not be as effective.

A low dose of oral aminosalicylate is given to maintain remission in children after a mild-to-moderate inflammatory exacerbation of *left-sided or extensive* ulcerative colitis. ⟨A⟩

Oral aminosalicylates are available in different preparations and release forms. EvGr The preparation and dosing schedule should be chosen taking into account the delivery characteristics and suitability for the child. When used to maintain remission single daily dosing of oral aminosalicylates can be more effective than multiple daily dosing, but may result in more side-effects.

Oral azathioprine or mercaptopurine [unlicensed indications] can be considered to maintain remission, if there has been two or more inflammatory exacerbations in a 12-month period that require treatment with systemic corticosteroids or if remission is not maintained by aminosalicylates, or following a single acute severe episode. ⟨A⟩ EvGr Oral azathioprine or mercaptopurine is usually required in these cases as an aminosalicylate alone may be ineffective in more severe disease. ⟨E⟩

There is no evidence to support the use of methotrexate p. 517 to induce or maintain remission in ulcerative colitis though its use is common in clinical practice.

Non-drug treatment

EvGr Surgery may be necessary as emergency treatment for severe ulcerative colitis that does not respond to drug treatment. Patients can also choose to have elective surgery for unresponsive or frequently relapsing disease that is affecting their quality of life. ⟨A⟩

Useful Resources

NICE. Ulcerative colitis: management in adults, children and young people. Clinical guideline 166. June 2013. www.nice.org.uk/guidance/CG166/

AMINOSALICYLATES

Aminosalicylates

- **SIDE-EFFECTS**
- **Rare** Acute pancreatitis · agranulocytosis · alopecia · aplastic anaemia · arthralgia · blood disorders · eosinophilia · fibrosing alveolitis · hepatitis · interstitial nephritis · leucopenia · lung disorders · lupus erythematosus-like syndrome · methaemoglobinaemia · myalgia · myocarditis · nephrotic syndrome · neutropenia · pericarditis · peripheral neuropathy · renal dysfunction · skin reactions · Stevens-Johnson syndrome · thrombocytopenia
- **Frequency not known** Abdominal pain · diarrhoea · exacerbation of symptoms of colitis · headache · hypersensitivity reactions · nausea · rash · urticaria · vomiting

SIDE-EFFECTS, FURTHER INFORMATION
- Blood Disorders A blood count should be performed and the drug stopped immediately if there is suspicion of a blood dyscrasia.
- **ALLERGY AND CROSS-SENSITIVITY** Contra-indicated in salicylate hypersensitivity.
- **RENAL IMPAIRMENT** Renal function should be monitored more frequently in renal impairment.
- **MONITORING REQUIREMENTS** Renal function should be monitored before starting an oral aminosalicylate, at 3 months of treatment, and then annually during treatment.
- **PATIENT AND CARER ADVICE**
  Blood disorders Patients receiving aminosalicylates, and their carers, should be advised to report any unexplained bleeding, bruising, purpura, sore throat, fever or malaise that occurs during treatment.

⤒ above

Balsalazide sodium

- **INDICATIONS AND DOSE**

Treatment of mild to moderate ulcerative colitis, acute attack
- BY MOUTH
  - Child 12–17 years: 2.25 g 3 times a day until remission occurs or for up to maximum of 12 weeks

Maintenance of remission of ulcerative colitis
- BY MOUTH
  - Child 12–17 years: 1.5 g twice daily (max. per dose 3 g), adjusted according to response; maximum 6 g per day

- **UNLICENSED USE** Not licensed for use in children under 18 years.
- **CAUTIONS** History of asthma
- **INTERACTIONS** → Appendix 1: balsalazide
- **SIDE-EFFECTS** Cholelithiasis
- **PREGNANCY** Manufacturer advises avoid.
- **BREAST FEEDING** Diarrhoea may develop in the infant. Monitor breast-fed infants for diarrhoea.
- **HEPATIC IMPAIRMENT** Avoid in severe impairment.
- **RENAL IMPAIRMENT** Manufacturer advises avoid in moderate to severe impairment.

- **MEDICINAL FORMS**
  There can be variation in the licensing of different medicines containing the same drug.
  Capsule
  CAUTIONARY AND ADVISORY LABELS 21, 25
  - Colazide (Almirall Ltd)
    Balsalazide disodium 750 mg Colazide 750mg capsules | 130 capsule PoM £30.42 DT price = £30.42

⤒ above

Mesalazine

- **INDICATIONS AND DOSE**

ASACOL® MR 400MG TABLETS

Treatment of mild to moderate ulcerative colitis, acute attack
- BY MOUTH
  - Child 12–17 years: 800 mg 3 times a day

Maintenance of remission of ulcerative colitis and Crohn's ileo-colitis
- BY MOUTH
  - Child 12–17 years: 400–800 mg 2–3 times a day

continued →

ASACOL® FOAM ENEMA

Treatment of acute attack of mild to moderate ulcerative colitis affecting the rectosigmoid region

▸ BY RECTUM

▸ Child 12–17 years: 1 g daily for 4–6 weeks, to be administered into the rectum

Treatment of acute attack of mild to moderate ulcerative colitis, affecting the descending colon

▸ BY RECTUM

▸ Child 12–17 years: 2 g once daily for 4–6 weeks, to be administered into the rectum

ASACOL® SUPPOSITORIES

Treatment and maintenance of remission of ulcerative colitis affecting the rectosigmoid region

▸ BY RECTUM

▸ Child 12–17 years: 250–500 mg 3 times a day, last dose to be administered at bedtime

IPOCOL®

Treatment of mild to moderate ulcerative colitis, acute attack

▸ BY MOUTH

▸ Child 6–17 years (body-weight 40 kg and above): 800 mg 3 times a day

Maintenance of remission of ulcerative colitis

▸ BY MOUTH

▸ Child 6–17 years (body-weight 40 kg and above): 1.2–2 g daily in divided doses

OCTASA®

Treatment of mild to moderate ulcerative colitis, acute attack

▸ BY MOUTH

▸ Child 6–17 years (body-weight 40 kg and above): 2.4–4 g daily in divided doses

Maintenance of remission of ulcerative colitis and Crohn's ileo-colitis

▸ BY MOUTH

▸ Child 6–17 years (body-weight 40 kg and above): 1.2–2 g once daily, alternatively daily in divided doses

PENTASA® GRANULES

Treatment of mild to moderate ulcerative colitis, acute attack

▸ BY MOUTH

▸ Child 5–17 years (body-weight up to 40 kg): 10–20 mg/kg 3 times a day

▸ Child 5–17 years (body-weight 40 kg and above): 1–2 g twice daily, total daily dose may alternatively be given in 3–4 divided doses

Maintenance of remission of ulcerative colitis

▸ BY MOUTH

▸ Child 5–17 years (body-weight up to 40 kg): 7.5–15 mg/kg twice daily, total daily dose may alternatively be given in 3 divided doses

▸ Child 5–17 years (body-weight 40 kg and above): 2 g once daily

PENTASA® RETENTION ENEMA

Treatment of acute attack of mild to moderate ulcerative colitis affecting the rectosigmoid region

▸ BY RECTUM

▸ Child 12–17 years: 1 g once daily, dose to be administered at bedtime

PENTASA® SUPPOSITORIES

Treatment of acute attack, ulcerative proctitis

▸ BY RECTUM

▸ Child 12–17 years: 1 g daily for 2–4 weeks

Maintenance, ulcerative proctitis

▸ BY RECTUM

▸ Child 12–17 years: 1 g daily

PENTASA® TABLETS

Treatment of mild to moderate ulcerative colitis, acute attack

▸ BY MOUTH

▸ Child 5–17 years (body-weight up to 40 kg): 10–20 mg/kg 3 times a day

▸ Child 5–17 years (body-weight 40 kg and above): 1–2 g twice daily, total daily dose may alternatively be given in 3 divided doses

Maintenance of remission of ulcerative colitis

▸ BY MOUTH

▸ Child 5–17 years (body-weight up to 40 kg): 7.5–15 mg/kg twice daily, total daily dose may alternatively be given in 3 divided doses

▸ Child 5–17 years (body-weight 40 kg and above): 2 g once daily

SALOFALK® ENEMA

Treatment of acute attack of mild to moderate ulcerative colitis or maintenance of remission

▸ BY RECTUM

▸ Child 12–17 years: 2 g once daily, dose to be administered at bedtime

SALOFALK® GRANULES

Treatment of mild to moderate ulcerative colitis, acute attack

▸ BY MOUTH

▸ Child 5–17 years (body-weight up to 40 kg): 30–50 mg/kg once daily, dose preferably given in the morning, alternatively 10–20 mg/kg 3 times a day

▸ Child 5–17 years (body-weight 40 kg and above): 1.5–3 g once daily, dose preferably given in the morning, alternatively 0.5–1 g 3 times a day

Maintenance of remission of ulcerative colitis

▸ BY MOUTH

▸ Child 5–17 years (body-weight up to 40 kg): 7.5–15 mg/kg twice daily, total daily dose may alternatively be given in 3 divided doses

▸ Child 5–17 years (body-weight 40 kg and above): 500 mg 3 times a day

SALOFALK® RECTAL FOAM

Treatment of mild ulcerative colitis affecting sigmoid colon and rectum

▸ BY RECTUM

▸ Child 12–17 years: 2 g once daily, dose to be administered into the rectum at bedtime, alternatively 2 g daily in 2 divided doses

SALOFALK® SUPPOSITORIES

Treatment of acute attack of mild to moderate ulcerative colitis affecting the rectum, sigmoid colon and descending colon

▸ BY RECTUM

▸ Child 12–17 years: 0.5–1 g 2–3 times a day, adjusted according to response, dose to be given using 500 mg suppositories

SALOFALK® TABLETS

Treatment of mild to moderate ulcerative colitis, acute attack

▸ BY MOUTH

▸ Child 5–17 years (body-weight up to 40 kg): 10–20 mg/kg 3 times a day

▸ Child 5–17 years (body-weight 40 kg and above): 0.5–1 g 3 times a day

Maintenance of remission of ulcerative colitis

▸ BY MOUTH

▸ Child 5–17 years (body-weight up to 40 kg): 7.5–15 mg/kg twice daily, total daily dose may alternatively be given in 3 divided doses

▸ Child 5-17 years (body-weight 40 kg and above): 500 mg 3 times a day

DOSE EQUIVALENCE AND CONVERSION
▸ There is no evidence to show that any one oral preparation of mesalazine is more effective than another; however, the delivery characteristics of oral mesalazine preparations may vary.

- UNLICENSED USE
▸ With oral use *Asacol*® (all preparations) not licensed for use in children under 18 years. *Pentasa*® tablets not licensed for use in children under 15 years. *Pentasa*® granules and *Salofalk*® tablets and granules not licensed for use in children under 6 years.
▸ With rectal use *Asacol*® (all preparations) and *Salofalk*® enema not licensed for use in children under 18 years. *Salofalk*® suppositories and *Pentasa*® suppositories not licensed for use in children under 15 years. *Salofalk*® rectal foam no dose recommendations for children (age range not specified by manufacturer).
- CONTRA-INDICATIONS Blood clotting abnormalities
- CAUTIONS Pulmonary disease
- INTERACTIONS → Appendix 1: mesalazine
- SIDE-EFFECTS
▸ Rare Dizziness
▸ Very rare Oligospermia (reversible)
- PREGNANCY Negligible quantities cross placenta.
- BREAST FEEDING Diarrhoea reported in breast-fed infants, but negligible amounts of mesalazine detected in breast milk. Monitor breast-fed infant for diarrhoea.
- HEPATIC IMPAIRMENT Avoid in severe impairment.
- RENAL IMPAIRMENT Use with caution. Avoid if estimated glomerular filtration rate less than 20 mL/minute/1.73 m².
- DIRECTIONS FOR ADMINISTRATION
PENTASA® TABLETS Tablets may be halved, quartered, or dispersed in water, but should not be chewed.
SALOFALK® GRANULES Granules should be placed on tongue and washed down with water without chewing.
PENTASA® GRANULES Granules should be placed on tongue and washed down with water or orange juice without chewing.
Contents of one sachet should be weighed and divided immediately before use; discard any remaining granules.
- PRESCRIBING AND DISPENSING INFORMATION There is no evidence to show that any one oral preparation of mesalazine is more effective than another; however, the delivery characteristics of oral mesalazine preparations may vary.
Flavours of granule formulations of *Salofalk*® may include vanilla.
- PATIENT AND CARER ADVICE
If it is necessary to switch a patient to a different brand of mesalazine, the patient should be advised to report any changes in symptoms.
Some products may require special administration advice; patients and carers should be informed.
Medicines for Children leaflet: Mesalazine (oral) for inflammatory bowel disease www.medicinesforchildren.org.uk/mesalazine-oral-for-inflammatory-bowel-disease
Medicines for Children leaflet: Mesalazine foam enema for inflammatory bowel disease www.medicinesforchildren.org.uk/mesalazine-foam-enema-for-inflammatory-bowel-disease
Medicines for Children leaflet: Mesalazine liquid enema for inflammatory bowel disease www.medicinesforchildren.org.uk/mesalazine-liquid-enema-for-inflammatory-bowel-disease
Medicines for Children leaflet: Mesalazine suppositories for inflammatory bowel disease www.medicinesforchildren.org.uk/mesalazine-suppositories-for-inflammatory-bowel-disease

- MEDICINAL FORMS
There can be variation in the licensing of different medicines containing the same drug.

Modified-release tablet
CAUTIONARY AND ADVISORY LABELS 21 (does not apply to Pentasa® tablets), 25 (does not apply to Pentasa® tablets)
▸ Pentasa (Ferring Pharmaceuticals Ltd)
   Mesalazine 500 mg Pentasa 500mg modified-release tablets | 100 tablet PoM £30.74 DT price = £30.74
   Mesalazine 1 gram Pentasa 1g modified-release tablets | 60 tablet PoM £36.89 DT price = £36.89

Foam
EXCIPIENTS: May contain Cetostearyl alcohol (including cetyl and stearyl alcohol), disodium edetate, hydroxybenzoates (parabens), polysorbates, propylene glycol, sodium metabisulfite
▸ Asacol (Allergan Ltd)
   Mesalazine 1 gram per 1 application Asacol 1g/application foam enema | 14 dose PoM £26.72 DT price = £30.17
▸ Salofalk (Dr. Falk Pharma UK Ltd)
   Mesalazine 1 gram per 1 application Salofalk 1g/application foam enema | 14 dose PoM £30.17 DT price = £30.17

Gastro-resistant tablet
CAUTIONARY AND ADVISORY LABELS 5 (does not apply to Octasa®), 25
▸ Asacol MR (Allergan Ltd)
   Mesalazine 400 mg Asacol 400mg MR gastro-resistant tablets | 84 tablet PoM £27.45 DT price = £27.45 | 168 tablet PoM £54.90
   Mesalazine 800 mg Asacol 800mg MR gastro-resistant tablets | 84 tablet PoM £54.90 DT price = £54.90
▸ Octasa MR (Tillotts Pharma Ltd)
   Mesalazine 400 mg Octasa 400mg MR gastro-resistant tablets | 90 tablet PoM £16.58 DT price = £16.58 | 120 tablet PoM £22.10
   Mesalazine 800 mg Octasa 800mg MR gastro-resistant tablets | 90 tablet PoM £40.38 DT price = £80.75 | 180 tablet PoM £80.75 DT price = £80.75
▸ Salofalk (Dr. Falk Pharma UK Ltd)
   Mesalazine 250 mg Salofalk 250mg gastro-resistant tablets | 100 tablet PoM £16.19
   Mesalazine 500 mg Salofalk 500mg gastro-resistant tablets | 100 tablet PoM £32.38

Suppository
▸ Asacol (Allergan Ltd)
   Mesalazine 250 mg Asacol 250mg suppositories | 20 suppository PoM £4.82 DT price = £4.82
   Mesalazine 500 mg Asacol 500mg suppositories | 10 suppository PoM £4.82 DT price = £4.82
▸ Pentasa (Ferring Pharmaceuticals Ltd)
   Mesalazine 1 gram Pentasa 1g suppositories | 28 suppository PoM £40.01 DT price = £40.01
▸ Salofalk (Dr. Falk Pharma UK Ltd)
   Mesalazine 500 mg Salofalk 500mg suppositories | 30 suppository PoM £14.81
   Mesalazine 1 gram Salofalk 1g suppositories | 30 suppository PoM £29.62

Modified-release granules
CAUTIONARY AND ADVISORY LABELS 25 (does not apply to Pentasa® granules)
EXCIPIENTS: May contain Aspartame
▸ Pentasa (Ferring Pharmaceuticals Ltd)
   Mesalazine 1 gram Pentasa 1g modified-release granules sachets sugar-free | 50 sachet PoM £30.74 DT price = £30.74
   Mesalazine 2 gram Pentasa 2g modified-release granules sachets sugar-free | 60 sachet PoM £73.78 DT price = £73.78
   Mesalazine 4 gram Pentasa 4g modified-release granules sachets sugar-free | 30 sachet PoM £73.78 DT price = £73.78
▸ Salofalk (Dr. Falk Pharma UK Ltd)
   Mesalazine 500 mg Salofalk 500mg gastro-resistant modified-release granules sachets sugar-free | 100 sachet PoM £28.74
   Mesalazine 1 gram Salofalk 1g gastro-resistant modified-release granules sachets sugar-free | 50 sachet PoM £28.74 DT price = £28.74
   Mesalazine 1.5 gram Salofalk 1.5g gastro-resistant modified-release granules sachets sugar-free | 60 sachet PoM £48.85 DT price = £48.85
   Mesalazine 3 gram Salofalk 3g gastro-resistant modified-release granules sachets sugar-free | 60 sachet PoM £97.70 DT price = £97.70

Enema

> Pentasa (Ferring Pharmaceuticals Ltd)
> **Mesalazine 10 mg per 1 ml** Pentasa Mesalazine 1g/100ml enema |
> 7 enema PoM £17.73 DT price = £17.73

> Salofalk (Dr. Falk Pharma UK Ltd)
> **Mesalazine 33.9 mg per 1 ml** Salofalk 2g/59ml enema |
> 7 enema PoM £29.92 DT price = £29.92

Olsalazine sodium

● INDICATIONS AND DOSE

Treatment of acute attack of mild ulcerative colitis
> BY MOUTH
> Child 2–17 years: 500 mg twice daily, dose to be taken
> after food, then increased if necessary up to 1 g 3 times
> a day, dose to be increased over 1 week

Maintenance of remission of mild ulcerative colitis
> BY MOUTH
> Child 2–17 years: Maintenance 250–500 mg twice daily,
> dose to be taken after food

● **UNLICENSED USE** Not licensed for use in children under
12 years.

● **INTERACTIONS** → Appendix 1: olsalazine

● **SIDE-EFFECTS**
> **Common or very common** Watery diarrhoea
> **Frequency not known** Blurred vision · palpitation ·
photosensitivity · pyrexia · tachycardia

● **PREGNANCY** Manufacturer advises avoid unless potential
benefit outweighs risk.

● **BREAST FEEDING** Monitor breast-fed infants for diarrhoea.

● **RENAL IMPAIRMENT** Use with caution; manufacturer
advises avoid in significant impairment.

● **DIRECTIONS FOR ADMINISTRATION** Capsules can be
opened and contents sprinkled on food.

● **MEDICINAL FORMS**
There can be variation in the licensing of different medicines
containing the same drug. Forms available from special-order
manufacturers include: oral suspension, oral solution
Tablet
CAUTIONARY AND ADVISORY LABELS 21
> Olsalazine sodium (Non-proprietary)
> **Olsalazine sodium 500 mg** Olsalazine 500mg tablets |
> 60 tablet PoM £161.00 DT price = £161.00
Capsule
CAUTIONARY AND ADVISORY LABELS 21
> Olsalazine sodium (Non-proprietary)
> **Olsalazine sodium 250 mg** Olsalazine 250mg capsules |
> 112 capsule PoM £144.00 DT price = £144.00

Sulfasalazine

(Sulphasalazine)

● INDICATIONS AND DOSE

**Treatment of acute attack of mild to moderate and severe
ulcerative colitis | Active Crohn's disease**
> BY MOUTH
> Child 2–11 years: 10–15 mg/kg 4–6 times a day (max. per
> dose 1 g) until remission occurs; increased if necessary
> up to 60 mg/kg daily in divided doses
> Child 12–17 years: 1–2 g 4 times a day until remission
> occurs
> BY RECTUM
> Child 5–7 years: 500 mg twice daily
> Child 8–11 years: 500 mg, dose to be administered in the
> morning and 1 g, dose to be administered at night
> Child 12–17 years: 0.5–1 g twice daily

**Maintenance of remission of mild to moderate and severe
ulcerative colitis**
> BY MOUTH
> Child 2–11 years: 5–7.5 mg/kg 4 times a day (max. per
> dose 500 mg)
> Child 12–17 years: 500 mg 4 times a day
> BY RECTUM
> Child 5–7 years: 500 mg twice daily
> Child 8–11 years: 500 mg, dose to be administered in the
> morning and 1 g, dose to be administered at night
> Child 12–17 years: 0.5–1 g twice daily

Juvenile idiopathic arthritis
> BY MOUTH
> Child 2–11 years: Initially 5 mg/kg twice daily for 1 week,
> then 10 mg/kg twice daily for 1 week, then 20 mg/kg
> twice daily for 1 week; maintenance 20–25 mg/kg twice
> daily; maximum 2 g per day
> Child 12–17 years: Initially 5 mg/kg twice daily for
> 1 week, then 10 mg/kg twice daily for 1 week, then
> 20 mg/kg twice daily for 1 week; maintenance
> 20–25 mg/kg twice daily; maximum 3 g per day

● **UNLICENSED USE** Not licensed for use in children for
juvenile idiopathic arthritis.

● **CONTRA-INDICATIONS** Child under 2 years of age

● **CAUTIONS** Acute porphyrias p. 577 · G6PD deficiency ·
history of allergy · history of asthma · maintain adequate
fluid intake · risk of haematological toxicity · risk of hepatic
toxicity · slow acetylator status

● **INTERACTIONS** → Appendix 1: sulfasalazine

● **SIDE-EFFECTS**
> **Common or very common** Blood disorders · cough ·
dizziness · fever · Heinz body anaemia · insomnia ·
megaloblastic anaemia · proteinuria · pruritus · stomatitis ·
taste disturbances · tinnitus
> **Uncommon** Alopecia · convulsions · depression · dyspnoea ·
vasculitis
> **Frequency not known** Anaphylaxis · aseptic meningitis ·
ataxia · crystalluria · disturbances of smell · epidermal
necrolysis · exfoliative dermatitis · gastro-intestinal
intolerance · hallucinations · hypersensitivity reactions ·
leucopenia (especially in patients with rheumatoid
arthritis) · loss of appetite · neutropenia (especially in
patients with rheumatoid arthritis) · oligospermia ·
parotitis · photosensitivity · rashes · serum sickness · some
soft contact lenses may be stained · thrombocytopenia
(especially in patients with rheumatoid arthritis) · yellow-
orange discoloration of other body fluids · yellow-orange
discoloration of skin · yellow-orange discoloration of urine
SIDE-EFFECTS, FURTHER INFORMATION
> Gastro-intestinal side-effects Upper gastro-intestinal side-
effects common over 4 g daily.
> Blood disorders Haematological abnormalities occur usually
in the first 3 to 6 months of treatment and are reversible
on cessation of treatment.

● **PREGNANCY** Theoretical risk of neonatal haemolysis in
third trimester; adequate folate supplements should be
given to mother.

● **BREAST FEEDING** Small amounts in milk (1 report of
bloody diarrhoea); theoretical risk of neonatal haemolysis
especially in G6PD-deficient infants.

● **HEPATIC IMPAIRMENT** Use with caution.

● **RENAL IMPAIRMENT** Risk of toxicity, including crystalluria,
in moderate impairment—ensure high fluid intake. Avoid
in severe impairment.

● **MONITORING REQUIREMENTS**
> Blood disorders Close monitoring of full blood counts
(including differential white cell count and platelet count)
is necessary initially, and at monthly intervals during the
first 3 months.

▸ **Renal function** Although the manufacturer recommends renal function tests in rheumatic diseases, evidence of practical value is unsatisfactory.

▸ **Liver function** Liver function tests should be performed at monthly intervals for first 3 months.

● **PATIENT AND CARER ADVICE**
Contact lenses Some soft contact lenses may be stained.

● **MEDICINAL FORMS**
There can be variation in the licensing of different medicines containing the same drug. Forms available from special-order manufacturers include: oral suspension

Oral suspension
CAUTIONARY AND ADVISORY LABELS 14
EXCIPIENTS: May contain Alcohol
▸ Sulfasalazine (Non-proprietary)
Sulfasalazine 50 mg per 1 ml Sulfasalazine 250mg/5ml oral suspension sugar free sugar-free | 500 ml PoM £42.92 DT price = £42.92

Gastro-resistant tablet
CAUTIONARY AND ADVISORY LABELS 5, 14, 25
▸ Sulfasalazine (Non-proprietary)
Sulfasalazine 500 mg Sulfasalazine 500mg gastro-resistant tablets | 100 tablet PoM no price available | 112 tablet PoM £11.18 DT price = £11.18
▸ Salazopyrin EN (Pfizer Ltd)
Sulfasalazine 500 mg Salazopyrin EN-Tabs 500mg | 112 tablet PoM £8.43 DT price = £11.18
▸ Sulazine EC (Genesis Pharmaceuticals Ltd)
Sulfasalazine 500 mg Sulazine EC 500mg tablets | 112 tablet PoM £8.00 DT price = £11.18

Tablet
CAUTIONARY AND ADVISORY LABELS 14
▸ Sulfasalazine (Non-proprietary)
Sulfasalazine 500 mg Sulfasalazine 500mg tablets | 112 tablet PoM £9.00 DT price = £7.37
▸ Salazopyrin (Pfizer Ltd)
Sulfasalazine 500 mg Salazopyrin 500mg tablets | 112 tablet PoM £6.97 DT price = £7.37

Suppository
CAUTIONARY AND ADVISORY LABELS 14
▸ Salazopyrin (Pfizer Ltd)
Sulfasalazine 500 mg Salazopyrin 500mg suppositories | 10 suppository PoM £3.30

CORTICOSTEROIDS

F 416

Budesonide

18-May-2017

● **INDICATIONS AND DOSE**
BUDENOFALK® CAPSULES
Mild to moderate Crohn's disease affecting the ileum or ascending colon | Chronic diarrhoea due to collagenous colitis
▸ BY MOUTH
▸ **Child 12–17 years:** 3 mg 3 times a day for up to 8 weeks, reduce dose for the last 2 weeks of treatment

ENTOCORT® CAPSULES
Mild to moderate Crohn's disease affecting the ileum or ascending colon
▸ BY MOUTH
▸ **Child 12–17 years:** 9 mg once daily for up to 8 weeks; reduce dose for the last 2–4 weeks of treatment, to be taken in the morning

ENTOCORT® ENEMA
Ulcerative colitis involving rectal and recto-sigmoid disease
▸ BY RECTUM
▸ **Child 12–17 years:** 1 enema daily for 4 weeks, to be administered at bedtime

● **UNLICENSED USE** Not licensed for use in children for Crohn's disease or ulcerative colitis.

● **INTERACTIONS** → Appendix 1: corticosteroids

● **HEPATIC IMPAIRMENT** When used in autoimmune hepatitis liver function tests should be monitored every 2 weeks for 1 month, then at least every 3 months.

● **DIRECTIONS FOR ADMINISTRATION** Capsules can be opened and the contents mixed with apple or orange juice.

● **PRESCRIBING AND DISPENSING INFORMATION**
ENTOCORT® CAPSULES Dispense modified-release capsules in original container (contains desiccant).

● **MEDICINAL FORMS**
There can be variation in the licensing of different medicines containing the same drug.

Gastro-resistant capsule
CAUTIONARY AND ADVISORY LABELS 5, 10, 22, 25
▸ Budenofalk (Dr. Falk Pharma UK Ltd)
Budesonide 3 mg Budenofalk 3mg gastro-resistant capsules | 100 capsule PoM £75.05 DT price = £75.05

Modified-release capsule
CAUTIONARY AND ADVISORY LABELS 5, 10, 25
▸ Entocort CR (Tillotts Pharma Ltd)
Budesonide 3 mg Entocort CR 3mg capsules | 100 capsule PoM £84.15 DT price = £84.15

Enema
▸ Entocort (Tillotts Pharma Ltd)
Budesonide 20 microgram per 1 ml Entocort 2mg/100ml enema | 7 enema PoM £33.66

IMMUNOSUPPRESSANTS ›TUMOR NECROSIS FACTOR ALPHA (TNF-α) INHIBITORS

Infliximab

31-May-2016

● **INDICATIONS AND DOSE**
Severe active Crohn's disease
▸ BY INTRAVENOUS INFUSION
▸ **Child 6–17 years:** Initially 5 mg/kg, then 5 mg/kg after 2 weeks, then 5 mg/kg after 4 weeks, then maintenance 5 mg/kg every 8 weeks, interval between maintenance doses adjusted according to response; discontinue if no response within 10 weeks of initial dose

Fistulating Crohn's disease
▸ BY INTRAVENOUS INFUSION
▸ **Child 6–17 years:** Initially 5 mg/kg, then 5 mg/kg after 2 weeks, followed by 5 mg/kg after 4 weeks, if condition has responded consult product literature for guidance on further doses

Severe active ulcerative colitis
▸ BY INTRAVENOUS INFUSION
▸ **Child 6–17 years:** Initially 5 mg/kg, then 5 mg/kg after 2 weeks, followed by 5 mg/kg after 4 weeks, then 5 mg/kg every 8 weeks, discontinue if no response within 8 weeks of initial dose

● **UNLICENSED USE** Not licensed for fistulating Crohn's disease in children.

IMPORTANT SAFETY INFORMATION
Adequate resuscitation facilities must be available when infliximab is used.

● **CONTRA-INDICATIONS** Moderate or severe heart failure · severe infections

● **CAUTIONS** Demyelinating disorders (risk of exacerbation) · dermatomyositis · development of malignancy · hepatitis B virus—monitor for active infection · history of malignancy · history of prolonged immunosuppressant or PUVA treatment in patients with psoriasis · mild heart failure (discontinue if symptoms develop or worsen) · predisposition to infection (discontinue if new serious infection develops) · risk of delayed hypersensitivity reactions if drug-free interval exceeds 16 weeks (re-administration after interval exceeding 16 weeks not recommended)

CAUTIONS, FURTHER INFORMATION

▸ Tuberculosis Manufacturer advises to evaluate patients for active and latent tuberculosis before treatment. Active tuberculosis should be treated with standard treatment for at least 2 months before starting infliximab. If latent tuberculosis is diagnosed, treatment should be started before commencing treatment with infliximab. Patients who have previously received adequate treatment for tuberculosis can start infliximab but should be monitored every 3 months for possible recurrence. In patients without active tuberculosis but who were previously not treated adequately, chemoprophylaxis should ideally be completed before starting infliximab. In patients at high risk of tuberculosis who cannot be assessed by tuberculin skin test, chemoprophylaxis can be given concurrently with infliximab. Patients should be advised to seek medical attention if symptoms suggestive of tuberculosis develop (e.g. persistent cough, weight loss and fever).

▸ Hypersensitivity reactions Hypersensitivity reactions (including fever, chest pain, hypotension, hypertension, dyspnoea, transient visual loss, pruritus, urticaria, serum sickness-like reactions, angioedema, anaphylaxis) reported during or within 1–2 hours after infusion (risk greatest during first or second infusion or in patients who discontinue other immunosuppressants). Manufacturer advises prophylactic antipyretics, antihistamines, or hydrocortisone may be administered.

● INTERACTIONS → Appendix 1: monoclonal antibodies

● SIDE-EFFECTS

▸ **Common or very common** Alopecia · arthralgia · constipation · diarrhoea · dizziness · dry skin · dyspepsia · ecchymosis · epistaxis · flushing · gastro-intestinal haemorrhage · gastro-oesophageal reflux · hyperhydrosis · hypertension · hypoaesthesia · hypotension · myalgia · new onset or worsening psoriasis · palpitation · paraesthesia · rash · sleep disturbances · tachycardia

▸ **Uncommon** Abnormal skin pigmentation · agitation · amnesia · arrhythmia · bradycardia · bullous eruption · cheilitis · cholecystitis · confusion · eye disorders · heart failure · hepatitis · hyperkeratosis · impaired healing · intestinal perforation · nervousness · neuropathy · pancreatitis · peripheral ischaemia · pleurisy · pulmonary oedema · rosacea · seborrhoea · seizures · syncope · vaginitis

▸ **Rare** Demyelinating disorders · interstitial lung disease · leukaemia · lymphoma · melanoma · pericardial effusion · Stevens-Johnson syndrome · toxic epidermal necrolysis · vasospasm

▸ **Frequency not known** Abdominal pain · anaemia · antibody formation · aplastic anaemia · blood disorders · depression · fever · headache · hepatic failure · hepatosplenic T-cell lymphoma (more likely in inflammatory bowel disease) · hypersensitivity reactions · injection-site reactions · leucopenia · lupus erythematosus-like syndrome · Merkel cell carcinoma · nausea · pancytopenia · pruritus · thrombocytopenia · worsening heart failure · worsening symptoms of dermatomyositis

SIDE-EFFECTS, FURTHER INFORMATION
Associated with infections, sometimes severe, including tuberculosis, septicaemia, and hepatitis B reactivation.

● CONCEPTION AND CONTRACEPTION Manufacturer advises adequate contraception during and for at least 6 months after last dose.

● PREGNANCY Use only if essential.

● BREAST FEEDING Amount probably too small to be harmful.

● PRE-TREATMENT SCREENING
Tuberculosis Patients should be evaluated for tuberculosis before treatment.

● MONITORING REQUIREMENTS
▸ Monitor for infection before, during, and for 6 months after treatment.
▸ All patients should be observed carefully for 1–2 hours after infusion and resuscitation equipment should be available for immediate use (risk of hypersensitivity reactions).
▸ Monitor for symptoms of delayed hypersensitivity if re-administered after a prolonged period.
▸ Manufacturer advises periodic skin examination for non-melanoma skin cancer, particularly in patients with risk factors.

● DIRECTIONS FOR ADMINISTRATION For *intravenous infusion* reconstitute each 100-mg vial of powder with 10 mL Water for Injections; to dissolve, gently swirl vial without shaking; allow to stand for 5 minutes; dilute required dose with Sodium Chloride 0.9% to a final volume of 250 mL and give through a low protein-binding filter (1.2 micron or less) over at least 2 hours; start infusion within 3 hours of reconstitution.

● PRESCRIBING AND DISPENSING INFORMATION Infliximab is a biological medicine. Biological medicines must be prescribed and dispensed by brand name, see *Biological medicines* and *Biosimilar medicines*, under Guidance on prescribing p. 1.

● PATIENT AND CARER ADVICE An alert card should be provided.
Tuberculosis Patients and carers should be advised to seek medical attention if symptoms suggestive of tuberculosis (e.g. persistent cough, weight loss, and fever) develop.
Blood disorders Patients and carers should be advised to seek medical attention if symptoms suggestive of blood disorders (such as fever, sore throat, bruising, or bleeding) develop.
Hypersensitivity reactions Patients and carers should be advised to keep Alert card with them at all times and seek medical advice if symptoms of delayed hypersensitivity develop.

● NATIONAL FUNDING/ACCESS DECISIONS
NICE technology appraisals (TAs)
▸ **Infliximab for Crohn's disease (May 2010)** NICE TA187
In children over 6 years of age, infliximab is recommended for the treatment of severe active Crohn's disease that has not responded to conventional therapy (including corticosteroids and other drugs affecting the immune response, and primary nutrition therapy) or when conventional therapy cannot be used because of intolerance or contra-indications.

Infliximab should be given as a planned course of treatment for 12 months or until treatment failure, whichever is shorter. Treatment should be continued beyond 12 months only if there is evidence of active disease—in these cases the need for treatment should be reviewed at least annually. If the disease relapses after stopping treatment, infliximab can be restarted.
www.nice.org.uk/TA187

▸ **Infliximab, adalimumab and golimumab for treating moderately to severely active ulcerative colitis after the failure of conventional therapy (February 2015)** NICE TA329
Infliximab is an option for treating severely active ulcerative colitis in children whose disease has responded inadequately to conventional therapy including corticosteroids and mercaptopurine or azathioprine.

Infliximab should be given as a planned course of treatment until treatment fails (including the need for surgery) or until 12 months after starting treatment, whichever is shorter. Treatment should be continued only if there is clear evidence of a response. Patients who continue treatment should be reassessed every 12 months

to determine whether ongoing treatment is still clinically appropriate.
www.nice.org.uk/TA329

● MEDICINAL FORMS
There can be variation in the licensing of different medicines containing the same drug.

Powder for solution for infusion
CAUTIONARY AND ADVISORY LABELS 10
▸ Flixabi (Biogen Idec Ltd) ▼
  Infliximab 100 mg Flixabi 100mg powder for concentrate for solution for infusion vials | 1 vial [PoM] £377.00 (Hospital only)
▸ Inflectra (Hospira UK Ltd) ▼
  Infliximab 100 mg Inflectra 100mg powder for concentrate for solution for infusion vials | 1 vial [PoM] £377.66 (Hospital only)
▸ Remicade (Merck Sharp & Dohme Ltd)
  Infliximab 100 mg Remicade 100mg powder for concentrate for solution for infusion vials | 1 vial [PoM] £419.62 (Hospital only)
▸ Remsima (Napp Pharmaceuticals Ltd) ▼
  Infliximab 100 mg Remsima 100mg powder for concentrate for solution for infusion vials | 1 vial [PoM] £377.66 (Hospital only)

1.2 Coeliac disease

Coeliac disease

25-Jul-2016

Description of condition
Coeliac disease is an autoimmune condition which is associated with chronic inflammation of the small intestine. Dietary proteins known as gluten, which are present in wheat, barley and rye, activate an abnormal immune response in the intestinal mucosa, which can lead to malabsorption of nutrients.

Aims of treatment
The management of coeliac disease is aimed at eliminating symptoms (such as diarrhoea, bloating and abdominal pain) and reducing the risk of complications, including those resulting from malabsorption.

Non-drug treatment
[EvGr] The only effective treatment for coeliac disease is a strict, life-long, gluten-free diet. A range of gluten-free products is available for prescription (see *Borderline substances*). Ⓐ

Drug treatment
[EvGr] Children who have coeliac disease are at an increased risk of malabsorption of key nutrients (such as calcium and vitamin D). Supplementation of key nutrients may be required if dietary intake is insufficient.

Carers of children who have coeliac disease should be advised **not** to medicate with over-the-counter vitamin or mineral supplements. Initiation of supplementation should involve a discussion with a member of the child's healthcare team in order to identify the individual needs of the patient and to allow for appropriate ongoing monitoring. Ⓐ

Useful Resources
Coeliac disease: recognition, assessment and management. National Institute for Health and Care Excellence. Clinical guideline 20. September 2015.
www.nice.org.uk/guidance/ng20

1.3 Irritable bowel syndrome

Irritable bowel syndrome

24-Feb-2016

Description of condition
Irritable bowel syndrome (IBS) is a gastrointestinal disorder characterised by abdominal pain or discomfort that may be relieved by defaecation. It can also be associated with the passage of mucus, bloating, and disordered defaecation; either diarrhoea, constipation, or alternating diarrhoea and constipation. Constipation presents with straining, urgency, and a sensation of incomplete evacuation. Before a diagnosis of IBS is made, the symptoms should be present at least once per week for at least 2 months and other potential pathological causes of the symptoms should be excluded. IBS symptoms are often aggravated by psychological factors, such as anxieties, emotional stress, and fear.

Aims of treatment
Treatment of IBS is focused on symptom control in order to improve quality of life, including minimising abdominal pain and normalising the frequency and consistency of stools.

Non-drug treatment
[EvGr] There is no evidence of the effectiveness of any form of dietary advice or increased fibre intake in children and it is not known whether dietary advice recommended to adult patients is of benefit to children. Ⓐ
[EvGr] Eating regularly, limiting fresh fruit intake, and, reducing intake of 'resistant starch' and insoluble fibre (e.g. bran) can be recommended. If an increase in dietary fibre is required, soluble fibre such as oats, ispaghula husk p. 39, or sterculia p. 40 can be recommended. Ensuring a sufficient intake of fluids can also be recommended. Ⓔ

Drug treatment
[EvGr] Clinicians should only prescribe drugs for children with IBS in cases of severe symptoms that have not responded to non-drug approaches. Treatment options include laxatives, antimotility drugs or antispasmodic drugs. Ⓐ
[EvGr] A laxative can be used to treat abdominal pain if the underlying cause is suspected to be constipation. An osmotic laxative, such as a macrogol or lactulose p. 40, is preferred; lactulose may cause flatulence during the first few days of treatment. Loperamide hydrochloride p. 47 may relieve diarrhoea and antispasmodic drugs may relieve pain. Ⓔ

> **Other drugs used for Irritable bowel syndrome** Alverine citrate p. 62 · Mebeverine hydrochloride, p. 62

ANTISPASMODICS

Mebeverine with ispaghula husk

04-Feb-2016

The properties listed below are those particular to the combination only. For the properties of the components please consider, mebeverine hydrochloride p. 62, ispaghula husk p. 39.

> ● INDICATIONS AND DOSE
> **Irritable bowel syndrome**
> ▸ BY MOUTH
> ▸ Child 12-17 years: 1 sachet twice daily, in water, morning and evening, 30 minutes before food and 1 sachet daily if required, taken 30 minutes before midday meal

● INTERACTIONS → Appendix 1: mebeverine

- **DIRECTIONS FOR ADMINISTRATION** Contents of one sachet should be stirred into a glass (approx. 150 mL) of cold water and drunk immediately.
- **PATIENT AND CARER ADVICE** Patients or carers should be given advice on how to administer ispaghula husk with mebeverine granules.

- **MEDICINAL FORMS**
  There can be variation in the licensing of different medicines containing the same drug.
  Effervescent granules
  CAUTIONARY AND ADVISORY LABELS 13, 22
  EXCIPIENTS: May contain Aspartame
  ELECTROLYTES: May contain Potassium
  ▸ Fybogel Mebeverine (Reckitt Benckiser Healthcare (UK) Ltd)
  Mebeverine hydrochloride 135 mg, Ispaghula husk 3.5 gram Fybogel Mebeverine effervescent granules sachets orange sugar-free | 10 sachet P £4.64 DT price = £4.64

Peppermint oil

- **INDICATIONS AND DOSE**

COLPERMIN®

Relief of abdominal colic and distension, particularly in irritable bowel syndrome
  ▸ BY MOUTH
  ▸ Child 15-17 years: 1-2 capsules 3 times a day for up to 3 months if necessary, capsule to be swallowed whole with water

- **CAUTIONS** Sensitivity to menthol
- **INTERACTIONS** → Appendix 1: peppermint oil
- **SIDE-EFFECTS**
  ▸ **Rare** Allergic reactions · ataxia · bradycardia · headache · muscle tremor · rash
  ▸ **Frequency not known** Heartburn · perianal irritation
- **PREGNANCY** Not known to be harmful.
- **BREAST FEEDING** Significant levels of menthol in breast milk unlikely.
- **DIRECTIONS FOR ADMINISTRATION** Capsules should not be broken or chewed because peppermint oil may irritate mouth or oesophagus.
- **MEDICINAL FORMS**
  There can be variation in the licensing of different medicines containing the same drug.
  Modified-release capsule
  CAUTIONARY AND ADVISORY LABELS 5, 22, 25
  EXCIPIENTS: May contain Arachis (peanut) oil
  ▸ Colpermin (McNeil Products Ltd)
  Peppermint oil 200 microlitre Colpermin gastro-resistant modified-release capsules | 20 capsule GSL £3.33 | 100 capsule GSL £12.18 DT price = £12.18

1.4 Short bowel syndrome

Short bowel syndrome

31-Aug-2016

Description of condition

Children with a shortened bowel due to large surgical resection (with or without stoma formation) may require medical management to ensure adequate absorption of nutrients and fluid. Absorption of oral medication is also often impaired.

Aims of treatment

The management of short bowel syndrome focuses on ensuring adequate nutrition and drug absorption, thereby reducing the risk of complications resulting from these effects.

Drug treatment

Nutritional deficiencies

EvGr Children with a short bowel may require replacement of vitamins and minerals depending on the extent and position of the bowel resection. Deficiencies in vitamins A, B_{12}, D, E, and K, essential fatty acids, zinc and selenium can occur.

Hypomagnesaemia is common and is treated with oral or intravenous magnesium supplementation (see Magnesium p. 570), though administration of oral magnesium may cause diarrhoea. Occasionally the use of oral alfacalcidol p. 603 and correction of sodium depletion may be useful. Nutritional support can range from oral supplements to parenteral nutrition, depending on the severity of intestinal failure. Ⓐ

Diarrhoea and high output stomas

Diarrhoea is a common symptom of short bowel syndrome and can be due to multiple factors. EvGr The use of oral rehydration salts can be considered in order to promote adequate hydration. Oral intake influences the volume of stool passed, so reducing food intake will lessen diarrhoea, but will also exacerbate the problems of undernutrition. A child may require parenteral nutrition to allow them to eat less if the extent of diarrhoea is unacceptable.

Pharmacological treatment may be necessary, with the choice of drug depending on the potential for side-effects and the degree of resection. Ⓐ

Antimotility drugs
EvGr Loperamide hydrochloride p. 47 reduces intestinal motility and thus exerts antidiarrhoeal actions. Loperamide hydrochloride is preferred over other antimotility drugs as it is not sedative and does not cause dependence or fat malabsorption. High doses of loperamide hydrochloride [unlicensed] may be required in children with a short bowel due to disrupted enterohepatic circulation and a rapid gastro-intestinal transit time.

Co-phenotrope p. 47 has traditionally been used alone or in combination with other medications to help decrease faecal output. Co-phenotrope crosses the blood–brain barrier and can produce central nervous system side-effects, which may limit its use; the potential for dependence and anticholinergic effects may also restrict its use. Ⓐ

Colestyramine
EvGr In children with an intact colon and less than 100 cm of ileum resected, colestyramine p. 125 can be used to bind the unabsorbed bile salts, which reduces diarrhoea. When colestyramine is given to these children, it is important to monitor for evidence of fat malabsorption (steatorrhoea) or fat-soluble vitamin deficiencies. Ⓐ

Antisecretory drugs
EvGr Drugs that reduce gastric acid secretion reduce jejunostomy output. Omeprazole p. 57 is readily absorbed in the duodenum and upper small bowel, but if less than 50 cm of jejunum remains, it may need to be given intravenously. Use of a proton pump inhibitor alone does not eliminate the need for further intervention for fluid control (such as antimotility agents, intravenous fluids, or oral rehydration salts). Ⓐ

Growth factors
Growth factors can be used to facilitate intestinal adaptation after surgery in children with short bowel syndrome, thus enhancing fluid, electrolyte, and micronutrient absorption.

Teduglutide p. 35 is an analogue of endogenous human glucagon-like peptide 2 (GLP-2) which is licensed for use in the management of short bowel syndrome in children aged one year and over. It may be considered after a period of stabilisation following surgery, during which intravenous fluids and nutritional support should have been optimised.

Drug absorption

For *Prescribing in children with stoma* see Stoma care p. 72.

EvGr Many drugs are incompletely absorbed by children with a short bowel and may need to be prescribed in much higher doses than usual (such as levothyroxine, warfarin, oral contraceptives, and digoxin) or may need to be given intravenously. ⟨Å⟩

Several factors can alter the absorption of drugs taken by mouth in children with a compromised gastrointestinal system. The most important factors are the length of intestine available for drug absorption, and which section has been removed. The small intestine, with its large surface area and high blood flow, is the most important site of drug absorption. The larger the amount of the small intestine that has been removed, the higher the possibility that drug absorption will be affected. Other factors such as gastric emptying and gastric transit time also affect drug handling.

EvGr Enteric-coated and modified-release preparations are unsuitable for use in patients with short bowel syndrome, particularly in children with an ileostomy, as there may not be sufficient release of the active ingredient.

Dosage forms with quick dissolution (such as soluble tablets) should be used. Uncoated tablets and liquid formulations may also be suitable. ⟨Å⟩ EvGr Before prescribing liquid formulations, prescribers should consider the osmolarity, excipient content, and volume required. Hyperosmolar liquids and some excipients (such as sorbitol) can result in fluid loss. The calorie density of oral supplements should also be considered, as it will influence the volume to be taken. ⟨Ɛ⟩

AMINO ACIDS AND DERIVATIVES

Teduglutide

01-Sep-2016

- **DRUG ACTION** Teduglutide is an analogue of human glucagon-like peptide-2 (GLP-2), which preserves mucosal integrity by promoting growth and repair of the intestine.

- **INDICATIONS AND DOSE**

Short bowel syndrome (initiated under specialist supervision)

▸ BY SUBCUTANEOUS INJECTION

▸ Child 1-17 years: 0.05 mg/kg once daily, dose to be administered to alternating quadrants of the abdomen; alternatively the thigh can be used, for optimal injection volume per body weight, consult product literature. Review treatment after 12 weeks

- **CONTRA-INDICATIONS** Active or suspected malignancy · history of gastro-intestinal malignancy (in previous 5 years)

- **CAUTIONS** Abrupt withdrawal of parenteral support (reduce gradually with concomitant monitoring of fluid status) · cardiac insufficiency · cardiovascular disease · colo-rectal polyps · hypertension

CAUTIONS, FURTHER INFORMATION

▸ Colo-rectal polyps Manufacturer recommends faecal occult blood testing in children before initiation of treatment and yearly thereafter. Manufacturer also advises colonoscopy or sigmoidoscopy in children aged 12 years and older before initiation of treatment, after 1 year of treatment and then every 5 years thereafter. Colonoscopy or sigmoidoscopy should be performed in all children with unexplained blood in stool.

- **SIDE-EFFECTS**

▸ **Common or very common** Abdominal distension · abdominal pain · allergic dermatitis · anxiety · arthralgia · chest pain · cholecystitis · cholestasis · congestive heart failure · cough · decreased appetite · dyspnoea · flushing · headache · intestinal obstruction · nausea · night sweats ·

pancreatitis · paraesthesia · peripheral oedema · rash · renal colic · sleep disorder · vomiting

▸ **Uncommon** Syncope

▸ **Frequency not known** Gastro-intestinal neoplasia · pancreatic duct stenosis · pancreatic infection

- **ALLERGY AND CROSS-SENSITIVITY** Manufacturer advises caution in patients with tetracycline hypersensitivity.

- **PREGNANCY** EvGr Specialist sources indicate use if necessary—no human data available. ⟨Đ⟩

- **BREAST FEEDING** Manufacturer advises avoid—toxicity in *animal* studies.

- **RENAL IMPAIRMENT** Manufacturer advises use half the daily dose in moderate or severe impairment and end-stage renal disease.

- **MONITORING REQUIREMENTS** Manufacturer advises monitoring of small bowel function, gall bladder, bile ducts and pancreas during treatment.

- **TREATMENT CESSATION** Caution when discontinuing treatment—risk of dehydration.

- **PATIENT AND CARER ADVICE** Patients with cardiovascular disease should seek medical attention if they notice sudden weight gain, swollen ankles or dyspnoea—may indicate increased fluid absorption.

- **MEDICINAL FORMS**
There can be variation in the licensing of different medicines containing the same drug.

Powder and solvent for solution for injection

▸ Revestive (Shire Pharmaceuticals Ltd) ▼
Teduglutide 5 mg Revestive 5mg powder and solvent for solution for injection vials | 28 vial PoM no price available

2 Constipation and bowel cleansing

2.1 Bowel cleansing

Other drugs used for Bowel cleansing Bisacodyl, p. 44 · Docusate sodium, p. 43

DIAGNOSTIC AGENTS ⟩ RADIOGRAPHIC CONTRAST MEDIA

Meglumine amidotrizoate with sodium amidotrizoate

(Diatrizoates)

- **DRUG ACTION** Meglumine amidotrizoate with sodium amidotrizoate is a radiological contrast medium with high osmolality.

- **INDICATIONS AND DOSE**

Uncomplicated meconium ileus

▸ BY RECTUM

▸ Neonate: 15–30 mL for 1 dose.

Distal intestinal obstruction syndrome in children with cystic fibrosis

▸ BY MOUTH, OR BY RECTUM

▸ Child 1-23 months: 15–30 mL for 1 dose

▸ Child (body-weight 15-25 kg): 50 mL for 1 dose

▸ Child (body-weight 26 kg and above): 100 mL for 1 dose

Radiological investigations

▸ Child: Dose to be recommended by radiologist

- **UNLICENSED USE** Not licensed for use in distal intestinal obstruction syndrome.

- **CONTRA-INDICATIONS** Hyperthyroidism
- **CAUTIONS** Asthma · benign nodular goitre · dehydration · electrolyte disturbance (correct first) · enteritis · history of allergy · in children with oesophageal fistulae (aspiration may lead to pulmonary oedema) · latent hyperthyroidism · risk of anaphylactoid reactions increased by concomitant administration of beta-blockers
- **SIDE-EFFECTS**
- ▶ **Common or very common** Diarrhoea · nausea · vomiting
- ▶ **Frequency not known** Abdominal pain · bowel necrosis · disturbances in consciousness · dizziness · electrolyte disturbances · headache · hypersensitivity reactions · hyperthyroidism · intestinal perforation · oral mucosal blistering · pyrexia · skin reactions · toxic epidermal necrolysis
- **ALLERGY AND CROSS-SENSITIVITY** Hypersensitivity to iodine.
- **PREGNANCY** Manufacturer advises caution.
- **BREAST FEEDING** Amount probably too small to be harmful.
- **DIRECTIONS FOR ADMINISTRATION** Intravenous prehydration is essential in neonates and infants. Fluid intake should be encouraged for 3 hours after administration. *By mouth*, for child bodyweight under 25 kg, dilute *Gastrografin*® with 3 times its volume of water or fruit juice; for child bodyweight over 25 kg, dilute *Gastrografin*® with twice its volume of water or fruit juice. *By rectum*, administration must be carried out slowly under radiological supervision to ensure required site is reached. For child under 5 years, dilute *Gastrografin*® with 5 times its volume of water; for child over 5 years dilute *Gastrografin*® with 4 times its volume of water.
- **MEDICINAL FORMS**
  There can be variation in the licensing of different medicines containing the same drug.
  Oral solution
  EXCIPIENTS: May contain Disodium edetate
  ▶ **Gastrografin** (Bayer Plc)
  Sodium amidotrizoate 100 mg per 1 ml, Meglumine amidotrizoate 660 mg per 1 ml Gastrografin oral solution sugar-free | 1000 ml ℗ £175.00 (Hospital only)

LAXATIVES 〉 OSMOTIC LAXATIVES

Citric acid with magnesium carbonate
(Formulated as a bowel cleansing preparation)

- **INDICATIONS AND DOSE**

Bowel evacuation for surgery, colonoscopy or radiological examination
▶ BY MOUTH
▶ Child 5–9 years: One-third of a sachet to be given at 8 a.m. the day before the procedure and, one-third of a sachet to be given between 2 and 4 p.m. the day before the procedure
▶ Child 10–17 years: 0.5–1 sachet, given at 8 a.m. the day before the procedure and 0.5–1 sachet, given between 2 and 4 p.m. the day before the procedure

- **CONTRA-INDICATIONS** Acute severe colitis · gastric retention · gastro-intestinal obstruction · gastro-intestinal perforation · toxic megacolon
- **CAUTIONS** Children · colitis (avoid if acute severe colitis) · debilitated · hypovolaemia (should be corrected before administration of bowel cleansing preparations) · impaired gag reflex or possibility of regurgitation or aspiration · patients with fluid and electrolyte disturbances

  CAUTIONS, FURTHER INFORMATION
  Adequate hydration should be maintained during treatment.

- **INTERACTIONS** → Appendix 1: bowel cleansing preparations
- **SIDE-EFFECTS**
- ▶ **Common or very common** Abdominal distention · abdominal pain · nausea · vomiting
- ▶ **Uncommon** Dehydration · dizziness · electrolyte disturbances · headache

  SIDE-EFFECTS, FURTHER INFORMATION
  ▶ **Abdominal pain** Abdominal pain is usually transient and can be reduced by taking preparation more slowly.

- **PREGNANCY** Use with caution.
- **BREAST FEEDING** Use with caution.
- ⊘ **HEPATIC IMPAIRMENT** Avoid in hepatic coma if risk of renal failure.
- **RENAL IMPAIRMENT** Avoid if estimated glomerular filtration rate less than 30 mL/minute/1.73 m² —risk of hypermagnesaemia.
- **MONITORING REQUIREMENTS** Renal function should be measured before starting treatment in patients at risk of fluid and electrolyte disturbances.
- **DIRECTIONS FOR ADMINISTRATION** One sachet should be reconstituted with 200 mL of hot water; the solution should be allowed to cool for approx. 30 minutes before drinking.
- **PRESCRIBING AND DISPENSING INFORMATION** Reconstitution of one sachet containing 11.57 g magnesium carbonate and 17.79 g anhydrous citric acid produces a solution containing magnesium citrate with 118 mmol Mg²⁺.
  Flavours of oral powders may include lemon and lime.
- **PATIENT AND CARER ADVICE** Low residue or fluid only diet (e.g. water, fruit squash, clear soup, black tea or coffee) recommended before procedure (according to prescriber's advice) and copious intake of clear fluids recommended until procedure. Patient or carers should be given advice on how to administer oral powder.

- **MEDICINAL FORMS**
  There can be variation in the licensing of different medicines containing the same drug.
  Effervescent powder
  CAUTIONARY AND ADVISORY LABELS 13, 10
  ELECTROLYTES: May contain Magnesium
  ▶ **Citramag** (Sanochemia Diagnostics UK Ltd)
  Magnesium carbonate heavy 11.57 gram, Citric acid anhydrous 17.79 gram Citramag effervescent powder sachets sugar-free | 10 sachet ℗ £18.92

Macrogol 3350 with anhydrous sodium sulfate, potassium chloride, sodium bicarbonate and sodium chloride
(Formulated as a bowel cleansing preparation)

- **INDICATIONS AND DOSE**

Bowel cleansing before radiological examination, colonoscopy, or surgery
▶ INITIALLY BY MOUTH
▶ Child 12–17 years: Initially 2 litres daily for 2 doses: first dose of reconstituted solution taken on the evening before procedure and the second dose on the morning of procedure, alternatively (by mouth) initially 250 mL every 10–15 minutes, reconstituted solution to be administered, alternatively (by nasogastric tube) initially 20–30 mL/minute, starting on the day before procedure until 4 litres have been consumed

Gastro-intestinal system

1

Distal intestinal obstruction syndrome
- ▸ BY MOUTH, OR BY NASOGASTRIC TUBE, OR BY GASTROSTOMY TUBE
- ▸ **Child 1-17 years:** 10 mL/kilogram/hour for 30 minutes, then increased to 20 mL/kilogram/hour for 30 minutes, then increased if tolerated to 25 mL/kilogram/hour, max. 100 mL/kg (or 4 litres) over 4 hours, repeat 4 hour treatment if necessary

- ● **UNLICENSED USE** *Klean-Prep* ® not licensed for use in children.
- ● **CONTRA-INDICATIONS** Acute severe colitis · gastric retention · gastro-intestinal obstruction · gastro-intestinal perforation · gastro-intestinal ulceration · toxic megacolon
- ● **CAUTIONS** Children · colitis (avoid if acute severe colitis) · debilitated patients · fluid and electrolyte disturbances · heart failure · hypovolaemia (should be corrected before administration of bowel cleansing preparations) · impaired gag reflex or possibility of regurgitation or aspiration
- ● **INTERACTIONS** → Appendix 1: bowel cleansing preparations
- ● **SIDE-EFFECTS**
- ▸ **Common or very common** Abdominal distention · abdominal pain · nausea · vomiting
- ▸ **Uncommon** Anal discomfort · dehydration · dizziness · electrolyte disturbances · headache
  SIDE-EFFECTS, FURTHER INFORMATION
- ▸ Abdominal pain Abdominal pain is usually transient and can be reduced by taking preparation more slowly.
- ● **PREGNANCY** Manufacturers advise use only if essential—no information available.
- ● **BREAST FEEDING** Manufacturers advise use only if essential—no information available.
- ● **MONITORING REQUIREMENTS** Renal function should be measured before starting treatment in patients at risk of fluid and electrolyte disturbances.
- ● **DIRECTIONS FOR ADMINISTRATION** 1 sachet should be reconstituted with 1 litre of water. Flavouring such as clear fruit cordials may be added if required. After reconstitution the solution should be kept in a refrigerator and discarded if unused after 24 hours.
- ● **PRESCRIBING AND DISPENSING INFORMATION** Each *Klean-Prep* ® sachet provides Na⁺ 125 mmol, K⁺ 10 mmol, Cl⁻ 35 mmol and HCO₃⁻ 20mmol when reconstituted with 1 litre of water.
- ● **PATIENT AND CARER ADVICE** Solid food should not be taken for 2 hours before starting treatment. Adequate hydration should be maintained during treatment. Treatment can be stopped if bowel motions become watery and clear.

- ● **MEDICINAL FORMS**
  There can be variation in the licensing of different medicines containing the same drug.
  Powder
  CAUTIONARY AND ADVISORY LABELS 10, 13
  EXCIPIENTS: May contain Aspartame
  ELECTROLYTES: May contain Bicarbonate, chloride, potassium, sodium
- ▸ **Klean-Prep** (Norgine Pharmaceuticals Ltd)
  Potassium chloride 742.5 mg, Sodium chloride 1.465 gram, Sodium bicarbonate 1.685 gram, Sodium sulfate anhydrous 5.685 gram, Polyethylene glycol 3350 59 gram Klean-Prep oral powder 69g sachets sugar-free | 4 sachet Ⓟ £9.98

LAXATIVES ⟩ STIMULANT LAXATIVES

Magnesium citrate with sodium picosulfate

(Formulated as a bowel cleansing preparation)

- ● **INDICATIONS AND DOSE**
  PICOLAX ® SACHETS
  Bowel evacuation on day before radiological procedure, endoscopy, or surgery
  - ▸ BY MOUTH
  - ▸ **Child 1 year:** 0.25 sachet taken before 8 a.m, then 0.25 sachet after 6–8 hours
  - ▸ **Child 2-3 years:** 0.5 sachet taken before 8 a.m, then 0.5 sachet after 6–8 hours
  - ▸ **Child 4-8 years:** 1 sachet taken before 8 a.m, then 0.5 sachet after 6–8 hours
  - ▸ **Child 9-17 years:** 1 sachet taken before 8 a.m, then 1 sachet after 6–8 hours
  PHARMACOKINETICS
  Acts within 3 hours of first dose.

- ● **CONTRA-INDICATIONS** Acute severe colitis · ascites · congestive cardiac failure · gastric retention · gastro-intestinal obstruction · gastro-intestinal perforation · gastro-intestinal ulceration · toxic megacolon
- ● **CAUTIONS** Cardiac disease (avoid in congestive cardiac failure) · children · colitis (avoid if acute severe colitis) · debilitated patients · fluid and electrolyte disturbances · hypovolaemia (should be corrected before administration) · impaired gag reflex or possibility of regurgitation or aspiration · recent gastro-intestinal surgery
- ● **SIDE-EFFECTS**
- ▸ **Common or very common** Abdominal distention · abdominal pain (usually transient—reduced by taking more slowly) · nausea · vomiting
- ▸ **Uncommon** Dehydration · dizziness · electrolyte disturbances · headache
- ▸ **Frequency not known** Anal discomfort · fatigue · rash · sleep disturbances
- ● **PREGNANCY** Caution.
- ● **BREAST FEEDING** Caution.
- ● **HEPATIC IMPAIRMENT** Avoid in hepatic coma if risk of renal failure.
- ● **RENAL IMPAIRMENT** Avoid if estimated glomerular filtration rate less than 30 mL/minute/1.73 m²—risk of hypermagnesaemia.
- ● **DIRECTIONS FOR ADMINISTRATION** One sachet of sodium picosulfate with magnesium citrate powder should be reconstituted with 150 mL (approx. half a glass) of cold water; patients should be warned that heat is generated during reconstitution and that the solution should be allowed to cool before drinking.
  PICOLAX ® SACHETS One sachet should be reconstituted with 150 mL (approx. half a glass) of cold water.
- ● **PRESCRIBING AND DISPENSING INFORMATION** Flavours of oral powder formulations may include lemon.
  PICOLAX ® SACHETS One reconstituted sachet contains K⁺ 5 mmol and Mg²⁺ 87 mmol.
- ● **PATIENT AND CARER ADVICE** Low residue diet recommended on the day before procedure and copious intake of water or other clear fluids recommended during treatment. Patients or carers should be given advice on how to administer sodium picosulfate with magnesium citrate oral powder.
  PICOLAX ® SACHETS Low residue diet recommended on the day before procedure and copious intake of water or other clear fluids recommended during treatment.

Patients and carers should be given advice on how to administer oral powder; they should be warned that heat is generated during reconstitution and that the solution should be allowed to cool before drinking.

● **MEDICINAL FORMS**
There can be variation in the licensing of different medicines containing the same drug.

Powder
CAUTIONARY AND ADVISORY LABELS 10, 13
ELECTROLYTES: May contain Magnesium, potassium
▸ Picolax (Ferring Pharmaceuticals Ltd)
Sodium picosulfate 10 mg, Magnesium oxide 3.5 gram, Citric acid anhydrous 12 gram Picolax oral powder 16.1g sachets sugar-free | 20 sachet [PoM] no price available

2.2 Constipation

Constipation

06-Jun-2017

Description of condition
Constipation is defaecation that is unsatisfactory because of infrequent stools, difficult stool passage, or seemingly incomplete defaecation. It can occur at any age and is common in childhood.

Overview
Before prescribing laxatives it is important to be sure that the child *is* constipated and that the constipation is not secondary to an underlying undiagnosed complaint. Early identification of constipation and effective treatment can improve outcomes for children. Without early diagnosis and treatment, an acute episode of constipation can lead to anal fissure and become chronic. In children with secondary constipation caused by a drug, the drug should be reviewed.

Laxatives
Bulk-forming laxatives
Bulk-forming laxatives include bran, ispaghula husk p. 39, methylcellulose p. 39 and sterculia p. 40. They are of particular value in children with small hard stools if fibre cannot be increased in the diet. [EvGr] They relieve constipation by increasing faecal mass, which stimulates peristalsis; children and their carers should be advised that the full effect may take some days to develop. Adequate fluid intake must be maintained to avoid intestinal obstruction, though this may be difficult for children. ⓐ

Methylcellulose, ispaghula husk and sterculia may be used in patients who cannot tolerate bran. Methylcellulose also acts as a faecal softener.

Stimulant laxative
Stimulant laxatives include bisacodyl p. 44, sodium picosulfate p. 46, and members of the anthraquinone group, senna p. 45, co-danthramer p. 44 and co-danthrusate p. 45. Stimulant laxatives increase intestinal motility and often cause abdominal cramp; they should be avoided in intestinal obstruction.

The use of co-danthramer and co-danthrusate is limited to constipation in terminally ill patients because of potential carcinogenicity (based on animal studies) and evidence of genotoxicity.

Docusate sodium p. 43 is believed to act as both a stimulant laxative and as a faecal softener (below). Glycerol suppositories act as a lubricant and as a rectal stimulant by virtue of the mildly irritant action of glycerol.

Faecal softeners
Faecal softeners are claimed to act by decreasing surface tension and increasing penetration of intestinal fluid into the faecal mass. Docusate sodium, and glycerol suppositories p. 45 have softening properties. Enemas containing arachis oil p. 43 (ground-nut oil, peanut oil) lubricate and soften impacted faeces and promote a bowel movement. Liquid paraffin has also been used as a lubricant for the passage of stool but manufacturer advises that it should be used with caution because of its adverse effects, which include anal seepage and the risks of granulomatous disease of the gastro-intestinal tract or of lipoid pneumonia on aspiration.

Osmotic laxatives
Osmotic laxatives increase the amount of water in the large bowel, either by drawing fluid from the body into the bowel or by retaining the fluid they were administered with. Lactulose p. 40 is a semi-synthetic disaccharide which is not absorbed from the gastro-intestinal tract. It produces an osmotic diarrhoea of low faecal pH, and discourages the proliferation of ammonia-producing organisms. It is therefore useful in the treatment of hepatic encephalopathy. Macrogols (such as macrogol 3350 with potassium chloride, sodium bicarbonate and sodium chloride p. 41) are inert polymers of ethylene glycol which sequester fluid in the bowel; giving fluid with macrogols may reduce the dehydrating effect sometimes seen with osmotic laxatives.

Macrogols are an effective non-traumatic means of evacuation in children with faecal impaction and can be used in the long-term management of chronic constipation.

Bowel cleansing preparations
Bowel cleansing preparations are used before colonic surgery, colonoscopy, or radiological examination to ensure the bowel is free of solid contents; examples include macrogol 3350 with anhydrous sodium sulfate, potassium chloride, sodium bicarbonate and sodium chloride p. 36, citric acid with magnesium carbonate p. 36, magnesium citrate with sodium picosulfate p. 37 and sodium acid phosphate with sodium phosphate p. 42. Bowel cleansing preparations are not treatments for constipation.

Management
[EvGr] The first-line treatment for children with constipation requires the use of a laxative in combination with dietary modification or with behavioural interventions. Diet modification alone is not recommended as first-line treatment.

In children, an increase in dietary fibre, adequate fluid intake and exercise is advised. Diet should be balanced and contain fruits, vegetables, high-fibre bread, baked beans and wholegrain breakfast cereals. Unprocessed bran (which may cause bloating and flatulence and reduces the absorption of micronutrients) is **not** recommended.

If faecal impaction is not present (or has been treated), the child should be treated promptly with a laxative. A macrogol (such as macrogol 3350 with potassium chloride, sodium bicarbonate and sodium chloride) is preferred as first-line management. If the response is inadequate, add a stimulant laxative or change to a stimulant laxative if the first-line therapy is not tolerated. If stools remain hard, lactulose or another laxative with softening effects, such as docusate sodium can be added.

In children with chronic constipation, laxatives should be continued for several weeks after a regular pattern of bowel movements or toilet training is established. The dose of laxatives should then be tapered gradually, over a period of months, according to response. Some children may require laxative therapy for several years.

A shorter duration of laxative treatment may be possible in some children with a short history of constipation.

Laxatives should be administered at a time that produces an effect that is likely to fit in with the child's toilet routine. ⓐ

Faecal impaction
[EvGr] Treatment of faecal impaction may initially increase symptoms of soiling and abdominal pain. In children over 1 year of age with faecal impaction, an oral preparation containing a macrogol (such as macrogol 3350 with potassium chloride, sodium bicarbonate and sodium

chloride) is used to clear faecal mass and to establish and maintain soft well-formed stools, using an escalating dose regimen depending on symptoms and response. If disimpaction does not occur after 2 weeks, a stimulant laxative can be added or if stools are hard, used in combination with an osmotic laxative such as lactulose. Long-term regular use of laxatives is essential to maintain well-formed stools and prevent recurrence of faecal impaction; intermittent use may provoke relapses.

Suppositories and enemas should not be used in primary care unless all oral medications have failed and preferably only then following specialist advice. If the impacted mass is not expelled following treatment with macrogols and a stimulant laxative, a sodium citrate p. 43 enema can be administered. Although rectal administration of laxatives may be effective, this route is frequently distressing for the child and may lead to persistence of withholding. A sodium acid phosphate with sodium phosphate enema may be administered under specialist supervision if disimpaction does not occur after a sodium citrate enema. Manual evacuation under anaesthetic may be necessary if disimpaction does not occur after oral and rectal treatment, or if the child is afraid. Children undergoing disimpaction should be reviewed within one week. Maintenance treatment should be started as soon as the bowel is disimpacted. ⒶΑ

Useful Resources

Constipation in children and young People: Diagnosis and management of idiopathic childhood constipation in primary and secondary care. National Institute for Health and Care Excellence. Clinical guideline 99. May 2010. www.nice.org.uk/guidance/cg99

LAXATIVES › BULK-FORMING LAXATIVES

Ispaghula husk

24-Feb-2016

- **DRUG ACTION** Bulk-forming laxatives relieve constipation by increasing faecal mass which stimulates peristalsis.

- **INDICATIONS AND DOSE**

Constipation
▸ BY MOUTH
▸ Child 1 month–5 years: 2.5–5 mL twice daily, dose to be taken only when prescribed by a doctor, as half or whole level spoonful in water, preferably after meals, morning and evening
▸ Child 6–11 years: 2.5–5 mL twice daily, dose to be given as a half or whole level spoonful in water, preferably after meals, morning and evening
▸ Child 12–17 years: 1 sachet twice daily, dose to be given in water preferably after meals, morning and evening

DOSE EQUIVALENCE AND CONVERSION
▸ 1 sachet equivalent to 2 level 5 ml spoonsful.

- **CONTRA-INDICATIONS** Colonic atony · faecal impaction · intestinal obstruction · reduced gut motility
- **CAUTIONS** Adequate fluid intake should be maintained to avoid intestinal obstruction
- **SIDE-EFFECTS** Abdominal distension · flatulence · gastro-intestinal impaction · gastro-intestinal obstruction · hypersensitivity
- **DIRECTIONS FOR ADMINISTRATION** Dose to be taken with at least 150 mL liquid.
- **PRESCRIBING AND DISPENSING INFORMATION** Flavours of soluble granules formulations may include plain, lemon, or orange.
- **HANDLING AND STORAGE** Ispaghula husk contains potent allergens. Individuals exposed to the product (including those handling the product) can develop hypersensitivity reactions such as rhinitis, conjunctivitis, bronchospasm and in some cases, anaphylaxis.

- **PATIENT AND CARER ADVICE** Manufacturer advises that preparations that swell in contact with liquid should always be carefully swallowed with water and should not be taken immediately before going to bed. Patients and their carers should be advised that the full effect may take some days to develop and should be given advice on how to administer ispaghula husk.

- **MEDICINAL FORMS**
There can be variation in the licensing of different medicines containing the same drug.

Effervescent granules
CAUTIONARY AND ADVISORY LABELS 13
EXCIPIENTS: May contain Aspartame
▸ Ispaghula husk (Non-proprietary)
Ispaghula husk 3.5 gram Ispaghula husk 3.5g effervescent granules sachets gluten free sugar free sugar-free | 30 sachet Ⓟ no price available DT price = £2.72
▸ Fybogel (Reckitt Benckiser Healthcare (UK) Ltd)
Ispaghula husk 3.5 gram Fybogel 3.5g effervescent granules sachets plain SF sugar-free | 30 sachet GSL £2.72 DT price = £2.72
Fybogel Orange 3.5g effervescent granules sachets SF sugar-free | 30 sachet GSL £2.72 DT price = £2.72
Fybogel Lemon 3.5g effervescent granules sachets SF sugar-free | 30 sachet GSL £2.72 DT price = £2.72
▸ Fybogel Hi-Fibre (Reckitt Benckiser Healthcare (UK) Ltd)
Ispaghula husk 3.5 gram Fybogel Hi-Fibre Orange 3.5g effervescent granules sachets sugar-free | 10 sachet GSL £2.26 sugar-free | 30 sachet GSL £4.85 DT price = £2.72
Fybogel Hi-Fibre Lemon 3.5g effervescent granules sachets sugar-free | 10 sachet GSL £2.26
▸ Ispagel (Bristol Laboratories Ltd)
Ispaghula husk 3.5 gram Ispagel Orange 3.5g effervescent granules sachets sugar-free | 10 sachet GSL £1.65 sugar-free | 30 sachet GSL £2.45 DT price = £2.72

Granules
CAUTIONARY AND ADVISORY LABELS 13
EXCIPIENTS: May contain Aspartame
▸ Ispaghula husk (Non-proprietary)
Ispaghula husk 3.5 gram Ispaghula husk 3.5g granules sachets gluten free | 30 sachet GSL £2.72

Powder
CAUTIONARY AND ADVISORY LABELS 13
EXCIPIENTS: May contain Aspartame
▸ Ispaghula husk (Non-proprietary)
Ispaghula husk 1 mg per 1 mg Husk oral powder sugar-free | 200 gram GSL £5.24

Combinations available: *Senna with ispaghula husk,* p. 46

Methylcellulose

- **DRUG ACTION** Bulk-forming laxatives relieve constipation by increasing faecal mass which stimulates peristalsis.

- **INDICATIONS AND DOSE**

Constipation | Diarrhoea
▸ BY MOUTH USING TABLETS
▸ Child 7–11 years: 2 tablets twice daily
▸ Child 12–17 years: 3–6 tablets twice daily

- **UNLICENSED USE** No age limit specified by manufacturer.
- **CONTRA-INDICATIONS** Colonic atony · difficulty in swallowing · faecal impaction · infective bowel disease · intestinal obstruction
- **CAUTIONS** Adequate fluid intake should be maintained to avoid intestinal obstruction
- **SIDE-EFFECTS** Abdominal distension (especially during the first few days of treatment) · flatulence (especially during the first few days of treatment) · gastro-intestinal impaction · gastro-intestinal obstruction · hypersensitivity
- **DIRECTIONS FOR ADMINISTRATION** In constipation the dose should be taken with at least 300 mL liquid. In diarrhoea, ileostomy, and colostomy control, avoid liquid intake for 30 minutes before and after dose.

Gastro-intestinal system

1

- **PATIENT AND CARER ADVICE** Patients and their carers should be advised that the full effect may take some days to develop. Preparations that swell in contact with liquid should always be carefully swallowed with water and should not be taken immediately before going to bed.

- **MEDICINAL FORMS**
There can be variation in the licensing of different medicines containing the same drug.
Tablet
 ▸ Celevac (AMCo)
   Methylcellulose "450" 500 mg Celevac 500mg tablets |
   112 tablet GSL £3.22 DT price = £3.22

Sterculia

19-Feb-2016

- **DRUG ACTION** Sterculia is a bulk-forming laxative. It relieves constipation by increasing faecal mass which stimulates peristalsis.

- **INDICATIONS AND DOSE**

Constipation
 ▸ BY MOUTH
  ▸ Child 6-11 years: 0.5-1 sachet 1-2 times a day, alternatively, half to one heaped 5-mL spoonful once or twice a day; washed down without chewing with plenty of liquid after meals
  ▸ Child 12-17 years: 1-2 sachets 1-2 times a day, alternatively, one to two heaped 5-mL spoonfuls once or twice a day; washed down without chewing with plenty of liquid after meals

- **CONTRA-INDICATIONS** Colonic atony · difficulty in swallowing · faecal impaction · intestinal obstruction
- **CAUTIONS** Adequate fluid intake should be maintained to avoid intestinal obstruction
- **SIDE-EFFECTS** Abdominal distension (especially during the first few days of treatment) · flatulence (especially during the first few days of treatment) · gastro-intestinal impaction · gastro-intestinal obstruction · hypersensitivity
- **DIRECTIONS FOR ADMINISTRATION** May be mixed with soft food (e.g. yoghurt) before swallowing, followed by plenty of liquid.
- **PATIENT AND CARER ADVICE** Patients and their carers should be advised that the full effect may take some days to develop. Preparations that swell in contact with liquid should always be carefully swallowed with water and should not be taken immediately before going to bed.

- **MEDICINAL FORMS**
There can be variation in the licensing of different medicines containing the same drug.
Granules
CAUTIONARY AND ADVISORY LABELS 25, 27
 ▸ Normacol (Norgine Pharmaceuticals Ltd)
   Sterculia 620 mg per 1 gram Normacol granules 7g sachets |
   60 sachet GSL £6.35 DT price = £6.35
   Normacol granules | 500 gram GSL £7.54 DT price = £7.54

Sterculia with frangula

The properties listed below are those particular to the combination only. For the properties of the components please consider, sterculia above.

- **INDICATIONS AND DOSE**

Constipation
 ▸ BY MOUTH
  ▸ Child 6-11 years: 0.5-1 sachet 1-2 times a day, alternatively, 0.5-1 heaped 5-mL spoonful once or twice a day; washed down without chewing with plenty of liquid after meals

  ▸ Child 12-17 years: 1-2 sachets 1-2 times a day, alternatively, 1-2 heaped 5 mL spoonfuls once or twice a day; washed down without chewing with plenty of liquid after meals

- **PREGNANCY** Manufacturer advises avoid.
- **BREAST FEEDING** Manufacturer advises avoid.
- **PATIENT AND CARER ADVICE** Patients and their carers should be advised that the full effect may take some days to develop. Preparations that swell in contact with liquid should always be carefully swallowed with water and should not be taken immediately before going to bed.

- **MEDICINAL FORMS**
There can be variation in the licensing of different medicines containing the same drug.
Granules
 ▸ Normacol Plus (Norgine Pharmaceuticals Ltd)
   Frangula 80 mg per 1 gram, Sterculia 620 mg per 1 gram Normacol Plus granules 7g sachets | 60 sachet GSL £6.78 DT price = £6.78
   Normacol Plus granules | 500 gram GSL £8.05 DT price = £8.05

LAXATIVES > OSMOTIC LAXATIVES

Lactulose

- **INDICATIONS AND DOSE**

Constipation
 ▸ BY MOUTH
  ▸ Child 1-11 months: 2.5 mL twice daily, adjusted according to response
  ▸ Child 1-4 years: 2.5-10 mL twice daily, adjusted according to response
  ▸ Child 5-17 years: 5-20 mL twice daily, adjusted according to response

Hepatic encephalopathy (portal systemic encephalopathy)
 ▸ BY MOUTH
  ▸ Child 12-17 years: Adjusted according to response to 30-50 mL 3 times a day, subsequently adjusted to produce 2-3 soft stools per day

PHARMACOKINETICS
Lactulose may take up to 48 hours to act.

- **UNLICENSED USE** Not licensed for use in children for hepatic encephalopathy.
- **CONTRA-INDICATIONS** Galactosaemia · intestinal obstruction
- **CAUTIONS** Lactose intolerance
- **SIDE-EFFECTS**
 ▸ **Common or very common** Abdominal discomfort · cramps · flatulence · nausea · vomiting
  SIDE-EFFECTS, FURTHER INFORMATION
 ▸ Nausea Nausea can be reduced by administration with water, fruit juice or meals.
- **PREGNANCY** Not known to be harmful.
- **PATIENT AND CARER ADVICE**
Medicines for Children leaflet: Lactulose for constipation www.medicinesforchildren.org.uk/lactulose-for-constipation

- **MEDICINAL FORMS**
There can be variation in the licensing of different medicines containing the same drug.
Oral solution
 ▸ Lactulose (Non-proprietary)
   Lactulose 666.667 mg per 1 ml Lactulose 10g/15ml oral solution 15ml sachets sugar free sugar-free | 10 sachet P £2.50 DT price = £2.50
   Lactulose 680 mg per 1 ml Lactulose 3.1-3.7g/5ml oral solution | 300 ml P £2.73 | 500 ml P £4.55 DT price = £2.52

▶ **Duphalac** (Mylan Ltd)
Lactulose 680 mg per 1 ml Duphalac 3.35g/5ml syrup | 200 ml P
£1.92
▶ **Lactugal** (Intrapharm Laboratories Ltd)
Lactulose 680 mg per 1 ml Lactugal 3.1-3.7g/5ml oral solution |
500 ml P £4.56 DT price = £2.52 | 2000 ml P £16.42

Macrogol 3350 with potassium chloride, sodium bicarbonate and sodium chloride

● **INDICATIONS AND DOSE**

Chronic constipation (dose for non-proprietary 'full-strength' sachets)

▶ BY MOUTH
▶ Child 12-17 years: 1–3 sachets daily in divided doses usually for up to 2 weeks; maintenance 1–2 sachets daily

Faecal impaction (dose for non-proprietary 'full-strength' sachets)

▶ BY MOUTH
▶ Child 12-17 years: 4 sachets on first day, then increased in steps of 2 sachets daily, total daily dose to be drunk within a 6 hour period, after disimpaction, switch to maintenance laxative therapy if required; maximum 8 sachets per day

MOVICOL-HALF®

Chronic constipation

▶ BY MOUTH
▶ Child 12-17 years: 2–6 sachets daily in divided doses usually for up to 2 weeks; maintenance 2–4 sachets daily

Faecal impaction

▶ BY MOUTH
▶ Child 12-17 years: Initially 8 sachets daily on first day, then increased in steps of 4 sachets daily, total daily dose to be drunk within 6 hours, after disimpaction, switch to maintenance laxative therapy; maximum 16 sachets per day

MOVICOL-PAEDIATRIC®

Chronic constipation | Prevention of faecal impaction

▶ BY MOUTH
▶ Child 1-11 months: 0.5–1 sachet daily
▶ Child 1 year: 1 sachet daily, adjust dose to produce regular soft stools; maximum 4 sachets per day
▶ Child 2-5 years: 1 sachet daily, adjust dose to produce regular soft stools; maximum 4 sachets per day
▶ Child 6-11 years: 2 sachets daily, adjust dose to produce regular soft stools; maximum 4 sachets per day

Faecal impaction

▶ BY MOUTH
▶ Child 1-11 months: 0.5–1 sachet daily
▶ Child 1-4 years: Initially 2 sachets daily on first day, then 4 sachets daily for 2 days, then 6 sachets daily for 2 days, then 8 sachets daily, total daily dose to be taken over a 12-hour period, after disimpaction, switch to maintenance laxative therapy
▶ Child 5-11 years: Initially 4 sachets daily on first day, then increased in steps of 2 sachets daily, total daily dose to be taken over a 12-hour period, after disimpaction, switch to maintenance laxative therapy; maximum 12 sachets per day

MOVICOL® LIQUID

Chronic constipation

▶ BY MOUTH
▶ Child 12-17 years: 25 mL 1–3 times a day usually for up to 2 weeks; maintenance 25 mL 1–2 times a day

MOVICOL® ORAL POWDER

Chronic constipation

▶ BY MOUTH
▶ Child 12-17 years: 1–3 sachets daily in divided doses usually for up to 2 weeks; maintenance 1–2 sachets daily

Faecal impaction

▶ BY MOUTH
▶ Child 12-17 years: Initially 4 sachets daily on first day, then increased in steps of 2 sachets daily, total daily dose to be drunk within a 6 hour period, after disimpaction, switch to maintenance laxative therapy if required; maximum 8 sachets per day

● **UNLICENSED USE**
MOVICOL-PAEDIATRIC® *Movicol® Paediatric* not licensed for use in faecal impaction in children under 5 years, or for chronic constipation in children under 2 years.

● **CONTRA-INDICATIONS** Crohn's disease · intestinal obstruction · intestinal perforation · paralytic ileus · severe inflammatory conditions of the intestinal tract · toxic megacolon · ulcerative colitis

MOVICOL-PAEDIATRIC® Cardiovascular impairment · renal impairment

● **CAUTIONS** Cardiovascular impairment (should not take more than 2 'full-strength' sachets or 4 'half-strength' sachets in any one hour) · discontinue if symptoms of fluid and electrolyte disturbance

MOVICOL-PAEDIATRIC® Impaired consciousness (with high doses) · impaired gag reflex (with high doses) · reflux oesophagitis (with high doses)

● **SIDE-EFFECTS** Abdominal distention · addominal pain · flatulence · nausea

● **PREGNANCY** Limited data, but manufacturer advises that it can be used.

● **BREAST FEEDING** Manufacturer advises that it can be used.

● **RENAL IMPAIRMENT**
MOVICOL-PAEDIATRIC® Contra-indicated in renal impairment.

● **DIRECTIONS FOR ADMINISTRATION** Contents of each 'full strength' sachet of oral powder to be dissolved in half a glass (approx. 125 mL) of water; after reconstitution the solution should be kept in a refrigerator and discarded if unused after 6 hours.

MOVICOL® LIQUID 25 mL of oral concentrate to be diluted with half a glass (approx. 100 mL) of water. After dilution the solution should be discarded if unused after 24 hours.

MOVICOL-PAEDIATRIC® Contents of each sachet to be dissolved in quarter of a glass (approx. 60–65 mL) of water; after reconstitution the solution should be kept in a refrigerator and discarded if unused after 24 hours.

MOVICOL® ORAL POWDER Contents of each sachet to be dissolved in half a glass (approx. 125 mL) of water; after reconstitution the solution should be kept in a refrigerator and discarded if unused after 6 hours.

MOVICOL-HALF® Contents of each sachet to be dissolved in quarter of a glass (approx. 60–65 mL) of water; after reconstitution the solution should be kept in a refrigerator and discarded if unused after 6 hours.

● **PRESCRIBING AND DISPENSING INFORMATION** Flavours of oral liquid formulations may include orange.
    Flavours of oral powder formulations may include chocolate, lime and lemon, or plain.

MOVICOL® LIQUID 25 mL of oral concentrate when diluted with 100 mL water provides K^+ 5.4 mmol/litre.

MOVICOL® ORAL POWDER Amount of potassium chloride varies according to flavour of *Movicol®* as follows:

plain-flavour (sugar-free) = 50.2 mg/sachet; lime and lemon flavour = 46.6 mg/sachet; chocolate flavour = 31.7 mg/sachet. 1 sachet when reconstituted with 125 mL water provides K⁺ 5.4 mmol/litre.

* **PATIENT AND CARER ADVICE**
Patients or carers should be counselled on how to take the oral powder and oral solution.
MOVICOL® LIQUID Patients or carers should be counselled on how to take *Movicol®* oral solution.
MOVICOL® ORAL POWDER Patients or carers should be counselled on how to take *Movicol®* oral powder.
MOVICOL-HALF® Patients or carers should be given advice on how to administer *Movicol-Half®* oral powder.
Medicines for Children leaflet: Movicol for constipation www.medicinesforchildren.org.uk/movicol-for-constipation

* **MEDICINAL FORMS**
There can be variation in the licensing of different medicines containing the same drug.
Oral solution
CAUTIONARY AND ADVISORY LABELS 13
ELECTROLYTES: May contain Bicarbonate, chloride, potassium, sodium
  ‣ Movicol (Norgine Pharmaceuticals Ltd)
    Macrogol '3350' 105 gram per 1 litre, Potassium 5.4 mmol per 1 litre, Bicarbonate 17 mmol per 1 litre, Chloride 53 mmol per 1 litre, Sodium 65 mmol per 1 litre Movicol Liquid sugar-free | 500 ml ℗ £5.15 DT price = £5.15
Powder
CAUTIONARY AND ADVISORY LABELS 13
ELECTROLYTES: May contain Bicarbonate, chloride, potassium, sodium
  ‣ **Macrogol 3350 with potassium chloride, sodium bicarbonate and sodium chloride (Non-proprietary)**
    Macrogol '3350' 105 gram per 1 litre, Potassium 5.4 mmol per 1 litre, Bicarbonate 17 mmol per 1 litre, Chloride 53 mmol per 1 litre, Sodium 65 mmol per 1 litre Macrogol compound oral powder sachets sugar free sugar-free | 20 sachet ℗ £4.45 sugar-free | 30 sachet ℗ £6.68 DT price = £4.27
    Macrogol compound oral powder sachets sugar free plain sugar-free | 20 sachet ℗ £3.42 sugar-free | 30 sachet ℗ £4.27 DT price = £4.27
  ‣ Movicol (Norgine Pharmaceuticals Ltd)
    Macrogol '3350' 52.5 gram per 1 litre, Potassium 5.4 mmol per 1 litre, Bicarbonate 17 mmol per 1 litre, Chloride 53 mmol per 1 litre, Sodium 65 mmol per 1 litre Movicol-Half oral powder 6.9g sachets sugar-free | 20 sachet ℗ £3.37 sugar-free | 30 sachet ℗ £5.06 DT price = £4.38
    Movicol Paediatric Plain oral powder 6.9g sachets sugar-free | 30 sachet [PoM] £4.38 DT price = £4.38
    Movicol Paediatric Chocolate oral powder 6.9g sachets sugar-free | 30 sachet [PoM] £4.38 DT price = £4.38
    Macrogol '3350' 105 gram per 1 litre, Potassium 5.4 mmol per 1 litre, Bicarbonate 17 mmol per 1 litre, Chloride 53 mmol per 1 litre, Sodium 65 mmol per 1 litre Movicol Plain oral powder 13.7g sachets sugar-free | 30 sachet ℗ £7.72 DT price = £4.27 sugar-free | 50 sachet ℗ £12.85
    Movicol Chocolate oral powder 13.9g sachets sugar-free | 30 sachet ℗ £7.72 DT price = £4.27
    Movicol oral powder 13.8g sachets lemon & lime sugar-free | 20 sachet ℗ £5.15 sugar-free | 30 sachet ℗ £7.72 DT price = £4.27 sugar-free | 50 sachet ℗ £12.85

Magnesium hydroxide

* **INDICATIONS AND DOSE**
Constipation
  ‣ BY MOUTH
  ‣ Child 3-11 years: 5-10 mL as required, dose to be given mixed with water at bedtime
  ‣ Child 12-17 years: 30-45 mL as required, dose to be given mixed with water at bedtime

* **CONTRA-INDICATIONS** Acute gastro-intestinal conditions
* **INTERACTIONS** → Appendix 1: magnesium
* **SIDE-EFFECTS** Colic

* **HEPATIC IMPAIRMENT** Avoid in hepatic coma if risk of renal failure.
* **RENAL IMPAIRMENT** Avoid or reduce dose. Increased risk of toxicity in renal impairment.
* **PRESCRIBING AND DISPENSING INFORMATION** When prepared extemporaneously, the BP states Magnesium Hydroxide Mixture, BP consists of an aqueous suspension containing about 8% hydrated magnesium oxide.

* **MEDICINAL FORMS**
There can be variation in the licensing of different medicines containing the same drug.
Oral suspension
  ‣ Phillips' Milk of Magnesia (Omega Pharma Ltd)
    Magnesium hydroxide 83 mg per 1 ml Phillips' Milk of Magnesia 415mg/5ml oral suspension sugar-free | 200 ml [GSL] £3.22 DT price = £3.22

Sodium acid phosphate with sodium phosphate

* **INDICATIONS AND DOSE**
Constipation (using Phosphates Enema BP Formula B) | **Bowel evacuation before abdominal radiological procedures, endoscopy, and surgery (using Phosphates Enema BP Formula B)**
  ‣ BY RECTUM
  ‣ Child 3-6 years: 45-65 mL once daily
  ‣ Child 7-11 years: 65-100 mL once daily
  ‣ Child 12-17 years: 100-128 mL once daily

FLEET® READY-TO-USE ENEMA

Constipation | Bowel evacuation before abdominal radiological procedures | Bowel evacuation before endoscopy | Bowel evacuation before surgery
  ‣ BY RECTUM
  ‣ Child 3-6 years: 40-60 mL once daily
  ‣ Child 7-11 years: 60-90 mL once daily
  ‣ Child 12-17 years: 90-118 mL once daily

* **CONTRA-INDICATIONS** Conditions associated with increased colonic absorption · gastro-intestinal obstruction · inflammatory bowel disease
* **CAUTIONS** Ascites · congestive heart failure · electrolyte disturbances · uncontrolled hypertension
* **SIDE-EFFECTS** Electrolyte disturbances · local irritation
* **HEPATIC IMPAIRMENT** Use with caution in cirrhosis.
* **RENAL IMPAIRMENT** Use with caution.
* **PRESCRIBING AND DISPENSING INFORMATION** When prepared extemporaneously, the BP states Phosphates Enema BP Formula B consists of sodium dihydrogen phosphate dihydrate 12.8 g, disodium phosphate dodecahydrate 10.24 g, purified water, freshly boiled and cooled, to 128 mL.

* **MEDICINAL FORMS**
There can be variation in the licensing of different medicines containing the same drug.
Enema
  ‣ **Sodium acid phosphate with sodium phosphate (Non-proprietary)**
    Disodium hydrogen phosphate dodecahydrate 80 mg per 1 ml, Sodium dihydrogen phosphate dihydrate 100 mg per 1 ml Phosphates enema (Formula B) 128ml long tube | 1 enema ℗ £27.93 DT price = £27.93
    Phosphates enema (Formula B) 128ml standard tube | 1 enema ℗ £3.98 DT price = £3.98
  ‣ Fleet Ready-to-use (Casen Recordati S.L.)
    Disodium hydrogen phosphate dodecahydrate 80 mg per 1 ml, Sodium dihydrogen phosphate dihydrate 181 mg per 1 ml Cleen Ready-to-use 133ml enema | 1 enema ℗ £0.68

Sodium citrate

● **INDICATIONS AND DOSE**

MICOLETTE®

Constipation
▸ BY RECTUM
- Child 3-17 years: 5–10 mL for 1 dose

MICRALAX®

Constipation
▸ BY RECTUM
- Child 3-17 years: 5 mL for 1 dose

RELAXIT®

Constipation
▸ BY RECTUM
- Child 1 month-2 years: 5 mL for 1 dose, insert only half the nozzle length
- Child 3-17 years: 5 mL for 1 dose

● **CONTRA-INDICATIONS** Acute gastro-intestinal conditions
● **CAUTIONS** Sodium and water retention in susceptible individuals
● **INTERACTIONS** → Appendix 1: sodium citrate

● **MEDICINAL FORMS**
There can be variation in the licensing of different medicines containing the same drug.

Enema
▸ Micolette Micro-enema (Pinewood Healthcare)
Sodium citrate 90 mg per 1 ml Micolette Micro-enema 5ml | 12 enema P £4.26
▸ Micralax Micro-enema (Focus Pharmaceuticals Ltd)
Sodium citrate 90 mg per 1 ml Micralax Micro-enema 5ml | 12 enema P £4.87
▸ Relaxit (Supra Enterprises Ltd)
Sodium citrate 90 mg per 1 ml Relaxit Micro-enema 5ml | 12 enema £5.21

LAXATIVES › SOFTENING LAXATIVES

Arachis oil

● **INDICATIONS AND DOSE**

To soften impacted faeces
▸ BY RECTUM
- Child 3-6 years (under close medical supervision): 45–65 mL as required
- Child 7-11 years (under close medical supervision): 65–100 mL as required
- Child 12-17 years (under close medical supervision): 100–130 mL as required

● **UNLICENSED USE** Licensed for use in children (age range not specified by manufacturer).
● **CONTRA-INDICATIONS** Inflammatory bowel disease
● **CAUTIONS** Hypersensitivity to soya · intestinal obstruction
● **ALLERGY AND CROSS-SENSITIVITY** Contra-indicated if history of hypersensitivity to arachis oil or peanuts.
● **DIRECTIONS FOR ADMINISTRATION** Warm enema in warm water before use.

● **MEDICINAL FORMS**
There can be variation in the licensing of different medicines containing the same drug.
Enema
▸ Arachis oil (Non-proprietary)
Arachis oil 1 ml per 1 ml Arachis oil 130ml enema | 1 enema P £47.50 DT price = £47.50

Docusate sodium   20-Apr-2016

(Dioctyl sodium sulphosuccinate)

● **INDICATIONS AND DOSE**

Chronic constipation
▸ BY MOUTH
- Child 6 months-1 year: 12.5 mg 3 times a day, adjusted according to response, use paediatric oral solution
- Child 2-11 years: 12.5–25 mg 3 times a day, adjusted according to response, use paediatric oral solution
- Child 12-17 years: Up to 500 mg daily in divided doses, adjusted according to response
▸ BY RECTUM
- Child 12-17 years: 120 mg for 1 dose

Adjunct in abdominal radiological procedures
▸ BY MOUTH
- Child 12-17 years: 400 mg, to be administered with barium meal
▸ BY RECTUM
- Child 12-17 years: 120 mg for 1 dose

PHARMACOKINETICS
Oral preparations act within 1–2 days; response to rectal administration usually occurs within 20 minutes.

● **UNLICENSED USE** *Adult oral solution and capsules* not licensed for use in children under 12 years.
● **CONTRA-INDICATIONS** Avoid in intestinal obstruction
● **CAUTIONS** Do not give with liquid paraffin · excessive use of stimulant laxatives can cause diarrhoea and related effects such as hypokalaemia · rectal preparations not indicated if haemorrhoids or anal fissure
● **INTERACTIONS** → Appendix 1: docusate sodium
● **SIDE-EFFECTS** Abdominal cramp · diarrhoea (excessive use) · hypokalaemia · rash
● **PREGNANCY** Not known to be harmful—manufacturer advises caution.
● **BREAST FEEDING**
▸ With oral use Present in milk following oral administration— manufacturer advises caution.
▸ With rectal use Rectal administration not known to be harmful.
● **DIRECTIONS FOR ADMINISTRATION** For administration *by mouth*, solution may be mixed with milk or squash.

● **MEDICINAL FORMS**
There can be variation in the licensing of different medicines containing the same drug.
Oral solution
▸ Docusate sodium (Non-proprietary)
Docusate sodium 2.5 mg per 1 ml Docusate 12.5mg/5ml oral solution sugar free sugar-free | 300 ml P £7.79 DT price = £5.29
Docusate sodium 10 mg per 1 ml Docusate 50mg/5ml oral solution sugar free sugar-free | 300 ml P £7.99 DT price = £7.99
▸ Docusol (Typharm Ltd)
Docusate sodium 2.5 mg per 1 ml Docusol Paediatric 12.5mg/5ml oral solution sugar-free | 300 ml P £5.29 DT price = £5.29
Enema
▸ Norgalax (Essential Pharma Ltd)
Docusate sodium 12 mg per 1 gram Norgalax 120mg/10g enema | 6 enema P £28.00
Capsule
▸ Dioctyl (UCB Pharma Ltd)
Docusate sodium 100 mg Dioctyl 100mg capsules | 30 capsule P £2.09 DT price = £2.09 | 100 capsule P £6.98

Combinations available: *Co-danthrusate,* p. 45

Gastro-intestinal system

1

LAXATIVES > STIMULANT LAXATIVES

Bisacodyl

● **INDICATIONS AND DOSE**

Constipation

▶ BY MOUTH
▸ Child 4–17 years: 5–20 mg once daily, adjusted according to response, dose to be taken at night
▶ BY RECTUM
▸ Child 2–17 years: 5–10 mg once daily, adjusted according to response

Bowel clearance before radiological procedures and surgery

▶ INITIALLY BY MOUTH
▸ Child 4–9 years: 5 mg once daily for 2 days before procedure, dose to be taken at bedtime and (by rectum) 5 mg if required, dose to be administered 1 hour before procedure
▸ Child 10–17 years: 10 mg once daily for 2 days before procedure, dose to be taken at bedtime and (by rectum) 10 mg if required, dose to be administered 1 hour before procedure

PHARMACOKINETICS
Tablets act in 10–12 hours; suppositories act in 20–60 minutes.

● **CONTRA-INDICATIONS** Acute abdominal conditions · acute inflammatory bowel disease · intestinal obstruction · severe dehydration

● **CAUTIONS** Excessive use of stimulant laxatives can cause diarrhoea and related effects such as hypokalaemia · risk of electrolyte imbalance with prolonged use

● **INTERACTIONS** → Appendix 1: bisacodyl

● **SIDE-EFFECTS**

GENERAL SIDE-EFFECTS
Abdominal cramp · colitis · nausea · vomiting

SPECIFIC SIDE-EFFECTS
▸ With rectal use Local irritation

● **PREGNANCY** May be suitable for constipation in pregnancy, if a stimulant effect is necessary.

● **MEDICINAL FORMS**
There can be variation in the licensing of different medicines containing the same drug. Forms available from special-order manufacturers include: oral suspension, suppository, enema

Gastro-resistant tablet
CAUTIONARY AND ADVISORY LABELS 5, 25
▸ Bisacodyl (Non-proprietary)
  Bisacodyl 5 mg Bisacodyl 5mg gastro-resistant tablets | 60 tablet Ⓟ £3.25 DT price = £1.96 | 100 tablet Ⓟ £5.40 | 500 tablet Ⓟ £25.73 | 1000 tablet Ⓟ £51.45
▸ Dulco-Lax (bisacodyl) (Boehringer Ingelheim Self-Medication Division)
  Bisacodyl 5 mg Dulcolax 5mg gastro-resistant tablets | 40 tablet Ⓟ £2.44 | 100 tablet Ⓟ £3.60

Enema
▸ Bisacodyl (Non-proprietary)
  Bisacodyl 333.333 microgram per 1 ml Bisacodyl 10mg/30ml enema | 1 enema PoM no price available

Suppository
▸ Bisacodyl (Non-proprietary)
  Bisacodyl 10 mg Bisacodyl 10mg suppositories | 12 suppository Ⓟ £3.53 DT price = £3.53
▸ Dulco-Lax (bisacodyl) (Boehringer Ingelheim Self-Medication Division)
  Bisacodyl 5 mg Dulcolax 5mg suppositories for children | 5 suppository Ⓟ £1.04 DT price = £1.04
  Bisacodyl 10 mg Dulcolax 10mg suppositories | 12 suppository Ⓟ £2.35 DT price = £3.53

Co-danthramer

● **INDICATIONS AND DOSE**

Constipation in terminally ill patients (standard strength capsules)

▶ BY MOUTH USING CAPSULES
▸ Child 6–11 years: 1 capsule once daily, dose should be taken at night
▸ Child 12–17 years: 1–2 capsules once daily, dose should be taken at night

Constipation in terminally ill patients (strong capsules)

▶ BY MOUTH USING CAPSULES
▸ Child 12–17 years: 1–2 capsules once daily, dose should be given at night

Constipation in terminally ill patients (standard strength suspension)

▶ BY MOUTH USING ORAL SUSPENSION
▸ Child 2–11 years: 2.5–5 mL once daily, dose should be taken at night
▸ Child 12–17 years: 5–10 mL once daily, dose should be taken at night

Constipation in terminally ill patients (strong suspension)

▶ BY MOUTH USING ORAL SUSPENSION
▸ Child 12–17 years: 5 mL once daily, dose should be taken at night

DOSE EQUIVALENCE AND CONVERSION
▸ Co-danthramer (standard strength) capsules contain dantron 25 mg with poloxamer '188' 200 mg per capsule.
▸ Co-danthramer (standard strength) oral suspension contains dantron 25 mg with poloxamer '188' 200 mg per 5 mL.
▸ Co-danthramer **strong** capsules contain dantron 37.5 mg with poloxamer '188' 500 mg.
▸ Co-danthramer **strong** oral suspension contains dantron 75 mg with poloxamer '188' 1 g per 5 mL.
▸ Co-danthramer suspension 5 mL = one co-danthramer capsule, **but** strong co-danthramer suspension 5 mL = two strong co-danthramer capsules.

● **CONTRA-INDICATIONS** Acute abdominal conditions · acute inflammatory bowel disease · intestinal obstruction · severe dehydration

● **CAUTIONS** Excessive use of stimulant laxatives can cause diarrhoea and related effects such as hypokalaemia · may cause local irritation · *rodent* studies indicate potential carcinogenic risk

CAUTIONS, FURTHER INFORMATION
▸ Local irritation Avoid prolonged contact with skin (as in incontinent patients or infants wearing nappies—risk of irritation and excoriation).

● **INTERACTIONS** → Appendix 1: dantron

● **SIDE-EFFECTS** Abdominal cramp · urine may be coloured red

● **PREGNANCY** Manufacturers advise avoid—limited information available.

● **BREAST FEEDING** Manufacturers advise avoid—no information available.

● **MEDICINAL FORMS**
There can be variation in the licensing of different medicines containing the same drug.

Oral suspension
CAUTIONARY AND ADVISORY LABELS 14 (urine red)
▸ Co-danthramer (Non-proprietary)
  Dantron 5 mg per 1 ml, Poloxamer 188 40 mg per 1 ml Co-danthramer 25mg/200mg/5ml oral suspension sugar free sugar-free | 300 ml PoM £146.39 DT price = £146.39
  Dantron 15 mg per 1 ml, Poloxamer 188 200 mg per 1 ml Co-danthramer 75mg/1000mg/5ml oral suspension sugar free sugar-free | 300 ml PoM £293.63 DT price = £293.63

Co-danthrusate

20-Apr-2016

- **INDICATIONS AND DOSE**

Constipation in terminally ill patients
- ▶ BY MOUTH USING CAPSULES
- ▶ Child 6-11 years: 1 capsule once daily, to be taken at night
- ▶ Child 12-17 years: 1-3 capsules once daily, to be taken at night
- ▶ BY MOUTH USING ORAL SUSPENSION
- ▶ Child 6-11 years: 5 mL once daily, to be taken at night
- ▶ Child 12-17 years: 5-15 mL once daily, to be taken at night

DOSE EQUIVALENCE AND CONVERSION
- ▶ Co-danthrusate suspension contains dantron 50 mg and docusate 60 mg per 5 mL.
- ▶ Co-danthrusate capsules contain dantron 50 mg and docusate 60 mg per capsule.

- **CONTRA-INDICATIONS** Acute abdominal conditions · acute inflammatory bowel disease · intestinal obstruction · severe dehydration
- **CAUTIONS** Excessive use of stimulant laxatives can cause diarrhoea and related effects such as hypokalaemia · may cause local irritation · *rodent* studies indicate potential carcinogenic risk

  CAUTIONS, FURTHER INFORMATION
- ▶ Local irritation Avoid prolonged contact with skin (as in incontinent patients or infants wearing nappies—risk of irritation and excoriation).
- **INTERACTIONS** → Appendix 1: dantron, docusate sodium
- **SIDE-EFFECTS** Abdominal cramp · urine may be coloured red
- **PREGNANCY** Manufacturers advise avoid—limited information available.
- **BREAST FEEDING** Manufacturers advise avoid—no information available.

- **MEDICINAL FORMS**
  There can be variation in the licensing of different medicines containing the same drug.
  Oral suspension
  CAUTIONARY AND ADVISORY LABELS 14 (urine red)
  - ▶ Co-danthrusate (Non-proprietary)
    Dantron 10 mg per 1 ml, Docusate sodium 12 mg per 1 ml Co-danthrusate 50mg/60mg/5ml oral suspension sugar free sugar-free | 200 ml PoM £89.92 DT price = £89.92
  Capsule
  CAUTIONARY AND ADVISORY LABELS 14 (urine red)
  - ▶ Co-danthrusate (Non-proprietary)
    Dantron 50 mg, Docusate sodium 60 mg Co-danthrusate 50mg/60mg capsules | 63 capsule PoM no price available DT price = £52.50

Glycerol

(Glycerin)

- **INDICATIONS AND DOSE**

Constipation
- ▶ BY RECTUM
- ▶ Child 1-11 months: 1 g as required
- ▶ Child 1-11 years: 2 g as required
- ▶ Child 12-17 years: 4 g as required

- **INTERACTIONS** → Appendix 1: glycerol
- **DIRECTIONS FOR ADMINISTRATION** Moisten suppositories with water before insertion.
- **PRESCRIBING AND DISPENSING INFORMATION** When prepared extemporaneously, the BP states Glycerol

Suppositories, BP consists of gelatin 140 mg, glycerol 700 mg, purified water to 1 g.
- **PATIENT AND CARER ADVICE**
  Medicines for Children leaflet: Glycerin (glycerol) suppositories for constipation www.medicinesforchildren.org.uk/glycerin-glycerol-suppositories-for-constipation

- **MEDICINAL FORMS**
  There can be variation in the licensing of different medicines containing the same drug. Forms available from special-order manufacturers include: suppository
  Suppository
  - ▶ Glycerol (Non-proprietary)
    Gelatin 140 mg per 1 gram, Glycerol 700 mg per 1 gram Glycerol 2g suppositories | 12 suppository GSL £1.75 DT price = £1.67
    Glycerol 1g suppositories | 12 suppository GSL £1.69 DT price = £1.04
    Glycerol 4g suppositories | 12 suppository GSL £1.31 DT price = £1.16

Senna

13-Jun-2016

- **DRUG ACTION** Senna is a stimulant laxative. After metabolism of sennosides in the gut the anthrone component stimulates peristalsis thereby increasing the motility of the large intestine.

- **INDICATIONS AND DOSE**

Constipation
- ▶ BY MOUTH USING TABLETS
- ▶ Child 2-3 years: 3.75-15 mg once daily, adjusted according to response
- ▶ Child 4-5 years: 3.75-30 mg once daily, adjusted according to response
- ▶ Child 6-17 years: 7.5-30 mg once daily, adjusted according to response
- ▶ BY MOUTH USING SYRUP
- ▶ Child 1 month-3 years: 3.75-15 mg once daily, adjusted according to response
- ▶ Child 4-17 years: 3.75-30 mg once daily, adjusted according to response

PHARMACOKINETICS
Onset of action 8-12 hours.

- **UNLICENSED USE** *Tablets* not licensed for use in children under 6 years. *Syrup* not licensed for use in children under 2 years.
  Doses in BNF Publications adhere to national guidelines and may differ from those in product literature.
- **CONTRA-INDICATIONS** Intestinal obstruction · undiagnosed abdominal pain
- **INTERACTIONS** → Appendix 1: senna
- **SIDE-EFFECTS** Abdominal spasm · discoloration of urine · pruritus
  SIDE-EFFECTS, FURTHER INFORMATION
  Prolonged or excessive use of stimulant laxatives can cause diarrhoea and related effects such as hypokalaemia.
- **PREGNANCY** EvGr Specialist sources indicate suitable for use in pregnancy. ⓓ
- **BREAST FEEDING** EvGr Specialist sources indicate suitable for use in breast-feeding in infants over 1 month. ⓓ
- **PATIENT AND CARER ADVICE**
  Medicines for Children leaflet: Senna for constipation www.medicinesforchildren.org.uk/senna-for-constipation
- **NATIONAL FUNDING/ACCESS DECISIONS**
  NHS restrictions *Senokot* ® tablets.
- **EXCEPTIONS TO LEGAL CATEGORY** Senna is on sale to the public for use in children over 12 years; doses on packs may vary from those in BNF Publications.

● MEDICINAL FORMS
There can be variation in the licensing of different medicines containing the same drug.

Oral solution
▸ Senokot (Forum Health Products Ltd, Reckitt Benckiser Healthcare (UK) Ltd)
Sennoside B (as Sennosides) 1.5 mg per 1 ml Senokot 7.5mg/5ml Syrup Pharmacy sugar free sugar-free | 500 ml P £4.76 DT price = £4.76

Tablet
▸ Senna (Non-proprietary)
Sennoside B (as Sennosides) 7.5 mg Senna 7.5mg tablets | 20 tablet P £1.00 | 60 tablet P £2.50 DT price = £2.01 | 100 tablet P £2.13
▸ Ex-Lax Senna (Novartis Consumer Health UK Ltd)
Sennoside B (as Sennosides) 12 mg Ex-Lax Senna 12mg pills | 20 tablet GSL £1.54
▸ Senokot (Reckitt Benckiser Healthcare (UK) Ltd, Forum Health Products Ltd)
Sennoside B (as Sennosides) 7.5 mg Senokot 7.5mg tablets | 20 tablet GSL £1.61 | 60 tablet GSL £4.20 DT price = £2.01 | 100 tablet GSL £5.49 | 500 tablet GSL £12.50
Sennoside B (as Sennosides) 15 mg Senokot Max Strength 15mg tablets | 24 tablet GSL £3.23 | 48 tablet GSL £5.69 DT price = £5.69

Senna with ispaghula husk
24-Feb-2016

The properties listed below are those particular to the combination only. For the properties of the components please consider, senna p. 45, ispaghula husk p. 39.

● INDICATIONS AND DOSE

Constipation
▸ BY MOUTH
▸ Child 12-17 years: 5-10 g once daily, to be taken at night, 5 g equivalent to one level spoonful of granules

● INTERACTIONS → Appendix 1: senna

● SIDE-EFFECTS Urine coloured yellow or red-brown

● PREGNANCY Manufacturer advises avoid during first trimester. To be used only intermittently and only if dietary and lifestyle changes fail.

● DIRECTIONS FOR ADMINISTRATION Take at night with at least 150 mL liquid..

● MEDICINAL FORMS
There can be variation in the licensing of different medicines containing the same drug.

Granules
CAUTIONARY AND ADVISORY LABELS 25
EXCIPIENTS: May contain Sucrose
▸ Manevac (Meda Pharmaceuticals Ltd)
Senna fruit 124 mg per 1 gram, Ispaghula 542 mg per 1 gram Manevac granules | 400 gram P £9.50 DT price = £9.50

Sodium picosulfate
06-May-2016

(Sodium picosulphate)

● DRUG ACTION Sodium picosulfate is a stimulant laxative. After metabolism in the colon it stimulates the mucosa thereby increasing the motility of the large intestine.

● INDICATIONS AND DOSE

Constipation
▸ BY MOUTH
▸ Child 1 month-3 years: 2.5-10 mg once daily, adjusted according to response
▸ Child 4-17 years: 2.5-20 mg once daily, adjusted according to response

PHARMACOKINETICS
Onset of action 6-12 hours.

● UNLICENSED USE Doses in BNF Publications adhere to national guidelines and may differ from those in product literature.

● CONTRA-INDICATIONS Intestinal obstruction · undiagnosed abdominal pain

● INTERACTIONS → Appendix 1: sodium picosulfate

● SIDE-EFFECTS
▸ Common or very common Abdominal cramp
▸ Uncommon Dizziness · nausea · vomiting
▸ Frequency not known Angioedema · pruritus · rash · syncope

SIDE-EFFECTS, FURTHER INFORMATION
Prolonged or excessive use can cause diarrhoea and related effects such as hypokalaemia.

● PREGNANCY Manufacturer states evidence limited but not known to be harmful.

● BREAST FEEDING EvGr Specialist sources indicate suitable for use in breast-feeding in infants over 1 month—not known to be present in milk. ⏞

● PATIENT AND CARER ADVICE
Medicines for Children leaflet: Sodium picosulfate for constipation www.medicinesforchildren.org.uk/sodium-picosulfate-for-constipation

● MEDICINAL FORMS
There can be variation in the licensing of different medicines containing the same drug.

Oral solution
EXCIPIENTS: May contain Alcohol
▸ Sodium picosulfate (Non-proprietary)
Sodium picosulfate 1 mg per 1 ml Sodium picosulfate 5mg/5ml oral solution sugar free sugar-free | 100 ml P £2.37 sugar-free | 300 ml P £7.10 DT price = £7.10
▸ Dulco-Lax (sodium picosulfate) (Boehringer Ingelheim Self-Medication Division)
Sodium picosulfate 1 mg per 1 ml Dulcolax Pico 5mg/5ml liquid sugar-free | 100 ml P £1.94 sugar-free | 300 ml P £4.62 DT price = £7.10

3   Diarrhoea

Acute diarrhoea

Management of acute diarrhoea

The priority in acute diarrhoea, as in gastro-enteritis, is the prevention or reversal of fluid and electrolyte depletion—this is particularly important in infants. **Oral rehydration preparations** are used in the prevention or reversal of fluid and electrolyte depletion. Severe dehydration requires immediate admission to hospital and urgent replacement of fluid and electrolytes.

Adsorbents and bulk-forming drugs

Adsorbents such as kaolin are **not** recommended for *acute diarrhoeas*. Bulk-forming drugs, such as ispaghula husk p. 39, methylcellulose p. 39, and sterculia p. 40 are rarely effective in controlling faecal consistency in ileostomy and colostomy.

Colestyramine p. 125 binds unabsorbed bile salts and provides symptomatic relief of diarrhoea following ileal disease or resection.

Antibacterial drugs

Antibacterial drugs are generally unnecessary in simple gastro-enteritis because the complaint usually resolves quickly without such treatment, and infective diarrhoeas in the UK often have a viral cause. Systemic bacterial infection does, however, need appropriate systemic treatment.

Antimotility drugs
Antimotility drugs relieve symptoms of diarrhoea. They prolong the duration of intestinal transit by binding to opioid receptors in the gastro-intestinal tract. Loperamide hydrochloride below is used due to its action on opioid receptors in the gastrointestinal tract and because it does not cross the blood-brain barrier readily. Antimotility drugs have a role in the management of uncomplicated *acute diarrhoea* in adults but not in children under 12 years.

Antimotility drugs have a role in Inflammatory bowel disease p. 24 and are also used in Stoma care p. 72.

Antispasmodics
Antispasmodics are occasionally of value in treating abdominal cramp associated with diarrhoea but they should **not** be used for primary treatment. Antispasmodics and antiemetics should be **avoided** in young children with gastro-enteritis since they are rarely effective and have troublesome side-effects.

Enkephalinase inhibitors
Racecadotril p. 48 is a pro-drug of thiorphan. Thiorphan is an enkephalinase inhibitor that inhibits the breakdown of endogenous opioids, thereby reducing intestinal secretions. Racecadotril is licensed, as an adjunct to rehydration, for the symptomatic treatment of uncomplicated acute diarrhoea; it should only be used in children over 3 months of age when usual supportive measures, including oral rehydration, are insufficient to control the condition. Racecadotril does not affect the duration of intestinal transit.

Other drugs used for Diarrhoea Codeine phosphate, p. 265

ANTIDIARRHOEALS > ANTIPROPULSIVES

⌐ 262

Co-phenotrope

● **INDICATIONS AND DOSE**
Adjunct to rehydration in acute diarrhoea
▸ BY MOUTH
▸ Child 2-3 years: 0.5 tablet 3 times a day
▸ Child 4-8 years: 1 tablet 3 times a day
▸ Child 9-11 years: 1 tablet 4 times a day
▸ Child 12-15 years: 2 tablets 3 times a day
▸ Child 16-17 years: Initially 4 tablets, followed by 2 tablets every 6 hours until diarrhoea controlled

Control of faecal consistency after colostomy or ileostomy
▸ BY MOUTH
▸ Child 2-3 years: 0.5 tablet 3 times a day
▸ Child 4-8 years: 1 tablet 3 times a day
▸ Child 9-11 years: 1 tablet 4 times a day
▸ Child 12-15 years: 2 tablets 3 times a day
▸ Child 16-17 years: Initially 4 tablets, then 2 tablets 4 times a day

● **UNLICENSED USE** Not licensed for use in children under 4 years.
● **CONTRA-INDICATIONS** Gastro-intestinal obstruction · intestinal atony · myasthenia gravis (but some antimuscarinics may be used to decrease muscarinic side-effects of anticholinesterases) · paralytic ileus · pyloric stenosis · severe ulcerative colitis · significant bladder outflow obstruction · toxic megacolon · urinary retention
● **CAUTIONS** Presence of subclinical doses of atropine may give rise to atropine side-effects in susceptible individuals or in overdosage · young children are particularly susceptible to **overdosage**; symptoms may be delayed and observation is needed for at least 48 hours after ingestion
● **INTERACTIONS** → Appendix 1: atropine, opioids
● **SIDE-EFFECTS**
▸ Very rare Angle-closure glaucoma

▸ **Frequency not known** Abdominal pain · anorexia · constipation · dilation of the pupils with loss of accomodation · dry mouth · dryness of the skin · fever · flushing · giddiness · nausea · photophobia · reduced bronchial secretions · transient bradycardia (followed by tachycardia, palpitation and arrhythmias) · urinary retention · urinary urgency · vomiting
● **PREGNANCY** Manufacturer advises caution.
● **BREAST FEEDING** May be present in milk.
● **HEPATIC IMPAIRMENT** Avoid in jaundice.
● **DIRECTIONS FOR ADMINISTRATION** For administration *by mouth* tablets may be crushed.
● **PRESCRIBING AND DISPENSING INFORMATION** A mixture of diphenoxylate hydrochloride and atropine sulfate in the mass proportions 100 parts to 1 part respectively.
● **EXCEPTIONS TO LEGAL CATEGORY** Co-phenotrope 2.5/0.025 can be sold to the public for children over 16 years (provided packs do not contain more than 20 tablets) as an adjunct to rehydration in acute diarrhoea (max. daily dose 10 tablets).

● **MEDICINAL FORMS**
There can be variation in the licensing of different medicines containing the same drug.
Tablet
▸ Co-phenotrope (Non-proprietary)
Atropine sulfate 25 microgram, Diphenoxylate hydrochloride 2.5 mg Lomotil 2.5mg/25microgram tablets | 100 tablet [PoM] no price available [CD5]

Loperamide hydrochloride

● **INDICATIONS AND DOSE**
Symptomatic treatment of acute diarrhoea
▸ BY MOUTH
▸ Child 4-7 years: 1 mg 3-4 times a day for up to 3 days only
▸ Child 8-11 years: 2 mg 4 times a day for up to 5 days
▸ Child 12-17 years: Initially 4 mg, followed by 2 mg for up to 5 days, dose to be taken after each loose stool; usual dose 6-8 mg daily; maximum 16 mg per day

Chronic diarrhoea
▸ BY MOUTH
▸ Child 1-11 months: 100-200 micrograms/kg twice daily, to be given 30 minutes before feeds; increased if necessary up to 2 mg/kg daily in divided doses
▸ Child 1-11 years: 100-200 micrograms/kg 3-4 times a day (max. per dose 2 mg), increased if necessary up to 1.25 mg/kg daily in divided doses; maximum 16 mg per day
▸ Child 12-17 years: 2-4 mg 2-4 times a day; maximum 16 mg per day

● **UNLICENSED USE** Not licensed for use in children for chronic diarrhoea. *Capsules* not licensed for use in children under 8 years. *Syrup* not licensed for use in children under 4 years.
● **CONTRA-INDICATIONS** Active ulcerative colitis · antibiotic-associated colitis · conditions where abdominal distension develops · conditions where inhibition of peristalsis should be avoided
● **CAUTIONS** Not recommended for children under 12 years
● **INTERACTIONS** → Appendix 1: loperamide
● **SIDE-EFFECTS**
▸ **Common or very common** Dizziness · flatulence · headache · nausea
▸ **Uncommon** Abdominal pain · drowsiness · dry mouth · dyspepsia · rash · vomiting

- **Rare** Fatigue · hypertonia · paralytic ileus · Stevens-Johnson syndrome · toxic epidermal necrolysis · urinary retention
- **PREGNANCY** Manufacturers advise avoid—no information available.
- **BREAST FEEDING** Amount probably too small to be harmful.
- **HEPATIC IMPAIRMENT** Risk of accumulation—manufacturer advises caution.
- **PRESCRIBING AND DISPENSING INFORMATION**
  Palliative care
  For further information on the use of loperamide in palliative care, see www.palliativedrugs.com/formulary/en/loperamide.html.
- **PATIENT AND CARER ADVICE**
  Medicines for Children leaflet. Loperamide for diarrhoea www.medicinesforchildren.org.uk/loperamide-for-diarrhoea
- **EXCEPTIONS TO LEGAL CATEGORY** Loperamide can be sold to the public, for use in children over 12 years, provided it is licensed and labelled for the treatment of acute diarrhoea.

- **MEDICINAL FORMS**
  There can be variation in the licensing of different medicines containing the same drug. Forms available from special-order manufacturers include: oral suspension, oral solution
  Tablet
  - Loperamide hydrochloride (Non-proprietary)
    Loperamide hydrochloride 2 mg Loperamide 2mg tablets | 30 tablet [PoM] £2.15 DT price = £2.15
  - Norimode (Tillomed Laboratories Ltd)
    Loperamide hydrochloride 2 mg Norimode 2mg tablets | 30 tablet [PoM] £2.15 DT price = £2.15
  Oral solution
  - Imodium (Janssen-Cilag Ltd)
    Loperamide hydrochloride 200 microgram per 1 ml Imodium 1mg/5ml oral solution sugar-free | 100 ml [PoM] £1.17 DT price = £1.17
  Capsule
  - Loperamide hydrochloride (Non-proprietary)
    Loperamide hydrochloride 2 mg Loperamide 2mg capsules | 30 capsule [PoM] £2.99 DT price = £0.96
  Orodispersible tablet
  - Imodium (McNeil Products Ltd)
    Loperamide hydrochloride 2 mg Imodium Instant Melts 2mg orodispersible tablets sugar-free | 12 tablet [P] £3.75 sugar-free | 18 tablet [P] £5.02 DT price = £5.02

Loperamide with simeticone

The properties listed below are those particular to the combination only. For the properties of the components please consider, loperamide hydrochloride p. 47, simeticone p. 51.

- **INDICATIONS AND DOSE**
  Acute diarrhoea with abdominal colic
  ▸ BY MOUTH
  - Child 12–17 years: Initially 1 tablet, then 1 tablet, after each loose stool, for up to 2 days; maximum 4 tablets per day

- **INTERACTIONS** → Appendix 1: loperamide

- **MEDICINAL FORMS**
  There can be variation in the licensing of different medicines containing the same drug.
  Tablet
  - Imodium Plus (McNeil Products Ltd)
    Loperamide hydrochloride 2 mg, Dimeticone (as Simeticone) 125 mg Imodium Plus caplets | 12 tablet [P] £3.66

ANTIDIARRHOEALS 〉 ENKEPHALINASE INHIBITORS

Racecadotril

11-Feb-2016

- **INDICATIONS AND DOSE**
  Adjunct to rehydration, for the symptomatic treatment of uncomplicated acute diarrhoea
  ▸ BY MOUTH USING GRANULES
  - Child 3 months–17 years (body-weight up to 9 kg): 10 mg 3 times a day until diarrhoea stops; maximum duration of treatment 7 days
  - Child 3 months–17 years (body-weight 9–12 kg): 20 mg 3 times a day until diarrhoea stops; maximum duration of treatment 7 days
  - Child 3 months–17 years (body-weight 13–27 kg): 30 mg 3 times a day until diarrhoea stops; maximum duration of treatment 7 days
  - Child 3 months–17 years (body-weight 28 kg and above): 60 mg 3 times a day until diarrhoea stops; maximum duration of treatment 7 days

- **CONTRA-INDICATIONS** Antibiotic-associated diarrhoea
- **SIDE-EFFECTS**
  ▸ **Uncommon** Erythema · rash
  ▸ **Frequency not known** Angioedema · pruritus · urticaria
  SIDE-EFFECTS, FURTHER INFORMATION
  ▸ Skin reactions Severe skin reactions have been reported—discontinue treatment immediately.
- **PREGNANCY** Manufacturer advises avoid—no information available.
- **BREAST FEEDING** Manufacturer advises avoid—no information available.
- **HEPATIC IMPAIRMENT** Manufacturer advises avoid.
- **RENAL IMPAIRMENT** Manufacturer advises avoid.
- **DIRECTIONS FOR ADMINISTRATION** Granules may be added to food or mixed with water or bottle feeds and then taken immediately.
- **PATIENT AND CARER ADVICE** Patients and carers should be given advice on how to administer racecadotril granules.
- **NATIONAL FUNDING/ACCESS DECISIONS**
  Scottish Medicines Consortium (SMC) Decisions
  The *Scottish Medicines Consortium*, has advised (July 2014) that racecadotril (*Hidrasec®*) is **not** recommended for use within NHS Scotland for the treatment of acute diarrhoea in children because there is insufficient evidence that it improves the recovery rate.

- **MEDICINAL FORMS**
  There can be variation in the licensing of different medicines containing the same drug.
  Granules
  EXCIPIENTS: May contain Sucrose
  ▸ Hidrasec (Lincoln Medical Ltd)
    Racecadotril 10 mg Hidrasec Infants 10mg granules sachets | 20 sachet [PoM] £8.42
    Racecadotril 30 mg Hidrasec Children 30mg granules sachets | 20 sachet [PoM] £8.42

4 Disorders of gastric acid and ulceration

4.1 Dyspepsia

Dyspepsia

Overview

Dyspepsia covers upper abdominal pain, fullness, early satiety, bloating, and nausea. It can occur with gastric and duodenal ulceration, gastro-oesophageal reflux disease, gastritis, and upper gastro-intestinal motility disorders, but most commonly it is of uncertain origin.

Patients with dyspepsia should be advised about lifestyle changes (avoidance of excess alcohol and of aggravating foods such as fats); other measures include weight reduction, smoking cessation, and raising the head of the bed. Some medications may cause dyspepsia—these should be stopped, if possible.

A compound alginate preparation may provide relief from dyspepsia; persistent dyspepsia requires investigation. Treatment with a H2-receptor antagonist or a proton pump inhibitor should be initiated only on the advice of a hospital specialist.

Helicobacter pylori may be present in children with dyspepsia. *H. pylori* eradication therapy should be considered for persistent dyspepsia if it is ulcer-like. However, most children with functional (investigated, non-ulcer) dyspepsia do not benefit symptomatically from *H. pylori* eradication.

ANTACIDS

Antacids

Overview

Antacids (usually containing aluminium or magnesium compounds) can often relieve symptoms in *ulcer dyspepsia* and in *non-erosive gastro-oesophageal reflux* ; they are also sometimes used in functional (non-ulcer) dyspepsia but the evidence of benefit is uncertain.

Aluminium- and **magnesium**-containing antacids, being relatively insoluble in water, are long-acting if retained in the stomach. They are suitable for most antacid purposes. Magnesium-containing antacids tend to be laxative whereas aluminium-containing antacids may be constipating; antacids containing both magnesium and aluminium may reduce these colonic side-effects.

Complexes such as **hydrotalcite** confer no special advantage.

Calcium-containing antacids can induce rebound acid secretion; with modest doses the clinical significance of this is doubtful, but prolonged high doses also cause hypercalcaemia and alkalosis.

Simeticone

Simeticone (activated dimeticone) p. 51 is used to treat infantile colic, but the evidence of benefit is uncertain.

Simeticone is added to an antacid as an antifoaming agent to relieve flatulence. These preparations may be useful for the relief of hiccup in palliative care.

Alginates

Alginates taken in combination with an antacid increases the viscosity of stomach contents and can protect the oesophageal mucosa from acid reflux. Some alginate-containing preparations form a viscous gel ('raft') that floats on the surface of the stomach contents, thereby reducing symptoms of reflux. Alginate-containing preparations are used in the management of mild symptoms of dyspepsia and gastro-oesophageal reflux disease.

The amount of additional ingredient or antacid in individual preparations varies widely, as does their sodium content, so that preparations may not be freely interchangeable.

ANTACIDS ⟩ ALGINATE

Alginic acid

- ● **INDICATIONS AND DOSE**

  GAVISCON INFANT® POWDER SACHETS

  Management of gastro-oesophageal reflux disease
  - ▸ BY MOUTH
    - ▸ Neonate (body-weight up to 4.5 kg): 1 dose as required, to be mixed with feeds (or water, for breast-fed infants); maximum 6 doses per day.

    - ▸ Neonate (body-weight 4.5 kg and above): 2 doses as required, to be mixed with feeds (or water, for breast-fed infants); maximum 12 doses per day.

    - ▸ Child 1–23 months (body-weight up to 4.5 kg): 1 dose as required, to be mixed with feeds (or water, for breast-fed infants); maximum 6 doses per day
    - ▸ Child 1–23 months (body-weight 4.5 kg and above): 2 doses as required, to be mixed with feeds (or water, for breast-fed infants); maximum 12 doses per day

- ● **CONTRA-INDICATIONS** Intestinal obstruction · preterm neonates · where excessive water loss likely (e.g. fever, diarrhoea, vomiting, high room temperature)

  GAVISCON INFANT® POWDER SACHETS Concurrent use of preparations containing thickening agents

- ● **HEPATIC IMPAIRMENT** In patients with fluid retention, avoid antacids containing large amounts of sodium. Avoid antacids containing magnesium salts in hepatic coma if there is a risk of renal failure.

- ● **RENAL IMPAIRMENT** In patients with fluid retention, avoid antacids containing large amounts of sodium.

- ● **PRESCRIBING AND DISPENSING INFORMATION** Each half of the dual-sachet is identified as 'one dose'.

  To avoid errors prescribe with directions in terms of 'dose'.

- ● **MEDICINAL FORMS**
  There can be variation in the licensing of different medicines containing the same drug.

  Powder
  ELECTROLYTES: May contain Sodium
  - ▸ Gaviscon Infant (Forum Health Products Ltd)
    Magnesium alginate 87.5 mg, Sodium alginate 225 mg Gaviscon Infant oral powder sachets sugar-free | 15 dual dose sachet GSL £4.82 DT price = £4.82

Sodium alginate with potassium bicarbonate

The properties listed below are those particular to the combination only. For the properties of the components please consider, alginic acid above.

- ● **INDICATIONS AND DOSE**

  Management of mild symptoms of dyspepsia and gastro-oesophageal reflux disease
  - ▸ BY MOUTH USING CHEWABLE TABLETS
    - ▸ Child 6–11 years (under medical advice only): 1 tablet, to be chewed after meals and at bedtime continued →

‣ Child 12-17 years: 1-2 tablets, to be chewed after meals and at bedtime
▸ BY MOUTH USING ORAL SUSPENSION
‣ Child 2-11 years (under medical advice only): 2.5-5 mL, to be taken after meals and at bedtime
‣ Child 12-17 years: 5-10 mL, to be taken after meals and at bedtime

● PRESCRIBING AND DISPENSING INFORMATION Flavours of oral liquid formulations may include aniseed or peppermint.

● MEDICINAL FORMS
There can be variation in the licensing of different medicines containing the same drug.
Oral suspension
ELECTROLYTES: May contain Potassium, sodium
▸ Acidex Advance (Pinewood Healthcare)
Potassium bicarbonate 20 mg per 1 ml, Sodium alginate 100 mg per 1 ml Acidex Advance oral suspension sugar-free |
250 ml P £2.21 sugar-free | 500 ml P £4.42 DT price = £5.12
Acidex Advance oral suspension aniseed sugar-free | 250 ml P £2.21 sugar-free | 500 ml P £4.42 DT price = £5.12
▸ Gaviscon Advance (Reckitt Benckiser Healthcare (UK) Ltd)
Potassium bicarbonate 20 mg per 1 ml, Sodium alginate 100 mg per 1 ml Gaviscon Advance oral suspension aniseed sugar-free |
150 ml P £3.23 sugar-free | 250 ml P £2.56 sugar-free |
300 ml P £5.82 sugar-free | 500 ml P £5.12 DT price = £5.12
Gaviscon Advance oral suspension peppermint sugar-free | 250 ml P £2.56 sugar-free | 300 ml P £5.82 sugar-free | 500 ml P £5.12 DT price = £5.12
Chewable tablet
EXCIPIENTS: May contain Aspartame
ELECTROLYTES: May contain Potassium, sodium
▸ Sodium alginate with potassium bicarbonate (Non-proprietary)
Potassium bicarbonate 100 mg, Sodium alginate 500 mg Sodium alginate 500mg / Potassium bicarbonate 100mg chewable tablets sugar free sugar-free | 60 tablet GSL no price available DT price = £3.07
▸ Brands may include Gaviscon Advance

ANTACIDS ⟩ ALUMINIUM AND MAGNESIUM

Co-magaldrox

The properties listed below are those particular to the combination only. For the properties of the components please consider, aluminium hydroxide p. 572, magnesium hydroxide p. 42.

● INDICATIONS AND DOSE
MAALOX®
Dyspepsia
▸ BY MOUTH
‣ Child 14-17 years: 10-20 mL, to be taken 20-60 minutes after meals, and at bedtime or when required
MUCOGEL®
Dyspepsia
▸ BY MOUTH
‣ Child 12-17 years: 10-20 mL 3 times a day, to be taken 20-60 minutes after meals, and at bedtime, or when required

● INTERACTIONS → Appendix 1: antacids
● PRESCRIBING AND DISPENSING INFORMATION Co-magaldrox is a mixture of aluminium hydroxide and magnesium hydroxide; the proportions are expressed in the form x/y where x and y are the strengths in milligrams per unit dose of magnesium hydroxide and aluminium hydroxide respectively.
MUCOGEL® Mucogel® suspension is low in sodium.
MAALOX® Maalox® suspension is low in sodium.

● MEDICINAL FORMS
There can be variation in the licensing of different medicines containing the same drug.
Oral suspension
▸ Maalox (Sanofi)
Magnesium hydroxide 39 mg per 1 ml, Aluminium hydroxide gel dried 44 mg per 1 ml Maalox oral suspension sugar-free |
500 ml GSL £3.35 DT price = £2.99
▸ Mucogel (Chemidex Pharma Ltd)
Magnesium hydroxide 39 mg per 1 ml, Aluminium hydroxide gel dried 44 mg per 1 ml Mucogel oral suspension sugar-free |
500 ml GSL £2.99 DT price = £2.99

Co-simalcite

● INDICATIONS AND DOSE
Dyspepsia
▸ BY MOUTH
‣ Child 8-11 years: 5 mL 4 times a day as required, to be taken between meals and at bedtime
‣ Child 12-17 years: 10 mL 4 times a day as required, to be taken between meals and at bedtime

● CONTRA-INDICATIONS Hypophosphataemia · infants · neonates

CONTRA-INDICATIONS, FURTHER INFORMATION
▸ Aluminium-containing antacids Aluminium-containing antacids should not be used in neonates and infants because accumulation may lead to increased plasma-aluminium concentrations.

● SIDE-EFFECTS

SIDE-EFFECTS, FURTHER INFORMATION
▸ Constipation and diarrhoea Magnesium-containing antacids tend to be laxative whereas aluminium-containing antacids may be constipating; antacids containing both magnesium and aluminium may reduce these colonic side-effects.

● HEPATIC IMPAIRMENT Avoid; can cause constipation which can precipitate coma. Avoid in hepatic coma; risk of renal failure.

● RENAL IMPAIRMENT Antacids containing magnesium salts should be avoided or used at a reduced dose because there is an increased risk of toxicity. Aluminium-containing antacids should not be used in children with renal impairment, because accumulation may lead to increased plasma-aluminium concentrations.

● PRESCRIBING AND DISPENSING INFORMATION Altacite Plus® is low in Na+.

● MEDICINAL FORMS
There can be variation in the licensing of different medicines containing the same drug.
Oral suspension
▸ Altacite Plus (Peckforton Pharmaceuticals Ltd)
Simeticone 25 mg per 1 ml, Hydrotalcite 100 mg per 1 ml Altacite Plus oral suspension sugar-free | 100 ml £4.00 sugar-free |
500 ml P £5.20 DT price = £5.20

Simeticone with aluminium hydroxide and magnesium hydroxide

The properties listed below are those particular to the combination only. For the properties of the components please consider, simeticone below, aluminium hydroxide p. 572.

- **INDICATIONS AND DOSE**
Dyspepsia
‣ BY MOUTH
  ‣ Child 2–4 years: 5 mL 3 times a day
  ‣ Child 5–11 years: 5–10 mL 3–4 times a day
  ‣ Child 12–17 years: 5–10 mL 4 times a day, to be taken after meals and at bedtime, or when required

- **INTERACTIONS** → Appendix 1: antacids

- **MEDICINAL FORMS**
There can be variation in the licensing of different medicines containing the same drug.
Oral suspension
‣ Maalox Plus (Sanofi)
  Simeticone 5 mg per 1 ml, Magnesium hydroxide 39 mg per 1 ml, Aluminium hydroxide gel dried 44 mg per 1 ml Maalox Plus oral suspension sugar-free | 180 ml GSL £2.01

ANTACIDS > MAGNESIUM

Magnesium trisilicate with magnesium carbonate and sodium bicarbonate

The properties listed below are those particular to the combination only. For the properties of the components please consider, magnesium trisilicate, magnesium carbonate, sodium bicarbonate p. 558.

- **INDICATIONS AND DOSE**
Dyspepsia
‣ BY MOUTH
  ‣ Child 5–11 years: 5–10 mL 3 times a day, alternatively as required, dose to be made up with water
  ‣ Child 12–17 years: 10–20 mL 3 times a day, alternatively as required, dose to be made up with water

- **CONTRA-INDICATIONS** Hypophosphataemia · Severe renal failure

- **CAUTIONS** Heart failure · hypermagnesaemia · hypertension · metabolic alkalosis · respiratory alkalosis

- **INTERACTIONS** → Appendix 1: antacids, sodium bicarbonate

- **SIDE-EFFECTS** Belching due to liberated carbon dioxide · diarrhoea

- **HEPATIC IMPAIRMENT** In patients with fluid retention avoid antacids containing large amounts of sodium. Avoid antacids containing magnesium salts in hepatic coma if there is a risk of renal failure.

- **RENAL IMPAIRMENT** Magnesium trisilicate and magnesium carbonate mixtures have high sodium content; avoid in patients with fluid retention.

- **PRESCRIBING AND DISPENSING INFORMATION** When prepared extemporaneously, the BP states Magnesium Trisilicate Mixture, BP consists of 5% each of magnesium trisilicate, light magnesium carbonate, and sodium bicarbonate in a suitable vehicle with a peppermint flavour.

- **MEDICINAL FORMS**
There can be variation in the licensing of different medicines containing the same drug.
Oral suspension
‣ Magnesium trisilicate with magnesium carbonate and sodium bicarbonate (Non-proprietary)
  Magnesium carbonate light 50 mg per 1 ml, Magnesium trisilicate 50 mg per 1 ml, Sodium bicarbonate 50 mg per 1 ml Magnesium trisilicate oral suspension | 200 ml GSL £1.65 DT price = £1.65

ANTIFOAMING DRUGS

Simeticone
(Activated dimeticone)

- **DRUG ACTION** Simeticone (activated dimeticone) is an antifoaming agent.

- **INDICATIONS AND DOSE**
DENTINOX®
Colic | Wind pains
‣ BY MOUTH
  ‣ Neonate: 2.5 mL, to be taken with or after each feed; may be added to bottle feed; maximum 6 doses per day.
  ‣ Child 1 month–1 year: 2.5 mL, to be taken with or after each feed; may be added to bottle feed; maximum 6 doses per day
INFACOL®
Colic | Wind pains
‣ BY MOUTH
  ‣ Neonate: 0.5–1 mL, to be taken before feeds.
  ‣ Child 1 month–1 year: 0.5–1 mL, to be taken before feeds

- **PRESCRIBING AND DISPENSING INFORMATION**
DENTINOX® The brand name *Dentinox®* is also used for other preparations including teething gel.

- **PATIENT AND CARER ADVICE**
INFACOL® Patients or carers should be given advice on use of the *Infacol®* dropper.

- **LESS SUITABLE FOR PRESCRIBING**
INFACOL® *Infacol®* is less suitable for prescribing (evidence of benefit in infantile colic uncertain).
DENTINOX® *Dentinox®* colic drops are less suitable for prescribing (evidence of benefit in infantile colic uncertain).

- **MEDICINAL FORMS**
There can be variation in the licensing of different medicines containing the same drug.
Oral suspension
‣ Infacol (Teva UK Ltd)
  Simeticone 40 mg per 1 ml Infacol 40mg/ml oral suspension sugar-free | 50 ml GSL £2.71 DT price = £2.71
Oral drops
‣ Dentinox Infant (Dendron Ltd)
  Simeticone 8.4 mg per 1 ml Dentinox Infant colic drops | 100 ml GSL £1.73

Combinations available: *Co-simalcite*, p. 50 · *Simeticone with aluminium hydroxide and magnesium hydroxide*, above

4.2 Gastric and duodenal ulceration

Peptic ulceration

Overview

Peptic ulceration commonly involves the stomach, duodenum, and lower oesophagus; after gastric surgery it involves the gastro-enterostomy stoma. Healing can be promoted by general measures, stopping smoking and taking antacids and by antisecretory drug treatment, but relapse is common when treatment ceases. Nearly all duodenal ulcers and most gastric ulcers not associated with NSAIDs are caused by *Helicobacter pylori*.

Helicobacter pylori infection

Eradication of *Helicobacter pylori* reduces the recurrence of gastric and duodenal ulcers and the risk of rebleeding. The presence of *H. pylori* should be confirmed before starting eradication treatment. If possible, the antibacterial sensitivity of the organism should be established at the time of endoscopy and biopsy. Acid inhibition combined with antibacterial treatment is highly effective in the eradication of *H. pylori*; reinfection is rare. Antibiotic-associated colitis is an uncommon risk.

Treatment to eradicate *H. pylori* infection in children should be initiated under specialist supervision. One week triple-therapy regimens that comprise omeprazole p. 57, amoxicillin p. 325, and either clarithromycin p. 315 or metronidazole p. 319 are recommended, see p. 53. Resistance to clarithromycin or to metronidazole is much more common than to amoxicillin and can develop during treatment. A regimen containing amoxicillin and clarithromycin is therefore recommended for initial therapy and one containing amoxicillin and metronidazole is recommended for eradication failure or for a child who has been treated with a macrolide for other infections. There is usually no need to continue antisecretory treatment (with a proton pump inhibitor or H$_2$-receptor antagonist); however, if the ulcer is large, or complicated by haemorrhage or perforation then antisecretory treatment is continued for a further 3 weeks. Lansoprazole p. 56 may be considered if omeprazole is unsuitable. Treatment failure usually indicates antibacterial resistance or poor compliance.

Two-week triple-therapy regimens offer the possibility of higher eradication rates compared to one-week regimens, but adverse effects are common and poor compliance is likely to offset any possible gain.

Two-week dual-therapy regimens using a proton pump inhibitor and a single antibacterial produce low rates of *H. pylori* eradication and are **not** recommended.

See under *NSAID-associated ulcers* for the role of *H. pylori* eradication therapy in children starting or taking NSAIDs.

Test for *Helicobacter pylori*

^{13}C-Urea breath test kits are available for confirming the presence of gastro-duodenal infection with *Helicobacter pylori*. The test involves collection of breath samples before and after ingestion of an oral solution of ^{13}C-urea; the samples are sent for analysis by an appropriate laboratory. The test should not be performed within 4 weeks of treatment with an antibacterial or within 2 weeks of treatment with an antisecretory drug. A specific ^{13}C-Urea breath test kit for children is available (*Helicobacter Test INFAI for children of the age* 3–11 ®). However the appropriateness of testing for *H. pylori* infection in children has not been established. Breath, saliva, faecal, and urine tests for *H. pylori* are frequently unreliable in children; the most accurate method of diagnosis is endoscopy with biopsy.

NSAID-associated ulcers

Gastro-intestinal bleeding and ulceration can occur with NSAID use. Whenever possible, NSAIDs should be **withdrawn** if an ulcer occurs.

Children at high risk of developing gastro-intestinal complications with a NSAID include those with a history of peptic ulcer disease or serious upper gastro-intestinal complication, those taking other medicines that increase the risk of upper gastro-intestinal side-effect, or those with serious co-morbidity. In children at risk of ulceration, a proton pump inhibitor can be considered for protection against gastric and duodenal ulcers associated with non-selective NSAIDs; high dose ranitidine p. 53 is an alternative.

NSAID use and *H. pylori* infection are independent risk factors for gastro-intestinal bleeding and ulceration. In children already taking a NSAID, eradication of *H. pylori* is unlikely to reduce the risk of NSAID-induced bleeding or ulceration. However, in children about to start long-term NSAID treatment who are *H. pylori* positive and have dyspepsia or a history of gastric or duodenal ulcer, eradication of *H. pylori* may reduce the overall risk of ulceration.

If the NSAID can be *discontinued* in a child who has developed an ulcer, a proton pump inhibitor usually produces the most rapid healing; alternatively the ulcer can be treated with an H$_2$-receptor antagonist.

If *NSAID treatment needs to continue*, the ulcer is treated with a proton pump inhibitor.

GASTROPROTECTIVE COMPLEXES AND CHELATORS

Chelates and complexes

Sucralfate

Sucralfate below is a complex of aluminium hydroxide and sulfated sucrose that appears to act by protecting the mucosa from acid-pepsin attack; it has minimal antacid properties.

▌ Sucralfate

● **INDICATIONS AND DOSE**

Benign gastric ulceration | Benign duodenal ulceration
▸ BY MOUTH
▸ Child 1 month–1 year: 250 mg 4–6 times a day
▸ Child 2–11 years: 500 mg 4–6 times a day
▸ Child 12–14 years: 1 g 4–6 times a day
▸ Child 15–17 years: 2 g twice daily, dose to be taken on rising and at bedtime, alternatively 1 g 4 times a day for 4–6 weeks, or in resistant cases up to 12 weeks, dose to be taken 1 hour before meals and at bedtime; maximum 8 g per day

Prophylaxis of stress ulceration in child under intensive care
▸ BY MOUTH
▸ Child 1 month–1 year: 250 mg 4–6 times a day
▸ Child 2–11 years: 500 mg 4–6 times a day
▸ Child 12–14 years: 1 g 4–6 times a day
▸ Child 15–17 years: 1 g 6 times a day; maximum 8 g per day

● **UNLICENSED USE** Not licensed for use in children under 15 years. Tablets not licensed for prophylaxis of stress ulceration.

● **CAUTIONS** Patients under intensive care (**Important:** reports of bezoar formation)

Recommended regimens for *Helicobacter pylori* eradication

Age range	Acid suppressant	Antibacterial		
		Amoxicillin	Clarithromycin	Metronidazole
Child 1–5 years	Omeprazole 1–2 mg/kg once daily (max. per dose 40 mg)	250 mg twice daily 125 mg 3 times a day –	7.5 mg/kg (max. 500 mg) twice daily – 7.5 mg/kg (max. 500 mg) twice daily	– 100 mg 3 times a day 100 mg twice daily
Child 6–11 years	Omeprazole 1–2 mg/kg once daily (max. per dose 40 mg)	500 mg twice daily 250 mg 3 times a day –	7.5 mg/kg (max. 500 mg) twice daily – 7.5 mg/kg (max. 500 mg) twice daily	– 200 mg 3 times a day 200 mg twice daily
Child 12–17 years	Omeprazole 40 mg once daily	1 g twice daily 500 mg 3 times a day –	500 mg twice daily – 500 mg twice daily	– 400 mg 3 times a day 400 mg twice daily

CAUTIONS, FURTHER INFORMATION
▸ **Bezoar formation** Following reports of bezoar formation associated with sucralfate, caution is advised in seriously ill patients, especially those receiving concomitant enteral feeds or those with predisposing conditions such as delayed gastric emptying.

● **INTERACTIONS** → Appendix 1: sucralfate

● **SIDE-EFFECTS**
▸ **Common or very common** Constipation
▸ **Uncommon** Back pain · bezoar formation · diarrhoea · dizziness · drowsiness · dry mouth · eadache · flatulence · gastric discomfort · indigestion · nausea · rash

● **PREGNANCY** No evidence of harm; absorption from gastro-intestinal tract negligible.

● **BREAST FEEDING** Amount probably too small to be harmful.

● **RENAL IMPAIRMENT** Use with caution; aluminium is absorbed and may accumulate.

● **DIRECTIONS FOR ADMINISTRATION** Administration of sucralfate and enteral feeds should be separated by 1 hour and for administration by *mouth*, sucralfate should be given 1 hour before meals. *Oral suspension* blocks fine-bore feeding tubes. Crushed *tablets* may be dispersed in water.

● **PRESCRIBING AND DISPENSING INFORMATION** Flavours of oral liquid formulations may include aniseed and caramel.

● **MEDICINAL FORMS**
There can be variation in the licensing of different medicines containing the same drug. Forms available from special-order manufacturers include: tablet, oral suspension

Tablet
CAUTIONARY AND ADVISORY LABELS 5
▸ Sucralfate (Non-proprietary)
Sucralfate 1 gram Sulcrate 1g tablets | 100 tablet no price available
Carafate 1g tablets | 100 tablet no price available

H₂-RECEPTOR ANTAGONISTS

H₂-receptor antagonists

Overview

Histamine H₂-receptor antagonists heal *gastric and duodenal ulcers* by reducing gastric acid output as a result of histamine H₂-receptor blockade; they are also used to relieve symptoms of *dyspepsia* and *gastro-oesophageal reflux disease*. H₂-receptor antagonists should not normally be used for *Zollinger–Ellison syndrome* because proton pump inhibitors are more effective.

Maintenance treatment with low doses has largely been replaced in *Helicobacter pylori* positive children by eradication regimens.

H₂-receptor antagonist therapy can promote healing of *NSAID-associated ulcers*.

Treatment with a H₂-receptor antagonist has not been shown to be beneficial in haematemesis and melaena, but prophylactic use reduces the frequency of bleeding from *gastroduodenal erosions in hepatic coma*, and possibly in other conditions requiring intensive care. Treatment also reduces the risk of *acid aspiration* in obstetric patients at delivery (Mendelson's syndrome).

H₂-receptor antagonists are also used to reduce the degradation of pancreatic enzyme supplements in children with cystic fibrosis.

H₂-receptor antagonists

● **SIDE-EFFECTS**
▸ **Common or very common** Diarrhoea · dizziness · headache
▸ **Uncommon** Erythema multiforme · rash · toxic epidermal necrolysis
▸ **Rare** Arthralgia · blood disorders · bradycardia · cholestatic jaundice · confusion · depression · hallucinations · hepatitis · leucopenia · myalgia · pancytopenia · psychiatric reactions · thrombocytopenia
▸ **Frequency not known** Gynaecomastia · impotence

SIDE-EFFECTS, FURTHER INFORMATION
▸ **Psychiatric reactions** Psychiatric reactions, including confusion, depression, and hallucinations occur particularly in the very ill.

◤ above

Ranitidine

● **INDICATIONS AND DOSE**
Benign gastric ulceration | Duodenal ulceration
▸ BY MOUTH

▸ **Neonate:** 2 mg/kg 3 times a day (max. per dose 3 mg/kg 3 times a day), oral absorption is unreliable.

▸ **Child 1–5 months:** 1 mg/kg 3 times a day (max. per dose 3 mg/kg 3 times a day)
▸ **Child 6 months–2 years:** 2–4 mg/kg twice daily
▸ **Child 3–11 years:** 2–4 mg/kg twice daily (max. per dose 150 mg)
▸ **Child 12–17 years:** 150 mg twice daily, alternatively 300 mg once daily, dose to be taken at night continued →

Prophylaxis of stress ulceration

▶ INITIALLY BY SLOW INTRAVENOUS INJECTION

▶ **Neonate:** 0.5–1 mg/kg every 6–8 hours.

▶ **Child 1 month-11 years:** 1 mg/kg every 6–8 hours (max. per dose 50 mg), may be given as an intermittent infusion at a rate of 25 mg/hour

▶ **Child 12-17 years:** 50 mg every 8 hours, dose to be diluted to 20 mL and given over at least 2 minutes, then (by mouth) 150 mg twice daily, may be given when oral feeding commences

Reflux oesophagitis and other conditions where gastric acid reduction is beneficial

▶ BY MOUTH

▶ **Neonate:** 2 mg/kg 3 times a day (max. per dose 3 mg/kg 3 times a day), oral absorption is unreliable.

▶ **Child 1-5 months:** 1 mg/kg 3 times a day (max. per dose 3 mg/kg 3 times a day)

▶ **Child 6 months-2 years:** 2–4 mg/kg twice daily

▶ **Child 3-11 years:** 2–4 mg/kg twice daily (max. per dose 150 mg); increased to up to 5 mg/kg twice daily (max. per dose 300 mg), dose increase for severe gastro-oesophageal disease

▶ **Child 12-17 years:** 150 mg twice daily, alternatively 300 mg once daily, dose to be taken at night, then increased if necessary to 300 mg twice daily for up to 12 weeks in moderate to severe gastro-oesophageal reflux disease, alternatively increased if necessary to 150 mg 4 times a day for up to 12 weeks in moderate to severe gastro-oesophageal reflux disease

▶ BY SLOW INTRAVENOUS INJECTION

▶ **Neonate:** 0.5–1 mg/kg every 6–8 hours.

▶ **Child:** 1 mg/kg every 6–8 hours (max. per dose 50 mg), may be given as an intermittent infusion at a rate of 25 mg/hour

● **UNLICENSED USE** *Oral* preparations not licensed for use in children under 3 years. *Injection* not licensed for use in children under 6 months.

● **INTERACTIONS** → Appendix 1: H$_2$ receptor antagonists

● **SIDE-EFFECTS**

▶ **Uncommon** Blurred vision

▶ **Frequency not known** Alopecia · interstitial nephritis · involuntary movement disorders · pancreatitis

● **PREGNANCY** Manufacturer advises avoid unless essential, but not known to be harmful.

● **BREAST FEEDING** Significant amount present in milk, but not known to be harmful.

● **RENAL IMPAIRMENT** Use half normal dose if estimated glomerular filtration rate less than 50 mL/minute/1.73 m^2.

● **DIRECTIONS FOR ADMINISTRATION** For *slow intravenous injection* dilute to a concentration of 2.5 mg/mL with Glucose 5% or Sodium Chloride 0.9%; give over at least 3 minutes.

● **PATIENT AND CARER ADVICE**
In fat malabsorption syndrome, give oral doses 1–2 hours before food to enhance effects of pancreatic enzyme replacement.
Medicines for Children leaflet: Ranitidine for acid reflux
www.medicinesforchildren.org.uk/ranitidine-for-acid-reflux

● **EXCEPTIONS TO LEGAL CATEGORY** Ranitidine can be sold to the public for children over 16 years (provided packs do not contain more than 2 weeks' supply) for the short-term symptomatic relief of heartburn, dyspepsia, and hyperacidity, and for the prevention of these symptoms when associated with consumption of food or drink (max. single dose 75 mg, max. daily dose 300 mg).

● MEDICINAL FORMS
There can be variation in the licensing of different medicines containing the same drug. Forms available from special-order manufacturers include: oral suspension, oral solution, infusion

Tablet

▶ Ranitidine (Non-proprietary)

Ranitidine (as Ranitidine hydrochloride) 150 mg Ranitidine 150mg tablets | 60 tablet [PoM] £1.27 DT price = £1.24

Ranitidine (as Ranitidine hydrochloride) 300 mg Ranitidine 300mg tablets | 30 tablet [PoM] £1.27 DT price = £1.27

▶ Ranitil (Tillomed Laboratories Ltd)

Ranitidine (as Ranitidine hydrochloride) 150 mg Ranitil 150mg tablets | 60 tablet [PoM] £18.13 DT price = £1.24

Ranitidine (as Ranitidine hydrochloride) 300 mg Ranitil 300mg tablets | 30 tablet [PoM] £17.64 DT price = £1.27

▶ Zantac (Omega Pharma Ltd, GlaxoSmithKline UK Ltd)

Ranitidine (as Ranitidine hydrochloride) 75 mg Zantac 75 tablets | 24 tablet [P] £5.16 | 48 tablet [P] £7.75

Ranitidine (as Ranitidine hydrochloride) 150 mg Zantac 150mg tablets | 60 tablet [PoM] £1.30 DT price = £1.24

Ranitidine (as Ranitidine hydrochloride) 300 mg Zantac 300mg tablets | 30 tablet [PoM] £1.30 DT price = 1.27

Solution for injection

▶ Ranitidine (Non-proprietary)

Ranitidine (as Ranitidine hydrochloride) 25 mg per 1 ml Ranitidine 50mg/2ml solution for injection ampoules | 5 ampoule [PoM] £2.69-£5.00 DT price = £2.69

▶ Zantac (GlaxoSmithKline UK Ltd)

Ranitidine (as Ranitidine hydrochloride) 25 mg per 1 ml Zantac 50mg/2ml solution for injection ampoules | 5 ampoule [PoM] £2.82 DT price = £2.69

Effervescent tablet

CAUTIONARY AND ADVISORY LABELS 13
ELECTROLYTES: May contain Sodium

▶ Ranitidine (Non-proprietary)

Ranitidine (as Ranitidine hydrochloride) 150 mg Ranitidine 150mg effervescent tablets | 60 tablet [PoM] £35.00 DT price = £34.93

Ranitidine (as Ranitidine hydrochloride) 300 mg Ranitidine 300mg effervescent tablets | 30 tablet [PoM] £35.00 DT price = £34.93

Oral solution

EXCIPIENTS: May contain Alcohol

▶ Ranitidine (Non-proprietary)

Ranitidine (as Ranitidine hydrochloride) 15 mg per 1 ml Ranitidine 75mg/5ml oral solution sugar free sugar-free | 100 ml [PoM] £2.07-£2.64 sugar-free | 300 ml [PoM] £21.55 DT price = £6.26

▶ Zantac (GlaxoSmithKline UK Ltd)

Ranitidine (as Ranitidine hydrochloride) 15 mg per 1 ml Zantac 150mg/10ml syrup sugar-free | 300 ml [PoM] £20.76 DT price = £6.26

PROTON PUMP INHIBITORS

Proton pump inhibitors

Overview

Omeprazole p. 57 is an effective short-term treatment for *gastric* and *duodenal ulcers*; it is also used in combination with antibacterials for the eradication of *Helicobacter pylori*. An initial short course of omeprazole is the treatment of choice in *gastro-oesophageal reflux disease* with severe symptoms; children with endoscopically confirmed *erosive, ulcerative, or stricturing oesophagitis* usually need to be maintained on omeprazole.

Omeprazole is also used for the prevention and treatment of NSAID-associated ulcers. In children who need to continue NSAID treatment after an ulcer has healed, the dose of omeprazole should not normally be reduced because asymptomatic ulcer deterioration may occur.

Omeprazole is effective in the treatment of the *Zollinger-Ellison syndrome* (including cases resistant to other treatment). It is also used to reduce the degradation of pancreatic enzyme supplements in children with cystic fibrosis.

Lansoprazole p. 56 is not licensed for use in children, but may be considered when the available formulations of omeprazole are unsuitable.

Esomeprazole below can be used for the management of gastro-oesophageal reflux disease when the available formulations of omeprazole and lansoprazole are unsuitable.

Proton pump inhibitors

● **DRUG ACTION** Proton pump inhibitors inhibit gastric acid secretion by blocking the hydrogen-potassium adenosine triphosphatase enzyme system (the 'proton pump') of the gastric parietal cell.

> **IMPORTANT SAFETY INFORMATION**
>
> MHRA ADVICE: PROTON PUMP INHIBITORS (PPIS): VERY LOW RISK OF SUBACUTE CUTANEOUS LUPUS ERYTHEMATOSUS (SEPTEMBER 2015)
>
> Very infrequent cases of subacute cutaneous lupus erythematosus (SCLE) have been reported in patients taking PPIs. Drug-induced SCLE can occur weeks, months or even years after exposure to the drug.
>
> If a patient treated with a PPI develops lesions—especially in sun-exposed areas of the skin—and it is accompanied by arthralgia:
> • advise them to avoid exposing the skin to sunlight;
> • consider SCLE as a possible diagnosis;
> • consider discontinuing PPI treatment unless it is imperative for a serious acid-related condition; a patient who develops SCLE with a particular PPI may be at risk of the same reaction with another;
> • in most cases, symptoms resolve on PPI withdrawal; topical or systemic steroids might be necessary for treatment of SCLE only if there are no signs of remission after a few weeks or months.

● **CAUTIONS** May increase the risk of gastro-intestinal infections (including *Clostridium difficile* infection) · patients at risk of osteoporosis

CAUTIONS, FURTHER INFORMATION
▸ Risk of osteoporosis Patients at risk of osteoporosis should maintain an adequate intake of calcium and vitamin D, and if necessary, receive other preventative therapy.

● **SIDE-EFFECTS**
▸ **Common or very common** Abdominal pain · constipation · diarrhoea · flatulence · gastro-intestinal disturbances · headache · nausea · vomiting
▸ **Uncommon** Arthralgia · dizziness · dry mouth · fatigue · myalgia · paraesthesia · peripheral oedema · pruritus · rash · sleep disturbances
▸ **Rare** Alopecia · anaphylaxis · blood disorders · bronchospasm · confusion · depression · fever · gynaecomastia · hallucinations · hepatitis · hypersensitivity reactions · hypomagnesaemia (usually after 1 year of treatment, but sometimes after 3 months of treatment) · hyponatraemia · interstitial nephritis · jaundice · leucocytosis · leucopenia · pancytopenia · photosensitivity · Stevens-Johnson syndrome · stomatitis · sweating · taste disturbance · thrombocytopenia · toxic epidermal necrolysis · visual disturbances

SIDE-EFFECTS, FURTHER INFORMATION
Rebound acid hypersecretion and protracted dyspepsia may occur after stopping prolonged treatment with a proton pump inhibitor.

● **MONITORING REQUIREMENTS** Measurement of serum-magnesium concentrations should be considered before and during prolonged treatment with a proton pump inhibitor, especially when used with other drugs that cause hypomagnesaemia or with digoxin.

● **PRESCRIBING AND DISPENSING INFORMATION** A proton pump inhibitor should be prescribed for appropriate indications at the lowest effective dose for the shortest period; the need for long-term treatment should be reviewed periodically.

▶ **above**

Esomeprazole

● **INDICATIONS AND DOSE**

Gastro-oesophageal reflux disease (in the presence of erosive reflux oesophagitis)
▸ BY MOUTH
▸ Child 1–11 years (body-weight 10–19 kg): 10 mg once daily for 8 weeks
▸ Child 1–11 years (body-weight 20 kg and above): 10–20 mg once daily for 8 weeks
▸ Child 12–17 years: Initially 40 mg once daily for 4 weeks, continued for further 4 weeks if not fully healed or symptoms persist; maintenance 20 mg daily
▸ BY INTRAVENOUS INJECTION, OR BY INTRAVENOUS INFUSION
▸ Child 1–11 years (body-weight up to 20 kg): 10 mg once daily, injection to be given over at least 3 minutes
▸ Child 1–11 years (body-weight 20 kg and above): 10–20 mg once daily, injection to be given over at least 3 minutes
▸ Child 12–17 years: 40 mg daily, injection to be given over at least 3 minutes

Symptomatic treatment of gastro-oesophageal reflux disease (in the absence of oesophagitis)
▸ BY MOUTH
▸ Child 1–11 years (body-weight 10 kg and above): 10 mg once daily for up to 8 weeks
▸ Child 12–17 years: 20 mg once daily for up to 4 weeks
▸ BY INTRAVENOUS INJECTION, OR BY INTRAVENOUS INFUSION
▸ Child 1–11 years: 10 mg once daily, injection to be given over at least 3 minutes
▸ Child 12–17 years: 20 mg once daily, injection to be given over at least 3 minutes

● **UNLICENSED USE** Tablets and capsules not licensed for use in children 1–11 years.

● **INTERACTIONS** → Appendix 1: proton pump inhibitors

● **PREGNANCY** Manufacturer advises caution—no information available.

● **BREAST FEEDING** Manufacturer advises avoid—no information available.

● **HEPATIC IMPAIRMENT** 1–11 years max. 10 mg daily in severe impairment. 12–17 years max. 20 mg daily in severe impairment.

● **RENAL IMPAIRMENT** Manufacturer advises caution in severe renal insufficiency.

● **DIRECTIONS FOR ADMINISTRATION**
▸ With intravenous use For *intravenous infusion*, dilute reconstituted solution to a concentration not exceeding 800 micrograms/mL with Sodium Chloride 0.9%; give over 10–30 minutes.
▸ With oral use Do not chew or crush capsules; swallow whole or mix capsule contents in water and drink within 30 minutes. Do not crush or chew tablets; swallow whole or disperse in water and drink within 30 minutes. Disperse the contents of each sachet of gastro-resistant granules in approx. 15 mL water. Stir and leave to thicken for a few minutes; stir again before administration and use within 30 minutes; rinse container with 15 mL water to obtain full dose. For administration through a gastric tube, consult product literature.

● **PATIENT AND CARER ADVICE** Counselling on administration of gastro-resistant capsules, tablets, and granules advised.

● MEDICINAL FORMS
There can be variation in the licensing of different medicines containing the same drug. Forms available from special-order manufacturers include: oral suspension

Gastro-resistant capsule

▸ Esomeprazole (Non-proprietary)
Esomeprazole (as Esomeprazole magnesium dihydrate)
20 mg Esomeprazole 20mg gastro-resistant capsules |
28 capsule [PoM] £12.95 DT price = £2.64
Esomeprazole (as Esomeprazole magnesium dihydrate)
40 mg Esomeprazole 40mg gastro-resistant capsules |
28 capsule [PoM] £17.63 DT price = £3.30
▸ Emozul (Consilient Health Ltd)
Esomeprazole (as Esomeprazole magnesium dihydrate)
20 mg Emozul 20mg gastro-resistant capsules | 28 capsule [PoM]
£2.64 DT price = £2.64
Esomeprazole (as Esomeprazole magnesium dihydrate)
40 mg Emozul 40mg gastro-resistant capsules | 28 capsule [PoM]
£3.30 DT price = £3.30
▸ Ventra (Ethypharm UK Ltd)
Esomeprazole (as Esomeprazole magnesium dihydrate)
20 mg Ventra 20mg gastro-resistant capsules | 28 capsule [PoM]
£2.55 DT price = £2.64
Esomeprazole (as Esomeprazole magnesium dihydrate)
40 mg Ventra 40mg gastro-resistant capsules | 28 capsule [PoM]
£2.97 DT price = £3.30

Gastro-resistant tablet

▸ Esomeprazole (Non-proprietary)
Esomeprazole (as Esomeprazole magnesium trihydrate)
20 mg Esomeprazole 20mg gastro-resistant tablets | 28 tablet [PoM]
£18.50 DT price = £2.65
Esomeprazole (as Esomeprazole magnesium trihydrate)
40 mg Esomeprazole 40mg gastro-resistant tablets | 28 tablet [PoM]
£25.19 DT price = £3.31
▸ Nexium (AstraZeneca UK Ltd, Pfizer Consumer Healthcare Ltd)
Esomeprazole (as Esomeprazole magnesium trihydrate)
20 mg Nexium 20mg gastro-resistant tablets | 28 tablet [PoM]
£18.50 DT price = £2.65
Esomeprazole (as Esomeprazole magnesium trihydrate)
40 mg Nexium 40mg gastro-resistant tablets | 28 tablet [PoM]
£25.19 DT price = £3.31

Powder for solution for injection

▸ Esomeprazole (Non-proprietary)
Esomeprazole (as Esomeprazole sodium) 40 mg Esomeprazole
40mg powder for solution for injection vials | 1 vial [PoM] £3.07–£3.13
(Hospital only)
▸ Nexium (AstraZeneca UK Ltd)
Esomeprazole (as Esomeprazole sodium) 40 mg Nexium I.V 40mg
powder for solution for injection vials | 1 vial [PoM] £4.25 (Hospital
only)

Gastro-resistant granules

CAUTIONARY AND ADVISORY LABELS 25
▸ Nexium (AstraZeneca UK Ltd)
Esomeprazole (as Esomeprazole magnesium trihydrate)
10 mg Nexium 10mg gastro-resistant granules sachets |
28 sachet [PoM] £25.19 DT price = £25.19

▶ 55

Lansoprazole

07-Jun-2017

● INDICATIONS AND DOSE

Benign gastric ulcer

▸ BY MOUTH
▸ Child (body-weight up to 30 kg): 0.5–1 mg/kg once daily
(max. per dose 15 mg once daily), doses to be taken in the
morning
▸ Child (body-weight 30 kg and above): 15–30 mg once
daily, doses to be taken in the morning

Duodenal ulcer

▸ BY MOUTH
▸ Child (body-weight up to 30 kg): 0.5–1 mg/kg once daily
(max. per dose 15 mg once daily), doses to be taken in the
morning
▸ Child (body-weight 30 kg and above): 15–30 mg once
daily, doses to be taken in the morning

**NSAID-associated duodenal ulcer | NSAID-associated
gastric ulcer**

▸ BY MOUTH
▸ Child (body-weight up to 30 kg): 0.5–1 mg/kg once daily
(max. per dose 15 mg once daily), doses to be taken in
the morning
▸ Child (body-weight 30 kg and above): 15–30 mg once
daily, doses to be taken in the morning

Gastro-oesophageal reflux disease

▸ BY MOUTH
▸ Child (body-weight up to 30 kg): 0.5–1 mg/kg once daily
(max. per dose 15 mg once daily), doses to be taken in
the morning
▸ Child (body-weight 30 kg and above): 15–30 mg once
daily, doses to be taken in the morning

Acid-related dyspepsia

▸ BY MOUTH
▸ Child (body-weight up to 30 kg): 0.5–1 mg/kg once daily
(max. per dose 15 mg once daily), doses to be taken in
the morning
▸ Child (body-weight 30 kg and above): 15–30 mg once
daily, doses to be taken in the morning

**Fat malabsorption despite pancreatic enzyme
replacement therapy in cystic fibrosis**

▸ BY MOUTH
▸ Child (body-weight up to 30 kg): 0.5–1 mg/kg once daily
(max. per dose 15 mg once daily), doses to be taken in
the morning
▸ Child (body-weight 30 kg and above): 15–30 mg once
daily, doses to be taken in the morning

● UNLICENSED USE Not licensed for use in children.
● INTERACTIONS → Appendix 1: proton pump inhibitors
● SIDE-EFFECTS
▸ Very rare Colitis · raised serum cholesterol · raised
triglycerides
▸ Frequency not known Anorexia · glossitis · impotence ·
pancreatitis · petechiae · purpura · restlessness · tremor
● PREGNANCY Manufacturer advises avoid.
● BREAST FEEDING Avoid—present in milk in *animal* studies.
● HEPATIC IMPAIRMENT Use half normal dose in moderate to
severe liver disease.
● DIRECTIONS FOR ADMINISTRATION Orodispersible tablets
should be placed on the tongue, allowed to disperse and
swallowed, or may be swallowed whole with a glass of
water. Alternatively, tablets can be dispersed in a small
amount of water and administered by an oral syringe or
nasogastric tube.
● PATIENT AND CARER ADVICE
Counselling on administration of orodispersible tablet
advised.
Medicines for Children leaflet: Lansoprazole for gastro-
oesophageal reflux disease (GORD) and ulcers
www.medicinesforchildren.org.uk/lansoprazole-for-gord-and-
ulcers

● MEDICINAL FORMS
There can be variation in the licensing of different medicines
containing the same drug. Forms available from special-order
manufacturers include: oral suspension, oral solution, powder

Gastro-resistant capsule

CAUTIONARY AND ADVISORY LABELS 5, 22, 25
▸ Lansoprazole (Non-proprietary)
Lansoprazole 15 mg Lansoprazole 15mg gastro-resistant capsules |
28 capsule [PoM] £12.92 DT price = £0.54
Lansoprazole 30 mg Lansoprazole 30mg gastro-resistant capsules |
28 capsule [PoM] £23.63 DT price = £1.11

Orodispersible tablet

CAUTIONARY AND ADVISORY LABELS 5, 22

EXCIPIENTS: May contain Aspartame

▸ **Lansoprazole (Non-proprietary)**
Lansoprazole 15 mg Lansoprazole 15mg orodispersible tablets | 28 tablet [PoM] £3.99 DT price = £2.10
Lansoprazole 30 mg Lansoprazole 30mg orodispersible tablets | 28 tablet [PoM] £6.99 DT price = £3.42

▸ **Zoton FasTab (Pfizer Ltd)**
Lansoprazole 15 mg Zoton FasTab 15mg | 28 tablet [PoM] £2.99 DT price = £2.10
Lansoprazole 30 mg Zoton FasTab 30mg | 28 tablet [PoM] £5.50 DT price = £3.42

F 55

Omeprazole

● **INDICATIONS AND DOSE**

Helicobacter pylori **eradication in combination with amoxicillin and clarithromycin; or in combination with amoxicillin and metronidazole; or in combination with clarithromycin and metronidazole**
▸ BY MOUTH

▸ Child 1–5 years: 1–2 mg/kg once daily (max. per dose 40 mg)
▸ Child 6–11 years: 1–2 mg/kg once daily (max. per dose 40 mg)
▸ Child 12–17 years: 40 mg once daily

Treatment of duodenal ulcers including those complicating NSAID therapy | Treatment of benign gastric ulcers including those complicating NSAID therapy
▸ BY MOUTH

▸ Neonate: 700 micrograms/kg once daily for 7–14 days, then increased if necessary to 1.4–2.8 mg/kg once daily.

▸ Child 1 month–1 year: 700 micrograms/kg once daily, increased if necessary to 3 mg/kg once daily (max. per dose 20 mg)
▸ Child 2–17 years (body-weight 10–19 kg): 10 mg once daily, increased if necessary to 20 mg once daily
▸ Child 2–17 years (body-weight 20 kg and above): 20 mg once daily, increased if necessary to 40 mg once daily
▸ BY INTRAVENOUS INJECTION, OR BY INTRAVENOUS INFUSION
▸ Child 1 month–11 years: Initially 500 micrograms/kg once daily (max. per dose 20 mg), increased if necessary to 2 mg/kg once daily (max. per dose 40 mg), injection to be given over 5 minutes
▸ Child 12–17 years: 40 mg once daily, injection to be given over 5 minutes

Zollinger–Ellison syndrome
▸ BY MOUTH

▸ Neonate: 700 micrograms/kg once daily for 7–14 days, then increased if necessary to 1.4–2.8 mg/kg once daily.

▸ Child 1 month–1 year: 700 micrograms/kg once daily, increased if necessary to 3 mg/kg once daily (max. per dose 20 mg)
▸ Child 2–17 years (body-weight 10–19 kg): 10 mg once daily, increased if necessary to 20 mg once daily
▸ Child 2–17 years (body-weight 20 kg and above): 20 mg once daily, increased if necessary to 40 mg once daily
▸ BY INTRAVENOUS INJECTION, OR BY INTRAVENOUS INFUSION
▸ Child 1 month–11 years: Initially 500 micrograms/kg once daily (max. per dose 20 mg), increased if necessary to 2 mg/kg once daily (max. per dose 40 mg), injection to be given over 5 minutes
▸ Child 12–17 years: 40 mg once daily, injection to be given over 5 minutes

Gastro-oesophageal reflux disease
▸ BY MOUTH

▸ Neonate: 700 micrograms/kg once daily for 7–14 days, then increased if necessary to 1.4–2.8 mg/kg once daily.

▸ Child 1 month–1 year: 700 micrograms/kg once daily, increased if necessary to 3 mg/kg once daily (max. per dose 20 mg)
▸ Child 2–17 years (body-weight 10–19 kg): 10 mg once daily, increased if necessary to 20 mg once daily, in severe ulcerating reflux oesophagitis, maximum 12 weeks at higher dose
▸ Child 2–17 years (body-weight 20 kg and above): 20 mg once daily, increased if necessary to 40 mg once daily, in severe ulcerating reflux oesophagitis, maximum 12 weeks at higher dose
▸ BY INTRAVENOUS INJECTION, OR BY INTRAVENOUS INFUSION
▸ Child 1 month–11 years: Initially 500 micrograms/kg once daily (max. per dose 20 mg), increased if necessary to 2 mg/kg once daily (max. per dose 40 mg), injection to be given over 5 minutes
▸ Child 12–17 years: 40 mg once daily, injection to be given over 5 minutes

Acid-related dyspepsia
▸ BY MOUTH

▸ Neonate: 700 micrograms/kg once daily for 7–14 days, then increased if necessary to 1.4–2.8 mg/kg once daily.

▸ Child 1 month–1 year: 700 micrograms/kg once daily, increased if necessary to 3 mg/kg once daily (max. per dose 20 mg)
▸ Child 2–17 years (initiated by a specialist) (body-weight 10–19 kg): 10 mg once daily, increased if necessary to 20 mg once daily
▸ Child 2–17 years (initiated by a specialist) (body-weight 20 kg and above): 20 mg once daily, increased if necessary to 40 mg once daily
▸ BY INTRAVENOUS INJECTION, OR BY INTRAVENOUS INFUSION
▸ Child 1 month–11 years: Initially 500 micrograms/kg once daily (max. per dose 20 mg), increased if necessary to 2 mg/kg once daily (max. per dose 40 mg), injection to be given over 5 minutes
▸ Child 12–17 years: 40 mg once daily, injection to be given over 5 minutes

Fat malabsorption despite pancreatic enzyme replacement therapy in cystic fibrosis
▸ BY MOUTH

▸ Neonate: 700 micrograms/kg once daily for 7–14 days, then increased if necessary to 1.4–2.8 mg/kg once daily.

▸ Child 1 month–1 year: 700 micrograms/kg once daily, increased if necessary to 3 mg/kg once daily (max. per dose 20 mg)
▸ Child 2–17 years (body-weight 10–19 kg): 10 mg once daily, increased if necessary to 20 mg once daily
▸ Child 2–17 years (body-weight 20 kg and above): 20 mg once daily, increased if necessary to 40 mg once daily
▸ BY INTRAVENOUS INJECTION, OR BY INTRAVENOUS INFUSION
▸ Child 1 month–11 years: Initially 500 micrograms/kg once daily (max. per dose 20 mg), increased if necessary to 2 mg/kg once daily (max. per dose 40 mg), injection to be given over 5 minutes
▸ Child 12–17 years: 40 mg once daily, injection to be given over 5 minutes

● **UNLICENSED USE** *Capsules and tablets* not licensed for use in children except for severe ulcerating reflux oesophagitis in children over 1 year. *Injection* not licensed for use in children under 12 years.

● **INTERACTIONS** → Appendix 1: proton pump inhibitors

● **SIDE-EFFECTS** Agitation · impotence

1

Gastro-intestinal system

- **PREGNANCY** Not known to be harmful.
- **BREAST FEEDING** Present in milk but not known to be harmful.
- **HEPATIC IMPAIRMENT** No more than 700 micrograms/kg (max. 20 mg) once daily.
- **DIRECTIONS FOR ADMINISTRATION** For administration by *mouth*, swallow whole, or disperse *Losec MUPS*® tablets in water, *or* mix capsule contents or *Losec MUPS*® tablets with fruit juice or yoghurt. Preparations consisting of an e/c tablet within a capsule should **not** be opened.

  For administration through an *enteral feeding tube*, use *Losec MUPS*® or the contents of a capsule containing omeprazole dispersed in a large volume of water, or in 10 mL Sodium Bicarbonate 8.4% (1 mmol Na⁺/mL). Allow to stand for 10 minutes before administration.
  - With intravenous use For *intermittent intravenous infusion*, dilute reconstituted solution to a concentration of 400 micrograms/mL with Glucose 5% or Sodium Chloride 0.9%; give over 20–30 minutes.
- **PATIENT AND CARER ADVICE**
  Medicines for Children leaflet: Omeprazole for gastro-oesophageal reflux disease (GORD) www.medicinesforchildren.org.uk/omeprazole-for-gord
  - With oral use Counselling on administration advised.
- **PROFESSION SPECIFIC INFORMATION**
  Dental practitioners' formulary
  Gastro-resistant omeprazole capsules may be prescribed.

- **MEDICINAL FORMS**
  There can be variation in the licensing of different medicines containing the same drug. Forms available from special-order manufacturers include: oral suspension, oral solution

  Gastro-resistant capsule
  - Omeprazole (Non-proprietary)
    Omeprazole 10 mg Omeprazole 10mg gastro-resistant capsules | 28 capsule [PoM] £9.30 DT price = £0.89
    Omeprazole 20 mg Omeprazole 20mg gastro-resistant capsules | 28 capsule [PoM] £13.50 DT price = £0.91
    Omeprazole 40 mg Omeprazole 40mg gastro-resistant capsules | 7 capsule [PoM] £6.96 DT price = £0.75 | 28 capsule [PoM] £19.72
  - Losec (AstraZeneca UK Ltd)
    Omeprazole 10 mg Losec 10mg gastro-resistant capsules | 28 capsule [PoM] £9.30 DT price = £0.89
    Omeprazole 20 mg Losec 20mg gastro-resistant capsules | 28 capsule [PoM] £13.92 DT price = £0.91
    Omeprazole 40 mg Losec 40mg gastro-resistant capsules | 7 capsule [PoM] £6.96 DT price = £0.75
  - Mepradec (Discovery Pharmaceuticals)
    Omeprazole 10 mg Mepradec 10mg gastro-resistant capsules | 28 capsule [PoM] £0.83 DT price = £0.89
    Omeprazole 20 mg Mepradec 20mg gastro-resistant capsules | 28 capsule [PoM] £0.83 DT price = £0.91

  Gastro-resistant tablet
  CAUTIONARY AND ADVISORY LABELS 25
  - Omeprazole (Non-proprietary)
    Omeprazole 10 mg Omeprazole 10mg gastro-resistant tablets | 28 tablet [PoM] £18.91 DT price = £7.90
    Omeprazole (as Omeprazole magnesium) 10 mg Omeprazole 10mg dispersible gastro-resistant tablets | 28 tablet [PoM] £8.06 DT price = £7.75
    Omeprazole 20 mg Omeprazole 20mg gastro-resistant tablets | 28 tablet [PoM] £28.56 DT price = £6.01
    Omeprazole (as Omeprazole magnesium) 20 mg Omeprazole 20mg dispersible gastro-resistant tablets | 28 tablet [PoM] £11.60 DT price = £11.60
    Omeprazole 40 mg Omeprazole 40mg gastro-resistant tablets | 7 tablet [PoM] £15.00 DT price = £6.02
    Omeprazole (as Omeprazole magnesium) 40 mg Omeprazole 40mg dispersible gastro-resistant tablets | 7 tablet [PoM] £6.30 DT price = £5.80
  - Losec (AstraZeneca UK Ltd)
    Omeprazole (as Omeprazole magnesium) 10 mg Losec MUPS 10mg gastro-resistant tablets | 28 tablet [PoM] £7.75 DT price = £7.75
    Omeprazole (as Omeprazole magnesium) 20 mg Losec MUPS 20mg gastro-resistant tablets | 28 tablet [PoM] £11.60 DT price = £11.60

Omeprazole (as Omeprazole magnesium) 40 mg Losec MUPS 40mg gastro-resistant tablets | 7 tablet [PoM] £5.80 DT price = £5.80
- Mezzopram (Sandoz Ltd)
  Omeprazole (as Omeprazole magnesium) 10 mg Mezzopram 10mg gastro-resistant tablets | 28 tablet [PoM] £6.58 DT price = £7.75
  Omeprazole (as Omeprazole magnesium) 20 mg Mezzopram 20mg gastro-resistant tablets | 28 tablet [PoM] £9.86 DT price = £11.60
  Omeprazole (as Omeprazole magnesium) 40 mg Mezzopram 40mg gastro-resistant tablets | 7 tablet [PoM] £4.93 DT price = £5.80

Powder for solution for infusion
- Omeprazole (Non-proprietary)
  Omeprazole (as Omeprazole sodium) 40 mg Omeprazole 40mg powder for solution for infusion vials | 5 vial [PoM] £32.45 (Hospital only) | 5 vial [PoM] £16.54

4.3 Gastro-oesophageal reflux disease

Gastro-oesophageal reflux disease

Management

Gastro-oesophageal reflux disease includes non-erosive gastro-oesophageal reflux and erosive oesophagitis. Uncomplicated gastro-oesophageal reflux is common in infancy and most symptoms, such as intermittent vomiting or repeated, effortless regurgitation, resolve without treatment between 12 and 18 months of age. Older children with gastro-oesophageal reflux disease may have heartburn, acid regurgitation and dysphagia. Oesophageal inflammation (oesophagitis), ulceration or stricture formation may develop in early childhood; gastro-oesophageal reflux disease may also be associated with chronic respiratory disorders including asthma.

Parents and carers of *neonates* and *infants* should be reassured that most symptoms of uncomplicated gastro-oesophageal reflux resolve without treatment. An increase in the frequency and a decrease in the volume of feeds may reduce symptoms. A feed thickener or pre-thickened formula feed can be used on the advice of a dietician. If necessary, a suitable alginate-containing preparation can be used instead of thickened feeds. A thickening agent should be tried for up to 2 weeks before considering other treatment.

Older children should be advised about life-style changes such as weight reduction if overweight, and the avoidance of alcohol and smoking. An alginate-containing antacid can be used to relieve symptoms.

Children who do not respond to these measures or who have problems such as respiratory disorders or suspected oesophagitis need to be referred to hospital. On the advice of a paediatrician, a **histamine H₂-receptor antagonist** can be used to relieve symptoms of gastro-oesophageal reflux disease, promote mucosal healing and permit reduction in antacid consumption. A **proton pump inhibitor** can be used for the treatment of moderate, non-erosive oesophagitis that is unresponsive to an H₂- receptor antagonist. Endoscopically confirmed *erosive*, *ulcerative*, or *stricturing* disease in children is usually treated with a proton pump inhibitor. Reassessment is necessary if symptoms persist despite 4–6 weeks of treatment; long-term use of an H₂-receptor antagonist or proton pump inhibitor should not be undertaken without full assessment of the underlying condition. For endoscopically confirmed *erosive*, *ulcerative*, or *stricturing* disease, the proton pump inhibitor usually needs to be maintained at the minimum effective dose.

Motility stimulants, such as erythromycin p. 316 may improve gastro-oesophageal sphincter contraction and accelerate gastric emptying. Evidence for the long-term efficacy of motility stimulants in the management of gastro-oesophageal reflux in children is unconvincing.

For advice on specialised formula feeds, see Enteral feeds.

Pregnancy

If dietary and lifestyle changes fail to control gastro-oesophageal reflux disease in pregnancy, an antacid or an alginate can be used. If this is ineffective, ranitidine p. 53 can be tried. Omeprazole p. 57 is reserved for women with severe or complicated reflux disease.

> **Other drugs used for Gastro-oesophageal reflux disease**
> Esomeprazole, p. 55 · Lansoprazole, p. 56

ANTACIDS > ALGINATE

Sodium alginate with calcium carbonate and sodium bicarbonate

The properties listed below are those particular to the combination only. For the properties of the components please consider, alginic acid p. 49, sodium bicarbonate p. 558, calcium carbonate p. 567.

- ● **INDICATIONS AND DOSE**

  Mild symptoms of gastro-oesophageal reflux disease
  - ▸ BY MOUTH
  - ▸ Child 6–11 years: 5–10 mL, to be taken after meals and at bedtime
  - ▸ Child 12–17 years: 10–20 mL, to be taken after meals and at bedtime

- ● **INTERACTIONS** → Appendix 1: calcium salts, sodium bicarbonate

- ● **PRESCRIBING AND DISPENSING INFORMATION** Flavours of oral liquid formulations may include aniseed or peppermint.

- ● **PATIENT AND CARER ADVICE**

  Medicines for Children leaflet: Gaviscon for gastro-oesophageal reflux disease www.medicinesforchildren.org.uk/gaviscon-gastro-oesophageal-reflux-disease

- ● **MEDICINAL FORMS**

  There can be variation in the licensing of different medicines containing the same drug.

  Oral suspension

  ELECTROLYTES: May contain Sodium
  - ▸ **Sodium alginate with calcium carbonate and sodium bicarbonate** (Non-proprietary)
    Calcium carbonate 16 mg per 1 ml, Sodium bicarbonate 26.7 mg per 1 ml, Sodium alginate 50 mg per 1 ml Alginate raft-forming oral suspension sugar-free peppermint sugar-free | 500 ml [GSL] no price available DT price = £1.95
    Alginate raft-forming oral suspension sugar free aniseed sugar-free | 500 ml [GSL] no price available DT price = £1.95
    Alginate raft-forming oral suspension sugar free sugar-free | 500 ml [GSL] no price available DT price = £1.95
  - ▸ Brands may include Acidex, Entrocalm Heartburn and Indigestion Relief, Gaviscon, Gaviscon Cool, Gaviscon Liquid Relief, Peptac

4.4 *Helicobacter pylori* diagnosis

DIAGNOSTIC AGENTS

Urea (13C)

- ● **INDICATIONS AND DOSE**

  Diagnosis of gastro-duodenal *Helicobacter pylori* infection
  - ▸ BY MOUTH
  - ▸ Child: (consult product literature)

- ● **MEDICINAL FORMS**

  There can be variation in the licensing of different medicines containing the same drug.

  Soluble tablet
  - ▸ **Pylobactell** (Torbet Laboratories Ltd)
    Urea [13-C] 100 mg Pylobactell breath test kit | 1 kit [PoM] £20.75

  Powder
  - ▸ **Helicobacter Test INFAI** (INFAI UK Ltd)
    Urea [13-C] 45 mg Helicobacter Test INFAI for children breath test kit sugar-free | 1 kit [PoM] £19.10
    Urea [13-C] 75 mg Helicobacter Test INFAI breath test kit sugar-free | 1 kit [PoM] £21.70

  Tablet
  - ▸ **Diabact UBT** (Seahorse Laboratories Ltd)
    Urea [13-C] 50 mg diabact UBT 50mg tablets | 1 tablet [PoM] £21.25 | 10 tablet [PoM] no price available (Hospital only)

5 Food allergy

Food allergy

15-Dec-2016

Description of condition

Food allergy is an adverse immune response to a food, commonly associated with cutaneous and gastro-intestinal reactions, and less frequently associated with respiratory reactions and anaphylaxis. It is distinct from food intolerance which is non-immunological. Cow's milk, hen's eggs, soy, wheat, peanuts, tree nuts, fish, and shellfish are the most common allergens. Cross-reactivity between similar foods can occur (e.g. allergy to other mammalian milk in patients with cow's milk allergy).

Management of food allergy

[EvGr] Allergy caused by specific foods should be managed by strict avoidance of the causal food. Sodium cromoglicate p. 161 is licensed as an adjunct to dietary avoidance in children with food allergy. Educating the child or their carer about appropriate nutrition, food preparation, and the risks of accidental exposure is recommended, such as food and drinks to avoid, ensuring adequate nutritional intake, and interpreting food labels. For children in whom elimination diets might affect growth, a consultation with a nutritionist is recommended to identify alternative dietary sources. [A]

Drug treatment

[EvGr] There is low quality evidence to support the use of antihistamines to treat acute, **non-life-threatening** symptoms (such as flushing and urticaria) if accidental ingestion of allergenic food has occurred (see *Antihistamines*, under Antihistamines, allergen immunotherapy and allergic emergencies p. 165). Chlorphenamine maleate p. 172 is licensed for the symptomatic control of food allergy. In case of food-induced anaphylaxis, adrenaline/epinephrine p. 132 is the first-line immediate treatment (see also *Allergic emergencies*, under Antihistamines, allergen immunotherapy and allergic emergencies p. 165). Carers and children (of an appropriate age) who are at risk of anaphylaxis should be trained to use self-injectable adrenaline/epinephrine. [A]

Cow's milk allergy

[EvGr] Parents of infants with suspected allergy to cow's milk should be informed about the most appropriate hypoallergenic formula or milk substitute. Cow's milk avoidance is recommended for the mothers of breast-fed infants who have cow's milk allergy. Children who are allergic to milk should receive alternative dietary sources of calcium and vitamin D. [A]

Useful Resources

Food allergy in under 19s: assessment and diagnosis. National Institute for Health and Care Excellence. Clinical guideline 116. February 2011
www.nice.org.uk/guidance/cg116

6 Gastro-intestinal smooth muscle spasm

Antispasmodics

Antimuscarinics

The intestinal smooth muscle relaxant properties of antimuscarinic and other antispasmodic drugs may be useful in *irritable bowel syndrome*.

Antimuscarinics (formerly termed 'anticholinergics') reduce intestinal motility. They are occasionally used for the management of *irritable bowel syndrome*.

Antimuscarinics that are used for gastro-intestinal smooth muscle spasm includes the tertiary amine dicycloverine hydrochloride below and the quaternary ammonium compounds propantheline bromide p. 61 and hyoscine butylbromide p. 61. The quaternary ammonium compounds are less lipid soluble than atropine and are less likely to cross the blood-brain barrier; they are also less well absorbed from the gastro-intestinal tract.

Dicycloverine hydrochloride, may also have some direct action on smooth muscle. Hyoscine butylbromide is advocated as a gastro-intestinal antispasmodic, but it is poorly absorbed; the injection may be useful in endoscopy and radiology.

Other indications for antimuscarinic drugs include asthma and airways disease, motion sickness, urinary frequency and enuresis, mydriasis and cycloplegia, premedication, palliative care and as an antidote to organophosphorus poisoning.

Other antispasmodics

Alverine citrate p. 62, mebeverine hydrochloride p. 62, and peppermint oil p. 34 are believed to be direct relaxants of intestinal smooth muscle and may relieve pain in *irritable bowel syndrome*, and *primary dysmenorrhoea*. They have no serious adverse effects but, like all antispasmodics, should be avoided in paralytic ileus.

Motility stimulants

Domperidone is a dopamine receptor antagonist which stimulates gastric emptying and small intestinal transit, and enhances the strength of oesophageal sphincter contraction. The MHRA/CHM has issued restrictions on its use because domperidone is associated with a small increased risk of serious cardiac side effects.

A low dose of erythromycin p. 316 stimulates gastro-intestinal motility and may be used on the advice of a paediatric gastroenterologist to promote tolerance of enteral feeds; erythromycin may be less effective as a prokinetic drug in preterm neonates than in older children.

ANTIMUSCARINICS

F 468

Dicycloverine hydrochloride

(Dicyclomine hydrochloride)

● **INDICATIONS AND DOSE**

Symptomatic relief of gastro-intestinal disorders characterised by smooth muscle spasm
▸ BY MOUTH
▸ Child 6-23 months: 5–10 mg 3–4 times a day, dose to be taken 15 minutes before feeds
▸ Child 2-11 years: 10 mg 3 times a day
▸ Child 12-17 years: 10–20 mg 3 times a day

● **CONTRA-INDICATIONS** Child under 6 months
● **INTERACTIONS** → Appendix 1: dicycloverine
● **PREGNANCY** Not known to be harmful; manufacturer advises use only if essential.
● **BREAST FEEDING** Avoid—present in milk; apnoea reported in infant.
● **EXCEPTIONS TO LEGAL CATEGORY** Dicycloverine hydrochloride can be sold to the public provided that max. single dose is 10 mg and max. daily dose is 60 mg.

● **MEDICINAL FORMS**
There can be variation in the licensing of different medicines containing the same drug.
Oral solution
▸ Dicycloverine hydrochloride (Non-proprietary)
Dicycloverine hydrochloride 2 mg per 1 ml Dicycloverine 10mg/5ml oral solution | 100 ml [PoM] no price available | 120 ml [PoM] £196.36 DT price = £178.79 | 300 ml [PoM] no price available
Tablet
▸ Dicycloverine hydrochloride (Non-proprietary)
Dicycloverine hydrochloride 10 mg Dicycloverine 10mg tablets | 100 tablet [PoM] £201.22 DT price = £184.25
Dicycloverine hydrochloride 20 mg D cycloverine 20mg tablets | 84 tablet [PoM] £203.42 DT price = £196.69

Dicycloverine hydrochloride with aluminium hydroxide, magnesium oxide and simeticone

The properties listed below are those particular to the combination only. For the properties of the components please consider, dicycloverine hydrochloride above, aluminium hydroxide p. 572, simeticone p. 51.

● **INDICATIONS AND DOSE**

Symptomatic relief of gastro-intestinal disorders characterised by smooth muscle spasm
▸ BY MOUTH
▸ Child 12-17 years: 10–20 mL every 4 hours as required

● **INTERACTIONS** → Appendix 1: antacids, dicycloverine

● **MEDICINAL FORMS**
There can be variation in the licensing of different medicines containing the same drug.
Oral suspension
▸ Kolanticon (Peckforton Pharmaceuticals Ltd)
Dicycloverine hydrochloride 500 microgram per 1 ml, Simeticone 4 mg per 1 ml, Magnesium oxide light 20 mg per 1 ml, Aluminium hydroxide dried 40 mg per 1 ml Kolanticon gel sugar-free | 200 ml [P] £4.00 sugar-free | 500 ml [P] £6.00

Hyoscine butylbromide

`F 468` 13-Mar-2017

● **INDICATIONS AND DOSE**

Symptomatic relief of gastro-intestinal or genito-urinary disorders characterised by smooth muscle spasm

▸ BY MOUTH

  ▸ Child 6–11 years: 10 mg 3 times a day
  ▸ Child 12–17 years: 20 mg 4 times a day

Acute spasm | Spasm in diagnostic procedures

▸ INITIALLY BY INTRAMUSCULAR INJECTION, OR BY SLOW INTRAVENOUS INJECTION

  ▸ Child 2–5 years: 5 mg, then (by intramuscular injection or by slow intravenous injection) 5 mg after 30 minutes if required, dose may be repeated more frequently in endoscopy; maximum 15 mg per day
  ▸ Child 6–11 years: 5–10 mg, then (by intramuscular injection or by intravenous injection) 5–10 mg after 30 minutes if required, dose may be repeated more frequently in endoscopy; maximum 30 mg per day
  ▸ Child 12–17 years: 20 mg, then (by intramuscular injection or by slow intravenous injection) 20 mg after 30 minutes if required, dose may be repeated more frequently in endoscopy; maximum 80 mg per day

Excessive respiratory secretions in palliative care

▸ BY MOUTH

  ▸ Child 1 month–1 year: 300–500 micrograms/kg 3–4 times a day (max. per dose 5 mg)
  ▸ Child 2–4 years: 5 mg 3–4 times a day
  ▸ Child 5–11 years: 10 mg 3–4 times a day
  ▸ Child 12–17 years: 10–20 mg 3–4 times a day

▸ BY INTRAMUSCULAR INJECTION, OR BY INTRAVENOUS INJECTION

  ▸ Child 1 month–4 years: 300–500 micrograms/kg 3–4 times a day (max. per dose 5 mg)
  ▸ Child 5–11 years: 5–10 mg 3–4 times a day
  ▸ Child 12–17 years: 10–20 mg 3–4 times a day

Bowel colic (in palliative care)

▸ BY MOUTH

  ▸ Child 1 month–1 year: 300–500 micrograms/kg 3–4 times a day (max. per dose 5 mg)
  ▸ Child 2–4 years: 5 mg 3–4 times a day
  ▸ Child 5–11 years: 10 mg 3–4 times a day
  ▸ Child 12–17 years: 10–20 mg 3–4 times a day

▸ BY INTRAMUSCULAR INJECTION, OR BY INTRAVENOUS INJECTION

  ▸ Child 1 month–4 years: 300–500 micrograms/kg 3–4 times a day (max. per dose 5 mg)
  ▸ Child 5–11 years: 5–10 mg 3–4 times a day
  ▸ Child 12–17 years: 10–20 mg 3–4 times a day

PHARMACOKINETICS

Administration by mouth is associated with poor absorption.

● **UNLICENSED USE** *Tablets* not licensed for use in children under 6 years. *Injection* not licensed for use in children (age range not specified by manufacturer).

IMPORTANT SAFETY INFORMATION

MHRA/CHM ADVICE: HYOSCINE BUTYLBROMIDE (*BUSCOPAN*®) INJECTION: RISK OF SERIOUS ADVERSE EFFECTS IN PATIENTS WITH UNDERLYING CARDIAC DISEASE (FEBRUARY 2017)

The MHRA advises that hyoscine butylbromide injection can cause serious adverse effects including tachycardia, hypotension, and anaphylaxis; several reports have noted that anaphylaxis is more likely to be fatal in patients with underlying coronary heart disease. Hyoscine butylbromide injection is contra-indicated in patients with tachycardia and should be used with caution in patients with cardiac disease; the MHRA recommends that these patients are monitored and that resuscitation equipment and trained personnel are readily available.

● **CONTRA-INDICATIONS**
▸ With intramuscular use or intravenous use Tachycardia

● **INTERACTIONS** → Appendix 1: hyoscine

● **SIDE-EFFECTS**

GENERAL SIDE-EFFECTS

Anaphylaxis

SPECIFIC SIDE-EFFECTS

▸ **Common or very common**
▸ With intramuscular use or intravenous use Tachycardia
▸ **Uncommon**
▸ With oral use Tachycardia
▸ **Frequency not known**
▸ With intramuscular use or intravenous use Hypotension

● **PREGNANCY** Manufacturer advises avoid.

● **BREAST FEEDING** Amount too small to be harmful.

● **DIRECTIONS FOR ADMINISTRATION**
▸ With oral use For administration by *mouth*, injection solution may be used; content of ampoule may be stored in a refrigerator for up to 24 hours after opening.
▸ With intravenous use For *intravenous injection*, may be diluted with Glucose 5% or Sodium Chloride 0.9%; give over at least 1 minute.

● **PRESCRIBING AND DISPENSING INFORMATION**

Palliative care

For further information on the use of hyoscine butylbromide in palliative care, see www.palliativedrugs.com/formulary/en/bnf-1-2.html.

● **MEDICINAL FORMS**

There can be variation in the licensing of different medicines containing the same drug. Forms available from special-order manufacturers include: oral suspension, oral solution

Solution for injection

▸ Buscopan (Boehringer Ingelheim Ltd)
  Hyoscine butylbromide 20 mg per 1 ml Buscopan 20mg/1ml solution for injection ampoules | 10 ampoule `PoM` £2.92 DT price = £2.92

Tablet

▸ Buscopan (Boehringer Ingelheim Self-Medication Division, Boehringer Ingelheim Ltd)
  Hyoscine butylbromide 10 mg Buscopan 10mg tablets | 56 tablet `PoM` £3.00 DT price = £3.00

`F 468`

Propantheline bromide

● **INDICATIONS AND DOSE**

Symptomatic relief of gastro-intestinal disorders characterised by smooth muscle spasm

▸ BY MOUTH

  ▸ Child 1 month–11 years: 300 micrograms/kg 3–4 times a day (max. per dose 15 mg), dose to be taken at least one hour before food
  ▸ Child 12–17 years: 15 mg 3 times a day, dose to be taken at least one hour before food and 30 mg, dose to be taken at night; maximum 120 mg per day

● **UNLICENSED USE** *Tablets* not licensed for use in children under 12 years.

● **INTERACTIONS** → Appendix 1: propantheline

● **SIDE-EFFECTS** Facial flushing

● **PREGNANCY** Manufacturer advises avoid unless essential—no information available.

● **BREAST FEEDING** May suppress lactation.

● **HEPATIC IMPAIRMENT** Manufacturer advises caution.

● **RENAL IMPAIRMENT** Manufacturer advises caution.

● **MEDICINAL FORMS**
There can be variation in the licensing of different medicines containing the same drug. Forms available from special-order manufacturers include: oral suspension, oral solution

Tablet

CAUTIONARY AND ADVISORY LABELS 23

▸ **Propantheline bromide (Non-proprietary)**
Propantheline bromide 15 mg Propantheline bromide 15mg tablets | 100 tablet PoM no price available

▸ **Pro-Banthine** (Kyowa Kirin Ltd)
Propantheline bromide 15 mg Pro-Banthine 15mg tablets | 112 tablet PoM £20.74 DT price = £20.74

ANTISPASMODICS

Alverine citrate

24-Feb-2016

● **INDICATIONS AND DOSE**

Symptomatic relief of gastro-intestinal disorders characterised by smooth muscle spasm | Dysmenorrhoea
▸ BY MOUTH
▸ Child 12–17 years: 60–120 mg 1–3 times a day

● **CONTRA-INDICATIONS** Intestinal obstruction · paralytic ileus

● **SIDE-EFFECTS** Dizziness · dyspnoea · headache · hepatitis · jaundice (resolves with cessation) · nausea · pruritus · wheezing

● **PREGNANCY** Manufacturer advises avoid—limited information available

● **BREAST FEEDING** Manufacturer advises avoid—limited information available.

● **PATIENT AND CARER ADVICE**

Driving and skilled tasks
Dizziness may affect performance of skilled tasks (e.g. driving).

● **MEDICINAL FORMS**
There can be variation in the licensing of different medicines containing the same drug.

Capsule

▸ **Alverine citrate (Non-proprietary)**
Alverine citrate 60 mg Alverine 60mg capsules | 100 capsule P £19.49 DT price = £19.48
Alverine citrate 120 mg Alverine 120mg capsules | 60 capsule P £23.28 DT price = £23.28

▸ **Audmonal** (Teva UK Ltd)
Alverine citrate 60 mg Audmonal 60mg capsules | 100 capsule P £14.80 DT price = £19.48
Alverine citrate 120 mg Audmonal Forte 120mg capsules | 60 capsule P £17.75 DT price = £23.28

▸ **Gielism** (HFA Healthcare Products Ltd)
Alverine citrate 60 mg Gielism 60mg capsules | 100 capsule P £19.48 DT price = £19.48

▸ **Spasmonal** (Meda Pharmaceuticals Ltd)
Alverine citrate 60 mg Spasmonal 60mg capsules | 100 capsule P £16.45 DT price = £19.48
Alverine citrate 120 mg Spasmonal Forte 120mg capsules | 60 capsule P £19.42 DT price = £23.28

Mebeverine hydrochloride

● **INDICATIONS AND DOSE**

Adjunct in gastro-intestinal disorders characterised by smooth muscle spasm
▸ BY MOUTH USING IMMEDIATE-RELEASE MEDICINES
▸ Child 3 years: 25 mg 3 times a day, dose preferably taken 20 minutes before meals
▸ Child 4–7 years: 50 mg 3 times a day, dose preferably taken 20 minutes before meals
▸ Child 8–9 years: 100 mg 3 times a day, dose preferably taken 20 minutes before meals

▸ Child 10–17 years: 135–150 mg 3 times a day, dose preferably taken 20 minutes before meals

Irritable bowel syndrome
▸ BY MOUTH USING MODIFIED-RELEASE MEDICINES
▸ Child 12–17 years: 200 mg twice daily

● **UNLICENSED USE** *Tablets and liquid* not licensed for use in children under 10 years. *Granules* not licensed for use in children under 12 years. *Modified-release capsules* not licensed for use in children under 18 years.

● **CONTRA-INDICATIONS** Paralytic ileus

● **INTERACTIONS** → Appendix 1: mebeverine

● **SIDE-EFFECTS** Allergic reactions · angioedema · rash · urticaria

● **PREGNANCY** Not known to be harmful—manufacturers advise avoid.

● **BREAST FEEDING** Manufacturers advise avoid—no information available.

● **PATIENT AND CARER ADVICE**
Patients or carers should be given advice on the timing of administration of mebeverine hydrochloride tablets and oral suspension.
Medicines for Children leaflet: Mebeverine for intestinal spasm www.medicinesforchildren.org.uk/mebeverine-for-intestinal-spasms

● **MEDICINAL FORMS**
There can be variation in the licensing of different medicines containing the same drug.

Oral suspension

▸ **Mebeverine hydrochloride (Non-proprietary)**
Mebeverine hydrochloride (as Mebeverine pamoate) 10 mg per 1 ml Mebeverine 50mg/5ml oral suspension sugar free sugar-free | 300 ml PoM £187.00 DT price = £187.00

Modified-release capsule

CAUTIONARY AND ADVISORY LABELS 25

▸ **Colofac MR** (Mylan Ltd)
Mebeverine hydrochloride 200 mg Colofac MR 200mg capsules | 60 capsule PoM £6.92 DT price = £6.92

Tablet

▸ **Mebeverine hydrochloride (Non-proprietary)**
Mebeverine hydrochloride 135 mg Mebeverine 135mg tablets | 100 tablet PoM £20.00 DT price = £5.22

▸ **Colofac** (Mylan Ltd)
Mebeverine hydrochloride 135 mg Colofac 135mg tablets | 100 tablet PoM £9.02 DT price = £5.22

7 Liver disorders and related conditions

7.1 Biliary disorders

Cholestasis

01-May-2017

Description of condition

Cholestasis is an impairment of bile formation and/or bile flow, which may clinically present with fatigue, pruritus, dark urine, pale stools and, in its most overt form, jaundice and signs of fat soluble vitamin deficiencies.

Treatment

EvGr Ursodeoxycholic acid p. 64 [unlicensed] and colestyramine p. 125 [unlicensed under 6 years] are used to relieve cholestatic pruritus in children, even if evidence to support their use is limited.

Colestyramine is an anion-exchange resin that is not absorbed from the gastro-intestinal tract. It relieves pruritus by forming an insoluble complex in the intestine with bile acids and other compounds—the reduction of serum bile acid levels reduces excess deposition in the dermal tissue with a resultant decrease in pruritus.

Under specialist supervision, other drugs which may be used as an alternative treatment for **intractable** cholestatic pruritus include rifampicin p. 349 [unlicensed indication], phenobarbital p. 208 [unlicensed indication] and opioid antagonists [unlicensed indication]. However, they should be used with caution and under expert guidance as these children usually have severe liver disease—careful monitoring is required. ⟨E⟩

Inborn errors of primary bile acid synthesis

01-May-2017

Description of condition

Inborn errors of primary bile acid synthesis are a group of diseases in which the liver does not produce enough primary bile acids due to enzyme deficiencies. These acids are the main components of the bile, and include cholic acid and chenodeoxycholic acid.

Treatment

Cholic acid p. 64 is licensed for the treatment of inborn errors of primary bile acid synthesis due to an inborn deficiency of two specific liver enzymes. It acts by replacing some of the missing bile acids, therefore relieving the symptoms of the disease.

Chenodeoxycholic acid below [unlicensed] and ursodeoxycholic acid p. 64 [unlicensed indication] have been used to treat inborn errors in primary bile acid synthesis, but there is an absence of evidence to recommend their use. Chenodeoxycholic acid and ursodeoxycholic acid are available from Special-order manufacturers p. 1029 or specialist importing companies.

Primary biliary cholangitis

30-May-2017

Description of condition

Primary biliary cholangitis (or primary biliary cirrhosis) is a chronic cholestatic disease which develops due to progressive destruction of small and intermediate bile ducts within the liver, subsequently evolving to fibrosis and cirrhosis.

Treatment

[EvGr] Ursodeoxycholic acid p. 64 is recommended for the management of primary biliary cholangitis, including those with asymptomatic disease. It slows disease progression, but the effect on overall survival is uncertain. ⟨A⟩

Smith-Lemli-Opitz syndrome

30-May-2017

Description of condition

Smith-Lemli-Opitz syndrome is an inborn error of cholesterol synthesis. It is characterised by multiple congenital anomalies, intellectual deficit, growth delay, microcephaly, and behavioural problems. The disease is present at birth, but may be detected in later childhood or adulthood in mild forms. Hypoglycaemia due to adrenal insufficiency can present as an acute manifestation.

Aims of treatment

There is currently no cure for Smith-Lemli-Opitz syndrome. Management is aimed at symptom relief and alleviation of functional disabilities.

Treatment

[EvGr] Children with Smith-Lemli-Opitz syndrome are treated with dietary cholesterol supplementation, including high cholesterol foods (such as egg yolks) or a suspension of pharmaceutical grade cholesterol p. 65 (available from Special-order manufacturers p. 1029 or specialist importing companies) to help improve growth failure and photosensitivity. ⟨E⟩ However, it is not clear who will benefit most from cholesterol treatment or how long it should continue.

[EvGr] In some cases bile acid supplements, such as chenodeoxycholic acid below [unlicensed] and ursodeoxycholic acid p. 64 [unlicensed indication] have been also used for this condition, but their use is not generally recommended. ⟨E⟩

BILE ACIDS

▌ Chenodeoxycholic acid

● **INDICATIONS AND DOSE**

Cerebrotendinous xanthomatosis

▶ BY MOUTH

▶ Neonate: 5 mg/kg 3 times a day.

▶ Child: 5 mg/kg 3 times a day

Defective synthesis of bile acid

▶ BY MOUTH

▶ Neonate: Initially 5 mg/kg 3 times a day, reduced to 2.5 mg/kg 3 times a day.

▶ Child: Initially 5 mg/kg 3 times a day, reduced to 2.5 mg/kg 3 times a day

Smith-Lemli-Opitz syndrome

▶ BY MOUTH

▶ Neonate: 7 mg/kg once daily, alternatively 7 mg/kg daily in divided doses.

▶ Child: 7 mg/kg once daily, alternatively 7 mg/kg daily in divided doses

● **UNLICENSED USE** Not licensed.

● **CONTRA-INDICATIONS** Non-functioning gall bladder · radio-opaque stones

● **INTERACTIONS** → Appendix 1: chenodeoxycholic acid

● **SIDE-EFFECTS**
▶ **Rare** Diarrhoea

● **PREGNANCY** Avoid—fetotoxicity reported in *animal* studies.

● **DIRECTIONS FOR ADMINISTRATION** For administration *by mouth*, add the contents of a 250 mg capsule to 25 mL of sodium bicarbonate solution 8.4% (1 mmol/mL) to produce a suspension containing chenodeoxycholic acid 10 mg/mL; use immediately after preparation, discard any remaining suspension.

● **MEDICINAL FORMS**
There can be variation in the licensing of different medicines containing the same drug. Forms available from special-order manufacturers include: tablet, capsule

Tablet
▶ Chenodeoxycholic acid (Non-proprietary)
Chenodeoxycholic acid 250 mg Chenodiol 250mg tablets | 100 tablet [PoM] no price available

Capsule
▶ Chenodeoxycholic acid (Non-proprietary)
Chenodeoxycholic acid 250 mg Xenbilox 250mg capsules | 100 capsule [PoM] no price available

Cholic acid

21-Mar-2016

- **DRUG ACTION** Cholic acid is the predominant primary bile acid in humans, which can be used to provide a source of bile acid in patients with inborn deficiencies in bile acid synthesis.

- **INDICATIONS AND DOSE**

Inborn errors of primary bile acid synthesis (initiated by a specialist)
▸ BY MOUTH
  ▸ Child (body-weight up to 10 kg): 50 mg daily, then increased in steps of 50 mg daily in divided doses; usual dose 5–15 mg/kg daily in divided doses, dose to be given with food at the same time each day
  ▸ Child (body-weight 10 kg and above): Usual dose 5–15 mg/kg daily; increased in steps of 50 mg daily in divided doses if required, dose to be given with food at the same time each day; Usual maximum 500 mg/24 hours

- **INTERACTIONS** → Appendix 1: cholic acid

- **SIDE-EFFECTS** Diarrhoea · gallstones (long term use) · pruritus

  SIDE-EFFECTS, FURTHER INFORMATION
  Patients presenting with pruritus and/or persistent diarrhoea should be investigated for potential overdose by a serum and/or urine bile acid assay.

- **PREGNANCY** Limited data available—not known to be harmful, manufacturer advises continue treatment.
  Manufacturer advises monitor patient parameters more frequently in pregnancy.

- **BREAST FEEDING** Present in milk but not known to be harmful.

- **HEPATIC IMPAIRMENT** Manufacturer advises monitor closely.

- **MONITORING REQUIREMENTS** Manufacturer advises monitor serum and/or urine bile-acid concentrations every 3 months for the first year, then every 6 months for three years, then annually; monitor liver function tests at the same or greater frequency.

- **DIRECTIONS FOR ADMINISTRATION** Manufacturer advises capsules may be opened and the content added to infant formula, juice, fruit compote, or yoghurt for administration.

- **PATIENT AND CARER ADVICE** Counselling advised on administration.

- **MEDICINAL FORMS**
  There can be variation in the licensing of different medicines containing the same drug.
  Capsule
  CAUTIONARY AND ADVISORY LABELS 25
  ▸ Kolbam (Retrophin Inc) ▼
  Cholic acid 50 mg Kolbam 50mg capsules | 90 capsule [PoM] £3,240.00
  Cholic acid 250 mg Kolbam 250mg capsules | 90 capsule [PoM] £11,340.00
  ▸ Orphacol (Laboratoires CTRS) ▼
  Cholic acid 50 mg Orphacol 50mg capsules | 30 capsule [PoM] £1,860.00 | 60 capsule [PoM] £3,720.00
  Cholic acid 250 mg Orphacol 250mg capsules | 30 capsule [PoM] £6,630.00

Ursodeoxycholic acid

- **INDICATIONS AND DOSE**

Cholestasis
▸ BY MOUTH
  ▸ Neonate: 5 mg/kg 3 times a day (max. per dose 10 mg/kg 3 times a day), adjusted according to response.

  ▸ Child 1-23 months: 5 mg/kg 3 times a day (max. per dose 10 mg/kg 3 times a day), adjusted according to response

Improvement of hepatic metabolism of essential fatty acids and bile flow, in children with cystic fibrosis
▸ BY MOUTH
  ▸ Child: 10–15 mg/kg twice daily, total daily dose may alternatively be given in 3 divided doses

Cholestasis associated with total parenteral nutrition
▸ BY MOUTH
  ▸ Neonate: 10 mg/kg 3 times a day.

  ▸ Child: 10 mg/kg 3 times a day

Sclerosing cholangitis
▸ BY MOUTH
  ▸ Child: 5–10 mg/kg 2–3 times a day (max. per dose 15 mg/kg 3 times a day), adjusted according to response

- **UNLICENSED USE** Not licensed for use in children for the treatment of cholestasis, sclerosing cholangitis, cholestasis associated with total parenteral nutrition or the improvement of hepatic metabolism of essential fatty acids and bile flow in cystic fibrosis.

- **CONTRA-INDICATIONS** Non-functioning gall bladder · radio-opaque stones

- **INTERACTIONS** → Appendix 1: ursodeoxycholic acid

- **SIDE-EFFECTS**
▸ Rare Diarrhoea

- **PREGNANCY** No evidence of harm but manufacturer advises avoid.

- **BREAST FEEDING** Not known to be harmful but manufacturer advises avoid.

- **HEPATIC IMPAIRMENT** Avoid in chronic liver disease (but used in primary biliary cirrhosis)

- **PATIENT AND CARER ADVICE**
  Patients should be given dietary advice (including avoidance of excessive cholesterol and calories).
  Medicines for Children leaflet: Ursodeoxycholic acid for cholestasis and sclerosing cholangitis www.medicinesforchildren.org.uk/ursodeoxycholic-acid-for-cholestasis-and-sclerosing-cholangitis

- **MEDICINAL FORMS**
  There can be variation in the licensing of different medicines containing the same drug. Forms available from special-order manufacturers include: oral suspension, oral solution
  Oral suspension
  CAUTIONARY AND ADVISORY LABELS 21
  ▸ Ursofalk (Dr. Falk Pharma UK Ltd)
  Ursodeoxycholic acid 50 mg per 1ml Ursofalk 250mg/5ml oral suspension sugar-free | 250 ml [PoM] £26.98 DT price = £26.98
  Tablet
  CAUTIONARY AND ADVISORY LABEL 21
  ▸ Ursodeoxycholic acid (Non-proprietary)
  Ursodeoxycholic acid 150 mg Ursodeoxycholic acid 150mg tablets | 60 tablet [PoM] £19.02 DT price = £19.02
  Ursodeoxycholic acid 300 mg Ursodeoxycholic acid 300mg tablets | 60 tablet [PoM] £47.63 DT price = £47.63
  ▸ Cholurso (HFA Healthcare Products Ltd)
  Ursodeoxycholic acid 250 mg Cholurso 250mg tablets | 60 tablet [PoM] £18.00
  Ursodeoxycholic acid 500 mg Cholurso 500mg tablets | 60 tablet [PoM] £45.00

- **Destolit** (Norgine Pharmaceuticals Ltd)
  Ursodeoxycholic acid 150 mg Destolit 150mg tablets |
  60 tablet PoM £18.39 DT price = £19.02
- **Ursofalk** (Dr. Falk Pharma UK Ltd)
  Ursodeoxycholic acid 500 mg Ursofalk 500mg tablets |
  100 tablet PoM £80.00

Capsule
CAUTIONARY AND ADVISORY LABELS 21
- **Ursodeoxycholic acid** (Non-proprietary)
  Ursodeoxycholic acid 250 mg Ursodeoxycholic acid 250mg capsules
  | 60 capsule PoM £31.50 DT price = £25.29
- **Ursofalk** (Dr. Falk Pharma UK Ltd)
  Ursodeoxycholic acid 250 mg Ursofalk 250mg capsules |
  60 capsule PoM £30.17 DT price = £25.29 | 100 capsule PoM
  £31.88

LIPIDS > STEROLS

Cholesterol

- **INDICATIONS AND DOSE**

Smith-Lemli-Opitz syndrome
- BY MOUTH

- Neonate: 5–10 mg/kg 3–4 times a day.

- Child: 5–10 mg/kg 3–4 times a day, doses up to
  15 mg/kg 4 times daily have been used

- **UNLICENSED USE** Not licensed.
- **CONTRA-INDICATIONS**

CONTRA-INDICATIONS, FURTHER INFORMATION
For contra-indications, consult product literature.
- **CAUTIONS**

CAUTIONS, FURTHER INFORMATION
For advice on cautions, consult product literature.
- **DIRECTIONS FOR ADMINISTRATION** Cholesterol powder can
  be mixed with vegetable oil before administration.

- **MEDICINAL FORMS**
  There can be variation in the licensing of different medicines
  containing the same drug. Forms available from special-order
  manufacturers include: oral suspension, powder

7.2 Oesophageal varices

**PITUITARY AND HYPOTHALAMIC HORMONES
AND ANALOGUES** > VASOPRESSIN AND
ANALOGUES

Terlipressin acetate

- **INDICATIONS AND DOSE**

GLYPRESSIN® INJECTION

**Adjunct in acute massive haemorrhage of gastro-
intestinal tract or oesophageal varices (specialist use
only)**
- BY INTRAVENOUS INJECTION

- Child 12-17 years (body-weight up to 50 kg): Initially 2 mg
  every 4 hours until bleeding controlled, then reduced
  to 1 mg every 4 hours if required, maximum duration
  48 hours
- Child 12-17 years (body-weight 50 kg and above): Initially
  2 mg every 4 hours until bleeding controlled, reduced if
  not tolerated to 1 mg every 4 hours, maximum duration
  48 hours

VARIQUEL® INJECTION

**Adjunct in acute massive haemorrhage of gastro-
intestinal tract or oesophageal varices (specialist use
only)**
- BY INTRAVENOUS INJECTION

- Child 12-17 years (body-weight up to 50 kg): Initially 1 mg,
  then 1 mg every 4–6 hours for up to 72 hours, to be
  administered over 1 minute
- Child 12-17 years (body-weight 50-69 kg): Initially 1.5 mg,
  then 1 mg every 4–6 hours for up to 72 hours, to be
  administered over 1 minute
- Child 12-17 years (body-weight 70 kg and above): Initially
  2 mg, then 1 mg every 4–6 hours for up to 72 hours, to
  be administered over 1 minute

- **UNLICENSED USE** Unlicensed for use in children.
- **CAUTIONS** Arrhythmia · electrolyte and fluid disturbances ·
  heart disease · history of QT-interval prolongation ·
  respiratory disease · septic shock · uncontrolled
  hypertension · vascular disease
- **INTERACTIONS** → Appendix 1: terlipressin
- **SIDE-EFFECTS**
- **Common or very common** Abdominal cramps · arrhythmia ·
  bradycardia · diarrhoea · headache · hypertension ·
  hypotension · pallor · peripheral ischaemia
- **Uncommon** Angina · bronchospasm · convulsions · hot
  flushes · hyponatraemia · intestinal ischaemia · myocardial
  infarction · nausea · pulmonary oedema · respiratory
  failure · tachycardia · vomiting
- **Rare** Dyspnoea
- **Very rare** Hyperglycaemia · stroke
- **Frequency not known** Heart failure · skin necrosis
- **PREGNANCY** Avoid unless benefits outweigh risk—uterine
  contractions and increased intra-uterine pressure in early
  pregnancy, and decreased uterine blood flow reported.
- **BREAST FEEDING** Avoid unless benefits outweigh risk—no
  information available.
- **RENAL IMPAIRMENT** Use with caution in chronic renal
  failure.

- **MEDICINAL FORMS**
  There can be variation in the licensing of different medicines
  containing the same drug.
  Solution for injection
  - **Glypressin** (Ferring Pharmaceuticals Ltd)
    Terlipressin acetate 120 microgram per 1 ml Glypressin 1mg/8.5ml
    solution for injection ampoules | 5 ampoule PoM no price available
  - **Variquel** (Sinclair IS Pharma Plc)
    Terlipressin acetate 200 microgram per 1 ml Variquel 1mg/5ml
    solution for injection vials | 5 vial PoM £89.98 (Hospital only)
  Powder and solvent for solution for injection
  - **Glypressin** (Ferring Pharmaceuticals Ltd)
    Terlipressin acetate 1 mg Glypressin 1mg powder and solvent for
    solution for injection vials | 5 vial PoM £92.33
  - **Variquel** (Alliance Pharmaceuticals Ltd)
    Terlipressin acetate 1 mg Variquel 1mg powder and solvent for
    solution for injection vials | 5 vial PoM £89.48

Vasopressin

- **INDICATIONS AND DOSE**

**Adjunct in acute massive haemorrhage of gastrointestinal
tract or oesophageal varices (specialist use only)**
- BY CONTINUOUS INTRAVENOUS INFUSION

- Child: Initially 0.3 unit/kg (max. per dose 20 units),
  dose to be administered over 20–30 minutes, then
  0.3 unit/kg/hour, adjusted according to response (max.
  per dose 1 unit/kg/hour), if bleeding stops, continue at
  same dose for 12 hours, then withdraw gradually over
  24–48 hours; max. duration of treatment 72 hours,
  dose may alternatively be infused directly into the
  superior mesenteric artery

- **UNLICENSED USE** Not licensed for use in children.
- **CONTRA-INDICATIONS** Chronic nephritis (until reasonable blood nitrogen concentrations attained) · vascular disease (especially disease of coronary arteries) unless extreme caution
- **CAUTIONS** Asthma · avoid fluid overload · conditions which might be aggravated by water retention · epilepsy · heart failure · hypertension · migraine
- **SIDE-EFFECTS**
  ► **Rare** Gangrene
  ► **Frequency not known** Abdominal cramps · anaphylaxis · anginal attacks · belching · constriction of coronary arteries · desire to defaecate · fluid retention · headache · hypersensitivity reactions · myocardial ischaemia · nausea · pallor · peripheral ischaemia · sweating · tremor · vertigo · vomiting
- **PREGNANCY** Oxytocic effect in third trimester.
- **BREAST FEEDING** Not known to be harmful.
- **DIRECTIONS FOR ADMINISTRATION** For *intravenous infusion* (argipressin); dilute with Glucose 5% or Sodium Chloride 0.9% to a concentration of 0.2–1 unit/mL.

- **MEDICINAL FORMS**
  There can be variation in the licensing of different medicines containing the same drug.
  Solution for injection
  ► Vasopressin (Non-proprietary)
  Argipressin 20 unit per 1 ml Argipressin 20units/1ml solution for injection ampoules | 10 ampoule (PoM) £800.00 (Hospital only)

8   Obesity

Obesity

01-Jun-2016

Description of condition

Obesity is directly linked to many health problems including cardiovascular disease, type 2 diabetes, and obstructive sleep apnoea syndrome. It can also contribute to psychological and psychiatric morbidities.

In children and adolescents, body mass index (BMI) should be used as a practical estimation of body fat. However, it should be interpreted with caution as it is not a direct measure of adiposity. Assessing the BMI of children is more complicated than for adults because it changes as they grow and mature, with different growth patterns seen between boys and girls.

Public Health England advises that the British 1990 (UK90) growth reference charts should be used to determine the weight status of children. A child ≥ the 91st centile is classified as overweight, and as obese if ≥ the 98th centile. Waist circumference is not recommended as a routine measure, but should be used as an additional predictor for risk of developing other long-term health problems. Children who are overweight or obese and have significant comorbidities or complex needs should be considered for specialist referral.

Aims of treatment

Children who are overweight or obese and are no longer growing taller will ultimately need to lose weight and maintain weight loss to improve their BMI. However, preventing further weight gain while making lifestyle changes, may be an appropriate short-term aim.

Overview

EvGr The goals of management of obesity should be agreed together with the child and their parents or carers; parents or carers should be encouraged to take responsibility for lifestyle changes of their children. Referral to a specialist can be considered for children who are overweight or obese and have significant comorbidities or complex needs (e.g. learning disabilities). Children should be assessed for comorbidities such as hypertension, hyperinsulinaemia, dyslipidaemia, type 2 diabetes, psychosocial dysfunction, and exacerbation of conditions such as asthma.

An initial assessment should consider potential underlying causes (e.g. hypothyroidism) and a review of the appropriateness of current medications, which are known to cause weight gain, e.g. atypical antipsychotics, beta-adrenoceptor blocking drugs, insulin (when used in the treatment of type 2 diabetes), sodium valproate, and tricyclic antidepressants. Ⓐ

Lifestyle changes

EvGr Obese children should be encouraged to engage in a sustainable weight management programme which includes strategies to change behaviour, increase physical activity and improve diet and eating behaviour. These changes should be encouraged within the whole family. Any dietary changes should be age appropriate and consistent with healthy eating recommendations. Surgical intervention is not generally recommended in children or adolescents. Ⓐ

Drug treatment

EvGr Drug treatment is not generally recommended for children younger than 12 years, unless there are exceptional circumstances, such as if severe comorbidities are present. In children over 12 years, drug treatment is only recommended if physical comorbidities, such as orthopaedic problems or sleep apnoea, or severe psychological comorbidities are present. Drug treatment should **never** be used as the sole element of treatment and should be used as part of an overall weight management plan. Orlistat below [unlicensed use] is the only drug currently available in the UK that is recommended specifically for the treatment of obesity; it acts by reducing the absorption of dietary fat. Treatment should be started and monitored in a specialist paediatric setting by experienced multidisciplinary teams. An initial 6–12 month trial is recommended, with regular review to assess effectiveness, adverse effects and adherence.

Treatment may also be used to maintain weight loss rather than to continue to lose weight. A vitamin and mineral supplement may also be considered if there is concern about inadequate micronutrient intake, particularly for younger children who need vitamins and minerals for growth and development. Ⓐ

Useful Resources

Obesity: identification, assessment and management. Clinical Guideline 189. National Institute for Health and Care Excellence. November 2014. www.nice.org.uk/guidance/cg189

Measuring and interpreting BMI in Children. Public Health England. www.noo.org.uk

PERIPHERALLY ACTING ANTIOBESITY DRUGS ›
LIPASE INHIBITORS

Orlistat

- **DRUG ACTION** Orlistat, a lipase inhibitor, reduces the absorption of dietary fat.

- **INDICATIONS AND DOSE**
  Adjunct in obesity
  ► BY MOUTH
  ► Child 12–17 years (initiated by a specialist): 120 mg up to 3 times a day, dose to be taken immediately before, during, or up to 1 hour after each main meal, continue treatment beyond 12 weeks only under specialist supervision, if a meal is missed or contains no fat, the dose of orlistat should be omitted

- **UNLICENSED USE** Not licensed for use in children.
- **CONTRA-INDICATIONS** Cholestasis · chronic malabsorption syndrome
- **CAUTIONS** Chronic kidney disease · may impair absorption of fat-soluble vitamins · volume depletion

  CAUTIONS, FURTHER INFORMATION
  Vitamin supplementation (especially of vitamin D) may be considered if there is concern about deficiency of fat-soluble vitamins.
- **INTERACTIONS** → Appendix 1: orlistat
- **SIDE-EFFECTS**
  ‣ **Common or very common** Abdominal distension (gastro-intestinal effects minimised by reduced fat intake) · abdominal pain (gastro-intestinal effects minimised by reduced fat intake) · anxiety · faecal incontinence · faecal urgency · flatulence · gingival disorders · headache · hypoglycaemia · liquid stools · malaise · menstrual disturbances · oily leakage from rectum · oily stools · respiratory infections · tooth disorders · urinary tract infection
  ‣ **Frequency not known** Bullous eruptions · cholelithiasis · diverticulitis · hepatitis · hypothyroidism · oxalate nephropathy · rectal bleeding
- **PREGNANCY** Use with caution.
- **BREAST FEEDING** Avoid—no information available.

- **MEDICINAL FORMS**
  There can be variation in the licensing of different medicines containing the same drug.
  Capsule
  ‣ **Orlistat (Non-proprietary)**
  Orlistat 120 mg Orlistat 120mg capsules | 84 capsule PoM £35.42
  DT price = £17.55
  ‣ **Alli** (GlaxoSmithKline Consumer Healthcare)
  Orlistat 60 mg Alli 60mg capsules | 84 capsule P £29.10
  ‣ **Beacita** (Actavis UK Ltd)
  Orlistat 120 mg Beacita 120mg capsules | 84 capsule PoM £31.63
  DT price = £17.55
  ‣ **Xenical** (Roche Products Ltd)
  Orlistat 120 mg Xenical 120mg capsules | 84 capsule PoM £31.63
  DT price = £17.55

9 Rectal and anal disorders

9.1 Anal fissures

Anal fissure

31-Aug-2016

Description of condition

An anal fissure is a tear or ulcer in the lining of the anal canal, immediately within the anal margin. Clinical features of anal fissure include bleeding and persistent pain on defecation, and a linear split in the anal mucosa. Constipation (passage of hard stools) is the most common cause in children. The majority of anal fissures are posterior, and an underlying cause should be considered (secondary anal fissure) if fissures are multiple, occur laterally, and are refractory to treatment.

EvGr Suspect sexual abuse if a child has an anal fissure, and if constipation, Crohn's disease or passing hard stools have been excluded as the cause (see also *Useful resources* below).◬

Aims of treatment

The aim of treatment is to relieve pain and promote healing of the fissure.

Drug treatment

EvGr Initial management of acute anal fissures should focus on ensuring that stools are soft and easily passed. Osmotic laxatives, such as lactulose p. 40 or macrogols (macrogol 3350 with potassium chloride, sodium bicarbonate and sodium chloride p. 41), are recommended. A simple analgesic (such as paracetamol p. 260 or ibuprofen p. 625, may be offered for prolonged burning pain following defecation.

Children should be referred to a paediatric specialist if the anal fissure has not healed following two weeks of initial management, or earlier if there is significant pain.◬

Useful Resources

Child maltreatment: when to suspect maltreatment in under 18s. National Institute for Health and Care Excellence. Clinical guideline 89. July 2009. www.nice.org.uk/guidance/cg89

9.2 Haemorrhoids

Haemorrhoids

01-Dec-2016

Description of condition

Haemorrhoids, or piles, are abnormal swellings of the vascular mucosal anal cushions around the anus. Internal haemorrhoids arise above the dentate line and are usually painless unless they become strangulated. External haemorrhoids originate below the dentate line and can be itchy or painful. Haemorrhoids in children are rare but may occur in infants with portal hypertension.

Aims of treatment

The aims of treatment are to reduce the symptoms (pain, bleeding and swelling), promote healing, and prevent recurrence.

Non-drug treatment

EvGr Stools should be kept soft and easy to pass (to minimise straining) by increasing dietary fibre and fluid intake. Advice about perianal hygiene is helpful to aid healing and reduce irritation and itching.◬

Drug treatment

EvGr If constipation is present, it should be treated, see Constipation p. 38.

A simple analgesic, such as paracetamol p. 260, can be used for pain relief. NSAIDs should be avoided if rectal bleeding is present.

Symptomatic treatment with a locally applied preparation is appropriate for short periods.◬ Manufacturer advises preparations containing local anaesthetics (lidocaine, cinchocaine, and pramocaine [unlicensed]) should only be used for a few days as they may cause sensitisation of the anal skin— local anaesthetic ointments can be absorbed through the rectal mucosa (with a theoretical risk of systemic effects) and very rarely may cause increased irritation; excessive application should be **avoided** in infants and children.

Topical preparations combining corticosteroids with local anaesthetics and soothing agents are available for the management of haemorrhoids. Manufacturer advises long-term use of corticosteroid creams can cause ulceration and permanent damage due to thinning of the perianal skin and should be avoided. Continuous or excessive use carries a risk of adrenal suppression and systemic corticosteroid effects (particularly in infants).

Gastro-intestinal system

EvGr Topical preparations containing corticosteroids must not be used if infection is present (such as perianal streptococcal infection, *herpes simplex* or perianal thrush).

Recurrent symptoms, should be referred to secondary care for further investigation and management. E

CORTICOSTEROIDS

Benzyl benzoate with bismuth oxide, bismuth subgallate, hydrocortisone acetate, peru balsam and zinc oxide

- ● **INDICATIONS AND DOSE**

Haemorrhoids | Pruritus ani
- ▸ BY RECTUM USING OINTMENT
- ▸ Child 12–17 years: Apply twice daily for no longer than 7 days, to be applied morning and night, an additional dose should be applied after a bowel movement
- ▸ BY RECTUM USING SUPPOSITORIES
- ▸ Child 12–17 years: 1 suppository twice daily for no longer than 7 days, to be inserted night and morning, additional dose after a bowel movement

- ● CAUTIONS Local anaesthetic component can be absorbed through the rectal mucosa (avoid excessive application, particularly in children and infants) · local anaesthetic component may cause sensitisation (use for short periods only—no longer than a few days)
- ● PRESCRIBING AND DISPENSING INFORMATION A proprietary brand *Anusol Plus HC*® (ointment and suppositories) is on sale to the public.

- ● MEDICINAL FORMS
There can be variation in the licensing of different medicines containing the same drug.
Ointment
- ▸ Anusol-Hc (McNeil Products Ltd)
Hydrocortisone acetate 2.5 mg per 1 gram, Bismuth oxide 8.75 mg per 1 gram, Benzyl benzoate 12.5 mg per 1 gram, Peru Balsam 18.75 mg per 1 gram, Bismuth subgallate 22.5 mg per 1 gram, Zinc oxide 107.5 mg per 1 gram Anusol HC ointment | 30 gram PoM £2.49
Suppository
- ▸ Anusol-Hc (McNeil Products Ltd)
Hydrocortisone acetate 10 mg, Bismuth oxide 24 mg, Benzyl benzoate 33 mg, Peru Balsam 49 mg, Bismuth subgallate 59 mg, Zinc oxide 296 mg Anusol HC suppositories | 12 suppository PoM £1.74

Benzyl benzoate with bismuth oxide, hydrocortisone acetate, peru balsam, pramocaine hydrochloride and zinc oxide

- ● **INDICATIONS AND DOSE**

Haemorrhoids | Pruritus ani
- ▸ BY RECTUM
- ▸ Child 12–17 years: Apply twice daily for no longer than 7 days, to be applied morning and night and after a bowel movement

- ● CAUTIONS Local anaesthetic component can be absorbed through the rectal mucosa (avoid excessive application) · local anaesthetic component may cause sensitisation (use for short periods only—no longer than a few days)

- ● MEDICINAL FORMS
There can be variation in the licensing of different medicines containing the same drug.
No licensed medicines listed.

Cinchocaine hydrochloride with fluocortolone caproate and fluocortolone pivalate

- ● **INDICATIONS AND DOSE**

Haemorrhoids | Pruritus ani
- ▸ BY RECTUM USING OINTMENT
- ▸ Child: Apply twice daily for 5–7 days, apply 3–4 times a day if required, on the first day of treatment, then apply once daily for a few days after symptoms have cleared
- ▸ BY RECTUM USING SUPPOSITORIES
- ▸ Child 12–17 years: Initially 1 suppository daily for 5–7 days, to be inserted after a bowel movement, then 1 suppository once daily on alternate days for 1 week

Haemorrhoids (severe cases) | Pruritus ani (severe cases)
- ▸ BY RECTUM USING SUPPOSITORIES
- ▸ Child 12–17 years: Initially 1 suppository 2–3 times a day for 5–7 days, then 1 suppository once daily on alternate days for 1 week

- ● CAUTIONS Local anaesthetic component can be absorbed through the rectal mucosa (avoid excessive application) · local anaesthetic component may cause sensitisation (use for short periods only—no longer than a few days)

- ● MEDICINAL FORMS
There can be variation in the licensing of different medicines containing the same drug.
Ointment
- ▸ Ultraproct (Meadow Laboratories Ltd)
Fluocortolone pivalate 920 microgram per 1 gram, Fluocortolone caproate 950 microgram per 1 gram, Cinchocaine hydrochloride 5 mg per 1 gram Ultraproct ointment | 30 gram PoM £8.27
Suppository
- ▸ Ultraproct (Meadow Laboratories Ltd)
Fluocortolone pivalate 610 microgram, Fluocortolone caproate 630 microgram, Cinchocaine hydrochloride 1 mg Ultraproct suppositories | 12 suppository PoM £4.06

Cinchocaine with hydrocortisone

- ● **INDICATIONS AND DOSE**

PROCTOSEDYL® OINTMENT

Haemorrhoids | Pruritus ani
- ▸ TO THE SKIN, OR BY RECTUM
- ▸ Child: Apply twice daily, to be administered morning and night and after a bowel movement. Apply externally or by rectum. Do not use for longer than 7 days

PROCTOSEDYL® SUPPOSITORIES

Haemorrhoids | Pruritus ani
- ▸ BY RECTUM
- ▸ Child 12–17 years: 1 suppository, insert suppository night and morning and after a bowel movement. Do not use for longer than 7 days

UNIROID-HC® OINTMENT

Haemorrhoids | Pruritus ani
- ▸ TO THE SKIN, OR BY RECTUM
- ▸ Child 1 month–11 years (under medical advice only): Apply twice daily, and apply after a bowel movement, apply externally or by rectum, do not use for longer than 7 days
- ▸ Child 12–17 years: Apply twice daily, and apply after a bowel movement, apply externally or by rectum, do not use for longer than 7 days

UNIROID-HC® SUPPOSITORIES

Haemorrhoids | Pruritus ani

▶ BY RECTUM

▸ **Child 12-17 years:** 1 suppository, insert twice daily and after a bowel movement. Do not use for longer than 7 days

● CAUTIONS Local anaesthetic component can be absorbed through the rectal mucosa (avoid excessive application, particularly in children and infants) · local anaesthetic component may cause sensitisation (use for short periods only—no longer than a few days)

● MEDICINAL FORMS
There can be variation in the licensing of different medicines containing the same drug.

Ointment

▸ Proctosedyl (Sanofi)
Cinchocaine hydrochloride 5 mg per 1 gram, Hydrocortisone 5 mg per 1 gram Proctosedyl ointment | 30 gram PoM £10.34

▸ Uniroid HC (Chemidex Pharma Ltd)
Cinchocaine hydrochloride 5 mg per 1 gram, Hydrocortisone 5 mg per 1 gram Uniroid HC ointment | 30 gram PoM £4.23

Suppository

▸ Cinchocaine with hydrocortisone (Non-proprietary)
Cinchocaine hydrochloride 5 mg, Hydrocortisone 5 mg Cinchocaine 5mg / Hydrocortisone 5mg suppositories | 12 suppository PoM no price available

▸ Proctosedyl (Sanofi)
Cinchocaine hydrochloride 5 mg, Hydrocortisone 5 mg Proctosedyl suppositories | 12 suppository PoM £5.08

▸ Uniroid HC (Chemidex Pharma Ltd)
Cinchocaine hydrochloride 5 mg, Hydrocortisone 5 mg Uniroid HC suppositories | 12 suppository PoM £1.91

Cinchocaine with prednisolone

● INDICATIONS AND DOSE

Haemorrhoids | Pruritus ani

▶ BY RECTUM USING OINTMENT

▸ **Child:** Apply twice daily for 5–7 days, apply 3–4 times a day on the first day if necessary, then apply once daily for a few days after symptoms have cleared

▶ BY RECTUM USING SUPPOSITORIES

▸ **Child 12-17 years:** 1 suppository daily for 5–7 days, to be inserted after a bowel movement

Haemorrhoids (severe cases) | Pruritus ani (severe cases)

▶ BY RECTUM USING SUPPOSITORIES

▸ **Child 12-17 years:** Initially 1 suppository 2–3 times a day, then 1 suppository daily for a total of 5–7 days, to be inserted after a bowel movement

● CAUTIONS Local anaesthetic component can be absorbed through the rectal mucosa (avoid excessive application) · local anaesthetic component may cause sensitisation (use for short periods only—no longer than a few days)

● MEDICINAL FORMS
There can be variation in the licensing of different medicines containing the same drug.

Ointment

▸ Scheriproct (Bayer Plc)
Prednisolone hexanoate 1.9 mg per 1 gram, Cinchocaine hydrochloride 5 mg per 1 gram Scheriproct ointment | 30 gram PoM £2.94 DT price = £2.94

Suppository

▸ Scheriproct (Bayer Plc)
Cinchocaine hydrochloride 1 mg, Prednisolone hexanoate 1.3 mg Scheriproct suppositories | 12 suppository PoM £1.38 DT price = £1.38

Hydrocortisone with lidocaine

● INDICATIONS AND DOSE

Haemorrhoids | Pruritus ani

▶ BY RECTUM USING AEROSOL SPRAY

▸ **Child 2-13 years (under medical advice only):** 1 spray up to 3 times a day, spray once over the affected area

▸ **Child 14-17 years:** 1 spray up to 3 times a day for no longer than 7 days without medical advice, spray once over the affected area

▶ BY RECTUM USING OINTMENT

▸ **Child:** Apply several times daily, for short term use only

● CAUTIONS Local anaesthetic component can be absorbed through the rectal mucosa (avoid excessive application) · local anaesthetic component may cause sensitisation (use for short periods only—no longer than a few days)

● MEDICINAL FORMS
There can be variation in the licensing of different medicines containing the same drug.

Ointment

▸ Hydrocortisone with lidocaine (Non-proprietary)
Hydrocortisone acetate 2.75 mg per 1 gram, Lidocaine 50 mg per 1 gram Lidocaine 5% / Hydrocortisone acetate 0.275% ointment | 20 gram PoM no price available DT price = £4.19

▸ Xyloproct (Aspen Pharma Trading Ltd)
Hydrocortisone acetate 2.75 mg per 1 gram, Lidocaine 50 mg per 1 gram Xyloproct 5%/0.275% ointment | 20 gram PoM £4.19 DT price = £4.19

Spray

▸ Perinal (Dermal Laboratories Ltd)
Hydrocortisone 2 mg per 1 gram, Lidocaine hydrochloride 10 mg per 1 gram Perinal spray | 30 ml P £6.11

Hydrocortisone with pramocaine

● INDICATIONS AND DOSE

Pain and irritation associated with local, non-infected anal or perianal conditions

▶ BY RECTUM

▸ **Child 12-17 years:** 1 applicatorful 2–3 times a day and 1 applicatorful, after a bowel movement, do not use for longer than 7 days; maximum 4 applicatorfuls per day

● CAUTIONS Local anaesthetic component can be absorbed through the rectal mucosa (avoid excessive application) · local anaesthetic component may cause sensitisation (use for short periods only—no longer than a few days)

● MEDICINAL FORMS
There can be variation in the licensing of different medicines containing the same drug.

Foam

▸ Proctofoam HC (Meda Pharmaceuticals Ltd)
Hydrocortisone acetate 10 mg per 1 gram, Pramocaine hydrochloride 10 mg per 1 gram Proctofoam HC foam enema | 40 dose PoM £6.07 DT price = £6.07

10 Reduced exocrine secretions

Exocrine pancreatic insufficiency

14-Dec-2016

Description of condition

Exocrine pancreatic insufficiency is characterised by reduced secretion of pancreatic enzymes into the duodenum.

The main clinical manifestations are maldigestion and malnutrition, associated with low circulating levels of

1

Gastro-intestinal system

micronutrients, fat-soluble vitamins and lipoproteins. Children also present with gastro-intestinal symptoms, such as diarrhoea, abdominal cramps and steatorrhoea.

Exocrine pancreatic insufficiency can result from cystic fibrosis, coeliac disease, Zollinger-Ellison syndrome, and gastro-intestinal or pancreatic surgical resection.

Aims of treatment

The aim of treatment is to relieve gastro-intestinal symptoms and to achieve a normal nutritional status.

Drug treatment

EvGr Pancreatic enzyme replacement therapy with pancreatin below is the mainstay of treatment for children with exocrine pancreatic insufficiency. ⟨A⟩

Pancreatin contains the three main groups of digestive enzymes: lipase, amylase and protease. These enzymes respectively digest fats, carbohydrates and proteins into their basic components so that they can be absorbed and utilised by the body. EvGr Pancreatin should be administered with meals and snacks. The dose should be adjusted, as necessary, to the lowest effective dose according to the symptoms of maldigestion and malabsorption. ⟨A⟩

Fibrosing colonopathy has been reported in children with cystic fibrosis taking high dose pancreatic enzyme replacement therapy (in excess of 10 000 units/kg/day of lipase). Possible risk factors are gender (boys are at greater risk than girls), more severe cystic fibrosis, and concomitant use of laxatives. The peak age for developing fibrosing colonopathy is between 2 and 8 years. Manufacturers of *Pancrease HL* ® and *Nutrizym 22* ® recommend that the total dose of pancreatin used in patients with cystic fibrosis should not usually exceed 10 000 units/kg/day of lipase. Manufacturers recommend that if a patient taking pancreatin develops new abdominal symptoms (or any change in existing abdominal symptoms) the patient should be reviewed to exclude the possibility of colonic damage.

There is limited evidence that acid suppression may improve the effectiveness of pancreatin. EvGr Acid-suppressing drugs (proton pump inhibitors or H₂-receptor antagonists) may be trialled in children who continue to experience symptoms despite high doses of pancreatin.

Levels of fat-soluble vitamins and micronutrients (such as zinc and selenium) should be routinely assessed and supplementation recommended whenever necessary. ⟨A⟩

Pancreatin preparations			
Preparation	Protease units	Amylase units	Lipase units
Creon® 10 000 capsule, e/c granules	600	8000	10 000
Creon® Micro e/c granules (per 100 mg)	200	3600	5000
Pancrex® granules (per gram)	300	4000	5000
Pancrex V® capsule, powder	430	9000	8000
Pancrex V '125'® capsule, powder	160	3300	2950
Pancrex V® e/c tablet	110	1700	1900
Pancrex V® Forte e/c tablet	330	5000	5600
Pancrex V® powder (per gram)	1400	30 000	25 000

Higher-strength pancreatin preparations			
Preparation	Protease units	Amylase units	Lipase units
Creon® 25 000 capsule, e/c pellets	1000	18 000	25 000
Creon® 40 000 capsule, e/c granules	1600	25 000	40 000
Nutrizym 22® capsule, e/c minitablets	1100	19 800	22 000
Pancrease HL® capsule, e/c minitablets	1250	22 500	25 000

Non-drug treatment

EvGr Dietary advice should be provided. Food intake should be distributed between three main meals per day, and two or three snacks. Food that is difficult to digest should be avoided, such as legumes (peas, beans lentils) and high-fibre foods. Alcohol should be avoided completely. Reduced fat diets are not recommended. ⟨A⟩

Medium-chain triglycerides (see MCT oil, in *Borderline substances*), which are directly absorbed by the intestinal mucosa, were thought to be useful in some children. However evidence has shown that MCT-enriched preparations offer no advantage over a normal balanced diet.

PANCREATIC ENZYMES

Pancreatin

08-Mar-2017

● **DRUG ACTION** Supplements of pancreatin are given to compensate for reduced or absent exocrine secretion. They assist the digestion of starch, fat, and protein.

● **INDICATIONS AND DOSE**

CREON® 10000

Pancreatic insufficiency
▸ BY MOUTH
▸ Child: Initially 1–2 capsules, dose to be taken with each meal either taken whole or contents mixed with acidic fluid or soft food (then swallowed immediately without chewing)

CREON® 25000

Pancreatic insufficiency
▸ BY MOUTH
▸ Child 2–17 years: Initially 1–2 capsules, dose to be taken with each meal either taken whole or contents mixed with acidic fluid or soft food (then swallowed immediately without chewing)

CREON® 40000

Pancreatic insufficiency
▸ BY MOUTH
▸ Child 2–17 years: Initially 1–2 capsules, dose to be taken with each meal either taken whole or contents mixed with acidic fluid or soft food (then swallowed immediately without chewing)

CREON® MICRO

Pancreatic insufficiency
▸ BY MOUTH
▸ Neonate: Initially 100 mg, for administration advice, see *Directions for administration.*

▸ Child: Initially 100 mg, for administration advice, see *Directions for administration*

DOSE EQUIVALENCE AND CONVERSION
▸ For *Creon*® Micro: 100 mg granules = one measured scoopful (scoop supplied with product).

NUTRIZYM 22® GASTRO-RESISTANT CAPSULES

Pancreatic insufficiency

▸ BY MOUTH

▸ **Child 15–17 years:** Initially 1–2 capsules, dose to be taken with meals and 1 capsule as required, dose to be taken with snacks, doses should be swallowed whole or contents taken with water, or mixed with acidic fluid or soft food (then swallowed immediately without chewing)

PANCREASE HL®

Pancreatic insufficiency

▸ BY MOUTH

▸ **Child 15–17 years:** Initially 1–2 capsules, dose to be taken during each meal and 1 capsule, to be taken with snacks, all doses either taken whole or contents mixed with slightly acidic liquid or soft food (then swallowed immediately without chewing)

PANCREX®

Pancreatic insufficiency

▸ BY MOUTH

▸ **Child 2–17 years:** 5–10 g, to be taken just before meals, washed down or mixed with milk or water

PANCREX® V

Pancreatic insufficiency

▸ BY MOUTH

▸ **Child 1–11 months:** 1–2 capsules, contents of capsule to be mixed with feeds

▸ **Child 1–17 years:** 2–6 capsules, dose to be taken with each meal either swallowed whole or sprinkled on food

PANCREX® V CAPSULES '125'

Pancreatic insufficiency

▸ BY MOUTH

▸ **Neonate:** 1–2 capsules, contents of capsule to be given in each feed (or mixed with feed and given by spoon).

PANCREX® V POWDER

Pancreatic insufficiency

▸ BY MOUTH

▸ **Neonate:** 250–500 mg, dose to be taken with each feed.

▸ **Child:** 0.5–2 g, to be taken before or with meals, washed down or mixed with milk or water

PANCREX® V TABLETS

Pancreatic insufficiency

▸ BY MOUTH

▸ **Child 2–17 years:** 5–15 tablets, to be taken before meals

PANCREX® V TABLETS FORTE

Pancreatic insufficiency

▸ BY MOUTH

▸ **Child 2–17 years:** 6–10 tablets, to be taken before meals

● CONTRA-INDICATIONS

PANCREASE HL® Should not be used in children aged 15 years or less with cystic fibrosis

NUTRIZYM 22® GASTRO-RESISTANT CAPSULES Should not be used in children aged 15 years or less with cystic fibrosis

● CAUTIONS Can irritate the perioral skin and buccal mucosa if retained in the mouth · excessive doses can cause perianal irritation

● INTERACTIONS → Appendix 1: pancreatin

● SIDE-EFFECTS Abdominal discomfort · hyperuricaemia (associated with very high doses) · hyperuricosuria (associated with very high doses) · mucosal irritation · nausea · skin irritation · vomiting

● PREGNANCY Not known to be harmful.

● DIRECTIONS FOR ADMINISTRATION Pancreatin is inactivated by gastric acid therefore manufacturer advises

pancreatin preparations are best taken with food (or immediately before or after food). Since pancreatin is inactivated by heat, excessive heat should be avoided if preparations are mixed with liquids or food; manufacturer advises the resulting mixtures should not be kept for more than one hour and any left-over food or liquid containing pancreatin should be discarded. Enteric-coated preparations deliver a higher enzyme concentration in the duodenum (provided the capsule contents are swallowed whole without chewing). Manufacturer advises gastro-resistant granules should be mixed with slightly acidic soft food or liquid such as apple juice, and then swallowed immediately without chewing. Capsules containing enteric-coated granules can be opened and the granules administered in the same way. For infants, *Creon Micro®* granules can be mixed with a small amount of milk on a spoon and administered immediately—granules should not be added to the baby's bottle. Manufacturer advises *Pancrex®* V powder may be administered via nasogastric tube or gastrostomy tube—consult local and national official guidelines.

● PRESCRIBING AND DISPENSING INFORMATION Preparations may contain pork pancreatin—consult product literature.

● HANDLING AND STORAGE Hypersensitivity reactions occur occasionally and may affect those handling the powder.

● PATIENT AND CARER ADVICE Patients or carers should be given advice on administration.

It is important to ensure adequate hydration at all times in patients receiving higher-strength pancreatin preparations.

Medicines for Children leaflet: Pancreatin for pancreatic insufficiency www.medicinesforchildren.org.uk/pancreatin-for-pancreatic-insufficiency

● MEDICINAL FORMS

There can be variation in the licensing of different medicines containing the same drug.

Gastro-resistant capsule

▸ Creon (Mylan Ltd)

Protease 600 unit, Amylase 8000 unit, Lipase 10000 unit Creon 10000 gastro-resistant capsules | 100 capsule P £12.93

Protease 1000 unit, Amylase 18000 unit, Lipase 25000 unit Creon 25000 gastro-resistant capsules | 100 capsule PoM £28.25

Protease 1600 unit, Amylase 25000 unit, Lipase 40000 unit Creon 40000 gastro-resistant capsules | 100 capsule PoM £41.80

▸ Nutrizym (Merck Serono Ltd)

Protease 1100 unit, Amylase 19800 unit, Lipase 22000 unit Nutrizym 22 gastro-resistant capsules | 100 capsule PoM £33.33

▸ Pancrease (Janssen-Cilag Ltd)

Protease 1250 unit, Amylase 22500 unit, Lipase 25000 unit Pancrease HL gastro-resistant capsules | 100 capsule PoM £40.38

Gastro-resistant tablet

CAUTIONARY AND ADVISORY LABELS 5, 25

▸ Pancrex (Essential Pharmaceuticals Ltd)

Protease 110 unit, Amylase 1700 unit, Lipase 1900 unit Pancrex V gastro-resistant tablets | 300 tablet P £38.79

Protease 330 unit, Amylase 5000 unit, Lipase 5600 unit Pancrex V Forte gastro-resistant tablets | 300 tablet P £48.11

Gastro-resistant granules

CAUTIONARY AND ADVISORY LABELS 25

▸ Creon (Mylan Ltd)

Protease 200 unit, Amylase 3600 unit, Lipase 5000 unit Creon Micro Pancreatin 60.12mg gastro-resistant granules | 20 gram P £31.50

▸ Pancrex (Essential Pharmaceuticals Ltd)

Protease 300 unit, Amylase 4000 unit, Lipase 5000 unit Pancrex gastro-resistant granules | 300 gram P £57.00

Powder

▶ Pancrex (Essential Pharmaceuticals Ltd)
Protease 1400 unit, Lipase 25000 unit, Amylase
30000 unit Pancrex V oral powder sugar-free | 300 gram P £58.88

Capsule

▶ Pancrex (Essential Pharmaceuticals Ltd)
Protease 160 unit, Lipase 2950 unit, Amylase 3300 unit Pancrex
V 125mg capsules | 300 capsule P £42.07
Protease 430 unit, Lipase 8000 unit, Amylase 9000 unit Pancrex
V capsules | 300 capsule P £53.20

11 Stoma care

Stoma care

24-Feb-2016

Description of condition

A stoma is an artificial opening on the abdomen to divert
flow of faeces or urine into an external pouch located outside
of the body. This procedure may be temporary or permanent.
Colostomy and ileostomy are the most common forms of
stoma but a gastrostomy, jejunostomy, duodenostomy or
caecostomy may also be performed. Understanding the type
and extent of surgical intervention in each patient is crucial
in managing the patient's pharmaceutical needs correctly.

Overview

Prescribing for patients with stoma calls for special care due
to modifications in drug delivery, resulting in a higher risk of
sub-optimal absorption. The following is a brief account of
some of the main points to be borne in mind.

Enteric-coated and modified-release medicines are
unsuitable, particularly in patients with an ileostomy, as
there may not be sufficient release of active ingredient.
Soluble tablets, liquids, capsules or uncoated tablets are
more suitable due to their quicker dissolution. When a solid-
dose form such as a capsule or a tablet is given, the contents
of the ostomy bag should be checked for any remnants.

Preparations containing sorbitol as an excipient should be
avoided, due to its laxative side effects.

Analgesics

Opioid analgesics may cause troublesome constipation in
colostomy patients. When a non-opioid analgesic is
required, paracetamol is usually suitable. Anti-inflammatory
analgesics may cause gastric irritation and bleeding; faecal
output should be monitored for traces of blood.

Antacids

The tendency to diarrhoea from magnesium salts or
constipation from aluminium or calcium salts may be
increased in patients with stoma.

Antisecretory drugs

The gastric acid secretion often increases stoma output.
Proton pump inhibitors and somatostatin analogues
(octreotide p. 445) are often used to reduce this risk.

Antidiarrhoeal drugs

Loperamide hydrochloride p. 47 and codeine phosphate
p. 265 reduce intestinal motility and decrease water and
sodium output from an ileostomy. Loperamide
hydrochloride circulates through the enterohepatic
circulation, which is disrupted in patients with a short bowel;
high doses of loperamide hydrochloride may be required.
Codeine phosphate can be added if response with
loperamide hydrochloride alone is inadequate.

Digoxin

Children with a stoma are particularly susceptible to
hypokalaemia. This predisposes children on digoxin p. 79 to
digoxin toxicity; potassium supplements or a potassium-
sparing diuretic may be advisable.

Diuretics

Diuretics should be used with caution in patients with an
ileostomy or with urostomy as they may become excessively
dehydrated and potassium depletion may easily occur. It is
usually advisable to use a potassium-sparing diuretic.

Iron preparations

Iron preparations may cause loose stools and sore skin in
these patients. If this is troublesome and if iron is definitely
indicated, an intramuscular iron preparation should be used.
Modified-release preparations should be avoided for the
reasons given above.

Laxatives

Laxatives should be used in children with stoma only under
specialist supervision; they should be prescribed with
caution for those with an ileostomy as they may cause rapid
and severe loss of water and electrolytes.

Colostomy patients may suffer from constipation and
whenever possible it should be treated by increasing fluid
intake or dietary fibre. If a laxative is required, it should
generally be used for short periods only.

Care of stoma

Patients and their carers are usually given advice about the
use of cleansing agents, protective creams, lotions,
deodorants, or sealants whilst in hospital, either by the
surgeon or by stoma care nurses. Voluntary organisations
offer help and support to patients with stoma.

Chapter 2
Cardiovascular system

CONTENTS

1   Arrhythmias

Arrhythmias

Overview

Management of an arrhythmia requires precise diagnosis of the type of arrhythmia; electrocardiography and referral to a paediatric cardiologist is essential; underlying causes such as heart failure require appropriate treatment.

Bradycardia

Adrenaline/epinephrine p. 132 is useful in the treatment of symptomatic bradycardia in an infant or child.

Supraventricular tachycardia

In supraventricular tachycardia adenosine p. 77 is given by rapid intravenous injection. If adenosine is ineffective, intravenous amiodarone hydrochloride p. 76, flecainide acetate p. 75, or a beta-blocker (such as esmolol hydrochloride p. 103) can be tried; verapamil hydrochloride p. 106 can also be considered in children over 1 year. Atenolol p. 103, sotalol hydrochloride p. 78 and flecainide acetateare used for the prophylaxis of paroxysmal supraventricular tachycardias.

The use of d.c. shock and vagal stimulation also have a role in the treatment of supraventricular tachycardia.

Syndromes associated with accessory conducting pathways

Amiodarone hydrochloride, flecainide acetate, or a beta-blocker is used to prevent recurrence of supraventricular tachycardia in infants and young children with these syndromes (e.g. Wolff-Parkinson-White syndrome).

Atrial flutter

In atrial flutter without structural heart defects, sinus rhythm is restored with d.c. shock or cardiac pacing; drug treatment is usually not necessary. Amiodarone hydrochloride is used in atrial flutter when structural heart defects are present or after heart surgery. Sotalol hydrochloride may also be considered.

Atrial fibrillation

Atrial fibrillation is very rare in children. To restore sinus rhythm d.c. shock is used; beta-blockers, alone or together with digoxin p. 79 may be useful for ventricular rate control.

Ectopic tachycardia

Intravenous amiodarone hydrochlorideis used in conjunction with body cooling and synchronised pacing in postoperative junctional ectopic tachycardia. Oral amiodarone hydrochloride or flecainide acetate are used in congenital junctional ectopic tachycardia.

Amiodarone hydrochloride, flecainide acetate, or a beta-blocker are used in atrial ectopic tachycardia; amiodarone hydrochloride is preferred in those with poor ventricular function.

Ventricular tachycardia and ventricular fibrillation

Pulseless ventricular tachycardia or ventricular fibrillation require resuscitation, see Paediatric Advanced Life Support algorithm. Amiodarone hydrochloride is used in resuscitation for pulseless ventricular tachycardia or ventricular fibrillation unresponsive to d.c. shock; lidocaine hydrochloride p. 796 can be used as an alternative only if amiodarone hydrochloride is not available.

Amiodarone hydrochloride is also used in a haemodynamically stable child when drug treatment is required; lidocaine hydrochloride can be used as an alternative only if amiodarone hydrochloride is not available.

Torsade de pointes

Torsade de pointes is a form of ventricular tachycardia associated with long QT syndrome, which may be congenital or drug induced. Episodes may be self-limiting, but are frequently recurrent and can cause impairment or loss of consciousness. If not controlled, the arrhythmia can progress to ventricular fibrillation and sometimes death. Intravenous magnesium sulfate can be used to treat torsade de pointes (dose recommendations vary—consult local guidelines). Anti-arrhythmics can further prolong the QT interval, thus worsening the condition.

Drugs for arrhythmias

Anti-arrhythmic drugs can be classified clinically into those that act on supraventricular arrhythmias (e.g. verapamil hydrochloride), those that act on both supraventricular and ventricular arrhythmias (e.g. amiodarone hydrochloride), and those that act on ventricular arrhythmias (e.g. lidocaine hydrochloride).

Anti-arrhythmic drugs can also be classified according to their effects on the electrical behaviour of myocardial cells during activity (the Vaughan Williams classification) although this classification is of less clinical significance:

Cardiovascular system

2

- Class I: membrane stabilising drugs (e.g. lidocaine, flecainide)
- Class II: beta-blockers
- Class III: amiodarone; sotalol (also Class II)
- Class IV: calcium-channel blockers (includes verapamil but not dihydropyridines)

The negative inotropic effects of anti-arrhythmic drugs tend to be additive. Therefore special care should be taken if two or more are used, especially if myocardial function is impaired. Most drugs that are effective in countering arrhythmias can also provoke them in some circumstances; moreover, hypokalaemia enhances the arrhythmogenic (pro-arrhythmic) effect of many drugs.

Adenosine is the treatment of choice for terminating supraventricular tachycardias, including those associated with accessory conducting pathways (e.g. Wolff-Parkinson-White syndrome). It is also used in the diagnosis of supraventricular arrhythmias. It is not negatively inotropic and does not cause significant hypotension. The injection should be administered by rapid intravenous injection into a central or large peripheral vein.

Amiodarone hydrochloride is useful in the management of both supraventricular and ventricular tachyarrhythmias. It can be given by intravenous infusion and by mouth, and causes little or no myocardial depression. Unlike oral amiodarone hydrochloride, intravenous amiodarone hydrochloride acts relatively rapidly. Intravenous amiodarone hydrochloride is also used in cardiopulmonary resuscitation for ventricular fibrillation or pulseless ventricular tachycardia unresponsive to d.c. shock.

Amiodarone hydrochloride has a very long half-life (extending to several weeks) and only needs to be given once daily (but high doses may cause nausea unless divided). Many weeks or months may be required to achieve steady state plasma-amiodarone concentration; this is particularly important when drug interactions are likely.

Beta-blockers act as anti-arrhythmic drugs principally by attenuating the effects of the sympathetic system on automaticity and conductivity within the heart. Sotalol hydrochloride has a role in the management of ventricular arrhythmias.

Oral administration of digoxin slows the ventricular rate in atrial fibrillation and in atrial flutter. However, intravenous infusion of digoxin is rarely effective for rapid control of ventricular rate.

Flecainide acetate is useful for the treatment of resistant re-entry supraventricular tachycardia, ventricular tachycardia, ventricular ectopic beats, arrhythmias associated with accessory conducting pathways (e.g. Wolff-Parkinson- White syndrome), and paroxysmal atrial fibrillation. Flecainide acetate crosses the placenta and can be used to control fetal supraventricular arrhythmias.

Lidocaine hydrochloride can be used in cardiopulmonary resuscitation in children with ventricular fibrillation or pulseless ventricular tachycardia unresponsive to d.c. shock, but only if amiodarone hydrochloride is not available. Doses may need to be reduced in children with persistently poor cardiac output and hepatic or renal failure.

Verapamil hydrochloride can cause severe haemodynamic compromise (refractory hypotension and cardiac arrest) when used for the acute treatment of arrhythmias in neonates and infants; it is contra-indicated in children under 1 year. It is also contra-indicated in those with congestive heart failure, syndromes associated with accessory conducting pathways (e.g. Wolff-Parkinson-White syndrome) and in most receiving concomitant beta-blockers. It can be useful in older children with supraventricular tachycardia.

Other drugs used for Arrhythmias Metoprolol tartrate, p. 103 · Propranolol hydrochloride, p. 101

ANTIARRHYTHMICS ⟩ CLASS IB

Lidocaine hydrochloride
(Lignocaine hydrochloride)

- **INDICATIONS AND DOSE**

Ventricular arrhythmias | Pulseless ventricular tachycardia | Ventricular fibrillation
▸ INITIALLY BY INTRAVENOUS INJECTION, OR BY INTRAOSSEOUS INJECTION

▸ Neonate: Initially 0.5–1 mg/kg, followed immediately by (by intravenous infusion) 0.6–3 mg/kg/hour, alternatively (by intravenous injection or by intraosseous injection) 0.5–1 mg/kg repeated at intervals of not less than 5 minutes if infusion is not immediately available following initial injection, until infusion can be initiated; maximum 3 mg/kg per course.

▸ Child 1 month–11 years: Initially 0.5–1 mg/kg, followed immediately by (by intravenous infusion) 0.6–3 mg/kg/hour, alternatively (by intravenous injection or by intraosseous injection) 0.5–1 mg/kg repeated at intervals of not less than 5 minutes if infusion is not immediately available following initial injection, until infusion can be initiated; maximum 3 mg/kg per course

▸ Child 12–17 years: Initially 50–100 mg, followed by (by intravenous infusion) 120 mg, dose to be given over 30 minutes, then (by intravenous infusion) 240 mg, dose to be given over 2 hours, then (by intravenous infusion) 60 mg/hour, reduce dose further if infusion is continued beyond 24 hours, if infusion not immediately available following initial injection, the initial injection dose may be repeated at intervals of not less than 5 minutes (to a maximum 300 mg dose in 1 hour) until infusion can be initiated

Neonatal seizures
▸ BY INTRAVENOUS INFUSION

▸ Neonate: Initially 2 mg/kg, dose to be given over 10 minutes, followed by 6 mg/kg/hour for 6 hours; reduced to 4 mg/kg/hour for 12 hours, then reduced to 2 mg/kg/hour for a further 12 hours, preterm neonates may require lower doses.

- **UNLICENSED USE** Not licensed for use in children under 1 year.

- **CONTRA-INDICATIONS** All grades of atrioventricular block · severe myocardial depression · sino-atrial disorders

- **CAUTIONS** Acute porphyria (consider infusion with glucose for its anti-porphyrinogenic effects) · congestive cardiac failure (consider lower dose) · post cardiac surgery (consider lower dose)

- **INTERACTIONS** → Appendix 1: antiarrhythmics

- **SIDE-EFFECTS**
▸ **Common or very common**
Bradycardia (may lead to cardiac arrest) · confusion · convulsions · dizziness (particularly if injection too rapid) · drowsiness (particularly if injection too rapid) · hypotension (may lead to cardiac arrest) · paraesthesia (particularly if injection too rapid) · respiratory depression
▸ **Rare** Anaphylaxis

- **PREGNANCY** Crosses the placenta but not known to be harmful in *animal* studies—use if benefit outweighs risk.

- **BREAST FEEDING** Present in milk but amount too small to be harmful.

- **HEPATIC IMPAIRMENT** Caution—increased risk of side-effects.

- **RENAL IMPAIRMENT** Possible accumulation of lidocaine and active metabolite; caution in severe impairment.

- **MONITORING REQUIREMENTS** Monitor ECG and have resuscitation facilities available.
- **DIRECTIONS FOR ADMINISTRATION** For *intravenous infusion*, dilute with Glucose 5% or Sodium Chloride 0.9%.
- **MEDICINAL FORMS**
  There can be variation in the licensing of different medicines containing the same drug. Forms available from special-order manufacturers include: solution for injection

Solution for injection

▸ **Lidocaine hydrochloride (Non-proprietary)**
  Lidocaine hydrochloride 5 mg per 1 ml Lidocaine 50mg/10ml (0.5%) solution for injection ampoules | 10 ampoule [PoM] £7.00
  Lidocaine hydrochloride 10 mg per 1 ml Lidocaine 100mg/10ml (1%) solution for injection Mini-Plasco ampoules | 20 ampoule [PoM] £10.89
  Lidocaine 100mg/10ml (1%) solution for injection ampoules | 10 ampoule [PoM] £4.40 DT price = £4.36
  Lidocaine 100mg/10ml (1%) solution for injection Sure-Amp ampoules | 20 ampoule [PoM] £8.80
  Lidocaine 200mg/20ml (1%) solution for injection vials | 10 vial [PoM] £19.00
  Lidocaine 200mg/20ml (1%) solution for injection ampoules | 10 ampoule [PoM] £7.00-£9.63 DT price = £9.63
  Lidocaine 50mg/5ml (1%) solution for injection ampoules | 10 ampoule [PoM] £2.57-£3.10 DT price = £2.57
  Lidocaine 20mg/2ml (1%) solution for injection ampoules | 10 ampoule [PoM] £3.50 DT price = £2.18
  Lidocaine 50mg/5ml (1%) solution for injection Sure-Amp ampoules | 20 ampoule [PoM] £6.00
  Lidocaine hydrochloride 20 mg per 1 ml Lidocaine 100mg/5ml (2%) solution for injection ampoules | 10 ampoule [PoM] £2.67-£3.80 DT price = £2.67
  Lidocaine 400mg/20ml (2%) solution for injection vials | 10 vial [PoM] £19.50
  Lidocaine 200mg/10ml (2%) solution for injection Mini-Plasco ampoules | 20 ampoule [PoM] £14.52
  Lidocaine 40mg/2ml (2%) solution for injection ampoules | 10 ampoule [PoM] £4.00 DT price = £2.34
  Lidocaine 100mg/5ml (2%) solution for injection Sure-Amp ampoules | 20 ampoule [PoM] £6.00
  Lidocaine 400mg/20ml (2%) solution for injection ampoules | 10 ampoule [PoM] £8.00-£9.90 DT price = £9.90

ANTIARRHYTHMICS ⟩ CLASS IC

Flecainide acetate

- **INDICATIONS AND DOSE**

Supraventricular arrhythmias

▸ BY MOUTH USING MODIFIED-RELEASE MEDICINES
▸ Child 12-17 years: 200 mg daily

Resistant re-entry supraventricular tachycardia | Ventricular ectopic beats or ventricular tachycardia | Arrhythmias associated with accessory conduction pathways (e.g. Wolff-Parkinson-White syndrome) | Paroxysmal atrial fibrillation

▸ BY MOUTH USING IMMEDIATE-RELEASE MEDICINES

▸ Neonate: 2 mg/kg 2-3 times a day, adjusted according to response, also adjust dose according to plasma-flecainide concentration.

▸ Child 1 month-11 years: 2 mg/kg 2-3 times a day, adjusted according to response, also adjust dose according to plasma-flecainide concentration,; maximum 8 mg/kg per day; maximum 300 mg per day
▸ Child 12-17 years: Initially 50-100 mg twice daily; increased if necessary up to 300 mg daily, maximum 400 mg daily for ventricular arrhythmias in heavily built children

▸ INITIALLY BY SLOW INTRAVENOUS INJECTION, OR BY INTRAVENOUS INFUSION

▸ Neonate: Initially 1-2 mg/kg, dose to be given over 10-30 minutes, followed by (by continuous intravenous infusion) 100-250 micrograms/kg/hour if required until arrhythmia controlled, transfer patient to oral treatment following intravenous treatment.

▸ Child 1 month-11 years: Initially 2 mg/kg, dose to be given over 10-30 minutes, followed by (by continuous intravenous infusion) 100-250 micrograms/kg/hour if required until arrhythmia controlled, maximum cumulative dose of 600 mg in the first 24 hours, transfer patient to oral treatment following intravenous treatment
▸ Child 12-17 years: Initially 2 mg/kg (max. per dose 150 mg), dose to be given over 10-30 minutes, followed by (by continuous intravenous infusion) 1.5 mg/kg/hour if required for 1 hour, then (by continuous intravenous infusion) reduced to 100-250 micrograms/kg/hour until arrhythmia controlled, maximum cumulative dose of 600 mg in the first 24 hours, transfer patient to oral treatment following intravenous treatment

DOSE ADJUSTMENTS DUE TO INTERACTIONS
Manufacturer advises reduce dose by half with concurrent use of amiodarone.

DOSE EQUIVALENCE AND CONVERSION
▸ Patients stabilised on 200 mg daily immediate-release flecainide may be transferred to modified-release medicines.

- **UNLICENSED USE** Not licensed for use in children under 12 years.
- **CONTRA-INDICATIONS** Abnormal left ventricular function · atrial conduction defects (unless pacing rescue available) · bundle branch block (unless pacing rescue available) · control of arrhythmias in acute situations (for modified-release forms only) · distal block (unless pacing rescue available) · haemodynamically significant valvular heart disease · heart failure · long-standing atrial fibrillation where conversion to sinus rhythm not attempted · second-degree or greater AV block (unless pacing rescue available) · sinus node dysfunction (unless pacing rescue available)
- **CAUTIONS** Atrial fibrillation following heart surgery · patients with pacemakers (especially those who may be pacemaker dependent because stimulation threshold may rise appreciably)
- **INTERACTIONS** → Appendix 1: antiarrhythmics
- **SIDE-EFFECTS**
  ▸ **Common or very common** Asthenia · dizziness · dyspnoea · fatigue · fever · oedema · pro-arrhythmic effects · visual disturbances
  ▸ **Rare** Amnesia · confusion · convulsions · depression · dyskinesia · hallucinations · peripheral neuropathy · pneumonitis
  ▸ **Frequency not known** Anaemia · anorexia · anxiety · ataxia · corneal deposits · drowsiness · flushing · gastrointestinal disturbances · headache · hepatic dysfunction · hypersensitivity reactions · hypoaesthesia · increased antinuclear antibodies · increased sweating · insomnia · leucopenia · paraesthesia · photosensitivity · rash · syncope · thrombocytopenia · tinnitus · tremor · urticaria · vertigo
- **PREGNANCY** Used in pregnancy to treat maternal and fetal arrhythmias in specialist centres; toxicity reported in *animal* studies; infant hyperbilirubinaemia also reported.
- **BREAST FEEDING** Significant amount present in milk but not known to be harmful.
- **HEPATIC IMPAIRMENT** Avoid or reduce dose in severe impairment. Monitor plasma-flecainide concentration.

2

Cardiovascular system

• **RENAL IMPAIRMENT** Reduce dose by 25–50% if estimated glomerular filtration rate less than 35 mL/minute/1.73 m². Monitor plasma-flecainide concentration.

• **MONITORING REQUIREMENTS**
‣ Plasma-flecainide concentration for optimal response 200–800 micrograms/litre; blood sample should be taken immediately before next dose.
‣ With intravenous use ECG monitoring and resuscitation facilities must be available.

• **DIRECTIONS FOR ADMINISTRATION**
‣ With oral use For administration *by mouth*, milk, infant formula, and dairy products may reduce absorption of flecainide—separate doses from feeds. Liquid has a local anaesthetic effect and should be given at least 30 minutes before or after food. Do not store liquid in refrigerator as precipitation occurs.
‣ With intravenous use For *intravenous administration* give initial dose over 30 minutes in children with sustained ventricular tachycardia or cardiac failure. Dilute injection using Glucose 5%; concentrations of more than 300 micrograms/mL are unstable in chloride-containing solutions.

• **PATIENT AND CARER ADVICE**
Medicines for Children leaflet: Flecainide for arrhythmias
www.medicinesforchildren.org.uk/flecainide-arrhythmias

• **MEDICINAL FORMS**
There can be variation in the licensing of different medicines containing the same drug. Forms available from special-order manufacturers include: oral suspension, oral solution

Tablet
‣ Flecainide acetate (Non-proprietary)
Flecainide acetate 50 mg Flecainide 50mg tablets | 60 tablet PoM £13.50 DT price = £8.64
Flecainide acetate 100 mg Flecainide 100mg tablets | 60 tablet PoM £19.83 DT price = £10.10
‣ Tambocor (Meda Pharmaceuticals Ltd)
Flecainide acetate 50 mg Tambocor 50mg tablets | 60 tablet PoM £11.57 DT price = £8.64
Flecainide acetate 100 mg Tambocor 100mg tablets | 60 tablet PoM £16.53 DT price = £10.10

Solution for injection
‣ Tambocor (Meda Pharmaceuticals Ltd)
Flecainide acetate 10 mg per 1 ml Tambocor 150mg/15ml solution for injection ampoules | 5 ampoule PoM £21.99

Modified-release capsule
CAUTIONARY AND ADVISORY LABELS 25
‣ Tambocor XL (Meda Pharmaceuticals Ltd)
Flecainide acetate 200 mg Tambocor XL 200mg capsules | 30 capsule PoM £14.77

ANTIARRHYTHMICS ⟩ CLASS III

Amiodarone hydrochloride

• **INDICATIONS AND DOSE**

Supraventricular and ventricular arrhythmias (initiated in hospital or under specialist supervision)
‣ BY MOUTH

‣ **Neonate:** Initially 5–10 mg/kg twice daily for 7–10 days, then reduced to 5–10 mg/kg daily.

‣ **Child 1 month–11 years:** Initially 5–10 mg/kg twice daily (max. per dose 200 mg) for 7–10 days, then reduced to 5–10 mg/kg once daily; maximum 200 mg per day

‣ **Child 12–17 years:** 200 mg 3 times a day for 1 week, then 200 mg twice daily for 1 week, then usually 200mg daily adjusted according to repsonse
‣ INITIALLY BY INTRAVENOUS INFUSION

‣ **Neonate:** Initially 5 mg/kg, then (by intravenous infusion) 5 mg/kg every 12–24 hours, dose to be given over 30 minutes.

‣ **Child:** Initially 5–10 mg/kg, dose to be given over 20 minutes to 2 hours, then (by continuous intravenous infusion) 300 micrograms/kg/hour, adjusted according to response; (by continuous intravenous infusion) increased if necessary up to 1.5 mg/kg/hour; maximum 1.2 g per day

Ventricular fibrillation or pulseless ventricular tachycardia refractory to defibrillation (for cardiopulmonary resuscitation)
‣ INITIALLY BY INTRAVENOUS INJECTION

‣ **Neonate:** 5 mg/kg, dose to be given over at least 3 minutes.

‣ **Child:** 5 mg/kg (max. per dose 300 mg), dose to be given over at least 3 minutes

• **UNLICENSED USE** Not licensed for use in children under 3 years.

• **CONTRA-INDICATIONS**
GENERAL CONTRA-INDICATIONS
Avoid in severe conduction disturbances (unless pacemaker fitted) · avoid in sinus node disease (unless pacemaker fitted) · avoid rapid loading after cardiac surgery · iodine sensitivity · sino-atrial heart block (except in cardiac arrest) · sinus bradycardia (except in cardiac arrest) · thyroid dysfunction
SPECIFIC CONTRA-INDICATIONS
‣ With intravenous use Avoid bolus injection in cardiomyopathy · avoid bolus injection in congestive heart failure · avoid in circulatory collapse · avoid in severe arterial hypotension · avoid in severe respiratory failure

• **CAUTIONS**
GENERAL CAUTIONS
Acute porphyrias p. 577 · conduction disturbances (in excessive dosage) · heart failure · hypokalaemia · severe bradycardia (in excessive dosage)
SPECIFIC CAUTIONS
‣ With intravenous use Avoid benzyl alcohol containing injections in neonates (in neonates) · moderate and transient fall in blood pressure (circulatory collapse precipitated by rapid administration or overdosage) · severe hepatocellular toxicity

• **INTERACTIONS** → Appendix 1: antiarrhythmics

• **SIDE-EFFECTS**
GENERAL SIDE-EFFECTS
‣ **Common or very common** Bradycardia · hyperthyroidism · hypothyroidism · jaundice · nausea · persistent slate grey skin discoloration · phototoxicity · pulmonary toxicity (including pneumonitis and fibrosis) · raised serum transaminases (may require dose reduction or withdrawal if accompanied by acute liver disorders) · reversible corneal microdeposits (sometimes with night glare) · sleep disorders · taste disturbances · tremor · vomiting
‣ **Uncommon** Conduction disturbances · onset or worsening of arrhythmia · peripheral myopathy (usually reversible on withdrawal) · peripheral neuropathy (usually reversible on withdrawal)
‣ **Very rare** Alopecia · aplastic anaemia · ataxia · benign intracranial hypertension · bronchospasm (in patients with severe respiratory failure) · chronic liver disease · cirrhosis · epididymo-orchitis · exfoliative dermatitis · haemolytic anaemia · headache · hypersensitivity · impaired vision due to optic neuritis or optic neuropathy (including blindness) · impotence · rash · sinus arrest · thrombocytopenia · vasculitis · vertigo
‣ **Frequency not known** Hot flushes · hypotension · respiratory distress syndrome · sweating
SPECIFIC SIDE-EFFECTS
‣ **Very rare**
‣ With intravenous use Anaphylaxis on rapid injection

SIDE-EFFECTS, FURTHER INFORMATION

▸ **Corneal microdeposits** Most patients taking amiodarone develop corneal microdeposits (reversible on withdrawal of treatment); these rarely interfere with vision, but drivers may be dazzled by headlights at night. However, if vision is impaired or if optic neuritis or optic neuropathy occur, amiodarone must be stopped to prevent blindness and expert advice sought.

▸ **Thyroid function** Amiodarone contains iodine and can cause disorders of thyroid function; both hypothyroidism and hyperthyroidism can occur. Thyrotoxicosis may be very refractory, and amiodarone should usually be withdrawn at least temporarily to help achieve control; treatment with carbimazole may be required. Hypothyroidism can be treated with replacement therapy without withdrawing amiodarone if it is essential; careful supervision is required.

▸ **Hepatotoxicity** Amiodarone is also associated with hepatotoxicity and treatment should be discontinued if severe liver function abnormalities or clinical signs of liver disease develop.

▸ **Pulmonary toxicity** Pneumonitis should always be suspected if new or progressive shortness of breath or cough develops in a patient taking amiodarone.

▸ **Peripheral neuropathy** Fresh neurological symptoms should raise the possibility of peripheral neuropathy.

● **PREGNANCY** Possible risk of neonatal goitre; use only if no alternative.

● **BREAST FEEDING** Avoid; present in milk in significant amounts; theoretical risk of neonatal hypothyroidism from release of iodine.

● **MONITORING REQUIREMENTS**

▸ Thyroid function tests should be performed before treatment and then every 6 months. Clinical assessment of thyroid function alone is unreliable. Thyroxine (T4) may be raised in the absence of hyperthyroidism; therefore tri-iodothyronine (T3), T4, and thyroid-stimulating hormone (thyrotrophin, TSH) should all be measured. A raised T3 and T4 with a very low or undetectable TSH concentration suggests the development of thyrotoxicosis.

▸ Liver function tests required before treatment and then every 6 months.

▸ Serum potassium concentration should be measured before treatment.

▸ Chest x-ray required before treatment.

▸ Pulmonary function tests required before treatment.

▸ With intravenous use ECG monitoring and resuscitation facilities must be available. Monitor liver transaminases closely.

● **DIRECTIONS FOR ADMINISTRATION**

▸ With intravenous use Intravenous administration via central venous catheter recommended if repeated or continuous infusion required, as infusion via peripheral veins may cause pain and inflammation. For *intravenous infusion*, dilute to a concentration of not less than 600 micrograms/mL with Glucose 5%. Incompatible with Sodium Chloride infusion fluids; avoid equipment containing the plasticizer di-2-ethylhexphthalate (DEHP).

▸ With oral use For administration *by mouth*, tablets may be crushed and dispersed in water; injection solution should **not** be given orally (irritant).

● **PATIENT AND CARER ADVICE**

Because of the possibility of phototoxic reactions, patients should be advised to shield the skin from light during treatment and for several months after discontinuing amiodarone; a wide-spectrum sunscreen to protect against both long-wave ultraviolet and visible light should be used.

Medicines for Children leaflet: Amiodarone for abnormal heart rhythms www.medicinesforchildren.org.uk/amiodarone-abnormal-heart-rhythms-0

● **MEDICINAL FORMS**

There can be variation in the licensing of different medicines containing the same drug. Forms available from special-order manufacturers include: oral suspension, oral solution

Tablet

CAUTIONARY AND ADVISORY LABELS 11

▸ **Amiodarone hydrochloride (Non-proprietary)**
Amiodarone hydrochloride 100 mg Amiodarone 100mg tablets | 28 tablet [PoM] £4.25 DT price = £1.53
Amiodarone hydrochloride 200 mg Amiodarone 200mg tablets | 28 tablet [PoM] £7.80 DT price = £1.91

▸ **Cordarone X** (Sanofi)
Amiodarone hydrochloride 100 mg Cordarone X 100 tablets | 28 tablet [PoM] £4.28 DT price = £1.53
Amiodarone hydrochloride 200 mg Cordarone X 200 tablets | 28 tablet [PoM] £6.99 DT price = £1.91

Solution for injection

EXCIPIENTS: May contain Benzyl alcohol

▸ **Amiodarone hydrochloride (Non-proprietary)**
Amiodarone hydrochloride 30 mg per 1 ml Amiodarone 300mg/10ml solution for injection pre-filled syringes | 1 pre-filled disposable injection [PoM] £13.80
Amiodarone hydrochloride 50 mg per 1 ml Amiodarone 150mg/3ml concentrate for solution for injection ampoules | 10 ampoule [PoM] £15.00

▸ **Cordarone X** (Sanofi)
Amiodarone hydrochloride 50 mg per 1 ml Cordarone X 150mg/3ml solution for injection ampoules | 6 ampoule [PoM] £9.60

ANTIARRHYTHMICS ⟩ OTHER

Adenosine

● **INDICATIONS AND DOSE**

Used in conjunction with radionuclide myocardial perfusion imaging in patients who cannot exercise adequately or for whom exercise is inappropriate

▸ BY INTRAVENOUS INFUSION

▸ Child: (consult product literature)

Termination of supraventricular tachycardias, including those associated with accessory conducting pathways (e.g. Wolff-Parkinson-White syndrome) | Diagnosis of supraventricular arrhythmias

▸ BY RAPID INTRAVENOUS INJECTION

▸ Neonate: Initially 150 micrograms/kg, then increased in steps of 50–100 micrograms/kg every 1–2 minutes (max. per dose 300 micrograms/kg) if required, dose to be repeated until tachycardia terminated or maximum single dose given.

▸ Child 1–11 months: Initially 150 micrograms/kg, then increased in steps of 50–100 micrograms/kg every 1–2 minutes (max. per dose 500 micrograms/kg) if required, dose to be repeated until tachycardia terminated or maximum single dose given

▸ Child 1–11 years: Initially 100 micrograms/kg, then increased in steps of 50–100 micrograms/kg every 1–2 minutes (max. per dose 12 mg) if required, dose to be repeated until tachycardia terminated or maximum single dose given

▸ Child 12-17 years: Initially 3 mg, followed by 6 mg after 1–2 minutes if required, followed by 12 mg after 1–2 minutes if required, in some children over 12 years 3 mg dose ineffective (e.g. if a small peripheral vein is used for administration) and higher initial dose sometimes used; however, those with *heart transplant* are **very sensitive** to the effects of adenosine, and should **not** receive higher initial doses

DOSE ADJUSTMENTS DUE TO INTERACTIONS

If essential to give with dipyridamole reduce adenosine dose to a quarter of the usual dose.

● **UNLICENSED USE** *Adenocor*® licensed for treatment of paroxysmal supraventricular tachycardia in children; not

2

Cardiovascular system

licensed for diagnosis in children; *Adenoscan*® not licensed in children.

- CONTRA-INDICATIONS Asthma · decompensated heart failure · long QT syndrome · second- or third-degree AV block and sick sinus syndrome (unless pacemaker fitted) · severe hypotension
- CAUTIONS Atrial fibrillation with accessory pathway (conduction down anomalous pathway may increase) · atrial flutter with accessory pathway (conduction down anomalous pathway may increase) · autonomic dysfunction · bundle branch block · first-degree AV block · heart transplant · left main coronary artery stenosis · left to right shunt · pericardial effusion · pericarditis · QT-interval prolongation · recent myocardial infarction · severe heart failure · stenotic carotid artery disease with cerebrovascular insufficiency · stenotic valvular heart disease · uncorrected hypovolaemia
- INTERACTIONS → Appendix 1: antiarrhythmics
- SIDE-EFFECTS
- ▸ **Common or very common** Angina (discontinue) · apprehension · arrhythmia (discontinue if asystole or severe bradycardia occur) · AV block · dizziness · dyspnoea · flushing · headache · nausea · sinus pause
- ▸ **Uncommon** Blurred vision · hyperventilation · metallic taste · palpitation · sweating · weakness
- ▸ **Very rare** Bronchospasm · injection-site reactions · transient worsening of intracranial hypertension
- ▸ **Frequency not known** Cardiac arrest · convulsions · hypotension (discontinue if severe) · respiratory failure (discontinue) · syncope · vomiting
- PREGNANCY Large doses may produce fetal toxicity; manufacturer advises use only if potential benefit outweighs risk.
- BREAST FEEDING No information available—unlikely to be present in milk owing to short half-life.
- MONITORING REQUIREMENTS Monitor ECG and have resuscitation facilities available.
- DIRECTIONS FOR ADMINISTRATION For *rapid intravenous injection* give over 2 seconds into central or large peripheral vein followed by rapid Sodium Chloride 0.9% flush; injection solution may be diluted with Sodium Chloride 0.9% if required.

- MEDICINAL FORMS
  There can be variation in the licensing of different medicines containing the same drug. Forms available from special-order manufacturers include: solution for injection, infusion, solution for infusion

  Solution for injection
  ELECTROLYTES: May contain Sodium
  ▸ **Adenosine (Non-proprietary)**
  Adenosine 3 mg per 1 ml Adenosine 6mg/2ml solution for injection vials | 6 vial [PoM] £26.70-£29.24 (Hospital only)
  ▸ **Adenocor (Sanofi)**
  Adenosine 3 mg per 1 ml Adenocor 6mg/2ml solution for injection vials | 6 vial [PoM] £29.94 (Hospital only)

  Solution for infusion
  ELECTROLYTES: May contain Sodium
  ▸ **Adenosine (Non-proprietary)**
  Adenosine 3 mg per 1 ml Adenosine 30mg/10ml solution for infusion vials | 6 vial [PoM] £70.00-£85.57 (Hospital only)
  ▸ **Adenoscan (Sanofi)**
  Adenosine 3 mg per 1 ml Adenoscan 30mg/10ml solution for infusion vials | 6 vial [PoM] £85.57

BETA-ADRENOCEPTOR BLOCKERS ›
NON-SELECTIVE

▰ Ⓕ **100**

| Sotalol hydrochloride

- **INDICATIONS AND DOSE**

Life-threatening arrhythmias including ventricular tachyarrhythmias
▸ BY MOUTH
- ▸ **Child 12-17 years:** Initially 80 mg once daily, alternatively initially 40 mg twice daily, then increased to 80–160 mg twice daily, dose to be increased gradually at intervals of 2–3 days; higher doses of 480–640 mg daily may be required for life-threatening ventricular arrhythmias (under specialist supervision)

Ventricular arrhythmias, life-threatening ventricular tachyarrhythmia and supraventricular arrhythmias (initiated under specialist supervision)
▸ BY MOUTH
- ▸ **Neonate:** Initially 1 mg/kg twice daily, increased if necessary up to 4 mg/kg twice daily, dose to be increased at intervals of 3–4 days.

Atrial flutter, ventricular arrhythmias, life-threatening ventricular tachyarrhythmia and supraventricular arrhythmias (initiated under specialist supervision)
▸ BY MOUTH
- ▸ **Child 1 month-11 years:** Initially 1 mg/kg twice daily, then increased if necessary up to 4 mg/kg twice daily (max. per dose 80 mg twice daily), dose to be increased at intervals of 2–3 days
- ▸ **Child 12-17 years:** Initially 80 mg once daily, alternatively initially 40 mg twice daily, increased to 80–160 mg twice daily, dose to be increased gradually at intervals of 2–3 days

- UNLICENSED USE Not licensed for use in children under 12 years.

IMPORTANT SAFETY INFORMATION
Sotalol may prolong the QT interval, and it occasionally causes life threatening ventricular arrhythmias (**important**: particular care is required to avoid hypokalaemia in patients taking sotalol—electrolyte disturbances, particularly hypokalaemia and hypomagnesaemia should be corrected before sotalol started and during use).
Reduce dose or discontinue if corrected QT interval exceeds 550 msec.

- CONTRA-INDICATIONS Long QT syndrome (congenital or acquired) · torsade de pointes
- CAUTIONS Diarrhoea (severe or prolonged)
- INTERACTIONS → Appendix 1: beta blockers (non-selective)
- SIDE-EFFECTS Arrhythmogenic (pro-arrhythmic) effect (torsade de pointes—increased risk in females)
- BREAST FEEDING Water soluble beta-blockers such as sotalol are present in breast milk in greater amounts than other beta blockers.
- RENAL IMPAIRMENT Halve normal dose if estimated glomerular filtration rate 30–60 mL/minute/1.73 m^2; use one-quarter normal dose if estimated glomerular filtration rate 10–30 mL/minute/1.73 m^2. Avoid if estimated glomerular filtration rate less than 10 mL/minute/1.73 m^2.
- MONITORING REQUIREMENTS Measurement of corrected QT interval, and monitoring of ECG and electrolytes required; correct hypokalaemia, hypomagnesaemia, or other electrolyte disturbances.

- **DIRECTIONS FOR ADMINISTRATION** For administration *by mouth*, tablets may be crushed and dispersed in water.

- **MEDICINAL FORMS**
There can be variation in the licensing of different medicines containing the same drug. Forms available from special-order manufacturers include: oral suspension, oral solution

Tablet
CAUTIONARY AND ADVISORY LABELS 8
▸ **Sotalol hydrochloride (Non-proprietary)**
Sotalol hydrochloride 40 mg Sotalol 40mg tablets |
28 tablet PoM £1.11 DT price = £1.02
Sotalol hydrochloride 80 mg Sotalol 80mg tablets |
28 tablet PoM £3.75 DT price = £1.10 | 56 tablet PoM no price available
Sotalol hydrochloride 160 mg Sotalol 160mg tablets |
28 tablet PoM £6.25 DT price = £5.93
▸ **Beta-Cardone** (Focus Pharmaceuticals Ltd)
Sotalol hydrochloride 200 mg Beta-Cardone 200mg tablets |
28 tablet PoM £2.40 DT price = £2.40
▸ **Sotacor** (Bristol-Myers Squibb Pharmaceuticals Ltd)
Sotalol hydrochloride 80 mg Sotacor 80mg tablets |
30 tablet PoM £3.28

CARDIAC GLYCOSIDES

Cardiac glycosides

Digoxin-specific antibody

Serious cases of digoxin toxicity should be discussed with the National Poisons Information Service (see further information, under Emergency treatment of poisoning p. 803). Digoxin-specific antibody p. 812 fragments are indicated for the treatment of known or strongly suspected life-threatening digoxin toxicity associated with ventricular arrhythmias or bradyarrhythmias unresponsive to atropine sulfate p. 779 and when measures beyond the withdrawal of digoxin below and correction of any electrolyte abnormalities are considered necessary.

Digoxin

Digoxin is most useful in the treatment of supraventricular tachycardias, especially for controlling ventricular response in persistent atrial fibrillation. Digoxin has a limited role in children with chronic heart failure.

For the management of atrial fibrillation, the maintenance dose of digoxin is determined on the basis of the ventricular rate at rest, which should not be allowed to fall below an acceptable level for the child.

Digoxin is now rarely used for rapid control of heart rate, even with intravenous administration, response may take many hours; persistence of tachycardia is therefore not an indication for exceeding the recommended dose. The intramuscular route is **not** recommended.

In children with heart failure who are in sinus rhythm, a loading dose may not be required.

Unwanted effects depend both on the concentration of digoxin in the plasma and on the sensitivity of the conducting system or of the myocardium, which is often increased in heart disease. It can sometimes be difficult to distinguish between toxic effects and clinical deterioration because the symptoms of both are similar. The plasma-digoxin concentration alone cannot indicate toxicity reliably, but the likelihood of toxicity increases progressively through the range 1.5 to 3 micrograms/litre for digoxin. Renal function is very important in determining digoxin dosage.

Hypokalaemia predisposes the child to digitalis toxicity and should be avoided; it is managed by giving a potassium-sparing diuretic or, if necessary, potassium supplements.

If toxicity occurs, digoxin should be withdrawn; serious manifestations require urgent specialist management. Digoxin-specific antibody fragments are available for reversal of life-threatening overdosage.

Digoxin
16-Jun-2017

- **DRUG ACTION** Digoxin is a cardiac glycoside that increases the force of myocardial contraction and reduces conductivity within the atrioventricular (AV) node.

- **INDICATIONS AND DOSE**

Supraventricular arrhythmias | Chronic heart failure
▸ BY MOUTH

▸ **Neonate (body-weight up to 1.5 kg):** Initially 25 micrograms/kg in 3 divided doses for 24 hours, then 4–6 micrograms/kg daily in 1–2 divided doses.

▸ **Neonate (body-weight 1.5-2.5 kg):** Initially 30 micrograms/kg in 3 divided doses for 24 hours, then 4–6 micrograms/kg daily in 1–2 divided doses.

▸ **Neonate (body-weight 2.6 kg and above):** Initially 45 micrograms/kg in 3 divided doses for 24 hours, then 10 micrograms/kg daily in 1–2 divided doses.

▸ **Child 1 month-1 year:** Initially 45 micrograms/kg in 3 divided doses for 24 hours, then 10 micrograms/kg daily in 1–2 divided doses
▸ **Child 2-4 years:** Initially 35 micrograms/kg in 3 divided doses for 24 hours, then 10 micrograms/kg daily in 1–2 divided doses
▸ **Child 5-9 years:** Initially 25 micrograms/kg in 3 divided doses (max. per dose 750 micrograms) for 24 hours, then 6 micrograms/kg daily in 1–2 divided doses; maximum 250 micrograms per day
▸ **Child 10-17 years:** Initially 0.75–1.5 mg in 3 divided doses for 24 hours, then 62.5–250 micrograms daily in 1–2 divided doses, higher doses may be necessary
▸ BY INTRAVENOUS INFUSION

▸ **Neonate (body-weight up to 1.5 kg):** Initially 20 micrograms/kg in 3 divided doses for 24 hours, then 4–6 micrograms/kg daily in 1–2 divided doses.

▸ **Neonate (body-weight 1.5-2.5 kg):** Initially 30 micrograms/kg in 3 divided doses for 24 hours, then 4–6 micrograms/kg daily in 1–2 divided doses.

▸ **Neonate (body-weight 2.6 kg and above):** Initially 35 micrograms/kg in 3 divided doses for 24 hours, then 10 micrograms/kg daily in 1–2 divided doses.

▸ **Child 1 month-1 year:** Initially 35 micrograms/kg in 3 divided doses for 24 hours, then 10 micrograms/kg daily in 1–2 divided doses
▸ **Child 2-4 years:** Initially 35 micrograms/kg in 3 divided doses for 24 hours, then 10 micrograms/kg daily in 1–2 divided doses
▸ **Child 5-9 years:** Initially 25 micrograms/kg in 3 divided doses (max. per dose 500 micrograms) for 24 hours, then 6 micrograms/kg daily in 1–2 divided doses; maximum 250 micrograms per day
▸ **Child 10-17 years:** Initially 0.5–1 mg in 3 divided doses for 24 hours, then 62.5–250 micrograms daily in 1–2 divided doses, higher doses may be necessary

DOSE ADJUSTMENTS DUE TO INTERACTIONS
Manufacturer advises reduce dose by half with concurrent use of amiodarone, dronedarone and quinine.

DOSE EQUIVALENCE AND CONVERSION
▸ Dose may need to be reduced if digoxin (or another cardiac glycoside) has been given in the preceding 2 weeks.
▸ When switching from intravenous to oral route may need to increase dose by 20–33% to maintain the same plasma-digoxin concentration.

Cardiovascular system

2

- **UNLICENSED USE** Digoxin is licensed for use in heart failure and supraventricular arrhythmias.
- **CONTRA-INDICATIONS** Constrictive pericarditis (unless to control atrial fibrillation or improve systolic dysfunction—but use with caution) · hypertrophic cardiomyopathy (unless concomitant atrial fibrillation and heart failure—but use with caution) · intermittent complete heart block · myocarditis · second degree AV block · supraventricular arrhythmias associated with accessory conducting pathways e.g. Wolff-Parkinson-White syndrome (although can be used in infancy) · ventricular tachycardia or fibrillation
- **CAUTIONS** Avoid hypercalcaemia (risk of digitalis toxicity) · avoid hypokalaemia (risk of digitalis toxicity) · avoid hypomagnesaemia (risk of digitalis toxicity) · avoid hypoxia (risk of digitalis toxicity) · severe respiratory disease · sick sinus syndrome · thyroid disease
- **INTERACTIONS** → Appendix 1: digoxin
- **SIDE-EFFECTS**
  - **Common or very common** Arrhythmias · blurred vision · conduction disturbances · diarrhoea · dizziness · eosinophilia · nausea · rash · vomiting · yellow vision
  - **Uncommon** Depression
  - **Very rare** Anorexia · apathy · confusion · fatigue · gynaecomastia on long-term use · headache · intestinal ischaemia and necrosis · psychosis · thrombocytopenia · weakness

  Overdose
  If toxicity occurs, digoxin should be withdrawn; serious manifestations require urgent specialist management.
- **PREGNANCY** May need dosage adjustment.
- **BREAST FEEDING** Amount too small to be harmful.
- **RENAL IMPAIRMENT** Use half normal dose if estimated glomerular filtration rate is 10–50 mL/minute/1.73 m^2 and use a quarter normal dose if estimated glomerular filtration rate is less than 10 mL/minute/1.73 m^2. Monitor plasma-digoxin concentration in renal impairment.
- **MONITORING REQUIREMENTS**
  - For plasma-digoxin concentration assay, blood should be taken at least 6 hours after a dose.
  - Plasma-digoxin concentration should be maintained in the range 0.8–2 micrograms/litre.
  - Monitor serum electrolytes and renal function. Toxicity increased by electrolyte disturbances.
- **DIRECTIONS FOR ADMINISTRATION**
  - With intravenous use Avoid rapid intravenous administration (risk of hypertension and reduced coronary flow). For *intravenous infusion*, dilute with Sodium Chloride 0.9% or Glucose 5% to a max. concentration of 62.5 micrograms/mL; loading doses should be given over 30–60 minutes and maintenance dose over 10–20 minutes.
  - With oral use For *oral* administration, oral solution must **not** be diluted.
- **PATIENT AND CARER ADVICE** Patient counselling is advised for digoxin elixir (use pipette).
- **MEDICINAL FORMS**
  There can be variation in the licensing of different medicines containing the same drug. Forms available from special-order manufacturers include: oral suspension, oral solution, solution for injection

  Tablet
  - Digoxin (Non-proprietary)
    Digoxin 62.5 microgram Digoxin 62.5microgram tablets | 28 tablet [PoM] £9.99 DT price = £1.82 | 500 tablet [PoM] no price available
    Digoxin 125 microgram Digoxin 125microgram tablets | 28 tablet [PoM] £4.99 DT price = £1.82
    Digoxin 250 microgram Digoxin 250microgram tablets | 28 tablet [PoM] £4.99 DT price = £1.83 | 500 tablet [PoM] no price available

- Lanoxin (Aspen Pharma Trading Ltd)
  Digoxin 62.5 microgram Lanoxin PG 62.5microgram tablets | 500 tablet [PoM] £8.09
  Digoxin 125 microgram Lanoxin 125 tablets | 500 tablet [PoM] £8.09
  Digoxin 250 microgram Lanoxin 250microgram tablets | 500 tablet [PoM] £8.09

Solution for injection
EXCIPIENTS: May contain Alcohol, propylene glycol
- Digoxin (Non-proprietary)
  Digoxin 100 microgram per 1 ml Lanoxin Injection Pediatric 100micrograms/1ml solution for injection ampoules | 10 ampoule [PoM] no price available

Solution for infusion
- Digoxin (Non-proprietary)
  Digoxin 250 microgram per 1 ml Digoxin 500micrograms/2ml solution for infusion ampoules | 10 ampoule [PoM] £7.00
- Lanoxin (Aspen Pharma Trading Ltd)
  Digoxin 250 microgram per 1 ml Lanoxin 500micrograms/2ml solution for infusion ampoules | 5 ampoule [PoM] £3.30

Oral solution
- Lanoxin (Aspen Pharma Trading Ltd)
  Digoxin 50 microgram per 1 ml Lanoxin PG 50micrograms/ml elixir | 60 ml [PoM] £5.35 DT price = £5.35

2 Bleeding disorders

Antifibrinolytic drugs and haemostatics

Overview

Fibrin dissolution can be impaired by the administration of tranexamic acid below, which inhibits fibrinolysis. It can be used to prevent bleeding or treat bleeding associated with excessive fibrinolysis (e.g. in surgery, dental extraction, obstetric disorders, and traumatic hyphaema) and in the management of menorrhagia; it may also be used in hereditary angioedema, epistaxis, and thrombolytic overdose. Tranexamic acid can also be used in cardiac surgery to reduce blood loss and to reduce the need for use of blood products.

Desmopressin p. 412 is used in the management of mild to moderate haemophilia and von Willebrand's disease. It is also used for fibrinolytic response testing.

ANTIHAEMORRHAGICS > ANTIFIBRINOLYTICS

Tranexamic acid

26-Apr-2017

- **INDICATIONS AND DOSE**
  Inhibition of fibrinolysis
  - BY MOUTH
  - Child: 15–25 mg/kg 2–3 times a day (max. per dose 1.5 g)
  - BY SLOW INTRAVENOUS INJECTION
  - Child: 10 mg/kg 2–3 times a day (max. per dose 1 g), dose to be given over at least 10 minutes
  - BY CONTINUOUS INTRAVENOUS INFUSION
  - Child: 45 mg/kg, dose to be given over 24 hours

  Menorrhagia
  - BY MOUTH
  - Child 12–17 years: 1 g 3 times a day for up to 4 days, to be initiated when menstruation has started; maximum 4 g per day

  Hereditary angioedema
  - BY MOUTH
  - Child: 15–25 mg/kg 2–3 times a day (max. per dose 1.5 g), for short-term prophylaxis of hereditary angioedema, tranexamic acid is started several days

before planned procedures which may trigger an acute attack of hereditary angioedema (e.g. dental work) and continued for 2–5 days afterwards
▸ BY SLOW INTRAVENOUS INJECTION
▸ Child: 10 mg/kg 2–3 times a day (max. per dose 1 g), dose to be given over at least 10 minutes
▸ BY CONTINUOUS INTRAVENOUS INFUSION
▸ Child: 45 mg/kg, dose to be given over 24 hours

Prevention of excessive bleeding after dental procedures (e.g. in haemophilia)
▸ BY INTRAVENOUS INJECTION
▸ Child 6-17 years: 10 mg/kg (max. per dose 1.5 g), dose to be given pre-operatively
▸ BY MOUTH
▸ Child 6-17 years: 15–25 mg/kg (max. per dose 1.5 g), dose to be given pre-operatively, then 15–25 mg/kg 2–3 times a day (max. per dose 1.5 g) for up to 8 days, dose to be given postoperatively

Prevention of excessive bleeding after dental procedures (e.g. in haemophilia) with mouthwash 5% solution (specialist use only)
▸ BY MOUTH
▸ Child 6-17 years: 5–10 mL 4 times a day for 2 days, rinse mouth with solution; the solution should not be swallowed

Reduction of blood loss during cardiac surgery
▸ BY SLOW INTRAVENOUS INJECTION, OR BY INTRAVENOUS INFUSION
▸ Child: (consult local protocol)

● UNLICENSED USE Not licensed for reduction of blood loss during cardiac surgery; injection not licensed for use in children under 1 year or for administration by intravenous infusion

● CONTRA-INDICATIONS Fibrinolytic conditions following disseminated intravascular coagulation (unless predominant activation of fibrinolytic system with severe bleeding) · history of convulsions · thromboembolic disease

● CAUTIONS Irregular menstrual bleeding (establish cause before initiating therapy) · massive haematuria (avoid if risk of ureteric obstruction) · patients receiving oral contraceptives (increased risk of thrombosis)

CAUTIONS, FURTHER INFORMATION
▸ Menorrhagia Before initiating treatment for menorrhagia, exclude structural or histological causes or fibroids causing distortion of uterine cavity.

● INTERACTIONS → Appendix 1: tranexamic acid

● SIDE-EFFECTS
▸ **Common or very common** Diarrhoea (reduce dose) · nausea · vomiting
▸ **Uncommon** Dermatitis
▸ **Rare** Impairment of colour vision (discontinue) · thromboembolic events · visual disturbances (discontinue)
▸ **Frequency not known** Convulsions (usually with high doses) · hypotension (on rapid intravenous injection) · malaise (on rapid intravenous injection)

● PREGNANCY No evidence of teratogenicity in *animal* studies; manufacturer advises use only if potential benefit outweighs risk—crosses the placenta.

● BREAST FEEDING Small amount present in milk— antifibrinolytic effect in infant unlikely.

● RENAL IMPAIRMENT Reduce dose in mild to moderate impairment. Avoid in severe impairment.

● MONITORING REQUIREMENTS Regular liver function tests in long-term treatment of hereditary angioedema.

● DIRECTIONS FOR ADMINISTRATION For *intravenous administration*, dilute with Glucose 5% *or* Sodium chloride 0.9%.

● PATIENT AND CARER ADVICE
Medicines for Children leaflet: Tranexamic acid for heavy bleeding during periods www.medicinesforchildren.org.uk/tranexamic-acid-for-heavy-bleeding-during-periods
Medicines for Children leaflet: Tranexamic acid for treatment for prevention of bleeding www.medicinesforchildren.org.uk/tranexamic-acid-for-treatment-or-prevention-of-bleeding

● MEDICINAL FORMS
There can be variation in the licensing of different medicines containing the same drug. Forms available from special-order manufacturers include: oral suspension, oral solution

Tablet
▸ **Tranexamic acid** (Non-proprietary)
  Tranexamic acid 500 mg Tranexamic acid 500mg tablets | 60 tablet [PoM] £32.10 DT price = £4.23
▸ **Cyklokapron** (Meda Pharmaceuticals Ltd)
  Tranexamic acid 500 mg Cyklokapron 500mg tablets | 60 tablet [PoM] £14.30 DT price = £4.23

Solution for injection
▸ **Tranexamic acid** (Non-proprietary)
  Tranexamic acid 100 mg per 1 ml Tranexamic acid 500mg/5ml solution for injection ampoules | 5 ampoule [PoM] £7.50 (Hospital only) | 10 ampoule [PoM] £15.47 (Hospital only)
▸ **Cyklokapron** (Pfizer Ltd)
  Tranexamic acid 100 mg per 1 ml Cyklokapron 500mg/5ml solution for injection ampoules | 10 ampoule [PoM] £15.47

2.1 Coagulation factor deficiencies

BLOOD AND RELATED PRODUCTS ›
COAGULATION PROTEINS

▌Dried prothrombin complex

(Human prothrombin complex)

● INDICATIONS AND DOSE
Treatment and peri-operative prophylaxis of haemorrhage in patients with congenital deficiency of factors II, VII, IX, or X if purified specific coagulation factors not available | Treatment and peri-operative prophylaxis of haemorrhage in patients with acquired deficiency of factors II, VII, IX, or X (e.g. during warfarin treatment)
▸ BY INTRAVENOUS INFUSION
▸ Child: (consult haematologist)

● CONTRA-INDICATIONS Angina · history of heparin induced thrombocytopenia · recent myocardial infarction (except in life-threatening haemorrhage following overdosage of oral anticoagulants, and before induction of fibrinolytic therapy)

● CAUTIONS Disseminated intravascular coagulation · history of myocardial infarction or coronary heart disease · postoperative use · risk of thrombosis · vaccination against hepatitis A and hepatitis B may be required

● SIDE-EFFECTS
▸ **Rare** Headache
▸ **Very rare** Anaphylaxis · antibody formation · hypersensitivity reactions · pyrexia
▸ **Frequency not known** Disseminated intravascular coagulation · nephrotic syndrome · thrombotic events

● HEPATIC IMPAIRMENT Monitor closely in hepatic impairment (risk of thromboembolic complications).

● PRESCRIBING AND DISPENSING INFORMATION Dried prothrombin complex is prepared from human plasma by a suitable fractionation technique, and contains factor IX, together with variable amounts of factors II, VII, and X.
Available from CSL Behring (*Beriplex® P/N*), Octapharma (*Octaplex®*).

Cardiovascular system

2

● **MEDICINAL FORMS**
There can be variation in the licensing of different medicines
containing the same drug.
No licensed medicines listed.

Factor IX fraction, dried

● **INDICATIONS AND DOSE**
**Treatment and prophylaxis of haemorrhage in congenital
factor IX deficiency (haemophilia B)**
▸ BY INTRAVENOUS INJECTION, OR BY CONTINUOUS
INTRAVENOUS INFUSION
▸ Child: (consult haematologist)

● **CONTRA-INDICATIONS** Disseminated intravascular
coagulation

● **CAUTIONS** Risk of thrombosis—principally with former low
purity products · vaccination against hepatitis A and
hepatitis B may be required (not necessary with
recombinant preparation)

● **SIDE-EFFECTS** Allergic reactions · chills · dizziness · fever ·
gastro-intestinal disturbances · headache

● **PRESCRIBING AND DISPENSING INFORMATION** Dried factor
IX fraction is prepared from human plasma by a suitable
fractionation technique; it may also contain clotting
factors II, VII, and X.

● **MEDICINAL FORMS**
There can be variation in the licensing of different medicines
containing the same drug.
Powder and solvent for solution for injection
▸ AlphaNine (Grifols UK Ltd)
Factor IX high purity 1000 unit AlphaNine 1,000unit powder and
solvent for solution for injection vials | 1 vial [PoM] £390.00
Factor IX high purity 1500 unit AlphaNine 1,500unit powder and
solvent for solution for injection vials | 1 vial [PoM] no price available
▸ Haemonine (Biotest (UK) Ltd)
Factor IX high purity 500 unit Haemonine 500unit powder and
solvent for solution for injection vials | 1 vial [PoM] £255.00 (Hospital
only)
Factor IX high purity 1000 unit Haemonine 1,000unit powder and
solvent for solution for injection vials | 1 vial [PoM] £510.00 (Hospital
only)
▸ Mononine (CSL Behring UK Ltd)
Factor IX high purity 1000 unit Mononine 1,000unit powder and
solvent for solution for injection vials | 1 vial [PoM] £478.43
▸ Replenine-VF (Bio Products Laboratory Ltd)
Factor IX high purity 500 unit Replenine-VF 500unit powder and
solvent for solution for injection vials | 1 vial [PoM] £180.00
Factor IX high purity 1000 unit Replenine-VF 1,000unit powder and
solvent for solution for injection vials | 1 vial [PoM] £360.00
Powder and solvent for solution for infusion
▸ BeneFIX (Pfizer Ltd)
Nonacog alfa 250 unit BeneFIX 250unit powder and solvent for
solution for infusion vials | 1 vial [PoM] £151.80 (Hospital only)
Nonacog alfa 500 unit BeneFIX 500unit powder and solvent for
solution for infusion vials | 1 vial [PoM] £303.60 (Hospital only)
Nonacog alfa 1000 unit BeneFIX 1,000unit powder and solvent for
solution for infusion vials | 1 vial [PoM] £607.20 (Hospital only)
Nonacog alfa 2000 unit BeneFIX 2,000unit powder and solvent for
solution for infusion vials | 1 vial [PoM] £1,214.40 (Hospital only)
Nonacog alfa 3000 unit BeneFIX 3,000unit powder and solvent for
solution for infusion vials | 1 vial [PoM] £1,821.60 (Hospital only)

Factor VIIa (recombinant)

(Eptacog alfa (activated))

● **INDICATIONS AND DOSE**
**Treatment and prophylaxis of haemorrhage in patients
with haemophilia A or B with inhibitors to factors VIII or
IX, acquired haemophilia, factor VII deficiency, or
Glanzmann's thrombasthenia**
▸ BY INTRAVENOUS INJECTION
▸ Child: (consult haematologist)

● **CAUTIONS** Disseminated intravascular coagulation · risk of
thrombosis

● **SIDE-EFFECTS**
▸ Very rare Allergic reactions · cerebrovascular accident ·
coagulation disorders · fever · myocardial infarction ·
nausea · pain · rash · thrombotic events

● **MEDICINAL FORMS**
There can be variation in the licensing of different medicines
containing the same drug.
Powder and solvent for solution for injection
▸ NovoSeven (Novo Nordisk Ltd)
Eptacog alfa activated 50000 unit NovoSeven 1mg (50,000units)
powder and solvent for solution for injection pre-filled syringes |
1 pre-filled disposable injection [PoM] £525.20 (Hospital only)
NovoSeven 1mg (50,000units) powder and solvent for solution for
injection vials | 1 vial [PoM] £525.20 (Hospital only)
Eptacog alfa activated 100000 unit NovoSeven 2mg (100,000units)
powder and solvent for solution for injection vials | 1 vial [PoM]
£1,050.40 (Hospital only)
NovoSeven 2mg (100,000units) powder and solvent for solution for
injection pre-filled syringes | 1 pre-filled disposable injection [PoM]
£1,050.40 (Hospital only)
Eptacog alfa activated 250000 unit NovoSeven 5mg (250,000units)
powder and solvent for solution for injection pre-filled syringes |
1 pre-filled disposable injection [PoM] 2,626.00 (Hospital only)
NovoSeven 5mg (250,000units) powder and solvent for solution for
injection vials | 1 vial [PoM] £2,626.00 (Hospital only)
Eptacog alfa activated 400000 unit NovoSeven 8mg
(400,000units) powder and solvent for solution for injection vials |
1 vial [PoM] £4,201.60 (Hospital only)
NovoSeven 8mg (400,000units) powder and solvent for solution for
injection pre-filled syringes | 1 pre-filled disposable injection [PoM]
£4,201.60 (Hospital only)

Factor VIII fraction, dried

(Human coagulation factor VIII, dried)

● **INDICATIONS AND DOSE**
**Treatment and prophylaxis of haemorrhage in congenital
factor VIII deficiency (haemophilia A), acquired factor
VIII deficiency | Von Willebrand's disease**
▸ BY INTRAVENOUS INJECTION, OR BY INTRAVENOUS INFUSION,
OR BY CONTINUOUS INTRAVENOUS INFUSION
▸ Child: (consult haematologist)

● **CAUTIONS** Intravascular haemolysis after large or
frequently repeated doses in patients with blood groups A,
B, or AB—less likely with high potency concentrates ·
vaccination against hepatitis A and hepatitis B may be
required (not necessary with recombinant preparation)

● **SIDE-EFFECTS** Anaphylaxis · angioedema · antibody
formation · blurred vision · chills · coughing · dizziness ·
drowsiness · dyspnoea · fever · flushing · gastro-intestinal
disturbances · headache · hypersensitivity reactions ·
hypotension · palpitation · paraesthesia · taste
disturbances · urticaria

● **MONITORING REQUIREMENTS** Monitor for development of
factor VIII inhibitors.

● **PRESCRIBING AND DISPENSING INFORMATION** Dried factor
VIII fraction is prepared from human plasma by a suitable

fractionation technique; it may also contain varying amounts of von Willebrand factor. *Optivate®*, *Fanhdi®*, and *Octanate®* are not indicated for use in von Willebrand's disease.

Recombinant human coagulation factor VIII including octocog alfa, moroctocog alfa, and simoctocog alfa are not indicated for use in von Willebrand's disease.

● MEDICINAL FORMS
There can be variation in the licensing of different medicines containing the same drug.
Powder and solvent for solution for injection
▸ Advate (Baxalta UK Ltd)
  Octocog alfa 250 unit Advate 250unit powder and solvent for solution for injection vials | 1 vial [PoM] no price available
  Octocog alfa 500 unit Advate 500unit powder and solvent for solution for injection vials | 1 vial [PoM] no price available
  Octocog alfa 1000 unit Advate 1,000unit powder and solvent for solution for injection vials | 1 vial [PoM] no price available
  Octocog alfa 2000 unit Advate 2,000unit powder and solvent for solution for injection vials | 1 vial [PoM] no price available
▸ Elocta (Swedish Orphan Biovitrum Ltd) ▼
  Efmoroctocog alfa 250 unit Elocta 250unit powder and solvent for solution for injection vials | 1 vial [PoM] no price available (Hospital only)
  Efmoroctocog alfa 500 unit Elocta 500unit powder and solvent for solution for injection vials | 1 vial [PoM] no price available (Hospital only)
  Efmoroctocog alfa 1000 unit Elocta 1,000unit powder and solvent for solution for injection vials | 1 vial [PoM] no price available (Hospital only)
  Efmoroctocog alfa 1500 unit Elocta 1,500unit powder and solvent for solution for injection vials | 1 vial [PoM] no price available (Hospital only)
  Efmoroctocog alfa 2000 unit Elocta 2,000unit powder and solvent for solution for injection vials | 1 vial [PoM] no price available (Hospital only)
  Efmoroctocog alfa 3000 unit Elocta 3,000unit powder and solvent for solution for injection vials | 1 vial [PoM] no price available (Hospital only)
▸ Fanhdi (Grifols UK Ltd)
  Factor VIII high purity 500 unit Fanhdi 500unit powder and solvent for solution for injection vials | 1 vial [PoM] £165.00 (Hospital only)
  Factor VIII high purity 1000 unit Fanhdi 1,000unit powder and solvent for solution for injection vials | 1 vial [PoM] £330.00 (Hospital only)
  Factor VIII high purity 1500 unit Fanhdi 1,500unit powder and solvent for solution for injection vials | 1 vial [PoM] £495.00
▸ Haemoctin (Biotest (UK) Ltd)
  Factor VIII high purity 250 unit Haemoctin 250unit powder and solvent for solution for injection vials | 1 vial [PoM] £127.50 (Hospital only)
  Factor VIII high purity 500 unit Haemoctin 500unit powder and solvent for solution for injection vials | 1 vial [PoM] £255.00 (Hospital only)
  Factor VIII high purity 1000 unit Haemoctin 1,000unit powder and solvent for solution for injection vials | 1 vial [PoM] £510.00 (Hospital only)
▸ Helixate NexGen (CSL Behring UK Ltd)
  Octocog alfa 250 unit Helixate NexGen 250unit powder and solvent for solution for injection vials | 1 vial [PoM] £118.57
  Octocog alfa 500 unit Helixate NexGen 500unit powder and solvent for solution for injection vials | 1 vial [PoM] £237.15
  Octocog alfa 1000 unit Helixate NexGen 1,000unit powder and solvent for solution for injection vials | 1 vial [PoM] £474.30
  Octocog alfa 2000 unit Helixate NexGen 2,000unit powder and solvent for solution for injection vials | 1 vial [PoM] £948.60
▸ Kogenate (Bayer Plc)
  Octocog alfa 250 unit Kogenate Bayer 250unit powder and solvent for solution for injection vials | 1 vial [PoM] £157.50
  Octocog alfa 500 unit Kogenate Bayer 500unit powder and solvent for solution for injection vials | 1 vial [PoM] £315.00
  Octocog alfa 1000 unit Kogenate Bayer 1,000unit powder and solvent for solution for injection vials | 1 vial [PoM] £630.00
  Octocog alfa 2000 unit Kogenate Bayer 2,000unit powder and solvent for solution for injection vials | 1 vial [PoM] £1,260.00
▸ Nuwiq (Octapharma Ltd) ▼
  Simoctocog alfa 250 unit Nuwiq 250unit powder and solvent for solution for injection vials | 1 vial [PoM] £190.00 (Hospital only)
  Simoctocog alfa 500 unit Nuwiq 500unit powder and solvent for solution for injection vials | 1 vial [PoM] £380.00 (Hospital only)
  Simoctocog alfa 1000 unit Nuwiq 1,000unit powder and solvent for solution for injection vials | 1 vial [PoM] £760.00 (Hospital only)
  Simoctocog alfa 2000 unit Nuwiq 2,000unit powder and solvent for solution for injection vials | 1 vial [PoM] £1,520.00 (Hospital only)
Powder and solvent for solution for infusion
▸ Advate (Baxalta UK Ltd)
  Octocog alfa 1500 unit Advate 1,500unit powder and solvent for solution for infusion vials | 1 vial [PoM] no price available
  Octocog alfa 3000 unit Advate 3,000unit powder and solvent for solution for infusion vials | 1 vial [PoM] no price available
▸ Kogenate (Bayer Plc)
  Octocog alfa 3000 unit Kogenate Bayer 3,000unit powder and solvent for solution for injection vials | 1 vial [PoM] £1,890.00

▌Factor XIII fraction, dried

(Human fibrin-stabilising factor, dried)

● INDICATIONS AND DOSE
Congenital factor XIII deficiency
▸ BY INTRAVENOUS INJECTION, OR BY INTRAVENOUS INFUSION
▸ Child: (consult haematologist)

● CAUTIONS Vaccination against hepatitis A and hepatitis B may be required

● SIDE-EFFECTS
▸ **Rare** Allergic reactions · fever

● MEDICINAL FORMS
There can be variation in the licensing of different medicines containing the same drug.
Powder and solvent for solution for injection
▸ Fibrogammin P (CSL Behring UK Ltd)
  Factor XIII 250 unit Fibrogammin 250unit powder and solvent for solution for injection vials | 1 vial [PoM] £90.59
  Factor XIII 1250 unit Fibrogammin 1,250unit powder and solvent for solution for injection vials | 1 vial [PoM] £452.95

▌Fibrinogen, dried

(Human fibrinogen)

● INDICATIONS AND DOSE
Treatment of haemorrhage in congenital hypofibrinogenaemia or afibrinogenaemia
▸ BY INTRAVENOUS INJECTION, OR BY INTRAVENOUS INFUSION
▸ Child: (consult haematologist)

● CAUTIONS Risk of thrombosis

● SIDE-EFFECTS
▸ **Rare** Allergic reactions · fever
▸ **Very rare** Myocardial infarction · pulmonary embolism · thromboembolic events

● PREGNANCY Manufacturer advises not known to be harmful—no information available.

● BREAST FEEDING Manufacturer advises avoid—no information available.

● PRESCRIBING AND DISPENSING INFORMATION Fibrinogen is prepared from human plasma.

● MEDICINAL FORMS
There can be variation in the licensing of different medicines containing the same drug.
Powder for solution for infusion
▸ Riastap (CSL Behring UK Ltd)
  Fibrinogen 1 gram Riastap 1g powder for solution for infusion vials | 1 vial [PoM] £340.00

Protein C concentrate

- **INDICATIONS AND DOSE**

Congenital protein C deficiency
- ▸ BY INTRAVENOUS INJECTION
- ▸ Child: (consult haematologist)

- **CAUTIONS** Hypersensitivity to heparins · vaccination against hepatitis A and hepatitis B may be required
- **SIDE-EFFECTS**
- ▸ **Very rare** Bleeding · dizziness · fever · hypersensitivity reactions
- **PRESCRIBING AND DISPENSING INFORMATION** Protein C is prepared from human plasma.

- **MEDICINAL FORMS**
There can be variation in the licensing of different medicines containing the same drug.
Powder and solvent for solution for injection
- ▸ Ceprotin (Baxalta UK Ltd)
Protein C 500 unit Ceprotin 500unit powder and solvent for solution for injection vials | 1 vial [PoM] no price available
Protein C 1000 unit Ceprotin 1000unit powder and solvent for solution for injection vials | 1 vial [PoM] no price available

BLOOD AND RELATED PRODUCTS ›
HAEMOSTATIC PRODUCTS

Factor VIII inhibitor bypassing fraction

- **INDICATIONS AND DOSE**

Treatment and prophylaxis of haemorrhage in patients with congenital factor VIII deficiency (haemophilia A) and factor VIII inhibitors | Treatment of haemorrhage in non-haemophiliac patients with acquired factor VIII inhibitors
- ▸ BY INTRAVENOUS INFUSION, OR BY INTRAVENOUS INJECTION
- ▸ Child: (consult haematologist)

- **CONTRA-INDICATIONS** Disseminated intravascular coagulation
- **CAUTIONS** Vaccination against hepatitis A and hepatitis B may be required
- **SIDE-EFFECTS** Anaphylaxis · disseminated intravascular coagulation · flushing · hypersensitivity · hypotension · myocardial infarction · paraesthesia · pyrexia · rash · thrombosis · urticaria
- **PRESCRIBING AND DISPENSING INFORMATION** Preparations with factor VIII inhibitor bypassing activity are prepared from human plasma.

- **MEDICINAL FORMS**
There can be variation in the licensing of different medicines containing the same drug.
Powder and solvent for solution for injection
- ▸ FEIBA Imuno (Baxalta UK Ltd)
Factor VIII inhibitor bypassing fraction 500 unit FEIBA 500unit powder and solvent for solution for injection vials | 1 vial [PoM] no price available
Powder and solvent for solution for infusion
- ▸ FEIBA Imuno (Baxalta UK Ltd)
Factor VIII inhibitor bypassing fraction 1000 unit FEIBA 1,000unit powder and solvent for solution for infusion vials | 1 vial [PoM] no price available

BLOOD AND RELATED PRODUCTS › PLASMA PRODUCTS

Fresh frozen plasma

- **INDICATIONS AND DOSE**

Replacement of coagulation factors or other plasma proteins where their concentration or functional activity is critically reduced
- ▸ BY INTRAVENOUS INFUSION
- ▸ Child: (consult haematologist)

- **CONTRA-INDICATIONS** Avoid use as a volume expander · IgA deficiency with confirmed antibodies to IgA
- **CAUTIONS** Cardiac decompensation · need for compatibility · pulmonary oedema · severe protein S deficiency (avoid products with low protein S activity e.g. *OctaplasLG®*) · vaccination against hepatitis A and hepatitis B may be required
- **SIDE-EFFECTS**
- ▸ **Common or very common** Nausea · pruritus · rash
- ▸ **Uncommon** Oedema · vomiting
- ▸ **Rare** Agitation · allergic reactions · bronchospasm · cardiorespiratory collapse · chills · fever · tachycardia
- ▸ **Very rare** Arrhythmia · hypertension · thromboembolism
- **PRESCRIBING AND DISPENSING INFORMATION** Fresh frozen plasma is prepared from the supernatant liquid obtained by centrifugation of one donation of whole blood.
   A preparation of solvent/detergent treated human plasma (frozen) from pooled donors is available from Octapharma (*OctaplasLG®*).
   Children under 16 years should only receive virucidally inactivated preparations of fresh frozen plasma, sourced from 'low prevalence BSE regions' such as the USA.

- **MEDICINAL FORMS**
There can be variation in the licensing of different medicines containing the same drug.
No licensed medicines listed.

2.2 Subarachnoid haemorrhage

CALCIUM-CHANNEL BLOCKERS

F 104

Nimodipine

- **DRUG ACTION** Nimodipine is a dihydropyridine calcium-channel blocker.

- **INDICATIONS AND DOSE**

Treatment of vasospasm following subarachnoid haemorrhage (specialist use only)
- ▸ BY INTRAVENOUS INFUSION
- ▸ Child 1 month–11 years: Initially 15 micrograms/kg/hour (max. per dose 500 micrograms/hour), increased after 2 hours if no severe decrease in blood pressure; increased to 30 micrograms/kg/hour (max. per dose 2 mg/hour), continue for at least 5 days (max. 14 days), use initial dose of 7.5 micrograms/kg/hour if blood pressure unstable
- ▸ Child 12–17 years (body-weight up to 70 kg): Initially 0.5 mg/hour, increased after 2 hours if no severe decrease in blood pressure; increased to 1–2 mg/hour, continue for at least 5 days (max. 14 days)
- ▸ Child 12–17 years (body-weight 70 kg and above): Initially up to 1 mg/hour, use dose if blood pressure stable; increased after 2 hours if no severe decrease in blood pressure; increased to 1–2 mg/hour, continue for at least 5 days (max. 14 days)

Prevention of vasospasm following subarachnoid haemorrhage

▶ BY MOUTH

▶ Child: 0.9–1.2 mg/kg 6 times a day (max. per dose 60 mg), started within 4 days of haemorrhage and continued for 21 days

● **UNLICENSED USE** Not licensed for use in children.

● **CONTRA-INDICATIONS** Acute porphyrias p. 577

● **CAUTIONS** Cerebral oedema · hypotension · severely raised intracranial pressure

● **INTERACTIONS** → Appendix 1: calcium channel blockers

● **SIDE-EFFECTS** Flushing · gastro-intestinal disorders · headache · hypotension · ileus · nausea · sweating and feeling of warmth · thrombocytopenia · variation in heart-rate

● **PREGNANCY** Manufacturer advises use only if potential benefit outweighs risk.

● **BREAST FEEDING** Manufacturer advises avoid—present in milk.

● **HEPATIC IMPAIRMENT** Elimination reduced in cirrhosis—monitor blood pressure.

● **RENAL IMPAIRMENT**

▶ With intravenous use Manufacturer advises monitor renal function closely in renal impairment.

● **DIRECTIONS FOR ADMINISTRATION** Avoid concomitant administration of nimodipine infusion and tablets.

▶ With oral use For administration *by mouth*, tablets may be crushed or halved but are light sensitive—administer immediately.

▶ With intravenous use For *continuous intravenous infusion*, administer undiluted *via* a Y-piece on a central venous catheter connected to a running infusion of Glucose 5%, or Sodium Chloride 0.9%; not to be added to an infusion container; incompatible with polyvinyl chloride giving sets or containers; protect infusion from light.

▶ With intravenous use Polyethylene, polypropylene, or glass apparatus should be used. PVC should be avoided.

● **MEDICINAL FORMS**
There can be variation in the licensing of different medicines containing the same drug. Forms available from special-order manufacturers include: oral suspension

Solution for infusion

▶ Nimotop (Bayer Plc)
Nimodipine 200 microgram per 1 ml Nimotop 0.02% solution for infusion 50ml vials | 5 vial PoM £68.00 (Hospital only)

Tablet

▶ Nimotop (Bayer Plc)
Nimodipine 30 mg Nimotop 30mg tablets | 100 tablet PoM £40.00

---

3 Blood clots
3.1 Blocked catheters and lines

ANTITHROMBOTIC DRUGS ⟩ TISSUE
PLASMINOGEN ACTIVATORS

Fibrinolytic drugs

Overview

Alteplase below, streptokinase p. 86 and urokinase p. 86 are used in children to dissolve intravascular thrombi and unblock occluded arteriovenous shunts, catheters, and indwelling central lines blocked with fibrin clots. Treatment should be started as soon as possible after a clot has formed and discontinued once a pulse in the affected limb is detected, or the shunt or catheter unblocked.

The safety and efficacy of treatment remains uncertain, especially in neonates. A fibrinolytic drug is probably only appropriate where arterial occlusion threatens ischaemic damage; an anticoagulant may stop the clot getting bigger. Alteplase is the preferred fibrinolytic in children and neonates; there is less risk of adverse effects including allergic reactions.

Fibrinolytics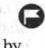

● **DRUG ACTION** Fibrinolytic drugs act as thrombolytics by activating plasminogen to form plasmin, which degrades fibrin and so breaks up thrombi.

● **CONTRA-INDICATIONS** Acute pancreatitis · aneurysm · arteriovenous malformation · bacterial endocarditis · bleeding diatheses · coagulation defects · neoplasm with risk of haemorrhage · pericarditis · recent haemorrhage · recent surgery (including dental extraction) · recent trauma · severe hypertension

● **CAUTIONS** Conditions with an increased risk of haemorrhage · hypertension · risk of bleeding (including that from venepuncture or invasive procedures)

● **SIDE-EFFECTS** Allergic reactions · anaphylaxis · back pain · bleeding · bleeding (usually limited to the site of injection, but can occur from other sites) · cerebral oedema (caused by reperfusion) · convulsions · fever · flushing · hypotension · intracerebral haemorrhage · nausea · pulmonary oedema (caused by reperfusion) · rash · uveitis · vomiting

SIDE-EFFECTS, FURTHER INFORMATION

▶ Bleeding Serious bleeding calls for discontinuation of the thrombolytic and may require administration of coagulation factors and antifibrinolytic drugs (e.g. tranexamic acid). Rarely further embolism may occur (either due to clots that break away from the original thrombus or to cholesterol crystal emboli).

▶ Hypotension Hypotension can usually be controlled by elevating the patient's legs, or by reducing the rate of infusion or stopping it temporarily.

● **PREGNANCY** Thrombolytic drugs can possibly lead to premature separation of the placenta in the first 18 weeks of pregnancy. There is also a risk of maternal haemorrhage throughout pregnancy and post-partum, and also a theoretical risk of fetal haemorrhage throughout pregnancy.

● **HEPATIC IMPAIRMENT** Avoid in severe hepatic impairment as there is an increased risk of bleeding.

☞ above

Alteplase

(rt-PA; Tissue-type plasminogen activator)

● **INDICATIONS AND DOSE**

Intravascular thrombosis

▶ BY INTRAVENOUS INFUSION

▶ Neonate: 100–500 micrograms/kg/hour for 3–6 hours, use ultrasound assessment to monitor effect before considering a second course of treatment (consult local protocol).

▶ Child: 100–500 micrograms/kg/hour for 3–6 hours, use ultrasound assessment to monitor effect before considering a second course of treatment; maximum 100 mg per day

ACTILYSE CATHFLO®

Thrombolytic treatment of occluded central venous access devices (including those used for haemodialysis)

▶ BY INTRAVENOUS INJECTION

▶ Child: (consult product literature)

- **UNLICENSED USE** *Actilyse*® not licensed for use in children.
- **CONTRA-INDICATIONS** Oesophageal varices · recent delivery · recent ulcerative gastro-intestinal disease · stroke
- **INTERACTIONS** → Appendix 1: alteplase
- **SIDE-EFFECTS** Risk of cerebral bleeding increased in acute stroke
- **ALLERGY AND CROSS-SENSITIVITY** Contra-indicated if history of hypersensitivity to gentamicin (residue from manufacturing process).
- **DIRECTIONS FOR ADMINISTRATION** For *intravenous infusion* (*Actilyse*®), dissolve in Water for Injections to a concentration of 1 mg/mL or 2 mg/mL and infuse intravenously; alternatively dilute further in Sodium Chloride 0.9% to a concentration of not less than 200 micrograms/mL; not to be diluted in Glucose.

- **MEDICINAL FORMS**
  There can be variation in the licensing of different medicines containing the same drug. Forms available from special-order manufacturers include: solution for injection
  Powder and solvent for solution for injection
  ▸ Actilyse (Boehringer Ingelheim Ltd)
    Alteplase 10 mg Actilyse 10mg powder and solvent for solution for injection vials | 1 vial [PoM] £172.80
    Alteplase 20 mg Actilyse 20mg powder and solvent for solution for injection vials | 1 vial [PoM] £259.20
  ▸ Actilyse Cathflo (Boehringer Ingelheim Ltd)
    Alteplase 2 mg Actilyse Cathflo 2mg powder and solvent for solution for injection vials | 5 vial [PoM] £225.00 (Hospital only)
  Powder and solvent for solution for infusion
  ▸ Actilyse (Boehringer Ingelheim Ltd)
    Alteplase 50 mg Actilyse 50mg powder and solvent for solution for infusion vials | 1 vial [PoM] £432.00

F 85

Streptokinase

- **INDICATIONS AND DOSE**
  Intravascular thrombosis
  ▸ INITIALLY BY INTRAVENOUS INFUSION
  ▸ Child 1 month–11 years: Initially 2500–4000 units/kg, dose to be given over 30 minutes, followed by (by continuous intravenous infusion) 500–1000 units/kg/hour for up to 3 days until reperfusion occurs
  ▸ Child 12–17 years: Initially 250 000 units, dose to be given over 30 minutes, followed by (by continuous intravenous infusion) 100 000 units/hour for up to 3 days until reperfusion occurs

- **UNLICENSED USE** Not licensed for use in children.
- **CONTRA-INDICATIONS** Avoid in children who have had streptococcal infection in the last 12 months
- **CAUTIONS** Atrial fibrillation · cavernous pulmonary disease · cerebrovascular disease · mitral valve defect · recent delivery or abortion · septic thrombotic disease
- **INTERACTIONS** → Appendix 1: streptokinase
- **SIDE-EFFECTS**
  ▸ Rare Guillain-Barré syndrome
- **ALLERGY AND CROSS-SENSITIVITY** Contra-indicated if previous allergic reaction to either streptokinase or anistreplase (no longer available). Prolonged persistence of antibodies to streptokinase and anistreplase (no longer available) can reduce the effectiveness of subsequent treatment; therefore, streptokinase should not be used again beyond 4 days of first administration of either streptokinase or anistreplase.
- **DIRECTIONS FOR ADMINISTRATION** For *intravenous infusion*, reconstitute with Sodium Chloride 0.9%, then dilute further with Glucose 5% or Sodium Chloride 0.9%

after reconstitution. Monitor fibrinogen concentration closely; if fibrinogen concentration less than 1 g/litre, stop streptokinase infusion and start unfractionated heparin; restart streptokinase once fibrinogen concentration reaches 1 g/litre.

- **MEDICINAL FORMS**
  There can be variation in the licensing of different medicines containing the same drug.
  No licensed medicines listed.

F 85

Urokinase

- **INDICATIONS AND DOSE**
  Occluded arteriovenous shunts, catheters, and indwelling central lines
  ▸ TO THE DEVICE AS A FLUSH
  ▸ Neonate: 5000–25 000 units, inject directly into occluded catheter or central line, dilute dose in sodium chloride 0.9% to fill catheter dead space **only**. Leave for 20–60 minutes then aspirate the lysate and flush with sodium chloride 0.9%.
  ▸ Child: 5000–25 000 units, inject directly into occluded catheter or central line, dilute dose in sodium chloride 0.9% to fill catheter dead space **only**. Leave for 20–60 minutes then aspirate the lysate and flush with sodium chloride 0.9%.

- **CONTRA-INDICATIONS** Recent stroke
- **CAUTIONS** Atrial fibrillation · cavernous pulmonary disease · mitral valve defect · recent delivery · septic thrombotic disease · severe cerebrovascular disease
- **INTERACTIONS** → Appendix 1: urokinase
- **BREAST FEEDING** Manufacturer advises avoid—no information available.
- **DIRECTIONS FOR ADMINISTRATION** May be diluted, after reconstitution, with Sodium Chloride 0.9%.

- **MEDICINAL FORMS**
  There can be variation in the licensing of different medicines containing the same drug.
  Powder for solution for injection
  ▸ Urokinase (Non-proprietary)
    Urokinase 10000 unit Urokinase 10,000unit powder for solution for injection vials | 1 vial [PoM] £33.79
    Urokinase 50000 unit Urokinase 50,000unit powder for solution for injection vials | 1 vial [PoM] £69.70
    Urokinase 100000 unit Urokinase 100,000unit powder for solution for injection vials | 1 vial [PoM] £106.17
    Urokinase 250000 unit Urokinase 250,000unit powder for solution for injection vials | 1 vial [PoM] £185.65
    Urokinase 500000 unit Urokinase 500,000unit powder for solution for injection vials | 1 vial [PoM] £365.00
  ▸ Syner-KINASE (Syner-Med (Pharmaceutical Products) Ltd)
    Urokinase 10000 unit Syner-KINASE 10,000unit powder for solution for injection vials | 1 vial [PoM] £35.95 (Hospital only)
    Urokinase 25000 unit Syner-KINASE 25,000unit powder for solution for injection vials | 1 vial [PoM] £45.95 (Hospital only)
    Urokinase 100000 unit Syner-KINASE 100,000unit powder for solution for injection vials | 1 vial [PoM] £112.95 (Hospital only)
    Urokinase 250000 unit Syner-KINASE 250,000unit powder for solution for injection vials | 1 vial [PoM] no price available (Hospital only)
    Urokinase 500000 unit Syner-KINASE 500,000unit powder for solution for injection vials | 1 vial [PoM] no price available (Hospital only)

3.2 Thromboembolism

Venous thromboembolism

Prophylaxis of venous thromboembolism

Low-dose heparin (unfractionated) p. 92 by subcutaneous injection is used to prevent thrombotic episodes in 'high-risk' patients; laboratory monitoring of APTT or anti-Factor Xa concentration is also required in prophylactic regimens in children. Low molecular weight heparins, aspirin (antiplatelet dose), and warfarin sodium p. 94 can also be used for prophylaxis.

Treatment of venous thromboembolism

For the initial treatment of thrombotic episodes heparin (unfractionated) is given as an intravenous loading dose, followed by continuous intravenous infusion (using an infusion pump) or by intermittent subcutaneous injection; the use of intermittent intravenous injection is no longer recommended. Alternatively, a low molecular weight heparin may be given for initial treatment. If an oral anticoagulant (usually warfarin sodium) is also required, it may be started at the same time as the heparin (the heparin needs to be continued for at least 5 days and until the INR has been in the therapeutic range for 2 consecutive days). Laboratory monitoring of coagulation activity, preferably on a daily basis, involves determination of the activated partial thromboplastin time (APTT) (for heparin (unfractionated) only) or of the anti-Factor Xa concentration (for low molecular weight heparins). Local guidelines on recommended APTT for neonates and children should be followed; monitoring of APTT should be discussed with a specialist prior to treatment for thrombotic episodes in neonates.

Management of venous thromboembolism in pregnancy

Heparins are used for the management of venous thromboembolism in pregnancy because they do not cross the placenta. Low molecular weight heparins are preferred because they have a lower risk of osteoporosis and of heparin-induced thrombocytopenia. Low molecular weight heparins are eliminated more rapidly in pregnancy, requiring alteration of the dosage regimen for drugs such as dalteparin sodium p. 91, enoxaparin sodium p. 92 and tinzaparin sodium p. 93; see also under individual drugs. Treatment should be stopped at the onset of labour and advice sought from a specialist on continuing therapy after birth.

Extracorporeal circuits

Heparin (unfractionated) is also used in the maintenance of extracorporeal circuits in cardiopulmonary bypass and haemodialysis.

Haemorrhage

If haemorrhage occurs it is usually sufficient to withdraw unfractionated or low molecular weight heparin (unfractionated), but if rapid reversal of the effects of the heparin (unfractionated) is required, protamine sulfate p. 812 is a specific antidote (but only partially reverses the effects of low molecular weight heparin (unfractionated)).

Oral anticoagulants

Overview

The main use of anticoagulants is to prevent thrombus formation or extension of an existing thrombus in the slower-moving venous side of the circulation, where the thrombus consists of a fibrin web enmeshed with platelets and red cells.

Anticoagulants are of less use in preventing thrombus formation in arteries, for in faster-flowing vessels thrombi are composed mainly of platelets with little fibrin.

Oral anticoagulants antagonise the effects of vitamin K and take at least 48 to 72 hours for the anticoagulant effect to develop fully; if an immediate effect is required, unfractionated or low molecular weight heparin must be given concomitantly.

Uses

Warfarin sodium p. 94 is the drug of choice for the treatment of systemic thromboembolism in children (not neonates) after initial heparinisation. It may also be used occasionally for the treatment of intravascular or intracardiac thrombi. Warfarin sodium is used prophylactically in those with chronic atrial fibrillation, dilated cardiomyopathy, certain forms of reconstructive heart surgery, mechanical prosthetic heart valves, and some forms of hereditary thrombophilia (e.g. homozygous protein C deficiency).

Unfractionated or a low molecular weight heparin (see under Parenteral anticoagulants p. 88) is usually preferred for the prophylaxis of venous thromboembolism in children undergoing surgery; alternatively warfarin sodium can be continued in selected children currently taking warfarin sodium and who are at a high risk of thromboembolism (seek expert advice).

Dose

The base-line prothrombin time should be determined but the initial dose should not be delayed whilst awaiting the result.

An induction dose is usually given over 4 days. The subsequent maintenance dose depends on the prothrombin time, reported as INR (international normalised ratio) and should be taken at the same time each day.

Target INR

The following indications and target INRs for adults for warfarin take into account recommendations of the British Society for Haematology Guidelines on Oral Anticoagulation with warfarin—fourth edition. *Br J Haematol* 2011; **154**: 311–324:

An INR which is within 0.5 units of the target value is generally satisfactory; larger deviations require dosage adjustment. Target values (rather than ranges) are now recommended.

INR 2.5 for:
- treatment of deep-vein thrombosis or pulmonary embolism (including those associated with antiphospholipid syndrome or for recurrence in patients no longer receiving warfarin sodium)
- atrial fibrillation
- cardioversion—target INR should be achieved at least 3 weeks before cardioversion and anticoagulation should continue for at least 4 weeks after the procedure (higher target values, such as an INR of 3, can be used for up to 4 weeks before the procedure to avoid cancellations due to low INR)
- dilated cardiomyopathy
- mitral stenosis or regurgitation in patients with either atrial fibrillation, a history of systemic embolism, a left atrial thrombus, or an enlarged left atrium
- bioprosthetic heart valves in the mitral position (treat for 3 months), or in patients with a history of systemic embolism (treat for at least 3 months), or with a left atrial thrombus at surgery (treat until clot resolves), or with other risk factors (e.g. atrial fibrillation or a low ventricular ejection fraction)
- acute arterial embolism requiring embolectomy (consider long-term treatment)
- myocardial infarction

INR 3.5 for:

- recurrent deep-vein thrombosis or pulmonary embolism in patients currently receiving anticoagulation and with an INR above 2;

Mechanical prosthetic heart valves:

- the recommended target INR depends on the type and location of the valve, and patient-related risk factors
- consider increasing the INR target or adding an antiplatelet drug, if an embolic event occurs whilst anticoagulated at the target INR.

Haemorrhage

The main adverse effect of all oral anticoagulants is haemorrhage. Checking the INR and omitting doses when appropriate is essential; if the anticoagulant is stopped but not reversed, the INR should be measured 2–3 days later to ensure that it is falling. The cause of an elevated INR should be investigated. The following recommendations (which take into account the recommendations of the British Society for Haematology Guidelines on Oral Anticoagulation with Warfarin—fourth edition. *Br J Haematol* 2011; **154**: 311–324) are based on the result of the INR and whether there is major or minor bleeding; the recommendations apply to adults taking warfarin:

- Major bleeding—stop warfarin sodium; give phytomenadione (vitamin K$_1$) p. 609 by slow intravenous injection; give dried prothrombin complex p. 81 (factors II, VII, IX, and X); if dried prothrombin complex unavailable, fresh frozen plasma can be given but is less effective; recombinant factor VIIa is not recommended for emergency anticoagulation reversal
- INR >8.0, minor bleeding—stop warfarin sodium; give phytomenadione (vitamin K$_1$) by slow intravenous injection; repeat dose of phytomenadione if INR still too high after 24 hours; restart warfarin sodium when INR <5.0
- INR >8.0, no bleeding—stop warfarin sodium; give phytomenadione (vitamin K$_1$) by mouth using the intravenous preparation orally [unlicensed use]; repeat dose of phytomenadione if INR still too high after 24 hours; restart warfarin sodium when INR <5.0
- INR 5.0–8.0, minor bleeding—stop warfarin sodium; give phytomenadione (vitamin K$_1$) by slow intravenous injection; restart warfarin sodium when INR <5.0
- INR 5.0–8.0, no bleeding—withhold 1 or 2 doses of warfarin sodium and reduce subsequent maintenance dose
- Unexpected bleeding at therapeutic levels—always investigate possibility of underlying cause e.g. unsuspected renal or gastro-intestinal tract pathology

Parenteral anticoagulants

Anticoagulants

Although thrombotic episodes are uncommon in childhood, anticoagulants may be required in children with congenital heart disease; in children undergoing haemodialysis; for preventing thrombosis in children requiring chemotherapy and following surgery; and for systemic venous thromboembolism secondary to inherited thrombophilias, systemic lupus erythematosus, or indwelling central venous catheters.

Heparin

Heparin initiates anticoagulation rapidly but has a short duration of action. It is now often referred to as being **standard** or heparin (unfractionated) p. 92 to distinguish it from the **low molecular weight heparins**, which have a longer duration of action. For children at high risk of bleeding, heparin (unfractionated) is more suitable than low

molecular weight heparin because its effect can be terminated rapidly by stopping the infusion.

Heparins are used in both the treatment and prophylaxis of thromboembolic disease, mainly to prevent further clotting rather than to lyse existing clots—surgery or a thrombolytic drug may be necessary if a thrombus obstructs major vessels.

Low molecular weight heparins

Dalteparin sodium p. 91, enoxaparin sodium p. 92, and tinzaparin sodium p. 93 are low molecular weight heparins used for treatment and prophylaxis of thrombotic episodes in children. Their duration of action is longer than that of heparin (unfractionated) and in adults and older children *once-daily subcutaneous* dosage is sometimes possible; however, younger children require relatively higher doses (possibly due to larger volume of distribution, altered heparin pharmacokinetics, or lower plasma concentrations of antithrombin) and twice daily dosage is sometimes necessary. Low molecular weight heparins are convenient to use, especially in children with poor venous access.

Heparinoids

Danaparoid sodium p. 90 is a heparinoid that has a role in children who develop heparin-induced thrombocytopenia, providing they have no evidence of cross-reactivity.

Heparin flushes

The use of heparin flushes should be kept to a minimum. For maintaining patency of peripheral venous catheters, sodium chloride injection 0.9% is as effective as heparin flushes. The role of heparin flushes in maintaining patency of arterial and central venous catheters is unclear.

Epoprostenol

Epoprostenol (prostacyclin) p. 115 can be given to inhibit platelet aggregation during renal dialysis when heparins are unsuitable or contra-indicated. It is a potent vasodilator and therefore its side-effects include flushing, headache and hypotension.

> **Other drugs used for Thromboembolism** Alteplase, p. 85 · Streptokinase, p. 86

ANTITHROMBOTIC DRUGS > ANTIPLATELET DRUGS

Antiplatelet drugs

Overview

Antiplatelet drugs decrease platelet aggregation and inhibit thrombus formation in the arterial circulation, because in faster-flowing vessels, thrombi are composed mainly of platelets with little fibrin.

Aspirin p. 89 has limited use in children because it has been associated with Reye's syndrome. Aspirin-containing preparations should not be given to children and adolescents under 16 years, unless specifically indicated, such as for Kawasaki disease, for prophylaxis of clot formation after cardiac surgery, or for prophylaxis of stroke in children at high risk.

If aspirin causes dyspepsia, or if the child is at a high risk of gastro-intestinal bleeding, a proton pump inhibitor or a H$_2$-receptor antagonist can be added.

Dipyridamole p. 90 is also used as an antiplatelet drug to prevent clot formation after cardiac surgery and may be used with specialist advice for treatment of persistent coronary artery aneurysms in Kawasaki disease.

Kawasaki disease

Initial treatment is with high dose aspirin and a single dose of intravenous normal immunoglobulin; this combination has an additive anti-inflammatory effect resulting in faster resolution of fever and a decreased incidence of coronary artery complications. After the acute phase, when the patient is afebrile, aspirin is continued at a lower dose to prevent coronary artery abnormalities.

| Aspirin

(Acetylsalicylic Acid)

- **INDICATIONS AND DOSE**

Antiplatelet | Prevention of thrombus formation after cardiac surgery
▸ BY MOUTH
▸ Neonate: 1–5 mg/kg once daily.

▸ Child 1 month–11 years: 1–5 mg/kg once daily (max. per dose 75 mg)
▸ Child 12–17 years: 75 mg once daily

Kawasaki disease
▸ BY MOUTH
▸ Neonate: Initially 8 mg/kg 4 times a day for 2 weeks *or* until afebrile, followed by 5 mg/kg once daily for 6–8 weeks, if no evidence of coronary lesions after 8 weeks, discontinue treatment or seek expert advice.

▸ Child 1 month–11 years: Initially 7.5–12.5 mg/kg 4 times a day for 2 weeks *or* until afebrile, then 2–5 mg/kg once daily for 6–8 weeks, if no evidence of coronary lesions after 8 weeks, discontinue treatment or seek expert advice

- **UNLICENSED USE** Not licensed for use in children under 16 years.
- **CONTRA-INDICATIONS** Active peptic ulceration · bleeding disorders (antiplatelet dose) · children under 16 years (risk of Reye's syndrome) · haemophilia · previous peptic ulceration (analgesic dose) · severe cardiac failure (analgesic dose)

  CONTRA-INDICATIONS, FURTHER INFORMATION
  ▸ Reye's syndrome Owing to an association with Reye's syndrome, aspirin-containing preparations should not be given to children under 16 years, unless specifically indicated, e.g. for Kawasaki disease.
- **CAUTIONS** Allergic disease · anaemia · asthma · dehydration · G6PD deficiency · preferably avoid during fever or viral infection in children (risk of Reye's syndrome) · previous peptic ulceration (but manufacturers may advise avoidance of low-dose aspirin in history of peptic ulceration) · thyrotoxicosis · uncontrolled hypertension
- **INTERACTIONS** → Appendix 1: aspirin
- **SIDE-EFFECTS** Blood disorders (with analgesic doses) · bronchospasm · confusion (with analgesic doses) · gastro-intestinal haemorrhage (occasionally major) · gastro-intestinal irritation (with slight asymptomatic blood loss at higher doses) · haemorrhage including subconjunctival haemorrhage (reported with antiplatelet doses) · increased bleeding time · skin reactions in hypersensitive patients · tinnitus (with analgesic doses)

Overdose

The main features of salicylate poisoning are hyperventilation, tinnitus, deafness, vasodilatation, and sweating. Coma is uncommon but indicates very severe poisoning.

For specific details on the management of poisoning, see *Aspirin*, under Emergency treatment of poisoning p. 803.

- **ALLERGY AND CROSS-SENSITIVITY** Aspirin is **contra-indicated** in history of hypersensitivity to aspirin or any other NSAID—which includes those in whom attacks of asthma, angioedema, urticaria, or rhinitis have been precipitated by aspirin or any other NSAID.
- **PREGNANCY** Use antiplatelet doses with caution during third trimester; impaired platelet function and risk of haemorrhage; delayed onset and increased duration of labour with increased blood loss; avoid analgesic doses if possible in last few weeks (low doses probably not harmful); high doses may be related to intra-uterine growth restriction, teratogenic effects, closure of fetal ductus arteriosus in utero and possibly persistent pulmonary hypertension of newborn; kernicterus may occur in jaundiced neonates.
- **BREAST FEEDING** Avoid—possible risk of Reye's syndrome; regular use of high doses could impair platelet function and produce hypoprothrombinaemia in infant if neonatal vitamin K stores low.
- **HEPATIC IMPAIRMENT** Avoid in severe impairment—increased risk of gastro-intestinal bleeding.
- **RENAL IMPAIRMENT** Use with caution; avoid in severe impairment; sodium and water retention; deterioration in renal function; increased risk of gastro-intestinal bleeding.
- **PATIENT AND CARER ADVICE**
  Medicines for Children leaflet: Aspirin for prevention of blood clots www.medicinesforchildren.org.uk/aspirin-prevention-blood-clots-0

- **MEDICINAL FORMS**
  There can be variation in the licensing of different medicines containing the same drug. Forms available from special-order manufacturers include: capsule, oral suspension, oral solution

Gastro-resistant tablet
CAUTIONARY AND ADVISORY LABELS 5, 25, 32
▸ Aspirin (Non-proprietary)
  Aspirin 75 mg Aspirin 75mg gastro-resistant tablets | 28 tablet Ⓟ £0.86 DT price = £0.86 | 56 tablet PoM no price available | 56 tablet Ⓟ £1.72
  Aspirin 300 mg Aspirin 300mg gastro-resistant tablets | 100 tablet PoM £20.34 DT price = £20.34
▸ Micropirin (Dexcel-Pharma Ltd)
  Aspirin 75 mg Micropirin 75mg gastro-resistant tablets | 28 tablet Ⓟ £1.45 DT price = £0.86 | 56 tablet Ⓟ £2.87
▸ Nu-Seals (Alliance Pharmaceuticals Ltd)
  Aspirin 75 mg Nu-Seals 75 gastro-resistant tablets | 56 tablet Ⓟ £3.12

Tablet
CAUTIONARY AND ADVISORY LABELS 21, 32
▸ Aspirin (Non-proprietary)
  Aspirin 75 mg Aspirin 75mg tablets | 28 tablet PoM £1.13 DT price = £1.13
  Aspirin 300 mg Aspirin 300mg tablets | 32 tablet Ⓟ £3.35 DT price = £3.35 | 100 tablet PoM £10.47

Dispersible tablet
CAUTIONARY AND ADVISORY LABELS 13, 21, 32
▸ Aspirin (Non-proprietary)
  Aspirin 75 mg Aspirin 75mg dispersible tablets | 28 tablet Ⓟ £0.70 DT price = £0.70 | 100 tablet Ⓟ £0.64 DT price = £2.50 | 1000 tablet Ⓟ £25.00
  Aspirin 300 mg Aspirin 300mg dispersible tablets | 32 tablet Ⓟ £1.12 DT price = £1.12 | 32 tablet PoM no price available DT price = £1.12 | 100 tablet PoM £3.50 DT price = £3.50 | 1000 tablet PoM £35.00
▸ Danamep (Ecogen Europe Ltd)
  Aspirin 75 mg Danamep 75mg dispersible tablets | 28 tablet PoM £0.50 DT price = £0.70
▸ Disprin (Reckitt Benckiser Healthcare (UK) Ltd)
  Aspirin 300 mg Disprin 300mg dispersible tablets | 32 tablet Ⓟ £1.87 DT price = £1.12

Cardiovascular system

2

Dipyridamole

- **INDICATIONS AND DOSE**

Kawasaki disease (initiated under specialist supervision)
- ▸ BY MOUTH USING IMMEDIATE-RELEASE MEDICINES
- ▸ Child 1 month–11 years: 1 mg/kg 3 times a day

Prevention of thrombus formation after cardiac surgery
- ▸ BY MOUTH USING IMMEDIATE-RELEASE MEDICINES
- ▸ Child 1 month–11 years: 2.5 mg/kg twice daily
- ▸ Child 12–17 years: 100–200 mg 3 times a day

- **UNLICENSED USE** Not licensed for use in children.
- **CAUTIONS** Aortic stenosis · coagulation disorders · heart failure · hypotension · left ventricular outflow obstruction · may exacerbate migraine · myasthenia gravis (risk of exacerbation)
- **INTERACTIONS** → Appendix 1: dipyridamole
- **SIDE-EFFECTS** Angioedema · dizziness · gastro-intestinal effects · hot flushes · hypersensitivity reactions · hypotension · increased bleeding after surgery · increased bleeding during surgery · myalgia · rash · severe bronchospasm · tachycardia · throbbing headache · thrombocytopenia · urticaria
- **PREGNANCY** Not known to be harmful.
- **BREAST FEEDING** Manufacturers advise use only if essential—small amount present in milk.
- **DIRECTIONS FOR ADMINISTRATION** Injection solution can be given orally.

- **MEDICINAL FORMS**
There can be variation in the licensing of different medicines containing the same drug. Forms available from special-order manufacturers include: oral suspension, oral solution
Oral suspension
- ▸ Dipyridamole (Non-proprietary)
Dipyridamole 10 mg per 1 ml Dipyridamole 50mg/5ml oral suspension sugar free sugar-free | 150 ml [PoM] £41.06 DT price = £41.06
Dipyridamole 40 mg per 1 ml Dipyridamole 200mg/5ml oral suspension sugar free sugar-free | 150 ml [PoM] £122.78–£133.53 DT price = £133.53
Tablet
CAUTIONARY AND ADVISORY LABELS 22
- ▸ Dipyridamole (Non-proprietary)
Dipyridamole 25 mg Dipyridamole 25mg tablets | 84 tablet [PoM] £9.40 DT price = £9.40
Dipyridamole 100 mg Dipyridamole 100mg tablets | 84 tablet [PoM] £12.50 DT price = £4.07
- ▸ Persantin (Boehringer Ingelheim Ltd)
Dipyridamole 100 mg Persantin 100mg tablets | 84 tablet [PoM] £6.30 DT price = £4.07

ANTITHROMBOTIC DRUGS > HEPARINOIDS

Danaparoid sodium

- **INDICATIONS AND DOSE**

Thromboembolic disease in patients with history of heparin-induced thrombocytopenia
- ▸ INITIALLY BY INTRAVENOUS INJECTION

- ▸ Neonate: Initially 30 units/kg, then (by continuous intravenous infusion) 1.2–2 units/kg/hour, infusion dose to be adjusted according to coagulation activity.

- ▸ Child 1 month–15 years (body-weight up to 55 kg): Initially 30 units/kg (max. per dose 1250 units), then (by continuous intravenous infusion) 1.2–2 units/kg/hour, infusion dose to be adjusted according to coagulation activity
- ▸ Child 1 month–15 years (body-weight 55 kg and above): Initially 30 units/kg (max. per dose 2500 units), then

(by continuous intravenous infusion) 1.2–2 units/kg/hour, infusion dose to be adjusted according to coagulation activity

- ▸ Child 16–17 years (body-weight up to 55 kg): Initially 1250 units, then (by continuous intravenous infusion) 400 units/hour for 2 hours, then (by continuous intravenous infusion) 300 units/hour for 2 hours, then (by continuous intravenous infusion) 200 units/hour for 5 days, infusion dose to be adjusted according to coagulation activity
- ▸ Child 16–17 years (body-weight 55–90 kg): Initially 2500 units, then (by continuous intravenous infusion) 400 units/hour for 2 hours, then (by continuous intravenous infusion) 300 units/hour for 2 hours, then (by continuous intravenous infusion) 200 units/hour for 5 days, infusion dose to be adjusted according to coagulation activity
- ▸ Child 16–17 years (body-weight 91 kg and above): Initially 3750 units, then (by continuous intravenous infusion) 400 units/hour for 2 hours, then (by continuous intravenous infusion) 300 units/hour for 2 hours, then (by continuous intravenous infusion) 200 units/hour for 5 days, infusion dose to be adjusted according to coagulation activity

- **UNLICENSED USE** Not licensed for use in children.
- **CONTRA-INDICATIONS** Active peptic ulcer (unless this is the reason for operation) · acute bacterial endocarditis · diabetic retinopathy · epidural anaesthesia (with treatment doses) · haemophilia and other haemorrhagic disorders · recent cerebral haemorrhage · severe hypertension · spinal anaesthesia (with treatment doses) · thrombocytopenia (unless patient has heparin-induced thrombocytopenia)
- **CAUTIONS** Antibodies to heparins (risk of antibody-induced thrombocytopenia) · body-weight over 90 kg · recent bleeding · risk of bleeding
- **INTERACTIONS** → Appendix 1: danaparoid
- **SIDE-EFFECTS** Bleeding · hypersensitivity reactions · rash
- **PREGNANCY** Manufacturer advises avoid—limited information available but not known to be harmful.
- **BREAST FEEDING** Amount probably too small to be harmful but manufacturer advises avoid.
- **HEPATIC IMPAIRMENT** Caution in moderate impairment (increased risk of bleeding). Avoid in severe impairment unless patient has heparin-induced thrombocytopenia and no alternative available.
- **RENAL IMPAIRMENT** Use with caution in moderate impairment. Avoid in severe impairment unless patient has heparin-induced thrombocytopenia and no alternative available. Increased risk of bleeding in renal impairment, monitor anti-Factor Xa activity.
- **MONITORING REQUIREMENTS** Monitor anti factor Xa activity in patients with body-weight over 90 kg.
- **DIRECTIONS FOR ADMINISTRATION** For *intravenous infusion*, dilute with Glucose 5% or Sodium Chloride 0.9%.

- **MEDICINAL FORMS**
There can be variation in the licensing of different medicines containing the same drug.
Solution for injection
- ▸ Danaparoid sodium (Non-proprietary)
Danaparoid sodium 1250 unit per 1 ml Danaparoid sodium 750units/0.6ml solution for injection ampoules | 10 ampoule [PoM] £599.99

ANTITHROMBOTIC DRUGS > HEPARINS

Heparins

- **CONTRA-INDICATIONS** Acute bacterial endocarditis · after major trauma · epidural anaesthesia with treatment doses · haemophilia and other haemorrhagic disorders · peptic ulcer · recent cerebral haemorrhage · recent surgery to eye · recent surgery to nervous system · severe hypertension · spinal anaesthesia with treatment doses · thrombocytopenia (including history of heparin-induced thrombocytopenia)

● SIDE-EFFECTS
▸ **Rare** Alopecia (on prolonged use) · anaphylaxis · angioedema · hyperkalaemia · hypersensitivity reactions · injection-site reactions · osteoporosis (risk lower with low molecular weight heparins) · priapism · rebound hyperlipidaemia (following unfractionated heparin withdrawal) · skin necrosis · urticaria
▸ **Frequency not known** Haemorrhage · thrombocytopenia

SIDE-EFFECTS, FURTHER INFORMATION
▸ Haemorrhage If haemorrhage occurs it is usually sufficient to withdraw unfractionated or low molecular weight heparin, but if rapid reversal of the effects of the heparin is required, protamine sulfate is a specific antidote (but only partially reverses the effects of low molecular weight heparins).
▸ Heparin-induced thrombocytopenia Clinically important heparin-induced thrombocytopenia is immune-mediated and does not usually develop until after 5–10 days; it can be complicated by thrombosis.

Signs of heparin-induced thrombocytopenia include a 30% reduction of platelet count, thrombosis, or skin allergy. If heparin-induced thrombocytopenia is strongly suspected or confirmed, the heparin should be **stopped** and an alternative anticoagulant, such as danaparoid, should be given. Ensure platelet counts return to normal range in those who require warfarin.
▸ Hyperkalaemia Inhibition of aldosterone secretion by unfractionated or low molecular weight heparin can result in hyperkalaemia; patients with diabetes mellitus, chronic renal failure, acidosis, raised plasma potassium or those taking potassium-sparing drugs seem to be more susceptible. The risk appears to increase with duration of therapy.

● ALLERGY AND CROSS-SENSITIVITY Hypersensitivity to unfractionated or low molecular weight heparin.

● MONITORING REQUIREMENTS
▸ Heparin-induced thrombocytopenia Platelet counts should be measured just before treatment with unfractionated or low molecular weight heparin, and regular monitoring of platelet counts may be required if given for longer than 4 days. See the British Society for Haematology's Guidelines on the diagnosis and management of heparin-induced thrombocytopenia: second edition. *Br J Haematol* 2012; **159**: 528–540.
▸ Hyperkalaemia Plasma-potassium concentration should be measured in patients at risk of hyperkalaemia before starting the heparin and monitored regularly thereafter, particularly if treatment is to be continued for longer than 7 days.

▸ 90

Dalteparin sodium

● INDICATIONS AND DOSE
Treatment of thrombotic episodes
▸ BY SUBCUTANEOUS INJECTION

▸ Neonate: 100 units/kg twice daily.

▸ Child 1 month–11 years: 100 units/kg twice daily
▸ Child 12–17 years: 200 units/kg once daily (max. per dose 18 000 units); reduced to 100 units/kg twice daily, dose reduced if increased risk of bleeding

Treatment of venous thromboembolism in pregnancy
▸ BY SUBCUTANEOUS INJECTION
▸ Child 12–17 years (body-weight up to 50 kg): 5000 units twice daily, use body-weight in early pregnancy to calculate the dose
▸ Child 12–17 years (body-weight 50–69 kg): 6000 units twice daily, use body-weight in early pregnancy to calculate the dose
▸ Child 12–17 years (body-weight 70–89 kg): 8000 units twice daily, use body-weight in early pregnancy to calculate the dose
▸ Child 12–17 years (body-weight 90 kg and above): 10 000 units twice daily, use body-weight in early pregnancy to calculate the dose

Prophylaxis of thrombotic episodes.
▸ BY SUBCUTANEOUS INJECTION
▸ Neonate: 100 units/kg once daily.

▸ Child 1 month–11 years: 100 units/kg once daily
▸ Child 12–17 years: 2500–5000 units once daily

● UNLICENSED USE Not licensed for treatment of venous thromboembolism in pregnancy. Not licensed for use in children.

● INTERACTIONS → Appendix 1: low molecular-weight heparins

● PREGNANCY Not known to be harmful, low molecular weight heparins do not cross the placenta. Multidose vial contains benzyl alcohol—manufacturer advises avoid.

● BREAST FEEDING Due to the relatively high molecular weight and inactivation in the gastro-intestinal tract, passage into breast-milk and absorption by the nursing infant are likely to be negligible, however manufacturers advise avoid.

● HEPATIC IMPAIRMENT Dose reduction may be required in severe impairment—risk of bleeding may be increased.

● RENAL IMPAIRMENT Risk of bleeding may be increased—dose reduction may be required. Use of unfractionated heparin may be preferable.

● MONITORING REQUIREMENTS Routine monitoring of anti-Factor Xa activity is not usually required during treatment with dalteparin, except in neonates; monitoring may also be necessary in severely ill children and those with renal or hepatic impairment.

● MEDICINAL FORMS
There can be variation in the licensing of different medicines containing the same drug.
Solution for injection
EXCIPIENTS: May contain Benzyl alcohol
▸ Dalteparin sodium (Non-proprietary)
Dalteparin sodium 10000 unit per 1 ml Dalteparin sodium 10,000units/1ml solution for injection pre-filled syringes | 5 pre-filled disposable injection [PoM] no price available DT price = £28.23 | 5 pre-filled disposable injection no price available DT price = £28.23
Dalteparin sodium 12500 unit per 1 ml Dalteparin sodium 2,500units/0.2ml solution for injection pre-filled syringes | 10 pre-filled disposable injection [PoM] no price available DT price = £18.58
Dalteparin sodium 25000 unit per 1 ml Dalteparin sodium 7,500units/0.3ml solution for injection pre-filled syringes | 10 pre-filled disposable injection [PoM] no price available DT price = £42.34
Dalteparin sodium 12,500units/0.5ml solution for injection pre-filled syringes | 5 pre-filled disposable injection [PoM] no price available DT price = £35.29
Dalteparin sodium 5,000units/0.2ml solution for injection pre-filled syringes | 5 pre-filled disposable injection [PoM] no price available DT price = £28.23
Dalteparin sodium 15,000units/0.6ml solution for injection pre-filled syringes | 5 pre-filled disposable injection [PoM] no price available DT price = £42.34
Dalteparin sodium 10,000units/0.4ml solution for injection pre-filled syringes | 5 pre-filled disposable injection [PoM] no price available DT price = £28.23

2

Cardiovascular system

Dalteparin sodium 18,000units/0.72ml solution for injection pre-filled syringes | 5 pre-filled disposable injection [PoM] no price available DT price = £50.82

▸ **Fragmin** (Pfizer Ltd)
Dalteparin sodium 2500 unit per 1 ml Fragmin 10,000units/4ml solution for injection ampoules | 10 ampoule [PoM] £51.22
Dalteparin sodium 10000 unit per 1 ml Fragmin 10,000units/1ml solution for injection pre-filled syringes | 5 pre-filled disposable injection [PoM] £28.23 DT price = £28.23
Fragmin 10,000units/1ml solution for injection ampoules | 10 ampoule [PoM] £51.22
Dalteparin sodium 12500 unit per 1 ml Fragmin 2,500units/0.2ml solution for injection pre-filled syringes | 10 pre-filled disposable injection [PoM] £18.58 DT price = £18.58
Dalteparin sodium 25000 unit per 1 ml Fragmin 18,000units/0.72ml solution for injection pre-filled syringes | 5 pre-filled disposable injection [PoM] £50.82 DT price = £50.82
Fragmin 15,000units/0.6ml solution for injection pre-filled syringes | 5 pre-filled disposable injection [PoM] £42.34 DT price = £42.34
Fragmin 5,000units/0.2ml solution for injection pre-filled syringes | 10 pre-filled disposable injection [PoM] £28.23 DT price = £28.23
Fragmin 12,500units/0.5ml solution for injection pre-filled syringes | 5 pre-filled disposable injection [PoM] £35.29 DT price = £35.29
Fragmin 7,500units/0.3ml solution for injection pre-filled syringes | 10 pre-filled disposable injection [PoM] £42.34 DT price = £42.34
Fragmin 100,000units/4ml solution for injection vials | 1 vial [PoM] £48.66
Fragmin 10,000units/0.4ml solution for injection pre-filled syringes | 5 pre-filled disposable injection [PoM] £28.23 DT price = £28.23

▸ 90

Enoxaparin sodium

● **INDICATIONS AND DOSE**
Treatment of thrombotic episodes
▸ BY SUBCUTANEOUS INJECTION

▸ Neonate: 1.5–2 mg/kg twice daily.

▸ Child 1 month: 1.5 mg/kg twice daily
▸ Child 2 months–17 years: 1 mg/kg twice daily

Treatment of venous thromboembolism in pregnancy
▸ BY SUBCUTANEOUS INJECTION
▸ Child 12–17 years (body-weight up to 50 kg): 40 mg twice daily, dose based on early pregnancy body-weight
▸ Child 12–17 years (body-weight 50–69 kg): 60 mg twice daily, dose based on early pregnancy body-weight
▸ Child 12–17 years (body-weight 70–89 kg): 80 mg twice daily, dose based on early pregnancy body-weight
▸ Child 12–17 years (body-weight 90 kg and above): 100 mg twice daily, dose based on early pregnancy body-weight

Prophylaxis of thrombotic episodes
▸ BY SUBCUTANEOUS INJECTION

▸ Neonate: 750 micrograms/kg twice daily.

▸ Child 1 month: 750 micrograms/kg twice daily
▸ Child 2 months–17 years: 500 micrograms/kg twice daily; maximum 40 mg per day
DOSE EQUIVALENCE AND CONVERSION
▸ 1 mg equivalent to 100 units.

● **UNLICENSED USE** Not licensed for treatment of venous thromboembolism in pregnancy. Not licensed for use in children.
● **INTERACTIONS** → Appendix 1: low molecular-weight heparins
● **PREGNANCY** Not known to be harmful, low molecular weight heparins do not cross the placenta. Multidose vial contains benzyl alcohol—avoid.
● **BREAST FEEDING** Due to the relatively high molecular weight of enoxaparin and inactivation in the gastro-intestinal tract, passage into breast-milk and absorption by the nursing infant are likely to be negligible; however manufacturers advise avoid.

● **HEPATIC IMPAIRMENT** Reduce dose in severe impairment—risk of bleeding may be increased.
● **RENAL IMPAIRMENT** Risk of bleeding increased; reduce dose if estimated glomerular filtration rate less than 30 mL/minute/1.73 m^2—consult product literature for details. Use of unfractionated heparin may be preferable.
● **MONITORING REQUIREMENTS** Routine monitoring of anti-Factor Xa activity is not usually required during treatment with enoxaparin, except in neonates; monitoring may also be necessary in severely ill children and those with renal or hepatic impairment.

● **MEDICINAL FORMS**
There can be variation in the licensing of different medicines containing the same drug.
Solution for injection
EXCIPIENTS: May contain Benzyl alcohol
▸ **Clexane** (Sanofi)
Enoxaparin sodium 100 mg per 1 ml Clexane 60mg/0.6ml solution for injection pre-filled syringes | 10 pre-filled disposable injection [PoM] £39.26 DT price = £39.26
Clexane 300mg/3ml solution for injection multidose vials | 1 vial [PoM] £21.33
Clexane 80mg/0.8ml solution for injection pre-filled syringes | 10 pre-filled disposable injection [PoM] £55.13 DT price = £55.13
Clexane 40mg/0.4ml solution for injection pre-filled syringes | 10 pre-filled disposable injection [PoM] £30.27 DT price = £30.27
Clexane 100mg/1ml solution for injection pre-filled syringes | 10 pre-filled disposable injection [PoM] £72.30 DT price = £72.30
Clexane 20mg/0.2ml solution for injection pre-filled syringes | 10 pre-filled disposable injection [PoM] £20.86 DT price = £20.86
Enoxaparin sodium 150 mg per 1 ml Clexane Forte 120mg/0.8ml solution for injection pre-filled syringes | 10 pre-filled disposable injection [PoM] £87.93 DT price = £87.93
Clexane Forte 150mg/1ml solution for injection pre-filled syringes | 10 pre-filled disposable injection [PoM] £99.91 DT price = £99.91

▸ 90

Heparin (unfractionated)

● **INDICATIONS AND DOSE**
Prevention of clotting in extracorporeal circuits
▸ TO THE DEVICE AS A FLUSH
▸ Child: (consult product literature)

Maintenance of neonatal umbilical arterial catheter
▸ BY INTRAVENOUS INFUSION
▸ Neonate: 0.5 unit/hour.

Treatment of thrombotic episodes
▸ INITIALLY BY INTRAVENOUS INJECTION

▸ Neonate up to 35 weeks corrected gestational age: Initially 50 units/kg, then (by continuous intravenous infusion) 25 units/kg/hour, adjusted according to APTT.

▸ Neonate: Initially 75 units/kg, then (by continuous intravenous infusion) 25 units/kg/hour, adjusted according to APTT.

▸ Child 1–11 months: Initially 75 units/kg, then (by continuous intravenous infusion) 25 units/kg/hour, adjusted according to APTT
▸ Child 1–17 years: Initially 75 units/kg, then (by continuous intravenous infusion) 20 units/kg/hour, adjusted according to APTT
▸ BY SUBCUTANEOUS INJECTION
▸ Child: 250 units/kg twice daily, adjusted according to APTT

Prophylaxis of thrombotic episodes
▸ BY SUBCUTANEOUS INJECTION
▸ Child: 100 units/kg twice daily (max. per dose 5000 units), adjusted according to APTT

Maintenance of cardiac shunts and critical stents
▸ TO THE DEVICE AS A FLUSH
▸ Child: (consult local protocol)

- **UNLICENSED USE** Check product literature for licensed use in children.
- **INTERACTIONS** → Appendix 1: heparin (unfractionated)
- **PREGNANCY** Does not cross the placenta; maternal osteoporosis reported after prolonged use; multidose vials may contain benzyl alcohol—some manufacturers advise avoid.
- **BREAST FEEDING** Not excreted into milk due to high molecular weight.
- **HEPATIC IMPAIRMENT** Risk of bleeding increased—reduce dose or avoid in severe impairment (including oesophageal varices).
- **RENAL IMPAIRMENT** Risk of bleeding increased in severe impairment—dose may need to be reduced.
- **DIRECTIONS FOR ADMINISTRATION** For *continuous intravenous infusion*, dilute with Glucose 5% or Sodium chloride 0.9%.
- In neonates For *maintenance of neonatal umbilical arterial catheter*, dilute 50 units to a final volume of 50 mL with Sodium Chloride 0.45% or use ready-made bag containing 500 units in 500 mL Sodium Chloride 0.9%; infuse at 0.5 mL/hour. For *neonatal intensive care (treatment of thrombosis)*, dilute 1250 units/kg body-weight to a final volume of 50 mL with infusion fluid; an intravenous infusion rate of 1 mL/hour provides a dose of 25 units/kg/hour.

- **MEDICINAL FORMS**
There can be variation in the licensing of different medicines containing the same drug. Forms available from special-order manufacturers include: solution for injection, solution for infusion
Solution for injection
EXCIPIENTS: May contain Benzyl alcohol
- **Heparin (unfractionated) (Non-proprietary)**
Heparin sodium 1000 unit per 1 ml Heparin sodium 1,000units/1ml solution for injection ampoules | 10 ampoule [PoM] £14.85
Heparin sodium 5,000units/5ml solution for injection vials | 10 vial [PoM] £16.50–£37.41
Heparin sodium 20,000units/20ml solution for injection ampoules | 10 ampoule [PoM] £70.80–£70.88
Heparin sodium 5,000units/5ml solution for injection ampoules | 10 ampoule [PoM] £37.45–£37.47
Heparin sodium 10,000units/10ml solution for injection ampoules | 10 ampoule [PoM] £64.50–£64.59
Heparin sodium 5000 unit per 1 ml Heparin sodium 5,000units/1ml solution for injection ampoules | 10 ampoule [PoM] £29.04
Heparin sodium 25,000units/5ml solution for injection vials | 10 vial [PoM] £45.00–£84.60
Heparin sodium 25,000units/5ml solution for injection ampoules | 10 ampoule [PoM] £75.78
Heparin calcium 25000 unit per 1 ml Heparin calcium 5,000units/0.2ml solution for injection ampoules | 10 ampoule [PoM] £44.70
Heparin sodium 25000 unit per 1 ml Heparin sodium 25,000units/1ml solution for injection ampoules | 10 ampoule [PoM] £76.95
Heparin sodium 5,000units/0.2ml solution for injection ampoules | 10 ampoule [PoM] £37.35
Intravenous flush
EXCIPIENTS: May contain Benzyl alcohol
- **Heparin (unfractionated) (Non-proprietary)**
Heparin sodium 10 unit per 1 ml Heparin sodium 50units/5ml patency solution ampoules | 10 ampoule [PoM] £14.96 DT price = £14.96
Heparin sodium 50units/5ml I.V. flush solution ampoules | 10 ampoule [PoM] £14.96 DT price = £14.96
Heparin sodium 100 unit per 1 ml Heparin sodium 200units/2ml I.V. flush solution ampoules | 10 ampoule [PoM] £15.68 DT price = £15.68
Heparin sodium 200units/2ml patency solution ampoules | 10 ampoule [PoM] £15.68 DT price = £15.68
Infusion
- **Heparin (unfractionated) (Non-proprietary)**
Heparin sodium 2 unit per 1 ml Heparin sodium 1,000units/500ml infusion Viaflex bags | 1 bag [PoM] no price available
Heparin sodium 2,000units/1,000ml infusion Viaflex bags | 1 bag [PoM] no price available
Heparin sodium 5 unit per 1 ml Heparin sodium 5,000units/1litre infusion Viaflex bags | 1 bag [PoM] no price available

---

F 90

Tinzaparin sodium

- **INDICATIONS AND DOSE**
Treatment of thrombotic episodes
  ▸ BY SUBCUTANEOUS INJECTION
  ▸ Child 1 month: 275 units/kg once daily
  ▸ Child 2–11 months: 250 units/kg once daily
  ▸ Child 1–4 years: 240 units/kg once daily
  ▸ Child 5–9 years: 200 units/kg once daily
  ▸ Child 10–17 years: 175 units/kg once daily
Treatment of venous thromboembolism in pregnancy
  ▸ BY SUBCUTANEOUS INJECTION
  ▸ Child 12–17 years: 175 units/kg once daily, dose based on early pregnancy body-weight
Prophylaxis of thrombotic episodes
  ▸ BY SUBCUTANEOUS INJECTION
  ▸ Child: 50 units/kg once daily

- **UNLICENSED USE** Not licensed for the treatment of venous thromboembolism in pregnancy. Not licensed for use in children.
- **INTERACTIONS** → Appendix 1: low molecular-weight heparins
- **SIDE-EFFECTS**
  ▸ Uncommon Headache
- **PREGNANCY** Not known to be harmful, low molecular weight heparins do not cross the placenta. Vials contain benzyl alcohol—manufacturer advises avoid.
- **BREAST FEEDING** Due to the relatively high molecular weight of tinzaparin and inactivation in the gastro-intestinal tract, passage into breast-milk and absorption by the nursing infant are likely to be negligible; however manufacturer advise avoid.
- **RENAL IMPAIRMENT** Manufacturer advises caution if estimated glomerular filtration rate less than 30 mL/minute/1.73 m^2. Risk of bleeding may be increased. Unfractionated heparin may be preferable. In renal impairment monitoring of anti-Factor Xa may be required if estimated glomerular filtration rate less than 30 mL/minute/1.73 m^2.
- **MONITORING REQUIREMENTS** Routine monitoring of anti-Factor Xa activity is not usually required except in neonates; monitoring may also be necessary in severely ill children and those with renal or hepatic impairment.

- **MEDICINAL FORMS**
There can be variation in the licensing of different medicines containing the same drug.
Solution for injection
EXCIPIENTS: May contain Benzyl alcohol, sulfites
- **Tinzaparin sodium (Non-proprietary)**
Tinzaparin sodium 10000 unit per 1 ml Tinzaparin sodium 3,500units/0.35ml solution for injection pre-filled syringes | 10 pre-filled disposable injection [PoM] £27.71 DT price = £27.71
Tinzaparin sodium 4,500units/0.45ml solution for injection pre-filled syringes | 10 pre-filled disposable injection [PoM] £35.63 DT price = £35.63
Tinzaparin sodium 2,500units/0.25ml solution for injection pre-filled syringes | 10 pre-filled disposable injection [PoM] £19.80 DT price = £19.80
- **Innohep** (LEO Pharma)
Tinzaparin sodium 10000 unit per 1 ml Innohep 20,000units/2ml solution for injection vials | 10 vial [PoM] £105.66 DT price = £105.66
Tinzaparin sodium 20000 unit per 1 ml Innohep 18,000units/0.9ml solution for injection pre-filled syringes | 6 pre-filled disposable injection [PoM] £64.25 | 10 pre-filled disposable injection [PoM] £107.08 DT price = £107.08
Innohep 8,000units/0.4ml solution for injection pre-filled syringes | 6 pre-filled disposable injection [PoM] £28.56 | 10 pre-filled disposable injection [PoM] £47.60 DT price = £47.60
Innohep 40,000units/2ml solution for injection vials | 1 vial [PoM] £34.20 DT price = £34.20

Cardiovascular system

2

Innohep 16,000units/0.8ml solution for injection pre-filled syringes |
6 pre-filled disposable injection [PoM] £57.12 | 10 pre-filled
disposable injection [PoM] £95.20 DT price = £95.20
Innohep 12,000units/0.6ml solution for injection pre-filled syringes |
6 pre-filled disposable injection [PoM] £42.84 | 10 pre-filled
disposable injection [PoM] £71.40 DT price = £71.40
Innohep 14,000units/0.7ml solution for injection pre-filled syringes |
6 pre-filled disposable injection [PoM] £49.98 | 10 pre-filled
disposable injection [PoM] £83.30 DT price = £83.30
Innohep 10,000units/0.5ml solution for injection pre-filled syringes |
6 pre-filled disposable injection [PoM] £35.70 | 10 pre-filled
disposable injection [PoM] £59.50 DT price = £59.50

ANTITHROMBOTIC DRUGS > VITAMIN K ANTAGONISTS

Vitamin K antagonists

IMPORTANT SAFETY INFORMATION

MHRA/CHM ADVICE: DIRECT-ACTING ANTIVIRALS TO TREAT
CHRONIC HEPATITIS C: RISK OF INTERACTION WITH VITAMIN K
ANTAGONISTS AND CHANGES IN INR (JANUARY 2017)

A EU-wide review has identified that changes in liver
function, secondary to hepatitis C treatment with direct-
acting antivirals, may affect the efficacy of vitamin K
antagonists; the MHRA has advised that INR should be
monitored closely in patients receiving concomitant
treatment.

- **CONTRA-INDICATIONS** Avoid use within 48 hours
postpartum · haemorrhagic stroke · significant bleeding
- **CAUTIONS** Bacterial endocarditis (use only if warfarin
otherwise indicated) · conditions in which risk of bleeding
is increased · history of gastrointestinal bleeding · peptic
ulcer · postpartum (delay warfarin until risk of
haemorrhage is low—usually 5–7 days after delivery) ·
recent ischaemic stroke · recent surgery · uncontrolled
hypertension
- **SIDE-EFFECTS** Alopecia · diarrhoea · haemorrhage · hepatic
dysfunction · jaundice · nausea · pancreatitis · purpura ·
pyrexia · rash · skin necrosis (increased risk in patients with
protein C or protein S deficiency) · vomiting · 'purple toes'
- **CONCEPTION AND CONTRACEPTION** Women of child-
bearing age should be warned of the danger of
teratogenicity.
- **PREGNANCY** Should not be given in the first trimester of
pregnancy. Warfarin, acenocoumarol, and phenindione
cross the placenta with risk of congenital malformations,
and placental, fetal, or neonatal haemorrhage, especially
during the last few weeks of pregnancy and at delivery.
Therefore, if at all possible, they should be avoided in
pregnancy, especially in the first and third trimesters
(difficult decisions may have to be made, particularly in
women with prosthetic heart valves, atrial fibrillation, or
with a history of recurrent venous thrombosis or
pulmonary embolism). Stopping these drugs before the
sixth week of gestation may largely avoid the risk of fetal
abnormality.
- **MONITORING REQUIREMENTS**
  - The base-line prothrombin time should be determined but
the initial dose should not be delayed whilst awaiting the
result.
  - It is essential that the INR be determined daily or on
alternate days in early days of treatment, then at longer
intervals (depending on response), then up to every
12 weeks.
  - Change in patient's clinical condition, particularly
associated with liver disease, intercurrent illness, or drug
administration, necessitates more frequent testing.

- **PATIENT AND CARER ADVICE** Anticoagulant treatment
booklets should be issued to all patients or their carers;
these booklets include advice for patients on
anticoagulant treatment, an alert card to be carried by the
patient at all times, and a section for recording of INR
results and dosage information. In **England, Wales**, and
Northern Ireland, they are available for purchase from:
  3M Security Print and Systems Limited
  Gorse Street, Chadderton
  Oldham
  OL9 9QH
  Tel: 0845 610 1112
GP practices can obtain supplies through their Local Area
Team stores. NHS Trusts can order supplies from
www.nhsforms.co.uk or by emailing nhsforms@spsl.uk.com.
  In **Scotland**, treatment booklets and starter information
packs can be obtained by emailing
stockorders.DPPAS@apsgroup.co.uk or by fax on
(0131) 6299 967
  Electronic copies of the booklets and further advice are
also available at www.npsa.nhs.uk/nrls/alerts-and-directives/
alerts/anticoagulant.

[F above]

Warfarin sodium

10-Oct-2016

- **INDICATIONS AND DOSE**

**Treatment and prophylaxis of thrombotic episodes
(induction)**
▶ BY MOUTH

- Neonate (initiated under specialist supervision): Initially
200 micrograms/kg for 1 dose on day 1, then reduced to
100 micrograms/kg once daily for the following 3 days,
subsequent doses dependent on INR levels, induction
dose may need to be altered according to condition (e.g.
abnormal liver function tests, cardiac failure),
concomitant interacting drugs, and if baseline INR
above 1.3.

- Child: Initially 200 micrograms/kg (max. per dose
10 mg) for 1 dose on day 1, then reduced to
100 micrograms/kg once daily (max. per dose 5 mg) for
the following 3 days, subsequent doses adjusted
according to INR levels, induction dose may need to be
altered according to condition (e.g. abnormal liver
function tests, cardiac failure), concomitant interacting
drugs, and if baseline INR above 1.3

**Treatment and prophylaxis of thrombotic episodes
following induction dose (if INR still below 1.4)**
▶ BY MOUTH

- Neonate (under expert supervision): 200 micrograms/kg
once daily.

- Child: 200 micrograms/kg once daily (max. per dose
10 mg)

**Treatment and prophylaxis of thrombotic episodes
following induction dose (if INR above 3.0)**
▶ BY MOUTH

- Neonate (under expert supervision): 50 micrograms/kg
once daily.

- Child: 50 micrograms/kg once daily (max. per dose
2.5 mg)

**Treatment and prophylaxis of thrombotic episodes
following induction dose (if INR above 3.5)**
▶ BY MOUTH

- Neonate (under expert supervision): Dose to be omitted.

- Child: Dose to be omitted

Treatment and prophylaxis of thrombotic episodes (usual maintenance)
▸ BY MOUTH

▸ Neonate (under expert supervision): Maintenance 100–300 micrograms/kg once daily, doses up to 400 micrograms/kg once daily may be required especially if bottle fed, to be adjusted according to INR.

▸ Child: Maintenance 100–300 micrograms/kg once daily, doses up to 400 micrograms/kg once daily may be required especially if bottle fed, to be adjusted according to INR

● UNLICENSED USE Not licensed for use in children.

> **IMPORTANT SAFETY INFORMATION**
> MHRA/CHM ADVICE: WARFARIN: REPORTS OF CALCIPHYLAXIS (JULY 2016)
> An EU-wide review has concluded that on rare occasions, warfarin use may lead to calciphylaxis—patients should be advised to consult their doctor if they develop a painful skin rash; if calciphylaxis is diagnosed, appropriate treatment should be started and consideration should be given to stopping treatment with warfarin. The MHRA has advised that calciphylaxis is most commonly observed in patients with known risk factors such as end-stage renal disease, however cases have also been reported in patients with normal renal function.

● INTERACTIONS → Appendix 1: coumarins

● SIDE-EFFECTS Calciphylaxis

● PREGNANCY Babies of mothers taking warfarin at the time of delivery need to be offered immediate prophylaxis with intramuscular phytomenadione (vitamin K₁).

● BREAST FEEDING Not present in milk in significant amounts and appears safe. Risk of haemorrhage which is increased by vitamin K deficiency.

● HEPATIC IMPAIRMENT Avoid in severe impairment, especially if prothrombin time is already prolonged.

● RENAL IMPAIRMENT Use with caution in mild to moderate impairment. In severe renal impairment, monitor INR more frequently.

● PRESCRIBING AND DISPENSING INFORMATION
Dietary differences Infant formula is supplemented with vitamin K, which makes formula-fed infants resistant to warfarin; they may therefore need higher doses. In contrast breast milk contains low concentrations of vitamin K making breast-fed infants more sensitive to warfarin.

● PATIENT AND CARER ADVICE Anticoagulant card to be provided.
Medicines for Children leaflet: Warfarin for the treatment and prevention of thrombosis www.medicinesforchildren.org.uk/warfarin-treatment-and-prevention-thrombosis

● MEDICINAL FORMS
There can be variation in the licensing of different medicines containing the same drug. Forms available from special-order manufacturers include: oral suspension, oral solution

Oral suspension
CAUTIONARY AND ADVISORY LABELS 10
▸ Warfarin sodium (Non-proprietary)
Warfarin sodium 1 mg per 1 ml Warfarin 1mg/ml oral suspension sugar free sugar-free | 150 ml [PoM] £108.00 DT price = £108.00

Tablet
CAUTIONARY AND ADVISORY LABELS 10
▸ Warfarin sodium (Non-proprietary)
Warfarin sodium 500 microgram Warfarin 500microgram tablets | 28 tablet [PoM] £1.70 DT price = £1.52
Warfarin sodium 1 mg Warfarin 1mg tablets | 28 tablet [PoM] £1.16 DT price = £0.71 | 500 tablet [PoM] no price available

Warfarin sodium 3 mg Warfarin 3mg tablets | 28 tablet [PoM] £1.20 DT price = £0.74 | 500 tablet [PoM] £13.21
Warfarin sodium 4 mg Coumadin 4mg tablets | 100 tablet [PoM] no price available
Warfarin sodium 5 mg Warfarin 5mg tablets | 28 tablet [PoM] £1.29 DT price = £0.78 | 500 tablet [PoM] no price available

4 Blood pressure conditions
4.1 Hypertension

Hypertension

Overview
Hypertension in children and adolescents can have a substantial effect on long-term health. Possible causes of hypertension (e.g. congenital heart disease, renal disease and endocrine disorders) and the presence of any complications (e.g. left ventricular hypertrophy) should be established. Treatment should take account of contributory factors and any factors that increase the risk of cardiovascular complications.

Serious hypertension is rare in *neonates* but it can present with signs of congestive heart failure; the cause is often renal and can follow embolic arterial damage.

Children (or their parents or carers) should be given advice on lifestyle changes to reduce blood pressure or cardiovascular risk; these include weight reduction (in obese children), reduction of dietary salt, reduction of total and saturated fat, increasing exercise, increasing fruit and vegetable intake, and not smoking.

Indications for antihypertensive therapy in children include symptomatic hypertension, secondary hypertension, hypertensive target-organ damage, diabetes mellitus, persistent hypertension despite lifestyle measures, and pulmonary hypertension. The effect of antihypertensive treatment on growth and development is not known; treatment should be started only if benefits are clear.

Antihypertensive therapy should be initiated with a single drug at the lowest recommended dose; the dose can be increased until the target blood pressure is achieved. Once the highest recommended dose is reached, or sooner if the patient begins to experience side-effects, a second drug may be added if blood pressure is not controlled. If more than one drug is required, these should be given as separate products to allow dose adjustment of individual drugs, but fixed-dose combination products may be useful in adolescents if compliance is a problem.

Acceptable drug classes for use in children with hypertension include **ACE inhibitors**, **alpha-blockers**, **beta-blockers**, **calcium-channel blockers**, and **thiazide diuretics**. There is limited information on the use of **angiotensin-II receptor antagonists** in children. Diuretics and beta-blockers have a long history of safety and efficacy in children. The newer classes of antihypertensive drugs, including ACE inhibitors and calcium-channel blockers have been shown to be safe and effective in short-term studies in children. Refractory hypertension may require additional treatment with agents such as minoxidil p. 114 or clonidine hydrochloride p. 99.

Other measures to reduce cardiovascular risk
Aspirin p. 89 may be used to reduce the risk of cardiovascular events; however, concerns about an increased risk of bleeding and Reye's syndrome need to be considered.

A **statin** can be of benefit in older children who have a high risk of cardiovascular disease and have hypercholesterolaemia.

Cardiovascular system

2

Hypertension in diabetes

Hypertension can occur in type 2 diabetes and treatment prevents both macrovascular and microvascular complications. ACE inhibitors may be considered in children with diabetes and microalbuminaemia or proteinuric renal disease. Beta-blockers are best avoided in children with, or at a high risk of developing, diabetes, especially when combined with a thiazide diuretic.

Hypertension in renal disease

ACE inhibitors may be considered in children with micro-albuminuria or proteinuric renal disease. High doses of loop diuretics may be required. Specific cautions apply to the use of ACE inhibitors in renal impairment, but ACE inhibitors may be effective. Dihydropyridine calcium-channel blockers may be added.

Hypertension in pregnancy

High blood pressure in pregnancy may usually be due to pre-existing essential hypertension or to pre-eclampsia. Methyldopa is safe in pregnancy. Beta-blockers are effective and safe in the third trimester. Modified-release preparations of nifedipine p. 106 [unlicensed] are also used for hypertension in pregnancy. Intravenous administration of labetalol hydrochloride p. 101 can be used to control hypertensive crises; alternatively hydralazine hydrochloride p. 113 can be given by the intravenous route.

Hypertensive emergencies

Hypertensive emergencies in children may be accompanied by signs of hypertensive encephalopathy, including seizures. Controlled reduction in blood pressure over 72–96 hours is essential; rapid reduction can reduce perfusion leading to organ damage. Treatment should be initiated with intravenous drugs; once blood pressure is controlled, oral therapy can be started. It may be necessary to infuse fluids particularly during the first 12 hours to expand plasma volume should the blood pressure drop too rapidly.

Controlled reduction of blood pressure is achieved by intravenous administration of labetalol hydrochloride or sodium nitroprusside p. 114. Esmolol hydrochloride p. 103 is useful for short-term use and has a short duration of action. Nicardipine hydrochloride p. 105 can be administered as a continuous intravenous infusion for life-threatening hypertension in paediatric intensive care settings. In less severe cases, nifedipine capsules can be used.

Other antihypertensive drugs which can be given intravenously include hydralazine hydrochloride and clonidine hydrochloride.

Hypertension in acute nephritis occurs as a result of sodium and water retention; it should be treated with sodium and fluid restriction, and with furosemide p. 136; antihypertensive drugs may be added if necessary.

Also see advice on short-term management of hypertensive episodes in phaeochromocytoma.

Phaeochromocytoma

Long-term management of phaeochromocytoma involves surgery. However, surgery should not take place until there is adequate blockade of both alpha- and beta-adrenoceptors. Alpha-blockers are used in the short-term management of hypertensive episodes in phaeochromocytoma. Once alpha blockade is established, tachycardia can be controlled by the cautious addition of a beta-blocker; a cardioselective beta-blocker is preferred. There is no nationwide consensus on the optimal drug regimen or doses used for the management of phaeochromocytoma.

Phenoxybenzamine hydrochloride p. 114, a powerful alpha-blocker, is effective in the management of phaeochromocytoma but it has many side-effects.

Pulmonary hypertension

Only pulmonary *arterial* hypertension is currently suitable for drug treatment. Pulmonary arterial hypertension includes persistent pulmonary hypertension of the newborn, idiopathic pulmonary arterial hypertension in children, and pulmonary hypertension related to congenital heart disease and cardiac surgery.

Some types of pulmonary hypertension are treated with vasodilator antihypertensive therapy and oxygen. Diuretics may also have a role in children with right-sided heart failure.

Initial treatment of *persistent pulmonary hypertension of the newborn* involves the administration of **nitric oxide**; epoprostenol p. 115 can be used until nitric oxide is available. Oral sildenafil p. 117 may be helpful in less severe cases. Epoprostenol and sildenafil can cause profound systemic hypotension. In rare circumstances either tolazoline p. 117 or magnesium sulfate p. 571 can be given by intravenous infusion when nitric oxide and epoprostenol have failed.

Treatment of *idiopathic pulmonary arterial hypertension* is determined by acute vasodilator testing; drugs used for treatment include calcium-channel blockers (usually nifedipine), long-term intravenous epoprostenol, nebulised iloprost p. 116, bosentan p. 116, or sildenafil. Anticoagulation (usually with warfarin sodium p. 94) may also be required to prevent secondary thrombosis.

Inhaled nitric oxide is a potent and selective pulmonary vasodilator. It acts on cyclic guanosine monophosphate (cGMP) resulting in smooth muscle relaxation. Inhaled nitric oxide is used in the treatment of persistent pulmonary hypertension of the newborn, and may also be useful in other forms of arterial pulmonary hypertension. Dependency can occur with high doses and prolonged use; to avoid rebound pulmonary hypertension the drug should be withdrawn gradually, often with the aid of sildenafil p. 117.

Excess nitric oxide can cause methaemoglobinaemia; therefore, methaemoglobin concentration should be measured regularly, particularly in neonates.

Nitric oxide increases the risk of haemorrhage by inhibiting platelet aggregation, but it does not usually cause bleeding.

Epoprostenol (prostacyclin) p. 115 is a prostaglandin and a potent vasodilator. It is used in the treatment of persistent pulmonary hypertension of the newborn, idiopathic pulmonary arterial hypertension, and in the acute phase following cardiac surgery. It is given by continuous 24-hour intravenous infusion.

Epoprostenol is a powerful inhibitor of platelet aggregation and there is a possible risk of haemorrhage. It is sometimes used as an antiplatelet in renal dialysis when heparins are unsuitable or contra-indicated. It can also cause serious systemic hypotension and, if withdrawn suddenly, can cause pulmonary hypertensive crisis.

Children on prolonged treatment can become tolerant to epoprostenol, and therefore require an increase in dose.

Iloprost p. 116 is a synthetic analogue of epoprostenol and is efficacious when nebulised in adults with pulmonary arterial hypertension, but experience in children is limited. It is more stable than epoprostenol and has a longer half-life.

Bosentan p. 116 is a dual endothelin receptor antagonist used orally in the treatment of pulmonary arterial hypertension. The concentration of endothelin, a potent vasoconstrictor, is raised in sustained pulmonary hypertension.

Sildenafil, a vasodilator developed for the treatment of erectile dysfunction, is also used for pulmonary arterial hypertension. It is used either alone or as an adjunct to other drugs.

Sildenafil is a selective phosphodiesterase type-5 inhibitor. Inhibition of this enzyme in the lungs enhances the vasodilatory effects of nitric oxide and promotes relaxation of vascular smooth muscle.

Sildenafil has also been used in pulmonary hypertension for weaning children off inhaled nitric oxide following cardiac surgery, and less successfully in idiopathic pulmonary arterial hypertension.

Tolazoline p. 117 is now rarely used to correct pulmonary artery vasospasm in pulmonary hypertension of the newborn as better alternatives are available. Tolazoline is an alpha-blocker and produces both pulmonary and systemic vasodilation.

Antihypertensive drugs

Vasodilator antihypertensive drugs

Vasodilators have a potent hypotensive effect, especially when used in combination with a beta-blocker and a thiazide. **Important:** see Hypertension (hypertensive emergencies) for a warning on the hazards of a very rapid fall in blood pressure.

Hydralazine hydrochloride p. 113 is given by mouth as an adjunct to other antihypertensives for the treatment of resistant hypertension but is rarely used; when used alone it causes tachycardia and fluid retention.

Sodium nitroprusside p. 114 is given by intravenous infusion to control severe hypertensive crisis when parenteral treatment is necessary. At low doses it reduces systemic vascular resistance and increases cardiac output; at high doses it can produce profound systemic hypotension—continuous blood pressure monitoring is therefore essential. Sodium nitroprusside may also be used to control paradoxical hypertension after surgery for coarctation of the aorta.

Minoxidil p. 114 should be reserved for the treatment of severe hypertension resistant to other drugs. Vasodilatation is accompanied by increased cardiac output and tachycardia and children develop fluid retention. For this reason the addition of a beta-blocker and a diuretic (usually furosemide p. 136, in high dosage) are mandatory. Hypertrichosis is troublesome and renders this drug unsuitable for females.

Prazosin p. 98 and doxazosin p. 470 have alpha-blocking and vasodilator properties.

Centrally acting antihypertensive drugs

Methyldopa, a centrally acting antihypertensive, is of little value in the management of refractory sustained hypertension in infants and children. On prolonged use it is associated with fluid retention (which may be alleviated by concomitant use of diuretics).

Methyldopa is also effective for the management of hypertension in pregnancy.

Clonidine hydrochloride p. 99 is also a centrally acting antihypertensive but has the disadvantage that sudden withdrawal may cause a hypertensive crisis. Clonidine hydrochloride is also used under specialist supervision for pain management, sedation, and opioid withdrawal, attention deficit hyperactivity disorder, and Tourette syndrome.

Adrenergic neurone blocking drugs

Adrenergic neurone blocking drugs prevent the release of noradrenaline from postganglionic adrenergic neurones. These drugs do not control supine blood pressure and may cause postural hypotension. For this reason they have largely fallen from use in adults and are rarely used in children.

Alpha-adrenoceptor blocking drugs

Doxazosin and prazosin have post-synaptic alpha-blocking and vasodilator properties and rarely cause tachycardia.

They can, however, reduce blood pressure rapidly after the first dose and should be introduced with caution.

Alpha-blockers can be used with other antihypertensive drugs in the treatment of resistant hypertension.

Drugs affecting the renin-angiotensin system

Angiotensin-converting enzyme inhibitors

Angiotensin-converting enzyme inhibitors (ACE inhibitors) inhibit the conversion of angiotensin I to angiotensin II. The main indications of ACE inhibitors in children are shown below. In infants and young children, captopril p. 109 is often considered first.

Initiation under specialist supervision

Treatment with ACE inhibitors should be initiated under specialist supervision and with careful clinical monitoring in children.

Heart failure

ACE inhibitors have a valuable role in all grades of heart failure, usually combined with a loop diuretic. Potassium supplements and potassium-sparing diuretics should be discontinued before introducing an ACE inhibitor because of the risk of hyperkalaemia. Profound first-dose hypotension can occur when ACE inhibitors are introduced to children with heart failure who are already taking a high dose of a loop diuretic. Temporary withdrawal of the loop diuretic reduces the risk, but can cause severe rebound pulmonary oedema.

Hypertension

ACE inhibitors may be considered for hypertension when thiazides and beta-blockers are contra-indicated, not tolerated, or fail to control blood pressure; they may be considered for hypertension in children with type 1 diabetes with nephropathy. ACE inhibitors can reduce blood pressure very rapidly in some patients particularly in those receiving diuretic therapy.

Diabetic nephropathy

ACE inhibitors also have a role in the management of diabetic nephropathy.

Renal effects

Renal function and electrolytes should be checked before starting ACE inhibitors (or increasing the dose) and monitored during treatment (more frequently if features mentioned below are present). Hyperkalaemia and other side-effects of ACE inhibitors are more common in children with impaired renal function and the dose may need to be reduced.

Concomitant treatment with NSAIDs increases the risk of renal damage, and potassium-sparing diuretics (or potassium-containing salt substitutes) increase the risk of hyperkalaemia.

In children with severe bilateral renal artery stenosis (or severe stenosis of the artery supplying a single functioning kidney), ACE inhibitors reduce or abolish glomerular filtration and are likely to cause severe and progressive renal failure. They are therefore contra-indicated in children known to have these forms of critical renovascular disease.

ACE inhibitor treatment is unlikely to have an adverse effect on overall renal function in children with severe unilateral renal artery stenosis and a normal contralateral kidney, but glomerular filtration is likely to be reduced (or even abolished) in the affected kidney and the long-term consequences are unknown.

ACE inhibitors are therefore best avoided in those with known or suspected renovascular disease, unless the blood pressure cannot be controlled by other drugs. If they are used in these circumstances renal function needs to be monitored.

ACE inhibitors should also be used with particular caution in children who may have undiagnosed and clinically silent renovascular disease. ACE inhibitors are useful for the management of hypertension and proteinuria in children with nephritis. They are thought to have a beneficial effect by reducing intra-glomerular hypertension and protecting the glomerular capillaries and membrane.

ACE inhibitors in combination with other drugs
Concomitant diuretics
ACE inhibitors can cause a very rapid fall in blood pressure in volume-depleted children; treatment should therefore be initiated with very low doses. In some children the diuretic dose may need to be reduced or the diuretic discontinued at least 24 hours beforehand (may not be possible in heart failure—risk of pulmonary oedema). If high-dose diuretic therapy cannot be stopped, close observation is recommended after administration of the first dose of ACE inhibitor, for at least 2 hours or until the blood pressure has stabilised.

Angiotensin-II receptor antagonists

Candesartan cilexetil p. 112, losartan potassium p. 112 and valsartan p. 113 are specific angiotensin-II receptor antagonists with many properties similar to those of the ACE inhibitors. However, unlike ACE inhibitors, they do not inhibit the breakdown of bradykinin and other kinins, and thus are less likely to cause the persistent dry cough which can complicate ACE inhibitor therapy. They are therefore a useful alternative for children who have to discontinue an ACE inhibitor because of persistent cough.

Candesartan cilexetil, losartan potassium or valsartan can be used as an alternative to an ACE inhibitor in the management of hypertension.

Renal effects
Angiotensin-II receptor antagonists should be used with caution in renal artery stenosis (see also Renal effects under ACE Inhibitors, above).

Neonates

The neonatal response to treatment with ACE inhibitors is very variable, and some neonates develop profound hypotension with even small doses; a test-dose should be used initially and increased cautiously. Adverse effects such as apnoea, seizures, renal failure, and severe unpredictable hypotension are very common in the first month of life and it is therefore recommended that ACE inhibitors are avoided whenever possible, particularly in preterm neonates.

> **Other drugs used for Hypertension** Chlortalidone, p. 138 · Diazoxide, p. 445

ALPHA-ADRENOCEPTOR BLOCKERS

Prazosin

- **INDICATIONS AND DOSE**

Hypertension
▸ BY MOUTH
▸ Child 1 month–11 years: Initially 10–15 micrograms/kg 2–4 times a day, initial dose to be taken at bedtime, then increased to 500 micrograms/kg daily in divided doses, dose to be increased gradually; maximum 20 mg per day
▸ Child 12–17 years: Initially 500 micrograms 2–3 times a day for 3-7 days, initial dose to be taken at bedtime, then increased to 1 mg 2–3 times a day for a further 3–7 days, then increased if necessary up to 20 mg daily in divided doses, dose should be increased gradually

Congestive heart failure (rarely used)
▸ BY MOUTH
▸ Child 1 month–11 years: 5 micrograms/kg twice daily, initial dose to be taken at bedtime, then increased to 100 micrograms/kg daily in divided doses, doses should be increased gradually
▸ Child 12–17 years: 500 micrograms 2–4 times a day, initial dose to be taken at bedtime, then increased to 4 mg daily in divided doses; maintenance 4–20 mg daily in divided doses

- **UNLICENSED USE** Not licensed for use in children under 12 years.

- **CONTRA-INDICATIONS** History of micturition syncope · history of postural hypotension · not recommended for congestive heart failure due to mechanical obstruction (e.g. aortic stenosis)

- **CAUTIONS** Cataract surgery (risk of intra-operative floppy iris syndrome) · first dose hypotension

- **INTERACTIONS** → Appendix 1: alpha blockers

- **SIDE-EFFECTS**
▸ **Common or very common** Blurred vision · depression · dizziness · drowsiness · dry mouth · dyspnoea · gastro-intestinal disturbances · headache · nasal congestion · nervousness · oedema · palpitations · syncope · urinary frequency · vertigo · weakness
▸ **Uncommon** Allergic reactions · arthralgia · epistaxis · eye disorders · impotence · insomnia · paraesthesia · pruritus · rash · sweating · tachycardia · tinnitus · urticaria
▸ **Rare** Alopecia · bradycardia · flushing · gynaecomastia · hallucinations · pancreatitis · priapism · urinary incontinence · vasculitis · worsening of narcolepsy
▸ **Frequency not known** Angioedema · asthenia · hypotension · postural hypotension

- **PREGNANCY** No evidence of teratogenicity; manufacturers advise use only when potential benefit outweighs risk.

- **BREAST FEEDING** Present in milk, amount probably too small to be harmful; manufacturer advises use with caution.

- **HEPATIC IMPAIRMENT** Start with low doses and adjust according to response.

- **RENAL IMPAIRMENT** Start with low doses in moderate to severe impairment; increase with caution.

- **DIRECTIONS FOR ADMINISTRATION** For administration *by mouth*, tablets may be dispersed in water.

- **PATIENT AND CARER ADVICE**
First dose effect First dose may cause collapse due to hypotensive effect (therefore should be taken on retiring to bed).

Driving and skilled tasks
May affect performance of skilled tasks e.g. driving.

- **MEDICINAL FORMS**
There can be variation in the licensing of different medicines containing the same drug. Forms available from special-order manufacturers include: tablet, oral suspension, oral solution
Tablet
▸ Prazosin (Non-proprietary)
 Prazosin (as Prazosin hydrochloride) 2 mg Minipress 2mg tablets | 100 tablet PoM no price available
 Prazosin (as Prazosin hydrochloride) 5 mg Minipress 5mg tablets | 100 tablet PoM no price available
▸ Hypovase (Pfizer Ltd)
 Prazosin (as Prazosin hydrochloride) 500 microgram Hypovase 500microgram tablets | 60 tablet PoM £2.69 DT price = £2.69
 Prazosin (as Prazosin hydrochloride) 1 mg Hypovase 1mg tablets | 60 tablet PoM £3.46 DT price = £3.46

ANTIHYPERTENSIVES, CENTRALLY ACTING

Clonidine hydrochloride

- **INDICATIONS AND DOSE**

Severe hypertension
- ▸ BY MOUTH
  - ▸ Child 2–17 years: Initially 0.5–1 microgram/kg 3 times a day, then increased if necessary up to 25 micrograms/kg daily in divided doses, increase dose gradually; maximum 1.2 mg per day
- ▸ BY SLOW INTRAVENOUS INJECTION
  - ▸ Child 2–17 years: 2–6 micrograms/kg (max. per dose 300 micrograms) for 1 dose

- **UNLICENSED USE** Not licensed for use in children.
- **CONTRA-INDICATIONS** Severe bradyarrhythmia secondary to second- or third-degree AV block or sick sinus syndrome
- **CAUTIONS** Cerebrovascular disease · constipation · heart failure · history of depression · mild to moderate bradyarrhythmia · polyneuropathy · Raynaud's syndrome or other occlusive peripheral vascular disease
- **INTERACTIONS** → Appendix 1: clonidine
- **SIDE-EFFECTS**
  - ▸ **Common or very common** Constipation · depression · dizziness · drowsiness · dry mouth · headache · malaise · nausea · postural hypotension · salivary gland pain · sexual dysfunction · sleep disturbances · vomiting
  - ▸ **Uncommon** Bradycardia · delusion · hallucination · paraesthesia · pruritus · rash · Raynaud's syndrome · urticaria
  - ▸ **Rare** Alopecia · AV block · colonic pseudo-obstruction · decreased lacrimation · gynaecomastia · nasal dryness
  - ▸ **Frequency not known** Bradyarrhythmia · confusion · fluid retention · hepatitis · impaired visual accommodation
- **PREGNANCY** May lower fetal heart rate. Avoid oral use unless potential benefit outweighs risk. Avoid using injection.
- **BREAST FEEDING** Avoid—present in milk.
- **RENAL IMPAIRMENT** Use with caution.
- **TREATMENT CESSATION** Must be withdrawn gradually to avoid hypertensive crisis.
- **DIRECTIONS FOR ADMINISTRATION**
  - ▸ With intravenous use For *intravenous injection*, give over 10–15 minutes; compatible with Sodium Chloride 0.9% or Glucose 5%.
  - ▸ With oral use For administration *by mouth*, tablets may be crushed and dissolved in water.
- **PATIENT AND CARER ADVICE**
  Medicines for Children leaflet: Clonidine for Tourette's syndrome, ADHD and sleep-onset disorder www.medicinesforchildren.org.uk/clonidine-tourettes-syndrome-adhd-and-sleep-onset-disorder

  Driving and skilled tasks
  Drowsiness may affect performance of skilled tasks (e.g. driving); effects of alcohol may be enhanced.
- **LESS SUITABLE FOR PRESCRIBING** Clonidine is less suitable for prescribing.

- **MEDICINAL FORMS**
  There can be variation in the licensing of different medicines containing the same drug. Forms available from special-order manufacturers include: oral suspension, oral solution, solution for injection

  Tablet
  CAUTIONARY AND ADVISORY LABELS 3, 8
  - ▸ **Clonidine hydrochloride** (Non-proprietary)
    Clonidine hydrochloride 25 microgram Clonidine 25microgram tablets | 112 tablet PoM £9.15 DT price = £5.08

  - ▸ **Catapres** (Boehringer Ingelheim Ltd)
    Clonidine hydrochloride 100 microgram Catapres 100microgram tablets | 100 tablet PoM £8.04 DT price = £8.04
  - ▸ **Dixarit** (Boehringer Ingelheim Ltd)
    Clonidine hydrochloride 25 microgram Dixarit 25microgram tablets | 112 tablet PoM £6.99 DT price = £5.08

  Solution for injection
  - ▸ **Catapres** (Boehringer Ingelheim Ltd)
    Clonidine hydrochloride 150 microgram per 1 ml Catapres 150micrograms/1ml solution for injection ampoules | 5 ampoule PoM £2.09

BETA-ADRENOCEPTOR BLOCKERS

Beta-adrenoceptor blocking drugs

Overview

Beta-adrenoceptor blocking drugs (beta-blockers) block the beta-adrenoceptors in the heart, peripheral vasculature, bronchi, pancreas, and liver.

Many beta-blockers are available but experience in children is limited to the use of only a few.

Differences between beta-blockers may affect choice. The water-soluble beta-blockers, atenolol p. 103 and sotalol hydrochloride p. 78, are less likely to enter the brain and may therefore cause less sleep disturbance and nightmares. Water-soluble beta-blockers are excreted by the kidneys and dosage reduction is often necessary in renal impairment.

Some beta-blockers, such as atenolol, have an intrinsically longer duration of action and need to be given only once daily. Carvedilol p. 122 and labetalol hydrochloride p. 101 are beta-blockers which have, in addition, an arteriolar vasodilating action and thus lower peripheral resistance. Although carvedilol and labetalol hydrochloride possess both alpha- and beta-blocking properties, these drugs have no important advantages over other beta-blockers in the treatment of hypertension.

Beta-blockers slow the heart and can depress the myocardium; they are contra-indicated in children with second- or third-degree heart block.

Beta-blockers can precipitate asthma and should usually be avoided in children with a history of asthma or bronchospasm. If there is no alternative, a child with well-controlled asthma can be treated for a co-existing condition (e.g. arrhythmia) with a cardioselective beta-blocker, which should be initiated with caution at a low dose by a specialist and the child monitored closely for adverse effects. Atenolol and metoprolol tartrate p. 103 have less effect on the beta$_2$ (bronchial) receptors and are, therefore, relatively *cardioselective*, but they are not *cardiospecific*; they have a lesser effect on airways resistance but are not free of this side-effect.

Beta-blockers are also associated with fatigue, coldness of the extremities, and sleep disturbances with nightmares (may be less common with the water-soluble beta-blockers).

Beta-blockers can affect carbohydrate metabolism causing hypoglycaemia or hyperglycaemia in children with or without diabetes; they can also interfere with metabolic and autonomic responses to hypoglycaemia thereby masking symptoms such as tachycardia. However, beta-blockers are not contra-indicated in diabetes, although the cardioselective beta-blockers (e.g. atenolol and metoprolol tartrate) may be preferred. Beta-blockers should be avoided altogether in those with frequent episodes of hypoglycaemia.

Hypertension

Beta-blockers are effective for reducing blood pressure, but their mode of action is not understood; they reduce cardiac output, alter baroceptor reflex sensitivity, and block peripheral adrenoceptors. Some beta-blockers depress plasma renin secretion. It is possible that a central effect may also partly explain their mode of action. Blood pressure

2

Cardiovascular system

Cardiovascular system

2

can usually be controlled with relatively few side-effects. In general the dose of beta-blocker does not have to be high.

Labetalol hydrochloride may be given intravenously for *hypertensive emergencies* in children; however, care is needed to avoid dangerous hypotension or beta-blockade, particularly in neonates. Esmolol hydrochloride p. 103 is also used intravenously for the treatment of hypertension particularly in the peri-operative period.

Beta-blockers can be used to control the pulse rate in children with *phaeochromocytoma*. However, they should never be used alone as beta-blockade without concurrent alpha-blockade may lead to a hypertensive crisis; phenoxybenzamine hydrochloride p. 114 should always be used together with the beta-blocker.

Arrhythmias

In arrhythmias, beta-blockers act principally by attenuating the effects of the sympathetic system on automaticity and conductivity within the heart. They can be used alone or in conjunction with digoxin p. 79 to control the ventricular rate in *atrial fibrillation*. Beta-blockers are also useful in the management of *supraventricular tachycardias* and *ventricular tachycardias* particularly to prevent recurrence of the tachycardia.

Esmolol hydrochloride is a relatively cardioselective beta-blocker with a very short duration of action, used intravenously for the short-term treatment of supraventricular arrhythmias and sinus tachycardia, particularly in the peri-operative period.

Sotalol hydrochloride is a non-cardioselective beta-blocker with additional class III anti-arrhythmic activity. Atenolol and sotalol hydrochloride suppress ventricular ectopic beats and non-sustained ventricular tachycardia. However, the pro-arrhythmic effects of sotalol hydrochloride, particularly in children with sick sinus syndrome, may prolong the QT interval and induce torsade de pointes.

Heart failure

Beta-blockers may produce benefit in heart failure by blocking sympathetic activity and the addition of a beta-blocker such as carvedilol to other treatment for heart failure may be beneficial. Treatment should be initiated by those experienced in the management of heart failure.

Thyrotoxicosis

Beta-blockers are used in the management of *thyrotoxicosis* including neonatal thyrotoxicosis; propranolol hydrochloride p. 101 can reverse clinical symptoms within 4 days. Beta-blockers are also used for the pre-operative preparation for thyroidectomy; the thyroid gland is rendered less vascular, thus facilitating surgery.

Other uses

In tetralogy of Fallot, esmolol hydrochloride or propranolol hydrochloride may be given intravenously in the initial management of *cyanotic spells*; propranolol hydrochloride is given by mouth for preventing cyanotic spells. If a severe cyanotic spell in a child with congenital heart disease persists despite optimal use of 100% oxygen, propranolol hydrochloride is given by intravenous infusion. If cyanosis is still present after 10 minutes, sodium bicarbonate p. 558 intravenous infusion is given in a dose to correct acidosis (or dose calculated according to arterial blood gas results); sodium bicarbonate 4.2% intravenous infusion is appropriate for a child under 1 year and sodium bicarbonate 8.4% intravenous infusion in children over 1 year. If blood-glucose concentration is less than 3 mmol/litre, glucose 10% intravenous infusion is given, followed by intravenous or intramuscular injection of morphine p. 271.

Beta-blockers are also used in the *prophylaxis of migraine*. Betaxolol p. 653, carteolol hydrochloride p. 654, levobunolol hydrochloride p. 654, and timolol maleate p. 654 are used topically in *glaucoma*.

Beta-adrenoceptor blockers (systemic)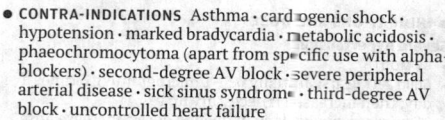

- **CONTRA-INDICATIONS** Asthma · cardiogenic shock · hypotension · marked bradycardia · metabolic acidosis · phaeochromocytoma (apart from specific use with alpha-blockers) · second-degree AV block · severe peripheral arterial disease · sick sinus syndrome · third-degree AV block · uncontrolled heart failure

  CONTRA-INDICATIONS, FURTHER INFORMATION
  ▸ Bronchospasm Beta-blockers, including those considered to be cardioselective, should usually be avoided in patients with a history of asthma, bronchospasm or a history of obstructive airways disease. However, when there is no alternative, a cardioselective beta-blocker can be given to these patients with caution and under specialist supervision. In such cases the risk of inducing bronchospasm should be appreciated and appropriate precautions taken.

- **CAUTIONS** Diabetes · first-degree AV block · history of obstructive airways disease (introduce cautiously) · myasthenia gravis · portal hypertension (risk of deterioration in liver function) · psoriasis · symptoms of thyrotoxicosis may be masked

- **SIDE-EFFECTS**
  ▸ **Rare** Dry eyes (reversible on withdrawal) · rashes (reversible on withdrawal)
  ▸ **Frequency not known** Alopecia · bradycardia · bronchospasm · coldness of the extremities · conduction disorders · dizziness · dyspnoea · exacerbation of intermittent claudication · exacerbation of psoriasis · exacerbation of Raynaud's phenomenon · fatigue · gastro-intestinal disturbances · headache · heart failure · hyperglycaemia (in patients with or without diabetes) · hypoglycaemia (in patients with or without diabetes) · hypotension · paraesthesia · peripheral vasoconstriction · psychoses · purpura · sexual dysfunction · sleep disturbances (with nightmares) · symptoms of hypoglycaemia masked · thrombocytopenia · vertigo · visual disturbances

  SIDE-EFFECTS, FURTHER INFORMATION
  ▸ Bradycardia With administration by intravenous injection, excessive bradycardia can occur and may be countered with **intravenous injection** of atropine sulfate.

  Overdose
  Therapeutic overdosages with beta-blockers may cause lightheadedness, dizziness, and possibly syncope as a result of bradycardia and hypotension; heart failure may be precipitated or exacerbated. For details on the management of poisoning, see Beta-blockers, under Emergency treatment of poisoning p. 803.

- **ALLERGY AND CROSS-SENSITIVITY** Caution is advised in patients with a history of hypersensitivity—may increase sensitivity to allergens and result in more serious hypersensitivity response. Furthermore beta-adrenoceptor blockers may reduce response to adrenaline (epinephrine).

- **PREGNANCY** Beta-blockers may cause intra-uterine growth restriction, neonatal hypoglycaemia, and bradycardia; the risk is greater in severe hypertension.

- **BREAST FEEDING** With systemic use in the mother, infants should be monitored as there is a risk of possible toxicity due to beta-blockade. However, the amount of most beta-blockers present in milk is too small to affect infants.

- **MONITORING REQUIREMENTS** Monitor lung function (in patients with a history of obstructive airway disease).

- **TREATMENT CESSATION** Avoid abrupt withdrawal.

BETA-ADRENOCEPTOR BLOCKERS 〉
ALPHA- AND BETA-ADRENOCEPTOR BLOCKERS

F 100

Labetalol hydrochloride

- **INDICATIONS AND DOSE**
Hypertensive emergencies
▸ BY INTRAVENOUS INFUSION

- **Neonate:** Initially 0.5 mg/kg/hour (max. per dose 4 mg/kg/hour), dose to be adjusted according to response at intervals of at least 15 minutes.

- **Child 1 month–11 years:** Initially 0.5–1 mg/kg/hour (max. per dose 3 mg/kg/hour), dose to be adjusted according to response at intervals of at least 15 minutes

- **Child 12–17 years:** Initially 30–120 mg/hour, dose to be adjusted according to response at intervals of at least 15 minutes

Hypertension
▸ BY MOUTH

- **Child 1 month–11 years:** 1–2 mg/kg 3–4 times a day
- **Child 12–17 years:** Initially 50–100 mg twice daily, dose to be increased if required at intervals of 3–14 days; usual dose 200–400 mg twice daily, higher doses to be given in 3–4 divided doses; maximum 2.4 g per day
▸ BY INTRAVENOUS INJECTION

- **Child 1 month–11 years:** 250–500 micrograms/kg (max. per dose 20 mg) for 1 dose
- **Child 12–17 years:** 50 mg, dose to be given over at least 1 minute, then 50 mg after 5 minutes if required; maximum 200 mg per course

- **UNLICENSED USE** Not licensed for use in children.

> **IMPORTANT SAFETY INFORMATION**
> ▸ With intravenous use
> Consult local guidelines. In hypertensive encephalopathy reduce blood pressure to normotensive level over 24–48 hours (more rapid reduction may lead to cerebral infarction, blindness, and death). If child fitting, reduce blood pressure rapidly, but not to normal levels.

- **CAUTIONS** Liver damage
- **INTERACTIONS** → Appendix 1: beta blockers (non-selective)
- **SIDE-EFFECTS**
▸ Rare Lichenoid rash
▸ **Frequency not known** Difficulty in micturition · epigastric pain · liver damage · nausea · postural hypotension · vomiting · weakness
- **PREGNANCY** The use of labetalol in maternal hypertension is not known to be harmful, except possibly in the first trimester. If labetalol is used close to delivery, infants should be monitored for signs of alpha-blockade (as well as beta blockade).
- **BREAST FEEDING** Infants should be monitored as there is a risk of possible toxicity due to alpha-blockade (in addition to beta-blockade).
- **HEPATIC IMPAIRMENT** Avoid—severe hepatocellular injury reported.
- **RENAL IMPAIRMENT** Dose reduction may be required.
- **MONITORING REQUIREMENTS**
▸ Liver damage Severe hepatocellular damage reported after both short-term and long-term treatment. Appropriate laboratory testing needed at first symptom of liver dysfunction and if laboratory evidence of damage (or if jaundice) labetalol should be stopped and not restarted.

- **EFFECT ON LABORATORY TESTS** Interferes with laboratory tests for catecholamines.
- **DIRECTIONS FOR ADMINISTRATION**
▸ With intravenous use For *intravenous infusion*, dilute to a concentration of 1 mg/mL in Glucose 5% or Sodium Chloride and Glucose 5%; if fluid restricted may be given undiluted, preferably through a central venous catheter. Avoid upright position during and for 3 hours after intravenous administration.
▸ With oral use For administration *by mouth*, injection may be given orally with squash or juice.
- **PATIENT AND CARER ADVICE**
Medicines for Children leaflet: Labetalol hydrochloride for hypertension www.medicinesforchildren.org.uk/labetalol-hydrochloride-for-hypertension

- **MEDICINAL FORMS**
There can be variation in the licensing of different medicines containing the same drug. Forms available from special-order manufacturers include: oral suspension, oral solution
Solution for injection
▸ **Labetalol hydrochloride** (Non-proprietary)
Labetalol hydrochloride 5 mg per 1 ml Labetalol 100mg/20ml solution for injection ampoules | 5 ampoule [PoM] £44.44–£53.33
Tablet
CAUTIONARY AND ADVISORY LABELS 8, 21
▸ **Labetalol hydrochloride** (Non-proprietary)
Labetalol hydrochloride 100 mg Labetalol 100mg tablets | 56 tablet [PoM] £7.21 DT price = £5.71
Labetalol hydrochloride 200 mg Labetalol 200mg tablets | 56 tablet [PoM] £9.97 DT price = £8.77
Labetalol hydrochloride 400 mg Labetalol 400mg tablets | 56 tablet [PoM] £23.14 DT price = £23.14
▸ **Trandate** (Focus Pharmaceuticals Ltd)
Labetalol hydrochloride 50 mg Trandate 50mg tablets | 56 tablet [PoM] £3.79 DT price = £3.79
Labetalol hydrochloride 100 mg Trandate 100mg tablets | 56 tablet [PoM] £4.64 DT price = £5.71 | 250 tablet [PoM] £15.62
Labetalol hydrochloride 200 mg Trandate 200mg tablets | 56 tablet [PoM] £7.41 DT price = £8.77 | 250 tablet [PoM] £24.76
Labetalol hydrochloride 400 mg Trandate 400mg tablets | 56 tablet [PoM] £10.15 DT price = £23.14

BETA-ADRENOCEPTOR BLOCKERS 〉
NON-SELECTIVE

F 100

Propranolol hydrochloride

- **INDICATIONS AND DOSE**
Hyperthyroidism with autonomic symptoms
▸ BY MOUTH

- **Neonate:** Initially 250–500 micrograms/kg every 6–8 hours, adjusted according to response.

- **Child:** Initially 250–500 micrograms/kg every 8 hours, adjusted according to response; increased if necessary up to 1 mg/kg every 8 hours (max. per dose 40 mg every 8 hours)
▸ BY INTRAVENOUS INJECTION

- **Neonate:** Initially 20–50 micrograms/kg every 6–8 hours, adjusted according to response, to be given over 10 minutes.

- **Child:** Initially 25–50 micrograms/kg every 6–8 hours (max. per dose 5 mg), adjusted according to response, to be given over 10 minutes

Thyrotoxicosis (adjunct)
▸ BY MOUTH

- **Neonate:** Initially 250–500 micrograms/kg every 6–8 hours, adjusted according to response.

- **Child:** Initially 250–500 micrograms/kg every 8 hours, adjusted according to response; increased continued →

if necessary up to 1 mg/kg every 8 hours (max. per dose 40 mg every 8 hours)

▸ BY INTRAVENOUS INJECTION

▸ Neonate: Initially 20–50 micrograms/kg every 6–8 hours, adjusted according to response, to be given over 10 minutes.

▸ Child: Initially 25–50 micrograms/kg every 6–8 hours (max. per dose 5 mg), adjusted according to response, to be given over 10 minutes

Thyrotoxic crisis

▸ BY MOUTH

▸ Neonate: Initially 250–500 micrograms/kg every 6–8 hours, adjusted according to response.

▸ Child: Initially 250–500 micrograms/kg every 8 hours, adjusted according to response; increased if necessary up to 1 mg/kg every 8 hours (max. per dose 40 mg every 8 hours)

▸ BY INTRAVENOUS INJECTION

▸ Neonate: Initially 20–50 micrograms/kg every 6–8 hours, adjusted according to response, to be given over 10 minutes.

▸ Child: Initially 25–50 micrograms/kg every 6–8 hours (max. per dose 5 mg), adjusted according to response, to be given over 10 minutes

Hypertension

▸ BY MOUTH

▸ Neonate: Initially 250 micrograms/kg 3 times a day, then increased if necessary up to 2 mg/kg 3 times a day.

▸ Child 1 month-11 years: Initially 0.25–1 mg/kg 3 times a day, then increased to 5 mg/kg daily in divided doses, dose should be increased at weekly intervals

▸ Child 12–17 years: Initially 80 mg twice daily, then increased if necessary up to 160–320 mg daily, dose should be increased at weekly intervals, slow-release preparations may be used for once daily administration

Migraine prophylaxis

▸ BY MOUTH

▸ Child 2–11 years: Initially 200–500 micrograms/kg twice daily; usual dose 10–20 mg twice daily (max. per dose 2 mg/kg twice daily)

▸ Child 12–17 years: Initially 20–40 mg twice daily; usual dose 40–80 mg twice daily (max. per dose 120 mg); maximum 4 mg/kg per day

Arrhythmias

▸ BY MOUTH

▸ Neonate: 250–500 micrograms/kg 3 times a day, adjusted according to response.

▸ Child: 250–500 micrograms/kg 3–4 times a day (max. per dose 1 mg/kg 4 times a day), adjusted according to response; maximum 160 mg per day

▸ BY SLOW INTRAVENOUS INJECTION

▸ Neonate: 20–50 micrograms/kg, then 20–50 micrograms/kg every 6–8 hours if required, eCG monitoring required.

▸ Child: 25–50 micrograms/kg, then 25–50 micrograms/kg every 6–8 hours if required, eCG monitoring required

Tetralogy of Fallot

▸ BY MOUTH

▸ Neonate: 0.25–1 mg/kg 2–3 times a day (max. per dose 2 mg/kg 3 times a day).

▸ Child 1 month-11 years: 0.25–1 mg/kg 3–4 times a day, maximum dose to be given in divided doses; maximum 5 mg/kg per day

▸ BY SLOW INTRAVENOUS INJECTION

▸ Neonate: Initially 15–20 micrograms/kg (max. per dose 100 micrograms/kg), then 15–20 micrograms/kg every 12 hours if required, eCG monitoring is required with administration.

▸ Child 1 month-11 years: Initially 15–20 micrograms/kg (max. per dose 100 micrograms/kg), higher doses are rarely necessary, then 15–20 micrograms/kg every 6–8 hours if required, eCG monitoring is required with administration

● UNLICENSED USE Not licensed for treatment of hypertension in children under 12 years.

● INTERACTIONS → Appendix 1: beta blockers (non-selective)

● SIDE-EFFECTS

▸ Rare Dry eyes (reversible on withdrawal)

● HEPATIC IMPAIRMENT Reduce oral dose.

● RENAL IMPAIRMENT Manufacturer advises caution; dose reduction may be required.

● DIRECTIONS FOR ADMINISTRATION For *slow intravenous injection*, give over at least 3–5 minutes; rate of administration should not exceed 1 mg/minute. May be diluted with Sodium Chloride 0.9% or Glucose 5%. Incompatible with bicarbonate.

● PRESCRIBING AND DISPENSING INFORMATION Modified-release preparations can be used for once daily administration.

● MEDICINAL FORMS
There can be variation in the licensing of different medicines containing the same drug. Forms available from special-order manufacturers include: oral suspension, oral solution

Oral solution
CAUTIONARY AND ADVISORY LABELS 8
▸ Propranolol hydrochloride (Non-proprietary)
Propranolol hydrochloride 1 mg per 1 ml Propranolol 5mg/5ml oral solution sugar free sugar-free | 150 ml PoM £18.50 DT price = £15.50

Propranolol hydrochloride 2 mg per 1 ml Propranolol 10mg/5ml oral solution sugar free sugar-free | 150 ml PoM £23.45 DT price = £20.45

Propranolol hydrochloride 8 mg per 1 ml Propranolol 40mg/5ml oral solution sugar free sugar-free | 150 ml PoM £31.50 DT price = £31.50

Propranolol hydrochloride 10 mg per 1 ml Propranolol 50mg/5ml oral solution sugar free sugar-free | 150 ml PoM £29.98 DT price = £24.98

Modified-release capsule
CAUTIONARY AND ADVISORY LABELS 8, 25
▸ Propranolol hydrochloride (Non-proprietary)
Propranolol hydrochloride 80 mg Propranolol 80mg modified-release capsules | 28 capsule PoM £4.95 DT price = £4.95
Propranolol hydrochloride 160 mg Propranolol 160mg modified-release capsules | 28 capsule PoM £4.88 DT price = £4.88
▸ Bedranol SR (Sandoz Ltd, Almus Pharmaceuticals Ltd)
Propranolol hydrochloride 80 mg Bedranol SR 80mg capsules | 28 capsule PoM £4.16 DT price = £4.95
Propranolol hydrochloride 160 mg Bedranol SR 160mg capsules | 28 capsule PoM £4.59–£5.09 DT price = £4.88
▸ Beta-Prograne (Tillomed Laboratories Ltd, Actavis UK Ltd, Teva UK Ltd)
Propranolol hydrochloride 160 mg Beta-Prograne 160mg modified-release capsules | 28 capsule PoM £6.11 DT price = £4.88
▸ Half Beta-Prograne (Teva UK Ltd, Tillomed Laboratories Ltd, Actavis UK Ltd)
Propranolol hydrochloride 80 mg Half Beta-Prograne 80mg modified-release capsules | 28 capsule PoM £4.95 DT price = £4.95

Tablet
CAUTIONARY AND ADVISORY LABELS 8
▸ Propranolol hydrochloride (Non-proprietary)
Propranolol hydrochloride 10 mg Propranolol 10mg tablets | 28 tablet PoM £1.47 DT price = £0.83

Propranolol hydrochloride **40 mg** Propranolol 40mg tablets |
28 tablet [PoM] £1.85 DT price = £0.85
Propranolol hydrochloride **80 mg** Propranolol 80mg tablets |
56 tablet [PoM] £9.33 DT price = £1.53
Propranolol hydrochloride **160 mg** Propranolol 160mg tablets |
56 tablet [PoM] £5.87 DT price = £5.87

BETA-ADRENOCEPTOR BLOCKERS ⟩
SELECTIVE

F 100

Atenolol

- **INDICATIONS AND DOSE**

Hypertension
▸ BY MOUTH

- Neonate: 0.5–2 mg/kg once daily, dose may be given in
2 divided doses.

- Child 1 month–11 years: 0.5–2 mg/kg once daily, dose
may be given in 2 divided doses, doses higher than
50 mg daily are rarely necessary
- Child 12–17 years: 25–50 mg once daily, dose may be
given in 2 divided doses, higher doses are rarely
necessary

Arrhythmias
▸ BY MOUTH

- Neonate: 0.5–2 mg/kg once daily, dose may be given in
2 divided doses.

- Child 1 month–11 years: 0.5–2 mg/kg once daily, dose
may be given in 2 divided doses; maximum 100 mg per
day
- Child 12–17 years: 50–100 mg once daily, dose may be
given in 2 divided doses

- **UNLICENSED USE** Not licensed for use in children under
12 years.
- **INTERACTIONS** → Appendix 1: beta blockers (selective)
- **BREAST FEEDING** Water soluble beta-blockers such as
atenolol are present in breast milk in greater amounts than
other beta blockers.
- **RENAL IMPAIRMENT** Initially use 50% of usual dose if
estimated glomerular filtration rate
10–35 mL/minute/1.73 m^2; initially use 30–50% of usual
dose if estimated glomerular filtration rate less than
10 mL/minute/1.73 m^2.
- **PATIENT AND CARER ADVICE**
Medicines for Children leaflet: Atenolol for hypertension
www.medicinesforchildren.org.uk/atenolol-hypertension-0

- **MEDICINAL FORMS**
There can be variation in the licensing of different medicines
containing the same drug. Forms available from special-order
manufacturers include: oral suspension, oral solution
Oral solution
▸ Atenolol (Non-proprietary)
Atenolol **5 mg per 1 ml** Atenolol 25mg/5ml oral solution sugar free
sugar-free | 300 ml [PoM] £6.72 DT price = £5.59
Tablet
CAUTIONARY AND ADVISORY LABELS 8
▸ Atenolol (Non-proprietary)
Atenolol **25 mg** Atenolol 25mg tablets | 28 tablet [PoM] £1.39 DT
price = £0.71
Atenolol **50 mg** Atenolol 50mg tablets | 28 tablet [PoM] £1.44 DT
price = £0.75
Atenolol **100 mg** Atenolol 100mg tablets | 28 tablet [PoM] £5.19 DT
price = £0.75
▸ Tenormin (AstraZeneca UK Ltd)
Atenolol **50 mg** Tenormin LS 50mg tablets | 28 tablet [PoM] £5.11
DT price = £0.73
Atenolol **100 mg** Tenormin 100mg tablets | 28 tablet [PoM] £6.49
DT price = £0.75

F 100

Esmolol hydrochloride

- **INDICATIONS AND DOSE**

Arrhythmias Hypertensive emergencies
▸ INITIALLY BY INTRAVENOUS INJECTION

- Child: Loading dose 500 micrograms/kg, to be given
over 1 minute, then (by intravenous infusion)
maintenance 50 micrograms/kg/minute for 4 minutes
(rate reduced if low blood pressure or low heart rate), if
inadequate response, repeat loading dose and increase
maintenance infusion, (by intravenous injection)
loading dose 500 micrograms/kg, given over 1 minute,
then (by intravenous infusion) maintenance
100 micrograms/kg/minute for 4 minutes, if response
still inadequate, repeat loading dose and increase
maintenance infusion, (by intravenous injection)
loading dose 500 micrograms/kg, given over 1 minute,
then (by intravenous infusion) maintenance
150 micrograms/kg/minute for 4 minutes, if response
still inadequate, repeat loading dose and increase
maintenance infusion, (by intravenous injection)
loading dose 500 micrograms/kg, given over 1 minute,
then (by intravenous infusion) maintenance
200 micrograms/kg/minute for 4 minutes, doses over
300 micrograms/kg/minute not recommended

Tetralogy of Fallot
▸ INITIALLY BY INTRAVENOUS INJECTION

- Neonate: Initially 600 micrograms/kg, dose to be given
over 1–2 minutes, then (by intravenous infusion)
300–900 micrograms/kg/minute if required.

- **UNLICENSED USE** Not licensed for use in children.
- **INTERACTIONS** → Appendix 1: beta blockers (selective)
- **SIDE-EFFECTS** Thrombophlebitis · venous irritation
- **BREAST FEEDING** Manufacturer advises avoidance.
- **RENAL IMPAIRMENT** Manufacturer advises caution.
- **DIRECTIONS FOR ADMINISTRATION** Give through a central
venous catheter; incompatible with bicarbonate.

- **MEDICINAL FORMS**
There can be variation in the licensing of different medicines
containing the same drug.
Solution for injection
▸ Brevibloc (Baxter Healthcare Ltd)
Esmolol hydrochloride **10 mg per 1 ml** Brevibloc Premixed
100mg/10ml solution for injection vials | 5 vial [PoM] no price
available
Solution for infusion
▸ Brevibloc (Baxter Healthcare Ltd)
Esmolol hydrochloride **10 mg per 1 ml** Brevibloc Premixed
2.5g/250ml infusion bags | 1 bag [PoM] £89.69

F 100

Metoprolol tartrate

- **INDICATIONS AND DOSE**

Hypertension
▸ BY MOUTH USING IMMEDIATE-RELEASE MEDICINES

- Child 1 month–11 years: Initially 1 mg/kg twice daily,
increased if necessary up to 8 mg/kg daily in
2–4 divided doses (max. per dose 400 mg)
- Child 12–17 years: Initially 50–100 mg daily, increased if
necessary to 200 mg daily in 1–2 divided doses, high
doses are rarely necessary; maximum 400 mg per day
▸ BY MOUTH USING MODIFIED-RELEASE MEDICINES
- Child 12–17 years: 200 mg once daily   continued →

Arrhythmias

▸ BY MOUTH USING IMMEDIATE-RELEASE MEDICINES

▸ Child 12-17 years: Usual dose 50 mg 2-3 times a day, then increased if necessary up to 300 mg daily in divided doses

● UNLICENSED USE Not licensed for use in children.

● INTERACTIONS → Appendix 1: beta blockers (selective)

● HEPATIC IMPAIRMENT Reduce dose in severe impairment.

● MEDICINAL FORMS
There can be variation in the licensing of different medicines containing the same drug. Forms available from special-order manufacturers include: capsule, oral suspension, oral solution

Modified-release tablet
CAUTIONARY AND ADVISORY LABELS 8, 25
▸ **Lopresor SR** (Recordati Pharmaceuticals Ltd)
Metoprolol tartrate 200 mg Lopresor SR 200mg tablets | 28 tablet PoM £9.80

Tablet
CAUTIONARY AND ADVISORY LABELS 8
▸ **Metoprolol tartrate** (Non-proprietary)
Metoprolol tartrate 50 mg Metoprolol 50mg tablets | 28 tablet PoM £3.00 DT price = £1.05 | 56 tablet PoM £2.44
Metoprolol tartrate 100 mg Metoprolol 100mg tablets | 28 tablet PoM £3.00 DT price = £1.17 | 56 tablet PoM £2.74
▸ **Lopresor** (Recordati Pharmaceuticals Ltd)
Metoprolol tartrate 50 mg Lopresor 50mg tablets | 56 tablet PoM £2.57
Metoprolol tartrate 100 mg Lopresor 100mg tablets | 56 tablet PoM £6.68

CALCIUM-CHANNEL BLOCKERS

Calcium-channel blockers

Overview

Calcium-channel blockers differ in their predilection for the various possible sites of action and, therefore, their therapeutic effects are disparate, with much greater variation than those of beta-blockers. There are important differences between verapamil hydrochloride p. 106, diltiazem hydrochloride p. 140, and the dihydropyridine calcium-channel blockers (amlodipine below, nicardipine hydrochloride p. 105, nifedipine p. 106, and nimodipine p. 84). Verapamil hydrochloride and diltiazem hydrochloride should usually be **avoided** in heart failure because they may further depress cardiac function and cause clinically significant deterioration.

Verapamil hydrochloride is used for the treatment of hypertension and arrhythmias. However, it is no longer first-line treatment for arrhythmias in children because it has been associated with fatal collapse especially in infants under 1 year; adenosine p. 77 is now recommended for first-line use.

Verapamil hydrochloride is a highly negatively inotropic calcium channel-blocker and it reduces cardiac output, slows the heart rate, and may impair atrioventricular conduction. It may precipitate heart failure, exacerbate conduction disorders, and cause hypotension at high doses and should **not** be used with beta-blockers. Constipation is the most common side-effect.

Nifedipine relaxes vascular smooth muscle and dilates coronary and peripheral arteries. It has more influence on vessels and less on the myocardium than does verapamil hydrochloride and unlike verapamil hydrochloride has no anti-arrhythmic activity. It rarely precipitates heart failure because any negative inotropic effect is offset by a reduction in left ventricular work. Short-acting formulations of nifedipine may be used if a modified-release preparation delivering the appropriate dose is not available or if a child is unable to swallow (a liquid preparation may be prepared using capsules). Nifedipine may also be used for the management of angina due to coronary artery disease in Kawasaki disease or progeria and in the management of Raynaud's syndrome.

Nicardipine hydrochloride has similar effects to those of nifedipine and may produce less reduction of myocardial contractility; it should only be used for the treatment of life-threatening hypertension in paediatric intensive care settings and in postoperative hypertension.

Amlodipine also resembles nifedipine and nicardipine hydrochloride in its effects and does not reduce myocardial contractility or produce clinical deterioration in heart failure. It has a longer duration of action and can be given once daily. Nifedipine and amlodipine are used for the treatment of hypertension. Side-effects associated with vasodilatation such as flushing and headache (which become less obtrusive after a few days), and ankle swelling (which may respond only partially to diuretics) are common.

Nimodipine is related to nifedipine but the smooth muscle relaxant effect preferentially acts on cerebral arteries. Its use is confined to prevention and treatment of vascular spasm following aneurysmal subarachnoid haemorrhage.

Diltiazem hydrochloride is a peripheral vasodilator and also has mild depressor effects on the myocardium. It is used in the treatment of Raynaud's syndrome.

Calcium-channel blockers

● DRUG ACTION Calcium-channel blockers (less correctly called 'calcium-antagonists') interfere with the inward displacement of calcium ions through the slow channels of active cell membranes. They influence the myocardial cells, the cells within the specialised conducting system of the heart, and the cells of vascular smooth muscle. Thus, myocardial contractility may be reduced, the formation and propagation of electrical impulses within the heart may be depressed, and coronary or systemic vascular tone may be diminished.

● SIDE-EFFECTS

Overdose
Features of calcium-channel blocker poisoning include nausea, vomiting, dizziness, agitation, confusion, and coma in severe poisoning. Metabolic acidosis and hyperglycaemia may occur.

For details on the management of poisoning, see Calcium-channel blockers, under Emergency treatment of poisoning p. 803.

● TREATMENT CESSATION There is some evidence that sudden withdrawal of calcium-channel blockers may be associated with an exacerbation of myocardial ischaemia.

▶ above

Amlodipine

● DRUG ACTION Amlodipine is a dihydropyridine calcium-channel blocker.

● INDICATIONS AND DOSE

Hypertension
▸ BY MOUTH
▸ Child 1 month-11 years: Initially 100-200 micrograms/kg once daily; increased if necessary up to 400 micrograms/kg once daily, adjusted at intervals of 1-2 weeks; maximum 10 mg per day
▸ Child 12-17 years: Initially 5 mg once daily, then increased if necessary up to 10 mg once daily, adjusted at intervals of 1-2 weeks

DOSE EQUIVALENCE AND CONVERSION
▸ Tablets from various suppliers may contain different salts (e.g. amlodipine besilate, amlodipine maleate, and amlodipine mesilate) but the strength is expressed in terms of amlodipine (base); tablets containing different salts are considered interchangeable.

- **UNLICENSED USE** Not licensed for use in children under 6 years.
- **CONTRA-INDICATIONS** Cardiogenic shock · significant aortic stenosis
- **INTERACTIONS** → Appendix 1: calcium channel blockers
- **SIDE-EFFECTS**
‣ **Common or very common** Abdominal pain · dizziness · fatigue · flushing · headache · nausea · oedema · palpitation · sleep disturbances
‣ **Uncommon** Alopecia · arthralgia · asthenia · back pain · chest pain · dry mouth · dyspnoea · gastro-intestinal disturbances · gynaecomastia · hypotension · impotence · mood changes · muscle cramps · myalgia · paraesthesia · pruritus · purpura · rashes · rhinitis · skin discolouration · sweating · syncope · taste disturbances · tinnitus · tremor · urinary disturbances · visual disturbances · weight changes
‣ **Very rare** Angioedema · arrhythmias · cholestasis · coughing · gastritis · gingival hyperplasia · hepatitis · hyperglycaemia · jaundice · myocardial infarction · pancreatitis · peripheral neuropathy · tachycardia · thrombocytopenia · urticaria · vasculitis
‣ **Frequency not known** Erythema multiforme

Overdose
In overdose, the dihydropyridine calcium-channel blockers cause severe hypotension secondary to profound peripheral vasodilatation.

- **PREGNANCY** No information available—manufacturer advises avoid, but risk to fetus should be balanced against risk of uncontrolled maternal hypertension.
- **BREAST FEEDING** Manufacturer advises avoid—no information available.
- **HEPATIC IMPAIRMENT** May need dose reduction—half-life prolonged.
- **DIRECTIONS FOR ADMINISTRATION** Tablets may be dispersed in water.
- **PATIENT AND CARER ADVICE**
Medicines for Children leaflet: Amlodipine for hypertension
www.medicinesforchildren.org.uk/amlodipine-for-hypertension

- **MEDICINAL FORMS**
There can be variation in the licensing of different medicines containing the same drug. Forms available from special-order manufacturers include: oral suspension, oral solution

Oral solution
‣ Amlodipine (Non-proprietary)
 Amlodipine 1 mg per 1 ml Amlodipine 5mg/5ml oral solution sugar free sugar-free | 150 ml [PoM] £75.76 DT price = £75.76
 Amlodipine 2 mg per 1 ml Amlodipine 10mg/5ml oral solution sugar free sugar-free | 150 ml [PoM] £115.73 DT price = £115.73

Tablet
‣ Amlodipine (Non-proprietary)
 Amlodipine 5 mg Amlodipine 5mg tablets | 28 tablet [PoM] £9.42 DT price = £0.73
 Amlodipine 10 mg Amlodipine 10mg tablets | 28 tablet [PoM] £14.07 DT price = £0.79
‣ Istin (Pfizer Ltd)
 Amlodipine 5 mg Istin 5mg tablets | 28 tablet [PoM] £11.08 DT price = £0.73
 Amlodipine 10 mg Istin 10mg tablets | 28 tablet [PoM] £16.55 DT price = £0.79

▸ 104

Nicardipine hydrochloride

- **DRUG ACTION** Nicardipine is a dihydropyridine calcium-channel blocker.

- **INDICATIONS AND DOSE**

Life-threatening hypertension (specialist use only) | Post-operative hypertension (specialist use only)
‣ BY CONTINUOUS INTRAVENOUS INFUSION
 ‣ Neonate: Initially 500 nanograms/kg/minute (max. per dose 5 micrograms/kg/minute), adjusted according to response; maintenance 1–4 micrograms/kg/minute.
 ‣ Child: Initially 500 nanograms/kg/minute (max. per dose 5 micrograms/kg/minute), adjusted according to response; maintenance 1–4 micrograms/kg/minute (max. per dose 250 micrograms/minute)

- **CONTRA-INDICATIONS** Acute porphyrias p. 577 · avoid within 8 days of myocardial infarction · cardiogenic shock · compensatory hypertension · significant or advanced aortic stenosis
- **CAUTIONS** Congestive heart failure · elevated intracranial pressure · increased risk of serious hypotension · portal hypertension · pulmonary oedema · significantly impaired left ventricular function · stroke
- **INTERACTIONS** → Appendix 1: calcium channel blockers
- **SIDE-EFFECTS** Atrioventricular block · dizziness · flushing · headache · hypotension · nausea · palpitations · paralytic ileus · peripheral oedema · pulmonary oedema · tachycardia · thrombocytopenia · vomiting
SIDE-EFFECTS, FURTHER INFORMATION
‣ Hypotension and reflex tachycardia Systemic hypotension and reflex tachycardia with rapid reduction of blood pressure may occur—during intravenous use consider stopping infusion or decreasing dose by half.

Overdose
In overdose, the dihydropyridine calcium-channel blockers cause severe hypotension secondary to profound peripheral vasodilatation.

- **PREGNANCY** May inhibit labour. Not to be used in multiple pregnancy (twins or more) unless there is no other acceptable alternative. Toxicity in *animal* studies. Risk of severe maternal hypotension and fatal foetal hypoxia—avoid excessive decrease in blood pressure.
- **BREAST FEEDING** Manufacturer advises avoid—present in breast milk.
- **HEPATIC IMPAIRMENT** Half-life prolonged in severe impairment—consider using low initial dose. Use with caution in hepatic impairment—increased risk of serious hypotension.
- **RENAL IMPAIRMENT** Use with caution—increased risk of serious hypotension; consider using low initial dose.
- **MONITORING REQUIREMENTS** Monitor blood pressure and heart rate at least every 5 minutes during intravenous infusion, and then until stable, and continue monitoring for at least 12 hours after end of infusion.
- **DIRECTIONS FOR ADMINISTRATION** Intravenous nicardipine should only be administered under the supervision of a specialist and in a hospital or intensive care setting in which patients can be closely monitored.
 For *continuous intravenous infusion*, dilute to a concentration of 100–200 micrograms/mL with Glucose 5% and give *via* volumetric infusion pump or syringe driver; protect from light; to minimise peripheral venous irritation, change site of infusion every 12 hours; risk of adsorption on to plastic in the presence of saline solutions; incompatible with bicarbonate or alkaline solutions—consult product literature.

- **MEDICINAL FORMS**
There can be variation in the licensing of different medicines containing the same drug.
Solution for infusion
‣ Nicardipine hydrochloride (Non-proprietary)
Nicardipine hydrochloride 1 mg per 1 ml Nicardipine 10mg/10ml solution for injection ampoules | 5 ampoule [PoM] £50.00
Nicardipine hydrochloride 2.5 mg per 1 ml Cardene I.V. 25mg/10ml solution for infusion ampoules | 10 ampoule [PoM] no price available

F 104

Nifedipine

21-Nov-2016

- **DRUG ACTION** Nifedipine is a dihydropyridine calcium-channel blocker.

- **INDICATIONS AND DOSE**

Hypertensive crisis | Acute angina in Kawasaki disease or progeria
‣ BY MOUTH USING IMMEDIATE-RELEASE MEDICINES
‣ Child: Initially 250–500 micrograms/kg (max. per dose 10 mg), then repeat once if necessary, may cause unpredictable and severe reduction of blood pressure— monitor closely following administration; if ineffective consider alternative treatment and seek specialist advice

Hypertension | Angina in Kawasaki disease or progeria
‣ BY MOUTH USING IMMEDIATE-RELEASE MEDICINES
‣ Child 1 month–11 years: 200–300 micrograms/kg 3 times a day, dose frequency depends on preparation used; maximum 3 mg/kg per day; maximum 90 mg per day
‣ Child 12–17 years: 5–20 mg 3 times a day, dose frequency depends on preparation used; maximum 90 mg per day

Raynaud's syndrome
‣ BY MOUTH USING IMMEDIATE-RELEASE MEDICINES
‣ Child 2–17 years: 2.5–10 mg 2–4 times a day, start with low doses at night and increase gradually to avoid postural hypotension, dose frequency depends on preparation used

Persistent hyperinsulinaemic hypoglycaemia
‣ BY MOUTH USING IMMEDIATE-RELEASE MEDICINES
‣ Neonate: 100–200 micrograms/kg 4 times a day (max. per dose 600 micrograms/kg).

- **UNLICENSED USE** Not licensed for use in children.
- **CONTRA-INDICATIONS** Cardiogenic shock · significant aortic stenosis
- **CAUTIONS** Diabetes mellitus · heart failure · poor cardiac reserve · severe hypotension · short-acting formulations are not recommended for angina or long-term management of hypertension; their use may be associated with large variations in blood pressure and reflex tachycardia · significantly impaired left ventricular function (heart failure deterioration observed)
- **INTERACTIONS** → Appendix 1: calcium channel blockers
- **SIDE-EFFECTS**
‣ **Common or very common** Asthenia · dizziness · gastro-intestinal disturbance · headache · hypotension · lethargy · oedema · palpitation · vasodilatation
‣ **Uncommon** Angioedema · anxiety · chills · dyspnoea · dysuria · epistaxis · erectile dysfunction · hypersensitivity reactions · jaundice · joint swelling · migraine · myalgia · nasal congestion · nocturia · paraesthesia · polyuria · pruritus · rash · sleep disturbance · sweating · syncope · tachycardia · tremor · urticaria · vertigo · visual disturbance
‣ **Rare** Anorexia · gum hyperplasia · hyperglycaemia · male infertility · mood disturbances · photosensitivity reactions · purpura

‣ **Frequency not known** Agranulocytosis · anaphylaxis · dysphagia · gynaecomastia · intestinal obstruction · intestinal ulcer

Overdose
In overdose, the dihydropyridine calcium-channel blockers cause severe hypotension secondary to profound peripheral vasodilatation.

- **PREGNANCY** May inhibit labour; manufacturer advises avoid before week 20, but risk to fetus should be balanced against risk of uncontrolled maternal hypertension. Use only if other treatment options are not indicated or have failed.
- **BREAST FEEDING** Amount too small to be harmful but manufacturers advise avoid.
- **HEPATIC IMPAIRMENT** Dose reduction may be required in severe liver disease.
- **DIRECTIONS FOR ADMINISTRATION** For rapid effect in *hypertensive crisis* or *acute angina*, bite capsules and swallow liquid or use liquid preparation if 5 mg or 10 mg dose inappropriate. If liquid unavailable, extract contents of capsule via a syringe and use immediately—cover syringe with foil to protect contents from light; capsule contents may be diluted with water if necessary.
- **PATIENT AND CARER ADVICE**
Medicines for Children leaflet: Nifedipine for high blood pressure www.medicinesforchildren.org.uk/nifedipine-for-high-blood-pressure

- **MEDICINAL FORMS**
There can be variation in the licensing of different medicines containing the same drug. Forms available from special-order manufacturers include: oral suspension, oral drops
Oral drops
‣ Nifedipine (Non-proprietary)
Nifedipine 20 mg per 1 ml Nifedipir-ratiopharm 20mg/ml oral drops | 30 ml [PoM] no price available | 100 ml [PoM] no price available
Capsule
‣ Nifedipine (Non-proprietary)
Nifedipine 5 mg Nifedipine 5mg capsules | 84 capsule [PoM] £19.99 DT price = £19.30
Nifedipine 10 mg Nifedipine 10mg capsules | 84 capsule [PoM] £21.00 DT price = £11.55
‣ Adalat (Bayer Plc)
Nifedipine 5 mg Adalat 5mg capsules | 90 capsule [PoM] £5.73
Nifedipine 10 mg Adalat 10mg capsules | 90 capsule [PoM] £7.30

F 104

Verapamil hydrochloride

- **INDICATIONS AND DOSE**

Treatment of supraventricular arrhythmias
‣ BY SLOW INTRAVENOUS INJECTION
‣ Child 1–17 years (administered on expert advice): 100–300 micrograms/kg (max. per dose 5 mg) for 1 dose, to be given over 2–3 minutes (with ECG and blood-pressure monitoring), dose can be repeated after 30 minutes if necessary

Hypertension
‣ BY MOUTH USING IMMEDIATE-RELEASE MEDICINES
‣ Child 12–23 months (administered on expert advice): 20 mg 2–3 times a day
‣ Child 2–17 years (administered on expert advice): 40–120 mg 2–3 times a day

Prophylaxis of supraventricular arrhythmias (administered on expert advice)
‣ BY MOUTH USING IMMEDIATE-RELEASE MEDICINES
‣ Child 12–23 months: 20 mg 2–3 times a day
‣ Child 2–17 years: 40–120 mg 2–3 times a day

- **CONTRA-INDICATIONS** Acute porphyrias p. 577 · atrial flutter or fibrillation associated with accessory conducting pathways (e.g. Wolff-Parkinson-White-syndrome) ·

bradycardia · cardiogenic shock · history of heart failure (even if controlled by therapy) · history of significantly impaired left ventricular function (even if controlled by therapy) · hypotension · second- and third-degree AV block · sick sinus syndrome · sino-atrial block

- **CAUTIONS** First-degree AV block
- **INTERACTIONS** → Appendix 1: calcium channel blockers
- **SIDE-EFFECTS**
▸ **Common or very common** Constipation
▸ **Uncommon** Ankle oedema · dizziness · fatigue · flushing · headache · nausea · vomiting
▸ **Rare** Allergic reactions · angioedema · arthralgia · asystole · bradycardia · erythema · erythromelalgia · gingival hyperplasia after long-term treatment · gynaecomastia after long-term treatment · heart block · heart failure · hypersensitivity reactions involving reversibly raised liver function tests · hypotension · increased prolactin concentration · myalgia · paraesthesia · pruritus · Stevens-Johnson syndrome · urticaria

SIDE-EFFECTS, FURTHER INFORMATION
▸ Intravenous administration or high doses Hypotension, heart failure, bradycardia, heart block, and asystole are side-effects associated with intravenous administration or high doses.

Overdose
In overdose, verapamil has a profound cardiac depressant effect causing hypotension and arrhythmias, including complete heart block and asystole.

- **PREGNANCY** May reduce uterine blood flow with fetal hypoxia. Manufacturer advises avoid in first trimester unless absolutely necessary. May inhibit labour.
- **BREAST FEEDING** Amount too small to be harmful.
- **HEPATIC IMPAIRMENT** Oral dose may need to be reduced.
- **DIRECTIONS FOR ADMINISTRATION** For *intravenous injection*, may be diluted with Glucose 5% *or* Sodium Chloride 0.9%. Incompatible with solutions of pH greater than 6.

- **MEDICINAL FORMS**
There can be variation in the licensing of different medicines containing the same drug. Forms available from special-order manufacturers include: oral suspension, oral solution

Tablet
▸ **Verapamil hydrochloride** (Non-proprietary)
Verapamil hydrochloride 40 mg Verapamil 40mg tablets | 84 tablet PoM £2.07 DT price = £1.63
Verapamil hydrochloride 80 mg Verapamil 80mg tablets | 84 tablet PoM £2.33 DT price = £1.98
Verapamil hydrochloride 120 mg Verapamil 120mg tablets | 28 tablet PoM £2.01 DT price = £1.48
Verapamil hydrochloride 160 mg Verapamil 160mg tablets | 56 tablet PoM £33.84 DT price = £28.20

Solution for injection
▸ **Securon** (Mylan Ltd)
Verapamil hydrochloride 2.5 mg per 1 ml Securon IV 5mg/2ml solution for injection ampoules | 5 ampoule PoM £5.41

Oral solution
▸ **Verapamil hydrochloride** (Non-proprietary)
Verapamil hydrochloride 8 mg per 1 ml Verapamil 40mg/5ml oral solution sugar free sugar-free | 150 ml PoM £39.00 DT price = £39.00

DIURETICS 〉THIAZIDES AND RELATED DIURETICS

Thiazides and related diuretics

- **CONTRA-INDICATIONS** Addison's disease · hypercalcaemia · hyponatraemia · refractory hypokalaemia · symptomatic hyperuricaemia
- **CAUTIONS** Diabetes · gout · hyperaldosteronism · malnourishment · nephrotic syndrome · systemic lupus erythematosus

CAUTIONS, FURTHER INFORMATION
▸ Potassium loss Hypokalaemia can occur with both thiazide and loop diuretics. The risk of hypokalaemia depends on the duration of action as well as the potency and is thus greater with thiazides than with an equipotent dose of a loop diuretic.

Hypokalaemia is particularly dangerous in children being treated with cardiac glycosides. In hepatic failure hypokalaemia caused by diuretics can precipitate encephalopathy.

The use of potassium-sparing diuretics avoids the need to take potassium supplements.

▸ Existing conditions Thiazides and related diuretics can exacerbate diabetes, gout, and systemic lupus erythematosus.

- **SIDE-EFFECTS**
▸ **Common or very common** Altered plasma-lipid concentrations · gout · hypercalcaemia · hyperglycaemia · hyperuricaemia · hypochloraemic alkalosis · hypokalaemia · hypomagnesaemia · hyponatraemia · metabolic and electrolyte disturbances · mild gastrointestinal disturbances · postural hypotension
▸ **Uncommon** Agranulocytosis · blood disorders · impotence · leucopenia · thrombocytopenia
▸ **Frequency not known** Cardiac arrhythmias · dizziness · headache · hypersensitivity reactions · intrahepatic cholestasis · pancreatitis · paraesthesia · photosensitivity · pneumonitis · pulmonary oedema · severe skin reactions · visual disturbances

- **PREGNANCY** Thiazides and related diuretics should not be used to treat gestational hypertension. They may cause neonatal thrombocytopenia, bone marrow suppression, jaundice, electrolyte disturbances, and hypoglycaemia; placental perfusion may also be reduced. Stimulation of labour, uterine inertia, and meconium staining have also been reported.

- **HEPATIC IMPAIRMENT** Caution in mild to moderate impairment. Avoid in severe liver disease. Hypokalaemia may precipitate coma in hepatic impairment, although hypokalaemia can be prevented by using a potassium-sparing diuretic.

- **RENAL IMPAIRMENT** Thiazides and related diuretics should be used with caution because they can further reduce renal function. They are ineffective if estimated glomerular filtration rate is less than 30 mL/minute/1.73 m^2 and should be avoided. Metolazone remains effective if estimated glomerular filtration rate is less than 30 mL/minute/1.73 m^2 but is associated with a risk of excessive diuresis. Electrolytes should be monitored in renal impairment.

- **MONITORING REQUIREMENTS** Electrolytes should be monitored, particularly with high doses and long-term use.

◤ above

Bendroflumethiazide

(Bendrofluazide)

- **INDICATIONS AND DOSE**

Hypertension
▸ BY MOUTH
▸ Child 1 month-1 year: 50–100 micrograms/kg daily, adjusted according to response
▸ Child 2-11 years: Initially 50–400 micrograms/kg daily (max. per dose 10 mg), then maintenance 50–100 micrograms/kg daily, adjusted according to response; maximum 10 mg per day
▸ Child 12-17 years: 2.5 mg once daily, dose to be taken as a single dose in the morning, higher doses are rarely necessary   continued →

2

Cardiovascular system

Oedema in heart failure, renal disease and hepatic disease | Pulmonary oedema
▸ BY MOUTH
▸ Child 1 month–1 year: 50–100 micrograms/kg daily, adjusted according to response
▸ Child 2–11 years: Initially 50–400 micrograms/kg daily (max. per dose 10 mg), then maintenance 50–100 micrograms/kg daily, adjusted according to response; maximum 10 mg per day
▸ Child 12–17 years: Initially 5–10 mg once daily or on alternate days, adjusted according to response, dose to be taken as a single dose in the morning; maximum 10 mg per day

● INTERACTIONS → Appendix 1: thiazide diuretics
● BREAST FEEDING The amount present in milk is too small to be harmful. Large doses may suppress lactation.

● MEDICINAL FORMS
There can be variation in the licensing of different medicines containing the same drug. Forms available from special-order manufacturers include: oral suspension, oral solution

Tablet
▸ Bendroflumethiazide (Non-proprietary)
Bendroflumethiazide 2.5 mg Bendroflumethiazide 2.5mg tablets | 28 tablet [PoM] £3.68 DT price = £0.66 | 500 tablet [PoM] £21.85
Bendroflumethiazide 5 mg Bendroflumethiazide 5mg tablets | 28 tablet [PoM] £9.80 DT price = £0.86 | 500 tablet [PoM] no price available
▸ Aprinox (AMCo)
Bendroflumethiazide 2.5 mg Aprinox 2.5mg tablets | 500 tablet [PoM] £27.31
▸ Neo-Naclex (AMCo)
Bendroflumethiazide 2.5 mg Neo-Naclex 2.5mg tablets | 28 tablet [PoM] £0.33 DT price = £0.66

◀ 107

Chlorothiazide

● INDICATIONS AND DOSE

Heart failure | Hypertension | Ascites
▸ BY MOUTH
▸ Neonate: 10–20 mg/kg twice daily.

▸ Child 1–5 months: 10–20 mg/kg twice daily
▸ Child 6 months–11 years: 10 mg/kg twice daily; maximum 1 g per day
▸ Child 12–17 years: 0.25–1 g once daily, alternatively 125–500 mg twice daily

Reduction of diazoxide-induced sodium and water retention in the management of chronic hypoglycaemia | Potentiating the glycaemic effect of diazoxide in the management of chronic hypoglycaemia
▸ BY MOUTH
▸ Child: 3–5 mg/kg twice daily

Nephrogenic and partial pituitary diabetes insipidus
▸ BY MOUTH
▸ Child: 10–20 mg/kg twice daily (max. per dose 500 mg)

● UNLICENSED USE Not licensed.
● CAUTIONS Neonate (theoretical risk of kernicterus if very jaundiced)
● BREAST FEEDING The amount present in milk is too small to be harmful. Large doses may suppress lactation.

● MEDICINAL FORMS
There can be variation in the licensing of different medicines containing the same drug. Forms available from special-order manufacturers include: tablet, oral suspension, oral solution

Oral suspension
▸ Chlorothiazide (Non-proprietary)
Chlorothiazide 50 mg per 1 ml Diuril 250mg/5ml oral suspension | 237 ml [PoM] no price available

Tablet
▸ Chlorothiazide (Non-proprietary)
Chlorothiazide 250 mg Diuril 250mg tablets | 100 tablet [PoM] no price available

DRUGS ACTING ON THE RENIN–ANGIOTENSIN SYSTEM ⟩ ACE INHIBITORS

Angiotensin-converting enzyme inhibitors

● CONTRA-INDICATIONS Bilateral renovascular disease
● CAUTIONS Afro-Caribbean patients (may respond less well to ACE inhibitors) · concomitant diuretics · diabetes (may lower blood glucose) · first dose hypotension (especially in patients taking high doses of diuretics, on a low-sodium diet, on dialysis, dehydrated, or with heart failure) · neonates (in neonates) · primary aldosteronism (patients may respond less well to ACE inhibitors) · the risk of agranulocytosis is possibly increased in collagen vascular disease (blood counts recommended) · use with care (or avoid) in those with a history of idiopathic or hereditary angioedema · use with care in patients with hypertrophic cardiomyopathy · use with care in patients with severe or symptomatic aortic stenosis (risk of hypotension)

CAUTIONS, FURTHER INFORMATION
▸ Anaphylactoid reactions To prevent anaphylactoid reactions, ACE inhibitors should be avoided during dialysis with high-flux polyacrylonitrile membranes and during low-density lipoprotein apheresis with dextran sulfate; they should also be withheld before desensitisation with wasp or bee venom.

● SIDE-EFFECTS
▸ Common or very common Apnoea (in neonates) · renal failure (in neonates) · seizures (in neonates) · severe unpredictable hypotension (in neonates)
▸ Frequency not known Pruritus · abdominal pain · altered liver function tests · angioedema (onset may be delayed; higher incidence reported in Afro-Caribbean patients) · arthralgia · blood disorders · bronchospasm · cholestatic jaundice · constipation · diarrhoea · dizziness · dyspepsia · eosinophilia · fatigue · fever · fulminant hepatic necrosis · haemolytic anaemia · headache · hepatic failure · hepatitis · hyperkalaemia · hypoglycaemia · leucocytosis · leucopenia · malaise · myalgia · nausea · neutropenia · pancreatitis · paraesthesia · persistent dry cough · photosensitivity · positive antinuclear antibody · profound hypotension · raised erythrocyte sedimentation rate · rash · renal impairment · rhinitis · serositis · sinusitis · sore throat · taste disturbance · thrombocytopenia · urticaria · vasculitis · vomiting

SIDE-EFFECTS, FURTHER INFORMATION
▸ Hepatic effects In light of reports of cholestatic jaundice, hepatitis, fulminant hepatic necrosis, and hepatic failure, ACE inhibitors should be discontinued if marked elevation of hepatic enzymes or jaundice occur.

● ALLERGY AND CROSS-SENSITIVITY ACE inhibitors are contra-indicated in patients with hypersensitivity to ACE inhibitors (including angioedema).
● PREGNANCY ACE inhibitors should be avoided in pregnancy unless essential. They may adversely affect fetal and neonatal blood pressure control and renal function; skull defects and oligohydramnios have also been reported.
● BREAST FEEDING Information on the use of ACE inhibitors in breast-feeding is limited.
● RENAL IMPAIRMENT Use with caution, starting with low dose, and adjust according to response. Hyperkalaemia and other side-effects of ACE inhibitors are more common

in those with impaired renal function and the dose may need to be reduced.

- **MONITORING REQUIREMENTS** Renal function and electrolytes should be checked before starting ACE inhibitors (or increasing the dose) and monitored during treatment (more frequently if side effects mentioned are present).
- **DIRECTIONS FOR ADMINISTRATION** For hypertension the first dose should preferably be given at bedtime.

F 108

Captopril

- **INDICATIONS AND DOSE**

Hypertension
▶ BY MOUTH

- ▸ Preterm neonate (initiated under specialist supervision): Test dose 10 micrograms/kg, monitor blood pressure carefully for 1–2 hours; usual dose 10–50 micrograms/kg 2–3 times a day, then increased if necessary up to 300 micrograms/kg daily in divided doses, ongoing doses should only be given if test dose tolerated.

- ▸ Neonate (initiated under specialist supervision): Test dose 10–50 micrograms/kg, monitor blood pressure carefully for 1–2 hours; usual dose 10–50 micrograms/kg 2–3 times a day, then increased if necessary up to 2 mg/kg daily in divided doses, ongoing doses should only be given if test dose tolerated.

- ▸ Child 1-11 months (initiated under specialist supervision): Test dose 100 micrograms/kg (max. per dose 6.25 mg), monitor blood pressure carefully for 1–2 hours; usual dose 100–300 micrograms/kg 2–3 times a day, then increased if necessary up to 4 mg/kg daily in divided doses, ongoing doses should only be given if test dose tolerated

- ▸ Child 1-11 years (initiated under specialist supervision): Test dose 100 micrograms/kg (max. per dose 6.25 mg), monitor blood pressure carefully for 1–2 hours; usual dose 100–300 micrograms/kg 2–3 times a day, then increased if necessary up to 6 mg/kg daily in divided doses, ongoing doses should only be given if test dose tolerated

- ▸ Child 12-17 years (initiated under specialist supervision): Test dose 100 micrograms/kg, alternatively test dose 6.25 mg, monitor blood pressure carefully for 1–2 hours; usual dose 12.5–25 mg 2–3 times a day, then increased if necessary up to 150 mg daily in divided doses, ongoing doses should only be given if test dose tolerated

Heart failure
▶ BY MOUTH

- ▸ Preterm neonate (initiated under specialist supervision): Test dose 10 micrograms/kg, monitor blood pressure carefully for 1–2 hours; usual dose 10–50 micrograms/kg 2–3 times a day, then increased if necessary up to 300 micrograms/kg daily in divided doses, ongoing doses should only be given if test dose tolerated.

- ▸ Neonate (initiated under specialist supervision): Test dose 10–50 micrograms/kg, monitor blood pressure carefully for 1–2 hours; usual dose 10–50 micrograms/kg 2–3 times a day, then increased if necessary up to 2 mg/kg daily in divided doses, ongoing doses should only be given if test dose tolerated.

- ▸ Child 1-11 months (initiated under specialist supervision): Test dose 100 micrograms/kg (max. per dose 6.25 mg),

monitor blood pressure carefully for 1–2 hours; usual dose 100–300 micrograms/kg 2–3 times a day, then increased if necessary up to 4 mg/kg daily in divided doses, ongoing doses should only be given if test dose tolerated

- ▸ Child 1-11 years (initiated under specialist supervision): Test dose 100 micrograms/kg (max. per dose 6.25 mg), monitor blood pressure carefully for 1–2 hours; usual dose 100–300 micrograms/kg 2–3 times a day, then increased if necessary up to 6 mg/kg daily in divided doses, ongoing doses should only be given if test dose tolerated

- ▸ Child 12-17 years (initiated under specialist supervision): Test dose 100 micrograms/kg, alternatively test dose 6.25 mg, monitor blood pressure carefully for 1–2 hours; usual dose 12.5–25 mg 2–3 times a day, then increased if necessary up to 150 mg daily in divided doses, ongoing doses should only be given if test dose tolerated

Proteinuria in nephritis (under expert supervision)
▶ BY MOUTH

- ▸ Preterm neonate: Test dose 10 micrograms/kg, monitor blood pressure carefully for 1–2 hours; usual dose 10–50 micrograms/kg 2–3 times a day, then increased if necessary up to 300 micrograms/kg daily in divided doses, ongoing doses should only be given if test dose tolerated.

- ▸ Neonate: Test dose 10–50 micrograms/kg, monitor blood pressure carefully for 1–2 hours; usual dose 10–50 micrograms/kg 2–3 times a day, then increased if necessary up to 2 mg/kg daily in divided doses, ongoing doses should only be given if test dose tolerated.

- ▸ Child 1-11 months: Test dose 100 micrograms/kg (max. per dose 6.25 mg), monitor blood pressure carefully for 1–2 hours; usual dose 100–300 micrograms/kg 2–3 times a day, then increased if necessary up to 4 mg/kg daily in divided doses, ongoing doses should only be given if test dose tolerated

- ▸ Child 1-11 years: Test dose 100 micrograms/kg (max. per dose 6.25 mg), monitor blood pressure carefully for 1–2 hours; usual dose 100–300 micrograms/kg 2–3 times a day, then increased if necessary up to 6 mg/kg daily in divided doses, ongoing doses should only be given if test dose tolerated

- ▸ Child 12-17 years: Test dose 100 micrograms/kg, alternatively test dose 6.25 mg, monitor blood pressure carefully for 1–2 hours; usual dose 12.5–25 mg 2–3 times a day, then increased if necessary up to 150 mg daily in divided doses, ongoing doses should only be given if test dose tolerated

Diabetic nephropathy in type 1 diabetes mellitus
▶ BY MOUTH

- ▸ Child 12-17 years (under expert supervision): Test dose 100 micrograms/kg, alternatively test dose 6.25 mg, monitor blood pressure carefully for 1– 2 hours; usual dose 12.5–25 mg 2–3 times a day, increased if necessary up to 100 mg daily in divided doses, ongoing doses should only be given if test dose tolerated

- **UNLICENSED USE** Not licensed for use in children under 18 years.
- **INTERACTIONS** → Appendix 1: ACE inhibitors
- **SIDE-EFFECTS**
- ▶ **Common or very common** Alopecia · dry mouth · dyspnoea · sleep disorder
- ▶ **Uncommon** Angina · arrhythmia · flushing · pallor · palpitation · Raynaud's syndrome · tachycardia
- ▶ **Rare** Anorexia · stomatitis
- ▶ **Very rare** Allergic alveolitis · blurred vision · cardiac arrest · cardiogenic shock · cerebrovascular events · confusion ·

depression · eosinophilic pneumonia · glossitis · gynaecomastia · hyponatraemia · impotence · peptic ulcer · photosensitivity · Stevens-Johnson syndrome · syncope

- **BREAST FEEDING** Avoid in first few weeks after delivery, particularly in preterm infants—risk of profound neonatal hypotension; can be used in mothers breast-feeding older infants if essential but monitor infant's blood pressure.

- **DIRECTIONS FOR ADMINISTRATION** Administer under close supervision. Give test dose whilst child supine. Tablets can be dispersed in water.

- **PATIENT AND CARER ADVICE**
Medicines for Children leaflet: Captopril for heart failure
www.medicinesforchildren.org.uk/captopril-heart-failure-0

- **MEDICINAL FORMS**
There can be variation in the licensing of different medicines containing the same drug. Forms available from special-order manufacturers include: tablet, capsule, oral suspension, oral solution

Tablet
- Captopril (Non-proprietary)
  Captopril 12.5 mg Captopril 12.5mg tablets | 56 tablet [PoM] £2.80 DT price = £2.44 | 100 tablet [PoM] £5.00
  Captopril 25 mg Captopril 25mg tablets | 56 tablet [PoM] £4.52 DT price = £0.92 | 100 tablet [PoM] £8.07
  Captopril 50 mg Captopril 50mg tablets | 56 tablet [PoM] £5.83 DT price = £2.47 | 100 tablet [PoM] £10.41
- Capoten (Bristol-Myers Squibb Pharmaceuticals Ltd)
  Captopril 25 mg Capoten 25mg tablets | 28 tablet [PoM] £5.26
- Ecopace (AMCo)
  Captopril 12.5 mg Ecopace 12.5mg tablets | 56 tablet [PoM] £0.48 DT price = £2.44
  Captopril 25 mg Ecopace 25mg tablets | 56 tablet [PoM] £0.60 DT price = £0.92
  Captopril 50 mg Ecopace 50mg tablets | 56 tablet [PoM] £0.72 DT price = £2.47

Oral solution
ELECTROLYTES: May contain Sodium
- Noyada (Martindale Pharmaceuticals Ltd)
  Captopril 1 mg per 1 ml Noyada 5mg/5ml oral solution sugar-free | 100 ml [PoM] £98.21 DT price = £98.21
  Captopril 5 mg per 1 ml Noyada 25mg/5ml oral solution sugar-free | 100 ml [PoM] £108.94 DT price = £108.94

F 108

Enalapril maleate

- **INDICATIONS AND DOSE**
Hypertension
▶ BY MOUTH

- Neonate (under expert supervision): Initially 10 micrograms/kg once daily, monitor blood pressure carefully for 1–2 hours, increased if necessary up to 500 micrograms/kg daily in 1–3 divided doses, limited information.

- Child 1 month-11 years (under expert supervision): Initially 100 micrograms/kg once daily, monitor blood pressure carefully for 1–2 hours, then increased if necessary up to 1 mg/kg daily in 1–2 divided doses

- Child 12–17 years (under expert supervision) (body-weight up to 50 kg): Initially 2.5 mg once daily, monitor blood pressure carefully for 1–2 hours, maintenance 10–20 mg daily in 1–2 divided doses

- Child 12–17 years (under expert supervision) (body-weight 50 kg and above): Initially 2.5 mg once daily, monitor blood pressure carefully for 1–2 hours, maintenance 10–20 mg daily in 1–2 divided doses; maximum 40 mg per day

Heart failure
▶ BY MOUTH

- Neonate (under expert supervision): Initially 10 micrograms/kg once daily, monitor blood pressure carefully for 1–2 hours, increased if necessary up to 500 micrograms/kg daily in 1–3 divided doses, limited information.

- Child 1 month-11 years (under expert supervision): Initially 100 micrograms/kg once daily, monitor blood pressure carefully for 1–2 hours, then increased if necessary up to 1 mg/kg daily in 1–2 divided doses

- Child 12–17 years (under expert supervision) (body-weight up to 50 kg): Initially 2.5 mg once daily, monitor blood pressure carefully for 1–2 hours, maintenance 10–20 mg daily in 1–2 divided doses

- Child 12–17 years (under expert supervision) (body-weight 50 kg and above): Initially 2.5 mg once daily, monitor blood pressure carefully for 1–2 hours, maintenance 10–20 mg daily in 1–2 divided doses; maximum 40 mg per day

Proteinuria in nephritis (under expert supervision)
▶ BY MOUTH

- Neonate: Initially 10 micrograms/kg once daily, monitor blood pressure carefully for 1–2 hours, increased if necessary up to 500 micrograms/kg daily in 1–3 divided doses, limited information.

- Child 1 month-11 years: Initially 100 micrograms/kg once daily, monitor blood pressure carefully for 1–2 hours, then increased if necessary up to 1 mg/kg daily in 1–2 divided doses

- Child 12–17 years (body-weight up to 50 kg): Initially 2.5 mg once daily, monitor blood pressure carefully for 1–2 hours, maintenance 10–20 mg daily in 1–2 divided doses

- Child 12–17 years (body-weight 50 kg and above): Initially 2.5 mg once daily, monitor blood pressure carefully for 1–2 hours, maintenance 10–20 mg daily in 1–2 divided doses; maximum 40 mg per day

Diabetic nephropathy (under expert supervision)
▶ BY MOUTH

- Child 12–17 years (body-weight up to 50 kg): Initially 2.5 mg once daily, monitor blood pressure carefully for 1–2 hours; maintenance 10–20 mg daily in 1–2 divided doses

- Child 12–17 years (body-weight 50 kg and above): Initially 2.5 mg once daily, monitor blood pressure carefully for 1–2 hours; maintenance 10–20 mg daily in 1–2 divided doses; maximum 40 mg per day

- **UNLICENSED USE** Not licensed for use in children for congestive heart failure, proteinuria in nephritis or diabetic nephropathy; not licensed for use in children less than 20 kg for hypertension.

- **INTERACTIONS** → Appendix 1: ACE inhibitors

- **SIDE-EFFECTS**
- **Common or very common** Asthenia · blurred vision · depression · dyspnoea
- **Uncommon** Alopecia · anorexia · arrhythmias · confusion · drowsiness · dry mouth · flushing · hyponatraemia · ileus · impotence · insomnia · muscle cramps · nervousness · palpitation · peptic ulcer · sweating · tinnitus · vertigo
- **Rare** Abnormal dreams · allergic alveolitis · exfoliative dermatitis · glossitis · gynaecomastia · pemphigus · pulmonary infiltrates · Raynaud's syndrome · Stevens-Johnson syndrome · stomatitis · toxic epidermal necrolysis
- **Very rare** Gastro-intestinal angioedema

- **BREAST FEEDING** Avoid in first few weeks after delivery, particularly in preterm infants—risk of profound neonatal hypotension; can be used in mothers breast-feeding older infants if essential but monitor infant's blood pressure.

- **HEPATIC IMPAIRMENT** Enalapril is a prodrug and requires close monitoring in patients with hepatic impairment.
- **DIRECTIONS FOR ADMINISTRATION** Tablets may be crushed and suspended in water immediately before use.
- **PATIENT AND CARER ADVICE**
Medicines for Children leaflet: Enalapril for high blood pressure www.medicinesforchildren.org.uk/enalapril-for-high-blood-pressure

- **MEDICINAL FORMS**
There can be variation in the licensing of different medicines containing the same drug. Forms available from special-order manufacturers include: oral suspension, oral solution

Tablet
▸ Enalapril maleate (Non-proprietary)
Enalapril maleate 2.5 mg Enalapril 2.5mg tablets | 28 tablet PoM £4.65 DT price = £3.46
Enalapril maleate 5 mg Enalapril 5mg tablets | 28 tablet PoM £4.13 DT price = £0.84
Enalapril maleate 10 mg Enalapril 10mg tablets | 28 tablet PoM £5.64 DT price = £0.90
Enalapril maleate 20 mg Enalapril 20mg tablets | 28 tablet PoM £6.63 DT price = £0.98
▸ Innovace (Merck Sharp & Dohme Ltd)
Enalapril maleate 2.5 mg Innovace 2.5mg tablets | 28 tablet PoM £5.35 DT price = £3.46
Enalapril maleate 5 mg Innovace 5mg tablets | 28 tablet PoM £7.51 DT price = £0.84
Enalapril maleate 10 mg Innovace 10mg tablets | 28 tablet PoM £10.53 DT price = £0.90
Enalapril maleate 20 mg Innovace 20mg tablets | 28 tablet PoM £12.51 DT price = £0.98

F 108

Lisinopril

- **INDICATIONS AND DOSE**

Hypertension
▸ BY MOUTH
▸ Child 6–11 years (under expert supervision): Initially 70 micrograms/kg once daily (max. per dose 5 mg), increased to up to 600 micrograms/kg once daily, alternatively increased to up to 40 mg once daily, dose to be increased in intervals of 1–2 weeks
▸ Child 12–17 years (under expert supervision): Initially 5 mg once daily; usual maintenance 10–20 mg once daily; maximum 80 mg per day

Proteinuria in nephritis (under expert supervision)
▸ BY MOUTH
▸ Child 6–11 years: Initially 70 micrograms/kg once daily (max. per dose 5 mg), increased to up to 600 micrograms/kg once daily, alternatively increased to up to 40 mg once daily, dose to be increased in intervals of 1–2 weeks
▸ Child 12–17 years: Initially 5 mg once daily; usual maintenance 10–20 mg once daily; maximum 80 mg per day

Diabetic nephropathy (under expert supervision)
▸ BY MOUTH
▸ Child 12–17 years: Initially 5 mg once daily; usual maintenance 10–20 mg once daily; maximum 80 mg per day

Heart failure (adjunct) (under close medical supervision)
▸ BY MOUTH
▸ Child 12–17 years: Initially 2.5 mg once daily; increased in steps of up to 10 mg at least every 2 weeks; maximum 35 mg per day

- **UNLICENSED USE** Not licensed for use in children.
- **INTERACTIONS** → Appendix 1: ACE inhibitors

- **SIDE-EFFECTS**
▸ **Uncommon** Raynaud's syndrome · vertigo · asthenia · cerebrovascular accident · confusion · impotence · mood changes · palpitation · sleep disturbances · tachycardia
▸ **Rare** Alopecia · dry mouth · gynaecomastia · psoriasis
▸ **Very rare** Allergic alveolitis · pemphigus · profuse sweating · pulmonary infiltrates · Stevens-Johnson syndrome · toxic epidermal necrolysis
- **BREAST FEEDING** Not recommended; alternative treatment options, with better established safety information during breast-feeding, are available.

- **PATIENT AND CARER ADVICE**
Medicines for Children leaflet: Lisinopril for high blood pressure www.medicinesforchildren.org.uk/lisinopril-for-high-blood-pressure

- **MEDICINAL FORMS**
There can be variation in the licensing of different medicines containing the same drug. Forms available from special-order manufacturers include: oral suspension, oral solution

Oral solution
▸ Lisinopril (Non-proprietary)
Lisinopril 1 mg per 1 ml Lisinopril 5mg/5ml oral solution sugar free sugar-free | 150 ml PoM £154.11 DT price = £154.11

Tablet
▸ Lisinopril (Non-proprietary)
Lisinopril 2.5 mg Lisinopril 2.5mg tablets | 28 tablet PoM £1.51 DT price = £0.71
Lisinopril 5 mg Lisinopril 5mg tablets | 28 tablet PoM £7.80 DT price = £0.73
Lisinopril 10 mg Lisinopril 10mg tablets | 28 tablet PoM £9.60 DT price = £0.79
Lisinopril 20 mg Lisinopril 20mg tablets | 28 tablet PoM £10.90 DT price = £0.83
▸ Zestril (AstraZeneca UK Ltd)
Lisinopril 5 mg Zestril 5mg tablets | 28 tablet PoM £4.71 DT price = £0.73
Lisinopril 10 mg Zestril 10mg tablets | 28 tablet PoM £7.38 DT price = £0.79
Lisinopril 20 mg Zestril 20mg tablets | 28 tablet PoM £6.51 DT price = £0.83

DRUGS ACTING ON THE RENIN-ANGIOTENSIN SYSTEM > ANGIOTENSIN II RECEPTOR ANTAGONISTS

Angiotensin II receptor antagonists

- **CAUTIONS** Afro-Caribbean patients—particularly those with left ventricular hypertrophy (may not benefit from an angiotensin-II receptor antagonist) · aortic or mitral valve stenosis · hypertrophic cardiomyopathy · patients with a history of angioedema · patients with primary aldosteronism (may not benefit from an angiotensin-II receptor antagonist) · renal artery stenosis
- **SIDE-EFFECTS** Hyperkalaemia · angioedema (may be delayed onset) · symptomatic hypotension including dizziness (particularly in children with hyponatraemia or intravascular volume depletion e.g. those taking high-dose diuretics)
- **PREGNANCY** Angiotensin-II receptor antagonists should be avoided in pregnancy unless essential. They may adversely affect fetal and neonatal blood pressure control and renal function; neonatal skull defects and oligohydramnios have also been reported.
- **BREAST FEEDING** Information on the use of angiotensin-II receptor antagonists in breast-feeding is limited. They are not recommended in breast-feeding and alternative treatment options, with better established safety information during breast-feeding, are available.

2

Cardiovascular system

- **RENAL IMPAIRMENT** Use with caution, starting with low dose, and adjust according to response.
- **MONITORING REQUIREMENTS** Monitor plasma-potassium concentration, particularly in children with renal impairment.

⇱ 111

Candesartan cilexetil

- **INDICATIONS AND DOSE**

Hypertension
- ▸ BY MOUTH
  - ▸ Child 6–17 years (under expert supervision) (body-weight up to 50 kg): Initially 4 mg once daily, adjusted according to response, lower dose may be used in intravascular volume depletion; maximum 8 mg per day
  - ▸ Child 6–17 years (under expert supervision) (body-weight 50 kg and above): Initially 4 mg once daily, adjusted according to response, lower dose may be used in intravascular volume depletion; maximum 16 mg per day

- **CONTRA-INDICATIONS** Cholestasis
- **INTERACTIONS** → Appendix 1: angiotensin-II receptor antagonists
- **SIDE-EFFECTS**
- ▸ **Common or very common** Cough · headache · rash · vertigo
- ▸ **Uncommon** Hyponatraemia
- ▸ **Very rare** Arthralgia · back pain · blood disorders · hepatitis · myalgia · nausea · pruritus · urticaria
- **HEPATIC IMPAIRMENT** Reduce initial dose in mild or moderate impairment. Avoid in severe hepatic impairment.
- **RENAL IMPAIRMENT** Reduce initial dose. Use with caution if estimated glomerular filtration rate is less than 30 mL/minute/1.73 m² —no information available.

- **MEDICINAL FORMS**
There can be variation in the licensing of different medicines containing the same drug. Forms available from special-order manufacturers include: oral suspension, oral solution

Tablet
- ▸ Candesartan cilexetil (Non-proprietary)
  Candesartan cilexetil 2 mg Candesartan 2mg tablets | 7 tablet [PoM] £3.40 DT price = £1.92
  Candesartan cilexetil 4 mg Candesartan 4mg tablets | 7 tablet [PoM] £7.82 DT price = £0.66 | 28 tablet [PoM] £9.78
  Candesartan cilexetil 8 mg Candesartan 8mg tablets | 28 tablet [PoM] £9.89 DT price = £0.98
  Candesartan cilexetil 16 mg Candesartan 16mg tablets | 28 tablet [PoM] £12.72 DT price = £1.15
  Candesartan cilexetil 32 mg Candesartan 32mg tablets | 28 tablet [PoM] £16.13 DT price = £1.59
- ▸ Amias (Takeda UK Ltd)
  Candesartan cilexetil 2 mg Amias 2mg tablets | 7 tablet [PoM] £3.58 DT price = £1.92
  Candesartan cilexetil 4 mg Amias 4mg tablets | 7 tablet [PoM] £3.88 DT price = £0.66 | 28 tablet [PoM] £9.78
  Candesartan cilexetil 8 mg Amias 8mg tablets | 28 tablet [PoM] £9.89 DT price = £0.98
  Candesartan cilexetil 16 mg Amias 16mg tablets | 28 tablet [PoM] £12.72 DT price = £1.15
  Candesartan cilexetil 32 mg Amias 32mg tablets | 28 tablet [PoM] £16.13 DT price = £1.59

⇱ 111

Losartan potassium

- **INDICATIONS AND DOSE**

Hypertension
- ▸ BY MOUTH
  - ▸ Child 6–17 years (under expert supervision) (body-weight 20–49 kg): Initially 700 micrograms/kg once daily (max.

per dose 25 mg), adjusted according to response to 50 mg daily, lower initial dose may be used in intravascular volume depletion; maximum 50 mg per day
  - ▸ Child 6–17 years (under expert supervision) (body-weight 50 kg and above): Initially 50 mg once daily, adjusted according to response to 1.4 mg/kg once daily; maximum 100 mg per day

Hypertension with intravascular volume depletion
- ▸ BY MOUTH
  - ▸ Child 6–17 years (under expert supervision) (body-weight 50 kg and above): Initially 25 mg once daily; adjusted according to response to 1.4 mg/kg once daily; maximum 100 mg per day

- **CAUTIONS** Severe heart failure
- **INTERACTIONS** → Appendix 1: angiotensin-II receptor antagonists
- **SIDE-EFFECTS**
- ▸ **Common or very common** Anaemia · malaise
- ▸ **Uncommon** Abdominal pain · angina · constipation · cough · diarrhoea · drowsiness · dyspnoea · headache · nausea · oedema · palpitation · pruritus · rash · sleep disorders · urticaria · vomiting
- ▸ **Rare** Atrial fibrillation · cerebrovascular accident · hepatitis · paraesthesia
- ▸ **Frequency not known** Arthralgia · depression · erectile dysfunction · Henoch-Schönlein purpura · hyponatraemia · myalgia · pancreatitis · photosensitivity · rhabdomyolysis · thrombocytopenia · tinnitus · vasculitis
- **HEPATIC IMPAIRMENT** Avoid—no information available.
- **RENAL IMPAIRMENT** Avoid if estimated glomerular filtration rate is less than 30 mL/minute/1.73 m² —no information available.
- **PRESCRIBING AND DISPENSING INFORMATION** Flavours of oral liquid formulations may include berry-citrus.

- **MEDICINAL FORMS**
There can be variation in the licensing of different medicines containing the same drug. Forms available from special-order manufacturers include: oral suspension, oral solution

Oral suspension
- ▸ Cozaar (Merck Sharp & Dohme Ltd)
  Losartan potassium 2.5 mg per 1 ml Cozaar 2.5mg/ml oral suspension sugar-free | 200 ml [PoM] £53.68 DT price = £53.68

Tablet
- ▸ Losartan potassium (Non-proprietary)
  Losartan potassium 12.5 mg Losartan 12.5mg tablets | 28 tablet [PoM] £30.00 DT price = £26.66
  Losartan potassium 25 mg Losartan 25mg tablets | 28 tablet [PoM] £16.18 DT price = £0.80
  Losartan potassium 50 mg Losartan 50mg tablets | 28 tablet [PoM] £12.80 DT price = £0.86
  Losartan potassium 100 mg Losartan 100mg tablets | 28 tablet [PoM] £16.18 DT price = £0.99
- ▸ Cozaar (Merck Sharp & Dohme Ltd)
  Losartan potassium 12.5 mg Cozaar 12.5mg tablets | 28 tablet [PoM] £9.70 DT price = £26.66
  Losartan potassium 25 mg Cozaar 25mg tablets | 28 tablet [PoM] £16.18 DT price = £0.80
  Losartan potassium 50 mg Cozaar 50mg tablets | 28 tablet [PoM] £12.80 DT price = £0.86
  Losartan potassium 100 mg Cozaar 100mg tablets | 28 tablet [PoM] £16.18 DT price = £0.99

Valsartan

F 111

- **INDICATIONS AND DOSE**

Hypertension

▸ BY MOUTH
- Child 6–17 years (under expert supervision) (body-weight 18–34 kg): Initially 40 mg once daily, adjusted according to response; maximum 80 mg per day
- Child 6–17 years (under expert supervision) (body-weight 35–79 kg): Initially 80 mg once daily, adjusted according to response; maximum 160 mg per day
- Child 6–17 years (under expert supervision) (body-weight 80 kg and above): Initially 80 mg once daily, adjusted according to response; maximum 320 mg per day

- **UNLICENSED USE** Capsules not licensed for use in children.
- **CONTRA-INDICATIONS** Biliary cirrhosis · cholestasis
- **INTERACTIONS** → Appendix 1: angiotensin-II receptor antagonists
- **SIDE-EFFECTS**
▸ **Uncommon** Abdominal pain · cough · diarrhoea · headache · malaise · nausea
▸ **Frequency not known** Anaemia · myalgia · neutropenia · pruritus · rash · renal failure · serum sickness · thrombocytopenia · vasculitis
- **HEPATIC IMPAIRMENT** Max. dose 80 mg daily in mild to moderate impairment. Avoid in severe hepatic impairment.
- **RENAL IMPAIRMENT** Avoid if estimated glomerular filtration rate is less than 30 mL/minute/1.73 m^2—no information available.

- **MEDICINAL FORMS**
There can be variation in the licensing of different medicines containing the same drug. Forms available from special-order manufacturers include: oral suspension, oral solution

Oral solution
▸ Diovan (Novartis Pharmaceuticals UK Ltd)
Valsartan 3 mg per 1 ml Diovan 3mg/1ml oral solution | 160 ml [PoM] £7.20

Tablet
▸ Valsartan (Non-proprietary)
Valsartan 40 mg Valsartan 40mg tablets | 7 tablet [PoM] £5.00 DT price = £3.11 | 28 tablet [PoM] no price available
Valsartan 80 mg Valsartan 80mg tablets | 28 tablet [PoM] £13.69 DT price = £13.69
Valsartan 160 mg Valsartan 160mg tablets | 28 tablet [PoM] £14.69 DT price = £14.69
Valsartan 320 mg Valsartan 320mg tablets | 28 tablet [PoM] £20.23 DT price = £13.01

Capsule
▸ Valsartan (Non-proprietary)
Valsartan 40 mg Valsartan 40mg capsules | 28 capsule [PoM] £13.97 DT price = £3.31
Valsartan 80 mg Valsartan 80mg capsules | 28 capsule [PoM] £13.97 DT price = £2.21
Valsartan 160 mg Valsartan 160mg capsules | 28 capsule [PoM] £18.41 DT price = £4.05

VASODILATORS ⟩ VASODILATOR ANTIHYPERTENSIVES

Hydralazine hydrochloride

- **INDICATIONS AND DOSE**

Resistant hypertension (adjunct)
▸ BY MOUTH
- Neonate: 250–500 micrograms/kg every 8–12 hours, increased if necessary to 2–3 mg/kg every 8 hours.

- Child 1 month–11 years: 250–500 micrograms/kg every 8–12 hours, increased if necessary to 7.5 mg/kg daily; maximum 200 mg per day
- Child 12–17 years: 25 mg twice daily, increased to 50–100 mg twice daily
▸ BY SLOW INTRAVENOUS INJECTION
- Neonate: 100–500 micrograms/kg, dose may be repeated if necessary every 4–6 hours; maximum 3 mg/kg per day.

- Child 1 month–11 years: 100–500 micrograms/kg, dose may be repeated if necessary every 4–6 hours; maximum 3 mg/kg per day; maximum 60 mg per day
- Child 12–17 years: 5–10 mg, dose may be repeated if necessary every 4–6 hours
▸ BY CONTINUOUS INTRAVENOUS INFUSION
- Neonate: 12.5–50 micrograms/kg/hour, continuous intravenous infusion is the preferred route in cardiac patients; maximum 2 mg/kg per day.

- Child 1 month–11 years: 12.5–50 micrograms/kg/hour, continuous intravenous infusion is the preferred route in cardiac patients; maximum 3 mg/kg per day
- Child 12–17 years: 3–9 mg/hour, continuous intravenous infusion is the preferred route in cardiac patients; maximum 3 mg/kg per day

- **UNLICENSED USE** Not licensed for use in children.
- **CONTRA-INDICATIONS** Acute porphyrias p. 577 · cor pulmonale · high output heart failure · idiopathic systemic lupus erythematosus · myocardial insufficiency due to mechanical obstruction · severe tachycardia
- **CAUTIONS** Cerebrovascular disease · occasionally blood pressure reduction too rapid even with low parenteral doses
- **INTERACTIONS** → Appendix 1: hydralazine
- **SIDE-EFFECTS**
▸ **Rare** Rashes
▸ **Frequency not known** Abnormal liver function · agitation · anorexia · anxiety · arthralgia · blood disorders · dizziness · dyspnoea · fever · fluid retention · flushing · gastro-intestinal disturbances · haematuria · haemolytic anaemia · headache · hypotension · increased lacrimation · jaundice · leucopenia · myalgia · nasal congestion · palpitation · paraesthesia · peripheral neuritis · polyneuritis · proteinuria · raised plasma creatinine · systemic lupus erythematosus-like syndrome after long-term therapy (especially in slow acetylator individuals) · tachycardia · thrombocytopenia
SIDE-EFFECTS, FURTHER INFORMATION
The incidence of side-effects is lower if the dose is kept low, but systemic lupus erythematosus should be suspected if there is unexplained weight loss, arthritis, or any other unexplained ill health.
- **PREGNANCY** Neonatal thrombocytopenia reported, but risk should be balanced against risk of uncontrolled maternal hypertension. Manufacturer advises avoid before third trimester.
- **BREAST FEEDING** Present in milk but not known to be harmful. Monitor infant in breast-feeding.
- **HEPATIC IMPAIRMENT** Reduce dose.
- **RENAL IMPAIRMENT** Reduce dose if estimated glomerular filtration rate less than 30 mL/minute/1.73 m^2.
- **MONITORING REQUIREMENTS** Manufacturer advises test for antinuclear factor and for proteinuria every 6 months and check acetylator status before increasing dose, but evidence of clinical value unsatisfactory.
- **DIRECTIONS FOR ADMINISTRATION**
▸ With oral use For administration *by mouth*, diluted injection may be given orally.

Cardiovascular system

▸ With intravenous use For *continuous intravenous infusion*, initially reconstitute 20 mg with 1 mL Water for Injections, then dilute with Sodium Chloride 0.9%. Incompatible with Glucose intravenous infusion. For *intravenous injection*, initially reconstitute 20 mg with 1 mL Water for Injections, then dilute to a concentration of 0.5–1 mg/mL with Sodium Chloride 0.9% and administer over 5–20 minutes.

● MEDICINAL FORMS
There can be variation in the licensing of different medicines containing the same drug. Forms available from special-order manufacturers include: oral suspension, oral solution

Tablet
EXCIPIENTS: May contain Gluten, propylene glycol
▸ **Hydralazine hydrochloride (Non-proprietary)**
Hydralazine hydrochloride 10 mg Apo-Hydralazine 10mg tablets | 100 tablet PoM no price available
Hydralazine hydrochloride 25 mg Hydralazine 25mg tablets | 56 tablet PoM £8.92 DT price = £6.60 | 84 tablet PoM £14.00
Hydralazine hydrochloride 50 mg Hydralazine 50mg tablets | 56 tablet PoM £16.82 DT price = £12.45
▸ **Apresoline (AMCo)**
Hydralazine hydrochloride 25 mg Apresoline 25mg tablets | 84 tablet PoM £3.38

Powder for solution for injection
▸ **Hydralazine hydrochloride (Non-proprietary)**
Hydralazine hydrochloride 20 mg Hydralazine 20mg powder for concentrate for solution for injection ampoules | 5 ampoule PoM £64.50
▸ **Apresoline (AMCo)**
Hydralazine hydrochloride 20 mg Apresoline 20mg powder for solution for injection ampoules | 5 ampoule PoM £11.09

Minoxidil

● INDICATIONS AND DOSE
Severe hypertension
▸ BY MOUTH
▸ Child 1 month–11 years: Initially 200 micrograms/kg daily in 1–2 divided doses, then increased in steps of 100–200 micrograms/kg, increased at intervals of at least 3 days; maximum 1 mg/kg per day
▸ Child 12–17 years: Initially 5 mg daily in 1–2 divided doses, then increased in steps of 5–10 mg daily, increased at intervals of at least 3 days, seldom necessary to exceed 50 mg daily; maximum 100 mg per day

● CONTRA-INDICATIONS Phaeochromocytoma
● CAUTIONS Acute porphyrias p. 577
● INTERACTIONS → Appendix 1: minoxidil
● PREGNANCY Avoid—possible toxicity including reduced placental perfusion. Neonatal hirsutism reported.
● BREAST FEEDING Present in milk but not known to be harmful.
● RENAL IMPAIRMENT Use with caution in significant impairment.

● MEDICINAL FORMS
There can be variation in the licensing of different medicines containing the same drug.
Tablet
▸ **Loniten (Pfizer Ltd)**
Minoxidil 2.5 mg Loniten 2.5mg tablets | 60 tablet PoM £8.88 DT price = £8.88
Minoxidil 5 mg Loniten 5mg tablets | 60 tablet PoM £15.83 DT price = £15.83
Minoxidil 10 mg Loniten 10mg tablets | 60 tablet PoM £30.68 DT price = £30.68

4.1a Hypertension associated with phaeochromocytoma

VASODILATORS ❭ PERIPHERAL VASODILATORS

Phenoxybenzamine hydrochloride

● INDICATIONS AND DOSE
Hypertension in phaeochromocytoma
▸ BY MOUTH
▸ Child: 0.5–1 mg/kg twice daily, adjusted according to response

● UNLICENSED USE Not licensed for use in children.
● CONTRA-INDICATIONS History of cerebrovascular accident
● CAUTIONS Avoid contact with skin (risk of contact sensitisation) · avoid in acute porphyrias p. 577 · carcinogenic in *animals* · cerebrovascular disease · congestive heart failure · severe ischaemic heart disease
● SIDE-EFFECTS
▸ Rare Gastro-intestinal disturbances
▸ Frequency not known Inhibition of ejaculation · lassitude · miosis · nasal congestion · postural hypotension (with dizziness and marked compensatory tachycardia)
● PREGNANCY Hypotension may occur in newborn.
● BREAST FEEDING May be present in milk.
● RENAL IMPAIRMENT Use with caution.
● DIRECTIONS FOR ADMINISTRATION For administration *by mouth*, capsules may be opened
● HANDLING AND STORAGE Owing to risk of contact sensitisation healthcare professionals should avoid contamination of hands.

● MEDICINAL FORMS
There can be variation in the licensing of different medicines containing the same drug. Forms available from special-order manufacturers include: oral suspension, oral solution
Capsule
▸ **Phenoxybenzamine hydrochloride (Non-proprietary)**
Phenoxybenzamine hydrochloride 10 mg Phenoxybenzamine 10mg capsules | 30 capsule PoM £97.38 DT price = £97.38

4.1b Hypertensive crises

Other drugs used for Hypertensive crises Esmolol hydrochloride, p. 103 · Labetalol hydrochloride, p. 101

VASODILATORS ❭ VASODILATOR ANTIHYPERTENSIVES

Sodium nitroprusside

● INDICATIONS AND DOSE
Hypertensive emergencies
▸ BY CONTINUOUS INTRAVENOUS INFUSION
▸ Neonate: Initially 500 nanograms/kg/minute, then increased in steps of 200 nanograms/kg/minute (max. per dose 8 micrograms/kg/minute) as required, max. 4 micrograms/kg/minute if used for longer than 24 hours.
▸ Child: Initially 500 nanograms/kg/minute, then increased in steps of 200 nanograms/kg/minute (max. per dose 8 micrograms/kg/minute) as required, max. 4 micrograms/kg/minute if used for longer than 24 hours

● UNLICENSED USE Not licensed for use in the UK.

- **CONTRA-INDICATIONS** Compensatory hypertension · Leber's optic atrophy · severe vitamin B$_{12}$ deficiency
- **CAUTIONS** Hyponatraemia · hypothermia · hypothyroidism · impaired cerebral circulation
- **INTERACTIONS** → Appendix 1: sodium nitroprusside
- **SIDE-EFFECTS** Abdominal pain · acute transient phlebitis · anxiety · dizziness · headache · nausea · palpitation · perspiration · reduced platelet count · retching · retrosternal discomfort

  SIDE-EFFECTS, FURTHER INFORMATION
- Side-effects associated with over rapid reduction in blood pressure: Headache, dizziness, nausea, retching, abdominal pain, perspiration, palpitation, anxiety, retrosternal discomfort—reduce infusion rate if any of these side-effects occur.

  Overdose
  Side-effects caused by excessive plasma concentration of the cyanide metabolite include tachycardia, sweating, hyperventilation, arrhythmias, marked metabolic acidosis (discontinue and give antidote, see cyanide in Emergency treatment of poisoning p. 803).
- **PREGNANCY** Avoid prolonged use—potential for accumulation of cyanide in fetus.
- **BREAST FEEDING** No information available. Caution advised due to thiocyanate metabolite.
- **HEPATIC IMPAIRMENT** Use with caution. Avoid in hepatic failure—cyanide or thiocyanate metabolites may accumulate.
- **RENAL IMPAIRMENT** Avoid prolonged use—cyanide or thiocyanate metabolites may accumulate.
- **MONITORING REQUIREMENTS** Monitor blood pressure (including intra-arterial blood pressure) and blood-cyanide concentration, and if treatment exceeds 3 days, also blood thiocyanate concentration.
- **TREATMENT CESSATION** Avoid sudden withdrawal—terminate infusion over 15–30 minutes.
- **DIRECTIONS FOR ADMINISTRATION** For *continuous intravenous infusion* in Glucose 5%, infuse *via* infusion device to allow precise control. For further details, consult product literature. Protect infusion from light.

- **MEDICINAL FORMS**
  There can be variation in the licensing of different medicines containing the same drug.
  Powder and solvent for solution for infusion
  - Sodium nitroprusside (Non-proprietary)
    Sodium nitroprusside dihydrate 50 mg Sodium nitroprusside 50mg powder and solvent for solution for infusion vials | 1 vial PoM no price available

4.1c Pulmonary hypertension

ANTITHROMBOTIC DRUGS > PROSTAGLANDINS, CARDIOVASCULAR

Epoprostenol

(Prostacyclin)

- **DRUG ACTION** Epoprostenol is a prostaglandin and a potent vasodilator. It is also a powerful inhibitor of platelet aggregation.

- **INDICATIONS AND DOSE**
  Persistent pulmonary hypertension of the newborn
  ▶ BY CONTINUOUS INTRAVENOUS INFUSION

  ▶ Neonate: Initially 2 nanograms/kg/minute (max. per dose 20 nanograms/kg/minute), adjusted according to response, rarely doses up to 40 nanograms/kg/minute are used.

  Idiopathic pulmonary arterial hypertension
  ▶ BY CONTINUOUS INTRAVENOUS INFUSION
  ▶ Child: Initially 2 nanograms/kg/minute, increased if necessary up to 40 nanograms/kg/minute

  PHARMACOKINETICS
  Short half-life of approximately 3 minutes, therefore it must be administered by continuous intravenous infusion.

- **UNLICENSED USE** Not licensed for use in children.
- **CONTRA-INDICATIONS** Pulmonary veno-occlusive disease · severe left ventricular dysfunction
- **CAUTIONS** Avoid abrupt withdrawal (risk of rebound pulmonary hypertension/pulmonary hypertensive crisis) · haemorrhagic diathesis
- **INTERACTIONS** → Appendix 1: epoprostenol
- **SIDE-EFFECTS**
  ▶ **Common or very common** Abdominal pain · anxiety · arthralgia · bleeding · bradycardia · chest pain · diarrhoea · flushing · headache · hypotension · jaw pain · nausea · sepsis · tachycardia · vomiting
  ▶ **Uncommon** Dry mouth · pulmonary oedema · sweating
  ▶ **Rare** Agitation · pallor
  ▶ **Frequency not known** Serious systemic hypotension
- **PREGNANCY** Manufacturer advises caution—no information available.
- **BREAST FEEDING** Manufacturer advises avoid—no information available.
- **MONITORING REQUIREMENTS**
  ▶ Anticoagulant monitoring required when given with anticoagulants.
  ▶ Monitor blood pressure.
- **TREATMENT CESSATION** Avoid abrupt withdrawal (risk of rebound pulmonary hypertension and pulmonary hypertensive crisis).
- **DIRECTIONS FOR ADMINISTRATION** Reconstitute using the glycine buffer diluent provided to make a concentrate (pH 10.5); filter the concentrate using the filter provided. The concentrate can be administered via a central venous catheter, alternatively it may be diluted further either with the glycine buffer diluent *or* to a minimum concentration of 1.43 micrograms/mL with Sodium Chloride 0.9%. Solution stable for 12 hours at room temperature, although some units use for 24 hours and allow for loss of potency; solution stable for 24 hours if prepared in glycine buffer diluent only and administered via an ambulatory cold pouch system (to maintain solution at 2–8°C). *Neonatal intensive care*, prepare a filtered concentrate of 10 micrograms/mL using the 500-microgram vial. *Neonate body-weight under 2 kg*, using the concentrate, dilute 150 micrograms/kg body-weight to a final volume of 50 mL with Sodium Chloride 0.9%; an intravenous infusion rate of 0.1 mL/hour provides a dose of 5 nanograms/kg/minute. *Neonate body-weight over 2 kg*, using the concentrate, dilute 60 micrograms/kg body-weight to a final volume of 50 mL with Sodium Chloride 0.9%; an intravenous infusion rate of 0.1 mL/hour provides a dose of 2 nanograms/kg/minute.

- **MEDICINAL FORMS**
  There can be variation in the licensing of different medicines containing the same drug.
  Powder for solution for infusion
  ▶ Veletri (Actelion Pharmaceuticals UK Ltd)
    Epoprostenol (as Epoprostenol sodium) 500 microgram Veletri 500microgram powder for solution for infusion vials | 1 vial PoM £24.44
    Epoprostenol (as Epoprostenol sodium) 1.5 mg Veletri 1.5mg powder for solution for infusion vials | 1 vial PoM £49.24

Cardiovascular system

2

Powder and solvent for solution for infusion

▸ Flolan (GlaxoSmithKline UK Ltd)
Epoprostenol (as Epoprostenol sodium) 500 microgram Flolan 500microgram powder and solvent (pH10.5) for solution for infusion vials | 1 vial [PoM] £22.22
Flolan 500microgram powder and solvent (pH12) for solution for infusion vials | 1 vial [PoM] £22.22
Epoprostenol (as Epoprostenol sodium) 1.5 mg Flolan 1.5mg powder and solvent (pH10.5) for solution for infusion vials | 1 vial [PoM] £44.76
Flolan 1.5mg powder and solvent (pH12) for solution for infusion vials | 1 vial [PoM] £44.76

Iloprost

● **INDICATIONS AND DOSE**

Idiopathic or familial pulmonary arterial hypertension (initiated under specialist supervision)

▸ BY INHALATION OF NEBULISED SOLUTION

▸ Child 8–17 years: Initially 2.5 micrograms for 1 dose, increased to 5 micrograms for 1 dose, increased if tolerated to 5 micrograms 6–9 times a day, adjusted according to response; reduced if not tolerated to 2.5 micrograms 6–9 times a day, reduce to lower maintenance dose if high dose not tolerated

Raynaud's syndrome

▸ BY INTRAVENOUS INFUSION

▸ Child 12–17 years: Initially 30 nanograms/kg/hour, increased to 60–120 nanograms/kg/hour daily for 3–5 days, dose to be given over 6 hours, dose increase should be performed gradually

● **UNLICENSED USE** Not licensed for use in children.

● **CONTRA-INDICATIONS** Conditions which increase risk of haemorrhage · congenital or acquired valvular defects of the myocardium · decompensated cardiac failure (unless under close medical supervision) · pulmonary veno-occlusive disease · severe arrhythmias · severe coronary heart disease

● **CAUTIONS**

GENERAL CAUTIONS
Hypotension (do not initiate if systolic blood pressure below 85 mmHg) · unstable pulmonary hypertension with advanced right heart failure
SPECIFIC CAUTIONS
▸ When used by inhalation Acute pulmonary infection · severe asthma

● **INTERACTIONS** → Appendix 1: iloprost

● **SIDE-EFFECTS**

▸ **Common or very common** Chest pain · cough · diarrhoea · dyspnoea · haemorrhage · headache · hypotension · jaw pain · nausea · oral irritation · rash · throat pain · vomiting
▸ **Frequency not known** Bronchospasm · taste disturbance · thrombocytopenia · wheezing

● **PREGNANCY**

▸ When used by inhalation Use if potential benefit outweighs risk.

● **BREAST FEEDING**

▸ When used by inhalation Manufacturer advises avoid—no information available.

● **HEPATIC IMPAIRMENT**
Dose may need to be halved in liver cirrhosis.
▸ When used by inhalation Initially 2.5 micrograms at intervals of 3–4 hours (max. 6 times daily), adjusted according to response (consult product literature).

● **DIRECTIONS FOR ADMINISTRATION**

▸ With intravenous use For intravenous infusion dilute to a concentration of 200 nanograms/mL with Glucose 5% or Sodium Chloride 0.9%; alternatively, may be diluted to a concentration of 2 micrograms/mL and given via syringe driver.

▸ When used by inhalation For inhaled treatment, to minimise accidental exposure use only with nebulisers listed in Ventavis® product literature in a well ventilated room.

● **PRESCRIBING AND DISPENSING INFORMATION**

▸ When used by inhalation Delivery characteristics of nebuliser devices may vary—only switch devices under medical supervision.
▸ With intravenous use Concentrate for infusion available on a named patient basis from Bayer Schering in 0.5 mL and 1 mL ampoules.

● **MEDICINAL FORMS**
There can be variation in the licensing of different medicines containing the same drug.

Nebuliser liquid

▸ Ventavis (Bayer Plc)
Iloprost (as Iloprost trometamol) 10 microgram per 1 ml Ventavis 10micrograms/ml nebuliser solution 1ml ampoules | 30 ampoule [PoM] £400.19 | 168 ampou e [PoM] £2,241.08

ENDOTHELIN RECEPTOR ANTAGONISTS

Bosentan

● **INDICATIONS AND DOSE**

Pulmonary arterial hypertension (initiated under specialist supervision)

▸ BY MOUTH
▸ Child 2–17 years (body-weight 10–20 kg): Initially 31.25 mg once daily for 4 weeks, then increased to 31.25 mg twice daily
▸ Child 2–17 years (body-weight 20–40 kg): Initially 31.25 mg twice daily for 4 weeks, then increased to 62.5 mg twice daily
▸ Child 12–17 years (body-weight 40 kg and above): Initially 62.5 mg twice daily for 4 weeks, then increased to 125 mg twice daily (max. per dose 250 mg)

● **CONTRA-INDICATIONS** Acute porphyrias p. 577

● **CAUTIONS** Not to be initiated if systemic systolic blood pressure is below 85 mmHg

● **INTERACTIONS** → Appendix 1: bosentan

● **SIDE-EFFECTS**

▸ **Common or very common** Anaemia · diarrhoea · flushing · gastro-oesophageal reflux · headache · hypotension · oedema · palpitation · syncope
▸ **Uncommon** Leucopenia · neutrcpenia · thrombocytopenia
▸ **Rare** Liver cirrhosis · liver failure

● **CONCEPTION AND CONTRACEPTION** Effective contraception required during administration (hormonal contraception not considered effective). Monthly pregnancy tests advised.

● **PREGNANCY** Avoid (teratogenic in animal studies).

● **BREAST FEEDING** Manufacturer advises avoid—no information available.

● **HEPATIC IMPAIRMENT** Avoid in moderate and severe impairment.

● **MONITORING REQUIREMENTS**

▸ Monitor haemoglobin before and during treatment (monthly for first 4 months, then 3-monthly).
▸ Monitor liver function before treatment, at monthly intervals during treatment, and 2 weeks after dose increase (reduce dose or suspend treatment if liver enzymes raised significantly)—discontinue if symptoms of liver impairment.

● **TREATMENT CESSATION** Avoid abrupt withdrawal—withdraw treatment gradually.

● **DIRECTIONS FOR ADMINISTRATION** Tablets may be cut, or suspended in water or non-acidic liquid. Suspension is stable at room-temperature (max. 25°C) for 24 hours.

- **MEDICINAL FORMS**
There can be variation in the licensing of different medicines containing the same drug.

Tablet
- Tracleer (Actelion Pharmaceuticals UK Ltd)
Bosentan (as Bosentan monohydrate) 62.5 mg Tracleer 62.5mg tablets | 56 tablet PoM £1,510.21
Bosentan (as Bosentan monohydrate) 125 mg Tracleer 125mg tablets | 56 tablet PoM £1,510.21

PHOSPHODIESTERASE TYPE-5 INHIBITORS

Sildenafil

- **INDICATIONS AND DOSE**

Pulmonary arterial hypertension (initiated under specialist supervision)
- BY MOUTH

- Neonate: Initially 250–500 micrograms/kg every 4–8 hours, adjusted according to response, start with the lower dose and frequency, especially if used with other vasodilators; maximum 30 mg per day.

- Child 1-11 months: Initially 250–500 micrograms/kg every 4–8 hours, adjusted according to response, start with the lower dose and frequency, especially if used with other vasodilators; maximum 30 mg per day
- Child 1-17 years (body-weight up to 20 kg): 10 mg 3 times a day
- Child 1-17 years (body-weight 20 kg and above): 20 mg 3 times a day

DOSE ADJUSTMENTS DUE TO INTERACTIONS
Manufacturer advises reduce dose with concurrent use of moderate and potent inhibitors of CYP3A4 (avoid with ketoconazole, itraconazole and ritonavir)—no specific recommendation made for children.

- **UNLICENSED USE** Not licensed for use in children under 1 year.
- **CONTRA-INDICATIONS** Hereditary degenerative retinal disorders · history of non-arteritic anterior ischaemic optic neuropathy · recent history of stroke · sickle-cell anaemia
- **CAUTIONS** Active peptic ulceration · anatomical deformation of the penis · autonomic dysfunction · bleeding disorders · cardiovascular disease · hypotension (avoid if severe) · intravascular volume depletion · left ventricular outflow obstruction · ocular disorders · predisposition to priapism · pulmonary veno-occlusive disease
- **INTERACTIONS** → Appendix 1: phosphodiesterase type-5 inhibitors
- **SIDE-EFFECTS**
- **Common or very common** Abdominal distension · alopecia · anaemia · anxiety · back pain · bronchitis · cellulitis · cough · diarrhoea · dry mouth · dyspepsia · epistaxis · fever · flushing · gastritis · gastro-oesophageal reflux · haemorrhoids · headache · influenza-like symptoms · insomnia · limb pain · migraine · myalgia · nasal congestion · night sweats · oedema · painful red eyes · paraesthesia · photophobia · retinal haemorrhage · tremor · vertigo · visual disturbances
- **Uncommon** Gynaecomastia · haematuria · penile haemorrhage · priapism
- **Frequency not known** Non-arteritic anterior ischaemic optic neuropathy (discontinue if sudden visual impairment occurs) · sudden hearing loss (advise patient to seek medical help) · rash · retinal vascular occlusion
- **PREGNANCY** Use only if potential benefit outweighs risk—no evidence of harm in *animal* studies.
- **BREAST FEEDING** Manufacturer advises avoid—no information available.

- **HEPATIC IMPAIRMENT** Reduce dose if not tolerated in mild to moderate impairment. Manufacturer advises avoid in severe impairment.
- **RENAL IMPAIRMENT** Reduce dose if not tolerated
- **TREATMENT CESSATION** Avoid abrupt withdrawal.
- **PATIENT AND CARER ADVICE**
Medicines for Children leaflet: Sildenafil for pulmonary hypertension www.medicinesforchildren.org.uk/sildenafil-for-pulmonary-hypertension
- **NATIONAL FUNDING/ACCESS DECISIONS**
Scottish Medicines Consortium (SMC) Decisions
The *Scottish Medicines Consortium* has advised (October 2012) that sildenafil (*Revatio*®) is accepted for restricted use within NHS Scotland for the treatment of pulmonary arterial hypertension in children aged 1–17 years; sildenafil should only be prescribed on the advice of specialists in the Scottish Pulmonary Vascular Unit or the Scottish Adult Congenital Cardiac Service.

- **MEDICINAL FORMS**
There can be variation in the licensing of different medicines containing the same drug. Forms available from special-order manufacturers include: oral suspension, oral solution

Tablet
- Sildenafil (Non-proprietary)
Sildenafil (as Sildenafil citrate) 20 mg Sildenafil 20mg tablets | 90 tablet PoM £379.38–£424.01
- Revatio (Pfizer Ltd)
Sildenafil (as Sildenafil citrate) 20 mg Revatio 20mg tablets | 90 tablet PoM £446.33

Oral suspension
- Revatio (Pfizer Ltd)
Sildenafil (as Sildenafil citrate) 10 mg per 1 ml Revatio 10mg/ml oral suspension sugar-free | 112 ml PoM £186.75

VASODILATORS > PERIPHERAL VASODILATORS

Tolazoline

- **DRUG ACTION** Tolazoline is an alpha-blocker and produces both pulmonary and systemic vasodilation.

- **INDICATIONS AND DOSE**

Correction of pulmonary vasospasm in neonates
- INITIALLY BY INTRAVENOUS INJECTION

- Neonate: Initially 1 mg/kg, to be given over 2–5 minutes, followed by (by continuous intravenous infusion) maintenance 200 micrograms/kg/hour if required, careful blood pressure monitoring should be carried out, doses above 300 micrograms/kg/hour associated with cardiotoxicity and renal failure.

- BY ENDOTRACHEAL TUBE

- Neonate: 200 micrograms/kg.

- **UNLICENSED USE** Not licensed for use in children.
- **CONTRA-INDICATIONS** Peptic ulcer disease
- **CAUTIONS** Cardiotoxic accumulation may occur with continuous infusion (particularly in renal impairment) · mitral stenosis
- **SIDE-EFFECTS** Blood dyscrasias · blotchy skin · cardiac arrhythmias · diarrhoea · epigastric pain · flushing · haematuria · haemorrhage (with high doses) · headache · marked hypertension (with high doses) · metabolic alkalosis · nausea · oliguria · renal failure (with high doses) · severe hypotension (with high doses) · shivering · sweating · tachycardia · thrombocytopenia · vomiting
- **RENAL IMPAIRMENT** Lower doses may be necessary. Accumulates in renal impairment. Risk of cardiotoxicity.
- **MONITORING REQUIREMENTS** Monitor blood pressure regularly for sustained systemic hypotension.

Cardiovascular system

2

● **DIRECTIONS FOR ADMINISTRATION** For *continuous intravenous infusion*, dilute with Glucose 5% or Sodium Chloride 0.9%. Prepare a fresh solution every 24 hours. For *endotracheal administration*, dilute with 0.5–1 mL of Sodium Chloride 0.9%.

● **MEDICINAL FORMS**
There can be variation in the licensing of different medicines containing the same drug. Forms available from special-order manufacturers include: solution for injection

4.2 Hypotension and shock

Sympathomimetics

Overview

The properties of sympathomimetics vary according to whether they act on alpha or on beta adrenergic receptors. Response to sympathomimetics can also vary considerably in children, particularly in neonates. It is important to titrate the dose to the desired effect and to monitor the child closely.

Inotropic sympathomimetics

Dopamine hydrochloride p. 119 has a variable, unpredictable, and dose dependent impact on vascular tone. Low dose infusion normally causes vasodilatation, but there is little evidence that this is clinically beneficial; moderate doses increase myocardial contractility and cardiac output in older children, but in neonates moderate doses may cause a reduction in cardiac output. High doses cause vasoconstriction and increase vascular resistance, and should therefore be used with caution following cardiac surgery, or where there is co-existing neonatal pulmonary hypertension.

In neonates the response to inotropic sympathomimetics varies considerably, particularly in those born prematurely; careful dose titration and monitoring are necessary.

Isoprenaline injection is available from 'special-order' manufacturers or specialist importing companies.

Shock

Shock is a medical emergency associated with a high mortality. The underlying causes of shock such as haemorrhage, sepsis or myocardial insufficiency should be corrected. Additional treatment is dependent on the type of shock.

Septic shock is associated with severe hypovolaemia (due to vasodilation and capillary leak) which should be corrected with crystalloids or colloids. If hypotension persists despite volume replacement, dopamine hydrochloride should be started. For shock refractory to treatment with dopamine hydrochloride, if cardiac output is high and peripheral vascular resistance is low (warm shock), noradrenaline/norepinephrine p. 120 should be added *or* if cardiac output is low and peripheral vascular resistance is high (cold shock), adrenaline/epinephrine p. 132 should be added. Additionally, in cold shock, a vasodilator such as milrinone p. 124, glyceryl trinitrate p. 132, or sodium nitroprusside p. 114 (on specialist advice only) can be used to reduce vascular resistance.

If the shock is resistant to volume expansion and catecholamines, and there is suspected or proven adrenal insufficiency, low dose hydrocortisone p. 420 can be used. ACTH-stimulated plasma-cortisol concentration should be measured; however, hydrocortisone can be started without such information. Alternatively, if the child is resistant to catecholamines, and vascular resistance is low, vasopressin p. 65 can be added.

Neonatal septic shock can be complicated by the transition from fetal to neonatal circulation. Treatment to reverse right ventricular failure, by decreasing pulmonary artery pressures, is commonly needed in neonates with fluid-refractory shock and persistent pulmonary hypertension of the newborn. Rapid administration of fluid in neonates with patent ductus arteriosus may cause left-to-right shunting and congestive heart failure induced by ventricular overload.

In *cardiogenic shock*, the aim is to improve cardiac output and to reduce the afterload on the heart. If central venous pressure is low, cautious volume expansion with a colloid or crystalloid can be used. An inotrope such as adrenaline/epinephrine or dopamine hydrochloride should be given to increase cardiac output. Dobutamine p. 119 is a peripheral vasodilator and is an alternative if hypotension is not significant.

Milrinone has both inotropic and vasodilatory effects and can be used when vascular resistance is high. Alternatively, glyceryl trinitrate or sodium nitroprusside (on specialist advice only) can be used to reduce vasoconstriction.

Hypovolaemic shock should be treated with a crystalloid or colloid solution (or whole or reconstituted blood if source of hypovolaemia is haemorrhage) and further steps to improve cardiac output and decrease vascular resistance can be taken, as in cardiogenic shock.

The use of sympathomimetic inotropes and vasoconstrictors should preferably be confined to the intensive care setting and undertaken with invasive haemodynamic monitoring.

See also advice on the management of anaphylactic shock in Antihistamines, allergen immunotherapy and allergic emergencies p. 165.

Vasoconstrictor sympathomimetics

Vasoconstrictor sympathomimetics raise blood pressure transiently by acting on alpha-adrenergic receptors to constrict peripheral vessels. They are sometimes used as an emergency method of elevating blood pressure where other measures have failed.

The danger of vasoconstrictors is that although they raise blood pressure they also reduce perfusion of vital organs such as the kidney.

Ephedrine hydrochloride p. 120 is used to reverse hypotension caused by spinal and epidural anaesthesia.

Metaraminol p. 120 is used as a vasopressor during cardiopulmonary bypass.

Phenylephrine hydrochloride p. 121 causes peripheral vasoconstriction and increases arterial pressure.

Ephedrine hydrochloride, metaraminol and phenylephrine hydrochloride are rarely needed in children and should be used under specialist supervision.

Noradrenaline/norepinephrine is reserved for children with low systemic vascular resistance that is unresponsive to fluid resuscitation following septic shock, spinal shock, and anaphylaxis.

Adrenaline/epinephrine is mainly used for its inotropic action. Low doses (acting on beta receptors) cause systemic and pulmonary vasodilation, with some increase in heart rate and stroke volume and an increase in contractility; high doses act predominantly on alpha receptors causing intense systemic vasoconstriction.

SYMPATHOMIMETICS ＞ INOTROPIC

Dobutamine

- **DRUG ACTION** Dobutamine is a cardiac stimulant which acts on beta$_1$ receptors in cardiac muscle, and increases contractility with little effect on rate.

- **INDICATIONS AND DOSE**

Inotropic support in low cardiac output states, after cardiac surgery, cardiomyopathies, shock
  - ▸ BY CONTINUOUS INTRAVENOUS INFUSION

  - ▸ Neonate: Initially 5 micrograms/kg/minute, then adjusted according to response to 2–20 micrograms/kg/minute, doses as low as 0.5–1 microgram/kg/minute have been used.

  - ▸ Child: Initially 5 micrograms/kg/minute, then adjusted according to response to 2–20 micrograms/kg/minute, doses as low as 0.5–1 microgram/kg/minute have been used

- **CONTRA-INDICATIONS** Phaeochromocytoma
- **CAUTIONS** Acute heart failure · acute myocardial infarction · arrhythmias · correct hypercapnia before starting and during treatment · correct hypovolaemia before starting and during treatment · correct hypoxia before starting and during treatment · correct metabolic acidosis before starting and during treatment · diabetes mellitus · extravasation may cause tissue necrosis · extreme caution or avoid in marked obstruction of cardiac ejection (such as idiopathic hypertrophic subaortic stenosis) · hyperthyroidism · ischaemic heart disease · occlusive vascular disease · severe hypotension · susceptibility to angle-closure glaucoma · tachycardia · tolerance may develop with continuous infusions longer than 72 hours
- **INTERACTIONS** → Appendix 1: Sympathomimetics, inotropic
- **SIDE-EFFECTS**
- ▸ **Rare** Psychosis
- ▸ **Very rare** Angle-closure glaucoma · AV block · bradycardia · cardiac arrest · coronary artery spasm · hypokalaemia · myocardial infarction · petechial bleeding
- ▸ **Frequency not known** Anxiety · arrhythmias · bronchospasm · cerebral haemorrhage · chest pain · dyspnoea · eosinophilia · fever · headache · hypertension (marked increase in systolic blood pressure indicates overdose) · hypotension · increased urinary urgency · myoclonic spasm · nausea · palpitation · paraesthesia · phlebitis · pruritus of scalp · pulmonary oedema · rash · reduced platelet aggregation (on prolonged use) · tachycardia · tremor · vomiting
- **PREGNANCY** No evidence of harm in *animal* studies—manufacturers advise use only if potential benefit outweighs risk.
- **BREAST FEEDING** Manufacturers advise avoid—no information available.
- **DIRECTIONS FOR ADMINISTRATION** Dobutamine injection should be diluted before use or given undiluted with syringe pump. Dobutamine concentrate for intravenous infusion should be diluted before use.
  For *continuous intravenous infusion*, using infusion pump, dilute to a concentration of 0.5–1 mg/mL (max. 5 mg/mL if fluid restricted) with Glucose 5% *or* Sodium Chloride 0.9%; infuse higher concentration solutions through central venous catheter only. Incompatible with bicarbonate and other strong alkaline solutions.
  Neonatal intensive care, dilute 30 mg/kg body-weight to a final volume of 50 mL with infusion fluid; an intravenous infusion rate of 0.5 mL/hour provides a dose of 5 micrograms/kg/minute; max. concentration of 5 mg/mL; infuse higher concentration solutions through central venous catheter only. Incompatible with bicarbonate and other strong alkaline solutions.

- **MEDICINAL FORMS**
  There can be variation in the licensing of different medicines containing the same drug.
  Solution for infusion
  EXCIPIENTS: May contain Sulfites
  - ▸ **Dobutamine (Non-proprietary)**
    Dobutamine (as Dobutamine hydrochloride) 5 mg per 1 ml Dobutamine 250mg/50ml solution for infusion vials | 1 vial PoM £7.50
    Dobutamine (as Dobutamine hydrochloride) 12.5 mg per 1 ml Dobutamine 250mg/20ml concentrate for solution for infusion ampoules | 5 ampoule PoM £26.00–£26.25

Dopamine hydrochloride

- **DRUG ACTION** Dopamine is a cardiac stimulant which acts on beta$_1$ receptors in cardiac muscle, and increases contractility with little effect on rate.

- **INDICATIONS AND DOSE**

To correct the haemodynamic imbalance due to acute hypotension, shock, cardiac failure, adjunct following cardiac surgery
  - ▸ BY CONTINUOUS INTRAVENOUS INFUSION

  - ▸ Neonate: Initially 3 micrograms/kg/minute (max. per dose 20 micrograms/kg/minute), adjusted according to response.

  - ▸ Child: Initially 5 micrograms/kg/minute (max. per dose 20 micrograms/kg/minute), adjusted according to response

- **UNLICENSED USE** Not licensed for use in children under 12 years.
- **CONTRA-INDICATIONS** Phaeochromocytoma · tachyarrhythmia
- **CAUTIONS** Correct hypovolaemia · hypertension (may raise blood pressure) · hyperthyroidism
- **INTERACTIONS** → Appendix 1: Sympathomimetics, inotropic
- **SIDE-EFFECTS**
- ▸ **Common or very common** Chest pain · dyspnoea · headache · hypotension · nausea · palpitation · tachycardia · vasoconstriction · vomiting
- ▸ **Uncommon** Bradycardia · gangrene · hypertension · mydriasis
- ▸ **Rare** Fatal ventricular arrhythmias
- **PREGNANCY** No evidence of harm in *animal* studies—manufacturer advises use only if potential benefit outweighs risk.
- **BREAST FEEDING** May suppress lactation—not known to be harmful.
- **DIRECTIONS FOR ADMINISTRATION** Dopamine concentrate for intravenous infusion to be diluted before use.
  For *continuous intravenous infusion*, dilute to a max. concentration of 3.2 mg/mL with Glucose 5% *or* Sodium Chloride 0.9%. Infuse higher concentrations through central venous catheter using a syringe pump to avoid extravasation and fluid overload. Incompatible with bicarbonate and other alkaline solutions.
  Neonatal intensive care, dilute 30 mg/kg body-weight to a final volume of 50 mL with infusion fluid; an intravenous infusion rate of 0.3 mL/hour provides a dose of 3 micrograms/kg/minute; max. concentration of 3.2 mg/mL; infuse higher concentrations through central venous catheter. Incompatible with bicarbonate and other alkaline solutions.

2

Cardiovascular system

- **MEDICINAL FORMS**
  There can be variation in the licensing of different medicines containing the same drug. Forms available from special-order manufacturers include: solution for infusion

  Solution for infusion
  ▸ Dopamine hydrochloride (Non-proprietary)
  Dopamine hydrochloride 40 mg per 1 ml Dopamine 200mg/5ml solution for infusion ampoules | 5 ampoule [PoM] £20.00 | 10 ampoule [PoM] £9.04
  Dopamine 200mg/5ml concentrate for solution for infusion ampoules | 10 ampoule [PoM] no price available
  Dopamine hydrochloride 160 mg per 1 ml Dopamine 800mg/5ml solution for infusion ampoules | 10 ampoule [PoM] £34.00

SYMPATHOMIMETICS ❭ VASOCONSTRICTOR

Ephedrine hydrochloride

- **INDICATIONS AND DOSE**

  Reversal of hypotension from spinal or epidural anaesthesia
  ▸ BY SLOW INTRAVENOUS INJECTION
  ▸ Child 1–11 years: 500–750 micrograms/kg every 3–4 minutes, adjusted according to response, alternatively 17–25 mg/m² every 3–4 minutes, adjusted according to response, injection solution to contain ephedrine hydrochloride 3 mg/ml; maximum 30 mg per course
  ▸ Child 12–17 years: 3–7.5 mg every 3–4 minutes (max. per dose 9 mg), adjusted according to response, injection solution to contain ephedrine hydrochloride 3 mg/ml; maximum 30 mg per course

- **CAUTIONS** Diabetes mellitus · hypertension · hyperthyroidism · susceptibility to angle-closure glaucoma
- **INTERACTIONS** → Appendix 1: sympathomimetics, vasoconstrictor
- **SIDE-EFFECTS**
  ▸ **Common or very common** Anginal pain · anorexia · anxiety · arrhythmias · changes in blood-glucose concentration · confusion · difficulty in micturition · dizziness · dyspnoea · flushing · headache · hypersalivation · insomnia · nausea · psychoses · restlessness · sweating · tachycardia · tremor · urine retention · vasoconstriction with hypertension · vasodilation with hypotension · vomiting ·
  ▸ **Very rare** Angle-closure glaucoma
  ▸ **Frequency not known** Bradycardia · increased lacrimation (can have adverse effects on contact lens wear)
- **PREGNANCY** Increased fetal heart rate reported with parenteral ephedrine.
- **BREAST FEEDING** Present in milk; manufacturer advises avoid—irritability and disturbed sleep reported.
- **RENAL IMPAIRMENT** Use with caution.
- **DIRECTIONS FOR ADMINISTRATION** For *slow intravenous injection*, give via central venous catheter using a solution containing ephedrine hydrochloride 3 mg/ml.

- **MEDICINAL FORMS**
  There can be variation in the licensing of different medicines containing the same drug.

  Solution for injection
  ▸ Ephedrine hydrochloride (Non-proprietary)
  Ephedrine hydrochloride 3 mg per 1 ml Ephedrine 30mg/10ml solution for injection ampoules | 10 ampoule [PoM] £76.87
  Ephedrine 30mg/10ml solution for injection pre-filled syringes | 1 pre-filled disposable injection [PoM] £7.59–£9.50 | 12 pre-filled disposable injection [PoM] £114.00
  Ephedrine hydrochloride 30 mg per 1 ml Ephedrine 30mg/1ml solution for injection ampoules | 10 ampoule [PoM] £4.98–£5.03

Metaraminol

- **INDICATIONS AND DOSE**

  Acute hypotension
  ▸ BY INTRAVENOUS INFUSION
  ▸ Child 12–17 years: 15–100 mg, adjusted according to response

  Emergency treatment of acute hypotension
  ▸ INITIALLY BY INTRAVENOUS INJECTION
  ▸ Child 12–17 years: Initially 0.5–5 mg, then (by intravenous infusion) 15–100 mg, adjusted according to response

- **UNLICENSED USE** Not licensed for use in children.
- **CONTRA-INDICATIONS** Hypertension
- **CAUTIONS** Cirrhosis · coronary vascular thrombosis · diabetes mellitus · extravasation at injection site may cause necrosis · following myocardial infarction · hypercapnia · hyperthyroidism · hypoxia · mesenteric vascular thrombosis · peripheral vascular thrombosis · Prinzmetal's variant angina · susceptibility to angle-closure glaucoma · uncorrected hypovolaemia

  CAUTIONS, FURTHER INFORMATION
  ▸ Hypertensive response Metaraminol has a longer duration of action than noradrenaline, and an excessive vasopressor response may cause a prolonged rise in blood pressure.
- **INTERACTIONS** → Appendix 1: sympathomimetics, vasoconstrictor
- **SIDE-EFFECTS** Angle-closure glaucoma · anorexia · anxiety · arrhythmias · bradycardia · confusion · dyspnoea · fatal ventricular arrhythmia reported in Laennec's cirrhosis · headache · hypertension · hypoxia · insomnia · nausea · palpitation · peripheral ischaemia · psychosis · tachycardia · tremor · urinary retention · vomiting · weakness
- **PREGNANCY** May reduce placental perfusion—manufacturer advises use only if potential benefit outweighs risk.
- **BREAST FEEDING** Manufacturer advises caution—no information available.
- **MONITORING REQUIREMENTS** Monitor blood pressure and rate of flow frequently.
- **DIRECTIONS FOR ADMINISTRATION** For *intravenous infusion*, dilute to a concentration of 30–200 micrograms/mL with Glucose 5% or Sodium Chloride 0.9% and give through a central venous catheter.

- **MEDICINAL FORMS**
  There can be variation in the licensing of different medicines containing the same drug. Forms available from special-order manufacturers include: solution for injection

  Solution for injection
  ▸ Metaraminol (Non-proprietary)
  Metaraminol (as Metaraminol tartrate) 10 mg per 1 ml Metaraminol 10mg/1ml solution for injection ampoules | 10 ampoule [PoM] £31.97

Noradrenaline/norepinephrine

- **INDICATIONS AND DOSE**

  Acute hypotension (septic shock) | Shock secondary to excessive vasodilation (as noradrenaline)
  ▸ BY CONTINUOUS INTRAVENOUS INFUSION

  ▸ Neonate: 20–100 nanograms/kg/minute (max. per dose 1 microgram/kg/minute), adjusted according to response.

  ▸ Child: 20–100 nanograms/kg/minute (max. per dose 1 microgram/kg/minute), adjusted according to response

DOSE EQUIVALENCE AND CONVERSION
▸ 1 mg of noradrenaline base is equivalent to 2 mg of noradrenaline acid tartrate. **Doses expressed as the base.**

● **UNLICENSED USE** Not licensed for use in children.
● **CONTRA-INDICATIONS** Hypertension
● **CAUTIONS** Coronary vascular thrombosis · diabetes mellitus · extravasation at injection site may cause necrosis · following myocardial infarction · hypercapnia · hyperthyroidism · hypoxia · mesenteric vascular thrombosis · peripheral vascular thrombosis · Prinzmetal's variant angina · susceptibility to angle-closure glaucoma · uncorrected hypovolaemia
● **INTERACTIONS** → Appendix 1: sympathomimetics, vasoconstrictor
● **SIDE-EFFECTS** Angle-closure glaucoma · anorexia · anxiety · arrhythmias · bradycardia · confusion · dyspnoea · headache · hypertension · hypoxia · insomnia · nausea · palpitation · peripheral ischaemia · psychosis · tachycardia · tremor · urinary retention · vomiting · weakness
● **PREGNANCY** Avoid—may reduce placental perfusion.
● **MONITORING REQUIREMENTS** Monitor blood pressure and rate of flow frequently.
● **DIRECTIONS FOR ADMINISTRATION**
For *continuous intravenous infusion*, dilute to a max. concentration of noradrenaline (base) 40 micrograms/mL (higher concentrations can be used if fluid-restricted) with Glucose 5% or Sodium Chloride and Glucose. Infuse through central venous catheter; discard if discoloured. Incompatible with bicarbonate or alkaline solutions.
Neonatal intensive care, dilute 600 micrograms(base)/kg body-weight to a final volume of 50 mL with infusion fluid; an intravenous infusion rate of 0.1 mL/hour provides a dose of 20 nanograms(base)/kg/minute; infuse through central venous catheter; max. concentration of noradrenaline (base) 40 micrograms/mL (higher concentrations can be used if fluid-restricted). Discard if discoloured. Incompatible with bicarbonate or alkaline solutions.
● **PRESCRIBING AND DISPENSING INFORMATION** For a period of time, preparations on the UK market may be described as either noradrenaline base or noradrenaline acid tartrate; doses in the BNF are expressed as the base.

● **MEDICINAL FORMS**
There can be variation in the licensing of different medicines containing the same drug. Forms available from special-order manufacturers include: infusion, solution for infusion

Solution for infusion
▸ **Noradrenaline/norepinephrine (Non-proprietary)**
Noradrenaline (as Noradrenaline acid tartrate) 1 mg per 1 ml Noradrenaline (Norepinephrine) 4mg/4ml concentrate for solution for infusion ampoules | 10 ampoule [PoM] £44.00
Noradrenaline (Norepinephrine) 8mg/8ml concentrate for solution for infusion ampoules | 10 ampoule [PoM] £116.00
Noradrenaline (base) 2mg/2ml solution for infusion ampoules | 5 ampoule [PoM] £12.00 (Hospital only)
Noradrenaline (base) 4mg/4ml solution for infusion ampoules | 5 ampoule [PoM] £22.00 (Hospital only)
Noradrenaline (base) 4mg/4ml concentrate for solution for infusion ampoules | 10 ampoule [PoM] £58.00
Noradrenaline (Norepinephrine) 2mg/2ml concentrate for solution for Infusion ampoules | 5 ampoule [PoM] £11.00

Phenylephrine hydrochloride

● **INDICATIONS AND DOSE**
Acute hypotension
▸ BY SUBCUTANEOUS INJECTION, OR BY INTRAMUSCULAR INJECTION
▸ Child 1–11 years: 100 micrograms/kg every 1–2 hours (max. per dose 5 mg) as required
▸ Child 12–17 years: Initially 2–5 mg (max. per dose 5 mg), followed by 1–10 mg, after at least 15 minutes if required
▸ BY SLOW INTRAVENOUS INJECTION
▸ Child 1–11 years: Initially 5–20 micrograms/kg (max. per dose 500 micrograms), repeated as necessary after at least 15 minutes
▸ Child 12–17 years: 100–500 micrograms, repeated as necessary after at least 15 minutes
▸ BY INTRAVENOUS INFUSION
▸ Child 1–15 years: Initially 100–500 nanograms/kg/minute, adjusted according to response
▸ Child 16–17 years: Initially up to 180 micrograms/minute, reduced to 30–60 micrograms/minute, adjusted according to response

● **UNLICENSED USE** Not licensed for use in children by intravenous infusion or injection.
● **CONTRA-INDICATIONS** Hypertension · severe hyperthyroidism
● **CAUTIONS** Coronary disease · coronary vascular thrombosis · diabetes · extravasation at injection site may cause necrosis · following myocardial infarction · hypercapnia · hyperthyroidism · hypoxia · mesenteric vascular thrombosis · peripheral vascular thrombosis · Prinzmetal's variant angina · susceptibility to angle-closure glaucoma · uncorrected hypovolaemia
CAUTIONS, FURTHER INFORMATION
▸ Hypertensive response Phenylephrine has a longer duration of action than noradrenaline (norepinephrine), and an excessive vasopressor response may cause a prolonged rise in blood pressure.
● **INTERACTIONS** → Appendix 1: sympathomimetics, vasoconstrictor
● **SIDE-EFFECTS** Angle-closure glaucoma · anorexia · anxiety · arrhythmias · bradycardia (also reflex bradycardia) · confusion · dyspnoea · headache · hypertension · hypoxia · insomnia · nausea · palpitation · peripheral ischaemia · psychosis · tachycardia · tremor · urinary retention · vomiting · weakness
● **PREGNANCY** Avoid if possible; malformations reported following use in first trimester; fetal hypoxia and bradycardia reported in late pregnancy and labour.
● **MONITORING REQUIREMENTS** Contra-indicated in hypertension—monitor blood pressure and rate of flow frequently.
● **DIRECTIONS FOR ADMINISTRATION** For *intravenous injection*, dilute to a concentration of 1 mg/mL with Water for Injections and administer slowly. For *intravenous infusion*, dilute to a concentration of 20 micrograms/mL with Glucose 5% or Sodium Chloride 0.9% and administer as a continuous infusion via a central venous catheter using a controlled infusion device.
● **PRESCRIBING AND DISPENSING INFORMATION** Intravenous administration preferred when managing acute hypotension in children.

● **MEDICINAL FORMS**
There can be variation in the licensing of different medicines containing the same drug. Forms available from special-order manufacturers include: solution for injection

Solution for injection

▸ Phenylephrine hydrochloride (Non-proprietary)
Phenylephrine (as Phenylephrine hydrochloride) 50 microgram per 1 ml Phenylephrine 500micrograms/10ml solution for injection pre-filled syringes | 1 pre-filled disposable injection PoM £15.00 | 10 pre-filled disposable injection PoM £150.00
Phenylephrine hydrochloride 100 microgram per 1 ml Phenylephrine 1mg/10ml solution for injection ampoules | 10 ampoule PoM £40.00
Phenylephrine hydrochloride 10 mg per 1 ml Phenylephrine 10mg/1ml solution for injection ampoules | 10 ampoule PoM £99.12

5   Heart failure

Other drugs used for Heart failure Bendroflumethiazide, p. 107 · Captopril, p. 109 · Chlorothiazide, p. 108 · Chlortalidone, p. 138 · Digoxin, p. 79 · Enalapril maleate, p. 110 · Glyceryl trinitrate, p. 132 · Lisinopril, p. 111

BETA-ADRENOCEPTOR BLOCKERS 〉
ALPHA- AND BETA-ADRENOCEPTOR BLOCKERS

F 100

Carvedilol

● **INDICATIONS AND DOSE**

Adjunct in heart failure (limited information available)

▸ BY MOUTH

▸ Child 2–17 years: Initially 50 micrograms/kg twice daily (max. per dose 3.125 mg) for at least 2 weeks, then increased to 100 micrograms/kg twice daily for at least 2 weeks, then increased to 200 micrograms/kg twice daily, then increased if necessary up to 350 micrograms/kg twice daily (max. per dose 25 mg)

● **UNLICENSED USE** Not licensed for use in children under 18 years.

● **CONTRA-INDICATIONS** Acute or decompensated heart failure requiring intravenous inotropes

● **INTERACTIONS** → Appendix 1: beta blockers (non-selective)

● **SIDE-EFFECTS** Allergic skin reactions · angina · AV block · changes in liver enzymes · depressed mood · disturbances of micturition · influenza-like symptoms · leucopenia · nasal stuffiness · postural hypotension · thrombocytopenia · wheezing

● **PREGNANCY** Information on the safety of carvedilol during pregnancy is lacking. If carvedilol is used close to delivery, infants should be monitored for signs of alpha-blockade (as well as beta-blockade).

● **BREAST FEEDING** Infants should be monitored as there is a risk of possible toxicity due to alpha-blockade (in addition to beta-blockade).

● **HEPATIC IMPAIRMENT** Avoid in hepatic impairment.

● **MONITORING REQUIREMENTS** Monitor renal function during dose titration in patients with heart failure who also have renal impairment, low blood pressure, ischaemic heart disease, or diffuse vascular disease.

● **PATIENT AND CARER ADVICE**
Medicines for Children leaflet: Carvedilol for heart failure www.medicinesforchildren.org.uk/carvedilol-heart-failure-0

● **MEDICINAL FORMS**
There can be variation in the licensing of different medicines containing the same drug. Forms available from special-order manufacturers include: oral suspension

Tablet

CAUTIONARY AND ADVISORY LABELS 8

▸ Carvedilol (Non-proprietary)
Carvedilol 3.125 mg Carvedilol 3.125mg tablets | 28 tablet PoM £8.00 DT price = £0.82
Carvedilol 6.25 mg Carvedilol 6.25mg tablets | 28 tablet PoM £8.99 DT price = £0.91
Carvedilol 12.5 mg Carvedilol 12.5mg tablets | 28 tablet PoM £9.99 DT price = £0.95
Carvedilol 25 mg Carvedilol 25mg tablets | 28 tablet PoM £12.50 DT price = £1.07

DIURETICS 〉 POTASSIUM-SPARING DIURETICS 〉 ALDOSTERONE ANTAGONISTS

Potassium canrenoate

● **INDICATIONS AND DOSE**

Short-term diuresis for oedema in heart failure and in ascites

▸ BY INTRAVENOUS INJECTION, OR BY INTRAVENOUS INFUSION

▸ Neonate: 1–2 mg/kg twice daily.

▸ Child 1 month–11 years: 1–2 mg/kg twice daily

▸ Child 12–17 years: 1–2 mg/kg twice daily (max. per dose 200 mg)

DOSE EQUIVALENCE AND CONVERSION

▸ To convert to equivalent oral spironolactone dose, multiply potassium canrenoate dose by 0.7.

● **UNLICENSED USE** Not licensed for use in the UK.

● **CONTRA-INDICATIONS** Hyperkalaemia · hyponatraemia

● **CAUTIONS** Acute porphyrias p. 577 · hypotension · potential metabolic products carcinogenic in *rodents*

● **INTERACTIONS** → Appendix 1: potassium canrenoate

● **SIDE-EFFECTS**

▸ **Common or very common** Ataxia · drowsiness · headache · hyperuricaemia · menstrual irregularities · pain at injection site on rapid administration

▸ **Uncommon** Eosinophilia · hyperkalaemia · thrombocytopenia

▸ **Rare** Agranulocytosis · alopecia · deepening of voice · erythema · hepatotoxicity · hoarseness · hypersensitivity reactions · osteomalacia · urticaria

▸ **Frequency not known** Gastro-intestinal disturbances · gynaecomastia · hirsutism · hypochloraemic acidosis · hyponatraemia · hypotension · mastalgia · transient confusion with high doses

● **PREGNANCY** Crosses placenta. Feminisation and undescended testes in male fetus in *animal* studies—manufacturer advises avoid.

● **BREAST FEEDING** Present in breast milk—manufacturer advises avoid.

● **RENAL IMPAIRMENT** Use with caution if estimated glomerular filtration rate 30–60 mL/minute/1.73 m^2. Avoid if estimated glomerular filtration rate less than 30 mL/minute/1.73 m^2. Monitor plasma-potassium concentration if estimated glomerular filtration rate 30–60 mL/minute/1.73 m^2.

● **MONITORING REQUIREMENTS** Monitor electrolytes (discontinue if hyperkalaemia occurs).

● **DIRECTIONS FOR ADMINISTRATION** Consult product literature. Intravenous injection to be given over at least 3 minutes.

● **PRESCRIBING AND DISPENSING INFORMATION** Potassium canrenoate injection is available from 'special-order' manufacturers or specialist importing companies.

● **MEDICINAL FORMS**
There can be variation in the licensing of different medicines containing the same drug.

Solution for injection
▸ Potassium canrenoate (Non-proprietary)
Potassium canrenoate 20 mg per 1 ml Aldactone 200mg/10ml solution for injection ampoules | 10 ampoule [PoM] no price available

Spironolactone

● **INDICATIONS AND DOSE**

Oedema in heart failure and in ascites | Nephrotic syndrome | Reduction of hypokalaemia induced by diuretics or amphotericin
▸ BY MOUTH

▸ Neonate: Initially 1–2 mg/kg daily in 1–2 divided doses; increased if necessary up to 7 mg/kg daily, in resistant ascites.

▸ Child 1 month–11 years: Initially 1–3 mg/kg daily in 1–2 divided doses; increased if necessary up to 9 mg/kg daily, in resistant ascites

▸ Child 12–17 years: Initially 50–100 mg daily in 1–2 divided doses; increased if necessary up to 9 mg/kg daily, in resistant ascites; maximum 400 mg per day

● **UNLICENSED USE** Not licensed for reduction of hypokalaemia induced by diuretics or amphotericin.

● **CONTRA-INDICATIONS** Addison's disease · anuria · hyperkalaemia

● **CAUTIONS** Acute porphyrias p. 577 · potential metabolic products carcinogenic in *rodents*

● **INTERACTIONS** → Appendix 1: aldosterone antagonists

● **SIDE-EFFECTS** Acute renal failure · agranulocytosis · alopecia · benign breast tumour · breast pain · changes in libido · confusion · dizziness · drowsiness · electrolyte disturbances · gastro-intestinal disturbances · gynaecomastia · hepatotoxicity · hyperkalaemia (discontinue) · hypertrichosis · hyperuricaemia · hyponatraemia · leg cramps · leucopenia · malaise · menstrual disturbances · rash · Stevens-Johnson syndrome · thrombocytopenia

● **PREGNANCY** Use only if potential benefit outweighs risk—feminisation of male fetus in *animal* studies.

● **BREAST FEEDING** Metabolites present in milk, but amount probably too small to be harmful.

● **RENAL IMPAIRMENT** Avoid in acute renal insufficiency or severe impairment. Monitor plasma-potassium concentration (high risk of hyperkalaemia in renal impairment).

● **MONITORING REQUIREMENTS** Monitor electrolytes—discontinue if hyperkalaemia occurs.

● **PATIENT AND CARER ADVICE**
Medicines for Children leaflet: Spironolactone for heart failure www.medicinesforchildren.org.uk/spironolactone-for-heart-failure

● **MEDICINAL FORMS**
There can be variation in the licensing of different medicines containing the same drug. Forms available from special-order manufacturers include: oral suspension, oral solution

Tablet
CAUTIONARY AND ADVISORY LABELS 21
▸ Spironolactone (Non-proprietary)
Spironolactone 25 mg Spironolactone 25mg tablets | 28 tablet [PoM] £3.50 DT price = £1.30
Spironolactone 50 mg Spironolactone 50mg tablets | 28 tablet [PoM] £6.00 DT price = £1.70
Spironolactone 100 mg Spironolactone 100mg tablets | 28 tablet [PoM] £6.24 DT price = £2.00 | 30 tablet [PoM] no price available

▸ Aldactone (Pfizer Ltd)
Spironolactone 25 mg Aldactone 25mg tablets | 100 tablet [PoM] £8.89
Spironolactone 50 mg Aldactone 50mg tablets | 100 tablet [PoM] £17.78
Spironolactone 100 mg Aldactone 100mg tablets | 28 tablet [PoM] £9.96 DT price = £2.00 | 100 tablet [PoM] £35.56

PHOSPHODIESTERASE TYPE-3 INHIBITORS

Enoximone

● **DRUG ACTION** Enoximone is a phosphodiesterase type-3 inhibitor that exerts most effect on the myocardium; it has positive inotropic properties and vasodilator activity.

● **INDICATIONS AND DOSE**

Congestive heart failure, low cardiac output following cardiac surgery
▸ INITIALLY BY SLOW INTRAVENOUS INJECTION

▸ Neonate: Loading dose 500 micrograms/kg, followed by (by continuous intravenous infusion) 5–20 micrograms/kg/minute, adjusted according to response, infusion to be given over 24 hours; maximum 24 mg/kg per day.

▸ Child: Loading dose 500 micrograms/kg, followed by (by continuous intravenous infusion) 5–20 micrograms/kg/minute, adjusted according to response, infusion dose to be given over 24 hours; maximum 24 mg/kg per day

● **UNLICENSED USE** Not licensed for use in children.

● **CAUTIONS** Heart failure associated with hypertrophic cardiomyopathy, stenotic or obstructive valvular disease or other outlet obstruction

● **SIDE-EFFECTS** Chills · diarrhoea · ectopic beats · fever · headache · hypotension · insomnia · nausea · oliguria · supraventricular arrhythmias (more likely in patients with pre-existing arrhythmias) · upper and lower limb pain · urinary retention · ventricular tachycardia (more likely in patients with pre-existing arrhythmias) · vomiting

● **PREGNANCY** Manufacturer advises use only if potential benefit outweighs risk.

● **BREAST FEEDING** Manufacturer advises caution—no information available.

● **HEPATIC IMPAIRMENT** Dose reduction may be required.

● **RENAL IMPAIRMENT** Consider dose reduction.

● **MONITORING REQUIREMENTS** Monitor blood pressure, heart rate, ECG, central venous pressure, fluid and electrolyte status, renal function, platelet count and hepatic enzymes.

● **DIRECTIONS FOR ADMINISTRATION** Incompatible with glucose solutions. Use only plastic containers or syringes; crystal formation if glass used. Avoid extravasation.
For *intravenous administration*, dilute to concentration of 2.5 mg/mL with Sodium Chloride 0.9% or Water for Injections; the initial loading dose should be given by slow intravenous injection over at least 15 minutes.

● **PRESCRIBING AND DISPENSING INFORMATION**
Phosphodiesterase type-3 inhibitors possess positive inotropic and vasodilator activity and are useful in infants and children with low cardiac output especially after cardiac surgery. Phosphodiesterase type-3 inhibitors should be limited to short-term use because long-term oral administration has been associated with increased mortality in adults with congestive heart failure.

● **PATIENT AND CARER ADVICE**
Medicines for Children leaflet: Enoximone for pulmonary hypertension www.medicinesforchildren.org.uk/enoximone-for-pulmonary-hypertension

- **MEDICINAL FORMS**
There can be variation in the licensing of different medicines containing the same drug.
Solution for injection
EXCIPIENTS: May contain Alcohol, propylene glycol
  ▸ **Perfan** (Myogen GmbH)
  Enoximone 5 mg per 1 ml Perfan 100mg/20ml solution for injection ampoules | 10 ampoule [PoM] no price available (Hospital only)

Milrinone

- **DRUG ACTION** Milrinone is a phosphodiesterase type-3 inhibitor that exerts most effect on the myocardium; it has positive inotropic properties and vasodilator activity.

- **INDICATIONS AND DOSE**
Congestive heart failure, low cardiac output following cardiac surgery, shock
  ▸ INITIALLY BY INTRAVENOUS INFUSION
  ▸ **Neonate:** Initially 50–75 micrograms/kg, given over 30-60 minutes, reduce or omit initial dose if at risk of hypotension, then (by continuous intravenous infusion) 30–45 micrograms/kg/hour for 2–3 days (usually for 12 hours after cardiac surgery).
  ▸ **Child:** Initially 50–75 micrograms/kg, given over 30-60 minutes, reduce or omit initial dose if at risk of hypotension, then (by continuous intravenous infusion) 30–45 micrograms/kg/hour for 2–3 days (usually for 12 hours after cardiac surgery)

- **UNLICENSED USE** Not licensed for use in children.
- **CONTRA-INDICATIONS** Severe hypovolaemia
- **CAUTIONS** Correct hypokalaemia · heart failure associated with hypertrophic cardiomyopathy, stenotic or obstructive valvular disease or other outlet obstruction
- **SIDE-EFFECTS**
  ▸ **Common or very common** Ectopic beats · headache · hypotension · supraventricular arrhythmias (more likely in patients with pre-existing arrhythmias) · ventricular tachycardia
  ▸ **Uncommon** Chest pain · hypokalaemia · thrombocytopenia · tremor · ventricular fibrillation
  ▸ **Very rare** Anaphylaxis · bronchospasm · rash
- **PREGNANCY** Manufacturer advises use only if potential benefit outweighs risk.
- **BREAST FEEDING** Manufacturer advises avoid—no information available.
- **RENAL IMPAIRMENT** Use half to three-quarters normal dose and monitor response if estimated glomerular filtration rate less than 50 mL/minute/1.73 m^2.
- **MONITORING REQUIREMENTS**
  ▸ Monitor blood pressure, heart rate, ECG, central venous pressure, fluid and electrolyte status, renal function, platelet count and hepatic enzymes.
  ▸ Monitor renal function.
- **DIRECTIONS FOR ADMINISTRATION** Avoid extravasation. For *intravenous infusion* dilute with Glucose 5% or Sodium Chloride 0.9% *or* Sodium Chloride and Glucose intravenous infusion to a concentration of 200 micrograms/mL (higher concentrations of 400 micrograms/mL have been used).
  Loading dose may be given undiluted if fluid-restricted.
- **PRESCRIBING AND DISPENSING INFORMATION**
Phosphodiesterase type-3 inhibitors possess positive inotropic and vasodilator activity and are useful in infants and children with low cardiac output especially after cardiac surgery. Phosphodiesterase type-3 inhibitors should be limited to short-term use because long-term oral administration has been associated with increased mortality in adults with congestive heart failure.

- **MEDICINAL FORMS**
There can be variation in the licensing of different medicines containing the same drug. Forms available from special-order manufacturers include: solution for infusion
Solution for injection
  ▸ **Primacor** (Sanofi)
  Milrinone 1 mg per 1 ml Primacor 10mg/10ml solution for injection ampoules | 10 ampoule [PoM] £199.06

6 Hyperlipidaemia

Lipid-regulating drugs

Risk factors for cardiovascular disease

Atherosclerosis begins in childhood and raised serum cholesterol in children is associated with cardiovascular disease in adulthood. Lowering the cholesterol, without hindering growth and development in children and adolescents, should reduce the risk of cardiovascular disease in later life.

The risk factors for developing cardiovascular disease include raised serum cholesterol concentration, smoking, hypertension, impaired glucose tolerance, male sex, ethnicity, obesity, triglyceride concentration, chronic kidney disease, and a family history of cardiovascular disease. Heterozygous familial hypercholesterolaemia is the most common cause of raised serum cholesterol in children; homozygous familial hypercholesterolaemia is very rare and its specialised management is not covered in *BNF for Children*. Familial hypercholesterolaemia can lead to a greater risk of early coronary heart disease and should be managed by a specialist.

Secondary causes of hypercholesterolaemia should be addressed, these include obesity, diet, diabetes mellitus, hypothyroidism, nephrotic syndrome, obstructive biliary disease, glycogen storage disease, and drugs such as corticosteroids.

Management

The aim of management of hypercholesterolaemia is to reduce the risk of atherosclerosis while ensuring adequate growth and development. Children with hypercholesterolaemia (or their carers) should receive advice on appropriate lifestyle changes such as improved diet, increased exercise, weight reduction, and not smoking; Hypertension p. 95 should also be managed appropriately. Drug therapy may also be necessary.

Hypothyroidism

Children with hypothyroidism should receive adequate thyroid replacement therapy before their requirement for lipid-regulating treatment is assessed because correction of hypothyroidism itself may resolve the lipid abnormality. Untreated hypothyroidism increases the risk of myositis with lipid regulating drugs.

Drug treatment in heterozygous familial hypercholesterolaemia

Lifestyle modifications alone are unlikely to lower cholesterol concentration adequately in heterozygous familial hypercholesterolaemia and drug treatment is often required. Lipid-regulating drugs should be considered by the age of 10 years. The decision to initiate drug treatment will depend on the child's age, the age of onset of coronary heart disease within the family, and the presence of other cardiovascular risk factors. In children with a family history of coronary heart disease in early adulthood, drug treatment before the age of 10 years, and a combination of lipid-regulating drugs may be necessary.

Drug treatment in secondary hypercholesterolaemia

If 6–12 months of dietary and other lifestyle interventions has failed to lower cholesterol concentration adequately, drug treatment may be indicated in children 10 years and older (rarely necessary in younger children) who are at a high risk of developing cardiovascular disease.

Choice of drugs

Experience in the use of lipid-regulating drugs in children is limited and they should be initiated on specialist advice.

Statins are more effective than other classes of drugs in lowering LDL-cholesterol but less effective than the fibrates in reducing triglycerides. Statins also increase concentrations of HDL-cholesterol. Statins reduce cardiovascular disease events and total mortality in adults, irrespective of the initial cholesterol concentration. They are the drugs of first choice in children and are generally well tolerated; atorvastatin p. 128 and simvastatin p. 130 are the preferred statins. Other lipid-regulating drugs can be used if statins are ineffective or are not tolerated.

Evolocumab p. 131 is licensed for the treatment of homozygous familial hypercholesterolaemia; it is used in combination with other lipid-lowering therapies.

Ezetimibe p. 126 can be used alone when statins are not tolerated, or in combination with a statin when a high dose statin fails to control cholesterol concentration adequately.

Bile acid sequestrants are also available but tolerability of and compliance with these drugs is poor, and their use is declining.

Fibrates may reduce the risk of coronary heart disease in those with low HDL-cholesterol or with raised triglycerides. Evidence for the use of a fibrate (bezafibrate p. 126 or fenofibrate p. 127) in children is limited; fibrates should be considered only if dietary intervention and treatment with a statin and a bile acid sequestrant is unsuccessful or contra-indicated.

In hypertriglyceridaemia which cannot be controlled by very strict diet, omega-3 fatty acid compounds can be considered.

LIPID MODIFYING DRUGS > BILE ACID SEQUESTRANTS

Bile acid sequestrants

- **DRUG ACTION** Bile acid sequestrants act by binding bile acids, preventing their reabsorption; this promotes hepatic conversion of cholesterol into bile acids; the resultant increased LDL-receptor activity of liver cells increases the clearance of LDL-cholesterol from the plasma.
- **CAUTIONS** Interference with the absorption of fat-soluble vitamins (supplements of vitamins A, D, K, and folic acid may be required when treatment is prolonged).
- **SIDE-EFFECTS** Constipation · diarrhoea · gastro-intestinal discomfort · hypertriglyceridaemia (aggravation) · hypoprothrombinaemia associated with vitamin K deficiency · increased risk of bleeding · nausea · vomiting
- **PREGNANCY** Bile acid sequestrants should be used with caution as although the drugs are not absorbed, they may cause fat-soluble vitamin deficiency on prolonged use.
- **BREAST FEEDING** Bile acid sequestrants should be used with caution as although the drugs are not absorbed, they may cause fat-soluble vitamin deficiency on prolonged use.
- **MONITORING REQUIREMENTS** A child's growth and development should be monitored.

☞ above

Colestipol hydrochloride

- **INDICATIONS AND DOSE**

Familial hypercholesterolaemia

▸ BY MOUTH

▸ Child 12–17 years: Initially 5 g 1–2 times a day, then increased in steps of 5 g every month, total daily dose may be given in 1–2 divided doses or as a single dose if tolerated; maximum 30 g per day

- **UNLICENSED USE** Not licensed for use in children.
- **INTERACTIONS** → Appendix 1: colestipol
- **DIRECTIONS FOR ADMINISTRATION** The contents of each sachet should be mixed with at least 100 mL of water or other suitable liquid such as fruit juice or skimmed milk; alternatively it can be mixed with thin soups, cereals, yoghurt, or pulpy fruits ensuring at least 100 mL of liquid is provided.

Other drugs should be taken at least 1 hour before or 4–6 hours after colestipol to reduce possible interference with absorption.

- **PATIENT AND CARER ADVICE** Patient counselling on administration is advised for colestipol hydrochloride granules (avoid other drugs at same time).
- **MEDICINAL FORMS**
There can be variation in the licensing of different medicines containing the same drug.

Granules
CAUTIONARY AND ADVISORY LABELS 13
▸ Colestid (Pfizer Ltd)
Colestipol hydrochloride 5 gram Colestid 5g granules sachets plain sugar-free | 30 sachet [PoM] £15.05
Colestid Orange 5g granules sachets sugar-free | 30 sachet [PoM] £15.05

Tablet
▸ Colestipol hydrochloride (Non-proprietary)
Colestipol hydrochloride 1 gram Colestid 1g tablets | 120 tablet [PoM] no price available

☞ above

Colestyramine

(Cholestyramine)

- **INDICATIONS AND DOSE**

Familial hypercholesterolaemia

▸ BY MOUTH

▸ Child 6–11 years: Initially 4 g once daily, then increased to 4 g up to 3 times a day, adjusted according to response

▸ Child 12–17 years: Initially 4 g once daily, then increased in steps of 4 g every week; increased to 12–24 g daily in 1–4 divided doses, adjusted according to response; maximum 36 g per day

Pruritus associated with partial biliary obstruction and primary biliary cirrhosis

▸ BY MOUTH

▸ Child 1–11 months: 1 g once daily, adjusted according to response, total daily dose may alternatively be given in 2–4 divided doses; maximum 9 g per day

▸ Child 1–5 years: 2 g once daily, adjusted according to response, total daily dose may alternatively be given in 2–4 divided doses; maximum 18 g per day

▸ Child 6–11 years: 4 g once daily, adjusted according to response, total daily dose may alternatively be given in 2–4 divided doses; maximum 24 g per day

▸ Child 12–17 years: 4–8 g once daily, adjusted according to response, total daily dose may alternatively be given in 2–4 divided doses; maximum 36 g per day continued →

Diarrhoea associated with Crohn's disease, ileal resection, vagotomy, diabetic vagal neuropathy, and radiation
▶ BY MOUTH
▶ **Child 1–11 months:** 1 g once daily, adjusted according to response, total daily dose may alternatively be given in 2–4 divided doses, if no response within 3 days an alternative therapy should be initiated; maximum 9 g per day
▶ **Child 1–5 years:** 2 g once daily, adjusted according to response, total daily dose may alternatively be given in 2–4 divided doses, if no response within 3 days an alternative therapy should be initiated; maximum 18 g per day
▶ **Child 6–11 years:** 4 g once daily, adjusted according to response, total daily dose may alternatively be given in 2–4 divided doses, if no response within 3 days an alternative therapy should be initiated; maximum 24 g per day
▶ **Child 12–17 years:** 4–8 g once daily, adjusted according to response, total daily dose may alternatively be given in 2–4 divided doses, if no response within 3 days an alternative therapy should be initiated; maximum 36 g per day

● **UNLICENSED USE** Not licensed for use in children under 6 years to reduce cholesterol.
● **CONTRA-INDICATIONS** Complete biliary obstruction (not likely to be effective)
● **INTERACTIONS** → Appendix 1: colestyramine
● **SIDE-EFFECTS**
▶ **Rare** Intestinal obstruction
▶ **Frequency not known** Hyperchloraemic acidosis (on prolonged use)
● **DIRECTIONS FOR ADMINISTRATION** The contents of each sachet should be mixed with at least 150 mL of water or other suitable liquid such as fruit juice, skimmed milk, thin soups, and pulpy fruits with a high moisture content.
Other drugs should be taken at least 1 hour before or 4–6 hours after colestyramine to reduce possible interference with absorption.
● **PATIENT AND CARER ADVICE** Patient counselling on administration is advised for colestyramine powder (avoid other drugs at same time).

● **MEDICINAL FORMS**
There can be variation in the licensing of different medicines containing the same drug. Forms available from special-order manufacturers include: oral suspension, oral solution
Powder
CAUTIONARY AND ADVISORY LABELS 13
EXCIPIENTS: May contain Aspartame, sucrose
▶ **Colestyramine** (Non-proprietary)
Colestyramine anhydrous 4 gram Colestyramine 4g oral powder sachets | 50 sachet PoM no price available DT price = £10.76
Colestyramine 4g oral powder sachets sugar-free | 50 sachet PoM £27.68–£30.00 DT price = £27.68
▶ **Questran** (Bristol-Myers Squibb Pharmaceuticals Ltd)
Colestyramine anhydrous 4 gram Questran 4g oral powder sachets | 50 sachet PoM £10.76 DT price = £10.76
▶ **Questran Light** (Bristol-Myers Squibb Pharmaceuticals Ltd)
Colestyramine anhydrous 4 gram Questran Light 4g oral powder sachets sugar-free | 50 sachet PoM £16.15 DT price = £27.68

LIPID MODIFYING DRUGS ❭ CHOLESTEROL ABSORPTION INHIBITORS

Ezetimibe
19-May-2016

● **DRUG ACTION** Ezetimibe inhibits the intestinal absorption of cholesterol.

● **INDICATIONS AND DOSE**

Adjunct to dietary measures and statin treatment in primary hypercholesterolaemia | Adjunct to dietary measures and statin in homozygous familial hypercholesterolaemia | Primary hypercholesterolaemia (if statin inappropriate or not tolerated) | Adjunct to dietary measures in homozygous sitosterolaemia
▶ BY MOUTH
▶ **Child 10–17 years:** 10 mg daily

● **INTERACTIONS** → Appendix 1: ezetimibe
● **SIDE-EFFECTS**
▶ **Common or very common** Fatigue · gastro-intestinal disturbances · headache · myalgia
▶ **Rare** Anaphylaxis · angioedema · arthralgia · hepatitis · hypersensitivity reactions · rash
▶ **Very rare** Cholecystitis · cholelithiasis · myopathy · pancreatitis · raised creatine kinase · rhabdomyolysis · thrombocytopenia
● **PREGNANCY** Manufacturer advises use only if potential benefit outweighs risk—no information available.
● **BREAST FEEDING** Manufacturer advises avoid—present in milk in *animal* studies.
● **HEPATIC IMPAIRMENT** Avoid in moderate and severe impairment—may accumulate.

● **MEDICINAL FORMS**
There can be variation in the licensing of different medicines containing the same drug.
Tablet
▶ **Ezetrol** (Merck Sharp & Dohme Ltd)
Ezetimibe 10 mg Ezetrol 10mg tablets | 28 tablet PoM £26.31 DT price = £26.31

Combinations available: *Simvastatin with ezetimibe,* p. 130

LIPID MODIFYING DRUGS ❭ FIBRATES

Bezafibrate

● **DRUG ACTION** Fibrates act by decreasing serum triglycerides; they have variable effect on LDL-cholestrol.

● **INDICATIONS AND DOSE**

Hyperlipidaemia including familial hypercholesterolaemia (administered on expert advice)
▶ BY MOUTH USING IMMEDIATE-RELEASE MEDICINES
▶ **Child 10–17 years:** 200 mg once daily (max. per dose 200 mg 3 times a day), adjusted according to response

● **UNLICENSED USE** Not licensed for use in children.
● **CONTRA-INDICATIONS** Gall bladder disease · hypoalbuminaemia · nephrotic syndrome · photosensitivity to fibrates
● **CAUTIONS** Correct hypothyroidism before initiating treatment
● **INTERACTIONS** → Appendix 1: fibrates
● **SIDE-EFFECTS**
▶ **Common or very common** Abdominal distension · anorexia · diarrhoea · nausea
▶ **Uncommon** Alopecia · cholestasis · dizziness · erectile dysfunction · headache · myotoxicity (with myasthenia, myalgia, or very rarely rhabdomyolysis)—special risk in renal impairment · photosensitivity reactions · pruritus · rash · renal failure · urticaria

▸ **Rare** Pancreatitis · peripheral neuropathy
▸ **Very rare** Anaemia · gallstones · increased platelet count ·
interstitial lung disease · leucopenia · pancytopenia ·
Stevens-Johnson syndrome · thrombocytopenic purpura ·
toxic epidermal necrolysis

● **PREGNANCY** Manufacturers advise avoid—no information
available.

● **BREAST FEEDING** Manufacturer advises avoid—no
information available.

● **HEPATIC IMPAIRMENT** Avoid in severe liver disease.

● **RENAL IMPAIRMENT** Reduce dose if estimated glomerular
filtration rate 15–60 mL/minute/1.73 m^2. Avoid if
estimated glomerular filtration rate less than
15 mL/minute/1.73 m^2.
Myotoxicity Special care needed in patients with renal
disease, as progressive increases in serum creatinine
concentration or failure to follow dosage guidelines may
result in myotoxicity (rhabdomyolysis); discontinue if
myotoxicity suspected or creatine kinase concentration
increases significantly.

● **MONITORING REQUIREMENTS** Consider monitoring of liver
function and creatine kinase when fibrates used in
combination with a statin.

● **PRESCRIBING AND DISPENSING INFORMATION** Fibrates are
mainly used in those whose serum-triglyceride
concentration is greater than 10 mmol/litre or in those
who cannot tolerate a statin (specialist use).

● **MEDICINAL FORMS**
There can be variation in the licensing of different medicines
containing the same drug. Forms available from special-order
manufacturers include: oral suspension
Tablet
CAUTIONARY AND ADVISORY LABELS 21
▸ **Bezafibrate (Non-proprietary)**
Bezafibrate 200 mg Bezafibrate 200mg tablets | 100 tablet [PoM]
£8.50 DT price = £4.36
▸ **Bezalip** (Teva UK Ltd)
Bezafibrate 200 mg Bezalip 200mg tablets | 100 tablet [PoM] £8.63
DT price = £4.36

Fenofibrate
14-Jun-2017

● **DRUG ACTION** Fibrates act by decreasing serum
triglycerides; they have variable effect on LDL-cholestrol.

● **INDICATIONS AND DOSE**
**Hyperlipidaemias including familial
hypercholesterolaemia (administered on expert advice)**
▸ BY MOUTH USING CAPSULES
▸ Child 4-14 years: One 67 mg (micronised) capsule per
20 kg body-weight daily, maximum four 67 mg capsules
daily, or max. three 67 mg capsules daily with
concomitant statin
▸ Child 15-17 years: Initially 3 capsules daily, then
increased if necessary to 4 capsules daily, max. 3
capsules daily with concomitant statin, dose relates to
67 mg (micronised) capsules

DOSE ADJUSTMENTS DUE TO INTERACTIONS
Manufacturer advises max. dose 200 mg daily with
concurrent use of a statin—no specific recommendation
made for children.

● **UNLICENSED USE** 200 mg and 267 mg capsules not licensed
in children.

● **CONTRA-INDICATIONS** Gall bladder disease · pancreatitis
(unless due to severe hypertriglyceridaemia) ·
photosensitivity to ketoprofen

● **CAUTIONS** Correct hypothyroidism before initiating
treatment

● **INTERACTIONS** → Appendix 1: fibrates

● SIDE-EFFECTS
▸ **Common or very common** Abdominal distension · anorexia ·
diarrhoea · nausea
▸ **Uncommon** Alopecia · cholestasis · dizziness · erectile
dysfunction · headache · myotoxicity (with myasthenia,
myalgia, or very rarely rhabdomyolysis)—special risk in
renal impairment · pancreatitis · photosensitivity reactions
· pruritus · pulmonary embolism · rash · renal failure ·
urticaria
▸ **Rare** Hepatitis · peripheral neuropathy
▸ **Very rare** Anaemia · gallstones · increased platelet count ·
interstitial lung disease · leucopenia · pancytopenia ·
Stevens-Johnson syndrome · thrombocytopenic purpura ·
toxic epidermal necrolysis
▸ **Frequency not known** Interstitial pneumopathies

● **PREGNANCY** Avoid—embryotoxicity in *animal* studies.

● **BREAST FEEDING** Manufacturers advise avoid—no
information available.

● **HEPATIC IMPAIRMENT** Avoid.

● **RENAL IMPAIRMENT** Manufacturer advises max. 67 mg
daily if estimated glomerular filtration rate
30–59 mL/minute/1.73 m^2.
    Manufacturer advises use with caution in mild-to-
moderate impairment; avoid if estimated glomerular
filtration rate less than 30 mL/minute/1.73 m^2.
Myotoxicity Special care needed in patients with renal
disease, as progressive increases in serum creatinine
concentration or failure to follow dosage guidelines may
result in myotoxicity (rhabdomyolysis); discontinue if
myotoxicity suspected or creatine kinase concentration
increases significantly.

● **MONITORING REQUIREMENTS** Manufacturer advises
monitor hepatic transaminases every 3 months during the
first 12 months of treatment and periodically thereafter—
discontinue treatment if levels increase to more than
3 times the upper limit of normal; monitor serum
creatinine levels during the first 3 months of treatment
and periodically thereafter—interrupt treatment if
creatinine level is 50% above the upper limit of normal.

● **PRESCRIBING AND DISPENSING INFORMATION** Fibrates are
mainly used in those whose serum-triglyceride
concentration is greater than 10 mmol/litre or in those
who cannot tolerate a statin (specialist use).

● **MEDICINAL FORMS**
There can be variation in the licensing of different medicines
containing the same drug.
Capsule
CAUTIONARY AND ADVISORY LABELS 21
▸ **Fenofibrate (Non-proprietary)**
Fenofibrate micronised 67 mg Fenofibrate micronised 67mg
capsules | 90 capsule [PoM] £23.30 DT price = £22.64
Fenofibrate micronised 200 mg Fenofibrate micronised 200mg
capsules | 28 capsule [PoM] £21.75 DT price = £4.54
Fenofibrate micronised 267 mg Fenofibrate micronised 267mg
capsules | 28 capsule [PoM] £21.75 DT price = £4.86
▸ **Lipantil Micro** (Mylan Ltd)
Fenofibrate micronised 67 mg Lipantil Micro 67 capsules |
90 capsule [PoM] £23.30 DT price = £22.64
Fenofibrate micronised 200 mg Lipantil Micro 200 capsules |
28 capsule [PoM] £14.23 DT price = £4.54
Fenofibrate micronised 267 mg Lipantil Micro 267 capsules |
28 capsule [PoM] £21.75 DT price = £4.86

LIPID MODIFYING DRUGS > STATINS

Statins

● **DRUG ACTION** Statins competitively inhibit 3-hydroxy-
3-methylglutaryl coenzyme A (HMG CoA) reductase, an
enzyme involved in cholesterol synthesis, especially in the
liver.

2

Cardiovascular system

- **CAUTIONS** High alcohol intake · history of liver disease · hypothyroidism · patients at increased risk of muscle toxicity, including myopathy or rhabdomyolysis (e.g. those with a personal or family history of muscular disorders, previous history of muscular toxicity, and a high alcohol intake)

CAUTIONS, FURTHER INFORMATION

▶ Muscle effects Muscle toxicity can occur with all statins, however the likelihood increases with higher doses and in certain patients (see below). Statins should be used with caution in patients at increased risk of muscle toxicity, including those with a personal or family history of muscular disorders, previous history of muscular toxicity, a high alcohol intake, renal impairment or hypothyroidism.

In patients at increased risk of muscle effects, a statin should not usually be started if the baseline creatine kinase concentration is more than 5 times the upper limit of normal (some patients may present with an extremely elevated baseline creatine kinase concentration, for example because of a physical occupation or rigorous exercise—specialist advice should be sought regarding consideration of statin therapy in these patients).

▶ Hypothyroidism Hypothyroidism should be managed adequately before starting treatment with a statin.

- **SIDE-EFFECTS**

▶ **Rare** Hepatitis · jaundice

▶ **Very rare** Hepatic failure. · interstitial lung disease · lupus erythematosus-like reactions · pancreatitis

▶ **Frequency not known** Alopecia · altered liver function tests · amnesia · arthralgia · asthenia · depression · dizziness · fatigue · gastro-intestinal disturbances · headache · hyperglycaemia · hypersensitivity reactions · may be associated with the development of diabetes mellitus (particularly in those already at risk of the condition) · myalgia · myopathy · myositis · paraesthesia · peripheral neuropathy · pruritus · rash · rhabdomyolysis · sexual dysfunction · sleep disturbance · thrombocytopenia · urticaria · visual disturbance

SIDE-EFFECTS, FURTHER INFORMATION

▶ Muscle effects The risk of myopathy, myositis, and rhabdomyolysis associated with statin use is rare. Although myalgia has been reported commonly in patients receiving statins, muscle toxicity truly attributable to statin use is rare. Muscle toxicity can occur with all statins, however the likelihood increases with higher doses.

If muscular symptoms or raised creatine kinase occur during treatment, other possible causes (e.g. rigorous physical activity, hypothyroidism, infection, recent trauma, and drug or alcohol addiction) should be excluded before statin therapy is implicated, particularly if statin treatment has previously been tolerated for more than 3 months. When a statin is suspected to be the cause of myopathy, and creatine kinase concentration is markedly elevated (more than 5 times upper limit of normal), or if muscular symptoms are severe, treatment should be discontinued. If symptoms resolve and creatine kinase concentrations return to normal, the statin should be reintroduced at a lower dose and the patient monitored closely; an alternative statin should be prescribed if unacceptable side-effects are experienced with a particular statin. Statins should not be discontinued in the event of small, asymptomatic elevations of creatine kinase. Routine monitoring of creatine kinase is unnecessary in asymptomatic patients.

▶ Interstitial lung disease If patients develop symptoms such as dyspnoea, cough, and weight loss, they should seek medical attention.

- **CONCEPTION AND CONTRACEPTION** Adequate contraception is required during treatment and for 1 month afterwards.

- **PREGNANCY** Statins should be avoided in pregnancy (discontinue 3 months before attempting to conceive) as congenital anomalies have been reported and the decreased synthesis of cholesterol possibly affects fetal development.

- **HEPATIC IMPAIRMENT** Statins should be used with caution in those with a history of liver disease. Avoid in active liver disease or when there are unexplained persistent elevations in serum transaminases.

- **MONITORING REQUIREMENTS**

▶ Before starting treatment with statins, at least one full lipid profile (non-fasting) should be measured, including total cholesterol, HDL-cholesterol, non-HDL-cholesterol (calculated as total cholesterol minus HDL-cholesterol), and triglyceride concentrations, thyroid-stimulating hormone, and renal function should also be assessed.

▶ Liver function There is little information available on a rational approach to liver-function monitoring; however, NICE suggests that liver enzymes should be measured before treatment, and repeated within 3 months and at 12 months of starting treatment, unless indicated at other times by signs or symptoms suggestive of hepatotoxicity (NICE clinical guideline 181 (July 2014). Lipid Modification—Cardiovascular risk assessment and the modification of blood lipids for the primary and secondary prevention of cardiovascular disease).

Those with serum transaminases that are raised, but less than 3 times the upper limit of the reference range, should **not** be routinely excluded from statin therapy. Those with serum transaminases of more than 3 times the upper limit of the reference range should discontinue statin therapy.

▶ Creatine kinase Creatine kinase concentration should be measured in children before treatment and if unexplained muscle pain occurs.

- **PATIENT AND CARER ADVICE** Advise patients to report promptly unexplained muscle pain, tenderness, or weakness.

⬛ 127

Atorvastatin

07-Jun-2017

- **INDICATIONS AND DOSE**

Hyperlipidaemia including familial hypercholesterolaemia

▶ BY MOUTH

▶ Child 10–17 years: Initially 1 mg once daily, then increased if necessary up to 20 mg once daily, dose to be adjusted at intervals of at least 4 weeks

Homozygous familial hypercholesterolaemia

▶ BY MOUTH

▶ Child 10–17 years: Initially 10 mg once daily, then increased if necessary up to 80 mg once daily, dose to be adjusted at intervals of at least 4 weeks

DOSE ADJUSTMENTS DUE TO INTERACTIONS

Manufacturer advises if concurrent use of ciclosporin is unavoidable, max. dose cannot exceed 10 mg daily.

- **CAUTIONS** Haemorrhagic stroke

- **INTERACTIONS** → Appendix 1: statins

- **SIDE-EFFECTS**

▶ **Common or very common** Back pain · epistaxis · hyperglycaemia · nasopharyngitis · pharyngeolaryngeal pain

▶ **Uncommon** Anorexia · blurred vision · chest pain · hypoglycaemia · malaise · neck pain · peripheral oedema · pyrexia · tinnitus · weight gain

▶ **Rare** Cholestasis · Stevens-Johnson syndrome · toxic epidermal necrolysis

▶ **Very rare** Gynaecomastia · hearing loss

- **BREAST FEEDING** Manufacturer advises avoid—no information available.

● **PATIENT AND CARER ADVICE**
Patient counselling is advised for atorvastatin tablets (muscle effects).

Medicines for Children leaflet: Atorvastatin for high cholesterol www.medicinesforchildren.org.uk/atorvastatin-high-cholesterol-0

● **MEDICINAL FORMS**
There can be variation in the licensing of different medicines containing the same drug. Forms available from special-order manufacturers include: oral suspension, oral solution

Tablet
▸ **Atorvastatin (Non-proprietary)**
Atorvastatin (as Atorvastatin calcium trihydrate)
10 mg Atorvastatin 10mg tablets | 28 tablet PoM £13.00 DT price = £0.88 | 90 tablet PoM £41.78
Atorvastatin (as Atorvastatin calcium trihydrate)
20 mg Atorvastatin 20mg tablets | 28 tablet PoM £24.64 DT price = £1.02 | 90 tablet PoM £79.20
Atorvastatin (as Atorvastatin calcium trihydrate)
30 mg Atorvastatin 30mg tablets | 28 tablet PoM £25.35 DT price = £25.35
Atorvastatin (as Atorvastatin calcium trihydrate)
40 mg Atorvastatin 40mg tablets | 28 tablet PoM £24.64 DT price = £1.19 | 90 tablet PoM £79.20
Atorvastatin (as Atorvastatin calcium trihydrate)
60 mg Atorvastatin 60mg tablets | 28 tablet PoM £28.97 DT price = £28.97
Atorvastatin (as Atorvastatin calcium trihydrate)
80 mg Atorvastatin 80mg tablets | 28 tablet PoM £28.21 DT price = £1.89 | 90 tablet PoM £90.67
▸ **Lipitor** (Pfizer Ltd)
Atorvastatin (as Atorvastatin calcium trihydrate) 10 mg Lipitor 10mg tablets | 28 tablet PoM £13.00 DT price = £0.88
Atorvastatin (as Atorvastatin calcium trihydrate) 20 mg Lipitor 20mg tablets | 28 tablet PoM £24.64 DT price = £1.02
Atorvastatin (as Atorvastatin calcium trihydrate) 40 mg Lipitor 40mg tablets | 28 tablet PoM £24.64 DT price = £1.19
Atorvastatin (as Atorvastatin calcium trihydrate) 80 mg Lipitor 80mg tablets | 28 tablet PoM £28.21 DT price = £1.89

Chewable tablet
CAUTIONARY AND ADVISORY LABELS 24
▸ **Lipitor** (Pfizer Ltd)
Atorvastatin (as Atorvastatin calcium trihydrate) 10 mg Lipitor 10mg chewable tablets sugar-free | 30 tablet PoM £13.80 DT price = £13.80
Atorvastatin (as Atorvastatin calcium trihydrate) 20 mg Lipitor 20mg chewable tablets sugar-free | 30 tablet PoM £26.40 DT price = £26.40

F 127

Fluvastatin

12-Apr-2017

● **INDICATIONS AND DOSE**
Heterozygous familial hypercholesterolaemia
▸ INITIALLY BY MOUTH USING IMMEDIATE-RELEASE MEDICINES
▸ Child 9–17 years: Initially 20 mg daily, dose to be taken in the evening, then (by mouth) adjusted in steps of 20 mg daily (max. per dose 40 mg twice daily), adjusted at intervals of at least 6 weeks; maximum 80 mg per day
▸ BY MOUTH USING MODIFIED-RELEASE MEDICINES
▸ Child 9–17 years: 80 mg daily, dose form is not appropriate for initial dose titration

● INTERACTIONS → Appendix 1: statins
● SIDE-EFFECTS
▸ **Very rare** Vasculitis
● **BREAST FEEDING** Manufacturer advises avoid—no information available.
● **RENAL IMPAIRMENT** Manufacturer advises doses above 40 mg daily should be initiated with caution if estimated glomerular filtration rate less than 30 mL/minute/1.73 m².
● **PATIENT AND CARER ADVICE** Patient counselling is advised for fluvastatin tablets/capsules (muscle effects).

● **MEDICINAL FORMS**
There can be variation in the licensing of different medicines containing the same drug.
Modified-release tablet
CAUTIONARY AND ADVISORY LABELS 25
▸ **Fluvastatin (Non-proprietary)**
Fluvastatin (as Fluvastatin sodium) 80 mg Fluvastatin 80mg modified-release tablets | 28 tablet PoM no price available DT price = £19.20
▸ **Dorisin XL** (Aspire Pharma Ltd)
Fluvastatin (as Fluvastatin sodium) 80 mg Dorisin XL 80mg tablets | 28 tablet PoM £19.20 DT price = £19.20
▸ **Lescol XL** (Novartis Pharmaceuticals UK Ltd)
Fluvastatin (as Fluvastatin sodium) 80 mg Lescol XL 80mg tablets | 28 tablet PoM £19.20 DT price = £19.20
▸ **Luvinsta XL** (Actavis UK Ltd)
Fluvastatin (as Fluvastatin sodium) 80 mg Luvinsta XL 80mg tablets | 28 tablet PoM £19.20 DT price = £19.20
▸ **Nandovar XL** (Sandoz Ltd)
Fluvastatin (as Fluvastatin sodium) 80 mg Nandovar XL 80mg tablets | 28 tablet PoM £16.32 DT price = £19.20
Capsule
▸ **Fluvastatin (Non-proprietary)**
Fluvastatin (as Fluvastatin sodium) 20 mg Fluvastatin 20mg capsules | 28 capsule PoM £6.96 DT price = £2.06
Fluvastatin (as Fluvastatin sodium) 40 mg Fluvastatin 40mg capsules | 28 capsule PoM £7.42 DT price = £2.30
▸ **Lescol** (Novartis Pharmaceuticals UK Ltd)
Fluvastatin (as Fluvastatin sodium) 20 mg Lescol 20mg capsules | 28 capsule PoM £15.26 DT price = £2.06
Fluvastatin (as Fluvastatin sodium) 40 mg Lescol 40mg capsules | 28 capsule PoM £15.26 DT price = £2.30

F 127

Pravastatin sodium

● **INDICATIONS AND DOSE**
Hyperlipidaemia including familial hypercholesterolaemia
▸ BY MOUTH
▸ Child 8–13 years: 10 mg daily, then increased if necessary up to 20 mg daily, dose to be taken at night, dose to be adjusted at intervals of at least 4 weeks
▸ Child 14–17 years: 10 mg daily, then increased if necessary up to 40 mg daily, dose to be taken at night, dose to be adjusted at intervals of at least 4 weeks

DOSE ADJUSTMENTS DUE TO INTERACTIONS
Manufacturer advises initial dose 20 mg daily with concurrent use of ciclosporin, increasing with caution to 40 mg daily—no specific recommendation made for children.

● INTERACTIONS → Appendix 1: statins
● SIDE-EFFECTS
▸ **Uncommon** Abnormal urination · dysuria · nocturia · urinary frequency
▸ **Very rare** Fulminant hepatic necrosis
● **BREAST FEEDING** Manufacturer advises avoid—small amount of drug present in breast milk.
● **RENAL IMPAIRMENT** Start with lower doses in moderate to severe impairment.
● **PATIENT AND CARER ADVICE** Patient counselling is advised for pravastatin tablets (muscle effects).

● **MEDICINAL FORMS**
There can be variation in the licensing of different medicines containing the same drug. Forms available from special-order manufacturers include: oral suspension, oral solution
Tablet
▸ **Pravastatin sodium (Non-proprietary)**
Pravastatin sodium 10 mg Pravastatin 10mg tablets | 28 tablet PoM £16.10 DT price = £0.87
Pravastatin sodium 20 mg Pravastatin 20mg tablets | 28 tablet PoM £29.60 DT price = £1.04
Pravastatin sodium 40 mg Pravastatin 40mg tablets | 28 tablet PoM £29.60 DT price = £1.26

Rosuvastatin

☞ 127

- **INDICATIONS AND DOSE**

Hyperlipidaemia including familial hypercholesterolaemia

▸ BY MOUTH
▸ **Child 10–17 years:** Initially 5 mg once daily, then increased if necessary to 20 mg once daily, dose to be increased at intervals of at least 4 weeks, use lower max. dose in children with risk factors for myopathy or rhabdomyolysis (including personal or family history of muscular disorders or toxicity)

- **CAUTIONS** Patients of Asian origin
- **INTERACTIONS** → Appendix 1: statins
- **SIDE-EFFECTS**
▸ **Common or very common** Proteinuria
▸ **Very rare** Gynaecomastia · haematuria
▸ **Frequency not known** Oedema · Stevens-Johnson syndrome
- **BREAST FEEDING** Manufacturer advises avoid—no information available.
- **RENAL IMPAIRMENT** Reduce dose if estimated glomerular filtration rate less than 60 mL/minute/1.73 m². Avoid if estimated glomerular filtration rate less than 30 mL/minute/1.73 m².
- **PATIENT AND CARER ADVICE** Patient counselling is advised for rosuvastatin tablets (muscle effects).

- **MEDICINAL FORMS**
There can be variation in the licensing of different medicines containing the same drug. Forms available from special-order manufacturers include: oral suspension

Tablet
▸ Crestor (AstraZeneca UK Ltd)
Rosuvastatin (as Rosuvastatin calcium) 5 mg Crestor 5mg tablets | 28 tablet PoM £18.03 DT price = £18.03
Rosuvastatin (as Rosuvastatin calcium) 10 mg Crestor 10mg tablets | 28 tablet PoM £18.03 DT price = £18.03
Rosuvastatin (as Rosuvastatin calcium) 20 mg Crestor 20mg tablets | 28 tablet PoM £26.02 DT price = £26.02
Rosuvastatin (as Rosuvastatin calcium) 40 mg Crestor 40mg tablets | 28 tablet PoM £29.69 DT price = £29.69

Simvastatin

☞ 127

- **INDICATIONS AND DOSE**

Hyperlipidaemia including familial hypercholesterolaemia

▸ BY MOUTH
▸ **Child 5–9 years:** Initially 10 mg once daily, then increased if necessary up to 20 mg once daily, dose to be taken at night, increased at intervals of at least 4 weeks
▸ **Child 10–17 years:** Initially 10 mg once daily, then increased if necessary up to 40 mg once daily, dose to be taken at night, increased at intervals of at least 4 weeks

DOSE ADJUSTMENTS DUE TO INTERACTIONS
Manufacturer advises max. dose 10 mg daily with concurrent use of bezafibrate—no specific recommendation made for children.
Manufacturer advises max. dose 20 mg daily with concurrent use of amiodarone or amlodipine—no specific recommendation made for children.
Manufacturer advises reduce dose with concurrent use of some moderate inhibitors of CYP3A4 (max. 20 mg daily with verapamil and diltiazem)—no specific recommendation made for children.

- **UNLICENSED USE** Not licensed for use in children under 10 years.
- **INTERACTIONS** → Appendix 1: statins

- **SIDE-EFFECTS**
▸ **Rare** Anaemia
▸ **Frequency not known** Tendinopathy
- **BREAST FEEDING** Manufacturer advises avoid—no information available.
- **RENAL IMPAIRMENT** Doses above 10 mg daily should be used with caution if estimated glomerular filtration rate less than 30 mL/minute/1.73 m².
- **PATIENT AND CARER ADVICE** Patient counselling is advised for simvastatin tablets/oral suspension (muscle effects).

- **MEDICINAL FORMS**
There can be variation in the licensing of different medicines containing the same drug. Forms available from special-order manufacturers include: oral suspension, oral solution

Oral suspension
EXCIPIENTS: May contain Propylene glycol
▸ Simvastatin (Non-proprietary)
Simvastatin 4 mg per 1 ml Simvastatin 20mg/5ml oral suspension sugar free sugar-free | 150 ml PoM £126.87 DT price = £126.41
Simvastatin 8 mg per 1 ml Simvastatin 40mg/5ml oral suspension sugar free sugar-free | 150 ml PoM £193.80 DT price = £193.09

Tablet
▸ Simvastatin (Non-proprietary)
Simvastatin 10 mg Simvastatin 10mg tablets | 28 tablet PoM £18.00 DT price = £0.68
Simvastatin 20 mg Simvastatin 20mg tablets | 28 tablet PoM £29.60 DT price = £0.80
Simvastatin 40 mg Simvastatin 40mg tablets | 28 tablet PoM £29.60 DT price = £0.86
Simvastatin 80 mg Simvastatin 80mg tablets | 28 tablet PoM £29.61 DT price = £1.74
▸ Simvador (Discovery Pharmaceuticals)
Simvastatin 10 mg Simvador 10mg tablets | 28 tablet PoM £0.60 DT price = £0.68
Simvastatin 20 mg Simvador 20mg tablets | 28 tablet PoM £0.69 DT price = £0.80
Simvastatin 40 mg Simvador 40mg tablets | 28 tablet PoM £0.77 DT price = £0.86
Simvastatin 80 mg Simvador 80mg tablets | 28 tablet PoM £1.54 DT price = £1.74
▸ Zocor (Merck Sharp & Dohme Ltd)
Simvastatin 10 mg Zocor 10mg tablets | 28 tablet PoM £18.03 DT price = £0.68
Simvastatin 20 mg Zocor 20mg tablets | 28 tablet PoM £29.69 DT price = £0.80
Simvastatin 40 mg Zocor 40mg tablets | 28 tablet PoM £29.69 DT price = £0.86
Simvastatin 80 mg Zocor 80mg tablets | 28 tablet PoM £29.69 DT price = £1.74

Simvastatin with ezetimibe

The properties listed below are those particular to the combination only. For the properties of the components please consider, simvastatin above, ezetimibe p. 126.

- **INDICATIONS AND DOSE**

Homozygous familial hypercholesterolaemia, primary hypercholesterolaemia, and mixed hyperlipidaemia in patients over 10 years stabilised on the individual components in the same proportions, or for patients not adequately controlled by statin alone
▸ BY MOUTH
▸ **Child (initiated by a specialist):** (consult product literature)

- **INTERACTIONS** → Appendix 1: ezetimibe, statins

- **MEDICINAL FORMS**
There can be variation in the licensing of different medicines containing the same drug.

Tablet
▸ Inegy (Merck Sharp & Dohme Ltd)
Ezetimibe 10 mg, Simvastatin 20 mg Inegy 10mg/20mg tablets | 28 tablet PoM £33.42 DT price = £33.42

Ezetimibe 10 mg, Simvastatin 40 mg Inegy 10mg/40mg tablets |
28 tablet [PoM] £38.98 DT price = £38.98
Ezetimibe 10 mg, Simvastatin 80 mg Inegy 10mg/80mg tablets |
28 tablet [PoM] £41.21 DT price = £41.21

LIPID MODIFYING DRUGS > OTHERS

Evolocumab

24-Apr-2017

- **DRUG ACTION** Evolocumab binds to a pro-protein involved in the regulation of LDL receptors on liver cells; receptor numbers are increased, which results in increased uptake of LDL-cholesterol from the blood.

- **INDICATIONS AND DOSE**

Homozygous familial hypercholesterolaemia (in combination with other lipid-lowering therapies)
▸ BY SUBCUTANEOUS INJECTION
▸ Child 12-17 years: Initially 420 mg every month; increased if necessary to 420 mg every 2 weeks, if inadequate response after 12 weeks of treatment, to be administered into the thigh, abdomen or upper arm

Homozygous familial hypercholesterolaemia in patients on apheresis (in combination with other lipid-lowering therapies)
▸ BY SUBCUTANEOUS INJECTION
▸ Child 12-17 years: 420 mg every 2 weeks, to correspond with apheresis schedule, to be administered into the thigh, abdomen or upper arm

- **INTERACTIONS** → Appendix 1: monoclonal antibodies
- **SIDE-EFFECTS**
▸ **Common or very common** Arthralgia · back pain · influenza · nasopharyngitis · nausea · rash · upper respiratory tract infection
▸ **Uncommon** Urticaria
- **PREGNANCY** Manufacturer advises avoid unless essential—limited information available.
- **BREAST FEEDING** Manufacturer advises avoid—no information available.
- **HEPATIC IMPAIRMENT** Manufacturer advises monitor in moderate impairment—possible reduced efficacy; use with caution in severe impairment—no information available.
- **RENAL IMPAIRMENT** Manufacturer advises caution if estimated glomerular filtration rate less than 30 mL/minute/1.73 m^2—no information available.
- **HANDLING AND STORAGE** Manufacturer advises store in a refrigerator (2–8°C)—consult product literature for further information regarding storage outside refrigerator.
- **PATIENT AND CARER ADVICE** Patients and their carers should be given training in subcutaneous injection technique.

- **MEDICINAL FORMS**
There can be variation in the licensing of different medicines containing the same drug.
Solution for injection
▸ Repatha (Amgen Ltd)
Evolocumab 140 mg per 1ml Repatha 140mg/1ml solution for injection pre-filled syringes | 1 pre-filled disposable injection [PoM] £170.00
▸ Repatha SureClick (Amgen Ltd)
Evolocumab 140 mg per 1ml Repatha SureClick 140mg/1ml solution for injection pre-filled disposable devices | 2 pre-filled disposable injection [PoM] £340.20

7 Myocardial ischaemia

Nitrates

Overview
Nitrates are potent coronary vasodilators, but their principal benefit follows from a reduction in venous return which reduces left ventricular work. Unwanted effects such as flushing, headache, and postural hypotension may limit therapy, especially if the child is unusually sensitive to the effects of nitrates or is hypovolaemic. Glyceryl trinitrate p. 132 is also used in extravasation.

Nitrates

- **CONTRA-INDICATIONS** Aortic stenosis · cardiac tamponade · constrictive pericarditis · hypertrophic cardiomyopathy · hypotensive conditions · hypovolaemia · marked anaemia · mitral stenosis · raised intracranial pressure due to cerebral haemorrhage · raised intracranial pressure due to head trauma · toxic pulmonary oedema
- **CAUTIONS** Heart failure due to obstruction · hypothermia · hypothyroidism · hypoxaemia · malnutrition · metal-containing transdermal systems should be removed before magnetic resonance imaging procedures, cardioversion, or diathermy · recent history of myocardial infarction · susceptibility to angle-closure glaucoma · tolerance · ventilation and perfusion abnormalities

CAUTIONS, FURTHER INFORMATION
▸ Tolerance Children receiving nitrates continuously throughout the day can develop tolerance (with reduced therapeutic effects). Reduction of blood-nitrate concentrations to low levels for 4 to 8 hours each day usually maintains effectiveness in such patients.

- **SIDE-EFFECTS**
GENERAL SIDE-EFFECTS
▸ **Common or very common** Dizziness · postural hypotension · tachycardia · throbbing headache
▸ **Uncommon** Flushing · heartburn · nausea · rash · syncope · temporary hypoxaemia · vomiting
▸ **Very rare** Angle-closure glaucoma
▸ **Frequency not known** Paradoxical bradycardia

SPECIFIC SIDE-EFFECTS
▸ With intravenous use Abdominal pain · apprehension · diaphoresis · muscle twitching · palpitation · prolonged administration has been associated with methaemoglobinaemia · restlessness · retrosternal discomfort · severe hypotension

SIDE-EFFECTS, FURTHER INFORMATION
▸ With intravenous use Specific side-effects following injection (particularly if given too rapidly) include severe hypotension, diaphoresis, apprehension, restlessness, muscle twitching, retrosternal discomfort, palpitation, abdominal pain; prolonged administration has been associated with methaemoglobinaemia.

- **ALLERGY AND CROSS-SENSITIVITY** Contra-indicated in nitrate hypersensitivity.
- **BREAST FEEDING** No information available— manufacturers advise use only if potential benefit outweighs risk.
- **HEPATIC IMPAIRMENT** Caution in severe impairment.
- **RENAL IMPAIRMENT** Manufacturers advise use with caution in severe impairment.
- **MONITORING REQUIREMENTS** Monitor blood pressure and heart rate during intravenous infusion.
- **TREATMENT CESSATION** Avoid abrupt withdrawal.

Cardiovascular system

2

Cardiovascular system

Glyceryl trinitrate

▶ 131

● INDICATIONS AND DOSE

Hypertension during and after cardiac surgery | Heart failure after cardiac surgery | Coronary vasoconstriction in myocardial ischaemia | Vasoconstriction in shock
▶ BY CONTINUOUS INTRAVENOUS INFUSION

▶ Neonate: 0.2–0.5 microgram/kg/minute, adjusted according to response, maintenance 1–3 micrograms/kg/minute (max. per dose 10 micrograms/kg/minute).

▶ Child: Initially 0.2–0.5 microgram/kg/minute, adjusted according to response, maintenance 1–3 micrograms/kg/minute (max. per dose 10 micrograms/kg/minute); maximum 200 micrograms/minute

● **UNLICENSED USE** Not licensed for use in children.
● **INTERACTIONS** → Appendix 1: nitrates
● **PREGNANCY** Not known to be harmful.
● **DIRECTIONS FOR ADMINISTRATION** For *continuous intravenous infusion*, dilute to max. concentration of 400 micrograms/mL (but concentration of 1 mg/mL has been used via a central venous catheter) with Glucose 5% or Sodium Chloride 0.9%. *Neonatal intensive care*, dilute 3 mg/kg body-weight to a final volume of 50 mL with Glucose 5% or Sodium Chloride 0.9%; an intravenous infusion rate of 1 mL/hour provides a dose of 1 microgram/kg/minute; max. concentration of 400 micrograms/mL (but concentration of 1 mg/mL has been used via a central venous catheter).

Glass or polyethylene apparatus is preferable; loss of potency will occur if PVC is used. Glyceryl trinitrate 1 mg/ml to be diluted before use or given undiluted with syringe pump. Glyceryl trinitrate 5 mg/ml to be diluted before use.

● **MEDICINAL FORMS**
There can be variation in the licensing of different medicines containing the same drug.
Solution for infusion
EXCIPIENTS: May contain Ethanol, propylene glycol
▶ Glyceryl trinitrate (Non-proprietary)
Glyceryl trinitrate 1 mg per 1 ml Glyceryl trinitrate 50mg/50ml solution for infusion vials | 1 vial [PoM] £15.90 | 25 vial [PoM] no price available
Glyceryl trinitrate 5 mg per 1 ml Glyceryl trinitrate 50mg/10ml solution for infusion ampoules | 5 ampoule [PoM] £64.90
Glyceryl trinitrate 25mg/5ml solution for infusion ampoules | 5 ampoule [PoM] £32.45
▶ Nitrocine (Aspire Pharma Ltd)
Glyceryl trinitrate 1 mg per 1 ml Nitrocine 10mg/10ml solution for infusion ampoules | 10 ampoule [PoM] £58.75 (Hospital only)
▶ Nitronal (Merck Serono Ltd)
Glyceryl trinitrate 1 mg per 1 ml Nitronal 5mg/5ml solution for infusion ampoules | 10 ampoule [PoM] £18.04
Nitronal 50mg/50ml solution for infusion vials | 1 vial [PoM] £14.76

7.1 Cardiac arrest

Cardiopulmonary resuscitation

Overview

The algorithms for cardiopulmonary resuscitation (Life support algorithm (image) p. 1063) reflect the recommendations of the Resuscitation Council (UK); they cover paediatric basic life support, paediatric advanced life support, and newborn life support. The guidelines are available at www.resus.org.uk.

Paediatric advanced life support

Cardiopulmonary (cardiac) arrest in children is rare and frequently represents the terminal event of progressive shock or respiratory failure.

During cardiopulmonary arrest in children without intravenous access, the intraosseous route is chosen because it provides rapid and effective response; if circulatory access cannot be gained, the endotracheal tube can be used. When the endotracheal route is used ten times the intravenous dose should be used; the drug should be injected quickly down a narrow bore suction catheter beyond the tracheal end of the tube and then flushed in with 1 or 2 mL of sodium chloride 0.9%. The endotracheal route is useful for lipid-soluble drugs, including lidocaine hydrochloride p. 74, adrenaline/epinephrine below, atropine sulfate p. 779, and naloxone hydrochloride p. 813. Drugs that are not lipid-soluble (e.g. sodium bicarbonate p. 558 and calcium chloride p. 567) should **not** be administered by this route because they will injure the airways.

For the management of acute anaphylaxis, see allergic emergencies under Antihistamines, allergen immunotherapy and allergic emergencies p. 165.

SYMPATHOMIMETICS ⟩ VASOCONSTRICTOR

Adrenaline/epinephrine

● **DRUG ACTION** Acts on both alpha and beta receptors and increases both heart rate and contractility (beta$_1$ effects); it can cause peripheral vasodilation (a beta$_2$ effect) or vasoconstriction (an alpha effect).

● INDICATIONS AND DOSE

Acute hypotension
▶ BY CONTINUOUS INTRAVENOUS INFUSION

▶ Neonate: Initially 100 nanograms/kg/minute, adjusted according to response, higher doses up to 1.5 micrograms/kg/minute have been used in acute hypotension.

▶ Child: Initially 100 nanograms/kg/minute, adjusted according to response, higher doses up to 1.5 micrograms/kg/minute have been used in acute hypotension

Croup (when not effectively controlled with corticosteroid treatment)
▶ BY INHALATION OF NEBULISED SOLUTION
▶ Child 1 month–11 years: 400 micrograms/kg (max. per dose 5 mg), dose to be repeated after 30 minutes if necessary

PHARMACOKINETICS
The effects of nebulised adrenaline for the treatment of croup lasts for 2–3 hours.

Emergency treatment of acute anaphylaxis (under expert supervision) | Angioedema (if laryngeal oedema is present) (under expert supervision)
▶ BY INTRAMUSCULAR INJECTION
▶ Child 1 month–5 years: 150 micrograms, doses may be repeated several times if necessary at 5 minute intervals according to blood pressure, pulse, and respiratory function, suitable syringe to be used for measuring small volume; injected preferably into the anterolateral aspect of the middle third of the thigh
▶ Child 6–11 years: 300 micrograms, doses may be repeated several times if necessary at 5 minute intervals according to blood pressure, pulse, and respiratory function, to be injected preferably into the anterolateral aspect of the middle third of the thigh
▶ Child 12–17 years: 500 micrograms, to be injected preferably into the anterolateral aspect of the middle third of the thigh, doses may be repeated several times

if necessary at 5 minute intervals according to blood pressure, pulse, and respiratory function, 300 micrograms (0.3 mL) to be administered if child small or prepubertal

Acute anaphylaxis when there is doubt as to the adequacy of the circulation (specialist use only) | Angioedema (if laryngeal oedema is present) (specialist use only)
▶ BY SLOW INTRAVENOUS INJECTION
▸ Child: 1 microgram/kg (max. per dose 50 micrograms), using dilute 1 in 10 000 adrenaline injection, dose to be repeated according to response, if multiple doses required, adrenaline should be given as a slow intravenous infusion stopping when a response has been obtained

EMERADE® 150 MICROGRAMS
Acute anaphylaxis (for self-administration)
▶ BY INTRAMUSCULAR INJECTION
▸ Child (body-weight up to 15 kg): 150 micrograms, then 150 micrograms after 5–15 minutes as required
▸ Child (body-weight 15–30 kg): 150 micrograms, then 150 micrograms after 5–15 minutes as required, on the basis of a dose of 10 micrograms/kg, 300 micrograms may be more appropriate for some children

EMERADE® 300 MICROGRAMS
Acute anaphylaxis (for self-administration)
▶ BY INTRAMUSCULAR INJECTION
▸ Child (body-weight 30 kg and above): 300 micrograms, then 300 micrograms after 5–15 minutes as required

EMERADE® 500 MICROGRAMS
Acute anaphylaxis (for self-administration for patients at risk of severe anaphylaxis)
▶ BY INTRAMUSCULAR INJECTION
▸ Child 12–17 years: 500 micrograms, then 500 micrograms after 5–15 minutes as required

EPIPEN® AUTO-INJECTOR 0.3MG
Acute anaphylaxis (for self-administration)
▶ BY INTRAMUSCULAR INJECTION
▸ Child (body-weight 30 kg and above): 300 micrograms, then 300 micrograms after 5–15 minutes as required

EPIPEN® JR AUTO-INJECTOR 0.15MG
Acute anaphylaxis (for self-administration)
▶ BY INTRAMUSCULAR INJECTION
▸ Child (body-weight up to 15 kg): 150 micrograms, then 150 micrograms after 5–15 minutes as required
▸ Child (body-weight 15–30 kg): 150 micrograms, then 150 micrograms after 5–15 minutes as required, on the basis of a dose of 10 micrograms/kg, 300 micrograms may be more appropriate for some children

JEXT® 150 MICROGRAMS
Acute anaphylaxis (for self-administration)
▶ BY INTRAMUSCULAR INJECTION
▸ Child (body-weight up to 15 kg): 150 micrograms, then 150 micrograms after 5–15 minutes as required
▸ Child (body-weight 15–30 kg): 150 micrograms, then 150 micrograms after 5–15 minutes as required, on the basis of a dose of 10 micrograms/kg, 300 micrograms may be more appropriate for some children

JEXT® 300 MICROGRAMS
Acute anaphylaxis (for self-administration)
▶ BY INTRAMUSCULAR INJECTION
▸ Child (body-weight 30 kg and above): 300 micrograms, then 300 micrograms after 5–15 minutes as required

● UNLICENSED USE
▸ With intramuscular use for acute anaphylaxis Auto-injectors delivering 150-microgram dose of adrenaline may not be licensed for use in children with body-weight under 15 kg.

▸ With intravenous use for acute hypotension Adrenaline 1 in 1000 (1 mg/mL) solution is not licensed for intravenous administration.

IMPORTANT SAFETY INFORMATION
SAFE PRACTICE
Intravenous route should be used with **extreme care** by specialists only.

● CAUTIONS Arrhythmias · cerebrovascular disease · cor pulmonale · diabetes mellitus · hypercalcaemia · hyperreflexia · hypertension · hyperthyroidism · hypokalaemia · ischaemic heart disease · obstructive cardiomyopathy · occlusive vascular disease · organic brain damage · phaeochromocytoma · prostate disorders · psychoneurosis · severe angina · susceptibility to angle-closure glaucoma

CAUTIONS, FURTHER INFORMATION
Cautions listed are only for non-life-threatening situations.

● INTERACTIONS → Appendix 1: sympathomimetics, vasoconstrictor

● SIDE-EFFECTS Angina · angle-closure glaucoma · anorexia · anxiety · arrhythmias · cold extremities · confusion · difficulty in micturition · dizziness · dry mouth · dyspnoea · headache · hyperglycaemia · hypersalivation · hypertension (risk of cerebral haemorrhage) · hypokalaemia · insomnia · metabolic acidosis · mydriasis · myocardial infarction · nausea · pallor · palpitation · psychosis · pulmonary oedema (on excessive dosage or extreme sensitivity) · restlessness · sweating · tachycardia · tissue necrosis at injection site · tissue necrosis of bowel · tissue necrosis of extremities · tissue necrosis of kidneys · tissue necrosis of liver · tremor · urinary retention · vomiting · weakness

● PREGNANCY May reduce placental perfusion and cause tachycardia, cardiac irregularities, and extrasystoles in fetus. Can delay second stage of labour. Manufacturers advise use only if benefit outweighs risk.

● BREAST FEEDING Present in milk but unlikely to be harmful as poor oral bioavailability.

● RENAL IMPAIRMENT Manufacturers advise use with caution in severe impairment.

● MONITORING REQUIREMENTS Monitor blood pressure and ECG.

● DIRECTIONS FOR ADMINISTRATION
▸ With intravenous use for acute hypotension For *continuous intravenous infusion*, dilute with Glucose 5% or Sodium Chloride 0.9% and give through a central venous catheter. Incompatible with bicarbonate and alkaline solutions. *Neonatal intensive care*, dilute 3 mg/kg body-weight to a final volume of 50 mL with infusion fluid; an intravenous infusion rate of 0.1 mL/hour provides a dose of 100 nanograms/kg/minute; infuse through a central venous catheter. Incompatible with bicarbonate and alkaline solutions. These infusions are usually made up with adrenaline 1 in 1000 (1 mg/mL) solution.
▸ When used by inhalation For nebulisation in croup, adrenaline 1 in 1000 solution may be diluted with sterile sodium chloride 0.9% solution.

● PRESCRIBING AND DISPENSING INFORMATION It is important, in acute anaphylaxis where intramuscular injection might still succeed, time should not be wasted seeking intravenous access.
Great vigilance is needed to ensure that the *correct strength* of adrenaline injection is used; anaphylactic shock kits need to make a *very clear distinction* between the 1 in 10 000 strength and the 1 in 1000 strength.
Patients with severe allergy should be instructed in the self-administration of adrenaline by intramuscular injection.

Packs for self-administration need to be **clearly labelled with instructions** on how to administer adrenaline (intramuscularly, preferably at the midpoint of the outer thigh, through light clothing if necessary) so that in the case of rapid collapse someone else is able to give it. It is important to ensure individuals at risk and their carers understand that:

- two injection devices should be carried at all times to treat symptoms until medical assistance is available; if, after the first injection, the individual does not start to feel better, the second injection should be given 5 to 15 minutes after the first;
- an ambulance should be called after every administration, even if symptoms improve;
- the individual should lie down with their legs raised (unless they have breathing difficulties, in which case they should sit up) and should not be left alone.

Adrenaline for administration by intramuscular injection is available in 'auto-injectors' (e.g. *Emerade*®, *EpiPen*®, or *Jext*®), pre-assembled syringes fitted with a needle suitable for very rapid administration (if necessary by a bystander or a healthcare provider if it is the only preparation available); injection technique is device specific.

To ensure patients receive the auto-injector device that they have been trained to use, prescribers should specify the brand to be dispensed.

- **PATIENT AND CARER ADVICE**
Individuals at considerable risk of anaphylaxis need to carry (or have available) adrenaline at all times and the patient, or their carers, need to be *instructed in advance* when and how to inject it.

JEXT® **300 MICROGRAMS** 1.1 mL of the solution remains in the auto-injector device after use.

JEXT® **150 MICROGRAMS** 1.25 mL of the solution remains in the auto-injector device after use.

EPIPEN® **JR AUTO-INJECTOR 0.15MG** 1.7 mL of the solution remains in the auto-injector device after use.

EMERADE® **300 MICROGRAMS** 0.2 mL of the solution remains in the auto-injector device after use.

EPIPEN® **AUTO-INJECTOR 0.3MG** 1.7 mL of the solution remains in the auto-injector device after use.

EMERADE® **500 MICROGRAMS** No solution remains in the auto-injector device after use.

EMERADE® **150 MICROGRAMS** 0.35 mL of the solution remains in the auto-injector device after use.
Medicines for Children leaflet: Adrenaline auto-injector for anaphylaxis www.medicinesforchildren.org.uk/adrenaline-auto-injector-anapylaxis-0

- **EXCEPTIONS TO LEGAL CATEGORY** POM restriction does not apply to the intramuscular administration of up to 1 mg of adrenaline injection 1 in 1000 (1 mg/mL) for the emergency treatment of anaphylaxis.

- **MEDICINAL FORMS**
There can be variation in the licensing of different medicines containing the same drug. Forms available from special-order manufacturers include: solution for injection

Solution for injection
EXCIPIENTS: May contain Sulfites

▸ **Adrenaline/epinephrine (Non-proprietary)**
Adrenaline 100 microgram per 1 ml Adrenaline (base) 100micrograms/1ml (1 in 10,000) dilute solution for injection ampoules | 10 ampoule PoM £63.09
Adrenaline (base) 1mg/10ml (1 in 10,000) dilute solution for injection pre-filled syringes | 1 pre-filled disposable injection PoM £6.87 | 1 pre-filled disposable injection PoM £18.00 (Hospital only) | 10 pre-filled disposable injection PoM £180.00 (Hospital only)
Adrenaline (as Adrenaline acid tartrate) 100 microgram per 1 ml Adrenaline (base) 1mg/10ml (1 in 10,000) dilute solution for injection ampoules | 1 ampoule PoM £43.53 | 10 ampoule PoM £73.13
Adrenaline (base) 500micrograms/5ml (1 in 10,000) dilute solution for injection ampoules | 10 ampoule PoM £67.22

Adrenaline 1 mg per 1 ml Adrenaline (base) 10mg/10ml (1 in 1,000) solution for injection ampoules | 10 ampoule PoM £79.65
Adrenaline (base) for anaphylaxis 1mg/1ml (1 in 1,000) solution for injection pre-filled syringes | 1 pre-filled disposable injection PoM £10.40
Adrenaline (base) 1mg/1ml (1 in 1,000) solution for injection pre-filled syringes | 1 pre-filled disposable injection PoM £10.40
Adrenaline (as Adrenaline acid tartrate) 1 mg per 1 ml Adrenaline (base) 5mg/5ml (1 in 1,000) solution for injection ampoules | 10 ampoule PoM £77.34
Adrenaline (base) 500micrograms/0.5ml (1 in 1,000) solution for injection ampoules | 10 ampoule PoM £59.87–£61.33 DT price = £59.87
Adrenaline (base) 1mg/1ml (1 in 1,000) solution for injection ampoules | 10 ampoule PoM £6.01 DT price = £6.01

▸ **Emerade** (Bausch & Lomb UK Ltd)
Adrenaline 1 mg per 1 ml Emerade 300micrograms/0.3ml (1 in 1,000) solution for injection auto-injectors | 1 pre-filled disposable injection PoM £25.99 DT price = £26.45
Adrenaline (as Adrenaline acid tartrate) 1 mg per 1 ml Emerade 150micrograms/0.15ml (1 in 1,000) solution for injection auto-injectors | 1 pre-filled disposable injection PoM £25.99
Emerade 500micrograms/0.5ml (1 in 1,000) solution for injection auto-injectors | 1 pre-filled disposable injection PoM £26.99

▸ **EpiPen** (Meda Pharmaceuticals Ltd)
Adrenaline 500 microgram per 1 ml EpiPen Jr. 150micrograms/0.3ml (1 in 2,000) solut on for injection auto-injectors | 1 pre-filled disposable injection PoM £26.45 | 2 pre-filled disposable injection PoM £52.90
Adrenaline 1 mg per 1 ml EpiPen 300micrograms/0.3ml (1 in 1,000) solution for injection auto-injectors | 1 pre-filled disposable injection PoM £26.45 DT price = £26.45 | 2 pre-filled disposable injection PoM £52.90

▸ **Jext** (ALK-Abello Ltd)
Adrenaline 1 mg per 1 ml Jext 300micrograms/0.3ml (1 in 1,000) solution for injection auto-injectors | 1 pre-filled disposable injection PoM £23.99 DT price = £26.45
Adrenaline (as Adrenaline acid tartrate) 1 mg per 1 ml Jext 150micrograms/0.15ml (1 in 1,000) solution for injection auto-injectors | 1 pre-filled disposable injection PoM £23.99

8 Oedema

Diuretics

Overview

Diuretics are used for a variety of conditions in children including pulmonary oedema (caused by conditions such as respiratory distress syndrome and bronchopulmonary dysplasia), congestive heart failure, and hypertension. Hypertension in children is often resistant to therapy and may require the use of several drugs in combination. Maintenance of fluid and electrolyte balance can be difficult in children on diuretics, particularly neonates whose renal function may be immature.

Loop diuretics are used for pulmonary oedema, congestive heart failure, and in renal disease.

Thiazides are used less commonly than loop diuretics but are often used in combination with loop diuretics or spironolactone p. 123 in the management of pulmonary oedema and, in lower doses, for hypertension associated with cardiac disease.

Aminophylline **infusion** p. 161; has been used with intravenous furosemide p. 136 to relieve fluid overload in critically ill children.

Heart failure

Heart failure is less common in children than in adults; it can occur as a result of congenital heart disease (e.g. septal defects), dilated cardiomyopathy, myocarditis, or cardiac surgery. Drug treatment of heart failure due to left ventricular systolic dysfunction is covered below; optimal management of heart failure with preserved left ventricular function has not been established.

Acute heart failure can occur after cardiac surgery or as a complication in severe acute infections with or without myocarditis. Therapy consists of volume loading, vasodilator or inotropic drugs.

Chronic heart failure is initially treated with a **loop diuretic**, usually furosemide supplemented with spironolactone, amiloride hydrochloride p. 138, or potassium chloride p. 575.

If diuresis with furosemide is insufficient, the addition of metolazone p. 138 or a **thiazide diuretic** can be considered. With metolazone the resulting diuresis can be profound and care is needed to avoid potentially dangerous electrolyte disturbance.

If diuretics are insufficient an ACE inhibitor, titrated to the maximum tolerated dose, can be used. **ACE inhibitors** are used for the treatment of all grades of heart failure in adults and can also be useful for children with heart failure. Addition of digoxin p. 79 can be considered in children who remain symptomatic despite treatment with a diuretic and an ACE inhibitor.

Some beta-blockers improve outcome in adults with heart failure, but data on beta-blockers in children are limited. Carvedilol p. 122 has vasodilatory properties and therefore (like ACE inhibitors) also lowers afterload.

In children receiving specialist cardiology care, the phosphodiesterase type-3 inhibitor enoximone p. 123 is sometimes used by mouth for its inotropic and vasodilator effects. Spironolactone is usually used as a potassium-sparing drug with a loop diuretic; in adults low doses of spironolactone are effective in the treatment of heart failure. Careful monitoring of serum potassium is necessary if spironolactone is used in combination with an ACE inhibitor.

Thiazides and related diuretics

Thiazides and related compounds are moderately potent diuretics; they inhibit sodium reabsorption at the beginning of the distal convoluted tubule. They are usually administered early in the day so that the diuresis does not interfere with sleep.

In the management of *hypertension* a low dose of a thiazide produces a maximal or near-maximal blood pressure lowering effect, with very little biochemical disturbance. Higher doses cause more marked changes in plasma potassium, sodium, uric acid, glucose, and lipids, with little advantage in blood pressure control. Thiazides also have a role in chronic heart failure.

Bendroflumethiazide p. 107 is licensed for use in children; chlorothiazide p. 108 is also used.

Chlortalidone p. 138, a thiazide-related compound, has a longer duration of action than the thiazides and may be given on alternate days in younger children.

Metolazone is particularly effective when combined with a loop diuretic (even in renal failure) and is most effective when given 30–60 minutes before furosemide profound diuresis can occur and the child should therefore be monitored carefully.

Loop diuretics

Loop diuretics inhibit reabsorption of sodium, potassium, and chloride from the ascending limb of the loop of Henlé in the renal tubule and are powerful diuretics.

Furosemide and bumetanide p. 136 are similar in activity; they produce dose-related diuresis. Furosemide is used extensively in children. It can be used for pulmonary oedema (e.g. in respiratory distress syndrome and bronchopulmonary dysplasia), congestive heart failure, and in renal disease.

Potassium-sparing diuretics and aldosterone antagonists

Spironolactone is the most commonly used potassium sparing diuretic in children; it is an aldosterone antagonist

and enhances potassium retention and sodium excretion in the distal tubule. Spironolactone is combined with other diuretics to reduce urinary potassium loss. It is also used in nephrotic syndrome, the long-term management of Bartter's syndrome, and high doses can help to control ascites in babies with chronic neonatal hepatitis. The clinical value of spironolactone in the management of pulmonary oedema in preterm neonates with chronic lung disease is uncertain.

Potassium canrenoate p. 122 given intravenously, is an alternative aldosterone antagonist that may be useful if a potassium-sparing diuretic is required and the child is unable to take oral medication. It is metabolised to canrenone, which is also a metabolite of spironolactone.

Amiloride hydrochloride on its own is a weak diuretic. It causes retention of potassium and is therefore given with thiazide or loop diuretics as an alternative to giving potassium supplements.

A potassium-sparing diuretic such as spironolactone or amiloride hydrochloride may also be used in the management of amphotericin-induced hypokalaemia.

Potassium supplements must **not** be given with potassium-sparing diuretics. Administration of a potassium-sparing diuretic to a child receiving an ACE inhibitor or an angiotensin-II receptor antagonist can also cause severe hyperkalaemia.

Potassium-sparing diuretics with other diuretics

Although it is preferable to prescribe diuretics separately in children, the use of fixed combinations may be justified in older children if compliance is a problem. (Some preparations may not be licensed for use in children— consult product literature).

Other diuretics

Mannitol p. 137 is used to treat cerebral oedema, raised intraocular pressure, peripheral oedema, and acites.

The carbonic anhydrase inhibitor acetazolamide p. 655 is a weak diuretic although it is little used for its diuretic effect. Acetazolamide and eye drops of dorzolamide p. 656 and brinzolamide p. 656 inhibit the formation of aqueous humour and are used in glaucoma. Acetazolamide is also used in the treatment of epilepsy, and raised intracranial pressure.

Diuretics with potassium

Diuretics and potassium supplements should be prescribed separately.

DIURETICS ⟩ LOOP DIURETICS

Loop diuretics

- **DRUG ACTION** Loop diuretics inhibit reabsorption from the ascending limb of the loop of Henlé in the renal tubule and are powerful diuretics.

- **CONTRA-INDICATIONS** Anuria · renal failure due to nephrotoxic or hepatotoxic drugs · severe hypokalaemia · severe hyponatraemia

- **CAUTIONS** Can cause acute urinary retention in children with obstruction of urinary outflow · can exacerbate diabetes (but hyperglycaemia less likely than with thiazides) · can excacerbate gout · comatose and precomatose states associated with liver cirrhosis · hypotension should be corrected before initiation of treatment · hypovolaemia should be corrected before initiation of treatment

 CAUTIONS, FURTHER INFORMATION
▸ Potassium loss Hypokalaemia can occur with both thiazide and loop diuretics. The risk of hypokalaemia depends on the duration of action as well as the potency and is thus greater with thiazides than with an equipotent dose of a

loop diuretic.

Hypokalaemia is particularly dangerous in children being treated with cardiac glycosides. In hepatic failure hypokalaemia caused by diuretics can precipitate encephalopathy.

The use of potassium-sparing diuretics avoids the need to take potassium supplements.

▸ Urinary retention Loop diuretics can cause acute urinary retention in children with obstruction of urinary outflow, therefore adequate urinary output should be established before initiating treatment.

● SIDE-EFFECTS
▸ Very rare Hyperuricaemia
▸ Frequency not known Acute urinary retention · blood disorders · bone-marrow depression · deafness (usually with high doses and rapid intravenous administration, and in renal impairment) · electrolyte disturbances · hepatic encephalopathy · hyperglycaemia (less common than with thiazides) · hypersensitivity reactions · hypochloraemia · hypokalaemia · hypomagnesaemia · hyponatraemia · increased calcium excretion (nephrocalcinosis and nephrolithiasis reported with long-term use of furosemide in preterm infants) · leucopenia · metabolic alkalosis · mild gastro-intestinal disturbances · pancreatitis · photosensitivity · postural hypotension · rash · temporary increase in serum-cholesterol and triglyceride concentration · thrombocytopenia · tinnitus (usually with high doses and rapid intravenous administration, and in renal impairment) · visual disturbances

● HEPATIC IMPAIRMENT Hypokalaemia induced by loop diuretics may precipitate hepatic encephalopathy and coma—potassium-sparing diuretics can be used to prevent this.

● RENAL IMPAIRMENT High doses of loop diuretics may occasionally be needed in renal impairment. High doses or rapid intravenous administration can cause tinnitus and deafness.

● MONITORING REQUIREMENTS Monitor electrolytes during treatment.

⚑ 135

Bumetanide

● INDICATIONS AND DOSE

Oedema in heart failure, renal disease, and hepatic disease | Pulmonary oedema
▸ BY MOUTH
▸ Child 1 month–11 years: 15–50 micrograms/kg 1–4 times a day (max. per dose 2 mg); maximum 5 mg per day
▸ Child 12–17 years: Initially 1 mg, dose to be taken in the morning, then 1 mg after 6–8 hours if required

Oedema in heart failure, renal disease, and hepatic disease (severe cases) | Pulmonary oedema (severe cases)
▸ BY MOUTH
▸ Child 12–17 years: Initially 5 mg daily, increased in steps of 5 mg every 12–24 hours, adjusted according to response

● UNLICENSED USE Not licensed for use in children under 12 years.

● INTERACTIONS → Appendix 1: loop diuretics

● SIDE-EFFECTS Breast pain · gynaecomastia · musculoskeletal pain (associated with high doses in renal failure)

● PREGNANCY Bumetanide should not be used to treat gestational hypertension because of the maternal hypovolaemia associated with this condition.

● BREAST FEEDING No information available. May inhibit lactation.

● MEDICINAL FORMS
There can be variation in the licensing of different medicines containing the same drug. Forms available from special-order manufacturers include: oral suspension

Oral solution
▸ Bumetanide (Non-proprietary)
Bumetanide 200 microgram per 1 ml Bumetanide 1mg/5ml oral solution sugar free sugar-free | 150 ml PoM £198.00 DT price = £198.00

Tablet
▸ Bumetanide (Non-proprietary)
Bumetanide 1 mg Bumetanide 1mg tablets | 28 tablet PoM £7.35 DT price = £1.64
Bumetanide 5 mg Bumetanide 5mg tablets | 28 tablet PoM £7.00 DT price = £6.98

⚑ 135

Furosemide

(Frusemide)

● INDICATIONS AND DOSE

Oedema in heart failure, renal disease, and hepatic disease | Pulmonary oedema
▸ BY MOUTH
▸ Neonate: 0.5–2 mg/kg every 12–24 hours, alternatively 0.5–2 mg/kg every 24 hours, if corrected gestational age under 31 weeks.
▸ Child 1 month–11 years: 0.5–2 mg/kg 2–3 times a day, alternatively 0.5–2 mg/kg every 24 hours, if corrected gestational age of under 31 weeks, higher doses may be required in resistant oedema; maximum 80 mg per day; maximum 12 mg/kg per day
▸ Child 12–17 years: 20–40 mg daily; increased to 80–120 mg daily, in resistant oedema
▸ BY SLOW INTRAVENOUS INJECTION
▸ Neonate: 0.5–1 mg/kg every 12–24 hours, alternatively 0.5–1 mg/kg every 24 hours, if corrected gestational age under 31 weeks.
▸ Child 1 month–11 years: 0.5–1 mg/kg every 8 hours (max. per dose 40 mg every 8 hours) as required; maximum 6 mg/kg per day
▸ Child 12–17 years: 20–40 mg every 8 hours as required, higher doses may be required in resistant cases
▸ BY CONTINUOUS INTRAVENOUS INFUSION
▸ Child: 0.1–2 mg/kg/hour

Oedema in heart failure, renal disease, and hepatic disease following cardiac surgery | Pulmonary oedema following cardiac surgery
▸ BY CONTINUOUS INTRAVENOUS INFUSION
▸ Child: Initially 100 micrograms/kg/hour, dose to be doubled every 2 hours until urine output exceeds 1 mL/kg/hour

Oliguria
▸ BY MOUTH
▸ Child 12–17 years: Initially 250 mg daily, then increased in steps of 250 mg every 4–6 hours (max. per dose 2 g) if required
▸ BY INTRAVENOUS INFUSION
▸ Child 1 month–11 years: 2–5 mg/kg up to 4 times a day; maximum 1 g per day
▸ Child 12–17 years: Initially 250 mg, dose to be administered over 1 hour, increased to 500 mg, increased dose is given if satisfactory urine output not obtained; dose administered over 2 hours, then increased to 1 g, increased dose given if satisfactory response not obtained within subsequent hour; dose to be administered over 4 hours. If no response obtained dialysis probably required;, effective dose of up to 1 g given at a maximum rate of 4 mg/minute can be repeated every 24 hours

- **CAUTIONS** Effect may be prolonged in neonates (in neonates) · hepatorenal syndrome · hypoproteinaemia may reduce diuretic effect and increase risk of side-effects
- **INTERACTIONS** → Appendix 1: loop diuretics
- **SIDE-EFFECTS** Gout · intrahepatic cholestasis
- **PREGNANCY** Furosemide should not be used to treat gestational hypertension because of the maternal hypovolaemia associated with this condition.
- **BREAST FEEDING** Amount too small to be harmful. May inhibit lactation.
- **DIRECTIONS FOR ADMINISTRATION**
▶ With intravenous use For *intravenous injection*, give over 5–10 minutes at a usual rate of 100 micrograms/kg/minute (not exceeding 500 micrograms/kg/minute), max. 4 mg/minute; lower rate of infusion may be necessary in renal impairment. For *intravenous infusion*, dilute with Sodium Chloride 0.9% to a concentration of 1–2 mg/mL. Glucose solutions unsuitable (infusion pH must be above 5.5).
▶ With oral use For administration by *mouth*, tablets can be crushed and mixed with water or injection solution diluted and given by mouth. Risk of ototoxicity may be reduced by giving high oral doses in 2 or more divided doses.
- **PRESCRIBING AND DISPENSING INFORMATION**
▶ With oral use Some liquid preparations contain alcohol, caution especially in neonates.

- **MEDICINAL FORMS**
There can be variation in the licensing of different medicines containing the same drug. Forms available from special-order manufacturers include: oral suspension, oral solution

Tablet
▶ **Furosemide (Non-proprietary)**
Furosemide 20 mg Furosemide 20mg tablets | 28 tablet PoM £1.02 DT price = £0.73
Furosemide 40 mg Furosemide 40mg tablets | 28 tablet PoM £1.03 DT price = £0.69 | 1000 tablet PoM £28.21
Furosemide 500 mg Furosemide 500mg tablets | 28 tablet PoM £70.00 DT price = £38.26
▶ **Diuresal** (Ennogen Pharma Ltd)
Furosemide 500 mg Diuresal 500mg tablets | 28 tablet PoM no price available DT price = £38.26

Solution for injection
▶ **Furosemide (Non-proprietary)**
Furosemide 10 mg per 1 ml Furosemide 250mg/25ml solution for injection ampoules | 10 ampoule PoM £25.00-£40.00
Furosemide 50mg/5ml solution for injection ampoules | 10 ampoule PoM £4.50-£7.60
Furosemide 20mg/2ml solution for injection ampoules | 10 ampoule PoM £3.60

Oral solution
EXCIPIENTS: May contain Alcohol
▶ **Furosemide (Non-proprietary)**
Furosemide 4 mg per 1 ml Furosemide 20mg/5ml oral solution sugar free sugar-free | 150 ml PoM £14.83 DT price = £14.78
Furosemide 8 mg per 1 ml Furosemide 40mg/5ml oral solution sugar free sugar-free | 150 ml PoM £18.69 DT price = £18.69
Furosemide 10 mg per 1 ml Furosemide 50mg/5ml oral solution sugar free sugar-free | 150 ml PoM £20.21 DT price = £20.21
▶ **Frusol** (Rosemont Pharmaceuticals Ltd)
Furosemide 4 mg per 1 ml Frusol 20mg/5ml oral solution sugar-free | 150 ml PoM £12.07 DT price = £14.78
Furosemide 8 mg per 1 ml Frusol 40mg/5ml oral solution sugar-free | 150 ml PoM £15.58 DT price = £18.69
Furosemide 10 mg per 1 ml Frusol 50mg/5ml oral solution sugar-free | 150 ml PoM £16.84 DT price = £20.21

DIURETICS > OSMOTIC DIURETICS

Mannitol

- **INDICATIONS AND DOSE**
Cerebral oedema
▶ BY INTRAVENOUS INFUSION
▶ Child 1 month-11 years: 0.25–1.5 g/kg, repeated if necessary, to be administered over 30–60 minutes, dose may be repeated 1–2 times after 4–8 hours
▶ Child 12-17 years: 0.25–2 g/kg, repeated if necessary, to be administered over 30-60 minutes, dose may be repeated 1–2 times after 4–8 hours
Peripheral oedema and ascites
▶ BY INTRAVENOUS INFUSION
▶ Child: 1–2 g/kg, to be given over 2–6 hours

- **UNLICENSED USE** Not for use in children under 12 years.
- **CONTRA-INDICATIONS** Anuria · intracranial bleeding (except during craniotomy) · severe cardiac failure · severe dehydration · severe pulmonary oedema
- **CAUTIONS** Extravasation causes inflammation and thrombophlebitis
- **SIDE-EFFECTS**
▶ **Uncommon** Electrolyte imbalance · fluid imbalance · hypotension · thrombophlebitis
▶ **Rare** Anaphylaxis · arrhythmia · blurred vision · chest pain · chills · convulsions · cramp · dehydration · dizziness · dry mouth · fever · focal osmotic nephrosis · headache · hypersensitivity reactions · hypertension · nausea · oedema · pulmonary oedema · raised intracranial pressure · rhinitis · skin necrosis · thirst · urinary retention · urticaria · vomiting
▶ **Very rare** Acute renal failure · congestive heart failure
- **PREGNANCY** Manufacturer advises avoid unless essential— no information available.
- **BREAST FEEDING** Manufacturer advises avoid unless essential—no information available.
- **RENAL IMPAIRMENT** Use with caution in severe impairment.
- **PRE-TREATMENT SCREENING** Assess cardiac function before treatment.
- **MONITORING REQUIREMENTS** Monitor fluid and electrolyte balance, serum osmolality, and cardiac, pulmonary and renal function.
- **DIRECTIONS FOR ADMINISTRATION** Examine infusion for crystals. If crystals present, dissolve by warming infusion fluid (allow to cool to body temperature before administration).
For mannitol 20%, an in-line filter is recommended (15-micron filters have been used).

- **MEDICINAL FORMS**
There can be variation in the licensing of different medicines containing the same drug. Forms available from special-order manufacturers include: infusion, solution for infusion

Infusion
▶ **Mannitol (Non-proprietary)**
Mannitol 100 mg per 1 ml Mannitol 50g/500ml (10%) infusion Viaflo bags | 1 bag PoM no price available | 20 bag PoM no price available
Mannitol 50g/500ml (10%) infusion Viaflex bags | 1 bag PoM no price available | 20 bag PoM no price available
Polyfusor K mannitol 10% infusion 500ml bottles | 1 bottle PoM £4.46 | 12 bottle PoM no price available
Mannitol 150 mg per 1 ml Mannitol 75g/500ml (15%) infusion Viaflo bags | 20 bag PoM no price available
Mannitol 200 mg per 1 ml Mannitol 100g/500ml (20%) infusion Viaflex bags | 1 bag PoM no price available | 20 bag PoM no price available

Cardiovascular system

2

Polyfusor M mannitol 20% infusion 500ml bottles | 1 bottle PoM
£5.86 | 12 bottle PoM no price available
Mannitol 50g/250ml (20%) infusion Viaflex bags | 1 bag PoM no
price available | 30 bag PoM no price available
Mannitol 100g/500ml (20%) infusion Viaflo bags | 1 bag PoM no
price available | 20 bag PoM no price available

DIURETICS > POTASSIUM-SPARING DIURETICS

Amiloride hydrochloride

● **INDICATIONS AND DOSE**
Adjunct to thiazide or loop diuretics for oedema in heart failure, and hepatic disease (where potassium conservation desirable)
▸ BY MOUTH
▸ Neonate: 100–200 micrograms/kg twice daily.

▸ Child 1 month–11 years: 100–200 micrograms/kg twice daily; maximum 20 mg per day
▸ Child 12–17 years: 5–10 mg twice daily

● **UNLICENSED USE** Not licensed for use in children.
● **CONTRA-INDICATIONS** Addison's disease · anuria · hyperkalaemia
● **CAUTIONS** Diabetes mellitus
● **INTERACTIONS** → Appendix 1: potassium-sparing diuretics
● **SIDE-EFFECTS** Abdominal pain · agitation · alopecia · angina · anorexia · arrhythmias · arthralgia · confusion · constipation · cough · diarrhoea · dizziness · dry mouth · dyspepsia · dyspnoea · encephalopathy · flatulence · gastro-intestinal bleeding · headache · hyperkalaemia · insomnia · jaundice · malaise · muscle cramp · nasal congestion · nausea · palpitation · paraesthesia · postural hypotension · pruritus · raised intra-ocular pressure · rash · sexual dysfunction · thirst · tinnitus · tremor · urinary disturbances · visual disturbance · vomiting · weakness
● **PREGNANCY** Not to be used to treat gestational hypertension.
● **BREAST FEEDING** Manufacturer advises avoid—no information available.
● **RENAL IMPAIRMENT** Manufacturers advise avoid in severe impairment. Monitor plasma-potassium concentration (high risk of hyperkalaemia in renal impairment).
● **MONITORING REQUIREMENTS** Monitor electrolytes.

● **MEDICINAL FORMS**
There can be variation in the licensing of different medicines containing the same drug. Forms available from special-order manufacturers include: oral suspension, oral solution
Oral solution
EXCIPIENTS: May contain Propylene glycol
▸ Amiloride hydrochloride (Non-proprietary)
 Amiloride hydrochloride 1 mg per 1 ml Amiloride 5mg/5ml oral solution sugar free sugar-free | 150 ml PoM no price available DT price = £37.35
▸ Amilamont (Rosemont Pharmaceuticals Ltd)
 Amiloride hydrochloride 1 mg per 1 ml Amilamont 5mg/5ml oral solution sugar free sugar-free | 150 ml PoM £37.35 DT price = £37.35
Tablet
▸ Amiloride hydrochloride (Non-proprietary)
 Amiloride hydrochloride 5 mg Amiloride 5mg tablets | 28 tablet PoM £1.21 DT price = £1.21

DIURETICS > THIAZIDES AND RELATED DIURETICS

⬛ 107

Chlortalidone

(Chlorthalidone)

● **INDICATIONS AND DOSE**
Ascites | Oedema in nephrotic syndrome
▸ BY MOUTH
▸ Child 5–11 years: 0.5–1 mg/kg every 48 hours (max. per dose 1.7 mg/kg every 48 hours), dose to be taken in the morning
▸ Child 12–17 years: Up to 50 mg daily
Hypertension
▸ BY MOUTH
▸ Child 5–11 years: 0.5–1 mg/kg every 48 hours (max. per dose 1.7 mg/kg every 48 hours), dose to be taken in the morning
▸ Child 12–17 years: 25 mg daily, dose to be taken in the morning, then increased if necessary to 50 mg daily
Stable heart failure
▸ BY MOUTH
▸ Child 5–11 years: 0.5–1 mg/kg every 48 hours (max. per dose 1.7 mg/kg every 48 hours), dose to be taken in the morning
▸ Child 12–17 years: 25–50 mg daily, dose to be taken in the morning, then increased if necessary to 100–200 mg daily, reduce to lowest effective dose for maintenance

● **INTERACTIONS** → Appendix 1: thiazide diuretics
● **SIDE-EFFECTS**
▸ Rare Jaundice
● **BREAST FEEDING** The amount present in milk is too small to be harmful. Large doses may suppress lactation.

● **MEDICINAL FORMS**
There can be variation in the licensing of different medicines containing the same drug. Forms available from special-order manufacturers include: oral suspension
Tablet
▸ Chlortalidone (Non-proprietary)
 Chlortalidone 25 mg Chlortalidone 25mg tablets | 100 tablet PoM no price available
 Chlortalidone 50 mg Chlortalidone 50mg tablets | 30 tablet PoM £90.55 DT price = £90.20

⬛ 107

Metolazone

● **INDICATIONS AND DOSE**
Oedema resistant to loop diuretics in heart failure, renal disease and hepatic disease | Pulmonary oedema | Adjunct to loop diuretics to induce diuresis
▸ BY MOUTH
▸ Child 1 month–11 years: 100–200 micrograms/kg 1–2 times a day
▸ Child 12–17 years: 5–10 mg once daily, dose to be taken in the morning; increased if necessary to 5–10 mg twice daily, dose increased in resistant oedema

● **UNLICENSED USE** Not licensed for use in children.
● **CAUTIONS** Acute porphyrias p. 577
● **INTERACTIONS** → Appendix 1: thiazide diuretics
● **SIDE-EFFECTS** Chest pain · chills
● **BREAST FEEDING** The amount present in milk is too small to be harmful. Large doses may suppress lactation.
● **DIRECTIONS FOR ADMINISTRATION** Tablets may be crushed and mixed with water immediately before use.

- **MEDICINAL FORMS**
  There can be variation in the licensing of different medicines containing the same drug. Forms available from special-order manufacturers include: tablet, oral suspension, oral solution

  Tablet
  ▸ Metolazone (Non-proprietary)
  Metolazone 2.5 mg Zaroxolyn 2.5mg tablets | 100 tablet PoM no price available
  Metolazone 5 mg Zaroxolyn 5mg tablets | 50 tablet PoM no price available

9 Patent ductus arteriosus

Drugs affecting the ductus arteriosus

> **Other drugs used for Patent ductus arteriosus not listed below** Ibuprofen, p. 625 · Indometacin, p. 628

Closure of the ductus arteriosus

Patent ductus arteriosus is a frequent problem in premature neonates with respiratory distress syndrome. Substantial left-to-right shunting through the ductus arteriosus may increase the risk of intraventricular haemorrhage, necrotising enterocolitis, bronchopulmonary dysplasia, and possibly death. Indometacin p. 628 or ibuprofen p. 625 can be used to close the ductus arteriosus. Indometacin has been used for many years and is effective but it reduces cerebral blood flow, and causes a transient fall in renal and gastro-intestinal blood flow. Ibuprofen may also be used; it has little effect on renal function (there may be a small reduction in sodium excretion) when used in doses for closure of the ductus arteriosus; gastro-intestinal problems are uncommon. If drug treatment fails to close the ductus arteriosus, surgery may be indicated.

Maintenance of patency

In the newborn with duct-dependent congenital heart disease it is often necessary to maintain the patency of the ductus arteriosus whilst awaiting surgery. Alprostadil below (prostaglandin E1) and dinoprostone below (prostaglandin E2) are potent vasodilators that are effective for maintaining the patency of the ductus arteriosus. They are usually given by continuous intravenous infusion, but oral dosing of dinoprostone is still used in some centres. During the infusion of a prostaglandin, the newborn requires careful monitoring of heart rate, blood pressure, respiratory rate, and core body temperature. In the event of complications such as apnoea, profound bradycardia, or severe hypotension, the infusion should be temporarily stopped and the complication dealt with; the infusion should be restarted at a lower dose. Recurrent or prolonged apnoea may require ventilatory support in order for the prostaglandin infusion to continue.

PROSTAGLANDIN ANALOGUES AND PROSTAMIDES > PROSTAGLANDINS

▍Alprostadil

- **INDICATIONS AND DOSE**
  Maintaining patency of the ductus arteriosus
  ▸ BY CONTINUOUS INTRAVENOUS INFUSION

  ▸ Neonate: Initially 5 nanograms/kg/minute, adjusted according to response, adjusted in steps of 5 nanograms/kg/minute (max. per dose 100 nanograms/kg/minute), maximum dose associated with increased side-effects.

- **UNLICENSED USE** Alprostadil doses in BNFC may differ from those in product literature.
- **CONTRA-INDICATIONS** Avoid in hyaline membrane disease
- **CAUTIONS** History of haemorrhage
- **INTERACTIONS** → Appendix 1: alprostadil
- **SIDE-EFFECTS** Apnoea (particularly in neonates under 2 kg) · bradycardia · cardiac arrest · convulsions · cortical proliferation of long bones · diarrhoea · disseminated intravascular coagulation · fever · flushing · gastric-outlet obstruction · hypokalaemia · hypotension · oedema · tachycardia · weakening of the wall of the ductus arteriosus and pulmonary artery (following prolonged use)
- **MONITORING REQUIREMENTS**
  ▸ During the infusion of a prostaglandin, the newborn requires careful monitoring of heart rate, blood pressure, respiratory rate, and core body temperature.
  ▸ Monitor arterial pressure, respiratory rate, heart rate, temperature, and venous blood pressure in arm and leg; facilities for intubation and ventilation must be immediately available
- **DIRECTIONS FOR ADMINISTRATION** Dilute 150 micrograms/kg body-weight to a final volume of 50 mL with Glucose 5% or Sodium Chloride 0.9%; an intravenous infusion rate of 0.1 mL/hour provides a dose of 5 nanograms/kg/minute. Undiluted solution must not come into contact with the barrel of the plastic syringe; add the required volume of alprostadil to a volume of infusion fluid in the syringe and then make up to final volume.

- **MEDICINAL FORMS**
  There can be variation in the licensing of different medicines containing the same drug.
  Solution for infusion
  ▸ Prostin VR (Pfizer Ltd)
  Alprostadil 500 microgram per 1 ml Prostin VR 500micrograms/1ml concentrate for solution for infusion ampoules | 5 ampoule PoM £375.96 (Hospital only)

▍Dinoprostone

- **INDICATIONS AND DOSE**
  Maintaining patency of the ductus arteriosus
  ▸ BY CONTINUOUS INTRAVENOUS INFUSION

  ▸ Neonate: Initially 5 nanograms/kg/minute, then increased in steps of 5 nanograms/kg/minute as required; increased to 20 nanograms/kg/minute, doses up to 100 nanogram/kg/minute have been used but are associated with increased side-effects.

  ▸ BY MOUTH

  ▸ Neonate: 20–25 micrograms/kg every 1–2 hours, then increased if necessary to 40–50 micrograms/kg every 1–2 hours, if treatment continues for more than 1 week gradually reduce the dose.

- **UNLICENSED USE** Not licensed for use in children.
- **CONTRA-INDICATIONS** Avoid in hyaline membrane disease
- **CAUTIONS** History of haemorrhage
- **SIDE-EFFECTS** Cortical hyperostosis (prolonged use) · apnoea (particularly with high doses and in low birth-weight neonates) · bradycardia · bronchospasm · cardiac arrest · diarrhoea · erythema · flushing · gastric outlet obstruction (if used for longer than 5 days) · hypotension · local reactions · nausea · pyrexia · raised white blood cell count · respiratory depression (particularly with high doses and in low birth-weight neonates) · shivering · temporary pyrexia · vomiting
- **HEPATIC IMPAIRMENT** Manufacturers advise avoid.

- **RENAL IMPAIRMENT** Manufacturers advise avoid.
- **MONITORING REQUIREMENTS** Monitor arterial oxygenation, heart rate, temperature, and blood pressure in arm and leg; facilities for intubation and ventilation must be immediately available. During infusion of dinoprostone, the newborn requires careful monitoring of heart rate, blood pressure, respiratory rate and core body temperature.
- **DIRECTIONS FOR ADMINISTRATION**
  ‣ With intravenous use For *continuous intravenous infusion*, dilute to a concentration of 1 microgram/mL with Glucose 5% or Sodium Chloride 0.9%.
  ‣ With oral use For administration by *mouth*, injection solution can be given orally; dilute with water.

- **MEDICINAL FORMS**
  There can be variation in the licensing of different medicines containing the same drug.
  Solution for infusion
  ‣ Prostin E2 (Pfizer Ltd)
  Dinoprostone 1 mg per 1 ml Prostin E2 750micrograms/0.75ml solution for infusion ampoules | 1 ampoule [PoM] £8.52 (Hospital only)
  Dinoprostone 10 mg per 1 ml Prostin E2 5mg/0.5ml solution for infusion ampoules | 1 ampoule [PoM] £18.40 (Hospital only)

10 Vascular disease

Peripheral vascular disease

Classification and management

Raynaud's syndrome, a vasospastic peripheral vascular disease, consists of recurrent, long-lasting, and episodic vasospasm of the fingers and toes often associated with exposure to cold. Management includes avoidance of exposure to cold and stopping smoking (if appropriate). More severe symptoms may require vasodilator treatment, which is most often successful in primary Raynaud's syndrome. Nifedipine p. 106 and diltiazem hydrochloride below are useful for reducing the frequency and severity of vasospastic attacks. In very severe cases, where digital infarction is likely, intravenous infusion of the prostacyclin analogue iloprost p. 116 may be helpful.

Vasodilator therapy is not established as being effective for *chilblains*.

CALCIUM-CHANNEL BLOCKERS

F 104

Diltiazem hydrochloride

- **INDICATIONS AND DOSE**
  Raynaud's syndrome
  ‣ BY MOUTH
  ‣ Child 12–17 years: 30–60 mg 2–3 times a day

- **UNLICENSED USE** Not licensed for use in children.
- **CONTRA-INDICATIONS** Acute porphyrias p. 577 · cardiogenic shock · left ventricular failure with pulmonary congestion · second- or third-degree AV block (unless pacemaker fitted) · severe bradycardia · sick sinus syndrome · significant aortic stenosis
- **CAUTIONS** Bradycardia (avoid if severe) · first degree AV block · heart failure · prolonged PR interval · significantly impaired left ventricular function
- **INTERACTIONS** → Appendix 1: calcium channel blockers
- **SIDE-EFFECTS**
  ‣ **Common or very common** Asthenia · AV block · bradycardia · dizziness · gastro-intestinal disturbances · headache · hot flushes · hypotension · malaise · oedema (notably of ankles) · palpitation · sino-atrial block
  ‣ **Rare** Erythema multiforme · exfoliative dermatitis · photosensitivity · rashes
  ‣ **Frequency not known** Depression · extrapyramidal symptoms · gum hyperplasia · gynaecomastia · hepatitis
  Overdose
  In overdose, diltiazem has a profound cardiac depressant effect causing hypotension and arrhythmias, including complete heart block and asystole.

- **PREGNANCY** Avoid.
- **BREAST FEEDING** Significant amount present in milk—no evidence of harm but avoid unless no safer alternative.
- **HEPATIC IMPAIRMENT** Reduce dose.
- **RENAL IMPAIRMENT** Start with smaller dose.

- **MEDICINAL FORMS**
  There can be variation in the licensing of different medicines containing the same drug. Forms available from special-order manufacturers include: oral suspension, oral solution
  Modified-release tablet
  CAUTIONARY AND ADVISORY LABELS 25
  ‣ Diltiazem hydrochloride (Non-proprietary)
  Diltiazem hydrochloride 60 mg Diltiazem 60mg modified-release tablets | 84 tablet [PoM] £41.59 DT price = £41.59 | 100 tablet [PoM] £49.51
  ‣ Tildiem (Sanofi)
  Diltiazem hydrochloride 60 mg Tildiem 60mg modified-release tablets | 90 tablet [PoM] £7.96

Chapter 3
Respiratory system

CONTENTS

Respiratory system, drug delivery

Inhalation

This route delivers the drug directly to the airways; the dose required is smaller than when given by mouth and side-effects are reduced.

Children and their carers should be advised to follow manufacturers' instructions on the care and cleansing of inhaler devices.

Inhaler devices

A *pressurised metered-dose inhaler* is an effective method of drug administration in mild to moderate chronic asthma; to deliver the drug effectively, particularly in children under 12 years, a spacer device should also be used (see also NICE guidance). By the age of 3 years, a child can usually be taught to use a spacer device without a mask. As soon as a child is able to use the mouthpiece, then this is the preferred delivery system. When a pressurised metered-dose inhaler with a spacer is unsuitable or inconvenient, a *dry-powder inhaler* or *breath-actuated inhaler* may be used instead if the child is able to use the device effectively.

Dry powder inhalers may be useful in children over 5 years, who are unwilling or unable to use a pressurised metered-dose inhaler with a spacer device; *breath-actuated inhalers* may be useful in older children if they are able to use the device effectively. The child or child's carer should be instructed carefully on the use of the inhaler. It is important to check that the inhaler is being used correctly; poor inhalation technique may be mistaken for a lack of response to the drug.

On changing from a pressurised metered-dose inhaler to a dry powder inhaler, the child may notice a lack of sensation in the mouth and throat previously associated with each actuation; coughing may occur more frequently following use of a dry-powder inhaler.

CFC-free metered-dose inhalers should be cleaned **weekly** according to the manufacturer's instructions.

Spacer devices

Spacer devices are particularly useful for infants, for children with poor inhalation technique, or for nocturnal asthma, because the device reduces the need for coordination between actuation of a pressurised metered-dose inhaler and inhalation. The spacer device reduces the velocity of the aerosol and subsequent impaction on the oropharynx and allows more time for evaporation of the propellant so that a larger proportion of the particles can be inhaled and deposited in the lungs. Smaller-volume spacers may be more manageable for pre-school children and infants. The spacer device used must be compatible with the prescribed metered-dose inhaler.

Use and care of spacer devices
The suitability of the spacer device should be carefully assessed; opening the one-way valve is dependent on the child's inspiratory flow. Some devices can be tipped to 45° to open the valve during inhaler actuation and inspiration to assist the child.

Inhalation from the spacer device should follow the actuation as soon as possible because the drug aerosol is very short-lived. The total dose (which may be more than a single puff) should be administered as single actuations (with tidal breathing for 10–20 seconds or 5 breaths for each actuation) for children with good inspiratory flow. Larger doses may be necessary for a child with acute bronchospasm.

The device should be cleansed once a month by washing in mild detergent and then allowed to dry in air without rinsing; the mouthpiece should be wiped clean of detergent before use. Some manufacturers recommend more frequent cleaning, but this should be avoided since any electrostatic charge may affect drug delivery. Spacer devices should be replaced every 6–12 months.

Nebulisers

Solutions for nebulisation for use in acute severe asthma are administered over 5–10 minutes from a nebuliser, usually driven by oxygen in hospital.

Children with a severe attack of asthma should preferably have oxygen during nebulisation since beta$_2$ agonists can increase arterial hypoxaemia.

A nebuliser converts a solution of a drug into an aerosol for inhalation. It is used to deliver higher doses of drug to the airways than is usual with standard inhalers. The main indications for use of a nebuliser are:

- to deliver a beta$_2$ agonist or ipratropium bromide p. 147 to a child with an *acute exacerbation* of asthma or of airways obstruction;
- to deliver *prophylactic medication* to a child unable to use other conventional devices;
- to deliver an antibacterial (such as colistimethate sodium p. 331 or tobramycin p. 300) to a child with chronic purulent infection (as in cystic fibrosis or bronchiectasis);
- to deliver budesonide p. 155 to a child with severe croup.

The proportion of a nebuliser solution that reaches the lungs depends on the type of nebuliser and although it can be as high as 30% it is more frequently close to 10% and sometimes below 10%. The remaining solution is left in the nebuliser as residual volume or it is deposited in the mouthpiece and tubing. The extent to which the nebulised solution is deposited in the airways or alveoli depends on particle size. Particles with a median diameter of 1–5 microns are deposited in the airways and are therefore appropriate for asthma whereas a particle size of 1–2 microns is needed for alveolar deposition. The type of nebuliser is therefore chosen according to the deposition required and according to the viscosity of the solution.

Nebulised bronchodilators are appropriate for children with chronic persistent asthma or those with severe acute asthma. In chronic asthma, nebulised bronchodilators should only be used to relieve persistent daily wheeze, however, with the development of spacers with facemasks, it is now unusual for a child to require long-term nebulised asthma therapy. The use of nebulisers in chronic persistent asthma should be considered only:

- after a review of the diagnosis and use of current inhaler devices;
- if the airflow obstruction is significantly reversible by bronchodilators without unacceptable side-effects;
- if the child does not benefit from use of conventional inhaler device, such as pressurised metered-dose inhaler plus spacer;
- if the child is complying with the prescribed dose and frequency of anti-inflammatory treatment including regular use of high-dose inhaled corticosteroid.

When a nebuliser is prescribed, the child or child's carer must:

- have clear instructions from a doctor, specialist nurse, physiotherapist, or pharmacist on the use of the nebuliser (and on peak-flow monitoring);
- be instructed not to treat acute attacks without also seeking medical help;
- have regular follow-up with doctor or specialist nurse.

Jet nebulisers
Jet nebulisers are more widely used than ultrasonic nebulisers. Most jet nebulisers require an optimum flow rate of 6–8 litres/minute and in hospital can be driven by piped air or oxygen; in acute asthma the nebuliser should always be driven by oxygen. Domiciliary oxygen cylinders do not provide an adequate flow rate therefore an electrical compressor is required for domiciliary use.

Some jet nebulisers are able to increase drug output during inspiration and hence increase efficiency.

Safe practice
The Department of Health has reminded users of the need to use the correct grade of tubing when connecting a nebuliser to a medical gas supply or compressor.

Nebuliser diluent
Nebulisation may be carried out using an undiluted nebuliser solution or it may require dilution beforehand. The usual diluent is sterile sodium chloride 0.9% (physiological saline).

In England and Wales nebulisers and compressors are not available on the NHS (but they are free of VAT); some nebulisers (but not compressors) are available on form GP10A in Scotland (for details consult Scottish Drug Tariff).

Oral

Systemic side-effects occur more frequently when a drug is given orally rather than by inhalation. Oral corticosteroids, theophylline p. 162, and leukotriene receptor antagonists are sometimes required for the management of asthma. Oral administration of a beta$_2$ agonist is generally not recommended for children, but may be necessary in infants and young children who are unable or unwilling to use an inhaler device.

Parenteral

Drugs such as beta$_2$ agonists, corticosteroids, and aminophylline p. 161 can be given by injection in acute severe asthma when drug administration by nebulisation is inadequate or inappropriate; in these circumstances the child should generally be treated in a high dependency or intensive care unit.

Peak flow meters

Peak flow meters may be used to assess lung function in children over 5 years with asthma, but symptom monitoring is the most reliable assessment of asthma control. They are best used for short periods to assess the severity of asthma and to monitor response to treatment: continuous use of peak flow meters may detract from compliance with inhalers.

Peak flow charts should be issued to patients where appropriate, and are available to purchase from:

3M Security Print and Systems Limited. Gorse Street, Chadderton, Oldham, OL9 9QH. Tel: 0845 610 1112

GP practices can obtain supplies through their Area Team stores.

NHS Hospitals can order supplies from www.nhsforms.co.uk/ or by emailing nhsforms@mmm.com.

In Scotland, peak flow charts can be obtained by emailing stockorders.dppas@apsgroup.co.uk.

NICE technology appraisals (TAs)
Inhaler devices for children under 5 years with chronic asthma (August 2000) NICE TA10
When selecting inhaler devices for children under 5 years with chronic asthma, a child's needs and likelihood of good compliance should govern the choice of inhaler and spacer device; only then should cost be considered.

- corticosteroid and bronchodilator therapy should be delivered by pressurised metered-dose inhaler and spacer device, with a facemask if necessary;
- if this is not effective, and depending on the child's condition, nebulised therapy may be considered and, in children over 3 years, a dry powder inhaler may also be considered.

www.nice.org.uk/TA10

Inhaler devices for children 5–15 years with chronic asthma (March 2002) NICE TA38
When selecting inhaler devices for children between 5–15 years with chronic asthma, a child's needs, ability to develop and maintain effective technique, and likelihood of good compliance should govern the choice of inhaler and spacer device; only then should cost be considered.

- corticosteroid therapy should be routinely delivered by a pressurised metered-dose inhaler and spacer device;
- for other inhaled drugs, particularly bronchodilators, a wider range of devices should be considered;
- children and their carers should be trained in the use of the chosen device; suitability of the device should be reviewed at least annually. Inhaler technique and compliance should be monitored.

www.nice.org.uk/TA38

1   Airways disease, obstructive

Asthma

31-Mar-2016

Description of condition

Asthma is a common chronic inflammatory condition of the airways characterised by bronchoconstriction. The most frequent symptoms are cough, wheezing, chest tightness, and shortness of breath. The bronchoconstriction is usually reversible (either spontaneously or with the aid of medication) leading to intermittent symptoms, but in some patients with chronic asthma the inflammation may result in irreversible airway obstruction. Occasionally, asthma symptoms can get gradually or suddenly worse provoking an acute asthma attack that, if severe, may require hospitalisation.

Aims of treatment

In clinical practice, patients may choose to balance the aims of asthma management against the potential side-effects or inconvenience of taking medication necessary to achieve perfect control. Complete control of asthma is defined as no daytime symptoms, no night-time awakening due to asthma, no asthma attacks, no need for rescue medication, no limitations on activity including exercise, and normal lung function (in practical terms FEV_1 and/or peak flow > 80% predicted or best).

Lifestyle changes

EvGr Weight loss in overweight patients may lead to an improvement in asthma symptoms. Parents with asthma should be advised about the danger to themselves and to their children with asthma, of smoking, and be offered appropriate support to stop smoking. Breathing exercise programmes (including physiotherapist-taught methods) can be offered as an adjuvant to drug treatment in order to improve quality of life and reduce symptoms. ⟨A⟩

Management of chronic asthma

EvGr A stepwise approach aims to stop symptoms quickly and to improve peak flow. Start at the step most appropriate to initial severity of asthma. The aim is to achieve early control and to maintain it by *stepping up* treatment as necessary and *stepping down* treatment when control is good. Before initiating a new drug consider whether diagnosis is correct, check compliance and inhaler technique, and eliminate trigger factors for acute attacks. ⟨A⟩

Child over 5 years
Step 1—Mild intermittent asthma

- EvGr Start inhaled short-acting beta₂ agonist (such as salbutamol p. 150 or terbutaline sulfate p. 152) as required

  Children using more than one short-acting bronchodilator inhaler a month should have their asthma urgently assessed and action taken to improve poorly controlled asthma. Inhaled ipratropium bromide p. 147 also acts as a short-acting bronchodilator but inhaled short-acting beta₂ agonists are preferred.

  Move to **step 2** if the child presents with any one of the following features; is using an inhaled beta₂ agonist three times a week or more, being symptomatic three times a week or more, experiencing night-time symptoms at least once a week, or has had an asthma attack in the last 2 years. ⟨A⟩

Step 2—Regular preventer therapy

- EvGr Consider adding regular inhaled standard-dose corticosteroid (alternatives to inhaled corticosteroid are leukotriene receptor antagonists, theophylline p. 162, inhaled sodium cromoglicate p. 161, or inhaled nedocromil sodium p. 161, but are less effective) ⟨A⟩

  Note, inhaled standard-dose corticosteroid
  Child over 12 years: 200–800 micrograms/day beclometasone dipropionate p. 154 or equivalent
  Child 5–12 years: 200–400 micrograms/day beclometasone dipropionate or equivalent
  EvGr Beclometasone dipropionate and budesonide p. 155 are approximately equivalent in clinical practice although there may be variations with different drug delivery devices. Fluticasone p. 156 provides equal clinical activity to beclometasone dipropionate and budesonide at half the dosage.

  Start the inhaled corticosteroid at a dose appropriate to severity of disease and adjust to the lowest effective dose at which control of asthma is maintained. Inhaled corticosteroids (except ciclesonide p. 156) should be initially taken twice daily, however, the same total daily dose can be considered once a day if good control is established. ⟨A⟩
  EvGr In children, administration of high doses of inhaled corticosteroids may be associated with systemic side-effects, including growth failure, reduced bone mineral density, and adrenal suppression, see individual drug monographs for monitoring information.

  If asthma is not adequately controlled, move to **step 3**. ⟨A⟩

Step 3—Initial add-on therapy

- EvGr Consider adding a regular inhaled long-acting beta₂ agonist (LABA) such as formoterol fumarate p. 148 or salmeterol p. 149 to be used in conjunction with an inhaled corticosteroid (see also CHM advice for formoterol fumarate and salmeterol)

  If the child is gaining some benefit from addition of a LABA but control is *inadequate* then continue the LABA and increase dose of inhaled corticosteroid to top end of inhaled standard-dose corticosteroid range. If there is *no response* to the LABA, discontinue and increase dose of inhaled corticosteroid. If control is still inadequate, start a trial of either a leukotriene receptor antagonist (montelukast p. 159, or zafirlukast p. 160 if over 12 years) or modified-release theophylline. ⟨A⟩

Step 4—Persistent poor control

Consider the following options:

- EvGr Increase dose of inhaled corticosteroid (a spacer should be used), *or*
- Add a leukotriene receptor antagonist, modified-release theophylline, or modified-release oral beta₂ agonist (caution in children already taking a LABA) ⟨A⟩

  Note, increased inhaled corticosteroid dose
  Child over 12 years: up to 2000 micrograms/day beclometasone dipropionate or equivalent
  Child 5–12 years: up to 800 micrograms/day beclometasone dipropionate or equivalent
  EvGr Beclometasone dipropionate and budesonide are approximately equivalent in clinical practice although there may be variations with different drug delivery devices. Fluticasone provides equal clinical activity to beclometasone dipropionate and budesonide at half the dosage.

  Before proceeding to **step 5**, refer children with inadequately controlled asthma to specialist care. ⟨A⟩

Step 5—Continuous or frequent use of oral corticosteroids

- EvGr Add regular oral corticosteroid (prednisolone p. 421, as single daily dose) at lowest dose to provide adequate control; continue high-dose inhaled corticosteroid (in exceptional cases, this may exceed licensed doses) ⟨A⟩

Child under 5 years
Step 1—Mild intermittent asthma

- EvGr Inhaled short-acting beta₂ agonist (such as salbutamol or terbutaline sulfate) as required

  Children identified to be using more than one short-acting bronchodilator inhaler a month should have their asthma urgently assessed and action taken to improve poorly controlled asthma.

  Move to **step 2** if the child presents with any one of the following features; is using an inhaled beta₂ agonist three times a week or more, being symptomatic three times a week or more, experiencing night-time symptoms at least once a week. ⟨A⟩

Step 2—Regular preventer therapy

- EvGr Consider adding regular standard-dose inhaled corticosteroid
- If child is unable to take an inhaled corticosteroid, a leukotriene receptor antagonist (such as montelukast) is an effective first-line preventer ⟨A⟩

  Note, inhaled standard-dose corticosteroid
  Child under 5 years: 200–400 micrograms/day beclometasone dipropionate or equivalent
  EvGr Beclometasone dipropionate and budesonide are approximately equivalent in clinical practice although there may be variations with different drug delivery devices.

Fluticasone provides equal clinical activity to beclometasone dipropionate and budesonide at half the dosage.

Start inhaled corticosteroid at a dose appropriate to severity of disease and adjust to the lowest effective dose at which control of asthma is maintained.

In children, administration of high doses of inhaled corticosteroids may be associated with systemic side-effects, including growth failure, reduced bone mineral density and adrenal suppression, see individual drug monographs for monitoring information.

If asthma is not adequately controlled, move to **step 3**. Ⓐ

Step 3—Initial add-on therapy

- [EvGr] In children 2–5 years, add a leukotriene receptor antagonist if not added during step 2. If a leukotriene receptor antagonist was added at step 2, reconsider addition of standard-dose inhaled corticosteroid.
- In children under 2 years, consider proceeding to **step 4** Ⓐ

Step 4—Persistent poor control

- [EvGr] Refer child to respiratory paediatrician Ⓐ

Stepping down

[EvGr] Once asthma is controlled, it is recommended to step down therapy and continue to regularly review the child. When deciding which drug to step down first and at what rate, the severity of asthma, the side-effects of treatment, duration on current dose, the beneficial effects achieved, and the child's preference, should be considered.

The child should be maintained at the lowest possible dose of inhaled corticosteroid. Reductions should be considered every three months, decreasing the dose by approximately 25–50% each time. Reduce the dose slowly as children deteriorate at different rates. Ⓐ

Pregnancy and breast-feeding

[EvGr] Women with asthma should be closely monitored during pregnancy. It is particularly important that asthma should be well controlled during pregnancy; when this is achieved asthma has no important effects on pregnancy, labour, or on the fetus. Women planning to become pregnant should be counselled about the importance of taking their asthma medication regularly to maintain good control. Drugs for asthma should preferably be administered by inhalation to minimise exposure of the fetus. Short-acting beta₂ agonists, long-acting beta₂ agonists, oral and inhaled corticosteroids, sodium cromoglicate p. 161, nedocromil sodium p. 161, and oral and intravenous theophyllines can be used as normal during pregnancy. There is limited information on use of leukotriene receptor antagonists during pregnancy, however they may be used if potential benefit outweighs risk. Drugs for asthma, including corticosteroid tablets, can be used as normal and in-line with manufacturers' recommendations in breast-feeding.

Severe acute attacks of asthma can have an adverse effect on pregnancy and should be treated promptly in hospital with conventional therapy, including nebulisation of a beta₂ agonist and oral or parenteral administration of a corticosteroid; prednisolone p. 421 is the preferred corticosteroid for oral administration since very little of the drug reaches the fetus. Oxygen should be given immediately to maintain arterial oxygen saturation of 94–98% and prevent maternal and fetal hypoxia. Ⓐ

Management of acute asthma

Child over 2 years

Levels of severity

The nature of treatment required for the management of acute asthma depends on the level of severity, described as follows:

Moderate acute asthma

- Able to talk in sentences
- Arterial oxygen saturation (SpO₂) ≥ 92%

- Peak flow ≥ 50% best or predicted
- Heart rate ≤ 140/minute in children aged 2–5 years; heart rate ≤ 125/minute in children over 5 years
- Respiratory rate ≤ 40/minute in children aged 2–5 years; respiratory rate ≤ 30/minute in children over 5 years

Severe acute asthma

- Can't complete sentences in one breath or too breathless to talk or feed
- SpO₂ < 92%
- Peak flow 33–50% best or predicted
- Heart rate > 140/minute in children aged 2–5 years; heart rate > 125/minute in children aged over 5 years
- Respiratory rate > 40/minute in children aged 2–5 years; respiratory rate > 30/minute in children aged over 5 years

Life-threatening acute asthma

Any one of the following in a child with severe asthma:

- SpO₂ < 92%
- Peak flow < 33% best or predicted
- Silent chest
- Cyanosis
- Poor respiratory effort
- Hypotension
- Exhaustion
- Confusion

Management of acute asthma in children over 2 years

[EvGr] Following initial assessment, supplementary high flow oxygen should be given to all children with life-threatening acute asthma or SpO₂ < 94% to achieve normal saturations of 94–98%.

First-line treatment for acute asthma is an inhaled short-acting beta₂ agonist (salbutamol p. 150 or terbutaline sulfate p. 152) given as soon as possible, ideally via a metered dose inhaler and spacer device in mild to moderate acute asthma. Children with severe or life-threatening acute asthma should be transferred to hospital urgently

In all cases of acute asthma, children should be prescribed an adequate once daily dose of oral prednisolone. Treatment for up to 3 days is usually sufficient, but the length of course should be tailored to the number of days necessary to bring about recovery. Intravenous hydrocortisone p. 420 should be reserved for severely affected children who are unable to retain oral medication.

Nebulised ipratropium bromide p. 147 can be combined with beta₂ agonist treatment for children with severe or life-threatening acute asthma or in those with a poor initial response to beta₂ agonist therapy to provide greater bronchodilation. Consider adding magnesium sulfate p. 571 to nebulised salbutamol and ipratropium bromide in the first hour in children with a short duration of acute severe asthma symptoms presenting with an oxygen saturation less than 92%.

Children with continuing severe asthma despite frequent nebulised beta₂ agonists and ipratropium bromide plus oral corticosteroids, and those with life-threatening features, need urgent review by a specialist with a view to transfer to a high dependency unit or paediatric intensive care unit (PICU) to receive second-line intravenous therapies. Ⓐ

[EvGr] In a severe asthma attack where the child has not responded to initial inhaled therapy, early addition of a single bolus dose of intravenous salbutamol may be an option. Continuous intravenous infusion of salbutamol, administered under specialist supervision with continuous ECG and electrolyte monitoring, should be considered in patients with unreliable inhalation or severe refractory asthma. Aminophylline p. 161 may be considered in children with severe or life-threatening acute asthma unresponsive to maximal doses of bronchodilators and corticosteroids. Aminophylline is not recommended in children with mild to moderate acute asthma. Intravenous magnesium sulfate has been used for acute asthma [unlicensed use] although its place in management is not yet established. Ⓐ

Child under 2 years

[EvGr] Inhaled short-acting beta$_2$ agonists are the initial treatment of choice for acute asthma in children under 2 years. For mild to moderate acute asthma attacks, a metered-dose inhaler with a spacer and mask is the optimal drug delivery device. In a hospital setting, consider oral prednisolone daily for up to 3 days, early in the management of severe asthma attacks. For more severe symptoms, inhaled ipratropium bromide p. 147 in combination with an inhaled beta$_2$ agonist is also an option. ⟨A⟩

Follow up in all cases

[EvGr] Episodes of acute asthma may be a failure of preventative therapy, review is required to prevent further episodes. A careful history should be taken to establish the reason for the asthma attack. Inhaler technique should be checked and regular treatment should be reviewed. Children and their carers should be given a written asthma action plan aimed at preventing relapse, optimising treatment, and preventing delay in seeking assistance in future attacks. It is essential that the child's GP practice is informed within 24 hours of discharge from the emergency department or hospital following an asthma attack. Children who have had a near-fatal asthma attack should be kept under specialist supervision indefinitely. A respiratory specialist should follow up all patients admitted with a severe asthma attack for at least one year after the admission. ⟨A⟩

Bronchodilators

Beta$_2$ agonists

Selective beta$_2$ agonists produce bronchodilation. A short-acting beta$_2$ agonist is used for immediate relief of asthma symptoms while a long-acting beta$_2$ agonist is used in addition to an inhaled corticosteroid in children requiring prophylactic treatment.

The selective beta$_2$ agonists (selective beta$_2$-adrenoceptor agonists, selective beta$_2$ stimulants) such as salbutamol p. 150 or terbutaline sulfate p. 152 are the safest and most effective short-acting beta$_2$ agonists for the treatment of asthma.

Adrenaline/epinephrine p. 132 (which has both alpha-and beta-adrenoceptor agonist properties) is used in the emergency management of acute allergic and anaphylactic reactions, in angioedema, and in cardiopulmonary resuscitation; it is also used as a nebuliser solution to treat severe croup.

Short-acting beta$_2$ agonists

Mild to moderate symptoms of asthma respond rapidly to the inhalation of a selective short-acting beta$_2$ agonist such as salbutamol or terbutaline sulfate. If beta$_2$ agonist inhalation is needed more often than twice a week, or if night-time symptoms occur at least once a week, or if the patient has suffered an exacerbation in the last 2 years, then prophylactic treatment should be considered using a stepped approach.

A short-acting beta$_2$ agonist inhaled immediately before exertion reduces *exercise-induced asthma*; however, frequent exercise-induced asthma probably reflects poor overall control and calls for reassessment of asthma treatment.

Long-acting beta$_2$ agonists

Formoterol fumarate p. 148 (eformoterol) and salmeterol p. 149 are longer-acting beta$_2$ agonists which are administered by inhalation. They should be used for asthma only in children who regularly use an inhaled corticosteroid. They have a role in the long-term management of chronic asthma and can be useful in nocturnal asthma.

Salmeterol should not be used for the relief of an asthma attack; it has a slower onset of action than salbutamol or terbutaline sulfate. Formoterol fumarate is licensed for

short-term symptom relief and for the prevention of exercise-induced bronchospasm; its speed of onset of action is similar to that of salbutamol.

Vilanterol is a long-acting beta$_2$ agonist available in a combination inhaler with fluticasone furoate.

Combination inhalers that contain a long-acting beta$_2$ agonist and a corticosteroid ensure that long-acting beta$_2$ agonists are not used without concomitant corticosteroids, but reduce the flexibility to adjust the dose of each component.

Oral

Oral preparations of beta$_2$ agonists may be used for children if an inhaler device cannot be used but inhaled beta$_2$ agonists are more effective and have fewer side-effects. A modified-release formulation of salbutamol may be of value in nocturnal asthma as an alternative to modified-release theophylline p. 162 preparations, but an inhaled long-acting beta$_2$ agonist is preferable.

Parenteral

Beta$_2$ agonists can be given intravenously in children with severe or life-threatening acute asthma. Chronic asthma unresponsive to stepwise treatment may benefit from continuous subcutaneous infusion of a beta$_2$ agonist, but this should be used only under the supervision of a respiratory specialist; the evidence of benefit is uncertain and it may be difficult to withdraw such treatment once started.

Antimuscarinic bronchodilators

Ipratropium bromide p. 147 by nebulisation can be added to other standard treatment in life-threatening acute asthma or if acute asthma fails to improve with standard therapy. Ipratropium bromide can be used to provide short-term relief in chronic asthma, but short-acting beta$_2$ agonists act more quickly and are preferred.

The aerosol inhalation of ipratropium bromide has a maximum effect 30–60 minutes after use; its duration of action is 3 to 6 hours.

Theophylline

Theophylline is a xanthine used as a bronchodilator in asthma. It may have an additive effect when used in conjunction with small doses of beta$_2$ agonists; the combination may increase the risk of side-effects, including hypokalaemia.

Theophylline is given by injection as aminophylline p. 161, a mixture of theophylline with ethylenediamine, which is 20 times more soluble than theophylline alone. Aminophylline injection is needed rarely for severe acute asthma.

Compound bronchodilator preparations

In general, children are best treated with single-ingredient preparations, such as a selective beta$_2$ agonist or ipratropium bromide, so that the dose of each drug can be adjusted. This flexibility is lost with compound bronchodilator preparations.

Croup

Management

Mild croup is largely self-limiting, but treatment with a single dose of a corticosteroid (e.g. dexamethasone p. 419) by mouth may be of benefit.

More severe croup (or mild croup that might cause complications) calls for hospital admission; a single dose of a corticosteroid (e.g. dexamethasone or prednisolone p. 421 by mouth) should be administered before transfer to hospital. In hospital, dexamethasone (by mouth or by injection) or budesonide p. 155 (by nebulisation) will often reduce symptoms; the dose may need to be repeated after 12 hours if necessary.

For severe croup not effectively controlled with corticosteroid treatment, nebulised adrenaline/epinephrine solution 1 in 1000 (1 mg/mL) p. 132 should be given with close clinical monitoring; the effects of nebulised adrenaline/epinephrine last 2–3 hours and the child needs to be monitored carefully for recurrence of the obstruction.

Oxygen

Overview

Oxygen should be regarded as a drug. It is prescribed for hypoxaemic patients to increase alveolar oxygen tension and decrease the work of breathing. The concentration of oxygen required depends on the condition being treated; administration of an inappropriate concentration of oxygen may have serious or even fatal consequences. High concentrations of oxygen can cause pulmonary epithelial damage (bronchopulmonary dysplasia), convulsions, and retinal damage, especially in preterm neonates.

Oxygen is probably the most common drug used in medical emergencies. It should be prescribed initially to achieve a normal or near-normal oxygen saturation. In most acutely ill children with an expected or known normal or low arterial carbon dioxide (P_aCO_2), oxygen saturation should be maintained above 92%; some clinicians may aim for a target of 94–98%. In some clinical situations, such as carbon monoxide poisoning, it is more appropriate to aim for the highest possible oxygen saturation until the child is stable. Hypercapnic respiratory failure is rare in children; in those children at risk, a lower oxygen saturation target of 88–92% is indicated.

High concentration oxygen therapy is safe in uncomplicated cases of conditions such as pneumonia, pulmonary thromboembolism, pulmonary fibrosis, shock, severe trauma, sepsis, or anaphylaxis. In such conditions low arterial oxygen (P_aO_2) is usually associated with low or normal arterial carbon dioxide (P_aCO_2), and therefore there is little risk of hypoventilation and carbon dioxide retention.

In severe acute asthma, the arterial carbon dioxide (P_aCO_2) is usually subnormal but as asthma deteriorates it may rise steeply (particularly in children). These patients usually require high concentrations of oxygen and if the arterial carbon dioxide (P_aCO_2) remains high despite other treatment, intermittent positive-pressure ventilation needs to be considered urgently.

Oxygen should not be given to neonates except under expert supervision. Particular care is required in preterm neonates because of the risk of hyperoxia.

Low concentration oxygen therapy (controlled oxygen therapy) is reserved for children at risk of hypercapnic respiratory failure, which is more likely in children with:

- advanced cystic fibrosis
- advanced non-cystic fibrosis bronchiectasis
- severe kyphoscoliosis or severe ankylosing spondylitis
- severe lung scarring caused by tuberculosis
- musculoskeletal disorders with respiratory weakness, especially if on home ventilation
- an overdose of opioids, benzodiazepines, or other drugs causing respiratory depression.

Until blood gases can be measured, initial oxygen should be given using a controlled concentration of 28% or less, titrated towards a target concentration of 88–92%. The aim is to provide the child with enough oxygen to achieve an acceptable arterial oxygen tension without worsening carbon dioxide retention and respiratory acidosis.

Domiciliary oxygen

Oxygen should only be prescribed for use in the home after careful evaluation in hospital by a respiratory care specialist.

Carers and children who smoke should be advised of the risks of smoking when receiving oxygen, including the risk of fire. Smoking cessation therapy should be recommended before home oxygen prescription.

Long-term oxygen therapy

The aim of long-term oxygen therapy is to maintain oxygen saturation of at least 92%. Children (especially those with chronic neonatal lung disease) often require supplemental oxygen, either for 24-hours a day or during periods of sleep; many children are eventually weaned off long-term oxygen therapy as their condition improves.

Long-term oxygen therapy should be considered for children with conditions such as:

- bronchopulmonary dysplasia (chronic neonatal lung disease);
- congenital heart disease with pulmonary hypertension;
- pulmonary hypertension secondary to pulmonary disease;
- idiopathic pulmonary hypertension;
- sickle-cell disease with persistent nocturnal hypoxia;
- interstitial lung disease and obliterative bronchiolitis;
- cystic fibrosis;
- obstructive sleep apnoea syndrome;
- neuromuscular or skeletal disease requiring non-invasive ventilation;
- pulmonary malignancy or other terminal disease with disabling dyspnoea.

Increased respiratory depression is seldom a problem in children with stable respiratory failure treated with low concentrations of oxygen although it may occur during exacerbations; children and their carers should be warned to call for medical help if drowsiness or confusion occurs.

Short-burst oxygen therapy

Oxygen is occasionally prescribed for short-burst (intermittent) use for episodes of breathlessness.

Ambulatory oxygen therapy

Ambulatory oxygen is prescribed for children on long-term oxygen therapy who need to be away from home on a regular basis.

Oxygen therapy equipment

Under the NHS oxygen may be supplied as **oxygen cylinders**. Oxygen flow can be adjusted as the cylinders are equipped with an oxygen flow meter. Oxygen delivered from a cylinder should be passed through a humidifier if used for long periods.

Oxygen concentrators are more economical for children who require oxygen for long periods, and in England and Wales can be ordered on the NHS on a regional tendering basis. A concentrator is recommended for a child who requires oxygen for more than 8 hours a day (or 21 cylinders per month). Exceptionally, if a higher concentration of oxygen is required the output of 2 oxygen concentrators can be combined using a 'Y' connection.

A nasal cannula is usually preferred to a face mask for long-term oxygen therapy from an oxygen concentrator. Nasal cannulas can, however, cause dermatitis and mucosal drying in sensitive individuals.

Giving oxygen by nasal cannula allows the child to talk, eat, and drink, but the concentration of oxygen is not controlled and the method may not be appropriate for acute respiratory failure. When oxygen is given through a nasal cannula at a rate of 1–2 litres/minute the inspiratory oxygen concentration is usually low, but it varies with ventilation and can be high if the patient is underventilating.

Arrangements for supplying oxygen

The following oxygen services may be ordered in England and Wales:

- emergency oxygen;

- short-burst (intermittent) oxygen therapy;
- long-term oxygen therapy;
- ambulatory oxygen.

The type of oxygen service (or combination of services) should be ordered on a Home Oxygen Order Form (HOOF); the amount of oxygen required (hours per day) and flow rate should be specified. The clinician will determine the appropriate equipment to be provided. Special needs or preferences should be specified on the HOOF.

The clinician should obtain the consent of the child or carers to pass on the child's details to the supplier, the fire brigade, and other relevant organisations. The supplier will contact the child or carer to make arrangements for delivery, installation, and maintenance of the equipment. The supplier will also train the child or carer to use the equipment.

The clinician should send the HOOF to the supplier who will continue to provide the service until a revised HOOF is received, or until notified that the child no longer requires the home oxygen service.

HOOF and further instructions are available at www.bprs.co.uk/oxygen.html.

- East of England, North East: BOC Medical: Tel: 0800 136 603 Fax: 0800 169 9989
- South West: Air Liquide: Tel: 0808 202 2229 Fax: 0191 497 4340
- London East, Midlands, North West:Air Liquide: Tel: 0500 823 773 Fax: 0800 781 4610
- Yorkshire and Humberside, West Midlands, Wales: Air Products: Tel: 0800 373 580 Fax: 0800 214 709
- South East Coast, South Central: Dolby Vivisol: Tel: 08443 814 402 Fax: 0800 781 4610

In **Scotland** refer the child for assessment by a paediatric respiratory consultant. If the need for a concentrator is confirmed the consultant will arrange for the provision of a concentrator through the Common Services Agency. Prescribers should complete a Scottish Home Oxygen Order Form (SHOOF) and email it to Health Facilities Scotland. Health Facilities Scotland will then liaise with their contractor to arrange the supply of oxygen. Further information can be obtained at www.dolbyvivisol.com/our-services/healthcare-professionals/home-oxygen-services-(sco).aspx.

In **Northern Ireland** oxygen concentrators and cylinders should be prescribed on form HS21; oxygen concentrators are supplied by a local contractor. Prescriptions for oxygen cylinders and accessories can be dispensed by pharmacists contracted to provide domiciliary oxygen services.

ANTIMUSCARINICS

Antimuscarinics (inhaled)

09-Feb-2016

- **CAUTIONS** Bladder outflow obstruction · paradoxical bronchospasm · prostatic hyperplasia · susceptibility to angle-closure glaucoma
- **SIDE-EFFECTS**
- ▶ **Common or very common** Constipation · cough · diarrhoea · dry mouth · gastro-intestinal motility disorder · headache · sinusitis
- ▶ **Uncommon** Angle-closure glaucoma · atrial fibrillation · blurred vision · dizziness · mydriasis · nasopharyngitis · nausea · palpitation · paradoxical bronchospasm · pharyngitis · rash · tachycardia · throat irritation · urinary retention
- ▶ **Rare** Dental caries

▶ above

Ipratropium bromide

24-Feb-2016

- **INDICATIONS AND DOSE**

Reversible airways obstruction
- ▶ BY INHALATION OF AEROSOL
- ▶ Child 1 month–5 years: 20 micrograms 3 times a day
- ▶ Child 6–11 years: 20–40 micrograms 3 times a day
- ▶ Child 12–17 years: 20–40 micrograms 3–4 times a day

Acute bronchospasm
- ▶ BY INHALATION OF NEBULISED SOLUTION
- ▶ Child 1 month–5 years: 125–250 micrograms as required; maximum 1 mg per day
- ▶ Child 6–11 years: 250 micrograms as required; maximum 1 mg per day
- ▶ Child 12–17 years: 500 micrograms as required, doses higher than max. can be given under medical supervision; maximum 2 mg per day

Severe or life-threatening acute asthma
- ▶ BY INHALATION OF NEBULISED SOLUTION
- ▶ Child 1 month–11 years: 250 micrograms every 20–30 minutes for the first 2 hours, then 250 micrograms every 4–6 hours as required
- ▶ Child 12–17 years: 500 micrograms every 4–6 hours as required

PHARMACOKINETICS
The maximal effect of inhaled ipratropium occurs 30–60 minutes after use; its duration of action is 3 to 6 hours and bronchodilation can usually be maintained with treatment 3 times a day.

- **UNLICENSED USE** EvGr The dose of ipratropium for severe or life-threatening acute asthma is unlicensed. ⟨A⟩
- **CAUTIONS** Cystic fibrosis
  CAUTIONS, FURTHER INFORMATION
- ▶ Glaucoma *Acute angle-closure glaucoma* has been reported with nebulised ipratropium, particularly when given with nebulised salbutamol (and possibly other beta₂ agonists); care needed to protect the patient's eyes from nebulised drug or from drug powder.
- **INTERACTIONS** → Appendix 1: ipratropium
- **SIDE-EFFECTS**
- ▶ **Uncommon** Laryngospasm · pharyngeal oedema · stomatitis · vomiting
- ▶ **Rare** Ocular accommodation disorder
- **PREGNANCY** Manufacturer advises only use if potential benefit outweighs the risk.
- **BREAST FEEDING** No information available—manufacturer advises only use if potential benefit outweighs risk.
- **DIRECTIONS FOR ADMINISTRATION** If dilution of ipratropium bromide nebuliser solution is necessary use only sterile sodium chloride 0.9%.
- **PATIENT AND CARER ADVICE** Patients or carers should be given advice on appropriate inhaler technique.

- **MEDICINAL FORMS**
  There can be variation in the licensing of different medicines containing the same drug.

Nebuliser liquid
- ▶ Ipratropium bromide (Non-proprietary)
  Ipratropium bromide 250 microgram per 1 ml Ipratropium bromide 500micrograms/2ml nebuliser liquid unit dose vials | 20 unit dose PoM £2.93 DT price = £2.60
  Ipratropium bromide 250micrograms/1ml nebuliser liquid unit dose vials | 20 unit dose PoM £4.58 DT price = £4.51
  Ipratropium 250micrograms/1ml nebuliser liquid Steri-Neb unit dose vials | 20 unit dose PoM £6.99 DT price = £4.51
  Ipratropium 500micrograms/2ml nebuliser liquid Steri-Neb unit dose vials | 20 unit dose PoM £15.99 DT price = £2.60

3

▸ **Atrovent UDV** (Boehringer Ingelheim Ltd)
Ipratropium bromide 250 microgram per 1 ml Atrovent
500micrograms/2ml nebuliser liquid UDVs | 20 unit dose PoM £4.87
DT price = £2.60 | 60 unit dose PoM £14.59
Atrovent 250micrograms/1ml nebuliser liquid UDVs | 20 unit
dose PoM £4.14 DT price = £4.51 | 60 unit dose PoM £12.44
▸ **Respontin** (GlaxoSmithKline UK Ltd)
Ipratropium bromide 250 microgram per 1 ml Respontin
500micrograms/2ml Nebules | 20 unit dose PoM £5.60 DT price =
£2.60

Pressurised inhalation

▸ **Ipratropium bromide** (Non-proprietary)
Ipratropium bromide 20 microgram per 1 dose Ipratropium
bromide 20micrograms/dose inhaler CFC free | 200 dose PoM no
price available DT price = £5.56
▸ **Atrovent** (Boehringer Ingelheim Ltd)
Ipratropium bromide 20 microgram per 1 dose Atrovent
20micrograms/dose inhaler CFC free | 200 dose PoM £5.56 DT price
= £5.56

BETA₂-ADRENOCEPTOR AGONISTS, SELECTIVE

Beta₂-adrenoceptor agonists, selective

12-Feb-2016

● **CONTRA-INDICATIONS** Severe pre-eclampsia

● **CAUTIONS** Arrhythmias · cardiovascular disease · diabetes
(risk of hyperglycaemia and ketoacidosis, especially with
intravenous use) · hypertension · hyperthyroidism ·
hypokalaemia · susceptibility to QT-interval prolongation

CAUTIONS, FURTHER INFORMATION
▸ **Hypokalaemia** Potentially serious hypokalaemia may result
from beta₂ agonist therapy. Particular caution is required
in severe asthma, because this effect may be potentiated
by concomitant treatment with theophylline and its
derivatives, corticosteroids, diuretics, and by hypoxia.

● **SIDE-EFFECTS** Angioedema · arrhythmias · behavioural
disturbances · collapse · fine tremor (particularly in the
hands) · headache · hyperglycaemia (especially when given
intravenously) · hypersensitivity reactions · hypokalaemia
(with high doses) · hypotension · ketoacidosis (especially
when given intravenously) · muscle cramps · myocardial
ischaemia · nervous tension · palpitation · paradoxical
bronchospasm (occasionally severe) · peripheral
vasodilation · rash · sleep disturbances · tachycardia ·
urticaria

● **PREGNANCY** Women planning to become pregnant should
be counselled about the importance of taking their asthma
medication regularly to maintain good control.

● **MONITORING REQUIREMENTS**
▸ In severe asthma, plasma-potassium concentration should
be monitored (risk of hypokalaemia).
▸ In patients with diabetes, monitor blood glucose (risk of
hyperglycaemia and ketoacidosis, especially when beta₂
agonist given intravenously).

● **PATIENT AND CARER ADVICE**
The **dose**, the frequency, and the maximum number of
inhalations in 24 hours of the beta₂ agonist should be
stated explicitly to the patient or their carer. The patient
or their carer should be advised to seek medical advice
when the prescribed dose of beta₂ agonist fails to provide
the usual degree of symptomatic relief because this usually
indicates a worsening of the asthma and the patient may
require a prophylactic drug. Patients or their carers should
be advised to follow manufacturers' instructions on the
care and cleansing of inhaler devices.

BETA₂-ADRENOCEPTOR AGONISTS, SELECTIVE › LONG-ACTING

⟟ above

Formoterol fumarate

(Eformoterol fumarate)

● **INDICATIONS AND DOSE**
**Reversible airways obstruction in patients requiring long-
term regular bronchodilator therapy | Nocturnal asthma
in patients requiring long-term regular bronchodilator
therapy | Prophylaxis of exercise-induced bronchospasm
in patients requiring long-term regular bronchodilator
therapy | Chronic asthma in patients who regularly use
an inhaled corticosteroid**

▸ BY INHALATION OF POWDER
▸ **Child 6–11 years:** 12 micrograms twice daily, a daily dose
of 24 micrograms of formoterol should be sufficient for
the majority of children, particularly for younger age-
groups; higher doses should be used rarely, and only
when control is not maintained on the lower dose
▸ **Child 12–17 years:** 12 micrograms twice daily, dose may
be increased in more severe airway obstruction;
increased to 24 micrograms twice daily, a daily dose of
24 micrograms of formoterol should be sufficient for
the majority of children, particularly for younger age-
groups; higher doses should be used rarely, and only
when control is not maintained on the lower dose
▸ BY INHALATION OF AEROSOL
▸ **Child 12–17 years:** 12 micrograms twice daily, dose may
be increased in more severe airway obstruction;
increased to 24 micrograms twice daily, a daily dose of
24 micrograms of formoterol should be sufficient for
the majority of children, particularly for younger age-
groups; higher doses should be used rarely, and only
when control is not maintained on the lower dose

OXIS®

Chronic asthma
▸ BY INHALATION OF POWDER
▸ **Child 6–17 years:** 6–12 micrograms 1–2 times a day
(max. per dose 12 micrograms), occasionally doses up
to the maximum daily may be needed, reassess
treatment if additional doses required on more than
2 days a week; maximum 48 micrograms per day

Relief of bronchospasm
▸ BY INHALATION OF POWDER
▸ **Child 6–17 years:** 6–12 micrograms

Prophylaxis of exercise-induced bronchospasm
▸ BY INHALATION OF POWDER
▸ **Child 6–17 years:** 6–12 micrograms, dose to be taken
before exercise

PHARMACOKINETICS
At recommended inhaled doses, the duration of action of
formoterol is about 12 hours.

IMPORTANT SAFETY INFORMATION
CHM ADVICE
To ensure safe use, the CHM has advised that for the
management of chronic asthma, long-acting beta₂
agonist (formoterol) should:
● be added only if regular use of standard-dose inhaled
corticosteroids has failed to control asthma
adequately;
● not be initiated in patients with rapidly deteriorating
asthma;
● be introduced at a low dose and the effect properly
monitored before considering dose increase;
● be discontinued in the absence of benefit;

- not be used for the relief of exercise-induced asthma symptoms unless regular inhaled corticosteroids are also used;
- be reviewed as clinically appropriate: stepping down therapy should be considered when good long-term asthma control has been achieved.

- **CAUTIONS** High doses of beta$_2$ agonists can be dangerous in some children
- **INTERACTIONS** → Appendix 1: beta$_2$ agonists
- **SIDE-EFFECTS**
- ▸ **Very rare** QT-interval prolongation
- ▸ **Frequency not known** Dizziness · nausea · pruritus · taste disturbances
- **PREGNANCY** Inhaled drugs for asthma can be taken as normal during pregnancy.
- **BREAST FEEDING** Inhaled drugs for asthma can be taken as normal during breast-feeding.
- **PATIENT AND CARER ADVICE** Advise patients not to exceed prescribed dose, and to follow manufacturer's directions; if a previously effective dose of inhaled formoterol fails to provide adequate relief, a doctor's advice should be obtained as soon as possible. Patients should be advised to report any deterioration in symptoms following initiation of treatment with a long-acting beta$_2$ agonist. Patient or carer should be given advice on how to administer formoterol fumarate inhalers.

- **MEDICINAL FORMS**
There can be variation in the licensing of different medicines containing the same drug.

Inhalation powder
- ▸ **Easyhaler (formoterol)** (Orion Pharma (UK) Ltd)
Formoterol fumarate dihydrate 12 microgram per 1 dose Formoterol Easyhaler 12micrograms/dose dry powder inhaler | 120 dose PoM £23.75 DT price = £23.75
- ▸ **Foradil** (Novartis Pharmaceuticals UK Ltd)
Formoterol fumarate dihydrate 12 microgram Foradil 12microgram inhalation powder capsules with device | 60 capsule PoM £28.06 DT price = £28.06
- ▸ **Oxis Turbohaler** (AstraZeneca UK Ltd)
Formoterol fumarate dihydrate 6 microgram per 1 dose Oxis 6 Turbohaler | 60 dose PoM £24.80 DT price = £24.80
Formoterol fumarate dihydrate 12 microgram per 1 dose Oxis 12 Turbohaler | 60 dose PoM £24.80 DT price = £24.80

Pressurised inhalation
- ▸ **Atimos Modulite** (Chiesi Ltd)
Formoterol fumarate dihydrate 12 microgram per 1 dose Atimos Modulite 12micrograms/dose inhaler | 100 dose PoM £30.06 DT price = £30.06

Combinations available: *Budesonide with formoterol*, p. 156 · *Fluticasone with formoterol*, p. 157

▶ 148

Salmeterol

- **INDICATIONS AND DOSE**

Reversible airways obstruction in patients requiring long-term regular bronchodilator therapy | Nocturnal asthma in patients requiring long-term regular bronchodilator therapy | Prevention of exercise-induced bronchospasm in patients requiring long-term regular bronchodilator therapy | Chronic asthma only in patients who regularly use an inhaled corticosteroid (not for immediate relief of acute asthma)
- ▶ BY INHALATION OF AEROSOL, OR BY INHALATION OF POWDER
- ▸ **Child 5-11 years:** 50 micrograms twice daily
- ▸ **Child 12-17 years:** 50 micrograms twice daily, dose may be increased in more severe airway obstruction; increased to 100 micrograms twice daily

PHARMACOKINETICS
At recommended inhaled doses, the duration of action of salmeterol is about 12 hours.

- **UNLICENSED USE** *Neovent* ® not licensed for use in children under 12 years.

> **IMPORTANT SAFETY INFORMATION**
> CHM ADVICE
> To ensure safe use, the CHM has advised that for the management of chronic asthma, long-acting beta$_2$ agonist (salmeterol) should:
> - be added only if regular use of standard-dose inhaled corticosteroids has failed to control asthma adequately;
> - not be initiated in patients with rapidly deteriorating asthma;
> - be introduced at a low dose and the effect properly monitored before considering dose increase;
> - be discontinued in the absence of benefit;
> - not be used for the relief of exercise-induced asthma symptoms unless regular inhaled corticosteroids are also used;
> - be reviewed as clinically appropriate: stepping down therapy should be considered when good long-term asthma control has been achieved.

- **CAUTIONS** High doses of beta$_2$ agonists can be dangerous in some children
- **INTERACTIONS** → Appendix 1: beta$_2$ agonists
- **SIDE-EFFECTS** Arthralgia · dizziness · nausea
- **PREGNANCY** Inhaled drugs for asthma can be taken as normal during pregnancy.
- **BREAST FEEDING** Inhaled drugs for asthma can be taken as normal during breast-feeding.
- **PATIENT AND CARER ADVICE**
Advise patients that salmeterol should **not** be used for relief of acute attacks, not to exceed prescribed dose, and to follow manufacturer's directions; if a previously effective dose of inhaled salmeterol fails to provide adequate relief, a doctor's advice should be obtained as soon as possible.
Patients should be advised to report any deterioration in symptoms following initiation of treatment with a long-acting beta$_2$ agonist.
Medicines for Children leaflet: Salmeterol inhaler for asthma prevention (prophylaxis) www.medicinesforchildren.org.uk/salmeterol-inhaler-for-asthma-prevention

- **MEDICINAL FORMS**
There can be variation in the licensing of different medicines containing the same drug.

Inhalation powder
- ▸ **Serevent Accuhaler** (GlaxoSmithKline UK Ltd)
Salmeterol (as Salmeterol xinafoate) 50 microgram per 1 dose Serevent 50micrograms/dose Accuhaler | 60 dose PoM £35.11 DT price = £35.11

Pressurised inhalation
- ▸ **Salmeterol (Non-proprietary)**
Salmeterol (as Salmeterol xinafoate) 25 microgram per 1 dose Salmeterol 25micrograms/dose inhaler CFC free | 120 dose PoM £29.26 DT price = £29.26
- ▸ **Neovent** (Kent Pharmaceuticals Ltd)
Salmeterol (as Salmeterol xinafoate) 25 microgram per 1 dose Neovent 25micrograms/dose inhaler CFC free | 120 dose PoM £29.26 DT price = £29.26
- ▸ **Serevent Evohaler** (GlaxoSmithKline UK Ltd)
Salmeterol (as Salmeterol xinafoate) 25 microgram per 1 dose Serevent 25micrograms/dose Evohaler | 120 dose PoM £29.26 DT price = £29.26
- ▸ **Soltel** (Kent Pharmaceuticals Ltd)
Salmeterol (as Salmeterol xinafoate) 25 microgram per 1 dose Soltel 25micrograms/dose inhaler CFC free | 120 dose PoM £19.95 DT price = £29.26
- ▸ **Vertine** (Teva UK Ltd)
Salmeterol (as Salmeterol xinafoate) 25 microgram per 1 dose Vertine 25micrograms/dose inhaler CFC free | 120 dose PoM £23.40 DT price = £29.26

Combinations available: *Fluticasone with salmeterol*, p. 157

BETA$_2$-ADRENOCEPTOR AGONISTS, SELECTIVE > SHORT-ACTING

F 148

Salbutamol

(Albuterol)

● INDICATIONS AND DOSE

Acute asthma

▸ BY INTRAVENOUS INJECTION

▸ Child 1–23 months: 5 micrograms/kg for 1 dose, dose to be administered over 5 minutes, reserve intravenous beta$_2$ agonists for those in whom inhaled therapy cannot be used reliably or there is no current effect

▸ Child 2–17 years: 15 micrograms/kg (max. per dose 250 micrograms) for 1 dose, dose to be administered over 5 minutes, reserve intravenous beta$_2$ agonists for those in whom inhaled therapy cannot be used reliably or there is no current effect

▸ BY CONTINUOUS INTRAVENOUS INFUSION

▸ Child: 1–2 micrograms/kg/minute, adjusted according to response and heart rate, increased if necessary up to 5 micrograms/kg/minute, doses above 2 micrograms/kg/minute should be given in an intensive care setting, reserve intravenous beta$_2$ agonists for those in whom inhaled therapy cannot be used reliably or there is no current effect

Moderate, severe, or life-threatening acute asthma

▸ BY INHALATION OF NEBULISED SOLUTION

▸ Child 1 month–4 years: 2.5 mg, repeat every 20–30 minutes or when required, give via oxygen-driven nebuliser if available

▸ Child 5–11 years: 2.5–5 mg, repeat every 20–30 minutes or when required, give via oxygen-driven nebuliser if available

▸ Child 12–17 years: 5 mg, repeat every 20–30 minutes or when required, give via oxygen-driven nebuliser if available

Moderate and severe acute asthma

▸ BY INHALATION OF AEROSOL

▸ Child: 2–10 puffs, each puff is to be inhaled separately, repeat every 10–20 minutes or when required, give via large volume spacer (and a close-fitting face mask in children under 3 years), each puff is equivalent to 100 micrograms

Exacerbation of reversible airways obstruction (including nocturnal asthma) | Prophylaxis of allergen- or exercise-induced bronchospasm

▸ BY INHALATION OF AEROSOL

▸ Child: 100–200 micrograms, up to 4 times a day for persistent symptoms

▸ BY MOUTH

▸ Child 1 month–1 year: 100 micrograms/kg 3–4 times a day (max. per dose 2 mg), inhalation route preferred over oral route

▸ Child 2–5 years: 1–2 mg 3–4 times a day, inhalation route preferred over oral route

▸ Child 6–11 years: 2 mg 3–4 times a day, inhalation route preferred over oral route

▸ Child 12–17 years: 2–4 mg 3–4 times a day, inhalation route preferred over oral route

Severe hyperkalaemia

▸ BY INTRAVENOUS INJECTION

▸ Neonate: 4 micrograms/kg, repeated if necessary, to be administered over 5 minutes.

▸ Child: 4 micrograms/kg, repeated if necessary, to be administered over 5 minutes

▸ BY INHALATION OF NEBULISED SOLUTION

▸ Neonate: 2.5–5 mg, repeated if necessary, intravenous injection route preferred over inhalation of nebulised solution.

▸ Child: 2.5–5 mg, repeated if necessary, intravenous injection route preferred over inhalation of nebulised solution

Chronic asthma

▸ BY MOUTH USING MODIFIED-RELEASE MEDICINES

▸ Child 3–11 years: 4 mg twice daily

▸ Child 12–17 years: 8 mg twice daily

ASMASAL CLICKHALER®

Acute bronchospasm

▸ BY INHALATION OF POWDER

▸ Child 5–17 years: 1–2 puffs, up to 4 times daily for persistent symptoms

Prophylaxis of allergen- or exercise-induced bronchospasm

▸ BY INHALATION OF POWDER

▸ Child 5–17 years: 1–2 puffs

EASYHALER® SALBUTAMOL

Acute bronchospasm

▸ BY INHALATION OF POWDER

▸ Child 5–11 years: 100–200 micrograms; maximum 800 micrograms per day

▸ Child 12–17 years: Initially 100–200 micrograms, increased if necessary to 400 micrograms; maximum 800 micrograms per day

Prophylaxis of allergen- or exercise-induced bronchospasm

▸ BY INHALATION OF POWDER

▸ Child 5–11 years: 100–200 micrograms

▸ Child 12–17 years: 200 micrograms

PULVINAL® SALBUTAMOL

Acute bronchospasm

▸ BY INHALATION OF POWDER

▸ Child 5–17 years: Initially 200 micrograms, up to 800 micrograms daily for persistent symptoms

Prophylaxis of allergen- or exercise-induced bronchospasm

▸ BY INHALATION OF POWDER

▸ Child 5–17 years: 200 micrograms

SALBULIN NOVOLIZER®

Acute bronchospasm

▸ BY INHALATION OF POWDER

▸ Child 6–11 years: 100–200 micrograms, up to 400 micrograms daily for persistent symptoms

▸ Child 12–17 years: Initially 100–200 micrograms, up to 800 micrograms daily for persistent symptoms

Prophylaxis of allergen- or exercise-induced bronchospasm

▸ BY INHALATION OF POWDER

▸ Child 6–11 years: 100–200 micrograms

▸ Child 12–17 years: 200 micrograms

VENTOLIN ACCUHALER®

Acute bronchospasm

▸ BY INHALATION OF POWDER

▸ Child 5–17 years: Initially 200 micrograms, up to 4 times daily for persistent symptoms

Prophylaxis of allergen- or exercise-induced bronchospasm

▸ BY INHALATION OF POWDER

▸ Child 5–17 years: 200 micrograms

PHARMACOKINETICS

At recommended inhaled doses, the duration of action of salbutamol is about 3 to 5 hours.

- **UNLICENSED USE** Not licensed for use in hyperkalaemia.
- With oral use Syrup and tablets not licensed for use in children under 2 years. Modified-release tablets not licensed for use in children under 3 years.
- With intravenous use Injection and solution for intravenous infusion not licensed for use in children under 12 years. Administration of undiluted salbutamol injection through a central venous catheter is not licensed.
- **CAUTIONS** High doses of beta$_2$ agonists can be dangerous in some children
- **INTERACTIONS** → Appendix 1: beta$_2$ agonists
- **SIDE-EFFECTS** Lactic acidosis (with high doses) · nausea
- **BREAST FEEDING** Inhaled drugs for asthma can be taken as normal during breast-feeding.
- **DIRECTIONS FOR ADMINISTRATION**
- With intravenous use For *continuous intravenous infusion*, dilute to a concentration of 200 micrograms/mL with Glucose 5% *or* Sodium Chloride 0.9%. If fluid-restricted, can be given undiluted through central venous catheter [unlicensed]. For *intravenous injection*, dilute to a concentration of 50 micrograms/mL with Glucose 5%, Sodium Chloride 0.9%, *or* Water for injections.
- When used by inhalation For *nebulisation*, dilute nebuliser solution with a suitable volume of sterile Sodium Chloride 0.9% solution according to nebuliser type and duration of administration; salbutamol and ipratropium bromide solutions are compatible and can be mixed for nebulisation.
- **PATIENT AND CARER ADVICE**
  For inhalation by aerosol or dry powder, advise patients and carers not to exceed prescribed dose and to follow manufacturer's directions; if a previously effective dose of inhaled salbutamol fails to provide at least 3 hours relief, a doctor's advice should be obtained as soon as possible. *For inhalation by nebuliser*, the dose given by nebuliser is substantially higher than that given by inhaler. Patients should therefore be warned that it is dangerous to exceed the prescribed dose and they should seek medical advice if they fail to respond to the usual dose of the respirator solution.
  Medicines for Children leaflet: Salbutamol inhaler for asthma and wheeze www.medicinesforchildren.org.uk/salbutamol-inhaler-for-asthma-and-wheeze

- **MEDICINAL FORMS**
  There can be variation in the licensing of different medicines containing the same drug.

Tablet

▸ **Salbutamol (Non-proprietary)**
  Salbutamol (as Salbutamol sulfate) 2 mg Salbutamol 2mg tablets | 28 tablet PoM £106.43 DT price = £104.95
  Salbutamol (as Salbutamol sulfate) 4 mg Salbutamol 4mg tablets | 28 tablet PoM £108.95 DT price = £107.43

Inhalation powder

▸ **Easyhaler (salbutamol)** (Orion Pharma (UK) Ltd)
  Salbutamol 100 microgram per 1 dose Easyhaler Salbutamol sulfate 100micrograms/dose dry powder inhaler | 200 dose PoM £3.31 DT price = £3.31
  Salbutamol 200 microgram per 1 dose Easyhaler Salbutamol sulfate 200micrograms/dose dry powder inhaler | 200 dose PoM £6.63 DT price = £6.63

▸ **Salbulin Novolizer** (Meda Pharmaceuticals Ltd)
  Salbutamol (as Salbutamol sulfate) 100 microgram per 1 dose Salbulin Novolizer 100micrograms/dose inhalation powder | 200 dose PoM £4.95
  Salbulin Novolizer 100micrograms/dose inhalation powder refill | 200 dose PoM £2.75

▸ **Ventolin Accuhaler** (GlaxoSmithKline UK Ltd)
  Salbutamol 200 microgram per 1 dose Ventolin 200micrograms/dose Accuhaler | 60 dose PoM £3.60 DT price = £3.60

Solution for injection

▸ **Ventolin** (GlaxoSmithKline UK Ltd)
  Salbutamol (as Salbutamol sulfate) 500 microgram per 1 ml Ventolin 500micrograms/1ml solution for injection ampoules | 5 ampoule PoM £1.91

Solution for infusion

▸ **Ventolin** (GlaxoSmithKline UK Ltd)
  Salbutamol (as Salbutamol sulfate) 1 mg per 1 ml Ventolin 5mg/5ml solution for infusion ampoules | 10 ampoule PoM £24.81

Oral solution

▸ **Salbutamol (Non-proprietary)**
  Salbutamol (as Salbutamol sulfate) 400 microgram per 1 ml Salbutamol 2mg/5ml oral solution sugar free sugar-free | 150 ml PoM no price available DT price = £1.15

▸ **Ventolin** (GlaxoSmithKline UK Ltd)
  Salbutamol (as Salbutamol sulfate) 400 microgram per 1 ml Ventolin 2mg/5ml syrup sugar-free | 150 ml PoM £1.15 DT price = £1.15

Pressurised inhalation

▸ **Salbutamol (Non-proprietary)**
  Salbutamol (as Salbutamol sulfate) 100 microgram per 1 dose Salbutamol 100micrograms/dose inhaler CFC free | 200 dose PoM £1.50 DT price = £1.50

▸ **AirSalb** (Sandoz Ltd)
  Salbutamol (as Salbutamol sulfate) 100 microgram per 1 dose AirSalb 100micrograms/dose inhaler CFC free | 200 dose PoM £1.50 DT price = £1.50

▸ **Airomir** (Teva UK Ltd)
  Salbutamol (as Salbutamol sulfate) 100 microgram per 1 dose Airomir 100micrograms/dose inhaler | 200 dose PoM £1.97 DT price = £1.50

▸ **Airomir Autohaler** (Teva UK Ltd)
  Salbutamol (as Salbutamol sulfate) 100 microgram per 1 dose Airomir 100micrograms/dose Autohaler | 200 dose PoM £6.02 DT price = £6.30

▸ **Salamol** (Teva UK Ltd)
  Salbutamol (as Salbutamol sulfate) 100 microgram per 1 dose Salamol 100micrograms/dose inhaler CFC free | 200 dose PoM £1.46 DT price = £1.50

▸ **Salamol Easi-Breathe** (Teva UK Ltd)
  Salbutamol (as Salbutamol sulfate) 100 microgram per 1 dose Salamol 100micrograms/dose Easi-Breathe inhaler | 200 dose PoM £6.30 DT price = £6.30

▸ **Ventolin Evohaler** (GlaxoSmithKline UK Ltd)
  Salbutamol (as Salbutamol sulfate) 100 microgram per 1 dose Ventolin 100micrograms/dose Evohaler | 200 dose PoM £1.50 DT price = £1.50

Nebuliser liquid

▸ **Salbutamol (Non-proprietary)**
  Salbutamol (as Salbutamol sulfate) 1 mg per 1 ml Salbutamol 2.5mg/2.5ml nebuliser liquid unit dose vials | 20 unit dose PoM £1.91 DT price = £1.91
  Salbutamol (as Salbutamol sulfate) 2 mg per 1 ml Salbutamol 5mg/2.5ml nebuliser liquid unit dose vials | 20 unit dose PoM £3.82 DT price = £3.82

▸ **Salamol Steri-Neb** (Teva UK Ltd)
  Salbutamol (as Salbutamol sulfate) 1 mg per 1 ml Salamol 2.5mg/2.5ml nebuliser liquid Steri-Neb unit dose vials | 20 unit dose PoM £1.91 DT price = £1.91
  Salbutamol (as Salbutamol sulfate) 2 mg per 1 ml Salamol 5mg/2.5ml nebuliser liquid Steri-Neb unit dose vials | 20 unit dose PoM £3.82 DT price = £3.82

▸ **Ventolin** (GlaxoSmithKline UK Ltd)
  Salbutamol (as Salbutamol sulfate) 5 mg per 1 ml Ventolin 5mg/ml respirator solution | 20 ml PoM £2.18 DT price = £2.18

▸ **Ventolin Nebules** (GlaxoSmithKline UK Ltd)
  Salbutamol (as Salbutamol sulfate) 1 mg per 1 ml Ventolin 2.5mg Nebules | 20 unit dose PoM £1.65 DT price = £1.91
  Salbutamol (as Salbutamol sulfate) 2 mg per 1 ml Ventolin 5mg Nebules | 20 unit dose PoM £2.78 DT price = £3.82

3

Respiratory system

Terbutaline sulfate

F 148

● **INDICATIONS AND DOSE**

Acute asthma

▶ BY SUBCUTANEOUS INJECTION, OR BY SLOW INTRAVENOUS INJECTION

▸ Child 2–14 years: 10 micrograms/kg up to 4 times a day (max. per dose 300 micrograms), reserve intravenous beta₂ agonists for those in whom inhaled therapy cannot be used reliably or there is no current effect

▸ Child 15–17 years: 250–500 micrograms up to 4 times a day, reserve intravenous beta₂ agonists for those in whom inhaled therapy cannot be used reliably or there is no current effect

▶ BY CONTINUOUS INTRAVENOUS INFUSION

▸ Child: Loading dose 2–4 micrograms/kg, then 1–10 micrograms/kg/hour, dose to be adjusted according to response and heart rate, close monitoring is required for doses above 10 micrograms/kg/hour, reserve intravenous beta₂ agonists for those in whom inhaled therapy cannot be used reliably or there is no current effect

Moderate, severe, or life-threatening acute asthma

▶ BY INHALATION OF NEBULISED SOLUTION

▸ Child 1 month–4 years: 5 mg, repeat every 20–30 minutes or when required, give via oxygen-driven nebuliser if available

▸ Child 5–11 years: 5–10 mg, repeat every 20–30 minutes or when required, give via oxygen-driven nebuliser if available

▸ Child 12–17 years: 10 mg, repeat every 20–30 minutes or when required, give via oxygen-driven nebuliser if available

Exacerbation of reversible airways obstruction (including nocturnal asthma) | Prevention of exercise-induced bronchospasm

▶ BY INHALATION OF POWDER

▸ Child 5–17 years: 500 micrograms up to 4 times a day, for occasional use only

▶ BY MOUTH

▸ Child 1 month–6 years: 75 micrograms/kg 3 times a day (max. per dose 2.5 mg), administration by mouth is not recommended

▸ Child 7–14 years: 2.5 mg 2–3 times a day, administration by mouth is not recommended

▸ Child 15–17 years: Initially 2.5 mg 3 times a day, then increased if necessary to 5 mg 3 times a day, administration by mouth is not recommended

PHARMACOKINETICS

At recommended inhaled doses, the duration of action of terbutaline is about 3 to 5 hours.

● **UNLICENSED USE** Tablets not licensed for use in children under 7 years. Injection not licensed for use in children under 2 years.

● **CAUTIONS** High doses of beta₂ agonists can be dangerous in some children

● **INTERACTIONS** → Appendix 1: beta₂ agonists

● **SIDE-EFFECTS** Nausea

● **PREGNANCY** Inhaled drugs for asthma can be taken as normal during pregnancy.

● **BREAST FEEDING** Inhaled drugs for asthma can be taken as normal during breast-feeding.

● **DIRECTIONS FOR ADMINISTRATION**

▸ With intravenous use For *continuous intravenous infusion*, dilute to a concentration of 5 micrograms/mL with Glucose 5% or Sodium Chloride 0.9%; if fluid-restricted, dilute to a concentration of 100 micrograms/mL.

▸ When used by inhalation For *nebulisation*, dilute nebuliser solution with sterile Sodium Chloride 0.9% solution

according to nebuliser type and duration of administration; terbutaline and ipratropium bromide solutions are compatible and may be mixed for nebulisation.

● **PATIENT AND CARER ADVICE**

For inhalation by dry powder, advise patients and carers not to exceed prescribed dose and to follow manufacturer's directions; if a previously effective dose of inhaled terbutaline fails to provide at least 3 hours relief, a doctor's advice should be obtained as soon as possible. *For inhalation by nebuliser*, the dose given by nebuliser is substantially higher than that given by inhaler. Patients should therefore be warned that it is dangerous to exceed the prescribed dose and they should seek medical advice if they fail to respond to the usual dose of the respirator solution.

● **MEDICINAL FORMS**

There can be variation in the licensing of different medicines containing the same drug. Forms available from special-order manufacturers include: solution for injection

Solution for injection

▸ Bricanyl (AstraZeneca UK Ltd)

Terbutaline sulfate 500 microgram per 1 ml Bricanyl 2.5mg/5ml solution for injection ampoules | 10 ampoule [PoM] £16.74 Bricanyl 500micrograms/1ml solution for injection ampoules | 5 ampoule [PoM] £2.16

Inhalation powder

▸ Bricanyl Turbohaler (AstraZeneca UK Ltd)

Terbutaline sulfate 500 microgram per 1 dose Bricanyl 500micrograms/dose Turbohaler | 100 dose [PoM] £6.92 DT price = £6.92

Nebuliser liquid

▸ Terbutaline sulfate (Non-proprietary)

Terbutaline sulfate 2.5 mg per 1 ml Terbutaline 5mg/2ml nebuliser liquid unit dose vials | 20 unit dose [PoM] £4.04 DT price = £4.04

▸ Bricanyl Respules (AstraZeneca UK Ltd)

Terbutaline sulfate 2.5 mg per 1 ml Bricanyl 5mg/2ml Respules | 20 unit dose [PoM] £5.82 DT price = £4.04

Tablet

▸ Bricanyl (AstraZeneca UK Ltd)

Terbutaline sulfate 5 mg Bricanyl 5mg tablets | 100 tablet [PoM] £4.91 DT price = £4.91

CORTICOSTEROIDS

Airways disease, use of corticosteroids

Asthma

Inhaled corticosteroids

Corticosteroids are effective in the management of *asthma*; they reduce airway inflammation.

An inhaled corticosteroid is used regularly for prophylaxis of asthma when a child requires a beta₂ agonist more than twice a week, or if symptoms disturb sleep at least once a week, or if the child has suffered an exacerbation in the last 2 years requiring a systemic corticosteroid.

Current or previous smoking reduces the effectiveness of inhaled corticosteroids and higher doses may be necessary.

Corticosteroid inhalers must be used regularly for maximum benefit; alleviation of symptoms usually occurs 3 to 7 days after initiation but may take longer. Beclometasone dipropionate p. 154, budesonide p. 155, fluticasone p. 156, and mometasone furoate p. 158 appear to be equally effective. A spacer device should be used for administering inhaled corticosteroids in children under 15 years); a spacer device is also useful in children over 15 years, particularly if high doses are required.

In children 12–18 years using an inhaled corticosteroid and a long-acting beta₂ agonist for the prophylaxis of asthma, but who are poorly controlled, *Symbicort®* (budesonide with formoterol p. 156) may be used as a reliever (instead of a short-acting beta$_2$ agonist), in addition to its regular use for the prophylaxis of asthma [unlicensed]. *Symbicort* ® can also be used in this way in children 12–18 years using an inhaled corticosteroid with a dose greater than 400 micrograms beclometasone dipropionate daily, but who are poorly controlled [unlicensed] (standard doses of other inhaled corticosteroids can be used). When starting this treatment, the total regular dose of inhaled corticosteroid should not be reduced. Children and their carers must be carefully instructed on the appropriate dose and management of exacerbations before initiating this treatment, preferably by a respiratory specialist. Children using budesonide with formoterol as a reliever once a day or more should have their treatment reviewed regularly. This management approach has not been investigated with combination inhalers containing other corticosteroids and long-acting beta$_2$ agonists.

High doses of inhaled corticosteroids can be prescribed for children who respond only partially to standard doses of an inhaled corticosteroid and a long-acting beta$_2$ agonist or to other long-acting bronchodilators. High doses should be continued only if there is clear benefit over the lower dose. The recommended maximum dose of an inhaled corticosteroid should not generally be exceeded; however, if a higher dose is required it should be initiated and supervised by a respiratory paediatrician. The use of high doses of an inhaled corticosteroid can minimise the requirement for an oral corticosteroid.

Oral corticosteroids

Systemic therapy may be required during periods of stress, such as during severe infections, or when airways obstruction or mucus prevent drug access to smaller airways.

An acute attack of asthma should be treated with a short course (3–5 days) of oral corticosteroid. The dose can usually be stopped abruptly but it should be reduced gradually in children under 12 years who have taken corticosteroids for more than 14 days. Tapering is not needed in children 12–18 years provided that the child receives an inhaled corticosteroid in an adequate dose (apart from those on maintenance oral corticosteroid treatment or where oral corticosteroids are required for 3 or more weeks).

In chronic continuing asthma, when the response to other drugs has been inadequate, longer term administration of an oral corticosteroid may be necessary; in such cases high doses of an inhaled corticosteroid should be continued to minimise oral corticosteroid requirements.

An oral corticosteroid should normally be taken as a single dose in the morning to reduce the disturbance to circadian cortisol secretion. Dosage should always be titrated to the lowest dose that controls symptoms. Some clinicians use alternate-day dosing of an oral corticosteroid.

Parenteral corticosteroids

Hydrocortisone injection p. 420 has a role in the emergency treatment of acute severe asthma.

Corticosteroids (inhaled)

- **SIDE-EFFECTS**
- ▸ **Very rare** Paradoxical bronchospasm
- ▸ **Frequency not known** Adrenal crisis (with prolonged high doses) · adrenal suppression (with prolonged high doses) · aggression · anxiety · behavioural changes · bruising · candidiasis of the mouth · candidiasis of the throat · cataracts · coma (with prolonged high doses) · Cushing's syndrome (with moon face, striae and acne) · depression · dysphonia · glaucoma (with prolonged high doses) · hoarseness · hyperactivity · hyperglycaemia (usually only with high doses) · irritability · reduced growth velocity · reduced mineral bone density (with long-term treatment of high doses) · side-effects applicable to systemic

corticosteroids may also apply if absorption occurs following inhaled use · sleep disturbances · throat irritation

SIDE-EFFECTS, FURTHER INFORMATION

- ▸ Candidiasis The risk of oral candidiasis can be reduced by using a spacer device with the corticosteroid inhaler; rinsing the mouth with water after inhalation of a dose may also be helpful. An anti-fungal oral suspension or oral gel can be used to treat oral candidiasis without discontinuing corticosteroid therapy.
- ▸ Paradoxical bronchospasm The potential for paradoxical bronchospasm (calling for discontinuation and alternative therapy) should be borne in mind—mild bronchospasm may be prevented by inhalation of a short-acting beta$_2$ agonist beforehand (or by transfer from an aerosol inhalation to a dry powder inhalation).

- **PREGNANCY** Inhaled drugs for asthma can be taken as normal during pregnancy.

- **BREAST FEEDING** Inhaled corticosteroids for asthma can be taken as normal during breast-feeding.

- **MONITORING REQUIREMENTS** The height and weight of children receiving prolonged treatment with inhaled corticosteroids should be monitored annually; if growth is slowed, referral to a paediatrician should be considered.

- **NATIONAL FUNDING/ACCESS DECISIONS**

NICE technology appraisals (TAs)

- ▸ **Inhaled corticosteroids for the treatment of chronic asthma in children under 12 years (November 2007)** NICE TA131

For children under 12 years with chronic asthma in whom treatment with an inhaled corticosteroid is considered appropriate, the least costly product that is suitable for an individual child (taking into consideration NICE TAs 38 and 10), within its marketing authorisation, is recommended.

For children under 12 years with chronic asthma in whom treatment with an inhaled corticosteroid and a long-acting beta$_2$ agonist is considered appropriate, the following apply:

- the use of a combination inhaler within its marketing authorisation is recommended as an option;
- the decision to use a combination inhaler or two agents in separate inhalers should be made on an individual basis, taking into consideration therapeutic need and the likelihood of treatment adherence;
- if a combination inhaler is chosen, then the least costly inhaler that is suitable for the individual child is recommended.

www.nice.org.uk/TA131

- ▸ **Inhaled corticosteroids for the treatment of chronic asthma in adults and children over 12 years (March 2008)** NICE TA138

For adults and children over 12 years with chronic asthma in whom treatment with an inhaled corticosteroid is considered appropriate, the least costly product that is suitable for an individual (taking into consideration NICE TAs 38 and 10), within its marketing authorisation is recommended.

For adults and children over 12 years with chronic asthma in whom treatment with an inhaled corticosteroid and a long-acting beta$_2$ agonist is considered appropriate, the following apply:

- the use of a combination inhaler within its marketing authorisation is recommended as an option;
- the decision to use a combination inhaler or two agents in separate inhalers should be made on an individual basis, taking into consideration therapeutic need, and the likelihood of treatment adherence;
- if a combination inhaler is chosen, then the least costly inhaler that is suitable for the individual is recommended.

www.nice.org.uk/TA138

3

Respiratory system

Beclometasone dipropionate

(Beclomethasone dipropionate)

● **INDICATIONS AND DOSE**

Prophylaxis of asthma

▸ BY INHALATION OF POWDER
▸ Child 5-11 years: 100–200 micrograms twice daily, dose to be adjusted as necessary
▸ Child 12-17 years: 200–400 micrograms twice daily; increased if necessary up to 800 micrograms twice daily, dose to be adjusted as necessary

ASMABEC CLICKHALER®

Prophylaxis of asthma

▸ BY INHALATION OF POWDER
▸ Child 6-11 years: 100–200 micrograms twice daily, dose to be adjusted as necessary
▸ Child 12-17 years: 100–400 micrograms twice daily (max. per dose 1 mg twice daily), dose to be adjusted as necessary

CLENIL MODULITE®

Prophylaxis of asthma

▸ BY INHALATION OF AEROSOL
▸ Child 2-11 years: 100–200 micrograms twice daily
▸ Child 12-17 years: 200–400 micrograms twice daily, adjusted according to response; increased if necessary up to 1 mg twice daily

QVAR® PREPARATIONS

Prophylaxis of asthma

▸ BY INHALATION OF AEROSOL
▸ Child 12-17 years: 50–200 micrograms twice daily; increased if necessary up to 400 micrograms twice daily

POTENCY

Qvar® has extra-fine particles, is more potent than traditional beclometasone dipropionate CFC-containing inhalers and is approximately twice as potent as *Clenil Modulite®*.

DOSE EQUIVALENCE AND CONVERSION

▸ Dose adjustments may be required for some inhaler devices, see under individual preparations.

● **UNLICENSED USE** *Easyhaler® Beclometasone Dipropionate* is not licensed for use in children under 18 years. *Clenil Modulite®* -200 and -250 are not licensed for use in children under 12 years.

IMPORTANT SAFETY INFORMATION

MHRA/CHM ADVICE (JULY 2008)
Beclometasone dipropionate CFC-free pressurised metered-dose inhalers (*Qvar®* and *Clenil Modulite®*) are **not** interchangeable and should be prescribed by brand name; *Qvar®* has extra-fine particles, is more potent than traditional beclometasone dipropionate CFC-containing inhalers, and is approximately twice as potent as *Clenil Modulite®*.

● **INTERACTIONS** → Appendix 1: corticosteroids
● **PRESCRIBING AND DISPENSING INFORMATION** The MHRA has advised (July 2008) that beclometasone dipropionate CFC-free inhalers should be prescribed by brand name.

CLENIL MODULITE® *Clenil Modulite®* is not interchangeable with other CFC-free beclometasone dipropionate inhalers.

QVAR® PREPARATIONS When switching a patient with well-controlled asthma from another corticosteroid inhaler, initially a 100-microgram metered dose of *Qvar®* should be prescribed for 200–250 micrograms of beclometasone dipropionate or budesonide and for 100 micrograms of fluticasone propionate. When

switching a patient with poorly controlled asthma from another corticosteroid inhaler, initially a 100-microgram metered dose of *Qvar®* should be prescribed for 100 micrograms of beclometasone dipropionate, budesonide, or fluticasone propionate; the dose of *Qvar®* should be adjusted according to response.

● **PATIENT AND CARER ADVICE** Steroid card should be issued with high doses of inhaled beclometasone dipropionate. Medicines for Children leaflet: Beclometasone for asthma prevention (prophylaxis) www.medicinesforchildren.org.uk/beclometasone-inhaler-asthma-prevention-prophylaxis-0

● **PROFESSION SPECIFIC INFORMATION**

Dental practitioners' formulary

Clenil Modulite® 50 micrograms/metered inhalation may be prescribed.

● **MEDICINAL FORMS**

There can be variation in the licensing of different medicines containing the same drug.

Inhalation powder

CAUTIONARY AND ADVISORY LABELS 8, 10

▸ **Asmabec Clickhaler** (Focus Pharmaceuticals Ltd)
Beclometasone dipropionate 100 microgram per 1 dose Asmabec 100 Clickhaler | 200 dose |PoM| £9.8□
▸ **Easyhaler (beclometasone)** (Orion Pharma (UK) Ltd)
Beclometasone dipropionate 200 microgram per
1 dose Easyhaler Beclometasone 200 micrograms/dose dry powder inhaler | 200 dose |PoM| £14.93

Pressurised inhalation

CAUTIONARY AND ADVISORY LABELS 8, 10

▸ **Beclometasone dipropionate (Non-proprietary)**
Beclometasone dipropionate 50 microgram per
1 dose Beclometasone 50micrograms/dose inhaler CFC free | 200 dose |PoM| no price available
Beclometasone dipropionate 100 microgram per
1 dose Beclometasone 100micrograms/dose inhaler CFC free | 200 dose |PoM| £54.20
Beclometasone dipropionate 200 microgram per
1 dose Beclometasone 200micrograms/dose inhaler CFC free | 200 dose |PoM| no price available
▸ **Clenil Modulite** (Chiesi Ltd)
Beclometasone dipropionate 50 microgram per 1 dose Clenil Modulite 50micrograms/dose inhaler | 200 dose |PoM| £3.70
Beclometasone dipropionate 100 microgram per 1 dose Clenil Modulite 100micrograms/dose inhaler | 200 dose |PoM| £7.42
Beclometasone dipropionate 200 microgram per 1 dose Clenil Modulite 200micrograms/dose inhaler | 200 dose |PoM| £16.17
Beclometasone dipropionate 250 microgram per 1 dose Clenil Modulite 250micrograms/dose inhaler | 200 dose |PoM| £16.29
▸ **Qvar** (Teva UK Ltd)
Beclometasone dipropionate 50 microgram per 1 dose Qvar 50 inhaler | 200 dose |PoM| £7.87
Beclometasone dipropionate 100 microgram per 1 dose Qvar 100 inhaler | 200 dose |PoM| £17.2□
▸ **Qvar Autohaler** (Teva UK Ltd)
Beclometasone dipropionate 50 microgram per 1 dose Qvar 50 Autohaler | 200 dose |PoM| £7.87 DT price = £7.87
Beclometasone dipropionate 100 microgram per 1 dose Qvar 100 Autohaler | 200 dose |PoM| £17.21 DT price = £17.21
▸ **Qvar Easi-Breathe** (Teva UK Ltd)
Beclometasone dipropionate 50 microgram per 1 dose Qvar 50micrograms/dose Easi-Breathe inhaler | 200 dose |PoM| £7.74 DT price = £7.87
Beclometasone dipropionate 100 microgram per 1 dose Qvar 100micrograms/dose Easi-Breathe inhaler | 200 dose |PoM| £16.95 DT price = £17.21

F 153

Budesonide

20-Nov-2016

● INDICATIONS AND DOSE

Bronchopulmonary dysplasia with spontaneous respiration

▶ BY INHALATION OF NEBULISED SUSPENSION

▸ Neonate: 500 micrograms twice daily.

▸ Child 1–4 months: 500 micrograms twice daily

Bronchopulmonary dysplasia with spontaneous respiration (severe symptoms)

▶ BY INHALATION OF NEBULISED SUSPENSION

▸ Child 1–4 months (body-weight 2.5 kg and above): 1 mg twice daily

Prophylaxis of mild to moderate asthma (in patients stabilised on twice daily dose)

▶ BY INHALATION OF POWDER

▸ Child 6–11 years: 200–400 micrograms once daily, dose to be given in the evening

▸ Child 12–17 years: 200–400 micrograms once daily (max. per dose 800 micrograms), dose to be given in the evening

Prophylaxis of asthma

▶ BY INHALATION OF POWDER

▸ Child 6–11 years: 100–400 micrograms twice daily, dose to be adjusted as necessary

▸ Child 12–17 years: 100–800 micrograms twice daily, dose to be adjusted as necessary

▶ BY INHALATION OF NEBULISED SUSPENSION

▸ Child 6 months–11 years: 125–500 micrograms twice daily, adjusted according to response; maximum 2 mg per day

▸ Child 12–17 years: Initially 0.25–1 mg twice daily, adjusted according to response, doses higher than recommended max. may be used in severe disease; maximum 2 mg per day

BUDELIN NOVOLIZER®

Prophylaxis of asthma

▶ BY INHALATION OF POWDER

▸ Child 6–11 years: 200–400 micrograms twice daily, dose is adjusted as necessary

▸ Child 12–17 years: 200–800 micrograms twice daily, dose is adjusted as necessary

Alternative in mild to moderate asthma, for patients previously stabilised on a twice daily dose

▶ BY INHALATION OF POWDER

▸ Child 6–11 years: 200–400 micrograms once daily, to be taken in the evening

▸ Child 12–17 years: 200–400 micrograms once daily (max. per dose 800 micrograms), to be taken in the evening

PULMICORT® RESPULES

Prophylaxis of asthma

▶ BY INHALATION OF NEBULISED SUSPENSION

▸ Child 3 months–11 years: Initially 0.5–1 mg twice daily, reduced to 250–500 micrograms twice daily

▸ Child 12–17 years: Initially 1–2 mg twice daily, reduced to 0.5–1 mg twice daily

Croup

▶ BY INHALATION OF NEBULISED SUSPENSION

▸ Child: 2 mg for 1 dose, alternatively 1 mg for 2 doses separated by a 30 minute interval, dose may be repeated every 12 hours until clinical improvement

PULMICORT® TURBOHALER

Prophylaxis of asthma

▶ BY INHALATION OF POWDER

▸ Child 5–11 years: 100–400 micrograms twice daily, dose to be adjusted as necessary

▸ Child 12–17 years: 100–800 micrograms twice daily, dose to be adjusted as necessary

Alternative in mild to moderate asthma, for patients previously stabilised on a twice daily dose

▶ BY INHALATION OF POWDER

▸ Child 5–11 years: 200–400 micrograms once daily, to be taken in the evening

▸ Child 12–17 years: 200–400 micrograms once daily (max. per dose 800 micrograms), to be taken in the evening

POTENCY

Dose adjustments may be required for some inhaler devices, see under individual preparations.

● UNLICENSED USE *Pulmicort®* nebuliser solution not licensed for use in children under 3 months; not licensed for use in bronchopulmonary dysplasia.

● INTERACTIONS → Appendix 1: corticosteroids

● DIRECTIONS FOR ADMINISTRATION Budesonide nebuliser suspension is not suitable for use in ultrasonic nebulisers.

● PATIENT AND CARER ADVICE With high doses, a steroid card should be supplied. Patients or carers should be given advice on how to administer budesonide dry powder inhaler and nebuliser suspension.
Medicines for Children leaflet: Budesonide inhaler for asthma prevention (prophylaxis) www.medicinesforchildren.org.uk/budesonide-inhaler-asthma-prevention-prophylaxis

BUDELIN NOVOLIZER® Patients or carers should be given advice on adminstration of *Budelin NovolizerA®*.

● MEDICINAL FORMS
There can be variation in the licensing of different medicines containing the same drug.

Inhalation powder

CAUTIONARY AND ADVISORY LABELS 8, 10

▶ Budelin Novolizer (Meda Pharmaceuticals Ltd)
Budesonide 200 microgram per 1 dose Budelin Novolizer 200micrograms/dose inhalation powder | 100 dose PoM £14.86
Budelin Novolizer 200micrograms/dose inhalation powder refill | 100 dose PoM £9.59

▶ Easyhaler (budesonide) (Orion Pharma (UK) Ltd)
Budesonide 100 microgram per 1 dose Easyhaler Budesonide 100micrograms/dose dry powder inhaler | 200 dose PoM £8.86 DT price = £11.84
Budesonide 200 microgram per 1 dose Easyhaler Budesonide 200micrograms/dose dry powder inhaler | 200 dose PoM £17.71
Budesonide 400 microgram per 1 dose Easyhaler Budesonide 400micrograms/dose dry powder inhaler | 100 dose PoM £17.71

▶ Pulmicort Turbohaler (AstraZeneca UK Ltd)
Budesonide 100 microgram per 1 dose Pulmicort 100 Turbohaler | 200 dose PoM £11.84 DT price = £11.84
Budesonide 200 microgram per 1 dose Pulmicort 200 Turbohaler | 100 dose PoM £11.84 DT price = £11.84
Budesonide 400 microgram per 1 dose Pulmicort 400 Turbohaler | 50 dose PoM £13.86 DT price = £13.86

Nebuliser liquid

CAUTIONARY AND ADVISORY LABELS 8, 10

▶ Budesonide (Non-proprietary)
Budesonide 250 microgram per 1 ml Budesonide 500micrograms/2ml nebuliser liquid unit dose vials | 20 unit dose PoM £30.40 DT price = £24.86
Budesonide 500 microgram per 1 ml Budesonide 1mg/2ml nebuliser liquid unit dose vials | 20 unit dose PoM £42.41 DT price = £38.60

▶ Pulmicort Respules (AstraZeneca UK Ltd)
Budesonide 250 microgram per 1 ml Pulmicort 0.5mg Respules | 20 unit dose PoM £26.42 DT price = £24.86
Budesonide 500 microgram per 1 ml Pulmicort 1mg Respules | 20 unit dose PoM £40.00 DT price = £38.60

3

Respiratory system

3

Respiratory system

Budesonide with formoterol

The properties listed below are those particular to the combination only. For the properties of the components please consider, budesonide p. 155, formoterol fumarate p. 148.

- **INDICATIONS AND DOSE**
SYMBICORT 100/6 TURBOHALER®
Asthma, maintenance therapy
▶ BY INHALATION OF POWDER
▸ Child 6–17 years: Initially 1–2 puffs twice daily; reduced to 1 puff daily, dose reduced only if control is maintained
Asthma, maintenance and reliever therapy
▶ BY INHALATION OF POWDER
▸ Child 12–17 years: Maintenance 2 puffs daily in 1–2 divided doses; 1 puff as required for relief of symptoms, increased if necessary up to 6 puffs as required; maximum 8 puffs per day
SYMBICORT 200/6 TURBOHALER®
Asthma, maintenance therapy
▶ BY INHALATION OF POWDER
▸ Child 12–17 years: Initially 1–2 puffs twice daily; reduced to 1 puff daily, dose reduced only if control is maintained
Asthma, maintenance and reliever therapy
▶ BY INHALATION OF POWDER
▸ Child 12–17 years: Maintenance 2 puffs daily in 1–2 divided doses, increased if necessary to 2 puffs twice daily; 1 puff as required for relief of symptoms, increased if necessary up to 6 puffs as required; maximum 8 puffs per day
SYMBICORT 400/12 TURBOHALER®
Asthma, maintenance therapy
▶ BY INHALATION OF POWDER
▸ Child 12–17 years: Initially 1 puff twice daily; reduced to 1 puff daily, dose reduced only if control is maintained

- **UNLICENSED USE**
SYMBICORT 100/6 TURBOHALER® *Symbicort®* not licensed for use in children for asthma maintenance and reliever therapy.
SYMBICORT 200/6 TURBOHALER® *Symbicort®* not licensed for use in children for asthma maintenance and reliever therapy.
- **INTERACTIONS** → Appendix 1: beta₂ agonists, corticosteroids
- **PATIENT AND CARER ADVICE** With high doses, a steroid card should be supplied.
Patients counselling is advised for budesonide with formoterol dry powder inhalation (administration).

- **MEDICINAL FORMS**
There can be variation in the licensing of different medicines containing the same drug.
Inhalation powder
CAUTIONARY AND ADVISORY LABELS 8, 10 (high doses)
▶ Symbicort Turbohaler (AstraZeneca UK Ltd)
Formoterol fumarate dihydrate 6 microgram per 1 dose, Budesonide 100 microgram per 1 dose Symbicort 100/6 Turbohaler | 120 dose [PoM] £33.00 DT price = £33.00
Formoterol fumarate dihydrate 6 microgram per 1 dose, Budesonide 200 microgram per 1 dose Symbicort 200/6 Turbohaler | 120 dose [PoM] £38.00 DT price = £38.00
Formoterol fumarate dihydrate 12 microgram per 1 dose, Budesonide 400 microgram per 1 dose Symbicort 400/12 Turbohaler | 60 dose [PoM] £38.00 DT price = £38.00

F 153
Ciclesonide

- **INDICATIONS AND DOSE**
Prophylaxis of asthma
▶ BY INHALATION OF AEROSOL
▸ Child 12–17 years: 160 micrograms once daily; reduced to 80 micrograms daily, if control maintained

- **INTERACTIONS** → Appendix 1: corticosteroids
- **SIDE-EFFECTS** Nausea · taste disturbance
- **PATIENT AND CARER ADVICE** Patients or carers should be given advice on how to administer ciclesonide aerosol inhaler.

- **MEDICINAL FORMS**
There can be variation in the licensing of different medicines containing the same drug.
Pressurised inhalation
CAUTIONARY AND ADVISORY LABELS 8
▶ Alvesco (Takeda UK Ltd)
Ciclesonide 80 microgram per 1 dose Alvesco 80 inhaler | 120 dose [PoM] £32.83 DT price = £32.83
Ciclesonide 160 microgram per 1 dose Alvesco 160 inhaler | 60 dose [PoM] £19.31 DT price = £19.31 | 120 dose [PoM] £38.62 DT price = £38.62

F 153
Fluticasone

04-Jan-2016

- **INDICATIONS AND DOSE**
Prophylaxis of asthma
▶ BY INHALATION OF POWDER
▸ Child 5–15 years: Initially 50–100 micrograms twice daily (max. per dose 200 micrograms twice daily), dose to be adjusted as necessary
▸ Child 16–17 years: Initially 100–500 micrograms twice daily (max. per dose 1 mg twice daily), dose may be increased according to severity of asthma. Doses above 500 micrograms twice daily initiated by a specialist
▶ BY INHALATION OF AEROSOL
▸ Child 4–15 years: Initially 50–100 micrograms twice daily (max. per dose 200 micrograms twice daily), dose to be adjusted as necessary
▸ Child 16–17 years: Initially 100–500 micrograms twice daily (max. per dose 1 mg twice daily), dose may be increased according to severity of asthma. Doses above 500 micrograms twice daily initiated by a specialist
▶ BY INHALATION OF NEBULISED SUSPENSION
▸ Child 4–15 years: 1 mg twice daily
▸ Child 16–17 years: 0.5–2 mg twice daily

- **INTERACTIONS** → Appendix 1: corticosteroids
- **SIDE-EFFECTS** Arthralgia · dyspepsia
- **DIRECTIONS FOR ADMINISTRATION** Fluticasone nebuliser liquid may be diluted with sterile sodium chloride 0.9%. It is not suitable for use in ultrasonic nebulisers.
- **PATIENT AND CARER ADVICE** With high doses, a steroid card should be supplied.
Patients or carers should be given advice on how to administer all fluticasone inhalations preparations. Medicines for Children leaflet: Fluticasone inhaler for asthma prevention (prophylaxis) www.medicinesforchildren.org.uk/fluticasone-inhaler-for-asthma-prevention

- **MEDICINAL FORMS**
There can be variation in the licensing of different medicines containing the same drug.
Inhalation powder
CAUTIONARY AND ADVISORY LABELS 8, 10
▶ Flixotide Accuhaler (GlaxoSmithKline UK Ltd)
Fluticasone propionate 50 microgram per 1 dose Flixotide 50micrograms/dose Accuhaler | 60 dose [PoM] £7.66 DT price = £7.66

Fluticasone propionate 100 microgram per 1 dose Flixotide
100micrograms/dose Accuhaler | 60 dose [PoM] £10.72 DT price =
£10.72
Fluticasone propionate 250 microgram per 1 dose Flixotide
250micrograms/dose Accuhaler | 60 dose [PoM] £25.51 DT price =
£25.51
Fluticasone propionate 500 microgram per 1 dose Flixotide
500micrograms/dose Accuhaler | 60 dose [PoM] £43.37 DT price =
£43.37

Pressurised inhalation
CAUTIONARY AND ADVISORY LABELS 8, 10
▸ Flixotide Evohaler (GlaxoSmithKline UK Ltd)
Fluticasone propionate 50 microgram per 1 dose Flixotide
50micrograms/dose Evohaler | 120 dose [PoM] £5.44 DT price = £5.44
Fluticasone propionate 125 microgram per 1 dose Flixotide
125micrograms/dose Evohaler | 120 dose [PoM] £21.26 DT price =
£21.26
Fluticasone propionate 250 microgram per 1 dose Flixotide
250micrograms/dose Evohaler | 120 dose [PoM] £36.14 DT price =
£36.14

Nebuliser liquid
CAUTIONARY AND ADVISORY LABELS 8, 10
▸ Flixotide Nebule (GlaxoSmithKline UK Ltd)
Fluticasone propionate 250 microgram per 1 ml Flixotide
0.5mg/2ml Nebules | 10 unit dose [PoM] £9.34
Fluticasone propionate 1 mg per 1 ml Flixotide 2mg/2ml Nebules |
10 unit dose [PoM] £37.35

Fluticasone furoate with vilanterol

● **INDICATIONS AND DOSE**

RELVAR ELLIPTA® 184 MICROGRAMS/22 MICROGRAMS
Prophylaxis of asthma
▸ BY INHALATION OF POWDER
▸ Child 12–17 years: 1 inhalation once daily

RELVAR ELLIPTA® 92 MICROGRAMS/22 MICROGRAMS
Prophylaxis of asthma
▸ BY INHALATION OF POWDER
▸ Child 12–17 years: 1 inhalation once daily

● **INTERACTIONS** → Appendix 1: beta$_2$ agonists,
corticosteroids

● **SIDE-EFFECTS** Abdominal pain · back pain

● **PREGNANCY** Manufacturer advises use only if potential
benefit outweighs risk.

● **BREAST FEEDING** Manufacturer advises avoid—no
information available.

● **HEPATIC IMPAIRMENT** Max. dose fluticasone furoate
92 micrograms, vilanterol 22 micrograms.
RELVAR ELLIPTA®
184 MICROGRAMS/22 MICROGRAMS Avoid in moderate to
severe impairment.

● **PATIENT AND CARER ADVICE** A steroid card should be
provided.
Patients or carers should be given advice on how to
administer fluticasone with vilanterol powder for
inhalation.

● **MEDICINAL FORMS**
There can be variation in the licensing of different medicines
containing the same drug.
Inhalation powder
CAUTIONARY AND ADVISORY LABELS 8, 10
▸ Relvar Ellipta (GlaxoSmithKline UK Ltd) ▼
Vilanterol 22 microgram per 1 dose, Fluticasone furoate
92 microgram per 1 dose Relvar Ellipta 92micrograms/dose /
22micrograms/dose dry powder inhaler | 30 dose [PoM] £22.00 DT
price = £22.00
Vilanterol 22 microgram per 1 dose, Fluticasone furoate
184 microgram per 1 dose Relvar Ellipta 184micrograms/dose /
22micrograms/dose dry powder inhaler | 30 dose [PoM] £29.50 DT
price = £29.50

Fluticasone with formoterol

The properties listed below are those particular to the
combination only. For the properties of the components
please consider, fluticasone p. 156, formoterol fumarate
p. 148.

● **INDICATIONS AND DOSE**

FLUTIFORM® 50
Prophylaxis of asthma
▸ BY INHALATION OF AEROSOL
▸ Child 12–17 years: 2 puffs twice daily

FLUTIFORM® 125
Prophylaxis of asthma
▸ BY INHALATION OF AEROSOL
▸ Child 12–17 years: 2 puffs twice daily

● **INTERACTIONS** → Appendix 1: beta$_2$ agonists,
corticosteroids

● **PATIENT AND CARER ADVICE** With high doses, a steroid
card should be provided.
Patients or carers should be given advice on how to
administer fluticasone with formoterol aerosol inhalation.

● **MEDICINAL FORMS**
There can be variation in the licensing of different medicines
containing the same drug.
Pressurised inhalation
CAUTIONARY AND ADVISORY LABELS 8, 10 (high doses)
▸ Flutiform (Napp Pharmaceuticals Ltd)
Formoterol fumarate dihydrate 5 microgram per 1 dose,
Fluticasone propionate 50 microgram per 1 dose Flutiform
50micrograms/dose / 5micrograms/dose inhaler | 120 dose [PoM]
£14.40 DT price = £14.40
Formoterol fumarate dihydrate 5 microgram per 1 dose,
Fluticasone propionate 125 microgram per 1 dose Flutiform
125micrograms/dose / 5micrograms/dose inhaler | 120 dose [PoM]
£28.00 DT price = £28.00

Fluticasone with salmeterol   13-Jun-2017

The properties listed below are those particular to the
combination only. For the properties of the components
please consider, fluticasone p. 156, salmeterol p. 149.

● **INDICATIONS AND DOSE**

SERETIDE 100 ACCUHALER®
Prophylaxis of asthma
▸ BY INHALATION OF POWDER
▸ Child 5–17 years: 1 inhalation twice daily, reduced to
1 inhalation daily, use reduced dose only if control
maintained

SERETIDE 250 ACCUHALER®
Prophylaxis of asthma
▸ BY INHALATION OF POWDER
▸ Child 12–17 years: 1 inhalation twice daily

SERETIDE 500 ACCUHALER®
Prophylaxis of asthma
▸ BY INHALATION OF POWDER
▸ Child 12–17 years: 1 inhalation twice daily

SERETIDE 50 EVOHALER®
Prophylaxis of asthma
▸ BY INHALATION OF AEROSOL
▸ Child 5–17 years: 2 puffs twice daily, reduced to 2 puffs
once daily, use reduced dose only if control maintained

SERETIDE 125 EVOHALER®
Prophylaxis of asthma
▸ BY INHALATION OF AEROSOL
▸ Child 12–17 years: 2 puffs twice daily continued →

Respiratory system

3

SERETIDE 250 EVOHALER®

Prophylaxis of asthma
▶ BY INHALATION OF AEROSOL
▶ Child 12–17 years: 2 puffs twice daily

● **INTERACTIONS** → Appendix 1: beta₂ agonists, corticosteroids

● **PATIENT AND CARER ADVICE** With preparations containing greater than 100 micrograms fluticasone, a steroid card should be provided.

Patients or carers should be given advice on how to administer fluticasone with salmeterol dry powder inhalation and aerosol inhalation.

● **MEDICINAL FORMS**
There can be variation in the licensing of different medicines containing the same drug.

Inhalation powder
CAUTIONARY AND ADVISORY LABELS 8, 10 (excluding Seretide 100 Accuhaler®)
▶ Seretide Accuhaler (GlaxoSmithKline UK Ltd)
  Salmeterol (as Salmeterol xinafoate) 50 microgram per 1 dose, Fluticasone propionate 100 microgram per 1 dose Seretide 100 Accuhaler | 60 dose PoM £18.00 DT price = £18.00
  Salmeterol (as Salmeterol xinafoate) 50 microgram per 1 dose, Fluticasone propionate 250 microgram per 1 dose Seretide 250 Accuhaler | 60 dose PoM £35.00 DT price = £35.00
  Salmeterol (as Salmeterol xinafoate) 50 microgram per 1 dose, Fluticasone propionate 500 microgram per 1 dose Seretide 500 Accuhaler | 60 dose PoM £40.92 DT price = £40.92

Pressurised inhalation
CAUTIONARY AND ADVISORY LABELS 8, 10 (excluding Seretide 50 Evohaler®)
▶ Seretide Evohaler (GlaxoSmithKline UK Ltd)
  Salmeterol (as Salmeterol xinafoate) 25 microgram per 1 dose, Fluticasone propionate 50 microgram per 1 dose Seretide 50 Evohaler | 120 dose PoM £18.00 DT price = £18.00
  Salmeterol (as Salmeterol xinafoate) 25 microgram per 1 dose, Fluticasone propionate 125 microgram per 1 dose Seretide 125 Evohaler | 120 dose PoM £35.00 DT price = £35.00
  Salmeterol (as Salmeterol xinafoate) 25 microgram per 1 dose, Fluticasone propionate 250 microgram per 1 dose Seretide 250 Evohaler | 120 dose PoM £59.48 DT price = £59.48

F 153

▌ Mometasone furoate

● **INDICATIONS AND DOSE**

Prophylaxis of asthma
▶ BY INHALATION OF POWDER
▶ Child 12–17 years: Initially 400 micrograms daily in 1–2 divided doses, single dose to be inhaled in the evening, reduced to 200 micrograms once daily, if control maintained

Prophylaxis of severe asthma
▶ BY INHALATION OF POWDER
▶ Child 12–17 years: Increased if necessary up to 400 micrograms twice daily

● **INTERACTIONS** → Appendix 1: corticosteroids

● **SIDE-EFFECTS**
▶ Common or very common Headache
▶ Uncommon Dyspepsia · palpitation · weight gain

● **PATIENT AND CARER ADVICE** Patients or carers should be given advice on how to administer mometasone by inhaler. With high doses, a steroid card should be supplied.
Medicines for Children leaflet: Mometasone furoate inhaler for asthma prevention (prophylaxis) www.medicinesforchildren.org.uk/mometasone-furoate-inhaler-for-asthma-prevention-prophylaxis

● **NATIONAL FUNDING/ACCESS DECISIONS**
Scottish Medicines Consortium (SMC) Decisions
The *Scottish Medicines Consortium* has advised (November 2003) that *Asmanex®* is restricted for use following failure of first-line inhaled corticosteroids.

● **MEDICINAL FORMS**
There can be variation in the licensing of different medicines containing the same drug.

Inhalation powder
CAUTIONARY AND ADVISORY LABELS 8, 10
▶ Asmanex Twisthaler (Merck Sharp & Dohme Ltd)
  Mometasone furoate 200 microgram per 1 dose Asmanex 200micrograms/dose Twisthaler | 30 dose PoM £15.70 DT price = £15.70 | 60 dose PoM £23.54 DT price = £23.54
  Mometasone furoate 400 microgram per 1 dose Asmanex 400micrograms/dose Twisthaler | 30 dose PoM £21.78 DT price = £21.78 | 60 dose PoM £36.05 DT price = £36.05

IMMUNOSUPPRESSANTS › MONOCLONAL ANTIBODIES

▌ Omalizumab

● **INDICATIONS AND DOSE**

Prophylaxis of severe persistent allergic asthma
▶ BY SUBCUTANEOUS INJECTION
▶ Child 6–17 years: Dose according to immunoglobulin E concentration and body-weight (consult product literature)

Add-on therapy for chronic spontaneous urticaria in patients who have had an inadequate response to H₁ antihistamine treatment
▶ BY SUBCUTANEOUS INJECTION
▶ Child 12–17 years: 300 mg every 4 weeks

● **CAUTIONS** Autoimmune disease · susceptibility to helminth infection—discontinue if infection does not respond to anthelmintic

● **INTERACTIONS** → Appendix 1: monoclonal antibodies

● **SIDE-EFFECTS**
▶ Common or very common Abdominal pain · arthralgia · headache · injection-site reactions · pyrexia · sinusitis · upper respiratory tract infection
▶ Uncommon Bronchospasm · cough · diarrhoea · dizziness · drowsiness · dyspepsia · flushing · influenza-like illness · malaise · nausea · paraesthesia · pharyngitis · photosensitivity · postural hypotension · pruritus · rash · syncope · urticaria · weight gain
▶ Rare Angioedema · antibody formation · laryngoedema · parasitic infection
▶ Frequency not known Alopecia · arterial thromboembolic events · Churg-Strauss syndrome · joint swelling · myalgia · serum sickness (including fever and lymphadenopathy) · thrombocytopenia

SIDE-EFFECTS, FURTHER INFORMATION
▶ Churg-Strauss syndrome Churg-Strauss syndrome has occurred rarely in patients given omalizumab; the reaction is usually associated with the reduction of oral corticosteroid therapy. Churg-Strauss syndrome can present as eosinophilia, vasculitic rash, cardiac complications, worsening pulmonary symptoms, or peripheral neuropathy.
▶ Hypersensitivity reactions Hypersensitivity reactions can also occur immediately following treatment with omalizumab or sometimes more than 24 hours after the first injection.

● **PREGNANCY** Manufacturer advises avoid unless essential—crosses the placenta.

● **BREAST FEEDING** Manufacturer advises avoid—present in milk in *animal* studies.

● **HEPATIC IMPAIRMENT** Manufacturer advises caution—no information available.

● **RENAL IMPAIRMENT** Manufacturer advises caution—no information available.

● **NATIONAL FUNDING/ACCESS DECISIONS**

NICE technology appraisals (TAs)

▸ **Omalizumab for severe persistent allergic asthma (April 2013)** NICE TA278

Omalizumab is recommended as an option for treating severe persistent confirmed allergic IgE-mediated asthma as an add-on to optimised standard therapy in patients aged 6 years and over:

● who need continuous or frequent treatment with oral corticosteroids (defined as 4 or more courses in the previous year), **and**

● only if the manufacturer makes omalizumab available with the discount agreed in the patient access scheme.

Optimised standard therapy is defined as a full trial of and, if tolerated, documented compliance with inhaled high-dose corticosteroids, long-acting beta$_2$ agonists, leukotriene receptor antagonists, theophyllines, oral corticosteroids, and smoking cessation if clinically appropriate.

Patients currently receiving omalizumab whose disease does not meet the criteria should be able to continue treatment until they and their clinician consider it appropriate to stop.

www.nice.org.uk/TA278

▸ **Omalizumab for previously treated chronic spontaneous urticaria (June 2015)** NICE TA339

Omalizumab is an option as add-on therapy for the treatment of severe chronic spontaneous urticaria in patients 12 years and over, only if:

● the severity of the condition is assessed objectively, for example, using a weekly urticaria activity score of 28 or more,

● the patient's condition has not responded to standard treatment with H$_1$-antihistamines and leukotriene receptor antagonists,

● omalizumab is stopped at or before the fourth dose if the condition has not responded,

● omalizumab is stopped at the end of a course of treatment (6 doses) if the condition has responded and is restarted only if the condition relapses,

● omalizumab is administered under the management of a secondary care specialist in dermatology, immunology or allergy,

● the manufacturer provides omalizumab with the discount agreed in the patient access scheme.

Patients currently receiving omalizumab whose disease does not meet the above criteria should have the option to continue treatment until they and their clinician consider it appropriate to stop.

www.nice.org.uk/TA339

Scottish Medicines Consortium (SMC) Decisions

The *Scottish Medicines Consortium* has advised (December 2014) that omalizumab (*Xolair*®) is accepted for restricted use within NHS Scotland for the treatment of chronic spontaneous urticaria in patients aged 12 years and over, who have had an inadequate response to combination therapy with H$_1$-antihistamines, leukotriene receptor antagonists and H$_2$-antihistamines, used according to current treatment guidelines.

● **MEDICINAL FORMS**
There can be variation in the licensing of different medicines containing the same drug.

Solution for injection

▸ **Xolair** (Novartis Pharmaceuticals UK Ltd)
Omalizumab 150 mg per 1 ml Xolair 150mg/1ml solution for injection pre-filled syringes | 1 pre-filled disposable injection PoM £256.15
Xolair 75mg/0.5ml solution for injection pre-filled syringes | 1 pre-filled disposable injection PoM £128.07

Leukotriene receptor antagonists

Overview

The leukotriene receptor antagonists, montelukast below and zafirlukast p. 160, block the effects of cysteinyl leukotrienes in the airways; they can be used in children for the management of chronic asthma with an inhaled corticosteroid or as an alternative if an inhaled corticosteroid cannot be used.

Montelukast has not been shown to be more effective than a standard dose of inhaled corticosteroid, but the two drugs appear to have an additive effect. The leukotriene receptor antagonists may be of benefit in exercise- induced asthma and in those with concomitant rhinitis, but they are less effective in children with severe asthma who are also receiving high doses of other drugs.

There is some limited evidence to support the intermittent use of montelukast in children under 12 years with episodic wheeze associated with viral infections [unlicensed use]. Treatment is started at the onset of either asthma symptoms or of coryzal symptoms and continued for 7 days; there is no evidence to support this use in moderate or severe asthma.

▌ Montelukast

● **INDICATIONS AND DOSE**

Prophylaxis of asthma

▸ BY MOUTH

▸ Child 6 months–5 years: 4 mg once daily, dose to be taken in the evening

▸ Child 6–14 years: 5 mg once daily, dose to be taken in the evening

▸ Child 15–17 years: 10 mg once daily, dose to be taken in the evening

Symptomatic relief of seasonal allergic rhinitis in patients with asthma.

▸ BY MOUTH

▸ Child 15–17 years: 10 mg once daily, dose to be taken in the evening

● **INTERACTIONS** → Appendix 1: montelukast

● **SIDE-EFFECTS**

▸ **Common or very common** Abdominal pain · headache · hyperkinesia (in young children) · thirst

▸ **Uncommon** Abnormal dreams · aggressive behaviour · agitation · anxiety · arthralgia · bruising · depression · dizziness · drowsiness · dry mouth · dyspepsia · epistaxis · hostility · hypoaesthesia · irritability · malaise · muscle cramps · myalgia · oedema · paraesthesia · psychomotor hyperactivity · restlessness · seizures · sleep disturbances · sleep-walking

▸ **Rare** Disturbance in attention · increased bleeding tendency · memory impairment · palpitation · tremor

▸ **Very rare** Churg-Strauss syndrome · disorientation · erythema multiforme · erythema nodosum · hallucinations · hepatic disorders · hepatic eosinophilic infiltration · suicidal behaviour · suicidal thoughts

SIDE-EFFECTS, FURTHER INFORMATION
Churg-Strauss syndrome has occurred very rarely in association with the use of montelukast; in many of the reported cases the reaction followed the reduction or withdrawal of oral corticosteroid therapy. Prescribers should be alert to the development of eosinophilia, vasculitic rash, worsening pulmonary symptoms, cardiac complications, or peripheral neuropathy.

● **PREGNANCY** Manufacturer advises avoid unless essential. There is limited evidence for the safe use of montelukast during pregnancy; however, it can be taken as normal in women who have shown a significant improvement in asthma not achievable with other drugs before becoming pregnant.

- **BREAST FEEDING** Manufacturer advises avoid unless essential.
- **DIRECTIONS FOR ADMINISTRATION** Granules may be swallowed or mixed with cold, soft food (not liquid) and taken immediately.
- **PRESCRIBING AND DISPENSING INFORMATION** Flavours of chewable tablet formulations may include cherry.
- **PATIENT AND CARER ADVICE** Patients or carers should be given advice on how to administer montelukast granules. Medicines for Children leaflet: Montelukast for asthma www.medicinesforchildren.org.uk/montelukast-for-asthma
- **NATIONAL FUNDING/ACCESS DECISIONS**

SINGULAIR® GRANULES

Scottish Medicines Consortium (SMC) Decisions
The *Scottish Medicines Consortium* has advised (June 2007) that *Singulair®* granules are restricted for use as an alternative to low-dose inhaled corticosteroids for children 2–14 years with mild persistent asthma who have not recently had serious asthma attacks that required oral corticosteroid use and who are not capable of using inhaled corticosteroids; *Singulair®* granules should be initiated by a specialist in paediatric asthma.

SINGULAIR® CHEWABLE TABLETS

Scottish Medicines Consortium (SMC) Decisions
The *Scottish Medicines Consortium* has advised (June 2007) that *Singulair®* chewable tablets are restricted for use as an alternative to low-dose inhaled corticosteroids for children 2–14 years with mild persistent asthma who have not recently had serious asthma attacks that required oral corticosteroid use and who are not capable of using inhaled corticosteroids; *Singulair®* chewable tablets should be initiated by a specialist in paediatric asthma.

- **MEDICINAL FORMS**
There can be variation in the licensing of different medicines containing the same drug.

Granules
- Montelukast (Non-proprietary)
  Montelukast (as Montelukast sodium) 4 mg Montelukast 4mg granules sachets sugar free sugar-free | 28 sachet [PoM] £4.21–£24.41 DT price = £4.26
- Singulair (Merck Sharp & Dohme Ltd)
  Montelukast (as Montelukast sodium) 4 mg Singulair Paediatric 4mg granules sachets sugar-free | 28 sachet [PoM] £25.69 DT price = £4.26

Tablet
- Montelukast (Non-proprietary)
  Montelukast (as Montelukast sodium) 10 mg Montelukast 10mg tablets | 28 tablet [PoM] £26.97 DT price = £1.61
- Singulair (Merck Sharp & Dohme Ltd)
  Montelukast (as Montelukast sodium) 10 mg Singulair 10mg tablets | 28 tablet [PoM] £26.97 DT price = £1.61

Chewable tablet
CAUTIONARY AND ADVISORY LABELS 23, 24
EXCIPIENTS: May contain Aspartame
- Montelukast (Non-proprietary)
  Montelukast (as Montelukast sodium) 4 mg Montelukast 4mg chewable tablets sugar free sugar-free | 28 tablet [PoM] £25.69 DT price = £1.34
  Montelukast (as Montelukast sodium) 5 mg Montelukast 5mg chewable tablets sugar free sugar-free | 28 tablet [PoM] £25.69 DT price = £1.50
- Singulair (Merck Sharp & Dohme Ltd)
  Montelukast (as Montelukast sodium) 4 mg Singulair Paediatric 4mg chewable tablets sugar-free | 28 tablet [PoM] £25.69 DT price = £1.34
  Montelukast (as Montelukast sodium) 5 mg Singulair Paediatric 5mg chewable tablets sugar-free | 28 tablet [PoM] £25.69 DT price = £1.50

Zafirlukast

- **INDICATIONS AND DOSE**

Prophylaxis of asthma
- BY MOUTH
- Child 12–17 years: 20 mg twice daily

- **SIDE-EFFECTS**
- **Common or very common** Gastro-intestinal disturbances · headache · respiratory infections
- **Uncommon** Insomnia · malaise
- **Rare** Angioedema · arthralgia · bleeding disorders · hepatitis · hyperbilirubinaemia · hypersensitivity reactions · myalgia · skin reactions · thrombocytopenia
- **Very rare** Agranulocytosis · Churg-Strauss syndrome

SIDE-EFFECTS, FURTHER INFORMATION
Churg-Strauss syndrome has occurred very rarely in association with the use of zafirlukast; in many of the reported cases the reaction followed the reduction or withdrawal of oral corticosteroid therapy. Prescribers should be alert to the development of eosinophilia, vasculitic rash, worsening pulmonary symptoms, cardiac complications, or peripheral neuropathy.
- Hepatic disorder Patients or their carers should be told how to recognise development of liver disorder and advised to seek medical attention if symptoms or signs such as persistent nausea, vomiting, malaise, or jaundice develop.
- **PREGNANCY** Manufacturer advises use only if potential benefit outweighs risk. There is limited evidence for the safe use of zafirlukast during pregnancy; however, it can be taken as normal in women who have shown a significant improvement in asthma not achievable with other drugs before becoming pregnant.
- **BREAST FEEDING** Present in milk—manufacturer advises avoid.
- **HEPATIC IMPAIRMENT** Manufacturer advises avoid.
- **RENAL IMPAIRMENT** Manufacturer advises caution.
- **PATIENT AND CARER ADVICE**
Medicines for Children leaflet: Zafirlukast for asthma prevention (prophylaxis) www.medicinesforchildren.org.uk/zafirlukast-for-asthma-prevention

- **MEDICINAL FORMS**
There can be variation in the licensing of different medicines containing the same drug.

Tablet
CAUTIONARY AND ADVISORY LABELS 23
- Accolate (AstraZeneca UK Ltd)
  Zafirlukast 20 mg Accolate 20mg tablets | 56 tablet [PoM] £17.75 DT price = £17.75

MAST-CELL STABILISERS

Cromoglicate and related therapy

Overview

The mode of action of sodium cromoglicate p. 161 and nedocromil sodium p. 161 is not completely understood; they may be of value as *prophylaxis* in asthma with an allergic basis, but the evidence for benefit of sodium cromoglicate in children is contentious. Prophylaxis with sodium cromoglicate or nedocromil sodium is less effective than with inhaled corticosteroids.

Nedocromil sodium may be of some benefit in the prophylaxis of exercise-induced asthma.

Sodium cromoglicate and nedocromil sodium may also have a role in allergic conjunctivitis; sodium cromoglicate is used also in allergic rhinitis and allergy-related diarrhoea.

Nedocromil sodium

- **INDICATIONS AND DOSE**

Prophylaxis of asthma
- BY INHALATION OF AEROSOL
- Child 5–17 years: Initially 4 mg 4 times a day, when control achieved may be possible to reduce to twice daily

DOSE EQUIVALENCE AND CONVERSION
- 2 puffs = 4 mg.

- **UNLICENSED USE** Not licensed for use in children under 6 years.
- **SIDE-EFFECTS**
- **Common or very common** Abdominal pain · dyspepsia · nausea · pharyngitis · vomiting
- **Rare** Taste disturbances
- **Frequency not known** Bronchospasm · cough · headache · paradoxical bronchospasm · throat irritation

SIDE-EFFECTS, FURTHER INFORMATION
- Paradoxical bronchospasm If paradoxical bronchospasm occurs, a short-acting beta₂ agonist such as salbutamol or terbutaline should be used to control symptoms; treatment with nedocromil should be discontinued.
- **PREGNANCY** Inhaled drugs can be taken as normal during pregnancy.
- **BREAST FEEDING** Inhaled drugs can be taken as normal during breast-feeding.
- **TREATMENT CESSATION** Withdrawal should be done gradually over a period of one week—symptoms of asthma may recur.
- **PRESCRIBING AND DISPENSING INFORMATION** Flavours of inhalers may include mint.
- **PATIENT AND CARER ADVICE** Regular use is necessary. Patient counselling is advised for Nedocromil aerosol for inhalation (administration).

- **MEDICINAL FORMS**
There can be variation in the licensing of different medicines containing the same drug.
Pressurised inhalation
CAUTIONARY AND ADVISORY LABELS 8
- Tilade (Sanofi)
Nedocromil sodium 2 mg per 1 dose Tilade 2mg/dose inhaler CFC free | 112 dose [PoM] £39.94

Sodium cromoglicate

(Sodium cromoglycate)

- **INDICATIONS AND DOSE**

Prophylaxis of asthma
- BY INHALATION OF AEROSOL
- Child 5–17 years: Initially 10 mg 4 times a day, additional dose may also be taken before exercise, increased if necessary to 10 mg 6–8 times a day; maintenance 5 mg 4 times a day, 5 mg is equivalent to 1 puff

Food allergy (in conjunction with dietary restriction)
- BY MOUTH
- Child 2–13 years: Initially 100 mg 4 times a day for 2–3 weeks, then increased if necessary up to 40 mg/kg daily, then reduced according to response, to be taken before meals
- Child 14–17 years: Initially 200 mg 4 times a day for 2–3 weeks, then increased if necessary up to 40 mg/kg daily, then reduced according to response, to be taken before meals

- **CAUTIONS**
- When used by inhalation Discontinue if eosinophilic pneumonia occurs
- **SIDE-EFFECTS**
- When used by inhalation Bronchospasm · cough · eosinophilic pneumonia · headache · paradoxical bronchospasm · rhinitis · throat irritation
- With oral use Joint pain · occasional nausea · rashes

SIDE-EFFECTS, FURTHER INFORMATION
- Paradoxical bronchospasm
- When used by inhalation If paradoxical bronchospasm occurs, a short-acting beta₂ agonist such as salbutamol or terbutaline should be used to control symptoms; treatment with sodium cromoglicate should be discontinued.
- **PREGNANCY** Not known to be harmful. Inhaled drugs can be taken as normal during pregnancy.
- **BREAST FEEDING** Unlikely to be present in milk. Inhaled drugs can be taken as normal during breast-feeding.
- **TREATMENT CESSATION**
- When used by inhalation Withdrawal of sodium cromoglicate should be done gradually over a period of one week—symptoms of asthma may recur.
- **DIRECTIONS FOR ADMINISTRATION** Capsules may be swallowed whole or the contents dissolved in hot water and diluted with cold water before taking.
- **PATIENT AND CARER ADVICE**
- With oral use Patient counselling is advised for sodium cromoglicate capsules (administration).
- When used by inhalation Patient counselling is advised for sodium cromoglicate pressurised inhalation (administration).

- **MEDICINAL FORMS**
There can be variation in the licensing of different medicines containing the same drug. Forms available from special-order manufacturers include: oral solution
Capsule
CAUTIONARY AND ADVISORY LABELS 22
- Nalcrom (Sanofi)
Sodium cromoglicate 100 mg Nalcrom 100mg capsules | 100 capsule [PoM] £41.14 DT price = £41.14
Pressurised inhalation
CAUTIONARY AND ADVISORY LABELS 8
- Intal (Sanofi)
Sodium cromoglicate 5 mg per 1 dose Intal 5mg/dose inhaler CFC free | 112 dose [PoM] £18.33

XANTHINES

Aminophylline

- **INDICATIONS AND DOSE**

Severe acute asthma in patients not previously treated with theophylline
- BY SLOW INTRAVENOUS INJECTION
- Child: 5 mg/kg (max. per dose 500 mg), to be followed by intravenous infusion

Severe acute asthma
- BY INTRAVENOUS INFUSION
- Child 1 month–11 years: 1 mg/kg/hour, adjusted according to plasma-theophylline concentration
- Child 12–17 years: 500–700 micrograms/kg/hour, adjusted according to plasma-theophylline concentration

Chronic asthma
- BY MOUTH USING MODIFIED-RELEASE MEDICINES
- Child (body-weight 40 kg and above): Initially 225 mg twice daily for 1 week, then increased if necessary to 450 mg twice daily, adjusted according to plasma-theophylline concentration

continued →

DOSE ADJUSTMENTS DUE TO INTERACTIONS
Dose adjustment may be necessary if smoking started or stopped during treatment.

DOSES AT EXTREMES OF BODY-WEIGHT
To avoid excessive dosage in obese patients, dose should be calculated on the basis of ideal weight for height.

PHARMACOKINETICS
Aminophylline is a stable mixture or combination of theophylline and ethylenediamine; the ethylenediamine confers greater solubility in water.
Theophylline is metabolised in the liver. The plasma-theophylline concentration is increased in heart failure, hepatic impairment, and in viral infections. The plasma-theophylline concentration is decreased in smokers, and by alcohol consumption. Differences in the half-life of aminophylline are important because the toxic dose is close to the therapeutic dose.

- **UNLICENSED USE** Aminophylline injection not licensed for use in children under 6 months.

- **CAUTIONS** Arrhythmias following rapid intravenous injection · cardiac arrhythmias or other cardiac disease · epilepsy · fever · hypertension · hyperthyroidism · peptic ulcer · risk of hypokalaemia

- **INTERACTIONS** → Appendix 1: aminophylline

- **SIDE-EFFECTS** Arrhythmias (especially if given rapidly by intravenous injection) · CNS stimulation · convulsions (especially if given rapidly by intravenous injection) · diarrhoea · gastric irritation · headache · hypotension (especially if given rapidly by intravenous injection) · insomnia · nausea · palpitation · tachycardia · vomiting

SIDE-EFFECTS, FURTHER INFORMATION

- Hypokalaemia Potentially serious hypokalaemia may result from beta$_2$ agonist therapy. Particular caution is required in severe asthma, because this effect may be potentiated by concomitant treatment with theophylline and its derivatives, corticosteroids, and diuretics, and by hypoxia. Plasma-potassium concentration should therefore be monitored in severe asthma.

Overdose
Theophylline and related drugs are often prescribed as modified-release formulations and toxicity can therefore be delayed. They cause vomiting (which may be severe and intractable), agitation, restlessness, dilated pupils, sinus tachycardia, and hyperglycaemia. More serious effects are haematemesis, convulsions, and supraventricular and ventricular arrhythmias. Severe hypokalaemia may develop rapidly.

For specific details on the management of poisoning, see *Theophylline*, under Emergency treatment of poisoning p. 803.

- **ALLERGY AND CROSS-SENSITIVITY** Allergy to ethylenediamine can cause urticaria, erythema, and exfoliative dermatitis.

- **PREGNANCY** Neonatal irritability and apnoea have been reported. Theophylline can be taken as normal during pregnancy as it is particularly important that asthma should be well controlled during pregnancy.

- **BREAST FEEDING** Present in milk—irritability in infant reported; modified-release preparations preferable. Theophylline can be taken as normal during breast-feeding.

- **HEPATIC IMPAIRMENT** Reduce dose.

- **MONITORING REQUIREMENTS**
- Aminophylline is monitored therapeutically in terms of plasma-theophylline concentrations.
- Measurement of plasma-theophylline concentration may be helpful and is **essential** if a loading dose of intravenous aminophylline is to be given to patients who are already taking theophylline, because serious side-effects such as

convulsions and arrhythmias can occasionally precede other symptoms of toxicity.

- In most individuals, a plasma-theophylline concentration of 10–20 mg/litre (55–110 micromol/litre) is required for satisfactory bronchodilation, although a lower plasma-theophylline concentration of 5–15 mg/litre may be effective. Adverse effects can occur within the range 10–20 mg/litre and both the frequency and severity increase at concentrations above 20 mg/litre.

- If aminophylline is given intravenously, a blood sample should be taken 4–6 hours after starting treatment.

- With oral use Plasma-theophylline concentration is measured 5 days after starting oral treatment and at least 3 days after any dose adjustment. A blood sample should usually be taken 4–6 hours after an oral dose of a modified-release preparation (sampling times may vary—consult local guidelines).

- **DIRECTIONS FOR ADMINISTRATION**
- With intravenous use For *intravenous injection*, give **very slowly** over at least 20 minutes (with close monitoring). For *intravenous infusion*, dilute to a concentration of 1 mg/mL with Glucose 5% *or* Sodium Chloride 0.9%.
- With intramuscular use Aminophylline is too irritant for intramuscular use.

- **PRESCRIBING AND DISPENSING INFORMATION** Patients taking oral theophylline or aminophylline should not normally receive a loading dose of intravenous aminophylline.

Consider intravenous aminophylline for treatment of severe and life-threatening acute asthma only after consultation with senior medical staff.
Modified release The rate of absorption from modified-release preparations can vary between brands. If a prescription for a modified-release oral aminophylline preparation does not specify a brand name, the pharmacist should contact the prescriber and agree the brand to be dispensed. Additionally, it is essential that a patient discharged from hospital should be maintained on the brand on which that patient was stabilised as an in-patient.

- **MEDICINAL FORMS**
There can be variation in the licensing of different medicines containing the same drug. Forms available from special-order manufacturers include: solution for infusion

Solution for injection
- **Aminophylline** (Non-proprietary)
  Aminophylline 25 mg per 1 ml Aminophylline 250mg/10ml solution for injection ampoules | 10 ampoule PoM £6.50 DT price = £6.50

Modified-release tablet
CAUTIONARY AND ADVISORY LABELS 25
- **Aminophylline** (Non-proprietary)
  Aminophylline hydrate 225 mg Aminophylline hydrate 225mg modified-release tablets | 56 tablet P no price available DT price = £2.40
- **Phyllocontin Continus** (Napp Pharmaceuticals Ltd)
  Aminophylline hydrate 225 mg Phyllocontin Continus 225mg tablets | 56 tablet P £2.40 DT price = £2.40

Theophylline

- **INDICATIONS AND DOSE**

NUELIN SA® 175MG TABLETS
Chronic asthma
- BY MOUTH USING MODIFIED-RELEASE MEDICINES
- Child 6–11 years: 175 mg every 12 hours
- Child 12–17 years: 175–350 mg every 12 hours

NUELIN SA® 250 TABLETS
Chronic asthma
- BY MOUTH USING MODIFIED-RELEASE MEDICINES
- Child 6–11 years: 125–250 mg every 12 hours
- Child 12–17 years: 250–500 mg every 12 hours

SLO-PHYLLIN®

Chronic asthma

▸ BY MOUTH USING MODIFIED-RELEASE MEDICINES

▸ Child 6 months-1 year: 12 mg/kg every 12 hours (max. per dose 120 mg)

▸ Child 2-5 years: 60–120 mg every 12 hours

▸ Child 6-11 years: 125–250 mg every 12 hours

▸ Child 12-17 years: 250–500 mg every 12 hours

UNIPHYLLIN CONTINUS®

Chronic asthma

▸ BY MOUTH USING MODIFIED-RELEASE MEDICINES

▸ Child 2-11 years: 9 mg/kg every 12 hours (max. per dose 200 mg), dose may be increased in some children with chronic asthma; increased to 10–16 mg/kg every 12 hours (max. per dose 400 mg), may be appropriate to give larger evening or morning dose to achieve optimum therapeutic effect when symptoms most severe; in patients whose night or daytime symptoms persist despite other therapy, who are not currently receiving theophylline, total daily requirement may be added as single evening or morning dose

▸ Child 12-17 years: 200 mg every 12 hours, adjusted according to response to 400 mg every 12 hours, may be appropriate to give larger evening or morning dose to achieve optimum therapeutic effect when symptoms most severe; in patients whose night or daytime symptoms persist despite other therapy, who are not currently receiving theophylline, total daily requirement may be added as single evening or morning dose

DOSE ADJUSTMENTS DUE TO INTERACTIONS
Dose adjustment may be necessary if smoking started or stopped during treatment.

PHARMACOKINETICS
Theophylline is metabolised in the liver. The plasma-theophylline concentration is increased in heart failure, hepatic impairment, and in viral infections. The plasma-theophylline concentration is decreased in smokers, and by alcohol consumption. Differences in the half-life of theophylline are important because the toxic dose is close to the therapeutic dose.

● UNLICENSED USE Slo-phyllin® capsules not licensed for use in children under 2 years.

● CAUTIONS Cardiac arrhythmias or other cardiac disease · epilepsy · fever · hypertension · hyperthyroidism · peptic ulcer · risk of hypokalaemia

● INTERACTIONS → Appendix 1: theophylline

● SIDE-EFFECTS Arrhythmias · CNS stimulation · convulsions · diarrhoea · gastric irritation · headache · insomnia · nausea · palpitation · tachycardia · vomiting
SIDE-EFFECTS, FURTHER INFORMATION

▸ Hypokalaemia Potentially serious hypokalaemia may result from beta₂ agonist therapy. Particular caution is required in severe asthma, because this effect may be potentiated by concomitant treatment with theophylline and its derivatives, corticosteroids, and diuretics, and by hypoxia. Plasma-potassium concentration should therefore be monitored in severe asthma.

Overdose

Theophylline in overdose can cause vomiting (which may be severe and intractable), agitation, restlessness, dilated pupils, sinus tachycardia, and hyperglycaemia. More serious effects are haematemesis, convulsions, and supraventricular and ventricular arrhythmias. Severe hypokalaemia may develop rapidly.

For details on the management of poisoning, see Theophylline, under Emergency treatment of poisoning p. 803.

● PREGNANCY Neonatal irritability and apnoea have been reported. Theophylline can be taken as normal during pregnancy as it is particularly important that asthma should be well controlled during pregnancy.

● BREAST FEEDING Present in milk—irritability in infant reported; modified-release preparations preferable. Theophylline can be taken as normal during breast-feeding.

● HEPATIC IMPAIRMENT Reduce dose.

● MONITORING REQUIREMENTS

▸ In most individuals, a plasma-theophylline concentration of 10–20 mg/litre (55–110 micromol/litre) is required for satisfactory bronchodilation, although a lower plasma-theophylline concentration of 5–15 mg/litre may be effective. Adverse effects can occur within the range 10–20 mg/litre and both the frequency and severity increase at concentrations above 20 mg/litre.

▸ Plasma-theophylline concentration is measured 5 days after starting oral treatment and at least 3 days after any dose adjustment. A blood sample should usually be taken 4–6 hours after an oral dose of a modified-release preparation (sampling times may vary—consult local guidelines).

● DIRECTIONS FOR ADMINISTRATION
SLO-PHYLLIN® Contents of the capsule (enteric-coated granules) may be sprinkled on to a spoonful of soft food (e.g. yoghurt) and swallowed without chewing.

● PRESCRIBING AND DISPENSING INFORMATION The rate of absorption from modified-release preparations can vary between brands. If a prescription for a modified-release oral theophylline preparation does not specify a brand name, the pharmacist should contact the prescriber and agree the brand to be dispensed. Additionally, it is essential that a patient discharged from hospital should be maintained on the brand on which that patient was stabilised as an in-patient.

● PATIENT AND CARER ADVICE
SLO-PHYLLIN® Patient or carer should be given advice on how to administer theophylline modified release capsules.

● MEDICINAL FORMS
There can be variation in the licensing of different medicines containing the same drug.

Modified-release tablet

CAUTIONARY AND ADVISORY LABELS 21, 25

▸ Nuelin SA (Meda Pharmaceuticals Ltd)
Theophylline 175 mg Nuelin SA 175mg tablets | 60 tablet P £6.38 DT price = £6.38
Theophylline 250 mg Nuelin SA 250 tablets | 60 tablet P £8.92 DT price = £8.92

▸ Uniphyllin Continus (Napp Pharmaceuticals Ltd)
Theophylline 200 mg Uniphyllin Continus 200mg tablets | 56 tablet P £2.96 DT price = £2.96
Theophylline 300 mg Uniphyllin Continus 300mg tablets | 56 tablet P £4.77 DT price = £4.77
Theophylline 400 mg Uniphyllin Continus 400mg tablets | 56 tablet P £5.65 DT price = £5.65

Modified-release capsule

CAUTIONARY AND ADVISORY LABELS 25

▸ Theophylline (Non-proprietary)
Theophylline 300 mg Theo-24 300mg modified-release capsules | 100 capsule no price available

▸ Slo-Phyllin (Merck Serono Ltd)
Theophylline 60 mg Slo-Phyllin 60mg capsules | 56 capsule P £2.76 DT price = £2.76
Theophylline 125 mg Slo-Phyllin 125mg capsules | 56 capsule P £3.48 DT price = £3.48
Theophylline 250 mg Slo-Phyllin 250mg capsules | 56 capsule P £4.34 DT price = £4.34

Nebuliser solutions

- **HYPERTONIC SODIUM CHLORIDE SOLUTIONS**

- **INDICATIONS AND DOSE**

MUCOCLEAR® 3%

Mobilise lower respiratory tract secretions in mucous consolidation (e.g. cystic fibrosis) | Mild to moderate acute viral bronchiolitis in infants

▸ BY INHALATION OF NEBULISED SOLUTION

▸ Child: 4 mL 2–4 times a day, temporary irritation, such as coughing, hoarseness, or reversible bronchoconstriction may occur; an inhaled bronchodilator can be used before treatment with hypertonic sodium chloride to reduce the risk of these adverse effects

MucoClear 3% inhalation solution 4ml ampoules (Pari Medical Ltd) **Sodium chloride 30 mg per 1 ml** | 20 ampoule · NHS indicative price = £12.98 · Drug Tariff (Part IXa) | 60 ampoule · NHS indicative price = £27.00 · Drug Tariff (Part IXa)

- **INDICATIONS AND DOSE**

MUCOCLEAR® 6%

Mobilise lower respiratory tract secretions in mucous consolidation (e.g. cystic fibrosis)

▸ BY INHALATION OF NEBULISED SOLUTION

▸ Child: 4 mL twice daily, temporary irritation, such as coughing, hoarseness, or reversible bronchoconstriction may occur; an inhaled bronchodilator can be used before treatment with hypertonic sodium chloride to reduce the risk of these adverse effects

MucoClear 6% inhalation solution 4ml ampoules (Pari Medical Ltd) **Sodium chloride 60 mg per 1 ml** | 20 ampoule · NHS indicative price = £12.98 · Drug Tariff (Part IXa) | 60 ampoule · NHS indicative price = £27.00 · Drug Tariff (Part IXa)

- **INDICATIONS AND DOSE**

NEBUSAL®

Mobilise lower respiratory tract secretions in mucous consolidation (e.g. cystic fibrosis)

▸ BY INHALATION OF NEBULISED SOLUTION

▸ Child: 4 mL up to twice daily, temporary irritation, such as coughing, hoarseness, or reversible bronchoconstriction may occur; an inhaled bronchodilator can be used before treatment with hypertonic sodium chloride to reduce the risk of these adverse effects

Nebusal 7% inhalation solution 4ml vials (Forest Laboratories UK Ltd) **Sodium chloride 70 mg per 1 ml** | 60 vial · NHS indicative price = £27.00 · Drug Tariff (Part IXa)

Peak flow meters

- **LOW RANGE PEAK FLOW METERS**

MEDI® LOW RANGE

Range 40–420 litres/minute.

Compliant to standard EN ISO 23747:2007 except for scale range.

Medi peak flow meter low range (Medicareplus International Ltd) | 1 device · NHS indicative price = £6.50 · Drug Tariff (Part IXa) price = £6.50

MINI-WRIGHT® LOW RANGE

Range 30–400 litres/minute.

Compliant to standard EN ISO 23747:2007 except for scale range.

Mini-Wright peak flow meter low range (Clement Clarke International Ltd) | 1 device · NHS indicative price = £7.14 · Drug Tariff (Part IXa) price = £6.50

POCKETPEAK® LOW RANGE

Range 50–400 litres/minute.

Compliant to standard EN ISO 23747:2007 except for scale range.

nSpire Pocket Peak peak flow meter low range (nSpire Health Ltd) | 1 device · NHS indicative price = £6.53 · Drug Tariff (Part IXa) price = £6.50

- **STANDARD RANGE PEAK FLOW METERS**

AIRZONE®

Range 60–720 litres/minute.

Conforms to standard EN ISO 23747:2007.

AirZone peak flow meter standard range (Clement Clarke International Ltd) | 1 device · NHS indicative price = £4.69 · Drug Tariff (Part IXa) price = £4.50

MEDI® STANDARD RANGE

Range 60–800 litres/minute.

Conforms to standard EN ISO 23747:2007.

Medi peak flow meter standard range (Medicareplus International Ltd) | 1 device · NHS indicative price = £4.50 · Drug Tariff (Part IXa) price = £4.50

MICROPEAK®

Range 60–900 litres/minute.

Conforms to standard EN ISO 23747:2007.

MicroPeak peak flow meter standard range (Micro Medical Ltd) | 1 device · NHS indicative price = £6.50 · Drug Tariff (Part IXa) price = £4.50

MINI-WRIGHT® STANDARD RANGE

Range 60–800 litres/minute.

Conforms to standard EN ISO 23747:2007.

Mini-Wright peak flow meter standard range (Clement Clarke International Ltd) | 1 device · NHS indicative price = £7.08 · Drug Tariff (Part IXa) price = £4.50

PIKO-1®

Range 15–999 litres/minute.

Conforms to standard EN ISO 23747:2007.

nSpire PiKo-1 peak flow meter standard range (nSpire Health Ltd) | 1 device · NHS indicative price = £9.50 · Drug Tariff (Part IXa) price = £4.50

PINNACLE®

Range 60–900 litres/minute.

Conforms to standard EN ISO 23747:2007.

Fyne Dynamics Pinnacle peak flow meter standard range (Fyne Dynamics Ltd) | 1 device · NHS indicative price = £6.50 · Drug Tariff (Part IXa) price = £4.50

POCKETPEAK® STANDARD RANGE

Range 60–800 litres/minute.

Conforms to standard EN ISO 23747:2007.

nSpire Pocket Peak peak flow meter standard range (nSpire Health Ltd) | 1 device · NHS indicative price = £6.53 · Drug Tariff (Part IXa) price = £4.50

VITALOGRAPH®

Range 50–800 litres/minute.

Conforms to standard EN ISO 23747:2007.

Vitalograph peak flow meter standard range (Vitalograph Ltd) | 1 device · NHS indicative price = £4.33 · Drug Tariff (Part IXa) price = £4.50

Spacers

- **SPACERS**

A2A SPACER®

For use with all pressurised (aerosol) inhalers.

A2A Spacer (Clement Clarke International Ltd) | 1 device · NHS indicative price = £4.15 · Drug Tariff (Part IXa)

A2A Spacer with medium mask (Clement Clarke International Ltd) | 1 device · NHS indicative price = £5.68 · Drug Tariff (Part IXa)

A2A Spacer with small mask (Clement Clarke International Ltd) | 1 device · NHS indicative price = £6.68 · Drug Tariff (Part IXa)

ABLE SPACER®

Small-volume device. For use with all pressurised (aerosol) inhalers.

Able Spacer (Clement Clarke International Ltd) | 1 device · NHS indicative price = £4.39 · Drug Tariff (Part IXa)

Able Spacer with medium mask (Clement Clarke International Ltd) | 1 device · NHS indicative price = £7.16 · Drug Tariff (Part IXa)

Able Spacer with small mask (Clement Clarke International Ltd) | 1 device · NHS indicative price = £7.16 · Drug Tariff (Part IXa)

AEROCHAMBER PLUS®

Medium-volume device. For use with all pressurised (aerosol) inhalers.

AeroChamber Plus (GlaxoSmithKline UK Ltd) | 1 device · NHS indicative price = £4.86 · Drug Tariff (Part IXa)

AeroChamber Plus with adult mask (GlaxoSmithKline UK Ltd) | 1 device · NHS indicative price = £8.11 · Drug Tariff (Part IXa)

AeroChamber Plus with child mask (GlaxoSmithKline UK Ltd) | 1 device · NHS indicative price = £8.11 · Drug Tariff (Part IXa)

AeroChamber Plus with infant mask (GlaxoSmithKline UK Ltd) | 1 device · NHS indicative price = £8.11 · Drug Tariff (Part IXa)

BABYHALER®

For paediatric use with *Flixotide*®, and *Ventolin*® inhalers.

● **PRESCRIBING AND DISPENSING INFORMATION**
Not available for NHS prescription.

Babyhaler (Allen & Hanburys Ltd) | 1 device · No NHS indicative price available · Drug Tariff (Part IXa)

HALERAID®

Device to place over pressurised (aerosol) inhalers to aid when strength in hands is impaired (e.g. in arthritis). For use with *Flixotide*®, *Seretide*®, *Serevent*®, and *Ventolin*® inhalers.

● **PRESCRIBING AND DISPENSING INFORMATION**
Not available for NHS prescription.

Haleraid-120 (Allen & Hanburys Ltd) | 1 device · No NHS indicative price available · Drug Tariff (Part IXa)

Haleraid-200 (Allen & Hanburys Ltd) | 1 device · No NHS indicative price available · Drug Tariff (Part IXa)

OPTICHAMBER®

For use with all pressurised (aerosol) inhalers.

OptiChamber (Respironics (UK) Ltd) | 1 device · NHS indicative price = £4.28 · Drug Tariff (Part IXa)

OPTICHAMBER® DIAMOND

For use with all pressurised (aerosol) inhalers.

OptiChamber Diamond (Respironics (UK) Ltd) | 1 device · NHS indicative price = £4.49 · Drug Tariff (Part IXa)

OptiChamber Diamond with large LiteTouch mask 5 years-adult (Respironics (UK) Ltd) | 1 device · NHS indicative price = £7.49 · Drug Tariff (Part IXa)

OptiChamber Diamond with medium LiteTouch mask 1-5 years (Respironics (UK) Ltd) | 1 device · NHS indicative price = £7.49 · Drug Tariff (Part IXa)

OptiChamber Diamond with small LiteTouch mask 0-18 months (Respironics (UK) Ltd) | 1 device · NHS indicative price = £7.49 · Drug Tariff (Part IXa)

POCKET CHAMBER®

Small volume device. For use with all pressurised (aerosol) inhalers.

Pocket Chamber (nSpire Health Ltd) | 1 device · NHS indicative price = £4.18 · Drug Tariff (Part IXa)

Pocket Chamber with adult mask (nSpire Health Ltd) | 1 device · NHS indicative price = £9.75 · Drug Tariff (Part IXa)

Pocket Chamber with child mask (nSpire Health Ltd) | 1 device · NHS indicative price = £9.75 · Drug Tariff (Part IXa)

Pocket Chamber with infant mask (nSpire Health Ltd) | 1 device · NHS indicative price = £9.75 · Drug Tariff (Part IXa)

Pocket Chamber with teenager mask (nSpire Health Ltd) | 1 device · NHS indicative price = £9.75 · Drug Tariff (Part IXa)

SPACE CHAMBER PLUS®

For use with all pressurised (aerosol) inhalers.

Space Chamber Plus (Medical Developments International Ltd) | 1 device · NHS indicative price = £4.26 · Drug Tariff (Part IXa)

Space Chamber Plus with large mask (Medical Developments International Ltd) | 1 device · NHS indicative price = £6.98 · Drug Tariff (Part IXa)

Space Chamber Plus with medium mask (Medical Developments International Ltd) | 1 device · NHS indicative price = £6.98 · Drug Tariff (Part IXa)

Space Chamber Plus with small mask (Medical Developments International Ltd) | 1 device · NHS indicative price = £6.98 · Drug Tariff (Part IXa)

VOLUMATIC®

Large-volume device. For use with *Clenil Modulite*®, *Flixotide*®, *Seretide*®, *Serevent*®, and *Ventolin*® inhalers.

Volumatic (GlaxoSmithKline UK Ltd) | 1 device · NHS indicative price = £3.85 · Drug Tariff (Part IXa)

Volumatic with paediatric mask (GlaxoSmithKline UK Ltd) | 1 device · NHS indicative price = £6.77 · Drug Tariff (Part IXa)

VORTEX®

Medium-volume device. For use with all pressurised (aerosol) inhalers.

Vortex Spacer (Pari Medical Ltd) | 1 device · NHS indicative price = £6.28 · Drug Tariff (Part IXa)

Vortex with child mask 0-2 years (Pari Medical Ltd) | 1 device · NHS indicative price = £7.99 · Drug Tariff (Part IXa)

Vortex with child mask 2 years+ (Pari Medical Ltd) | 1 device · NHS indicative price = £7.99 · Drug Tariff (Part IXa)

2   Allergic conditions

Antihistamines, allergen immunotherapy and allergic emergencies

Antihistamines

Antihistamines (histamine H_1-receptor antagonists) are classified as *sedating* or *non-sedating*, according to their relative potential for CNS depression. Antihistamines differ in their duration of action, incidence of drowsiness, and antimuscarinic effects; the response to an antihistamine may vary from child to child. Either a sedating or a non-sedating antihistamine may be used to treat an acute allergic reaction; for conditions with more persistent symptoms which require regular treatment, a non-sedating antihistamine should be used to minimise the risk of sedation and psychomotor impairment associated with sedating antihistamines.

Oral antihistamines are used in the treatment of nasal allergies, particularly seasonal allergic rhinitis (hay fever), and may be of some value in vasomotor rhinitis; rhinorrhoea and sneezing is reduced, but antihistamines are usually less effective for nasal congestion. Antihistamines are used topically to treat allergic reactions in the eye and in the nose. Topical application of antihistamines to the skin is not recommended.

An oral antihistamine may be used to prevent urticaria, and for the treatment of acute urticarial rashes, pruritus, insect bites, and stings. Antihistamines are also used in the management of nausea and vomiting, of migraine, and the adjunctive management of anaphylaxis and angioedema.

The *non-sedating* antihistamine cetirizine hydrochloride p. 168 is safe and effective in children. Other non-sedating antihistamines that are used include acrivastine p. 167, bilastine p. 167, desloratadine p. 168 (an active metabolite of loratadine p. 170), fexofenadine hydrochloride p. 169 (an active metabolite of terfenadine), levocetirizine hydrochloride p. 169 (an isomer of cetirizine hydrochloride), loratadine, and mizolastine p. 170. Most non-sedating antihistamines are long-acting (usually 12–24 hours). There is little evidence that desloratadine or levocetirizine hydrochloride confer any additional benefit—they should be reserved for children who cannot tolerate other therapies.

Sedating antihistamines are occasionally useful when insomnia is associated with urticaria and pruritus. Most of the sedating antihistamines are relatively short-acting, but promethazine may be effective for up to 12 hours. Alimemazine tartrate p. 171 and **promethazine** have a more sedative effect than chlorphenamine maleate p. 172 and cyclizine p. 250. Chlorphenamine maleate is used as an adjunct to adrenaline/epinephrine p. 132 in the emergency treatment of anaphylaxis and angioedema.

Allergen immunotherapy

Immunotherapy using allergen vaccines containing house dust mite, animal dander (cat or dog), or extracts of grass and tree pollen can improve symptoms of asthma and allergic rhinoconjunctivitis in children. A vaccine containing extracts of wasp and bee venom is used to reduce the risk of severe anaphylaxis and systemic reactions in children with hypersensitivity to wasp and bee stings. An oral preparation of grass pollen extract (*Grazax*®) is also licensed for disease-modifying treatment of grass pollen-induced rhinitis and conjunctivitis. Children requiring immunotherapy must be referred to a hospital specialist for accurate diagnosis, assessment, and treatment.

Omalizumab p. 158 is a monoclonal antibody that binds to immunoglobulin E (IgE). It is licensed for use as additional therapy in children over 6 years with proven IgE-mediated sensitivity to inhaled allergens, whose severe persistent allergic asthma cannot be controlled adequately with high-dose inhaled corticosteroid together with a long-acting beta$_2$ agonist. Omalizumab should be initiated by physicians experienced in the treatment of severe persistent asthma. Omalizumab is also indicated as add-on therapy for the treatment of chronic spontaneous urticaria in patients who have had an inadequate response to H$_1$ antihistamine treatment.

Allergic emergencies

Anaphylaxis

Anaphylaxis is a severe, life-threatening, generalised or systemic hypersensitivity reaction. It is characterised by the rapid onset of respiratory and/or circulatory problems and is usually associated with skin and mucosal changes; prompt treatment is required. Children with pre-existing asthma, especially poorly controlled asthma, are at particular risk of life-threatening reactions. Insect stings are a recognised risk (in particular wasp and bee stings). Latex and certain foods, including eggs, fish, cow's milk protein, peanuts, sesame, shellfish, soy, and tree nuts may also precipitate anaphylaxis (see Food allergy p. 59). Medicinal products particularly associated with anaphylaxis include blood products, vaccines, allergen immunotherapy preparations, antibacterials, aspirin p. 89 and other NSAIDs, and neuromuscular blocking drugs. In the case of drugs, anaphylaxis is more likely after parenteral administration; resuscitation facilities must always be available for injections associated with special risk. Refined arachis (peanut) oil, which may be present in some medicinal products, is unlikely to cause an allergic reaction—nevertheless it is wise to check the full formula of preparations which may contain allergens.

Treatment of anaphylaxis

Adrenaline/epinephrine provides physiological reversal of the immediate symptoms associated with hypersensitivity reactions such as *anaphylaxis* and *angioedema*.

First-line treatment includes:

- securing the airway, restoration of blood pressure (laying the child flat and raising the legs, or in the recovery position if unconscious or nauseous and at risk of vomiting);

- administering adrenaline/epinephrine by **intramuscular** injection; the dose should be repeated if necessary at 5-minute intervals according to blood pressure, pulse, and respiratory function;
- administering high-flow **oxygen** and **intravenous fluids**;
- administering an antihistamine, such as chlorphenamine maleate, by slow intravenous injection or intramuscular injection as adjunctive treatment given after adrenaline.
- Administering an intravenous corticosteroid such as hydrocortisone p. 420 (preferably as sodium succinate) is of secondary value in the initial management of anaphylaxis because the onset of action is delayed for several hours, but should be given to prevent further deterioration in severely affected children.

Continuing respiratory deterioration requires further treatment with **bronchodilators** including inhaled or intravenous salbutamol p. 150, inhaled ipratropium bromide p. 147, intravenous aminophylline p. 161, or intravenous magnesium sulfate p. 571 [unlicensed indication] (as for acute severe asthma); in addition to oxygen, assisted respiration and possibly emergency tracheotomy may be necessary.

When a child is so ill that there is doubt about the adequacy of the circulation, the initial injection of adrenaline/epinephrine may need to be given as a *dilute solution by the intravenous route*, or by the *intraosseous route* if venous access is difficult; for details see adrenaline/epinephrine.

On discharge, the child should be considered for further treatment with an oral antihistamine and an oral corticosteroid for up to 3 days to reduce the risk of further reaction. The child, or carer, should be instructed to return to hospital if symptoms recur and to contact their general practitioner for follow-up.

Children who are suspected of having had an anaphylactic reaction should be referred to a specialist for specific allergy diagnosis. Avoidance of the allergen is the principal treatment; if appropriate, an adrenaline/epinephrine auto-injector should be given for self-administration or a replacement supplied.

Intramuscular adrenaline (epinephrine)

The *intramuscular route is the first choice route* for the administration of adrenaline/epinephrine p. 132 in the management of anaphylaxis. Adrenaline/epinephrine is best given as an intramuscular injection into the anterolateral aspect of the middle third of the thigh; it has a rapid onset of action after intramuscular administration and in the shocked patient its absorption from the intramuscular site is faster and more reliable than from the subcutaneous site.

Children with severe allergy, and their carers, should ideally be instructed in the self-administration of adrenaline/epinephrine by intramuscular injection.

Prompt injection of adrenaline/epinephrine is of paramount importance. The adrenaline/epinephrine doses recommended for the emergency treatment of anaphylaxis by appropriately trained healthcare professionals are based on the revised recommendations of the Working Group of the Resuscitation Council (UK).

Respiratory system

3

Dose of intramuscular injection of adrenaline (epinephrine) for the emergency treatment of anaphylaxis by healthcare professionals

Age	Dose	Volume of adrenaline
▶ Child 1 month–5 years	150 micrograms	0.15 mL 1 in 1000 (1 mg/mL) adrenaline[1]
▶ Child 6–11 years	300 micrograms	0.3 mL 1 in 1000 (1 mg/mL) adrenaline
▶ Child 12–17 years	500 micrograms	0.5 mL 1 in 1000 (1 mg/mL) adrenaline[2]

These doses may be repeated several times if necessary at 5-minute intervals according to blood pressure, pulse and respiratory function.

1. Use suitable syringe for measuring small volume
2. 300 micrograms (0.3 mL) if child is small or prepubertal

Intravenous adrenaline (epinephrine)
Intravenous adrenaline/epinephrine should be given only by those experienced in its use, in a setting where patients can be carefully monitored.

Where the child is severely ill and there is real doubt about adequacy of the circulation and absorption from the intramuscular injection site, adrenaline/epinephrine may be given by **slow** *intravenous injection*, repeated according to response; if multiple doses are required consider giving adrenaline by slow intravenous infusion.

It is also important that, where intramuscular injection might still succeed, time should not be wasted seeking intravenous access.

Adrenaline/epinephrine is also given by the intravenous route for *acute hypotension*.

Angioedema
Angioedema is dangerous if *laryngeal oedema* is present. In this circumstance adrenaline/epinephrine injection, oxygen, antihistamines and corticosteroids should be given as described under **Anaphylaxis**. Tracheal intubation may be necessary. In some children with laryngeal oedema, adrenaline 1 in 1000 (1 mg/mL) solution may be given by nebuliser. However, nebulised adrenaline/epinephrine cannot be relied upon for a systemic effect—intramuscular adrenaline/epinephrine should be used.

Hereditary angioedema
The treatment of hereditary angioedema should be under specialist supervision. Unlike allergic angioedema, adrenaline/epinephrine, corticosteroids, and antihistamines should not be used for the treatment of acute attacks, including attacks involving laryngeal oedema, as they are ineffective and may delay appropriate treatment—intubation may be necessary p. 177. The administration of C1-esterase inhibitor p. 177 (in fresh frozen plasma or in partially purified form) can terminate acute attacks of *hereditary angioedema*; it can also be used for short-term prophylaxis before dental, medical, or surgical procedures. Tranexamic acid p. 80 is used for short-term or long-term prophylaxis of hereditary angioedema; short-term prophylaxis is started several days before planned procedures which may trigger an acute attack of hereditary angioedema (e.g. dental work) and continued for 2–5 days afterwards. Danazol [unlicensed indication] is best avoided in children because of its androgenic effects, but it can be used for short-term prophylaxis of hereditary angioedema.

ANTIHISTAMINES ⟩ NON-SEDATING

❘ Acrivastine
19-May-2017

● **INDICATIONS AND DOSE**
Symptomatic relief of allergy such as hayfever, chronic idiopathic urticaria
▶ BY MOUTH
▶ Child 12–17 years: 8 mg 3 times a day

● **CONTRA-INDICATIONS** Avoid in acute porphyrias p. 577 (some antihistamines are thought to be safe)

● **INTERACTIONS** → Appendix 1: antihistamines (non-sedating)

● **SIDE-EFFECTS**
▶ **Uncommon** Antimuscarinic effects · gastro-intestinal disturbances · headache · psychomotor impairment
▶ **Rare** Anaphylaxis · angioedema · arrhythmias · blood disorders · bronchospasm · confusion · convulsions · depression · dizziness · extrapyramidal effects · hypersensitivity reactions · hypotension · liver dysfunction · palpitation · photosensitivity reactions · rashes · sleep disturbances · tremor
▶ **Frequency not known** Blurred vision · drowsiness · dry mouth · urinary retention
SIDE-EFFECTS, FURTHER INFORMATION
Non-sedating antihistamines such as acrivastine cause less sedation and psychomotor impairment than the older antihistamines because they penetrate the blood brain barrier only to a slight extent.

If drowsiness occurs, it may diminish after a few days of treatment.

Children are more susceptible to side-effects.

● **ALLERGY AND CROSS-SENSITIVITY** Contra-indicated if history of hypersensitivity to triprolidine.

● **PREGNANCY** Most manufacturers of antihistamines advise avoiding their use during pregnancy; however, there is no evidence of teratogenicity.

● **BREAST FEEDING** Most antihistamines are present in breast milk in varying amounts; although not known to be harmful, most manufacturers advise avoiding their use in mothers who are breast-feeding.

● **RENAL IMPAIRMENT** Avoid in severe impairment.

● **PATIENT AND CARER ADVICE**
Driving and skilled tasks
Although drowsiness is rare, nevertheless children and their carers should be advised that it can occur and may affect performance of skilled tasks (e.g. cycling or driving); alcohol should be avoided.

● **MEDICINAL FORMS**
There can be variation in the licensing of different medicines containing the same drug.
Capsule
▶ **Benadryl Allergy Relief** (McNeil Products Ltd)
Acrivastine 8 mg Benadryl Allergy Relief 8mg capsules |
24 capsule Ⓟ £4.95

❘ Bilastine
22-May-2017

● **INDICATIONS AND DOSE**
Symptomatic relief of allergic rhinoconjunctivitis and urticaria
▶ BY MOUTH
▶ Child 12–17 years: 20 mg once daily

● **CONTRA-INDICATIONS** Avoid in acute porphyrias p. 577 (some antihistamines are thought to be safe)

● **INTERACTIONS** → Appendix 1: antihistamines (non-sedating)

- SIDE-EFFECTS
  - ▶ **Common or very common** Headache · malaise
  - ▶ **Uncommon** Abdominal pain · anxiety · diarrhoea · dizziness · dyspnoea · gastritis · increased appetite · insomnia · oral herpes · prolongation of the QT interval · pyrexia · thirst · tinnitus · vertigo · weight gain

  SIDE-EFFECTS, FURTHER INFORMATION
  Children are more susceptible to side-effects.

  Non-sedating antihistamines such as bilastine cause less sedation and psychomotor impairment than the older antihistamines because they penetrate the blood brain barrier only to a slight extent.
- PREGNANCY Avoid—limited information available. Most manufacturers of antihistamines advise avoiding their use during pregnancy; however, there is no evidence of teratogenicity.
- BREAST FEEDING Avoid—no information available. Most antihistamines are present in breast milk in varying amounts; although not known to be harmful, most manufacturers advise avoiding their use in mothers who are breast-feeding.
- DIRECTIONS FOR ADMINISTRATION Take tablet 1 hour before or 2 hours after food or fruit juice.
- PATIENT AND CARER ADVICE
  Patients or carers should be given advice on how to administer bilastine tablets.

  Driving and skilled tasks
  Although drowsiness is rare, nevertheless patients should be advised that it can occur and may affect performance of skilled tasks (e.g. cycling or driving); alcohol should be avoided.

- MEDICINAL FORMS
  There can be variation in the licensing of different medicines containing the same drug.
  Tablet
  CAUTIONARY AND ADVISORY LABELS 23
  ▶ Ilaxten (A. Menarini Farmaceutica Internazionale SRL)
  Bilastine 20 mg Ilaxten 20mg tablets | 30 tablet PoM £15.09

Cetirizine hydrochloride

- **INDICATIONS AND DOSE**

  Symptomatic relief of allergy such as hay fever, chronic idiopathic urticaria, atopic dermatitis
  - ▶ BY MOUTH
  - ▶ Child 1 year: 250 micrograms/kg twice daily
  - ▶ Child 2–5 years: 2.5 mg twice daily
  - ▶ Child 6–11 years: 5 mg twice daily
  - ▶ Child 12–17 years: 10 mg once daily

- UNLICENSED USE Not licensed for use in children under 2 years.
- CONTRA-INDICATIONS Avoid in acute porphyrias p. 577 (some antihistamines are thought to be safe)
- CAUTIONS Epilepsy
- INTERACTIONS → Appendix 1: antihistamines (non-sedating)
- SIDE-EFFECTS
  - ▶ **Uncommon** Antimuscarinic effects · blurred vision · dry mouth · gastro-intestinal disturbances · headache · psychomotor impairment · urinary retention
  - ▶ **Rare** Anaphylaxis · angioedema · arrhythmias · blood disorders · bronchospasm · confusion · convulsions · depression · dizziness · extrapyramidal effects · hypersensitivity reactions · hypotension · liver dysfunction · palpitation · photosensitivity reactions · rashes · sleep disturbances · tremor
  - ▶ **Frequency not known** Drowsiness

SIDE-EFFECTS, FURTHER INFORMATION
Non-sedating antihistamines such as cetirizine cause less sedation and psychomotor impairment than the older antihistamines because they penetrate the blood brain barrier only to a slight extent.

If drowsiness occurs, it may diminish after a few days of treatment.

Children are more susceptible to side-effects.

- PREGNANCY Most manufacturers of antihistamines advise avoiding their use during pregnancy; however, there is no evidence of teratogenicity.
- BREAST FEEDING Most antihistamines are present in breast milk in varying amounts; although not known to be harmful, most manufacturers advise avoiding their use in mothers who are breast-feeding.
- RENAL IMPAIRMENT Use half normal dose if estimated glomerular filtration rate 30–50 mL/minute/1.73 m². Use half normal dose and reduce dose frequency to alternate days if estimated glomerular filtration rate 10–30 mL/minute/1.73 m². Avoid if estimated glomerular filtration rate less than 10 mL/minute/1.73 m².
- PATIENT AND CARER ADVICE
  Medicines for Children leaflet: Cetirizine hydrochloride for hay fever www.medicinesforchildren.org.uk/cetirizine-hay-fever-0
  Driving and skilled tasks
  Although drowsiness is rare, nevertheless patients should be advised that it can occur and may affect performance of skilled tasks (e.g. cycling or driving); alcohol should be avoided.
- PROFESSION SPECIFIC INFORMATION
  Dental practitioners' formulary
  Cetirizine Tablets 10 mg may be prescribed.
  Cetirizine Oral Solution 5 mg/5 mL may be prescribed.
- MEDICINAL FORMS
  There can be variation in the licensing of different medicines containing the same drug.
  Oral solution
  EXCIPIENTS: May contain Propylene glycol
  ▶ Cetirizine hydrochloride (Non-proprietary)
  Cetirizine hydrochloride 1 mg per 1 ml Cetirizine 1mg/ml oral solution sugar free sugar-free | 200 ml PoM £1.55 DT price = £1.55
  Tablet
  ▶ Cetirizine hydrochloride (Non-proprietary)
  Cetirizine hydrochloride 10 mg Cetirizine 10mg tablets | 30 tablet PoM £0.83 DT price = £0.76
  Capsule
  ▶ Benadryl Allergy (McNeil Products Ltd)
  Cetirizine hydrochloride 10 mg Benadryl Allergy Liquid Release 10mg capsules | 7 capsule GSL £2.91 DT price = £2.91

Desloratadine
23-May-2017

- **INDICATIONS AND DOSE**

  Symptomatic relief of allergy such as allergic rhinitis, urticaria, chronic idiopathic urticaria
  - ▶ BY MOUTH
  - ▶ Child 1–5 years: 1.25 mg once daily
  - ▶ Child 6–11 years: 2.5 mg once daily
  - ▶ Child 12–17 years: 5 mg once daily

  PHARMACOKINETICS
  Desloratadine is a metabolite of loratadine.

- CAUTIONS Acute porphyrias p. 577
- INTERACTIONS → Appendix 1: antihistamines (non-sedating)
- SIDE-EFFECTS
  - ▶ **Uncommon** Antimuscarinic effects · blurred vision · dry mouth · gastro-intestinal disturbances · headache · psychomotor impairment · urinary retention

▸ **Rare** Anaphylaxis · angioedema · arrhythmias · blood disorders · bronchospasm · confusion · convulsions · depression · dizziness · extrapyramidal effects · hypersensitivity reactions · hypotension · liver dysfunction · myalgia · palpitation · photosensitivity reactions · rashes · sleep disturbances · tremor
▸ **Very rare** Hallucinations
▸ **Frequency not known** Drowsiness

SIDE-EFFECTS, FURTHER INFORMATION

Non-sedating antihistamines such as desloratadine cause less sedation and psychomotor impairment than the older antihistamines because they penetrate the blood brain barrier only to a slight extent. If drowsiness occurs, it may diminish after a few days of treatment.

Children are more susceptible to side-effects.

● **ALLERGY AND CROSS-SENSITIVITY** Contra-indicated if history of hypersensitivity to loratadine.

● **PREGNANCY** Most manufacturers of antihistamines advise avoiding their use during pregnancy; however, there is no evidence of teratogenicity.

● **BREAST FEEDING** Most antihistamines are present in breast milk in varying amounts; although not known to be harmful, most manufacturers advise avoiding their use in mothers who are breast-feeding.

● **RENAL IMPAIRMENT** Use with caution in severe impairment.

● **PRESCRIBING AND DISPENSING INFORMATION** Flavours of oral liquid formulations may include bubblegum.

● **PATIENT AND CARER ADVICE**

Driving and skilled tasks

Although drowsiness is rare, nevertheless patients should be advised that it can occur and may affect performance of skilled tasks (e.g. cycling or driving); excess alcohol should be avoided.

● **MEDICINAL FORMS**

There can be variation in the licensing of different medicines containing the same drug.

Oral solution

EXCIPIENTS: May contain Propylene glycol, sorbitol

▸ **Desloratadine** (Non-proprietary)
Desloratadine 500 microgram per 1 ml Desloratadine 2.5mg/5ml oral solution sugar free sugar-free | 100 ml PoM £6.77 sugar-free | 150 ml £6.40–£10.15 DT price = £10.15

▸ **Neoclarityn** (Merck Sharp & Dohme Ltd)
Desloratadine 500 microgram per 1 ml Neoclarityn 2.5mg/5ml oral solution sugar-free | 100 ml PoM £6.77 sugar-free | 150 ml £10.15 DT price = £10.15

Tablet

▸ **Desloratadine** (Non-proprietary)
Desloratadine 5 mg Desloratadine 5mg tablets | 30 tablet PoM £6.77 DT price = £0.95

▸ **Neoclarityn** (Merck Sharp & Dohme Ltd)
Desloratadine 5 mg Neoclarityn 5mg tablets | 30 tablet PoM £6.77 DT price = £0.95

Fexofenadine hydrochloride   22-May-2017

● **INDICATIONS AND DOSE**

Symptomatic relief of seasonal allergic rhinitis
▸ BY MOUTH
▸ **Child 6–11 years:** 30 mg twice daily
▸ **Child 12–17 years:** 120 mg once daily

Symptomatic relief of chronic idiopathic urticaria
▸ BY MOUTH
▸ **Child 12–17 years:** 180 mg once daily

PHARMACOKINETICS
Fexofenadine is a metabolite of terfenadine.

● **INTERACTIONS** → Appendix 1: antihistamines (non-sedating)

● **SIDE-EFFECTS**
▸ **Uncommon** Antimuscarinic effects · blurred vision · dry mouth · gastro-intestinal disturbances · headache · psychomotor impairment · urinary retention
▸ **Rare** Anaphylaxis · angioedema · arrhythmias · blood disorders · bronchospasm · confusion · convulsions · depression · dizziness · extrapyramidal effects · hypersensitivity reactions · hypotension · liver dysfunction · palpitation · photosensitivity reactions · rashes · sleep disturbances · tremor
▸ **Frequency not known** Drowsiness

SIDE-EFFECTS, FURTHER INFORMATION

Non-sedating antihistamines such as fexofenadine cause less sedation and psychomotor impairment than the older antihistamines because they penetrate the blood brain barrier only to a slight extent.

If drowsiness occurs, it may diminish after a few days of treatment.

Children are more susceptible to side-effects.

● **PREGNANCY** Most manufacturers of antihistamines advise avoiding their use during pregnancy; however, there is no evidence of teratogenicity.

● **BREAST FEEDING** Most antihistamines are present in breast milk in varying amounts; although not known to be harmful, most manufacturers advise avoiding their use in mothers who are breast-feeding.

● **PATIENT AND CARER ADVICE**

Driving and skilled tasks

Although drowsiness is rare, nevertheless patients should be advised that it can occur and may affect performance of skilled tasks (e.g. cycling or driving); alcohol should be avoided.

● **MEDICINAL FORMS**

There can be variation in the licensing of different medicines containing the same drug. Forms available from special-order manufacturers include: oral suspension, oral solution

Tablet

CAUTIONARY AND ADVISORY LABELS 5

▸ **Fexofenadine hydrochloride** (Non-proprietary)
Fexofenadine hydrochloride 120 mg Fexofenadine 120mg tablets | 30 tablet PoM £7.15 DT price = £1.69
Fexofenadine hydrochloride 180 mg Fexofenadine 180mg tablets | 30 tablet PoM £9.65 DT price = £2.50

▸ **Telfast** (Sanofi)
Fexofenadine hydrochloride 30 mg Telfast 30mg tablets | 60 tablet PoM £5.46 DT price = £5.46
Fexofenadine hydrochloride 120 mg Telfast 120mg tablets | 30 tablet PoM £5.99 DT price = £1.69
Fexofenadine hydrochloride 180 mg Telfast 180mg tablets | 30 tablet PoM £7.58 DT price = £2.50

Levocetirizine hydrochloride   24-May-2017

● **INDICATIONS AND DOSE**

Symptomatic relief of allergy such as hay fever, urticaria
▸ BY MOUTH
▸ **Child 2–5 years:** 1.25 mg twice daily
▸ **Child 6–17 years:** 5 mg once daily

PHARMACOKINETICS
Levocetirizine is an isomer of cetirizine.

● **UNLICENSED USE** Tablets not licensed for use in children under 6 years.

● **CONTRA-INDICATIONS** Avoid in acute porphyrias p. 577 (some antihistamines are thought to be safe)

● **INTERACTIONS** → Appendix 1: antihistamines (non-sedating)

3

Respiratory system

Respiratory system

3

● SIDE-EFFECTS
▸ **Uncommon** Antimuscarinic effects · blurred vision · dry mouth · gastro-intestinal disturbances · headache · psychomotor impairment · urinary retention
▸ **Rare** Anaphylaxis · angioedema · arrhythmias · blood disorders · bronchospasm · confusion · convulsions · depression · dizziness · extrapyramidal effects · hypersensitivity reactions · hypotension · liver dysfunction · palpitation · photosensitivity reactions · rashes · sleep disturbances · tremor
▸ **Very rare** Weight gain
▸ **Frequency not known** Drowsiness

SIDE-EFFECTS, FURTHER INFORMATION
Non-sedating antihistamines such as levocetirizine cause less sedation and psychomotor impairment than the older antihistamines because they penetrate the blood brain barrier only to a slight extent.

If drowsiness occurs, it may diminish after a few days of treatment.

Children are more susceptible to side-effects.

● **PREGNANCY** Most manufacturers of antihistamines advise avoiding their use during pregnancy; however, there is no evidence of teratogenicity.

● **BREAST FEEDING** Most antihistamines are present in breast milk in varying amounts; although not known to be harmful, most manufacturers advise avoiding their use in mothers who are breast-feeding.

● **RENAL IMPAIRMENT** Reduce dose frequency to alternate days if estimated glomerular filtration rate 30–50 mL/minute/1.73 m². Reduce dose frequency to every 3 days if estimated glomerular filtration rate 10–30 mL/minute/1.73 m². Avoid if estimated glomerular filtration rate less than 10 mL/minute/1.73 m².

● **PATIENT AND CARER ADVICE**
Driving and skilled tasks
Although drowsiness is rare, nevertheless patients should be advised that it can occur and may affect performance of skilled tasks (e.g. cycling or driving); alcohol should be avoided.

● MEDICINAL FORMS
There can be variation in the licensing of different medicines containing the same drug.
Oral solution
▸ Xyzal (UCB Pharma Ltd)
  Levocetirizine dihydrochloride 500 microgram per 1 ml Xyzal 0.5mg/ml oral solution sugar-free | 200 ml [PoM] £6.00 DT price = £6.00
Tablet
▸ Levocetirizine hydrochloride (Non-proprietary)
  Levocetirizine dihydrochloride 5 mg Levocetirizine 5mg tablets | 30 tablet [PoM] £4.39 DT price = £4.36
▸ Xyzal (UCB Pharma Ltd)
  Levocetirizine dihydrochloride 5 mg Xyzal 5mg tablets | 30 tablet [PoM] £4.39 DT price = £4.36

Loratadine

22-May-2017

● **INDICATIONS AND DOSE**
Symptomatic relief of allergy such as hay fever, chronic idiopathic urticaria
▸ BY MOUTH
▸ Child 2–11 years (body-weight up to 31 kg): 5 mg once daily
▸ Child 2–11 years (body-weight 31 kg and above): 10 mg once daily
▸ Child 12–17 years: 10 mg once daily

● **CAUTIONS** Acute porphyrias p. 577
● **INTERACTIONS** → Appendix 1: antihistamines (non-sedating)

● SIDE-EFFECTS
▸ **Uncommon** Antimuscarinic effects · blurred vision · dry mouth · gastro-intestinal disturbances · Headache · psychomotor impairment · urinary retention
▸ **Rare** Anaphylaxis · angioedema · arrhythmias · blood disorders · bronchospasm · confusion · convulsions · depression · dizziness · extrapyramidal effects · hypersensitivity reactions · hypotension · liver dysfunction · palpitation · photosensitivity reactions · rashes · sleep disturbances · tremor
▸ **Frequency not known** Drowsiness

SIDE-EFFECTS, FURTHER INFORMATION
Non-sedating antihistamines such as loratadine cause less sedation and psychomotor impairment than the older antihistamines because they penetrate the blood brain barrier only to a slight extent.

If drowsiness occurs, it may diminish after a few days of treatment.

Children are more susceptible to side-effects.

● **PREGNANCY** Most manufacturers of antihistamines advise avoiding their use during pregnancy; however, there is no evidence of teratogenicity.

● **BREAST FEEDING** Most antihistamines are present in breast milk in varying amounts; although not known to be harmful, most manufacturers advise avoiding their use in mothers who are breast-feeding.

● **HEPATIC IMPAIRMENT** Reduce dose frequency to alternate days in severe impairment.

● **PATIENT AND CARER ADVICE**
Driving and skilled tasks
Although drowsiness is rare, nevertheless patients and their carers should be advised that it can occur and may affect performance of skilled tasks (e.g. cycling or driving); alcohol should be avoided.

● **PROFESSION SPECIFIC INFORMATION**
Dental practitioners' formulary
Loratadine 10 mg tablets may be prescribed.
Loratadine syrup 5 mg/5 mL may be prescribed.

● MEDICINAL FORMS
There can be variation in the licensing of different medicines containing the same drug.
Oral solution
EXCIPIENTS: May contain Propylene glycol
▸ Loratadine (Non-proprietary)
  Loratadine 1 mg per 1 ml Loratadine 5mg/5ml oral solution | 100 ml [PoM] £2.63 DT price = £1 86
Tablet
▸ Loratadine (Non-proprietary)
  Loratadine 10 mg Loratadine 10mg tablets | 30 tablet [P] £1.44 DT price = £0.84
▸ Clarityn (Loratadine) (Bayer Plc)
  Loratadine 10 mg Clarityn Allergy 10mg tablets | 60 tablet [P] £8.85
Oral lyophilisate
▸ Clarityn (Loratadine) (Bayer P c)
  Loratadine 10 mg Clarityn Rapide Allergy 10mg tablets sugar-free | 10 tablet [GSL] £3.24

Mizolastine

22-May-2017

● **INDICATIONS AND DOSE**
Symptomatic relief of allergy such as hay fever, urticaria
▸ BY MOUTH
▸ Child 12–17 years: 10 mg once daily

● **CONTRA-INDICATIONS** Avoid in acute porphyrias p. 577 (some antihistamines are thought to be safe) · cardiac disease · hypokalaemia · susceptibility to QT-interval prolongation

- **INTERACTIONS** → Appendix 1: antihistamines (non-sedating)
- **SIDE-EFFECTS**
- ▸ **Common or very common** Anxiety · asthenia · weight gain
- ▸ **Uncommon** Antimuscarinic effects · arthralgia · blurred vision · dry mouth · gastro-intestinal disturbances · headache · myalgia · psychomotor impairment · urinary retention
- ▸ **Rare** Anaphylaxis · angioedema · arrhythmias · blood disorders · bronchospasm · confusion · convulsions · depression · dizziness · extrapyramidal effects · hypersensitivity reactions · hypotension · liver dysfunction · palpitation · photosensitivity reactions · rashes · sleep disturbances · tremor
- ▸ **Frequency not known** Drowsiness

SIDE-EFFECTS, FURTHER INFORMATION
Non-sedating antihistamines such as mizolastine cause less sedation and psychomotor impairment than the older antihistamines because they penetrate the blood brain barrier only to a slight extent.

If drowsiness occurs, it may diminish after a few days of treatment.

Children are more susceptible to side-effects.

- **PREGNANCY** Most manufacturers of antihistamines advise avoiding their use during pregnancy; however, there is no evidence of teratogenicity.
- **BREAST FEEDING** Most antihistamines are present in breast milk in varying amounts; although not known to be harmful, most manufacturers advise avoiding their use in mothers who are breast-feeding.
- **HEPATIC IMPAIRMENT** Manufacturer advises avoid in significant impairment.
- **PATIENT AND CARER ADVICE**

Driving and skilled tasks
Although drowsiness is rare, nevertheless patients and their carers should be advised that it can occur and may affect performance of skilled tasks (e.g. cycling or driving); alcohol should be avoided.

- **MEDICINAL FORMS**
There can be variation in the licensing of different medicines containing the same drug.
Modified-release tablet
CAUTIONARY AND ADVISORY LABELS 25
- ▸ **Mizollen** (Sanofi)
Mizolastine 10 mg Mizollen 10mg modified-release tablets | 30 tablet [PoM] £6.92 DT price = £6.92

ANTIHISTAMINES ⟩ SEDATING

Alimemazine tartrate

(Trimeprazine tartrate)

- ● **INDICATIONS AND DOSE**

Urticaria | Pruritus
- ▸ BY MOUTH
- ▸ **Child 6 months–1 year** (specialist use only): 250 micrograms/kg 3–4 times a day (max. per dose 2.5 mg)
- ▸ **Child 2–4 years:** 2.5 mg 3–4 times a day
- ▸ **Child 5–11 years:** 5 mg 3–4 times a day
- ▸ **Child 12–17 years:** 10 mg 2–3 times a day, in severe cases up to maximum daily dose has been used; maximum 100 mg per day

Premedication to anaesthesia
- ▸ BY MOUTH
- ▸ **Child 2–6 years:** Up to 2 mg/kg, to be given 1–2 hours before operation

- **UNLICENSED USE** Not licensed for use in children under 2 years.

- **CONTRA-INDICATIONS** Children under 2 years except on specialist advice (safety of such use has not been established) · epilepsy · hepatic dysfunction · history of narrow angle glaucoma · hypothyroidism · many antihistamines should be avoided in acute porphyrias p. 577 but alimemazine is thought to be safe · myasthenia gravis · neonate (due to significant antimuscarinic activity) · phaeochromocytoma · renal dysfunction
- **CAUTIONS** Cardiovascular diseases (due to tachycardia-inducing and hypotensive effects of phenothiazines) · exposure to sunlight should be avoided during treatment with high doses · pyloroduodenal obstruction · urinary retention · volume depleted patients who are more susceptible to orthostatic hypotension
- **INTERACTIONS** → Appendix 1: antihistamines (sedating)
- **SIDE-EFFECTS**
- ▸ **Rare** Anaphylaxis · angioedema · bronchospasm · hypersensitivity reactions
- ▸ **Frequency not known** Acute dystonia · agitation · agranulocytosis · akathisia · akinesia · angle-closure glaucoma · anti-muscarinic effects · arrhythmias (may be predisposed by hypokalaemia and cardiac disease) · blurred vision · contact sensitisation · convulsions · drowsiness · dry mouth · dyskinesia · gastro-intestinal disturbances · headache · hyperprolactinaemia · hypotension · insomnia · jaundice · leukopenia (on prolonged high dose) · nasal stuffiness · neuroleptic malignant syndrome · ocular changes · pallor · paradoxical excitement · parkinsonism · photosensitivity · postural hypotension (in volume depletion) · rashes · respiratory depression · rigidity · tardive dyskinesia (usually after prolonged high doses) · tremor · urinary retention

SIDE-EFFECTS, FURTHER INFORMATION
Patients on high dosage may develop photosensitivity and should avoid exposure to direct sunlight.

Children are more susceptible to side-effects.

Drowsiness is a significant side-effect with most of the older antihistamines although paradoxical stimulation may occur rarely in children, especially with high doses. Drowsiness may diminish after a few days of treatment and is considerably less of a problem with the newer antihistamines.

- **PREGNANCY** Most manufacturers of antihistamines advise avoiding their use during pregnancy; however, there is no evidence of teratogenicity. Use in the latter part of the third trimester may cause adverse effects in neonates such as irritability, paradoxical excitability, and tremor.
- **BREAST FEEDING** Most antihistamines are present in breast milk in varying amounts; although not known to be harmful, most manufacturers advise avoiding their use in mothers who are breast-feeding.
- **HEPATIC IMPAIRMENT** Avoid in severe liver disease—increased risk of coma.
- **RENAL IMPAIRMENT** Avoid.
- **PATIENT AND CARER ADVICE**

Driving and skilled tasks
Drowsiness may affect performance of skilled tasks (e.g. cycling or driving); sedating effects enhanced by alcohol.

- **MEDICINAL FORMS**
There can be variation in the licensing of different medicines containing the same drug. Forms available from special-order manufacturers include: oral solution
Oral solution
CAUTIONARY AND ADVISORY LABELS 2
- ▸ **Alimemazine tartrate** (Non-proprietary)
Alimemazine tartrate 1.5 mg per 1 ml Alimemazine 7.5mg/5ml oral solution | 100 ml [PoM] £179.54 DT price = £179.54
Alimemazine tartrate 6 mg per 1 ml Alimemazine 30mg/5ml oral solution | 100 ml [PoM] £243.51 DT price = £243.51

Respiratory system

3

Tablet

CAUTIONARY AND ADVISORY LABELS 2
▶ **Alimemazine tartrate (Non-proprietary)**
Alimemazine tartrate 10 mg Alimemazine 10mg tablets |
25 tablet PoM no price available | 28 tablet PoM £112.85 DT price
= £112.85

Chlorphenamine maleate

(Chlorpheniramine maleate)

● **INDICATIONS AND DOSE**

Symptomatic relief of allergy such as hay fever, urticaria, food allergy, drug reactions | Relief of itch associated with chickenpox
▶ BY MOUTH
▶ Child 1-23 months: 1 mg twice daily
▶ Child 2-5 years: 1 mg every 4–6 hours; maximum 6 mg per day
▶ Child 6-11 years: 2 mg every 4–6 hours; maximum 12 mg per day
▶ Child 12-17 years: 4 mg every 4–6 hours; maximum 24 mg per day
▶ BY INTRAMUSCULAR INJECTION, OR BY INTRAVENOUS INJECTION
▶ Child 1-5 months: 250 micrograms/kg (max. per dose 2.5 mg), repeated if necessary; maximum 4 doses per day
▶ Child 6 months-5 years: 2.5 mg, repeated if necessary; maximum 4 doses per day
▶ Child 6-11 years: 5 mg, repeated if necessary; maximum 4 doses per day
▶ Child 12-17 years: 10 mg, repeated if necessary; maximum 4 doses per day

Emergency treatment of anaphylactic reactions
▶ BY INTRAMUSCULAR INJECTION, OR BY INTRAVENOUS INJECTION
▶ Child 1-5 months: 250 micrograms/kg (max. per dose 2.5 mg), repeated if necessary; maximum 4 doses per day
▶ Child 6 months-5 years: 2.5 mg, repeated if necessary; maximum 4 doses per day
▶ Child 6-11 years: 5 mg, repeated if necessary; maximum 4 doses per day
▶ Child 12-17 years: 10 mg, repeated if necessary; maximum 4 doses per day

● **UNLICENSED USE** *Injection* not licensed for use in neonates. *Tablets* not licensed for use in children under 6 years. *Syrup* not licensed for use in children under 1 year.

> **IMPORTANT SAFETY INFORMATION**
>
> MHRA/CHM ADVICE (MARCH 2008 AND FEBRUARY 2009) OVER-THE-COUNTER COUGH AND COLD MEDICINES FOR CHILDREN
> Children under 6 years should not be given over-the-counter cough and cold medicines containing chlorphenamine.

● **CONTRA-INDICATIONS** Many antihistamines should be avoided in acute porphyrias p. 577 but chlorphenamine is thought to be safe · neonate (due to significant antimuscarinic activity)
● **CAUTIONS** Epilepsy · pyloroduodenal obstruction · susceptibility to angle-closure glaucoma · urinary retention
● **INTERACTIONS** → Appendix 1: antihistamines (sedating)
● **SIDE-EFFECTS**
GENERAL SIDE-EFFECTS
▶ **Common or very common** Blurred vision · dry mouth · gastro-intestinal disturbances · headache · psychomotor impairment · urinary retention

▶ **Rare** Anaphylaxis · angioedema · arrhythmias · bronchospasm · confusion · convulsions · depression · dizziness · extrapyramidal effects · hypersensitivity reactions · hypotension · liver dysfunction · palpitation · photosensitivity reactions · sleep disturbances · tremor
▶ **Frequency not known** Antimuscarinic effects · blood disorders · exfoliative dermatitis · rashes · tinnitus
SPECIFIC SIDE-EFFECTS
▶ With intramuscular use or intravenous use CNS stimulation · irritant effects · transient hypotension
SIDE-EFFECTS, FURTHER INFORMATION
Children are more susceptible to side-effects.
  Drowsiness is a significant side-effect with most of the older antihistamines although paradoxical stimulation may occur rarely in children, especially with high doses. Drowsiness may diminish after a few days of treatment and is considerably less of a problem with the newer antihistamines.

● **PREGNANCY** Most manufacturers of antihistamines advise avoiding their use during pregnancy; however, there is no evidence of teratogenicity. Use in the latter part of the third trimester may cause adverse effects in neonates such as irritability, paradoxical excitability, and tremor.

● **BREAST FEEDING** Most antihistamines are present in breast milk in varying amounts; although not known to be harmful, most manufacturers advise avoiding their use in mothers who are breast-feeding.

● **HEPATIC IMPAIRMENT** Avoid in severe liver disease—increased risk of coma.

● **DIRECTIONS FOR ADMINISTRATION** For *intravenous injection*, give over 1 minute; if small dose required, dilute with Sodium Chloride 0.9%.

● **PATIENT AND CARER ADVICE**
Driving and skilled tasks
Drowsiness may affect performance of skilled tasks (e.g. cycling or driving); sedating effects enhanced by alcohol.
Medicines for Children leaflet: Chlorphenamine maleate for allergy symptoms www.medicinesforchildren.org.uk/chlorphenamine-maleate-allergy-symptoms-0

● **PROFESSION SPECIFIC INFORMATION**
Dental practitioners' formulary Chlorphenamine tablets may be prescribed. Chlorphenamine oral solution may be prescribed.

● **EXCEPTIONS TO LEGAL CATEGORY**
Prescription only medicine restriction does not apply to chlorphenamine injection where administration is for saving life in emergency.

● **MEDICINAL FORMS**
There can be variation in the licensing of different medicines containing the same drug. Forms available from special-order manufacturers include: oral solution
Solution for injection
▶ **Chlorphenamine maleate (Non-proprietary)**
Chlorphenamine maleate 10 mg per 1 ml Chlorphenamine 10mg/1ml solution for injection ampoules | 5 ampoule PoM £22.48-£22.50 DT price = £22.50
Oral solution
CAUTIONARY AND ADVISORY LABELS 2
▶ **Chlorphenamine maleate (Non-proprietary)**
Chlorphenamine maleate 400 microgram per 1 ml Chlorphenamine 2mg/5ml oral solution sugar free sugar-free | 150 ml P £2.62 DT price = £2.62
▶ **Allerief** (Orbis Consumer Products Ltd)
Chlorphenamine maleate 400 microgram per 1 ml Allerief 2mg/5ml oral solution sugar-free | 150 ml P £2.22 DT price = £2.62
▶ **Piriton** (GlaxoSmithKline Consumer Healthcare)
Chlorphenamine maleate 400 microgram per 1 ml Piriton 2mg/5ml syrup | 150 ml P £2.78 DT price = £2.62

Tablet
CAUTIONARY AND ADVISORY LABELS 2
▶ **Chlorphenamine maleate (Non-proprietary)**
  Chlorphenamine maleate 4 mg Chlorphenamine 4mg tablets |
  28 tablet P £1.00 DT price = £0.76
▶ **Hayleve** (Genesis Pharmaceuticals Ltd)
  Chlorphenamine maleate 4 mg Hayleve 4mg tablets | 28 tablet P
  £0.76 DT price = £0.76
▶ **Piriton** (GlaxoSmithKline Consumer Healthcare)
  Chlorphenamine maleate 4 mg Piriton Allergy 4mg tablets |
  30 tablet P £2.06 | 60 tablet P £3.73
▶ **Pollenase (chlorphenamine)** (E M Pharma)
  Chlorphenamine maleate 4 mg Pollenase Antihistamine 4mg
  tablets | 30 tablet P £1.00

Hydroxyzine hydrochloride   22-Feb-2016

● **DRUG ACTION** Hydroxyzine is a sedating antihistamine
which exerts its actions by antagonising the effects of
histamine.

● **INDICATIONS AND DOSE**
Pruritus
▶ BY MOUTH
▶ Child 6 months–5 years: 5–15 mg daily in divided doses,
  dose adjusted according to weight; maximum 2 mg/kg
  per day
▶ Child 6–17 years (body-weight up to 40 kg): Initially
  15–25 mg daily in divided doses, dose increased as
  necessary, adjusted according to weight; maximum
  2 mg/kg per day
▶ Child 6–17 years (body-weight 40 kg and above): Initially
  15–25 mg daily in divided doses, increased if necessary
  to 50–100 mg daily in divided doses, dose adjusted
  according to weight

● **UNLICENSED USE** *Ucerax*® preparations not licensed for
use in children under 1 year.

> **IMPORTANT SAFETY INFORMATION**
> MHRA/CHM ADVICE: RISK OF QT-INTERVAL PROLONGATION AND
> TORSADE DE POINTES (APRIL 2015)
> Following concerns of heart rhythm abnormalities, the
> safety and efficacy of hydroxyzine has been reviewed by
> the European Medicines Agency. The review concludes
> that hydroxyzine is associated with a small risk of QT-
> interval prolongation and torsade de pointes; these
> events are most likely to occur in patients who have risk
> factors for QT prolongation, e.g. concomitant use of
> drugs that prolong the QT-interval, cardiovascular
> disease, family history of sudden cardiac death,
> significant electrolyte imbalance (low plasma-potassium
> or plasma-magnesium concentrations), or significant
> bradycardia.
>   To minimise the risk of such adverse effects, the
> following dose restrictions have been made and new
> cautions and contra-indications added:
> ● Hydroxyzine is contra-indicated in patients with
>   prolonged QT-interval or who have risk factors for QT-
>   interval prolongation;
> ● Consider the risks of QT-interval prolongation and
>   torsade de pointes before prescribing to patients
>   taking drugs that lower heart rate or plasma-
>   potassium concentration;
> ● In children with body-weight up to 40 kg, the
>   maximum daily dose is 2 mg/kg;
> ● The lowest effective dose for the shortest period of
>   time should be prescribed.

● **CONTRA-INDICATIONS** Acquired or congenital QT interval
prolongation · avoid in acute porphyrias p. 577 (some
antihistamines are thought to be safe) · predisposition to
QT interval prolongation

CONTRA-INDICATIONS, FURTHER INFORMATION
▶ QT interval prolongation Risk factors for QT interval
  prolongation include significant electrolyte imbalance,
  bradycardia, cardiovascular disease, and family history of
  sudden cardiac death.
● **CAUTIONS** Bladder outflow obstruction · breathing
  problems · cardiovascular disease · children · decreased
  gastrointestinal motility · dementia · epilepsy ·
  hypertension · hyperthyroidism · myasthenia gravis ·
  pyloroduodenal obstruction · stenosing peptic ulcer ·
  susceptibility to angle-closure glaucoma · urinary
  retention
CAUTIONS, FURTHER INFORMATION
Children have an increased susceptibility to side-effects,
particularly CNS effects.
● **INTERACTIONS** → Appendix 1: antihistamines (sedating)
● **SIDE-EFFECTS**
▶ **Common or very common** Dry mouth · fatigue · headache
▶ **Uncommon** Constipation · dizziness · insomnia · nausea
▶ **Rare** Blood disorders · bronchospasm · liver dysfunction ·
  rashes
▶ **Frequency not known** Agitation · alopecia · anorexia ·
  anxiety · blurred vision · coma · confusion · convulsions
  (with high doses) · depression · diarrhoea · dizziness ·
  dyskinesia (after stopping use) · extrapyramidal effects ·
  flushing · hallucinations · hypotension · impotence ·
  labrynthitis · menstrual disturbances · myalgia · palpitation
  · priapsim · psychomotor impairment · sleep disturbances ·
  tachycardia · tinnitus · tremor (with high doses) · urinary
  retention · ventricular arrhythmias · vertigo · vomiting
SIDE-EFFECTS, FURTHER INFORMATION
Drowsiness is a significant side-effect with most of the
older antihistamines although paradoxical stimulation
may occur rarely, especially with high doses. Drowsiness
may diminish after a few days of treatment and is
considerably less of a problem with the newer
antihistamines.
● **ALLERGY AND CROSS-SENSITIVITY** Manufacturer advises
  hydroxyzine should be avoided in patients with previous
  hypersensitivity to cetirizine or other piperazine
  derivatives, and aminophylline.
● **PREGNANCY** Manufacturers advise avoid—toxicity in
  animal studies with higher doses. Use in the latter part of
  the third trimester may cause irritability, paradoxical
  excitability, and tremor in the neonate.
● **BREAST FEEDING** Manufacturer advises avoid—expected
  to be present in milk but effect unknown.
● **HEPATIC IMPAIRMENT** Manufacturer advises reduce daily
  dose by one-third. Manufacturer advises avoid in severe
  liver disease—increased risk of coma.
● **RENAL IMPAIRMENT** Manufacturers advise reduce daily
  dose by half in moderate to severe renal impairment.
● **EFFECT ON LABORATORY TESTS** May interfere with
  methacholine test—manufacturer advises stop treatment
  96 hours prior to test. May interfere with skin testing for
  allergy—manufacturer advises stop treatment one week
  prior to test.
● **PATIENT AND CARER ADVICE**
Driving and skilled tasks
Drowsiness may affect performance of skilled tasks (e.g.
cycling or driving); sedating effects enhanced by alcohol.
● **MEDICINAL FORMS**
There can be variation in the licensing of different medicines
containing the same drug. Forms available from special-order
manufacturers include: oral suspension, oral solution
Tablet
CAUTIONARY AND ADVISORY LABELS 2
▶ **Atarax** (Alliance Pharmaceuticals Ltd)
  Hydroxyzine hydrochloride 10 mg Atarax 10mg tablets |
  84 tablet PoM £1.20 DT price = £1.20
  Hydroxyzine hydrochloride 25 mg Atarax 25mg tablets |
  28 tablet PoM £0.62 DT price = £0.62

Ketotifen

- ● **INDICATIONS AND DOSE**
Allergic rhinitis
  - ▸ BY MOUTH
  - ▸ Child 3-17 years: 1 mg twice daily

- ● **CONTRA-INDICATIONS** Avoid in acute porphyrias p. 577 (some antihistamines are thought to be safe) · neonate (due to significant antimuscarinic activity)
- ● **CAUTIONS** Epilepsy · pyloroduodenal obstruction · susceptibility to angle-closure glaucoma · urinary retention
- ● **INTERACTIONS** → Appendix 1: antihistamines (sedating)
- ● **SIDE-EFFECTS**
  - ▸ **Common or very common** Irritability · nervousness
  - ▸ **Uncommon** Cystitis
  - ▸ **Rare** Weight gain
  - ▸ **Very rare** Stevens-Johnson syndrome
  - ▸ **Frequency not known** Anaphylaxis · angioedema · antimuscarinic effects · arrhythmias · blood disorders · blurred vision · bronchospasm · confusion · convulsions · depression · dizziness · dry mouth · extrapyramidal effects · gastro-intestinal disturbances · headache · hypersensitivity reactions · hypotension · liver dysfunction · palpitation · photosensitivity reactions · psychomotor impairment · rashes · sleep disturbances · tremor · urinary retention

  SIDE-EFFECTS, FURTHER INFORMATION
  Drowsiness is a significant side-effect with most of the older antihistamines although paradoxical stimulation may occur rarely, especially with high doses. Drowsiness may diminish after a few days of treatment and is considerably less of a problem with the newer antihistamines.
- ● **PREGNANCY** Most manufacturers of antihistamines advise avoiding their use during pregnancy; however, there is no evidence of teratogenicity. Use in the latter part of the third trimester may cause adverse effects in neonates such as irritability, paradoxical excitability, and tremor.
- ● **BREAST FEEDING** Most antihistamines are present in breast milk in varying amounts; although not known to be harmful, most manufacturers advise avoiding their use in mothers who are breast-feeding.
- ● **HEPATIC IMPAIRMENT** Avoid in severe liver disease—increased risk of coma.
- ● **PATIENT AND CARER ADVICE**
Driving and skilled tasks
Drowsiness may affect performance of skilled tasks (e.g. driving or cycling); sedating effects enhanced by alcohol.

- ● **MEDICINAL FORMS**
There can be variation in the licensing of different medicines containing the same drug.
  Oral solution
  CAUTIONARY AND ADVISORY LABELS 2, 21
  - ▸ Zaditen (CD Pharma AB)
    Ketotifen (as Ketotifen fumarate) 200 microgram per 1 ml Zaditen 1mg/5ml elixir sugar-free | 300 ml [PoM] £8.91 DT price = £8.91
  Tablet
  CAUTIONARY AND ADVISORY LABELS 2, 21
  - ▸ Zaditen (CD Pharma AB)
    Ketotifen (as Ketotifen fumarate) 1 mg Zaditen 1mg tablets | 60 tablet [PoM] £7.53

Promethazine hydrochloride

- ● **INDICATIONS AND DOSE**
Symptomatic relief of allergy such as hay fever and urticaria | Insomnia associated with urticaria and pruritus
  - ▸ BY MOUTH
  - ▸ Child 2-4 years: 5 mg twice daily, alternatively 5–15 mg once daily, dose to be taken at night
  - ▸ Child 5-9 years: 5–10 mg twice daily, alternatively 10–25 mg once daily, dose to be taken at night
  - ▸ Child 10-17 years: 10–20 mg 2–3 times a day, alternatively 25 mg once daily, dose to be taken at night, increased if necessary to 25 mg twice daily

Sedation (short-term use)
  - ▸ BY MOUTH
  - ▸ Child 2-4 years: 15–20 mg
  - ▸ Child 5-9 years: 20–25 mg
  - ▸ Child 10-17 years: 25–50 mg

Sedation in intensive care
  - ▸ BY MOUTH, OR BY SLOW INTRAVENOUS INJECTION, OR BY DEEP INTRAMUSCULAR INJECTION
  - ▸ Child 1 month-11 years: 0.5–1 mg/kg 4 times a day (max. per dose 25 mg), adjusted according to response
  - ▸ Child 12-17 years: 25–50 mg 4 times a day, adjusted according to response

Nausea | Vomiting | Vertigo | Labyrinthine disorders | Motion sickness
  - ▸ BY MOUTH
  - ▸ Child 2-4 years: 5 mg, to be taken at bedtime on night before travel, repeat following morning if necessary
  - ▸ Child 5-9 years: 10 mg, to be taken at bedtime on night before travel, repeat following morning if necessary
  - ▸ Child 10-17 years: 20–25 mg, to be taken at bedtime on night before travel, repeat following morning if necessary

- ● **UNLICENSED USE** Not licensed for use for sedation in children under 2 years.

> **IMPORTANT SAFETY INFORMATION**
> MHRA/CHM ADVICE (MARCH 2008 AND FEBRUARY 2009) OVER-THE-COUNTER COUGH AND COLD MEDICINES FOR CHILDREN
> Children under 6 years should not be given over-the-counter cough and cold medicines containing promethazine.

- ● **CONTRA-INDICATIONS** Many antihistamines should be avoided in acute porphyrias p. 577 but promethazine is thought to be safe · neonate (due to significant antimuscarinic activity) · should not be given to children under 2 years, except on specialist advice, because the safety of such use has not been established
- ● **CAUTIONS**
GENERAL CAUTIONS
Epilepsy · pyloroduodenal obstruction · severe coronary artery disease · susceptibility to angle-closure glaucoma · urinary retention
SPECIFIC CAUTIONS
  - ▸ With intravenous use Avoid extravasation with intravenous injection
- ● **INTERACTIONS** → Appendix 1: antihistamines (sedating)
- ● **SIDE-EFFECTS**
  - ▸ **Rare** Anaphylaxis · angioedema · angle-closure glaucoma · arrhythmias · blood disorders · bronchospasm · confusion · convulsions · depression · dizziness · extrapyramidal effects · hypersensitivity reactions · hypotension · liver dysfunction · palpitation · photosensitivity reactions · rashes · sleep disturbances · tremor

▶ **Frequency not known** Antimuscarinic effects · blurred vision · drowsiness · dry mouth · gastro-intestinal disturbances · headache · psychomotor impairment · restlessness · urinary retention

SIDE-EFFECTS, FURTHER INFORMATION
Children are more susceptible to side-effects.

Drowsiness is a significant side-effect with most of the older antihistamines although paradoxical stimulation may occur rarely in children, especially with high doses. Drowsiness may diminish after a few days of treatment and is considerably less of a problem with the newer antihistamines.

● **PREGNANCY** Most manufacturers of antihistamines advise avoiding their use during pregnancy; however, there is no evidence of teratogenicity. Use in the latter part of the third trimester may cause adverse effects in neonates such as irritability, paradoxical excitability, and tremor.

● **BREAST FEEDING** Most antihistamines are present in breast milk in varying amounts; although not known to be harmful, most manufacturers advise avoiding their use in mothers who are breast-feeding.

● **HEPATIC IMPAIRMENT** Avoid in severe liver disease—increased risk of coma.

● **RENAL IMPAIRMENT** Use with caution.

● **PATIENT AND CARER ADVICE**
Driving and skilled tasks
Drowsiness may affect the performance of skilled tasks (e.g. cycling or driving); sedating effects enhanced by alcohol.

● **PROFESSION SPECIFIC INFORMATION**
Dental practitioners' formulary
Promethazine Hydrochloride Tablets 10 mg or 25 mg may be prescribed.
Promethazine Hydrochloride Oral Solution (elixir) 5 mg/5 mL may be prescribed.

● **LESS SUITABLE FOR PRESCRIBING** Promethazine is less suitable for prescribing for sedation.

● **EXCEPTIONS TO LEGAL CATEGORY** Prescription only medicine restriction does not apply to promethazine hydrochloride injection where administration is for saving life in emergency.

● **MEDICINAL FORMS**
There can be variation in the licensing of different medicines containing the same drug. Forms available from special-order manufacturers include: oral suspension, oral solution

Solution for injection
EXCIPIENTS: May contain Sulfites
▶ **Phenergan** (Sanofi)
Promethazine hydrochloride 25 mg per 1 ml Phenergan 25mg/1ml solution for injection ampoules | 10 ampoule PoM £6.74

Oral solution
CAUTIONARY AND ADVISORY LABELS 2
EXCIPIENTS: May contain Sulfites
ELECTROLYTES: May contain Sodium
▶ **Phenergan** (Sanofi)
Promethazine hydrochloride 1 mg per 1 ml Phenergan 5mg/5ml elixir sugar-free | 100 ml Ⓟ £2.85 DT price = £2.85

Tablet
CAUTIONARY AND ADVISORY LABELS 2
▶ **Promethazine hydrochloride (Non-proprietary)**
Promethazine hydrochloride 10 mg Promethazine hydrochloride 10mg tablets | 56 tablet PoM £2.96 DT price = £2.96
▶ **Phenergan** (Sanofi)
Promethazine hydrochloride 10 mg Phenergan 10mg tablets | 56 tablet Ⓟ £2.96 DT price = £2.96
Promethazine hydrochloride 25 mg Phenergan 25mg tablets | 56 tablet Ⓟ £4.65 DT price = £4.65
▶ **Sominex** (Teva UK Ltd)
Promethazine hydrochloride 20 mg Sominex 20mg tablets | 8 tablet Ⓟ £1.89 | 16 tablet Ⓟ £2.69

VACCINES ⟩ ALLERGEN-TYPE VACCINES

Bee venom extract

● **INDICATIONS AND DOSE**
Hypersensitivity to bee venom
▶ BY SUBCUTANEOUS INJECTION
▶ Child: (consult product literature)

IMPORTANT SAFETY INFORMATION
DESENSITISING VACCINES
In view of concerns about the safety of desensitising vaccines, it is recommended that they are used by specialists and only for the following indications:
● seasonal allergic hay fever (caused by pollen) that has not responded to anti-allergic drugs;
● hypersensitivity to wasp and bee venoms.
Desensitising vaccines should generally be avoided or used with particular care in patients with asthma.

● **CONTRA-INDICATIONS** Children under 5 years · consult product literature

● **CAUTIONS** Consult product literature

● **INTERACTIONS** → Appendix 1: bee venom extract

● **SIDE-EFFECTS**

SIDE-EFFECTS, FURTHER INFORMATION
Consult product literature.
▶ Hypersensitivity reactions Hypersensitivity reactions to immunotherapy (especially to wasp and bee venom extracts) can be life-threatening; bronchospasm usually develops within 1 hour and anaphylaxis within 30 minutes of injection. Therefore, cardiopulmonary resuscitation must be immediately available and patients need to be monitored for at least 1 hour after injection. If symptoms or signs of hypersensitivity develop (e.g. rash, urticaria, bronchospasm, faintness), **even when mild**, the patient should be observed until these have **resolved completely**.

● **PREGNANCY** Avoid.

● **PRESCRIBING AND DISPENSING INFORMATION** Each set of allergen extracts usually contains vials for the administration of graded amounts of allergen to patients undergoing hyposensitisation. Maintenance sets containing vials at the highest strength are also available. Product literature must be consulted for details of allergens, vial strengths, and administration.

● **NATIONAL FUNDING/ACCESS DECISIONS**
NICE technology appraisals (TAs)
▶ *Pharmalgen*® for bee and wasp venom allergy (February 2012) NICE TA246
Pharmalgen® is an option for the treatment of IgE-mediated bee and wasp venom allergy in those who have had:
● a severe systemic reaction to bee or wasp venom;
● a moderate systemic reaction to bee or wasp venom and who have a raised baseline serum-tryptase concentration, a high risk of future stings, or anxiety about future stings.
Treatment with *Pharmalgen*® should be initiated and monitored in a specialist centre experienced in venom immunotherapy.
www.nice.org.uk/TA246

● **MEDICINAL FORMS**
There can be variation in the licensing of different medicines containing the same drug.
Powder and solvent for solution for injection
▶ **Bee Venom** (ALK-Abello Ltd)
Bee venom 120 nanogram Pharmalgen Bee Venom 120nanogram powder and solvent for solution for injection vials | 1 vial PoM no price available

Bee venom 1.2 microgram Pharmalgen Bee Venom 1.2microgram powder and solvent for solution for injection vials | 1 vial [PoM] no price available

Bee venom 12 microgram Pharmalgen Bee Venom 12microgram powder and solvent for solution for injection vials | 1 vial [PoM] no price available

Bee venom 120 microgram Pharmalgen Bee Venom maintenance set 120microgram powder and solvent for solution for injection vials | 1 vial [PoM] no price available | 4 vial [PoM] £150.00

Grass pollen extract

● **INDICATIONS AND DOSE**

Treatment of seasonal allergic hay fever due to grass pollen in patients who have failed to respond to anti-allergy drugs

▸ BY SUBCUTANEOUS INJECTION
▸ Child: (consult product literature)

Treatment of seasonal allergic hay fever due to grass pollen in patients who have failed to respond to anti-allergy drugs (initiated under specialist supervision)

▸ BY MOUTH
▸ Child 5-17 years: 1 tablet daily, treatment to be started at least 4 months before start of pollen season and continue for up to 3 years

> **IMPORTANT SAFETY INFORMATION**
> DESENSITISING VACCINES
> In view of concerns about the safety of desensitising vaccines, it is recommended that they are used by specialists and only for the following indications:
> ● seasonal allergic hay fever (caused by pollen) that has not responded to anti-allergic drugs;
> ● hypersensitivity to wasp and bee venoms.
> Desensitising vaccines should generally be avoided or used with particular care in patients with asthma.

● **CONTRA-INDICATIONS** Children under 5 years · consult product literature
● **CAUTIONS** Consult product literature
● **INTERACTIONS** → Appendix 1: grass pollen extract
● **SIDE-EFFECTS**

SIDE-EFFECTS, FURTHER INFORMATION
Consult product literature.

▸ Hypersensitivity reactions Hypersensitivity reactions to immunotherapy can be life-threatening; bronchospasm usually develops within 1 hour and anaphylaxis within 30 minutes of injection. Therefore, cardiopulmonary resuscitation must be immediately available and patients need to be monitored for at least 1 hour after injection. If symptoms or signs of hypersensitivity develop (e.g. rash, urticaria, bronchospasm, faintness), **even when mild**, the patient should be observed until these have **resolved completely**.

● **PREGNANCY** Should be avoided in pregnant women—consult product literature.
● **MONITORING REQUIREMENTS** The first dose of grass pollen extract should be (Grazax®) should be taken under medical supervision and the patient should be monitored for 20-30 minutes.
● **DIRECTIONS FOR ADMINISTRATION** Oral lyophylisates should be placed under the tongue and allowed to disperse. Advise patient not to swallow for 1 minute, or eat or drink for 5 minutes after taking the tablet. The first should be taken under medical supervision and the patient should be monitored for 20-30 minutes.
● **PRESCRIBING AND DISPENSING INFORMATION** Each set of allergen extracts usually contains vials for the administration of graded amounts of allergen to patients undergoing hyposensitisation. Maintenance sets

containing vials at the highest strength are also available. Product literature must be consulted for details of allergens, vial strengths, and administration.

● **PATIENT AND CARER ADVICE**
▸ With oral use Patients or carers should be given advice on how to administer oral lyophilisate.

● **MEDICINAL FORMS**
There can be variation in the licensing of different medicines containing the same drug.

Suspension for injection
▸ **Pollinex Grasses + Rye** (Allergy Therapeutics (UK) Ltd)
Pollinex Grasses + Rye suspension for injection treatment and extension course vials | 4 vial [PoM] £450.00

Oral lyophilisate
▸ **Grazax** (ALK-Abello Ltd)
Phleum pratense 75000 SQ-T Grazax 75,000 SQ-T oral lyophilisates sugar-free | 30 tablet [PoM] £80.12

Tree pollen extract

● **INDICATIONS AND DOSE**

Treatment of seasonal allergic hay fever due to tree pollen in patients who have failed to respond to anti-allergy drugs

▸ BY SUBCUTANEOUS INJECTION
▸ Child: (consult product literature)

> **IMPORTANT SAFETY INFORMATION**
> DESENSITISING VACCINES
> In view of concerns about the safety of desensitising vaccines, it is recommended that they are used by specialists and only for the following indications:
> ● seasonal allergic hay fever (caused by pollen) that has not responded to anti-allergic drugs;
> ● hypersensitivity to wasp and bee venoms.
> Desensitising vaccines should generally be avoided or used with particular care in patients with asthma.

● **CONTRA-INDICATIONS** Children under 5 years · consult product literature
● **CAUTIONS** Consult product literature
● **INTERACTIONS** → Appendix 1: tree pollen extract
● **SIDE-EFFECTS**

SIDE-EFFECTS, FURTHER INFORMATION
Consult product literature.

▸ Hypersensitivity reactions Hypersensitivity reactions to immunotherapy (especially to wasp and bee venom extracts) can be life-threatening; bronchospasm usually develops within 1 hour and anaphylaxis within 30 minutes of injection. Therefore, cardiopulmonary resuscitation must be immediately available and patients need to be monitored for at least 1 hour after injection. If symptoms or signs of hypersensitivity develop (e.g. rash, urticaria, bronchospasm, faintness), **even when mild**, the patient should be observed until these have **resolved completely**.

● **PREGNANCY** Should be avoided in pregnant women—consult product literature.
● **PRESCRIBING AND DISPENSING INFORMATION** Each set of allergen extracts usually contains vials for the administration of graded amounts of allergen to patients undergoing hyposensitisation. Maintenance sets containing vials at the highest strength are also available. Product literature must be consulted for details of allergens, vial strengths, and administration.

- **MEDICINAL FORMS**
There can be variation in the licensing of different medicines containing the same drug.
Suspension for injection
‣ Pollinex Trees (Allergy Therapeutics (UK) Ltd)
Pollinex Trees No 3 suspension for injection 1ml vials | 1 vial PoM no price available
Pollinex Trees No 2 suspension for injection 1ml vials | 1 vial PoM no price available
Pollinex Trees No 1 suspension for injection 1ml vials | 1 vial PoM no price available
Pollinex Trees suspension for injection treatment and extension course vials | 4 vial PoM £450.00

Wasp venom extract

- **INDICATIONS AND DOSE**
Hypersensitivity to wasp venom
‣ BY SUBCUTANEOUS INJECTION
‣ Child: (consult product literature)

IMPORTANT SAFETY INFORMATION
DESENSITISING VACCINES
In view of concerns about the safety of desensitising vaccines, it is recommended that they are used by specialists and only for the following indications:
- seasonal allergic hay fever (caused by pollen) that has not responded to anti-allergic drugs;
- hypersensitivity to wasp and bee venoms.
Desensitising vaccines should generally be avoided or used with particular care in patients with asthma.

- **CONTRA-INDICATIONS** Children under 5 years · consult product literature
- **CAUTIONS** Consult product literature
- **INTERACTIONS** → Appendix 1: wasp venom extract
- **SIDE-EFFECTS**
SIDE-EFFECTS, FURTHER INFORMATION
Consult product literature.
‣ Hypersensitivity reactions Hypersensitivity reactions to immunotherapy (especially to wasp and bee venom extracts) can be life-threatening; bronchospasm usually develops within 1 hour and anaphylaxis within 30 minutes of injection. Therefore, cardiopulmonary resuscitation must be immediately available and patients need to be monitored for at least 1 hour after injection. If symptoms or signs of hypersensitivity develop (e.g. rash, urticaria, bronchospasm, faintness), **even when mild**, the patient should be observed until these have **resolved completely**.
- **PREGNANCY** Avoid.
- **PRESCRIBING AND DISPENSING INFORMATION** Each set of allergen extracts usually contains vials for the administration of graded amounts of allergen to patients undergoing hyposensitisation. Maintenance sets containing vials at the highest strength are also available. Product literature must be consulted for details of allergens, vial strengths, and administration.
- **NATIONAL FUNDING/ACCESS DECISIONS**
NICE technology appraisals (TAs)
‣ *Pharmalgen*® for bee and wasp venom allergy (February 2012) NICE TA246
Pharmalgen® is an option for the treatment of IgE-mediated bee and wasp venom allergy in those who have had:
- a severe systemic reaction to bee or wasp venom;
- a moderate systemic reaction to bee or wasp venom and who have a raised baseline serum-tryptase concentration, a high risk of future stings, or anxiety about future stings.

Treatment with *Pharmalgen*® should be initiated and monitored in a specialist centre experienced in venom immunotherapy.
www.nice.org.uk/TA246

- **MEDICINAL FORMS**
There can be variation in the licensing of different medicines containing the same drug.
Powder and solvent for solution for injection
‣ Wasp Venom (ALK-Abello Ltd)
Wasp venom 120 nanogram Pharmalgen Wasp Venom 120nanogram powder and solvent for solution for injection vials | 1 vial PoM no price available
Wasp venom 1.2 microgram Pharmalgen Wasp Venom 1.2microgram powder and solvent for solution for injection vials | 1 vial PoM no price available
Wasp venom 12 microgram Pharmalgen Wasp Venom 12microgram powder and solvent for solution for injection vials | 1 vial PoM no price available
Wasp venom 120 microgram Pharmalgen Wasp Venom maintenance set 120microgram vaccine powder and solvent for solution for injection vials | 1 vial PoM no price available | 4 vial PoM £150.00

2.1 Angioedema

Other drugs used for Angioedema Adrenaline/epinephrine p. 132

DRUGS USED IN HEREDITARY ANGIOEDEMA ›
COMPLEMENT REGULATORY PROTEINS

C1-esterase inhibitor

- **INDICATIONS AND DOSE**
BERINERT®
Acute attacks of hereditary angioedema (under expert supervision)
‣ BY SLOW INTRAVENOUS INJECTION, OR BY INTRAVENOUS INFUSION
‣ Child: 20 units/kg
Short-term prophylaxis of hereditary angioedema before dental, medical, or surgical procedures (under expert supervision)
‣ BY SLOW INTRAVENOUS INJECTION, OR BY INTRAVENOUS INFUSION
‣ Child: 15–30 units/kg (max. per dose 1000 units) for 1 dose, to be administered less than 6 hours before procedure
CINRYZE®
Acute attacks of hereditary angioedema (under expert supervision)
‣ BY SLOW INTRAVENOUS INJECTION
‣ Child 12–17 years: 1000 units for 1 dose, dose may be repeated if necessary
Short-term prophylaxis of hereditary angioedema before dental, medical, or surgical procedures (under expert supervision)
‣ BY SLOW INTRAVENOUS INJECTION
‣ Child 12–17 years: 1000 units for 1 dose, to be administered up to 24 hours before procedure
Long-term prophylaxis of severe, recurrent attacks of hereditary angioedema where acute treatment is inadequate, or when oral prophylaxis is inadequate or not tolerated (under expert supervision)
‣ BY SLOW INTRAVENOUS INJECTION
‣ Child 12–17 years: 1000 units every 3–4 days, interval between doses to be adjusted according to response

3

Respiratory system

- **CAUTIONS** Vaccination against hepatitis A and hepatitis B may be required
- **SIDE-EFFECTS** Fever · headache · thrombosis (with high doses)
- **PREGNANCY** Manufacturer advises avoid unless essential.
- **DIRECTIONS FOR ADMINISTRATION**
  CINRYZE® For *slow intravenous injection*, reconstitute (with solvent provided) to a concentration of 100 units/mL; give at a rate of 1 mL/minute.
- **PRESCRIBING AND DISPENSING INFORMATION** C1-esterase inhibitor is prepared from human plasma.

- **MEDICINAL FORMS**
  There can be variation in the licensing of different medicines containing the same drug.
  Powder and solvent for solution for injection
  ELECTROLYTES: May contain Sodium
  ▸ **Berinert P** (CSL Behring UK Ltd)
  C1-esterase inhibitor 500 unit Berinert 500unit powder and solvent for solution for injection vials | 1 vial (PoM) £467.50
  C1-esterase inhibitor 1500 unit Berinert 1,500unit powder and solvent for solution for injection vials | 1 vial (PoM) £1,402.50
  ▸ **Cinryze** (Shire Pharmaceuticals Ltd) ▼
  C1-esterase inhibitor 500 unit Cinryze 500unit powder and solvent for solution for injection vials | 2 vial (PoM) £1,336.00

3 Conditions affecting sputum viscosity

Mucolytics for cystic fibrosis

Overview

Mucolytics, such as carbocisteine below are used to facilitate mucociliary clearance and expectoration by reducing sputum viscosity but evidence of efficacy is limited.

Dornase alfa below is used to reduce sputum viscosity in children with cystic fibrosis.

Nebulised hypertonic sodium chloride (3–7%) is used to mobilise lower respiratory tract secretions in mucus consolidation (e.g cystic fibrosis). Nebulised hypertonic sodium chloride solution (3%) is used for mild to moderate acute viral bronchiolitis in infants.

Mesna p. 527 (*Mistabron*®) is used in some children with cystic fibrosis when other mucolytics have failed to reduce sputum viscosity.

Acetylcysteine p. 814 has been used to treat meconium ileus in neonates and distal intestinal obstruction syndrome in children with cystic fibrosis, but evidence of efficacy is lacking. *Gastrografin*®, or a bowel cleansing preparation containing macrogols, is usually more effective. Acetylcysteine may be used as a mucolytic to prevent further obstruction.

MUCOLYTICS

❘ Carbocisteine

- **INDICATIONS AND DOSE**
  Reduction of sputum viscosity
  ▸ BY MOUTH
  ▸ Child 2-4 years: 62.5–125 mg 4 times a day
  ▸ Child 5-11 years: 250 mg 3 times a day
  ▸ Child 12-17 years: Initially 2.25 g daily in divided doses, then reduced to 1.5 g daily in divided doses, as condition improves

IMPORTANT SAFETY INFORMATION
Mucodyne Paediatric® syrup 250 mg/5 mL has replaced the 125 mg/5 mL formulation—take care to ensure the appropriate dose is administered.

- **CONTRA-INDICATIONS** Active peptic ulceration
- **CAUTIONS** History of peptic ulceration (may disrupt the gastric mucosal barrier)
- **SIDE-EFFECTS**
- ▸ **Rare** Gastro-intestinal bleeding
- ▸ **Frequency not known** Erythema multiforme · Stevens-Johnson syndrome
- **PREGNANCY** Manufacturer advises avoid in first trimester.
- **BREAST FEEDING** No information available.
- **PRESCRIBING AND DISPENSING INFORMATION** Flavours of oral liquid formulations may include cherry, raspberry, cinnamon, or rum.

- **MEDICINAL FORMS**
  There can be variation in the licensing of different medicines containing the same drug.
  Oral solution
  ▸ **Carbocisteine** (Non-proprietary)
  Carbocisteine 75 mg per 1 ml Carbocisteine 750mg/10ml oral solution 10ml sachets sugar free sugar-free | 15 sachet (PoM) £3.85 DT price = £3.85
  ▸ **Mucodyne** (Sanofi)
  Carbocisteine 50 mg per 1 ml Mucodyne Paediatric 250mg/5ml syrup | 125 ml (PoM) £12.60
  Mucodyne 250mg/5ml syrup | 300 ml (PoM) £8.39 DT price = £8.39
  Capsule
  ▸ **Carbocisteine** (Non-proprietary)
  Carbocisteine 375 mg Carbocisteine 375mg capsules | 120 capsule (PoM) £18.98 DT price = £9.36
  ▸ **Mucodyne** (Sanofi)
  Carbocisteine 375 mg Mucodyne 375mg capsules | 120 capsule (PoM) £18.98 DT price = £9.36

3.1 Cystic fibrosis

MUCOLYTICS

❘ Dornase alfa

(Phosphorylated glycosylated recombinant human deoxyribonuclease 1 (rhDNase))

- **DRUG ACTION** Dornase alfa is a genetically engineered version of a naturally occurring human enzyme which cleaves extracellular deoxyribonucleic acid (DNA).

- **INDICATIONS AND DOSE**
  Management of cystic fibrosis patients with a forced vital capacity (FVC) of greater than 40% of predicted to improve pulmonary function
  ▸ BY INHALATION OF NEBULISED SOLUTION
  ▸ Child 5-17 years: 2500 units once daily, administered by jet nebuliser

  DOSE EQUIVALENCE AND CONVERSION
  ▸ Dornase alfa 1000 units is equivalent to 1 mg

- **SIDE-EFFECTS**
- ▸ **Rare** Chest pain · conjunctivitis · dyspepsia · dysphonia · dyspnoea · laryngitis · pharyngitis · pyrexia · rash · rhinitis · urticaria
- **PREGNANCY** No evidence of teratogenicity; manufacturer advises use only if potential benefit outweighs risk.
- **BREAST FEEDING** Amount probably too small to be harmful—manufacturer advises caution.
- **DIRECTIONS FOR ADMINISTRATION** Dornase alfa is administered by inhalation using a jet nebuliser, usually

once daily at least 1 hour before physiotherapy; however, alternate-day therapy may be as effective as daily treatment.

For use undiluted with jet nebulisers only; ultrasonic nebulisers are unsuitable.

- **PRESCRIBING AND DISPENSING INFORMATION** Not all children benefit from treatment with dornase alfa; improvement occurs within 2 weeks, but in more severely affected children a trial of 6–12 weeks may be required.

- **PATIENT AND CARER ADVICE**
Medicines for Children leaflet: Dornase alfa for cystic fibrosis
www.medicinesforchildren.org.uk/dornase-alfa-for-cystic-fibrosis

- **MEDICINAL FORMS**
There can be variation in the licensing of different medicines containing the same drug.
Nebuliser liquid
  - Pulmozyme (Roche Products Ltd)
  Dornase alfa 1 mg per 1 ml Pulmozyme 2.5mg nebuliser liquid 2.5ml ampoules | 30 ampoule PoM £496.43 DT price = £496.43

Ivacaftor
22-Mar-2017

- **INDICATIONS AND DOSE**
Treatment of cystic fibrosis in patients who have a G551D mutation in the cystic fibrosis transmembrane conductance regulator (CFTR) gene (under expert supervision)
  - BY MOUTH
  - Child 6-17 years: 150 mg every 12 hours

DOSE ADJUSTMENTS DUE TO INTERACTIONS
Manufacturer advises reduce dose to 150 mg twice a week with concurrent use of potent inhibitors of CYP3A4. Manufacturer advises reduce dose to 150 mg once daily with concurrent use of moderate inhibitors of CYP3A4.

- **CONTRA-INDICATIONS** Organ transplantation (no information available)
- **INTERACTIONS** → Appendix 1: ivacaftor
- **SIDE-EFFECTS**
  - **Common or very common** Abdominal pain · diarrhoea · dizziness · ear discomfort · headache · nasal congestion · nasopharyngitis · oropharyngeal pain · pharyngeal erythema · pharyngeal oedema · rash · rhinitis · tinnitus · upper respiratory-tract infection
  - **Uncommon** Gynaecomastia · nipple disorders · vestibular disorder
- **PREGNANCY** Manufacturer advises use only if potential benefit outweighs risk—no information available.
- **BREAST FEEDING** Manufacturer advises use only if potential benefit outweighs risk—no information available.
- **HEPATIC IMPAIRMENT** Max. 150 mg once daily in moderate impairment; in severe impairment, manufacturer recommends use only if potential benefit outweighs risk—starting dose 150 mg on alternate days, dosing interval adjusted according to clinical response and tolerability.
- **RENAL IMPAIRMENT** Caution in severe impairment.
- **PRE-TREATMENT SCREENING** If the patient's genotype is unknown, a validated genotyping method should be performed to confirm the presence of the G551D mutation in at least one allele of the CFTR gene before starting treatment.
- **MONITORING REQUIREMENTS**
  - Manufacturer advises monitor liver function before treatment, every 3 months during the first year of treatment, then annually thereafter (more frequent monitoring should be considered in patients with a history of transaminase elevations).

- Manufacturer advises baseline and follow-up ophthalmic examinations in children.
- **DIRECTIONS FOR ADMINISTRATION** Tablets should be taken with fat-containing food.
- **PRESCRIBING AND DISPENSING INFORMATION** Ivacaftor should be prescribed by a physician experienced in the treatment of cystic fibrosis.
- **PATIENT AND CARER ADVICE**
Patients or carers should be given advice on how to administer ivacaftor tablets.

Driving and skilled tasks
Manufacturer advises that patients and their carers should be counselled on the effects on driving and skilled tasks—increased risk of dizziness.

- **MEDICINAL FORMS**
There can be variation in the licensing of different medicines containing the same drug.
Tablet
CAUTIONARY AND ADVISORY LABELS 25
  - Kalydeco (Vertex Pharmaceuticals (UK) Ltd) ▼
  Ivacaftor 150 mg Kalydeco 150mg tablets | 56 tablet PoM £14,000.00

Lumacaftor with ivacaftor
22-Nov-2016

The properties listed below are those particular to the combination only. For the properties of the components please consider, ivacaftor above.

- **INDICATIONS AND DOSE**
Treatment of cystic fibrosis in patients who are homozygous for the F508del mutation in the cystic fibrosis transmembrane conductance regulator (CFTR) gene (under expert supervision)
  - BY MOUTH
  - Child 12-17 years: 400/250 mg every 12 hours

DOSE ADJUSTMENTS DUE TO INTERACTIONS
Manufacturer advises reduce initial dose to 200/125 mg daily for the first week in those also taking a potent inhibitor of CYP3A4.

DOSE EQUIVALENCE AND CONVERSION
  - Dose expressed as x/y mg of lumacaftor/ivacaftor.

- **CAUTIONS** Forced expiratory volume in 1 second (FEV_1) less than 40% of the predicted normal value—additional monitoring required at initiation of treatment · pulmonary exacerbation—no information available
- **INTERACTIONS** → Appendix 1: ivacaftor, lumacaftor
- **SIDE-EFFECTS**
  - **Common or very common** Dyspnoea · elevated transaminases (clinically significant) · flatulence · menstrual disturbances · metrorrhagia · nausea · rhinorrhoea · vomiting
  - **Uncommon** Cholestatic hepatitis · hepatic encephalopathy · hypertension
- **BREAST FEEDING** Manufacturer advises avoid—present in milk in *animal* studies.
- **HEPATIC IMPAIRMENT** Manufacturer advises reduce dose to 400/250 mg in the morning and 200/125 mg in the evening (600/375 mg total daily dose) in moderate impairment; reduce dose to 200/125 mg every 12 hours (400/250 mg total daily dose) in severe impairment. Manufacturer advises use with caution in severe impairment.
- **PRE-TREATMENT SCREENING** If the patient's genotype is unknown, a validated genotyping method should be performed to confirm the presence of the F508del mutation on both alleles of the CFTR gene before starting treatment.

- **MONITORING REQUIREMENTS** Manufacturer advises monitor blood pressure periodically during treatment.
- **DIRECTIONS FOR ADMINISTRATION** Tablets should be taken with fat-containing food.
- **PATIENT AND CARER ADVICE**
  Patients or carers should be given advice on how to administer tablets.

  Missed doses
  Manufacturer advises if a dose is more than 6 hours late, the missed dose should not be taken and the next dose should be taken at the normal time.
- **NATIONAL FUNDING/ACCESS DECISIONS**

  NICE technology appraisals (TAs)
  ▶ **Lumacaftor with ivacaftor for treating cystic fibrosis homozygous for the F508del mutation (July 2016)** NICE TA398
  Lumacaftor with ivacaftor is **not** recommended, within its marketing authorisation, for treating cystic fibrosis in patients who are homozygous for the F508del mutation in the cystic fibrosis transmembrane conductance regulator (CFTR) gene.

  Patients whose treatment was started before this guidance was published may continue treatment until they (or their carers) and their clinician consider it appropriate to stop.
  www.nice.org.uk/TA398

  Scottish Medicines Consortium (SMC) Decisions
  The *Scottish Medicines Consortium* has advised (May 2016) that lumacaftor with ivacaftor (*Orkambi*®) is **not** recommended within NHS Scotland for the treatment of cystic fibrosis in patients who are homozygous for the F508del mutation in the cystic fibrosis transmembrane conductance regulator (CFTR) gene.

- **MEDICINAL FORMS**
  There can be variation in the licensing of different medicines containing the same drug.
  Tablet
  CAUTIONARY AND ADVISORY LABELS 25
  EXCIPIENTS: May contain Propylene glycol
  ▶ **Orkambi** (Vertex Pharmaceuticals (UK) Ltd) ▼
  Ivacaftor 125 mg, Lumacaftor 200 mg Orkambi 200mg/125mg
  tablets | 112 tablet [PoM] £8,000.00

4 Cough and congestion

Aromatic inhalations, cough preparations and systemic nasal decongestants

Aromatic inhalations
Inhalations containing volatile substances such as eucalyptus oil are traditionally used to relieve congestion and ease breathing. Although the vapour may contain little of the additive it encourages deliberate inspiration of warm moist air which is often comforting. Boiling water should not be used owing to the risk of scalding.

Strong aromatic decongestants (applied as rubs or to pillows) are not recommended for infants under the age of 3 months. Sodium chloride 0.9% solution p. 561 given as nasal drops can be used to liquefy mucous secretions and relieve nasal congestion in infants and young children; administration before feeds may ease feeding difficulties caused by nasal congestion.

Cough preparations

Cough suppressants
Cough may be a symptom of an underlying disorder such as asthma, gastro-oesophageal reflux disease, or rhinitis, which should be addressed before prescribing cough suppressants. Cough may be associated with smoking or environmental pollutants. Cough can also result from bronchiectasis including that associated with cystic fibrosis; cough can also have a significant habit component. There is little evidence of any significant benefit from the use of cough suppressants in children with acute cough in ambulatory settings. Cough suppressants may cause sputum retention and this can be harmful in children with bronchiectasis.

The use of cough suppressants containing pholcodine p. 181 or similar opioid analgesics is not generally recommended in children and should be avoided in children under 6 years; the use of over-the-counter cough suppressants containing codeine phosphate p. 265 should be avoided in children under 12 years and in children of any age known to be CYP2D6 ultra-rapid metabolisers.

Sedating antihistamines are used as the cough suppressant component of many compound cough preparations on sale to the public; all tend to cause drowsiness which may reflect their main mode of action.

Demulcent and expectorant cough preparations
Simple linctus and other demulcent cough preparations containing soothing substances, such as syrup or glycerol, may temporarily relieve a dry irritating cough. These preparations have the advantage of being harmless and inexpensive and sugar-free versions are available.

Expectorants are claimed to promote expulsion of bronchial secretions, but there is no evidence that any drug can specifically facilitate expectoration.

Compound cough preparations for children are on sale to the public but should not be used in children under 6 years; the rationale for some is dubious. Care should be taken to give the correct dose and to not use more than one preparation at a time.

MHRA/CHM advice (March 2008 and February 2009)
Children under 6 years should not be given over-the-counter cough and cold medicines containing the following ingredients:

- brompheniramine, chlorphenamine maleate p. 172, diphenhydramine, doxylamine, promethazine, or triprolidine (antihistamines);
- dextromethorphan or pholcodine (cough suppressants);
- guaifenesin or ipecacuanha (expectorants);
- phenylephrine hydrochloride p. 121, pseudoephedrine hydrochloride p. 667, ephedrine hydrochloride p. 120, oxymetazoline, or xylometazoline hydrochloride p. 667 (decongestants).

Over-the-counter cough and cold medicines can be considered for children aged 6–12 years after basic principles of best care have been tried, but treatment should be restricted to five days or less. Children should not be given more than 1 cough or cold preparation at a time because different brands may contain the same active ingredient; care should be taken to give the correct dose.

Systemic nasal decongestants
Nasal congestion in children due to allergic or vasomotor rhinitis should be treated with oral antihistamines, topical nasal preparations containing corticosteroids, or topical decongestants.

There is little evidence to support the use of systemic decongestants in children.

Pseudoephedrine hydrochloride has few sympathomimetic effects, and is commonly combined with other ingredients (including antihistamines) in preparations intended for the relief of cough and cold symptoms.

3

COUGH AND COLD PREPARATIONS 〉 COUGH SUPPRESSANTS

Pholcodine

● **INDICATIONS AND DOSE**

Dry cough
▸ BY MOUTH USING LINCTUS
▸ Child 6–11 years: 2–5 mg 3–4 times a day
▸ Child 12–17 years: 5–10 mg 3–4 times a day

IMPORTANT SAFETY INFORMATION

MHRA/CHM ADVICE (MARCH 2008 AND FEBRUARY 2009) OVER-THE-COUNTER COUGH AND COLD MEDICINES FOR CHILDREN

Children under 6 years should not be given over-the-counter cough and cold medicines containing pholcodine (cough suppressant).

Over-the-counter cough and cold medicines can be considered for children aged 6–12 years after basic principles of best care have been tried, but treatment should be restricted to 5 days or less. Children should not be given more than 1 cough or cold preparation at a time because different brands may contain the same active ingredient; care should be taken to give the correct dose.

● **CONTRA-INDICATIONS** Bronchiectasis · bronchiolitis · chronic bronchitis · patients at risk of respiratory failure
● **CAUTIONS** Asthma · chronic cough · persistent cough · productive cough
● **INTERACTIONS** → Appendix 1: pholcodine
● **SIDE-EFFECTS** Confusion · constipation · dizziness · drowsiness · excitation · nausea · rash · sputum retention · vomiting
● **PREGNANCY** Manufacturer advises avoid unless potential benefit outweighs risk.
● **BREAST FEEDING** Manufacturer advises avoid unless potential benefit outweighs risk—no information available.
● **HEPATIC IMPAIRMENT** Avoid in hepatic impairment.
● **RENAL IMPAIRMENT** Use with caution in renal impairment. Avoid in severe renal impairment.
● **PRESCRIBING AND DISPENSING INFORMATION** Pholcodine is not generally recommended for children.

Flavours of oral liquid formulations may include orange.

When prepared extemporaneously, the BP states Pholcodine Linctus, BP consists of pholcodine 5 mg/5 mL in a suitable flavoured vehicle, containing citric acid monohydrate 1% and Pholcodine Linctus, Strong, BP consists of pholcodine 10 mg/5 mL in a suitable flavoured vehicle, containing citric acid monohydrate 2%

● **MEDICINAL FORMS**
There can be variation in the licensing of different medicines containing the same drug.

Oral solution
▸ Pholcodine (Non-proprietary)
  Pholcodine 1 mg per 1 ml Pholcodine 5mg/5ml linctus | 200 ml P £1.32 DT price = £1.32 CD5
  Pholcodine 5mg/5ml linctus sugar free sugar-free | 200 ml £1.34 DT price = £1.34 CD5 sugar-free | 2000 ml P £13.40 CD5
  Pholcodine 2 mg per 1 ml Pholcodine 10mg/5ml linctus strong sugar free sugar-free | 2000 ml P £10.88 DT price = £9.88 CD5
  Pholcodine 10mg/5ml linctus strong | 200 ml P £1.61 CD5
▸ Galenphol (Thornton & Ross Ltd)
  Pholcodine 400 microgram per 1 ml Galenphol Paediatric 2mg/5ml linctus sugar-free | 2000 ml P £4.50 DT price = £4.50 CD5
  Pholcodine 1 mg per 1 ml Galenphol 5mg/5ml linctus sugar-free | 2000 ml P £8.50 CD5
  Pholcodine 2 mg per 1 ml Galenphol Strong 10mg/5ml linctus sugar-free | 2000 ml P £9.88 DT price = £9.88 CD5

▸ Pavacol-D (Alliance Pharmaceuticals Ltd)
  Pholcodine 1 mg per 1 ml Pavacol-D 5mg/5ml mixture sugar-free | 150 ml P £1.69 CD5 sugar-free | 300 ml P £2.55 CD5

COUGH AND COLD PREPARATIONS 〉 OTHER

Citric acid
(Formulated as Simple Linctus)

● **INDICATIONS AND DOSE**

Cough
▸ BY MOUTH
▸ Child 1 month–11 years: 5–10 mL 3–4 times a day, this dose is for Simple Linctus, Paediatric, BP (0.625%)

Cough
▸ BY MOUTH
▸ Child 12–17 years: 5 mL 3–4 times a day, this dose is for Simple Linctus, BP (2.5%)

● **PRESCRIBING AND DISPENSING INFORMATION** Flavours of oral liquid formulations may include anise.

When prepared extemporaneously, the BP states Simple Linctus, Paediatric, BP consists of citric acid monohydrate 0.625% and Simple Linctus, BP consists of citric acid monohydrate 2.5%, both in a suitable vehicle with an anise flavour.

● **MEDICINAL FORMS**
There can be variation in the licensing of different medicines containing the same drug.

Oral solution
▸ Citric acid (Non-proprietary)
  Citric acid monohydrate 6.25 mg per 1 ml Simple linctus paediatric sugar free sugar-free | 2000 ml GSL £12.50
  Simple linctus paediatric | 200 ml GSL £1.05–£1.13 DT price = £1.05
  Citric acid monohydrate 25 mg per 1 ml Simple linctus sugar free sugar-free | 200 ml GSL £1.25 DT price = £0.89 sugar-free | 2000 ml GSL £8.90
  Simple linctus | 200 ml GSL £0.93 DT price = £0.93

MENTHOL AND DERIVATIVES

Eucalyptus with menthol

● **INDICATIONS AND DOSE**

Aromatic inhalation for relief of nasal congestion
▸ BY INHALATION
▸ Child: Add one teaspoonful to a pint of hot, **not** boiling, water and inhale the vapour

● **PRESCRIBING AND DISPENSING INFORMATION** When prepared extemporaneously, the BP states Menthol and Eucalyptus Inhalation, BP 1980 consists of racementhol or levomenthol 2 g, eucalyptus oil 10 mL, light magnesium carbonate 7 g, water to 100 mL.

Not recommended (applied as a rub or to pillows) for infants under the age of 3 months.

● **PROFESSION SPECIFIC INFORMATION**

Dental practitioners' formulary
Menthol and Eucalyptus Inhalation BP, 1980 may be prescribed.

● **MEDICINAL FORMS**
There can be variation in the licensing of different medicines containing the same drug.

Inhalation vapour
▸ Eucalyptus with menthol (Non-proprietary)
  Menthol 20 mg per 1 ml, Magnesium carbonate light 70 mg per 1 ml, Eucalyptus oil 100 microlitre per 1 ml Menthol and Eucalyptus inhalation | 100 ml GSL £1.36 DT price = £1.36

RESINS

Benzoin tincture

(Friars' Balsam)

- ● **INDICATIONS AND DOSE**
  Aromatic inhalation for relief of nasal congestion
  - ▶ BY INHALATION
  - ▶ Child: Add 5 mL to a pint of hot, **not** boiling, water and inhale the vapour; repeat after 4 hours if necessary

- ● SIDE-EFFECTS Allergic contact dermatitis
- ● PRESCRIBING AND DISPENSING INFORMATION Not recommended (applied as a rub or to pillows) for infants under 3 months.
  When prepared extemporaneously, the BP states Benzoin Tincture, Compound, BP consists of balsamic acids approx. 4.5%.

- ● MEDICINAL FORMS
  There can be variation in the licensing of different medicines containing the same drug.
  Liquid
  CAUTIONARY AND ADVISORY LABELS 15
  - ▶ Benzoin tincture (Non-proprietary)
    Balsamic acids 16.5 mg per 1 ml Benzoin tincture | 500 ml [GSL]
    £9.95 DT price = £9.95

5 Respiratory depression, respiratory distress syndrome and apnoea

Respiratory stimulants

Respiratory stimulants

Respiratory stimulants (analeptic drugs), such as caffeine citrate p. 183, reduce the frequency of neonatal apnoea, and the need for mechanical ventilation during the first 7 days of treatment. They are typically used in the management of very preterm neonates, and continued until a corrected gestational age of 34 to 35 weeks is reached (or longer if necessary). They should only be given under **expert supervision** in hospital; it is important to rule out any underlying disorder, such as seizures, hypoglycaemia, or infection, causing respiratory exhaustion before starting treatment with a respiratory stimulant.

Pulmonary surfactants

Pulmonary surfactants derived from animal lungs, beractant below and poractant alfa below are used to prevent and treat respiratory distress syndrome (hyaline membrane disease) in neonates and preterm neonates. Prophylactic use of a pulmonary surfactant may reduce the need for mechanical ventilation and is more effective than 'rescue treatment' in preterm neonates of 29 weeks or less corrected gestational age. Pulmonary surfactants may also be of benefit in neonates with meconium aspiration syndrome or intrapartum streptococcal infection. Pulmonary immaturity with surfactant deficit is the commonest reason for respiratory failure in the neonate, especially in those of less than 30 weeks corrected gestational age. Betamethasone p. 418 given to the mother (at least 12 hours but preferably 48 hours) before delivery substantially enhances pulmonary maturity in the neonate.

PULMONARY SURFACTANTS

Beractant

- ● **INDICATIONS AND DOSE**
  Treatment of respiratory distress syndrome in preterm neonates, birth-weight over 700 g (specialist use only)
  - ▶ BY ENDOTRACHEAL TUBE
  - ▶ Preterm neonate: 100 mg/kg, preferably administer within 8 hours of birth; dose may be repeated within 48 hours at intervals of at least 6 hours for up to 4 doses.

  Prophylaxis of respiratory distress syndrome in preterm neonates (specialist use only)
  - ▶ BY ENDOTRACHEAL TUBE
  - ▶ Neonate up to 32 weeks corrected gestational age: 100 mg/kg, preferably administer within 15 minutes of birth; dose may be repeated within 48 hours at intervals of at least 6 hours for up to 4 doses.

  DOSE EQUIVALENCE AND CONVERSION
  - ▶ Phospholipid 100 mg/kg is equivalent to a volume of 4 mL/kg.

- ● CAUTIONS Consult product literature
- ● SIDE-EFFECTS
  - ▶ Rare Bradycardia · decreased oxygen saturation · pulmonary haemorrhage
  - ▶ Frequency not known Hyperoxia · intracranial haemorrhage · obstruction of the endotracheal tube by mucous secretions

- ● MEDICINAL FORMS
  There can be variation in the licensing of different medicines containing the same drug.
  Liquid
  - ▶ Survanta (AbbVie Ltd)
    Phospholipids (as Beractant) 25 mg per 1 ml Survanta 200mg/8ml endotracheopulmonary suspension bottles | 1 bottle [PoM] £306.43

Poractant alfa

- ● **INDICATIONS AND DOSE**
  Treatment of respiratory distress syndrome in neonates, birth weight over 700 g (specialist use only)
  - ▶ BY ENDOTRACHEAL TUBE
  - ▶ Neonate: 100–200 mg/kg, then 100 mg/kg every 12 hours if required, maximum 300–400 mg/kg per course.

  Prophylaxis of respiratory distress syndrome (specialist use only)
  - ▶ BY ENDOTRACHEAL TUBE
  - ▶ Neonate 24 weeks to 31 weeks corrected gestational age: 100–200 mg/kg, administer soon after birth, preferably within 15 minutes, then 100 mg/kg after 6–12 hours if required, then 100 mg/kg after 12 hours if required, and if neonate still intubated. Max 300–400 mg/kg per course.

- ● CAUTIONS Consult product literature
- ● SIDE-EFFECTS
  - ▶ Rare Bradycardia · decreased oxygen saturation · hypotension · pulmonary haemorrhage
  - ▶ Frequency not known Hyperoxia · intracranial haemorrhage · obstruction of the endotracheal tube by mucous secretions

- **MEDICINAL FORMS**
  There can be variation in the licensing of different medicines containing the same drug.
  Liquid
  ▸ Curosurf (Chiesi Ltd)
    Phospholipids (as Poractant alfa) 80 mg per 1 ml Curosurf 240mg/3ml endotracheopulmonary suspension vials | 1 vial [PoM] £547.40 (Hospital only)
    Curosurf 120mg/1.5ml endotracheopulmonary suspension vials | 1 vial [PoM] £281.64 (Hospital only)

5.1 Neonatal apnoea

XANTHINES

Caffeine citrate

24-Feb-2016

- **INDICATIONS AND DOSE**
  Neonatal apnoea (specialist supervision in hospital)
  ▸ BY MOUTH, OR BY INTRAVENOUS INFUSION
  ▸ Neonate: Initially 20 mg/kg, administered over 30 minutes if given by intravenous infusion, then 5 mg/kg once daily, administered over 10 minutes if given by intravenous infusion, started 24 hours after initial dose; increased if necessary to 10 mg/kg daily.

  DOSE EQUIVALENCE AND CONVERSION
  ▸ Caffeine citrate 2 mg ≡ caffeine base 1 mg
  PHARMACOKINETICS
  Caffeine citrate is well absorbed when given orally.

- **UNLICENSED USE** [EvGr] Caffeine citrate loading doses in the BNF *for children* may differ to those in product literature. ⟨E⟩

  > **IMPORTANT SAFETY INFORMATION**
  > MHRA/CHM ADVICE: SAFE PRACTICE
  > From August 2013, all licensed preparations of caffeine are required to be labelled as caffeine citrate. To minimise the risk of dosing errors, **always state dose in terms of caffeine citrate when prescribing caffeine**. Some stock packaged as caffeine base.

- **CAUTIONS** Cardiovascular disease · gastro-oesophageal reflux · rhythm disorder · seizure disorders
- **INTERACTIONS** → Appendix 1: caffeine citrate
- **SIDE-EFFECTS**
- **Common or very common** Fluid and electrolyte imbalance · hyperglycaemia · hypertension · hypoglycaemia · irritability · restlessness · tachycardia
- **Frequency not known** Gastro-oesophageal reflux
- **HEPATIC IMPAIRMENT** Manufacturer advises caution with impaired hepatic function.
- **RENAL IMPAIRMENT** Reduced daily maintenance dose required—consult product literature. Manufacturer advises caution with impaired renal function—potential for accumulation of caffeine.
- **MONITORING REQUIREMENTS**
- [EvGr] The therapeutic range for plasma-caffeine concentration is usually 10–20 mg/litre (50–100 micromol/litre), but a concentration of 25–35 mg/litre (130–180 micromol/litre) may be required. Signs of toxicity only normally occur at concentrations greater than 50 mg/litre (260 micromol/litre). ⟨D⟩
- Monitor for recurrence of apnoea for 1 week after stopping treatment.
- **DIRECTIONS FOR ADMINISTRATION** Caffeine citrate injection may be administered *by mouth* or *by intravenous infusion*.

- **NATIONAL FUNDING/ACCESS DECISIONS**
  Scottish Medicines Consortium (SMC) Decisions
  The *Scottish Medicines Consortium* has advised (September 2013) that *Peyona*® is accepted for use within NHS Scotland for the treatment of primary apnoea of premature newborns only whilst *Peyona*® is available at the price agreed in the patient access scheme.

- **MEDICINAL FORMS**
  There can be variation in the licensing of different medicines containing the same drug. Forms available from special-order manufacturers include: oral suspension, oral solution
  Solution for injection
  ▸ Caffeine citrate (Non-proprietary)
    Caffeine citrate 10 mg per 1 ml Caffeine citrate 10mg/1ml solution for injection ampoules | 10 ampoule [PoM] £48.82
  Solution for infusion
  ▸ Peyona (Chiesi Ltd)
    Caffeine citrate 20 mg per 1 ml Peyona 20mg/ml solution for infusion ampoules | 10 ampoule [PoM] £172.50 (Hospital only)
  Oral solution
  ▸ Caffeine citrate (Non-proprietary)
    Caffeine citrate 10 mg per 1 ml Caffeine citrate 50mg/5ml oral solution | 5 ml [PoM] £24.41-£25.85 DT price = £25.13

Chapter 4
Nervous system

CONTENTS

1 Epilepsy and other seizure disorders

Epilepsy

26-May-2017

Control of the epilepsies

The object of treatment is to prevent the occurrence of seizures by maintaining an effective dose of one or more antiepileptic drugs. Careful adjustment of doses is necessary, starting with low doses and increasing gradually until seizures are controlled or there are significant adverse effects.

When choosing an antiepileptic drug, the presenting epilepsy syndrome should first be considered. If the syndrome is not clear, the seizure type should determine the choice of treatment. Concomitant medication, co-morbidity, age, and sex should be taken into account.

The frequency of administration is often determined by the plasma-drug half-life, and should be kept as low as possible to encourage better adherence. Most antiepileptics, when used in usual dosage, can be given twice daily. Lamotrigine p. 203, perampanel p. 197, phenobarbital p. 208 and phenytoin p. 198, which have long half-lives, can be given as a daily dose at bedtime. However, with large doses, some antiepileptics may need to be given three times daily to avoid adverse effects associated with high peak plasma-drug concentrations. Young children metabolise some antiepileptics more rapidly than adults and therefore may require more frequent doses and a higher amount per kilogram body-weight.

Management

When monotherapy with a first-line antiepileptic drug has failed, monotherapy with a second drug should be tried; the diagnosis should be checked before starting an alternative drug if the first drug showed lack of efficacy. The change from one antiepileptic drug to another should be cautious, slowly withdrawing the first drug only when the new regimen has been established. Combination therapy with two or more antiepileptic drugs may be necessary, but the concurrent use of antiepileptic drugs increases the risk of adverse effects and drug interactions. If combination therapy does not bring about worthwhile benefits, revert to the regimen (monotherapy or combination therapy) that provided the best balance between tolerability and efficacy. A single antiepileptic drug should be prescribed wherever possible and will achieve seizure control for the majority of children.

MHRA/CHM advice: Antiepileptic drugs: new advice on switching between different manufacturers' products for a particular drug (November 2013)
The CHM has reviewed spontaneous adverse reactions received by the MHRA and publications that reported potential harm arising from switching of antiepileptic drugs in patients previously stabilised on a branded product to a generic. The CHM concluded that reports of loss of seizure control and/or worsening of side-effects around the time of switching between products could be explained as chance associations, but that a causal role of switching could not be ruled out in all cases. The following guidance has been issued to help minimise risk:

- Different antiepileptic drugs vary considerably in their characteristics, which influences the risk of whether switching between different manufacturers' products of a particular drug may cause adverse effects or loss of seizure control;
- Antiepileptic drugs have been divided into three risk-based categories to help healthcare professionals decide whether it is necessary to maintain continuity of supply of a specific manufacturer's product. These categories are listed below;
- If it is felt desirable for a patient to be maintained on a specific manufacturer's product this should be prescribed either by specifying a brand name, or by using the generic drug name and name of the manufacturer (otherwise known as the Marketing Authorisation Holder);
- This advice relates only to antiepileptic drug use for treatment of epilepsy; it does not apply to their use in other indications (e.g. mood stabilisation, neuropathic pain);
- Please report on a Yellow Card any suspected adverse reactions to antiepileptic drugs;
- Dispensing pharmacists should ensure the continuity of supply of a particular product when the prescription specifies it. If the prescribed product is unavailable, it may be necessary to dispense a product from a different manufacturer to maintain continuity of treatment of that antiepileptic drug. Such cases should be discussed and agreed with both the prescriber and patient (or carer);
- Usual dispensing practice can be followed when a specific product is not stated.

Category 1

Phenytoin, carbamazepine p. 189, phenobarbital, primidone p. 209. For these drugs, doctors are advised to ensure that their patient is maintained on a specific manufacturer's product.

Category 2

Valproate, lamotrigine, perampanel, rufinamide, clobazam p. 210, clonazepam p. 211, oxcarbazepine p. 197, eslicarbazepine acetate, zonisamide p. 207, topiramate p. 204. For these drugs, the need for continued supply of a particular manufacturer's product should be based on clinical judgement and consultation with the patient and/or carer taking into account factors such as seizure frequency and treatment history.

Category 3

Levetiracetam p. 196, lacosamide p. 193, tiagabine p. 203, gabapentin p. 192, pregabalin, ethosuximide p. 191, vigabatrin p. 206. For these drugs, it is usually unnecessary to ensure that patients are maintained on a specific manufacturer's product unless there are specific concerns such as patient anxiety, and risk of confusion or dosing errors Interactions.

Antiepileptic hypersensitivity syndrome

Antiepileptic hypersensitivity syndrome is a rare but potentially fatal syndrome associated with some antiepileptic drugs (carbamazepine, lacosamide, lamotrigine, oxcarbazepine, phenobarbital, phenytoin, primidone, and rufinamide p. 200); rarely cross-sensitivity occurs between some of these antiepileptic drugs. Some other antiepileptics (eslicarbazepine acetate, stiripentol p. 203, and zonisamide) have a theoretical risk. The symptoms usually start between 1 and 8 weeks of exposure; fever, rash, and lymphadenopathy are most commonly seen. Other systemic signs include liver dysfunction, haematological, renal, and pulmonary abnormalities, vasculitis, and multi-organ failure. If signs or symptoms of hypersensitivity syndrome occur, the drug should be withdrawn immediately, the child should not be re-exposed, and expert advice should be sought.

Risk of suicidal thoughts and behaviour

The MHRA has advised (August 2008) that all antiepileptic drugs are associated with a small increased risk of suicidal thoughts and behaviour. Symptoms may occur as early as one week after starting treatment. Children and their parents or carers should be advised to seek medical advice if the child develops any mood changes, distressing thoughts, or feelings about suicide or harming themselves, and should be referred for appropriate treatment if necessary.

Interactions

Interactions between antiepileptics are complex and may increase toxicity without a corresponding increase in antiepileptic effect. Interactions are usually caused by hepatic enzyme induction or inhibition; displacement from protein binding sites is not usually a problem. These interactions are highly variable and unpredictable.

Withdrawal

Antiepileptic drugs should be withdrawn under specialist supervision. Avoid abrupt withdrawal, particularly of barbiturates and benzodiazepines, because this can precipitate severe rebound seizures. Reduction in dosage should be gradual and, in the case of barbiturates, withdrawal of the drug may take months.

The decision to withdraw antiepileptic drugs from a seizure-free child, and its timing, is often difficult and depends on individual circumstances. Even in children who have been seizure-free for several years, there is a significant risk of seizure recurrence on drug withdrawal.

Drugs should be gradually withdrawn over at least 2–3 months by reducing the daily dose by 10–25% at intervals of 1–2 weeks. Benzodiazepines may need to be withdrawn over 6 months or longer.

In children receiving several antiepileptic drugs, only one drug should be withdrawn at a time.

Monitoring

Routine measurement of plasma concentrations of antiepileptic drugs is not usually justified, because the target concentration ranges are arbitrary and often vary between individuals. However, plasma-drug concentrations may be measured in children with worsening seizures, status epilepticus, suspected non-compliance, or suspected toxicity. Similarly, haematological and biochemical monitoring should not be undertaken unless clinically indicated.

Plasma concentration of some medications may change during pregnancy and monitoring may be required (see under *Pregnancy*).

Driving

If a driver has a seizure (of any type) they must stop driving immediately and inform the Driver and Vehicle Licensing Agency (DVLA).

Patients who have had a first unprovoked epileptic seizure or a single isolated seizure must not drive for 6 months; driving may then be resumed, provided the patient has been assessed by a specialist as fit to drive and investigations do not suggest a risk of further seizures.

Patients with established epilepsy may drive a motor vehicle provided they are not a danger to the public and are compliant with treatment and follow up. To continue driving, these patients must be seizure-free for at least one year (or have a pattern of seizures established for one year where there is no influence on their level of consciousness or the ability to act); also, they must not have a history of unprovoked seizures.

Patients who have had a *seizure while asleep* are not permitted to drive for one year from the date of each seizure unless:

- a history or pattern of sleep seizures occurring **only** ever while asleep has been established over the course of at least one year from the date of the first sleep seizure; or
- an established pattern of purely asleep seizures can be demonstrated over the course of three years if the patient has previously had seizures whilst awake (or awake and asleep).

The DVLA recommends that patients should not drive during medication changes or withdrawal of antiepileptic drugs, and for 6 months after their last dose. If a seizure occurs due to a prescribed change or withdrawal of epilepsy treatment, the patient will have their driving license revoked for 1 year; relicensing may be considered earlier if treatment has been reinstated for 6 months and no further seizures have occurred.

Pregnancy

Young women of child-bearing potential should discuss with a specialist the impact of both epilepsy, and its treatment, on the outcome of pregnancy.

There is an increased risk of teratogenicity associated with the use of antiepileptic drugs (especially if used during the first trimester and particularly if the patient takes two or more antiepileptic drugs). Valproate is associated with the highest risk of major and minor congenital malformations (in particular neural tube defects), and long-term developmental disorders. There is also an increased risk of teratogenicity with phenytoin, primidone, phenobarbital, lamotrigine, and carbamazepine. Topiramate carries an increased risk of cleft palate if taken in the first trimester of pregnancy. There is not enough evidence to establish the risk of teratogenicity with other antiepileptic drugs.

Prescribers should also consider carefully the choice of antiepileptic therapy in pre-pubescent girls who may later become pregnant. Young women of child-bearing potential who take antiepileptic drugs should be given advice about the need for an effective contraception method to avoid unplanned pregnancy. Some antiepileptic drugs can reduce the efficacy of hormonal contraceptives, and the efficacy of some antiepileptics may be affected by hormonal contraception.

Young women who want to become pregnant should be referred to a specialist for advice in advance of conception. For some women, the severity of seizure or the seizure type may not pose a serious threat, and drug withdrawal may be considered; therapy may be resumed after the first trimester. If treatment with antiepileptic drugs must continue throughout pregnancy, then monotherapy is preferable at the lowest effective dose.

Once an unplanned pregnancy is discovered it is usually too late for changes to be made to the treatment regimen; the risk of harm to the mother and fetus from convulsive seizures outweighs the risk of continued therapy. The likelihood of a woman who is taking antiepileptic drugs having a baby with no malformations is at least 90%, and it is important that women do not stop taking essential treatment because of concern over harm to the fetus. To reduce the risk of neural tube defects, folate supplementation is advised before conception and throughout the first trimester. In the case of sodium valproate p. 200 and valproic acid p. 205 an urgent consultation is required to reconsider the benefits and risks of valproate therapy.

The concentration of antiepileptic drugs in the plasma can change during pregnancy. Doses of phenytoin, carbamazepine, and lamotrigine should be adjusted on the basis of plasma-drug concentration monitoring; the dose of other antiepileptic drugs should be monitored carefully during pregnancy and after birth, and adjustments made on a clinical basis. Plasma-drug concentration monitoring during pregnancy is also useful to check compliance. Additionally, in patients taking topiramate or levetiracetam, it is recommended that fetal growth should be monitored. Women who have seizures in the second half of pregnancy should be assessed for eclampsia before any change is made to antiepileptic treatment. Status epilepticus should be treated according to the standard protocol.

Routine injection of vitamin K at birth minimises the risk of neonatal haemorrhage associated with antiepileptics.

Withdrawal effects in the newborn may occur with some antiepileptic drugs, in particular benzodiazepines and phenobarbital, and can take several days to diminish.

Epilepsy and Pregnancy Register
All pregnant women with epilepsy, whether taking medication or not, should be encouraged to notify the UK Epilepsy and Pregnancy Register (Tel: 0800 389 1248).

Breast-feeding
Young women taking antiepileptic monotherapy should generally be encouraged to breast-feed; if a woman is on combination therapy or if there are other risk factors, such as premature birth, specialist advice should be sought.

All infants should be monitored for sedation, feeding difficulties, adequate weight gain, and developmental milestones. Infants should also be monitored for adverse effects associated with the antiepileptic drug particularly with newer antiepileptics, if the antiepileptic is readily transferred into breast-milk causing high infant serum-drug concentrations (e.g. ethosuximide, lamotrigine, primidone, and zonisamide), or if slower metabolism in the infant causes drugs to accumulate (e.g. phenobarbital and lamotrigine). Serum-drug concentration monitoring should be undertaken in breast-fed infants if suspected adverse reactions develop; if toxicity develops it may be necessary to introduce formula feeds to limit the infant's drug exposure, or to wean the infant off breast-milk altogether.

Primidone, phenobarbital, and the benzodiazepines are associated with an established risk of drowsiness in breast-fed babies and caution is required.

Withdrawal effects may occur in infants if a mother suddenly stops breast-feeding, particularly if she is taking phenobarbital, primidone, or lamotrigine.

Focal seizures with or without secondary generalisation

Carbamazepine p. 189 and lamotrigine p. 203 are the drugs of choice for focal seizures; levetiracetam p. 196, oxcarbazepine p. 197 and sodium valproate p. 200 can be considered if these are unsuitable. These drugs may also be used as adjunctive treatment. Other adjunctive options include clobazam p. 210, gabapentin p. 192, and topiramate p. 204. If adjunctive treatment is ineffective or not tolerated, a tertiary specialist should be consulted who may consider eslicarbazepine acetate, lacosamide p. 193, phenobarbital p. 208, phenytoin p. 198, pregabalin tiagabine p. 203, vigabatrin p. 206, and zonisamide p. 207.

Generalised seizures

Tonic-clonic seizures
The drug of choice for newly diagnosed tonic-clonic seizures in children is sodium valproate (except in female patients, see *Valproate* below), or lamotrigine where sodium valproate is unsuitable (but may exacerbate myoclonic seizures). In children with established epilepsy with generalised tonic-clonic seizures only, lamotrigine may be prescribed as the first-line choice. Carbamazepine or oxcarbazepine can also be considered but may exacerbate myoclonic or absence seizures. Clobazam, lamotrigine, levetiracetam, sodium valproate, or topiramate may be used as adjunctive treatment if monotherapy is ineffective or not tolerated.

Absence seizures
Ethosuximide p. 191 and sodium valproate (except in female patients, see *Valproate* below) are the drugs of choice for absence seizures and syndromes; lamotrigine can be used if these are unsuitable, ineffective or not tolerated. Sodium valproate should be used as the first choice if there is a high risk of generalised tonic-clonic seizures. A combination of any two of these drugs may be used if monotherapy is ineffective. Second-line therapy includes clobazam, clonazepam p. 211, levetiracetam, topiramate or zonisamide which may be considered by a tertiary specialist if adjunctive treatment fails. Carbamazepine, gabapentin, oxcarbazepine, phenytoin, pregabalin, tiagabine, and vigabatrin are not recommended in absence seizures or syndromes.

Myoclonic seizures
Myoclonic seizures (myoclonic jerks) occur in a variety of syndromes, and response to treatment varies considerably. Sodium valproate is the drug of choice (except in female patients, see *Valproate* below); consider levetiracetam or topiramate if sodium valproate is unsuitable (but consider the less favourable side-effect profile of topiramate). A combination of two of these drugs may be used if monotherapy is ineffective or poorly tolerated. Second-line therapy includes clobazam, clonazepam, piracetam or zonisamide which should be prescribed under the supervision of a tertiary specialist. Carbamazepine, gabapentin, oxcarbazepine, phenytoin, pregabalin, tiagabine, and vigabatrin are not recommended for the treatment of myoclonic seizures.

Tonic and atonic seizures
Tonic or atonic seizures are treated with sodium valproate (except in female patients, see *Valproate* below); lamotrigine can be considered as adjunctive treatment if sodium valproate is ineffective or not tolerated. If adjunctive treatment fails, a tertiary specialist should be consulted who may consider rufinamide p. 200 or topiramate. Carbamazepine, gabapentin, oxcarbazepine, pregabalin,

tiagabine, and vigabatrin are not recommended in atonic or tonic seizures.

Epilepsy syndromes

Infantile spasms

Vigabatrin is the drug of choice for infantile spasms associated with tuberous sclerosis. Corticosteroids, such as prednisolone p. 421 or tetracosactide p. 452, are second-line options if vigabatrin is ineffective. In spasms of other causes, vigabatrin, prednisolone or tetracosactide can be considered as first-line options. A tertiary specialist should be consulted before treating infantile spasms.

Dravet syndrome

Sodium valproate (except in female patients, see *Valproate* below) or topiramate is the treatment of choice in Dravet syndrome. Clobazam or stiripentol p. 203 may be considered as adjunctive treatment. Carbamazepine, gabapentin, lamotrigine, oxcarbazepine, phenytoin, pregabalin, tiagabine, and vigabatrin should not be used as they may exacerbate myoclonic seizures. A tertiary specialist should be involved in decisions regarding treatment of Dravet syndrome.

Lennox-Gastaut syndrome

Sodium valproate is the first-line drug for treating Lennox-Gastaut syndrome (except in female patients, see *Valproate* below); lamotrigine can be used as adjunctive treatment if sodium valproate is ineffective or not tolerated. Rufinamide and topiramate may be considered by tertiary epilepsy specialists. Carbamazepine, gabapentin, oxcarbazepine, pregabalin, tiagabine, and vigabatrin should not be used. Felbamate [unlicensed] may be used in tertiary specialist centres when all other treatment options have failed.

Landau-Kleffner syndrome

Always discuss with or refer to tertiary epilepsy specialists.

Neonatal seizures

Seizures can occur before delivery, but they are most common up to 24 hours after birth. Seizures in neonates occur as a result of biochemical disturbances, inborn errors of metabolism, hypoxic ischaemic encephalopathy, drug withdrawal, meningitis, stroke, cerebral haemorrhage or malformation, or severe jaundice (kernicterus).

Seizures caused by biochemical imbalance and those in neonates with inherited abnormal pyridoxine or biotin metabolism should be corrected by treating the underlying cause. Seizures caused by drug withdrawal following intra-uterine exposure are treated with a drug withdrawal regimen.

Phenobarbital can be used to manage neonatal seizures where there is a risk of recurrence; phenytoin is an alternative. Midazolam p. 215 and **rectal** paraldehyde p. 215 may also be useful in the management of acute neonatal seizures. Lidocaine hydrochloride p. 796 may be used if other treatments are unsuccessful; lidocaine hydrochloride should not be given to neonates who have received phenytoin infusion because of the risk of cardiac toxicity.

Antiepileptic drugs

Carbamazepine and related antiepileptics

Carbamazepine is a drug of choice for simple and complex focal seizures and is a first-line treatment option for generalised tonic-clonic seizures. It can be used as adjunctive treatment for focal seizures when monotherapy has been ineffective. It is essential to initiate carbamazepine therapy at a low dose and build this up slowly in small increments every 3–7 days. Carbamazepine may exacerbate tonic, atonic, myoclonic and absence seizures and is therefore not recommended if these seizures are present.

Oxcarbazepine is not recommended in tonic, atonic, absence or myoclonic seizures due to the risk of seizure exacerbation.

Ethosuximide

Ethosuximide is a first-line treatment option for absence seizures, and may be used as adjunctive treatment when monotherapy has failed.

Gabapentin

Gabapentin p. 192 is used as adjunctive therapy for the treatment of focal seizures with or without secondary generalisation; it is licensed as monotherapy in children over 12 years. It is not recommended if tonic, atonic, absence or myoclonic seizures are present.

Lamotrigine

Lamotrigine p. 203 is an antiepileptic drug recommended as a first-line treatment for focal seizures and primary and secondary generalised tonic-clonic seizures. It is also licensed as monotherapy for typical absence seizures in children (but efficacy may not be maintained in all children). It may be tried as an adjunctive treatment for atonic and tonic seizures if first-line treatment has failed [unlicensed]. Myoclonic seizures may be exacerbated by lamotrigine and it can cause serious rashes; dose recommendations should be adhered to closely.

Lamotrigine is used either as sole treatment or as an adjunct to treatment with other antiepileptic drugs. Valproate increases plasma-lamotrigine concentration, whereas the enzyme-inducing antiepileptics reduce it; care is therefore required in choosing the appropriate initial dose and subsequent titration. When the potential for interaction is not known, treatment should be initiated with lower doses, such as those used with valproate.

Levetiracetam and brivaracetam

Levetiracetam p. 196 is used for monotherapy and adjunctive treatment of focal seizures with or without secondary generalisation, and for adjunctive treatment of myoclonic seizures in children with juvenile myoclonic epilepsy and primary generalised tonic-clonic seizures. Levetiracetam may be prescribed alone and in combination for the treatment of myoclonic seizures, and under specialist supervision for absence seizures [both unlicensed].

Brivaracetam p. 188 is used as adjunctive therapy in the treatment of partial-onset seizures with or without secondary generalisation.

Phenobarbital and primidone

Phenobarbital p. 208 is effective for tonic-clonic, focal seizures and neonatal seizures but may cause behavioural disturbances and hyperkinesia. It may be tried for atypical absence, atonic, and tonic seizures. For therapeutic purposes phenobarbital and *phenobarbital sodium* should be considered equivalent in effect. Rebound seizures may be a problem on withdrawal.

Primidone p. 209 is largely converted to phenobarbital and this is probably responsible for its antiepileptic action. It is used rarely in children. A low initial dose of primidone is essential.

Phenytoin

Phenytoin p. 198 is licensed for tonic-clonic and focal seizures but may exacerbate absence or myoclonic seizures and should be avoided if theses seizures are present. It has a narrow therapeutic index and the relationship between dose and plasma-drug concentration is non-linear; small dosage increases in some patients may produce large increases in plasma concentration with acute toxic side-effects. Similarly, a few missed doses or a small change in drug absorption may result in a marked change in plasma-drug concentration. Monitoring of plasma-drug concentration improves dosage adjustment.

When only parenteral administration is possible, fosphenytoin sodium p. 191, a pro-drug of phenytoin, may be convenient to give. Whereas phenytoin should be given intravenously only, fosphenytoin sodium may also be given by intramuscular injection.

4

Nervous system

Rufinamide

Rufinamide p. 200 is licensed for the adjunctive treatment of seizures in Lennox-Gastaut syndrome. It may be considered by a tertiary specialist for the treatment of refractory tonic or atonic seizures [unlicensed].

Topiramate

Topiramate p. 204 can be given alone or as adjunctive treatment in generalised tonic-clonic seizures or focal seizures. It can also be used for absence, tonic and atonic seizures under specialist supervision and as an option in myoclonic seizures [all unlicensed]. Topiramate is also licensed for prophylaxis of migraine.

Valproate

Valproate (as either sodium valproate p. 200 or valproic acid p. 205) is effective in controlling tonic-clonic seizures, particularly in primary generalised epilepsy. It is a drug of choice in primary generalised tonic-clonic seizures, focal seizures, generalised absences and myoclonic seizures, and can be tried in atypical absence seizures. It is recommended as a first-line option in atonic and tonic seizures. Valproate should generally be avoided in children under 2 years especially with other antiepileptics, but it may be required in infants with continuing epileptic tendency. Sodium valproate has widespread metabolic effects, and monitoring of liver function tests and full blood count is essential. Valproate should not be used in female children, in females of childbearing potential, and pregnant females, unless alternative treatments are ineffective or not tolerated, becuase of its high teratogenic potential; the benefits and risks of valproate therapy should be carefully reconsidered at regular treatment reviews, see *Important safety information* in the sodium valproate and valproic acid drug monographs. Plasma-valproate concentrations are not a useful index of efficacy, therefore routine monitoring is unhelpful.

Zonisamide

Zonisamide p. 207 can be used as an adjunctive treatment for refractory focal seizures with or without secondary generalisation in children and adolescents aged 6 years and above. It can also be used under the supervision of a specialist for refractory absence and myoclonic seizures [unlicensed indications].

Benzodiazepines

Clobazam p. 210 may be used as adjunctive therapy in the treatment of generalised tonic-clonic and refractory focal seizures. It may be prescribed under the care of a specialist for refractory absence and myoclonic seizures. Clonazepam p. 211 may be prescribed by a specialist for refractory absence and myoclonic seizures, but its sedative side-effects may be prominent.

Other drugs

Acetazolamide p. 655, a carbonic anhydrase inhibitor, has a specific role in treating epilepsy associated with menstruation. Piracetam is used as adjunctive treatment for cortical myoclonus.

Status epilepticus

Convulsive status epilepticus

Immediate measures to manage status epilepticus include positioning the child to avoid injury, supporting respiration including the provision of oxygen, maintaining blood pressure, and the correction of any hypoglycaemia. Pyridoxine hydrochloride p. 600 should be administered if the status epilepticus is caused by pyridoxine deficiency.

Seizures lasting 5 minutes should be treated urgently with buccal midazolam p. 215 or intravenous lorazepam p. 214 (repeated once after 10 minutes if seizures recur or fail to respond). Intravenous diazepam p. 212 is effective but it carries a high risk of venous thrombophlebitis (reduced by using an emulsion formulation of diazepam injection).

Patients should be monitored for respiratory depression and hypotension.

Important

If, after initial treatment with benzodiazepines, seizures recur or fail to respond 25 minutes after onset, phenytoin sodium should be used, or if the child is on regular phenytoin, give phenobarbital sodium intravenously over 5 minutes; the paediatric intensive care unit should be contacted. Paraldehyde p. 215 can be given after starting phenytoin infusion.

If these measures fail to control seizures 45 minutes after onset, anaesthesia with thiopental sodium p. 214 should be instituted with full intensive care support.

Phenytoin sodium can be given by intravenous infusion over 20 minutes, followed by the maintenance dosage if appropriate.

Paraldehyde given rectally causes little respiratory depression and is therefore useful where facilities for resuscitation are poor.

Non-convulsive status epilepticus

The urgency to treat non-convulsive status epilepticus depends on the severity of the childs condition. If there is incomplete loss of awareness, oral antiepileptic therapy should be continued or restarted. Children who fail to respond to oral antiepileptic therapy or have complete lack of awareness can be treated in the same way as for convulsive status epilepticus, although anaesthesia is rarely needed.

Febrile convulsions

Brief febrile convulsions need no specific treatment; antipyretic medication (e.g. paracetamol p. 260), is commonly used to reduce fever and prevent further convulsions but evidence to support this practice is lacking. *Prolonged febrile convulsions* (those lasting 5 minutes or longer), or *recurrent febrile convulsions* without recovery must be treated actively (as for convulsive status epilepticus).

Long-term anticonvulsant prophylaxis for febrile convulsions is rarely indicated.

ANTIEPILEPTICS

Brivaracetam

13-Feb-2017

> ● **INDICATIONS AND DOSE**

> **Adjunctive therapy of partial-onset seizures with or without secondary generalisation**
> ▶ BY MOUTH, OR BY INTRAVENOUS INJECTION, OR BY INTRAVENOUS INFUSION
> ▶ Child 16–17 years: Initially 25–50 mg twice daily, adjusted according to response; usual maintenance 25–100 mg twice daily

● **INTERACTIONS** → Appendix 1: antiepileptics

● **SIDE-EFFECTS**
▶ **Common or very common** Anxiety · constipation · decreased appetite · depression · dizziness · insomnia · irritability · malaise · nausea · somnolence · vertigo · vomiting
▶ **Uncommon** Aggression · agitation · neutropenia · psychotic disorder · suicidal ideation

● **PREGNANCY** Manufacturer advises avoid unless potential benefit outweighs risk—limited information available.

● **BREAST FEEDING** Manufacturer advises avoid—present in milk in *animal* studies.

● **HEPATIC IMPAIRMENT** Manufacturer advises consider a starting dose of 25 mg twice daily in chronic liver disease; max. maintenance dose 75 mg twice daily in all stages of impairment.

● **TREATMENT CESSATION** Manufacturer advises avoid abrupt withdrawal—reduce daily dose in steps of 50 mg at weekly intervals, then reduce to 20 mg daily for a final week.

- **DIRECTIONS FOR ADMINISTRATION**
▸ With intravenous use For intermittent *intravenous infusion*, manufacturer advises dilute in Glucose 5% *or* Sodium Chloride 0.9% *or* Lactated Ringer's solution; give over 15 minutes.
▸ With oral use Manufacturer advises oral solution can be diluted in water or juice shortly before swallowing.

- **PRESCRIBING AND DISPENSING INFORMATION**
Manufacturer advises if switching between oral therapy and intravenous therapy (for those temporarily unable to take oral medication), the total daily dose and the frequency of administration should be maintained.

- **PATIENT AND CARER ADVICE**
Missed doses
Manufacturer advises if one or more doses are missed, a single dose should be taken as soon as possible and the next dose should be taken at the usual time.

Driving and skilled tasks
Manufacturer advises patients and carers should be cautioned on the effects on driving and performance of skilled tasks—increased risk of dizziness.

- **NATIONAL FUNDING/ACCESS DECISIONS**
Scottish Medicines Consortium (SMC) Decisions
The *Scottish Medicines Consortium* has advised (July 2016) that brivaracetam (*Briviact®*) is accepted for restricted use within NHS Scotland as adjunctive therapy in the treatment of partial-onset seizures with or without secondary generalisation in patients with refractory epilepsy. Treatment should be initiated by physicians who have appropriate experience in the treatment of epilepsy.

All Wales Medicines Strategy Group (AWMSG) Decisions
The *All Wales Medicines Strategy Group* has advised (October 2016) that Brivaracetam (*Briviact®*) is recommended as an option for restricted use within NHS Wales. Brivaracetam (*Briviact®*) should be restricted to use in the treatment of patients with refractory epilepsy, who remain uncontrolled with, or are intolerant to, other adjunctive anti-epileptic medicines, within its licensed indication as adjunctive therapy in the treatment of partial-onset seizures (POS) with or without secondary generalisation in adult and adolescent patients from 16 years of age with epilepsy. Brivaracetam (*Briviact®*) is not recommended for use within NHS Wales outside of this subpopulation.

- **MEDICINAL FORMS**
There can be variation in the licensing of different medicines containing the same drug.
Solution for injection
CAUTIONARY AND ADVISORY LABELS 2
ELECTROLYTES: May contain Sodium
▸ **Briviact** (UCB Pharma Ltd) ▼
  Brivaracetam 10 mg per 1 ml Briviact 50mg/5ml solution for injection vials | 10 vial [PoM] £222.75
Oral solution
CAUTIONARY AND ADVISORY LABELS 2, 8
EXCIPIENTS: May contain Sorbitol
ELECTROLYTES: May contain Sodium
▸ **Briviact** (UCB Pharma Ltd) ▼
  Brivaracetam 10 mg per 1 ml Briviact 10mg/ml oral solution sugar-free | 300 ml [PoM] £115.83
Tablet
CAUTIONARY AND ADVISORY LABELS 2, 8, 25
▸ **Briviact** (UCB Pharma Ltd) ▼
  Brivaracetam 10 mg Briviact 10mg tablets | 14 tablet [PoM] £34.64
  Brivaracetam 25 mg Briviact 25mg tablets | 56 tablet [PoM] £129.64
  Brivaracetam 50 mg Briviact 50mg tablets | 56 tablet [PoM] £129.64
  Brivaracetam 75 mg Briviact 75mg tablets | 56 tablet [PoM] £129.64
  Brivaracetam 100 mg Briviact 100mg tablets | 56 tablet [PoM] £129.64

Carbamazepine

- **INDICATIONS AND DOSE**
Trigeminal neuralgia
▸ BY MOUTH USING IMMEDIATE-RELEASE MEDICINES
▸ Child 1 month–11 years: Initially 5 mg/kg once daily, dose to be taken at night, alternatively initially 2.5 mg/kg twice daily, then increased in steps of 2.5–5 mg/kg every 3–7 days as required; maintenance 5 mg/kg 2–3 times a day, increased if necessary up to 20 mg/kg daily
▸ Child 12–17 years: Initially 100–200 mg 1–2 times a day, then increased to 200–400 mg 2–3 times a day, increased if necessary up to 1.8 g daily, dose should be increased slowly

Prophylaxis of bipolar disorder
▸ BY MOUTH USING IMMEDIATE-RELEASE MEDICINES
▸ Child 1 month–11 years: Initially 5 mg/kg once daily, dose to be taken at night, alternatively initially 2.5 mg/kg twice daily, then increased in steps of 2.5–5 mg/kg every 3–7 days as required; maintenance 5 mg/kg 2–3 times a day, increased if necessary up to 20 mg/kg daily
▸ Child 12–17 years: Initially 100–200 mg 1–2 times a day, then increased to 200–400 mg 2–3 times a day, increased if necessary up to 1.8 g daily, dose should be increased slowly

Focal and generalised tonic-clonic seizures
▸ BY MOUTH USING IMMEDIATE-RELEASE MEDICINES
▸ Child 1 month–11 years: Initially 5 mg/kg once daily, dose to be taken at night, alternatively initially 2.5 mg/kg twice daily, then increased in steps of 2.5–5 mg/kg every 3–7 days as required; maintenance 5 mg/kg 2–3 times a day, increased if necessary up to 20 mg/kg daily
▸ Child 12–17 years: Initially 100–200 mg 1–2 times a day, then increased to 200–400 mg 2–3 times a day, increased if necessary up to 1.8 g daily, dose should be increased slowly
▸ BY RECTUM
▸ Child: Up to 250 mg up to 4 times a day, to be used for short-term use (max. 7 days) when oral therapy temporarily not possible, use approx. 25% more than the oral dose

DOSE EQUIVALENCE AND CONVERSION
▸ Suppositories of 125 mg may be considered to be approximately equivalent in therapeutic effect to tablets of 100 mg but final adjustment should always depend on clinical response (plasma concentration monitoring recommended).

CARBAGEN® SR
Trigeminal neuralgia
▸ BY MOUTH
▸ Child 5–11 years: Initially 5 mg/kg daily in 1–2 divided doses, then increased in steps of 2.5–5 mg/kg every 3–7 days as required; maintenance 10–15 mg/kg daily in 1–2 divided doses, increased if necessary up to 20 mg/kg daily in 1–2 divided doses
▸ Child 12–17 years: Initially 100–400 mg daily in 1–2 divided doses, then increased to 400–1200 mg daily in 1–2 divided doses, increased if necessary up to 1.8 g daily in 1–2 divided doses, dose should be increased slowly

Focal and generalised tonic-clonic seizures | Prophylaxis of bipolar disorder
▸ BY MOUTH
▸ Child 5–11 years: Initially 5 mg/kg daily in 1–2 divided doses, then increased in steps of 2.5–5 mg/kg every 3–7 days as required, dose should be increased slowly; maintenance 10–15 mg/kg daily in continued →

1–2 divided doses, increased if necessary up to 20 mg/kg daily in 1–2 divided doses
▸ Child 12–17 years: Initially 100–400 mg daily in 1–2 divided doses, then increased to 400–1200 mg daily in 1–2 divided doses, increased if necessary up to 1.8 g daily in 1–2 divided doses, dose should be increased slowly

TEGRETOL® PROLONGED RELEASE

Focal and generalised tonic-clonic seizures | Prophylaxis of bipolar disorder
▸ BY MOUTH
▸ Child 5–11 years: Initially 5 mg/kg daily in 2 divided doses, then increased in steps of 2.5–5 mg/kg every 3–7 days as required; maintenance 10–15 mg/kg daily in 2 divided doses, increased if necessary up to 20 mg/kg daily in 2 divided doses
▸ Child 12–17 years: Initially 100–400 mg daily in 2 divided doses, dose should be increased slowly; maintenance 400–1200 mg daily in 2 divided doses, increased if necessary up to 1.8 g daily in 2 divided doses

Trigeminal neuralgia
▸ BY MOUTH
▸ Child 5–11 years: Initially 5 mg/kg daily in 2 divided doses, then increased in steps of 2.5–5 mg/kg every 3–7 days as required; maintenance 10–15 mg/kg daily in 2 divided doses, increased if necessary up to 20 mg/kg daily in 2 divided doses
▸ Child 12–17 years: Initially 100–400 mg daily in 2 divided doses, dose should be increased slowly; maintenance 400–1200 mg daily in 2 divided doses, increased if necessary up to 1.8 g daily in 2 divided doses, dose should be increased slowly

● CONTRA-INDICATIONS Acute porphyrias p. 577 · AV conduction abnormalities (unless paced) · history of bone-marrow depression
● CAUTIONS Cardiac disease · history of haematological reactions to other drugs · may exacerbate absence and myoclonic seizures · skin reactions · susceptibility to angle-closure glaucoma
CAUTIONS, FURTHER INFORMATION
Consider vitamin D supplementation in patients who are immobilised for long periods or who have inadequate sun exposure or dietary intake of calcium.
▸ Blood, hepatic, or skin disorders Carbamazepine should be withdrawn immediately in cases of aggravated liver dysfunction or acute liver disease. Leucopenia that is severe, progressive, or associated with clinical symptoms requires withdrawal (if necessary under cover of a suitable alternative).
● INTERACTIONS → Appendix 1: antiepileptics
● SIDE-EFFECTS
▸ Common or very common Allergic skin reactions · aplastic anaemia · ataxia · blood disorders · blurring of vision · dermatitis · dizziness · drowsiness · dry mouth · eosinophilia · fatigue · haemolytic anaemia · headache · hyponatraemia (leading in rare cases to water intoxication) · leucopenia · nausea · oedema · thrombocytopenia · unsteadiness · urticaria · vomiting
▸ Uncommon Constipation · diarrhoea · involuntary movements (including nystagmus) · visual disturbances
▸ Rare Abdominal pain · aggression · agitation · anorexia · cardiac conduction disorders · confusion · delayed multi-organ hypersensitivity disorder · depression · dysarthria · hallucinations · hepatitis · hypertension · hypotension · jaundice · lymph node enlargement · muscle weakness · paraesthesia · peripheral neuropathy · restlessness · systemic lupus erythematosus · vanishing bile duct syndrome
▸ Very rare Arthralgia · muscle spasm · acne · alopecia · alterations in skin pigmentation · angle-closure glaucoma ·

aseptic meningitis · AV block with syncope · circulatory collapse · conjunctivitis · dyspnoea · exacerbation of coronary artery disease · galactorrhoea · gynaecomastia · hearing disorders · hepatic failure · hirsutism · hypercholesterolaemia · impaired male fertility · interstitial nephritis · muscle pain · neuroleptic malignant syndrome · osteomalacia · osteoporosis · pancreatitis · photosensitivity · pneumonia · pneumonitis · psychosis · pulmonary hypersensitivity · purpura · renal failure · sexual dysfunction · Stevens-Johnson syndrome · stomatitis · sweating · taste disturbance · thromboembolism · thrombophlebitis · toxic epidermal necrolysis · urinary frequency · urinary retention
▸ Frequency not known Suicidal ideation
SIDE-EFFECTS, FURTHER INFORMATION
Some side-effects (such as headache, ataxia, drowsiness, nausea, vomiting, blurring of vision, dizziness, unsteadiness, and allergic skin reactions) are dose-related, and may be dose-limiting. These side-effects are more common at the start of treatment. Children should be offered a modified-release preparation to reduce the risk of side-effects; altering the timing of medication may also be beneficial.
Overdose
For details on the management of poisoning, see Active elimination techniques, under Emergency treatment of poisoning p. 803.
● ALLERGY AND CROSS-SENSITIVITY Antiepileptic hypersensitivity syndrome associated with carbamazepine. See under Epilepsy p. 184 for more information. Caution—cross-sensitivity reported with oxcarbazepine and with phenytoin.
● PREGNANCY Doses should be adjusted on the basis of plasma-drug concentration monitoring.
● BREAST FEEDING Amount probably too small to be harmful. Monitor infant for possible adverse reactions.
● HEPATIC IMPAIRMENT Metabolism impaired in advanced liver disease.
● RENAL IMPAIRMENT Use with caution.
● PRE-TREATMENT SCREENING Test for HLA-B*1502 allele in individuals of Han Chinese or Thai origin (avoid unless no alternative—risk of Stevens-Johnson syndrome in presence of HLA-B*1502 allele).
● MONITORING REQUIREMENTS
▸ Plasma concentration for optimum response 4–12 mg/litre (20–50 micromol/litre) measured after 1–2 weeks.
▸ Manufacturer recommends blood counts and hepatic and renal function tests (but evidence of practical value uncertain).
● TREATMENT CESSATION When stopping treatment with carbamazepine for bipolar disorder, reduce the dose gradually over a period of at least 4 weeks.
● DIRECTIONS FOR ADMINISTRATION Oral liquid has been used rectally—should be retained for at least 2 hours (but may have laxative effect).
TEGRETOL® PROLONGED RELEASE *Tegretol® Prolonged Release* tablets can be halved but should not be chewed.
● PRESCRIBING AND DISPENSING INFORMATION
Switching between formulations Different formulations of oral preparations may vary in bioavailability. Patients being treated for epilepsy should be maintained on a specific manufacturer's product.
● PATIENT AND CARER ADVICE
Medicines for Children leaflet: Carbamazepine (oral) for preventing seizures www.medicinesforchildren.org.uk/carbamazepine-oral-preventing-seizures-0
Blood, hepatic, or skin disorders Patients or their carers should be told how to recognise signs of blood, liver, or skin disorders, and advised to seek immediate medical

attention if symptoms such as fever, rash, mouth ulcers, bruising, or bleeding develop.

● **PROFESSION SPECIFIC INFORMATION**

Dental practitioners' formulary
Carbamazepine Tablets may be prescribed.

● **MEDICINAL FORMS**
There can be variation in the licensing of different medicines containing the same drug. Forms available from special-order manufacturers include: oral suspension, oral solution

Modified-release tablet
CAUTIONARY AND ADVISORY LABELS 3, 8, 25
▸ **Carbagen SR** (Mylan Ltd)
Carbamazepine 200 mg Carbagen SR 200mg tablets | 56 tablet [PoM] £4.16 DT price = £5.20
Carbamazepine 400 mg Carbagen SR 400mg tablets | 56 tablet [PoM] £8.20 DT price = £10.24
▸ **Tegretol Retard** (Novartis Pharmaceuticals UK Ltd)
Carbamazepine 200 mg Tegretol Prolonged Release 200mg tablets | 56 tablet [PoM] £5.20 DT price = £5.20
Carbamazepine 400 mg Tegretol Prolonged Release 400mg tablets | 56 tablet [PoM] £10.24 DT price = £10.24

Tablet
CAUTIONARY AND ADVISORY LABELS 3, 8
▸ **Carbamazepine (Non-proprietary)**
Carbamazepine 100 mg Carbamazepine 100mg tablets | 28 tablet [PoM] no price available | 84 tablet [PoM] no price available DT price = £2.07
Carbamazepine 200 mg Carbamazepine 200mg tablets | 28 tablet [PoM] no price available | 84 tablet [PoM] no price available DT price = £3.83
Carbamazepine 400 mg Carbamazepine 400mg tablets | 28 tablet [PoM] no price available | 56 tablet [PoM] no price available DT price = £5.02
▸ **Carbagen** (Mylan Ltd)
Carbamazepine 100 mg Carbagen 100mg tablets | 28 tablet [PoM] £5.74 | 84 tablet [PoM] no price available DT price = £2.07 (Hospital only)
Carbamazepine 200 mg Carbagen 200mg tablets | 28 tablet [PoM] £4.99 | 84 tablet [PoM] no price available DT price = £3.83 (Hospital only)
Carbamazepine 400 mg Carbagen 400mg tablets | 28 tablet [PoM] £4.27 | 56 tablet [PoM] no price available DT price = £5.02 (Hospital only)
▸ **Tegretol** (Novartis Pharmaceuticals UK Ltd)
Carbamazepine 100 mg Tegretol 100mg tablets | 84 tablet [PoM] £2.07 DT price = £2.07
Carbamazepine 200 mg Tegretol 200mg tablets | 84 tablet [PoM] £3.83 DT price = £3.83
Carbamazepine 400 mg Tegretol 400mg tablets | 56 tablet [PoM] £5.02 DT price = £5.02

Suppository
CAUTIONARY AND ADVISORY LABELS 3, 8
▸ **Carbamazepine (Non-proprietary)**
Carbamazepine 125 mg Carbamazepine 125mg suppositories | 5 suppository [PoM] £120.00 DT price = £120.00
Carbamazepine 250 mg Carbamazepine 250mg suppositories | 5 suppository [PoM] £140.00 DT price = £140.00

Oral suspension
CAUTIONARY AND ADVISORY LABELS 3, 8
▸ **Carbamazepine (Non-proprietary)**
Carbamazepine 20 mg per 1 ml Carbamazepine 100mg/5ml oral suspension sugar free sugar-free | 300 ml [PoM] £7.13 DT price = £6.12
▸ **Tegretol** (Novartis Pharmaceuticals UK Ltd)
Carbamazepine 20 mg per 1 ml Tegretol 100mg/5ml liquid sugar-free | 300 ml [PoM] £6.12 DT price = £6.12

Ethosuximide

● **INDICATIONS AND DOSE**

Absence seizures | Atypical absence seizures (adjunct) | Myoclonic seizures
▸ BY MOUTH
▸ **Child 1 month–5 years:** Initially 5 mg/kg twice daily (max. per dose 125 mg), dose to be increased every

5–7 days; maintenance 10–20 mg/kg twice daily (max. per dose 500 mg), total daily dose may rarely be given in 3 divided doses
▸ **Child 6-17 years:** Initially 250 mg twice daily, then increased in steps of 250 mg every 5–7 days; usual dose 500–750 mg twice daily, increased if necessary up to 1 g twice daily

● **CAUTIONS** Avoid in acute porphyrias p. 577

● **INTERACTIONS** → Appendix 1: antiepileptics

● **SIDE-EFFECTS**
▸ **Common or very common** Anorexia · abdominal pain · diarrhoea · gastro-intestinal disturbances · nausea · vomiting · weight loss
▸ **Uncommon** Aggression · ataxia · dizziness · drowsiness · euphoria · fatigue · headache · hiccup · impaired concentration · irritability
▸ **Rare** Depression · dyskinesia · gingival hypertrophy · increased libido · myopia · photophobia · psychosis · rash · sleep disturbances · tongue swelling · vaginal bleeding
▸ **Frequency not known** Agranulocytosis · aplastic anaemia · blood disorders · hyperactivity · increase in seizure frequency · leucopenia · pancytopenia · Stevens-Johnson syndrome · suicidal ideation · systemic lupus erythematosus
SIDE-EFFECTS, FURTHER INFORMATION
▸ **Blood disorders** Blood counts required if features of infection.

● **PREGNANCY** The dose should be monitored carefully during pregnancy and after birth, and adjustments made on a clinical basis.

● **BREAST FEEDING** Present in milk. Hyperexcitability and sedation reported.

● **HEPATIC IMPAIRMENT** Use with caution.

● **RENAL IMPAIRMENT** Use with caution.

● **PATIENT AND CARER ADVICE**
Blood disorders Patients or their carers should be told how to recognise signs of blood disorders, and advised to seek immediate medical attention if symptoms such as fever, mouth ulcers, bruising, or bleeding develop.
Medicines for Children leaflet: Ethosuximide for preventing seizures www.medicinesforchildren.org.uk/ethosuximide-for-preventing-seizures

● **MEDICINAL FORMS**
There can be variation in the licensing of different medicines containing the same drug.

Oral solution
CAUTIONARY AND ADVISORY LABELS 8
▸ **Ethosuximide (Non-proprietary)**
Ethosuximide 50 mg per 1 ml Ethosuximide 250mg/5ml syrup | 200 ml [PoM] £173.00 DT price = £4.22

Capsule
CAUTIONARY AND ADVISORY LABELS 8
▸ **Ethosuximide (Non-proprietary)**
Ethosuximide 250 mg Ethosuximide 250mg capsules | 56 capsule [PoM] £173.00 DT price = £173.00

Fosphenytoin sodium

● **DRUG ACTION** Fosphenytoin is a pro-drug of phenytoin.

● **INDICATIONS AND DOSE**

Status epilepticus
▸ BY INTRAVENOUS INFUSION
▸ **Child 5-17 years:** Initially 20 mg(PE)/kg, dose to be administered at a rate of 3 mg(PE)/kg/minute, maximum 150 mg(PE)/kg/minute, then 4–5 mg(PE)/kg daily in 1–4 divided doses, dose to be administered at a rate of 1–2 mg(PE)/kg/minute, maximum continued →

4

Nervous system

100 mg(PE)/minute, dose to be adjusted according to response and trough plasma-phenytoin concentration

Prophylaxis or treatment of seizures associated with neurosurgery or head injury
▶ BY INTRAVENOUS INFUSION
▶ Child 5–17 years: Initially 10–15 mg(PE)/kg, then 4–5 mg(PE)/kg daily in 1–4 divided doses, dose to be administered at a rate of 1–2 mg(PE)/kg/minute, maximum 100 mg(PE)/minute, dose to be adjusted according to response and trough plasma-phenytoin concentration

Temporary substitution for oral phenytoin
▶ BY INTRAVENOUS INFUSION
▶ Child 5–17 years: Same dose and same dosing frequency as oral phenytoin therapy, intravenous infusion to be administered at a rate of 1–2 mg(PE)/kg/minute, maximum 100 mg(PE)/minute

DOSE EQUIVALENCE AND CONVERSION
▶ Doses are expressed as phenytoin sodium equivalent (PE); fosphenytoin sodium 1.5 mg ≡ phenytoin sodium 1 mg.

● **UNLICENSED USE** Fosphenytoin sodium doses in BNFC may differ from those in product literature.
● **CONTRA-INDICATIONS** Acute porphyrias p. 577 · second-degree heart block · sino-atrial block · sinus bradycardia · Stokes-Adams syndrome · third-degree heart block
● **CAUTIONS** Heart failure · hypotension · injection solutions alkaline (irritant to tissues) · respiratory depression · resuscitation facilities must be available
● **INTERACTIONS** → Appendix 1: antiepileptics
● **SIDE-EFFECTS**
▶ **Common or very common** Alterations in respiratory function · arrhythmias · asthenia · cardiovascular collapse · cardiovascular depression (particularly if injection too rapid) · chills · CNS depression (particularly if injection too rapid) · dry mouth · dysarthria · ecchymosis · euphoria · hypotension · incoordination · pruritus · respiratory arrest · taste disturbance · tinnitus · vasodilatation · visual disturbances
▶ **Uncommon** Decreased reflexes · hypoacusis · hypoaesthesia · increased reflexes · muscle spasm · muscle weakness · pain · stupor
▶ **Frequency not known** Confusion · extrapyramidal disorder · hyperglycaemia · purple glove syndrome · tonic seizures · twitching

SIDE-EFFECTS, FURTHER INFORMATION
▶ Cardiovascular reactions Intravenous infusion of fosphenytoin has been associated with severe cardiovascular reactions including asystole, ventricular fibrillation, and cardiac arrest. Hypotension, bradycardia, and heart block have also been reported. The following are recommended:
  ● monitor heart rate, blood pressure, and respiratory function for duration of infusion;
  ● observe patient for at least 30 minutes after infusion;
  ● if hypotension occurs, reduce infusion rate or discontinue;
  ● reduce dose or infusion rate in elderly, and in renal or hepatic impairment.
● **ALLERGY AND CROSS-SENSITIVITY** Cross-sensitivity reported with carbamazepine.
● **PREGNANCY** Changes in plasma-protein binding make interpretation of plasma-phenytoin concentrations difficult—monitor unbound fraction. The dose should be monitored carefully during pregnancy and after birth, and adjustments made on a clinical basis.
● **BREAST FEEDING** Small amounts present in milk, but not known to be harmful.

● **HEPATIC IMPAIRMENT** Consider 10–25% reduction in dose or infusion rate (except initial dose for status epilepticus).
● **RENAL IMPAIRMENT** Consider 10–25% reduction in dose or infusion rate (except initial dose for status epilepticus).
● **PRE-TREATMENT SCREENING** HLA-B*1502 allele in individuals of Han Chinese or Thai origin—avoid unless essential (increased risk of Stevens-Johnson syndrome).
● **MONITORING REQUIREMENTS**
▶ Manufacturer recommends blood counts (but evidence of practical value uncertain).
▶ Monitor heart rate, blood pressure, ECG, and respiratory function during infusion.
● **DIRECTIONS FOR ADMINISTRATION** For intermittent intravenous infusion (Pro-Epanutin®), give in Glucose 5% or Sodium chloride 0.9%; dilute to a concentration of 1.5–25 mg (phenytoin sodium equivalent (PE))/mL.
● **PRESCRIBING AND DISPENSING INFORMATION** Prescriptions for fosphenytoin sodium should state the dose in terms of phenytoin sodium equivalent (PE); fosphenytoin sodium 1.5 mg ≡ phenytoin sodium 1 mg.

● **MEDICINAL FORMS**
There can be variation in the licensing of different medicines containing the same drug.
Solution for injection
ELECTROLYTES: May contain Phosphate
▶ **Pro-Epanutin** (Pfizer Ltd)
   Fosphenytoin sodium 75 mg per 1 ml Pro-Epanutin 750mg/10ml concentrate for solution for injection vials | 10 vial [PoM] £400.00 (Hospital only)

Gabapentin

● **INDICATIONS AND DOSE**

Adjunctive treatment of focal seizures with or without secondary generalisation
▶ BY MOUTH
▶ Child 2–5 years: 10 mg/kg once daily on day 1, then 10 mg/kg twice daily on day 2, then 10 mg/kg 3 times a day on day 3, then increased to 30–70 mg/kg daily in 3 divided doses, adjusted according to response, some children may not tolerate daily increments; longer intervals (up to weekly) may be more appropriate
▶ Child 6–11 years: 10 mg/kg once daily on day 1, then 10 mg/kg twice daily (max. per dose 300 mg) on day 2, then 10 mg/kg 3 times a day (max. per dose 300 mg) on day 3, usual dose 25–35 mg/kg daily in 3 divided doses, some children may not tolerate daily increments; longer intervals (up to weekly) may be more appropriate, daily dose maximum to be given in 3 divided doses; maximum 70 mg/kg per day
▶ Child 12–17 years: Initially 300 mg once daily on day 1, then 300 mg twice daily on day 2, then 300 mg 3 times a day on day 3, alternatively initially 300 mg 3 times a day on day 1, then increased in steps of 300 mg every 2–3 days in 3 divided doses, adjusted according to response; usual dose 0.9–3.6 g daily in 3 divided doses (max. per dose 1.6 g 3 times a day), some children may not tolerate daily increments; longer intervals (up to weekly) may be more appropriate

Monotherapy for focal seizures with or without secondary generalisation
▶ BY MOUTH
▶ Child 12–17 years: Initially 300 mg once daily on day 1, then 300 mg twice daily on day 2, then 300 mg 3 times a day on day 3, alternatively initially 300 mg 3 times a day on day 1, then increased in steps of 300 mg every 2–3 days in 3 divided doses, adjusted according to

response; usual dose 0.9–3.6 g daily in 3 divided doses (max. per dose 1.6 g 3 times a day), some children may not tolerate daily increments; longer intervals (up to weekly) may be more appropriate

- **UNLICENSED USE** Not licensed for use in children under 6 years. Not licensed at doses over 50 mg/kg daily in children under 12 years.

> **IMPORTANT SAFETY INFORMATION**
> The levels of propylene glycol, acesulfame K and saccharin sodium may exceed the recommended WHO daily intake limits if high doses of gabapentin oral solution (Rosemont brand) are given to adolescents or adults with low body-weight (39–50 kg)—consult product literature.

- **CAUTIONS** Diabetes mellitus · high doses of oral solution in adolescents and adults with low body-weight · history of psychotic illness · mixed seizures (including absences)
- **INTERACTIONS** → Appendix 1: antiepileptics
- **SIDE-EFFECTS**
▸ **Common or very common** Abdominal pain · abnormal reflexes · abnormal thoughts · acne · amnesia · anorexia · anxiety · arthralgia · ataxia · confusion · constipation · convulsions · cough · depression · diarrhoea · dizziness · drowsiness · dry mouth · dry throat · dyspepsia · dyspnoea · emotional lability · fever · flatulence · flu syndrome · gingivitis · headache · hostility · hypertension · impotence · increased appetite · insomnia · leucopenia · malaise · movement disorders · myalgia · nausea · nervousness · nystagmus · oedema · paraesthesia · pruritus · rash · rhinitis · speech disorder · tremor · twitching · vasodilatation · vertigo · visual disturbances · vomiting · weight gain
▸ **Uncommon** Palpitations
▸ **Frequency not known** Acute renal failure · alopecia · blood glucose fluctuations in patients with diabetes · breast hypertrophy · gynaecomastia · hallucinations · hepatitis · hypersensitivity syndrome · incontinence · pancreatitis · Stevens-Johnson syndrome · suicidal ideation · thrombocytopenia · tinnitus
- **PREGNANCY** The dose should be monitored carefully during pregnancy and after birth, and adjustments made on a clinical basis.
- **BREAST FEEDING** Present in milk—manufacturer advises use only if potential benefit outweighs risk.
- **RENAL IMPAIRMENT** Reduce dose if estimated glomerular filtration rate less than 80 mL/minute/1.73 m^2; consult product literature.
- **EFFECT ON LABORATORY TESTS** False positive readings with some urinary protein tests.
- **DIRECTIONS FOR ADMINISTRATION** Capsules can be opened but the bitter taste is difficult to mask.
- **PATIENT AND CARER ADVICE**
Medicines for Children leaflet: Gabapentin for preventing seizures www.medicinesforchildren.org.uk/gabapentin-for-preventing-seizures

- **MEDICINAL FORMS**
There can be variation in the licensing of different medicines containing the same drug. Forms available from special-order manufacturers include: oral suspension, oral solution

Tablet
CAUTIONARY AND ADVISORY LABELS 3, 5, 8
▸ **Gabapentin (Non-proprietary)**
Gabapentin 600 mg Gabapentin 600mg tablets | 100 tablet PoM £106.00 DT price = £8.72
Gabapentin 800 mg Gabapentin 800mg tablets | 100 tablet PoM £98.13 DT price = £29.29
▸ **Neurontin** (Pfizer Ltd)
Gabapentin 600 mg Neurontin 600mg tablets | 100 tablet PoM £84.80 DT price = £8.72
Gabapentin 800 mg Neurontin 800mg tablets | 100 tablet PoM £98.13 DT price = £29.29

Oral solution
CAUTIONARY AND ADVISORY LABELS 3, 5, 8
EXCIPIENTS: May contain Propylene glycol
ELECTROLYTES: May contain Potassium, sodium
▸ **Gabapentin (Non-proprietary)**
Gabapentin 50 mg per 1 ml Gabapentin 50mg/ml oral solution sugar free sugar-free | 150 ml PoM £69.00 DT price = £69.00
Capsule
CAUTIONARY AND ADVISORY LABELS 3, 5, 8
▸ **Gabapentin (Non-proprietary)**
Gabapentin 100 mg Gabapentin 100mg capsules | 100 capsule PoM £18.29 DT price = £1.91
Gabapentin 300 mg Gabapentin 300mg capsules | 100 capsule PoM £42.40 DT price = £2.82
Gabapentin 400 mg Gabapentin 400mg capsules | 100 capsule PoM £49.06 DT price = £3.24
▸ **Neurontin** (Pfizer Ltd)
Gabapentin 100 mg Neurontin 100mg capsules | 100 capsule PoM £18.29 DT price = £1.91
Gabapentin 300 mg Neurontin 300mg capsules | 100 capsule PoM £42.40 DT price = £2.82
Gabapentin 400 mg Neurontin 400mg capsules | 100 capsule PoM £49.06 DT price = £3.24

Lacosamide

- **INDICATIONS AND DOSE**

Adjunctive treatment of focal seizures with or without secondary generalisation
▸ BY MOUTH, OR BY INTRAVENOUS INFUSION
▸ **Child 16–17 years:** Initially 50 mg twice daily, infusion to be administered over 15–60 minutes (for up to 5 days), then increased, if tolerated, in steps of 50 mg twice daily, adjusted according to response, dose to be increased in weekly intervals; maintenance 100 mg twice daily (max. per dose 200 mg twice daily)

Adjunctive treatment of focal seizures with or without secondary generalisation (alternative loading dose regimen when it is necessary to rapidly attain therapeutic plasma concentrations) (under close medical supervision)
▸ BY MOUTH, OR BY INTRAVENOUS INFUSION
▸ **Child 16–17 years:** Loading dose 200 mg, infusion to be administered over 15–60 minutes (for up to 5 days), followed by maintenance 100 mg twice daily, to be given 12 hours after initial dose, then increased, if tolerated, in steps of 50 mg twice daily (max. per dose 200 mg twice daily), adjusted according to response, dose to be increased in weekly intervals

- **CONTRA-INDICATIONS** Second- or third-degree AV block
- **CAUTIONS** Conduction problems · risk of PR-interval prolongation · severe cardiac disease
- **INTERACTIONS** → Appendix 1: antiepileptics
- **SIDE-EFFECTS**
▸ **Common or very common** Abnormal gait · blurred vision · cognitive disorder · constipation · depression · dizziness · drowsiness · fatigue · flatulence · headache · impaired coordination · nausea · nystagmus · pruritus · tremor · vomiting
▸ **Rare** Multi-organ hypersensitivity reaction
▸ **Frequency not known** Aggression · agitation · agranulocytosis · atrial fibrillation · atrial flutter · AV block · bradycardia · confusion · dry mouth · dysarthria · dyspepsia · euphoria · hypoesthesia · irritability · muscle spasm · PR-interval prolongation · psychosis · rash · suicidal ideation · tinnitus
- **ALLERGY AND CROSS-SENSITIVITY** Antiepileptic hypersensitivity syndrome associated with lacosamide. See under Epilepsy p. 184 for more information.

4

Nervous system

- **PREGNANCY** The dose should be monitored carefully during pregnancy and after birth, and adjustments made on a clinical basis.
- **BREAST FEEDING** Manufacturer advises avoid—present in milk in *animal* studies.
- **HEPATIC IMPAIRMENT** Titrate with caution in mild to moderate impairment if co-existing renal impairment. Caution in severe impairment—no information available.
- **RENAL IMPAIRMENT** Loading dose regimen can be considered in mild to moderate impairment—titrate above 200 mg with caution. Titrate with caution in severe impairment, max. 250 mg daily.

  Consult product literature for loading dose if estimated glomerular filtration rate is less than 30 mL/minute/1.73 m^2.
- **DIRECTIONS FOR ADMINISTRATION** For *intravenous infusion*, give undiluted or dilute with Glucose 5% *or* Sodium Chloride 0.9%.
- **PRESCRIBING AND DISPENSING INFORMATION** Flavours of syrup may include strawberry.
- **PATIENT AND CARER ADVICE**
  Medicines for Children leaflet: Lacosamide for preventing seizures www.medicinesforchildren.org.uk/lacosamide-for-preventing-seizures
- **NATIONAL FUNDING/ACCESS DECISIONS**
  Scottish Medicines Consortium (SMC) Decisions
  The *Scottish Medicines Consortium* has advised (January 2009) that lacosamide (*Vimpat®*) is accepted for restricted use within NHS Scotland as adjunctive treatment for focal seizures with or without secondary generalisation in patients from 16 years. It is restricted for specialist use in refractory epilepsy.
- **MEDICINAL FORMS**
  There can be variation in the licensing of different medicines containing the same drug.
  Solution for infusion
  ELECTROLYTES: May contain Sodium
  ▸ Vimpat (UCB Pharma Ltd)
  Lacosamide 10 mg per 1 ml Vimpat 200mg/20ml solution for infusion vials | 1 vial [PoM] £29.70
  Oral solution
  CAUTIONARY AND ADVISORY LABELS 8
  EXCIPIENTS: May contain Aspartame, propylene glycol
  ELECTROLYTES: May contain Sodium
  ▸ Vimpat (UCB Pharma Ltd)
  Lacosamide 10 mg per 1 ml Vimpat 10mg/ml syrup sugar-free | 200 ml [PoM] £25.74 DT price = £25.74
  Tablet
  CAUTIONARY AND ADVISORY LABELS 8
  ▸ Vimpat (UCB Pharma Ltd)
  Lacosamide 50 mg Vimpat 50mg tablets | 14 tablet [PoM] £10.81 DT price = £10.81
  Lacosamide 100 mg Vimpat 100mg tablets | 14 tablet [PoM] £21.62 | 56 tablet [PoM] £86.50 DT price = £86.50
  Lacosamide 150 mg Vimpat 150mg tablets | 14 tablet [PoM] £32.44 | 56 tablet [PoM] £129.74 DT price £129.74
  Lacosamide 200 mg Vimpat 200mg tablets | 56 tablet [PoM] £144.16 DT price = £144.16

Lamotrigine

- **INDICATIONS AND DOSE**

Monotherapy of focal seizures | Monotherapy of primary and secondary generalised tonic-clonic seizures | Monotherapy of seizures associated with Lennox-Gastaut syndrome
▸ BY MOUTH
▸ Child 12–17 years: Initially 25 mg once daily for 14 days, then increased to 50 mg once daily for further 14 days, then increased in steps of up to 100 mg every

7–14 days; maintenance 100–200 mg daily in 1–2 divided doses; increased if necessary up to 500 mg daily, dose titration should be repeated if restarting after interval of more than 5 days

Monotherapy of typical absence seizures
▸ BY MOUTH
▸ Child 2–11 years: Initially 300 micrograms/kg daily in 1–2 divided doses, for 14 days, then 600 micrograms/kg daily in 1–2 divided doses, for further 14 days, then increased in steps of up to 600 micrograms/kg every 7–14 days; maintenance 1–10 mg/kg daily in 1–2 divided doses, increased if necessary up to 15 mg/kg daily, dose titration should be repeated if restarting after interval of more than 5 days

Adjunctive therapy of focal seizures with valproate | Adjunctive therapy of primary and secondary generalised tonic-clonic seizures with valproate | Adjunctive therapy of seizures associated with Lennox-Gastaut syndrome with valproate
▸ BY MOUTH
▸ Child 2–11 years (body-weight up to 13 kg): Initially 2 mg once daily on alternate days for first 14 days, then 300 micrograms/kg once daily for further 14 days, then increased in steps of up to 300 micrograms/kg every 7–14 days; maintenance 1–5 mg/kg daily in 1–2 divided doses, dose titration should be repeated if restarting after interval of more than 5 days; maximum 200 mg per day
▸ Child 2–11 years (body-weight 13 kg and above): Initially 150 micrograms/kg once daily for 14 days, then 300 micrograms/kg once daily for further 14 days, then increased in steps of up to 300 micrograms/kg every 7–14 days; maintenance 1–5 mg/kg daily in 1–2 divided doses, dose titration should be repeated if restarting after interval of more than 5 days; maximum 200 mg per day
▸ Child 12–17 years: Initially 25 mg once daily on alternate days for 14 days, then 25 mg once daily for further 14 days, then increased in steps of up to 50 mg every 7–14 days; maintenance 100–200 mg daily in 1–2 divided doses, dose titration should be repeated if restarting after interval of more than 5 days

Adjunctive therapy of focal seizures (with enzyme inducing drugs) without valproate | Adjunctive therapy of primary and secondary generalised tonic-clonic seizures (with enzyme inducing drugs) without valproate | Adjunctive therapy of seizures associated with Lennox-Gastaut syndromes (with enzyme inducing drugs) without valproate
▸ BY MOUTH
▸ Child 2–11 years: Initially 300 micrograms/kg twice daily for 14 days, then 600 micrograms/kg twice daily for further 14 days, then increased in steps of up to 1.2 mg/kg every 7–14 days; maintenance 5–15 mg/kg daily in 1–2 divided doses, dose titration should be repeated if restarting after interval of more than 5 days; maximum 400 mg per day
▸ Child 12–17 years: Initially 50 mg once daily for 14 days, then 50 mg twice daily for further 14 days, then increased in steps of up to 100 mg every 7–14 days; maintenance 200–400 mg daily in 2 divided doses, increased if necessary up to 700 mg daily, dose titration should be repeated if restarting after interval of more than 5 days

Adjunctive therapy of focal seizures (without enzyme inducing drugs) without valproate | Adjunctive therapy of primary and secondary generalised tonic-clonic seizures (without enzyme inducing drugs) without valproate | Adjunctive therapy of seizures associated with Lennox-Gastaut syndromes (without enzyme inducing drugs) without valproate

▶ BY MOUTH

▶ **Child 2–11 years:** Initially 300 micrograms/kg daily in 1–2 divided doses for 14 days, then 600 micrograms/kg daily in 1–2 divided doses for further 14 days, then increased in steps of up to 600 micrograms/kg every 7–14 days; maintenance 1–10 mg/kg daily in 1–2 divided doses, dose titration should be repeated if restarting after interval of more than 5 days; maximum 200 mg per day

▶ **Child 12–17 years:** Initially 25 mg once daily for 14 days, then increased to 50 mg once daily for further 14 days, then increased in steps of up to 100 mg every 7–14 days; maintenance 100–200 mg daily in 1–2 divided doses, dose titration should be repeated if restarting after interval of more than 5 days

---

IMPORTANT SAFETY INFORMATION

SAFE PRACTICE

Do not confuse the different combinations or indications.

● **CAUTIONS** Myoclonic seizures (may be exacerbated)

● **INTERACTIONS** → Appendix 1: antiepileptics

● **SIDE-EFFECTS**

▶ **Common or very common** Blurred vision · aggression · agitation · arthralgia · ataxia · back pain · diarrhoea · diplopia · dizziness · drowsiness · dry mouth · headache · insomnia · nausea · nystagmus · rash · tremor · vomiting

▶ **Rare** Conjunctivitis

▶ **Very rare** Anaemia · blood disorders · confusion · hallucination · hepatic failure · hypersensitivity syndrome · increase in seizure frequency · leucopenia · lupus erythematosus-like reactions · movement disorders · pancytopenia · thrombocytopenia · unsteadiness

▶ **Frequency not known** Aseptic meningitis · suicidal ideation

SIDE-EFFECTS, FURTHER INFORMATION

▶ **Skin reactions** Serious skin reactions including Stevens-Johnson syndrome and toxic epidermal necrolysis have developed (especially in children); most rashes occur in the first 8 weeks. Rash is sometimes associated with hypersensitivity syndrome and is more common in patients with history of allergy or rash from other antiepileptic drugs. Consider withdrawal if rash or signs of hypersensitivity syndrome develop. Factors associated with increased risk of serious skin reactions include concomitant use of valproate, initial lamotrigine dosing higher than recommended, and more rapid dose escalation than recommended.

● **ALLERGY AND CROSS-SENSITIVITY** Antiepileptic hypersensitivity syndrome associated with lamotrigine. See under Epilepsy p. 184 for more information.

● **PREGNANCY** Doses should be adjusted on the basis of plasma-drug concentration monitoring.

● **BREAST FEEDING** Present in milk, but limited data suggest no harmful effect on infant.

● **HEPATIC IMPAIRMENT** Halve dose in moderate impairment. Quarter dose in severe impairment.

● **RENAL IMPAIRMENT** Consider reducing maintenance dose in significant impairment. Caution in renal failure; metabolite may accumulate.

● **TREATMENT CESSATION** Avoid abrupt withdrawal (taper off over 2 weeks or longer) unless serious skin reaction occurs.

● **PRESCRIBING AND DISPENSING INFORMATION** Patients being treated for epilepsy may need to be maintained on a specific manufacturer's branded or generic lamotrigine product.

Switching between formulations Care should be taken when switching between oral formulations in the treatment of epilepsy. The need for continued supply of a particular manufacturer's product should be based on clinical judgement and consultation with the patient or their carer, taking into account factors such as seizure frequency and treatment history.

● **PATIENT AND CARER ADVICE**

Skin reactions Warn patients and carers to see their doctor immediately if rash or signs or symptoms of hypersensitivity syndrome develop.

Blood disorders Patients and their carers should be alert for symptoms and signs suggestive of bone-marrow failure, such as anaemia, bruising, or infection. Aplastic anaemia, bone-marrow depression, and pancytopenia have been associated rarely with lamotrigine.

Medicines for Children leaflet: Lamotrigine for preventing seizures www.medicinesforchildren.org.uk/lamotrigine-for-preventing-seizures

---

● **MEDICINAL FORMS**

There can be variation in the licensing of different medicines containing the same drug. Forms available from special-order manufacturers include: oral suspension, oral solution

Dispersible tablet

CAUTIONARY AND ADVISORY LABELS 8, 13

▶ **Lamotrigine (Non-proprietary)**

Lamotrigine 5 mg Lamotrigine 5mg dispersible tablets sugar free sugar-free | 28 tablet [PoM] £15.00 DT price = £7.00

Lamotrigine 25 mg Lamotrigine 25mg dispersible tablets sugar free sugar-free | 56 tablet [PoM] £20.41 DT price = £2.09

Lamotrigine 100 mg Lamotrigine 100mg dispersible tablets sugar free sugar-free | 56 tablet [PoM] £58.68 DT price = £3.57

▶ **Lamictal (GlaxoSmithKline UK Ltd)**

Lamotrigine 2 mg Lamictal 2mg dispersible tablets sugar-free | 30 tablet [PoM] £18.81 DT price = £18.81

Lamotrigine 5 mg Lamictal 5mg dispersible tablets sugar-free | 28 tablet [PoM] £9.38 DT price = £7.00

Lamotrigine 25 mg Lamictal 25mg dispersible tablets sugar-free | 56 tablet [PoM] £23.53 DT price = £2.09

Lamotrigine 100 mg Lamictal 100mg dispersible tablets sugar-free | 56 tablet [PoM] £69.04 DT price = £3.57

Tablet

CAUTIONARY AND ADVISORY LABELS 8

▶ **Lamotrigine (Non-proprietary)**

Lamotrigine 25 mg Lamotrigine 25mg tablets | 56 tablet [PoM] £20.41 DT price = £1.18

Lamotrigine 50 mg Lamotrigine 50mg tablets | 56 tablet [PoM] £3.94 DT price = £1.31

Lamotrigine 100 mg Lamotrigine 100mg tablets | 56 tablet [PoM] £5.87 DT price = £1.64

Lamotrigine 200 mg Lamotrigine 200mg tablets | 56 tablet [PoM] £12.00 DT price = £2.51

▶ **Lamictal (GlaxoSmithKline UK Ltd)**

Lamotrigine 25 mg Lamictal 25mg tablets | 56 tablet [PoM] £23.53 DT price = £1.18

Lamotrigine 50 mg Lamictal 50mg tablets | 56 tablet [PoM] £40.02 DT price = £1.31

Lamotrigine 100 mg Lamictal 100mg tablets | 56 tablet [PoM] £69.04 DT price = £1.64

Lamotrigine 200 mg Lamictal 200mg tablets | 56 tablet [PoM] £117.35 DT price = £2.51

Levetiracetam

- **INDICATIONS AND DOSE**

Monotherapy of focal seizures with or without secondary generalisation
▶ BY MOUTH, OR BY INTRAVENOUS INFUSION
▶ Child 16-17 years: Initially 250 mg once daily for 1 week, then increased to 250 mg twice daily, then increased in steps of 250 mg twice daily (max. per dose 1.5 g twice daily), adjusted according to response, dose to be increased every 2 weeks

Adjunctive therapy of focal seizures with or without secondary generalisation
▶ BY MOUTH
▶ Child 1-5 months: Initially 7 mg/kg once daily, then increased in steps of up to 7 mg/kg twice daily (max. per dose 21 mg/kg twice daily), dose to be increased every 2 weeks
▶ Child 6 months-17 years (body-weight up to 50 kg): Initially 10 mg/kg once daily, then increased in steps of up to 10 mg/kg twice daily (max. per dose 30 mg/kg twice daily), dose to be increased every 2 weeks
▶ Child 12-17 years (body-weight 50 kg and above): Initially 250 mg twice daily, then increased in steps of 500 mg twice daily (max. per dose 1.5 g twice daily), dose to be increased every 2-4 weeks
▶ BY INTRAVENOUS INFUSION
▶ Child 4-17 years (body-weight up to 50 kg): Initially 10 mg/kg once daily, then increased in steps of up to 10 mg/kg twice daily (max. per dose 30 mg/kg twice daily), dose to be increased every 2 weeks
▶ Child 12-17 years (body-weight 50 kg and above): Initially 250 mg twice daily, then increased in steps of 500 mg twice daily (max. per dose 1.5 g twice daily), dose to be increased every 2 weeks

Adjunctive therapy of myoclonic seizures and tonic-clonic seizures
▶ BY MOUTH, OR BY INTRAVENOUS INFUSION
▶ Child 12-17 years (body-weight up to 50 kg): Initially 10 mg/kg once daily, then increased in steps of up to 10 mg/kg twice daily (max. per dose 30 mg/kg twice daily), dose to be increased every 2 weeks
▶ Child 12-17 years (body-weight 50 kg and above): Initially 250 mg twice daily, then increased in steps of 500 mg twice daily (max. per dose 1.5 g twice daily), dose to be increased every 2 weeks

- **UNLICENSED USE** *Granules* not licensed for use in children under 6 years, for initial treatment in children with body-weight less than 25 kg, or for the administration of doses below 250 mg.
- **INTERACTIONS** → Appendix 1: antiepileptics
- **SIDE-EFFECTS**
▶ **Common or very common** Abdominal pain · aggression · anorexia · anxiety · ataxia · convulsion · cough · depression · diarrhoea · dizziness · drowsiness · dyspepsia · headache · insomnia · irritability · malaise · nasopharyngitis · nausea · rash · tremor · vertigo · vomiting
▶ **Uncommon** Agitation · alopecia · amnesia · blurred vision · confusion · diplopia · eczema · impaired attention · leucopenia · myalgia · paraesthesia · pruritus · psychosis · suicidal ideation · thrombocytopenia · weight changes
▶ **Rare** Agranulocytosis · choreoathetosis · drug reaction with eosinophilia and systemic symptoms (DRESS) · dyskinesia · erythema multiforme · hepatic failure · hyponatraemia · neutropenia · pancreatitis · pancytopenia · Stevens-Johnson syndrome · toxic epidermal necrolysis
▶ **Frequency not known** Completed suicide · pancytopenia
- **PREGNANCY** The dose should be monitored carefully during pregnancy and after birth, and adjustments made

on a clinical basis. It is recommended that the fetal growth should be monitored.
- **BREAST FEEDING** Present in milk—manufacturer advises avoid.
- **HEPATIC IMPAIRMENT** Halve dose in severe hepatic impairment if estimated glomerular filtration rate less than 60 mL/minute/1.73 m².
- **RENAL IMPAIRMENT** Reduce dose if estimated glomerular filtration rate less than 80 mL/minute/1.73 m² (consult product literature).
- **DIRECTIONS FOR ADMINISTRATION**
▶ With intravenous use For *intravenous infusion* (*Keppra®*), dilute requisite dose with at least 100 mL Glucose 5% or Sodium Chloride 0.9%; give over 15 minutes.
▶ With oral use For administration of *oral solution*, requisite dose may be diluted in a glass of water.
- **PRESCRIBING AND DISPENSING INFORMATION** If switching between oral therapy and intravenous therapy (for those temporarily unable to take oral medication), the intravenous dose should be the same as the established oral dose.
- **PATIENT AND CARER ADVICE** Medicines for Children leaflet: Levetiracetam for preventing seizures www.medicinesforchildren.org.uk/levetiracetam-for-preventing-seizures
- **MEDICINAL FORMS** There can be variation in the licensing of different medicines containing the same drug. Forms available from special-order manufacturers include: oral suspension, oral solution

Granules
CAUTIONARY AND ADVISORY LABELS 8
▶ **Desitrend** (Desitin Pharma Ltd)
Levetiracetam 250 mg Desitrend 250mg granules sachets sugar-free | 60 sachet PoM £22.41
Levetiracetam 500 mg Desitrend 500mg granules sachets sugar-free | 60 sachet PoM £39.46
Levetiracetam 1 gram Desitrend 1000mg granules sachets sugar-free | 60 sachet PoM £76.27

Tablet
CAUTIONARY AND ADVISORY LABELS 8
▶ **Levetiracetam** (Non-proprietary)
Levetiracetam 250 mg Levetiracetam 250mg tablets | 60 tablet PoM £28.01 DT price = £1.98
Levetiracetam 500 mg Levetiracetam 500mg tablets | 60 tablet PoM £49.32 DT price = £2.49
Levetiracetam 750 mg Levetiracetam 750mg tablets | 60 tablet PoM £84.02 DT price = £4.06
Levetiracetam 1 gram Levetiracetam 1g tablets | 60 tablet PoM £95.34 DT price = £5.50
▶ **Keppra** (UCB Pharma Ltd)
Levetiracetam 250 mg Keppra 250mg tablets | 60 tablet PoM £28.01 DT price = £1.98
Levetiracetam 500 mg Keppra 500mg tablets | 60 tablet PoM £49.32 DT price = £2.49
Levetiracetam 750 mg Keppra 750mg tablets | 60 tablet PoM £84.02 DT price = £4.06
Levetiracetam 1 gram Keppra 1g tablets | 60 tablet PoM £95.34 DT price = £5.50

Solution for infusion
ELECTROLYTES: May contain Sodium
▶ **Levetiracetam** (Non-proprietary)
Levetiracetam 100 mg per 1 ml Levetiracetam 500mg/5ml concentrate for solution for infusion vials | 1 vial PoM £127.31 | 10 vial PoM £114.57-£127.31
Levetiracetam 500mg/5ml solution for infusion vials | 10 vial PoM £127.31
▶ **Desitrend** (Desitin Pharma Ltd)
Levetiracetam 100 mg per 1 ml Desitrend 500mg/5ml concentrate for solution for infusion ampoules | 10 ampoule PoM £127.31
▶ **Keppra** (UCB Pharma Ltd)
Levetiracetam 100 mg per 1 ml Keppra 500mg/5ml concentrate for solution for infusion vials | 10 vial PoM £127.31

Oral solution

CAUTIONARY AND ADVISORY LABELS 8
- ▸ Levetiracetam (Non-proprietary)
  Levetiracetam 100 mg per 1 ml Levetiracetam 100mg/ml oral solution sugar free sugar-free | 150 ml PoM £27.00 sugar-free | 300 ml PoM £66.95 DT price = £5.33
- ▸ Desitrend (Desitin Pharma Ltd)
  Levetiracetam 100 mg per 1 ml Desitrend 100mg/ml oral solution sugar-free | 300 ml PoM £15.90 DT price = £5.33
- ▸ Keppra (UCB Pharma Ltd)
  Levetiracetam 100 mg per 1 ml Keppra 100mg/ml oral solution sugar-free | 150 ml PoM £33.48 sugar-free | 300 ml PoM £66.95 DT price = £5.33

Oxcarbazepine

- ● **INDICATIONS AND DOSE**

Monotherapy for the treatment of focal seizures with or without secondary generalised tonic-clonic seizures
- ▸ BY MOUTH
- ▸ Child 6–17 years: Initially 4–5 mg/kg twice daily (max. per dose 300 mg), then increased in steps of up to 5 mg/kg twice daily, adjusted according to response, dose to be adjusted at weekly intervals; maximum 46 mg/kg per day

Adjunctive therapy for the treatment of focal seizures with or without secondary generalised tonic-clonic seizures
- ▸ BY MOUTH
- ▸ Child 6-17 years: Initially 4–5 mg/kg twice daily (max. per dose 300 mg), then increased in steps of up to 5 mg/kg twice daily, adjusted according to response, dose to be adjusted at weekly intervals; maintenance 15 mg/kg twice daily; maximum 46 mg/kg per day

DOSE ADJUSTMENTS DUE TO INTERACTIONS
In adjunctive therapy, the dose of concomitant antiepileptics may need to be reduced when using high doses of oxcarbazepine.

- ● **CAUTIONS** Avoid in acute porphyrias p. 577 · cardiac conduction disorders · heart failure · hyponatraemia
- ● **INTERACTIONS** → Appendix 1: antiepileptics
- ● **SIDE-EFFECTS**
- ▸ **Common or very common** Abdominal pain · acne · agitation · alopecia · amnesia · asthenia · ataxia · confusion · constipation · depression · diarrhoea · diplopia · dizziness · drowsiness · headache · hyponatraemia · impaired concentration · nausea · nystagmus · rash · tremor · visual disorders · vomiting
- ▸ **Uncommon** Leucopenia · urticaria
- ▸ **Very rare** Arrhythmias · atrioventricular block · hepatitis · multi-organ hypersensitivity disorders · pancreatitis · Stevens-Johnson syndrome · systemic lupus erythematosus · thrombocytopenia · toxic epidermal necrolysis
- ▸ **Frequency not known** Aplastic anaemia · bone marrow depression · hypertension · hypothyroidism · neutropenia · osteoporotic bone disorders · pancytopenia · suicidal ideation
- ● **ALLERGY AND CROSS-SENSITIVITY** Caution in patients with hypersensitivity to carbamazepine. Antiepileptic hypersensitivity syndrome associated with oxcarbazepine. See under Epilepsy p. 184 for more information.
- ● **PREGNANCY** The dose should be monitored carefully during pregnancy and after birth, and adjustments made on a clinical basis.
- ● **BREAST FEEDING** Amount probably too small to be harmful but manufacturer advises avoid.
- ● **HEPATIC IMPAIRMENT** Caution in severe impairment—no information available.

- ● **RENAL IMPAIRMENT** Halve initial dose if estimated glomerular filtration rate less than 30 mL/minute/1.73 m^2, increase according to response at intervals of at least 1 week.
- ● **PRE-TREATMENT SCREENING** Test for HLA-B*1502 allele in individuals of Han Chinese or Thai origin (avoid unless no alternative—risk of Stevens-Johnson syndrome in presence of HLA-B*1502 allele).
- ● **MONITORING REQUIREMENTS**
- ▸ Monitor plasma-sodium concentration in patients at risk of hyponatraemia.
- ▸ Monitor body-weight in patients with heart failure.
- ● **PRESCRIBING AND DISPENSING INFORMATION** Patients may need to be maintained on a specific manufacturer's branded or generic oxcarbazepine product.
  Switching between formulations Care should be taken when switching between oral formulations. The need for continued supply of a particular manufacturer's product should be based on clinical judgement and consultation with the patient or their carer, taking into account factors such as seizure frequency and treatment history.
- ● **PATIENT AND CARER ADVICE**
  Blood, hepatic, or skin disorders Patients or their carers should be told how to recognise signs of blood, liver, or skin disorders, and advised to seek immediate medical attention if symptoms such as lethargy, confusion, muscular twitching, fever, rash, blistering, mouth ulcers, bruising, or bleeding develop.
  Medicines for Children: Oxcarbazepine for preventing seizures www.medicinesforchildren.org.uk/oxcarbazepine-for-preventing-seizures

- ● **MEDICINAL FORMS**
  There can be variation in the licensing of different medicines containing the same drug. Forms available from special-order manufacturers include: oral suspension

Oral suspension
CAUTIONARY AND ADVISORY LABELS 3, 8
EXCIPIENTS: May contain Propylene glycol
- ▸ Trileptal (Novartis Pharmaceuticals UK Ltd)
  Oxcarbazepine 60 mg per 1 ml Trileptal 60mg/ml oral suspension sugar-free | 250 ml PoM £48.96 DT price = £48.96

Tablet
CAUTIONARY AND ADVISORY LABELS 3, 8
- ▸ Oxcarbazepine (Non-proprietary)
  Oxcarbazepine 150 mg Oxcarbazepine 150mg tablets | 50 tablet PoM £11.14 DT price = £8.42
  Oxcarbazepine 300 mg Oxcarbazepine 300mg tablets | 50 tablet PoM £22.61 DT price = £5.89
  Oxcarbazepine 600 mg Oxcarbazepine 600mg tablets | 50 tablet PoM £45.19 DT price = £38.76
- ▸ Trileptal (Novartis Pharmaceuticals UK Ltd)
  Oxcarbazepine 150 mg Trileptal 150mg tablets | 50 tablet £12.24 DT price = £8.42
  Oxcarbazepine 300 mg Trileptal 300mg tablets | 50 tablet PoM £24.48 DT price = £5.89
  Oxcarbazepine 600 mg Trileptal 600mg tablets | 50 tablet PoM £48.96 DT price = £38.76

Perampanel

- ● **INDICATIONS AND DOSE**

Adjunctive treatment of focal seizures with or without secondary generalised seizures
- ▸ BY MOUTH
- ▸ Child 12-17 years: Initially 2 mg once daily, dose to be taken before bedtime, then increased, if tolerated, in steps of 2 mg at intervals of at least every 2 weeks, adjusted according to response; maintenance 4–8 mg once daily; maximum 12 mg per day continued →

4

Nervous System

DOSE ADJUSTMENTS DUE TO INTERACTIONS
Titrate at intervals of at least 1 week with concomitant carbamazepine, fosphenytoin, oxcarbazepine, or phenytoin.

- **INTERACTIONS** → Appendix 1: antiepileptics
- **SIDE-EFFECTS** Aggression · anxiety · ataxia · back pain · blurred vision · changes in appetite · confusion · diplopia · dizziness · drowsiness · dysarthria · gait disturbance · irritability · malaise · nausea · suicidal behaviour · suicidal ideation · vertigo · weight increase
- **PREGNANCY** Manufacturer advises avoid. The dose should be monitored carefully during pregnancy and after birth, and adjustments made on a clinical basis.
- **BREAST FEEDING** Avoid—present in milk in *animal* studies.
- **HEPATIC IMPAIRMENT** Increase at intervals of at least 2 weeks, up to max. 8 mg daily in mild or moderate impairment. Avoid in severe impairment.
- **RENAL IMPAIRMENT** Avoid in moderate or severe impairment.
- **PRESCRIBING AND DISPENSING INFORMATION**
Switching between formulations Care should be taken when switching between oral formulations. The need for continued supply of a particular manufacturer's product should be based on clinical judgement and consultation with the patient or their carer, taking into account factors such as seizure frequency and treatment history.
  Patients may need to be maintained on a specific manufacturer's branded or generic perampanel product.

- **MEDICINAL FORMS**
There can be variation in the licensing of different medicines containing the same drug.
Tablet
CAUTIONARY AND ADVISORY LABELS 3, 8, 25
- Fycompa (Eisai Ltd) ▼
  Perampanel 2 mg Fycompa 2mg tablets | 7 tablet [PoM] £35.00 | 28 tablet [PoM] £140.00
  Perampanel 4 mg Fycompa 4mg tablets | 28 tablet [PoM] £140.00
  Perampanel 6 mg Fycompa 6mg tablets | 28 tablet [PoM] £140.00
  Perampanel 8 mg Fycompa 8mg tablets | 28 tablet [PoM] £140.00
  Perampanel 10 mg Fycompa 10mg tablets | 28 tablet [PoM] £140.00
  Perampanel 12 mg Fycompa 12mg tablets | 28 tablet [PoM] £140.00

Phenytoin

19-Apr-2017

- **INDICATIONS AND DOSE**
Tonic-clonic seizures | Focal seizures
  ▶ BY MOUTH
  - Child 1 month–11 years: Initially 1.5–2.5 mg/kg twice daily, then adjusted according to response to 2.5–5 mg/kg twice daily (max. per dose 7.5 mg/kg twice daily), dose also adjusted according to plasma-phenytoin concentration; maximum 300 mg per day
  - Child 12–17 years: Initially 75–150 mg twice daily, then adjusted according to response to 150–200 mg twice daily (max. per dose 300 mg twice daily), dose also adjusted according to plasma-phenytoin concentration
  ▶ INITIALLY BY SLOW INTRAVENOUS INJECTION
  - Neonate: Loading dose 18 mg/kg, dose to be administered over 20–30 minutes, then (by mouth) 2.5–5 mg/kg twice daily (max. per dose 7.5 mg/kg twice daily), adjusted according to response, dose also adjusted according to plasma-phenytoin concentration.

Prevention and treatment of seizures during or following neurosurgery or severe head injury
  ▶ BY MOUTH
  - Child: Initially 2.5 mg/kg twice daily, then adjusted according to response to 4–8 mg/kg daily, dose also

adjusted according to plasma-phenytoin concentration; maximum 300 mg per day

Status epilepticus | Acute symptomatic seizures associated with head trauma or neurosurgery
  ▶ INITIALLY BY SLOW INTRAVENOUS INJECTION, OR BY INTRAVENOUS INFUSION
  - Neonate: Loading dose 20 mg/kg, then (by slow intravenous injection or by intravenous infusion) 2.5–5 mg/kg twice daily.
  - Child 1 month–11 years: Loading dose 20 mg/kg, then (by slow intravenous injection or by intravenous infusion) 2.5–5 mg/kg twice daily
  - Child 12–17 years: Loading dose 20 mg/kg, then (by intravenous infusion or by slow intravenous injection) up to 100 mg 3–4 times a day
DOSE EQUIVALENCE AND CONVERSION
  - Preparations containing phenytoin sodium are **not** bioequivalent to those containing phenytoin base (such as *Epanutin Infatabs*® and *Epanutin*® suspension); 100 mg of phenytoin sodium is approximately equivalent in therapeutic effect to 92 mg phenytoin base. The dose is the same for all phenytoin products when initiating therapy. However, if switching between these products the difference in phenytoin content may be clinically significant. Care is needed when making changes between formulations and plasma-phenytoin concentration monitoring is recommended.

- **UNLICENSED USE**
  - With oral use Licensed for use in children (age range not specified by manufacturer).
  - With intravenous use Phenytoin doses in BNF publications may differ from those in product literature.

IMPORTANT SAFETY INFORMATION

NHS IMPROVEMENT PATIENT SAFETY ALERT: RISK OF DEATH AND SEVERE HARM FROM ERROR WITH INJECTABLE PHENYTOIN (NOVEMBER 2016)
Use of injectable phenytoin is error-prone throughout the prescribing, preparation, administration and monitoring processes; all relevant staff should be made aware of appropriate guidance on the safe use of injectable phenytoin to reduce the risk of error.

- **CONTRA-INDICATIONS**
GENERAL CONTRA-INDICATIONS
Acute porphyrias p. 577
SPECIFIC CONTRA-INDICATIONS
  - With intravenous use Second- and third-degree heart block · sino-atrial block · sinus bradycardia · Stokes-Adams syndrome
- **CAUTIONS**
GENERAL CAUTIONS
Enteral feeding (interrupt feeding for 2 hours before and after dose; more frequent monitoring may be necessary)
SPECIFIC CAUTIONS
  - With intravenous use Heart failure · hypotension · injection solutions alkaline (irritant to tissues) · respiratory depression · resuscitation facilities must be available
CAUTIONS, FURTHER INFORMATION
Consider vitamin D supplementation in patients who are immobilised for long periods or who have inadequate sun exposure or dietary intake of calcium.
  Intramuscular phenytoin should not be used (absorption is slow and erratic).
- **INTERACTIONS** → Appendix 1: antiepileptics

● **SIDE-EFFECTS**

GENERAL SIDE-EFFECTS

▸ **Common or very common** Acne · anorexia · coarsening of facial appearance · constipation · dizziness · drowsiness · gingival hypertrophy and tenderness (maintain good oral hygiene) · headache · hirsutism · insomnia · nausea · paraesthesia · rash · transient nervousness · tremor · vomiting

▸ **Rare** Leucopenia · aplastic anaemia · blood disorders · dyskinesia · hepatotoxicity · lupus erythematosus · lymphadenopathy · megaloblastic anaemia · osteomalacia · peripheral neuropathy · polyarteritis nodosa · Stevens-Johnson syndrome · thrombocytopenia · toxic epidermal necrolysis

▸ **Frequency not known** Hypersensitivity syndrome · interstitial nephritis · pneumonitis · polyarthropathy · suicidal ideation

SPECIFIC SIDE-EFFECTS

▸ **Common or very common**

▸ **With intravenous use** Alterations in respiratory function · arrhythmias · cardiovascular collapse · cardiovascular depression (particularly if injection too rapid) · CNS depression (particularly if injection too rapid) · hypotension · respiratory arrest

▸ **Frequency not known**

▸ **With intravenous use** Purple glove syndrome · tonic seizures

SIDE-EFFECTS, FURTHER INFORMATION

▸ **Hepatotoxicity** Discontinue immediately and do not re-administer.

▸ **Rash** Discontinue; if mild re-introduce cautiously but discontinue immediately if recurrence.

▸ **Use in adolescents** Phenytoin may cause coarsening of facial appearance, acne, hirsutism, and gingival hyperplasia and so may be particularly undesirable in adolescent patients.

▸ **Bradycardia and hypotension**

▸ **With intravenous use** Reduce rate of administration if bradycardia or hypotension occurs.

Overdose

Symptoms of phenytoin toxicity include nystagmus, diplopia, slurred speech, ataxia, confusion, and hyperglycaemia.

● **ALLERGY AND CROSS-SENSITIVITY** Cross-sensitivity reported with carbamazepine. Antiepileptic hypersensitivity syndrome associated with phenytoin. See under Epilepsy p. 184 for more information.

● **PREGNANCY** Changes in plasma-protein binding make interpretation of plasma-phenytoin concentrations difficult—monitor unbound fraction. Doses should be adjusted on the basis of plasma-drug concentration monitoring.

● **BREAST FEEDING** Small amounts present in milk, but not known to be harmful.

● **HEPATIC IMPAIRMENT** Reduce dose to avoid toxicity.

● **PRE-TREATMENT SCREENING** HLAB* 1502 allele in individuals of Han Chinese or Thai origin—avoid unless essential (increased risk of Stevens- Johnson syndrome).

● **MONITORING REQUIREMENTS**

▸ Therapeutic plasma-phenytoin concentrations reduced in first 3 months of life because of reduced protein binding.

▸ Trough plasma concentration for optimum response: neonate–3 months, 6–15 mg/litre (25–60 micromol/litre); child 3 months–18 years, 10–20 mg/litre (40–80 micromol/litre).

▸ Manufacturer recommends blood counts (but evidence of practical value uncertain).

▸ With intravenous use Monitor ECG and blood pressure.

● **DIRECTIONS FOR ADMINISTRATION** Manufacturer advises each injection or infusion should be preceded and followed by an injection of Sodium Chloride 0.9% through the same needle or catheter to avoid local venous irritation.

▸ With intravenous use EvGr For *intravenous injection*, give into a large vein at a rate not exceeding 1 mg/kg/minute (max. 50 mg/minute). ◈ Manufacturer advises for *intravenous infusion*, dilute to a concentration not exceeding 10 mg/mL with Sodium Chloride 0.9% and give into a large vein through an in-line filter (0.22–0.50 micron). EvGr Give at a rate not exceeding 1 mg/kg/minute (max. 50 mg/minute). ◈ Complete administration within 1 hour of preparation.

● **PRESCRIBING AND DISPENSING INFORMATION** Switching between formulations Different formulations of oral preparations may vary in bioavailability. Patients being treated for epilepsy should be maintained on a specific manufacturer's product.

● **PATIENT AND CARER ADVICE** Blood or skin disorders Patients or their carers should be told how to recognise signs of blood or skin disorders, and advised to seek immediate medical attention if symptoms such as fever, rash, mouth ulcers, bruising, or bleeding develop. Leucopenia that is severe, progressive, or associated with clinical symptoms requires withdrawal (if necessary under cover of a suitable alternative). Medicines for Children leaflet: Phenytoin for preventing seizures www.medicinesforchildren.org.uk/phenytoin-for-preventing-seizures

● **MEDICINAL FORMS** There can be variation in the licensing of different medicines containing the same drug. Forms available from special-order manufacturers include: oral suspension, oral solution

Tablet

CAUTIONARY AND ADVISORY LABELS 8

▸ Phenytoin (Non-proprietary)

Phenytoin sodium 100 mg Phenytoin sodium 100mg tablets | 28 tablet [PoM] £32.95 DT price = £23.00 | 100 tablet [PoM] no price available

Solution for injection

EXCIPIENTS: May contain Alcohol, propylene glycol

ELECTROLYTES: May contain Sodium

▸ Phenytoin (Non-proprietary)

Phenytoin sodium 50 mg per 1 ml Phenytoin sodium 250mg/5ml solution for injection ampoules | 5 ampoule [PoM] £15.50–£24.40 | 10 ampoule [PoM] no price available

▸ Epanutin (Phenytoin sodium) (Pfizer Ltd)

Phenytoin sodium 50 mg per 1 ml Epanutin Ready-Mixed Parenteral 250mg/5ml solution for injection ampoules | 10 ampoule [PoM] £48.79

Oral suspension

CAUTIONARY AND ADVISORY LABELS 8

▸ Epanutin (Phenytoin) (Pfizer Ltd)

Phenytoin 6 mg per 1 ml Epanutin 30mg/5ml oral suspension | 500 ml [PoM] £4.27 DT price = £4.27

Chewable tablet

CAUTIONARY AND ADVISORY LABELS 8, 24

▸ Epanutin (Phenytoin) (Pfizer Ltd)

Phenytoin 50 mg Epanutin Infatabs 50mg chewable tablets | 200 tablet [PoM] £13.18

Capsule

CAUTIONARY AND ADVISORY LABELS 8

▸ Phenytoin (Non-proprietary)

Phenytoin sodium 25 mg Phenytoin sodium 25mg capsules | 28 capsule [PoM] £7.24–£7.26 DT price = £7.26

Phenytoin sodium 50 mg Phenytoin sodium 50mg capsules | 28 capsule [PoM] £7.07 DT price = £9.37

Phenytoin sodium 100 mg Phenytoin sodium 100mg capsules | 84 capsule [PoM] £68.76 DT price = £42.88

Phenytoin sodium 300 mg Phenytoin sodium 300mg capsules | 28 capsule [PoM] £9.11–£41.94 DT price = £41.94

Nervous system

4

Rufinamide

- **INDICATIONS AND DOSE**

Adjunctive treatment of seizures in Lennox-Gastaut syndrome
▶ BY MOUTH

- Child 4–17 years (body-weight up to 30 kg): Initially 100 mg twice daily, then increased in steps of 100 mg twice daily (max. per dose 500 mg twice daily), adjusted according to response, dose to be increased at intervals of not less than 2 days
- Child 4–17 years (body-weight 30–49 kg): Initially 200 mg twice daily, then increased in steps of 200 mg twice daily (max. per dose 900 mg twice daily), adjusted according to response, dose to be increased at intervals of not less than 2 days
- Child 4–17 years (body-weight 50–69 kg): Initially 200 mg twice daily, then increased in steps of 200 mg twice daily (max. per dose 1.2 g twice daily), adjusted according to response, dose to be increased at intervals of not less than 2 days
- Child 4–17 years (body-weight 70 kg and above): Initially 200 mg twice daily, then increased in steps of 200 mg twice daily (max. per dose 1.6 g twice daily), adjusted according to response, dose to be increased at intervals of not less than 2 days

Adjunctive treatment of seizures in Lennox-Gastaut syndrome with valproate
▶ BY MOUTH

- Child 4–17 years (body-weight up to 30 kg): Initially 100 mg twice daily, then increased in steps of 100 mg twice daily (max. per dose 300 mg twice daily), adjusted according to response, dose to be increased at intervals of not less than 2 days

- **INTERACTIONS** → Appendix 1: antiepileptics
- **SIDE-EFFECTS** Abdominal pain · acne · anorexia · anxiety · back pain · blurred vision · constipation · diarrhoea · diplopia · dizziness · drowsiness · dyspepsia · epistaxis · fatigue · gait disturbances · headache · hyperactivity · hypersensitivity syndrome · impaired coordination · increase in seizure frequency · influenza-like symptoms · insomnia · nausea · nystagmus · oligomenorrhoea · rash · rhinitis · tremor · vomiting · weight loss
- **ALLERGY AND CROSS-SENSITIVITY** Antiepileptic hypersensitivity syndrome associated with rufinamide. See under Epilepsy p. 184 for more information.
- **PREGNANCY** The dose should be monitored carefully during pregnancy and after birth, and adjustments made on a clinical basis.
- **BREAST FEEDING** Manufacturer advises avoid—no information available.
- **HEPATIC IMPAIRMENT** Caution and careful dose titration in mild to moderate impairment. Avoid in severe impairment.
- **DIRECTIONS FOR ADMINISTRATION** Tablets may be crushed and given in half a glass of water.
- **PRESCRIBING AND DISPENSING INFORMATION** Switching between formulations Care should be taken when switching between oral formulations. The need for continued supply of a particular manufacturer's product should be based on clinical judgement and consultation with the patient or their carer, taking into account factors such as seizure frequency and treatment history.
  Patients may need to be maintained on a specific manufacturer's branded or generic rufinamide product.
- **PATIENT AND CARER ADVICE** Counselling on antiepileptic hypersensitivity syndrome is advised.

Medicines for Children leaflet: Rufinamide for preventing seizures www.medicinesforchildren.org.uk/rufinamide-for-preventing-seizures

- **NATIONAL FUNDING/ACCESS DECISIONS**
Scottish Medicines Consortium (SMC) Decisions
The *Scottish Medicines Consortium* has advised (October 2008) that rufinamide (*Inovelon*®) is accepted for restricted use within NHS Scotland as adjunctive therapy in the treatment of seizures associated with Lennox-Gastaut syndrome in patients 4 years and above. It is restricted for use when alternative traditional antiepileptic drugs are unsatisfactory.

- **MEDICINAL FORMS**
There can be variation in the licensing of different medicines containing the same drug.

Oral suspension
CAUTIONARY AND ADVISORY LABELS 8, 21
EXCIPIENTS: May contain Propylene glycol
▶ Inovelon (Eisai Ltd)
  Rufinamide 40 mg per 1 ml Inovelon 40mg/ml oral suspension sugar-free | 460 ml POM £94.71 DT price = £94.71

Tablet
CAUTIONARY AND ADVISORY LABELS 8, 21
▶ Inovelon (Eisai Ltd)
  Rufinamide 100 mg Inovelon 100mg tablets | 10 tablet POM £5.15
  Rufinamide 200 mg Inovelon 200mg tablets | 60 tablet POM £61.77
  Rufinamide 400 mg Inovelon 400mg tablets | 60 tablet POM £102.96

Sodium valproate

13-Apr-2017

- **INDICATIONS AND DOSE**
All forms of epilepsy
▶ BY MOUTH USING IMMEDIATE-RELEASE MEDICINES

- Neonate: Initially 20 mg/kg once daily; maintenance 10 mg/kg twice daily.

- Child 1 month–11 years: Initially 10–15 mg/kg daily in 1–2 divided doses (max. per dose 600 mg); maintenance 25–30 mg/kg daily in 2 divided doses, doses up to 60 mg/kg daily in 2 divided doses may be used in infantile spasms; monitor clinical chemistry and haematological parameters if dose exceeds 40 mg/kg daily
- Child 12–17 years: Initially 600 mg daily in 1–2 divided doses, increased in steps of 150–300 mg every 3 days; maintenance 1–2 g daily in 2 divided doses; maximum 2.5 g per day
▶ BY RECTUM

- Neonate: Initially 20 mg/kg once daily; maintenance 10 mg/kg twice daily.

- Child 1 month–11 years: Initially 10–15 mg/kg daily in 1–2 divided doses (max. per dose 600 mg); maintenance 25–30 mg/kg daily in 2 divided doses, doses up to 60 mg/kg daily in 2 divided doses may be used in infantile spasms; monitor clinical chemistry and haematological parameters if dose exceeds 40 mg/kg daily
- Child 12–17 years: Initially 600 mg daily in 1–2 divided doses, increased in steps of 150–300 mg every 3 days; maintenance 1–2 g daily in 2 divided doses; maximum 2.5 g per day

Initiation of valproate treatment
▶ INITIALLY BY INTRAVENOUS INJECTION

- Neonate: 10 mg/kg twice daily.

- Child 1 month–11 years: Initially 10 mg/kg, then (by intravenous infusion or by intravenous injection) increased to 20–40 mg/kg daily in 2–4 divided doses, alternatively (by continuous intravenous infusion) increased to 20–40 mg/kg daily, monitor clinical chemistry and haematological parameters if dose exceeds 40 mg/kg daily

▸ Child 12–17 years: Initially 10 mg/kg, followed by (by intravenous infusion or by intravenous injection) up to 2.5 g daily in 2–4 divided doses, alternatively (by continuous intravenous infusion) up to 2.5 g daily; (by intravenous injection or by intravenous infusion or by continuous intravenous infusion) usual dose 1–2 g daily, alternatively (by intravenous injection or by intravenous infusion or by continuous intravenous infusion) usual dose 20–30 mg/kg daily, intravenous injection to be administered over 3–5 minutes

Continuation of valproate treatment
▸ BY INTRAVENOUS INJECTION, OR BY INTRAVENOUS INFUSION, OR BY CONTINUOUS INTRAVENOUS INFUSION
▸ Child: If switching from oral therapy to intravenous therapy give the same dose as current oral daily dose, give over 3–5 minutes by intravenous injection *or* in 2–4 divided doses by intravenous infusion

EPILIM CHRONOSPHERE®

All forms of epilepsy
▸ BY MOUTH
▸ Child: Total daily dose to be given in 1–2 divided doses (consult product literature)

EPILIM CHRONO®

All forms of epilepsy
▸ BY MOUTH
▸ Child (body-weight 20 kg and above): Total daily dose to be given in 1–2 divided doses (consult product literature)

EPISENTA® CAPSULES

All forms of epilepsy
▸ BY MOUTH
▸ Child: Total daily dose to be given in 1–2 divided doses (consult product literature)

EPISENTA® GRANULES

All forms of epilepsy
▸ BY MOUTH
▸ Child: Total daily dose to be given in 1–2 divided doses (consult product literature)

EPIVAL®

All forms of epilepsy
▸ BY MOUTH
▸ Child: Total daily dose to be given in 1–2 divided doses (consult product literature)

IMPORTANT SAFETY INFORMATION
MHRA/CHM ADVICE: VALPROATE AND RISK OF ABNORMAL PREGNANCY OUTCOMES
Infants exposed to valproate in utero are at a high risk of serious developmental disorders (up to 30–40% risk) and congenital malformations (approx. 11% risk). Valproate should not be used in female children, females of childbearing potential or during pregnancy unless alternative treatments are ineffective or not tolerated.

NHS IMPROVEMENT PATIENT SAFETY ALERT: RESOURCES TO SUPPORT THE SAFETY OF GIRLS AND WOMEN WHO ARE BEING TREATED WITH VALPROATE (APRIL 2017)
The MHRA has published a set of resources, the valproate toolkit, to emphasise the need to avoid the use of valproate in girls and women of childbearing potential, warn women of the very high risks to the unborn child of valproate in pregnancy, and emphasise the need for effective contraception planning and specialist oversight of changes to medication when planning a pregnancy, as abrupt changes to medication can be harmful.

All organisations providing NHS-funded care where valproate is prescribed or dispensed should undertake systematic identification of girls and women who are taking valproate and ensure the MHRA resources are used to support them to make informed choices.

● CONTRA-INDICATIONS Acute porphyrias p. 577 · known or suspected mitochondrial disorders (higher rate of acute liver failure and liver-related deaths) · personal or family history of severe hepatic dysfunction

● CAUTIONS Systemic lupus erythematosus

CAUTIONS, FURTHER INFORMATION
Consider vitamin D supplementation in patients that are immobilised for long periods or who have inadequate sun exposure or dietary intake of calcium.

▸ Liver toxicity Liver dysfunction (including fatal hepatic failure) has occurred in association with valproate (especially in children under 3 years and in those with metabolic or degenerative disorders, organic brain disease or severe seizure disorders associated with mental retardation) usually in first 6 months and usually involving multiple antiepileptic therapy. Raised liver enzymes during valproate treatment are usually transient but patients should be reassessed clinically and liver function (including prothrombin time) monitored until return to normal—discontinue if abnormally prolonged prothrombin time (particularly in association with other relevant abnormalities).

● INTERACTIONS → Appendix 1: antiepileptics

● SIDE-EFFECTS
▸ Common or very common Aggression · anaemia · confusion · convulsion · deafness · diarrhoea · extrapyramidal disorders · gastric irritation · haemorrhage · headache · hyponatraemia · memory impairment · menstrual disturbance · nausea · nystagmus · somnolence · stupor · thrombocytopenia · transient hair loss (regrowth may be curly) · tremor · weight gain
▸ Uncommon Angioedema · ataxia · coma · encephalopathy · increased alertness · lethargy · leucopenia · pancytopenia · paraesthesia · peripheral oedema · rash · reduced bone mineral density · syndrome of inappropriate secretion of antidiuretic hormone · vasculitis
▸ Rare Behavioural disturbance · blood disorders · bone marrow failure · drowsiness · drug rash with eosinophilia and systemic symptoms (DRESS) syndrome · enuresis · Fanconi's syndrome · hallucinations · hearing loss · hyperactivity · hyperammonaemia · hypothyroidism · learning disorders · male infertility · myelodysplastic syndrome · polycystic ovaries · Stevens-Johnson syndrome · systemic lupus erythematosus · toxic epidermal necrolysis
▸ Very rare Acne · gynaecomastia · hepatic dysfunction · hirsutism · increase in bleeding time · pancreatitis
▸ Frequency not known Hypersensitivity reactions · suicidal ideation

SIDE-EFFECTS, FURTHER INFORMATION
▸ Hepatic dysfunction Withdraw treatment immediately if persistent vomiting and abdominal pain, anorexia, jaundice, oedema, malaise, drowsiness, or loss of seizure control.
▸ Pancreatitis Discontinue treatment if symtoms of pancreatitis develop.

● CONCEPTION AND CONTRACEPTION Valproate is associated with teratogenic risks and should not be used in females of child-bearing potential unless there is no safer alternative—this should be fully considered and discussed before prescribing for females of child-bearing age. Exclude pregnancy before treatment—effective contraception advised in females of child-bearing potential. In females planning to become pregnant, all efforts should be made to switch to appropriate alternative treatment prior to conception.

- **PREGNANCY** Valproate is associated with the highest risk of major and minor congenital malformations (in particular neural tube defects), and long-term neurodevelopmental effects. Valproate should not be used during pregnancy unless there is no safer alternative and only after a careful discussion of the risks. If valproate is to be used during pregnancy, the lowest effective dose should be prescribed in divided doses or as modified-release tablets to avoid peaks in plasma-valproate concentrations; doses greater than 1 g daily are associated with an increased risk of teratogenicity. Neonatal bleeding (related to hypofibrinaemia) reported. Neonatal hepatotoxicity also reported.

  Specialist prenatal monitoring should be instigated when valproate has been taken in pregnancy.

  The dose should be monitored carefully during pregnancy and after birth, and adjustments made on a clinical basis.

- **BREAST FEEDING** Present in milk—risk of haematological disorders in breast-fed newborns and infants.

- **HEPATIC IMPAIRMENT** Avoid if possible—hepatotoxicity and hepatic failure may occasionally occur (usually in first 6 months). Avoid in active liver disease.

- **RENAL IMPAIRMENT** Reduce dose.

- **MONITORING REQUIREMENTS**
  - Plasma-valproate concentrations are not a useful index of efficacy, therefore routine monitoring is unhelpful.
  - Monitor liver function before therapy and during first 6 months especially in patients most at risk.
  - Measure full blood count and ensure no undue potential for bleeding before starting and before surgery.

- **EFFECT ON LABORATORY TESTS** False-positive urine tests for ketones.

- **TREATMENT CESSATION** [EvGr] Avoid abrupt withdrawal; if treatment with valproate is stopped, reduce the dose gradually over at least 4 weeks. ⓐ

- **DIRECTIONS FOR ADMINISTRATION**
  - With intravenous use For *intravenous injection*, may be diluted in Glucose 5% *or* Sodium Chloride 0.9% and given over 3–5 minutes. For *intravenous infusion*, dilute injection solution with Glucose 5% *or* Sodium Chloride 0.9%.
  - With rectal use For *rectal administration*, sodium valproate oral solution may be given rectally and retained for 15 minutes (may require dilution with water to prevent rapid expulsion).

  EPIVAL® Tablets may be halved but not crushed or chewed.

  EPISENTA® CAPSULES Contents of capsule may be mixed with cold soft food or drink and swallowed immediately without chewing.

  EPILIM® SYRUP May be diluted, preferably in Syrup BP; use within 14 days.

  EPISENTA® GRANULES Granules may be mixed with cold soft food or drink and swallowed immediately without chewing.

  EPILIM CHRONOSPHERE® Granules may be mixed with soft food or drink that is cold or at room temperature, and swallowed immediately without chewing.

- **PRESCRIBING AND DISPENSING INFORMATION**
  Switching between formulations Care should be taken when switching between oral formulations in the treatment of epilepsy. The need for continued supply of a particular manufacturer's product should be based on clinical judgement and consultation with the patient or their carer, taking into account factors such as seizure frequency and treatment history.

Patients being treated for epilepsy may need to be maintained on a specific manufacturer's branded or generic oral sodium valproate product.

EPILIM CHRONOSPHERE® Prescribe close to the nearest whole 50-mg sachet.

- **PATIENT AND CARER ADVICE**
  Risk of abnormal pregnancy outcomes A patient guide and card should be provided to all female patients.
  Blood or hepatic disorders Patients or their carers should be told how to recognise signs and symptoms of blood or liver disorders and advised to seek immediate medical attention if symptoms develop.
  Pancreatitis Patients or their carers should be told how to recognise signs and symptoms of pancreatitis and advised to seek immediate medical attention if symptoms such as abdominal pain, nausea, or vomiting develop.
  Medicines for Children leaflet: Sodium valproate for preventing seizures www.medicinesforchildren.org.uk/sodium-valproate-for-preventing-seizures

  MHRA advice: Valproate and the risk of abnormal pregnancy outcomes Female patients and their carers should be counselled on the risk of valproate treatment during pregnancy. Ensure female patients are provided with relevant resources, to support their understanding of the risks. In particular the prescriber must ensure the patient understands:
  - the risks associated with valproate during pregnancy;
  - the need to use effective contraception;
  - the need for regular review of treatment;
  - the need to rapidly consult if she is planning a pregnancy or becomes pregnant.

  EPISENTA® CAPSULES Patients and carers should be counselled on the administration of capsules.

  EPISENTA® GRANULES Patients and carers should be counselled on the administration of granules.

  EPILIM CHRONOSPHERE® Patients and carers should be counselled on the administration of granules.

- **MEDICINAL FORMS**
  There can be variation in the licensing of different medicines containing the same drug. Forms available from special-order manufacturers include: oral suspension, oral solution, suppository

Modified-release tablet
CAUTIONARY AND ADVISORY LABELS 8, 10, 21, 25
- Epilim Chrono (Sanofi) ▼
  Sodium valproate 200 mg Epilim Chrono 200 tablets | 100 tablet [PoM] £11.65 DT price = £11.65
  Sodium valproate 300 mg Epilim Chrono 300 tablets | 100 tablet [PoM] £17.47 DT price = £17.47
  Sodium valproate 500 mg Epilim Chrono 500 tablets | 100 tablet [PoM] £29.10 DT price = £29.10
- Epival CR (Chanelle Medical UK Ltd) ▼
  Sodium valproate 300 mg Epival CR 300mg tablets | 100 tablet [PoM] £12.13 DT price = £17.47
  Sodium valproate 500 mg Epival CR 500mg tablets | 100 tablet [PoM] £20.21 DT price = £29.10

Gastro-resistant tablet
CAUTIONARY AND ADVISORY LABELS 5, 8, 10, 25
- **Sodium valproate (non-proprietary)** ▼
  Sodium valproate 200 mg Sodium valproate 200mg gastro-resistant tablets | 100 tablet [PoM] £7.70 DT price = £4.64
  Sodium valproate 500 mg Sodium valproate 500mg gastro-resistant tablets | 100 tablet [PoM] £19.25 DT price = £8.80
- Epilim (Sanofi) ▼
  Sodium valproate 200 mg Epilim 200 gastro-resistant tablets | 100 tablet [PoM] £7.70 DT price = £4.64
  Sodium valproate 500 mg Epilim 500 gastro-resistant tablets | 100 tablet [PoM] £19.25 DT price = £8.80

Tablet
CAUTIONARY AND ADVISORY LABELS 8, 10, 21
- Epilim (Sanofi) ▼
  Sodium valproate 100 mg Epilim 100mg crushable tablets | 100 tablet [PoM] £5.60 DT price = £5.60

Powder and solvent for solution for injection

▸ **Sodium valproate** (non-proprietary) ▼
  Sodium valproate 400 mg Sodium valproate 400mg powder and solvent for solution for injection vials | 4 vial [PoM] £49.00

▸ **Epilim** (Sanofi) ▼
  Sodium valproate 400 mg Epilim Intravenous 400mg powder and solvent for solution for injection vials | 1 vial [PoM] £13.32

Solution for injection

▸ **Sodium valproate** (non-proprietary) ▼
  Sodium valproate 100 mg per 1 ml Sodium valproate 400mg/4ml solution for injection ampoules | 5 ampoule [PoM] £57.90

▸ **Episenta** (Desitin Pharma Ltd) ▼
  Sodium valproate 100 mg per 1 ml Episenta 300mg/3ml solution for injection ampoules | 5 ampoule [PoM] £35.00

Modified-release capsule

CAUTIONARY AND ADVISORY LABELS 8, 10, 21, 25

▸ **Episenta** (Desitin Pharma Ltd) ▼
  Sodium valproate 150 mg Episenta 150mg modified-release capsules | 100 capsule [PoM] £7.00
  Sodium valproate 300 mg Episenta 300mg modified-release capsules | 100 capsule [PoM] £13.00 DT price = £13.00

Oral solution

CAUTIONARY AND ADVISORY LABELS 8, 10, 21

▸ **Sodium valproate** (non-proprietary) ▼
  Sodium valproate 40 mg per 1 ml Sodium valproate 200mg/5ml oral solution sugar free sugar-free | 300 ml [PoM] £5.01–£7.78 DT price = £5.01

▸ **Epilim** (Sanofi) ▼
  Sodium valproate 40 mg per 1 ml Epilim 200mg/5ml liquid sugar-free | 300 ml [PoM] £7.78 DT price = £5.01
  Epilim 200mg/5ml syrup | 300 ml [PoM] £9.33 DT price = £9.33

Modified-release granules

CAUTIONARY AND ADVISORY LABELS 8, 10, 21, 25

▸ **Epilim Chronosphere MR** (Sanofi) ▼
  Sodium valproate 50 mg Epilim Chronosphere MR 50mg granules sachets sugar-free | 30 sachet [PoM] £30.00
  Sodium valproate 100 mg Epilim Chronosphere MR 100mg granules sachets sugar-free | 30 sachet [PoM] £30.00 DT price = £30.00
  Sodium valproate 250 mg Epilim Chronosphere MR 250mg granules sachets sugar-free | 30 sachet [PoM] £30.00 DT price = £30.00
  Sodium valproate 500 mg Epilim Chronosphere MR 500mg granules sachets sugar-free | 30 sachet [PoM] £30.00 DT price = £30.00
  Sodium valproate 750 mg Epilim Chronosphere MR 750mg granules sachets sugar-free | 30 sachet [PoM] £30.00 DT price = £30.00
  Sodium valproate 1 gram Epilim Chronosphere MR 1000mg granules sachets sugar-free | 30 sachet [PoM] £30.00 DT price = £30.00

▸ **Episenta** (Desitin Pharma Ltd) ▼
  Sodium valproate 500 mg Episenta 500mg modified-release granules sachets sugar-free | 100 sachet [PoM] £21.00 DT price = £21.00
  Sodium valproate 1 gram Episenta 1000mg modified-release granules sachets sugar-free | 100 sachet [PoM] £41.00 DT price = £41.00

Stiripentol

● **INDICATIONS AND DOSE**

Adjunctive therapy of refractory generalised tonic-clonic seizures in children with severe myoclonic epilepsy in infancy (Dravet Syndrome) in combination with clobazam and valproate (under expert supervision)
▸ BY MOUTH
▸ **Child 3-17 years:** Initially 10 mg/kg daily in 2–3 divided doses, increased to up to 50 mg/kg daily in 2–3 divided doses, titrated over minimum of 3 days

● **CONTRA-INDICATIONS** History of psychosis

● **INTERACTIONS** → Appendix 1: antiepileptics

● **SIDE-EFFECTS**
▸ **Common or very common** Aggression · anorexia · ataxia · drowsiness · dystonia · hyperexcitability · hyperkinesia · hypotonia · irritability · nausea · neutropenia · sleep disorders · vomiting · weight loss
▸ **Uncommon** Fatigue · photosensitivity · rash · urticaria

● **ALLERGY AND CROSS-SENSITIVITY** Antiepileptic hypersensitivity syndrome theoretically associated with stiripentol. See under Epilepsy p. 184 for more information.

● **PREGNANCY** The dose should be monitored carefully during pregnancy and after birth, and adjustments made on a clinical basis.

● **BREAST FEEDING** Present in milk in *animal* studies.

● **HEPATIC IMPAIRMENT** Avoid—no information available.

● **RENAL IMPAIRMENT** Avoid—no information available.

● **MONITORING REQUIREMENTS**
▸ Perform full blood count and liver function tests prior to initiating treatment and every 6 months thereafter.
▸ Monitor growth.

● **DIRECTIONS FOR ADMINISTRATION** Do not take with milk, dairy products, carbonated drinks, fruit juice, or with food or drinks that contains caffeine.

● **PATIENT AND CARER ADVICE**
Medicines for Children leaflet: Stiripentol for preventing seizures www.medicinesforchildren.org.uk/stiripentol-for-preventing-seizures

● **MEDICINAL FORMS**
There can be variation in the licensing of different medicines containing the same drug.

Powder
CAUTIONARY AND ADVISORY LABELS 1, 8, 13, 21
EXCIPIENTS: May contain Aspartame
▸ **Diacomit** (Alan Pharmaceuticals)
  Stiripentol 250 mg Diacomit 250mg oral powder sachets | 60 sachet [PoM] £284.00 DT price = £284.00
  Stiripentol 500 mg Diacomit 500mg oral powder sachets | 60 sachet [PoM] £493.00

Capsule
CAUTIONARY AND ADVISORY LABELS 1, 8, 21
▸ **Diacomit** (Alan Pharmaceuticals)
  Stiripentol 250 mg Diacomit 250mg capsules | 60 capsule [PoM] £284.00 DT price = £284.00
  Stiripentol 500 mg Diacomit 500mg capsules | 60 capsule [PoM] £493.00

Tiagabine

● **INDICATIONS AND DOSE**

Adjunctive treatment for focal seizures with or without secondary generalisation that are not satisfactorily controlled by other antiepileptics (with enzyme-inducing drugs)
▸ BY MOUTH
▸ **Child 12-17 years:** Initially 5–10 mg daily in 1–2 divided doses, then increased in steps of 5–10 mg/24 hours every week; maintenance 30–45 mg daily in 2–3 divided doses

Adjunctive treatment for focal seizures with or without secondary generalisation that are not satisfactorily controlled by other antiepileptics (without enzyme-inducing drugs)
▸ BY MOUTH
▸ **Child 12-17 years:** Initially 5–10 mg daily in 1–2 divided doses, then increased in steps of 5–10 mg/24 hours every week; maintenance 15–30 mg daily in 2–3 divided doses

● **CAUTIONS** Avoid in acute porphyrias p. 577
CAUTIONS, FURTHER INFORMATION
Tiagabine should be avoided in absence, myoclonic, tonic and atonic seizures due to risk of seizure exacerbation.

● **INTERACTIONS** → Appendix 1: antiepileptics

Nervous system

4

- **SIDE-EFFECTS**
- ▶ **Common or very common** Diarrhoea · dizziness · emotional lability · impaired concentration · nervousness · speech impairment · tiredness · tremor
- ▶ **Rare** Bruising · confusion · depression · drowsiness · non-convulsive status epilepticus · psychosis · suicidal ideation · visual disturbances
- ▶ **Frequency not known** Leucopenia
- **PREGNANCY** The dose should be monitored carefully during pregnancy and after birth, and adjustments made on a clinical basis.
- **HEPATIC IMPAIRMENT** In mild to moderate impairment reduce dose, prolong the dose interval, or both. Avoid in severe impairment.
- **PATIENT AND CARER ADVICE**
  Driving and skilled tasks
  May impair performance of skilled tasks (e.g. driving). Medicines for Children leaflet: Tiagibine for preventing seizures www.medicinesforchildren.org.uk/tiagibine-for-preventing-seizures
- **MEDICINAL FORMS**
  There can be variation in the licensing of different medicines containing the same drug. Forms available from special-order manufacturers include: oral suspension
  Tablet
  CAUTIONARY AND ADVISORY LABELS 21
  ▶ Gabitril (Teva UK Ltd)
  Tiagabine (as Tiagabine hydrochloride monohydrate)
  5 mg Gabitril 5mg tablets | 100 tablet PoM £52.04
  Tiagabine (as Tiagabine hydrochloride monohydrate)
  10 mg Gabitril 10mg tablets | 100 tablet PoM £104.09
  Tiagabine (as Tiagabine hydrochloride monohydrate)
  15 mg Gabitril 15mg tablets | 100 tablet PoM £156.13

Topiramate

- **INDICATIONS AND DOSE**

Monotherapy of generalised tonic-clonic seizures or focal seizures with or without secondary generalisation
▶ BY MOUTH
▶ Child 6-17 years: Initially 0.5–1 mg/kg once daily (max. per dose 25 mg) for 1 week, dose to be taken at night, then increased in steps of 250–500 micrograms/kg twice daily, dose to be increased by a maximum of 25 mg twice daily at intervals of 1–2 weeks; usual dose 50 mg twice daily (max. per dose 7.5 mg/kg twice daily), if child cannot tolerate titration regimens recommended above then smaller steps or longer interval between steps may be used; maximum 500 mg per day

Adjunctive treatment of generalised tonic-clonic seizures or focal seizures with or without secondary generalisation | Adjunctive treatment for seizures associated with Lennox-Gastaut syndrome
▶ BY MOUTH
▶ Child 2-17 years: Initially 1–3 mg/kg once daily (max. per dose 25 mg) for 1 week, dose to be taken at night, then increased in steps of 0.5–1.5 mg/kg twice daily, dose to be increased by a maximum of 25 mg twice daily at intervals of 1–2 weeks; usual dose 2.5–4.5 mg/kg twice daily (max. per dose 7.5 mg/kg twice daily), if child cannot tolerate recommended titration regimen then smaller steps or longer interval between steps may be used; maximum 400 mg per day

Migraine prophylaxis
▶ BY MOUTH
▶ Child 16-17 years: Initially 25 mg once daily for 1 week, dose to be taken at night, then increased in steps of 25 mg every week; usual dose 50–100 mg daily in 2 divided doses, if child cannot tolerate recommended

titration regimen then smaller steps or longer interval between steps may be used; maximum 200 mg per day

- **UNLICENSED USE** Not licensed for use in children for migraine prophylaxis.
- **CAUTIONS** Avoid in acute porphyrias p. 577 · risk of metabolic acidosis · risk of nephrolithiasis—ensure adequate hydration (especially in strenuous activity or warm environment)
- **INTERACTIONS** → Appendix 1: antiepileptics
- **SIDE-EFFECTS**
- ▶ **Common or very common** Abdominal pain · aggression · agitation · alopecia · anaemia · anxiety · appetite changes · arthralgia · cognitive impairment · confusion · constipation · depression · diarrhoea · dizziness · drowsiness · dry mouth · dyspepsia · dyspnoea · epistaxis · gastritis · impaired attention · impaired coordination · irritability · malaise · mood changes · movement disorders · muscle spasm · muscular weakness · myalgia · nausea · nephrolithiasis · nystagmus · paraesthesia · pruritus · rash · seizures · sleep disturbance · speech disorder · taste disturbance · tinnitus · tremor · urinary disorders · visual disturbances · vomiting
- ▶ **Uncommon** Abdominal distension · altered sense of smell · blepharospasm · blood disorders · bradycardia · dry eye · flatulence · flushing · gingival bleeding · glossodynia · haematuria · halitosis · hearing loss · hypokalaemia · hypotension · increased lacrimation · influenza-like symptoms · leucopenia · metabolic acidosis · mydriasis · neutropenia · palpitation · pancreatitis · panic attack · peripheral neuropathy · photophobia · postural hypotension · psychosis · reduced sweating · salivation · sexual dysfunction · skin discoloration · suicidal ideation · thirst · thrombocytopenia · urinary calculus
- ▶ **Rare** Abnormal skin odour · calcinosis · hepatic failure · hepatitis · periorbital oedema · Raynaud's syndrome · Stevens-Johnson syndrome · unilateral blindness
- ▶ **Very rare** Angle-closure glaucoma
- ▶ **Frequency not known** Encephalopathy · hyperammonaemia · maculopathy · toxic epidermal necrolysis
  SIDE-EFFECTS, FURTHER INFORMATION
- ▶ Acute myopia with secondary angle-closure glaucoma Topiramate has been associated with acute myopia with secondary angle-closure glaucoma, typically occurring within 1 month of starting treatment. Choroidal effusions resulting in anterior displacement of the lens and iris have also been reported. If raised intra-ocular pressure occurs:
  - seek specialist ophthalmological advice;
  - use appropriate measures to reduce intra-ocular pressure;
  - stop topiramate as rapidly as feasible
- **PREGNANCY** Increased risk of cleft palate if taken in the first trimester of pregnancy. The dose should be monitored carefully during pregnancy and after birth, and adjustments made on a clinical basis. It is recommended that the fetal growth should be monitored.
- **BREAST FEEDING** Manufacturer advises avoid—present in milk.
- **HEPATIC IMPAIRMENT** Use with caution in moderate to severe impairment—clearance may be reduced.
- **RENAL IMPAIRMENT** Half usual starting and maintenance dose if estimated glomerular filtration less than 70 mL/minute/1.73 m^2—reduced clearance and longer time to steady-state plasma concentration. Use with caution.
- **DIRECTIONS FOR ADMINISTRATION**
  TOPAMAX® CAPSULES Swallow whole or sprinkle contents of capsule on soft food and swallow immediately without chewing.

● **PRESCRIBING AND DISPENSING INFORMATION**
Switching between formulations Care should be taken when switching between oral formulations in the treatment of epilepsy. The need for continued supply of a particular manufacturer's product should be based on clinical judgement and consultation with the patient or their carer, taking into account factors such as seizure frequency and treatment history.

Patients being treated for epilepsy may need to be maintained on a specific manufacturer's branded or generic topiramate product.

● **PATIENT AND CARER ADVICE**
Medicines for Children leaflet: Topiramate for preventing seizures www.medicinesforchildren.org.uk/topiramate-for-preventing-seizures

TOPAMAX® CAPSULES Patients or carers should be given advice on how to administer *Topamax*® capsules.

● **MEDICINAL FORMS**
There can be variation in the licensing of different medicines containing the same drug. Forms available from special-order manufacturers include: oral suspension, oral solution

Tablet
CAUTIONARY AND ADVISORY LABELS 3, 8
▸ **Topiramate (Non-proprietary)**
   Topiramate 25 mg Topiramate 25mg tablets | 60 tablet PoM £7.62 DT price = £1.66
   Topiramate 50 mg Topiramate 50mg tablets | 60 tablet PoM £12.83 DT price = £1.87
   Topiramate 100 mg Topiramate 100mg tablets | 60 tablet PoM £15.20 DT price = £2.52
   Topiramate 200 mg Topiramate 200mg tablets | 60 tablet PoM £19.99 DT price = £14.00
▸ **Topamax (Janssen-Cilag Ltd)**
   Topiramate 25 mg Topamax 25mg tablets | 60 tablet PoM £19.29 DT price = £1.66
   Topiramate 50 mg Topamax 50mg tablets | 60 tablet PoM £31.69 DT price = £1.87
   Topiramate 100 mg Topamax 100mg tablets | 60 tablet PoM £56.76 DT price = £2.52
   Topiramate 200 mg Topamax 200mg tablets | 60 tablet PoM £110.23 DT price = £14.00

Capsule
CAUTIONARY AND ADVISORY LABELS 3, 8
▸ **Topiramate (Non-proprietary)**
   Topiramate 15 mg Topiramate 15mg capsules | 60 capsule PoM £28.11 DT price = £25.14
   Topiramate 25 mg Topiramate 25mg capsules | 60 capsule PoM £25.95 DT price = £14.83
   Topiramate 50 mg Topiramate 50mg capsules | 60 capsule PoM £62.81 DT price = £56.06
▸ **Topamax (Janssen-Cilag Ltd)**
   Topiramate 15 mg Topamax 15mg sprinkle capsules | 60 capsule PoM £14.79 DT price = £25.14
   Topiramate 25 mg Topamax 25mg sprinkle capsules | 60 capsule PoM £22.18 DT price = £14.83
   Topiramate 50 mg Topamax 50mg sprinkle capsules | 60 capsule PoM £36.45 DT price = £56.06

Valproic acid

18-Apr-2017

● **INDICATIONS AND DOSE**

CONVULEX®

Epilepsy
▸ BY MOUTH
   ▸ **Child 1 month–11 years:** Initially 10–15 mg/kg daily in 2–4 divided doses, max. 600 mg daily; usual maintenance 25–30 mg/kg daily in 2–4 divided doses, doses up to 60 mg/kg daily in 2–4 divided doses in infantile spasms; monitor clinical chemistry and haematological parameters if dose exceeds 40 mg/kg daily
   ▸ **Child 12–17 years:** Initially 600 mg daily in 2–4 divided doses, increased in steps of 150–300 mg every 3 days;

usual maintenance 1–2 g daily in 2–4 divided doses, max. 2.5 g daily in 2–4 divided doses

DOSE EQUIVALENCE AND CONVERSION
▸ *Convulex*® has a 1:1 dose relationship with products containing sodium valproate, but nevertheless care is needed if switching or making changes.

IMPORTANT SAFETY INFORMATION
MHRA/CHM ADVICE: VALPROATE AND RISK OF ABNORMAL PREGNANCY OUTCOMES
Infants exposed to valproate in utero are at a high risk of serious developmental disorders (up to 30–40% risk) and congenital malformations (approx. 11% risk). Valproate should not be used in female children, females of childbearing potential or during pregnancy unless alternative treatments are ineffective or not tolerated.

NHS IMPROVEMENT PATIENT SAFETY ALERT: RESOURCES TO SUPPORT THE SAFETY OF GIRLS AND WOMEN WHO ARE BEING TREATED WITH VALPROATE (APRIL 2017)
The MHRA has published a set of resources, the valproate toolkit, to emphasise the need to avoid the use of valproate in girls and women of childbearing potential, warn women of the very high risks to the unborn child of valproate in pregnancy, and emphasise the need for effective contraception planning and specialist oversight of changes to medication when planning a pregnancy, as abrupt changes to medication can be harmful.

All organisations providing NHS-funded care where valproate is prescribed or dispensed should undertake systematic identification of girls and women who are taking valproate and ensure the MHRA resources are used to support them to make informed choices.

● **CONTRA-INDICATIONS** Acute porphyrias p. 577 · known or suspected mitochondrial disorders (higher rate of acute liver failure and liver-related deaths) · personal or family history of severe hepatic dysfunction

● **CAUTIONS** Systemic lupus erythematosus
CAUTIONS, FURTHER INFORMATION
Consider vitamin D supplementation in patients that are immobilised for long periods or who have inadequate sun exposure or dietary intake of calcium.
▸ Liver toxicity Liver dysfunction (including fatal hepatic failure) has occurred in association with valproate (especially in children under 3 years and in those with metabolic or degenerative disorders, organic brain disease or severe seizure disorders associated with mental retardation) usually in first 6 months and usually involving multiple antiepileptic therapy. Raised liver enzymes during valproate treatment are usually transient but patients should be reassessed clinically and liver function (including prothrombin time) monitored until return to normal—discontinue if abnormally prolonged prothrombin time (particularly in association with other relevant abnormalities).

● **INTERACTIONS** → Appendix 1: antiepileptics

● **SIDE-EFFECTS**
▸ **Common or very common** Diarrhoea · gastric irritation · hyperammonaemia · nausea · thrombocytopenia · transient hair loss (regrowth may be curly) · weight gain
▸ **Uncommon** Aggression · ataxia · behavioural disturbances · hyperactivity · increased alertness · tremor · vasculitis
▸ **Rare** Anaemia · blood disorders · confusion · drowsiness · hallucinations · hearing loss · hepatic dysfunction · lethargy · leucopenia · pancytopenia · rash · stupor
▸ **Very rare** Acne · coma · dementia · encephalopathy · enuresis · extrapyramidal symptoms · Fanconi's syndrome · gynaecomastia · hirsutism · hyponatraemia · increase in bleeding time · pancreatitis · peripheral oedema · reduced

bone mineral density · Stevens-Johnson syndrome · suicidal ideation · toxic epidermal necrolysis

▸ **Frequency not known** Drug rash with eosinophilia and systemic symptoms (DRESS) syndrome · hypersensitivity reactions · male infertility · menstrual disturbances · syndrome of inappropriate secretion of antidiuretic hormone

SIDE-EFFECTS, FURTHER INFORMATION

▸ Hepatic dysfunction Withdraw treatment immediately if persistent vomiting and abdominal pain, anorexia, jaundice, oedema, malaise, drowsiness, or loss of seizure control.

▸ Pancreatitis Discontinue treatment if symptoms of pancreatitis develop.

● CONCEPTION AND CONTRACEPTION Valproate is associated with teratogenic risks and should not be used in females of child-bearing potential unless there is no safer alternative—this should be fully considered and discussed before prescribing for females of child-bearing age. Effective contraception advised in females of child-bearing potential. In females planning to become pregnant, all efforts should be made to switch to appropriate alternative treatment prior to conception.

● PREGNANCY Valproate is associated with the highest risk of major and minor congenital malformations (in particular neural tube defects), and long-term neurodevelopmental effects. Valproate should not be used during pregnancy unless there is no safer alternative and only after a careful discussion of the risks. If valproate is to be used during pregnancy, the lowest effective dose should be prescribed in divided doses to avoid peaks in plasma-valproate concentrations; doses greater than 1 g daily are associated with an increased risk of teratogenicity. Neonatal bleeding (related to hypofibrinaemia). Neonatal hepatotoxicity also reported.

Specialist prenatal monitoring should be instigated when valproate has been taken in pregnancy. The dose should be monitored carefully during pregnancy and after birth, and adjustments made on a clinical basis.

● BREAST FEEDING Present in milk—risk of haematological disorders in breast-fed newborns and infants.

● HEPATIC IMPAIRMENT Avoid if possible—hepatotoxicity and hepatic failure may occasionally occur (usually in first 6 months). Avoid in active liver disease.

● RENAL IMPAIRMENT Reduce dose.

● MONITORING REQUIREMENTS

▸ Monitor closely if dose greater than 45 mg/kg daily.

▸ Monitor liver function before therapy and during first 6 months especially in patients most at risk.

▸ Measure full blood count and ensure no undue potential for bleeding before starting and before surgery.

● EFFECT ON LABORATORY TESTS False-positive urine tests for ketones.

● TREATMENT CESSATION [EvGr] Avoid abrupt withdrawal; if treatment with valproate is stopped, reduce the dose gradually over at least 4 weeks. ⓐ

● PRESCRIBING AND DISPENSING INFORMATION

CONVULEX® Patients being treated for epilepsy may need to be maintained on a specific manufacturer's branded or generic oral valproic acid product.

● PATIENT AND CARER ADVICE

Risk of abnormal pregnancy outcomes A patient guide and card should be provided to all female patients.

Blood or hepatic disorders Patients or their carers should be told how to recognise signs and symptoms of blood or liver disorders and advised to seek immediate medical attention if symptoms develop.

Pancreatitis Patients or their carers should be told how to recognise signs and symptoms of pancreatitis and advised

to seek immediate medical attention if symptoms such as abdominal pain, nausea, or vomiting develop.

MHRA advice: Valproate and the risk of abnormal pregnancy outcomes Female patients and their carers should be counselled on the risk of valproate treatment during pregnancy. Ensure female patients are provided with relevant resources, to support their understanding of the risks. In particular the prescriber must ensure the patient understands:
● the risks associated with valproate during pregnancy;
● the need to use effective contraception;
● the need for regular review of treatment;
● the need to rapidly consult if she is planning a pregnancy or becomes pregnant

● MEDICINAL FORMS
There can be variation in the licensing of different medicines containing the same drug.

Gastro-resistant capsule

CAUTIONARY AND ADVISORY LABELS 8, 21, 25, 10

▸ Convulex (Pfizer Ltd) ▼
Valproic acid 150 mg Convulex 150mg gastro-resistant capsules | 100 capsule [PoM] £3.68
Valproic acid 300 mg Convulex 300mg gastro-resistant capsules | 100 capsule [PoM] £7.35
Valproic acid 500 mg Convulex 500mg gastro-resistant capsules | 100 capsule [PoM] £12.25

Vigabatrin

● INDICATIONS AND DOSE

Adjunctive treatment of focal seizures with or without secondary generalisation not satisfactorily controlled with other antiepileptics (under expert supervision)

▸ BY MOUTH

▸ **Neonate:** Initially 15–20 mg/kg twice daily, to be increased over 2–3 weeks to usual maintenance dose, usual maintenance 30–40 mg/kg twice daily (max. per dose 75 mg/kg).

▸ Child 1–23 months: Initially 15–20 mg/kg twice daily (max. per dose 250 mg), to be increased over 2–3 weeks to usual maintenance dose, usual maintenance 30–40 mg/kg twice daily (max. per dose 75 mg/kg)

▸ Child 2–11 years: Initially 15–20 mg/kg twice daily (max. per dose 250 mg), to be increased over 2–3 weeks to usual maintenance dose, usual maintenance 30–40 mg/kg twice daily (max. per dose 1.5 g)

▸ Child 12–17 years: Initially 250 mg twice daily, to be increased over 2–3 weeks to usual maintenance dose, usual maintenance 1–1.5 g twice daily

▸ BY RECTUM

▸ Child 1–23 months: Initially 15–20 mg/kg twice daily (max. per dose 250 mg), to be increased over 2–3 weeks to usual maintenance dose, usual maintenance 30–40 mg/kg twice daily (max. per dose 75 mg/kg)

▸ Child 2–11 years: Initially 15–20 mg/kg twice daily (max. per dose 250 mg), to be increased over 2–3 weeks to usual maintenance dose, usual maintenance 30–40 mg/kg twice daily (max. per dose 1.5 g)

▸ Child 12–17 years: Initially 250 mg twice daily, to be increased over 2–3 weeks to usual maintenance dose, usual maintenance 1–1.5 g twice daily

Monotherapy in the management of infantile spasms in West's syndrome (under expert supervision)

▸ BY MOUTH

▸ **Neonate:** Initially 15–25 mg/kg twice daily, to be adjusted according to response over 7 days to usual maintenance dose; usual maintenance 40–50 mg/kg twice daily (max. per dose 75 mg/kg).

▸ **Child 1 month-1 year:** Initially 15–25 mg/kg twice daily, to be adjusted according to response over 7 days to usual maintenance dose; usual maintenance 40–50 mg/kg twice daily (max. per dose 75 mg/kg)

● **UNLICENSED USE** Granules not licensed for rectal use. Tablets not licensed to be crushed and dispersed in liquid. Vigabatrin doses in BNF publications may differ from those in product literature.

● **CONTRA-INDICATIONS** Visual field defects

● **CAUTIONS** History of behavioural problems · history of depression · history of psychosis

CAUTIONS, FURTHER INFORMATION
Vigabatrin may worsen absence, myoclonic, tonic and atonic seizures.

▸ **Visual field defects** Vigabatrin is associated with visual field defects. The onset of symptoms varies from 1 month to several years after starting. In most cases, visual field defects have persisted despite discontinuation, and further deterioration after discontinuation cannot be excluded. Product literature advises visual field testing before treatment and at 6-month intervals. Patients and their carers should be warned to report any new visual symptoms that develop and those with symptoms should be referred for an urgent ophthalmological opinion. Gradual withdrawal of vigabatrin should be considered.

● **INTERACTIONS** → Appendix 1: antiepileptics

● **SIDE-EFFECTS**

▸ **Common or very common** Abdominal pain · aggression · agitation · blurred vision · depression · diplopia · dizziness · drowsiness · excitation · fatigue · headache · impaired concentration · impaired memory · irritability · nausea · nervousness · nystagmus · oedema · paraesthesia · paranoia · speech disorder · tremor · visual field defects · vomiting · weight gain

▸ **Uncommon** Ataxia · mania · occasional increase in seizure frequency (especially if myoclonic) · psychosis · rash

▸ **Rare** Peripheral retinal neuropathy · retinal disorders · suicidal ideation

▸ **Very rare** Hepatitis · optic atrophy · optic neuritis

▸ **Frequency not known** Movement disorders in infantile spasms

SIDE-EFFECTS, FURTHER INFORMATION

▸ **Encephalopathic symptoms** Encephalopathic symptoms including marked sedation, stupor, and confusion with non-specific slow wave EEG can occur *rarely*—reduce dose or withdraw.

▸ **Visual field defects** About one-third of patients treated with vigabatrin have suffered visual field defects; counselling and **careful monitoring** for this side-effect are required.

● **PREGNANCY** The dose should be monitored carefully during pregnancy and after birth, and adjustments made on a clinical basis.

● **BREAST FEEDING** Present in milk—manufacturer advises avoid.

● **RENAL IMPAIRMENT** Consider reduced dose or increased dose interval if estimated glomerular filtration rate less than 60 mL/minute/1.73 m^2.

● **MONITORING REQUIREMENTS** Closely monitor neurological function.

● **DIRECTIONS FOR ADMINISTRATION**

▸ **With oral use** The contents of a sachet should be dissolved in water or a soft drink immediately before taking. Tablets may be crushed and dispersed in liquid.

▸ **With rectal use** Dissolve contents of sachet in small amount of water and administer rectally [unlicensed use].

● **PATIENT AND CARER ADVICE**
Patients and their carers should be warned to report any new visual symptoms that develop.

Medicines for Children leaflet: Vigabatrin for preventing seizures www.medicinesforchildren.org.uk/vigabatrin-for-preventing-seizures

● **MEDICINAL FORMS**
There can be variation in the licensing of different medicines containing the same drug. Forms available from special-order manufacturers include: oral solution

Powder
CAUTIONARY AND ADVISORY LABELS 3, 8, 13
▸ Sabril (Sanofi)
Vigabatrin 500 mg Sabril 500mg oral powder sachets sugar-free | 50 sachet [PoM] £24.60 DT price = £24.60

Tablet
CAUTIONARY AND ADVISORY LABELS 3, 8
▸ Sabril (Sanofi)
Vigabatrin 500 mg Sabril 500mg tablets | 100 tablet [PoM] £44.41 DT price = £44.41

Zonisamide

● **INDICATIONS AND DOSE**

Adjunctive treatment for refractory focal seizures with or without secondary generalisation

▸ BY MOUTH

▸ **Child 6-17 years (body-weight 20-54 kg):** Initially 1 mg/kg once daily for 7 days, then increased in steps of 1 mg/kg every 7 days, usual maintenance 6–8 mg/kg once daily (max. per dose 500 mg once daily), dose to be increased at 2-week intervals in patients who are **not** receiving concomitant carbamazepine, phenytoin, phenobarbital or other potent inducers of cytochrome P450 enzyme CYP3A4

▸ **Child 6-17 years (body-weight 55 kg and above):** Initially 1 mg/kg once daily for 7 days, then increased in steps of 1 mg/kg every 7 days, usual maintenance 300–500 mg once daily, dose to be increased at 2-week intervals in patients who are **not** receiving concomitant carbamazepine, phenytoin, phenobarbital or other potent inducers of cytochrome P450 enzyme CYP3A4

● **CAUTIONS** Low body-weight or poor appetite—monitor weight throughout treatment (fatal cases of weight loss reported in children) · metabolic acidosis—monitor serum bicarbonate concentration in children and those with other risk factors (consider dose reduction or discontinuation if metabolic acidosis develops) · risk factors for renal stone formation (particularly predisposition to nephrolithiasis)

CAUTIONS, FURTHER INFORMATION
Avoid overheating and ensure adequate hydration especially in children, during strenuous activity or if in warm environment (fatal cases of heat stroke reported in children).

● **INTERACTIONS** → Appendix 1: antiepileptics

● **SIDE-EFFECTS**

▸ **Common or very common** Abdominal pain · agitation · alopecia · anorexia · ataxia · confusion · constipation · depression · diarrhoea · diplopia · dizziness · drowsiness · ecchymosis · fatigue · impaired attention · impaired memory · insomnia · irritability · nausea · nystagmus · paraesthesia · peripheral oedema · pruritus · psychosis · pyrexia · rash (consider withdrawal) · speech disorder · tremor · weight loss

▸ **Uncommon** Aggression · cholecystitis · cholelithiasis · dyspepsia · hypokalaemia · pneumonia · seizures · suicidal ideation · urinary calculus · urinary tract infection · vomiting

▸ **Very rare** Amnesia · aspiration · blood disorders · coma · dyspnoea · hallucinations · heat stroke · hepatitis · hydronephrosis · impaired sweating · metabolic acidosis ·

myasthenic syndrome · neuroleptic malignant syndrome · pancreatitis · renal failure · renal tubular acidosis · rhabdomyolysis · Stevens-Johnson syndrome · toxic epidermal necrolysis

- **ALLERGY AND CROSS-SENSITIVITY** Contra-indicated in sulfonamide hypersensitivity. Antiepileptic hypersensitivity syndrome theoretically associated with zonisamide. See under Epilepsy p. 184 for more information.
- **CONCEPTION AND CONTRACEPTION** Manufacturer advises women of childbearing potential should use adequate contraception during treatment and for 4 weeks after last dose.
- **PREGNANCY** The dose should be monitored carefully during pregnancy and after birth, and adjustments made on a clinical basis.
- **BREAST FEEDING** Manufacturer advises avoid for 4 weeks after last dose.
- **HEPATIC IMPAIRMENT** Initially increase dose at 2-week intervals if mild or moderate impairment. Avoid in severe impairment.
- **RENAL IMPAIRMENT** Initially increase dose at 2-week intervals; discontinue if renal function deteriorates.
- **TREATMENT CESSATION** Avoid abrupt withdrawal (consult product literature for recommended withdrawal regimens in children).
- **PRESCRIBING AND DISPENSING INFORMATION**
  Switching between formulations Care should be taken when switching between oral formulations. The need for continued supply of a particular manufacturer's product should be based on clinical judgement and consultation with the patient or their carer, taking into account factors such as seizure frequency and treatment history.
  Patients may need to be maintained on a specific manufacturer's branded or generic zonisamide product.
- **PATIENT AND CARER ADVICE**
  Children and their carers should be made aware of how to prevent and recognise overheating and dehydration. Medicines for Children leaflet: Zonisamide for preventing seizures www.medicinesforchildren.org.uk/zonisamide-for-preventing-seizures
- **NATIONAL FUNDING/ACCESS DECISIONS**
  Scottish Medicines Consortium (SMC) Decisions
  The *Scottish Medicines Consortium* has advised (February 2014) that zonisamide (*Zonegran* ®) is accepted for restricted use within NHS Scotland as adjunctive treatment of focal seizures, with or without secondary generalisation, in adolescents and children aged 6 years and above. It is restricted to use on advice from specialists in paediatric neurology or epilepsy.

- **MEDICINAL FORMS**
  There can be variation in the licensing of different medicines containing the same drug. Forms available from special-order manufacturers include: oral suspension, oral solution
  Capsule
  CAUTIONARY AND ADVISORY LABELS 3, 8, 10
  ▸ Zonisamide (Non-proprietary)
  Zonisamide 25 mg Zonisamide 25mg capsules | 14 capsule [PoM] £7.83–£8.82 DT price = £8.66
  Zonisamide 50 mg Zonisamide 50mg capsules | 56 capsule [PoM] £41.74–£47.04 DT price = £46.16
  Zonisamide 100 mg Zonisamide 100mg capsules | 56 capsule [PoM] £56.07–£62.72 DT price = £62.20
  ▸ Zonegran (Eisai Ltd)
  Zonisamide 25 mg Zonegran 25mg capsules | 14 capsule [PoM] £8.82 DT price = £8.66
  Zonisamide 50 mg Zonegran 50mg capsules | 56 capsule [PoM] £47.04 DT price = £46.16
  Zonisamide 100 mg Zonegran 100mg capsules | 56 capsule [PoM] £62.72 DT price = £62.20

ANTIEPILEPTICS > BARBITURATES

Phenobarbital

(Phenobarbitone)

- **INDICATIONS AND DOSE**
  All forms of epilepsy except typical absence seizures
  ▸ BY MOUTH
  ▸ Child 1 month–11 years: Initially 1–1.5 mg/kg twice daily, then increased in steps of 2 mg/kg daily as required; maintenance 2.5–4 mg/kg 1–2 times a day
  ▸ Child 12–17 years: 60–180 mg once daily
  ▸ INITIALLY BY SLOW INTRAVENOUS INJECTION
  ▸ Neonate: Initially 20 mg/kg, then (by slow intravenous injection or by mouth) 2.5–5 mg/kg once daily, adjusted according to response.

  Status epilepticus
  ▸ BY SLOW INTRAVENOUS INJECTION
  ▸ Neonate: Initially 20 mg/kg, dose to be administered at a rate no faster than 1 mg/kg/minute, then 2.5–5 mg/kg 1–2 times a day.
  ▸ Child 1 month–11 years: Initially 20 mg/kg, dose to be administered at a rate no faster than 1 mg/kg/minute, then 2.5–5 mg/kg 1–2 times a day
  ▸ Child 12–17 years: Initially 20 mg/kg (max. per dose 1 g), dose to be administered at a rate no faster than 1 mg/kg/minute, then 300 mg twice daily

  DOSE EQUIVALENCE AND CONVERSION
  ▸ For therapeutic purposes phenobarbital and phenobarbital sodium may be considered equivalent in effect.

- **CAUTIONS** Avoid in acute porphyrias p. 577 · children · debilitated · history of alcohol abuse · history of drug abuse · respiratory depression (avoid if severe)
  CAUTIONS, FURTHER INFORMATION
  Consider vitamin D supplementation in patients who are immobilised for long periods or who have inadequate sun exposure or dietary intake of calcium.
- **INTERACTIONS** → Appendix 1: antiepileptics
- **SIDE-EFFECTS**
  ▸ Common or very common Agranulocytosis · allergic skin reactions · ataxia · behavioural disturbances · cholestasis · depression · drowsiness · hallucinations · hepatitis · hyperactivity particularly in the elderly and in children · hypotension · impaired cognition · impaired memory · irritability · lethargy · megaloblastic anaemia (may be treated with folic acid) · nystagmus · osteomalacia · respiratory depression · thrombocytopenia
  ▸ Very rare Antiepileptic hypersensitivity syndrome · Stevens-Johnson syndrome · suicidal ideation · toxic epidermal necrolysis
  ▸ Frequency not known Hyperkinesia
  Overdose
  For details on the management of poisoning, see Active elimination techniques, under Emergency treatment of poisoning p. 803.
- **ALLERGY AND CROSS-SENSITIVITY** Antiepileptic hypersensitivity syndrome associated with phenobarbital. See under Epilepsy p. 184 for more information.
- **PREGNANCY** The dose should be monitored carefully during pregnancy and after birth, and adjustments made on a clinical basis.
- **BREAST FEEDING** Avoid if possible; drowsiness may occur.
- **HEPATIC IMPAIRMENT** May precipitate coma. Avoid in severe impairment.
- **RENAL IMPAIRMENT** Use with caution.

● **MONITORING REQUIREMENTS**
▶ Plasma-phenobarbital concentration for optimum response is 15–40 mg/litre (60–180 micromol/litre); however, monitoring the plasma-drug concentration is less useful than with other drugs because tolerance occurs.

● **TREATMENT CESSATION** Avoid abrupt withdrawal (dependence with prolonged use).

● **DIRECTIONS FOR ADMINISTRATION**
▶ With oral use For administration by *mouth*, tablets may be crushed.
▶ With intravenous use For *intravenous injection*, dilute to a concentration of 20 mg/mL with Water for Injections; give over 20 minutes (no faster than 1 mg/kg/minute).

● **PRESCRIBING AND DISPENSING INFORMATION** Some hospitals supply **alcohol-free** formulations of varying phenobarbital strengths.
Switching between formulations Different formulations of oral preparations may vary in bioavailability. Patients should be maintained on a specific manufacturer's product.

● **PATIENT AND CARER ADVICE**
Medicines for Children leaflet: Phenobarbital for preventing seizures www.medicinesforchildren.org.uk/phenobarbital-for-preventing-seizures

● **MEDICINAL FORMS**
There can be variation in the licensing of different medicines containing the same drug. Forms available from special-order manufacturers include: tablet, capsule, oral suspension, oral solution

Tablet
CAUTIONARY AND ADVISORY LABELS 2, 8
▶ Phenobarbital (Non-proprietary)
Phenobarbital 15 mg Phenobarbital 15mg tablets | 28 tablet [PoM] £24.95 DT price = £17.29 [CD3]
Phenobarbital 30 mg Phenobarbital 30mg tablets | 28 tablet [PoM] £5.99 DT price = £0.78 [CD3]
Phenobarbital 60 mg Phenobarbital 60mg tablets | 28 tablet [PoM] £7.99 DT price = £6.03 [CD3]

Solution for injection
EXCIPIENTS: May contain Propylene glycol
▶ Phenobarbital (Non-proprietary)
Phenobarbital sodium 30 mg per 1 ml Phenobarbital 30mg/1ml solution for injection ampoules | 10 ampoule [PoM] £80.71–£81.42 [CD3]
Phenobarbital sodium 60 mg per 1 ml Phenobarbital 60mg/1ml solution for injection ampoules | 10 ampoule [PoM] £85.82 [CD3]
Phenobarbital sodium 200 mg per 1 ml Phenobarbital 200mg/1ml solution for injection ampoules | 10 ampoule [PoM] £66.63–£69.96 [CD3]

Oral solution
CAUTIONARY AND ADVISORY LABELS 2, 8
▶ Phenobarbital (Non-proprietary)
Phenobarbital 3 mg per 1 ml Phenobarbital 15mg/5ml elixir | 500 ml [PoM] £83.00 DT price = £83.00 [CD3]

Primidone

● **INDICATIONS AND DOSE**

All forms of epilepsy except typical absence seizures
▶ BY MOUTH
▶ Child 1 month–1 year: Initially 125 mg daily, dose to be taken at bedtime, then increased in steps of 125 mg every 3 days, adjusted according to response; maintenance 125–250 mg twice daily
▶ Child 2–4 years: Initially 125 mg once daily, dose to be taken at bedtime, then increased in steps of 125 mg every 3 days, adjusted according to response; maintenance 250–375 mg twice daily
▶ Child 5–8 years: Initially 125 mg once daily, dose to be taken at bedtime, then increased in steps of 125 mg every 3 days, adjusted according to response; maintenance 375–500 mg twice daily

▶ Child 9–17 years: Initially 125 mg once daily, dose to be taken at bedtime, then increased in steps of 125 mg every 3 days, increased to 250 mg twice daily, then increased in steps of 250 mg every 3 days (max. per dose 750 mg twice daily), adjusted according to response

● **CAUTIONS** Avoid in acute porphyria p. 577 · children · debilitated · history of alcohol abuse · history of drug abuse · respiratory depression (avoid if severe)
CAUTIONS, FURTHER INFORMATION
Consider vitamin D supplementation in patients who are immobilised for long periods or who have inadequate sun exposure or dietary intake of calcium.

● **INTERACTIONS** → Appendix 1: antiepileptics

● **SIDE-EFFECTS**
▶ **Common or very common** Agranulocytosis · allergic skin reactions · ataxia · behavioural disturbances · cholestasis · depression · drowsiness · hallucinations · hepatitis · hyperactivity · hypotension · impaired cognition · impaired memory · irritability · lethargy · megaloblastic anaemia (may be treated with folic acid) · nausea · nystagmus · osteomalacia · respiratory depression · thrombocytopenia · visual disturbances
▶ **Uncommon** Dizziness · headache · vomiting
▶ **Rare** Arthralgia · lupus erythematosus · psychosis
▶ **Very rare** Antiepileptic Hypersensitivity Syndrome · Stevens-Johnson syndrome · suicidal ideation · toxic epidermal necrolysis
▶ **Frequency not known** Dupuytren's contracture

● **ALLERGY AND CROSS-SENSITIVITY** Antiepileptic hypersensitivity syndrome associated with primidone. See under Epilepsy p. 184 for more information.

● **PREGNANCY** The dose should be monitored carefully during pregnancy and after birth, and adjustments made on a clinical basis.

● **HEPATIC IMPAIRMENT** Reduce dose. May precipitate coma.

● **RENAL IMPAIRMENT** Use with caution.

● **MONITORING REQUIREMENTS**
▶ Monitor plasma concentrations of derived phenobarbital; plasma concentration for optimum response is 15–40 mg/litre (60–180 micromol/litre).

● **TREATMENT CESSATION** Avoid abrupt withdrawal (dependence with prolonged use).

● **PRESCRIBING AND DISPENSING INFORMATION**
Switching between formulations Different formulations of oral preparations may vary in bioavailability. Patients being treated for epilepsy should be maintained on a specific manufacturer's product.

● **MEDICINAL FORMS**
There can be variation in the licensing of different medicines containing the same drug. Forms available from special-order manufacturers include: capsule, oral suspension

Oral suspension
▶ Primidone (Non-proprietary)
Primidone 25 mg per 1 ml Liskantin Saft 125mg/5ml oral suspension | 250 ml [PoM] no price available

Tablet
CAUTIONARY AND ADVISORY LABELS 2, 8
▶ Primidone (Non-proprietary)
Primidone 50 mg Primidone 50mg tablets | 100 tablet [PoM] £110.00–£112.37 DT price = £111.46
Primidone 250 mg Primidone 250mg tablets | 90 tablet [PoM] no price available | 100 tablet [PoM] £99.65–£121.94 DT price = £114.51

HYPNOTICS, SEDATIVES AND ANXIOLYTICS ›
BENZODIAZEPINES

Benzodiazepines

- **CONTRA-INDICATIONS** Acute pulmonary insufficiency · marked neuromuscular respiratory weakness · sleep apnoea syndrome · unstable myasthenia gravis
- **CAUTIONS** Avoid prolonged use (and abrupt withdrawal thereafter) · history of alcohol dependence or abuse · history of drug dependence or abuse · myasthenia gravis · respiratory disease

  CAUTIONS, FURTHER INFORMATION
  ▸ Paradoxical effects A paradoxical increase in hostility and aggression may be reported by patients taking benzodiazepines. The effects range from talkativeness and excitement to aggressive and antisocial acts. Adjustment of the dose (up or down) sometimes attenuates the impulses. Increased anxiety and perceptual disorders are other paradoxical effects.

- **SIDE-EFFECTS**

  Overdose
  Benzodiazepines taken alone cause drowsiness, ataxia, dysarthria, nystagmus, and occasionally respiratory depression, and coma. For details on the management of poisoning, see Benzodiazepines, under Emergency treatment of poisoning p. 803.

- **PREGNANCY** Risk of neonatal withdrawal symptoms when used during pregnancy. Avoid regular use and use only if there is a clear indication such as seizure control. High doses administered during late pregnancy or labour may cause neonatal hypothermia, hypotonia, and respiratory depression.

- **RENAL IMPAIRMENT** Increased cerebral sensitivity to benzodiazepines.

- **PATIENT AND CARER ADVICE**

  Driving and skilled tasks
  Drowsiness may persist the next day and affect performance of skilled tasks (e.g. driving); effects of alcohol enhanced.

  For information on 2015 legislation regarding driving whilst taking certain controlled drugs, including benzodiazepines, see *Drugs and Skilled Tasks* under Guidance on prescribing p. 1.

  ╔ above

Clobazam

- **INDICATIONS AND DOSE**

  Adjunct in epilepsy
  ▸ BY MOUTH
  ▸ **Child 1 month–5 years:** Initially 125 micrograms/kg twice daily, dose to be increased if necessary every 5 days, maintenance 250 micrograms/kg twice daily (max. per dose 500 micrograms/kg twice daily); maximum 30 mg per day
  ▸ **Child 6–17 years:** Initially 5 mg daily, dose to be increased if necessary at intervals of 5 days, maintenance 0.3–1 mg/kg daily, daily doses of up to 30 mg may be given as a single dose at bedtime, higher doses should be divided; maximum 60 mg per day

  Monotherapy for catamenial (menstruation) seizures (usually for 7–10 days each month, just before and during menstruation) (under expert supervision) |
  Cluster seizures
  ▸ BY MOUTH
  ▸ **Child 1 month–5 years:** Initially 125 micrograms/kg twice daily, dose to be increased if necessary every 5 days, maintenance 250 micrograms/kg twice daily (max. per

dose 500 micrograms/kg twice daily); maximum 30 mg per day
- **Child 6–17 years:** Initially 5 mg daily, dose to be increased if necessary at intervals of 5 days, maintenance 0.3–1 mg/kg daily, daily doses of up to 30 mg may be given as a single dose at bedtime, higher doses should be divided; maximum 60 mg per day

- **UNLICENSED USE** Not licensed for use in children under 6 years. Not licensed as monotherapy.

> **IMPORTANT SAFETY INFORMATION**
> Do **not** confuse with clonazepam.

- **CONTRA-INDICATIONS** Hyperkinesis · obsessional states · phobic states · respiratory depression
- **CAUTIONS** Muscle weakness · organic brain changes · personality disorder (within the fearful group—dependent, avoidant, obsessive-compulsive) may increase risk of dependence

  CAUTIONS, FURTHER INFORMATION
  The effectiveness of clobazam may decrease significantly after weeks or months of continuous therapy.

- **INTERACTIONS** → Appendix 1: clobazam
- **SIDE-EFFECTS**
  ▸ **Common or very common** Amnesia · ataxia (especially in the elderly) · confusion (especially in the elderly) · dependence · drowsiness the next day · lightheadedness the next day · muscle weakness · paradoxical increase in aggression
  ▸ **Uncommon** Dizziness · dysarthria · gastro-intestinal disturbances · gynaecomastia · incontinence · salivation changes · tremor · visual disturbances
  ▸ **Rare** Apnoea · blood disorders · changes in libido · headache · hypotension · jaundice · respiratory depression · skin reactions · urinary retention · vertigo
  ▸ **Frequency not known** Delusions · excitement · hallucinations · irritability · psychosis · restlessness
- **BREAST FEEDING** Benzodiazepines are present in milk, and should be avoided if possible during breast-feeding.

  All infants should be monitored for sedation, feeding difficulties, adequate weight gain, and developmental milestones.
- **HEPATIC IMPAIRMENT** Start with smaller initial doses or reduce dose. Can precipitate coma. Avoid in severe impairment.
- **RENAL IMPAIRMENT** Start with small doses in severe impairment.
- **MONITORING REQUIREMENTS** Routine measurement of plasma concentrations of antiepileptic drugs is not usually justified, because the target concentration ranges are arbitrary and often vary between individuals. However, plasma drug concentrations may be measured in children with worsening seizures, status epilepticus, suspected noncompliance, or suspected toxicity. Similarly, haematological and biochemical monitoring should not be undertaken unless clinically indicated.
- **PRESCRIBING AND DISPENSING INFORMATION**
  Switching between formulations Care should be taken when switching between oral formulations in the treatment of epilepsy. The need for continued supply of a particular manufacturer's product should be based on clinical judgement and consultation with the patient or their carer, taking into account factors such as seizure frequency and treatment history.

  Patients being treated for epilepsy may need to be maintained on a specific manufacturer's branded or generic clobazam product.

● **PATIENT AND CARER ADVICE**
Medicines for Children leaflet: Clobazam for preventing seizures www.medicinesforchildren.org.uk/clobazam-preventing-seizures-0

● **NATIONAL FUNDING/ACCESS DECISIONS**
NHS restrictions Clobazam is not prescribable under the NHS except for epilepsy and endorsed 'SLS'.

● **MEDICINAL FORMS**
There can be variation in the licensing of different medicines containing the same drug. Forms available from special-order manufacturers include: capsule, oral suspension

Oral suspension
CAUTIONARY AND ADVISORY LABELS 2, 19, 8
▸ **Clobazam (Non-proprietary)**
Clobazam 1 mg per 1 ml Clobazam 5mg/5ml oral suspension sugar free sugar-free | 150 ml [PoM] £90.00 DT price = £90.00 [CD4-1] sugar-free | 250 ml [PoM] £150.00 [CD4-1]
Clobazam 2 mg per 1 ml Clobazam 10mg/5ml oral suspension sugar free sugar-free | 150 ml [PoM] £95.00–£97.50 DT price = £95.00 [CD4-1] sugar-free | 250 ml [PoM] £162.50 [CD4-1]
▸ **Perizam** (Rosemont Pharmaceuticals Ltd)
Clobazam 1 mg per 1 ml Perizam 1mg/ml oral suspension sugar-free | 150 ml [PoM] £90.00 DT price = £90.00 [CD4-1]
Clobazam 2 mg per 1 ml Perizam 2mg/ml oral suspension sugar-free | 150 ml [PoM] £95.00 DT price = £95.00 [CD4-1]
▸ **Tapclob** (Martindale Pharmaceuticals Ltd)
Clobazam 1 mg per 1 ml Tapclob 5mg/5ml oral suspension sugar-free | 150 ml [PoM] £90.00 DT price = £90.00 [CD4-1] sugar-free | 250 ml [PoM] £150.00 [CD4-1]
Clobazam 2 mg per 1 ml Tapclob 10mg/5ml oral suspension sugar-free | 150 ml [PoM] £95.00 DT price = £95.00 [CD4-1] sugar-free | 250 ml [PoM] £158.34 [CD4-1]

Tablet
CAUTIONARY AND ADVISORY LABELS 2, 19, 8
▸ **Clobazam (Non-proprietary)**
Clobazam 10 mg Clobazam 10mg tablets | 30 tablet [PoM] £3.36 DT price = £3.27 [CD4-1]
▸ **Frisium** (Sanofi)
Clobazam 10 mg Frisium 10mg tablets | 30 tablet [PoM] £2.51 DT price = £3.27 [CD4-1]

F 210

Clonazepam

● **INDICATIONS AND DOSE**
All forms of epilepsy
▸ BY MOUTH
▸ **Child 1-11 months:** Initially 250 micrograms once daily for 4 nights, dose to be increased over 2–4 weeks, usual dose 0.5–1 mg daily, dose to be taken at night; may be given in 3 divided doses if necessary
▸ **Child 1-4 years:** Initially 250 micrograms once daily for 4 nights, dose to be increased over 2–4 weeks, usual dose 1–3 mg daily, dose to be taken at night; may be given in 3 divided doses if necessary
▸ **Child 5-11 years:** Initially 500 micrograms once daily for 4 nights, dose to be increased over 2–4 weeks, usual dose 3–6 mg daily, dose to be taken at night; may be given in 3 divided doses if necessary
▸ **Child 12-17 years:** Initially 1 mg once daily for 4 nights, dose to be increased over 2–4 weeks, usual dose 4–8 mg daily, dose usually taken at night; may be given in 3–4 divided doses if necessary

● **UNLICENSED USE** Clonazepam doses in BNFC may differ from those in product literature.

> **IMPORTANT SAFETY INFORMATION**
> Do **not** confuse with clobazam.

● **CONTRA-INDICATIONS** Coma · current alcohol abuse · current drug abuse · respiratory depression

● **CAUTIONS** Acute porphyrias p. 577 · airways obstruction · brain damage · cerebellar ataxia · depression · spinal ataxia · suicidal ideation
CAUTIONS, FURTHER INFORMATION
The effectiveness of clonazepam may decrease significantly after weeks or months of continuous therapy.

● **INTERACTIONS** → Appendix 1: clonazepam

● **SIDE-EFFECTS**
▸ **Common or very common** Amnesia · bronchial hypersecretion in infants and small children · co-ordination disturbances · confusion · dependence · dizziness · drowsiness · fatigue · muscle hypotonia · nystagmus · poor concentration · restlessness · salivary hypersecretion in infants and small children · withdrawal symptoms
▸ **Rare** Aggression · anxiety · blood disorders · dysarthria · gastro-intestinal symptoms · headache · paradoxical effects · pruritus · respiratory depression · reversible hair loss · sexual dysfunction · skin pigmentation changes · urinary incontinence · urticaria · visual disturbances on long-term treatment
▸ **Very rare** Increase in seizure frequency

● **BREAST FEEDING** Present in milk, and should be avoided if possible during breast-feeding.
All infants should be monitored for sedation, feeding difficulties, adequate weight gain, and developmental milestones.

● **HEPATIC IMPAIRMENT** Start with smaller initial doses or reduce dose. Can precipitate coma. Avoid in severe impairment.

● **RENAL IMPAIRMENT** Start with small doses in severe impairment.

● **MONITORING REQUIREMENTS** Routine measurement of plasma concentrations of antiepileptic drugs is not usually justified, because the target concentration ranges are arbitrary and often vary between individuals. However, plasma drug concentrations may be measured in children with worsening seizures, status epilepticus, suspected noncompliance, or suspected toxicity. Similarly, haematological and biochemical monitoring should not be undertaken unless clinically indicated.

● **PRESCRIBING AND DISPENSING INFORMATION**
Switching between formulations Care should be taken when switching between oral formulations in the treatment of epilepsy. The need for continued supply of a particular manufacturer's product should be based on clinical judgement and consultation with the patient or their carer, taking into account factors such as seizure frequency and treatment history.
Patients being treated for epilepsy may need to be maintained on a specific manufacturer's branded or generic oral clonazepam product.

● **PATIENT AND CARER ADVICE**
Medicines for Children leaflet: Clonazepam for preventing seizures www.medicinesforchildren.org.uk/clonazepam-preventing-seizures-0

● **MEDICINAL FORMS**
There can be variation in the licensing of different medicines containing the same drug. Forms available from special-order manufacturers include: orodispersible tablet, oral suspension, oral solution, oral drops

Tablet
CAUTIONARY AND ADVISORY LABELS 2, 8
▸ **Clonazepam (Non-proprietary)**
Clonazepam 500 microgram Clonazepam 500microgram tablets | 100 tablet [PoM] £30.11 DT price = £28.39 [CD4-1]
Clonazepam 2 mg Clonazepam 2mg tablets | 100 tablet [PoM] £33.41 DT price = £31.11 [CD4-1]

4

Nervous system

4

Nervous system

Oral drops

▸ Clonazepam (Non-proprietary)

Clonazepam 2.5 mg per 1 ml Rivotril 2.5mg/1ml drops sugar-free | 10 ml PoM no price available CD4-1

Oral solution

CAUTIONARY AND ADVISORY LABELS 2, 8
EXCIPIENTS: May contain Ethanol

▸ Clonazepam (Non-proprietary)

Clonazepam 100 microgram per 1 ml Clonazepam 500micrograms/5ml oral solution sugar free sugar-free | 150 ml PoM £83.40 DT price = £69.50 CD4-1

Clonazepam 400 microgram per 1 ml Clonazepam 2mg/5ml oral solution sugar free sugar-free | 150 ml PoM £108.36 DT price = £108.36 CD4-1

Oral lyophilisate

▸ Clonazepam (Non-proprietary)

Clonazepam 500 microgram Klonopin 0.5mg oral lyophilisates sugar-free | 60 tablet PoM no price available CD4-1

▰ 210

Diazepam

21-Nov-2016

● **INDICATIONS AND DOSE**

Tetanus

▸ BY INTRAVENOUS INJECTION

▸ Child: 100–300 micrograms/kg every 1–4 hours

▸ BY INTRAVENOUS INFUSION, OR BY NASODUODENAL TUBE

▸ Child: 3–10 mg/kg, adjusted according to response, to be given over 24 hours

Muscle spasm in cerebral spasticity or in postoperative skeletal muscle spasm

▸ BY MOUTH

▸ Child 1–11 months: Initially 250 micrograms/kg twice daily

▸ Child 1–4 years: Initially 2.5 mg twice daily

▸ Child 5–11 years: Initially 5 mg twice daily

▸ Child 12–17 years: Initially 10 mg twice daily; maximum 40 mg per day

Status epilepticus | Febrile convulsions | Convulsions due to poisoning

▸ BY INTRAVENOUS INJECTION

▸ Neonate: 300–400 micrograms/kg, then 300–400 micrograms/kg after 10 minutes if required, to be given over 3–5 minutes.

▸ Child 1 month–11 years: 300–400 micrograms/kg (max. per dose 10 mg), then 300–400 micrograms/kg after 10 minutes if required, to be given over 3–5 minutes

▸ Child 12–17 years: 10 mg, then 10 mg after 10 minutes if required, to be given over 3–5 minutes

▸ BY RECTUM

▸ Neonate: 1.25–2.5 mg, then 1.25–2.5 mg after 10 minutes if required.

▸ Child 1 month–1 year: 5 mg, then 5 mg after 10 minutes if required

▸ Child 2–11 years: 5–10 mg, then 5–10 mg after 10 minutes if required

▸ Child 12–17 years: 10–20 mg, then 10–20 mg after 10 minutes if required

Life-threatening acute drug-induced dystonic reactions

▸ BY INTRAVENOUS INJECTION

▸ Child 1 month–11 years: 100 micrograms/kg, repeated if necessary, to be given over 3–5 minutes

▸ Child 12–17 years: 5–10 mg, repeated if necessary, to be given over 3–5 minutes

● **UNLICENSED USE** *Diazepam Desitin®*, *Diazepam Rectubes®*, and *Stesolid Rectal Tubes®* not licensed for use in children under 1 year.

> **IMPORTANT SAFETY INFORMATION**
> ANAESTHESIA
> Benzodiazepines should only be administered for anaesthesia by, or under the direct supervision of, personnel experienced in their use, with adequate training in anaesthesia and airway management.

● **CONTRA-INDICATIONS** Avoid injections containing benzyl alcohol in neonates · CNS depression · compromised airway · hyperkinesis · obsessional states · phobic states · respiratory depression

● **CAUTIONS**

GENERAL CAUTIONS

Muscle weakness · organic brain changes · parenteral administration (close observation required until full recovery from sedation) · personality disorder (within the fearful group—dependent, avoidant, obsessive-compulsive) may increase risk of dependence

SPECIFIC CAUTIONS

▸ With intravenous use High risk of venous thrombophlebitis with intravenous use (reduced by using an emulsion formulation)

CAUTIONS, FURTHER INFORMATION

▸ Special precautions for intravenous injection When given intravenously facilities for reversing respiratory depression with mechanical ventilation must be immediately available.

● **INTERACTIONS** → Appendix 1: diazepam

● **SIDE-EFFECTS**

GENERAL SIDE-EFFECTS

▸ Common or very common Amnesia · ataxia · confusion · dependence · drowsiness the next day · lightheadedness the next day · muscle weakness   paradoxical increase in aggression

▸ Uncommon Dizziness · dysarthria · gastro-intestinal disturbances · gynaecomastia · incontinence · salivation changes · tremor · visual disturbances

▸ Rare Apnoea · blood disorders   changes in libido · headache · hypotension · jaundice · respiratory depression · skin reactions · urinary retention · vertigo

▸ Frequency not known Delusions · excitement · hallucinations · hypotonia (when used for muscle spasm) · irritability · marked respiratory depression, particularly with high dose (facilities for its treatment are essential) · psychosis · restlessness

SPECIFIC SIDE-EFFECTS

▸ With intravenous use Pain · thrombophlebitis

● **PREGNANCY** Women who have seizures in the second half of pregnancy should be assessed for eclampsia before any change is made to antiepileptic treatment. Status epilepticus should be treated according to the standard protocol.
Epilepsy and Pregnancy Register All pregnant women with epilepsy, whether taking medication or not, should be encouraged to notify the UK Epilepsy and Pregnancy Register (Tel: 0800 389 1248).

● **BREAST FEEDING** Present in milk, and should be avoided if possible during breast-feeding.

● **HEPATIC IMPAIRMENT** Start with smaller initial doses or reduce dose. Can precipitate coma. If treatment is necessary, benzodiazepines with shorter half lives are safer, such as temazepam or oxazepam.
    Avoid in severe impairment.

● **RENAL IMPAIRMENT** Start with small doses in severe impairment.

4

● **DIRECTIONS FOR ADMINISTRATION**

▸ With intravenous use Diazepam is adsorbed by plastics of infusion bags and giving sets. Emulsion formulation preferred for intravenous injection.

For *continuous intravenous infusion* of diazepam emulsion, dilute to a concentration of max. 400 micrograms/mL with Glucose 5% or 10%; max. 6 hours between addition and completion of infusion. For *continuous intravenous infusion* of diazepam solution, dilute to a concentration of max. 50 micrograms/mL with Glucose 5% or Sodium Chloride 0.9%.

● **PATIENT AND CARER ADVICE**

Driving and skilled tasks

May impair judgement and increase reaction time, and so affect ability to drive or perform skilled tasks; they increase the effects of alcohol. Moreover the hangover effects of a night dose may impair performance on the following day.

Patients given sedatives and analgesics during minor outpatient procedures should be very carefully warned about the risks of undertaking skilled tasks (e.g. driving) afterwards. For intravenous benzodiazepines the risk extends to **at least 24 hours** after administration. Responsible persons should be available to take patients home afterwards. The dangers of taking **alcohol** should be emphasised.

Medicines for Children leaflet: Diazepam (rectal) for stopping seizures www.medicinesforchildren.org.uk/diazepam-rectal-stopping-seizures-0

Medicines for Children leaflet: Diazepam for muscle spasm www.medicinesforchildren.org.uk/diazepam-for-muscle-spasm

● **PROFESSION SPECIFIC INFORMATION**

Dental practitioners' formulary

Diazepam Tablets may be prescribed.

Diazepam Oral Solution 2 mg/5 mL may be prescribed.

● **MEDICINAL FORMS**

There can be variation in the licensing of different medicines containing the same drug. Forms available from special-order manufacturers include: oral suspension, oral solution, suppository

Tablet

CAUTIONARY AND ADVISORY LABELS 2, 19

▸ **Diazepam (Non-proprietary)**

Diazepam 2 mg Diazepam 2mg tablets | 28 tablet PoM £1.10 DT price = £0.73 CD4-1 | 1000 tablet PoM £160.71 CD4-1

Diazepam 5 mg Diazepam 5mg tablets | 28 tablet PoM £1.12 DT price = £0.76 CD4-1 | 1000 tablet PoM £210.71 CD4-1

Diazepam 10 mg Diazepam 10mg tablets | 28 tablet PoM £4.99 DT price = £0.85 CD4-1 | 500 tablet PoM £113.04 CD4-1

Emulsion for injection

▸ **Diazemuls (Actavis UK Ltd)**

Diazepam 5 mg per 1 ml Diazemuls 10mg/2ml emulsion for injection ampoules | 10 ampoule PoM £9.05 CD4-1

Solution for injection

EXCIPIENTS: May contain Benzyl alcohol, ethanol, propylene glycol

▸ **Diazepam (Non-proprietary)**

Diazepam 5 mg per 1 ml Diazepam 10mg/2ml solution for injection ampoules | 10 ampoule PoM £5.50 DT price = £5.50 CD4-1

Oral suspension

▸ **Diazepam (Non-proprietary)**

Diazepam 400 microgram per 1 ml Diazepam 2mg/5ml oral suspension | 100 ml PoM £31.75–£39.00 DT price = £31.75 CD4-1

Diazepam 1 mg per 1 ml Diazepam 5mg/5ml oral suspension | 100 ml PoM £55.00–£66.00 CD4-1

Oral solution

CAUTIONARY AND ADVISORY LABELS 2, 19

▸ **Diazepam (Non-proprietary)**

Diazepam 400 microgram per 1 ml Diazepam 2mg/5ml oral solution sugar free sugar-free | 100 ml PoM £31.75–£38.10 DT price = £31.75 CD4-1

Enema

CAUTIONARY AND ADVISORY LABELS 2, 19

▸ **Diazepam (Non-proprietary)**

Diazepam 2 mg per 1 ml Diazepam 5mg RecTubes | 5 tube PoM £5.85 DT price = £5.85 CD4-1

Diazepam 2.5mg/1.25ml rectal solution tube | 5 tube PoM no price available CD4-1

Diazepam 2.5mg RecTubes | 5 tube PoM £5.65 CD4-1

Diazepam 5mg/2.5ml rectal solution tube | 5 tube PoM £5.85 DT price = £5.85 CD4-1

Diazepam 4 mg per 1 ml Diazepam 10mg RecTubes | 5 tube PoM £7.35 DT price = £7.35 CD4-1

Diazepam 10mg/2.5ml rectal solution tube | 5 tube PoM £7.35 DT price = £7.35 CD4-1

▸ **Stesolid (Actavis UK Ltd)**

Diazepam 2 mg per 1 ml Stesolid 5mg rectal tube | 5 tube PoM £6.89 DT price = £5.85 CD4-1

Diazepam 4 mg per 1 ml Stesolid 10mg rectal tube | 5 tube PoM £8.78 DT price = £7.35 CD4-1

1.1 Status epilepticus

Other drugs used for Status epilepticus Diazepam, p. 212 · Fosphenytoin sodium,p. 191 · Phenobarbital, p. 208 · Phenytoin, p. 198

ANTIEPILEPTICS

Paraldehyde

● **INDICATIONS AND DOSE**

Status epilepticus

▸ BY RECTUM

▸ Neonate: 0.8 mL/kilogram for 1 dose, the dose is based on the use of a premixed solution of paraldehyde in olive oil in equal volumes.

▸ Child: 0.8 mL/kilogram (max. per dose 20 mL) for 1 dose, the dose is based on the use of a premixed solution of paraldehyde in olive oil in equal volumes

● **UNLICENSED USE** Not licensed for use in children as an enema.

● **CONTRA-INDICATIONS** Gastric disorders · rectal administration in colitis

● **CAUTIONS** Bronchopulmonary disease

● **INTERACTIONS** → Appendix 1: antiepileptics

● **SIDE-EFFECTS** Rash

● **PREGNANCY** Avoid unless essential—crosses placenta.

● **BREAST FEEDING** Avoid unless essential—present in milk.

● **HEPATIC IMPAIRMENT** Use with caution.

● **PATIENT AND CARER ADVICE**

Medicines for Children leaflet: Paraldehyde for seizures www.medicinesforchildren.org.uk/paraldehyde-for-seizures

● **MEDICINAL FORMS**

There can be variation in the licensing of different medicines containing the same drug. Forms available from special-order manufacturers include: enema

ANTIEPILEPTICS › BARBITURATES

Thiopental sodium

(Thiopentone sodium)

● **INDICATIONS AND DOSE**

Prolonged status epilepticus

▸ INITIALLY BY SLOW INTRAVENOUS INJECTION

▸ Neonate: Initially up to 2 mg/kg, then (by continuous intravenous infusion) up to 8 mg/kg/hour, adjusted according to response

▸ Child: Initially up to 4 mg/kg, then (by continuous intravenous infusion) up to 8 mg/kg/hour, adjusted according to response

Induction of anaesthesia

▸ BY SLOW INTRAVENOUS INJECTION

▸ Neonate: Initially up to 2 mg/kg, then 1 mg/kg, repeated if necessary; maximum 4 mg/kg per course.

▸ Child: Initially up to 4 mg/kg, then 1 mg/kg, repeated if necessary; maximum 7 mg/kg per course

● **UNLICENSED USE** Not licensed for use in status epilepticus. Not licensed for use by intravenous infusion.

> **IMPORTANT SAFETY INFORMATION**
> Thiopental sodium should only be administered by, or under the direct supervision of, personnel experienced in its use, with adequate training in anaesthesia and airway management, and when resuscitation equipment is available.

● **CONTRA-INDICATIONS** Acute porphyrias p. 577 · myotonic dystrophy

● **CAUTIONS** Acute circulatory failure (shock) · avoid intra-arterial injection · cardiovascular disease · fixed cardiac output · hypovolaemia · reconstituted solution is highly alkaline (extravasation causes tissue necrosis and severe pain)

● **INTERACTIONS** → Appendix 1: thiopental

● **SIDE-EFFECTS** Arrhythmias · cough · headache · hypersensitivity reactions · hypotension · laryngeal spasm · myocardial depression · rash · sneezing

● **PREGNANCY** May depress neonatal respiration when used during delivery.

● **BREAST FEEDING** Breast-feeding can be resumed as soon as mother has recovered sufficiently from anaesthesia.

● **HEPATIC IMPAIRMENT** Use with caution—reduce dose.

● **RENAL IMPAIRMENT** Caution in severe impairment.

● **DIRECTIONS FOR ADMINISTRATION** For *intravenous injection*, reconstitute 500-mg vial with 20 mL Water for Injections to give 25 mg/mL solution; give over at least 10–15 seconds; for *intravenous infusion* reconstituted solution may be further diluted with Sodium Chloride 0.9%.

● **PATIENT AND CARER ADVICE**

Driving and skilled tasks

Patients given sedatives and analgesics during minor outpatient procedures should be very carefully warned about the risk of driving or undertaking skilled tasks afterwards. For a short general anaesthetic the risk extends to **at least 24 hours** after administration. Responsible persons should be available to take patients home. The dangers of taking **alcohol** should also be emphasised.

● **MEDICINAL FORMS**

There can be variation in the licensing of different medicines containing the same drug. Forms available from special-order manufacturers include: solution for injection

Powder for solution for injection

▸ Thiopental sodium (Non-proprietary)

Thiopental sodium 500 mg Thiopental 500mg powder for solution for injection vials | 25 vial [PoM] £172.50

HYPNOTICS, SEDATIVES AND ANXIOLYTICS › BENZODIAZEPINES

F 210

Lorazepam

● **INDICATIONS AND DOSE**

Premedication

▸ BY MOUTH

▸ Child 1 month–11 years: 50–100 micrograms/kg (max. per dose 4 mg), to be given at least 1 hour before procedure, same dose may be given the night before procedure in addition to, or to replace, dose before procedure

▸ Child 12-17 years: 1–4 mg, to be given at least 1 hour before procedure, same dose may be given the night before procedure in addition to, or to replace, dose before procedure

▸ BY INTRAVENOUS INJECTION

▸ Child: 50–100 micrograms/kg (max. per dose 4 mg), to be administered 30–45 minutes before procedure

Status epilepticus | Febrile convulsions | Convulsions caused by poisoning

▸ BY SLOW INTRAVENOUS INJECTION

▸ Neonate: 100 micrograms/kg for 1 dose, then 100 micrograms/kg after 10 minutes if required for 1 dose, to be administered into a large vein.

▸ Child 1 month-11 years: 100 micrograms/kg (max. per dose 4 mg) for 1 dose, then 100 micrograms/kg after 10 minutes (max. per dose 4 mg) if required for 1 dose, to be administered into a large vein

▸ Child 12-17 years: 4 mg for 1 dose, then 4 mg after 10 minutes if required for 1 dose, to be administered into a large vein

● **UNLICENSED USE** Not licensed for use in febrile convulsions. Not licensed for use in convulsions caused by poisoning. Not licensed for use as intravenous premedication in children under 12 years. Not licensed for use as oral premedication in children under 5 years.

> **IMPORTANT SAFETY INFORMATION**
> ANAESTHESIA
> Benzodiazepines should only be administered for anaesthesia by, or under the direct supervision of, personnel experienced in their use, with adequate training in anaesthesia and airway management.

● **CONTRA-INDICATIONS** Avoid injections containing benzyl alcohol in neonates · CNS depression · compromised airway · hyperkinesis · obsessional states · phobic states · respiratory depression

● **CAUTIONS** Personality disorder (within the fearful group—dependent, avoidant, obsessive-compulsive) may increase risk of dependence · muscle weakness · organic brain changes · parenteral administration

CAUTIONS, FURTHER INFORMATION

▸ Paradoxical effects A paradoxical increase in hostility and aggression may be reported by patients taking benzodiazepines. The effects range from talkativeness and excitement to aggressive and antisocial acts. Adjustment of the dose (up or down) sometimes attenuates the impulses. Increased anxiety and perceptual disorders are other paradoxical effects.

▸ **Special precautions for parenteral administration** When given parenterally, facilities for managing respiratory depression with mechanical ventilation must be available. Close observation required until full recovery from sedation.

● **INTERACTIONS** → Appendix 1: lorazepam

● **SIDE-EFFECTS**

▸ **Common or very common** Amnesia · ataxia · confusion · dependence · drowsiness the next day · lightheadedness the next day · muscle weakness · paradoxical increase in aggression

▸ **Uncommon** Dizziness · dysarthria · gastro-intestinal disturbances · gynaecomastia · incontinence · salivation changes · tremor · visual disturbances

▸ **Rare** Apnoea · blood disorders · changes in libido · headache · hypotension · jaundice · respiratory depression · skin reactions · urinary retention · vertigo

▸ **Frequency not known** Delusions · excitement · hallucinations · irritability · marked respiratory depression, particularly with high dose and intravenous use (facilities for its treatment are essential) · pain (on intravenous injection) · psychosis · restlessness · thrombophlebitis (on intravenous injection)

● **BREAST FEEDING** Benzodiazepines are present in milk, and should be avoided if possible during breast-feeding.

● **HEPATIC IMPAIRMENT** Start with smaller initial doses or reduce dose. Can precipitate coma. Avoid in severe impairment.

● **RENAL IMPAIRMENT** Start with small doses in severe impairment.

● **DIRECTIONS FOR ADMINISTRATION** For *intravenous injection*, dilute with an equal volume of Sodium Chloride 0.9% (for neonates, dilute injection solution to a concentration of 100 micrograms/mL). Give over 3–5 minutes; max. rate 50 micrograms/kg over 3 minutes.

● **PATIENT AND CARER ADVICE**

Driving and skilled tasks
May impair judgement and increase reaction time, and so affect ability to drive or operate machinery; they increase the effects of alcohol. Moreover the hangover effects of a night dose may impair driving on the following day.

Patients given sedatives and analgesics during minor outpatient procedures should be very carefully warned about the risks of undertaking skilled tasks (e.g. driving) afterwards. For intravenous benzodiazepines the risk extends to **at least 24 hours** after administration. Responsible persons should be available to take patients home afterwards. The dangers of taking **alcohol** should be emphasised.

● **MEDICINAL FORMS**
There can be variation in the licensing of different medicines containing the same drug. Forms available from special-order manufacturers include: oral suspension, oral solution, solution for injection

Solution for injection
EXCIPIENTS: May contain Benzyl alcohol, propylene glycol

▸ **Ativan** (Pfizer Ltd)
Lorazepam 4 mg per 1 ml Ativan 4mg/1ml solution for injection ampoules | 10 ampoule [PoM] £3.54 [CD4-1]

Tablet
CAUTIONARY AND ADVISORY LABELS 2, 19

▸ **Lorazepam** (Non-proprietary)
Lorazepam 1 mg Lorazepam 1mg tablets | 28 tablet [PoM] £6.90 DT price = £4.41 [CD4-1] | 30 tablet [PoM] no price available [CD4-1]
Lorazepam 2.5 mg Lorazepam 2.5mg tablets | 28 tablet [PoM] £12.20 DT price = £12.20 [CD4-1] | 30 tablet [PoM] no price available [CD4-1]

F 210

Midazolam

21-Nov-2016

● **INDICATIONS AND DOSE**

Status epilepticus | Febrile convulsions

▸ BY BUCCAL ADMINISTRATION

▸ **Neonate:** 300 micrograms/kg, then 300 micrograms/kg after 10 minutes if required.

▸ **Child 1-2 months:** 300 micrograms/kg (max. per dose 2.5 mg), then 300 micrograms/kg after 10 minutes (max. per dose 2.5 mg) if required

▸ **Child 3-11 months:** 2.5 mg, then 2.5 mg after 10 minutes if required

▸ **Child 1-4 years:** 5 mg, then 5 mg after 10 minutes if required

▸ **Child 5-9 years:** 7.5 mg, then 7.5 mg after 10 minutes if required

▸ **Child 10-17 years:** 10 mg, then 10 mg after 10 minutes if required

▸ INITIALLY BY INTRAVENOUS INJECTION

▸ **Neonate:** Initially 150–200 micrograms/kg, followed by (by continuous intravenous infusion) 60 micrograms/kg/hour, (by continuous intravenous infusion) increased in steps of 60 micrograms/kg/hour every 15 minutes (max. per dose 300 micrograms/kg/hour) until seizure controlled.

▸ **Child:** Initially 150–200 micrograms/kg, followed by (by continuous intravenous infusion) 60 micrograms/kg/hour, (by continuous intravenous infusion) increased in steps of 60 micrograms/kg/hour every 15 minutes (max. per dose 300 micrograms/kg/hour) until seizure controlled

Conscious sedation for procedures

▸ BY MOUTH

▸ **Child:** 500 micrograms/kg (max. per dose 20 mg), to be administered 30–60 minutes before procedure

▸ BY BUCCAL ADMINISTRATION

▸ **Child 6 months-9 years:** 200–300 micrograms/kg (max. per dose 5 mg)

▸ **Child 10-17 years (body-weight up to 70 kg):** 6–7 mg

▸ **Child 10-17 years (body-weight 70 kg and above):** 6–7 mg (max. per dose 8 mg)

▸ BY RECTUM

▸ **Child 6 months-11 years:** 300–500 micrograms/kg, to be administered 15–30 minutes before procedure

▸ BY INTRAVENOUS INJECTION

▸ **Child 1 month-5 years:** Initially 25–50 micrograms/kg, to be administered over 2–3 minutes, 5–10 minutes before procedure, dose can be increased if necessary in small steps to maximum total dose per course; maximum 6 mg per course

▸ **Child 6-11 years:** Initially 25–50 micrograms/kg, to be administered over 2–3 minutes, 5–10 minutes before procedure, dose can be increased if necessary in small steps to maximum total dose per course; maximum 10 mg per course

▸ **Child 12-17 years:** Initially 25–50 micrograms/kg, to be administered over 2–3 minutes, 5–10 minutes before procedure, dose can be increased if necessary in small steps to maximum total dose per course; maximum 7.5 mg per course

Premedication

▸ BY MOUTH

▸ **Child:** 500 micrograms/kg (max. per dose 20 mg), to be taken 15–30 minutes before the procedure

▸ BY RECTUM

▸ **Child 6 months-11 years:** 300–500 micrograms/kg, to be administered 15–30 minutes before induction

continued →

Induction of anaesthesia (but rarely used)
▸ BY SLOW INTRAVENOUS INJECTION
▸ Child 7-17 years: Initially 150 micrograms/kg (max. per dose 7.5 mg), dose to be given in steps of 50 micrograms/kg (max. 2.5 mg) over 2–5 minutes; wait for 2–5 minutes before subsequent dosing, then 50 micrograms/kg every 2 minutes (max. per dose 2.5 mg) if required; maximum 500 micrograms/kg per course; maximum 25 mg per course

Sedation of patient receiving intensive care
▸ INITIALLY BY SLOW INTRAVENOUS INJECTION
▸ Child 6 months-11 years: Initially 50–200 micrograms/kg, to be administered over at least 3 minutes, followed by (by continuous intravenous infusion) 30–120 micrograms/kg/hour, adjusted according to response, initial dose may not be required and lower maintenance doses needed if opioid analgesics also used; reduce dose (or reduce or omit initial dose) in hypovolaemia, vasoconstriction, or hypothermia
▸ Child 12-17 years: Initially 30–300 micrograms/kg, dose to be given in steps of 1–2.5 mg every 2 minutes, followed by (by continuous intravenous infusion) 30–200 micrograms/kg/hour, adjusted according to response, initial dose may not be required and lower maintenance doses needed if opioid analgesics also used; reduce dose (or reduce or omit initial dose) in hypovolaemia, vasoconstriction, or hypothermia
▸ BY CONTINUOUS INTRAVENOUS INFUSION
▸ Neonate up to 32 weeks corrected gestational age: 60 micrograms/kg/hour for 24 hours, then reduced to 30 micrograms/kg/hour, adjusted according to response for maximum treatment duration of 4 days.
▸ Neonate 32 weeks corrected gestational age and above: 60 micrograms/kg/hour, adjusted according to response for maximum treatment duration of 4 days.
▸ Child 1-5 months: 60 micrograms/kg/hour, adjusted according to response

● UNLICENSED USE Oromucosal solution not licensed for use in children under 3 months. Unlicensed oromucosal formulations are also available and may have different doses—refer to product literature. Injection not licensed for use in status epilepticus or febrile convulsions.
  Not licensed for use in children under 6 months for premedication and conscious sedation.
  Not licensed for use by mouth. Not licensed for use by buccal administration for conscious sedation.

> **IMPORTANT SAFETY INFORMATION**
> ANAESTHESIA
> Benzodiazepines should only be administered for anaesthesia by, or under the direct supervision of, personnel experienced in their use, with adequate training in anaesthesia and airway management.
>
> PRESCRIBING OF MIDAZOLAM IN PALLIATIVE CARE
> The use of high-strength midazolam (5 mg/mL in 2 mL and 10 mL ampoules, or 2 mg/mL in 5 mL ampoules) should be considered in palliative care and other situations where a higher strength may be more appropriate to administer the prescribed dose, and where the risk of overdosage has been assessed. It is advised that flumazenil is available when midazolam is used, to reverse the effects if necessary.

● CONTRA-INDICATIONS CNS depression · compromised airway · severe respiratory depression
● CAUTIONS Cardiac disease · children (particularly if cardiovascular impairment) · concentration of midazolam in children under 15 kg not to exceed 1 mg/mL · debilitated

patients (reduce dose) · hypothermia · hypovolaemia (risk of severe hypotension) · neonates · risk of airways obstruction and hypoventilation in children under 6 months (monitor respiratory rate and oxygen saturation) · vasoconstriction

CAUTIONS, FURTHER INFORMATION
▸ Recovery when used for sedation Midazolam has a fast onset of action, recovery is faster than for other benzodiazepines such as diazepam, but may be significantly longer in the elderly, in patients with a low cardiac output, or after repeated dosing.

● INTERACTIONS → Appendix 1: midazolam
● SIDE-EFFECTS Amnesia · anaphylaxis · ataxia · blood disorders · bronchospasm · cardiac arrest · confusion · convulsions (more common in neonates) · depression of consciousness · dizziness · drowsiness · dry mouth · dysarthria · euphoria · fatigue · gastro-intestinal disturbances · hallucinations · headache · heart rate changes · hiccups · hypotension · incontinence · increased appetite · injection-site reactions · involuntary movements · jaundice · laryngospasm · muscle weakness · paradoxical aggression · paradoxical excitement · respiratory arrest (particularly with high doses or on rapid injection) · respiratory depression (may be severe with sedative and peri-operative use—facilities for its treatment are essential) · respiratory depression (particularly with high doses or on rapid injection) · restlessness (with sedative and peri-operative use) · salivation changes · severe disinhibition (with sedative and peri-operative use) · skin reactions · thrombosis · urinary retention · vertigo · visual disturbances

SIDE-EFFECTS, FURTHER INFORMATION
▸ Sedation Midazolam is associated with profound sedation when high doses are given or when it is used with certain other drugs. Midazolam is not recommended for prolonged sedation in neonates; drug accumulation is likely to occur.
Overdose
There have been reports of overdosage when high strength midazolam has been used for conscious sedation. The use of high-strength midazolam (5 mg/mL in 2 mL and 10 mL ampoules, or 2 mg/mL in 5 mL ampoules) should be restricted to general anaesthesia, intensive care, palliative care, or other situations where the risk has been assessed. It is advised that flumazenil is available when midazolam is used, to reverse the effects if necessary.

● BREAST FEEDING Small amount present in milk—avoid breast-feeding for 24 hours after administration (although amount probably too small to be harmful after single doses).

● HEPATIC IMPAIRMENT Use with caution particularly in sedative doses; can precipitate coma. For status epilepticus and febrile convulsions: use with caution in mild to moderate impairment; avoid in severe impairment.

● RENAL IMPAIRMENT Use with caution in chronic renal failure.

● DIRECTIONS FOR ADMINISTRATION
▸ With intravenous use For *intravenous infusion* (Hypnovel®), give continuously *in* Glucose 5% *or* Sodium chloride 0.9%. For *intravenous injection* in status epilepticus and febrile convulsions, dilute with Glucose 5% or Sodium Chloride 0.9%; rapid intravenous injection (less than 2 minutes) may cause seizure-like myoclonus in preterm neonate. For neonate and children under 15 kg dilute to a max. concentration of 1 mg/mL. *Neonatal intensive care*, dilute 15 mg/kg body-weight to a final volume of 50 mL with infusion fluid; an intravenous infusion rate of 0.1 mL/hour provides a dose of 30 micrograms/kg/hour.
▸ With oral use For administration *by mouth* for sedation and premedication, injection solution may be diluted with apple or black currant juice, chocolate sauce, or cola.

● PATIENT AND CARER ADVICE

Patients or carers should be given advice on how to administer midazolam oromucosal solution.

Patients given sedatives and analgesics during minor outpatient procedures should be very carefully warned about the risks of undertaking skilled tasks (e.g. driving) afterwards. For intravenous benzodiazepines the risk extends to **at least 24 hours** after administration. Responsible persons should be available to take patients home afterwards. The dangers of taking **alcohol** should be emphasised.

Medicines for Children leaflet: Midazolam for stopping seizures www.medicinesforchildren.org.uk/midazolam-for-stopping-seizures

● MEDICINAL FORMS

There can be variation in the licensing of different medicines containing the same drug. Forms available from special-order manufacturers include: oral suspension, oral solution, oromucosal solution, solution for injection, infusion, solution for infusion

Solution for injection

▸ Midazolam (Non-proprietary)

Midazolam (as Midazolam hydrochloride) 1 mg per
1 ml Midazolam 5mg/5ml solution for injection ampoules | 10 ampoule PoM £6.00 DT price = £6.00 CD3
Midazolam 2mg/2ml solution for injection ampoules | 10 ampoule PoM £5.00 CD3

Midazolam (as Midazolam hydrochloride) 2 mg per
1 ml Midazolam 10mg/5ml solution for injection ampoules | 10 ampoule PoM £8.09 DT price = £8.09 CD3 | 10 ampoule PoM no price available DT price = £8.09 (Hospital only) CD3

Midazolam (as Midazolam hydrochloride) 5 mg per
1 ml Midazolam 50mg/10ml solution for injection ampoules | 10 ampoule PoM £78.00 CD3
Midazolam 10mg/2ml solution for injection ampoules | 10 ampoule PoM £7.97 DT price = £6.90 CD3

▸ Hypnovel (Roche Products Ltd)

Midazolam (as Midazolam hydrochloride) 5 mg per 1 ml Hypnovel 10mg/2ml solution for injection ampoules | 10 ampoule PoM £7.11 DT price = £6.90 CD3

Solution for infusion

▸ Midazolam (Non-proprietary)

Midazolam (as Midazolam hydrochloride) 1 mg per
1 ml Midazolam 50mg/50ml solution for infusion vials | 1 vial PoM £9.56–£11.00 CD3

Midazolam (as Midazolam hydrochloride) 2 mg per
1 ml Midazolam 100mg/50ml solution for infusion vials | 1 vial PoM £9.05–£12.50 CD3

Oral solution

▸ Midazolam (Non-proprietary)

Midazolam (as Midazolam hydrochloride) 2 mg per
1 ml Midazolam 2mg/ml oral solution sugar free sugar-free | 118 ml PoM no price available CD3

Oromucosal solution

CAUTIONARY AND ADVISORY LABELS 2

▸ Buccolam (Shire Pharmaceuticals Ltd)

Midazolam (as Midazolam hydrochloride) 5 mg per
1 ml Buccolam 7.5mg/1.5ml oromucosal solution pre-filled syringes sugar-free | 4 unit dose PoM £89.00 DT price = £89.00 CD3
Buccolam 10mg/2ml oromucosal solution pre-filled oral syringes sugar-free | 4 unit dose PoM £91.50 DT price = £91.50 CD3
Buccolam 5mg/1ml oromucosal solution pre-filled oral syringes sugar-free | 4 unit dose PoM £85.50 DT price = £85.50 CD3
Buccolam 2.5mg/0.5ml oromucosal solution pre-filled oral syringes sugar-free | 4 unit dose PoM £82.00 DT price = £82.00 CD3

2   Mental health disorders

2.1   Attention deficit hyperactivity disorder

Attention deficit hyperactivity disorder

Management

CNS stimulants should be prescribed for children with severe and persistent symptoms of *attention deficit hyperactivity disorder* (ADHD), when the diagnosis has been confirmed by a specialist; children with moderate symptoms of ADHD can be treated with CNS stimulants when psychological interventions have been unsuccessful or are unavailable. Prescribing of CNS stimulants may be continued by general practitioners, under a shared-care arrangement. Treatment of ADHD often needs to be continued into adolescence, and may need to be continued into adulthood.

Drug treatment of ADHD should be part of a comprehensive treatment programme. The choice of medication should take into consideration co-morbid conditions (such as tic disorders, Tourette syndrome, and epilepsy), the adverse effect profile, potential for drug misuse, tolerance and dependance; and preferences of the child and carers. Methylphenidate hydrochloride p. 218 and atomoxetine below are used for the management of ADHD; dexamfetamine sulfate p. 220 and lisdexamfetamine mesilate p. 221 are an alternative in children who do not respond to these drugs. Guanfacine p. 222, a non-stimulant alpha$_2$-adrenoceptor agonist, can be used in children for whom stimulants are not suitable, not tolerated, or ineffective. Therapeutic response to guanfacine should be evaluated every 3 months for the first year and then at least yearly, when prescribed for extended periods.

The need to continue drug treatment for ADHD should be reviewed at least annually. This may involve suspending treatment.

A tricyclic antidepressant such as imipramine hydrochloride p. 231 is sometimes used in the treatment of ADHD; it should not be prescribed concomitantly with a CNS stimulant.

CNS STIMULANTS ⟩ CENTRALLY ACTING SYMPATHOMIMETICS

Atomoxetine

28-Sep-2016

● INDICATIONS AND DOSE

Attention deficit hyperactivity disorder (initiated by a specialist)

▸ BY MOUTH

- Child 6–17 years (body-weight up to 70 kg): Initially 500 micrograms/kg daily for 7 days, dose is increased according to response; maintenance 1.2 mg/kg daily, total daily dose may be given either as a single dose in the morning or in 2 divided doses with last dose no later than early evening, high daily doses to be given under the direction of a specialist; maximum 1.8 mg/kg per day; maximum 120 mg per day

▸ Child 6–17 years (body-weight 70 kg and above): Initially 40 mg daily for 7 days, dose is increased according to response; maintenance 80 mg daily, total daily dose may be given either as a single dose in the morning or in 2 divided doses with last dose no later than early evening, high daily doses to be given under the direction of a specialist; maximum 120 mg per day

- **UNLICENSED USE** Doses above 100 mg daily not licensed. Atomoxetine doses in BNF Publications may differ from those in product literature.
- **CONTRA-INDICATIONS** Phaeochromocytoma · severe cardiovascular disease · severe cerebrovascular disease
- **CAUTIONS** QT-interval prolongation · aggressive behaviour · cardiovascular disease · cerebrovascular disease · emotional lability · history of seizures · hostility · hypertension · mania · psychosis · structural cardiac abnormalities · susceptibility to angle-closure glaucoma · tachycardia
- **INTERACTIONS** → Appendix 1: atomoxetine
- **SIDE-EFFECTS**
  - **Common or very common** Abdominal pain · anorexia · anxiety · chills · constipation · depression · dermatitis · dizziness · drowsiness · dry mouth · dyspepsia · flatulence · flushing · headache · increased blood pressure · irritability · lethargy · malaise · mydriasis · nausea · palpitation · paraesthesia · prostatitis · rash · sexual dysfunction · sleep disturbances · sweating · tachycardia · taste disturbances · tremor · urinary dysfunction · vomiting
  - **Uncommon** Aggression · cold extremities · emotional lability · hostility · hypoaesthesia · menstrual disturbances · muscle spasms · pruritus · psychosis · QT-interval prolongation · suicidal ideation · syncope · tics
  - **Rare** Raynaud's phenomenon · seizures
  - **Very rare** Angle-closure glaucoma · hepatic disorders
- **PREGNANCY** Manufacturer advises avoid unless potential benefit outweighs risk.
- **BREAST FEEDING** Avoid-present in milk in *animal* studies.
- **HEPATIC IMPAIRMENT** Halve dose in moderate impairment. Quarter dose in severe impairment.
- **MONITORING REQUIREMENTS**
  - Monitor for appearance or worsening of anxiety, depression or tics.
  - Pulse, blood pressure, psychiatric symptoms, appetite, weight and height should be recorded at initiation of therapy, following each dose adjustment, and at least every 6 months thereafter.
- **PATIENT AND CARER ADVICE**
  Suicidal ideation Following reports of suicidal thoughts and behaviour, patients and their carers should be informed about the risk and told to report clinical worsening, suicidal thoughts or behaviour, irritability, agitation, or depression.

  Hepatic impairment Following rare reports of hepatic disorders, patients and carers should be advised of the risk and be told how to recognise symptoms; prompt medical attention should be sought in case of abdominal pain, unexplained nausea, malaise, darkening of the urine, or jaundice.

  Medicines for Children leaflet: Atomoxetine for attention deficit hyperactivity disorder (ADHD) www.medicinesforchildren.org.uk/atomoxetine-attention-deficit-hyperactivity-disorder-adhd
- **NATIONAL FUNDING/ACCESS DECISIONS**

  NICE technology appraisals (TAs)
  - Methylphenidate, atomoxetine and dexamfetamine for attention deficit hyperactivity disorder (ADHD) (March 2006) NICE TA98
  Atomoxetine is recommended, within its licensed indications, as an option for the management of ADHD in children and adolescents.
  www.nice.org.uk/TA98

  Scottish Medicines Consortium (SMC) Decisions
  The *Scottish Medicines Consortium* has advised (December 2015) that atomoxetine oral solution (*Strattera*®) is accepted for restricted use, within its licensed indications, for treating patients who are unable to swallow capsules.

- **MEDICINAL FORMS**
  There can be variation in the licensing of different medicines containing the same drug. Forms available from special-order manufacturers include: oral suspension, oral solution

  Oral solution
  CAUTIONARY AND ADVISORY LABELS 3
  - Strattera (Eli Lilly and Company Ltd)
    Atomoxetine (as Atomoxetine hydrochloride) 4 mg per 1 ml Strattera 4mg/1ml oral solution sugar-free | 300 ml [PoM] £85.00 DT price = £85.00

  Capsule
  CAUTIONARY AND ADVISORY LABELS 3
  - Strattera (Eli Lilly and Company Ltd)
    Atomoxetine (as Atomoxetine hydrochloride) 10 mg Strattera 10mg capsules | 7 capsule [PoM] £13.25 | 28 capsule [PoM] £53.09 DT price = £53.09
    Atomoxetine (as Atomoxetine hydrochloride) 18 mg Strattera 18mg capsules | 7 capsule [PoM] £13.25 | 28 capsule [PoM] £53.09 DT price = £53.09
    Atomoxetine (as Atomoxetine hydrochloride) 25 mg Strattera 25mg capsules | 7 capsule [PoM] £13.28 | 28 capsule [PoM] £53.09 DT price = £53.09
    Atomoxetine (as Atomoxetine hydrochloride) 40 mg Strattera 40mg capsules | 7 capsule [PoM] £13.28 | 28 capsule [PoM] £53.09 DT price = £53.09
    Atomoxetine (as Atomoxetine hydrochloride) 60 mg Strattera 60mg capsules | 28 capsule [PoM] £53.09 DT price = £53.09
    Atomoxetine (as Atomoxetine hydrochloride) 80 mg Strattera 80mg capsules | 28 capsule [PoM] £70.79 DT price = £70.79
    Atomoxetine (as Atomoxetine hydrochloride) 100 mg Strattera 100mg capsules | 28 capsule [PoM] £70.79 DT price = £70.79

Methylphenidate hydrochloride

06-Jun-2017

- **INDICATIONS AND DOSE**

  Attention deficit hyperactivity disorder (initiated under specialist supervision)
  - BY MOUTH USING IMMEDIATE-RELEASE MEDICINES
  - Child 4-5 years: Initially 2.5 mg twice daily, increased in steps of 2.5 mg daily if required, at weekly intervals, increased if necessary up to 1.4 mg/kg daily in 2-3 divided doses, discontinue if no response after 1 month, if effect wears off in evening (with rebound hyperactivity) a dose at bedtime may be appropriate (establish need with trial bedtime dose). Treatment may be started using a modified-release preparation
  - Child 6-17 years: Initially 5 mg 1-2 times a day, increased in steps of 5-10 mg daily if required, at weekly intervals, increased if necessary up to 60 mg daily in 2-3 divided doses, increased if necessary up to 2.1 mg/kg daily in 2-3 divided doses, the licensed maximum dose is 60 mg daily in 2-3 doses, higher dose (up to a maximum of 90 mg daily) under the direction of a specialist, discontinue if no response after 1 month, if effect wears off in evening (with rebound hyperactivity) a dose at bedtime may be appropriate (establish need with trial bedtime dose). Treatment may be started using a modified-release preparation

  DOSE EQUIVALENCE AND CONVERSION
  - When switching from *immediate-release* preparations to *modified-release* preparations—consult product literature.

  CONCERTA® XL

  Attention deficit hyperactivity disorder
  - BY MOUTH
  - Child 6-17 years: Initially 18 mg once daily, dose to be taken in the morning, increased in steps of 18 mg every week, adjusted according to response; increased if necessary up to 2.1 mg/kg daily, licensed max. dose is 54 mg once daily, to be increased to higher dose only under direction of specialist; discontinue if no response after 1 month, maximum 108 mg per day

DOSE EQUIVALENCE AND CONVERSION

‣ Total daily dose of 15 mg of standard-release formulation is considered equivalent to *Concerta*® XL 18 mg once daily.

DELMOSART® PROLONGED-RELEASE TABLET

Attention deficit hyperactivity disorder (under expert supervision)

▶ BY MOUTH

‣ Child 6–17 years: Initially 18 mg once daily, dose to be taken in the morning, then increased in steps of 18 mg every week if required, discontinue if no response after 1 month; maximum 54 mg per day

DOSE EQUIVALENCE AND CONVERSION

‣ Total daily dose of 15 mg of standard-release formulation is considered equivalent to *Delmosart*® 18 mg once daily.

EQUASYM® XL

Attention deficit hyperactivity disorder

▶ BY MOUTH

‣ Child 6–17 years: Initially 10 mg once daily, dose to be taken in the morning before breakfast; increased gradually at weekly intervals if necessary; increased if necessary up to 2.1 mg/kg daily, licensed max. dose is 60 mg daily, to be increased to higher dose only under direction of specialist; discontinue if no response after 1 month; maximum 90 mg per day

MEDIKINET® XL

Attention deficit hyperactivity disorder

▶ BY MOUTH

‣ Child 6–17 years: Initially 10 mg once daily, dose to be taken in the morning with breakfast; adjusted at weekly intervals according to response; increased if necessary up to 2.1 mg/kg daily, licensed max. dose is 60 mg daily, to be increased to higher dose only under direction of specialist; discontinue if no response after 1 month; maximum 90 mg per day

● UNLICENSED USE Doses over 60 mg daily not licensed; doses of *Concerta XL* over 54 mg daily not licensed. Not licensed for use in children under 6 years.

● CONTRA-INDICATIONS Anorexia nervosa · arrhythmias · cardiomyopathy, · cardiovascular disease · cerebrovascular disorders · heart failure · hyperthyroidism · phaeochromocytoma · psychosis · severe depression · severe hypertension · structural cardiac abnormalities · suicidal ideation · uncontrolled bipolar disorder · vasculitis

● CAUTIONS Agitation · alcohol dependence · anxiety · drug dependence · epilepsy (discontinue if increased seizure frequency) · family history of Tourette syndrome · susceptibility to angle-closure glaucoma · tics

CONCERTA® XL, DELMOSART® Dysphagia (dose form not appropriate) · restricted gastro-intestinal lumen (dose form not appropriate)

● INTERACTIONS → Appendix 1: methylphenidate

● SIDE-EFFECTS

▶ Common or very common Abdominal pain · aggression · alopecia · anorexia · arrhythmias · arthralgia · asthenia · changes in blood pressure · cough · depression · diarrhoea · dizziness · drowsiness · dry mouth · dyspepsia · fever · growth restriction · headache · insomnia · irritability · movement disorders · nasopharyngitis · nausea · nervousness · palpitation · pruritus · rash · reduced weight gain · tachycardia · tics · vomiting

▶ Uncommon Abnormal dreams · confusion · constipation · dyspnoea · epistaxis · haematuria · muscle cramps · suicidal ideation · urinary frequency

▶ Rare Angina · sweating · visual disturbances;

▶ Very rare Angle-closure glaucoma · blood disorders · cerebral arteritis · dependence · erythema multiforme ·

exfoliative dermatitis · hepatic dysfunction · leucopenia · myocardial infarction · neuroleptic malignant syndrome · psychosis · seizures · thrombocytopenia · tolerance · Tourette syndrome

▶ Frequency not known Bradycardia · convulsions · supraventricular tachycardia

● PREGNANCY Limited experience—avoid unless potential benefit outweighs risk.

● BREAST FEEDING Limited information available—avoid.

● MONITORING REQUIREMENTS

▶ Monitor for psychiatric disorders.

▶ Pulse, blood pressure, psychiatric symptoms, appetite, weight and height should be recorded at initiation of therapy, following each dose adjustment, and at least every 6 months thereafter.

● TREATMENT CESSATION Avoid abrupt withdrawal.

● DIRECTIONS FOR ADMINISTRATION

MEDIKINET® XL Contents of capsule can be sprinkled on a tablespoon of apple sauce or yoghurt (then swallowed immediately without chewing).

EQUASYM® XL Contents of capsule can be sprinkled on a tablespoon of apple sauce (then swallowed immediately without chewing).

● PRESCRIBING AND DISPENSING INFORMATION Different versions of modified-release preparations may not have the same clinical effect. To avoid confusion between these different formulations of methylphenidate, prescribers should specify the brand to be dispensed.

CONCERTA® XL Consists of an immediate-release component (22% of the dose) and a modified-release component (78% of the dose).

MEDIKINET® XL Consists of an immediate-release component (50% of the dose) and a modified-release component (50% of the dose).

EQUASYM® XL Consists of an immediate-release component (30% of the dose) and a modified-release component (70% of the dose).

● PATIENT AND CARER ADVICE

Drugs and Driving Prescribers and other healthcare professionals should advise patients if treatment is likely to affect their ability to perform skilled tasks (e.g. driving). This applies especially to drugs with sedative effects; patients should be warned that these effects are increased by alcohol. General information about a patient's fitness to drive is available from the Driver and Vehicle Licensing Agency at www.dvla.gov.uk.

2015 legislation regarding driving whilst taking certain drugs, may also apply to methylphenidate, see *Drugs and Skilled Tasks* under Guidance on prescribing p. 1.

CONCERTA® XL, DELMOSART® Tablet membrane may pass through gastro-intestinal tract unchanged.

● NATIONAL FUNDING/ACCESS DECISIONS

NICE technology appraisals (TAs)

▶ Methylphenidate, atomoxetine and dexamfetamine for attention deficit hyperactivity disorder (ADHD) (March 2006) NICE TA98

Methylphenidate is recommended, within its licensed indications, as an option for the management of ADHD in children and adolescents.

www.nice.org.uk/TA98

● MEDICINAL FORMS
There can be variation in the licensing of different medicines containing the same drug. Forms available from special-order manufacturers include: oral suspension, oral solution

Modified-release tablet

CAUTIONARY AND ADVISORY LABELS 25

▶ Concerta XL (Janssen-Cilag Ltd)

Methylphenidate hydrochloride 18 mg Concerta XL 18mg tablets | 30 tablet PoM £31.19 DT price = £31.19 CD2

4

Nervous system

Methylphenidate hydrochloride 27 mg Concerta XL 27mg tablets | 30 tablet [PoM] £36.81 DT price = £36.81 [CD2]
Methylphenidate hydrochloride 36 mg Concerta XL 36mg tablets | 30 tablet [PoM] £42.45 DT price = £42.45 [CD2]
Methylphenidate hydrochloride 54 mg Concerta XL 54mg tablets | 30 tablet [PoM] £73.62 DT price = £60.48 [CD2]

▸ **Delmosart** (Actavis UK Ltd)
Methylphenidate hydrochloride 18 mg Delmosart 18mg modified-release tablets | 30 tablet [PoM] £15.59 DT price = £31.19 [CD2]
Methylphenidate hydrochloride 27 mg Delmosart 27mg modified-release tablets | 30 tablet [PoM] £18.41 DT price = £36.81 [CD2]
Methylphenidate hydrochloride 36 mg Delmosart 36mg modified-release tablets | 30 tablet [PoM] £21.23 DT price = £42.45 [CD2]
Methylphenidate hydrochloride 54 mg Delmosart 54mg modified-release tablets | 30 tablet [PoM] £36.81 DT price = £60.48 [CD2]

Tablet
▸ **Methylphenidate hydrochloride** (Non-proprietary)
Methylphenidate hydrochloride 5 mg Methylphenidate 5mg tablets | 30 tablet [PoM] £3.03 DT price = £3.03 [CD2]
Methylphenidate hydrochloride 10 mg Methylphenidate 10mg tablets | 30 tablet [PoM] £5.49 DT price = £5.49 [CD2]
Methylphenidate hydrochloride 20 mg Methylphenidate 20mg tablets | 30 tablet [PoM] £10.92 DT price = £10.92 [CD2]

▸ **Medikinet** (Flynn Pharma Ltd)
Methylphenidate hydrochloride 5 mg Medikinet 5mg tablets | 30 tablet [PoM] £3.03 DT price = £3.03 [CD2]
Methylphenidate hydrochloride 10 mg Medikinet 10mg tablets | 30 tablet [PoM] £5.49 DT price = £5.49 [CD2]
Methylphenidate hydrochloride 20 mg Medikinet 20mg tablets | 30 tablet [PoM] £10.92 DT price = £10.92 [CD2]

▸ **Ritalin** (Novartis Pharmaceuticals UK Ltd)
Methylphenidate hydrochloride 10 mg Ritalin 10mg tablets | 30 tablet [PoM] £6.68 DT price = £5.49 [CD2]

▸ **Tranquilyn** (Genesis Pharmaceuticals Ltd)
Methylphenidate hydrochloride 5 mg Tranquilyn 5mg tablets | 30 tablet [PoM] £3.03 DT price = £3.03 [CD2]
Methylphenidate hydrochloride 10 mg Tranquilyn 10mg tablets | 30 tablet [PoM] £5.49 DT price = £5.49 [CD2]
Methylphenidate hydrochloride 20 mg Tranquilyn 20mg tablets | 30 tablet [PoM] £10.92 DT price = £10.92 [CD2]

Modified-release capsule
CAUTIONARY AND ADVISORY LABELS 25
▸ **Equasym XL** (Shire Pharmaceuticals Ltd)
Methylphenidate hydrochloride 10 mg Equasym XL 10mg capsules | 30 capsule [PoM] £25.00 DT price = £25.00 [CD2]
Methylphenidate hydrochloride 20 mg Equasym XL 20mg capsules | 30 capsule [PoM] £30.00 DT price = £30.00 [CD2]
Methylphenidate hydrochloride 30 mg Equasym XL 30mg capsules | 30 capsule [PoM] £35.00 DT price = £35.00 [CD2]

▸ **Medikinet XL** (Flynn Pharma Ltd)
Methylphenidate hydrochloride 5 mg Medikinet XL 5mg capsules | 30 capsule [PoM] £24.04 [CD2]
Methylphenidate hydrochloride 10 mg Medikinet XL 10mg capsules | 30 capsule [PoM] £24.04 DT price = £25.00 [CD2]
Methylphenidate hydrochloride 20 mg Medikinet XL 20mg capsules | 30 capsule [PoM] £28.86 DT price = £30.00 [CD2]
Methylphenidate hydrochloride 30 mg Medikinet XL 30mg capsules | 30 capsule [PoM] £33.66 DT price = £35.00 [CD2]
Methylphenidate hydrochloride 40 mg Medikinet XL 40mg capsules | 30 capsule [PoM] £57.72 DT price = £57.72 [CD2]
Methylphenidate hydrochloride 50 mg Medikinet XL 50mg capsules | 30 capsule [PoM] £62.52 [CD2]
Methylphenidate hydrochloride 60 mg Medikinet XL 60mg capsules | 30 capsule [PoM] £67.32 [CD2]

CNS STIMULANTS > CENTRALLY ACTING SYMPATHOMIMETICS > AMFETAMINES

Dexamfetamine sulfate

(Dexamphetamine sulfate)

● **INDICATIONS AND DOSE**

Refractory attention deficit hyperactivity disorder (initiated under specialist supervision)
▸ BY MOUTH
▸ Child 6–17 years: Initially 2.5 mg 2–3 times a day, increased in steps of 5 mg once weekly if required, increased if necessary up to 1 mg/kg daily, maintenance dose to be given in 2–4 divided doses, up to 20 mg daily (40 mg daily has been required in some children)

● **CONTRA-INDICATIONS** Agitated states · cardiovascular disease · history of alcohol abuse · history of drug abuse · hyperexcitability · hyperthyroidism · moderate hypertension · severe hypertension · structural cardiac abnormalities

● **CAUTIONS** Anorexia · bipolar disorder · history of epilepsy (discontinue if seizures occur) · mild hypertension · psychosis · susceptibility to angle-closure glaucoma · tics · Tourette syndrome
CAUTIONS, FURTHER INFORMATION
▸ Tics and Tourette syndrome Discontinue use if tics occur.
▸ Growth restriction in children Monitor height and weight as growth restriction may occur during prolonged therapy (drug-free periods may allow catch-up in growth but withdraw slowly to avoid inducing depression or renewed hyperactivity).

● **INTERACTIONS** → Appendix 1: amfetamines

● **SIDE-EFFECTS**
▸ **Common or very common** Abdominal cramps · acidosis · aggression · alopecia · anhedonia · anorexia · anxiety · ataxia · cardiomyopathy · cardiovascular collapse · cerebral vasculitis · chest pain · confusion · depression · diarrhoea · dizziness · dry mouth · dysphoria · euphoria · growth restriction in children · headache · hyperactivity · hyperpyrexia · hyperreflexia · hypertension · hypotension · impaired concentration · irritability · ischaemic colitis · malaise · mydriasis · myocardial infarction · nausea · nervousness · neuroleptic malignant syndrome · obsessive-compulsive behaviour · palpitations · panic attack · paranoia · psychosis · rash · renal impairment · restlessness · rhabdomyolysis · seizures · sexual dysfunction · sleep disturbances · stroke · sweating · tachycardia · taste disturbance · Tourette syndrome (in predisposed individuals) · tremor · urticaria · visual disturbances · weight loss
▸ **Very rare** Angle-closure glaucoma
▸ **Frequency not known** Choreoathetoid movements (in predisposed individuals) · dyskinesia (in predisposed individuals) · increased appetite · tics (in predisposed individuals)

Overdose
Amfetamines cause wakefulness, excessive activity, paranoia, hallucinations, and hypertension followed by exhaustion, convulsions, hyperthermia, and coma. See Stimulants under Emergency treatment of poisoning p. 803.

● **PREGNANCY** Avoid retrospective evidence of uncertain significance suggesting possible embryotoxicity).

● **BREAST FEEDING** Significant amount in milk—avoid.

● **RENAL IMPAIRMENT** Use with caution.

● **MONITORING REQUIREMENTS**
▸ Monitor growth in children.

- ▸ Monitor for aggressive behaviour or hostility during initial treatment.
- ▸ Pulse, blood pressure, psychiatric symptoms, appetite, weight and height should be recorded at initiation of therapy, following each dose adjustment, and at least every 6 months thereafter.
- ● **TREATMENT CESSATION** Avoid abrupt withdrawal.
- ● **DIRECTIONS FOR ADMINISTRATION** Tablets can be halved.
- ● **PRESCRIBING AND DISPENSING INFORMATION** Data on safety and efficacy of long-term use not complete.
- ● **PATIENT AND CARER ADVICE**
  Drugs and Driving Prescribers and other healthcare professionals should advise patients if treatment is likely to affect their ability to perform skilled tasks (e.g. driving). This applies especially to drugs with sedative effects; patients should be warned that these effects are increased by alcohol. General information about a patient's fitness to drive is available from the Driver and Vehicle Licensing Agency at www.dvla.gov.uk.
      For information on 2015 legislation regarding driving whilst taking certain controlled drugs, including amfetamines, see *Drugs and Skilled Tasks* under Guidance on prescribing p. 1.
- ● **NATIONAL FUNDING/ACCESS DECISIONS**
  NICE technology appraisals (TAs)
- ▸ Methylphenidate, atomoxetine and dexamfetamine for attention deficit hyperactivity disorder (ADHD) (March 2006) NICE TA98
  Dexamfetamine is recommended, within its licensed indications, as an option for the management of ADHD in children and adolescents.
  www.nice.org.uk/TA98

- ● **MEDICINAL FORMS**
  There can be variation in the licensing of different medicines containing the same drug. Forms available from special-order manufacturers include: modified-release capsule, oral suspension, oral solution

  Oral solution
  - ▸ Dexamfetamine sulfate (Non-proprietary)
    Dexamfetamine sulfate 1 mg per 1 ml Dexamfetamine 5mg/5ml oral solution sugar free sugar-free | 150 ml [PoM] £29.44–£34.35 [CD2] sugar-free | 500 ml [PoM] £114.49 DT price = £114.49 [CD2]

  Modified-release capsule
  - ▸ Dexedrine Spansules (Imported (United States))
    Dexamfetamine sulfate 5 mg Dexedrine 5mg Spansules | 100 capsule [PoM] no price available [CD2]
    Dexamfetamine sulfate 10 mg Dexedrine 10mg Spansules | 100 capsule [PoM] no price available [CD2]
    Dexamfetamine sulfate 15 mg Dexedrine 15mg Spansules | 100 capsule [PoM] no price available [CD2]

  Tablet
  - ▸ Dexamfetamine sulfate (Non-proprietary)
    Dexamfetamine sulfate 5 mg Dexamfetamine 5mg tablets | 28 tablet [PoM] £24.75 DT price = £24.75 [CD2]
  - ▸ Amfexa (Flynn Pharma Ltd)
    Dexamfetamine sulfate 5 mg Amfexa 5mg tablets | 30 tablet [PoM] £19.89 [CD2]
    Dexamfetamine sulfate 10 mg Amfexa 10mg tablets | 30 tablet [PoM] £39.78 [CD2]
    Dexamfetamine sulfate 20 mg Amfexa 20mg tablets | 30 tablet [PoM] £79.56 [CD2]

Lisdexamfetamine mesilate

- ● **DRUG ACTION** Lisdexamfetamine is a prodrug of dexamfetamine.

- ● **INDICATIONS AND DOSE**
  Attention deficit hyperactivity disorder refractory to methylphenidate (initiated by a specialist)
  - ▸ BY MOUTH
    - ▸ Child 6–17 years: Initially 30 mg once daily, increased in steps of 20 mg every week if required, dose to be taken in the morning, discontinue if response insufficient after 1 month; maximum 70 mg per day

- ● **CONTRA-INDICATIONS** Advanced arteriosclerosis · agitated states · hyperexcitability · hyperthyroidism · moderate hypertension · severe hypertension · symptomatic cardiovascular disease

- ● **CAUTIONS** Anorexia · bipolar disorder · history of alcohol abuse · history of cardiac abnormalities · history of cardiovascular disease · history of drug abuse · may lower seizure threshold (discontinue if seizures occur) · psychosis · susceptibility to angle-closure glaucoma · tics · Tourette syndrome

  CAUTIONS, FURTHER INFORMATION
  - ▸ Tics and Tourette syndrome Discontinue use if tics occur.
  - ▸ Growth restriction in children Monitor height and weight as growth restriction may occur during prolonged therapy (drug-free periods may allow catch-up in growth but withdraw slowly to avoid inducing depression or renewed hyperactivity).

- ● **INTERACTIONS** → Appendix 1: amfetamines

- ● **SIDE-EFFECTS**
  - ▸ **Common or very common** Abdominal cramps · aggression · decreased appetite · diarrhoea · dizziness · drowsiness · dry mouth · dyspnoea · growth restriction in children · headache · labile mood · malaise · mydriasis · nausea · pyrexia · sleep disturbances · tics · vomiting · weight loss
  - ▸ **Uncommon** Anorexia · anxiety · depression · dermatillomania · dysphoria · hallucination · hypertension · logorrhoea · mania · palpitation · paranoia · rash · restlessness · sexual dysfunction · sweating · tachycardia · tremor · visual disturbances
  - ▸ **Very rare** Angle-closure glaucoma
  - ▸ **Frequency not known** Cardiomyopathy · choreoathetoid movements (in predisposed individuals) · dyskinesia (in predisposed individuals) · euphoria · seizures · Tourette syndrome (in predisposed individuals)

  Overdose
  Amfetamines cause wakefulness, excessive activity, paranoia, hallucinations, and hypertension followed by exhaustion, convulsions, hyperthermia, and coma. See Stimulants under Emergency treatment of poisoning p. 803.

- ● **PREGNANCY** Manufacturer advises use only if potential benefit outweighs risk.

- ● **BREAST FEEDING** Manufacturer advises avoid—present in human milk.

- ● **RENAL IMPAIRMENT** Max. dose 50 mg daily in severe impairment.

- ● **MONITORING REQUIREMENTS**
  - ▸ Monitor for aggressive behaviour or hostility during initial treatment.
  - ▸ Monitor growth in children.
  - ▸ Pulse, blood pressure, psychiatric symptoms, appetite, weight and height should be recorded at initiation of therapy, following each dose adjustment, and at least every 6 months thereafter.

- ● **TREATMENT CESSATION** Avoid abrupt withdrawal.

- **DIRECTIONS FOR ADMINISTRATION** Swallow whole or mix contents of capsule in yoghurt or a glass of water or orange juice; contents should be dispersed completely and consumed immediately.
- **PATIENT AND CARER ADVICE**
Patients and carers should be counselled on the administration of capsules.
Drugs and Driving Prescribers and other healthcare professionals should advise patients if treatment is likely to affect their ability to perform skilled tasks (e.g. driving). This applies especially to drugs with sedative effects; patients should be warned that these effects are increased by alcohol. General information about a patient's fitness to drive is available from the Driver and Vehicle Licensing Agency at www.dvla.gov.uk.

  For information on 2015 legislation regarding driving whilst taking certain controlled drugs, including amfetamines, see *Drugs and Skilled Tasks* under Guidance on prescribing p. 1.

- **MEDICINAL FORMS**
There can be variation in the licensing of different medicines containing the same drug.
Capsule
CAUTIONARY AND ADVISORY LABELS 3, 25
  ‣ Elvanse (Shire Pharmaceuticals Ltd) ▼
    Lisdexamfetamine dimesylate 20 mg Elvanse 20mg capsules |
    28 capsule [PoM] £54.62 DT price = £54.62 [CD2]
    Lisdexamfetamine dimesylate 30 mg Elvanse Adult 30mg capsules
    | 28 capsule [PoM] £58.24 DT price = £58.24 [CD2]
    Elvanse 30mg capsules | 28 capsule [PoM] £58.24 DT price =
    £58.24 [CD2]
    Lisdexamfetamine dimesylate 40 mg Elvanse 40mg capsules |
    28 capsule [PoM] £62.82 DT price = £62.82 [CD2]
    Lisdexamfetamine dimesylate 50 mg Elvanse Adult 50mg capsules
    | 28 capsule [PoM] £68.60 DT price = £68.60 [CD2]
    Elvanse 50mg capsules | 28 capsule [PoM] £68.60 DT price =
    £68.60 [CD2]
    Lisdexamfetamine dimesylate 60 mg Elvanse 60mg capsules |
    28 capsule [PoM] £75.18 DT price = £75.18 [CD2]
    Lisdexamfetamine dimesylate 70 mg Elvanse 70mg capsules |
    28 capsule [PoM] £83.16 DT price = £83.16 [CD2]
    Elvanse Adult 70mg capsules | 28 capsule [PoM] £83.16 DT price =
    £83.16 [CD2]

SYMPATHOMIMETICS > ALPHA$_2$-ADRENOCEPTOR AGONISTS

Guanfacine
26-May-2016

- **INDICATIONS AND DOSE**

Attention deficit hyperactivity disorder in children for whom stimulants are not suitable, not tolerated or ineffective (initiated under specialist supervision)
  ‣ BY MOUTH
  ‣ Child 6–12 years (body-weight 25 kg and above): Initially 1 mg once daily; adjusted in steps of 1 mg every week if necessary and if tolerated; maintenance 0.05–0.12 mg/kg once daily (max. per dose 4 mg), for optimal weight-adjusted dose titrations, consult product literature
  ‣ Child 13–17 years (body-weight 34–41.4 kg): Initially 1 mg once daily; adjusted in steps of 1 mg every week if necessary and if tolerated; maintenance 0.05–0.12 mg/kg once daily (max. per dose 4 mg), for optimal weight-adjusted dose titrations, consult product literature
  ‣ Child 13–17 years (body-weight 41.5–49.4 kg): Initially 1 mg once daily; adjusted in steps of 1 mg every week if necessary and if tolerated; maintenance 0.05–0.12 mg/kg once daily (max. per dose 5 mg), for optimal weight-adjusted dose titrations, consult product literature

  ‣ Child 13–17 years (body-weight 49.5–58.4 kg): Initially 1 mg once daily; adjusted in steps of 1 mg every week if necessary and if tolerated; maintenance 0.05–0.12 mg/kg once daily (max. per dose 6 mg), for optimal weight-adjusted dose titrations, consult product literature
  ‣ Child 13–17 years (body-weight 58.5 kg and above): Initially 1 mg once daily; adjusted in steps of 1 mg every week if necessary and if tolerated; maintenance 0.05–0.12 mg/kg once daily (max. per dose 7 mg), for optimal weight-adjusted dose titrations, consult product literature

DOSE ADJUSTMENTS DUE TO INTERACTIONS
Manufacturer advises reduce dose by half with concurrent use of moderate and potent inhibitors of CYP3A4.
Manufacturer advises increase dose up to max. 7 mg daily with concurrent use of potent inducers of CYP3A4—no specific recommendation made for children.

- **CAUTIONS** Bradycardia (risk of torsade de pointes) · heart block (risk of torsade de pointes) · history of cardiovascular disease · history of QT-interval prolongation · hypokalaemia (risk of torsade de pointes)
- **INTERACTIONS** → Appendix 1: guanfacine
- **SIDE-EFFECTS**
  ‣ **Common or very common** Abdominal pain · anxiety · bradycardia · constipation · decreased appetite · depression · diarrhoea · dizziness · dry mouth · enuresis · headache · hypotension · irritability · malaise · mood lability · nausea · rash · sleep disturbance · somnolence · vomiting · weight increase
  ‣ **Uncommon** Agitation · chest pain · convulsion · dyspepsia · first-degree AV block · hallucination · pallor · pollakiuria · pruritus · sinus arrhythmia · syncope · tachycardia
  ‣ **Rare** Hypertension
  ‣ **Frequency not known** Suicidal ideation
  SIDE-EFFECTS, FURTHER INFORMATION
  ‣ Somnolence and sedation Somnolence and sedation may occur, predominantly during the first 2-3 weeks of treatment and with dose increases; manufacturer advises to consider dose reduction or discontinuation of treatment if symptoms are clinically significant or persistent.
  Overdose
  Features may include hypotension, initial hypertension, bradycardia, lethargy, and respiratory depression. Manufacturer advises that patients who develop lethargy should be observed for development of more serious toxicity for up to 24 hours.

- **CONCEPTION AND CONTRACEPTION** Manufacturer recommends effective contraception in females of childbearing potential.
- **PREGNANCY** Manufacturer advises avoid—toxicity in *animal* studies.
- **BREAST FEEDING** Manufacturer advises avoid—present in milk in *animal* studies.
- **HEPATIC IMPAIRMENT** Manufacturer advises consider dose reduction.
- **RENAL IMPAIRMENT** Manufacturer advises consider dose reduction in severe impairment and end-stage renal disease.

- **MONITORING REQUIREMENTS**
  ‣ Manufacturer advises to conduct a baseline evaluation to identify patients at risk of somnolence, sedation, hypotension, bradycardia, QT-prolongation, and arrhythmia; this should include assessment of cardiovascular status. Monitor for signs of these adverse effects weekly during dose titration and then every 3 months during the first year of treatment, and every 6 months thereafter. Monitor BMI prior to treatment and

then every 3 months for the first year of treatment, and every 6 months thereafter. More frequent monitoring is advised following dose adjustments.
▸ Monitor blood pressure and pulse during dose downward titration and following discontinuation of treatment.

● TREATMENT CESSATION Manufacturer advises avoid abrupt withdrawal; consider dose tapering to minimise potential withdrawal effects.

● DIRECTIONS FOR ADMINISTRATION Manufacturer advises avoid administration with high fat meals (may increase absorption).

● PATIENT AND CARER ADVICE
Patients or carers should be counselled on administration of guanfacine modified-release tablets.

Missed doses
Manufacturer advises that patients and carers should inform their prescriber if more than one dose is missed; consider dose re-titration.

Driving and skilled tasks
Manufacturer advises patients and carers should be counselled about the effects on driving and performance of skilled tasks—increased risk of dizziness and syncope.

● MEDICINAL FORMS
There can be variation in the licensing of different medicines containing the same drug.
Modified-release tablet
CAUTIONARY AND ADVISORY LABELS 25, 2
▸ Intuniv (Shire Pharmaceuticals Ltd) ▼
  Guanfacine (as Guanfacine hydrochloride) 1 mg Intuniv 1mg modified-release tablets | 28 tablet [PoM] £56.00
  Guanfacine (as Guanfacine hydrochloride) 2 mg Intuniv 2mg modified-release tablets | 28 tablet [PoM] £58.52
  Guanfacine (as Guanfacine hydrochloride) 3 mg Intuniv 3mg modified-release tablets | 28 tablet [PoM] £65.52
  Guanfacine (as Guanfacine hydrochloride) 4 mg Intuniv 4mg modified-release tablets | 28 tablet [PoM] £76.16

2.2 Bipolar disorder and mania

Drugs for mania and hypomania

Overview
Antimanic drugs are used to control acute attacks and to prevent recurrence of episodes of mania or hypomania. Long-term treatment of bipolar disorder should continue for at least two years from the last manic episode and up to five years if the patient has risk factors for relapse.
An antidepressant drug may also be required for the treatment of co-existing depression, but should be avoided in patients with rapid-cycling bipolar disorder, a recent history of hypomania, or with rapid mood fluctuations.

Benzodiazepines
Use of benzodiazepines may be helpful in the initial stages of treatment for behavioural disturbance or agitation; they should not be used for long periods because of the risk of dependence.

Antipsychotic drugs
Antipsychotic drugs (normally olanzapine p. 242, quetiapine p. 243, or risperidone p. 244) are useful in acute episodes of mania and hypomania; if the response to antipsychotic drugs is inadequate, lithium or valproate may be added. An antipsychotic drug may be used concomitantly with lithium or valproate in the initial treatment of severe acute mania.
Atypical antipsychotics are the treatment of choice for the long-term management of bipolar disorder in children and adolescents; if the patient has frequent relapses or continuing functional impairment, consider concomitant therapy with lithium or valproate. An atypical antipsychotic

that causes less weight gain and does not increase prolactin levels is preferred.
When discontinuing antipsychotics, the dose should be reduced gradually over at least 4 weeks if the child is continuing on other antimanic drugs; if the child is not continuing on other antimanic drugs, or has a history of manic relapse, a withdrawal period of up to 3 months is required.

Carbamazepine
Carbamazepine p. 189 may be used under specialist supervision for the prophylaxis of bipolar disorder (manic-depressive disorder) in children unresponsive to a combination of other prophylactic drugs; it is used in patients with rapid-cycling manic-depressive illness (4 or more affective episodes per year). The dose of carbamazepine should not normally be increased if an acute episode of mania occurs.

Valproate
Valproic acid p. 205 (as the semisodium salt) is licensed in adults for the treatment of manic episodes associated with bipolar disorder. Sodium valproate p. 200 is unlicensed for the treatment of bipolar disorder. Valproate (valproic acid and sodium valproate) can also be used for the prophylaxis of bipolar disorder [unlicensed use]. It must be started and supervised by a specialist experienced in managing bipolar disorder.
Valproate (valproic acid and sodium valproate) should not be used in female children, in females of childbearing potential and pregnant females, unless alternative treatments are ineffective or not tolerated, because of its high teratogenic potential; the benefits and risks of valproate therapy should be carefully reconsidered at regular treatment reviews. In patients with frequent relapse or continuing functional impairment, consider switching therapy to lithium or an atypical antipsychotic, or adding lithium or an atypical antipsychotic to valproate. If a patient taking valproate experiences an acute episode of mania that is not ameliorated by increasing the valproate dose, consider concomitant therapy with olanzapine, quetiapine, or risperidone.

Lithium
Lithium salts are used in the prophylaxis and treatment of mania, in the prophylaxis of bipolar disorder (manic-depressive disorder), and bipolar depression, and as concomitant therapy with antidepressant medication in children who have had an incomplete response to treatment for acute depression in bipolar disorder [unlicensed indication]. It is also used for the treatment of aggressive or self-harming behaviour [unlicensed indication].
The decision to give prophylactic lithium requires specialist advice, and must be based on careful consideration of the likelihood of recurrence in the individual child, and the benefit of treatment weighed against the risks. The full prophylactic effect of lithium may not occur for six to twelve months after the initiation of therapy. An atypical antipsychotic or valproate (given alone or as adjunctive therapy with lithium) are alternative prophylactic treatments in patients who experience frequent relapses or continued functional impairment.

> **Other drugs used for Bipolar disorder and mania**
> Aripiprazole, p. 240 · Perphenazine, p. 238

4

Nervous system

Lithium salts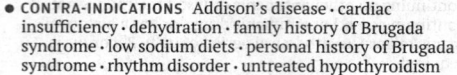

- **CONTRA-INDICATIONS** Addison's disease · cardiac insufficiency · dehydration · family history of Brugada syndrome · low sodium diets · personal history of Brugada syndrome · rhythm disorder · untreated hypothyroidism
- **CAUTIONS** Avoid abrupt withdrawal · cardiac disease · concurrent ECT (may lower seizure threshold) · diuretic treatment (risk of toxicity) · epilepsy (may lower seizure threshold) · myasthenia gravis · psoriasis (risk of exacerbation) · QT interval prolongation · review dose as necessary in diarrhoea · review dose as necessary in intercurrent infection (especially if sweating profusely) · review dose as necessary in vomiting · surgery

CAUTIONS, FURTHER INFORMATION

▸ Long-term use Long-term use of lithium has been associated with thyroid disorders and mild cognitive and memory impairment. Long-term treatment should therefore be undertaken only with careful assessment of risk and benefit, and with monitoring of thyroid function every 6 months (more often if there is evidence of deterioration).

   The need for continued therapy should be assessed regularly and patients should be maintained on lithium after 3–5 years only if benefit persists.

- **SIDE-EFFECTS**
- ▸ **Very rare** Nystagmus
- ▸ **Frequency not known** Acneiform eruptions · alopecia · anorexia · arrhythmia · arthralgia · AV block · benign intracranial hypertension · bradycardia · cardiomyopathy · cognitive impairment · dry mouth · dysgeusia · ECG changes · electrolyte imbalance · encephalopathy · euthyroid goitre · extrapyramidal side-effects · fine tremor · gastritis · gastro-intestinal disturbances · hallucinations · hyperparathyroidism · hypersalivation · hyperthyroidism · hypothyroidism · kidney changes · leucocytosis · malaise · memory loss · myalgia · myasthenia gravis · nephrogenic diabetes insipidus · nephrotic syndrome · oedema · other skin disorders · parathyroid adenoma · peripheral neuropathy · polydipsia · psoriasis exacerbation · QT interval prolongation · Raynaud's phenomena · renal impairment · sexual dysfunction · sinus node dysfunction · speech disorder · thyroid changes · vertigo · weight changes

Overdose

Signs of intoxication require withdrawal of treatment and include increasing gastro-intestinal disturbances (vomiting, diarrhoea), visual disturbances, polyuria, muscle weakness, fine tremor increasing to coarse tremor, CNS disturbances (confusion and drowsiness increasing to lack of coordination, restlessness, stupor); abnormal reflexes, myoclonus, incontinence, hypernatraemia. With severe overdosage seizures, cardiac arrhythmias (including sino-atrial block, bradycardia and first-degree heart block), blood pressure changes, circulatory failure, renal failure, coma and sudden death reported.

   For details on the management of poisoning, see Lithium, under Emergency treatment of poisoning p. 803.

- **CONCEPTION AND CONTRACEPTION** Manufacturer advises effective contraception during treatment for women of child bearing potential.
- **PREGNANCY** Dose requirements increased during the second and third trimesters (but on delivery return abruptly to normal). Avoid if possible, particularly in the first trimester (risk of teratogenicity, including cardiac abnormalities).

   Close monitoring of serum-lithium concentration advised in pregnancy (risk of toxicity in neonate).
- **BREAST FEEDING** Present in milk and risk of toxicity in infant—avoid.

- **RENAL IMPAIRMENT** Caution in mild to moderate impairment. Avoid in severe impairment. In renal impairment monitor serum-lithium concentration closely and adjust dose accordingly.
- **MONITORING REQUIREMENTS**
- ▸ Serum concentrations Lithium salts have a narrow therapeutic/toxic ratio and should therefore not be prescribed unless facilities for monitoring serum-lithium concentrations are available.

   Samples should be taken 12 hours after the dose to achieve a serum-lithium concentration of 0.4–1 mmol/litre (lower end of the range for maintenance therapy and elderly patients).

   A target serum-lithium concentration of 0.8–1 mmol/litre is recommended for acute episodes of mania, and for patients who have previously relapsed or have sub-syndromal symptoms. It is important to determine the optimum range for each individual patient.

   Routine serum-lithium monitoring should be performed weekly after initiation and after each dose change until concentrations are stable, then every 3 months thereafter. Additional serum-lithium measurements should be made if a patient develops significant intercurrent disease or if there is a significant change in a patient's sodium or fluid intake.
- ▸ Renal function should be monitored at baseline and every 6 months thereafter (more often if there is evidence of deterioration or if the patient has other risk factors, such as starting ACE inhibitors, NSAIDs, or diuretics).
- ▸ Assess cardiac and thyroid function before initiating, and thereafter every 6 months on stabilised regimens.
- **TREATMENT CESSATION** While there is no clear evidence of withdrawal or rebound psychosis, abrupt discontinuation of lithium increases the risk of relapse. If lithium is to be discontinued, the dose should be reduced gradually over a period of at least 4 weeks (preferably over a period of up to 3 months). Patients and their carers should be warned of the risk of relapse if lithium is discontinued abruptly. If lithium is stopped or is to be discontinued abruptly, consider changing therapy to an atypical antipsychotic or valproate.
- **PATIENT AND CARER ADVICE**
   Patients should be advised to report signs and symptoms of lithium toxicity, hypothyroidism, renal dysfunction (including polyuria and polydipsia), and benign intracranial hypertension (persistent headache and visual disturbance).

   Maintain adequate fluid intake and avoid dietary changes which reduce or increase sodium intake.

Driving and skilled tasks

May impair performance of skilled tasks (e.g. driving, operating machinery).

Lithium treatment packs A lithium treatment pack should be given to patients on initiation of treatment with lithium. The pack consists of a patient information booklet, lithium alert card, and a record book for tracking serum-lithium concentration. Packs may be purchased from

   3M

   0845 610 1112

   nhsforms@mmm.uk.com

⌐ 224

Lithium carbonate

- **INDICATIONS AND DOSE**

Treatment and prophylaxis of mania | Treatment and prophylaxis of bipolar disorder | Treatment and prophylaxis of recurrent depression | Treatment and prophylaxis of aggressive or self-harming behaviour
▸ BY MOUTH
▸ Child 12–17 years: Dose adjusted to achieve a serum-lithium concentration of 0.4–1 mmol/litre 12 hours after a dose on days 4–7 of treatment, then every week until dosage has remained constant for 4 weeks and every 3 months thereafter, doses are initially divided throughout the day, but once daily administration is preferred when serum-lithium concentration stabilised

CAMCOLIT® IMMEDIATE-RELEASE TABLET

Treatment of mania | Treatment of bipolar disorder | Treatment of recurrent depression | Treatment of aggressive or self-harming behaviour
▸ BY MOUTH
▸ Child 12–17 years: Initially 1–1.5 g daily, dose adjusted to achieve a serum-lithium concentration of 0.4–1 mmol/litre 12 hours after a dose on days 4–7 of treatment, then every week until dosage has remained constant for 4 weeks and every 3 months thereafter, doses are initially divided throughout the day, but once daily administration is preferred when serum-lithium concentration stabilised

Prophylaxis of mania | Prophylaxis of bipolar disorder | Prophylaxis of recurrent depression | Prophylaxis of aggressive or self-harming behaviour
▸ BY MOUTH
▸ Child 12–17 years: Initially 300–400 mg daily, dose adjusted to achieve a serum-lithium concentration of 0.4–1 mmol/litre 12 hours after a dose on days 4–7 of treatment, then every week until dosage has remained constant for 4 weeks and every 3 months thereafter, doses are initially divided throughout the day, but once daily administration is preferred when serum-lithium concentration stabilised

CAMCOLIT® MODIFIED-RELEASE TABLET

Treatment of mania | Treatment of bipolar disorder | Treatment of recurrent depression | Treatment of aggressive or self-harming behaviour
▸ BY MOUTH
▸ Child 12–17 years: Initially 1–1.5 g daily, dose adjusted to achieve a serum-lithium concentration of 0.4–1 mmol/litre 12 hours after a dose on days 4–7 of treatment, then every week until dosage has remained constant for 4 weeks and every 3 months thereafter, doses are initially divided throughout the day, but once daily administration is preferred when serum-lithium concentration stabilised

Prophylaxis of mania | Prophylaxis of bipolar disorder | Prophylaxis of recurrent depression | Prophylaxis of aggressive or self-harming behaviour
▸ BY MOUTH
▸ Child 12–17 years: Initially 300–400 mg daily, dose adjusted to achieve a serum-lithium concentration of 0.4–1 mmol/litre 12 hours after a dose on days 4–7 of treatment, then every week until dosage has remained constant for 4 weeks and every 3 months thereafter, doses are initially divided throughout the day, but once daily administration is preferred when serum-lithium concentration stabilised

LISKONUM®

Treatment of mania | Treatment of bipolar disorder | Treatment of recurrent depression | Treatment of aggressive or self-harming behaviour
▸ BY MOUTH
▸ Child 12–17 years: Initially 225–675 mg twice daily, dose adjusted to achieve a serum-lithium concentration of 0.4–1 mmol/litre 12 hours after a dose on days 4–7 of treatment, then every week until dosage has remained constant for 4 weeks and every 3 months thereafter, doses are initially divided throughout the day, but once daily administration is preferred when serum-lithium concentration stabilised

Prophylaxis of mania | Prophylaxis of bipolar disorder | Prophylaxis of recurrent depression | Prophylaxis of aggressive or self-harming behaviour
▸ BY MOUTH
▸ Child 12–17 years: Initially 225–450 mg twice daily, dose adjusted to achieve a serum-lithium concentration of 0.4–1 mmol/litre 12 hours after a dose on days 4–7 of treatment, then every week until dosage has remained constant for 4 weeks and every 3 months thereafter, doses are initially divided throughout the day, but once daily administration is preferred when serum-lithium concentration stabilised

DOSE EQUIVALENCE AND CONVERSION
▸ **Preparations vary widely in bioavailability**; changing the preparation requires the same precautions as initiation of treatment.

- **UNLICENSED USE** Not licensed for aggressive or self-harming behaviour. Not licensed for concomitant therapy with antidepressant medication in children who have had an incomplete response to treatment for acute depression in bipolar disorder. *Camcolit®* brand not licensed for use in children.

- **INTERACTIONS** → Appendix 1: lithium

- **MEDICINAL FORMS**
There can be variation in the licensing of different medicines containing the same drug. Forms available from special-order manufacturers include: oral suspension

Modified-release tablet
CAUTIONARY AND ADVISORY LABELS 10, 25
▸ Lithium carbonate (Non-proprietary)
   Lithium carbonate 400 mg Lithium carbonate 400mg modified-release tablets | 100 tablet [PoM] no price available DT price = £4.02
▸ Camcolit (Essential Pharma Ltd)
   Lithium carbonate 400 mg Camcolit 400 modified-release tablets | 100 tablet [PoM] £48.18 DT price = £4.02
▸ Liskonum (Teofarma)
   Lithium carbonate 450 mg Liskonum 450mg modified-release tablets | 60 tablet [PoM] £11.84 DT price = £11.84
▸ Priadel (lithium carbonate) (Sanofi)
   Lithium carbonate 200 mg Priadel 200mg modified-release tablets | 100 tablet [PoM] £2.76 DT price = £2.76
   Lithium carbonate 400 mg Priadel 400mg modified-release tablets | 100 tablet [PoM] £4.02 DT price = £4.02

Tablet
CAUTIONARY AND ADVISORY LABELS 10
▸ Lithium carbonate (Non-proprietary)
   Lithium carbonate 250 mg Lithium carbonate 250mg tablets | 100 tablet [PoM] £87.00 DT price = £87.00

4

Nervous system

4

Nervous system

Lithium citrate

☞ 224

● INDICATIONS AND DOSE

Treatment and prophylaxis of mania | Treatment and prophylaxis of bipolar disorder | Treatment and prophylaxis of recurrent depression | Treatment and prophylaxis of aggressive or self-harming behaviour

▸ BY MOUTH

▸ Child: Dose adjusted to achieve a serum-lithium concentration of 0.4–1 mmol/litre 12 hours after a dose on days 4–7 of treatment, then every week until dosage has remained constant for 4 weeks and every 3 months thereafter; doses are initially divided throughout the day, but once daily administration is preferred when serum-lithium concentration stabilised

DOSE EQUIVALENCE AND CONVERSION

▸ **Preparations vary widely in bioavailability**; changing the preparation requires the same precautions as initiation of treatment.

LI-LIQUID®

Treatment and prophylaxis of mania | Treatment and prophylaxis of bipolar disorder | Treatment and prophylaxis of recurrent depression | Treatment and prophylaxis of aggressive or self-harming behaviour

▸ BY MOUTH

▸ Child: Dose adjusted to achieve a serum-lithium concentration of 0.4–1 mmol/litre 12 hours after a dose on days 4–7 of treatment, then every week until dosage has remained constant for 4 weeks and every 3 months thereafter

DOSE EQUIVALENCE AND CONVERSION

▸ For Li-Liquid®: Lithium citrate tetrahydrate 509 mg is equivalent to lithium carbonate 200 mg.
▸ **Preparations vary widely in bioavailability**; changing the preparation requires the same precautions as initiation of treatment.

PRIADEL® LIQUID

Treatment and prophylaxis of mania | Treatment and prophylaxis of bipolar disorder | Treatment and prophylaxis of recurrent depression | Treatment and prophylaxis of aggressive or self-harming behaviour

▸ BY MOUTH

▸ Child: Dose adjusted to achieve a serum-lithium concentration of 0.4–1 mmol/litre 12 hours after a dose on days 4–7 of treatment, then every week until dosage has remained constant for 4 weeks and every 3 months thereafter, doses are initially divided throughout the day, but once daily administration is preferred when serum-lithium concentration stabilised

DOSE EQUIVALENCE AND CONVERSION

▸ For Priadel® liquid: Lithium citrate tetrahydrate 520 mg is equivalent to lithium carbonate 204 mg.
▸ **Preparations vary widely in bioavailability**; changing the preparation requires the same precautions as initiation of treatment.

● UNLICENSED USE Not licensed for use in children.

● INTERACTIONS → Appendix 1: lithium

● MEDICINAL FORMS
There can be variation in the licensing of different medicines containing the same drug.

Oral solution
CAUTIONARY AND ADVISORY LABELS 10
▸ Lithium citrate (Non-proprietary)
Lithium citrate 101.8 mg per 1 ml Lithium citrate 509mg/5ml oral solution | 150 ml [PoM] no price available DT price = £5.79
Lithium citrate 104 mg per 1 ml Lithium citrate 520mg/5ml oral solution sugar free sugar-free | 150 ml [PoM] no price available

Lithium citrate 203.6 mg per 1 ml Lithium citrate 1.018g/5ml oral solution | 150 ml [PoM] no price available DT price = £11.58
▸ Li-Liquid (Rosemont Pharmaceuticals Ltd)
Lithium citrate 101.8 mg per 1 ml Li-Liquid 509mg/5ml oral solution | 150 ml [PoM] £5.79 DT price = £5.79
Lithium citrate 203.6 mg per 1 ml Li-Liquid 1.018g/5ml oral solution | 150 ml [PoM] £11.58 DT price = £11.58
▸ Priadel (lithium citrate) (Sanofi)
Lithium citrate 104 mg per 1 ml Priadel 520mg/5ml liquid sugar-free | 150 ml [PoM] £6.73

2.3 Depression

Antidepressant drugs

Overview

Depression in children should be managed by an appropriate specialist and treatment should involve psychological therapy.

Choice

The major classes of antidepressant drugs include the tricyclics and related antidepressant drugs, the selective serotonin re-uptake inhibitors (SSRIs), and the monoamine oxidase inhibitors (MAOIs).

Antidepressant drugs should not be used routinely in mild depression, and psychological therapy should be considered initially; however, a trial of antidepressant therapy may be considered in cases refractory to psychological treatments or in those associated with psychosocial or medical problems. Drug treatment of mild depression may also be considered in children with a history of moderate or severe depression.

Choice of antidepressant drug should be based on the individual child's requirements, including the presence of concomitant disease, existing therapy, suicide risk, and previous response to antidepressant therapy.

When drug treatment of depression is considered necessary in children, the SSRIs should be considered first-line treatment; following a safety and efficacy review, fluoxetine p. 228 is licensed to treat depression in children.

Tricyclic antidepressant drugs should be avoided for the treatment of depression in children.

St John's wort (Hypericum perforatum) is a popular herbal remedy on sale to the public for treating mild depression in adults. It should not be used for the treatment of depression in children because St John's wort can induce drug metabolising enzymes and a number of important interactions with conventional drugs, including conventional antidepressants, have been identified. Furthermore, the amount of active ingredient varies between different preparations of St John's wort and switching from one to another can change the degree of enzyme induction. If a child stops taking St John's wort, the concentration of interacting drugs may increase, leading to toxicity.

Management

Children should be reviewed every 1–2 weeks at the start of antidepressant treatment. Treatment should be continued for at least 4 weeks before considering whether to switch antidepressant due to lack of efficacy. In cases of partial response, continue for a further 2–4 weeks. Following remission, antidepressant treatment should be continued at the same dose for at least 6 months. Children with a history of recurrent depression should continue treatment for at least 2 years.

Hyponatraemia and antidepressant therapy

Hyponatraemia (possibly due to inappropriate secretion of antidiuretic hormone) has been associated with all types of antidepressants; however, it has been reported more frequently with SSRIs than with other antidepressant drugs. Hyponatraemia should be considered in all children who develop drowsiness, confusion, or convulsions while taking an antidepressant.

Suicidal behaviour and antidepressant therapy
The use of antidepressant drugs has been linked with suicidal thoughts and behaviour. Where necessary, children should be monitored for suicidal behaviour, self-harm, and hostility, particularly at the beginning of treatment or if the dose is changed.

Serotonin syndrome
Serotonin syndrome or serotonin toxicity is a relatively uncommon adverse drug reaction caused by excessive central and peripheral serotonergic activity. Onset of symptoms, which range from mild to life-threatening, can occur within hours or days following the initiation, dose escalation, or overdose of a serotonergic drug, the addition of a new serotonergic drug, or the replacement of one serotonergic drug by another without allowing a long enough washout period in-between, particularly when the first drug is an irreversible MAOI or a drug with a long half-life. Severe toxicity, which is a medical emergency, usually occurs with a combination of serotonergic drugs, one of which is generally an MAOI.

The characteristic symptoms of serotonin syndrome fall into 3 main areas, although features from each group may not be seen in all patients—neuromuscular hyperactivity (such as tremor, hyperreflexia, clonus, myoclonus, rigidity), autonomic dysfunction (tachycardia, blood pressure changes, hyperthermia, diaphoresis, shivering, diarrhoea), and altered mental state (agitation, confusion, mania).

Treatment consists of withdrawal of the serotonergic medication and supportive care; specialist advice should be sought.

Important safety information: Depressive illness in children and adolescents
The balance of risks and benefits for the treatment of depressive illness in individuals under 18 years is considered unfavourable for the SSRIs citalopram, escitalopram, paroxetine, and sertraline, and for mirtazapine and venlafaxine. Clinical trials have failed to show efficacy and have shown an increase in harmful outcomes. However, it is recognised that specialists may sometimes decide to use these drugs in response to individual clinical need; children and adolescents should be monitored carefully for suicidal behaviour, self-harm or hostility, particularly at the beginning of treatment. Only fluoxetine has been shown in clinical trials to be effective for treating depressive illness in children and adolescents. However, it is possible that, in common with the other SSRIs, it is associated with a small risk of self-harm and suicidal thoughts. Overall, the balance of risks and benefits for fluoxetine in the treatment of depressive illness in individuals under 18 years is considered favourable, but children and adolescents must be carefully monitored as above.

Anxiety
Management of *acute anxiety* in children with drug treatment is contentious. For *chronic anxiety* (of longer than 4 weeks' duration), it may be appropriate to use an antidepressant drug before a benzodiazepine.

Tricyclic antidepressants are not effective for treating depression in children.

Some tricyclic antidepressant drugs may have a role in some forms of *neuralgia*, and in *nocturnal enuresis* in children.

Dosage
It is important to use doses that are sufficiently high for effective treatment but not so high as to cause toxic effects. Low doses should be used for initial treatment.

In most children the long half-life of tricyclic antidepressant drugs allows **once-daily** administration,

usually at night; the use of modified-release preparations is therefore unnecessary.

> **Other drugs used for Depression** Lithium carbonate, p. 225 · Lithium citrate, p. 226

ANTIDEPRESSANTS › SELECTIVE SEROTONIN RE-UPTAKE INHIBITORS

Selective serotonin re-uptake inhibitors

- **DRUG ACTION** Selectively inhibit the re-uptake of serotonin (5-hydroxytryptamine, 5-HT).
- **CONTRA-INDICATIONS** Poorly controlled epilepsy · SSRIs should not be used if the patient enters a manic phase.
- **CAUTIONS** Cardiac disease · concurrent electroconvulsive therapy · diabetes mellitus · epilepsy (discontinue if convulsions develop) · history of bleeding disorders (especially gastro-intestinal bleeding) · history of mania · susceptibility to angle-closure glaucoma
- **SIDE-EFFECTS**
  - **Common or very common** Abdominal pain (dose-related) · constipation (dose-related) · diarrhoea (dose-related) · dyspepsia (dose-related) · gastro-intestinal effects (dose-related) · nausea (dose-related) · vomiting (dose-related)
  - **Uncommon** Serotonin syndrome
  - **Very rare** Angle-closure glaucoma
  - **Frequency not known** Anaphylaxis · angioedema · anorexia with weight loss · anxiety · arthralgia · asthenia · bleeding disorders · convulsions · dizziness · drowsiness · dry mouth · dyskinesias · ecchymoses · galactorrhoea · hallucinations · headache · hypersensitivity reactions · hypomania · hyponatraemia · increased appetite · insomnia · mania · movement disorders · myalgia · nervousness · photosensitivity · purpura · rash · sexual dysfunction · suicidal behaviour · sweating · tremor · urinary retention · urticaria · visual disturbances · weight gain

  SIDE-EFFECTS, FURTHER INFORMATION
  - Hypersensitivity reactions If hypersensitivity reactions (including rash) occur, consider discontinuation—may be sign of impending serious systemic reaction, possibly associated with vasculitis.

  Overdose
  Symptoms of poisoning by selective serotonin re-uptake inhibitors include nausea, vomiting, agitation, tremor, nystagmus, drowsiness, and sinus tachycardia; convulsions may occur. Rarely, severe poisoning results in the serotonin syndrome, with marked neuropsychiatric effects, neuromuscular hyperactivity, and autonomic instability; hyperthermia, rhabdomyolysis, renal failure, and coagulopathies may develop.

  For details on the management of poisoning, see Selective serotonin re-uptake inhibitors, under Emergency treatment of poisoning p. 803.

- **PREGNANCY** Manufacturers advise avoid during pregnancy unless the potential benefit outweighs the risk. There is a small increased risk of congenital heart defects when taken during early pregnancy. If used during the third trimester there is a risk of neonatal withdrawal symptoms, and persistent pulmonary hypertension in the newborn has been reported.

- **TREATMENT CESSATION** Gastro-intestinal disturbances, headache, anxiety, dizziness, paraesthesia, electric shock sensation in the head, neck, and spine, tinnitus, sleep disturbances, fatigue, influenza-like symptoms, and sweating are the most common features of abrupt withdrawal of an SSRI or marked reduction of the dose; palpitation and visual disturbances can occur less commonly. The dose should be tapered over at least a few weeks to avoid these effects. For some patients, it may be necessary to withdraw treatment over a longer period; consider obtaining specialist advice if symptoms persist.

Withdrawal effects may occur within 5 days of stopping treatment with antidepressant drugs; they are usually mild and self-limiting, but in some cases may be severe. The risk of withdrawal symptoms is increased if the antidepressant is stopped suddenly after regular administration for 8 weeks or more. The dose should preferably be reduced gradually over about 4 weeks, or longer if withdrawal symptoms emerge (6 months in patients who have been on long-term maintenance treatment).

- **PATIENT AND CARER ADVICE**
Driving and skilled tasks
May also impair performance of skilled tasks (e.g. driving, operating machinery).

☞ 227

Citalopram

- **INDICATIONS AND DOSE**
Major depression
  - BY MOUTH USING TABLETS
  - Child 12–17 years: Initially 10 mg once daily, increased if necessary to 20 mg once daily, dose to be increased over 2–4 weeks; maximum 40 mg per day
  - BY MOUTH USING ORAL DROPS
  - Child 12–17 years: Initially 8 mg once daily, increased if necessary to 16 mg once daily, dose to be increased over 2–4 weeks; maximum 32 mg per day

DOSE EQUIVALENCE AND CONVERSION
  - 4 oral drops (8 mg) is equivalent in therapeutic effect to 10 mg tablet.

- **UNLICENSED USE** Not licensed for use in children.
- **CONTRA-INDICATIONS** QT-interval prolongation
- **CAUTIONS** Susceptibility to QT-interval prolongation
- **INTERACTIONS** → Appendix 1: SSRIs
- **SIDE-EFFECTS** Taste disturbance · abnormal dreams · aggression · amnesia · bradycardia · confusion · coughing · euphoria · haemorrhage · hepatitis · hypokalaemia · impaired concentration · increased salivation · malaise · micturition disorders · migraine · mydriasis · oedema · palpitation · paraesthesia · polyuria · postural hypotension · pruritus · QT-interval prolongation · rhinitis · tachycardia · tinnitus · yawning
- **BREAST FEEDING** Present in milk—use with caution.
- **HEPATIC IMPAIRMENT** Use doses at lower end of range; for *tablets* up to maximum 20 mg; for *oral solution* up to maximum 16 mg.
- **RENAL IMPAIRMENT** No information available for estimated glomerular filtration rate less than 20 mL/minute/1.73 m^2.
- **DIRECTIONS FOR ADMINISTRATION** *Cipramil*® oral drops should be mixed with water, orange juice, or apple juice before taking.
- **PATIENT AND CARER ADVICE**
Driving and skilled tasks
Patients should be advised of the effects of citalopram on driving and skilled tasks.
  Counselling on administration of oral drops is advised.

- **MEDICINAL FORMS**
There can be variation in the licensing of different medicines containing the same drug.
Oral drops
EXCIPIENTS: May contain Alcohol
  - Citalopram (Non-proprietary)
    Citalopram (as Citalopram hydrochloride) 40 mg per 1 ml Citalopram 40mg/ml oral drops sugar free sugar-free | 15 ml [PoM] £20.16 DT price = £4.74
  - Cipramil (Lundbeck Ltd)
    Citalopram (as Citalopram hydrochloride) 40 mg per 1 ml Cipramil 40mg/ml drops sugar-free | 15 ml [PoM] £10.08 DT price = £4.74
Tablet
  - Citalopram (Non-proprietary)
    Citalopram (as Citalopram hydrobromide) 10 mg Citalopram 10mg tablets | 28 tablet [PoM] £8.90 DT price = £0.77
    Citalopram (as Citalopram hydrobromide) 20 mg Citalopram 20mg tablets | 28 tablet [PoM] £15.99 DT price = £0.81
    Citalopram (as Citalopram hydrobromide) 40 mg Citalopram 40mg tablets | 28 tablet [PoM] £27.00 DT price = £1.01
  - Cipramil (Lundbeck Ltd)
    Citalopram (as Citalopram hydrobromide) 20 mg Cipramil 20mg tablets | 28 tablet [PoM] £8.95 DT price = £0.81

☞ 227

Fluoxetine

- **INDICATIONS AND DOSE**
Major depression
  - BY MOUTH
  - Child 8–17 years: Initially 10 mg daily, increased if necessary up to 20 mg daily, dose to be increased after 1–2 weeks of initial dose, daily dose may be administered as a single or divided dose

PHARMACOKINETICS
Consider the long half-life of fluoxetine when adjusting dosage (or in overdosage).

- **INTERACTIONS** → Appendix 1: SSRIs
- **SIDE-EFFECTS** Alopecia · changes in blood sugar · chills · confusion · dysphagia · dyspnoea · euphoria · flushing · haemorrhage · hepatitis · hypotension · impaired concentration · malaise · neuroleptic malignant syndrome-like event · palpitation · pharyngitis · priapism · pulmonary fibrosis · pulmonary inflammation · sleep disturbances · taste disturbance · toxic epidermal necrolysis · urinary frequency · vasodilatation · yawning
- **BREAST FEEDING** Present in milk—avoid.
- **HEPATIC IMPAIRMENT** Reduce dose or increase dose interval.
- **DIRECTIONS FOR ADMINISTRATION** Dispersible tablets can be dispersed in water for administration or swallowed whole with plenty of water.
- **PATIENT AND CARER ADVICE**
Patients and carers should be counselled on the administration of dispersible tablets.

Driving and skilled tasks
Patients should be counselled about the effects on driving and skilled tasks.
Medicines for Children leaflet: Fluoxetine for depression, obsessive compulsive disorder and bulimia nervosa
www.medicinesforchildren.org.uk/fluoxetine-depression-obsessive-compulsive-disorder-and-bulimia-nervosa

- **MEDICINAL FORMS**
There can be variation in the licensing of different medicines containing the same drug. Forms available from special-order manufacturers include: tablet, oral suspension, oral solution
Dispersible tablet
CAUTIONARY AND ADVISORY LABELS 10
  - Olena (AMCo)
    Fluoxetine (as Fluoxetine hydrochloride) 20 mg Olena 20mg dispersible tablets sugar-free | 28 tablet [PoM] £3.44 DT price = £3.44

Oral solution

- ▶ Fluoxetine (Non-proprietary)
  Fluoxetine (as Fluoxetine hydrochloride) 4 mg per 1 ml Fluoxetine 20mg/5ml oral solution | 70 ml [PoM] £2.81 DT price = £2.81
  Fluoxetine 20mg/5ml oral solution sugar free sugar-free | 70 ml [PoM] £12.95 DT price = £12.95
- ▶ Prozac (Eli Lilly and Company Ltd)
  Fluoxetine (as Fluoxetine hydrochloride) 4 mg per 1 ml Prozac 20mg/5ml liquid | 70 ml [PoM] £11.12 DT price = £2.81
- ▶ Prozep (Chemidex Pharma Ltd)
  Fluoxetine (as Fluoxetine hydrochloride) 4 mg per 1 ml Prozep 20mg/5ml oral solution sugar-free | 70 ml [PoM] £12.95 DT price = £12.95

Capsule

- ▶ Fluoxetine (Non-proprietary)
  Fluoxetine (as Fluoxetine hydrochloride) 10 mg Fluoxetine 10mg capsules | 30 capsule [PoM] £55.00–£72.00 DT price = £66.16
  Fluoxetine (as Fluoxetine hydrochloride) 20 mg Fluoxetine 20mg capsules | 30 capsule [PoM] £20.00 DT price = £0.87
  Fluoxetine (as Fluoxetine hydrochloride) 30 mg Fluoxetine 30mg capsules | 30 capsule [PoM] £1.80–£2.12 DT price = £2.12
  Fluoxetine (as Fluoxetine hydrochloride) 40 mg Fluoxetine 40mg capsules | 30 capsule [PoM] £1.80–£2.16 DT price = £2.12
  Fluoxetine (as Fluoxetine hydrochloride) 60 mg Fluoxetine 60mg capsules | 30 capsule [PoM] £54.36 DT price = £6.74
- ▶ Oxactin (Discovery Pharmaceuticals)
  Fluoxetine (as Fluoxetine hydrochloride) 20 mg Oxactin 20mg capsules | 30 capsule [PoM] £0.83 DT price = £0.87
- ▶ Prozac (Eli Lilly and Company Ltd)
  Fluoxetine (as Fluoxetine hydrochloride) 20 mg Prozac 20mg capsules | 30 capsule [PoM] £1.50 DT price = £0.87

F 227

Fluvoxamine maleate

● **INDICATIONS AND DOSE**

Obsessive-compulsive disorder
▶ BY MOUTH
- ▶ Child 8–17 years: Initially 25 mg daily, then increased in steps of 25 mg every 4–7 days (max. per dose 100 mg twice daily) if required, dose to be increased according to response, doses above 50 mg should be given in 2 divided doses, if no improvement in obsessive-compulsive disorder within 10 weeks, treatment should be reconsidered

● **INTERACTIONS** → Appendix 1: SSRIs
● **SIDE-EFFECTS**
- ▶ **Common or very common** Malaise · palpitation · tachycardia
- ▶ **Uncommon** Ataxia · confusion · postural hypotension
- ▶ **Rare** Abnormal liver function, usually symptomatic (discontinue treatment)
- ▶ **Frequency not known** Neuroleptic malignant syndrome-like event · paraesthesia · taste disturbance
● **BREAST FEEDING** Present in milk—avoid.
● **HEPATIC IMPAIRMENT** Start with low dose.
● **RENAL IMPAIRMENT** Start with low dose.
● **PATIENT AND CARER ADVICE**

Driving and skilled tasks
Patients should be counselled about the effects on driving and skilled tasks.

● **MEDICINAL FORMS**
There can be variation in the licensing of different medicines containing the same drug. Forms available from special-order manufacturers include: oral suspension

Tablet

- ▶ Fluvoxamine maleate (Non-proprietary)
  Fluvoxamine maleate 50 mg Fluvoxamine 50mg tablets | 60 tablet [PoM] £25.32 DT price = £20.34
  Fluvoxamine maleate 100 mg Fluvoxamine 100mg tablets | 30 tablet [PoM] £25.32 DT price = £20.34
- ▶ Faverin (BGP Products Ltd)
  Fluvoxamine maleate 50 mg Faverin 50mg tablets | 60 tablet [PoM] £17.10 DT price = £20.34
  Fluvoxamine maleate 100 mg Faverin 100mg tablets | 30 tablet [PoM] £17.10 DT price = £20.34

F 227

Sertraline

● **INDICATIONS AND DOSE**

Obsessive-compulsive disorder
▶ BY MOUTH
- ▶ Child 6–11 years: Initially 25 mg daily for 1 week, then increased to 50 mg daily, then increased in steps of 50 mg at intervals of at least 1 week if required; maximum 200 mg per day
- ▶ Child 12–17 years: Initially 50 mg daily, then increased in steps of 50 mg at intervals of at least 1 week if required; maximum 200 mg per day

Major depression
▶ BY MOUTH
- ▶ Child 12–17 years: Initially 50 mg once daily, then increased in steps of 50 mg at intervals of at least 1 week if required; maximum 200 mg per day

● **UNLICENSED USE** Not licensed for use in children for depression.
● **INTERACTIONS** → Appendix 1: SSRIs
● **SIDE-EFFECTS** Aggression · amnesia · bronchospasm · hepatitis · hypercholesterolaemia · hyperprolactinaemia · hypertension · hypoglycaemia · hypothyroidism · jaundice · leucopenia · liver failure · menstrual irregularities · palpitation · pancreatitis · paraesthesia · postural hypotension · stomatitis · tachycardia · tinnitus · urinary incontinence
● **BREAST FEEDING** Not known to be harmful but consider discontinuing breast-feeding.
● **HEPATIC IMPAIRMENT** Reduce dose or increase dose interval in mild or moderate impairment. Avoid in severe impairment.
● **RENAL IMPAIRMENT** Use with caution.
● **PATIENT AND CARER ADVICE**

Driving and skilled tasks
Patients should be counselled on the effects on driving and skilled tasks.
Medicines for Children leaflet: Sertraline for OCD (obsessive compulsive disorder) and depression www.medicinesforchildren.org.uk/sertraline-for-ocd-obsessive-compulsive-disorder-and-depression

● **MEDICINAL FORMS**
There can be variation in the licensing of different medicines containing the same drug. Forms available from special-order manufacturers include: oral suspension

Tablet

- ▶ Sertraline (Non-proprietary)
  Sertraline (as Sertraline hydrochloride) 50 mg Sertraline 50mg tablets | 28 tablet [PoM] £19.25 DT price = £1.13
  Sertraline (as Sertraline hydrochloride) 100 mg Sertraline 100mg tablets | 28 tablet [PoM] £29.09 DT price = £1.26
- ▶ Lustral (Pfizer Ltd)
  Sertraline (as Sertraline hydrochloride) 50 mg Lustral 50mg tablets | 28 tablet [PoM] £17.82 DT price = £1.13
  Sertraline (as Sertraline hydrochloride) 100 mg Lustral 100mg tablets | 28 tablet [PoM] £29.16 DT price = £1.26

ANTIDEPRESSANTS > TRICYCLIC ANTIDEPRESSANTS

Amitriptyline hydrochloride

● **INDICATIONS AND DOSE**

Depressive illness (not recommended—increased risk of fatality in overdose)
▶ BY MOUTH
- ▶ Child 16–17 years: Initially 10–25 mg 3 times a day, alternatively initially 30–75 mg once daily, dose to be taken at bedtime, increased if necessary to 150–200 mg daily, dose to be increased gradually continued →

Nervous system

4

Neuropathic pain

▶ BY MOUTH

▶ **Child 2-11 years:** Initially 200–500 micrograms/kg once daily (max. per dose 10 mg), dose to be taken at night, increased if necessary up to 1 mg/kg twice daily, to be given on specialist advice

▶ **Child 12-17 years:** Initially 10 mg once daily, increased if necessary to 75 mg once daily, dose to be taken at night, dose to be increased gradually, higher doses to be given on specialist advice

● **UNLICENSED USE** Not licensed for use in neuropathic pain.

● **CONTRA-INDICATIONS** Acute porphyrias p. 577 · arrhythmias · during manic phase of bipolar disorder · heart block

● **CAUTIONS** Cardiovascular disease · chronic constipation · diabetes · epilepsy · history of bipolar disorder · history of psychosis · hyperthyroidism (risk of arrhythmias) · patients with a significant risk of suicide · phaeochromocytoma (risk of arrhythmias) · susceptibility to angle-closure glaucoma · urinary retention

CAUTIONS, FURTHER INFORMATION
Treatment should be stopped if the patient enters a manic phase.

● **INTERACTIONS** → Appendix 1: tricyclic antidepressants

● **SIDE-EFFECTS**

▶ **Common or very common** Abdominal pain · fatigue · hypertension · mydriasis · oedema · palpitation · restlessness · stomatitis

▶ **Rare** Dysarthria · extrapyramidal symptoms · paralytic ileus · tremor

▶ **Very rare** Neuroleptic malignant syndrome · precipitation of angle-closure glaucoma

▶ **Frequency not known** Agitation · alopecia · anorexia · anxiety · arrhythmia · blurred vision · breast enlargement · changes in blood sugar · chills (on withdrawal) · confusion · constipation · convulsions · delusions · dizziness · drowsiness · dry mouth · ECG changes · galactorrhoea · gynaecomastia · haematological reactions · hallucinations · headache (on withdrawal) · heart block · hepatic reactions · hypomania · hyponatraemia · increased appetite · increased intra-ocular pressure · influenza-like symptoms (on withdrawal) · Insomnia (on withdrawal) · irritability · mania · movement disorders (on withdrawal) · myalgia (on withdrawal) · nausea · nausea (on withdrawal) · paraesthesia · photosensitivity · postural hypotension · pruritus · rash · sexual dysfunction · sleep disturbances · sudden death of patients with cardiac disease · suicidal behaviour · sweating · sweating (on withdrawal) · tachycardia · taste disturbance · tinnitus · urinary retention · urticaria · vivid dreams (on withdrawal) · vomiting · weight gain · weight loss

Overdose

Overdosage with amitriptyline is associated with a relatively high rate of fatality. Symptoms of overdosage may include dry mouth, coma of varying degree, hypotension, hypothermia, hyperreflexia, extensor plantar responses, convulsions, respiratory failure, cardiac conduction defects, and arrhythmias. Dilated pupils and urinary retention also occur. For details on the management of poisoning, see Tricyclic and related antidepressants, under Emergency treatment of poisoning p. 803.

● **PREGNANCY** Use only if potential benefit outweighs risk.

● **BREAST FEEDING** The amount secreted into breast milk is too small to be harmful.

● **HEPATIC IMPAIRMENT** Sedative effects are increased in hepatic impairment. Avoid in severe liver disease.

● **TREATMENT CESSATION** Withdrawal effects may occur within 5 days of stopping treatment with antidepressant

drugs; they are usually mild and self-limiting, but in some cases may be severe. The risk of withdrawal symptoms is increased if the antidepressant is stopped suddenly after regular administration for 8 weeks or more. The dose should preferably be reduced gradually over about 4 weeks, or longer if withdrawal symptoms emerge (6 months in patients who have been on long-term maintenance treatment). If possible tricyclic and related antidepressants should be withdrawn slowly.

● **PRESCRIBING AND DISPENSING INFORMATION** Limited quantities of tricyclic antidepressants should be prescribed at any one time because their cardiovascular and epileptogenic effects are dangerous in overdosage.

● **PATIENT AND CARER ADVICE**

Driving and skilled tasks
Drowsiness may affect the performance of skilled tasks (e.g. driving). Effects of alcohol enhanced.
Medicines for Children leaflet: Amitriptyline for neuropathic pain www.medicinesforchildren.org.uk/amitriptyline-for-neuropathic-pain

● **LESS SUITABLE FOR PRESCRIBING** Amitriptyline hydrochloride is less suitable for prescribing, see Antidepressant drugs p. 226.

● **MEDICINAL FORMS**
There can be variation in the licensing of different medicines containing the same drug. Forms available from special-order manufacturers include: oral suspension, oral solution

Oral solution
CAUTIONARY AND ADVISORY LABELS 2

▶ **Amitriptyline hydrochloride** (Non-proprietary)
Amitriptyline hydrochloride 2 mg per 1 ml Amitriptyline 10mg/5ml oral solution sugar free sugar-free | 150 ml [PoM] £122.76 DT price = £114.57

Amitriptyline hydrochloride 5 mg per 1 ml Amitriptyline 25mg/5ml oral solution sugar free sugar-free | 150 ml [PoM] £18.00 DT price = £18.00

Amitriptyline hydrochloride 10 mg per 1 ml Amitriptyline 50mg/5ml oral solution sugar free sugar-free | 150 ml [PoM] £19.20 DT price = £19.20

Tablet
CAUTIONARY AND ADVISORY LABELS 2

▶ **Amitriptyline hydrochloride** (Non-proprietary)
Amitriptyline hydrochloride 10 mg Amitriptyline 10mg tablets | 28 tablet [PoM] £1.12 DT price = £1.09
Amitriptyline hydrochloride 25 mg Amitriptyline 25mg tablets | 28 tablet [PoM] £1.13 DT price = £0.79
Amitriptyline hydrochloride 50 mg Amitriptyline 50mg tablets | 28 tablet [PoM] £5.99 DT price = £2.77

Doxepin

● **INDICATIONS AND DOSE**

Depressive illness (particularly where sedation is required)

▶ BY MOUTH

▶ **Child 12-17 years:** Initially 75 mg daily in divided doses, alternatively 75 mg once daily, adjusted according to response, dose to be taken at bedtime; maintenance 25–300 mg daily, doses above 100 mg given in 3 divided doses

● **CONTRA-INDICATIONS** Acute porphyrias p. 577 · arrhythmias · during manic phase of bipolar disorder · heart block

● **CAUTIONS** Cardiovascular disease · chronic constipation · diabetes · epilepsy · history of bipolar disorder · history of psychosis · hyperthyroidism (risk of arrhythmias) · patients with significant risk of suicide · phaeochromocytoma (risk of arrhythmias) · susceptibility to angle-closure glaucoma · urinary retention

CAUTIONS, FURTHER INFORMATION
Treatment should be stopped if the patient enters a manic phase.

- **INTERACTIONS** → Appendix 1: tricyclic antidepressants
- **SIDE-EFFECTS**
  - ▸ **Common or very common** Agitation · anxiety · confusion · dizziness · drowsiness · irritability · paraesthesia · sleep disturbances
  - ▸ **Rare** Dysarthria · extrapyramidal symptoms · paralytic ileus · tremor
  - ▸ **Very rare** Neuroleptic malignant syndrome · precipitation of angle-closure glaucoma
  - ▸ **Frequency not known** Abdominal pain · alopecia · anorexia · arrhythmia · blurred vision · breast enlargement · changes in blood sugar · constipation · convulsions · delusions · diarrhoea · dry mouth · flushing · galactorrhoea · gynaecomastia · haematological reactions · hallucinations · headache (on withdrawal) · heart block · hepatic reactions · hypomania · hyponatraemia · increased appetite · influenza-like symptoms (on withdrawal) · insomnia (on withdrawal) · mania · movement disorders (on withdrawal) · myalgia (on withdrawal) · nausea · nausea (on withdrawal) · oedema · photosensitivity · pruritus · rash · sexual dysfunction · stomatitis · sudden death of patients with cardiac disease · suicidal behaviour · sweating · sweating (on withdrawal) · taste disturbance · tinnitus · urinary retention · urticaria · vivid dreams (on withdrawal) · vomiting · weight gain · weight loss

SIDE-EFFECTS, FURTHER INFORMATION
The patient should be encouraged to persist with treatment as some tolerance to these side-effects seems to develop. They are reduced if low doses are given initially and then gradually increased, but this must be balanced against the need to obtain a full therapeutic effect as soon as possible.

Overdose
Tricyclic and related antidepressants cause dry mouth, coma of varying degree, hypotension, hypothermia, hyperreflexia, extensor plantar responses, convulsions, respiratory failure, cardiac conduction defects, and arrhythmias. Dilated pupils and urinary retention also occur. For details on the management of poisoning see Tricyclic and related antidepressants under Emergency treatment of poisoning p. 803.

- **PREGNANCY** Use with caution—limited information available.
- **BREAST FEEDING** The amount secreted into breast milk is too small to be harmful. Accumulation of metabolite may cause sedation and respiratory depression in neonate.
- **HEPATIC IMPAIRMENT** Sedative effects are increased in hepatic impairment. Avoid in severe liver disease.
- **RENAL IMPAIRMENT** Use with caution.
- **TREATMENT CESSATION** Withdrawal effects may occur within 5 days of stopping treatment with antidepressant drugs; they are usually mild and self-limiting, but in some cases may be severe. The risk of withdrawal symptoms is increased if the antidepressant is stopped suddenly after regular administration for 8 weeks or more. The dose should preferably be reduced gradually over about 4 weeks, or longer if withdrawal symptoms emerge (6 months in patients who have been on long-term maintenance treatment). If possible tricyclic and related antidepressants should be withdrawn slowly.
- **PRESCRIBING AND DISPENSING INFORMATION** Limited quantities of tricyclic antidepressants should be prescribed at any one time because their cardiovascular and epileptogenic effects are dangerous in overdosage.

- **PATIENT AND CARER ADVICE**
  Driving and skilled tasks
  Drowsiness may affect performance of skilled tasks (e.g. driving). Effects of alcohol enhanced.

- **MEDICINAL FORMS**
  There can be variation in the licensing of different medicines containing the same drug. Forms available from special-order manufacturers include: capsule, oral suspension, oral solution
  Capsule
  CAUTIONARY AND ADVISORY LABELS 2
  ▸ Doxepin (Non-proprietary)
  Doxepin (as Doxepin hydrochloride) 25 mg Doxepin 25mg capsules | 28 capsule PoM £97.00 DT price = £97.00
  Doxepin (as Doxepin hydrochloride) 50 mg Doxepin 50mg capsules | 28 capsule PoM £154.00 DT price = £154.00

Imipramine hydrochloride

- **INDICATIONS AND DOSE**
  Nocturnal enuresis
  ▸ BY MOUTH
  ▸ Child 6-7 years: 25 mg once daily, to be taken at bedtime, initial period of treatment (including gradual withdrawal) 3 months—full physical examination before further course
  ▸ Child 8-10 years: 25–50 mg once daily, to be taken at bedtime, initial period of treatment (including gradual withdrawal) 3 months—full physical examination before further course
  ▸ Child 11-17 years: 50–75 mg once daily, to be taken at bedtime, initial period of treatment (including gradual withdrawal) 3 months—full physical examination before further course

  Attention deficit hyperactivity disorder (under expert supervision)
  ▸ BY MOUTH
  ▸ Child 6-17 years: 10–30 mg twice daily

- **UNLICENSED USE** Not licensed for use for attention deficit hyperactivity disorder.
- **CONTRA-INDICATIONS** Acute porphyrias p. 577 · arrhythmia · during the manic phase of bipolar disorder · heart block
- **CAUTIONS** Cardiovascular disease · chronic constipation · diabetes · epilepsy · history of bipolar disorder · history of psychosis · hyperthyroidism (risk of arrhythmias) · patients with a significant risk of suicide · phaeochromocytoma (risk of arrhythmias) · susceptibility to angle-closure glaucoma · urinary retention

  CAUTIONS, FURTHER INFORMATION
  Treatment should be stopped if the patient enters a manic phase.

- **INTERACTIONS** → Appendix 1: tricyclic antidepressants
- **SIDE-EFFECTS**
  - ▸ **Common or very common** Fatigue · flushing · headache · palpitation · restlessness
  - ▸ **Rare** Extrapyramidal symptoms · paralytic ileus
  - ▸ **Very rare** Abdominal pain · aggression · allergic alveolitis · cardiac decompensation · diarrhoea · hypertension · mydriasis · myoclonus · neuroleptic malignant syndrome · oedema · peripheral vasospasm · precipitation of angle-closure glaucoma · stomatitis
  - ▸ **Frequency not known** Agitation · alopecia · anorexia · anxiety · arrhythmia · blurred vision · breast enlargement · changes in blood sugar · chills (on withdrawal) · confusion · constipation · convulsions · delusions · dizziness · drowsiness · dry mouth · dysarthria · ECG changes · galactorrhoea · gynaecomastia · haematological reactions · hallucinations · headache (on withdrawal) · heart block · hepatic reactions · hypomania · hyponatraemia · increased

appetite · influenza-like symptoms (on withdrawal) · insomnia (on withdrawal) · irritability · mania · movement disorders (on withdrawal) · myalgia (on withdrawal) · nausea · nausea (on withdrawal) · paraesthesia · photosensitivity · postural hypotension · pruritus · rash · sexual dysfunction · sleep disturbances · sudden death of patients with cardiac disease · suicidal behaviour · sweating · sweating (on withdrawal) · tachycardia · taste disturbance · tinnitus · tremor · urinary retention · urticaria · vivid dreams (on withdrawal) · vomiting · weight gain · weight loss

Overdose
Tricyclic and related antidepressants cause dry mouth, coma of varying degree, hypotension, hypothermia, hyperreflexia, extensor plantar responses, convulsions, respiratory failure, cardiac conduction defects, and arrhythmias. Dilated pupils and urinary retention also occur. For details on the management of poisoning see Tricyclic and related antidepressants under Emergency treatment of poisoning p. 803.

- **PREGNANCY** Colic, tachycardia, dyspnoea, irritability, muscle spasms, respiratory depression and withdrawal symptoms reported in neonates when used in the third trimester.

- **BREAST FEEDING** The amount secreted into breast milk is too small to be harmful.

- **HEPATIC IMPAIRMENT** Sedative effects are increased in hepatic impairment. Avoid in severe liver disease.

- **RENAL IMPAIRMENT** Use with caution in severe impairment.

- **TREATMENT CESSATION** Withdrawal effects may occur within 5 days of stopping treatment with antidepressant drugs; they are usually mild and self-limiting, but in some cases may be severe. The risk of withdrawal symptoms is increased if the antidepressant is stopped suddenly after regular administration for 8 weeks or more. The dose should preferably be reduced gradually over about 4 weeks, or longer if withdrawal symptoms emerge (6 months in patients who have been on long-term maintenance treatment). If possible tricyclic antidepressants should be withdrawn slowly.

- **PRESCRIBING AND DISPENSING INFORMATION** Limited quantities of tricyclic antidepressants should be prescribed at any one time because their cardiovascular and epileptogenic effects are dangerous in overdosage.

- **PATIENT AND CARER ADVICE**
Driving and skilled tasks
Drowsiness may affect the performance of skilled tasks (e.g. driving). Effects of alcohol enhanced.
Medicines for Children leaflet:
Imipramine www.medicinesforchildren.org.uk/imipramine

- **MEDICINAL FORMS**
There can be variation in the licensing of different medicines containing the same drug. Forms available from special-order manufacturers include: oral suspension, oral solution

Oral solution
CAUTIONARY AND ADVISORY LABELS 2
- **Imipramine hydrochloride (Non-proprietary)**
Imipramine hydrochloride 5 mg per 1 ml Imipramine 25mg/5ml oral solution sugar free sugar-free | 150 ml PoM £42.00 DT price = £40.38

Tablet
CAUTIONARY AND ADVISORY LABELS 2
- **Imipramine hydrochloride (Non-proprietary)**
Imipramine hydrochloride 10 mg Imipramine 10mg tablets | 28 tablet PoM £1.01 DT price = £1.01
Imipramine hydrochloride 25 mg Imipramine 25mg tablets | 28 tablet PoM £1.01 DT price = £1.01

Nortriptyline

- **INDICATIONS AND DOSE**
Depressive illness
▶ BY MOUTH
- Child 12-17 years: To be initiated at a low dose, then increased if necessary to 30–50 mg daily in divided doses, alternatively increased if necessary to 30–50 mg once daily; maximum 150 mg per day

- **CONTRA-INDICATIONS** Acute porphyrias p. 577 · arrhythmias · during the manic phase of bipolar disorder · heart block

- **CAUTIONS** Cardiovascular disease · chronic constipation · diabetes · epilepsy · history of bipolar disorder · history of psychosis · hyperthyroidism (risk of arrhythmias) · patients with a significant risk of suicide · phaeochromocytoma (risk of arrhythmias) · susceptibility to angle-closure glaucoma · urinary retention

CAUTIONS, FURTHER INFORMATION
Treatment should be stopped if the patient enters a manic phase.

- **INTERACTIONS** → Appendix 1: tricyclic antidepressants

- **SIDE-EFFECTS**
▶ **Common or very common** Fatigue · hypertension · mydriasis · restlessness
▶ **Rare** Extrapyramidal symptoms · paralytic ileus
▶ **Very rare** Neuroleptic malignant syndrome · precipitation of angle-closure glaucoma
▶ **Frequency not known** Abdominal pain · agitation · alopecia · anorexia · anxiety · arrhythmia · blurred vision · breast enlargement · changes in blood sugar · chills (on withdrawal) · confusion · constipation · convulsions · delusions · diarrhoea · dizziness · drowsiness · dry mouth · dysarthria · ECG changes · flushing · galactorrhoea · gynaecomastia · haematological reactions · hallucinations · headache (on withdrawal) · heart block · hepatic reactions · hypomania · hyponatraemia · increased appetite · influenza-like symptoms (on withdrawal) · insomnia (on withdrawal) · irritability · mania · movement disorders (on withdrawal) · myalgia (on withdrawal) · nausea · nausea (on withdrawal) · oedema · paraesthesia · photosensitivity · postural hypotension · pruritus · rash · sexual dysfunction · sleep disturbances · stomatitis · sudden death of patients with cardiac disease · suicidal behaviour · sweating · sweating (on withdrawal) · tachycardia · taste disturbance · tinnitus · tremor · urinary retention · urticaria · vivid dreams (on withdrawal) · vomiting · weight gain · weight loss

Overdose
Tricyclic and related antidepressants cause dry mouth, coma of varying degree, hypotension, hypothermia, hyperreflexia, extensor plantar responses, convulsions, respiratory failure, cardiac conduction defects, and arrhythmias. Dilated pupils and urinary retention also occur. For details on the management of poisoning see Tricyclic and related antidepressants under Emergency treatment of poisoning p 803.

- **PREGNANCY** Use only if potential benefit outweighs risk.

- **BREAST FEEDING** The amount secreted into breast milk is too small to be harmful.

- **HEPATIC IMPAIRMENT** Sedative effects are increased in hepatic impairment. Avoid in severe liver disease.

- **MONITORING REQUIREMENTS**
▶ Manufacturer advises plasma-nortriptyline concentration monitoring if dose above 100 mg daily, but evidence of practical value uncertain.

- **TREATMENT CESSATION** Withdrawal effects may occur within 5 days of stopping treatment with antidepressant drugs; they are usually mild and self-limiting, but in some cases may be severe. The risk of withdrawal symptoms is increased if the antidepressant is stopped suddenly after regular administration for 8 weeks or more. The dose should preferably be reduced gradually over about 4 weeks, or longer if withdrawal symptoms emerge (6 months in patients who have been on long-term maintenance treatment). If possible tricyclic and related antidepressants should be withdrawn slowly.

- **PRESCRIBING AND DISPENSING INFORMATION** Limited quantities of tricyclic antidepressants should be prescribed at any one time because their cardiovascular and epileptogenic effects are dangerous in overdosage.
- **PATIENT AND CARER ADVICE** Drowsiness may affect the performance of skilled tasks (e.g. driving). Effects of alcohol enhanced.

- **MEDICINAL FORMS**
There can be variation in the licensing of different medicines containing the same drug. Forms available from special-order manufacturers include: oral suspension, oral solution

Tablet
CAUTIONARY AND ADVISORY LABELS 2
▶ Nortriptyline (Non-proprietary)
Nortriptyline (as Nortriptyline hydrochloride) 10 mg Nortriptyline 10mg tablets | 30 tablet [PoM] £11.79 | 100 tablet [PoM] £31.50-£68.41 DT price = £31.50
Nortriptyline (as Nortriptyline hydrochloride) 25 mg Nortriptyline 25mg tablets | 30 tablet [PoM] £12.43 | 100 tablet [PoM] £31.72-£111.06 DT price = £31.72
Nortriptyline (as Nortriptyline hydrochloride) 50 mg Nortriptyline 50mg tablets | 30 tablet [PoM] £24.86

2.4 Psychoses and schizophrenia

Psychoses and related disorders

06-Mar-2017

Advice on doses of antipsychotic drugs above BNF for Children upper limit

- Consider alternative approaches including adjuvant therapy.
- Bear in mind risk factors, including obesity. Consider potential for drug interactions—see interactions: Appendix 1 (antipsychotics).
- Carry out ECG to exclude untoward abnormalities such as prolonged QT interval; repeat ECG periodically **and** reduce dose if prolonged QT interval or other adverse abnormality develops.
- Increase dose slowly and not more often than once weekly.
- Carry out regular pulse, blood pressure, and temperature checks; ensure that patient maintains adequate fluid intake.
- Consider high-dose therapy to be for limited period and review regularly; abandon if no improvement after 3 months (return to standard dosage).

Important: When prescribing an antipsychotic for administration on an emergency basis, the intramuscular dose should be **lower** than the corresponding oral dose (owing to absence of first-pass effect), particularly if the child is very active (increased blood flow to muscle considerably increases the rate of absorption). The prescription should specify the dose for **each route** and should not imply that the same dose can be given by mouth or by intramuscular injection. The dose of antipsychotic for emergency use should be reviewed at least **daily**.

Antipsychotic drugs

There is little information on the efficacy and safety of antipsychotic drugs in children and adolescents and much of the information available has been extrapolated from adult data; in particular, little is known about the long-term effects of antipsychotic drugs on the developing nervous system. Antipsychotic drugs should be initiated and managed under the close supervision of an appropriate specialist.

Antipsychotic drugs are also known as 'neuroleptics' and (misleadingly) as 'major tranquillisers'.

In the short term they are used to calm disturbed children whatever the underlying psychopathology, which may be schizophrenia, brain damage, mania, toxic delirium, or agitated depression. Antipsychotic drugs are used to alleviate severe anxiety but this too should be a short-term measure.

Schizophrenia

The aim of treatment is to alleviate the suffering of the child (and carer) and to improve social and cognitive functioning. Many children require life-long treatment with antipsychotic medication. Antipsychotic drugs relieve positive psychotic symptoms such as thought disorder, hallucinations, and delusions, and prevent relapse; they are usually less effective on negative symptoms such as apathy and social withdrawal. In many patients, negative symptoms persist between episodes of treated positive symptoms, but earlier treatment of psychotic illness may protect against the development of negative symptoms over time. Children with acute schizophrenia generally respond better than those with chronic symptoms.

Long-term treatment of a child with a definitive diagnosis of schizophrenia is usually required after the first episode of illness in order to prevent relapses. Doses that are effective in acute episodes should generally be continued as prophylaxis.

First-generation antipsychotic drugs

The first-generation antipsychotic drugs act predominantly by blocking dopamine D_2 receptors in the brain. First-generation antipsychotic drugs are not selective for any of the four dopamine pathways in the brain and so can cause a range of side-effects, particularly extrapyramidal symptoms and elevated prolactin. The **phenothiazine** derivatives can be divided into 3 main groups:

- *Group* 1: chlorpromazine hydrochloride p. 236, levomepromazine p. 257, and promazine hydrochloride, generally characterised by pronounced sedative effects and moderate antimuscarinic and extrapyramidal side-effects.
- *Group* 2: pericyazine p. 240, generally characterised by moderate sedative effects, but fewer extrapyramidal side-effects than groups 1 or 3.
- *Group* 3: perphenazine p. 238, prochlorperazine p. 258, and trifluoperazine p. 239, generally characterised by fewer sedative and antimuscarinic effects, but more pronounced extrapyramidal side-effects than groups 1 and 2.

Butyrophenones (e.g. haloperidol p. 237) resemble the group 3 phenothiazines in their clinical properties. **Diphenylbutylpiperidines** (pimozide p. 238) and the **substituted benzamides** (sulpiride p. 244) have reduced sedative, antimuscarinic, and extrapyramidal effects.

Second-generation antipsychotic drugs

The second-generation antipsychotic drugs (also referred to as atypical antipsychotic drugs) act on a range of receptors in comparison to first-generation antipsychotic drugs and have more distinct clinical profiles, particularly with regard to side-effects.

Prescribing of antipsychotic drugs in children with learning disabilities

[EvGr] When prescribing for children with learning disabilities who are prescribed antipsychotic drugs and who are not experiencing psychotic symptoms, the following considerations should be taken into account ⟨A⟩:

4

Nervous system

- [EvGr] A reduction in dose or the discontinuation of long-term antipsychotic treatment;
- Review of the child's condition after dose reduction or discontinuation of an antipsychotic agent;
- Referral to a psychiatrist experienced in working with children who have learning disabilities and mental health problems;
- Annual documentation of the reasons for continuing a prescription if the antipsychotic is not reduced in dose or discontinued ⒶＡ.

Side effects of antipsychotic drugs
Side-effects caused by antipsychotic drugs are common and contribute significantly to non-adherence to therapy.

Extrapyramidal symptoms
Extrapyramidal symptoms occur most frequently with the piperazine phenothiazines (fluphenazine, perphenazine, prochlorperazine, and trifluoperazine), the butyrophenones (benperidol and haloperidol), and the first-generation depot preparations. They are easy to recognise but cannot be predicted accurately because they depend on the dose, the type of drug, and on individual susceptibility.

Extrapyramidal symptoms consist of:

- *parkinsonian symptoms* (including tremor), which may occur more commonly in adults or the elderly and may appear gradually;
- *dystonia* (abnormal face and body movements) and dyskinesia, which occur more commonly in children or young adults and appear after only a few doses;
- *akathisia* (restlessness), which characteristically occurs after large initial doses and may resemble an exacerbation of the condition being treated;
- *tardive dyskinesia* (rhythmic, involuntary movements of tongue, face, and jaw), which usually develops on long-term therapy or with high dosage, but it may develop on short-term treatment with low doses—short-lived tardive dyskinesia may occur after withdrawal of the drug.

Parkinsonian symptoms remit if the drug is withdrawn and may be suppressed by the administration of antimuscarinic drugs. However, routine administration of such drugs is not justified because not all patients are affected and they may unmask or worsen tardive dyskinesia.

Tardive dyskinesia is the most serious manifestation of extrapyramidal symptoms; it is of particular concern because it may be irreversible on withdrawing therapy and treatment is usually ineffective. In children, tardive dyskinesia is more likely to occur when the antipsychotic drug is withdrawn. However, some manufacturers suggest that drug withdrawal at the earliest signs of tardive dyskinesia (fine vermicular movements of the tongue) may halt its full development. Tardive dyskinesia occurs fairly frequently, especially in the elderly, and treatment must be carefully and regularly reviewed.

Hyperprolactinaemia
Most antipsychotic drugs, both first- and second-generation, increase prolactin concentration to some extent because dopamine inhibits prolactin release. Aripiprazole reduces prolactin because it is a dopamine-receptor partial agonist. Risperidone, amisulpride, and first-generation antipsychotic drugs are most likely to cause symptomatic hyperprolactinaemia. The clinical symptoms of hyperprolactinaemia include sexual dysfunction, reduced bone mineral density, menstrual disturbances, breast enlargement, and galactorrhoea.

Sexual dysfunction
Sexual dysfunction is one of the main causes of non-adherence to antipsychotic medication; physical illness, psychiatric illness, and substance misuse are contributing factors. Antipsychotic-induced sexual dysfunction is caused by more than one mechanism. Reduced dopamine transmission and hyperprolactinaemia decrease libido; antimuscarinic effects can cause disorders of arousal; and

alpha₁-adrenoceptor antagonists are associated with erection and ejaculation problems in men. Risperidone and haloperidol commonly cause sexual dysfunction. If sexual dysfunction is thought to be antipsychotic-induced, dose reduction or switching medication should be considered.

Cardiovascular side-effects
Antipsychotic drugs have been associated with cardiovascular side-effects such as tachycardia, arrhythmias, and hypotension. QT-interval prolongation is a particular concern with pimozide and haloperidol. There is also a higher probability of QT-interval prolongation in patients using any intravenous antipsychotic drug, or any antipsychotic drug or combination of antipsychotic drugs with doses exceeding the recommended maximum. Cases of sudden death have occurred.

Hyperglycaemia and weight gain
Hyperglycaemia, and sometimes diabetes, can occur with antipsychotic drugs, particularly clozapine, olanzapine, quetiapine, and risperidone. All antipsychotic drugs may cause weight gain, but the risk and extent varies. Clozapine and olanzapine commonly cause weight gain. Olanzapine is associated with more weight gain than other second generation antipsychotic drugs. Weight gain happens soon after treatment with olanzapine has started.

Hypotension and interference with temperature regulation
Hypotension and interference with temperature regulation are dose-related side-effects. Clozapine, chlorpromazine, and quetiapine can cause postural hypotension (especially during initial dose titration) which may be associated with syncope or reflex tachycardia in some children.

Neuroleptic malignant syndrome
Neuroleptic malignant syndrome (hyperthermia, fluctuating level of consciousness, muscle rigidity, and autonomic dysfunction with pallor, tachycardia, labile blood pressure, sweating, and urinary incontinence) is a rare but potentially fatal side-effect of all antipsychotic drugs. Discontinuation of the antipsychotic drug is essential because there is no proven effective treatment, but bromocriptine and dantrolene have been used. The syndrome, which usually lasts for 5–7 days after drug discontinuation, may be unduly prolonged if depot preparations have been used.

Blood dyscrasias
Perform blood counts if unexplained infection or fever develops.

Choice
The antipsychotic drugs most commonly used in children are haloperidol p. 237, risperidone p. 244, and olanzapine p. 242. There is little meaningful difference in efficacy between each of the antipsychotic drugs (other than clozapine p. 241), and response and tolerability to each antipsychotic drug varies. There is no first-line antipsychotic drug which is suitable for all children. Choice of antipsychotic medication is influenced by the child's medication history, the degree of sedation required (although tolerance to this usually develops), and consideration of individual patient factors such as risk of extrapyramidal side-effects, weight gain, impaired glucose tolerance, QT-interval prolongation, or the presence of negative symptoms.

Negative symptoms
Second generation antipsychotic drugs may be better at treating the negative symptoms of schizophrenia.

Extrapyramidal side-effects
Second-generation antipsychotic drugs may be prescribed if extrapyramidal side-effects are a particular concern. Of these, aripiprazole p. 240, clozapine, olanzapine, and quetiapine p. 243 are least likely to cause extrapyramidal side-effects. Although amisulpride p. 239 is a dopamine-receptor antagonist, extrapyramidal side-effects are less common than with the first-generation antipsychotic drugs because amisulpride selectively blocks mesolimbic dopamine

receptors, and extrapyramidal symptoms are caused by blockade of the striatal dopamine pathway.

QT interval
Aripiprazole has negligible effect on the QT interval. Other antipsychotic drugs with a reduced tendency to prolong QT interval include amisulpride, clozapine, olanzapine, perphenazine p. 238, risperidone, and sulpiride p. 244.

Diabetes
Schizophrenia is associated with insulin resistance and diabetes; the risk of diabetes is increased in children with schizophrenia who take antipsychotic drugs. First-generation antipsychotic drugs are less likely to cause diabetes than second-generation antipsychotic drugs, and of the first-generation antipsychotic drugs, haloperidol has the lowest risk. Amisulpride and aripiprazole have the lowest risk of diabetes of the second-generation antipsychotic drugs. Amisulpride, aripiprazole, haloperidol, sulpiride, and trifluoperazine p. 239 are least likely to cause weight gain.

Sexual dysfunction and prolactin
The antipsychotic drugs with the lowest risk of sexual dysfunction are aripiprazole and quetiapine. Olanzapine may be considered if sexual dysfunction is judged to be secondary to hyperprolactinaemia. Hyperprolactinaemia is usually not clinically significant with aripiprazole, clozapine, olanzapine, and quetiapine treatment. When changing from other antipsychotic drugs, a reduction in prolactin concentration may increase fertility.

Children should receive an antipsychotic drug for 4–6 weeks before it is deemed ineffective. Prescribing more than one antipsychotic drug at a time should be avoided except in exceptional circumstances (e.g. clozapine augmentation or when changing medication during titration) because of the increased risk of adverse effects such as extrapyramidal symptoms, QT-interval prolongation, and sudden cardiac death.

Clozapine is used for the treatment of schizophrenia in children unresponsive to, or intolerant of, other antipsychotic drugs. Clozapine should be introduced if schizophrenia is not controlled despite the sequential use of two or more antipsychotic drugs (one of which should be a second-generation antipsychotic drug), each for at least 6–8 weeks. If symptoms do not respond adequately to an optimised dose of clozapine, plasma-clozapine concentration should be checked before adding a second antipsychotic drug to augment clozapine; allow 8–10 weeks' treatment to assess response. Children must be registered with a clozapine patient monitoring service.

Monitoring
Full blood count, urea and electrolytes, and liver function test monitoring is required at the start of therapy with antipsychotic drugs, and then annually thereafter.

Blood lipids and weight should be measured at baseline, at 3 months (weight should be measured at frequent intervals during the first 3 months), and then yearly.

Fasting blood glucose should be measured at baseline, at 4–6 months, and then yearly.

Before initiating antipsychotic drugs, an ECG may be required, particularly if physical examination identifies cardiovascular risk factors, if there is a personal history of cardiovascular disease, or if the child is being admitted as an inpatient.

Blood pressure monitoring is advised before starting therapy and frequently during dose titration of antipsychotic drugs.

Other uses
Nausea and vomiting, choreas, motor tics, and intractable hiccup.

Equivalent doses of oral antipsychotics
These equivalences are intended **only** as an approximate guide; individual dosage instructions should **also** be checked; children should be carefully monitored after **any**

change in medication. Equivalent daily dose of antipsychotic drug:
- Chlorpromazine 100 mg
- Clozapine 50 mg
- Haloperidol 2–3 mg
- Pimozide 2 mg
- Risperidone 0.5–1 mg
- Sulpiride 200 mg
- Trifluoperazine 5 mg

Important: These equivalences must **not** be extrapolated beyond the maximum dose for the drug. Higher doses require careful titration in specialist units and the equivalences shown here may not be appropriate.

Dosage
After an initial period of stabilisation, the total daily oral dose of antipsychotic drugs can be given as a single dose in most children.

Antipsychotic depot injections
There is limited information on the use of antipsychotic depot injections in children and use should be restricted to specialist centres.

ANTIPSYCHOTICS

Antipsychotic drugs

- **CAUTIONS** Blood dyscrasias · cardiovascular disease · conditions predisposing to seizures · depression · diabetes (may raise blood glucose) · epilepsy · history of jaundice · myasthenia gravis · photosensitisation (may occur with higher dosages) · severe respiratory disease · susceptibility to angle-closure glaucoma
  CAUTIONS, FURTHER INFORMATION
  ‣ Cardiovascular disease An ECG may be required, particularly if physical examination identifies cardiovascular risk factors, personal history of cardiovascular disease, or if the patient is being admitted as an inpatient.
- **SIDE-EFFECTS**
  ‣ **Rare** Neuroleptic malignant syndrome—discontinue (potentially fatal)
  ‣ **Very rare** Precipitation of angle-closure glaucoma
  ‣ **Frequency not known** Agitation · agranulocytosis · akathisia · antimuscarinic symptoms · apathy · blood dyscrasias · blurred vision · cardiovascular side-effects · confusion · constipation · contact sensitisation · convulsions · corneal and lens opacities · diabetes · difficulty with micturition · dizziness · drowsiness · dry mouth · dystonia · excitement · extrapyramidal symptoms · gastro-intestinal disturbances · headache · hyperglycaemia · hyperprolactineamia · hypotension (dose related) · insomnia · interference with temperature regulation (dose related) · jaundice (including cholestatic) · leucopenia · nasal congestion · parkinsonian symptoms · photosensitisation · purplish pigmentation of the conjunctiva · purplish pigmentation of the cornea · purplish pigmentation of the retina · purplish pigmentation of the skin · rashes · sexual dysfunction · tardive dyskinesia · venous thromboembolism · weight gain

Overdose
Phenothiazines cause less depression of consciousness and respiration than other sedatives. Hypotension, hypothermia, sinus tachycardia, and arrhythmias may complicate poisoning. For details on the management of poisoning see Antipsychotics under Emergency treatment of poisoning p. 803.

- **PREGNANCY** Extrapyramidal effects and withdrawal syndrome have been reported occasionally in the neonate when antipsychotic drugs are taken during the third trimester of pregnancy. Following maternal use of antipsychotic drugs in the third trimester, neonates should be monitored for symptoms including agitation, hypertonia, hypotonia, tremor, drowsiness, feeding problems, and respiratory distress.

● **BREAST FEEDING** There is limited information available on the short- and long-term effects of antipsychotic drugs on the breast-fed infant. *Animal studies* indicate possible adverse effects of antipsychotic medicines on the developing nervous system. Chronic treatment with antipsychotic drugs whilst breast-feeding should be avoided unless absolutely necessary. Phenothiazine derivatives are sometimes used in breast-feeding women for short-term treatment of nausea and vomiting.

● **MONITORING REQUIREMENTS**
‣ It is advisable to monitor prolactin concentration at the start of therapy, at 6 months, and then yearly. Patients taking antipsychotic drugs not normally associated with symptomatic hyperprolactinaemia should be considered for prolactin monitoring if they show symptoms of hyperprolactinaemia (such as breast enlargement and galactorrhoea).
‣ Patients with schizophrenia should have physical health monitoring (including cardiovascular disease risk assessment) at least once per year.
‣ Regular clinical monitoring of endocrine function should be considered when children are taking an antipsychotic drug known to increase prolactin levels; this includes measuring weight and height, assessing sexual maturation, and monitoring menstrual function.

● **TREATMENT CESSATION** There is a high risk of relapse if medication is stopped after 1–2 years. Withdrawal of antipsychotic drugs after long-term therapy should always be gradual and closely monitored to avoid the risk of acute withdrawal syndromes or rapid relapse. Patients should be monitored for 2 years after withdrawal of antipsychotic medication for signs and symptoms of relapse.

● **PATIENT AND CARER ADVICE**
As photosensitisation may occur with higher dosages, patients should avoid direct sunlight.

Driving and skilled tasks
Drowsiness may affect performance of skilled tasks (e.g. driving or operating machinery), especially at start of treatment; effects of alcohol are enhanced.

ANTIPSYCHOTICS > FIRST-GENERATION

F 235

Chlorpromazine hydrochloride

● **INDICATIONS AND DOSE**

Childhood schizophrenia and other psychoses (under expert supervision)
‣ BY MOUTH
‣ Child 1-5 years: 500 micrograms/kg every 4–6 hours, adjusted according to response; maximum 40 mg per day
‣ Child 6-11 years: 10 mg 3 times a day, adjusted according to response; maximum 75 mg per day
‣ Child 12-17 years: Initially 25 mg 3 times a day, adjusted according to response, alternatively initially 75 mg once daily, adjusted according to response, dose to be taken at night; maintenance 75–300 mg daily, increased if necessary up to 1 g daily

Relief of acute symptoms of psychoses (under expert supervision)
‣ BY DEEP INTRAMUSCULAR INJECTION
‣ Child 1-5 years: 500 micrograms/kg every 6–8 hours; maximum 40 mg per day
‣ Child 6-11 years: 500 micrograms/kg every 6–8 hours; maximum 75 mg per day
‣ Child 12-17 years: 25–50 mg every 6–8 hours

Nausea and vomiting of terminal illness (where other drugs have failed or are not available)
‣ BY MOUTH
‣ Child 1-5 years: 500 micrograms/kg every 4–6 hours; maximum 40 mg per day
‣ Child 6-11 years: 500 micrograms/kg every 4–6 hours; maximum 75 mg per day
‣ Child 12-17 years: 10–25 mg every 4–6 hours
‣ BY DEEP INTRAMUSCULAR INJECTION
‣ Child 1-5 years: 500 micrograms/kg every 6–8 hours; maximum 40 mg per day
‣ Child 6-11 years: 500 micrograms/kg every 6–8 hours; maximum 75 mg per day
‣ Child 12-17 years: Initially 25 mg, then 25–50 mg every 3–4 hours until vomiting stops

DOSE ADJUSTMENTS DUE TO INTERACTIONS
‣ Dose adjustment may be necessary if smoking started or stopped during treatment.

DOSE EQUIVALENCE AND CONVERSION
‣ For equivalent therapeutic effect 100 mg chlorpromazine base given *rectally* as a suppository ≡ 20–25 mg chlorpromazine hydrochloride *by intramuscular injection* ≡ 40–50 mg of chlorpromazine base or hydrochloride given *by mouth*.

● **CONTRA-INDICATIONS** CNS depression · comatose states · hypothyroidism · phaeochromocytoma

● **INTERACTIONS** → Appendix 1: phenothiazines

● **SIDE-EFFECTS**

SIDE-EFFECTS, FURTHER INFORMATION
‣ Acute dystonic reactions Phenothiazines can induce acute dystonic reactions such as facial and skeletal muscle spasms and oculogyric crises; children (especially girls, young women, and those under 10 kg) are particularly susceptible.

● **HEPATIC IMPAIRMENT** Can precipitate coma; phenothiazines are hepatotoxic.

● **RENAL IMPAIRMENT** Start with small doses in severe renal impairment because of increased cerebral sensitivity.

● **MONITORING REQUIREMENTS**
‣ Patients should remain supine with blood pressure monitoring for 30 minutes after intramuscular injection.

● **HANDLING AND STORAGE** Owing to the risk of contact sensitisation, pharmacists, nurses, and other health workers should avoid direct contact with chlorpromazine; tablets should not be crushed and solutions should be handled with care.

● **MEDICINAL FORMS**
There can be variation in the licensing of different medicines containing the same drug. Forms available from special-order manufacturers include: tablet, capsule, oral suspension, oral solution

Tablet
CAUTIONARY AND ADVISORY LABELS 2, 11
‣ Chlorpromazine hydrochloride (Non-proprietary)
  Chlorpromazine hydrochloride 25 mg Chlorpromazine 25mg tablets | 28 tablet [PoM] £4.92 CT price = £1.70
  Chlorpromazine hydrochloride 50 mg Chlorpromazine 50mg tablets | 28 tablet [PoM] £5.28 CT price = £1.74
  Chlorpromazine hydrochloride 100 mg Chlorpromazine 100mg tablets | 28 tablet [PoM] £5.70 MT price = £1.78

Solution for injection
‣ Largactil (Sanofi)
  Chlorpromazine hydrochloride 25 mg per 1 ml Largactil 50mg/2ml solution for injection ampoules | 10 ampoule [PoM] £7.51

Oral solution
CAUTIONARY AND ADVISORY LABELS 2, 11
‣ Chlorpromazine hydrochloride (Non-proprietary)
  Chlorpromazine hydrochloride 5 mg per 1 ml Chlorpromazine 25mg/5ml syrup | 150 ml [PoM] £2.35 DT price = £2.35
  Chlorpromazine 25mg/5ml oral solution sugar free sugar-free | 150 ml [PoM] £2.35 DT price = £2.35

Chlorpromazine 25mg/5ml oral solution | 150 ml [PoM] £2.35 DT price = £2.35
Chlorpromazine hydrochloride 20 mg per 1 ml Chlorpromazine 100mg/5ml oral solution | 150 ml [PoM] £5.50 DT price = £5.50

⯌ 235

Haloperidol

12-Dec-2016

● **INDICATIONS AND DOSE**
Schizophrenia (under expert supervision)
▶ BY MOUTH
▶ **Child 3–12 years:** Initially 500 micrograms daily in 2–3 divided doses; usual dose 1–4 mg daily in 2–3 divided doses, daily maximum to be given in 2–3 divided doses; maximum 6 mg per day
▶ **Child 13-17 years:** Initially 500 micrograms daily in 2–3 divided doses; usual dose 1–6 mg daily in 2–3 divided doses, daily maximum to be given in 2–3 divided doses; maximum 10 mg per day

Childhood behavioural disorders, especially when associated with hyperactivity and aggression (under expert supervision) | Gilles de la Tourette syndrome (under expert supervision)
▶ BY MOUTH
▶ **Child 3–12 years:** Initially 250 micrograms daily in 2–3 divided doses; usual dose 0.5–3 mg daily in 2–3 divided doses, daily maximum to be given in 2–3 divided doses; maximum 3 mg per day
▶ **Child 13-17 years:** Initially 250 micrograms daily in 2–3 divided doses; usual dose 2–6 mg daily in 2–3 divided doses, daily maximum to be given in 2–3 divided doses; maximum 6 mg per day

Nausea and vomiting in palliative care
▶ BY MOUTH
▶ **Child 12-17 years:** 1.5 mg once daily, dose to be taken at night, increased if necessary to 1.5 mg twice daily (max. per dose 5 mg twice daily)
▶ BY CONTINUOUS INTRAVENOUS INFUSION, OR BY CONTINUOUS SUBCUTANEOUS INFUSION
▶ **Child 1 month-11 years:** 25–85 micrograms/kg, to be administered over 24 hours
▶ **Child 12-17 years:** 1.5–5 mg, to be administered over 24 hours

Restlessness and confusion in palliative care
▶ BY MOUTH
▶ **Child 1-17 years:** 10–20 micrograms/kg every 8–12 hours

DOSE ADJUSTMENTS DUE TO INTERACTIONS
Dose adjustment may be necessary if smoking started or stopped during treatment.

● **UNLICENSED USE** Not licensed for use in children for nausea and vomiting in palliative care.

IMPORTANT SAFETY INFORMATION
When prescribing, dispensing or administering, check that this injection is the correct preparation—this preparation is usually used in hospital for the rapid control of an *acute episode* and should not be confused with depot preparations which are usually used in the community or clinics for *maintenance* treatment.

● **CONTRA-INDICATIONS** Bradycardia · CNS depression · comatose states · lesions of the basal ganglia · phaeochromocytoma · QT-interval prolongation
● **CAUTIONS** Hypocalcaemia · hypokalaemia · hypomagnesaemia · metabolic disturbances · subarachnoid haemorrhage
● **INTERACTIONS** → Appendix 1: haloperidol
● **SIDE-EFFECTS**
▶ **Common or very common** Depression · weight loss
▶ **Uncommon** Dyspnoea · oedema

▶ **Rare** Bronchospasm · hypoglycaemia · inappropriate antidiuretic hormone secretion
▶ **Frequency not known** Stevens-Johnson syndrome · toxic epidermal necrolysis
SIDE-EFFECTS, FURTHER INFORMATION
Less sedating and fewer antimuscarinic or hypotensive symptoms.
● **PREGNANCY** Avoid unless benefits outweigh risks.
● **HEPATIC IMPAIRMENT** Can precipitate coma.
● **RENAL IMPAIRMENT** Start with small doses in severe renal impairment because of increased cerebral sensitivity.
● **MONITORING REQUIREMENTS** Baseline ECG required before treatment—assess need for further ECGs during treatment on an individual basis.
● **PRESCRIBING AND DISPENSING INFORMATION**
Palliative care
For further information on the use of haloperidol in palliative care, see www.palliativedrugs.com/formulary/en/haloperidol.html.

● **MEDICINAL FORMS**
There can be variation in the licensing of different medicines containing the same drug. Forms available from special-order manufacturers include: oral suspension, oral solution
Tablet
CAUTIONARY AND ADVISORY LABELS 2
▶ **Haloperidol (Non-proprietary)**
Haloperidol 500 microgram Haloperidol 500microgram tablets | 28 tablet [PoM] £22.05 DT price = £22.05
Haloperidol 1.5 mg Haloperidol 1.5mg tablets | 28 tablet [PoM] £5.99 DT price = £1.78
Haloperidol 5 mg Haloperidol 5mg tablets | 28 tablet [PoM] £3.80 DT price = £2.10
Haloperidol 10 mg Haloperidol 10mg tablets | 28 tablet [PoM] £12.99 DT price = £12.96
Solution for injection
▶ **Haloperidol (Non-proprietary)**
Haloperidol 5 mg per 1 ml Haloperidol 5mg/1ml solution for injection ampoules | 10 ampoule [PoM] £35.00 DT price = £35.00
Oral solution
CAUTIONARY AND ADVISORY LABELS 2
▶ **Haloperidol (Non-proprietary)**
Haloperidol 200 microgram per 1 ml Haloperidol 200micrograms/ml oral solution sugar free sugar-free | 200 ml [PoM] £195.00
Haloperidol 1 mg per 1 ml Haloperidol 5mg/5ml oral solution sugar free sugar-free | 100 ml [PoM] £35.99 DT price = £6.47 sugar-free | 500 ml [PoM] £32.35
Haloperidol 2 mg per 1 ml Haloperidol 10mg/5ml oral solution sugar free sugar-free | 100 ml [PoM] £46.75 DT price = £7.10 sugar-free | 500 ml [PoM] £35.50
▶ **Haldol** (Janssen-Cilag Ltd)
Haloperidol 2 mg per 1 ml Haldol 2mg/ml oral solution sugar-free | 100 ml [PoM] £4.45 DT price = £7.10
Capsule
CAUTIONARY AND ADVISORY LABELS 2
▶ **Serenace** (Teva UK Ltd)
Haloperidol 500 microgram Serenace 500microgram capsules | 30 capsule [PoM] £1.18 DT price = £1.18

⯌ 235

Pericyazine

(Periciazine)

● **INDICATIONS AND DOSE**
Schizophrenia (under expert supervision) | Psychoses (severe mental or behavioural disorders only) (under expert supervision)
▶ BY MOUTH
▶ **Child 1-11 years:** Initially 500 micrograms daily for 10-kg child, increased by 1 mg for each additional 5 kg; dose may be gradually increased according to response but maintenance should not exceed twice initial dose; maximum 10 mg per day continued →

4

Nervous system

4

Nervous system

▸ Child 12–17 years: Initially 25 mg 3 times a day, increased in steps of 25 mg every week, adjusted according to response, increased if necessary up to 100 mg 3 times a day, total daily dose may alternatively be given in 2 divided doses

● **UNLICENSED USE** Tablets not licensed for use in children.

● **CONTRA-INDICATIONS** CNS depression · comatose states · phaeochromocytoma

● **INTERACTIONS** → Appendix 1: phenothiazines

● **SIDE-EFFECTS**

▸ **Common or very common** Hypotension (when treatment initiated)

▸ **Frequency not known** Respiratory depression

SIDE-EFFECTS, FURTHER INFORMATION
More sedating.

● **HEPATIC IMPAIRMENT** Can precipitate coma; phenothiazines are hepatotoxic.

● **RENAL IMPAIRMENT** Avoid in renal impairment.

● **MEDICINAL FORMS**
There can be variation in the licensing of different medicines containing the same drug. Forms available from special-order manufacturers include: oral suspension, oral solution

Oral solution
CAUTIONARY AND ADVISORY LABELS 2
▸ Pericyazine (Non-proprietary)
   Pericyazine 2 mg per 1 ml Pericyazine 10mg/5ml oral solution | 100 ml [PoM] £46.00–£46.01 DT price = £46.01

Tablet
CAUTIONARY AND ADVISORY LABELS 2
▸ Pericyazine (Non-proprietary)
   Pericyazine 2.5 mg Pericyazine 2.5mg tablets | 84 tablet [PoM] £15.87 DT price = £15.87
   Pericyazine 10 mg Pericyazine 10mg tablets | 84 tablet [PoM] £40.12 DT price = £40.12

F 235

Perphenazine

● **INDICATIONS AND DOSE**

Schizophrenia and other psychoses | Mania | Short-term adjunctive management of anxiety | Severe psychomotor agitation, excitement, and violent or dangerously impulsive behaviour | Severe nausea and vomiting unresponsive to other anti-emetics

▸ BY MOUTH

▸ Child 14–17 years (under close medical supervision): Initially 4 mg 3 times a day, adjusted according to response; maximum 24 mg per day

● **CONTRA-INDICATIONS** CNS depression · comatose states · phaeochromocytoma

● **CAUTIONS** Hypothyroidism

● **INTERACTIONS** → Appendix 1: phenothiazines

● **SIDE-EFFECTS**

▸ **Rare** Systemic lupus erythematosus

▸ **Frequency not known** Dystonic reactions

SIDE-EFFECTS, FURTHER INFORMATION
Less sedating.

▸ Acute dystonic reactions Phenothiazines can all induce acute dystonic reactions such as facial and skeletal muscle spasms and oculogyric crises; children (especially girls, young women, and those under 10 kg) are particularly susceptible.

● **HEPATIC IMPAIRMENT** Can precipitate coma; phenothiazines are hepatotoxic.

● **RENAL IMPAIRMENT** Start with small doses in severe renal impairment because of increased cerebral sensitivity.

● **MEDICINAL FORMS**
There can be variation in the licensing of different medicines containing the same drug. Forms available from special-order manufacturers include: tablet, oral suspension

F 235

Pimozide

● **INDICATIONS AND DOSE**

Schizophrenia

▸ BY MOUTH

▸ Child 12–17 years (under expert supervision): Initially 1 mg daily, adjusted according to response, then increased in steps of 2–4 mg at intervals of not less than 1 week; usual dose 2–20 mg daily

Tourette syndrome (under expert supervision)

▸ BY MOUTH

▸ Child 2–11 years: 1–4 mg daily

▸ Child 12–17 years: 2–10 mg daily

● **UNLICENSED USE** Not licensed for use in Tourette syndrome.

● **CONTRA-INDICATIONS** CNS depression · comatose states · history of arrhythmias · history or family history of congenital QT prolongation · phaeochromocytoma

● **INTERACTIONS** → Appendix 1: pimozide

● **SIDE-EFFECTS**

▸ **Rare** Hyponatraemia

▸ **Frequency not known** Glycosuria · serious arrhythmias · venous thromboembolism

SIDE-EFFECTS, FURTHER INFORMATION
Less sedating.

● **HEPATIC IMPAIRMENT** Can precipitate coma.

● **RENAL IMPAIRMENT** Start with small doses in severe renal impairment because of increased cerebral sensitivity.

● **MONITORING REQUIREMENTS**

▸ ECG monitoring Following reports of sudden unexplained death, an ECG is recommended before treatment. It is also recommended that patients taking pimozide should have an annual ECG (if the QT interval is prolonged, treatment should be reviewed and either withdrawn or dose reduced under close supervision) and that pimozide should not be given with other antipsychotic drugs (including depot preparations), tricyclic antidepressants or other drugs which prolong the QT interval, such as certain antimalarials, antiarrhythmic drugs and certain antihistamines and should not be given with drugs which cause electrolyte disturbances (especially diuretics).

● **MEDICINAL FORMS**
There can be variation in the licensing of different medicines containing the same drug. Forms available from special-order manufacturers include: oral suspension

Tablet
CAUTIONARY AND ADVISORY LABELS 2
▸ Pimozide (Non-proprietary)
   Pimozide 4 mg Pimozide 4mg tablets | 100 tablet [PoM] no price available DT price = £40.31
▸ Orap (Eumedica Pharmaceuticals)
   Pimozide 1 mg Orap 1mg tablets | 100 tablet [PoM] no price available
   Pimozide 4 mg Orap 4mg tablets | 100 tablet [PoM] £40.31 DT price = £40.31

F 235

Sulpiride

● **INDICATIONS AND DOSE**

Schizophrenia with predominantly negative symptoms

▸ BY MOUTH

▸ Child 14–17 years (under expert supervision): 200–400 mg twice daily; maximum 800 mg per day

Schizophrenia with mainly positive symptoms
▶ BY MOUTH
▶ Child 14–17 years (under expert supervision): 200–400 mg twice daily; maximum 2.4 g per day

Tourette syndrome (under expert supervision)
▶ BY MOUTH
▶ Child 2–11 years: 50–400 mg twice daily
▶ Child 12–17 years: 100–400 mg twice daily

● UNLICENSED USE Not licensed for use in Tourette syndrome.

● CONTRA-INDICATIONS CNS depression · comatose states · phaeochromocytoma

● CAUTIONS Aggressive patients (even low doses may aggravate symptoms) · agitated patients (even low doses may aggravate symptoms) · excited patients (even low doses may aggravate symptoms)

● INTERACTIONS → Appendix 1: sulpiride

● SIDE-EFFECTS Hepatitis · venous thromboembolism

● HEPATIC IMPAIRMENT Can precipitate coma.

● RENAL IMPAIRMENT Start with small doses in severe renal impairment because of increased cerebral sensitivity.

● MONITORING REQUIREMENTS Sulpiride does not affect blood pressure to the same extent as other antipsychotic drugs and so blood pressure monitoring is not mandatory for this drug.

● PRESCRIBING AND DISPENSING INFORMATION Flavours of oral liquid formulations may include lemon and aniseed.

● PATIENT AND CARER ADVICE
Medicines for Children leaflet: Sulpiride for schizophrenia and Tourette's syndrome www.medicinesforchildren.org.uk/sulpiride-for-schizophrenia-and-tourettes-syndrome

● MEDICINAL FORMS
There can be variation in the licensing of different medicines containing the same drug. Forms available from special-order manufacturers include: oral suspension, oral solution

Oral solution
CAUTIONARY AND ADVISORY LABELS 2
▶ Sulpiride (Non-proprietary)
 Sulpiride 40 mg per 1 ml Sulpiride 200mg/5ml oral solution sugar free sugar-free | 150 ml PoM £28.00 DT price = £27.00

Tablet
CAUTIONARY AND ADVISORY LABELS 2
▶ Sulpiride (Non-proprietary)
 Sulpiride 200 mg Sulpiride 200mg tablets | 30 tablet PoM £9.49 DT price = £3.56
 Sulpiride 400 mg Sulpiride 400mg tablets | 30 tablet PoM £18.80 DT price = £18.80
▶ Dolmatil (Sanofi)
 Sulpiride 200 mg Dolmatil 200mg tablets | 100 tablet PoM £6.00
 Sulpiride 400 mg Dolmatil 400mg tablets | 100 tablet PoM £19.00

F 235

Trifluoperazine

● INDICATIONS AND DOSE

Schizophrenia and other psychoses | Short-term adjunctive management of psychomotor agitation, excitement, and violent or dangerously impulsive behaviour
▶ BY MOUTH
▶ Child 12–17 years (under expert supervision): Initially 5 mg twice daily, increased by 5 mg daily after 1 week, then at intervals of 3 days, according to response

Short-term adjunctive management of severe anxiety
▶ BY MOUTH
▶ Child 3–5 years (under expert supervision): Up to 500 micrograms twice daily
▶ Child 6–11 years (under expert supervision): Up to 2 mg twice daily

▶ Child 12–17 years (under expert supervision): 1–2 mg twice daily, increased if necessary to 3 mg twice daily

Severe nausea and vomiting unresponsive to other antiemetics
▶ BY MOUTH
▶ Child 3–5 years: Up to 500 micrograms twice daily
▶ Child 6–11 years: Up to 2 mg twice daily
▶ Child 12–17 years: 1–2 mg twice daily (max. per dose 3 mg twice daily)

● CONTRA-INDICATIONS CNS depression · comatose states · phaeochromocytoma

● INTERACTIONS → Appendix 1: phenothiazines

● SIDE-EFFECTS Anorexia · dystonic reactions · muscle weakness

SIDE-EFFECTS, FURTHER INFORMATION
Extrapyramidal symptoms are more frequent, especially at doses exceeding 6 mg daily.
 Phenothiazines can all induce acute dystonic reactions such as facial and skeletal muscle spasms and oculogyric crises; children (especially girls, young women, and those under 10 kg) are particularly susceptible.

● HEPATIC IMPAIRMENT Can precipitate coma; phenothiazines are hepatotoxic.

● RENAL IMPAIRMENT Start with small doses in severe renal impairment because of increased cerebral sensitivity.

● MONITORING REQUIREMENTS Trifluoperazine does not affect blood pressure to the same extent as other antipsychotic drugs and so blood pressure monitoring is not mandatory for this drug.

● MEDICINAL FORMS
There can be variation in the licensing of different medicines containing the same drug.

Oral solution
CAUTIONARY AND ADVISORY LABELS 2
▶ Trifluoperazine (Non-proprietary)
 Trifluoperazine (as Trifluoperazine hydrochloride) 200 microgram per 1 ml Trifluoperazine 1mg/5ml oral solution sugar free sugar-free | 200 ml PoM £102.53 DT price = £102.53
 Trifluoperazine (as Trifluoperazine hydrochloride) 1 mg per 1 ml Trifluoperazine 5mg/5ml oral solution sugar free sugar-free | 150 ml PoM £25.50 DT price = £25.50

Tablet
CAUTIONARY AND ADVISORY LABELS 2
▶ Trifluoperazine (Non-proprietary)
 Trifluoperazine (as Trifluoperazine hydrochloride) 1 mg Trifluoperazine 1mg tablets | 112 tablet PoM £54.00 DT price = £54.00
 Trifluoperazine (as Trifluoperazine hydrochloride) 5 mg Trifluoperazine 5mg tablets | 112 tablet PoM £123.20 DT price = £123.20

ANTIPSYCHOTICS › SECOND-GENERATION

F 235

Amisulpride

● DRUG ACTION Amisulpride is a selective dopamine receptor antagonist with high affinity for mesolimbic D_2 and D_3 receptors.

● INDICATIONS AND DOSE

Acute psychotic episode in schizophrenia
▶ BY MOUTH
▶ Child 15–17 years (under expert supervision): 200–400 mg twice daily, adjusted according to response; maximum 1.2 g per day

Schizophrenia with predominantly negative symptoms
▶ BY MOUTH
▶ Child 15–17 years (under expert supervision): 50–300 mg daily

● UNLICENSED USE Not licensed for use in children.

Nervous system

4

- **CONTRA-INDICATIONS** CNS depression · comatose states · phaeochromocytoma · pre-pubertal children · prolactin-dependent tumours
- **INTERACTIONS** → Appendix 1: amisulpride
- **SIDE-EFFECTS**
  - **Common or very common** Anxiety
  - **Uncommon** Bradycardia
- **PREGNANCY** Avoid.
- **BREAST FEEDING** Avoid—no information available.
- **RENAL IMPAIRMENT** Halve dose if estimated glomerular filtration rate 30–60 mL/minute/1.73 m². Use one-third dose if estimated glomerular filtration rate 10–30 mL/minute/1.73 m². No information available if estimated glomerular filtration rate less than 10 mL/minute/1.73 m².
- **MONITORING REQUIREMENTS** Amisulpride does not affect blood pressure to the same extent as other antipsychotic drugs and so blood pressure monitoring is not mandatory for this drug.
- **PRESCRIBING AND DISPENSING INFORMATION** Flavours of oral liquid formulations may include caramel.

- **MEDICINAL FORMS**
  There can be variation in the licensing of different medicines containing the same drug. Forms available from special-order manufacturers include: oral suspension, oral solution
  Oral solution
  CAUTIONARY AND ADVISORY LABELS 2
  - Amisulpride (Non-proprietary)
    Amisulpride 100 mg per 1 ml Amisulpride 100mg/ml oral solution sugar free sugar-free | 60 ml |PoM| £36.00 DT price = £36.00
  - Solian (Sanofi)
    Amisulpride 100 mg per 1 ml Solian 100mg/ml oral solution sugar-free | 60 ml |PoM| £33.76 DT price = £36.00
  Tablet
  CAUTIONARY AND ADVISORY LABELS 2
  - Amisulpride (Non-proprietary)
    Amisulpride 50 mg Amisulpride 50mg tablets | 60 tablet |PoM| £22.76 DT price = £2.06
    Amisulpride 100 mg Amisulpride 100mg tablets | 60 tablet |PoM| £39.48 DT price = £3.59
    Amisulpride 200 mg Amisulpride 200mg tablets | 60 tablet |PoM| £66.00 DT price = £5.44
    Amisulpride 400 mg Amisulpride 400mg tablets | 60 tablet |PoM| £132.00 DT price = £35.21
  - Solian (Sanofi)
    Amisulpride 50 mg Solian 50 tablets | 60 tablet |PoM| £22.76 DT price = £2.06
    Amisulpride 100 mg Solian 100 tablets | 60 tablet |PoM| £35.29 DT price = £3.59
    Amisulpride 200 mg Solian 200 tablets | 60 tablet |PoM| £58.99 DT price = £5.44
    Amisulpride 400 mg Solian 400 tablets | 60 tablet |PoM| £117.97 DT price = £35.21

☞ 235

Aripiprazole

- **DRUG ACTION** Aripiprazole is a dopamine D_2 partial agonist with weak 5-HT$_{1a}$ partial agonism and 5-HT$_{2A}$ receptor antagonism.

- **INDICATIONS AND DOSE**
  Schizophrenia
  - BY MOUTH
    - Child 15–17 years (under expert supervision): Initially 2 mg once daily for 2 days, increased to 5 mg once daily for 2 days, then increased to 10 mg once daily, then increased in steps of 5 mg if required; maximum 30 mg per day

  Treatment of mania (under expert supervision)
  - BY MOUTH
    - Child 13–17 years: Initially 2 mg once daily for 2 days, increased to 5 mg once daily for 2 days, then increased

to 10 mg once daily, increased in steps of 5 mg if required, maximum duration of treatment 12 weeks, doses above 10 mg daily should only be used in exceptional cases; maximum 30 mg per day

DOSE ADJUSTMENTS DUE TO INTERACTIONS
Manufacturer advises double the dose with concurrent use of potent inducers of CYP3A4—no specific recommendation made for children. Manufacturer advises reduce dose by half with concurrent use of potent inhibitors of CYP3A4 or CYP2D6—no specific recommendation made for children.

- **CONTRA-INDICATIONS** CNS depression · comatose state · phaeochromocytoma
- **CAUTIONS** Cerebrovascular disease
- **INTERACTIONS** → Appendix 1: aripiprazole
- **SIDE-EFFECTS**
  - **Common or very common** Anxiety · hypersalivation · malaise
  - **Uncommon** Depression · dry mouth
  - **Frequency not known** Alopecia · anorexia · bradycardia · hepatitis · hyponatraemia · infection · laryngospasm · myalgia · oedema · oropharyngeal spasm · pancreatitis · pathological gambling · respiratory disorders · rhabdomyolysis · suicidal ideation · sweating · urinary disorders

  SIDE-EFFECTS, FURTHER INFORMATION
  Increased incidence of side-effects associated with doses of 30 mg daily; doses above 10 mg daily should only be used in exceptional cases and with close clinical monitoring.
- **PREGNANCY** Use only if potential benefit outweighs risk.
- **BREAST FEEDING** Manufacturer advises avoid—present in milk.
- **HEPATIC IMPAIRMENT** Use with caution in severe impairment.
- **MONITORING REQUIREMENTS** Aripiprazole does not affect blood pressure to the same extent as other antipsychotic drugs and so blood pressure monitoring is not mandatory for this drug.
- **DIRECTIONS FOR ADMINISTRATION** Orodispersible tablets should be placed on the tongue and allowed to dissolve, or be dispersed in water and swallowed.
- **PATIENT AND CARER ADVICE**
  Patients or carers should be given advice on how to administer aripiprazole orodispersible tablets.
  Medicines for Children leaflet: Aripiprazole for schizophrenia, bipolar disorder and movement disorders
  www.medicinesforchildren.org.uk/aripiprazole-schizophrenia-bipolar-disorder-and-movement-disorders
- **NATIONAL FUNDING/ACCESS DECISIONS**
  NICE technology appraisals (TAs)
  - **Aripiprazole for the treatment of schizophrenia in people aged 15 to 17 years (January 2011)**
    Aripiprazole is recommended as an option for the treatment of schizophrenia in adolescents aged 15 to 17 years who have not responded adequately to, or who are intolerant of, risperidone, or for whom risperidone is contra-indicated.
    www.nice.org.uk/TA213
  - **Aripiprazole for the treatment of moderate to severe manic episodes in adolescents with bipolar I disorder (July 2013)**
    Aripiprazole is recommended as an option for the treatment of moderate to severe manic episodes for up to 12 weeks in adolescents aged over 13 years with bipolar I disorder.
    www.nice.org.uk/TA292

ABILIFY® ORAL SOLUTION

Scottish Medicines Consortium (SMC) Decisions

The *Scottish Medicines Consortium*, has advised (August 2013) that oral aripiprazole (*Abilify®*) is accepted for restricted use within NHS Scotland for the treatment of moderate to severe manic episodes in Bipolar I Disorder in adolescents aged 13 years and older for a period of up to 12 weeks. It is restricted to initiation and management under the supervision of a child/adolescent psychiatrist.

● **MEDICINAL FORMS**

There can be variation in the licensing of different medicines containing the same drug. Forms available from special-order manufacturers include: oral solution

Tablet

CAUTIONARY AND ADVISORY LABELS 2

▸ **Aripiprazole (Non-proprietary)**
Aripiprazole 5 mg Aripiprazole 5mg tablets | 28 tablet [PoM] £96.04 DT price = £1.60
Aripiprazole 10 mg Aripiprazole 10mg tablets | 28 tablet [PoM] £96.04 DT price = £1.76
Aripiprazole 15 mg Aripiprazole 15mg tablets | 28 tablet [PoM] £96.04 DT price = £1.86
Aripiprazole 30 mg Aripiprazole 30mg tablets | 28 tablet [PoM] £192.08 DT price = £20.65

▸ **Abilify** (Otsuka Pharmaceuticals (U.K.) Ltd)
Abilify 5 mg Abilify 5mg tablets | 28 tablet [PoM] £96.04 DT price = £1.60
Abilify 10 mg Abilify 10mg tablets | 28 tablet [PoM] £96.04 DT price = £1.76
Abilify 15 mg Abilify 15mg tablets | 28 tablet [PoM] £96.04 DT price = £1.86
Abilify 30 mg Abilify 30mg tablets | 28 tablet [PoM] £192.08 DT price = £20.65

Oral solution

CAUTIONARY AND ADVISORY LABELS 2

▸ **Aripiprazole (Non-proprietary)**
Aripiprazole 1 mg per 1 ml Aripiprazole 1mg/ml oral solution | 150 ml [PoM] £102.90 DT price = £102.90

▸ **Abilify** (Otsuka Pharmaceuticals (U.K.) Ltd)
Aripiprazole 1 mg per 1 ml Abilify 1mg/ml oral solution | 150 ml [PoM] £102.90 DT price = £102.90

Orodispersible tablet

CAUTIONARY AND ADVISORY LABELS 2
EXCIPIENTS: May contain Aspartame

▸ **Aripiprazole (Non-proprietary)**
Aripiprazole 10 mg Aripiprazole 10mg orodispersible tablets sugar free sugar-free | 28 tablet [PoM] £91.24 DT price = £78.89
Aripiprazole 15 mg Aripiprazole 15mg orodispersible tablets sugar free sugar-free | 28 tablet [PoM] £91.24 DT price = £78.89

▸ **Abilify** (Otsuka Pharmaceuticals (U.K.) Ltd)
Aripiprazole 10 mg Abilify 10mg orodispersible tablets sugar-free | 28 tablet [PoM] £96.04 DT price = £78.89
Aripiprazole 15 mg Abilify 15mg orodispersible tablets sugar-free | 28 tablet [PoM] £96.04 DT price = £78.89

F 235

┃ Clozapine

● **DRUG ACTION** Clozapine is a dopamine D_1, dopamine D_2, 5-HT_{2A}, alpha$_1$-adrenoceptor, and muscarinic-receptor antagonist.

● **INDICATIONS AND DOSE**

Schizophrenia in patients unresponsive to, or intolerant of, conventional antipsychotic drugs

▸ BY MOUTH

▸ Child 12–17 years (under expert supervision): 12.5 mg 1–2 times a day for day 1, then 25–50 mg for day 2, then increased, if tolerated, in steps of 25–50 mg daily, dose to be increased gradually over 14–21 days, increased to up to 300 mg daily in divided doses, larger dose to be taken at night, up to 200 mg daily may be taken as a single dose at bedtime; increased in steps of 50–100 mg 1–2 times a week if required, it is preferable to increase once a week; usual dose 200–450 mg daily,

max. 900 mg per day, if restarting after interval of more than 48 hours, 12.5 mg once or twice on first day (but may be feasible to increase more quickly than on initiation)—extreme caution if previous respiratory or cardiac arrest with initial dosing

DOSE ADJUSTMENTS DUE TO INTERACTIONS
Dose adjustment may be necessary if smoking started or stopped during treatment.

● **UNLICENSED USE** Not licensed for use in children under 16 years.

● **CONTRA-INDICATIONS** Alcoholic and toxic psychoses · bone-marrow disorders · coma · drug intoxication · history of agranulocytosis · history of circulatory collapse · history of neutropenia · paralytic ileus · severe cardiac disorders (e.g. myocarditis) · severe CNS depression · uncontrolled epilepsy

● **CAUTIONS** Susceptibility to angle-closure glaucoma · taper off other antipsychotics before starting

CAUTIONS, FURTHER INFORMATION

▸ Agranulocytosis Neutropenia and potentially fatal agranulocytosis reported. Leucocyte and differential blood counts must be normal before starting; monitor counts every week for 18 weeks then at least every 2 weeks and if clozapine continued and blood count stable after 1 year at least every 4 weeks (and 4 weeks after discontinuation); if leucocyte count below 3000 /mm^3 or if absolute neutrophil count below 1500 /mm^3 discontinue permanently and refer to haematologist. Patients who have a low white blood cell count because of benign ethnic neutropenia may be started on clozapine with the agreement of a haematologist. Avoid drugs which depress leucopoiesis; patients should report immediately symptoms of infection, especially influenza-like illness.

▸ Myocarditis and cardiomyopathy Fatal myocarditis (most commonly in first 2 months) and cardiomyopathy reported.
  • Perform physical examination and take full medical history before starting
  • Specialist examination required if cardiac abnormalities or history of heart disease found—clozapine initiated only in absence of severe heart disease and if benefit outweighs risk
  • Persistent tachycardia especially in first 2 months should prompt observation for other indicators for myocarditis or cardiomyopathy
  • If myocarditis or cardiomyopathy suspected clozapine should be stopped and patient evaluated urgently by cardiologist
  • Discontinue permanently in clozapine-induced myocarditis or cardiomyopathy

▸ Intestinal obstruction Impairment of intestinal peristalsis, including constipation, intestinal obstruction, faecal impaction, and paralytic ileus, (including fatal cases) reported. Clozapine should be used with caution in patients receiving drugs that may cause constipation (e.g. antimuscarinic drugs) or in those with a history of colonic disease or lower abdominal surgery. It is essential that constipation is recognised and actively treated.

● **INTERACTIONS** → Appendix 1: clozapine

● **SIDE-EFFECTS**

▸ **Common or very common** Anorexia · constipation · hypersalivation · malaise · speech disorders · urinary incontinence

▸ **Uncommon** Agranulocytosis

▸ **Rare** Circulatory collapse · dysphagia · hepatitis · myocarditis · pancreatitis · pericarditis · pneumonia · pulmonary aspiration

▸ **Very rare** Cardiomyopathy · hypercholesterolaemia · hypertriglyceridaemia · interstitial nephritis · intestinal obstruction (including fatal cases) · myocardial infarction ·

obsessive compulsive disorder · parotid gland enlargement · respiratory depression

▶ **Frequency not known** Hepatic disorders · hepatic failure · muscle disorders · renal failure

SIDE-EFFECTS, FURTHER INFORMATION

▶ Hypersalivation Hypersalivation associated with clozapine therapy can be treated with hyoscine hydrobromide [unlicensed indication], provided that the patient is not at particular risk from the additive antimuscarinic side-effects of hyoscine and clozapine.

● **PREGNANCY** Use with caution.

● **BREAST FEEDING** Avoid.

● **HEPATIC IMPAIRMENT** Avoid in symptomatic liver disease. Avoid in progressive liver disease. Avoid in hepatic failure. Monitor hepatic function regularly.

● **RENAL IMPAIRMENT** Avoid in severe impairment.

● **MONITORING REQUIREMENTS**
▶ Monitor leucocyte and differential blood counts. Clozapine requires differential white blood cell monitoring weekly for 18 weeks, then fortnightly for up to one year, and then monthly as part of the clozapine patient monitoring service.
▶ Close medical supervision during initiation (risk of collapse because of hypotension and convulsions).
▶ Blood lipids and weight should be measured at baseline, at 3 months (weight should be measured at frequent intervals during the first 3 months), and then yearly with antipsychotics. Patients taking clozapine require more frequent monitoring of these parameters: every 3 months for the first year, then yearly.
▶ Fasting blood glucose should be measured at baseline, at 4–6 months, and then yearly. Patients taking clozapine should have fasting blood glucose tested at baseline, after one months' treatment, then every 4–6 months.
▶ Patient, prescriber, and supplying pharmacist must be registered with the appropriate Patient Monitoring Service—it takes several days to do this.

● **TREATMENT CESSATION** On planned withdrawal reduce dose over 1–2 weeks to avoid risk of rebound psychosis. If abrupt withdrawal necessary observe patient carefully.

● **DIRECTIONS FOR ADMINISTRATION** Shake oral suspension well for 90 seconds when dispensing or if visibly settled and stand for 24 hours before use; otherwise shake well for 10 seconds before use. May be diluted with water.

● **PRESCRIBING AND DISPENSING INFORMATION** Clozapine has been used for psychosis in Parkinson's disease in children aged 16 years and over.

● **PATIENT AND CARER ADVICE** Patients or carers should be given advice on how to administer clozapine oral suspension.

● **MEDICINAL FORMS**
There can be variation in the licensing of different medicines containing the same drug. Forms available from special-order manufacturers include: oral suspension, oral solution

Oral suspension
CAUTIONARY AND ADVISORY LABELS 2, 10
▶ Denzapine (Britannia Pharmaceuticals Ltd)
Clozapine 50 mg per 1 ml Denzapine 50mg/ml oral suspension sugar-free | 100 ml [PoM] £39.60

Tablet
CAUTIONARY AND ADVISORY LABELS 2, 10
▶ Clozaril (Mylan Ltd)
Clozapine 25 mg Clozaril 25mg tablets | 28 tablet [PoM] £2.95 | 84 tablet [PoM] £6.30 (Hospital only) | 100 tablet [PoM] £7.50 (Hospital only)
Clozapine 100 mg Clozaril 100mg tablets | 28 tablet [PoM] £11.76 | 84 tablet [PoM] £25.21 (Hospital only) | 100 tablet [PoM] £30.01 (Hospital only)
▶ Denzapine (Britannia Pharmaceuticals Ltd)
Clozapine 25 mg Denzapine 25mg tablets | 84 tablet [PoM] £16.64 | 100 tablet [PoM] £19.80

Clozapine 100 mg Denzapine 100mg tablets | 84 tablet [PoM] £66.53 | 100 tablet [PoM] £79.20
▶ Zaponex (Leyden Delta B.V.)
Clozapine 25 mg Zaponex 25mg tablets 84 tablet [PoM] £8.28 | 500 tablet [PoM] £48.39
Clozapine 100 mg Zaponex 100mg tablets | 84 tablet [PoM] £33.88 | 500 tablet [PoM] £196.43

F 235

Olanzapine

● **DRUG ACTION** Olanzapine is a dopamine D_1, D_2, D_4, 5-HT_2, histamine-1, and muscarinic-receptor antagonist.

● **INDICATIONS AND DOSE**

Schizophrenia | Combination therapy for mania
▶ BY MOUTH
▶ Child 12-17 years (under expert supervision): Initially 5–10 mg daily, adjusted according to response, usual dose 5–20 mg daily, doses greater than 10 mg daily only after reassessment, when one or more factors present that might result in slower metabolism (e.g. female gender, non-smoker) consider lower initial dose and more gradual dose increase, maximum 20 mg per day

Monotherapy for mania
▶ BY MOUTH
▶ Child 12-17 years (under expert supervision): 15 mg daily, adjusted according to response, usual dose 5–20 mg daily, doses greater than 15 mg daily only after reassessment, when one or more factors present that might result in slower metabolism (e.g. female gender, non-smoker) consider lower initial dose and more gradual dose increase; maximum 20 mg per day

DOSE ADJUSTMENTS DUE TO INTERACTIONS
Dose adjustment may be necessary if smoking started or stopped during treatment.

● **UNLICENSED USE** Not licensed for use in children.

● **CAUTIONS** Bone-marrow depression · diabetes mellitus (risk of exacerbation or ketoacidosis) · hypereosinophilic disorders · low leucocyte count low neutrophil count · myeloproliferative disease · paralytic ileus

● **INTERACTIONS** → Appendix 1: olanzapine

● **SIDE-EFFECTS**
▶ **Common or very common** Arthralgia · hypercholesterolaemia · hypertriglyceridaemia · increased appetite · malaise · oedema
▶ **Uncommon** Alopecia · amnesia · bradycardia · epistaxis
▶ **Rare** Hepatitis · pancreatitis · rhabdomyolysis

● **PREGNANCY** Use only if potential benefit outweighs risk; neonatal lethargy, tremor, and hypertonia reported when used in third trimester.

● **BREAST FEEDING** Avoid—present in milk.

● **HEPATIC IMPAIRMENT** Consider initial dose of 5 mg daily.

● **RENAL IMPAIRMENT** Consider initial dose of 5 mg daily.

● **MONITORING REQUIREMENTS**
▶ Blood lipids and weight should be measured at baseline, at 3 months (weight should be measured at frequent intervals during the first 3 months), and then yearly with antipsychotic drugs. Patients taking olanzapine require more frequent monitoring of these parameters: every 3 months for the first year, then yearly.
▶ Fasting blood glucose should be measured at baseline, at 4–6 months, and then yearly. Patients taking olanzapine should have fasting blood glucose tested at baseline, after one months' treatment, then every 4–6 months.

● **DIRECTIONS FOR ADMINISTRATION** Olanzapine orodispersible tablet may be placed on the tongue and allowed to dissolve, or dispersed in water, orange juice, apple juice, milk, or coffee.

● **PATIENT AND CARER ADVICE**
Patients or carers should be given advice on how to
administer orodispersible tablets.
Medicines for Children leaflet: Olanzapine for schizophrenia,
bipolar disorder, mania and agitation www.medicinesforchildren.
org.uk/olanzapine-schizophrenia-bipolar-disorder-mania-and-
agitation

● **MEDICINAL FORMS**
There can be variation in the licensing of different medicines
containing the same drug. Forms available from special-order
manufacturers include: oral suspension, oral solution

Tablet
CAUTIONARY AND ADVISORY LABELS 2
▶ **Olanzapine (Non-proprietary)**
Olanzapine 2.5 mg Olanzapine 2.5mg tablets | 28 tablet [PoM]
£21.85 DT price = £0.87
Olanzapine 5 mg Olanzapine 5mg tablets | 28 tablet [PoM] £43.70
DT price = £0.95
Olanzapine 7.5 mg Olanzapine 7.5mg tablets | 28 tablet [PoM]
£62.27 DT price = £0.92 | 56 tablet [PoM] £131.10
Olanzapine 10 mg Olanzapine 10mg tablets | 28 tablet [PoM] £87.40
DT price = £1.05
Olanzapine 15 mg Olanzapine 15mg tablets | 28 tablet [PoM]
£119.18 DT price = £1.28
Olanzapine 20 mg Olanzapine 20mg tablets | 28 tablet [PoM]
£158.90 DT price = £1.54
▶ **Zalasta** (Consilient Health Ltd)
Olanzapine 2.5 mg Zalasta 2.5mg tablets | 28 tablet [PoM] £18.57
DT price = £0.87
Olanzapine 5 mg Zalasta 5mg tablets | 28 tablet [PoM] £37.14 DT
price = £0.95
Olanzapine 7.5 mg Zalasta 7.5mg tablets | 56 tablet [PoM] £111.43
Olanzapine 10 mg Zalasta 10mg tablets | 28 tablet [PoM] £74.29 DT
price = £1.05
Olanzapine 15 mg Zalasta 15mg tablets | 28 tablet [PoM] £101.30
DT price = £1.28
Olanzapine 20 mg Zalasta 20mg tablets | 28 tablet [PoM] £135.06
DT price = £1.54
▶ **Zyprexa** (Eli Lilly and Company Ltd)
Olanzapine 2.5 mg Zyprexa 2.5mg tablets | 28 tablet [PoM] £21.85
DT price = £0.87
Olanzapine 5 mg Zyprexa 5mg tablets | 28 tablet [PoM] £43.70 DT
price = £0.95
Olanzapine 7.5 mg Zyprexa 7.5mg tablets | 56 tablet [PoM] £131.10
Olanzapine 10 mg Zyprexa 10mg tablets | 28 tablet [PoM] £87.40 DT
price = £1.05
Olanzapine 15 mg Zyprexa 15mg tablets | 28 tablet [PoM] £119.18
DT price = £1.28
Olanzapine 20 mg Zyprexa 20mg tablets | 28 tablet [PoM] £158.90
DT price = £1.54

Oral lyophilisate
▶ **Zyprexa Velotabs** (Eli Lilly and Company Ltd)
Olanzapine 5 mg Zyprexa 5mg Velotabs sugar-free | 28 tablet [PoM]
£48.07 DT price = £48.07
Olanzapine 10 mg Zyprexa 10mg Velotabs sugar-free |
28 tablet [PoM] £87.40 DT price = £87.40
Olanzapine 15 mg Zyprexa 15mg Velotabs sugar-free |
28 tablet [PoM] £131.10 DT price = £131.10
Olanzapine 20 mg Zyprexa 20mg Velotabs sugar-free |
28 tablet [PoM] £174.79 DT price = £174.79

Orodispersible tablet
CAUTIONARY AND ADVISORY LABELS 2
EXCIPIENTS: May contain Aspartame
▶ **Olanzapine (Non-proprietary)**
Olanzapine 5 mg Olanzapine 5mg orodispersible tablets sugar free
sugar-free | 28 tablet [PoM] £1.72 DT price = £1.70
Olanzapine 5mg orodispersible tablets | 28 tablet [PoM] £4.99 DT
price = £2.82
Olanzapine 10 mg Olanzapine 10mg orodispersible tablets |
28 tablet [PoM] £5.99 DT price = £3.50
Olanzapine 10mg orodispersible tablets sugar free sugar-free |
28 tablet [PoM] £2.24 DT price = £2.23
Olanzapine 15 mg Olanzapine 15mg orodispersible tablets sugar free
sugar-free | 28 tablet [PoM] £2.76 DT price = £2.75
Olanzapine 15mg orodispersible tablets | 28 tablet [PoM] £6.99 DT
price = £4.18
Olanzapine 20 mg Olanzapine 20mg orodispersible tablets sugar
free sugar-free | 28 tablet [PoM] £3.79 DT price = £3.73

Olanzapine 20mg orodispersible tablets | 28 tablet [PoM] £7.99 DT
price = £5.26
▶ **Zalasta** (Consilient Health Ltd)
Olanzapine 5 mg Zalasta 5mg orodispersible tablets sugar-free |
28 tablet [PoM] £40.85 DT price = £1.70
Olanzapine 10 mg Zalasta 10mg orodispersible tablets sugar-free |
28 tablet [PoM] £74.29 DT price = £2.23
Olanzapine 15 mg Zalasta 15mg orodispersible tablets sugar-free |
28 tablet [PoM] £111.43 DT price = £2.75
Olanzapine 20 mg Zalasta 20mg orodispersible tablets sugar-free |
28 tablet [PoM] £148.57 DT price = £3.73

F 235

Quetiapine

● **DRUG ACTION** Quetiapine is a dopamine D_1, dopamine D_2,
5-HT_2, alpha$_1$-adrenoceptor, and histamine-1 receptor
antagonist.

● **INDICATIONS AND DOSE**
Schizophrenia
▶ BY MOUTH USING IMMEDIATE-RELEASE MEDICINES
▶ Child 12–17 years (under expert supervision): Initially
25 mg twice daily, adjusted according to response.
adjusted in steps of 25–50 mg; maximum 750 mg per
day
▶ BY MOUTH USING MODIFIED-RELEASE MEDICINES
▶ Child 12–17 years (under expert supervision): Initially
50 mg once daily, adjusted according to response.
adjusted in steps of 50 mg daily, usual dose
400–800 mg once daily; maximum 800 mg per day

Treatment of mania in bipolar disorder
▶ BY MOUTH USING IMMEDIATE-RELEASE MEDICINES
▶ Child 12–17 years (under expert supervision): 25 mg twice
daily for day 1, then 50 mg twice daily for day 2, then
100 mg twice daily for day 3, then 150 mg twice daily
for day 4, then 200 mg twice daily for day 5, then
adjusted in steps of up to 100 mg daily, adjusted
according to response, usual dose 400–600 mg daily in
2 divided doses

DOSE EQUIVALENCE AND CONVERSION
▶ Patients can be switched from immediate-release to
modified-release tablets at the equivalent daily dose;
to maintain clinical response, dose titration may be
required.

● **UNLICENSED USE** Not licensed for use in children.
● **CAUTIONS** Cerebrovascular disease · patients at risk of
aspiration pneumonia · treatment of depression in patients
under 25 years (increased risk of suicide)
● **INTERACTIONS** → Appendix 1: quetiapine
● **SIDE-EFFECTS**
▶ **Common or very common** Asthenia · dysarthria · dyspnoea ·
elevated plasma-cholesterol concentrations · elevated
plasma-triglyceride concentrations · increased appetite ·
irritability · peripheral oedema · sleep disorders
▶ **Uncommon** Hyponatraemia · hypothyroidism · restless legs
syndrome · rhinitis
▶ **Rare** Hepatitis · pancreatitis
▶ **Very rare** Angioedema · inappropriate secretion of
antidiuretic hormone · rhabdomyolysis · Stevens-Johnson
syndrome
▶ **Frequency not known** Suicidal behaviour (particularly on
initiation) · toxic epidermal necrolysis
● **PREGNANCY** Use only if potential benefit outweighs risk.
● **BREAST FEEDING** Manufacturer advises avoid.
● **HEPATIC IMPAIRMENT** For *immediate-release tablets*,
initially 25 mg daily, increased daily in steps of 25–50 mg.
For *modified-release tablets*, initially 50 mg daily, increased
daily in steps of 50 mg.

4

Nervous system

● MEDICINAL FORMS
There can be variation in the licensing of different medicines containing the same drug. Forms available from special-order manufacturers include: oral suspension, oral solution, powder

Modified-release tablet
CAUTIONARY AND ADVISORY LABELS 2, 23, 25
▸ Atrolak XL (Accord Healthcare Ltd)
Quetiapine (as Quetiapine fumarate) 50 mg Atrolak XL 50mg tablets | 60 tablet [PoM] £67.65 DT price = £67.66
Quetiapine (as Quetiapine fumarate) 200 mg Atrolak XL 200mg tablets | 60 tablet [PoM] £113.09 DT price = £113.10
Quetiapine (as Quetiapine fumarate) 300 mg Atrolak XL 300mg tablets | 60 tablet [PoM] £169.99 DT price = £170.00
Quetiapine (as Quetiapine fumarate) 400 mg Atrolak XL 400mg tablets | 60 tablet [PoM] £226.19 DT price = £226.20
▸ Biquelle XL (Aspire Pharma Ltd)
Quetiapine (as Quetiapine fumarate) 50 mg Biquelle XL 50mg tablets | 60 tablet [PoM] £29.45 DT price = £67.66
Quetiapine (as Quetiapine fumarate) 150 mg Biquelle XL 150mg tablets | 60 tablet [PoM] £49.45 DT price = £113.10
Quetiapine (as Quetiapine fumarate) 200 mg Biquelle XL 200mg tablets | 60 tablet [PoM] £49.45 DT price = £113.10
Quetiapine (as Quetiapine fumarate) 300 mg Biquelle XL 300mg tablets | 60 tablet [PoM] £74.45 DT price = £170.00
Quetiapine (as Quetiapine fumarate) 400 mg Biquelle XL 400mg tablets | 60 tablet [PoM] £98.95 DT price = £226.20
▸ Brancico XL (Zentiva)
Quetiapine (as Quetiapine fumarate) 50 mg Brancico XL 50mg tablets | 60 tablet [PoM] £20.00 DT price = £67.66
Quetiapine (as Quetiapine fumarate) 150 mg Brancico XL 150mg tablets | 60 tablet [PoM] £46.95 DT price = £113.10
Quetiapine (as Quetiapine fumarate) 200 mg Brancico XL 200mg tablets | 60 tablet [PoM] £40.00 DT price = £113.10
Quetiapine (as Quetiapine fumarate) 300 mg Brancico XL 300mg tablets | 60 tablet [PoM] £60.00 DT price = £170.00
Quetiapine (as Quetiapine fumarate) 400 mg Brancico XL 400mg tablets | 60 tablet [PoM] £80.00 DT price = £226.20
▸ Ebesque XL (Ethypharm UK Ltd)
Quetiapine (as Quetiapine fumarate) 50 mg Ebesque XL 50mg tablets | 60 tablet [PoM] £31.80 DT price = £67.66
Quetiapine (as Quetiapine fumarate) 200 mg Ebesque XL 200mg tablets | 60 tablet [PoM] £53.16 DT price = £113.10
Quetiapine (as Quetiapine fumarate) 300 mg Ebesque XL 300mg tablets | 60 tablet [PoM] £79.90 DT price = £170.00
Quetiapine (as Quetiapine fumarate) 400 mg Ebesque XL 400mg tablets | 60 tablet [PoM] £106.31 DT price = £226.20
▸ Mintreleq XL (Aristo Pharma Ltd)
Quetiapine (as Quetiapine fumarate) 50 mg Mintreleq XL 50mg tablets | 60 tablet [PoM] £29.45 DT price = £67.66
Quetiapine (as Quetiapine fumarate) 150 mg Mintreleq XL 150mg tablets | 60 tablet [PoM] £49.45 DT price = £113.10
Quetiapine (as Quetiapine fumarate) 200 mg Mintreleq XL 200mg tablets | 60 tablet [PoM] £49.45 DT price = £113.10
Quetiapine (as Quetiapine fumarate) 300 mg Mintreleq XL 300mg tablets | 60 tablet [PoM] £74.45 DT price = £170.00
Quetiapine (as Quetiapine fumarate) 400 mg Mintreleq XL 400mg tablets | 60 tablet [PoM] £98.95 DT price = £226.20
▸ Psyquet XL (Sandoz Ltd)
Quetiapine (as Quetiapine fumarate) 50 mg Psyquet XL 50mg tablets | 60 tablet [PoM] £27.97 DT price = £67.66
Quetiapine (as Quetiapine fumarate) 150 mg Psyquet XL 150mg tablets | 60 tablet [PoM] £46.97 DT price = £113.10
Quetiapine (as Quetiapine fumarate) 200 mg Psyquet XL 200mg tablets | 60 tablet [PoM] £46.97 DT price = £113.10
Quetiapine (as Quetiapine fumarate) 300 mg Psyquet XL 300mg tablets | 60 tablet [PoM] £70.72 DT price = £170.00
Quetiapine (as Quetiapine fumarate) 400 mg Psyquet XL 400mg tablets | 60 tablet [PoM] £93.99 DT price = £226.20
▸ Seroquel XL (AstraZeneca UK Ltd)
Quetiapine (as Quetiapine fumarate) 50 mg Seroquel XL 50mg tablets | 60 tablet [PoM] £67.66 DT price = £67.66
Quetiapine (as Quetiapine fumarate) 150 mg Seroquel XL 150mg tablets | 60 tablet [PoM] £113.10 DT price = £113.10
Quetiapine (as Quetiapine fumarate) 200 mg Seroquel XL 200mg tablets | 60 tablet [PoM] £113.10 DT price = £113.10
Quetiapine (as Quetiapine fumarate) 300 mg Seroquel XL 300mg tablets | 60 tablet [PoM] £170.00 DT price = £170.00
Quetiapine (as Quetiapine fumarate) 400 mg Seroquel XL 400mg tablets | 60 tablet [PoM] £226.20 DT price = £226.20

▸ Sondate XL (Teva UK Ltd)
Quetiapine (as Quetiapine fumarate) 50 mg Sondate XL 50mg tablets | 60 tablet [PoM] £19.99 DT price = £67.66
Quetiapine (as Quetiapine fumarate) 150 mg Sondate XL 150mg tablets | 60 tablet [PoM] £39.99 DT price = £113.10
Quetiapine (as Quetiapine fumarate) 200 mg Sondate XL 200mg tablets | 60 tablet [PoM] £39.99 DT price = £113.10
Quetiapine (as Quetiapine fumarate) 300 mg Sondate XL 300mg tablets | 60 tablet [PoM] £59.99 DT price = £170.00
Quetiapine (as Quetiapine fumarate) 400 mg Sondate XL 400mg tablets | 60 tablet [PoM] £79.99 DT price = £226.20
▸ Tenprolide XL (Actavis UK Ltd)
Quetiapine (as Quetiapine fumarate) 50 mg Tenprolide XL 50mg tablets | 60 tablet [PoM] £67.66 DT price = £67.66
Quetiapine (as Quetiapine fumarate) 200 mg Tenprolide XL 200mg tablets | 60 tablet [PoM] £113.10 DT price = £113.10
Quetiapine (as Quetiapine fumarate) 300 mg Tenprolide XL 300mg tablets | 60 tablet [PoM] £170.00 DT price = £170.00
Quetiapine (as Quetiapine fumarate) 400 mg Tenprolide XL 400mg tablets | 60 tablet [PoM] £226.20 DT price = £226.20
▸ Zaluron XL (Fontus Health Ltd)
Quetiapine (as Quetiapine fumarate) 50 mg Zaluron XL 50mg tablets | 60 tablet [PoM] £27.96 DT price = £67.66
Quetiapine (as Quetiapine fumarate) 150 mg Zaluron XL 150mg tablets | 60 tablet [PoM] £46.96 DT price = £113.10
Quetiapine (as Quetiapine fumarate) 200 mg Zaluron XL 200mg tablets | 60 tablet [PoM] £46.96 DT price = £113.10
Quetiapine (as Quetiapine fumarate) 300 mg Zaluron XL 300mg tablets | 60 tablet [PoM] £70.71 DT price = £170.00
Quetiapine (as Quetiapine fumarate) 400 mg Zaluron XL 400mg tablets | 60 tablet [PoM] £93.98 DT price = £226.20

Tablet
CAUTIONARY AND ADVISORY LABELS 2
▸ Quetiapine (Non-proprietary)
Quetiapine (as Quetiapine fumarate) 25 mg Quetiapine 25mg tablets | 60 tablet [PoM] £38.05 DT price = £1.01
Quetiapine (as Quetiapine fumarate) 100 mg Quetiapine 100mg tablets | 60 tablet [PoM] £107.45 DT price = £1.62
Quetiapine (as Quetiapine fumarate) 150 mg Quetiapine 150mg tablets | 60 tablet [PoM] £107.45 DT price = £2.04
Quetiapine (as Quetiapine fumarate) 200 mg Quetiapine 200mg tablets | 60 tablet [PoM] £107.45 DT price = £2.36
Quetiapine (as Quetiapine fumarate) 300 mg Quetiapine 300mg tablets | 60 tablet [PoM] £161.50 DT price = £3.07
▸ Seroquel (AstraZeneca UK Ltd)
Quetiapine (as Quetiapine fumarate) 25 mg Seroquel 25mg tablets | 60 tablet [PoM] £40.50 DT price = £1.01
Quetiapine (as Quetiapine fumarate) 100 mg Seroquel 100mg tablets | 60 tablet [PoM] £113.10 DT price = £1.62
Quetiapine (as Quetiapine fumarate) 200 mg Seroquel 200mg tablets | 60 tablet [PoM] £113.10 DT price = £2.36
Quetiapine (as Quetiapine fumarate) 300 mg Seroquel 300mg tablets | 60 tablet [PoM] £170.00 DT price = £3.07

F 235

Risperidone

● DRUG ACTION Risperidone is a dopamine D_2, 5-HT_{2A}, alpha$_1$-adrenoceptor, and histamine-1 receptor antagonist.

● INDICATIONS AND DOSE
Acute and chronic psychosis
▸ BY MOUTH
▸ Child 12-17 years (under expert supervision): 2 mg daily in 1-2 divided doses for day 1, then 4 mg daily in 1-2 divided doses for day 2, slower titration is appropriate in some patients; usual dose 4-6 mg daily, doses above 10 mg daily only if benefit considered to outweigh risk; maximum 16 mg per day

Short-term monotherapy of mania in bipolar disorder (under expert supervision)
▸ BY MOUTH
▸ Child 12-17 years: Initially 500 micrograms once daily, then adjusted in steps of 0.5-1 mg daily, adjusted according to response; usual dose 2.5 mg daily in 1-2 divided doses; maximum 6 mg per day

Short-term treatment (up to 6 weeks) of persistent aggression in conduct disorder (under expert supervision)
▶ BY MOUTH
▶ Child 5-17 years (body-weight up to 50 kg): Initially 250 micrograms once daily, then increased in steps of 250 micrograms once daily on alternate days, adjusted according to response; usual dose 500 micrograms once daily; maximum 750 micrograms per day
▶ Child 5-17 years (body-weight 50 kg and above): Initially 500 micrograms once daily, then increased in steps of 500 micrograms once daily on alternate days, adjusted according to response; usual dose 1 mg once daily; maximum 1.5 mg per day

Short-term treatment of severe aggression in autism (under expert supervision)
▶ BY MOUTH
▶ Child 5-17 years (body-weight 15-20 kg): Initially 250 micrograms daily for at least 4 days, then increased if necessary to 500 micrograms daily, then increased in steps of 250 micrograms daily, dose to be increased at intervals of 2 weeks, review effectiveness and any side-effects after 3–4 weeks; stop if no response at 6 weeks; maximum 1 mg per day
▶ Child 5-17 years (body-weight 20-45 kg): Initially 500 micrograms daily for at least 4 days, then increased if necessary to 1 mg daily, then increased in steps of 500 micrograms daily, dose to be increased at intervals of 2 weeks, review effectiveness and any side-effects after 3–4 weeks; stop if no response at 6 weeks; maximum 2.5 mg per day
▶ Child 5-17 years (body-weight 45 kg and above): Initially 500 micrograms daily for at least 4 days, then increased if necessary to 1 mg daily, then increased in steps of 500 micrograms daily, dose to be increased at intervals of 2 weeks, review effectiveness and any side-effects after 3–4 weeks; stop if no response at 6 weeks; maximum 3 mg per day

● **UNLICENSED USE** Not licensed for use in children for psychosis, mania, or autism.

● **CAUTIONS** Avoid in acute porphyrias p. 577 · cataract surgery (risk of intra-operative floppy iris syndrome) · dehydration · family history of sudden cardiac death (perform ECG) · prolactin-dependent tumours

● **INTERACTIONS** → Appendix 1: risperidone

● **SIDE-EFFECTS**
▶ **Common or very common** Anxiety · appetite changes · arthralgia · depression · epistaxis · hypertension · infection · malaise · myalgia · oedema · respiratory disorders · sleep disorders · toothache · urinary disorders
▶ **Uncommon** Alopecia · elevated plasma-cholesterol concentrations · elevated plasma-triglyceride concentrations · hypoaesthesia · paraesthesia · taste disturbances · tinnitus · visual disorders
▶ **Rare** Inappropriate antidiuretic hormone secretion · intestinal obstruction · intra-operative floppy iris syndrome · pancreatitis · pulmonary embolism · rhabdomyolysis

● **PREGNANCY** Use only if potential benefit outweighs risk.

● **BREAST FEEDING** Use only if potential benefit outweighs risk—small amount present in milk.

● **HEPATIC IMPAIRMENT** Initial and subsequent oral doses should be halved.

● **RENAL IMPAIRMENT** Initial and subsequent oral doses should be halved.

● **DIRECTIONS FOR ADMINISTRATION** Orodispersible tablets should be placed on the tongue, allowed to dissolve and swallowed. Oral liquid may be diluted with any non-alcoholic drink, except tea.

● **PATIENT AND CARER ADVICE**
Patients or carers should be given advice on how to administer risperidone orodispersible tablets and oral liquid (counselling on use of dose syringe advised). Medicines for Children leaflet: Risperidone for psychological disorders www.medicinesforchildren.org.uk/risperidone-for-psychological-disorders

● **MEDICINAL FORMS**
There can be variation in the licensing of different medicines containing the same drug. Forms available from special-order manufacturers include: oral solution

Oral solution
CAUTIONARY AND ADVISORY LABELS 2
▶ **Risperidone (Non-proprietary)**
Risperidone 1 mg per 1 ml Risperidone 1mg/ml oral solution sugar free sugar-free | 100 ml PoM £58.22 DT price = £4.16
▶ **Risperdal** (Janssen-Cilag Ltd)
Risperidone 1 mg per 1 ml Risperdal 1mg/ml oral solution sugar-free | 100 ml PoM £37.01 DT price = £4.16

Orodispersible tablet
CAUTIONARY AND ADVISORY LABELS 2
EXCIPIENTS: May contain Aspartame
▶ **Risperidone (Non-proprietary)**
Risperidone 500 microgram Risperidone 500microgram orodispersible tablets sugar free sugar-free | 28 tablet PoM £23.88 DT price = £23.86
Risperidone 1 mg Risperidone 1mg orodispersible tablets sugar free sugar-free | 28 tablet PoM £21.09 DT price = £21.07
Risperidone 2 mg Risperidone 2mg orodispersible tablets sugar free sugar-free | 28 tablet PoM £38.79 DT price = £38.77
Risperidone 3 mg Risperidone 3mg orodispersible tablets sugar free sugar-free | 28 tablet PoM £33.50 DT price = £33.50
Risperidone 4 mg Risperidone 4mg orodispersible tablets sugar free sugar-free | 28 tablet PoM £37.95 DT price = £37.95
▶ **Risperdal Quicklet** (Janssen-Cilag Ltd)
Risperidone 500 microgram Risperdal Quicklet 500microgram orodispersible tablets sugar-free | 28 tablet PoM £8.23 DT price = £23.86

Tablet
CAUTIONARY AND ADVISORY LABELS 2
▶ **Risperidone (Non-proprietary)**
Risperidone 500 microgram Risperidone 500microgram tablets | 20 tablet PoM £6.18 DT price = £0.78
Risperidone 1 mg Risperidone 1mg tablets | 20 tablet PoM £0.84 DT price = £0.76 | 60 tablet PoM £25.07
Risperidone 2 mg Risperidone 2mg tablets | 60 tablet PoM £60.10 DT price = £1.41
Risperidone 3 mg Risperidone 3mg tablets | 60 tablet PoM £88.38 DT price = £1.57
Risperidone 4 mg Risperidone 4mg tablets | 60 tablet PoM £116.67 DT price = £1.78
Risperidone 6 mg Risperidone 6mg tablets | 28 tablet PoM £82.50 DT price = £3.21 | 60 tablet PoM no price available
▶ **Risperdal** (Janssen-Cilag Ltd)
Risperidone 500 microgram Risperdal 500microgram tablets | 20 tablet PoM £5.08 DT price = £0.78
Risperidone 1 mg Risperdal 1mg tablets | 20 tablet PoM £8.36 DT price = £0.76 | 60 tablet PoM £17.56
Risperidone 2 mg Risperdal 2mg tablets | 60 tablet PoM £34.62 DT price = £1.41
Risperidone 3 mg Risperdal 3mg tablets | 60 tablet PoM £50.91 DT price = £1.57
Risperidone 4 mg Risperdal 4mg tablets | 60 tablet PoM £67.20 DT price = £1.78
Risperidone 6 mg Risperdal 6mg tablets | 28 tablet PoM £67.88 DT price = £3.21

4 Nervous system

3 Movement disorders

3.1 Dystonias and other involuntary movements

Dystonias and related disorders

Dystonias

Dystonias may result from conditions such as cerebral palsy or may be related to a deficiency of the neurotransmitter dopamine as in Segawa syndrome.

Dopaminergic drugs used in dystonias

Levodopa, the amino-acid precursor of dopamine, acts by replenishing depleted striatal dopamine. It is given with an extracerebral **dopa-decarboxylase inhibitor**, which reduces the peripheral conversion of levodopa to dopamine, thereby limiting side-effects such as nausea, vomiting, and cardiovascular effects; additionally, effective brain-dopamine concentrations are achieved with lower doses of levodopa. The extracerebral dopa-decarboxylase inhibitor most commonly used in children is carbidopa (in co-careldopa p. 247).

Levodopa therapy should be initiated at a low dose and increased in small steps; the final dose should be as low as possible. Intervals between doses should be chosen to suit the needs of the individual child.

In severe dystonias related to cerebral palsy, improvement can be expected within 2 weeks. Children with Segawa syndrome are particularly sensitive to levodopa; they may even become symptom free on small doses. Levodopa also has a role in treating metabolic disorders such as defects in tetrahydrobiopterin synthesis and dihydrobiopterin reductase deficiency. Tetrahydrobiopterin may have a role in metabolic disorders.

Children may experience nausea within 2 hours of taking a dose; nausea and vomiting with co-careldopa is rarely dose-limiting.

In dystonic cerebral palsy, treatment with larger doses of levodopa is associated with the development of potentially troublesome motor complications (including response fluctuations and dyskinesias). Response fluctuations are characterised by large variations in motor performance, with normal function during the 'on' period, and weakness and restricted mobility during the 'off' period.

Antimuscarinic drugs used in dystonias

The antimuscarinic drugs procyclidine hydrochloride below and trihexyphenidyl hydrochloride p. 247 reduce the symptoms of dystonias, including those induced by antipsychotic drugs; there is no justification for giving them routinely in the absence of dystonic symptoms. Tardive dyskinesia is not improved by antimuscarinic drugs and may be made worse.

There are no important differences between the antimuscarinic drugs, but some children tolerate one better than another.

Procyclidine hydrochloride can be given parenterally and is effective emergency treatment for acute drug-induced dystonic reactions.

If treatment with an antimuscarinic is ineffective, intravenous diazepam p. 212 can be given for life-threatening acute drug-induced dystonic reactions.

Drugs used in essential tremor, chorea, tics, and related disorders

Haloperidol p. 237 can also improve motor tics and symptoms of Tourette syndrome and related choreas. Other treatments for Tourette syndrome include pimozide p. 238

[unlicensed indication] (**important**: ECG monitoring required), and sulpiride p. 244 [unlicensed indication].

Propranolol hydrochloride p. 101 or another beta-adrenoceptor blocking drug may be useful in treating essential tremor or tremor associated with anxiety or thyrotoxicosis.

Botulinum toxin type A p. 248 should be used under specialist supervision. Treatment with botulinum toxin type A can be considered after an acquired non-progressive brain injury if rapid-onset spasticity causes postural or functional difficulties, and in children with spasticity in whom focal dystonia causes postural or functional difficulties or pain.

> **Other drugs used for Dystonias and other involuntary movements** Trifluoperazine, p. 239

ANTIMUSCARINICS

▌Procyclidine hydrochloride

- **DRUG ACTION** Procyclidine exerts its antiparkinsonian action by reducing the effects of the relative central cholinergic excess that occurs as a result of dopamine deficiency.

- **INDICATIONS AND DOSE**

  Acute dystonia
  ▸ BY INTRAMUSCULAR INJECTION, OR BY INTRAVENOUS INJECTION
  ▸ Child 1 month–1 year: 0.5–2 mg for 1 dose, dose usually effective in 5–10 minutes but may need 30 minutes for relief
  ▸ Child 2–9 years: 2–5 mg for 1 dose, dose usually effective in 5–10 minutes but may need 30 minutes for relief
  ▸ Child 10–17 years: 5–10 mg, occasionally, more than 10 mg, dose usually effective in 5–10 minutes but may need 30 minutes for relief

  Dystonia
  ▸ BY MOUTH
  ▸ Child 7–11 years: 1.25 mg 3 times a day
  ▸ Child 12–17 years: 2.5 mg 3 times a day

- **UNLICENSED USE** Not licensed for use in children.

- **CONTRA-INDICATIONS** Gastro-intestinal obstruction · myasthenia gravis

- **CAUTIONS** Cardiovascular disease · hypertension · liable to abuse · psychotic disorder · pyrexia · those susceptible to angle-closure glaucoma

- **INTERACTIONS** → Appendix 1: procyclidine

- **SIDE-EFFECTS** Angle-closure glaucoma · anxiety · blurred vision · confusion · constipation · dizziness · dry mouth · euphoria · gingivitis · hallucinations · impaired memory · nausea · rash · restlessness · tachycardia · urinary retention · vomiting

- **PREGNANCY** Use only if potential benefit outweighs risk.

- **BREAST FEEDING** No information available.

- **HEPATIC IMPAIRMENT** Use with caution.

- **RENAL IMPAIRMENT** Use with caution.

- **TREATMENT CESSATION** Avoid abrupt withdrawal in patients taking long-term treatment.

- **PATIENT AND CARER ADVICE**
  Driving and skilled tasks
  May affect performance of skilled tasks (e.g. driving).

● **MEDICINAL FORMS**
There can be variation in the licensing of different medicines containing the same drug. Forms available from special-order manufacturers include: oral suspension, oral solution

Solution for injection
▸ **Procyclidine hydrochloride (Non-proprietary)**
  Procyclidine hydrochloride 5 mg per 1 ml Procyclidine 10mg/2ml solution for injection ampoules | 5 ampoule PoM £60.00–£78.75 DT price = £72.50

Oral solution
▸ **Procyclidine hydrochloride (Non-proprietary)**
  Procyclidine hydrochloride 500 microgram per 1 ml Procyclidine 2.5mg/5ml oral solution sugar free sugar-free | 150 ml PoM £7.94–£8.22 DT price = £7.08
  Procyclidine hydrochloride 1 mg per 1 ml Procyclidine 5mg/5ml oral solution sugar free sugar-free | 150 ml PoM £14.54–£14.72 DT price = £13.13

Tablet
▸ **Procyclidine hydrochloride (Non-proprietary)**
  Procyclidine hydrochloride 5 mg Procyclidine 5mg tablets | 28 tablet PoM DT price = £12.24 | 100 tablet PoM £43.71 | 500 tablet PoM £218.57
▸ **Kemadrin** (Aspen Pharma Trading Ltd)
  Procyclidine hydrochloride 5 mg Kemadrin 5mg tablets | 100 tablet PoM £4.72 | 500 tablet PoM £23.62

Trihexyphenidyl hydrochloride

(Benzhexol hydrochloride)

● **DRUG ACTION** Trihexyphenidyl exerts its effects by reducing the effects of the relative central cholinergic excess that occurs as a result of dopamine deficiency.

● **INDICATIONS AND DOSE**

Dystonia
▸ BY MOUTH
▸ **Child 3 months–17 years:** Initially 1–2 mg daily in 1–2 divided doses, then increased in steps of 1 mg every 3–7 days, dose to be adjusted according to response and side-effects; maximum 2 mg/kg per day

● **UNLICENSED USE** Not licensed for use in children.

● **CONTRA-INDICATIONS** Gastro-intestinal obstruction · myasthenia gravis

● **CAUTIONS** Cardiovascular disease · hypertension · liable to abuse · psychotic disorders · pyrexia · those susceptible to angle-closure glaucoma

● **INTERACTIONS** → Appendix 1: trihexyphenidyl

● **SIDE-EFFECTS**
▸ **Very rare** Angle-closure glaucoma
▸ **Frequency not known** Anxiety · blurred vision · confusion · constipation · dizziness · dry mouth · euphoria · hallucinations · impaired memory · nausea · rash · restlessness · tachycardia · urinary retention · vomiting

● **PREGNANCY** Use only if potential benefit outweighs risk.

● **BREAST FEEDING** Avoid.

● **HEPATIC IMPAIRMENT** Use with caution.

● **RENAL IMPAIRMENT** Use with caution.

● **TREATMENT CESSATION** Avoid abrupt withdrawal in patients taking long-term treatment.

● **DIRECTIONS FOR ADMINISTRATION** Tablets should be taken with or after food.

● **PATIENT AND CARER ADVICE**
  Driving and skilled tasks
  May affect performance of skilled tasks (e.g. driving). Medicines for Children leaflet: Trihexyphenidyl hydrochloride for dystonia www.medicinesforchildren.org.uk/trihexyphenidyl-hydrochloride-for-dystonia

● **MEDICINAL FORMS**
There can be variation in the licensing of different medicines containing the same drug. Forms available from special-order manufacturers include: oral suspension, oral solution

Oral solution
EXCIPIENTS: May contain Propylene glycol
▸ **Trihexyphenidyl hydrochloride (Non-proprietary)**
  Trihexyphenidyl hydrochloride 1 mg per 1 ml Trihexyphenidyl 5mg/5ml oral solution | 200 ml PoM £22.00–£24.00 DT price = £22.00

Tablet
▸ **Trihexyphenidyl hydrochloride (Non-proprietary)**
  Trihexyphenidyl hydrochloride 2 mg Trihexyphenidyl 2mg tablets | 84 tablet PoM £5.56 DT price = £4.20
  Trihexyphenidyl hydrochloride 5 mg Trihexyphenidyl 5mg tablets | 84 tablet PoM £17.91 DT price = £17.91

DOPAMINERGIC DRUGS > DOPAMINE PRECURSORS

Co-careldopa   28-Sep-2016

● **INDICATIONS AND DOSE**

Dopamine-sensitive dystonias including Segawa syndrome and dystonias related to cerebral palsy (dose expressed as levodopa)
▸ BY MOUTH
▸ **Child 3 months–17 years:** Initially 250 micrograms/kg 2–3 times a day, dose to be increased according to response every 2–3 days, increased if necessary up to 1 mg/kg 3 times a day, preparation containing 1:4 ratio of carbidopa:levodopa is to be used

Treatment of defects in tetrahydrobiopterin synthesis and dihydrobiopterin reductase deficiency (dose expressed as levodopa)
▸ BY MOUTH
▸ **Neonate:** Initially 250–500 micrograms/kg 4 times a day, dose to be increased every 4–5 days according to response, a preparation containing 1:4 carbidopa: levodopa to be administered; maintenance 2.5–3 mg/kg 4 times a day, at higher doses consider preparation containing 1:10 carbidopa:levodopa, review regularly (every 3–6 months).
▸ **Child:** Initially 250–500 micrograms/kg 4 times a day, dose to be increased every 4–5 days according to response, a preparation containing 1:4 carbidopa: levodopa to be administered; maintenance 2.5–3 mg/kg 4 times a day, at higher doses consider preparation containing 1:10 carbidopa:levodopa, review regularly (every 3–6 months in early childhood)

DOSE EQUIVALENCE AND CONVERSION
▸ The proportions are expressed in the form x/y where x and y are the strengths in milligrams of carbidopa and levodopa respectively.
▸ 2 tablets *Sinemet*® 12.5 mg/50 mg is equivalent to 1 tablet *Sinemet*® Plus 25 mg/100 mg.

● **UNLICENSED USE** Not licensed for use in children.

● **CAUTIONS** Cardiovascular disease · diabetes mellitus · history of myocardial infarction with residual arrhythmia · history of peptic ulcer · history of skin melanoma (risk of activation) · osteomalacia · psychiatric illness (avoid if severe and discontinue if deterioration) · pulmonary disease · susceptibility to angle-closure glaucoma

● **INTERACTIONS** → Appendix 1: carbidopa, levodopa

● **SIDE-EFFECTS**
▸ **Common or very common** Agitation · anorexia · arrhythmias · dizziness · insomnia · nausea · postural hypotension · reddish discoloration of urine and other body fluids · tachycardia · vomiting

Nervous system

4

‣ **Rare** Abnormal involuntary movements (may be dose-limiting) · Henoch-Schönlein purpura · hypersensitivity · labile hypertension · psychiatric symptoms (including hypomania, may be dose-limiting)
‣ **Very rare** Angle-closure glaucoma
‣ **Frequency not known** Depression · drowsiness · flushing · gastro-intestinal bleeding · headache · liver enzyme changes · peripheral neuropathy · pruritus · rash · sweating · syndrome resembling neuroleptic malignant syndrome (on withdrawal) · taste disturbance

● **PREGNANCY** Use with caution—toxicity has occurred in *animal* studies.

● **BREAST FEEDING** May suppress lactation; present in milk—avoid.

● **MONITORING REQUIREMENTS** In prolonged therapy, psychiatric, hepatic, haematological, renal, and cardiovascular monitoring is advisable; warn patients to resume normal activities gradually.

● **EFFECT ON LABORATORY TESTS** False positive tests for urinary ketones have been reported.

● **TREATMENT CESSATION** Avoid abrupt withdrawal.

● **PRESCRIBING AND DISPENSING INFORMATION** Co-careldopa is a mixture of carbidopa and levodopa; the proportions are expressed in the form x/y where x and y are the strengths in milligrams of carbidopa and levodopa respectively.

● **PATIENT AND CARER ADVICE**
Sudden onset of sleep Excessive daytime sleepiness and sudden onset of sleep can occur with co-careldopa.
Patients starting treatment with these drugs should be warned of the risk and of the need to exercise caution when driving or operating machinery. Those who have experienced excessive sedation or sudden onset of sleep should refrain from driving or operating machines until these effects have stopped occurring.
Management of excessive daytime sleepiness should focus on the identification of an underlying cause, such as depression or concomitant medication. Patients should be counselled on improving sleep behaviour.
Warn patients to resume normal activity gradually.

● **NATIONAL FUNDING/ACCESS DECISIONS**
DUODOPA®

Scottish Medicines Consortium (SMC) Decisions
The *Scottish Medicines Consortium* has advised (June 2016) that *Duodopa®* intestinal gel is accepted for restricted use within NHS Scotland, within its licensed indication, only in patients not eligible for deep brain stimulation. This advice is contingent upon the continuing availability of the Patient Access Scheme in NHS Scotland or a list price that is equivalent or lower.

● **MEDICINAL FORMS**
There can be variation in the licensing of different medicines containing the same drug. Forms available from special-order manufacturers include: oral suspension, oral solution
Modified-release tablet
CAUTIONARY AND ADVISORY LABELS 10, 14, 25
‣ Co-careldopa (Non-proprietary)
Carbidopa (as Carbidopa monohydrate) 25 mg, Levodopa 100 mg Co-careldopa 25mg/100mg modified-release tablets | 50 tablet [PoM] no price available | 60 tablet [PoM] no price available DT price = £11.60 | 100 tablet [PoM] no price available
Carbidopa (as Carbidopa monohydrate) 50 mg, Levodopa 200 mg Co-careldopa 50mg/200mg modified-release tablets | 60 tablet [PoM] no price available DT price = £11.60
‣ Apodespan PR (Accord Healthcare Ltd)
Carbidopa (as Carbidopa monohydrate) 50 mg, Levodopa 200 mg Apodespan PR 50mg/200mg tablets | 60 tablet [PoM] £11.59 DT price = £11.60

‣ Caramet CR (Teva UK Ltd)
Carbidopa (as Carbidopa monohydrate) 25 mg, Levodopa 100 mg Caramet 25mg/100mg CR tablets | 60 tablet [PoM] £11.47 DT price = £11.60
Carbidopa (as Carbidopa monohydrate 50 mg, Levodopa 200 mg Caramet 50mg/200mg CR tablets | 60 tablet [PoM] £11.47 DT price = £11.60
‣ Half Sinemet CR (Merck Sharp & Dohme Ltd)
Carbidopa (as Carbidopa monohydrate) 25 mg, Levodopa 100 mg Half Sinemet CR 25mg/100mg tablets | 60 tablet [PoM] £11.60 DT price = £11.60
‣ Lecado (Sandoz Ltd)
Carbidopa (as Carbidopa monohydrate) 25 mg, Levodopa 100 mg Lecado 100mg/25mg modified-release tablets | 60 tablet [PoM] £9.86 DT price = £11.60
Carbidopa (as Carbidopa monohydrate) 50 mg, Levodopa 200 mg Lecado 200mg/50mg modified-release tablets | 60 tablet [PoM] £9.86 DT price = £11.60
‣ Sinemet CR (Merck Sharp & Dohme Ltd)
Carbidopa (as Carbidopa monohydrate) 50 mg, Levodopa 200 mg Sinemet CR 50mg/200mg tablets | 60 tablet [PoM] £11.60 DT price = £11.60

Tablet
CAUTIONARY AND ADVISORY LABELS 10, 14
‣ Co-careldopa (Non-proprietary)
Carbidopa (as Carbidopa monohydrate) 12.5 mg, Levodopa 50 mg Co-careldopa 12.5mg/50mg tablets | 90 tablet [PoM] £6.28 DT price = £6.28
Carbidopa (as Carbidopa monohydrate) 10 mg, Levodopa 100 mg Co-careldopa 10mg/100mg tablets | 100 tablet [PoM] £8.29 DT price = £7.95
Carbidopa (as Carbidopa monohydrate) 25 mg, Levodopa 100 mg Co-careldopa 25mg/100mg tablets | 100 tablet [PoM] £26.99 DT price = £14.75
Carbidopa (as Carbidopa monohydrate) 25 mg, Levodopa 250 mg Co-careldopa 25mg/250mg tablets | 100 tablet [PoM] £35.00 DT price = £34.98
‣ Sinemet (Merck Sharp & Dohme Ltd)
Carbidopa (as Carbidopa monohydrate) 12.5 mg, Levodopa 50 mg Sinemet 12.5mg/50mg tablets | 90 tablet [PoM] £6.28 DT price = £6.28
Carbidopa (as Carbidopa monohydrate) 10 mg, Levodopa 100 mg Sinemet 10mg/100mg tablets | 100 tablet [PoM] £7.30 DT price = £7.95
Carbidopa (as Carbidopa monohydrate) 25 mg, Levodopa 250 mg Sinemet 25mg/250mg tablets | 100 tablet [PoM] £18.29 DT price = £34.98
‣ Sinemet Plus (Merck Sharp & Dohme Ltd)
Carbidopa (as Carbidopa monohydrate) 25 mg, Levodopa 100 mg Sinemet Plus 25mg/100mg tablets | 100 tablet [PoM] £12.88 DT price = £14.75

MUSCLE RELAXANTS > PERIPHERALLY ACTING > NEUROTOXINS (BOTULINUM TOXINS)

Botulinum toxin type A

24-Apr-2017

● **INDICATIONS AND DOSE**
Dynamic equinus foot deformity caused by spasticity in ambulant paediatric cerebral palsy
‣ **Child 2–17 years:** (consult product literature)
DOSE EQUIVALENCE AND CONVERSION
‣ **Important:** information is specific to each individual preparation.

● **CONTRA-INDICATIONS** Generalised disorders of muscle activity · infection at injection site · myasthenia gravis

● **CAUTIONS** Atrophy in target muscle · chronic respiratory disorder · excessive weakness in target muscle · history of aspiration · history of dysphagia · inflammation in target muscle · neurological disorders · neuromuscular disorders · off-label use (fatal adverse events reported)
CAUTIONS, FURTHER INFORMATION
Neuromuscular or neurological disorders can lead to increased sensitivity and exaggerated muscle weakness including dysphagia and respiratory compromise.

- **INTERACTIONS** → Appendix 1: botulinum toxin type A
- **SIDE-EFFECTS**
  GENERAL SIDE-EFFECTS
  ▸ **Common or very common** Excessive doses may paralyse distant muscles · increased electrophysiologic jitter in some distant muscles · influenza-like symptoms · misplaced injections may paralyse nearby muscle groups
  ▸ **Rare** Anaphylaxis · antibody formation (substantial deterioration in response) · arrhythmias · hypersensitivity reactions · myocardial infarction · pruritus · rash · seizures
  ▸ **Very rare** Aspiration · dysphagia · dysphonia · exaggerated muscle weakness · respiratory disorders
  SPECIFIC SIDE-EFFECTS
  ▸ **Common or very common**
  ▸ **When used for paediatric cerebral palsy** Abnormal gait · drowsiness · malaise · myalgia · pain in extremities · paraesthesia · urinary incontinence
  ▸ **When used for spasmodic torticollis** Weakness
- **CONCEPTION AND CONTRACEPTION** Avoid in women of child-bearing age unless using effective contraception.
- **PREGNANCY** Avoid unless essential—toxicity in *animal* studies (manufacturer of *Botox*® advises avoid).
- **BREAST FEEDING** Low risk of systemic absorption but avoid unless essential.
- **PRESCRIBING AND DISPENSING INFORMATION** Preparations are not interchangeable.
- **PATIENT AND CARER ADVICE**
  Medicines for Children leaflet: Botulinum toxin for muscle spasticity www.medicinesforchildren.org.uk/botulinum-toxin-muscle-spasticity-0
  Patients and carers should be warned of the signs and symptoms of toxin spread, such as muscle weakness and breathing difficulties; they should be advised to seek immediate medical attention if swallowing, speech or breathing difficulties occur.

- **MEDICINAL FORMS**
  There can be variation in the licensing of different medicines containing the same drug.
  Powder for solution for injection
  ▸ **Azzalure** (Galderma (UK) Ltd)
  Botulinum toxin type A 125 unit Azzalure 125unit powder for solution for injection vials | 1 vial PoM £64.00 | 2 vial PoM £128.00
  ▸ **Bocouture** (Merz Pharma UK Ltd)
  Botulinum toxin type A 50 unit Bocouture 50unit powder for solution for injection vials | 1 vial PoM £72.00
  Botulinum toxin type A 100 unit Bocouture 100unit powder for solution for injection vials | 1 vial PoM £229.90
  ▸ **Botox** (Allergan Ltd)
  Botulinum toxin type A 50 unit Botox 50unit powder for solution for injection vials | 1 vial PoM £77.50
  Botulinum toxin type A 100 unit Botox 100unit powder for solution for injection vials | 1 vial PoM £138.20
  Botulinum toxin type A 200 unit Botox 200unit powder for solution for injection vials | 1 vial PoM £276.40
  ▸ **Dysport** (Ipsen Ltd)
  Botulinum toxin type A 300 unit Dysport 300unit powder for solution for injection vials | 1 vial PoM £92.40
  Botulinum toxin type A 500 unit Dysport 500unit powder for solution for injection vials | 2 vial PoM £308.00
  ▸ **Xeomin** (Merz Pharma UK Ltd)
  Botulinum toxin type A 50 unit Xeomin 50unit powder for solution for injection vials | 1 vial PoM £72.00
  Botulinum toxin type A 100 unit Xeomin 100unit powder for solution for injection vials | 1 vial PoM £129.90
  Botulinum toxin type A 200 unit Xeomin 200unit powder for solution for injection vials | 1 vial PoM £259.80 (Hospital only)

4 Nausea and labyrinth disorders

Nausea and labyrinth disorders

Drug treatment

Antiemetics should be prescribed only when the cause of vomiting is known because otherwise they may delay diagnosis, particularly in children. Antiemetics are unnecessary and sometimes harmful when the cause can be treated, such as in diabetic ketoacidosis, or in digoxin p. 79 or antiepileptic overdose.

If antiemetic drug treatment is indicated, the drug is chosen according to the aetiology of vomiting.

Antihistamines are effective against nausea and vomiting resulting from many underlying conditions. There is no evidence that any one antihistamine is superior to another but their duration of action and incidence of adverse effects (drowsiness and antimuscarinic effects) differ.

The **phenothiazines** are dopamine antagonists and act centrally by blocking the chemoreceptor trigger zone. They are of considerable value for the prophylaxis and treatment of nausea and vomiting associated with diffuse neoplastic disease, radiation sickness, and the emesis caused by drugs such as opioids, general anaesthetics, and cytotoxics. Prochlorperazine p. 258, perphenazine p. 238, and trifluoperazine p. 239 are less sedating than chlorpromazine hydrochloride p. 236; severe dystonic reactions sometimes occur with phenothiazines. Some phenothiazines are available as rectal suppositories, which can be useful in children with persistent vomiting or with severe nausea; for children over 12 years prochlorperazine can also be administered as a buccal tablet which is placed between the upper lip and the gum.

Other antipsychotic drugs including haloperidol p. 237 and levomepromazine p. 257 are used for the relief of nausea in palliative care.

Metoclopramide hydrochloride p. 252 is an effective antiemetic and its activity closely resembles that of the phenothiazines. Metoclopramide hydrochloride also acts directly on the gastro-intestinal tract and it may be superior to the phenothiazines for emesis associated with gastroduodenal, hepatic, and biliary disease. Due to the risk of neurological side effects, metoclopramide hydrochloride should only be used in children as second line therapy in postoperative and cytotoxic induced nausea and vomiting.

Domperidone p. 251 acts at the chemoreceptor trigger zone; it has the advantage over metoclopramide hydrochloride and the phenothiazines of being less likely to cause central effects such as sedation and dystonic reactions because it does not readily cross the blood-brain barrier.

Granisetron p. 253 and ondansetron p. 253 are specific $5HT_3$-receptor antagonists which block $5HT_3$ receptors in the gastro-intestinal tract and in the CNS. They are of value in the management of nausea and vomiting in children receiving cytotoxics and in postoperative nausea and vomiting.

Nabilone p. 251 is a synthetic cannabinoid with antiemetic properties. It may be used for nausea and vomiting caused by cytotoxic chemotherapy that is unresponsive to conventional antiemetics.

Dexamethasone p. 419 has antiemetic effects. Dexamethasone may also have a role in cytotoxic-induced nausea and vomiting.

Vomiting during pregnancy

Nausea in the first trimester of pregnancy is generally mild and does not require drug therapy. On rare occasions if vomiting is severe, short-term treatment with an antihistamine, such as **promethazine**, may be required. Prochlorperazine or metoclopramide hydrochloride are alternatives. If symptoms do not settle in 24 to 48 hours then specialist opinion should be sought. Hyperemesis gravidarum is a more serious condition, which requires regular antiemetic therapy, intravenous fluid and electrolyte replacement and sometimes nutritional support. Supplementation with thiamine p. 601 must be considered in order to reduce the risk of Wernicke's encephalopathy.

Postoperative nausea and vomiting

The incidence of postoperative nausea and vomiting depends on many factors including the anaesthetic used, and the type and duration of surgery. Other risk factors include female sex, non-smokers, a history of postoperative nausea and vomiting or motion sickness, and intraoperative and postoperative use of opioids. Therapy to prevent postoperative nausea and vomiting should be based on the assessed risk. Drugs used include **5HT₃-receptor antagonists**, droperidol p. 257, dexamethasone, some **phenothiazines** (e.g. prochlorperazine), and **antihistamines** (e.g. cyclizine below). A combination of two or more antiemetic drugs that have different mechanisms of action is often indicated in those at high risk of postoperative nausea and vomiting or where postoperative vomiting presents a particular danger (e.g. in some types of surgery). When a prophylactic antiemetic drug has failed, postoperative nausea and vomiting should be treated with one or more drugs from a different class.

Opioid-induced nausea and vomiting

Cyclizine, ondansetron, and prochlorperazine are used to relieve opioid-induced nausea and vomiting; ondansetron has the advantage of not producing sedation.

Motion sickness

Antiemetics should be given to prevent motion sickness rather than after nausea or vomiting develop. The most effective drug for the prevention of motion sickness is hyoscine hydrobromide p. 256. For children over 10 years old, a transdermal hyoscine patch provides prolonged activity but it needs to be applied several hours before travelling. The sedating antihistamines are slightly less effective against motion sickness, but are generally better tolerated than hyoscine. If a sedative effect is desired **promethazine** is useful, but generally a slightly less sedating antihistamine such as cyclizine or cinnarizine p. 255 is preferred. Domperidone, metoclopramide hydrochloride, 5HT₃-receptor antagonists, and the phenothiazines (except the antihistamine phenothiazine promethazine) are **ineffective** in motion sickness.

Other vestibular disorders

Management of vestibular diseases is aimed at treating the underlying cause as well as treating symptoms of the balance disturbance and associated nausea and vomiting. **Antihistamines** (such as cinnarizine), and **phenothiazines** (such as prochlorperazine) are effective for prophylaxis and treatment of nausea and vertigo resulting from vestibular disorders; however, when nausea and vertigo are associated with middle ear surgery, treatment can be difficult.

Cytotoxic chemotherapy, palliative care, and migraine

Antiemetics have a role in the management of nausea and vomiting induced by cytotoxic chemotherapy, in palliative care, and associated with migraine.

Other drugs used for Nausea and labyrinth disorders
Promethazine hydrochloride, p. 174

ANTIEMETICS AND ANTINAUSEANTS ›
ANTIHISTAMINES

Cyclizine

● **INDICATIONS AND DOSE**

Nausea and vomiting of known cause | Nausea and vomiting associated with vestibular disorders and palliative care

▸ BY MOUTH, OR BY INTRAVENOUS INJECTION
- Child 1 month–5 years: 0.5–1 mg/kg up to 3 times a day (max. per dose 25 mg), intravenous injection to be given over 3–5 minutes, for motion sickness, take 1–2 hours before departure
- Child 6–11 years: 25 mg up to 3 times a day, intravenous injection to be given over 3–5 minutes, for motion sickness, take 1–2 hours before departure
- Child 12–17 years: 50 mg up to 3 times a day, intravenous injection to be given over 3–5 minutes, for motion sickness, take 1–2 hours before departure

▸ BY RECTUM
- Child 2–5 years: 12.5 mg up to 3 times a day
- Child 6–11 years: 25 mg up to 3 times a day
- Child 12–17 years: 50 mg up to 3 times a day

▸ BY CONTINUOUS INTRAVENOUS INFUSION, OR BY SUBCUTANEOUS INFUSION
- Child 1–23 months: 3 mg/kg, dose to be given over 24 hours
- Child 2–5 years: 50 mg, dose to be given over 24 hours
- Child 6–11 years: 75 mg, dose to be given over 24 hours
- Child 12–17 years: 150 mg, dose to be given over 24 hours

● **UNLICENSED USE** Tablets not licensed for use in children under 6 years. Injection not licensed for use in children.

● **CONTRA-INDICATIONS** Avoid in acute porphyrias p. 577 (some antihistamines are thought to be safe) · neonate (due to significant antimuscarinic activity)

● **CAUTIONS** Epilepsy · glaucoma · may counteract haemodynamic benefits of opioids · neuromuscular disorders—increased risk of transient paralysis with intravenous use · pyloroduodenal obstruction · severe heart failure—may cause fall in cardiac output and associated increase in heart rate, mean arterial pressure and pulmonary wedge pressure · urinary retention

● **INTERACTIONS** → Appendix 1: antihistamines (sedating)

● **SIDE-EFFECTS**

GENERAL SIDE-EFFECTS
▸ **Common or very common** Drowsiness
▸ **Rare** Anaphylaxis · angioedema · angle-closure glaucoma · arrhythmias · blood disorders · bronchospasm · confusion · convulsions · depression · dizziness · extrapyramidal effects · hypersensitivity reactions · hypotension · liver dysfunction · palpitation · paradoxical stimulation (especially with high doses in children) · photosensitivity reactions · rashes · sleep disturbances · tremor
▸ **Frequency not known** Antimuscarinic effects · blurred vision · dry mouth · gastro-intestinal disturbances · hallucinations · headache · hypertension · movement disorders · oculogyric crisis · paraesthesia · psychomotor impairment · tachycardia · transient speech disorders · twitching · urinary retention

SPECIFIC SIDE-EFFECTS
▸ **Rare**
▸ With intravenous use Transient paralysis
▸ **Frequency not known**
▸ With subcutaneous use Local irritation

SIDE-EFFECTS, FURTHER INFORMATION
Children are more susceptible to side-effects.

Drowsiness is a significant side-effect with most of the older antihistamines although paradoxical stimulation may occur rarely in children, especially with high doses. Drowsiness may diminish after a few days of treatment and is considerably less of a problem with the newer antihistamines.

- **PREGNANCY** Manufacturer advises avoid; however, there is no evidence of teratogenicity. The use of sedating antihistamines in the latter part of the third trimester may cause adverse effects in neonates such as irritability, paradoxical excitability, and tremor.
- **BREAST FEEDING** No information available. Most antihistamines are present in breast milk in varying amounts; although not known to be harmful, most manufacturers advise avoiding their use in mothers who are breast-feeding.
- **HEPATIC IMPAIRMENT** Avoid in severe liver disease—increased risk of coma.
- **DIRECTIONS FOR ADMINISTRATION** For administration *by mouth*, tablets may be crushed.
  Mixing and compatibility for the use of syringe drivers in palliative care Cyclizine may precipitate at concentrations above 10 mg/mL or in the presence of sodium chloride 0.9% *or* as the concentration of diamorphine relative to cyclizine increases; mixtures of diamorphine and cyclizine are also likely to precipitate after 24 hours.
- **PATIENT AND CARER ADVICE**
  Driving and skilled tasks
  Drowsiness may affect performance of skilled tasks (e.g. cycling, driving); effects of alcohol enhanced.

- **MEDICINAL FORMS**
  There can be variation in the licensing of different medicines containing the same drug. Forms available from special-order manufacturers include: oral suspension, oral solution, suppository
  Tablet
  CAUTIONARY AND ADVISORY LABELS 2
  ▸ Cyclizine (Non-proprietary)
  Cyclizine hydrochloride 50 mg Cyclizine 50mg tablets |
  30 tablet P £2.19–£5.00 | 100 tablet P £13.64 DT price = £7.29
  Solution for injection
  ▸ Cyclizine (Non-proprietary)
  Cyclizine lactate 50 mg per 1 ml Cyclizine 50mg/1ml solution for injection ampoules | 5 ampoule PoM £13.54 DT price = £13.54

ANTIEMETICS AND ANTINAUSEANTS ⟩
CANNIBINOIDS

Nabilone

- **INDICATIONS AND DOSE**
  Nausea and vomiting caused by cytotoxic chemotherapy, unresponsive to conventional antiemetics (preferably in hospital setting) (under close medical supervision)
  ▸ BY MOUTH
  ▸ Child: (consult local protocol)

- **UNLICENSED USE** Not licensed for use in children.
- **CAUTIONS** Adverse effects on mental state can persist for 48–72 hours after stopping · heart disease · history of psychiatric disorder · hypertension
- **INTERACTIONS** → Appendix 1: nabilone
- **SIDE-EFFECTS**
- ▸ Common or very common Ataxia · concentration difficulties · drowsiness · dry mouth · dysphoria · euphoria · headache · hypotension · nausea · sleep disturbance · vertigo · visual disturbance
- ▸ Frequency not known Abdominal pain · confusion · decreased appetite · decreased coordination · depression ·

disorientation · hallucinations · psychosis · tachycardia · tremors

SIDE-EFFECTS, FURTHER INFORMATION
Drowsiness and dizziness occur frequently with standard doses.

- **PREGNANCY** Avoid unless essential.
- **BREAST FEEDING** Avoid—no information available.
- **HEPATIC IMPAIRMENT** Avoid in severe impairment.
- **PATIENT AND CARER ADVICE**
  Behavioural effects Patients should be made aware of possible changes of mood and other adverse behavioural effects.

  Driving and skilled tasks
  Drowsiness may affect performance of skilled tasks (e.g. driving). Effects of alcohol enhanced.
  For information on 2015 legislation regarding driving whilst taking certain controlled drugs, including nabilone, see *Drugs and skilled tasks* under Guidance on prescribing p. 1.

- **MEDICINAL FORMS**
  There can be variation in the licensing of different medicines containing the same drug. Forms available from special-order manufacturers include: capsule
  Capsule
  CAUTIONARY AND ADVISORY LABELS 2
  ▸ Nabilone(Non-proprietary)
    Nabilone 250 microgram Nabilone 250 microgram capsules |
    20 capsule PoM £185.00 CD2 Nabilone 1 mg capsule |
    20 capsule PoM £196.00 CD2

ANTIEMETICS AND ANTINAUSEANTS ⟩
DOPAMINE RECEPTOR ANTAGONISTS

Domperidone
17-Oct-2016

- **INDICATIONS AND DOSE**
  Relief of nausea and vomiting
  ▸ BY MOUTH
  ▸ Child (body-weight up to 35 kg): 250 micrograms/kg up to 3 times a day; maximum 750 micrograms/kg per day
  ▸ Child 12-17 years (body-weight 35 kg and above): 10 mg up to 3 times a day; maximum 30 mg per day

  Gastro-oesophageal reflux disease (but efficacy not proven)
  ▸ BY MOUTH

  ▸ Neonate: 250 micrograms/kg 3 times a day, dose can be increased if response inadequate, increased if necessary up to 400 micrograms/kg 3 times a day, interrupt treatment occasionally to assess recurrence—consider restarting if symptoms recur, discontinue if response inadequate at higher dose.

  ▸ Child: 250 micrograms/kg 3 times a day (max. per dose 10 mg), dose can be increased if response inadequate, increased if necessary up to 400 micrograms/kg 3 times a day (max. per dose 20 mg), interrupt treatment occasionally to assess recurrence—consider restarting if symptoms recur, if response inadequate at higher dose

- **UNLICENSED USE** Not licensed for use in children for gastro-oesophageal reflux disease.

IMPORTANT SAFETY INFORMATION
MHRA/CHM ADVICE—DOMPERIDONE: RISK OF CARDIAC SIDE-EFFECTS—RESTRICTED INDICATION, NEW CONTRA-INDICATIONS, REDUCED DOSE AND DURATION OF USE
The benefits and risks of domperidone have been reviewed. As domperidone is associated with a small increased risk of serious cardiac side-effects, the following restrictions to indication, dose and duration of

4

Nervous system

treatment have been made, and new contra-indications added:

- Domperidone should only be used for the relief of the symptoms of nausea and vomiting;
- Domperidone should be used at the lowest effective dose for the shortest possible duration (max. treatment duration should not normally exceed 1 week);
- Domperidone is contra-indicated for use in conditions where cardiac conduction is, or could be impaired, or where there is underlying cardiac disease, when administered concomitantly with drugs that prolong the QT interval or potent CYP3A4 inhibitors, and in severe hepatic impairment;
- The recommended dose in adults and adolescents over 12 years and over 35 kg is 10 mg up to 3 times daily;
- The recommended dose in children under 35 kg is 250 micrograms/kg up to 3 times daily;
- Oral liquid formulations should be given via an appropriately designed, graduated oral syringe to ensure dose accuracy.

This advice does not apply to unlicensed uses of domperidone (e.g. palliative care).

- **CONTRA-INDICATIONS** Cardiac disease · gastro-intestinal haemorrhage · mechanical obstruction · mechanical perforation · predisposition to cardiac conduction disorders · prolactinoma
- **CAUTIONS** Children · if there are cardiac concerns, obtain ECG before and during treatment
- **INTERACTIONS** → Appendix 1: domperidone
- **SIDE-EFFECTS**
- **Common or very common** Drowsiness · dry mouth · malaise
- **Uncommon** Anxiety · breast pain · decreased libido · diarrhoea · galactorrhoea · headache · pruritus · rash
- **Frequency not known** Agitation · amenorrhoea · convulsions · extrapyramidal disorders · gynaecomastia · nervousness · oculogyric crisis · QT-interval prolongation · sudden cardiac death · urinary retention · ventricular arrhythmias
- **PREGNANCY** Use only if potential benefit outweighs risk.
- **BREAST FEEDING** Amount too small to be harmful.
- **HEPATIC IMPAIRMENT** Avoid in moderate or severe impairment.
- **RENAL IMPAIRMENT** Reduce frequency.
- **PATIENT AND CARER ADVICE**
Arrhythmia Patients and their carers should be told how to recognise signs of arrhythmia and advised to seek medical attention if symptoms such as palpitation or syncope develop.
Medicines for Children leaflet: Domperidone for gastro-oesophageal reflux www.medicinesforchildren.org.uk/domperidone-for-gastro-oesophageal-reflux

- **MEDICINAL FORMS**
There can be variation in the licensing of different medicines containing the same drug. Forms available from special-order manufacturers include: oral suspension

Oral suspension
CAUTIONARY AND ADVISORY LABELS 22
- Domperidone (non-proprietary) ▼
Domperidone 1 mg per 1 ml Domperidone 5mg/5ml oral suspension sugar free sugar-free | 200 ml [PoM] £13.43 DT price = £13.43

Tablet
CAUTIONARY AND ADVISORY LABELS 22
- Domperidone (non-proprietary) ▼
Domperidone (as Domperidone maleate) 10 mg Domperidone 10mg tablets | 30 tablet [PoM] £2.71 DT price = £0.71 | 100 tablet [PoM] £9.04 DT price = £2.37

- Motilium (Zentiva) ▼
Domperidone (as Domperidone maleate 10 mg Motilium 10mg tablets | 30 tablet [PoM] £2.71 DT price = £0.71 | 100 tablet [PoM] £9.04 DT price = £2.37

Metoclopramide hydrochloride   21-Nov-2016

- **INDICATIONS AND DOSE**

Second-line option for treatment of established postoperative nausea and vomiting; Prevention of delayed chemotherapy-induced nausea and vomiting
- BY MOUTH, OR BY INTRAMUSCULAR INJECTION, OR BY INTRAVENOUS INJECTION
- Child: 100–150 micrograms/kg up to 3 times a day (max. per dose 10 mg), when administered by slow intravenous injection, to be given over at least 3 minutes

- **UNLICENSED USE** Maxolon® tablets not licensed for use in children.

> **IMPORTANT SAFETY INFORMATION**
>
> MHRA/CHM ADVICE—METOCLOPRAMIDE: RISK OF NEUROLOGICAL ADVERSE EFFECTS—RESTRICTED DOSE AND DURATION OF USE (AUGUST 2013)
>
> The benefits and risks of metoclopramide have been reviewed by the European Medicines Agency's Committee on Medicinal Products for Human Use, which concluded that the risk of neurological effects such as extrapyramidal disorders and tardive dyskinesia outweigh the benefits in long-term or high-dose treatment. To help minimise the risk of potentially serious neurological adverse effects, the following restrictions to indications, dose and duration of use have been made:
>
> - In children aged 1–18 years, metoclopramide should only be used as a second-line option for prevention of delayed chemotherapy-induced nausea and vomiting and for treatment of established postoperative nausea and vomiting;
> - Use of metoclopramide is contra-indicated in children aged under 1 year;
> - Metoclopramide should only be prescribed for short-term use (up to 5 days);
> - Recommended dose is 100–150 micrograms/kg (max. 10 mg), repeated up to 3 times daily;
> - Intravenous doses should be administered as a slow bolus over at least 3 minutes;
> - Oral liquid formulations should be given via an appropriately designed, graduated oral syringe to ensure dose accuracy.
>
> This advice does not apply to unlicensed uses of metoclopramide (e.g. palliative care).

- **CONTRA-INDICATIONS** 3–4 days after gastrointestinal surgery · gastro-intestinal haemorrhage · gastro-intestinal obstruction · gastro-intestinal perforation · phaeochromocytoma
- **CAUTIONS** Asthma · atopic allergy · bradycardia · cardiac conduction disturbances · epilepsy · may mask underlying disorders such as cerebral irritation · uncorrected electrolyte imbalance
- **INTERACTIONS** → Appendix 1: metoclopramide
- **SIDE-EFFECTS**
GENERAL SIDE-EFFECTS
- **Common or very common** Extrapyramidal effects · galactorrhoea · gynaecomastia · hyperprolactinaemia · menstrual changes
- **Very rare** Depression · methaemoglobinaemia (more severe in G6PD deficiency) · neuroleptic malignant syndrome

▸ **Frequency not known** Anxiety · confusion · diarrhoea · dizziness · drowsiness · dyspnoea · hypotension · oedema · pruritus · rash · restlessness · tardive dyskinesia on prolonged administration · tremor · urticaria · visual disturbances

SPECIFIC SIDE-EFFECTS
▸ **Very rare**
▸ **With intravenous use** Cardiac conduction abnormalities

SIDE-EFFECTS, FURTHER INFORMATION
▸ Acute dystonic reactions Metoclopramide can induce acute dystonic reactions such as facial and skeletal muscle spasms and oculogyric crises; children (especially girls, young women, and those under 10 kg) are particularly susceptible. With metoclopramide, dystonic effects usually occur shortly after starting treatment and subside within 24 hours of stopping it. An antimuscarinic drug such as procyclidine is used to abort dystonic attacks.

● **PREGNANCY** Not known to be harmful.
● **BREAST FEEDING** Small amount present in milk; avoid.
● **HEPATIC IMPAIRMENT** Reduce dose.
● **RENAL IMPAIRMENT** Avoid or use small dose in severe impairment; increased risk of extrapyramidal reactions.
● **DIRECTIONS FOR ADMINISTRATION** Oral liquid preparation to be given via a graduated oral dosing syringe.
● **PATIENT AND CARER ADVICE** Counselling on use of pipette advised with oral solution.

● **MEDICINAL FORMS**
There can be variation in the licensing of different medicines containing the same drug. Forms available from special-order manufacturers include: oral solution

Solution for injection
▸ **Metoclopramide hydrochloride (Non-proprietary)**
  Metoclopramide hydrochloride 5 mg per 1 ml Metoclopramide 10mg/2ml solution for injection ampoules | 5 ampoule PoM £1.31 | 10 ampoule PoM £3.30 DT price = £3.30
▸ **Maxolon (AMCo)**
  Metoclopramide hydrochloride 5 mg per 1 ml Maxolon 10mg/2ml solution for injection ampoules | 12 ampoule PoM £3.21
  Maxolon High Dose 100mg/20ml solution for injection ampoules | 10 ampoule PoM £26.68

Oral solution
▸ **Metoclopramide hydrochloride (Non-proprietary)**
  Metoclopramide hydrochloride 1 mg per 1 ml Metoclopramide 5mg/5ml oral solution sugar free sugar-free | 150 ml PoM £19.77 DT price = £19.77

Tablet
▸ **Metoclopramide hydrochloride (Non-proprietary)**
  Metoclopramide hydrochloride 10 mg Metoclopramide 10mg tablets | 28 tablet PoM £1.40 DT price = £0.72
▸ **Maxolon (AMCo)**
  Metoclopramide hydrochloride 10 mg Maxolon 10mg tablets | 84 tablet PoM £5.24

ANTIEMETICS AND ANTINAUSEANTS ⟩
SEROTONIN (5HT₃) RECEPTOR ANTAGONISTS

▮ Granisetron

● **DRUG ACTION** Granisetron is a specific $5HT_3$-receptor antagonist which blocks $5HT_3$ receptors in the gastro-intestinal tract and in the CNS.

● **INDICATIONS AND DOSE**
Management of nausea and vomiting induced by cytotoxic chemotherapy
▸ BY MOUTH
▸ Child 12–17 years: 1–2 mg, to be taken within 1 hour before start of treatment, then 2 mg daily in 1–2 divided doses for up to 1 week following chemotherapy

▸ BY INTRAVENOUS INFUSION
▸ Child 2–17 years: 10–40 micrograms/kg (max. per dose 3 mg), repeated if necessary, to be given before start of chemotherapy, for treatment, dose may be repeated within 24 hours if necessary, not less than 10 minutes after initial dose; maximum 2 doses per day

● **UNLICENSED USE** Tablets not licensed in children (age range not specified by manufacturer).
● **CAUTIONS** Subacute intestinal obstruction · susceptibility to QT-interval prolongation (including electrolyte disturbances)
● **INTERACTIONS** → Appendix 1: granisetron
● **SIDE-EFFECTS**
▸ **Common or very common** Constipation · diarrhoea · headache · insomnia
▸ **Uncommon** Extrapyramidal reactions · QT-interval prolongation · rash
● **PREGNANCY** Manufacturer advises avoid.
● **BREAST FEEDING** Avoid—no information available.
● **HEPATIC IMPAIRMENT** Manufacturer advises use with caution.
● **DIRECTIONS FOR ADMINISTRATION** For *intravenous infusion*, dilute up to 3 mL of granisetron injection in Glucose 5% or Sodium Chloride 0.9% to a total volume of 10–30 mL; give over 5 minutes.

● **MEDICINAL FORMS**
There can be variation in the licensing of different medicines containing the same drug.
Solution for injection
▸ Granisetron (Non-proprietary)
  Granisetron (as Granisetron hydrochloride) 1 mg per 1 ml Granisetron 3mg/3ml concentrate for solution for injection ampoules | 5 ampoule PoM £24.00
  Granisetron 1mg/1ml concentrate for solution for injection ampoules | 5 ampoule PoM £8.00
Tablet
▸ Granisetron (Non-proprietary)
  Granisetron (as Granisetron hydrochloride) 1 mg Granisetron 1mg tablets | 10 tablet PoM £51.20 DT price = £40.77
  Granisetron (as Granisetron hydrochloride) 2 mg Granisetron 2mg tablets | 5 tablet PoM no price available DT price = £52.39
▸ Kytril (Roche Products Ltd)
  Granisetron (as Granisetron hydrochloride) 1 mg Kytril 1mg tablets | 10 tablet PoM £52.39 DT price = £40.77
  Granisetron (as Granisetron hydrochloride) 2 mg Kytril 2mg tablets | 5 tablet PoM £52.39 DT price = £52.39

▮ Ondansetron

● **DRUG ACTION** Ondansetron is a specific $5HT_3$-receptor antagonist which blocks $5HT_3$ receptors in the gastro-intestinal tract and in the CNS.

● **INDICATIONS AND DOSE**
Prevention of postoperative nausea and vomiting
▸ BY SLOW INTRAVENOUS INJECTION
▸ Child: 100 micrograms/kg (max. per dose 4 mg) for 1 dose, dose to be given over at least 30 seconds before, during, or after induction of anaesthesia
Treatment of postoperative nausea and vomiting
▸ BY SLOW INTRAVENOUS INJECTION
▸ Child: 100 micrograms/kg (max. per dose 4 mg) for 1 dose, dose to be given over at least 30 seconds
Prevention and treatment of chemotherapy- and radiotherapy-induced nausea and vomiting—initial dose
▸ BY INTRAVENOUS INFUSION
▸ Child 6 months–17 years (body surface area up to 1.3 m²): 5 mg/m² for 1 dose then give orally, alternatively 150 micrograms/kg continued →

4

Nervous system

(max. per dose 8 mg), dose to be administered immediately before chemotherapy, then 150 micrograms/kg every 4 hours (max. per dose 8 mg) for 2 further doses then give orally; maximum 32 mg per day
▸ Child 6 months-17 years (body surface area 1.3 m² and above): 8 mg for 1 dose then give orally, alternatively 150 micrograms/kg (max. per dose 8 mg), dose to be administered immediately before chemotherapy, then 150 micrograms/kg every 4 hours (max. per dose 8 mg) for 2 further doses then give orally, intravenous infusion to be administered over at least 15 minutes; maximum 32 mg per day

Prevention and treatment of chemotherapy- and radiotherapy-induced nausea and vomiting–(follow-on dose based on body surface area)
▸ BY MOUTH
▸ Child 6 months-17 years (body surface area up to 0.6 m²): 2 mg every 12 hours for up to 5 days (dose can be started 12 hours after intravenous administration); maximum 32 mg per day
▸ Child 6 months-17 years (body surface area 0.6-1.2 m²): 4 mg every 12 hours for up to 5 days (dose can be started 12 hours after intravenous administration); maximum 32 mg per day
▸ Child 6 months-17 years (body surface area 1.3 m² and above): 8 mg every 12 hours for up to 5 days (dose can be started 12 hours after intravenous administration); maximum 32 mg per day

Prevention and treatment of chemotherapy- and radiotherapy-induced nausea and vomiting–(follow-on dose based on body-weight)
▸ BY MOUTH
▸ Child 6 months-17 years (body-weight up to 10.1 kg): 2 mg every 12 hours for up to 5 days (dose can be started 12 hours after intravenous administration); maximum 32 mg per day
▸ Child 6 months-17 years (body-weight 10.1-40 kg): 4 mg every 12 hours for up to 5 days (dose can be started 12 hours after intravenous administration); maximum 32 mg per day
▸ Child 6 months-17 years (body-weight 41 kg and above): 8 mg every 12 hours for up to 5 days (dose can be started 12 hours after intravenous administration); maximum 32 mg per day

● UNLICENSED USE Not licensed for radiotherapy-induced nausea and vomiting in children.
● CONTRA-INDICATIONS Congenital long QT syndrome
● CAUTIONS Adenotonsillar surgery · subacute intestinal obstruction · susceptibility to QT-interval prolongation (including electrolyte disturbances)
● INTERACTIONS → Appendix 1: ondansetron
● SIDE-EFFECTS
GENERAL SIDE-EFFECTS
▸ **Common or very common** Constipation · flushing · headache · injection site-reactions
▸ **Uncommon** Arrhythmias · bradycardia · chest pain · hiccups · hypotension · movement disorders · seizures
SPECIFIC SIDE-EFFECTS
▸ **Rare**
▸ With intravenous use Dizziness · transient visual disturbances
▸ **Very rare**
▸ With intravenous use Transient blindness
● PREGNANCY No information available; avoid unless potential benefit outweighs risk.
● BREAST FEEDING Present in milk in *animal* studies—avoid.
● HEPATIC IMPAIRMENT Reduce dose in moderate or severe impairment.

● DIRECTIONS FOR ADMINISTRATION
▸ With intravenous use For *intravenous infusion*, dilute to a concentration of 320–640 micrograms/mL with Glucose 5% or Sodium Chloride 0.9%; give over at least 15 minutes.
▸ With oral use Orodispersible films and lyophilisates should be placed on the tongue, allowed to disperse and swallowed.
● PRESCRIBING AND DISPENSING INFORMATION Flavours of oral liquid formulations may include strawberry.
● PATIENT AND CARER ADVICE Patients or carers should be given advice on how to administer orodispersible films and lyophilisates.

● MEDICINAL FORMS
There can be variation in the licensing of different medicines containing the same drug. Forms available from special-order manufacturers include: oral suspension, oral solution

Tablet
▸ Ondansetron (Non-proprietary)
Ondansetron (as Ondansetron hydrochloride) 4 mg Ondansetron 4mg tablets | 10 tablet [PoM] £25.46 DT price = £1.04 | 30 tablet [PoM] £76.38
Ondansetron (as Ondansetron hydrochloride) 8 mg Ondansetron 8mg tablets | 10 tablet [PoM] £47.99 DT price = £1.90
▸ Ondemet (Alliance Pharmaceuticals Ltd)
Ondansetron (as Ondansetron hydrochloride) 4 mg Ondemet 4mg tablets | 30 tablet [PoM] £81.15
Ondansetron (as Ondansetron hydrochloride) 8 mg Ondemet 8mg tablets | 10 tablet [PoM] £54.36 DT price = £1.90 (Hospital only)
▸ Zofran (Novartis Pharmaceuticals UK Ltd)
Ondansetron (as Ondansetron hydrochloride) 4 mg Zofran 4mg tablets | 30 tablet [PoM] £107.91
Ondansetron (as Ondansetron hydrochloride) 8 mg Zofran 8mg tablets | 10 tablet [PoM] £71.94 DT price = £1.90

Solution for injection
▸ Ondansetron (Non-proprietary)
Ondansetron (as Ondansetron hydrochloride) 2 mg per 1 ml Ondansetron 8mg/4ml solution for injection ampoules | 5 ampoule [PoM] £58.45
Ondansetron 4mg/2ml solution for injection ampoules | 5 ampoule [PoM] £38.33 | 10 ampoule [PoM] £7.50
▸ Zofran Flexi-amp (Novartis Pharmaceuticals UK Ltd)
Ondansetron (as Ondansetron hydrochloride) 2 mg per 1 ml Zofran Flexi-amp 8mg/4ml solution for injection | 5 ampoule [PoM] £59.95
Zofran Flexi-amp 4mg/2ml solution for injection | 5 ampoule [PoM] £29.97

Oral solution
▸ Ondansetron (Non-proprietary)
Ondansetron (as Ondansetron hydrochloride) 800 microgram per 1 ml Ondansetron 4mg/5ml oral solution sugar free sugar-free | 50 ml [PoM] £39.00 DT price = £3.68
▸ Zofran (Novartis Pharmaceuticals UK Ltd)
Ondansetron (as Ondansetron hydrochloride) 800 microgram per 1 ml Zofran 4mg/5ml syrup sugar-free | 50 ml [PoM] £35.97 DT price = £38.68

Orodispersible film
▸ Setofilm (Norgine Pharmaceuticals Ltd)
Ondansetron 4 mg Setofilm 4mg orodispersible films sugar-free | 10 film [PoM] £28.50
Ondansetron 8 mg Setofilm 8mg orodispersible films sugar-free | 10 film [PoM] £57.00

Oral lyophilisate
EXCIPIENTS: May contain Aspartame
▸ Zofran Melt (Novartis Pharmaceuticals UK Ltd)
Ondansetron 4 mg Zofran Melt 4mg oral lyophilisates sugar-free | 10 tablet [PoM] £35.97 DT price = £35.97
Ondansetron 8 mg Zofran Melt 8mg oral lyophilisates sugar-free | 10 tablet [PoM] £71.94 DT price = £71.94

Orodispersible tablet
▸ Ondansetron (Non-proprietary)
Ondansetron 4 mg Ondansetron 4mg orodispersible tablets | 10 tablet [PoM] £43.46 DT price = £43.46
Ondansetron 8 mg Ondansetron 8mg orodispersible tablets | 10 tablet [PoM] £85.43 DT price = £85.43

ANTIHISTAMINES > SEDATING

Cinnarizine

- **INDICATIONS AND DOSE**

Relief of symptoms of vestibular disorders, such as vertigo, tinnitus, nausea, and vomiting in Ménière's disease
- BY MOUTH
  - Child 5–11 years: 15 mg 3 times a day
  - Child 12–17 years: 30 mg 3 times a day

Motion sickness
- BY MOUTH
  - Child 5–11 years: Initially 15 mg, dose to be taken 2 hours before travel, then 7.5 mg every 8 hours if required, dose to be taken during journey
  - Child 12–17 years: Initially 30 mg, dose to be taken 2 hours before travel, then 15 mg every 8 hours if required, dose to be taken during journey

- **CONTRA-INDICATIONS** Avoid in acute porphyrias p. 577 (some antihistamines are thought to be safe) · neonate (due to significant antimuscarinic activity)
- **CAUTIONS** Epilepsy · glaucoma · pyloroduodenal obstruction · urinary retention
- **INTERACTIONS** → Appendix 1: antihistamines (sedating)
- **SIDE-EFFECTS**
- **Common or very common** Drowsiness
- **Rare** Anaphylaxis · angioedema · angle-closure glaucoma · arrhythmias · blood disorders · bronchospasm · confusion · convulsions · depression · dizziness · extrapyramidal effects · hypersensitivity reactions · hypotension · lichen planus · liver dysfunction · lupus-like skin reactions · palpitation · paradoxical stimulation (especially with high doses in children) · photosensitivity reactions · rashes · sleep disturbances · sweating · tremor · weight gain
- **Frequency not known** Antimuscarinic effects · blurred vision · dry mouth · gastro-intestinal disturbances · headache · psychomotor impairment · urinary retention
SIDE-EFFECTS, FURTHER INFORMATION
Children are more susceptible to side-effects.
  Drowsiness is a significant side-effect with most of the older antihistamines although paradoxical stimulation may occur rarely in children, especially with high doses. Drowsiness may diminish after a few days of treatment and is considerably less of a problem with the newer antihistamines.
- **PREGNANCY** Manufacturer advises avoid; however, there is no evidence of teratogenicity. The use of sedating antihistamines in the latter part of the third trimester may cause adverse effects in neonates such as irritability, paradoxical excitability, and tremor.
- **BREAST FEEDING** Most antihistamines are present in breast milk in varying amounts; although not known to be harmful, most manufacturers advise avoiding their use in mothers who are breast-feeding.
- **HEPATIC IMPAIRMENT** Avoid in severe liver disease— increased risk of coma.
- **RENAL IMPAIRMENT** Use with caution—no information available.
- **PATIENT AND CARER ADVICE**
  Driving and skilled tasks
  Drowsiness may affect performance of skilled tasks (e.g. cycling, driving); sedating effects enhanced by alcohol.

- **MEDICINAL FORMS**
There can be variation in the licensing of different medicines containing the same drug. Forms available from special-order manufacturers include: oral suspension

Tablet
CAUTIONARY AND ADVISORY LABELS 2
- Cinnarizine (Non-proprietary)
  Cinnarizine 15 mg Cinnarizine 15mg tablets | 84 tablet P £15.40
  DT price = £4.57
- Stugeron (McNeil Products Ltd, Janssen-Cilag Ltd)
  Cinnarizine 15 mg Stugeron 15mg tablets | 15 tablet P £1.84 | 100 tablet P £4.18

Promethazine teoclate

- **INDICATIONS AND DOSE**

Nausea | Vomiting | Labyrinthine disorders
- BY MOUTH
  - Child 5–9 years: 12.5–37.5 mg daily
  - Child 10–17 years: 25–75 mg daily; maximum 100 mg per day

Motion sickness prevention (acts longer than promethazine hydrochloride)
- BY MOUTH
  - Child 5–9 years: 12.5 mg once daily, dose to be taken at bedtime on night before travel or 1–2 hours before travel
  - Child 10–17 years: 25 mg once daily, dose to be taken at bedtime on night before travel or 1–2 hours before travel

Motion sickness treatment (acts longer than promethazine hydrochloride)
- BY MOUTH
  - Child 5–9 years: 12.5 mg, dose to be taken at onset of motion sickness, then 12.5 mg daily for 2 days, dose to be taken at bedtime
  - Child 10–17 years: 25 mg, dose to be taken at onset of motion sickness, then 25 mg once daily for 2 days, dose to be taken at bedtime

> **IMPORTANT SAFETY INFORMATION**
> MHRA/CHM ADVICE (MARCH 2008 AND FEBRUARY 2009) OVER-THE-COUNTER COUGH AND COLD MEDICINES FOR CHILDREN
> Children under 6 years should not be given over-the-counter cough and cold medicines containing promethazine.

- **CONTRA-INDICATIONS** Neonate (due to significant antimuscarinic activity) · should not be given to children under 2 years, except on specialist advice, because the safety of such use has not been established
- **CAUTIONS** Acute porphyrias p. 577 · asthma · bronchiectasis · bronchitis · epilepsy · pyloroduodenal obstruction · Reye's syndrome · severe coronary artery disease · susceptibility to angle-closure glaucoma · urinary retention
- **INTERACTIONS** → Appendix 1: antihistamines (sedating)
- **SIDE-EFFECTS**
- **Rare** Anaphylaxis · angioedema · angle-closure glaucoma · arrhythmias · blood disorders · bronchospasm · confusion · convulsions · depression · dizziness · extrapyramidal effects · hypersensitivity reactions · hypotension · liver dysfunction · palpitation · photosensitivity reactions · rashes · sleep disturbances · tremor
- **Frequency not known** Antimuscarinic effects · blurred vision · drowsiness · dry mouth · gastro-intestinal disturbances · headache · injection pain · psychomotor impairment · restlessness · urinary retention
SIDE-EFFECTS, FURTHER INFORMATION
Children are more susceptible to side-effects.

Drowsiness is a significant side-effect with most of the older antihistamines although paradoxical stimulation may occur rarely in children, especially with high doses. Drowsiness may diminish after a few days of treatment and is considerably less of a problem with the newer antihistamines.

- **PREGNANCY** Most manufacturers of antihistamines advise avoiding their use during pregnancy; however, there is no evidence of teratogenicity. Use in the latter part of the third trimester may cause adverse effects in neonates such as irritability, paradoxical excitability, and tremor.
- **BREAST FEEDING** Most antihistamines are present in breast milk in varying amounts; although not known to be harmful, most manufacturers advise avoiding their use in mothers who are breast-feeding.
- **HEPATIC IMPAIRMENT** Avoid in severe liver disease—increased risk of coma.
- **RENAL IMPAIRMENT** Use with caution.
- **PATIENT AND CARER ADVICE**
  Driving and skilled tasks
  Drowsiness may affect performance of skilled tasks (e.g. cycling or driving); sedating effects enhanced by alcohol.

- **MEDICINAL FORMS**
  There can be variation in the licensing of different medicines containing the same drug.
  Tablet
  CAUTIONARY AND ADVISORY LABELS 2
  ▸ **Avomine** (Manx Healthcare Ltd)
  Promethazine teoclate 25 mg Avomine 25mg tablets |
  10 tablet P £1.13 | 28 tablet P £3.13 DT price = £3.13

ANTIMUSCARINICS

▸ 468

Hyoscine hydrobromide
(Scopolamine hydrobromide)

17-Oct-2016

- **INDICATIONS AND DOSE**
  Motion sickness
  ▸ BY MOUTH
  ▸ Child 4–9 years: 75–150 micrograms, dose to be taken up to 30 minutes before the start of journey, then 75–150 micrograms every 6 hours if required; maximum 450 micrograms per day
  ▸ Child 10–17 years: 150–300 micrograms, dose to be taken up to 30 minutes before the start of journey, then 150–300 micrograms every 6 hours if required; maximum 900 micrograms per day
  ▸ BY TRANSDERMAL APPLICATION
  ▸ Child 10–17 years: Apply 1 patch, apply behind ear 5–6 hours before journey, then apply 1 patch after 72 hours if required, remove old patch and site replacement patch behind the other ear

  Hypersalivation associated with clozapine therapy
  ▸ BY MOUTH
  ▸ Child 12–17 years: 300 micrograms up to 3 times a day; maximum 900 micrograms per day

  Excessive respiratory secretions
  ▸ BY MOUTH, OR BY SUBLINGUAL ADMINISTRATION
  ▸ Child 2–11 years: 10 micrograms/kg 4 times a day (max. per dose 300 micrograms)
  ▸ Child 12–17 years: 300 micrograms 4 times a day
  ▸ BY TRANSDERMAL APPLICATION
  ▸ Child 1 month–2 years: 250 micrograms every 72 hours, dose equates to a quarter patch
  ▸ Child 3–9 years: 500 micrograms every 72 hours, dose equates to a half patch
  ▸ Child 10–17 years: 1 mg every 72 hours, dose equates to one patch

  Excessive respiratory secretion (in palliative care)
  ▸ BY SUBCUTANEOUS INJECTION, OR BY INTRAVENOUS INJECTION
  ▸ Child: 10 micrograms/kg every 4–8 hours (max. per dose 600 micrograms)
  ▸ BY CONTINUOUS SUBCUTANEOUS INFUSION, OR BY INTRAVENOUS INFUSION
  ▸ Child: 40–60 micrograms/kg over 24 hours

  Bowel colic pain in palliative care
  ▸ BY MOUTH USING SUBLINGUAL TABLETS
  ▸ Child: 10 micrograms/kg 3 times a day (max. per dose 300 micrograms), as *Kwells®*.

  Premedication
  ▸ BY SUBCUTANEOUS INJECTION, OR BY INTRAMUSCULAR INJECTION
  ▸ Child 1–11 years: 15 micrograms/kg (max. per dose 600 micrograms), to be administered 30–60 minutes before induction of anaesthesia
  ▸ Child 12–17 years: 200–600 micrograms, to be administered 30–60 minutes before induction of anaesthesia
  ▸ BY INTRAVENOUS INJECTION
  ▸ Child 1–11 years: 15 micrograms/kg (max. per dose 600 micrograms), to be administered immediately before induction of anaesthesia
  ▸ Child 12–17 years: 200–600 micrograms, to be administered immediately before induction of anaesthesia

- **UNLICENSED USE** Not licensed for use in excessive respiratory secretions or hypersalivation associated with clozapine therapy.

> **IMPORTANT SAFETY INFORMATION**
> Antimuscarininc drugs used for premedication to general anaesthesia should only be administered by, or under the direct supervision of, personnel experienced in their use.

- **CAUTIONS** Epilepsy
  CAUTIONS, FURTHER INFORMATION
  ▸ Anticholinergic syndrome
  ▸ With systemic use In some children hyoscine may cause the central anticholinergic syndrome (excitement, ataxia, hallucinations, behavioural abnormalities, and drowsiness).
- **INTERACTIONS** → Appendix 1: hyoscine
- **PREGNANCY** Use only if potential benefit outweighs risk. Injection may depress neonatal respiration.
- **BREAST FEEDING** Amount too small to be harmful.
- **HEPATIC IMPAIRMENT** Use with caution.
- **RENAL IMPAIRMENT** Use with caution.
- **DIRECTIONS FOR ADMINISTRATION**
  ▸ With transdermal use *Patch* applied to hairless area of skin behind ear; if less than whole patch required **either** cut with scissors along full thickness ensuring membrane is not peeled away **or** cover portion to prevent contact with skin.
  ▸ With oral use For administration by *mouth*, injection solution may be given orally.
- **PRESCRIBING AND DISPENSING INFORMATION** Flavours of chewable tablet formulations may include raspberry.
  Palliative care
  For further information on the use of hyoscine hydrobromide in palliative care, see www.palliativedrugs.com/formulary/en/hyoscine-hydrobromide.html.
- **PATIENT AND CARER ADVICE**
  ▸ With transdermal use Explain accompanying instructions to patient and in particular emphasise advice to wash hands after handling and to wash application site after removing, and to use one patch at a time.

Driving and skilled tasks
‣ With transdermal use Drowsiness may persist for up to 24 hours or longer after removal of patch; effects of alcohol enhanced.

● MEDICINAL FORMS
There can be variation in the licensing of different medicines containing the same drug. Forms available from special-order manufacturers include: oral suspension, oral solution

Tablet
CAUTIONARY AND ADVISORY LABELS 2
‣ Hyoscine hydrobromide (Non-proprietary)
  Hyoscine hydrobromide 300 microgram Hyoscine hydrobromide 300microgram tablets | 12 tablet P no price available DT price = £1.67
‣ Kwells (Bayer Plc)
  Hyoscine hydrobromide 150 microgram Kwells Kids 150microgram tablets | 12 tablet P £1.67 DT price = £1.67
  Hyoscine hydrobromide 300 microgram Kwells 300microgram tablets | 12 tablet P £1.67 DT price = £1.67
‣ Travel Calm (The Boots Company Plc)
  Hyoscine hydrobromide 300 microgram Travel Calm 300microgram tablets | 12 tablet P no price available DT price = £1.67

Solution for injection
‣ Hyoscine hydrobromide (Non-proprietary)
  Hyoscine hydrobromide 400 microgram per 1 ml Hyoscine hydrobromide 400micrograms/1ml solution for injection ampoules | 10 ampoule PoM £25.00–£47.21 DT price = £47.21
  Hyoscine hydrobromide 600 microgram per 1 ml Hyoscine hydrobromide 600micrograms/1ml solution for injection ampoules | 10 ampoule PoM £53.93 DT price = £53.93

Transdermal patch
CAUTIONARY AND ADVISORY LABELS 19
‣ Scopoderm (GlaxoSmithKline Consumer Healthcare)
  Hyoscine 1 mg per 72 hour Scopoderm 1.5mg patches | 2 patch P £5.72 DT price = £4.97

Chewable tablet
CAUTIONARY AND ADVISORY LABELS 2, 24
‣ Joy-Rides (Forest Laboratories UK Ltd)
  Hyoscine hydrobromide 150 microgram Joy-rides 150microgram chewable tablets sugar-free | 12 tablet P £1.55

ANTIPSYCHOTICS › FIRST-GENERATION

◤ F 235

Droperidol

● DRUG ACTION Droperidol is a butyrophenone, structurally related to haloperidol, which blocks dopamine receptors in the chemoreceptor trigger zone.

● INDICATIONS AND DOSE
Prevention and treatment of postoperative nausea and vomiting
‣ BY INTRAVENOUS INJECTION
‣ Child 2-17 years: 20–50 micrograms/kg (max. per dose 1.25 mg), dose to be given 30 minutes before end of surgery, then 20–50 micrograms/kg every 6 hours (max. per dose 1.25 mg) if required

● CONTRA-INDICATIONS Bradycardia · CNS depression · comatose states · hypokalaemia · hypomagnesaemia · phaeochromocytoma · QT-interval prolongation
● CAUTIONS Chronic obstructive pulmonary disease · electrolyte disturbances · history of alcohol abuse · respiratory failure
● INTERACTIONS → Appendix 1: droperidol
● SIDE-EFFECTS Anxiety · cardiac arrest · hallucinations · inappropriate antidiuretic hormone secretion
● BREAST FEEDING Limited information available—avoid repeated administration.
● HEPATIC IMPAIRMENT In postoperative nausea and vomiting, max. 625 micrograms repeated every 6 hours as required.

● RENAL IMPAIRMENT In postoperative nausea and vomiting, max. 625 micrograms repeated every 6 hours as required.
● MONITORING REQUIREMENTS Continuous pulse oximetry required if risk of ventricular arrhythmia—continue for 30 minutes following administration.

● MEDICINAL FORMS
There can be variation in the licensing of different medicines containing the same drug.
Solution for injection
‣ Droperidol (Non-proprietary)
  Droperidol 2.5 mg per 1 ml Droperidol 2.5mg/1ml solution for injection ampoules | 10 ampoule PoM no price available
‣ Xomolix (Kyowa Kirin Ltd)
  Droperidol 2.5 mg per 1 ml Xomolix 2.5mg/1ml solution for injection ampoules | 10 ampoule PoM £39.40

◤ F 235

Levomepromazine
12-Dec-2016

(Methotrimeprazine)

● INDICATIONS AND DOSE
Restlessness and confusion in palliative care
‣ BY CONTINUOUS SUBCUTANEOUS INFUSION
‣ Child 1-11 years: 0.35–3 mg/kg, to be administered over 24 hours
‣ Child 12-17 years: 12.5–200 mg, to be administered over 24 hours

Nausea and vomiting in palliative care
‣ BY CONTINUOUS INTRAVENOUS INFUSION, OR BY SUBCUTANEOUS INFUSION
‣ Child 1 month-11 years: 100–400 micrograms/kg, to be administered over 24 hours
‣ Child 12-17 years: 5–25 mg, to be administered over 24 hours

● CONTRA-INDICATIONS CNS depression · comatose states · phaeochromocytoma
● CAUTIONS Patients receiving large initial doses should remain supine
● INTERACTIONS → Appendix 1: phenothiazines
● SIDE-EFFECTS Raised erythrocyte sedimentation rate
● HEPATIC IMPAIRMENT Can precipitate coma; phenothiazines are hepatotoxic.
● RENAL IMPAIRMENT Start with small doses in severe renal impairment because of increased cerebral sensitivity.
● DIRECTIONS FOR ADMINISTRATION For administration by *subcutaneous infusion* dilute with a suitable volume of Sodium Chloride 0.9%.
● PRESCRIBING AND DISPENSING INFORMATION
Palliative care
For further information on the use of levomepromazine in palliative care, see www.palliativedrugs.com/formulary/en/levomepromazine.html.

● MEDICINAL FORMS
There can be variation in the licensing of different medicines containing the same drug.
Solution for injection
‣ Levomepromazine (Non-proprietary)
  Levomepromazine hydrochloride 25 mg per 1 ml Levomepromazine 25mg/1ml solution for injection ampoules | 10 ampoule PoM £20.13 DT price = £20.13
‣ Nozinan (Sanofi)
  Levomepromazine hydrochloride 25 mg per 1 ml Nozinan 25mg/1ml solution for injection ampoules | 10 ampoule PoM £20.13 DT price = £20.13

4

Nervous system

Prochlorperazine

F 235

● **INDICATIONS AND DOSE**

Prevention and treatment of nausea and vomiting
▸ BY MOUTH
▸ Child 1–11 years (body-weight 10 kg and above): 250 micrograms/kg 2–3 times a day
▸ Child 12–17 years: 5–10 mg up to 3 times a day if required
▸ BY INTRAMUSCULAR INJECTION
▸ Child 2–4 years: 1.25–2.5 mg up to 3 times a day if required
▸ Child 5–11 years: 5–6.25 mg up to 3 times a day if required
▸ Child 12–17 years: 12.5 mg up to 3 times a day if required

Nausea and vomiting in previously diagnosed migraine
▸ BY MOUTH USING BUCCAL TABLET
▸ Child 12–17 years: 3–6 mg twice daily, tablets to be placed high between upper lip and gum and left to dissolve

DOSE EQUIVALENCE AND CONVERSION
▸ Doses are expressed as prochlorperazine maleate or mesilate; 1 mg prochlorperazine maleate ≡ 1 mg prochlorperazine mesilate.

● **UNLICENSED USE** Injection not licensed for use in children. Buccal tablets not licensed for use in children.

● **CONTRA-INDICATIONS** Avoid oral route in child under 10 kg · children (in psychotic disorders) · CNS depression · comatose states · phaeochromocytoma

● **CAUTIONS** Hypotension (more likely after intramuscular injection)

● **INTERACTIONS** → Appendix 1: phenothiazines

● **SIDE-EFFECTS** Dystonic reactions · respiratory depression may occur in susceptible patients

SIDE-EFFECTS, FURTHER INFORMATION
▸ Acute dystonic reactions Phenothiazines can all induce acute dystonic reactions such as facial and skeletal muscle spasms and oculogyric crises; children (especially girls, young women, and those under 10 kg) are particularly susceptible.

● **HEPATIC IMPAIRMENT** Can precipitate coma; phenothiazines are hepatotoxic.

● **RENAL IMPAIRMENT** Start with small doses in severe renal impairment because of increased cerebral sensitivity.

● **DIRECTIONS FOR ADMINISTRATION** Buccal tablets are placed high between upper lip and gum and left to dissolve.

● **PATIENT AND CARER ADVICE** Patients or carers should be given advice on how to administer prochlorperazine buccal tablets.

● **MEDICINAL FORMS**
There can be variation in the licensing of different medicines containing the same drug.

Tablet
CAUTIONARY AND ADVISORY LABELS 2
▸ Prochlorperazine (Non-proprietary)
Prochlorperazine maleate 5 mg Prochlorperazine 5mg tablets | 28 tablet PoM £1.31 DT price = £0.97 | 84 tablet PoM £3.93
▸ Stemetil (Sanofi)
Prochlorperazine maleate 5 mg Stemetil 5mg tablets | 28 tablet PoM £1.98 DT price = £0.97 | 84 tablet PoM £5.94

Solution for injection
▸ Prochlorperazine (Non-proprietary)
Prochlorperazine mesilate 12.5 mg per 1 ml Prochlorperazine 12.5mg/1ml solution for injection ampoules | 10 ampoule PoM no price available DT price = £5.23

▸ Stemetil (Sanofi)
Prochlorperazine mesilate 12.5 mg per 1 ml Stemetil 12.5mg/1ml solution for injection ampoules | 10 ampoule PoM £5.23 DT price = £5.23

Buccal tablet
CAUTIONARY AND ADVISORY LABELS 2
▸ Prochlorperazine (Non-proprietary)
Prochlorperazine maleate 3 mg Prochlorperazine 3mg buccal tablets | 50 tablet PoM £35.94–£43.13 DT price = £43.13
▸ Buccastem (Alliance Pharmaceuticals Ltd)
Prochlorperazine maleate 3 mg Buccastem M 3mg tablets | 8 tablet P £3.66

Oral solution
CAUTIONARY AND ADVISORY LABELS 2
▸ Stemetil (Sanofi)
Prochlorperazine mesilate 1 mg per 1 ml Stemetil 5mg/5ml syrup | 100 ml PoM £3.34 DT price = £3.34

5   Pain

Analgesics

Drugs used for pain

The non-opioid drugs, paracetamol p. 260 and ibuprofen p. 625 (and other NSAIDs), are particularly suitable for pain in musculoskeletal conditions, whereas the opioid analgesics are more suitable for moderate to severe pain, particularly of visceral origin.

Pain in sickle-cell disease
The pain of mild sickle-cell crises is managed with paracetamol, an NSAID, codeine phosphate p. 265, or dihydrocodeine tartrate p. 268. Severe crises may require the use of morphine p. 271 or diamorphine hydrochloride p. 267; concomitant use of an NSAID may potentiate analgesia and allow lower doses of the opioid to be used. A mixture of nitrous oxide and oxygen (*Entonox®*, *Equanox®*) may also be used.

Dental and orofacial pain
Analgesics should be used judiciously in dental care as a **temporary** measure until the cause of the pain has been dealt with.

Dental pain of inflammatory origin, such as that associated with pulpitis, apical infection, localised osteitis or pericoronitis is usually best managed by treating the infection, providing drainage, restorative procedures, and other local measures. Analgesics provide temporary relief of pain (usually for about 1 to 7 days) until the causative factors have been brought under control. In the case of pulpitis, intra-osseous infection or abscess, reliance on analgesics alone is usually inappropriate.

Similarly the pain and discomfort associated with acute problems of the oral mucosa (e.g. acute herpetic gingivostomatitis, erythema multiforme) may be relieved by benzydamine hydrochloride p. 677 or topical anaesthetics until the cause of the mucosal disorder has been dealt with. However, where a child is febrile, the antipyretic action of paracetamol or ibuprofen is often helpful.

The *choice* of an analgesic for dental purposes should be based on its suitability for the child. Most dental pain is relieved effectively by non-steroidal anti-inflammatory drugs (NSAIDs) e.g. ibuprofen. Paracetamol has analgesic and antipyretic effects but no anti-inflammatory effect.

Opioid analgesics such as dihydrocodeine tartrate act on the central nervous system and are traditionally used for *moderate to severe pain*. However, opioid analgesics are relatively ineffective in dental pain and their side-effects can be unpleasant.

Combining a non-opioid with an opioid analgesic can provide greater relief of pain than either analgesic given alone. However, this applies only when an adequate dose of each analgesic is used. Most combination analgesic preparations have not been shown to provide greater relief of pain than an adequate dose of the non-opioid component given alone. Moreover, combination preparations have the disadvantage of an increased number of side-effects.

Any analgesic given before a dental procedure should have a low risk of increasing postoperative bleeding. In the case of pain after the dental procedure, taking an analgesic before the effect of the local anaesthetic has worn off can improve control. Postoperative analgesia with ibuprofen is usually continued for about 24 to 72 hours.

Dysmenorrhoea

Paracetamol or a NSAID will generally provide adequate relief of pain from dysmenorrhoea. Alternatively use of a combined hormonal contraceptive in adolescent girls may prevent the pain.

Non-opioid analgesics and compound analgesic preparations

Paracetamol has analgesic and antipyretic properties but no demonstrable anti-inflammatory activity; unlike opioid analgesics, it does not cause respiratory depression and is less irritant to the stomach than the NSAIDs. **Overdosage** with paracetamol is particularly dangerous as it may cause hepatic damage which is sometimes not apparent for 4 to 6 days.

Non-steroidal anti-inflammatory analgesics (NSAIDs) are particularly useful for the treatment of children with chronic disease accompanied by pain and inflammation. Some of them are also used in the short-term treatment of mild to moderate pain including transient musculoskeletal pain but paracetamol is now often preferred. They are also suitable for the relief of pain in *dysmenorrhoea* and to treat pain caused by *secondary bone tumours*, many of which produce lysis of bone and release prostaglandins. Due to an association with Reye's syndrome, aspirin p. 89 should be avoided in children under 16 years except in Kawasaki disease or for its antiplatelet action. Several NSAIDs are also used for postoperative analgesia.

Compound analgesic preparations

Compound analgesic preparations that contain a simple analgesic (such as paracetamol) with an opioid component reduce the scope for effective titration of the individual components in the management of pain of varying intensity.

Compound analgesic preparations containing paracetamol with a *low dose* of an opioid analgesic (e.g. 8 mg of codeine phosphate per compound tablet) may be used in older children but the advantages have not been substantiated. The low dose of the opioid may be enough to cause opioid side-effects (in particular, constipation) and can complicate the treatment of **overdosage** yet may not provide significant additional relief of pain.

A *full dose* of the opioid component (e.g. 60 mg codeine phosphate) in compound analgesic preparations effectively augments the analgesic activity but is associated with the full range of opioid side-effects (including nausea, vomiting, severe constipation, drowsiness, respiratory depression, and risk of dependence on long-term administration).

In general, when assessing pain, it is necessary to weigh up carefully whether there is a need for a non-opioid and an opioid analgesic to be taken simultaneously.

Opioid analgesics

Opioid analgesics are usually used to relieve moderate to severe pain particularly of visceral origin. Repeated administration may cause tolerance, but this is no deterrent in the control of pain in terminal illness. Regular use of a potent opioid may be appropriate for certain cases of chronic non-malignant pain; treatment should be supervised by a specialist and the child should be assessed at regular intervals.

Strong opioids

Morphine remains the most valuable opioid analgesic for severe pain although it frequently causes nausea and vomiting. It is the standard against which other opioid analgesics are compared. In addition to relief of pain, morphine also confers a state of euphoria and mental detachment.

Morphine is the opioid of choice for the oral treatment of *severe pain in palliative care*. It is given regularly every 4 hours (or every 12 or 24 hours as modified-release preparations).

Buprenorphine p. 263 has both opioid agonist and antagonist properties and may precipitate withdrawal symptoms, including pain, in children dependent on other opioids. It has abuse potential and may itself cause dependence. It has a much longer duration of action than morphine and sublingually is an effective analgesic for 6 to 8 hours. Unlike most opioid analgesics, the effects of buprenorphine are only partially reversed by naloxone hydrochloride p. 813. It is rarely used in children.

Diamorphine hydrochloride (heroin) p. 267 is a powerful opioid analgesic. It may cause less nausea and hypotension than morphine p. 271. In *palliative care* the greater solubility of diamorphine hydrochloride allows effective doses to be injected in smaller volumes and this is important in the emaciated child. Diamorphine hydrochloride is sometimes given by the intranasal route to treat acute pain in children and is available as a nasal spray; intranasal administration of diamorphine injection has been used [unlicensed].

Alfentanil p. 788, fentanyl p. 268 and remifentanil p. 789 are used by injection for intra-operative analgesia. Fentanyl is available in a transdermal drug delivery system as a self-adhesive patch which is changed every 72 hours.

Methadone hydrochloride p. 286 is less sedating than morphine and acts for longer periods. In prolonged use, methadone hydrochloride should not be administered more often than twice daily to avoid the risk of accumulation and opioid overdosage. Methadone hydrochloride may be used instead of morphine when excitation (or exacerbation of pain) occurs with morphine. Methadone hydrochloride may also be used to treat children with neonatal abstinence syndrome.

Papaveretum p. 275 should not be used in children; morphine is easier to prescribe and less prone to error with regard to the strength and dose.

Pethidine hydrochloride p. 276 produces prompt but short-lasting analgesia; it is less constipating than morphine, but even in high doses is a less potent analgesic. Its use in children is not recommended. Pethidine hydrochloride is used for analgesia in labour; however, other opioids, such as morphine or diamorphine hydrochloride, are often preferred for obstetric pain.

Tramadol hydrochloride p. 276 is used in older children and produces analgesia by two mechanisms: an opioid effect and an enhancement of serotonergic and adrenergic pathways. It has fewer of the typical opioid side-effects (notably, less respiratory depression, less constipation and less addiction potential); psychiatric reactions have been reported.

Weak opioids

Codeine phosphate p. 265 can be used for the relief of short-term acute moderate pain in children older than 12 years where other painkillers such as paracetamol p. 260 or ibuprofen p. 625 have proved ineffective.

Dihydrocodeine tartrate p. 268 has an analgesic efficacy similar to that of codeine phosphate.

Postoperative analgesia

A combination of opioid and non-opioid analgesics is used to treat postoperative pain. The use of intra-operative opioids affects the prescribing of postoperative analgesics. A postoperative opioid analgesic should be given with care since it may potentiate any residual respiratory depression.

4

Nervous system

Morphine is used most widely. Tramadol hydrochloride is not as effective in severe pain as other opioid analgesics. Buprenorphine p. 263 may antagonise the analgesic effect of previously administered opioids and is generally not recommended. Pethidine hydrochloride is generally not recommended for postoperative pain because it is metabolised to norpethidine which may accumulate, particularly in neonates and in renal impairment; norpethidine stimulates the central nervous system and may cause convulsions.

Opioids are also given epidurally [unlicensed route] in the postoperative period but are associated with side-effects such as pruritus, urinary retention, nausea and vomiting; respiratory depression can be delayed, particularly with morphine.

Patient-controlled analgesia (PCA) and nurse-controlled analgesia (NCA) can be used to relieve postoperative pain—consult hospital protocols.

Pain management and opioid dependence
Although caution is necessary, patients who are dependent on opioids or have a history of drug dependence may be treated with opioid analgesics when there is a clinical need. Treatment with opioid analgesics in this patient group should normally be carried out with the advice of specialists. However, doctors do not require a special licence to prescribe opioid analgesics to patients with opioid dependence for relief of pain due to organic disease or injury.

> **Other drugs used for Pain** Diclofenac potassium, p. 622 · Mefenamic acid, p. 629

ANALGESICS ⟩ NON-OPIOID

Paracetamol
05-May-2016
(Acetaminophen)

● **INDICATIONS AND DOSE**

Pain | Pyrexia with discomfort
▸ BY MOUTH

▸ Neonate 28 weeks to 32 weeks corrected gestational age: 20 mg/kg for 1 dose, then 10–15 mg/kg every 8–12 hours as required, maximum daily dose to be given in divided doses; maximum 30 mg/kg per day.

▸ Neonate 32 weeks corrected gestational age and above: 20 mg/kg for 1 dose, then 10–15 mg/kg every 6–8 hours as required, maximum daily dose to be given in divided doses; maximum 60 mg/kg per day.

▸ Child 1-2 months: 30–60 mg every 8 hours as required, maximum daily dose to be given in divided doses; maximum 60 mg/kg per day
▸ Child 3-5 months: 60 mg every 4–6 hours; maximum 4 doses per day
▸ Child 6 months-1 year: 120 mg every 4–6 hours; maximum 4 doses per day
▸ Child 2-3 years: 180 mg every 4–6 hours; maximum 4 doses per day
▸ Child 4-5 years: 240 mg every 4–6 hours; maximum 4 doses per day
▸ Child 6-7 years: 240–250 mg every 4–6 hours; maximum 4 doses per day
▸ Child 8-9 years: 360–375 mg every 4–6 hours; maximum 4 doses per day
▸ Child 10-11 years: 480–500 mg every 4–6 hours; maximum 4 doses per day
▸ Child 12-15 years: 480–750 mg every 4–6 hours; maximum 4 doses per day
▸ Child 16-17 years: 0.5–1 g every 4–6 hours; maximum 4 doses per day

▸ BY RECTUM

▸ Neonate 28 weeks to 32 weeks corrected gestational age: 20 mg/kg for 1 dose, then 10–15 mg/kg every 12 hours as required, maximum daily dose to be given in divided doses; maximum 30 mg/kg per day.

▸ Neonate 32 weeks corrected gestational age and above: 30 mg/kg for 1 dose, then 15–20 mg/kg every 8 hours as required, maximum daily dose to be given in divided doses; maximum 60 mg/kg per day.

▸ Child 1-2 months: 30–60 mg every 8 hours as required, maximum daily dose to be given in divided doses; maximum 60 mg/kg per day
▸ Child 3-11 months: 60–125 mg every 4–6 hours as required; maximum 4 doses per day
▸ Child 1-4 years: 125–250 mg every 4–6 hours as required; maximum 4 doses per day
▸ Child 5-11 years: 250–500 mg every 4–6 hours as required; maximum 4 doses per day
▸ Child 12-17 years: 500 mg every 4–6 hours
▸ BY INTRAVENOUS INFUSION

▸ Neonate 32 weeks corrected gestational age and above: 7.5 mg/kg every 8 hours, dose to be administered over 15 minutes.

▸ Neonate: 10 mg/kg every 4–6 hours, dose to be administered over 15 minutes; maximum 30 mg/kg per day.

▸ Child (body-weight up to 10 kg): 10 mg/kg every 4–6 hours, dose to be administered over 15 minutes; maximum 30 mg/kg per day
▸ Child (body-weight 10-50 kg): 15 mg/kg every 4–6 hours, dose to be administered over 15 minutes; maximum 60 mg/kg per day
▸ Child (body-weight 50 kg and above): 1 g every 4–6 hours, dose to be administered over 15 minutes; maximum 4 g per day

Pain in children with risk factors for hepatotoxicity | Pyrexia with discomfort in children with risk factors for hepatotoxicity
▸ BY INTRAVENOUS INFUSION

▸ Neonate 32 weeks corrected gestational age and above: 7.5 mg/kg every 8 hours, dose to be administered over 15 minutes.

▸ Neonate: 10 mg/kg every 4–6 hours, dose to be administered over 15 minutes; maximum 30 mg/kg per day.

▸ Child (body-weight up to 10 kg): 10 mg/kg every 4–6 hours, dose to be administered over 15 minutes; maximum 30 mg/kg per day
▸ Child (body-weight 10-50 kg): 15 mg/kg every 4–6 hours, dose to be administered over 15 minutes; maximum 60 mg/kg per day
▸ Child (body-weight 50 kg and above): 1 g every 4–6 hours, dose to be administered over 15 minutes; maximum 3 g per day

Post-operative pain
▸ BY MOUTH

▸ Child 1 month-5 years: 20–30 mg/kg for 1 dose, then 15–20 mg/kg every 4–6 hours, maximum daily dose to be given in divided doses; maximum 75 mg/kg per day
▸ Child 6-11 years: 20–30 mg/kg (max. per dose 1 g) for 1 dose, then 15–20 mg/kg every 4–6 hours, maximum daily dose to be given in divided doses; maximum 75 mg/kg per day; maximum 4 g per day
▸ Child 12-17 years: 1 g every 4–6 hours; maximum 4 doses per day

▸ BY RECTUM
▸ Child 1-2 months: 30 mg/kg for 1 dose, then
15–20 mg/kg every 4–6 hours, maximum daily dose to
be given in divided doses; maximum 75 mg/kg per day
▸ Child 3 months-5 years: 30–40 mg/kg for 1 dose, then
15–20 mg/kg every 4–6 hours, maximum daily dose to
be given in divided doses; maximum 75 mg/kg per day
▸ Child 6-11 years: 30–40 mg/kg (max. per dose 1 g) for
1 dose, then 15–20 mg/kg every 4–6 hours, maximum
daily dose to be given in divided doses; maximum
75 mg/kg per day; maximum 4 g per day
▸ Child 12-17 years: 1 g every 4–6 hours; maximum
4 doses per day

**Prophylaxis of post-immunisation pyrexia following
immunisation with meningococcal group B vaccine**
▸ BY MOUTH
▸ Child 2 months: 60 mg, first dose to be given at the time
of vaccination, then 60 mg after 4–6 hours, then 60 mg
after 4–6 hours
▸ Child 4 months: 60 mg, first dose to be given at the time
of vaccination, then 60 mg after 4–6 hours, then 60 mg
after 4–6 hours

Post-immunisation pyrexia in infants
▸ BY MOUTH
▸ Child 2-3 months: 60 mg for 1 dose, then 60 mg after
4–6 hours if required
▸ Child 4 months: 60 mg for 1 dose, then 60 mg after
4–6 hours; maximum 4 doses per day

PANADOL OA®
Mild to moderate pain | Pyrexia
▸ BY MOUTH
▸ Child 12-17 years: 1 g up to 4 times a day, dose not to be
taken more often than every 4 hours

● UNLICENSED USE Paracetamol oral suspension
500 mg/5 mL not licensed for use in children under
16 years. Not licensed for use in children under 2 months
by mouth; under 3 months by rectum. EvGr Not licensed
for use as prophylaxis of post-immunisation pyrexia
following immunisation with meningococcal group B
vaccine. ⓔ Intravenous infusion not licensed in pre-term
neonates. Intravenous infusion dose not licensed in
children and neonates with body-weight under 10 kg.

● CAUTIONS Before administering, check when paracetamol
last administered and cumulative paracetamol dose over
previous 24 hours · body-weight under 50 kg · chronic
alcohol consumption · chronic dehydration · chronic
malnutrition · hepatocellular insufficiency · long-term use
(especially in those who are malnourished)
CAUTIONS, FURTHER INFORMATION
EvGr Some patients may be at increased risk of
experiencing toxicity at therapeutic doses, particularly
those with a body-weight under 50 kg and those with risk
factors for hepatotoxicity. Clinical judgement should be
used to adjust the dose of oral and intravenous
paracetamol in these patients. ⓔ
EvGr Co-administration of enzyme-inducing
antiepileptic medications may increase toxicity; doses
should be reduced. ⓔ

● INTERACTIONS → Appendix 1: paracetamol

● SIDE-EFFECTS
GENERAL SIDE-EFFECTS
▸ Rare Acute generalised exanthematous pustulosis ·
malaise · skin reactions · Stevens-Johnson syndrome · toxic
epidermal necrolysis
▸ Frequency not known Blood disorders · leucopenia ·
neutropenia · thrombocytopenia
SPECIFIC SIDE-EFFECTS
▸ Rare
▸ With intravenous use Flushing · tachycardia

▸ Frequency not known
▸ With intravenous use Hypotension
Overdose
Important: liver damage and less frequently renal damage
can occur following overdose.
Nausea and vomiting, the only early features of
poisoning, usually settle within 24 hours. Persistence
beyond this time, often associated with the onset of right
subcostal pain and tenderness, usually indicates
development of hepatic necrosis.
For specific details on the management of poisoning, see
Paracetamol, under Emergency treatment of poisoning
p. 803

● PREGNANCY Not known to be harmful.

● BREAST FEEDING Amount too small to be harmful.

● HEPATIC IMPAIRMENT Dose-related toxicity—avoid large
doses.

● RENAL IMPAIRMENT Increase infusion dose interval to
every 6 hours if estimated glomerular filtration rate less
than 30 mL/minute/1.73 m².

● DIRECTIONS FOR ADMINISTRATION For *intravenous infusion*
(*Perfalgan*®), give in Glucose 5% *or* Sodium Chloride 0.9%;
dilute to a concentration of not less than 1 mg/mL and use
within an hour; may also be given undiluted. For children
under 33 kg, use 50 mL-vial.

● PRESCRIBING AND DISPENSING INFORMATION BP directs
that when Paediatric Paracetamol Oral Suspension or
Paediatric Paracetamol Mixture is prescribed Paracetamol
Oral Suspension 120 mg/5 mL should be dispensed.

● PATIENT AND CARER ADVICE
Medicines for Children leaflet: Paracetamol for mild-to-moderate
pain www.medicinesforchildren.org.uk/paracetamol-for-
mildtomoderate-pain

● PROFESSION SPECIFIC INFORMATION
Dental practitioners' formulary
Paracetamol Tablets may be prescribed.
Paracetamol Soluble Tablets 500 mg may be prescribed.
Paracetamol Oral Suspension may be prescribed.

● EXCEPTIONS TO LEGAL CATEGORY Paracetamol capsules or
tablets can be sold to the public provided packs contain no
more than 32 capsules or tablets; pharmacists can sell
multiple packs up to a total quantity of 100 capsules or
tablets in justifiable circumstances.

● MEDICINAL FORMS
There can be variation in the licensing of different medicines
containing the same drug. Forms available from special-order
manufacturers include: oral suspension, oral solution,
suppository
Tablet
CAUTIONARY AND ADVISORY LABELS 29(does not apply to 1 g
tablet), 30
▸ **Paracetamol (Non-proprietary)**
Paracetamol 500 mg Paracetamol 500mg caplets |
100 tablet PoM £3.18 DT price = £2.19
Paracetamol 500mg tablets | 100 tablet PoM £2.56 DT price = £2.19
| 1000 tablet PoM £21.90 | 5000 tablet PoM no price available
▸ **Paravict** (Ecogen Europe Ltd)
Paracetamol 500 mg Paravict 500mg tablets | 100 tablet PoM
£1.62 DT price = £2.19
Suppository
CAUTIONARY AND ADVISORY LABELS 30
▸ **Paracetamol (Non-proprietary)**
Paracetamol 80 mg Paracetamol 80mg suppositories |
10 suppository Ⓟ £10.00
Paracetamol 120 mg Paracetamol 120mg suppositories |
10 suppository Ⓟ £11.26 DT price = £11.26
Paracetamol 125 mg Paracetamol 125mg suppositories |
10 suppository Ⓟ £15.00 DT price = £13.80
Paracetamol 240 mg Paracetamol 240mg suppositories |
10 suppository Ⓟ £22.01 DT price = £22.01
Paracetamol 250 mg Paracetamol 250mg suppositories |
10 suppository Ⓟ £24.15 DT price = £27.60

4

Nervous system

Paracetamol 500 mg Paracetamol 500mg suppositories |
10 suppository P £36.50 DT price = £36.50
Paracetamol 1 gram Paracetamol 1g suppositories |
10 suppository P £59.50 | 12 suppository P no price available
▸ **Alvedon** (Intrapharm Laboratories Ltd)
Paracetamol 60 mg Alvedon 60mg suppositories |
10 suppository P £11.95 DT price = £11.95
Paracetamol 125 mg Alvedon 125mg suppositories |
10 suppository P £13.80 DT price = £13.80
Paracetamol 250 mg Alvedon 250mg suppositories |
10 suppository P £27.60 DT price = £27.60

Oral suspension
CAUTIONARY AND ADVISORY LABELS 30
▸ **Paracetamol (Non-proprietary)**
Paracetamol 24 mg per 1 ml Paracetamol 120mg/5ml oral
suspension paediatric | 100 ml P £0.72 | 500 ml P £3.11 DT price
= £3.11
Paracetamol 120mg/5ml oral suspension paediatric sugar free sugar-
free | 100 ml P £1.29 DT price = £1.29 sugar-free | 200 ml P £2.58
sugar-free | 500 ml P £6.45 sugar-free | 1000 ml P £12.90
Paracetamol 50 mg per 1 ml Paracetamol 250mg/5ml oral
suspension | 100 ml P £1.12 DT price = £1.12 | 500 ml P £5.60
Paracetamol 250mg/5ml oral suspension sugar free sugar-free |
100 ml P £1.10 sugar-free | 200 ml P £2.00 DT price = £2.02
sugar-free | 500 ml P £5.18 sugar-free | 1000 ml P £9.85
Paracetamol 100 mg per 1 ml Paracetamol 500mg/5ml oral
suspension sugar free sugar-free | 150 ml PoM £24.00 DT price =
£24.00
▸ **Calpol** (McNeil Products Ltd)
Paracetamol 24 mg per 1 ml Calpol Infant 120mg/5ml oral
suspension | 200 ml P £3.35
Paracetamol 50 mg per 1 ml Calpol Six Plus 250mg/5ml oral
suspension | 200 ml P £3.88
Calpol Six Plus 250mg/5ml oral suspension sugar free sugar-free |
100 ml P £2.40 sugar-free | 200 ml P £3.88 DT price = £2.02

Effervescent tablet
CAUTIONARY AND ADVISORY LABELS 29, 30
▸ **Paracetamol (Non-proprietary)**
Paracetamol 500 mg Paracetamol 500mg soluble tablets |
100 tablet PoM £8.33 DT price = £9.21

Solution for infusion
CAUTIONARY AND ADVISORY LABELS 30
▸ **Paracetamol (Non-proprietary)**
Paracetamol 10 mg per 1 ml Paracetamol 1g/100ml solution for
infusion vials | 10 vial PoM £12.00
▸ **Perfalgan** (Bristol-Myers Squibb Pharmaceuticals Ltd)
Paracetamol 10 mg per 1 ml Perfalgan 1g/100ml solution for
infusion vials | 12 vial PoM £14.96
Perfalgan 500mg/50ml solution for infusion vials | 12 vial PoM
£13.60

Oral solution
CAUTIONARY AND ADVISORY LABELS 30
▸ **Paracetamol (Non-proprietary)**
Paracetamol 24 mg per 1 ml Paracetamol 120mg/5ml oral solution
paediatric sugar free sugar-free | 500 ml P £2.86 DT price = £2.86
sugar-free | 2000 ml P £25.80
Paracetamol 100 mg per 1 ml Paracetamol 500mg/5ml oral
solution sugar free sugar-free | 150 ml P £24.00 sugar-free |
200 ml PoM £18.00 DT price = £18.00

Capsule
CAUTIONARY AND ADVISORY LABELS 29, 30
▸ **Paracetamol (Non-proprietary)**
Paracetamol 500 mg Paracetamol 500mg capsules |
100 capsule PoM £3.84 DT price = £2.91

Orodispersible tablet
CAUTIONARY AND ADVISORY LABELS 30
▸ **Calpol Fastmelts** (McNeil Products Ltd)
Paracetamol 250 mg Calpol Six Plus Fastmelts 250mg tablets sugar-
free | 24 tablet P £3.59

Combinations available: *Co-codamol,* p. 264 · *Co-dydramol,*
p. 266

Paracetamol with tramadol

The properties listed below are those particular to the
combination only. For the properties of the components
please consider, paracetamol p. 260, tramadol hydrochloride
p. 276.

● **INDICATIONS AND DOSE**
Moderate to severe pain
▸ BY MOUTH
▸ **Child 12–17 years:** 2 tablets up to every 6 hours;
maximum 8 tablets per day

● **INTERACTIONS** → Appendix 1: opioids, paracetamol

● **MEDICINAL FORMS**
There can be variation in the licensing of different medicines
containing the same drug.
Effervescent tablet
CAUTIONARY AND ADVISORY LABELS 2, 13, 29, 30
ELECTROLYTES: May contain Sodium
▸ **Tramacet** (Grunenthal Ltd)
Tramadol hydrochloride 37.5 mg, Paracetamol 325 mg Tramacet
37.5mg/325mg effervescent tablets sugar-free | 60 tablet PoM £9.68
DT price = £9.68 CD3
Tablet
CAUTIONARY AND ADVISORY LABELS 2, 25, 29, 30
▸ **Paracetamol with tramadol (Non-proprietary)**
Tramadol hydrochloride 37.5 mg, Paracetamol 325 mg Tramadol
37.5mg / Paracetamol 325mg tablets | 60 tablet PoM £9.20–£9.68 DT
price = £9.22 CD3
Tramadol hydrochloride 75 mg, Paracetamol 650 mg Tramadol
75mg / Paracetamol 650mg tablets | 30 tablet PoM £19.50 CD3
▸ **Tramacet** (Grunenthal Ltd)
Tramadol hydrochloride 37.5 mg, Paracetamol 325 mg Tramacet
37.5mg/325mg tablets | 60 tablet PoM £9.68 DT price = £9.22 CD3

ANALGESICS > OPIOIDS

Opioids

● **CONTRA-INDICATIONS** Acute respiratory depression ·
comatose patients · head injury (opioid analgesics interfere
with pupillary responses vital for neurological assessment)
· raised intracranial pressure (opioid analgesics interfere
with pupillary responses vital for neurological assessment)
· risk of paralytic ileus
● **CAUTIONS** Adrenocortical insufficiency (reduced dose is
recommended) · asthma (avoid during an acute attack) ·
convulsive disorders · diseases of the biliary tract ·
hypotension · hypothyroidism (reduced dose is
recommended) · impaired respiratory function (avoid in
chronic obstructive pulmonary disease) · inflammatory
bowel disorders · myasthenia gravis · obstructive bowel
disorders · shock

CAUTIONS, FURTHER INFORMATION
▸ Dependence Repeated use of opioid analgesics is associated
with the development of psychological and physical
dependence; although this is rarely a problem with
therapeutic use, caution is advised if prescribing for
patients with a history of drug dependence.
▸ Palliative care In the control of pain in terminal illness, the
cautions listed should not necessarily be a deterrent to the
use of opioid analgesics.

● **SIDE-EFFECTS**
▸ Common or very common Biliary spasm · bradycardia ·
confusion · constipation · dependence · difficulty with
micturition · dizziness ·drowsiness · dry mouth · dysphoria
· euphoria · flushing · hallucinations · headache ·
hypotension (larger doses) · miosis · mood changes ·
muscle rigidity (larger doses) · nausea (particularly in
initial stages) · oedema · palpitation · postural hypotension
· pruritus · rash · respiratory depression (larger doses) ·
sexual dysfunction · sleep disturbances · sweating ·

tachycardia · ureteric spasm · urinary retention · urticaria · vertigo · visual disturbances · vomiting (particularly in initial stages)

▸ **Frequency not known** Adrenal insufficiency (long-term use) · hyperalgesia (long-term use) · hypogonadism (long-term use)

SIDE-EFFECTS, FURTHER INFORMATION

▸ Hypogonadism and adrenal insufficiency Long-term use of opioid analgesics can cause hypogonadism and adrenal insufficiency in both males and females. This is thought to be dose related and can lead to amenorrhoea, reduced libido, infertility, depression, and erectile dysfunction.

▸ Hyperalgesia Long-term use of opioid analgesics has also been associated with a state of abnormal pain sensitivity (hyperalgesia). Pain associated with hyperalgesia is usually distinct from pain associated with disease progression or breakthrough pain, and is often more diffuse and less defined. Treatment of hyperalgesia involves reducing the dose of opioid medication or switching therapy; cases of suspected hyperalgesia should be referred to a specialist pain team.

▸ Respiratory depression Respiratory depression is a major concern with opioid analgesics; neonates (particularly if pre-term) may be more susceptible. It may be treated by artificial ventilation or be reversed by naloxone.

▸ Dependence and withdrawal Psychological dependence rarely occurs when opioids are used therapeutically (e.g. for pain relief) but tolerance can develop during long-term treatment.

Overdose
Opioids (narcotic analgesics) cause coma, respiratory depression, and pinpoint pupils. For details on the management of poisoning, see Opioids, under Emergency treatment of poisoning p. 803 and consider the specific antidote, naloxone hydrochloride p. 813.

● **PREGNANCY** Respiratory depression and withdrawal symptoms can occur in the neonate if opioid analgesics are used during delivery; also gastric stasis and inhalation pneumonia has been reported in the mother if opioid analgesics are used during labour.

● **HEPATIC IMPAIRMENT** Avoid use or reduce dose; may precipitate coma in patients with hepatic impairment.

● **TREATMENT CESSATION** Avoid abrupt withdrawal after long-term treatment; they should be withdrawn gradually to avoid abstinence symptoms.

● **PATIENT AND CARER ADVICE**
Driving and skilled tasks
Drowsiness may affect performance of skilled tasks (e.g. driving); effects of alcohol enhanced. Driving at the start of therapy with opioid analgesics, and following dose changes, should be avoided.

For information on 2015 legislation regarding driving whilst taking certain controlled drugs, including opioids, see *Drugs and Skilled Tasks* under Guidance on prescribing p. 1.

🔖 262

Buprenorphine

27-Apr-2017

● **DRUG ACTION** Buprenorphine is an opioid-receptor partial agonist (it has opioid agonist and antagonist properties).

● **INDICATIONS AND DOSE**
Moderate to severe pain
▸ BY SUBLINGUAL ADMINISTRATION
▸ Child (body-weight 16-25 kg): 100 micrograms every 6–8 hours
▸ Child (body-weight 25-37.5 kg): 100–200 micrograms every 6–8 hours
▸ Child (body-weight 37.5-50 kg): 200–300 micrograms every 6–8 hours

▸ Child (body-weight 50 kg and above): 200–400 micrograms every 6–8 hours
▸ BY INTRAMUSCULAR INJECTION, OR BY SLOW INTRAVENOUS INJECTION
▸ Child 6 months-11 years: 3–6 micrograms/kg every 6–8 hours (max. per dose 9 micrograms/kg)
▸ Child 12-17 years: 300–600 micrograms every 6–8 hours

● **UNLICENSED USE** Sublingual tablets not licensed for use in children under 6 years.

● **CAUTIONS** Impaired consciousness

● **INTERACTIONS** → Appendix 1: opioids

● **SIDE-EFFECTS**
▸ **Common or very common** Abdominal pain · agitation · anorexia · anxiety · asthenia · diarrhoea · dyspepsia · dyspnoea · fatigue · mild withdrawal symptoms in patients dependent on opioids · paraesthesia · vasodilatation
▸ **Uncommon** Cough · depersonalisation · dry eye · dry skin · dysarthria · flatulence · hypertension · hypoaesthesia · hypoxia · impaired memory · influenza-like symptoms · muscle cramp · myalgia · pyrexia · restlessness · rhinitis · rigors · syncope · taste disturbance · tinnitus · tremor · wheezing
▸ **Rare** Diverticulitis · dysphagia · impaired concentration · paralytic ileus · psychosis
▸ **Very rare** Hiccups · hyperventilation · muscle fasciculation · retching
▸ **Frequency not known** Hepatic necrosis · hepatitis

Overdose
The effects of buprenorphine are only partially reversed by naloxone.

● **BREAST FEEDING** Present in low levels in breast milk. Neonates should be monitored for drowsiness, adequate weight gain, and developmental milestones.

● **RENAL IMPAIRMENT** Avoid use or reduce dose; opioid effects increased and prolonged and increased cerebral sensitivity occurs.

● **PRE-TREATMENT SCREENING** Documentation of viral hepatitis status is recommended before commencing therapy for opioid dependence.

● **MONITORING REQUIREMENTS** Monitor liver function; when used in opioid dependence baseline liver function test is recommended before commencing therapy, and regular liver function tests should be performed throughout treatment.

● **DIRECTIONS FOR ADMINISTRATION** For administration by *mouth*, tablets may be halved.

● **MEDICINAL FORMS**
There can be variation in the licensing of different medicines containing the same drug.

Solution for injection
▸ Temgesic (RB Pharmaceuticals Ltd)
Buprenorphine (as Buprenorphine hydrochloride)
300 microgram per 1 ml Temgesic 300micrograms/1ml solution for injection ampoules | 5 ampoule PoM £2.46 CD3

Sublingual tablet
CAUTIONARY AND ADVISORY LABELS 2, 26
▸ Buprenorphine (Non-proprietary)
Buprenorphine (as Buprenorphine hydrochloride)
200 microgram Buprenorphine 200microgram sublingual tablets sugar free sugar-free | 50 tablet PoM £6.05 DT price = £5.04 CD3
Buprenorphine (as Buprenorphine hydrochloride)
400 microgram Buprenorphine 400microgram sublingual tablets sugar free sugar-free | 7 tablet PoM £1.60 DT price = £1.60 CD3
Buprenorphine (as Buprenorphine hydrochloride)
2 mg Buprenorphine 2mg sublingual tablets sugar free sugar-free | 7 tablet PoM £8.35 DT price = £1.33 CD3
Buprenorphine (as Buprenorphine hydrochloride)
8 mg Buprenorphine 8mg sublingual tablets sugar free sugar-free | 7 tablet PoM £22.50 DT price = £2.21 CD3

4

Nervous system

- **Natzon** (Morningside Healthcare Ltd)
  Buprenorphine (as Buprenorphine hydrochloride)
  400 microgram Natzon 0.4mg sublingual tablets sugar-free |
  7 tablet [PoM] £1.60 DT price = £1.60 [CD3]
  Buprenorphine (as Buprenorphine hydrochloride) 2 mg Natzon
  2mg sublingual tablets sugar-free | 7 tablet [PoM] £6.35 DT price =
  £1.33 [CD3]
  Buprenorphine (as Buprenorphine hydrochloride) 8 mg Natzon
  8mg sublingual tablets sugar-free | 7 tablet [PoM] £19.05 DT price =
  £2.21 [CD3]
- **Prefibin** (Sandoz Ltd)
  Buprenorphine (as Buprenorphine hydrochloride)
  400 microgram Prefibin 0.4mg sublingual tablets sugar-free |
  7 tablet [PoM] £1.60 DT price = £1.60 [CD3]
  Buprenorphine (as Buprenorphine hydrochloride) 2 mg Prefibin
  2mg sublingual tablets sugar-free | 7 tablet [PoM] £5.38 DT price =
  £1.33 [CD3]
  Buprenorphine (as Buprenorphine hydrochloride) 8 mg Prefibin
  8mg sublingual tablets sugar-free | 7 tablet [PoM] £16.15 DT price =
  £2.21 [CD3]
- **Subutex** (RB Pharmaceuticals Ltd)
  Buprenorphine (as Buprenorphine hydrochloride)
  400 microgram Subutex 0.4mg sublingual tablets sugar-free |
  7 tablet [PoM] £1.60 DT price = £1.60 [CD3]
  Buprenorphine (as Buprenorphine hydrochloride) 2 mg Subutex
  2mg sublingual tablets sugar-free | 7 tablet [PoM] £6.35 DT price =
  £1.33 [CD3]
  Buprenorphine (as Buprenorphine hydrochloride) 8 mg Subutex
  8mg sublingual tablets sugar-free | 7 tablet [PoM] £19.05 DT price =
  £2.21 [CD3]
- **Temgesic** (RB Pharmaceuticals Ltd)
  Buprenorphine (as Buprenorphine hydrochloride)
  200 microgram Temgesic 200microgram sublingual tablets sugar-
  free | 50 tablet [PoM] £5.04 DT price = £5.04 [CD3]
  Buprenorphine (as Buprenorphine hydrochloride)
  400 microgram Temgesic 400microgram sublingual tablets sugar-
  free | 50 tablet [PoM] £10.07 DT price = £10.07 [CD3]
- **Tephine** (Sandoz Ltd)
  Buprenorphine (as Buprenorphine hydrochloride)
  200 microgram Tephine 200microgram sublingual tablets sugar-free
  | 50 tablet [PoM] £4.27 DT price = £5.04 [CD3]
  Buprenorphine (as Buprenorphine hydrochloride)
  400 microgram Tephine 400microgram sublingual tablets sugar-free
  | 50 tablet [PoM] £8.54 DT price = £10.07 [CD3]

⇲ 262

Co-codamol

- **INDICATIONS AND DOSE**

**Short-term treatment of acute moderate pain (using
co-codamol 8/500 preparations only)**
- ▸ BY MOUTH
- ▸ Child 12-17 years: 8/500-16/1000 mg every 6 hours as
  required for maximum 3 days; maximum 64/4000 mg
  per day

**Short-term treatment of acute moderate pain (using
co-codamol 15/500 preparations only)**
- ▸ BY MOUTH
- ▸ Child 12-17 years: 15/500-30/1000 mg every 6 hours as
  required for maximum 3 days; maximum 120/4000 mg
  per day

**Short-term treatment of acute moderate pain (using
co-codamol 30/500 preparations only)**
- ▸ BY MOUTH
- ▸ Child 12-17 years: 30/500-60/1000 mg every 6 hours as
  required for maximum 3 days; maximum 240/4000 mg
  per day

KAPAKE® 15/500

Short-term treatment of acute pain
- ▸ BY MOUTH
- ▸ Child 12-15 years: 1 tablet every 6 hours as required for
  maximum 3 days; maximum 4 tablets per day

- ▸ Child 16-17 years: 2 tablets every 6 hours as required for
  maximum 3 days; maximum 8 tablets per day

> **IMPORTANT SAFETY INFORMATION**
> See codeine phosphate p. 265 for MHRA/CHM advice for
> restrictions on the use of codeine as an analgesic in
> children.

- **CONTRA-INDICATIONS** Acute ulcerative colitis · antibiotic-
  associated colitis · children who undergo the removal of
  tonsils or adenoids for the treatment of obstructive sleep
  apnoea · conditions where abdominal distention develops ·
  conditions where inhibition of peristalsis should be
  avoided · known ultra-rapid codeine metabolisers
- **CAUTIONS** Acute abdomen · alcohol dependence · avoid
  abrupt withdrawal after long-term treatment · cardiac
  arrhythmias · chronic alcoholism · chronic dehydration ·
  chronic malnutrition · convulsive disorders · gallstones ·
  hepatocellular insufficiency

  CAUTIONS, FURTHER INFORMATION
- ▸ Variation in metabolism The capacity to metabolise codeine
  to morphine can vary considerably between individuals;
  there is a marked increase in morphine toxicity in patients
  who are ultra-rapid codeine metabolisers (CYP2D6 ultra-
  rapid metabolisers) and a reduced therapeutic effect in
  poor codeine metabolisers.
- **INTERACTIONS** → Appendix 1: opioids, paracetamol
- **SIDE-EFFECTS** Abdominal pain · anorexia · blood disorders
  · depression (with larger doses) · hypothermia · leucopenia
  · malaise · muscle fasciculation · neutropenia · pancreatitis
  · seizures · thrombocytopenia

  Overdose
  Important: liver damage (and less frequently renal
  damage) following overdosage with paracetamol.
- **BREAST FEEDING** Avoid—although amount of codeine
  usually too small to be harmful, mothers vary considerably
  in their capacity to metabolise codeine—risk of morphine
  overdose in infant.
- **HEPATIC IMPAIRMENT** Dose-related toxicity with
  paracetamol—avoid large doses.
- **RENAL IMPAIRMENT** Reduce dose or avoid codeine;
  increased and prolonged effect; increased cerebral
  sensitivity.
- **PRESCRIBING AND DISPENSING INFORMATION** Co-codamol
  is a mixture of codeine phosphate and paracetamol; the
  proportions are expressed in the form x/y, where x and y
  are the strengths in milligrams of codeine phosphate and
  paracetamol respectively.
  When co-codamol tablets, dispersible (or effervescent)
  tablets, or capsules are prescribed and **no strength is
  stated**, tablets, dispersible (or effervescent) tablets, or
  capsules, respectively, containing codeine phosphate 8 mg
  and paracetamol 500 mg should be dispensed.
  The Drug Tariff allows tablets of co-codamol labelled
  'dispersible' to be dispensed against an order for
  'effervescent' and *vice versa*.
- **LESS SUITABLE FOR PRESCRIBING** Co-codamol is less
  suitable for prescribing.
- **EXCEPTIONS TO LEGAL CATEGORY** Co-codamol 8/500 can
  be sold to the public in certain circumstances; for
  exemptions see *Medicines, Ethics and Practice,* London,
  Pharmaceutical Press (always consult latest edition).

4

- **MEDICINAL FORMS**
There can be variation in the licensing of different medicines containing the same drug. Forms available from special-order manufacturers include: oral suspension, oral solution

Tablet
CAUTIONARY AND ADVISORY LABELS 2(does not apply to the 8/500 tablet), 29, 30

▸ **Co-codamol** (Non-proprietary)
Codeine phosphate 8 mg, Paracetamol 500 mg Co-codamol 8mg/500mg tablets | 100 tablet [PoM] £4.43 DT price = £2.97 [CD5] | 500 tablet [PoM] £14.85 [CD5] | 1000 tablet [PoM] £29.70 [CD5]
Codeine phosphate 15 mg, Paracetamol 500 mg Co-codamol 15mg/500mg tablets | 100 tablet [PoM] £15.00 DT price = £9.58 [CD5]
Codeine phosphate 30 mg, Paracetamol 500 mg Co-codamol 30mg/500mg caplets | 100 tablet [PoM] £3.97 DT price = £3.97 [CD5] Co-codamol 30mg/500mg tablets | 30 tablet [PoM] £1.19 DT price = £1.19 [CD5] | 100 tablet [PoM] £7.53 DT price = £3.97 [CD5]

▸ **Codipar** (AMCo)
Codeine phosphate 15 mg, Paracetamol 500 mg Codipar 15mg/500mg tablets | 100 tablet [PoM] £8.25 DT price = £9.58 [CD5]

▸ **Kapake** (Galen Ltd)
Codeine phosphate 30 mg, Paracetamol 500 mg Kapake 30mg/500mg tablets | 100 tablet [PoM] £6.04 DT price = £3.97 [CD5]

▸ **Migraleve Yellow** (McNeil Products Ltd)
Codeine phosphate 8 mg, Paracetamol 500 mg Migraleve Yellow tablets | 16 tablet [PoM] no price available [CD5]

▸ **Panadol Ultra** (GlaxoSmithKline Consumer Healthcare)
Codeine phosphate 12.8 mg, Paracetamol 500 mg Panadol Ultra 12.8mg/500mg tablets | 20 tablet [P] £2.61 DT price = £3.48 [CD5]

▸ **Solpadeine Max** (Omega Pharma Ltd)
Codeine phosphate 12.8 mg, Paracetamol 500 mg Solpadeine Max 12.8mg/500mg tablets | 20 tablet [P] £3.48 DT price = £3.48 [CD5] | 30 tablet [P] £4.52 DT price = £4.52 [CD5]

▸ **Solpadol** (Sanofi)
Codeine phosphate 30 mg, Paracetamol 500 mg Solpadol 30mg/500mg caplets | 30 tablet [PoM] £2.02 DT price = £1.19 [CD5] | 100 tablet [PoM] £6.74 DT price = £3.97 [CD5]

▸ **Zapain** (AMCo)
Codeine phosphate 30 mg, Paracetamol 500 mg Zapain 30mg/500mg tablets | 100 tablet [PoM] £3.03 DT price = £3.97 [CD5]

Effervescent tablet
CAUTIONARY AND ADVISORY LABELS 2(does not apply to the 8/500 tablet), 13, 29, 30
EXCIPIENTS: May contain Aspartame
ELECTROLYTES: May contain Sodium

▸ **Co-codamol** (Non-proprietary)
Codeine phosphate 8 mg, Paracetamol 500 mg Co-codamol 8mg/500mg effervescent tablets | 100 tablet [PoM] £12.97 DT price = £6.88 [CD5]
Codeine phosphate 30 mg, Paracetamol 500 mg Co-codamol 30mg/500mg effervescent tablets | 32 tablet [PoM] £4.78 DT price = £2.77 [CD5] | 100 tablet [PoM] £13.95 DT price = £8.66 [CD5]

▸ **Codipar** (AMCo)
Codeine phosphate 15 mg, Paracetamol 500 mg Codipar 15mg/500mg effervescent tablets sugar-free | 100 tablet [PoM] £8.25 DT price = £8.25 [CD5]

▸ **Solpadol** (Sanofi)
Codeine phosphate 30 mg, Paracetamol 500 mg Solpadol 30mg/500mg effervescent tablets | 32 tablet [PoM] £2.59 DT price = £2.77 [CD5] | 100 tablet [PoM] £8.90 DT price = £8.66 [CD5]

▸ **Tylex** (UCB Pharma Ltd)
Codeine phosphate 30 mg, Paracetamol 500 mg Tylex 30mg/500mg effervescent tablets | 100 tablet [PoM] £9.06 DT price = £8.66 [CD5]

Capsule
CAUTIONARY AND ADVISORY LABELS 2(does not apply to the 8/500 capsule), 29, 30
EXCIPIENTS: May contain Sulfites

▸ **Co-codamol** (Non-proprietary)
Codeine phosphate 8 mg, Paracetamol 500 mg Co-codamol 8mg/500mg capsules | 100 capsule [PoM] £14.48 DT price = £12.66 [CD5]
Codeine phosphate 30 mg, Paracetamol 500 mg Co-codamol 30mg/500mg capsules | 100 capsule [PoM] £7.01 DT price = £3.50 [CD5]

▸ **Codipar** (AMCo)
Codeine phosphate 15 mg, Paracetamol 500 mg Codipar 15mg/500mg capsules | 100 capsule [PoM] £7.25 DT price = £7.25 [CD5]

▸ **Kapake** (Galen Ltd)
Codeine phosphate 30 mg, Paracetamol 500 mg Kapake 30mg/500mg capsules | 100 capsule [PoM] £6.04 DT price = £3.50 [CD5]

▸ **Paracodol** (Bayer Plc)
Codeine phosphate 8 mg, Paracetamol 500 mg Paracodol 8mg/500mg capsules | 20 capsule [P] £1.71 [CD5] | 32 capsule [P] £2.69 DT price = £4.05 [CD5]

▸ **Solpadol** (Sanofi)
Codeine phosphate 30 mg, Paracetamol 500 mg Solpadol 30mg/500mg capsules | 100 capsule [PoM] £6.74 DT price = £3.50 [CD5]

▸ **Tylex** (UCB Pharma Ltd)
Codeine phosphate 30 mg, Paracetamol 500 mg Tylex 30mg/500mg capsules | 100 capsule [PoM] £7.93 DT price = £3.50 [CD5]

▸ **Zapain** (AMCo)
Codeine phosphate 30 mg, Paracetamol 500 mg Zapain 30mg/500mg capsules | 100 capsule [PoM] £3.85 DT price = £3.50 [CD5]

◀ 262

Codeine phosphate

- **INDICATIONS AND DOSE**

Acute diarrhoea
▸ BY MOUTH
▸ **Child 12–17 years:** 30 mg 3–4 times a day; usual dose 15–60 mg 3–4 times a day

Short-term treatment of acute moderate pain
▸ BY MOUTH, OR BY INTRAMUSCULAR INJECTION
▸ **Child 12–17 years:** 30–60 mg every 6 hours if required for maximum 3 days; maximum 240 mg per day

---

IMPORTANT SAFETY INFORMATION
MHRA/CHM ADVICE (JULY 2013) CODEINE FOR ANALGESIA: RESTRICTED USE IN CHILDREN DUE TO REPORTS OF MORPHINE TOXICITY
Codeine should only be used to relieve acute moderate pain in children older than 12 years and only if it cannot be relieved by other painkillers such as paracetamol or ibuprofen alone. A significant risk of serious and life-threatening adverse reactions has been identified in children with obstructive sleep apnoea who received codeine after tonsillectomy or adenoidectomy:
- in children aged 12–18 years, the maximum daily dose of codeine should not exceed 240 mg. Doses may be taken up to four times a day at intervals of no less than 6 hours. The lowest effective dose should be used and duration of treatment should be limited to 3 days
- codeine is contra-indicated in all children (under 18 years) who undergo the removal of tonsils or adenoids for the treatment of obstructive sleep apnoea
- codeine is not recommended for use in children whose breathing may be compromised, including those with neuromuscular disorders, severe cardiac or respiratory conditions, respiratory infections, multiple trauma or extensive surgical procedures
- codeine is contra-indicated in patients of any age who are known to be ultra-rapid metabolisers of codeine (CYP2D6 ultra-rapid metabolisers)
- codeine should not be used in breast-feeding mothers because it can pass to the baby through breast milk
- parents and carers should be advised on how to recognise signs and symptoms of morphine toxicity, and to stop treatment and seek medical attention if signs or symptoms of toxicity occur (including reduced consciousness, lack of appetite, somnolence, constipation, respiratory depression, 'pin-point' pupils, nausea, vomiting)

MHRA/CHM ADVICE (APRIL 2015) CODEINE FOR COUGH AND COLD: RESTRICTED USE IN CHILDREN
Do not use codeine in children under 12 years as it is associated with a risk of respiratory side effects. Codeine

Nervous system

4

is not recommended for adolescents (12–18 years) who have problems with breathing. When prescribing or dispensing codeine-containing medicines for cough and cold, consider that codeine is contra-indicated in:
- children younger than 12 years old
- patients of any age known to be CYP2D6 ultra-rapid metabolisers
- breastfeeding mothers

- **CONTRA-INDICATIONS** Acute ulcerative colitis · antibiotic-associated colitis · children under 18 years who undergo the removal of tonsils or adenoids for the treatment of obstructive sleep apnoea · conditions where abdominal distension develops · conditions where inhibition of peristalsis should be avoided · known ultra-rapid codeine metabolisers

- **CAUTIONS** Acute abdomen · cardiac arrhythmias · gallstones · not recommended for adolescents aged 12–18 years with breathing problems

  CAUTIONS, FURTHER INFORMATION
  ▶ Variation in metabolism The capacity to metabolise codeine to morphine can vary considerably between individuals; there is a marked increase in morphine toxicity in patients who are ultra-rapid codeine metabolisers (CYP2D6 ultra-rapid metabolisers) and a reduced therapeutic effect in poor codeine metabolisers.

- **INTERACTIONS** → Appendix 1: opioids

- **SIDE-EFFECTS** Abdominal pain · anorexia · antidiuretic effect · hypothermia · malaise · muscle fasciculation · pancreatitis · seizures

- **BREAST FEEDING** Avoid—although amount usually too small to be harmful, mothers vary considerably in their capacity to metabolise codeine—risk of morphine overdose in infant.

- **RENAL IMPAIRMENT** Avoid use or reduce dose; opioid effects increased and prolonged and increased cerebral sensitivity occurs.

- **PRESCRIBING AND DISPENSING INFORMATION** BP directs that when Diabetic Codeine Linctus is prescribed, Codeine Linctus formulated with a vehicle appropriate for administration to diabetics, whether or not labelled 'Diabetic Codeine Linctus', shall be dispensed or supplied.

- **PATIENT AND CARER ADVICE**
  Medicines for Children leaflet: Codeine phosphate for pain
  www.medicinesforchildren.org.uk/codeine-phosphate-pain-0

- **MEDICINAL FORMS**
  There can be variation in the licensing of different medicines containing the same drug. Forms available from special-order manufacturers include: oral suspension, oral solution, solution for injection

  Tablet
  CAUTIONARY AND ADVISORY LABELS 2
  ▶ Codeine phosphate (Non-proprietary)
  Codeine phosphate 15 mg Codeine 15mg tablets | 28 tablet PoM £1.40 DT price = £0.95 CD5 | 30 tablet PoM no price available CD5 | 100 tablet PoM £3.39 DT price = £3.39 CD5 | 500 tablet PoM no price available CD5
  Codeine phosphate 30 mg Codeine 30mg tablets | 28 tablet PoM £1.59 DT price = £1.10 CD5 | 30 tablet PoM no price available CD5 | 100 tablet PoM £5.68 DT price = £3.93 CD5 | 500 tablet PoM £19.65 CD5
  Codeine phosphate 60 mg Codeine 60mg tablets | 28 tablet PoM £5.95 DT price = £1.67 CD5

  Solution for injection
  ▶ Codeine phosphate (Non-proprietary)
  Codeine phosphate 60 mg per 1 ml Codeine 60mg/1ml solution for injection ampoules | 10 ampoule PoM £23.70–£25.70 CD2

Oral solution
CAUTIONARY AND ADVISORY LABELS 2
▶ Codeine phosphate (Non-proprietary)
Codeine phosphate 3 mg per 1 ml Codeine 15mg/5ml linctus sugar free sugar-free | 200 ml P £1.90 DT price = £1.62 CD5 sugar-free | 2000 ml P £16.20 CD5
Codeine 15mg/5ml linctus | 200 ml P £1.90 DT price = £1.90 CD5 | 2000 ml P no price available CD5
Codeine phosphate 5 mg per 1 ml Codeine 25mg/5ml oral solution | 500 ml PoM £6.46 DT price = £6.46 CD5
▶ Galcodine (Thornton & Ross Ltd)
Codeine phosphate 3 mg per 1 ml Galcodine 15mg/5ml linctus sugar-free | 2000 ml P £9.90 CD5

⯈ 262

Co-dydramol

- **INDICATIONS AND DOSE**
  Mild to moderate pain (using co-dydramol 10/500 preparations only)
  ▶ BY MOUTH
  ▶ Child 12–17 years: 10/500–20/1000 mg every 4–6 hours as required; maximum 80/4000 mg per day

  Severe pain (using co-dydramol 20/500 preparations only)
  ▶ BY MOUTH
  ▶ Child 12–17 years: 20/500–40/1000 mg every 4–6 hours as required; maximum 160/4000 mg per day

  Severe pain (using co-dydramol 30/500 preparations only)
  ▶ BY MOUTH
  ▶ Child 12–17 years: 30/500–60/1000 mg every 4–6 hours as required; maximum 240/4000 mg per day

  DOSE EQUIVALENCE AND CONVERSION
  ▶ A mixture of dihydrocodeine tartrate and paracetamol; the proportions are expressed in the form x/y, where x and y are the strengths in milligrams of dihydrocodeine and paracetamol respectively.

- **CAUTIONS** Alcohol dependence · before administering, check when paracetamol last administered and cumulative paracetamol dose over previous 24 hours · chronic alcoholism · chronic dehydration · chronic malnutrition · hepatocellular insufficiency · pancreatitis · severe cor pulmonale

- **INTERACTIONS** → Appendix 1: opioids, paracetamol

- **SIDE-EFFECTS** Abdominal pain · acute generalised exanthematous pustulosis · blood disorders · leucopenia · malaise · neutropenia · pancreatitis · paraesthesia · paralytic ileus · skin reactions · Stevens-Johnson syndrome · thrombocytopenia · toxic epidermal necrolysis
  Overdose
  Important: liver damage (and less frequently renal damage) following overdosage with paracetamol.

- **BREAST FEEDING** Amount of dihydrocodeine too small to be harmful but use only if potential benefit outweighs risk.

- **HEPATIC IMPAIRMENT** Dose-related toxicity with paracetamol—avoid large doses.

- **RENAL IMPAIRMENT** Reduce dose or avoid dihydrocodeine; increased and prolonged effect; increased cerebral sensitivity.

- **PRESCRIBING AND DISPENSING INFORMATION** When co-dydramol tablets are prescribed and **no strength is stated**, tablets containing dihydrocodeine tartrate 10 mg and paracetamol 500 mg should be dispensed.

- **LESS SUITABLE FOR PRESCRIBING** Co-dydramol is less suitable for prescribing.

● **MEDICINAL FORMS**
There can be variation in the licensing of different medicines containing the same drug. Forms available from special-order manufacturers include: oral suspension, oral solution

Tablet
CAUTIONARY AND ADVISORY LABELS 2(does not apply to the 10/500 tablet), 29, 30

▸ **Co-dydramol (Non-proprietary)**
Dihydrocodeine tartrate 10 mg, Paracetamol 500 mg Co-dydramol 10mg/500mg tablets | 30 tablet [PoM] £1.14 DT price = £0.94 [CD5] | 100 tablet [PoM] £3.27 DT price = £3.13 [CD5] | 500 tablet [PoM] £15.65 [CD5]

F 262

Diamorphine hydrochloride   10-Jun-2016

(Heroin hydrochloride)

● **INDICATIONS AND DOSE**

Acute or chronic pain

▸ BY MOUTH

▸ Child 1 month–11 years: 100–200 micrograms/kg every 4 hours (max. per dose 10 mg), adjusted according to response

▸ Child 12–17 years: 5–10 mg every 4 hours, adjusted according to response

▸ BY CONTINUOUS INTRAVENOUS INFUSION

▸ Child 1 month–11 years: 12.5–25 micrograms/kg/hour, adjusted according to response

▸ BY INTRAVENOUS INJECTION

▸ Child 1–2 months: 20 micrograms/kg every 6 hours, adjusted according to response

▸ Child 3–5 months: 25–50 micrograms/kg every 6 hours, adjusted according to response

▸ Child 6–11 months: 75 micrograms/kg every 4 hours, adjusted according to response

▸ Child 1–11 years: 75–100 micrograms/kg every 4 hours (max. per dose 5 mg), adjusted according to response

▸ Child 12–17 years: 2.5–5 mg every 4 hours, adjusted according to response

▸ BY INTRAMUSCULAR INJECTION, OR BY SUBCUTANEOUS INJECTION

▸ Child 12–17 years: 5 mg every 4 hours, adjusted according to response

Acute or chronic pain in ventilated neonates

▸ INITIALLY BY INTRAVENOUS INJECTION

▸ Neonate: Initially 50 micrograms/kg, dose to be administered over 30 minutes, followed by (by continuous intravenous infusion) 15 micrograms/kg/hour, adjusted according to response.

Acute or chronic pain in non-ventilated neonates

▸ BY CONTINUOUS INTRAVENOUS INFUSION

▸ Neonate: 2.5–7 micrograms/kg/hour, adjusted according to response.

Acute severe nociceptive pain in an emergency setting (specialist supervision in hospital)

▸ BY INTRANASAL ADMINISTRATION

▸ Child 2–15 years (body-weight 12–17 kg): 1.44 mg for 1 dose, spray into alternate nostrils

▸ Child 2–15 years (body-weight 18–23 kg): 2.16 mg for 1 dose, spray into alternate nostrils

▸ Child 2–15 years (body-weight 24–29 kg): 2.88 mg for 1 dose, spray into alternate nostrils

▸ Child 2–15 years (body-weight 30–39 kg): 3.2 mg for 1 dose, spray into alternate nostrils

▸ Child 2–15 years (body-weight 40–50 kg): 4.8 mg for 1 dose, spray into alternate nostrils

● **CONTRA-INDICATIONS** Delayed gastric emptying · phaeochromocytoma

● **CAUTIONS** CNS depression · severe cor pulmonale · severe diarrhoea · toxic psychosis

● **INTERACTIONS** → Appendix 1: opioids

● **SIDE-EFFECTS** Anorexia · asthenia · myocardial infarction · raised intracranial pressure · syncope · taste disturbance

● **BREAST FEEDING** Therapeutic doses unlikely to affect infant; withdrawal symptoms in infants of dependent mothers; breast-feeding not best method of treating dependence in offspring.

● **RENAL IMPAIRMENT** Avoid use or reduce dose; opioid effects increased and prolonged; increased cerebral sensitivity.

● **MONITORING REQUIREMENTS**

▸ With intranasal use Manufacturer advises monitor for at least 30 minutes following administration.

● **DIRECTIONS FOR ADMINISTRATION**

▸ With intravenous use For *intravenous infusion*, dilute in Glucose 5% or Sodium Chloride 0.9%; Glucose 5% is preferable as an infusion fluid.

▸ With intranasal use Manufacturer advises spray should be directed at the nasal side wall whilst the patient is in a semi-recumbent position.

● **PRESCRIBING AND DISPENSING INFORMATION** Intranasal administration of diamorphine hydrochloride injection has been used [unlicensed]—no dose recommendation.

● **MEDICINAL FORMS**
There can be variation in the licensing of different medicines containing the same drug. Forms available from special-order manufacturers include: capsule, oral solution, solution for injection, powder for solution for injection

Tablet
CAUTIONARY AND ADVISORY LABELS 2

▸ **Diamorphine hydrochloride (Non-proprietary)**
Diamorphine hydrochloride 10 mg Diamorphine 10mg tablets | 100 tablet [PoM] £30.07–£30.76 DT price = £29.56 [CD2]

Powder for solution for injection

▸ **Diamorphine hydrochloride (Non-proprietary)**
Diamorphine hydrochloride 5 mg Diamorphine 5mg powder for solution for injection vials | 5 vial [PoM] £15.00 [CD2] Diamorphine 5mg powder for solution for injection ampoules | 5 ampoule [PoM] £11.36 DT price = £11.36 [CD2]
Diamorphine hydrochloride 10 mg Diamorphine 10mg powder for solution for injection ampoules | 5 ampoule [PoM] £15.06–£16.56 DT price = £13.56 [CD2] Diamorphine 10mg powder for solution for injection vials | 5 vial [PoM] £19.00 [CD2]
Diamorphine hydrochloride 30 mg Diamorphine 30mg powder for solution for injection vials | 5 vial [PoM] £21.00 [CD2] Diamorphine 30mg powder for solution for injection ampoules | 5 ampoule [PoM] £14.59–£16.52 DT price = £12.65 [CD2]
Diamorphine hydrochloride 100 mg Diamorphine 100mg powder for solution for injection vials | 5 vial [PoM] £40.00–£54.00 [CD2] Diamorphine 100mg powder for solution for injection ampoules | 5 ampoule [PoM] £42.39 DT price = £42.39 [CD2]
Diamorphine hydrochloride 500 mg Diamorphine 500mg powder for solution for injection vials | 5 vial [PoM] £190.00–£235.00 DT price = £205.00 [CD2] Diamorphine 500mg powder for solution for injection ampoules | 5 ampoule [PoM] £187.70 DT price = £187.70 [CD2]

Spray
EXCIPIENTS: May contain Benzalkonium chloride, disodium edetate

▸ **Ayendi (Wockhardt UK Ltd)**
Diamorphine (as Diamorphine hydrochloride) 720 microgram per 1 dose Ayendi 720micrograms/actuation nasal spray | 68 dose [PoM] £107.90 (Hospital only) [CD2] | 160 dose [PoM] £112.50 (Hospital only) [CD2]
Diamorphine (as Diamorphine hydrochloride) 1.6 mg per 1 dose Ayendi 1600micrograms/actuation nasal spray | 68 dose [PoM] £113.52 (Hospital only) [CD2] | 160 dose [PoM] £123.75 (Hospital only) [CD2]

F 262

Dihydrocodeine tartrate

● **INDICATIONS AND DOSE**

Moderate to severe pain

▸ BY MOUTH USING IMMEDIATE-RELEASE MEDICINES

▸ Child 1–3 years: 500 micrograms/kg every 4–6 hours

▸ Child 4–11 years: 0.5–1 mg/kg every 4–6 hours (max. per dose 30 mg)

▸ Child 12–17 years: 30 mg every 4–6 hours

▸ BY INTRAMUSCULAR INJECTION, OR BY SUBCUTANEOUS INJECTION

▸ Child 1–3 years: 500 micrograms/kg every 4–6 hours

▸ Child 4–11 years: 0.5–1 mg/kg every 4–6 hours (max. per dose 30 mg)

▸ Child 12–17 years: 30 mg every 4–6 hours (max. per dose 50 mg)

Chronic severe pain

▸ BY MOUTH USING MODIFIED-RELEASE MEDICINES

▸ Child 12–17 years: 60–120 mg every 12 hours

DF118 FORTE®

Severe pain

▸ BY MOUTH

▸ Child 12–17 years: 40–80 mg 3 times a day; maximum 240 mg per day

● **UNLICENSED USE** Most preparations not licensed for use in children under 4 years.

● **CAUTIONS** Pancreatitis · severe cor pulmonale

● **INTERACTIONS** → Appendix 1: opioids

● **SIDE-EFFECTS** Abdominal pain · diarrhoea · paraesthesia · paralytic ileus · seizures

● **BREAST FEEDING** Use only if potential benefit outweighs risk.

● **RENAL IMPAIRMENT** Avoid use or reduce dose; opioid effects increased and prolonged and increased cerebral sensitivity occurs.

● **PROFESSION SPECIFIC INFORMATION**

Dental practitioners' formulary
Dihydrocodeine tablets 30 mg may be prescribed.

● **MEDICINAL FORMS**
There can be variation in the licensing of different medicines containing the same drug. Forms available from special-order manufacturers include: oral suspension, oral solution

Modified-release tablet
CAUTIONARY AND ADVISORY LABELS 2, 25
▸ DHC Continus (Napp Pharmaceuticals Ltd)
Dihydrocodeine tartrate 60 mg DHC Continus 60mg tablets | 56 tablet [PoM] £5.20 DT price = £5.20 [CD5]
Dihydrocodeine tartrate 90 mg DHC Continus 90mg tablets | 56 tablet [PoM] £8.66 DT price = £8.66 [CD5]
Dihydrocodeine tartrate 120 mg DHC Continus 120mg tablets | 56 tablet [PoM] £10.95 DT price = £10.95 [CD5]

Tablet
CAUTIONARY AND ADVISORY LABELS 2
▸ Dihydrocodeine tartrate (Non-proprietary)
Dihydrocodeine tartrate 30 mg Dihydrocodeine 30mg tablets | 28 tablet [PoM] £1.33 DT price = £1.15 [CD5] | 30 tablet [PoM] £1.56 [CD5] | 100 tablet [PoM] £4.11 DT price = £4.11 [CD5] | 500 tablet [PoM] £20.55 [CD5]
▸ DF 118 (Martindale Pharmaceuticals Ltd)
Dihydrocodeine tartrate 40 mg DF 118 Forte 40mg tablets | 100 tablet [PoM] £9.78 DT price = £9.78 [CD5]

Solution for injection
▸ Dihydrocodeine tartrate (Non-proprietary)
Dihydrocodeine tartrate 50 mg per 1 ml Dihydrocodeine 50mg/1ml solution for injection ampoules | 10 ampoule [PoM] £95.70 DT price = £95.70 [CD2]

Oral solution
CAUTIONARY AND ADVISORY LABELS 2
▸ Dihydrocodeine tartrate (Non-proprietary)
Dihydrocodeine tartrate 2 mg per 1 ml Dihydrocodeine 10mg/5ml oral solution | 150 ml [PoM] £7.92 DT price = £7.61 [CD5]

F 262

Fentanyl

● **INDICATIONS AND DOSE**

Chronic intractable pain not currently treated with a strong opioid analgesic

▸ BY TRANSDERMAL APPLICATION

▸ Child 16–17 years: Initially 12 micrograms/hour every 72 hours, alternatively initially 25 micrograms/hour every 72 hours, when starting, evaluation of the analgesic effect should not be made before the system has been worn for 24 hours (to allow for the gradual increase in plasma-fentanyl concentration)—previous analgesic therapy should be phased out gradually from time of first patch application, dose should be adjusted at 48–72 hour intervals in steps of 12–25 micrograms/hour if necessary, more than one patch may be used at a time (but applied at the same time to avoid confusion)—consider additional or alternative analgesic therapy if dose required exceeds 300 micrograms/hour (important: it takes 17 hours or more for the plasma-fentanyl concentration to decrease by 50%—replacement opioid therapy should be initiated at a low dose and increased gradually)

Chronic intractable pain currently treated with a strong opioid analgesic

▸ BY TRANSDERMAL APPLICATION

▸ Child 2–17 years: Initial dose based on previous 24-hour opioid requirement (consult product literature), for evaluating analgesic efficacy and dose increments, see under *Chronic intractable pain not currently treated with a strong opioid analgesic*, for conversion from long term oral morphine to transdermal fentanyl, see *Pain management with opioids* under p. 19.

Spontaneous respiration: analgesia and enhancement of anaesthesia, during operation

▸ BY INTRAVENOUS INJECTION

▸ Child 1 month–11 years: Initially 1–3 micrograms/kg, then 1 microgram/kg as required, dose to be administered over at least 30 seconds

▸ Child 12–17 years: Initially 50–100 micrograms (max. per dose 200 micrograms), dose maximum on specialist advice, then 25–50 micrograms as required, dose to be administered over at least 30 seconds

Assisted ventilation: analgesia and enhancement of anaesthesia during operation

▸ BY INTRAVENOUS INJECTION

▸ Neonate: Initially 1–5 micrograms/kg, then 1–3 micrograms/kg as required, dose to be administered over at least 30 seconds

▸ Child 1 month–11 years: Initially 1–5 micrograms/kg, then 1–3 micrograms/kg as required, dose to be administered over at least 30 seconds

▸ Child 12–17 years: Initially 1–5 micrograms/kg, then 50–200 micrograms as required, dose to be administered over at least 30 seconds

Assisted ventilation: analgesia and respiratory depression in intensive care

▸ INITIALLY BY INTRAVENOUS INJECTION

▸ Neonate: Initially 1–5 micrograms/kg, then (by intravenous infusion) 1.5 micrograms/kg/hour, adjusted according to response

▸ **Child:** Initially 1–5 micrograms/kg, then (by intravenous infusion) 1–6 micrograms/kg/hour, adjusted according to response

Breakthrough pain in patients receiving opioid therapy for chronic cancer pain
▸ BY BUCCAL ADMINISTRATION USING LOZENGES
▸ **Child 16-17 years:** Initially 200 micrograms, dose to be given over 15 minutes, then 200 micrograms after 15 minutes if required, no more than 2 dose units for each pain episode; if adequate pain relief not achieved with 1 dose unit for consecutive breakthrough pain episodes, increase the strength of the dose unit until adequate pain relief achieved with 4 lozenges or less daily, if more than 4 episodes of breakthrough pain each day, adjust background analgesia

DOSE EQUIVALENCE AND CONVERSION
▸ Fentanyl preparations for the treatment of breakthrough pain are not interchangeable; if patients are switched from another fentanyl-containing preparation, a new dose titration is required.

DOSES AT EXTREMES OF BODY-WEIGHT
To avoid excessive dosage in obese patients, weight-based doses may need to be calculated on the basis of ideal bodyweight.

● **UNLICENSED USE**
▸ With intravenous use Not licensed for use in children under 2 years; infusion not licensed for use in children under 12 years.
● **CAUTIONS** Cerebral tumour · diabetes mellitus (with *Actiq*® lozenges) · impaired consciousness
CAUTIONS, FURTHER INFORMATION
▸ With transdermal use Transdermal fentanyl patches are not suitable for acute pain or in those patients whose analgesic requirements are changing rapidly because the long time to steady state prevents rapid titration of the dose. Risk of fatal respiratory depression, particularly in patients not previously treated with a strong opioid analgesic; manufacturer recommends use only in opioid tolerant patients.
▸ With intravenous use Repeated intra-operative doses should be given with care since the resulting respiratory depression can persist postoperatively and occasionally it may become apparent for the first time postoperatively when monitoring of the patient might be less intensive.
● **INTERACTIONS** → Appendix 1: opioids
● **SIDE-EFFECTS**
GENERAL SIDE-EFFECTS
▸ **Common or very common** Abdominal pain · aesthenia · anorexia · anxiety · appetite changes · application-site reactions · diarrhoea · dyspepsia · dyspnoea · gastro-oesophageal reflux disease · hypertension · myoclonus · paraesthesia · pharyngitis · rhinitis · stomatitis · tremor · vasodilation
▸ **Uncommon** Amnesia · arthralgia · blood disorders · chills · depressed level of consciousness · dysgeusia · flatulence · hypoventilation · ileus · impaired concentration · impaired coordination · loss of consciousness · malaise · parosmia · pyrexia · seizures · speech disorder · thirst · thrombocytopenia
▸ **Rare** Hiccups
▸ **Very rare** Apnoea · arrhythmia · ataxia · bladder pain · delusions · haemoptysis
SPECIFIC SIDE-EFFECTS
▸ **Common or very common**
▸ With intravenous use Myoclonic movements
▸ **Uncommon**
▸ With intravenous use Laryngospasm
▸ **Rare**
▸ With intravenous use Asystole · insomnia

SIDE-EFFECTS, FURTHER INFORMATION
▸ Fever or external heat Monitor patients using patches for increased side-effects if fever present (increased absorption possible); and avoid exposing application site to external heat, for example a hot bath or sauna (may also increase absorption).
▸ Muscle rigidity Intravenous administration of fentanyl can cause muscle rigidity, particularly of the chest wall or jaw; this can be managed by the use of neuromuscular blocking drugs.
● **BREAST FEEDING** Monitor infant for opioid-induced side-effects.
● **RENAL IMPAIRMENT** Avoid use or reduce dose; opioid effects increased and prolonged and increased cerebral sensitivity occurs.
● **DIRECTIONS FOR ADMINISTRATION**
▸ With transdermal use For *patches*, apply to dry, non-irritated, non-irradiated, non-hairy skin on torso or upper arm, removing after 72 hours and siting replacement patch on a different area (avoid using the same area for several days).
▸ With intravenous use For *intravenous infusion*, injection solution may be diluted in Glucose 5% or Sodium Chloride 0.9%.
▸ With buccal use Patients should be advised to place the lozenge in the mouth against the cheek and move it around the mouth using the applicator; each lozenge should be sucked over a 15 minute period. In patients with a dry mouth, water may be used to moisten the buccal mucosa. Patients with diabetes should be advised each lozenge contains approximately 2 g glucose.
● **PRESCRIBING AND DISPENSING INFORMATION**
▸ With transdermal use Prescriptions for fentanyl patches can be written to show the strength in terms of the release rate and it is acceptable to write *'Fentanyl 25 patches'* to prescribe patches that release fentanyl 25 micrograms per hour. The dosage should be expressed in terms of the interval between applying a patch and replacing it with a new one, e.g. *'one patch to be applied every 72 hours'*. The total quantity of patches to be supplied should be written in words and figures.
● **PATIENT AND CARER ADVICE**
▸ With transdermal use Patients and carers should be informed about safe use, including correct administration and disposal, strict adherence to dosage instructions, and the symptoms and signs of opioid overdosage. Patches should be removed immediately in case of breathing difficulties, marked drowsiness, confusion, dizziness, or impaired speech, and patients and carers should seek prompt medical attention.
Medicines for Children leaflet: Fentanyl lozenges for pain www.medicinesforchildren.org.uk/fentanyl-lozenges-for-pain
Medicines for Children leaflet: Fentanyl patches for pain www.medicinesforchildren.org.uk/fentanyl-patches-for-pain

● **MEDICINAL FORMS**
There can be variation in the licensing of different medicines containing the same drug. Forms available from special-order manufacturers include: solution for injection, infusion, solution for infusion
Solution for injection
▸ Fentanyl (Non-proprietary)
Fentanyl (as Fentanyl citrate) 50 microgram per 1 ml Fentanyl 100micrograms/2ml solution for injection ampoules | 10 ampoule [PoM] £13.95 [CD2]
Fentanyl 500micrograms/10ml solution for injection ampoules | 10 ampoule [PoM] £13.95 [CD2]
▸ Sublimaze (Janssen-Cilag Ltd)
Fentanyl (as Fentanyl citrate) 50 microgram per 1 ml Sublimaze 500micrograms/10ml solution for injection ampoules | 5 ampoule [PoM] £6.53 [CD2]

Solution for infusion

▸ Fentanyl (Non-proprietary)

Fentanyl (as Fentanyl citrate) 50 microgram per 1 ml Fentanyl 2.5mg/50ml solution for infusion vials | 1 vial [PoM] £5.00 [CD2]

Transdermal patch

CAUTIONARY AND ADVISORY LABELS 2

▸ Fentanyl (Non-proprietary)

Fentanyl 12 microgram per 1 hour Fentanyl 12micrograms/hour transdermal patches | 5 patch [PoM] no price available DT price = £12.59 [CD2]

Fentanyl 25 microgram per 1 hour Fentanyl 25micrograms/hour transdermal patches | 5 patch [PoM] no price available DT price = £17.99 [CD2]

Fentanyl 50 microgram per 1 hour Fentanyl 50micrograms/hour transdermal patches | 5 patch [PoM] no price available DT price = £33.66 [CD2]

Fentanyl 75 microgram per 1 hour Fentanyl 75micrograms/hour transdermal patches | 5 patch [PoM] no price available DT price = £46.99 [CD2]

Fentanyl 100 microgram per 1 hour Fentanyl 100micrograms/hour transdermal patches | 5 patch [PoM] no price available DT price = £57.86 [CD2]

▸ Durogesic DTrans (Janssen-Cilag Ltd)

Fentanyl 12 microgram per 1 hour Durogesic DTrans 12micrograms transdermal patches | 5 patch [PoM] £12.59 DT price = £12.59 [CD2]

Fentanyl 25 microgram per 1 hour Durogesic DTrans 25micrograms transdermal patches | 5 patch [PoM] £17.99 DT price = £17.99 [CD2]

Fentanyl 50 microgram per 1 hour Durogesic DTrans 50micrograms transdermal patches | 5 patch [PoM] £33.66 DT price = £33.66 [CD2]

Fentanyl 75 microgram per 1 hour Durogesic DTrans 75micrograms transdermal patches | 5 patch [PoM] £46.99 DT price = £46.99 [CD2]

Fentanyl 100 microgram per 1 hour Durogesic DTrans 100micrograms transdermal patches | 5 patch [PoM] £57.86 DT price = £57.86 [CD2]

▸ Fencino (Ethypharm UK Ltd)

Fentanyl 12 microgram per 1 hour Fencino 12micrograms/hour transdermal patches | 5 patch [PoM] £8.46 DT price = £12.59 [CD2]

Fentanyl 25 microgram per 1 hour Fencino 25micrograms/hour transdermal patches | 5 patch [PoM] £12.10 DT price = £17.99 [CD2]

Fentanyl 50 microgram per 1 hour Fencino 50micrograms/hour transdermal patches | 5 patch [PoM] £22.62 DT price = £33.66 [CD2]

Fentanyl 75 microgram per 1 hour Fencino 75micrograms/hour transdermal patches | 5 patch [PoM] £31.54 DT price = £46.99 [CD2]

Fentanyl 100 microgram per 1 hour Fencino 100micrograms/hour transdermal patches | 5 patch [PoM] £38.88 DT price = £57.86 [CD2]

▸ Fentalis (Sandoz Ltd)

Fentanyl 25 microgram per 1 hour Fentalis Reservoir 25micrograms/hour transdermal patches | 5 patch [PoM] £22.89 DT price = £17.99 [CD2]

Fentanyl 50 microgram per 1 hour Fentalis Reservoir 50micrograms/hour transdermal patches | 5 patch [PoM] £42.77 DT price = £33.66 [CD2]

Fentanyl 75 microgram per 1 hour Fentalis Reservoir 75micrograms/hour transdermal patches | 5 patch [PoM] £59.62 DT price = £46.99 [CD2]

Fentanyl 100 microgram per 1 hour Fentalis Reservoir 100micrograms/hour transdermal patches | 5 patch [PoM] £73.49 DT price = £57.86 [CD2]

▸ Matrifen (Teva UK Ltd)

Fentanyl 12 microgram per 1 hour Matrifen 12micrograms/hour transdermal patches | 5 patch [PoM] £7.52 DT price = £12.59 [CD2]

Fentanyl 25 microgram per 1 hour Matrifen 25micrograms/hour transdermal patches | 5 patch [PoM] £10.76 DT price = £17.99 [CD2]

Fentanyl 50 microgram per 1 hour Matrifen 50micrograms/hour transdermal patches | 5 patch [PoM] £20.12 DT price = £33.66 [CD2]

Fentanyl 75 microgram per 1 hour Matrifen 75micrograms/hour transdermal patches | 5 patch [PoM] £28.06 DT price = £46.99 [CD2]

Fentanyl 100 microgram per 1 hour Matrifen 100micrograms/hour transdermal patches | 5 patch [PoM] £34.59 DT price = £57.86 [CD2]

▸ Mezolar Matrix (Sandoz Ltd)

Fentanyl 12 microgram per 1 hour Mezolar Matrix 12micrograms/hour transdermal patches | 5 patch [PoM] £7.53 DT price = £12.59 [CD2]

Fentanyl 25 microgram per 1 hour Mezolar Matrix 25micrograms/hour transdermal patches | 5 patch [PoM] £10.77 DT price = £17.99 [CD2]

Fentanyl 37.5 microgram per 1 hour Mezolar Matrix 37.5micrograms/hour transdermal patches | 5 patch [PoM] £15.46 [CD2]

Fentanyl 50 microgram per 1 hour Mezolar Matrix 50micrograms/hour transdermal patches | 5 patch [PoM] £20.13 DT price = £33.66 [CD2]

Fentanyl 75 microgram per 1 hour Mezolar Matrix 75micrograms/hour transdermal patches | 5 patch [PoM] £28.07 DT price = £46.99 [CD2]

Fentanyl 100 microgram per 1 hour Mezolar Matrix 100micrograms/hour transdermal patches | 5 patch [PoM] £34.60 DT price = £57.86 [CD2]

▸ Mylafent (Mylan Ltd)

Fentanyl 12 microgram per 1 hour Mylafent 12micrograms/hour transdermal patches | 5 patch [PoM] £7.53 DT price = £12.59 [CD2]

Fentanyl 25 microgram per 1 hour Mylafent 25micrograms/hour transdermal patches | 5 patch [PoM] £10.77 DT price = £17.99 [CD2]

Fentanyl 50 microgram per 1 hour Mylafent 50micrograms/hour transdermal patches | 5 patch [PoM] £20.13 DT price = £33.66 [CD2]

Fentanyl 75 microgram per 1 hour Mylafent 75micrograms/hour transdermal patches | 5 patch [PoM] £28.07 DT price = £46.99 [CD2]

Fentanyl 100 microgram per 1 hour Mylafent 100micrograms/hour transdermal patches | 5 patch [PoM] £34.60 DT price = £57.86 [CD2]

▸ Osmanil (Zentiva)

Fentanyl 12 microgram per 1 hour Osmanil 12micrograms/hour transdermal patches | 5 patch [PoM] £18.11 DT price = £12.59 [CD2]

Fentanyl 25 microgram per 1 hour Osmanil 25micrograms/hour transdermal patches | 5 patch [PoM] £26.94 DT price = £17.99 [CD2]

Fentanyl 50 microgram per 1 hour Osmanil 50micrograms/hour transdermal patches | 5 patch [PoM] £50.32 DT price = £33.66 [CD2]

Fentanyl 75 microgram per 1 hour Osmanil 75micrograms/hour transdermal patches | 5 patch [PoM] £70.15 DT price = £46.99 [CD2]

Fentanyl 100 microgram per 1 hour Osmanil 100micrograms/hour transdermal patches | 5 patch [PoM] £86.46 DT price = £57.86 [CD2]

▸ Tilofyl (Tillomed Laboratories Ltd)

Fentanyl 25 microgram per 1 hour Tilofyl 25micrograms/hour transdermal patches | 5 patch [PoM] £27.00 DT price = £17.99 [CD2]

Fentanyl 50 microgram per 1 hour Tilofyl 50micrograms/hour transdermal patches | 5 patch [PoM] £51.00 DT price = £33.66 [CD2]

Fentanyl 75 microgram per 1 hour Tilofyl 75micrograms/hour transdermal patches | 5 patch [PoM] £71.00 DT price = £46.99 [CD2]

Fentanyl 100 microgram per 1 hour Tilofyl 100micrograms/hour transdermal patches | 5 patch [PoM] £88.00 DT price = £57.86 [CD2]

▸ Victanyl (Actavis UK Ltd)

Fentanyl 12 microgram per 1 hour Victanyl 12micrograms/hour transdermal patches | 5 patch [PoM] £12.58 DT price = £12.59 [CD2]

Fentanyl 25 microgram per 1 hour Victanyl 25micrograms/hour transdermal patches | 5 patch [PoM] £25.89 DT price = £17.99 [CD2]

Fentanyl 50 microgram per 1 hour Victanyl 50micrograms/hour transdermal patches | 5 patch [PoM] £48.36 DT price = £33.66 [CD2]

Fentanyl 75 microgram per 1 hour Victanyl 75micrograms/hour transdermal patches | 5 patch [PoM] £67.41 DT price = £46.99 [CD2]

Fentanyl 100 microgram per 1 hour Victanyl 100micrograms/hour transdermal patches | 5 patch [PoM] £83.09 DT price = £57.86 [CD2]

▸ Yemex (Sandoz Ltd)

Fentanyl 12 microgram per 1 hour Yemex 12micrograms/hour transdermal patches | 5 patch [PoM] £12.59 DT price = £12.59 [CD2]

Fentanyl 25 microgram per 1 hour Yemex 25micrograms/hour transdermal patches | 5 patch [PoM] £17.99 DT price = £17.99 [CD2]

Fentanyl 50 microgram per 1 hour Yemex 50micrograms/hour transdermal patches | 5 patch [PoM] £33.66 DT price = £33.66 [CD2]

Fentanyl 75 microgram per 1 hour Yemex 75micrograms/hour transdermal patches | 5 patch [PoM] £46.99 DT price = £46.99 [CD2]

Fentanyl 100 microgram per 1 hour Yemex 100micrograms/hour transdermal patches | 5 patch [PoM] £57.86 DT price = £57.86 [CD2]

Lozenge

CAUTIONARY AND ADVISORY LABELS 2
EXCIPIENTS: May contain Propylene glycol

▸ Actiq (Teva UK Ltd)

Fentanyl (as Fentanyl citrate) 200 microgram Actiq 200microgram lozenges with integral oromucosal applicator | 3 lozenge [PoM] £21.05 [CD2] | 30 lozenge [PoM] £210.41 [CD2]

Fentanyl (as Fentanyl citrate) 400 microgram Actiq 400microgram lozenges with integral oromucosal applicator | 3 lozenge [PoM] £21.05 [CD2] | 30 lozenge [PoM] £210.41 [CD2]

Fentanyl (as Fentanyl citrate) 600 microgram Actiq 600microgram lozenges with integral oromucosal applicator | 3 lozenge [PoM] £21.05 [CD2] | 30 lozenge [PoM] £210.41 [CD2]

Fentanyl (as Fentanyl citrate) 800 microgram Actiq 800microgram lozenges with integral oromucosal applicator | 3 lozenge [PoM] £21.05 [CD2] | 30 lozenge [PoM] £210.41 [CD2]

Fentanyl (as Fentanyl citrate) 1.2 mg Actiq 1.2mg lozenges with integral oromucosal applicator | 3 lozenge PoM £21.05 CD2 | 30 lozenge PoM £210.41 CD2
Fentanyl (as Fentanyl citrate) 1.6 mg Actiq 1.6mg lozenges with integral oromucosal applicator | 3 lozenge PoM £21.05 CD2 | 30 lozenge PoM £210.41 CD2

▶ 262

Hydromorphone hydrochloride

● **INDICATIONS AND DOSE**

Severe pain in cancer
▶ BY MOUTH USING IMMEDIATE-RELEASE MEDICINES
▶ Child 12–17 years: 1.3 mg every 4 hours, dose to be increased if necessary according to severity of pain
▶ BY MOUTH USING MODIFIED-RELEASE MEDICINES
▶ Child 12–17 years: 4 mg every 12 hours, dose to be increased if necessary according to severity of pain

● CONTRA-INDICATIONS Acute abdomen

● CAUTIONS Pancreatitis · toxic psychosis

● INTERACTIONS → Appendix 1: opioids

● SIDE-EFFECTS
▶ **Common or very common** Abdominal pain · anorexia · anxiety
▶ **Uncommon** Agitation · diarrhoea · dysgeusia · dyskinesia · myoclonus · paraesthesia · paralytic ileus · peripheral oedema · seizures · tremor

● BREAST FEEDING Avoid—no information available.

● RENAL IMPAIRMENT Avoid use or reduce dose; opioid effects increased and prolonged and increased cerebral sensitivity occurs.

● DIRECTIONS FOR ADMINISTRATION For *immediate-release* capsules, swallow whole capsule or sprinkle contents on soft food. For *modified-release* capsules, swallow whole or open capsule and sprinkle contents on soft cold food (swallow the pellets within the capsule whole; do not crush or chew).

● PATIENT AND CARER ADVICE Patients or carers should be given advice on how to administer hydromorphone hydrochloride capsules and modified-release capsules.

● MEDICINAL FORMS
There can be variation in the licensing of different medicines containing the same drug. Forms available from special-order manufacturers include: oral solution

Modified-release capsule
CAUTIONARY AND ADVISORY LABELS 2
▶ Palladone SR (Napp Pharmaceuticals Ltd)
Hydromorphone hydrochloride 2 mg Palladone SR 2mg capsules | 56 capsule PoM £20.98 CD2
Hydromorphone hydrochloride 4 mg Palladone SR 4mg capsules | 56 capsule PoM £28.75 CD2
Hydromorphone hydrochloride 8 mg Palladone SR 8mg capsules | 56 capsule PoM £56.08 CD2
Hydromorphone hydrochloride 16 mg Palladone SR 16mg capsules | 56 capsule PoM £106.53 CD2
Hydromorphone hydrochloride 24 mg Palladone SR 24mg capsules | 56 capsule PoM £159.82 CD2

Capsule
CAUTIONARY AND ADVISORY LABELS 2
▶ Palladone (Napp Pharmaceuticals Ltd)
Hydromorphone hydrochloride 1.3 mg Palladone 1.3mg capsules | 56 capsule PoM £8.82 CD2
Hydromorphone hydrochloride 2.6 mg Palladone 2.6mg capsules | 56 capsule PoM £17.64 CD2

▶ 262

Morphine

12-Dec-2016

● **INDICATIONS AND DOSE**

Pain
▶ BY SUBCUTANEOUS INJECTION
▶ Neonate: Initially 100 micrograms/kg every 6 hours, adjusted according to response.
▶ Child 1–5 months: Initially 100–200 micrograms/kg every 6 hours, adjusted according to response
▶ Child 6 months–1 year: Initially 100–200 micrograms/kg every 4 hours, adjusted according to response
▶ Child 2–11 years: Initially 200 micrograms/kg every 4 hours, adjusted according to response
▶ Child 12–17 years: Initially 2.5–10 mg every 4 hours, adjusted according to response
▶ INITIALLY BY INTRAVENOUS INJECTION
▶ Neonate: 50 micrograms/kg every 6 hours, adjusted according to response, dose to be administered over at least 5 minutes, alternatively (by intravenous injection) initially 50 micrograms/kg, dose to be administered over at least 5 minutes, followed by (by continuous intravenous infusion) 5–20 micrograms/kg/hour, adjusted according to response.
▶ Child 1–5 months: 100 micrograms/kg every 6 hours, adjusted according to response, dose to be administered over at least 5 minutes, alternatively (by intravenous injection) initially 100 micrograms/kg, dose to be administered over at least 5 minutes, followed by (by continuous intravenous infusion) 10–30 micrograms/kg/hour, adjusted according to response
▶ Child 6 months–11 years: 100 micrograms/kg every 4 hours, adjusted according to response, dose to be administered over at least 5 minutes, alternatively (by intravenous injection) initially 100 micrograms/kg, dose to be administered over at least 5 minutes, followed by (by continuous intravenous infusion) 20–30 micrograms/kg/hour, adjusted according to response
▶ Child 12–17 years: 5 mg every 4 hours, adjusted according to response, dose to be administered over at least 5 minutes, alternatively (by intravenous injection) initially 5 mg, dose to be administered over at least 5 minutes, followed by (by continuous intravenous infusion) 20–30 micrograms/kg/hour, adjusted according to response
▶ BY MOUTH, OR BY RECTUM
▶ Child 1–2 months: Initially 50–100 micrograms/kg every 4 hours, adjusted according to response
▶ Child 3–5 months: 100–150 micrograms/kg every 4 hours, adjusted according to response
▶ Child 6–11 months: 200 micrograms/kg every 4 hours, adjusted according to response
▶ Child 1 year: Initially 200–300 micrograms/kg every 4 hours, adjusted according to response
▶ Child 2–11 years: Initially 200–300 micrograms/kg every 4 hours (max. per dose 10 mg), adjusted according to response
▶ Child 12–17 years: Initially 5–10 mg every 4 hours, adjusted according to response
▶ BY CONTINUOUS SUBCUTANEOUS INFUSION
▶ Child 1–2 months: 10 micrograms/kg/hour, adjusted according to response
▶ Child 3 months–17 years: 20 micrograms/kg/hour, adjusted according to response continued →

4

Nervous system

4

Nervous system

Pain (with modified-release 12-hourly preparations)
▶ BY MOUTH USING MODIFIED-RELEASE MEDICINES
▶ Child: Every 12 hours, dose adjusted according to daily morphine requirements, dosage requirements should be reviewed if the brand is altered

Pain (with modified-release 24-hourly preparations)
▶ BY MOUTH USING MODIFIED-RELEASE MEDICINES
▶ Child: Every 24 hours, dose adjusted according to daily morphine requirements, dosage requirements should be reviewed if the brand is altered

Neonatal opioid withdrawal (under expert supervision)
▶ BY MOUTH
▶ Neonate: Initially 40 micrograms/kg every 4 hours until symptoms controlled, dose to be increased if necessary; reduce frequency gradually over 6–10 days, stop when 40 micrograms/kg once daily achieved, dose may vary—consult local guidelines.

Persistent cyanosis in congenital heart disease when blood glucose less than 3 mmol/litre (following glucose)
▶ BY INTRAVENOUS INJECTION, OR BY INTRAMUSCULAR INJECTION
▶ Child: 100 micrograms/kg

DOSE EQUIVALENCE AND CONVERSION
▶ The doses stated refer equally to morphine hydrochloride and sulfate.

● **UNLICENSED USE**
▶ With oral use *Oramorph*® solution and *MXL*® capsules not licensed for use in children under 1 year. *Sevredol*® tablets not licensed for use in children under 3 years. *Oramorph*® unit dose vials and *Filnarine*® SR tablets not licensed for use in children under 6 years. *MST Continus*® preparations licensed to treat children with cancer pain (age-range not specified by manufacturer).
▶ With rectal use Suppositories are not licensed for use in children.

> **IMPORTANT SAFETY INFORMATION**
> Do not confuse modified-release 12-hourly preparations with 24-hourly preparations, see *Prescribing and dispensing information*.

● **CONTRA-INDICATIONS** Acute abdomen · delayed gastric emptying · heart failure secondary to chronic lung disease · phaeochromocytoma
● **CAUTIONS** Cardiac arrhythmias · pancreatitis · severe cor pulmonale
● **INTERACTIONS** → Appendix 1: opioids
● **SIDE-EFFECTS** Abdominal pain · agitation · amenorrhoea · anorexia · asthenia · bronchospasm · delirium · disorientation · dyspepsia · exacerbation of pancreatitis · excitation · hypertension · hypothermia · inhibition of cough reflex · malaise · muscle fasciculation · myoclonus · nystagmus · paraesthesia · paralytic ileus · raised intracranial pressure · restlessness · rhabdomyolysis · seizures · syncope · taste disturbance
● **BREAST FEEDING** Therapeutic doses unlikely to affect infant.
● **RENAL IMPAIRMENT** Avoid use or reduce dose; opioid effects increased and prolonged; increased cerebral sensitivity.
● **DIRECTIONS FOR ADMINISTRATION**
▶ With intravenous use For *continuous intravenous infusion*, dilute with Glucose 5% or 10% or Sodium Chloride 0.9%.
▶ With intravenous use in neonates *Neonatal intensive care*, dilute 2.5 mg/kg body-weight to a final volume of 50 mL with infusion fluid; an intravenous infusion rate of 0.1 mL/hour provides a dose of 5 micrograms/kg/hour.

▶ With oral use For *modified release capsules*—swallow whole or open capsule and sprinkle contents on soft food.
● **PRESCRIBING AND DISPENSING INFORMATION** Modified-release preparations are available as 12-hourly or 24-hourly formulations; prescribers must ensure that the correct preparation is prescribed. Preparations that should be given 12-hourly include *Filnarine*® SR, *MST Continus*®, *Morphgesic*® SR and *Zomorph*®. Preparations that should be given 24-hourly include *MXL*®.
Prescriptions must specify the 'form'.
▶ With rectal use Both the strength of the suppositories and the morphine salt contained in them must be specified by the prescriber.
● **PATIENT AND CARER ADVICE**
Patients or carers should be given advice on how to administer morphine modified-release capsules.
Medicines for Children leaflet: Morphine for pain www.medicinesforchildren.org.uk/morphine-for-pain
● **EXCEPTIONS TO LEGAL CATEGORY** Morphine Oral Solutions Prescription-only medicines or schedule 2 controlled drug. The proportion of morphine hydrochloride may be altered when specified by the prescriber; if above 13 mg per 5 mL the solution becomes a schedule 2 controlled drug. It is usual to adjust the strength so that the dose volume is 5 or 10 mL. Oral solutions of morphine can be prescribed by writing the formula:
Morphine hydrochloride 5 mg
Chloroform water to 5 mL

● **MEDICINAL FORMS**
There can be variation in the licensing of different medicines containing the same drug. Forms available from special-order manufacturers include: capsule, oral solution, solution for injection, infusion, solution for infusion, suppository

Modified-release tablet
CAUTIONARY AND ADVISORY LABELS 2, 25
▶ **MST Continus** (Napp Pharmaceuticals Ltd)
Morphine sulfate 5 mg MST Continus 5mg tablets | 60 tablet [PoM] £3.29 DT price = £3.29 [CD2]
Morphine sulfate 10 mg MST Continus 10mg tablets | 60 tablet [PoM] £5.20 DT price = £5.20 [CD2]
Morphine sulfate 15 mg MST Continus 15mg tablets | 60 tablet [PoM] £9.10 DT price = £9.10 [CD2]
Morphine sulfate 30 mg MST Continus 30mg tablets | 60 tablet [PoM] £12.47 DT price = £12.47 [CD2]
Morphine sulfate 60 mg MST Continus 60mg tablets | 60 tablet [PoM] £24.32 DT price = £24.32 [CD2]
Morphine sulfate 100 mg MST Continus 100mg tablets | 60 tablet [PoM] £38.50 DT price = £38.50 [CD2]
Morphine sulfate 200 mg MST Continus 200mg tablets | 60 tablet [PoM] £81.34 DT price = £81.34 [CD2]
▶ **Morphgesic SR** (AMCo)
Morphine sulfate 10 mg Morphgesic SR 10mg tablets | 60 tablet [PoM] £3.85 DT price = £5.20 [CD2]
Morphine sulfate 30 mg Morphgesic SR 30mg tablets | 60 tablet [PoM] £9.24 DT price = £12.47 [CD2]
Morphine sulfate 60 mg Morphgesic SR 60mg tablets | 60 tablet [PoM] £18.04 DT price = £24.32 [CD2]
Morphine sulfate 100 mg Morphgesic SR 100mg tablets | 60 tablet [PoM] £28.54 DT price = £38.50 [CD2]

Tablet
CAUTIONARY AND ADVISORY LABELS 2
▶ **Sevredol** (Napp Pharmaceutical Ltd)
Morphine sulfate 10 mg Sevredol 10mg tablets | 56 tablet [PoM] £5.31 DT price = £5.31 [CD2]
Morphine sulfate 20 mg Sevredol 20mg tablets | 56 tablet [PoM] £10.61 DT price = £10.61 [CD2]
Morphine sulfate 50 mg Sevredol 50mg tablets | 56 tablet [PoM] £28.02 DT price = £28.02 [CD2]

Suppository
CAUTIONARY AND ADVISORY LABELS 2
▶ **Morphine (Non-proprietary)**
Morphine sulfate 10 mg Morphine sulfate 10mg suppositories | 12 suppository [PoM] £18.62 DT price = £18.62 [CD2]

Solution for injection

▶ **Morphine (Non-proprietary)**

Morphine sulfate 1 mg per 1 ml Morphine sulfate 5mg/5ml solution for injection ampoules | 10 ampoule [PoM] £35.90 [CD2]
Morphine sulfate 1mg/1ml solution for injection ampoules | 10 ampoule [PoM] £26.10 [CD2]
Morphine sulfate 10mg/10ml solution for injection ampoules | 10 ampoule [PoM] £15.00–£38.00 [CD2]

Morphine sulfate 10 mg per 1 ml Morphine sulfate 10mg/1ml solution for injection ampoules | 10 ampoule [PoM] £9.36 DT price = £9.36 [CD2]

Morphine sulfate 15 mg per 1 ml Morphine sulfate 15mg/1ml solution for injection ampoules | 10 ampoule [PoM] £8.95 DT price = £8.95 [CD2]

Morphine sulfate 20 mg per 1 ml Morphine sulfate 20mg/1ml solution for injection ampoules | 10 ampoule [PoM] £54.27 [CD2]

Morphine sulfate 30 mg per 1 ml Morphine sulfate 30mg/1ml solution for injection ampoules | 10 ampoule [PoM] £9.04 DT price = £8.84 [CD2]
Morphine sulfate 60mg/2ml solution for injection ampoules | 5 ampoule [PoM] £10.07 [CD2]

Modified-release capsule

CAUTIONARY AND ADVISORY LABELS 2

▶ **MXL** (Napp Pharmaceuticals Ltd)

Morphine sulfate 30 mg MXL 30mg capsules | 28 capsule [PoM] £10.91 [CD2]

Morphine sulfate 60 mg MXL 60mg capsules | 28 capsule [PoM] £14.95 [CD2]

Morphine sulfate 90 mg MXL 90mg capsules | 28 capsule [PoM] £22.04 [CD2]

Morphine sulfate 120 mg MXL 120mg capsules | 28 capsule [PoM] £29.15 [CD2]

Morphine sulfate 150 mg MXL 150mg capsules | 28 capsule [PoM] £36.43 [CD2]

Morphine sulfate 200 mg MXL 200mg capsules | 28 capsule [PoM] £46.15 [CD2]

▶ **Zomorph** (Ethypharm UK Ltd)

Morphine sulfate 10 mg Zomorph 10mg modified-release capsules | 60 capsule [PoM] £3.47 DT price = £3.47 [CD2]

Morphine sulfate 30 mg Zomorph 30mg modified-release capsules | 60 capsule [PoM] £8.30 DT price = £8.30 [CD2]

Morphine sulfate 60 mg Zomorph 60mg modified-release capsules | 60 capsule [PoM] £16.20 DT price = £16.20 [CD2]

Morphine sulfate 100 mg Zomorph 100mg modified-release capsules | 60 capsule [PoM] £21.80 [CD2]

Morphine sulfate 200 mg Zomorph 200mg modified-release capsules | 60 capsule [PoM] £43.60 DT price = £43.60 [CD2]

Solution for infusion

▶ **Morphine (Non-proprietary)**

Morphine sulfate 1 mg per 1 ml Morphine sulfate 50mg/50ml solution for infusion vials | 1 vial [PoM] £5.78 DT price = £5.78 [CD2] | 10 vial [PoM] £28.90 [CD2]

Morphine sulfate 2 mg per 1 ml Morphine sulfate 100mg/50ml solution for infusion vials | 1 vial [PoM] £6.48 [CD2] | 10 vial [PoM] £57.60 [CD2]

Oral solution

CAUTIONARY AND ADVISORY LABELS 2

▶ **Morphine (Non-proprietary)**

Morphine sulfate 2 mg per 1 ml Morphine sulfate 10mg/5ml oral solution unit dose vials sugar free sugar-free | 1 unit dose [PoM] no price available [CD5]
Morphine sulfate 10mg/5ml oral solution | 100 ml [PoM] £2.01 [CD5] | 300 ml [PoM] £6.54 DT price = £5.45 [CD5] | 500 ml [PoM] £9.08 [CD5]

▶ **Oramorph** (Boehringer Ingelheim Ltd)

Morphine sulfate 2 mg per 1 ml Oramorph 10mg/5ml oral solution | 100 ml [PoM] £1.89 [CD5] | 300 ml [PoM] £5.45 DT price = £5.45 [CD5] | 500 ml [PoM] £8.50 [CD5]

Morphine sulfate 20 mg per 1 ml Oramorph 20mg/ml concentrated oral solution sugar-free | 30 ml [PoM] £4.98 [CD2] sugar-free | 120 ml [PoM] £19.50 DT price = £19.50 [CD2]

Modified-release granules

CAUTIONARY AND ADVISORY LABELS 2, 13

▶ **MST Continus** (Napp Pharmaceuticals Ltd)

Morphine sulfate 20 mg MST Continus Suspension 20mg granules sachets sugar-free | 30 sachet [PoM] £24.58 [CD2]

Morphine sulfate 30 mg MST Continus Suspension 30mg granules sachets sugar-free | 30 sachet [PoM] £25.54 [CD2]

Morphine sulfate 60 mg MST Continus Suspension 60mg granules sachets sugar-free | 30 sachet [PoM] £51.09 [CD2]

Morphine sulfate 100 mg MST Continus Suspension 100mg granules sachets sugar-free | 30 sachet [PoM] £85.15 [CD2]

Morphine sulfate 200 mg MST Continus Suspension 200mg granules sachets sugar-free | 30 sachet [PoM] £170.30 [CD2]

Morphine with cyclizine

The properties listed below are those particular to the combination only. For the properties of the components please consider, morphine p. 271, cyclizine p. 250.

● **INDICATIONS AND DOSE**

CYCLIMORPH-10®

Moderate to severe pain (short-term use only)
▶ BY SUBCUTANEOUS INJECTION, OR BY INTRAMUSCULAR INJECTION, OR BY INTRAVENOUS INJECTION
▶ Child 12-17 years: 1 mL, do not repeat dose more often than every 4 hours; maximum 3 doses per day

CYCLIMORPH-15®

Moderate to severe pain (short-term use only)
▶ BY SUBCUTANEOUS INJECTION, OR BY INTRAMUSCULAR INJECTION, OR BY INTRAVENOUS INJECTION
▶ Child 12-17 years: 1 mL, do not repeat dose more often than every 4 hours; maximum 3 doses per day

● **CAUTIONS** Myocardial infarction (cyclizine may aggravate severe heart failure and counteract the haemodynamic benefits of opioids) · not recommended in palliative care

● **INTERACTIONS** → Appendix 1: antihistamines (sedating), opioids

● **MEDICINAL FORMS**
There can be variation in the licensing of different medicines containing the same drug.

Solution for injection

▶ **Cyclimorph** (AMCo)

Morphine tartrate 15 mg per 1 ml, Cyclizine tartrate 50 mg per 1 ml Cyclimorph 15 solution for injection 1ml ampoules | 5 ampoule [PoM] £9.12 [CD2]

Morphine tartrate 10 mg per 1 ml, Cyclizine tartrate 50 mg per 1 ml Cyclimorph 10 solution for injection 1ml ampoules | 5 ampoule [PoM] £8.77 [CD2]

F 262

Oxycodone hydrochloride

19-May-2017

● **INDICATIONS AND DOSE**

Moderate to severe pain in palliative care
▶ BY MOUTH USING IMMEDIATE-RELEASE MEDICINES
▶ Child 1 month–11 years: Initially 200 micrograms/kg every 4–6 hours (max. per dose 5 mg), dose to be increased if necessary according to severity of pain
▶ Child 12-17 years: Initially 5 mg every 4–6 hours, dose to be increased if necessary according to severity of pain
▶ BY MOUTH USING MODIFIED-RELEASE MEDICINES
▶ Child 8-11 years: Initially 5 mg every 12 hours, dose to be increased if necessary according to severity of pain
▶ Child 12-17 years: Initially 10 mg every 12 hours, dose to be increased if necessary according to severity of pain

DOSE EQUIVALENCE AND CONVERSION
▶ 2 mg oral oxycodone is approximately equivalent to 1 mg parenteral oxycodone.

ONEXILA XL®

Severe pain
▶ BY MOUTH
▶ Child 12-17 years: Initially 10 mg every 24 hours, dose to be increased if necessary according to severity of pain, some patients may require higher doses than the maximum daily dose; maximum 400 mg per day

● **UNLICENSED USE** Oral solution, *Oxynorm*®, *Longtec*®, and *Oxycontin*® not licensed for use in children. Capsules and

Dolcodon® PR not licensed for use in children under 12 years.

IMPORTANT SAFETY INFORMATION
Do not confuse modified-release 12-hourly preparations with 24-hourly preparations, see *Prescribing and dispensing information*.

- **CONTRA-INDICATIONS** Acute abdomen · chronic constipation · cor pulmonale · delayed gastric emptying
- **CAUTIONS** Pancreatitis · toxic psychosis
- **INTERACTIONS** → Appendix 1: opioids
- **SIDE-EFFECTS**
  ► **Common or very common** Abdominal pain · anorexia · anxiety · asthenia · bronchospasm · chills · diarrhoea · dyspepsia · dyspnoea · impaired cough reflex
  ► **Uncommon** Agitation · amenorrhoea · amnesia · belching · cholestasis · dehydration · disorientation · dry skin · dysphagia · flatulence · gastritis · hiccups · hypoaesthesia · hypotonia · malaise · muscle fasciculation · paraesthesia · paralytic ileus · pyrexia · restlessness · seizures · speech disorder · supraventricular tachycardia · syncope · taste disturbance · thirst · tremor · vasodilatation
- **BREAST FEEDING** Present in milk—avoid.
- **HEPATIC IMPAIRMENT** Max. initial dose 2.5 mg every 6 hours in patients not currently treated with an opioid with mild impairment. Avoid in moderate to severe impairment.
- **RENAL IMPAIRMENT** Max. initial dose 2.5 mg every 6 hours in patients not currently treated with an opioid with mild to moderate impairment. Opioid effects increased and prolonged and increased cerebral sensitivity occurs.
  Avoid if estimated glomerular filtration rate less than 10 mL/minute/1.73 m².
- **PRESCRIBING AND DISPENSING INFORMATION** Modified-release preparations are available as 12-hourly or 24-hourly formulations. Preparations that should be given 12-hourly include *Abtard*®, *Carexil*®, *Leveraxo*®, *Longtec*®, *Oxeltra*®, *OxyContin*®, *Oxylan*®, *Reltebon*®, and *Zomestine*®. Preparations that should be given 24-hourly include *Onexila*® XL.

Palliative care
For further information on the use of oxycodone in palliative care, see www.palliativedrugs.com/formulary/en/oxycodone.html.

- **MEDICINAL FORMS**
  There can be variation in the licensing of different medicines containing the same drug. Forms available from special-order manufacturers include: oral solution

Modified-release tablet
CAUTIONARY AND ADVISORY LABELS 2, 25
► **Oxycodone hydrochloride (Non-proprietary)**
Oxycodone hydrochloride 5 mg Oxycodone 5mg modified-release tablets | 28 tablet [PoM] £12.52 DT price = £12.52 [CD2]
Oxycodone hydrochloride 10 mg Oxycodone 10mg modified-release tablets | 56 tablet [PoM] £25.04 DT price = £25.04 [CD2]
Oxycodone hydrochloride 20 mg Oxycodone 20mg modified-release tablets | 56 tablet [PoM] £50.08 DT price = £50.08 [CD2]
Oxycodone hydrochloride 40 mg Oxycodone 40mg modified-release tablets | 56 tablet [PoM] £100.19 DT price = £100.19 [CD2]
Oxycodone hydrochloride 80 mg Oxycodone 80mg modified-release tablets | 56 tablet [PoM] £200.39 DT price = £200.39 [CD2]
► **Abtard** (Ethypharm UK Ltd)
Oxycodone hydrochloride 5 mg Abtard 5mg modified-release tablets | 28 tablet [PoM] £6.26 DT price = £12.52 [CD2]
Oxycodone hydrochloride 10 mg Abtard 10mg modified-release tablets | 56 tablet [PoM] £12.52 DT price = £25.04 [CD2]
Oxycodone hydrochloride 15 mg Abtard 15mg modified-release tablets | 56 tablet [PoM] £19.06 DT price = £38.12 [CD2]
Oxycodone hydrochloride 20 mg Abtard 20mg modified-release tablets | 56 tablet [PoM] £25.04 DT price = £50.08 [CD2]
Oxycodone hydrochloride 30 mg Abtard 30mg modified-release tablets | 56 tablet [PoM] £38.11 DT price = £76.23 [CD2]
Oxycodone hydrochloride 40 mg Abtard 40mg modified-release tablets | 56 tablet [PoM] £50.09 DT price = £100.19 [CD2]
Oxycodone hydrochloride 60 mg Abtard 60mg modified-release tablets | 56 tablet [PoM] £76.24 DT price = £152.49 [CD2]
Oxycodone hydrochloride 80 mg Abtard 80mg modified-release tablets | 56 tablet [PoM] £100.19 DT price = £200.39 [CD2]
► **Carexil** (Sandoz Ltd)
Oxycodone hydrochloride 5 mg Carexil 5mg modified-release tablets | 28 tablet [PoM] £6.26 DT price = £12.52 [CD2]
Oxycodone hydrochloride 10 mg Carexil 10mg modified-release tablets | 56 tablet [PoM] £12.52 DT price = £25.04 [CD2]
Oxycodone hydrochloride 20 mg Carexil 20mg modified-release tablets | 56 tablet [PoM] £25.04 DT price = £50.08 [CD2]
Oxycodone hydrochloride 40 mg Carexil 40mg modified-release tablets | 56 tablet [PoM] £60.11 DT price = £100.19 [CD2]
Oxycodone hydrochloride 80 mg Carexil 80mg modified-release tablets | 56 tablet [PoM] £120.23 DT price = £200.39 [CD2]
► **Leveraxo** (Mylan Ltd)
Oxycodone hydrochloride 5 mg Leveraxo 5mg modified-release tablets | 28 tablet [PoM] £12.39 DT price = £12.52 [CD2]
Oxycodone hydrochloride 10 mg Leveraxo 10mg modified-release tablets | 56 tablet [PoM] £24.79 DT price = £25.04 [CD2]
Oxycodone hydrochloride 20 mg Leveraxo 20mg modified-release tablets | 56 tablet [PoM] £49.58 DT price = £50.08 [CD2]
Oxycodone hydrochloride 30 mg Leveraxo 30mg modified-release tablets | 56 tablet [PoM] £75.47 DT price = £76.23 [CD2]
Oxycodone hydrochloride 40 mg Leveraxo 40mg modified-release tablets | 56 tablet [PoM] £99.19 DT price = £100.19 [CD2]
Oxycodone hydrochloride 60 mg Leveraxo 60mg modified-release tablets | 56 tablet [PoM] £150.97 DT price = £152.49 [CD2]
Oxycodone hydrochloride 80 mg Leveraxo 80mg modified-release tablets | 56 tablet [PoM] £198.39 DT price = £200.39 [CD2]
► **Longtec** (Qdem Pharmaceuticals Ltd)
Oxycodone hydrochloride 5 mg Longtec 5mg modified-release tablets | 28 tablet [PoM] £6.26 DT price = £12.52 [CD2]
Oxycodone hydrochloride 10 mg Longtec 10mg modified-release tablets | 56 tablet [PoM] £12.52 DT price = £25.04 [CD2]
Oxycodone hydrochloride 15 mg Longtec 15mg modified-release tablets | 56 tablet [PoM] £19.06 DT price = £38.12 [CD2]
Oxycodone hydrochloride 20 mg Longtec 20mg modified-release tablets | 56 tablet [PoM] £25.04 DT price = £50.08 [CD2]
Oxycodone hydrochloride 30 mg Longtec 30mg modified-release tablets | 56 tablet [PoM] £38.11 DT price = £76.23 [CD2]
Oxycodone hydrochloride 40 mg Longtec 40mg modified-release tablets | 56 tablet [PoM] £50.09 DT price = £100.19 [CD2]
Oxycodone hydrochloride 60 mg Longtec 60mg modified-release tablets | 56 tablet [PoM] £76.24 DT price = £152.49 [CD2]
Oxycodone hydrochloride 80 mg Longtec 80mg modified-release tablets | 56 tablet [PoM] £100.19 DT price = £200.39 [CD2]
Oxycodone hydrochloride 120 mg Longtec 120mg modified-release tablets | 56 tablet [PoM] £152.51 DT price = £305.02 [CD2]
► **Onexila XL** (Aspire Pharma Ltd)
Oxycodone hydrochloride 10 mg Onexila XL 10mg tablets | 28 tablet [PoM] £12.52 [CD2]
Oxycodone hydrochloride 20 mg Onexila XL 20mg tablets | 28 tablet [PoM] £12.52 [CD2]
Oxycodone hydrochloride 40 mg Onexila XL 40mg tablets | 28 tablet [PoM] £25.04 [CD2]
Oxycodone hydrochloride 80 mg Onexila XL 80mg tablets | 28 tablet [PoM] £50.09 [CD2]
► **Oxeltra** (Wockhardt UK Ltd)
Oxycodone hydrochloride 5 mg Oxeltra 5mg modified-release tablets | 28 tablet [PoM] £11.27 DT price = £12.52 [CD2]
Oxycodone hydrochloride 10 mg Oxeltra 10mg modified-release tablets | 56 tablet [PoM] £22.54 DT price = £25.04 [CD2]
Oxycodone hydrochloride 15 mg Oxeltra 15mg modified-release tablets | 56 tablet [PoM] £34.31 DT price = £38.12 [CD2]
Oxycodone hydrochloride 20 mg Oxeltra 20mg modified-release tablets | 56 tablet [PoM] £45.07 DT price = £50.08 [CD2]
Oxycodone hydrochloride 30 mg Oxeltra 30mg modified-release tablets | 56 tablet [PoM] £68.61 DT price = £76.23 [CD2]
Oxycodone hydrochloride 40 mg Oxeltra 40mg modified-release tablets | 56 tablet [PoM] £90.17 DT price = £100.19 [CD2]
Oxycodone hydrochloride 60 mg Oxeltra 60mg modified-release tablets | 56 tablet [PoM] £137.24 DT price = £152.49 [CD2]
Oxycodone hydrochloride 80 mg Oxeltra 80mg modified-release tablets | 56 tablet [PoM] £180.35 DT price = £200.39 [CD2]
► **OxyContin** (Napp Pharmaceuticals Ltd)
Oxycodone hydrochloride 5 mg OxyContin 5mg modified-release tablets | 28 tablet [PoM] £12.52 DT price = £12.52 [CD2]

Oxycodone hydrochloride 10 mg OxyContin 10mg modified-release tablets | 56 tablet [PoM] £25.04 DT price = £25.04 [CD2]
Oxycodone hydrochloride 15 mg OxyContin 15mg modified-release tablets | 56 tablet [PoM] £38.12 DT price = £38.12 [CD2]
Oxycodone hydrochloride 20 mg OxyContin 20mg modified-release tablets | 56 tablet [PoM] £50.08 DT price = £50.08 [CD2]
Oxycodone hydrochloride 30 mg OxyContin 30mg modified-release tablets | 56 tablet [PoM] £76.23 DT price = £76.23 [CD2]
Oxycodone hydrochloride 40 mg OxyContin 40mg modified-release tablets | 56 tablet [PoM] £100.19 DT price = £100.19 [CD2]
Oxycodone hydrochloride 60 mg OxyContin 60mg modified-release tablets | 56 tablet [PoM] £152.49 DT price = £152.49 [CD2]
Oxycodone hydrochloride 80 mg OxyContin 80mg modified-release tablets | 56 tablet [PoM] £200.39 DT price = £200.39 [CD2]
Oxycodone hydrochloride 120 mg OxyContin 120mg modified-release tablets | 56 tablet [PoM] £305.02 DT price = £305.02 [CD2]

▸ **Oxylan** (Chanelle Medical UK Ltd)
Oxycodone hydrochloride 5 mg Oxylan 5mg modified-release tablets | 28 tablet [PoM] £12.50 DT price = £12.52 [CD2]
Oxycodone hydrochloride 10 mg Oxylan 10mg modified-release tablets | 56 tablet [PoM] £24.99 DT price = £25.04 [CD2]
Oxycodone hydrochloride 20 mg Oxylan 20mg modified-release tablets | 56 tablet [PoM] £49.98 DT price = £50.08 [CD2]
Oxycodone hydrochloride 40 mg Oxylan 40mg modified-release tablets | 56 tablet [PoM] £99.98 DT price = £100.19 [CD2]
Oxycodone hydrochloride 80 mg Oxylan 80mg modified-release tablets | 56 tablet [PoM] £199.97 DT price = £200.39 [CD2]

▸ **Reltebon** (Actavis UK Ltd)
Oxycodone hydrochloride 5 mg Reltebon 5mg modified-release tablets | 28 tablet [PoM] £6.26 DT price = £12.52 [CD2]
Oxycodone hydrochloride 10 mg Reltebon 10mg modified-release tablets | 56 tablet [PoM] £12.52 DT price = £25.04 [CD2]
Oxycodone hydrochloride 15 mg Reltebon 15mg modified-release tablets | 56 tablet [PoM] £19.06 DT price = £38.12 [CD2]
Oxycodone hydrochloride 20 mg Reltebon 20mg modified-release tablets | 56 tablet [PoM] £25.04 DT price = £50.08 [CD2]
Oxycodone hydrochloride 30 mg Reltebon 30mg modified-release tablets | 56 tablet [PoM] £38.11 DT price = £76.23 [CD2]
Oxycodone hydrochloride 40 mg Reltebon 40mg modified-release tablets | 56 tablet [PoM] £50.09 DT price = £100.19 [CD2]
Oxycodone hydrochloride 60 mg Reltebon 60mg modified-release tablets | 56 tablet [PoM] £76.24 DT price = £152.49 [CD2]
Oxycodone hydrochloride 80 mg Reltebon 80mg modified-release tablets | 56 tablet [PoM] £100.19 DT price = £200.39 [CD2]

▸ **Zomestine** (Accord Healthcare Ltd)
Oxycodone hydrochloride 5 mg Zomestine 5mg modified-release tablets | 28 tablet [PoM] £5.01 DT price = £12.52 [CD2]
Oxycodone hydrochloride 10 mg Zomestine 10mg modified-release tablets | 56 tablet [PoM] £10.02 DT price = £25.04 [CD2]
Oxycodone hydrochloride 20 mg Zomestine 20mg modified-release tablets | 56 tablet [PoM] £20.03 DT price = £50.08 [CD2]
Oxycodone hydrochloride 40 mg Zomestine 40mg modified-release tablets | 56 tablet [PoM] £40.08 DT price = £100.19 [CD2]
Oxycodone hydrochloride 80 mg Zomestine 80mg modified-release tablets | 56 tablet [PoM] £80.16 DT price = £200.39 [CD2]

Oral solution
CAUTIONARY AND ADVISORY LABELS 2
▸ **Oxycodone hydrochloride (Non-proprietary)**
Oxycodone hydrochloride 1 mg per 1 ml Oxycodone 5mg/5ml oral solution sugar free sugar-free | 250 ml [PoM] £9.71 DT price = £9.71 [CD2]
Oxycodone hydrochloride 10 mg per 1 ml Oxycodone 10mg/ml oral solution sugar free sugar-free | 120 ml [PoM] £46.63 DT price = £46.63 [CD2]

▸ **OxyNorm** (Napp Pharmaceuticals Ltd)
Oxycodone hydrochloride 1 mg per 1 ml OxyNorm liquid 5mg/5ml oral solution sugar-free | 250 ml [PoM] £9.71 DT price = £9.71 [CD2]
Oxycodone hydrochloride 10 mg per 1 ml OxyNorm 10mg/ml concentrate oral solution sugar-free | 120 ml [PoM] £46.63 DT price = £46.63 [CD2]

▸ **Shortec** (Qdem Pharmaceuticals Ltd)
Oxycodone hydrochloride 1 mg per 1 ml Shortec liquid 5mg/5ml oral solution sugar-free | 250 ml [PoM] £8.25 DT price = £9.71 [CD2]
Oxycodone hydrochloride 10 mg per 1 ml Shortec 10mg/ml concentrate oral solution sugar-free | 120 ml [PoM] £39.64 DT price = £46.63 [CD2]

Capsule
CAUTIONARY AND ADVISORY LABELS 2
▸ **Lynlor** (Actavis UK Ltd)
Oxycodone hydrochloride 5 mg Lynlor 5mg capsules | 56 capsule [PoM] £6.86 DT price = £11.43 [CD2]
Oxycodone hydrochloride 10 mg Lynlor 10mg capsules | 56 capsule [PoM] £13.72 DT price = £22.86 [CD2]
Oxycodone hydrochloride 20 mg Lynlor 20mg capsules | 56 capsule [PoM] £27.43 DT price = £45.71 [CD2]

▸ **OxyNorm** (Napp Pharmaceuticals Ltd)
Oxycodone hydrochloride 5 mg OxyNorm 5mg capsules | 56 capsule [PoM] £11.43 DT price = £11.43 [CD2]
Oxycodone hydrochloride 10 mg OxyNorm 10mg capsules | 56 capsule [PoM] £22.86 DT price = £22.86 [CD2]
Oxycodone hydrochloride 20 mg OxyNorm 20mg capsules | 56 capsule [PoM] £45.71 DT price = £45.71 [CD2]

▸ **Shortec** (Qdem Pharmaceuticals Ltd)
Oxycodone hydrochloride 5 mg Shortec 5mg capsules | 56 capsule [PoM] £6.86 DT price = £11.43 [CD2]
Oxycodone hydrochloride 10 mg Shortec 10mg capsules | 56 capsule [PoM] £13.72 DT price = £22.86 [CD2]
Oxycodone hydrochloride 20 mg Shortec 20mg capsules | 56 capsule [PoM] £27.43 DT price = £45.71 [CD2]

[F 262]

Papaveretum

● **INDICATIONS AND DOSE**
Postoperative analgesia | Severe chronic pain
▸ BY SUBCUTANEOUS INJECTION, OR BY INTRAMUSCULAR INJECTION
▸ Neonate: 115 micrograms/kg every 4 hours if required.
▸ Child 1–11 months: 154 micrograms/kg every 4 hours if required
▸ Child 1–5 years: 1.93–3.85 mg every 4 hours if required
▸ Child 6–11 years: 3.85–7.7 mg every 4 hours if required
▸ Child 12–17 years: 7.7–15.4 mg every 4 hours if required
▸ BY INTRAVENOUS INJECTION
▸ Child: Use 25 to 50% of the corresponding subcutaneous/intramuscular dose

Premedication
▸ BY SUBCUTANEOUS INJECTION, OR BY INTRAMUSCULAR INJECTION
▸ Neonate: 115 micrograms/kg every 4 hours if required.
▸ Child 1–11 months: 154 micrograms/kg every 4 hours if required
▸ Child 1–5 years: 1.93–3.85 mg every 4 hours if required
▸ Child 6–11 years: 3.85–7.7 mg every 4 hours if required
▸ Child 12–17 years: 7.7–15.4 mg every 4 hours if required
▸ BY INTRAVENOUS INJECTION
▸ Child: Use 25 to 50% of the corresponding subcutaneous/intramuscular dose

> IMPORTANT SAFETY INFORMATION
> Do **not** confuse with papaverine.

● **CONTRA-INDICATIONS** Heart failure secondary to chronic lung disease · phaeochromocytoma
● **CAUTIONS** Supraventricular tachycardia
● **INTERACTIONS** → Appendix 1: opioids
● **SIDE-EFFECTS** Hypothermia
● **BREAST FEEDING** Therapeutic doses unlikely to affect infant.
● **RENAL IMPAIRMENT** Avoid use or reduce dose; opioid effects increased and prolonged and increased cerebral sensitivity occurs.
● **PRESCRIBING AND DISPENSING INFORMATION** The name *Omnopon*® was formerly used for papaveretum preparations.

Papaveretum is a mixture of 253 parts of morphine hydrochloride, 23 parts of papaverine hydrochloride and 20 parts of codeine hydrochloride.

- **LESS SUITABLE FOR PRESCRIBING** Papaveretum is less suitable for prescribing.

- **MEDICINAL FORMS**
There can be variation in the licensing of different medicines containing the same drug. Forms available from special-order manufacturers include: solution for injection
Solution for injection
  - Papaveretum (Non-proprietary)
  Papaveretum 15.4 mg per 1 ml Papaveretum 15.4mg/1ml solution for injection ampoules | 10 ampoule [PoM] £48.96 [CD2]

F 262

Pethidine hydrochloride

(Meperidine)

- **INDICATIONS AND DOSE**
Obstetric analgesia
  - BY SUBCUTANEOUS INJECTION, OR BY INTRAMUSCULAR INJECTION
  - Child 12-17 years: 1 mg/kg (max. per dose 100 mg), then 1 mg/kg after 1-3 hours if required; maximum 400 mg per day

- **CONTRA-INDICATIONS** Phaeochromocytoma
- **CAUTIONS** Accumulation of metabolites may result in neurotoxicity · cardiac arrhythmias · not suitable for severe continuing pain · severe cor pulmonale
- **INTERACTIONS** → Appendix 1: opioids
- **SIDE-EFFECTS** Hypothermia · restlessness · tremor
Overdose
Convulsions reported in overdosage.
- **BREAST FEEDING** Present in milk but not known to be harmful.
- **RENAL IMPAIRMENT** Avoid use or reduce dose; opioid effects increased and prolonged and increased cerebral sensitivity occurs.

- **MEDICINAL FORMS**
There can be variation in the licensing of different medicines containing the same drug. Forms available from special-order manufacturers include: solution for injection
Solution for injection
  - Pethidine hydrochloride (Non-proprietary)
  Pethidine hydrochloride 10 mg per 1 ml Pethidine 50mg/5ml solution for injection ampoules | 10 ampoule [PoM] £52.91 [CD2]
  Pethidine hydrochloride 50 mg per 1 ml Pethidine 50mg/1ml solution for injection ampoules | 10 ampoule [PoM] £4.97 DT price = £4.97 [CD2]
  Pethidine 100mg/2ml solution for injection ampoules | 10 ampoule [PoM] £4.66 DT price = £4.66 [CD2]

F 262

Tramadol hydrochloride

- **INDICATIONS AND DOSE**
Moderate to severe pain
  - BY INTRAMUSCULAR INJECTION, OR BY INTRAVENOUS INJECTION, OR BY INTRAVENOUS INFUSION
  - Child 12-17 years: 50-100 mg every 4-6 hours, intravenous injection to be given over 2-3 minutes
Moderate to severe acute pain
  - BY MOUTH USING IMMEDIATE-RELEASE MEDICINES
  - Child 12-17 years: Initially 100 mg, then 50-100 mg every 4-6 hours; Usual maximum 400 mg/24 hours

Moderate to severe chronic pain
  - BY MOUTH USING IMMEDIATE-RELEASE MEDICINES
  - Child 12-17 years: Initially 50 mg, then, adjusted according to response; Usual maximum 400 mg/24 hours
Postoperative pain
  - BY INTRAVENOUS INJECTION
  - Child 12-17 years: Initially 100 mg, then 50 mg every 10-20 minutes if required up to total maximum 250 mg (including initial dose) in first hour, then 50-100 mg every 4-6 hours, intravenous injection to be given over 2-3 minutes; maximum 600 mg per day

Moderate to severe pain (with modified-release 12-hourly preparations)
  - BY MOUTH USING MODIFIED-RELEASE MEDICINES
  - Child 12-17 years: 50-100 mg twice daily, increased if necessary to 150-200 mg twice daily, doses exceeding the usual maximum not generally required; Usual maximum 400 mg/24 hours

Moderate to severe pain (with modified-release 24-hourly preparations)
  - BY MOUTH USING MODIFIED-RELEASE MEDICINES
  - Child 12-17 years: Initially 100-150 mg once daily, increased if necessary up to 400 mg once daily; Usual maximum 400 mg/24 hours

ZYDOL® XL
Moderate to severe pain
  - BY MOUTH USING MODIFIED-RELEASE TABLETS
  - Child 12-17 years: Initially 150 mg once daily, increased if necessary up to 400 mg once daily

> **IMPORTANT SAFETY INFORMATION**
> Do not confuse modified-release 12-hourly preparations with 24-hourly preparations, see *Prescribing and dispensing information.*

- **CONTRA-INDICATIONS** Acute intoxication with alcohol · acute intoxication with analgesics · acute intoxication with hypnotics · acute intoxication with opioids · not suitable for narcotic withdrawal treatment · uncontrolled epilepsy
- **CAUTIONS** Excessive bronchial secretions · history of epilepsy—use tramadol only if compelling reasons · impaired consciousness · not suitable as a substitute in opioid-dependent patients · not suitable in some types of general anaesthesia · susceptibility to seizures—use tramadol only if compelling reasons
  CAUTIONS, FURTHER INFORMATION
  - General anaesthesia Not recommended for analgesia during potentially light planes of general anaesthesia (possibly increased intra-operative recall reported).
- **INTERACTIONS** → Appendix 1: opioids
- **SIDE-EFFECTS**
  - Common or very common Malaise
  - Uncommon Diarrhoea · flatulence · gastritis · retching
  - Rare Abnormal coordination · anorexia · anxiety · bronchospasm · changes in appetite · delirium · dyspnoea · hypertension · muscle weakness · nightmares · paraesthesia · seizures · syncope · tremor · wheezing
  - Frequency not known Blood disorders · hypoglycaemia · speech disorders
- **PREGNANCY** Embryotoxic in *animal* studies—manufacturers advise avoid.
- **BREAST FEEDING** Amount probably too small to be harmful, but manufacturer advises avoid.
- **HEPATIC IMPAIRMENT** Caution (avoid for *oral drops*) in severe impairment.
- **RENAL IMPAIRMENT** Avoid use or reduce dose; opioid effects increased and prolonged and increased cerebral

sensitivity occurs. Caution (avoid for *oral drops*) in severe impairment.

● **DIRECTIONS FOR ADMINISTRATION** Tramadol hydrochloride *orodispersible tablets* should be sucked and then swallowed. May also be dispersed in water. Some tramadol hydrochloride modified-release capsule preparations may be opened and the contents swallowed immediately without chewing—check individual preparations.

For *intravenous infusion*, dilute in Glucose 5% or Sodium Chloride 0.9%.

● **PRESCRIBING AND DISPENSING INFORMATION** Modified-release preparations are available as 12-hourly or 24-hourly formulations. Non-proprietary preparations of modified-release tramadol may be available as either 12-hourly or 24-hourly formulations; prescribers and dispensers must ensure that the correct formulation is prescribed and dispensed. Branded preparations that should be given 12-hourly include *Invodol*® *SR*, *Mabron*®, *Maneo*®, *Marol*®, *Maxitram*® *SR*, *Oldaram*®, *Tilodol*® *SR*, *Tramquel*® *SR*, *Tramulief*® *SR*, *Zamadol*® *SR*, *Zeridame*® *SR* and *Zydol SR*®. Preparations that should be given 24-hourly include *Tradorec XL*®, *Zamadol*® 24hr, and *Zydol XL*®.

● **PATIENT AND CARER ADVICE**
Patients or carers should be given advice on how to administer tramadol hydochloride orodispersible tablets.
Medicines for Children leaflet: Tramadol for pain
www.medicinesforchildren.org.uk/tramadol-for-pain

● **MEDICINAL FORMS**
There can be variation in the licensing of different medicines containing the same drug. Forms available from special-order manufacturers include: oral suspension

Modified-release tablet
CAUTIONARY AND ADVISORY LABELS 2, 25
▸ **Tramadol hydrochloride (Non-proprietary)**
Tramadol hydrochloride 50 mg Tramadol 50mg modified-release tablets | 60 tablet [PoM] no price available DT price = £4.60 [CD3]
Tramadol hydrochloride 100 mg Tramadol 100mg modified-release tablets | 60 tablet [PoM] £44.80 [CD3]
Tramadol hydrochloride 150 mg Tramadol 150mg modified-release tablets | 60 tablet [PoM] £57.85 [CD3]
Tramadol hydrochloride 200 mg Tramadol 200mg modified-release tablets | 30 tablet [PoM] no price available [CD3] | 60 tablet [PoM] £69.60 [CD3]
Tramadol hydrochloride 300 mg Tramadol 300mg modified-release tablets | 30 tablet [PoM] no price available [CD3]
Tramadol hydrochloride 400 mg Tramadol 400mg modified-release tablets | 28 tablet [PoM] no price available [CD3] | 30 tablet [PoM] no price available [CD3]
▸ **Invodol SR** (Ennogen Healthcare Ltd)
Tramadol hydrochloride 100 mg Invodol SR 100mg tablets | 60 tablet [PoM] £14.61 [CD3]
Tramadol hydrochloride 150 mg Invodol SR 150mg tablets | 60 tablet [PoM] £21.91 [CD3]
Tramadol hydrochloride 200 mg Invodol SR 200mg tablets | 60 tablet [PoM] £29.22 [CD3]
▸ **Mabron** (Morningside Healthcare Ltd)
Tramadol hydrochloride 100 mg Mabron 100mg modified-release tablets | 60 tablet [PoM] £18.26 [CD3]
Tramadol hydrochloride 150 mg Mabron 150mg modified-release tablets | 60 tablet [PoM] £27.39 [CD3]
Tramadol hydrochloride 200 mg Mabron 200mg modified-release tablets | 60 tablet [PoM] £36.52 [CD3]
▸ **Maneo** (Mylan Ltd)
Tramadol hydrochloride 100 mg Maneo 100mg modified-release tablets | 60 tablet [PoM] £6.95 [CD3]
Tramadol hydrochloride 150 mg Maneo 150mg modified-release tablets | 60 tablet [PoM] £10.40 [CD3]
Tramadol hydrochloride 200 mg Maneo 200mg modified-release tablets | 60 tablet [PoM] £14.20 [CD3]
▸ **Marol** (Teva UK Ltd)
Tramadol hydrochloride 100 mg Marol 100mg modified-release tablets | 60 tablet [PoM] £6.94 [CD3]

Tramadol hydrochloride 150 mg Marol 150mg modified-release tablets | 60 tablet [PoM] £10.39 [CD3]
Tramadol hydrochloride 200 mg Marol 200mg modified-release tablets | 60 tablet [PoM] £14.19 [CD3]
▸ **Oldaram** (Ranbaxy (UK) Ltd)
Tramadol hydrochloride 100 mg Oldaram 100mg modified-release tablets | 60 tablet [PoM] £18.80 [CD3]
Tramadol hydrochloride 150 mg Oldaram 150mg modified-release tablets | 60 tablet [PoM] £28.21 [CD3]
Tramadol hydrochloride 200 mg Oldaram 200mg modified-release tablets | 60 tablet [PoM] £37.62 [CD3]
▸ **Tilodol SR** (Sandoz Ltd)
Tramadol hydrochloride 100 mg Tilodol SR 100mg tablets | 60 tablet [PoM] £15.52 [CD3]
Tramadol hydrochloride 150 mg Tilodol SR 150mg tablets | 60 tablet [PoM] £23.28 [CD3]
Tramadol hydrochloride 200 mg Tilodol SR 200mg tablets | 60 tablet [PoM] £31.04 [CD3]
▸ **Tradorec XL** (Endo Ventures Ltd)
Tramadol hydrochloride 100 mg Tradorec XL 100mg tablets | 30 tablet [PoM] £14.10 [CD3]
Tramadol hydrochloride 200 mg Tradorec XL 200mg tablets | 30 tablet [PoM] £14.98 [CD3]
Tramadol hydrochloride 300 mg Tradorec XL 300mg tablets | 30 tablet [PoM] £22.47 [CD3]
▸ **Tramulief SR** (AMCo)
Tramadol hydrochloride 100 mg Tramulief SR 100mg tablets | 60 tablet [PoM] £6.98 [CD3]
Tramadol hydrochloride 150 mg Tramulief SR 150mg tablets | 60 tablet [PoM] £10.48 [CD3]
Tramadol hydrochloride 200 mg Tramulief SR 200mg tablets | 60 tablet [PoM] £14.28 [CD3]
▸ **Zamadol 24hr** (Meda Pharmaceuticals Ltd)
Tramadol hydrochloride 150 mg Zamadol 24hr 150mg modified-release tablets | 28 tablet [PoM] £10.70 [CD3]
Tramadol hydrochloride 200 mg Zamadol 24hr 200mg modified-release tablets | 28 tablet [PoM] £14.26 [CD3]
Tramadol hydrochloride 300 mg Zamadol 24hr 300mg modified-release tablets | 28 tablet [PoM] £21.39 [CD3]
Tramadol hydrochloride 400 mg Zamadol 24hr 400mg modified-release tablets | 28 tablet [PoM] £28.51 [CD3]
▸ **Zeridame SR** (Actavis UK Ltd)
Tramadol hydrochloride 100 mg Zeridame SR 100mg tablets | 60 tablet [PoM] £17.21 [CD3]
Tramadol hydrochloride 150 mg Zeridame SR 150mg tablets | 60 tablet [PoM] £25.82 [CD3]
Tramadol hydrochloride 200 mg Zeridame SR 200mg tablets | 60 tablet [PoM] £34.43 [CD3]
▸ **Zydol SR** (Grunenthal Ltd)
Tramadol hydrochloride 50 mg Zydol SR 50mg tablets | 60 tablet [PoM] £4.60 DT price = £4.60 [CD3]
Tramadol hydrochloride 100 mg Zydol SR 100mg tablets | 60 tablet [PoM] £18.26 [CD3]
Tramadol hydrochloride 150 mg Zydol SR 150mg tablets | 60 tablet [PoM] £27.39 [CD3]
Tramadol hydrochloride 200 mg Zydol SR 200mg tablets | 60 tablet [PoM] £36.52 [CD3]
▸ **Zydol XL** (Grunenthal Ltd)
Tramadol hydrochloride 150 mg Zydol XL 150mg tablets | 30 tablet [PoM] £12.18 [CD3]
Tramadol hydrochloride 200 mg Zydol XL 200mg tablets | 30 tablet [PoM] £17.98 [CD3]
Tramadol hydrochloride 300 mg Zydol XL 300mg tablets | 30 tablet [PoM] £24.94 [CD3]
Tramadol hydrochloride 400 mg Zydol XL 400mg tablets | 30 tablet [PoM] £32.47 [CD3]

Soluble tablet
CAUTIONARY AND ADVISORY LABELS 2, 13
▸ **Zydol** (Grunenthal Ltd)
Tramadol hydrochloride 50 mg Zydol 50mg soluble tablets sugar-free | 20 tablet [PoM] £2.79 Schedule 3 (CD No Register Exempt Safe Custody) sugar-free | 100 tablet [PoM] £13.33 DT price = £13.33 [CD3]

Solution for injection
▸ **Tramadol hydrochloride (Non-proprietary)**
Tramadol hydrochloride 50 mg per 1 ml Tramadol 100mg/2ml solution for injection ampoules | 5 ampoule [PoM] £4.90–£5.65 [CD3] | 10 ampoule [PoM] £10.00 [CD3]
▸ **Zamadol** (Meda Pharmaceuticals Ltd)
Tramadol hydrochloride 50 mg per 1 ml Zamadol 100mg/2ml solution for injection ampoules | 5 ampoule [PoM] £5.49 [CD3]

▸ **Zydol** (Grunenthal Ltd)

Tramadol hydrochloride 50 mg per 1 ml Zydol 100mg/2ml solution for injection ampoules | 5 ampoule [PoM] £4.00 [CD3]

Modified-release capsule

CAUTIONARY AND ADVISORY LABELS 2, 25

▸ **Tramadol hydrochloride (Non-proprietary)**

Tramadol hydrochloride 50 mg Tramadol 50mg modified-release capsules | 60 capsule [PoM] £7.24 DT price = £7.24 [CD3]
Tramadol hydrochloride 100 mg Tramadol 100mg modified-release capsules | 60 capsule [PoM] £14.47 DT price = £14.47 [CD3]
Tramadol hydrochloride 150 mg Tramadol 150mg modified-release capsules | 60 capsule [PoM] £21.71 DT price = £21.71 [CD3]
Tramadol hydrochloride 200 mg Tramadol 200mg modified-release capsules | 60 capsule [PoM] £28.93 DT price = £28.93 [CD3]

▸ **Maxitram SR** (Chiesi Ltd)

Tramadol hydrochloride 50 mg Maxitram SR 50mg capsules | 60 capsule [PoM] £4.55 DT price = £7.24 [CD3]
Tramadol hydrochloride 100 mg Maxitram SR 100mg capsules | 60 capsule [PoM] £12.14 DT price = £14.47 [CD3]
Tramadol hydrochloride 150 mg Maxitram SR 150mg capsules | 60 capsule [PoM] £18.21 DT price = £21.71 [CD3]
Tramadol hydrochloride 200 mg Maxitram SR 200mg capsules | 60 capsule [PoM] £24.28 DT price = £28.93 [CD3]

▸ **Tramquel SR** (Beechmere Pharmaceuticals Ltd)

Tramadol hydrochloride 50 mg Tramquel SR 50mg capsules | 60 capsule [PoM] £7.24 DT price = £7.24 [CD3]
Tramadol hydrochloride 100 mg Tramquel SR 100mg capsules | 60 capsule [PoM] £14.47 DT price = £14.47 [CD3]
Tramadol hydrochloride 150 mg Tramquel SR 150mg capsules | 60 capsule [PoM] £21.71 DT price = £21.71 [CD3]
Tramadol hydrochloride 200 mg Tramquel SR 200mg capsules | 60 capsule [PoM] £28.93 DT price = £28.93 [CD3]

▸ **Zamadol SR** (Meda Pharmaceuticals Ltd)

Tramadol hydrochloride 50 mg Zamadol SR 50mg capsules | 60 capsule [PoM] £7.24 DT price = £7.24 [CD3]
Tramadol hydrochloride 100 mg Zamadol SR 100mg capsules | 60 capsule [PoM] £14.47 DT price = £14.47 [CD3]
Tramadol hydrochloride 150 mg Zamadol SR 150mg capsules | 60 capsule [PoM] £21.71 DT price = £21.71 [CD3]
Tramadol hydrochloride 200 mg Zamadol SR 200mg capsules | 60 capsule [PoM] £28.93 DT price = £28.93 [CD3]

Oral drops

CAUTIONARY AND ADVISORY LABELS 2, 13

▸ **Tramadol hydrochloride (Non-proprietary)**

Tramadol hydrochloride 100 mg per 1 ml Tramadol (as Tramadol hydrochloride) 100mg/ml oral drops | 10 ml [PoM] £3.50 DT price = £3.50 [CD3]

Capsule

CAUTIONARY AND ADVISORY LABELS 2

▸ **Tramadol hydrochloride (Non-proprietary)**

Tramadol hydrochloride 50 mg Tramadol 50mg capsules | 30 capsule [PoM] £4.71 DT price = £0.86 [CD3] | 100 capsule [PoM] £14.40 DT price = £2.87 [CD3]

▸ **Zamadol** (Meda Pharmaceuticals Ltd)

Tramadol hydrochloride 50 mg Zamadol 50mg capsules | 100 capsule [PoM] £8.00 DT price = £2.87 [CD3]

▸ **Zydol** (Grunenthal Ltd)

Tramadol hydrochloride 50 mg Zydol 50mg capsules | 30 capsule [PoM] £2.29 DT price = £0.86 [CD3] | 100 capsule [PoM] £7.63 DT price = £2.87 [CD3]

Orodispersible tablet

CAUTIONARY AND ADVISORY LABELS 2

▸ **Tramadol hydrochloride (Non-proprietary)**

Tramadol hydrochloride 50 mg Tramadol 50mg orodispersible tablets sugar free sugar-free | 60 tablet [PoM] no price available [CD3]

▸ **Zamadol Melt** (Meda Pharmaceuticals Ltd)

Tramadol hydrochloride 50 mg Zamadol Melt 50mg tablets sugar-free | 60 tablet [PoM] £7.12 [CD3]

Combinations available: *Paracetamol with tramadol*, p. 262

5.1 Migraine

Migraine

Treatment of acute migraine

Treatment of a migraine attack should be guided by response to previous treatment and the severity of the attacks. A **simple analgesic** such as paracetamol p. 260 (preferably in a soluble or dispersible form) or an NSAID, usually ibuprofen p. 625, is often effective; concomitant antiemetic treatment may be required. If treatment with an analgesic is inadequate, an attack may be treated with a specific antimigraine compound such as the 5HT$_1$- receptor agonist sumatriptan p. 279. **Ergot alkaloids** are associated with many side-effects and should be avoided.

Excessive use of acute treatments for migraine (opioid and non-opioid analgesics, 5HT$_1$-receptor agonists, and ergotamine) is associated with medication-overuse headache (analgesic-induced headache); therefore, increasing consumption of these medicines needs careful management.

5HT$_1$-receptor agonists

5HT$_1$-receptor agonists are used in the treatment of acute migraine attacks; treatment of children should be initiated by a specialist. A 5HT$_1$-receptor agonist may be used during the established headache phase of an attack and is the preferred treatment in those who fail to respond to conventional analgesics. 5HT$_1$-receptor agonists are **not** indicated for the treatment of hemiplegic, basilar, or opthalmoplegic migraine.

If a child does not respond to one 5HT$_1$-receptor agonist, an alternative 5HT$_1$-receptor agonist should be tried. For children who have prolonged attacks that frequently recur despite treatment with a 5HT$_1$-receptor agonist, combination therapy with an NSAID such as naproxen p. 631 can be considered. Sumatriptan and zolmitriptan p. 280 are used for migraine in children. They may also be of value in cluster headache.

Antiemetics

Antiemetics, including domperidone p. 251, phenothiazines, and antihistamines, relieve the nausea associated with migraine attacks. Antiemetics may be given by intramuscular injection or rectally if vomiting is a problem. Domperidone has the added advantage of promoting gastric emptying and normal peristalsis; a single dose should be given at the onset of symptoms.

Prophylaxis of migraine

Where migraine attacks are frequent, possible provoking factors such as stress should be sought; combined oral contraceptives may also provoke migraine. Preventive treatment should be considered if migraine attacks interfere with school and social life, particularly for children who:

• suffer at least two attacks a month;
• suffer an increasing frequency of headaches;
• suffer significant disability despite suitable treatment for migraine attacks;
• cannot take suitable treatment for migraine attacks.

In children it is often possible to stop prophylaxis after a period of treatment.

Propranolol hydrochloride p. 101 may be effective in preventing migraine in children but it is contra-indicated in those with asthma. Side-effects such as depression and postural hypotension can further limit its use.

Pizotifen p. 279, an antihistamine and a serotonin-receptor antagonist, may also be used but its efficacy in children has not been clearly established. Common side-effects include drowsiness and weight gain.

Topiramate is licensed for migraine prophylaxis.

Cluster headache and the trigeminal autonomic cephalalgias

Cluster headache rarely responds to standard analgesics. Sumatriptan given by subcutaneous injection is the drug of choice for the treatment of cluster headache. If an injection is unsuitable, sumatriptan nasal spray or zolmitriptan nasal spray may be used. Treatment should be initiated by a specialist. Alternatively, 100% oxygen at a rate of 10-15 litres/minute for 10-20 minutes is useful in aborting an attack.

The other trigeminal autonomic cephalalgias, paroxysmal hemicrania (sensitive to indometacin p. 628), and short-lasting unilateral neuralgiform headache attacks with conjunctival injection and tearing, are seen rarely and are best managed by a specialist.

ANTIHISTAMINES > SEDATING

Paracetamol with buclizine hydrochloride and codeine phosphate

The properties listed below are those particular to the combination only. For the properties of the components please consider, paracetamol p. 260, codeine phosphate p. 265.

● **INDICATIONS AND DOSE**

MIGRALEVE®

Acute migraine
▸ BY MOUTH
  ▸ Child 12-14 years: Initially 1 tablet, (pink tablet) to be taken at onset of attack, or if it is imminent, followed by 1 tablet every 4 hours if required, (yellow tablet) to be taken following initial dose; maximum 1 pink and 3 yellow tablets in 24 hours
  ▸ Child 15-17 years: Initially 2 tablets, (pink tablets) to be taken at onset of attack or if it is imminent, followed by 2 tablets every 4 hours if required, (yellow tablets) to be taken following initial dose; maximum 2 pink and 6 yellow tablets in 24 hours

● **INTERACTIONS** → Appendix 1: antihistamines (sedating), opioids, paracetamol
● **LESS SUITABLE FOR PRESCRIBING**
MIGRALEVE® *Migraleve*® is less suitable for prescribing.

● **MEDICINAL FORMS**
There can be variation in the licensing of different medicines containing the same drug.
Tablet
CAUTIONARY AND ADVISORY LABELS 2, 17, 30
  ▸ Migraleve (McNeil Products Ltd)
    Migraleve tablets | 48 tablet [PoM] £3.64 [CD5]
  ▸ Migraleve Pink (McNeil Products Ltd)
    Buclizine hydrochloride 6.25 mg, Codeine phosphate 8 mg, Paracetamol 500 mg Migraleve Pink tablets | 32 tablet [PoM] no price available [CD5] | 48 tablet [PoM] £3.97 [CD5]

Pizotifen

● **INDICATIONS AND DOSE**

Prophylaxis of migraine
▸ BY MOUTH
  ▸ Child 5-17 years: Initially 500 micrograms once daily, dose to be taken at night, then increased to up to 1.5 mg daily in divided doses, dose to be increased gradually, max. single dose (at night) 1 mg

● **UNLICENSED USE** 1.5 mg tablets not licensed for use in children.

● **CAUTIONS** Avoid abrupt withdrawal · history of epilepsy · susceptibility to angle-closure glaucoma · urinary retention
● **INTERACTIONS** → Appendix 1: antihistamines (sedating)
● **SIDE-EFFECTS**
  ▸ **Common or very common** Dizziness · drowsiness · dry mouth · increased appetite · nausea · weight gain
  ▸ **Uncommon** Constipation
  ▸ **Rare** Aggression · anxiety · arthralgia · depression · hallucination · insomnia · myalgia · paraesthesia
  ▸ **Very rare** Seizures
  ▸ **Frequency not known** Hepatitis · jaundice · muscle cramps
● **PREGNANCY** Avoid unless potential benefit outweighs risk.
● **BREAST FEEDING** Amount probably too small to be harmful, but manufacturer advises avoid.
● **HEPATIC IMPAIRMENT** Use with caution.
● **RENAL IMPAIRMENT** Use with caution.
● **PATIENT AND CARER ADVICE**
  Driving and skilled tasks
  Drowsiness may affect performance of skilled tasks (e.g. driving); effects of alcohol enhanced.
  Medicines for Children leaflet: Pizotifen to prevent migraine headaches www.medicinesforchildren.org.uk/pizotifen-to-prevent-migraine-headaches

● **MEDICINAL FORMS**
There can be variation in the licensing of different medicines containing the same drug. Forms available from special-order manufacturers include: oral solution
Tablet
CAUTIONARY AND ADVISORY LABELS 2
  ▸ Pizotifen (Non-proprietary)
    Pizotifen (as Pizotifen hydrogen malate)
    500 microgram Pizotifen 500microgram tablets | 28 tablet [PoM] £8.50 DT price = £2.03
    Pizotifen (as Pizotifen hydrogen malate) 1.5 mg Pizotifen 1.5mg tablets | 28 tablet [PoM] £8.50 DT price = £2.01

TRIPTANS

Sumatriptan

● **INDICATIONS AND DOSE**

Treatment of acute migraine
▸ BY MOUTH
  ▸ Child 6-9 years: Initially 25 mg for 1 dose, followed by 25 mg after at least 2 hours if required, to be taken only if migraine recurs (patient not responding to initial dose should not take second dose for same attack)
  ▸ Child 10-11 years: Initially 50 mg for 1 dose, followed by 50 mg after at least 2 hours, to be taken only if migraine recurs (patient not responding to initial dose should not take second dose for same attack)
  ▸ Child 12-17 years: Initially 50-100 mg for 1 dose, followed by 50-100 mg after at least 2 hours if required, to be taken only if migraine recurs (patient not responding to initial dose should not take second dose for same attack)
▸ BY SUBCUTANEOUS INJECTION
  ▸ Child 10-17 years: Initially 6 mg for 1 dose, followed by 6 mg after at least 1 hour if required, to be taken only if migraine recurs (patient not responding to initial dose should not take second dose for same attack), dose to be administered using an auto-injector; maximum 12 mg per day
▸ BY INTRANASAL ADMINISTRATION
  ▸ Child 12-17 years: Initially 10-20 mg for 1 dose, followed by 10-20 mg after at least 2 hours if required, to be taken only if migraine recurs (patient not responding to initial dose should not take second dose for same attack); maximum 40 mg per day continued →

Nervous system

4

Treatment of acute cluster headache
▶ BY SUBCUTANEOUS INJECTION
▶ Child 10–17 years (under expert supervision): Initially 6 mg for 1 dose, followed by 6 mg after at least 1 hour if required, to be taken only if headache recurs (patient not responding to initial dose should not take second dose for same attack), dose to be administered using auto-injector; maximum 12 mg per day
▶ BY INTRANASAL ADMINISTRATION
▶ Child 12–17 years (under expert supervision): Initially 10–20 mg for 1 dose, followed by 10–20 mg after at least 2 hours if required, to be taken only if headache recurs (patient not responding to initial dose should not take second dose for same attack); maximum 40 mg per day

● UNLICENSED USE Tablets and injection not licensed for use in children. Not licensed for treating cluster headache in children. Intranasal doses for treating acute migraine in children may differ from those in product literature.

● CONTRA-INDICATIONS Coronary vasospasm · ischaemic heart disease · mild uncontrolled hypertension · moderate and severe hypertension · peripheral vascular disease · previous cerebrovascular accident · previous myocardial infarction · previous transient ischaemic attack · Prinzmetal's angina

● CAUTIONS Conditions which predispose to coronary artery disease · history of seizures · mild, controlled hypertension · pre-existing cardiac disease · risk factors for seizures

● INTERACTIONS → Appendix 1: sumatriptan

● SIDE-EFFECTS

GENERAL SIDE-EFFECTS
▶ Common or very common Dizziness · drowsiness · dyspnoea · fatigue · flushing · myalgia · nausea · sensory disturbances · transient increase in blood pressure · vomiting · weakness
▶ Frequency not known Arrhythmias · angina · anxiety · arthralgia · bradycardia · diarrhoea · dystonia · hypersensitivity reactions · hypotension · ischaemic colitis · myocardial infarction · neck stiffness · nystagmus · palpitation · Raynaud's syndrome · seizures · sweating · tachycardia · transient ischaemic ECG changes · tremor · visual disturbances

SPECIFIC SIDE-EFFECTS
▶ Common or very common
▶ With intranasal use Dysgeusia · epistaxis

SIDE-EFFECTS, FURTHER INFORMATION
Sensations of tingling, heat, heaviness, pressure, or tightness of any part of the body may occur (including throat and chest—discontinue if intense, may be due to coronary vasoconstriction or to anaphylaxis).

● ALLERGY AND CROSS-SENSITIVITY Caution in patients with sensitivity to sulfonamides.

● PREGNANCY There is limited experience of using 5HT$_1$-receptor agonists during pregnancy; manufacturers advise that they should be avoided unless the potential benefit outweighs the risk.

● BREAST FEEDING Present in milk but amount probably too small to be harmful; withhold breast-feeding for 12 hours after treatment.

● HEPATIC IMPAIRMENT Reduce dose of oral therapy. Avoid in severe impairment.

● RENAL IMPAIRMENT Use with caution.

● PATIENT AND CARER ADVICE

Driving and skilled tasks
Drowsiness may affect performance of skilled tasks (e.g. driving).

● MEDICINAL FORMS
There can be variation in the licensing of different medicines containing the same drug.
Solution for injection
CAUTIONARY AND ADVISORY LABELS 3, 10
▶ Sumatriptan (Non-proprietary)
Sumatriptan (as Sumatriptan succinate) 12 mg per 1 ml Sumatriptan 6mg/0.5ml solution for injection pre-filled pen | 2 pre-filled disposable injection PoM £43.00 DT price = £39.50
▶ Imigran Subject (GlaxoSmithKline UK Ltd)
Sumatriptan (as Sumatriptan succinate) 12 mg per 1 ml Imigran Subject 6mg/0.5ml solution for injection syringe refill pack | 2 pre-filled disposable injection PoM £40.41 DT price = £40.41
Imigran Subject 6mg/0.5ml solution for injection pre-filled syringes with device | 2 pre-filled disposable injection PoM £50.96 DT price = £50.96

Spray
CAUTIONARY AND ADVISORY LABELS 3 10
▶ Imigran (GlaxoSmithKline UK Ltd)
Sumatriptan 100 mg per 1 ml Imigran 10mg nasal spray | 2 unit dose PoM £11.80 DT price = £11.80
Sumatriptan 200 mg per 1 ml Imigran 20mg nasal spray | 2 unit dose PoM £14.16 | 6 unit dose PoM £42.47 DT price = £42.47

Tablet
CAUTIONARY AND ADVISORY LABELS 3, 10
▶ Sumatriptan (Non-proprietary)
Sumatriptan (as Sumatriptan succinate) 50 mg Sumatriptan 50mg tablets | 6 tablet PoM £22.56 DT price = £1.25
Boots Migraine Relief 50mg tablets | 2 tablet P no price available
Sumatriptan (as Sumatriptan succinate) 100 mg Sumatriptan 100mg tablets | 6 tablet PoM £36.47 DT price = £1.43
▶ Imigran (GlaxoSmithKline UK Ltd, Forest Laboratories UK Ltd)
Sumatriptan (as Sumatriptan succinate) 50 mg Imigran Radis 50mg tablets | 6 tablet PoM £23.90 DT price = £1.25
Imigran 50mg tablets | 6 tablet PoM £31.85 DT price = £1.25
Imigran Recovery 50mg tablets | 2 tablet P £4.76
Sumatriptan (as Sumatriptan succinate) 100 mg Imigran 100mg tablets | 6 tablet PoM £51.48 DT price = £1.43
Imigran Radis 100mg tablets | 6 tablet PoM £42.90 DT price = £1.43
▶ Migraitan (Bristol Laboratories Ltd)
Sumatriptan (as Sumatriptan succinate) 50 mg Migraitan 50mg tablets | 2 tablet P £4.24

Zolmitriptan

● INDICATIONS AND DOSE

Treatment of acute migraine
▶ BY MOUTH
▶ Child 12–17 years: 2.5 mg, followed by 2.5 mg after at least 2 hours if required, dose to be taken only if migraine recurs, if response unsatisfactory after 3 attacks consider increasing dose to 5 mg or switching to alternative treatment; maximum 10 mg per day
▶ BY INTRANASAL ADMINISTRATION
▶ Child 12–17 years: 5 mg, dose to be administered as soon as possible after onset into one nostril, followed by 5 mg after at least 2 hours if required, dose to be administered only if migraine recurs; maximum 10 mg per day

Treatment of acute cluster headache
▶ BY INTRANASAL ADMINISTRATION
▶ Child 12–17 years: 5 mg, dose to be administered as soon as possible after onset into one nostril only, followed by 5 mg after at least 2 hours if required, dose to be administered only if migraine recurs; maximum 10 mg per day

DOSE ADJUSTMENTS DUE TO INTERACTIONS
Manufacturer advises max. dose 5 mg in 24 hours with concurrent use of moderate and potent inhibitors of CYP1A2, cimetidine and moclobemide.

DOSE EQUIVALENCE AND CONVERSION
▶ 1 spray of Zomig® nasal spray = 5 mg zolmitriptan.

● UNLICENSED USE Not licensed for use in children.

- **CONTRA-INDICATIONS** Arrhythmias associated with accessory cardiac conduction pathways · ischaemic heart disease · previous cerebrovascular accident · transient ischaemic attack · uncontrolled hypertension · vasospasm · Wolff-Parkinson-White syndrome
- **CAUTIONS** Should not be taken within 24 hours of any other 5HT₁-receptor agonist
- **INTERACTIONS** → Appendix 1: zolmitriptan
- **SIDE-EFFECTS**
  GENERAL SIDE-EFFECTS
- ▸ **Common or very common** Abdominal pain · drowsiness · dry mouth · dysphagia · headache · muscle weakness · myalgia · palpitation · paraesthesia
- ▸ **Uncommon** Polyuria · tachycardia · transient increase in blood pressure
- ▸ **Rare** Urticaria
- ▸ **Very rare** Angina · gastro-intestinal infarction · ischaemic colitis · myocardial infarction · splenic infarction
- ▸ **Frequency not known** Asthenia · dizziness
  SPECIFIC SIDE-EFFECTS
- ▸ **With intranasal use** Epistaxis · taste disturbance
  SIDE-EFFECTS, FURTHER INFORMATION
  Sensations of tingling, heat, heaviness, pressure, or tightness of any part of the body may occur (including throat and chest—discontinue if intense, may be due to coronary vasoconstriction or to anaphylaxis).
- **PREGNANCY** There is limited experience of using 5HT₁-receptor agonists during pregnancy; manufacturers advise that they should be avoided unless the potential benefit outweighs the risk.
- **BREAST FEEDING** Use with caution—present in milk in *animal* studies.
- **HEPATIC IMPAIRMENT** Max. 5 mg in 24 hours in moderate or severe impairment.
- **DIRECTIONS FOR ADMINISTRATION** Zolmitriptan orodispersible tablets should be placed on the tongue, allowed to disperse and swallowed.
- **PATIENT AND CARER ADVICE** Patients or carers should be given advice on how to administer zolmitriptan orodispersible tablets.

- **MEDICINAL FORMS**
  There can be variation in the licensing of different medicines containing the same drug.
  Spray
  ▸ Zomig (AstraZeneca UK Ltd)
  Zolmitriptan 50 mg per 1 ml Zomig 5mg/0.1ml nasal spray 0.1ml unit dose | 6 unit dose [PoM] £36.50 DT price = £36.50
  Orodispersible tablet
  EXCIPIENTS: May contain Aspartame
  ▸ Zolmitriptan (Non-proprietary)
  Zolmitriptan 2.5 mg Zolmitriptan 2.5mg orodispersible tablets sugar free sugar-free | 6 tablet [PoM] £20.35 DT price = £1.69
  Zolmitriptan 5 mg Zolmitriptan 5mg orodispersible tablets sugar free sugar-free | 6 tablet [PoM] £20.35 DT price = £12.70
  ▸ Zomig Rapimelt (AstraZeneca UK Ltd)
  Zolmitriptan 2.5 mg Zomig Rapimelt 2.5mg orodispersible tablets sugar-free | 6 tablet [PoM] £23.99 DT price = £1.69
  Zolmitriptan 5 mg Zomig Rapimelt 5mg orodispersible tablets sugar-free | 6 tablet [PoM] £23.94 DT price = £12.70
  Tablet
  ▸ Zolmitriptan (Non-proprietary)
  Zolmitriptan 2.5 mg Zolmitriptan 2.5mg tablets | 6 tablet [PoM] £18.36 DT price = £1.48 | 12 tablet [PoM] £30.60
  Zolmitriptan 5 mg Zolmitriptan 5mg tablets | 6 tablet [PoM] £3.60 | 12 tablet [PoM] £7.20
  ▸ Zomig (AstraZeneca UK Ltd)
  Zolmitriptan 2.5 mg Zomig 2.5mg tablets | 6 tablet [PoM] £23.94 DT price = £1.48

5.2 Neuropathic pain

Neuropathic pain

Overview and management

Neuropathic pain, which occurs as a result of damage to neural tissue, includes *compression neuropathies, peripheral neuropathies* (e.g. due to Diabetic complications p. 429, HIV infection p. 391, chemotherapy), *trauma, idiopathic neuropathy, central pain* (e.g. pain following spinal cord injury and syringomyelia), *postherpetic neuralgia*, and *phantom limb pain*. The pain may occur in an area of sensory deficit and may be described as burning, shooting or scalding; it may be accompanied by pain that is evoked by a nonnoxious stimulus (allodynia).

Children with chronic neuropathic pain require multidisciplinary management, which may include physiotherapy and psychological support. Neuropathic pain is generally managed with a **tricyclic antidepressant** such as amitriptyline hydrochloride p. 229 or **antiepileptic drugs** such as carbamazepine p. 189. Children with localised pain may benefit from **topical local anaesthetic** preparations, particularly while awaiting specialist review. Neuropathic pain may respond only partially to **opioid analgesics**. A corticosteroid may help to relieve pressure in compression neuropathy and thereby reduce pain.

Chronic facial pain

Chronic oral and facial pain including *persistent idiopathic facial pain* (also termed 'atypical facial pain') and *temporomandibular dysfunction* (previously termed temporomandibular joint pain dysfunction syndrome) may call for prolonged use of analgesics or for other drugs. **Tricyclic antidepressants** may be useful for facial pain [unlicensed indication], but are not on the Dental Practitioners' List. Disorders of this type require specialist referral and psychological support to accompany drug treatment. Children on long-term therapy need to be monitored both for progress and for side-effects.

6 Sleep disorders
6.1 Insomnia

Hypnotics and anxiolytics

Overview

Most anxiolytics ('sedatives') will induce sleep when given at night and most hypnotics will sedate when given during the day. Hypnotics and anxiolytics should be reserved for short courses to alleviate acute conditions after causal factors have been established.

The role of drug therapy in the management of anxiety disorders in children and adolescents is uncertain; drug therapy should be initiated only by specialists after psychosocial interventions have failed. Benzodiazepines and tricyclic antidepressants have been used but adverse effects may be problematic.

Hypnotics

The prescribing of hypnotics to children, except for occasional use such as for sedation for procedures is not justified. There is a risk of habituation with prolonged use. Problems settling children at night should be managed with behavioural therapy.

Dental procedures

Some anxious children may benefit from the use of a hypnotic the night before a dental appointment.

Chloral and derivatives

Chloral hydrate below and derivatives were formerly popular hypnotics for children. Chloral hydrate is now mainly used for sedation during diagnostic procedures.

Antihistamines

Some **antihistamines** such as promethazine hydrochloride p. 174 are used for occasional insomnia in adults; their prolonged duration of action can often cause drowsiness the following day. The sedative effect of antihistamines may diminish after a few days of continued treatment; antihistamines are associated with headache, psychomotor impairment and antimuscarinic effects. The use of hypnotics in children is not usually justified.

Melatonin

Melatonin p. 283 is a pineal hormone that may affect sleep pattern. Clinical experience suggests that when appropriate behavioural sleep interventions fail, melatonin may be of value for treating sleep onset insomnia and delayed sleep phase syndrome in children with conditions such as visual impairment, cerebral palsy, attention deficit hyperactivity disorder, autism, and learning difficulties. It is also sometimes used before magnetic resonance imaging (MRI), computed tomography (CT), or EEG investigations. Little is known about its long-term effects in children, and there is uncertainty as to the effect on other circadian rhythms including endocrine or reproductive hormone secretion. The need to continue melatonin therapy should be reviewed every 6 months.

Anxiolytics

Anxiolytic treatment should be used in children only to relieve acute anxiety (and related insomnia) caused by fear (e.g. before surgery). Anxiolytic treatment should be limited to the lowest possible dose for the shortest possible time.

Buspirone

Buspirone hydrochloride is thought to act at specific serotonin ($5HT_{1A}$) receptors; safety and efficacy in children have yet to be determined.

HYPNOTICS, SEDATIVES AND ANXIOLYTICS ›
NON-BENZODIAZEPINE

Chloral hydrate

- **INDICATIONS AND DOSE**

Sedation for painless procedures

▶ BY MOUTH, OR BY RECTUM

▸ Neonate: 30–50 mg/kg, to be given 45–60 minutes before procedure, doses up to 100 mg/kg may be used with respiratory monitoring, administration by rectum only if oral route not available.

▸ Child 1 month–11 years: 30–50 mg/kg (max. per dose 1 g), to be given 45–60 minutes before procedure, administration by rectum only if oral route not available, increased if necessary up to 100 mg/kg (max. per dose 2 g)

▸ Child 12–17 years: 1–2 g, to be given 45–60 minutes before procedure, administration by rectum only if oral route not available

Insomnia (short-term use), using chloral hydrate 143.3 mg/5 ml oral solution

▶ BY MOUTH USING ORAL SOLUTION

▸ Child 2–11 years: 1–1.75 mL/kilogram, alternatively 30–50 mg/kg once daily, dose to be taken with water or milk at bedtime; maximum 35 mL per day; maximum 1 g per day

▸ Child 12–17 years: 15–30 mL, alternatively 430–860 mg once daily, dose to be taken with water or milk at bedtime; maximum 70 mL per day; maximum 2 g per day

Insomnia (short-term use), using chloral betaine 707 mg (≡ 414 mg chloral hydrate) tablets

▶ BY MOUTH USING TABLETS

▸ Child 12–17 years: 1–2 tablets, alternatively 414–828 mg once daily, dose to be taken with water or milk at bedtime; maximum 4 tablets per day; maximum 2 g per day

● **UNLICENSED USE** Not licensed for sedation for painless procedures.

● **CONTRA-INDICATIONS** Acute porphyrias p. 577 · gastritis · severe cardiac disease

● **CAUTIONS** Avoid contact with mucous membranes · avoid contact with skin · avoid prolonged use (and abrupt withdrawal thereafter) · reduce dose in debilitated

● **INTERACTIONS** → Appendix 1: chloral hydrate

● **SIDE-EFFECTS** Abdominal distension · delirium (especially on abrupt withdrawal) · dependence · excitement · flatulence · gastric irritation · headache · ketonuria · nausea · rash · tolerance · vomiting

● **PREGNANCY** Avoid.

● **BREAST FEEDING** Risk of sedation in infant—avoid.

● **HEPATIC IMPAIRMENT** Reduce dose in mild to moderate impairment. Can precipitate coma. Avoid in severe impairment.

● **RENAL IMPAIRMENT** Avoid in severe impairment.

● **DIRECTIONS FOR ADMINISTRATION** For administration *by mouth* dilute liquid with plenty of water or juice to mask unpleasant taste.

● **PRESCRIBING AND DISPENSING INFORMATION** Flavours of oral liquid formulations may include black currant.

When prepared extemporaneously, the BP states Chloral Mixture, BP 2000 consists of chloral hydrate 500 mg/5 mL in a suitable vehicle.

● **PATIENT AND CARER ADVICE**

Driving and skilled tasks

Drowsiness may persist the next day and affect performance of skilled tasks (e.g. driving); effects of alcohol enhanced.

● **MEDICINAL FORMS**

There can be variation in the licensing of different medicines containing the same drug. Forms available from special-order manufacturers include: oral suspension, oral solution, suppository, enema

Tablet

CAUTIONARY AND ADVISORY LABELS 19, 27

▸ Chloral betaine (Non-proprietary)

Chloral betaine 707 mg Cloral betaine 707mg tablets | 30 tablet [PoM] £138.59 DT price = £138.59

Oral solution

CAUTIONARY AND ADVISORY LABELS 1(paediatric solution only), 19 (solution other than paediatric only), 27

▸ Chloral hydrate (Non-proprietary)

Chloral hydrate 28.66 mg per 1 ml Chloral hydrate 143.3mg/5ml oral solution BP | 150 ml [PoM] £244.25 DT price = £244.25

4

Nervous system

Melatonin

- **INDICATIONS AND DOSE**

Sleep onset insomnia (initiated under specialist supervision) | Delayed sleep phase syndrome (initiated under specialist supervision)
- ▶ BY MOUTH USING MODIFIED-RELEASE TABLETS
- ▶ Child: Initially 2–3 mg daily for 1–2 weeks, then increased if necessary to 4–6 mg daily, dose to be taken before bedtime; maximum 10 mg per day

- **UNLICENSED USE** Not licensed for use in children.
- **CAUTIONS** Autoimmune disease (manufacturer advises avoid—no information available)
- **INTERACTIONS** → Appendix 1: melatonin
- **SIDE-EFFECTS**
- ▶ **Uncommon** Abdominal pain · abnormal dreams · anxiety · chest pain · dizziness · dry mouth · dry skin · dyspepsia · glycosuria · headache · hypertension · irritability · malaise · mouth ulceration · nausea · nervousness · proteinuria · pruritus · rash · restlessness · weight gain
- ▶ **Rare** Aggression · arthritis · electrolyte disturbances · flatulence · gastritis · haematuria · halitosis · hot flushes · hypersalivation · hypertriglyceridaemia · impaired memory · increased libido · lacrimation · leucopenia · mood changes · muscle spasm · nail disorder · palpitation · paraesthesia · polyuria · priapism · prostatitis · restless legs syndrome · syncope · thirst · thrombocytopenia · visual disturbances · vomiting
- ▶ **Frequency not known** Galactorrhoea · mouth oedema · tongue oedema
- **PREGNANCY** No information available—avoid.
- **BREAST FEEDING** Present in milk—avoid.
- **HEPATIC IMPAIRMENT** Clearance reduced—avoid.
- **RENAL IMPAIRMENT** No information available—use with caution.
- **PRESCRIBING AND DISPENSING INFORMATION** Treatment with melatonin should be initiated and supervised by a specialist, but may be continued by general practitioners under a shared-care arrangement. The need to continue melatonin therapy should be reviewed every 6 months.

  Melatonin is available as a modified-release tablet (*Circadin*®) and also as unlicensed formulations. Unlicensed immediate-release preparations are available; the manufacturer should be specified in the shared-care guideline because of variability in clinical effect of unlicensed formulations.
- **PATIENT AND CARER ADVICE**
  Medicines for Children leaflet: Melatonin for sleep problems www.medicinesforchildren.org.uk/melatonin-for-sleep-disorders

- **MEDICINAL FORMS**
  There can be variation in the licensing of different medicines containing the same drug.

  Modified-release tablet
  CAUTIONARY AND ADVISORY LABELS 2, 21, 25
  - ▶ Melatonin (Non-proprietary)
    Melatonin 3 mg Melatonin 3mg modified-release tablets | 120 tablet [PoM] no price available
  - ▶ Circadin (Flynn Pharma Ltd)
    Melatonin 2 mg Circadin 2mg modified-release tablets | 30 tablet [PoM] £15.39 DT price = £15.39

7 **Substance dependence**

Substance dependence

Guidance on treatment of drug misuse

Treatment of alcohol or opioid dependence in children requires specialist management. The UK health departments have produced guidance on the treatment of drug misuse in the UK. *Drug Misuse and Dependence: UK Guidelines on Clinical Management* (2007) is available at www.nta.nhs.uk/uploads/clinical_guidelines_2007.pdf.

Nicotine dependence

Smoking cessation interventions are a cost-effective way of reducing ill health and prolonging life. Smokers should be advised to stop and offered help with follow-up when appropriate. If possible, smokers should have access to smoking cessation services for behavioural support.

Therapy to aid smoking cessation is chosen according to the smoker's likely adherence, availability of counselling and support, previous experience of smoking-cessation aids, contra-indications and adverse effects of the preparations, and the smoker's preferences. **Nicotine replacement therapy** is an effective aid to smoking cessation. The use of nicotine p. 284 replacement therapy in an individual who is already accustomed to nicotine introduces few new risks and it is widely accepted that there are no circumstances in which it is safer to smoke than to use nicotine replacement therapy.

Some individuals benefit from having more than one type of nicotine replacement therapy prescribed, such as a combination of transdermal and oral preparations.

Concomitant medication

Cigarette smoking increases the metabolism of some medicines by stimulating the hepatic enzyme CYP1A2. When smoking is discontinued, the dose of these drugs, in particular theophylline p. 162, and some antipsychotics (including clozapine p. 241, olanzapine p. 242, chlorpromazine hydrochloride p. 236, and haloperidol p. 237, may need to be reduced. Regular monitoring for adverse effects is advised.

Nicotine replacement therapy

Nicotine replacement therapy can be used in place of cigarettes after abrupt cessation of smoking, or alternatively to reduce the amount of cigarettes used in advance of making a quit attempt. Nicotine replacement therapy can also be used to minimise passive smoking, and to treat cravings and reduce compensatory smoking after enforced abstinence in smoke-free environments. Smokers who find it difficult to achieve abstinence should consult a healthcare professional for advice.

Choice

Nicotine patches are a prolonged-release formulation and are applied for 16 hours (with the patch removed overnight) or for 24 hours. If the individual experiences strong cravings for cigarettes on waking, a 24-hour patch may be more suitable. Immediate-release nicotine preparations (gum, lozenges, sublingual tablets, inhalator, nasal spray, and oral spray) are used whenever the urge to smoke occurs or to prevent cravings.

The choice of nicotine replacement preparation depends largely on patient preference, and should take into account what preparations, if any, have been tried before. Patients with a high level of nicotine dependence, or who have failed with nicotine replacement therapy previously, may benefit from using a combination of an immediate-release preparation and patches to achieve abstinence.

Side-effects of specific nicotine preparations

Mild local reactions at the beginning of treatment are common because of the irritant effect of nicotine. Oral

4

Nervous system

preparations and *inhalation cartridges* can cause irritation of the throat, *gum*, *lozenges*, and *oral spray* can cause increased salivation, and *patches* can cause minor skin irritation. The *nasal spray* commonly causes coughing, nasal irritation, epistaxis, sneezing, and watery eyes; the *oral spray* can cause watery eyes and blurred vision.

Gastro-intestinal disturbances are common and may be caused by swallowed nicotine. Nausea, vomiting, dyspepsia, and hiccup occur most frequently. Ulcerative stomatitis has also been reported. Dry mouth is a common side-effect of *lozenges*, *patches*, *oral spray*, and *sublingual tablets*. *Lozenges* cause diarrhoea, constipation, dysphagia, oesophagitis, gastritis, mouth ulcers, bloating, flatulence, and less commonly, taste disturbance, thirst, gingival bleeding, and halitosis. The *oral spray* may also cause abdominal pain, flatulence, and taste disturbance.

Palpitations may occur with nicotine replacement therapy and rarely *patches* and *oral spray* can cause arrhythmia. *Patches*, *lozenges*, and *oral spray* can cause chest pain. The *inhalator* can very rarely cause reversible atrial fibrillation.

Paraesthesia is a common side-effect of *oral spray*. Abnormal dreams can occur with *patches*; removal of the patch before bed may help. *Lozenges* and *oral spray* may cause rash and hot flushes. Sweating and myalgia can occur with *patches* and *oral spray*; the *patches* can also cause arthralgia.

Neonatal abstinence syndrome

Neonatal abstinence syndrome occurs at birth as a result of intra-uterine exposure to opioids or high-dose benzodiazepines. Treatment is usually initiated if:

- feeding becomes a problem and tube feeding is required;
- there is profuse vomiting or watery diarrhoea;
- the baby remains very unsettled after two consecutive feeds despite gentle swaddling and the use of a pacifier.

Treatment involves weaning the baby from the drug on which it is dependent. Morphine p. 271 or methadone hydrochloride p. 286 can be used in babies of mothers who have been taking opioids. Morphine is widely used because the dose can be easily adjusted, but methadone hydrochloride may provide smoother control of symptoms. Weaning babies from opioids usually takes 7–10 days. Weaning babies from benzodiazepines that have a long half-life is difficult to manage; chlorpromazine hydrochloride may be used in these situations but excessive sedation may occur. For babies who are dependent on barbiturates, phenobarbital p. 208 may be tried, although it does not control gastro-intestinal symptoms.

7.1 Nicotine dependence

NICOTINIC RECEPTOR AGONISTS

Nicotine

- **INDICATIONS AND DOSE**

Nicotine replacement therapy in individuals who smoke fewer than 20 cigarettes each day

‣ BY MOUTH USING CHEWING GUM
‣ Child 12-17 years: 2 mg as required, chew 1 piece of gum when the urge to smoke occurs or to prevent cravings, if attempting smoking cessation, treatment should continue for 3 months before reducing the dose
‣ BY SUBLINGUAL ADMINISTRATION USING SUBLINGUAL TABLETS
‣ Child 12-17 years: 1 tablet every 1 hour, increased to 2 tablets every 1 hour if required, if attempting smoking cessation, treatment should continue for up to 3 months before reducing the dose; maximum 40 tablets per day

Nicotine replacement therapy in individuals who smoke more than 20 cigarettes each day or who require more than 15 pieces of 2-mg strength gum each day

‣ BY MOUTH USING CHEWING GUM
‣ Child 12-17 years: 4 mg as required, chew 1 piece of gum when the urge to smoke occurs or to prevent cravings, individuals should not exceed 15 pieces of 4-mg strength gum daily, if attempting smoking cessation, treatment should continue for 3 months before reducing the dose

Nicotine replacement therapy in individuals who smoke more than 20 cigarettes each day

‣ BY SUBLINGUAL ADMINISTRATION USING SUBLINGUAL TABLETS
‣ Child 12-17 years: 2 tablets every 1 hour, if attempting smoking cessation, treatment should continue for up to 3 months before reducing the dose; maximum 40 tablets per day

Nicotine replacement therapy

‣ BY INHALATION USING INHALATOR
‣ Child 12-17 years: As required, the cartridges can be used when the urge to smoke occurs or to prevent cravings, individuals should not exceed 12 cartridges of the 10-mg strength daily, or 6 cartridges of the 15-mg strength daily
‣ BY MOUTH USING LOZENGES
‣ Child 12-17 years: 1 lozenge every 1–2 hours as required, one lozenge should be used when the urge to smoke occurs, individuals who smoke less than 20 cigarettes each day should usually use the lower-strength lozenges; individuals who smoke more than 20 cigarettes each day and those who fail to stop smoking with the low-strength lozenges should use the higher-strength lozenges; If attempting smoking cessation, treatment should continue for 6–12 weeks before attempting a reduction in dose; maximum 15 lozenges per day
‣ BY MOUTH USING OROMUCOSAL SPRAY
‣ Child 12-17 years: 1–2 sprays as required, individuals can spray in the mouth when the urge to smoke occurs or to prevent cravings, individuals should not exceed 2 sprays per episode (up to 4 sprays every hour); maximum 64 sprays per day
‣ BY INTRANASAL ADMINISTRATION USING NASAL SPRAY
‣ Child 12-17 years: 1 spray as required, individuals can spray into each nostril when the urge to smoke occurs, up to twice every hour for 16 hours daily, if attempting smoking cessation, treatment should continue for 8 weeks before reducing the dose; maximum 64 sprays per day
‣ BY TRANSDERMAL APPLICATION USING PATCHES
‣ Child 12-17 years: Individuals who smoke more than 10 cigarettes daily should apply a high-strength patch daily for 6–8 weeks, followed by the medium-strength patch for 2 weeks, and then the low-strength patch for the final 2 weeks; individuals who smoke fewer than 10 cigarettes daily can usually start with the medium-strength patch for 6–8 weeks, followed by the low-strength patch for 2–4 weeks; a slower titration schedule can be used in individuals who are not ready to quit but want to reduce cigarette consumption before a quit attempt; if abstinence is not achieved, or if withdrawal symptoms are experienced, the strength of the patch used should be maintained or increased until the patient is stabilised; individuals using the high-strength patch who experience excessive side-effects, that do not resolve within a few days, should change to a medium-strength patch for the remainder of the initial period and then use the low-strength patch for 2–4 weeks

- **UNLICENSED USE** All preparations are licensed for children over 12 years (with the exception of *Nicotinell*® lozenges which are licensed for children under 18 years only when recommended by a doctor).

- **CAUTIONS**
  GENERAL CAUTIONS
  Diabetes mellitus—blood-glucose concentration should be monitored closely when initiating treatment · haemodynamically unstable patients hospitalised with cerebrovascular accident · haemodynamically unstable patients hospitalised with myocardial infarction · haemodynamically unstable patients hospitalised with severe arrhythmias · phaeochromocytoma · uncontrolled hyperthyroidism

  SPECIFIC CAUTIONS
  ‣ When used by inhalation Bronchospastic disease · chronic throat disease · obstructive lung disease
  ‣ With intranasal use Bronchial asthma (may exacerbate)
  ‣ With oral use Gastritis (can be aggravated by swallowed nicotine) · gum may also stick to and damage dentures · oesophagitis (can be aggravated by swallowed nicotine) · peptic ulcers (can be aggravated by swallowed nicotine)
  ‣ With transdermal use patches should not be placed on broken skin · patients with skin disorders

  CAUTIONS, FURTHER INFORMATION
  Most warnings for nicotine replacement therapy also apply to continued cigarette smoking, but the risk of continued smoking outweighs any risks of using nicotine preparations.
  Specific cautions for individual preparations are usually related to the local effect of nicotine.

- **SIDE-EFFECTS**
  ‣ **Common or very common** Bloating · blurred vision · constipation · coughing · diarrhoea · dry mouth · dyspepsia · dysphagia · epistaxis · flatulence · gastritis · gastro-intestinal disturbances (may be caused by swallowed nicotine) · hiccup · increased salivation · irritation of the throat · mild local reactions at the beginning of treatment are common because of the irritant effect of nicotine · minor skin irritation · mouth ulcers · nasal irritation · nausea · oesophagitis · paraesthesia · sneezing · vomiting · watery eyes
  ‣ **Uncommon** Gingival bleeding · halitosis · thirst
  ‣ **Rare** Arrhythmia
  ‣ **Very rare** Reversible atrial fibrillation
  ‣ **Frequency not known** Abdominal pain · abnormal dreams (may occur with patches, removal of the patch before bed may help) · arthralgia · chest pain · flatulence · hot flushes · myalgia · palpitations · rash · sweating · taste disturbance · ulcerative stomatitis

  SIDE-EFFECTS, FURTHER INFORMATION
  Side-effects listed have been reported with use of various nicotine replacement therapy preparations. See *Nicotine replacement therapy*, under Substance dependence p. 283 for further details on individual preparations.
  ‣ Nicotine withdrawal Some systemic effects occur on initiation of therapy, particularly if the patient is using high-strength preparations; however, the patient may confuse side-effects of the nicotine-replacement preparation with nicotine withdrawal symptoms.
  Common symptoms of nicotine withdrawal include malaise, headache, dizziness, sleep disturbance, coughing, influenza–like symptoms, depression, irritability, increased appetite, weight gain, restlessness, anxiety, drowsiness, aphthous ulcers, decreased heart rate, and impaired concentration.

- **PREGNANCY** The use of nicotine replacement therapy in pregnancy is preferable to the continuation of smoking, but should be used only if smoking cessation without nicotine replacement fails. Intermittent therapy is preferable to patches but should avoid liquorice-flavoured nicotine products. Patches are useful, however, if the patient is experiencing pregnancy-related nausea and

vomiting. If patches are used, they should be removed before bed.

- **BREAST FEEDING** Nicotine is present in milk; however, the amount to which the infant is exposed is small and less hazardous than second-hand smoke. Intermittent therapy is preferred.

- **HEPATIC IMPAIRMENT** Use with caution in moderate to severe hepatic impairment.

- **RENAL IMPAIRMENT** Use with caution in severe renal impairment.

- **DIRECTIONS FOR ADMINISTRATION** Acidic beverages, such as coffee or fruit juice, may decrease the absorption of nicotine through the buccal mucosa and should be avoided for 15 minutes before the use of oral nicotine replacement therapy.
  Administration by transdermal patch Patches should be applied on waking to dry, non-hairy skin on the hip, trunk, or upper arm and held in position for 10–20 seconds to ensure adhesion; place next patch on a different area and avoid using the same site for several days.
  Administration by nasal spray Initially 1 spray should be used in both nostrils but when withdrawing from therapy, the dose can be gradually reduced to 1 spray in 1 nostril.
  Administration by oral spray The oral spray should be released into the mouth, holding the spray as close to the mouth as possible and avoiding the lips. The patient should not inhale while spraying and avoid swallowing for a few seconds after use. If using the oral spray for the first time, or if unit not used for 2 or more days, prime the unit before administration.
  Administration by sublingual tablet Each tablet should be placed under the tongue and allowed to dissolve.
  Administration by lozenge Slowly allow each lozenge to dissolve in the mouth; periodically move the lozenge from one side of the mouth to the other. Lozenges last for 10–30 minutes, depending on their size.
  Administration by inhalation Insert the cartridge into the device and draw in air through the mouthpiece; each session can last for approximately 5 minutes. The amount of nicotine from 1 puff of the cartridge is less than that from a cigarette, therefore it is necessary to inhale more often than when smoking a cigarette. A single 10 mg cartridge lasts for approximately 20 minutes of intense use; a single 15 mg cartridge lasts for approximately 40 minutes of intense use.
  Administration by medicated chewing gum Chew the gum until the taste becomes strong, then rest it between the cheek and gum; when the taste starts to fade, repeat this process. One piece of gum lasts for approximately 30 minutes.

- **PRESCRIBING AND DISPENSING INFORMATION** Flavours of chewing gum and lozenges may include mint, freshfruit, freshmint, icy white, or cherry.

- **PATIENT AND CARER ADVICE** Patient or carers should be given advice on how to administer nicotine chewing gum, inhalators, lozenges, sublingual tablets, oral spray, nasal spray and patches.

- **MEDICINAL FORMS**
  There can be variation in the licensing of different medicines containing the same drug.

  Spray
  EXCIPIENTS: May contain Ethanol
  ‣ **Nicotine (Non-proprietary)**
    Nicotine 500 microgram per 1 actuation Nicotine 10mg/ml nasal spray | 10 ml GSL no price available DT price = £13.80
  ‣ Brands may include NicAssist, Nicorette, Nicorette QuickMist

  Sublingual tablet
  CAUTIONARY AND ADVISORY LABELS 26
  ‣ **Nicotine (Non-proprietary)**
    Nicotine (as Nicotine cyclodextrin complex) 2 mg Nicotine 2mg sublingual tablets sugar-free | 100 tablet GSL no price available DT price = £13.12
  ‣ Brands may include NicAssist, Nicorette Microtab

4

Nervous system

Transdermal patch
▸ Nicotine (Non-proprietary)

Nicotine 7 mg per 24 hour Nicotine 7mg/24hours transdermal patches | 7 patch GSL no price available

Nicotine 14 mg per 24 hour Nicotine 14mg/24hours transdermal patches | 7 patch GSL no price available

Nicotine 10 mg per 16 hour Nicotine 10mg/16hours patches | 7 patch GSL no price available DT price = £10.37

Nicotine 21 mg per 24 hour Nicotine 21mg/24hours transdermal patches | 7 patch GSL no price available DT price = £9.97

Nicotine 15 mg per 16 hour Nicotine 15mg/16hours patches | 7 patch GSL no price available DT price = £10.37

Nicotine 25 mg per 16 hour Nicotine 25mg/16hours patches | 7 patch GSL no price available DT price = £10.37

▸ Brands may include NicAssist, NiQuitin, NiQuitin Clear, Nicorette invisi, Nicotinell TTS

Medicated chewing-gum
▸ Nicotine (Non-proprietary)

Nicotine 2 mg Nicotine 2mg medicated chewing gum sugar-free | 30 piece GSL no price available sugar-free | 105 piece GSL no price available sugar-free | 210 piece GSL no price available

Nicotine 4 mg Nicotine 4mg medicated chewing gum sugar-free | 105 piece GSL no price available sugar-free | 210 piece GSL no price available

▸ Brands may include NicAssist, NiQuitin, Nicorette, Nicorette Icy White, Nicotinell

Lozenge
EXCIPIENTS: May contain Aspartame
ELECTROLYTES: May contain Sodium
▸ Nicotine (Non-proprietary)

Nicotine (as Nicotine bitartrate) 1 mg Nicotine1mg lozenges sugar-free | 96 lozenge GSL no price available DT price = £9.12

Nicotine (as Nicotine bitartrate) 2 mg Nicotine 2mg lozenges sugar-free | 96 lozenge GSL no price available

▸ Brands may include NicAssist, NiQuitin, Nicorette, Nicotinell

Inhalation vapour
▸ Nicotine (Non-proprietary)

Nicotine 15 mg Nicotine 15mg Inhalator | 4 cartridge GSL no price available DT price = £4.27 | 20 cartridge GSL no price available DT price = £15.11

▸ Brands may include NicAssist, Nicorette

7.2 Opioid dependence

OPIOIDS

☞ 262

▌Methadone hydrochloride

● **INDICATIONS AND DOSE**

Neonatal opioid withdrawal
▸ BY MOUTH

▸ Neonate: Initially 100 micrograms/kg, then increased in steps of 50 micrograms/kg every 6 hours until symptoms are controlled, doses may vary, consult local guidelines, for maintenance, total daily dose that controls symptoms to be given in 2 divided doses.

● **UNLICENSED USE** Not licensed for use in children.

IMPORTANT SAFETY INFORMATION
Methadone oral solution 1 mg/mL is 2½ times the strength of Methadone Linctus (2 mg/5mL). Many preparations of Methadone oral solution are licensed for opioid drug addiction only but some are also licensed for analgesia in severe pain.

● **CONTRA-INDICATIONS** Phaeochromocytoma

● **CAUTIONS** Family history of sudden death (ECG monitoring recommended) · history of cardiac conduction abnormalities

CAUTIONS, FURTHER INFORMATION
▸ QT-interval prolongation Patients with the following risk factors for QT-interval prolongation should be carefully

monitored while taking methadone: heart or liver disease, electrolyte abnormalities, or concomitant treatment with drugs that can prolong QT interval; patients requiring more than 100 mg daily should also be monitored.

● **INTERACTIONS** → Appendix 1: opioids

● **SIDE-EFFECTS** Dry eyes · dysmenorrhoea · hyperprolactinaemia · hypothermia · QT-interval prolongation · raised intracranial pressure · restlessness · torsade de pointes

SIDE-EFFECTS, FURTHER INFORMATION
Methadone is a long-acting opioid therefore effects may be cumulative.

Methadone, even in low doses is a **special hazard** for children; non-dependent adults are also at risk of toxicity; dependent adults are at risk if tolerance is incorrectly assessed during induction.

Overdose
Methadone has a very long duration of action; patients may need to be monitored for long periods following large overdoses.

● **BREAST FEEDING** Withdrawal symptoms in infant; breast-feeding permissible during maintenance but dose should be as low as possible and infant monitored to avoid sedation (high doses of methadone carry an increased risk of sedation and respiratory depression in the neonate).

● **RENAL IMPAIRMENT** Avoid use or reduce dose; opioid effects increased and prolonged and increased cerebral sensitivity occurs.

● **TREATMENT CESSATION** Avoid abrupt withdrawal. When used for neonatal opioid withdraw, reduce dose over 7–10 days.

● **DIRECTIONS FOR ADMINISTRATION** Syrup preserved with hydroxybenzoate (parabens) esters may be incompatible with methadone hydrochloride.

● **PRESCRIBING AND DISPENSING INFORMATION** Flavours of oral liquid formulations may include tolu.

● **MEDICINAL FORMS**
There can be variation in the licensing of different medicines containing the same drug. Forms available from special-order manufacturers include: oral suspension, oral solution

Oral solution
CAUTIONARY AND ADVISORY LABELS 2
▸ Methadone hydrochloride (Non-proprietary)

Methadone hydrochloride 1 mg per 1 ml Methadone 1mg/ml oral solution | 100 ml PoM £1.00–£1.30 DT price = £1.00 CD2 | 500 ml PoM £6.18 DT price = £5.00 CD2 | 2500 ml PoM £25.00–£32.10 CD2

Methadone 1mg/ml oral solution sugar free sugar-free | 50 ml PoM £1.04 DT price = £1.04 CD2 sugar-free | 100 ml PoM £2.08 DT price = £2.08 CD2 sugar-free | 500 ml PoM £6.30 DT price = £6.30 sugar-free | 2500 ml PoM £31.50–£32.50 CD2

▸ Methadose (Rosemont Pharmaceuticals Ltd)

Methadone hydrochloride 10 mg per 1 ml Methadose 10mg/ml oral solution concentrate sugar-free | 150 ml PoM £12.01 CD2

Methadone hydrochloride 20 mg per 1 ml Methadose 20mg/ml oral solution concentrate sugar-free | 150 ml PoM £24.02 CD2

▸ Metharose (Rosemont Pharmaceuticals Ltd)

Methadone hydrochloride 1 mg per 1 ml Metharose 1mg/ml oral solution sugar free sugar-free | 500 ml PoM £6.82 DT price = £6.30 CD2

▸ Physeptone (Martindale Pharmaceuticals Ltd)

Methadone hydrochloride 1 mg per 1 ml Physeptone 1mg/ml mixture | 100 ml PoM £1.08 DT price = £1.00 CD2 | 500 ml PoM £5.46 DT price = £5.00 CD2 | 2500 ml PoM £27.29 CD2

Physeptone 1mg/ml mixture sugar free sugar-free | 100 ml PoM £1.08 DT price = £2.08 CD2 sugar-free | 500 ml PoM £5.46 DT price = £6.30 CD2 sugar-free | 2500 ml PoM £27.29 CD2

Chapter 5
Infection

CONTENTS

1 Amoebic infection

Other drugs used for Amoebic infection Metronidazole, p. 319 · Tinidazole, p. 320

ANTIPROTOZOALS

Diloxanide furoate

- **INDICATIONS AND DOSE**

  Chronic amoebiasis | Acute amoebiasis as adjunct to metronidazole or tinidazole
  - BY MOUTH
  - Child 1 month–11 years: 6.6 mg/kg 3 times a day for 10 days
  - Child 12–17 years: 500 mg 3 times a day for 10 days

- **UNLICENSED USE** Not licensed for use in children under 25 kg body-weight.
- **SIDE-EFFECTS** Flatulence · pruritus · urticaria · vomiting
- **PREGNANCY** Manufacturer advises avoid—no information available.
- **BREAST FEEDING** Manufacturer advises avoid.

- **MEDICINAL FORMS**
  There can be variation in the licensing of different medicines containing the same drug. Forms available from special-order manufacturers include: oral suspension, oral solution

  Tablet
  CAUTIONARY AND ADVISORY LABELS 9
  - Diloxanide furoate (Non-proprietary)
    Diloxanide furoate 500 mg Diloxanide 500mg tablets |
    30 tablet PoM £93.50

2 Bacterial infection

Antibacterials, principles of therapy

07-Mar-2017

Choice of a suitable drug

Before selecting an antibacterial the clinician must first consider two factors— the patient and the known or likely causative organism. Factors related to the patient which must be considered include history of allergy, renal and hepatic function, susceptibility to infection (i.e. whether immunocompromised), ability to tolerate drugs by mouth, severity of illness, ethnic origin, age, whether taking other medication and, if female, whether pregnant, breast-feeding or taking an oral contraceptive.

The known or likely organism and its antibacterial sensitivity, in association with the above factors, will suggest one or more antibacterials, the final choice depending on the microbiological, pharmacological, and toxicological properties.

The principles involved in selection of an antibacterial must allow for a number of variables including changing renal and hepatic function, increasing bacterial resistance, and information on side-effects. Duration of therapy, dosage, and route of administration depend on site, type and severity of infection and response.

Antibacterial policies

Local policies often limit the antibacterials that may be used to achieve reasonable economy consistent with adequate cover, and to reduce the development of resistant organisms. A policy may indicate a range of drugs for general use, and permit other drugs only on the advice of the microbiologist or paediatric infectious diseases specialist.

Before starting therapy

The following precepts should be considered before starting:
- Viral infections should not be treated with antibacterials. However, antibacterials may be used to treat secondary bacterial infection (e.g. bacterial pneumonia secondary to influenza);

- Samples should be taken for culture and sensitivity testing; 'blind' antibacterial prescribing for unexplained pyrexia usually leads to further difficulty in establishing the diagnosis;
- Knowledge of **prevalent organisms** and their current sensitivity is of great help in choosing an antibacterial before bacteriological confirmation is available. Generally, narrow-spectrum antibacterials are preferred to broad-spectrum antibacterials unless there is a clear clinical indication (e.g. life-threatening sepsis);
- The **dose** of an antibacterial varies according to a number of factors including age, weight, hepatic function, renal function, and severity of infection. The prescribing of the so-called 'standard' dose in serious infections may result in failure of treatment or even death of the patient; therefore it is important to prescribe a dose appropriate to the condition. An inadequate dose may also increase the likelihood of antibacterial resistance. On the other hand, for an antibacterial with a narrow margin between the toxic and therapeutic dose (e.g. an aminoglycoside) it is also important to avoid an excessive dose and the concentration of the drug in the plasma may need to be monitored;
- The **route** of administration of an antibacterial often depends on the severity of the infection. Life-threatening infections often require intravenous therapy. Antibacterials that are well absorbed may be given by mouth even for some serious infections. Parenteral administration is also appropriate when the oral route cannot be used (e.g. because of vomiting) or if absorption is inadequate (e.g. in neonates and young children). Whenever possible, painful intramuscular injections should be avoided in children;
- **Duration** of therapy depends on the nature of the infection and the response to treatment. Courses should not be unduly prolonged because they encourage resistance, they may lead to side-effects and they are costly. However, in certain infections such as tuberculosis or osteomyelitis it may be necessary to treat for prolonged periods. Conversely a single dose of an antibacterial may cure uncomplicated urinary-tract infections. The prescription for an antibacterial should specify the duration of treatment or the date when treatment is to be reviewed.

Superinfection

In general, broad-spectrum antibacterial drugs such as the cephalosporins are more likely to be associated with adverse reactions related to the selection of resistant organisms e.g. *fungal infections* or *antibiotic-associated colitis* (pseudomembranous colitis); other problems associated with superinfection include vaginitis and pruritus ani.

Therapy

When the pathogen has been isolated treatment may be changed to a more appropriate antibacterial if necessary. If no bacterium is cultured the antibacterial can be continued or stopped on clinical grounds.

Switching from parenteral to oral treatment

The ongoing parenteral administration of an antibacterial should be reviewed regularly. In older children it may be possible to switch to an oral antibacterial; in neonates and infants this should be done more cautiously because of the relatively high incidence of bacteraemia and the possibility of variable oral absorption.

Prophylaxis

In most situations, only a short course of prophylactic antibacterial is needed. Longer-term antibacterial prophylaxis is appropriate in specific indications such as vesico-ureteric reflux.

Notifiable diseases

Doctors must notify the Proper Officer of the local authority (usually the consultant in communicable disease control) when attending a patient suspected of suffering from any of the diseases listed below; a form is available from the Proper Officer.

Anthrax	Mumps
Botulism	Paratyphoid fever
Brucellosis	Plague
Cholera	Poliomyelitis, acute
Diarrhoea (infectious bloody)	Rabies
Diphtheria	Rubella
Encephalitis, acute	SARS
Food poisoning	Scarlet fever
Haemolytic uraemic syndrome	Smallpox
Haemorrhagic fever (viral)	Streptococcal disease (Group A,
Hepatitis, viral	invasive)
Legionnaires' disease	Tetanus
Leprosy	Tuberculosis
Malaria	Typhoid fever
Measles	Typhus
Meningitis	Whooping cough
Meningococcal septicaemia	Yellow fever

Note It is good practice for doctors to also inform the consultant in communicable disease control of instances of other infections (e.g. psittacosis) where there could be a public health risk.

Sepsis, early management

[EvGr] Children identified as being at high risk of severe illness or death due to suspected sepsis should be given a broad-spectrum antibacterial at the maximum recommended dose without delay (ideally within one hour). Microbiological samples and blood cultures must be taken prior to administration of antibiotics; the prescription should be adjusted subsequently according to susceptibility results.

A thorough clinical examination should be carried out to identify sources of infection. If the cause of infection is identified, treat in line with local antibacterial guidance or susceptibility results.

Children aged up to 17 years with suspected community-acquired sepsis of any cause should be treated with ceftriaxone p. 308. If the child is already in hospital or is known to have previously been infected or colonised with ceftriaxone-resistant bacteria, an alternative antibiotic should be chosen following local guidelines. Children younger than 3 months should also receive an additional antibiotic that is active against *listeria* (such as ampicillin p. 326 or amoxicillin p. 325).

Neonates who are in hospital with suspected sepsis within 72 hours of birth, should be treated with intravenous benzylpenicillin sodium p. 323 and gentamicin p. 299. Community-acquired sepsis in neonates (who are more than 40 weeks corrected gestational age) should be treated with ceftriaxone p. 308, unless already receiving an intravenous calcium infusion. Neonates aged 40 weeks corrected gestational age or below, or receiving an intravenous calcium infusion, should receive cefotaxime p. 307, dosed according to age.

The need for intravenous fluids, inotropes, vasopressors and oxygen should also be assessed without delay, taking into consideration the child's lactate concentration, systolic blood pressure (in children over 12 years) and their risk of severe illness or death. Children at high risk should be monitored continuously if possible, and no less than every 30 minutes.

Children with suspected sepsis who are not immediately deemed to be at high risk of severe illness or death, should be re-assessed regularly for the need for empirical treatment, taking into consideration all risk factors including lactate concentration and evidence of acute kidney injury. ⒶⒷ

Antibacterials, use for prophylaxis

16-Mar-2017

Prevention of recurrence of rheumatic fever

- Phenoxymethylpenicillin p. 324 by mouth *or* erythromycin p. 316 by mouth.

Prevention of secondary case of invasive group A streptococcal infection

- Phenoxymethylpenicillin by mouth.

   If child penicillin allergic, *either* erythromycin by mouth or azithromycin p. 314 by mouth [unlicensed indication].

   For details of those who should receive chemoprophylaxis contact a consultant in communicable disease control (or a consultant in infectious diseases or the local Public Health England Laboratory).

Prevention of secondary case of meningococcal meningitis

- Ciprofloxacin p. 333 by mouth [unlicensed indication] *or* rifampicin p. 349 by mouth *or* ceftriaxone p. 308 by intramuscular injection [unlicensed indication].

   For details of those who should receive chemoprophylaxis contact a consultant in communicable disease control (or a consultant in infectious diseases or the local Public Health England laboratory). Unless there has been direct exposure of the mouth or nose to infectious droplets from a patient with meningococcal disease who has received less than 24 hours of antibacterial treatment, healthcare workers do not generally require chemoprophylaxis.

Prevention of secondary case of *Haemophilus influenzae* type b disease

- Rifampicin by mouth *or* (if rifampicin cannot be used) ceftriaxone by intramuscular injection, or by intravenous injection, or by intravenous infusion [unlicensed indication].

   For details of those who should receive chemoprophylaxis contact a consultant in communicable disease control (or a consultant in infectious diseases or the local Public Health England laboratory). Unless there has been direct exposure of the mouth or nose to infectious droplets from a patient with meningococcal disease who has received less than 24 hours of antibacterial treatment, healthcare workers do not generally require chemoprophylaxis.

   Within 4 weeks of illness onset in an index case with confirmed or suspected invasive *Haemophilus influenzae* type b disease, give antibacterial prophylaxis to all household contacts if there is a vulnerable individual in the household. Also, give antibacterial prophylaxis to the index case if they are in contact with vulnerable household contacts or if they are under 10 years of age. Vulnerable individuals include the immunocompromised, those with asplenia, or children under 10 years of age. If there are 2 or more cases of invasive *Haemophilus influenzae* type b disease within 120 days in a pre-school or primary school, antibacterial prophylaxis should also be given to all room contacts (including staff). Also see immunisation against *Haemophilus influenzae* type b disease.

Prevention of secondary case of diphtheria in non-immune patient

- Erythromycin (*or* another macrolide e.g. azithromycin *or* clarithromycin p. 315) by mouth.

Treat for further 10 days if nasopharyngeal swabs positive after first 7 days' treatment.

Prevention of pertussis

- Clarithromycin (*or* azithromycin *or* erythromycin) by mouth.

   Within 3 weeks of onset of cough in the index case, give antibacterial prophylaxis to all close contacts if amongst them there is at least one unimmunised or partially immunised child under 1 year of age, *or* if there is at least one individual who has not received a pertussis-containing vaccine more than 1 week and less than 5 years ago (so long as that individual lives or works with children under 4 months of age, is pregnant at over 32 weeks gestation, or is a healthcare worker who works with children under 1 year of age or with pregnant women).

Prevention of pneumococcal infection in asplenia or in patients with sickle-cell disease

- Phenoxymethylpenicillin by mouth.

   If cover also needed for *H. influenzae* in child give amoxicillin p. 325 instead.

   If penicillin-allergic, erythromycin by mouth.

   Antibacterial prophylaxis is not fully reliable. Antibacterial prophylaxis may be discontinued in children over 5 years of age with sickle-cell disease who have received pneumococcal immunisation and who do not have a history of severe pneumococcal infection.

Prevention of *Staphylococcus aureus* lung infection in cystic fibrosis

- *Primary prevention*, flucloxacillin p. 330 by mouth.
- *Secondary prevention*, flucloxacillin by mouth.

Prevention of tuberculosis in susceptible close contacts or those who have become tuberculin positive

- See *Close contacts* and *Chemoprophylaxis for latent tuberculosis* under Tuberculosis p. 345.

Prevention of urinary-tract infection

- Trimethoprim p. 344 by mouth *or* nitrofurantoin p. 354 by mouth.

   Antibacterial prophylaxis can be considered for recurrent infection, significant urinary-tract anomalies, or significant kidney damage.

Prevention of infection from animal and human bites

- Co-amoxiclav p. 328 alone (*or* clindamycin p. 313 if penicillin-allergic).

   Cleanse wound thoroughly. For tetanus-prone wound, give human tetanus immunoglobulin p. 745 (with a tetanus-containing vaccine if necessary, according to immunisation history and risk of infection).

   Consider rabies prophylaxis for bites from animals in endemic countries. Assess risk of blood-borne viruses (including HIV, hepatitis B and C) and give appropriate prophylaxis to prevent viral spread. Antibacterial prophylaxis recommended for wounds less than 48–72 hours old when the risk of infection is high (e.g. bites from humans or cats; bites to the hand, foot, face, or genital area; bites involving oedema, crush or puncture injury, or other moderate to severe injury; wounds that cannot be debrided adequately; patients with diabetes mellitus, cirrhosis, asplenia, prosthetic joints or valves, or those who are immunocompromised). Give antibacterial prophylaxis for up to 5 days.

Prevention of infection in gastro-intestinal procedures

Operations on stomach or oesophagus

- Single dose of i/v gentamicin p. 299 *or* i/v cefuroxime p. 306 *or* i/v co-amoxiclav (additional intra-operative or postoperative doses may be given for prolonged procedures or if there is major blood loss).

  Intravenous antibacterial prophylaxis should be given up to 30 minutes before the procedure.

  Add i/v teicoplanin p. 311 (*or* vancomycin p. 312) if high risk of meticillin-resistant *Staphylococcus aureus*.

Open biliary surgery

- Single dose of i/v cefuroxime + i/v metronidazole p. 319 *or* i/v gentamicin + i/v metronidazole *or* i/v co-amoxiclav alone (additional intra-operative or postoperative doses may be given for prolonged procedures or if there is major blood loss).

  Intravenous antibacterial prophylaxis should be given up to 30 minutes before the procedure.

  Where i/v metronidazole is suggested, it may alternatively be given by suppository but to allow adequate absorption, it should be given 2 hours before surgery.

  Add i/v teicoplanin (*or* vancomycin) if high risk of meticillin-resistant *Staphylococcus aureus*.

Resections of colon and rectum, and resections in inflammatory bowel disease, and appendicectomy

- Single dose of i/v gentamicin + i/v metronidazole *or* i/v cefuroxime + i/v metronidazole *or* i/v co-amoxiclav alone (additional intra-operative or postoperative doses may be given for prolonged procedures or if there is major blood loss).

  Intravenous antibacterial prophylaxis should be given up to 30 minutes before the procedure.

  Where i/v metronidazole is suggested, it may alternatively be given by suppository but to allow adequate absorption, it should be given 2 hours before surgery.

  Add i/v teicoplanin p. 311 (*or* vancomycin p. 312) if high risk of meticillin-resistant *Staphylococcus aureus*.

Endoscopic retrograde cholangiopancreatography

- Single dose of i/v gentamicin p. 299 *or* oral *or* i/v ciprofloxacin p. 333.

  Intravenous antibacterial prophylaxis should be given up to 30 minutes before the procedure.

  Prophylaxis recommended if pancreatic pseudocyst, immunocompromised, history of liver transplantation, or risk of incomplete biliary drainage. For biliary complications following liver transplantation, add i/v amoxicillin p. 325 or i/v teicoplanin (*or* vancomycin).

Percutaneous endoscopic gastrostomy or jejunostomy

- Single dose of i/v co-amoxiclav p. 328 or i/v cefuroxime p. 306.

  Intravenous antibacterial prophylaxis should be given up to 30 minutes before the procedure.

  Use single dose of i/v teicoplanin (*or* vancomycin) if history of allergy to penicillins or cephalosporins, or if high risk of meticillin-resistant *Staphylococcus aureus*.

Prevention of infection in orthopaedic surgery

Closed fractures

- Single dose of i/v cefuroxime *or* i/v flucloxacillin p. 330 (additional intra-operative or postoperative doses may be given for prolonged procedures or if there is major blood loss).

  Intravenous antibacterial prophylaxis should be given up to 30 minutes before the procedure.

  If history of allergy to penicillins or to cephalosporins or if high risk of meticillin-resistant *Staphylococcus aureus*, use single dose of i/v teicoplanin (*or* vancomycin) (additional intra-operative or postoperative doses may be given for prolonged procedures or if there is major blood loss).

Open fractures

- Use i/v co-amoxiclav alone *or* i/v cefuroxime + i/v metronidazole p. 319 (*or* i/v clindamycin p. 313 alone if history of allergy to penicillins or to cephalosporins).

  Add i/v teicoplanin (*or* vancomycin) if high risk of meticillin-resistant *Staphylococcus aureus*. Start prophylaxis within 3 hours of injury and continue until soft tissue closure (max. 72 hours).

  At first debridement also use a single dose of i/v cefuroxime + i/v metronidazole + i/v gentamicin *or* i/v co-amoxiclav + i/v gentamicin *or* i/v clindamycin + i/v gentamicin if history of allergy to penicillins or to cephalosporins).

  At time of skeletal stabilisation and definitive soft tissue closure use a single dose of i/v gentamicin and i/v teicoplanin (*or* vancomycin) (intravenous antibacterial prophylaxis should be given up to 30 minutes before the procedure.

High lower-limb amputation

- Use i/v co-amoxiclav alone *or* i/v cefuroxime + i/v metronidazole.

  Intravenous antibacterial prophylaxis should be given up to 30 minutes before the procedure.

  Continue antibacterial prophylaxis for at least 2 doses after procedure (max. duration of prophylaxis 5 days). If history of allergy to penicillin or to cephalosporins, or if high risk of meticillin-resistant *Staphylococcus aureus*, use i/v teicoplanin (*or* vancomycin) + i/v gentamicin + i/v metronidazole.

  Where i/v metronidazole is suggested, it may alternatively be given by suppository but to allow adequate absorption, it should be given 2 hours before surgery.

Prevention of infection in obstetric surgery

Termination of pregnancy

- Single dose of oral metronidazole (additional intra-operative or postoperative doses may be given for prolonged procedures or if there is major blood loss).

  If genital chlamydial infection cannot be ruled out, give doxycycline p. 338 postoperatively.

Prevention of infective endocarditis

NICE guidance: Antimicrobial prophylaxis against infective endocarditis in adults and children undergoing interventional procedures (March 2008, updated 2016)

- Chlorhexidine mouthwash is not recommended for the prevention of infective endocarditis in at risk children undergoing dental procedures.

  Antibacterial prophylaxis is not *routinely* recommended for the prevention of infective endocarditis in children undergoing the following procedures:
  - dental;
  - upper and lower respiratory tract (including ear, nose, and throat procedures and bronchoscopy);
  - genito-urinary tract (including urological, gynaecological, and obstetric procedures);
  - upper and lower gastro-intestinal tract.

  While these procedures can cause bacteraemia, there is no clear association with the development of infective endocarditis. Prophylaxis may expose children to the adverse effects of antimicrobials when the evidence of benefit has not been proven.

  Any infection in children at risk of endocarditis should be investigated promptly and treated appropriately to reduce the risk of endocarditis.

  If children at risk of infective endocarditis are undergoing a gastro-intestinal or genito-urinary tract procedure at a site where infection is suspected, they should receive appropriate antibacterial therapy that includes cover against organisms that cause endocarditis.

Children at risk of infective endocarditis should be:
▸ advised to maintain good oral hygiene;
▸ told how to recognise signs of infective endocarditis, and advised when to seek expert advice.

Patients at risk of infective endocarditis include those with valve replacement, acquired valvular heart disease with stenosis or regurgitation, structural congenital heart disease (including surgically corrected or palliated structural conditions, but excluding isolated atrial septal defect, fully repaired ventricular septal defect, fully repaired patent ductus arteriosus, and closure devices considered to be endothelialised), hypertrophic cardiomyopathy, or a previous episode of infective endocarditis.

Dermatological procedures

Advice of a Working Party of the British Society for Antimicrobial Chemotherapy is that patients who undergo dermatological procedures do not require antibacterial prophylaxis against endocarditis.

The British Association of Dermatologists Therapy Guidelines and Audit Subcommittee advise that such dermatological procedures include skin biopsies and excision of moles or of malignant lesions.

Joint prostheses and dental treatment

Advice of a Working Party of the British Society for Antimicrobial Chemotherapy is that patients with prosthetic joint implants (including total hip replacements) do not require antibacterial prophylaxis for dental treatment. The Working Party considers that it is unacceptable to expose patients to the adverse effects of antibacterials when there is no evidence that such prophylaxis is of any benefit, but that those who develop any intercurrent infection require prompt treatment with antibacterials to which the infecting organisms are sensitive.

The Working Party has commented that joint infections have rarely been shown to follow dental procedures and are even more rarely caused by oral streptococci.

Immunosuppression and indwelling intraperitoneal catheters

Advice of a Working Party of the British Society for Antimicrobial Chemotherapy is that patients who are immunosuppressed (including transplant patients) and patients with indwelling intraperitoneal catheters do not require antibacterial prophylaxis for dental treatment provided there is no other indication for prophylaxis.

The Working Party has commented that there is little evidence that dental treatment is followed by infection in immunosuppressed and immunodeficient patients nor is there evidence that dental treatment is followed by infection in patients with indwelling intraperitoneal catheters.

Blood infections, bacterial

Antibacterial therapy for septicaemia: community-acquired

● *Child 1 month–18 years*, aminoglycoside + amoxicillin p. 325 (*or* ampicillin p. 326) *or* cefotaxime p. 307 (*or* ceftriaxone p. 308) alone
▸ If pseudomonas or resistant micro-organisms suspected, use a broad-spectrum antipseudomonal beta-lactam antibacterial.
▸ If anaerobic infection suspected, add metronidazole p. 319.
▸ If Gram-positive infection suspected, add flucloxacillin p. 330 *or* vancomycin p. 312 (*or* teicoplanin p. 311).
▸ *Suggested duration of treatment* at least 5 days.

Antibacterial therapy for septicaemia: hospital-acquired

● *Child 1 month–18 years*, a broad-spectrum antipseudomonal beta-lactam antibacterial (e.g. piperacillin with tazobactam p. 322, ticarcillin with clavulanic acid p. 323, imipenem with cilastatin p. 302, *or* meropenem p. 302)
▸ If pseudomonas suspected, or if multiple-resistant organisms suspected, or if severe sepsis, add aminoglycoside.
▸ If meticillin-resistant *Staphylococcus aureus* suspected, add vancomycin (*or* teicoplanin).
▸ If anaerobic infection suspected, add metronidazole to a broad-spectrum cephalosporin.
▸ *Suggested duration of treatment* at least 5 days.

Septicaemia related to vascular catheter

● Vancomycin (*or* teicoplanin)
▸ If Gram-negative sepsis suspected, especially in the immunocompromised, add a broad-spectrum antipseudomonal beta-lactam.
▸ Consider removing vascular catheter, particularly if infection caused by *Staphylococcus aureus*, pseudomonas, or *Candida* species.

Meningococcal septicaemia

If meningococcal disease suspected, a single dose of benzylpenicillin sodium p. 323 should be given before urgent transfer to hospital, so long as this does not delay the transfer; cefotaxime may be an alternative in penicillin allergy; chloramphenicol p. 340 may be used if history of immediate hypersensitivity reaction to penicillin or to cephalosporins.

● Benzylpenicillin sodium or cefotaxime (*or* ceftriaxone)
● *If history of immediate hypersensitivity reaction to penicillin or to cephalosporins*, chloramphenicol

To eliminate nasopharyngeal carriage, ciprofloxacin p. 333, or rifampicin p. 349, or ceftriaxone may be used.

Antibacterial therapy for septicaemia in neonates

● *Neonate less than 72 hours old*, benzylpenicillin sodium + gentamicin p. 299
▸ If Gram-negative septicaemia suspected, use benzylpenicillin sodium + gentamicin + cefotaxime; stop benzylpenicillin sodium if Gram-negative infection confirmed.
▸ *Suggested duration of treatment* usually 7 days.
● *Neonate more than 72 hours old*, flucloxacillin + gentamicin *or* amoxicillin (*or* ampicillin) + cefotaxime
▸ *Suggested duration of treatment* usually 7 days.

Cardiovascular system infections, bacterial

Antibacterial therapy for endocarditis: initial 'blind' therapy

● Flucloxacillin p. 330 (*or* benzylpenicillin sodium p. 323 if symptoms less severe) + gentamicin p. 299
● *If cardiac prostheses present, or if penicillin-allergic, or if meticillin-resistant Staphylococcus aureus suspected*, vancomycin p. 312 + rifampicin p. 349 + gentamicin

Antibacterial therapy for endocarditis caused by staphylococci

● Flucloxacillin
▸ Add rifampicin for at least 2 weeks in prosthetic valve endocarditis
▸ *Suggested duration of treatment* at least 4 weeks (at least

6 weeks for prosthetic valve endocarditis)

- *If penicillin-allergic or if meticillin-resistant Staphylococcus aureus*, vancomycin + rifampicin
  - *Suggested duration of treatment* at least 4 weeks (at least 6 weeks for prosthetic valve endocarditis)

Antibacterial therapy for native-valve endocarditis caused by fully-sensitive streptococci (e.g. viridans streptococci)

- Benzylpenicillin sodium
  - *Suggested duration of treatment* 4 weeks
- *Alternative if a large vegetation, intracardial abscess, or infected emboli are absent*, benzylpenicillin sodium + gentamicin
  - *Suggested duration of treatment* 2 weeks
- *If penicillin-allergic*, vancomycin
  - *Suggested duration of treatment* 4 weeks

Antibacterial therapy for native-valve endocarditis caused by less-sensitive streptococci

- Benzylpenicillin sodium + gentamicin
  - *Suggested duration of treatment* 4–6 weeks (stop gentamicin after 2 weeks for micro-organisms moderately sensitive to penicillin)
- *If aminoglycoside cannot be used and if streptococci moderately sensitive to penicillin*, benzylpenicillin sodium
  - *Suggested duration of treatment* 4 weeks
- *If penicillin-allergic or highly penicillin-resistant*, vancomycin (*or* teicoplanin p. 311) + gentamicin
  - *Suggested duration of treatment* 4–6 weeks (stop gentamicin after 2 weeks for micro-organisms moderately sensitive to penicillin)

Antibacterial therapy for prosthetic valve endocarditis caused by streptococci

- Benzylpenicillin sodium + gentamicin
  - *Suggested duration of treatment* at least 6 weeks (stop gentamicin after 2 weeks if micro-organisms fully sensitive to penicillin)
- *If penicillin-allergic or highly penicillin-resistant*, vancomycin (*or* teicoplanin) + gentamicin
  - *Suggested duration of treatment* at least 6 weeks (stop gentamicin after 2 weeks if micro-organisms fully sensitive to penicillin)

Antibacterial therapy for endocarditis caused by enterococci (e.g. *Enterococcus faecalis*)

- Amoxicillin p. 325 (*or* ampicillin p. 326) + gentamicin
- *If gentamicin-resistant*, substitute gentamicin with streptomycin p. 299
  - *Suggested duration of treatment* at least 4 weeks (at least 6 weeks for prosthetic valve endocarditis)
- *If penicillin-allergic or penicillin-resistant*, vancomycin (*or* teicoplanin) + gentamicin
- If gentamicin-resistant, substitute gentamicin with streptomycin
  - *Suggested duration of treatment* at least 4 weeks (at least 6 weeks for prosthetic valve endocarditis)

Antibacterial therapy for endocarditis caused by *Haemophilus, Actinobacillus, Cardiobacterium, Eikenella*, and *Kingella* species ('HACEK' micro-organisms)

- Amoxicillin (*or* ampicillin) + gentamicin
  - *Suggested duration of treatment* 4 weeks (6 weeks for

prosthetic valve endocarditis); stop gentamicin after 2 weeks

- *If amoxicillin-resistant*, ceftriaxone p. 308 + gentamicin
  - *Suggested duration of treatment* 4 weeks (6 weeks for prosthetic valve endocarditis); stop gentamicin after 2 weeks

Central nervous system infections, bacterial

Antibacterial therapy for meningitis: initial empirical therapy

- Transfer patient to hospital urgently.
- If *meningococcal disease* (meningitis with non-blanching rash or meningococcal septicaemia) suspected, benzylpenicillin sodium p. 323 should be given before transfer to hospital, so long as this does not delay the transfer. If a patient with suspected bacterial meningitis without non-blanching rash cannot be transferred to hospital urgently, benzylpenicillin sodium should be given before the transfer. Cefotaxime p. 307 may be an alternative in penicillin allergy; chloramphenicol p. 340 may be used if history of immediate hypersensitivity reaction to penicillin or to cephalosporins.
- In hospital, consider adjunctive treatment with dexamethasone p. 419, preferably starting before or with first dose of antibacterial, but no later than 12 hours after starting antibacterial; avoid dexamethasone in septic shock, meningococcal septicaemia, or if immunocompromised, or in meningitis following surgery.

  In hospital, if aetiology unknown:

- *Neonate and child 1–3 months*, cefotaxime (*or* ceftriaxone p. 308) + amoxicillin p. 325 (*or* ampicillin p. 326)
  - Consider adding vancomycin p. 312 if prolonged or multiple use of other antibacterials in the last 3 months, or if travelled, in the last 3 months, to areas outside the UK with highly penicillin- and cephalosporin-resistant pneumococci
  - *Suggested duration of treatment* at least 14 days
- *Child 3 months–18 years* cefotaxime (*or* ceftriaxone)
  - Consider adding vancomycin if prolonged or multiple use of other antibacterials in the last 3 months, or if travelled, in the last 3 months, to areas outside the UK with highly penicillin- and cephalosporin-resistant pneumococci
  - *Suggested duration of treatment* at least 10 days

Antibacterial therapy for meningitis caused by group B streptococcus

- Benzylpenicillin sodium + gentamicin p. 299 *or* cefotaxime (*or* ceftriaxone) alone
  - *Suggested duration of treatment* at least 14 days; stop gentamicin after 5 days

Antibacterial therapy for meningitis caused by meningococci

- Benzylpenicillin sodium *or* cefotaxime (*or* ceftriaxone)
  - *Suggested duration of treatment* 7 days.
- *If history of immediate hypersensitivity reaction to penicillin or to cephalosporins*, chloramphenicol
  - *Suggested duration of treatment* 7 days.

Antibacterial therapy for meningitis caused by pneumococci

- Cefotaxime (*or* ceftriaxone)
  - Consider adjunctive treatment with dexamethasone, preferably starting before or with first dose of

antibacterial, but no later than 12 hours after starting antibacterial (may reduce penetration of vancomycin into cerebrospinal fluid).

▶ If micro-organism penicillin-sensitive, replace cefotaxime with benzylpenicillin sodium.

▶ If micro-organism highly penicillin- and cephalosporin-resistant, add vancomycin and if necessary rifampicin p. 349.

▶ *Suggested duration of antibacterial treatment* 14 days.

Antibacterial therapy for meningitis caused by *Haemophilus influenzae*

● Cefotaxime (*or* ceftriaxone)

▶ Consider adjunctive treatment with dexamethasone, preferably starting before or with first dose of antibacterial, but no later than 12 hours after starting antibacterial.

▶ *Suggested duration of antibacterial treatment* 10 days.

▶ For *H. influenzae* type b give rifampicin for 4 days before hospital discharge to those under 10 years of age or to those in contact with vulnerable household contacts

● *If history of immediate hypersensitivity reaction to penicillin or to cephalosporins, or if micro-organism resistant to* cefotaxime, chloramphenicol

▶ Consider adjunctive treatment with dexamethasone, preferably starting before or with first dose of antibacterial, but no later than 12 hours after starting antibacterial.

▶ *Suggested duration of antibacterial treatment* 10 days.

▶ For *H. influenzae* type b give rifampicin for 4 days before hospital discharge to those under 10 years of age or to those in contact with vulnerable household contacts

Antibacterial therapy for meningitis caused by Listeria

● Amoxicillin (*or* ampicillin) + gentamicin

▶ *Suggested duration of treatment* 21 days.

▶ Consider stopping gentamicin after 7 days

● *If history of immediate hypersensitivity reaction to penicillin,* co-trimoxazole p. 335

▶ *Suggested duration of treatment* 21 days.

Ear infections, bacterial

Antibacterial therapy for otitis externa

For topical treatments, consider *Otitis externa*, under Ear p. 660.

Consider systemic antibacterial if spreading cellulitis or patient systemically unwell.

● Flucloxacillin p. 330

▶ *If penicillin-allergic*, clarithromycin p. 315 (*or* azithromycin p. 314 *or* erythromycin p. 316)

▶ *If pseudomonas suspected*, ciprofloxacin p. 333 (*or* an aminoglycoside)

Antibacterial therapy for otitis media

Many infections are caused by viruses. Most uncomplicated cases resolve without antibacterial treatment. In children without systemic features, antibacterial treatment may be started after 72 hours if no improvement. Consider earlier treatment if deterioration, if systemically unwell, if at high risk of serious complications (e.g. in immunosuppression, cystic fibrosis), if mastoiditis present, or in children under 2 years of age with bilateral otitis media.

● Amoxicillin p. 325 (*or* ampicillin p. 326)

▶ Consider co-amoxiclav p. 328 if no improvement after 48 hours.

▶ In severe infection, initial parenteral therapy with co-amoxiclav or cefuroxime p. 306.

▶ *Suggested duration of treatment* 5 days (longer if severely ill).

● *If penicillin-allergic*, clarithromycin (*or* azithromycin *or* erythromycin)

▶ *Suggested duration of treatment* 5 days (longer if severely ill)

Eye infections, bacterial

Antibacterial therapy for purulent conjunctivitis

● Chloramphenicol eye drops p. 648.

Antibacterial therapy for congenital chlamydial conjunctivitis

● Erythromycin p. 316 (by mouth)

▶ *Suggested duration of treatment* 14 days

Antibacterial therapy for congenital gonococcal conjunctivitis

● Cefotaxime p. 307 (*or* ceftriaxone p. 308)

▶ *Suggested duration of treatment* single dose.

Gastro-intestinal system infections, bacterial

Antibacterial therapy for gastro-enteritis

Frequently self-limiting and may not be bacterial.

● Antibacterial not usually indicated.

Antibacterial therapy for campylobacter enteritis

Frequently self-limiting; treat if immunocompromised or if severe infection.

● Clarithromycin p. 315 (*or* azithromycin p. 314 *or* erythromycin p. 316)

● *Alternative*, ciprofloxacin p. 333

▶ Strains with decreased sensitivity to ciprofloxacin isolated frequently

Antibacterial therapy for salmonella (non-typhoid)

Treat invasive or severe infection. Do not treat less severe infection unless there is a risk of developing invasive infection (e.g. immunocompromised children, those with haemoglobinopathy, or children under 6 months of age).

● Ciprofloxacin *or* cefotaxime p. 307

Antibacterial therapy for shigellosis

Antibacterial not indicated for mild cases.

● Azithromycin *or* ciprofloxacin

● *Alternatives if micro-organism sensitive*, amoxicillin p. 325 *or* trimethoprim p. 344

Antibacterial therapy for typhoid fever

Infections from Middle-East, South Asia, and South-East Asia may be multiple-antibacterial-resistant and sensitivity should be tested.

● Cefotaxime (*or* ceftriaxone p. 308)

▶ azithromycin may be an alternative in mild or moderate disease caused by multiple-antibacterial-resistant micro-organisms

● *Alternative if micro-organism sensitive*, ciprofloxacin *or* chloramphenicol p. 340

Antibacterial therapy for *Clostridium difficile* infection

- *For first episode of mild to moderate infection*, oral metronidazole p. 319
  - *Suggested duration of treatment* 10–14 days
- *For second or subsequent episode of infection, for severe infection, for infection not responding to metronidazole, or in children intolerant of metronidazole*, oral vancomycin p. 312
  - *Suggested duration of treatment* 10–14 days
- *For infection not responding to vancomycin, or for life-threatening infection, or in patients with ileus*, oral vancomycin + i/v metronidazole
  - *Suggested duration of treatment* 10–14 days

Antibacterial therapy for peritonitis

- A cephalosporin + metronidazole *or* amoxicillin + gentamicin p. 299 + metronidazole *or* piperacillin with tazobactam p. 322 alone

Antibacterial therapy for peritonitis: peritoneal dialysis-associated

- Vancomycin (*or* teicoplanin p. 311) + ceftazidime p. 307 added to dialysis fluid *or* vancomycin added to dialysis fluid + ciprofloxacin by mouth
  - *Suggested duration of treatment* 14 days or longer

Antibacterial therapy for necrotising enterocolitis in neonates

- In neonates
- Benzylpenicillin sodium p. 323 + gentamicin + metronidazole *or* amoxicillin (*or* ampicillin p. 326) + gentamicin + metronidazole *or* amoxicillin (*or* ampicillin) + cefotaxime + metronidazole

Genital system infections, bacterial

Antibacterial therapy for uncomplicated genital chlamydial infection, non-gonococcal urethritis, and non-specific genital infection

Contact tracing recommended.

- *Child under 12 years*, erythromycin p. 316
  - *Suggested duration of treatment* 14 days
- *Child 12–18 years*, azithromycin p. 314 as a single dose *or* doxycycline p. 338 for 7 days
- *Alternatively*, erythromycin for 14 days

Antibacterial therapy for gonorrhoea: uncomplicated

Contact tracing recommended. Consider chlamydia co-infection. Choice of antibacterial depends on locality where infection acquired.

- *Child under 12 years*, single-dose of ceftriaxone p. 308
- *Child 12–18 years*, single-dose of cefixime p. 307
- *Alternatively, if micro-organism sensitive*, single-dose of ciprofloxacin p. 333
- *Child 12–18 years with pharyngeal infection*, single-dose of ceftriaxone

Antibacterial therapy for pelvic inflammatory disease

Contact tracing recommended.

- *Child 2–12 years*, erythromycin + metronidazole p. 319 + single-dose of i/m ceftriaxone
  - *Suggested duration of treatment* 14 days (except i/m ceftriaxone)

- *Child 12–18 years*, doxycycline + metronidazole + single-dose of i/m ceftriaxone
  - If severely ill, seek specialist advice.
  - *Suggested duration of treatment* 14 days (except i/m ceftriaxone)

Antibacterial therapy for syphilis

Contact tracing recommended.

- *Child under 12 years*, benzylpenicillin sodium p. 323 *or* procaine benzylpenicillin [unlicensed]
  - *Suggested duration of treatment* 10 days

Early syphilis (infection of less than 2 years)

- *Child 12–18 years*, benzathine benzylpenicillin [unlicensed]
  - *Suggested duration of treatment* single-dose (repeat dose after 7 days for females in the third trimester of pregnancy)
- *Alternatively*, doxycycline or erythromycin
  - *Suggested duration of treatment* 14 days

Late latent syphilis (asymptomatic infection of more than 2 years)

- *Child 12–18 years*, benzathine benzylpenicillin [unlicensed].
  - *Suggested duration of treatment* once weekly for 2 weeks
- *Alternatively*, doxycycline
  - *Suggested duration of treatment* 28 days

Asymptomatic contacts of patients with infectious syphilis

- *Child 12–18 years*, doxycycline
  - *Suggested duration of treatment* 14 days

Antibacterial therapy for neonatal congenital syphilis

- Benzylpenicillin sodium
  - Also consider treating neonates with suspected congenital syphilis whose mothers were treated inadequately for syphilis, or whose mothers were treated for syphilis in the 4 weeks before delivery, or whose mothers were treated with non-penicillin antibacterials for syphilis.
  - *Suggested duration of treatment* 10 days.

Musculoskeletal system infections, bacterial

Antibacterial therapy for osteomyelitis

Seek specialist advice if chronic infection or prostheses present.

- Flucloxacillin p. 330
  - Consider adding fusidic acid p. 342 or rifampicin p. 349 for initial 2 weeks.
  - *Suggested duration of treatment* 6 weeks for acute infection
- *If penicillin-allergic*, clindamycin p. 313
  - Consider adding fusidic acid or rifampicin for initial 2 weeks.
  - *Suggested duration of treatment* 6 weeks for acute infection
- *If meticillin-resistant Staphylococcus aureus suspected*, vancomycin p. 312 (*or* teicoplanin p. 311)
  - Consider adding fusidic acid or rifampicin for initial 2 weeks.
  - *Suggested duration of treatment* 6 weeks for acute infection

Antibacterial therapy for septic arthritis

Seek specialist advice if prostheses present.

- Flucloxacillin
▸ *Suggested duration of treatment* 4–6 weeks (longer if infection complicated).
- If *penicillin-allergic*, clindamycin
▸ *Suggested duration of treatment* 4–6 weeks (longer if infection complicated).
- If *meticillin-resistant Staphylococcus aureus suspected*, vancomycin (*or* teicoplanin)
▸ *Suggested duration of treatment* 4–6 weeks (longer if infection complicated).
- If *gonococcal arthritis or Gram-negative infection suspected*, cefotaxime p. 307 (*or* ceftriaxone p. 308)
▸ *Suggested duration of treatment* 4–6 weeks (longer if infection complicated; treat gonococcal infection for 2 weeks).

Nose infections, bacterial

Antibacterial therapy for sinusitis

Antibacterial therapy should usually be used only for persistent symptoms and purulent discharge lasting at least 7 days or if severe symptoms. Also, consider antibacterial for those at high risk of serious complications (e.g. in immunosuppression, cystic fibrosis).

- Amoxicillin p. 325 (*or* ampicillin p. 326) or clarithromycin p. 315 (*or* azithromycin p. 314 *or* erythromycin p. 316)
▸ *Suggested duration of treatment* 7 days.
▸ Consider oral co-amoxiclav p. 328 if no improvement after 48 hours.
▸ In severe infection, initial parenteral therapy with co-amoxiclav or cefuroxime p. 306 may be required.

Oral bacterial infections

Antibacterial drugs

Antibacterial drugs should only be prescribed for the *treatment* of oral infections on the basis of defined need. They may be used in conjunction with (but not as an alternative to) other appropriate measures, such as providing drainage or extracting a tooth.

The 'blind' prescribing of an antibacterial for unexplained pyrexia, cervical lymphadenopathy, or facial swelling can lead to difficulty in establishing the diagnosis. In severe oral infections, a sample should always be taken for bacteriology.

Oral infections which may require antibacterial treatment include acute periapical or periodontal abscess, cellulitis, acutely created oral-antral communication (and acute sinusitis), severe pericoronitis, localised osteitis, acute necrotising ulcerative gingivitis, and destructive forms of chronic periodontal disease. Most of these infections are readily resolved by the early establishment of drainage and removal of the cause (typically an infected necrotic pulp). Antibacterials may be required if treatment has to be delayed, in immunocompromised patients, or in those with conditions such as diabetes. Certain rarer infections including bacterial sialadenitis, osteomyelitis, actinomycosis, and infections involving fascial spaces such as Ludwig's angina, require antibiotics and specialist hospital care.

Antibacterial drugs may also be useful after dental surgery in some cases of spreading infection. Infection may spread to involve local lymph nodes, to fascial spaces (where it can cause airway obstruction), or into the bloodstream (where it can lead to cavernous sinus thrombosis and other serious complications). Extension of an infection can also lead to maxillary sinusitis; osteomyelitis is a complication, which usually arises when host resistance is reduced.

If the oral infection fails to respond to antibacterial treatment within 48 hours the antibacterial should be changed, preferably on the basis of bacteriological investigation. Failure to respond may also suggest an incorrect diagnosis, lack of essential additional measures (such as drainage), poor host resistance, or poor patient compliance.

Combination of a penicillin (or a macrolide) with metronidazole p. 319 may sometimes be helpful for the treatment of severe oral infections or oral infections.

Penicillins

Phenoxymethylpenicillin p. 324 is effective for dentoalveolar abscess.

Broad-spectrum penicillins

Amoxicillin p. 325 is as effective as phenoxymethylpenicillin but is better absorbed; however, it may encourage emergence of resistant organisms.

Like phenoxymethylpenicillin, amoxicillin is ineffective against bacteria that produce beta-lactamases.

Co-amoxiclav p. 328 is active against beta-lactamase-producing bacteria that are resistant to amoxicillin. Co-amoxiclav may be used for severe dental infection with spreading cellulitis or dental infection not responding to first-line antibacterial treatment.

Cephalosporins

The cephalosporins offer little advantage over the penicillins in dental infections, often being less active against anaerobes. Infections due to oral streptococci (often termed viridans streptococci) which become resistant to penicillin are usually also resistant to cephalosporins. This is of importance in the case of patients who have had rheumatic fever and are on long-term penicillin therapy. Cefalexin p. 304 and cefradine p. 305 have been used in the treatment of oral infections.

Tetracyclines

In children over 12 years of age, tetracyclines can be effective against oral anaerobes but the development of resistance (especially by oral streptococci) has reduced their usefulness for the treatment of acute oral infections; they may still have a role in the treatment of destructive (refractory) forms of periodontal disease. Doxycycline p. 338 has a longer duration of action than tetracycline p. 339 or oxytetracycline p. 339 and need only be given once daily; it is reported to be more active against anaerobes than some other tetracyclines.

Doxycycline may have a role in the treatment of recurrent aphthous ulceration, or as an adjunct to gingival scaling and root planing for periodontitis.

Macrolides

The macrolides are an alternative for oral infections in penicillin-allergic patients or where a beta-lactamase producing organism is involved. However, many organisms are now resistant to macrolides or rapidly develop resistance; their use should therefore be limited to short courses.

Clindamycin

Clindamycin p. 313 should not be used routinely for the treatment of oral infections because it may be no more effective than penicillins against anaerobes and there may be cross-resistance with erythromycin p. 316-resistant bacteria. Clindamycin can be used for the treatment of dentoalveolar abscess that has not responded to penicillin or to metronidazole.

Metronidazole and tinidazole

Metronidazole is an alternative to a penicillin for the treatment of many oral infections where the patient is allergic to penicillin or the infection is due to beta-lactamase-producing anaerobes. It is the drug of first choice for the treatment of acute necrotising ulcerative gingivitis (Vincent's infection) and pericoronitis; amoxicillin is a suitable alternative. For these purposes metronidazole for 3 days is sufficient, but the duration of treatment may need to be longer in pericoronitis. Tinidazole p. 320 is licensed for the treatment of acute ulcerative gingivitis.

Respiratory system infections, bacterial

Antibacterial therapy for *Haemophilus influenzae* epiglottitis

- Cefotaxime p. 307 (*or* ceftriaxone p. 308)
- *If history of immediate hypersensitivity reaction to penicillin or to cephalosporins*, chloramphenicol p. 340

Antibacterial therapy for pneumonia: community-acquired

Children under 2 years with mild symptoms of lower respiratory tract infection (particularly those vaccinated with pneumococcal polysaccharide conjugate vaccine (adsorbed) p. 763 and haemophilus type b conjugate vaccine) are unlikely to have pneumonia; antibacterial treatment may be considered if symptoms persist.

- *Neonate*, benzylpenicillin sodium p. 323 + gentamicin p. 299
- *Child* 1 *month*–18 *years*, amoxicillin p. 325 (*or* ampicillin p. 326) by mouth
- Pneumococci with decreased penicillin sensitivity have been isolated in the UK, but are not common.
- If no response to treatment, add clarithromycin p. 315 (*or* azithromycin p. 314 *or* erythromycin p. 316)
- If staphylococci suspected (e.g. in influenza or measles), give by mouth amoxicillin + flucloxacillin p. 330 *or* co-amoxiclav p. 328 alone
- If septicaemia, complicated pneumonia, or if oral administration not possible, initiate treatment with i/v amoxicillin *or* i/v co-amoxiclav *or* i/v cefuroxime p. 306 *or* i/v cefotaxime (*or* ceftriaxone)
- *Suggested duration of treatment* 7 days (may extend treatment to 14 days in some cases e.g. if staphylococci suspected)
- *Child* 1 *month*–18 *years, if penicillin-allergic*, clarithromycin (*or* azithromycin *or* erythromycin)
- *Suggested duration of treatment* 7 days (may extend treatment to 14 days in some cases e.g. if staphylococci suspected)

Antibacterial therapy for pneumonia possibly caused by atypical pathogens

- Clarithromycin (*or* azithromycin *or* erythromycin)
- *Suggested duration of treatment* 10–14 days
- *Alternative for chlamydial or mycoplasma infections in children over 12 years*, doxycycline p. 338
- *Suggested duration of treatment* 10–14 days

Antibacterial therapy for pneumonia: hospital-acquired

- *Early-onset infection* (less than 5 days after admission to hospital), treat as for severe community-acquired pneumonia of unknown aetiology; if life-threatening infection, or if recent history of antibacterial treatment, or if resistant organisms suspected, treat as for late-onset hospital-acquired pneumonia
- *Late-onset infection* (more than 5 days after admission to hospital), an antipseudomonal penicillin (e.g. piperacillin

with tazobactam p. 322) *or* another antipseudomonal beta-lactam

- If meticillin-resistant *Staphylococcus aureus* suspected, add vancomycin p. 312.
- If severe illness caused by *Pseudomonas aeruginosa*, add an aminoglycoside.
- *Suggested duration of treatment* 7 days (longer if *Pseudomonas aeruginosa* confirmed)

Antibacterial therapy for staphylococcal lung infection in cystic fibrosis

- Flucloxacillin
- If child already taking flucloxacillin prophylaxis or if severe exacerbation, add fusidic acid p. 342 or rifampicin p. 349; use flucloxacillin at treatment dose
- *If penicillin-allergic*, clarithromycin (*or* azithromycin *or* erythromycin) or clindamycin p. 313
- Use clarithromycin only if micro-organism sensitive

Antibacterial therapy for *Haemophilus influenzae* lung infection in cystic fibrosis

- Amoxicillin *or* a broad-spectrum cephalosporin
- In severe exacerbation use a third-generation cephalosporin (e.g. cefotaxime)

Antibacterial therapy for pseudomonal lung infection in cystic fibrosis

- Ciprofloxacin p. 333 + *nebulised* colistimethate sodium p. 331
- *For severe exacerbation*, an antipseudomonal beta-lactam antibacterial + parenteral tobramycin p. 300

Skin infections, bacterial

Antibacterial therapy for impetigo: small areas of skin infected

Seek local microbiology advice before using topical treatment in hospital.

- Topical fusidic acid p. 342
- *Suggested duration of treatment* 7 days is usually adequate (max. 10 days).
- *Alternatively, if meticillin-resistant Staphylococcus aureus*, topical mupirocin p. 668
- *Suggested duration of treatment* 7 days is usually adequate (max. 10 days).

Impetigo: widespread infection

- Oral flucloxacillin p. 330
- If streptococci suspected in severe infection, add phenoxymethylpenicillin p. 324
- *Suggested duration of treatment* 7 days.
- *If penicillin-allergic*, oral clarithromycin p. 315 (*or* azithromycin p. 314 *or* erythromycin p. 316)
- *Suggested duration of treatment* 7 days.

Antibacterial therapy for erysipelas

- Phenoxymethylpenicillin *or* benzylpenicillin sodium p. 323
- If severe infection, replace phenoxymethylpenicillin or benzylpenicillin sodium with high-dose flucloxacillin
- *Suggested duration of treatment* at least 7 days
- *If penicillin-allergic*, clindamycin p. 313 or clarithromycin (*or* azithromycin *or* erythromycin)
- *Suggested duration of treatment* at least 7 days.

Antibacterial therapy for cellulitis

- Flucloxacillin (high dose)
- ‣ If streptococcal infection confirmed, replace flucloxacillin with phenoxymethylpenicillin or benzylpenicillin sodium
- ‣ If Gram-negative bacteria or anaerobes suspected (e.g. facial infection, orbital infection, or infection caused by animal or human bites), use broad-spectrum antibacterials; if periumbilical cellulitis, use flucloxacillin + gentamicin p. 299
- *If penicillin-allergic*, clindamycin *or* clarithromycin (*or* azithromycin *or* erythromycin)
- ‣ If Gram-negative bacteria suspected, use broad-spectrum antibacterials.

Antibacterial therapy for staphylococcal scalded skin syndrome

- Flucloxacillin
- ‣ *Suggested duration of treatment* 7–10 days.
- *If penicillin-allergic*, clarithromycin (*or* azithromycin *or* erythromycin)
- ‣ *Suggested duration of treatment* 7–10 days.

Antibacterial therapy for animal and human bites

Cleanse wound thoroughly. For tetanus-prone wound, give human tetanus immunoglobulin p. 745 (with a tetanus-containing vaccine if necessary, according to immunisation history and risk of infection). Consider rabies prophylaxis for bites from animals in endemic countries; assess risk of blood-borne viruses (including HIV, hepatitis B and C) and give appropriate prophylaxis to prevent viral spread.

- Co-amoxiclav p. 328
- *If penicillin-allergic*, clindamycin

Antibacterial therapy for surgical wound infection

- Flucloxacillin *or* co-amoxiclav

Antibacterial therapy for paronychia or 'septic spots' in neonate

- Flucloxacillin
- ‣ If systemically unwell, add an aminoglycoside.

ANTIBACTERIALS › AMINOGLYCOSIDES

Aminoglycosides

Overview

These include amikacin p. 298, gentamicin p. 299, neomycin sulfate p. 662, streptomycin p. 299, and tobramycin p. 300. All are bactericidal and active against some Gram-positive and many Gram-negative organisms. Amikacin, gentamicin, and tobramycin are also active against *Pseudomonas aeruginosa*; streptomycin is active against *Mycobacterium tuberculosis* and is now almost entirely reserved for tuberculosis.

The aminoglycosides are not absorbed from the gut (although there is a risk of absorption in inflammatory bowel disease and liver failure) and must therefore be given by injection for systemic infections.

Gentamicin is the aminoglycoside of choice in the UK and is used widely for the treatment of serious infections. It has a broad spectrum but is inactive against anaerobes and has poor activity against haemolytic streptococci and pneumococci. When used for the 'blind' therapy of undiagnosed serious infections it is usually given in conjunction with a penicillin or metronidazole p. 319 (or both). Gentamicin is used together with another antibiotic for the treatment of endocarditis. Streptomycin may be used as an alternative in gentamicin-resistant enterococcal endocarditis.

Loading and maintenance doses of gentamicin may be calculated on the basis of the patient's weight and renal function (e.g. using a nomogram); adjustments are then made according to serum-gentamicin concentrations. High doses are occasionally indicated for serious infections, especially in the neonate, in the patient with cystic fibrosis, or in the immunocompromised patient. Whenever possible treatment should not exceed 7 days.

Amikacin is more stable than gentamicin to enzyme inactivation. Amikacin is used in the treatment of serious infections caused by gentamicin-resistant Gram-negative bacilli.

Tobramycin has similar activity to gentamicin. It is slightly more active against *Ps. aeruginosa* but shows less activity against certain other Gram-negative bacteria..

Neomycin sulfate is too toxic for parenteral administration and can only be used for infections of the skin or mucous membranes or to reduce the bacterial population of the colon prior to bowel surgery or in hepatic failure. Oral administration may lead to malabsorption. Small amounts of neomycin sulfate may be absorbed from the gut in patients with hepatic failure and, as these patients may also be uraemic, cumulation may occur with resultant ototoxicity.

Cystic fibrosis

A higher dose of parenteral aminoglycoside is often required in children with cystic fibrosis because renal clearance of the aminoglycoside is increased. Aminoglycosides have a role in the treatment of pseudomonal lung infections in cystic fibrosis. Tobramycin can be administered by nebuliser or by inhalation of powder on a cyclical basis (28 days of tobramycin followed by a 28-day tobramycin-free interval) for the treatment of chronic pulmonary *Ps. aeruginosa* infection in cystic fibrosis; however, resistance may develop and some patients do not respond to treatment.

Once daily dosage

Once daily administration of aminoglycosides is more convenient, provides adequate serum concentrations, and has largely superseded *multiple- daily dose regimens* (given in 2–3 divided doses during the 24 hours). Local guidelines on dosage and serum concentrations should be consulted. A once-daily, high-dose regimen of an aminoglycoside should be avoided in children with endocarditis or burns of more than 20% of the total body surface area. There is insufficient evidence to recommend a once daily, high-dose regimen of an aminoglycoside in pregnancy.

Serum concentrations

Serum concentration monitoring avoids both excessive and subtherapeutic concentrations thus preventing toxicity and ensuring efficacy. Serum-aminoglycoside concentrations should be monitored in patients receiving parenteral aminoglycosides and **must** be determined in obesity, and in cystic fibrois, or if high doses are being given, or if there is renal impairment.

Neonates

As aminoglycosides are eliminated principally via the kidney, neonatal treatment must reflect the changes in glomerular filtration that occur with increasing gestational and postnatal age. The *extended interval dose regimen* is used in neonates, and serum-aminoglycoside concentrations **must** be measured. In patients on single daily dose regimens it may become necessary to prolong the dose interval to more than 24 hours if the trough concentration is high.

Aminoglycosides (by injection)

- **CONTRA-INDICATIONS** Myasthenia gravis (aminoglycosides may impair neuromuscular transmission)
- **CAUTIONS** Care must be taken with dosage (the main side-

effects of the aminoglycosides are dose-related) · conditions characterised by muscular weakness (aminoglycosides may impair neuromuscular transmission) · if possible, dehydration should be corrected before starting an aminoglycoside · whenever possible, parenteral treatment should not exceed 7 days

- SIDE-EFFECTS
- ► **Rare** Antibiotic-associated colitis · electrolyte disturbances · hypocalcaemia · hypokalaemia · hypomagnesaemia on prolonged therapy · nausea · peripheral neuropathy · stomatitis · vomiting
- ► **Very rare** Blood disorders · CNS effects · convulsions · encephalopathy · headache
- ► **Frequency not known** Auditory damage · impaired neuromuscular transmission · irreversible ototoxicity · nephrotoxicity · transient myasthenic syndrome in patients with normal neuromuscular function with large doses given during surgery · vestibular damage
  SIDE-EFFECTS, FURTHER INFORMATION
- ► **Nephrotoxicity** Occurs most commonly in children with renal failure.

- **PREGNANCY** There is a risk of auditory or vestibular nerve damage in the infant when aminoglycosides are used in the second and third trimesters of pregnancy. The risk is greatest with streptomycin. The risk is probably very small with gentamicin and tobramycin, but their use should be avoided unless essential.
    If given during pregnancy, serum-aminoglycoside concentration monitoring is essential.

- **RENAL IMPAIRMENT** If there is impairment of renal function, the interval between doses must be increased; if the renal impairment is severe, the dose itself should be reduced as well. Excretion of aminoglycosides is principally via the kidney and accumulation occurs in renal impairment.
    A once-daily, high-dose regimen of an aminoglycoside should be avoided in children over 1 month of age with a creatinine clearance less than 20 mL/minute/1.73 m^2.
    Ototoxicity and nephrotoxicity occur commonly in patients with renal failure. Serum-aminoglycoside concentrations **must** be monitored in patients with renal impairment; earlier and more frequent measurement of aminoglycoside concentration may be required.

- MONITORING REQUIREMENTS
- ► **Serum concentrations** Serum concentration monitoring avoids both excessive and subtherapeutic concentrations thus preventing toxicity and ensuring efficacy. Serum-aminoglycoside concentrations should be measured in all patients receiving parenteral aminoglycosides and **must** be determined in obesity, if high doses are being given and in cystic fibrosis.
    Serum aminoglycoside concentrations **must** be determined in neonates.
    In children with normal renal function, aminoglycoside concentrations should be measured after 3 or 4 doses of a multiple daily dose regimen.
    Blood samples should be taken just before the next dose is administered ('trough') concentration. If the pre-dose ('trough') concentration is high, the interval between doses must be increased. For multiple daily dose regimens, blood samples should also be taken approximately 1 hour after intramuscular or intravenous administration ('peak' concentration). If the post-dose ('peak') concentration is high, the dose must be decreased.
- ► Renal function should be assessed before starting an aminoglycoside and during treatment.
- ► Auditory and vestibular function should also be monitored during treatment.

F 297

Amikacin

- INDICATIONS AND DOSE

Serious Gram-negative infections resistant to gentamicin (multiple daily dose regimen)
- ► BY SLOW INTRAVENOUS INJECTION
- ► Child 1 month–11 years: 7.5 mg/kg every 12 hours, to be administered over 3–5 minutes
- ► Child 12–17 years: 7.5 mg/kg every 12 hours; increased to 7.5 mg/kg every 8 hours (max. per dose 500 mg every 8 hours) for up to 10 days, higher dose to be used in severe infection, to be administered over 3–5 minutes; maximum 15 g per course

Serious Gram-negative infections resistant to gentamicin (once daily dose regimen)
- ► BY INTRAVENOUS INFUSION, OR BY INTRAVENOUS INJECTION
- ► Child: Initially 15 mg/kg adjusted according to plasma-concentration monitoring, not to be used for endocarditis or meningitis, dose to be adjusted according to serum-amikacin concentration, intravenous injection to be administered over 3–5 minutes

Neonatal sepsis (extended interval dose regimen)
- ► BY SLOW INTRAVENOUS INJECTION, OR BY INTRAVENOUS INFUSION
- ► Neonate: 15 mg/kg every 24 hours, intravenous injection to be administered over 3–5 minutes.

Neonatal sepsis (multiple daily dose regimen)
- ► BY INTRAMUSCULAR INJECTION, OR BY SLOW INTRAVENOUS INJECTION, OR BY INTRAVENOUS INFUSION
- ► Neonate: Loading dose 10 mg/kg, then 7.5 mg/kg every 12 hours, intravenous injection to be administered over 3–5 minutes.

Pseudomonal lung infection in cystic fibrosis
- ► BY SLOW INTRAVENOUS INJECTION, OR BY INTRAVENOUS INFUSION
- ► Child: 10 mg/kg every 8 hours (max. per dose 500 mg every 8 hours), intravenous injection to be administered over 3–5 minutes

DOSES AT EXTREMES OF BODY-WEIGHT
To avoid excessive dosage in obese patients, use ideal weight for height to calculate dose and monitor serum-amikacin concentration closely

- **UNLICENSED USE** Dose for cystic fibrosis not licensed.
- **INTERACTIONS** → Appendix 1: aminoglycosides
- SIDE-EFFECTS
- ► **Uncommon** Rash
- MONITORING REQUIREMENTS
- ► *Multiple daily dose regimen*: one-hour ('peak') serum concentration should not exceed 30 mg/litre; pre-dose ('trough') concentration should be less than 10 mg/litre.
- ► *Once daily dose regimen*: pre-dose ('trough') concentration should be less than 5 mg/litre.
- **DIRECTIONS FOR ADMINISTRATION** For *intravenous infusion*, dilute with Glucose 5% or Sodium Chloride 0.9%; give over 30–60 minutes.
- **PRESCRIBING AND DISPENSING INFORMATION** Local guidelines may vary in the dosing advice provided.

- MEDICINAL FORMS
  There can be variation in the licensing of different medicines containing the same drug.
  Solution for injection
- ► Amikacin (Non-proprietary)
  Amikacin (as Amikacin sulfate) 250 mg per 1 ml Amikacin 500mg/2ml solution for injection vials | 5 vial [PoM] £60.00
- ► Amikin (Bristol-Myers Squibb Pharmaceuticals Ltd)
  Amikacin (as Amikacin sulfate) 50 mg per 1 ml Amikin 100mg/2ml solution for injection vials | 5 vial [PoM] £10.33

5

Infection

Gentamicin

F 297

- ● **INDICATIONS AND DOSE**

Septicaemia | Meningitis and other CNS infections | Biliary-tract infection | Acute pyelonephritis | Endocarditis | Pneumonia in hospital patients | Adjunct in listerial meningitis
- ▸ BY INTRAVENOUS INFUSION
- ▸ Child: Initially 7 mg/kg, to be given in a once daily regimen (not suitable for endocarditis or meningitis), subsequent doses adjusted according to serum-gentamicin concentration
- ▸ BY INTRAMUSCULAR INJECTION, OR BY SLOW INTRAVENOUS INJECTION
- ▸ Child 1 month–11 years: 2.5 mg/kg every 8 hours, to be given in a multiple daily dose regimen, intravenous injection to be administered over at least 3 minutes
- ▸ Child 12–17 years: 2 mg/kg every 8 hours, to be given in a multiple daily dose regimen, intravenous injection to be administered over at least 3 minutes

Neonatal sepsis
- ▸ BY SLOW INTRAVENOUS INJECTION, OR BY INTRAVENOUS INFUSION
- ▸ Neonate up to 7 days: 5 mg/kg every 36 hours, to be given in an extended interval dose regimen.
- ▸ Neonate 7 days to 28 days: 5 mg/kg every 24 hours, to be given in an extended interval dose regimen.

Pseudomonal lung infection in cystic fibrosis
- ▸ BY SLOW INTRAVENOUS INJECTION, OR BY INTRAVENOUS INFUSION
- ▸ Child: 3 mg/kg every 8 hours, to be given in a multiple daily dose regimen, intravenous injection to be administered over at least 3 minutes

Bacterial ventriculitis and CNS infection (supplement to systemic therapy) (administered on expert advice)
- ▸ BY INTRATHECAL INJECTION, OR BY INTRAVENTRICULAR INJECTION
- ▸ Neonate: (consult local protocol).
- ▸ Child: Initially 1 mg daily, then increased if necessary to 5 mg daily, seek specialist advice

DOSES AT EXTREMES OF BODY-WEIGHT
To avoid excessive dosage in obese patients, use ideal weight for height to calculate parenteral dose and monitor serum-gentamicin concentration closely.

- ● **INTERACTIONS** → Appendix 1: aminoglycosides

- ● **SIDE-EFFECTS**
- ▸ **Uncommon** Rash

- ● **MONITORING REQUIREMENTS**
- ▸ Extended interval dose regimen in neonates: pre-dose ('trough') concentration should be less than 2 mg/litre (less than 1 mg/litre if more than 3 doses administered); consider monitoring one hour ('peak') concentration in neonates with poor response to treatment, with oedema, with Gram-negative infection, or with birth-weight greater than 4.5 kg (consider increasing dose if 'peak' concentration less than 8 mg/litre in severe sepsis).
- ▸ Once daily dose regimen: pre-dose ('trough') concentration should be less than 1 mg/litre.
- ▸ Multiple daily dose regimen: one hour ('peak') serum concentration should be 5–10 mg/litre; pre-dose ('trough') concentration should be less than 2 mg/litre.
- ▸ Multiple daily dose regimen for endocarditis: one hour ('peak') serum concentration should be 3–5 mg/litre; pre-dose ('trough') concentration should be less than 1 mg/litre. Serum-gentamicin concentration should be

determined twice each week (more often in renal impairment).
- ▸ Multiple daily dose regimen for cystic fibrosis: one hour ('peak') serum concentration should be 8–12 mg/litre; pre-dose ('trough') concentration should be less than 2 mg/litre.
- ▸ Intrathecal/intraventricular injection: cerebrospinal fluid concentration should not exceed 10 mg/litre.

- ● **DIRECTIONS FOR ADMINISTRATION** For *intrathecal* or *intraventricular* injection, use preservative-free intrathecal preparations only.
    For *intravenous infusion*, dilute in Glucose 5% or Sodium Chloride 0.9%; give over 30 minutes.

- ● **PRESCRIBING AND DISPENSING INFORMATION** Local guidelines may vary in the dosing advice provided. Only preservative-free intrathecal preparation should be used.

- ● **MEDICINAL FORMS**
There can be variation in the licensing of different medicines containing the same drug.

Solution for injection
- ▸ Gentamicin (Non-proprietary)
    Gentamicin (as Gentamicin sulfate) 5 mg per 1 ml Gentamicin Intrathecal 5mg/1ml solution for injection ampoules | 5 ampoule [PoM] £36.28 (Hospital only)
    Gentamicin (as Gentamicin sulfate) 10 mg per 1 ml Gentamicin 20mg/2ml solution for injection ampoules | 5 ampoule [PoM] £11.25
    Gentamicin Paediatric 20mg/2ml solution for injection vials | 5 vial [PoM] £11.25 DT price = £11.25
    Gentamicin (as Gentamicin sulfate) 40 mg per 1 ml Gentamicin 80mg/2ml solution for injection vials | 5 vial [PoM] £20.00
    Gentamicin 80mg/2ml solution for injection ampoules | 5 ampoule [PoM] £6.88 | 10 ampoule [PoM] £10.00
- ▸ Cidomycin (Sanofi)
    Gentamicin (as Gentamicin sulfate) 40 mg per 1 ml Cidomycin Adult Injectable 80mg/2ml solution for injection vials | 5 vial [PoM] £6.88
    Cidomycin Adult Injectable 80mg/2ml solution for injection ampoules | 5 ampoule [PoM] £6.88

Infusion
- ▸ Gentamicin (Non-proprietary)
    Gentamicin (as Gentamicin sulfate) 1 mg per 1 ml Gentamicin 80mg/80ml infusion bags | 20 bag [PoM] £39.00
    Gentamicin (as Gentamicin sulfate) 3 mg per 1 ml Gentamicin 240mg/80ml infusion bags | 20 bag [PoM] £119.00
    Gentamicin 360mg/120ml infusion bags | 20 bag [PoM] £169.00

F 297

Streptomycin

- ● **INDICATIONS AND DOSE**

Tuberculosis, resistant to other treatment, in combination with other drugs
- ▸ BY DEEP INTRAMUSCULAR INJECTION
- ▸ Child: 15 mg/kg once daily (max. per dose 1 g)

Adjunct to doxycycline in brucellosis (administered on expert advice)
- ▸ BY DEEP INTRAMUSCULAR INJECTION
- ▸ Child: 5–10 mg/kg every 6 hours, total daily dose may alternatively be given in 2–3 divided doses

- ● **UNLICENSED USE** Not licensed for use in children.

IMPORTANT SAFETY INFORMATION
Side-effects increase after a cumulative dose of 100 g, which should only be exceeded in exceptional circumstances.

- ● **INTERACTIONS** → Appendix 1: aminoglycosides
- ● **SIDE-EFFECTS**
- ▸ **Common or very common** Rash
- ▸ **Frequency not known** Hypersensitivity reactions · paraesthesia of mouth

- **RENAL IMPAIRMENT** Should preferably be avoided. If essential, use with great care and consider dose reduction.
- **MONITORING REQUIREMENTS**
- One-hour ('peak') concentration should be 15–40 mg/litre; pre-dose ('trough') concentration should be less than 5 mg/litre (less than 1 mg/litre in renal impairment).

- **MEDICINAL FORMS**
  There can be variation in the licensing of different medicines containing the same drug. Forms available from special-order manufacturers include: powder for solution for injection

F 297

Tobramycin

30-Nov-2016

- **INDICATIONS AND DOSE**

Chronic *Pseudomonas aeruginosa* infection in patients with cystic fibrosis
- BY INHALATION OF NEBULISED SOLUTION
- Child 6–17 years: 300 mg every 12 hours for 28 days, subsequent courses repeated after 28-day interval without tobramycin nebuliser solution
- BY INHALATION OF POWDER
- Child 6–17 years: 112 mg every 12 hours for 28 days, subsequent courses repeated after 28-day interval without tobramycin inhalation powder

Pseudomonal lung infection in cystic fibrosis
- BY SLOW INTRAVENOUS INJECTION
- Child: 8–10 mg/kg daily in 3 divided doses, to be given as a multiple daily dose regimen over 3–5 minutes
- BY INTRAVENOUS INFUSION
- Child: Initially 10 mg/kg once daily (max. per dose 660 mg), to be given over 30 minutes, subsequent doses adjusted according to serum-tobramycin concentration

Septicaemia | Meningitis and other CNS infections | Biliary-tract infection | Acute pyelonephritis | Pneumonia in hospital patients
- BY SLOW INTRAVENOUS INJECTION
- Child 1 month-11 years: 2–2.5 mg/kg every 8 hours, to be given as a multiple daily dose regimen over 3–5 minutes
- Child 12–17 years: 1 mg/kg every 8 hours, to be given as a multiple daily dose regimen over 3–5 minutes; increased if necessary up to 5 mg/kg daily in 3–4 divided doses, to be given in severe infections as a multiple daily dose regimen over 3–5 minutes, dose to be reduced back to 3 mg/kg as soon as clinically indicated
- BY INTRAVENOUS INFUSION
- Child: Initially 7 mg/kg, to be given as a once daily dose regimen, subsequent doses adjusted according to serum-tobramycin concentration

Neonatal sepsis
- BY INTRAVENOUS INJECTION, OR BY INTRAVENOUS INFUSION

- Neonate up to 32 weeks corrected gestational age: 4–5 mg/kg every 36 hours, to be given as an extended interval dose regimen, intravenous injection to be given over 3–5 minutes.

- Neonate 32 weeks corrected gestational age and above: 4–5 mg/kg every 24 hours, to be given as an extended interval dose regimen, intravenous injection to be given over 3–5 minutes.

- BY SLOW INTRAVENOUS INJECTION, OR BY INTRAVENOUS INFUSION

- Neonate up to 7 days: 2 mg/kg every 12 hours, to be given as a multiple daily dose regimen.

- Neonate 7 days to 28 days: 2–2.5 mg/kg every 8 hours, to be given as a multiple daily dose regimen.

DOSES AT EXTREMES OF BODY-WEIGHT
To avoid excessive dosage in obese patients, use ideal weight for height to calculate parenteral dose and monitor serum-tobramycin concentration closely.

VANTOBRA® NEBULISER SOLUTION
Chronic pulmonary *Pseudomonas aeruginosa* infection in patients with cystic fibrosis
- BY INHALATION OF NEBULISED SOLUTION
- Child 6–17 years: 170 mg every 12 hours for 28 days, subsequent courses repeated after 28-day interval without tobramycin nebuliser solution

- **CAUTIONS**
- When used by inhalation Conditions characterised by muscular weakness—may impair neuromuscular transmission · history of prolonged previous or concomitant intravenous aminoglycosides—increased risk of ototoxicity · renal impairment—limited information available · severe haemoptysis—risk of further haemorrhage
- **INTERACTIONS** → Appendix 1: aminoglycosides
- **SIDE-EFFECTS**
- **Common or very common**
- When used by inhalation Malaise · rhinitis · tinnitus
- **Uncommon**
- With intravenous use Rash
- **Rare**
- When used by inhalation Aphonia · hearing loss
- **Very rare**
- When used by inhalation Pruritus · urticaria
- **Frequency not known**
- When used by inhalation Bronchospasm cough (more frequent by inhalation of powder) · dysphonia · epistaxis · haemoptysis · laryngitis · mouth ulcers · pharyngitis · salivary hypersecretion · taste disturbances

SIDE-EFFECTS, FURTHER INFORMATION
- Ear effects
- When used by inhalation Manufacturer advises monitor serum-tobramycin concentration in patients with known or suspected signs of auditory dysfunction; if ototoxicity develops—discontinue treatment until serum concentration falls below 2 mg/litre.

VANTOBRA® NEBULISER SOLUTION
- **Uncommon** Dyspnoea
- **Rare** Anorexia · asthenia · asthma · chest discomfort · dizziness · headache · nausea · pyrexia · vomiting
- **Very rare** Abdominal pain · back pain diarrhoea · ear pain · fungal infection · hyperventilation · hypoxia · lymphadenopathy · sinusitis · somnolence

- **RENAL IMPAIRMENT**
- When used by inhalation Manufacturer advises monitor serum-tobramycin concentration; if nephrotoxicity develops—discontinue treatment until serum concentration falls below 2 mg/litre.

- **MONITORING REQUIREMENTS**
- With intravenous use in neonates *Extended interval dose regimen in neonates*: pre-dose ('trough') concentration should be less than 2 mg/litre.
- With intravenous use *Once daily dose regimen*: pre-dose ('trough') concentration should be less than 1 mg/litre. *Multiple daily dose regimen*: one-hour ('peak') serum concentration should not exceed 10 mg/litre (8–12 mg/litre in cystic fibrosis); pre-dose ('trough') concentration should be less than 2 mg/litre.

▸ When used by inhalation Measure lung function before and after initial dose of tobramycin and monitor for bronchospasm; if bronchospasm occurs in a patient not using a bronchodilator, repeat test using bronchodilator. Manufacturer advises monitor renal function before treatment and then annually.

● DIRECTIONS FOR ADMINISTRATION
▸ With intravenous use For *intravenous infusion*, dilute with Glucose 5% or Sodium Chloride 0.9%; give over 20–60 minutes.
▸ When used by inhalation Other inhaled drugs should be administered before tobramycin.

● PRESCRIBING AND DISPENSING INFORMATION Local guidelines may vary in dosing advice provided.

● PATIENT AND CARER ADVICE Patient counselling is advised for Tobramycin dry powder for inhalation (administration).

VANTOBRA® NEBULISER SOLUTION

Missed doses
Manufacturer advises if a dose is more than 6 hours late, the missed dose should not be taken and the next dose should be taken at the normal time.

● NATIONAL FUNDING/ACCESS DECISIONS

NICE technology appraisals (TAs)
▸ Tobramycin by dry powder inhalation for pseudomonal lung infection in cystic fibrosis (March 2013) NICE TA276
Tobramycin dry powder for inhalation is recommended for chronic pulmonary infection caused by *Pseudomonas aeruginosa* in patients with cystic fibrosis only if there is an inadequate response to colistimethate sodium, or if colistimethate sodium cannot be used because of contraindications or intolerance. The manufacturer must provide tobramycin dry powder for inhalation at the discount agreed as part of the patient access scheme to primary, secondary and tertiary care in the NHS. Patients currently receiving tobramycin dry powder for inhalation can continue treatment until they and their clinician consider it appropriate to stop.
www.nice.org.uk/TA276

● MEDICINAL FORMS
There can be variation in the licensing of different medicines containing the same drug.

Solution for injection
▸ Tobramycin (Non-proprietary)
Tobramycin (as Tobramycin sulfate) **40 mg per 1 ml** Tobramycin 40mg/1ml solution for injection vials | 10 vial PoM £37.00 (Hospital only)
Tobramycin 80mg/2ml solution for injection vials | 5 vial PoM £20.80 | 10 vial PoM £37.72 | 10 vial PoM £47.00 (Hospital only)
Tobramycin 240mg/6ml solution for injection vials | 1 vial PoM £19.20
▸ Nebcin (Flynn Pharma Ltd)
Tobramycin (as Tobramycin sulfate) **40 mg per 1 ml** Nebcin 80mg/2ml solution for injection vials | 1 vial PoM £5.37

Nebuliser liquid
▸ Bramitob (Chiesi Ltd)
Tobramycin **75 mg per 1 ml** Bramitob 300mg/4ml nebuliser solution 4ml ampoules | 56 ampoule PoM £1,187.00
▸ TOBI (Novartis Pharmaceuticals UK Ltd)
Tobramycin **60 mg per 1 ml** Tobi 300mg/5ml nebuliser solution 5ml ampoules | 56 ampoule PoM £1,305.92 DT price = £1,305.92
▸ Tymbrineb (Teva UK Ltd)
Tobramycin **60 mg per 1 ml** Tymbrineb 300mg/5ml nebuliser solution 5ml ampoules | 56 ampoule PoM £1,127.84 DT price = £1,305.92
▸ Vantobra (Pari Medical Ltd)
Tobramycin **100 mg per 1 ml** Vantobra 170mg/1.7ml nebuliser solution 1.7ml ampoules | 56 ampoule PoM £1,305.00

Carbapenems

Overview

The carbapenems are beta-lactam antibacterials with a broad-spectrum of activity which includes many Grampositive and Gram-negative bacteria, and anaerobes; **imipenem** (imipenem with cilastatin p. 302) and meropenem p. 302 have good activity against *Pseudomonas aeruginosa*. The carbapenems are not active against meticillin-resistant *Staphylococcus aureus* and *Enterococcus faecium*.

Imipenem (imipenem with cilastatin) and meropenem are used for the treatment of severe hospital-acquired infections and polymicrobial infections caused by multipleantibacterial resistant organisms (including septicaemia, hospital-acquired pneumonia, intra-abdominal infections, skin and soft-tissue infections, and complicated urinary-tract infections).

Ertapenem below is licensed for treating abdominal and gynaecological infections and for community-acquired pneumonia, but it is not active against atypical respiratory pathogens and it has limited activity against penicillin-resistant pneumococci. Unlike the other carbapenems, ertapenem is not active against *Pseudomonas* or against *Acinetobacter spp.*

Imipenem is partially inactivated in the kidney by enzymatic activity and is therefore administered in combination with **cilastatin** (imipenem with cilastatin), a specific enzyme inhibitor, which blocks its renal metabolism. Meropenem and ertapenem are stable to the renal enzyme which inactivates imipenem and therefore can be given without cilastatin.

Side-effects of imipenem with cilastatin are similar to those of other beta-lactam antibiotics. Meropenem has less seizure-inducing potential and can be used to treat central nervous system infection.

Ertapenem

● INDICATIONS AND DOSE

Abdominal infections | Acute gynaecological infections | Community-acquired pneumonia
▸ BY INTRAVENOUS INFUSION
▸ Child 3 months–12 years: 15 mg/kg every 12 hours; maximum 1 g per day
▸ Child 13–17 years: 1 g once daily

Diabetic foot infections of the skin and soft-tissue
▸ BY INTRAVENOUS INFUSION
▸ Child 13–17 years: 1 g once daily

● CAUTIONS CNS disorders—risk of seizures

● INTERACTIONS → Appendix 1: carbapenems

● SIDE-EFFECTS
▸ **Common or very common** Diarrhoea · headache · injection-site reactions · nausea · pruritus · raised platelet count · rash (also reported with eosinophilia and systemic symptoms) · vomiting
▸ **Uncommon** Abdominal pain · anorexia · antibiotic-associated colitis · asthenia · bradycardia · chest pain · confusion · constipation · dizziness · dry mouth · dyspepsia · dyspnoea · hypotension · melaena · oedema · petechiae · pharyngeal discomfort · raised glucose · seizures · sleep disturbances · taste disturbances
▸ **Rare** Agitation · anxiety · arrhythmia · blood disorders · cholecystitis · cough · depression · dysphagia · electrolyte disturbances · haemorrhage · hypoglycaemia · increase in blood pressure · jaundice · liver disorder · muscle cramp · nasal congestion · neutropenia · pelvic peritonitis · renal

5

Infection

impairment · scleral disorder · syncope · thrombocytopenia · tremor · wheezing
▸ **Frequency not known** Dyskinesia · hallucinations · muscular weakness
● **ALLERGY AND CROSS-SENSITIVITY** Avoid if history of **immediate hypersensitivity** reaction to beta-lactam antibacterials.
   Use with caution in patients with sensitivity to beta-lactam antibacterials.
● **PREGNANCY** Manufacturer advises avoid unless potential benefit outweighs risk.
● **BREAST FEEDING** Present in milk—manufacturer advises avoid.
● **RENAL IMPAIRMENT** Use with caution (risk of seizures); avoid if estimated glomerular filtration rate less than 30 mL/minute/1.73 m².
● **DIRECTIONS FOR ADMINISTRATION** For *intravenous infusion* (*Invanz®*), give intermittently *in* Sodium chloride 0.9%. Reconstitute 1 g with 10 mL Water for injections *or* Sodium chloride 0.9%; dilute requisite dose in infusion fluid to a final concentration not exceeding 20 mg/mL; give over 30 minutes; incompatible with glucose solutions.

● **MEDICINAL FORMS**
There can be variation in the licensing of different medicines containing the same drug.
Powder for solution for infusion
ELECTROLYTES: May contain Sodium
▸ **Invanz** (Merck Sharp & Dohme Ltd)
   Ertapenem (as Ertapenem sodium) 1 gram Invanz 1g powder for solution for infusion vials | 1 vial [PoM] £31.65

Imipenem with cilastatin

● **INDICATIONS AND DOSE**

Aerobic and anaerobic Gram-positive and Gram-negative infections (not indicated for CNS infections) | Hospital-acquired septicaemia
▸ BY INTRAVENOUS INFUSION

▸ Neonate up to 7 days: 20 mg/kg every 12 hours.

▸ Neonate 7 days to 20 days: 20 mg/kg every 8 hours.

▸ Neonate 21 days to 28 days: 20 mg/kg every 6 hours.

▸ Child 1-2 months: 20 mg/kg every 6 hours
▸ Child 3 months-17 years: 15 mg/kg every 6 hours (max. per dose 500 mg)

Infection caused by *Pseudomonas* or other less sensitive organisms | Empirical treatment of infection in febrile patients with neutropenia | Life-threatening infection
▸ BY INTRAVENOUS INFUSION
▸ Child 3 months-17 years: 25 mg/kg every 6 hours (max. per dose 1 g)

Cystic fibrosis
▸ BY INTRAVENOUS INFUSION
▸ Child: 25 mg/kg every 6 hours (max. per dose 1 g)

DOSE EQUIVALENCE AND CONVERSION
▸ Dose expressed in terms of imipenem.

● **UNLICENSED USE** Not licensed for use in children under 1 year; not licensed for use in children with renal impairment.
● **CAUTIONS** CNS disorders · epilepsy
● **SIDE-EFFECTS**
▸ **Common or very common** Diarrhoea · eosinophilia · nausea (may reduce rate of infusion) · rash · vomiting
▸ **Uncommon** Confusion · dizziness · drowsiness · hallucinations · hypotension · leucopenia · myoclonic activity · seizures · thrombocytopenia · thrombocytosis

▸ **Rare** Acute renal failure · anaphylactic reactions · antibiotic-associated colitis · encephalopathy · hearing loss · hepatitis · paraesthesia · polyuria · Stevens-Johnson syndrome · taste disturbances · tooth, tongue or urine discoloration · toxic epidermal necrolysis · tremor
▸ **Very rare** Abdominal pain · aggravation of myasthenia gravis · asthenia · cyanosis · dyspnoea · flushing · glossitis · haemolytic anaemia · headache · heartburn · hyperhidrosis · hypersalivation · hyperventilation · palpitation · polyarthralgia · tachycardia · tinnitus
▸ **Frequency not known** Neurotoxicity (at high dose, renal failure, CNS disease)
● **ALLERGY AND CROSS-SENSITIVITY** Avoid if history of **immediate hypersensitivity** reaction to beta-lactam antibacterials.
   Use with caution in patients with sensitivity to beta-lactam antibacterials.
● **PREGNANCY** Manufacturer advises avoid unless potential benefit outweighs risk (toxicity in *animal* studies).
● **BREAST FEEDING** Present in milk but unlikely to be absorbed.
● **RENAL IMPAIRMENT** Reduce dose if estimated glomerular filtration rate less than 70 mL/minute/1.73 m², risk of CNS side-effects.
● **EFFECT ON LABORATORY TESTS** Positive Coombs' test.
● **DIRECTIONS FOR ADMINISTRATION** For *intravenous infusion* dilute to a concentration of 5 mg (as imipenem)/mL in Sodium chloride 0.9%; give up to 500 mg (as imipenem) over 20–30 minutes, give dose greater than 500 mg (as imipenem) over 40–60 minutes.

● **MEDICINAL FORMS**
There can be variation in the licensing of different medicines containing the same drug.
Powder for solution for infusion
ELECTROLYTES: May contain Sodium
▸ **Imipenem with cilastatin** (Non-proprietary)
   Cilastatin (as Cilastatin sodium) 500 mg, Imipenem (as Imipenem monohydrate) 500 mg Imipenem 500mg / Cilastatin 500mg powder for solution for infusion vials | 1 vial [PoM] £12.00 (Hospital only) | 5 vial [PoM] £60.00 (Hospital only) | 10 vial [PoM] £75.45
▸ **Primaxin I.V.** (Merck Sharp & Dohme Ltd)
   Cilastatin (as Cilastatin sodium) 500 mg, Imipenem (as Imipenem monohydrate) 500 mg Primaxin IV 500mg powder for solution for infusion vials | 1 vial [PoM] £12.00

Meropenem

● **INDICATIONS AND DOSE**

Aerobic and anaerobic Gram-positive and Gram-negative infections | Hospital-acquired septicaemia
▸ BY INTRAVENOUS INFUSION, OR BY INTRAVENOUS INJECTION
▸ Neonate up to 7 days: 20 mg/kg every 12 hours.

▸ Neonate 7 days to 28 days: 20 mg/kg every 8 hours.

▸ Child 1 month-11 years (body-weight up to 50 kg): 10–20 mg/kg every 8 hours
▸ Child 1 month-11 years (body-weight 50 kg and above): 0.5–1 g every 8 hours
▸ Child 12-17 years: 0.5–1 g every 8 hours

Severe aerobic and anaerobic Gram-positive and Gram-negative infections
▸ BY INTRAVENOUS INFUSION, OR BY INTRAVENOUS INJECTION
▸ Neonate up to 7 days: 40 mg/kg every 12 hours.

▸ Neonate 7 days to 28 days: 40 mg/kg every 8 hours.

Exacerbations of chronic lower respiratory-tract infection in cystic fibrosis

▸ BY INTRAVENOUS INFUSION

▸ Child 1 month–11 years (body-weight up to 50 kg): 40 mg/kg every 8 hours
▸ Child 1 month–11 years (body-weight 50 kg and above): 2 g every 8 hours
▸ Child 12–17 years: 2 g every 8 hours

Meningitis

▸ BY INTRAVENOUS INFUSION

▸ Neonate up to 7 days: 40 mg/kg every 12 hours.

▸ Neonate 7 days to 28 days: 40 mg/kg every 8 hours.

▸ Child 1 month–11 years (body-weight up to 50 kg): 40 mg/kg every 8 hours
▸ Child 1 month–11 years (body-weight 50 kg and above): 2 g every 8 hours
▸ Child 12–17 years: 2 g every 8 hours

● **UNLICENSED USE** Not licensed for use in children under 3 months.

● **INTERACTIONS** → Appendix 1: carbapenems

● **SIDE-EFFECTS**

▸ **Common or very common** Abdominal pain · diarrhoea · disturbances in liver function tests · headache · nausea · pruritus · rash · thrombocythaemia · vomiting
▸ **Uncommon** Eosinophilia · leucopenia · paraesthesia · thrombocytopenia
▸ **Rare** Convulsions
▸ **Frequency not known** Antibiotic-associated colitis · haemolytic anaemia · Stevens-Johnson syndrome · toxic epidermal necrolysis

● **ALLERGY AND CROSS-SENSITIVITY** Avoid if history of **immediate hypersensitivity** reaction to beta-lactam antibacterials.
Use with caution in patients with sensitivity to beta-lactam antibacterials.

● **PREGNANCY** Use only if potential benefit outweighs risk—no information available.

● **BREAST FEEDING** Unlikely to be absorbed (however, manufacturer advises avoid).

● **HEPATIC IMPAIRMENT** Monitor liver function in hepatic impairment.

● **RENAL IMPAIRMENT** Use normal dose every 12 hours if estimated glomerular filtration rate 26–50 mL/minute/1.73 m^2. Use half normal dose every 12 hours if estimated glomerular filtration rate 10–25 mL/minute/1.73 m^2. Use half normal dose every 24 hours if estimated glomerular filtration rate less than 10 mL/minute/1.73 m^2.

● **EFFECT ON LABORATORY TESTS** Positive Coombs' test.

● **DIRECTIONS FOR ADMINISTRATION** *Intravenous injection* to be administered over 5 minutes.
Displacement value may be significant when reconstituting injection, consult local guidelines. For *intravenous infusion*, dilute reconstituted solution further to a concentration of 1–20 mg/mL *in* Glucose 5% *or* Sodium Chloride 0.9%; give over 15–30 minutes.

● **MEDICINAL FORMS**
There can be variation in the licensing of different medicines containing the same drug.
Powder for solution for injection
ELECTROLYTES: May contain Sodium
▸ **Meropenem (Non-proprietary)**
Meropenem (as Meropenem trihydrate) 500 mg Meronem 500mg powder for solution for injection vials | 10 vial PoM £80.75–£103.10 DT price = £80.75
Meropenem (as Meropenem trihydrate) 1 gram Meronem 1g powder for solution for injection vials | 10 vial PoM £206.28–£206.30

DT price = £161.18 (Hospital only) | 10 vial PoM £161.18–£190.00 DT price = £161.18
▸ **Meronem** (Pfizer Ltd)
Meropenem (as Meropenem trihydrate) 500 mg Meronem 500mg powder for solution for injection vials | 10 vial PoM £103.14 DT price = £80.75
Meropenem (as Meropenem trihydrate) 1 gram Meronem 1g powder for solution for injection vials | 10 vial PoM £206.28 DT price = £161.18

ANTIBACTERIALS ⟩ CEPHALOSPORINS

Cephalosporins

Overview

The cephalosporins are broad-spectrum antibiotics which are used for the treatment of septicaemia, pneumonia, meningitis, biliary-tract infections, peritonitis, and urinary-tract infections. The pharmacology of the cephalosporins is similar to that of the penicillins, excretion being principally renal. Cephalosporins penetrate the cerebrospinal fluid poorly unless the meninges are inflamed; cefotaxime p. 307 and ceftriaxone p. 308 are suitable cephalosporins for infections of the CNS (e.g meningitis).

The principal side-effect of the cephalosporins is hypersensitivity and about 0.5–6.5% of penicillin-sensitive patients will also be allergic to the cephalosporins. If a cephalosporin is essential in patients with a history of immediate hypersensitivity to penicillin, because a suitable alternative antibacterial is not available, then cefixime p. 307, cefotaxime, ceftazidime p. 307, ceftriaxone, or cefuroxime p. 306 can be used with caution; cefaclor p. 305, cefadroxil p. 304, cefalexin p. 304, and cefradine p. 305 should be avoided.

The orally active 'first generation' cephalosporins, cefalexin, cefradine, and cefadroxil and the 'second generation' cephalosporin, cefaclor have a similar antimicrobial spectrum. They are useful for urinary-tract infections which do not respond to other drugs or which occur in pregnancy, respiratory-tract infections, otitis media, sinusitis, and skin and soft-tissue infections. Cefaclor has good activity against *H. influenzae*. Cefadroxil has a long duration of action and can be given twice daily; it has poor activity against *H. influenzae*. **Cefuroxime axetil**, an ester of the 'second generation' cephalosporin cefuroxime, has the same antibacterial spectrum as the parent compound; it is poorly absorbed and needs to be given with food to maximise absorption.

Cefixime is an orally active 'third generation' cephalosporin. It has a longer duration of action than the other cephalosporins that are active by mouth. It is only licensed for acute infections.

Cefuroxime is a 'second generation' cephalosporin that is less susceptible than the earlier cephalosporins to inactivation by beta-lactamases. It is, therefore, active against certain bacteria which are resistant to the other drugs and has greater activity against *Haemophilus influenzae*.

Cefotaxime, ceftazidime and ceftriaxone are 'third generation' cephalosporins with greater activity than the 'second generation' cephalosporins against certain Gram-negative bacteria. However, they are less active than cefuroxime against Gram-positive bacteria, most notably *Staphylococcus aureus*. Their broad antibacterial spectrum may encourage superinfection with resistant bacteria or fungi.

Ceftazidime has good activity against pseudomonas. It is also active against other Gram-negative bacteria.

Ceftriaxone has a longer half-life and therefore needs to be given only once daily. Indications include serious infections such as septicaemia, pneumonia, and meningitis. The calcium salt of ceftriaxone forms a precipitate in the gall bladder which may rarely cause symptoms but these usually resolve when the antibacterial is stopped. In neonates, ceftriaxone may displace bilirubin from plasma-albumin and should be avoided in neonates with unconjugated hyperbilirubinaemia, hypoalbuminaemia, acidosis or impaired bilirubin binding.

Cephalosporins

- **DRUG ACTION** Cephalosporins are antibacterials that attach to penicillin binding proteins to interrupt cell wall biosynthesis, leading to bacterial cell lysis and death.
- **SIDE-EFFECTS**
- ▸ **Rare** Antibiotic-associated colitis
- ▸ **Frequency not known** Abdominal discomfort · agranulocytosis · allergic reactions · anaphylaxis · aplastic anaemia · blood disorders · confusion · diarrhoea · disturbances in liver enzymes · dizziness · eosinophilia · haemolytic anaemia · hallucinations · headache · hyperactivity · hypertonia · leucopenia · nausea · nervousness · pruritus · rashes · reversible interstitial nephritis · serum sickness-like reactions with rashes, fever and arthralgia · sleep disturbances · Stevens-Johnson syndrome · thrombocytopenia · toxic epidermal necrolysis · transient cholestatic jaundice · transient hepatitis · urticaria · vomiting

  SIDE-EFFECTS, FURTHER INFORMATION
- ▸ Antibiotic-associated colitis Antibiotic-associated colitis may occur more commonly with second- and third-generation cephalosporins.
- **ALLERGY AND CROSS-SENSITIVITY** Contra-indicated in patients with cephalosporin hypersensitivity.
- ▸ Cross-sensitivity with other beta-lactam antibacterials About 0.5–6.5% of penicillin-sensitive patients will also be allergic to the cephalosporins. Patients with a history of **immediate hypersensitivity** to penicillin and other beta-lactams should not receive a cephalosporin. Cephalosporins should be used with caution in patients with sensitivity to penicillin and other beta-lactams.
- **EFFECT ON LABORATORY TESTS** False positive urinary glucose (if tested for reducing substances). False positive Coombs' test.

ANTIBACTERIALS > CEPHALOSPORINS, FIRST-GENERATION

Cefadroxil

- **INDICATIONS AND DOSE**

Susceptible infections due to sensitive Gram-positive and Gram-negative bacteria
- ▸ BY MOUTH
- ▸ Child 6–17 years (body-weight up to 40 kg): 0.5 g twice daily
- ▸ Child 6–17 years (body-weight 40 kg and above): 0.5–1 g twice daily

Skin infections | Soft-tissue infections | Uncomplicated urinary-tract infections
- ▸ BY MOUTH
- ▸ Child 6–17 years (body-weight 40 kg and above): 1 g once daily

- **INTERACTIONS** → Appendix 1: cephalosporins
- **PREGNANCY** Not known to be harmful.
- **BREAST FEEDING** Present in milk in low concentration, but appropriate to use.
- **RENAL IMPAIRMENT** Reduce dose if estimated glomerular filtration rate less than 50 mL/minute/1.73 m².

- **MEDICINAL FORMS**
  There can be variation in the licensing of different medicines containing the same drug.
  Capsule
  CAUTIONARY AND ADVISORY LABELS 9
- ▸ Cefadroxil (Non-proprietary)
  Cefadroxil (as Cefadroxil monohydrate) 500 mg Cefadroxil 500mg capsules | 20 capsule [PoM] £22.38 DT price = £22.38 | 100 capsule [PoM] £111.90

Cefalexin

(Cephalexin)

- **INDICATIONS AND DOSE**

Susceptible infections due to sensitive Gram-positive and Gram-negative bacteria
- ▸ BY MOUTH
- ▸ Neonate up to 7 days: 25 mg/kg twice daily (max. per dose 125 mg).
- ▸ Neonate 7 days to 20 days: 25 mg/kg 3 times a day (max. per dose 125 mg).
- ▸ Neonate 21 days to 28 days: 25 mg/kg 4 times a day (max. per dose 125 mg).
- ▸ Child 1–11 months: 12.5 mg/kg twice daily, alternatively 125 mg twice daily
- ▸ Child 1–4 years: 12.5 mg/kg twice daily, alternatively 125 mg 3 times a day
- ▸ Child 5–11 years: 12.5 mg/kg twice daily, alternatively 250 mg 3 times a day
- ▸ Child 12–17 years: 500 mg 2–3 times a day

Serious susceptible infections due to sensitive Gram-positive and Gram-negative bacteria
- ▸ BY MOUTH
- ▸ Child 1 month–11 years: 25 mg/kg 2–4 times a day (max. per dose 1 g 4 times a day)
- ▸ Child 12–17 years: 1–1.5 g 3–4 times a day

Prophylaxis of recurrent urinary-tract infection
- ▸ BY MOUTH
- ▸ Child: 12.5 mg/kg once daily (max. per dose 125 mg), dose to be taken at night

- **INTERACTIONS** → Appendix 1: cephalosporins
- **PREGNANCY** Not known to be harmful.
- **BREAST FEEDING** Present in milk in low concentration, but appropriate to use.
- **RENAL IMPAIRMENT** Reduce dose in moderate impairment.
- **PATIENT AND CARER ADVICE**
  Medicines for Children leaflet: Cefalexin for bacterial infections www.medicinesforchildren.org.uk/cefalexin-bacterial-infections-0
- **PROFESSION SPECIFIC INFORMATION**
  Dental practitioners' formulary
  Cefalexin Capsules may be prescribed.
  Cefalexin Tablets may be prescribed.
  Cefalexin Oral Suspension may be prescribed.
- **MEDICINAL FORMS**
  There can be variation in the licensing of different medicines containing the same drug.
  Oral suspension
  CAUTIONARY AND ADVISORY LABELS 9
- ▸ Cefalexin (Non-proprietary)
  Cefalexin 25 mg per 1 ml Cefalexin 125mg/5ml oral suspension sugar free sugar-free | 100 ml [PoM] no price available
  Cefalexin 125mg/5ml oral suspension | 100 ml [PoM] £4.90 DT price = £0.84
  Cefalexin 50 mg per 1 ml Cefalexin 250mg/5ml oral suspension sugar free sugar-free | 100 ml [PoM] no price available

Cefalexin 250mg/5ml oral suspension | 100 ml [PoM] £5.25 DT price = £2.56

Cefalexin 100 mg per 1 ml Cefalexin 500mg/5ml oral suspension | 100 ml [PoM] no price available
- **Keflex** (Flynn Pharma Ltd)

Cefalexin 25 mg per 1 ml Keflex 125mg/5ml oral suspension | 100 ml [PoM] £0.84 DT price = £0.84

Cefalexin 50 mg per 1 ml Keflex 250mg/5ml oral suspension | 100 ml [PoM] £1.40 DT price = £2.56

Tablet
CAUTIONARY AND ADVISORY LABELS 9
- **Cefalexin (Non-proprietary)**

Cefalexin 250 mg Cefalexin 250mg tablets | 28 tablet [PoM] £5.02 DT price = £1.79

Cefalexin 500 mg Cefalexin 500mg tablets | 21 tablet [PoM] £5.88 DT price = £1.84
- **Keflex** (Flynn Pharma Ltd)

Cefalexin 250 mg Keflex 250mg tablets | 28 tablet [PoM] £1.60 DT price = £1.79

Cefalexin 500 mg Keflex 500mg tablets | 21 tablet [PoM] £2.08 DT price = £1.84

Capsule
CAUTIONARY AND ADVISORY LABELS 9
- **Cefalexin (Non-proprietary)**

Cefalexin 250 mg Cefalexin 250mg capsules | 28 capsule [PoM] £4.01 DT price = £1.31

Cefalexin 500 mg Cefalexin 500mg capsules | 21 capsule [PoM] £5.88 DT price = £1.43 | 100 capsule [PoM] £9.43
- **Keflex** (Flynn Pharma Ltd)

Cefalexin 250 mg Keflex 250mg capsules | 28 capsule [PoM] £1.46 DT price = £1.31

Cefalexin 500 mg Keflex 500mg capsules | 21 capsule [PoM] £1.98 DT price = £1.43

F 304

Cefradine

(Cephradine)

● INDICATIONS AND DOSE
Susceptible infections due to sensitive Gram-positive and Gram-negative bacteria | Surgical prophylaxis
- BY MOUTH
- Child 7–11 years: 25–50 mg/kg daily in 2–4 divided doses
- Child 12–17 years: 250–500 mg 4 times a day, alternatively 0.5–1 g twice daily; increased if necessary up to 1 g 4 times a day, increased dose may be used in severe infections

Prevention of *Staphylococcus aureus* lung infection in cystic fibrosis
- BY MOUTH
- Child 7–17 years: 2 g twice daily

- ● **UNLICENSED USE** Not licensed for use in children for prevention of *Staphylococcus aureus* lung infection in cystic fibrosis.
- ● **INTERACTIONS** → Appendix 1: cephalosporins
- ● **PREGNANCY** Not known to be harmful.
- ● **BREAST FEEDING** Present in milk in low concentration, but appropriate to use.
- ● **RENAL IMPAIRMENT** Reduce dose if estimated glomerular filtration rate less than 20 mL/minute/1.73 m^2.
- ● **PROFESSION SPECIFIC INFORMATION**

Dental practitioners' formulary
Cefradine Capsules may be prescribed.

- ● **MEDICINAL FORMS**
There can be variation in the licensing of different medicines containing the same drug.

Capsule
CAUTIONARY AND ADVISORY LABELS 9
- **Cefradine (Non-proprietary)**

Cefradine 250 mg Cefradine 250mg capsules | 20 capsule [PoM] £6.00 DT price = £1.81 | 100 capsule [PoM] no price available

Cefradine 500 mg Cefradine 500mg capsules | 20 capsule [PoM] £8.75 DT price = £2.73 | 100 capsule [PoM] no price available
- **Nicef** (Strides Shasun (UK) Ltd)

Cefradine 250 mg Nicef 250mg capsules | 20 capsule [PoM] £3.55 DT price = £1.81 | 100 capsule [PoM] £9.39

Cefradine 500 mg Nicef 500mg capsules | 20 capsule [PoM] £5.58 DT price = £2.73 | 100 capsule [PoM] £33.72

ANTIBACTERIALS ⟩ CEPHALOSPORINS, SECOND-GENERATION

F 304

Cefaclor

● INDICATIONS AND DOSE
Susceptible infections due to sensitive Gram-positive and Gram-negative bacteria
- BY MOUTH USING IMMEDIATE-RELEASE MEDICINES
- Child 1–11 months: 20 mg/kg daily in 3 divided doses, alternatively 62.5 mg 3 times a day
- Child 1–4 years: 20 mg/kg daily in 3 divided doses, alternatively 125 mg 3 times a day
- Child 5–11 years: 20 mg/kg daily in 3 divided doses, usual max. 1 g daily, alternatively 250 mg 3 times a day
- Child 12–17 years: 250 mg 3 times a day; maximum 4 g per day
- BY MOUTH USING MODIFIED-RELEASE MEDICINES
- Child 12–17 years: 375 mg every 12 hours, dose to be taken with food

Severe susceptible infections due to sensitive Gram-positive and Gram-negative bacteria
- BY MOUTH USING IMMEDIATE-RELEASE MEDICINES
- Child 1–11 months: 40 mg/kg daily in 3 divided doses, usual max. 1 g daily, alternatively 125 mg 3 times a day
- Child 1–4 years: 40 mg/kg daily in 3 divided doses, usual max. 1 g daily, alternatively 250 mg 3 times a day
- Child 5–11 years: 40 mg/kg daily in 3 divided doses, usual max. 1 g daily
- Child 12–17 years: 500 mg 3 times a day; maximum 4 g per day

Pneumonia
- BY MOUTH USING MODIFIED-RELEASE TABLETS
- Child 12–17 years: 750 mg every 12 hours, dose to be taken with food

Lower urinary-tract infections
- BY MOUTH USING MODIFIED-RELEASE MEDICINES
- Child 12–17 years: 375 mg every 12 hours, dose to be taken with food

Asymptomatic carriage of *Haemophilus influenzae* or mild exacerbations in cystic fibrosis
- BY MOUTH USING IMMEDIATE-RELEASE MEDICINES
- Child 1–11 months: 125 mg every 8 hours
- Child 1–6 years: 250 mg 3 times a day
- Child 7–17 years: 500 mg 3 times a day

- ● **INTERACTIONS** → Appendix 1: cephalosporins
- ● **SIDE-EFFECTS**

SIDE-EFFECTS, FURTHER INFORMATION
- Skin reactions Cefaclor is associated with protracted skin reactions, especially in children.
- ● **PREGNANCY** Not known to be harmful.
- ● **BREAST FEEDING** Present in milk in low concentration, but appropriate to use.
- ● **RENAL IMPAIRMENT** No dose adjustment required. Manufacturer advises caution.

● MEDICINAL FORMS
There can be variation in the licensing of different medicines containing the same drug.

Oral suspension
CAUTIONARY AND ADVISORY LABELS 9

▶ Cefaclor (Non-proprietary)

Cefaclor (as Cefaclor monohydrate) 25 mg per 1 ml Cefaclor 125mg/5ml oral suspension | 100 ml [PoM] no price available

Cefaclor (as Cefaclor monohydrate) 50 mg per 1 ml Cefaclor 250mg/5ml oral suspension | 100 ml [PoM] no price available

▶ Distaclor (Flynn Pharma Ltd)

Cefaclor (as Cefaclor monohydrate) 25 mg per 1 ml Distaclor 125mg/5ml oral suspension | 100 ml [PoM] £4.13

Cefaclor (as Cefaclor monohydrate) 50 mg per 1 ml Distaclor 250mg/5ml oral suspension | 100 ml [PoM] £8.26

▶ Keftid (Strides Shasun (UK) Ltd)

Cefaclor (as Cefaclor monohydrate) 25 mg per 1 ml Keftid 125mg/5ml oral suspension sugar-free | 100 ml [PoM] £5.16 DT price = £5.16

Cefaclor (as Cefaclor monohydrate) 50 mg per 1 ml Keftid 250mg/5ml oral suspension sugar-free | 100 ml [PoM] £10.32 DT price = £10.32

Modified-release tablet
CAUTIONARY AND ADVISORY LABELS 9, 21, 25

▶ Distaclor MR (Flynn Pharma Ltd)

Cefaclor (as Cefaclor monohydrate) 375 mg Distaclor MR 375mg tablets | 14 tablet [PoM] £9.10 DT price = £9.10

Capsule
CAUTIONARY AND ADVISORY LABELS 9

▶ Cefaclor (Non-proprietary)

Cefaclor (as Cefaclor monohydrate) 250 mg Cefaclor 250mg capsules | 21 capsule [PoM] no price available DT price = £6.80

Cefaclor (as Cefaclor monohydrate) 500 mg Cefaclor 500mg capsules | 50 capsule [PoM] no price available

▶ Distaclor (Flynn Pharma Ltd)

Cefaclor (as Cefaclor monohydrate) 500 mg Distaclor 500mg capsules | 21 capsule [PoM] £7.50 DT price = £7.50

▶ Keftid (Strides Shasun (UK) Ltd)

Cefaclor (as Cefaclor monohydrate) 250 mg Keftid 250mg capsules | 21 capsule [PoM] £6.80 DT price = £6.80

Cefaclor (as Cefaclor monohydrate) 500 mg Keftid 500mg capsules | 50 capsule [PoM] £31.99

◤ 304

Cefuroxime

17-Mar-2017

● INDICATIONS AND DOSE

Susceptible infections due to Gram-positive and Gram-negative bacteria

▶ BY MOUTH

▶ Child 3 months-1 year: 10 mg/kg twice daily (max. per dose 125 mg)

▶ Child 2-11 years: 15 mg/kg twice daily (max. per dose 250 mg)

▶ Child 12-17 years: 250 mg twice daily, dose may be doubled in severe lower respiratory-tract infections or if pneumonia is suspected

▶ BY INTRAVENOUS INFUSION, OR BY INTRAVENOUS INJECTION

▶ Neonate up to 7 days: 25 mg/kg every 12 hours, increased if necessary to 50 mg/kg every 12 hours, increased dose used in severe infection.

▶ Neonate 7 days to 20 days: 25 mg/kg every 8 hours, increased if necessary to 50 mg/kg every 8 hours, increased dose used in severe infection.

▶ Neonate 21 days to 28 days: 25 mg/kg every 6 hours, increased if necessary to 50 mg/kg every 6 hours, increased dose used in severe infection.

▶ BY INTRAVENOUS INFUSION, OR BY INTRAVENOUS INJECTION, OR BY INTRAMUSCULAR INJECTION

▶ Child: 20 mg/kg every 8 hours (max. per dose 750 mg); increased to 50–60 mg/kg every 6–8 hours (max. per dose 1.5 g), increased dose used for severe infection and cystic fibrosis

Lyme disease

▶ BY MOUTH

▶ Child 3 months-11 years: 15 mg/kg twice daily (max. per dose 500 mg) for 14–21 days (for 28 days in Lyme arthritis)

▶ Child 12-17 years: 500 mg twice daily for 14–21 days (for 28 days in Lyme arthritis)

Lower urinary-tract infection

▶ BY MOUTH

▶ Child 12-17 years: 125 mg twice daily

Surgical prophylaxis

▶ INITIALLY BY INTRAVENOUS INJECTION

▶ Child: 50 mg/kg (max. per dose 1.5 g, to be administered up to 30 minutes before the procedure, then (by intravenous injection or by intramuscular injection) 30 mg/kg every 8 hours (max. per dose 750 mg) if required for up to 3 doses (for high-risk procedures)

● UNLICENSED USE

▶ With oral use Not licensed for treatment of Lyme disease in children under 12 years. Duration of treatment in Lyme disease is unlicensed.

● INTERACTIONS → Appendix 1: cephalosporins

● PREGNANCY Not known to be harmful.

● BREAST FEEDING Present in milk in low concentration, but appropriate to use.

● RENAL IMPAIRMENT Reduce parenteral dose if estimated glomerular filtration rate less than 20 mL/minute/1.73 m².

● DIRECTIONS FOR ADMINISTRATION Single doses over 750 mg should be administered by the intravenous route only.

▶ With intravenous use Displacement value may be significant when reconstituting injection, consult local guidelines. For intermittent intravenous infusion, dilute reconstituted solution further in glucose 5% or sodium chloride 0.9%; give over 30 minutes.

● MEDICINAL FORMS
There can be variation in the licensing of different medicines containing the same drug. Forms available from special-order manufacturers include: solution for injection, infusion

Tablet
CAUTIONARY AND ADVISORY LABELS 9, 21, 25

▶ Cefuroxime (Non-proprietary)

Cefuroxime (as Cefuroxime axetil) 50 mg Cefuroxime 250mg tablets | 14 tablet [PoM] £17.72 DT price = £17.72

▶ Zinnat (GlaxoSmithKline UK Ltd)

Cefuroxime (as Cefuroxime axetil) 125 mg Zinnat 125mg tablets | 14 tablet [PoM] £4.56 DT price = £4.56

Cefuroxime (as Cefuroxime axetil) 250 mg Zinnat 250mg tablets | 14 tablet [PoM] £9.11 DT price = £11.72

Powder for injection
ELECTROLYTES: May contain Sodium

▶ Cefuroxime (Non-proprietary)

Cefuroxime (as Cefuroxime sodium) 750 mg Cefuroxime 750mg powder for injection vials | 1 vial [PoM] £2.52 | 10 vial [PoM] £25.20

Cefuroxime (as Cefuroxime sodium) 1.5 gram Cefuroxime 1.5g powder for injection vials | 1 vial [PoM] £5.05 | 10 vial [PoM] £50.50

▶ Zinacef (GlaxoSmithKline UK Ltd)

Cefuroxime (as Cefuroxime sodium) 250 mg Zinacef 250mg powder for injection vials | 5 vial [PoM] £4.70

Cefuroxime (as Cefuroxime sodium) 750 mg Zinacef 750mg powder for injection vials | 5 vial [PoM] £11.72 (Hospital only)

Cefuroxime (as Cefuroxime sodium) 1.5 gram Zinacef 1.5g powder for injection vials | 1 vial [PoM] £5.70

Oral suspension
CAUTIONARY AND ADVISORY LABELS 9, 21
EXCIPIENTS: May contain Aspartame, sucrose

▶ Zinnat (GlaxoSmithKline UK Ltd)

Cefuroxime (as Cefuroxime axetil) 25 mg per 1 ml Zinnat 125mg/5ml oral suspension | 70 ml [PoM] £5.20

ANTIBACTERIALS ⟩ CEPHALOSPORINS,
THIRD-GENERATION

⚑ 304

Cefixime

- **INDICATIONS AND DOSE**

Acute infections due to sensitive Gram-positive and Gram-negative bacteria
▸ BY MOUTH
- Child 6–11 months: 75 mg daily
- Child 1–4 years: 100 mg daily
- Child 5–9 years: 200 mg daily
- Child 10–17 years: 200–400 mg daily, alternatively 100–200 mg twice daily

Uncomplicated gonorrhoea
▸ BY MOUTH
- Child 12–17 years: 400 mg for 1 dose

- **UNLICENSED USE** Use of cefixime for uncomplicated gonorrhoea is an unlicensed indication.
- **INTERACTIONS** → Appendix 1: cephalosporins
- **PREGNANCY** Not known to be harmful.
- **BREAST FEEDING** Manufacturer advises avoid unless essential—no information available.
- **RENAL IMPAIRMENT** Reduce dose if estimated glomerular filtration rate less than 20 mL/minute/1.73 m².

- **MEDICINAL FORMS**
There can be variation in the licensing of different medicines containing the same drug.
Tablet
CAUTIONARY AND ADVISORY LABELS 9
▸ Suprax (Sanofi)
Cefixime 200 mg Suprax 200mg tablets | 7 tablet [PoM] £13.23 DT price = £13.23

⚑ 304

Cefotaxime

- **INDICATIONS AND DOSE**

Uncomplicated gonorrhoea
▸ BY INTRAMUSCULAR INJECTION
- Child 12–17 years: 500 mg for 1 dose

Severe exacerbations of *Haemophilus influenzae* infection in cystic fibrosis
▸ BY INTRAVENOUS INJECTION, OR BY INTRAVENOUS INFUSION
- Child: 50 mg/kg every 6–8 hours; maximum 12 g per day

Congenital gonococcal conjunctivitis
▸ BY INTRAMUSCULAR INJECTION
- Neonate: 100 mg/kg (max. per dose 1 g) for 1 dose.

Infections due to sensitive Gram-positive and Gram-negative bacteria | Surgical prophylaxis | Haemophilus epiglottitis
▸ BY INTRAMUSCULAR INJECTION, OR BY INTRAVENOUS INJECTION, OR BY INTRAVENOUS INFUSION
- Neonate up to 7 days: 25 mg/kg every 12 hours.
- Neonate 7 days to 20 days: 25 mg/kg every 8 hours.
- Neonate 21 days to 28 days: 25 mg/kg every 6–8 hours.
- Child: 50 mg/kg every 8–12 hours

Severe susceptible infections due to sensitive Gram-positive and Gram-negative bacteria | Meningitis
▸ BY INTRAMUSCULAR INJECTION, OR BY INTRAVENOUS INJECTION, OR BY INTRAVENOUS INFUSION
- Neonate up to 7 days: 50 mg/kg every 12 hours.
- Neonate 7 days to 20 days: 50 mg/kg every 8 hours.
- Neonate 21 days to 28 days: 50 mg/kg every 6–8 hours.
- Child: 50 mg/kg every 6 hours; maximum 12 g per day

Emergency treatment of suspected bacterial meningitis or meningococcal disease, before urgent transfer to hospital, in patients who cannot be given benzylpenicillin (e.g. because of an allergy)
▸ BY INTRAVENOUS INJECTION, OR BY INTRAMUSCULAR INJECTION
- Child 1 month-11 years: 50 mg/kg for 1 dose
- Child 12–17 years: 1 g for 1 dose

- **INTERACTIONS** → Appendix 1: cephalosporins
- **SIDE-EFFECTS**
▸ **Rare** Arrhythmias (following rapid injection)
- **PREGNANCY** Not known to be harmful.
- **BREAST FEEDING** Present in milk in low concentration, but appropriate to use.
- **RENAL IMPAIRMENT** Usual initial dose, then use half normal dose if estimated glomerular filtration rate less than 5 mL/minute/1.73 m².
- **DIRECTIONS FOR ADMINISTRATION**
▸ With intravenous use Displacement value may be significant, consult local guidelines. For intermittent *intravenous infusion* dilute in glucose 5% *or* sodium chloride 0.9%; administer over 20–60 minutes; incompatible with alkaline solutions.

- **MEDICINAL FORMS**
There can be variation in the licensing of different medicines containing the same drug.
Powder for solution for injection
▸ Cefotaxime (Non-proprietary)
Cefotaxime (as Cefotaxime sodium) 500 mg Cefotaxime 500mg powder for solution for injection vials | 1 vial [PoM] £1.50 | 10 vial [PoM] £25.50–£30.00
Cefotaxime (as Cefotaxime sodium) 1 gram Cefotaxime 1g powder for solution for injection vials | 1 vial [PoM] £3.00 | 10 vial [PoM] £35.00
Cefotaxime (as Cefotaxime sodium) 2 gram Cefotaxime 2g powder for solution for injection vials | 1 vial [PoM] £8.00 | 10 vial [PoM] £37.50

⚑ 304

Ceftazidime

- **INDICATIONS AND DOSE**

Pseudomonal lung infection in cystic fibrosis
▸ BY INTRAVENOUS INFUSION, OR BY INTRAVENOUS INJECTION, OR BY DEEP INTRAMUSCULAR INJECTION
- Child: 50 mg/kg every 8 hours; maximum 9 g per day

Febrile neutropenia
▸ BY INTRAVENOUS INFUSION, OR BY INTRAVENOUS INJECTION
- Child: 50 mg/kg every 8 hours; maximum 6 g per day

Meningitis
▸ BY INTRAVENOUS INJECTION, OR BY INTRAVENOUS INFUSION
- Neonate up to 7 days: 50 mg/kg every 24 hours.
- Neonate 7 days to 20 days: 50 mg/kg every 12 hours.
- Neonate 21 days to 28 days: 50 mg/kg every 8 hours.
- Child: 50 mg/kg every 8 hours; maximum 6 g per day

continued →

Susceptible infections due to sensitive Gram-positive and Gram-negative bacteria

▶ BY INTRAVENOUS INJECTION, OR BY INTRAVENOUS INFUSION

▸ Neonate up to 7 days: 25 mg/kg every 24 hours.

▸ Neonate 7 days to 20 days: 25 mg/kg every 12 hours.

▸ Neonate 21 days to 28 days: 25 mg/kg every 8 hours.

▸ Child: 25 mg/kg every 8 hours; maximum 6 g per day

Severe susceptible infections due to sensitive Gram-positive and Gram-negative bacteria

▶ BY INTRAVENOUS INJECTION, OR BY INTRAVENOUS INFUSION

▸ Neonate up to 7 days: 50 mg/kg every 24 hours.

▸ Neonate 7 days to 20 days: 50 mg/kg every 12 hours.

▸ Neonate 21 days to 28 days: 50 mg/kg every 8 hours.

▸ Child: 50 mg/kg every 8 hours; maximum 6 g per day

Chronic *Burkholderia cepacia* infection in cystic fibrosis

▶ BY INHALATION OF NEBULISED SOLUTION

▸ Child: 1 g twice daily

● **UNLICENSED USE** Nebulised route unlicensed.

● **INTERACTIONS** → Appendix 1: cephalosporins

● **SIDE-EFFECTS** Paraesthesia · taste disturbances

● **PREGNANCY** Not known to be harmful.

● **BREAST FEEDING** Present in milk in low concentration, but appropriate to use.

● **HEPATIC IMPAIRMENT** Manufacturer advises caution in severe impairment.

● **RENAL IMPAIRMENT** Reduce dose if estimated glomerular filtration rate less than 50 mL/minute/1.73 m^2—consult product literature.

● **DIRECTIONS FOR ADMINISTRATION** Intramuscular administration used when intravenous administration not possible; single doses over 1 g by intravenous route only.

▸ With intravenous use Displacement value may be significant, consult local guidelines. For intermittent intravenous infusion dilute reconstituted solution further to a concentration of not more than 40 mg/mL in Glucose 5% or Glucose 10% *or* Sodium chloride 0.9%; give over 20–30 minutes.

▸ When used by inhalation For nebulisation, dissolve dose in 3 mL of water for injection.

● **MEDICINAL FORMS**
There can be variation in the licensing of different medicines containing the same drug. Forms available from special-order manufacturers include: infusion, solution for infusion

Powder for solution for injection

ELECTROLYTES: May contain Sodium

▶ Ceftazidime (Non-proprietary)
Ceftazidime (as Ceftazidime pentahydrate) 500 mg Ceftazidime 500mg powder for solution for injection vials | 1 vial PoM £4.25
Ceftazidime (as Ceftazidime pentahydrate) 1 gram Ceftazidime 1g powder for solution for injection vials | 1 vial PoM £8.20 | 5 vial PoM £39.55 | 10 vial PoM £13.90
Ceftazidime (as Ceftazidime pentahydrate) 2 gram Ceftazidime 2g powder for solution for injection vials | 1 vial PoM £18.50 | 5 vial PoM £79.15 | 10 vial PoM £27.70

▶ Fortum (GlaxoSmithKline UK Ltd)
Ceftazidime (as Ceftazidime pentahydrate) 500 mg Fortum 500mg powder for solution for injection vials | 1 vial PoM £4.40 (Hospital only)
Ceftazidime (as Ceftazidime pentahydrate) 1 gram Fortum 1g powder for solution for injection vials | 1 vial PoM £8.79 (Hospital only)
Ceftazidime (as Ceftazidime pentahydrate) 2 gram Fortum 2g powder for solution for injection vials | 1 vial PoM £17.59 (Hospital only)
Ceftazidime (as Ceftazidime pentahydrate) 3 gram Fortum 3g powder for solution for injection vials | 1 vial PoM £25.76 (Hospital only)

F 304

Ceftriaxone

15-Jun-2016

● **INDICATIONS AND DOSE**

Community-acquired pneumonia | Hospital-acquired pneumonia | Intra-abdominal infections | Complicated urinary-tract infections

▶ BY INTRAVENOUS INFUSION

▸ Neonate up to 15 days: 20–50 mg/kg once daily, doses at the higher end of the recommended range used in severe cases.

▸ Neonate 15 days to 28 days: 50–80 mg/kg once daily, doses at the higher end of the recommended range used in severe cases.

▸ Child 1 month-11 years (body-weight up to 50 kg): 50–80 mg/kg once daily, doses at the higher end of the recommended range used in severe cases; maximum 4 g per day

▸ Child 9-11 years (body-weight 50 kg and above): 1–2 g once daily, 2 g dose to be used for hospital-acquired pneumonia and severe cases

▸ Child 12-17 years: 1–2 g once daily, 2 g dose to be used for hospital-acquired pneumonia and severe cases

▶ BY INTRAVENOUS INJECTION

▸ Child 9-11 years (body-weight 50 kg and above): 1–2 g once daily, 2 g dose to be used for hospital-acquired pneumonia and severe cases

▸ Child 12-17 years: 1–2 g once daily 2 g dose to be used for hospital-acquired pneumonia and severe cases

▶ BY DEEP INTRAMUSCULAR INJECTION

▸ Child 1 month-11 years (body-weight up to 50 kg): 50–80 mg/kg once daily, doses at the higher end of the recommended range used in severe cases; maximum 4 g per day

▸ Child 9-11 years (body-weight 50 kg and above): 1–2 g once daily, 2 g dose to be used for hospital-acquired pneumonia and severe cases

▸ Child 12-17 years: 1–2 g once daily, 2 g dose to be used for hospital-acquired pneumonia and severe cases

Complicated skin and soft tissue infections | Infections of bones and joints

▶ BY INTRAVENOUS INFUSION

▸ Neonate up to 15 days: 20–50 mg/kg once daily, doses at the higher end of the recommended range used in severe cases.

▸ Neonate 15 days to 28 days: 50–100 mg/kg once daily, doses at the higher end of the recommended range used in severe cases.

▸ Child 1 month-11 years (body-weight up to 50 kg): 50–100 mg/kg once daily, doses at the higher end of the recommended range used in severe cases; maximum 4 g per day

▸ Child 9-11 years (body-weight 50 kg and above): 2 g once daily

▸ Child 12-17 years: 2 g once daily

▶ BY INTRAVENOUS INJECTION

▸ Child 9-11 years (body-weight 50 kg and above): 2 g once daily

▸ Child 12-17 years: 2 g once daily

▶ BY DEEP INTRAMUSCULAR INJECTION

▸ Child 1 month-11 years (body-weight up to 50 kg): 50–100 mg/kg once daily, doses at the higher end of the recommended range used in severe cases; maximum 4 g per day

▸ Child 9-11 years (body-weight 50 kg and above): 2 g once daily

▸ Child 12-17 years: 2 g once daily

Suspected bacterial infection in neutropenic patients

▶ BY INTRAVENOUS INFUSION

▸ Neonate up to 15 days: 20–50 mg/kg once daily, doses at the higher end of the recommended range used in severe cases.

▸ Neonate 15 days to 28 days: 50–100 mg/kg once daily, doses at the higher end of the recommended range used in severe cases.

▸ Child 1 month–11 years (body-weight up to 50 kg): 50–100 mg/kg once daily, doses at the higher end of the recommended range used in severe cases; maximum 4 g per day

▸ Child 9–11 years (body-weight 50 kg and above): 2–4 g once daily, doses at the higher end of the recommended range used in severe cases

▸ Child 12–17 years: 2–4 g once daily, doses at the higher end of the recommended range used in severe cases

▶ BY INTRAVENOUS INJECTION

▸ Child 9–11 years (body-weight 50 kg and above): 2–4 g once daily, doses at the higher end of the recommended range used in severe cases

▸ Child 12–17 years: 2–4 g once daily, doses at the higher end of the recommended range used in severe cases

▶ BY DEEP INTRAMUSCULAR INJECTION

▸ Child 1 month–11 years (body-weight up to 50 kg): 50–100 mg/kg once daily, doses at the higher end of the recommended range used in severe cases; maximum 4 g per day

▸ Child 9–11 years (body-weight 50 kg and above): 2–4 g once daily, doses at the higher end of the recommended range used in severe cases

▸ Child 12–17 years: 2–4 g once daily, doses at the higher end of the recommended range used in severe cases

Bacterial meningitis | Bacterial endocarditis

▶ BY INTRAVENOUS INFUSION

▸ Neonate up to 15 days: 50 mg/kg once daily.

▸ Neonate 15 days to 28 days: 80–100 mg/kg once daily, 100 mg/kg once daily dose should be used for bacterial endocarditis.

▸ Child 1 month–11 years (body-weight up to 50 kg): 80–100 mg/kg once daily, 100 mg/kg once daily dose should be used for bacterial endocarditis; maximum 4 g per day

▸ Child 9–11 years (body-weight 50 kg and above): 2–4 g once daily, doses at the higher end of the recommended range used in severe cases

▸ Child 12–17 years: 2–4 g once daily, doses at the higher end of the recommended range used in severe cases

▶ BY INTRAVENOUS INJECTION

▸ Child 9–11 years (body-weight 50 kg and above): 2–4 g once daily, doses at the higher end of the recommended range used in severe cases

▸ Child 12–17 years: 2–4 g once daily, doses at the higher end of the recommended range used in severe cases

▶ BY DEEP INTRAMUSCULAR INJECTION

▸ Child 1 month–11 years (body-weight up to 50 kg): 80–100 mg/kg once daily, 100 mg/kg once daily dose should be used for bacterial endocarditis; maximum 4 g per day

▸ Child 9–11 years (body-weight 50 kg and above): 2–4 g once daily, doses at the higher end of the recommended range used in severe cases

▸ Child 12–17 years: 2–4 g once daily, doses at the higher end of the recommended range used in severe cases

Surgical prophylaxis

▶ BY INTRAVENOUS INFUSION

▸ Neonate up to 15 days: 20–50 mg/kg for 1 dose, dose to be administered 30–90 minutes before procedure.

▸ Neonate 15 days to 28 days: 50–80 mg/kg for 1 dose, dose to be administered 30–90 minutes before procedure.

▸ Child 1 month–11 years (body-weight up to 50 kg): 50–80 mg/kg (max. per dose 4 g) for 1 dose, dose to be administered 30–90 minutes before procedure

▸ Child 9–11 years (body-weight 50 kg and above): 2 g for 1 dose, dose to be administered 30–90 minutes before procedure

▸ Child 12–17 years: 2 g for 1 dose, dose to be administered 30–90 minutes before procedure

▶ BY INTRAVENOUS INJECTION

▸ Child 9–11 years (body-weight 50 kg and above): 2 g for 1 dose, dose to be administered 30–90 minutes before procedure

▸ Child 12–17 years: 2 g for 1 dose, dose to be administered 30–90 minutes before procedure

▶ BY DEEP INTRAMUSCULAR INJECTION

▸ Child 1 month–11 years (body-weight up to 50 kg): 50–80 mg/kg (max. per dose 4 g) for 1 dose, dose to be administered 30–90 minutes before procedure

▸ Child 9–11 years (body-weight 50 kg and above): 2 g for 1 dose, dose to be administered 30–90 minutes before procedure

▸ Child 12–17 years: 2 g for 1 dose, dose to be administered 30–90 minutes before procedure

Uncomplicated gonorrhoea | Pelvic inflammatory disease

▶ BY DEEP INTRAMUSCULAR INJECTION

▸ Child 1 month–11 years (body-weight up to 45 kg): 125 mg for 1 dose

▸ Child 9–11 years (body-weight 45 kg and above): 250 mg for 1 dose

▸ Child 12–17 years: 500 mg for 1 dose

Syphilis

▶ BY INTRAVENOUS INFUSION

▸ Neonate up to 15 days: 50 mg/kg once daily for 10–14 days.

▸ Neonate 15 days to 28 days: 75–100 mg/kg once daily for 10–14 days.

▸ Child 1 month–11 years (body-weight up to 50 kg): 75–100 mg/kg once daily for 10–14 days; maximum 4 g per day

▸ Child 9–11 years (body-weight 50 kg and above): 0.5–1 g once daily for 10–14 days, dose increased to 2 g once daily for neurosyphilis

▸ Child 12–17 years: 0.5–1 g once daily for 10–14 days, dose increased to 2 g once daily for neurosyphilis

▶ BY INTRAVENOUS INJECTION

▸ Child 9–11 years (body-weight 50 kg and above): 0.5–1 g once daily for 10–14 days, dose increased to 2 g once daily for neurosyphilis

▸ Child 12–17 years: 0.5–1 g once daily for 10–14 days, dose increased to 2 g once daily for neurosyphilis

▶ BY DEEP INTRAMUSCULAR INJECTION

▸ Child 1 month–11 years (body-weight up to 50 kg): 75–100 mg/kg once daily for 10–14 days; maximum 4 g per day

▸ Child 9–11 years (body-weight 50 kg and above): 0.5–1 g once daily for 10–14 days, dose increased to 2 g once daily for neurosyphilis

▸ Child 12–17 years: 0.5–1 g once daily for 10–14 days, dose increased to 2 g once daily for neurosyphilis

continued →

5

Infection

Infection

5

Disseminated Lyme borreliosis (early [Stage II] and late [Stage III])

▶ BY INTRAVENOUS INFUSION

▸ Neonate 15 days to 28 days: 50–80 mg/kg once daily for 14–21 days, the recommended treatment durations vary and national or local guidelines should be taken into consideration.

▸ Child 1 month–11 years (body-weight up to 50 kg): 50–80 mg/kg once daily for 14–21 days, the recommended treatment durations vary and national or local guidelines should be taken into consideration; maximum 4 g per day

▸ Child 9–11 years (body-weight 50 kg and above): 2 g once daily for 14–21 days, the recommended treatment durations vary and national or local guidelines should be taken into consideration

▸ Child 12–17 years: 2 g once daily for 14–21 days, the recommended treatment durations vary and national or local guidelines should be taken into consideration

▶ BY INTRAVENOUS INJECTION

▸ Child 9–11 years (body-weight 50 kg and above): 2 g once daily for 14–21 days, the recommended treatment durations vary and national or local guidelines should be taken into consideration

▸ Child 12–17 years: 2 g once daily for 14–21 days, the recommended treatment durations vary and national or local guidelines should be taken into consideration

▶ BY DEEP INTRAMUSCULAR INJECTION

▸ Child 1 month–11 years (body-weight up to 50 kg): 50–80 mg/kg once daily for 14–21 days, the recommended treatment durations vary and national or local guidelines should be taken into consideration; maximum 4 g per day

▸ Child 9–11 years (body-weight 50 kg and above): 2 g once daily for 14–21 days, the recommended treatment durations vary and national or local guidelines should be taken into consideration

▸ Child 12–17 years: 2 g once daily for 14–21 days, the recommended treatment durations vary and national or local guidelines should be taken into consideration

Congenital gonococcal conjunctivitis

▶ BY DEEP INTRAMUSCULAR INJECTION, OR BY INTRAVENOUS INFUSION

▸ Neonate: 25–50 mg/kg (max. per dose 125 mg) for 1 dose, intravenous infusion to be administered over 60 minutes.

Prevention of secondary case of meningococcal meningitis

▶ BY INTRAMUSCULAR INJECTION

▸ Child 1 month–11 years: 125 mg for 1 dose

▸ Child 12–17 years: 250 mg for 1 dose

Prevention of secondary case of *Haemophilus influenzae* type b disease

▶ BY INTRAVENOUS INFUSION

▸ Child 1 month–11 years: 50 mg/kg daily (max. per dose 1 g) for 2 days

▶ BY INTRAMUSCULAR INJECTION, OR BY INTRAVENOUS INJECTION, OR BY INTRAVENOUS INFUSION

▸ Child 12–17 years: 1 g daily for 2 days

Acute otitis media

▶ BY DEEP INTRAMUSCULAR INJECTION

▸ Child 1 month–11 years (body-weight up to 50 kg): 50 mg/kg for 1 dose, dose can be given for 3 days if severely ill or previous therapy failed

▸ Child 9–11 years (body-weight 50 kg and above): 1–2 g for 1 dose, dose can be given for 3 days if severely ill or previous therapy failed

▸ Child 12–17 years: 1–2 g for 1 dose, dose can be given for 3 days if severely ill or previous therapy failed

● UNLICENSED USE [EvGr] Not licensed for prophylaxis of *Haemophilus influenzae* type b disease. ⟨E⟩ Not licensed for prophylaxis of meningococcal meningitis.
[EvGr] Not licensed for congenital gonococcal conjunctivitis. Not licensed for use in children under 12 years of age for uncomplicated gonorrhoea. Not licensed for use in children for pelvic inflammatory disease. ⟨E⟩

● CONTRA-INDICATIONS Concomitant treatment with intravenous calcium (including total parenteral nutrition containing calcium) in premature and full-term neonates—risk of precipitation in urine and lungs (fatal reactions) · full-term neonates with jaundice, hypoalbuminaemia, acidosis, unconjugated hyperbilirubinaemia, or impaired bilirubin binding—risk of developing bilirubin encephalopathy · premature neonates less than 41 weeks corrected gestational age

● CAUTIONS History of hypercalciuria · history of kidney stones · use with caution in neonates

● INTERACTIONS → Appendix 1: cephalosporins

● SIDE-EFFECTS

▸ **Common or very common** Calcium ceftriaxone precipitates in gall bladder—consider discontinuation if symptomatic · calcium ceftriaxone precipitates in urine (particularly in very young, dehydrated or those who are immobilised)—consider discontinuation if symptomatic

▸ **Uncommon** Genital fungal infection

▸ **Rare** Bronchospasm · glycosuria · haematuria · prolongation of prothrombin time

▸ **Frequency not known** Convulsion · glossitis · oliguria · pancreatitis · stomatitis · toxic epidermal necrolysis · vertigo

● PREGNANCY Manufacturer advises use only if benefit outweighs risk—limited data available but not known to be harmful in *animal* studies. [EvGr] Specialist sources indicate suitable for use in pregnancy. ⟨D⟩

● BREAST FEEDING [EvGr] Specialist sources advise ceftriaxone is compatible with breastfeeding—present in milk in low concentration but limited effects to breast-fed infant. ⟨D⟩

● RENAL IMPAIRMENT Manufacturer advises reduce dose and monitor efficacy in patients with severe renal impairment in combination with hepatic impairment—no information available.
Manufacturer advises reduce dose if estimated glomerular filtration rate less than 10 mL/minute/1.73 m^2 max. 50 mg/kg daily or max. 2 g daily).

● MONITORING REQUIREMENTS Manufacturer advises to monitor full blood count regularly during prolonged treatment.

● DIRECTIONS FOR ADMINISTRATION

▸ With intravenous use For *intravenous infusion* (preferred route), dilute reconstituted solution with Glucose 5% (or 10% in neonates) *or* Sodium Chloride 0.9%; give over at least 30 minutes (60 minutes in neonates—may displace bilirubin from serum albumin). Not to be given simultaneously with parenteral nutrition or infusion fluids containing calcium, even by different infusion lines; in children, may be infused sequentially with infusion fluids containing calcium if flush with sodium chloride 0.9% between infusions or give infusions by different infusion lines at different sites. Displacement value may be significant, consult local guidelines.
For *intravenous injection*, give over 5 minutes; intravenous doses of 50 mg/kg or more in children under 12 years should be given by infusion.

▸ With intramuscular use or intravenous use Twice daily dosing may be considered for doses greater than 2 g daily.

▸ With intramuscular use For *intramuscular injection*, may be mixed with 1% Lidocaine Hydrochloride Injection to reduce pain at intramuscular injection site. Intramuscular injection should only be considered when the intravenous route is not possible or less appropriate. If administered by intramuscular injection, the lower end of the dose range should be used for the shortest time possible; volume depends on the age and size of the child, but doses over 1 g must be divided between more than one site. The maximum intramuscular dose is 2 g, doses greater than 2 g must be given by intravenous infusion or intravenous injection (see above). Displacement value may be significant, consult local guidelines.

- MEDICINAL FORMS
  There can be variation in the licensing of different medicines containing the same drug. Forms available from special-order manufacturers include: infusion
  Powder for solution for injection
  ELECTROLYTES: May contain Sodium
  ▸ Ceftriaxone (Non-proprietary)
    Ceftriaxone (as Ceftriaxone sodium) 250 mg Ceftriaxone 250mg powder for solution for injection vials | 1 vial PoM £1.80 DT price = £2.40
    Ceftriaxone (as Ceftriaxone sodium) 1 gram Ceftriaxone 1g powder for solution for injection vials | 1 vial PoM no price available DT price = £9.58 | 10 vial PoM £95.80
    Ceftriaxone (as Ceftriaxone sodium) 2 gram Ceftriaxone 2g powder for solution for injection vials | 1 vial PoM no price available DT price = £19.18 | 10 vial PoM £191.80
    Ceftriaxone 2g powder for solution for infusion vials | 1 vial PoM £17.70 DT price = £19.18
  ▸ Rocephin (Roche Products Ltd)
    Ceftriaxone (as Ceftriaxone sodium) 250 mg Rocephin 250mg powder for solution for injection vials | 1 vial PoM £2.40 DT price = £2.40
    Ceftriaxone (as Ceftriaxone sodium) 1 gram Rocephin 1g powder for solution for injection vials | 1 vial PoM £9.58 DT price = £9.58
    Ceftriaxone (as Ceftriaxone sodium) 2 gram Rocephin 2g powder for solution for injection vials | 1 vial PoM £19.18 DT price = £19.18

ANTIBACTERIALS > GLYCOPEPTIDE ANTIBACTERIALS

Teicoplanin

- DRUG ACTION The glycopeptide antibiotic teicoplanin has bactericidal activity against aerobic and anaerobic Gram-positive bacteria including multi-resistant staphylococci. However, there are reports of *Staphylococcus aureus* with reduced susceptibility to glycopeptides and increasing reports of glycopeptide-resistant enterococci. Teicoplanin is similar to vancomycin, but has a significantly longer duration of action, allowing once daily administration after the loading dose.

- INDICATIONS AND DOSE
  Surgical prophylaxis
  ▸ BY INTRAVENOUS INJECTION
  ▸ Child: (consult local protocol)
  Potentially serious Gram-positive infections including endocarditis, and serious infections due to *Staphylococcus aureus*
  ▸ INITIALLY BY INTRAVENOUS INJECTION, OR BY INTRAVENOUS INFUSION
  ▸ Neonate: Initially 16 mg/kg for 1 dose, followed by (by intravenous infusion) 8 mg/kg once daily, subsequent dose to be administered 24 hours after initial dose.

  ▸ Child: Initially 10 mg/kg every 12 hours (max. per dose 400 mg) for 3 doses, then (by intravenous injection or by intravenous infusion or by intramuscular injection) 6 mg/kg once daily (max. per dose 400 mg), (After initial 3 doses subsequent doses can be given by intramuscular route, if necessary, although, intravenous route is preferable)

Severe Gram-positive infections (including burns, septicaemia, septic arthritis and osteomyelitis)
▸ BY INTRAVENOUS INJECTION, OR BY INTRAVENOUS INFUSION
▸ Child: Initially 10 mg/kg every 12 hours for 3 doses, then 10 mg/kg once daily
PHARMACOKINETICS
Teicoplanin should **not** be given by mouth for systemic infections because it is not absorbed significantly.

- UNLICENSED USE Not licensed for surgical prophylaxis.
- INTERACTIONS → Appendix 1: teicoplanin
- SIDE-EFFECTS
- Common or very common Pruritus · rash
- Uncommon Bronchospasm · diarrhoea · dizziness · eosinophilia · fever · headache · leucopenia · mild hearing loss · nausea · thrombocytopenia · thrombophlebitis · tinnitus · vestibular disorders · vomiting
- Frequency not known Exfoliative dermatitis · nephrotoxicity · renal failure · Stevens-Johnson syndrome · toxic epidermal necrolysis
  SIDE-EFFECTS, FURTHER INFORMATION
- Nephrotoxicity Teicoplanin is associated with a lower incidence of nephrotoxicity than vancomycin.
- ALLERGY AND CROSS-SENSITIVITY Caution if history of vancomycin sensitivity.
- PREGNANCY Manufacturer advises use only if potential benefit outweighs risk.
- BREAST FEEDING No information available.
- RENAL IMPAIRMENT Use normal dose regimen on days 1–4, then use normal maintenance dose every 48 hours if estimated glomerular filtration rate 30–80 mL/minute/1.73 m^2 and use normal maintenance dose every 72 hours if estimated glomerular filtration rate less than 30 mL/minute/1.73 m^2. Plasma-teicoplanin concentration should be monitored during parenteral maintenance treatment. Also monitor renal and auditory function during prolonged treatment in renal impairment.
- MONITORING REQUIREMENTS
- Plasma-teicoplanin concentration is not measured routinely because a relationship between plasma concentration and toxicity has not been established. However, the plasma-teicoplanin concentration can be used to optimise parenteral treatment in severe sepsis or burns, deep-seated staphylococcal infection (including bone and joint infection), endocarditis and in intravenous drug abusers. Pre-dose ('trough') concentrations should be greater than 15 mg/litre (greater than 20 mg/litre in endocarditis or deep-seated infection such as bone and joint infection), but less than 60 mg/litre.
- Blood counts and liver and kidney function tests required.
- DIRECTIONS FOR ADMINISTRATION For intermittent intravenous infusion, dilute reconstituted solution further in sodium chloride 0.9% or glucose 5%; give over 30 minutes. Intermittent intravenous infusion preferred in neonates.

- MEDICINAL FORMS
  There can be variation in the licensing of different medicines containing the same drug. Forms available from special-order manufacturers include: solution for injection
  Powder and solvent for solution for injection
  ELECTROLYTES: May contain Sodium
  ▸ Targocid (Sanofi) ▼
    Teicoplanin 200 mg Targocid 200mg powder and solvent for solution for injection vials | 1 vial PoM £3.93
    Teicoplanin 400 mg Targocid 400mg powder and solvent for solution for injection vials | 1 vial PoM £7.32

5

Infection

Vancomycin

- **DRUG ACTION** The glycopeptide antibiotic vancomycin has bactericidal activity against aerobic and anaerobic Gram-positive bacteria including multi-resistant staphylococci. However, there are reports of *Staphylococcus aureus* with reduced susceptibility to glycopeptides. There are increasing reports of glycopeptide-resistant enterococci. Penetration into cerebrospinal fluid is poor.

- **INDICATIONS AND DOSE**

Clostridium difficile infection

▶ BY MOUTH

▸ Child 1 month–4 years: 5 mg/kg 4 times a day for 10–14 days, dose may be increased if infection fails to respond or is life-threatening, increased if necessary up to 10 mg/kg 4 times a day

▸ Child 5–11 years: 62.5 mg 4 times a day for 10–14 days, dose may be increased if infection fails to respond or is life-threatening, increased if necessary up to 250 mg 4 times a day

▸ Child 12–17 years: 125 mg 4 times a day for 10–14 days, dose may be increased if infection fails to respond or is life-threatening, increased if necessary up to 500 mg 4 times a day

Infections due to Gram-positive bacteria including endocarditis, osteomyelitis, septicaemia and soft-tissue infections

▶ BY INTRAVENOUS INFUSION

▸ Neonate up to 29 weeks corrected gestational age: 15 mg/kg every 24 hours adjusted according to plasma-concentration monitoring.

▸ Neonate 29 weeks to 35 weeks corrected gestational age: 15 mg/kg every 12 hours adjusted according to plasma-concentration monitoring.

▸ Neonate 35 weeks corrected gestational age and above: 15 mg/kg every 8 hours adjusted according to plasma-concentration monitoring.

▸ Child: 15 mg/kg every 8 hours adjusted according to plasma-concentration monitoring; maximum 2 g per day

Surgical prophylaxis (when high risk of MRSA)

▶ BY INTRAVENOUS INFUSION

▸ Child: (consult local protocol)

CNS infection e.g. ventriculitis (administered on expert advice)

▶ BY INTRAVENTRICULAR ADMINISTRATION

▸ Neonate: 10 mg every 24 hours.

▸ Child: 10 mg every 24 hours, for all children reduce to 5 mg daily if ventricular size reduced or increase to 15–20 mg once daily if ventricular size increased, adjust dose according to CSF concentration after 3–4 days; aim for pre-dose ('trough') concentration less than 10 mg/litre. If CSF not draining free reduce dose frequency to once every 2–3 days

Peritonitis associated with peritoneal dialysis

▶ BY INTRAPERITONEAL ADMINISTRATION

▸ Child: Add to each bag of dialysis fluid to achieve a concentration of 20–25 mg/litre

Eradication of meticillin-resistant *Staphylococcus aureus* from the respiratory tract in cystic fibrosis

▶ BY INHALATION OF NEBULISED SOLUTION

▸ Child: 4 mg/kg twice daily (max. per dose 250 mg) for 5 days, alternatively 4 mg/kg 4 times a day (max. per dose 250 mg) for 5 days

PHARMACOKINETICS

Vancomycin should **not** be given by mouth for systemic infections because it is not absorbed significantly.

- **UNLICENSED USE** Vancomycin doses in BNF publications may differ from those in product literature. Use of vancomycin (added to dialysis fluid) for the treatment of peritonitis associated with peritoneal dialysis is an unlicensed route. Not licensed for intraventricular use or inhalation. Not licensed for use by the intrathecal route for the treatment of meningitis.

> **IMPORTANT SAFETY INFORMATION**
>
> SAFE PRACTICE
> For intraventricular administration, seek specialist advice.

- **CAUTIONS**
  GENERAL CAUTIONS
  Avoid if history of deafness
  SPECIFIC CAUTIONS
  ▸ With oral use Systemic absorption may follow oral administration especially in inflammatory bowel disorders or following multiple doses

- **INTERACTIONS** → Appendix 1: vancomycin

- **SIDE-EFFECTS**
- **Common or very common**
  ▸ With intravenous use Blood disorders, including neutropenia (usually after 1 week or high cumulative dose) · interstitial nephritis · nephrotoxicity · ototoxicity (discontinue if tinnitus occurs) · renal failure
- **Rare**
  ▸ With intravenous use Agranulocytosis thrombocytopenia
- **Frequency not known**
  ▸ With intravenous use Anaphylaxis · cardiac arrest on rapid infusion · chills · dyspnoea · eosinophilia · exfoliative dermatitis · fever · flushing of the upper body ('red man' syndrome) · nausea · pain and muscle spasm of back and chest · phlebitis (irritant to tissue) · pruritus · rashes · severe hypotension on rapid infusion · shock on rapid infusion · Stevens-Johnson syndrome · toxic epidermal necrolysis · urticaria · vasculitis · wheezing

  SIDE-EFFECTS, FURTHER INFORMATION
  ▸ Nephrotoxicity Vancomycin is associated with a higher incidence of nephrotoxicity than teicoplanin.

- **ALLERGY AND CROSS-SENSITIVITY** Caution if teicoplanin sensitivity.

- **PREGNANCY** Manufacturer advises use only if potential benefit outweighs risk.
  Plasma-vancomycin concentration monitoring essential to reduce risk of fetal toxicity.

- **BREAST FEEDING** Present in milk—significant absorption following oral administration unlikely.

- **RENAL IMPAIRMENT** Reduce dose. In renal impairment monitor plasma-vancomycin concentration and renal function regularly. Also monitor auditory function.

- **MONITORING REQUIREMENTS**
  ▸ All patients require plasma-vancomycin measurement (after 3 or 4 doses if renal function normal, earlier if renal impairment).
  ▸ All patients require blood counts, urinalysis, and renal function tests.
  ▸ With intravenous use Pre-dose ('trough') concentration should be 10–15 mg/litre (15–20 mg/litre for less sensitive strains of meticillin-resistant *Staphylococcus aureus*).
  ▸ With intraventricular use Aim for pre-dose ('trough') concentration less than 10 mg/litre.
  ▸ When used by inhalation Measure lung function before and after initial dose of vancomycin and monitor for bronchospasm.

- **DIRECTIONS FOR ADMINISTRATION**
  ▸ With intravenous use Avoid rapid infusion (risk of anaphylactoid reactions) and rotate infusion sites.
  Displacement value may be significant, consult product

literature and local guidelines. For intermittent intravenous infusion, the reconstituted preparation should be further diluted in sodium chloride 0.9% *or* glucose 5% to a concentration of up to 5 mg/mL; give over at least 60 minutes (rate not to exceed 10 mg/minute for doses over 500 mg); use continuous infusion only if intermittent not available (limited evidence); 10 mg/mL can be used if infused via a central venous line over at least 1 hour.

▸ With oral use Injection can be used to prepare solution for oral administration; flavouring syrups may be added to the solution at the time of administration.

▸ When used by inhalation *For nebulisation* administer required dose in 4 mL of sodium chloride 0.9% (or water for injections). Administer inhaled bronchodilator before vancomycin.

● **MEDICINAL FORMS**
There can be variation in the licensing of different medicines containing the same drug. Forms available from special-order manufacturers include: oral suspension, oral solution, pastille, solution for injection, infusion

Powder for solution for infusion
▸ Vancomycin (Non-proprietary)
Vancomycin (as Vancomycin hydrochloride) 500 mg Vancomycin 500mg powder for solution for infusion vials | 1 vial PoM £7.25 | 10 vial PoM £62.50
Vancomycin 500mg powder for concentrate for solution for infusion vials | 1 vial PoM £8.50 | 10 vial PoM £62.50
Vancomycin (as Vancomycin hydrochloride) 1 gram Vancomycin 1g powder for solution for infusion vials | 1 vial PoM £14.50 | 10 vial PoM £125.00
Vancomycin 1g powder for concentrate for solution for infusion vials | 1 vial PoM £17.25 | 10 vial PoM £120.50
▸ Vancocin (Flynn Pharma Ltd)
Vancomycin (as Vancomycin hydrochloride) 500 mg Vancocin 500mg powder for solution for infusion vials | 1 vial PoM £6.25
Vancomycin (as Vancomycin hydrochloride) 1 gram Vancocin 1g powder for solution for infusion vials | 1 vial PoM £12.50

Capsule
CAUTIONARY AND ADVISORY LABELS 9
▸ Vancomycin (Non-proprietary)
Vancomycin (as Vancomycin hydrochloride) 125 mg Vancomycin 125mg capsules | 28 capsule PoM £132.47 DT price = £132.47
Vancomycin (as Vancomycin hydrochloride) 250 mg Vancomycin 250mg capsules | 28 capsule PoM £140.08 DT price = £140.08
▸ Vancocin Matrigel (Flynn Pharma Ltd)
Vancomycin (as Vancomycin hydrochloride) 125 mg Vancocin Matrigel 125mg capsules | 28 capsule PoM £88.31 DT price = £132.47

ANTIBACTERIALS > LINCOSAMIDES

Clindamycin

● **DRUG ACTION** Clindamycin is active against Gram-positive cocci, including streptococci and penicillin-resistant staphylococci, and also against many anaerobes, especially *Bacteroides fragilis*. It is well concentrated in bone and excreted in bile and urine.

● **INDICATIONS AND DOSE**

Staphylococcal bone and joint infections such as osteomyelitis | Peritonitis | Intra-abdominal sepsis | Meticillin-resistant *Staphylococcus aureus* (MRSA) in bronchiectasis, bone and joint infections, and skin and soft-tissue infections | Erysipelas or cellulitis in penicillin-allergic patients (alternative to macrolides)
▸ BY MOUTH

▸ Neonate up to 14 days: 3–6 mg/kg 3 times a day.

▸ Neonate 14 days to 28 days: 3–6 mg/kg 4 times a day.

▸ Child: 3–6 mg/kg 4 times a day (max. per dose 450 mg)

▸ BY DEEP INTRAMUSCULAR INJECTION, OR BY INTRAVENOUS INFUSION

▸ Child: 3.75–6.25 mg/kg 4 times a day; increased if necessary up to 10 mg/kg 4 times a day (max. per dose 1.2 g), increased dose used for severe infections, total daily dose may alternatively be given in 3 divided doses, single doses above 600 mg to be administered by intravenous infusion only, single doses by intravenous infusion not to exceed 1.2 g

Staphylococcal lung infection in cystic fibrosis
▸ BY MOUTH

▸ Child: 5–7 mg/kg 4 times a day (max. per dose 600 mg)

Treatment of falciparum malaria (to be given with or following quinine)
▸ BY MOUTH

▸ Child: 7–13 mg/kg every 8 hours (max. per dose 450 mg) for 7 days

● **UNLICENSED USE** Not licensed for treatment of falciparum malaria.

● **CONTRA-INDICATIONS** Avoid injections containing benzyl alcohol in neonates · diarrhoeal states

● **CAUTIONS** Avoid in acute porphyrias p. 577

● **INTERACTIONS** → Appendix 1: clindamycin

● **SIDE-EFFECTS** Abdominal discomfort · anaphylactoid reactions · antibiotic-associated colitis · diarrhoea (discontinue treatment) · eosinophilia · exfoliative dermatitis · jaundice · leucopenia · nausea · oesophageal ulcers · oesophagitis · polyarthritis · pruritus · rash · Stevens-Johnson syndrome · taste disturbances · thrombocytopenia · toxic epidermal necrolysis · urticaria · vesiculobullous dermatitis · vomiting
▸ With intramuscular use Abscess · induration · pain
▸ With intravenous use Thrombophlebitis

SIDE-EFFECTS, FURTHER INFORMATION
▸ Antibiotic-associated colitis Clindamycin has been associated with antibiotic-associated colitis, which may be fatal. Although antibiotic-associated colitis can occur with most antibacterials, it occurs more frequently with clindamycin. Patients should therefore discontinue treatment immediately if diarrhoea develops.

● **PREGNANCY** Not known to be harmful.

● **BREAST FEEDING** Amount probably too small to be harmful but bloody diarrhoea reported in 1 infant.

● **MONITORING REQUIREMENTS** Monitor liver and renal function if treatment exceeds 10 days. Monitor liver and renal function in neonates and infants.

● **DIRECTIONS FOR ADMINISTRATION** Avoid rapid intravenous administration. For *intravenous infusion*, dilute to a concentration of not more than 18 mg/mL with Glucose 5% *or* Sodium Chloride 0.9%; give over 10–60 minutes at a max. rate of 20 mg/kg/hour.

● **PATIENT AND CARER ADVICE** Capsules should be swallowed with a glass of water. Patients and their carers should be advised to discontinue immediately and contact doctor if diarrhoea develops.

● **PROFESSION SPECIFIC INFORMATION**

Dental practitioners' formulary
Clindamycin capsules may be prescribed.

● **MEDICINAL FORMS**
There can be variation in the licensing of different medicines containing the same drug. Forms available from special-order manufacturers include: oral suspension, oral solution

Solution for injection
EXCIPIENTS: May contain Benzyl alcohol
▸ Clindamycin (Non-proprietary)
Clindamycin (as Clindamycin phosphate) 150 mg per 1 ml Clindamycin 600mg/4ml solution for injection ampoules | 5 ampoule PoM £61.75

5

Infection

Clindamycin 300mg/2ml solution for injection ampoules |
5 ampoule [PoM] £28.50–£31.01

▸ **Dalacin C** (Pfizer Ltd)
Clindamycin (as Clindamycin phosphate) 150 mg per 1 ml Dalacin
C Phosphate 300mg/2ml solution for injection ampoules |
5 ampoule [PoM] £31.01
Dalacin C Phosphate 600mg/4ml solution for injection ampoules |
5 ampoule [PoM] £61.75

Capsule

CAUTIONARY AND ADVISORY LABELS 9, 27

▸ **Clindamycin** (Non-proprietary)
Clindamycin (as Clindamycin hydrochloride) 150 mg Clindamycin
150mg capsules | 24 capsule [PoM] £13.72 DT price = £3.81 |
100 capsule [PoM] £55.21
Clindamycin (as Clindamycin hydrochloride) 300 mg Clindamycin
300mg capsules | 30 capsule [PoM] £46.00 DT price = £39.65

▸ **Dalacin C** (Pfizer Ltd)
Clindamycin (as Clindamycin hydrochloride) 75 mg Dalacin C
75mg capsules | 24 capsule [PoM] £7.45 DT price = £7.45
Clindamycin (as Clindamycin hydrochloride) 150 mg Dalacin C
150mg capsules | 24 capsule [PoM] £13.72 DT price = £3.81 |
100 capsule [PoM] £55.08

ANTIBACTERIALS › MACROLIDES

Macrolides

Overview

The macrolides have an antibacterial spectrum that is similar
but not identical to that of penicillin; they are thus an
alternative in penicillin-allergic patients. They are active
against many-penicillin-resistant staphylococci, but some
are now also resistant to the macrolides.

Indications for the macrolides include campylobacter
enteritis, respiratory infections (including pneumonia,
whooping cough, Legionella, chlamydia, and mycoplasma
infection), and skin infections.

Erythromycin p. 316 is also used in the treatment of early
syphilis, uncomplicated genital chlamydial infection, and
non-gonococcal urethritis. Erythromycin has poor activity
against *Haemophilus influenzae*. Erythromycin causes nausea,
vomiting, and diarrhoea in some patients; in mild to
moderate infections this can be avoided by giving a lower
dose or the total dose in 4 divided doses, but if a more
serious infection, such as Legionella pneumonia, is
suspected higher doses are needed.

Azithromycin below is a macrolide with slightly less
activity than erythromycin against Gram-positive bacteria,
but enhanced activity against some Gram-negative
organisms including *H. influenzae*. Plasma concentrations
are very low, but tissue concentrations are much higher. It
has a long tissue half-life and once daily dosage is
recommended. Azithromycin is also used in the treatment of
uncomplicated genital chlamydial infection, non-gonococcal
urethritis, typhoid [unlicensed indication], and trachoma
[unlicensed indication].

Clarithromycin p. 315 is an erythromycin derivative with
slightly greater activity than the parent compound. Tissue
concentrations are higher than with erythromycin. It is given
twice daily. Clarithromycin is also used in regimens for
Helicobacter pylori eradication.

Erythromycin, azithromycin, and clarithromycin have a
role in the treatment of Lyme disease p. 345.

Spiramycin is also a macrolide which is used for the
treatment of toxoplasmosis.

Macrolides

● **CAUTIONS** Electrolyte disturbances (predisposition to QT
interval prolongation) · may aggravate myasthenia gravis ·
predisposition to QT interval prolongation

● **SIDE-EFFECTS**
▸ **Common or very common** Abdominal discomfort · diarrhoea
· nausea · vomiting
▸ **Uncommon** Cholestatic jaundice · hepatotoxicity · rash
▸ **Rare** Antibiotic-associated colitis · arrhythmias ·
pancreatitis · QT interval prolongation · Stevens-Johnson
syndrome · toxic epidermal necrolysis
▸ **Frequency not known** Reversible hearing loss (sometimes
with tinnitus) can occur after large doses
▸ **With intravenous use** Local tenderness · phlebitis

SIDE-EFFECTS, FURTHER INFORMATION
Gastro-intestinal side-effects are mild and less frequent
with azithromycin and clarithromycin than with
erythromycin.

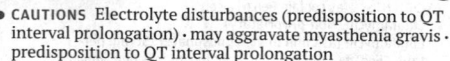
⌐ above

Azithromycin

● **INDICATIONS AND DOSE**

**Prevention of secondary case of invasive group A
streptococcal infection in patients who are allergic to
penicillin**
▸ BY MOUTH
▸ Child 6 months–11 years: 12 mg/kg once daily (max. per
dose 500 mg) for 5 days
▸ Child 12–17 years: 500 mg once daily for 5 days

**Respiratory-tract infections, otitis media, skin and soft-
tissue infections**
▸ BY MOUTH
▸ Child 6 months–17 years: 10 mg/kg once daily (max. per
dose 500 mg) for 3 days
▸ Child 6 months–17 years (body-weight 15–25 kg): 200 mg
once daily for 3 days
▸ Child 6 months–17 years (body-weight 26–35 kg): 300 mg
once daily for 3 days
▸ Child 6 months–17 years (body-weight 36–45 kg): 400 mg
once daily for 3 days
▸ Child 6 months–17 years (body-weight 46 kg and
above): 500 mg once daily for 3 days

Infection in cystic fibrosis
▸ BY MOUTH
▸ Child 6 months–17 years: 10 mg/kg once daily (max. per
dose 500 mg) for 3 days, repeated after 1 week to
complete course, treatment may be repeated as
necessary

**Chronic *Pseudomonas aeruginosa* infection in cystic
fibrosis**
▸ BY MOUTH
▸ Child 6–17 years (body-weight 25–40 kg): 250 mg 3 times a
week
▸ Child 6–17 years (body-weight 41 kg and above): 500 mg
3 times a week

**Uncomplicated genital chlamydial infections | Non-
gonococcal urethritis**
▸ BY MOUTH
▸ Child 12–17 years: 1 g for 1 dose

Lyme disease (under expert supervision)
▸ BY MOUTH
▸ Child 6 months–17 years: 10 mg/kg once daily (max. per
dose 500 mg) for 7–10 days

**Mild to moderate typhoid due to multiple-antibacterial
resistant organisms**
▸ BY MOUTH
▸ Child 6 months–17 years: 10 mg/kg once daily (max. per
dose 500 mg) for 7 days

● **UNLICENSED USE** Not licensed for typhoid fever, Lyme
disease, chronic *Pseudomonas aeruginosa* infection in
cystic fibrosis, or prophylaxis of group A streptococcal
infection.

● **INTERACTIONS** → Appendix 1: macrolides

- **SIDE-EFFECTS**
- ▶ **Common or very common** Anorexia · arthralgia · disturbances in taste · disturbances in vision · dizziness · dyspepsia · flatulence · headache · malaise · paraesthesia · reversible hearing loss (sometimes with tinnitus) after long-term therapy
- ▶ **Uncommon** Anxiety · chest pain · constipation · gastritis · hypoaesthesia · leucopenia · oedema · photosensitivity · sleep disturbances
- ▶ **Rare** Agitation
- ▶ **Frequency not known** Acute renal failure · convulsions · haemolytic anaemia · interstitial nephritis · smell disturbances · syncope · thrombocytopenia · tongue discoloration
- **PREGNANCY** Manufacturers advise use only if adequate alternatives not available.
- **BREAST FEEDING** Present in milk; use only if no suitable alternatives.
- **HEPATIC IMPAIRMENT** Manufacturers advise avoid in severe liver disease–no information available.
- **RENAL IMPAIRMENT** Use with caution if estimated glomerular filtration rate less than $10 \, \text{mL/minute}/1.73 \, \text{m}^2$.
- **PRESCRIBING AND DISPENSING INFORMATION** Flavours of oral liquid formulations may include cherry or banana.
- **PATIENT AND CARER ADVICE**
  Medicines for Children leaflet: Azithromycin for bacterial infections www.medicinesforchildren.org.uk/azithromycin-bacterial-infections-0
- **PROFESSION SPECIFIC INFORMATION**
  Dental practitioners' formulary
  Azithromycin Capsules may be prescribed.
  Azithromycin Tablets may be prescribed.
  Azithromycin Oral Suspension 200 mg/5 mL may be prescribed.
- **EXCEPTIONS TO LEGAL CATEGORY** Azithromycin tablets can be sold to the public for the treatment of confirmed, asymptomatic *Chlamydia trachomatis* genital infection in those over 16 years of age, and for the epidemiological treatment of their sexual partners, subject to maximum single dose of 1 g, maximum daily dose 1 g, and a pack size of 1 g.

- **MEDICINAL FORMS**
  There can be variation in the licensing of different medicines containing the same drug. Forms available from special-order manufacturers include: oral suspension

Tablet
CAUTIONARY AND ADVISORY LABELS 5, 9
- ▶ **Azithromycin (Non-proprietary)**
  Azithromycin 250 mg Azithromycin 250mg tablets | 4 tablet PoM £10.11 DT price = £1.36 | 6 tablet PoM £14.46
  Azithromycin 500 mg Azithromycin 500mg tablets | 3 tablet PoM £9.80 DT price = £1.25

Oral suspension
CAUTIONARY AND ADVISORY LABELS 5, 9
- ▶ **Azithromycin (Non-proprietary)**
  Azithromycin 40 mg per 1 ml Azithromycin 200mg/5ml oral suspension | 15 ml PoM £6.18 DT price = £4.06 | 30 ml PoM £11.04 DT price = £11.04
- ▶ **Zithromax** (Pfizer Ltd)
  Azithromycin 40 mg per 1 ml Zithromax 200mg/5ml oral suspension | 15 ml PoM £4.06 DT price = £4.06 | 22.5 ml PoM £6.10 DT price = £6.10 | 30 ml PoM £11.04 DT price = £11.04

Capsule
CAUTIONARY AND ADVISORY LABELS 5, 9, 23
- ▶ **Azithromycin (Non-proprietary)**
  Azithromycin (as Azithromycin dihydrate) 250 mg Azithromycin 250mg capsules | 4 capsule PoM £10.10 | 6 capsule PoM £15.15 DT price = £15.13
- ▶ **Zithromax** (Pfizer Ltd)
  Azithromycin (as Azithromycin dihydrate) 250 mg Zithromax 250mg capsules | 4 capsule PoM £7.16 | 6 capsule PoM £10.74 DT price = £15.13

▶ 314

Clarithromycin

- **INDICATIONS AND DOSE**
  Respiratory-tract infections | Mild to moderate skin and soft-tissue infections | Otitis media
  - ▶ BY MOUTH USING IMMEDIATE-RELEASE MEDICINES
  - ▶ Neonate: 7.5 mg/kg twice daily.
  - ▶ Child 1 month–11 years (body-weight up to 8 kg): 7.5 mg/kg twice daily
  - ▶ Child 1 month–11 years (body-weight 8–11 kg): 62.5 mg twice daily
  - ▶ Child 1 month–11 years (body-weight 12–19 kg): 125 mg twice daily
  - ▶ Child 1 month–11 years (body-weight 20–29 kg): 187.5 mg twice daily
  - ▶ Child 1 month–11 years (body-weight 30–40 kg): 250 mg twice daily
  - ▶ Child 12–17 years: 250 mg twice daily usually for 7–14 days, increased to 500 mg twice daily, if required in severe infections (e.g. pneumonia)
  - ▶ BY MOUTH USING MODIFIED-RELEASE MEDICINES
  - ▶ Child 12–17 years: 500 mg once daily usually for 7–14 days, increased to 1 g once daily, if required in severe infections (e.g. pneumonia)
  - ▶ BY INTRAVENOUS INFUSION
  - ▶ Child 1 month–11 years: 7.5 mg/kg every 12 hours (max. per dose 500 mg every 12 hours) maximum duration 5 days, switch to oral route when appropriate, to be administered into a large proximal vein
  - ▶ Child 12–17 years: 500 mg every 12 hours maximum duration 5 days, switch to oral route when appropriate, to be administered into a large proximal vein

  Lyme disease
  - ▶ BY MOUTH
  - ▶ Child 1 month–11 years: 7.5 mg/kg twice daily (max. per dose 500 mg) for 14–21 days
  - ▶ Child 12–17 years: 500 mg twice daily for 14–21 days

  Prevention of pertussis
  - ▶ BY MOUTH
  - ▶ Neonate: 7.5 mg/kg twice daily for 7 days.
  - ▶ Child 1 month–11 years (body-weight up to 8 kg): 7.5 mg/kg twice daily for 7 days
  - ▶ Child 1 month–11 years (body-weight 8–11 kg): 62.5 mg twice daily for 7 days
  - ▶ Child 1 month–11 years (body-weight 12–19 kg): 125 mg twice daily for 7 days
  - ▶ Child 1 month–11 years (body-weight 20–29 kg): 187.5 mg twice daily for 7 days
  - ▶ Child 1 month–11 years (body-weight 30–40 kg): 250 mg twice daily for 7 days
  - ▶ Child 12–17 years: 500 mg twice daily for 7 days

  ***Helicobacter pylori* eradication in combination with omeprazole, and amoxicillin or metronidazole**
  - ▶ BY MOUTH
  - ▶ Child 1–5 years: 7.5 mg/kg twice daily (max. per dose 500 mg)
  - ▶ Child 6–11 years: 7.5 mg/kg twice daily (max. per dose 500 mg)
  - ▶ Child 12–17 years: 500 mg twice daily

- **UNLICENSED USE** Tablets not licensed for use in children under 12 years; oral suspension not licensed for use in infants under 6 months. Intravenous infusion not licensed for use in children under 12 years.

- **INTERACTIONS** → Appendix 1: macrolides

- **SIDE-EFFECTS**
  - ▶ **Common or very common** Dyspepsia · headache · hyperhidrosis · insomnia · taste disturbances

- **Uncommon** Anorexia · anxiety · blood disorders · chest pain · constipation · dizziness · dry mouth · flatulence · gastritis · glossitis · hepatic dysfunction including jaundice · leucopenia · malaise · myalgia · stomatitis · tinnitus · tremor
- **Frequency not known** Abnormal dreams · confusion · convulsions · depression · hypoglycaemia · interstitial nephritis · myopathy · paraesthesia · psychotic disorders · renal failure · smell disturbances · tongue discoloration · tooth discoloration
- **PREGNANCY** Manufacturer advises avoid, particularly in the first trimester, unless potential benefit outweighs risk.
- **BREAST FEEDING** Manufacturer advises avoid unless potential benefit outweighs risk—present in milk.
- **HEPATIC IMPAIRMENT** Avoid in severe impairment if renal impairment also present.
- **RENAL IMPAIRMENT** Use half normal dose if estimated glomerular filtration rate less than 30 mL/minute/1.73 m^2, max. duration 14 days. Avoid if severe hepatic impairment also present. Avoid *Klaricid XL*® or clarithromyin m/r preparations if estimated glomerular filtration rate less than 30 mL/minute/1.73 m^2.
- **DIRECTIONS FOR ADMINISTRATION** For intermittent intravenous infusion dilute reconstituted solution further in Glucose 5% *or* Sodium chloride 0.9% to a concentration of 2 mg/mL; give into large proximal vein over 60 minutes.
- **PATIENT AND CARER ADVICE**
  Medicines for Children leaflet: Clarithromycin for bacterial infections www.medicinesforchildren.org.uk/clarithromycin-bacterial-infections
- **PROFESSION SPECIFIC INFORMATION**

  Dental practitioners' formulary
  Clarithromycin Tablets may be prescribed. Clarithromycin Oral Suspension may be prescribed.

- **MEDICINAL FORMS**
  There can be variation in the licensing of different medicines containing the same drug. Forms available from special-order manufacturers include: infusion

  Modified-release tablet
  CAUTIONARY AND ADVISORY LABELS 9, 21, 25
  - Clarie XL (Teva UK Ltd)
    Clarithromycin 500 mg Clarie XL 500mg tablets | 7 tablet [PoM] £6.72 DT price = £6.72 | 14 tablet [PoM] £13.23
  - Klaricid XL (Mylan Ltd)
    Clarithromycin 500 mg Klaricid XL 500mg tablets | 7 tablet [PoM] £6.72 DT price = £6.72 | 14 tablet [PoM] £13.23
  - Xetinin XL (Morningside Healthcare Ltd)
    Clarithromycin 500 mg Xetinin XL 500mg tablets | 7 tablet [PoM] £6.72 DT price = £6.72 | 14 tablet [PoM] £13.23

  Granules
  CAUTIONARY AND ADVISORY LABELS 9, 13
  - Klaricid (Mylan Ltd)
    Clarithromycin 250 mg Klaricid Adult 250mg granules sachets | 14 sachet [PoM] £11.68

  Tablet
  CAUTIONARY AND ADVISORY LABELS 9
  - Clarithromycin (Non-proprietary)
    Clarithromycin 250 mg Clarithromycin 250mg tablets | 14 tablet [PoM] £10.50 DT price = £1.36
    Clarithromycin 500 mg Clarithromycin 500mg tablets | 14 tablet [PoM] £21.50 DT price = £2.21

  Oral suspension
  CAUTIONARY AND ADVISORY LABELS 9
  - Clarithromycin (Non-proprietary)
    Clarithromycin 25 mg per 1 ml Clarithromycin 125mg/5ml oral suspension | 70 ml [PoM] £4.88 DT price = £4.06
    Clarithromycin 50 mg per 1 ml Clarithromycin 250mg/5ml oral suspension | 70 ml [PoM] £7.08 DT price = £5.43
  - Klaricid (Mylan Ltd)
    Clarithromycin 25 mg per 1 ml Klaricid Paediatric 125mg/5ml oral suspension | 70 ml [PoM] £5.26 DT price = £4.06 | 100 ml [PoM] £9.04
    Clarithromycin 50 mg per 1 ml Klaricid Paediatric 250mg/5ml oral suspension | 70 ml [PoM] £10.51 DT price = £5.43

Powder for solution for infusion
ELECTROLYTES: May contain Sodium
- Clarithromycin (Non-proprietary)
  Clarithromycin 500 mg Clarithromycin 500mg powder for solution for infusion vials | 1 vial [PoM] £11.25 DT price = £9.45
  Clarithromycin 500mg powder for concentrate for solution for infusion vials | 1 vial [PoM] £8.98 DT price = £9.45
- Klaricid (Mylan Ltd)
  Clarithromycin 500 mg Klaricid IV 500mg powder for solution for infusion vials | 1 vial [PoM] £9.45 DT price = £9.45

F 314

Erythromycin

- **INDICATIONS AND DOSE**

Susceptible infections in patients with penicillin hypersensitivity (e.g. respiratory-tract infections (including Legionella infection), skin and oral infections, and campylobacter enteritis)
▸ BY MOUTH

▸ Neonate: 12.5 mg/kg every 6 hours.

▸ Child 1 month–1 year: 125 mg 4 times a day, total daily dose may alternatively be given in two divided doses, increased to 250 mg 4 times a day, dose increase may be used in severe infections
▸ Child 2–7 years: 250 mg 4 times a day, total daily dose may alternatively be given in two divided doses, increased to 500 mg 4 times a day, dose increase may be used in severe infections
▸ Child 8–17 years: 250–500 mg 4 times a day, total daily dose may alternatively be given in two divided doses, increased to 500–1000 mg 4 times a day, dose increase may be used in severe infections
▸ BY INTRAVENOUS INFUSION

▸ Neonate: 10–12.5 mg/kg every 6 hours.

▸ Child: 12.5 mg/kg every 6 hours (max. per dose 1 g)

Lyme disease (under expert supervision)
▸ BY MOUTH
▸ Child: 12.5 mg/kg 4 times a day (max. per dose 500 mg) for 14–21 days

Chlamydial ophthalmia
▸ BY MOUTH

▸ Neonate: 12.5 mg/kg every 6 hours.

▸ Child 1 month–1 year: 125 mg 4 times a day, increased to 250 mg every 6 hours, dose increase for severe infections, total daily dose may alternatively be given in two divided doses
▸ Child 2–7 years: 250 mg 4 times a day, increased to 500 mg every 6 hours, dose increase for severe infections, total daily dose may alternatively be given in two divided doses
▸ Child 8–17 years: 250–500 mg 4 times a day, increased to 500–1000 mg every 6 hours, dose increase for severe infections, total daily dose may alternatively be given in two divided doses
▸ BY INTRAVENOUS INFUSION

▸ Neonate: 10–12.5 mg/kg every 6 hours.

▸ Child: 12.5 mg/kg every 6 hours (max. per dose 1 g)

Early syphilis
▸ BY MOUTH
▸ Child 12–17 years: 500 mg 4 times a day for 14 days

Uncomplicated genital chlamydia | Non-gonococcal urethritis
▸ BY MOUTH
▸ Child 1 month–1 year: 12.5 mg/kg 4 times a day for 14 days
▸ Child 2–11 years: 250 mg twice daily for 14 days
▸ Child 12–17 years: 500 mg twice daily for 14 days

Pelvic inflammatory disease
► BY MOUTH
▸ Child 1 month–1 year: 12.5 mg/kg 4 times a day for 14 days
▸ Child 2–11 years: 250 mg twice daily for 14 days
▸ Child 12–17 years: 500 mg twice daily for 14 days

Prevention and treatment of pertussis
► BY MOUTH
▸ Neonate: 12.5 mg/kg every 6 hours.
▸ Child 1 month–1 year: 125 mg 4 times a day, total daily dose may alternatively be given in two divided doses, increased to 250 mg 4 times a day, dose increase may be used in severe infections
▸ Child 2–7 years: 250 mg 4 times a day, total daily dose may alternatively be given in two divided doses, increased to 500 mg 4 times a day, dose increase may be used in severe infections
▸ Child 8–17 years: 250–500 mg 4 times a day, total daily dose may alternatively be given in two divided doses, increased to 500–1000 mg 4 times a day, dose increase may be used in severe infections
► BY INTRAVENOUS INFUSION
▸ Neonate: 10–12.5 mg/kg every 6 hours.
▸ Child: 12.5 mg/kg every 6 hours (max. per dose 1 g)

Prevention of secondary case of diphtheria in non-immune patient
► BY MOUTH
▸ Child 1 month–1 year: 125 mg every 6 hours for 7 days, treat for further 10 days if nasopharyngeal swabs positive after first 7 days' treatment
▸ Child 2–7 years: 250 mg every 6 hours for 7 days, treat for further 10 days if nasopharyngeal swabs positive after first 7 days' treatment
▸ Child 8–17 years: 500 mg every 6 hours for 7 days, treat for further 10 days if nasopharyngeal swabs positive after first 7 days' treatment

Prevention of secondary case of invasive group A streptococcal infection in penicillin allergic patients
► BY MOUTH
▸ Child 1 month–1 year: 125 mg every 6 hours for 10 days
▸ Child 2–7 years: 250 mg every 6 hours for 10 days
▸ Child 8–17 years: 250–500 mg every 6 hours for 10 days

Prevention of pneumococcal infection in asplenia or in patients with sickle-cell disease (if penicillin-allergic)
► BY MOUTH
▸ Child 1 month–1 year: 125 mg twice daily, antibiotic prophylaxis is not fully reliable
▸ Child 2–7 years: 250 mg twice daily, antibiotic prophylaxis is not fully reliable. It may be discontinued in those over 5 years of age with sickle-cell disease who have received pneumococcal immunisation and who do not have a history of severe pneumococcal infection
▸ Child 8–17 years: 500 mg twice daily, antibiotic prophylaxis is not fully reliable. It may be discontinued in those with sickle-cell disease who have received pneumococcal immunisation and who do not have a history of severe pneumococcal infection

Prevention of recurrence of rheumatic fever
► BY MOUTH
▸ Child 1 month–1 year: 125 mg twice daily
▸ Child 2–17 years: 250 mg twice daily

Acne
► BY MOUTH
▸ Child 1–23 months: 250 mg once daily, alternatively 125 mg twice daily
▸ Child 12–17 years: 500 mg twice daily

Gastro-intestinal stasis
► BY MOUTH
▸ Neonate: 3 mg/kg 4 times a day.
▸ Child: 3 mg/kg 4 times a day
► BY INTRAVENOUS INFUSION
▸ Neonate: 3 mg/kg 4 times a day.
▸ Child 1–11 months: 3 mg/kg 4 times a day

● **UNLICENSED USE** Not licensed for use in gastro-intestinal stasis.

● **CAUTIONS** Avoid in acute porphyrias p. 577 · neonate under 2 weeks (risk of hypertrophic pyloric stenosis)

● **INTERACTIONS** → Appendix 1: macrolides

● **PREGNANCY** Not known to be harmful.

● **BREAST FEEDING** Only small amounts in milk—not known to be harmful.

● **HEPATIC IMPAIRMENT** May cause idiosyncratic hepatotoxicity.

● **RENAL IMPAIRMENT** Reduce dose in severe renal impairment (ototoxicity).

● **DIRECTIONS FOR ADMINISTRATION** Dilute reconstituted solution further in glucose 5% (neutralised with Sodium bicarbonate) or sodium chloride 0.9% to a concentration of 1–5 mg/mL; give over 20–60 minutes. Concentration of up to 10 mg/mL may be used in fluid-restriction if administered via a central venous catheter.

● **PRESCRIBING AND DISPENSING INFORMATION** Flavours of oral liquid formulations may include banana.

● **PATIENT AND CARER ADVICE**
Medicines for Children leaflet: Erythromycin for bacterial infections www.medicinesforchildren.org.uk/erythromycin-for-bacterial-infections

● **PROFESSION SPECIFIC INFORMATION**
Dental practitioners' formulary
Erythromycin tablets e/c may be prescribed. Erythromycin ethyl succinate oral suspension may be prescribed. Erythromycin stearate tablets may be prescribed. Erythromycin ethyl succinate tablets may be prescribed.

● **MEDICINAL FORMS**
There can be variation in the licensing of different medicines containing the same drug.

Gastro-resistant capsule
CAUTIONARY AND ADVISORY LABELS 5, 9, 25
► Erythromycin (Non-proprietary)
Erythromycin 250 mg Erythromycin 250mg gastro-resistant capsules | 28 capsule [PoM] no price available DT price = £5.61 | 30 capsule [PoM] no price available
► Erymax (Teva UK Ltd)
Erythromycin 250 mg Erymax 250mg gastro-resistant capsules | 28 capsule [PoM] £5.61 DT price = £5.61 | 112 capsule [PoM] £22.44
► Tiloryth (Tillomed Laboratories Ltd)
Erythromycin 250 mg Tiloryth 250mg gastro-resistant capsules | 30 capsule [PoM] £5.65 | 100 capsule [PoM] £18.66

Gastro-resistant tablet
CAUTIONARY AND ADVISORY LABELS 5, 9, 25
► Erythromycin (Non-proprietary)
Erythromycin 250 mg Erythromycin 250mg gastro-resistant tablets | 28 tablet [PoM] £2.25 DT price = £1.45 | 500 tablet [PoM] £27.20

Tablet
CAUTIONARY AND ADVISORY LABELS 9
► Erythromycin (Non-proprietary)
Erythromycin (as Erythromycin ethyl succinate) 500 mg Erythromycin ethyl succinate 500mg tablets | 28 tablet [PoM] £15.95–£19.50 DT price = £10.78
► Erythrocin (AMCo)
Erythromycin (as Erythromycin stearate) 250 mg Erythrocin 250 tablets | 100 tablet [PoM] £18.20 DT price = £18.20
Erythromycin (as Erythromycin stearate) 500 mg Erythrocin 500 tablets | 100 tablet [PoM] £36.40 DT price = £36.40

5

Infection

5

Infection

▸ **Erythrolar** (Ennogen Pharma Ltd)
Erythromycin (as Erythromycin stearate) 250 mg Erythrolar
250mg tablets | 100 tablet [PoM] £22.80 DT price = £18.20
Erythromycin (as Erythromycin stearate) 500 mg Erythrolar
500mg tablets | 100 tablet [PoM] £45.60 DT price = £36.40
▸ **Erythroped A** (AMCo)
Erythromycin (as Erythromycin ethyl succinate)
500 mg Erythroped A 500mg tablets | 28 tablet [PoM] £10.78 DT
price = £10.78

Oral suspension
CAUTIONARY AND ADVISORY LABELS 9
▸ **Erythromycin (Non-proprietary)**
Erythromycin (as Erythromycin ethyl succinate) 25 mg per
1 ml Erythromycin ethyl succinate 125mg/5ml oral suspension |
100 ml [PoM] £4.05 DT price = £4.05
Erythromycin ethyl succinate 125mg/5ml oral suspension sugar free
sugar-free | 100 ml [PoM] £4.99 DT price = £3.56
Erythromycin (as Erythromycin ethyl succinate) 50 mg per
1 ml Erythromycin ethyl succinate 250mg/5ml oral suspension |
100 ml [PoM] £6.38 DT price = £6.38
Erythromycin ethyl succinate 250mg/5ml oral suspension sugar free
sugar-free | 100 ml [PoM] £7.99 DT price = £5.32
Erythromycin (as Erythromycin ethyl succinate) 100 mg per
1 ml Erythromycin ethyl succinate 500mg/5ml oral suspension |
100 ml [PoM] £11.24 DT price = £11.24
Erythromycin ethyl succinate 500mg/5ml oral suspension sugar free
sugar-free | 100 ml [PoM] no price available
▸ **Erythroped** (AMCo)
Erythromycin (as Erythromycin ethyl succinate) 25 mg per
1 ml Erythroped PI SF 125mg/5ml oral suspension sugar-free |
140 ml [PoM] £3.06
Erythromycin (as Erythromycin ethyl succinate) 50 mg per
1 ml Erythroped SF 250mg/5ml oral suspension sugar-free |
140 ml [PoM] £5.95
Erythromycin (as Erythromycin ethyl succinate) 100 mg per
1 ml Erythroped Forte SF 500mg/5ml oral suspension sugar-free |
140 ml [PoM] £10.56 DT price = £10.56

Powder for solution for infusion
▸ **Erythromycin (Non-proprietary)**
Erythromycin (as Erythromycin lactobionate)
1 gram Erythromycin 1g powder for solution for infusion vials |
1 vial [PoM] £18.45–£22.92

ANTIBACTERIALS › MONOBACTAMS

Aztreonam

● **DRUG ACTION** Aztreonam is a monocyclic beta-lactam
('monobactam') antibiotic with an antibacterial spectrum
limited to Gram-negative aerobic bacteria including
Pseudomonas aeruginosa, *Neisseria meningitidis*, and
Haemophilus influenzae; it should not be used alone for
'blind' treatment since it is not active against Gram-
positive organisms. Aztreonam is also effective against
Neisseria gonorrhoeae (but not against concurrent
chlamydial infection).

● **INDICATIONS AND DOSE**

Gram-negative infections including *Pseudomonas*
aeruginosa*, *Haemophilus influenzae*, and *Neisseria
meningitidis
▸ BY INTRAVENOUS INJECTION, OR BY INTRAVENOUS INFUSION
▸ Neonate up to 7 days: 30 mg/kg every 12 hours.

▸ Neonate 7 days to 28 days: 30 mg/kg every 6–8 hours.

▸ Child 1 month-11 years: 30 mg/kg every 6–8 hours
▸ Child 12-17 years: 1 g every 8 hours, alternatively 2 g
every 12 hours

Severe gram-negative infections including *Pseudomonas*
aeruginosa*, *Haemophilus influenzae*, *Neisseria
***meningitidis*, and lung infections in cystic fibrosis**
▸ BY INTRAVENOUS INFUSION, OR BY INTRAVENOUS INJECTION
▸ Child 2-11 years: 50 mg/kg every 6–8 hours (max. per
dose 2 g 4 times a day)
▸ Child 12-17 years: 2 g every 6–8 hours

Chronic pulmonary *Pseudomonas aeruginosa* infection in
patients with cystic fibrosis
▸ BY INHALATION OF NEBULISED SOLUTION
▸ Child 6-17 years: 75 mg 3 times a day for 28 days, doses
to be administered at least 4 hours apart, subsequent
courses repeated after 28-day interval without
aztreonam nebuliser solution

● **UNLICENSED USE** Injection not licensed for use in children
under 7 days.

● **CAUTIONS**
▸ When used by inhalation Haemoptysis— risk of further
haemorrhage

● **SIDE-EFFECTS**
GENERAL SIDE-EFFECTS
Bronchospasm · rash
SPECIFIC SIDE-EFFECTS
▸ **Rare**
▸ With intravenous use Antibiotic-associated colitis · asthenia ·
blood disorders · breast tenderness · chest pain · confusion
· diplopia · dizziness · dyspnoea · gastro-intestinal bleeding
· halitosis · headache · hepatitis · hypotension · insomnia ·
jaundice · myalgia · neutropenia · paraesthesia · seizures ·
thrombocytopenia · tinnitus
▸ **Frequency not known**
▸ When used by inhalation Arthralgia · cough · haemoptysis ·
pharyngolaryngeal pain · pyrexia · rhinorrhoea · wheezing
▸ With intravenous use Abdominal pain · diarrhoea · erythema
multiforme · flushing · mouth ulcers · nausea · taste
disturbances · toxic epidermal necrolysis · vomiting

● **ALLERGY AND CROSS-SENSITIVITY** Contra-indicated in
aztreonam hypersensitivity.
Use with caution in patients with hypersensitivity to
other beta-lactam antibiotics (although aztreonam may be
less likely than other beta-lactams to cause
hypersensitivity in penicillin-sensitive patients).

● **PREGNANCY**
▸ With intravenous use No information available;
manufacturer of injection advises avoid.
▸ When used by inhalation No information available;
manufacturer of powder for nebuliser solution advises
avoid unless essential.

● **BREAST FEEDING** Amount in milk probably too small to be
harmful.

● **HEPATIC IMPAIRMENT**
▸ With intravenous use Use injection with caution. Monitor
liver function.

● **RENAL IMPAIRMENT**
▸ With intravenous use If estimated glomerular filtration rate
10–30 mL/minute/1.73 m^2, usual initial dose of injection,
then half normal dose. If estimated glomerular filtration
rate less than 10 mL/minute/1.73 m^2, usual initial dose of
injection, then one-quarter normal dose.

● **MONITORING REQUIREMENTS**
▸ When used by inhalation Measure lung function before and
after initial dose of aztreonam and monitor for
bronchospasm.

● **DIRECTIONS FOR ADMINISTRATION**
▸ With intravenous use For *intravenous injection*, give over
3–5 minutes. Displacement value of injection may be
significant, consult local guidelines. For intermittent
intravenous infusion, dilute reconstituted solution further
in Glucose 5% *or* Sodium chloride 0.9% to a concentration
of less than 20 mg/mL; to be given over 20–60 minutes.
▸ When used by inhalation Other inhaled drugs should be
administered before aztreonam a bronchodilator should
be administered before each dose.

Scottish Medicines Consortium (SMC) Decisions
The *Scottish Medicines Consortium* has advised (December 2014) that aztreonam powder for nebuliser solution (*Cayston*®) is accepted for restricted use within NHS Scotland when inhaled colistimethate sodium and inhaled tobramycin are not tolerated or are not providing satisfactory therapeutic benefit (measured as ≥2% decline in forced expiratory volume in 1 second).

● MEDICINAL FORMS
There can be variation in the licensing of different medicines containing the same drug.
Powder and solvent for nebuliser solution
▸ Cayston (Gilead Sciences International Ltd)
 Aztreonam (as Aztreonam lysine) 75 mg Cayston 75mg powder and solvent for nebuliser solution vials with Altera Nebuliser Handset
 | 84 vial PoM £2,181.53

Powder for solution for injection
▸ Azactam (Bristol-Myers Squibb Pharmaceuticals Ltd)
 Aztreonam 1 gram Azactam 1g powder for solution for injection vials
 | 1 vial PoM £9.40 (Hospital only)
 Aztreonam 2 gram Azactam 2g powder for solution for injection vials
 | 1 vial PoM £18.82 (Hospital only)

ANTIBACTERIALS 〉 NITROIMIDAZOLE DERIVATIVES

Metronidazole

● **DRUG ACTION** Metronidazole is an antimicrobial drug with high activity against anaerobic bacteria and protozoa.

● **INDICATIONS AND DOSE**
Anaerobic infections
▸ BY MOUTH
▸ Child 1 month: 7.5 mg/kg every 12 hours usually treated for 7 days (for 10–14 days in *Clostridium difficile* infection)
▸ Child 2 months-11 years: 7.5 mg/kg every 8 hours (max. per dose 400 mg) usually treated for 7 days (for 10–14 days in *Clostridium difficile* infection)
▸ Child 12-17 years: 400 mg every 8 hours usually treated for 7 days (for 10–14 days in *Clostridium difficile* infection)
▸ BY RECTUM
▸ Child 1-11 months: 125 mg 3 times a day for 3 days, then 125 mg twice daily, for usual total treatment duration of 7 days
▸ Child 1-4 years: 250 mg 3 times a day for 3 days, then 250 mg twice daily, for usual total treatment duration of 7 days
▸ Child 5-9 years: 500 mg 3 times a day for 3 days, then 500 mg twice daily, for usual total treatment duration of 7 days
▸ Child 10-17 years: 1 g 3 times a day for 3 days, then 1 g twice daily, for usual total treatment duration of 7 days
▸ BY INTRAVENOUS INFUSION
▸ Neonate up to 26 weeks corrected gestational age: Loading dose 15 mg/kg, followed by 7.5 mg/kg after 24 hours, then 7.5 mg/kg daily usually treated for a total duration of 7 days (for 10–14 days in *Clostridium difficile* infection).
▸ Neonate 26 weeks to 34 weeks corrected gestational age: Loading dose 15 mg/kg, followed by 7.5 mg/kg after 12 hours, then 7.5 mg/kg every 12 hours usually treated for a total duration of 7 days (for 10–14 days in *Clostridium difficile* infection).
▸ Neonate 34 weeks corrected gestational age and above: Loading dose 15 mg/kg, followed by 7.5 mg/kg after 8 hours, then 7.5 mg/kg every 8 hours usually treated for a total duration of 7 days (for 10–14 days in *Clostridium difficile* infection).
▸ Child 1 month: Loading dose 15 mg/kg, followed by 7.5 mg/kg after 8 hours, then 7.5 mg/kg every 8 hours usually treated for a total duration of 7 days (for 10–14 days in *Clostridium difficile* infection)
▸ Child 2 months-17 years: 7.5 mg/kg every 8 hours (max. per dose 500 mg) usually treated for 7 days (for 10–14 days in *Clostridium difficile* infection)

Helicobacter pylori **eradication; in combination with clarithromycin and omeprazole**
▸ BY MOUTH
▸ Child 1-5 years: 100 mg twice daily
▸ Child 6-11 years: 200 mg twice daily
▸ Child 12-17 years: 400 mg twice daily

Helicobacter pylori **eradication; in combination with amoxicillin and omeprazole**
▸ BY MOUTH
▸ Child 1-5 years: 100 mg 3 times a day
▸ Child 6-11 years: 200 mg 3 times a day
▸ Child 12-17 years: 400 mg 3 times a day

Fistulating Crohn's disease
▸ BY MOUTH
▸ Child: 7.5 mg/kg 3 times a day usually given for 1 month but should not be used for longer than 3 months because of concerns about peripheral neuropathy

Pelvic inflammatory disease
▸ BY MOUTH
▸ Child 12-17 years: 400 mg twice daily for 14 days

Acute ulcerative gingivitis
▸ BY MOUTH
▸ Child 1-2 years: 50 mg every 8 hours for 3 days
▸ Child 3-6 years: 100 mg every 12 hours for 3 days
▸ Child 7-9 years: 100 mg every 8 hours for 3 days
▸ Child 10-17 years: 200–250 mg every 8 hours for 3 days

Acute oral infections
▸ BY MOUTH
▸ Child 1-2 years: 50 mg every 8 hours for 3–7 days
▸ Child 3-6 years: 100 mg every 12 hours for 3–7 days
▸ Child 7-9 years: 100 mg every 8 hours for 3–7 days
▸ Child 10-17 years: 200–250 mg every 8 hours for 3–7 days

Surgical prophylaxis
▸ BY MOUTH
▸ Child 1 month-11 years: 30 mg/kg (max. per dose 500 mg), to be administered 2 hours before surgery
▸ Child 12-17 years: 400–500 mg, to be administered 2 hours before surgery, then 400–500 mg every 8 hours if required for up to 3 doses (in high-risk procedures)
▸ BY RECTUM
▸ Child 5-9 years: 500 mg, to be administered 2 hours before surgery, then 500 mg every 8 hours if required for up to 3 doses (in high-risk procedures)
▸ Child 10-17 years: 1 g, to be administered 2 hours before surgery, then 1 g every 8 hours if required for up to 3 doses (in high-risk procedures)
▸ BY INTRAVENOUS INFUSION
▸ Neonate up to 40 weeks corrected gestational age: 10 mg/kg, to be administered up to 30 minutes before the procedure.
▸ Neonate 40 weeks corrected gestational age and above: 20–30 mg/kg, to be administered up to 30 minutes before the procedure.

continued →

5

Infection

- Child 1 month-11 years: 30 mg/kg (max. per dose 500 mg), to be administered up to 30 minutes before the procedure
- Child 12-17 years: 500 mg, to be administered up to 30 minutes before the procedure, then 500 mg every 8 hours if required for up to 3 further doses (in high-risk procedures)

Invasive intestinal amoebiasis | Extra-intestinal amoebiasis (including liver abscess)
▸ BY MOUTH
- Child 1-2 years: 200 mg 3 times a day for 5 days in intestinal infection (for 5–10 days in extra-intestinal infection)
- Child 3-6 years: 200 mg 4 times a day for 5 days in intestinal infection (for 5–10 days in extra-intestinal infection)
- Child 7-9 years: 400 mg 3 times a day for 5 days in intestinal infection (for 5–10 days in extra-intestinal infection)
- Child 10-17 years: 800 mg 3 times a day for 5 days in intestinal infection (for 5–10 days in extra-intestinal infection)

Urogenital trichomoniasis
▸ BY MOUTH
- Child 1-2 years: 50 mg 3 times a day for 7 days
- Child 3-6 years: 100 mg twice daily for 7 days
- Child 7-9 years: 100 mg 3 times a day for 7 days
- Child 10-17 years: 200 mg 3 times a day for 7 days, alternatively 400–500 mg twice daily for 5–7 days, alternatively 2 g for 1 dose

Giardiasis
▸ BY MOUTH
- Child 1-2 years: 500 mg once daily for 3 days
- Child 3-6 years: 600–800 mg once daily for 3 days
- Child 7-9 years: 1 g once daily for 3 days
- Child 10-17 years: 2 g once daily for 3 days, alternatively 400 mg 3 times a day for 5 days, alternatively 500 mg twice daily for 7–10 days

Established case of tetanus
▸ BY INTRAVENOUS INFUSION
- Child: (consult product literature)

● INTERACTIONS → Appendix 1: metronidazole

● SIDE-EFFECTS
▸ **Very rare** Arthralgia · ataxia · darkening of urine · dizziness · drowsiness · erythema multiforme · headache · hepatitis · jaundice · leucopenia (on prolonged or intensive therapy) · myalgia · pancreatitis · pancytopenia · peripheral neuropathy (on prolonged or intensive therapy) · pruritus · psychotic disorders · rash · thrombocytopenia · transient epileptiform seizures (on prolonged or intensive therapy) · visual disturbances
▸ **Frequency not known** Anorexia · aseptic meningitis · furred tongue · gastro-intestinal disturbances · nausea · optic neuropathy · oral mucositis · taste disturbances · vomiting

● PREGNANCY Manufacturer advises avoidance of high-dose regimens; use only if potential benefit outweighs risk.

● BREAST FEEDING Significant amount in milk; manufacturer advises avoid large single doses though otherwise compatible; may give milk a bitter taste.

● HEPATIC IMPAIRMENT In severe liver disease reduce total daily dose to one-third, and give once daily. Use with caution in hepatic encephalopathy.

● MONITORING REQUIREMENTS Clinical and laboratory monitoring advised if treatment exceeds 10 days.

● DIRECTIONS FOR ADMINISTRATION For *intravenous infusion*, give over 20–30 minutes.

● PRESCRIBING AND DISPENSING INFORMATION Metronidazole is well absorbed orally and the intravenous route is normally reserved for severe infections.

Metronidazole by the rectal route is an effective alternative to the intravenous route when oral administration is not possible.

● PATIENT AND CARER ADVICE
Medicines for Children leaflet: Metronidazole for bacterial infections www.medicinesforchildren.org.uk/metronidazole-bacterial-infections

● PROFESSION SPECIFIC INFORMATION
Dental practitioners' formulary Metronidazole Tablets may be prescribed. Metronidazole Oral Suspension may be prescribed.

● MEDICINAL FORMS
There can be variation in the licensing of different medicines containing the same drug. Forms available from special-order manufacturers include: oral suspension, oral solution

Tablet
CAUTIONARY AND ADVISORY LABELS 4, 9, 21, 25, 27
▸ **Metronidazole (Non-proprietary)**
Metronidazole 200 mg Metronidazole 200mg tablets | 21 tablet [PoM] £4.99 DT price = £2.65 | 250 tablet [PoM] £19.69
Metronidazole 400 mg Metronidazole 400mg tablets | 21 tablet [PoM] £7.95 DT price = £5.57
Metronidazole 500 mg Metronidazole 500mg tablets | 21 tablet [PoM] £37.82 DT price = £37.82
▸ **Flagyl (Zentiva)**
Metronidazole 200 mg Flagyl 200mg tablets | 21 tablet [PoM] £4.49 DT price = £2.65
Metronidazole 400 mg Flagyl 400mg tablets | 14 tablet [PoM] £6.34

Suppository
CAUTIONARY AND ADVISORY LABELS 4, 9
▸ **Flagyl (Zentiva)**
Metronidazole 500 mg Flagyl 500mg suppositories | 10 suppository [PoM] £15.18
Metronidazole 1 gram Flagyl 1g suppositories | 10 suppository [PoM] £23.06

Oral suspension
CAUTIONARY AND ADVISORY LABELS 4, 9
▸ **Metronidazole (Non-proprietary)**
Metronidazole (as Metronidazole benzoate) 40 mg per 1 ml Metronidazole 200mg/5ml oral suspension | 100 ml [PoM] £32.93 DT price = £32.93

Infusion
ELECTROLYTES: May contain Sodium
▸ **Metronidazole (Non-proprietary)**
Metronidazole 5 mg per 1 ml Metronidazole 500mg/100ml infusion 100ml bags | 20 bag [PoM] £60.00
Metronidazole 500mg/100ml infusion 100ml Macoflex bags | 1 bag [PoM] no price available | 60 bag [PoM] no price available

Tinidazole

● DRUG ACTION Tinidazole is an antimicrobial drug with high activity against anaerobic bacteria and protozoa; it has a longer duration of action than metronidazole.

● INDICATIONS AND DOSE
Intestinal amoebiasis
▸ BY MOUTH
- Child 1 month-11 years 50–60 mg/kg once daily (max. per dose 2 g) for 3 days
- Child 12-17 years: 2 g once daily for 2–3 days

Amoebic involvement of liver
▸ BY MOUTH
- Child 1 month-11 years: 50–60 mg/kg once daily (max. per dose 2 g) for 5 days
- Child 12-17 years: 1.5–2 g once daily for 3–6 days

Urogenital trichomoniasis | Giardiasis
▸ BY MOUTH
- Child 1 month-11 years: 50–75 mg/kg (max. per dose 2 g) for 1 single dose, dose may be repeated once if necessary

Medicines for Children leaflet: Penicillin V for prevention of pneumococcal infection www.medicinesforchildren.org.uk/penicillin-v-for-prevention-of-pneumococcal-infection

- **PROFESSION SPECIFIC INFORMATION**
Dental practitioners' formulary
Phenoxymethylpenicillin Tablets may be prescribed.
Phenoxymethylpenicillin Oral Solution may be prescribed.

- **MEDICINAL FORMS**
There can be variation in the licensing of different medicines containing the same drug.

Oral solution
CAUTIONARY AND ADVISORY LABELS 9, 23
▸ Phenoxymethylpenicillin (Non-proprietary)
Phenoxymethylpenicillin (as Phenoxymethylpenicillin potassium)
25 mg per 1 ml Phenoxymethylpenicillin 125mg/5ml oral solution | 100 ml [PoM] £34.00 DT price = £14.73
Phenoxymethylpenicillin 125mg/5ml oral solution sugar free sugar-free | 100 ml [PoM] £25.00 DT price = £16.02
Phenoxymethylpenicillin (as Phenoxymethylpenicillin potassium)
50 mg per 1 ml Phenoxymethylpenicillin 250mg/5ml oral solution | 100 ml [PoM] £35.00 DT price = £14.66
Phenoxymethylpenicillin 250mg/5ml oral solution sugar free sugar-free | 100 ml [PoM] £35.00 DT price = £16.02

Tablet
CAUTIONARY AND ADVISORY LABELS 9, 23
▸ Phenoxymethylpenicillin (Non-proprietary)
Phenoxymethylpenicillin (as Phenoxymethylpenicillin potassium)
250 mg Phenoxymethylpenicillin 250mg tablets | 28 tablet [PoM] £5.00 DT price = £1.04

ANTIBACTERIALS ❯ PENICILLINS, BROAD-SPECTRUM

⏴ 322

Amoxicillin

(Amoxicillin)

- **INDICATIONS AND DOSE**
Susceptible infections (including urinary-tract infections, otitis media, sinusitis, uncomplicated community acquired pneumonia, salmonellosis, oral infections)
▸ BY MOUTH

- Neonate 7 days to 28 days: 30 mg/kg 3 times a day (max. per dose 125 mg).

- Child 1–11 months: 125 mg 3 times a day; increased if necessary up to 30 mg/kg 3 times a day
- Child 1–4 years: 250 mg 3 times a day; increased if necessary up to 30 mg/kg 3 times a day
- Child 5–11 years: 500 mg 3 times a day; increased if necessary up to 30 mg/kg 3 times a day (max. per dose 1 g)
- Child 12–17 years: 500 mg 3 times a day; increased if necessary up to 1 g 3 times a day, use increased dose in severe infections
▸ BY INTRAVENOUS INJECTION, OR BY INTRAVENOUS INFUSION

- Neonate up to 7 days: 30 mg/kg every 12 hours, increased if necessary to 60 mg/kg every 12 hours, increased dose used in severe infection, community-acquired pneumonia or salmonellosis.

- Neonate 7 days to 28 days: 30 mg/kg every 8 hours, increased if necessary to 60 mg/kg every 8 hours, increased dose used in severe infection, community-acquired pneumonia or salmonellosis.

- Child: 20–30 mg/kg every 8 hours (max. per dose 500 mg), increased if necessary to 40–60 mg/kg every 8 hours (max. per dose 1 g every 8 hours), increased dose used in severe infection

Cystic fibrosis (treatment of asymptomatic *Haemophilus influenzae* carriage or mild exacerbation)
▸ BY MOUTH

- Neonate 7 days to 28 days: 30 mg/kg 3 times a day (max. per dose 125 mg).

- Child 1–11 months: 125 mg 3 times a day; increased if necessary up to 30 mg/kg 3 times a day
- Child 1–4 years: 250 mg 3 times a day; increased if necessary up to 30 mg/kg 3 times a day
- Child 5–11 years: 500 mg 3 times a day; increased if necessary up to 30 mg/kg 3 times a day (max. per dose 1 g)
- Child 12–17 years: 500 mg 3 times a day; increased if necessary up to 1 g 3 times a day, use increased dose in severe infections
▸ BY INTRAVENOUS INJECTION, OR BY INTRAVENOUS INFUSION

- Neonate up to 7 days: 30 mg/kg every 12 hours, increased if necessary to 60 mg/kg every 12 hours, increased dose used in severe infection.

- Neonate 7 days to 28 days: 30 mg/kg every 8 hours, increased if necessary to 60 mg/kg every 8 hours, increased dose used in severe infection.

- Child: 20–30 mg/kg every 8 hours (max. per dose 500 mg), increased if necessary to 40–60 mg/kg every 8 hours (max. per dose 1 g every 8 hours), increased dose used in severe infection

Lyme disease (under expert supervision)
▸ BY MOUTH

- Neonate 7 days to 28 days: 30 mg/kg 3 times a day (max. per dose 125 mg 3 times a day) usual duration 2–4 weeks

- Child 1–11 months: 125 mg 3 times a day; increased if necessary up to 30 mg/kg 3 times a day usual duration 2–4 weeks
- Child 1–4 years: 250 mg 3 times a day; increased if necessary up to 30 mg/kg 3 times a day usual duration 2–4 weeks
- Child 5–17 years: 500 mg 3 times a day for 14–21 days (for 28 days in Lyme arthritis)

Anthrax (treatment and post-exposure prophylaxis)
▸ BY MOUTH
- Child (body-weight up to 20 kg): 80 mg/kg daily in 3 divided doses
- Child (body-weight 20 kg and above): 500 mg 3 times a day

Listerial meningitis (in combination with another antibiotic)
▸ BY INTRAVENOUS INFUSION

- Neonate up to 7 days: 50–100 mg/kg every 12 hours.

- Neonate 7 days to 28 days: 50–100 mg/kg every 8 hours.

- Child: 50 mg/kg every 4–6 hours (max. per dose 2 g every 4 hours)

Group B streptococcal infection | Enterococcal endocarditis (in combination with another antibiotic)
▸ BY INTRAVENOUS INFUSION

- Neonate up to 7 days: 50 mg/kg every 12 hours.

- Neonate 7 days to 28 days: 50 mg/kg every 8 hours.

- Child: 50 mg/kg every 4–6 hours (max. per dose 2 g every 4 hours)

continued →

Prevention of pneumococcal infection in asplenia or in patients with sickle-cell disease—if cover also needed for *Haemophilus influenzae*
▶ BY MOUTH
- Child 1 month–4 years: 125 mg twice daily
- Child 5–11 years: 250 mg twice daily
- Child 12–17 years: 500 mg twice daily

***Helicobacter pylori* eradication in combination with clarithromycin and omeprazole**
▶ BY MOUTH
- Child 1–5 years: 250 mg twice daily
- Child 6–11 years: 500 mg twice daily
- Child 12–17 years: 1 g twice daily

***Helicobacter pylori* eradication in combination with metronidazole and omeprazole**
▶ BY MOUTH
- Child 1–5 years: 125 mg 3 times a day
- Child 6–11 years: 250 mg 3 times a day
- Child 12–17 years: 500 mg 3 times a day

- **UNLICENSED USE** Amoxicillin doses in BNF Publications may differ from those in product literature.

- **CAUTIONS**
  GENERAL CAUTIONS
  Acute lymphocytic leukaemia (increased risk of erythematous rashes) · chronic lymphocytic leukaemia (increased risk of erythematous rashes) · cytomegalovirus infection (increased risk of erythematous rashes) · glandular fever (erythematous rashes common) · maintain adequate hydration with high doses (particularly during parenteral therapy)
  SPECIFIC CAUTIONS
  ▶ With intravenous use Accumulation of sodium can occur with high parenteral doses

- **INTERACTIONS** → Appendix 1: penicillins

- **SIDE-EFFECTS**
  ▶ Common or very common Nausea · vomiting
  SIDE-EFFECTS, FURTHER INFORMATION
  ▶ Rash If rash occurs, discontinue treatment.

- **PREGNANCY** Not known to be harmful.

- **BREAST FEEDING** Trace amount in milk, but appropriate to use.

- **RENAL IMPAIRMENT** Reduce dose in severe impairment; rashes more common. Risk of crystalluria with high doses (particularly during parenteral therapy). Accumulation of sodium from injection can occur in patients with renal failure.

- **DIRECTIONS FOR ADMINISTRATION** Displacement value may be significant when reconstituting injection, consult local guidelines. Dilute intravenous injection to a concentration of 50 mg/mL (100 mg/mL for neonates). May be further diluted with Glucose 5% *or* Glucose 10% *or* Sodium chloride 0.9% *or* 0.45% for intravenous infusion. Give intravenous infusion over 30 minutes when using doses over 30 mg/kg.

- **PRESCRIBING AND DISPENSING INFORMATION** Flavours of oral liquid formulations and sachets may include peach, strawberry, or lemon.

- **PATIENT AND CARER ADVICE**
  Patient counselling is advised for Amoxicillin (*Amoxil*®) paediatric suspension (use of pipette).
  Medicines for Children leaflet: Amoxicillin for bacterial infections www.medicinesforchildren.org.uk/amoxicillin-bacterial-infections-0

- **PROFESSION SPECIFIC INFORMATION**
  Dental practitioners' formulary
  Amoxicillin capsules may be prescribed. Amoxicillin sachets may be prescribed as Amoxicillin Oral Powder. Amoxicillin Oral Suspension may be prescribed.

- **MEDICINAL FORMS**
  There can be variation in the licensing of different medicines containing the same drug.

Powder for solution for injection
ELECTROLYTES: May contain Sodium
▶ Amoxicillin (Non-proprietary)
Amoxicillin (as Amoxicillin sodium) 250 mg Amoxicillin 250mg powder for solution for injection vials | 10 vial ⓟoM £4.80
Amoxicillin (as Amoxicillin sodium) 500 mg Amoxicillin 500mg powder for solution for injection vials | 10 vial ⓟoM £9.60 DT price = £5.48
Amoxicillin (as Amoxicillin sodium) 1 gram Amoxicillin 1g powder for solution for injection vials | 1 vial ⓟoM £1.92
▶ Amoxil (GlaxoSmithKline UK Ltd)
Amoxicillin (as Amoxicillin sodium) 500 mg Amoxil 500mg powder for solution for injection vials | 10 vial ⓟoM £5.48 DT price = £5.48
Amoxicillin (as Amoxicillin sodium) 1 gram Amoxil 1g powder for solution for injection vials | 10 vial ⓟoM £10.96 DT price = £10.96

Oral suspension
CAUTIONARY AND ADVISORY LABELS 9
EXCIPIENTS: May contain Sucrose
▶ Amoxicillin (Non-proprietary)
Amoxicillin (as Amoxicillin trihydrate) 25 mg per 1 ml Amoxicillin 125mg/5ml oral suspension sugar free sugar-free | 100 ml ⓟoM £25.00 DT price = £1.03
Amoxicillin 125mg/5ml oral suspension | 100 ml ⓟoM £25.00 DT price = £0.96
Amoxicillin (as Amoxicillin trihydrate) 50 mg per 1 ml Amoxicillin 250mg/5ml oral suspension sugar free sugar-free | 100 ml ⓟoM £35.00 DT price = £1.18
Amoxicillin 250mg/5ml oral suspension | 100 ml ⓟoM £35.00 DT price = £1.13
▶ Amoxil (GlaxoSmithKline UK Ltd)
Amoxicillin (as Amoxicillin trihydrate) 100 mg per 1 ml Amoxil 125mg/1.25ml paediatric oral suspension | 20 ml ⓟoM £3.18 DT price = £3.18

Powder
CAUTIONARY AND ADVISORY LABELS 9, 13
▶ Amoxicillin (Non-proprietary)
Amoxicillin (as Amoxicillin trihydrate) 3 gram Amoxicillin 3g oral powder sachets sugar free sugar-free | 2 sachet ⓟoM £15.00 DT price = £9.98

Capsule
CAUTIONARY AND ADVISORY LABELS 9
▶ Amoxicillin (Non-proprietary)
Amoxicillin (as Amoxicillin trihydrate) 250 mg Amoxicillin 250mg capsules | 15 capsule ⓟoM £5.00 DT price = £0.78 | 21 capsule ⓟoM £8.99 DT price = £1.09 | 500 capsule ⓟoM £120.00
Amoxicillin (as Amoxicillin trihydrate) 500 mg Amoxicillin 500mg capsules | 15 capsule ⓟoM £7.50 DT price = £0.91 | 21 capsule ⓟoM £15.00 DT price = £1.27 | 100 capsule ⓟoM £75.00
▶ Amoxil (GlaxoSmithKline UK Ltd)
Amoxicillin (as Amoxicillin trihydrate) 250 mg Amoxil 250mg capsules | 21 capsule ⓟoM £0.92 DT price = £1.09
Amoxicillin (as Amoxicillin trihydrate) 500 mg Amoxil 500mg capsules | 21 capsule ⓟoM £0.89 DT price = £1.27

Combinations available: *Co-amoxiclav,* p. 328

▶ 322

Ampicillin

- **INDICATIONS AND DOSE**

Susceptible infections (including bronchitis, urinary-tract infections, otitis media, sinusitis, uncomplicated community-acquired pneumonia, salmonellosis)
▶ BY MOUTH

▶ Neonate 7 days to 20 days: 30 mg/kg 3 times a day (max. per dose 125 mg).

▶ Neonate 21 days to 28 days: 30 mg/kg 4 times a day (max. per dose 125 mg).

▶ Child 1–11 months: 125 mg 4 times a day; increased if necessary up to 30 mg/kg 4 times a day
▶ Child 1–4 years: 250 mg 4 times a day; increased if necessary up to 30 mg/kg 4 times a day

▸ Child 5–11 years: 500 mg 4 times a day; increased if necessary up to 30 mg/kg 4 times a day (max. per dose 1 g)

▸ Child 12–17 years: 500 mg 4 times a day; increased if necessary to 1 g 4 times a day, use increased dose in severe infection

▸ **BY INTRAVENOUS INJECTION, OR BY INTRAVENOUS INFUSION**

▸ Neonate up to 7 days: 30 mg/kg every 12 hours, increased if necessary to 60 mg/kg every 12 hours, increased dose used in severe infection, community-acquired pneumonia or salmonellosis.

▸ Neonate 7 days to 20 days: 30 mg/kg every 8 hours, increased if necessary to 60 mg/kg every 8 hours, increased dose used in severe infection, community-acquired pneumonia or salmonellosis.

▸ Neonate 21 days to 28 days: 30 mg/kg every 6 hours, increased if necessary to 60 mg/kg every 6 hours, increased dose used in severe infection, community-acquired pneumonia or salmonellosis.

▸ Child: 25 mg/kg every 6 hours (max. per dose 500 mg every 6 hours), increased if necessary to 50 mg/kg every 6 hours (max. per dose 1 g every 6 hours), increased dose used in severe infection

Group B streptococcal infection | Enterococcal endocarditis (in combination with another antibacterial)

▸ **BY INTRAVENOUS INFUSION**

▸ Neonate up to 7 days: 50 mg/kg every 12 hours.

▸ Neonate 7 days to 20 days: 50 mg/kg every 8 hours.

▸ Neonate 21 days to 28 days: 50 mg/kg every 6 hours.

▸ Child: 50 mg/kg every 4–6 hours (max. per dose 2 g every 4 hours)

Listerial meningitis

▸ **BY INTRAVENOUS INFUSION**

▸ Neonate up to 7 days: 100 mg/kg every 12 hours.

▸ Neonate 7 days to 20 days: 100 mg/kg every 8 hours.

▸ Neonate 21 days to 28 days: 100 mg/kg every 6 hours.

▸ Child: 50 mg/kg every 4–6 hours (max. per dose 2 g every 4 hours)

● **CAUTIONS**

GENERAL CAUTIONS

Acute lymphocytic leukaemia (increased risk of erythematous rashes) · chronic lymphocytic leukaemia (increased risk of erythematous rashes) · cytomegalovirus infection (increased risk of erythematous rashes) · glandular fever (erythematous rashes common)

SPECIFIC CAUTIONS

▸ With intravenous use Accumulation of electrolytes contained in parenteral preparations can occur with high doses

● **INTERACTIONS** → Appendix 1: penicillins

● **SIDE-EFFECTS**

▸ **Common or very common** Nausea · vomiting

SIDE-EFFECTS, FURTHER INFORMATION

▸ Rash If rash occurs, discontinue treatment.

● **PREGNANCY** Not known to be harmful.

● **BREAST FEEDING** Trace amounts in milk, but appropriate to use.

● **RENAL IMPAIRMENT** If estimated glomerular filtration rate less than 10 mL/minute/1.73 m² reduce dose or frequency; rashes more common. Accumulation of electrolytes

contained in parenteral preparations can occur in patients with renal failure.

● **DIRECTIONS FOR ADMINISTRATION**

▸ With oral use Administer at least 30 minutes before food.

▸ With intravenous use Displacement value may be significant when reconstituting injection, consult local guidelines. Dilute intravenous injection to a concentration of 50–100 mg/mL. May be further diluted with glucose 5% or 10% or sodium chloride 0.9% or 0.45% for infusion. Give over 30 minutes when using doses of greater than 50 mg/kg to avoid CNS toxicity including convulsions.

● **PATIENT AND CARER ADVICE**

Medicines for Children leaflet: Ampicillin for bacterial infection www.medicinesforchildren.org.uk/ampicillin-bacterial-infection

● **MEDICINAL FORMS**

There can be variation in the licensing of different medicines containing the same drug.

Oral suspension

CAUTIONARY AND ADVISORY LABELS 9, 23

▸ Ampicillin (Non-proprietary)

Ampicillin 25 mg per 1 ml Ampicillin 125mg/5ml oral suspension | 100 ml [PoM] £29.86 DT price = £29.86

Ampicillin 50 mg per 1 ml Ampicillin 250mg/5ml oral suspension | 100 ml [PoM] £38.86 DT price = £38.86

Powder for solution for injection

▸ Ampicillin (Non-proprietary)

Ampicillin (as Ampicillin sodium) 500 mg Ampicillin 500mg powder for solution for injection vials | 10 vial [PoM] £78.30 DT price = £78.30

Capsule

CAUTIONARY AND ADVISORY LABELS 9, 23

▸ Ampicillin (Non-proprietary)

Ampicillin 250 mg Ampicillin 250mg capsules | 28 capsule [PoM] £20.50 DT price = £20.50

Ampicillin 500 mg Ampicillin 500mg capsules | 28 capsule [PoM] £40.30 DT price = £40.30

◣ F 322

Co-fluampicil

● **INDICATIONS AND DOSE**

Mixed infections involving beta-lactamase-producing staphylococci

▸ **BY MOUTH**

▸ Child 1 month–9 years: 125/125 mg every 6 hours

▸ Child 10–17 years: 250/250 mg every 6 hours

▸ **BY INTRAMUSCULAR INJECTION, OR BY SLOW INTRAVENOUS INJECTION, OR BY INTRAVENOUS INFUSION**

▸ Child 1 month–1 year: 62.5/62.5 mg every 6 hours

▸ Child 2–9 years: 125/125 mg every 6 hours

▸ Child 10–17 years: 250/250 mg every 6 hours

Severe mixed infections involving beta-lactamase-producing staphylococci

▸ **BY MOUTH**

▸ Child 1 month–9 years: 250/250 mg every 6 hours

▸ Child 10–17 years: 500/500 mg every 6 hours

▸ **BY INTRAMUSCULAR INJECTION, OR BY SLOW INTRAVENOUS INJECTION, OR BY INTRAVENOUS INFUSION**

▸ Child 1 month–1 year: 125/125 mg every 6 hours

▸ Child 2–9 years: 250/250 mg every 6 hours

▸ Child 10–17 years: 500/500 mg every 6 hours

IMPORTANT SAFETY INFORMATION

HEPATIC DISORDERS

Cholestatic jaundice and hepatitis may occur very rarely, up to two months after treatment with flucloxacillin has been stopped. Administration for more than 2 weeks and increasing age are risk factors. Healthcare professionals are reminded that:

● flucloxacillin should not be used in patients with a history of hepatic dysfunction associated with flucloxacillin;

- flucloxacillin should be used with caution in patients with hepatic impairment;
- careful enquiry should be made about hypersensitivity reactions to beta-lactam antibacterials.

● CAUTIONS

GENERAL CAUTIONS

Acute lymphocytic leukaemia (increased risk of erythematous rashes) · chronic lymphocytic leukaemia (increased risk of erythematous rashes) · cytomegalovirus infection (increased risk of erythematous rashes) · glandular fever (erythematous rashes common)

SPECIFIC CAUTIONS

▸ With intravenous use Accumulation of electrolytes contained in parenteral preparations can occur with high doses · risk of kernicterus in jaundiced neonates when high doses given parenterally

● INTERACTIONS → Appendix 1: penicillins

● SIDE-EFFECTS

▸ **Common or very common** Gastro-intestinal disturbances · nausea · vomiting

▸ **Very rare** Cholestatic jaundice · hepatitis

SIDE-EFFECTS, FURTHER INFORMATION

▸ Rash If rash occurs, discontinue treatment.

● PREGNANCY Not known to be harmful.

● BREAST FEEDING Trace amount in milk, but appropriate to use.

● HEPATIC IMPAIRMENT Use with caution.

● RENAL IMPAIRMENT Reduce dose or frequency if estimated glomerular filtration rate less than 10 mL/minute/1.73 m^2; rashes more common. Accumulation of electrolytes contained in parenteral preparations can occur in patients with renal failure.

● EFFECT ON LABORATORY TESTS False-positive urinary glucose (if tested for reducing substances).

● PRESCRIBING AND DISPENSING INFORMATION Dose expressed as a combination of equal parts by mass of flucloxacillin and ampicillin.

● MEDICINAL FORMS

There can be variation in the licensing of different medicines containing the same drug.

Oral suspension

CAUTIONARY AND ADVISORY LABELS 9, 22

▸ Co-fluampicil (Non-proprietary)

Ampicillin (as Ampicillin trihydrate) 25 mg per 1 ml, Flucloxacillin (as Flucloxacillin magnesium) 25 mg per 1 ml Co-fluampicil 125mg/125mg/5ml oral suspension | 100 ml [PoM] £23.93 DT price = £23.93

Powder for solution for injection

ELECTROLYTES: May contain Sodium

▸ Co-fluampicil (Non-proprietary)

Ampicillin (as Ampicillin sodium) 250 mg, Flucloxacillin (as Flucloxacillin sodium) 250 mg Co-fluampicil 250mg/250mg powder for solution for injection vials | 10 vial [PoM] £13.33

Capsule

CAUTIONARY AND ADVISORY LABELS 9, 22

▸ Co-fluampicil (Non-proprietary)

Ampicillin (as Ampicillin trihydrate) 250 mg, Flucloxacillin (as Flucloxacillin sodium) 250 mg Co-fluampicil 250mg/250mg capsules | 28 capsule [PoM] £10.31 DT price = £2.18 | 100 capsule [PoM] £7.79–£42.99

ANTIBACTERIALS > PENICILLINS, BROAD-SPECTRUM WITH BETA-LACTAMASE INHIBITOR

F 322

Co-amoxiclav

● INDICATIONS AND DOSE

Infections due to beta-lactamase-producing strains (where amoxicillin alone not appropriate), including respiratory tract infections, bone and joint infections, genito-urinary and abdominal infections, cellulitis and animal bites

▸ BY MOUTH USING TABLETS

▸ Child 12–17 years: 250/125 mg every 8 hours; increased to 500/125 mg every 8 hours, increased dose used for severe infection

▸ BY INTRAVENOUS INJECTION, OR BY INTRAVENOUS INFUSION

▸ Neonate: 30 mg/kg every 12 hours.

▸ Child 1–2 months: 30 mg/kg every 12 hours

▸ Child 3 months–17 years: 30 mg/kg every 8 hours (max. per dose 1.2 g every 8 hours)

Infections due to beta-lactamase-producing strains (where amoxicillin alone not appropriate) including respiratory-tract infections, bone and joint infections, genito-urinary and abdominal infections, cellulitis, animal bites (doses for 125/31 suspension)

▸ BY MOUTH USING ORAL SUSPENSION

▸ Neonate: 0.25 mL/kilogram 3 times a day.

▸ Child 1–11 months: 0.25 mL/kilogram 3 times a day, dose doubled in severe infection

▸ Child 1–5 years: 0.25 mL/kilogram 3 times a day, alternatively 5 mL 3 times a day, dose doubled in severe infection

Infections due to beta-lactamase-producing strains (where amoxicillin alone not appropriate) including respiratory-tract infections, bone and joint infections, genito-urinary and abdominal infections, cellulitis, animal bites (doses for 250/62 suspension)

▸ BY MOUTH USING ORAL SUSPENSION

▸ Child 6–11 years: 0.15 mL/kilogram 3 times a day, alternatively 5 mL 3 times a day, dose doubled in severe infection

Infections due to beta-lactamase-producing strains (where amoxicillin alone not appropriate) including respiratory-tract infections, bone and joint infections, genito-urinary and abdominal infections, cellulitis, animal bites (doses for 400/57 suspension)

▸ BY MOUTH USING ORAL SUSPENSION

▸ Child 2 months–1 year: 0.15 mL/kilogram twice daily, doubled in severe infection

▸ Child 2–6 years (body-weight 13–21 kg): 2.5 mL twice daily, doubled in severe infection

▸ Child 7–12 years (body-weight 22–40 kg): 5 mL twice daily, doubled in severe infection

▸ Child 12–17 years (body-weight 41 kg and above): 10 mL twice daily; increased if necessary to 10 mL 3 times a day, increased frequency to be used in severe infection

Severe dental infection with spreading cellulitis | Dental infection not responding to first-line antibacterial

▸ BY MOUTH USING TABLETS

▸ Child 12–17 years: 250/125 mg every 8 hours for 5 days

DOSE EQUIVALENCE AND CONVERSION

▸ Doses are expressed as co-amoxiclav.

▸ A mixture of amoxicillin (as the trihydrate or as the sodium salt) and clavulanic acid (as potassium clavulanate); the proportions are expressed in the form x/y where x and y are the strengths in milligrams of amoxicillin and clavulanic acid respectively.

- **CONTRA-INDICATIONS** History of co-amoxiclav-associated jaundice or hepatic dysfunction · history of penicillin-associated jaundice or hepatic dysfunction
- **CAUTIONS**
  GENERAL CAUTIONS
  Acute lymphocytic leukaemia (increased risk of erythematous rashes) · chronic lymphocytic leukaemia (increased risk of erythematous rashes) · cytomegalovirus infection (increased risk of erythematous rashes) · glandular fever (erythematous rashes common) · maintain adequate hydration with high doses (particularly during parental therapy)
  SPECIFIC CAUTIONS
  ▸ With intravenous use Accumulation of electrolytes contained in parenteral preparations can occur with high doses
  CAUTIONS, FURTHER INFORMATION
  ▸ Cholestatic jaundice Cholestatic jaundice can occur either during or shortly after the use of co-amoxiclav. An epidemiological study has shown that the risk of acute liver toxicity was about 6 times greater with co-amoxiclav than with amoxicillin. Cholestatic jaundice is more common in patients above the age of 65 years and in men; these reactions have only rarely been reported in children. Jaundice is usually self-limiting and very rarely fatal. The duration of treatment should be appropriate to the indication and should not usually exceed 14 days.
- **INTERACTIONS** → Appendix 1: penicillins
- **SIDE-EFFECTS**
  GENERAL SIDE-EFFECTS
  ▸ **Common or very common** Cholestatic jaundice · hepatitis · nausea · vomiting
  ▸ **Rare** Dizziness · headache · prolongation of bleeding time
  ▸ **Frequency not known** Exfoliative dermatitis · Steven-Johnson syndrome · toxic epidermal necrolysis · vasculitis
  SPECIFIC SIDE-EFFECTS
  ▸ **Rare**
  ▸ With intravenous use Phlebitis at injection site
  ▸ With oral use Superficial staining of teeth with suspension
  SIDE-EFFECTS, FURTHER INFORMATION
  ▸ Rash If rash occurs, discontinue treatment.
- **PREGNANCY** Not known to be harmful.
- **BREAST FEEDING** Trace amount in milk, but appropriate to use.
- **HEPATIC IMPAIRMENT** Monitor liver function in liver disease.
- **RENAL IMPAIRMENT**
  ▸ With oral use *Co-amoxiclav 125/31 suspension*, *250/62 suspension*, *250/125 tablets, or 500/125 tablets* : use normal dose every 12 hours if estimated glomerular filtration rate 10–30 mL/minute/1.73 m^2. Use the normal dose recommended for mild or moderate infections every 12 hours if estimated glomerular filtration rate less than 10 mL/minute/1.73 m^2.
    Co-amoxiclav 400/57 suspension : avoid if estimated glomerular filtration rate less than 30 mL/minute/1.73 m^2.
  ▸ With intravenous use *Co-amoxiclav injection* : use normal initial dose and then use half normal dose every 12 hours if estimated glomerular filtration rate 10–30 mL/minute/1.73 m^2; use normal initial dose and then use half normal dose every 24 hours if estimated glomerular filtration rate less than 10 mL/minute/1.73 m^2. Risk of crystalluria with high doses (particularly during parenteral therapy).
    Accumulation of electrolytes contained in parenteral preparations can occur in patients with renal failure.
- **DIRECTIONS FOR ADMINISTRATION** For *intravenous infusion*, dilute reconstituted solution to a concentration of 10 mg/mL with Sodium Chloride 0.9%; give

intermittently over 30–40 minutes. For *intravenous injection*, administer over 3–4 minutes.
- **PRESCRIBING AND DISPENSING INFORMATION** Doses are expressed as co-amoxiclav: a mixture of amoxicillin (as the trihydrate or as the sodium salt) and clavulanic acid (as potassium clavulanate); the proportions are expressed in the form x/y where x and y are the strengths in milligrams of amoxicillin and clavulanic acid respectively.
  Flavours of oral liquid formulations may include raspberry and orange.
- **PATIENT AND CARER ADVICE**
  Medicines for Children leaflet: Co-amoxiclav for bacterial infections www.medicinesforchildren.org.uk/co-amoxiclav-bacterial-infections-0
- **PROFESSION SPECIFIC INFORMATION**
  Dental practitioners' formulary
  Co-amoxiclav 250/125 Tablets may be prescribed.
  Co-amoxiclav 125/31 Suspension may be prescribed.
  Co-amoxiclav 250/62 Suspension may be prescribed.
- **MEDICINAL FORMS**
  There can be variation in the licensing of different medicines containing the same drug. Forms available from special-order manufacturers include: infusion
  Oral suspension
  CAUTIONARY AND ADVISORY LABELS 9
  EXCIPIENTS: May contain Aspartame
  ▸ **Co-amoxiclav** (Non-proprietary)
  Clavulanic acid (as Potassium clavulanate) 6.25 mg per 1 ml, Amoxicillin (as Amoxicillin trihydrate) 25 mg per 1 ml Co-amoxiclav 125mg/31mg/5ml oral suspension | 100 ml PoM £5.00 DT price = £5.00
  Co-amoxiclav 125mg/31mg/5ml oral suspension sugar free sugar-free | 100 ml PoM £25.00 DT price = £1.94
  Clavulanic acid (as Potassium clavulanate) 12.5 mg per 1 ml, Amoxicillin (as Amoxicillin trihydrate) 50 mg per 1 ml Co-amoxiclav 250mg/62mg/5ml oral suspension | 100 ml PoM £5.00 DT price = £5.00
  Co-amoxiclav 250mg/62mg/5ml oral suspension sugar free sugar-free | 100 ml PoM £35.00 DT price = £1.73
  Clavulanic acid (as Potassium clavulanate) 11.4 mg per 1 ml, Amoxicillin (as Amoxicillin trihydrate) 80 mg per 1 ml Co-amoxiclav 400mg/57mg/5ml oral suspension sugar free sugar-free | 35 ml PoM £4.13 DT price = £4.13 sugar-free | 70 ml PoM £6.97 DT price = £5.79
  ▸ **Augmentin** (GlaxoSmithKline UK Ltd)
  Clavulanic acid (as Potassium clavulanate) 6.25 mg per 1 ml, Amoxicillin (as Amoxicillin trihydrate) 25 mg per 1 ml Augmentin 125/31 SF oral suspension sugar-free | 100 ml PoM £3.54 DT price = £1.94
  Clavulanic acid (as Potassium clavulanate) 12.5 mg per 1 ml, Amoxicillin (as Amoxicillin trihydrate) 50 mg per 1 ml Augmentin 250/62 SF oral suspension sugar-free | 100 ml PoM £3.60 DT price = £1.73
  ▸ **Augmentin-Duo** (GlaxoSmithKline UK Ltd)
  Clavulanic acid (as Potassium clavulanate) 11.4 mg per 1 ml, Amoxicillin (as Amoxicillin trihydrate) 80 mg per 1 ml Augmentin-Duo 400/57 oral suspension sugar-free | 35 ml PoM £4.13 DT price = £4.13 sugar-free | 70 ml PoM £5.79 DT price = £5.79
  Tablet
  CAUTIONARY AND ADVISORY LABELS 9
  ▸ **Co-amoxiclav** (Non-proprietary)
  Clavulanic acid (as Potassium clavulanate) 125 mg, Amoxicillin (as Amoxicillin trihydrate) 250 mg Co-amoxiclav 250mg/125mg tablets | 21 tablet PoM £6.00 DT price = £1.86 | 100 tablet PoM no price available
  Clavulanic acid (as Potassium clavulanate) 125 mg, Amoxicillin (as Amoxicillin trihydrate) 500 mg Co-amoxiclav 500mg/125mg tablets | 21 tablet PoM £12.00 DT price = £1.88
  Clavulanic acid (as Potassium clavulanate) 125 mg, Amoxicillin (as Amoxicillin trihydrate) 875 mg Co-amoxiclav 875mg/125mg tablets | 14 tablet PoM £18.00 DT price = £8.60
  ▸ **Augmentin** (GlaxoSmithKline UK Ltd)
  Clavulanic acid (as Potassium clavulanate) 125 mg, Amoxicillin (as Amoxicillin trihydrate) 250 mg Augmentin 375mg tablets | 21 tablet PoM £5.03 DT price = £1.86

5

Infection

Clavulanic acid (as Potassium clavulanate) 125 mg, Amoxicillin (as Amoxicillin trihydrate) 500 mg Augmentin 625mg tablets | 21 tablet PoM £9.60 DT price = £1.88

Powder for solution for injection
ELECTROLYTES: May contain Potassium, sodium
▸ Co-amoxiclav (Non-proprietary)
Clavulanic acid (as Potassium clavulanate) 100 mg, Amoxicillin (as Amoxicillin sodium) 500 mg Co-amoxiclav 500mg/100mg powder for solution for injection vials | 10 vial PoM £14.90
Clavulanic acid (as Potassium clavulanate) 200 mg, Amoxicillin (as Amoxicillin sodium) 1000 mg Co-amoxiclav 1000mg/200mg powder for solution for injection vials | 10 vial PoM £29.70
▸ Augmentin Intravenous (GlaxoSmithKline UK Ltd)
Clavulanic acid (as Potassium clavulanate) 100 mg, Amoxicillin (as Amoxicillin sodium) 500 mg Augmentin Intravenous 600mg powder for solution for injection vials | 10 vial PoM £10.60
Clavulanic acid (as Potassium clavulanate) 200 mg, Amoxicillin (as Amoxicillin sodium) 1000 mg Augmentin Intravenous 1.2g powder for solution for injection vials | 10 vial PoM £10.60

ANTIBACTERIALS > PENICILLINS, MECILLINAM-TYPE

F 322

Pivmecillinam hydrochloride

● **INDICATIONS AND DOSE**
Acute uncomplicated cystitis
▸ BY MOUTH
▸ Child (body-weight 40 kg and above): Initially 400 mg for 1 dose, then 200 mg every 8 hours for 3 days

Chronic or recurrent bacteriuria
▸ BY MOUTH
▸ Child (body-weight 40 kg and above): 400 mg every 6–8 hours

Urinary-tract infections
▸ BY MOUTH
▸ Child (body-weight up to 40 kg): 5–10 mg/kg every 6 hours, alternatively 20–40 mg/kg daily in 3 divided doses

● **UNLICENSED USE** Not licensed for use in children under 3 months.
● **CONTRA-INDICATIONS** Carnitine deficiency · gastro-intestinal obstruction · infants under 3 months · oesophageal strictures
● **CAUTIONS** Avoid in acute porphyrias p. 577
● **INTERACTIONS** → Appendix 1: penicillins
● **SIDE-EFFECTS**
▸ **Common or very common** Abdominal pain · dizziness · headache · nausea · vomiting
▸ **Frequency not known** Mouth ulcers · oesophagitis · reduced serum and total body carnitine (especially with long-term or repeated use)
● **PREGNANCY** Not known to be harmful, but manufacturer advises avoid.
● **BREAST FEEDING** Trace amount in milk, but appropriate to use.
● **MONITORING REQUIREMENTS** Liver and renal function tests required in long-term use.
● **EFFECT ON LABORATORY TESTS** False-positive urinary glucose (if tested for reducing substances).
● **DIRECTIONS FOR ADMINISTRATION** Tablets should be swallowed whole with plenty of fluid during meals while sitting or standing.
● **PATIENT AND CARER ADVICE** Patient counselling is advised on administration of pivmecillinam hydrochloride tablets (posture).

● **MEDICINAL FORMS**
There can be variation in the licensing of different medicines containing the same drug.
Tablet
CAUTIONARY AND ADVISORY LABELS 9, 21, 27
▸ Selexid (LEO Pharma)
Pivmecillinam hydrochloride 200 mg Selexid 200mg tablets | 10 tablet PoM £5.40 DT price = £5.40 | 18 tablet PoM £9.72

ANTIBACTERIALS > PENICILLINS, PENICILLINASE-RESISTANT

F 322

Flucloxacillin

● **INDICATIONS AND DOSE**
Infections due to beta-lactamase-producing staphylococci including otitis externa | Adjunct in pneumonia | Adjunct in impetigo | Adjunct in cellulitis
▸ BY MOUTH
▸ Neonate up to 7 days: 25 mg/kg twice daily.
▸ Neonate 7 days to 20 days: 25 mg/kg 3 times a day.
▸ Neonate 21 days to 28 days: 25 mg/kg 4 times a day.
▸ Child 1 month-1 year: 62.5–125 mg 4 times a day
▸ Child 2–9 years: 125–250 mg 4 times a day
▸ Child 10–17 years: 250–500 mg 4 times a day
▸ BY INTRAMUSCULAR INJECTION
▸ Child: 12.5–25 mg/kg every 6 hours (max. per dose 500 mg every 6 hours)
▸ BY SLOW INTRAVENOUS INJECTION, OR BY INTRAVENOUS INFUSION
▸ Neonate up to 7 days: 25 mg/kg every 12 hours.
▸ Neonate 7 days to 20 days: 25 mg/kg every 8 hours.
▸ Neonate 21 days to 28 days: 25 mg/kg every 6 hours.
▸ Child: 12.5–25 mg/kg every 6 hours (max. per dose 1 g every 6 hours)

Severe infections due to beta-lactamase-producing staphylococci including otitis externa | Adjunct in pneumonia (severe infection) | Adjunct in impetigo (severe infection) | Adjunct in cellulitis (severe infection)
▸ BY SLOW INTRAVENOUS INJECTION, OR BY INTRAVENOUS INFUSION
▸ Neonate up to 7 days: 50 mg/kg every 12 hours.
▸ Neonate 7 days to 20 days: 50 mg/kg every 8 hours.
▸ Neonate 21 days to 28 days: 50 mg/kg every 6 hours.
▸ Child: 25–50 mg/kg every 6 hours (max. per dose 2 g every 6 hours)

Endocarditis (in combination with other antibacterial if necessary)
▸ BY SLOW INTRAVENOUS INJECTION, OR BY INTRAVENOUS INFUSION
▸ Child: 50 mg/kg every 6 hours (max. per dose 2 g every 6 hours)

Osteomyelitis
▸ BY SLOW INTRAVENOUS INJECTION, OR BY INTRAVENOUS INFUSION
▸ Neonate up to 7 days: 50–100 mg/kg every 12 hours.
▸ Neonate 7 days to 20 days: 50–100 mg/kg every 8 hours.
▸ Neonate 21 days to 28 days: 50–100 mg/kg every 6 hours.
▸ Child: 50 mg/kg every 6 hours (max. per dose 2 g every 6 hours)

Cerebral abscess | Staphylococcal meningitis
▶ BY SLOW INTRAVENOUS INJECTION, OR BY INTRAVENOUS INFUSION
▸ Neonate up to 7 days: 50–100 mg/kg every 12 hours.
▸ Neonate 7 days to 20 days: 50–100 mg/kg every 8 hours.
▸ Neonate 21 days to 28 days: 50–100 mg/kg every 6 hours.
▸ Child: 50 mg/kg every 6 hours (max. per dose 2 g every 6 hours)

Staphylococcal lung infection in cystic fibrosis
▶ BY MOUTH
▸ Child: 25 mg/kg 4 times a day (max. per dose 1 g), alternatively 100 mg/kg daily in 3 divided doses; maximum 4 g per day
▶ BY SLOW INTRAVENOUS INJECTION, OR BY INTRAVENOUS INFUSION
▸ Child: 50 mg/kg every 6 hours (max. per dose 2 g every 6 hours)

Prevention of *Staphylococcus aureus* lung infection in cystic fibrosis—primary prevention
▶ BY MOUTH
▸ Neonate: 125 mg twice daily.
▸ Child 1 month–3 years: 125 mg twice daily

Prevention of *Staphylococcus aureus* lung infection in cystic fibrosis—secondary prevention
▶ BY MOUTH
▸ Child: 50 mg/kg twice daily (max. per dose 1 g twice daily)

IMPORTANT SAFETY INFORMATION

HEPATIC DISORDERS
Cholestatic jaundice and hepatitis may occur very rarely, up to two months after treatment with flucloxacillin has been stopped. Administration for more than 2 weeks and increasing age are risk factors. Healthcare professionals are reminded that:
• flucloxacillin should not be used in patients with a history of hepatic dysfunction associated with flucloxacillin
• flucloxacillin should be used with caution in patients with hepatic impairment
• careful enquiry should be made about hypersensitivity reactions to beta-lactam antibacterials

● CAUTIONS
▶ With intravenous use Accumulation of electrolytes can occur with high doses · risk of kernicterus in jaundiced neonates when high doses given parenterally
● INTERACTIONS → Appendix 1: penicillins
● SIDE-EFFECTS
▶ Common or very common Gastrointestinal disturbances
▶ Very rare Cholestatic jaundice · hepatitis
● PREGNANCY Not known to be harmful.
● BREAST FEEDING Trace amounts in milk, but appropriate to use.
● HEPATIC IMPAIRMENT Use with caution.
● RENAL IMPAIRMENT Use normal dose every 8 hours if estimated glomerular filtration rate less than 10 mL/minute/1.73 m^2.
▶ With intravenous use Accumulation of electrolytes can occur in patients with renal failure.
● EFFECT ON LABORATORY TESTS False-positive urinary glucose (if tested for reducing substances).
● DIRECTIONS FOR ADMINISTRATION For *intravenous infusion*, dilute reconstituted solution *in* Glucose 5% *or*

Sodium Chloride 0.9% and give intermittently over 30–60 minutes.
● PATIENT AND CARER ADVICE
Medicines for Children leaflet: Flucloxacillin for bacterial infections
www.medicinesforchildren.org.uk/flucloxacillin-for-bacterial-infections
● MEDICINAL FORMS
There can be variation in the licensing of different medicines containing the same drug. Forms available from special-order manufacturers include: infusion

Oral solution
CAUTIONARY AND ADVISORY LABELS 9, 23
▶ **Flucloxacillin (Non-proprietary)**
Flucloxacillin (as Flucloxacillin sodium) 25 mg per 1 ml Flucloxacillin 125mg/5ml oral solution | 100 ml [PoM] £20.99 DT price = £6.58
Flucloxacillin 125mg/5ml oral solution sugar free sugar-free | 100 ml [PoM] £31.41 DT price = £22.31
Flucloxacillin (as Flucloxacillin sodium) 50 mg per 1 ml Flucloxacillin 250mg/5ml oral solution sugar free sugar-free | 100 ml [PoM] £36.27 DT price = £26.91
Flucloxacillin 250mg/5ml oral solution | 100 ml [PoM] £26.04 DT price = £26.04

Powder for solution for injection
▶ **Flucloxacillin (Non-proprietary)**
Flucloxacillin (as Flucloxacillin sodium) 250 mg Flucloxacillin 250mg powder for solution for injection vials | 10 vial [PoM] £10.43–£12.25
Flucloxacillin (as Flucloxacillin sodium) 500 mg Flucloxacillin 500mg powder for solution for injection vials | 10 vial [PoM] £20.85–£24.50
Flucloxacillin (as Flucloxacillin sodium) 1 gram Flucloxacillin 1g powder for solution for injection vials | 10 vial [PoM] £41.75–£49.00

Capsule
CAUTIONARY AND ADVISORY LABELS 9, 23
▶ **Flucloxacillin (Non-proprietary)**
Flucloxacillin (as Flucloxacillin sodium) 250 mg Flucloxacillin 250mg capsules | 20 capsule [PoM] £3.58 | 28 capsule [PoM] £5.00 DT price = £1.31 | 100 capsule [PoM] £17.80
Flucloxacillin (as Flucloxacillin sodium) 500 mg Flucloxacillin 500mg capsules | 20 capsule [PoM] £7.50 | 28 capsule [PoM] £10.50 DT price = £2.17 | 100 capsule [PoM] £37.50

Combinations available: *Co-fluampicil*, p. 327

ANTIBACTERIALS > POLYMYXINS

Colistimethate sodium
18-Dec-2016
(Colistin sulfomethate sodium)

● DRUG ACTION The polymyxin antibiotic, **colistimethate sodium** (colistin sulfomethate sodium), is active against Gram-negative organisms including *Pseudomonas aeruginosa*, *Acinetobacter baumanii* and *Klebsiella pneumoniae*. It is not absorbed by mouth and thus needs to be given by injection for a systemic effect.

● INDICATIONS AND DOSE

Gram-negative infections resistant to other antibacterials, including those caused by *Pseudomonas aeruginosa*, *Acinetobacter baumanii* and *Klebsiella pneumoniae*
▶ BY SLOW INTRAVENOUS INJECTION, OR BY INTRAVENOUS INFUSION
▸ Child (body-weight up to 60 kg): 50 000–75 000 units/kg daily in 3 divided doses, to be administered into a totally implantable venous access device when giving via slow intravenous injection
▸ Child (body-weight 60 kg and above): 1–2 million units 3 times a day, to be administered into a totally implantable venous access device when giving via slow intravenous injection; maximum 6 million units per day continued →

5

Infection

Adjunct to standard antibacterial therapy for Pseudomonas aeruginosa infection in cystic fibrosis
▶ BY INHALATION OF NEBULISED SOLUTION
▶ Child 1 month–1 year: 0.5–1 million units twice daily, adjusted according to response, increased to 1 million units 3 times daily for subsequent respiratory isolates of Pseudomonas aeruginosa
▶ Child 2–17 years: 1–2 million units twice daily, adjusted according to response, increased to 2 million units 3 times daily for subsequent respiratory isolates of Pseudomonas aeruginosa
▶ BY INHALATION OF POWDER
▶ Child 6–17 years: 1.66 million units twice daily

PROMIXIN® INJECTION

Gram-negative infections resistant to other antibacterials, including those caused by Pseudomonas aeruginosa, Acinetobacter baumanii , Klebsiella pneumoniae
▶ BY SLOW INTRAVENOUS INJECTION, OR BY INTRAVENOUS INFUSION
▶ Child (body-weight up to 40 kg): 75 000–150 000 units/kg daily in 3 divided doses, to be administered into a totally implantable venous access device when giving via slow intravenous injection
▶ Child (body-weight 40 kg and above): 9 million units daily in 2–3 divided doses, to be administered into a totally implantable venous access device when giving via slow intravenous injection

PROMIXIN® NEBULISER SOLUTION

Management of chronic pulmonary infections due to Pseudomonas aeruginosa in patients with cystic fibrosis
▶ BY INHALATION OF NEBULISED SOLUTION
▶ Child 1 month–1 year: 0.5–1 million units twice daily, for specific advice on administration using nebulisers—consult product literature; maximum 2 million units per day
▶ Child 2–17 years: 1–2 million units 2–3 times a day, for specific advice on administration using nebulisers—consult product literature; maximum 6 million units per day

● CONTRA-INDICATIONS Myasthenia gravis
● CAUTIONS
GENERAL CAUTIONS
Acute porphyrias p. 577
SPECIFIC CAUTIONS
▶ When used by inhalation Severe haemoptysis—risk of further haemorrhage
● INTERACTIONS → Appendix 1: colistimethate
● SIDE-EFFECTS
▶ Common or very common
▶ When used by inhalation Bronchospasm · cough · dysphonia · nausea · sore mouth · Sore throat · taste disturbances · vomiting
▶ Uncommon
▶ When used by inhalation Hypersalivation · thirst
▶ Rare
▶ With intravenous use Vasomotor instability
▶ Frequency not known
▶ With intravenous use Apnoea · confusion · headache · muscle weakness · nephrotoxicity · neurotoxicity reported especially with excessive doses · perioral paraesthesia · peripheral paraesthesia · psychosis · rash · slurred speech · vertigo · visual disturbances
SIDE-EFFECTS, FURTHER INFORMATION
▶ Dose-related side-effects The major adverse effects are dose-related neurotoxicity and nephrotoxicity.
● PREGNANCY
▶ When used by inhalation Clinical use suggests probably safe.

▶ With intravenous use Use only if potential benefit outweighs risk.
● BREAST FEEDING Present in milk but poorly absorbed from gut; manufacturers advise avoid (or use only if potential benefit outweighs risk).
● RENAL IMPAIRMENT
▶ With intravenous use Reduce dose. Monitor plasma colistimethate sodium concentration during parenteral treatment—consult product literature. Recommended 'peak' plasma colistimethate sodium concentration (approx. 1 hour after intravenous injection or infusion) 5–15 mg/litre; pre-dose ('trough') concentration 2–6 mg/litre.
● MONITORING REQUIREMENTS
▶ With intravenous use Monitor renal function.
▶ When used by inhalation Measure lung function before and after initial dose of colistimethate sodium and monitor for bronchospasm; if bronchospasm occurs in a patient not using a bronchodilator, repeat test using a bronchodilator before the dose of colistimethate sodium.
● DIRECTIONS FOR ADMINISTRATION
▶ When used by inhalation Other inhaled drugs should be administered before colistimethate sodium. For nebulisation administer required dose in 2–4 mL of sodium chloride 0.9% (or water for injections) or a 1:1 mixture of sodium chloride 0.9% and water for injection.
▶ With intravenous use For intravenous infusion, dilute to a concentration of 40 000 units/mL with Sodium Chloride 0.9%; give over 30 minutes. For slow intravenous injection into a totally implantable venous access device, dilute to a concentration of 90 000 units/mL with Sodium Chloride 0.9% for child under 12 years (200 000 units/mL for child over 12 years).

COLOMYCIN® Colomycin® Injection may be used for nebulisation; administer required dose in 2–4 mL of sodium chloride 0.9%, (or water for injections) or a 1:1 mixture of sodium chloride 0.9% and water for injection.
● PRESCRIBING AND DISPENSING INFORMATION
Colistimethate sodium is included in some preparations for topical application.
● PATIENT AND CARER ADVICE
Driving and skilled tasks
Manufacturer advises patients and carers should be counselled on the effects on driving and performance of skilled tasks—increased risk of dizziness, confusion and visual disturbances.
▶ When used by inhalation Patient should be advised to rinse mouth with water after each dose of dry powder inhalation. Patients or carers should be given advice on how to administer colistimethate sodium; first dose should be given under medical supervision.
● NATIONAL FUNDING/ACCESS DECISIONS
NICE technology appraisals (TAs)
▶ Colistimethate sodium by dry powder inhalation for pseudomonal lung infection in cystic fibrosis (March 2013) NICE TA276
Colistimethate sodium dry powder for inhalation is recommended for chronic pulmonary infection caused by Pseudomonas aeruginosa in patients with cystic fibrosis who would benefit from continued treatment, but do not tolerate the drug in its nebulised form. The manufacturer must provide colistimethate sodium dry powder for inhalation at the discount agreed as part of the patient access scheme to primary, secondary and tertiary care in the NHS. Patients currently receiving colistimethate sodium dry powder for inhalation can continue treatment until they and their clinician consider it appropriate to stop.
www.nice.org.uk/TA276

- **MEDICINAL FORMS**
  There can be variation in the licensing of different medicines containing the same drug.

Powder for solution for injection
ELECTROLYTES: May contain Sodium
▸ Colistimethate sodium (Non-proprietary)
Colistimethate sodium 1000000 unit Colistimethate 1million unit powder for solution for injection vials | 10 vial [PoM] £19.75 | 10 vial [PoM] £16.79 (Hospital only)
▸ Colomycin (Teva UK Ltd)
Colistimethate sodium 1000000 unit Colomycin 1million unit powder for solution for injection vials | 10 vial [PoM] £18.00
Colistimethate sodium 2000000 unit Colomycin 2million unit powder for solution for injection vials | 10 vial [PoM] £32.40
▸ Promixin (Profile Pharma Ltd)
Colistimethate sodium 1000000 unit Promixin 1million unit powder for solution for injection vials | 10 vial [PoM] £30.00 (Hospital only)

Powder for nebuliser solution
▸ ColiFin (Pari Medical Ltd)
Colistimethate sodium 1000000 unit ColiFin 1 MIU powder for nebuliser solution unit dose vials | 56 unit dose [PoM] £180.53
Colistimethate sodium 2000000 unit ColiFin 2 MIU powder for nebuliser solution unit dose vials | 56 unit dose [PoM] £261.72
▸ Promixin (Profile Pharma Ltd)
Colistimethate sodium 1000000 unit Promixin 1million unit powder for nebuliser solution unit dose vials | 30 unit dose [PoM] £168.00 DT price = £168.00

ANTIBACTERIALS > QUINOLONES

Quinolones

Overview

Ciprofloxacin below is active against both Gram-positive and Gram-negative bacteria. It is particularly active against Gram-negative bacteria, including salmonella, shigella, campylobacter, neisseria, and pseudomonas. Ciprofloxacin has only moderate activity against Gram-positive bacteria such as *Streptococcus pneumoniae* and *Enterococcus faecalis*; it should not be used for pneumococcal pneumonia. It is active against chlamydia and some mycobacteria. Most anaerobic organisms are not susceptible. Ciprofloxacin is licensed in children over 1 year of age for pseudomonal infections in cystic fibrosis, for complicated urinary-tract infections, and for treatment and prophylaxis of inhalation anthrax. When the benefits of treatment outweigh the risks, ciprofloxacin is licensed in children over 1 year of age for severe infections of the respiratory tract and of the gastro-intestinal system (including typhoid fever). It is also used in the treatment of septicaemia caused by multi-resistant organisms (usually hospital acquired) and gonorrhoea (although resistance is increasing). Ciprofloxacin is also used in the prophylaxis of meningococcal disease.

Nalidixic acid p. 335 may be used in uncomplicated urinary-tract infections that are resistant to other antibiotics in children over 3 months of age.

Many staphylococci are resistant to quinolones and their use should be avoided in MRSA infections.

Ofloxacin eye drops p. 648 are used in ophthalmic infections.

There is much less experience of the other quinolones in children; expert advice should be sought.

Quinolones

TENDON DAMAGE
Tendon damage (including rupture) has been reported rarely in patients receiving quinolones. Tendon rupture may occur within 48 hours of starting treatment; cases have also been reported several months after stopping a quinolone. Healthcare professionals are reminded that:
- quinolones are contra-indicated in patients with a history of tendon disorders related to quinolone use;
- the risk of tendon damage is increased by the concomitant use of corticosteroids;
- if tendinitis is suspected, the quinolone should be discontinued immediately.

- **CONTRA-INDICATIONS** History of tendon disorders related to quinolone use
- **CAUTIONS** Can prolong the QT interval · children or adolescents (arthropathy has developed in weight-bearing joints in young *animals*) · conditions that predispose to seizures · diabetes (may affect blood glucose) · exposure to excessive sunlight should be avoided (discontinue if photosensitivity occurs) · G6PD deficiency · history of epilepsy · myasthenia gravis (risk of exacerbation)

  CAUTIONS, FURTHER INFORMATION Quinolones cause arthropathy in the weight-bearing joints of immature *animals* and are therefore generally not recommended in children and growing adolescents. However, the significance of this effect in humans is uncertain and in some specific circumstances short-term use of either ciprofloxacin or nalidixic acid may be justified in children.

- **SIDE-EFFECTS**
▸ **Common or very common** Diarrhoea · dizziness · headache · nausea · vomiting
▸ **Uncommon** Abdominal pain · anorexia · anxiety · arthralgia · asthenia · blood disorders · confusion · depression · disturbances in taste · disturbances in vision · dyspepsia · eosinophilia · hallucinations · leucopenia · myalgia · rash · sleep disturbances · thrombocytopenia · tremor
▸ **Rare** Antibiotic-associated colitis · convulsions · disturbances in hearing · disturbances in smell · dyspnoea · hepatic dysfunction · hepatitis · hypotension · interstitial nephritis · jaundice · photosensitivity · psychoses · renal failure · symptoms of peripheral neuropathy (sometimes irreversible) · tendon damage · tendon inflammation · vasculitis
▸ **Very rare** Stevens-Johnson syndrome · toxic epidermal necrolysis

  SIDE-EFFECTS, FURTHER INFORMATION
  The drug should be **discontinued** if psychiatric, neurological, or hypersensitivity reactions (including severe rash) occur.

- **ALLERGY AND CROSS-SENSITIVITY** Use of quinolones contra-indicated in quinolone hypersensitivity.
- **PREGNANCY** Avoid in pregnancy—shown to cause arthropathy in *animal* studies; safer alternatives are available.

 above

Ciprofloxacin

- **INDICATIONS AND DOSE**
Fistulating Crohn's disease
▸ BY MOUTH
▸ Child: 5 mg/kg twice daily
Severe respiratory-tract infections, gastro-intestinal infection
▸ BY MOUTH
▸ Neonate: 15 mg/kg twice daily.

▸ Child: 20 mg/kg twice daily (max. per dose 750 mg)

continued →

Infection

5

▸ BY INTRAVENOUS INFUSION
▸ Neonate: 10 mg/kg every 12 hours, to be given over 60 minutes.

▸ Child: 10 mg/kg every 8 hours (max. per dose 400 mg), to be given over 60 minutes

Pseudomonal lower respiratory-tract infection in cystic fibrosis
▸ BY MOUTH
▸ Child: 20 mg/kg twice daily (max. per dose 750 mg)
▸ BY INTRAVENOUS INFUSION
▸ Child: 10 mg/kg every 8 hours (max. per dose 400 mg), to be given over 60 minutes

Complicated urinary-tract infections
▸ BY MOUTH
▸ Neonate: 10 mg/kg twice daily.

▸ Child: 10 mg/kg twice daily, dose to be doubled in severe infection (max. 750 mg twice daily)
▸ BY INTRAVENOUS INFUSION
▸ Neonate: 6 mg/kg every 12 hours, to be given over 60 minutes.

▸ Child: 6 mg/kg every 8 hours; increased to 10 mg/kg every 8 hours (max. per dose 400 mg), in severe infection

Gonorrhoea
▸ BY MOUTH
▸ Child 12–17 years: 500 mg for 1 dose

Anthrax (treatment and post-exposure prophylaxis)
▸ BY MOUTH
▸ Child: 15 mg/kg twice daily (max. per dose 500 mg)
▸ BY INTRAVENOUS INFUSION
▸ Child: 10 mg/kg every 12 hours (max. per dose 400 mg)

Prevention of secondary case of meningococcal meningitis
▸ BY MOUTH
▸ Neonate: 30 mg/kg (max. per dose 125 mg) for 1 dose.

▸ Child 1 month–4 years: 30 mg/kg (max. per dose 125 mg) for 1 dose
▸ Child 5–11 years: 250 mg for 1 dose
▸ Child 12–17 years: 500 mg for 1 dose

● **UNLICENSED USE** Not licensed for use in children under 1 year of age. Licensed for use in children over 1 year for complicated urinary-tract infections, for pseudomonal lower respiratory-tract infections in cystic fibrosis, for prophylaxis and treatment of inhalational anthrax. Licensed for use in children over 1 year for other infections where the benefit is considered to outweigh the potential risks. Not licensed for use in children for gastro-intestinal anthrax. Not licensed for use in children for prophylaxis of meningococcal meningitis.

● **CAUTIONS** Acute myocardial infarction (risk factor for QT interval prolongation) · avoid excessive alkalinity of urine (risk of crystalluria) · bradycardia (risk factor for QT interval prolongation) · congenital long QT syndrome (risk factor for QT interval prolongation) · electrolyte disturbances (risk factor for QT interval prolongation) · ensure adequate fluid intake (risk of crystalluria) · heart failure with reduced left ventricular ejection fraction (risk factor for QT interval prolongation) · history of symptomatic arrhythmias (risk factor for QT interval prolongation)

● **INTERACTIONS** → Appendix 1: quinolones
● **SIDE-EFFECTS**
▸ **Common or very common** Flatulence
▸ **With intravenous use** Pain at injection site · phlebitis at injection site
▸ **Rare** Abnormal dreams · chest pain · dysphagia · dyspnoea · erythema nodosum · hot flushes · hyperglycaemia ·

hypoglycaemia · oedema · pancreatitis · sweating · syncope · tachycardia
▸ **Very rare** Intracranial hypertension · movement disorders · tenosynovitis · tinnitus · vasculitis
▸ **Frequency not known** Peripheral neuropathy · polyneuropathy

● **PREGNANCY** A single dose of ciprofloxacin may be used for the prevention of a secondary case of meningococcal meningitis.

● **BREAST FEEDING** Amount too small to be harmful but manufacturer advises avoid.

● **RENAL IMPAIRMENT** Reduce dose if estimated glomerular filtration rate less than 30 mL/minute/1.73 m² — consult product literature.

● **PRESCRIBING AND DISPENSING INFORMATION** Flavours of oral liquid formulations may include strawberry.

● **PATIENT AND CARER ADVICE**
Driving and skilled tasks
May impair performance of skilled tasks (e.g. driving); effects enhanced by alcohol.
Medicines for Children leaflet: Ciprofloxacin for bacterial infections www.medicinesforchildren.org.uk/ciprofloxacin-bacterial-infections-0

● **MEDICINAL FORMS**
There can be variation in the licensing of different medicines containing the same drug. Forms available from special-order manufacturers include: oral suspension

Tablet
CAUTIONARY AND ADVISORY LABELS 7, 9, 25
▸ Ciprofloxacin (Non-proprietary)
Ciprofloxacin (as Ciprofloxacin hydrochloride)
100 mg Ciprofloxacin 100mg tablets | 6 tablet [PoM] £4.50 DT price = £1.90
Ciprofloxacin (as Ciprofloxacin hydrochloride)
250 mg Ciprofloxacin 250mg tablets | 10 tablet [PoM] £7.25 DT price = £0.75 | 20 tablet [PoM] £11.20 | 100 tablet [PoM] no price available
Ciprofloxacin (as Ciprofloxacin hydrochloride)
500 mg Ciprofloxacin 500mg tablets | 10 tablet [PoM] £14.00 DT price = £0.89 | 20 tablet [PoM] £21.23 | 100 tablet [PoM] no price available
Ciprofloxacin (as Ciprofloxacin hydrochloride)
750 mg Ciprofloxacin 750mg tablets | 10 tablet [PoM] £20.00 DT price = £8.00 | 20 tablet [PoM] no price available
▸ Ciproxin (Bayer Plc)
Ciprofloxacin (as Ciprofloxacin hydrochloride) 250 mg Ciproxin 250mg tablets | 10 tablet [PoM] £6.59 DT price = £0.75
Ciprofloxacin (as Ciprofloxacin hydrochloride) 500 mg Ciproxin 500mg tablets | 10 tablet [PoM] £12.49 DT price = £0.89
Ciprofloxacin (as Ciprofloxacin hydrochloride) 750 mg Ciproxin 750mg tablets | 10 tablet [PoM] £17.78 DT price = £8.00

Oral suspension
CAUTIONARY AND ADVISORY LABELS 7, 9 25
▸ Ciproxin (Bayer Plc)
Ciproxin 50 mg per 1 ml Ciproxin 250mg/5ml oral suspension | 100 ml [PoM] £21.29 DT price = £21.29

Solution for infusion
ELECTROLYTES: May contain Sodium
▸ Ciprofloxacin (Non-proprietary)
Ciprofloxacin (as Ciprofloxacin lactate 2 mg per 1 ml Ciprofloxacin 400mg/200ml solution for infusion bottles | 5 bottle [PoM] £19.59
Ciprofloxacin 400mg/200ml solution for infusion vials | 1 vial [PoM] £19.79 (Hospital only)
Ciprofloxacin 200mg/100ml solution for infusion bottles | 10 bottle [PoM] £14.45
▸ Ciproxin (Bayer Plc)
Ciprofloxacin (as Ciprofloxacin lactate) 2 mg per 1 ml Ciproxin Infusion 100mg/50ml solution for infusion bottles | 1 bottle [PoM] £7.61 (Hospital only)
Ciproxin Infusion 400mg/200ml solution for infusion bottles | 5 bottle [PoM] £114.23 (Hospital only)
Ciproxin Infusion 200mg/100ml solution for infusion bottles | 5 bottle [PoM] £75.06 (Hospital only)

Infusion

▸ Ciprofloxacin (Non-proprietary)
  Ciprofloxacin (as Ciprofloxacin lactate) 2 mg per
  1 ml Ciprofloxacin 400mg/200ml infusion bags | 10 bag PoM
  £200.00

F 333

Nalidixic acid

- **INDICATIONS AND DOSE**

Treatment of urinary tract infection resistant to other antibiotics

▸ BY MOUTH

- Child 3 months–11 years: 12.5 mg/kg 4 times a day for 7 days, then reduced to 7.5 mg/kg 4 times a day for prolonged therapy in chronic infections
- Child 12–17 years: 900 mg 4 times a day for 7 days, then reduced to 600 mg 4 times a day for prolonged therapy in chronic infections

Prophylaxis of urinary tract infections resistant to other antibiotics

▸ BY MOUTH

- Child 3 months–11 years: 15 mg/kg twice daily

- **CAUTIONS** Acute myocardial infarction (risk factor for QT interval prolongation) · avoid in acute porphyrias p. 577 · bradycardia (risk factor for QT interval prolongation) · congenital long QT syndrome (risk factor for QT interval prolongation) · electrolyte disturbances (risk factor for QT interval prolongation) · heart failure with reduced left ventricular ejection fraction (risk factor for QT interval prolongation) · history of symptomatic arrhythmias (risk factor for QT interval prolongation)

- **INTERACTIONS** → Appendix 1: quinolones

- **SIDE-EFFECTS** Cranial nerve palsy · increased intracranial pressure · metabolic acidosis · peripheral neuropathy · toxic psychosis

- **BREAST FEEDING** Risk to infant very small but one case of haemolytic anaemia reported.

- **HEPATIC IMPAIRMENT** Manufacturer advises caution in liver disease.

- **RENAL IMPAIRMENT** Use with caution; avoid if estimated glomerular filtration rate less than 20 mL/minute/1.73 m².

- **MONITORING REQUIREMENTS** Monitor blood counts, renal and liver function if treatment exceeds 2 weeks.

- **EFFECT ON LABORATORY TESTS** False positive urinary glucose (if tested for reducing substances).

- **PRESCRIBING AND DISPENSING INFORMATION** Flavours of oral liquid formulations may include raspberry and strawberry.

- **MEDICINAL FORMS**
  There can be variation in the licensing of different medicines containing the same drug.
  No licensed medicines listed.

ANTIBACTERIALS ⟩ SULFONAMIDES

Co-trimoxazole

- **DRUG ACTION** Sulfamethoxazole and trimethoprim are used in combination (as **co-trimoxazole**) because of their synergistic activity (the importance of the sulfonamides has decreased as a result of increasing bacterial resistance and their replacement by antibacterials which are generally more active and less toxic).

- **INDICATIONS AND DOSE**

Treatment of susceptible infections

▸ BY MOUTH

- Child 6 weeks–5 months: 120 mg twice daily, alternatively 24 mg/kg twice daily
- Child 6 months–5 years: 240 mg twice daily, alternatively 24 mg/kg twice daily
- Child 6–11 years: 480 mg twice daily, alternatively 24 mg/kg twice daily
- Child 12–17 years: 960 mg twice daily

▸ BY INTRAVENOUS INFUSION

- Child 6 weeks–17 years: 18 mg/kg every 12 hours; increased to 27 mg/kg every 12 hours (max. per dose 1.44 g), increased dose used in severe infection

Treatment of *Pneumocystis jirovecii* (*Pneumocystis carinii*) infections (undertaken where facilities for appropriate monitoring available—consult microbiologist and product literature)

▸ BY MOUTH, OR BY INTRAVENOUS INFUSION

- Child: 120 mg/kg daily in 2–4 divided doses for 14–21 days, oral route preferred for children

Prophylaxis of *Pneumocystis jirovecii* (*Pneumocystis carinii*) infections

▸ BY MOUTH

- Child: 450 mg/m² twice daily (max. per dose 960 mg twice daily) for 3 days of the week (either consecutively or on alternate days), dose regimens may vary, consult local guidelines

DOSE EQUIVALENCE AND CONVERSION

▸ 480 mg of co-trimoxazole consists of sulfamethoxazole 400 mg and trimethoprim 80 mg.

- **UNLICENSED USE** Not licensed for *Burkholderia cepacia* infections in cystic fibrosis. Not licensed for *Stenotrophomonas maltophilia* infections. Not licensed for use in children under 6 weeks.

> **IMPORTANT SAFETY INFORMATION**
> RESTRICTIONS ON THE USE OF CO-TRIMOXAZOLE
> Co-trimoxazole is the drug of choice in the prophylaxis and treatment of *Pneumocystis jirovecii* (*Pneumocystis carinii*) pneumonia; it is also indicated for nocardiasis, *Stenotrophomonas maltophilia* infection [unlicensed indication], and toxoplasmosis. It should only be considered for use in acute exacerbations of chronic bronchitis and infections of the urinary tract when there is bacteriological evidence of sensitivity to co-trimoxazole and good reason to prefer this combination to a single antibacterial; similarly it should only be used in acute otitis media in children when there is good reason to prefer it. Co-trimoxazole is also used for the treatment of infections caused by *Burkholderia cepacia* in cystic fibrosis [unlicensed indication].

- **CONTRA-INDICATIONS** Acute porphyrias p. 577

- **CAUTIONS** Asthma · avoid in blood disorders (unless under specialist supervision) · avoid in infants under 6 weeks (except for treatment or prophylaxis of pneumocystis pneumonia) because of the risk of kernicterus · G6PD deficiency (risk of haemolytic anaemia) · maintain adequate fluid intake · predisposition to folate deficiency

5

Infection

- **INTERACTIONS** → Appendix 1: sulfamethoxazole, trimethoprim
- **SIDE-EFFECTS**
  ‣ **Common or very common** Diarrhoea · headache · hyperkalaemia · nausea · rash
  ‣ **Uncommon** Vomiting
  ‣ **Rare** Agranulocytosis · bone marrow depression
  ‣ **Very rare** Anorexia · antibiotic-associated colitis · arthralgia · aseptic meningitis · ataxia · blood disorders · convulsions · cough · depression · eosinophilia · glossitis · hallucinations · hepatic necrosis · hypoglycaemia · hyponatraemia · interstitial nephritis · jaundice · leucopenia · liver damage · megaloblastic anaemia · myalgia · myocarditis · pancreatitis · peripheral neuropathy · photosensitivity · pulmonary infiltrates · renal disorders · shortness of breath · Stevens-Johnson syndrome · stomatitis · systemic lupus erythematosus · thrombocytopenia · tinnitus · toxic epidermal necrolysis · uveitis · vasculitis · vertigo
  ‣ **Frequency not known** Rhabdomyolysis reported in HIV-infected patients
  SIDE-EFFECTS, FURTHER INFORMATION
  ‣ **Blood disorders or rash** Co-trimoxazole is associated with rare but serious side effects. Discontinue immediately if blood disorders (including leucopenia, thrombocytopenia, megaloblastic anaemia, eosinophilia) or rash (including Stevens-Johnson syndrome, toxic epidermal necrolysis, photosensitivity) develop.
- **PREGNANCY** Teratogenic risk in first trimester (trimethoprim a folate antagonist). Neonatal haemolysis and methaemoglobinaemia in third trimester; fear of increased risk of kernicterus in neonates appears to be unfounded.
- **BREAST FEEDING** Small risk of kernicterus in jaundiced infants and of haemolysis in G6PD-deficient infants (due to sulfamethoxazole).
- **HEPATIC IMPAIRMENT** Manufacturer advises avoid in severe liver disease.
- **RENAL IMPAIRMENT** Use half normal dose if estimated glomerular filtration rate 15–30 mL/minute/1.73 m^2. Avoid if estimated glomerular filtration rate less than 15 mL/minute/1.73 m^2 and if plasma-sulfamethoxazole concentration cannot be monitored. Plasma concentration monitoring may be required in patients with moderate to severe renal impairment; seek expert advice.
- **MONITORING REQUIREMENTS**
  ‣ Plasma concentration monitoring may be required with high doses; seek expert advice.
  ‣ Monitor blood counts on prolonged treatment.
- **DIRECTIONS FOR ADMINISTRATION** For intermittent *intravenous infusion*, may be further diluted in glucose 5% and 10% or sodium chloride 0.9%. Dilute contents of 1 ampoule (5 mL) to 125 mL, 2 ampoules (10 mL) to 250 mL or 3 ampoules (15 mL) to 500 mL; suggested duration of infusion 60–90 minutes (but may be adjusted according to fluid requirements); if fluid restriction necessary, 1 ampoule (5 mL) may be diluted with 75 mL glucose 5% and the required dose infused over max. 60 minutes; check container for haze or precipitant during administration. In severe fluid restriction may be given undiluted via a central venous line.
- **PRESCRIBING AND DISPENSING INFORMATION** Co-trimoxazole is a mixture of trimethoprim and sulfamethoxazole (sulphamethoxazole) in the proportions of 1 part to 5 parts.
  Flavours of oral liquid formulations may include banana, or vanilla.

- **MEDICINAL FORMS**
  There can be variation in the licensing of different medicines containing the same drug.
  Solution for infusion
  EXCIPIENTS: May contain Alcohol, propylene glycol, sulfites
  ELECTROLYTES: May contain Sodium
  ‣ Co-trimoxazole (Non-proprietary)
    Trimethoprim 16 mg per 1 ml, Sulfamethoxazole 80 mg per 1 ml Co-trimoxazole 80mg/400mg/5ml solution for infusion ampoules | 10 ampoule [PoM] £35.00
  ‣ Septrin (Aspen Pharma Trading Ltd)
    Trimethoprim 16 mg per 1 ml, Sulfamethoxazole 80 mg per 1 ml Septrin for Infusion 80mg/400mg/5ml solution for infusion ampoules | 10 ampoule [PoM] £17.76
  Oral suspension
  CAUTIONARY AND ADVISORY LABELS 9
  ‣ Co-trimoxazole (Non-proprietary)
    Trimethoprim 8 mg per 1 ml, Sulfamethoxazole 40 mg per 1 ml Co-trimoxazole 40mg/200mg/5ml oral suspension sugar free sugar-free | 100 ml [PoM] £9.95 DT price = £9.95
    Trimethoprim 16 mg per 1 ml, Sulfamethoxazole 80 mg per 1 ml Co-trimoxazole 80mg/400mg/5ml oral suspension | 100 ml [PoM] £10.95 DT price = £10.95
  Tablet
  CAUTIONARY AND ADVISORY LABELS 9
  ‣ Co-trimoxazole (Non-proprietary)
    Trimethoprim 80 mg, Sulfamethoxazole 400 mg Co-trimoxazole 80mg/400mg tablets | 28 tablet [PoM] £15.50 DT price = £2.51 | 100 tablet [PoM] £8.96-£10.91
    Trimethoprim 160 mg, Sulfamethoxazole 300 mg Co-trimoxazole 160mg/800mg tablets | 100 tablet [PoM] £23.40-£24.00 DT price = £23.46

Sulfadiazine

(Sulphadiazine)

- **DRUG ACTION** Sulfadiazine is a short-acting sulphonamide with bacteriostatic activity against a broad spectrum of organisms. The importance of the sulphonamides has decreased as a result of increasing bacterial resistance and their replacement by antibacterials which are generally more active and less toxic.

- **INDICATIONS AND DOSE**
  Toxoplasmosis in pregnancy (in combination with pyrimethamine and folinic acid)
  ‣ BY MOUTH
  ‣ Child 12-17 years: 1 g 3 times a day until delivery
  Congenital toxoplasmosis (in combination with pyrimethamine and folinic acid)
  ‣ BY MOUTH
  ‣ Neonate: 50 mg/kg twice daily for 12 months.

- **UNLICENSED USE** Not licensed for use in toxoplasmosis.
- **CONTRA-INDICATIONS** Acute porphyrias p. 577
- **CAUTIONS** Asthma · avoid in blood disorders (unless under specialist supervision) · avoid in infants under 6 weeks (except for treatment or prophylaxis of *pneumocystis pneumonia*) because of the risk of kernicterus · G6PD deficiency (risk of haemolytic anaemia) · maintain adequate fluid intake · predisposition to folate deficiency
- **INTERACTIONS** → Appendix 1: sulfonamides
- **SIDE-EFFECTS**
  ‣ **Common or very common** Diarrhoea · headache · hyperkalaemia · nausea · rash
  ‣ **Uncommon** Vomiting
  ‣ **Rare** Agranulocytosis · bone marrow depression
  ‣ **Very rare** Anorexia · antibiotic-associated colitis · arthralgia · aseptic meningitis · ataxia · blood disorders · convulsions · cough · depression · eosinophilia · glossitis · hallucinations · hepatic necrosis · hypoglycaemia · hyponatraemia · interstitial nephritis · jaundice ·

leucopenia · liver damage · megaloblastic anaemia · myalgia · myocarditis · pancreatitis · peripheral neuropathy · photosensitivity · pulmonary infiltrates · renal disorders · shortness of breath · Stevens-Johnson syndrome · stomatitis · systemic lupus erythematosus · thrombocytopenia · tinnitus · toxic epidermal necrolysis · uveitis · vasculitis · vertigo
▸ **Frequency not known** Benign intracranial hypertension · hypothyroidism · optic neuropathy · rhabdomyolysis reported in HIV-infected patients
SIDE-EFFECTS, FURTHER INFORMATION
▸ Blood disorders or rash Discontinue immediately if blood disorders (including leucopenia, thrombocytopenia, megaloblastic anaemia, eosinophilia) or rash (including Stevens-Johnson syndrome, toxic epidermal necrolysis, photosensitivity) develop.
● **PREGNANCY** Risk of neonatal haemolysis and methaemoglobinaemia in third trimester; fear of increased risk of kernicterus in neonates appears to be unfounded.
● **BREAST FEEDING** Small risk of kernicterus in jaundiced infants and of haemolysis in G6PD-deficient infants.
● **HEPATIC IMPAIRMENT** Use with caution in mild to moderate impairment; avoid in severe impairment.
● **RENAL IMPAIRMENT** Use with caution in mild to moderate impairment; avoid in severe impairment; high risk of crystalluria.
● **MONITORING REQUIREMENTS** Monitor blood counts on prolonged treatment.

● **MEDICINAL FORMS**
There can be variation in the licensing of different medicines containing the same drug. Forms available from special-order manufacturers include: oral suspension
Tablet
CAUTIONARY AND ADVISORY LABELS 9, 27
▸ **Sulfadiazine (Non-proprietary)**
Sulfadiazine 500 mg Sulfadiazine 500mg tablets | 56 tablet [PoM] £139.62 DT price = £114.27

ANTIBACTERIALS › TETRACYCLINES AND RELATED DRUGS

Tetracyclines

Overview

The tetracyclines are broad-spectrum antibiotics whose value has decreased owing to increasing bacterial resistance. In children over 12 years of age they are useful for infections caused by chlamydia (trachoma, psittacosis, salpingitis, urethritis, and lymphogranuloma venereum), rickettsia (including Q-fever), brucella (doxycycline p. 338 with either streptomycin p. 299 or rifampicin p. 349), and the spirochaete, *Borrelia burgdorferi* (See Lyme disease). They are also used in respiratory and genital mycoplasma infections, in acne, in destructive (refractory) periodontal disease, in exacerbations of chronic respiratory diseases (because of their activity against *Haemophilus influenzae*), and for leptospirosis in penicillin hypersensitivity (as an alternative to erythromycin p. 316).

Microbiologically, there is little to choose between the various tetracyclines, the only exception being minocycline p. 339 which has a broader spectrum; it is active against *Neisseria meningitidis* and has been used for meningococcal prophylaxis but is no longer recommended because of side-effects including dizziness and vertigo. Compared to other tetracyclines, minocycline is associated with a greater risk of lupus-erythematosus-like syndrome. Minocycline sometimes causes irreversible pigmentation.

Tetracyclines have a role in the management of meticillin-resistant *Staphylococcus aureus* (MRSA) infections.

Tetracyclines

● **CONTRA-INDICATIONS** Children under 12 years (deposition in growing bone and teeth, by binding to calcium, causes staining and occasionally dental hypoplasia)
● **CAUTIONS** Myasthenia gravis (muscle weakness may be increased) · systemic lupus erythematosus (may be exacerbated)
● **SIDE-EFFECTS**
▸ **Rare** Anaphylaxis · angioedema · blood disorders · exfoliative dermatitis · hepatotoxicity · hypersensitivity reactions · pancreatitis · pericarditis · photosensitivity (particularly with demeclocycline) · rash · Stevens-Johnson syndrome · urticaria
▸ **Frequency not known** Antibiotic-associated colitis · benign intracranial hypertension · bulging fontanelles (in infants) · diarrhoea · dysphagia · headache · nausea · oesophageal irritation · visual disturbances · vomiting
SIDE-EFFECTS, FURTHER INFORMATION
▸ Benign intracranial hypertension Headache and visual disturbances may indicate benign intracranial hypertension (discontinue treatment).
● **PREGNANCY** Should **not** be given to pregnant women; effects on skeletal development have been documented in the first trimester in *animal* studies. Administration during the second or third trimester may cause discoloration of the child's teeth, and maternal hepatotoxicity has been reported with large parenteral doses.
● **BREAST FEEDING** Should **not** be given to women who are breast-feeding (although absorption and therefore discoloration of teeth in the infant is probably usually prevented by chelation with calcium in milk).
● **HEPATIC IMPAIRMENT** Should be avoided or used with caution in patients with hepatic impairment.

☛ above

Demeclocycline hydrochloride

● **INDICATIONS AND DOSE**
Susceptible infections (e.g. chlamydia, rickettsia and mycoplasma)
▸ BY MOUTH
▸ Child 12–17 years: 150 mg 4 times a day, alternatively 300 mg twice daily

● **CAUTIONS** Photosensitivity more common than with other tetracyclines
● **INTERACTIONS** → Appendix 1: tetracyclines
● **SIDE-EFFECTS** Acute renal failure · reversible nephrogenic diabetes insipidus
● **HEPATIC IMPAIRMENT** Max. 1 g daily in divided doses.
● **RENAL IMPAIRMENT** May exacerbate renal failure and should **not** be given to patients with renal impairment.
● **PATIENT AND CARER ADVICE** Patients should be advised to avoid exposure to sunlight or sun lamps.

● **MEDICINAL FORMS**
There can be variation in the licensing of different medicines containing the same drug. Forms available from special-order manufacturers include: oral suspension, oral solution
Tablet
▸ **Demeclocycline hydrochloride (Non-proprietary)**
Demeclocycline hydrochloride 150 mg Demeclocycline 150mg tablets | 100 tablet [PoM] no price available
Capsule
CAUTIONARY AND ADVISORY LABELS 7, 9, 11, 23
▸ **Demeclocycline hydrochloride (Non-proprietary)**
Demeclocycline hydrochloride 150 mg Demeclocycline 150mg capsules | 28 capsule [PoM] £160.89 DT price = £160.89

5

Infection

Doxycycline

F 337

- **INDICATIONS AND DOSE**

Susceptible infections (e.g. chlamydia, rickettsia and mycoplasma)
▸ BY MOUTH USING IMMEDIATE-RELEASE MEDICINES
▸ Child 12–17 years: Initially 200 mg daily for 1 dose, then maintenance 100 mg once daily

Severe infections (including refractory urinary-tract infections)
▸ BY MOUTH USING IMMEDIATE-RELEASE MEDICINES
▸ Child 12–17 years: 200 mg daily

Acne
▸ BY MOUTH USING IMMEDIATE-RELEASE MEDICINES
▸ Child 12–17 years: 100 mg once daily

Early syphilis
▸ BY MOUTH USING IMMEDIATE-RELEASE MEDICINES
▸ Child 12–17 years: 100 mg twice daily for 14 days

Late latent syphilis
▸ BY MOUTH USING IMMEDIATE-RELEASE MEDICINES
▸ Child 12–17 years: 100 mg twice daily for 28 days

Uncomplicated genital chlamydia | Non-gonococcal urethritis
▸ BY MOUTH USING IMMEDIATE-RELEASE MEDICINES
▸ Child 12–17 years: 100 mg twice daily for 7 days

Pelvic inflammatory disease
▸ BY MOUTH USING IMMEDIATE-RELEASE MEDICINES
▸ Child 12–17 years: 100 mg twice daily for 14 days

Lyme disease (under expert supervision)
▸ BY MOUTH USING IMMEDIATE-RELEASE MEDICINES
▸ Child 12–17 years: 100 mg twice daily for 10–14 days (for 28 days in Lyme arthritis)

Anthrax (treatment or post-exposure prophylaxis)
▸ BY MOUTH USING IMMEDIATE-RELEASE MEDICINES
▸ Child 1 month–11 years: 2.5 mg/kg twice daily (max. per dose 100 mg twice daily), only to be used in children under 12 years if alternative antibacterial cannot be given
▸ Child 12–17 years: 100 mg twice daily

Prophylaxis of malaria
▸ BY MOUTH USING IMMEDIATE-RELEASE MEDICINES
▸ Child 12–17 years: 100 mg once daily, to be started 1–2 days before entering endemic area and continued for 4 weeks after leaving, can be used for up to 2 years

Adjunct to quinine in treatment of *Plasmodium falciparum* malaria
▸ BY MOUTH USING IMMEDIATE-RELEASE MEDICINES
▸ Child 12–17 years: 200 mg daily for 7 days

Periodontitis (as an adjunct to gingival scaling and root planing)
▸ BY MOUTH USING IMMEDIATE-RELEASE MEDICINES
▸ Child 12–17 years: 20 mg twice daily for 3 months

- **UNLICENSED USE** Not licensed for use in children under 12 years. Doxycycline doses in BNF Publications may differ from those in product literature. Not licensed for severe recurrent aphthous ulceration. Not licensed for malaria prophylaxis during pregnancy. Not licensed for treatment or post-exposure prophylaxis of anthrax.
- **CAUTIONS** Alcohol dependence
- **INTERACTIONS** → Appendix 1: tetracyclines
- **SIDE-EFFECTS** Anorexia · anxiety · dry mouth · flushing · fungal superinfection (when used for periodontitis) · tinnitus
- **PREGNANCY** When travel to malarious areas is unavoidable during pregnancy, doxycycline can be used for malaria prophylaxis if other regimens are unsuitable,

and if the entire course of doxycycline can be completed before 15 weeks' gestation.
- **RENAL IMPAIRMENT** Use with caution (avoid excessive doses).
- **MONITORING REQUIREMENTS** When used for periodontitis, monitor for superficial fungal infection particularly if predisposition to oral candidiasis.
- **DIRECTIONS FOR ADMINISTRATION** Capsules and Tablets should be swallowed whole with plenty of fluid, while sitting or standing. Capsules should be taken during meals.
- **PATIENT AND CARER ADVICE** Counselling on administration advised (posture).
Photosensitivity Patients should be advised to avoid exposure to sunlight or sun lamps.
- **PROFESSION SPECIFIC INFORMATION**
Dental practitioners' formulary
Doxycycline Capsules 100 mg may be prescribed. Dispersible tablets may be prescribed as Dispersible Doxycycline Tablets. Tablets may be prescribed as Doxycycline Tablets 20 mg.

- **MEDICINAL FORMS**
There can be variation in the licensing of different medicines containing the same drug. Forms available from special-order manufacturers include: oral suspension, oral solution

Tablet
CAUTIONARY AND ADVISORY LABELS 6, 11, 27
▸ Periostat (Alliance Pharmaceuticals Ltd)
Doxycycline (as Doxycycline hyclate) 20 mg Periostat 20mg tablets | 56 tablet [PoM] £17.30 DT price = £17.30

Dispersible tablet
CAUTIONARY AND ADVISORY LABELS 6, 9, 11, 13
▸ Vibramycin-D (Pfizer Ltd)
Doxycycline (as Doxycycline monohydrate) 100 mg Vibramycin-D 100mg dispersible tablets sugar-free | 8 tablet [PoM] £4.91 DT price = £4.91

Capsule
CAUTIONARY AND ADVISORY LABELS 6, 9, 11, 27
▸ Doxycycline (Non-proprietary)
Doxycycline (as Doxycycline hyclate) 50 mg Doxycycline 50mg capsules | 28 capsule [PoM] £2.26 DT price = £1.29
Doxycycline (as Doxycycline hyclate) 100 mg Doxycycline 100mg capsules | 8 capsule [PoM] £1.44 DT price = £0.87 | 50 capsule [PoM] £5.44

Lymecycline

F 337

- **INDICATIONS AND DOSE**

Susceptible infections (e.g. chlamydia, rickettsia and mycoplasma)
▸ BY MOUTH
▸ Child 12–17 years: 408 mg twice daily, increased to 1.224–1.632 g daily, (in severe infection)

Acne
▸ BY MOUTH
▸ Child 12–17 years: 408 mg daily for at least 8 weeks

- **INTERACTIONS** → Appendix 1: tetracyclines
- **RENAL IMPAIRMENT** May exacerbate renal failure and should **not** be given to patients with renal impairment.

- **MEDICINAL FORMS**
There can be variation in the licensing of different medicines containing the same drug.

Capsule
CAUTIONARY AND ADVISORY LABELS 6, 9
▸ Lymecycline (Non-proprietary)
Lymecycline 408 mg Lymecycline 408mg capsules | 28 capsule [PoM] £6.95 DT price = £5.14 | 56 capsule [PoM] £11.66
▸ Tetralysal (Galderma (UK) Ltd)
Lymecycline 408 mg Tetralysal 300 capsules | 28 capsule [PoM] £6.95 DT price = £5.14 | 56 capsule [PoM] £11.53

☞ 337

Minocycline

● **INDICATIONS AND DOSE**

Susceptible infections (e.g. chlamydia, rickettsia and mycoplasma)
▶ BY MOUTH USING IMMEDIATE-RELEASE MEDICINES
▶ Child 12–17 years: 100 mg twice daily

Acne
▶ BY MOUTH USING IMMEDIATE-RELEASE MEDICINES
▶ Child 12–17 years: 100 mg once daily, alternatively 50 mg twice daily
▶ BY MOUTH USING MODIFIED-RELEASE MEDICINES
▶ Child 12–17 years: 100 mg daily

● **CAUTIONS** Systemic lupus erythematosus
● **INTERACTIONS** → Appendix 1: tetracyclines
● **SIDE-EFFECTS**
▶ **Rare** Acute renal failure · alopecia · anorexia · hyperaesthesia · impaired hearing · paraesthesia · pigmentation (sometimes irreversible) · tinnitus
▶ **Very rare** Discoloration of conjunctiva · discoloration of sweat · discoloration of tears · systemic lupus erythematosus
▶ **Frequency not known** Dizziness (more common in women) · vertigo (more common in women)
● **RENAL IMPAIRMENT** Use with caution (avoid excessive doses).
● **MONITORING REQUIREMENTS** If treatment continued for longer than 6 months, monitor every 3 months for hepatotoxicity, pigmentation and for systemic lupus erythematosus—discontinue if these develop or if pre-existing systemic lupus erythematosus worsens.
● **DIRECTIONS FOR ADMINISTRATION** Tablets or capsules should be swallowed whole with plenty of fluid while sitting or standing.
● **PATIENT AND CARER ADVICE** Counselling on administration advised (posture).
● **LESS SUITABLE FOR PRESCRIBING** Less suitable for prescribing (compared with other tetracyclines, minocycline is associated with a greater risk of lupus-erythematosus-like syndrome; it sometimes causes irreversible pigmentation).

● **MEDICINAL FORMS**
There can be variation in the licensing of different medicines containing the same drug. Forms available from special-order manufacturers include: oral suspension, oral solution
Tablet
CAUTIONARY AND ADVISORY LABELS 6, 9
▶ Minocycline (Non-proprietary)
Minocycline (as Minocycline hydrochloride) 50 mg Minocycline 50mg tablets | 28 tablet PoM £8.50 DT price = £6.19
Minocycline (as Minocycline hydrochloride) 100 mg Minocycline 100mg tablets | 28 tablet PoM £14.50 DT price = £14.01
Modified-release capsule
CAUTIONARY AND ADVISORY LABELS 6, 25
▶ Minocycline (Non-proprietary)
Minocycline (as Minocycline hydrochloride) 100 mg Minocycline 100mg modified-release capsules | 56 capsule PoM £24.75 DT price = £20.08
▶ Acnamino MR (Dexcel-Pharma Ltd)
Minocycline (as Minocycline hydrochloride) 100 mg Acnamino MR 100mg capsules | 56 capsule PoM £21.14 DT price = £20.08
▶ Minocin MR (Meda Pharmaceuticals Ltd)
Minocycline (as Minocycline hydrochloride) 100 mg Minocin MR 100mg capsules | 56 capsule PoM £20.08 DT price = £20.08
Capsule
CAUTIONARY AND ADVISORY LABELS 6, 9
▶ Aknemin (Almirall Ltd)
Minocycline (as Minocycline hydrochloride) 50 mg Aknemin 50 capsules | 56 capsule PoM £15.27 DT price = £15.27
Minocycline (as Minocycline hydrochloride) 100 mg Aknemin 100mg capsules | 28 capsule PoM £13.09 DT price = £13.09

☞ 337

Oxytetracycline

● **INDICATIONS AND DOSE**

Susceptible infections (e.g. chlamydia, rickettsia and mycoplasma)
▶ BY MOUTH
▶ Child 12–17 years: 250–500 mg 4 times a day

Acne
▶ BY MOUTH
▶ Child 12–17 years: 500 mg twice daily for at least 3 months, if there is no improvement after the first 3 months another oral antibacterial should be used, maximum improvement usually occurs after 4 to 6 months but in more severe cases treatment may need to be continued for 2 years or longer

● **INTERACTIONS** → Appendix 1: tetracyclines
● **RENAL IMPAIRMENT** May exacerbate renal failure and should **not** be given to patients with renal impairment.
● **PROFESSION SPECIFIC INFORMATION**
Dental practitioners' formulary
Oxytetracycline Tablets may be prescribed.

● **MEDICINAL FORMS**
There can be variation in the licensing of different medicines containing the same drug. Forms available from special-order manufacturers include: oral suspension
Tablet
CAUTIONARY AND ADVISORY LABELS 7, 9, 23
▶ Oxytetracycline (Non-proprietary)
Oxytetracycline (as Oxytetracycline dihydrate)
250 mg Oxytetracycline 250mg tablets | 28 tablet PoM £3.45 DT price = £1.07 | 1000 tablet PoM no price available

☞ 337

Tetracycline

● **INDICATIONS AND DOSE**

Susceptible infections (e.g. chlamydia, rickettsia, mycoplasma)
▶ BY MOUTH
▶ Child 12–17 years: 250 mg 4 times a day, increased if necessary to 500 mg 3–4 times a day, increased dose used in severe infections

Acne
▶ BY MOUTH
▶ Child 12–17 years: 500 mg twice daily for at least 3 months, if there is no improvement after the first 3 months another oral antibacterial should be used, maximum improvement usually occurs after 4 to 6 months but in more severe cases treatment may need to be continued for 2 years or longer

Non-gonococcal urethritis
▶ BY MOUTH
▶ Child 12–17 years: 500 mg 4 times a day for 7–14 days (21 days if failure or relapse after first course)

● **INTERACTIONS** → Appendix 1: tetracyclines
● **SIDE-EFFECTS** Acute renal failure · skin discoloration
● **HEPATIC IMPAIRMENT** Max. 1 g daily in divided doses.
● **RENAL IMPAIRMENT** May exacerbate renal failure and should **not** be given to patients with renal impairment.
● **DIRECTIONS FOR ADMINISTRATION** Tablets should be swallowed whole with plenty of fluid while sitting or standing.
● **PATIENT AND CARER ADVICE** Counselling on administration advised.
● **PROFESSION SPECIFIC INFORMATION**
Dental practitioners' formulary
Tetracycline Tablets may be prescribed.

● **MEDICINAL FORMS**
There can be variation in the licensing of different medicines containing the same drug. Forms available from special-order manufacturers include: capsule, oral solution

Tablet
CAUTIONARY AND ADVISORY LABELS 7, 9, 23
▸ Tetracycline (Non-proprietary)
Tetracycline hydrochloride 250 mg Tetracycline 250mg tablets | 28 tablet [PoM] £13.90 DT price = £1.82

ANTIBACTERIALS > OTHER

Chloramphenicol

● **DRUG ACTION** Chloramphenicol is a potent broad-spectrum antibiotic.

● **INDICATIONS AND DOSE**

Life threatening infections particularly those caused by *Haemophilus infuenzae* | Typhoid fever
▸ BY MOUTH, OR BY INTRAVENOUS INJECTION, OR BY INTRAVENOUS INFUSION
▸ Child: 12.5 mg/kg every 6 hours, dose may be doubled in severe infections such as septicaemia, meningitis and epiglottitis providing plasma-chloramphenicol concentrations are measured and high doses reduced as soon as indicated
▸ BY INTRAVENOUS INJECTION
▸ Neonate up to 14 days: 12.5 mg/kg twice daily, doses should be checked carefully as overdosage can be fatal.

▸ Neonate 14 days to 28 days: 12.5 mg/kg 2–4 times a day, doses should be checked carefully as overdosage can be fatal.

Cystic fibrosis for the treatment of respiratory *Burkholderia cepacia* infection resistant to other antibacterials
▸ BY MOUTH, OR BY INTRAVENOUS INFUSION, OR BY INTRAVENOUS INJECTION
▸ Child: (consult product literature)

● **CONTRA-INDICATIONS** Acute porphyrias p. 577
● **CAUTIONS** Avoid repeated courses and prolonged treatment
● **INTERACTIONS** → Appendix 1: chloramphenicol
● **SIDE-EFFECTS**
Blood disorders · depression · diarrhoea · dry mouth · erythema multiforme · glossitis · grey syndrome (in neonates) · headache · nausea · nocturnal haemoglobinuria · optic neuritis · peripheral neuritis · reversible and irreversible aplastic anaemia (with reports of resulting leukaemia) · stomatitis · urticaria · vomiting
SIDE-EFFECTS, FURTHER INFORMATION
Associated with serious haematological side-effects when given systemically and should therefore be reserved for the treatment of life-threatening infections.
▸ With intravenous use in neonates Grey syndrome (abdominal distension, pallid cyanosis, circulatory collapse) may follow excessive doses in neonates with immature hepatic metabolism.
● **PREGNANCY** Manufacturer advises avoid; neonatal 'grey-baby syndrome' if used in third trimester.
● **BREAST FEEDING** Manufacturer advises avoid; use another antibiotic; may cause bone-marrow toxicity in infant; concentration in milk usually insufficient to cause 'grey syndrome'.
● **HEPATIC IMPAIRMENT** Reduce dose. Avoid if possible— increased risk of bone-marrow depression. Monitor plasma-chloramphenicol concentration in hepatic impairment.

● **RENAL IMPAIRMENT** Avoid in severe renal impairment unless no alternative; dose-related depression of haematopoiesis.
● **MONITORING REQUIREMENTS**
▸ Plasma concentration monitoring preferred in those under 4 years of age.
▸ Plasma concentration monitoring required in neonates. Grey baby syndrome may follow excessive doses in neonates with immature hepatic metabolism.
▸ Recommended peak plasma concentration (approx. 2 hours after administration by mouth, intravenous injection or infusion) 10–25 mg/litre; pre-dose ('trough') concentration should not exceed 15 mg/litre.
▸ Blood counts required before and periodically during treatment.
● **DIRECTIONS FOR ADMINISTRATION** Displacement value may be significant for injection, consult local guidelines. For intermittent intravenous infusion dilute reconstituted solution further in glucose 5% or sodium chloride 0.9%.
● **MEDICINAL FORMS**
There can be variation in the licensing of different medicines containing the same drug.
Powder for solution for injection
ELECTROLYTES: May contain Sodium
▸ Chloramphenicol (Non-proprietary)
Chloramphenicol (as Chloramphenicol sodium succinate)
1 gram Chloramphenicol 1g powder for solution for injection vials | 1 vial [PoM] £22.00
Capsule
▸ Chloramphenicol (Non-proprietary)
Chloramphenicol 250 mg Chloramphenicol 250mg capsules | 60 capsule [PoM] £377.00 DT price = £377.00

Fosfomycin

22-Mar-2017

● **DRUG ACTION** Fosfomycin, a phosphonic acid antibacterial, is active against a range of Gram-positive and Gram-negative bacteria including *Staphylococcus aureus* and Enterobacteriaceae.

● **INDICATIONS AND DOSE**

Acute uncomplicated lower urinary-tract infections (in females)
▸ BY MOUTH USING GRANULES
▸ Child 12–17 years (female): 3 g for 1 dose.

Osteomyelitis when first-line treatments are inappropriate or ineffective | Hospital-acquired lower respiratory-tract infections when first-line treatments are inappropriate or ineffective
▸ BY INTRAVENOUS INFUSION
▸ Neonate up to 40 weeks corrected gestational age: 100 mg/kg daily in 2 divided doses.

▸ Neonate 40 weeks to 44 weeks corrected gestational age: 200 mg/kg daily in 3 divided doses.

▸ Child 1–11 months (body-weight up to 10 kg): 200–300 mg/kg daily in 3 divided doses, consider using the high-dose regimen in severe infection, particularly when suspected or known to be caused by less sensitive organisms
▸ Child 1–11 years (body-weight 10–39 kg): 200–400 mg/kg daily in 3–4 divided doses, consider using the high-dose regimen in severe infection, particularly when suspected or known to be caused by less sensitive organisms
▸ Child 12–17 years (body-weight 40 kg and above): 12–24 g daily in 2–3 divided doses (max. per dose 8 g), use the high-dose regimen in severe infection, particularly when suspected or known to be caused by less sensitive organisms

Complicated urinary-tract infections when first-line treatment ineffective or inappropriate
▶ BY INTRAVENOUS INFUSION

▸ Neonate up to 40 weeks corrected gestational age: 100 mg/kg daily in 2 divided doses.

▸ Neonate 40 weeks to 44 weeks corrected gestational age: 200 mg/kg daily in 3 divided doses.

▸ Child 1-11 months (body-weight up to 10 kg): 200–300 mg/kg daily in 3 divided doses, consider using the high-dose regimen in severe infection, particularly when suspected or known to be caused by less sensitive organisms

▸ Child 1-11 years (body-weight 10-39 kg): 200–400 mg/kg daily in 3–4 divided doses, consider using the high-dose regimen in severe infection, particularly when suspected or known to be caused by less sensitive organisms

▸ Child 12-17 years (body-weight 40 kg and above): 12–16 g daily in 2–3 divided doses (max. per dose 8 g), use the high-dose regimen in severe infection, particularly when suspected or known to be caused by less sensitive organisms

Bacterial meningitis when first-line treatment ineffective or inappropriate
▶ BY INTRAVENOUS INFUSION

▸ Neonate up to 40 weeks corrected gestational age: 100 mg/kg daily in 2 divided doses.

▸ Neonate 40 weeks to 44 weeks corrected gestational age: 200 mg/kg daily in 3 divided doses.

▸ Child 1-11 months (body-weight up to 10 kg): 200–300 mg/kg daily in 3 divided doses, consider using the high-dose regimen in severe infection, particularly when suspected or known to be caused by less sensitive organisms

▸ Child 1-11 years (body-weight 10-39 kg): 200–400 mg/kg daily in 3–4 divided doses, consider using the high-dose regimen in severe infection, particularly when suspected or known to be caused by less sensitive organisms

▸ Child 12-17 years (body-weight 40 kg and above): 16–24 g daily in 3–4 divided doses (max. per dose 8 g), use the high-dose regimen in severe infection suspected or known to be caused by less sensitive organisms

● CAUTIONS
▸ With intravenous use Cardiac insufficiency · hyperaldosteronism · hypernatraemia · hypertension · pulmonary oedema
● SIDE-EFFECTS
  GENERAL SIDE-EFFECTS
▶ **Common or very common** Gastro-intestinal disturbances
▶ **Uncommon** Diarrhoea · nausea · rash · vomiting
▶ **Frequency not known** Abdominal pain · antibiotic-associated colitis
  SPECIFIC SIDE-EFFECTS
● **Common or very common**
▶ With oral use Diarrhoea · dizziness · headache
▶ **Uncommon**
▶ With intravenous use Decreased appetite · dyspnoea · fatigue · headache · hypernatraemia · hypokalaemia · taste disturbances · vertigo
▶ **Rare**
▶ With intravenous use Aplastic anaemia · blood disorders · eosinophilia
▶ **Very rare**
▶ With intravenous use Fatty liver · visual impairment

▶ **Frequency not known**
▶ With intravenous use Bronchospasm · confusion · hepatitis · jaundice · tachycardia
● PREGNANCY Manufacturer advises use only if potential benefit outweighs risk.
● BREAST FEEDING Manufacturer advises use only if potential benefit outweighs risk—present in milk.
● RENAL IMPAIRMENT
▶ With oral use Avoid *oral* treatment if estimated glomerular filtration rate less than 10 mL/minute/1.73 m^2.
▶ With intravenous use Age under 12 years (body-weight under 40 kg)—no information available. Age 12–18 years (body-weight over 40 kg)—use with caution if estimated glomerular filtration rate 40–80 mL/minute/1.73 m^2, and consult product literature for dose if estimated glomerular filtration rate less than 40 mL/minute/1.73 m^2.
● MONITORING REQUIREMENTS
▶ With intravenous use Monitor electrolytes and fluid balance.
● DIRECTIONS FOR ADMINISTRATION
▶ With intravenous use Displacement value may be significant when reconstituting injection, consult local guidelines. Reconstitute each 2-g vial with 50 mL Glucose 5% *or* Glucose 10% *or* Water for Injections; do not exceed infusion rate of 133 mg/minute.
▶ With oral use Manufacturer advises granules should be taken on an empty stomach (about 2–3 hours before or after a meal), preferably before bedtime and after emptying the bladder. The granules should be dissolved into a glass of water and taken immediately.
● PRESCRIBING AND DISPENSING INFORMATION Doses expressed as fosfomycin base.
● NATIONAL FUNDING/ACCESS DECISIONS
Scottish Medicines Consortium (SMC) Decisions
The *Scottish Medicines Consortium* has advised (February 2015) that fosfomycin (*Fomicyt*®) is accepted for restricted use within NHS Scotland; initiation should be restricted to microbiologists or infectious disease specialists.
  The *Scottish Medicines Consortium* has advised (September 2016) that fosfomycin trometamol (*Monuril*®) is accepted for use within NHS Scotland for the treatment of acute lower uncomplicated urinary tract infections, caused by pathogens sensitive to fosfomycin in adult and adolescent females and for prophylaxis in diagnostic and surgical transurethral procedures.

● MEDICINAL FORMS
There can be variation in the licensing of different medicines containing the same drug.
Powder for solution for infusion
ELECTROLYTES: May contain Sodium
▶ **Fomicyt** (Nordic Pharma Ltd)
  Fosfomycin (as Fosfomycin sodium) 2 gram Fomicyt 2g powder for solution for infusion vials | 10 vial PoM £150.00
  Fosfomycin (as Fosfomycin sodium) 4 gram Fomicyt 4g powder for solution for infusion vials | 10 vial PoM £300.00
Granules
CAUTIONARY AND ADVISORY LABELS 9, 13, 23
EXCIPIENTS: May contain Sucrose
▶ **Fosfomycin** (Non-proprietary)
  Fosfomycin (as Fosfomycin trometamol) 3 gram Fosfomycin 3g granules sachets | 1 sachet PoM £75.45
▶ **Monuril** (Zambon S.p.A.)
  Fosfomycin (as Fosfomycin trometamol) 3 gram Monuril 3g granules sachets | 1 sachet PoM £4.86
Capsule
▶ **Fosfomycin** (Non-proprietary)
  Fosfomycin calcium 500 mg Fosfocina 500mg capsules | 24 capsule PoM no price available

5

Infection

5

Infection

Fusidic acid

16-Jun-2017

- **DRUG ACTION** Fusidic acid and its salts are narrow-spectrum antibiotics used for staphylococcal infections.

- **INDICATIONS AND DOSE**

Staphylococcal skin infection
- BY MOUTH USING TABLETS
- Child 12–17 years: 250 mg every 12 hours for 5–10 days, dose expressed as sodium fusidate
- TO THE SKIN
- Child: Apply 3–4 times a day usually for 7 days

Penicillin-resistant staphylococcal infection including osteomyelitis | Staphylococcal endocarditis in combination with other antibacterials
- BY MOUTH USING ORAL SUSPENSION
- Neonate: 15 mg/kg 3 times a day.

- Child 1–11 months: 15 mg/kg 3 times a day
- Child 1–4 years: 250 mg 3 times a day
- Child 5–11 years: 500 mg 3 times a day
- Child 12–17 years: 750 mg 3 times a day
- BY MOUTH USING TABLETS
- Child 12–17 years: 500 mg every 8 hours, increased to 1 g every 8 hours, increased dose can be used for severe infections, dose expressed as sodium fusidate

Staphylococcal infections due to susceptible organisms
- BY INTRAVENOUS INFUSION
- Child (body-weight up to 50 kg): 6–7 mg/kg 3 times a day, dose expressed as sodium fusidate
- Child (body-weight 50 kg and above): 500 mg 3 times a day, dose expressed as sodium fusidate

DOSE EQUIVALENCE AND CONVERSION
- Fusidic acid is incompletely absorbed and doses recommended for suspension are proportionally higher than those for sodium fusidate tablets. 500 mg of sodium fusidate is equivalent to 480 mg fusidic acid.

- **CAUTIONS**
- With systemic use Impaired transport and metabolism of bilirubin
- With topical use Avoid contact of cream or ointment with eyes

CAUTIONS, FURTHER INFORMATION
- Avoiding resistance
- With topical use To avoid the development of resistance, fusidic acid should not be used for longer than 10 days and local microbiology advice should be sought before using it in hospital.

- **INTERACTIONS** → Appendix 1: fusidic acid

- **SIDE-EFFECTS**
- **Common or very common**
- With intravenous use Hepatic disorders · venous intolerance (reduced if given via central vein)
- With oral use Abdominal pain · diarrhoea · dyspepsia · nausea · vomiting
- With systemic use Dizziness · drowsiness
- **Uncommon**
- With systemic use Anorexia · headache · malaise · pruritus · rash · urticaria
- **Rare**
- With topical use Hypersensitivity reactions
- **Frequency not known**
- With oral use Hepatic disorders
- With systemic use Acute renal failure (usually with jaundice) · blood disorders · cholestasis · hepatorenal syndrome

SIDE-EFFECTS, FURTHER INFORMATION
- Hepatic disorders
- With systemic use Elevated liver enzymes, hyperbilirubinaemia and jaundice can occur—these effects are usually reversible following withdrawal of therapy.

- **PREGNANCY**
- With systemic use Not known to be harmful; manufacturer advises use only if potential benefit outweighs risk.

- **BREAST FEEDING**
- With systemic use Present in milk—manufacturer advises caution.

- **HEPATIC IMPAIRMENT**
- With systemic use Manufacturer advises caution—monitor liver function periodically during treatment.

- **MONITORING REQUIREMENTS**
- With systemic use Manufacturer advises monitor liver function with high doses or on prolonged therapy; monitoring also advised for patients with biliary tract obstruction, those taking potentially hepatotoxic medication, or those taking concurrent medication with a similar excretion pathway.

- **DIRECTIONS FOR ADMINISTRATION** Manufacturer advises *for intravenous infusion*, give intermittently in Sodium chloride 0.9% or Glucose 5%; reconstitute each vial with 10 mL buffer solution, then add contents of vial to 500 mL infusion fluid to give a solution containing approximately 1 mg/mL. Give requisite dose via a central line over 2 hours (give over at least 6 hours if administered via a large peripheral vein).

- **PRESCRIBING AND DISPENSING INFORMATION** Flavours of oral liquid formulations may include banana and orange.

- **PROFESSION SPECIFIC INFORMATION**

Dental practitioners' formulary
May be prescribed as Sodium Fusidate ointment.

- **MEDICINAL FORMS**
There can be variation in the licensing of different medicines containing the same drug.

Tablet
CAUTIONARY AND ADVISORY LABELS 9
- Fucidin (Sodium fusidate) (LEO Pharma)
  Sodium fusidate 250 mg Fucidin 250mg tablets | 10 tablet [PoM] £6.02 DT price = £6.02 | 100 tablet [PoM] £54.99

Oral suspension
CAUTIONARY AND ADVISORY LABELS 9, 21
- Fucidin (Fusidic acid) (LEO Pharma)
  Fusidic acid 50 mg per 1 ml Fucidin 250mg/5ml oral suspension | 50 ml [PoM] £6.73 DT price = £6.73

Powder and solvent for solution for infusion
ELECTROLYTES: May contain Sodium
- Fusidic acid (Non-proprietary)
  Sodium fusidate 500 mg Sodium fusidate 500mg powder and solvent for solution for infusion vials | 1 vial [PoM] £38.00

Cream
EXCIPIENTS: May contain Butylated hydroxyanisole, cetostearyl alcohol (including cetyl and stearyl alcohol)
- Fusidic acid (Non-proprietary)
  Fusidic acid 20 mg per 1 gram Fusidic acid 2% cream | 15 gram [PoM] £1.92 DT price = £1.80 | 30 gram [PoM] £3.60 DT price = £3.60
- Fucidin (Fusidic acid) (LEO Pharma)
  Fusidic acid 20 mg per 1 gram Fucidin 20mg/g cream | 15 gram [PoM] £1.92 DT price = £1.80 | 30 gram [PoM] £3.59 DT price = £3.60

Ointment
EXCIPIENTS: May contain Cetostearyl alcohol (including cetyl and stearyl alcohol), wool fat and related substances including lanolin
- Fucidin (Sodium fusidate) (LEO Pharma)
  Sodium fusidate 20 mg per 1 gram Fucidin 20mg/g ointment | 15 gram [PoM] £2.68 DT price = £2.68 | 30 gram [PoM] £4.55 DT price = £4.55

Linezolid

- **DRUG ACTION** Linezolid, an oxazolidinone antibacterial, is active against Gram-positive bacteria including meticillin-resistant *Staphylococcus aureus* (MRSA), and glycopeptide-resistant enterococci. Resistance to linezolid can develop with prolonged treatment or if the dose is less than that recommended. Linezolid is **not** active against common Gram-negative organisms; it must be given in combination with other antibacterials for mixed infections that also involve Gram-negative organisms.

- **INDICATIONS AND DOSE**

Pneumonia (when other antibacterials e.g. a glycopetide, such as vancomycin, cannot be used) (initiated under specialist supervision) | Complicated skin and soft-tissue infections caused by Gram-positive bacteria, when other antibacterials cannot be used (initiated under specialist supervision)

  - ► BY MOUTH, OR BY INTRAVENOUS INFUSION

  - ► Neonate up to 7 days: 10 mg/kg every 12 hours, increased if necessary to 10 mg/kg every 8 hours, increased dose can be used if poor response.

  - ► Neonate 7 days to 28 days: 10 mg/kg every 8 hours.

  - ► Child 1 month–11 years: 10 mg/kg every 8 hours (max. per dose 600 mg)

  - ► Child 12–17 years: 600 mg every 12 hours

- **UNLICENSED USE** Not licensed for use in children.

IMPORTANT SAFETY INFORMATION

CHM ADVICE (OPTIC NEUROPATHY)

Severe optic neuropathy may occur rarely, particularly if linezolid is used for longer than 28 days. The CHM recommends that:

- patients should be warned to report symptoms of visual impairment (including blurred vision, visual field defect, changes in visual acuity and colour vision) immediately;
- patients experiencing new visual symptoms (regardless of treatment duration) should be evaluated promptly, and referred to an ophthalmologist if necessary;
- visual function should be monitored regularly if treatment is required for longer than 28 days.

BLOOD DISORDERS

Haematopoietic disorders (including thrombocytopenia, anaemia, leucopenia, and pancytopenia) have been reported in patients receiving linezolid. It is recommended that full blood counts are monitored weekly. Close monitoring is recommended in patients who:

- receive treatment for more than 10–14 days;
- have pre-existing myelosuppression;
- are receiving drugs that may have adverse effects on haemoglobin, blood counts, or platelet function;
- have severe renal impairment.

If significant myelosuppression occurs, treatment should be stopped unless it is considered essential, in which case intensive monitoring of blood counts and appropriate management should be implemented.

- **CAUTIONS** Acute confusional states · bipolar depression · carcinoid tumour · phaeochromocytoma · schizophrenia · thyrotoxicosis · uncontrolled hypertension

  CAUTIONS, FURTHER INFORMATION

  ► Close observation Unless close observation and blood pressure monitoring possible, linezolid should be avoided in uncontrolled hypertension, phaeochromocytoma,

carcinoid tumour, thyrotoxicosis, bipolar depression, schizophrenia, or acute confusional states.

- **INTERACTIONS** → Appendix 1: linezolid

- **SIDE-EFFECTS**

  GENERAL SIDE-EFFECTS

  - ► **Common or very common** Diarrhoea · eosinophilia · headache · nausea · taste disturbances · vomiting
  - ► **Uncommon** Abdominal pain · blurred vision · constipation · diaphoresis · dizziness · dry mouth · dyspepsia · electrolyte disturbances · fatigue · fever · gastritis · glossitis · hypertension · hypoaesthesia · insomnia · leucopenia · pancreatitis · paraesthesia · polyuria · pruritus · rash · stomatitis · thirst · thrombocytopenia · tinnitus · tongue discoloration
  - ► **Rare** Renal failure · tachycardia · transient ischaemic attacks
  - ► **Frequency not known** Anaemia · antibiotic-associated colitis · convulsions · hyponatraemia · lactic acidosis · optic neuropathy reported on prolonged therapy · pancytopenia · peripheral neuropathy reported on prolonged therapy · Stevens-Johnson syndrome · tooth discoloration · toxic epidermal necrolysis

  SPECIFIC SIDE-EFFECTS

  - ► **Uncommon**
  - ► With intravenous medium Injection-site reactions

- **PREGNANCY** Manufacturer advises use only if potential benefit outweighs risk—no information available.

- **BREAST FEEDING** Manufacturer advises avoid—present in milk in *animal* studies.

- **HEPATIC IMPAIRMENT** No dose adjustment necessary but in severe hepatic impairment use only if potential benefit outweighs risk.

- **RENAL IMPAIRMENT** No dose adjustment necessary but metabolites may accumulate if estimated glomerular filtration rate less than 30 mL/minute/1.73 m^2.

- **MONITORING REQUIREMENTS** Monitor full blood count (including platelet count) weekly.

- **DIRECTIONS FOR ADMINISTRATION** Infusion to be administered over 30–120 minutes.

- **PRESCRIBING AND DISPENSING INFORMATION** Flavours of oral liquid formulations may include orange.

  There is limited information on use in children and expert advice should be sought.

- **PATIENT AND CARER ADVICE** Patients should be advised to read the patient information leaflet given with linezolid.

- **MEDICINAL FORMS**

  There can be variation in the licensing of medicines containing the same drug.

  Infusion

  EXCIPIENTS: May contain Glucose

  ELECTROLYTES: May contain Sodium

  - ► Linezolid (Non-proprietary)

    Linezolid 2 mg per 1 ml Linezolid 600mg/300ml infusion bags | 10 bag PoM £445.00 (Hospital only)

  - ► Zyvox (Pfizer Ltd)

    Linezolid 2 mg per 1 ml Zyvox 600mg/300ml infusion bags | 10 bag PoM £445.00

  Oral suspension

  CAUTIONARY AND ADVISORY LABELS 9, 10

  EXCIPIENTS: May contain Aspartame

  - ► Zyvox (Pfizer Ltd)

    Linezolid 20 mg per 1 ml Zyvox 100mg/5ml granules for oral suspension | 150 ml PoM £222.50

  Tablet

  CAUTIONARY AND ADVISORY LABELS 9, 10

  - ► Linezolid (Non-proprietary)

    Linezolid 600 mg Linezolid 600mg tablets | 10 tablet PoM £82.12–£445.00 DT price = £323.32

  - ► Zyvox (Pfizer Ltd)

    Linezolid 600 mg Zyvox 600mg tablets | 10 tablet PoM £445.00 DT price = £323.32

Infection

5

Trimethoprim

- **INDICATIONS AND DOSE**

Urinary-tract infections | Respiratory tract infections
- ▶ BY MOUTH

- ▸ Neonate: Initially 3 mg/kg for 1 dose, then 1–2 mg/kg twice daily.

- ▸ Child 4–5 weeks: 4 mg/kg twice daily (max. per dose 200 mg)
- ▸ Child 6 weeks–5 months: 4 mg/kg twice daily (max. per dose 200 mg), alternatively 25 mg twice daily
- ▸ Child 6 months–5 years: 4 mg/kg twice daily (max. per dose 200 mg), alternatively 50 mg twice daily
- ▸ Child 6–11 years: 4 mg/kg twice daily (max. per dose 200 mg), alternatively 100 mg twice daily
- ▸ Child 12–17 years: 200 mg twice daily

Prophylaxis of urinary-tract infection (considered for recurrent infection, significant urinary-tract anomalies, or significant kidney damage)
- ▶ BY MOUTH

- ▸ Neonate: 2 mg/kg once daily, dose to be taken at night.

- ▸ Child 4–5 weeks: 2 mg/kg once daily (max. per dose 100 mg), dose to be taken at night
- ▸ Child 6 weeks–5 months: 2 mg/kg once daily (max. per dose 100 mg), dose to be taken at night, alternatively 12.5 mg once daily, dose to be taken at night
- ▸ Child 6 months–5 years: 2 mg/kg once daily (max. per dose 100 mg), dose to be taken at night, alternatively 25 mg once daily, dose to be taken at night
- ▸ Child 6–11 years: 2 mg/kg once daily (max. per dose 100 mg), dose to be taken at night, alternatively 50 mg once daily, dose to be taken at night
- ▸ Child 12–17 years: 100 mg once daily, dose to be taken at night

Treatment of mild to moderate *Pneumocystis jirovecii* (*Pneumocystis carinii*) pneumonia in patients who cannot tolerate co-trimoxazole (in combination with dapsone)
- ▶ BY MOUTH
- ▸ Child: 5 mg/kg every 6–8 hours

Shigellosis | Invasive salmonella infection
- ▶ BY MOUTH
- ▸ Child: (consult product literature)

- **UNLICENSED USE** Not licensed for treatment of pneumocystis pneumonia. Not licensed for use in children under 6 weeks.
- **CONTRA-INDICATIONS** Blood dyscrasias
- **CAUTIONS** Acute porphyrias p. 577 · neonates (specialist supervision required) · predisposition to folate deficiency
- **INTERACTIONS** → Appendix 1: trimethoprim
- **SIDE-EFFECTS**
- ▸ **Rare** Allergic reactions · anaphylaxis · angioedema · erythema multiforme · photosensitivity · toxic epidermal necrolysis
- ▸ **Frequency not known** Aseptic meningitis · depression of haematopoiesis · gastro-intestinal disturbances · hyperkalaemia · nausea · pruritus · rashes · vomiting

SIDE-EFFECTS, FURTHER INFORMATION
Trimethoprim has side-effects similar to co-trimoxazole but they are less severe and occur less frequently.
- **PREGNANCY** Teratogenic risk in first trimester (folate antagonist). Manufacturers advise avoid during pregnancy.
- **BREAST FEEDING** Present in milk—short-term use not known to be harmful.
- **RENAL IMPAIRMENT** Use half normal dose after 3 days if estimated glomerular filtration rate

15–30 mL/minute/1.73 m². Use half normal dose if estimated glomerular filtration rate less than 15 mL/minute/1.73 m². Monitor plasma-trimethoprim concentration if estimated glomerular filtration rate less than 10 mL/minute/1.73 m².
- **MONITORING REQUIREMENTS** Manufacturer recommends blood counts on long-term therapy (but evidence of practical value unsatisfactory).
- **PATIENT AND CARER ADVICE**
Blood disorders On long-term treatment, patients and their carers should be told how to recognise signs of blood disorders and advised to seek immediate medical attention if symptoms such as fever, sore throat, rash, mouth ulcers, purpura, bruising or bleeding develop.
Medicines for Children leaflet: Trimethoprim for bacterial infections www.medicinesforchildren.org.uk/trimethoprim-for-bacterial-infections

- **MEDICINAL FORMS**
There can be variation in the licensing of different medicines containing the same drug. Forms available from special-order manufacturers include: oral suspension, oral solution
Oral suspension
CAUTIONARY AND ADVISORY LABELS 9
- ▸ **Trimethoprim** (Non-proprietary)
Trimethoprim 10 mg per 1 ml Trimethoprim 50mg/5ml oral suspension sugar free sugar-free | 100 ml [PoM] £2.69 DT price = £2.12
- ▸ **Monotrim** (Chemidex Pharma Ltd)
Trimethoprim 10 mg per 1 ml Monotrim 50mg/5ml oral suspension sugar-free | 100 ml [PoM] £1.77 DT price = £2.12
Tablet
CAUTIONARY AND ADVISORY LABELS 9
- ▸ **Trimethoprim** (Non-proprietary)
Trimethoprim 100 mg Trimethoprim 100mg tablets | 28 tablet [PoM] £9.99 DT price = £0.85
Trimethoprim 200 mg Trimethoprim 200mg tablets | 6 tablet [PoM] £2.15 DT price = £0.49 | 14 tablet [PoM] £9.99 DT price = £1.15

Combinations available: Co-trimoxazole, p. 335

2.1 Anthrax

Anthrax

Treatment and post-exposure prophylaxis

Inhalation or *gastro-intestinal anthrax* should be treated initially with either ciprofloxacin p. 333 or, in patients over 12 years, doxycycline p. 338 [unlicensed indication] combined with one or two other antibacterials (such as amoxicillin p. 325, benzylpenicillin sodium p. 323, chloramphenicol p. 340, clarithromycin p. 315, clindamycin p. 313, imipenem with cilastatin p. 302, rifampicin p. 349 [unlicensed indication], and vancomycin p. 312). When the condition improves and the sensitivity of the *Bacillus anthracis* strain is known, treatment may be switched to a single antibacterial. Treatment should continue for 60 days because germination may be delayed.

Cutaneous anthrax should be treated with either ciprofloxacin [unlicensed indication] or doxycycline [unlicensed indication] for 7 days. Treatment may be switched to amoxicillin if the infecting strain is susceptible. Treatment may need to be extended to 60 days if exposure is due to aerosol. A combination of antibacterials for 14 days is recommended for cutaneous anthrax with systemic features, extensive oedema, or lesions of the head or neck.

Ciprofloxacin or doxycycline may be given for *post-exposure prophylaxis*. If exposure is confirmed, antibacterial prophylaxis should continue for 60 days. Antibacterial prophylaxis may be switched to amoxicillin after 10–14 days if the strain of *B. anthracis* is susceptible. Vaccination against

attention if symptoms such as persistent nausea, vomiting, malaise or jaundice develop.

● **MEDICINAL FORMS**
There can be variation in the licensing of different medicines containing the same drug. Forms available from special-order manufacturers include: oral suspension, oral solution
Capsule
CAUTIONARY AND ADVISORY LABELS 8, 14
▸ Mycobutin (Pfizer Ltd)
   Rifabutin 150 mg Mycobutin 150mg capsules | 30 capsule PoM
   £90.38

Rifampicin

● **INDICATIONS AND DOSE**
Brucellosis in combination with other antibacterials | Legionnaires disease in combination with other antibacterials | Serious staphylococcal infections in combination with other antibacterials
▸ BY MOUTH, OR BY INTRAVENOUS INFUSION
▸ Neonate: 5–10 mg/kg twice daily.

▸ Child 1–11 months: 5–10 mg/kg twice daily
▸ Child 1–17 years: 10 mg/kg twice daily (max. per dose 600 mg)
Tuberculosis, in combination with other drugs (intermittent supervised 6-month treatment) (under expert supervision)
▸ BY MOUTH
▸ Child: 15 mg/kg 3 times a week (max. per dose 900 mg) for 6 months (initial and continuation phases)
Tuberculosis, in combination with other drugs (standard unsupervised 6-month treatment)
▸ BY MOUTH
▸ Child (body-weight up to 50 kg): 15 mg/kg once daily for 6 months (initial and continuation phases); maximum 450 mg per day
▸ Child (body-weight 50 kg and above): 15 mg/kg once daily for 6 months (initial and continuation phases); maximum 600 mg per day
Congenital tuberculosis
▸ BY MOUTH
▸ Neonate: 15 mg/kg once daily for 6 months (initial and continuation phases).

Prevention of tuberculosis in susceptible close contacts or those who have become tuberculin positive, in combination with isoniazid
▸ BY MOUTH
▸ Child 1 month–11 years (body-weight up to 50 kg): 15 mg/kg daily for 3 months; maximum 450 mg per day
▸ Child 1 month–11 years (body-weight 50 kg and above): 15 mg/kg daily for 3 months; maximum 600 mg per day
▸ Child 12–17 years (body-weight up to 50 kg): 450 mg daily for 3 months
▸ Child 12–17 years (body-weight 50 kg and above): 600 mg daily for 3 months
Prevention of tuberculosis in susceptible close contacts or those who have become tuberculin positive, who are isoniazid-resistant
▸ BY MOUTH
▸ Child 1 month–11 years (body-weight up to 50 kg): 15 mg/kg daily for 6 months; maximum 450 mg per day
▸ Child 1 month–11 years (body-weight 50 kg and above): 15 mg/kg daily for 6 months; maximum 600 mg per day

▸ Child 12–17 years (body-weight up to 50 kg): 450 mg daily for 6 months
▸ Child 12–17 years (body-weight 50 kg and above): 600 mg daily for 6 months
Prevention of secondary case of *Haemophilus influenzae* type b disease
▸ BY MOUTH
▸ Child 1–2 months: 10 mg/kg once daily for 4 days
▸ Child 3 months–11 years: 20 mg/kg once daily (max. per dose 600 mg) for 4 days
▸ Child 12–17 years: 600 mg once daily for 4 days
Prevention of secondary case of meningococcal meningitis
▸ BY MOUTH
▸ Neonate: 5 mg/kg every 12 hours for 2 days.

▸ Child 1–11 months: 5 mg/kg every 12 hours for 2 days
▸ Child 1–11 years: 10 mg/kg every 12 hours (max. per dose 600 mg), for 2 days
▸ Child 12–17 years: 600 mg every 12 hours for 2 days
Pruritus due to cholestasis
▸ BY MOUTH
▸ Child: 5–10 mg/kg once daily (max. per dose 600 mg)

● **UNLICENSED USE** Not licensed for use in children for pruritus due to cholestasis.
● **CONTRA-INDICATIONS** Acute porphyrias p. 577 · jaundice
● **CAUTIONS** Discolours soft contact lenses
● **INTERACTIONS** → Appendix 1: rifampicin
● **SIDE-EFFECTS**
GENERAL SIDE-EFFECTS
Acute renal failure · adrenal insufficiency · alterations of liver function · anorexia · antibiotic-associated colitis · body secretions coloured orange-red · collapse and shock · diarrhoea · disseminated intravascular coagulation · drowsiness · eosinophilia · exfoliative dermatitis · flushing · gastro-intestinal symptoms · haemolytic anaemia · headache · influenza-like symptoms (with chills, fever, dizziness, bone pain) · jaundice · leucopenia · menstrual disturbances · muscular weakness · myopathy · nausea · oedema · pemphigoid reactions · psychoses · rashes · respiratory symptoms · saliva coloured orange-red · shortness of breath · Stevens-Johnson syndrome · thrombocytopenic purpura · toxic epidermal necrolysis · urine coloured orange-red · urticaria · vomiting

SPECIFIC SIDE-EFFECTS
▸ With intravenous use Thrombophlebitis reported if infusion used for prolonged period
SIDE-EFFECTS, FURTHER INFORMATION
Discontinue permanently if serious side-effects develop.
▸ Intermittent therapy Side-effects that mainly occur with intermittent therapy include influenza-like symptoms (with chills, fever, dizziness, bone pain), respiratory symptoms (including shortness of breath), collapse and shock, haemolytic anaemia, thrombocytopenic purpura, disseminated intravascular coagulation, and acute renal failure
● **ALLERGY AND CROSS-SENSITIVITY** Contra-indicated in patients with rifamycin hypersensitivity.
● **CONCEPTION AND CONTRACEPTION** Important Effectiveness of hormonal contraceptives is reduced and alternative family planning advice should be offered.
● **PREGNANCY** Manufacturers advise very high doses teratogenic in *animal* studies in first trimester; risk of neonatal bleeding may be increased in third trimester.
● **BREAST FEEDING** Amount too small to be harmful.
● **HEPATIC IMPAIRMENT** Avoid or do not exceed 8 mg/kg daily. Impaired elimination. In patients with pre-existing liver disease or hepatic impairment, monitor liver function

regularly and particularly frequently in the first 2 months; blood counts should also be monitored in these patients.

- **RENAL IMPAIRMENT** Use with caution if doses above 10 mg/kg daily.
- **MONITORING REQUIREMENTS**
  - ▸ *Renal function* should be checked before treatment.
  - ▸ *Hepatic function* should be checked before treatment. If there is no evidence of liver disease (and pre-treatment liver function is normal), further checks are only necessary if the patient develops fever, malaise, vomiting, jaundice or unexplained deterioration during treatment. However, liver function should be monitored on prolonged therapy.
  - ▸ Blood counts should be monitored in patients on prolonged therapy.
- **DIRECTIONS FOR ADMINISTRATION** Displacement value may be significant, consult local reconstitution guidelines; reconstitute with solvent provided. May be further diluted with Glucose 5% *or* Sodium chloride 0.9% to a final concentration of 1.2 mg/mL. Infuse over 2–3 hours.
- **PRESCRIBING AND DISPENSING INFORMATION** If treatment interruption occurs, re-introduce with low dosage and increase gradually.
  - ▸ With oral use In general, doses should be rounded up to facilitate administration of suitable volumes of liquid or an appropriate strength of tablet. Doses may also need to be recalculated to allow for weight gain in younger children. Flavours of syrup may include raspberry.
- **PATIENT AND CARER ADVICE**
  Soft contact lenses Patients or their carers should be advised that rifampicin discolours soft contact lenses.
  Hepatic disorders Patients or their carers should be told how to recognise signs of liver disorder, and advised to discontinue treatment and seek immediate medical attention if symptoms such as persistent nausea, vomiting, malaise or jaundice develop.
  Medicines for Children leaflet: Rifampicin for meningococcal prophylaxis www.medicinesforchildren.org.uk/rifampicin-for-meningococcal-prophylaxis
  Medicines for Children leaflet: Rifampicin for the treatment of tuberculosis www.medicinesforchildren.org.uk/rifampicin-for-treatment-of-tuberculosis

- **MEDICINAL FORMS**
  There can be variation in the licensing of different medicines containing the same drug. Forms available from special-order manufacturers include: oral suspension, oral solution

Powder and solvent for solution for injection
- ▸ Rifampicin (Non-proprietary)
  Rifampicin 300 mg RIFA parenteral 300mg powder and solvent for solution for injection vials | 1 vial [PoM] no price available

Oral suspension
CAUTIONARY AND ADVISORY LABELS 8, 14, 23
EXCIPIENTS: May contain Sucrose
- ▸ Rifadin (Sanofi)
  Rifampicin 20 mg per 1 ml Rifadin 100mg/5ml syrup | 120 ml [PoM] £4.27

Capsule
CAUTIONARY AND ADVISORY LABELS 8, 14, 23
- ▸ Rifampicin (Non-proprietary)
  Rifampicin 150 mg Rifampicin 150mg capsules | 100 capsule [PoM] £44.83 DT price = £44.83
  Rifampicin 300 mg Rifampicin 300mg capsules | 100 capsule [PoM] £103.25 DT price = £103.22
- ▸ Rifadin (Sanofi)
  Rifampicin 150 mg Rifadin 150mg capsules | 100 capsule [PoM] £18.32 DT price = £44.83
  Rifampicin 300 mg Rifadin 300mg capsules | 100 capsule [PoM] £36.63 DT price = £103.22
- ▸ Rimactane (Sandoz Ltd)
  Rifampicin 300 mg Rimactane 300mg capsules | 60 capsule [PoM] £21.98

Powder and solvent for solution for infusion
ELECTROLYTES: May contain Sodium
- ▸ Rifadin (Sanofi)
  Rifampicin 600 mg Rifadin 600mg powder and solvent for solution for infusion vials | 1 vial [PoM] £9.20

Rifampicin with isoniazid

The properties listed below are those particular to the combination only. For the properties of the components please consider, rifampicin p. 349, isoniazid p. 352.

- **INDICATIONS AND DOSE**
  Treatment of tuberculosis (continuation phase)
  - ▸ BY MOUTH
    - ▸ Child: Although not licensed in children, consideration may be given to use of *Rifinah* ® in older children, provided the respective dose of each drug is appropriate for the weight of the child (consult local protocol).

  DOSE EQUIVALENCE AND CONVERSION
  - ▸ *Rifinah* ® Tablets contain rifampicin and isoniazid; the proportions are expressed in the form x/y where x and y are the strengths in milligrams of rifampicin and isoniazid respectively.
  - ▸ Each *Rifinah* ® 150/100 Tablet contains rifampicin 150 mg and isoniazid 100 mg.
  - ▸ Each *Rifinah* ® 300/150 Tablet contains rifampicin 300 mg and isoniazid 150 mg.

- **UNLICENSED USE** Not licensed for use in children.
- **INTERACTIONS** → Appendix 1: isoniazid, rifampicin
- **PATIENT AND CARER ADVICE**
  Medicines for Children leaflet: Isoniazid and rifampicin combination for latent tuberculosis www.medicinesforchildren.org.uk/isoniazid-and-rifampicin-combination-latent-tuberculosis

- **MEDICINAL FORMS**
  There can be variation in the licensing of different medicines containing the same drug.
  Tablet
  CAUTIONARY AND ADVISORY LABELS 8, 14, 23
  - ▸ Rifinah (Sanofi)
    Isoniazid 100 mg, Rifampicin 150 mg Rifinah 150mg/100mg tablets | 84 tablet [PoM] £19.09
    Isoniazid 150 mg, Rifampicin 300 mg Rifinah 300mg/150mg tablets | 56 tablet [PoM] £25.22

Rifampicin with isoniazid and pyrazinamide

The properties listed below are those particular to the combination only. For the properties of the components please consider, rifampicin p. 349, isoniazid p. 352, pyrazinamide p. 353.

- **INDICATIONS AND DOSE**
  Initial treatment of tuberculosis (in combination with ethambutol)
  - ▸ Child: Although not licensed in children, consideration may be given to use of *Rifater* ® in older children, provided the respective dose of each drug is appropriate for the weight of the child (consult local protocol).

  DOSE EQUIVALENCE AND CONVERSION
  - ▸ Tablet quantities refer to the number of *Rifater* ® Tablets which should be taken. Each *Rifater* ® Tablet contains isoniazid 50 mg, pyrazinamide 300 mg and rifampicin 120 mg.

- **UNLICENSED USE** Not licensed for use in children.

- **INTERACTIONS** → Appendix 1: isoniazid, pyrazinamide, rifampicin

- **MEDICINAL FORMS**
There can be variation in the licensing of different medicines containing the same drug.
Tablet
CAUTIONARY AND ADVISORY LABELS 8, 14, 22
▸ Rifater (Sanofi)
Isoniazid 50 mg, Rifampicin 120 mg, Pyrazinamide 300 mg Rifater tablets | 100 tablet PoM £26.34

ANTIMYCOBACTERIALS > OTHER

Cycloserine

- **INDICATIONS AND DOSE**
Tuberculosis resistant to first-line drugs, in combination with other drugs
▸ BY MOUTH
▸ Child 2–11 years: Initially 5 mg/kg twice daily (max. per dose 250 mg), then increased if necessary up to 10 mg/kg twice daily (max. per dose 500 mg), dose to be increased according to blood concentration and response
▸ Child 12–17 years: Initially 250 mg every 12 hours for 2 weeks, then increased if necessary up to 500 mg every 12 hours, dose to be increased according to blood concentration and response

PHARMACOKINETICS
Cycloserine penetrates the CNS.

- **UNLICENSED USE** Licensed for use in children (age range not specified by manufacturer).
- **CONTRA-INDICATIONS** Alcohol dependence · depression · epilepsy · psychotic states · severe anxiety
- **INTERACTIONS** → Appendix 1: cycloserine
- **SIDE-EFFECTS** Allergic dermatitis · changes in liver function tests · confusion · convulsions · depression · dizziness · drowsiness · headache · heart failure at high doses · megaloblastic anaemia · psychosis · rashes · tremor · vertigo

SIDE-EFFECTS, FURTHER INFORMATION
▸ CNS toxicity Discontinue or reduce dose if symptoms of CNS toxicity occur.
▸ Rashes or allergic dermatitis Discontinue or reduce dose if rashes or allergic dermatitis develops.
- **PREGNANCY** Manufacturer advises use only if potential benefit outweighs risk—crosses the placenta.
- **BREAST FEEDING** Present in milk—amount too small to be harmful.
- **RENAL IMPAIRMENT** Increase interval between doses if creatinine clearance less than 50 mL/minute/1.73 m². Monitor blood-cycloserine concentration if creatinine clearance less than 50 mL/minute/1.73 m².
- **MONITORING REQUIREMENTS**
▸ Blood concentration should not exceed a peak concentration of 30 mg/litre (measured 3–4 hours after the dose).
▸ Monitor haematological, renal, and hepatic function.

- **MEDICINAL FORMS**
There can be variation in the licensing of different medicines containing the same drug.
Capsule
CAUTIONARY AND ADVISORY LABELS 2, 8
▸ Cycloserine (Non-proprietary)
Cycloserine 250 mg Cycloserine 250mg capsules | 100 capsule PoM £402.63 DT price = £402.63

Ethambutol hydrochloride

- **INDICATIONS AND DOSE**
Tuberculosis, in combination with other drugs (standard unsupervised 6-month treatment)
▸ BY MOUTH
▸ Child: 20 mg/kg once daily for 2 months (initial phase)
Tuberculosis, in combination with other drugs (intermittent supervised 6-month treatment) (under expert supervision)
▸ BY MOUTH
▸ Child: 30 mg/kg 3 times a week for 2 months (initial phase)
Congenital tuberculosis, in combination with other drugs
▸ BY MOUTH
▸ Neonate: 20 mg/kg once daily for 2 months (initial phase).

- **CONTRA-INDICATIONS** Optic neuritis · poor vision
- **CAUTIONS** Young children
CAUTIONS, FURTHER INFORMATION
▸ Understanding warnings Patients who cannot understand warnings about visual side-effects should, if possible, be given an alternative drug. In particular, ethambutol should be used with caution in children until they are at least 5 years old and capable of reporting symptomatic visual changes accurately.
- **INTERACTIONS** → Appendix 1: ethambutol
- **SIDE-EFFECTS**
▸ **Rare** Pruritus · rash · thrombocytopenia · urticaria
▸ **Frequency not known** Colour blindness · loss of visual acuity · optic neuritis · peripheral neuritis · red/green colour blindness · restriction of visual fields · visual disturbances

SIDE-EFFECTS, FURTHER INFORMATION
▸ Ocular toxicity Ocular toxicity is more common where excessive dosage is used or if the patient's renal function is impaired. Early discontinuation of the drug is almost always followed by recovery of eyesight.
- **PREGNANCY** Not known to be harmful.
- **BREAST FEEDING** Amount too small to be harmful.
- **RENAL IMPAIRMENT** If creatinine clearance less than 30 mL/minute/1.73 m², use 15–25 mg/kg (max. 2.5 g) 3 times a week. Risk of optic nerve damage. Should preferably be avoided in patients with renal impairment. If creatinine clearance less than 30 mL/minute/1.73 m², monitor plasma-ethambutol concentration.
- **MONITORING REQUIREMENTS**
▸ 'Peak' concentration (2–2.5 hours after dose) should be 2–6 mg/litre (7–22 micromol/litre); 'trough' (pre-dose) concentration should be less than 1 mg/litre (4 micromol/litre).
▸ Renal function should be checked before treatment.
▸ Visual acuity should be tested by Snellen chart before treatment with ethambutol.
▸ In young children, routine ophthalmological monitoring recommended.
- **PATIENT AND CARER ADVICE**
Ocular toxicity The earliest features of ocular toxicity are subjective and patients should be advised to discontinue therapy immediately if they develop deterioration in vision and promptly seek further advice.
Medicines for Children leaflet: Ethambutol for the treatment of tuberculosis www.medicinesforchildren.org.uk/ethambutol-for-the-treatment-of-tuberculosis

5

Infection

- **MEDICINAL FORMS**
There can be variation in the licensing of different medicines containing the same drug. Forms available from special-order manufacturers include: oral suspension, oral solution

Tablet
CAUTIONARY AND ADVISORY LABELS 8
‣ Ethambutol hydrochloride (Non-proprietary)
Ethambutol hydrochloride 100 mg Ethambutol 100mg tablets | 56 tablet [PoM] £11.51 DT price = £11.51
Ethambutol hydrochloride 400 mg Ethambutol 400mg tablets | 56 tablet [PoM] £42.74 DT price = £42.74

Isoniazid

- **INDICATIONS AND DOSE**
Tuberculosis, in combination with other drugs (standard unsupervised 6-month treatment)
▸ BY MOUTH, OR BY INTRAMUSCULAR INJECTION, OR BY INTRAVENOUS INJECTION
▸ Child: 10 mg/kg once daily (max. per dose 300 mg) for 6 months (initial and continuation phases)

Tuberculosis, in combination with other drugs (intermittent supervised 6-month treatment) (under expert supervision)
▸ BY MOUTH, OR BY INTRAMUSCULAR INJECTION, OR BY INTRAVENOUS INJECTION
▸ Child: 15 mg/kg 3 times a week (max. per dose 900 mg) for 6 months (initial and continuation phases)

Congenital tuberculosis, in combination with other drugs
▸ BY MOUTH, OR BY INTRAMUSCULAR INJECTION, OR BY INTRAVENOUS INJECTION
▸ Neonate: 10 mg/kg daily for 6 months (initial and continuation phases).

Prevention of tuberculosis in susceptible close contacts or those who have become tuberculin positive
▸ BY MOUTH, OR BY INTRAMUSCULAR INJECTION, OR BY INTRAVENOUS INJECTION
▸ Neonate: 10 mg/kg daily for 6 months.
▸ Child 1 month–11 years: 10 mg/kg daily (max. per dose 300 mg) for 6 months, alternatively 10 mg/kg daily (max. per dose 300 mg) for 3 months, to be taken in combination with rifampicin
▸ Child 12–17 years: 300 mg daily for 6 months, alternatively 300 mg daily for 3 months, to be taken in combination with rifampicin

- **CONTRA-INDICATIONS** Drug-induced liver disease
- **CAUTIONS** Acute porphyrias p. 577 · alcohol dependence · diabetes mellitus · epilepsy · history of psychosis · HIV infection · malnutrition · slow acetylator status (increased risk of side-effects)

CAUTIONS, FURTHER INFORMATION
▸ Peripheral neuropathy Peripheral neuropathy is more likely to occur where there are pre-existing risk factors such as diabetes, alcohol dependence, chronic renal failure, pregnancy, malnutrition and HIV infection. In patients at increased risk of peripheral neuropathy, pyridoxine hydrochloride p. 600 should be given prophylactically from the start of treatment.

- **INTERACTIONS** → Appendix 1: isoniazid
- **SIDE-EFFECTS**
▸ **Common or very common** Peripheral neuropathy
▸ **Rare** Hepatitis · psychotic episodes
▸ **Frequency not known** Agranulocytosis · aplastic anaemia · blood disorders · constipation · convulsions · difficulty with micturition · dry mouth · fever · gynaecomastia · haemolytic anaemia · hearing loss (in patients with end-stage renal impairment) · hyperglycaemia · hyperreflexia · hypersensitivity reactions · interstitial pneumonitis ·

nausea · optic neuritis · pancreatitis · pellagra · peripheral neuritis with high doses · purpura · Stevens-Johnson syndrome · systemic lupus erythematosus-like syndrome · tinnitus (in patients with end-stage renal impairment) · vertigo · vomiting

- **PREGNANCY** Not known to be harmful; prophylactic pyridoxine recommended.
- **BREAST FEEDING** Theoretical risk of convulsions and neuropathy; prophylactic pyridoxine advisable in mother. Monitor infant for possible toxicity.
- **HEPATIC IMPAIRMENT** Use with caution. In patients with pre-existing liver disease or hepatic impairment monitor liver function regularly and particularly frequently in the first 2 months.
- **RENAL IMPAIRMENT** Risk of ototoxicity and peripheral neuropathy; prophylactic pyridoxine hydrochloride p. 600 recommended.
- **MONITORING REQUIREMENTS**
▸ *Renal function* should be checked before treatment.
▸ *Hepatic function* should be checked before treatment. If there is no evidence of liver disease (and pre-treatment liver function is normal), further checks are only necessary if the patient develops fever, malaise, vomiting, jaundice or unexplained deterioration during treatment.
- **PRESCRIBING AND DISPENSING INFORMATION**
Doses may need to be recalculated to allow for weight gain in younger children.
▸ With oral use In general, doses should be rounded up to facilitate administration of suitable volumes of liquid or an appropriate strength of tablet.
- **PATIENT AND CARER ADVICE**
Hepatic disorders Patients or their carers should be told how to recognise signs of liver disorder, and advised to discontinue treatment and seek immediate medical attention if symptoms such as persistent nausea, vomiting, malaise or jaundice develop.
Medicines for Children leaflet: Isoniazid for latent tuberculosis www.medicinesforchildren.org.uk/isoniazid-for-latent-tuberculosis
Medicines for Children leaflet: Isoniazid for treatment of tuberculosis www.medicinesforchildren.org.uk/isoniazid-for-the-treatment-of-tuberculosis
- **MEDICINAL FORMS**
There can be variation in the licensing of different medicines containing the same drug. Forms available from special-order manufacturers include: oral suspension, oral solution

Solution for injection
▸ Isoniazid (Non-proprietary)
Isoniazid 20 mg per 1 ml Tebesium-S 100mg/5ml solution for injection ampoules | 12 ampoule [PoM] no price available
Isoniazid 25 mg per 1 ml Isoniazid 50mg/2ml solution for injection ampoules | 10 ampoule [PoM] £329.08

Tablet
CAUTIONARY AND ADVISORY LABELS 8, 22
▸ Isoniazid (Non-proprietary)
Isoniazid 50 mg Isoniazid 50mg tablets | 56 tablet [PoM] £19.24 DT price = £19.24
Isoniazid 100 mg Isoniazid 100mg tablets | 28 tablet [PoM] £19.24 DT price = £19.24
Isoniazid 300 mg Isoniazid 300mg tablets | 30 tablet [PoM] no price available

Combinations available: *Rifampicin with isoniazid*, p. 350 · *Rifampicin with isoniazid and pyrazinamide*, p. 350

Pyrazinamide

- **INDICATIONS AND DOSE**

Tuberculosis, in combination with other drugs (standard unsupervised 6-month treatment)
▸ BY MOUTH
- Child (body-weight up to 50 kg): 35 mg/kg once daily for 2 months (initial phase); maximum 1.5 g per day
- Child (body-weight 50 kg and above): 35 mg/kg once daily for 2 months (initial phase); maximum 2 g per day

Tuberculosis, in combination with other drugs (intermittent supervised 6-month treatment) (under expert supervision)
▸ BY MOUTH
- Child (body-weight up to 50 kg): 50 mg/kg 3 times a week (max. per dose 2 g 3 times a week) for 2 months (initial phase)
- Child (body-weight 50 kg and above): 50 mg/kg 3 times a week (max. per dose 2.5 g 3 times a week) for 2 months (initial phase)

Congenital tuberculosis, in combination with other drugs
▸ BY MOUTH
- Neonate: 35 mg/kg once daily for 2 months (initial phase).

- **CAUTIONS** Diabetes
- **INTERACTIONS** → Appendix 1: pyrazinamide
- **SIDE-EFFECTS** Anorexia · arthralgia · dysuria · fever · hepatomegaly · hepatotoxicity · jaundice · liver failure · nausea · photosensitivity · rash · sideroblastic anaemia · splenomegaly · thrombocytopenia · vomiting
- **PREGNANCY** Manufacturer advises use only if potential benefit outweighs risk.
- **BREAST FEEDING** Amount too small to be harmful.
- **HEPATIC IMPAIRMENT** Idiosyncratic hepatotoxicity more common; avoid in severe hepatic impairment. In patients with pre-existing liver disease or hepatic impairment monitor liver function regularly and particularly frequently in the first 2 months.
- **RENAL IMPAIRMENT** If estimated glomerular filtration rate less than 30 mL/minute/1.73 m^2, use 25–30 mg/kg 3 times a week.
- **MONITORING REQUIREMENTS**
▸ *Renal function* should be checked before treatment.
▸ *Hepatic function* should be checked before treatment. If there is no evidence of liver disease (and pre-treatment liver function is normal), further checks are only necessary if the patient develops fever, malaise, vomiting, jaundice or unexplained deterioration during treatment.
- **PRESCRIBING AND DISPENSING INFORMATION** In general, doses should be rounded up to facilitate administration of suitable volumes of liquid or an appropriate strength of tablet. Doses may also need to be recalculated to allow for weight gain in younger children.
- **PATIENT AND CARER ADVICE**
Hepatic disorders Patients or their carers should be told how to recognise signs of liver disorder, and advised to discontinue treatment and seek immediate medical attention if symptoms such as persistent nausea, vomiting, malaise or jaundice develop.
Medicines for Children leaflet: Pyrazinamide for treatment of tuberculosis www.medicinesforchildren.org.uk/pyrazinamide-for-tuberculosis

- **MEDICINAL FORMS**
There can be variation in the licensing of different medicines containing the same drug. Forms available from special-order manufacturers include: oral suspension, oral solution

Tablet
CAUTIONARY AND ADVISORY LABELS 8
▸ **Pyrazinamide** (Non-proprietary)
Pyrazinamide 500 mg Pyrazinamide 500mg tablets |
30 tablet POM £31.35–£38.34 | 50 tablet POM no price available
▸ **Zinamide** (Thornton & Ross Ltd)
Pyrazinamide 500 mg Zinamide 500mg tablets | 30 tablet POM
£31.35

Combinations available: *Rifampicin with isoniazid and pyrazinamide*, p. 350

2.5 Urinary tract infections

Urinary-tract infections

Overview

Urinary-tract infection is more common in adolescent girls than in boys; when it occurs in adolescent boys there is frequently an underlying abnormality of the renal tract. Recurrent episodes of infection are an indication for radiological investigation especially in children in whom untreated pyelonephritis may lead to permanent kidney damage.

Escherichia coli is the most common cause of urinary-tract infection; *Staphylococcus saprophyticus* is also common in sexually active young women. Less common causes include *Proteus* and *Klebsiella spp. Pseudomonas aeruginosa* infections usually occur in the hospital setting and may be associated with functional or anatomical abnormalities of the renal tract. *Staphylococcus epidermidis* and *Enterococcus faecalis* infection may complicate catheterisation or instrumentation.

A specimen of urine should be collected for culture and sensitivity testing before starting antibacterial therapy;

- in children under 3 years of age;
- in children with suspected upper urinary-tract infection, complicated infection, or recurrent infection;
- if resistant organisms are suspected;
- if urine dipstick testing gives a single positive result for leucocyte esterase or nitrite;
- if clinical symptoms are not consistent with results of dipstick testing;
- in pregnant women.

Treatment should not be delayed while waiting for results. The antibacterial chosen should reflect current local bacterial sensitivity to antibacterials.

Antibacterial therapy for urinary-tract infections

Urinary-tract infections in children require prompt antibacterial treatment to minimise the risk of renal scarring.

Children under 3 months of age should be transferred to hospital and treated initially with intravenous antibacterials such as amoxicillin p. 325 (*or* ampicillin p. 326) with gentamicin p. 299, or a cephalosporin (such as cefotaxime p. 307) alone, until the infection responds; full doses of oral antibacterials are then given for a further period.

Children over 3 months of age with uncomplicated lower urinary-tract infection, can be treated with trimethoprim p. 344 or nitrofurantoin p. 354. *Suggested duration of treatment* 3 days. Re-assess child if they remain unwell 24–48 hours after initial assessment.

Alternatively, *children over 3 months of age, with uncomplicated lower urinary-tract infection,* may be treated with amoxicillin (*or* ampicillin) *or* oral first generation cephalosporin (e.g. cefalexin p. 304). Use amoxicillin only if micro-organism sensitive. *Suggested duration of treatment* 3 days. Re-assess child if unwell 24–48 hours after initial assessment.

Acute pyelonephritis in children over 3 months of age can be treated with a first generation cephalosporin or co-amoxiclav p. 328 for 7–10 days.

If the patient is severely ill, then the infection is best treated initially by intravenous injection of a broad-spectrum antibacterial such as cefotaxime or co-amoxiclav; gentamicin is an alternative.

Resistant infections

Widespread bacterial resistance to ampicillin, amoxicillin, and trimethoprim has been reported. Alternatives for resistant organisms include co-amoxiclav (amoxicillin with clavulanic acid), an oral cephalosporin, pivmecillinam hydrochloride p. 330, or a quinolone.

Antibacterial prophylaxis

Recurrent episodes of infection are an indication for imaging tests. *Antibacterial prophylaxis* with low doses of trimethoprim or nitrofurantoin may be considered for children with recurrent infection, significant urinary-tract anomalies, or significant kidney damage. Nitrofurantoin is contra-indicated in children under 3 months of age because of the theoretical possibility of haemolytic anaemia.

Pregnancy

Urinary-tract infection in *pregnancy* may be asymptomatic and requires prompt treatment to prevent progression to acute pyelonephritis. Penicillins and cephalosporins are suitable for treating urinary-tract infection during pregnancy. Nitrofurantoin may also be used but it should be avoided at term. Sulfonamides, quinolones, and tetracyclines should be avoided during pregnancy; trimethoprim should also preferably be avoided particularly in the first trimester.

Renal impairment

In *renal failure* antibacterials normally excreted by the kidney accumulate with resultant toxicity unless the dose is reduced. This applies especially to the aminoglycosides which should be used with great caution; tetracyclines, methenamine hippurate, and nitrofurantoin should be avoided altogether.

ANTIBACTERIALS

| Nitrofurantoin

- ● **INDICATIONS AND DOSE**
  Acute uncomplicated urinary-tract infections
  ▸ BY MOUTH USING IMMEDIATE-RELEASE MEDICINES
  ▸ Child 3 months–11 years: 750 micrograms/kg 4 times a day for 3–7 days
  ▸ Child 12–17 years: 50 mg 4 times a day for 3–7 days
  ▸ BY MOUTH USING MODIFIED-RELEASE MEDICINES
  ▸ Child 12–17 years: 100 mg twice daily, dose to be taken with food

  Severe chronic recurrent urinary-tract infections
  ▸ BY MOUTH USING IMMEDIATE-RELEASE MEDICINES
  ▸ Child 12–17 years: 100 mg 4 times a day for 3–7 days

  Prophylaxis of urinary-tract infection (considered for recurrent infection, significant urinary-tract anomalies, or significant kidney damage)
  ▸ BY MOUTH USING IMMEDIATE-RELEASE MEDICINES
  ▸ Child 3 months–11 years: 1 mg/kg once daily, dose to be taken at night
  ▸ Child 12–17 years: 50–100 mg once daily, dose to be taken at night

Genito-urinary surgical prophylaxis
▸ BY MOUTH USING MODIFIED-RELEASE MEDICINES
▸ Child 12–17 years: 100 mg twice daily on day of procedure and for 3 days after

- ● **CONTRA-INDICATIONS** Acute porphyrias p. 577 · G6PD deficiency · infants less than 3 months old
- ● **CAUTIONS** Anaemia · diabetes mellitus · electrolyte imbalance · folate deficiency · pulmonary disease · susceptibility to peripheral neuropathy · urine may be coloured yellow or brown · vitamin B deficiency
- ● **INTERACTIONS** → Appendix 1: nitrofurantoin
- ● **SIDE-EFFECTS**
  ▸ **Rare** Agranulocytosis · aplastic anaemia · arthralgia · benign intracranial hypertension · blood disorders · cholestatic jaundice · erythema multiforme · exfoliative dermatitis · hepatitis · pancreatitis · thrombocytopenia · transient alopecia
  ▸ **Frequency not known** Acute pulmonary reactions · anaphylaxis · angioedema · anorexia chronic pulmonary reactions (pulmonary fibrosis reported; possible association with lupus erythematosus-like syndrome) · diarrhoea · hypersensitivity reaction · nausea · peripheral neuropathy · pruritus · rash · sialadenitis · urticaria · vomiting
- ● **PREGNANCY** Avoid at term—may produce neonatal haemolysis.
- ● **BREAST FEEDING** Avoid; only small amounts in milk but enough to produce haemolysis in G6PD-deficient infants.
- ● **HEPATIC IMPAIRMENT** Use with caution; cholestatic jaundice and chronic active hepatitis reported.
- ● **RENAL IMPAIRMENT** Risk of peripheral neuropathy; antibacterial efficacy depends on renal secretion of the drug into urinary tract. Avoid if estimated glomerular filtration rate less than 45 mL/minute/1.73 m^2; may be used with caution if estimated glomerular filtration rate 30–44 mL/minute/1.73 m^2 as a short-course only (3 to 7 days), to treat uncomplicated lower urinary-tract infection caused by suspected or proven multidrug resistant bacteria and only if potential benefit outweighs risk.
- ● **MONITORING REQUIREMENTS** On long-term therapy, monitor liver function and monitor for pulmonary symptoms (discontinue if deterioration in lung function).
- ● **EFFECT ON LABORATORY TESTS** False positive urinary glucose (if tested for reducing substances).
- ● **PATIENT AND CARER ADVICE**
  Medicines for Children leaflet: Nitrofurantoin for urinary tract infections www.medicinesforchildren.org.uk/nitrofurantoin-for-urinary-tract-infections
- ● **MEDICINAL FORMS**
  There can be variation in the licensing of different medicines containing the same drug. Forms available from special-order manufacturers include: oral suspension, oral solution
  Tablet
  CAUTIONARY AND ADVISORY LABELS 9, 14, 21
  ▸ **Nitrofurantoin** (Non-proprietary)
  Nitrofurantoin 50 mg Nitrofurantoin 50mg tablets | 28 tablet [PoM] £35.00 DT price = £11.66 | 100 tablet [PoM] £111.89
  Nitrofurantoin 100 mg Nitrofurantoin 100mg tablets | 28 tablet [PoM] £16.80 DT price = £7.03 | 100 tablet [PoM] £60.00
  ▸ **Genfura** (Genesis Pharmaceuticals Ltd)
  Nitrofurantoin 50 mg Genfura 50mg tablets | 28 tablet [PoM] £23.57 DT price = £11.66
  Nitrofurantoin 100 mg Genfura 100mg tablets | 28 tablet [PoM] £18.76 DT price = £7.03 | 100 tablet [PoM] £67.02

Oral suspension

CAUTIONARY AND ADVISORY LABELS 9, 14, 21

▸ **Nitrofurantoin (Non-proprietary)**
Nitrofurantoin 5 mg per 1 ml Nitrofurantoin 25mg/5ml oral
suspension sugar free sugar-free | 300 ml [PoM] £446.95 DT price =
£446.95

Modified-release capsule

CAUTIONARY AND ADVISORY LABELS 9, 14, 21, 25

▸ **Macrobid** (AMCo)
Nitrofurantoin 100 mg Macrobid 100mg modified-release capsules
| 14 capsule [PoM] £9.50 DT price = £9.50

Capsule

CAUTIONARY AND ADVISORY LABELS 9, 14, 21

▸ **Nitrofurantoin (Non-proprietary)**
Nitrofurantoin 50 mg Nitrofurantoin 50mg capsules |
30 capsule [PoM] £15.42 DT price = £15.42
Nitrofurantoin 100 mg Nitrofurantoin 100mg capsules |
30 capsule [PoM] £10.42 DT price = £10.42

3 Fungal infection

Antifungals, systemic use

Common fungal infections

The systemic treatment of common fungal infections is
outlined below; specialist treatment is required in most
forms of systemic or disseminated fungal infections. Local
treatment is suitable for a number of fungal infections
(genital, bladder, eye, ear, oropharynx, and skin).

Aspergillosis

Aspergillosis most commonly affects the respiratory tract
but in severely immunocompromised patients, invasive
forms can affect the heart, brain, and skin. Voriconazole
p. 361 is the treatment of choice for aspergillosis; liposomal
amphotericin p. 357 is an alternative first-line treatment
when voriconazole cannot be used. Caspofungin p. 361 or
itraconazole p. 360 can be used in patients who are
refractory to, or intolerant of voriconazole and liposomal
amphotericin. Itraconazole is also used for the treatment of
chronic pulmonary aspergillosis or as an adjunct in the
treatment of allergic bronchopulmonary aspergillosis
[unlicensed indication].

Candidiasis

Many superficial candidal infections, including infections of
the skin, are treated locally. Systemic antifungal treatment is
required in widespread or intractable infection. Vaginal
candidiasis can be treated with locally acting antifungals;
alternatively, fluconazole p. 358 can be given by mouth.

Oropharyngeal candidiasis generally responds to topical
therapy. Fluconazole is given by mouth for unresponsive
infections; it is reliably absorbed and is effective.
Itraconazole may be used for infections that do not respond
to fluconazole. Topical therapy may not be adequate in
immunocompromised children and an oral triazole
antifungal is preferred.

For *invasive or disseminated candidiasis*, either
amphotericin by intravenous infusion or an **echinocandin**
can be used. Fluconazole is an alternative for *Candida
albicans* infection in clinically stable children who have not
received an azole antifungal recently. Amphotericin should
be considered for the initial treatment of CNS candidiasis.
Voriconazole can be used for infections caused by
fluconazole-resistant *Candida* spp. when oral therapy is
required, or in children intolerant of amphotericin or an
echinocandin. In refractory cases, flucytosine p. 363 can be
used with intravenous amphotericin.

Cryptococcosis

Cryptococcosis is uncommon but infection in the
immunocompromised, especially in HIV-positive patients,
can be life-threatening; cryptococcal meningitis is the most
common form of fungal meningitis. The treatment of choice
in cryptococcal meningitis is amphotericin by intravenous
infusion and flucytosine by intravenous infusion for 2 weeks,
followed by fluconazole by mouth for 8 weeks or until
cultures are negative. In cryptococcosis, fluconazole is
sometimes given alone as an alternative in HIV-positive
patients with mild, localised infections or in those who
cannot tolerate amphotericin. Following successful
treatment, fluconazole can be used for prophylaxis against
relapse until immunity recovers.

Histoplasmosis

Histoplasmosis is rare in temperate climates; it can be life-
threatening, particularly in HIV-infected persons.
Itraconazole can be used for the treatment of
immunocompetent patients with indolent non-meningeal
infection, including chronic pulmonary histoplasmosis.
Amphotericin by intravenous infusion is used for the initial
treatment of fulminant or severe infections, followed by a
course of itraconazole by mouth. Following successful
treatment, itraconazole can be used for prophylaxis against
relapse until immunity recovers.

Skin and nail infections

Mild localised fungal infections of the skin (including tinea
corporis, tinea cruris, and tinea pedis) respond to topical
therapy. Systemic therapy is appropriate if topical therapy
fails, if many areas are affected, or if the site of infection is
difficult to treat such as in infections of the nails
(onychomycosis) and of the scalp (tinea capitis).

Oral imidazole or triazole antifungals (particularly
itraconazole) and terbinafine p. 696 are used more
frequently than griseofulvin p. 363 because they have a
broader spectrum of activity and require a shorter duration
of treatment.

Tinea capitis is treated systemically; additional topical
application of an antifungal may reduce transmission.
Griseofulvin is used for tinea capitis in adults and children; it
is effective against infections caused by *Trichophyton
tonsurans* and *Microsporum* spp. Terbinafine is used for tinea
capitis caused by *T. tonsurans* [unlicensed indication]. The
role of terbinafine in the management of *Microsporum*
infections is uncertain. Fluconazole and itraconazole are
alternatives in the treatment of tinea capitis caused by
T. tonsurans or *Microsporum* spp. [both unlicensed
indications].

Pityriasis versicolor may be treated with itraconazole by
mouth if topical therapy is ineffective; fluconazole by mouth
is an alternative. Oral terbinafine is **not** effective for
pityriasis versicolor.

Antifungal treatment may not be necessary in
asymptomatic patients with tinea infection of the nails. If
treatment is necessary, a systemic antifungal is more
effective than topical therapy. Terbinafine and itraconazole
have largely replaced griseofulvin for the systemic treatment
of *onychomycosis*, particularly of the toenail; they should be
used under specialist advice in children. Although
terbinafine is not licensed for use in children, it is considered
to be the drug of choice for onychomycosis. Itraconazole can
be administered as intermittent 'pulse' therapy. Topical
antifungals also have a role in the treatment of
onychomycosis.

Immunocompromised children

Immunocompromised children are at particular risk of
fungal infections and may receive antifungal drugs
prophylactically; oral triazole antifungals are the drugs of
choice for prophylaxis. Fluconazole is more reliably absorbed
than itraconazole, but fluconazole is not effective against
Aspergillus spp. Itraconazole is preferred in patients at risk of
invasive aspergillosis. Micafungin p. 357 can be used for
prophylaxis of candidiasis in patients undergoing

haematopoietic stem cell transplantation when fluconazole or itraconazole cannot be used.

Amphotericin by intravenous infusion or caspofungin is used for the empirical *treatment* of serious fungal infections in immunocompromised children; caspofungin is not effective against fungal infections of the CNS.

Triazole antifungals

Triazole antifungal drugs have a role in the prevention and systemic treatment of fungal infections.

Fluconazole is very well absorbed after oral administration. It also achieves good penetration into the cerebrospinal fluid to treat fungal meningitis. Fluconazole is excreted largely unchanged in the urine and can be used to treat candiduria.

Itraconazole is active against a wide range of dermatophytes. There is limited information available on use in children. Itraconazole capsules require an acid environment in the stomach for optimal absorption. Itraconazole has been associated with liver damage and should be avoided or used with caution in patients with liver disease; fluconazole is less frequently associated with hepatotoxicity.

Voriconazole is a broad-spectrum antifungal drug which is licensed in adults for use in life-threatening infections.

Imidazole antifungals

The imidazole antifungals include clotrimazole p. 492, econazole nitrate p. 492, ketoconazole p. 695, and tioconazole p. 696. They are used for the local treatment of vaginal candidiasis and for dermatophyte infections. Miconazole p. 493 can be used locally for oral infections; it is also effective in intestinal infections. Systemic absorption may follow use of miconazole oral gel and may result in significant drug interactions.

Polyene antifungals

The polyene antifungals include amphotericin and nystatin p. 680; neither drug is absorbed when given by mouth. Nystatin p. 680 is used for oral, oropharyngeal, and perioral infections by local application in the mouth. Nystatin is also used for *Candida albicans* infection of the skin.

Amphotericin p. 357 by intravenous infusion is used for the treatment of systemic fungal infections and is active against most fungi and yeasts. It is highly protein bound and penetrates poorly into body fluids and tissues. When given parenterally amphotericin is toxic and side-effects are common. Lipid formulations of amphotericin (*Abelcet*® and *AmBisome*®) are significantly less toxic and are recommended when the conventional formulation of amphotericin is contra-indicated because of toxicity, especially nephrotoxicity or when response to conventional amphotericin is inadequate; lipid formulations are more expensive.

Echinocandin antifungals

The echinocandin antifungals include caspofungin below and micafungin p. 357. They are only active against *Aspergillus* spp. and *Candida* spp.; however, micafungin is not used for the treatment of aspergillosis. Echinocandins are not effective against fungal infections of the CNS. Echinocandin antifungals have a role in the prevention and systemic treatment of fungal infections.

Other antifungals

Flucytosine p. 363 is used with amphotericin in a synergistic combination. Bone marrow depression can occur which limits its use, particularly in HIV-positive patients; weekly blood counts are necessary during prolonged therapy. Resistance to flucytosine can develop during therapy and sensitivity testing is essential before and during treatment.

Flucytosine has a role in the treatment of systemic candidiasis and cryptococcal meningitis.

Griseofulvin p. 363 is effective for widespread or intractable dermatophyte infections but has been superseded by newer antifungals, particularly for nail infections. Griseofulvin is used in the treatment of tinea capitis. It is the drug of choice for trichophyton infections in children. Duration of therapy is dependent on the site of the infection and may extend to a number of months.

Terbinafine p. 696 is the drug of choice for fungal nail infections and is also used for ringworm infections where oral treatment is considered appropriate.

ANTIFUNGALS > ECHINOCANDIN ANTIFUNGALS

Caspofungin

● **INDICATIONS AND DOSE**

Invasive aspergillosis | Invasive candidiasis | Empirical treatment of systemic fungal infections in patients with neutropenia

▸ BY INTRAVENOUS INFUSION

▸ Neonate: 25 mg/m^2 once daily.

▸ Child 1–2 months: 25 mg/m^2 once daily.
▸ Child 3–11 months: 50 mg/m^2 once daily
▸ Child 1–17 years: 70 mg/m^2 once daily (max. per dose 70 mg) for 1 day, then 50 mg/m^2 once daily (max. per dose 70 mg); increased to 70 mg/m^2 once daily (max. per dose 70 mg), dose may be increased if lower dose tolerated but inadequate response

DOSE ADJUSTMENTS DUE TO INTERACTIONS
Manufacturer advises increase dose to 70 mg/m^2 daily (max. 70 mg daily) with concurrent use of some enzyme inducers (such as carbamazepine, dexamethasone, phenytoin, and rifampicin).

● INTERACTIONS → Appendix 1: caspofungin

● SIDE-EFFECTS

▸ **Common or very common** Arthralgia · diarrhoea · dyspnoea · flushing · headache · hypokalaemia · hypomagnesaemia · hypotension · injection-site reactions · nausea · pruritus · rash · sweating · tachycardia · vomiting

▸ **Uncommon** Abdominal pain · anaemia · anorexia · anxiety · arrhythmia · ascites · blurred vision · bronchospasm · chest pain · cholestasis · constipation · cough · disorientation · dizziness · dry mouth · dyspepsia · dysphagia · erythema multiforme · fatigue · flatulence · heart failure · hepatic dysfunction · hyperglycaemia · hypertension · hypoaesthesia · hypocalcaemia · leucopenia · metabolic acidosis · muscular weakness · myalgia · palpitation · paraesthesia · renal failure · sleep disturbances · taste disturbances · thrombocytopenia · thrombophlebitis · tremor

▸ **Frequency not known** Acute respiratory distress syndrome · anaphylaxis · hypercalcaemia

● PREGNANCY Manufacturer advises avoid unless essential—toxicity in *animal* studies.

● BREAST FEEDING Present in milk in *animal* studies— manufacturer advises avoid.

● HEPATIC IMPAIRMENT Usual initial dose, then use 70% of normal maintenance dose in moderate impairment. No information available for severe impairment.

● DIRECTIONS FOR ADMINISTRATION For *intravenous infusion* (*Candidas*®), allow vial to reach room temperature; initially reconstitute 50 mg with 10.5 mL Water for Injections to produce a 5.2 mg/mL solution, or reconstitute 70 mg with 10.5 mL Water for Injections to produce a 7.2 mg/mL solution; mix gently to dissolve; dilute requisite dose to a final concentration not exceeding

500 micrograms/mL with Sodium Chloride 0.9%; give over 60 minutes; incompatible with glucose solutions.

- **MEDICINAL FORMS**
  There can be variation in the licensing of different medicines containing the same drug.
  Powder for solution for infusion
  ‣ Cancidas (Merck Sharp & Dohme Ltd)
    Caspofungin (as Caspofungin acetate) 50 mg Cancidas 50mg powder for solution for infusion vials | 1 vial [PoM] £327.67
    Caspofungin (as Caspofungin acetate) 70 mg Cancidas 70mg powder for solution for infusion vials | 1 vial [PoM] £416.78

Micafungin

- **INDICATIONS AND DOSE**
  Invasive candidiasis
  ‣ BY INTRAVENOUS INFUSION

  ‣ Neonate (administered on expert advice): 2 mg/kg once daily for at least 14 days; increased if necessary to 4 mg/kg once daily, increase dose if response inadequate.

  ‣ Child (body-weight up to 40 kg): 2 mg/kg once daily for at least 14 days; increased if necessary to 4 mg/kg once daily, increase dose if response inadequate

  ‣ Child (body-weight 40 kg and above): 100 mg once daily for at least 14 days; increased if necessary to 200 mg once daily, increase dose if response inadequate

  Oesophageal candidiasis
  ‣ BY INTRAVENOUS INFUSION

  ‣ Child 16–17 years (body-weight up to 40 kg): 3 mg/kg once daily

  ‣ Child 16–17 years (body-weight 40 kg and above): 150 mg once daily

  Prophylaxis of candidiasis in patients undergoing bone-marrow transplantation or who are expected to become neutropenic for over 10 days
  ‣ BY INTRAVENOUS INFUSION

  ‣ Neonate: 1 mg/kg once daily continue for at least 7 days after neutrophil count is in desirable range.

  ‣ Child (body-weight up to 40 kg): 1 mg/kg once daily continue for at least 7 days after neutrophil count is in desirable range

  ‣ Child (body-weight 40 kg and above): 50 mg once daily continue for at least 7 days after neutrophil count is in desirable range

- **INTERACTIONS** → Appendix 1: micafungin
- **SIDE-EFFECTS**
  ‣ **Common or very common** Abdominal pain · anaemia · blood pressure changes · diarrhoea · fever · headache · hepatomegaly · hypocalcaemia · hypokalaemia · hypomagnesaemia · leucopenia · nausea · phlebitis · rash · renal failure · tachycardia · thrombocytopenia · vomiting
  ‣ **Uncommon** Anorexia · anxiety · bradycardia · cholestasis · confusion · constipation · dizziness · dyspepsia · dyspnoea · eosinophilia · flushing · hepatitis · hyperhidrosis · hyperkalaemia · hyponatraemia · hypophosphataemia · palpitation · pancytopenia · pruritus · sleep disturbances · tachycardia · taste disturbances · tremor
  ‣ **Rare** Haemolytic anaemia
  ‣ **Frequency not known** Disseminated intravascular coagulation · hepatotoxicity (potentially life-threatening; more common in children under 1 year) · Stevens-Johnson syndrome · toxic epidermal necrolysis

- **PREGNANCY** Manufacturer advises avoid unless essential—toxicity in *animal* studies.

- **BREAST FEEDING** Manufacturer advises use only if potential benefit outweighs risk—present in milk in *animal* studies.

- **HEPATIC IMPAIRMENT** Use with caution in mild to moderate impairment. Avoid in severe impairment.
- **RENAL IMPAIRMENT** Use with caution; renal function may deteriorate.
- **MONITORING REQUIREMENTS**
  ‣ Monitor renal function.
  ‣ Monitor liver function—discontinue if significant and persistent abnormalities in liver function tests develop.
- **DIRECTIONS FOR ADMINISTRATION** For *intravenous infusion* reconstitute each vial with 5 mL Glucose 5% *or* Sodium Chloride 0.9%; gently rotate vial, without shaking, to dissolve; dilute requisite dose to a concentration of 0.5–2 mg/mL with Glucose 5% *or* Sodium Chloride 0.9%; protect infusion from light; give over 60 minutes.

- **MEDICINAL FORMS**
  There can be variation in the licensing of different medicines containing the same drug.
  Powder for solution for infusion
  ‣ Mycamine (Astellas Pharma Ltd)
    Micafungin (as Micafungin sodium) 50 mg Mycamine 50mg powder for solution for infusion vials | 1 vial [PoM] £196.08
    Micafungin (as Micafungin sodium) 100 mg Mycamine 100mg powder for solution for infusion vials | 1 vial [PoM] £341.00

ANTIFUNGALS › POLYENE ANTIFUNGALS

Amphotericin

(Amphotericin B)

- **INDICATIONS AND DOSE**
  ABELCET®

  Severe invasive candidiasis | Severe systemic fungal infections in patients not responding to conventional amphotericin or to other antifungal drugs or where toxicity or renal impairment precludes conventional amphotericin, including invasive aspergillosis, cryptococcal meningitis and disseminated cryptococcosis in HIV patients
  ‣ BY INTRAVENOUS INFUSION
  ‣ Child: Test dose 100 micrograms/kg (max. per dose 1 mg), then 5 mg/kg once daily

  AMBISOME®

  Severe systemic or deep mycoses where toxicity (particularly nephrotoxicity) precludes use of conventional amphotericin | Suspected or proven infection in febrile neutropenic patients unresponsive to broad-spectrum antibacterials
  ‣ BY INTRAVENOUS INFUSION

  ‣ Neonate: 1 mg/kg once daily, increased if necessary to 3 mg/kg once daily; maximum 5 mg/kg per day.

  ‣ Child: Test dose 100 micrograms/kg (max. per dose 1 mg), to be given over 10 minutes, then 3 mg/kg once daily; maximum 5 mg/kg per day

  Visceral leishmaniasis (unresponsive to the antimonial alone)
  ‣ BY INTRAVENOUS INFUSION
  ‣ Child: 1–3 mg/kg daily for 10–21 days to a cumulative dose of 21–30 mg/kg, alternatively 3 mg/kg for 5 consecutive days, followed by 3 mg/kg after 6 days for 1 dose

  FUNGIZONE®

  Systemic fungal infections
  ‣ BY INTRAVENOUS INFUSION

  ‣ Neonate: 1 mg/kg once daily, increased if necessary to 1.5 mg/kg daily for 7 days, then reduced to 1–1.5 mg/kg once daily on alternate days if required.

continued →

5

Infection

▸ **Child:** Test dose 100 micrograms/kg (max. per dose 1 mg), included as part of first dose of 250 micrograms/kg daily, then increased if tolerated to 1 mg/kg daily, dose is gradually increased over 2–4 days; in severe infection max. 1.5 mg/kg daily or on alternate days. Prolonged treatment usually necessary; if interrupted for longer than 7 days recommence at 250 micrograms/kg daily and increase gradually

● **UNLICENSED USE**
AMBISOME® *Ambisome*® not licensed for use in children under 1 month.
FUNGIZONE® Intravenous conventional formulation amphotericin (*Fungizone*®) is licensed for use in children (age range not specified by manufacturer).

● **CAUTIONS** Avoid rapid infusion (risk of arrhythmias) · when given parenterally, toxicity common (close supervision necessary and close observation required for at least 30 minutes after test dose)
CAUTIONS, FURTHER INFORMATION
▸ Anaphylaxis Anaphylaxis can occur with any intravenous amphotericin product and a test dose is advisable before the first infusion in children over 1 month of age; the patient should be carefully observed for at least 30 minutes after the test dose. Prophylactic antipyretics or hydrocortisone should only be used in patients who have previously experienced acute adverse reactions (in whom continued treatment with amphotericin is essential).

● **INTERACTIONS** → Appendix 1: amphotericin

● **SIDE-EFFECTS**
▸ **Common or very common** Abdominal pain · abnormal liver function (discontinue treatment) · anaemia · arrhythmias · blood disorders · blood pressure changes · cardiovascular effects · chest pain · diarrhoea · disturbances in renal function · dyspnoea · electrolyte disturbances · febrile reactions · headache · hypokalaemia · hypomagnesaemia · nausea · rash · renal tubular acidosis · thrombocytopenia · vomiting
▸ **Uncommon** Anaphylactoid reactions · bronchospasm · convulsions · diplopia · encephalopathy · hearing loss · neurological disorders · peripheral neuropathy · tremor
▸ **Frequency not known** Anorexia · arthralgia · myalgia · Stevens-Johnson syndrome · toxic epidermal necrolysis

● **PREGNANCY** Not known to be harmful but manufacturers advise avoid unless potential benefit outweighs risk.

● **BREAST FEEDING** No information available.

● **RENAL IMPAIRMENT** Use only if no alternative; nephrotoxicity may be reduced with use of lipid formulation.

● **MONITORING REQUIREMENTS** Hepatic and renal function tests, blood counts, and plasma electrolyte (including plasma-potassium and magnesium concentration) monitoring required.

● **DIRECTIONS FOR ADMINISTRATION**
ABELCET® **Amphotericin (lipid complex)**
For *intravenous infusion*, allow suspension to reach room temperature, shake gently to ensure no yellow settlement, withdraw requisite dose (using 17–19 gauge needle) into one or more 20-mL syringes; replace needle on syringe with a 5-micron filter needle provided (fresh needle for each syringe) and dilute in Glucose 5% to a concentration of 2 mg/mL; preferably give *via* an infusion pump at a rate of 2.5 mg/kg/hour (initial test dose given over 15 minutes); an in-line filter (pore size no less than 15 micron) may be used; do not use sodium chloride or other electrolyte solutions—flush existing intravenous line with Glucose 5% or use separate line.
AMBISOME® **Amphotericin (liposomal)**
For *intravenous infusion,*, reconstitute each vial with 12 mL Water for Injections and shake vigorously to

produce a preparation containing 4 mg/mL; withdraw requisite dose from vial and introduce into Glucose 5% or 10% through the 5-micron filter provided, to produce a final concentration of 0.2–2 mg/mL; infuse over 30–60 minutes, or if non-anaphylactic infusion-related reactions occur infuse over 2 hours (initial test dose given over 10 minutes); an in-line filter (pore size no less than 1 micron) may be used; incompatible with sodium chloride solutions—flush existing intravenous line with Glucose 5% or 10%, or use separate line.

FUNGIZONE® **Amphotericin (as sodium deoxycholate complex)**
For *intravenous infusion*, reconstitute each vial with 10 mL Water for Injections and shake immediately to produce a 5 mg/mL colloidal solution; dilute further in Glucose 5% to a concentration of 100 micrograms/mL (in fluid-restricted children, up to 400 micrograms/mL given via a central line); pH of glucose solution must not be below 4.2 (check each container—consult product literature for details of buffer); infuse over 4–6 hours, or if tolerated over a minimum of 2 hours (initial test dose given over 20–30 minutes); begin infusion immediately after dilution and protect from light; incompatible with Sodium Chloride solutions—flush existing intravenous line with Glucose 5% or use separate line; an in-line filter (pore size no less than 1 micron) may be used.

● **PRESCRIBING AND DISPENSING INFORMATION** Different preparations of intravenous amphotericin vary in their pharmacodynamics, pharmacokinetics, dosage, and administration; these preparations should **not** be considered interchangeable. To avoid confusion, prescribers should specify the brand to be dispensed.

● **MEDICINAL FORMS**
There can be variation in the licensing of different medicines containing the same drug.
Suspension for infusion
ELECTROLYTES: May contain Sodium
▸ Abelcet (Teva UK Ltd)
Amphotericin B (as Amphotericin B phospholipid complex) 5 mg per 1 ml Abelcet 100mg/20ml concentrate for suspension for infusion vials | 10 vial [PoM] £775.04 (Hospital only)
Powder for solution for infusion
EXCIPIENTS: May contain Sucrose
ELECTROLYTES: May contain Sodium
▸ AmBisome (Gilead Sciences International Ltd)
Amphotericin B liposomal 50 mg AmBisome 50mg powder for solution for infusion vials | 10 vial [PoM] £821.87
▸ Fungizone (Bristol-Myers Squibb Pharmaceuticals Ltd)
Amphotericin B 50 mg Fungizone Intravenous 50mg powder for solution for infusion vials | 1 vial [PoM] £3.88

ANTIFUNGALS ⟩ TRIAZOLE ANTIFUNGALS

Fluconazole

● **INDICATIONS AND DOSE**
Candidal balanitis
▸ BY MOUTH
▸ **Child 16–17 years:** 150 mg for 1 dose
Vaginal candidiasis
▸ BY MOUTH
▸ **Child 1 month–15 years:** 150 mg for 1 dose, for use in patients who are post-puberty
▸ **Child 16–17 years:** 150 mg for 1 dose
Vulvovaginal candidiasis (recurrent)
▸ BY MOUTH
▸ **Child:** Initially 150 mg every 72 hours for 3 doses, then 150 mg once weekly for 6 months, for use in patients who are post-puberty

Mucosal candidiasis (except genital)
▸ BY MOUTH, OR BY INTRAVENOUS INFUSION

▸ Neonate up to 14 days: 3–6 mg/kg, dose to be given on first day, then 3 mg/kg every 72 hours.

▸ Neonate 14 days to 28 days: 3–6 mg/kg, dose to be given on first day, then 3 mg/kg every 48 hours.

▸ Child 1 month–11 years: 3–6 mg/kg, dose to be given on first day, then 3 mg/kg daily (max. per dose 100 mg) for 7–14 days in oropharyngeal candidiasis (max. 14 days except in severely immunocompromised patients); for 14–30 days in other mucosal infections (e.g. oesophagitis, candiduria, non-invasive bronchopulmonary infections)

▸ Child 12–17 years: 50 mg daily for 7–14 days in oropharyngeal candidiasis (max. 14 days except in severely immunocompromised patients); for 14–30 days in other mucosal infections (e.g. oesophagitis, candiduria, non-invasive bronchopulmonary infections); increased to 100 mg daily, increased dose only for unusually difficult infections

Tinea capitis
▸ BY MOUTH

▸ Child 1–17 years: 6 mg/kg daily (max. per dose 300 mg) for 2–4 weeks

Tinea pedis, corporis, cruris, pityriasis versicolor | Dermal candidiasis
▸ BY MOUTH

▸ Child: 3 mg/kg daily (max. per dose 50 mg) for 2–4 weeks (for up to 6 weeks in tinea pedis); max. duration of treatment 6 weeks

Invasive candidal infections (including candidaemia and disseminated candidiasis) and cryptococcal infections (including meningitis)
▸ BY MOUTH, OR BY INTRAVENOUS INFUSION

▸ Neonate up to 14 days: 6–12 mg/kg every 72 hours, treatment continued according to response (at least 8 weeks for cryptococcal meningitis).

▸ Neonate 14 days to 28 days: 6–12 mg/kg every 48 hours, treatment continued according to response (at least 8 weeks for cryptococcal meningitis).

▸ Child: 6–12 mg/kg daily (max. per dose 800 mg), treatment continued according to response (at least 8 weeks for cryptococcal meningitis)

Prevention of fungal infections in immunocompromised patients
▸ BY MOUTH, OR BY INTRAVENOUS INFUSION

▸ Neonate up to 14 days: 3–12 mg/kg every 72 hours, dose given according to extent and duration of neutropenia.

▸ Neonate 14 days to 28 days: 3–12 mg/kg every 48 hours, dose given according to extent and duration of neutropenia.

▸ Child: 3–12 mg/kg daily (max. per dose 400 mg), commence treatment before anticipated onset of neutropenia and continue for 7 days after neutrophil count in desirable range, dose given according to extent and duration of neutropenia

Prevention of fungal infections in immunocompromised patients (for patients with high risk of systemic infections e.g. following bone-marrow transplantation)
▸ BY MOUTH, OR BY INTRAVENOUS INFUSION

▸ Child: 12 mg/kg daily (max. per dose 400 mg), commence treatment before anticipated onset of neutropenia and continue for 7 days after neutrophil count in desirable range

Prevention of relapse of cryptococcal meningitis in HIV-infected patients after completion of primary therapy
▸ BY MOUTH, OR BY INTRAVENOUS INFUSION

▸ Child: 6 mg/kg daily (max. per dose 200 mg)

● **UNLICENSED USE** Not licensed for tinea infections in children, or for vaginal candidiasis in girls under 16 years, or for prevention of relapse of cryptococcal meningitis after completion of primary therapy in children with AIDS.

● **CONTRA-INDICATIONS** Acute porphyrias p. 577

● **CAUTIONS** Susceptibility to QT interval prolongation

● **INTERACTIONS** → Appendix 1: antifungals, azoles

● **SIDE-EFFECTS**

▸ **Common or very common** Abdominal discomfort · diarrhoea · flatulence · headache · nausea · rash

▸ **Uncommon** Alopecia · anaphylaxis · angioedema · dizziness · dyspepsia · hepatic disorders · hyperlipidaemia · pruritus · seizures · Stevens-Johnson syndrome · taste disturbance · toxic epidermal necrolysis · vomiting

▸ **Frequency not known** Hypokalaemia · leucopenia · thrombocytopenia

SIDE-EFFECTS, FURTHER INFORMATION
If rash occurs, discontinue treatment (or monitor closely if infection invasive or systemic); severe cutaneous reactions are more likely in patients with AIDS.

● **PREGNANCY** Manufacturer advises avoid—multiple congenital abnormalities reported with long-term high doses.

● **BREAST FEEDING** Present in milk but amount probably too small to be harmful.

● **HEPATIC IMPAIRMENT** Toxicity with related drugs.

● **RENAL IMPAIRMENT** Usual initial dose then halve subsequent doses if estimated glomerular filtration rate less than 50 mL/minute/1.73 m².

● **MONITORING REQUIREMENTS** Monitor liver function with high doses or extended courses—discontinue if signs or symptoms of hepatic disease (risk of hepatic necrosis).

● **DIRECTIONS FOR ADMINISTRATION** For *intravenous infusion*, give over 10–30 minutes; do not exceed an infusion rate of 5–10 mL/minute.

● **PRESCRIBING AND DISPENSING INFORMATION** Flavours of oral liquid formulations may include orange.

● **PROFESSION SPECIFIC INFORMATION**

Dental practitioners' formulary
Fluconazole Capsules 50 mg may be prescribed.
Fluconazole Oral Suspension 50 mg/5 mL may be prescribed.

● **EXCEPTIONS TO LEGAL CATEGORY** Fluconazole capsules can be sold to the public for vaginal candidiasis and associated candidal balanitis in those aged 16–60 years, in a container or packaging containing not more than 150 mg and labelled to show a max. dose of 150 mg.

● **MEDICINAL FORMS**
There can be variation in the licensing of different medicines containing the same drug.

Solution for infusion
ELECTROLYTES: May contain Sodium
▸ **Fluconazole (Non-proprietary)**
　Fluconazole 2 mg per 1 ml Fluconazole 100mg/50ml solution for infusion bottles | 5 bottle PoM £12.60
　Fluconazole 200mg/100ml solution for infusion vials | 1 vial PoM £29.28
　Fluconazole 50mg/25ml solution for infusion vials | 1 vial PoM £7.31–£7.32
　Fluconazole 200mg/100ml solution for infusion bottles | 5 bottle PoM £274.50
▸ **Diflucan** (Pfizer Ltd)
　Fluconazole 2 mg per 1 ml Diflucan 200mg/100ml solution for infusion vials | 1 vial PoM £29.28

5

Infection

Oral suspension

CAUTIONARY AND ADVISORY LABELS 9

▸ Fluconazole (Non-proprietary)

Fluconazole 10 mg per 1 ml Fluconazole 50mg/5ml oral suspension | 35 ml [PoM] £20.51 DT price = £20.51

▸ Diflucan (Pfizer Ltd)

Fluconazole 10 mg per 1 ml Diflucan 50mg/5ml oral suspension | 35 ml [PoM] £16.61 DT price = £20.51

Fluconazole 40 mg per 1 ml Diflucan 200mg/5ml oral suspension | 35 ml [PoM] £66.42 DT price = £66.42

Capsule

CAUTIONARY AND ADVISORY LABELS 9 (50 mg and 200 mg strengths only)

▸ Fluconazole (Non-proprietary)

Fluconazole 50 mg Fluconazole 50mg capsules | 7 capsule [PoM] £5.00 DT price = £0.91

Fluconazole 150 mg Fluconazole 150mg capsules | 1 capsule [P] no price available DT price = £0.84 | 1 capsule [PoM] £8.50 DT price = £0.84

Fluconazole 200 mg Fluconazole 200mg capsules | 7 capsule [PoM] £6.02 DT price = £6.02

▸ Diflucan (Pfizer Ltd)

Fluconazole 50 mg Diflucan 50mg capsules | 7 capsule [PoM] £16.61 DT price = £0.91

Fluconazole 150 mg Diflucan 150mg capsules | 1 capsule [PoM] £7.12 DT price = £0.84

Fluconazole 200 mg Diflucan 200mg capsules | 7 capsule [PoM] £66.42 DT price = £6.02

Itraconazole

● **INDICATIONS AND DOSE**

Oropharyngeal candidiasis

▸ BY MOUTH

▸ Child 1 month–11 years: 3–5 mg/kg once daily for 15 days; maximum 100 mg per day

▸ Child 12–17 years: 100 mg once daily for 15 days

Oropharyngeal candidiasis in patients with AIDS or neutropenia

▸ BY MOUTH

▸ Child 1 month–11 years: 3–5 mg/kg once daily for 15 days; maximum 200 mg per day

▸ Child 12–17 years: 200 mg once daily for 15 days

Systemic candidiasis where other antifungal drugs inappropriate or ineffective

▸ BY MOUTH

▸ Child: 5 mg/kg once daily (max. per dose 200 mg), dose increased in invasive or disseminated disease and in cryptococcal meningitis, increased to 5 mg/kg twice daily (max. per dose 200 mg)

▸ BY INTRAVENOUS INFUSION

▸ Child: 2.5 mg/kg every 12 hours (max. per dose 200 mg) for 2 days, then 2.5 mg/kg once daily (max. per dose 200 mg) for max. 12 days

Pityriasis versicolor

▸ BY MOUTH

▸ Child 1 month–11 years: 3–5 mg/kg once daily (max. per dose 200 mg) for 7 days

▸ Child 12–17 years: 200 mg once daily for 7 days

Tinea pedis | Tinea manuum

▸ BY MOUTH

▸ Child 1 month–11 years: 3–5 mg/kg once daily (max. per dose 100 mg) for 30 days

▸ Child 12–17 years: 100 mg once daily for 30 days, alternatively 200 mg twice daily for 7 days

Tinea corporis | Tinea cruris

▸ BY MOUTH

▸ Child 1 month–11 years: 3–5 mg/kg once daily (max. per dose 100 mg) for 15 days

▸ Child 12–17 years: 100 mg once daily for 15 days, alternatively 200 mg once daily for 7 days

Tinea capitis

▸ BY MOUTH

▸ Child 1–17 years: 3–5 mg/kg once daily (max. per dose 200 mg) for 2–6 weeks

Onychomycosis

▸ BY MOUTH

▸ Child 1–11 years: 5 mg/kg daily (max. per dose 200 mg) for 7 days, subsequent courses repeated after 21-day intervals; fingernails 2 courses, toenails 3 courses

▸ Child 12–17 years: 200 mg once daily for 3 months, alternatively 200 mg twice daily for 7 days, subsequent courses repeated after 21-day intervals; fingernails 2 courses, toenails 3 courses

Systemic aspergillosis where other antifungal drugs inappropriate or ineffective

▸ BY INTRAVENOUS INFUSION

▸ Child: 2.5 mg/kg every 12 hours (max. per dose 200 mg) for 2 days, then 2.5 mg/kg once daily (max. per dose 200 mg) for max. 12 days

▸ BY MOUTH

▸ Child: 5 mg/kg once daily (max. per dose 200 mg), increased to 5 mg/kg twice daily (max. per dose 200 mg), dose increased in invasive or disseminated disease and in cryptococcal meningitis

Histoplasmosis

▸ BY MOUTH

▸ Child: 5 mg/kg 1–2 times a day (max. per dose 200 mg)

Systemic cryptococcosis including cryptococcal meningitis where other antifungal drugs inappropriate or ineffective

▸ BY MOUTH

▸ Child: 5 mg/kg once daily (max. per dose 200 mg), dose increased in invasive or disseminated disease and in cryptococcal meningitis, increased to 5 mg/kg twice daily (max. per dose 200 mg)

▸ BY INTRAVENOUS INFUSION

▸ Child: 2.5 mg/kg every 12 hours (max. per dose 200 mg) for 2 days, then 2.5 mg/kg once daily (max. per dose 200 mg) for max. 12 days

Maintenance in HIV-infected patients to prevent relapse of underlying fungal infection and prophylaxis in neutropenia when standard therapy inappropriate

▸ BY MOUTH

▸ Child: 5 mg/kg once daily (max. per dose 200 mg), then increased to 5 mg/kg twice daily (max. per dose 200 mg), dose increased only if low plasma-itraconazole concentration

Prophylaxis of deep fungal infections (when standard therapy inappropriate) in patients with haematological malignancy or undergoing bone-marrow transplantation who are expected to become neutropenic

▸ BY MOUTH USING ORAL SOLUTION

▸ Child: 2.5 mg/kg twice daily, to be started before transplantation or before chemotherapy (taking care to avoid interaction with cytotoxic drugs) and continued until neutrophil count recovers, safety and efficacy not established

● **UNLICENSED USE** Not licensed for use in children (age range not specified by manufacturer).

IMPORTANT SAFETY INFORMATION

HEART FAILURE

Following reports of heart failure, caution is advised when prescribing itraconazole to patients at high risk of heart failure. Those at risk include:

● patients receiving high doses and longer treatment courses;

● older adults and those with cardiac disease;

- patients with chronic lung disease (including chronic obstructive pulmonary disease) associated with pulmonary hypertension;
- patients receiving treatment with negative inotropic drugs, e.g. calcium channel blockers.

Itraconazole should be avoided in patients with ventricular dysfunction or a history of heart failure unless the infection is serious.

- **CONTRA-INDICATIONS** Acute porphyrias p. 577
- **CAUTIONS** Active liver disease · history of hepatotoxicity with other drugs · susceptibility to congestive heart failure
- **INTERACTIONS** → Appendix 1: antifungals, azoles
- **SIDE-EFFECTS**

  GENERAL SIDE-EFFECTS
  - **Common or very common** Abdominal pain · blood pressure changes · cough · diarrhoea · dyspnoea · headache · hepatitis · hypokalaemia · nausea · rash · taste disturbances · vomiting
  - **Uncommon** Constipation · dizziness · dyspepsia · flatulence · menstrual disorder · myalgia · oedema · peripheral neuropathy (discontinue treatment)
  - **Rare** Alopecia · deafness · erectile dysfunction · heart failure · hypertriglyceridaemia · leucopenia · pancreatitis · photosensitivity · Stevens-Johnson syndrome · tinnitus · toxic epidermal necrolysis · urinary frequency · visual disturbances
  - **Frequency not known** Arthralgia · confusion · drowsiness · hepatotoxicity · renal impairment · thrombocytopenia · tremor

  SPECIFIC SIDE-EFFECTS
  - With intravenous use Hyperglycaemia

  SIDE-EFFECTS, FURTHER INFORMATION
  - Hepatotoxicity Potentially life-threatening hepatotoxicity reported very rarely—discontinue if signs of hepatitis develop.
- **CONCEPTION AND CONTRACEPTION** Ensure effective contraception during treatment and until the next menstrual period following end of treatment.
- **PREGNANCY** Manufacturer advises use only in life-threatening situations (toxicity at high doses in *animal* studies).
- **BREAST FEEDING** Small amounts present in milk—may accumulate; manufacturer advises avoid.
- **HEPATIC IMPAIRMENT** Dose reduction may be necessary. Use only if potential benefit outweighs risk of hepatotoxicity.
- **RENAL IMPAIRMENT** Risk of congestive heart failure.
  - With oral use Bioavailability of oral formulations possibly reduced.
  - With intravenous use Use intravenous infusion with caution if estimated glomerular filtration rate 30–80 mL/minute/1.73 m^2 (monitor renal function); avoid intravenous infusion if estimated golmerular filtration rate less than 30 mL/minute/1.73 m^2.
- **MONITORING REQUIREMENTS**
  - Absorption reduced in AIDS and neutropenia (monitor plasma-itraconazole concentration and increase dose if necessary).
  - Monitor liver function if treatment continues for longer than one month, if receiving other hepatotoxic drugs, if history of hepatotoxicity with other drugs, or in hepatic impairment.
- **DIRECTIONS FOR ADMINISTRATION**
  - With intravenous use For *intravenous infusion*, dilute 250 mg with 50 mL Sodium Chloride 0.9% and give requisite dose through an in-line filter (0.2 micron) over 60 minutes.
  - With oral use For *oral liquid*, do not take with food; swish around mouth and swallow, do not rinse afterwards.

- **PRESCRIBING AND DISPENSING INFORMATION** Flavours of oral liquid formulations may include cherry.
- **PATIENT AND CARER ADVICE** Patients should be told how to recognise signs of liver disorder and advised to seek prompt medical attention if symptoms such as anorexia, nausea, vomiting, fatigue, abdominal pain or dark urine develop.
  - With oral use Patients or carers should be given advice on how to administer itraconazole oral liquid.

- **MEDICINAL FORMS**
  There can be variation in the licensing of different medicines containing the same drug. Forms available from special-order manufacturers include: oral suspension, oral solution

  Solution for infusion
  EXCIPIENTS: May contain Propylene glycol
  - Sporanox (Janssen-Cilag Ltd)
    Itraconazole 10 mg per 1 ml Sporanox I.V. 250mg/25ml solution for infusion ampoules and diluent | 1 ampoule PoM £79.71

  Oral solution
  CAUTIONARY AND ADVISORY LABELS 9, 23
  - Itraconazole (Non-proprietary)
    Itraconazole 10 mg per 1 ml Itraconazole 50mg/5ml oral solution sugar free sugar-free | 150 ml PoM £58.34 DT price = £58.34
  - Sporanox (Janssen-Cilag Ltd)
    Itraconazole 10 mg per 1 ml Sporanox 50mg/5ml oral solution sugar-free | 150 ml PoM £58.34 DT price = £58.34

  Capsule
  CAUTIONARY AND ADVISORY LABELS 5, 9, 21, 25
  - Itraconazole (Non-proprietary)
    Itraconazole 100 mg Itraconazole 100mg capsules | 15 capsule PoM £13.77 DT price = £3.19 | 60 capsule PoM £56.21
  - Sporanox (Janssen-Cilag Ltd)
    Itraconazole 100 mg Sporanox-Pulse 100mg capsules | 28 capsule PoM £25.72
    Sporanox 100mg capsules | 4 capsule PoM £3.67 | 15 capsule PoM £13.77 DT price = £3.19 | 60 capsule PoM £55.10

Voriconazole

- **INDICATIONS AND DOSE**

Invasive aspergillosis | **Serious infections caused by *Scedosporium* spp., *Fusarium* spp., or invasive fluconazole-resistant *Candida* spp. (including *C. krusei*)**
  - BY MOUTH
  - Child 2–11 years: Treatment should be initiated with intravenous regimen, and oral regimen should be considered only after there is a significant clinical improvement; maintenance 9 mg/kg every 12 hours, adjusted in steps of 1 mg/kg and increased if necessary up to 350 mg every 12 hours, then adjusted in steps of 50 mg as required
  - Child 12–14 years (body-weight up to 50 kg): Treatment should be initiated with intravenous regimen, and oral regimen should be considered only after there is a significant clinical improvement; maintenance 9 mg/kg every 12 hours, adjusted in steps of 1 mg/kg and increased if necessary up to 350 mg every 12 hours, then adjusted in steps of 50 mg as required
  - Child 12–14 years (body-weight 50 kg and above): Initially 400 mg every 12 hours for 2 doses, then 200 mg every 12 hours, increased if necessary to 300 mg every 12 hours
  - Child 15–17 years (body-weight up to 40 kg): Initially 200 mg every 12 hours for 2 doses, then 100 mg every 12 hours, increased if necessary to 150 mg every 12 hours
  - Child 15–17 years (body-weight 40 kg and above): Initially 400 mg every 12 hours for 2 doses, then 200 mg every 12 hours, increased if necessary to 300 mg every 12 hours

continued →

5

Infection

▸ BY INTRAVENOUS INFUSION
‣ Child 2–11 years: Initially 9 mg/kg every 12 hours for 2 doses, then 8 mg/kg every 12 hours; adjusted in steps of 1 mg/kg as required; for max. 6 months
‣ Child 12–14 years (body-weight up to 50 kg): Initially 9 mg/kg every 12 hours for 2 doses, then 8 mg/kg every 12 hours; adjusted in steps of 1 mg/kg as required; for max. 6 months
‣ Child 12–14 years (body-weight 50 kg and above): Initially 6 mg/kg every 12 hours for 2 doses, then 4 mg/kg every 12 hours; reduced if not tolerated to 3 mg/kg every 12 hours; for max. 6 months
‣ Child 15–17 years: Initially 6 mg/kg every 12 hours for 2 doses, then 4 mg/kg every 12 hours; reduced if not tolerated to 3 mg/kg every 12 hours; for max. 6 months

DOSE ADJUSTMENTS DUE TO INTERACTIONS
Manufacturer advises increasing the maintenance dose with concurrent use of fosphenytoin, phenytoin, or rifabutin—no specific recommendations made for children.

● **CONTRA-INDICATIONS** Acute porphyrias p. 577
● **CAUTIONS** Avoid exposure to sunlight · bradycardia · cardiomyopathy · electrolyte disturbances · history of QT interval prolongation · patients at risk of pancreatitis · symptomatic arrhythmias
● **INTERACTIONS** → Appendix 1: antifungals, azoles
● **SIDE-EFFECTS**
GENERAL SIDE-EFFECTS
‣ **Common or very common** Abdominal pain · acute renal failure · agitation · alopecia · altered perception · anaemia · anxiety · asthenia · blood disorders · blurred vision · cheilitis · chest pain · confusion · depression · diarrhoea · dizziness · haematuria · hallucinations · headache · hypoglycaemia · hypokalaemia · hypotension · influenza-like symptoms · jaundice · leucopenia · nausea · oedema · pancytopenia · paraesthesia · photophobia · photosensitivity · pruritus · rash · respiratory distress syndrome · sinusitis · thrombocytopenia · tremor · visual disturbances · vomiting
‣ **Uncommon** Adrenocortical insufficiency · arrhythmias · arthritis · ataxia · blepharitis · cholecystitis · constipation · duodenitis · dyspepsia · flushing · fulminant hepatic failure · gingivitis · glossitis · hepatitis · hypersensitivity reactions · hypoaesthesia · hyponatraemia · nystagmus · optic neuritis · pancreatitis · psoriasis · QT interval prolongation · raised serum cholesterol · scleritis · Stevens-Johnson syndrome · syncope
‣ **Rare** Convulsions · discoid lupus erythematosus · extrapyramidal effects · hearing disturbances · hyperthyroidism · hypertonia · hypothyroidism · insomnia · optic atrophy · pseudomembranous colitis · pseudoporphyria · retinal haemorrhage · taste disturbances (more common with oral suspension) · tinnitus · toxic epidermal necrolysis
‣ **Frequency not known** On long term treatment, squamous cell carcinoma of skin (particularly in presence of phototoxicity) · periostitis (particularly in transplant patients)
SPECIFIC SIDE-EFFECTS
‣ **Common or very common**
‣ With intravenous use Injection-site reactions
SIDE-EFFECTS, FURTHER INFORMATION
‣ **Hepatotoxicity** Hepatitis, cholestasis, and fulminant hepatic failure usually occur in the first 10 days; risk of hepatotoxicity increased in patients with haematological malignancy. Consider treatment discontinuation if severe abnormalities in liver function tests.
‣ **Phototoxicity** Phototoxicity occurs commonly. If phototoxicity occurs, consider treatment discontinuation; if treatment is continued, monitor for pre-malignant skin

lesions and squamous cell carcinoma, and discontinue treatment if they occur.

● **CONCEPTION AND CONTRACEPTION** Effective contraception required during treatment.
● **PREGNANCY** Toxicity in *animal* studies—manufacturer advises avoid unless potential benefit outweighs risk.
● **BREAST FEEDING** Manufacturer advises avoid—no information available.
● **HEPATIC IMPAIRMENT**
Child 12–17 years In mild to moderate hepatic cirrhosis use usual initial dose then halve subsequent doses. No information available for severe hepatic cirrhosis—manufacturer advises use only if potential benefit outweighs risk.
● **RENAL IMPAIRMENT**
Child 2-12 years No information available.
Child 12-17 years Intravenous vehicle may accumulate if estimated glomerular filtration rate less than 50 mL/minute/1.73 m^2—use intravenous infusion only if potential benefit outweighs risk, and monitor renal function; alternatively, use tablets or oral suspension (no dose adjustment required).
● **MONITORING REQUIREMENTS**
‣ Monitor renal function.
‣ Monitor liver function before starting treatment, then at least weekly for 1 month, and then monthly during treatment.
● **DIRECTIONS FOR ADMINISTRATION** For *intravenous infusion*, reconstitute each 200 mg with 19 mL Water for Injections *or* Sodium Chloride 0.9% to produce a 10 mg/mL solution; dilute dose to concentration of 0.5–5 mg/mL with Glucose 5% or Sodium Chloride 0.9% and give intermittently at a rate not exceeding 3 mg/kg/hour.
● **PRESCRIBING AND DISPENSING INFORMATION** Flavours of oral liquid formulations may include orange.
● **PATIENT AND CARER ADVICE** Patients and their carers should be advised to keep the alert card with them at all times.

Patients and their carers should be told how to recognise symptoms of liver disorder, and advised to seek immediate medical attention if symptoms such as persistent nausea, vomiting, malaise or jaundice develop.

Patients and their carers should be advised that patients should avoid intense or prolonged exposure to direct sunlight, and to avoid the use of sunbeds. In sunlight, patients should cover sun-exposed areas of skin and use a sunscreen with a high sun protection factor. Patients should seek medical attention if they experience sunburn or a severe skin reaction following exposure to light or sun.

● **MEDICINAL FORMS**
There can be variation in the licensing of different medicines containing the same drug.
Tablet
CAUTIONARY AND ADVISORY LABELS 9, 11, 23
‣ **Voriconazole (Non-proprietary)**
Voriconazole 50 mg Voriconazole 50mg tablets | 28 tablet [PoM] £45.43–£275.68 DT price = £118.99
Voriconazole 200 mg Voriconazole 200mg tablets | 28 tablet [PoM] £157.49–£1,102.74 DT price = £460.32
‣ **VFEND (Pfizer Ltd)**
Voriconazole 50 mg VFEND 50mg tablets | 28 tablet [PoM] £275.68 DT price = £118.99
Voriconazole 200 mg VFEND 200mg tablets | 28 tablet [PoM] £1,102.74 DT price = £460.32
Oral suspension
CAUTIONARY AND ADVISORY LABELS 9, 11, 23
‣ **VFEND (Pfizer Ltd)**
Voriconazole 40 mg per 1 ml VFEND 40mg/ml oral suspension | 75 ml [PoM] £551.37

Drugs for cutaneous larva migrans (creeping eruption)

Dog and cat hookworm larvae may enter human skin where they produce slowly extending itching tracks usually on the foot. Single tracks can be treated with topical tiabendazole (no commercial preparation available). Multiple infections respond to ivermectin, albendazole or **tiabendazole** (thiabendazole) by mouth [all unlicensed] (available from 'special-order' manufacturers or specialist importing companies).

Drugs for strongyloidiasis

Adult *Strongyloides stercoralis* live in the gut and produce larvae which penetrate the gut wall and invade the tissues, setting up a cycle of auto-infection. Ivermectin [unlicensed] (available from 'special-order' manufacturers or specialist importing companies) is the treatment of choice for chronic *Strongyloides* infection in adults and children over 5 years. Albendazole [unlicensed] (available from 'special order' manufacturers or specialist importing companies) is an alternative given to adults and children over 2 years.

ANTHELMINTICS

Albendazole

- **INDICATIONS AND DOSE**

Chronic *Strongyloides* infection
▸ BY MOUTH
▸ Child 2–17 years: 400 mg twice daily for 3 days, dose may be repeated after 3 weeks if necessary

Hydatid disease, in conjunction with surgery to reduce the risk of recurrence or as primary treatment in inoperable cases
▸ BY MOUTH
▸ Child 2–17 years: 7.5 mg/kg twice daily (max. per dose 400 mg twice daily) for 28 days followed by 14-day break, repeated for up to 2–3 cycles

Hookworm infections
▸ BY MOUTH
▸ Child 2–17 years: 400 mg for 1 dose

- **UNLICENSED USE** Albendazole is an unlicensed drug.
- **INTERACTIONS** → Appendix 1: albendazole

- **MEDICINAL FORMS**
There can be variation in the licensing of different medicines containing the same drug. Forms available from special-order manufacturers include: tablet, chewable tablet, oral suspension
Tablet
CAUTIONARY AND ADVISORY LABELS 9
▸ Albendazole (Non-proprietary)
  Albendazole 400 mg Eskazole 400mg tablets | 60 tablet [PoM] no price available
Chewable tablet
CAUTIONARY AND ADVISORY LABELS 9
▸ Albendazole (Non-proprietary)
  Albendazole 200 mg Zentel 200mg chewable tablets | 6 tablet [PoM] no price available
  Albendazole 400 mg Zentel 400mg chewable tablets | 1 tablet [PoM] no price available | 3 tablet [PoM] no price available

Diethylcarbamazine

- **INDICATIONS AND DOSE**

***Wuchereria bancrofti* infections | *Brugia malayi* infections**
▸ BY MOUTH
▸ Child 1 month–9 years: Initially 1 mg/kg daily in divided doses on the first day, then increased to 3 mg/kg daily in divided doses, dose to be increased gradually over 3 days

▸ Child 10–17 years: Initially 1 mg/kg daily in divided doses on the first day, then increased to 6 mg/kg daily in divided doses, dose to be increased gradually over 3 days

***Loa loa* infections**
▸ BY MOUTH
▸ Child 1 month–9 years: Initially 1 mg/kg daily in divided doses on the first day, then increased to 3 mg/kg daily in divided doses, dose to be increased gradually over 3 days
▸ Child 10–17 years: Initially 1 mg/kg daily in divided doses on the first day, then increased to 6 mg/kg daily in divided doses, dose to be increased gradually over 3 days

- **UNLICENSED USE** Diethylcarbamazine is an unlicensed drug.

- **MEDICINAL FORMS**
There can be variation in the licensing of different medicines containing the same drug.
No licensed medicines listed.

Ivermectin

17-May-2017

- **INDICATIONS AND DOSE**

Chronic *Strongyloides* infection
▸ BY MOUTH
▸ Child 5–17 years: 200 micrograms/kg daily for 2 days

Onchocerciasis
▸ BY MOUTH
▸ Child 5–17 years: 150 micrograms/kg for 1 dose, retreatment at intervals of 6 to12 months, depending on symptoms, must be given until adult worms die out

Scabies, in combination with topical drugs, for the treatment of hyperkeratotic (crusted or 'Norwegian') scabies that does not respond to topical treatment alone
▸ BY MOUTH
▸ Child: (consult product literature)

- **UNLICENSED USE** Ivermectin is unlicensed.
- **INTERACTIONS** → Appendix 1: ivermectin
- **SIDE-EFFECTS** Aggravation of itching · aggravation of rash

- **MEDICINAL FORMS**
There can be variation in the licensing of different medicines containing the same drug. Forms available from special-order manufacturers include: tablet
Tablet
▸ Ivermectin (Non-proprietary)
  Ivermectin 3 mg Stromectol 3mg tablets | 4 tablet [PoM] no price available | 20 tablet [PoM] no price available

Levamisole

- **INDICATIONS AND DOSE**

Roundworm infections
▸ BY MOUTH
▸ Child: 2.5–3 mg/kg (max. per dose 150 mg) for 1 dose

Hookworm infections
▸ BY MOUTH
▸ Child: 2.5 mg/kg (max. per dose 150 mg) for 1 dose, dose to be repeated after 7 days if severe

Nephrotic syndrome (initiated under specialist supervision)
▸ BY MOUTH
▸ Child: 2.5 mg/kg once daily on alternate days (max. per dose 150 mg)

- **UNLICENSED USE** Not licensed.

- **CONTRA-INDICATIONS** Blood disorders
- **CAUTIONS** Epilepsy · juvenile idiopathic arthritis · Sjögren's syndrome
- **INTERACTIONS** → Appendix 1: levamisole
- **SIDE-EFFECTS** Arthralgia (on *prolonged treatment*) · blood disorders (on *prolonged treatment*) · convulsions (on *prolonged treatment*) · diarrhoea · dizziness · headache · influenza-like syndrome (on *prolonged treatment*) · insomnia (on *prolonged treatment*) · myalgia (on *prolonged treatment*) · nausea · rash (on *prolonged treatment*) · taste disturbances (on *prolonged treatment*) · vasculitis (on *prolonged treatment*) · vomiting
- **PREGNANCY** Embryotoxic in *animal* studies, avoid if possible.
- **BREAST FEEDING** No information available.
- **HEPATIC IMPAIRMENT** Use with caution—dose adjustment may be necessary.
- **PATIENT AND CARER ADVICE**
  Medicines for Children leaflet: Levamisole for nephrotic syndrome www.medicinesforchildren.org.uk/levamisole-for-nephrotic-syndrome

- **MEDICINAL FORMS**
  There can be variation in the licensing of different medicines containing the same drug. Forms available from special-order manufacturers include: tablet
  Tablet
  CAUTIONARY AND ADVISORY LABELS 4
  ▸ **Ergamisol** (Imported (Belgium))
    Levamisole (as Levamisole hydrochloride) 50 mg Ergamisol 50mg tablets | 20 tablet P̲o̲M̲ no price available

Mebendazole

- **INDICATIONS AND DOSE**
  Threadworm infections
  ▸ BY MOUTH
  ▸ Child 6 months–17 years: 100 mg for 1 dose, if reinfection occurs, second dose may be needed after 2 weeks
  Whipworm infections | Hookworm infections
  ▸ BY MOUTH
  ▸ Child 1–17 years: 100 mg twice daily for 3 days
  Roundworm infections
  ▸ BY MOUTH
  ▸ Child 1 year: 100 mg twice daily for 3 days
  ▸ Child 2–17 years: 100 mg twice daily for 3 days, alternatively 500 mg for 1 dose

- **UNLICENSED USE** Not licensed for use as a single dose of 500 mg in roundworm infections. Not licensed for use in children under 2 years.
- **INTERACTIONS** → Appendix 1: mebendazole
- **SIDE-EFFECTS**
  ▸ **Common or very common** Abdominal pain
  ▸ **Uncommon** Diarrhoea · flatulence
  ▸ **Rare** Alopecia · convulsions · dizziness · hepatitis · neutropenia · rash · Stevens-Johnson syndrome · toxic epidermal necrolysis · urticaria
- **PREGNANCY** Manufacturer advises avoid—toxicity in *animal* studies.
- **BREAST FEEDING** Amount present in milk too small to be harmful but manufacturer advises avoid.
- **PRESCRIBING AND DISPENSING INFORMATION** Flavours of oral liquid formulations may include banana.
- **PATIENT AND CARER ADVICE**
  Medicines for Children leaflet: Mebendazole for worm infections www.medicinesforchildren.org.uk/mebendazole-for-worm-infections

- **EXCEPTIONS TO LEGAL CATEGORY** Mebendazole tablets can be sold to the public if supplied for oral use in the treatment of enterobiasis in adults and children over 2 years provided its container or package is labelled to show a max. single dose of 100 mg and it is supplied in a container or package containing not more than 800 mg.

- **MEDICINAL FORMS**
  There can be variation in the licensing of different medicines containing the same drug.
  Oral suspension
  ▸ **Ovex** (McNeil Products Ltd)
    Mebendazole 20 mg per 1 ml Ovex 100mg/5ml oral suspension | 30 ml P̲ £6.03 DT price = £1.55
  ▸ **Vermox** (Janssen-Cilag Ltd)
    Mebendazole 20 mg per 1 ml Vermox 100mg/5ml oral suspension | 30 ml P̲o̲M̲ £1.55 DT price = £1.55
  Chewable tablet
  ▸ **Ovex** (McNeil Products Ltd)
    Mebendazole 100 mg Ovex 100mg chewable tablets sugar-free | 1 tablet P̲ £2.03 sugar-free | 4 tablet P̲ £4.74
  ▸ **Vermox** (Janssen-Cilag Ltd)
    Mebendazole 100 mg Vermox 100mg chewable tablets sugar-free | 6 tablet P̲o̲M̲ £1.34 DT price = £1.34

Praziquantel

- **INDICATIONS AND DOSE**
  Tapeworm infections (*Taenia solium*)
  ▸ BY MOUTH
  ▸ Child 4–17 years: 5–10 mg/kg for 1 dose, to be taken after a light breakfast
  Tapeworm infections (*Hymenolepis nana*)
  ▸ BY MOUTH
  ▸ Child 4–17 years: 25 mg/kg for 1 dose, to be taken after a light breakfast
  ***Schistosoma haematobium* worm infections | *Schistosoma mansoni* worm infections**
  ▸ BY MOUTH
  ▸ Child 4–17 years: 20 mg/kg, followed by 20 mg/kg after 4–6 hours
  ***Schistosoma japonicum* worm infections**
  ▸ BY MOUTH
  ▸ Child 4–17 years: 20 mg/kg 3 times a day for 1 day

- **UNLICENSED USE** Praziquantel is an unlicensed drug.
- **INTERACTIONS** → Appendix 1: praziquantel

- **MEDICINAL FORMS**
  There can be variation in the licensing of different medicines containing the same drug. Forms available from special-order manufacturers include: tablet
  Tablet
  ▸ **Praziquantel** (Non-proprietary)
    Praziquantel 150 mg Cesol 150mg tablets | 6 tablet P̲o̲M̲ no price available
    Praziquantel 600 mg Biltricide 600mg tablets | 6 tablet P̲o̲M̲ no price available
  ▸ **Cysticide** (Imported (Germany))
    Praziquantel 500 mg Cysticide 500mg tablets | 90 tablet P̲o̲M̲ no price available

5 Protozoal infection

Antiprotozoal drugs

Amoebicides

Metronidazole p. 319 is the drug of choice for *acute invasive amoebic dysentery* since it is very effective against vegetative forms of *Entamoeba histolytica* in ulcers. Tinidazole p. 320 is also effective. Metronidazole and tinidazole are also active against amoebae which may have migrated to the liver. Treatment with metronidazole (or tinidazole) is followed by a 10-day course of diloxanide furoate p. 287.

Diloxanide furoate is the drug of choice for asymptomatic patients with *E. histolytica* cysts in the faeces; metronidazole and tinidazole are relatively ineffective. Diloxanide furoate is relatively free from toxic effects and the usual course is of 10 days, given alone for chronic infections or following metronidazole or tinidazole treatment.

For *amoebic abscesses* of the liver metronidazole is effective; tinidazole is an alternative. Aspiration of the abscess is indicated where it is suspected that it may rupture or where there is no improvement after 72 hours of metronidazole; the aspiration may need to be repeated. Aspiration aids penetration of metronidazole and, for abscesses with large volumes of pus, if carried out in conjunction with drug therapy, may reduce the period of disability.

Diloxanide furoate is not effective against hepatic amoebiasis, but a 10-day course should be given at the completion of metronidazole or tinidazole treatment to destroy any amoebae in the gut.

Trichomonacides

Metronidazole is the treatment of choice for *Trichomonas vaginalis* infection. Contact tracing is recommended and sexual contacts should be treated simultaneously. If metronidazole is ineffective, tinidazole may be tried.

Antigiardial drugs

Metronidazole is the treatment of choice for *Giardia lamblia* infections. Tinidazole may be used as an alternative to metronidazole.

Leishmaniacides

Cutaneous leishmaniasis frequently heals spontaneously but if skin lesions are extensive or unsightly, treatment is indicated, as it is in visceral leishmaniasis (kala-azar). Leishmaniasis should be treated under specialist supervision.

Sodium stibogluconate below, an organic pentavalent antimony compound, is used for visceral leishmaniasis. The dosage varies with different geographical regions and expert advice should be obtained. Skin lesions can also be treated with sodium stibogluconate.

Amphotericin p. 357 is used with or after an antimony compound for visceral leishmaniasis unresponsive to the antimonial alone; side-effects may be reduced by using liposomal amphotericin (*AmBisome®*). *Abelcet®*, a lipid formulation of amphotericin is also likely to be effective but less information is available.

Pentamidine isetionate p. 365 (pentamidine isethionate) has been used in antimony-resistant visceral leishmaniasis, but although the initial response is often good, the relapse rate is high; it is associated with serious side-effects. Other treatments include paromomycin [unlicensed] (available from 'special-order' manufacturers or specialist importing companies).

Trypanocides

The prophylaxis and treatment of trypanosomiasis is difficult and differs according to the strain of organism. Expert advice should therefore be obtained.

Drugs for toxoplasmosis

Most infections caused by *Toxoplasma gondii* are self-limiting, and treatment is not necessary. Exceptions are patients with eye involvement (toxoplasma choroidoretinitis), and those who are immunosuppressed. Toxoplasmic encephalitis is a common complication of AIDS. The treatment of choice is a combination of

pyrimethamine p. 382 and sulfadiazine p. 336, given for several weeks (expert advice **essential**). Pyrimethamine is a folate antagonist, and adverse reactions to this combination are relatively common (folinic acid supplements and weekly blood counts needed). Alternative regimens use combinations of pyrimethamine with clindamycin p. 313 or clarithromycin p. 315 or azithromycin p. 314. Long-term secondary prophylaxis is required after treatment of toxoplasmosis in immunocompromised patients; prophylaxis should continue until immunity recovers.

If toxoplasmosis is acquired in pregnancy, transplacental infection may lead to severe disease in the fetus; specialist advice should be sought on management. Spiramycin [unlicensed] (available from 'special-order' manufacturers or specialist importing companies) may reduce the risk of transmission of maternal infection to the fetus. When there is evidence of placental or fetal infection, pyrimethamine may be given with sulfadiazine and folinic acid p. 528 after the first trimester.

In neonates without signs of toxoplasmosis, but born to mothers known to have become infected, spiramycin is given while awaiting laboratory results. If toxoplasmosis is confirmed in the infant, pyrimethamine and sulfadiazine are given for 12 months, together with folinic acid.

5.1 Leishmaniasis

ANTIPROTOZOALS

Sodium stibogluconate

- **INDICATIONS AND DOSE**
Visceral leishmaniasis (specialist use only)
▶ BY INTRAVENOUS INJECTION, OR BY INTRAMUSCULAR INJECTION
▸ Child: 20 mg/kg daily for at least 20 days

- **UNLICENSED USE**
▸ With intravenous injection Licensed for use in children (age range not specified by manufacturer).

- **CAUTIONS** Heart disease (withdraw if conduction disturbances occur) · mucocutaneous disease · predisposition to QT interval prolongation · treat intercurrent infection (e.g. pneumonia)
CAUTIONS, FURTHER INFORMATION
▸ Mucocutaneous disease Successful treatment of mucocutaneous leishmaniasis may induce severe inflammation around the lesions (may be life-threatening if pharyngeal or tracheal involvement)—may require corticosteroid.

- **INTERACTIONS** → Appendix 1: sodium stibogluconate
- **SIDE-EFFECTS**
▸ **Rare** Bleeding from gums · bleeding from nose · fever · flushing · jaundice · rash · substernal pain · sweating · vertigo
▸ **Frequency not known** Abdominal pain · anaphylaxis · anorexia · arthralgia · coughing · diarrhoea · ECG changes · headache · lethargy · myalgia · nausea · pain on intramuscular injection · pain on intravenous administration · pancreatitis · thrombosis on intravenous administration · vomiting

- **PREGNANCY** Manufacturer advises use only if potential benefit outweighs risk.
- **BREAST FEEDING** Amount probably too small to be harmful.
- **HEPATIC IMPAIRMENT** Use with caution.
- **RENAL IMPAIRMENT** Avoid in significant impairment.
- **MONITORING REQUIREMENTS** Monitor ECG before and during treatment.

Infection

5

- DIRECTIONS FOR ADMINISTRATION Intravenous injections must be given slowly over 5 minutes (to reduce risk of local thrombosis) and stopped if coughing or substernal pain occur. Injection should be filtered immediately before administration using a filter of 5 microns or less.

- MEDICINAL FORMS
There can be variation in the licensing of different medicines containing the same drug.
Solution for injection
▸ Pentostam (GlaxoSmithKline UK Ltd)
Antimony pentavalent (as Sodium stibogluconate) 100 mg per 1 ml Pentostam 10g/100ml solution for injection vials | 1 vial PoM £66.43

5.2 Malaria

Antimalarials

Artemether with lumefantrine

Artemether with lumefantrine p. 377 is licensed for the *treatment of acute non-complicated falciparum malaria.*

Chloroquine

Chloroquine p. 379 is used for the *prophylaxis of malaria* in areas of the world where the *risk of chloroquine-resistant falciparum malaria is still low.* It is also used with proguanil hydrochloride p. 381 when chloroquine-resistant falciparum malaria is present but this regimen may not give optimal protection (see Recommended regimens for prophylaxis against malaria p. 372).

Chloroquine is **no longer recommended** for the *treatment of falciparum malaria* owing to widespread resistance, nor is it recommended if the infective species is *not known* or if the infection is *mixed*; in these cases treatment should be with quinine p. 382, *Malarone*®, or *Riamet*®. It is still recommended for the *treatment of non-falciparum malaria.*

Mefloquine

Mefloquine p. 380 is used for the *prophylaxis of malaria* in areas of the world where there is a *high risk of chloroquine resistant falciparum malaria* (for details, see Recommended regimens for prophylaxis against malaria p. 372).

Mefloquine is now rarely used for the *treatment of falciparum malaria* because of increased resistance. It is rarely used for the *treatment of non-falciparum malaria* because better tolerated alternatives are available. Mefloquine should not be used for treatment if it has been used for prophylaxis.

Piperaquine with artenimol

Artenimol with piperaquine phosphate p. 377 is not recommended for the first-line treatment of acute uncomplicated falciparum malaria because there is limited experience of its use in travellers who usually reside in areas where malaria is not endemic. Piperaquine has a long half-life.

Primaquine

Primaquine p. 381 is used to eliminate the liver stages of *P. vivax* or *P. ovale* following chloroquine treatment.

Proguanil

Proguanil hydrochloride is used (usually *with chloroquine*, but occasionally *alone*) for the *prophylaxis of malaria*, (for details, see Recommended regimens for prophylaxis against malaria p. 372).

Proguanil hydrochloride used alone is not suitable for the *treatment of malaria*; however, *Malarone*® (a combination of atovaquone with proguanil hydrochloride p. 378) is licensed for the treatment of acute uncomplicated falciparum malaria. *Malarone*® is also used for the *prophylaxis of falciparum malaria* in areas of *widespread mefloquine or chloroquine resistance. Malarone*® is also used as an alternative to mefloquine or doxycycline p. 338. *Malarone*® is particularly suitable for short trips to highly chloroquine-resistant areas because it needs to be taken only for 7 days after leaving an endemic area.

Pyrimethamine

Pyrimethamine p. 382 should not be used alone, but is used with sulfadoxine.

Pyrimethamine with sulfadoxine p. 382 is not recommended for the *prophylaxis of malaria*, but can be used in the *treatment of falciparum malaria with (or following) quinine*.

Quinine

Quinine is not suitable for the *prophylaxis of malaria.*

Quinine is used for the *treatment of falciparum malaria* or if the infective species is *not known* or if the infection is mixed (for details see Malaria, treatment p. 371).

Tetracyclines

Doxycycline is used in adults and children over 12 years for the *prophylaxis of malaria* in areas of widespread mefloquine or *chloroquine resistance*. Doxycycline is also used as an alternative to mefloquine or *Malarone*® (for details, see Recommended regimens for prophylaxis against malaria p. 372).

Malaria, prophylaxis

Prophylaxis against malaria

The recommendations on prophylaxis reflect guidelines agreed by UK malaria specialists; the advice is aimed at residents of the UK who travel to endemic areas. The choice of drug for a particular individual should take into account:

- risk of exposure to malaria
- extent of drug resistance
- efficacy of the recommended drugs
- side-effects of the drugs
- patient-related factors (e.g. age, pregnancy, renal or hepatic impairment, compliance with prophylactic regimen)

Prophylactic doses are based on guidelines agreed by UK malaria experts and may differ from advice in product literature. **Weight is a better guide than age.** If in doubt obtain advice from specialist centre (see under Malaria, treatment p. 371).

Protection against bites

Prophylaxis is not absolute, and breakthrough infection can occur with any of the drugs recommended. Personal protection against being bitten is very important. Mosquito nets impregnated with permethrin p. 699 provide the most effective barrier protection against insects (infants should sleep with a mosquito net stretched over the cot or baby carrier); mats and vaporised insecticides are also useful. Diethyltoluamide (DEET) 20–50% in lotions, sprays, or roll-on formulations is safe and effective when applied to the skin of adults and children over 2 months of age. It can also be used during pregnancy and breast-feeding. The duration of protection varies according to the concentration of DEET and is longest for DEET 50%. When sunscreen is also required, DEET should be applied after the sunscreen. DEET reduces the SPF of sunscreen, so a sunscreen of SPF 30-50 should be applied. Long sleeves and trousers worn after dusk also provide protection against bites.

Length of prophylaxis
In order to determine tolerance and to establish habit, prophylaxis should generally be started one week (2–3 weeks in the case of mefloquine p. 380) before travel into an endemic area; *Malarone*® or doxycycline p. 338 prophylaxis should be started 1–2 days before travel. Prophylaxis should be continued for **4 weeks after leaving** (except for *Malarone*® prophylaxis which should be stopped 1 week after leaving). For extensive journeys across different regions, the traveller must be protected in all areas of risk.

In those requiring long-term prophylaxis, chloroquine p. 379 and proguanil hydrochloride p. 381 may be used for periods of over 5 years. Mefloquine is licensed for up to 1 year (although, if it is tolerated in the short term, there is no evidence of harm when it is used for up to 3 years). Doxycycline can be used for up to 2 years. *Malarone*® can be used for up to 1 year. Prophylaxis with mefloquine, doxycycline, or *Malarone*® may be considered for longer durations if it is justified by the risk of exposure to malaria. Specialist advice should be sought for long-term prophylaxis.

Return from malarial region
It is important to be aware that **any illness** that occurs within 1 year and **especially within 3 months of return** might be malaria even if all recommended precautions against malaria were taken. Travellers should be **warned** of this and told that if they develop any illness **particularly within 3 months** of their return they should go **immediately** to a doctor and specifically mention their exposure to malaria.

Epilepsy
Both chloroquine and mefloquine are unsuitable for malaria prophylaxis in individuals with a history of epilepsy. In areas *without chloroquine resistance* proguanil alone is recommended; in areas *with chloroquine resistance*, doxycycline or *Malarone*® may be considered.

Asplenia
Asplenic individuals (or those with severe splenic dysfunction) are at particular risk of severe malaria. If travel to malarious areas is unavoidable, rigorous precautions are required against contracting the disease.

Renal impairment
Avoidance (or dosage reduction) of proguanil hydrochloride is recommended since it is excreted by the kidneys. *Malarone*® should not be used for prophylaxis in patients with estimated glomerular filtration rate less than 30 mL/minute/1.73m². Chloroquine is only partially excreted by the kidneys and reduction of the dose for prophylaxis is not required except in severe impairment. Mefloquine is considered to be appropriate to use in renal impairment and does not require dosage reduction. Doxycycline is also considered to be appropriate.

Pregnancy
Travel to malarious areas should be avoided during pregnancy; if travel is unavoidable, effective prophylaxis must be used. Chloroquine and proguanil hydrochloride can be given in the usual doses during pregnancy, but these drugs are not appropriate for most areas because their effectiveness has declined, particularly in Sub-Saharan Africa; in the case of proguanil hydrochloride, folic acid p. 546 (in doses greater than standard pregnancy prophylaxis) should be given for at least the first trimester. The centres listed (see Malaria, treatment, below) should be consulted for advice on prophylaxis in chloroquine-resistant areas. Although the manufacturer advises that mefloquine should not be used during pregnancy, particularly in the first trimester, unless the potential benefit outweighs the risk, studies of mefloquine in pregnancy (including use in the first trimester) indicate that it can be considered for travel to chloroquine-resistant areas. Doxycycline is contra-indicated during pregnancy; however, it can be used for malaria prophylaxis if other regimens are unsuitable, and if the entire course of doxycycline can be completed before 15 weeks' gestation [unlicensed]. *Malarone*® should be avoided during pregnancy, however, it can be considered during the second and third trimesters if there is no suitable alternative.

Breast-feeding
Prophylaxis is required in **breast-fed infants**; although antimalarials are present in milk, the amounts are too variable to give reliable protection.

Anticoagulants
Travellers taking warfarin sodium p. 94 should begin chemoprophylaxis 2–3 weeks before departure. The INR should be stable before departure. It should be measured before starting chemoprophylaxis, 7 days after starting, and after completing the course. For prolonged stays, the INR should be checked at regular intervals.

Standby treatment
Children and their carers visiting remote, malarious areas for prolonged periods should carry standby treatment if they are likely to be more than 24 hours away from medical care. Self-medication should be **avoided** if medical help is accessible.

In order to avoid excessive self-medication, the traveller should be provided with **written instructions** that urgent medical attention should be sought if fever (38°C or more) develops 7 days (or more) after arriving in a malarious area and that self-treatment is indicated if medical help is not available within 24 hours of fever onset.

In view of the continuing emergence of resistant strains and of the different regimens required for different areas expert advice should be sought on the best treatment course for an individual traveller. A drug used for chemoprophylaxis should not be considered for standby treatment for the same traveller.

Specific recommendations
Where a journey requires two regimens, the regimen for the higher risk area should be used for the whole journey. Those travelling to remote or little-visited areas may require expert advice. See also *Recommended regimens for prophylaxis against malaria* .

Important
Settled immigrants (or long-term visitors) to the UK may be unaware that **any immunity they may have acquired while living in malarious areas is lost rapidly** after migration to the UK, or that any non-malarious areas where they lived previously **may now be malarious**.

Malaria, treatment

Advice for healthcare professionals
A number of specialist centres are able to provide advice on specific problems.

PHE (Public Health England) Malaria Reference Laboratory (020) 7637 0248 (fax) (prophylaxis only)
www.malaria-reference.co.uk
National Travel Health Network and Centre 0845 602 6712
Travel Medicine Team, Health Protection Scotland (registered users of Travax only) www.travax.nhs.uk (for registered users of the NHS Travax website only)
(0141) 300 1100 (weekdays 2–4 p.m. only)
Birmingham (0121) 424 2358
Liverpool (0151) 705 3100
London 0845 155 5000 (treatment)
Oxford (01865) 225 430

Key to recommended regimens for prophylaxis against malaria

Codes for regimens	Details of regimens for prophylaxis against malaria
-	No risk
1	Chemoprophylaxis not recommended, but avoid mosquito bites and consider malaria if fever presents
2	Chloroquine only
3	Chloroquine with proguanil
4	Atovaquone with proguanil hydrochloride or doxycycline or mefloquine
5	Atovaquone with proguanil hydrochloride or doxycycline

Specific recommendations

Country	Comments on risk of malaria and regional or seasonal variation	Codes for regimens
Afghanistan	Risk below 2000 m from May–November	3
	Low risk below 2000 m from December–April	1
Algeria	Very low risk in Illizi department only	1
Andaman and Nicobar Islands (India)	Risk present	1
Angola	High risk	4
Argentina	Low risk in low altitude areas of Salta provinces bordering Bolivia and in Chaco, Corrientes, and Misiones provinces close to border with Paraguay and Brazil	2
	No risk in Iguaçu Falls and areas other than those above	1
Armenia	No risk	1
Azerbaijan	Low to no risk	1
Bangladesh	High risk in Chittagong Hill Tract districts (but not Chittagong city)	4
	Low to no risk in Chittagong city and other areas, except Chittagong Hill Tract districts	1
Belize	Low risk in rural areas	2
	No risk in Belize district (including Belize city and islands)	1
Benin	High risk	4
Bhutan	Risk in southern belt districts, along border with India: Chukha, Geyleg-phug, Samchi, Samdrup Jonkhar, and Shemgang	3
	Low to no risk in areas other than those above	1
Bolivia	High risk in Amazon basin	4
	Risk in rural areas below 2500 m (other than above)	2
	No risk above 2500 m	1
Botswana	High risk from November–June in northern half, including Okavango Delta area	4
	Low risk from July–October in northern half; low to no risk all year in southern half	1
Brazil	Risk in Amazon basin, including city of Manaus	4
	Very low risk in areas other than those above, and no risk in Iguaçu Falls	1
Brunei Darussalam	Very low risk	1
Burkina Faso	High risk	4
Burundi	High risk	4
Cambodia	High risk, with widespread chloroquine and mefloquine resistance, in western provinces bordering Thailand	5
	High risk in areas other than those above and below	4
	Very low risk in Angkor Wat and Lake Tonle Sap, including Siem Reap; no risk in Phnom Penh	1
Cameroon	High risk	4
Cape Verde	Very low risk on island of Santiago (Sao Tiago) and Boa Vista	1
Central African Republic	High risk	4
Chad	High risk	4
China	High risk in Yunnan and Hainan provinces	4
	Very low risk in areas other than those above and below	1
	No risk in Hong Kong	-
Colombia	High risk in rural areas below 1600 m	4
	Low to no risk above 1600 m and in Cartagena	1

Country	Comments on risk of malaria and regional or seasonal variation	Codes for regimens
Comoros	High risk	4
Congo	High risk	4
Costa Rica	Risk in Limon province (but not city of Limon)	2
	Very low risk in areas other than those above	1
Cote d'Ivoire (Ivory Coast)	High risk	4
Democratic Republic of the Congo	High risk	4
Djibouti	High risk	4
Dominican Republic	Risk in all areas except cities of Santiago and Santo Domingo	2
	Cities of Santiago and Santo Domingo	1
East Timor (Timor-Leste)	High risk	4
Ecuador	Risk in areas below 1500 m including coastal provinces and Amazon basin (no risk in Galapagos islands or city of Guayaquil)	4
Egypt	No risk	1
El Salvador	Low risk in rural areas of Santa Ana, Ahuachapán, and La Unión provinces in western part of country; low to no risk in other areas	1
Equatorial Guinea	High risk	4
Eritrea	High risk below 2200 m	4
Ethiopia	High risk below 2000 m	4
French Guiana	High risk (particularly in border areas) except city of Cayenne or Devil's Island (Ile du Diable)	4
	No risk in city of Cayenne or Devil's Island (Ile du Diable)	1
Gabon	High risk	4
Gambia	High risk	4
Georgia	Very low risk in rural south east from June–October	1
Ghana	High risk	4
Guatemala	Low risk below 1500 m	2
	No risk in Guatemala City, Antigua, or Lake Atitlan	-
Guinea	High risk	4
Guinea-Bissau	High risk	4
Guyana	High risk in all interior regions	4
	Very low risk in Georgetown and coastal region	1
Haiti	Risk present	2
Honduras	Risk below 1000 m and in Roatán and other Bay Islands (no risk in San Pedro Sula or Tegucigalpa)	2
India	High risk in states of Assam and Orissa, districts of East Godavari, Srikakulam, Vishakhapatnam, and Vizianagaram in the state of Andhra Pradesh, and districts of Balaghat, Dindori, Mandla, and Seoni in the state of Madhya Pradesh	4
	Risk in areas other than those above or below (including Goa, Andaman and Nicobar islands)	1
	No risk in Lakshadweep islands	-
Indonesia	High risk in Lombok and Irian Jaya (Papua)	4
	Risk in areas other than those above or below	3
	Very low risk in Bali, and cities on islands of Java and Sumatra	1
	No risk in city of Jakarta	-
Indonesia (Borneo)	High risk	4
Iran	Risk from March–November in rural south eastern provinces and in north, along Azerbaijan border in Ardabil, and near Turkmenistan border in North Khorasan	3
	Low to no risk in areas other than those above	1
Iraq	Very low risk from May–November in rural northern area below 1500 m	1
Kenya	High risk below 2500 m (except city of Nairobi)	4
	Very low risk in the highlands above 2500 m and in city of Nairobi	1
Kyrgyzstan	Very low risk from June–October in southwest areas bordering Tajikistan and Uzbekistan	1

Infection

5

Key to recommended regimens for prophylaxis against malaria

Codes for regimens	Details of regimens for prophylaxis against malaria
-	No risk
1	Chemoprophylaxis not recommended, but avoid mosquito bites and consider malaria if fever presents
2	Chloroquine only
3	Chloroquine with proguanil
4	Atovaquone with proguanil hydrochloride or doxycycline or mefloquine
5	Atovaquone with proguanil hydrochloride or doxycycline

Specific recommendations

Country	Comments on risk of malaria and regional or seasonal variation	Codes for regimens
Laos	High risk along the border with Myanmar in the provinces of Bokeo and Louang Namtha, and along the border with Thailand in the province of Champasak and Saravan	5
	High risk in areas other than those above or below	4
	Low to no risk in city of Vientiane	1
Liberia	High risk	4
Libya	No risk	1
Madagascar	High risk	4
Malawi	High risk	4
Malaysia	Risk in inland forested areas of peninsular Malaysia	4
	Very low risk in rest of peninsular Malaysia, including Cameron Highlands and city of Kuala Lumpur	1
Malaysia (Borneo)	High risk in inland areas of eastern Sabah and in inland, forested areas of Sarawak	4
	Very low risk in areas other than those above, including coastal areas of Sabah and Sarawak	1
Mali	High risk	4
Mauritania	High risk all year in southern provinces, and from July–October in the northern provinces	4
	Low risk from November–June in the northern provinces	1
Mauritius	No risk	1
Mayotte	Risk present	4
Mexico	Low risk in Oaxaca and Chiapas	2
	Very low risk in areas other than those above	1
Mozambique	High risk	4
Myanmar	High risk (but not in cities of Mandalay and Yangon)	5
	No risk in cities of Mandalay and Yangon	1
Namibia	High risk all year in regions of Caprivi Strip, Kavango, and Kunene river, and from November–June in northern third of country	4
	Low to no risk in areas other than those above; low risk from July–October in northern third of country	1
Nepal	Risk below 1500 m, particularly in Terai district	3
	No risk in city of Kathmandu and on typical Himalayan treks	1
Nicaragua	Low risk (except Managua)	2
	Very low risk in Managua	1
Niger	High risk	4
Nigeria	High risk	4
North Korea	Very low risk in some southern areas	1
Pakistan	Risk below 2000 m	3
	Low to no risk above 2000 m	1
Panama	Risk east of Canal Zone	3
	Low risk west of Canal Zone	2
	No risk in Panama City or Canal Zone itself	1
Papua New Guinea	High risk below 1800 m	4
	Low to no risk above 1800 m	1

Country	Comments on risk of malaria and regional or seasonal variation	Codes for regimens
Paraguay	Low risk in departments of Alto Paraná and Caaguazú	2
	Very low risk in areas other than those above	1
Peru	High risk in Amazon basin along border with Brazil, particularly in Loreto province	4
	Risk in rural areas below 2000 m (other than those above and below) including in Amazon basin along border with Bolivia	2
	No risk in city of Lima and coastal region south of Chiclayo	1
Philippines	Risk in rural areas below 600 m and on islands of Luzon, Mindanao, Mindoro, and Palawan	3
	No risk in cities or on islands of Boracay, Bohol, Catanduanes, Cebu, or Leyte	1
Rwanda	High risk	4
São Tomé and Principe	High risk	4
Saudi Arabia	Risk in south-western provinces along border with Yemen, including below 2000 m in Asir province	3
	No risk in cities of Jeddah, Makkah (Mecca), Medina, Riyadh, or Ta'if, or above 2000 m in Asir province	1
Senegal	High risk	4
Sierra Leone	High risk	4
Solomon Islands	High risk	4
Somalia	High risk	4
South Africa	Moderate risk from September–May in low altitude areas of Mpumalanga and Limpopo, which border Mozambique and Zimbabwe (including Kruger National Park)	4
	Low risk in north-east KwaZulu-Natal	1
	Low risk in areas bordering those above	1
South Korea	Very low risk in northern areas, in Gangwon-do and Gyeonggi-do provinces, and Incheon city (towards Demilitarized Zone)	1
South Sudan	High risk	4
Sri Lanka	Low risk north of Vavuniya	1
	Very low risk in areas other than those above and below	1
	No risk in Colombo or Kandy	-
Sudan	High risk in central and southern areas; risk also present in rest of country (except Khartoum)	4
	Very low risk in Khartoum	1
Suriname	High risk (except coastal districts or city of Paramaribo)	4
	Very low risk in coastal districts; no risk in city of Paramaribo	1
Swaziland	High risk in northern and eastern regions bordering Mozambique and South Africa, including all of Lubombo district and Big Bend, Mhlume, Simunye, and Tshaneni regions	4
	Very low risk in the areas other than those above	1
Syria	Very low risk in small, remote foci of El Hasakah	1
Tajikistan	Risk below 2000 m from June–October	3
	Low risk below 2000 m from November–May	1
Tanzania	High risk below 1800 m; risk also in Zanzibar	4
Thailand	High risk, with chloroquine and mefloquine resistance, in rural forested borders with Cambodia, Laos, and Myanmar	5
	Very low risk in areas other than those above, including Kanchanaburi (Kwai Bridge); no risk in cities of Bangkok, Chiang Mai, Chiang Rai, Koh Phangan, Koh Samui, and Pattaya	1
Togo	High risk	4
Turkey	Low risk from May–October along the border plain with Syria, around Adana and east of Adana	2
	Very low risk from November–April along the border plain with Syria, around Adana and east of Adana; very low risk all year in rest of country	1
Uganda	High risk	4
Uzbekistan	Very low risk in extreme south-east	1
Vanuatu	Risk present	4

Key to recommended regimens for prophylaxis against malaria

Codes for regimens	Details of regimens for prophylaxis against malaria
-	No risk
1	Chemoprophylaxis not recommended, but avoid mosquito bites and consider malaria if fever presents
2	Chloroquine only
3	Chloroquine with proguanil
4	Atovaquone with proguanil hydrochloride or doxycycline or mefloquine
5	Atovaquone with proguanil hydrochloride or doxycycline

Specific recommendations

Country	Comments on risk of malaria and regional or seasonal variation	Codes for regimens
Venezuela	High risk in all areas south of, and including, the Orinoco river and Angel Falls	4
	Risk in rural areas of Apure, Monagas, Sucre, and Zulia states	3
	No risk in city of Caracas or on Margarita Island	1
Vietnam	Risk in rural areas, and in southern provinces of Tay Ninh, Lam Dong, Dac Lac, Gia Lai, and Kon Tum	5
	Very low risk in Mekong river delta until border area with Cambodia; no risk in large cities (including Ho Chi Minh (Saigon) and Hanoi), Red river delta, and coastal areas north of Nha Trang and Phu Quoc Island	1
Western Sahara	No risk	1
Yemen	Risk below 2000 m	3
	Very low risk on Socrota Island; no risk above 2000 m, including Sana'a city	1
Zambia	High risk	4
Zimbabwe	High risk all year in Zambezi valley, and from November–June in areas below 1200 m	4
	Low risk from July–October in areas below 1200 m; very low risk all year in Harare and Bulawayo	1

Advice for travellers

Hospital for Tropical Diseases Travel Healthline
(020) 7950 7799 www.fitfortravel.nhs.uk
WHO advice on international travel and health
www.who.int/ith
National Travel Health Network and Centre (NaTHNaC)
www.nathnac.net

Treatment

Recommendations on the prophylaxis and treatment of malaria reflect guidelines agreed by UK malaria specialists. Choice will depend on the age of the child.

If the infective species is **not known**, or if the infection is **mixed**, initial treatment should be as for *falciparum malaria* with quinine p. 382, *Malarone*® (atovaquone with proguanil hydrochloride p. 378), or *Riamet*® (artemether with lumefantrine p. 377). Falciparum malaria can progress rapidly in unprotected individuals and antimalarial treatment should be considered in those with features of severe malaria and possible exposure, even if the initial blood tests for the organism are negative.

Falciparum malaria (treatment)

Falciparum malaria (malignant malaria) is caused by *Plasmodium falciparum*. In most parts of the world *P. falciparum* is now resistant to chloroquine p. 379 which should not therefore be given for treatment. Quinine, *Malarone*® (atovaquone with proguanil hydrochloride), or *Riamet*® (artemether with lumefantrine) can be given by mouth if the child can swallow and retain tablets and there are no serious manifestations (e.g. impaired consciousness); quinine should be given by intravenous infusion if the child is seriously ill or unable to take tablets. Mefloquine p. 380 is now rarely used for treatment because of concerns about resistance.

Oral quinine is well tolerated by children although the salts are bitter. Quinine is given by mouth together with or followed by clindamycin p. 313 [unlicensed indication] or, in children over 12 doxycycline p. 338.

If the parasite is likely to be sensitive, pyrimethamine with sulfadoxine p. 382 as a single dose [un icensed] may be given (instead of either clindamycin or doxycycline) together with, or after, a course of quinine.

Alternatively, *Malarone*®, or *Riamet*® may be given instead of quinine. It is not necessary to give clindamycin, doxycycline, or pyrimethamine with sulfadoxine after *Malarone*® or *Riamet*® treatment.

If the child is seriously ill or unable to swallow tablets, or if more than 2% of red blood cell are parasitized, quinine should be given by *intravenous infusion* [unlicensed] (until patient can swallow tablets to complete the 7-day course *together with* or *followed by either* doxycycline in children over 12 years, or clindamycin).

Specialist advice should be sought in difficult cases (e.g. very high parasite count, deterioration on optimal doses of quinine, infection acquired in quinine-resistant areas of south east Asia) because intravenous **artesunate** may be available for 'named-patient' use.

Pregnancy

Falciparum malaria is particularly dangerous in pregnancy, especially in the last trimester. The treatment doses of oral and intravenous quinine (including the loading dose) can safely be given in pregnancy. Clindamycin [unlicensed indication] should be given for 7 days with or after quinine. Doxycycline should be avoided in pregnancy (affects teeth and skeletal development in fetus); pyrimethamine with sulfadoxine, *Malarone*®, and Riamet® are also best avoided until more information is available. Specialist advice should be sought in difficult cases (e.g. very high parasite count, deterioration on optimal doses of quinine, infection acquired in quinine-resistant areas of south east Asia) because intravenous artesunate may be available for 'named patient' use.

Non-falciparum malaria (treatment)
Non-falciparum malaria is usually caused by *Plasmodium vivax* and less commonly by *P. ovale* and *P. malariae*. *P. knowlesi* is also present in the Asia-Pacific region. Chloroquine is the drug of choice for the treatment of non-falciparum malaria (but chloroquine-resistant *P. vivax* has been reported in the Indonesian archipelago, the Malay Peninsula, including Myanmar, and eastward to Southern Vietnam).

For the treatment of chloroquine-resistant non-falciparum malaria, *Malarone*® [unlicensed indication], quinine, or *Riamet*® [unlicensed indication] can be used; as with chloroquine, primaquine p. 381 should be given for radical cure.

Chloroquine alone is adequate for *P. malariae* and *P. knowlesi* infections but in the case of *P. vivax* and *P. ovale*, a radical cure (to destroy parasites in the liver and thus prevent relapses) is required. This is achieved with primaquine [unlicensed] given after chloroquine.

For a radical cure, primaquine [unlicensed] is then given to children over 6 months of age; specialist advice should be sought for children under 6 months of age.

Parenteral
If the child is unable to take oral therapy, quinine can be given by intravenous infusion, changed to oral chloroquine as soon as the patient's condition permits.

Pregnancy
Treatment doses of chloroquine can be given for non-falciparum malaria. In the case of *P.vivax* or *P.ovale*, however, the radical cure with primaquine should be **postponed** until the pregnancy is over; instead chloroquine should be continued, given weekly, during the pregnancy.

ANTIPROTOZOALS > ANTIMALARIALS

Artemether with lumefantrine

- **INDICATIONS AND DOSE**
 **Treatment of acute uncomplicated falciparum malaria |
 Treatment of chloroquine-resistant non-falciparum malaria**
 ▸ BY MOUTH
 ▸ Child (body-weight 5–14 kg): Initially 1 tablet, followed by 1 tablet for 5 doses each given at 8, 24, 36, 48, and 60 hours (total 6 tablets over 60 hours)
 ▸ Child (body-weight 15–24 kg): Initially 2 tablets, followed by 2 tablets for 5 doses each given at 8, 24, 36, 48, and 60 hours (total 12 tablets over 60 hours)
 ▸ Child (body-weight 25–34 kg): Initially 3 tablets, followed by 3 tablets for 5 doses each given at 8, 24, 36, 48, and 60 hours (total 18 tablets over 60 hours)
 ▸ Child 12–17 years (body-weight 35 kg and above): Initially 4 tablets, followed by 4 tablets for 5 doses each given at 8, 24, 36, 48, and 60 hours (total 24 tablets over 60 hours)

- **UNLICENSED USE** Use in treatment of non-falciparum malaria is an unlicensed indication.
- **CONTRA-INDICATIONS** Family history of congenital QT interval prolongation · family history of sudden death · history of arrhythmias · history of clinically relevant bradycardia · history of congestive heart failure accompanied by reduced left ventricular ejection fraction
- **CAUTIONS** Avoid in acute porphyrias p. 577 · electrolyte disturbances
- **SIDE-EFFECTS**
- Common or very common Abdominal pain · anorexia · arthralgia · asthenia · cough · diarrhoea · dizziness ·

headache · myalgia · nausea · palpitation · paraesthesia · prolonged QT interval · pruritus · rash · sleep disturbances · vomiting
▸ Uncommon Ataxia · clonus · hypoaesthesia
- **PREGNANCY** Toxicity in *animal* studies with artemether. Manufacturer advises use only if potential benefit outweighs risk.
- **BREAST FEEDING** Manufacturer advises avoid breastfeeding for at least 1 week after last dose. Present in milk in *animal* studies.
- **HEPATIC IMPAIRMENT** Manufacturer advises caution in severe impairment.
- **RENAL IMPAIRMENT** Manufacturer advises caution in severe impairment. In severe renal impairment monitor ECG and plasma potassium concentration.
- **MONITORING REQUIREMENTS** Monitor patients unable to take food (greater risk of recrudescence).
- **DIRECTIONS FOR ADMINISTRATION** Tablets may be crushed just before administration.
- **PATIENT AND CARER ADVICE**
 Driving and skilled tasks
 Dizziness may affect performance of skilled tasks (e.g. driving).

- **MEDICINAL FORMS**
 There can be variation in the licensing of different medicines containing the same drug.
 Tablet
 CAUTIONARY AND ADVISORY LABELS 21
 ▸ Riamet (Novartis Pharmaceuticals UK Ltd)
 Artemether 20 mg, Lumefantrine 120 mg Riamet tablets | 24 tablet [PoM] £22.50

Artenimol with piperaquine phosphate

(Piperaquine tetraphosphate with dihydroartemisinin)

- **INDICATIONS AND DOSE**
 Treatment of uncomplicated falciparum malaria
 ▸ BY MOUTH
 ▸ Child 6 months–17 years (body-weight 7–12 kg): 0.5 tablet once daily for 3 days, max. 2 courses in 12 months; second course given at least 2 months after first course
 ▸ Child 6 months–17 years (body-weight 13–23 kg): 1 tablet once daily for 3 days, max. 2 courses in 12 months; second course given at least 2 months after first course
 ▸ Child 6 months–17 years (body-weight 24–35 kg): 2 tablets once daily for 3 days, max. 2 courses in 12 months; second course given at least 2 months after first course
 ▸ Child 6 months–17 years (body-weight 36–74 kg): 3 tablets once daily for 3 days, max. 2 courses in 12 months; second course given at least 2 months after first course
 ▸ Child 6 months–17 years (body-weight 75–99 kg): 4 tablets once daily for 3 days, max. 2 courses in 12 months; second course given at least 2 months after first course

- **CONTRA-INDICATIONS** Acute myocardial infarction · bradycardia · congenital long QT syndrome · electrolyte disturbances · family history of sudden death · heart failure with reduced left ventricular ejection fraction · history of symptomatic arrhythmias · left ventricular hypertrophy · risk factors for QT interval prolongation · severe hypertension
- **INTERACTIONS** → Appendix 1: antimalarials
- **SIDE-EFFECTS**
- Common or very common Abdominal pain · anaemia · blood disorders · conjunctivitis · cough · diarrhoea · irregular

heart rate · leucopenia · malaise · QT interval prolonged · rash · thrombocytopenia · vomiting

▶ **Uncommon** Acanthosis · arrhythmias · arthralgia · convulsions · headache · heart murmur · hepatitis · hepatomegaly · influenza-like symptoms · jaundice · nausea · stomatitis

● **PREGNANCY** Teratogenic in *animal* studies—manufacturer advises use only if other antimalarials cannot be used.

● **BREAST FEEDING** Manufacturer advises avoid—present in milk in *animal* studies.

● **HEPATIC IMPAIRMENT** No information available in moderate to severe impairment. Manufacturer advises monitor ECG and plasma-potassium concentration in moderate to severe hepatic impairment.

● **RENAL IMPAIRMENT** No information available in moderate to severe impairment. Manufacturer advises monitor ECG and plasma-potassium concentration in moderate to severe renal impairment.

● **MONITORING REQUIREMENTS**
▶ Consider obtaining ECG in all patients before third dose and 4–6 hours after third dose. If QT_C interval more than 500 milliseconds, discontinue treatment and monitor ECG for a further 24–48 hours.
▶ Obtain ECG as soon as possible after starting treatment then continue monitoring in those taking medicines that increase plasma-piperaquine concentration, in children who are vomiting or in females.

● **DIRECTIONS FOR ADMINISTRATION** Tablets to be taken at least 3 hours before and at least 3 hours after food. Tablets may be crushed and mixed with water immediately before administration.

● **PATIENT AND CARER ADVICE** Patients or carers should be given advice on how to administer tablets containing piperaquine phosphate with artenimol.

● **MEDICINAL FORMS**
There can be variation in the licensing of different medicines containing the same drug.

Tablet
▶ **Eurartesim** (Logixx Pharma Solutions Ltd) ▼
Artenimol 40 mg, Piperaquine phosphate 320 mg Eurartesim 320mg/40mg tablets | 12 tablet [PoM] £40.00

Atovaquone with proguanil hydrochloride

● **INDICATIONS AND DOSE**

MALARONE®

Prophylaxis of falciparum malaria, particularly where resistance to other antimalarial drugs suspected
▶ BY MOUTH
▶ Child (body-weight 41 kg and above): 1 tablet daily, to be started 1–2 days before entering endemic area and continued for 1 week after leaving

Treatment of acute uncomplicated falciparum malaria | Treatment of non-falciparum malaria
▶ BY MOUTH
▶ Child (body-weight 11-20 kg): 1 tablet once daily for 3 days
▶ Child (body-weight 21-30 kg): 2 tablets once daily for 3 days
▶ Child (body-weight 31-40 kg): 3 tablets once daily for 3 days
▶ Child (body-weight 41 kg and above): 4 tablets once daily for 3 days

MALARONE® PAEDIATRIC

Prophylaxis of falciparum malaria, particularly where resistance to other antimalarial drugs suspected
▶ BY MOUTH
▶ Child (body-weight 5-8 kg): 0.5 tablet once daily, to be started 1–2 days before entering endemic area and continued for 1 week after leaving
▶ Child (body-weight 9-10 kg): 0.75 tablet once daily, to be started 1–2 days before entering endemic area and continued for 1 week after leaving
▶ Child (body-weight 11-20 kg): 1 tablet once daily, to be started 1–2 days before entering endemic area and continued for 1 week after leaving
▶ Child (body-weight 21-30 kg): 2 tablets once daily, to be started 1–2 days before entering endemic area and continued for 1 week after leaving
▶ Child (body-weight 31-40 kg): 3 tablets once daily, to be started 1–2 days before entering endemic area and continued for 1 week after leaving
▶ Child (body-weight 41 kg and above): Use *Malarone®* (standard) tablets.

Treatment of acute uncomplicated falciparum malaria | Treatment of non-falciparum malaria
▶ BY MOUTH
▶ Child (body-weight 5-8 kg): 2 tablets once daily for 3 days
▶ Child (body-weight 9-10 kg): 3 tablets once daily for 3 days
▶ Child (body-weight 11 kg and above): Use *Malarone®* (standard) tablets.

● **UNLICENSED USE** Not licensed for treatment of non-falciparum malaria. Not licensed for prophylaxis of malaria in children under 11 kg.

● **CAUTIONS** Diarrhoea or vomiting (reduced absorption of atovaquone) · efficacy not evaluated in cerebral or complicated malaria (including hyperparasitaemia, pulmonary oedema or renal failure)

● **INTERACTIONS** → Appendix 1: antimalarials

● **SIDE-EFFECTS**
▶ **Common or very common** Abdominal pain · abnormal dreams · anorexia · cough · depression · diarrhoea · dizziness · fever · headache · insomnia · nausea · pruritus · rash · vomiting
▶ **Uncommon** Anxiety · blood disorders · hair loss · hyponatraemia · palpitation · stomatitis
▶ **Frequency not known** Cholestasis · hallucinations · hepatitis · mouth ulcers · photosensitivity · seizures · Stevens-Johnson syndrome · tachycardia · vasculitis

● **PREGNANCY** Manufacturer advises avoid unless essential.

● **BREAST FEEDING** Use only if no suitable alternative available.

● **RENAL IMPAIRMENT** Avoid for malaria prophylaxis and, if possible, for treatment if estimated glomerular filtration rate less than 30 mL/minute/1.73 m^2.

● **DIRECTIONS FOR ADMINISTRATION**
MALARONE® PAEDIATRIC Tablets may be crushed and mixed with food or milky drink just before administration.

● **PATIENT AND CARER ADVICE** Warn travellers about **importance** of avoiding mosquito bites, **importance** of taking prophylaxis regularly, and **importance** of immediate visit to doctor if ill within 1 year and **especially** within 3 months of return.
Medicines for Children leaflet: Malarone for prevention of malaria www.medicinesforchildren.org.uk/malarone-for-prevention-of-malaria

● **NATIONAL FUNDING/ACCESS DECISIONS**
NHS restrictions Drugs for malaria prophylaxis not prescribable on the NHS; health authorities may investigate circumstances under which antimalarials prescribed.

- **MEDICINAL FORMS**
  There can be variation in the licensing of different medicines containing the same drug.
  Tablet
  CAUTIONARY AND ADVISORY LABELS 21
  ▸ **Malarone** (GlaxoSmithKline UK Ltd)
    Proguanil hydrochloride 25 mg, Atovaquone 62.5 mg Malarone Paediatric tablets | 12 tablet PoM £6.26
    Proguanil hydrochloride 100 mg, Atovaquone 250 mg Malarone tablets | 12 tablet PoM £25.21 DT price = £25.21

Chloroquine

- **INDICATIONS AND DOSE**
  Prophylaxis of malaria
  ▸ INITIALLY BY MOUTH USING SYRUP
  ▸ **Child 4–5 weeks (body-weight up to 4.5 kg):** 25 mg once weekly, started 1 week before entering endemic area and continued for 4 weeks after leaving
  ▸ **Child 6 weeks–5 months (body-weight 4.5–7 kg):** 50 mg once weekly, started 1 week before entering endemic area and continued for 4 weeks after leaving
  ▸ **Child 6–11 months (body-weight 8–10 kg):** 75 mg once weekly, started 1 week before entering endemic area and continued for 4 weeks after leaving
  ▸ **Child 1–2 years (body-weight 11–14 kg):** 100 mg once weekly, started 1 week before entering endemic area and continued for 4 weeks after leaving
  ▸ **Child 3–4 years (body-weight 15–16.4 kg):** 125 mg once weekly, started 1 week before entering endemic area and continued for 4 weeks after leaving
  ▸ **Child 5–7 years (body-weight 16.5–24 kg):** 150 mg once weekly, alternatively (by mouth using tablets) 155 mg once weekly, started 1 week before entering endemic area and continued for 4 weeks after leaving
  ▸ **Child 8–13 years (body-weight 25–44 kg):** 225 mg once weekly, alternatively (by mouth using tablets) 232.5 mg once weekly, started 1 week before entering endemic area and continued for 4 weeks after leaving
  ▸ INITIALLY BY MOUTH USING TABLETS
  ▸ **Child 14–17 years (body-weight 45 kg and above):** 310 mg once weekly, alternatively (by mouth using syrup) 300 mg once weekly, started 1 week before entering endemic area and continued for 4 weeks after leaving

  Treatment of non-falciparum malaria
  ▸ BY MOUTH
  ▸ **Child:** Initially 10 mg/kg (max. per dose 620 mg), then 5 mg/kg after 6–8 hours (max. per dose 310 mg), then 5 mg/kg daily (max. per dose 310 mg) for 2 days

  P. vivax or P. ovale infection during pregnancy while radical cure is postponed
  ▸ BY MOUTH
  ▸ **Child:** 10 mg/kg once weekly (max. per dose 310 mg)

  DOSE EQUIVALENCE AND CONVERSION
  ▸ Doses expressed as chloroquine base. Chloroquine base 150 mg = chloroquine sulfate 200 mg = chloroquine phosphate 250 mg (approx).

- **UNLICENSED USE** Chloroquine doses for the treatment and prophylaxis of malaria in BNF publications may differ from those in product literature.

- **CAUTIONS** Acute porphyrias p. 577 · diabetes (may lower blood glucose) · G6PD deficiency · long-term therapy (regular ophthalmic examination recommended by manufacturers) · may aggravate myasthenia gravis · may exacerbate psoriasis · neurological disorders, especially epilepsy (avoid for prophylaxis of malaria if history of epilepsy) · severe gastro-intestinal disorders

- **INTERACTIONS** → Appendix 1: antimalarials

- **SIDE-EFFECTS**
  GENERAL SIDE-EFFECTS
  ▸ **Common or very common** Gastro-intestinal disturbances · headache · pruritus · rashes · skin reactions
  ▸ **Uncommon** Convulsions · discoloration of mucous membranes · discoloration of nails · discoloration of skin · ECG changes · hair depigmentation · hair loss · keratopathy · ototoxicity · retinal damage · visual changes
  ▸ **Rare** Acute generalised exanthematous pustulosis · agranulocytosis · angioedema · aplastic anaemia · blood disorders · bone marrow suppression · cardiomyopathy · emotional disturbances · exfoliative dermatitis · hepatic damage · hypersensitivity reactions · mental changes · myopathy · neuromyopathy · photosensitivity · psychosis · Stevens-Johnson syndrome · thrombocytopenia · urticaria
  ▸ **Frequency not known** Bronchospasm · diffuse parenchymal lung disease · drug rash with eosinophilia and systemic symptoms · extrapyramidal symptoms (associated with use in malaria) · hypotension · visual disturbances

  SIDE-EFFECTS, FURTHER INFORMATION
  ▸ Malaria prophylaxis and treatment Serious skin reactions, ECG changes, visual effects, ototoxicity, blood disorders, mental changes, myopathies and hepatic damage are not usually associated with malaria prophylaxis or treatment.

  Overdose
  Chloroquine is very toxic in overdosage; overdosage is extremely hazardous and difficult to treat. Urgent advice from the National Poisons Information Service is essential. Life-threatening features include arrhythmias (which can have a very rapid onset) and convulsions (which can be intractable).

- **PREGNANCY** Benefit of use in prophylaxis and treatment in malaria outweighs risk. For rheumatoid disease, it is not necessary to withdraw an antimalarial drug during pregnancy if the disease is well controlled.

- **BREAST FEEDING** Present in breast milk and breast-feeding should be avoided when used to treat rheumatic disease. Amount in milk probably too small to be harmful when used for malaria.

- **HEPATIC IMPAIRMENT** Use with caution in moderate to severe impairment.

- **RENAL IMPAIRMENT** Only partially excreted by the kidneys and reduction of the dose is not required for prophylaxis of malaria except in severe impairment. For rheumatoid arthritis and lupus erythematosus, reduce dose. Manufacturers advise caution.

- **MONITORING REQUIREMENTS** Ophthalmic examination with long-term therapy.

- **PATIENT AND CARER ADVICE** Warn travellers going to malarious areas about **importance** of avoiding mosquito bites, **importance** of taking prophylaxis regularly, and **importance** of immediate visit to doctor if ill within 1 year and **especially** within 3 months of return.

- **NATIONAL FUNDING/ACCESS DECISIONS**
  NHS restrictions Drugs for malaria prophylaxis not prescribable on the NHS; health authorities may investigate circumstances under which antimalarials are prescribed.

- **EXCEPTIONS TO LEGAL CATEGORY** Can be sold to the public provided it is licensed and labelled for the prophylaxis of malaria.

- **MEDICINAL FORMS**
  There can be variation in the licensing of different medicines containing the same drug. Forms available from special-order manufacturers include: oral solution
  Oral solution
  CAUTIONARY AND ADVISORY LABELS 5
  ▸ **Malarivon** (Wallace Manufacturing Chemists Ltd)
    Chloroquine phosphate 16 mg per 1 ml Malarivon 80mg/5ml syrup | 75 ml PoM £30.00

Tablet
CAUTIONARY AND ADVISORY LABELS 5
▸ Avloclor (Alliance Pharmaceuticals Ltd)
  Chloroquine phosphate 250 mg Avloclor 250mg tablets |
  20 tablet PoM £7.95 DT price = £7.95

Chloroquine with proguanil

The properties listed below are those particular to the combination only. For the properties of the components please consider, chloroquine p. 379, proguanil hydrochloride p. 381.

● **INDICATIONS AND DOSE**
Prophylaxis of malaria
▸ BY MOUTH
▸ Child: (consult product literature)

● INTERACTIONS → Appendix 1: antimalarials

● EXCEPTIONS TO LEGAL CATEGORY Can be sold to the public provided it is licensed and labelled for the prophylaxis of malaria.

● MEDICINAL FORMS
There can be variation in the licensing of different medicines containing the same drug.
Tablets
▸ Paludrine/Avloclor (Alliance Pharmaceuticals Ltd)
  Paludrine/Avloclor tablets anti-malarial travel pack | 112 tablet P
  £13.50

Mefloquine

● **INDICATIONS AND DOSE**
Treatment of malaria
▸ BY MOUTH
▸ Child: (consult product literature)
Prophylaxis of malaria
▸ BY MOUTH
▸ Child (body-weight 5-15 kg): 62.5 mg once weekly, dose to be started 2–3 weeks before entering endemic area and continued for 4 weeks after leaving
▸ Child (body-weight 16-24 kg): 125 mg once weekly, dose to be started 2–3 weeks before entering endemic area and continued for 4 weeks after leaving
▸ Child (body-weight 25-44 kg): 187.5 mg once weekly, dose to be started 2–3 weeks before entering endemic area and continued for 4 weeks after leaving
▸ Child (body-weight 45 kg and above): 250 mg once weekly, dose to be started 2–3 weeks before entering endemic area and continued for 4 weeks after leaving

● UNLICENSED USE Mefloquine doses in BNF Publications may differ from those in product literature. Not licensed for use in children under 5 kg body-weight and under 3 months.

● CONTRA-INDICATIONS Avoid for prophylaxis if history of psychiatric disorders (including depression) or convulsions · avoid for standby treatment if history of convulsions · history of blackwater fever

● CAUTIONS Cardiac conduction disorders · epilepsy (avoid for prophylaxis) · not recommended in infants under 3 months (5 kg) · traumatic brain injury
CAUTIONS, FURTHER INFORMATION
▸ Neuropsychiatric reactions Mefloquine is associated with potentially serious neuropsychiatric reactions. Abnormal dreams, insomnia, anxiety, and depression occur commonly. Psychosis, suicidal ideation, and suicide have also been reported. Psychiatric symptoms such as nightmares, acute anxiety, depression, restlessness, or confusion should be regarded as potentially prodromal for

a more serious event. Adverse reactions may occur and persist up to several months after discontinuation because mefloquine has a long half-life. For a prescribing checklist, and further information on side-effects, particularly neuropsychiatric side-effects, which may be associated with the use of mefloquine for malaria prophylaxis, see the *Guide for Healthcare Professionals* provided by the manufacturer.

● INTERACTIONS → Appendix 1: antimalarials

● SIDE-EFFECTS
▸ **Common or very common** Abdominal pain · diarrhoea · dizziness · headache · nausea · neuropsychiatric reactions · pruritus · visual disturbances · vomiting
▸ **Very rare** Optic neuropathy
▸ **Frequency not known** Alopecia · amnesia · anorexia · arrhythmias · arthralgia · ataxia · blood disorders · bradycardia · cataract · chest pain · confusion · drowsiness · dyspepsia · dyspnoea · encephalopathy · fever · flushing · hepatic failure · hyperhidrosis · hypertension · hypotension · leucocytosis · leucopenia · malaise · motor neuropathies · muscle weakness · myalgia · oedema - palpitation · panic attacks · pneumonitis · rash · seizures · sensory neuropathies · speech disturbances Stevens-Johnson syndrome · syncope · tachycardia · thrombocytopenia · tremor · vestibular disorders

● ALLERGY AND CROSS-SENSITIVITY Contra-indicated in patients with hypersensitivity to quinine.

● CONCEPTION AND CONTRACEPTION Manufacturer advises adequate contraception during prophylaxis and for 3 months after stopping (teratogenicity in *animal* studies).

● PREGNANCY Manufacturer advises avoid (particularly in the first trimester) unless the potential benefit outweighs the risk; however, studies of mefloquine in pregnancy (including use in the first trimester) indicate that it can be considered for travel to chloroquine-resistant areas.

● BREAST FEEDING Present in milk but risk to infant minimal.

● HEPATIC IMPAIRMENT Elimination may be prolonged; avoid in severe impairment.

● RENAL IMPAIRMENT Manufacturer advises caution.

● DIRECTIONS FOR ADMINISTRATION Tablet may be crushed and mixed with food such as jam or honey just before administration.

● PATIENT AND CARER ADVICE A patient alert card should be provided. Manufacturer advises that patients receiving mefloquine for malaria prophylaxis should be informed to discontinue its use if neuropsychiatric symptoms occur and seek immediate medical advice so that mefloquine can be replaced with an alternative antimalarial. Travellers should also be warned about **importance** of avoiding mosquito bites, **importance** of taking prophylaxis regularly, and **importance** of immediate visit to doctor if ill within 1 year and especially within 3 months of return.
Driving and skilled tasks
Dizziness or a disturbed sense of balance may affect performance of skilled tasks (e.g. driving); effects may occur and persist up to several months after stopping mefloquine.

● NATIONAL FUNDING/ACCESS DECISIONS
NHS restrictions Drugs for malaria prophylaxis not prescribable on the NHS; health authorities may investigate circumstances under which antimalarials prescribed.

- **MEDICINAL FORMS**
  There can be variation in the licensing of different medicines containing the same drug.

Tablet
CAUTIONARY AND ADVISORY LABELS 10, 21, 27
▸ **Lariam** (Roche Products Ltd)
  Mefloquine (as Mefloquine hydrochloride) 250 mg Lariam 250mg tablets | 8 tablet PoM £14.53

Primaquine

- **INDICATIONS AND DOSE**

Adjunct in the treatment of non-falciparum malaria caused by *P.vivax* infection
▸ BY MOUTH
  ▸ Child 6 months–17 years: 500 micrograms/kg daily (max. per dose 30 mg) for 14 days

Adjunct in the treatment of non-falciparum malaria caused by *P.ovale* infection
▸ BY MOUTH
  ▸ Child 6 months–17 years: 250 micrograms/kg daily (max. per dose 15 mg) for 14 days

Adjunct in the treatment of non-falciparum malaria caused by *P.vivax* infection in patients with mild G6PD deficiency (administered on expert advice) | Adjunct in the treatment of non-falciparum malaria caused by *P.ovale* infection in patients with mild G6PD deficiency (administered on expert advice)
▸ BY MOUTH
  ▸ Child: 750 micrograms/kg once weekly for 8 weeks; maximum 45 mg per week

Treatment of mild to moderate pneumocystis infection (in combination with clindamycin)
▸ BY MOUTH
  ▸ Child: This combination is associated with considerable toxicity (consult product literature)

- **UNLICENSED USE** Not licensed.
- **CAUTIONS** G6PD deficiency · systemic diseases associated with granulocytopenia (e.g. juvenile idiopathic arthritis, rheumatoid arthritis, lupus erythematosus)
- **INTERACTIONS** → Appendix 1: antimalarials
- **SIDE-EFFECTS**
▸ **Common or very common** Abdominal pain · anorexia · nausea · vomiting
▸ **Uncommon** Haemolytic anaemia especially in G6PD deficiency · leucopenia · methaemoglobinaemia
- **PREGNANCY** Risk of neonatal haemolysis and methaemoglobinaemia in third trimester.
- **BREAST FEEDING** No information available; theoretical risk of haemolysis in G6PD-deficient infants.
- **PRE-TREATMENT SCREENING** Before starting primaquine, blood should be tested for glucose-6-phosphate dehydrogenase (G6PD) activity since the drug can cause haemolysis in G6PD-deficient patients. Specialist advice should be obtained in G6PD deficiency.
- **MEDICINAL FORMS**
  There can be variation in the licensing of different medicines containing the same drug. Forms available from special-order manufacturers include: oral suspension

Tablet
▸ **Primaquine** (Non-proprietary)
  Primaquine (as Primaquine phosphate) 15 mg Primaquine 15mg tablets | 100 tablet PoM no price available

Proguanil hydrochloride

- **INDICATIONS AND DOSE**

Prophylaxis of malaria
▸ BY MOUTH
  ▸ Child 4–11 weeks (body-weight up to 6 kg): 25 mg once daily, dose to be started 1 week before entering endemic area and continued for 4 weeks after leaving
  ▸ Child 3–11 months (body-weight 6–9 kg): 50 mg once daily, dose to be started 1 week before entering endemic area and continued for 4 weeks after leaving
  ▸ Child 1–3 years (body-weight 10–15 kg): 75 mg once daily, dose to be started 1 week before entering endemic area and continued for 4 weeks after leaving
  ▸ Child 4–7 years (body-weight 16–24 kg): 100 mg once daily, dose to be started 1 week before entering endemic area and continued for 4 weeks after leaving
  ▸ Child 8–12 years (body-weight 25–44 kg): 150 mg once daily, dose to be started 1 week before entering endemic area and continued for 4 weeks after leaving
  ▸ Child 13–17 years (body-weight 45 kg and above): 200 mg once daily, dose to be started 1 week before entering endemic area and continued for 4 weeks after leaving

- **UNLICENSED USE** Proguanil doses in BNF Publications may differ from those in product literature.
- **INTERACTIONS** → Appendix 1: antimalarials
- **SIDE-EFFECTS**
▸ **Common or very common** Constipation · diarrhoea · mild gastric intolerance
▸ **Very rare** Cholestasis · hair loss · skin reactions · vasculitis
▸ **Frequency not known** Mouth ulcers · stomatitis
- **PREGNANCY** Benefit of prophylaxis in malaria outweighs risk. Adequate folate supplements should be given to mother.
- **BREAST FEEDING** Amount in milk probably too small to be harmful when used for malaria prophylaxis.
- **RENAL IMPAIRMENT** Use half normal dose if estimated glomerular filtration rate 20–60 mL/minute/1.73m². Use one-quarter normal dose on alternate days if estimated glomerular filtration rate 10–20 mL/minute/1.73m². Use one-quarter normal dose once weekly if estimated glomerular filtration rate less than 10 mL/minute/1.73m²; increased risk of haematological toxicity in severe impairment.
- **DIRECTIONS FOR ADMINISTRATION** Tablet may be crushed and mixed with food such as milk, jam, or honey just before administration.
- **PATIENT AND CARER ADVICE** Warn travellers about **importance** of avoiding mosquito bites, **importance** of taking prophylaxis regularly, and **importance** of immediate visit to doctor if ill within 1 year and **especially** within 3 months of return.
- **NATIONAL FUNDING/ACCESS DECISIONS**
  NHS restrictions Drugs for malaria prophylaxis not prescribable on the NHS; health authorities may investigate circumstances under which antimalarials are prescribed.
- **EXCEPTIONS TO LEGAL CATEGORY** Can be sold to the public provided it is licensed and labelled for the prophylaxis of malaria.
- **MEDICINAL FORMS**
  There can be variation in the licensing of different medicines containing the same drug. Forms available from special-order manufacturers include: oral suspension, oral solution

Tablet
CAUTIONARY AND ADVISORY LABELS 21
▸ **Paludrine** (Alliance Pharmaceuticals Ltd)
  Proguanil hydrochloride 100 mg Paludrine 100mg tablets | 98 tablet P £11.95 DT price = £11.95

Pyrimethamine

● **INDICATIONS AND DOSE**

Toxoplasmosis in pregnancy (in combination with sulfadiazine and folinic acid)
▸ BY MOUTH
▸ Child 12-17 years: 50 mg once daily until delivery

Congenital toxoplasmosis (in combination with sulfadiazine and folinic acid)
▸ BY MOUTH
▸ Neonate: 1 mg/kg twice daily for 2 days, then 1 mg/kg once daily for 6 months, then 1 mg/kg 3 times a week for 6 months.

Malaria
▸ BY MOUTH
▸ Child: No dose stated because not recommended alone

● **UNLICENSED USE** Not licensed for use in children under 5 years.
● **CAUTIONS** History of seizures—avoid large loading doses · predisposition to folate deficiency
● **INTERACTIONS** → Appendix 1: antimalarials
● **SIDE-EFFECTS**
▸ **Common or very common** Anaemia (with high doses) · blood disorders (with high doses) · diarrhoea · dizziness · headache · leucopenia (with high doses) · nausea · rash · thrombocytopenia (with high doses) · vomiting
▸ **Uncommon** Abnormal skin pigmentation · fever
▸ **Very rare** Buccal ulceration · colic · convulsions
● **PREGNANCY** Theoretical teratogenic risk in *first trimester* (folate antagonist). Adequate folate supplements should be given to the mother.
● **BREAST FEEDING** Significant amount in milk—avoid administration of other folate antagonists to infant. Avoid breast-feeding during toxoplasmosis treatment.
● **HEPATIC IMPAIRMENT** Manufacturer advises caution.
● **RENAL IMPAIRMENT** Manufacturer advises caution.
● **MONITORING REQUIREMENTS** Blood counts required with prolonged treatment.
● **LESS SUITABLE FOR PRESCRIBING** Pyrimethamine should not be used alone for malaria, but is used with sulfadoxine.

● **MEDICINAL FORMS**
There can be variation in the licensing of different medicines containing the same drug. Forms available from special-order manufacturers include: oral suspension
Tablet
▸ Daraprim (GlaxoSmithKline UK Ltd)
Pyrimethamine 25 mg Daraprim 25mg tablets | 30 tablet [PoM]
£13.00

Pyrimethamine with sulfadoxine

● **INDICATIONS AND DOSE**

Adjunct to quinine in treatment of Plasmodium falciparum malaria
▸ BY MOUTH
▸ Child 1 month-4 years (body-weight 5 kg and above): 12.5/250 mg for 1 dose
▸ Child 5-6 years: 25/500 mg for 1 dose
▸ Child 7-9 years: 37.5/750 mg for 1 dose
▸ Child 10-13 years: 50/1000 mg for 1 dose
▸ Child 14-17 years: 75/1500 mg for 1 dose

Malaria prophylaxis
▸ BY MOUTH
▸ Child: Not recommended by UK malaria experts

DOSE EQUIVALENCE AND CONVERSION
▸ Dose quantities are expressed in the form x/y where x and y are the strengths in milligrams of pyrimethamine and sulfadoxine respectively.

● **UNLICENSED USE** Not licensed for use in children of body-weight under 5 kg.
● **CONTRA-INDICATIONS** Acute porphyrias p. 577
● **CAUTIONS** Asthma · avoid in blood disorders (unless under specialist supervision) · avoid in infants under 6 weeks · G6PD deficiency · history of seizures—avoid large loading doses · not recommended for prophylaxis (severe side-effects on long-term use) · predisposition to folate deficiency
● **INTERACTIONS** → Appendix 1: antimalarials
● **SIDE-EFFECTS**
▸ **Common or very common** Diarrhoea · headache · hyperkalaemia · nausea · rash
▸ **Uncommon** Vomiting
▸ **Very rare** Anorexia · antibiotic-associated colitis · arthralgia · aseptic meningitis · ataxia · blood disorders · convulsions · cough · depression · eosinophilia · glossitis · hallucinations · hepatic necrosis · hypoglycaemia · hyponatraemia · interstitial nephritis · jaundice · leucopenia · liver damage · megaloblastic anaemia · myalgia · myocarditis · pancreatitis · peripheral neuropathy · photosensitivity · renal disorders · rhabdomyolysis reported in HIV-infected patients · shortness of breath · Stevens-Johnson syndrome · stomatitis · systemic lupus erythematosus · thrombocytopenia · tinnitus · toxic epidermal necrolysis · uveitis · vasculitis · vertigo
▸ **Frequency not known** Allergic alveolitis · eosinophilic alveolitis · pulmonary infiltrates

SIDE-EFFECTS, FURTHER INFORMATION
Discontinue immediately if blood disorders or rash occur. Discontinue if cough or shortness of breath occur.

● **ALLERGY AND CROSS-SENSITIVITY** Contra-indicated in patients with sulfonamide allergy.
● **PREGNANCY** Possible teratogenic risk in *first trimester* (pyrimethamine a folate antagonist); in *third trimester*— risk of neonatal haemolysis and methaemoglobinaemia. Fear of increased risk of kernicterus in neonates appears to be unfounded.
● **BREAST FEEDING** Small risk of kernicterus in jaundiced infants; risk of haemolysis in G6PD-deficient infants (due to sulfadoxine).
● **MONITORING REQUIREMENTS** Monitor blood counts on prolonged treatment.
● **PRESCRIBING AND DISPENSING INFORMATION** Also known as *Fansidar*®.
● **PATIENT AND CARER ADVICE** Patients should be advised to maintain adequate fluid intake.

● **MEDICINAL FORMS**
There can be variation in the licensing of different medicines containing the same drug.
No licensed medicines listed.

Quinine

● **INDICATIONS AND DOSE**

Non-falciparum malaria
▸ BY INTRAVENOUS INFUSION
▸ Child: 10 mg/kg every 8 hours (max. per dose 700 mg), infused over 4 hours, given if patient is unable to take oral therapy. Changed to oral chloroquine as soon as the patient's condition permits

Falciparum malaria

▸ BY MOUTH

▸ **Child:** 10 mg/kg every 8 hours (max. per dose 600 mg) for 7 days, together with or followed by either doxycycline (in children over 12 years), or clindamycin

▸ BY INTRAVENOUS INFUSION

▸ **Neonate:** Loading dose 20 mg/kg (max. per dose 1.4 g), infused over 4 hours, the loading dose of 20 mg/kg should **not** be used if the patient has received quinine or mefloquine during the previous 12 hours, then maintenance 10 mg/kg every 8 hours (max. per dose 700 mg) until patient can tolerate oral medication to complete the 7-day course, maintenance dose to be given 8 hours after the start of the loading dose and infused over 4 hours, the quinine should be given together with or followed by clindamycin.

▸ **Child:** Loading dose 20 mg/kg (max. per dose 1.4 g), infused over 4 hours, the loading dose of 20 mg/kg should **not** be used if the patient has received quinine or mefloquine during the previous 12 hours, then maintenance 10 mg/kg every 8 hours (max. per dose 700 mg) until patient can swallow tablets to complete the 7-day course, maintenance dose to be given 8 hours after the start of the loading dose and infused over 4 hours, the quinine should be given together with or followed by either doxycycline (in children over 12 years), or clindamycin

Falciparum malaria (in intensive care unit)

▸ BY INTRAVENOUS INFUSION

▸ **Neonate:** Loading dose 7 mg/kg, infused over 30 minutes, followed immediately by 10 mg/kg, infused over 4 hours, then maintenance 10 mg/kg every 8 hours (max. per dose 700 mg) until patient can swallow tablets to complete the 7-day course, maintenance dose to be given 8 hours after the start of the loading dose and infused over 4 hours, the quinine should be given together with or followed by clindamycin.

▸ **Child:** Loading dose 7 mg/kg, infused over 30 minutes, followed immediately by 10 mg/kg, infused over 4 hours, then maintenance 10 mg/kg every 8 hours (max. per dose 700 mg) until patient can swallow tablets to complete the 7-day course, maintenance dose to be given 8 hours after the start of the loading dose and infused over 4 hours, the quinine should be given together with or followed by either doxycycline (in children over 12 years), or clindamycin

DOSE EQUIVALENCE AND CONVERSION

▸ When using quinine for malaria, doses are valid for quinine hydrochloride, dihydrochloride, and sulfate; they are **not** valid for quinine bisulfate which contains a correspondingly smaller amount of quinine.

▸ Quinine (anhydrous base) 100 mg = quinine bisulfate 169 mg; quinine dihydrochloride 122 mg; quinine hydrochloride 122 mg; and quinine sulfate 121 mg. Quinine bisulfate 300 mg tablets are available but provide less quinine than 300 mg of the dihydrochloride, hydrochloride, or sulfate.

● **UNLICENSED USE** Injection not licensed.

● **CONTRA-INDICATIONS** Haemoglobinuria · myasthenia gravis · optic neuritis · tinnitus

● **CAUTIONS** Atrial fibrillation (monitor ECG during parenteral treatment) · cardiac disease (monitor ECG during parenteral treatment) · conduction defects (monitor ECG during parenteral treatment) · G6PD deficiency · heart block (monitor ECG during parenteral treatment)

● **INTERACTIONS** → Appendix 1: antimalarials

● **SIDE-EFFECTS** Agitation · tinnitus · abdominal pain · acute renal failure · angioedema · blood disorders · cardiovascular effects · cinchonism · confusion · diarrhoea · dyspnoea · flushed skin · headache · hearing impairment · hot skin · hypersensitivity reactions · hypoglycaemia (especially after parenteral administration) · intravascular coagulation · muscle weakness · nausea · photosensitivity · rashes · temporary blindness · thrombocytopenia · vertigo · visual disturbances · vomiting

Overdose
Quinine is very toxic in overdosage; life-threatening features include arrhythmias (which can have a very rapid onset) and convulsions (which can be intractable).
  For details on the management of poisoning, see Emergency treatment of poisoning p. 803.

● **PREGNANCY** High doses are teratogenic in *first trimester*, but in malaria benefit of treatment outweighs risk.

● **BREAST FEEDING** Present in milk but not known to be harmful.

● **HEPATIC IMPAIRMENT** For treatment of malaria in severe impairment, reduce parenteral maintenance dose to 5–7 mg/kg of quinine salt.

● **RENAL IMPAIRMENT** For treatment of malaria in severe impairment, reduce parenteral maintenance dose to 5–7 mg/kg of quinine salt.

● **MONITORING REQUIREMENTS** Monitor blood glucose and electrolyte concentration during parenteral treatment.

● **DIRECTIONS FOR ADMINISTRATION** For *intravenous infusion*, dilute to a concentration of 2 mg/mL (max. 30 mg/mL in fluid restriction) with Glucose 5% *or* Sodium Chloride 0.9% and give over 4 hours.

● **PRESCRIBING AND DISPENSING INFORMATION** Intravenous injection of quinine is so hazardous that it has been superseded by infusion.

● **MEDICINAL FORMS**
There can be variation in the licensing of different medicines containing the same drug. Forms available from special-order manufacturers include: capsule, oral suspension, oral solution, solution for infusion

Tablet
▸ **Quinine (Non-proprietary)**
  Quinine sulfate 200 mg Quinine sulfate 200mg tablets |
  28 tablet PoM £2.90 DT price = £1.61
  Quinine bisulfate 300 mg Quinine bisulfate 300mg tablets |
  28 tablet PoM £4.80 DT price = £1.82
  Quinine sulfate 300 mg Quinine sulfate 300mg tablets |
  28 tablet PoM £5.05 DT price = £1.86 | 500 tablet PoM no price available

5.3 Toxoplasmosis

Other drugs used for Toxoplasmosis Pyrimethamine, p. 382

ANTIBACTERIALS ⟩ MACROLIDES

Spiramycin

● **INDICATIONS AND DOSE**

Toxoplasmosis in pregnancy
▸ BY MOUTH
▸ **Child 12–17 years:** 1.5 g twice daily until delivery

Chemoprophylaxis of congenital toxoplasmosis
▸ BY MOUTH
▸ **Neonate:** 50 mg/kg twice daily.

● **DOSE EQUIVALENCE AND CONVERSION**
▸ 3000 units ≡ 1 mg spiramycin.

● **UNLICENSED USE** Not licensed.

- **CAUTIONS** Arrhythmias · cardiac disease · predisposition to QT interval prolongation
- **SIDE-EFFECTS**
  ▸ **Rare** Prolongation of QT interval · thrombocytopenia · vasculitis
  ▸ **Frequency not known** Diarrhoea · dizziness · gastro-intestinal disturbances · headache · hepatotoxicity · nausea · rash · vomiting
- **ALLERGY AND CROSS-SENSITIVITY** Sensitivity to other macrolides.
- **BREAST FEEDING** Present in breast milk.
- **HEPATIC IMPAIRMENT** Use with caution.

- **MEDICINAL FORMS**
  There can be variation in the licensing of different medicines containing the same drug.
  Powder for solution for infusion
  ▸ Spiramycin (Non-proprietary)
  Spiramycin (as Spiramycin adipate) 1.5 mega u Rovamycine 1.5million unit powder for solution for infusion vials | 1 vial PoM no price available
  Tablet
  ▸ Spiramycin (Non-proprietary)
  Spiramycin 1.5 mega u Rovamycine 1.5million unit tablets | 16 tablet PoM no price available
  Spiramycin 3 mega u Rovamycine 3million unit tablets | 10 tablet PoM no price available | 16 tablet PoM no price available

6 Viral infection
6.1 Hepatitis

Hepatitis

Overview

Treatment for viral hepatitis should be initiated by a specialist in hepatology or infectious diseases. The management of uncomplicated acute viral hepatitis is largely symptomatic. Hepatitis B and hepatitis C viruses are major causes of chronic hepatitis. Active or passive immunisation against hepatitis A and B infections can be given.

Chronic hepatitis B

Interferon alfa p. 529, peginterferon alfa-2a, lamivudine p. 401, adefovir dipivoxil, entecavir, and tenofovir disoproxil p. 402 have a role in the treatment of chronic hepatitis B in adults, but their role in children has not been well established. Specialist supervision is required for the management of chronic hepatitis B.

Tenofovir disoproxil, or a combination of tenofovir disoproxil with either emtricitabine p. 400 or lamivudine, may be used with other antiretrovirals, as part of 'highly active antiretroviral therapy' in children who require treatment for both HIV and chronic hepatitis B. If children infected with both HIV and chronic hepatitis B only require treatment for chronic hepatitis B, they should receive antivirals that are not active against HIV. Management of these children should be co-ordinated between HIV and hepatology specialists.

Chronic hepatitis C

Treatment should be considered for children with moderate or severe liver disease. Specialist supervision is required and the regimen is chosen according to the genotype of the infecting virus and the viral load. A combination of ribavirin below with either interferon alfa or peginterferon alfa-2b is licensed for use in children over 3 years with chronic hepatitis C. A combination of peginterferon alfa p. 386 and ribavirin is preferred.

6.2 Hepatitis infections
6.2a Chronic hepatitis C

> **Other drugs used for Chronic hepatitis C** Interferon alfa, p. 529

ANTIVIRALS > NUCLEOSIDE ANALOGUES

Ribavirin

(Tribavirin)

- **INDICATIONS AND DOSE**
Bronchiolitis
▸ BY INHALATION OF AEROSOL, OR BY INHALATION OF NEBULISED SOLUTION
  ▸ Child 1–23 months: Inhale a solution containing 20 mg/mL for 12–18 hours for at least 3 days, maximum of 7 days, to be administered via small particle aerosol generator

Life-threatening RSV, parainfluenza virus, and adenovirus infection in immunocompromised children (administered on expert advice)
▸ BY INTRAVENOUS INFUSION
  ▸ Child: 33 mg/kg for 1 dose, to be administered over 15 minutes, then 16 mg/kg every 6 hours for 4 days, then 8 mg/kg every 8 hours for 3 days

REBETOL® CAPSULES
Chronic hepatitis C (in combination with interferon alfa or peginterferon alfa) in previously untreated children without liver decompensation
▸ BY MOUTH
  ▸ Child 3–17 years (body-weight up to 47 kg): 15 mg/kg daily in 2 divided doses
  ▸ Child 3–17 years (body-weight 47–49 kg): 200 mg, dose to be given in the morning and 400 mg, dose to be given in the evening
  ▸ Child 3–17 years (body-weight 50–64 kg): 400 mg twice daily
  ▸ Child 3–17 years (body-weight 65–80 kg): 400 mg, dose to be given in the morning and 600 mg, dose to be given in the evening
  ▸ Child 3–17 years (body-weight 81–104 kg): 600 mg twice daily
  ▸ Child 3–17 years (body-weight 105 kg and above): 600 mg, dose to be given in the morning and 800 mg, dose to be given in the evening

REBETOL® ORAL SOLUTION
Chronic hepatitis C (in combination with interferon alfa or peginterferon alfa) in previously untreated children without liver decompensation
▸ BY MOUTH
  ▸ Child 3–17 years (body-weight up to 47 kg): 15 mg/kg daily in 2 divided doses
  ▸ Child 3–17 years (body-weight 47–49 kg): 200 mg daily, dose to be given in the morning and 400 mg daily, dose to be given in the evening
  ▸ Child 3–17 years (body-weight 50–64 kg): 400 mg twice daily
  ▸ Child 3–17 years (body-weight 65–80 kg): 400 mg daily, dose to be given in the morning and 600 mg daily, dose to be given in the evening
  ▸ Child 3–17 years (body-weight 81–104 kg): 600 mg twice daily
  ▸ Child 3–17 years (body-weight 105 kg and above): 600 mg daily, dose to be given in the morning and 800 mg daily, dose to be given in the evening

- **UNLICENSED USE** Inhalation licensed for use in children (age range not specified by manufacturer). Intravenous preparation not licensed.
- **CONTRA-INDICATIONS**
▸ With systemic use Active severe psychiatric condition · autoimmune disease · autoimmune hepatitis · consult product literature for specific contra-indications when ribavirin used in combination with other medicinal products · haemoglobinopathies · history of severe psychiatric condition · severe debilitating medical conditions · severe, uncontrolled cardiac disease in children with chronic hepatitis C
- **CAUTIONS**
▸ When used by inhalation Maintain standard supportive respiratory and fluid management therapy
▸ With systemic use Cardiac disease (assessment including ECG recommended before and during treatment—discontinue if deterioration) · consult product literature for specific cautions when ribavirin used in combination with other medicinal products · patients with a transplant—risk of rejection · risk of growth retardation in children, the reversibility of which is uncertain—if possible, consider starting treatment after pubertal growth spurt
- **INTERACTIONS** → Appendix 1: ribavirin
- **SIDE-EFFECTS**
▸ When used by inhalation Bacterial pneumonia · haemolysis · non-specific anaemia · pneumothorax · worsening respiration
▸ With oral use Abdominal pain · abnormal dreams · acne · alopecia · anxiety · aplastic anaemia · arrhythmias · arthralgia · asthenia · asthenia · ataxia · breast pain · cardiomyopathy · changes in blood pressure · cheilitis · chest pain · colitis · constipation · cough · dehydration · depression · diarrhoea · dizziness · dry eyes · dry mouth · dry skin · dyspepsia · dysphagia · dysphonia · dyspnoea · earache · epistaxis · eye pain · flatulence · flushing · gastro-intestinal bleeding · gastroesophageal reflux · gingivitis · glossitis · growth retardation (including decrease in height and weight) · haemolytic anaemia (anaemia may be improved by epoetin) · hallucination · headache · hearing impairment · hyperaesthesia · hyperglycaemia · hyperkinesia · hypertonia · hypertriglyceridaemia · hyperuricaemia · hypoaesthesia · hypocalcaemia · impaired concentration and memory · increased sweating · influenza-like symptoms · interstitial pneumonitis · leucopenia · loose stools · lymphadenopathy · menstrual disturbance · micturition disorders · mood disorders · mouth ulcers · musculoskeletal pain · myalgia · myocardial infarction · nasal congestion · nausea · neutropenia · optic neuropathy · oral candidiasis · pallor · palpitation · pancreatitis · panic attack · paraesthesia · peptic ulcer · pericarditis · peripheral ischaemia · peripheral neuropathy · peripheral oedema · photosensitivity · pruritus · psoriasis · psychotic disorders · pulmonary embolism · rash · renal failure · respiratory infections · retinal haemorrhage · rheumatoid arthritis · sarcoidosis · seizures · sexual dysfunction · sinus congestion · skin discoloration · sleep disturbances · sore throat · Stevens-Johnson syndrome · stomatitis · stroke · suicidal ideation (more frequent in children) · syncope · systemic lupus erythematosus · tachycardia · tachypnoea · taste disturbance · testicular pain · thrombocytopenia · thyroid disorders · tinnitus · tooth disorder · toxic epidermal necrolysis · urinary tract infections · vertigo · virilism · visual disturbances · vomiting · weight loss · wheezing

SIDE-EFFECTS, FURTHER INFORMATION
▸ With oral use Side effects listed are reported when oral ribavirin is used in combination with peginterferon alfa or interferon alfa, consult product literature for details.

- **CONCEPTION AND CONTRACEPTION**
▸ With systemic use Exclude pregnancy before treatment in females of childbearing age. Effective contraception essential during treatment and for 4 months after treatment in females and for 7 months after treatment in males of childbearing age. Routine monthly pregnancy tests recommended. Condoms must be used if partner of male patient is pregnant (ribavirin excreted in semen).
▸ When used by inhalation Women planning pregnancy should avoid exposure to aerosol.
- **PREGNANCY** Avoid; teratogenicity in *animal* studies.
▸ When used by inhalation Pregnant women should avoid exposure to aerosol.
- **BREAST FEEDING** Avoid—no information available.
- **HEPATIC IMPAIRMENT** No dosage adjustment required. Avoid oral ribavirin in severe hepatic dysfunction or decompensated cirrhosis.
- **RENAL IMPAIRMENT** Plasma-ribavirin concentration increased. Manufacturer advises avoid oral ribavirin if estimated glomerular filtration rate less than $50 \, \text{mL/minute}/1.73 \, \text{m}^2$—monitor haemoglobin concentration closely.
  Manufacturer advises use intravenous preparation with caution if estimated glomerular filtration rate less than $30 \, \text{mL/minute}/1.73 \, \text{m}^2$.
- **MONITORING REQUIREMENTS**
▸ When used by inhalation Monitor electrolytes closely. Monitor equipment for precipitation.
▸ With systemic use Determine full blood count, platelets, electrolytes, serum creatinine, liver function tests and uric acid before starting treatment and then on weeks 2 and 4 of treatment, then as indicated clinically—adjust dose if adverse reactions or laboratory abnormalities develop (consult product literature). Test thyroid function before treatment and then every 3 months.
▸ With oral use Eye examination recommended before treatment. Eye examination also recommended during treatment if pre-existing ophthalmological disorder or if decrease in vision reported—discontinue treatment if ophthalmological disorder deteriorates or if new ophthalmological disorder develops.
- **PRESCRIBING AND DISPENSING INFORMATION** Flavours of oral liquid formulations may include bubble-gum.
- **NATIONAL FUNDING/ACCESS DECISIONS**
  NICE technology appraisals (TAs)
▸ **Peginterferon alfa and ribavirin for chronic hepatitis C (November 2013)** NICE TA300
  Peginterferon alfa in combination with ribavirin is recommended (within the marketing authorisation) as an option for treating chronic hepatitis C in children.
  www.nice.org.uk/TA300
- **LESS SUITABLE FOR PRESCRIBING** Ribavirin inhalation is less suitable for prescribing.

- **MEDICINAL FORMS**
  There can be variation in the licensing of different medicines containing the same drug.

  Oral solution
  CAUTIONARY AND ADVISORY LABELS 21
▸ **Rebetol** (Merck Sharp & Dohme Ltd)
  Ribavirin 40 mg per 1 ml Rebetol 40mg/ml oral solution | 100 ml PoM £67.08

  Capsule
  CAUTIONARY AND ADVISORY LABELS 21
▸ **Rebetol** (Merck Sharp & Dohme Ltd)
  Ribavirin 200 mg Rebetol 200mg capsules | 84 capsule PoM £160.69 | 140 capsule PoM £267.81 | 168 capsule PoM £321.38

  Solution for injection
▸ **Virazole** (Meda Pharmaceuticals Ltd)
  Ribavirin 100 mg per 1 ml Virazole 1.2g/12ml solution for injection vials | 5 vial PoM £3600.00

5

Infection

IMMUNOSTIMULANTS ⟩ INTERFERONS

Peginterferon alfa

- **DRUG ACTION** Polyethylene glycol-conjugated ('pegylated') derivatives of interferon alfa (peginterferon alfa-2a and peginterferon alfa-2b) are available; pegylation increases the persistence of the interferon in the blood.

- **INDICATIONS AND DOSE**

PEGASYS®

Chronic hepatitis C (in combination with ribavirin) in previously untreated children without liver decompensation
- ► BY SUBCUTANEOUS INJECTION
- ► Child 5-17 years: (consult product literature)

VIRAFERONPEG®

Chronic hepatitis C (in combination with ribavirin) in previously untreated children without liver decompensation
- ► BY SUBCUTANEOUS INJECTION
- ► Child 3-17 years: (consult product literature)

- **CONTRA-INDICATIONS** Severe psychiatric illness
  CONTRA-INDICATIONS, FURTHER INFORMATION
  For contra-indications consult product literature.

- **CAUTIONS**
  CAUTIONS, FURTHER INFORMATION
  For cautions consult product literature.

- **INTERACTIONS** → Appendix 1: interferons

- **SIDE-EFFECTS**
- ► **Common or very common** Anorexia · influenza-like symptoms · lethargy · nausea
- ► **Frequency not known** Alopecia · arrhythmias · cardiovascular problems · coma · confusion · depression · hepatotoxicity · hyperglycaemia · hypersensitivity reactions · hypertension · hypertriglyceridaemia (sometimes severe) · hypotension · myelosuppression (particularly affecting granulocyte counts) · nephrotoxicity · ocular side-effects · pneumonia · pneumonitis · psoriasiform rash · pulmonary infiltrates · reversible motor problems in young children · seizures · suicidal behaviour · thyroid abnormalities

  SIDE-EFFECTS, FURTHER INFORMATION
  For information on side effects consult product literature.
- ► Respiratory symptoms Respiratory symptoms should be investigated and if pulmonary infiltrates are suspected or lung function is impaired the discontinuation of peginterferon alfa should be considered.

- **CONCEPTION AND CONTRACEPTION** Effective contraception required during treatment—consult product literature.

- **PREGNANCY** Manufacturers recommend avoid unless potential benefit outweighs risk (toxicity in *animal* studies).

- **BREAST FEEDING** Manufacturers advise avoid—no information available.

- **HEPATIC IMPAIRMENT** Avoid in severe impairment.

- **RENAL IMPAIRMENT** Reduce dose in moderate to severe impairment. For information on peginterferon alfa use in renal impairment consult product literature. Close monitoring required in renal impairment.

- **MONITORING REQUIREMENTS**
- ► Monitoring of lipid concentration is recommended.
- ► Monitoring of hepatic function is recommended.

- **NATIONAL FUNDING/ACCESS DECISIONS**
  NICE technology appraisals (TAs)
- ► Peginterferon alfa and ribavirin for chronic hepatitis C (November 2013) NICE TA300
  Peginterferon alfa in combination with ribavirin is recommended (within the marketing authorisation) as an option for treating chronic hepatitis C in children.
  www.nice.org.uk/TA300

- **MEDICINAL FORMS**
  There can be variation in the licensing of different medicines containing the same drug.
  Solution for injection
  EXCIPIENTS: May contain Benzyl alcohol
- ► **Pegasys** (Roche Products Ltd)
  Peginterferon alfa-2a 180 microgram per 1 ml Pegasys 90micrograms/0.5ml solution for injection pre-filled syringes | 1 pre-filled disposable injection [PoM] £76.51
  Peginterferon alfa-2a 270 microgram per 1 ml Pegasys 135micrograms/0.5ml solution for injection pre-filled syringes | 1 pre-filled disposable injection [PoM] £107.76 CT price = £107.76
  Pegasys 135micrograms/0.5ml solution for injection pre-filled pen | 1 pre-filled disposable injection [PoM] £107.76
  Peginterferon alfa-2a 360 microgram per 1 ml Pegasys 180micrograms/0.5ml solution for injection pre-filled syringes | 4 pre-filled disposable injection [PoM] £497.60
  Pegasys 180micrograms/0.5ml solution for injection pre-filled pen | 4 pre-filled disposable injection [PoM] £497.60
  Powder and solvent for solution for injection
- ► **ViraferonPeg CLEARCLICK** (Merck Sharp & Dohme Ltd)
  Peginterferon alfa-2b 50 microgram ViraferonPeg 50microgram powder and solvent for solution for injection pre-filled disposable devices CLEARCLICK | 1 pre-filled disposable injection [PoM] £66.46
  Peginterferon alfa-2b 80 microgram ViraferonPeg 80microgram powder and solvent for solution for injection pre-filled disposable devices CLEARCLICK | 1 pre-filled disposable injection [PoM] £106.34
  Peginterferon alfa-2b 100 microgram ViraferonPeg 100microgram powder and solvent for solution for injection pre-filled disposable devices CLEARCLICK | 1 pre-filled disposable injection [PoM] £132.92
  Peginterferon alfa-2b 120 microgram ViraferonPeg 120microgram powder and solvent for solution for injection pre-filled disposable devices CLEARCLICK | 1 pre-filled disposable injection [PoM] £159.51
  Peginterferon alfa-2b 150 microgram ViraferonPeg 150microgram powder and solvent for solution for injection pre-filled disposable devices CLEARCLICK | 1 pre-filled disposable injection [PoM] £199.38

6.3 Herpesvirus infections

Herpesvirus infections

Herpes simplex and varicella-zoster infection

The two most important herpesvirus pathogens are herpes simplex virus (herpesvirus hominis) and varicella-zoster virus.

Herpes simplex infections

Herpes infection of the mouth and lips and in the eye is generally associated with herpes simplex virus serotype 1 (HSV-1); other areas of the skin may also be infected, especially in immunodeficiency. Genital infection is most often associated with HSV-2 and also HSV-1. Treatment of herpes simplex infection should start as early as possible and usually within 5 days of the appearance of the infection.

In individuals with good immune function, mild infection of the eye (ocular herpes) or of the lips (herpes labialis or cold sores) is treated with a topical antiviral drug. Primary herpetic gingivostomatitis is managed by changes to diet and with analgesics. Severe infection, neonatal herpes infection or infection in immunocompromised individuals requires treatment with a systemic antiviral drug. After completing parenteral treatment of neonatal herpes simplex encephalitis, oral suppression therapy with aciclovir p. 387 for 6 months can be considered on specialist advice. Primary or recurrent genital herpes simplex infection is treated with an antiviral drug given by mouth. Persistence of a lesion or recurrence in an immunocompromised patient may signal the development of resistance.

Specialist advice should be sought for systemic treatment of herpes simplex infection in pregnancy.

Varicella-zoster infections

Regardless of immune function and the use of any immunoglobulins, neonates with *chickenpox* should be treated with a parenteral antiviral to reduce the risk of severe disease. Oral therapy in children is not recommended as absorption is variable. Chickenpox in otherwise healthy children between 1 month and 12 years is usually mild and antiviral treatment is not usually required.

Chickenpox is more severe in adolescents than in children; antiviral treatment started within 24 hours of the onset of rash may reduce the duration and severity of symptoms in otherwise healthy adolescents. Antiviral treatment is generally recommended in immunocompromised patients and those at special risk (e.g. because of severe cardiovascular or respiratory disease or chronic skin disorder); in such cases, an antiviral is given for 10 days with at least 7 days of parenteral treatment.

In pregnancy severe chickenpox may cause complications, especially varicella pneumonia. Specialist advice should be sought for the treatment of chickenpox during pregnancy.

Neonates and children who have been exposed to chickenpox and are at special risk of complications may require prophylaxis with varicella-zoster immunoglobulin (see under Disease-specific Immunoglobulins). Prophylactic intravenous aciclovir should be considered for neonates whose mothers develop chickenpox 4 days before to 2 days after delivery.

In *herpes zoster* (shingles) systemic antiviral treatment can reduce the severity and duration of pain, reduce complications, and reduce viral shedding. Treatment with the antiviral should be started within 72 hours of the onset of rash and is usually continued for 7–10 days. Immunocompromised patients at high risk of disseminated or severe infection should be treated with a parenteral antiviral drug.

Chronic pain which persists after the rash has healed (postherpetic neuralgia) requires specific management.

Choice

Aciclovir is active against herpesviruses but does not eradicate them. Uses of aciclovir include systemic treatment of varicella–zoster and the systemic and topical treatment of herpes simplex infections of the skin and mucous membranes. It is used by mouth for severe herpetic stomatitis. Aciclovir eye ointment is used for herpes simplex infections of the eye; it is combined with systemic treatment for ophthalmic zoster.

Famciclovir, a prodrug of penciclovir, is similar to aciclovir and is licensed in adults for use in herpes zoster and genital herpes; there is limited information available on use in children.

Valaciclovir p. 389 is an ester of aciclovir, licensed in adults for herpes zoster and herpes simplex infections of the skin and mucous membranes (including genital herpes); it is also licensed in children over 12 years for preventing cytomegalovirus disease following solid organ transplantation. Valaciclovir may be used for the treatment of mild herpes zoster in immunocompromised children over 12 years; treatment should be initiated under specialist supervision.

Cytomegalovirus infection

Ganciclovir p. 390 is related to aciclovir but it is more active against cytomegalovirus (CMV); it is also much more toxic than aciclovir and should therefore be prescribed under specialist supervision and only when the potential benefit outweighs the risks. Ganciclovir is administered by intravenous infusion for the *initial treatment* of CMV

infection. The use of ganciclovir may also be considered for symptomatic congenital CMV infection. Ganciclovir causes profound myelosuppression when given with zidovudine p. 403; the two should not normally be given together particularly during initial ganciclovir therapy. The likelihood of ganciclovir resistance increases in patients with a high viral load or in those who receive the drug over a long duration.

Valaciclovir is licensed for use in children over 12 years for prevention of cytomegalovirus disease following renal transplantation.

Foscarnet sodium p. 390 is also active against cytomegalovirus; it is toxic and can cause renal impairment. It is deposited in teeth, bone and cartilage, and *animal* studies have shown that deposition is greater in young animals. Its effect on skeletal development in children is not known. Foscarnet sodium should be prescribed under specialist supervision.

ANTIVIRALS > NUCLEOSIDE ANALOGUES

▌Aciclovir

(Acyclovir)

● **INDICATIONS AND DOSE**

Herpes simplex, suppression

▸ BY MOUTH

▸ **Child 12-17 years:** 400 mg twice daily, alternatively 200 mg 4 times a day; increased to 400 mg 3 times a day, dose may be increased if recurrences occur on standard suppressive therapy or for suppression of genital herpes during late pregnancy (from 36 weeks gestation), therapy interrupted every 6–12 months to reassess recurrence frequency—consider restarting after two or more recurrences

Herpes simplex, prophylaxis in the immunocompromised

▸ BY MOUTH

▸ **Child 1-23 months:** 100–200 mg 4 times a day

▸ **Child 2-17 years:** 200–400 mg 4 times a day

Herpes Simplex, treatment

▸ BY MOUTH

▸ **Child 1-23 months:** 100 mg 5 times a day usually for 5 days (longer if new lesions appear during treatment or if healing incomplete)

▸ **Child 2-17 years:** 200 mg 5 times a day usually for 5 days (longer if new lesions appear during treatment or if healing incomplete)

▸ BY INTRAVENOUS INFUSION

▸ **Neonate:** 20 mg/kg every 8 hours for 14 days (for at least 21 days if CNS involvement—confirm cerebrospinal fluid negative for herpes simplex virus before stopping treatment).

▸ **Child 1-2 months:** 20 mg/kg every 8 hours for 14 days (for at least 21 days if CNS involvement—confirm cerebrospinal fluid negative for herpes simplex virus before stopping treatment)

▸ **Child 3 months-11 years:** 250 mg/m² every 8 hours usually for 5 days

▸ **Child 12-17 years:** 5 mg/kg every 8 hours usually for 5 days

Herpes Simplex, treatment, in immunocompromised or if absorption impaired

▸ BY MOUTH

▸ **Child 1-23 months:** 200 mg 5 times a day usually for 5 days (longer if new lesions appear during treatment or if healing incomplete)

▸ **Child 2-17 years:** 400 mg 5 times a day usually for 5 days (longer if new lesions appear during treatment or if healing incomplete) continued →

Herpes Simplex, treatment, in immunocompromised or in simplex encephalitis

▶ BY INTRAVENOUS INFUSION
▶ Child 3 months-11 years: 500 mg/m^2 every 8 hours usually for 5 days (given for at least 21 days in encephalitis—confirm cerebrospinal fluid negative for herpes simplex virus before stopping treatment)
▶ Child 12-17 years: 10 mg/kg every 8 hours usually for 5 days (given for at least 14 days in encephalitis and for at least 21 days if also immunocompromised—confirm cerebrospinal fluid negative for herpes simplex virus before stopping treatment)

Varicella zoster (chickenpox), treatment | Herpes zoster (shingles), treatment

▶ BY MOUTH
▶ Child 1-23 months: 200 mg 4 times a day for 5 days
▶ Child 2-5 years: 400 mg 4 times a day for 5 days
▶ Child 6-11 years: 800 mg 4 times a day for 5 days
▶ Child 12-17 years: 800 mg 5 times a day for 7 days
▶ BY INTRAVENOUS INFUSION
▶ Neonate: 10–20 mg/kg every 8 hours for at least 7 days.
▶ Child 1-2 months: 10–20 mg/kg every 8 hours for at least 7 days
▶ Child 3 months-11 years: 250 mg/m^2 every 8 hours usually for 5 days
▶ Child 12-17 years: 5 mg/kg every 8 hours usually for 5 days

Varicella zoster (chickenpox), treatment in immunocompromised | Herpes zoster (shingles), treatment in immunocompromised

▶ BY INTRAVENOUS INFUSION
▶ Child 3 months-11 years: 500 mg/m^2 every 8 hours usually for 5 days
▶ Child 12-17 years: 10 mg/kg every 8 hours usually for 5 days

Herpes zoster (shingles), treatment in immunocompromised

▶ BY MOUTH
▶ Child 1-23 months: 200 mg 4 times a day continued for 2 days after crusting of lesions
▶ Child 2-5 years: 400 mg 4 times a day continued for 2 days after crusting of lesions
▶ Child 6-11 years: 800 mg 4 times a day continued for 2 days after crusting of lesions
▶ Child 12-17 years: 800 mg 5 times a day continued for 2 days after crusting of lesions

Herpes zoster, treatment in encephalitis | Varicella zoster, treatment in encephalitis

▶ BY INTRAVENOUS INFUSION
▶ Neonate: 10–20 mg/kg every 8 hours given for 10–14 days in encephalitis, possibly longer if also immunocompromised
▶ Child 1-2 months: 10–20 mg/kg every 8 hours given for 10–14 days in encephalitis, possibly longer if also immunocompromised
▶ Child 3 months-11 years: 500 mg/m^2 every 8 hours given for 10–14 days in encephalitis, possibly longer if also immunocompromised
▶ Child 12-17 years: 10 mg/kg every 8 hours given for 10–14 days in encephalitis, possibly longer if also immunocompromised

Varicella zoster (chickenpox), attenuation of infection if varicella–zoster immunoglobulin not indicated

▶ BY MOUTH
▶ Child: 10 mg/kg 4 times a day for 7 days, to be started 1 week after exposure

Varicella zoster (chickenpox), prophylaxis after delivery

▶ BY INTRAVENOUS INFUSION
▶ Neonate: 10 mg/kg every 8 hours continued until serological tests confirm absence of virus.

DOSES AT EXTREMES OF BODY-WEIGHT
▶ With intravenous use To avoid excessive dosage in obese patients parenteral dose should be calculated on the basis of ideal weight for height

● **UNLICENSED USE**
▶ With oral use Tablets and suspension not licensed for suppression of herpes simplex or for treatment of herpes zoster in children (age range not specified by manufacturer). Aciclovir doses in BNF may differ from those in product literature. Attenuation of chickenpox is an unlicensed indication.
▶ With intravenous use Intravenous infusion not licensed for herpes zoster in children under 18 years.

● **CAUTIONS** Maintain adequate hydration (especially with infusion or high doses)

● **INTERACTIONS** → Appendix 1: aciclovir

● **SIDE-EFFECTS**
▶ **Common or very common** Abdominal pain · diarrhoea · fatigue · headache · nausea · photosensitivity · pruritus · rash · urticaria · vomiting
▶ **Very rare** Acute renal failure · anaemia · ataxia · confusion · convulsions · dizziness · drowsiness · dysarthria · dyspnoea · hallucinations · hepatitis · jaundice · leucopenia · neurological reactions · thrombocytopenia
▶ With intravenous use Agitation · fever · psychosis · severe local inflammation (sometimes leading to ulceration) · tremors

● **PREGNANCY** Not known to be harmful—manufacturers advise use only when potential benefit outweighs risk.

● **BREAST FEEDING** Significant amount in milk after systemic administration—not known to be harmful but manufacturer advises caution.

● **RENAL IMPAIRMENT**
▶ With intravenous use Use *normal intravenous dose* every 12 hours if estimated glomerular filtration rate 25–50 mL/minute/1.73 m^2 (every 24 hours if estimated glomerular filtration rate 10–25 mL/minute/1.73 m^2. Consult product literature for intravenous dose if estimated glomerular filtration rate less than 10 mL/minute/1.73 m^2.
▶ With oral use For *herpes zoster*, use normal oral dose every 8 hours if estimated glomerular filtration rate 10–25 mL/minute/1.73 m^2 (every 12 hours if estimated glomerular filtration rate less than 10 mL/minute/1.73 m^2. For *herpes simplex*, use normal dose every 12 hours if estimated glomerular filtration rate less than 10 mL/minute/1.73 m^2.
▶ With systemic use Risk of neurological reactions increased. Maintain adequate hydration (especially during renal impairment).

● **DIRECTIONS FOR ADMINISTRATION** For *intravenous infusion*, reconstitute to 25 mg/mL with Water for Injections or Sodium Chloride 0.9% then dilute to concentration of 5 mg/mL with Sodium Chloride 0.9% or Sodium Chloride and Glucose and give over 1 hour; alternatively, may be administered in a concentration of 25 mg/mL using a suitable infusion pump and central venous access and given over 1 hour.

● **PRESCRIBING AND DISPENSING INFORMATION** Flavours of oral liquid preparations may include banana, or orange.

● **PATIENT AND CARER ADVICE**
Medicines for Children leaflet: Aciclovir (oral) for viral infections www.medicinesforchildren.org.uk/aciclovir-for-viral-infections

● **PROFESSION SPECIFIC INFORMATION**

Dental practitioners' formulary
Aciclovir Tablets 200 mg or 800 mg may be prescribed.
Aciclovir Oral Suspension 200 mg/5mL may be prescribed.

● **MEDICINAL FORMS**
There can be variation in the licensing of different medicines
containing the same drug.

Tablet
CAUTIONARY AND ADVISORY LABELS 9
▸ **Aciclovir (Non-proprietary)**
Aciclovir 200 mg Aciclovir 200mg tablets | 25 tablet PoM £10.00
DT price = £1.36
Aciclovir 400 mg Aciclovir 400mg tablets | 56 tablet PoM £15.00
DT price = £2.96
Aciclovir 800 mg Aciclovir 800mg tablets | 35 tablet PoM £20.00
DT price = £3.36

Dispersible tablet
CAUTIONARY AND ADVISORY LABELS 9
▸ **Aciclovir (Non-proprietary)**
Aciclovir 200 mg Aciclovir 200mg dispersible tablets |
25 tablet PoM £17.50 DT price = £1.47
Aciclovir 400 mg Aciclovir 400mg dispersible tablets |
56 tablet PoM £20.00 DT price = £11.98
Aciclovir 800 mg Aciclovir 800mg dispersible tablets |
35 tablet PoM £65.00 DT price = £10.98
▸ **Zovirax (GlaxoSmithKline UK Ltd)**
Aciclovir 200 mg Zovirax 200mg dispersible tablets |
25 tablet PoM £2.85 DT price = £1.47
Aciclovir 800 mg Zovirax 800mg dispersible tablets |
35 tablet PoM £10.50 DT price = £10.98

Oral suspension
CAUTIONARY AND ADVISORY LABELS 9
▸ **Aciclovir (Non-proprietary)**
Aciclovir 40 mg per 1 ml Aciclovir 200mg/5ml oral suspension sugar
free sugar-free | 125 ml PoM £35.76 DT price = £35.76
Aciclovir 80 mg per 1 ml Aciclovir 400mg/5ml oral suspension sugar
free sugar-free | 100 ml PoM £39.47 DT price = £39.47
▸ **Zovirax (GlaxoSmithKline UK Ltd)**
Aciclovir 40 mg per 1 ml Zovirax 200mg/5ml oral suspension sugar-
free | 125 ml PoM £29.56 DT price = £35.76
Aciclovir 80 mg per 1 ml Zovirax Double Strength 400mg/5ml oral
suspension sugar-free | 100 ml PoM £33.02 DT price = £39.47

Solution for infusion
ELECTROLYTES: May contain Sodium
▸ **Aciclovir (Non-proprietary)**
Aciclovir (as Aciclovir sodium) 25 mg per 1 ml Aciclovir 1g/40ml
solution for infusion vials | 1 vial PoM £40.00
Aciclovir 500mg/20ml solution for infusion vials | 5 vial PoM £7.15-
£100.00
Aciclovir 250mg/10ml solution for infusion vials | 5 vial PoM £16.25-
£50.00
Aciclovir 500mg/20ml concentrate for solution for infusion vials |
5 vial PoM no price available (Hospital only)

Powder for solution for infusion
ELECTROLYTES: May contain Sodium
▸ **Aciclovir (Non-proprietary)**
Aciclovir (as Aciclovir sodium) 250 mg Aciclovir 250mg powder for
solution for infusion vials | 5 vial PoM £49.30
▸ **Zovirax (GlaxoSmithKline UK Ltd)**
Aciclovir (as Aciclovir sodium) 250 mg Zovirax I.V. 250mg powder
for solution for infusion vials | 5 vial PoM £16.70
Aciclovir (as Aciclovir sodium) 500 mg Zovirax I.V. 500mg powder
for solution for infusion vials | 5 vial PoM £17.00

Valaciclovir

● **INDICATIONS AND DOSE**

**Herpes zoster infection, treatment in
immunocompromised patients**
▸ BY MOUTH
▸ Child 12–17 years: 1 g 3 times a day for at least 7 days
and continued for 2 days after crusting of lesions

Herpes simplex, treatment of first infective episode
▸ BY MOUTH
▸ Child 12–17 years: 500 mg twice daily for 5 days (longer if
new lesions appear during treatment or healing is
incomplete)

**Herpes simplex infections treatment of first episode in
immunocompromised or HIV-positive patients**
▸ BY MOUTH
▸ Child 12–17 years: 1 g twice daily for 10 days

Herpes simplex, treatment of recurrent infections
▸ BY MOUTH
▸ Child 12–17 years: 500 mg twice daily for 3–5 days

**Treatment of recurrent herpes simplex infections in
immunocompromised or HIV-positive patients**
▸ BY MOUTH
▸ Child 12–17 years: 1 g twice daily for 5–10 days

Herpes labialis treatment
▸ BY MOUTH
▸ Child 12–17 years: Initially 2 g, then 2 g after 12 hours

Herpes simplex, suppression of infections
▸ BY MOUTH
▸ Child 12–17 years: 500 mg daily in 1–2 divided doses,
therapy to be interrupted every 6–12 months to
reassess recurrence frequency—consider restarting
after two or more recurrences

**Herpes simplex, suppression of infections in
immunocompromised or HIV-positive patients**
▸ BY MOUTH
▸ Child 12–17 years: 500 mg twice daily, therapy to be
interrupted every 6–12 months to reassess recurrence
frequency—consider restarting after two or more
recurrences

**Prevention of cytomegalovirus disease following solid
organ transplantation when valganciclovir or ganciclovir
cannot be used**
▸ BY MOUTH
▸ Child 12–17 years: 2 g 4 times a day usually for 90 days,
preferably starting within 72 hours of transplantation

● **UNLICENSED USE** Not licensed for treatment of herpes
zoster in children. Not licensed for treatment or
suppression of herpes simplex infection in
immunocompromised or HIV-positive children.

● **CAUTIONS** Maintain adequate hydration (especially with
high doses)

● **INTERACTIONS** → Appendix 1: valaciclovir

● **SIDE-EFFECTS**
▸ **Very rare** Acute renal failure · anaemia · ataxia · confusion
· convulsions · dizziness · drowsiness · dysarthria · dyspnoea
· hallucinations · hepatitis · jaundice · leucopenia ·
neurological reactions · thrombocytopenia
▸ **Frequency not known** Abdominal pain · diarrhoea · fatigue ·
headache · nausea · photosensitivity · pruritus · rash ·
urticaria · vomiting

SIDE-EFFECTS, FURTHER INFORMATION
▸ Neurological reactions Neurological reactions (including
dizziness, confusion, hallucinations, convulsions, ataxia,
dysarthria, and drowsiness) more frequent with higher
doses.

● **PREGNANCY** Not known to be harmful—manufacturers
advise use only when potential benefit outweighs risk.

● **BREAST FEEDING** Significant amount in milk after systemic
administration—not known to be harmful but
manufacturer advises caution.

● **HEPATIC IMPAIRMENT** Manufacturer advises caution with
high doses used for preventing cytomegalovirus disease—
no information available in children.

● **RENAL IMPAIRMENT** For *herpes zoster*, 1 g every 12 hours if
estimated glomerular filtration rate

Infection

5

30–50 mL/minute/1.73 m² (1 g every 24 hours if estimated glomerular filtration rate 10–30 mL/minute/1.73 m²; 500 mg every 24 hours if estimated glomerular filtration rate less than 10 mL/minute/1.73 m²).

For *treatment of herpes simplex*, 500 mg (1 g in immunocompromised or HIV-positive children) every 24 hours if estimated glomerular filtration rate less than 30 mL/minute/1.73 m².

For *treatment of herpes labialis*, if estimated glomerular filtration rate 30–50 mL/minute/1.73 m², initially 1 g, then 1 g 12 hours after initial dose (if estimated glomerular filtration rate 10–30 mL/minute/1.73 m², initially 500 mg, then 500 mg 12 hours after initial dose; if estimated glomerular filtration rate less than 10 mL/minute/1.73 m², 500 mg as a single dose).

For *suppression of herpes simplex*, 250 mg (500 mg in immunocompromised or HIV-positive children) every 24 hours if estimated glomerular filtration rate less than 30 mL/minute/1.73 m².

Reduce dose according to estimated glomerular filtration rate for *cytomegalovirus prophylaxis* following solid organ transplantation (consult product literature). Maintain adequate hydration.

● **PRESCRIBING AND DISPENSING INFORMATION** Valaciclovir is a pro-drug of aciclovir.

● **MEDICINAL FORMS**
There can be variation in the licensing of different medicines containing the same drug. Forms available from special-order manufacturers include: oral suspension
Tablet
CAUTIONARY AND ADVISORY LABELS 9
▸ Valaciclovir (Non-proprietary)
 Valaciclovir (as Valaciclovir hydrochloride) 500 mg Valaciclovir 500mg tablets | 10 tablet PoM £20.59 DT price = £2.80 | 42 tablet PoM £86.30
▸ Valtrex (GlaxoSmithKline UK Ltd)
 Valaciclovir (as Valaciclovir hydrochloride) 250 mg Valtrex 250mg tablets | 60 tablet PoM £123.28 DT price = £123.28
 Valaciclovir (as Valaciclovir hydrochloride) 500 mg Valtrex 500mg tablets | 10 tablet PoM £20.59 DT price = £2.80 | 42 tablet PoM £86.30

6.3a Cytomegalovirus infections

ANTIVIRALS ⟩ NUCLEOSIDE ANALOGUES

Ganciclovir

● **INDICATIONS AND DOSE**

Prevention of cytomegalovirus disease during immunosuppressive therapy following organ transplantation
▸ BY INTRAVENOUS INFUSION
▸ Child: 5 mg/kg every 12 hours for 7–14 days

Treatment of life-threatening or sight-threatening cytomegalovirus infections in immunocompromised patients only
▸ BY INTRAVENOUS INFUSION
▸ Child: Initially 5 mg/kg every 12 hours for 14–21 days, followed by maintenance 6 mg/kg daily on 5 days of the week, alternatively 5 mg/kg daily until adequate recovery of immunity, maintenance only for patients at risk of relapse of retinitis, if retinitis progresses initial induction treatment may be repeated

Congenital cytomegalovirus infection of the CNS
▸ BY INTRAVENOUS INFUSION
▸ Neonate: 6 mg/kg every 12 hours for 6 weeks.

● **UNLICENSED USE** Not licensed for use in children.

● **CONTRA-INDICATIONS** Abnormally low haemoglobin count (consult product literature) · abnormally low neutrophil count (consult product literature) · abnormally low platelet count (consult product literature)

● **CAUTIONS** Children (possible risk of long-term carcinogenic or reproductive toxicity) · ensure adequate hydration · history of cytopenia · potential carcinogen · potential teratogen · radiotherapy · vesicant

● **INTERACTIONS** → Appendix 1: ganciclovir

● **SIDE-EFFECTS**
▸ **Common or very common** Abdominal pain · abnormal thinking · anaemia · anorexia · anxiety · arthralgia · chest pain · confusion · constipation · convulsions · cough · depression · dermatitis · diarrhoea · dizziness · dyspepsia · dysphagia · dyspnoea · ear pain · eye pain · fatigue · flatulence · headache · hepatic dysfunction · infection · injection-site reactions · insomnia · leucopenia · macular oedema · myalgia · nausea · night sweats · pancytopenia · peripheral neuropathy · pruritus · pyrexia · renal impairment · retinal detachment · taste disturbance · thrombocytopenia · vitreous floaters · vomiting · weight loss
▸ **Uncommon** Alopecia · anaphylactic reactions · arrhythmias · disturbances in hearing and vision · haematuria · hypotension · male infertility · mouth ulcers · pancreatitis · psychosis · tremor

● **ALLERGY AND CROSS-SENSITIVITY** Contra-indicated in patients hypersensitive to valganciclovir, aciclovir, or valaciclovir.

● **CONCEPTION AND CONTRACEPTION** Ensure effective contraception during treatment and barrier contraception for men during and for at least 90 days after treatment.

● **PREGNANCY** Avoid—teratogenic risk.

● **BREAST FEEDING** Avoid—no information available.

● **RENAL IMPAIRMENT** Reduce dose if estimated glomerular filtration rate less than 70 mL/minute/1.73 m²; consult product literature.

● **MONITORING REQUIREMENTS** Monitor full blood count closely (severe deterioration may require correction and possibly treatment interruption).

● **DIRECTIONS FOR ADMINISTRATION** Infuse into vein with adequate flow preferably using plastic cannula. For *intravenous infusion*, reconstitute with Water for Injections (500 mg/10 mL) then dilute to concentration of not more than 10 mg/mL with Glucose 5% or Sodium Chloride 0.9% and give over 1 hour.

● **HANDLING AND STORAGE** Caution in handling Ganciclovir is toxic and personnel should be adequately protected during handling and administration; if solution comes into contact with skin or mucosa, wash off immediately with soap and water.

● **MEDICINAL FORMS**
There can be variation in the licensing of different medicines containing the same drug.
Powder for solution for infusion
ELECTROLYTES: May contain Sodium
▸ Cymevene (Roche Products Ltd)
 Ganciclovir (as Ganciclovir sodium) 500 mg Cymevene 500mg powder for solution for infusion vials | 5 vial PoM £148.83

ANTIVIRALS ⟩ OTHER

Foscarnet sodium

● **INDICATIONS AND DOSE**

Cytomegalovirus disease
▸ BY INTRAVENOUS INFUSION
▸ Child (under expert supervision): Initially 60 mg/kg every 8 hours 2–3 weeks, then maintenance 60 mg/kg daily,

increased if tolerated to 90–120 mg/kg daily, if disease progresses on maintenance dose, repeat induction regimen

Mucocutaneous herpes simplex virus infections unresponsive to aciclovir in immunocompromised patients
▶ BY INTRAVENOUS INFUSION
▶ Child (under expert supervision): 40 mg/kg every 8 hours for 2–3 weeks or until lesions heal

● **UNLICENSED USE** Not licensed for use in children.
● **CAUTIONS** Ensure adequate hydration
● **INTERACTIONS** → Appendix 1: foscarnet
● **SIDE-EFFECTS**
▶ **Common or very common** Abdominal pain · acute renal failure · aggression · agitation · anaemia · anorexia · anxiety · changes in blood pressure · changes in ECG · confusion · constipation · convulsions · depression · diarrhoea · dizziness · dyspepsia · dysuria · electrolyte disturbances · genital irritation and ulceration (due to high concentrations excreted in urine) · granulocytopenia · headache · hepatic dysfunction · hypocalcaemia · hypokalaemia · hypomagnesaemia · leucopenia · malaise · myalgia · nausea (reduce infusion rate) · neurological disorders · oedema · palpitation · pancreatitis · paraesthesia (reduce infusion rate) · polyuria · pruritus · rash · renal impairment · thrombocytopenia · thrombophlebitis if given undiluted by peripheral vein · tremor · vomiting
▶ **Uncommon** Acidosis
▶ **Frequency not known** Diabetes insipidus · myasthenia · myositis · oesophageal ulceration · rhabdomyolysis · ventricular arrhythmias
● **CONCEPTION AND CONTRACEPTION** Men should avoid fathering a child during and for 6 months after treatment.
● **PREGNANCY** Manufacturer advises avoid.
● **BREAST FEEDING** Avoid—present in milk in *animal* studies.
● **RENAL IMPAIRMENT** Reduce dose; consult product literature.
● **MONITORING REQUIREMENTS**
▶ Monitor electrolytes, particularly calcium and magnesium.
▶ Monitor serum creatinine every second day during induction and every week during maintenance.
● **DIRECTIONS FOR ADMINISTRATION** Avoid rapid infusion. For *intravenous infusion*, give undiluted solution via a central venous catheter; alternatively dilute to a concentration of 12 mg/mL with Glucose 5% *or* Sodium Chloride 0.9% for administration via a peripheral vein; give over at least 1 hour (give doses greater than 60 mg/kg over 2 hours).

● **MEDICINAL FORMS**
There can be variation in the licensing of different medicines containing the same drug.
Solution for infusion
ELECTROLYTES: May contain Sodium
▶ Foscavir (Clinigen Healthcare Ltd)
Foscarnet sodium 24 mg per 1 ml Foscavir 6g/250ml solution for infusion bottles | 1 bottle [PoM] £119.85 (Hospital only)

6.4 HIV infection

HIV infection

Overview

There is no cure for infection caused by the human immunodeficiency virus (HIV) but a number of drugs slow or halt disease progression. Drugs for HIV infection (antiretrovirals) may be associated with serious side-effects. Although antiretrovirals increase life expectancy considerably and decrease the risk of complications associated with premature ageing, mortality and morbidity remain slightly higher than in uninfected individuals.

The natural progression of HIV disease is different in children compared to adults; drug treatment should only be undertaken by specialists within a formal paediatric HIV clinical network. Guidelines and dose regimens are under constant review and for this reason some dose recommendations have not been included in *BNF for Children*.

Further information on the management of children with HIV can be obtained from the Children's HIV Association (CHIVA) www.chiva.org.uk; and further information on antiretroviral use and toxicity can be obtained from the Paediatric European Network for Treatment of AIDS (PENTA) website penta-id.org/.

Principles of treatment

Treatment is aimed at suppressing viral replication for as long as possible; it should be started before the immune system is irreversibly damaged. The need for early drug treatment should, however, be balanced against the risk of toxicity. Commitment to treatment and strict adherence over many years are required; the regimen chosen should take into account convenience and the child's tolerance of treatment. The development of drug resistance is reduced by using a combination of drugs; such combinations should have synergistic or additive activity while ensuring that their toxicity is not additive. It is recommended that viral sensitivity to antiretroviral drugs is established before starting treatment or before switching drugs if the infection is not responding.

Initiation of treatment

Treatment is started in all HIV infected children under 1 year of age regardless of clinical and immunological parameters. In children over 1 year of age, treatment is based on the child's age, CD4 cell count, viral load, and symptoms. The choice of antiviral treatment for children should take into account the method and frequency of administration, risk of side-effects, compatibility of drugs with food, palatability, and the appropriateness of the formulation. Initiating treatment with a combination of drugs ('highly active antiretroviral therapy' which includes 2 nucleoside reverse transcriptase inhibitors with *either* a non-nucleoside reverse transcriptase inhibitor *or* a boosted protease inhibitor) is recommended. Abacavir p. 397 and lamivudine p. 401 are the nucleoside reverse transcriptase inhibitors of choice for initial therapy; however, zidovudine p. 403 and lamivudine are used in children who are positive for the HLA-B*5701 allele. Nevirapine p. 395 is the preferred non-nucleoside reverse transcriptase inhibitor in children under 3 years of age, but efavirenz p. 394 is preferred in older children. Lopinavir with ritonavir p. 405 is the preferred boosted protease inhibitor for initial therapy. The metabolism of many antiretrovirals varies in young children; it may therefore be necessary to adjust the dose according to the plasma-drug concentration. Children who require treatment for both HIV and chronic hepatitis B should receive antivirals that are active against both diseases.

Switching therapy

Deterioration of the condition (including clinical, virological changes, and CD4 cell changes) may require a complete change of therapy. The choice of an alternative regimen depends on factors such as the response to previous treatment, tolerance, and the possibility of cross-resistance.

Pregnancy

Treatment of HIV infection in pregnancy aims to reduce the risk of toxicity to the fetus (although information on the teratogenic potential of most antiretroviral drugs is limited),

5

Infection

to minimise the viral load and disease progression in the mother, and to prevent transmission of infection to the neonate. **All treatment options require careful assessment by a specialist**. Combination antiretroviral therapy maximises the chance of preventing transmission and represents optimal therapy for the mother. However, it may be associated with a greater risk of preterm delivery. Local protocols and national guidelines (www.bhiva.org) should be consulted for recommendations on treatment during pregnancy and the perinatal period. Pregnancies in HIV-positive women and babies born to them should be reported prospectively to the National Study of HIV in Pregnancy and Childhood at www.ucl.ac.uk/nshpc/ and to the Antiretroviral Pregnancy Registry at www.apregistry.com.

Breast-feeding

Breast-feeding by HIV-positive mothers may cause HIV infection in the infant and should be avoided.

Post-exposure prophylaxis

Children exposed to HIV infection through needlestick injury or by another route should be sent immediately to an accident and emergency department for post-exposure prophylaxis [unlicensed indication]. Antiretrovirals for prophylaxis are chosen on the basis of efficacy and potential for toxicity. Recommendations have been developed by the Children's HIV Association, www.chiva.org.uk.

Drugs used for HIV infection

Zidovudine, a nucleoside reverse transcriptase inhibitor (or 'nucleoside analogue'), was the first anti-HIV drug to be introduced. Other nucleoside reverse transcriptase inhibitors include abacavir, didanosine p. 398, emtricitabine p. 400, lamivudine, stavudine p. 402, and tenofovir disoproxil p. 402. There are concerns about renal toxicity and effects on bone mineralisation when tenofovir disoproxil is used in prepubertal children.

The protease inhibitors include atazanavir p. 404, darunavir p. 404, fosamprenavir p. 405 (a pro-drug of amprenavir), indinavir, lopinavir (available as lopinavir with ritonavir), ritonavir p. 406, and tipranavir p. 406. Indinavir is no longer recommended because it is associated with nephrolithiasis. Ritonavir in low doses boosts the activity of atazanavir, darunavir, fosamprenavir, lopinavir (available as lopinavir with ritonavir), and tipranavir increasing the persistence of plasma concentrations of these drugs; at such a low dose, ritonavir has no intrinsic antiviral activity. The protease inhibitors are metabolised by cytochrome P450 enzyme systems and therefore have a significant potential for drug interactions. Protease inhibitors are associated with lipodystrophy and metabolic effects.

The non-nucleoside reverse transcriptase inhibitors efavirenz, etravirine p. 395 nevirapine and rilpivirine p. 396 are active against the subtype HIV-1 but not HIV-2, a subtype that is rare in the UK. These drugs may interact with a number of drugs metabolised in the liver. Nevirapine is associated with a high incidence of rash (including Stevens-Johnson syndrome) and rarely fatal hepatitis. Rash is also associated with efavirenz and etravirine but it is usually milder. Psychiatric or CNS disturbances are common with efavirenz. CNS disturbances are often self-limiting and can be reduced by taking the dose at bedtime (especially in the first 2–4 weeks of treatment). Efavirenz has also been associated with an increased plasma cholesterol concentration. Etravirine is used in regimens containing a boosted protease inhibitor for HIV infection resistant to other non-nucleoside reverse transcriptase inhibitors and protease inhibitors.

Enfuvirtide below, which inhibits the fusion of HIV to the host cell, is licensed for managing infection that has failed to respond to a regimen of other antiretroviral drugs. Enfuvirtide below should be combined with other potentially active antiretroviral drugs; it is given by subcutaneous injection.

Maraviroc p. 407 is an antagonist of the CCR5 chemokine receptor. It is used in patients exclusively infected with CCR5−tropic HIV.

Dolutegravir p. 393 and raltegravir p. 393 are inhibitors of HIV integrase. They are used for the treatment of HIV infection when non-nucleoside reverse transcriptase inhibitors or protease inhibitors cannot be used because of intolerance, drug interactions, or resistance.

Immune reconstitution syndrome

Improvement in immune function as a result of antiretroviral treatment may provoke a marked inflammatory reaction against residual opportunistic organisms; these reactions may occur within the first few weeks or months of initiating treatment. Autoimmune disorders (such as Graves' disease) have also been reported many months after initiation of treatment.

Osteonecrosis

Osteonecrosis has been reported in children with advanced HIV disease or following long-term exposure to combination antiretroviral therapy.

Neonates

In order to prevent transmission of infection, neonates born to HIV-positive mothers should be given post-exposure prophylaxis as soon as possible after birth, but starting no later than 72 hours after birth. Zidovudine p. 403 alone should be given to neonates whose mothers had a viral load less than 50 HIV RNA copies/mL between 36 weeks' gestation and delivery, or whose mothers underwent caesarean section while taking zidovudine monotherapy. Combination antiretroviral therapy should be given to neonates whose mothers had a viral load over 50 HIV RNA copies/mL at delivery or whose mothers are found to be HIV positive after delivery. Prophylaxis is continued for 4 weeks.

ANTIVIRALS > HIV-FUSION INHIBITORS

Enfuvirtide

● **DRUG ACTION** Enfuvirtide inhibits the fusion of HIV to the host cell.

● **INDICATIONS AND DOSE**

HIV infection in combination with other antiretroviral drugs for resistant infection or for patients intolerant to other antiretroviral regimens

▸ BY SUBCUTANEOUS INJECTION

▸ Child 6-15 years: 2 mg/kg twice daily (max. per dose 90 mg)
▸ Child 16-17 years: 90 mg twice daily

● **SIDE-EFFECTS**

▸ **Common or very common** Acne · anorexia · anxiety · asthenia · conjunctivitis · diabetes mellitus · dry skin · erythema · gastro-oesophageal reflux disease · haematuria · hypertriglyceridaemia · impaired concentration · influenza-like illness · injection-site reactions · irritability · lymphadenopathy · myalgia · nightmares · pancreatitis · peripheral neuropathy · pneumonia · renal calculi · sinusitis · skin papilloma · tremor · vertigo · weight loss
▸ **Uncommon** Hypersensitivity reactions
▸ **Frequency not known** Osteonecrosis

SIDE-EFFECTS, FURTHER INFORMATION

▸ Hypersensitivity reactions Hypersensitivity reactions including rash, fever, nausea, vomiting, chills, rigors, low blood pressure, respiratory distress, glomerulonephritis, and raised liver enzymes reported; discontinue immediately if any signs or symptoms of systemic hypersensitivity develop and do not rechallenge.

- Osteonecrosis For further information see HIV infection p. 391.
- **PREGNANCY** Manufacturer advises use only if potential benefit outweighs risk.
- **HEPATIC IMPAIRMENT** Manufacturer advises caution— no information available; chronic hepatitis B or C (possibly greater risk of hepatic side-effects).
- **DIRECTIONS FOR ADMINISTRATION** For *subcutaneous injection*, reconstitute with 1.1 mL Water for Injections and allow to stand (for up to 45 minutes) to dissolve; do **not** shake or invert vial.
- **PATIENT AND CARER ADVICE**
  Hypersensitivity reactions Patients or carers should be told how to recognise signs of hypersensitivity, and advised to discontinue treatment and seek immediate medical attention if symptoms develop.

- **MEDICINAL FORMS**
  There can be variation in the licensing of different medicines containing the same drug.
  Powder and solvent for solution for injection
  ELECTROLYTES: May contain Sodium
  ▸ **Fuzeon** (Roche Products Ltd)
  Enfuvirtide 108 mg Fuzeon 108mg powder and solvent for solution for injection vials | 60 vial [PoM] £1,081.57

ANTIVIRALS > HIV-INTEGRASE INHIBITORS

Dolutegravir

20-Nov-2015

- **DRUG ACTION** Dolutegravir is an inhibitor of HIV integrase.

- **INDICATIONS AND DOSE**
  HIV infection without resistance to other inhibitors of HIV integrase, in combination with other antiretroviral drugs
  ▸ BY MOUTH
  ‣ Child 12-17 years (body-weight 40 kg and above): 50 mg once daily

  HIV infection in combination with other antiretroviral drugs (with concomitant carbamazepine, efavirenz, etravirine (without boosted protease inhibitors, but see also Interactions), fosphenytoin, phenobarbital, phenytoin, primidone, nevirapine, oxcarbazepine, St John's wort, rifampicin, or tipranavir)
  ▸ BY MOUTH
  ‣ Child 12-17 years (body-weight 40 kg and above): 50 mg twice daily, avoid concomitant use with these drugs if resistance to other inhibitors of HIV integrase suspected

- **INTERACTIONS** → Appendix 1: dolutegravir

- **SIDE-EFFECTS**
  ▸ **Common or very common** Abdominal pain · abnormal dreams · diarrhoea · dizziness · fatigue · flatulence · headache · insomnia · nausea · pruritus · raised creatine kinase · rash · vomiting
  ▸ **Uncommon** Hepatitis · hypersensitivity reactions
  ▸ **Frequency not known** Osteonecrosis
  SIDE-EFFECTS, FURTHER INFORMATION
  ▸ Hypersensitivity reactions Hypersensitivity reactions (including severe rash, or rash accompanied by fever, malaise, arthralgia, myalgia, blistering, oral lesions, conjunctivitis, angioedema, eosinophilia, or raised liver enzymes) reported uncommonly. Discontinue immediately if any sign or symptoms of hypersensitivity reactions develop.
  ▸ Osteonecrosis For further information see HIV infection p. 391.

- **PREGNANCY** Manufacturer advises use only if potential benefit outweighs risk.

- **HEPATIC IMPAIRMENT** Manufacturer advises caution in severe impairment—no information available.
- **DIRECTIONS FOR ADMINISTRATION** Avoid antacids 6 hours before or 2 hours after taking dolutegravir.
- **PATIENT AND CARER ADVICE**
  Patients or carers should be given advice on how to administer dolutegravir tablets.
  Missed doses
  If a dose is more than 20 hours late on the once daily regimen (or more than 8 hours late on the twice daily regimen), the missed dose should not be taken and the next dose should be taken at the normal time.

- **MEDICINAL FORMS**
  There can be variation in the licensing of different medicines containing the same drug.
  Tablet
  ▸ **Tivicay** (ViiV Healthcare UK Ltd) ▼
  Dolutegravir (as Dolutegravir sodium) 10 mg Tivicay 10mg tablets | 30 tablet [PoM] £99.75
  Dolutegravir (as Dolutegravir sodium) 25 mg Tivicay 25mg tablets | 30 tablet [PoM] £249.38
  Dolutegravir (as Dolutegravir sodium) 50 mg Tivicay 50mg tablets | 30 tablet [PoM] £498.75

  Combinations available: *Abacavir with dolutegravir and lamivudine,* p. 398

Raltegravir

- **DRUG ACTION** Raltegravir is an inhibitor of HIV integrase.

- **INDICATIONS AND DOSE**
  HIV infection resistant to multiple antiretrovirals, in combination with other antiretroviral drugs
  ▸ BY MOUTH USING TABLETS
  ‣ Child 6-17 years (body-weight 25 kg and above): 400 mg twice daily
  ▸ BY MOUTH USING CHEWABLE TABLETS
  ‣ Child 2-11 years (body-weight 12-13 kg): 75 mg twice daily
  ‣ Child 2-11 years (body-weight 14-19 kg): 100 mg twice daily
  ‣ Child 2-11 years (body-weight 20-27 kg): 150 mg twice daily
  ‣ Child 2-11 years (body-weight 28-39 kg): 200 mg twice daily
  ‣ Child 2-11 years (body-weight 40 kg and above): 300 mg twice daily
  DOSE EQUIVALENCE AND CONVERSION
  ▸ The bioavailability of *Isentress*® chewable tablets is higher than that of the 'standard' 400 mg tablets; the chewable tablets are **not** interchangeable with the 'standard' tablets on a milligram-for-milligram basis.

- **CAUTIONS** Psychiatric illness (may exacerbate underlying illness including depression) · risk factors for myopathy · risk factors for rhabdomyolysis

- **INTERACTIONS** → Appendix 1: raltegravir

- **SIDE-EFFECTS**
  ▸ **Common or very common** Abdominal pain · abnormal dreams · asthenia · depression · diarrhoea · dizziness · dyspepsia · flatulence · headache · hyperactivity · hypertriglyceridaemia · insomnia · nausea · rash · vomiting
  ▸ **Uncommon** Acne · alopecia · anaemia · anxiety · appetite changes · arthralgia · bradycardia · carpal tunnel syndrome · chest pain · chills · confusion · constipation · drowsiness · dry mouth · dry skin · dysphonia · epistaxis · erectile dysfunction · flushing · gastritis · gingivitis · glossitis · gynaecomastia · hepatitis · hyperhidrosis · hypertension · impaired memory and attention · lipodystrophy · Lipodystrophy Syndrome · menopausal symptoms · myalgia · nasal congestion · neutropenia · nocturia · oedema · osteopenia · pain on swallowing · palpitation ·

pancreatitis · peptic ulcer · peripheral neuropathy · polydipsia · pruritus · pyrexia · rash with eosinophilia and systemic symptoms · rectal bleeding · renal failure · rhabdomyolysis · skin papilloma · Stevens-Johnson syndrome · suicidal ideation · taste disturbances · thrombocytopenia · tinnitus · tremor · ventricular extrasystoles · visual disturbances
‣ **Frequency not known** Osteonecrosis

SIDE-EFFECTS, FURTHER INFORMATION
‣ **Rash** Rash occurs commonly. Discontinue if severe rash or rash accompanied by fever, malaise, arthralgia, myalgia, blistering, mouth ulceration, conjunctivitis, angioedema, hepatitis, or eosinophilia.
‣ **Osteonecrosis** For further information see HIV infection p. 391.

● **PREGNANCY** Manufacturer advises avoid—toxicity in *animal* studies.

● **HEPATIC IMPAIRMENT** Manufacturer advises caution in severe impairment—no information available. Use with caution in patients with chronic hepatitis B or C (at greater risk of hepatic side-effects).

● **PRESCRIBING AND DISPENSING INFORMATION** Dispense raltegravir chewable tablets in original container (contains desiccant).

● **MEDICINAL FORMS**
There can be variation in the licensing of different medicines containing the same drug.

Tablet
CAUTIONARY AND ADVISORY LABELS 25
‣ **Isentress** (Merck Sharp & Dohme Ltd)
Raltegravir 400 mg Isentress 400mg tablets | 60 tablet [PoM] £471.41

Chewable tablet
CAUTIONARY AND ADVISORY LABELS 24
EXCIPIENTS: May contain Aspartame
‣ **Isentress** (Merck Sharp & Dohme Ltd)
Raltegravir 25 mg Isentress 25mg chewable tablets | 60 tablet [PoM] £29.46 DT price = £29.46
Raltegravir 100 mg Isentress 100mg chewable tablets | 60 tablet [PoM] £117.85 DT price = £117.85

ANTIVIRALS › NON-NUCLEOSIDE REVERSE TRANSCRIPTASE INHIBITORS

Efavirenz

● **INDICATIONS AND DOSE**

HIV infection in combination with other antiretroviral drugs
‣ BY MOUTH USING CAPSULES
‣ Child 3 months–17 years (body-weight 3.5–4 kg): 100 mg once daily
‣ Child 3 months–17 years (body-weight 5–7.4 kg): 150 mg once daily
‣ Child 3 months–17 years (body-weight 7.5–14 kg): 200 mg once daily
‣ Child 3 months–17 years (body-weight 15–19 kg): 250 mg once daily
‣ Child 3 months–17 years (body-weight 20–24 kg): 300 mg once daily
‣ Child 3 months–17 years (body-weight 25–32.4 kg): 350 mg once daily
‣ Child 3 months–17 years (body-weight 32.5–39 kg): 400 mg once daily
‣ Child 3 months–17 years (body-weight 40 kg and above): 600 mg once daily
‣ BY MOUTH USING TABLETS
‣ Child (body-weight 40 kg and above): 600 mg once daily
‣ BY MOUTH USING ORAL SOLUTION
‣ Child 3–4 years (body-weight 13–14 kg): 360 mg once daily
‣ Child 3–4 years (body-weight 15–19 kg): 390 mg once daily

‣ Child 3–4 years (body-weight 20–24 kg): 450 mg once daily
‣ Child 3–4 years (body-weight 25–32.5 kg): 510 mg once daily
‣ Child 5–17 years (body-weight 13–14 kg): 270 mg once daily
‣ Child 5–17 years (body-weight 15–19 kg): 300 mg once daily
‣ Child 5–17 years (body-weight 20–24 kg): 360 mg once daily
‣ Child 5–17 years (body-weight 25–32.4 kg): 450 mg once daily
‣ Child 5–17 years (body-weight 32.5–39 kg): 510 mg once daily
‣ Child 5–17 years (body-weight 40 kg and above): 720 mg once daily

DOSE EQUIVALENCE AND CONVERSION
‣ The bioavailability of *Sustiva*® oral solution is lower than that of the capsules and tablets; the oral solution is **not** interchangeable with either capsules or tablets on a milligram-for-milligram basis.

● **UNLICENSED USE** Opening capsules and adding contents to food is an unlicensed method of administration.

● **CAUTIONS** Acute porphyrias p. 577 · history of psychiatric disorders · history of seizures

● **INTERACTIONS** → Appendix 1: efavirenz

● **SIDE-EFFECTS**
‣ **Common or very common** Abdominal pain · abnormal dreams · anxiety · depression · diarrhoea · dizziness · fatigue · headache · impaired concentration · nausea · pruritus · rash · sleep disturbances · Stevens-Johnson syndrome · vomiting
‣ **Uncommon** Amnesia · ataxia · blurred vision · convulsions · flushing · gynaecomastia · hepatitis · hypersensitivity · mania · pancreatitis · psychosis · suicidal ideation · tinnitus · tremor · vertigo
‣ **Rare** Hepatic failure · photosensitivity · suicide
‣ **Frequency not known** Lipodystrophy syndrome · osteonecrosis · raised serum cholesterol

SIDE-EFFECTS, FURTHER INFORMATION
‣ **Rash** Rash, usually in the first 2 weeks, is the most common side-effect; discontinue if severe rash with blistering, desquamation, mucosal involvement or fever; if rash mild or moderate, may continue without interruption—usually resolves within 1 month.
‣ **CNS effects** Administration at bedtime especially in first 2–4 weeks reduces CNS effects.
‣ **Osteonecrosis** For further information see HIV infection p. 391.
‣ **Immune Reconstitution Syndrome** For further information see HIV infection p. 391.

● **PREGNANCY** Reports of neural tube defects when used in first trimester.

● **HEPATIC IMPAIRMENT** Greater risk of hepatic side-effects in chronic hepatitis B or C. Avoid in severe impairment. In mild to moderate liver disease, monitor for dose-related side-effects (e.g. CNS effects) and liver function.

● **RENAL IMPAIRMENT** Manufacturer advises caution in severe renal failure—no information available.

● **MONITORING REQUIREMENTS** Monitor liver function if receiving other hepatotoxic drugs.

● **DIRECTIONS FOR ADMINISTRATION** Capsules may be opened and contents added to food (contents have a peppery taste).

● **PRESCRIBING AND DISPENSING INFORMATION** Flavours of oral liquid formulations may include strawberry and mint.

● **PATIENT AND CARER ADVICE**
Psychiatric disorders Patients or their carers should be advised to seek immediate medical attention if symptoms

such as severe depression, psychosis or suicidal ideation occur.

- **MEDICINAL FORMS**
There can be variation in the licensing of different medicines containing the same drug.

Tablet

CAUTIONARY AND ADVISORY LABELS 23

▸ **Efavirenz (Non-proprietary)**
Efavirenz 600 mg Efavirenz 600mg tablets | 30 tablet PoM
£200.27-£452.94 | 30 tablet PoM £18.33 (Hospital only)

▸ **Sustiva** (Bristol-Myers Squibb Pharmaceuticals Ltd)
Efavirenz 600 mg Sustiva 600mg tablets | 30 tablet PoM £200.27 (Hospital only)

Capsule

CAUTIONARY AND ADVISORY LABELS 23

▸ **Sustiva** (Bristol-Myers Squibb Pharmaceuticals Ltd)
Efavirenz 50 mg Sustiva 50mg capsules | 30 capsule PoM £16.73 (Hospital only)
Efavirenz 100 mg Sustiva 100mg capsules | 30 capsule PoM £33.41 (Hospital only)
Efavirenz 200 mg Sustiva 200mg capsules | 90 capsule PoM £200.27 (Hospital only)

Etravirine

- **INDICATIONS AND DOSE**

HIV infection resistant to other non-nucleoside reverse transcriptase inhibitor and protease inhibitors in combination with other antiretroviral drugs (including a boosted protease inhibitor)

▸ BY MOUTH

▸ Child 6-17 years (body-weight 16-19 kg): 100 mg twice daily

▸ Child 6-17 years (body-weight 20-24 kg): 125 mg twice daily

▸ Child 6-17 years (body-weight 25-29 kg): 150 mg twice daily

▸ Child 6-17 years (body-weight 30 kg and above): 200 mg twice daily

- **CONTRA-INDICATIONS** Acute porphyrias p. 577
- **INTERACTIONS** → Appendix 1: etravirine
- **SIDE-EFFECTS**

▸ **Common or very common** Abdominal pain · anaemia · diabetes · flatulence · gastritis · gastro-oesophageal reflux · hyperlipidaemia · hypertension · Lipodystrophy Syndrome · nausea · peripheral neuropathy · rash · renal failure

▸ **Uncommon** Blurred vision · bronchospasm · chest pain · drowsiness · dry mouth · gynaecomastia · haematemesis · hepatitis · malaise · pancreatitis · sweating

▸ **Rare** Stevens-Johnson syndrome

▸ **Very rare** Toxic epidermal necrolysis

▸ **Frequency not known** Haemorrhagic stroke · hypersensitivity reactions · osteonecrosis

SIDE-EFFECTS, FURTHER INFORMATION

▸ Hypersensitivity reactions Rash, usually in the second week, is the most common side-effect and appears more frequently in females. Life-threatening hypersensitivity reactions reported usually during week 3–6 of treatment and characterised by rash, eosinophilia, and systemic symptoms (including fever, general malaise, myalgia, arthralgia, blistering, oral lesions, conjunctivitis, and hepatitis). Discontinue permanently if hypersensitivity reaction or severe rash develop. If rash mild or moderate (without signs of hypersensitivity reaction), may continue without interruption—usually resolves within 2 weeks.

▸ Osteonecrosis For further information see HIV infection p. 391.

- **HEPATIC IMPAIRMENT** Manufacturer advises caution in moderate impairment; avoid in severe impairment— no information available; greater risk of hepatic side-effects in chronic hepatitis B or C.

- **DIRECTIONS FOR ADMINISTRATION** Patients with swallowing difficulties may disperse tablets in a glass of water just before administration.

- **PRESCRIBING AND DISPENSING INFORMATION** Dispense in original container (contains desiccant).

- **PATIENT AND CARER ADVICE**
Hypersensitivity reactions Patients or carers should be told how to recognise hypersensitivity reactions and advised to seek immediate medical attention if hypersensitivity reaction or severe rash develop.

Missed doses
If a dose is more than 6 hours late, the missed dose should not be taken and the next dose should be taken at the normal time.

- **MEDICINAL FORMS**
There can be variation in the licensing of different medicines containing the same drug.

Tablet

CAUTIONARY AND ADVISORY LABELS 21

▸ **Intelence** (Janssen-Cilag Ltd)
Etravirine 25 mg Intelence 25mg tablets | 120 tablet PoM £75.32
Etravirine 100 mg Intelence 100mg tablets | 120 tablet PoM £301.27
Etravirine 200 mg Intelence 200mg tablets | 60 tablet PoM £301.27

Nevirapine

- **INDICATIONS AND DOSE**

HIV infection in combination with other antiretroviral drugs (initial dose)

▸ BY MOUTH USING IMMEDIATE-RELEASE MEDICINES

▸ Child: Initially 150–200 mg/m² once daily (max. per dose 200 mg) for first 14 days, initial dose titration using 'immediate-release' preparation should not exceed 28 days; if rash occurs and is not resolved within 28 days, alternative treatment should be sought. If treatment interrupted for more than 7 days, restart using the lower dose of the 'immediate-release' preparation for the first 14 days as for new treatment

HIV infection in combination with other antiretroviral drugs (maintenance dose following initial dose titration if no rash present)

▸ BY MOUTH USING IMMEDIATE-RELEASE MEDICINES

▸ Child 1 month-2 years: 150–200 mg/m² twice daily (max. per dose 200 mg), alternatively 300–400 mg/m² once daily (max. per dose 400 mg)

▸ Child 3-17 years: 150–200 mg/m² twice daily (max. per dose 200 mg)

HIV infection in combination with other antiretroviral drugs (maintenance dose following initial dose titration if no rash present)

▸ BY MOUTH USING IMMEDIATE-RELEASE MEDICINES

▸ Child 3-17 years (body surface area 0.58-0.83 m²): 200 mg once daily

▸ Child 3-17 years (body surface area 0.84-1.17 m²): 300 mg once daily

▸ Child 3-17 years (body surface area 1.18 m² and above): 400 mg once daily

▸ BY MOUTH USING MODIFIED-RELEASE MEDICINES

▸ Child 3-17 years (body surface area 0.58-0.83 m²): 200 mg once daily

▸ Child 3-17 years (body surface area 0.84-1.17 m²): 300 mg once daily

▸ Child 3-17 years (body surface area 1.18 m² and above): 400 mg once daily

- **UNLICENSED USE** 'Immediate-release' tablets not licensed for use in children weighing less than 50 kg or with body surface area less than 1.25 m^2; 'immediate-release' tablets and suspension not licensed for once daily dose after the initial dose titration.
- **CONTRA-INDICATIONS** Acute porphyrias p. 577 · post-exposure prophylaxis
- **CAUTIONS** Females (at greater risk of hepatic side-effects) · high CD4 cell count (at greater risk of hepatic side-effects)
- **INTERACTIONS** → Appendix 1: nevirapine
- **SIDE-EFFECTS**
  - **Common or very common** Abdominal pain · diarrhoea · fatigue · fever · granulocytopenia · headache · hepatitis · hypersensitivity reactions (may involve hepatic reactions and rash) · nausea · rash · Stevens-Johnson syndrome · toxic epidermal necrolysis · vomiting
  - **Uncommon** Anaemia · arthralgia · myalgia
  - **Frequency not known** Osteonecrosis

  SIDE-EFFECTS, FURTHER INFORMATION
  - Hepatic effects Potentially life-threatening hepatotoxicity including fatal fulminant hepatitis reported usually in first 6 weeks; discontinue permanently if abnormalities in liver function tests accompanied by hypersensitivity reaction (rash, fever, arthralgia, myalgia, lymphadenopathy, hepatitis, renal impairment, eosinophilia, granulocytopenia); suspend if severe abnormalities in liver function tests but no hypersensitivity reaction—discontinue permanently if significant liver function abnormalities recur; monitor patient closely if mild to moderate abnormalities in liver function tests with no hypersensitivity reaction.
  - Rash Rash, usually in first 6 weeks, is most common side-effect; incidence reduced if introduced at low dose and dose increased gradually (after 14 days); Discontinue permanently if severe rash or if rash accompanied by blistering, oral lesions, conjunctivitis, facial oedema, general malaise or hypersensitivity reactions; if rash mild or moderate may continue without interruption but dose should not be increased until rash resolves.
  - Osteonecrosis For more information see HIV infection p. 391.
- **HEPATIC IMPAIRMENT** Manufacturer advises avoid modified-release preparation—no information available; use 'immediate-release' preparation with caution in moderate impairment and avoid in severe impairment. Use with caution in patients with chronic hepatitis B or C (at greater risk of hepatic side-effects).
- **RENAL IMPAIRMENT** Manufacturer advises avoid modified-release preparation—no information available.
- **MONITORING REQUIREMENTS**
  - Hepatic disease Close monitoring of liver function required during first 18 weeks; monitor liver function before treatment then every 2 weeks for 2 months then after 1 month and then regularly.
  - Rash Monitor closely for skin reactions during first 18 weeks.
- **PATIENT AND CARER ADVICE**
  Hypersensitivity reactions Patients or carers should be told how to recognise hypersensitivity reactions and advised to discontinue treatment and seek immediate medical attention if severe skin reaction, hypersensitivity reactions, or symptoms of hepatitis develop.
- **MEDICINAL FORMS**
  There can be variation in the licensing of different medicines containing the same drug.
  Oral suspension
  - Viramune (Boehringer Ingelheim Ltd)
    Nevirapine (as Nevirapine hemihydrate) 10 mg per 1 ml Viramune 50mg/5ml oral suspension | 240 ml [PoM] £50.40

Modified-release tablet
CAUTIONARY AND ADVISORY LABELS 5
- Nevirapine (Non-proprietary)
  Nevirapine 400 mg Nevirapine 400 mg modified-release tablets | 30 tablet [PoM] £52.13–£161.50
- Viramune (Boehringer Ingelheim Ltd)
  Nevirapine 100 mg Viramune 100mg modified-release tablets | 90 tablet [PoM] £127.50 (Hospital only)
  Nevirapine 400 mg Viramune 400mg modified-release tablets | 30 tablet [PoM] £170.00 (Hospital only)

Tablet
- Nevirapine (Non-proprietary)
  Nevirapine 200 mg Nevirapine 200mg tablets | 14 tablet [PoM] £33.69 | 60 tablet [PoM] £21.45–£170.□
- Viramune (Boehringer Ingelheim Ltd)
  Nevirapine 200 mg Viramune 200mg tablets | 14 tablet [PoM] £39.67 | 60 tablet [PoM] £170.00

Rilpivirine

28-Sep-2016

- **INDICATIONS AND DOSE**

  HIV infection in combination with other antiretroviral drugs in patients not previously treated with antiretroviral therapy and if plasma HIV-1 RNA concentration less than or equal to 100 000 copies/mL
  - BY MOUTH
  - Child 12–17 years: 25 mg once daily

- **INTERACTIONS** → Appendix 1: rilpivirine
- **SIDE-EFFECTS** Abdominal pain · abnormal dreams · anorexia · depression · dizziness · dry mouth · headache · hyperlipidaemia · Lipodystrophy Syndrome · malaise · nausea · osteonecrosis · raised serum amylase · raised serum lipase · rash · sleep disturbance · vomiting

  SIDE-EFFECTS, FURTHER INFORMATION
  - Osteonecrosis For further information see HIV infection p. 391.
- **PREGNANCY** Manufacturer advises avoid unless essential— no information available.
- **HEPATIC IMPAIRMENT** Manufacturer advises caution in moderate impairment; avoid in severe impairment— no information available; greater risk of hepatic side-effects in chronic hepatitis B or C.
- **RENAL IMPAIRMENT** Manufacturer advises caution in severe impairment.
- **DIRECTIONS FOR ADMINISTRATION** Avoid antacids 2 hours before or 4 hours after taking rilpivirine.
- **PATIENT AND CARER ADVICE**
  Patients or carers should be given advice on how to administer rilpivirine tablets.
  Missed doses
  If a dose is more than 12 hours late, the missed dose should not be taken and the next dose should be taken at the normal time.
- **NATIONAL FUNDING/ACCESS DECISIONS**

  All Wales Medicines Strategy Group (AWMSG) Decisions
  The *All Wales Medicines Strategy Group* has advised (October 2016) that Rilpivirine (*Edurant*®) is recommended as an option for use within NHS Wales in combination with other antiretroviral medicinal products for the treatment of human immunodeficiency virus type 1 (HIV-1) infection in antiretroviral treatment-naive patients from 12 years old to < 18 years old with a viral load ≤ 100,000 HIV-1 RNA copies/ml.

● **MEDICINAL FORMS**
There can be variation in the licensing of different medicines containing the same drug.

Tablet
CAUTIONARY AND ADVISORY LABELS 21, 25
▸ Edurant (Janssen-Cilag Ltd)
Rilpivirine (as Rilpivirine hydrochloride) **25 mg** Edurant 25mg tablets | 30 tablet [PoM] £200.27

Combinations available: *Emtricitabine with rilpivirine and tenofovir alafenamide*, p. 400

ANTIVIRALS ❭ NUCLEOSIDE REVERSE TRANSCRIPTASE INHIBITORS

Nucleoside reverse transcriptase inhibitors

● **SIDE-EFFECTS** Abdominal pain · anaemia · anorexia · arthralgia · blood disorders · cough · diarrhoea · dizziness · dyspnoea · fatigue · fever · flatulence · gastro-intestinal disturbances · headache · insomnia · liver damage · metabolic effects · myalgia · nausea · neutropenia · osteonecrosis · pancreatitis · rash · thrombocytopenia · urticaria · vomiting

SIDE-EFFECTS, FURTHER INFORMATION
▸ Osteonecrosis For further information see HIV infection p. 391.
● **PREGNANCY** Mitochondrial dysfunction has been reported in infants exposed to nucleoside reverse transcriptase inhibitors in utero; the main effects include haematological, metabolic, and neurological disorders; all infants whose mothers received nucleoside reverse transcriptase inhibitors during pregnancy should be monitored for relevant signs or symptoms.
● **HEPATIC IMPAIRMENT** Use with caution in children with hepatic impairment (greater risk of hepatic side effects). However, some nucleoside reverse transcriptase inhibitors are used in children who also have chronic hepatitis B.

▸ above

Abacavir

● **INDICATIONS AND DOSE**
HIV infection in combination with other antiretroviral drugs
▸ BY MOUTH
▸ Child 3 months–11 years: 8 mg/kg twice daily (max. per dose 300 mg), alternatively 16 mg/kg once daily (max. per dose 600 mg)
▸ Child 3 months–11 years (body-weight 14–20 kg): 150 mg twice daily, alternatively 300 mg once daily
▸ Child 3 months–11 years (body-weight 21–29 kg): 150 mg, taken in the morning and 300 mg, taken in the evening, alternatively 450 mg once daily
▸ Child 3 months–11 years (body-weight 30 kg and above): 300 mg twice daily, alternatively 600 mg once daily
▸ Child 12–17 years: 300 mg twice daily, alternatively 600 mg once daily

● **INTERACTIONS** → Appendix 1: abacavir
● **SIDE-EFFECTS**
▸ **Very rare** Stevens-Johnson syndrome · toxic epidermal necrolysis
▸ **Frequency not known** Hypersensitivity reactions

SIDE-EFFECTS, FURTHER INFORMATION
▸ Hypersensitivity reactions Life-threatening hypersensitivity reactions reported—characterised by fever or rash and possibly nausea, vomiting, diarrhoea, abdominal pain, dyspnoea, cough, lethargy, malaise, headache, and

myalgia; less frequently mouth ulceration, oedema, hypotension, sore throat, acute respiratory distress syndrome, anaphylaxis, paraesthesia, arthralgia, conjunctivitis, lymphadenopathy, lymphocytopenia and renal failure; rarely myolysis; laboratory abnormalities may include raised liver function tests and creatine kinase; symptoms usually appear in the first 6 weeks, but may occur at any time.

Discontinue immediately if any symptom of hypersensitivity develops and do not rechallenge (risk of more severe hypersensitivity reaction); discontinue if hypersensitivity cannot be ruled out, even when other diagnoses possible—if rechallenge necessary it must be carried out in hospital setting; if abacavir is stopped for any reason other than hypersensitivity, exclude hypersensitivity reaction as the cause and rechallenge only if medical assistance is readily available; care needed with concomitant use of drugs which cause skin toxicity.
▸ Gastro-intestinal disturbances More common in children.
▸ Rash More common in children.
● **ALLERGY AND CROSS-SENSITIVITY** Caution—increased risk of hypersensitivity reaction in presence of HLA-B*5701 allele.
● **HEPATIC IMPAIRMENT** Monitor closely in mild impairment (combination preparations not recommended as reduced abacavir dose may be required). Avoid in moderate impairment unless essential—close monitoring recommended. Avoid in severe impairment.
● **RENAL IMPAIRMENT** Manufacturer advises avoid in end-stage renal disease.
● **PRE-TREATMENT SCREENING** Test for HLA-B*5701 allele before treatment or if restarting treatment and HLA-B*5701 status not known.
● **MONITORING REQUIREMENTS** Monitor for symptoms of hypersensitivity reaction every 2 weeks for 2 months.
● **PRESCRIBING AND DISPENSING INFORMATION** Flavours of oral liquid formulations may include banana, or strawberry.
● **PATIENT AND CARER ADVICE** Patients should be provided with an alert card and advised to keep it with them at all times.
Patients and their carers should be told the importance of regular dosing (intermittent therapy may increase the risk of sensitisation), how to recognise signs of hypersensitivity, and advised to seek immediate medical attention if symptoms develop or before re-starting treatment.

● **MEDICINAL FORMS**
There can be variation in the licensing of different medicines containing the same drug.

Oral solution
EXCIPIENTS: May contain Propylene glycol
▸ Ziagen (ViiV Healthcare UK Ltd)
Abacavir (as Abacavir sulfate) **20 mg per 1 ml** Ziagen 20mg/ml oral solution sugar-free | 240 ml [PoM] £47.36
Tablet
▸ Ziagen (ViiV Healthcare UK Ltd)
Abacavir (as Abacavir sulfate) **300 mg** Ziagen 300mg tablets | 60 tablet [PoM] £177.60

Abacavir with dolutegravir and lamivudine

The properties listed below are those particular to the combination only. For the properties of the components please consider, abacavir p. 397, lamivudine p. 401, dolutegravir p. 393.

- **INDICATIONS AND DOSE**
  HIV infection
  ▶ BY MOUTH
  ▶ Child 12–17 years (body-weight 40 kg and above): 1 tablet once daily

- **INTERACTIONS** → Appendix 1: abacavir, dolutegravir, lamivudine

- **RENAL IMPAIRMENT** Avoid *Triumeq*® if estimated glomerular filtration rate less than 50 mL/minute/1.73 m².

- **PATIENT AND CARER ADVICE**
  Missed doses
  If a dose is more than 20 hours late, the missed dose should not be taken and the next dose should be taken at the normal time.

- **MEDICINAL FORMS**
  There can be variation in the licensing of different medicines containing the same drug.
  Tablet
  ▶ Triumeq (ViiV Healthcare UK Ltd) ▼
  Dolutegravir (as Dolutegravir sodium) 50 mg, Lamivudine 300 mg, Abacavir (as Abacavir sulfate) 600 mg Triumeq 50mg/600mg/300mg tablets | 30 tablet [PoM] £798.16

Abacavir with lamivudine

The properties listed below are those particular to the combination only. For the properties of the components please consider, abacavir p. 397, lamivudine p. 401.

- **INDICATIONS AND DOSE**
  HIV infection in combination with other antiretrovirals
  ▶ BY MOUTH
  ▶ Child 12–17 years (body-weight 40 kg and above): 1 tablet once daily

- **INTERACTIONS** → Appendix 1: abacavir, lamivudine

- **RENAL IMPAIRMENT** Avoid *Kivexa*® if estimated glomerular filtration rate less than 50 mL/minute/1.73 m².

- **MEDICINAL FORMS**
  There can be variation in the licensing of different medicines containing the same drug.
  Tablet
  ▶ Abacavir with lamivudine (Non-proprietary)
  Lamivudine 300 mg, Abacavir 600 mg Abacavir 600mg / Lamivudine 300mg tablets | 30 tablet [PoM] £150.83–£299.41 | 30 tablet [PoM] £224.56 (Hospital only)
  ▶ Kivexa (ViiV Healthcare UK Ltd)
  Lamivudine 300 mg, Abacavir 600 mg Kivexa 600mg/300mg tablets | 30 tablet [PoM] £299.41

Abacavir with lamivudine and zidovudine

The properties listed below are those particular to the combination only. For the properties of the components please consider, abacavir p. 397, lamivudine p. 401, zidovudine p. 403.

- **INDICATIONS AND DOSE**
  HIV infection (use only if patient is stabilised for 6–8 weeks on the individual components in the same proportions)
  ▶ BY MOUTH
  ▶ Child (body-weight 30 kg and above): 1 tablet twice daily

- **UNLICENSED USE** *Trizivir*® not licensed for use in children.

- **INTERACTIONS** → Appendix 1: abacavir, lamivudine, zidovudine

- **RENAL IMPAIRMENT** Avoid *Trizivir*® if estimated glomerular filtration rate less than 50 mL/minute/1.73 m².

- **MEDICINAL FORMS**
  There can be variation in the licensing of different medicines containing the same drug.
  Tablet
  ▶ Trizivir (ViiV Healthcare UK Ltd)
  Lamivudine 150 mg, Abacavir (as Abacavir sulfate) 300 mg, Zidovudine 300 mg Trizivir tablets | 60 tablet [PoM] £432.70

Didanosine

(ddI; DDI)

01-Sep-2016

- **INDICATIONS AND DOSE**
  HIV infection in combination with other antiretroviral drugs
  ▶ BY MOUTH
  ▶ Child 1–7 months: 50–100 mg/m² twice daily
  ▶ Child 8 months–17 years: 180–240 mg/m² once daily; usual dose 200 mg/m² once daily; maximum 400 mg per day

- **UNLICENSED USE** Tablets not licensed for use in children under 3 months. EC capsules not licensed for use in children under 6 years.

- **CAUTIONS** History of pancreatitis (preferably avoid, otherwise extreme caution) · hyperuricaemia · lactic acidosis · peripheral neuropathy
  CAUTIONS, FURTHER INFORMATION
  ▶ Lactic acidosis Lactic acidosis associated with hepatomegaly and hepatic steatosis has been reported with didanosine. Use with caution in patients with hepatomegaly, hepatitis, or other risk factors for liver disease and hepatic steatosis (including obesity and alcohol abuse). Discontinue treatment if symptoms of hyperlactataemia, lactic acidosis, progressive hepatomegaly or rapid deterioration of liver function become apparent.

- **INTERACTIONS** → Appendix 1: didanosine

- **SIDE-EFFECTS** Acute renal failure · alopecia · anaphylactic reactions · diabetes mellitus · dry eyes · dry mouth · hyperuricaemia (suspend if raised significantly) · hypoglycaemia · lactic acidosis · lipodystrophy · liver failure · non-cirrhotic portal hypertension · optic nerve changes · pancreatitis (less common in children) · parotid gland enlargement · peripheral neuropathy (switch to another antiretroviral if peripheral neuropathy develops) · retinal changes · rhabdomyolysis · sialadenitis
  SIDE-EFFECTS, FURTHER INFORMATION
  ▶ Pancreatitis Suspend treatment if serum lipase raised (even if asymptomatic) or if symptoms of pancreatitis develop; discontinue if pancreatitis confirmed. Whenever possible

F 397

avoid concomitant treatment with other drugs known to cause pancreatic toxicity (e.g. intravenous pentamidine isetionate); monitor closely if concomitant therapy unavoidable. Since significant elevations of triglycerides cause pancreatitis monitor closely if elevated.

▸ Lipodystrophy syndrome Metabolic effects may occur with antiretroviral regimens containing didanosine; these include fat redistribution, insulin resistance, and dyslipidaemia—collectively termed lipodystrophy syndrome. The usual risk factors for cardiovascular disease should be taken into account before starting therapy and patients should be advised about lifestyle changes to reduce their cardiovascular risk. Plasma lipids and blood glucose should be measured before starting treatment, after 3–6 months of treatment, and then annually.

● PREGNANCY Manufacturer advises use only if potential benefit outweighs risk.

● HEPATIC IMPAIRMENT In hepatic impairment, monitor for toxicity.

● RENAL IMPAIRMENT Reduce dose if estimated glomerular filtration rate less than 60 mL/minute/1.73 m^2; consult product literature.

● MONITORING REQUIREMENTS Ophthalmological examination (including visual acuity, colour vision, and dilated fundus examination) recommended annually or if visual changes occur.

● DIRECTIONS FOR ADMINISTRATION Capsules should be swallowed whole and taken at least 2 hours before or 2 hours after food.

  With chewable tablets, to ensure sufficient antacid, each dose to be taken as at least 2 tablets (child under 1 year 1 tablet) chewed thoroughly, crushed or dispersed in water; clear apple juice may be added for flavouring; tablets to be taken 2 hours after lopinavir with ritonavir capsules and oral solution or atazanavir with ritonavir.

● PATIENT AND CARER ADVICE Patients or carers should be given advice on how to administer didanosine capsules and chewable tablets.

● MEDICINAL FORMS
There can be variation in the licensing of different medicines containing the same drug.

Gastro-resistant capsule
CAUTIONARY AND ADVISORY LABELS 25
▸ Videx EC (Bristol-Myers Squibb Pharmaceuticals Ltd)
  Didanosine 125 mg Videx EC 125mg capsules | 30 capsule [PoM] £48.18 (Hospital only)
  Didanosine 200 mg Videx EC 200mg capsules | 30 capsule [PoM] £77.09 (Hospital only)
  Didanosine 250 mg Videx EC 250mg capsules | 30 capsule [PoM] £96.37 (Hospital only)
  Didanosine 400 mg Videx EC 400mg capsules | 30 capsule [PoM] £154.19 (Hospital only)

Chewable tablet
CAUTIONARY AND ADVISORY LABELS 23
EXCIPIENTS: May contain Aspartame
▸ Videx (Bristol-Myers Squibb Pharmaceuticals Ltd)
  Didanosine 25 mg Videx 25mg chewable dispersible tablets sugar-free | 60 tablet [PoM] £25.06 (Hospital only)

Elvitegravir with cobicistat, emtricitabine and tenofovir alafenamide
02-Jun-2017

The properties listed below are those particular to the combination only. For the properties of the components please consider, emtricitabine p. 400, elvitegravir, cobicistat.

● INDICATIONS AND DOSE

HIV infection (specialist use only)
▸ BY MOUTH
  ▸ Child 12–17 years (body-weight 35 kg and above): 1 tablet once daily

● INTERACTIONS → Appendix 1: cobicistat, elvitegravir, tenofovir

● SIDE-EFFECTS
▸ Uncommon Angioedema

● CONCEPTION AND CONTRACEPTION Manufacturer advises effective contraception in women of childbearing potential; if using a hormonal contraceptive, it must contain norgestimate as the progestogen and at least 30 micrograms ethinylestradiol—no information available on progestogens other than norgestimate.

● HEPATIC IMPAIRMENT Manufacturer advises use with caution in mild-to-moderate impairment (greater risk of hepatic side-effects); avoid in severe impairment—no information available.

● RENAL IMPAIRMENT Manufacturer advises avoid if creatinine clearance less than 30 mL/minute—limited information available.

● PRESCRIBING AND DISPENSING INFORMATION Dispense in original container—contains desiccant.

● PATIENT AND CARER ADVICE
Driving and skilled tasks
Manufacturer advises patients and carers should be counselled on the effects on driving and performance of skilled tasks—increased risk of dizziness.

● NATIONAL FUNDING/ACCESS DECISIONS

Scottish Medicines Consortium (SMC) Decisions
The *Scottish Medicines Consortium* has advised (May 2016) that elvitegravir with cobicistat, emtricitabine and tenofovir alafenamide (*Genvoya®*) is accepted for use within NHS Scotland for the treatment of human immunodeficiency virus type 1 (HIV-1), without known mutations associated with resistance to the integrase inhibitor class, emtricitabine or tenofovir. This advice is contingent upon the continuing availability of the patient access scheme in NHS Scotland or a list price that is equivalent or lower.

All Wales Medicines Strategy Group (AWMSG) Decisions
The *All Wales Medicines Strategy Group* has advised (July 2016) that elvitegravir with cobicistat, emtricitabine and tenofovir alafenamide (*Genvoya®*) is recommended as an option for use within NHS Wales for the treatment of human immunodeficiency virus type 1 (HIV-1), without known mutations associated with resistance to the integrase inhibitor class, emtricitabine or tenofovir. The recommendation applies only if the approved Wales Patient Access Scheme (WPAS) is used or where the list price is equivalent or lower.

● MEDICINAL FORMS
There can be variation in the licensing of different medicines containing the same drug.

Tablet
CAUTIONARY AND ADVISORY LABELS 21
▸ Genvoya (Gilead Sciences International Ltd) ▼
  Tenofovir alafenamide 10 mg, Cobicistat 150 mg, Elvitegravir 150 mg, Emtricitabine 200 mg Genvoya 150mg/150mg/200mg/10mg tablets | 30 tablet [PoM] £879.51

Emtricitabine
(FTC)

◉ **INDICATIONS AND DOSE**

HIV infection in combination with other antiretroviral drugs
▸ BY MOUTH USING CAPSULES
▸ Child (body-weight 33 kg and above): 200 mg once daily
▸ BY MOUTH USING ORAL SOLUTION
▸ Child 4 months–17 years (body-weight up to 33 kg): 6 mg/kg once daily
▸ Child 4 months–17 years (body-weight 33 kg and above): 240 mg once daily

DOSE EQUIVALENCE AND CONVERSION
▸ 240 mg oral solution ≡ 200 mg capsule; where appropriate the capsule may be used instead of the oral solution.

◉ **SIDE-EFFECTS** Abnormal dreams · hyperpigmentation · pruritus

◉ **HEPATIC IMPAIRMENT** On discontinuation, monitor patients with hepatitis B (risk of exacerbation of hepatitis).

◉ **RENAL IMPAIRMENT** Reduce dose or increase dosage interval if estimated glomerular filtration rate less than 50 mL/minute/1.73 m^2; consult product literature.

◉ **PRESCRIBING AND DISPENSING INFORMATION** Flavours of oral liquid formulations may include candy.

◉ **PATIENT AND CARER ADVICE**
Missed doses
If a dose is more than 12 hours late, the missed dose should not be taken and the next dose should be taken at the normal time.

◉ **MEDICINAL FORMS**
There can be variation in the licensing of different medicines containing the same drug.
Oral solution
ELECTROLYTES: May contain Sodium
▸ **Emtriva** (Gilead Sciences International Ltd)
Emtricitabine 10 mg per 1 ml Emtriva 10mg/ml oral solution sugar-free | 170 ml [PoM] £39.53
Capsule
▸ **Emtriva** (Gilead Sciences International Ltd)
Emtricitabine 200 mg Emtriva 200mg capsules | 30 capsule [PoM] £138.98

Emtricitabine with rilpivirine and tenofovir alafenamide
05-Jun-2017

The properties listed below are those particular to the combination only. For the properties of the components please consider, emtricitabine above, rilpivirine p. 396.

◉ **INDICATIONS AND DOSE**

HIV infection in patients with plasma HIV-1 RNA concentration of 100 000 copies/mL or less (specialist use only)
▸ BY MOUTH
▸ Child 12–17 years (body-weight 35 kg and above): 1 tablet once daily

◉ **INTERACTIONS** → Appendix 1: rilpivirine, tenofovir

◉ **SIDE-EFFECTS**
▸ Common or very common Raised bilirubin
▸ Uncommon Angioedema · dyspepsia · severe skin reactions (with systemic symptoms)
SIDE-EFFECTS, FURTHER INFORMATION
▸ Severe skin reactions Systemic symptoms reported with severe skin reactions include fever, blisters, conjunctivitis,

angioedema, elevated liver function tests, and eosinophilia.

◉ **HEPATIC IMPAIRMENT** Manufacturer advises use with caution in moderate impairment (greater risk of hepatic side-effects); avoid in severe impairment—no information available.

◉ **RENAL IMPAIRMENT** Manufacturer advises avoid if creatinine clearance less than 30 mL/minute—no information available.

◉ **PATIENT AND CARER ADVICE**
Vomiting Manufacturer advises if vomiting occurs within 4 hours of taking a dose, a replacement dose should be taken.
Driving and skilled tasks
Manufacturer advises patients and carers should be counselled on the effects on driving and performance of skilled tasks—increased risk of dizziness.

◉ **NATIONAL FUNDING/ACCESS DECISIONS**
Scottish Medicines Consortium (SMC) Decisions
The *Scottish Medicines Consortium* has advised (October 2016) that emtricitabine with rilpivirine and tenofovir alafenamide (*Odefsey*®) is accepted for use within NHS Scotland for the treatment of human immunodeficiency virus type 1 (HIV-1), without known mutations associated with resistance to the non-nucleoside reverse transcriptase inhibitor (NNRTI) class, tenofovir or emtricitabine, and with viral load HIV-1 RNA of 100 000 copies/mL or less.

All Wales Medicines Strategy Group (AWMSG) Decisions
The *All Wales Medicines Strategy Group* has advised (November 2016) that emtricitabine with rilpivirine and tenofovir alafenamide (*Odefsey*®) is recommended as an option for use within NHS Wales for the treatment of human immunodeficiency virus type 1, without known mutations associated with resistance to the non-nucleoside reverse transcriptase inhibitor (NNRTI) class, tenofovir or emtricitabine, and with viral load HIV-1 RNA of 100 000 copies/mL or less.

◉ **MEDICINAL FORMS**
There can be variation in the licensing of different medicines containing the same drug.
Tablet
CAUTIONARY AND ADVISORY LABELS 3, 21
▸ **Odefsey** (Gilead Sciences International Ltd) ▼
Rilpivirine (as Rilpivirine hydrochloride) 25 mg, Tenofovir alafenamide (as Tenofovir alafenamide fumarate) 25 mg, Emtricitabine 200 mg Odefsey 200mg/25mg/25mg tablets | 30 tablet [PoM] £525.95

Emtricitabine with tenofovir alafenamide
05-Jun-2017

The properties listed below are those particular to the combination only. For the properties of the components please consider, emtricitabine above.

◉ **INDICATIONS AND DOSE**

HIV infection in combination with other antiretroviral drugs (specialist use only)
▸ BY MOUTH
▸ Child 12–17 years (body-weight 35 kg and above): 200/10–200/25 mg once daily, dose is dependent on drug regimen—consult product literature

DOSE EQUIVALENCE AND CONVERSION
▸ Dose expressed as x/y mg emtricitabine/tenofovir alafenamide.

◉ **INTERACTIONS** → Appendix 1: tenofovir

- **SIDE-EFFECTS**
▶ **Uncommon** Angioedema · dyspepsia
- **HEPATIC IMPAIRMENT** Manufacturer advises use with caution (greater risk of hepatic side-effects).
- **RENAL IMPAIRMENT** Manufacturer advises avoid if creatinine clearance less than 30 mL/minute—limited information available.
- **PATIENT AND CARER ADVICE**
Vomiting Manufacturer advises if vomiting occurs within 1 hour of taking a dose, a replacement dose should be taken.

Missed doses
Manufacturer advises if a dose is more than 18 hours late, the missed dose should not be taken and the next dose should be taken at the normal time.

Driving and skilled tasks
Manufacturer advises patients and carers should be counselled on the effects on driving and performance of skilled tasks—increased risk of dizziness.

- **NATIONAL FUNDING/ACCESS DECISIONS**
Scottish Medicines Consortium (SMC) Decisions
The *Scottish Medicines Consortium* has advised (August 2016) that emtricitabine with tenofovir alafenamide (*Descovy*®) is accepted for use within NHS Scotland for the treatment of human immunodeficiency virus type 1 in combination with other antiretroviral agents.

All Wales Medicines Strategy Group (AWMSG) Decisions
The *All Wales Medicines Strategy Group* has advised (September 2016) that emtricitabine with tenofovir alafenamide (*Descovy*®) is recommended as an option for use within NHS Wales for the treatment of human immunodeficiency virus type 1 in combination with other antiretroviral agents.

- **MEDICINAL FORMS**
There can be variation in the licensing of different medicines containing the same drug.

Tablet
▶ Descovy (Gilead Sciences International Ltd) ▼
Tenofovir alafenamide (as Tenofovir alafenamide fumarate) 25 mg, Emtricitabine 200 mg Descovy 200mg/25mg tablets | 30 tablet [PoM] £355.73
Tenofovir alafenamide (as Tenofovir alafenamide fumarate) 10 mg, Emtricitabine 200 mg Descovy 200mg/10mg tablets | 30 tablet [PoM] £355.73

☞ 397

Lamivudine

(3TC)

- **INDICATIONS AND DOSE**

EPIVIR® ORAL SOLUTION

HIV infection in combination with other antiretroviral drugs
▶ BY MOUTH
▶ Child 1–2 months: 4 mg/kg twice daily
▶ Child 3 months–11 years (body-weight up to 14 kg): 4 mg/kg twice daily (max. per dose 150 mg), alternatively 8 mg/kg once daily (max. per dose 300 mg)
▶ Child 3 months–11 years (body-weight 14–20 kg): 4 mg/kg twice daily (max. per dose 150 mg), alternatively 8 mg/kg once daily (max. per dose 300 mg), alternatively 75 mg twice daily, alternatively 150 mg once daily
▶ Child 3 months–11 years (body-weight 21–29 kg): 4 mg/kg twice daily (max. per dose 150 mg), alternatively 8 mg/kg once daily (max. per dose 300 mg), alternatively 75 mg daily, dose to be taken in the morning and 150 mg daily, dose to be taken in the evening, alternatively 225 mg once daily

▶ Child 3 months–11 years (body-weight 30 kg and above): 4 mg/kg twice daily (max. per dose 150 mg), alternatively 8 mg/kg once daily (max. per dose 300 mg), alternatively 150 mg twice daily, alternatively 300 mg once daily
▶ Child 12–17 years: 150 mg twice daily, alternatively 300 mg once daily

EPIVIR® TABLETS

HIV infection in combination with other antiretroviral drugs
▶ BY MOUTH
▶ Child 1–2 months: 4 mg/kg twice daily
▶ Child 3 months–11 years (body-weight up to 14 kg): 4 mg/kg twice daily, alternatively 8 mg/kg once daily
▶ Child 3 months–11 years (body-weight 14–20 kg): 4 mg/kg twice daily (max. per dose 150 mg), alternatively 8 mg/kg once daily (max. per dose 300 mg), alternatively 75 mg twice daily, alternatively 150 mg once daily
▶ Child 3 months–11 years (body-weight 21–29 kg): 4 mg/kg twice daily (max. per dose 150 mg), alternatively 8 mg/kg once daily (max. per dose 300 mg), alternatively 75 mg daily, dose to be taken in the morning and 150 mg daily, dose to be taken in the evening, alternatively 225 mg once daily
▶ Child 3 months–11 years (body-weight 30 kg and above): 4 mg/kg twice daily (max. per dose 150 mg), alternatively 8 mg/kg once daily (max. per dose 300 mg), alternatively 150 mg twice daily, alternatively 300 mg once daily
▶ Child 12–17 years: 150 mg twice daily, alternatively 300 mg once daily

ZEFFIX®

Chronic hepatitis B infection either with compensated liver disease (with evidence of viral replication and histology of active liver inflammation or fibrosis) when first-line treatments cannot be used, or (in combination with another antiviral drug without cross-resistance to lamivudine) with decompensated liver disease
▶ BY MOUTH
▶ Child 2–11 years: 3 mg/kg once daily (max. per dose 100 mg), children receiving lamivudine for concomitant HIV infection should continue to receive lamivudine in a dose appropriate for HIV infection
▶ Child 12–17 years: 100 mg once daily, patients receiving lamivudine for concomitant HIV infection should continue to receive lamivudine in a dose appropriate for HIV infection

- **UNLICENSED USE**
EPIVIR® ORAL SOLUTION Not licensed for use in children under 3 months.
ZEFFIX® Not licensed for use in children.
EPIVIR® TABLETS Not licensed for use in children under 3 months.
- **CAUTIONS** Recurrent hepatitis in patients with chronic hepatitis B may occur on discontinuation of lamivudine
- **INTERACTIONS** → Appendix 1: lamivudine
- **SIDE-EFFECTS** Alopecia · muscle disorders · nasal symptoms · peripheral neuropathy · rhabdomyolysis
- **BREAST FEEDING** Can be used with caution in women infected with chronic hepatitis B alone, providing that adequate measures are taken to prevent hepatitis B infection in infants.
- **RENAL IMPAIRMENT** Reduce dose if estimated glomerular filtration rate less than 50 mL/minute/1.73 m²; consult product literature.
- **MONITORING REQUIREMENTS** When treating chronic hepatitis B with lamivudine, monitor liver function tests every 3 months, and viral markers of hepatitis B every

3–6 months, more frequently in patients with advanced liver disease or following transplantation (monitoring to continue for at least 1 year after discontinuation—recurrent hepatitis may occur on discontinuation).

- **PRESCRIBING AND DISPENSING INFORMATION** Flavours of oral liquid formulations may include banana and strawberry.

- **MEDICINAL FORMS**
There can be variation in the licensing of different medicines containing the same drug.
Oral solution
EXCIPIENTS: May contain Sucrose
- ▸ Epivir (ViiV Healthcare UK Ltd)
Lamivudine 10 mg per 1 ml Epivir 50mg/5ml oral solution | 240 ml [PoM] £33.16
Tablet
- ▸ Epivir (ViiV Healthcare UK Ltd)
Lamivudine 150 mg Epivir 150mg tablets | 60 tablet [PoM] £121.82 DT price = £121.82
Lamivudine 300 mg Epivir 300mg tablets | 30 tablet [PoM] £133.89 DT price = £133.89
- ▸ Zeffix (GlaxoSmithKline UK Ltd)
Lamivudine 100 mg Zeffix 100mg tablets | 28 tablet [PoM] £78.09 DT price = £71.41

▶ 397

Stavudine

01-Sep-2016

(d4T)

- **INDICATIONS AND DOSE**

HIV infection in combination with other antiretroviral drugs when no suitable alternative available and when prescribed for shortest period possible
- ▸ BY MOUTH
- ▸ Child (body-weight up to 30 kg): 1 mg/kg twice daily, to be taken preferably at least 1 hour before food
- ▸ Child (body-weight 30–59 kg): 30 mg twice daily, to be taken preferably at least 1 hour before food
- ▸ Child (body-weight 60 kg and above): 40 mg twice daily, to be taken preferably at least 1 hour before food

- **UNLICENSED USE** Capsules not licensed for use in children under 3 months.

- **CAUTIONS** Excessive alcohol intake · history of pancreatitis · history of peripheral neuropathy · lactic acidosis (especially when used in combination with didanosine)—use only if alternative regimens are not suitable
CAUTIONS, FURTHER INFORMATION
- ▸ Lactic acidosis Lactic acidosis associated with hepatomegaly and hepatic steatosis has been reported with stavudine. Use with caution in patients with hepatomegaly, hepatitis, or other risk factors for liver disease and hepatic steatosis (including obesity and alcohol abuse). Discontinue treatment if symptoms of hyperlactataemia, lactic acidosis, progressive hepatomegaly or rapid deterioration of liver function become apparent.

- **INTERACTIONS** → Appendix 1: stavudine

- **SIDE-EFFECTS**
- ▸ Common or very common Abnormal dreams · cognitive dysfunction · depression · drowsiness · peripheral neuropathy (switch to another antiretroviral if peripheral neuropathy develops) · pruritus
- ▸ Uncommon Anxiety · gynaecomastia
- ▸ Frequency not known Lactic acidosis · lipodystrophy
SIDE-EFFECTS, FURTHER INFORMATION
- ▸ Lipodystrophy syndrome Metabolic effects may occur with antiretroviral regimens containing stavudine; these include fat redistribution, insulin resistance, and dyslipidaemia—collectively termed lipodystrophy syndrome. The usual risk factors for cardiovascular disease should be taken into account before starting therapy and

patients should be advised about lifestyle changes to reduce their cardiovascular risk. Plasma lipids and blood glucose should be measured before starting treatment, after 3–6 months of treatment, and then annually.

- **PREGNANCY** Manufacturer advises use only if potential benefit outweighs risk.

- **RENAL IMPAIRMENT** Reduce dose to 50% if estimated glomerular filtration rate 25–50 mL/minute/1.73 m^2; reduce dose to 25% if estimated glomerular filtration rate less than 25 mL/minute/1.73 m^2. Risk of peripheral neuropathy.

- **PRESCRIBING AND DISPENSING INFORMATION** Flavours of oral liquid formulations may include cherry.

- **LESS SUITABLE FOR PRESCRIBING** Stavudine (especially in combination with didanosine) is associated with a higher risk of lipoatrophy and should be used only if alternative regimens are not suitable; it is considered to be less suitable for prescribing.

- **MEDICINAL FORMS**
There can be variation in the licensing of different medicines containing the same drug.
Oral solution
- ▸ Zerit (Bristol-Myers Squibb Pharmaceuticals Ltd)
Stavudine 1 mg per 1 ml Zerit 1mg/ml oral solution | 200 ml [PoM] £22.94 (Hospital only)
Capsule
- ▸ Zerit (Bristol-Myers Squibb Pharmaceuticals Ltd)
Stavudine 20 mg Zerit 20mg capsules | 56 capsule [PoM] £139.46 (Hospital only)
Stavudine 30 mg Zerit 30mg capsules | 56 capsule [PoM] £146.25 (Hospital only)
Stavudine 40 mg Zerit 40mg capsules | 56 capsule [PoM] £150.66 (Hospital only)

▶ 397

Tenofovir disoproxil

- **INDICATIONS AND DOSE**

HIV infection in combination with other antiretroviral drugs when first-line nucleoside reverse transcriptase inhibitors cannot be used because of resistance or contra-indications
- ▸ BY MOUTH
- ▸ Child 2-17 years: 6.5 mg/kg once daily (max. per dose 245 mg)
- ▸ Child 6-17 years (body-weight 17–21 kg): 123 mg once daily
- ▸ Child 6-17 years (body-weight 22–27 kg): 163 mg once daily
- ▸ Child 6-17 years (body-weight 28–34 kg): 204 mg once daily
- ▸ Child 6-17 years (body-weight 35 kg and above): 245 mg once daily

Chronic hepatitis B infection with compensated liver disease (with evidence of viral replication, and histology of active liver inflammation or fibrosis)
- ▸ BY MOUTH
- ▸ Child 12-17 years (body-weight 35 kg and above): 245 mg once daily

DOSE EQUIVALENCE AND CONVERSION
- ▸ 7.5 scoops of granules contains approx. 245 mg tenofovir disoproxil (as fumarate).

- **INTERACTIONS** → Appendix 1: tenofovir

- **SIDE-EFFECTS**
- ▸ Rare Nephrogenic diabetes insipidus · proximal renal tubulopathy · renal failure
- ▸ Frequency not known Hypophosphataemia · reduced bone density

- **RENAL IMPAIRMENT** Manufacturer advises avoid—no information available.

- **MONITORING REQUIREMENTS**
- ► Test renal function and serum phosphate before treatment, then every 4 weeks (more frequently if at increased risk of renal impairment) for 1 year and then every 3 months, interrupt treatment if renal function deteriorates or serum phosphate decreases.
- ► When treating chronic hepatitis B with tenofovir, monitor liver function tests every 3 months and viral markers for hepatitis B every 3–6 months during treatment (continue monitoring for at least 1 year after discontinuation—recurrent hepatitis may occur on discontinuation).

- **DIRECTIONS FOR ADMINISTRATION** *Granules*: mix 1 scoop of granules with 1 tablespoon of soft food (e.g. yoghurt, apple sauce) and take immediately without chewing. Do **not** mix granules with liquids.

- **PATIENT AND CARER ADVICE**
  Patients or carers should be given advice on how to administer tenofovir granules.

  Missed doses
  If a dose is more than 12 hours late, the missed dose should not be taken and the next dose should be taken at the normal time.

- **MEDICINAL FORMS**
  There can be variation in the licensing of different medicines containing the same drug.

  Granules
  CAUTIONARY AND ADVISORY LABELS 21
  ► Viread (Gilead Sciences International Ltd)
  Tenofovir disoproxil (as Tenofovir disoproxil fumarate) 33 mg per 1 gram Viread 33mg/g granules | 60 gram PoM £54.50

  Tablet
  CAUTIONARY AND ADVISORY LABELS 21
  ► Viread (Gilead Sciences International Ltd)
  Tenofovir disoproxil (as Tenofovir disoproxil fumarate)
  123 mg Viread 123mg tablets | 30 tablet PoM £102.60
  Tenofovir disoproxil (as Tenofovir disoproxil fumarate)
  163 mg Viread 163mg tablets | 30 tablet PoM £135.98
  Tenofovir disoproxil (as Tenofovir disoproxil fumarate)
  204 mg Viread 204mg tablets | 30 tablet PoM £170.19
  Tenofovir disoproxil (as Tenofovir disoproxil fumarate)
  245 mg Viread 245mg tablets | 30 tablet PoM £204.39

  ► 397

Zidovudine

01-Sep-2016

(Azidothymidine; AZT)

- **INDICATIONS AND DOSE**
  HIV infection in combination with other antiretroviral drugs
  ► BY MOUTH
  ► Child: 180 mg/m^2 twice daily (max. per dose 300 mg)
  ► Child (body-weight 8–13 kg): 100 mg twice daily
  ► Child (body-weight 14–20 kg): 100 mg, to be taken in the morning and 200 mg, to be taken in the evening
  ► Child (body-weight 21–27 kg): 200 mg twice daily
  ► Child (body-weight 28–29 kg): 200–250 mg twice daily
  ► Child (body-weight 30 kg and above): 250–300 mg twice daily

  HIV infection in combination with other antiretroviral drugs (dose expressed in mg/kg)
  ► BY MOUTH
  ► Child (body-weight 4–8 kg): 12 mg/kg twice daily
  ► Child (body-weight 9–29 kg): 9 mg/kg twice daily

  Prevention of maternal-fetal HIV transmission
  ► BY MOUTH, OR BY INTRAVENOUS INFUSION
  ► Child: Seek specialist advice (combination therapy preferred) (consult local protocol)

  HIV infection in combination with other antiretroviral drugs in patients temporarily unable to take zidovudine by mouth
  ► BY INTRAVENOUS INFUSION
  ► Child 3 months–11 years: 60–80 mg/m^2 every 6 hours usually for not more than 2 weeks, dose approximating to 9–12 mg/kg twice daily by mouth
  ► Child 12–17 years: 0.8–1 mg/kg every 4 hours usually for not more than 2 weeks, dose approximating to 1.2–1.5 mg/kg every 4 hours by mouth

- **CONTRA-INDICATIONS** Abnormally low haemoglobin concentration (consult product literature) · abnormally low neutrophil counts (consult product literature) · acute porphyrias p. 577 · neonates with hyperbilirubinaemia requiring treatment other than phototherapy, or with raised transaminase (consult product literature)

- **CAUTIONS** Lactic acidosis · risk of haematological toxicity particularly with high dose and advanced disease · vitamin B$_{12}$ deficiency (increased risk of neutropenia)
  CAUTIONS, FURTHER INFORMATION
  ► Lactic acidosis Lactic acidosis associated with hepatomegaly and hepatic steatosis has been reported with zidovudine. Use with caution in patients with hepatomegaly, hepatitis, or other risk factors for liver disease and hepatic steatosis (including obesity and alcohol abuse). Discontinue treatment if symptoms of hyperlactataemia, lactic acidosis, progressive hepatomegaly or rapid deterioration of liver function become apparent.

- **INTERACTIONS** → Appendix 1: zidovudine

- **SIDE-EFFECTS** Anaemia (may require transfusion) · anxiety · chest pain · convulsions · depression · dizziness · drowsiness · gynaecomastia · influenza-like symptoms · lactic acidosis · lipodystrophy · loss of mental acuity · myopathy · neuropathy · paraesthesia · pigmentation of nails · pigmentation of oral mucosa · pigmentation of skin · pruritus · sweating · taste disturbance · urinary frequency
  SIDE-EFFECTS, FURTHER INFORMATION
  ► Anaemia and myelosuppression If anaemia or myelosuppression occur, reduce dose or interrupt treatment according to product literature, or consider other treatment.
  ► Lipodystrophy syndrome Metabolic effects may occur with antiretroviral regimens containing zidovudine; these include fat redistribution, insulin resistance, and dyslipidaemia—collectively termed lipodystrophy syndrome. The usual risk factors for cardiovascular disease should be taken into account before starting therapy and patients should be advised about lifestyle changes to reduce their cardiovascular risk. Plasma lipids and blood glucose should be measured before starting treatment, after 3–6 months of treatment, and then annually.

- **HEPATIC IMPAIRMENT** Accumulation may occur.

- **RENAL IMPAIRMENT** Reduce dose if estimated glomerular filtration rate less than 10 mL/minute/1.73 m^2—consult product literature.

- **MONITORING REQUIREMENTS** Monitor full blood count after 4 weeks of treatment, then every 3 months.

- **DIRECTIONS FOR ADMINISTRATION** For *intermittent intravenous infusion*, dilute to a concentration of 2 mg/mL or 4 mg/mL with Glucose 5% and give over 1 hour.

- **PRESCRIBING AND DISPENSING INFORMATION** The abbreviation AZT which is sometimes used for zidovudine has also been used for another drug.

- **MEDICINAL FORMS**
There can be variation in the licensing of different medicines containing the same drug.

Solution for infusion
‣ Retrovir (ViiV Healthcare UK Ltd)
 Zidovudine 10 mg per 1 ml Retrovir IV 200mg/20ml concentrate for solution for infusion vials | 5 vial [PoM] £44.61

Oral solution
‣ Retrovir (ViiV Healthcare UK Ltd)
 Zidovudine 10 mg per 1 ml Retrovir 50mg/5ml oral solution sugar-free | 200 ml [PoM] £17.78

Capsule
‣ Zidovudine (Non-proprietary)
 Zidovudine 100 mg Zidovudine 100mg capsules | 60 capsule [PoM] no price available
 Zidovudine 250 mg Zidovudine 250mg capsules | 60 capsule [PoM] no price available
‣ Retrovir (ViiV Healthcare UK Ltd)
 Zidovudine 100 mg Retrovir 100mg capsules | 100 capsule [PoM] £88.86
 Zidovudine 250 mg Retrovir 250mg capsules | 40 capsule [PoM] £88.86

Zidovudine with lamivudine

The properties listed below are those particular to the combination only. For the properties of the components please consider, zidovudine p. 403, lamivudine p. 401.

- **INDICATIONS AND DOSE**

 HIV infection in combination with other antiretroviral drugs
 ‣ BY MOUTH
 ‣ Child (body-weight 14–20 kg): 0.5 tablet twice daily
 ‣ Child (body-weight 21–29 kg): 0.5 tablet daily, to be given in the morning and 1 tablet daily, to be given in the evening
 ‣ Child (body-weight 30 kg and above): 1 tablet twice daily

- **INTERACTIONS** → Appendix 1: lamivudine, zidovudine
- **RENAL IMPAIRMENT** Avoid if estimated glomerular filtration rate less than 50 mL/minute/1.73 m^2.

- **DIRECTIONS FOR ADMINISTRATION**
COMBIVIR® TABLETS Tablets may be crushed and mixed with semi-solid food or liquid just before administration.

- **MEDICINAL FORMS**
There can be variation in the licensing of different medicines containing the same drug.

Tablet
‣ Zidovudine with lamivudine (Non-proprietary)
 Lamivudine 150 mg, Zidovudine 300 mg Zidovudine 300mg / Lamivudine 150mg tablets | 60 tablet [PoM] £240.10–£285.11
‣ Combivir (ViiV Healthcare UK Ltd)
 Lamivudine 150 mg, Zidovudine 300 mg Combivir 150mg/300mg tablets | 60 tablet [PoM] £255.10

ANTIVIRALS > PROTEASE INHIBITORS

Protease inhibitors

- **CONTRA-INDICATIONS** Acute porphyrias p. 577
- **CAUTIONS** Haemophilia (increased risk of bleeding)
- **SIDE-EFFECTS** Abdominal pain · anaemia · anaphylaxis · anorexia · blood disorders · diarrhoea · dizziness · fatigue · flatulence · gastro-intestinal disturbances · headache · hepatic dysfunction · hypersensitivity reactions · metabolic effects · myalgia · myositis · nausea · neutropenia · osteonecrosis · pancreatitis · paraesthesia · pruritus · rash · rhabdomyolysis · sleep disturbances · Stevens-Johnson syndrome · taste disturbances · thrombocytopenia · vomiting

SIDE-EFFECTS, FURTHER INFORMATION
‣ Osteonecrosis For further information see HIV infection p. 391.
- **HEPATIC IMPAIRMENT** Use with caution in patients with chronic hepatitis B or C (increased risk of hepatic side-effects).

 above

Atazanavir

- **INDICATIONS AND DOSE**

 HIV infection in combination with other antiretroviral drugs—with low-dose ritonavir
 ‣ BY MOUTH
 ‣ Child 6–17 years (body-weight 15–19 kg): 150 mg once daily
 ‣ Child 6–17 years (body-weight 20–39 kg): 200 mg once daily
 ‣ Child 6–17 years (body-weight 40 kg and above): 300 mg once daily

- **CAUTIONS** Cardiac conduction disorders · electrolyte disturbances · predisposition to QT interval prolongation
- **INTERACTIONS** → Appendix 1: HIV-protease inhibitors
- **SIDE-EFFECTS**
‣ **Common or very common** AV block
‣ **Uncommon** Abnormal dreams · alopecia · amnesia · anxiety · arthralgia · chest pain · cholelithiasis · depression · disorientation · dry mouth · dyspnoea · gynaecomastia · haematuria · hypertension · increased appetite · mouth ulcers · nephrolithiasis · peripheral neuropathy · proteinuria · syncope · torsade de pointes · urinary frequency · weight changes
‣ **Rare** Abnormal gait · cholecystitis · hepatosplenomegaly · oedema · palpitation

SIDE-EFFECTS, FURTHER INFORMATION
‣ Rash Mild to moderate rash occurs commonly, usually within the first 3 weeks of therapy. Severe rash occurs less frequently and may be accompanied by systemic symptoms. Discontinue if severe rash develops.

- **PREGNANCY** Theoretical risk of hyperbilirubinaemia in neonate if used at term. Monitor viral load and plasma-atazanavir concentration during third trimester.
- **HEPATIC IMPAIRMENT** Manufacturer advises caution in mild impairment; avoid in moderate to severe impairment.

- **MEDICINAL FORMS**
There can be variation in the licensing of different medicines containing the same drug.

Capsule
CAUTIONARY AND ADVISORY LABELS 5, 21
‣ Reyataz (Bristol-Myers Squibb Pharmaceuticals Ltd)
 Atazanavir (as Atazanavir sulfate) 150 mg Reyataz 150mg capsules | 60 capsule [PoM] £303.38 (Hospital only)
 Atazanavir (as Atazanavir sulfate) 200 mg Reyataz 200mg capsules | 60 capsule [PoM] £303.38 (Hospital only)
 Atazanavir (as Atazanavir sulfate) 300 mg Reyataz 300mg capsules | 30 capsule [PoM] £303.38 (Hospital only)

above

Darunavir

- **INDICATIONS AND DOSE**

 HIV infection in combination with other antiretroviral drugs in patients previously treated with antiretroviral therapy—with low-dose ritonavir
 ‣ BY MOUTH
 ‣ Child 3–17 years (body-weight 15–29 kg): 375 mg twice daily
 ‣ Child 3–17 years (body-weight 30–39 kg): 450 mg twice daily

5

Infection

- Child 3-17 years (body-weight 40 kg and above): 600 mg twice daily
- Child 12-17 years: 800 mg once daily, once daily dose only to be used if no resistance to darunavir, if plasma HIV-RNA concentration less than 100 000 copies/mL, and if CD4 cell count greater than 100 cells × 10^6/litre

HIV infection in combination with other antiretroviral drugs in patients not previously treated with antiretroviral therapy—with low-dose ritonavir
▸ BY MOUTH
- Child 12-17 years (body-weight 40 kg and above): 800 mg once daily

● INTERACTIONS → Appendix 1: HIV-protease inhibitors
● SIDE-EFFECTS
▸ **Common or very common** Peripheral neuropathy · rash
▸ **Uncommon** Abnormal dreams · acne · alopecia · anxiety · arthralgia · chest pain · conjunctival hyperaemia · cough · depression · dry eyes · dry mouth · dyspnoea · dysuria · eczema · erectile dysfunction · flushing · gynaecomastia · hypertension · hypothyroidism · increased appetite · increased sweating · memory impairment · myocardial infarction · nail discoloration · nephrolithiasis · osteoporosis · peripheral oedema · polyuria · pyrexia · QT interval prolongation · reduced libido · renal failure · severe skin rash · Stevens-Johnson syndrome · stomatitis · tachycardia · throat irritation · toxic epidermal necrolysis · weight changes
▸ **Rare** Bradycardia · confusion · convulsions · haematemesis · palpitation · rhinorrhoea · seborrhoeic dermatits · syncope · visual disturbances
SIDE-EFFECTS, FURTHER INFORMATION
▸ Rash Mild to moderate rash occurs commonly, usually within the first 4 weeks of therapy and resolves without stopping treatment. Severe skin rash (including Stevens-Johnson syndrome and toxic epidermal necrolysis) occurs less frequently and may be accompanied by fever, malaise, arthralgia, myalgia, oral lesions, conjunctivitis, hepatitis, or eosinophilia; treatment should be stopped if severe rash develops.

● ALLERGY AND CROSS-SENSITIVITY Use with caution in patients with sulfonamide sensitivity.
● PREGNANCY Manufacturer advises use only if potential benefit outweighs risk; if required, use the twice daily dose regimen.
● HEPATIC IMPAIRMENT Manufacturer advises caution in mild to moderate impairment; avoid in severe impairment—no information available.
● MONITORING REQUIREMENTS Monitor liver function before and during treatment.
● PRESCRIBING AND DISPENSING INFORMATION Flavours of oral liquid formulations may include strawberry.
● PATIENT AND CARER ADVICE
Missed doses
If a dose is more than 6 hours late on the twice daily regimen (or more than 12 hours late on the once daily regimen), the missed dose should not be taken and the next dose should be taken at the normal time.

● MEDICINAL FORMS
There can be variation in the licensing of different medicines containing the same drug.
Oral suspension
CAUTIONARY AND ADVISORY LABELS 21
▸ Prezista (Janssen-Cilag Ltd)
 Darunavir (as Darunavir ethanolate) 100 mg per 1 ml Prezista 100mg/ml oral suspension sugar-free | 200 ml [PoM] £248.17
Tablet
CAUTIONARY AND ADVISORY LABELS 21
▸ Prezista (Janssen-Cilag Ltd)
 Darunavir (as Darunavir ethanolate) 75 mg Prezista 75mg tablets | 480 tablet [PoM] £446.70

Darunavir (as Darunavir ethanolate) 150 mg Prezista 150mg tablets | 240 tablet [PoM] £446.70
Darunavir (as Darunavir ethanolate) 400 mg Prezista 400mg tablets | 60 tablet [PoM] £297.80
Darunavir (as Darunavir ethanolate) 600 mg Prezista 600mg tablets | 60 tablet [PoM] £446.70
Darunavir (as Darunavir ethanolate) 800 mg Prezista 800mg tablets | 30 tablet [PoM] £297.80

F 404

Fosamprenavir
● DRUG ACTION Fosamprenavir is a pro-drug of amprenavir.

● INDICATIONS AND DOSE
HIV infection in combination with other antiretroviral drugs—with low-dose ritonavir
▸ BY MOUTH
- Child 6-17 years (body-weight 25-39 kg): 18 mg/kg twice daily (max. per dose 700 mg)
- Child 6-17 years (body-weight 40 kg and above): 700 mg twice daily
DOSE EQUIVALENCE AND CONVERSION
▸ 700 mg fosamprenavir is equivalent to approximately 600 mg amprenavir.

● INTERACTIONS → Appendix 1: HIV-protease inhibitors
● SIDE-EFFECTS
▸ **Rare** Stevens-Johnson syndrome
▸ **Frequency not known** Rash
SIDE-EFFECTS, FURTHER INFORMATION
▸ Rash Rash may occur, usually in the second week of therapy; discontinue permanently if severe rash with systemic or allergic symptoms or, mucosal involvement; if rash mild or moderate, may continue without interruption—usually resolves within 2 weeks and may respond to antihistamines.
● PREGNANCY Toxicity in *animal* studies; manufacturer advises use only if potential benefit outweighs risk.
● HEPATIC IMPAIRMENT Reduce dose in moderate to severe impairment. Manufacturer advises caution in mild impairment.
● DIRECTIONS FOR ADMINISTRATION In children, oral suspension should be taken with food.
● PRESCRIBING AND DISPENSING INFORMATION Flavours of oral liquid formulations may include grape, bubblegum, or peppermint.
● PATIENT AND CARER ADVICE Patients or carers should be given advice on how to administer fosamprenavir oral suspension.

● MEDICINAL FORMS
There can be variation in the licensing of different medicines containing the same drug.
Oral suspension
EXCIPIENTS: May contain Propylene glycol
▸ Telzir (ViiV Healthcare UK Ltd)
 Fosamprenavir (as Fosamprenavir calcium) 50 mg per 1 ml Telzir 50mg/ml oral suspension | 225 ml [PoM] £58.70
Tablet
▸ Telzir (ViiV Healthcare UK Ltd)
 Fosamprenavir (as Fosamprenavir calcium) 700 mg Telzir 700mg tablets | 60 tablet [PoM] £220.13

F 404

Lopinavir with ritonavir
● INDICATIONS AND DOSE
HIV infection in combination with other antiretroviral drugs
▸ BY MOUTH USING TABLETS
- Child 2-17 years (body-weight up to 40 kg and body surface area 0.5-0.7 m^2): 200/50 mg twice daily   continued →

- Child 2-17 years (body-weight up to 40 kg and body surface area 0.8-1.1 m²): 300/75 mg twice daily
- Child 2-17 years (body-weight 40 kg and above and body surface area 1.2 m² and above): 400/100 mg twice daily
- BY MOUTH USING ORAL SOLUTION
- Child 2-17 years: 2.9 mL/m² twice daily (max. per dose 5 mL), to be taken with food, oral solution contains 400 mg lopinavir, 100 mg ritonavir/5 mL

- **CAUTIONS** Cardiac conduction disorders · pancreatitis · structural heart disease
- **INTERACTIONS** → Appendix 1: HIV-protease inhibitors
- **SIDE-EFFECTS**
- **Common or very common** Amenorrhoea · anxiety · arthralgia · colitis · hypertension · menorrhagia · neuropathy · night sweats · sexual dysfunction · weight changes
- **Uncommon** Abnormal dreams · alopecia · artherosclerosis · AV block · cerebrovascular accident · convulsions · deep vein thrombosis · dry mouth · gastro-intestinal ulcer · haematuria · nephritis · rectal bleeding · stomatitis · tinnitus · tremor · visual disturbances

  SIDE-EFFECTS, FURTHER INFORMATION
- Pancreatitis Signs and symptoms suggestive of pancreatitis (including raised serum lipase) should be evaluated—discontinue if pancreatitis diagnosed
- **PREGNANCY** Avoid oral solution due to high propylene glycol content; use tablets only if potential benefit outweighs risk (toxicity in *animal* studies).
- **HEPATIC IMPAIRMENT** Avoid oral solution due to propylene glycol content; manufacturer advises avoid tablets in severe impairment.
- **RENAL IMPAIRMENT** Avoid oral solution due to high propylene glycol content.
- **MONITORING REQUIREMENTS** Monitor liver function before and during treatment.
- **PATIENT AND CARER ADVICE** Oral solution tastes bitter.

- **MEDICINAL FORMS**
  There can be variation in the licensing of different medicines containing the same drug.
  Oral solution
  CAUTIONARY AND ADVISORY LABELS 21
  EXCIPIENTS: May contain Alcohol, propylene glycol
- **Kaletra** (AbbVie Ltd)
  Ritonavir 20 mg per 1 ml, Lopinavir 80 mg per 1 ml Kaletra 80mg/20mg/1ml oral solution | 300 ml [PoM] £307.39
  Tablet
  CAUTIONARY AND ADVISORY LABELS 25
- **Kaletra** (AbbVie Ltd)
  Ritonavir 25 mg, Lopinavir 100 mg Kaletra 100mg/25mg tablets | 60 tablet [PoM] £76.85
  Ritonavir 50 mg, Lopinavir 200 mg Kaletra 200mg/50mg tablets | 120 tablet [PoM] £285.41

  F 404

Ritonavir

- **INDICATIONS AND DOSE**

HIV infection in combination with other antiretroviral drugs (high-dose ritonavir)
- BY MOUTH
- Child 2-17 years: Initially 250 mg/m² twice daily, increased in steps of 50 mg/m² every 2–3 days; increased to 350 mg/m² twice daily (max. per dose 600 mg twice daily), tolerability of this regimen is poor

Low-dose ritonavir to increase the effect of atazanavir
- BY MOUTH
- Child 6-17 years (body-weight 15-19 kg): 80–100 mg once daily

- Child 6-17 years (body-weight 20 kg and above): 100 mg once daily

Low-dose ritonavir to increase the effect of darunavir
- BY MOUTH
- Child 3-17 years (body-weight 15-29 kg): 50 mg twice daily
- Child 3-17 years (body-weight 30-39 kg): 60 mg twice daily
- Child 3-17 years (body-weight 40 kg and above): 100 mg twice daily
- Child 12-17 years (body-weight 40 kg and above): 100 mg once daily for use in patients taking darunavir once daily

Low-dose ritonavir to increase the effect of fosamprenavir
- BY MOUTH
- Child 6-17 years (body-weight 25-32 kg): 3 mg/kg twice daily
- Child 6-17 years (body-weight 33 kg and above): 100 mg twice daily

Low-dose ritonavir to increase the effect of tipranavir
- BY MOUTH
- Child 2-11 years: 150 mg/m² twice daily (max. per dose 200 mg)
- Child 12-17 years: 200 mg twice daily

- **CAUTIONS** Cardiac conduction disorders · pancreatitis · structural heart disease
- **INTERACTIONS** → Appendix 1: HIV-protease inhibitors
- **SIDE-EFFECTS**
- **Common or very common** Acne · anxiety · arthralgia · blood pressure changes · blurred vision · confusion · cough · decreased blood thyroxine concentration · fever · flushing · gastro-intestinal haemorrhage · menorrhagia · mouth ulcers · oedema · peripheral neuropathy · pharyngitis · renal impairment · seizures · syncope
- **Uncommon** Electrolyte disturbances · myocardial infarction
- **Rare** Toxic epidermal necrolysis

  SIDE-EFFECTS, FURTHER INFORMATION
- Pancreatitis Signs and symptoms suggestive of pancreatitis (including raised serum lipase) should be evaluated—discontinue if pancreatitis diagnosed
- **PREGNANCY** Only use low-dose booster to increase the effect of other protease inhibitors.
- **HEPATIC IMPAIRMENT** Avoid in decompensated liver disease; in severe impairment without decompensation, use 'booster' doses with caution (avoid treatment doses).
- **DIRECTIONS FOR ADMINISTRATION** Bitter taste of oral solution can be masked by mixing with chocolate milk; do not mix with water, measuring cup must be dry.
- **PATIENT AND CARER ADVICE** Patients or carers should be given advice on how to administer ritonavir oral solution.

- **MEDICINAL FORMS**
  There can be variation in the licensing of different medicines containing the same drug.
  Tablet
  CAUTIONARY AND ADVISORY LABELS 21, 25
- **Norvir** (AbbVie Ltd)
  Ritonavir 100 mg Norvir 100mg tablets | 30 tablet [PoM] £19.44

  F 404

Tipranavir

- **INDICATIONS AND DOSE**

HIV infection resistant to other protease inhibitors, in combination with other antiretroviral drugs in patients previously treated with antiretrovirals–with low-dose ritonavir
- BY MOUTH USING CAPSULES
- Child 12-17 years: 500 mg twice daily

‣ BY MOUTH USING ORAL SOLUTION
‣ Child 2-11 years: 375 mg/m^2 twice daily (max. per dose 500 mg)

DOSE EQUIVALENCE AND CONVERSION
‣ The bioavailability of tipranavir oral solution is higher than that of the capsules; the oral solution is not interchangeable with the capsules on a milligram-for-milligram basis.

● **CAUTIONS** Patients at risk of increased bleeding from trauma, surgery or other pathological conditions
● **INTERACTIONS** → Appendix 1: HIV-protease inhibitors
● **SIDE-EFFECTS**
‣ **Rare** Dehydration
‣ **Frequency not known** Anorexia · dyspnoea · influenza-like symptoms · peripheral neuropathy · photosensitivity · renal impairment
SIDE-EFFECTS, FURTHER INFORMATION
‣ **Hepatotoxicity** Potentially life-threatening hepatotoxicity reported. Discontinue if signs or symptoms of hepatitis develop or if liver-function abnormality develops (consult product literature).
● **PREGNANCY** Manufacturer advises use only if potential benefit outweighs risk—toxicity in *animal* studies.
● **HEPATIC IMPAIRMENT** Manufacturer advises caution in mild impairment; avoid in moderate or severe impairment—no information available.
● **MONITORING REQUIREMENTS** Monitor liver function before treatment then every 2 weeks for 1 month, then every 3 months.
● **PRESCRIBING AND DISPENSING INFORMATION** Flavours of oral liquid formulations may include toffee and mint.
● **PATIENT AND CARER ADVICE** Patients or carers should be told to observe the oral solution for crystallisation; the bottle should be replaced if more than a thin layer of crystals form (doses should continue to be taken at the normal time until the bottle is replaced).

● **MEDICINAL FORMS**
There can be variation in the licensing of different medicines containing the same drug.
Oral solution
CAUTIONARY AND ADVISORY LABELS 5, 21
EXCIPIENTS: May contain Vitamin e
‣ **Aptivus** (Boehringer Ingelheim Ltd)
Tipranavir 100 mg per 1 ml Aptivus 100mg/ml oral solution sugar-free | 95 ml PoM £129.65
Capsule
CAUTIONARY AND ADVISORY LABELS 5, 21
EXCIPIENTS: May contain Ethanol
‣ **Aptivus** (Boehringer Ingelheim Ltd)
Tipranavir 250 mg Aptivus 250mg capsules | 120 capsule PoM £441.00

ANTIVIRALS ⟩ OTHER

Maraviroc

● **DRUG ACTION** Maraviroc is an antagonist of the CCR5 chemokine receptor.

● **INDICATIONS AND DOSE**
CCR5-tropic HIV infection in combination with other antiretroviral drugs in patients previously treated with antiretrovirals
‣ BY MOUTH
‣ Child: (consult local protocol)

● **UNLICENSED USE** Not licensed for use in children.
● **CAUTIONS** Cardiovascular disease
● **INTERACTIONS** → Appendix 1: maraviroc

● **SIDE-EFFECTS**
‣ **Common or very common** Abdominal pain · anaemia · anorexia · depression · diarrhoea · flatulence · headache · insomnia · malaise · nausea · rash
‣ **Uncommon** Myositis · proteinuria · renal failure · seizures
‣ **Rare** Angina · granulocytopenia · hepatitis · pancytopenia · Stevens-Johnson syndrome · toxic epidermal necrolysis
‣ **Frequency not known** Eosinophilia · fever · hepatic reactions · hypersensitivity reactions · osteonecrosis · rash
SIDE-EFFECTS, FURTHER INFORMATION
‣ **Osteonecrosis** For further information see HIV infection p. 391.
● **PREGNANCY** Manufacturer advises use only if potential benefit outweighs risk—toxicity in *animal* studies.
● **HEPATIC IMPAIRMENT** Manufacturer advises caution in hepatic impairment, including patients with chronic hepatitis B or C.
● **RENAL IMPAIRMENT** If estimated glomerular filtration rate less than 80 mL/minute/1.73 m^2, consult product literature.

● **MEDICINAL FORMS**
There can be variation in the licensing of different medicines containing the same drug.
Tablet
‣ **Celsentri** (ViiV Healthcare UK Ltd)
Maraviroc 150 mg Celsentri 150mg tablets | 60 tablet PoM £441.27
Maraviroc 300 mg Celsentri 300mg tablets | 60 tablet PoM £441.27

6.5 Influenza

Influenza

Management

Oseltamivir p. 408 and zanamivir p. 409 are most effective for the treatment of influenza if started within a few hours of the onset of symptoms; oseltamivir is licensed for use within 48 hours of the first symptoms while zanamivir is licensed for use within 36 hours of the first symptoms. In otherwise healthy individuals they reduce the duration of symptoms by about 1–1.5 days.

Oseltamivir and zanamivir are licensed for post-exposure prophylaxis of influenza when influenza is circulating in the community. Oseltamivir should be given within 48 hours of exposure to influenza while zanamivir should be given within 36 hours of exposure to influenza. However, in children with severe influenza or in those who are immunocompromised, antivirals may still be effective after this time if viral shedding continues [unlicensed use]. Oseltamivir and zanamivir are also licensed for use in exceptional circumstances (e.g. when vaccination does not cover the infecting strain) to prevent influenza in an epidemic.

There is evidence that some strains of influenza A virus have reduced susceptibility to oseltamivir, but may retain susceptibility to zanamivir. Resistance to oseltamivir may be greater in severely immunocompromised children.

Zanamivir should be reserved for patients who are severely immunocompromised, or when oseltamivir cannot be used, or when resistance to oseltamivir is suspected. For those unable to use the dry powder for inhalation, zanamivir is available as a solution that can be administered by nebuliser or intravenously [unlicensed].

Information on pandemic influenza, avian influenza, and swine influenza may be found at www.gov.uk/phe.

Immunisation against influenza is recommended for persons at high risk, and to reduce transmission of infection.

Oseltamivir in children under 1 year of age

Data on the use of oseltamivir in children under 1 year of age is limited. Furthermore, oseltamivir may be ineffective in neonates because they may not be able to metabolise oseltamivir to its active form. However, oseltamivir can be used (under specialist supervision) for the treatment or post-exposure prophylaxis of influenza in children under 1 year of age. The Department of Health has advised (May 2009) that during a pandemic, treatment with oseltamivir can be overseen by healthcare professionals experienced in assessing children.

Amantadine hydrochloride is licensed for prophylaxis and treatment of influenza A in children over 10 years of age, but it is no longer recommended.

ANTIVIRALS › NEURAMINIDASE INHIBITORS

Oseltamivir

- **DRUG ACTION** Reduces replication of influenza A and B viruses by inhibiting viral neuraminidase.

- **INDICATIONS AND DOSE**

Prevention of influenza
▸ BY MOUTH

▸ Neonate: 3 mg/kg once daily for 10 days for post-exposure prophylaxis.

▸ Child 1-11 months: 3 mg/kg once daily for 10 days for post-exposure prophylaxis

▸ Child 1-12 years (body-weight 10-15 kg): 30 mg once daily for 10 days for post-exposure prophylaxis; for up to 6 weeks during an epidemic

▸ Child 1-12 years (body-weight 15-23 kg): 45 mg once daily for 10 days for post-exposure prophylaxis; for up to 6 weeks during an epidemic

▸ Child 1-12 years (body-weight 23-40 kg): 60 mg once daily for 10 days for post-exposure prophylaxis; for up to 6 weeks during an epidemic

▸ Child 1-12 years (body-weight 40 kg and above): 75 mg once daily for 10 days for post-exposure prophylaxis; for up to 6 weeks during an epidemic

▸ Child 13-17 years: 75 mg once daily for 10 days for post-exposure prophylaxis; for up to 6 weeks during an epidemic

Treatment of influenza
▸ BY MOUTH

▸ Neonate: 3 mg/kg twice daily for 5 days.

▸ Child 1-11 months: 3 mg/kg twice daily for 5 days
▸ Child 1-12 years (body-weight 10-15 kg): 30 mg twice daily for 5 days
▸ Child 1-12 years (body-weight 15-23 kg): 45 mg twice daily for 5 days
▸ Child 1-12 years (body-weight 23-40 kg): 60 mg twice daily for 5 days
▸ Child 1-12 years (body-weight 40 kg and above): 75 mg twice daily for 5 days
▸ Child 13-17 years: 75 mg twice daily for 5 days

- **UNLICENSED USE** Not licensed for use in premature infants.

- **SIDE-EFFECTS**
▸ **Common or very common** Abdominal pain · dyspepsia · headache · nausea · vomiting
▸ **Uncommon** Altered consciousness · arrhythmias · convulsions · eczema · rash
▸ **Rare** Gastro-intestinal bleeding · hepatitis · neuropsychiatric disorders · Stevens-Johnson syndrome · thrombocytopenia · toxic epidermal necrolysis · visual disturbances

- **PREGNANCY** Although safety data are limited, oseltamivir can be used in women who are pregnant when the potential benefit outweighs the risk (e.g. during a pandemic). Use only if potential benefit outweighs risk (e.g. during a pandemic).

- **BREAST FEEDING** Although safety data are limited, oseltamivir can be used in women who are breast-feeding when the potential benefit outweighs the risk (e.g. during a pandemic). Oseltamivir is the preferred drug in women who are breast-feeding. Amount probably too small to be harmful; use only if potential benefit outweighs risk (e.g. during a pandemic).

- **RENAL IMPAIRMENT**
For *treatment*, use 40% of normal dose twice daily if estimated glomerular filtration rate 30-60 mL/minute/1.73 m^2 (40% of normal dose once daily if estimated glomerular filtration rate 10-30 mL/minute/1.73 m^2).

For *prevention*, use 40% of normal dose once daily if estimated glomerular filtration rate 30-60 mL/minute/1.73 m^2 (40% of normal dose every 48 hours if estimated glomerular filtration rate 10-30 mL/minute/1.73 m^2).

Avoid for *treatment* and *prevention* if estimated glomerular filtration rate less than 10 mL/minute/1.73 m^2.

- **DIRECTIONS FOR ADMINISTRATION** If suspension not available, capsules can be opened and the contents mixed with a small amount of sweetened food, such as sugar water or chocolate syrup, just before administration.

- **PRESCRIBING AND DISPENSING INFORMATION** Flavours of oral liquid formulations may include tutti-frutti.

- **PATIENT AND CARER ADVICE**
Medicines for Children leaflet: Oseltamivir for influenza (flu) www.medicinesforchildren.org.uk/oseltamivir-for-influenza

- **NATIONAL FUNDING/ACCESS DECISIONS**
NICE technology appraisals (TAs)
▸ Oseltamivir, zanamivir, and amantadine for prophylaxis of influenza (September 2008) NICE TA158
Oseltamivir is **not** a substitute for vaccination, which remains the most effective way of preventing illness from influenza.
- Oseltamivir is **not** recommended for seasonal prophylaxis against influenza.
- When influenza is circulating in the community, oseltamivir is a treatment option recommended (in accordance with UK licensing) for post-exposure prophylaxis in at-risk patients who are not effectively protected by influenza vaccine, and who have been in close contact with someone suffering from influenza-like illness in the same household or residential setting. Oseltamivir should be given within 48 hours of exposure to influenza. (National surveillance schemes, including those run by Public Health England, should be used to indicate when influenza is circulating in the community.)
- During local outbreaks of influenza-like illness, when there is a high level of certainty that influenza is present, oseltamivir may be used for post-exposure prophylaxis in at-risk patients (regardless of influenza vaccination) living in long-term residential or nursing homes.
At risk patients are those who have one or more of the following conditions:
- chronic respiratory disease (including asthma);
- chronic heart disease;
- chronic renal disease;
- chronic liver disease;
- chronic neurological disease;
- immunosuppression;
- diabetes mellitus.

The Department of Health in England has advised (November 2010 and April 2011) that 'at risk patients' also includes children who are at risk of developing medical complications from influenza (treatment only) or females who are pregnant.

This guidance does not cover the circumstances of a pandemic, an impending pandemic, or a widespread epidemic of a new strain of influenza to which there is little or no immunity in the community.
www.nice.org.uk/TA158

▸ **Oseltamivir, zanamivir, and amantadine for treatment of influenza (February 2009)** NICE TA168

Oseltamivir is **not** a substitute for vaccination, which remains the most effective way of preventing illness from influenza.

- When influenza is circulating in the community, oseltamivir is an option recommended (in accordance with UK licensing) for the treatment of influenza in at-risk patients who can start treatment within 48 hours of the onset of symptoms. (National surveillance schemes, including those run by Public Health England, should be used to indicate when influenza is circulating in the community.)
- During local outbreaks of influenza-like illness, when there is a high level of certainty that influenza is present, oseltamivir may be used for treatment in at-risk patients living in long-term residential or nursing homes.

At risk patients are those who have one or more of the following conditions:

- chronic respiratory disease (including asthma and chronic obstructive pulmonary disease);
- chronic heart disease;
- chronic renal disease;
- chronic liver disease;
- chronic neurological disease;
- immunosuppression;
- diabetes mellitus.

The Department of Health in England has advised (November 2010 and April 2011) that 'at risk patients' also includes children who are at risk of developing medical complications from influenza (treatment only) or females who are pregnant.

This guidance does not cover the circumstances of a pandemic, an impending pandemic, or a widespread epidemic of a new strain of influenza to which there is little or no immunity in the community.
www.nice.org.uk/TA168

NHS restrictions Except for the treatment and prophylaxis of influenza as indicated in the NICE guidance; endorse prescription 'SLS'.

- **MEDICINAL FORMS**
There can be variation in the licensing of different medicines containing the same drug. Forms available from special-order manufacturers include: oral suspension, oral solution

Oral solution
CAUTIONARY AND ADVISORY LABELS 9
▸ **Oseltamivir (Non-proprietary)**
Oseltamivir (as Oseltamivir phosphate) 15 mg per 1 ml Oseltamivir 15mg/ml oral solution sugar free sugar-free | 20 ml [PoM] £10.00

Oral suspension
CAUTIONARY AND ADVISORY LABELS 9
EXCIPIENTS: May contain Sorbitol
▸ **Tamiflu** (Roche Products Ltd)
Oseltamivir (as Oseltamivir phosphate) 6 mg per 1 ml Tamiflu 6mg/ml oral suspension sugar-free | 65 ml [PoM] £10.27

Capsule
CAUTIONARY AND ADVISORY LABELS 9
▸ **Tamiflu** (Roche Products Ltd)
Oseltamivir (as Oseltamivir phosphate) 30 mg Tamiflu 30mg capsules | 10 capsule [PoM] £7.71

Oseltamivir (as Oseltamivir phosphate) 45 mg Tamiflu 45mg capsules | 10 capsule [PoM] £15.41
Oseltamivir (as Oseltamivir phosphate) 75 mg Tamiflu 75mg capsules | 10 capsule [PoM] £15.41

Zanamivir

- **DRUG ACTION** Reduces replication of influenza A and B viruses by inhibiting viral neuraminidase.

- **INDICATIONS AND DOSE**

Post-exposure prophylaxis of influenza
▸ BY INHALATION OF POWDER
▸ Child 5–17 years: 10 mg once daily for 10 days

Prevention of influenza during an epidemic
▸ BY INHALATION OF POWDER
▸ Child 5–17 years: 10 mg once daily for up to 28 days

Treatment of influenza
▸ BY INHALATION OF POWDER
▸ Child 5–17 years: 10 mg twice daily for 5 days (for up to 10 days if resistance to oseltamivir suspected)

- **UNLICENSED USE** Use of zanamivir for up to 10 days if resistance to oseltamivir suspected is an unlicensed duration.

- **CAUTIONS** Asthma · chronic pulmonary disease · uncontrolled chronic illness
CAUTIONS, FURTHER INFORMATION
▸ Asthma and chronic pulmonary disease Risk of bronchospasm—short-acting bronchodilator should be available. Avoid in severe asthma unless close monitoring possible and appropriate facilities available to treat bronchospasm.

- **SIDE-EFFECTS**
▸ **Common or very common** Rash
▸ **Uncommon** Angioedema · bronchospasm · dyspnoea · urticaria
▸ **Rare** Neuropsychiatric disorders · Stevens-Johnson syndrome · toxic epidermal necrolysis

- **PREGNANCY** Although safety data are limited, zanamivir can be used in women who are pregnant when the potential benefit outweighs the risk (e.g. during a pandemic). Use only if potential benefit outweighs risk (e.g. during a pandemic).

- **BREAST FEEDING** Although safety data are limited, zanamivir can be used in women who are breast-feeding when the potential benefit outweighs the risk (e.g. during a pandemic). Amount probably too small to be harmful; use only if potential benefit outweighs risk (e.g. during a pandemic).

- **DIRECTIONS FOR ADMINISTRATION** Other inhaled drugs should be administered before zanamivir.

- **PRESCRIBING AND DISPENSING INFORMATION** Except for the treatment and prophylaxis of influenza as indicated in the NICE guidance; endorse prescription 'SLS'.

- **NATIONAL FUNDING/ACCESS DECISIONS**

NICE technology appraisals (TAs)
▸ **Oseltamivir, zanamivir, and amantadine for prophylaxis of influenza (September 2008)** NICE TA158
Zanamivir is not a substitute for vaccination, which remains the most effective way of preventing illness from influenza.
- Zanamivir is not recommended for seasonal prophylaxis against influenza.
- When influenza is circulating in the community, zanamivir is an option recommended (in accordance with UK licensing) for post-exposure prophylaxis in at-risk patients who are not effectively protected by influenza vaccine, and who have been in close contact with someone suffering from influenza-like illness in the

same household or residential setting. Zanamivir should be given within 36 hours of exposure to influenza. (National surveillance schemes, including those run by Public Health England, should be used to indicate when influenza is circulating in the community.)

- During local outbreaks of influenza-like illness, when there is a high level of certainty that influenza is present, zanamivir may be used for post-exposure prophylaxis in at-risk patients (regardless of influenza vaccination) living in long-term residential or nursing homes.

At risk patients are those who have one or more of the following conditions:
- chronic respiratory disease (including asthma and chronic obstructive pulmonary disease);
- chronic heart disease;
- chronic renal disease;
- chronic liver disease;
- chronic neurological disease;
- immunosuppression;
- diabetes mellitus.

The Department of Health in England has advised (November 2010 and April 2011) that 'at risk patients' also includes children who are at risk of developing medical complications from influenza (treatment only) or females who are pregnant.

This guidance does not cover the circumstances of a pandemic, an impending pandemic, or a widespread epidemic of a new strain of influenza to which there is little or no immunity in the community.
www.nice.org.uk/TA158

▶ **Oseltamivir, zanamivir, and amantadine for treatment of influenza (February 2009)** NICE TA168

Zanamivir is not a substitute for vaccination, which remains the most effective way of preventing illness from influenza.

- When influenza is circulating in the community, zanamivir is an option recommended (in accordance with UK licensing) for the treatment of influenza in at-risk patients who can start treatment within 36 hours of the onset of symptoms. (National surveillance schemes, including those run by Public Health England, should be used to indicate when influenza is circulating in the community.)
- During local outbreaks of influenza-like illness, when there is a high level of certainty that influenza is present, zanamivir may be used for treatment in at-risk patients living in long-term residential or nursing homes.

At risk patients are those who have one or more of the following conditions:
- chronic respiratory disease (including asthma and chronic obstructive pulmonary disease);
- chronic heart disease;
- chronic renal disease;
- chronic liver disease;
- chronic neurological disease;
- immunosuppression;
- diabetes mellitus.

The Department of Health in England has advised (November 2010 and April 2011) that 'at risk patients' also includes children who are at risk of developing medical complications from influenza (treatment only) or females who are pregnant.

This guidance does not cover the circumstances of a pandemic, an impending pandemic, or a widespread epidemic of a new strain of influenza to which there is little or no immunity in the community.
www.nice.org.uk/TA168

- **MEDICINAL FORMS**
  There can be variation in the licensing of different medicines containing the same drug.

Inhalation powder
- ▶ Relenza (GlaxoSmithKline UK Ltd)
  Zanamivir 5 mg Relenza 5mg inhalation powder blisters with Diskhaler | 20 blister [PoM] £16.36

6.6 Respiratory syncytial virus

Respiratory syncytial virus

Management

Ribavirin p. 384 inhibits a wide range of DNA and RNA viruses. It is licensed for administration by inhalation for the treatment of severe bronchiolitis caused by the respiratory syncytial virus (RSV) in infants, especially when they have other serious diseases. However, there is no evidence that ribavirin produces clinically relevant benefit in RSV bronchiolitis. Ribavirin is effective in Lassa fever and has also been used parenterally in the treatment of life-threatening RSV, parainfluenza virus, and adenovirus infections in immunocompromised children [unlicensed indications].

Palivizumab p. 410 is a monoclonal antibody licensed for preventing serious lower respiratory-tract disease caused by respiratory syncytial virus in children at high risk of the disease; it should be prescribed under specialist supervision and on the basis of the likelihood of hospitalisation. Palivizumab is recommended for:

- children under 9 months of age with chronic lung disease (defined as requiring oxygen for at least 28 days from birth) and who were born preterm;
- children under 6 months of age with haemodynamically significant, acyanotic congenital heart disease who were born preterm;

Palivizumab should be considered for

- children under 2 years of age with severe combined immunodeficiency syndrome;
- children under 1 year of age who require long-term ventilation;
- children 1–2 years of age who require long-term ventilation and have an additional co-morbidity (including cardiac disease or pulmonary hypertension).

For details of the preterm age groups included in the recommendations, see *Immunisation against Infectious Disease* (2006), available at www.gov.uk/dh.

DRUGS FOR RESPIRATORY DISEASES ⟩
MONOCLONAL ANTIBODIES

Palivizumab

- **INDICATIONS AND DOSE**

Prevention of serious lower respiratory-tract disease caused by respiratory syncytial virus in children at high risk of the disease (under expert supervision)
▶ BY INTRAMUSCULAR INJECTION

- ▶ Neonate: 15 mg/kg once a month, preferably injected in the anterolateral thigh, to be administered during season of RSV risk.

- ▶ Child 1–23 months: 15 mg/kg once a month, preferably injected in the anterolateral thigh, to be administered during season of RSV risk, injection volume over 1 mL should be divided between 2 or more sites

Prevention of serious lower respiratory-tract disease caused by respiratory syncytial virus in children at high risk of the disease and undergoing cardiac bypass surgery (under expert supervision)
▶ BY INTRAMUSCULAR INJECTION
▶ Child 1–23 months: Initially 15 mg/kg, to be administered as soon as stable after surgery, preferably in the anterolateral thigh, then 15 mg/kg once a month, preferably injected in the anterolateral thigh, to be administered during season of RSV risk, injection volume over 1 mL should be divided between 2 or more sites

● **UNLICENSED USE** Licensed for the prevention of serious lower respiratory-tract disease caused by respiratory syncytial virus (RSV) in children under 6 months of age (at the start of the RSV season) and born at less than 35 weeks corrected gestational age, or in children under 2 years of age who have received treatment for bronchopulmonary dysplasia in the last 6 months, or in children under 2 years of age with haemodynamically significant congenital heart disease.

● **CAUTIONS** Moderate to severe acute infection · moderate to severe febrile illness · serum-palivizumab concentration may be reduced after cardiac surgery · thrombocytopenia

● **SIDE-EFFECTS**
▶ **Common or very common** Fever · injection-site reactions · nervousness
▶ **Uncommon** Asthenia · constipation · cough · diarrhoea · drowsiness · haemorrhage · hyperkinesia · leucopenia · pain · rash · rhinitis · vomiting · wheeze
▶ **Frequency not known** Anaphylaxis · apnoea · convulsions · hypersensitivity reactions · thrombocytopenia

● **ALLERGY AND CROSS-SENSITIVITY** Hypersensitivity to humanised monoclonal antibodies.

● **MEDICINAL FORMS**
There can be variation in the licensing of different medicines containing the same drug.
Solution for injection
▶ **Synagis** (AbbVie Ltd)
Palivizumab 100 mg per 1 ml Synagis 100mg/1ml solution for injection vials | 1 vial PoM £563.64
Synagis 50mg/0.5ml solution for injection vials | 1 vial PoM £306.34
Powder and solvent for solution for injection
▶ **Synagis** (AbbVie Ltd)
Palivizumab 50 mg Synagis 50mg powder and solvent for solution for injection vials | 1 vial PoM £306.34
Palivizumab 100 mg Synagis 100mg powder and solvent for solution for injection vials | 1 vial PoM £563.64

5

Infection

Chapter 6
Endocrine system

CONTENTS

1   Antidiuretic hormone disorders

Posterior pituitary hormones and antagonists

Posterior pituitary hormones

Diabetes insipidus

Diabetes insipidus is caused by either a deficiency of anti-diuretic hormone (ADH, vasopressin p. 65) secretion (cranial, neurogenic, or pituitary diabetes insipidus) or by failure of the renal tubules to react to secreted antidiuretic hormone (nephrogenic diabetes insipidus).

Vasopressin (antidiuretic hormone, ADH) is used in the treatment of *pituitary diabetes insipidus* as is its analogue desmopressin below. Dosage is tailored to produce a regular diuresis every 24 hours to avoid water intoxication. Treatment may be required permanently or for a limited period only in diabetes insipidus following trauma or pituitary surgery.

Desmopressin is more potent and has a longer duration of action than vasopressin; unlike vasopressin it has no vasoconstrictor effect. It is given by mouth or intranasally for maintenance therapy, and by injection in the postoperative period or in unconscious patients. Desmopressin is also used in the differential diagnosis of diabetes insipidus; following an intramuscular or intranasal dose, restoration of the ability to concentrate urine after water deprivation confirms a diagnosis of pituitary diabetes insipidus. Failure to respond suggests nephrogenic diabetes insipidus. Fluid input must be managed carefully to avoid hyponatraemia; this test is not usually recommended in young children.

In *nephrogenic* and *partial pituitary diabetes insipidus* benefit may be gained from the paradoxical antidiuretic effect of thiazides.

Other uses

Desmopressin is also used to boost factor VIII concentration in mild to moderate haemophilia and in von Willebrand's disease; it is also used to test fibrinolytic response. Desmopressin also has a role in nocturnal enuresis.

Vasopressin infusion is used to control variceal bleeding in portal hypertension, before introducing more definitive treatment. Terlipressin acetate, a derivative of vasopressin with reportedly less pressor and antidiuretic activity, and octreotide are used similarly but experience in children is limited.

1.1   Diabetes insipidus

> **Other drugs used for Diabetes insipidus** Chlorothiazide, p. 108

PITUITARY AND HYPOTHALAMIC HORMONES AND ANALOGUES > VASOPRESSIN AND ANALOGUES

Desmopressin

09-Jun-2017

- **DRUG ACTION** Desmopressin is an analogue of vasopressin.

- **INDICATIONS AND DOSE**

Diabetes insipidus, treatment
▶ BY MOUTH

▶ Neonate: Initially 1–4 micrograms 2–3 times a day, adjusted according to response.

▶ Child 1–23 months: Initially 10 micrograms 2–3 times a day, adjusted according to response; usual dose 30–150 micrograms daily

▶ Child 2–11 years: Initially 50 micrograms 2–3 times a day, adjusted according to response; usual dose 100–800 micrograms daily

▶ Child 12–17 years: Initially 100 micrograms 2–3 times a day, adjusted according to response; usual dose 0.2–1.2 mg daily

▸ BY SUBLINGUAL ADMINISTRATION
▸ Child 2–17 years: Initially 60 micrograms 3 times a day, adjusted according to response; usual dose 40–240 micrograms 3 times a day
▸ BY INTRANASAL ADMINISTRATION
▸ Neonate: Initially 100–500 nanograms, adjusted according to response; usual dose 1.25–10 micrograms daily in 1–2 divided doses.

▸ Child 1–23 months: Initially 2.5–5 micrograms 1–2 times a day, adjusted according to response
▸ Child 2–11 years: Initially 5–20 micrograms 1–2 times a day, adjusted according to response
▸ Child 12–17 years: Initially 10–20 micrograms 1–2 times a day, adjusted according to response
▸ BY INTRAMUSCULAR INJECTION
▸ Neonate: Initially 100 nanograms once daily, adjusted according to response.

▸ BY SUBCUTANEOUS INJECTION, OR BY INTRAMUSCULAR INJECTION
▸ Child 1 month–11 years: Initially 400 nanograms once daily, adjusted according to response
▸ Child 12–17 years: Initially 1–4 micrograms once daily, adjusted according to response

Primary nocturnal enuresis
▸ BY MOUTH
▸ Child 5–17 years: 200 micrograms once daily, only increased to 400 micrograms if lower dose not effective; withdraw for at least 1 week for reassessment after 3 months, dose to be taken at bedtime, limit fluid intake from 1 hour before to 8 hours after administration
▸ BY SUBLINGUAL ADMINISTRATION
▸ Child 5–17 years: 120 micrograms once daily, increased if necessary to 240 micrograms once daily, dose to be taken at bedtime, limit fluid intake from 1 hour before to 8 hours after administration, dose to be increased only if lower dose not effective, reassess after 3 months by withdrawing treatment for at least 1 week

Diabetes insipidus, diagnosis (water deprivation test)
▸ BY INTRANASAL ADMINISTRATION
▸ Neonate: Not recommended, use trial of treatment.

▸ Child 1–23 months: 5–10 micrograms for 1 dose, manage fluid input carefully to avoid hyponatraemia, not usually recommended
▸ Child 2–11 years: 10–20 micrograms for 1 dose, manage fluid input carefully to avoid hyponatraemia
▸ Child 12–17 years: 20 micrograms for 1 dose, manage fluid input carefully to avoid hyponatraemia
▸ BY INTRAMUSCULAR INJECTION, OR BY SUBCUTANEOUS INJECTION
▸ Neonate: Not recommended, use trial of treatment.

▸ Child 1–23 months: 400 nanograms for 1 dose, manage fluid input carefully to avoid hyponatraemia, not usually recommended
▸ Child 2–11 years: 0.5–1 microgram for 1 dose, manage fluid input carefully to avoid hyponatraemia
▸ Child 12–17 years: 1–2 micrograms for 1 dose, manage fluid input carefully to avoid hyponatraemia

Renal function testing
▸ BY INTRANASAL ADMINISTRATION
▸ Child 1–11 months: 10 micrograms, empty bladder at time of administration and restrict fluid intake to 50% at next 2 feeds to avoid fluid overload
▸ Child 1–14 years: 20 micrograms, empty bladder at time of administration and restrict fluid intake to 500 mL from 1 hour before until 8 hours after administration to avoid fluid overload

▸ Child 15–17 years: 40 micrograms, empty bladder at time of administration and limit fluid intake to 500 mL from 1 hour before until 8 hours after administration to avoid fluid overload
▸ BY SUBCUTANEOUS INJECTION, OR BY INTRAMUSCULAR INJECTION
▸ Child 1–11 months: 400 nanograms, empty bladder at time of administration and restrict fluid intake to 50% at next 2 feeds to avoid fluid overload
▸ Child 1–17 years: 2 micrograms, empty bladder at time of administration and restrict fluid intake to 500 mL from 1 hour before until 8 hours after administration to avoid fluid overload

Mild to moderate haemophilia and von Willebrand's disease
▸ BY INTRANASAL ADMINISTRATION
▸ Child 1–17 years: 4 micrograms/kg for 1 dose, for pre-operative use give 2 hours before procedure
▸ BY INTRAVENOUS INFUSION, OR BY SUBCUTANEOUS INJECTION
▸ Child: 300 nanograms/kg for 1 dose, to be administered immediately before surgery or after trauma; may be repeated at intervals of 12 hours if no tachycardia

Fibrinolytic response testing
▸ BY SUBCUTANEOUS INJECTION, OR BY INTRAVENOUS INJECTION
▸ Child 2–17 years: 300 nanograms/kg for 1 dose, blood to be sampled after 20 minutes for fibrinolytic activity

Assessment of antidiuretic hormone secretion (congenital deficiency suspected) (specialist use only)
▸ BY INTRANASAL ADMINISTRATION
▸ Child 1–23 months: Initially 100–500 nanograms for 1 dose

Assessment of antidiuretic hormone secretion (congenital deficiency not suspected) (specialist use only)
▸ BY INTRANASAL ADMINISTRATION
▸ Child 1–23 months: 1–5 micrograms for 1 dose

● **UNLICENSED USE** Consult product literature for individual preparations. Not licensed for assessment of antidiuretic hormone secretion. Oral use of *DDAVP* intravenous injection is not licensed.
● **CONTRA-INDICATIONS** Cardiac insufficiency · conditions treated with diuretics · history of hyponatraemia · polydipsia in alcohol dependence · psychogenic polydipsia
● **CAUTIONS**
GENERAL CAUTIONS
Asthma · avoid fluid overload · cardiovascular disease (not indicated for nocturnal enuresis or nocturia) · conditions which might be aggravated by water retention · cystic fibrosis · epilepsy · heart failure · hypertension (not indicated for nocturnal enuresis or nocturia) · migraine · nocturia—limit fluid intake to minimum from 1 hour before dose until 8 hours afterwards · nocturnal enuresis—limit fluid intake to minimum from 1 hour before dose until 8 hours afterwards
SPECIFIC CAUTIONS
Should not be given intranasally for nocturnal enuresis due to an increased incidence of side-effects
● **INTERACTIONS** → Appendix 1: desmopressin
● **SIDE-EFFECTS**
GENERAL SIDE-EFFECTS
▸ **Common or very common** Hyponatraemia (in more serious cases with convulsions) on administration without restricting fluid intake · nausea
▸ **Frequency not known** Allergic reactions · emotional disturbance in children · epistaxis · fluid retention · headache · nasal congestion · stomach pain · vomiting
SPECIFIC SIDE-EFFECTS
▸ With intranasal use Rhinitis

SIDE-EFFECTS, FURTHER INFORMATION

▸ Hyponatraemic convulsions The risk of hyponatraemic convulsions can be minimised by keeping to the recommended starting doses and by avoiding concomitant use of drugs which increase secretion of vasopressin (e.g. tricyclic antidepressants).

● **PREGNANCY** Small oxytocic effect in third trimester; increased risk of pre-eclampsia.

● **BREAST FEEDING** Amount too small to be harmful.

● **RENAL IMPAIRMENT** Use with caution; antidiuretic effect may be reduced.

● **MONITORING REQUIREMENTS** In *nocturia*, periodic blood pressure and weight checks are needed to monitor for fluid overload.

● **DIRECTIONS FOR ADMINISTRATION** *DDVAP*® and *Desmotabs*® tablets may be crushed.

   DDAVP® intranasal solution may be diluted with Sodium Chloride 0.9% to a concentration of 10 micrograms/mL.

   DDAVP® injection may be administered orally. Desmopressin oral lyophilisates are for sublingual administration.

▸ With intravenous use Higher doses of *DDAVP*® by *intravenous infusion*, used in mild to moderate haemophilia and von Willebrand's disease, may be diluted with 30–50 mL Sodium Chloride 0.9% intravenous infusion.

   For *intravenous infusion (Octim*®*)*, dilute with 50 mL of Sodium Chloride 0.9% and give over 20 minutes.

● **PRESCRIBING AND DISPENSING INFORMATION** Oral, intranasal, intravenous, subcutaneous and intramuscular doses are expressed as desmopressin acetate; sublingual doses are expressed as desmopressin base.

   Children requiring an intranasal dose of less than 10 micrograms should be given *DDAVP*® intranasal solution.

● **PATIENT AND CARER ADVICE**

Hyponatraemic convulsions Patients being treated for primary nocturnal enuresis should be warned to avoid fluid overload (including during swimming) and to stop taking desmopressin during an episode of vomiting or diarrhoea (until fluid balance normal).

Medicines for Children leaflet: Desmopressin for bedwetting www.medicinesforchildren.org.uk/desmopressin-bedwetting-0

● **MEDICINAL FORMS**

There can be variation in the licensing of different medicines containing the same drug. Forms available from special-order manufacturers include: capsule, oral suspension, oral solution, spray, nasal drops

Tablet

▸ **Desmopressin (Non-proprietary)**
Desmopressin acetate 100 microgram Desmopressin 100microgram tablets | 90 tablet [PoM] £76.62 DT price = £63.08
Desmopressin acetate 200 microgram Desmopressin 200microgram tablets | 30 tablet [PoM] £35.23 DT price = £7.25 | 90 tablet [PoM] no price available

▸ **DDAVP** (Ferring Pharmaceuticals Ltd)
Desmopressin acetate 100 microgram DDAVP 0.1mg tablets | 90 tablet [PoM] £44.12 DT price = £63.08
Desmopressin acetate 200 microgram DDAVP 0.2mg tablets | 90 tablet [PoM] £88.23

▸ **Desmotabs** (Ferring Pharmaceuticals Ltd)
Desmopressin acetate 200 microgram Desmotabs 0.2mg tablets | 30 tablet [PoM] £29.43 DT price = £7.25

Solution for injection

▸ **DDAVP** (Ferring Pharmaceuticals Ltd)
Desmopressin acetate 4 microgram per 1 ml DDAVP 4micrograms/1ml solution for injection ampoules | 10 ampoule [PoM] £13.16

▸ **Octim** (Ferring Pharmaceuticals Ltd)
Desmopressin acetate 15 microgram per 1 ml Octim 15micrograms/1ml solution for injection ampoules | 10 ampoule [PoM] £192.20

Spray

▸ **Desmopressin (Non-proprietary)**
Desmopressin acetate 2.5 microgram per 1 dose Minirin 2.5micrograms/dose nasal spray | 50 dose [PoM] no price available
Desmopressin acetate 10 microgram per 1 dose Desmopressin 10micrograms/dose nasal spray | 60 dose [PoM] £31.50 DT price = £23.25

▸ **Desmospray** (Ferring Pharmaceuticals Ltd)
Desmopressin acetate 2.5 microgram per 1 dose Desmospray 2.5micrograms/dose nasal spray | 50 dose no price available
Desmopressin acetate 10 microgram per 1 dose Desmospray 10micrograms/dose nasal spray | 60 dose [PoM] £25.02 DT price = £23.25

▸ **Octim** (Ferring Pharmaceuticals Ltd)
Desmopressin acetate 150 microgram per 1 dose Octim 150micrograms/dose nasal spray | 25 dose [PoM] £576.60

Oral solution

▸ **Desmopressin (Non-proprietary)**
Desmopressin (as Desmopressin acetate) 360 microgram per 1 ml Desmopressin 360micrograms/ml oral solution | 15 ml [PoM] £30.00 DT price = £30.00

Oral lyophilisate

CAUTIONARY AND ADVISORY LABELS 26

▸ **Desmopressin (Non-proprietary)**
Desmopressin (as Desmopressin acetate)
120 microgram Desmopressin 120microgram oral lyophilisates sugar free sugar-free | 30 tablet [PoM] no price available DT price = £30.34
Desmopressin (as Desmopressin acetate)
240 microgram Desmopressin 240microgram oral lyophilisates sugar free sugar-free | 30 tablet [PoM] no price available DT price = £60.68

▸ **DDAVP** (Ferring Pharmaceuticals Ltd)
Desmopressin (as Desmopressin acetate) 60 microgram DDAVP Melt 60microgram oral lyophilisates sugar-free | 100 tablet [PoM] £50.53 DT price = £50.53
Desmopressin (as Desmopressin acetate) 120 microgram DDAVP Melt 120microgram oral lyophilisates sugar-free | 100 tablet [PoM] £101.07 DT price = £101.07
Desmopressin (as Desmopressin acetate) 240 microgram DDAVP Melt 240microgram oral lyophilisates sugar-free | 100 tablet [PoM] £202.14

▸ **DesmoMelt** (Ferring Pharmaceuticals Ltd)
Desmopressin (as Desmopressin acetate)
120 microgram DesmoMelt 120microgram oral lyophilisates sugar-free | 30 tablet [PoM] £30.34 DT price = £33.34
Desmopressin (as Desmopressin acetate)
240 microgram DesmoMelt 240microgram oral lyophilisates sugar-free | 30 tablet [PoM] £60.68 DT price = £66.68

▸ **Noqdirna** (Ferring Pharmaceuticals Ltd)
Desmopressin (as Desmopressin acetate 25 microgram Noqdirna 25microgram oral lyophilisates sugar-free | 30 tablet [PoM] £15.16 DT price = £15.16
Desmopressin (as Desmopressin acetate)
50 microgram Noqdirna 50microgram oral lyophilisates sugar-free | 30 tablet [PoM] £15.16 DT price = £15.16

Nasal drops

▸ **DDAVP** (Ferring Pharmaceuticals Ltd)
Desmopressin acetate 100 microgram per 1 ml DDAVP 100micrograms/ml intranasal solution | 2.5 ml [PoM] £9.72 DT price = £9.72

2 Corticosteroid responsive conditions

CORTICOSTEROIDS

Corticosteroids, general use

Overview

Dosages of corticosteroids vary widely in different diseases and in different patients. If the use of a corticosteroid can save or prolong life, as in exfoliative dermatitis, pemphigus, acute leukaemia or acute transplant rejection, high doses may need to be given, because the complications of therapy are likely to be less serious than the effects of the disease itself.

When long-term corticosteroid therapy is used in some chronic diseases, the adverse effects of treatment may become greater than the disabilities caused by the disease. To minimise side-effects the maintenance dose should be kept as low as possible.

When potentially less harmful measures are ineffective corticosteroids are used topically for the treatment of inflammatory conditions of the skin. Corticosteroids should be avoided or used only under specialist supervision in psoriasis.

Corticosteroids are used both topically (by rectum) and systemically (by mouth or intravenously) in the management of ulcerative colitis and Crohn's disease.

Use can be made of the mineralocorticoid activity of fludrocortisone acetate p. 420 to treat postural hypotension in autonomic neuropathy.

High-dose corticosteroids should be avoided for the management of septic shock. However, low-dose hydrocortisone p. 420 can be used in septic shock that is resistant to volume expansion and catecholamines, and is accompanied by suspected or proven adrenal insufficiency.

The suppressive action of glucocorticoids on the hypothalamic-pituitary-adrenal axis is greatest and most prolonged when they are given at night. In most adults a single dose of dexamethasone p. 419 at night is sufficient to inhibit corticotropin secretion for 24 hours. This is the basis of the 'overnight dexamethasone suppression test' for diagnosing Cushing's syndrome.

Betamethasone p. 418 and dexamethasone are also appropriate for conditions where water retention would be a disadvantage.

A corticosteroid may be used in the management of raised intracranial pressure or cerebral oedema that occurs as a result of malignancy (see Prescribing in palliative care p. 19); high doses of betamethasone or dexamethasone are generally used. However, a corticosteroid should **not** be used for the management of head injury or stroke because it is unlikely to be of benefit and may even be harmful.

In acute hypersensitivity reactions, such as angioedema of the upper respiratory tract and anaphylaxis, corticosteroids are indicated as an adjunct to emergency treatment with adrenaline/epinephrine p. 132. In such cases hydrocortisone (as sodium succinate) by intravenous injection may be required.

In the management of asthma, corticosteroids are preferably used by inhalation but systemic therapy along with bronchodilators is required for the emergency treatment of severe acute asthma.

Betamethasone is used in women at risk of preterm delivery to reduce the incidence of neonatal respiratory distress syndrome [unlicensed use].

Dexamethasone should not be used routinely for the prophylaxis and treatment of chronic lung disease in neonates because of an association with adverse neurological effects.

Corticosteroids may be useful in conditions such as auto-immune hepatitis, rheumatoid arthritis, and sarcoidosis; they may also lead to remissions of acquired haemolytic anaemia and thrombocytopenic purpura.

High doses of a corticosteroid (usually prednisolone p. 421) are used in the treatment of *glomerular kidney disease*, including *nephrotic syndrome*. The condition frequently recurs; a corticosteroid given in high doses and for prolonged periods may delay relapse but the higher incidence of adverse effects limits the overall benefit. Those who suffer frequent relapses may be treated with prednisolone given in a low dose (daily or on alternate days) for 3–6 months; the dose should be adjusted to minimise effects on growth and development. Other drugs used in the treatment of glomerular kidney disease include levamisole

p. 367, cyclophosphamide p. 509, chlorambucil p. 508, and ciclosporin p. 496. *Congenital nephrotic syndrome* may be resistant to corticosteroids and immunosuppressants; indometacin p. 628 and an ACE inhibitor such as captopril p. 109 have been used.

Corticosteroids can improve the prognosis of serious conditions such as systemic lupus erythematosus and polyarteritis nodosa; the effects of the disease process may be suppressed and symptoms relieved, but the underlying condition is not cured, although it may ultimately remit. It is usual to begin therapy in these conditions at fairly high dose and then to reduce the dose to the lowest commensurate with disease control.

For other references to the use of corticosteroids see: Prescribing in Palliative Care, immunosuppression, rheumatic diseases, eye, otitis externa, allergic rhinitis, and aphthous ulcers.

Side-effects

Overdosage or prolonged use can exaggerate some of the normal physiological actions of corticosteroids leading to mineralocorticoid and glucocorticoid side-effects.

Mineralocorticoid side effects

- hypertension
- sodium retention
- water retention
- potassium loss
- calcium loss

Mineralocorticoid side effects are most marked with fludrocortisone acetate, but are significant with hydrocortisone, corticotropin, and tetracosactide p. 452. Mineralocorticoid actions are negligible with the high potency glucocorticoids, betamethasone and dexamethasone, and occur only slightly with methylprednisolone p. 421, prednisolone, and triamcinolone.

Glucocorticoid side effects

- diabetes
- osteoporosis
- in addition high doses are associated with avascular necrosis of the femoral head.
- Muscle wasting (proximal myopathy) can also occur.
- Corticosteroid therapy is also weakly linked with peptic ulceration and perforation.
- Psychiatric reactions may also occur.

Managing side-effects

Side-effects can be minimised by using lowest effective dose for minimum period possible. The suppressive action of a corticosteroid on cortisol secretion is least when it is given as a single dose in the morning. In an attempt to reduce pituitary-adrenal suppression further, the total dose for two days can sometimes be taken as a single dose on alternate days; alternate-day administration has not been very successful in the management of asthma. Pituitary-adrenal suppression can also be reduced by means of intermittent therapy with short courses. In some conditions it may be possible to reduce the dose of corticosteroid by adding a small dose of an immunosuppressive drug.

Whenever possible *local treatment* with creams, intra-articular injections, inhalations, eye-drops, or enemas should be used in preference to *systemic treatment*.

Inhaled corticosteroids have considerably fewer systemic effects than oral corticosteroids, but adverse effects including adrenal suppression have been reported. Use of other corticosteroid therapy (including topical) or concurrent use of drugs which inhibit corticosteroid metabolism should be taken into account when assessing systemic risk. In children, growth restriction associated with systemic corticosteroid therapy does not seem to occur with recommended doses of inhaled therapy; although initial growth velocity may be reduced, there appears to be no

6

Endocrine system

effect on achieving normal adult height. Large-volume spacer devices should be used for administering inhaled corticosteroids in children under 15 years; they are also useful in older children and adults, particularly if high doses are required. Spacer devices increase airway deposition and reduce oropharyngeal deposition.

Corticosteroids, replacement therapy

Overview

The adrenal cortex normally secretes hydrocortisone p. 420 (cortisol) which has glucocorticoid activity and weak mineralocorticoid activity. It also secretes the mineralocorticoid aldosterone.

In deficiency states, physiological replacement is best achieved with a combination of hydrocortisone and the mineralocorticoid fludrocortisone acetate p. 420; hydrocortisone alone does not usually provide sufficient mineralocorticoid activity for complete replacement.

In *Addison's disease* or following adrenalectomy, hydrocortisone by mouth is usually required. This is given in 2–3 divided doses, the larger in the morning and the smaller in the evening, mimicking the normal diurnal rhythm of cortisol secretion. The optimum daily dose is determined on the basis of clinical response. Glucocorticoid therapy is supplemented by fludrocortisone acetate.

In *acute adrenocortical insufficiency*, hydrocortisone is given intravenously (preferably as sodium succinate) every 6 to 8 hours in sodium chloride intravenous infusion 0.9% p. 561.

In *hypopituitarism*, glucocorticoids should be given as in adrenocortical insufficiency, but since production of aldosterone is also regulated by the renin-angiotensin system a mineralocorticoid is not usually required. Additional replacement therapy with levothyroxine sodium p. 464 and sex hormones should be given as indicated by the pattern of hormone deficiency.

In *congenital adrenal hyperplasia*, the pituitary gland increases production of corticotropin to compensate for reduced formation of cortisol; this results in excessive adrenal androgen production. Treatment is aimed at suppressing corticotropin using hydrocortisone. Careful and continual dose titration is required to avoid growth retardation and toxicity; for this reason potent, synthetic glucocorticoids such as dexamethasone are usually reserved for use in adolescents. The dose is adjusted according to clinical response and measurement of adrenal androgens and 17-hydroxyprogesterone. Salt-losing forms of congenital adrenal hyperplasia (where there is a lack of aldosterone production) also require mineralocorticoid replacement and salt supplementation (particularly in early life). The dose of mineralocorticoid is adjusted according to electrolyte concentration and plasma-renin activity.

Glucocorticoid therapy

Glucocorticoid and mineralocorticoid activity

In comparing the relative potencies of corticosteroids in terms of their anti-inflammatory (glucocorticoid) effects it should be borne in mind that high glucocorticoid activity in itself is of no advantage unless it is accompanied by relatively low mineralocorticoid activity (see Disadvantages of Corticosteroids). The mineralocorticoid activity of fludrocortisone acetate p. 420 is so high that its anti-inflammatory activity is of no clinical relevance.

Equivalent anti-inflammatory doses of corticosteroids

This table takes no account of mineralocorticoid effects, nor does it take account of variations in duration of action

Prednisolone 1 mg		
	≡	Betamethasone 150 micrograms
	≡	Deflazacort 1.2 mg
	≡	Dexamethasone 150 micrograms
	≡	Hydrocortisone 4 mg
	≡	Methylprednisolone 800 micrograms
	≡	Triamcinolone 800 micrograms

The relatively high mineralocorticoid activity of hydrocortisone p. 420, and the resulting fluid retention, makes it unsuitable for disease suppression on a long-term basis. However, hydrocortisone can be used for adrenal replacement therapy. Hydrocortisone is used on a short-term basis by intravenous injection for the emergency management of some conditions. The relatively moderate anti-inflammatory potency of hydrocortisone also makes it a useful topical corticosteroid for the management of inflammatory skin conditions because side-effects (both topical and systemic) are less marked.

Prednisolone p. 421 has predominantly glucocorticoid activity and is the corticosteroid most commonly used by mouth for long-term disease suppression.

Betamethasone p. 418 and dexamethasone p. 419 have very high glucocorticoid activity in conjunction with insignificant mineralocorticoid activity. This makes them particularly suitable for high-dose therapy in conditions where fluid retention would be a disadvantage.

Betamethasone and dexamethasone also have a long duration of action and this, coupled with their lack of mineralocorticoid action makes them particularly suitable for conditions which require suppression of corticotropin (corticotrophin) secretion.

Some esters of betamethasone and of beclometasone dipropionate p. 154 (beclometasone) exert a considerably more marked topical effect (e.g. on the skin or the lungs) than when given by mouth; use is made of this to obtain topical effects whilst minimising systemic side-effects (e.g. for skin applications and asthma inhalations).

Deflazacort p. 418 has a high glucocorticoid activity; it is derived from prednisolone.

Corticosteroids (systemic)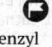

- **CONTRA-INDICATIONS** Avoid injections containing benzyl alcohol in neonates · avoid live virus vaccines in those receiving immunosuppressive doses (serum antibody response diminished) · systemic infection (unless specific therapy given)

  CONTRA-INDICATIONS, FURTHER INFORMATION
  For further information on contra-indications associated with intra-articular, intradermal and intralesional preparations, consult product literature.

- **CAUTIONS** Congestive heart failure · diabetes mellitus (including a family history of) · diverticulitis · epilepsy · glaucoma (including a family history of or susceptibility to) · history of steroid myopathy · history of tuberculosis or X-ray changes (frequent monitoring required) · hypertension · hypothyroidism · infection (particularly untreated) · myasthenia gravis · ocular herpes simplex (risk of corneal perforation) · osteoporosis · peptic ulcer · psychiatric reactions · recent intestinal anastomoses · recent myocardial infarction (rupture reported) · severe affective disorders (particularly if history of steroid-induced psychosis) · should not be used long-term · thromboembolic disorders · ulcerative colitis

CAUTIONS, FURTHER INFORMATION
For further information on cautions associated with intra-articular, intradermal and intralesional preparations, consult product literature.

● **SIDE-EFFECTS**

GENERAL SIDE-EFFECTS
Abdominal distension · acute pancreatitis · aggravation of epilepsy · aggravation of schizophrenia · amenorrhoea · anaphylaxis · bruising · candidiasis · congestive heart failure · corneal thinning · Cushing's syndrome (with moon face, striae and acne) · dyspepsia · ecchymoses · exacerbation of ophthalmic fungal disease · exacerbation of ophthalmic viral disease · exophthalmos · facial erythema · glaucoma · headache · hiccups · hirsutism · hypercholesterolaemia · hyperglycaemia · hyperhidrosis · hyperlipidaemia · hypersensitivity reactions · impaired healing · increased appetite · increased intra-ocular pressure · increased intracranial pressure with papilloedema (usually after withdrawal) · increased susceptibility to and severity of infection · insomnia · leucocytosis · long bone fractures · malaise · menstrual irregularities · muscle weakness · myocardial rupture following recent myocardial infarction · nausea · negative calcium balance · negative nitrogen balance · oesophageal ulceration · petechiae · posterior subcapsular cataracts · potassium loss · psychological dependence · reactivation of dormant tuberculosis · scleral thinning · skin atrophy · sodium retention · suppression of growth · telangiectasia · tendon rupture · thromboembolism · urticaria · vertebral fractures · vertigo · water retention · weight gain

SPECIFIC SIDE-EFFECTS
▸ With intra-articular use Flushing · may affect the hyaline cartilage

SIDE-EFFECTS, FURTHER INFORMATION
Side effects can be managed by choice of route and duration of course. For further detail see Corticosteroids, general use p. 414

▸ Adrenal suppression During prolonged therapy with corticosteroids, particularly with systemic use, adrenal atrophy develops and can persist for years after stopping. Abrupt withdrawal after a prolonged period can lead to acute adrenal insufficiency, hypotension, or death.

To compensate for a diminished adrenocortical response caused by prolonged corticosteroid treatment, any significant intercurrent illness, trauma, or surgical procedure requires a temporary increase in corticosteroid dose, or if already stopped, a temporary reintroduction of corticosteroid treatment. To avoid a precipitous fall in blood pressure during anaesthesia or in the immediate postoperative period, anaesthetists **must** know whether a patient is taking or has been taking a corticosteroid. A suitable regimen for corticosteroid replacement, in patients who have taken more than 10 mg prednisolone daily (or equivalent) within 3 months of surgery, is:

● Minor surgery under general anaesthesia—usual oral corticosteroid dose on the morning of surgery or hydrocortisone (usually the sodium succinate) intravenously at induction; the usual oral corticosteroid dose is recommenced after surgery.

● Moderate or major surgery—usual oral corticosteroid dose on the morning of surgery and hydrocortisone intravenously at induction, followed by hydrocortisone 3 times a day by intravenous injection for 24 hours after moderate surgery or for 48–72 hours after major surgery; the usual pre-operative oral corticosteroid dose is recommenced on stopping hydrocortisone injections.

Patients on long-term corticosteroid treatment should carry a steroid treatment card which gives guidance on minimising risk and provides details of prescriber, drug, dosage and duration of treatment.

▸ Infections Prolonged courses of corticosteroids increase susceptibility to infections and severity of infections;

clinical presentation of infections may also be atypical. Serious infections e.g. *septicaemia* and *tuberculosis* may reach an advanced stage before being recognised, and *amoebiasis* or *strongyloidiasis* may be activated or exacerbated (exclude before initiating a corticosteroid in those at risk or with suggestive symptoms). Fungal or viral *ocular infections* may also be exacerbated.

▸ Chickenpox Unless they have had chickenpox, patients receiving oral or parenteral corticosteroids for purposes other than replacement should be regarded as being *at risk of severe chickenpox* (see Steroid Treatment Card). Manifestations of fulminant illness include pneumonia, hepatitis and disseminated intravascular coagulation; rash is not necessarily a prominent feature.

Passive immunisation with varicella–zoster immunoglobulin is needed for exposed non–immune patients receiving systemic corticosteroids or for those who have used them within the previous 3 months. Confirmed chickenpox warrants specialist care and urgent treatment. Corticosteroids should not be stopped and dosage may need to be increased.

Topical, inhaled or rectal corticosteroids are less likely to be associated with an increased risk of severe chickenpox.

▸ Measles Patients taking corticosteroids should be advised to take particular care to avoid exposure to measles and to seek immediate medical advice if exposure occurs. Prophylaxis with intramuscular normal immunoglobulin may be needed.

▸ Psychiatric reactions Systemic corticosteroids, particularly in high doses, are linked to psychiatric reactions including euphoria, nightmares, insomnia, irritability, mood lability, suicidal thoughts, psychotic reactions, and behavioural disturbances. A serious paranoid state or depression with risk of suicide can be induced, particularly in patients with a history of mental disorder. These reactions frequently subside on reducing the dose or discontinuing the corticosteroid but they may also require specific management. Patients should be advised to seek medical advice if psychiatric symptoms (especially depression and suicidal thoughts) occur and they should also be alert to the rare possibility of such reactions during withdrawal of corticosteroid treatment.

Systemic corticosteroids should be prescribed with care in those predisposed to psychiatric reactions, including those who have previously suffered corticosteroid–induced psychosis, or who have a personal or family history of psychiatric disorders.

● **PREGNANCY** The benefit of treatment with corticosteroids during pregnancy outweighs the risk. Corticosteroid cover is required during labour. Following a review of the data on the safety of systemic corticosteroids used in pregnancy and breast-feeding the CSM (May 1998) concluded that corticosteroids vary in their ability to cross the placenta but there is no convincing evidence that systemic corticosteroids increase the incidence of congenital abnormalities such as cleft palate or lip. When administration is prolonged or repeated during pregnancy, systemic corticosteroids increase the risk of intra-uterine growth restriction; there is no evidence of intra-uterine growth restriction following short-term treatment (e.g. prophylactic treatment for neonatal respiratory distress syndrome). Any adrenal suppression in the neonate following prenatal exposure usually resolves spontaneously after birth and is rarely clinically important.

Pregnant women with fluid retention should be monitored closely when given systemic corticosteroids.

● **BREAST FEEDING** The benefit of treatment with corticosteroids during breast-feeding outweighs the risk.

● **HEPATIC IMPAIRMENT** The plasma-drug concentration may be increased (particularly on systemic use). Oral and parenteral use should be undertaken with caution.

6

Endocrine system

- **RENAL IMPAIRMENT** Use by oral and injectable routes should be undertaken with caution.

- **MONITORING REQUIREMENTS** The height and weight of children receiving prolonged treatment with corticosteroids should be monitored annually; if growth is slowed, referral to a paediatrician should be considered.

- **EFFECT ON LABORATORY TESTS** Suppression of skin test reactions.

- **TREATMENT CESSATION** The magnitude and speed of dose reduction in corticosteroid withdrawal should be determined on a case–by–case basis, taking into consideration the underlying condition that is being treated, and individual patient factors such as the likelihood of relapse and the duration of corticosteroid treatment. *Gradual* withdrawal of systemic corticosteroids should be considered in those whose disease is unlikely to relapse and have:
  - received more than 40 mg prednisolone (or equivalent) daily for more than 1 week *or* 2 mg/kg daily for 1 week *or* 1 mg/kg daily for 1 month;
  - been given repeat doses in the evening;
  - received more than 3 weeks' treatment;
  - recently received repeated courses (particularly if taken for longer than 3 weeks);
  - taken a short course within 1 year of stopping long-term therapy;
  - other possible causes of adrenal suppression.

  Systemic corticosteroids may be stopped abruptly in those whose disease is unlikely to relapse *and* who have received treatment for 3 weeks or less *and* who are not included in the patient groups described above.

  During corticosteroid withdrawal the dose may be reduced rapidly down to physiological doses (equivalent to prednisolone 2–2.5 mg/m² daily) and then reduced more slowly. Assessment of the disease may be needed during withdrawal to ensure that relapse does not occur.

- **PATIENT AND CARER ADVICE**

  Advice for patients Patients on long-term corticosteroid treatment should carry a Steroid Treatment Card which gives guidance on minimising risk and provides details of prescriber, drug, dosage and duration of treatment.

  A patient information leaflet should be supplied to every patient when a systemic corticosteroid is prescribed. Patients should especially be advised of the following:
  - **Immunosuppression** Prolonged courses of corticosteroids can increase susceptibility to infection and serious infections can go unrecognised. Unless already immune, patients are at risk of severe **chickenpox** and should avoid close contact with people who have chickenpox or shingles. Similarly, precautions should also be taken against contracting **measles**;
  - **Adrenal suppression** If the corticosteroid is given for longer than 3 weeks, treatment must not be stopped abruptly. Adrenal suppression can last for a year or more after stopping treatment and the patient must mention the course of corticosteroid when receiving treatment for any illness or injury;
  - **Mood and behaviour changes** Corticosteroid treatment, especially with high doses, can alter mood and behaviour early in treatment—the patient can become confused, irritable and suffer from delusion and suicidal thoughts. These effects can also occur when corticosteroid treatment is being withdrawn. Medical advice should be sought if worrying psychological changes occur;
  - **Other serious effects** Serious gastro-intestinal, musculoskeletal, and ophthalmic effects which require medical help can also occur.

  Steroid treatment cards Steroid treatment cards should be issued where appropriate. Consider giving a 'steroid card' to support communication of the risks associated with treatment, and specific written advice to consider

corticosteroid replacement during an episode of stress, such as severe intercurrent illness or an operation, to patients using greater than maximum licensed doses of inhaled corticosteroids. Steroid treatment cards are available for purchase from the NHS Print online ordering portal www.nhsforms.co.uk

GP practices can obtain supplies through Primary Care Support England. NHS Trusts can order supplies via the online ordering portal.

In **Scotland**, steroid treatment cards can be obtained from APS Group Scotland by emailing stockorders.dppas@apsgroup.co.uk or by fax on 0131 629 9967.

Betamethasone
F 416

- **INDICATIONS AND DOSE**

Suppression of inflammatory and allergic disorders | Congenital adrenal hyperplasia

▶ BY SLOW INTRAVENOUS INJECTION, OR BY INTRAVENOUS INFUSION

▶ Child 1-11 months: Initially 1 mg, repeated up to 4 times in 24 hours according to response

▶ Child 1-5 years: Initially 2 mg, repeated up to 4 times in 24 hours according to response

▶ Child 6-11 years: Initially 4 mg, repeated up to 4 times in 24 hours according to response

▶ Child 12-17 years: 4–20 mg, repeated up to 4 times in 24 hours according to response

- **INTERACTIONS** → Appendix 1: corticosteroids

- **PREGNANCY** Readily crosses the placenta. Transient effect on fetal movements and heart rate.

- **DIRECTIONS FOR ADMINISTRATION** For *intravenous infusion*, dilute with Glucose 5% or Sodium Chloride 0.9%.

- **MEDICINAL FORMS**
  There can be variation in the licensing of different medicines containing the same drug.
  Solution for injection
  CAUTIONARY AND ADVISORY LABELS 10
  ▶ **Betamethasone (Non-proprietary)**
  Betamethasone (as Betamethasone sodium phosphate) 4 mg per 1 ml Betamethasone 4mg/1ml solution for injection ampoules | 5 ampoule [PoM] £13.06–£15.68

Deflazacort
F 416

- **INDICATIONS AND DOSE**

Inflammatory and allergic disorders

▶ BY MOUTH

▶ Child 1 month-11 years: 0.25–1.5 mg/kg once daily or on alternate days; increased if necessary up to 2.4 mg/kg daily (max. per dose 120 mg), in emergency situations

▶ Child 12-17 years: 3–18 mg once daily or on alternate days; increased if necessary up to 2.4 mg/kg daily (max. per dose 120 mg), in emergency situations

Nephrotic syndrome

▶ BY MOUTH

▶ Child: Initially 1.5 mg/kg once daily (max. per dose 120 mg), reduced to the lowest effective dose for maintenance

- **INTERACTIONS** → Appendix 1: corticosteroids

- **PATIENT AND CARER ADVICE** Patient counselling is advised for deflazacort tablets (steroid card).

- **MEDICINAL FORMS**
There can be variation in the licensing of different medicines containing the same drug. Forms available from special-order manufacturers include: tablet

Tablet
CAUTIONARY AND ADVISORY LABELS 5, 10
▸ Calcort (Sanofi)
Deflazacort 6 mg Calcort 6mg tablets | 60 tablet [PoM] £15.82

[F 416]

Dexamethasone

06-Jun-2016

- **INDICATIONS AND DOSE**
Physiological replacement
▸ BY MOUTH, OR BY SLOW INTRAVENOUS INJECTION
▸ Child: 250–500 micrograms/m² every 12 hours, adjusted according to response

Suppression of inflammatory and allergic disorders
▸ BY MOUTH
▸ Child: 10–100 micrograms/kg daily in 1–2 divided doses, adjusted according to response; up to 300 micrograms/kg daily may be required in emergency situations
▸ BY INTRAMUSCULAR INJECTION, OR BY SLOW INTRAVENOUS INJECTION, OR BY INTRAVENOUS INFUSION
▸ Child 1 month-11 years: 83–333 micrograms/kg daily in 1–2 divided doses; maximum 20 mg per day
▸ Child 12-17 years: Initially 0.4–20 mg daily

Mild croup
▸ BY MOUTH
▸ Child: 150 micrograms/kg for 1 dose

Severe croup (or mild croup that might cause complications)
▸ INITIALLY BY MOUTH
▸ Child: Initially 150 micrograms/kg for 1 dose, to be given before transfer to hospital, then (by mouth or by intravenous injection) 150 micrograms/kg, then (by mouth or by intravenous injection) 150 micrograms/kg after 12 hours if required

Adjunctive treatment of bacterial meningitis (starting before or with first dose of antibacterial)
▸ BY SLOW INTRAVENOUS INJECTION
▸ Child 3 months-17 years: 150 micrograms/kg every 6 hours (max. per dose 10 mg) for 4 days

Life-threatening cerebral oedema
▸ BY INTRAVENOUS INJECTION
▸ Child (body-weight up to 35 kg): Initially 16.7 mg, then 3.3 mg every 3 hours for 3 days, then 3.3 mg every 6 hours for 1 day, then 1.7 mg every 6 hours for 4 days, then reduced in steps of 0.8 mg daily
▸ Child (body-weight 35 kg and above): Initially 20.8 mg, then 3.3 mg every 2 hours for 3 days, then 3.3 mg every 4 hours for 1 day, then 3.3 mg every 6 hours for 4 days, then reduced in steps of 1.7 mg daily

- **UNLICENSED USE**
▸ With intravenous use Consult product literature; not licensed for use in bacterial meningitis.

- **INTERACTIONS** → Appendix 1: corticosteroids

- **SIDE-EFFECTS** Perineal irritation may follow intravenous administration of the phosphate ester

- **PREGNANCY** Dexamethasone readily crosses the placenta.

- **DIRECTIONS FOR ADMINISTRATION**
For administration *by mouth* tablets may be dispersed in water or injection solution given by mouth.
For *intravenous infusion* dilute with Glucose 5% or Sodium Chloride 0.9%; give over 15–20 minutes.

- **PRESCRIBING AND DISPENSING INFORMATION**
Dexamethasone 3.8 mg/mL Injection has replaced Dexamethasone 4 mg/mL Injection. All dosage recommendations for intravenous, intramuscular,

intrarticular use or local infiltration; are given in units of dexamethasone base.

- **PATIENT AND CARER ADVICE** Patient counselling is advised for dexamethasone tablet, oral solution and injection (steroid card).
Medicines for Children leaflet: Dexamethasone for croup
www.medicinesforchildren.org.uk/dexamethasone-croup-0

- **MEDICINAL FORMS**
There can be variation in the licensing of different medicines containing the same drug. Forms available from special-order manufacturers include: capsule, oral suspension, oral solution

Soluble tablet
▸ Dexamethasone (Non-proprietary)
Dexamethasone (as Dexamethasone sodium phosphate)
2 mg Dexamethasone 2mg soluble tablets sugar free sugar-free | 50 tablet [PoM] £30.00–£31.03 DT price = £31.03
Dexamethasone (as Dexamethasone sodium phosphate)
4 mg Dexamethasone 4mg soluble tablets sugar free sugar-free | 50 tablet [PoM] £60.00–£62.06 DT price = £62.06
Dexamethasone (as Dexamethasone sodium phosphate)
8 mg Dexamethasone 8mg soluble tablets sugar free sugar-free | 50 tablet [PoM] £120.00–£123.70 DT price = £123.70

Tablet
CAUTIONARY AND ADVISORY LABELS 10, 21
▸ Dexamethasone (Non-proprietary)
Dexamethasone 500 microgram Dexamethasone 500microgram tablets | 28 tablet [PoM] £54.25 DT price = £54.25 | 30 tablet [PoM] £64.82
Dexamethasone 2 mg Dexamethasone 2mg tablets | 50 tablet [PoM] £49.00 DT price = £42.85 | 100 tablet [PoM] £98.00 | 500 tablet [PoM] £490.00
Dexamethasone 4 mg Dexamethasone 4mg tablets | 50 tablet [PoM] £85.00–£98.00

Solution for injection
CAUTIONARY AND ADVISORY LABELS 10
▸ Dexamethasone (Non-proprietary)
Dexamethasone (as Dexamethasone sodium phosphate) 3.3 mg per 1 ml Dexamethasone 6.6mg/2ml solution for injection vials | 5 vial [PoM] £24.00 DT price = £24.00
Dexamethasone 6.6mg/2ml solution for injection ampoules | 5 ampoule [PoM] £11.00 DT price = £11.00 | 10 ampoule [PoM] £22.00
Dexamethasone 3.3mg/1ml solution for injection ampoules | 5 ampoule [PoM] £12.00 | 10 ampoule [PoM] £12.00 DT price = £12.00
Dexamethasone (as Dexamethasone sodium phosphate) 3.8 mg per 1 ml Dexamethasone 3.8mg/1ml solution for injection vials | 10 vial [PoM] £19.99 DT price = £19.99

Oral solution
CAUTIONARY AND ADVISORY LABELS 10, 21
▸ Dexamethasone (Non-proprietary)
Dexamethasone (as Dexamethasone sodium phosphate)
400 microgram per 1 ml Dexamethasone 2mg/5ml oral solution sugar free sugar-free | 75 ml [PoM] no price available sugar-free | 150 ml [PoM] £42.30 DT price = £42.30
Dexamethasone (as Dexamethasone sodium phosphate) 2 mg per 1 ml Dexamethasone 10mg/5ml oral solution sugar free sugar-free | 50 ml [PoM] £24.50–£24.95 sugar-free | 150 ml [PoM] £101.40 DT price = £94.44
Dexamethasone (as Dexamethasone sodium phosphate) 4 mg per 1 ml Dexamethasone 20mg/5ml oral solution sugar free sugar-free | 50 ml [PoM] £49.50 DT price = £49.50
▸ Dexsol (Rosemont Pharmaceuticals Ltd)
Dexamethasone (as Dexamethasone sodium phosphate)
400 microgram per 1 ml Dexsol 2mg/5ml oral solution sugar-free | 75 ml [PoM] £21.15 sugar-free | 150 ml [PoM] £42.30 DT price = £42.30
▸ Martapan (Martindale Pharmaceuticals Ltd)
Dexamethasone (as Dexamethasone sodium phosphate)
400 microgram per 1 ml Martapan 2mg/5ml oral solution sugar-free | 150 ml [PoM] £42.30 DT price = £42.30

6

Endocrine system

Fludrocortisone acetate

F 416

INDICATIONS AND DOSE

Mineralocorticoid replacement in adrenocortical insufficiency
▶ BY MOUTH

▸ Neonate: Initially 50 micrograms once daily, adjusted according to response; usual dose 50–200 micrograms once daily, higher doses may be required, dose adjustment may be required if salt supplements are administered

▸ Child: Initially 50–100 micrograms once daily; maintenance 50–300 micrograms once daily, adjusted according to response, dose adjustment may be required if salt supplements are administered

INTERACTIONS → Appendix 1: corticosteroids

HEPATIC IMPAIRMENT Monitor patient closely in hepatic impairment.

PATIENT AND CARER ADVICE
Medicines for Children leaflet: Fludrocortisone for hormone replacement www.medicinesforchildren.org.uk/fludrocortisone-for-hormone-replacement

MEDICINAL FORMS
There can be variation in the licensing of different medicines containing the same drug. Forms available from special-order manufacturers include: capsule, oral suspension

Tablet
CAUTIONARY AND ADVISORY LABELS 10
▸ Fludrocortisone acetate (Non-proprietary)
Fludrocortisone acetate 100 microgram Fludrocortisone 100microgram tablets | 30 tablet PoM £30.00 DT price = £26.77 | 100 tablet PoM £55.00

Hydrocortisone

F 416

18-May-2017

INDICATIONS AND DOSE

Acute adrenocortical insufficiency (Addisonian crisis)
▶ INITIALLY BY SLOW INTRAVENOUS INJECTION

▸ Neonate: Initially 10 mg, then (by continuous intravenous infusion) 100 mg/m^2 daily, alternatively (by intravenous infusion) 100 mg/m^2 daily in divided doses, to be given every 6–8 hours; adjusted according to response, when stable reduce over 4–5 days to oral maintenance dose.

▶ BY SLOW INTRAVENOUS INJECTION, OR BY INTRAVENOUS INFUSION

▸ Child 1 month–11 years: Initially 2–4 mg/kg, then 2–4 mg/kg every 6 hours, adjusted according to response, when stable reduce over 4–5 days to oral maintenance dose

▸ Child 12–17 years: 100 mg every 6–8 hours

Congenital adrenal hyperplasia
▶ BY MOUTH USING IMMEDIATE-RELEASE MEDICINES

▸ Neonate: 9–15 mg/m^2 in 3 divided doses, adjusted according to response.

▸ Child: 9–15 mg/m^2 in 3 divided doses, adjusted according to response

Adrenal hypoplasia | Addison's disease, chronic maintenance or replacement therapy
▶ BY MOUTH USING IMMEDIATE-RELEASE MEDICINES

▸ Neonate: 8–10 mg/m^2 daily in 3 divided doses, the larger dose to be given in the morning and the smaller in the evening, higher doses may be needed.

▸ Child: 8–10 mg/m^2 daily in 3 divided doses, the larger dose to be given in the morning and the smaller in the evening, higher doses may be needed

Inflammatory bowel disease—induction of remission
▶ BY INTRAVENOUS INJECTION

▸ Child 2–17 years: 2.5 mg/kg every 6 hours (max. per dose 100 mg)

▶ BY CONTINUOUS INTRAVENOUS INFUSION

▸ Child 2–17 years: 10 mg/kg daily, maximum 400 mg per day

Ulcerative colitis | Proctitis | Proctosigmoiditis
▶ BY RECTUM USING RECTAL FOAM

▸ Child 2–17 years: Initially 1 metered application 1–2 times a day for 2–3 weeks, then reduced to 1 metered application once daily on alternate days, to be inserted into the rectum

Acute hypersensitivity reactions | angioedema
▶ BY INTRAMUSCULAR INJECTION, OR BY INTRAVENOUS INJECTION

▸ Child 1–5 months: Initially 25 mg 3 times a day, adjusted according to response

▸ Child 6 months–5 years: Initially 50 mg 3 times a day, adjusted according to response

▸ Child 6–11 years: Initially 100 mg 3 times a day, adjusted according to response

▸ Child 12–17 years: Initially 200 mg 3 times a day, adjusted according to response

Hypotension resistant to inotropic treatment and volume replacement (limited evidence)
▶ BY INTRAVENOUS INJECTION

▸ Neonate: Initially 2.5 mg/kg, then 2.5 mg/kg after 4 hours if required, followed by 2.5 mg/kg every 6 hours for 48 hours or until blood pressure recovers, dose to then be reduced gradually over at least 48 hours.

▸ Child: 1 mg/kg every 6 hours (max. per dose 100 mg)

Severe acute asthma | Life-threatening acute asthma
▶ BY INTRAVENOUS INJECTION

▸ Child 1 month–1 year: 4 mg/kg every 6 hours (max. per dose 100 mg), alternatively 25 mg every 6 hours until conversion to oral prednisolone is possible, dose given, preferably, as sodium succinate

▸ Child 2–4 years: 4 mg/kg every 6 hours (max. per dose 100 mg), alternatively 50 mg every 6 hours until conversion to oral prednisolone is possible, dose given, preferably, as sodium succinate

▸ Child 5–11 years: 4 mg/kg every 6 hours (max. per dose 100 mg), alternatively 100 mg every 6 hours until conversion to oral prednisolone is possible, dose given, preferably, as sodium succinate

▸ Child 12–17 years: 4 mg/kg every 6 hours (max. per dose 100 mg), alternatively 100 mg every 6 hours until conversion to oral prednisolone is possible, dose given, preferably, as sodium succinate

UNLICENSED USE Use of injection by mouth is unlicensed.

CONTRA-INDICATIONS
With rectal use Bowel perforation · extensive fistulas · intestinal obstruction · recent intestinal anastomoses

CAUTIONS
With rectal use Systemic absorption may occur

INTERACTIONS → Appendix 1: corticosteroids

SIDE-EFFECTS
▸ With intravenous use Phosphate ester associated with pain and paraesthesia (particularly in the perineal region)
▸ With rectal use Local irritation

DIRECTIONS FOR ADMINISTRATION
▸ With intravenous use For *intravenous administration*, dilute with Glucose 5% or Sodium Chloride 0.9%. For *intermittent infusion* give over 20–30 minutes.

6

Endocrine system

▸ With oral use For administration *by mouth*, injection solution may be swallowed [unlicensed use] but consider phosphate content.

● **PATIENT AND CARER ADVICE** Patient counselling is advised for hydrocortisone tablets and injections (steroid card).

● **LESS SUITABLE FOR PRESCRIBING**

▸ With intravenous use Hydrocortisone as the sodium phosphate is less suitable for prescribing as paraesthesia and pain (particularly in the perineal region) may follow intravenous injection.

● **EXCEPTIONS TO LEGAL CATEGORY** Prescription only medicine restriction does not apply where administration is for saving life in emergency.

● **MEDICINAL FORMS**
There can be variation in the licensing of different medicines containing the same drug. Forms available from special-order manufacturers include: capsule, oral suspension, oral solution

Tablet
CAUTIONARY AND ADVISORY LABELS 10, 21
▸ Hydrocortisone (Non-proprietary)
  Hydrocortisone 10 mg Hydrocortisone 10mg tablets |
  30 tablet PoM £85.11 DT price = £68.67
  Hydrocortisone 20 mg Hydrocortisone 20mg tablets |
  30 tablet PoM £147.26 DT price = £99.96

Powder for solution for injection
▸ Solu-Cortef (Pfizer Ltd)
  Hydrocortisone (as Hydrocortisone sodium succinate)
  100 mg Solu-Cortef 100mg powder for solution for injection vials |
  10 vial PoM £9.17

Powder and solvent for solution for injection
CAUTIONARY AND ADVISORY LABELS 10
▸ Solu-Cortef (Pfizer Ltd)
  Hydrocortisone (as Hydrocortisone sodium succinate)
  100 mg Solu-Cortef 100mg powder and solvent for solution for injection vials | 1 vial PoM £1.16 DT price = £1.16

Solution for injection
CAUTIONARY AND ADVISORY LABELS 10
▸ Hydrocortisone (Non-proprietary)
  Hydrocortisone (as Hydrocortisone sodium phosphate) 100 mg per 1 ml Hydrocortisone sodium phosphate 100mg/1ml solution for injection ampoules | 5 ampoule PoM £8.33
  Hydrocortisone sodium phosphate 500mg/5ml solution for injection ampoules | 5 ampoule PoM £36.45

Foam
EXCIPIENTS: May contain Cetostearyl alcohol (including cetyl and stearyl alcohol), hydroxybenzoates (parabens), propylene glycol
▸ Colifoam (Meda Pharmaceuticals Ltd)
  Hydrocortisone acetatae 100mg per 1 gram Colifoam 10% aerosol | 14 dose PoM £9.33 DT price = £9.33

F 416

Methylprednisolone
10-Aug-2016

● **INDICATIONS AND DOSE**

Inflammatory and allergic disorders
▸ BY MOUTH, OR BY SLOW INTRAVENOUS INJECTION, OR BY INTRAVENOUS INFUSION
▸ Child: 0.5–1.7 mg/kg daily in 2–4 divided doses, divide doses depending on condition and response

Treatment of graft rejection reactions
▸ BY INTRAVENOUS INJECTION
▸ Child: 10–20 mg/kg once daily for 3 days, alternatively 400–600 mg/m² once daily (max. per dose 1 g) for 3 days

Severe erythema multiforme | Lupus nephritis | Systemic onset juvenile idiopathic arthritis
▸ BY INTRAVENOUS INJECTION
▸ Child: 10–30 mg/kg once daily or on alternate days (max. per dose 1 g) for up to 3 doses

DEPO-MEDRONE®

Suppression of inflammatory and allergic disorders
▸ BY DEEP INTRAMUSCULAR INJECTION
▸ Child: Seek specialist advice, to be injected into the gluteal muscle

● **CAUTIONS** Rapid intravenous administration of large doses associated with cardiovascular collapse

● **INTERACTIONS** → Appendix 1: corticosteroids

● **DIRECTIONS FOR ADMINISTRATION** Intravenous injection given over 30 minutes. For intravenous infusion, may be diluted with sodium chloride intravenous infusion 0.9% or 0.45%, or glucose intravenous infusion 5% or 10%.

● **PATIENT AND CARER ADVICE** Patient counselling is advised for methylprednisolone tablets and injections (steroid card).

● **MEDICINAL FORMS**
There can be variation in the licensing of different medicines containing the same drug.

Powder and solvent for solution for injection
CAUTIONARY AND ADVISORY LABELS 10
▸ Methylprednisolone (Non-proprietary)
  Methylprednisolone (as Methylprednisolone sodium succinate)
  500 mg Methylprednisolone sodium succinate 500mg powder and solvent for solution for injection vials | 1 vial PoM £9.60
  Methylprednisolone (as Methylprednisolone sodium succinate)
  1 gram Methylprednisolone sodium succinate 1g powder and solvent for solution for injection vials | 1 vial PoM £17.30
▸ Solu-Medrone (Pfizer Ltd)
  Methylprednisolone (as Methylprednisolone sodium succinate)
  40 mg Solu-Medrone 40mg powder and solvent for solution for injection vials | 1 vial PoM £1.58
  Methylprednisolone (as Methylprednisolone sodium succinate)
  125 mg Solu-Medrone 125mg powder and solvent for solution for injection vials | 1 vial PoM £4.75
  Methylprednisolone (as Methylprednisolone sodium succinate)
  500 mg Solu-Medrone 500mg powder and solvent for solution for injection vials | 1 vial PoM £9.60
  Methylprednisolone (as Methylprednisolone sodium succinate)
  1 gram Solu-Medrone 1g powder and solvent for solution for injection vials | 1 vial PoM £17.30
  Methylprednisolone (as Methylprednisolone sodium succinate)
  2 gram Solu-Medrone 2g powder and solvent for solution for injection vials | 1 vial PoM £32.86

Tablet
CAUTIONARY AND ADVISORY LABELS 10, 21
▸ Medrone (Pfizer Ltd)
  Methylprednisolone 2 mg Medrone 2mg tablets | 30 tablet PoM £3.88
  Methylprednisolone 4 mg Medrone 4mg tablets | 30 tablet PoM £6.19
  Methylprednisolone 16 mg Medrone 16mg tablets | 30 tablet PoM £17.17
  Methylprednisolone 100 mg Medrone 100mg tablets | 20 tablet PoM £48.32

Suspension for injection
CAUTIONARY AND ADVISORY LABELS 10
▸ Depo-Medrone (Pfizer Ltd)
  Methylprednisolone acetate 40 mg per 1 ml Depo-Medrone 40mg/1ml suspension for injection vials | 1 vial PoM £3.44 DT price = £3.44 | 10 vial PoM £34.04
  Depo-Medrone 80mg/2ml suspension for injection vials | 1 vial PoM £6.18 DT price = £6.18 | 10 vial PoM £61.39
  Depo-Medrone 120mg/3ml suspension for injection vials | 1 vial PoM £8.96 DT price = £8.96 | 10 vial PoM £88.81

F 416

Prednisolone

● **INDICATIONS AND DOSE**

Severe croup (before transfer to hospital) | Mild croup that might cause complications (before transfer to hospital)
▸ BY MOUTH
▸ Child: 1–2 mg/kg

continued →

Mild to moderate acute asthma (when oral corticosteroid taken for more than a few days) | Severe or life-threatening acute asthma (when oral corticosteroid taken for more than a few days)
- BY MOUTH
- Child 1 month–11 years: 2 mg/kg once daily (max. per dose 60 mg) for up to 3 days, longer if necessary

Mild to moderate acute asthma | Severe or life-threatening acute asthma
- BY MOUTH
- Child 1 month–11 years: 1–2 mg/kg once daily (max. per dose 40 mg) for up to 3 days, longer if necessary
- Child 12–17 years: 40–50 mg daily for at least 5 days

Autoimmune inflammatory disorders (including juvenile idiopathic arthritis, connective tissue disorders and systemic lupus erythematosus)
- BY MOUTH
- Child: Initially 1–2 mg/kg once daily, to be reduced after a few days if appropriate; maximum 60 mg per day

Autoimmune hepatitis
- BY MOUTH
- Child: Initially 2 mg/kg once daily, to then be reduced to minimum effective dose; maximum 40 mg per day

Corticosteroid replacement therapy
- BY MOUTH
- Child 12–17 years: 2–2.5 mg/m^2 daily in 1–2 divided doses, adjusted according to response

Infantile spasms
- BY MOUTH
- Child 1 month–1 year: Initially 10 mg 4 times a day for 14 days; increased to 20 mg 3 times a day for 7 days if seizures not controlled after initial 7 days, reduce dose gradually over 15 days until stopped

Infantile spasms (dose reduction in patient taking 40 mg daily)
- BY MOUTH
- Child 1 month–1 year: Reduced in steps of 10 mg every 5 days, then stop

Infantile spasms (dose reduction in patient taking 60 mg daily)
- BY MOUTH
- Child 1 month–1 year: Reduced to 40 mg daily for 5 days, then reduced to 20 mg daily for 5 days, then reduced to 10 mg daily for 5 days and then stop

Idiopathic thrombocytopenic purpura
- BY MOUTH
- Child 1–9 years: 1–2 mg/kg daily for maximum of 14 days, alternatively 4 mg/kg daily for a maximum of 4 days

Nephrotic syndrome
- BY MOUTH
- Child: Initially 60 mg/m^2 once daily for 4–6 weeks until proteinuria ceases, then reduced to 40 mg/m^2 once daily on alternate days for 4–6 weeks, then withdraw by reducing dose gradually; maximum 80 mg per day

Nephrotic syndrome (prevention of relapse)
- BY MOUTH
- Child: 0.5–1 mg/kg once daily or on alternate days for 3–6 months

Ulcerative colitis | Crohn's disease
- BY MOUTH
- Child 2–17 years: 2 mg/kg once daily (max. per dose 60 mg) until remission occurs, followed by reducing doses

Pneumocystis pneumonia in moderate to severe infections associated with HIV infection
- BY MOUTH
- Child: 2 mg/kg daily for 5 days, the dose is then reduced over the next 16 days and then stopped, corticosteroid treatment should ideally be started at the same time as the anti-pneumocystis therapy and certainly no later than 24–72 hours afterwards, the corticosteroid should be withdrawn before anti-pneumocystis treatment is complete; maximum 80 mg per day

Proctitis
- BY RECTUM USING RECTAL FOAM
- Child 12–17 years: 1 metered application 1–2 times a day for 2 weeks, continued for further 2 weeks if good response, to be inserted into the rectum, 1 metered application contains 20 mg prednisolone
- BY RECTUM USING SUPPOSITORIES
- Child 2–17 years: 5 mg twice daily, to be inserted in to the rectum morning and night, after a bowel movement

Distal ulcerative colitis
- BY RECTUM USING RECTAL FOAM
- Child 12–17 years: 1 metered application 1–2 times a day for 2 weeks, continued for further 2 weeks if good response, to be inserted into the rectum, 1 metered application contains 20 mg prednisolone

Rectal complications of Crohn's disease
- BY RECTUM USING SUPPOSITORIES
- Child 2–17 years: 5 mg twice daily, to be inserted in to the rectum morning and night, after a bowel movement

- ● UNLICENSED USE Prednisolone rectal foam not licensed for use in children (age range not specified by manufacturer).
- ● CONTRA-INDICATIONS
- With rectal use Bowel perforation · extensive fistulas · intestinal obstruction · recent intestinal anastomoses
- ● CAUTIONS
- With rectal use Systemic absorption may occur with rectal preparations
- With systemic use Duchenne's muscular dystrophy (possible transient rhabdomyolysis and myoglobinuria following strenuous physical activity)
- ● INTERACTIONS → Appendix 1: corticosteroids
- ● PREGNANCY As it crosses the placenta 88% of prednisolone is inactivated.
- With systemic use Pregnant women with fluid retention should be monitored closely.
- ● BREAST FEEDING Prednisolone appears in small amounts in breast milk but maternal doses of up to 40 mg daily are unlikely to cause systemic effects in the infant.
- With systemic use Infant should be monitored for adrenal suppression if mother is taking a dose higher than 40 mg.
- ● PATIENT AND CARER ADVICE Patient counselling is advised for prednisolone tablets (steroid card).
  Prednisolone (oral) for nephrotic syndrome
  www.medicinesforchildren.org.uk/prednisolone-oral-for-nephrotic-syndrome
  Medicines for Children leaflet: Prednisolone for asthma
  www.medicinesforchildren.org.uk/prednisolone-for-asthma

- ● MEDICINAL FORMS
  There can be variation in the licensing of different medicines containing the same drug. Forms available from special-order manufacturers include: oral suspension, oral solution

Foam
- Prednisolone (Non-proprietary)
  Prednisolone (as Prednisolone sodium metasulfobenzoate) 20 mg per 1 application Prednisolone 20mg/application foam enema | 14 dose [PoM] £187.00 DT price = £187.00

Gastro-resistant tablet
CAUTIONARY AND ADVISORY LABELS 5, 10, 25
- Prednisolone (Non-proprietary)
  Prednisolone 1 mg Prednisolone 1mg gastro-resistant tablets | 30 tablet [PoM] £1.60–£1.92 DT price = £1.84

Prednisolone 2.5 mg Prednisolone 2.5mg gastro-resistant tablets |
28 tablet PoM £1.20 DT price = £1.17 | 30 tablet PoM £6.15 |
100 tablet PoM £4.29
Prednisolone 5 mg Prednisolone 5mg gastro-resistant tablets |
28 tablet PoM £1.21 DT price = £1.20 | 30 tablet PoM £6.29
▸ **Deltacortril Enteric** (Alliance Pharmaceuticals Ltd)
Prednisolone 2.5 mg Deltacortril 2.5mg gastro-resistant tablets |
30 tablet PoM £1.16
Prednisolone 5 mg Deltacortril 5mg gastro-resistant tablets |
30 tablet PoM £1.19
▸ **Dilacort** (Crescent Pharma Ltd, Teva UK Ltd)
Prednisolone 2.5 mg Dilacort 2.5mg gastro-resistant tablets |
28 tablet PoM £1.14-£1.85 DT price = £1.17
Prednisolone 5 mg Dilacort 5mg gastro-resistant tablets |
28 tablet PoM £1.45-£1.95 DT price = £1.20

Soluble tablet
CAUTIONARY AND ADVISORY LABELS 10, 13, 21
▸ **Prednisolone (Non-proprietary)**
Prednisolone (as Prednisolone sodium phosphate)
5 mg Prednisolone 5mg soluble tablets | 30 tablet PoM £60.00 DT
price = £53.48

Tablet
CAUTIONARY AND ADVISORY LABELS 10, 21
▸ **Prednisolone (Non-proprietary)**
Prednisolone 1 mg Prednisolone 1mg tablets | 28 tablet PoM
£4.00 DT price = £0.78
Prednisolone 2.5 mg Prednisolone 2.5mg tablets | 28 tablet PoM
£1.33
Prednisolone 5 mg Prednisolone 5mg tablets | 28 tablet PoM
£9.86 DT price = £0.87
Prednisolone 10 mg Prednisolone 10mg tablets | 28 tablet PoM
£2.72
Prednisolone 20 mg Prednisolone 20mg tablets | 28 tablet PoM
£5.43
Prednisolone 25 mg Prednisolone 25mg tablets | 56 tablet PoM
£75.00 DT price = £75.00
Prednisolone 30 mg Prednisolone 30mg tablets | 28 tablet PoM
£8.15
▸ **Pevanti** (AMCo)
Prednisolone 2.5 mg Pevanti 2.5mg tablets | 30 tablet PoM £1.42
DT price = £1.42
Prednisolone 5 mg Pevanti 5mg tablets | 30 tablet PoM £0.95
Prednisolone 10 mg Pevanti 10mg tablets | 30 tablet PoM £1.90
DT price = £1.90
Prednisolone 20 mg Pevanti 20mg tablets | 30 tablet PoM £3.80
DT price = £3.80
Prednisolone 25 mg Pevanti 25mg tablets | 56 tablet PoM £40.00
DT price = £75.00

Suppository
▸ **Prednisolone (Non-proprietary)**
Prednisolone (as Prednisolone sodium phosphate)
5 mg Prednisolone sodium phosphate 5mg suppositories |
10 suppository PoM £38.63 DT price = £38.63

Oral solution
CAUTIONARY AND ADVISORY LABELS 10
▸ **Prednisolone (Non-proprietary)**
Prednisolone 1 mg per 1 ml Prednisolone 5mg/5ml oral solution unit
dose | 10 unit dose PoM £11.41 DT price = £11.41
Prednisolone 10 mg per 1 ml Prednisolone 10mg/ml oral solution
sugar free sugar-free | 30 ml PoM £55.00-£55.50 DT price = £55.50

2.1 Cushing's syndrome and disease

Cushing's Syndrome

Management
Most types of *Cushing's syndrome* are treated surgically.
Metyrapone p. 424 may be useful to control the symptoms of
the disease or to prepare the child for surgery. The dosages
of metyrapone used are either low, and tailored to cortisol
production, or high, in which case corticosteroid
replacement therapy is also needed.

Ketoconazole below may have a direct effect on corticotropic
tumour cells in patients with Cushing's disease. It is used
under specialist supervision in children over 12 years for
treatment of endogenous Cushing's syndrome.

ENZYME INHIBITORS

Ketoconazole
16-Jun-2017

● **DRUG ACTION** An imidazole derivative which acts as a
potent inhibitor of cortisol and aldosterone synthesis by
inhibiting the activity of 17α-hydroxylase,
11-hydroxylation steps and at higher doses the cholesterol
side-chain cleavage enzyme. It also inhibits the activity of
adrenal C17-20 lyase enzymes resulting in androgen
synthesis inhibition, and may have a direct effect on
corticotropic tumour cells in patients with Cushing's
disease.

● **INDICATIONS AND DOSE**
Endogenous Cushing's syndrome (specialist use only)
▸ BY MOUTH
▸ **Child 12-17 years:** Initially 400–600 mg daily in
2–3 divided doses, increased to 800–1200 mg daily;
maintenance 400–800 mg daily in 2–3 divided doses,
for dose titrations in patients with established dose,
adjustments in adrenal insufficiency, or concomitant
corticosteroid replacement therapy, consult product
literature; maximum 1200 mg per day

● **CONTRA-INDICATIONS** Acquired QTc prolongation · avoid
concomitant use of hepatotoxic drugs · congenital QTc
prolongation

● **CAUTIONS** Risk of adrenal insufficiency

● **INTERACTIONS** → Appendix 1: antifungals, azoles

● **SIDE-EFFECTS**
▸ **Common or very common** Abdominal pain · adrenal
insufficiency · diarrhoea · hepatic enzymes increased ·
nausea · pruritus · rash · vomiting
▸ **Uncommon** Alopecia · dizziness · headache · malaise ·
somnolence · thrombocytopenia · urticaria
▸ **Rare** Hepatic failure · hepatitis · jaundice · liver damage
▸ **Very rare** Pyrexia
▸ **Frequency not known** Alcohol intolerance · anorexia ·
arthralgia · azoospermia · dermatitis · dry mouth ·
dysgeusia · dyspepsia · epistaxis · erectile dysfunction ·
erythema · flatulence · gynaecomastia · hot flush ·
increased appetite · insomnia · menstrual disorder ·
myalgia · nervousness · paraesthesia · peripheral oedema ·
photophobia · photosensitivity · raised intracranial
pressure · reduced testosterone concentrations · tongue
discoloration · xeroderma

SIDE-EFFECTS, FURTHER INFORMATION
▸ Hepatotoxicity Potentially life-threatening hepatotoxicity
reported rarely.

● **CONCEPTION AND CONTRACEPTION** Effective
contraception must be used in women of child-bearing
potential.

● **PREGNANCY** Manufacturer advises avoid—teratogenic in
animal studies.

● **BREAST FEEDING** Manufacturer advises avoid—present in
breast milk.

● **HEPATIC IMPAIRMENT** Avoid in acute or chronic
impairment. Do not initiate treatment if liver enzymes
greater than 2 times the normal upper limit.

● **MONITORING REQUIREMENTS**
▸ Monitor ECG before and one week after initiation, and
then as clinically indicated thereafter.
▸ Adrenal insufficiency Monitor adrenal function within one
week of initiation, then regularly thereafter. When cortisol
levels are normalised or close to target and effective dose

Endocrine system

6

established, monitor every 3–6 months as there is a risk of autoimmune disease development or exacerbation after normalisation of cortisol levels. If symptoms suggestive of adrenal insufficiency such as fatigue, anorexia, nausea, vomiting, hypotension, hyponatraemia, hyperkalaemia, and/or hypoglycaemia occur, measure cortisol levels and discontinue treatment temporarily (can be resumed thereafter at lower dose) or reduce dose and if necessary, initiate corticosteroid substitution.

▶ Hepatotoxicity Monitor liver function before initiation of treatment, then weekly for 1 month after initiation, then monthly for 6 months—more frequently if dose adjusted or abnormal liver function detected. Reduce dose if liver enzymes increase less than 3 times the normal upper limit—consult product literature; if liver enzymes are raised to 3 times or greater the normal upper limit, discontinue treatment permanently.

● PATIENT AND CARER ADVICE
Patients or their carers should be told how to recognise signs of liver disorder, and advised to discontinue treatment and seek prompt medical attention if symptoms such as anorexia, nausea, vomiting, fatigue, jaundice, abdominal pain, or dark urine develop.

Patients or their carers should also be told how to recognise signs of adrenal insufficiency.

Driving and skilled tasks
Dizziness and somnolence may affect the performance of skilled tasks (e.g. driving).

● MEDICINAL FORMS
There can be variation in the licensing of different medicines containing the same drug. Forms available from special-order manufacturers include: oral suspension
Tablet
CAUTIONARY AND ADVISORY LABELS 2, 5, 21
▶ Ketoconazole (non-proprietary) ▼
Ketoconazole 200 mg Ketoconazole 200mg tablets |
60 tablet PoM £480.00

Metyrapone

● DRUG ACTION Metyrapone is a competitive inhibitor of 11β-hydroxylation in the adrenal cortex; the resulting inhibition of cortisol (and to a lesser extent aldosterone) production leads to an increase in ACTH production which, in turn, leads to increased synthesis and release of cortisol precursors. Metyrapone may be used as a test of anterior pituitary function.

● INDICATIONS AND DOSE

Differential diagnosis of ACTH-dependent Cushing's syndrome (specialist supervision in hospital)
▶ BY MOUTH
▶ Child: 15 mg/kg every 4 hours for 6 doses, alternatively 300 mg/m² every 4 hours for 6 doses; usual dose 250–750 mg every 4 hours

Management of Cushing's syndrome (specialist supervision in hospital)
▶ BY MOUTH
▶ Child: Usual dose 0.25–6 g daily, dose to be tailored to cortisol production, dose is either low, and tailored to cortisol production, or high, in which case corticosteroid replacement therapy is also needed

● CONTRA-INDICATIONS Adrenocortical insufficiency
● CAUTIONS Avoid in acute porphyrias p. 577 · gross hypopituitarism (risk of precipitating acute adrenal failure) · hypertension on long-term administration · hypothyroidism (delayed response)
● INTERACTIONS → Appendix 1: metyrapone

● SIDE-EFFECTS
▶ Rare Abdominal pain · allergic skin reactions · hirsutism · hypoadrenalism
▶ Frequency not known Dizziness - headache · hypotension · nausea · sedation · vomiting
● PREGNANCY Avoid (may impair biosynthesis of fetal-placental steroids).
● BREAST FEEDING Avoid—no information available.
● HEPATIC IMPAIRMENT Use with caution in hepatic impairment (delayed response).
● PATIENT AND CARER ADVICE
Driving and skilled tasks
Drowsiness may affect the performance of skilled tasks (e.g. driving).

● MEDICINAL FORMS
There can be variation in the licensing of different medicines containing the same drug.
Capsule
CAUTIONARY AND ADVISORY LABELS 21
▶ Metopirone (HRA Pharma UK Ltd)
Metyrapone 250 mg Metopirone 250mg capsules |
100 capsule PoM £363.66

3 Diabetes mellitus and hypoglycaemia
3.1 Diabetes mellitus

Diabetes

05-Jun-2017

Description of condition

Diabetes mellitus is a group of metabolic disorders in which persistent hyperglycaemia is caused by deficient insulin secretion or by resistance to the action of insulin. This leads to the abnormalities of carbohydrate, fat and protein metabolism that are characteristic of diabetes mellitus.

Type 1 diabetes mellitus p. 425 and Type 2 diabetes mellitus p. 428 are the two most common classifications of diabetes. Other common types of diabetes are gestational diabetes (develops during pregnancy and resolves after delivery) and secondary diabetes (may be caused by pancreatic damage, hepatic cirrhosis, or endocrinological disease). Treatment with endocrine, antiviral or antipsychotic drugs may also cause secondary diabetes. In children, conditions such as cystic fibrosis can lead to diabetes; monogenic diabetes (previously known as maturity onset diabetes in the young) can also occur due to a single gene defect.

Driving

Information on the requirements for driving vehicles by young people receiving treatment for diabetes is available in the BNF or from the DVLA at www.gov.uk/guidance/diabetes-mellitus-assessing-fitness-to-drive

Alcohol

Adolescents and their carers should be made aware that alcohol can make the signs of hypoglycaemia less clear, and can cause delayed hypoglycaemia; (note: specialist sources recommend that **adult** patients with diabetes should drink alcohol only in moderation, and when accompanied by food).

Oral glucose tolerance tests

The oral glucose tolerance test is used mainly for diagnosis of impaired glucose tolerance; it is **not** recommended or necessary for routine diagnostic use of diabetes when severe symptoms of hyperglycaemia are present. In children who have less severe symptoms and blood glucose levels that do not establish or exclude diabetes (e.g. impaired fasting glycaemia), an oral glucose tolerance test may be required. It may be useful for diagnosis of monogenic diabetes or cystic fibrosis related diabetes, and is used to establish the presence of gestational diabetes.

An oral glucose tolerance test involves measuring the blood-glucose concentration after fasting, and then 2 hours after drinking a standard anhydrous glucose drink. Anhydrous glucose may alternatively be given as the appropriate amount of *Polycal*® or as *Rapilose*® OGTT oral solution.

HbA1c measurement

Glycated haemoglobin (HbA1c) forms when red blood cells are exposed to glucose in the plasma. The HbA1c test reflects average plasma glucose over the previous 2 to 3 months and provides a good indicator of glycaemic control. Unlike the oral glucose tolerance test, an HbA1c test can be performed at any time of the day and does not require any special preparation such as fasting.

HbA1c values are expressed in *mmol of glycated haemoglobin per mol of haemoglobin (mmol/mol)*, a standardised unit specific for HbA1c created by the International Federation of Clinical Chemistry and Laboratory Medicine (IFCC). HbA1c values were previously aligned to the assay used in the Diabetes Control and Complications Trial (DCCT) and expressed as a percentage.

Equivalent values	
IFCC-HbA1c (mmol/mol)	DCCT-HbA1c (%)
42	6.0
48	6.5
53	7.0
59	7.5
64	8.0
69	8.5
75	9.0

The HbA1c test is used for monitoring glycaemic control in both Type 1 diabetes below and Type 2 diabetes p. 428 in children, and for diagnosis of Type 2 diabetes in adults. [EvGr] HbA1c should not be used to diagnose diabetes in children. ⟨A⟩

HbA1c is also a reliable predictor of microvascular and macrovascular complications and mortality. Lower HbA1c is associated with a lower risk of long term vascular complications, and children and their carers should be supported to aim for an individualised HbA1c target (see Type 1 diabetes below and Type 2 diabetes p. 428). [EvGr] HbA1c should usually be measured in children with type 1 and type 2 diabetes every 3 months; and more frequently in children with type 1 diabetes if blood glucose is poorly controlled. ⟨A⟩

HbA1c monitoring is invalid in children with disturbed erythrocyte turnover or in children with a lack of, or abnormal haemoglobin (for example, any anaemia, a recent blood transfusion, or an altered red cell lifespan). In these cases, quality-controlled plasma glucose profiles, total glycated haemoglobin estimation (if there is abnormal haemoglobin), or fructosamine estimation can be used.

Laboratory measurement of fructosamine concentration measures the glycated fraction of all plasma proteins over the previous 14 to 21 days but is a less accurate measure of glycaemic control than HbA1c.

Type 1 diabetes

05-Jun-2017

Description of condition

Type 1 diabetes describes an absolute insulin deficiency in which there is little or no endogenous insulin secretory capacity due to destruction of insulin-producing beta-cells in the pancreatic islets of Langerhans. This form of the disease has an auto-immune basis in most cases, and it can occur at any age, but most commonly before adulthood.

Loss of insulin secretion results in hyperglycaemia and other metabolic abnormalities. If poorly managed, the resulting tissue damage has both short-term and long-term adverse effects on health; this can result in retinopathy, nephropathy, premature cardiovascular disease, and peripheral artery disease.

Typical features in children presenting with type 1 diabetes are hyperglycaemia, polyuria, polydipsia, weight loss, and excessive tiredness.

Aims of treatment

Treatment is aimed at using insulin regimens to achieve as optimal a level of blood-glucose control as is feasible, while avoiding or reducing the frequency of hypoglycaemic episodes, in order to minimise the risk of long-term microvascular and macrovascular complications. Disability from complications can often be prevented by early detection and active management of the disease (Diabetic complications p. 429).

[EvGr] The target for glycaemic control should be individualised for each child, considering factors such as daily activities, aspirations, likelihood of complications, adherence to treatment, comorbidities, and history of hypoglycaemia. Tighter control of blood-glucose is now recommended for children with type 1 diabetes and treatment should attempt to reach near normal HbA1c and blood-glucose concentration. A target HbA1c concentration of 48 mmol/mol (6.5 %) or lower is recommended in children to minimise the risk of long-term complications. The optimal plasma glucose targets for children are: ⟨A⟩

- [EvGr] Fasting blood-glucose concentration of 4–7 mmol/litre on waking;
- A blood-glucose concentration of 4–7 mmol/litre before meals at other times of the day;
- A blood-glucose concentration of 5–9 mmol/litre after meals;
- A blood-glucose concentration of at least 5 mmol/litre in young people when driving. ⟨A⟩

Overview

[EvGr] Type 1 diabetes requires insulin replacement, supported when necessary by active management of other associated cardiovascular risk factors such as hypertension. Tight glycaemic control may be achieved by intensive insulin management (multiple daily injections or insulin pump therapy) from diagnosis, accompanied by carbohydrate counting.

The effectiveness of metformin in combination with insulin is not yet known in children, and so should not be used; other oral antidiabetic drugs should not be used in combination with insulin as their use may increase the risk of hypoglycaemia.

Dietary control is important in both type 1 and type 2 diabetes and children (with their families) should be encouraged to develop good knowledge of nutrition and how it affects their diabetes and insulin requirements. Healthy eating, regular exercise, and control of body-weight can reduce cardiovascular risk and help improve glycaemic control.

Children with type 1 diabetes over the age of 6 months should receive immunisation against influenza and

6

Endocrine system

pneumococcal infection (in children treated with antidiabetic drugs)—see Vaccines p. 747. Ⓐ

Management of type 1 diabetes with insulin

EvGr All children with type 1 diabetes require insulin therapy (**see also Insulin p. 427**). Treatment should be initiated and managed by clinicians with relevant expertise; there are three basic types of insulin regimen, although each regimen should be individualised.

Children should also be offered carbohydrate-counting training as part of a structured education programme. Ⓐ

Multiple daily injection basal-bolus insulin regimens

One or more separate daily injections of intermediate-acting insulin or long-acting insulin analogue as the basal insulin; alongside multiple bolus injections of short-acting insulin before meals. This regimen offers flexibility to tailor insulin therapy with the carbohydrate load of each meal.

Mixed (biphasic) regimen

One, two, or three insulin injections per day of short-acting insulin mixed with intermediate-acting insulin. The insulin preparations may be mixed by the patient at the time of injection, or a premixed product can be used.

Continuous subcutaneous insulin infusion (insulin pump)

A regular or continuous amount of insulin (usually in the form of a rapid-acting insulin analogue or soluble insulin), delivered by a programmable pump and insulin storage reservoir via a subcutaneous needle or cannula.

Recommended insulin regimens

EvGr Children should be offered multiple daily injection basal-bolus regimens initiated at diagnosis, considering personal and family circumstances, and personal preferences. Children and their carers should be encouraged to adjust the insulin dose as appropriate after each blood-glucose measurement, and to inject rapid-acting insulin analogues before eating (rather than after eating); this reduces blood-glucose concentrations after meals and helps to optimise blood-glucose control.

If a multiple daily injection basal-bolus insulin regimen is unsuitable, or the child does not have optimal blood-glucose control, it may be necessary to offer an alternative insulin regimen (either continuous subcutaneous insulin infusion or once-, twice- or three-times daily mixed injections) as well as additional support (such as increased contact with their specialist diabetes team).

Continuous subcutaneous insulin infusion (or insulin pump) therapy may be considered under the care of a specialist team. It should only be offered to children over 12 years who suffer disabling hypoglycaemia, or, who have high HbA1c concentrations (69 mmol/mol [8.5 %] or above) with multiple daily injection therapy (including, if appropriate, the use of long-acting insulin analogues) despite a high level of care. Children under 12 years may be offered insulin pump therapy if a multiple daily injection regimen is impractical or inappropriate, but they should undergo a trial of a multiple dose injection regimen between the ages of 12 and 18 years.

If the chosen regimen is a twice daily injection regimen, the insulin dose should be adjusted according to the general trend in pre-meal, bedtime and occasional night-time blood-glucose concentration. Ⓐ

Insulin requirements

EvGr The dosage of insulin must be determined individually for each child and should be adjusted as necessary according to the results of regular monitoring of blood-glucose concentrations.

Prescribers and patients should be aware that initiation of insulin may be followed by a **temporary** partial remission phase or 'honeymoon period' when lower doses of insulin are required than are subsequently necessary to maintain

glycaemic control with an HbA1c concentration of less than 48 mmol/mol (6.5 %). Ⓐ

EvGr Insulin doses should be reviewed after puberty (around 1 year after menarche or after the growth spurt in boys) as insulin resistance falls after puberty, and maintenance of pubertal doses may increase the risk for excessive weight gain. Ⓔ

EvGr Persistent poor glucose control, leading to erratic insulin requirements or episodes of hypoglycaemia, may be due to many factors, including adherence, injection technique, injection site problems, blood-glucose monitoring skills, lifestyle issues (including diet and exercise), psychological issues, and organic causes such as renal disease, thyroid disorders, coeliac disease, Addison's disease or gastroparesis. A review of the child's injection sites should be offered at each clinic visit. Ⓐ

Infection, stress, accidental or surgical trauma, and puberty may all increase the required insulin dose. Insulin requirements may be decreased (and therefore susceptibility to hypoglycaemia increased) by physical activity, intercurrent illness, reduced food intake, and in certain endocrine disorders, such as anterior pituitary or adrenocortical insufficiency and hypothyroidism.

EvGr Rapid-acting insulin analogues should be supplied for use during intercurrent illness and episodes of hyperglycaemia. Ⓐ

Risks of hypoglycaemia with insulin

EvGr Hypoglycaemia is an inevitable adverse effect of insulin treatment, and children and their carers should be advised of the warning signs and actions to take (for guidance on management, see Hypoglycaemia p. 443). Ⓐ

Impaired awareness of hypoglycaemia can occur, when the ability to recognise usual symptoms is lost, or when the symptoms are blunted or no longer present. EvGr Awareness of hypoglycaemia should be discussed and assessed with the child and their carer approximately every 3 months. Ⓔ

An increase in the frequency of hypoglycaemic episodes may reduce the warning symptoms experienced by the child. Impaired awareness of symptoms below 3 mmol/litre is associated with a significantly increased risk of severe hypoglycaemia. Beta-blockers can also blunt hypoglycaemic awareness, by reducing warning signs such as tremor. Loss of warning of hypoglycaemia among insulin-treated children can be a serious hazard, especially for adolescents who are drivers, cyclists, or in dangerous occupations. Advice should be given in line with the Driver and Vehicle Licensing Agency (DVLA) guidance (see *Driving*, under Diabetes p. 424).

EvGr To restore the warning signs, episodes of hypoglycaemia must be minimised. Insulin regimens, doses and blood-glucose targets should be reviewed and continuous subcutaneous insulin infusion therapy and real-time continuous glucose monitoring should be considered. Ⓐ

EvGr Children and their carers should receive structured education to ensure they are following the principles of a flexible insulin regimen correctly, with additional education regarding avoiding and treating hypoglycaemia for those who continue to have impaired awareness. If recurrent severe episodes of hypoglycaemia continue despite appropriate interventions, the child should be referred to a specialist centre. Ⓔ

Manufacturers advise any switch between brands or formulation of insulin (including switching from animal to human insulin) should be done under strict supervision; a change in dose may be required.

Hypodermic equipment

EvGr Children and their carers should be advised on the safe disposal of lancets, single-use syringes, and needles, and should be provided with suitable disposal containers.

Arrangements should be made for the suitable disposal of these containers. Ⓐ

Lancets, needles, syringes, and accessories are listed under Hypodermic Equipment in Part IXA of the Drug Tariff (Part III of the Northern Ireland Drug Tariff, Part 3 of the Scottish Drug Tariff). The drug Tariffs can be accessed online at:

- National Health Service Drug Tariff for England and Wales: www.nhsbsa.nhs.uk/pharmacies-gp-practices-and-appliance-contractors/drug-tariff

- Health and Personal Social Services for Northern Ireland Drug Tariff: www.hscbusiness.hscni.net/services/2034.htm

- Scottish Drug Tariff: www.isdscotland.org/Health-Topics/Prescribing-and-Medicines/Scottish-Drug-Tariff

Useful Resources

Diabetes (type 1 and type 2) in children and young people: diagnosis and management. National Institute for Health and Care Excellence. Clinical guideline NG18. August 2015. www.nice.org.uk/guidance/ng18

Insulin

05-Jun-2017

Overview

For recommended insulin regimens see Type 1 diabetes p. 425 and Type 2 diabetes p. 428.

Insulin is a polypeptide hormone secreted by pancreatic beta-cells. Insulin increases glucose uptake by adipose tissue and muscles, and suppresses hepatic glucose release. The role of insulin is to lower blood-glucose concentrations in order to prevent hyperglycaemia and its associated microvascular, macrovascular and metabolic complications.

The natural profile of insulin secretion in the body consists of basal insulin (a low and steady secretion of background insulin that controls the glucose continuously released from the liver) and meal-time bolus insulin (secreted in response to glucose absorbed from food and drink).

Sources of insulin

Three types of insulin are available in the UK: human insulin, human insulin analogues, and animal insulin. Animal insulins are extracted and purified from animal sources (bovine or porcine insulin). Although widely used in the past, animal insulins are no longer initiated in people with diabetes but may still be used by some adult patients who cannot, or do not wish to, change to human insulins.

Human insulins are produced by recombinant DNA technology and have the same amino acid sequence as endogenous human insulin. Human insulin analogues are produced in the same way as human insulins, but the insulin is modified to produce a desired kinetic characteristic, such as an extended duration of action or faster absorption and onset of action.

Immunological resistance to insulin is uncommon and true insulin allergy is rare. Human insulin and insulin analogues are less immunogenic than animal insulins.

Administration of insulin

Insulin is inactivated by gastro-intestinal enzymes and must therefore be given by injection; the subcutaneous route is ideal in most circumstances. Insulin should be injected into a body area with plenty of subcutaneous fat—usually the abdomen (fastest absorption rate) or outer thighs/buttocks (slower absorption compared with the abdomen or inner thighs).

Absorption from a limb site can vary considerably (by as much as 20–40 %) day-to-day, particularly in children. Local tissue reactions, changes in insulin sensitivity, injection site, blood flow, depth of injection, and the amount of insulin injected can all affect the rate of absorption. Increased blood flow around the injection site due to exercise can also increase insulin absorption.

EvGr Lipohypertrophy can occur due to repeatedly injecting into the same small area, and can cause erratic absorption of insulin, and contribute to poor glycaemic control. Patients should be advised not to use affected areas for further injection until the skin has recovered. Lipohypertrophy can be minimised by using different injection sites in rotation. Injection sites should be checked for signs of infection, swelling, bruising, and lipohypertrophy before administration. Ⓐ

Insulin preparations

Insulin preparations can be broadly categorised into three groups based on their time-action profiles: short-acting insulins (including soluble insulin and rapid-acting insulins), intermediate-acting insulins and long-acting insulins. The duration of action of each particular type of insulin varies considerably from one patient to another, and needs to be assessed individually.

Short-acting insulins

Short-acting insulins have a short duration and a relatively rapid onset of action, to replicate the insulin normally produced by the body in response to glucose absorbed from a meal. These are available as soluble Insulin (human and, bovine or porcine—both rarely used), and the rapid-acting insulin analogues (insulin aspart p. 437, insulin glulisine p. 438 and insulin lispro p. 438).

Soluble insulin

Soluble insulin is usually given subcutaneously but some preparations can be given intravenously and intramuscularly. For maintenance regimens, it is usual to inject the insulin 15 to 30 minutes before meals, depending on the insulin preparation used.

When injected subcutaneously, soluble insulin has a rapid onset of action (30 to 60 minutes), a peak action between 1 and 4 hours, and a duration of action of up to 9 hours.

When injected intravenously, soluble insulin has a short half-life of only a few minutes and its onset of action is instantaneous.

Soluble insulin administered intravenously is the most appropriate form of insulin for use in diabetic emergencies e.g. Diabetic ketoacidosis p. 430 and peri-operatively.

Rapid-acting insulin

Insulin aspart, insulin glulisine, and insulin lispro have a faster onset of action (within 15 minutes) and shorter duration of action (approximately 2–5 hours) than soluble insulin, and are usually given by subcutaneous injection.

EvGr For maintenance regimens, these insulins should ideally be injected immediately before meals. Rapid-acting insulin, administered before meals, has an advantage over short-acting soluble insulin in terms of improved glucose control, reduction of HbA1c, and reduction in the incidence of severe hypoglycaemia, including nocturnal hypoglycaemia.

The routine use of *post-meal* injections of rapid-acting insulin should be avoided—when given during or after meals, they are associated with poorer glucose control, an increased risk of high postprandial-glucose concentration, and subsequent hypoglycaemia. Ⓐ

Intermediate-acting insulin

Intermediate-acting insulins (isophane insulin p. 434) have an intermediate duration of action, designed to mimic the effect of endogenous basal insulin. When given by subcutaneous injection, they have an onset of action of approximately 1–2 hours, a maximal effect at 3–12 hours, and a duration of action of 11–24 hours.

Isophane insulin is a suspension of insulin with protamine; it may be given as one or more daily injections alongside separate meal-time short-acting insulin injections, or mixed with a short-acting (soluble or rapid-

6

Endocrine system

acting) insulin in the same syringe—for recommended insulin regimens see Type 1 diabetes p. 425 and Type 2 diabetes p. 428. Isophane insulin may be mixed with a short-acting insulin by the patient, or a pre-mixed biphasic insulin can be supplied (biphasic isophane insulin p. 433, biphasic insulin aspart p. 434 and biphasic insulin lispro p. 434).

Biphasic insulins (biphasic isophane insulin, biphasic insulin aspart, biphasic insulin lispro) are pre-mixed insulin preparations containing various combinations of short-acting insulin (soluble insulin or rapid-acting analogue insulin) and an intermediate-acting insulin.

The percentage of short-acting insulin varies from 15 % to 50 %. These preparations should be administered by subcutaneous injection immediately before a meal.

Long-acting insulin

Like intermediate-acting insulins, the long-acting insulins (protamine zinc insulin p. 436, insulin zinc suspension p. 436, insulin detemir p. 435, insulin glargine p. 435, insulin degludec p. 435) mimic endogenous basal insulin secretion, but their duration of action may last up to 36 hours. They achieve a steady-state level after 2–4 days to produce a constant level of insulin.

Insulin glargine and insulin degludec are given once daily and insulin detemir is given once or twice daily according to individual requirements. The older long-acting insulins, (insulin zinc suspension and protamine zinc insulin) are now rarely prescribed.

Type 2 diabetes

05-Jun-2017

Description of condition

Type 2 diabetes is a chronic metabolic condition characterised by insulin resistance. Insufficient pancreatic insulin production also occurs progressively over time, resulting in hyperglycaemia.

Type 2 diabetes in children is associated with increased body-weight, increased risk of renal complications, hypertension, and dyslipidaemia; therefore it increases cardiovascular risk. It is associated with long-term microvascular and macrovascular complications, together with reduced quality of life and life expectancy.

Type 2 diabetes typically develops later in life but is increasingly diagnosed in children, despite previously being considered a disease of adulthood.

Aims of treatment

Treatment is aimed at minimising the risk of long-term microvascular and macrovascular complications by effective blood-glucose control and maintenance of HbA1c at or below the target value set for each individual child.

Overview

EvGr Lifestyle modifications (including weight loss, smoking cessation and regular exercise) can help to reduce hyperglycaemia and reduce cardiovascular risk and should be encouraged where appropriate. Children and their carers should also receive advice from a paediatric dietitian to help optimise body-weight and blood-glucose control.

Lifestyle modifications alone are often unsuccessful at achieving glycaemic control in children, therefore antidiabetic drugs should be offered and initiated alongside lifestyle interventions such as diet and exercise, from the time of diagnosis.

Children with type 2 diabetes should receive immunisation against influenza (over the age of 6 months) and pneumococcal infection—see Vaccines p. 747. ⟨A⟩

Antidiabetic drugs

In children, type 2 diabetes does not usually occur until adolescence and information on the use of oral antidiabetic

drugs in children is limited. For recommended treatment regimens and the place in therapy of each drug, see *Treatment of type 2 diabetes.*

EvGr Treatment with antidiabetic drugs should be initiated under specialist supervision **only**. ⟨E⟩

Metformin hydrochloride p. 430 is the only oral antidiabetic drug licensed for use in children. It has an anti-hyperglycaemic effect, lowering both basal and postprandial blood-glucose concentrations. Metformin hydrochloride does not stimulate insulin secretion and therefore, when given alone, does not cause hypoglycaemia.

EvGr The dose of standard-release metformin hydrochloride should be increased gradually to minimise the risk of gastro-intestinal side-effects. ⟨A⟩

There is little experience of the use of other non-insulin antidiabetic drugs in children, with most evidence extrapolated from adult studies.

Several **sulfonylureas** (such as gliclazide p. 432, glibenclamide p. 431 and tolbutamide p. 432) are available but experience in children is limited; they are not the recommended choice of treatment in children; therefore treatment should be initiated by a specialist. The sulfonylureas may cause hypoglycaemia which may be more common in children than in adults. Hypoglycaemia is more likely with long-acting sulfonylureas such as glibenclamide, which has been associated with severe, prolonged and sometimes fatal cases—for this reason sulfonylureas are usually avoided in children.

Treatment of type 2 diabetes

EvGr A target HbA1c concentration of 48 mmol/mol (6.5 %) or lower is ideal to minimise the risk of long-term complications, however an individualised lowest achievable target should be agreed with each child and their carers taking into account factors such as daily activities, individual life goals, complications, and comorbidities. HbA1c concentrations should be monitored every 3 months.

Note: Consider relaxing the target HbA1c level on a case-by-case basis, with particular consideration for children where tight blood-glucose control is not appropriate or poses a high risk of the consequences of hypoglycaemia.

Standard-release metformin hydrochloride is the first-line choice for initial treatment in children and should be offered from diagnosis, alongside nutrition and lifestyle advice.

If the combination of lifestyle changes and metformin hydrochloride fails to reduce HbA1c to the agreed target within 3 to 4 months of therapy, addition of a long-acting insulin or once-daily human isophane insulin p. 434 should be considered (see also, Insulin p. 427). ⟨A⟩

EvGr Initiation of insulin should be under specialist care. ⟨E⟩

EvGr Metformin hydrochloride should be continued alongside insulin, to improve insulin sensitivity. The combination of metformin hydrochloride and once-daily insulin is usually an effective treatment for maintaining glycaemic control in the majority of children for extended periods of time. ⟨A⟩

EvGr If the combination of basal insulin and metformin does not achieve the HbA1c target (and postprandial hyperglycaemia persists) addition of prandial rapid- or short-acting insulin should be initiated and titrated until the target HbA1c is met. ⟨A⟩ Weight gain may occur and can be particularly problematic in children with type 2 diabetes when insulin therapy is initiated, unless there is careful attention and adherence to dietary measures. EvGr The importance of diet and exercise should be emphasised. ⟨A⟩

Useful Resources

Diabetes (type 1 and type 2) in children and young people: diagnosis and management. National Institute for Health and Care Excellence. Clinical guideline NG18. August 2015 www.nice.org.uk/guidance/ng18.

Diabetic complications

Cardiovascular disease

Diabetes is a strong risk factor for cardiovascular disease later in life. Other risk factors for cardiovascular disease (smoking, hypertension, obesity and hyperlipidaemia) should be addressed. The use of an ACE inhibitor and of a lipid-regulating drug can be beneficial in children with diabetes and a high cardiovascular disease risk. (ACE inhibitors may also have a role in the management of diabetic nephropathy).

Diabetic nephropathy

Regular review of diabetic children over 12 years of age should include an annual test for microalbuminuria (the earliest sign of nephropathy). If reagent strip tests (*Micral-Test II®* or *Microbumintest®*) are used and prove positive, the result should be confirmed by laboratory analysis of a urine sample. Microalbuminuria can occur transiently during puberty; if it persists (at least 3 positive tests) treatment with an ACE inhibitor or an angiotensin-II receptor antagonist under specialist guidance should be considered; to minimise the risk of renal deterioration, blood pressure should be carefully controlled.

ACE inhibitors can potentiate the hypoglycaemic effect of insulin and oral antidiabetic drugs; this effect is more likely during the first weeks of combined treatment and in children with renal impairment.

See also treatment of hypertension in diabetes.

Neuropathy

Clinical neuropathy is rare in children whose diabetes is well controlled.

Diabetes, pregnancy and breast-feeding

Pregnancy and breast-feeding

During pregnancy, women with *pre-existing diabetes* can be treated with metformin hydrochloride p. 430 [unlicensed use], either alone or in combination with insulin p. 436. Metformin hydrochloride can be continued, or glibenclamide p. 431 resumed, during breast-feeding for those with pre-existing diabetes. Women with *gestational diabetes* may be treated, with or without concomitant insulin, with glibenclamide from 11 weeks gestation (after organogenesis) [unlicensed use] or with metformin hydrochloride [unlicensed use]. Women with gestational diabetes should discontinue hypoglycaemic treatment after giving birth.

Diabetes, surgery and medical illness

EvGr Children with diabetes should undergo surgery in centres with facilities and expertise for the care of children with diabetes. Detailed local protocols should be available to all healthcare professionals involved in the treatment of these children. All surgery requiring general anaesthesia in children with type 1 and type 2 diabetes requires hospital admission. Ⓐ

Note: The following recommendations provide general guidance for the management of diabetes during surgery. **Local protocols and guidelines should be referred to where they exist.**

Use of insulin during surgery

Elective surgery—minor procedures

EvGr *Minor procedures* (procedures of less than 2 hours requiring either general anaesthesia or heavy sedation) in children who have type 1 or type 2 diabetes should not have a major impact on glycaemic control, and a slight modification of the usual regimen may be all that is necessary—adjustments should be made following local protocol; taking into consideration the type of insulin or antidiabetic drugs the child usually takes, whether fasting is required, the time of day of the operation, and requirement for intravenous fluids and glucose. All children who are usually prescribed insulin require intravenous insulin during surgery, to avoid ketoacidosis. Ⓐ

Elective surgery—major procedures

EvGr *Major procedures* (procedures requiring general anaesthesia for more than 2 hours) in children who have type 1 or type 2 diabetes, should ideally be performed when diabetes is under optimal control. If glycaemic control is poor, the procedure should be delayed if possible; otherwise it is advisable to admit the child well in advance of surgery for stabilisation of glycaemic control.

Blood glucose concentration should be maintained within the usual target range of 5–10 mmol/litre throughout the peri-operative period for all surgical procedures.

Children usually prescribed insulin for type 1 or type 2 diabetes require an intravenous insulin infusion p. 436 during surgery (even if fasting) to avoid ketoacidosis. Detailed local protocols should be consulted. In general, the following steps should be followed:

- On the *evening before surgery*, the usual insulin regimen should be given as normal; the usual bedtime snack should be given and hourly capillary blood glucose monitoring should be initiated to detect hypoglycaemia or hyperglycaemia before the procedure. Ketones should also be checked if blood glucose is above 14 mmol/litre, and an appropriate dose of short-acting insulin should be administered to restore blood glucose to the target range;
- On the *morning of surgery* the **usual** insulin dose should be omitted;
- At least 2 *hours before the procedure*, a maintenance fluid infusion of sodium chloride 0.45 % and glucose 5 % (sodium chloride with glucose p. 563) intravenous infusion should be started. A switch to sodium chloride 0.9 % infusion p. 561 may be required if sodium concentration falls and there is risk of hyponatraemia. After surgery, potassium chloride p. 575 should be added to the intravenous fluid, according to the child's body weight and fluid requirements. Electrolytes must be measured frequently throughout, and adjustments to the infusion made as necessary;
- Soluble human insulin 1 unit/mL in sodium chloride 0.9 % intravenous infusion should be started with the maintenance fluids at an infusion rate appropriate to the blood glucose concentration, to maintain a concentration between 5 and 10 mmol/litre, adjusted according to hourly blood glucose monitoring;
- If the blood glucose concentration falls below 6 mmol/litre the insulin infusion should **not** be stopped as this will cause rebound hyperglycaemia; instead the rate should be reduced; however, if blood-glucose concentration drops below 4 mmol/litre the insulin infusion can be stopped temporarily for 10–15 minutes. Ⓐ

EvGr After surgery, continue the glucose infusion, and the intravenous insulin infusion or additional short-acting insulin as necessary, until the child can eat and drink normally and their usual treatment regimen can resume. A short-acting insulin can also be given if required to reduce hyperglycaemia. Ⓐ

Emergency surgery

EvGr Children with diabetes (type 1 and 2) requiring emergency surgery, should always have their blood glucose, blood or urinary ketone concentration, and serum electrolytes checked before surgery. If ketones are high, blood gases should also be checked. If ketoacidosis is present, recommendations for Diabetic ketoacidosis, below, should be followed immediately, and surgery delayed if possible. If there is no acidosis, intravenous fluids and an insulin infusion should be started and managed as for *major elective surgery* (above). Ⓐ

Use of antidiabetic drugs during surgery

EvGr If elective *minor surgical procedures* only require a short-fasting period (just one missed meal), it may be possible to adjust antidiabetic drugs to avoid a switch to a variable rate intravenous insulin infusion; normal drug treatment can continue.

Children who usually take **sulfonylureas** should have their medication stopped on the day of surgery. Ⓐ

EvGr **Sulfonylureas** are associated with hypoglycaemia in the fasted state and therefore should not be recommenced until the child is eating and drinking normally. Ⓔ

EvGr Children undergoing *minor procedures* require hourly blood glucose monitoring and, if blood glucose concentration rises above 10 mmol/litre, should be treated with subcutaneous rapid-acting insulin no more frequently than every 3 hours.

Children undergoing a *major surgical* procedure expected to last at least 2 hours should be managed on an intravenous insulin infusion following the recommendations for *Elective surgery* (above). Ⓐ

EvGr Insulin is almost always required in medical and surgical emergencies. Ⓔ

EvGr **Metformin hydrochloride below** is renally excreted; renal impairment may lead to accumulation and lactic acidosis during surgery. In children undergoing *major surgery* lasting more than 2 hours, metformin hydrochloride should be discontinued 24 hours before the procedure. Children having minor surgery lasting less than 2 hours may stop their metformin on the day of surgery. Metformin hydrochloride should not be restarted until at least 48 hours after surgery or after the child is eating again, and only once normal renal function has been established. Ⓐ

The manufacturer advises that metformin should also be omitted if contrast medium is administered during surgery to reduce the risk of contrast-induced nephropathy. It should be stopped prior to, or at the time of the test, and not to be restarted until 48 hours afterwards, and only once normal renal function has been established.

Use of antidiabetic drugs during medical illness

Manufacturers of some antidiabetic drugs recommend that they may need to be replaced temporarily with insulin during intercurrent illness when the drug is unlikely to control hyperglycaemia (such as coma, severe infection, trauma and other medical emergencies). Consult individual product literature.

Diabetic ketoacidosis

Management

The management of diabetic ketoacidosis involves the replacement of fluid and electrolytes and the administration of insulin. Guidelines for the Management of Diabetic Ketoacidosis, published by the British Society of Paediatric Endocrinology and Diabetes, (available at www.bsped.org.uk) should be followed. Clinically well children with mild ketoacidosis who are dehydrated up to 5% usually respond to oral rehydration and subcutaneous insulin. For those who do not respond, or are clinically unwell, or are dehydrated by more than 5%, insulin and replacement fluids are best given by intravenous infusion.

- To restore circulating volume for children in *shock*, give 10 mL/kg **sodium chloride 0.9%** as a rapid infusion, repeat as necessary up to a maximum of 30 mL/kg.
- Further fluid should be given by intravenous infusion at a rate that replaces deficit and provides replacement over 48 hours; initially use **sodium chloride 0.9%**, changing to **sodium chloride 0.45%** and **glucose 5%** after 12 hours if response is adequate and plasma-sodium concentration is stable.
- Include **potassium chloride** in the fluids unless anuria is suspected, adjust according to plasma-potassium concentration.
- Insulin infusion is necessary to switch off ketogenesis and reverse acidosis; it should not be started until at least 1 hour after the start of intravenous rehydration fluids.
- **Soluble insulin** should be diluted (and **mixed thoroughly**) with **sodium chloride 0.9%** intravenous infusion to a concentration of 1 unit/mL and infused at a rate of 0.1 units/kg/hour.
- **Sodium bicarbonate** infusion (1.26% or 2.74%) is rarely necessary and is used only in cases of extreme acidosis (blood pH less than 6.9) and shock, since the acid-base disturbance is normally corrected by treatment with insulin.
- Once blood glucose falls to 14 mmol/litre, **glucose intravenous infusion 5%** *or* **10%** should be added to the fluids.
- The insulin infusion rate can be reduced to no less than 0.05 units/kg/hour when blood-glucose concentration has fallen to 14 mmol/litre *and* blood pH is greater than 7.3 *and* a glucose infusion has been started; it is continued until the child is ready to take food by mouth. Subcutaneous insulin can then be started.
- The insulin infusion should not be stopped until 1 hour after starting subcutaneous soluble or long acting insulin, or 10 minutes after starting subcutaneous insulin aspart p. 437, or insulin glulisine p. 438, or insulin lispro p. 438.

Hyperosmolar hyperglycaemic state or hyperosmolar hyperglycaemic nonketotic coma occurs rarely in children. Treatment is similar to that of diabetic ketoacidosis, although lower rates of insulin infusion and slower rehydration may be required.

BLOOD GLUCOSE LOWERING DRUGS ›
BIGUANIDES

Metformin hydrochloride

06-Jun-2017

- **DRUG ACTION** Metformin exerts its effect mainly by decreasing gluconeogenesis and by increasing peripheral utilisation of glucose; since it acts only in the presence of endogenous insulin it is effective only if there are some residual functioning pancreatic islet cells.

- **INDICATIONS AND DOSE**

Diabetes mellitus

▸ BY MOUTH USING IMMEDIATE-RELEASE MEDICINES

▸ Child 8-9 years (specialist use only): Initially 200 mg once daily, dose to be adjusted according to response at intervals of at least 1 week, maximum daily dose to be given in 2–3 divided doses; maximum 2 g per day

▸ Child 10-17 years (specialist use only): Initially 500 mg once daily, dose to be adjusted according to response at intervals of at least 1 week, maximum daily dose to be given in 2–3 divided doses; maximum 2 g per day

- **UNLICENSED USE** Not licensed for use in children under 10 years.

- **CONTRA-INDICATIONS** Acute metabolic acidosis (including lactic acidosis and diabetic ketoacidosis)
- **CAUTIONS** Risk factors for lactic acidosis

  CAUTIONS, FURTHER INFORMATION
- Risk factors for lactic acidosis Manufacturer advises caution in chronic stable heart failure (monitor cardiac function), and concomitant use of drugs that can acutely impair renal function; interrupt treatment if dehydration occurs, and avoid in conditions that can acutely worsen renal function, or cause tissue hypoxia.
- **INTERACTIONS** → Appendix 1: metformin
- **SIDE-EFFECTS**
- **Common or very common** Abdominal pain · anorexia · diarrhoea (usually transient) · nausea · taste disturbance · vomiting
- **Rare** Decreased vitamin-B$_{12}$ absorption · erythema · lactic acidosis (withdraw treatment) · pruritus · urticaria
- **Frequency not known** Hepatitis

  SIDE-EFFECTS, FURTHER INFORMATION
- Gastro-intestinal effects Gastro-intestinal side-effects are initially common with metformin, and may persist in some patients, particularly when very high doses are given. A slow increase in dose may improve tolerability.
- **PREGNANCY** Can be used in pregnancy for both pre-existing and gestational diabetes. Women with gestational diabetes should discontinue treatment after giving birth.
- **BREAST FEEDING** May be used during breast-feeding in women with pre-existing diabetes.
- **HEPATIC IMPAIRMENT** Withdraw if tissue hypoxia likely.
- **RENAL IMPAIRMENT** Manufacturer advises consider dose reduction in moderate impairment. Manufacturer advises avoid if estimated glomerular filtration rate is less than 30 mL/minute/1.73 m^2.
- **MONITORING REQUIREMENTS** Determine renal function before treatment and at least annually (at least twice a year in patients with additional risk factors for renal impairment, or if deterioration suspected).
- **PATIENT AND CARER ADVICE**
  Manufacturer advises that patients and their carers should be informed of the risk of lactic acidosis and told to seek immediate medical attention if symptoms such as dyspnoea, muscle cramps, abdominal pain, hypothermia, or asthenia occur.
  Medicines for Children leaflet: Metformin for diabetes
  www.medicinesforchildren.org.uk/metformin-diabetes

- **MEDICINAL FORMS**
  There can be variation in the licensing of different medicines containing the same drug. Forms available from special-order manufacturers include: capsule, oral suspension, oral solution

  Tablet
  CAUTIONARY AND ADVISORY LABELS 21
- **Metformin hydrochloride (Non-proprietary)**
  Metformin hydrochloride 500 mg Metformin 500mg tablets | 28 tablet [PoM] £1.55 DT price = £0.86 | 84 tablet [PoM] £2.58 | 500 tablet [PoM] £15.36
  Metformin hydrochloride 850 mg Metformin 850mg tablets | 56 tablet [PoM] £2.48 DT price = £1.23 | 60 tablet [PoM] no price available | 300 tablet [PoM] £6.59
- **Glucophage** (Merck Serono Ltd)
  Metformin hydrochloride 500 mg Glucophage 500mg tablets | 84 tablet [PoM] £2.88
  Metformin hydrochloride 850 mg Glucophage 850mg tablets | 56 tablet [PoM] £3.20 DT price = £1.23

  Oral solution
  CAUTIONARY AND ADVISORY LABELS 21
- **Metformin hydrochloride (Non-proprietary)**
  Metformin hydrochloride 100 mg per 1 ml Metformin 500mg/5ml oral solution sugar free sugar-free | 100 ml [PoM] £10.51 sugar-free | 150 ml [PoM] £60.00 DT price = £15.77
  Metformin hydrochloride 170 mg per 1 ml Metformin 850mg/5ml oral solution sugar free sugar-free | 150 ml [PoM] £19.95

Metformin hydrochloride 200 mg per 1 ml Metformin 1g/5ml oral solution sugar free sugar-free | 150 ml [PoM] £23.48–£24.00

Powder
- **Metformin hydrochloride (Non-proprietary)**
  Metformin hydrochloride 1 gram Metformin 1g oral powder sachets sugar free sugar-free | 30 sachet [PoM] no price available

BLOOD GLUCOSE LOWERING DRUGS ›
SULFONYLUREAS

Sulfonylureas

- **DRUG ACTION** The sulfonylureas act mainly by augmenting insulin secretion and consequently are effective only when some residual pancreatic beta-cell activity is present; during long-term administration they also have an extrapancreatic action.
- **CONTRA-INDICATIONS** Presence of ketoacidosis
- **CAUTIONS** Can encourage weight gain (should be prescribed only if poor control and symptoms persist despite adequate attempts at dieting) · G6PD deficiency
- **SIDE-EFFECTS**
- **Uncommon** Hypoglycaemia
- **Rare** Agranulocytosis · aplastic anaemia · blood disorders · cholestatic jaundice · haemolytic anaemia · hepatic failure · hepatitis · leucopenia · pancytopenia · thrombocytopenia
- **Frequency not known** Allergic skin reactions (usually in the first 6–8 weeks of therapy) · constipation · diarrhoea · disturbance in liver function · erythema multiforme (usually in the first 6–8 weeks of therapy) · exfoliative dermatitis (usually in the first 6–8 weeks of therapy) · fever (usually in the first 6–8 weeks of therapy) · gastro-intestinal disturbances · hypersensitivity reactions (usually in the first 6–8 weeks of therapy) · jaundice (usually in the first 6–8 weeks of therapy) · nausea · vomiting

  SIDE-EFFECTS, FURTHER INFORMATION
- Hypoglycaemia This is uncommon and usually indicates excessive dosage. Sulfonylurea-induced hypoglycaemia may persist for many hours and must always be treated in hospital.
- **HEPATIC IMPAIRMENT** Sulfonylureas should be avoided or a reduced dose should be used in severe hepatic impairment, because there is an increased risk of hypoglycaemia. Jaundice may occur.
- **RENAL IMPAIRMENT** Sulfonylureas should be used with care in those with mild to moderate renal impairment, because of the hazard of hypoglycaemia. Care is required to use the lowest dose that adequately controls blood glucose. Avoid where possible in severe renal impairment.
- **PATIENT AND CARER ADVICE**
  Driving and skilled tasks
  Drivers need to be particularly careful to avoid hypoglycaemia and should be warned of the problems.

  ☞ above

▌Glibenclamide

- **INDICATIONS AND DOSE**
  Type 2 diabetes mellitus
- BY MOUTH
- Child 12–17 years: Initially 2.5 mg daily, adjusted according to response, dose to be taken with or immediately after breakfast; maximum 15 mg per day

  Maturity-onset diabetes of the young (specialist use only)
- BY MOUTH
- Child 12–17 years: Initially 2.5 mg daily, adjusted according to response, dose to be taken with or immediately after breakfast; maximum 15 mg per day

◀ 431

- **UNLICENSED USE** Not licensed for use in breast feeding females with pre-existing diabetes. Not licensed for use in gestational diabetes.
  Not licensed for use in children.
- **CONTRA-INDICATIONS** Avoid where possible in acute porphyrias p. 577
- **INTERACTIONS** → Appendix 1: sulfonylureas
- **PREGNANCY** The use of sulfonylureas in pregnancy should generally be avoided because of the risk of neonatal hypoglycaemia; however, glibenclamide can be used during the second and third trimesters of pregnancy in women with gestational diabetes.
- **BREAST FEEDING** Glibenclamide can be used during breast-feeding in women with pre-existing diabetes.

- **MEDICINAL FORMS**
  There can be variation in the licensing of different medicines containing the same drug. Forms available from special-order manufacturers include: oral suspension, oral solution
  Tablet
  ▸ Glibenclamide (Non-proprietary)
  Glibenclamide 2.5 mg Glibenclamide 2.5mg tablets | 28 tablet [PoM] £11.46 DT price = £8.91
  Glibenclamide 5 mg Glibenclamide 5mg tablets | 28 tablet [PoM] £14.72 DT price = £1.39

◀ 431

Gliclazide

- **INDICATIONS AND DOSE**

  Type 2 diabetes mellitus
  ▸ BY MOUTH USING IMMEDIATE-RELEASE MEDICINES
  ▸ Child 12-17 years: Initially 20 mg once daily, adjusted according to response, increased if necessary up to 160 mg once daily (max. per dose 160 mg twice daily), dose to be taken with breakfast

  Maturity-onset diabetes of the young (specialist use only)
  ▸ BY MOUTH USING IMMEDIATE-RELEASE MEDICINES
  ▸ Child 12-17 years: Initially 20 mg once daily, adjusted according to response, increased if necessary up to 160 mg once daily (max. per dose 160 mg twice daily), dose to be taken with breakfast

- **UNLICENSED USE** Not licensed for use in children.
- **CONTRA-INDICATIONS** Avoid where possible in acute porphyrias p. 577
- **INTERACTIONS** → Appendix 1: sulfonylureas
- **PREGNANCY** The use of sulfonylureas in pregnancy should generally be avoided because of the risk of neonatal hypoglycaemia.
- **BREAST FEEDING** Avoid—theoretical possibility of hypoglycaemia in the infant.
- **RENAL IMPAIRMENT** If necessary, gliclazide which is principally metabolised in the liver, can be used in renal impairment but careful monitoring of blood-glucose concentration is essential.

- **MEDICINAL FORMS**
  There can be variation in the licensing of different medicines containing the same drug. Forms available from special-order manufacturers include: oral suspension
  Tablet
  ▸ Gliclazide (Non-proprietary)
  Gliclazide 40 mg Gliclazide 40mg tablets | 28 tablet [PoM] £3.36 DT price = £3.36
  Gliclazide 80 mg Gliclazide 80mg tablets | 28 tablet [PoM] £7.22 DT price = £0.82 | 60 tablet [PoM] £9.32
  ▸ Diamicron (Servier Laboratories Ltd)
  Gliclazide 80 mg Diamicron 80mg tablets | 60 tablet [PoM] £4.38
  ▸ Zicron (Bristol Laboratories Ltd)
  Gliclazide 40 mg Zicron 40mg tablets | 28 tablet [PoM] £3.36 DT price = £3.36

Tolbutamide

- **INDICATIONS AND DOSE**

  Type 2 diabetes mellitus
  ▸ BY MOUTH
  ▸ Child 12-17 years (specialist use only): 0.5–1.5 g daily in divided doses, dose to be taken with or immediately after meals, alternatively 0.5–1.5 g once daily, dose to be taken with or immediately after breakfast; maximum 2 g per day

- **UNLICENSED USE** Not licensed for use in children.
- **CONTRA-INDICATIONS** Avoid where possible in acute porphyrias p. 577
- **INTERACTIONS** → Appendix 1: sulfonylureas
- **SIDE-EFFECTS** Headache · tinnitus
- **PREGNANCY** The use of sulfonylureas in pregnancy should generally be avoided because of the risk of neonatal hypoglycaemia.
- **BREAST FEEDING** The use of sulfonylureas in breast-feeding should be avoided because there is a theoretical possibility of hypoglycaemia in the infant.
- **RENAL IMPAIRMENT** If necessary, the short-acting drug tolbutamide can be used in renal impairment but careful monitoring of blood-glucose concentration is essential.

- **MEDICINAL FORMS**
  There can be variation in the licensing of different medicines containing the same drug. Forms available from special-order manufacturers include: oral suspension
  Tablet
  ▸ Tolbutamide (Non-proprietary)
  Tolbutamide 500 mg Tolbutamide 500mg tablets | 28 tablet [PoM] £34.88 DT price = £6.71 | 112 tablet [PoM] £27.00

INSULINS

Insulins

> **IMPORTANT SAFETY INFORMATION**
>
> NHS IMPROVEMENT PATIENT SAFETY ALERT: RISK OF SEVERE HARM AND DEATH DUE TO WITHDRAWING INSULIN FROM PEN DEVICES (NOVEMBER 2016)
> Insulin should not be extracted from insulin pen devices.
>   The strength of insulin in pen devices can vary by multiples of 100 units/mL. Insulin syringes have graduations only suitable for calculating doses of standard 100 units/mL. If insulin extracted from a pen or cartridge is of a higher strength, and that is not considered in determining the volume required, it can lead to a significant and potentially fatal overdose.

- **SIDE-EFFECTS**
  ▸ **Common or very common** Fat hypertrophy at injection site · local reactions at injection site · transient oedema
  ▸ **Rare** Hypersensitivity reactions · rash · urticaria
  Overdose
  Overdose causes hypoglycaemia.
- **PREGNANCY** During pregnancy, insulin requirements may alter and doses should be assessed frequently by an experienced diabetes physician. The dose of insulin generally needs to be increased in the second and third trimesters of pregnancy.
- **BREAST FEEDING** During breast-feeding, insulin requirements may alter and doses should be assessed frequently by an experienced diabetes physician.
- **HEPATIC IMPAIRMENT** Insulin requirements may be decreased in patients with hepatic impairment.

● **RENAL IMPAIRMENT** Insulin requirements may decrease in patients with renal impairment and therefore dose reduction may be necessary. The compensatory response to hypoglycaemia is impaired in renal impairment.

● **MONITORING REQUIREMENTS**

▸ Many patients now monitor their own blood-glucose concentrations; all carers and children need to be trained to do this.

▸ Since blood-glucose concentration varies substantially throughout the day, 'normoglycaemia' cannot always be achieved throughout a 24-hour period without causing damaging hypoglycaemia.

▸ It is therefore best to recommend that children should maintain a blood-glucose concentration of between 4 and 10 mmol/litre for most of the time (4–8 mmol/litre before meals and less than 10 mmol/litre after meals).

▸ While accepting that on occasions, for brief periods, the blood-glucose concentration will be above these values; strenuous efforts should be made to prevent it from falling below 4 mmol/litre. Patients using multiple injection regimens should understand how to adjust their insulin dose according to their carbohydrate intake. With fixed-dose insulin regimens, the carbohydrate intake needs to be regulated, and should be distributed throughout the day to match the insulin regimen. The intake of energy and of simple and complex carbohydrates should be adequate to allow normal growth and development but obesity must be avoided.

● **DIRECTIONS FOR ADMINISTRATION** Insulin is generally given by *subcutaneous injection*; the injection site should be rotated to prevent lipodystrophy. Injection devices ('pens'), which hold the insulin in a cartridge and meter the required dose, are convenient to use. Insulin syringes (for use with needles) are required for insulins not available in cartridge form, but are less popular with children and carers. For intensive insulin regimens multiple subcutaneous injections (3 or more times daily) are usually recommended.

● **PRESCRIBING AND DISPENSING INFORMATION**

Units The word 'unit' should **not** be abbreviated.

Show container to patient or carer and confirm the expected version is dispensed.

● **PATIENT AND CARER ADVICE**

Insulin Passport Insulin Passports and patient information booklets should be offered to patients receiving insulin. The Insulin Passport provides a record of the patient's current insulin preparations and contains a section for emergency information. The patient information booklet provides advice on the safe use of insulin. They are available for purchase from:

3M Security Print and Systems Limited
Gorse Street, Chadderton
Oldham
OL9 9QH
Tel: 0845 610 1112

GP practices can obtain supplies through their Local Area Team stores.

NHS Trusts can order supplies from www.nhsforms.co.uk/ or by emailing nhsforms@mmm.com. Further information is available at www.npsa.nhs.uk.

Hypoglycaemia Hypoglycaemia is a potential problem with insulin therapy. All patients must be carefully instructed on how to avoid it; this involves appropriate adjustment of insulin type, dose and frequency together with suitable timing and quantity of meals and snacks.

Driving and skilled tasks

Drivers need to be particularly careful to avoid hypoglycaemia and should be warned of the problems.

INSULINS ＞ INTERMEDIATE-ACTING

☞ 432

Biphasic isophane insulin

(Biphasic Isophane Insulin Injection– intermediate acting)

● **INDICATIONS AND DOSE**

Diabetes mellitus

▸ BY SUBCUTANEOUS INJECTION

▸ Child: According to requirements

● **INTERACTIONS** → Appendix 1: insulins

● **SIDE-EFFECTS** Protamine may cause allergic reactions

● **PRESCRIBING AND DISPENSING INFORMATION** A sterile buffered suspension of either porcine or human insulin complexed with protamine sulfate (or another suitable protamine) in a solution of insulin of the same species.

Check product container—the proportions of the two components should be checked carefully (the order in which the proportions are stated may not be the same in other countries).

● **MEDICINAL FORMS**

There can be variation in the licensing of different medicines containing the same drug.

Suspension for injection

▸ Humulin M3 (Eli Lilly and Company Ltd)

Insulin human (as Insulin soluble human) 30 unit per 1 ml, Insulin human (as Insulin isophane human) 70 unit per 1 ml Humulin M3 100units/ml suspension for injection 3ml cartridges | 5 cartridge PoM £19.08 DT price = £19.08

Humulin M3 100units/ml suspension for injection 10ml vials | 1 vial PoM £15.68

▸ Humulin M3 KwikPen (Eli Lilly and Company Ltd)

Insulin human (as Insulin soluble human) 30 unit per 1 ml, Insulin human (as Insulin isophane human) 70 unit per 1 ml Humulin M3 KwikPen 100units/ml suspension for injection 3ml pre-filled pen | 5 pre-filled disposable injection PoM £21.70 DT price = £21.70

▸ Hypurin Porcine 30/70 Mix (Wockhardt UK Ltd)

Insulin porcine (as Insulin soluble porcine) 30 unit per 1 ml, Insulin porcine (as Insulin isophane porcine) 70 unit per 1 ml Hypurin Porcine 30/70 Mix 100units/ml suspension for injection 3ml cartridges | 5 cartridge PoM £37.80

Hypurin Porcine 30/70 Mix 100units/ml suspension for injection 10ml vials | 1 vial PoM £25.20

▸ Insuman Comb 15 (Sanofi)

Insulin human (as Insulin soluble human) 15 unit per 1 ml, Insulin human (as Insulin isophane human) 85 unit per 1 ml Insuman Comb 15 100units/ml suspension for injection 3ml cartridges | 5 cartridge PoM £17.50

▸ Insuman Comb 25 (Sanofi)

Insulin human (as Insulin soluble human) 25 unit per 1 ml, Insulin human (as Insulin isophane human) 75 unit per 1 ml Insuman Comb 25 100units/ml suspension for injection 5ml vials | 1 vial PoM £5.61

Insuman Comb 25 100units/ml suspension for injection 3ml cartridges | 5 cartridge PoM £17.50

▸ Insuman Comb 25 SoloStar (Sanofi)

Insulin human (as Insulin soluble human) 25 unit per 1 ml, Insulin human (as Insulin isophane human) 75 unit per 1 ml Insuman Comb 25 100units/ml suspension for injection 3ml pre-filled SoloStar pen | 5 pre-filled disposable injection PoM £19.80

▸ Insuman Comb 50 (Sanofi)

Insulin human (as Insulin isophane human) 50 unit per 1 ml, Insulin human (as Insulin soluble human) 50 unit per 1 ml Insuman Comb 50 100units/ml suspension for injection 3ml cartridges | 5 cartridge PoM £17.50

6

Endocrine system

Isophane insulin

F 432

(Isophane Insulin Injection; Isophane Protamine Insulin Injection; Isophane Insulin (NPH)—intermediate acting)

● **INDICATIONS AND DOSE**
Diabetes mellitus
▸ BY SUBCUTANEOUS INJECTION
▸ Child: According to requirements

● **INTERACTIONS** → Appendix 1: insulins

● **SIDE-EFFECTS** Protamine may cause allergic reactions

● **PREGNANCY** Recommended where longer-acting insulins are needed.

● **PRESCRIBING AND DISPENSING INFORMATION** A sterile suspension of bovine or porcine insulin or of human insulin in the form of a complex obtained by the addition of protamine sulfate or another suitable protamine.

● **MEDICINAL FORMS**
There can be variation in the licensing of different medicines containing the same drug.
Suspension for injection
▸ Humulin I (Eli Lilly and Company Ltd)
Insulin human (as Insulin isophane human) 100 unit per 1 ml Humulin I 100units/ml suspension for injection 10ml vials | 1 vial PoM £15.68
Humulin I 100units/ml suspension for injection 3ml cartridges | 5 cartridge PoM £19.08 DT price = £19.08
▸ Humulin I KwikPen (Eli Lilly and Company Ltd)
Insulin human (as Insulin isophane human) 100 unit per 1 ml Humulin I KwikPen 100units/ml suspension for injection 3ml pre-filled pen | 5 pre-filled disposable injection PoM £21.70 DT price = £21.70
▸ Hypurin Bovine Isophane (Wockhardt UK Ltd)
Insulin bovine (as Insulin isophane bovine) 100 unit per 1 ml Hypurin Bovine Isophane 100units/ml suspension for injection 10ml vials | 1 vial PoM £27.72
Hypurin Bovine Isophane 100units/ml suspension for injection 3ml cartridges | 5 cartridge PoM £41.58
▸ Hypurin Porcine Isophane (Wockhardt UK Ltd)
Insulin porcine (as Insulin isophane porcine) 100 unit per 1 ml Hypurin Porcine Isophane 100units/ml suspension for injection 3ml cartridges | 5 cartridge PoM £37.80
Hypurin Porcine Isophane 100units/ml suspension for injection 10ml vials | 1 vial PoM £25.20
▸ Insulatard (Novo Nordisk Ltd)
Insulin human (as Insulin isophane human) 100 unit per 1 ml Insulatard 100units/ml suspension for injection 10ml vials | 1 vial PoM £7.48
▸ Insulatard InnoLet (Novo Nordisk Ltd)
Insulin human (as Insulin isophane human) 100 unit per 1 ml Insulatard InnoLet 100units/ml suspension for injection 3ml pre-filled pen | 5 pre-filled disposable injection PoM £20.40 DT price = £21.70
▸ Insulatard Penfill (Novo Nordisk Ltd)
Insulin human (as Insulin isophane human) 100 unit per 1 ml Insulatard Penfill 100units/ml suspension for injection 3ml cartridges | 5 cartridge PoM £22.90 DT price = £19.08
▸ Insuman Basal (Sanofi)
Insulin human (as Insulin isophane human) 100 unit per 1 ml Insuman Basal 100units/ml suspension for injection 5ml vials | 1 vial PoM £5.61
Insuman Basal 100units/ml suspension for injection 3ml cartridges | 5 cartridge PoM £17.50 DT price = £19.08
▸ Insuman Basal SoloStar (Sanofi)
Insulin human (as Insulin isophane human) 100 unit per 1 ml Insuman Basal 100units/ml suspension for injection 3ml pre-filled SoloStar pen | 5 pre-filled disposable injection PoM £19.80 DT price = £21.70

INSULINS › INTERMEDIATE-ACTING COMBINED WITH RAPID-ACTING

Biphasic insulin aspart

F 432

(Intermediate-acting insulin)

● **INDICATIONS AND DOSE**
Diabetes mellitus
▸ BY SUBCUTANEOUS INJECTION
▸ Child: Administer up to 10 minutes before or soon after a meal, according to requirements

● **INTERACTIONS** → Appendix 1: insulins

● **SIDE-EFFECTS** Protamine may cause allergic reactions

● **PRESCRIBING AND DISPENSING INFORMATION** Check product container—the proportions of the two components should be checked carefully (the order in which the proportions are stated may not be the same in other countries).

● **MEDICINAL FORMS**
There can be variation in the licensing of different medicines containing the same drug.
Suspension for injection
▸ NovoMix 30 FlexPen (Novo Nordisk Ltd)
Insulin aspart 30 unit per 1 ml, Insulin aspart (as Insulin aspart protamine) 70 unit per 1 ml NovoMix 30 FlexPen 100units/ml suspension for injection 3ml pre-filled pen | 5 pre-filled disposable injection PoM £29.89 DT price = £29.89
▸ NovoMix 30 Penfill (Novo Nordisk Ltd)
Insulin aspart 30 unit per 1 ml, Insulin aspart (as Insulin aspart protamine) 70 unit per 1 ml NovoMix 30 Penfill 100units/ml suspension for injection 3ml cartridges | 5 cartridge PoM £28.79 DT price = £28.79

Biphasic insulin lispro

F 432

(Intermediate-acting insulin)

● **INDICATIONS AND DOSE**
Diabetes mellitus
▸ BY SUBCUTANEOUS INJECTION
▸ Child: Administer up to 15 minutes before or soon after a meal, according to requirements

● **CAUTIONS** Children under 12 years (use only if benefit likely compared to soluble insulin)

● **INTERACTIONS** → Appendix 1: insulins

● **SIDE-EFFECTS** Protamine may cause allergic reactions

● **PRESCRIBING AND DISPENSING INFORMATION** Check product container—the proportions of the two components should be checked carefully (the order in which the proportions are stated may not be the same in other countries).

● **MEDICINAL FORMS**
There can be variation in the licensing of different medicines containing the same drug.
Suspension for injection
▸ Humalog Mix25 (Eli Lilly and Company Ltd)
Insulin lispro 25 unit per 1 ml, Insulin lispro (as Insulin lispro protamine) 75 unit per 1 ml Humalog Mix25 100units/ml suspension for injection 10ml vials | 1 vial PoM £16.61
Humalog Mix25 100units/ml suspension for injection 3ml cartridges | 5 cartridge PoM £29.46 DT price = £29.46
▸ Humalog Mix25 KwikPen (Eli Lilly and Company Ltd)
Insulin lispro 25 unit per 1 ml, Insulin lispro (as Insulin lispro protamine) 75 unit per 1 ml Humalog Mix25 KwikPen 100units/ml suspension for injection 3ml pre-filled pen | 5 pre-filled disposable injection PoM £30.98 DT price = £30.98

- Humalog Mix50 (Eli Lilly and Company Ltd)
  Insulin lispro 50 unit per 1 ml, Insulin lispro (as Insulin lispro protamine) 50 unit per 1 ml Humalog Mix50 100units/ml suspension for injection 3ml cartridges | 5 cartridge [PoM] £29.46
- Humalog Mix50 KwikPen (Eli Lilly and Company Ltd)
  Insulin lispro 50 unit per 1 ml, Insulin lispro (as Insulin lispro protamine) 50 unit per 1 ml Humalog Mix50 KwikPen 100units/ml suspension for injection 3ml pre-filled pen | 5 pre-filled disposable injection [PoM] £30.98 DT price = £30.98

INSULINS > LONG-ACTING

F 432

Insulin degludec

14-Mar-2017

(Recombinant human insulin analogue—long acting)

- **INDICATIONS AND DOSE**

Diabetes mellitus
- BY SUBCUTANEOUS INJECTION
- Child 1–17 years: Dose to be given according to requirements

- **INTERACTIONS** → Appendix 1: insulins

- **PREGNANCY** Evidence of the safety of long-acting insulin analogues in pregnancy is limited, therefore isophane insulin is recommended where longer-acting insulins are needed; insulin detemir may also be considered.

- **PRESCRIBING AND DISPENSING INFORMATION** Insulin degludec (*Tresiba*®) is available in strengths of 100 units/mL (allows 1-unit dose adjustment) and 200 units/mL (allows 2-unit dose adjustment)—ensure correct strength prescribed.

- **NATIONAL FUNDING/ACCESS DECISIONS**

All Wales Medicines Strategy Group (AWMSG) Decisions
The *All Wales Medicines Strategy Group* has advised (October 2016) that insulin degludec (*Tresiba*®) is **not** recommended for use within NHS Wales for the treatment of diabetes mellitus in adolescents and children from the age of 1 year.

- **MEDICINAL FORMS**
There can be variation in the licensing of different medicines containing the same drug.
Solution for injection
- Tresiba FlexTouch (Novo Nordisk Ltd) ▼
  Insulin human (as Insulin degludec) 100 unit per 1 ml Tresiba FlexTouch 100units/ml solution for injection 3ml pre-filled pen | 5 pre-filled disposable injection [PoM] £46.60
  Insulin human (as Insulin degludec) 200 unit per 1 ml Tresiba FlexTouch 200units/ml solution for injection 3ml pre-filled pen | 3 pre-filled disposable injection [PoM] £55.92
- Tresiba Penfill (Novo Nordisk Ltd) ▼
  Insulin human (as Insulin degludec) 100 unit per 1 ml Tresiba Penfill 100units/ml solution for injection 3ml cartridges | 5 cartridge [PoM] £46.60

F 432

Insulin detemir

(Recombinant human insulin analogue—long acting)

- **INDICATIONS AND DOSE**

Diabetes mellitus
- BY SUBCUTANEOUS INJECTION
- Child 2–17 years: According to requirements

- **INTERACTIONS** → Appendix 1: insulins

- **PREGNANCY** Evidence of the safety of long-acting insulin analogues in pregnancy is limited, therefore isophane insulin p. 434 is recommended where longer-acting insulins are needed; insulin detemir may also be considered where longer-acting insulins are needed.

- **MEDICINAL FORMS**
There can be variation in the licensing of different medicines containing the same drug.
Solution for injection
- Levemir FlexPen (Novo Nordisk Ltd)
  Insulin human (as Insulin detemir) 100 unit per 1 ml Levemir FlexPen 100units/ml solution for injection 3ml pre-filled disposable injection [PoM] £42.00 DT price = £42.00
- Levemir InnoLet (Novo Nordisk Ltd)
  Insulin human (as Insulin detemir) 100 unit per 1 ml Levemir InnoLet 100units/ml solution for injection 3ml pre-filled pen | 5 pre-filled disposable injection [PoM] £44.85 DT price = £42.00
- Levemir Penfill (Novo Nordisk Ltd)
  Insulin human (as Insulin detemir) 100 unit per 1 ml Levemir Penfill 100units/ml solution for injection 3ml cartridges | 5 cartridge [PoM] £42.00 DT price = £42.00

F 432

Insulin glargine

(Recombinant human insulin analogue—long acting)

- **INDICATIONS AND DOSE**

Diabetes mellitus
- BY SUBCUTANEOUS INJECTION
- Child 2–17 years: According to requirements

- **INTERACTIONS** → Appendix 1: insulins

- **PREGNANCY** Evidence of the safety of long-acting insulin analogues in pregnancy is limited, therefore isophane insulin is recommended where longer-acting insulins are needed; insulin detemir may also be considered.

- **PRESCRIBING AND DISPENSING INFORMATION** Insulin glargine is a biological medicine. Biological medicines must be prescribed and dispensed by brand name, see *Biological medicines* and *Biosimilar medicines*, under Guidance on prescribing p. 1. Dose adjustments and close metabolic monitoring is recommended if switching between insulin glargine preparations.

- **NATIONAL FUNDING/ACCESS DECISIONS**

Scottish Medicines Consortium (SMC) Decisions
The *Scottish Medicines Consortium* has advised that *Lantus*® preparations (April 2013) and *Toujeo*® (August 2015) are accepted for restricted use within NHS Scotland for the treatment of type 1 diabetes:

- in those who are at risk of or experience unacceptable frequency or severity of nocturnal hypoglycaemia on attempting to achieve better hypoglycaemic control during treatment with other insulins
- as a once daily insulin therapy for patients who require a carer to administer their insulin

It is **not** recommended for routine use in patients with type 2 diabetes unless they suffer from recurrent episodes of hypoglycaemia or require assistance with their insulin injections.

- **MEDICINAL FORMS**
There can be variation in the licensing of different medicines containing the same drug.
Solution for injection
- Abasaglar (Eli Lilly and Company Ltd) ▼
  Insulin human (as Insulin glargine) 100 unit per 1 ml Abasaglar 100units/ml solution for injection 3ml cartridges | 5 cartridge [PoM] £35.28 DT price = £41.50
- Abasaglar KwikPen (Eli Lilly and Company Ltd) ▼
  Insulin human (as Insulin glargine) 100 unit per 1 ml Abasaglar KwikPen 100units/ml solution for injection 3ml pre-filled pen | 5 pre-filled disposable injection [PoM] £35.28 DT price = £41.50
- Lantus (Sanofi)
  Insulin human (as Insulin glargine) 100 unit per 1 ml Lantus 100units/ml solution for injection 3ml cartridges | 5 cartridge [PoM] £41.50 DT price = £41.50
  Lantus 100units/ml solution for injection 10ml vials | 1 vial [PoM] £30.68

▸ **Lantus SoloStar** (Sanofi)
Insulin human (as Insulin glargine) 100 unit per 1 ml Lantus 100units/ml solution for injection 3ml pre-filled SoloStar pen | 5 pre-filled disposable injection PoM £41.50 DT price = £41.50

▸ **Toujeo** (Sanofi)
Insulin human (as Insulin glargine) 300 unit per 1 ml Toujeo 300units/ml solution for injection 1.5ml pre-filled SoloStar pen | 3 pre-filled disposable injection PoM £33.13

F 432

Insulin zinc suspension

(Insulin zinc suspension (mixed)–long acting)

● **INDICATIONS AND DOSE**
Diabetes mellitus
▸ BY SUBCUTANEOUS INJECTION
▸ Child: According to requirements

● **INTERACTIONS** → Appendix 1: insulins

● **PREGNANCY** Evidence of the safety of long-acting insulin analogues in pregnancy is limited, therefore isophane insulin p. 434 is recommended where longer-acting insulins are needed; insulin detemir p. 435 may also be considered.

● **PRESCRIBING AND DISPENSING INFORMATION** A sterile neutral suspension of bovine and/or porcine insulin or of human insulin in the form of a complex obtained by the addition of a suitable zinc salt; consists of rhombohedral crystals (10–40 microns) and of particles of no uniform shape (not exceeding 2 microns).

● **MEDICINAL FORMS**
There can be variation in the licensing of different medicines containing the same drug.
Suspension for injection
▸ **Hypurin Bovine Lente** (Wockhardt UK Ltd)
Insulin bovine (as Insulin zinc suspension mixed bovine) 100 unit per 1 ml Hypurin Bovine Lente 100units/ml suspension for injection 10ml vials | 1 vial PoM £27.72

F 432

Protamine zinc insulin

(Protamine zinc insulin injection–long acting)

● **INDICATIONS AND DOSE**
Diabetes mellitus
▸ BY SUBCUTANEOUS INJECTION
▸ Child: According to requirements

● **INTERACTIONS** → Appendix 1: insulins

● **SIDE-EFFECTS** Protamine may cause allergic reactions

● **PREGNANCY** Evidence of the safety of long-acting insulin analogues in pregnancy is limited, therefore isophane insulin p. 434 is recommended where longer-acting insulins are needed; insulin detemir p. 435 may also be considered.

● **PRESCRIBING AND DISPENSING INFORMATION** A sterile suspension of insulin in the form of a complex obtained by the addition of a suitable protamine and zinc chloride; this preparation was included in BP 1980 but is not included in BP 1988.

● **MEDICINAL FORMS**
There can be variation in the licensing of different medicines containing the same drug.
Suspension for injection
▸ **Hypurin Bovine Protamine Zinc** (Wockhardt UK Ltd)
Insulin bovine (as Insulin protamine zinc bovine) 100 unit per 1 ml Hypurin Bovine Protamine Zinc 100units/ml suspension for injection 10ml vials | 1 vial PoM £27.72

INSULINS ⟩ RAPID-ACTING

F 432

Insulin

(Insulin Injection; Neutral Insulin; Soluble Insulin–short acting)

● **INDICATIONS AND DOSE**
Diabetes mellitus
▸ BY SUBCUTANEOUS INJECTION
▸ Child: According to requirements
Hyperglycaemia during illness
▸ BY INTRAVENOUS INFUSION

▸ Neonate: 0.02–0.125 unit/kg/hour, dose to be adjusted according to blood-glucose concentration.

▸ Child: 0.025–0.1 unit/kg/hour, dose to be adjusted according to blood-glucose concentration.

Neonatal hyperglycaemia | Neonatal diabetes
▸ BY INTRAVENOUS INFUSION

▸ Neonate: 0.02–0.125 unit/kg/hour, dose to be adjusted according to blood-glucose concentration.

Diabetic ketoacidosis | Diabetes during surgery
▸ BY INTRAVENOUS INFUSION
▸ Child: (consult local protocol)

● **INTERACTIONS** → Appendix 1: insulins

● **DIRECTIONS FOR ADMINISTRATION** Short-acting injectable insulins can be given by continuous subcutaneous infusion using a portable infusion pump. This device delivers a continuous basal insulin infusion and patient-activated bolus doses at meal times. This technique can be useful for patients who suffer recurrent hypoglycaemia or marked morning rise in blood-glucose concentration despite optimised multiple-injection regimens. Patients on subcutaneous insulin infusion must be highly motivated, able to monitor their blood-glucose concentration, and have expert training, advice and supervision from an experienced healthcare team. Some insulin preparations are not recommended for use in subcutaneous insulin infusion pumps—may precipitate in catheter or needle—consult product literature.

▸ With intravenous use For *intravenous infusion*, dilute to a concentration of 1 unit/mL with Sodium Chloride 0.9% and mix thoroughly; insulin may be adsorbed by plastics, flush giving set with 5 mL of infusion fluid containing insulin. *For intravenous infusion in neonatal intensive care*, dilute 5 units to a final volume of 50 mL with Sodium Chloride 0.9% and mix thoroughly; an intravenous infusion rate of 0.1 mL/kg/hour provides a dose of 0.01 units/kg/hour.

● **PRESCRIBING AND DISPENSING INFORMATION** A sterile solution of insulin (i.e. bovine or porcine) or of human insulin; pH 6.6–8.0.

● **NATIONAL FUNDING/ACCESS DECISIONS**
NICE technology appraisals (TAs)
▸ **Continuous subcutaneous insulin infusion for the treatment of diabetes mellitus (type 1) (July 2008)** NICE TA151
Continuous subcutaneous insulin infusion is recommended as an option in children over 12 years with type 1 diabetes:
  ● who suffer repeated or unpredictable hypoglycaemia, whilst attempting to achieve optimal glycaemic control with multiple-injection regimens, or
  ● whose glycaemic control remains inadequate (HbA$_{1c}$ over 8.5% [69 mmol/mol]) despite optimised multiple-injection regimens (including the use of long-acting insulin analogues where appropriate).
Continuous subcutaneous insulin infusion is also recommended as an option for children under 12 years with type 1 diabetes for whom multiple-injection regimens

are considered impractical or inappropriate. Children on insulin pumps should undergo a trial of multiple-injection therapy between the ages of 12 and 18 years. www.nice.org.uk/TA151

● **MEDICINAL FORMS**
There can be variation in the licensing of different medicines containing the same drug. Forms available from special-order manufacturers include: solution for injection, solution for infusion

Solution for injection
▸ **Actrapid** (Novo Nordisk Ltd)
Insulin human (as Insulin soluble human) 100 unit per 1 ml Actrapid 100units/ml solution for injection 10ml vials | 1 vial PoM £7.48
▸ **Humulin S** (Eli Lilly and Company Ltd)
Insulin human (as Insulin soluble human) 100 unit per 1 ml Humulin S 100units/ml solution for injection 10ml vials | 1 vial PoM £15.68
Humulin S 100units/ml solution for injection 3ml cartridges | 5 cartridge PoM £19.08
▸ **Hypurin Bovine Neutral** (Wockhardt UK Ltd)
Insulin bovine (as Insulin soluble bovine) 100 unit per 1 ml Hypurin Bovine Neutral 100units/ml solution for injection 10ml vials | 1 vial PoM £27.72
Hypurin Bovine Neutral 100units/ml solution for injection 3ml cartridges | 5 cartridge PoM £41.58
▸ **Hypurin Porcine Neutral** (Wockhardt UK Ltd)
Insulin porcine (as Insulin soluble porcine) 100 unit per 1 ml Hypurin Porcine Neutral 100units/ml solution for injection 10ml vials | 1 vial PoM £25.20
Hypurin Porcine Neutral 100units/ml solution for injection 3ml cartridges | 5 cartridge PoM £37.80
▸ **Insuman Infusat** (Sanofi)
Insulin human 100 unit per 1 ml Insuman Infusat 100units/ml solution for injection 3.15ml cartridges | 5 cartridge PoM £250.00
Insuman Infusat 100units/ml solution for injection 10ml vials | 3 vial PoM £250.00
▸ **Insuman Rapid** (Sanofi)
Insulin human (as Insulin soluble human) 100 unit per 1 ml Insuman Rapid 100units/ml solution for injection 3ml cartridges | 5 cartridge PoM £17.50

▸ **F 432**

Insulin aspart

16-Jun-2017

(Recombinant human insulin analogue—short acting)

● **INDICATIONS AND DOSE**
Diabetes mellitus
▸ BY SUBCUTANEOUS INJECTION
▸ Child 1 month-1 year: Administer immediately before meals or when necessary shortly after meals, according to requirements
▸ Child 2-17 years: Administer immediately before meals or when necessary shortly after meals, according to requirements
▸ BY SUBCUTANEOUS INFUSION, OR BY INTRAVENOUS INFUSION, OR BY INTRAVENOUS INJECTION
▸ Child 1 month-1 year: According to requirements
▸ Child 2-17 years: According to requirements

● **UNLICENSED USE** Not licensed for use in children under 2 years.
● **INTERACTIONS** → Appendix 1: insulins
● **PREGNANCY** Not known to be harmful—may be used during pregnancy.
● **BREAST FEEDING** Not known to be harmful—may be used during lactation.
● **DIRECTIONS FOR ADMINISTRATION** Short-acting injectable insulins can be given by continuous subcutaneous infusion using a portable infusion pump. This device delivers a continuous basal insulin infusion and patient-activated bolus doses at meal times. This technique can be useful for patients who suffer recurrent hypoglycaemia or marked

morning rise in blood-glucose concentration despite optimised multiple-injection regimens. Patients on subcutaneous insulin infusion must be highly motivated, able to monitor their blood-glucose concentration, and have expert training, advice and supervision from an experienced healthcare team.
▸ With intravenous use For *intravenous infusion*, dilute to a concentration of 0.05–1 unit/mL with Glucose 5% or Sodium Chloride 0.9% and mix thoroughly; insulin may be adsorbed by plastics, flush giving set with 5 mL of infusion fluid containing insulin.

● **NATIONAL FUNDING/ACCESS DECISIONS**
NICE technology appraisals (TAs)
▸ **Continuous subcutaneous insulin infusion for the treatment of diabetes mellitus (type 1) (July 2008)** NICE TA151
Continuous subcutaneous insulin infusion is recommended as an option in children over 12 years with type 1 diabetes:
● who suffer repeated or unpredictable hypoglycaemia, whilst attempting to achieve optimal glycaemic control with multiple-injection regimens, **or**
● whose glycaemic control remains inadequate (HbA$_{1c}$ over 8.5% [69 mmol/mol]) despite optimised multiple-injection regimens (including the use of long-acting insulin analogues where appropriate).
Continuous subcutaneous insulin infusion is also recommended as an option for children under 12 years with type 1 diabetes for whom multiple-injection regimens are considered impractical or inappropriate. Children on insulin pumps should undergo a trial of multiple-injection therapy between the ages of 12 and 18 years. www.nice.org.uk/TA151

● **MEDICINAL FORMS**
There can be variation in the licensing of different medicines containing the same drug.

Solution for injection
▸ **Fiasp** (Novo Nordisk Ltd) ▼
Insulin aspart 100 unit per 1 ml Fiasp 100units/ml solution for injection 10ml vials | 1 vial PoM £14.08 DT price = £14.08
▸ **Fiasp FlexTouch** (Novo Nordisk Ltd) ▼
Insulin aspart 100 unit per 1 ml Fiasp FlexTouch 100units/ml solution for injection 3ml pre-filled pen | 5 pre-filled disposable injection PoM £30.60 DT price = £30.60
▸ **Fiasp Penfill** (Novo Nordisk Ltd) ▼
Insulin aspart 100 unit per 1 ml Fiasp Penfill 100units/ml solution for injection 3ml cartridges | 5 cartridge PoM £28.31 DT price = £28.31
▸ **NovoRapid** (Novo Nordisk Ltd)
Insulin aspart 100 unit per 1 ml NovoRapid 100units/ml solution for injection 10ml vials | 1 vial PoM £14.08 DT price = £14.08
▸ **NovoRapid FlexPen** (Novo Nordisk Ltd)
Insulin aspart 100 unit per 1 ml NovoRapid FlexPen 100units/ml solution for injection 3ml pre-filled pen | 5 pre-filled disposable injection PoM £30.60 DT price = £30.60
▸ **NovoRapid FlexTouch** (Novo Nordisk Ltd)
Insulin aspart 100 unit per 1 ml NovoRapid FlexTouch 100units/ml solution for injection 3ml pre-filled pen | 5 pre-filled disposable injection PoM £32.13 DT price = £30.60
▸ **NovoRapid Penfill** (Novo Nordisk Ltd)
Insulin aspart 100 unit per 1 ml NovoRapid Penfill 100units/ml solution for injection 3ml cartridges | 5 cartridge PoM £28.31 DT price = £28.31
▸ **NovoRapid PumpCart** (Novo Nordisk Ltd)
Insulin aspart 100 unit per 1 ml NovoRapid PumpCart 100units/ml solution for injection 1.6ml cartridges | 5 cartridge PoM £15.10

6

Endocrine system

F 432

Insulin glulisine

(Recombinant human insulin analogue–short acting)

● **INDICATIONS AND DOSE**

Diabetes mellitus

▶ BY SUBCUTANEOUS INJECTION
▶ Child: Administer immediately before meals or when necessary shortly after meals, according to requirements
▶ BY SUBCUTANEOUS INFUSION, OR BY INTRAVENOUS INFUSION
▶ Child: According to requirements

● **UNLICENSED USE** Not licensed for children under 6 years.

● **INTERACTIONS** → Appendix 1: insulins

● **DIRECTIONS FOR ADMINISTRATION** Short-acting injectable insulins can be given by continuous subcutaneous infusion using a portable infusion pump. This device delivers a continuous basal insulin infusion and patient-activated bolus doses at meal times. This technique can be useful for patients who suffer recurrent hypoglycaemia or marked morning rise in blood-glucose concentration despite optimised multiple-injection regimens. Patients on subcutaneous insulin infusion must be highly motivated, able to monitor their blood-glucose concentration, and have expert training, advice and supervision from an experienced healthcare team.

● **NATIONAL FUNDING/ACCESS DECISIONS**

NICE technology appraisals (TAs)

▶ Continuous subcutaneous insulin infusion for the treatment of diabetes mellitus (type 1) (July 2008) NICE TA151
Continuous subcutaneous insulin infusion is recommended as an option in children over 12 years with type 1 diabetes:

• who suffer repeated or unpredictable hypoglycaemia, whilst attempting to achieve optimal glycaemic control with multiple-injection regimens, **or**
• whose glycaemic control remains inadequate (HbA_{1c} over 8.5% [69 mmol/mol]) despite optimised multiple-injection regimens (including the use of long-acting insulin analogues where appropriate).

Continuous subcutaneous insulin infusion is also recommended as an option for children under 12 years with type 1 diabetes for whom multiple-injection regimens are considered impractical or inappropriate. Children on insulin pumps should undergo a trial of multiple-injection therapy between the ages of 12 and 18 years.
www.nice.org.uk/TA151

Scottish Medicines Consortium (SMC) Decisions

The *Scottish Medicines Consortium* has advised (October 2008) that *Apidra®* is accepted for restricted use within NHS Scotland for the treatment of children over 6 years with diabetes mellitus in whom the use of a short-acting insulin analogue is appropriate.

● **MEDICINAL FORMS**

There can be variation in the licensing of different medicines containing the same drug.

Solution for injection

▶ Apidra (Sanofi)
Insulin glulisine 100 unit per 1 ml Apidra 100units/ml solution for injection 10ml vials | 1 vial PoM £16.00
Apidra 100units/ml solution for injection 3ml cartridges | 5 cartridge PoM £28.30

▶ Apidra SoloStar (Sanofi)
Insulin glulisine 100 unit per 1 ml Apidra 100units/ml solution for injection 3ml pre-filled SoloStar pen | 5 pre-filled disposable injection PoM £28.30 DT price = £28.30

F 432

Insulin lispro

(Recombinant human insulin analogue–short acting)

● **INDICATIONS AND DOSE**

Diabetes mellitus

▶ BY SUBCUTANEOUS INJECTION
▶ Child 1 month–1 year: Administer shortly before meals or when necessary shortly after meals, according to requirements
▶ Child 2–17 years: Administer shortly before meals or when necessary shortly after meals, according to requirements
▶ BY SUBCUTANEOUS INFUSION, OR BY INTRAVENOUS INFUSION, OR BY INTRAVENOUS INJECTION
▶ Child 1 month–1 year: According to requirements
▶ Child 2–17 years: According to requirements

● **UNLICENSED USE** Not licensed for use in children under 2 years.

● **CAUTIONS** Children under 12 years (use only if benefit likely compared to soluble insulin)

● **INTERACTIONS** → Appendix 1: insulins

● **PREGNANCY** Not known to be harmful—may be used during pregnancy.

● **BREAST FEEDING** Not known to be harmful—may be used during lactation.

● **DIRECTIONS FOR ADMINISTRATION** Short-acting injectable insulins can be given by continuous subcutaneous infusion using a portable infusion pump. This device delivers a continuous basal insulin infusion and patient-activated bolus doses at meal times. This technique can be useful for patients who suffer recurrent hypoglycaemia or marked morning rise in blood-glucose concentration despite optimised multiple-injection regimens (see also NICE guidance, below). Patients on subcutaneous insulin infusion must be highly motivated, able to monitor their blood-glucose concentration, and have expert training, advice and supervision from an experienced healthcare team.

▶ With intravenous use For *intravenous infusion*, dilute to a concentration of 0.1–1 unit/mL with Glucose 5% or Sodium Chloride 0.9% and mix thoroughly; insulin may be adsorbed by plastics, flush giving set with 5 mL of infusion fluid containing insulin.

● **NATIONAL FUNDING/ACCESS DECISIONS**

NICE technology appraisals (TAs)

▶ Continuous subcutaneous insulin infusion for the treatment of diabetes mellitus (type 1) (July 2008) NICE TA151
Continuous subcutaneous insulin infusion is recommended as an option in children over 12 years with type 1 diabetes:

• who suffer repeated or unpredictable hypoglycaemia, whilst attempting to achieve optimal glycaemic control with multiple-injection regimens, **or**
• whose glycaemic control remains inadequate (HbA_{1c} over 8.5% [69 mmol/mol]) despite optimised multiple-injection regimens (including the use of long-acting insulin analogues where appropriate).

Continuous subcutaneous insulin infusion is also recommended as an option for children under 12 years with type 1 diabetes for whom multiple-injection regimens are considered impractical or inappropriate. Children on insulin pumps should undergo a trial of multiple-injection therapy between the ages of 12 and 18 years.
www.nice.org.uk/TA151

● MEDICINAL FORMS
There can be variation in the licensing of different medicines containing the same drug.

Solution for injection

▶ Humalog (Eli Lilly and Company Ltd)
Insulin lispro 100 unit per 1 ml Humalog 100units/ml solution for injection 10ml vials | 1 vial [PoM] £16.61 DT price = £16.61
Humalog 100units/ml solution for injection 3ml cartridges | 5 cartridge [PoM] £28.31 DT price = £28.31

▶ Humalog KwikPen (Eli Lilly and Company Ltd)
Insulin lispro 100 unit per 1 ml Humalog KwikPen 100units/ml solution for injection 3ml pre-filled pen | 5 pre-filled disposable injection [PoM] £29.46 DT price = £29.46
Insulin lispro 200 unit per 1 ml Humalog KwikPen 200units/ml solution for injection 3ml pre-filled pen | 5 pre-filled disposable injection [PoM] £58.92

3.1a Diabetes, diagnosis and monitoring

Diabetes mellitus, diagnostic and monitoring devices

Urinalysis

Reagent strips are available for measuring for glucose in the urine. Tests for ketones by patients are rarely required unless they become unwell—see Blood Monitoring.

Microalbuminuria can be detected with *Micral-Test II*® but this should be followed by confirmation in the laboratory, since false positive results are common.

Blood monitoring

Blood glucose monitoring using a meter gives a direct measure of the glucose concentration at the time of the test and can detect hypoglycaemia as well as hyperglycaemia. Carers and children should be properly trained in the use of blood glucose monitoring systems and the appropriate action to take on the results obtained. Inadequate understanding of the normal fluctuations in blood glucose can lead to confusion and inappropriate action.

Children using multiple injection regimens should understand how to adjust their insulin dose according to their carbohydrate intake. With fixed-dose insulin regimens, the carbohydrate intake needs to be regulated, and should be distributed throughout the day to match the insulin regimen.

In the UK blood-glucose concentration is expressed in mmol/litre and Diabetes UK advises that these units should be used for self-monitoring of blood glucose. In other European countries units of mg/100 mL (or mg/dL) are commonly used.

It is advisable to check that the meter is pre-set in the correct units.

If the blood glucose level is high or if the child is unwell, blood **ketones** should be measured according to local guidelines in order to detect diabetic ketoacidosis. Children and their carers should be trained in the use of blood ketone monitoring systems and to take appropriate action on the results obtained, including when to seek medical attention.

> **Other drugs used for Diabetes, diagnosis and monitoring**
> Glucose, p. 564

▐ Blood monitoring test strips

● BLOOD GLUCOSE TESTING STRIPS

Accu-Chek Inform II testing strips (Roche Diagnostics Ltd)
50 strip · No NHS indicative price available · Drug Tariff (Part IXr)

Active testing strips (Roche Diabetes Care Ltd)
50 strip · NHS indicative price = £9.95 · Drug Tariff (Part IXr)

Advocate Redi-Code+ testing strips (Diabetes Care Technology Ltd)
50 strip · NHS indicative price = £9.95 · Drug Tariff (Part IXr)

AutoSense testing strips (Advance Diagnostic Products (NI) Ltd)
25 strip · NHS indicative price = £4.50 · Drug Tariff (Part IXr)

Aviva testing strips (Roche Diabetes Care Ltd)
50 strip · NHS indicative price = £15.96 · Drug Tariff (Part IXr)

BGStar testing strips (Sanofi)
50 strip · NHS indicative price = £14.73 · Drug Tariff (Part IXr)

Betachek C50 cassette (National Diagnostic Products)
100 device · NHS indicative price = £29.98 · Drug Tariff (Part IXr)

Betachek G5 testing strips (National Diagnostic Products)
50 strip · NHS indicative price = £14.19 · Drug Tariff (Part IXr)

Betachek Visual testing strips (National Diagnostic Products)
50 strip · NHS indicative price = £6.80 · Drug Tariff (Part IXr)

Breeze 2 testing discs (Bayer Plc)
50 strip · NHS indicative price = £15.00 · Drug Tariff (Part IXr)

CareSens N testing strips (Spirit Healthcare Ltd)
50 strip · NHS indicative price = £12.75 · Drug Tariff (Part IXr)

CareSens PRO testing strips (Spirit Healthcare Ltd)
50 strip · NHS indicative price = £9.95 · Drug Tariff (Part IXr)

Compact testing strips (Roche Diabetes Care Ltd)
51 strip · NHS indicative price = £16.39 · Drug Tariff (Part IXr)

Contour Next testing strips (Bayer Diagnostics Manufacturing Ltd)
50 strip · NHS indicative price = £15.04 · Drug Tariff (Part IXr)

Contour TS testing strips (Bayer Diagnostics Manufacturing Ltd)
50 strip · NHS indicative price = £9.50 · Drug Tariff (Part IXr)

Contour testing strips (Bayer Diagnostics Manufacturing Ltd)
50 strip · NHS indicative price = £9.95 · Drug Tariff (Part IXr)

Dario Lite testing strips (LabStyle Innovations Ltd)
50 strip · NHS indicative price = £9.95 · Drug Tariff (Part IXr)

Dario testing strips (LabStyle Innovations Ltd)
50 strip · NHS indicative price = £14.95 · Drug Tariff (Part IXr)

Diastix testing strips (Bayer Diagnostics Manufacturing Ltd)
50 strip · NHS indicative price = £2.89 · Drug Tariff (Part IXr)

Element testing strips (Neon Diagnostics Ltd)
50 strip · NHS indicative price = £9.89 · Drug Tariff (Part IXr)

Finetest Lite testing strips (Neon Diagnostics Ltd)
50 strip · NHS indicative price = £5.95 · Drug Tariff (Part IXr)

FreeStyle Lite testing strips (Abbott Laboratories Ltd)
50 strip · NHS indicative price = £15.97 · Drug Tariff (Part IXr)

FreeStyle Optium testing strips (Abbott Laboratories Ltd)
50 strip · NHS indicative price = £15.87 · Drug Tariff (Part IXr)

FreeStyle testing strips (Abbott Laboratories Ltd)
50 strip · NHS indicative price = £15.97 · Drug Tariff (Part IXr)

GluNEO testing strips (Neon Diagnostics Ltd)
50 strip · NHS indicative price = £9.89 · Drug Tariff (Part IXr)

GlucoDock testing strips (Medisana Healthcare (UK) Ltd)
50 strip · NHS indicative price = £14.90 · Drug Tariff (Part IXr)

GlucoLab testing strips (Neon Diagnostics Ltd)
50 strip · NHS indicative price = £9.89 · Drug Tariff (Part IXr)

GlucoMen GM testing strips (A Menarini Diagnostics Ltd)
50 strip · NHS indicative price = £9.95 · Drug Tariff (Part IXr)

GlucoMen LX Sensor testing strips (A Menarini Diagnostics Ltd)
50 strip · NHS indicative price = £15.76 · Drug Tariff (Part IXr)

GlucoMen Sensor testing strips (A Menarini Diagnostics Ltd)
50 strip · NHS indicative price = £14.83 · Drug Tariff (Part IXr)

GlucoMen Visio testing strips (A Menarini Diagnostics Ltd)
50 strip · NHS indicative price = £15.75 · Drug Tariff (Part IXr)

GlucoMen areo Sensor testing strips (A Menarini Diagnostics Ltd)
50 strip · NHS indicative price = £9.95 · Drug Tariff (Part IXr)

GlucoNavii testing strips (Neon Diagnostics Ltd)
50 strip · NHS indicative price = £8.95 · Drug Tariff (Part IXr)

GlucoRx GO testing strips (GlucoRx Ltd)
50 strip · NHS indicative price = £9.95 · Drug Tariff (Part IXr)

GlucoRx HCT Glucose testing strips (GlucoRx Ltd)
50 strip · NHS indicative price = £9.95 · Drug Tariff (Part IXr)

GlucoRx Nexus testing strips (GlucoRx Ltd)
50 strip · NHS indicative price = £9.95 · Drug Tariff (Part IXr)

GlucoRx Q testing strips (GlucoRx Ltd)
50 strip · NHS indicative price = £5.45 · Drug Tariff (Part IXr)

Endocrine system

6

Meters and test strips

Meter (all NHS)	Type of monitoring	Compatible test strips	Test strip net price	Sensitivity range (mmol/litre)	Manufacturer
Accu-Chek® Active	Blood glucose	Active®	50 strip= £9.95	0.6-33.3 mmol/litre	Roche Diabetes Care Ltd
Accu-Chek® Advantage Meter no longer available	Blood glucose	Advantage Plus®	50 strip= £0.00	0.6-33.3 mmol/litre	Roche Diabetes Care Ltd
Accu-Chek® Aviva	Blood glucose	Aviva®	50 strip= £15.96	0.6-33.3 mmol/litre	Roche Diabetes Care Ltd
Accu-Chek® Aviva Expert	Blood glucose	Aviva®	50 strip= £15.96	0.6-33.3 mmol/litre	Roche Diabetes Care Ltd
Accu-Chek® Compact Plus Meter no longer available	Blood glucose	Compact®	3 × 17 strips= £16.39	0.6-33.3 mmol/litre	Roche Diabetes Care Ltd
Accu-Chek® Mobile	Blood glucose	Mobile®	100 device= £0.00	0.3-33.3 mmol/litre	Roche Diabetes Care Ltd
Accu-Chek® Aviva Nano	Blood glucose	Aviva®	50 strip= £15.96	0.6-33.3 mmol/litre	Roche Diabetes Care Ltd
BGStar® Free of charge from diabetes healthcare professionals	Blood glucose	BGStar®	50 strip= £14.73	1.1-33.3 mmol/litre	Sanofi
Breeze 2®	Blood glucose	Breeze 2®	50 strip= £15.00	0.6-33.3 mmol/litre	Bayer Plc
CareSens N® Free of charge from diabetes healthcare professionals	Blood glucose	CareSens N®	50 strip= £12.75	1.1-33.3 mmol/litre	Spirit Healthcare Ltd
Contour®	Blood glucose	Contour®	50 strip= £9.95	0.6-33.3 mmol/litre	Bayer Diagnostics Manufacturing Ltd
Contour® XT	Blood glucose	Contour® Next	50 strip= £15.04	0.6-33.3 mmol/litre	Bayer Diagnostics Manufacturing Ltd
Element®	Blood glucose	Element®	50 strip= £9.89	0.55-33.3 mmol/litre	Neon Diagnostics Ltd
FreeStyle® Meter no longer available	Blood glucose	FreeStyle®	50 strip= £15.97	1.1-27.8 mmol/litre	Abbott Laboratories Ltd
FreeStyle Freedom® Meter no longer available	Blood glucose	FreeStyle®	50 strip= £15.97	1.1-27.8 mmol/litre	Abbott Laboratories Ltd
FreeStyle Freedom Lite®	Blood glucose	FreeStyle Lite®	50 strip= £15.97	1.1-27.8 mmol/litre	Abbott Laboratories Ltd
FreeStyle InsuLinx®	Blood glucose	FreeStyle Lite®	50 strip= £15.97	1.1-27.8 mmol/litre	Abbott Laboratories Ltd
FreeStyle Lite®	Blood glucose	FreeStyle Lite®	50 strip= £15.97	1.1-27.8 mmol/litre	Abbott Laboratories Ltd
FreeStyle Mini® Meter no longer available	Blood glucose	FreeStyle®	50 strip= £15.97	1.1-27.8 mmol/litre	Abbott Laboratories Ltd
FreeStyle Optium®	Blood glucose	FreeStyle Optium®	50 strip= £15.87	1.1-27.8 mmol/litre	Abbott Laboratories Ltd
FreeStyle Optium®	Blood ketones	FreeStyle Optium® β-ketone	10 strip= £21.36	0-8.0 mmol/litre	Abbott Laboratories Ltd
FreeStyle Optium Neo®	Blood glucose	FreeStyle Optium®	50 strip= £15.87	1.1-27.8 mmol/litre	Abbott Laboratories Ltd
FreeStyle Optium Neo®	Blood ketones	FreeStyle Optium® β-ketone	10 strip= £21.36	0-8.0 mmol/litre	Abbott Laboratories Ltd
GlucoDock® module For use with iPhone®, iPod touch®, and iPad®	Blood glucose	GlucoDock®	50 strip= £14.90	1.1-33.3 mmol/litre	Medisana Healthcare (UK) Ltd

Meter (all NHS)	Type of monitoring	Compatible test strips	Test strip net price	Sensitivity range (mmol/litre)	Manufacturer
GlucoLab®	Blood glucose	GlucoLab®	50 strip= £9.89	0.55–33.3 mmol/litre	Neon Diagnostics Ltd
GlucoMen® GM	Blood glucose	GlucoMen® GM	50 strip= £9.95	0.6–33.3 mmol/litre	A Menarini Diagnostics Ltd
GlucoMen® LX	Blood glucose	GlucoMen® LX Sensor	50 strip= £15.76	1.1–33.3 mmol/litre	A Menarini Diagnostics Ltd
GlucoMen® LX Plus	Blood glucose	GlucoMen® LX Sensor	50 strip= £15.76	1.1–33.3 mmol/litre	A Menarini Diagnostics Ltd
GlucoMen® LX Plus	Blood ketones	GlucoMen® LX Ketone	10 strip= £21.06	0–0.8 mmol/litre	A Menarini Diagnostics Ltd
GlucoMen® Visio	Blood glucose	GlucoMen® Visio Sensor	50 strip= £15.75	1.1–33.3 mmol/litre	A Menarini Diagnostics Ltd
GlucoRx® Free of charge from diabetes healthcare professionals	Blood glucose	GlucoRx®	50 strip= £5.45	1.1–33.3 mmol/litre	GlucoRx Ltd
GlucoRx Nexus® Free of charge from diabetes healthcare professionals	Blood glucose	GlucoRx Nexus®	50 strip= £9.95	1.1–33.3 mmol/litre	GlucoRx Ltd
Glucotrend® Meter no longer available	Blood glucose	Active®	50 strip= £9.95	0.6–33.3 mmol/litre	Roche Diabetes Care Ltd
iBGStar®	Blood glucose	BGStar®	50 strip= £14.73	1.1–33.3 mmol/litre	Sanofi
IME-DC®	Blood glucose	IME-DC®	50 strip= £14.10	1.1–33.3 mmol/litre	Arctic Medical Ltd
Mendor Discreet®	Blood glucose	Mendor Discreet®	50 strip= £14.75	1.1–33.3 mmol/litre	SpringMed Solutions Ltd
Microdot®+ Free of charge from diabetes healthcare professionals	Blood glucose	Microdot®+	50 strip= £9.49	1.1–29.2 mmol/litre	Cambridge Sensors Ltd
MyGlucoHealth®	Blood glucose	MyGlucoHealth®	50 strip= £15.50	0.6–33.3 mmol/litre	Entra Health Systems Ltd
Omnitest® 3	Blood glucose	Omnitest® 3	50 strip= £9.89	0.6–33.3 mmol/litre	B.Braun Medical Ltd
One Touch Ultra® Meter no longer available	Blood glucose	One Touch Ultra®	50 strip= £9.99	1.1–33.3 mmol/litre	LifeScan
One Touch Ultra 2® Free of charge from diabetes healthcare professionals	Blood glucose	One Touch Ultra®	50 strip= £9.99	1.1–33.3 mmol/litre	LifeScan
One Touch UltraEasy® Free of charge from diabetes healthcare professionals	Blood glucose	One Touch Ultra®	50 strip= £9.99	1.1–33.3 mmol/litre	LifeScan
One Touch UltraSmart® Free of charge from diabetes healthcare professionals	Blood glucose	One Touch Ultra®	50 strip= £9.99	1.1–33.3 mmol/litre	LifeScan
One Touch® VerioPro Free of charge from diabetes healthcare professionals	Blood glucose	One Touch® Verio	50 strip= £15.12	1.1–33.3 mmol/litre	LifeScan
One Touch® Vita Free of charge from diabetes healthcare professionals	Blood glucose	One Touch® Vita	50 strip= £15.07	1.1–33.3 mmol/litre	LifeScan
SD CodeFree®	Blood glucose	SD CodeFree®	50 strip= £6.99	0.6–33.3 mmol/litre	SD Biosensor Inc
Sensocard Plus® Meter no longer available	Blood glucose	Sensocard®	50 strip= £16.30	1.1–33.3 mmol/litre	BBI Healthcare Ltd

Meter (all NHS)	Type of monitoring	Compatible test strips	Test strip net price	Sensitivity range (mmol/litre)	Manufacturer
SuperCheck2® Free of charge from diabetes healthcare professionals	Blood glucose	SuperCheck2®	50 strip= £8.49	1.1-33.3 mmol/litre	Apollo Medical Technologies Ltd
TRUEone® All-in-one test strips and meter	Blood glucose	TRUEone®	50 strip= £0.00	1.1-33.3 mmol/litre	Nipro Diagnostics (UK) Ltd
TRUEresult® Free of charge from diabetes healthcare professionals	Blood glucose	TRUEresult®	50 strip= £14.99	1.1-33.3 mmol/litre	Nipro Diagnostics (UK) Ltd
TRUEresult twist® Free of charge from diabetes healthcare professionals	Blood glucose	TRUEresult®	50 strip= £14.99	1.1-33.3 mmol/litre	Nipro Diagnostics (UK) Ltd
TRUEtrack® Free of charge from diabetes healthcare professionals	Blood glucose	TRUEtrack®	50 strip= £14.99	1.1-33.3 mmol/litre	Nipro Diagnostics (UK) Ltd
TRUEyou mini®	Blood glucose	TRUEyou®	50 strip= £9.92	1.1-33.3 mmol/litre	Nipro Diagnostics (UK) Ltd
WaveSense JAZZ® Free of charge from diabetes healthcare professionals	Blood glucose	WaveSense JAZZ®	50 strip= £9.87	1.1-33.3 mmol/litre	AgaMatrix Europe Ltd

GlucoZen.auto testing strips (GlucoZen Ltd)
50 strip · NHS indicative price = £7.64 · Drug Tariff (Part IXr)

Glucoflex-R testing strips (Bio-Diagnostics Ltd)
50 strip · NHS indicative price = £6.75 · Drug Tariff (Part IXr)

IME-DC testing strips (Arctic Medical Ltd)
50 strip · NHS indicative price = £14.10 · Drug Tariff (Part IXr)

MODZ testing strips (Modz Oy)
50 strip · NHS indicative price = £14.00 · Drug Tariff (Part IXr)

Medi-Test Glucose testing strips (BHR Pharmaceuticals Ltd)
50 strip · NHS indicative price = £2.33 · Drug Tariff (Part IXr)

MediSense SoftSense testing strips (Abbott Laboratories Ltd)
50 strip · NHS indicative price = £15.05 · Drug Tariff (Part IXr)

MediTouch 2 testing strips (Medisana Healthcare (UK) Ltd)
50 strip · NHS indicative price = £12.49 · Drug Tariff (Part IXr)

MediTouch testing strips (Medisana Healthcare (UK) Ltd)
50 strip · NHS indicative price = £14.90 · Drug Tariff (Part IXr)

Mendor Discreet testing strips (SpringMed Solutions Ltd)
50 strip · NHS indicative price = £14.75 · Drug Tariff (Part IXr)

Microdot+ testing strips (Cambridge Sensors Ltd)
50 strip · NHS indicative price = £9.49 · Drug Tariff (Part IXr)

Mission Glucose testing strips (Spirit Healthcare Ltd)
50 strip · NHS indicative price = £2.29 · Drug Tariff (Part IXr)

Mobile cassette (Roche Diabetes Care Ltd)
50 device · NHS indicative price = £16.24 · Drug Tariff (Part IXr)

Myglucohealth testing strips (Entra Health Systems Ltd)
50 strip · NHS indicative price = £15.50 · Drug Tariff (Part IXr)

Mylife Pura testing strips (Ypsomed Ltd)
50 strip · NHS indicative price = £9.50 · Drug Tariff (Part IXr)

Mylife Unio testing strips (Ypsomed Ltd)
50 strip · NHS indicative price = £9.50 · Drug Tariff (Part IXr)

Omnitest 3 testing strips (B.Braun Medical Ltd)
50 strip · NHS indicative price = £9.89 · Drug Tariff (Part IXr)

Omnitest 5 testing strips (B.Braun Medical Ltd)
50 strip · NHS indicative price = £9.89 · Drug Tariff (Part IXr)

On-Call Advanced testing strips (Point Of Care Testing Ltd)
50 strip · NHS indicative price = £13.65 · Drug Tariff (Part IXr)

OneTouch Select Plus testing strips (LifeScan)
50 strip · NHS indicative price = £9.99 · Drug Tariff (Part IXr)

OneTouch Ultra testing strips (LifeScan)
50 strip · NHS indicative price = £9.99 · Drug Tariff (Part IXr)

OneTouch Verio testing strips (LifeScan)
50 strip · NHS indicative price = £15.12 · Drug Tariff (Part IXr)

OneTouch Vita testing strips (LifeScan)
50 strip · NHS indicative price = £15.07 · Drug Tariff (Part IXr)

Performa testing strips (Roche Diabetes Care Ltd)
50 strip · NHS indicative price = £9.95 · Drug Tariff (Part IXr)

SD CodeFree testing strips (SD Biosensor Inc)
50 strip · NHS indicative price = £6.99 · Drug Tariff (Part IXr)

SURESIGN Resure testing strips (Ciga Healthcare Ltd)
50 strip · NHS indicative price = £8.49 · Drug Tariff (Part IXr)

Sensocard testing strips (BBI Healthcare Ltd)
50 strip · NHS indicative price = £16.30 · Drug Tariff (Part IXr)

SuperCheck 2 testing strips (Apollo Medical Technologies Ltd)
50 strip · NHS indicative price = £8.49 · Drug Tariff (Part IXr)

SuperCheck Plus testing strips (Apollo Medical Technologies Ltd)
50 strip · NHS indicative price = £9.45 · Drug Tariff (Part IXr)

TEE2 testing strips (Spirit Healthcare Ltd)
50 strip · NHS indicative price = £7.75 · Drug Tariff (Part IXr)

TRUEresult testing strips (Nipro Diagnostics (UK) Ltd)
50 strip · NHS indicative price = £14.99 · Drug Tariff (Part IXr)

TRUEyou testing strips (Nipro Diagnostics (UK) Ltd)
50 strip · NHS indicative price = £9.92 · Drug Tariff (Part IXr)

TrueTrack System testing strips (Nipro Diagnostics (UK) Ltd)
50 strip · NHS indicative price = £14.99 · Drug Tariff (Part IXr)

VivaChek Ino testing strips (JR Biomedical Ltd)
50 strip · NHS indicative price = £8.99 · Drug Tariff (Part IXr)

WaveSense JAZZ Duo testing strips (AgaMatrix Europe Ltd)
50 strip · NHS indicative price = £9.95 · Drug Tariff (Part IXr)

WaveSense JAZZ testing strips (AgaMatrix Europe Ltd)
50 strip · NHS indicative price = £9.87 · Drug Tariff (Part IXr)

eBchek testing strips (IRASCO Ltd)
50 strip · NHS indicative price = £15.89 · Drug Tariff (Part IXr)

iHealth testing strips (Technomed Ltd)
50 strip · NHS indicative price = £9.49 · Drug Tariff (Part IXr)

palmdoc iCare Advanced Solo testing strips (Palmdoc Ltd)
50 strip · NHS indicative price = £13.50 · Drug Tariff (Part IXr)

palmdoc iCare Advanced testing strips (Palmdoc Ltd)
50 strip · NHS indicative price = £9.70 · Drug Tariff (Part IXr)

palmdoc testing strips (Palmdoc Ltd)
50 strip · NHS indicative price = £9.40 · Drug Tariff (Part IXr)

- **BLOOD KETONES TESTING STRIPS**

FreeStyle Optium beta-ketone testing strips (Abbott Laboratories Ltd) | 10 strip · NHS indicative price = £21.36 · Drug Tariff (Part IXr)

GlucoMen LX beta-ketone testing strips (A Menarini Diagnostics Ltd) | 10 strip · NHS indicative price = £21.06 · Drug Tariff (Part IXr)

GlucoMen areo Ketone Sensor testing strips (A Menarini Diagnostics Ltd) | 10 strip · NHS indicative price = £9.95 · Drug Tariff (Part IXr)

GlucoRx HCT Ketone testing strips (GlucoRx Ltd) | 10 strip · NHS indicative price = £9.95 · Drug Tariff (Part IXr)

KetoSens testing strips (Spirit Healthcare Ltd) | 10 strip · NHS indicative price = £9.95 · Drug Tariff (Part IXr)

Hypodermic insulin injection pens

- **HYPODERMIC INSULIN INJECTION PENS**
AUTOPEN® 24
Autopen® 24 (for use with Sanofi- Aventis 3-mL insulin cartridges), allowing 1-unit dosage adjustment, max. 21 units (single-unit version) or 2-unit dosage adjustment, max. 42 units (2- unit version).

Autopen 24 hypodermic insulin injection pen reusable for 3ml cartridge 1 unit dial up / range 1-21 units (Owen Mumford Ltd)
1 device · NHS indicative price = £16.58 · Drug Tariff (Part IXa)

Autopen 24 hypodermic insulin injection pen reusable for 3ml cartridge 2 unit dial up / range 2-42 units (Owen Mumford Ltd)
1 device · NHS indicative price = £16.58 · Drug Tariff (Part IXa)

AUTOPEN® CLASSIC
Autopen® *Classic* (for use with Lilly and Wockhardt 3-mL insulin cartridges), allowing 1-unit dosage adjustment, max. 21 units (single-unit version) or 2-unit dosage adjustment, max. 42 units (2-unit version).

Autopen Classic hypodermic insulin injection pen reusable for 3ml cartridge 1 unit dial up / range 1-21 units (Owen Mumford Ltd)
1 device · NHS indicative price = £16.84 · Drug Tariff (Part IXa)

Autopen Classic hypodermic insulin injection pen reusable for 3ml cartridge 2 unit dial up / range 2-42 units (Owen Mumford Ltd)
1 device · NHS indicative price = £16.84 · Drug Tariff (Part IXa)

CLIKSTAR®
For use with *Lantus*®, *Apidra*®, and *Insuman*® 3-mL insulin cartridges; allowing 1-unit dose adjustment, max. 80 units.

ClikSTAR hypodermic insulin injection pen reusable for 3ml cartridge 1 unit dial up / range 1-80 units (Sanofi)
1 device · NHS indicative price = £25.00 · Drug Tariff (Part IXa)

ClikSTAR hypodermic insulin injection pen reusable for 3ml cartridge 1 unit dial up / range 1-80 units (Sanofi)
1 device · NHS indicative price = £25.00 · Drug Tariff (Part IXa)

HUMAPEN® LUXURA HD
For use with *Humulin*® and *Humalog*® 3-mL cartridges; allowing 0.5-unit dosage adjustment, max. 30 units.

HumaPen Luxura HD hypodermic insulin injection pen reusable for 3ml cartridge 0.5 unit dial up / range 1-30 units (Eli Lilly and Company Ltd)
1 device · NHS indicative price = £27.01 · Drug Tariff (Part IXa)

NOVOPEN® 4
For use with *Penfill*® 3-mL insulin cartridges; allowing 1-unit dosage adjustment, max. 60 units.

NovoPen 4 hypodermic insulin injection pen reusable for 3ml cartridge 1 unit dial up / range 1-60 units (Novo Nordisk Ltd)
1 device · NHS indicative price = £26.86 · Drug Tariff (Part IXa)

NovoPen 4 hypodermic insulin injection pen reusable for 3ml cartridge 1 unit dial up / range 1-60 units (Novo Nordisk Ltd)
1 device · NHS indicative price = £26.86 · Drug Tariff (Part IXa)

Needle free Insulin delivery systems

- **NEEDLE FREE INSULIN DELIVERY SYSTEMS**
INSUJET®
For use with any 10-mL vial or 3-mL cartridge of insulin, allowing 1-unit dosage adjustment, max 40 units.
Available as *starter set* (*InsuJet*® device, nozzle cap, nozzle and piston, 1 × 10-mL adaptor, 1 × 3-mL adaptor, 1 cartridge cap removal key), *nozzle pack* (15 nozzles), *cartridge adaptor pack* (15 adaptors), or *vial adaptor pack* (15 adaptors).

InsuJet starter set (Spirit Healthcare Ltd)
1 pack · NHS indicative price = £90.00 · Drug Tariff (Part IXa)

Urinanalysis reagent strips

- **PRESCRIBING AND DISPENSING INFORMATION**
Other reagent strips available for urinalysis
Include: *Combur-3 Test*® (glucose and protein—Roche Diagnostics); *Clinitek Microalbumin*® (albumin and creatinine—Siemens); *Ketodiastix*® (glucose and ketones—Bayer Diagnostics); *Medi-Test Combi* 2® (glucose and protein—BHR); *Micral-Test II*®, used to detect microalbuminuria but this should be followed by confirmation in the laboratory—false positive results are common (albumin—Roche Diagnostics); *Microbustix*® (albumin and creatinine—Siemens); *Uristix*® (glucose and protein—Siemens).
These reagent strips are not prescribable under National Health Service (NHS).

- **URINE GLUCOSE TESTING STRIPS**

Diastix testing strips (Bayer Diagnostics Manufacturing Ltd)
50 strip · NHS indicative price = £2.89 · Drug Tariff (Part IXr)

Medi-Test Glucose testing strips (BHR Pharmaceuticals Ltd)
50 strip · NHS indicative price = £2.33 · Drug Tariff (Part IXr)

Mission Glucose testing strips (Spirit Healthcare Ltd)
50 strip · NHS indicative price = £2.29 · Drug Tariff (Part IXr)

- **URINE PROTEIN TESTING STRIPS**

Albustix testing strips (Siemens Medical Solutions Diagnostics Ltd)
50 strip · NHS indicative price = £4.10 · Drug Tariff (Part IXr)

Medi-Test Protein 2 testing strips (BHR Pharmaceuticals Ltd)
50 strip · NHS indicative price = £3.27 · Drug Tariff (Part IXr)

- **URINE KETONES TESTING STRIPS**

GlucoRx KetoRx Sticks 2GK testing strips (GlucoRx Ltd)
50 strip · NHS indicative price = £2.25 · Drug Tariff (Part IXr)

Ketostix testing strips (Bayer Diagnostics Manufacturing Ltd)
50 strip · NHS indicative price = £3.06 · Drug Tariff (Part IXr)

Mission Ketone testing strips (Spirit Healthcare Ltd)
50 strip · NHS indicative price = £2.50 · Drug Tariff (Part IXr)

3.2 Hypoglycaemia

Hypoglycaemia   02-Jun-2017

Treatment of hypoglycaemia

Prompt treatment of hypoglycaemia in children from any cause is essential as severe hypoglycaemia may cause subsequent neurological damage. Hyperinsulinism, fatty acid oxidation disorders and glycogen storage disease are less common causes of acute hypoglycaemia in children.

Initially glucose 10–20 g is given by mouth either in liquid form or as granulated sugar or sugar lumps. If necessary this may be repeated after 10–15 minutes. After initial treatment, a snack providing sustained availability of carbohydrate (e.g. a sandwich, fruit, milk, or biscuits) or the next meal (if it is due) can prevent blood-glucose concentration from falling again.

Proprietary products of quick-acting carbohydrate (e.g. *GlucoGel®, Dextrogel®, GSF-Syrup®, Rapilose®* gel) are available on prescription for patients to keep on hand in case of hypoglycaemia.

Alternatively, approximately 10 g of glucose is available from 2 teaspoons of sugar, or from 3 sugar lumps, and also from non-diet versions of the following soft drinks: 110 mL of *Lucozade® Energy Original* (also, see note below), 100 mL of *Coca-Cola®*, 19 mL of *Ribena® Blackcurrant* (to be diluted).

Note: the carbohydrate content of commercially available glucose-containing drinks is currently subject to change—individual product labels should be checked. Patients should be aware that for a time, both old and new bottles and cans may be available—individual product labels should be checked.

Hypoglycaemia which causes unconsciousness or seizures is an emergency. Glucagon below, a polypeptide hormone produced by the alpha cells of the islets of Langerhans, increases blood-glucose concentration by mobilising glycogen stored in the liver. In hypoglycaemia, if sugar cannot be given by mouth, glucagon can be given by injection. Carbohydrates should be given as soon as possible to restore liver glycogen; glucagon is not appropriate for chronic hypoglycaemia. Glucagon can be issued to parents or carers of insulin-treated children for emergency use in hypoglycaemic attacks. It is often advisable to prescribe it on an 'if necessary' basis for hospitalised insulin-treated children, so that it can be given rapidly by the nurses during a hypoglycaemic emergency. If not effective in 10 minutes intravenous glucose should be given.

Alternatively, glucose intravenous infusion 10% can be given intravenously into a large vein through a large-gauge needle; care is required since this concentration is irritant especially if extravasation occurs. Glucose intravenous infusion 50% is **not** recommended, as it is very viscous and hypertonic. Close monitoring is necessary, particularly in the case of an overdose with a long-acting insulin because further administration of glucose may be required. Children whose hypoglycaemia is caused by an oral antidiabetic drug should be transferred to hospital because the hypoglycaemic effects of these drugs can persist for many hours.

Glucagon is not effective in the treatment of hypoglycaemia due to fatty acid oxidation or glycogen storage disorders.

Chronic hypoglycaemia

Diazoxide p. 445 is useful in the management of chronic hypoglycaemia due to excessive insulin secretion, either from a tumour involving the islets of Langerhans or from persisting hyperinsulinaemic hypoglycaemia of infancy (nesidioblastosis). Diazoxide has no place in the management of acute hypoglycaemia. Chlorothiazide p. 108 reduces diazoxide-induced sodium and water retention and has the added benefit of potentiating the glycaemic effect of diazoxide.

If diazoxide and chlorothiazide fail to suppress excessive glucose requirements in chronic hypoglycaemia then octreotide p. 445 or nifedipine p. 106 can be added. Octreotide suppresses secretion of growth hormone, but growth is unlikely to be affected in the long term.

Neonatal hypoglycaemia

Neonatal hypoglycaemia at birth is treated with glucose **intravenous infusion 10%**. Mild asymptomatic persistent hypoglycaemia may respond to a single dose of glucagon. Glucagon has also been used in the short-term management of endogenous hyperinsulinism.

GLYCOGENOLYTIC HORMONES

Glucagon

- **INDICATIONS AND DOSE**

Insulin-induced hypoglycaemia
▸ BY SUBCUTANEOUS INJECTION, OR BY INTRAMUSCULAR INJECTION
▸ Neonate: 20 micrograms/kg.

▸ Child 1 month–1 year: 500 micrograms
▸ Child 2–17 years (body-weight up to 25 kg): 500 micrograms, if no response within 10 minutes intravenous glucose must be given
▸ Child 2–17 years (body-weight 25 kg and above): 1 mg, if no response within 10 minutes intravenous glucose must be given

Endogenous hyperinsulinism
▸ BY INTRAMUSCULAR INJECTION, OR BY INTRAVENOUS INJECTION
▸ Neonate: 200 micrograms/kg (max. per dose 1 mg) for 1 dose.

▸ Child 1 month–1 year: 1 mg for 1 dose
▸ BY CONTINUOUS INTRAVENOUS INFUSION
▸ Neonate: 1–18 micrograms/kg/hour (max. per dose 50 micrograms/kg/hour), adjusted according to response.

▸ Child 1 month–1 year: 1–10 micrograms/kg/hour, dose to be adjusted as necessary

Diagnosis of growth hormone secretion (specialist use only)
▸ BY INTRAMUSCULAR INJECTION
▸ Child: 100 micrograms/kg (max. per dose 1 mg) for 1 dose, dose may vary, consult local guidelines

Beta-blocker poisoning (cardiogenic shock unresponsive to atropine)
▸ INITIALLY BY INTRAVENOUS INJECTION
▸ Child: 50–150 micrograms/kg (max. per dose 10 mg), to be administered in glucose 5% (with precautions to protect the airway in case of vomiting), followed by (by intravenous infusion) 50 micrograms/kg/hour

DOSE EQUIVALENCE AND CONVERSION
▸ 1 unit of glucagon = 1 mg of glucagon.

- **UNLICENSED USE** Dose and indication for cardiogenic shock unresponsive to atropine in beta-blocker overdose not licensed. Unlicensed for growth hormone test and hyperinsulinism.
- **CONTRA-INDICATIONS** Phaeochromocytoma
- **CAUTIONS** Glucagonoma · ineffective in chronic hypoglycaemia, starvation, and adrenal insufficiency · insulinoma · when used in the diagnosis of growth hormone secretion, delayed hypoglycaemia may result—deaths reported (ensure a meal is eaten before discharge)
- **INTERACTIONS** → Appendix 1: glucagon
- **SIDE-EFFECTS**
▸ **Rare** Hypersensitivity reactions
▸ **Frequency not known** Diarrhoea · hypokalaemia · nausea · vomiting
- **DIRECTIONS FOR ADMINISTRATION**
▸ With intravenous use When administered by *continuous intravenous infusion*, do not add to infusion fluids containing calcium—precipitation may occur.
- **PATIENT AND CARER ADVICE**
Medicines for Children leaflet: Glucagon for hypoglycaemia
www.medicinesforchildren.org.uk/glucagon-for-hypoglycaemia

- **EXCEPTIONS TO LEGAL CATEGORY** Prescription-only medicine restriction does not apply where administration is for saving life in emergency.

- **MEDICINAL FORMS**
  There can be variation in the licensing of different medicines containing the same drug.
  Powder and solvent for solution for injection
  ▸ GlucaGen Hypokit (Novo Nordisk Ltd)
  Glucagon hydrochloride 1 mg GlucaGen Hypokit 1mg powder and solvent for solution for injection | 1 vial PoM £11.52 DT price = £11.52

3.2a Chronic hypoglycaemia

Other drugs used for Chronic hypoglycaemia
Chlorothiazide, p. 108

GLYCOGENOLYTIC HORMONES

Diazoxide

- **INDICATIONS AND DOSE**
  Resistant hypertension
  ▸ BY MOUTH

  ▸ Neonate: Initially 1.7 mg/kg 3 times a day, adjusted according to response; maximum 15 mg/kg per day.

  ▸ Child: Initially 1.7 mg/kg 3 times a day, adjusted according to response; maximum 15 mg/kg per day

  Chronic intractable hypoglycaemia
  ▸ BY MOUTH

  ▸ Neonate: Initially 5 mg/kg twice daily, adjusted according to response, initial dose used to establish response; maintenance 1.5–3 mg/kg 2–3 times a day; increased if necessary up to 7 mg/kg 3 times a day, higher doses are unlikely to be beneficial, but may be required in some cases.

  ▸ Child: Initially 1.7 mg/kg 3 times a day, adjusted according to response; maintenance 1.5–3 mg/kg 2–3 times a day, increased if necessary up to 5 mg/kg 3 times a day, doses up to 5 mg/kg may be required in some cases, but higher doses are unlikely to be beneficial

- **UNLICENSED USE** Not licensed for resistant hypertension.

- **CAUTIONS** Aortic coarctation · aortic stenosis · arteriovenous shunt · heart failure · hyperuricaemia · impaired cardiac circulation · impaired cerebral circulation

- **INTERACTIONS** → Appendix 1: diazoxide

- **SIDE-EFFECTS** Taste disturbance · abdominal pain · anaemia · anorexia (prolonged use) · bleeding · constipation · decreased libido · dermatitis · diarrhoea · dizziness · dyspnoea · eosinophilia · extrapyramidal effects · galactorrhoea · headache · heart failure · hyperglycaemia · hyperosmolar non-ketotic coma · hypertrichosis · hyperuricaemia (prolonged use) · hypotension · ileus · lacrimation · leucopenia · lichenoid eruption · musculoskeletal pain · nausea · pancreatitis · pruritus · pulmonary hypertension · raised serum creatinine · raised serum urea · reversible nephritic syndrome · sodium and fluid retention · thrombocytopenia · tinnitus · transient cataracts · visual disturbances · voice changes (prolonged use) · vomiting

- **PREGNANCY** Use only if essential; alopecia and hypertrichosis reported in neonates with prolonged use; may inhibit uterine activity during labour.

- **BREAST FEEDING** Manufacturer advises avoid—no information available.

- **RENAL IMPAIRMENT** Dose reduction may be required.

- **MONITORING REQUIREMENTS**
  ▸ Monitor blood pressure.
  ▸ Monitor white cell and platelet count during prolonged use.
  ▸ Regularly assess growth, bone, and psychological development during prolonged use.

- **MEDICINAL FORMS**
  There can be variation in the licensing of different medicines containing the same drug. Forms available from special-order manufacturers include: capsule, oral suspension, oral solution
  Oral suspension
  ▸ Diazoxide (Non-proprietary)
  Diazoxide 50 mg per 1 ml Proglycem 250mg/5ml oral suspension | 30 ml PoM no price available DT price = £136.65
  Tablet
  ▸ Eudemine (Focus Pharmaceuticals Ltd)
  Diazoxide 50 mg Eudemine 50mg tablets | 100 tablet PoM £46.45
  Capsule
  ▸ Diazoxide (Non-proprietary)
  Diazoxide 25 mg Proglycem 25 capsules | 100 capsule PoM no price available

PITUITARY AND HYPOTHALAMIC HORMONES AND ANALOGUES ⟩ SOMATOSTATIN ANALOGUES

Somatostatin analogues

- **CAUTIONS** Diabetes mellitus (antidiabetic requirements may be reduced) · insulinoma (increased depth and duration of hypoglycaemia may occur—observe patients and monitor blood glucose levels when initiating treatment and changing doses)

- **SIDE-EFFECTS**
  ▸ **Rare** Pancreatitis (shortly after administration)
  ▸ **Frequency not known** Abdominal pain · anorexia · bloating · diarrhoea · flatulence · gallstones (after long-term treatment) · gastro-intestinal disturbances · hyperglycaemia (with chronic administration) · hypoglycaemia · impaired postprandial glucose tolerance (with chronic administration) · irritation at the injection site · nausea · pain at the injection site · steatorrhoea · vomiting

- **DIRECTIONS FOR ADMINISTRATION** Injection sites should be rotated.

⌐ above

Octreotide
17-Oct-2016

- **INDICATIONS AND DOSE**
  Persistent hyperinsulinaemic hypoglycaemia unresponsive to diazoxide and glucose
  ▸ BY SUBCUTANEOUS INJECTION

  ▸ Neonate: Initially 2–5 micrograms/kg every 6–8 hours, adjusted according to response; increased if necessary up to 7 micrograms/kg every 4 hours, dosing up to 7 micrograms/kg may rarely be required.

  ▸ Child: Initially 1–2 micrograms/kg every 4–6 hours, adjusted according to response; increased if necessary up to 7 micrograms/kg every 4 hours, dosing up to 7 micrograms/kg may rarely be required

  Bleeding from oesophageal or gastric varices
  ▸ BY CONTINUOUS INTRAVENOUS INFUSION
  ▸ Child: 1 microgram/kg/hour, higher doses may be required initially, when no active bleeding reduce dose over 24 hours; Usual maximum 50 micrograms/hour

- **UNLICENSED USE** Not licensed in children.

- **INTERACTIONS** → Appendix 1: octreotide

6

Endocrine system

- **SIDE-EFFECTS** Alopecia · arrhythmias · biliary colic (associated with abrupt withdrawal of subcutaneous octreotide) · bradycardia · constipation · dizziness · dyspnoea · headache · hepatitis · pancreatitis (associated with abrupt withdrawal of subcutaneous octreotide) · rash · reduced bile flow · reduced gall bladder motility

  SIDE-EFFECTS, FURTHER INFORMATION
- ▸ Gastro-intestinal side-effects Administering non-depot injections of octreotide between meals and at bedtime may reduce gastro-intestinal side-effects.
- **CONCEPTION AND CONTRACEPTION** Effective contraception required during treatment.
- **PREGNANCY** Possible effect on fetal growth; manufacturer advises use only if potential benefit outweighs risk.
- **BREAST FEEDING** Manufacturer advises avoid—present in milk in *animal* studies.
- **MONITORING REQUIREMENTS**
- ▸ Monitor thyroid function on long-term therapy.
- ▸ Monitor liver function.
- **TREATMENT CESSATION** Avoid abrupt withdrawal of short-acting subcutaneous octreotide (associated with biliary colic and pancreatitis).
- **DIRECTIONS FOR ADMINISTRATION** For *intravenous injection* or *intravenous infusion*, dilute with Sodium Chloride 0.9% to a concentration of 10–50%.
- **MEDICINAL FORMS**
  There can be variation in the licensing of different medicines containing the same drug.
  Solution for injection
  - ▸ Octreotide (Non-proprietary)
    Octreotide (as Octreotide acetate) 50 microgram per
    1 ml Octreotide 50micrograms/1ml solution for injection pre-filled syringes | 5 pre-filled disposable injection [PoM] £18.85 DT price = £18.85
    Octreotide 50micrograms/1ml solution for injection ampoules | 5 ampoule [PoM] £14.85–£18.60
    Octreotide 50micrograms/1ml solution for injection vials | 5 vial [PoM] £14.87–£22.00 DT price = £22.00
    Octreotide (as Octreotide acetate) 100 microgram per
    1 ml Octreotide 100micrograms/1ml solution for injection ampoules | 5 ampoule [PoM] £32.65 DT price = £27.97
    Octreotide 100micrograms/1ml solution for injection pre-filled syringes | 5 pre-filled disposable injection [PoM] £28.90–£32.90
    Octreotide 100micrograms/1ml solution for injection vials | 5 vial [PoM] £27.97–£32.65
    Octreotide (as Octreotide acetate) 200 microgram per
    1 ml Octreotide 1mg/5ml solution for injection vials | 1 vial [PoM] £65.00–£69.66
    Octreotide (as Octreotide acetate) 500 microgram per
    1 ml Octreotide 500micrograms/1ml solution for injection vials | 5 vial [PoM] £135.47–£158.25
    Octreotide 500micrograms/1ml solution for injection ampoules | 5 ampoule [PoM] £169.35 DT price = £135.47
    Octreotide 500micrograms/1ml solution for injection pre-filled syringes | 5 pre-filled disposable injection [PoM] £139.43–£169.00
  - ▸ Sandostatin (Novartis Pharmaceuticals UK Ltd)
    Octreotide (as Octreotide acetate) 50 microgram per
    1 ml Sandostatin 50micrograms/1ml solution for injection ampoules | 5 ampoule [PoM] £14.87
    Octreotide (as Octreotide acetate) 100 microgram per
    1 ml Sandostatin 100micrograms/1ml solution for injection ampoules | 5 ampoule [PoM] £27.97 DT price = £27.97
    Octreotide (as Octreotide acetate) 200 microgram per
    1 ml Sandostatin 1mg/5ml solution for injection vials | 1 vial [PoM] £55.73
    Octreotide (as Octreotide acetate) 500 microgram per
    1 ml Sandostatin 500micrograms/1ml solution for injection ampoules | 5 ampoule [PoM] £135.47 DT price = £135.47
  Powder and solvent for suspension for injection
  - ▸ Sandostatin LAR (Novartis Pharmaceuticals UK Ltd)
    Octreotide (as Octreotide acetate) 10 mg Sandostatin LAR 10mg powder and solvent for suspension for injection vials | 1 vial [PoM] £549.71

Octreotide (as Octreotide acetate) 20 mg Sandostatin LAR 20mg powder and solvent for suspension for injection vials | 1 vial [PoM] £799.33
Octreotide (as Octreotide acetate) 30 mg Sandostatin LAR 30mg powder and solvent for suspension for injection vials | 1 vial [PoM] £998.41

4 Disorders of bone metabolism

Bone metabolism

Disorders of bone metabolism

The two main disorders of bone metabolism that occur in children are rickets and osteoporosis. The two most common forms of rickets are Vitamin D deficiency rickets and hypophosphataemic rickets. See also calcium.

Osteoporosis

Osteoporosis in children may be primary (e.g. *osteogenesis imperfecta* and *idiopathic juvenile osteoporosis*), or secondary (e.g. due to inflammatory disorders, immobilisation, or corticosteroids); specialist management is required.

Corticosteroid-induced osteoporosis
To reduce the risk of osteoporosis doses of oral corticosteroids should be as low as possible and courses of treatment as short as possible.

Calcitonin

Calcitonin is involved with parathyroid hormone in the regulation of bone turnover and hence in the maintenance of calcium balance and homoeostasis. Calcitonin (salmon) p. 450 (synthetic or recombinant salmon calcitonin) is used by specialists to lower the plasma-calcium concentration in children with hypercalcaemia associated with malignancy.

Bisphosphonates

A bisphosphonate such as pamidronate disodium p. 448 is used in the management of severe forms of *osteogenesis imperfecta* and other causes of osteoporosis in children to reduce the number of fractures; the long-term effects of bisphosphonates in children have not been established. Single doses of bisphosphonates are also used to manage hypercalaemia. Treatment should be initiated under specialist advice **only**.

BISPHOSPHONATES

Bisphosphonates

- **DRUG ACTION** Bisphosphonates are adsorbed onto hydroxyapatite crystals in bone, slowing both their rate of growth and dissolution, and therefore reducing the rate of bone turnover.

  IMPORTANT SAFETY INFORMATION
  MHRA/CHM ADVICE: BISPHOSPHONATES: ATYPICAL FEMORAL FRACTURES (JUNE 2011)
  Atypical femoral fractures have been reported rarely with bisphosphonate treatment, mainly in patients receiving long-term treatment for osteoporosis.
  The need to continue bisphosphonate treatment for osteoporosis should be re-evaluated periodically based on an assessment of the benefits and risks of treatment for individual patients, particularly after 5 or more years of use.
  Patients should be advised to report any thigh, hip, or groin pain during treatment with a bisphosphonate.

Discontinuation of bisphosphonate treatment in patients suspected to have an atypical femoral fracture should be considered after an assessment of the benefits and risks of continued treatment.

MHRA/CHM ADVICE: BISPHOSPHONATES: OSTEONECROSIS OF THE JAW (NOVEMBER 2009) AND INTRAVENOUS BISPHOSPHONATES: OSTEONECROSIS OF THE JAW—FURTHER MEASURES TO MINIMISE RISK (JULY 2015)

The risk of osteonecrosis of the jaw is substantially greater for patients receiving intravenous bisphosphonates in the treatment of cancer than for patients receiving oral bisphosphonates for osteoporosis or Paget's disease.

Risk factors for developing osteonecrosis of the jaw that should be considered are: potency of bisphosphonate (highest for zoledronate), route of administration, cumulative dose, duration and type of malignant disease, concomitant treatment, smoking, comorbid conditions, and history of dental disease.

All patients should have a dental check-up (and any necessary remedial work should be performed) before bisphosphonate treatment, or as soon as possible after starting treatment. Patients should also maintain good oral hygiene, receive routine dental check-ups, and report any oral symptoms such as dental mobility, pain, or swelling, non-healing sores or discharge to a doctor and dentist during treatment.

Before prescribing an intravenous bisphosphonate, patients should be given a patient reminder card and informed of the risk of osteonecrosis of the jaw. Advise patients to tell their doctor if they have any problems with their mouth or teeth before starting treatment, and if the patient wears dentures, they should make sure their dentures fit properly. Patients should tell their doctor and dentist that they are receiving an intravenous bisphosphonate if they need dental treatment or dental surgery.

Guidance for dentists in primary care is included in *Oral Health Management of Patients Prescribed Bisphosphonates: Dental Clinical Guidance*, Scottish Dental Clinical Effectiveness Programme, April 2011 (available at www.sdcep.org.uk).

MHRA/CHM ADVICE: BISPHOSPHONATES: OSTEONECROSIS OF THE EXTERNAL AUDITORY CANAL (DECEMBER 2015)

Benign idiopathic osteonecrosis of the external auditory canal has been reported very rarely with bisphosphonate treatment, mainly in patients receiving long-term therapy (2 years or longer).

The possibility of osteonecrosis of the external auditory canal should be considered in patients receiving bisphosphonates who present with ear symptoms, including chronic ear infections, or suspected cholesteatoma.

Risk factors for developing osteonecrosis of the external auditory canal include: steroid use, chemotherapy, infection, an ear operation, or cotton-bud use.

Patients should be advised to report any ear pain, discharge from the ear, or an ear infection during treatment with a bisphosphonate.

● **PATIENT AND CARER ADVICE**
Atypical femoral fractures Patients should be advised to report any thigh, hip, or groin pain during treatment with a bisphosphonate.
Osteonecrosis of the jaw During bisphosphonate treatment patients should maintain good oral hygiene, receive routine dental check-ups, and report any oral symptoms.
Osteonecrosis of the external auditory canal Patients should be advised to report any ear pain, discharge from ear or an ear infection during treatment with a bisphosphonate.

F 446

Alendronic acid
14-Dec-2016
(Alendronate)

● **INDICATIONS AND DOSE**
Osteoporosis (due to osteogenesis imperfecta and other causes) (initiated under specialist supervision) | **Hypercalcaemia (initiated under specialist supervision)**
▸ BY MOUTH
▸ **Child:** (consult local protocol)

● **UNLICENSED USE** Not licensed for use in children.
● **CONTRA-INDICATIONS** Abnormalities of oesophagus · hypocalcaemia · other factors which delay emptying (e.g. stricture or achalasia)
● **CAUTIONS** Active gastro-intestinal bleeding · atypical femoral fractures · duodenitis · dysphagia · exclude other causes of osteoporosis · gastritis · history (within 1 year) of ulcers · surgery of the upper gastro-intestinal tract · symptomatic oesophageal disease · ulcers · upper gastro-intestinal disorders
● **INTERACTIONS** → Appendix 1: bisphosphonates
● **SIDE-EFFECTS**
▸ **Common or very common** Abdominal distension · abdominal pain · constipation · diarrhoea · dyspepsia · flatulence · headache · oesophageal reactions · regurgitation
▸ **Uncommon** Episcleritis · erythema · gastritis · nausea · rash · scleritis · uveitis · vomiting
▸ **Rare** Atypical femoral fractures with long-term use · hypocalcaemia · osteonecrosis of the jaw · photosensitivity · severe skin reactions · Stevens-Johnson syndrome · toxic epidermal necrolysis · upper gastro-intestinal ulcers
▸ **Very rare** Osteonecrosis of the external auditory canal
▸ **Frequency not known** Musculoskeletal pain
SIDE-EFFECTS, FURTHER INFORMATION
▸ Oesophageal reactions Severe oesophageal reactions (oesophagitis, oesophageal ulcers, oesophageal stricture and oesophageal erosions) have been reported; patients should be advised to stop taking the tablets and to seek medical attention if they develop symptoms of oesophageal irritation such as dysphagia, new or worsening heartburn, pain on swallowing or retrosternal pain.
● **PREGNANCY** Avoid.
● **BREAST FEEDING** Manufacturer advises avoid—no information available.
● **RENAL IMPAIRMENT** Avoid if estimated glomerular filtration rate is less than 35 mL/minute/1.73 m^2.
● **MONITORING REQUIREMENTS** Correct disturbances of calcium and mineral metabolism (e.g. vitamin-D deficiency, hypocalcaemia) before starting treatment. Monitor serum-calcium concentration during treatment.
● **DIRECTIONS FOR ADMINISTRATION** Tablets should be swallowed whole and oral solution should be swallowed as a single 100 mL dose. Doses should be taken with plenty of water while sitting or standing, on an empty stomach at least 30 minutes before breakfast (or another oral medicine); patient should stand or sit upright for at least 30 minutes after administration.
● **PATIENT AND CARER ADVICE** Patients or their carers should be given advice on how to administer alendronic acid tablets and oral solution.
Oesophageal reactions Patients (or their carers) should be advised to stop taking alendronic acid and to seek medical attention if they develop symptoms of oesophageal irritation such as dysphagia, new or worsening heartburn, pain on swallowing or retrosternal pain.

6

Endocrine system

6

● NATIONAL FUNDING/ACCESS DECISIONS

Scottish Medicines Consortium (SMC) Decisions

The *Scottish Medicines Consortium* has advised (April 2016) that alendronic acid (*Binosto*®) is accepted for restricted use within NHS Scotland for the treatment of postmenopausal osteoporosis where alendronic acid is the appropriate treatment choice, but the patient is unable to swallow tablets.

● MEDICINAL FORMS

There can be variation in the licensing of different medicines containing the same drug. Forms available from special-order manufacturers include: oral solution

Oral solution

▸ Alendronic acid (Non-proprietary)

  Alendronic acid 700 microgram per 1 ml Alendronic acid 70mg/100ml oral solution unit dose sugar free sugar-free | 4 unit dose [PoM] £27.36 DT price = £27.36

Effervescent tablet

▸ Binosto (Internis Pharmaceuticals Ltd)

  Alendronic acid (as Alendronate sodium) 70 mg Binosto 70mg effervescent tablets sugar-free | 4 tablet [PoM] £22.80 DT price = £22.80

Tablet

▸ Alendronic acid (Non-proprietary)

  Alendronic acid (as Alendronate sodium) 10 mg Alendronic acid 10mg tablets | 28 tablet [PoM] £3.25 DT price = £1.83

  Alendronic acid (as Alendronate sodium) 70 mg Alendronic acid 70mg tablets | 4 tablet [PoM] £22.80 DT price = £0.74

▸ Fosamax (Merck Sharp & Dohme Ltd)

  Alendronic acid (as Alendronate sodium) 10 mg Fosamax 10mg tablets | 28 tablet [PoM] £23.12 DT price = £1.83

  Alendronic acid (as Alendronate sodium) 70 mg Fosamax Once Weekly 70mg tablets | 4 tablet [PoM] £22.80 DT price = £0.74

F 446

Pamidronate disodium

(Formerly called aminohydroxypropylidenediphosphonate disodium (APD))

● INDICATIONS AND DOSE

Osteoporosis (due to osteogenesis imperfecta and other causes) (specialist use only) | Hypercalcaemia (specialist use only)

▸ BY INTRAVENOUS INFUSION

▸ Child: (consult product literature)

● UNLICENSED USE Not licensed for use in children.

● CAUTIONS Atypical femoral fractures · cardiac disease · ensure adequate hydration · previous thyroid surgery (risk of hypocalcaemia)

● INTERACTIONS → Appendix 1: bisphosphonates

● SIDE-EFFECTS

▸ Common or very common Arthralgia · bone pain · fever · headache · hypomagnesaemia · hypophosphataemia · influenza- like symptoms (sometimes accompanied by malaise, rigors, fatigue and flushes) · lymphocytopenia · myalgia · nausea · transient rise in body temperature · vomiting

▸ Rare Abdominal pain · acute renal failure · agitation · anaemia · anorexia · atypical femoral fractures · confusion · conjunctivitis · constipation · deterioration of renal disease · diarrhoea · dizziness · dyspepsia · haematuria · hallucinations · hyperkalaemia · hypernatraemia · hypertension · hypokalaemia · hypotension · insomnia · isolated cases of seizures · lethargy · leucopenia · muscle cramps · osteonecrosis of the jaw · other ocular symptoms · paraesthesia · pruritus · rash · somnolence · symptomatic hypocalcaemia · tetany · thrombocytopenia

▸ Very rare Osteonecrosis of the external auditory canal

▸ Frequency not known Atrial fibrillation · injection-site reactions · reactivation of herpes simplex · reactivation of herpes zoster

● PREGNANCY Avoid—toxicity in *animal* studies.

● BREAST FEEDING Avoid.

● HEPATIC IMPAIRMENT Caution in severe hepatic impairment—no information available.

● RENAL IMPAIRMENT Monitor renal function in renal disease or predisposition to renal impairment (e.g. in tumour-induced hypercalcaemia).

● DIRECTIONS FOR ADMINISTRATION For *slow intravenous infusion* (*Aredia*®; *Pamidronate disodium*, Hospira, Medac, Wockhardt), give intermittently in Glucose 5% or Sodium chloride 0.9%; give at a rate not exceeding 1 mg/minute; not to be given with infusion fluids containing calcium. For *Aredia*®, reconstitute initially with water for injections (15 mg in 5 mL, 30 mg or 90 mg in 10mL), then dilute with infusion fluid to a concentration of not more than 90 mg in 250 mL. For *Pamidronate disodium* (Medac, Hospira, Wockhardt) dilute with infusion fluid to a concentration of not more than 90 mg in 250 mL

● PATIENT AND CARER ADVICE A patient reminder card should be provided (risk of osteonecrosis of the jaw).

Driving and skilled tasks

Patients should be warned against performing skilled tasks (e.g. cycling, driving or operating machinery) immediately after treatment (somnolence or dizziness can occur).

● MEDICINAL FORMS

There can be variation in the licensing of different medicines containing the same drug.

Solution for infusion

▸ Pamidronate disodium (Non-proprietary)

  Pamidronate disodium 3 mg per 1 ml Pamidronate disodium 15mg/5ml solution for infusion vials | 1 vial [PoM] £27.50 (Hospital only) | 5 vial [PoM] £149.15

  Pamidronate disodium 30mg/10ml solution for infusion vials | 1 vial [PoM] £55.00 (Hospital only) | 1 vial [PoM] £59.66

  Pamidronate disodium 60mg/20ml solution for infusion vials | 1 vial [PoM] £110.00 (Hospital only)

  Pamidronate disodium 90mg/30ml solution for infusion vials | 1 vial [PoM] £165.00 (Hospital only)

  Pamidronate disodium 9 mg per 1 ml Pamidronate disodium 90mg/10ml solution for infusion vials | 1 vial [PoM] £170.45

  Pamidronate disodium 15 mg per 1 ml Pamidronate disodium 60mg/4ml solution for infusion ampoules | 1 ampoule [PoM] £119.32

  Pamidronate disodium 15mg/1ml solution for infusion ampoules | 4 ampoule [PoM] £119.32

  Pamidronate disodium 90mg/6ml solution for infusion ampoules | 1 ampoule [PoM] £170.46

  Pamidronate disodium 30mg/2ml solution for infusion ampoules | 2 ampoule [PoM] £119.32

F 446

Risedronate sodium

● INDICATIONS AND DOSE

Osteoporosis (due to osteogenesis imperfecta and other causes) (specialist use only) | Hypercalcaemia (specialist use only)

▸ BY MOUTH

▸ Child: (consult local protocol)

● UNLICENSED USE Not licensed for use in children.

● CONTRA-INDICATIONS Hypocalcaemia

● CAUTIONS Atypical femoral fractures · oesophageal abnormalities · other factors which delay transit or emptying (e.g. stricture or achalasia)

● INTERACTIONS → Appendix 1: bisphosphonates

● SIDE-EFFECTS

▸ Common or very common Abdominal pain · constipation · diarrhoea · dyspepsia · headache · musculoskeletal pain · nausea

▶ **Uncommon** Duodenitis · dysphagia · gastritis · oesophageal ulcer · oesophagitis · uveitis
▶ **Rare** Atypical femoral fractures · glossitis · oesophageal stricture
▶ **Very rare** Osteonecrosis of the external auditory canal
▶ **Frequency not known** Cutaneous vasculitis · gastroduodenal ulceration · hair loss · hepatic disorders · osteonecrosis of the jaw · Stevens-Johnson syndrome · toxic epidermal necrolysis

● **PREGNANCY** Avoid.

● **BREAST FEEDING** Avoid.

● **RENAL IMPAIRMENT** Avoid if estimated glomerular filtration rate is less than 30 mL/minute/1.73 m^2.

● **MONITORING REQUIREMENTS**
▶ Correct hypocalcaemia before starting.
▶ Correct other disturbances of bone and mineral metabolism (e.g. vitamin-D deficiency) at onset of treatment.

● **DIRECTIONS FOR ADMINISTRATION** Swallow tablets whole with full glass of water; on rising, take on an empty stomach at least 30 minutes before first food or drink of the day **or**, if taking at any other time of the day, avoid food and drink for at least 2 hours before or after risedronate (particularly avoid calcium-containing products e.g. milk; also avoid iron and mineral supplements and antacids); stand or sit upright for at least 30 minutes; do not take tablets at bedtime or before rising.

● **PATIENT AND CARER ADVICE** Patients or carers should be given advice on how to administer risedronate sodium tablets.
Oesophageal reactions Patients should be advised to stop taking the tablets and seek medical attention if they develop symptoms of oesophageal irritation such as dysphagia, pain on swallowing, retrosternal pain, or heartburn.
Medicines for Children leaflet: Risedronate for brittle bones www.medicinesforchildren.org.uk/risedronate-for-brittle-bones

● **MEDICINAL FORMS**
There can be variation in the licensing of different medicines containing the same drug. Forms available from special-order manufacturers include: oral suspension, oral solution

Tablet
▶ **Risedronate sodium (Non-proprietary)**
Risedronate sodium 5 mg Risedronate sodium 5mg tablets | 28 tablet [PoM] £24.78 DT price = £18.85
Risedronate sodium 30 mg Risedronate sodium 30mg tablets | 28 tablet [PoM] £143.95 DT price = £143.83
Risedronate sodium 35 mg Risedronate sodium 35mg tablets | 4 tablet [PoM] £19.12 DT price = £0.85
▶ **Actonel** (Warner Chilcott UK Ltd, Teva UK Ltd)
Risedronate sodium 5 mg Actonel 5mg tablets | 28 tablet [PoM] £17.99 DT price = £18.85
Risedronate sodium 30 mg Actonel 30mg tablets | 28 tablet [PoM] £143.95 DT price = £143.83
Risedronate sodium 35 mg Actonel Once a Week 35mg tablets | 4 tablet [PoM] £19.12 DT price = £0.85
Actonel 35mg tablets | 4 tablet [PoM] no price available DT price = £0.85

◤ 446

Sodium clodronate

● **INDICATIONS AND DOSE**
Osteoporosis (due to osteogenesis imperfecta or other causes) (specialist use only) | Hypercalcaemia (specialist use only)
▶ BY MOUTH
▶ Child: (consult local protocol)

● **UNLICENSED USE** Not licensed for use in children.

● **CONTRA-INDICATIONS** Acute gastro-intestinal inflammatory conditions

● **CAUTIONS** Atypical femoral fractures · maintain adequate fluid intake during treatment

● **INTERACTIONS** → Appendix 1: bisphosphonates

● **SIDE-EFFECTS**
▶ **Common or very common** Bronchospasm · diarrhoea · nausea · skin reactions · vomiting
▶ **Rare** Atypical femoral fractures
▶ **Very rare** Osteonecrosis of the external auditory canal · osteonecrosis of the jaw
▶ **Frequency not known** Renal impairment · uveitis

● **PREGNANCY** Avoid.

● **BREAST FEEDING** Manufacturer advises avoid—no information available.

● **RENAL IMPAIRMENT** Reduce dose if estimated glomerular filtration rate 30—50 mL/minute/1.73m^2. Use half normal dose if estimated glomerular filtration rate 10–30 mL/minute/1.73 m^2. Avoid if estimated glomerular filtration rate less than 10 mL/minute/1.73 m^2.

● **MONITORING REQUIREMENTS** Monitor renal function, serum calcium and serum phosphate before and during treatment.

● **DIRECTIONS FOR ADMINISTRATION** Avoid food for 2 hours before and 1 hour after treatment, particularly calcium-containing products e.g. milk; also avoid iron and mineral supplements and antacids; maintain adequate fluid intake.

● **PATIENT AND CARER ADVICE** Patients or carers should be given advice on how to administer sodium clodronate capsules and tablets.

● **MEDICINAL FORMS**
There can be variation in the licensing of different medicines containing the same drug.
Tablet
CAUTIONARY AND ADVISORY LABELS 10
▶ **Sodium clodronate (Non-proprietary)**
Sodium clodronate 800 mg Sodium clodronate 800mg tablets | 60 tablet [PoM] £116.72 DT price = £146.43
▶ **Bonefos** (Bayer Plc)
Sodium clodronate 800 mg Bonefos 800mg tablets | 60 tablet [PoM] £146.43 DT price = £146.43
▶ **Clasteon** (Beacon Pharmaceuticals Ltd)
Sodium clodronate 800 mg Clasteon 800mg tablets | 60 tablet [PoM] £146.43 DT price = £146.43
▶ **Loron** (Intrapharm Laboratories Ltd)
Sodium clodronate 520 mg Loron 520mg tablets | 60 tablet [PoM] £152.59 DT price = £152.59

Capsule
▶ **Sodium clodronate (Non-proprietary)**
Sodium clodronate 400 mg Sodium clodronate 400mg capsules | 30 capsule [PoM] £40.49 | 120 capsule [PoM] £161.97 DT price = £139.83
▶ **Bonefos** (Bayer Plc)
Sodium clodronate 400 mg Bonefos 400mg capsules | 120 capsule [PoM] £139.83 DT price = £139.83
▶ **Clasteon** (Beacon Pharmaceuticals Ltd)
Sodium clodronate 400 mg Clasteon 400mg capsules | 30 capsule [PoM] £34.96 | 120 capsule [PoM] £139.83 DT price = £139.83

6

Endocrine system

CALCIUM REGULATING DRUGS > BONE
RESORPTION INHIBITORS

Calcitonin (salmon)

(Salcatonin)

- **INDICATIONS AND DOSE**

Hypercalcaemia (limited experience in children) (specialist use only)

▶ BY SUBCUTANEOUS INJECTION, OR BY INTRAMUSCULAR INJECTION

▸ Child: 2.5–5 units/kg every 12 hours (max. per dose 400 units every 6–8 hours), adjusted according to response, no additional benefit with doses over 8 units/kg every 6 hours

▶ BY INTRAVENOUS INFUSION

▸ Child: 5–10 units/kg, to be administered by slow intravenous infusion over at least 6 hours

Osteoporosis (specialist use only)

▶ BY INTRAMUSCULAR INJECTION, OR BY SUBCUTANEOUS INJECTION

▸ Child: Refer for specialist advice, experience very limited

- **UNLICENSED USE** Not licensed in children.
- **CONTRA-INDICATIONS** Hypocalcaemia
- **CAUTIONS** Heart failure · history of allergy (skin test advised) · risk of malignancy—avoid prolonged use (use lowest effective dose for shortest possible time)
- **INTERACTIONS** → Appendix 1: calcitonin (salmon)
- **SIDE-EFFECTS**
▶ **Common or very common** Abdominal pain · diarrhoea · dizziness · fatigue · flushing · headache · malignancy (with long-term use) · musculoskeletal pain · nausea · taste disturbances · vomiting
▶ **Uncommon** Cough · hypersensitivity reactions · hypertension · injection-site reactions · oedema · polyuria · pruritus · rash · visual disturbances
▶ **Frequency not known** Tremor
- **PREGNANCY** Avoid unless potential benefit outweighs risk (toxicity in *animal* studies).
- **BREAST FEEDING** Avoid; inhibits lactation in *animals*.
- **RENAL IMPAIRMENT** Use with caution.
- **MONITORING REQUIREMENTS** Monitor bone growth.
- **DIRECTIONS FOR ADMINISTRATION** For *intravenous infusion*, dilute injection solution (e.g. 400 units in 500 mL) with Sodium Chloride 0.9% and give over at least 6 hours; glass or hard plastic containers should not be used; some loss of potency on dilution and administration—use diluted solution without delay.

- **MEDICINAL FORMS**
There can be variation in the licensing of different medicines containing the same drug.

Solution for injection

▸ Calcitonin (salmon) (Non-proprietary)
Calcitonin (salmon) 50 unit per 1 ml Calcitonin (salmon) 50units/1ml solution for injection ampoules | 5 ampoule PoM £167.50
Calcitonin (salmon) 100 unit per 1 ml Calcitonin (salmon) 100units/1ml solution for injection ampoules | 5 ampoule PoM £220.00
Calcitonin (salmon) 200 unit per 1 ml Calcitonin (salmon) 400units/2ml solution for injection vials | 1 vial PoM £352.00

5 Gonadotrophin responsive conditions

PITUITARY AND HYPOTHALAMIC HORMONES AND ANALOGUES > GONADOTROPIN-RELEASING HORMONES

Goserelin

- **DRUG ACTION** Administration of gonadorelin analogues produces an initial phase of stimulation; continued administration is followed by down-regulation of gonadotrophin-releasing hormone receptors, thereby reducing the release of gonadotrophins (follicle stimulating hormone and luteinising hormone) which in turn leads to inhibition of androgen and oestrogen production.

- **INDICATIONS AND DOSE**

ZOLADEX LA®

Gonadotrophin-dependent precocious puberty

▶ BY SUBCUTANEOUS INJECTION

▸ Child: 10.8 mg every 12 weeks, to be administered into the anterior abdominal wall, injections may be required more frequently in some cases

ZOLADEX®

Gonadotrophin-dependent precocious puberty

▶ BY SUBCUTANEOUS INJECTION

▸ Child: 3.6 mg every 28 days, to be administered into the anterior abdominal wall, injections may be required more frequently in some cases

- **UNLICENSED USE** Not licensed for use in children.
- **CONTRA-INDICATIONS** Undiagnosed vaginal bleeding
- **CAUTIONS** Depression · patients with metabolic bone disease (decrease in bone mineral density can occur)
- **SIDE-EFFECTS** Anaphylaxis · asthma · breast tenderness · changes in blood pressure · changes in breast size · changes in scalp and body hair · depression · headache · hypersensitivity reactions · local reactions at injection site · mood changes · ovarian cysts (may require withdrawal) · paraesthesia · pruritus · rash · urticaria · vaginal bleeding · visual disturbances · weight change · withdrawal bleeding
- **CONCEPTION AND CONTRACEPTION** Non-hormonal, barrier methods of contraception should be used during entire treatment period. Pregnancy should be excluded before treatment, the first injection should be given during menstruation or shortly afterwards or use barrier contraception for 1 month beforehand.
- **PREGNANCY** Avoid.
- **BREAST FEEDING** Avoid.
- **MONITORING REQUIREMENTS** Monitor bone mineral density.
- **DIRECTIONS FOR ADMINISTRATION** Rotate injection site to prevent atrophy and nodule formation.

- **MEDICINAL FORMS**
There can be variation in the licensing of different medicines containing the same drug.

Implant

▸ Zoladex (AstraZeneca UK Ltd)
Goserelin (as Goserelin acetate) 3.6 mg Zoladex 3.6mg implant SafeSystem pre-filled syringes | 1 pre-filled disposable injection PoM £65.00 DT price = £65.00
▸ Zoladex LA (AstraZeneca UK Ltd)
Goserelin (as Goserelin acetate) 10.8 mg Zoladex LA 10.8mg implant SafeSystem pre-filled syringes | 1 pre-filled disposable injection PoM £235.00 DT price = £235.00

Leuprorelin acetate

- **DRUG ACTION** Administration of gonadorelin analogues produces an initial phase of stimulation; continued administration is followed by down-regulation of gonadotrophin-releasing hormone receptors, thereby reducing the release of gonadotrophins (follicle stimulating hormone and luteinising hormone) which in turn leads to inhibition of androgen and oestrogen production.

- **INDICATIONS AND DOSE**

PROSTAP 3 DCS®

Gonadotrophin-dependent precocious puberty
▸ BY SUBCUTANEOUS INJECTION, OR BY INTRAMUSCULAR INJECTION
  ▸ Child: 11.25 mg every 12 weeks, injections may be required more frequently in some cases

PROSTAP SR DCS®

Gonadotrophin-dependent precocious puberty
▸ BY SUBCUTANEOUS INJECTION, OR BY INTRAMUSCULAR INJECTION
  ▸ Child: 3.75 mg every 4 weeks, half this dose is sometimes used in children with body-weight under 20 kg, injections may be required more frequently in some cases

- **UNLICENSED USE** Not licensed for use in children.
- **CONTRA-INDICATIONS** Undiagnosed vaginal bleeding
- **CAUTIONS** Patients with metabolic bone disease (decrease in bone mineral density can occur)
- **INTERACTIONS** → Appendix 1: leuprolelin
- **SIDE-EFFECTS** Abdominal pain · acne · anaphylaxis · asthma · breast tenderness (males and females) · changes in blood pressure · changes in breast size · changes in scalp and body hair · depression · headache · hypersensitivity reactions · local reactions at injection site · mood changes · paraesthesia · pruritus · rash · urticaria · visual disturbances · weight changes · withdrawal bleeding
- **PREGNANCY** Avoid—teratogenic in *animal* studies.
- **BREAST FEEDING** Avoid.
- **MONITORING REQUIREMENTS** Monitor bone mineral density.
- **DIRECTIONS FOR ADMINISTRATION** Rotate injection site to prevent atrophy and nodule formation.

- **MEDICINAL FORMS**
  There can be variation in the licensing of different medicines containing the same drug.
  Powder and solvent for suspension for injection
  ▸ Prostap 3 DCS (Takeda UK Ltd)
    Leuprorelin acetate 11.25 mg Prostap 3 DCS 11.25mg powder and solvent for suspension for injection pre-filled syringes | 1 pre-filled disposable injection PoM £225.72 DT price = £225.72
  ▸ Prostap SR DCS (Takeda UK Ltd)
    Leuprorelin acetate 3.75 mg Prostap SR DCS 3.75mg powder and solvent for suspension for injection pre-filled syringes | 1 pre-filled disposable injection PoM £75.24 DT price = £75.24

Triptorelin

27-Apr-2017

- **DRUG ACTION** Administration of gonadorelin analogues produces an initial phase of stimulation; continued administration is followed by down-regulation of gonadotrophin-releasing hormone receptors, thereby reducing the release of gonadotrophins (follicle stimulating hormone and luteinising hormone) which in turn leads to inhibition of androgen and oestrogen production.

- **INDICATIONS AND DOSE**

DECAPEPTYL® SR 11.25MG

Gonadotrophin-dependent precocious puberty
▸ BY INTRAMUSCULAR INJECTION
  ▸ Child: 11.25 mg every 3 months, discontinue when bone maturation consistent with age of 12 years in girls or 13–14 years in boys

GONAPEPTYL DEPOT®

Gonadotrophin-dependent precocious puberty
▸ BY SUBCUTANEOUS INJECTION, OR BY DEEP INTRAMUSCULAR INJECTION
  ▸ Child (body-weight up to 20 kg): Initially 1.875 mg every 2 weeks for 3 doses, to be administered on days 0, 14, and 28 of treatment, then 1.875 mg every 3–4 weeks, discontinue when bone maturation consistent with age over 12 years in girls and over 13 years in boys
  ▸ Child (body-weight 20–30 kg): Initially 2.5 mg every 2 weeks for 3 doses, to be administered on days 0, 14, and 28 of treatment, then 2.5 mg every 3–4 weeks, discontinue when bone maturation consistent with age over 12 years in girls and over 13 years in boys
  ▸ Child (body-weight 31 kg and above): Initially 3.75 mg every 2 weeks for 3 doses, to be administered on days 0, 14, and 28 of treatment, then 3.75 mg every 3–4 weeks, discontinue when bone maturation consistent with age over 12 years in girls and over 13 years in boys

- **CONTRA-INDICATIONS** Undiagnosed vaginal bleeding
- **SIDE-EFFECTS** Anaphylaxis · arthralgia · asthenia · asthma · breast tenderness (males and females) · changes in blood pressure · changes in breast size · changes in scalp and body hair · depression · gastro-intestinal disturbances · headache · hypersensitivity reactions · local reactions at injection site · mood changes · ovarian cysts (may require withdrawal) · paraesthesia · pruritus · rash · urticaria · visual disturbances · weight changes · withdrawal bleeding (may occur in the first month of treatment)
- **CONCEPTION AND CONTRACEPTION** Non-hormonal, barrier methods of contraception should be used during entire treatment period. Pregnancy should be excluded before treatment, the first injection should be given during menstruation or shortly afterwards or use barrier contraception for 1 month beforehand.
- **PREGNANCY** Avoid.
- **BREAST FEEDING** Avoid.
- **MONITORING REQUIREMENTS** Monitor bone mineral density.
- **DIRECTIONS FOR ADMINISTRATION** Rotate injection site to prevent atrophy and nodule formation.
- **PRESCRIBING AND DISPENSING INFORMATION**
  DECAPEPTYL® SR 11.25MG Each vial includes an overage to allow accurate administration of an 11.25 mg dose.

6

Endocrine system

- **MEDICINAL FORMS**
There can be variation in the licensing of different medicines containing the same drug.

Powder and solvent for suspension for injection

▸ **Decapeptyl SR** (Ipsen Ltd)
  Triptorelin (as Triptorelin acetate) 3 mg Decapeptyl SR 3mg powder and solvent for suspension for injection vials | 1 vial PoM £69.00 DT price = £69.00
  Triptorelin (as Triptorelin acetate) 11.25 mg Decapeptyl SR 11.25mg powder and solvent for suspension for injection vials | 1 vial PoM £207.00 DT price = £207.00
  Triptorelin (as Triptorelin embonate) 22.5 mg Decapeptyl SR 22.5mg powder and solvent for suspension for injection vials | 1 vial PoM £414.00 DT price = £414.00

▸ **Gonapeptyl Depot** (Ferring Pharmaceuticals Ltd)
  Triptorelin (as Triptorelin acetate) 3.75 mg Gonapeptyl Depot 3.75mg powder and solvent for suspension for injection pre-filled disposable devices | 1 pre-filled disposable injection PoM £81.69

6 Hypothalamic and anterior pituitary hormone related disorders

Hypothalamic and anterior pituitary hormones

Anterior pituitary hormones

Corticotrophins

Tetracosactide below (tetracosactrin), an analogue of corticotropin (adrenocorticotrophic hormone, ACTH), is used to test adrenocortical function; failure of plasma-cortisol concentration to rise after administration of tetracosactide indicates adrenocortical insufficiency. A low-dose test is considered by some clinicians to be more sensitive when used to confirm established, partial adrenal suppression.

Tetracosactide should be given only if no other ACTH preparations have been given previously. Tetracosactide depot injection (*Synacthen Depot*®) is also used in the treatment of infantile spasms but it is contra-indicated in neonates because of the presence of benzyl alcohol in the injection. Corticotropin-releasing factor, corticorelin p. 453, (also known as corticotropin-releasing hormone, CRH) is used to test anterior pituitary function and secretion of corticotropin.

Gonadotrophins

Gonadotrophins are occasionally used in the treatment of hypogonadotrophic hypogonadism and associated oligospermia. There is no justification for their use in primary gonadal failure.

Chorionic gonadotrophin p. 454 is used in the investigation of testicular function in suspected primary hypogonadism and incomplete masculinisation. It has also been used in delayed puberty in boys to stimulate endogenous testosterone production, but it has little advantage over testosterone.

Growth hormone

Growth hormone is used to treat proven deficiency of the hormone, Prader-Willi syndrome, Turner's syndrome, growth disturbance in children born small for corrected gestational age, chronic renal insufficiency, and short stature homeobox-containing gene (SHOX) deficiency. Growth hormone is also used in Noonan syndrome and idiopathic short stature [unlicensed indications] under specialist management. Treatment should be initiated and monitored by a paediatrician with expertise in managing growth-hormone disorders; treatment can be continued under a shared-care protocol by a general practitioner.

Growth hormone of human origin (HGH; somatotrophin) has been replaced by a growth hormone of human sequence, somatropin p. 454, produced using recombinant DNA technology.

Mecasermin p. 456, a human insulin-like growth factor-I (rhIGF-I), is licensed to treat growth failure in children with severe primary insulin-like growth factor-I deficiency.

Hypothalamic hormones

Gonadorelin p. 453 when injected intravenously in post-pubertal girls leads to a rapid rise in plasma concentrations of both luteinising hormone (LH) and follicle-stimulating hormone (FSH). It has not proved to be very helpful, however, in distinguishing hypothalamic from pituitary lesions. It is used in the assessment of delayed or precocious puberty.

Other growth hormone stimulation tests involve the use of insulin, glucagon p. 444, arginine p. 56, and clonidine hydrochloride p. 99 [all unlicensed use]. The tests should be carried out in specialist centres.

6.1 Adrenocortical function testing

PITUITARY AND HYPOTHALAMIC HORMONES AND ANALOGUES 〉 CORTICOTROPHINS

Tetracosactide

(Tetracosactrin)

- **INDICATIONS AND DOSE**

Diagnosis of adrenocortical insufficiency (diagnostic 30-minute test), standard-dose test
▸ BY INTRAMUSCULAR INJECTION, OR BY INTRAVENOUS INJECTION
▸ Child: 145 micrograms/m^2 (max. per dose 250 micrograms) for 1 dose

Diagnosis of adrenocortical insufficiency (diagnostic 30-minute test), low-dose test
▸ BY INTRAMUSCULAR INJECTION, OR BY INTRAVENOUS INJECTION
▸ Child: 0.3 microgram/m^2 for 1 dose

Infantile spasm
▸ BY INTRAMUSCULAR INJECTION USING DEPOT INJECTION
▸ Child 1-23 months: Initially 500 micrograms once daily on alternate days, adjusted according to response

- **UNLICENSED USE** Not licensed for low-dose test for adrenocortical insufficiency. Not licensed for treatment of infantile spasms.

- **CONTRA-INDICATIONS** Acute psychosis · adrenogenital syndrome · allergic disorders · asthma · avoid injections containing benzyl alcohol in neonates · Cushing's syndrome · infectious diseases · peptic ulcer · primary adrenocortical insufficiency · refractory heart failure

- **CAUTIONS** Active infectious diseases (should not be used unless disease-specific therapy is being given) · active systemic diseases (should not be used unless adequate disease-specific therapy is being given) · diabetes mellitus · diverticulitis · history of asthma · history of atopic allergy · history of eczema · history of hayfever · history of hypersensitivity · hypertension · latent amoebiasis (may become activated) · latent tuberculosis (may become activated) · myasthenia gravis · ocular herpes simplex · osteoporosis · predisposition to thromboembolic · psychological disturbances may be triggered · recent intestinal anastomosis · reduced immune response (should not be used unless adequate disease-specific therapy is being given) · ulcerative colitis

CAUTIONS, FURTHER INFORMATION
▸ Risk of anaphylaxis Should only be administered under medical supervision. Consult product literature.
▸ Hypertension Patients already receiving medication for moderate to severe hypertension must have their dosage adjusted if treatment started.
▸ Diabetes mellitus Patients already receiving medication for diabetes mellitus must have their dosage adjusted if treatment started.
● SIDE-EFFECTS Abdominal distention · abscess · acne · anaphylactic shock · anaphylactoid reactions in children aged under 3 years (benzyl alcohol-containing injections) · angioneurotic oedema · aseptic necrosis of femoral and humeral heads · benign intracranial pressure increased with papilloedema · calcium deficiency · cardiac disorders · convulsions · Cushing's syndrome · decreased carbohydrate tolerance · dizziness · dysponea · ecchymosis · erythema · euphoria · fluid retention · flushing · glaucoma · growth retardation · headache · hirsutism · hyperglycaemia · hyperhidrosis · hypersensitivity reactions (tend to be more severe in patients susceptible to allergies, especially asthma) · hypertension · hypokalaemia · hypokalaemic alkalosis · impaired healing · increased appetite · increased intraocular pressure · infection susceptibility increased · insomnia · irregular menstruation · leukocytosis · malaise · manifestations of latent diabetes mellitus · mood swings · muscle atrophy · muscular weakness · myopathy · nausea · necrotising vasculitis · negative nitrogen balance · osteoporosis · pancreatitis · pathological fracture of long bones · peptic ulcer · personality changes · petechiae · posterior subcapsular cataracts · pruritus · psychotic manifestations · Quincke's oedema · secondary adrenocortical unresponsiveness · secondary pituitary unresponsiveness · severe depression · skin atrophy · skin hyperpigmentation · skin reactions at injection site · sodium retention · spinal compression fractures · tendon rupture · thromboembolism · toxic reactions in children aged under 3 years (benzyl alcohol-containing injections) · ulcerative oesophagitis · urticaria · vertigo · vomiting · weight increase
● ALLERGY AND CROSS-SENSITIVITY Contra-indicated in patients with history of hypersensitivity to tetracosactide/corticotrophins or excipients.
● PREGNANCY Avoid (but may be used diagnostically if essential).
● BREAST FEEDING Avoid (but may be used diagnostically if essential).
● HEPATIC IMPAIRMENT An enhanced effect of tetracosactide therapy may occur in patients with cirrhosis of the liver. Use with caution in hepatic impairment. Monitor hepatic function closely during treatment.
● RENAL IMPAIRMENT Use with caution in patients with renal impairment.
● EFFECT ON LABORATORY TESTS May suppress skin test reactions.
  Post administration total plasma cortisol levels during 30-minute test for diagnosis of adrenocotical insufficiency might be misleading due to altered cortisol binding globulin levels in some special clinical situations including, patients on oral contraceptives, post-operative patients, critical illness, severe liver disease and nephrotic syndrome.
● DIRECTIONS FOR ADMINISTRATION For *intramuscular* or *intravenous injection*, may be diluted in sodium chloride 0.9% to 250 nanograms/mL.

● MEDICINAL FORMS
There can be variation in the licensing of different medicines containing the same drug.
Solution for injection
▸ Synacthen (Mallinckrodt Specialty Pharmaceuticals Ireland Ltd)
  Tetracosactide acetate 250 microgram per 1 ml Synacthen 250micrograms/1ml solution for injection ampoules | 1 ampoule [PoM] £38.00
Suspension for injection
EXCIPIENTS: May contain Benzyl alcohol
▸ Synacthen Depot (Mallinckrodt Specialty Pharmaceuticals Ireland Ltd)
  Tetracosactide acetate 1 mg per 1 ml Synacthen Depot 1mg/1ml suspension for injection ampoules | 1 ampoule [PoM] £346.28

6.2 Assessment of pituitary function

DIAGNOSTIC AGENTS

Corticorelin

(Corticotrophin-releasing hormone; CRH)

● INDICATIONS AND DOSE
Test of anterior pituitary function
▸ BY INTRAVENOUS INJECTION
▸ Child: 1 microgram/kg (max. per dose 100 micrograms) for 1 dose, to be administered over 30 seconds

● UNLICENSED USE Not licensed.
● SIDE-EFFECTS Flushing of face · flushing of neck · flushing of upper body · hypotension · mild sensation of smell · mild sensation of taste
● PREGNANCY Avoid.
● BREAST FEEDING Avoid.
● MEDICINAL FORMS
There can be variation in the licensing of different medicines containing the same drug.
No licensed medicines listed.

Gonadorelin

(Gonadotrophin-releasing hormone; GnRH; LH–RH)

● INDICATIONS AND DOSE
Assessment of anterior pituitary function | Assessment of delayed puberty
▸ BY INTRAVENOUS INJECTION, OR BY SUBCUTANEOUS INJECTION
▸ Child 1–17 years: 2.5 micrograms/kg (max. per dose 100 micrograms) for 1 dose

● CAUTIONS Pituitary adenoma
● SIDE-EFFECTS Abdominal pain · headache · hypersensitivity reaction on repeated administration of large doses · increased menstrual bleeding · irritation at injection site · nausea
● PREGNANCY Avoid.
● BREAST FEEDING Avoid.
● MEDICINAL FORMS
There can be variation in the licensing of different medicines containing the same drug.
Powder and solvent for solution for injection
EXCIPIENTS: May contain Benzyl alcohol
▸ Gonadorelin (Non-proprietary)
  Gonadorelin (as Gonadorelin hydrochloride)
  100 microgram Gonadorelin 100microgram powder and solvent for solution for injection vials | 1 vial [PoM] £75.00 (Hospital only)

Endocrine system

6

6.3 Gonadotrophin replacement therapy

GONADOTROPHINS

Chorionic gonadotrophin

(Human chorionic gonadotrophin; HCG)

- **DRUG ACTION** A preparation of a glycoprotein fraction secreted by the placenta and obtained from the urine of pregnant women having the action of the pituitary luteinising hormone.

- **INDICATIONS AND DOSE**

Delayed puberty in the male to stimulate endogenous testosterone production
- ▸ BY INTRAMUSCULAR INJECTION, OR BY SUBCUTANEOUS INJECTION
- ▸ Child: (consult product literature)

Test of testicular function, short stimulation test
- ▸ BY INTRAMUSCULAR INJECTION
- ▸ Child: 1500–2000 units once daily for 3 days

Test of testicular function, prolonged stimulation test
- ▸ BY INTRAMUSCULAR INJECTION
- ▸ Child: 1500–2000 units twice weekly for 3 weeks

Hypogonadotrophic hypogonadism
- ▸ BY INTRAMUSCULAR INJECTION
- ▸ Child: 1000–2000 units twice weekly, adjusted according to response

Undescended testes
- ▸ BY INTRAMUSCULAR INJECTION
- ▸ Child 7–16 years: Initially 500 units 3 times a week, adjusted according to response to up to 4000 units 3 times a week continue for 1–2 months after testicular descent
- ▸ Child 17 years: Initially 1000 units twice weekly, adjusted according to response to up to 4000 units 3 times a week continue for 1–2 months after testicular descent

- **UNLICENSED USE** Unlicensed in children for test of testicular function.
- **CONTRA-INDICATIONS** Androgen-dependent tumours
- **CAUTIONS** Asthma · cardiac impairment · epilepsy · migraine · prepubertal boys (risk of premature epiphyseal closure or precocious puberty)
- **SIDE-EFFECTS** Gynaecomastia · headache · local reactions · mood changes · oedema (particularly in males—reduce dose) · tiredness
- **RENAL IMPAIRMENT** Use with caution.
- **MEDICINAL FORMS**
  There can be variation in the licensing of different medicines containing the same drug.

  Powder and solvent for solution for injection
  - ▸ Choragon (Ferring Pharmaceuticals Ltd)
    Chorionic gonadotrophin human 5000 unit Choragon 5,000unit powder and solvent for solution for injection ampoules |
    3 ampoule [PoM] £9.77 [CD4-2]
  - ▸ Pregnyl (Merck Sharp & Dohme Ltd)
    Chorionic gonadotrophin human 1500 unit Pregnyl 1,500unit powder and solvent for solution for injection ampoules |
    1 ampoule [PoM] £2.12 [CD4-2]
    Chorionic gonadotrophin human 5000 unit Pregnyl 5,000unit powder and solvent for solution for injection ampoules |
    1 ampoule [PoM] £3.15 [CD4-2]

6.4 Growth hormone disorders

PITUITARY AND HYPOTHALAMIC HORMONES AND ANALOGUES 〉 HUMAN GROWTH HORMONES

Somatropin

(Recombinant Human Growth Hormone)

- **INDICATIONS AND DOSE**

Gonadal dysgenesis (Turner syndrome)
- ▸ BY SUBCUTANEOUS INJECTION
- ▸ Child: 1.4 mg/m^2 daily, alternatively 45–50 micrograms/kg daily

Deficiency of growth hormone
- ▸ BY SUBCUTANEOUS INJECTION, OR BY INTRAMUSCULAR INJECTION
- ▸ Child: 23–39 micrograms/kg daily, alternatively 0.7–1 mg/m^2 daily

Growth disturbance in children born small for gestational age whose growth has not caught up by 4 years or later | Noonan syndrome
- ▸ BY SUBCUTANEOUS INJECTION
- ▸ Child 4-17 years: 35 micrograms/kg daily, alternatively 1 mg/m^2 daily

Prader-Willi syndrome, in children with growth velocity greater than 1 cm/year, in combination with energy-restricted diet
- ▸ BY SUBCUTANEOUS INJECTION
- ▸ Child: 1 mg/m^2 daily, alternatively 35 micrograms/kg daily; maximum 2.7 mg per day

Chronic renal insufficiency (renal function decreased to less than 50%)
- ▸ BY SUBCUTANEOUS INJECTION
- ▸ Child: 45–50 micrograms/kg daily, alternatively 1.4 mg/m^2 daily, higher doses may be needed, adjust if necessary after 6 months

SHOX deficiency
- ▸ BY SUBCUTANEOUS INJECTION
- ▸ Child: 45–50 micrograms/kg daily

DOSE EQUIVALENCE AND CONVERSION
- ▸ Dose formerly expressed in units; somatropin 1 mg ≡ 3 units.

- **UNLICENSED USE** Not licensed for use in Noonan syndrome.
- **CONTRA-INDICATIONS** Avoid injections containing benzyl alcohol in neonates · evidence of tumour activity (complete antitumour therapy and ensure intracranial lesions inactive before starting) · not to be used after renal transplantation · not to be used for growth promotion in children with closed epiphyses (or near closure in Prader-Willi syndrome) · severe obesity in Prader-Willi syndrome · severe respiratory impairment in Prader-Willi syndrome
- **CAUTIONS** Diabetes mellitus (adjustment of antidiabetic therapy may be necessary) · disorders of the epiphysis of the hip (monitor for limping) · history of malignant disease · hypothyroidism—manufacturers recommend periodic thyroid function tests but limited evidence of clinical value · initiation of treatment close to puberty not recommended in child born small for corrected gestational age · papilloedema · relative deficiencies of other pituitary hormones · resolved intracranial hypertension (monitor closely) · Silver-Russell syndrome
- **INTERACTIONS** → Appendix 1: somatropin
- **SIDE-EFFECTS** Antibody formation · arthralgia · benign intracranial hypertension · carpal tunnel syndrome · fluid retention (peripheral oedema) · headache · hyperglycaemia · hypoglycaemia · hypothyroidism · insulin resistance ·

▸ Breast cancer risk with contraceptive use There is a small increase in the risk of having breast cancer diagnosed in women using, or who have recently used, a progestogen-only contraceptive pill; this relative risk may be due to an earlier diagnosis. The most important risk factor appears to be the age at which the contraceptive is stopped rather than the duration of use; the risk disappears gradually during the 10 years after stopping and there is no excess risk by 10 years. A possible small increase in the risk of breast cancer should be weighed against the benefits.

● **INTERACTIONS** → Appendix 1: norethisterone

● **SIDE-EFFECTS**

GENERAL SIDE-EFFECTS
Acne · alopecia · anaphylactoid reactions · breast tenderness · change in libido · depression · disturbance of appetite · dizziness · fluid retention · headache · hirsutism · insomnia (non-contraceptive indications) · jaundice · menstrual disturbances · nausea · premenstrual-like syndrome · pruritus · rash · skin reactions · urticaria · vomiting · weight change

SPECIFIC SIDE-EFFECTS
▸ With intramuscular use Injection-site reactions

SIDE-EFFECTS, FURTHER INFORMATION
▸ Cervical cancer Use of injectable progestogen-only contraceptives may be associated with a small increased risk of cervical cancer, similar to that seen with combined oral contraceptives (use of combined oral contraceptives for 5 years or longer is associated with a small increased risk of cervical cancer; the risk diminishes after stopping and disappears by about 10 years). The risk of cervical cancer with other progestogen-only contraceptives is not yet known.

● **PREGNANCY** Not known to be harmful in contraceptive doses. Avoid in other indications.

● **BREAST FEEDING** Progestogen-only contraceptives do not affect lactation.
▸ With intramuscular use Withhold breast-feeding for neonates with severe or persistent jaundice requiring medical treatment.

● **HEPATIC IMPAIRMENT** When used as a contraceptive; caution in severe liver disease and recurrent cholestatic jaundice, avoid in liver tumour. Caution when used for sexual maturation and to postpone menstruation; avoid if severe.

● **RENAL IMPAIRMENT** Use with caution in non-contraceptive indications.

● **PATIENT AND CARER ADVICE**
Missed oral contraceptive pill The following advice is recommended: 'If you forget a pill, take it as soon as you remember and carry on with the next pill at the right time. If the pill was more than 3 hours overdue you are not protected. Continue normal pill-taking but you must also use another method, such as the condom, for the next 2 days.'
    The Faculty of Sexual and Reproductive Healthcare recommends emergency contraception if one or more progestogen-only contraceptive tablets are missed or taken more than 3 hours late and unprotected intercourse has occurred before 2 further tablets have been correctly taken.
Diarrhoea and vomiting with oral contraceptives Vomiting and persistent, severe diarrhoea can interfere with the absorption of oral progestogen-only contraceptives. If vomiting occurs within 2 hours of taking an oral progestogen-only contraceptive, another pill should be taken as soon as possible. If a replacement pill is not taken within 3 hours of the normal time for taking the progestogen-only pill, or in cases of persistent vomiting or very severe diarrhoea, additional precautions should be used during illness and for 2 days after recovery.

Starting routine for oral contraceptives One tablet daily, on a continuous basis, starting on day 1 of cycle and taken at the same time each day (if delayed by longer than 3 hours contraceptive protection may be lost). Additional contraceptive precautions are not required if norethisterone is started up to and including day 5 of the menstrual cycle; if started after this time, additional contraceptive precautions are required for 2 days.
Changing from a combined oral contraceptive Start on the day following completion of the combined oral contraceptive course without a break (or in the case of ED tablets omitting the inactive ones).
After childbirth Oral progestogen-only contraceptives can be started up to and including day 21 postpartum without the need for additional contraceptive precautions. If started more than 21 days postpartum, additional contraceptive precautions are required for 2 days.
Contraceptives by injection Full counselling backed by *patient information leaflet* required before administration— likelihood of menstrual disturbance and the potential for a delay in return to full fertility. Delayed return of fertility and irregular cycles may occur after discontinuation of treatment but there is no evidence of permanent infertility.

● **MEDICINAL FORMS**
There can be variation in the licensing of different medicines containing the same drug. Forms available from special-order manufacturers include: oral suspension

Solution for injection
▸ **Noristerat** (Bayer Plc)
  Norethisterone enantate 200 mg per 1 ml Noristerat 200mg/1ml solution for injection ampoules | 1 ampoule [PoM] £4.05

Tablet
▸ **Norethisterone (Non-proprietary)**
  Norethisterone 5 mg Norethisterone 5mg tablets | 30 tablet [PoM] £2.48 DT price = £2.18
▸ **Noriday** (Pfizer Ltd)
  Norethisterone 350 microgram Noriday 350microgram tablets | 84 tablet [PoM] £2.10 DT price = £1.80
▸ **Primolut N** (Bayer Plc)
  Norethisterone 5 mg Primolut N 5mg tablets | 30 tablet [PoM] £2.26 DT price = £2.18
▸ **Utovlan** (Pfizer Ltd)
  Norethisterone 5 mg Utovlan 5mg tablets | 30 tablet [PoM] £1.40 DT price = £2.18 | 90 tablet [PoM] £4.21

7.2 Male sex hormone responsive conditions

Androgens, anti-androgens and anabolic steroids

Androgens

Androgens cause masculinisation; they are used as replacement therapy in androgen deficiency, in delayed puberty, and in those who are hypogonadal due to either pituitary or testicular disease.
    When given to patients with hypopituitarism androgens can lead to normal sexual development and potency but not to fertility. If fertility is desired, the usual treatment is with gonadotrophins or pulsatile gonadotrophin-releasing hormone which stimulates spermatogenesis as well as androgen production.
    Intramuscular depot preparations of **testosterone esters** are preferred for replacement therapy. Testosterone enantate or propionate or alternatively *Sustanon®*, which consists of a mixture of testosterone esters and has a longer duration of action, can be used. For induction of puberty, depot testosterone injections are given monthly and the

doses increased every 6 to 12 months according to response. Single ester testosterone injections may need to be given more frequently.

Oral **testosterone undecanoate** is used for induction of puberty. An alternative approach that promotes growth rather than sexual maturation uses oral oxandrolone below.

Chorionic gonadotrophin has also been used in delayed puberty in the male to stimulate endogenous testosterone production, but has little advantage over testosterone.

Testosterone topical gel is also available but experience of use in children under 15 years is limited. Topical testosterone is applied to the penis in the treatment of microphallus; an extemporaneously prepared cream should be used because the alcohol in proprietary gel formulations causes irritation.

Anti-androgens and precocious puberty

The gonadorelin stimulation test is used to distinguish between *gonadotrophin-dependent (central) precocious puberty* and *gonadotrophin-independent precocious puberty*. Treatment requires specialist management.

Gonadorelin analogues, used in the management of gonadotrophin-dependent precocious puberty, delay development of secondary sexual characteristics and growth velocity.

Testolactone p. 462 and cyproterone acetate p. 461 are used in the management of gonadotrophin-independent precocious puberty, resulting from McCune-Albright syndrome, familial male precocious puberty (testotoxicosis), hormone-secreting tumours, and ovarian and testicular disorders. Testolactone inhibits the aromatisation of testosterone, the rate limiting step in oestrogen synthesis. Cyproterone acetate is a progestogen with anti-androgen properties.

Spironolactone p. 123 is sometimes used in combination with testolactone because it has some androgen receptor blocking properties.

High blood concentration of sex hormones may activate release of gonadotrophin releasing hormone, leading to development of secondary, central gonadotrophin-dependent precocious puberty. This may require the addition of gonadorelin analogues to prevent progression of pubertal development and skeletal maturation.

Anabolic steroids have some androgenic activity but they cause less virilisation than androgens in girls. They are used in the treatment of some *aplastic anaemias*.

Oxandrolone is used to stimulate late pre-pubertal growth prior to induction of sexual maturation in boys with short stature and in girls with Turner's syndrome; specialist management is required.

ANABOLIC STEROIDS > ANDROSTAN DERIVATIVES

Oxandrolone

● **INDICATIONS AND DOSE**

Stimulation of late pre-pubertal growth in boys (of appropriate age) with short stature
▸ BY MOUTH
▸ Child 10–17 years (male): 1.25–2.5 mg daily for 3–6 months.

Stimulation of late pre-pubertal growth in girls with Turner's syndrome
▸ BY MOUTH
▸ Child (female): 0.625–2.5 mg daily, to be taken in combination with growth hormone.

● **CONTRA-INDICATIONS** History of primary liver tumours · hypercalcaemia · nephrosis

● **CAUTIONS** Cardiac impairment · diabetes mellitus · epilepsy · hypertension · migraine · skeletal metastases (risk of hypercalcaemia)

● **SIDE-EFFECTS**
▸ **Common or very common** Virilism in females · acne · androgenic effects · anxiety · asthenia · changes in libido · cholestatic jaundice · depression · electrolyte disturbances · excessive duration of penile erection · excessive frequency of penile erection · gastro-intestinal bleeding · gynaecomastia · headache · hirsutism · hypercalcaemia · hypertension · increased bone growth · male-pattern baldness · nausea · oedema · paraesthesia · polycythaemia · precocious sexual development in pre-pubertal males · premature closure of epiphyses in pre-pubertal males · pruritus · seborrhoea · sodium retention · suppression of spermatogenesis in males · weight gain
▸ **Rare** Liver tumours
▸ **Frequency not known** Sleep apnoea

● **PREGNANCY** Avoid—causes masculinisation of female fetus.

● **BREAST FEEDING** Avoid; may cause masculinisation in the female infant or precocious development in the male infant. High doses suppress lactation.

● **HEPATIC IMPAIRMENT** Avoid if possible—fluid retention and dose-related toxicity.

● **RENAL IMPAIRMENT** Use with caution—potential for fluid retention.

● **MEDICINAL FORMS**
There can be variation in the licensing of different medicines containing the same drug. Forms available from special-order manufacturers include: tablet
Tablet
▸ **Oxandrolone (Non-proprietary)**
Oxandrolone 2.5 mg Oxandrin 2.5mg tablets | 100 tablet [PoM] no price available [CD4–2]

ANDROGENS

Androgens

● **CONTRA-INDICATIONS** Breast cancer in males · history of liver tumours · hypercalcaemia · prostate cancer

● **CAUTIONS** Cardiac impairment · diabetes mellitus · epilepsy · hypertension · migraine · pre-pubertal boys (fusion of epiphyses is hastened and may result in short stature)—statural growth and sexual development should be monitored · skeletal metastases—risk of hypercalcaemia or hypercalciuria (if this occurs, treat appropriately and restart treatment once normal serum calcium concentration restored) · sleep apnoea · stop treatment or reduce dose if severe polycythaemia occurs · tumours—risk of hypercalcaemia or hypercalciuria (if this occurs, treat appropriately and restart treatment once normal serum calcium concentration restored)

● **SIDE-EFFECTS**
▸ **Common or very common** Acne · androgenic effects (to be assessed regularly in women) · anxiety · asthenia · changes in libido · cholestatic jaundice · depression · electrolyte disturbances · excessive duration of penile erection · excessive frequency of penile erection · gastro-intestinal bleeding · gynaecomastia · headache · hirsutism · hypercalcaemia · hypertension · increased bone growth · male-pattern baldness · nausea · oedema · paraesthesia · polycythaemia · precocious sexual development in pre-pubertal males · premature closure of epiphyses in pre-pubertal males · pruritus · seborrhoea · sodium retention · suppression of virilism in women · weight gain
▸ **Rare** Liver tumours
▸ **Frequency not known** Sleep apnoea

SIDE-EFFECTS, FURTHER INFORMATION

▸ **Polycythaemia** Stop treatment or reduce dose if severe polycythaemia occurs.

● **PREGNANCY** Avoid—causes masculinisation of female fetus.

● **BREAST FEEDING** Avoid.

● **HEPATIC IMPAIRMENT** Avoid if possible—fluid retention and dose-related toxicity.

● **RENAL IMPAIRMENT** Caution—potential for fluid retention.

● **MONITORING REQUIREMENTS** Monitor haematocrit and haemoglobulin before treatment, every three months for the first year, and yearly thereafter.

F 460

Testosterone enantate

● **INDICATIONS AND DOSE**

Induction and maintenance of sexual maturation in males (specialist use only)

▸ BY DEEP INTRAMUSCULAR INJECTION

▸ Child 12–17 years: 25–50 mg/m^2 every month, increase dose every 6–12 months according to response

● **UNLICENSED USE** Not licensed for use in children.

● **SIDE-EFFECTS** Suppression of spermatogenesis

● **MEDICINAL FORMS**
There can be variation in the licensing of different medicines containing the same drug.

Solution for injection

▸ **Testosterone enantate (Non-proprietary)**
Testosterone enantate 250 mg per 1 ml Testosterone enantate 250mg/1ml solution for injection ampoules | 3 ampoule PoM £79.75 DT price = £79.75 CD4-2

F 460

Testosterone propionate

● **INDICATIONS AND DOSE**

Delayed puberty in males

▸ BY INTRAMUSCULAR INJECTION

▸ Child: 50 mg once weekly

Treatment of microphallus (specialist use only)

▸ TO THE SKIN USING CREAM

▸ Child: Apply 3 times a day for 3 weeks

● **SIDE-EFFECTS** Suppression of spermatogenesis

● **MEDICINAL FORMS**
There can be variation in the licensing of different medicines containing the same drug. Forms available from special-order manufacturers include: solution for injection, cream

F 460

Testosterone undecanoate

● **INDICATIONS AND DOSE**

Induction and maintenance of sexual maturation in males (specialist use only)

▸ BY MOUTH

▸ Child 12–17 years: 40 mg once daily on alternate days, adjusted according to response to 120 mg daily

● **SIDE-EFFECTS** Suppression of spermatogenesis

● **MEDICINAL FORMS**
There can be variation in the licensing of different medicines containing the same drug.

Capsule

CAUTIONARY AND ADVISORY LABELS 21, 25

▸ **Restandol** (Merck Sharp & Dohme Ltd)
Testosterone undecanoate 40 mg Restandol 40mg Testocaps | 30 capsule PoM £8.55 CD4-2 | 60 capsule PoM £17.10 DT price = £17.10 CD4-2

7.2a Precocious puberty

Other drugs used for Precocious puberty Goserelin, p. 450
· Leuprorelin acetate, p. 451 · Triptorelin, p. 451

ANTI-ANDROGENS

Cyproterone acetate

● **INDICATIONS AND DOSE**

Gonadotrophin-independent precocious puberty (specialist use only)

▸ BY MOUTH

▸ Child: Initially 25 mg twice daily, adjusted according to response

● **UNLICENSED USE** Unlicensed for use in children.

● **CONTRA-INDICATIONS** Dubin-Johnson syndrome · history of thromboembolic disorders · liver-disease · malignant diseases · meningioma or history of meningioma · previous or existing liver tumours · Rotor syndrome · severe depression · severe diabetes (with vascular changes) · sickle-cell anaemia · wasting diseases · youths under 18 years (may arrest bone maturation and testicular development)

● **CAUTIONS** Diabetes mellitus · in prostate cancer, severe depression · in prostate cancer, sickle-cell anaemia · ineffective for male hypersexuality in chronic alcoholism (relevance to prostate cancer not known)

● **INTERACTIONS** → Appendix 1: cyproterone

● **SIDE-EFFECTS**

▸ **Rare** Hypersensitivity reactions · osteoporosis · rash

▸ **Frequency not known** Breathlessness · changes in hair pattern · fatigue · gynaecomastia (rarely leading to galactorrhoea and benign breast nodules) · hepatic failure · hepatitis · hepatotoxicity · inhibition of spermatogenesis · jaundice · lassitude · reduced sebum production (may clear acne) · risk of recurrence of thromboembolic disease · weight changes

SIDE-EFFECTS, FURTHER INFORMATION

▸ **Hepatotoxicity** Direct hepatic toxicity including jaundice, hepatitis and hepatic failure have been reported (fatalities reported, usually after several months, at dosages of 100 mg and above). If hepatotoxicity is confirmed, cyproterone should normally be withdrawn unless the hepatotoxicity can be explained by another cause such as metastatic disease (in which case cyproterone should be continued only if the perceived benefit exceeds the risk).

● **HEPATIC IMPAIRMENT** Avoid—dose-related toxicity.

● **MONITORING REQUIREMENTS**

▸ Monitor blood counts initially and throughout treatment.

▸ Monitor adrenocortical function regularly.

▸ Monitor hepatic function regularly—liver function tests should be performed before and regularly during treatment and whenever symptoms suggestive of hepatotoxicity occur.

6

Endocrine system

6

Endocrine system

- **PATIENT AND CARER ADVICE**
Driving and skilled tasks
Fatigue and lassitude may impair performance of skilled tasks (e.g. driving).

- **MEDICINAL FORMS**
There can be variation in the licensing of different medicines containing the same drug. Forms available from special-order manufacturers include: tablet, capsule, oral suspension, oral solution
Tablet
CAUTIONARY AND ADVISORY LABELS 21
▸ **Cyproterone acetate (Non-proprietary)**
Cyproterone acetate 50 mg Cyproterone 50mg tablets |
56 tablet [PoM] £48.95 | 168 tablet [PoM] £87.00 DT price = £87.00
Cyproterone acetate 100 mg Cyproterone 100mg tablets |
84 tablet [PoM] £132.57 DT price = £55.19
▸ **Androcur (Bayer Plc)**
Cyproterone acetate 50 mg Androcur 50mg tablets |
56 tablet [PoM] £29.25
▸ **Cyprostat (Bayer Plc)**
Cyproterone acetate 50 mg Cyprostat 50mg tablets |
168 tablet [PoM] £87.00 DT price = £87.00
Cyproterone acetate 100 mg Cyprostat 100mg tablets |
84 tablet [PoM] £87.00 DT price = £55.19

HORMONE ANTAGONISTS AND RELATED AGENTS > AROMATASE INHIBITORS

Testolactone

- **INDICATIONS AND DOSE**
Gonadotrophin-independent precocious puberty (specialist use only)
▸ BY MOUTH
▸ Child: 5 mg/kg 3–4 times a day; increased if necessary up to 10 mg/kg 4 times a day

- **SIDE-EFFECTS**
▸ **Common or very common** Anorexia · changes in hair pattern · diarrhoea · hypertension · nausea · peripheral neuropathy · vomiting · weight changes
▸ **Rare** Hypersensitivity reactions · rash
- **PREGNANCY** Avoid.
- **BREAST FEEDING** No information available.
- **MEDICINAL FORMS**
There can be variation in the licensing of different medicines containing the same drug.
Tablet
▸ **Testolactone (Non-proprietary)**
Testolactone 50 mg Teslac 50mg tablets | 100 tablet [PoM] no price available

8 Thyroid disorders
8.1 Hyperthyroidism

Antithyroid drugs

Overview

Antithyroid drugs are used for hyperthyroidism either to prepare children for thyroidectomy or for long-term management. In the UK carbimazole p. 463 is the most commonly used drug. Propylthiouracil p. 463 should be reserved for children who are intolerant of, or for those who experience sensitivity reactions to carbimazole (sensitivity is not necessarily displayed to both drugs), and for whom other treatments are inappropriate. Both drugs act primarily by interfering with the synthesis of thyroid hormones.

Treatment in children should be undertaken by a specialist.

Carbimazole or propylthiouracil are initially given in large doses to block thyroid function. This dose is continued until the child becomes euthyroid, usually after 4 to 8 weeks, and is then gradually reduced to a maintenance dose of 30–60% of the initial dose. Alternatively high-dose treatment is continued in combination with levothyroxine sodium p. 464 replacement (*blocking-replacement regimen*); this is particularly useful when dose adjustment proves difficult. Treatment is usually continued for 12 to 24 months. The blocking-replacement regimen is **not** suitable during pregnancy. Hypothyroidism should be avoided particularly during pregnancy as it can cause fetal goitre.

Iodine has been used as an adjunct to antithyroid drugs for 10 to 14 days before partial thyroidectomy; however, there is little evidence of a beneficial effect. Iodine should not be used for long-term treatment because its antithyroid action tends to diminish.

Radioactive sodium iodide (^{131}I) solution is used increasingly for the treatment of thyrotoxicosis at all ages, particularly where medical therapy or compliance is a problem, in patients with cardiac disease, and in patients who relapse after thyroidectomy.

Propranolol hydrochloride p. 101 is useful for rapid relief of thyrotoxic symptoms and can be used in conjunction with antithyroid drugs or as an adjunct to radioactive iodine. Beta-blockers are also useful in neonatal thyrotoxicosis and in supraventricular arrhythmias due to hyperthyroidism. Propranolol hydrochloride has been used in conjunction with iodine to prepare mildly thyrotoxic patients for surgery but it is preferable to make the patient euthyroid with carbimazole. Laboratory tests of thyroid function are not altered by beta-blockers. Most experience in treating thyrotoxicosis has been gained with propranolol but atenolol p. 103 is also used.

Thyrotoxic crisis ('thyroid storm') requires emergency treatment with intravenous administration of fluids, propranolol hydrochloride and hydrocortisone p. 420 as sodium succinate, as well as oral iodine solution and carbimazole or propylthiouracil which may need to be administered by nasogastric tube.

Pregnancy

Radioactive iodine therapy is contra-indicated during pregnancy. Propylthiouracil and carbimazole can be given but the blocking-replacement regimen is **not** suitable. Rarely, carbimazole has been associated with congenital defects, including aplasia cutis of the neonate, therefore propylthiouracil remains the drug of choice during the first trimester of pregnancy. In the second trimester, consider switching to carbimazole because of the potential risk of hepatotoxicity with propylthiouracil. Both propylthiouracil and carbimazole cross the placenta and in high doses may cause fetal goitre and hypothyroidism—the lowest dose that will control the hyperthyroid state should be used (requirements in Graves' disease tend to fall during pregnancy).

Neonates

Neonatal hyperthyroidism is treated with carbimazole or propylthiouracil, usually for 8 to 12 weeks. In severe symptomatic disease iodine may be needed to block the thyroid and propranolol required to treat peripheral symptoms.

Chapter 7
Genito-urinary system

CONTENTS

7

Genito-urinary system

1　Bladder and urinary disorders

1.1　Urinary frequency, enuresis, and incontinence

Urinary frequency, enuresis and incontinence

Urinary incontinence

Antimuscarinic drugs reduce symptoms of urgency and urge incontinence and increase bladder capacity; oxybutynin hydrochloride p. 468 also has a direct relaxant effect on urinary smooth muscle. Oxybutynin hydrochloride can be considered first for children under 12 years. Side-effects limit the use of oxybutynin hydrochloride, but they may be reduced by starting at a lower dose and then slowly titrating upwards; alternatively oxybutynin hydrochloride can be given by intravesicular instillation. Tolterodine tartrate p. 469 is also effective for urinary incontinence; it can be considered for children over 12 years, or for younger children who have failed to respond to oxybutynin hydrochloride. Modified-release preparations of oxybutynin hydrochloride and tolterodine tartrate are available; they may have fewer side-effects. Antimuscarinic treatment should be reviewed soon after it is commenced, and then at regular intervals; a response generally occurs within 6 months but occasionally may take longer. Children with nocturnal enuresis may require specific additional measures if night-time symptoms also need to be controlled.

Nocturnal enuresis in children

23-May-2017

Description of condition

Nocturnal enuresis is the involuntary discharge of urine during sleep, which is common in young children. Children are generally expected to be dry by a developmental age of 5 years, and historically it has been common practice to consider children for treatment only when they reach 7 years; however, symptoms may still persist in a small proportion by the age of 10 years.

Treatment

Children under 5 years
EvGr For children under 5 years, treatment is usually unnecessary as the condition is likely to resolve spontaneously. Reassurance and advice can be useful for some families. ◇

Non Drug Treatment
EvGr Initially, advice should be given on fluid intake, diet, toileting behaviour, and use of reward systems. For children who do not respond to this advice (more than 1–2 wet beds per week), an enuresis alarm should be the recommended treatment for motivated, well-supported children. Alarms in children under 7 years should be considered depending on the child's maturity, motivation and understanding of the alarm. Alarms have a lower relapse rate than drug treatment when discontinued.

Treatment using an alarm should be reviewed after 4 weeks and continued until a minimum of 2 weeks' uninterrupted dry nights have been achieved. If complete dryness is not achieved after 3 months but the condition is still improving and the child remains motivated to use the alarm, it is recommended to continue the treatment. Combined treatment with desmopressin p. 412, or the use of desmopressin alone, is recommended if the initial alarm treatment is unsuccessful or it is no longer appropriate or desirable. ◇

Drug Treatment
EvGr Treatment with oral or sublingual desmopressin is recommended for children over 5 years of age when alarm use is inappropriate or undesirable, or when rapid or short-term results are the priority (for example, to cover periods away from home). Desmopressin alone can also be used if there has been a partial response to a combination of desmopressin and an alarm following initial treatment with an alarm alone. Treatment should be assessed after 4 weeks and continued for 3 months if there are signs of response. Repeated courses of desmopressin can be used in responsive children who experience repeated recurrences of bedwetting, but should be withdrawn **gradually** at regular intervals (for 1 week every 3 months) for full reassessment.

Under specialist supervision, nocturnal enuresis associated with daytime symptoms (overactive bladder) can be managed with desmopressin alone or in combination with an antimuscarinic drug (such as oxybutynin hydrochloride p. 468 or tolterodine tartrate p. 469 [unlicensed indication]). Treatment should be continued for 3 months; the course can be repeated if necessary.

The tricyclic antidepressant imipramine hydrochloride p. 231 can be considered for children who have not responded to all other treatments and have undergone specialist assessment, however relapse is common after withdrawal and children and their carers should be aware of the dangers of overdose. Initial treatment should continue for 3 months; further courses can be considered following a medical review every 3 months. Tricyclic antidepressants should be withdrawn gradually. Ⓐ

Useful Resources

Bedwetting in under 19s. National Institute for Health and Care Excellence. Clinical guideline CG111. October 2010. www.nice.org.uk/guidance/cg111

ANTIMUSCARINICS

Antimuscarinics (systemic)

- **CONTRA-INDICATIONS** Gastro-intestinal obstruction · intestinal atony · myasthenia gravis (but some antimuscarinics may be used to decrease muscarinic side-effects of anticholinesterases) · paralytic ileus · pyloric stenosis · severe ulcerative colitis · significant bladder outflow obstruction · toxic megacolon · urinary retention
- **CAUTIONS** Arrhythmias (may be worsened) · autonomic neuropathy · cardiac insufficiency (due to association with tachycardia) · cardiac surgery (due to association with tachycardia) · children (increased risk of side-effects) · conditions characterised by tachycardia · congestive heart failure (may be worsened) · coronary artery disease (may be worsened) · diarrhoea · gastro-oesophageal reflux disease · hiatus hernia with reflux oesophagitis · hypertension · hyperthyroidism (due to association with tachycardia) · individuals susceptible to angle-closure glaucoma · pyrexia · ulcerative colitis
- **SIDE-EFFECTS**
- **Common or very common** Constipation · dilation of pupils with loss of accommodation · dry mouth · photophobia · reduced bronchial secretions · skin dryness · skin flushing · transient bradycardia (followed by tachycardia, palpitation and arrhythmias) · urinary retention · urinary urgency
- **Uncommon** Confusion · giddiness · nausea · vomiting
- **Very rare** Angle-closure glaucoma
- **Frequency not known** Angioedema · blurred vision · blurred vision · central nervous system stimulation · convulsion · diarrhoea · difficulty in micturition · disorientation · dizziness · drowsiness · dry eyes · euphoria · fatigue · flatulence · hallucinations · headache · impaired memory · palpitation · photosensitivity · rash · reduced sweating (may lead to heat sensations and fainting in hot environments or patients with fever) · restlessness · taste disturbances
- **PATIENT AND CARER ADVICE**
- **Driving and skilled tasks**
  Antimuscarinics can affect the performance of skilled tasks (e.g. driving).

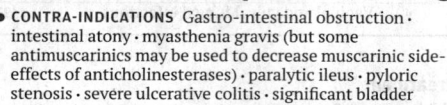

Oxybutynin hydrochloride

- **INDICATIONS AND DOSE**

Urinary frequency | Urinary urgency | Urinary incontinence | Neurogenic bladder instability

- ▸ BY MOUTH USING IMMEDIATE-RELEASE MEDICINES
- ▸ Child 2–4 years: 1.25–2.5 mg 2–3 times a day
- ▸ Child 5–11 years: Initially 2.5–3 mg twice daily, increased to 5 mg 2–3 times a day
- ▸ Child 12–17 years: Initially 5 mg 2–3 times a day, increased if necessary up to 5 mg 4 times a day

- ▸ BY INTRAVESICAL INSTILLATION
- ▸ Child 2–17 years: 5 mg 2–3 times a day
- ▸ BY MOUTH USING MODIFIED-RELEASE TABLETS
- ▸ Child 5–17 years: Initially 5 mg once daily, adjusted in steps of 5 mg every week, adjusted according to response; maximum 15 mg per day

Nocturnal enuresis associated with overactive bladder

- ▸ BY MOUTH USING IMMEDIATE-RELEASE MEDICINES
- ▸ Child 5–17 years: 2.5–3 mg twice daily, increased to 5 mg 2–3 times a day, last dose to be taken before bedtime
- ▸ BY MOUTH USING MODIFIED-RELEASE TABLETS
- ▸ Child 5–17 years: Initially 5 mg once daily, adjusted in steps of 5 mg every week, adjusted according to response; maximum 15 mg per day

DOSE EQUIVALENCE AND CONVERSION

- ▸ Patients taking immediate-release oxybutynin may be transferred to the nearest equivalent daily dose of *Lyrinel* ® *XL*

- **UNLICENSED USE** Not licensed for use in children under 5 years. Intravesical instillation not licensed for use in children.
- **CAUTIONS** Acute porphyrias p. 577
- **INTERACTIONS** → Appendix 1: oxybutynin
- **SIDE-EFFECTS**
- **Uncommon** Anorexia · facial flushing
- **Rare** Night terrors
- **PREGNANCY** Manufacturers advise avoid unless essential—toxicity in *animal* studies.
- **BREAST FEEDING** Manufacturers advise avoid—present in milk in *animal* studies.
- **HEPATIC IMPAIRMENT** Manufacturer advises caution.
- **RENAL IMPAIRMENT** Manufacturer advises caution.
- **PRESCRIBING AND DISPENSING INFORMATION** The need for therapy for urinary indications should be reviewed soon after it has been commenced and then at regular intervals; a response usually occurs within 6 months but may take longer.

  Intravesical instillation may be available from 'special-order' manufacturers or specialist importing companies.
- **PATIENT AND CARER ADVICE**
  Medicines for Children leaflet: Oxybutynin for daytime urinary symptoms www.medicinesforchildren.org.uk/oxybutynin-for-daytime-urinary-symptoms

- **MEDICINAL FORMS**
  There can be variation in the licensing of different medicines containing the same drug. Forms available from special-order manufacturers include: oral suspension, oral solution, bladder irrigation

Modified-release tablet
CAUTIONARY AND ADVISORY LABELS 3, 25
- ▸ Lyrinel XL (Janssen-Cilag Ltd)
  Oxybutynin hydrochloride 5 mg Lyrinel XL 5mg tablets | 30 tablet PoM £13.77 DT price = £13.77
  Oxybutynin hydrochloride 10 mg Lyrinel XL 10mg tablets | 30 tablet PoM £27.54 DT price = £27.54

Tablet
CAUTIONARY AND ADVISORY LABELS 3
- ▸ Oxybutynin hydrochloride (Non-proprietary)
  Oxybutynin hydrochloride 2.5 mg Oxybutynin 2.5mg tablets | 56 tablet PoM £6.58 DT price = £1.15 | 84 tablet PoM £7.71
  Oxybutynin hydrochloride 3 mg Oxybutynin 3mg tablets | 56 tablet PoM £16.80 DT price = £16.80
  Oxybutynin hydrochloride 5 mg Oxybutynin 5mg tablets | 56 tablet PoM £13.85 DT price = £1.49 | 84 tablet PoM £20.77
- ▸ Cystrin (Zentiva)
  Oxybutynin hydrochloride 5 mg Cystrin 5mg tablets | 84 tablet PoM £21.99
- ▸ Ditropan (Sanofi)
  Oxybutynin hydrochloride 2.5 mg Ditropan 2.5mg tablets | 84 tablet PoM £1.60

☞ above

7 Genito-urinary system

Oxybutynin hydrochloride 5 mg Ditropan 5mg tablets |
84 tablet [PoM] £2.90
Oral solution
CAUTIONARY AND ADVISORY LABELS 3
▸ Oxybutynin hydrochloride (Non-proprietary)
Oxybutynin hydrochloride 500 microgram per 1 ml Oxybutynin
2.5mg/5ml oral solution sugar free sugar-free | 150 ml [PoM]
£144.50–£173.40 DT price = £144.50
Oxybutynin hydrochloride 1 mg per 1 ml Oxybutynin 5mg/5ml oral
solution sugar free sugar-free | 150 ml [PoM] £199.20–£239.04 DT
price = £199.20

F 468

Tolterodine tartrate

● **INDICATIONS AND DOSE**
Urinary frequency | Urinary urgency | Urinary incontinence
▸ BY MOUTH USING IMMEDIATE-RELEASE MEDICINES
▸ Child 2–17 years: 1 mg once daily, then increased if
necessary up to 2 mg twice daily, adjusted according to
response
▸ BY MOUTH USING MODIFIED-RELEASE CAPSULES
▸ Child 2–17 years: 4 mg once daily
Nocturnal enuresis associated with overactive bladder
▸ BY MOUTH USING IMMEDIATE-RELEASE MEDICINES
▸ Child 5–17 years: 1 mg once daily, dose to be taken at
bedtime, then increased if necessary up to 2 mg twice
daily, adjusted according to response
DOSE EQUIVALENCE AND CONVERSION
▸ Children stabilised on immediate-release tolterodine
tartrate 2 mg twice daily may be transferred to
modified-release tolterodine tartrate 4 mg once daily.

● **UNLICENSED USE** Not licensed for use in children.
● **CAUTIONS** History of QT-interval prolongation
● **INTERACTIONS** → Appendix 1: tolterodine
● **SIDE-EFFECTS**
▸ **Common or very common** Bronchitis · chest pain · fatigue ·
paraesthesia · peripheral oedema · sinusitis · vertigo ·
weight gain
▸ **Uncommon** Memory impairment
▸ **Frequency not known** Flushing
● **PREGNANCY** Manufacturer advises avoid—toxicity in
animal studies.
● **BREAST FEEDING** Manufacturer advises avoid—no
information available.
● **HEPATIC IMPAIRMENT** Reduce dose. Avoid modified-
release preparations.
● **RENAL IMPAIRMENT** Reduce dose if estimated glomerular
filtration less than 30 mL/minute/1.73m^2. Avoid modified-
release preparations if estimated glomerular filtration rate
less than 30 mL/minute/1.73m^2.
● **PRESCRIBING AND DISPENSING INFORMATION** The need for
therapy for urinary indications should be reviewed soon
after it has been commenced and then at regular intervals;
a response usually occurs within 6 months but may take
longer.

● **MEDICINAL FORMS**
There can be variation in the licensing of different medicines
containing the same drug. Forms available from special-order
manufacturers include: oral suspension, oral solution, powder
Tablet
CAUTIONARY AND ADVISORY LABELS 3
▸ **Tolterodine tartrate (Non-proprietary)**
Tolterodine tartrate 1 mg Tolterodine 1mg tablets | 56 tablet [PoM]
£29.03 DT price = £1.85
Tolterodine tartrate 2 mg Tolterodine 2mg tablets | 56 tablet [PoM]
£30.56 DT price = £1.81
▸ **Detrusitol** (Pfizer Ltd)
Tolterodine tartrate 1 mg Detrusitol 1mg tablets | 56 tablet [PoM]
£29.03 DT price = £1.85

Tolterodine tartrate 2 mg Detrusitol 2mg tablets | 56 tablet [PoM]
£30.56 DT price = £1.81
Modified-release capsule
CAUTIONARY AND ADVISORY LABELS 3, 25
▸ **Tolterodine tartrate (Non-proprietary)**
Tolterodine tartrate 2 mg Tolterodine 2mg modified-release
capsules | 28 capsule [PoM] no price available DT price = £11.60
▸ **Blerone XL** (Zentiva)
Tolterodine tartrate 4 mg Blerone XL 4mg capsules |
28 capsule [PoM] £25.78 DT price = £25.78
▸ **Detrusitol XL** (Pfizer Ltd)
Tolterodine tartrate 4 mg Detrusitol XL 4mg capsules |
28 capsule [PoM] £25.78 DT price = £25.78
▸ **Efflosomyl XL** (Mylan Ltd)
Tolterodine tartrate 4 mg Efflosomyl XL 4mg capsules |
28 capsule [PoM] £20.62 DT price = £25.78
▸ **Inconex XL** (Sandoz Ltd)
Tolterodine tartrate 4 mg Inconex XL 4mg capsules |
28 capsule [PoM] £21.91 DT price = £25.78
▸ **Mariosea XL** (Teva UK Ltd)
Tolterodine tartrate 2 mg Mariosea XL 2mg capsules |
28 capsule [PoM] £11.59 DT price = £11.60
Tolterodine tartrate 4 mg Mariosea XL 4mg capsules |
28 capsule [PoM] £12.88 DT price = £25.78
▸ **Neditol XL** (Aspire Pharma Ltd)
Tolterodine tartrate 2 mg Neditol XL 2mg capsules |
28 capsule [PoM] £11.60 DT price = £11.60
Tolterodine tartrate 4 mg Neditol XL 4mg capsules |
28 capsule [PoM] £12.89 DT price = £25.78
▸ **Preblacon XL** (Actavis UK Ltd)
Tolterodine tartrate 4 mg Preblacon XL 4mg capsules |
28 capsule [PoM] £25.78 DT price = £25.78
▸ **Santizor XL** (Pfizer Ltd)
Tolterodine tartrate 4 mg Santizor XL 4mg capsules |
28 capsule [PoM] £25.78 DT price = £25.78

1.2 Urinary retention

Urinary retention

31-May-2017

Description of condition

Urinary retention is the inability to voluntarily urinate.
Causes in children can include severe voiding dysfunction,
urethral blockage, drug treatment (such as opioids and
antimuscarinic drugs), conditions that reduce detrusor
contractions or interfere with relaxation of the urethra, and
neurogenic causes.

Acute urinary retention is a medical emergency
characterised by the abrupt (over a period of hours)
development of the inability to pass urine, associated with
increasing pain and the presence of a distended bladder,
which can be palpated on examination.

Chronic urinary retention is the gradual (over months or
years) development of the inability to empty the bladder
completely, characterised by difficulties with initiating and
maintaining urinary stream, urinary overflow, no sensation
for needing to void and a post-void residual.

Treatment

[EvGr] Treatment of urinary retention depends on the
underlying condition. Catheterisation is used as an effective
initial management strategy, which should be followed by
diagnostic evaluation and appropriate treatment of the
underlying cause. Clean intermittent catheterisation on a
long-term basis is effective for children with idiopathic or
neurogenic bladder dysfunction.

The selective alpha-adrenoceptor blockers, doxazosin
p. 470 and tamsulosin hydrochloride p. 470, have been
shown to be of use in primary bladder neck dysfunction and
dysfunctional voiding; they reduce urethral sphincter
pressure, thereby improving bladder emptying in children.
Treatment should be under specialist advice only. ⟨E⟩

7

Genito-urinary system

ALPHA-ADRENOCEPTOR BLOCKERS

Doxazosin

- **INDICATIONS AND DOSE**

Hypertension

▸ BY MOUTH USING IMMEDIATE-RELEASE MEDICINES

▸ Child 6-11 years: Initially 500 micrograms once daily, then increased to 2–4 mg once daily, dose should be increased at intervals of 1 week

▸ Child 12-17 years: Initially 1 mg once daily for 1–2 weeks, then increased to 2 mg once daily, then increased if necessary to 4 mg once daily, rarely doses of up to 16 mg daily may be required

Dysfunctional voiding (initiated under specialist supervision)

▸ BY MOUTH USING IMMEDIATE-RELEASE MEDICINES

▸ Child 4-11 years: Initially 0.5 mg daily, adjusted according to response, dose should be increased at monthly intervals; maximum 2 mg per day

▸ Child 12-17 years: Initially 1 mg daily, adjusted according to response, dose may be doubled at intervals of 1 month; usual maintenance 2–4 mg daily; maximum 8 mg per day

DOSE EQUIVALENCE AND CONVERSION

▸ Patients stabilised on immediate-release doxazosin can be transferred to the equivalent dose of modified-release doxazosin.

- **UNLICENSED USE** Not licensed for use in children.

- **CONTRA-INDICATIONS** History of postural hypotension

- **CAUTIONS** Care with initial dose (postural hypotension) · cataract surgery (risk of intra-operative floppy iris syndrome) · heart failure · pulmonary oedema due to aortic or mitral stenosis

- **INTERACTIONS** → Appendix 1: alpha blockers

- **SIDE-EFFECTS**

▸ **Common or very common** Anxiety · back pain · coughing · dyspnoea · fatigue · influenza-like symptoms · myalgia · paraesthesia · sleep disturbance · vertigo

▸ **Uncommon** Agitation · angina · arthralgia · epistaxis · gout · hypoaesthesia · impotence · micturition disturbance · myocardial infarction · purpura · tinnitus · tremor · weight changes

▸ **Very rare** Abnormal ejaculation · alopecia · arrhythmias · bradycardia · bronchospasm · cholestasis · gynaecomastia · hepatitis · hot flushes · jaundice · leucopenia · thrombocytopenia

▸ **Frequency not known** Asthenia · blurred vision · depression · dizziness · gastro-intestinal disturbances · headache · hypersensitivity · hypotension · oedema · palpitations · postural hypotension · priapism · pruritus · rash · rhinitis · syncope · tachycardia

- **PREGNANCY** No evidence of teratogenicity; manufacturers advise use only when potential benefit outweighs risk.

- **BREAST FEEDING** Accumulates in milk in *animal* studies—manufacturer advises avoid.

- **HEPATIC IMPAIRMENT** Use with caution. Manufacturer advises avoid in severe impairment—no information available.

- **PATIENT AND CARER ADVICE**

Patient counselling is advised for doxazosin tablets (initial dose).

Driving and skilled tasks

May affect performance of skilled tasks e.g. driving.

- **MEDICINAL FORMS**

There can be variation in the licensing f different medicines containing the same drug. Forms available from special-order manufacturers include: capsule, oral suspension, oral solution

Tablet

▸ Doxazosin (Non-proprietary)

Doxazosin (as Doxazosin mesilate) 1 mg Doxazosin 1mg tablets | 28 tablet (PoM) £10.56 DT price = £0.71

Doxazosin (as Doxazosin mesilate) 2 mg Doxazosin 2mg tablets | 28 tablet (PoM) £14.08 DT price = £0.74

Doxazosin (as Doxazosin mesilate) 4 mg Doxazosin 4mg tablets | 28 tablet (PoM) £14.08 DT price = £0.84

▸ Cardura (Pfizer Ltd)

Doxazosin (as Doxazosin mesilate) 1 mg Cardura 1mg tablets | 28 tablet (PoM) £10.56 DT price = £0.71

Doxazosin (as Doxazosin mesilate) 2 mg Cardura 2mg tablets | 28 tablet (PoM) £14.08 DT price = £0.74

▸ Doxadura (Discovery Pharmaceuticals)

Doxazosin (as Doxazosin mesilate) 1 mg Doxadura 1mg tablets | 28 tablet (PoM) £0.64 DT price = £0.71

Doxazosin (as Doxazosin mesilate) 2 mg Doxadura 2mg tablets | 28 tablet (PoM) £0.66 DT price = £0.74

Doxazosin (as Doxazosin mesilate) 4 mg Doxadura 4mg tablets | 28 tablet (PoM) £0.73 DT price = £0.84

Tamsulosin hydrochloride

- **INDICATIONS AND DOSE**

Dysfunctional voiding (administered on expert advice)

▸ BY MOUTH USING MODIFIED-RELEASE MEDICINES

▸ Child 12-17 years: 400 micrograms once daily

- **UNLICENSED USE** Not licensed for use in children.

- **CONTRA-INDICATIONS** History of postural hypotension

- **CAUTIONS** Care with initial dose (postural hypotension) · cataract surgery (risk of intra-operative floppy iris syndrome)

- **INTERACTIONS** → Appendix 1: alpha blockers

- **SIDE-EFFECTS** Abnormal ejaculation · angioedema · asthenia · blurred vision · constipation · diarrhoea · dizziness · drowsiness · dry mouth · headache · hypersensitivity reactions · hypotension (notably postural hypotension) · intra-operative floppy iris syndrome · nausea · oedema · palpitations · priapism · pruritus · rash · rhinitis · syncope · urticaria · vomiting

- **HEPATIC IMPAIRMENT** Avoid in severe impairment.

- **RENAL IMPAIRMENT** Use with caution if estimated glomerular filtration rate less than 10 mL/minute/1.73 m^2.

- **PATIENT AND CARER ADVICE**

Driving and skilled tasks

May affect performance of skilled tasks e.g. driving.

- **MEDICINAL FORMS**

There can be variation in the licensing of different medicines containing the same drug.

Modified-release tablet

CAUTIONARY AND ADVISORY LABELS 25

▸ Tamsulosin hydrochloride (Non-proprietary)

Tamsulosin hydrochloride 400 microgram Tamsulosin 400microgram modified-release tablets | 30 tablet (PoM) £10.47 DT price = £10.47

▸ Cositam XL (Consilient Health Ltd)

Tamsulosin hydrochloride 400 microgram Cositam XL 400microgram tablets | 30 tablet (PoM) £8.89 DT price = £10.47

▸ Faramsil (Sandoz Ltd)

Tamsulosin hydrochloride 400 microgram Faramsil 400microgram modified-release tablets | 30 tablet (PoM) £8.89 DT price = £10.47

▸ Flectone XL (Teva UK Ltd)

Tamsulosin hydrochloride 400 microgram Flectone XL 400microgram tablets | 30 tablet (PoM) £9.95 DT price = £10.47

▸ Flomaxtra XL (Astellas Pharma Ltd)

Tamsulosin hydrochloride 400 microgram Flomaxtra XL 400microgram tablets | 30 tablet (PoM) £10.47 DT price = £10.47

Modified-release capsule
CAUTIONARY AND ADVISORY LABELS 25

▸ **Tamsulosin hydrochloride (Non-proprietary)**
Tamsulosin hydrochloride 400 microgram Tamsulosin 400microgram modified-release capsules | 30 capsule $\boxed{\text{PoM}}$ £5.08 DT price = £3.89

▸ **Contiflo XL** (Ranbaxy (UK) Ltd)
Tamsulosin hydrochloride 400 microgram Contiflo XL 400microgram capsules | 30 capsule $\boxed{\text{PoM}}$ £7.44 DT price = £3.89

▸ **Diffundox XL** (Zentiva)
Tamsulosin hydrochloride 400 microgram Diffundox XL 400microgram capsules | 30 capsule $\boxed{\text{PoM}}$ £9.55 DT price = £3.89

▸ **Flomax MR** (Boehringer Ingelheim Self-Medication Division)
Tamsulosin hydrochloride 400 microgram Flomax Relief MR 400microgram capsules | 14 capsule $\boxed{\text{P}}$ £5.58 | 28 capsule $\boxed{\text{P}}$ £10.55

▸ **Galebon** (Consilient Health Ltd)
Tamsulosin hydrochloride 400 microgram Galebon 400microgram modified-release capsules | 30 capsule $\boxed{\text{PoM}}$ £3.78 DT price = £3.89

▸ **Losinate MR** (Aspire Pharma Ltd)
Tamsulosin hydrochloride 400 microgram Losinate MR 400microgram capsules | 30 capsule $\boxed{\text{PoM}}$ £10.14 DT price = £3.89

▸ **Pamsvax XL** (Almus Pharmaceuticals Ltd, Actavis UK Ltd)
Tamsulosin hydrochloride 400 microgram Pamsvax XL 400microgram capsules | 30 capsule $\boxed{\text{PoM}}$ £1.31 DT price = £3.89

▸ **Petyme MR** (Teva UK Ltd)
Tamsulosin hydrochloride 400 microgram Petyme 400microgram MR capsules | 30 capsule $\boxed{\text{PoM}}$ £4.06 DT price = £3.89

▸ **Pinexel PR** (Wockhardt UK Ltd)
Tamsulosin hydrochloride 400 microgram Pinexel PR 400microgram capsules | 30 capsule $\boxed{\text{PoM}}$ £2.50 DT price = £3.89

▸ **Prosurin XL** (Mylan Ltd)
Tamsulosin hydrochloride 400 microgram Prosurin XL 400microgram capsules | 30 capsule $\boxed{\text{PoM}}$ £4.28 DT price = £3.89

▸ **Tabphyn MR** (Genus Pharmaceuticals Ltd)
Tamsulosin hydrochloride 400 microgram Tabphyn MR 400microgram capsules | 30 capsule $\boxed{\text{PoM}}$ £4.45 DT price = £3.89

▸ **Tamfrex XL** (Milpharm Ltd)
Tamsulosin hydrochloride 400 microgram Tamfrex XL 400microgram capsules | 30 capsule $\boxed{\text{PoM}}$ no price available DT price = £3.89

▸ **Tamurex** (Somex Pharma)
Tamsulosin hydrochloride 400 microgram Tamurex 400microgram modified-release capsules | 30 capsule $\boxed{\text{PoM}}$ £3.50 DT price = £3.89

1.3 Urological pain

Urological pain

Treatment
Lidocaine hydrochloride **gel** p. 796 is a useful topical application in *urethral pain* or to relieve the discomfort of catheterisation.

Alkalinisation of urine
Alkalinisation of urine can be undertaken with potassium citrate. The alkalinising action may relieve the discomfort of *cystitis* caused by lower urinary tract infections.

ALKALISING DRUGS

❙ Citric acid with potassium citrate

● **INDICATIONS AND DOSE**
Relief of discomfort in mild urinary-tract infections |
Alkalinisation of urine
▸ BY MOUTH USING ORAL SOLUTION
  ▸ Child 1–5 years: 5 mL 3 times a day, diluted well with water
  ▸ Child 6–17 years: 10 mL 3 times a day, diluted well with water

● **CAUTIONS** Cardiac disease

● **INTERACTIONS** → Appendix 1: potassium citrate

● **SIDE-EFFECTS** Hyperkalaemia on prolonged high dosage · mild diuresis

● **RENAL IMPAIRMENT** Avoid in severe impairment. Close monitoring required in renal impairment—high risk of hyperkalaemia.

● **PRESCRIBING AND DISPENSING INFORMATION** When prepared extemporaneously, the BP states Potassium Citrate Mixture BP consists of potassium citrate 30%, citric acid monohydrate 5% in a suitable vehicle with a lemon flavour. Extemporaneous preparations should be recently prepared according to the following formula: potassium citrate 3 g, citric acid monohydrate 500 mg, syrup 2.5 mL, quillaia tincture 0.1 mL, lemon spirit 0.05 mL, double-strength chloroform water 3 mL, water to 10 mL. Contains about 28 mmol K^+/10 mL.

● **EXCEPTIONS TO LEGAL CATEGORY** Proprietary brands of potassium citrate are on sale to the public for the relief of discomfort in mild urinary-tract infections.

● **MEDICINAL FORMS**
There can be variation in the licensing of different medicines containing the same drug.

Oral solution
CAUTIONARY AND ADVISORY LABELS 27

▸ **Citric acid with potassium citrate (Non-proprietary)**
Citric acid monohydrate 50 mg per 1 ml, Potassium citrate 300 mg per 1 ml Potassium citrate mixture | 200 ml $\boxed{\text{P}}$ £1.33 DT price = £1.33

2 Bladder instillations and urological surgery

Bladder instillations and urological surgery

Bladder infection
Various solutions are available as irrigations or washouts.

Aqueous chlorhexidine p. 673 can be used in the management of common infections of the bladder but it is ineffective against most *Pseudomonas spp*. Solutions containing chlorhexidine 1 in 5000 (0.02%) are used but they may irritate the mucosa and cause burning and haematuria (in which case they should be discontinued); sterile sodium chloride **solution 0.9%** (physiological saline) p. 561 is usually adequate and is preferred as a mechanical irrigant.

Dissolution of blood clots
Clot retention is usually treated by irrigation with sterile sodium chloride solution 0.9% but sterile sodium citrate solution for bladder irrigation 3% may also be helpful.

Maintenance of indwelling urinary catheters
The deposition which occurs in catheterised patients is usually chiefly composed of phosphate and to minimise this the catheter (if latex) should be changed at least as often as every 6 weeks. If the catheter is to be left for longer periods a silicone catheter should be used together with the appropriate use of catheter maintenance solutions. Repeated blockage usually indicates that the catheter needs to be changed.

❙ Catheter maintenance solutions

● **CATHETER MAINTENANCE SOLUTIONS**
OptiFlo R citric acid 6% catheter maintenance solution (Bard Ltd) 50 ml · NHS indicative price = £3.60 · Drug Tariff (Part IXa)100 ml · NHS indicative price = £3.60 · Drug Tariff (Part IXa)

7

Genito-urinary system

Uro-Tainer Twin Solutio R citric acid 6% catheter maintenance solution (B.Braun Medical Ltd) 60 ml · NHS indicative price = £4.81 · Drug Tariff (Part IXa)

OptiFlo S saline 0.9% catheter maintenance solution (Bard Ltd)
Sodium chloride 9 mg per 1 ml 50 ml · NHS indicative price = £3.39 · Drug Tariff (Part IXa) 100 ml · NHS indicative price = £3.39 · Drug Tariff (Part IXa)

Uro-Tainer M sodium chloride 0.9% catheter maintenance solution (B.Braun Medical Ltd)
Sodium chloride 9 mg per 1 ml 50 ml · No NHS indicative price available · Drug Tariff (Part IXa)100 ml · No NHS indicative price available · Drug Tariff (Part IXa)

Uro-Tainer sodium chloride 0.9% catheter maintenance solution (B.Braun Medical Ltd)
Sodium chloride 9 mg per 1 ml 50 ml · NHS indicative price = £3.51 · Drug Tariff (Part IXa)100 ml · NHS indicative price = £3.51 · Drug Tariff (Part IXa)

3 Contraception

Contraceptives, hormonal

Overview

The Fraser Guidelines (Department of Health Guidance (July 2004): Best practice guidance for doctors and other health professionals on the provision of advice and treatment to young people under 16 on contraception, sexual and reproductive health, available at www.tinyurl.com/bpg16) should be followed when prescribing contraception for women under 16 years. The UK Medical Eligibility Criteria for Contraceptive Use (available at www.fsrh.org) is published by the Faculty of Sexual and Reproductive Healthcare; it categorises the risks of using contraceptive methods with pre-existing medical conditions.

Hormonal contraception is the most effective method of fertility control, but can have major and minor side-effects, especially for certain groups of women. Hormonal contraception should only be used by adolescents after menarche.

Intra-uterine devices are a highly effective method of contraception but may produce undesirable local side-effects. They may be used in women of all ages irrespective of parity, but are less appropriate for those with an increased risk of pelvic inflammatory disease.

Barrier methods alone (condoms, diaphragms, and caps) are less effective but can be reliable for well-motivated couples if used in conjunction with a **spermicide**. Occasionally sensitivity reactions occur. A female condom (*Femidom®*) is also available; it is pre-lubricated but does not contain a spermicide.

Combined hormonal contraceptives

Oral contraceptives containing an oestrogen and a progestogen ('combined oral contraceptives') are effective preparations for general use. Advantages of combined oral contraceptives include:

- reliable and reversible;
- reduced dysmenorrhoea and menorrhagia;
- reduced incidence of premenstrual tension;
- less symptomatic fibroids and functional ovarian cysts;
- less benign breast disease;
- reduced risk of ovarian and endometrial cancer;
- reduced risk of pelvic inflammatory disease.

Combined oral contraceptives containing a fixed amount of an oestrogen and a progestogen in each active tablet are termed 'monophasic'; those with varying amounts of the two hormones are termed 'phasic'. A transdermal patch and a vaginal ring, both containing an oestrogen with a progestogen, are also available.

Combined Oral Contraceptives Monophasic 21-day preparations

Oestrogen content	Progestogen content	Brand
Ethinylestradiol 20 micrograms	Desogestrel 150 micrograms	Gedarel® 20/150
Ethinylestradiol 20 micrograms	Desogestrel 150 micrograms	Mercilon®
Ethinylestradiol 20 micrograms	Gestodene 75 micrograms	Femodette®
Ethinylestradiol 20 micrograms	Gestodene 75 micrograms	Millinette® 20/75
Ethinylestradiol 20 micrograms	Gestodene 75 micrograms	Sunya 20/75®
Ethinylestradiol 20 micrograms	Norethisterone acetate 1 mg	Loestrin 20®
Ethinylestradiol 30 micrograms	Desogestrel 150 micrograms	Gedarel® 30/150
Ethinylestradiol 30 micrograms	Desogestrel 150 micrograms	Marvelon®
Ethinylestradiol 30 micrograms	Drospirenone 3 mg	Yasmin®
Ethinylestradiol 30 micrograms	Gestodene 75 micrograms	Femodene®
Ethinylestradiol 30 micrograms	Gestodene 75 micrograms	Katya 30/75®
Ethinylestradiol 30 micrograms	Gestodene 75 micrograms	Millinette® 30/75
Ethinylestradiol 30 micrograms	Levonorgestrel 150 micrograms	Levest®
Ethinylestradiol 30 micrograms	Levonorgestrel 150 micrograms	Microgynon 30®
Ethinylestradiol 30 micrograms	Levonorgestrel 150 micrograms	Ovranette®
Ethinylestradiol 30 micrograms	Levonorgestrel 150 micrograms	Rigevidon®
Ethinylestradiol 30 micrograms	Norethisterone acetate 1.5 mg	Loestrin 30®
Ethinylestradiol 35 micrograms	Norgestimate 250 micrograms	Cilest®
Ethinylestradiol 35 micrograms	Norethisterone 500 micrograms	Brevinor®
Ethinylestradiol 35 micrograms	Norethisterone 1 mg	Norimin®
Mestranol 50 micrograms	Norethisterone 1 mg	Norinyl-1®

Combined Oral Contraceptives Monophasic 28-day preparations

Oestrogen content	Progestogen content	Brand
Ethinylestradiol 30 micrograms	Gestodene 75 micrograms	Femodene® ED
Ethinylestradiol 30 micrograms	Levonorgestrel 150 micrograms	Microgynon 30 ED®
Estradiol (as hemihydrate) 1.5 mg	Nomegestrol acetate 2.5 mg	Zoely®

Combined Oral Contraceptives Phasic 21-day preparations

Oestrogen content	Progestogen content	Brand
Ethinylestradiol 30 micrograms	Gestodene 50 micrograms	
Ethinylestradiol 40 micrograms	Gestodene 70 micrograms	Triadene®
Ethinylestradiol 30 micrograms	Gestodene 100 micrograms	
Ethinylestradiol 30 micrograms	Levonorgestrel 50 micrograms	
Ethinylestradiol 40 micrograms	Levonorgestrel 75 micrograms	Logynon®
Ethinylestradiol 30 micrograms	Levonorgestrel 125 micrograms	
Ethinylestradiol 30 micrograms	Levonorgestrel 50 micrograms	
Ethinylestradiol 40 micrograms	Levonorgestrel 75 micrograms	TriRegol®
Ethinylestradiol 30 micrograms	Levonorgestrel 125 micrograms	
Ethinylestradiol 35 micrograms	Norethisterone 500 micrograms	
Ethinylestradiol 35 micrograms	Norethisterone 1 mg	Synphase®
Ethinylestradiol 35 micrograms	Norethisterone 500 micrograms	

Combined Oral Contraceptives Phasic 28-day preparations

Oestrogen content	Progestogen content	Brand
Ethinylestradiol 30 micrograms	Levonorgestrel 50 micrograms	
Ethinylestradiol 40 micrograms	Levonorgestrel 75 micrograms	Logynon ED®
Ethinylestradiol 30 micrograms	Levonorgestrel 125 micrograms	
Estradiol valerate 3 mg		
Estradiol valerate 2 mg	Dienogest 2 mg	
Estradiol valerate 2 mg	Dienogest 3 mg	Qlaira®
Estradiol valerate 1 mg		

Choice

The majority of combined oral contraceptives contain ethinylestradiol as the oestrogen component; mestranol and estradiol are also used. The ethinylestradiol content of combined oral contraceptives ranges from 20 to 40 micrograms. Generally a preparation with the lowest oestrogen and progestogen content which gives good cycle control and minimal side-effects in the individual woman is chosen. It is recommended that combined hormonal contraceptives are not continued beyond 50 years of age since more suitable alternatives exist.

- *Low strength preparations* (containing ethinylestradiol 20 micrograms) are particularly appropriate for women with risk factors for circulatory disease, provided a combined oral contraceptive is otherwise suitable.
- *Standard strength preparations* (containing ethinylestradiol 30 or 35 micrograms or in 30–40 microgram *phased*

preparations) are appropriate for standard use. Phased preparations are generally reserved for women who *either* do not have withdrawal bleeding or who have breakthrough bleeding with monophasic products.

The progestogens ethinylestradiol with desogestrel p. 478, ethinylestradiol with drospirenone p. 479, and ethinylestradiol with gestodene p. 480 may be considered for women who have side-effects (such as acne, headache, depression, breast symptoms, and breakthrough bleeding) with other progestogens. Drospirenone, a derivative of spironolactone, has anti-androgenic and anti-mineralocorticoid activity; it should be used with care if an increased plasma-potassium concentration might be hazardous.

Dienogest with estradiol valerate p. 478 is in the combined oral contraceptive *Qlaira®*. Nomegestrol is the progestogen contained in the combined oral contraceptive *Zoely®*, in combination with estradiol.

The progestogen norelgestromin is combined with ethinylestradiol in a transdermal patch (*Evra®*). The vaginal contraceptive ring contains the progestogen etonogestrel combined with ethinylestradiol (*NuvaRing®*).

Surgery

Oestrogen-containing contraceptives should preferably be discontinued (and adequate alternative contraceptive arrangements made) 4 weeks before major elective surgery and all surgery to the legs or surgery which involves prolonged immobilisation of a lower limb; they should normally be recommenced at the first menses occurring at least 2 weeks after full mobilisation. A progestogen-only contraceptive may be offered as an alternative and the oestrogen-containing contraceptive restarted after mobilisation. When discontinuation of an oestrogen-containing contraceptive is not possible, e.g. after trauma or if a patient admitted for an elective procedure is still on an oestrogen-containing contraceptive, thromboprophylaxis (with unfractionated or low molecular weight heparin and graduated compression hosiery) is advised. These recommendations do not apply to minor surgery with short duration of anaesthesia, e.g. laparoscopic sterilisation or tooth extraction, or to women using oestrogen-free hormonal contraceptives.

Reason to stop immediately

Combined hormonal contraceptives or hormone replacement therapy (HRT) should be stopped (pending investigation and treatment), if any of the following occur:

- sudden severe chest pain (even if not radiating to left arm);
- sudden breathlessness (or cough with blood-stained sputum);
- unexplained swelling or severe pain in calf of one leg;
- severe stomach pain;
- serious neurological effects including unusual severe, prolonged headache especially if first time or getting progressively worse *or* sudden partial *or* complete loss of vision *or* sudden disturbance of hearing or other perceptual disorders *or* dysphasia *or* bad fainting attack or collapse *or* first unexplained epileptic seizure *or* weakness, motor disturbances, very marked numbness suddenly affecting one side or one part of body;
- hepatitis, jaundice, liver enlargement;
- blood pressure above systolic 160 mmHg or diastolic 95 mmHg; (in adolescents stop if blood pressure very high);
- prolonged immobility after surgery or leg injury;
- detection of a risk factor which contra-indicates treatment.

7

Genito-urinary system

Genito-urinary system

7

Progestogen-only contraceptives

Oral progestogen-only contraceptives

Oral progestogen-only preparations alter cervical mucus to prevent sperm penetration and may inhibit ovulation in some women; oral desogestrel-only preparations consistently inhibit ovulation and this is their primary mechanism of action. There is insufficient clinical trial evidence to compare the efficacy of oral progestogen-only contraceptives with each other or with combined hormonal contraceptives. Progestogen-only contraceptives offer a suitable alternative to combined hormonal contraceptives when oestrogens are contra-indicated (including those with venous thrombosis or a past history or predisposition to venous thrombosis, heavy smokers, those with hypertension above systolic 160 mmHg or diastolic 95 mmHg, valvular heart disease, diabetes mellitus with complications, and migraine with aura).

Parenteral progestogen-only contraceptives

Medroxyprogesterone acetate (*Depo-Provera*®, *SAYANA PRESS*®) p. 489 is a long-acting progestogen given by injection; it is at least as effective as the combined oral preparations but because of its prolonged action it should never be given without *full counselling backed by the patient information leaflet*. It may be used as a short-term or long-term contraceptive for women who have been counselled about the likelihood of menstrual disturbance and the potential for a delay in return to full fertility. Delayed return of fertility and irregular cycles may occur after discontinuation of treatment but there is no evidence of permanent infertility. Troublesome bleeding has been reported in patients given medroxyprogesterone acetate in the immediate puerperium; delaying the first injection until 6 weeks after birth may minimise bleeding problems. If the woman is not breast-feeding, the first injection may be given within 5 days postpartum (she should be warned that the risk of troublesome bleeding may be increased).

- In adolescents, medroxyprogesterone acetate (*Depo-Provera*®, *SAYANA PRESS*®) should be used only when other methods of contraception are inappropriate;
- in all women, the benefits of using medroxyprogesterone acetate beyond 2 years should be evaluated against the risks;
- in women with risk factors for osteoporosis, a method of contraception other than medroxyprogesterone acetate should be considered.

Norethisterone enantate (*Noristerat*®) is a long-acting progestogen given as an oily injection which provides contraception for 8 weeks; it is used as short-term interim contraception e.g. before vasectomy becomes effective.

An **etonogestrel-releasing implant** (*Nexplanon*®) is also available. It is a highly effective long-acting contraceptive, consisting of a single flexible rod that is inserted subdermally into the lower surface of the upper arm and provides contraception for up to 3 years. The manufacturer advises that in heavier women, blood-etonogestrel concentrations are lower and therefore the implant may not provide effective contraception during the third year; they advise that earlier replacement may be considered in such patients—however, evidence to support this recommendation is lacking. Local reactions such as bruising and itching can occur at the insertion site. The contraceptive effect of etonogestrel is rapidly reversed on removal of the implant.

Intra-uterine progestogen-only device

The progestogen-only intra-uterine systems *Mirena*®, *Jaydess*® and *Levosert*® release levonorgestrel p. 486 directly into the uterine cavity. *Mirena*® is licensed for use as a contraceptive, for the treatment of primary menorrhagia and for the prevention of endometrial hyperplasia during oestrogen replacement therapy. *Jaydess*® and *Levosert*® are licensed for contraception, and *Levosert*® is additionally licensed for the treatment of menorrhagia. These may therefore be a contraceptive method of choice for women who have excessively heavy menses.

The effects of the progestogen-only intra-uterine system are mainly local and hormonal including prevention of endometrial proliferation, thickening of cervical mucus, and suppression of ovulation in some women (in some cycles). In addition to the progestogenic activity, the intra-uterine system itself may contribute slightly to the contraceptive effect. Return of fertility after removal is rapid and appears to be complete.

Advantages of the progestogen-only intra-uterine system over copper intra-uterine devices are that there may be an improvement in any dysmenorrhoea and a reduction in blood loss; there is also evidence that the frequency of pelvic inflammatory disease may be reduced particularly in the youngest age groups who are most at risk).

In primary menorrhagia, menstrual bleeding is reduced significantly within 3–6 months of inserting the progestogen-only intra-uterine system, probably because it prevents endometrial proliferation. Another treatment should be considered if menorrhagia does not improve within this time.

Surgery

All progestogen-only contraceptives (including those given by injection) are suitable for use as an alternative to combined hormonal contraceptives before major elective surgery, before all surgery to the legs, or before surgery which involves prolonged immobilisation of a lower limb.

Emergency contraception

Hormonal methods

Hormonal emergency contraceptives include levonorgestrel and ulipristal acetate p. 484; either drug should be taken as soon as possible after unprotected intercourse to increase efficacy.

Levonorgestrel is effective if taken within 72 hours (3 days) of unprotected intercourse and may also be used between 72 and 96 hours after unprotected intercourse [unlicensed use], but efficacy decreases with time. Ulipristal acetate, a progesterone receptor modulator, is effective if taken within 120 hours (5 days) of unprotected intercourse.

Levonorgestrel is less effective than insertion of an intra-uterine device. Ulipristal acetate is as effective as levonorgestrel, but its efficacy compared to an intra-uterine device is not yet known.

Intra-uterine device

Insertion of an intra-uterine device is more effective than oral levonorgestrel for emergency contraception. A copper intra-uterine contraceptive device can be inserted up to 120 hours (5 days) after unprotected intercourse; sexually transmitted infections should be tested for and insertion of the device should usually be covered by antibacterial prophylaxis (e.g. azithromycin p. 314). If intercourse has occurred more than 5 days previously, the device can still be inserted up to 5 days after the earliest likely calculated ovulation (i.e. within the minimum period before implantation), regardless of the number of episodes of unprotected intercourse earlier in the cycle.

Contraceptives, interactions

06-Jun-2017

Overview

The effectiveness of *combined* oral contraceptives, *progestogen-only* oral contraceptives, contraceptive patches, vaginal rings, and emergency hormonal contraception can be considerably reduced by interaction with drugs that induce hepatic enzyme activity (e.g. carbamazepine p. 189, eslicarbazepine acetate, nevirapine p. 355, oxcarbazepine p. 197, phenytoin p. 198, phenobarbital p. 208, primidone p. 209, ritonavir p. 406, St John's Wort, topiramate p. 204 and, above all, rifabutin p. 348 and rifampicin p. 349) and possibly also griseofulvin p. 363. [EvGr] A condom together with a long-acting method (such as an injectable contraceptive) may be more suitable for patients with HIV infection or at risk of HIV infection; advice on the possibility of interaction with antiretroviral drugs should be sought from HIV specialists. ⟨ẞ⟩

Combined hormonal contraceptives interactions

[EvGr] Women using combined hormonal contraceptive patches, vaginal rings or oral tablets who require enzyme-inducing drugs or griseofulvin should be advised to change to a reliable contraceptive method that is unaffected by enzyme-inducers, such as some parenteral progestogen-only contraceptives (medroxyprogesterone acetate p. 489 and norethisterone p. 458) or intra-uterine devices (levonorgestrel p. 486; see also Contraceptives, non-hormonal p. 476). This should be continued for the duration of treatment and for four weeks after stopping. If a change in contraceptive method is undesirable or inappropriate the following options should be discussed ⟨ẞ⟩:

Short course (2 months or less) of an enzyme-inducing drug
[EvGr] Continuing the combined hormonal contraceptive method may be appropriate if used in combination with consistent and careful use of condoms for the duration of treatment and for four weeks after stopping the enzyme-inducing drug. ⟨ẞ⟩

Long-term course (over 2 months) of an enzyme-inducing drug (except rifampicin or rifabutin) or a course of griseofulvin
[EvGr] Use a monophasic combined oral contraceptive at a dose of ethinylestradiol 50 micrograms or more daily [unlicensed use] and use either an extended or a 'tricycling' regimen (i.e. taking three packets of monophasic tablets without a break followed by a shortened tablet-free interval of four days [unlicensed use]); continue for the duration of treatment with the interacting drug and for four weeks after stopping.

If breakthrough bleeding occurs (and all other causes are ruled out) it is recommended that the dose of ethinylestradiol is increased by increments of 10 micrograms up to a maximum of 70 micrograms daily [unlicensed use] on specialist advice, or to use additional precautions, or to change to a method unaffected by the interacting drugs.

Use of contraceptive patches and vaginal rings (including concurrent use of two patches or two vaginal rings) is not recommended for women taking enzyme-inducing drugs over a long period. ⟨ẞ⟩

Long-term course (over 2 months) of rifampicin or rifabutin
An alternative method of contraception (such as an IUD) is **always** recommended because they are such potent enzyme-inducing drugs; the alternative method of contraception should be continued for four weeks after stopping the enzyme-inducing drug.

Antibacterials that do not induce liver enzymes
[EvGr] It is recommended that no additional contraceptive precautions are required when *combined* oral contraceptives, contraceptive patches or vaginal rings are used with antibacterials that do not induce liver enzymes, unless diarrhoea or vomiting occur. These recommendations should be discussed with the woman. ⟨ẞ⟩

There had been concerns that some antibacterials that do not induce liver enzymes (e.g. ampicillin p. 326, doxycycline p. 338) reduce the efficacy of *combined* oral contraceptives by impairing the bacterial flora responsible for recycling ethinylestradiol from the large bowel. However, there is a lack of evidence to support this interaction.

Oral progestogen-only contraceptives interactions
Effectiveness of oral progestogen-only preparations is not affected by antibacterials that do not induce liver enzymes. [EvGr] The efficacy of oral progestogen-only preparations is, however, reduced by enzyme-inducing drugs or griseofulvin

and an alternative contraceptive method, unaffected by the interacting drug, is recommended during treatment with an interacting drug and for at least 4 weeks afterwards.

For a short course of an enzyme-inducing drug (less than two months), continuing the progestogen-only oral method may be appropriate if used in combination with consistent and careful use of condoms for the duration of treatment and for four weeks after stopping the enzyme-inducing drug. ⟨ẞ⟩

Parenteral progestogen-only contraceptives interactions

Effectiveness of parenteral progestogen-only contraceptives is not affected by antibacterials that do not induce liver enzymes. [EvGr] The effectiveness of intramuscular norethisterone injection and intramuscular and subcutaneous medroxyprogesterone acetate injections is not affected by enzyme-inducing drugs and they may be continued as normal during courses of these drugs.

Effectiveness of the etonogestrel-releasing implant p. 489 may be reduced by enzyme-inducing drugs or griseofulvin and an alternative contraceptive method, unaffected by the interacting drug, is recommended during treatment with the interacting drug and for at least 4 weeks after stopping.

For a short course of an enzyme-inducing drug, if a change in contraceptive method is undesirable or inappropriate, continued contraception with the implant may be appropriate if used in combination with consistent and careful use of condoms for the duration of treatment and for 4 weeks after stopping the enzyme-inducing drug. ⟨ẞ⟩

Hormonal emergency contraception interactions

The effectiveness of levonorgestrel and ulipristal acetate p. 484 is reduced in women taking enzyme-inducing drugs or griseofulvin (and for at least 4 weeks after stopping). [EvGr] A copper intra-uterine device can be offered instead. If the copper intra-uterine device is declined or unsuitable, the dose of levonorgestrel should be increased (See *Dose adjustments due to interactions* under levonorgestrel). There is no need to increase the dose for emergency contraception if the patient is taking antibacterials that are not enzyme inducers. ⟨ẞ⟩

The effectiveness of ulipristal acetate for emergency contraception may be reduced by drugs that increase gastric pH (such as regular use of antacids, H_2 receptor antagonists and proton pump inhibitors). [EvGr] Levonorgestrel or a copper intra-uterine device should be considered as alternatives.

Hormonal contraception should not be newly initiated in a patient until five days after administration of ulipristal acetate as emergency hormonal contraception—the contraceptive effect of ulipristal acetate will be reduced. Consistent and careful use of condoms is recommended.

Ulipristal acetate can be used as emergency hormonal contraception more than once in the same cycle. ⟨ẞ⟩ Conversely, manufacturer advises that use of levonorgestrel as emergency contraception more than once in the same cycle is not advisable due to increased risk of side-effects (such as menstrual irregularities).

[EvGr] Levonorgestrel should not be used (as emergency hormonal contraception) within 5 days of administration of ulipristal acetate (as emergency hormonal contraception), as the contraceptive effect of ulipristal acetate may be reduced by progestogens.

Ulipristal acetate is not recommend for use in women who have severe asthma treated by oral corticosteroids, due to the antiglucocorticoid effect of ulipristal acetate. ⟨ẞ⟩

Useful Resources

Drug interactions with hormonal contraception. The Faculty of Sexual and Reproductive Healthcare. Clinical guidance. January 2017.
www.fsrh.org/standards-and-guidance/current-clinical-guidance/drug-interactions

Contraceptives, non-hormonal

Spermicidal contraceptives

Spermicidal contraceptives are useful additional safeguards but do **not** give adequate protection if used alone unless fertility is already significantly diminished. They have two components: a spermicide and a vehicle which itself may have some inhibiting effect on sperm activity. They are suitable for use with barrier methods, such as diaphragms or caps; however, spermicidal contraceptives are not generally recommended for use with condoms, as there is no evidence of any additional protection compared with non-spermicidal lubricants.

Spermicidal contraceptives are not suitable for use in those with or at high risk of sexually transmitted infections (including HIV); high frequency use of the spermicide nonoxinol '9' p. 490 has been associated with genital lesions, which may increase the risk of acquiring these infections.

Contraceptive devices

Intra-uterine devices

The intra-uterine device (IUD) is a suitable contraceptive for young women irrespective of parity; however, it is less appropriate for those with an increased risk of pelvic inflammatory disease e.g. women under 25 years.

The most effective intra-uterine devices have at least 380 mm^2 of copper and have banded copper on the arms. Smaller devices have been introduced to minimise side-effects; these consist of a plastic carrier wound with copper wire or fitted with copper bands; some also have a central core of silver to prevent fragmentation of the copper.

A frameless, copper-bearing intra-uterine device (*Gyne Fix*®) is also available. It consists of a knotted, polypropylene thread with 6 copper sleeves; the device is anchored in the uterus by inserting the knot into the uterine fundus.

Caution with oil-based lubricants

Products such as petroleum jelly (*Vaseline*®), baby oil and oil-based vaginal and rectal preparations are likely to damage condoms and contraceptive diaphragms made from latex rubber, and may render them less effective as a barrier method of contraception and as a protection from sexually transmitted infections (including HIV).

3.1 Contraception, combined

OESTROGENS COMBINED WITH PROGESTOGENS

Combined hormonal contraceptives

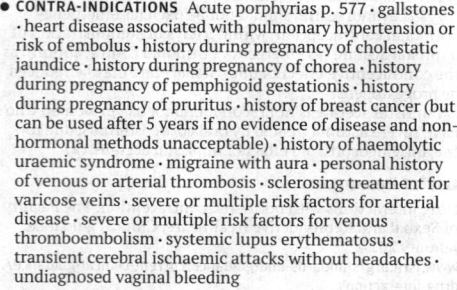

- **CONTRA-INDICATIONS** Acute porphyrias p. 577 · gallstones · heart disease associated with pulmonary hypertension or risk of embolus · history during pregnancy of cholestatic jaundice · history during pregnancy of chorea · history during pregnancy of pemphigoid gestationis · history during pregnancy of pruritus · history of breast cancer (but can be used after 5 years if no evidence of disease and non-hormonal methods unacceptable) · history of haemolytic uraemic syndrome · migraine with aura · personal history of venous or arterial thrombosis · sclerosing treatment for varicose veins · severe or multiple risk factors for arterial disease · severe or multiple risk factors for venous thromboembolism · systemic lupus erythematosus · transient cerebral ischaemic attacks without headaches · undiagnosed vaginal bleeding
- **CAUTIONS** Active trophoblastic disease (until return to normal of urine- and plasma-gonadotrophin

concentration)—seek specialist advice · Crohn's disease · gene mutations associated with breast cancer (e.g. BRCA 1) · history of severe depression especially if induced by hormonal contraceptive · hyperprolactinaemia (seek specialist advice) · inflammatory bowel disease · migraine · personal or family history of hypertriglyceridaemia (increased risk of pancreatitis) · risk factors for arterial disease · risk factors for venous thromboembolism · sickle-cell disease · undiagnosed breast mass

CAUTIONS, FURTHER INFORMATION

▶ Risk of venous thromboembolism There is an increased risk of venous thromboembolic disease in users of combined hormonal contraceptives particularly during the first year and possibly after restarting combined hormonal contraceptives following a break of four weeks or more. This risk is considerably smaller than that associated with pregnancy (about 60 cases of venous thromboembolic disease per 100 000 pregnancies). In all cases the risk of venous thromboembolism increases with age and in the presence of other risk factors, such as obesity. The risk also varies depending on the type of progestogen.

Provided that women are informed of the relative risks of venous thromboembolism and accept them, the choice of oral contraceptive is for the woman together with the prescriber jointly to make in light of her individual medical history and any contra-indications.

Combined hormonal contraceptives also slightly increase the risk of *arterial* thromboembolism; however, there is no evidence to suggest that this risk varies between different preparations.

▶ Risk factors for venous thromboembolism Use with **caution** if any of following factors present but **avoid** if two or more factors present:
- *family history of venous thromboembolism* in first-degree relative aged under 45 years (avoid contraceptive containing desogestrel or gestodene, *or* avoid if known prothrombotic coagulation abnormality e.g. factor V Leiden or antiphospholipid antibodies (including lupus anticoagulant));
- *obesity*; body mass index ≥ 30 kg/m^2 (avoid if body mass index ≥ 35 kg/m^2 unless no suitable alternative); (in adolescents, caution if obese according to BMI (adjusted for age and gender); in those who are markedly obese, avoid unless no suitable alternative);
- *long-term immobilisation* e.g. in a wheelchair (avoid if confined to bed or leg in plaster cast);
- *history of superficial thrombophlebitis*;
- *age* over 35 years (avoid if over 50 years);
- *smoking*.

Combined Hormonal Contraception and Risk of Venous Thromboembolism

Progestogen in Combined Hormonal Contraceptive	Estimated incidence per 10 000 women per year of use
Non-pregnant, not using combined hormonal contraception	2
Levonorgesterol[1]	5-7
Norgestimate[1]	5-7
Norethisterone[1]	5-7
Etonogestrel[1]	6-12
Norelgestromin[1]	6-12
Gestodene[1]	9-12
Desogestrel[1]	9-12
Drospirenone[1]	9-12
Dienogest[2]	Not known—insufficient data
Nomegestrol[2]	Not known—insufficient data

[1]Combined with ethinylestradiol [2]Combined with estradiol

▸ Risk factors for arterial disease Use with **caution** if any one of following factors present but **avoid** if two or more factors present:
- *family history of arterial disease* in first degree relative aged under 45 years (avoid if atherogenic lipid profile);
- *diabetes mellitus* (avoid if diabetes complications present);
- *hypertension*; blood pressure above *systolic* 140 *mmHg* or *diastolic* 90 *mmHg* (avoid if blood pressure above *systolic* 160 *mmHg* or *diastolic* 95 *mmHg*); (in adolescents, avoid if blood pressure very high);
- *smoking* (avoid if smoking 40 or more cigarettes daily);
- *age* over 35 years (avoid if over 50 years);
- *obesity* (avoid if body mass index $\geq$ 35 kg/m^2 unless no suitable alternative); (in adolescents, caution if obese according to BMI (adjusted for age and gender); in those who are markedly obese, avoid unless no suitable alternative);
- *migraine without aura* (avoid if *migraine with aura* (focal symptoms), *or* severe migraine frequently lasting over 72 hours despite treatment, *or* migraine treated with ergot derivatives).

▸ Migraine Women should report any increase in headache frequency or onset of focal symptoms (discontinue immediately and refer urgently to neurology expert if focal neurological symptoms not typical of aura persist for more than 1 hour).

Combined hormonal contraceptives should be stopped (pending investigation and treatment), if serious neurological effects occur, including unusual severe, prolonged headache especially if first time or getting progressively worse *or* sudden partial or complete loss of vision *or* sudden disturbance of hearing or other perceptual disorders *or* dysphasia *or* bad fainting attack or collapse *or* first unexplained epileptic seizure *or* weakness, motor disturbances, very marked numbness suddenly affecting one side or one part of body.

● INTERACTIONS → Appendix 1 combined hormonal contraceptives.

● SIDE-EFFECTS
▸ **Rare** Gallstones · systemic lupus erythematosus
▸ **Frequency not known** Abdominal cramps · absence of withdrawal bleeding · amenorrhoea after discontinuation · breast enlargement · breast secretion · breast tenderness · cervical erosion · changes in libido · changes in lipid metabolism · changes in vaginal discharge · chloasma · chorea · contact lenses may irritate · depression · fluid retention · headache · hepatic tumours · hypertension ·

irritability · leg cramps · liver impairment · nausea · nervousness · photosensitivity · reduced menstrual loss · skin reactions · thrombosis (more common when factor V Leiden present or in blood groups A, B, and AB) · visual disturbances · vomiting · 'spotting' in early cycles

SIDE-EFFECTS, FURTHER INFORMATION
▸ Breast cancer There is a small increase in the risk of having breast cancer diagnosed in women taking the combined oral contraceptive pill; this relative risk may be due to an earlier diagnosis. In users of combined oral contraceptive pills the cancers are more likely to be localised to the breast. The most important factor for diagnosing breast cancer appears to be the age at which the contraceptive is stopped rather than the duration of use; any increase in the rate of diagnosis diminishes gradually during the 10 years after stopping and disappears by 10 years.
▸ Cervical cancer Use of combined oral contraceptives for 5 years or longer is associated with a small increased risk of cervical cancer; the risk diminishes after stopping and disappears by about 10 years.

The possible small increase in the risk of breast cancer and cervical cancer should be weighed against the protective effect against cancers of the ovary and endometrium.

● PREGNANCY Not known to be harmful.

● BREAST FEEDING Avoid until weaning or for 6 months after birth (adverse effects on lactation).

● HEPATIC IMPAIRMENT Avoid in active liver disease including disorders of hepatic excretion (e.g. Dubin-Johnson or Rotor syndromes), infective hepatitis (until liver function returns to normal), liver tumours.

● DIRECTIONS FOR ADMINISTRATION
▸ With oral use Each tablet should be taken at approximately same time each day; if delayed, contraceptive protection may be lost. 21-*day combined preparations*, 1 tablet daily for 21 days; subsequent courses repeated after a 7-day interval (during which withdrawal bleeding occurs); if reasonably certain woman is not pregnant, first course can be started on any day of cycle—if starting on day 6 of cycle or later, additional precautions (barrier methods) necessary during first 7 days. *Every day (ED) combined preparations*, 1 *active* tablet daily for 21 days, followed by 1 *inactive* tablet daily for 7 days; subsequent courses repeated without interval (withdrawal bleeding occurs when *inactive* tablets being taken); if reasonably certain woman is not pregnant, first course can be started on any day of cycle—if starting on day 6 of cycle or later, additional precautions (barrier methods) necessary during first 7 days.
Changing to combined preparation containing different progestogen If previous contraceptive used correctly, or pregnancy can reasonably be excluded, start the first active tablet of new brand immediately. See individual monographs for requirements of specific preparations.
Changing from progestogen-only tablet If previous contraceptive used correctly, or pregnancy can reasonably be excluded, start new brand immediately, additional precautions (barrier methods) necessary for first 7 days.
Secondary amenorrhoea (exclude pregnancy) Start any day, additional precautions (barrier methods) necessary during first 7 days (9 days for *Qlaira*®).
After childbirth (not breast-feeding) Start 3 weeks after birth (increased risk of thrombosis if started earlier); later than 3 weeks postpartum additional precautions (barrier methods) necessary for first 7 days (9 days for *Qlaira*®).
After abortion or miscarriage Start same day.

● PATIENT AND CARER ADVICE
Missed pill The critical time for loss of contraceptive protection is when a pill is omitted at the *beginning* or *end* of a cycle (which lengthens the pill-free interval).
If a woman forgets to take a pill, it should be taken as

soon as she remembers, and the next one taken at the normal time (even if this means taking 2 pills together). A missed pill is one that is 24 or more hours late. If a woman misses only one pill, she should take an active pill as soon as she remembers and then resume normal pill-taking. No additional precautions are necessary.

If a woman misses 2 or more pills (especially from the first 7 in a packet), she may not be protected. She should take an active pill as soon as she remembers and then resume normal pill-taking. In addition, she must either abstain from sex or use an additional method of contraception such as a condom for the next 7 days. If these 7 days run beyond the end of the packet, the next packet should be started at once, omitting the pill-free interval (or, in the case of *everyday* (ED) pills, omitting the 7 inactive tablets).

Emergency contraception is recommended if 2 or more combined oral contraceptive tablets are missed from the first 7 tablets in a packet and unprotected intercourse has occurred since finishing the last packet.

Travel Women taking oral contraceptives are at an increased risk of deep vein thrombosis during travel involving long periods of immobility (over 3 hours). The risk may be reduced by appropriate exercise during the journey and possibly by wearing graduated compression hosiery.

Diarrhoea and vomiting Vomiting and persistent, severe diarrhoea can interfere with the absorption of combined oral contraceptives. If vomiting occurs within 2 hours of taking a combined oral contraceptive another pill should be taken as soon as possible. In cases of persistent vomiting or severe diarrhoea lasting more than 24 hours, additional precautions should be used during and for 7 days after recovery. If the vomiting and diarrhoea occurs during the last 7 tablets, the next pill-free interval should be omitted (in the case of ED tablets the inactive ones should be omitted).

F 476

Dienogest with estradiol valerate

● **INDICATIONS AND DOSE**

Contraception with 28-day combined preparations | **Menstrual symptoms with 28-day combined preparations**

▸ BY MOUTH

▸ Females of childbearing potential: 1 active tablet once daily for 26 days, followed by 1 inactive tablet daily for 2 days, withdrawal bleeding may occur during the 2-day interval of *inactive* tablets, tablets should be taken at approximately the same time each day

● **UNLICENSED USE** Consult product literature for the licensing status.

● **DIRECTIONS FOR ADMINISTRATION**
  ● Changing to *Qlaira®*: start the first active *Qlaira®* tablet on the day after taking the last active tablet of the previous brand

● **PATIENT AND CARER ADVICE**

Missed doses
A missed pill for a patient taking *Qlaira®* is one that is 12 hours or more late; for information on how to manage missed pills in women taking *Qlaira®*, refer to product literature.

Diarrhoea and vomiting In cases of persistent vomiting or severe diarrhoea lasting more than 12 hours in women taking *Qlaira®*, refer to product literature.

● **MEDICINAL FORMS**
There can be variation in the licensing of different medicines containing the same drug.

Tablet
▸ Dienogest with estradiol valerate (Non-proprietary)
  Dienogest 2 mg, Estradiol valerate 2 mg Estradiol valerate 2mg / Dienogest 2mg tablets | 15 tablet [PoM] no price available
  Estradiol valerate 2 mg, Dienogest 3 mg Estradiol valerate 2mg / Dienogest 3mg tablets | 51 tablet [PoM] no price available
▸ Qlaira (Bayer Plc)
  Qlaira tablets | 84 tablet [PoM] £25.18

F 476

Estradiol with nomegestrol

● **INDICATIONS AND DOSE**

Contraception

▸ BY MOUTH

▸ Females of childbearing potential: 1 active tablet daily for 24 days, followed by 1 inactive tablet daily for 4 days, to be started on day 1 of cycle with first active tablet (withdrawal bleeding occurs when inactive tablets being taken); subsequent courses repeated without interval

● **PREGNANCY** Toxicity in *animal* studies.

● **DIRECTIONS FOR ADMINISTRATION**
  ● Changing to *Zoely®*: start the first active *Zoely®* tablet on the day after taking the last active tablet of the previous brand or, at the latest, the day after the tablet-free or inactive tablet interval of the previous brand

● **PATIENT AND CARER ADVICE**
Diarrhoea and vomiting In cases of persistent vomiting or severe diarrhoea lasting more than 12 hours in women taking *Zoely®*, refer to product literature.

Missed doses
A missed pill for a patient taking *Zoely®* is one that is 12 hours or more late; for information on how to manage missed pills in women taking *Zoely®*, refer to product literature.

● **MEDICINAL FORMS**
There can be variation in the licensing of different medicines containing the same drug.

Tablet
▸ Zoely (Merck Sharp & Dohme Ltd) ▼
  Estradiol (as Estradiol hemihydrate) 1.5 mg, Nomegestrol 2.5 mg Zoely 2.5mg/1.5mg tablets | 84 tablet [PoM] £19.80 DT price = £19.80

F 476

Ethinylestradiol with desogestrel

● **INDICATIONS AND DOSE**

Contraception with 21-day combined preparations | **Menstrual symptoms with 21-day combined preparations**

▸ BY MOUTH

▸ Females of childbearing potential: 1 tablet once daily for 21 days; subsequent courses repeated after 7-day interval, withdrawal bleeding occurs during the 7-day interval, if reasonably certain woman is not pregnant, first course can be started on any day of cycle—if starting on day 6 of cycle or later, additional precautions (barrier methods) necessary during first 7 days, tablets should be taken at approximately the same time each day

● **UNLICENSED USE** Consult product literature for the licensing status.

- **MEDICINAL FORMS**
There can be variation in the licensing of different medicines containing the same drug.

Tablet
▸ Norinyl-1 (Pfizer Ltd)
  Mestranol 50 microgram, Norethisterone 1 mg Norinyl-1 tablets | 63 tablet [PoM] £2.19 DT price = £2.19

3.2 Contraception, devices

Other drugs used for Contraceptive devices
Levonorgestrel, p. 486

CONTRACEPTIVE DEVICES

Intra-uterine contraceptive devices (copper)

- **INDICATIONS AND DOSE**

Contraception
▸ BY INTRA-UTERINE ADMINISTRATION
▸ Females of childbearing potential: (consult product literature)

IMPORTANT SAFETY INFORMATION

MHRA/CHM ADVICE (JUNE 2015) INTRA-UTERINE CONTRACEPTION: UTERINE PERFORATION—UPDATED INFORMATION ON RISK FACTORS

Uterine perforation most often occurs during insertion, but might not be detected until sometime later. The risk of uterine perforation is increased when the device is inserted up to 36 weeks postpartum or in patients who are breastfeeding. Before inserting an intra-uterine contraceptive device, inform patients that perforation occurs in approximately 1 in every 1000 insertions and signs and symptoms include:

- severe pelvic pain after insertion (worse than period cramps);
- pain or increased bleeding after insertion which continues for more than a few weeks;
- sudden changes in periods;
- pain during intercourse;
- unable to feel the threads.

Patients should be informed on how to check their threads and to arrange a check-up if threads cannot be felt, especially if they also have significant pain. Partial perforation may occur even if the threads can be seen; consider this if there is severe pain following insertion and perform an ultrasound.

- **CONTRA-INDICATIONS** Active trophoblastic disease (until return to normal of urine and plasma-gonadotrophin concentration) · distorted uterine cavity · established or marked immunosuppression · genital malignancy · medical diathermy · pelvic inflammatory disease · recent sexually transmitted infection (if not fully investigated and treated) · severe anaemia · small uterine cavity · unexplained uterine bleeding · Wilson's disease
- **CAUTIONS** Anaemia · anticoagulant therapy (avoid if possible) · diabetes · disease-induced immunosuppression (risk of infection—avoid if marked immunosuppression) · drug-induced immunosuppression (risk of infection—avoid if marked immunosuppression) · endometriosis · epilepsy (risk of seizure at time of insertion) · fertility problems · history of pelvic inflammatory disease · increased risk of expulsion if inserted before uterine involution · menorrhagia (progestogen intra-uterine system might be preferable) · nulliparity · severe cervical

stenosis · severe primary dysmenorrhoea · severely scarred uterus (including after endometrial resection) · young age

CAUTIONS, FURTHER INFORMATION
An intra-uterine device should not be removed in mid-cycle unless an additional contraceptive was used for the previous 7 days. If removal is essential post-coital contraception should be considered.

▸ Risk of infection The main excess risk of infection occurs in the first 20 days after insertion and is believed to be related to existing carriage of a sexually transmitted infection. Women are considered to be at a higher risk of sexually transmitted infections if:
  - they are under 25 years old *or*
  - they are over 25 years old *and* • have a new partner *or*
  - have had more than one partner in the past year *or*
  - their regular partner has other partners.
In these women, pre-insertion screening (for chlamydia and, depending on sexual history and local prevalence of disease, *Neisseria gonorrhoeae*) should be performed. If results are unavailable at the time of fitting an intra-uterine device for emergency contraception, appropriate prophylactic antibacterial cover should be given. The woman should be advised to attend *as an emergency* if she experiences sustained pain during the next 20 days.

- **SIDE-EFFECTS** Allergy · bleeding (on insertion) · cervical perforation · displacement · dysmenorrhoea · expulsion · menorrhagia · occasionally epileptic seizure (on insertion) · pain (on insertion, alleviated by NSAID such as ibuprofen 30 minutes before insertion) · pelvic infection may be exacerbated · uterine perforation · vasovagal attack (on insertion)

SIDE-EFFECTS, FURTHER INFORMATION
▸ Presence of significant symptoms (especially pain) Advise the patient to seek medical attention promptly in case of significant symptoms.

- **ALLERGY AND CROSS-SENSITIVITY** Contra-indicated if patient has a copper allergy.
- **PREGNANCY** If an intra-uterine device fails and the woman wishes to continue to full-term the device should be removed in the first trimester if possible. Remove device; if pregnancy occurs, increased likelihood that it may be ectopic.
- **BREAST FEEDING** Not known to be harmful.
- **MONITORING REQUIREMENTS** Gynaecological examination before insertion, 6–8 weeks after insertion, then annually.
- **DIRECTIONS FOR ADMINISTRATION** The timing and technique of fitting an intra-uterine device are critical for its subsequent performance. *The healthcare professional inserting (or removing) the device should be fully trained in the technique and should provide full counselling backed, where available, by the patient information leaflet.* Devices should not be fitted during the heavy days of the period; they are best fitted after the end of menstruation and before the calculated time of implantation.
- **PRESCRIBING AND DISPENSING INFORMATION**
  UT380 STANDARD® For uterine length 6.5–9 cm; replacement every 5 years.

  NOVAPLUS T 380® AG '*Mini*' size for minimum uterine length 5 cm; '*Normal*' size for uterine length 6.5–9 cm; replacement every 5 years.

  GYNEFIX® Suitable for all uterine sizes; replacement every 5 years.

  UT380 SHORT® For uterine length 5–7 cm; replacement every 5 years.

  NOVA-T® 380 For uterine length 6.5–9 cm; replacement every 5 years.

  FLEXI-T®+ 380 For uterine length over 6 cm; replacement every 5 years.

NOVAPLUS T 380® CU 'Mini' size for minimum uterine length 5 cm; 'Normal' size for uterine length 6.5–9 cm; replacement every 5 years.

LOAD® 375 For uterine length over 7 cm; replacement every 5 years.

ANCORA® 375 CU For uterine length over 6.5 cm; replacement every 5 years.

T-SAFE® 380A QL For uterine length 6.5–9 cm; replacement every 10 years.

MULTILOAD® CU375 For uterine length 6–9 cm; replacement every 5 years.

MINI TT380® SLIMLINE For minimum uterine length 5 cm; replacement every 5 years.

COPPER T380 A® For uterine length 6.5–9 cm; replacement every 10 years.

TT380® SLIMLINE For uterine length 6.5–9 cm; replacement every 10 years.

NEO-SAFE® T380 For uterine length 6.5–9 cm; replacement every 5 years.

MULTI-SAFE® 375 For uterine length 6–9 cm; replacement every 5 years.

FLEXI-T® 300 For uterine length over 5 cm; replacement every 5 years.

● **MEDICINAL FORMS**
There can be variation in the licensing of different medicines containing the same drug.

Intra-uterine devices
▸ Intra-uterine contraceptive devices (R.F. Medical Supplies Ltd, Farla Medical Ltd, Durbin Plc, Williams Medical Supplies Ltd, Bayer Plc, Organon Laboratories Ltd)
Copper T380 A intra-uterine contraceptive device | 1 device £8.95
Steriload intra-uterine contraceptive device | 1 device £9.65
Load 375 intra-uterine contraceptive device | 1 device £8.52
Novaplus T 380 Ag intra-uterine contraceptive device mini | 1 device £12.50
T-Safe 380A QL intra-uterine contraceptive device | 1 device £10.55
UT380 Standard intra-uterine contraceptive device | 1 device £11.22
Nova-T 380 intra-uterine contraceptive device | 1 device £15.20
Flexi-T+ 380 intra-uterine contraceptive device | 1 device £10.06
Mini TT380 Slimline intra-uterine contraceptive device | 1 device £12.46
Flexi-T 300 intra-uterine contraceptive device | 1 device £9.47
Multi-Safe 375 intra-uterine contraceptive device | 1 device £8.96
Multiload Cu375 intra-uterine contraceptive device | 1 device £9.24
Optima TCu 380A intra-uterine contraceptive device | 1 device £9.65
Novaplus T 380 Ag intra-uterine contraceptive device normal | 1 device £12.50
GyneFix intra-uterine contraceptive device | 1 device £27.11
Novaplus T 380 Cu intra-uterine contraceptive device mini | 1 device £10.95
TT380 Slimline intra-uterine contraceptive device | 1 device £12.46
Ancora 375 Cu intra-uterine contraceptive device | 1 device £7.95
Novaplus T 380 Cu intra-uterine contraceptive device normal | 1 device £10.95
Neo-Safe T380 intra-uterine contraceptive device | 1 device £13.40
UT380 Short intra-uterine contraceptive device | 1 device £11.22

Vaginal contraceptives

● **SILICONE CONTRACEPTIVE DIAPHRAGMS**
Milex arcing spring silicone diaphragm 60mm (Durbin Plc)
1 device · NHS indicative price = £10.21 · Drug Tariff (Part IXa)

Milex arcing spring silicone diaphragm 65mm (Durbin Plc)
1 device · NHS indicative price = £10.21 · Drug Tariff (Part IXa)

Milex arcing spring silicone diaphragm 70mm (Durbin Plc)
1 device · NHS indicative price = £10.21 · Drug Tariff (Part IXa)

Milex arcing spring silicone diaphragm 75mm (Durbin Plc)
1 device · NHS indicative price = £10.21 · Drug Tariff (Part IXa)

Milex arcing spring silicone diaphragm 80mm (Durbin Plc)
1 device · NHS indicative price = £10.21 · Drug Tariff (Part IXa)

Milex arcing spring silicone diaphragm 85mm (Durbin Plc)
1 device · NHS indicative price = £10.21 · Drug Tariff (Part IXa)

Milex arcing spring silicone diaphragm 90mm (Durbin Plc)
1 device · NHS indicative price = £10.21 · Drug Tariff (Part IXa)

Milex omniflex coil spring silicone diaphragm 60mm (Durbin Plc)
1 device · NHS indicative price = £10.21 · Drug Tariff (Part IXa)

Milex omniflex coil spring silicone diaphragm 65mm (Durbin Plc)
1 device · NHS indicative price = £10.21 · Drug Tariff (Part IXa)

Milex omniflex coil spring silicone diaphragm 70mm (Durbin Plc)
1 device · NHS indicative price = £10.21 · Drug Tariff (Part IXa)

Milex omniflex coil spring silicone diaphragm 75mm (Durbin Plc)
1 device · NHS indicative price = £10.21 · Drug Tariff (Part IXa)

Milex omniflex coil spring silicone diaphragm 80mm (Durbin Plc)
1 device · NHS indicative price = £10.21 · Drug Tariff (Part IXa)

Milex omniflex coil spring silicone diaphragm 85mm (Durbin Plc)
1 device · NHS indicative price = £10.21 · Drug Tariff (Part IXa)

Milex omniflex coil spring silicone diaphragm 90mm (Durbin Plc)
1 device · NHS indicative price = £10.21 · Drug Tariff (Part IXa)

Ortho All-Flex arcing spring silicone diaphragm 65mm (Janssen-Cilag Ltd)
1 device · NHS indicative price = £8.35 · Drug Tariff (Part IXa)

Ortho All-Flex arcing spring silicone diaphragm 70mm (Janssen-Cilag Ltd)
1 device · NHS indicative price = £8.35 · Drug Tariff (Part IXa)

Ortho All-Flex arcing spring silicone diaphragm 75mm (Janssen-Cilag Ltd)
1 device · NHS indicative price = £8.35 · Drug Tariff (Part IXa)

Ortho All-Flex arcing spring silicone diaphragm 80mm (Janssen-Cilag Ltd)
1 device · NHS indicative price = £8.35 · Drug Tariff (Part IXa)

● **SILICONE CONTRACEPTIVE PESSARIES**
FemCap 22mm (Durbin Plc)
1 device · NHS indicative price = £15.29 · Drug Tariff (Part IXa)

FemCap 26mm (Durbin Plc)
1 device · NHS indicative price = £15.29 · Drug Tariff (Part IXa)

FemCap 30mm (Durbin Plc)
1 device · NHS indicative price = £15.29 · Drug Tariff (Part IXa)

3.3 Contraception, emergency

Other drugs used for Contraception, emergency Intra-uterine contraceptive devices (copper), p. 483 · Levonorgestrel, p. 486

PROGESTERONE RECEPTOR MODULATORS

Ulipristal acetate

● **DRUG ACTION** Ulipristal acetate is a progesterone receptor modulator with a partial progesterone antagonist effect.

● **INDICATIONS AND DOSE**
Emergency contraception
▸ BY MOUTH
▸ Females of childbearing potential: 30 mg for 1 dose, to be taken as soon as possible after coitus, but no later than after 120 hours

● **CONTRA-INDICATIONS** Repeated use as an emergency contraceptive within a menstrual cycle

● **CAUTIONS** Uncontrolled severe asthma

● **INTERACTIONS** → Appendix 1: ulipristal

● **SIDE-EFFECTS**
▸ **Common or very common** Abdominal pain · back pain · diarrhoea · dizziness · fatigue · gastro-intestinal disturbances · headache · menstrual irregularities · muscle spasms · nausea · vomiting

▸ **Uncommon** Blurred vision · breast tenderness · dry mouth · hot flushes · pruritus · rash · tremor · uterine spasm

● **CONCEPTION AND CONTRACEPTION** When ulipristal is given as an emergency contraceptive the effectiveness of combined hormonal and progestogen-only contraceptives may be reduced—additional precautions (barrier methods) required for 14 days for combined and parenteral progestogen-only hormonal contraceptives (16 days for *Qlaira*®) and 9 days for oral progestogen-only contraceptives.

● **PREGNANCY** Limited information available when used as an emergency contraceptive.

● **BREAST FEEDING** In emergency contraception manufacturer advises avoid for 1 week after administration—present in milk.

● **HEPATIC IMPAIRMENT** Manufacturer advises avoid in severe impairment—no information available.

● **MEDICINAL FORMS**
There can be variation in the licensing of different medicines containing the same drug.

Tablet
▸ **Ellaone** (HRA Pharma UK Ltd)
  Ulipristal acetate 30 mg EllaOne 30mg tablets | 1 tablet Ⓟ £14.05
▸ **Esmya** (Gedeon Richter (UK) Ltd)
  Ulipristal acetate 5 mg Esmya 5mg tablets | 28 tablet PoM £114.13

3.4 Contraception, oral progestogen-only

Other drugs used for Contraception, oral progestogen-only Norethisterone, p. 458

PROGESTOGENS

Desogestrel

● **INDICATIONS AND DOSE**

Contraception
▸ BY MOUTH
▸ Females of childbearing potential: 75 micrograms daily, dose to be taken at same time each day, starting on day 1 of cycle then continuously, if administration delayed for 12 hours or more it should be regarded as a 'missed pill'

● **UNLICENSED USE** Consult product literature for the licensing status of individual preparations.

● **CONTRA-INDICATIONS** Acute porphyrias p. 577 · history of breast cancer but can be used after 5 years if no evidence of disease and non-hormonal contraceptive methods unacceptable · severe arterial disease · undiagnosed vaginal bleeding

● **CAUTIONS** Active trophoblastic disease (until return to normal of urine- and plasma-gonadotrophin concentration)—seek specialist advice · arterial disease · functional ovarian cysts · history of jaundice in pregnancy · malabsorption syndromes · past ectopic pregnancy · sex-steroid dependent cancer · systemic lupus erythematosus with positive (or unknown) antiphospholipid antibodies
CAUTIONS, FURTHER INFORMATION
▸ Other conditions The product literature advises caution in patients with history of thromboembolism, hypertension, diabetes mellitus and migraine; evidence for caution in these conditions is unsatisfactory.

● **INTERACTIONS** → Appendix 1: desogestrel

● **SIDE-EFFECTS** Breast discomfort · changes in libido · depression · disturbance of appetite · dizziness · headache · menstrual irregularities · nausea · skin disorders · vomiting
SIDE-EFFECTS, FURTHER INFORMATION
▸ Breast cancer There is a small increase in the risk of having breast cancer diagnosed in women using, or who have recently used, a progestogen-only contraceptive pill; this relative risk may be due to an earlier diagnosis. The most important risk factor appears to be the age at which the contraceptive is stopped rather than the duration of use; the risk disappears gradually during the 10 years after stopping and there is no excess risk by 10 years. A possible small increase in the risk of breast cancer should be weighed against the benefits.

● **PREGNANCY** Not known to be harmful.

● **BREAST FEEDING** Progestogen-only contraceptives do not affect lactation.

● **HEPATIC IMPAIRMENT** Caution in severe liver disease and recurrent cholestatic jaundice. Avoid in liver tumour.

● **PATIENT AND CARER ADVICE**
Surgery All progestogen-only contraceptives are suitable for use as an alternative to combined hormonal contraceptives before major elective surgery, before all surgery to the legs, or before surgery which involves prolonged immobilisation of a lower limb.
Starting routine One tablet daily, on a continuous basis, starting on day 1 of cycle and taken at the same time each day (if delayed by longer than 12 hours contraceptive protection may be lost). Additional contraceptive precautions are not required if desogestrel is started up to and including day 5 of the menstrual cycle; if started after this time, additional contraceptive precautions are required for 2 days.
Changing from a combined oral contraceptive Start on the day following completion of the combined oral contraceptive course without a break (or in the case of ED tablets omitting the inactive ones).
After childbirth Oral progestogen-only contraceptives can be started up to and including day 21 postpartum without the need for additional contraceptive precautions. If started more than 21 days postpartum, additional contraceptive precautions are required for 2 days.
Diarrhoea and vomiting Vomiting and persistent, severe diarrhoea can interfere with the absorption of oral progestogen-only contraceptives. If vomiting occurs within 2 hours of taking desogestrel, another pill should be taken as soon as possible. If a replacement pill is not taken within 12 hours of the normal time for taking desogestrel, or in cases of persistent vomiting or very severe diarrhoea, additional precautions should be used during illness and for 2 days after recovery.

Missed doses
The following advice is recommended: 'If you forget a pill, take it as soon as you remember and carry on with the next pill at the right time. If the pill was more than 12 hours overdue you are not protected. Continue normal pill-taking but you must also use another method, such as the condom, for the next 2 days'.
  The Faculty of Sexual and Reproductive Healthcare recommends emergency contraception if one or more tablets are missed or taken more than 12 hours late and unprotected intercourse has occurred before 2 further tablets have been correctly taken.

● **NATIONAL FUNDING/ACCESS DECISIONS**
Scottish Medicines Consortium (SMC) Decisions
The *Scottish Medicines Consortium* has advised (September 2003) that *Cerazette*® should be restricted for use in women who cannot tolerate oestrogen-containing contraceptives or in whom such preparations are contra-indicated.

7

Genito-urinary system

Genito-urinary system

7

● MEDICINAL FORMS
There can be variation in the licensing of different medicines
containing the same drug.

Tablet

▸ **Desogestrel (Non-proprietary)**
Desogestrel 75 microgram Desogestrel 75microgram tablets |
84 tablet [PoM] £9.55 DT price = £2.17

▸ **Aizea** (Besins Healthcare (UK) Ltd)
Desogestrel 75 microgram Aizea 75microgram tablets |
84 tablet [PoM] £5.21 DT price = £2.17

▸ **Cerazette** (Merck Sharp & Dohme Ltd)
Desogestrel 75 microgram Cerazette 75microgram tablets |
84 tablet [PoM] £9.55 DT price = £2.17

▸ **Cerelle** (Consilient Health Ltd)
Desogestrel 75 microgram Cerelle 75microgram tablets |
84 tablet [PoM] £3.50 DT price = £2.17

▸ **Desomono** (MedRx Licences Ltd)
Desogestrel 75 microgram Desomono 75microgram tablets |
84 tablet [PoM] £7.49 DT price = £2.17

▸ **Desorex** (Somex Pharma)
Desogestrel 75 microgram Desorex 75microgram tablets |
84 tablet [PoM] £6.70 DT price = £2.17

▸ **Feanolla** (Lupin (Europe) Ltd)
Desogestrel 75 microgram Feanolla 75microgram tablets |
84 tablet [PoM] £3.49 DT price = £2.17

▸ **Nacrez** (Teva UK Ltd)
Desogestrel 75 microgram Nacrez 75microgram tablets |
84 tablet [PoM] £3.50 DT price = £2.17

▸ **Zelleta** (Morningside Healthcare Ltd)
Desogestrel 75 microgram Zelleta 75microgram tablets |
84 tablet [PoM] £3.35 DT price = £2.17

Levonorgestrel

18-Feb-2016

● INDICATIONS AND DOSE

Emergency contraception

▸ BY MOUTH

▸ Females of childbearing potential: 1.5 mg for 1 dose,
taken as soon as possible after coitus, preferably within
12 hours but no later than after 72 hours

Contraception

▸ BY MOUTH

▸ Females of childbearing potential: 1 tablet daily starting
on day 1 of the cycle then continuously, dose is to be
taken at the same time each day, if administration
delayed for 3 hours or more it should be regarded as a
"missed pill"

JAYDESS ® 13.5MG INTRA-UTERINE DEVICE

Contraception

▸ BY VAGINA

▸ Females of childbearing potential: Insert into uterine
cavity within 7 days of onset of menstruation, or any
time if replacement, or immediately after first-
trimester termination; postpartum insertions should
be delayed until at least 6 weeks after delivery
(12 weeks if uterus involution is substantially delayed);
effective for 3 years

LEVOSERT ® 20MICROGRAMS/24HOURS INTRA-UTERINE DEVICE

Contraception | Menorrhagia

▸ BY INTRA-UTERINE ADMINISTRATION

▸ Females of childbearing potential: Insert into uterine
cavity within 7 days of onset of menstruation, or any
time if replacement, or immediately after first-
trimester abortion; postpartum insertions should be
delayed until at least 6 weeks after delivery; effective
for 3 years

MIRENA® 20MICROGRAMS/24HOURS INTRA-UTERINE DEVICE

Contraception | Menorrhagia

▸ BY INTRA-UTERINE ADMINISTRATION

▸ Females of childbearing potential: Insert into uterine
cavity within 7 days of onset of menstruation, or any
time if replacement, or any time if reasonably certain
woman is not pregnant and there is no risk of
conception (additional precautions (e.g. barrier
methods) necessary for next 7 days), or immediately
after first-trimester termination by curettage;
postpartum insertions should be delayed until at least
4 weeks after delivery; effective for 5 years

Prevention of endometrial hyperplasia during oestrogen replacement therapy

▸ BY INTRA-UTERINE ADMINISTRATION

▸ Females of childbearing potential: Insert during last days
of menstruation or withdrawal bleeding or at any time
if amenorrhoeic; effective for 4 years

DOSE ADJUSTMENTS DUE TO INTERACTIONS

When used orally as an emergency contraceptive, the
effectiveness of levonorgestrel is reduced in women
taking enzyme-inducing drugs (and for up to 4 weeks
after stopping); a copper intra-uterine device should
preferably be used instead. If the copper intra-uterine
device is undesirable or inappropriate, the dose of
levonorgestrel should be increased to a total of 3 mg
taken as a single dose [unlicensed dose—advise women
accordingly]; pregnancy should be excluded following
use, and medical advice sought if pregnancy occurs.
There is no need to increase the dose for emergency
contraception if the patient is taking antibacterials that
are not enzyme inducers.

With the progestogen-only intra-uterine device,
levonorgestrel is released close to the site of the main
contraceptive action (on cervical mucus and
endometrium) and therefore progestogenic side-effects
and interactions are less likely; in particular, enzyme-
inducing drugs are unlikely to significantly reduce the
contraceptive effect of the progestogen-only intra-
uterine system and additional contraceptive precautions
are not required.

● UNLICENSED USE

▸ With oral use Consult product literature for licensing status
of individual preparations.

▸ With vaginal use Not licensed for use in women under
18 years.

IMPORTANT SAFETY INFORMATION

MHRA/CHM ADVICE (JUNE 2015) INTRA-UTERINE
CONTRACEPTION: UTERINE PERFORATION—UPDATED
INFORMATION ON RISK FACTORS

Uterine perforation most often occurs during insertion,
but might not be detected until some time later. The risk
of uterine perforation is increased when the device is
inserted up to 36 weeks postpartum or in patients who
are breastfeeding. Before inserting an intra-uterine
contraceptive device, inform patients that perforation
occurs in approximately 1 in every 1000 insertions and
signs and symptoms include:
● severe pelvic pain after insertion (worse than period
cramps);
● pain or increased bleeding after insertion which
continues for more than a few weeks;
● sudden changes in periods;
● pain during intercourse;
● unable to feel the threads.
Patients should be informed on how to check their
threads and to arrange a check-up if threads cannot be
felt, especially if they also have significant pain. Partial
perforation may occur even if the threads can be seen;

consider this if there is severe pain following insertion and perform an ultrasound.

● **CONTRA-INDICATIONS**

▸ With intra-uterine use Active trophoblastic disease (until return to normal of urine- and plasma-gonadotrophin concentration · acute cervicitis · acute vaginitis · distorted uterine cavity · established immunosuppression · genital malignancy · history of breast cancer but can be considered for a woman in long-term remission who has menorrhagia and requires effective contraception · infected abortion during the previous three months · marked immunosuppression · not suitable for emergency contraception · pelvic inflammatory disease · postpartum endometritis · recent sexually transmitted infection (if not fully investigated and treated) · severe anaemia · small uterine cavity · unexplained uterine bleeding

▸ With oral use Acute porphyrias p. 577

▸ With oral use for contraception History of breast cancer but can be used after 5 years if no evidence of disease and non-hormonal contraceptive methods unacceptable · severe arterial disease · undiagnosed vaginal bleeding

● **CAUTIONS**

▸ With intra-uterine use Disease-induced immunosuppression (risk of infection—avoid if marked immunosuppression) · anaemia · anticoagulant therapy (avoid if possible) · diabetes · drug-induced immunosuppression (risk of infection—avoid if marked immunosuppression) · endometriosis · epilepsy (risk of seizure at time of insertion) · fertility problems · history of pelvic inflammatory disease · increased risk of expulsion if inserted before uterine involution · menorrhagia (progestogen intra-uterine system might be preferable) · nulliparity · severe cervical stenosis · severe primary dysmenorrhoea · severely scarred uterus (including after endometrial resection) · young age

▸ With oral use for contraception Active trophoblastic disease (until return to normal of urine- and plasma-gonadotrophin concentration)—seek specialist advice · arterial disease · functional ovarian cysts · history of jaundice in pregnancy · malabsorption syndromes · past ectopic pregnancy · sex-steroid dependent cancer · systemic lupus erythematosus with positive (or unknown) antiphospholipid antibodies

▸ When used for emergency contraception Active trophoblastic disease (until return to normal of urine- and plasma-gonadotrophin concentration)—seek specialist advice · past ectopic pregnancy · severe malabsorption syndromes

CAUTIONS, FURTHER INFORMATION

An intra-uterine device should not be removed in mid-cycle unless an additional contraceptive was used for the previous 7 days. If removal is essential post-coital contraception should be considered.

▸ Risk of infection with intra-uterine devices The main excess risk of infection occurs in the first 20 days after insertion and is believed to be related to existing carriage of a sexually transmitted infection. Women are considered to be at a higher risk of sexually transmitted infections if:

● they are under 25 years old *or*
● they are over 25 years old *and*
● have a new partner *or*
● have had more than one partner in the past year *or*
● their regular partner has other partners.

In these women, pre-insertion screening (for chlamydia and, depending on sexual history and local prevalence of disease, *Neisseria gonorrhoeae*) should be performed. If results are unavailable at the time of fitting an intra-uterine device for emergency contraception, appropriate prophylactic antibacterial cover should be given. The woman should be advised to attend *as an emergency* if she experiences sustained pain during the next 20 days.

▸ Use as a contraceptive in co-morbidities

▸ With oral use The product literature advises caution in patients with history of thromboembolism, hypertension, diabetes meillitus and migraine; evidence for caution in these conditions is unsatisfactory.

MIRENA®20MICROGRAMS/24HOURS INTRA-UTERINE DEVICE Advanced uterine atrophy

● **INTERACTIONS** → Appendix 1: levonorgestrel

● **SIDE-EFFECTS**

GENERAL SIDE-EFFECTS

▸ **Common or very common** Depression (sometimes severe) · headache · nausea

▸ **Frequency not known** Vomiting

SPECIFIC SIDE-EFFECTS

▸ **Common or very common**

▸ With intra-uterine use Changes in the pattern and duration of menstrual bleeding (spotting or prolonged bleeding) · abdominal pain · acne · alopecia · back pain · breast pain · expulsion · hirsutism · migraine · nervousness · pelvic pain · peripheral oedema · salpingitis

▸ **Uncommon**

▸ With intra-uterine use Abdominal distension · cervicitis · eczema · pelvic inflammatory disease · pruritus · skin hyperpigmentation

▸ **Rare**

▸ With intra-uterine use Rash · uterine perforation

▸ **Frequency not known**

▸ With intra-uterine use Functional ovarian cysts (usually asymptomatic and usually resolve spontaneously—ultrasound monitoring recommended) · allergy · bleeding (on insertion) · cervical perforation · displacement · dysmenorrhoea · epileptic seizures (on insertion) · menorrhagia · pain (on insertion, alleviated by NSAID such as ibuprofen 30 minutes before insertion) · pelvic infection may be exacerbated · vasovagal attack (on insertion)

▸ With oral use Breast discomfort · breast tenderness · changes in libido · disturbances of appetite · dizziness · fatigue · menstrual irregularities · skin disorders

SIDE-EFFECTS, FURTHER INFORMATION

▸ Breast cancer There is a small increase in the risk of having breast cancer diagnosed in women using, or who have recently used, a progestogen-only contraceptive pill; this relative risk may be due to an earlier diagnosis. The most important risk factor appears to be the age at which the contraceptive is stopped rather than the duration of use; the risk disappears gradually during the 10 years after stopping and there is no excess risk by 10 years. A possible small increase in the risk of breast cancer should be weighed against the benefits.

Although the progestogen-only intra-uterine system produces little systemic progestogenic activity, it is usually avoided for 5 years after any evidence of breast cancer. However, the system can be considered for a woman in long-term remission from breast cancer who has menorrhagia and requires effective contraception.

▸ With intra-uterine use Endometrial disorders should be ruled out before insertion and the patient should be fully counselled (and provided with a patient information leaflet). Improvement in progestogenic side-effects, such as mastalgia and in the bleeding pattern may often become very light or absent.

▸ With intra-uterine use Removal of the intra-uterine system should be considered if the patient experiences migraine or severe headache, jaundice, marked increase of blood pressure, or severe arterial disease.

● **PREGNANCY**

▸ With oral use Not known to be harmful.

▸ With vaginal use If an intra-uterine device fails and the woman wishes to continue to full-term the device should be removed in the first trimester if possible. Avoid; if pregnancy occurs remove intra-uterine system.

7

Genito-urinary system

- **BREAST FEEDING** Progestogen-only contraceptives do not affect lactation.
- **HEPATIC IMPAIRMENT** Caution in severe liver disease and recurrent cholestatic jaundice. Avoid in liver tumour.
- **MONITORING REQUIREMENTS**
▸ With intra-uterine use Gynaecological examination before insertion, 4–6 weeks after insertion, then annually.
- **DIRECTIONS FOR ADMINISTRATION**
▸ With intra-uterine use *The doctor or nurse administering (or removing) the system should be fully trained in the technique and should provide full counselling reinforced by the patient information leaflet.*
- **PRESCRIBING AND DISPENSING INFORMATION**
▸ With intra-uterine use Levonorgestrel-releasing intra-uterine devices vary in licensed indication, duration of use and insertion technique—the MHRA recommends to prescribe and dispense by brand name to avoid inadvertent switching.

MIRENA®20MICROGRAMS/24HOURS INTRA-UTERINE DEVICE When system is removed (and not immediately replaced) and pregnancy is not desired, remove during the first few days of menstruation, otherwise additional precautions (e.g. barrier methods) should be used for at least 7 days before removal.

JAYDESS® 13.5MG INTRA-UTERINE DEVICE When system is removed (and not immediately replaced) and pregnancy is not desired, remove within 7 days of the onset of menstruation; additional precautions (e.g. barrier methods) should be used if the system is removed at some other time during the cycle and there is intercourse within 7 days.

LEVONELLE® ONE STEP Can be sold to women over 16 years; when supplying emergency contraception to the public, pharmacists should refer to guidance issued by the Royal Pharmaceutical Society.

- **PATIENT AND CARER ADVICE**
Diarrhoea and vomiting with use as an oral contraceptive
Vomiting and persistent, severe diarrhoea can interfere with the absorption of oral progestogen-only contraceptives. If vomiting occurs within 2 hours of taking an oral progestogen-only contraceptive, another pill should be taken as soon as possible. If a replacement pill is not taken within 3 hours of the normal time for taking the progestogen-only pill, or in cases of persistent vomiting or very severe diarrhoea, additional precautions should be used during illness and for 2 days after recovery.

Missed doses
When used as an oral contraceptive, the following advice is recommended 'If you forget a pill, take it as soon as you remember and carry on with the next pill at the right time. If the pill was more than 3 hours overdue you are not protected. Continue normal pill-taking but you must also use another method, such as the condom, for the next 2 days'.

The Faculty of Sexual and Reproductive Healthcare recommends emergency contraception if one or more progestogen-only contraceptive tablets are missed or taken more than 3 hours late and unprotected intercourse has occurred before 2 further tablets have been correctly taken.

Starting routine
▸ With oral use for Contraception One tablet daily, on a continuous basis, starting on day 1 of cycle and taken at the same time each day (if delayed by longer than 3 hours contraceptive protection may be lost). Additional contraceptive precautions are not required if levonorgestrel is started up to and including day 5 of the menstrual cycle; if started after this time, additional contraceptive precautions are required for 2 days.
Changing from a combined oral contraceptive Start on the day following completion of the combined oral contraceptive

course without a break (or in the case of ED tablets omitting the inactive ones).
After childbirth Oral progestogen-only contraceptives can be started up to and including day 21 postpartum without the need for additional contraceptive precautions. If started more than 21 days postpartum, additional contraceptive precautions are required for 2 days.
▸ With intra-uterine use Counsel women to seek medical attention promptly in case of significant symptoms, especially pain. Patient counselling advised. Patient information leaflet to be provided.
▸ With oral use for Emergency contraception If vomiting occurs within 2 hours of taking levonorgestrel, a replacement dose should be given.
▸ With oral use for Emergency contraception
When prescribing or supplying hormonal emergency contraception, women should be advised:
- that their next period may be early or late;
- that a barrier method of contraception needs to be used until the next period;
- to seek medical attention promptly if any lower abdominal pain occurs because this could signify an ectopic pregnancy;
- to return in 3 to 4 weeks if the subsequent menstrual bleed is abnormally light, heavy or brief, or is absent, or if she is otherwise concerned (if there is any doubt as to whether menstruation has occurred, a pregnancy test should be performed at least 3 weeks after unprotected intercourse).

- **EXCEPTIONS TO LEGAL CATEGORY** *Levonelle® One Step* can be sold to women over 16 years; when supplying emergency contraception to the public, pharmacists should refer to guidance issued by the Royal Pharmaceutical Society.

- **MEDICINAL FORMS**
There can be variation in the licensing of different medicines containing the same drug.
Intra-uterine device
▸ Jaydess (Bayer Plc) ▼
Levonorgestrel 13.5 mg Jaydess 13.5mg intra-uterine device | 1 device [PoM] £69.22
▸ Levosert (Allergan Ltd)
Levonorgestrel 20 microgram per 24 hour Levosert 20micrograms/24hours intra-uterine device | 1 device [PoM] £66.00 DT price = £88.00
▸ Mirena (Bayer Plc)
Levonorgestrel 20 microgram per 24 hour Mirena 20micrograms/24hours intra-uterine device | 1 device [PoM] £88.00 DT price = £88.00
Tablet
▸ Levonorgestrel (Non-proprietary)
Levonorgestrel 1.5 mg Levonorgestrel 1.5mg tablets | 1 tablet [P] £13.83 DT price = £5.20 | 1 tablet [PoM] £3.74–£5.20 DT price = £5.20
▸ Emerres (Morningside Healthcare Ltd)
Levonorgestrel 1.5 mg Emerres Una 1.5mg tablets | 1 tablet [P] £13.83 DT price = £5.20
Emerres 1.5mg tablets | 1 tablet [PoM] £3.35 DT price = £5.20
▸ Ezinelle (Mylan Ltd)
Levonorgestrel 1.5 mg Ezinelle 1.5mg tablets | 1 tablet [PoM] £9.64 DT price = £5.20
▸ Levonelle (Bayer Plc)
Levonorgestrel 1.5 mg Levonelle 1500microgram tablets | 1 tablet [PoM] £5.20 DT price = £5.20
Levonelle One Step 1.5mg tablets | 1 tablet [P] £13.83 DT price = £5.20
▸ Norgeston (Bayer Plc)
Levonorgestrel 30 microgram Norgeston 30microgram tablets | 35 tablet [PoM] £0.92 DT price = £0.92
▸ Upostelle (Consilient Health Ltd)
Levonorgestrel 1.5 mg Upostelle 1500microgram tablets | 1 tablet [PoM] £3.75 DT price = £5.20

3.5 Contraception, parenteral progestogen-only

Other drugs used for Contraception, parenteral progestogen-only Norethisterone, p. 458

PROGESTOGENS

Etonogestrel
27-Sep-2016

- **INDICATIONS AND DOSE**

Contraception (no hormonal contraceptive use in previous month)
▶ BY SUBDERMAL IMPLANTATION
▸ Females of childbearing potential: 1 implant inserted during first 5 days of cycle, implant should be removed within 3 years of insertion

Contraception (postpartum)
▶ BY SUBDERMAL IMPLANTATION
▸ Females of childbearing potential: 1 implant to be inserted 21–28 days after delivery (delay until 28 days postpartum if breast-feeding), implant should be removed within 3 years of insertion

Contraception following abortion or miscarriage in the second trimester
▶ BY SUBDERMAL IMPLANTATION
▸ Females of childbearing potential: 1 implant to be inserted 21–28 days after abortion or miscarriage, implant should be removed within 3 years of insertion

Contraception following abortion or miscarriage in the first trimester
▶ BY SUBDERMAL IMPLANTATION
▸ Females of childbearing potential: 1 implant to be inserted within 5 days after abortion or miscarriage, implant should be removed within 3 years of insertion

Contraception (changing from other hormonal contraceptive)
▶ BY SUBDERMAL IMPLANTATION
▸ Females of childbearing potential: Implant should be removed within 3 years of insertion (consult product literature)

- **UNLICENSED USE** *Nexplanon*® not licensed for use in females outside of the age range 18–40 years.

> **IMPORTANT SAFETY INFORMATION**
> MHRA/CHM ADVICE (JUNE 2016): *NEXPLANON*® (ETONOGESTREL) CONTRACEPTIVE IMPLANTS: REPORTS OF DEVICE IN VASCULATURE AND LUNG
> There have been rare reports of *Nexplanon*® implants reaching the lung via the pulmonary artery. An implant that cannot be palpated at its insertion site should be located and removed as soon as possible; if unable to locate implant within the arm, the MHRA recommends using chest imaging. Correct subdermal insertion reduces the risk of these events.

- **CONTRA-INDICATIONS** Acute porphyria · history of breast cancer but can be used after 5 years if no evidence of disease and non-hormonal contraceptive methods unacceptable · severe arterial disease · undiagnosed vaginal bleeding
- **CAUTIONS** Active trophoblastic disease (until return to normal of urine- and plasma-gonadotrophin concentration)—seek specialist advice · arterial disease · disturbances of lipid metabolism · history during pregnancy of deterioration of otosclerosis · history during pregnancy of pruritus · history of jaundice in pregnancy ·

malabsorption syndromes · possible risk of breast cancer · sex-steroid dependent cancer · systemic lupus erythematosus with positive (or unknown) antiphospholipid antibodies
- **INTERACTIONS** → Appendix 1: etonogestrel
- **SIDE-EFFECTS** Breast discomfort · changes in libido · depression · disturbance of appetite · dizziness · headache · injection-site reactions · menstrual irregularities · nausea · vomiting

SIDE-EFFECTS, FURTHER INFORMATION
▸ Cervical cancer Use of injectable progestogen-only contraceptives may be associated with a small increased risk of cervical cancer, similar to that seen with combined oral contraceptives. The risk of cervical cancer with other progestogen-only contraceptives is not yet known.
▸ Breast cancer There is a small increase in the risk of having breast cancer diagnosed in women using, or who have recently used, a progestogen-only contraceptive pill; this relative risk may be due to an earlier diagnosis. The most important risk factor appears to be the age at which the contraceptive is stopped rather than the duration of use; the risk disappears gradually during the 10 years after stopping and there is no excess risk by 10 years. A possible small increase in the risk of breast cancer should be weighed against the benefits.

- **PREGNANCY** Not known to be harmful, remove implant if pregnancy occurs.
- **BREAST FEEDING** Progestogen-only contraceptives do not affect lactation.
- **DIRECTIONS FOR ADMINISTRATION** The doctor or nurse administering (or removing) the system should be fully trained in the technique and should provide full counselling reinforced by the patient information leaflet.
- **PATIENT AND CARER ADVICE** Full counselling backed by patient information leaflet required before administration.

- **MEDICINAL FORMS**
There can be variation in the licensing of different medicines containing the same drug.
Implant
▸ Etonogestrel (Non-proprietary)
   Etonogestrel 68 mg Etonogestrel 68mg implant | 1 device [PoM] no price available DT price = £83.43
▸ Nexplanon (Merck Sharp & Dohme Ltd)
   Etonogestrel 68 mg Nexplanon 68mg implant | 1 device [PoM] £83.43 DT price = £83.43

Medroxyprogesterone acetate
24-May-2017

- **INDICATIONS AND DOSE**

Contraception
▶ BY DEEP INTRAMUSCULAR INJECTION
▸ Females of childbearing potential: 150 mg, to be administered within the first 5 days of cycle or within first 5 days after parturition (delay until 6 weeks after parturition if breast-feeding)
▶ BY SUBCUTANEOUS INJECTION
▸ Females of childbearing potential: 104 mg, to be administered within first 5 days of cycle or within 5 days postpartum (delay until 6 weeks postpartum if breast-feeding), injected into anterior thigh or abdomen, dose only suitable if no hormonal contraceptive use in previous month

Long-term contraception
▶ BY DEEP INTRAMUSCULAR INJECTION
▸ Females of childbearing potential: 150 mg every 12 weeks, first dose to be administered within the first 5 days of cycle or within first 5 days after parturition (delay until 6 weeks after parturition if breast-feeding)
continued →

7

Genito-urinary system

▶ BY SUBCUTANEOUS INJECTION
▶ Females of childbearing potential: 104 mg every 13 weeks, first dose to be administered within first 5 days of cycle or within 5 days postpartum (delay until 6 weeks postpartum if breast-feeding), injected into anterior thigh or abdomen, dose only suitable if no hormonal contraceptive use in previous month

Contraception (when patient changing from other hormonal contraceptive)
▶ BY SUBCUTANEOUS INJECTION
▶ Females of childbearing potential: (consult product literature)

● **UNLICENSED USE** EvGr Not licensed for the treatment of hot flushes caused by long-term androgen suppression in men. ⒶA

● **CONTRA-INDICATIONS** Acute porphyrias p. 577 · history of breast cancer but can be used after 5 years if no evidence of disease and non-hormonal contraceptive methods unacceptable · severe arterial disease · undiagnosed vaginal bleeding

● **CAUTIONS** History during pregnancy in disturbances of lipid metabolism · history during pregnancy of deterioration of otosclerosis · history during pregnancy of pruritus · possible risk of breast cancer

● **INTERACTIONS** → Appendix 1: medroxyprogesterone

● **SIDE-EFFECTS**
▶ **Rare** Osteoporosis · osteoporotic fractures
▶ **Frequency not known** Breast discomfort · changes in libido · depression · Disturbance of appetite · dizziness · headache · indigestion · injection site-reactions · loss of vision during treatment (discontinue treatment if papilloedema or retinal vascular lesions) · menstrual irregularities · nausea · reduced bone mineral density · skin disorders · vomiting · weight gain

SIDE-EFFECTS, FURTHER INFORMATION
Reduction in bone mineral density occurs in the first 2–3 years of use then stabilises.
▶ Cervical cancer Use of injectable progestogen-only contraceptives may be associated with a small increased risk of cervical cancer, similar to that seen with combined oral contraceptives. The risk of cervical cancer with other progestogen-only contraceptives is not yet known.

● **CONCEPTION AND CONTRACEPTION**
▶ With intramuscular use If interval between dose is greater than 12 weeks and 5 days (in long-term contraception), rule out pregnancy before next injection and advise patient to use additional contraceptive measures (e.g. barrier) for 14 days after the injection.
▶ With subcutaneous use If interval between dose is greater than 13 weeks and 7 days (in long-term contraception), rule out pregnancy before next injection.

● **PREGNANCY** Not known to be harmful.

● **BREAST FEEDING** Present in milk—no adverse effects reported. Progestogen-only contraceptives do not affect lactation.
The manufacturers advise that in women who are breast-feeding, the first dose should be delayed until 6 weeks after birth; however, evidence suggests no harmful effect to infant if given earlier. The benefits of using medroxyprogesterone acetate in breast-feeding women outweigh any risks.

● **HEPATIC IMPAIRMENT** Avoid in liver tumour. Caution in severe liver disease and recurrent cholestatic jaundice.

● **PATIENT AND CARER ADVICE** Full counselling backed by *patient information leaflet* required before administration—likelihood of menstrual disturbance and the potential for a delay in return to full fertility. Delayed return of fertility and irregular cycles may occur after discontinuation of

treatment but there is no evidence of permanent infertility.

● **MEDICINAL FORMS**
There can be variation in the licensing of different medicines containing the same drug.
Suspension for injection
▶ Depo-Provera (Pfizer Ltd)
   Medroxyprogesterone acetate 150 mg per 1 ml Depo-Provera 150mg/1ml suspension for injection pre-filled syringes | 1 pre-filled disposable injection PoM £6.01 DT price £6.01
▶ Sayana Press (Pfizer Ltd)
   Medroxyprogesterone acetate 160 mg per 1 ml Sayana Press 104mg/0.65 ml suspension for injection pre-filled disposable devices | 1 pre-filled disposable injection PoM £6.90

3.6 Contraception, spermicidal

SPERMICIDALS

Nonoxinol

● **INDICATIONS AND DOSE**

Spermicidal contraceptive in conjunction with barrier methods of contraception such as diaphragms or caps
▶ BY VAGINA
▶ Females of childbearing potential: (consult product literature)

● **SIDE-EFFECTS** Genital lesions

SIDE-EFFECTS, FURTHER INFORMATION
High frequency use of the spermicide nonoxinol '9' has been associated with genital lesions, which may increase the risk of acquiring these infections.

● **CONCEPTION AND CONTRACEPTION** No evidence of harm to latex condoms and diaphragms.

● **PREGNANCY** Toxicity in *animal studies*.

● **BREAST FEEDING** Present in milk in *animal* studies.

● **MEDICINAL FORMS**
There can be variation in the licensing of different medicines containing the same drug.
Gel
EXCIPIENTS: May contain Hydroxybenzoates (parabens), propylene glycol, sorbic acid
▶ Gygel (Marlborough Pharmaceuticals Ltd)
   Nonoxinol-9 20 mg per 1 ml Gygel 2% contraceptive jelly | 30 gram GSL £4.25 | 81 gram GSL £11.00

4 Vaginal and vulval conditions

Vaginal and vulval conditions

Management

Pre-pubertal girls may be particularly susceptible to vulvovaginitis. Barrier preparations applied after cleansing can be useful when the symptoms are due to non-specific irritation, but systemic drugs are required in the treatment of bacterial infection or threadworm infestation. Intravaginal preparations, particularly those that require the use of an applicator, are not generally suitable for young girls; topical preparations may be useful in some adolescent girls.

In older girls symptoms are often restricted to the vulva, but infections almost invariably involve the vagina, which should also be treated; treatment should be as for adults.

Preparations for vaginal and vulval changes

Topical oestrogen creams containing **estriol** 0.01% (*Gynest®*) are used in the treatment of labial adhesions; treatment is usually restricted to symptomatic cases. Estriol cream should be applied to the adhesions once or twice daily for 2–6 weeks; adhesions may recur following treatment.

Vaginal and vulval infections

Effective specific treatments are available for the common vaginal infections.

Fungal infections

Vaginal fungal infections are not normally a problem in younger girls but can occur in adolescents. *Candidal vulvitis* can be treated locally with cream, but is almost invariably associated with vaginal infection which should also be treated. *Vaginal candidiasis*, rare in girls before puberty, can be treated with antifungal pessaries or cream inserted high into the vagina (including during menstruation), however, these are not recommended for pre-pubertal girls and treatment with an external cream may be more appropriate. Single-dose intravaginal preparations offer an advantage when compliance is a problem. Local irritation can occur on application of vaginal antifungal products.

Imidazole drugs (clotrimazole p. 492, econazole nitrate p. 492, fenticonazole nitrate p. 493, and miconazole p. 493) are effective against candida in short courses of 1 to 3 days according to the preparation used; treatment can be repeated if initial course fails to control symptoms or if symptoms recur. Vaginal applications may be supplemented with antifungal cream for vulvitis and to treat other superficial sites of infection.

Oral treatment of vaginal infection with fluconazole p. 358 may be considered for girls post-puberty.

Vulvovaginal candidiasis in pregnancy

Vulvovaginal candidiasis is common during pregnancy and can be treated with vaginal application of an imidazole (such as clotrimazole), and a topical imidazole cream for vulvitis. Pregnant women need a longer duration of treatment, usually about 7 days, to clear the infection. There is limited absorption of imidazoles from the skin and vagina. Oral antifungal treatment should be avoided during pregnancy.

Recurrent vulvovaginal candidiasis

Recurrent vulvovaginal candidiasis is very rare in children, but can occur if there are predisposing factors such as antibacterial therapy, pregnancy, diabetes mellitus, or possibly oral contraceptive use. Reservoirs of infection can also lead to recontamination and should be treated; these include other skin sites such as the digits, nail beds, and umbilicus, as well as the gastro-intestinal tract and the bladder. The sexual partner may also be the source of re-infection and, if symptomatic, should be treated with a topical imidazole cream at the same time.

Treatment against candida may need to be extended for 6 months in recurrent vulvovaginal candidiasis.

Other infections

Trichomonal infections commonly involve the lower urinary tract as well as the genital system and need systemic treatment with metronidazole p. 319 or tinidazole p. 320.

Bacterial infections with Gram-negative organisms are particularly common in association with gynaecological operations and trauma. Metronidazole is effective against certain Gram-negative organisms, especially *Bacteroides* spp. and can be used prophylactically in gynaecological surgery.

Clindamycin cream, below, and metronidazole gel, below, are indicated for bacterial vaginosis.

The antiviral drugs aciclovir p. 387 and valaciclovir p. 389 can be used in the treatment of genital infection due to *herpes simplex virus*, the HSV type 2 being a major cause of genital ulceration. They have a beneficial effect on virus shedding and healing, generally giving relief from pain and other symptoms.

4.1 Vaginal and vulval infections

4.1a Vaginal and vulval bacterial infections

ANTIBACTERIALS › LINCOSAMIDES

Clindamycin

- **INDICATIONS AND DOSE**

DALACIN® 2% CREAM
Bacterial vaginosis
▸ BY VAGINA
▸ Child: 1 applicatorful daily for 3–7 nights, dose to be administered at night

DOSE EQUIVALENCE AND CONVERSION
▸ 1 applicatorful delivers a 5 g dose of clindamycin 2%.

- **UNLICENSED USE** Not licensed for use in children.

- **CAUTIONS** Avoid intravaginal preparations (particularly those that require the use of an applicator) in young girls who are not sexually active, unless there is no alternative

- **SIDE-EFFECTS** Cervicitis · irritation · vaginitis
  SIDE-EFFECTS, FURTHER INFORMATION Clindamycin 2% cream is poorly absorbed into the blood—low risk of systemic effects.

- **CONCEPTION AND CONTRACEPTION** Damages latex condoms and diaphragms.

- **MEDICINAL FORMS**
  There can be variation in the licensing of different medicines containing the same drug.
  Cream
  EXCIPIENTS: May contain Benzyl alcohol, cetostearyl alcohol (including cetyl and stearyl alcohol), polysorbates, propylene glycol
  ▸ Dalacin (Pfizer Ltd)
  Clindamycin (as Clindamycin phosphate) 20 mg per
  1 gram Dalacin 2% cream | 40 gram [PoM] £10.86 DT price = £10.86

ANTIBACTERIALS › NITROIMIDAZOLE DERIVATIVES

Metronidazole

- **DRUG ACTION** Metronidazole is an antimicrobial drug with high activity against anaerobic bacteria and protozoa.

- **INDICATIONS AND DOSE**

Bacterial vaginosis
▸ BY VAGINA USING VAGINAL GEL
▸ Child: 1 applicatorful daily for 5 days, dose to be administered at night

DOSE EQUIVALENCE AND CONVERSION
▸ 1 applicatorful delivers a 5g dose of metronidazole 0.75%

- **UNLICENSED USE** Metronidazole vaginal gel not licensed for use in children under 18 years.

- **CAUTIONS** Avoid intravaginal preparations (particularly those that require the use of an applicator) in young girls who are not sexually active, unless there is no alternative · not recommended during menstruation · some systemic absorption may occur with vaginal gel

- **INTERACTIONS** → Appendix 1: metronidazole

7

Genito-urinary system

- **SIDE-EFFECTS** Abnormal vaginal discharge · local irritation · pelvic discomfort · vaginal candidiasis
- **PATIENT AND CARER ADVICE**
  Medicines for Children leaflet: Metronidazole for bacterial infections www.medicinesforchildren.org.uk/metronidazole-bacterial-infections
- **MEDICINAL FORMS**
  There can be variation in the licensing of different medicines containing the same drug.
  Vaginal gel
  EXCIPIENTS: May contain Disodium edetate, hydroxybenzoates (parabens), propylene glycol
  ‣ **Metronidazole (Non-proprietary)**
  Metronidazole 7.5 mg per 1 gram Metronidazole 0.75% vaginal gel | 40 gram PoM no price available DT price = £4.31
  ‣ **Zidoval** (Meda Pharmaceuticals Ltd)
  Metronidazole 7.5 mg per 1 gram Zidoval 0.75% vaginal gel | 40 gram PoM £4.31 DT price = £4.31

CARBOXYLIC ACIDS

Lactic acid

- **INDICATIONS AND DOSE**
  BALANCE ACTIV RX® GEL
  Prevention of bacterial vaginosis
  ‣ BY VAGINA
  ‣ Child: 5 mL 1–2 times a week, insert the content of 1 tube (5 mL)

- **MEDICINAL FORMS**
  There can be variation in the licensing of different medicines containing the same drug.
  Vaginal gel
  EXCIPIENTS: May contain Propylene glycol
  ‣ **Balance Activ** (BBI Healthcare Ltd)
  Balance Activ BV vaginal pH correction gel | 7 device £5.25

4.1b Vaginal and vulval fungal infections

> **Other drugs used for Vaginal and vulval fungal infections**
> Fluconazole, p. 358

ANTIFUNGALS > IMIDAZOLE ANTIFUNGALS

Clotrimazole

- **INDICATIONS AND DOSE**
  Superficial sites of infection in vaginal and vulval candidiasis (dose for 1% or 2% cream)
  ‣ BY VAGINA USING CREAM
  ‣ Child: Apply 2–3 times a day, to be applied to anogenital area
  Vaginal candidiasis (dose for 10% intravaginal cream)
  ‣ BY VAGINA USING VAGINAL CREAM
  ‣ Child: 5 g for 1 dose, one applicatorful to be inserted into the vagina at night, dose can be repeated once if necessary
  Vaginal candidiasis
  ‣ BY VAGINA USING PESSARIES
  ‣ Child: 200 mg for 3 nights, course can be repeated once if necessary, alternatively 500 mg for 1 night, dose can be repeated once if necessary

Recurrent vulvovaginal candidiasis
‣ BY VAGINA USING PESSARIES
‣ Child: 500 mg every week for 6 months, dose to be administered following topical imidazole for 10–14 days

- **UNLICENSED USE** Consult product literature for individual preparations.
- **CAUTIONS** Avoid intravaginal preparations (particularly those that require use of an applicator) in young girls who are not sexually active, unless there is no alternative
- **INTERACTIONS** → Appendix 1: antifungals, azoles
- **SIDE-EFFECTS** Local irritation
- **CONCEPTION AND CONTRACEPTION** Cream and pessaries may damage latex condoms and diaphragms.
- **PREGNANCY** Pregnant women need a longer duration of treatment, usually about 7 days, to clear the infection. Oral antifungal treatment should be avoided during pregnancy.
- **EXCEPTIONS TO LEGAL CATEGORY** Brands for sale to the public include *Canesten*® Internal Cream.
- **MEDICINAL FORMS**
  There can be variation in the licensing of different medicines containing the same drug.
  Pessary
  EXCIPIENTS: May contain Benzyl alcohol, cetostearyl alcohol (including cetyl and stearyl alcohol), polysorbates
  ‣ **Clotrimazole (Non-proprietary)**
  Clotrimazole 500 mg Clotrimazole 500mg pessaries | 1 pessary P £3.75 DT price = £2.88
  ‣ **Canesten (clotrimazole)** (Bayer Plc)
  Clotrimazole 100 mg Canesten 100mg pessaries | 6 pessary P £3.50 DT price = £3.50
  Clotrimazole 200 mg Canesten 200mg pessaries | 3 pessary P £3.10 DT price = £3.10
  Clotrimazole 500 mg Canesten 500mg Soft Gel pessaries | 1 pessary P £6.41 DT price = £2.88
  Canesten 500mg pessaries | 1 pessary P no price available DT price = £2.88
  Canesten Vaginal 500mg pessaries | 1 pessary PoM £2.00 DT price = £2.88
  Cream
  EXCIPIENTS: May contain Benzyl alcohol, cetostearyl alcohol (including cetyl and stearyl alcohol), polysorbates
  ‣ **Clotrimazole (Non-proprietary)**
  Clotrimazole 10 mg per 1 gram Clotrimazole 1% cream | 20 gram P £2.06 DT price = £1.12 | 50 gram P £5.45 DT price = £2.80
  ‣ **Canesten (clotrimazole)** (Bayer Plc)
  Clotrimazole 10 mg per 1 gram Canesten 1% cream | 20 gram P £2.14 DT price = £1.12 | 50 gram P £3.50 DT price = £2.80
  Canesten Antifungal 1% cream | 20 gram P £1.85 DT price = £1.12
  Clotrimazole 20 mg per 1 gram Canesten 2% thrush cream | 10 gram P no price available | 20 gram P £4.46 DT price = £4.46
  Clotrimazole 100 mg per 1 gram Canesten Internal 10% cream | 5 gram P £6.23 DT price = £6.23
  Canesten 10% VC cream | 5 gram PoM £4.50 DT price = £6.23

Econazole nitrate

- **INDICATIONS AND DOSE**
  GYNO-PEVARYL® ONCE
  Vaginal and vulval candidiasis
  ‣ BY VAGINA
  ‣ Child: 1 pessary for 1 dose, pessary to be inserted at night, dose to be repeated once if necessary
  GYNO-PEVARYL® PESSARY
  Vaginal and vulval candidiasis
  ‣ BY VAGINA
  ‣ Child: 1 pessary daily for 3 days, pessary to be inserted at night, course can be repeated once if necessary

- **CAUTIONS** Avoid intravaginal preparations (particularly those that require use of an applicator) in young girls who are not sexually active, unless there is no alternative
- **SIDE-EFFECTS** Occasional local irritation
- **CONCEPTION AND CONTRACEPTION** Cream and pessaries damage latex condoms and diaphragms.
- **PREGNANCY** Pregnant women need a longer duration of treatment, usually about 7 days, to clear the infection.

- **MEDICINAL FORMS**
  There can be variation in the licensing of different medicines containing the same drug.
  Pessary
  ▸ Gyno-Pevaryl (Janssen-Cilag Ltd)
  Econazole nitrate 150 mg Gyno-Pevaryl Once 150mg vaginal pessary | 1 pessary PoM £3.69
  Gyno-Pevaryl 150mg vaginal pessaries | 3 pessary PoM £4.17

Fenticonazole nitrate

- **INDICATIONS AND DOSE**
  Vaginal and vulva candidiasis
  ▸ BY VAGINA USING CAPSULES
  ▸ Child: 200 mg daily for 3 days, alternatively 600 mg daily for 1 dose, to be inserted at night
  ▸ BY VAGINA USING CREAM
  ▸ Child: 1 applicatorful twice daily for 3 days
  DOSE EQUIVALENCE AND CONVERSION
  ▸ 1 applicatorful delivers a 5 g dose of fenticonazole 2 %.

- **CAUTIONS** Avoid intravaginal preparations (particularly those that require use of an applicator) in young girls who are not sexually active, unless there is no alternative
- **SIDE-EFFECTS** Local irritation
- **CONCEPTION AND CONTRACEPTION** Intravaginal cream and vaginal capsules damage latex condoms and diaphragms.

- **MEDICINAL FORMS**
  There can be variation in the licensing of different medicines containing the same drug.
  Cream
  EXCIPIENTS: May contain Cetostearyl alcohol (including cetyl and stearyl alcohol), propylene glycol, wool fat and related substances including lanolin
  ▸ Gynoxin (Recordati Pharmaceuticals Ltd)
  Fenticonazole nitrate 20 mg per 1 gram Gynoxin 2% vaginal cream | 30 gram PoM £3.74
  Capsule
  EXCIPIENTS: May contain Hydroxybenzoates (parabens)
  ▸ Gynoxin (Recordati Pharmaceuticals Ltd)
  Fenticonazole nitrate 200 mg Gynoxin 200mg vaginal capsules | 3 capsule PoM £2.42
  Fenticonazole nitrate 600 mg Gynoxin 600mg vaginal capsules | 1 capsule PoM £2.62

Miconazole

- **INDICATIONS AND DOSE**
  Vaginal and vulval candidiasis
  ▸ BY VAGINA USING CAPSULES
  ▸ Child: 1 capsule daily, ovule to be inserted at night as a single dose, dose can be repeated once if necessary

- **CAUTIONS** Avoid in acute porphyrias p. 577 · avoid intravaginal preparations (particularly those that require use of an applicator) in young girls who are not sexually active, unless there is no alternative
- **INTERACTIONS** → Appendix 1: antifungals, azoles
- **SIDE-EFFECTS**
- **Common or very common** Nausea · rash · vomiting
- **Frequency not known** Occasional local irritation

- **CONCEPTION AND CONTRACEPTION** *Gyno-Daktarin®* damages latex condoms and diaphragms.
- **PREGNANCY** Pregnant women need a longer duration of treatment, usually about 7 days, to clear the infection.
- **BREAST FEEDING** Manufacturer advises caution—no information available.

- **MEDICINAL FORMS**
  There can be variation in the licensing of different medicines containing the same drug.
  Capsule
  EXCIPIENTS: May contain hydroxybenzoates (parabens)
  ▸ Gyno-Daktarin (Janssen-Cilag Ltd)
  Miconazole nitrate 1.2 gram Gyno-Daktarin 1200mg vaginal capsules | 1 capsule PoM £2.94 DT price = £2.94

Chapter 8
Immune system and malignant disease

CONTENTS

Immune system

1 Immune system disorders and transplantation

Immune response

Inflammatory bowel disease

Azathioprine p. 495, mercaptopurine p. 516, or once weekly methotrexate p. 517 are used to induce remission in unresponsive or chronically active Crohn's disease. Azathioprine or mercaptopurine may also be helpful for retaining remission in frequently relapsing inflammatory bowel disease; once weekly methotrexate is used in Crohn's disease when azathioprine or mercaptopurine are ineffective or not tolerated. Response to azathioprine or mercaptopurine may not become apparent for several months. Folic acid p. 546 should be given to reduce the possibility of methotrexate toxicity. Folic acid is usually given weekly on a different day to the methotrexate; alternative regimens may be used in some settings.

Ciclosporin (cyclosporin) p. 496 is a potent immunosuppressant and is markedly nephrotoxic. In children with severe ulcerative colitis unresponsive to other treatment, ciclosporin may reduce the need for urgent colorectal surgery.

Immunosuppressant therapy

Immunosuppressants are used to suppress rejection in organ transplant recipients and to treat a variety of chronic inflammatory and autoimmune diseases. Solid organ transplant patients are maintained on drug regimens, which may include antiproliferative drugs (azathioprine or mycophenolate mofetil p. 503), calcineurin inhibitors (ciclosporin or tacrolimus p. 499), corticosteroids, or sirolimus p. 498. Choice is dependent on the type of organ, time after transplant, and clinical condition of the patient. Specialist management is required and other immunomodulators may be used to initiate treatment or to treat rejection.

Impaired immune responsiveness

Infections in the immunocompromised child can be severe and show atypical features. Specific local protocols should be followed for the management of infection. Corticosteroids may suppress clinical signs of infection and allow diseases such as septicaemia or tuberculosis to reach an advanced stage before being recognised. Children should be up-to-date with their childhood vaccinations before initiation of immunosuppressant therapy (e.g. before transplantation); vaccination with varicella-zoster vaccine is also necessary during this period—**important**: normal immunoglobulin administration should be considered as soon as possible after measles exposure, and varicella–zoster immunoglobulin (VZIG) is recommended for individuals who have significant chickenpox (varicella) exposure. Specialist advice should be sought on the use of live vaccines for those being treated with immunosuppressive drugs.

Antiproliferative immunosuppressants

Azathioprine is widely used for transplant recipients and it is also used to treat a number of auto-immune conditions, usually when corticosteroid therapy alone provides inadequate control. It is metabolised to mercaptopurine, and doses should be reduced (to one quarter of the original dose in children) when allopurinol p. 521 is given concurrently.

Mycophenolate mofetil is metabolised to mycophenolic acid which has a more selective mode of action than azathioprine.

There is evidence that compared with similar regimens incorporating azathioprine, mycophenolate mofetil may reduce the risk of acute rejection episodes; the risk of opportunistic infections (particularly due to tissue-invasive cytomegalovirus) and the occurrence of blood disorders such as leucopenia may be higher. Children may suffer a high incidence of side-effects, particularly gastrointestinal effects, calling for temporary reduction in dose or interruption of treatment.

Cyclophosphamide p. 509 is less commonly prescribed as an immunosuppressant.

Corticosteroids and other immunosuppressants

The corticosteroids prednisolone p. 421 and dexamethasone p. 419 are widely used in paediatric oncology; they have a marked antitumour effect. Dexamethasone is preferred for acute lymphoblastic leukaemia whilst prednisolone may be used for Hodgkin's disease, non-Hodgkin's lymphoma, and B-cell lymphoma and leukaemia.

Dexamethasone is the corticosteroid of choice in paediatric supportive and palliative care. For children who are not receiving a corticosteroid as a component of their chemotherapy, dexamethasone may be used to reduce raised intracranial pressure, or to help control emesis when combined with an appropriate anti-emetic.

The corticosteroids are also powerful immunosuppressants. They are used to prevent organ transplant rejection, and in high dose to treat rejection episodes.

Ciclosporin (cyclosporin), a calcineurin inhibitor, is a potent immunosuppressant which is virtually non-myelotoxic but markedly nephrotoxic. It may be used in organ and tissue transplantation, for prevention of graft rejection following bone marrow, kidney, liver, pancreas, heart, lung, and heart-lung transplantation, and for prophylaxis and treatment of graft-versus-host disease. Ciclosporin also has a role in steroid-sensitive and steroid-resistant nephrotic syndrome; in corticosteroid-sensitive nephrotic syndrome it may be given with prednisolone.

Tacrolimus is also a calcineurin inhibitor. Although not chemically related to ciclosporin it has a similar mode of action and side-effects.

Immunosuppressive therapy for renal transplantation in children and adolescents (April 2006) NICE TA99
When selecting immunosuppressive therapy for renal transplantation in children and adolescents, NICE has recommended that for induction therapy in the prophylaxis of organ rejection, either basiliximab or daclizumab [discontinued] are options for combining with a calcineurin inhibitor. For each individual, ciclosporin or tacrolimus is chosen as the calcineurin inhibitor on the basis of side-effects. Mycophenolate mofetil is recommended as part of an immunosuppressive regimen **only if**:

- the calcineurin inhibitor is not tolerated, particularly if nephrotoxicity endangers the transplanted kidney; *or*
- there is very high risk of nephrotoxicity from the calcineurin inhibitor, requiring a reduction in the dose of the calcineurin inhibitor or its avoidance.

Mycophenolic acid is not recommended as part of an immunosuppressive regimen for renal transplantation in children or adolescents.

Sirolimus [not licensed for use in children] is recommended as a component of immunosuppressive regimen **only if** intolerance necessitates the withdrawal of a calcineurin inhibitor.

These recommendations may not be consistent with the marketing authorisation of some of the products.
www.nice.org.uk/TA99

> **Other drugs used for Immune system disorders and transplantation** Hydroxychloroquine sulfate, p. 612 · Rituximab, p. 505

IMMUNE SERA AND IMMUNOGLOBULINS > IMMUNOGLOBULINS

Antithymocyte immunoglobulin (rabbit)

● INDICATIONS AND DOSE

Prophylaxis of organ rejection in heart allograft recipients
▸ BY INTRAVENOUS INFUSION
▸ Child: 1–2.5 mg/kg daily for 3–5 days, start treatment on day of transplantation, to be given over at least 6 hours

Prophylaxis of organ rejection in renal allograft recipients
▸ BY INTRAVENOUS INFUSION
▸ Child 1–17 years: 1–1.5 mg/kg daily for 3–9 days, start treatment on day of transplantation, to be given over at least 6 hours

Treatment of corticosteroid-resistant allograft rejection in renal transplantation
▸ BY INTRAVENOUS INFUSION
▸ Child 1–17 years: 1.5 mg/kg daily for 7–14 days, to be given over at least 6 hours

DOSES AT EXTREMES OF BODY-WEIGHT
To avoid excessive dosage in obese patients, calculate dose on the basis of ideal body weight.

● CONTRA-INDICATIONS Infection

● SIDE-EFFECTS Anaphylaxis · cytokine release syndrome · diarrhoea · dysphagia · fever · hypotension · increased susceptibility to infection · increased susceptibility to malignancy · infusion-related reactions · lymphopenia · myalgia · nausea · neutropenia · pruritus · rash · serum sickness · shivering · thrombocytopenia · vomiting

SIDE-EFFECTS, FURTHER INFORMATION
Tolerability is increased by pretreatment with an intravenous corticosteroid and antihistamine; an antipyretic drug such as paracetamol may also be beneficial.

● PREGNANCY Manufacturer advises use only if potential benefit outweighs risk—no information available.

● BREAST FEEDING Manufacturer advises avoid—no information available.

● MONITORING REQUIREMENTS Monitor blood count.

● DIRECTIONS FOR ADMINISTRATION For *continuous intravenous infusion* reconstitute each vial with 5 mL water for injections to produce a solution of 5 mg/mL; gently rotate to dissolve. Dilute requisite dose with Glucose 5% *or* Sodium Chloride 0.9% to an approx. concentration of 0.5 mg/mL; begin infusion immediately after dilution; give through an in-line filter (pore size 0.22 micron); incompatible with unfractionated heparin and hydrocortisone in glucose infusion—precipitation reported.

● MEDICINAL FORMS
There can be variation in the licensing of different medicines containing the same drug.

Solution for infusion
▸ Antithymocyte immunoglobulin (rabbit) (Non-proprietary)
Antithymocyte immunoglobulin (rabbit) 20 mg per 1 ml Grafalon 100mg/5ml concentrate for solution for infusion vials | 1 vial [PoM] no price available

Powder and solvent for solution for infusion
▸ Thymoglobulin (Sanofi)
Antithymocyte immunoglobulin (rabbit) 25 mg Thymoglobuline 25mg powder and solvent for solution for infusion vials | 1 vial [PoM] £158.77 (Hospital only)

IMMUNOSUPPRESSANTS > ANTIMETABOLITES

Azathioprine
11-May-2017

● DRUG ACTION Azathioprine is metabolised to mercaptopurine.

● INDICATIONS AND DOSE

Severe ulcerative colitis | Severe Crohn's disease
▸ BY MOUTH
▸ Child 2–17 years: Initially 2 mg/kg once daily, then increased if necessary up to 2.5 mg/kg once daily

Systemic lupus erythematosus | Vasculitis | Autoimmune conditions usually when corticosteroid therapy alone has proved inadequate
▸ BY MOUTH
▸ Child: Initially 1 mg/kg daily, then adjusted according to response to 3 mg/kg daily, consider withdrawal if no improvement within 3 months; maximum 3 mg/kg per day

Suppression of transplant rejection
▸ BY MOUTH, OR BY INTRAVENOUS INFUSION
▸ Child: Maintenance 1–3 mg/kg daily, adjusted according to response, consult local treatment protocol for details, oral route preferred, but if oral route is not possible then can be given by intravenous infusion, the total daily dose may alternatively be given in 2 divided doses

DOSE ADJUSTMENTS DUE TO INTERACTIONS
Manufacturer advises reduce dose to one-quarter of the usual dose with concurrent use of allopurinol.

8

Immune system and malignant disease

8

Immune system and malignant disease

- **CAUTIONS** Reduced thiopurine methyltransferase activity
- **INTERACTIONS** → Appendix 1: azathioprine
- **SIDE-EFFECTS**
  - ▸ **Rare** Hepatic veno-occlusive disease · lymphoma · pancreatitis · pneumonitis · red cell aplasia
  - ▸ **Frequency not known** Arthralgia · cholestatic jaundice · colitis in patients also receiving corticosteroids · diarrhoea · dizziness · dose-related bone marrow suppression · fever · hair loss · herpes zoster infection · hypersensitivity reactions · hypotension · increased susceptibility to infections in patients also receiving corticosteroids · interstitial nephritis · liver impairment · malaise · myalgia · nausea · neutropenia · rash · rigors · thrombocytopenia · vomiting

  SIDE-EFFECTS, FURTHER INFORMATION
  - ▸ Red cell aplasia Cases of pure red cell aplasia have been reported with azathioprine; dose reduction or discontinuation should be considered under specialist supervision.
  - ▸ Neutropenia and thrombocytopenia Usually resolved by reducing the dose.
  - ▸ Hypersensitivity reactions Hypersensitivity reactions (including malaise, dizziness, vomiting, diarrhoea, fever, rigors, myalgia, arthralgia, rash, hypotension and interstitial nephritis) call for immediate withdrawal.

- **ALLERGY AND CROSS-SENSITIVITY** Contra-indicated in hypersensitivity to mercaptopurine.

- **PREGNANCY** Transplant patients immunosuppressed with azathioprine should not discontinue it on becoming pregnant. However, there have been reports of premature birth and low-birth-weight following exposure to azathioprine, particularly in combination with corticosteroids. Spontaneous abortion has been reported following maternal or paternal exposure. Azathioprine is teratogenic in *animal* studies. The use of azathioprine during pregnancy needs to be supervised in specialist units. Treatment should not generally be initiated during pregnancy.

- **BREAST FEEDING** Present in milk in low concentration. No evidence of harm in small studies—use if potential benefit outweighs risk.

- **HEPATIC IMPAIRMENT** Reduce dose. Monitor liver function.

- **RENAL IMPAIRMENT** Reduce dose.

- **PRE-TREATMENT SCREENING**
  Thiopurine methyltransferase The enzyme thiopurine methyltransferase (TPMT) metabolises thiopurine drugs (azathioprine, mercaptopurine, tioguanine); the risk of myelosuppression is increased in patients with reduced activity of the enzyme, particularly for the few individuals in whom TPMT activity is undetectable. Consider measuring TPMT activity before starting azathioprine, mercaptopurine, or tioguanine therapy. Patients with absent TPMT activity should not receive thiopurine drugs; those with reduced TPMT activity may be treated under specialist supervision.

- **MONITORING REQUIREMENTS**
  - ▸ Monitor for toxicity throughout treatment.
  - ▸ Monitor full blood count weekly (more frequently with higher doses or if severe hepatic or renal impairment) for first 4 weeks (manufacturer advises weekly monitoring for 8 weeks but evidence of practical value unsatisfactory), thereafter reduce frequency of monitoring to at least every 3 months.
  - ▸ Blood tests and monitoring for signs of myelosuppression are essential in long-term treatment.

- **DIRECTIONS FOR ADMINISTRATION**
  - ▸ With intravenous use Consult local treatment protocol for details. For *intravenous injection*, reconstitute 50 mg with 5–15 mL Water for Injections; give over at least 1 minute.

For *intravenous infusion*, reconstitute 50 mg with 5–15 mL Water for Injections; dilute requisite dose to a concentration of 0.25–2.5 mg/mL in Glucose 5% or Sodium Chloride 0.9%. Intravenous injection is alkaline and very irritant. Intravenous route should therefore be used **only** if oral route not feasible and discontinued as soon as oral route can be tolerated. To reduce irritation flush line with infusion fluid.

- **PATIENT AND CARER ADVICE**
  Bone marrow suppression Patients and their carers should be warned to report immediately any signs or symptoms of bone marrow suppression e.g. inexplicable bruising or bleeding, infection.
  Medicines for Children leaflet: Azathioprine for inflammatory bowel disease www.medicinesforchildren.org.uk/azathioprine-inflammatory-bowel-disease-0
  Medicines for Children leaflet: Azathioprine for renal (kidney) transplant www.medicinesforchildren.org.uk/azathioprine-renal-kidney-transplant-0
  Medicines for Children leaflet: Azathioprine for severe atopic eczema www.medicinesforchildren.org.uk/azathioprine-severe-atopic-eczema-0

- **MEDICINAL FORMS**
  There can be variation in the licensing of different medicines containing the same drug. Forms available from special-order manufacturers include: capsule, oral suspension, oral solution

  Tablet
  CAUTIONARY AND ADVISORY LABELS 21
  - ▸ **Azathioprine (Non-proprietary)**
    Azathioprine 25 mg Azathioprine 25mg tablets | 28 tablet [PoM] £8.41 DT price = £1.66 | 100 tablet [PoM] £33.26
    Azathioprine 50 mg Azathioprine 50mg tablets | 56 tablet [PoM] £7.28 DT price = £2.21 | 100 tablet [PoM] £6.55
  - ▸ **Azapress (Ennogen Pharma Ltd)**
    Azathioprine 50 mg Azapress 50mg tablets | 56 tablet [PoM] £2.83 DT price = £2.21
  - ▸ **Imuran (Aspen Pharma Trading Ltd)**
    Azathioprine 25 mg Imuran 25mg tablets | 100 tablet [PoM] £10.99
    Azathioprine 50 mg Imuran 50mg tablets | 100 tablet [PoM] £7.99

  Powder for solution for injection
  - ▸ **Imuran (Aspen Pharma Trading Ltd)**
    Azathioprine 50 mg Imuran 50mg powder for solution for injection vials | 1 vial [PoM] £15.38

IMMUNOSUPPRESSANTS ⟩ CALCINEURIN INHIBITORS AND RELATED DRUGS

Ciclosporin

01-Sep-2016

(Cyclosporin)

- **DRUG ACTION** Ciclosporin inhibits production and release of lymphokines, thereby suppressing cell-mediated immune response.

- **INDICATIONS AND DOSE**
  Refractory ulcerative colitis
  - ▸ **BY MOUTH**
  - ▸ **Child 2–17 years:** Initially 2 mg/kg twice daily (max. per dose 5 mg/kg twice daily), dose adjusted according to blood-ciclosporin concentration and response
  - ▸ **BY INTRAVENOUS INFUSION**
  - ▸ **Child 3–17 years:** Initially 0.5–1 mg/kg twice daily, dose adjusted according to blood-ciclosporin concentration and response

  Short-term treatment of severe atopic dermatitis where conventional therapy ineffective or inappropriate (administered on expert advice)
  - ▸ **BY MOUTH**
  - ▸ **Child:** Initially 1.25 mg/kg twice daily (max. per dose 2.5 mg/kg twice daily) usual maximum duration of 8 weeks but may be used for longer under specialist

supervision, if good initial response not achieved within 2 weeks, increase dose rapidly up to maximum

Short-term treatment of very severe atopic dermatitis where conventional therapy ineffective or inappropriate (administered on expert advice)

▸ BY MOUTH

▸ Child: 2.5 mg/kg twice daily usual maximum duration of 8 weeks but may be used for longer under specialist supervision

Severe psoriasis where conventional therapy ineffective or inappropriate (administered on expert advice)

▸ BY MOUTH

▸ Child: Initially 1.25 mg/kg twice daily (max. per dose 2.5 mg/kg twice daily), increased gradually to maximum if no improvement within 1 month, initial dose of 2.5 mg/kg twice daily justified if treatment requires rapid improvement; discontinue if inadequate response after 3 months at the optimum dose; max. duration of treatment usually 1 year unless other treatments cannot be used

Prevention of graft rejection following bone-marrow, kidney, liver, pancreas, heart, lung, and heart-lung transplantation | Prevention and treatment of graft-versus-host disease

▸ BY MOUTH, OR BY INTRAVENOUS INFUSION

▸ Child: (consult local protocol)

Nephrotic syndrome

▸ BY MOUTH

▸ Child: 3 mg/kg twice daily, dose can be increased if necessary in corticosteroid-resistant disease; for maintenance reduce to lowest effective dose according to whole blood-ciclosporin concentrations, proteinuria, and renal function

DOSE ADJUSTMENTS DUE TO INTERACTIONS

▸ With oral use Manufacturer advises increase dose by 50% or switch to intravenous administration with concurrent use of octreotide.

● UNLICENSED USE Not licensed for use in children under 3 months. Not licensed for use in children under 16 years for atopic eczema (dermatitis) or psoriasis. Not licensed for use in ulcerative colitis.

IMPORTANT SAFETY INFORMATION

MHRA/CHM ADVICE: CICLOSPORIN MUST BE PRESCRIBED AND DISPENSED BY BRAND NAME (DECEMBER 2009)
Patients should be stabilised on a particular brand of oral ciclosporin because switching between formulations without close monitoring may lead to clinically important changes in blood-ciclosporin concentration.

● CONTRA-INDICATIONS Abnormal baseline renal function (in non-transplant indications) · malignancy (in non-transplant indications) · uncontrolled hypertension (in non-transplant indications) · uncontrolled infections (in non-transplant indications)

● CAUTIONS Hyperuricaemia · in atopic dermatitis, active herpes simplex infections—allow infection to clear before starting (if they occur during treatment withdraw if severe) · in atopic dermatitis, *Staphylococcus aureus* skin infections—not absolute contra-indication providing controlled (but avoid erythromycin unless no other alternative) · in psoriasis treat, patients with malignant or pre-malignant conditions of skin only after appropriate treatment (and if no other option) · in uveitis, Behcet's syndrome (monitor neurological status) · lymphoproliferative disorders (discontinue treatment) · malignancy

CAUTIONS, FURTHER INFORMATION

▸ Malignancy In psoriasis, exclude malignancies (including those of skin and cervix) before starting (biopsy any

lesions not typical of psoriasis) and treat patients with malignant or pre-malignant conditions of skin only after appropriate treatment (and if no other option); discontinue if lymphoproliferative disorder develops.

● INTERACTIONS → Appendix 1: ciclosporin

● SIDE-EFFECTS

▸ **Common or very common** Abdominal pain · acne · anorexia · convulsion · diarrhoea · fatigue · flushing · gingival hyperplasia · headache · hepatic dysfunction · hirsutism · hyperglycaemia · hyperkalaemia · hyperlipidaemia · hypertension · hypertrichosis · hyperuricaemia · hypomagnesaemia · leucopenia · muscle cramps · myalgia · nausea · paraesthesia · peptic ulcer · pyrexia · renal dysfunction (renal structural changes on long-term administration) · tremor · vomiting

▸ **Uncommon** Anaemia · oedema · signs of encephalopathy · thrombocytopenia · weight gain

▸ **Rare** Gynaecomastia · haemolytic uraemic syndrome · menstrual disturbances · micro-angiopathic haemolytic anaemia · motor polyneuropathy · muscle weakness · myopathy · pancreatitis

▸ **Very rare** Visual disturbances secondary to benign intracranial hypertension

▸ **Frequency not known** Migraine · pain in lower extremities

▸ **With intravenous use** Anaphylaxis

● PREGNANCY Crosses placenta; manufacturer advises avoid unless potential benefit outweighs risk—toxicity in *animal* studies.

● BREAST FEEDING Manufacturer advises avoid—present in milk.

● HEPATIC IMPAIRMENT Extensively metabolised by the liver—manufacturer advises dose adjustment based on bilirubin and liver enzyme levels.

● RENAL IMPAIRMENT In non-transplant indications, manufacturer advises establishing baseline renal function before initiation of treatment; if baseline function is impaired in non-transplant indications, except nephrotic syndrome—avoid. In nephrotic syndrome, manufacturer advises initial dose should not exceed 2.5 mg/kg daily in patients with baseline renal impairment. *During treatment* for non-transplant indications, manufacturer recommends if the estimated glomerular filtration rate decreases by more than 25% below baseline on more than one measurement, reduce dose by 25–50%. If the estimated glomerular filtration rate decrease from baseline exceeds 35%, further dose reduction should be considered (even if within normal range); discontinue if reduction not successful within 1 month.

● MONITORING REQUIREMENTS Monitor whole blood ciclosporin concentration (trough level dependent on indication—consult local treatment protocol for details).

▸ In long-term management of nephrotic syndrome, perform renal biopsies every 1–2 years.

● DIRECTIONS FOR ADMINISTRATION

▸ With oral use Mix solution with orange or apple juice, or other soft drink (to improve taste) immediately before taking (and rinse with more to ensure total dose). Do not mix with grapefruit juice. Total daily dose should be taken in 2 divided doses.

▸ With intravenous use For intermittent *intravenous infusion*, dilute to a concentration of 0.5–2.5 mg/mL with Glucose 5% *or* Sodium Chloride 0.9%; give over 2–6 hours; not to be used with PVC equipment. Observe patient for signs of anaphylaxis for at least 30 minutes after starting infusion and at frequent intervals thereafter.

● PRESCRIBING AND DISPENSING INFORMATION

Brand name prescribing Prescribing and dispensing of ciclosporin should be by brand name to avoid inadvertent switching. If it is necessary to switch a patient to a different brand of ciclosporin, the patient should be monitored closely for changes in blood-ciclosporin concentration, serum creatinine, blood pressure, and transplant function (for transplant indications). *Sandimmun®* capsules and oral solution are available direct from Novartis for patients who cannot be transferred to a different oral preparation.

- **PATIENT AND CARER ADVICE**
Patients and carers should be counselled on the administration of different formulations of ciclosporin.

Manufacturer advises avoid excessive exposure to UV light, including sunlight. In psoriasis and atopic dermatitis, avoid use of UVB or PUVA.

Medicines for Children leaflet: Ciclosporin for nephrotic syndrome www.medicinesforchildren.org.uk/ciclosporin-nephrotic-syndrome-0

- **MEDICINAL FORMS**
There can be variation in the licensing of different medicines containing the same drug.

Solution for infusion
EXCIPIENTS: May contain Alcohol, polyoxyl castor oils
▸ **Sandimmun** (Novartis Pharmaceuticals UK Ltd)
Ciclosporin 50 mg per 1 ml Sandimmun 250mg/5ml concentrate for solution for infusion ampoules | 10 ampoule [PoM] £110.05
Sandimmun 50mg/1ml concentrate for solution for infusion ampoules | 10 ampoule [PoM] £23.23

Oral solution
EXCIPIENTS: May contain Alcohol, propylene glycol
▸ **Neoral** (Novartis Pharmaceuticals UK Ltd)
Ciclosporin 100 mg per 1 ml Neoral 100mg/ml oral solution sugar-free | 50 ml [PoM] £102.30

Capsule
EXCIPIENTS: May contain Ethanol, ethyl lactate, propylene glycol
▸ **Ciclosporin** (Non-proprietary)
Ciclosporin 25 mg Ciclosporin 25mg capsules | 30 capsule [PoM] no price available DT price = £18.37
Ciclosporin 50 mg Ciclosporin 50mg capsules | 30 capsule [PoM] no price available DT price = £35.97
Ciclosporin 100 mg Ciclosporin 100mg capsules | 30 capsule [PoM] no price available DT price = £68.28
▸ **Capimune** (Mylan Ltd)
Ciclosporin 25 mg Capimune 25mg capsules | 30 capsule [PoM] £13.05 DT price = £18.37
Ciclosporin 50 mg Capimune 50mg capsules | 30 capsule [PoM] £25.50 DT price = £35.97
Ciclosporin 100 mg Capimune 100mg capsules | 30 capsule [PoM] £48.50 DT price = £68.28
▸ **Capsorin** (Morningside Healthcare Ltd)
Ciclosporin 25 mg Capsorin 25mg capsules | 30 capsule [PoM] £13.05 DT price = £18.37
Ciclosporin 50 mg Capsorin 50mg capsules | 30 capsule [PoM] £25.59 DT price = £35.97
Ciclosporin 100 mg Capsorin 100mg capsules | 30 capsule [PoM] £48.89 DT price = £68.28
▸ **Deximune** (Dexcel-Pharma Ltd)
Ciclosporin 25 mg Deximune 25mg capsules | 30 capsule [PoM] £13.06 DT price = £18.37
Ciclosporin 50 mg Deximune 50mg capsules | 30 capsule [PoM] £25.60 DT price = £35.97
Ciclosporin 100 mg Deximune 100mg capsules | 30 capsule [PoM] £48.90 DT price = £68.28
▸ **Neoral** (Novartis Pharmaceuticals UK Ltd)
Ciclosporin 10 mg Neoral 10mg capsules | 60 capsule [PoM] £18.25 DT price = £18.25
Ciclosporin 25 mg Neoral 25mg capsules | 30 capsule [PoM] £18.37 DT price = £18.37
Ciclosporin 50 mg Neoral 50mg capsules | 30 capsule [PoM] £35.97 DT price = £35.97
Ciclosporin 100 mg Neoral 100mg capsules | 30 capsule [PoM] £68.28 DT price = £68.28
▸ **Vanquoral** (Teva UK Ltd)
Ciclosporin 10 mg Vanquoral 10mg capsules | 30 capsule [PoM] £12.75 | 60 capsule [PoM] £12.75 DT price = £18.25
Ciclosporin 25 mg Vanquoral 25mg capsules | 30 capsule [PoM] £13.05 DT price = £18.37
Ciclosporin 50 mg Vanquoral 50mg capsules | 30 capsule [PoM] £25.59 DT price = £35.97
Ciclosporin 100 mg Vanquoral 100mg capsules | 30 capsule [PoM] £48.89 DT price = £68.28

Sirolimus

- **DRUG ACTION** Sirolimus is a non-calcineurin inhibiting immunosuppressant.

- **INDICATIONS AND DOSE**

As a component of immunosuppressive therapy for renal transplantation in children and adolescents only if intolerance necessitates the withdrawal of a calcineurin inhibitor
▸ BY MOUTH
  ▸ Child: (consult local protocol)
DOSE EQUIVALENCE AND CONVERSION
▸ The 500 microgram tablet is not bioequivalent to the 1 mg and 2 mg tablets. Multiples of 500 microgram tablets should **not** be used as a substitute for other tablet strengths.

- **UNLICENSED USE** Not licensed for use in children.
- **CAUTIONS** Hyperlipidaemia · increased susceptibility to infection (especially urinary-tract infection) · increased susceptibility to lymphoma and other malignancies, particularly of the skin (limit exposure to UV light)
- **INTERACTIONS** → Appendix 1: sirolimus
- **SIDE-EFFECTS**
▸ **Common or very common** Abdominal pain · acne · anaemia · arthralgia · ascites · constipation · diarrhoea · epistaxis · haemolytic uraemic syndrome · headache · hypercholesterolaemia · hyperglycaemia · hypertension · hypertriglyceridaemia · hypokalaemia · hypophosphataemia · impaired healing · leucopenia · lymphocele · nausea · neutropenia · oedema · osteonecrosis · pleural effusion · pneumonitis · proteinuria · pyrexia · rash · stomatitis · tachycardia · thrombocytopenia · thrombotic thrombocytopenic purpura · venous thromboembolism
▸ **Uncommon** Nephrotic syndrome · pancreatitis · pancytopenia · pericardial effusion · pulmonary embolism · pulmonary haemorrhage
▸ **Rare** Alveolar proteinosis · anaphylactic reactions · angioedema · exfoliative dermatitis · hepatic necrosis · hypersensitivity reactions · hypersensitivity vasculitis · interstitial lung disease · lymphoedema
▸ **Frequency not known** Focal segmental glomerulosclerosis · reversible impairment of male fertility
- **CONCEPTION AND CONTRACEPTION** Effective contraception must be used during treatment and for 12 weeks after stopping.
- **PREGNANCY** Avoid unless essential—toxicity in *animal* studies.
- **BREAST FEEDING** Discontinue breast-feeding.
- **HEPATIC IMPAIRMENT** Dose reduction may be necessary, consult local treatment protocols for details. Monitor whole blood-sirolimus level closely and consult local treatment protocol in hepatic impairment.
- **MONITORING REQUIREMENTS**
▸ Monitor whole blood-sirolimus trough concentration (Afro-Caribbean patients may require higher doses).
▸ Monitor kidney function when given with ciclosporin; monitor lipids; monitor urine proteins.
- **DIRECTIONS FOR ADMINISTRATION** Food may affect absorption (take at the same time with respect to food). Sirolimus oral solution should be mixed with at least 60 mL water or orange juice in a glass or plastic container immediately before taking; refill container with at least 120 mL of water or orange juice and drink immediately (to ensure total dose). Do not mix with any other liquids.
- **PATIENT AND CARER ADVICE** Patient or carers should be given advice on how to administer sirolimus.

Patients should be advised to avoid excessive exposure to UV light.

● **MEDICINAL FORMS**
There can be variation in the licensing of different medicines containing the same drug.

Oral solution
EXCIPIENTS: May contain Ethanol
▸ **Rapamune** (Pfizer Ltd)
Sirolimus 1 mg per 1 ml Rapamune 1mg/ml oral solution sugar-free | 60 ml [PoM] £162.41

Tablet
▸ **Rapamune** (Pfizer Ltd)
Sirolimus 500 microgram Rapamune 0.5mg tablets | 30 tablet [PoM] £69.00 DT price = £69.00
Sirolimus 1 mg Rapamune 1mg tablets | 30 tablet [PoM] £86.49 DT price = £86.49
Sirolimus 2 mg Rapamune 2mg tablets | 30 tablet [PoM] £172.98 DT price = £172.98

Tacrolimus

● **DRUG ACTION** Tacrolimus is a calcineurin inhibitor.

● **INDICATIONS AND DOSE**

ADOPORT®

Prophylaxis of graft rejection following liver transplantation, starting 12 hours after transplantation
▸ BY MOUTH
▸ Neonate: Initially 150 micrograms/kg twice daily.

▸ Child: Initially 150 micrograms/kg twice daily

Prophylaxis of graft rejection following kidney transplantation, starting within 24 hours of transplantation
▸ BY MOUTH
▸ Neonate: Initially 150 micrograms/kg twice daily.

▸ Child: Initially 150 micrograms/kg twice daily, a lower initial dose of 100 micrograms/kg twice daily has been used in adolescents to prevent very high 'trough' concentrations

Prophylaxis of graft rejection following heart transplantation following antibody induction, starting within 5 days of transplantation
▸ BY MOUTH
▸ Neonate: Initially 50–150 micrograms/kg twice daily.

▸ Child: Initially 50–150 micrograms/kg twice daily

Prophylaxis of graft rejection following heart transplantation without antibody induction, starting within 12 hours of transplantation
▸ BY MOUTH
▸ Neonate: Initially 150 micrograms/kg twice daily, dose to be given as soon as clinically possible (8–12 hours after discontinuation of intravenous infusion).

▸ Child: Initially 150 micrograms/kg twice daily, dose to be given as soon as clinically possible (8–12 hours after discontinuation of intravenous infusion)

Allograft rejection resistant to conventional immunosuppressive therapy
▸ BY MOUTH
▸ Child: Seek specialist advice

CAPEXION®

Prophylaxis of graft rejection following liver transplantation, starting 12 hours after transplantation
▸ BY MOUTH
▸ Neonate: Initially 150 micrograms/kg twice daily.

▸ Child: Initially 150 micrograms/kg twice daily

Prophylaxis of graft rejection following kidney transplantation, starting within 24 hours of transplantation
▸ BY MOUTH
▸ Neonate: Initially 150 micrograms/kg twice daily.

▸ Child: Initially 150 micrograms/kg twice daily, a lower initial dose of 100 micrograms/kg twice daily has been used in adolescents to prevent very high 'trough' concentrations

Prophylaxis of graft rejection following heart transplantation following antibody induction, starting within 5 days of transplantation
▸ BY MOUTH
▸ Neonate: Initially 50–150 micrograms/kg twice daily.

▸ Child: Initially 50–150 micrograms/kg twice daily

Prophylaxis of graft rejection following heart transplantation without antibody induction, starting within 12 hours of transplantation
▸ BY MOUTH
▸ Neonate: Initially 150 micrograms/kg twice daily, dose to be given as soon as clinically possible (8–12 hours after discontinuation of intravenous infusion).

▸ Child: Initially 150 micrograms/kg twice daily, dose to be given as soon as clinically possible (8–12 hours after discontinuation of intravenous infusion)

Allograft rejection resistant to conventional immunosuppressive therapy
▸ BY MOUTH
▸ Child: Seek specialist advice

MODIGRAF®

Prophylaxis of graft rejection following liver transplantation, starting 12 hours after transplantation
▸ BY MOUTH
▸ Neonate: Initially 150 micrograms/kg twice daily.

▸ Child: Initially 150 micrograms/kg twice daily

Prophylaxis of graft rejection following kidney transplantation, starting within 24 hours of transplantation
▸ BY MOUTH
▸ Neonate: Initially 150 micrograms/kg twice daily.

▸ Child: Initially 150 micrograms/kg twice daily, a lower initial dose of 100 micrograms/kg twice daily has been used in adolescents to prevent very high 'trough' concentrations

Prophylaxis of graft rejection following heart transplantation following antibody induction, starting within 5 days of transplantation
▸ BY MOUTH
▸ Neonate: Initially 50–150 micrograms/kg twice daily.

▸ Child: Initially 50–150 micrograms/kg twice daily

Prophylaxis of graft rejection following heart transplantation without antibody induction, starting within 12 hours of transplantation
▸ BY MOUTH
▸ Neonate: Initially 150 micrograms/kg twice daily, dose to be given as soon as clinically possible (8–12 hours after discontinuation of intravenous infusion).

▸ Child: Initially 150 micrograms/kg twice daily, dose to be given as soon as clinically possible (8–12 hours after discontinuation of intravenous infusion)   continued →

8

Immune system and malignant disease

Allograft rejection resistant to conventional immunosuppressive therapy
► BY MOUTH
► Child: Seek specialist advice

PROGRAF® CAPSULES

Prophylaxis of graft rejection following liver transplantation, starting 12 hours after transplantation
► BY MOUTH

► Neonate: Initially 150 micrograms/kg twice daily.

► Child: Initially 150 micrograms/kg twice daily

Prophylaxis of graft rejection following kidney transplantation, starting within 24 hours of transplantation
► BY MOUTH

► Neonate: Initially 150 micrograms/kg twice daily.

► Child: Initially 150 micrograms/kg twice daily, a lower initial dose of 100 micrograms/kg twice daily has been used in adolescents to prevent very high 'trough' concentrations

Prophylaxis of graft rejection following heart transplantation following antibody induction, starting within 5 days of transplantation
► BY MOUTH

► Neonate: Initially 50–150 micrograms/kg twice daily.

► Child: Initially 50–150 micrograms/kg twice daily

Prophylaxis of graft rejection following heart transplantation without antibody induction, starting within 12 hours of transplantation
► BY MOUTH

► Neonate: Initially 150 micrograms/kg twice daily, dose to be given as soon as clinically possible (8–12 hours after discontinuation of intravenous infusion).

► Child: Initially 150 micrograms/kg twice daily, dose to be given as soon as clinically possible (8–12 hours after discontinuation of intravenous infusion)

Allograft rejection resistant to conventional immunosuppressive therapy
► BY MOUTH
► Child: Seek specialist advice

PROGRAF® INFUSION

Prophylaxis of graft rejection following liver transplantation, starting 12 hours after transplantation when oral route not appropriate
► BY CONTINUOUS INTRAVENOUS INFUSION

► Neonate: Initially 50 micrograms/kg daily for up to 7 days (then transfer to oral therapy), dose to be administered over 24 hours.

► Child: Initially 50 micrograms/kg daily for up to 7 days (then transfer to oral therapy), dose to be administered over 24 hours

Prophylaxis of graft rejection following kidney transplantation, starting within 24 hours of transplantation when oral route not appropriate
► BY CONTINUOUS INTRAVENOUS INFUSION

► Neonate: Initially 75–100 micrograms/kg daily for up to 7 days (then transfer to oral therapy), dose to be administered over 24 hours.

► Child: Initially 75–100 micrograms/kg daily for up to 7 days (then transfer to oral therapy), dose to be administered over 24 hours

Prophylaxis of graft rejection following heart transplantation without antibody induction, starting within 12 hours of transplantation
► BY CONTINUOUS INTRAVENOUS INFUSION

► Neonate: Initially 30–50 micrograms/kg daily for up to 7 days (then transfer to oral therapy), dose to be administered over 24 hours.

► Child: Initially 30–50 micrograms/kg daily for up to 7 days (then transfer to oral therapy), dose to be administered over 24 hours

Allograft rejection resistant to conventional immunosuppressive therapy
► BY CONTINUOUS INTRAVENOUS INFUSION
► Child: Seek specialist advice (consult local protocol)

TACNI®

Prophylaxis of graft rejection following liver transplantation, starting 12 hours after transplantation
► BY MOUTH

► Neonate: Initially 150 micrograms/kg twice daily.

► Child: Initially 150 micrograms/kg twice daily

Prophylaxis of graft rejection following kidney transplantation, starting within 24 hours of transplantation
► BY MOUTH

► Neonate: Initially 150 micrograms/kg twice daily.

► Child: Initially 150 micrograms/kg twice daily, a lower initial dose of 100 micrograms/kg twice daily has been used in adolescents to prevent very high 'trough' concentrations

Prophylaxis of graft rejection following heart transplantation following antibody induction, starting within 5 days of transplantation
► BY MOUTH

► Neonate: Initially 50–150 micrograms/kg twice daily.

► Child: Initially 50–150 micrograms/kg twice daily

Prophylaxis of graft rejection following heart transplantation without antibody induction, starting within 12 hours of transplantation
► BY MOUTH

► Neonate: Initially 150 micrograms/kg twice daily, dose to be given as soon as clinically possible (8–12 hours after discontinuation of intravenous infusion).

► Child: Initially 150 micrograms/kg twice daily, dose to be given as soon as clinically possible (8–12 hours after discontinuation of intravenous infusion)

Allograft rejection resistant to conventional immunosuppressive therapy
► BY MOUTH
► Child: Seek specialist advice

VIVADEX®

Prophylaxis of graft rejection following liver transplantation, starting 12 hours after transplantation
► BY MOUTH

► Neonate: Initially 150 micrograms/kg twice daily.

► Child: Initially 150 micrograms/kg twice daily

Prophylaxis of graft rejection following kidney transplantation, starting within 24 hours of transplantation
► BY MOUTH

► Neonate: Initially 150 micrograms/kg twice daily.

► Child: Initially 150 micrograms/kg twice daily, a lower initial dose of 100 micrograms/kg twice daily has been used in adolescents to prevent very high 'trough' concentrations

Prophylaxis of graft rejection following heart transplantation following antibody induction, starting within 5 days of transplantation
▸ BY MOUTH

▸ Neonate: Initially 50–150 micrograms/kg twice daily.

▸ Child: Initially 50–150 micrograms/kg twice daily

Prophylaxis of graft rejection following heart transplantation without antibody induction, starting within 12 hours of transplantation
▸ BY MOUTH

▸ Neonate: Initially 150 micrograms/kg twice daily, dose to be given as soon as clinically possible (8–12 hours after discontinuation of intravenous infusion).

▸ Child: Initially 150 micrograms/kg twice daily, dose to be given as soon as clinically possible (8–12 hours after discontinuation of intravenous infusion)

Allograft rejection resistant to conventional immunosuppressive therapy
▸ BY MOUTH
▸ Child: Seek specialist advice

● UNLICENSED USE
  ADVAGRAF® *Advagraf*® not licensed for use in children.

IMPORTANT SAFETY INFORMATION

MHRA/CHM ADVICE: ORAL TACROLIMUS PRODUCTS: PRESCRIBE AND DISPENSE BY BRAND NAME ONLY, TO MINIMISE THE RISK OF INADVERTENT SWITCHING BETWEEN PRODUCTS, WHICH HAS BEEN ASSOCIATED WITH REPORTS OF TOXICITY AND GRAFT REJECTION (JUNE 2012)

Inadvertent switching between oral tacrolimus products has been associated with reports of toxicity and graft rejection. To ensure maintenance of therapeutic response when a patient is stabilised on a particular brand, oral tacrolimus products should be prescribed and dispensed by brand name only.
● *Adoport*®, *Prograf*®, *Capexion*®, *Tacni*®, and *Vivadex*® are immediate-release capsules that are taken twice daily, once in the morning and once in the evening;
● *Modigraf*® granules are used to prepare an immediate-release oral suspension which is taken twice daily, once in the morning and once in the evening;
● *Advagraf*® is a prolonged-release capsule that is taken once daily in the morning.
Switching between tacrolimus brands requires careful supervision and therapeutic monitoring by an appropriate specialist.
Important: *Envarsus*® is not interchangeable with other oral tacrolimus containing products; the MHRA has advised (June 2012) that oral tacrolimus products should be prescribed and dispensed by brand only.

● CAUTIONS Increased risk of infections · lymphoproliferative disorders · malignancies · neurotoxicity · QT-interval prolongation · UV light (avoid excessive exposure to sunlight and sunlamps)

● INTERACTIONS → Appendix 1: tacrolimus

● SIDE-EFFECTS
▸ Common or very common Acne · alopecia · anaemia · anorexia · anxiety · arthralgia · ascites · bile-duct abnormalities · bloating · blood disorders · cholestasis · confusion · constipation · depression · diarrhoea · dizziness · dyspepsia · dyspnoea · electrolyte disturbances · flatulence · gastro-intestinal inflammation · gastro-intestinal perforation · gastro-intestinal ulceration · haemorrhage · headache · hepatic dysfunction · hyperglycaemia · hyperkalaemia · hypertension · hyperuricaemia · hypokalaemia · impaired hearing ·

ischaemic events · jaundice · leucopenia · mood changes · muscle cramp · nausea · oedema · pancytopenia · paraesthesia · parenchymal lung disorders · peripheral neuropathy · photophobia · pleural effusion · psychosis · renal failure · renal impairment · renal tubular necrosis · seizures · sleep disturbances · sweating · tachycardia · thrombocytopenia · thromboembolic events · tinnitus · tremor · urinary abnormalities · visual disturbances · vomiting · weight changes
▸ Uncommon Amnesia · arrhythmia · cardiac arrest · cardiomyopathy · cataract · cerebrovascular accident · coagulation disorders · coma · dermatitis · dysmenorrhoea · encephalopathy · gastro-intestinal reflux disease · heart failure · hypertonia · hypoglycaemia · influenza-like symptoms · palpitation · pancreatitis · paralysis · paralytic ileus · peritonitis · photosensitivity · respiratory failure · speech disorder
▸ Rare Blindness · dehydration · hirsutism · pericardial effusion · posterior reversible encephalopathy syndrome · respiratory distress syndrome · thrombotic thrombocytopenic purpura · toxic epidermal necrolysis
▸ Very rare Haemorrhagic cystitis · myasthenia · Stevens-Johnson syndrome
▸ Frequency not known Agranulocytosis · haemolytic anaemia · pure red cell aplasia

SIDE-EFFECTS, FURTHER INFORMATION
▸ Cardiomyopathy Cardiomyopathy has been reported in children. Patients should be monitored by echocardiography for hypertrophic changes—consider dose reduction or discontinuation if these occur.

● ALLERGY AND CROSS-SENSITIVITY Contra-indicated if history of hypersensitivity to macrolides.

● CONCEPTION AND CONTRACEPTION Exclude pregnancy before treatment.

● PREGNANCY Avoid unless potential benefit outweighs risk—crosses the placenta and risk of premature delivery, intra-uterine growth restriction, and hyperkalaemia.

● BREAST FEEDING Avoid—present in breast milk (following systemic administration).

● HEPATIC IMPAIRMENT Dose reduction may be necessary in severe impairment.

● MONITORING REQUIREMENTS
▸ After initial dosing, and for maintenance treatment, tacrolimus doses should be adjusted according to whole-blood concentration. Monitor whole blood-tacrolimus trough concentration (especially during episodes of diarrhoea)—consult local treatment protocol for details.
▸ Monitor blood pressure, ECG (for hypertrophic changes—risk of cardiomyopathy), fasting blood-glucose concentration, haematological and neurological (including visual) and coagulation parameters, electrolytes, hepatic and renal function.

● DIRECTIONS FOR ADMINISTRATION For *continuous intravenous infusion* over 24 hours, dilute to a concentration of 4–100 micrograms/mL with Glucose 5% *or* Sodium Chloride 0.9%, to a total volume between 20–500mL. Tacrolimus is incompatible with PVC.

● PRESCRIBING AND DISPENSING INFORMATION
PROGRAF® INFUSION Intravenous route should only be used if oral route is inappropriate.

● PATIENT AND CARER ADVICE
Avoid excessive exposure to UV light including sunlight.
Driving and skilled tasks   May affect performance of skilled tasks (e.g. driving).
Medicines for Children leaflet: Tacrolimus for prevention of transplant rejection www.medicinesforchildren.org.uk/tacrolimus-for-prevention-of-transplant-rejection

8

Immune system and malignant disease

● NATIONAL FUNDING/ACCESS DECISIONS

Scottish Medicines Consortium (SMC) Decisions

The *Scottish Medicines Consortium* has advised (November 2010) that tacrolimus granules for oral suspension (*Modigraf*®) are accepted for restricted use within NHS Scotland in patients for whom tacrolimus is an appropriate choice of immunosuppressive therapy and where small changes (less than 500 micrograms) in dosing increments are required (such as, in paediatric patients) or in seriously ill patients who are unable to swallow tacrolimus capsules.

● MEDICINAL FORMS

There can be variation in the licensing of different medicines containing the same drug.

Granules

CAUTIONARY AND ADVISORY LABELS 13, 23

▸ **Modigraf** (Astellas Pharma Ltd)
Tacrolimus (as Tacrolimus monohydrate)
200 microgram Modigraf 0.2mg granules sachets sugar-free | 50 sachet [PoM] £71.30 DT price = £71.30
Tacrolimus (as Tacrolimus monohydrate) 1 mg Modigraf 1mg granules sachets sugar-free | 50 sachet [PoM] £356.65 DT price = £356.65

Solution for infusion

EXCIPIENTS: May contain Polyoxyl castor oils

▸ **Prograf** (Astellas Pharma Ltd)
Tacrolimus 5 mg per 1 ml Prograf 5mg/1ml solution for infusion ampoules | 10 ampoule [PoM] £584.51

Capsule

CAUTIONARY AND ADVISORY LABELS 23

▸ **Adoport** (Sandoz Ltd)
Tacrolimus 500 microgram Adoport 0.5mg capsules | 50 capsule [PoM] £42.92 DT price = £61.88
Tacrolimus 750 microgram Adoport 0.75mg capsules | 50 capsule [PoM] £51.75
Tacrolimus 1 mg Adoport 1mg capsules | 50 capsule [PoM] £55.69 DT price = £80.28 | 100 capsule [PoM] £111.36
Tacrolimus 2 mg Adoport 2mg capsules | 50 capsule [PoM] £111.00
Tacrolimus 5 mg Adoport 5mg capsules | 50 capsule [PoM] £205.74 DT price = £296.58

▸ **Capexion** (Mylan Ltd)
Tacrolimus 500 microgram Capexion 0.5mg capsules | 50 capsule [PoM] £52.50 DT price = £61.88

▸ **Prograf** (Astellas Pharma Ltd)
Tacrolimus 500 microgram Prograf 500microgram capsules | 50 capsule [PoM] £61.88 DT price = £61.88
Tacrolimus 1 mg Prograf 1mg capsules | 50 capsule [PoM] £80.28 DT price = £80.28 | 100 capsule [PoM] £160.54
Tacrolimus 5 mg Prograf 5mg capsules | 50 capsule [PoM] £296.58 DT price = £296.58

▸ **Tacni** (Teva Uk Ltd)
Tacrolimus 500 microgram Tacni 0.5mg capsules | 50 capsule [PoM] £50.48 DT price = £61.88
Tacrolimus 1 mg Tacni 1mg capsules | 50 capsule [PoM] £65.49 DT price = £80.28 | 100 capsule [PoM] £130.99
Tacrolimus 5 mg Tacni 5mg capsules | 50 capsule [PoM] £242.01 DT price = £296.58

IMMUNOSUPPRESSANTS ⟩ MONOCLONAL ANTIBODIES

Canakinumab

● DRUG ACTION Canakinumab is a recombinant human monoclonal antibody that selectively inhibits interleukin-1 beta receptor binding.

● INDICATIONS AND DOSE

Treatment of cryopyrin-associated periodic syndromes, including severe forms of familial cold auto-inflammatory syndrome (or familial cold urticaria), Muckle-Wells syndrome, and neonatal-onset multisystem inflammatory disease (also known as chronic infantile neurological cutaneous and articular syndrome)

▸ BY SUBCUTANEOUS INJECTION

▸ Child: (consult product literature

Active systemic juvenile idiopathic arthritis (in combination with methotrexate or alone) in children who have had an inadequate response to NSAIDs and systemic corticosteroids

▸ BY SUBCUTANEOUS INJECTION

▸ Child 2-17 years (body-weight 7.5 kg and above): 4 mg/kg every 4 weeks (max. per dose 300 mg)

● CONTRA-INDICATIONS Active infection · leucopenia · neutropenia

● CAUTIONS History of recurrent infection · latent and active tuberculosis · predisposition to infection

CAUTIONS, FURTHER INFORMATION

▸ Vaccinations Patients should receive all recommended vaccinations (including pneumococcal and inactivated influenza vaccine) before starting treatment; avoid live vaccines unless potential benefit outweighs risk—consult product literature for further information.

● INTERACTIONS → Appendix 1: monoclonal antibodies

● SIDE-EFFECTS

GENERAL SIDE-EFFECTS

▸ Common or very common Back pain · increased susceptibility to infection (including serious infection) · injection-site reactions · malaise · neutropenia · vertigo

▸ Uncommon Gastro-oesophageal reflux

▸ Frequency not known Malignancy · vomiting

SPECIFIC SIDE-EFFECTS

▸ When used for active systemic juvenile idiopathic arthritis Abdominal pain · arthralgia · musculoskeletal pain · rhinitis

● CONCEPTION AND CONTRACEPTION Effective contraception required during treatment and for up to 3 months after last dose.

● PREGNANCY Manufacturer advises avoid unless potential benefit outweighs risk.

● BREAST FEEDING Consider if benefit outweighs risk—not known if present in human milk.

● HEPATIC IMPAIRMENT No information available.

● RENAL IMPAIRMENT Limited information available but manufacturer advises no dose adjustment required.

● PRE-TREATMENT SCREENING Patients should be evaluated for latent and active tuberculosis before starting treatment.

● MONITORING REQUIREMENTS

▸ Monitor full blood count including neutrophil count before starting treatment, 1–2 months after starting treatment, and periodically thereafter.

▸ Monitor for signs and symptoms of tuberculosis during and after treatment.

Prevention of acute symptoms: For patients at low risk of emesis, pretreatment with a 5HT$_3$-receptor antagonist may be of benefit.

For patients at high risk of *emesis* or when other treatment is inadequate, a 5HT$_3$-receptor antagonist is often highly effective. The addition of dexamethasone p. 419 and other anti-emetics may also be required.

Prevention of delayed symptoms: dexamethasone, given by mouth, is the drug of choice for preventing delayed symptoms; it is used alone or with metoclopramide hydrochloride p. 252. Due to the risks of neurological side-effects, metoclopramide hydrochloride should only be used in children as a second-line option. The 5HT$_3$-receptor antagonists may have a role in preventing uncontrolled symptoms.

Prevention of anticipatory symptoms: Good symptom control is the best way to prevent anticipatory symptoms. Lorazepam p. 214 can be helpful for its amnesiac, sedative, and anxiolytic effects.

Bone-marrow suppression

All cytotoxic drugs except vincristine sulfate p. 523 and bleomycin p. 520 cause bone-marrow suppression. This commonly occurs 7 to 10 days after administration, but is delayed for certain drugs, such as melphalan p. 511. Peripheral blood counts must be checked before each treatment. The duration and severity of neutropenia can be reduced by the use of granulocyte-colony stimulating factors; their use should be reserved for children who have previously experienced severe neutropenia.

Cytotoxic drugs may be contra-indicated in children with acute infection; any infection should be treated before, or when starting, cytotoxic drugs.

Infection in a child with neutropenia requires immediate broad-spectrum antibacterial treatment that covers all likely pathogens. Appropriate bacteriological investigations should be conducted as soon as possible. Children taking cytotoxic drugs who have signs or symptoms of infection (or their carers) should be advised to seek prompt medical attention. All children should be investigated and treated under the supervision of an appropriate oncology or haematology specialist. Antifungal treatment may be required in a child with prolonged neutropenia or fever lasting longer than 4–5 days. Chickenpox and measles can be particularly hazardous in immunocompromised children. Varicella-zoster immunoglobulin p. 746 is indicated if the child does not have immunity against varicella and has had close contact with infectious chickenpox or herpes zoster. Antiviral prophylaxis can be considered in addition to varicella–zoster immunoglobulin or as an alternative if varicella–zoster immunoglobulin is inappropriate. If an immunocompromised child has come into close contact with an infectious individual with measles, normal immunoglobulin p. 743 should be given.

For advice on the use of live vaccines in individuals with impaired immune response, see Vaccines.

Alopecia

Reversible hair loss is a common complication, although it varies in degree between drugs and individual patients.

Long-term and delayed toxicity

Cytotoxic drugs may produce specific organ-related toxicity in children (e.g. cardiotoxicity with doxorubicin hydrochloride p. 513 or nephrotoxicity with cisplatin p. 521 and ifosfamide p. 510). Manifestations of such toxicity may not appear for several months or even years after cancer treatment. Careful follow-up of survivors of childhood cancer is therefore vital; national and local guidelines have been developed to facilitate this.

Thromboembolism

Venous thromboembolism can be a complication of cancer itself, but chemotherapy increases the risk.

Tumour lysis syndrome

Tumour lysis syndrome occurs secondary to spontaneous or treatment related rapid destruction of malignant cells. Patients at risk of tumour lysis syndrome include those with non- Hodgkin's lymphoma (especially if high grade and bulky disease), Burkitt's lymphoma, acute lymphoblastic leukaemia and acute myeloid leukaemia (particularly if high white blood cell counts or bulky disease), and occasionally those with solid tumours. Pre-existing hyperuricaemia, dehydration and renal impairment are also predisposing factors. Features, include hyperkalaemia, hyperuricaemia, and hyperphosphataemia with hypocalcaemia; renal damage and arrhythmias can follow. Early recognition of patients at risk, and initiation of prophylaxis or therapy for tumour lysis syndrome, is essential.

Treatment for cytotoxic-induced side effects

Hyperuricaemia

Hyperuricaemia, which may be present in high-grade lymphoma and leukaemia, can be markedly worsened by chemotherapy and is associated with acute renal failure.

Allopurinol p. 529 is used routinely in children at low to moderate risk of hyperuricaemia. It should be started 24 hours before treatment; patients should be adequately hydrated (consideration should be given to omitting phosphate and potassium from hydration fluids). The dose of mercaptopurine p. 516 or azathioprine p. 495 should be reduced if allopurinol is given concomitantly.

Rasburicase p. 529 is a recombinant urate oxidase used in children who are at high-risk of developing hyperuricaemia. It rapidly reduces plasma-uric acid concentration and may be of particular value in preventing complications following treatment of leukaemias or bulky lymphomas.

Methotrexate-induced mucositis and myelosuppression

Folinic acid p. 528 (given as calcium folinate) is used to counteract the folate-antagonist action of methotrexate and thus speed recovery from methotrexate-induced mucositis or myelosuppression ('folinic acid rescue').

The calcium salt of levofolinic acid p. 528, a single isomer of folinic acid, is also used following methotrexate administration. The dose of calcium levofolinate is generally half that of calcium folinate.

The disodium salts of folinic acid and levofolinic acid are also used for rescue therapy following methotrexate administration.

The efficacy of high dose methotrexate is enhanced by delaying initiation of folinic acid for at least 24 hours, local protocols define the correct time. Folinic acid is normally continued until the plasma-methotrexate concentration falls to 45–90 nanograms/mL (100–200 nanomol/litre).

In the treatment of methotrexate p. 517 overdose, folinate should be administered immediately; other measures to enhance the elimination of methotrexate are also necessary.

Urothelial toxicity

Haemorrhagic cystitis is a common manifestation of urothelial toxicity which occurs with the oxazaphosphorines, cyclophosphamide p. 509 and ifosfamide p. 510; it is caused by the metabolite acrolein. Adequate hydration is essential to reduce the risk of urothelial toxicity. Mesna p. 527 reacts specifically with acrolein in the urinary tract, preventing toxicity. Mesna is given for the same duration as cyclophosphamide or ifosfamide. It is generally given intravenously; the dose of mesna is equal to or greater than that of the oxazaphosphorine. See the role of nebulised mesna as a mucolytic in cystic fibrosis.

Cytotoxic antibiotics

Cytotoxic antibiotics are widely used. Many act as radiomimetics and simultaneous use of radiotherapy should be **avoided** because it may markedly increase toxicity.

Daunorubicin p. 516, doxorubicin hydrochloride p. 513, and epirubicin hydrochloride p. 513 are anthracycline

8

Immune system and malignant disease

antibiotics. Mitoxantrone p. 514 (mitozantrone) is an anthracycline derivative.

Epirubicin hydrochloride and mitoxantrone are considered less toxic than the other anthracycline antibiotics, and may be suitable for children who have received high cumulative doses of other anthracyclines.

Vinca alkaloids

The vinca alkaloids, vinblastine sulfate p. 522 and vincristine sulfate p. 523 are used to treat a variety of cancers including leukaemias, lymphomas, and some solid tumours.

Antimetabolites

Antimetabolites are incorporated into new nuclear material or they combine irreversibly with cellular enzymes and prevent normal cellular division. Cytarabine p. 515, fludarabine phosphate p. 515, mercaptopurine p. 516, methotrexate p. 517, and tioguanine p. 519 are commonly used in paediatric chemotherapy.

Other antineoplastic drugs

Asparaginase

Asparaginase is used almost exclusively in the treatment of acute lymphoblastic leukaemia. Hypersensitivity reactions may occur and facilities for the management of anaphylaxis should be available. A number of different preparations of asparaginase exist and only the product specified in the treatment protocol should be used.

ANTINEOPLASTIC DRUGS > ALKYLATING AGENTS

Busulfan

(Busulphan)

● **INDICATIONS AND DOSE**

Conditioning treatment before haematopoietic progenitor cell transplantation

▶ BY MOUTH, OR BY INTRAVENOUS INFUSION

▶ Child: (consult local protocol)

DOSES AT EXTREMES OF BODY-WEIGHT

Dose may need to be calculated based on body surface area or adjusted ideal body weight in obese patients—consult product literature.

IMPORTANT SAFETY INFORMATION

RISKS OF INCORRECT DOSING OF ORAL ANTI-CANCER MEDICINES
See Cytotoxic drugs p. 505.

● CAUTIONS Avoid in acute porphyrias p. 577 · high dose (antiepileptic prophylaxis required) · history of seizures (antiepileptic prophylaxis required) · ineffective once in blast crisis phase · previous progenitor cell transplant (increased risk of hepatic veno-occlusive disease) · previous radiation therapy (increased risk of hepatic veno-occlusive disease) · risk of second malignancy · three or more cycles of chemotherapy (increased risk of hepatic veno-occlusive disease)

● INTERACTIONS → Appendix 1: alkylating agents

● SIDE-EFFECTS

GENERAL SIDE-EFFECTS

▶ **Common or very common** Cardiac tamponade in thalassaemia · hepatic fibrosis · hepatic veno-occlusive disease · hepatotoxicity · hyperbilirubinaemia · jaundice · pneumonia · skin hyperpigmentation

▶ **Rare** Aplastic anaemia · erythema · hypersensitivity reactions · progressive pulmonary fibrosis · seizures · urticaria · visual disturbances

▶ **Very rare** Gynaecomastia · myasthenia gravis

▶ **Frequency not known** Alopecia · amenorrhoea (may be reversible) · bone-marrow suppression · dilutional

hyponatraemia · fluid retention · gastro-intestinal effects · hyperuricaemia · irreversible bone-marrow aplasia · lung toxicity · male sterility · nausea · oedema · oral mucositis · organ-related toxicity (long-term and delayed) · premature menopause · secondary malignancy · thromboembolism · tumour lysis syndrome · vomiting

SPECIFIC SIDE-EFFECTS

▶ With intravenous use Extravasation

SIDE-EFFECTS, FURTHER INFORMATION

▶ Lung toxicity Discontinue if lung toxicity develops.

▶ Secondary malignancy Alkylating drugs are associated with a marked increase in the incidence of secondary tumours and leukaemia, particularly when they are combined with extensive irradiation.

▶ Fluid retention Alkylating drugs can cause fluid retention with oedema and dilutional hyponatraemia in younger children; the risk of this complication is higher in the first 2 days and also when given with concomitant vinca alkaloids.

● CONCEPTION AND CONTRACEPTION Manufacturers advise effective contraception during and for 6 months after treatment in men or women. See also *Pregnancy and reproductive function* in Cytotoxic drugs p. 505.

● PREGNANCY Avoid (teratogenic in *animals*). See also *Pregnancy and reproductive function* in Cytotoxic drugs p. 505.

● BREAST FEEDING Discontinue breast-feeding.

● HEPATIC IMPAIRMENT Manufacturer advises caution. In patients with hepatic impairment, manufacturer advises regular liver function tests—consult product literature.

● MONITORING REQUIREMENTS

▶ Monitor cardiac and liver function.

▶ Monitor full blood count regularly throughout treatment.

● MEDICINAL FORMS

There can be variation in the licensing of different medicines containing the same drug. Forms available from special-order manufacturers include: capsule, oral suspension, oral solution

Tablet

▶ Busulfan (Non-proprietary)
Busulfan 2 mg Busulfan 2mg tablets | ⊂ tablet PoM £69.02

Solution for infusion

▶ Busilvex (Pierre Fabre Ltd)
Busulfan 6 mg per 1 ml Busilvex 60mg/10ml concentrate for solution for infusion ampoules | 8 ampoule PoM £1,610.00 (Hospital only)

Chlorambucil

● **INDICATIONS AND DOSE**

Hodgkin's disease | Non-Hodgkin's lymphoma

▶ BY MOUTH

▶ Child: (consult local protocol)

Relapsing steroid-sensitive nephrotic syndrome (initiated in specialist centres)

▶ BY MOUTH

▶ Child 3 months–17 years: 200 micrograms/kg daily for 8 weeks

● UNLICENSED USE Not licensed for use in nephrotic syndrome.

IMPORTANT SAFETY INFORMATION

RISKS OF INCORRECT DOSING OF ORAL ANTI-CANCER MEDICINES
See Cytotoxic drugs p. 505.

● CAUTIONS Avoid in acute porphyrias p. 577 · children with nephrotic syndrome (increased seizure risk) · history of epilepsy (increased seizure risk)

● INTERACTIONS → Appendix 1: alkylating agents

- **SIDE-EFFECTS**
- **Uncommon** Skin rash
- **Rare** Hepatotoxicity · jaundice · seizures
- **Very rare** Irreversible bone-marrow suppression · male sterility (in prepubertal and pubertal males) · peripheral neuropathy · pulmonary fibrosis · sterile cystitis · tremor
- **Frequency not known** Alopecia · amenorrhoea · bone-marrow suppression · dilutional hyponatraemia · fluid retention · gastro-intestinal effects · hyperuricaemia · nausea · oedema · oral mucositis · organ-related toxicity (long-term and delayed) · premature menopause · secondary malignancy · Stevens-Johnson syndrome · thromboembolism · toxic epidermal necrolysis · tumour lysis syndrome · vomiting

SIDE-EFFECTS, FURTHER INFORMATION
- Secondary malignancy Alkylating drugs are associated with a marked increase in the incidence of secondary tumours and leukaemia, particularly when they are combined with extensive irradiation.
- Fluid retention Alkylating drugs can cause fluid retention with oedema and dilutional hyponatraemia in younger children; the risk of this complication is higher in the first 2 days and also when given with concomitant vinca alkaloids.

- **CONCEPTION AND CONTRACEPTION** Contraceptive advice required, see *Pregnancy and reproductive function* in Cytotoxic drugs p. 505.
- **PREGNANCY** Avoid. See also *Pregnancy and reproductive function* in Cytotoxic drugs p. 505.
- **BREAST FEEDING** Discontinue breast-feeding.
- **HEPATIC IMPAIRMENT** Manufacturer advises consider dose reduction in severe impairment—limited information available.
- **MONITORING REQUIREMENTS** Monitor full blood count regularly throughout treatment.
- **PATIENT AND CARER ADVICE**
  Medicines for Children leaflet: Chlorambucil for nephrotic syndrome www.medicinesforchildren.org.uk/chlorambucil-nephrotic-syndrome-0

- **MEDICINAL FORMS**
  There can be variation in the licensing of different medicines containing the same drug.
  Tablet
  - Chlorambucil (Non-proprietary)
    Chlorambucil 2 mg Chlorambucil 2mg tablets | 25 tablet PoM
    £42.87 DT price = £42.87

Cyclophosphamide

- **INDICATIONS AND DOSE**

Acute lymphoblastic leukaemia, non-Hodgkin's lymphoma, retinoblastoma, neuroblastoma, rhabdomyosarcoma, soft-tissue sarcomas, Ewing tumour, neuroectodermal tumours (including medulloblastoma), infant brain tumours, ependymona, high-dose conditioning for bone marrow transplantation, lupus nephritis
- BY MOUTH, OR BY INTRAVENOUS INFUSION
- Child: (consult local protocol)

Steroid-sensitive nephrotic syndrome
- BY MOUTH
- Child 3 months-17 years: 2–3 mg/kg daily for 8 weeks
- BY INTRAVENOUS INFUSION
- Child 3 months-17 years: 500 mg/m^2 once a month for 6 months

- **UNLICENSED USE** Not licensed for use in children.

> **IMPORTANT SAFETY INFORMATION**
> RISKS OF INCORRECT DOSING OF ORAL ANTI-CANCER MEDICINES
> See Cytotoxic drugs p. 505.

- **CONTRA-INDICATIONS** Haemorrhagic cystitis
- **CAUTIONS** Avoid in acute porphyrias p. 577 · diabetes mellitus · previous or concurrent mediastinal irradiation—risk of cardiotoxicity
- **INTERACTIONS** → Appendix 1: alkylating agents
- **SIDE-EFFECTS**
  GENERAL SIDE-EFFECTS
- **Common or very common** Anorexia · cardiotoxicity at high doses · disturbances of carbohydrate metabolism · inappropriate secretion of anti-diuretic hormone · interstitial pulmonary fibrosis · pancreatitis · pigmentation of nails · pigmentation of palms · pigmentation of soles · urothelial toxicity
- **Rare** Hepatotoxicity · renal dysfunction
- **Frequency not known** Alopecia · amenorrhoea · bone-marrow suppression · dilutional hyponatraemia · fluid retention · gastro-intestinal effects · haemorrhagic cystitis · hyperuricaemia · male sterility · nausea · oedema · oral mucositis · organ-related toxicity (long-term and delayed) · premature menopause · secondary malignancy · thromboembolism · tumour lysis syndrome · vomiting
  SPECIFIC SIDE-EFFECTS
- With intravenous use Extravasation
  SIDE-EFFECTS, FURTHER INFORMATION
- Haemorrhagic cystitis and urothelial toxicity Haemorrhagic cystitis is a common manifestation of urothelial toxicity; adequate hydration is essential to reduce the risk of urothelial toxicity with intravenous use of cyclophosphamide; mesna provides further protection against urotoxic effects.
- Secondary malignancy Alkylating drugs are associated with a marked increase in the incidence of secondary tumours and leukaemia, particularly when they are combined with extensive irradiation.
- Fluid retention Alkylating drugs can cause fluid retention with oedema and dilutional hyponatraemia in younger children; the risk of this complication is higher in the first 2 days and also when given with concomitant vinca alkaloids.

- **CONCEPTION AND CONTRACEPTION** Manufacturer advises effective contraception during and for at least 3 months after treatment in men or women. See also *Pregnancy and reproductive function* in Cytotoxic drugs p. 505.
- **PREGNANCY** Avoid. See also *Pregnancy and reproductive function* in Cytotoxic drugs p. 505.
- **BREAST FEEDING** Discontinue breast-feeding during and for 36 hours after stopping treatment.
- **HEPATIC IMPAIRMENT** Reduce dose—consult local treatment protocol for details.
- **RENAL IMPAIRMENT** Reduce dose—consult local treatment protocol for details.
- **DIRECTIONS FOR ADMINISTRATION** Consult local treatment protocol for details.
- **PATIENT AND CARER ADVICE**
  Medicines for Children leaflet: Cyclophosphamide for nephrotic syndrome www.medicinesforchildren.org.uk/cyclophosphamide-nephrotic-syndrome-0

8

Immune system and malignant disease

● MEDICINAL FORMS
There can be variation in the licensing of different medicines containing the same drug. Forms available from special-order manufacturers include: tablet, oral suspension, oral solution, solution for injection, solution for infusion

Tablet
CAUTIONARY AND ADVISORY LABELS 25, 27
▸ Cyclophosphamide (Non-proprietary)
Cyclophosphamide (as Cyclophosphamide monohydrate)
50 mg Cyclophosphamide 50mg tablets | 100 tablet PoM £139.00 DT price = £139.00
▸ Cytoxan (Imported (United States))
Cyclophosphamide 25 mg Cytoxan 25mg tablets | 100 tablet PoM no price available

Powder for solution for injection
▸ Cyclophosphamide (Non-proprietary)
Cyclophosphamide (as Cyclophosphamide monohydrate)
500 mg Cyclophosphamide 500mg powder for solution for injection vials | 1 vial PoM £9.66 (Hospital only) | 1 vial PoM £9.66
Cyclophosphamide (as Cyclophosphamide monohydrate)
1 gram Cyclophosphamide 1g powder for solution for injection vials | 1 vial PoM £17.06 (Hospital only) | 1 vial PoM £17.91
Cyclophosphamide (as Cyclophosphamide monohydrate)
2 gram Cyclophosphamide 2g powder for solution for injection vials | 1 vial PoM £34.12 (Hospital only)

Dacarbazine

● INDICATIONS AND DOSE
Hodgkin's disease | Paediatric solid tumours
▸ BY INTRAVENOUS INJECTION, OR BY INTRAVENOUS INFUSION
▹ Child: (consult local protocol)

● CAUTIONS Caution in handling—irritant to tissues
● INTERACTIONS → Appendix 1: alkylating agents
● SIDE-EFFECTS
▸ Common or very common Anorexia
▸ Uncommon Blurred vision · confusion · facial flushing · facial paraesthesia · headache · influenza-like symptoms · rash · renal impairment · seizures
▸ Rare Diarrhoea · hepatic vein thrombosis · hepatotoxicity · injection-site reactions · irritant to skin · irritant to tissues · liver necrosis · photosensitivity
▸ Frequency not known Alopecia · bone-marrow suppression · extravasation · gastro-intestinal effects · hyperuricaemia · nausea · oral mucositis · organ-related toxicity (long-term and delayed) · thromboembolism · tumour lysis syndrome · vomiting
● CONCEPTION AND CONTRACEPTION Ensure effective contraception during and for at least 6 months after treatment in men or women. See also *Pregnancy and reproductive function* in Cytotoxic drugs p. 505.
● PREGNANCY Avoid (carcinogenic and teratogenic in *animal* studies). See also *Pregnancy and reproductive function* in Cytotoxic drugs p. 505.
● BREAST FEEDING Discontinue breast-feeding.
● HEPATIC IMPAIRMENT Dose reduction may be required in combined renal and hepatic impairment. Avoid in severe impairment.
● RENAL IMPAIRMENT Dose reduction may be required in combined renal and hepatic impairment. Avoid in severe impairment.
● PRESCRIBING AND DISPENSING INFORMATION Dacarbazine is a component of a commonly used combination for Hodgkin's disease (ABVD—doxorubicin [previously *Adriamycin*®], bleomycin, vinblastine, and dacarbazine).

● MEDICINAL FORMS
There can be variation in the licensing of different medicines containing the same drug.

Powder for solution for infusion
▸ Dacarbazine (Non-proprietary)
Dacarbazine (as Dacarbazine citrate) 500 mg Dacarbazine 500mg powder for solution for infusion vials | 1 vial PoM £37.50
Dacarbazine (as Dacarbazine citrate) 1 gram Dacarbazine 1g powder for solution for infusion vials | 1 vial PoM £70.00

Powder for solution for injection
▸ Dacarbazine (Non-proprietary)
Dacarbazine (as Dacarbazine citrate) 100 mg Dacarbazine 100mg powder for solution for injection vials | 10 vial PoM £90.00
Dacarbazine (as Dacarbazine citrate) 200 mg Dacarbazine 200mg powder for solution for injection vials | 10 vial PoM £160.00

Ifosfamide

● INDICATIONS AND DOSE
Rhabdomyosarcoma | Soft-tissue sarcomas | Ewing tumour | Germ cell tumour | Osteogenic sarcoma
▸ BY INTRAVENOUS INFUSION
▹ Child: (consult local protocol)

● CONTRA-INDICATIONS Acute infection · urinary-tract infection · urinary-tract obstruction · urothelial damage
● CAUTIONS Avoid in acute porphyrias p. 577
● INTERACTIONS → Appendix 1: alkylating agents
● SIDE-EFFECTS
▸ Common or very common Confusion · disorientation · drowsiness · psychosis · renal toxicity (may lead to tubular dysfunction, Fanconi's syndrome, or diabetes insipidus) · restlessness · urothelial toxicity causing haemorrhagic cystitis and dysuria
▸ Uncommon Severe encephalopathy
▸ Rare Anorexia · constipation · convulsions · diarrhoea
▸ Very rare Jaundice · syndrome of inappropriate antidiuretic hormone secretion · thrombophlebitis
▸ Frequency not known Alopecia · amenorrhoea · bone-marrow suppression · dilutional hyponatraemia · extravasation · fluid retention · gastro-intestinal effects · hyperuricaemia · male sterility · nausea · oedema · oral mucositis · organ-related toxicity (long-term and delayed) · premature menopause · secondary malignancy · thromboembolism · tumour lysis syndrome · vomiting
SIDE-EFFECTS, FURTHER INFORMATION
▸ Urothelial toxicity Adequate hydration may reduce the risk of urothelial toxicity with intravenous use of ifosfamide; mesna provides further protection against urotoxic effects.
▸ Secondary malignancy Alkylating drugs are associated with a marked increase in the incidence of secondary tumours and leukaemia, particularly when they are combined with extensive irradiation.
▸ Fluid retention Alkylating drugs can cause fluid retention with oedema and dilutional hyponatraemia in younger children; the risk of this complication is higher in the first 2 days and also when given with concomitant vinca alkaloids.
● CONCEPTION AND CONTRACEPTION Manufacturer advises adequate contraception during and for at least 6 months after treatment in men or women. See also *Pregnancy and reproductive function* in Cytotoxic drugs p. 505.
● PREGNANCY Avoid (teratogenic and carcinogenic in *animals*). See also *Pregnancy and reproductive function* in Cytotoxic drugs p. 505.
● BREAST FEEDING Discontinue breast-feeding.
● HEPATIC IMPAIRMENT Avoid.
● RENAL IMPAIRMENT Avoid.
● MONITORING REQUIREMENTS Ensure satisfactory electrolyte balance and renal function before each course

(risk of tubular dysfunction, Fanconi's syndrome or diabetes insipidus if renal toxicity not treated promptly).

- **MEDICINAL FORMS**
There can be variation in the licensing of different medicines containing the same drug.
Powder for solution for injection
▸ Ifosfamide (Non-proprietary)
Ifosfamide 1 gram Ifosfamide 1g powder for concentrate for solution for injection vials | 1 vial [PoM] £91.32
Ifosfamide 2 gram Ifosfamide 2g powder for concentrate for solution for injection vials | 1 vial [PoM] £179.88

Melphalan

- **INDICATIONS AND DOSE**

High intravenous dose with haematopoietic stem cell transplantation in the treatment of childhood neuroblastoma and some other advanced embryonal tumours
▸ BY INTRAVENOUS INFUSION
▸ Child: (consult local protocol)

- **UNLICENSED USE** Not licensed for use in embryonal tumours.

IMPORTANT SAFETY INFORMATION
RISKS OF INCORRECT DOSING OF ORAL ANTI-CANCER MEDICINES
See Cytotoxic drugs p. 505.

- **CAUTIONS** Avoid in acute porphyrias p. 577 · consider use of prophylactic anti-infective agents · for high-dose intravenous administration establish adequate hydration · haematopoietic stem cell transplantation essential for high dose treatment (consult local treatment protocol for details)
- **INTERACTIONS** → Appendix 1: alkylating agents
- **SIDE-EFFECTS**
GENERAL SIDE-EFFECTS
▸ **Rare** Interstitial pneumonitis · life threatening pulmonary fibrosis
▸ **Frequency not known** Alopecia · amenorrhoea · bone-marrow suppression (delayed) · dilutional hyponatraemia · fluid retention · gastro-intestinal effects · hyperuricaemia · male sterility · nausea · oedema · oral mucositis · organ-related toxicity (long-term and delayed) · premature menopause · secondary malignancy · thromboembolism · tumour lysis syndrome · vomiting
SPECIFIC SIDE-EFFECTS
▸ With intravenous use Extravasation
SIDE-EFFECTS, FURTHER INFORMATION
▸ Secondary malignancy Alkylating drugs are associated with a marked increase in the incidence of secondary tumours and leukaemia, particularly when they are combined with extensive irradiation.
▸ Fluid retention Alkylating drugs can cause fluid retention with oedema and dilutional hyponatraemia in younger children; the risk of this complication is higher in the first 2 days and also when given with concomitant vinca alkaloids.
- **CONCEPTION AND CONTRACEPTION** Manufacturer advises adequate contraception during treatment in men or women. See also *Pregnancy and reproductive function* in Cytotoxic drugs p. 505.
- **PREGNANCY** Avoid. See also *Pregnancy and reproductive function* in Cytotoxic drugs p. 505.
- **BREAST FEEDING** Discontinue breast-feeding.
- **RENAL IMPAIRMENT** Reduce dose initially (consult product literature).

- **MONITORING REQUIREMENTS** Monitor full blood count before and throughout treatment.

- **MEDICINAL FORMS**
There can be variation in the licensing of different medicines containing the same drug.
Powder and solvent for solution for injection
▸ Melphalan (Non-proprietary)
Melphalan (as Melphalan hydrochloride) 50 mg Melphalan 50mg powder and solvent for solution for injection vials | 1 vial [PoM] £137.37

Temozolomide

- **DRUG ACTION** Temozolomide is structurally related to dacarbazine.

- **INDICATIONS AND DOSE**

Treatment of recurrent or progressive malignant glioma
▸ BY MOUTH
▸ Child 3-17 years: (consult local protocol)

IMPORTANT SAFETY INFORMATION
RISKS OF INCORRECT DOSING OF ORAL ANTI-CANCER MEDICINES
See Cytotoxic drugs p. 505.

- **CAUTIONS** *Pneumocystis jirovecii* pneumonia—consult product literature for monitoring and prophylaxis requirements
- **INTERACTIONS** → Appendix 1: alkylating agents
- **SIDE-EFFECTS** Alopecia · bone-marrow suppression · gastro-intestinal effects · hyperuricaemia · nausea · oral mucositis · organ-related toxicity (long-term and delayed) · thromboembolism · tumour lysis syndrome · vomiting
SIDE-EFFECTS, FURTHER INFORMATION
For further information on side-effects consult product literature.
- **CONCEPTION AND CONTRACEPTION** Manufacturer advises adequate contraception during treatment. Men should avoid fathering a child during and for at least 6 months after treatment. See also *Pregnancy and reproductive function* in Cytotoxic drugs p. 505.
- **PREGNANCY** Avoid (teratogenic and embryotoxic in *animal* studies). See also *Pregnancy and reproductive function* in Cytotoxic drugs p. 505.
- **BREAST FEEDING** Discontinue breast-feeding.
- **HEPATIC IMPAIRMENT** Use with caution in severe impairment—no information available.
- **RENAL IMPAIRMENT** Manufacturer advises caution—no information available.
- **MONITORING REQUIREMENTS**
▸ Monitor liver function before treatment initiation, after each treatment cycle and midway through 42-day treatment cycles—consider the balance of benefits and risks of treatment if results are abnormal at any point (fatal liver injury reported).
▸ Monitor for myelodysplastic syndrome.
▸ Monitor for secondary malignancies.

- **MEDICINAL FORMS**
There can be variation in the licensing of different medicines containing the same drug. Forms available from special-order manufacturers include: oral suspension
Capsule
CAUTIONARY AND ADVISORY LABELS 23, 25
▸ Temozolomide (Non-proprietary)
Temozolomide 5 mg Temozolomide 5mg capsules | 5 capsule [PoM] £16.00
Temozolomide 20 mg Temozolomide 20mg capsules | 5 capsule [PoM] £65.00
Temozolomide 100 mg Temozolomide 100mg capsules | 5 capsule [PoM] £325.00

8

Immune system and malignant disease

8

Immune system and malignant disease

Temozolomide **140 mg** Temozolomide 140mg capsules |
5 capsule [PoM] £465.00
Temozolomide **180 mg** Temozolomide 180mg capsules |
5 capsule [PoM] £586.00
Temozolomide **250 mg** Temozolomide 250mg capsules |
5 capsule [PoM] £821.75

▸ **Temodal** (Merck Sharp & Dohme Ltd)
Temozolomide **5 mg** Temodal 5mg capsules | 5 capsule [PoM]
£10.59 (Hospital only)
Temozolomide **20 mg** Temodal 20mg capsules | 5 capsule [PoM]
£42.35 (Hospital only)
Temozolomide **100 mg** Temodal 100mg capsules | 5 capsule
£211.77 (Hospital only)
Temozolomide **140 mg** Temodal 140mg capsules | 5 capsule [PoM]
£296.48 (Hospital only)
Temozolomide **180 mg** Temodal 180mg capsules | 5 capsule [PoM]
£381.19 (Hospital only)
Temozolomide **250 mg** Temodal 250mg capsules | 5 capsule [PoM]
£529.43 (Hospital only)

▸ **Temomedac** (medac UK)
Temozolomide **5 mg** Temomedac 5mg capsules | 5 capsule [PoM]
£16.12
Temozolomide **20 mg** Temomedac 20mg capsules | 5 capsule [PoM]
£64.49
Temozolomide **100 mg** Temomedac 100mg capsules |
5 capsule [PoM] £322.43
Temozolomide **140 mg** Temomedac 140mg capsules |
5 capsule [PoM] £451.40
Temozolomide **180 mg** Temomedac 180mg capsules |
5 capsule [PoM] £580.37
Temozolomide **250 mg** Temomedac 250mg capsules |
5 capsule [PoM] £806.08

Thiotepa

● **INDICATIONS AND DOSE**

Conditioning treatment before haematopoietic stem cell transplantation in the treatment of haematological disease or solid tumours, in combination with other chemotherapy
▸ BY INTRAVENOUS INFUSION
▸ Child: (consult local protocol)

● CAUTIONS Avoid in acute porphyrias p. 577
● INTERACTIONS → Appendix 1: alkylating agents
● SIDE-EFFECTS Alopecia · amenorrhoea · bone-marrow suppression · dilutional hyponatraemia · extravasation · fluid retention · gastro-intestinal effects · hyperuricaemia · male sterility · nausea · oedema · oral mucositis · organ-related toxicity (long-term and delayed) · premature menopause · secondary malignancy · thromboembolism · tumour lysis syndrome · vomiting

SIDE-EFFECTS, FURTHER INFORMATION
▸ Secondary malignancy Alkylating drugs are associated with a marked increase in the incidence of secondary tumours and leukaemia, particularly when they are combined with extensive irradiation.
▸ Fluid retention Alkylating drugs can cause fluid retention with oedema and dilutional hyponatraemia in younger children; the risk of this complication is higher in the first 2 days and also when given with concomitant vinca alkaloids.

● CONCEPTION AND CONTRACEPTION Contraceptive advice required, see *Pregnancy and reproductive function* in Cytotoxic drugs p. 505.
● PREGNANCY Avoid (teratogenic and embryotoxic in *animals*). See also *Pregnancy and reproductive function* in Cytotoxic drugs p. 505.
● BREAST FEEDING Discontinue breast-feeding.
● NATIONAL FUNDING/ACCESS DECISIONS

Scottish Medicines Consortium (SMC) Decisions
The *Scottish Medicines Consortium* has advised (June 2012) that thiotepa (*Tepadina* ®) is **not** recommended for use

within NHS Scotland in combination with other chemotherapy as conditioning treatment in adults or children with haematological diseases, or solid tumours prior to haematopoietic stem cell transplantation.

● MEDICINAL FORMS
There can be variation in the licensing of different medicines containing the same drug.
Powder for solution for infusion
▸ **Tepadina** (Adienne Pharma & Biotech)
Thiotepa **15 mg** Tepadina 15mg powder for concentrate for solution for infusion vials | 1 vial [PoM] no price available
Thiotepa **100 mg** Tepadina 100mg powder for concentrate for solution for infusion vials | 1 vial [PoM] no price available

ANTINEOPLASTIC DRUGS > ANTHRACYCLINES AND RELATED DRUGS

Daunorubicin

● **INDICATIONS AND DOSE**

Acute myelogenous leukaemia | Acute lymphocytic leukaemia
▸ BY INTRAVENOUS INFUSION
▸ Child: (consult local protocol)

● UNLICENSED USE *DaunoXome* ® is not licensed for use in children.
● CONTRA-INDICATIONS Myocardial insufficiency · previous treatment with maximum cumulative doses of daunorubicin or other anthracycline · recent myocardial infarction · severe arrhythmia

CONTRA-INDICATIONS, FURTHER INFORMATION
Anthracycline antibiotics should not normally be used in children with left ventricular dysfunction.

● CAUTIONS Caution in handling—irritant to tissues
● INTERACTIONS → Appendix 1: anthracyclines
● SIDE-EFFECTS
▸ Common or very common Leucopenia
▸ Uncommon Mucositis
▸ Frequency not known Alopecia · bone-marrow suppression · cardiac toxicity (usually 1–6 months after initiation of therapy) · extravasation · fever · gastro-intestinal effects · hyperuricaemia · nausea · oral mucositis · organ-related toxicity (long-term and delayed) · red urine discolouration · thromboembolism · tumour lysis syndrome · vomiting

SIDE-EFFECTS, FURTHER INFORMATION
▸ Cardiotoxicity All anthracycline antibiotics have been associated with varying degrees of cardiac toxicity—this may be idiosyncratic and reversible, but is commonly related to total cumulative dose and is irreversible.

● CONCEPTION AND CONTRACEPTION Contraceptive advice required, see *Pregnancy and reproductive function* in Cytotoxic drugs p. 505.
● PREGNANCY Avoid (teratogenic and carcinogenic in *animal* studies). See also *Pregnancy and reproductive function* in Cytotoxic drugs p. 505.
● BREAST FEEDING Discontinue breast-feeding.
● HEPATIC IMPAIRMENT Reduce dose according to serum bilirubin concentration—consult local protocol for details. Avoid in severe impairment.
● RENAL IMPAIRMENT Reduce dose—consult local treatment protocol for details. Avoid in severe impairment.
● MONITORING REQUIREMENTS
▸ Cardiac monitoring essential.
▸ Cardiac function should be monitored before and at regular intervals throughout treatment and afterwards.

- **BREAST FEEDING** Discontinue breast-feeding.
- **HEPATIC IMPAIRMENT** Dose reduction may be necessary—consult local treatment protocol for details.

- **MEDICINAL FORMS**
  There can be variation in the licensing of different medicines containing the same drug.
  Solution for injection
  ‣ Vinblastine sulfate (Non-proprietary)
    Vinblastine sulfate 1 mg per 1 ml   Vinblastine 10mg/10ml solution for injection vials | 5 vial [PoM] £85.00

Vincristine sulfate

- **INDICATIONS AND DOSE**
  Acute leukaemias | Lymphomas | Paediatric solid tumours
  ‣ BY INTRAVENOUS INJECTION
  ‣ Child: (consult local protocol)

- **UNLICENSED USE** Licensed for use in children (age range not specified by manufacturer).

> **IMPORTANT SAFETY INFORMATION**
> Vincristine injections are for **intravenous administration only**. Inadvertent intrathecal administration can cause severe neurotoxicity, which is usually fatal.
>   The National Patient Safety Agency has advised (August 2008) that adult and teenage patients treated in an adult or adolescent unit should receive their vinca alkaloid dose in a 50 mL minibag. Teenagers and children treated in a child unit may receive their vinca alkaloid dose in a syringe.

- **CONTRA-INDICATIONS**
  CONTRA-INDICATIONS, FURTHER INFORMATION
  Intrathecal injection **contra-indicated**.
- **CAUTIONS** Caution in handling—irritant to tissues · ileus · neuromuscular disease
- **INTERACTIONS** → Appendix 1: vinca alkaloids
- **SIDE-EFFECTS**
  ‣ **Common or very common** Constipation
  ‣ **Rare** Convulsions followed by coma · inappropriate secretion of antidiuretic hormone
  ‣ **Frequency not known** Abdominal pain · alopecia (reversible) · autonomic neuropathy · diarrhoea · extravasation · gastro-intestinal effects · hyperuricaemia · intestinal necrosis · loss of deep tendon reflexes · motor weakness · myelosuppression (negligible) · nausea · neuromuscular effects (dose-limiting) · neurotoxicity · oral mucositis · organ-related toxicity (long-term and delayed) · ototoxicity · paralytic ileus (in young children) · peripheral neuropathy · peripheral paraesthesia · severe local irritation (care must be taken to avoid extravasation) · thromboembolism · tumour lysis syndrome · urinary retention · vomiting

  SIDE-EFFECTS, FURTHER INFORMATION
  ‣ Neurotoxicity Neurotoxicity, usually as peripheral or autonomic neuropathy, occurs with all vinca alkaloids and is a limiting side-effect of vincristine. Children with neurotoxicity commonly have peripheral paraesthesia, loss of deep tendon reflexes, abdominal pain, and constipation; ototoxicity has been reported. If symptoms of neurotoxicity are severe, doses should be reduced, but children generally tolerate vincristine better than adults.
     Motor weakness can also occur and dose reduction or discontinuation of therapy may be appropriate if motor weakness increases. Recovery from neurotoxic effects is usually slow but complete.
  ‣ Constipation Prophylactic use of laxatives may be considered.

- **CONCEPTION AND CONTRACEPTION** Contraceptive advice required, see *Pregnancy and reproductive function* in Cytotoxic drugs p. 505.
- **PREGNANCY** Avoid (teratogenicity and fetal loss in *animal* studies). See also *Pregnancy and reproductive function* in Cytotoxic drugs p. 505.
- **BREAST FEEDING** Discontinue breast-feeding.
- **HEPATIC IMPAIRMENT** Dose reduction may be necessary—consult local treatment protocol for details.

- **MEDICINAL FORMS**
  There can be variation in the licensing of different medicines containing the same drug.
  Solution for injection
  ‣ Vincristine sulfate (Non-proprietary)
    Vincristine sulfate 1 mg per 1 ml   Vincristine 1mg/1ml solution for injection vials | 1 vial [PoM] £13.47 (Hospital only) | 5 vial [PoM] £67.35
    Vincristine 2mg/2ml solution for injection vials | 1 vial [PoM] £26.66 (Hospital only) | 5 vial [PoM] £133.30
    Vincristine 5mg/5ml solution for injection vials | 5 vial [PoM] £329.50

ANTINEOPLASTIC DRUGS ⟩ OTHER

Asparaginase
16-Mar-2017

- **DRUG ACTION** Asparaginase is an enzyme which acts by breaking down L-asparagine to aspartic acid and ammonia, this disrupts protein synthesis of tumour cells.

- **INDICATIONS AND DOSE**
  Acute lymphoblastic leukaemia (in combination with other antineoplastic drugs) (specialist use only)
  ‣ BY INTRAVENOUS INFUSION
  ‣ Neonate: (consult product literature or local protocols).
  ‣ Child 1-11 months: (consult product literature or local protocols)
  ‣ Child 1-17 years: 5000 units/m^2 every 3 days

- **CONTRA-INDICATIONS** History of pancreatitis related to asparaginase therapy · history of serious haemorrhage related to asparaginase therapy · history of serious thrombosis related to asparaginase therapy · pancreatitis · pre-existing known coagulopathy
- **CAUTIONS** Diabetes (may raise blood glucose) · hypersensitivity reactions · hypertriglyceridaemia (severe)—increased risk of acute pancreatitis

  CAUTIONS, FURTHER INFORMATION
  ‣ Hypersensitivity reactions Serious hypersensitivity reactions, including life-threatening anaphylaxis, can occur—asparaginase should only be administered when appropriately trained staff and resuscitation facilities are immediately available; in the event of a hypersensitivity reaction, treatment should be stopped immediately and appropriate management initiated. Manufacturer advises an intracutaneous or small intravenous test dose can be used but is of limited value for predicting which patients will experience an allergic reaction.
- **INTERACTIONS** → Appendix 1: asparaginase
- **SIDE-EFFECTS**
  ‣ **Common or very common** Abdominal pain · acute pancreatitis—discontinue if suspected and do not re-start if confirmed · agitation · anaemia · confusion · decreased appetite · decreased clotting factors · decreased fibrinogen · depression · diarrhoea · dizziness · elevated blood lipids · haemorrhage · hallucination · hyperglycaemia · hypersensitivity reactions · hypoalbuminaemia · hypoglycaemia · myelosuppression · nausea · oedema · pain · somnolence · thrombosis · vomiting · weight loss
  ‣ **Uncommon** Headache · hyperammonaemia · hyperuricaemia

▸ **Rare** Convulsion · diabetic ketoacidosis · disturbances in consciousness (including coma) · hepatotoxicity · ischaemic stroke · parotitis · reversible posterior leucoencephalopathy syndrome

▸ **Very rare** Hypoparathyroidism · hypothyroidism (secondary) · tremor

SIDE-EFFECTS, FURTHER INFORMATION

▸ **Hepatotoxicity** There have been rare reports of cholestasis, icterus, hepatic cell necrosis and hepatic failure with fatal outcome; manufacturer advises interrupt treatment if these symptoms develop.

● **CONCEPTION AND CONTRACEPTION** Manufacturer advises effective contraception in men and women of child-bearing potential during treatment and for at least 3 months after last dose; asparaginase may reduce effectiveness of oral contraceptives—additional precautions (e.g. barrier method) are required, see also *Pregnancy and reproductive function* in Cytotoxic drugs p. 505.

● **PREGNANCY** Manufacturer advises avoid unless essential—toxicity in *animal* studies. See also *Pregnancy and reproductive function* in Cytotoxic drugs p. 505.

● **BREAST FEEDING** Manufacturer advises avoid—no information available.

● **HEPATIC IMPAIRMENT** Manufacturer advises avoid in severe impairment—no information available.

● **MONITORING REQUIREMENTS**

▸ Manufacturer advises monitor trough serum asparaginase levels 3 days after administration; consider switching to a different asparaginase preparation if target levels not reached—seek expert advice.

▸ Manufacturer advises monitor bilirubin, hepatic transaminases, and coagulation parameters before and during treatment; in addition, monitor plasma and urinary glucose, amylase, lipase, triglycerides, cholesterol and serum protein levels during treatment.

● **HANDLING AND STORAGE** Manufacturer advises store in a refrigerator (2–8°C)—consult product literature for storage conditions after reconstitution and dilution.

● **PATIENT AND CARER ADVICE**

Driving and skilled tasks
Manufacturer advises asparaginase has moderate influence on driving and performance of skilled tasks—increased risk of dizziness and somnolence.

● **MEDICINAL FORMS**
There can be variation in the licensing of different medicines containing the same drug.

Powder for solution for infusion

▸ Spectrila (medac UK) ▼
Asparaginase 10000 unit Spectrila 10,000unit powder for concentrate for solution for infusion vials | 1 vial [PoM] £450.00 (Hospital only)

Crisantaspase
16-Mar-2017

● **DRUG ACTION** Crisantaspase is the enzyme asparaginase produced by *Erwinia chrysanthemi*.

● **INDICATIONS AND DOSE**

Acute lymphoblastic leukaemia | Acute myeloid leukaemia | Non-Hodgkin's lymphoma

▸ BY INTRAVENOUS INJECTION, OR BY INTRAMUSCULAR INJECTION, OR BY SUBCUTANEOUS INJECTION

▸ **Child:** (consult local protocol)

● **UNLICENSED USE** Preparations of asparaginase derived from *Escherichia coli* are available but they are not licensed, they include: *Medac*® asparaginase and *Elspar*® asparaginase.

● **CONTRA-INDICATIONS** History of pancreatitis related to asparaginase therapy

● **CAUTIONS** Diabetes (may raise blood glucose)

● **INTERACTIONS** → Appendix 1: crisantaspase

● **SIDE-EFFECTS**

▸ **Common or very common** Coagulation disorders · confusion · convulsions · diarrhoea · dizziness · drowsiness · headache · lethargy · liver dysfunction · neurotoxicity · pancreatitis

▸ **Uncommon** Anaphylaxis · changes in blood lipids · hyperglycaemia

▸ **Rare** CNS depression

▸ **Very rare** Abdominal pain · hypertension · myalgia

▸ **Frequency not known** Alopecia · bone-marrow suppression · extravasation · gastro-intestinal effects · hyperuricaemia · nausea · oral mucositis · organ-related toxicity (long-term and delayed) · thromboembolism · tumour lysis syndrome · vomiting

● **ALLERGY AND CROSS-SENSITIVITY** Children who are hypersensitive to asparaginase derived from one organism may tolerate asparaginase derived from another organism but cross-sensitivity occurs in about 20–30% of individuals.

● **CONCEPTION AND CONTRACEPTION** Contraceptive advice required, see *Pregnancy and reproductive function* in Cytotoxic drugs p. 505.

● **PREGNANCY** Avoid. See also, *Pregnancy and reproductive function* in Cytotoxic drugs p. 505.

● **BREAST FEEDING** Discontinue breast-feeding.

● **DIRECTIONS FOR ADMINISTRATION** Facilities for the management of anaphylaxis should be available.

● **MEDICINAL FORMS**
There can be variation in the licensing of different medicines containing the same drug.

Powder for solution for injection

▸ Erwinase (EUSA Pharma Ltd)
Crisantaspase 10000 unit Erwinase 10,000unit powder for solution for injection vials | 5 vial [PoM] £3,065.00

Hydroxycarbamide

(Hydroxyurea)

● **INDICATIONS AND DOSE**

Sickle-cell disease in children who have recurrent episodes of acute pain (more than 3 admissions in the previous 12 months, or who are very symptomatic in the community) or who have had 2 or more episodes of acute sickle chest syndrome in the last 2 years (or 1 episode requiring ventilatory support)—consult with a specialist centre

▸ BY MOUTH

▸ **Child 2–17 years:** Initially 10–15 mg/kg once daily, increased in steps of 2.5–5 mg/kg daily, dose to be increased every 12 weeks according to response; usual dose 15–30 mg/kg daily; maximum 35 mg/kg per day

---

IMPORTANT SAFETY INFORMATION

RISKS OF INCORRECT DOSING OF ORAL ANTI-CANCER MEDICINES
See Cytotoxic drugs p. 505.

● **CAUTIONS** Leg ulcers (review treatment if cutaneous vasculitic ulcerations develop)

● **INTERACTIONS** → Appendix 1: hydroxycarbamide

● **SIDE-EFFECTS**

▸ **Common or very common** Headache · myelosuppression · skin reactions

▸ **Rare** Amenorrhoea (in sickle-cell disease) · fever (in sickle-cell disease)

▶ **Frequency not known** Alopecia · bleeding (in sickle-cell disease) · bone-marrow suppression · dizziness · hyperuricaemia · hypomagnesaemia (in sickle-cell disease) · nausea · oral mucositis · rash · reduced sperm count and activity · thromboembolism · tumour lysis syndrome · vomiting

● **CONCEPTION AND CONTRACEPTION** Manufacturer advises effective contraception before and during treatment.

● **PREGNANCY** Avoid (teratogenic in *animal* studies). See also *Pregnancy and reproductive function* in Cytotoxic drugs p. 505.

● **BREAST FEEDING** Discontinue breast-feeding.

● **HEPATIC IMPAIRMENT** Manufacturer advises caution in mild to moderate impairment. Avoid in severe impairment, unless used for malignant conditions.

● **RENAL IMPAIRMENT** In sickle-cell disease, reduce initial dose by 50% if estimated glomerular filtration rate less than 60 mL/minute/1.73 m^2. In sickle-cell disease, avoid if estimated glomerular filtration rate less than 30 mL/minute/1.73 m^2.

● **MONITORING REQUIREMENTS**
▶ Monitor renal and hepatic function before and during treatment.
▶ Monitor full blood count before treatment, and repeatedly throughout use; in sickle-cell disease monitor every 2 weeks for the first 2 months and then every 2 months thereafter (or every 2 weeks if on maximum dose).
▶ Patients receiving long-term therapy for malignant disease should be monitored for secondary malignancies.

● **PATIENT AND CARER ADVICE**
Patients receiving long-term therapy with hydroxycarbamide should be advised to protect skin from sun exposure.
Medicines for Children leaflet: Hydroxycarbamide for sickle cell disease www.medicinesforchildren.org.uk/hydroxycarbamide-for-sickle-cell-disease

● **MEDICINAL FORMS**
There can be variation in the licensing of different medicines containing the same drug. Forms available from special-order manufacturers include: capsule, oral suspension, oral solution

Tablet
▶ **Siklos** (Nordic Pharma Ltd)
  Hydroxycarbamide 100 mg Siklos 100mg tablets | 60 tablet [PoM] £100.00 DT price = £100.00
  Hydroxycarbamide 1 gram Siklos 1000mg tablets | 30 tablet [PoM] £500.00

Capsule
▶ **Hydroxycarbamide** (Non-proprietary)
  Hydroxycarbamide 500 mg Hydroxycarbamide 500mg capsules | 100 capsule [PoM] £86.00 DT price = £12.12
▶ **Droxia** (Imported (United States))
  Hydroxycarbamide 300 mg Droxia 300mg capsules | 60 capsule [PoM] no price available
▶ **Hydrea** (Bristol-Myers Squibb Pharmaceuticals Ltd)
  Hydroxycarbamide 500 mg Hydrea 500mg capsules | 100 capsule [PoM] £10.47 DT price = £12.12

Mitotane

● **DRUG ACTION** Mitotane selectively inhibits the activity of the adrenal cortex, necessitating corticosteroid replacement therapy.

● **INDICATIONS AND DOSE**
Symptomatic treatment of advanced or inoperable adrenocortical carcinoma
▶ BY MOUTH
▶ Child: (consult local protocol)

● **UNLICENSED USE** Not licensed for use in children.

IMPORTANT SAFETY INFORMATION
RISKS OF INCORRECT DOSING OF ORAL ANTI-CANCER MEDICINES
See Cytotoxic drugs p. 505.

● **CAUTIONS** Avoid in acute porphyrias p. 577 · risk of accumulation in overweight patients

● **INTERACTIONS** → Appendix 1: mitotane

● **SIDE-EFFECTS**
▶ **Common or very common** Anaemia · anorexia · asthenia · ataxia · cognitive impairment · confusion · diarrhoea · dizziness · drowsiness · epigastric discomfort · gastro-intestinal disturbances · gynaecomastia · headache · hypercholesterolaemia · hypertriglyceridaemia · leucopenia · liver disorders · movement disorder · myasthenia · nausea · neuropathy · paraesthesia · prolonged bleeding time · rash · thrombocytopenia · vomiting
▶ **Rare** Flushing · haematuria · haemorrhagic cystitis · hypersalivation · hypertension · hypouricaemia · ocular disorders · postural hypotension · proteinuria · pyrexia · visual disturbances
▶ **Frequency not known** Alopecia · bone-marrow suppression · gastro-intestinal effects · hyperuricaemia · nausea · neuropsychological impairment (possibly secondary to hypothyroidism, and growth retardation) · oral mucositis · organ-related toxicity (long-term and delayed) · thromboembolism · tumour lysis syndrome · vomiting

● **CONCEPTION AND CONTRACEPTION** Contraceptive advice required, see *Pregnancy and reproductive* function in Cytotoxic drugs p. 505.

● **PREGNANCY** Manufacturer advises avoid. See also *Pregnancy and reproductive function* in Cytotoxic drugs p. 505.

● **BREAST FEEDING** Discontinue breast-feeding.

● **HEPATIC IMPAIRMENT** Manufacturer advises caution in mild to moderate impairment. Avoid in severe impairment. In mild to moderate hepatic impairment, monitoring of plasma-mitotane concentration is recommended.

● **RENAL IMPAIRMENT** Manufacturer advises caution in mild to moderate impairment. Avoid in severe impairment. In mild to moderate renal impairment, monitoring of plasma-mitotane concentration is recommended.

● **MONITORING REQUIREMENTS**
▶ Monitor plasma-mitotane concentration—consult product literature.

● **PRESCRIBING AND DISPENSING INFORMATION**
Corticosteroid replacement therapy Corticosteroid replacement therapy is necessary with treatment with mitotane. The dose of glucocorticoid should be increased in case of shock, trauma, or infection.

● **PATIENT AND CARER ADVICE**
Patients should be warned to contact doctor immediately if injury, infection, or illness occurs (because of risk of acute adrenal insufficiency).

Driving and skilled tasks
Central nervous system toxicity may affect performance of skilled tasks (e.g. driving).

● **MEDICINAL FORMS**
There can be variation in the licensing of different medicines containing the same drug.
Tablet
CAUTIONARY AND ADVISORY LABELS 2, 10, 21
▶ **Lysodren** (HRA Pharma UK Ltd)
  Mitotane 500 mg Lysodren 500mg tablets | 100 tablet [PoM] £590.97

8

Immune system and malignant disease

Immune system and malignant disease

8

Pegaspargase

16-Mar-2017

- **DRUG ACTION** Pegaspargase breaks down the amino acid L-asparagine, thereby interfering with the growth of malignant cells, which are unable to synthesise L-asparagine.

● INDICATIONS AND DOSE

Acute lymphoblastic leukaemia (in combination with other antineoplastic drugs) (specialist use only)

▶ BY INTRAMUSCULAR INJECTION, OR BY INTRAVENOUS INFUSION

- ▶ Neonate: 82.5 units/kg every 14 days.
- ▶ Child (body surface area up to 0.6 m²): 82.5 units/kg every 14 days
- ▶ Child (body surface area 0.6 m² and above): 2500 units/m² every 14 days

---

IMPORTANT SAFETY INFORMATION
Be aware that doses are calculated either using units/kg or units/m², depending on the size of the child.

- **CONTRA-INDICATIONS** History of pancreatitis · history of serious haemorrhagic event with previous L-asparaginase therapy · history of serious thrombosis with previous L-asparaginase therapy
- **CAUTIONS** Concomitant use of other hepatotoxic drugs (particularly in pre-existing hepatic impairment)—monitor hepatic function · diabetes (may raise blood glucose) · hypersensitivity reactions · marked decrease of leukocyte count at start of treatment is possible—may be associated with significant rise in serum uric acid and development of uric acid nephropathy

CAUTIONS, FURTHER INFORMATION
- ▶ Hypersensitivity reactions Serious hypersensitivity reactions, including life-threatening anaphylaxis, can occur—pegaspargase should only be administered when appropriately trained staff and resuscitation facilities are immediately available; manufacturer advises patients should be closely monitored for signs of hypersensitivity during treatment and for an hour after administration. In the event of a hypersensitivity reaction, treatment should be stopped immediately and appropriate management initiated.

- **INTERACTIONS** → Appendix 1: pegaspargase
- **SIDE-EFFECTS**
- ▶ **Common or very common** Abdominal pain · convulsion · diarrhoea · elevated blood lipids · hyperglycaemia · hypersensitivity reactions · hypoxia · myelosuppression · pain in extremities · pancreatitis—discontinue if suspected and do not re-start if confirmed · peripheral motor neuropathy · rash · stomatitis · syncope · thrombosis—discontinue treatment · vomiting
- ▶ **Rare** Acute renal failure · reversible posterior leukoencephalopathy syndrome
- ▶ **Very rare** Tremor
- ▶ **Frequency not known** Confusion · decreased clotting factors · decreased fibrinogen · diabetic ketoacidosis · hepatobiliary disorders · hyperammonaemia—monitor if symptoms present · somnolence · toxic epidermal necrolysis

SIDE-EFFECTS, FURTHER INFORMATION
- ▶ Hepatobiliary disorders There have been rare reports of cholestasis, icterus, hepatic cell necrosis and hepatic failure with fatal outcome.

- **CONCEPTION AND CONTRACEPTION** Manufacturer advises effective contraception in men and women of child-bearing potential during treatment and for at least 6 months after discontinuing treatment; pegaspargase may reduce effectiveness of oral contraceptives—additional precautions (e.g. barrier method) are required,

see also *Pregnancy and reproductive function* in Cytotoxic drugs p. 505.

- **PREGNANCY** Manufacturer advises avoid unless essential. See also *Pregnancy and reproductive function* in Cytotoxic drugs p. 505.
- **BREAST FEEDING** Manufacturer advises avoid—no information available.
- **HEPATIC IMPAIRMENT** Manufacturer advises avoid in severe impairment.
- **MONITORING REQUIREMENTS**
- ▶ Manufacturer advises trough serum asparaginase activity levels may be measured before the next administration of pegaspargase; consider switching to a different asparaginase preparation if target levels not reached—seek expert advice.
- ▶ Manufacturer advises monitor plasma and urine glucose levels during treatment; monitor coagulation profile at baseline and periodically during and after treatment (particularly with concomitant use of other drugs that inhibit coagulation; monitor serum amylase.
- **DIRECTIONS FOR ADMINISTRATION** Manufacturer advises *for intramuscular injection*, volume over 2 mL must be divided between more than one site.
- **HANDLING AND STORAGE** Manufacturer advises store in a refrigerator between 2–8°C.
- **PATIENT AND CARER ADVICE**
Pancreatitis Manufacturer advises patients and carers should be told how to recognise signs and symptoms of pancreatitis and advised to seek medical attention if symptoms such as persistent, severe abdominal pain develop.

Driving and skilled tasks
Manufacturer advises patients and carers should be counselled on the effects on driving and performance of skilled tasks—increased risk of confusion and somnolence.

- **NATIONAL FUNDING/ACCESS DECISIONS**

NICE technology appraisals (TAs)
- ▶ Pegaspargase for treating acute lymphoblastic leukaemia (September 2016) NICE TA408
Pegaspargase, as part of antineoplastic combination therapy, is recommended as an option for treating acute lymphoblastic leukaemia only in patients with untreated newly diagnosed disease.
  Patients whose treatment was started within the NHS before this guidance was published may continue treatment until they and their clinician consider it appropriate to stop.
www.nice.org.uk/guidance/ta408

Scottish Medicines Consortium (SMC) Decisions
The *Scottish Medicines Consortium* has advised (October 2016) that pegaspargase (*Oncaspar®*) is accepted for use within NHS Scotland as a component of antineoplastic combination therapy in acute lymphoblastic leukaemia.

- **MEDICINAL FORMS**
There can be variation in the licensing of different medicines containing the same drug.

Solution for injection
- ▶ Pegaspargase (non-proprietary) ▼
  Pegaspargase 750 unit per 1 ml Oncaspar 3,750units/5ml solution for injection vials | 1 vial POM £ no price available

Procarbazine

- **DRUG ACTION** Procarbazine is a mild monoamine-oxidase inhibitor.

- **INDICATIONS AND DOSE**
Hodgkin's lymphoma
  ► BY MOUTH
    ► Child: (consult local protocol)

IMPORTANT SAFETY INFORMATION
RISKS OF INCORRECT DOSING OF ORAL ANTI-CANCER MEDICINES
See Cytotoxic drugs p. 505.

- **CONTRA-INDICATIONS** Pre-existing severe leucopenia · pre-existing severe thrombocytopenia

- **CAUTIONS** Cardiovascular disease · cerebrovascular disease · epilepsy · phaeochromocytoma · procarbazine is a mild monoamineoxidase inhibitor (dietary restriction is rarely considered necessary)

- **INTERACTIONS** → Appendix 1: procarbazine

- **SIDE-EFFECTS**
  ► **Common or very common** Loss of appetite
  ► **Frequency not known** Alopecia · bone-marrow suppression · gastro-intestinal effects · hypersensitivity rash (discontinue treatment) · hyperuricaemia · jaundice · nausea · oral mucositis · organ-related toxicity (long-term and delayed) · thromboembolism · tumour lysis syndrome · vomiting

- **CONCEPTION AND CONTRACEPTION** Contraceptive advice required, see *Pregnancy and reproductive function* in Cytotoxic drugs p. 505.

- **PREGNANCY** Avoid (teratogenic in *animal* studies and isolated reports in humans). See also *Pregnancy and reproductive function* in Cytotoxic drugs p. 505.

- **BREAST FEEDING** Discontinue breast-feeding.

- **HEPATIC IMPAIRMENT** Caution in mild to moderate impairment. Avoid in severe impairment.

- **RENAL IMPAIRMENT** Caution in mild to moderate impairment. Avoid in severe impairment.

- **MEDICINAL FORMS**
There can be variation in the licensing of different medicines containing the same drug.
Capsule
CAUTIONARY AND ADVISORY LABELS 4
  ► **Procarbazine (Non-proprietary)**
    Procarbazine (as Procarbazine hydrochloride)
    50 mg Procarbazine 50mg capsules | 50 capsule PoM £373.95

RETINOID AND RELATED DRUGS

Tretinoin

- **INDICATIONS AND DOSE**
Induction of remission in acute promyelocytic leukaemia (used in previously untreated patients as well as in those who have relapsed after standard chemotherapy or who are refractory to it)
  ► BY MOUTH
    ► Child: (consult local protocol)

- **CAUTIONS** Increased risk of thromboembolism during first month of treatment

- **INTERACTIONS** → Appendix 1: retinoids

- **SIDE-EFFECTS** Alopecia · anxiety · arrhythmias · benign intracranial hypertension (children particularly susceptible—consider dose reduction if intractable headache in children) · bone pain · cheilitis · chest pain · confusion · depression · dizziness · dry mucous membranes

· dry skin · erythema · flushing · gastro-intestinal disturbances · genital ulceration · headache · hearing disturbances · hypercalcaemia · insomnia · oedema · pancreatitis · paraesthesia · pruritus · raised lipids · raised liver enzymes · raised serum creatinine · rash · retinoic acid syndrome · shivering · sweating · thromboembolism · visual disturbances

SIDE-EFFECTS, FURTHER INFORMATION
  ► Retinoic acid syndrome Fever, dyspnoea, acute respiratory distress, pulmonary infiltrates, pleural effusion, hyperleucocytosis, hypotension, oedema, weight gain, hepatic, renal and multi-organ failure requires immediate treatment—consult product literature.
  ► Nervous system effects Children particularly susceptible to nervous system effects.

- **CONCEPTION AND CONTRACEPTION** Effective contraception must be used for at least 1 month before oral treatment, during treatment and for at least 1 month after stopping (oral progestogen-only contraceptives not considered effective).

- **PREGNANCY** Teratogenic. See *Pregnancy and reproductive function* in Cytotoxic drugs p. 505.

- **BREAST FEEDING** Avoid (discontinue breast-feeding).

- **HEPATIC IMPAIRMENT** Reduce dose—consult local treatment protocol for details.

- **RENAL IMPAIRMENT** Reduce dose—consult local treatment protocol for details.

- **MONITORING REQUIREMENTS** Monitor haematological and coagulation profile, liver function, serum calcium and plasma lipids before and during treatment.

- **PRESCRIBING AND DISPENSING INFORMATION** Tretinoin is the acid form of vitamin A.

- **MEDICINAL FORMS**
There can be variation in the licensing of different medicines containing the same drug.
Capsule
CAUTIONARY AND ADVISORY LABELS 21, 25
  ► **Tretinoin (Non-proprietary)**
    Tretinoin 10 mg Tretinoin 10mg capsules | 100 capsule PoM £240.00–£256.80 DT price = £240.00

2.1 Cytotoxic drug-induced side effects

DETOXIFYING DRUGS ⟩ UROPROTECTIVE DRUGS

Mesna

- **INDICATIONS AND DOSE**
Urothelial toxicity following oxazaphosphorine therapy
  ► BY INTRAVENOUS INJECTION, OR BY CONTINUOUS INTRAVENOUS INFUSION
    ► Child: (consult local protocol)
Mucolytic in cystic fibrosis
  ► BY INHALATION OF NEBULISED SOLUTION
    ► Child: 3–6 mL twice daily, use a 20% solution

- **UNLICENSED USE** Not licensed for use in children.

- **SIDE-EFFECTS**
  ► **Common or very common** Colic · depression · diarrhoea · fatigue · headache · hypotension · irritability · joint pains · limb pains · nausea · rash · tachycardia · vomiting
  ► **Rare** Hypersensitivity reactions (more common in patients with auto-immune disorders)

- **ALLERGY AND CROSS-SENSITIVITY** Contra-indicated if history of hypersensitivity to thiol-containing compounds.

8

Immune system and malignant disease

- **PREGNANCY** Not known to be harmful. See also *Pregnancy and reproductive function* in Cytotoxic drugs p. 505.
- **DIRECTIONS FOR ADMINISTRATION** For oral administration of the injection, contents of ampoule are taken in a flavoured drink such as orange juice or cola which may be stored in a refrigerator for up to 24 hours in a sealed container.

- **MEDICINAL FORMS**
There can be variation in the licensing of different medicines containing the same drug.
Solution for injection
  ▸ Mesna (Non-proprietary)
    Mesna 100 mg per 1 ml Mesna 1g/10ml solution for injection ampoules | 15 ampoule [PoM] £441.15
    Mesna 400mg/4ml solution for injection ampoules | 5 ampoule [PoM] no price available | 15 ampoule [PoM] £201.15

VITAMINS AND TRACE ELEMENTS > FOLATES

Folinic acid

- **INDICATIONS AND DOSE**

Reduction of methotrexate-induced toxicity
  ▸ BY MOUTH, OR BY INTRAVENOUS INFUSION, OR BY INTRAVENOUS INJECTION
  ▸ Child: (consult local protocol)

Methotrexate overdose
  ▸ BY INTRAVENOUS INFUSION, OR BY INTRAVENOUS INJECTION
  ▸ Child: (consult local protocol)

Megaloblastic anaemia due to folate deficiency
  ▸ BY MOUTH
  ▸ Child 1 month–11 years: 250 micrograms/kg once daily
  ▸ Child 12–17 years: 15 mg once daily

Metabolic disorders leading to folate deficiency
  ▸ BY MOUTH, OR BY INTRAVENOUS INFUSION
  ▸ Child: 15 mg once daily, larger doses may be required in older children

Prevention of megaloblastic anaemia associated with pyrimethamine and sulfadiazine treatment of congenital toxoplasmosis
  ▸ BY MOUTH
  ▸ Neonate: 5 mg 3 times a week; increased if necessary up to 20 mg 3 times a week, if the patient is neutropenic.
  ▸ Child 1–11 months: 10 mg 3 times a week

SODIOFOLIN®

As an antidote to methotrexate
  ▸ BY INTRAVENOUS INFUSION, OR BY INTRAVENOUS INJECTION
  ▸ Child: (consult product literature)

- **UNLICENSED USE** Consult product literature for licensing status of individual preparations.
- **CONTRA-INDICATIONS** Intrathecal injection
- **CAUTIONS** Avoid simultaneous administration of methotrexate · **not** indicated for pernicious anaemia or other megaloblastic anaemias caused by vitamin B_{12} deficiency
- **INTERACTIONS** → Appendix 1: folates
- **SIDE-EFFECTS**
  ▸ **Rare** Agitation (after high doses) · depression (after high doses) · gastro-intestinal disturbances (after high doses) · insomnia (after high doses) · pyrexia (after parenteral use)
- **PREGNANCY** Not known to be harmful; benefit outweighs risk.
- **BREAST FEEDING** Presence in milk unknown but benefit outweighs risk.

- **MEDICINAL FORMS**
There can be variation in the licensing of different medicines containing the same drug. Forms available from special-order manufacturers include: oral suspension, oral solution
Solution for injection
  ▸ Folinic acid (Non-proprietary)
    Folinic acid (as Calcium folinate) 7.5 mg per 1 ml Calcium folinate 15mg/2ml solution for injection ampoules | 5 ampoule [PoM] £39.00 DT price = £39.00
    Folinic acid (as Calcium folinate) 10 mg per 1 ml Calcium folinate 50mg/5ml solution for injection vials | 1 vial [PoM] £20.00 (Hospital only) | 1 vial [PoM] £20.00
    Calcium folinate 300mg/30ml solution for injection vials | 1 vial [PoM] £100.00 (Hospital only) | 1 vial [PoM] £100.00
    Calcium folinate 100mg/10ml solution for injection vials | 1 vial [PoM] £37.50 (Hospital only) | 1 vial [PoM] £37.50
    Folinic acid (as Disodium folinate) 50 mg per 1 ml Disodium folinate 50mg/1ml solution for injection vials | 1 vial [PoM] £24.70 Disodium folinate 200mg/4ml solution for injection vials | 1 vial [PoM] £80.40
  ▸ Refolinon (Pfizer Ltd)
    Folinic acid (as Calcium folinate) 3 mg per 1 ml Refolinon 30mg/10ml solution for injection ampoules | 5 ampoule [PoM] £23.12
  ▸ Sodiofolin (medac UK)
    Folinic acid (as Disodium folinate) 50 mg per 1 ml Sodiofolin 400mg/8ml solution for injection vials | 1 vial [PoM] £126.25 (Hospital only)
    Sodiofolin 100mg/2ml solution for injection vials | 1 vial [PoM] £35.09 (Hospital only)
Tablet
  ▸ Folinic acid (Non-proprietary)
    Folinic acid (as Calcium folinate) 15 mg Calcium folinate 15mg tablets | 10 tablet [PoM] £49.06 DT price = £49.05
  ▸ Refolinon (Pfizer Ltd)
    Folinic acid (as Calcium folinate) 15 mg Refolinon 15mg tablets | 30 tablet [PoM] £85.74

Levofolinic acid

- **DRUG ACTION** Levofolinic acid is an isomer of folinic acid.

- **INDICATIONS AND DOSE**

Reduction of methotrexate-induced toxicity
  ▸ BY INTRAMUSCULAR INJECTION, OR BY INTRAVENOUS INJECTION, OR BY INTRAVENOUS INFUSION
  ▸ Child: (consult local protocol)

Methotrexate overdose
  ▸ BY INTRAMUSCULAR INJECTION, OR BY INTRAVENOUS INJECTION, OR BY INTRAVENOUS INFUSION
  ▸ Child: (consult local protocol)

- **CONTRA-INDICATIONS** Intrathecal injection
- **CAUTIONS** Avoid simultaneous administration of methotrexate · **not** indicated for pernicious anaemia or other megaloblastic anaemias caused by vitamin B_{12} deficiency
- **INTERACTIONS** → Appendix 1: folates
- **SIDE-EFFECTS**
  ▸ **Rare** Agitation (after high doses) · depression (after high doses) · gastro-intestinal disturbances (after high doses) · insomnia (after high doses) · pyrexia (after parenteral use)
- **PREGNANCY** Not known to be harmful benefit outweighs risk.
- **BREAST FEEDING** Presence in milk unknown but benefit outweighs risk.

- **MEDICINAL FORMS**
There can be variation in the licensing of different medicines containing the same drug.
Solution for injection
  ▸ Isovorin (Pfizer Ltd)
    Levofolinic acid (as Calcium levofolinate) 10 mg per 1 ml Isovorin 175mg/17.5ml solution for injection vials | 1 vial [PoM] £81.33 (Hospital only)
    Isovorin 25mg/2.5ml solution for injection vials | 1 vial [PoM] £11.62 (Hospital only)

2.1a Hyperuricaemia associated with cytotoxic drugs

DETOXIFYING DRUGS > URATE OXIDASES

Rasburicase

- **INDICATIONS AND DOSE**

Prophylaxis and treatment of acute hyperuricaemia with initial chemotherapy for haematological malignancy
  - ▸ BY INTRAVENOUS INFUSION
  - ▸ Child: (consult local protocol)

- **UNLICENSED USE** Not licensed for use in children.
- **CONTRA-INDICATIONS** G6PD deficiency
- **CAUTIONS** Atopic allergies
- **SIDE-EFFECTS**
  - ▸ **Common or very common** Fever · nausea · vomiting
  - ▸ **Uncommon** Anaphylaxis · bronchospasm · diarrhoea · haemolytic anaemia · headache · hypersensitivity reactions · methaemoglobinaemia · rash
- **PREGNANCY** Manufacturer advises avoid—no information available.
- **BREAST FEEDING** Manufacturer advises avoid—no information available.
- **MONITORING REQUIREMENTS** Monitor closely for hypersensitivity.
- **EFFECT ON LABORATORY TESTS** May interfere with test for uric acid—consult product literature.

- **MEDICINAL FORMS**
  There can be variation in the licensing of different medicines containing the same drug.
  Powder and solvent for solution for infusion
  - ▸ Fasturtec (Sanofi)
    Rasburicase 1.5 mg Fasturtec 1.5mg powder and solvent for solution for infusion vials | 3 vial PoM £208.39 (Hospital only)
    Rasburicase 7.5 mg Fasturtec 7.5mg powder and solvent for solution for infusion vials | 1 vial PoM £347.32 (Hospital only)

XANTHINE OXIDASE INHIBITORS

Allopurinol

- **INDICATIONS AND DOSE**

Prophylaxis of hyperuricaemia associated with cancer chemotherapy | Prophylaxis of hyperuricaemic nephropathy, enzyme disorders causing increased serum urate e.g Lesch-Nyhan syndrome
  - ▸ BY MOUTH
  - ▸ Child 1 month-14 years: 10–20 mg/kg daily, dose to be taken preferably after food; maximum 400 mg per day
  - ▸ Child 15-17 years: Initially 100 mg daily, taken preferably after food; dose to be increased according to response, up to 900 mg daily in divided doses (max. per dose 300 mg)

- **CAUTIONS** Ensure adequate fluid intake · for hyperuricaemia associated with cancer therapy, allopurinol treatment should be started before cancer therapy
- **INTERACTIONS** → Appendix 1: allopurinol
- **SIDE-EFFECTS**
  - ▸ **Common or very common** Gastro-intestinal disorders · rashes (**withdraw** therapy; if rash mild re-introduce cautiously but **discontinue** immediately if recurrence)
  - ▸ **Rare** Alopecia · aplastic anaemia · arthralgia · blood disorders · drowsiness · eosinophilia resembling Stevens-Johnson syndrome · eosinophilia resembling toxic

epidermal necrolysis · exfoliation · fever · haemolytic anaemia · headache · hepatitis · hepatotoxicity · hypersensitivity reactions · hypertension · leucopenia · lymphadenopathy · malaise · neuropathy · paraesthesia · renal impairment · taste disturbances · thrombocytopenia · vasculitis · vertigo · visual disturbances
  - ▸ **Very rare** Seizures
- **PREGNANCY** Toxicity not reported. Manufacturer advises use only if no safer alternative and disease carries risk for mother or child.
- **BREAST FEEDING** Present in milk—not known to be harmful.
- **HEPATIC IMPAIRMENT** Reduce dose. Monitor hepatic function.
- **RENAL IMPAIRMENT** Manufacturer advises reduce dose or increase dose interval in severe impairment; adjust dose to maintain plasma-oxipurinol concentration below 100 micromol/litre.
- **PATIENT AND CARER ADVICE**
  Medicines for Children leaflet: Allopurinol for hyperuricaemia www.medicinesforchildren.org.uk/allopurinol-for-hyperuricaemia

- **MEDICINAL FORMS**
  There can be variation in the licensing of different medicines containing the same drug. Forms available from special-order manufacturers include: oral suspension, oral solution, mouthwash
  Tablet
  CAUTIONARY AND ADVISORY LABELS 8, 21, 27
  - ▸ Allopurinol (Non-proprietary)
    Allopurinol 100 mg Allopurinol 100mg tablets | 28 tablet PoM £8.15 DT price = £0.77
    Allopurinol 300 mg Allopurinol 300mg tablets | 28 tablet PoM £5.85 DT price = £0.85
  - ▸ Uricto (Ennogen Pharma Ltd)
    Allopurinol 100 mg Uricto 100mg tablets | 28 tablet PoM £1.25 DT price = £0.77
    Allopurinol 300 mg Uricto 300mg tablets | 28 tablet PoM £0.94 DT price = £0.85
  - ▸ Zyloric (Aspen Pharma Trading Ltd)
    Allopurinol 100 mg Zyloric 100mg tablets | 100 tablet PoM £10.19
    Allopurinol 300 mg Zyloric 300mg tablets | 28 tablet PoM £7.31 DT price = £0.85

3   Immunotherapy responsive malignancy

IMMUNOSTIMULANTS > INTERFERONS

Interferon alfa

- **DRUG ACTION** Interferon alfa has shown some antitumour effect in certain lymphomas and solid tumours.

- **INDICATIONS AND DOSE**

Induction of early regression of life-threatening corticosteroid resistant haemangiomata of infancy
  - ▸ BY SUBCUTANEOUS INJECTION
  - ▸ Child: (consult local protocol)

INTRONA® PEN

Chronic active hepatitis B
  - ▸ BY SUBCUTANEOUS INJECTION
  - ▸ Child 2-17 years: 5 000 000–10 000 000 units/m^2 3 times a week

Chronic active hepatitis C (in combination with oral ribavirin)
  - ▸ BY SUBCUTANEOUS INJECTION
  - ▸ Child 3-17 years: 3 000 000 units/m^2 3 times a week

continued →

8

Immune system and malignant disease

INTRONA® VIALS

Chronic active hepatitis B
▸ BY SUBCUTANEOUS INJECTION
▸ Child 2–17 years: 5 000 000–10 000 000 units/m² 3 times a week

Chronic active hepatitis C (in combination with ribavirin)
▸ BY SUBCUTANEOUS INJECTION
▸ Child 3–17 years: 3 000 000 units/m² 3 times a week

ROFERON-A®

Chronic active hepatitis B
▸ BY SUBCUTANEOUS INJECTION
▸ Child 2–17 years: 2 500 000–5 000 000 units/m² 3 times a week, up to 10 000 000 units/m² has been used 3 times a week

● **UNLICENSED USE** Not licensed for use in children for chronic active hepatitis B.
ROFERON-A® *Roferon-A®* not licensed for use in children.

● **CONTRA-INDICATIONS** Avoid injections containing benzyl alcohol in neonates · history of severe psychiatric illness
CONTRA-INDICATIONS, FURTHER INFORMATION
For contra-indications consult product literature and local treatment protocol.

● **CAUTIONS**
CAUTIONS, FURTHER INFORMATION
For cautions consult product literature and local treatment protocol.
 Interferon alfa should always be used under the close supervision of a specialist; the decision to treat should be made only after careful assessment of the expected benefits versus the potential risks, in particular the risk of growth inhibition caused by combination therapy.

● **INTERACTIONS** → Appendix 1: interferons

● **SIDE-EFFECTS**
▸ **Common or very common** Anorexia · influenza-like symptoms · lethargy · nausea
▸ **Rare** Pneumonia · pneumonitis · pulmonary infiltrates
▸ **Frequency not known** Alopecia · arrhythmias · cardiovascular problems · coma · confusion · depression · hepatotoxicity · hyperglycaemia · hypersensitivity reactions · hypertension · hypertriglyceridaemia (sometimes severe) · hypotension · myelosuppression (particularly affecting granulocyte counts) · nephrotoxicity · ocular side-effects · psoriasiform rash · reversible motor problems in young children · seizures · suicidal behaviour · thyroid abnormalities

SIDE-EFFECTS, FURTHER INFORMATION
Consult product literature and local treatment protocols for information on side-effects.
 Respiratory symptoms should be investigated and if pulmonary infiltrates are suspected or lung function is impaired the discontinuation of interferon alfa should be considered.

● **CONCEPTION AND CONTRACEPTION** Effective contraception required during treatment—consult product literature.

● **PREGNANCY** Avoid unless potential benefit outweighs risk (toxicity in *animal* studies).

● **BREAST FEEDING** Unlikely to be harmful.

● **HEPATIC IMPAIRMENT** Avoid in severe hepatic impairment. Close monitoring required in mild to moderate hepatic impairment.

● **RENAL IMPAIRMENT** Avoid in severe renal impairment. Close monitoring required in mild to moderate renal impairment.

● **MONITORING REQUIREMENTS**
▸ Monitoring of lipid concentration is recommended.
▸ Monitoring of hepatic function is recommended.

● **DIRECTIONS FOR ADMINISTRATION**
ROFERON-A® *Roferon-A®* injection for subcutaneous injection.
INTRONA® VIALS *IntronA®* injection vials for subcutaneous injection or intravenous infusion.

● **MEDICINAL FORMS**
There can be variation in the licensing of different medicines containing the same drug.
Solution for injection
EXCIPIENTS: May contain Benzyl alcohol
▸ **IntronA** (Merck Sharp & Dohme Ltd)
Interferon alfa-2b 10 mega u per 1 ml IntronA 10million units/1ml solution for injection vials | 1 vial PoM no price available
IntronA 25million units/2.5ml solution for injection multidose vials | 1 vial PoM £103.94
Interferon alfa-2b 15 mega u per 1 ml IntronA 18million units/1.2ml solution for injection multidose pens | 1 pre-filled disposable injection PoM £74.83
Interferon alfa-2b 25 mega u per 1 ml IntronA 30million units/1.2ml solution for injection multidose pens | 1 pre-filled disposable injection PoM £124.72
Interferon alfa-2b 50 mega u per 1 ml IntronA 60million units/1.2ml solution for injection multidose pens | 1 pre-filled disposable injection PoM £249.45
▸ **Roferon-A** (Roche Products Ltd)
Interferon alfa-2a 6 mega u per 1 ml Roferon-A 3million units/0.5ml solution for injection pre-filled syringes | 1 pre-filled disposable injection PoM £14.20
Interferon alfa-2a 9 mega u per 1 ml Roferon-A 4.5million units/0.5ml solution for injection pre-filled syringes | 1 pre-filled disposable injection PoM £21.29
Interferon alfa-2a 12 mega u per 1 ml Roferon-A 6million units/0.5ml solution for injection pre-filled syringes | 1 pre-filled disposable injection PoM £28.37
Interferon alfa-2a 18 mega u per 1 ml Roferon-A 9million units/0.5ml solution for injection pre-filled syringes | 1 pre-filled disposable injection PoM £42.57

Interferon gamma-1b

(Immune interferon)

● **INDICATIONS AND DOSE**

To reduce the frequency of serious infection in chronic granulomatous disease
▸ BY SUBCUTANEOUS INJECTION
▸ Child 6 months–17 years (body surface area up to 0.6 m²): 1.5 micrograms/kg 3 times a week
▸ Child 6 months–17 years (body surface area 0.6 m² and above): 50 micrograms/m² 3 times a week

To reduce the frequency of serious infection in severe malignant osteopetrosis
▸ BY SUBCUTANEOUS INJECTION
▸ Child (body surface area up to 0.6 m²): 1.5 micrograms/kg 3 times a week
▸ Child (body surface area 0.6 m² and above): 50 micrograms/m² 3 times a week

● **CONTRA-INDICATIONS** Simultaneous administration of foreign proteins including immunological products (such as vaccines)—risk of exaggerated immune response

● **CAUTIONS** Arrhythmias · cardiac disease · congestive heart failure · ischaemia · seizure disorders (including seizures associated with fever)

● **SIDE-EFFECTS**
▸ **Common or very common** Abdominal pain · arthralgia · chills · depression · diarrhoea · fatigue · fever · headache · injection-site reactions · myalgia · nausea · rash · vomiting
▸ **Rare** Confusion · systemic lupus erythematosus
▸ **Frequency not known** Neutropenia · proteinuria · raised liver enzymes · thrombocytopenia

- **CONCEPTION AND CONTRACEPTION** Effective contraception required during treatment—consult product literature.
- **PREGNANCY** Manufacturers recommend avoid unless potential benefit outweighs risk (toxicity in *animal* studies).
- **BREAST FEEDING** Manufacturers advise avoid—no information available.
- **HEPATIC IMPAIRMENT** Manufacturer advises caution in severe impairment—risk of accumulation.
- **RENAL IMPAIRMENT** Manufacturer advises caution in severe impairment—risk of accumulation.
- **MONITORING REQUIREMENTS** Monitor before and during treatment: haematological tests (including full blood count, differential white cell count, and platelet count), blood chemistry tests (including renal and liver function tests) and urinalysis.
- **MEDICINAL FORMS**
  There can be variation in the licensing of different medicines containing the same drug.
  Solution for injection
  ▸ Immukin (Boehringer Ingelheim Ltd)
  Interferon gamma-1b (recombinant human) 200 microgram per 1 ml Immukin 100micrograms/0.5ml solution for injection vials | 6 vial PoM £450.00

IMMUNOSTIMULANTS > OTHER

Mifamurtide

- **INDICATIONS AND DOSE**
  Treatment of high-grade, resectable, non-metastatic osteosarcoma after complete surgical resection (in combination with chemotherapy)
  ▸ BY INTRAVENOUS INFUSION
  ▸ Child 2-17 years: Infusion to be given over 1 hour (consult product literature or local protocols)

- **UNLICENSED USE** Not licensed for use in patients under 2 years of age at initial diagnosis.
- **CAUTIONS** Asthma—consider prophylactic bronchodilator therapy · chronic obstructive pulmonary disease—consider prophylactic bronchodilator therapy · history of autoimmune disease · history of collagen disease · history of inflammatory disease
- **INTERACTIONS** → Appendix 1: mifamurtide
- **SIDE-EFFECTS** Abdominal pain · alopecia · anaemia · anorexia · anxiety · blurred vision · confusion · constipation · cough · depression · diarrhoea · dizziness · drowsiness · dry skin · dyspepsia · dyspnoea · dysuria · epistaxis · flushing · gastro-intestinal disturbances · granulocytopenia · haematuria · haemoptysis · headache · hearing loss · hypertension · hypoaesthesia · hypokalaemia · hypotension · insomnia · leucopenia · musculoskeletal pain · nausea · oedema · palpitations · paraesthesia · phlebitis · pleural effusion · pollakiuria · rash · respiratory disorders · sweating · tachycardia · tachypnoea · thrombocytopenia · tinnitus · tremor · vertigo · vomiting
- **CONCEPTION AND CONTRACEPTION** Effective contraception required.
- **PREGNANCY** Avoid.
- **BREAST FEEDING** Avoid—no information available.
- **HEPATIC IMPAIRMENT** Use with caution—no information available.
- **RENAL IMPAIRMENT** Use with caution—no information available.
- **MONITORING REQUIREMENTS**
  ▸ Monitor renal function, hepatic function and clotting parameters.

▸ Monitor patients with history of venous thrombosis, vasculitis, or unstable cardiovascular disorders for persistent or worsening symptoms during administration—consult product literature.
- **NATIONAL FUNDING/ACCESS DECISIONS**
  NICE technology appraisals (TAs)
  ▸ **Mifamurtide for the treatment of osteosarcoma (October 2011)** NICE TA235
  Mifamurtide in combination with postoperative multi-agent chemotherapy is recommended (within its licensed indication), as an option for the treatment of high-grade resectable non-metastatic osteosarcoma after macroscopically complete surgical resection in children, adolescents and young adults and when mifamurtide is made available at a reduced cost to the NHS under the patient access scheme.
  www.nice.org.uk/TA235
- **MEDICINAL FORMS**
  There can be variation in the licensing of different medicines containing the same drug.
  Powder for suspension for infusion
  ▸ Mepact (Takeda UK Ltd)
  Mifamurtide 4 mg Mepact 4mg powder for suspension for infusion vials | 1 vial PoM £2,375.00

4　Targeted therapy responsive malignancy

ANTINEOPLASTIC DRUGS > PROTEIN KINASE INHIBITORS

Everolimus
09-Jun-2017

- **DRUG ACTION** Everolimus is a protein kinase inhibitor.

- **INDICATIONS AND DOSE**
  VOTUBIA® DISPERSIBLE TABLETS
  Subependymal giant cell astrocytoma associated with tuberous sclerosis complex
  ▸ BY MOUTH USING DISPERSIBLE TABLETS
  ▸ Child 1-17 years: (consult product literature)
  Adjunctive treatment of refractory partial-onset seizures, with or without secondary generalisation, associated with tuberous sclerosis complex
  ▸ BY MOUTH USING DISPERSIBLE TABLETS
  ▸ Child 2-17 years: (consult product literature)
  VOTUBIA® TABLETS
  Subependymal giant cell astrocytoma associated with tuberous sclerosis complex
  ▸ BY MOUTH USING TABLETS
  ▸ Child 1-17 years: (consult product literature)

> **IMPORTANT SAFETY INFORMATION**
> RISKS OF INCORRECT DOSING OF ORAL ANTI-CANCER MEDICINES
> See Cytotoxic drugs p. 505.

- **CAUTIONS** History of bleeding disorders
- **INTERACTIONS** → Appendix 1: everolimus
- **SIDE-EFFECTS**
  ▸ **Common or very common** Abdominal pain · anorexia · arthralgia · asthenia · chest pain · convulsions · dehydration · diarrhoea · dry mouth · dysphagia · electrolyte disturbance · epistaxis · eyelid oedema · fatigue · hand-foot syndrome · headache · hypercholesterolaemia · hyperglycaemia · hyperlipidaemia · hypertension · hypoglycaemia · increased susceptibility to aspergillosis · increased susceptibility to candidiasis · increased

Immune system and malignant disease

8

susceptibility to infections · increased susceptibility to pneumonia · insomnia · interstitial lung disease · irritability · nail disorders · peripheral oedema · pneumonitis · renal failure · skin disorders · taste disturbance

▸ **Uncommon** Aggression · agitation · congestive heart failure · flushing · impaired wound healing · rhabdomyolysis
▸ **Frequency not known** Alopecia · bone-marrow suppression · gastro-intestinal effects · haemorrhage · hepatitis B reactivation · hyperuricaemia · nausea · oral mucositis · organ-related toxicity (long-term and delayed) · thromboembolism · tumour lysis syndrome · vomiting

SIDE-EFFECTS, FURTHER INFORMATION
Reduce dose or discontinue if severe side-effects occur—consult product literature.

● **CONCEPTION AND CONTRACEPTION** Effective contraception must be used during and for up to 8 weeks after treatment.

● **PREGNANCY** Manufacturer advises avoid (toxicity in *animal* studies). See also *Pregnancy and reproductive function* in Cytotoxic drugs p. 505.

● **BREAST FEEDING** Manufacturer advises avoid.

● **HEPATIC IMPAIRMENT** Consult product literature.

● **MONITORING REQUIREMENTS**
▸ For *Votubia*® preparations: manufacturer advises everolimus blood concentration monitoring is required—consult product literature.
▸ Monitor blood-glucose concentration, serum-triglycerides and serum-cholesterol before treatment and periodically thereafter.
▸ Monitor renal function before treatment and periodically thereafter.

● **DIRECTIONS FOR ADMINISTRATION**
VOTUBIA® DISPERSIBLE TABLETS Manufacturer advises tablets must be dispersed in water before administration—consult product literature for details.

VOTUBIA® TABLETS Tablets may be dispersed in approximately 30 mL of water by gently stirring, immediately before drinking. After solution has been swallowed, any residue must be re-dispersed in the same volume of water and swallowed.

● **PRESCRIBING AND DISPENSING INFORMATION** *Votubia*® is available as both *tablets* and *dispersible tablets*. These formulations vary in their licensed indications and are not interchangeable—consult product literature for information on switching between formulations.

● **PATIENT AND CARER ADVICE**
Pneumonitis Non-infectious pneumonitis reported. Patients should be advised to seek urgent medical advice if new or worsening respiratory symptoms occur.

● **MEDICINAL FORMS**
There can be variation in the licensing of different medicines containing the same drug.

Dispersible tablet
CAUTIONARY AND ADVISORY LABELS 13
▸ Votubia (Novartis Pharmaceuticals UK Ltd)
Everolimus 2 mg Votubia 2mg dispersible tablets sugar-free | 30 tablet [PoM] £960.00
Everolimus 3 mg Votubia 3mg dispersible tablets sugar-free | 30 tablet [PoM] £1,440.00
Everolimus 5 mg Votubia 5mg dispersible tablets sugar-free | 30 tablet [PoM] £2,250.00

Tablet
CAUTIONARY AND ADVISORY LABELS 25
▸ Votubia (Novartis Pharmaceuticals UK Ltd)
Everolimus 2.5 mg Votubia 2.5mg tablets | 30 tablet [PoM] £1,200.00
Everolimus 5 mg Votubia 5mg tablets | 30 tablet [PoM] £2,250.00
Everolimus 10 mg Votubia 10mg tablets | 30 tablet [PoM] £2,970.00

Imatinib

21-Jul-2016

● **DRUG ACTION** Imatinib is a tyrosine kinase inhibitor.

● **INDICATIONS AND DOSE**
Treatment of newly diagnosed Philadelphia-chromosome-positive chronic myeloid leukaemia when bone marrow transplantation is not considered first line treatment | Treatment of Philadelphia-chromosome-positive chronic myeloid leukaemia in chronic phase after failure of interferon alfa, or in accelerated phase, or in blast crisis | Treatment of newly diagnosed Philadelphia-chromosome-positive acute lymphoblastic leukaemia in combination with chemotherapy
▸ BY MOUTH
▸ Child: (consult local protocol)

IMPORTANT SAFETY INFORMATION

RISKS OF INCORRECT DOSING OF ORAL ANTI-CANCER MEDICINES
See Cytotoxic drugs p. 505.

MHRA/CHM ADVICE (MAY 2016): RISK OF HEPATITIS B VIRUS REACTIVATION WITH BCR-ABL TYROSINE KINASE INHIBITORS
An EU wide review has concluded that imatinib can cause hepatitis B reactivation; the MHRA recommends establishing hepatitis B virus status in all patients before initiation of treatment.

● **CAUTIONS** Cardiac disease · hepatitis B infection · history of renal failure · risk factors for heart failure
CAUTIONS, FURTHER INFORMATION
▸ Hepatitis B infection The MHRA advises that patients who are carriers of hepatitis B virus should be closely monitored for signs and symptoms of active infection throughout treatment and for several months after stopping treatment; expert advice should be sought for patients who test positive for hepatitis B virus and in those with active infection.

● **INTERACTIONS** → Appendix 1: matinib

● **SIDE-EFFECTS**
▸ **Common or very common** Abdominal pain · appetite changes · arthralgia · ascites · conjunctivitis · constipation · cough · cramps · diarrhoea · dizziness · dry eyes · dry mouth · dry skin · dyspnoea · epistaxis · fatigue · flatulence · flushing · gastro-oesophageal reflux · haemorrhage · headache · hypoaesthesia · increased lacrimation · influenza-like symptoms · insomnia · oedema · paraesthesia · photosensitivity · pleural effusion · pruritus · pulmonary oedema · rash · sweating · taste disturbance · visual disturbances · weight changes
▸ **Uncommon** Acute respiratory failure · anxiety · cold extremities · cough · depression · drowsiness · dysphagia · electrolyte disturbances · gastric ulceration · gout · gynaecomastia · haematoma · hearing loss · heart failure · hepatic dysfunction · hepatitis · hypertension · hypotension · impaired memory · irregular menstruation · menorrhagia · migraine · palpitation · pancreatitis · peripheral neuropathy · renal failure · sexual dysfunction · skin hyperpigmentation · syncope · tachycardia · tinnitus · tremor · urinary frequency · vertigo
▸ **Rare** Angina · angioedema · arrhythmia · aseptic necrosis of bone · atrial fibrillation · cataract · confusion · convulsions · exfoliative dermatitis · gastro-intestinal perforation · glaucoma · haemolytic anaemia · hepatic failure · hepatic failure (fatal cases reported) · hepatic necrosis · increased intracranial pressure · inflammatory bowel disease · intestinal obstruction · myocardial infarction · myopathy · pulmonary fibrosis · pulmonary hypertension · rhabdomyolysis · Stevens-Johnson syndrome
▸ **Frequency not known** Alopecia · bone-marrow suppression · drug rash with eosinophilia and systemic symptoms

(DRESS) · gastro-intestinal effects · growth retardation in children · hepatitis B reactivation · hyperuricaemia · nausea · oral mucositis · organ-related toxicity (long-term and delayed) · thromboembolism · tumour lysis syndrome · vomiting

- **CONCEPTION AND CONTRACEPTION** Effective contraception required during treatment.
- **PREGNANCY** Manufacturer advises avoid unless potential benefit outweighs risk. See also *Pregnancy and reproductive function* in Cytotoxic drugs p. 505.
- **BREAST FEEDING** Discontinue breast-feeding.
- **HEPATIC IMPAIRMENT** Start with minimum recommended dose; reduce dose further if not tolerated; consult local treatment protocol.
- **RENAL IMPAIRMENT** Start with minimum recommended dose; reduce dose further if not tolerated; consult local treatment protocol.
- **MONITORING REQUIREMENTS**
- ▸ Monitor for gastrointestinal haemorrhage.
- ▸ Monitor complete blood counts regularly.
- ▸ Monitor for fluid retention.
- ▸ Monitor liver function.
- ▸ Monitor growth in children (may cause growth retardation).
- **DIRECTIONS FOR ADMINISTRATION** Tablets may be dispersed in water or apple juice.
- **PATIENT AND CARER ADVICE** Patients or carers should be given advice on how to administer imatinib tablets.

- **MEDICINAL FORMS**
There can be variation in the licensing of different medicines containing the same drug.

Tablet
CAUTIONARY AND ADVISORY LABELS 21, 27
- ▸ **Imatinib (Non-proprietary)**
  Imatinib (as Imatinib mesilate) 100 mg Imatinib 100mg tablets | 30 tablet PoM £486.66 | 60 tablet PoM £99.99–£973.32
  Imatinib (as Imatinib mesilate) 400 mg Imatinib 400mg tablets | 30 tablet PoM £199.98–£1,946.67 DT price = £1,946.67 | 60 tablet PoM £3,893.34
- ▸ **Glivec** (Novartis Pharmaceuticals UK Ltd) ▼
  Imatinib (as Imatinib mesilate) 100 mg Glivec 100mg tablets | 60 tablet PoM £973.32
  Imatinib (as Imatinib mesilate) 400 mg Glivec 400mg tablets | 30 tablet PoM £1,946.67 DT price = £1,946.67

Chapter 9
Blood and nutrition

CONTENTS

Blood and blood-forming organs

1 Anaemias

Anaemias

Initiation of treatment

Before initiating treatment for anaemia it is essential to determine which type is present. Iron salts may be harmful and result in iron overload if given alone to patients with anaemias other than those due to iron deficiency.

Sickle-cell anaemia

Sickle-cell disease is caused by a structural abnormality of haemoglobin resulting in deformed, less flexible red blood cells. Acute complications in the more severe forms include sickle-cell crisis, where infarction of the microvasculature and blood supply to organs results in severe pain. Sickle-cell crisis requires hospitalisation, intravenous fluids, analgesia and treatment of any concurrent infection. Chronic complications include skin ulceration, renal failure, and increased susceptibility to infection. Pneumococcal vaccine, haemophilus influenzae type b vaccine, an annual influenza vaccine and prophylactic penicillin reduce the risk of

infection. Hepatitis B vaccine should be considered if the patient is not immune.

In most forms of sickle-cell disease, varying degrees of haemolytic anaemia are present accompanied by increased erythropoiesis; this may increase folate requirements and folate supplementation may be necessary.

Hydroxycarbamide p. 524 can reduce the frequency of crises and the need for blood transfusions in sickle-cell disease. The beneficial effects of hydroxycarbamide may not become evident for several months.

G6PD deficiency

Glucose 6-phosphate dehydrogenase (G6PD) deficiency is highly prevalent in individuals originating from most parts of Africa, from most parts of Asia, from Oceania, and from Southern Europe; it can also occur, rarely, in any other individuals. G6PD deficiency is more common in males than it is in females.

Individuals with G6PD deficiency are susceptible to developing acute haemolytic anaemia when they take a number of common drugs. They are also susceptible to developing acute haemolytic anaemia when they eat fava beans (broad beans, *Vicia faba*); this is termed *favism* and can be more severe in children or when the fresh fava beans are eaten raw.

When prescribing drugs for patients with G6PD deficiency, the following three points should be kept in mind:

- G6PD deficiency is genetically heterogeneous; susceptibility to the haemolytic risk from drugs varies;

thus, a drug found to be safe in some G6PD-deficient individuals may not be equally safe in others;
- manufacturers do not routinely test drugs for their effects in G6PD-deficient individuals;
- the risk and severity of haemolysis is almost always dose-related.

The lists below should be read with these points in mind. Ideally, information about G6PD deficiency should be available before prescribing a drug listed below. However, in the absence of this information, the possibility of haemolysis should be considered, especially if the patient belongs to a group in which G6PD deficiency is common.

A very few G6PD-deficient individuals with chronic non-spherocytic haemolytic anaemia have haemolysis even in the absence of an exogenous trigger. These patients must be regarded as being at high risk of severe exacerbation of haemolysis following administration of any of the drugs listed below.

Drugs with definite risk of haemolysis in most G6PD-deficient individuals

- Dapsone and other sulfones (higher doses for dermatitis herpetiformis more likely to cause problems)
- Methylthioninium chloride
- Niridazole [not on UK market]
- Nitrofurantoin
- Pamaquin [not on UK market]
- Primaquine (30 mg weekly for 8 weeks has been found to be without undue harmful effects in African and Asian people)
- Quinolones (including ciprofloxacin, moxifloxacin, nalidixic acid, norfloxacin, and ofloxacin)
- Rasburicase
- Sulfonamides (including co-trimoxazole; some sulfonamides, e.g. sulfadiazine, have been tested and found not to be haemolytic in many G6PD-deficient individuals)

Drugs with possible risk of haemolysis in some G6PD-deficient individuals

- Aspirin (acceptable up to a dose of at least 1 g daily in most G6PD-deficient individuals)
- Chloroquine (acceptable in acute malaria and malaria chemoprophylaxis)
- Menadione, water-soluble derivatives (e.g. menadiol sodium phosphate)
- Quinidine (acceptable in acute malaria) [not on UK market]
- Quinine (acceptable in acute malaria)
- Sulfonylureas

Naphthalene in mothballs also causes haemolysis in individuals with Gana6PD deficiency.

Drugs used in hypoplastic, haemolytic, and renal anaemias

Anabolic steroids, pyridoxine hydrochloride p. 600, antilymphocyte immunoglobulin, and various corticosteroids are used in hypoplastic and haemolytic anaemias.

Antilymphocyte immunoglobulin given intravenously through a central line over 12–18 hours each day for 5 days produces a response in about 50% of cases of acquired *aplastic anaemia*; the response rate may be increased when ciclosporin p. 496 is given as well. Severe reactions are common in the first 2 days and profound immunosuppression can occur; antilymphocyte immunoglobulin should be given under specialist supervision with appropriate resuscitation facilities. Alternatively, oxymetholone tablets (available from 'special order' manufacturers or specialist importing companies) can be used in aplastic anaemia for 3 to 6 months.

It is unlikely that dietary deprivation of pyridoxine hydrochloride produces clinically relevant haematological effects. However, certain forms of *sideroblastic anaemia*

respond to pharmacological doses, possibly reflecting its role as a co-enzyme during haemoglobin synthesis. Pyridoxine hydrochloride is indicated in both *idiopathic acquired* and *hereditary sideroblastic anaemias*. Although complete cures have not been reported, some increase in haemoglobin can occur with high doses. *Reversible sideroblastic anaemias* respond to treatment of the underlying cause but pyridoxine hydrochloride is indicated in pregnancy, haemolytic anaemias, or during isoniazid p. 352 treatment.

Corticosteroids have an important place in the management of haematological disorders including *autoimmune haemolytic anaemia*, *idiopathic thrombocytopenias* and *neutropenias*, and *major transfusion reactions*. They are also used in chemotherapy schedules for many types of *lymphoma*, *lymphoid leukaemias*, and *paraproteinaemias*, including *multiple myeloma*.

Erythropoietins
Epoetins (recombinant human erythropoietins) are used to treat the anaemia associated with erythropoietin deficiency in chronic renal failure.

Epoetin beta p. 538 is also used for the prevention of anaemia in preterm neonates of low birth-weight; a therapeutic response may take several weeks.

There is insufficient information to support the use of erythropoietins in children with leukaemia or in those receiving cancer chemotherapy.

Darbepoetin is a glycosylated derivative of epoetin; it persists longer in the body and can be administered less frequently than epoetin.

1.1 Hypoplastic, haemolytic, and renal anaemias

ANABOLIC STEROIDS > ANDROSTAN DERIVATIVES

Oxymetholone

- **INDICATIONS AND DOSE**

Aplastic anaemia
▶ BY MOUTH
  ▶ Child: 1–5 mg/kg daily for 3 to 6 months

- **INTERACTIONS** → Appendix 1: oxymetholone

- **MEDICINAL FORMS**
There can be variation in the licensing of different medicines containing the same drug. Forms available from special-order manufacturers include: oral suspension

Capsule
▶ Oxymetholone (Non-proprietary)
  Oxymetholone **50 mg** Oxymetholone 50mg capsules | 50 capsule PoM £475.00 CD4–2

EPOETINS

Epoetins

IMPORTANT SAFETY INFORMATION
ERYTHROPOIETINS—HAEMOGLOBIN CONCENTRATION
In chronic kidney disease, the use of erythropoietins can be considered in a child with anaemia. The aim of treatment is to relieve symptoms of anaemia and to avoid the need for blood transfusion. The optimum haemoglobin concentration is dependent on the child's age and factors such as symptoms, comorbidities, and patient preferences. The haemoglobin concentration should not be increased beyond that which provides adequate control of symptoms of anaemia. In *adults*, overcorrection of haemoglobin concentration with

erythropoietins in those with chronic kidney disease may increase the risk of serious cardiovascular events and death; haemoglobin concentrations higher than 12 g/100 mL should be avoided in children.

- **CONTRA-INDICATIONS** Avoid injections containing benzyl alcohol in neonates · pure red cell aplasia following erythropoietin therapy · uncontrolled hypertension
- **CAUTIONS** Aluminium toxicity (can impair the response to erythropoietin) · concurrent infection (can impair the response to erythropoietin) · correct factors that contribute to the anaemia of chronic renal failure, such as iron or folate deficiency, before treatment. · during dialysis (increase in unfractionated or low molecular weight heparin dose may be needed) · epilepsy · inadequately treated or poorly controlled blood pressure—interrupt treatment if blood pressure uncontrolled · ischaemic vascular disease · malignant disease · other inflammatory disease (can impair the response to erythropoietin) · sickle-cell disease (lower target haemoglobin concentration may be appropriate) · sudden stabbing migraine-like pain (warning of a hypertensive crisis) · thrombocytosis (monitor platelet count for first 8 weeks)
- **SIDE-EFFECTS**
- ▶ **Common or very common** Aggravation of hypertension (dose-dependent) · cardiovascular events · diarrhoea · dose-dependent increase in platelet count regressing during treatment (but thrombocytosis rare) · headache · hypertensive crisis (in isolated patients with normal or low blood pressure) · increase in blood pressure (dose-dependent) · influenza-like symptoms (may be reduced if intravenous injection given over 5 minutes) · nausea · shunt thrombosis especially if tendency to hypotension or arteriovenous shunt complications · vomiting
- ▶ **Very rare** Sudden loss of efficacy because of pure red cell aplasia, particularly following subcutaneous administration in patients with chronic renal failure
- ▶ **Frequency not known** Anaphylaxis · angioedema · hyperkalaemia · hypersensitivity reactions · injection-site reactions · peripheral oedema · skin reactions
  SIDE-EFFECTS, FURTHER INFORMATION
- ▶ Hypertensive crisis In isolated patients with normal or low blood pressure, hypertensive crisis with encephalopathy-like symptoms and generalised tonic-clonic seizures requiring immediate medical attention has occured with epoetin.
- ▶ Pure red cell aplasia There have been very rare reports of pure red cell aplasia in patients treated with erythropoietins. In patients who develop a lack of efficacy with erythropoietin therapy and with a diagnosis of pure red cell aplasia, treatment with erythropoietins must be discontinued and testing for erythropoietin antibodies considered. Patients who develop pure red cell aplasia should **not** be switched to another form of erythropoietin.
- **MONITORING REQUIREMENTS**
- ▶ Monitor closely blood pressure, reticulocyte counts, haemoglobin, and electrolytes—interrupt treatment if blood pressure uncontrolled.
- ▶ Other factors, such as iron or folate deficiency, that contribute to the anaemia of chronic renal failure should be corrected before treatment and monitored during therapy. Supplemental iron may improve the response in resistant patients and in preterm neonates.

F 535

Darbepoetin alfa

- **INDICATIONS AND DOSE**

Symptomatic anaemia associated with chronic renal failure in patients on dialysis
- ▶ BY SUBCUTANEOUS INJECTION, OR BY INTRAVENOUS INJECTION
- ▶ Child 11–17 years: Initially 450 nanograms/kg once weekly, dose to be adjusted according to response by approximately 25% at intervals of at least 4 weeks, maintenance dose to be given once weekly or once every 2 weeks, reduce dose by approximately 25% if rise in haemoglobin concentration exceeds 2 g/100 mL over 4 weeks or if haemoglobin concentration exceeds 12 g/100 mL; if haemoglobin concentration continues to rise, despite dose reduction, suspend treatment until haemoglobin concentration decreases and then restart at a dose approximately 25% lower than the previous dose, when changing route give same dose then adjust according to weekly or fortnightly haemoglobin measurements, adjust doses not more frequently than every 2 weeks during maintenance treatment

Symptomatic anaemia associated with chronic renal failure in patients not on dialysis
- ▶ BY SUBCUTANEOUS INJECTION
- ▶ Child 11–17 years: Initially 450 nanograms/kg once weekly, alternatively initially 750 nanograms/kg every 2 weeks, dose to be adjusted according to response by approximately 25% at intervals of at least 4 weeks, maintenance dose can be given once weekly, every 2 weeks, or once a month, subcutaneous route preferred in patients not on haemodialysis, reduce dose by approximately 25% if rise in haemoglobin concentration exceeds 2 g/100 mL over 4 weeks or if haemoglobin concentration exceeds 12 g/100 mL; if haemoglobin concentration continues to rise, despite dose reduction, suspend treatment until haemoglobin concentration decreases and then restart at a dose approximately 25% lower than the previous dose, when changing route give same dose then adjust according to weekly or fortnightly haemoglobin measurements, adjust doses not more frequently than every 2 weeks during maintenance treatment

Symptomatic anaemia associated with chronic renal failure in patients not on dialysis
- ▶ BY INTRAVENOUS INJECTION
- ▶ Child 11–17 years: Initially 450 nanograms/kg once weekly, dose to be adjusted according to response by approximately 25% at intervals of at least 4 weeks, maintenance dose given once weekly, subcutaneous route preferred in patients not on haemodialysis, reduce dose by approximately 25% if rise in haemoglobin concentration exceeds 2 g/100 mL over 4 weeks or if haemoglobin concentration exceeds 12 g/100 mL; if haemoglobin concentration continues to rise, despite dose reduction, suspend treatment until haemoglobin concentration decreases and then restart at a dose approximately 25% lower than the previous dose, when changing route give same dose then adjust according to weekly or fortnightly haemoglobin measurements, adjust doses not more frequently than every 2 weeks during maintenance treatment

- **INTERACTIONS** → Appendix 1: darbepoetin alfa
- **SIDE-EFFECTS** Injection-site pain · oedema
- **PREGNANCY** No evidence of harm in *animal* studies—manufacturer advises caution.
- **BREAST FEEDING** Manufacturer advises avoid—no information available.
- **HEPATIC IMPAIRMENT** Manufacturer advises caution.

● MEDICINAL FORMS
There can be variation in the licensing of different medicines containing the same drug.

Solution for injection

▸ Aranesp (Amgen Ltd)

Darbepoetin alfa 25 microgram per 1 ml Aranesp
10micrograms/0.4ml solution for injection pre-filled syringes | 4 pre-filled disposable injection PoM £58.72

Darbepoetin alfa 40 microgram per 1 ml Aranesp
20micrograms/0.5ml solution for injection pre-filled syringes | 4 pre-filled disposable injection PoM £117.45

Darbepoetin alfa 100 microgram per 1 ml Aranesp
50micrograms/0.5ml solution for injection pre-filled syringes | 4 pre-filled disposable injection PoM £293.62
Aranesp 40micrograms/0.4ml solution for injection pre-filled syringes | 4 pre-filled disposable injection PoM £234.90
Aranesp 30micrograms/0.3ml solution for injection pre-filled syringes | 4 pre-filled disposable injection PoM £176.17

Darbepoetin alfa 200 microgram per 1 ml Aranesp
100micrograms/0.5ml solution for injection pre-filled syringes | 4 pre-filled disposable injection PoM £587.24
Aranesp 130micrograms/0.65ml solution for injection pre-filled syringes | 4 pre-filled disposable injection PoM £763.42
Aranesp 80micrograms/0.4ml solution for injection pre-filled syringes | 4 pre-filled disposable injection PoM £469.79
Aranesp 60micrograms/0.3ml solution for injection pre-filled syringes | 4 pre-filled disposable injection PoM £352.35

Darbepoetin alfa 500 microgram per 1 ml Aranesp
300micrograms/0.6ml solution for injection pre-filled syringes | 1 pre-filled disposable injection PoM £440.43
Aranesp 500micrograms/1ml solution for injection pre-filled syringes | 1 pre-filled disposable injection PoM £734.05
Aranesp 150micrograms/0.3ml solution for injection pre-filled syringes | 4 pre-filled disposable injection PoM £880.86

▸ Aranesp SureClick (Amgen Ltd)

Darbepoetin alfa 40 microgram per 1 ml Aranesp SureClick
20micrograms/0.5ml solution for injection pre-filled disposable devices | 1 pre-filled disposable injection PoM £29.36

Darbepoetin alfa 100 microgram per 1 ml Aranesp SureClick
40micrograms/0.4ml solution for injection pre-filled disposable devices | 1 pre-filled disposable injection PoM £58.72
Aranesp SureClick 80micrograms/0.4ml solution for injection pre-filled disposable devices | 1 pre-filled disposable injection PoM £117.45

Darbepoetin alfa 200 microgram per 1 ml Aranesp SureClick
60micrograms/0.3ml solution for injection pre-filled disposable devices | 1 pre-filled disposable injection PoM £88.09
Aranesp SureClick 100micrograms/0.5ml solution for injection pre-filled disposable devices | 1 pre-filled disposable injection PoM £146.81

Darbepoetin alfa 500 microgram per 1 ml Aranesp SureClick
150micrograms/0.3ml solution for injection pre-filled disposable devices | 1 pre-filled disposable injection PoM £220.22
Aranesp SureClick 300micrograms/0.6ml solution for injection pre-filled disposable devices | 1 pre-filled disposable injection PoM £440.43
Aranesp SureClick 500micrograms/1ml solution for injection pre-filled disposable devices | 1 pre-filled disposable injection PoM £734.05

F 535

Epoetin alfa

● INDICATIONS AND DOSE

BINOCRIT® PRE-FILLED SYRINGES

Symptomatic anaemia associated with chronic renal failure in patients on haemodialysis
▸ BY INTRAVENOUS INJECTION
▸ Child (body-weight up to 10 kg): Initially 50 units/kg 3 times a week, adjusted in steps of 25 units/kg 3 times a week, dose adjusted according to response at intervals of at least 4 weeks; maintenance 75–150 units/kg 3 times a week, intravenous injection to be given over 1–5 minutes, reduce dose by approximately 25% if rise in haemoglobin concentration exceeds 2 g/100 mL over 4 weeks or if haemoglobin concentration exceeds 12 g/100 mL; if haemoglobin concentration continues to rise, despite dose reduction, suspend treatment until haemoglobin

concentration decreases and then restart at a dose approximately 25% lower than the previous dose
▸ Child (body-weight 10–30 kg): Initially 50 units/kg 3 times a week, adjusted in steps of 25 units/kg 3 times a week, dose adjusted according to response at intervals of at least 4 weeks; maintenance 60–150 units/kg 3 times a week, intravenous injection to be given over 1–5 minutes, reduce dose by approximately 25% if rise in haemoglobin concentration exceeds 2 g/100 mL over 4 weeks or if haemoglobin concentration exceeds 12 g/100 mL; if haemoglobin concentration continues to rise, despite dose reduction, suspend treatment until haemoglobin concentration decreases and then restart at a dose approximately 25% lower than the previous dose
▸ Child (body-weight 31 kg and above): Initially 50 units/kg 3 times a week, adjusted in steps of 25 units/kg 3 times a week, dose adjusted according to response at intervals of at least 4 weeks; maintenance 30–100 units/kg 3 times a week, intravenous injection to be given over 1–5 minutes, reduce dose by approximately 25% if rise in haemoglobin concentration exceeds 2 g/100 mL over 4 weeks or if haemoglobin concentration exceeds 12 g/100 mL; if haemoglobin concentration continues to rise, despite dose reduction, suspend treatment until haemoglobin concentration decreases and then restart at a dose approximately 25% lower than the previous dose

EPREX® PRE-FILLED SYRINGES

Symptomatic anaemia associated with chronic renal failure in patients on haemodialysis
▸ BY INTRAVENOUS INJECTION
▸ Child (body-weight up to 10 kg): Initially 50 units/kg 3 times a week, adjusted in steps of 25 units/kg 3 times a week, dose adjusted according to response at intervals of at least 4 weeks; maintenance 75–150 units/kg 3 times a week, intravenous injection to be given over 1–5 minutes, reduce dose by approximately 25% if rise in haemoglobin concentration exceeds 2 g/100 mL over 4 weeks or if haemoglobin concentration exceeds 12 g/100 mL; if haemoglobin concentration continues to rise, despite dose reduction, suspend treatment until haemoglobin concentration decreases and then restart at a dose approximately 25% lower than the previous dose
▸ Child (body-weight 10–30 kg): Initially 50 units/kg 3 times a week, adjusted in steps of 25 units/kg 3 times a week, dose adjusted according to response at intervals of at least 4 weeks; maintenance 60–150 units/kg 3 times a week, intravenous injection to be given over 1–5 minutes, reduce dose by approximately 25% if rise in haemoglobin concentration exceeds 2 g/100 mL over 4 weeks or if haemoglobin concentration exceeds 12 g/100 mL; if haemoglobin concentration continues to rise, despite dose reduction, suspend treatment until haemoglobin concentration decreases and then restart at a dose approximately 25% lower than the previous dose
▸ Child (body-weight 31–60 kg): Initially 50 units/kg 3 times a week, adjusted in steps of 25 units/kg 3 times a week, dose adjusted according to response at intervals of at least 4 weeks; maintenance 30–100 units/kg 3 times a week, intravenous injection to be given over 1–5 minutes, reduce dose by approximately 25% if rise in haemoglobin concentration exceeds 2 g/100 mL over 4 weeks or if haemoglobin concentration exceeds 12 g/100 mL; if haemoglobin concentration continues to rise, despite dose reduction, suspend treatment until haemoglobin concentration decreases and then restart at a dose approximately 25% lower than the previous dose

continued →

▸ **Child (body-weight 61 kg and above):** Initially 50 units/kg 3 times a week, adjusted in steps of 25 units/kg 3 times a week, dose adjusted according to response at intervals of at least 4 weeks; maintenance 75–300 units/kg once weekly, maintenance dose can be given as a single dose or in divided doses, intravenous injection to be given over 1–5 minutes, reduce dose by approximately 25% if rise in haemoglobin concentration exceeds 2 g/100 mL over 4 weeks or if haemoglobin concentration exceeds 12 g/100 mL; if haemoglobin concentration continues to rise, despite dose reduction, suspend treatment until haemoglobin concentration decreases and then restart at a dose approximately 25% lower than the previous dose

● **INTERACTIONS** → Appendix 1: epoetin alfa

● **PREGNANCY** No evidence of harm. Benefits probably outweigh risk of anaemia and of blood transfusion in pregnancy.

● **BREAST FEEDING** Unlikely to be present in milk. Minimal effect on infant.

● **HEPATIC IMPAIRMENT** Manufacturers advise caution in chronic hepatic failure.

● **PRESCRIBING AND DISPENSING INFORMATION** Epoetin alfa is a biological medicine. Biological medicines must be prescribed and dispensed by brand name, see *Biological medicines* and *Biosimilar medicines*, under Guidance on prescribing p. 1.

● **MEDICINAL FORMS**
There can be variation in the licensing of different medicines containing the same drug.

Solution for injection
▸ Eprex (Janssen-Cilag Ltd)

Epoetin alfa 2000 unit per 1 ml Eprex 1,000units/0.5ml solution for injection pre-filled syringes | 6 pre-filled disposable injection [PoM] £33.18

Epoetin alfa 4000 unit per 1 ml Eprex 2,000units/0.5ml solution for injection pre-filled syringes | 6 pre-filled disposable injection [PoM] £66.37

Epoetin alfa 10000 unit per 1 ml Eprex 6,000units/0.6ml solution for injection pre-filled syringes | 6 pre-filled disposable injection [PoM] £199.11
Eprex 4,000units/0.4ml solution for injection pre-filled syringes | 6 pre-filled disposable injection [PoM] £132.74
Eprex 5,000units/0.5ml solution for injection pre-filled syringes | 6 pre-filled disposable injection [PoM] £165.92
Eprex 3,000units/0.3ml solution for injection pre-filled syringes | 6 pre-filled disposable injection [PoM] £99.55
Eprex 10,000units/1ml solution for injection pre-filled syringes | 6 pre-filled disposable injection [PoM] £331.85
Eprex 8,000units/0.8ml solution for injection pre-filled syringes | 6 pre-filled disposable injection [PoM] £265.48

Epoetin alfa 40000 unit per 1 ml Eprex 20,000units/0.5ml solution for injection pre-filled syringes | 1 pre-filled disposable injection [PoM] £110.62
Eprex 30,000units/0.75ml solution for injection pre-filled syringes | 1 pre-filled disposable injection [PoM] £199.11
Eprex 40,000units/1ml solution for injection pre-filled syringes | 1 pre-filled disposable injection [PoM] £265.48

⌐ 535

Epoetin beta

● **INDICATIONS AND DOSE**

Symptomatic anaemia associated with chronic renal failure
▸ BY SUBCUTANEOUS INJECTION

▸ **Neonate:** Initially 20 units/kg 3 times a week for 4 weeks, increased in steps of 20 units/kg 3 times a week, according to response at intervals of 4 weeks, total weekly dose may be divided into daily doses; maintenance dose, initially reduce dose by half then adjust according to response at intervals of 1–2 weeks, total weekly maintenance dose may be given as a single dose or in 3 or 7 divided doses. Subcutaneous route preferred in patients not on haemodialysis. Reduce dose by approximately 25% if rise in haemoglobin concentration exceeds 2 g/100 mL over 4 weeks or if haemoglobin concentration approaches or exceeds 12 g/100 mL; if haemoglobin concentration continues to rise, despite dose reduction, suspend treatment until haemoglobin concentration decreases and then restart at a dose approximately 25% lower than the previous dose; maximum 720 units/kg per week.

▸ **Child:** Initially 20 units/kg 3 times a week for 4 weeks, increased in steps of 20 units/kg 3 times a week, according to response at intervals of 4 weeks, total weekly dose may be divided into daily doses; maintenance dose, initially reduce dose by half then adjust according to response at intervals of 1–2 weeks, total weekly maintenance dose may be given as a single dose or in 3 or 7 divided doses. Subcutaneous route preferred in patients not on haemodialysis. Reduce dose by approximately 25% if rise in haemoglobin concentration exceeds 2 g/100 mL over 4 weeks or if haemoglobin concentration approaches or exceeds 12 g/100 mL; if haemoglobin concentration continues to rise, despite dose reduction, suspend treatment until haemoglobin concentration decreases and then restart at a dose approximately 25% lower than the previous dose; maximum 720 units/kg per week

▸ BY INTRAVENOUS INJECTION

▸ **Neonate:** Initially 40 units/kg 3 times a week for 4 weeks, then increased to 80 units/kg 3 times a week, then increased in steps of 20 units/kg 3 times a week if required, at intervals of 4 weeks; maintenance dose, initially reduce dose by half then adjust according to response at intervals of 1–2 weeks. Intravenous injection to be administered over 2 minutes. Subcutaneous route preferred in patients not on haemodialysis. Reduce dose by approximately 25% if rise in haemoglobin concentration exceeds 2 g/100 mL over 4 weeks or if haemoglobin concentration approaches or exceeds 12 g/100 mL; if haemoglobin concentration continues to rise, despite dose reduction, suspend treatment until haemoglobin concentration decreases and then restart at a dose approximately 25% lower than the previous dose; maximum 720 units/kg per week.

▸ **Child:** Initially 40 units/kg 3 times a week for 4 weeks, then increased to 80 units/kg 3 times a week, then increased in steps of 20 units/kg 3 times a week if required, at intervals of 4 weeks; maintenance dose, initially reduce dose by half then adjust according to response at intervals of 1–2 weeks. Intravenous injection to be administered over 2 minutes. Subcutaneous route preferred in patients not on haemodialysis. Reduce dose by approximately 25% if rise in haemoglobin concentration exceeds 2 g/100 mL over 4 weeks or if haemoglobin concentration approaches or exceeds 12 g/100 mL; if haemoglobin concentration continues to rise, despite dose reduction, suspend treatment until haemoglobin concentration decreases and then restart at a dose approximately 25% lower than the previous dose; maximum 720 units/kg per week

Prevention of anaemias of prematurity in neonates
▶ BY SUBCUTANEOUS INJECTION

▸ Neonate up to 33 weeks corrected gestational age (body-weight 0.75–1.5 kg): 250 units/kg 3 times a week preferably started within 3 days of birth and continued for 6 weeks, using single-dose unpreserved injection.

IMPORTANT SAFETY INFORMATION
MHRA/CHM ADVICE (MAY 2015) EPOETIN BETA (NEORECORMON): INCREASED RISK OF RETINOPATHY IN PRETERM INFANTS CANNOT BE EXCLUDED
There is a possible increased risk of retinopathy in premature infants, when epoetin beta is used for preventing anaemia of prematurity. When using epoetin beta in preterm infants:
- consider the benefits and risks of treatment, including the possible risk of retinopathy,
- monitor the infant for features of retinopathy, and
- advise parents or carers that their baby's eyes will be carefully monitored for any ill effects.

● INTERACTIONS → Appendix 1: epoetin beta
● PREGNANCY No evidence of harm. Benefits probably outweigh risk of anaemia and of blood transfusion in pregnancy.
● BREAST FEEDING Unlikely to be present in milk. Minimal effect on infant.
● HEPATIC IMPAIRMENT Manufacturers advise caution in chronic hepatic failure.

● MEDICINAL FORMS
There can be variation in the licensing of different medicines containing the same drug.
Solution for injection
EXCIPIENTS: May contain Phenylalanine
▶ NeoRecormon (Roche Products Ltd)
  Epoetin beta 1667 unit per 1 ml NeoRecormon 500units/0.3ml solution for injection pre-filled syringes | 6 pre-filled disposable injection PoM £21.05
  Epoetin beta 6667 unit per 1 ml NeoRecormon 2,000units/0.3ml solution for injection pre-filled syringes | 6 pre-filled disposable injection PoM £84.17
  Epoetin beta 10000 unit per 1 ml NeoRecormon 3,000units/0.3ml solution for injection pre-filled syringes | 6 pre-filled disposable injection PoM £126.25
  Epoetin beta 13333 unit per 1 ml NeoRecormon 4,000units/0.3ml solution for injection pre-filled syringes | 6 pre-filled disposable injection PoM £168.34
  Epoetin beta 16667 unit per 1 ml NeoRecormon 10,000units/0.6ml solution for injection pre-filled syringes | 6 pre-filled disposable injection PoM £420.85
  NeoRecormon 5,000units/0.3ml solution for injection pre-filled syringes | 6 pre-filled disposable injection PoM £210.42
  Epoetin beta 20000 unit per 1 ml NeoRecormon 6,000units/0.3ml solution for injection pre-filled syringes | 6 pre-filled disposable injection PoM £252.50
  Epoetin beta 33333 unit per 1 ml NeoRecormon 20,000units/0.6ml solution for injection pre-filled syringes | 6 pre-filled disposable injection PoM £841.71
  Epoetin beta 50000 unit per 1 ml NeoRecormon 30,000units/0.6ml solution for injection pre-filled syringes | 4 pre-filled disposable injection PoM £841.71

☞ 535

Epoetin zeta

● INDICATIONS AND DOSE
Symptomatic anaemia associated with chronic renal failure in patients on haemodialysis
▶ BY INTRAVENOUS INJECTION
▸ Child (body-weight up to 10 kg): Initially 50 units/kg 3 times a week, adjusted according to response, adjusted in steps of 25 units/kg 3 times a week, dose to be adjusted at intervals of at least 4 weeks; maintenance 75–150 units/kg 3 times a week, to be administered over 1–5 minutes, avoid increasing haemoglobin concentration at a rate exceeding 2 g/100 mL over 4 weeks
▸ Child (body-weight 10–30 kg): Initially 50 units/kg 3 times a week, adjusted according to response, adjusted in steps of 25 units/kg 3 times a week, dose to be adjusted at intervals of at least 4 weeks; maintenance 60–150 units/kg 3 times a week, to be administered over 1–5 minutes, avoid increasing haemoglobin concentration at a rate exceeding 2 g/100 mL over 4 weeks
▸ Child (body-weight 31 kg and above): Initially 50 units/kg 3 times a week, adjusted according to response, adjusted in steps of 25 units/kg 3 times a week, dose to be adjusted at intervals of at least 4 weeks; maintenance 30–100 units/kg 3 times a week, to be administered over 1–5 minutes, avoid increasing haemoglobin concentration at a rate exceeding 2 g/100 mL over 4 weeks

● INTERACTIONS → Appendix 1: epoetin zeta
● PREGNANCY No evidence of harm. Benefits probably outweigh risk of anaemia and of blood transfusion in pregnancy.
● BREAST FEEDING Unlikely to be present in milk. Minimal effect on infant.
● HEPATIC IMPAIRMENT Manufacturers advise caution in chronic hepatic failure.
● PRESCRIBING AND DISPENSING INFORMATION Epoetin zeta is a biological medicine. Biological medicines must be prescribed and dispensed by brand name, see *Biological medicines* and *Biosimilar medicines*, under Guidance on prescribing p. 1.

● MEDICINAL FORMS
There can be variation in the licensing of different medicines containing the same drug.
Solution for injection
EXCIPIENTS: May contain Phenylalanine
▶ Retacrit (Pfizer Ltd)
  Epoetin zeta 3333 unit per 1 ml Retacrit 2,000units/0.6ml solution for injection pre-filled syringes | 6 pre-filled disposable injection PoM £57.70 (Hospital only)
  Retacrit 3,000units/0.9ml solution for injection pre-filled syringes | 6 pre-filled disposable injection PoM £86.55 (Hospital only)
  Retacrit 1,000units/0.3ml solution for injection pre-filled syringes | 6 pre-filled disposable injection PoM £28.85 (Hospital only)
  Epoetin zeta 10000 unit per 1 ml Retacrit 6,000units/0.6ml solution for injection pre-filled syringes | 6 pre-filled disposable injection PoM £173.09 (Hospital only)
  Retacrit 10,000units/1ml solution for injection pre-filled syringes | 6 pre-filled disposable injection PoM £288.48 (Hospital only)
  Retacrit 8,000units/0.8ml solution for injection pre-filled syringes | 6 pre-filled disposable injection PoM £230.79 (Hospital only)
  Retacrit 4,000units/0.4ml solution for injection pre-filled syringes | 6 pre-filled disposable injection PoM £115.40 (Hospital only)
  Retacrit 5,000units/0.5ml solution for injection pre-filled syringes | 6 pre-filled disposable injection PoM £144.25 (Hospital only)
  Epoetin zeta 40000 unit per 1 ml Retacrit 20,000units/0.5ml solution for injection pre-filled syringes | 1 pre-filled disposable injection PoM £96.16 (Hospital only)
  Retacrit 40,000units/1ml solution for injection pre-filled syringes | 1 pre-filled disposable injection PoM £193.32 (Hospital only)

9

Blood and nutrition

Retacrit 30,000units/0.75ml solution for injection pre-filled syringes |
1 pre-filled disposable injection [PoM] £144.25 (Hospital only)

1.1a Atypical haemolytic uraemic syndrome and paroxysmal nocturnal haemoglobinuria

IMMUNOSUPPRESSANTS > MONOCLONAL ANTIBODIES

Eculizumab

- **DRUG ACTION** Eculizumab, a recombinant monoclonal antibody, inhibits terminal complement activation at the C5 protein and thereby reduces haemolysis and thrombotic microangiopathy.

- **INDICATIONS AND DOSE**

  Reduce haemolysis in paroxysmal nocturnal haemoglobinuria (PNH), in those with a history of blood transfusions (under expert supervision)
  - ► BY INTRAVENOUS INFUSION
  - ▸ Child: Refer for specialist advice, experience very limited

  Reduce thrombotic microangiopathy in atypical haemolytic uraemic syndrome (aHUS) (specialist use only)
  - ► BY INTRAVENOUS INFUSION
  - ▸ Child 2 months-17 years (body-weight 5-9 kg): Initially 300 mg once weekly for 2 weeks, followed by 300 mg every 3 weeks
  - ▸ Child 2 months-17 years (body-weight 10-19 kg): Initially 600 mg once weekly for 1 week, then reduced to 300 mg once weekly for 1 week, followed by 300 mg every 2 weeks
  - ▸ Child 2 months-17 years (body-weight 20-29 kg): Initially 600 mg once weekly for 3 weeks, followed by 600 mg every 2 weeks
  - ▸ Child 2 months-17 years (body-weight 30-39 kg): Initially 600 mg once weekly for 2 weeks, then increased to 900 mg once weekly for 1 week, followed by 900 mg every 2 weeks
  - ▸ Child 2 months-17 years (body-weight 40 kg and above): Initially 900 mg once weekly for 4 weeks, then increased to 1.2 g once weekly for 1 week, followed by 1.2 g every 2 weeks

- **UNLICENSED USE** Not licensed for use in children for paroxysmal nocturnal haemoglobinuria.

- **CONTRA-INDICATIONS** Patients unvaccinated against *Neisseria meningitidis* · unresolved *Neisseria meningitidis* infection

- **CAUTIONS** Active systemic infection
  CAUTIONS, FURTHER INFORMATION
  - ▸ Meningococcal infection Vaccinate against *Neisseria meningitidis* at least 2 weeks before treatment (tetravalent vaccine against serotypes A, C, W135 and Y recommended); revaccinate according to current medical guidelines. Patients receiving eculizumab less than 2 weeks after receiving meningococcal vaccine must be given prophylactic antibiotics until 2 weeks after vaccination. Advise patient to report promptly any signs of meningococcal infection. Other immunisations should also be up to date.

- **INTERACTIONS** → Appendix 1: monoclonal antibodies

- **SIDE-EFFECTS**
  - ▸ Common or very common Alopecia · arthralgia · blood disorders · cough · dizziness · dysgeusia · dysuria · fatigue · gastro-intestinal disturbances · headache · infection

(including meningococcal infection · influenza-like symptoms · infusion-related reactions · leucopenia · myalgia · nasopharyngitis · oedema paraesthesia · pruritus · rash · spontaneous erection · thrombocytopenia · vertigo
- ▸ Uncommon Anorexia · anxiety · chest pain · depression · epistaxis · gingival pain · Graves' disease · haematoma · hot flushing · hyperhidrosis · hypotension · jaundice · malignant melanoma · menstrual disorders · mood changes · muscle spasms · myelodysplastic syndrome · palpitation · petechiae · renal impairment · skin depigmentation · sleep disturbances · syncope · tinnitus · tremor · visual disturbances

- **CONCEPTION AND CONTRACEPTION** Manufacturer advises effective contraception during and for 5 months after treatment.

- **PREGNANCY** No information available—use only if potential benefit outweighs risk. Human IgG antibodies known to cross placenta.

- **BREAST FEEDING** No information available—manufacturer advises avoid breast-feeding during and for 5 months after treatment.

- **MONITORING REQUIREMENTS**
  - ▸ Monitor for 1 hour after infusion
  - ▸ For *paroxysmal nocturnal haemoglobinuria*, monitor for intravascular haemolysis (including serum-lactate dehydrogenase concentration) during treatment and for at least 8 weeks after discontinuation.
  - ▸ For *atypical haemolytic uraemic syndrome*, monitor for thrombotic microangiopathy (measure platelet count, serum-lactate dehydrogenase concentration, and serum creatinine) during treatment and for at least 12 weeks after discontinuation.

- **DIRECTIONS FOR ADMINISTRATION** Dilute requisite dose to a concentration of 5 mg/mL with Glucose 5% or Sodium Chloride 0.9% and mix gently; give over 25–45 minutes. If infusion-related reactions occur, infusion time may be increased to 4 hours in child under 12 years or 2 hours in child over 12 years.

- **PRESCRIBING AND DISPENSING INFORMATION** Consult product literature for details of supplemental doses with concomitant plasmapheresis, plasma exchange, or plasma infusion.

- **PATIENT AND CARER ADVICE** A patient information card should be provided.
  Patient or carers should be advised to report promptly any signs of meningococcal infection.

- **MEDICINAL FORMS**
  There can be variation in the licensing of different medicines containing the same drug.
  Solution for infusion
  ELECTROLYTES: May contain Sodium
  - ▸ Soliris (Alexion Pharma UK Ltd)
  Eculizumab 10 mg per 1 ml Soliris 300mg/30ml concentrate for solution for infusion vials | 1 vial [PoM] £3,150.00 (Hospital only)

1.2 Iron deficiency anaemia

Anaemia, iron deficiency

Treatment and prophylaxis

Treatment with an iron preparation is justified only in the presence of a demonstrable iron-deficiency state. Before starting treatment, it is important to exclude any serious underlying cause of the anaemia (e.g. gastro-intestinal bleeding). The possibility of thalassaemia should be considered in children of Mediterranean or Indian subcontinent descent.

Prophylaxis with an iron preparation may be appropriate in those with a poor diet, malabsorption, menorrhagia, pregnancy, in haemodialysis patients, and in the management of low birth-weight infants such as preterm neonates.

Oral iron
Iron salts should be given by mouth unless there are good reasons for using another route.

Ferrous salts show only marginal differences between one another in efficiency of absorption of iron. Haemoglobin regeneration rate is little affected by the type of salt used provided sufficient iron is given, and in most patients the speed of response is not critical. Choice of preparation is thus usually decided by formulation, palatability, incidence of side-effects, and cost.

Treatment of iron-deficiency anaemia
The oral dose of elemental iron to treat deficiency is 3–6 mg/kg (max. 200 mg) daily given in 2–3 divided doses. Iron supplementation may also be required to produce an optimum response to erythropoietins in iron-deficient children with chronic renal failure or in preterm neonates.

When prescribing, express the dose in terms of elemental iron and iron salt and select the most appropriate preparation; specify both the iron salt and formulation on the prescription. The iron content of artificial formula feeds should also be considered.

Iron content of different iron salts

Iron salt/amount	Content of ferrous iron
ferrous fumarate 200 mg	65 mg
ferrous gluconate 300 mg	35 mg
ferrous sulfate 300 mg	60 mg
ferrous sulfate, dried 200 mg	65 mg
sodium feredetate 190 mg	27.5 mg

Prophylaxis of iron deficiency
In neonates, haemoglobin and haematocrit concentrations change rapidly. These changes are not due to iron deficiency and cannot be corrected by iron supplementation. Similarly, neonatal anaemia resulting from repeated blood sampling does not respond to iron therapy.

All babies, including preterm neonates, are born with substantial iron stores but these stores can become depleted unless dietary intake is adequate. All babies require an iron intake of 400–700 nanograms daily to maintain body stores. Iron in breast milk is well absorbed but that in artificial feeds or in cow's milk is less so. Most artificial formula feeds are sufficiently fortified with iron to prevent deficiency and their iron content should be taken into account when considering further iron supplementation.

Prophylactic iron supplementation may be required in babies of low birth-weight who are solely breast-fed; supplementation is started 4–6 weeks after birth and continued until mixed feeding is established.

Infants with a poor diet may become anaemic in the second year of life, particularly if cow's milk, rather than fortified formula feed, is a major part of the diet.

Compound preparations
Some oral preparations contain ascorbic acid p. 602 to aid absorption of the iron, but the therapeutic advantage of such preparations is minimal and cost may be increased.

There is no justification for the inclusion of other ingredients, such as the **B group of vitamins**, except folic acid p. 546 for pregnant women.

Parenteral iron
Iron can be administered parenterally as iron dextran p. 542, iron sucrose p. 542 or ferric carboxymaltose p. 542. Parenteral iron is generally reserved for use when oral therapy is unsuccessful because the child cannot tolerate oral iron, or does not take it reliably, or if there is continuing blood loss, or in malabsorption.

Many children with chronic renal failure who are receiving haemodialysis (and some who are receiving peritoneal dialysis) also require iron by the intravenous route on a regular basis.

With the exception of children with severe renal failure receiving haemodialysis, parenteral iron does not produce a faster haemoglobin response than oral iron provided that the oral iron preparation is taken reliably and is absorbed adequately. If parenteral iron is necessary, the dose should be calculated according to the child's body-weight and total iron deficit. Depending on the preparation used, parenteral iron is given as a total dose or in divided doses. Further treatment should be guided by monitoring haemoglobin and serum iron concentrations.

MINERALS AND TRACE ELEMENTS ⟩
IRON, INJECTABLE

Iron (injectable)

IMPORTANT SAFETY INFORMATION
MHRA/CHM ADVICE: SERIOUS HYPERSENSITIVITY REACTIONS WITH INTRAVENOUS IRON (AUGUST 2013)
Serious hypersensitivity reactions, including life-threatening and fatal anaphylactic reactions, have been reported in patients receiving intravenous iron. These reactions can occur even when a previous administration has been tolerated (including a negative test dose). Test doses are no longer recommended and caution is needed with every dose of intravenous iron.

Intravenous iron products should only be administered when appropriately trained staff and resuscitation facilities are immediately available; patients should be closely monitored for signs of hypersensitivity during and for at least 30 minutes after every administration. In the event of a hypersensitivity reaction, treatment should be stopped immediately and appropriate management initiated.

The risk of hypersensitivity is increased in patients with known allergies, immune or inflammatory conditions, or those with a history of severe asthma, eczema, or other atopic allergy; in these patients, intravenous iron should only be used if the benefits outweigh the risks.

Intravenous iron should be avoided in the first trimester of pregnancy and used in the second or third trimesters only if the benefit outweighs the potential risks for both mother and fetus.

● **SIDE-EFFECTS** Hypersensitivity reactions
SIDE-EFFECTS, FURTHER INFORMATION
▸ Anaphylactic reactions Anaphylactic reactions can occur with parenteral administration of iron complexes and facilities for cardiopulmonary resuscitation must be available. If children complain of acute symptoms particularly nausea, back pain, breathlessness, or develop hypotension, the infusion should be stopped.

Overdose
For details on the management of poisoning, see Iron salts, under Emergency treatment of poisoning p. 803.

Blood and nutrition

9

Ferric carboxymaltose

▶ 541

- **INDICATIONS AND DOSE**

Iron-deficiency anaemia
- ▶ BY SLOW INTRAVENOUS INJECTION, OR BY INTRAVENOUS INFUSION
- ▸ Child: Dose calculated according to body-weight and iron deficit (consult product literature)

- **UNLICENSED USE** Not licensed for use in children under 14 years.
- **CAUTIONS** Allergic disorders · asthma · eczema · hypersensitivity can occur with parenteral iron and facilities for cardiopulmonary resuscitation must be available · infection (discontinue if ongoing bacteraemia) · oral iron should not be given until 5 days after last injection
- **INTERACTIONS** → Appendix 1: iron (injectable)
- **SIDE-EFFECTS**
- ▸ **Common or very common** Dizziness · gastro-intestinal disturbances · headache · injection-site reactions · rash
- ▸ **Uncommon** Anaphylaxis · arthralgia · back pain · chest pain · fatigue · flushing · hypertension · hypotension · malaise · myalgia · paraesthesia · peripheral oedema · pruritus · pyrexia · rigors · urticaria
- ▸ **Rare** Dyspnoea
- **PREGNANCY** Avoid in first trimester; crosses the placenta in *animal* studies. May influence skeletal development.
- **HEPATIC IMPAIRMENT** Use with caution. Avoid in conditions where iron overload increases risk of impairment.
- **PRESCRIBING AND DISPENSING INFORMATION** A ferric carboxymaltose complex containing 5% (50 mg/mL) of iron.

- **MEDICINAL FORMS**
There can be variation in the licensing of different medicines containing the same drug.
Solution for injection
ELECTROLYTES: May contain Sodium
- ▸ **Ferinject** (Vifor Pharma UK Ltd) ▼
Iron (as Ferric carboxymaltose) 50 mg per 1 ml Ferinject 1000mg/20ml solution for injection vials | 1 vial PoM £154.23
Ferinject 100mg/2ml solution for injection vials | 5 vial PoM £81.18
Ferinject 500mg/10ml solution for injection vials | 5 vial PoM £405.88

Iron dextran

▶ 541

- **INDICATIONS AND DOSE**

Iron-deficiency anaemia
- ▶ BY DEEP INTRAMUSCULAR INJECTION
- ▸ Child 14–17 years: Intramuscular injection to be administered into the gluteal muscle, doses calculated according to body-weight and iron deficit (consult product literature)
- ▶ BY SLOW INTRAVENOUS INJECTION, OR BY INTRAVENOUS INFUSION
- ▸ Child: Doses calculated according to body-weight and iron deficit (consult product literature)

- **UNLICENSED USE** Not licensed for use in children under 14 years.
- **CONTRA-INDICATIONS** Active rheumatoid arthritis · asthma · eczema · history of allergic disorders · infection
- **CAUTIONS** Hypersensitivity can occur with parenteral iron and facilities for cardiopulmonary resuscitation must be available · oral iron should not be given until 5 days after last injection
- **INTERACTIONS** → Appendix 1: iron (injectable)

- **SIDE-EFFECTS**
- ▸ **Uncommon** Abdominal pain · anaphylaxis · blurred vision · cramps · dyspnoea · flushing · nausea · numbness · pruritus · rash · vomiting
- ▸ **Rare** Angioedema · arrhythmias · arthralgia · chest pain · diarrhoea · dizziness · fatigue · hypotension · impaired consciousness · injection-site reactions · myalgia · restlessness · seizures · sweating · tachycardia · tremor
- ▸ **Very rare** Haemolysis · headache · hypertension · palpitation · paraesthesia · transient deafness
- **PREGNANCY** Avoid in first trimester.
- **HEPATIC IMPAIRMENT** Avoid in severe impairment.
- **RENAL IMPAIRMENT** Avoid in acute renal failure.
- **PRESCRIBING AND DISPENSING INFORMATION** A complex of ferric hydroxide with dextran containing 5% (50 mg/mL) of iron.

- **MEDICINAL FORMS**
There can be variation in the licensing of different medicines containing the same drug.
Solution for injection
- ▸ **CosmoFer** (Pharmacosmos UK Ltd) ▼
Iron (as Iron dextran) 50 mg per 1 ml CosmoFer 500mg/10ml solution for injection ampoules | 2 ampoule PoM £79.70
CosmoFer 100mg/2ml solution for injection ampoules | 5 ampoule PoM £39.85

Iron sucrose

▶ 541

- **INDICATIONS AND DOSE**

Iron-deficiency anaemia
- ▶ BY SLOW INTRAVENOUS INJECTION, OR BY INTRAVENOUS INFUSION
- ▸ Child (body-weight up to 67 kg): Dose calculated according to body-weight and iron deficit, each divided dose should not exceed 3 mg/kg/dose (consult product literature)
- ▸ Child (body-weight 67 kg and above): Dose calculated according to body-weight and iron deficit, each divided dose should not exceed max. 200 mg/dose (consult product literature)

- **UNLICENSED USE** Not licensed for use in children.
- **CONTRA-INDICATIONS** Anaphylaxis · asthma · eczema · history of allergic disorders
- **CAUTIONS** Hypersensitivity reactions can occur with parenteral iron and facilities for cardiopulmonary resuscitation must be available · infection (discontinue if ongoing bacteraemia · oral iron should not be given until 5 days after last injection
- **INTERACTIONS** → Appendix 1: iron (injectable)
- **SIDE-EFFECTS**
- ▸ **Common or very common** Taste disturbances
- ▸ **Uncommon** Abdominal pain · bronchospasm · chest pain · diarrhoea · dizziness · dyspnoea · fever · flushing · headache · hypotension · injection-site reactions · myalgia · nausea · palpitation · pruritus · rash · tachycardia · vomiting
- ▸ **Rare** Anaphylaxis · asthenia · fatigue · hypertension · paraesthesia · peripheral oedema
- ▸ **Frequency not known** Arthralgia · bradycardia · confusion · increased sweating
- **PREGNANCY** Avoid in first trimester.
- **HEPATIC IMPAIRMENT** Use with caution. Avoid in conditions where iron overload increases risk of impairment.
- **PRESCRIBING AND DISPENSING INFORMATION** A complex of ferric hydroxide with sucrose containing 2% (20 mg/mL) of iron.

- **MEDICINAL FORMS**
There can be variation in the licensing of different medicines containing the same drug.

Solution for injection
- Venofer (Vifor Pharma UK Ltd, Imported (United States)) ▼
  Iron (as Iron sucrose) 20 mg per 1 ml Venofer 100mg/5ml solution for injection vials | 5 vial PoM £43.52
  Venofer 50mg/2.5ml solution for injection vials | 5 vial PoM no price available

MINERALS AND TRACE ELEMENTS > IRON >
IRON, ORAL

Iron (oral) 🔘

- **SIDE-EFFECTS** Constipation · diarrhoea · epigastric pain (dose related) · faecal impaction · gastro-intestinal irritation · nausea (dose related)

  SIDE-EFFECTS, FURTHER INFORMATION
- **Managing side-effects** If side-effects occur, the dose may be reduced; alternatively, another iron salt may be used, but an improvement in tolerance may simply be a result of a lower content of elemental iron. The incidence of side-effects due to ferrous sulfate is no greater than with other iron salts when compared on the basis of equivalent amounts of elemental iron.
- **Altered bowel habit** Iron preparations taken orally can be constipating and occasionally lead to faecal impaction.

  Oral iron, particularly modified-release preparations, can exacerbate diarrhoea in patients with inflammatory bowel disease; care is also needed in patients with intestinal strictures and diverticular disease.

  The relationship between dose and altered bowel habit (constipation or diarrhoea) is less clear than for nausea and epigastric pain.

  Overdose
  For details on the management of poisoning, see Iron salts, under Emergency treatment of poisoning p. 803.

  Iron preparations are an important cause of accidental overdose in children and as little as 20 mg/kg of elemental iron can lead to symptoms of toxicity.

- **MONITORING REQUIREMENTS**
- **Therapeutic response** The haemoglobin concentration should rise by about 100–200 mg/100 mL (1–2 g/litre) per day *or* 2 g/100 mL (20 g/litre) over 3–4 weeks. When the haemoglobin is in the normal range, treatment should be continued for a further 3 months to replenish the iron stores. Epithelial tissue changes such as atrophic glossitis and koilonychia are usually improved, but the response is often slow.

- **PRESCRIBING AND DISPENSING INFORMATION** Express the dose in terms of elemental iron and iron salt and select the most appropriate preparation; specify both the iron salt and formulation on the prescription.

  The iron content of artificial formula feeds should also be considered.

  The most common reason for lack of response in children is poor compliance; poor absorption is rare in children.

- **PATIENT AND CARER ADVICE** Although iron preparations are best absorbed on an empty stomach they can be taken after food to reduce gastro-intestinal side-effects. May discolour stools.

▶ above

Ferrous fumarate

- **INDICATIONS AND DOSE**
Iron-deficiency anaemia (prophylactic)
- BY MOUTH USING TABLETS
- Child 12–17 years: 210 mg 1–2 times a day

- BY MOUTH USING SYRUP
- Child 12–17 years: 140 mg twice daily

Iron-deficiency anaemia (therapeutic)
- BY MOUTH USING TABLETS
- Child 12–17 years: 210 mg 2–3 times a day
- BY MOUTH USING SYRUP
- Child 12–17 years: 280 mg twice daily

FERSADAY®
Iron-deficiency anaemia (prophylactic)
- BY MOUTH
- Child 12–17 years: 322 mg daily

Iron-deficiency anaemia (therapeutic)
- BY MOUTH
- Child 12–17 years: 322 mg twice daily

GALFER® CAPSULES
Iron-deficiency anaemia (prophylactic)
- BY MOUTH
- Child 12–17 years: 305 mg daily

Iron-deficiency anaemia (therapeutic)
- BY MOUTH
- Child 12–17 years: 305 mg twice daily

GALFER® SYRUP
Iron-deficiency anaemia (prophylaxis)
- BY MOUTH

- Neonate up to 36 weeks corrected gestational age (body-weight up to 3 kg): 0.5 mL daily, prophylactic iron supplementation may be required in babies of low birth-weight who are solely breast-fed; supplementation is started 4–6 weeks after birth and continued until mixed feeding is established.

- Neonate: 0.25 mL/kilogram twice daily, the total daily dose may alternatively be given in 3 divided doses, prophylactic iron supplementation may be required in babies of low birth-weight who are solely breast-fed; supplementation is started 4–6 weeks after birth and continued until mixed feeding is established.

- Child 1 month–11 years: 0.25 mL/kilogram twice daily, the total daily dose may alternatively be given in 3 divided doses, prophylactic iron supplementation may be required in babies of low birth-weight who are solely breast-fed; supplementation is started 4–6 weeks after birth and continued until mixed feeding is established; maximum 20 mL per day
- Child 12–17 years: 10 mL once daily

Iron-deficiency anaemia (therapeutic)
- BY MOUTH
- Neonate: 0.25 mL/kilogram twice daily, the total daily dose may alternatively be given in 3 divided doses.

- Child 1 month–11 years: 0.25 mL/kilogram twice daily, the total daily dose may alternatively be given in 3 divided doses; maximum 20 mL per day
- Child 12–17 years: 10 mL 1–2 times a day

- **INTERACTIONS** → Appendix 1: iron (oral)

- **PRESCRIBING AND DISPENSING INFORMATION** Non-proprietary ferrous fumarate tablets may contain 210 mg (68 mg iron), syrup may contain approx. 140 mg (45 mg iron)/5 mL; *Galfer*® capsules contain ferrous fumarate 305 mg (100 mg iron); *Fersaday*® tablets contain ferrous fumarate 322 mg (100 mg iron).

- **PATIENT AND CARER ADVICE**
Medicines for Children leaflet: Ferrous fumarate for iron-deficiency anaemia www.medicinesforchildren.org.uk/ferrous-fumarate-for-iron-deficiency-anaemia

9

Blood and nutrition

- MEDICINAL FORMS
There can be variation in the licensing of different medicines containing the same drug.

Oral solution
- Ferrous fumarate (Non-proprietary)
Ferrous fumarate 28 mg per 1 ml Ferrous fumarate 140mg/5ml oral solution | 200 ml P £3.73 DT price = £3.73
- Galfer (Thornton & Ross Ltd)
Ferrous fumarate 28 mg per 1 ml Galfer 140mg/5ml syrup sugar-free | 300 ml P £5.33 DT price = £5.33

Tablet
- Ferrous fumarate (Non-proprietary)
Ferrous fumarate 210 mg Ferrous fumarate 210mg tablets | 84 tablet P £3.50 DT price = £3.50 | 84 tablet no price available DT price = £3.50
Ferrous fumarate 322 mg Ferrous fumarate 322mg tablets | 28 tablet P £1.00 DT price = £1.00

Capsule
- Galfer (Thornton & Ross Ltd)
Ferrous fumarate 305 mg Galfer 305mg capsules | 100 capsule P £2.33 DT price = £2.33 | 250 capsule P £5.00

F 543

Ferrous gluconate

- INDICATIONS AND DOSE

Prophylaxis of iron-deficiency anaemia
▶ BY MOUTH USING TABLETS
- Child 6–11 years: 300–900 mg daily
- Child 12–17 years: 600 mg daily

Treatment of iron-deficiency anaemia
▶ BY MOUTH USING TABLETS
- Child 6–11 years: 300–900 mg daily
- Child 12–17 years: 1.2–1.8 g daily in divided doses

- INTERACTIONS → Appendix 1: iron (oral)
- PRESCRIBING AND DISPENSING INFORMATION Ferrous gluconate 300 mg contains 35 mg iron.
- PATIENT AND CARER ADVICE
Medicines for Children leaflet: Ferrous gluconate for iron-deficiency anaemia www.medicinesforchildren.org.uk/ferrous-gluconate-for-iron-deficiency-anaemia

- MEDICINAL FORMS
There can be variation in the licensing of different medicines containing the same drug.

Tablet
- Ferrous gluconate (Non-proprietary)
Ferrous gluconate 300 mg Ferrous gluconate 300mg tablets | 28 tablet P £3.35 DT price = £1.95 | 1000 tablet P £119.64

F 543

Ferrous sulfate

- INDICATIONS AND DOSE

Iron-deficiency anaemia (prophylactic)
▶ BY MOUTH USING TABLETS
- Child 6–17 years: 200 mg daily

Iron-deficiency anaemia (therapeutic)
▶ BY MOUTH USING TABLETS
- Child 6–17 years: 200 mg 2–3 times a day

FEOSPAN®

Iron-deficiency anaemia
▶ BY MOUTH
- Child 1–17 years: 1 capsule daily, capsule can be opened and sprinkled on food

FERROGRAD®

Iron-deficiency anaemia (prophylactic and therapeutic)
▶ BY MOUTH
- Child 12–17 years: 1 tablet daily

IRONORM® DROPS

Iron-deficiency anaemia (prophylactic)
▶ BY MOUTH
- Child 1 month–5 years: 0.2 mL daily until mixed feeding established, higher doses up to max. 0.08 mL/kg daily may be needed, then 0.5–1.2 mL daily
- Child 6–11 years: 2.4 mL daily
- Child 12–17 years: 2.4–4.8 mL daily

Iron-deficiency anaemia (therapeutic)
▶ BY MOUTH
- Child 1 month–5 years: 0.12–0.24 mL/kilogram daily in 2–3 divided doses (max. per dose 8 mL)
- Child 6–11 years: 0.12–0.24 mL/kilogram daily in 2–3 divided doses (max. per dose 8 mL)
- Child 12–17 years: 4 mL 1–2 times a day

- INTERACTIONS → Appendix 1: iron (oral)
- PRESCRIBING AND DISPENSING INFORMATION
Iron content Ferrous sulfate 200 mg is equivalent to 65 mg iron; *Ironorm*® drops contain ferrous sulfate 125 mg (equivalent to 25 mg iron)/mL; *Feospan*® spansules contains ferrous sulfate 150 mg (47 mg iron) (spansule (= capsules m/r)); *Ferrograd*® tablets contain ferrous sulfate 325 mg (105 mg iron).
- PATIENT AND CARER ADVICE
Medicines for Children leaflet: Ferrous sulfate for iron-deficiency anaemia www.medicinesforchildren.org.uk/ferrous-sulfate-iron-deficiency-anaemia
- NATIONAL FUNDING/ACCESS DECISIONS
NHS restrictions *Feospan*® is not prescribable under the National Health Service.
- LESS SUITABLE FOR PRESCRIBING *Feospan*® is less suitable for prescribing. *Ferrograd*® is less suitable for prescribing.

- MEDICINAL FORMS
There can be variation in the licensing of different medicines containing the same drug.

Modified-release tablet
CAUTIONARY AND ADVISORY LABELS 25
- Ferrograd (Teofarma)
Ferrous sulfate dried 325 mg Ferrograd 325mg modified-release tablets | 30 tablet P £2.58 DT price = £2.58

Tablet
- Ferrous sulfate (Non-proprietary)
Ferrous sulfate dried 200 mg Ferrous sulfate 200mg tablets | 28 tablet P £8.15 DT price = £1.84 | 60 tablet P £1.78 | 100 tablet P £10.80 | 1000 tablet P £108.00

Modified-release capsule
CAUTIONARY AND ADVISORY LABELS 25
- Feospan Spansules (Intrapharm Laboratories Ltd)
Ferrous sulfate dried 150 mg Feospan 150mg Spansules | 30 capsule P £3.95

Oral drops
- Ironorm (Wallace Manufacturing Chemists Ltd)
Ferrous sulfate 125 mg per 1 ml Ironorm 125mg/ml oral drops sugar-free | 15 ml P £30.00

Ferrous sulfate with folic acid

The properties listed below are those particular to the combination only. For the properties of the components please consider, ferrous sulfate above, folic acid p. 546.

- INDICATIONS AND DOSE

Iron-deficiency anaemia
▶ BY MOUTH USING MODIFIED-RELEASE TABLETS
- Child 12–17 years: 1 tablet daily, to be taken before food

- INTERACTIONS → Appendix 1: folates, iron (oral)
- LESS SUITABLE FOR PRESCRIBING *Ferrograd Folic*® is less suitable for prescribing.

● **MEDICINAL FORMS**
There can be variation in the licensing of different medicines containing the same drug.

Modified-release tablet
CAUTIONARY AND ADVISORY LABELS 25
▸ Ferrograd Folic (Teofarma)
Folic acid 350 microgram, Ferrous sulfate dried
325 mg Ferrograd Folic 325mg/350microgram modified-release tablets | 30 tablet P £2.64 DT price = £2.64

F 543

Polysaccharide-iron complex

● **INDICATIONS AND DOSE**
Iron-deficiency anaemia (prophylactic)
▸ BY MOUTH

▸ Neonate: 1 drop (approximately 500 micrograms iron) per 450 g body-weight to be given 3 times a daily, dose to be administered from dropper bottle, prophylactic iron supplementation may be required in babies of low birth-weight who are solely breast-fed; supplementation is started 4–6 weeks after birth and continued until mixed feeding is established.

▸ Child 1 month-1 year: 1 drop (approximately 500 micrograms iron) per 450 g body-weight to be to be given 3 times a daily, dose to be administered from dropper bottle, prophylactic iron supplementation may be required in babies of low birth-weight who are solely breast-fed; supplementation is started 4–6 weeks after birth and continued until mixed feeding is established
▸ Child 12–17 years: 2.5 mL daily

Iron-deficiency anaemia (therapeutic)
▸ BY MOUTH
▸ Child 2–5 years: 2.5 mL daily
▸ Child 6–11 years: 5 mL daily
▸ Child 12–17 years: 5 mL 1–2 times a day

Iron-deficiency anaemia (therapeutic) if required during second and third trimester of pregnancy
▸ BY MOUTH
▸ Child 12–17 years: 5 mL once daily

● **INTERACTIONS** → Appendix 1: iron (oral)
● **PATIENT AND CARER ADVICE** Counselling on the use of the dropper advised.
● **NATIONAL FUNDING/ACCESS DECISIONS**
NHS restrictions *Niferex* is not available on prescription under NHS, except 30-mL paediatric dropper bottle for prophylaxis and treatment of iron deficiency in infants born prematurely; endorse prescription 'SLS'.

● **MEDICINAL FORMS**
There can be variation in the licensing of different medicines containing the same drug.

Oral solution
▸ Niferex (Tillomed Laboratories Ltd)
Iron (as Polysaccharide-iron complex) 100 mg Niferex 100mg/5ml elixir sugar-free | 30 mL P £2.16 sugar-free | 240 ml P £6.06

F 543

Sodium feredetate

(Sodium ironedetate)

● **INDICATIONS AND DOSE**
Iron-deficiency anaemia (therapeutic)
▸ BY MOUTH USING ORAL SOLUTION
▸ Neonate: Up to 2.5 mL twice daily, smaller doses to be used initially.

▸ Child 1–11 months: Up to 2.5 mL twice daily, smaller doses to be used initially
▸ Child 1–4 years: 2.5 mL 3 times a day

▸ Child 5–11 years: 5 mL 3 times a day
▸ Child 12–17 years: 5 mL 3 times a day, increased to 10 mL 3 times a day, dose to be increased gradually

Iron-deficiency anaemia (prophylactic)
▸ BY MOUTH USING ORAL SOLUTION

▸ Neonate: 1 mL daily, prophylactic iron supplementation may be required in babies of low birth-weight who are solely breast-fed; supplementation is started 4–6 weeks after birth and continued until mixed feeding is established

▸ Child 1–11 months: 1 mL daily, prophylactic iron supplementation may be required in babies of low birth-weight who are solely breast-fed; supplementation is started 4–6 weeks after birth and continued until mixed feeding is established

● **UNLICENSED USE** Not licensed for prophylaxis of iron deficiency.
● **INTERACTIONS** → Appendix 1: iron (oral)
● **PRESCRIBING AND DISPENSING INFORMATION** *Sytron* contains 190 mg sodium feredetate, which is equivalent to 27.5 mg of iron/5 mL.
● **PATIENT AND CARER ADVICE**
Medicines for Children leaflet: Sytron (sodium feredetate) for the prevention of anaemia www.medicinesforchildren.org.uk/sytron-sodium-feredetate-for-prevention-of-anaemia
Medicines for Children leaflet: Sytron (sodium feredetate) for the treatment of anaemia www.medicinesforchildren.org.uk/sytron-sodium-feredetate-for-treatment-of-anaemia

● **MEDICINAL FORMS**
There can be variation in the licensing of different medicines containing the same drug.

Oral solution
▸ Sodium feredetate (Non-proprietary)
Sodium feredetate 38 mg per 1 ml Sodium feredetate 190mg/5ml oral solution sugar free sugar-free | 500 ml PoM £14.95 DT price = £14.95
▸ Sytron (Forum Health Products Ltd)
Sodium feredetate 38 mg per 1 ml Sytron oral solution sugar-free | 500 ml P £14.95 DT price = £14.95

1.3 Megaloblastic anaemia

Anaemia, megaloblastic

Overview

Megaloblastic anaemias are rare in children; they may result from a lack of either vitamin B_{12} or folate and it is essential to establish in every case which deficiency is present and the underlying cause. In emergencies, when delay might be dangerous, it is sometimes necessary to administer both substances after the bone marrow test while plasma assay results are awaited. Normally, however, appropriate treatment should not be instituted until the results of tests are available.

Vitamin B_{12} is used in the treatment of megaloblastosis caused by *prolonged nitrous oxide anaesthesia*, which inactivates the vitamin, and in the rare disorders of *congenital transcobalamin II deficiency* and *homocystinuria*.

Vitamin B_{12} should be given prophylactically after *total ileal resection*.

Apart from dietary deficiency, all other causes of vitamin B_{12} deficiency are attributable to malabsorption. There is little place for the use of low-dose vitamin B_{12} orally and none for vitamin B_{12} intrinsic factor complexes given by mouth. Vitamin B_{12} in large oral doses [unlicensed] may be effective.

Hydroxocobalamin p. 547 has completely replaced

cyanocobalamin p. 547 as the form of vitamin B_{12} of choice for therapy; it is retained in the body longer than cyanocobalamin and thus for maintenance therapy can be given at intervals of up to 3 months. Treatment is generally initiated with frequent administration of intramuscular injections to replenish the depleted body stores. Thereafter, maintenance treatment, which is usually for life, can be instituted. There is no evidence that doses larger than those recommended provide any additional benefit in vitamin B^{12} neuropathy.

Folic acid below has few indications for long-term therapy since most causes of folate deficiency are self-limiting or will yield to a short course of treatment. It should not be used in undiagnosed megaloblastic anaemia unless vitamin B_{12} is administered concurrently otherwise neuropathy may be precipitated.

In *folate-deficient megaloblastic anaemia* (e.g. because of poor nutrition, pregnancy, or antiepileptic drugs), daily folic acid supplementation for 4 months brings about haematological remission and replenishes body stores; higher doses may be necessary in malabsorption states. In pregnancy, folic acid daily is continued to term.

For prophylaxis in *chronic haemolytic states, malabsorption,* or *in renal dialysis*, folic acid is given daily or sometimes weekly, depending on the diet and the rate of haemolysis.

Folic acid is also used for the prevention of methotrexate-induced side-effects in juvenile idiopathic arthritis, severe Crohn's disease and severe psoriasis.

Folic acid is actively excreted in breast milk and is well absorbed by the infant. It is also present in cow's milk and artificial formula feeds but is heat labile. Serum and red cell folate concentrations fall after delivery and urinary losses are high, particularly in low birth-weight neonates. Although symptomatic deficiency is rare in the absence of malabsorption or prolonged diarrhoea, it is common for neonatal units to give supplements of folic acid to all preterm neonates from 2 weeks of age until full-term corrected age is reached, particularly if heated breast milk is used without an artificial formula fortifier.

Folinic acid p. 528 is also effective in the treatment of folate deficient megaloblastic anaemia but it is normally only used in association with cytotoxic drugs; it is given as calcium folinate.

There is **no** justification for prescribing multiple ingredient vitamin preparations containing vitamin B_{12} or folic acid.

For the use of folic acid before and during pregnancy, see Neural tube defects (prevention in pregnancy) p. 610.

VITAMINS AND TRACE ELEMENTS > FOLATES

▌ Folic acid

09-Jun-2016

● **INDICATIONS AND DOSE**

Folate-deficient megaloblastic anaemia
▸ BY MOUTH
▸ Neonate: Initially 500 micrograms/kg once daily for up to 4 months.

▸ Child 1–11 months: Initially 500 micrograms/kg once daily (max. per dose 5 mg) for up to 4 months, doses up to 10 mg daily may be required in malabsorption states
▸ Child 1–17 years: 5 mg daily for 4 months (until term in pregnant women), doses up to 15 mg daily may be required in malabsorption states

Folate supplementation in neonates
▸ BY MOUTH
▸ Neonate: 50 micrograms once daily.

Prevention of neural tube defects (in those at a low risk of conceiving a child with a neural tube defect see p. 610)
▸ BY MOUTH
▸ Females of childbearing potential: 400 micrograms daily, to be taken before conception and until week 12 of pregnancy

Prevention of neural tube defects (in those in the high-risk group who wish to become pregnant or who are at risk of becoming pregnant see p. 610)
▸ BY MOUTH
▸ Females of childbearing potential: 5 mg daily, to be taken before conception and until week 12 of pregnancy

Prevention of neural tube defects (in those with sickle-cell disease)
▸ BY MOUTH
▸ Females of childbearing potential: 5 mg daily, patient should continue taking their normal dose of folic acid 5 mg daily (or increase the dose to 5 mg daily) before conception and continue this throughout pregnancy

Prevention of methotrexate side-effects in severe Crohn's disease | Prevention of methotrexate side-effects in severe psoriasis
▸ BY MOUTH
▸ Child: 5 mg once weekly, dose to be taken on a different day to methotrexate dose

Prophylaxis of folate deficiency in dialysis
▸ BY MOUTH
▸ Child 1 month–11 years: 250 micrograms/kg once daily (max. per dose 10 mg)
▸ Child 12–17 years: 5–10 mg once daily

Haemolytic anaemia | Metabolic disorders
▸ BY MOUTH
▸ Child 1 month–11 years: 2.5–5 mg once daily
▸ Child 12–17 years: 5–10 mg once daily

Prevention of methotrexate side-effects in juvenile idiopathic arthritis
▸ BY MOUTH
▸ Child: 1 mg daily, alternatively 5 mg once weekly, dose to be adjusted according to local guidelines, weekly dose to be taken on a different day to methotrexate dose

● **UNLICENSED USE** Unlicensed for limiting methotrexate toxicity.

● **CAUTIONS** Should never be given alone for pernicious anaemia (may precipitate subacute combined degeneration of the spinal cord)

● **INTERACTIONS** → Appendix 1: folates

● **SIDE-EFFECTS**
▸ Rare Gastro-intestinal disturbances

● **PATIENT AND CARER ADVICE**
Medicines for Children leaflet: Folic acid for megaloblastic anaemia caused by folate deficiency and haemolytic anaemia www.medicinesforchildren.org.uk/folic-acid-megaloblastic-anaemia-caused-folate-deficiency-and-haemolytic-anaemia

● **EXCEPTIONS TO LEGAL CATEGORY** Can be sold to the public provided daily doses do not exceed 500 micrograms.

● **MEDICINAL FORMS**
There can be variation in the licensing of different medicines containing the same drug. Forms available from special-order manufacturers include: capsule, oral suspension, oral solution

Tablet
▸ Folic acid (Non-proprietary)
Folic acid 400 microgram Folic acid 400microgram tablets | 90 tablet [PoM] no price available DT price = £2.71
Folic acid 5 mg Folic acid 5mg tablets | 28 tablet [PoM] £1.17 DT price = £0.90 | 1000 tablet [PoM] £32.14

Oral solution
▸ Folic acid (Non-proprietary)
  Folic acid 500 microgram per 1 ml Folic acid 2.5mg/5ml oral
  solution sugar free sugar-free | 150 ml [PoM] £9.16 DT price = £9.16
  sugar-free | 150 ml £9.16 DT price = £9.16
  Folic acid 1 mg per 1 ml Folic acid 5mg/5ml oral solution sugar free
  sugar-free | 150 ml [PoM] £13.74
▸ Lexpec (Rosemont Pharmaceuticals Ltd)
  Folic acid 500 microgram per 1 ml Lexpec Folic Acid 2.5mg/5ml
  oral solution sugar-free | 150 ml [PoM] £9.16 DT price = £9.16

VITAMINS AND TRACE ELEMENTS › VITAMIN B GROUP

Cyanocobalamin

● **INDICATIONS AND DOSE**

Vitamin B$_{12}$ deficiency of dietary origin
▸ BY MOUTH
▸ **Child:** 50–105 micrograms daily in 1–3 divided doses

● **PRESCRIBING AND DISPENSING INFORMATION** The BP
directs that when vitamin B$_{12}$ injection is prescribed or
demanded hydroxocobalamin injection shall be dispensed
or supplied.
  Currently available brands of the tablet may not be
suitable for vegans.

● **NATIONAL FUNDING/ACCESS DECISIONS**
NHS restrictions *Cyanocobalamin* liquid, *Cytacon*® tablets,
and *Cytamen*® injection are not available on prescription
under the NHS.

● **LESS SUITABLE FOR PRESCRIBING** Cyanocobalamin is less
suitable for prescribing.

● **MEDICINAL FORMS**
There can be variation in the licensing of different medicines
containing the same drug. Forms available from special-order
manufacturers include: tablet

Tablet
▸ Cyanocobalamin (Non-proprietary)
  Cyanocobalamin 50 microgram Cyanocobalamin 50microgram
  tablets | 50 tablet [P] £6.24 DT price = £8.99 | 50 tablet £8.99 DT
  price = £8.99 | 100 tablet no price available
  Cyanocobalamin 100 microgram Vitamin B12 100microgram
  tablets | 100 tablet £3.88
▸ Cytacon (AMCo)
  Cyanocobalamin 50 microgram Cytacon 50microgram tablets |
  50 tablet [P] £8.99 DT price = £8.99

Oral solution
▸ Cyanocobalamin (Non-proprietary)
  Cyanocobalamin 7 microgram per 1 ml Cyanocobalamin
  35micrograms/5ml oral solution | 200 ml [P] £8.75

Hydroxocobalamin

● **INDICATIONS AND DOSE**

Macrocytic anaemia without neurological involvement
▸ BY INTRAMUSCULAR INJECTION
▸ **Child:** Initially 0.25–1 mg 3 times a week for 2 weeks,
  then 0.25 mg once weekly until blood count normal,
  then 1 mg every 3 months

Macrocytic anaemia with neurological involvement
▸ BY INTRAMUSCULAR INJECTION
▸ **Child:** Initially 1 mg once daily on alternate days until
  no further improvement, then 1 mg every 2 months

**Prophylaxis of macrocytic anaemias associated with
vitamin B$_{12}$ deficiency**
▸ BY INTRAMUSCULAR INJECTION
▸ **Child:** 1 mg every 2–3 months

Leber's optic atrophy
▸ BY INTRAMUSCULAR INJECTION
▸ **Child:** Initially 1 mg daily for 2 weeks, then 1 mg twice
  weekly until no further improvement, then 1 mg every
  1–3 months

Congenital transcobalamin II deficiency
▸ BY INTRAMUSCULAR INJECTION
▸ **Neonate:** 1 mg 3 times a week for 1 year, then reduced to
  1 mg once weekly, adjusted as appropriate.
▸ **Child:** 1 mg 3 times a week for 1 year, then reduced to
  1 mg once weekly, adjusted as appropriate

Methylmalonic acidaemia and homocystinuria
▸ BY INTRAMUSCULAR INJECTION
▸ **Child:** Initially 1 mg daily for 5–7 days, then adjusted
  according to response to up to 1 mg 1–2 times a week,
  this is the maintenance dose

**Methylmalonic acidaemia, maintenance once
intramuscular response established**
▸ BY MOUTH
▸ **Child:** 5–10 mg 1–2 times a week, some children do not
  respond to oral route

CYANOKIT®
Poisoning with cyanides
▸ BY INTRAVENOUS INFUSION
▸ **Child (body-weight 5 kg and above):** Initially 70 mg/kg
  (max. per dose 5 g), to be given over 15 minutes, then
  70 mg/kg (max. per dose 5 g) if required, this second
  dose can be given over 15 minutes–2 hours depending
  on severity of poisoning and patient stability

● **UNLICENSED USE**
▸ With intramuscular use or oral use Licensed for use in children
  (age not specified by manufacturers). Not licensed for use
  in inborn errors of metabolism.

● **CAUTIONS**
▸ With intramuscular use or oral use Should not be given before
  diagnosis fully established

● **SIDE-EFFECTS**
GENERAL SIDE-EFFECTS
Dizziness · headache · pruritus

SPECIFIC SIDE-EFFECTS
▸ With intramuscular use Hypokalaemia (during initial
  treatment) · injection-site reactions · rash · thrombocytosis
  (during initial treatment)
▸ With intramuscular use or oral use Chromaturia · fever ·
  hypersensitivity reactions · nausea
▸ With intravenous use Dyspnoea · eye disorders · gastro-
  intestinal disturbances · hot flush · lymphocytopenia ·
  memory impairment · peripheral oedema · pustular rashes ·
  red coloration of urine · restlessness · reversible red
  coloration of skin and mucous membranes · throat
  disorders · transient hypertension

● **BREAST FEEDING** Present in milk but not known to be
harmful.

● **EFFECT ON LABORATORY TESTS**
▸ With intravenous use Deep red colour of hydroxocobalamin
  may interfere with laboratory tests.

● **DIRECTIONS FOR ADMINISTRATION**
▸ With intravenous use For *intravenous infusion (Cyanokit)*®,
  given intermittently *in* Sodium chloride 0.9%, reconstitute
  5 g vial with 200 mL Sodium Chloride 0.9%; gently invert
  vial for at least 1 minute to mix (do not shake).
▸ With oral use For administration by *mouth*, injection
  solution may be given orally; it will not have prolonged
  effect via this route.

9

Blood and nutrition

● **PRESCRIBING AND DISPENSING INFORMATION**
▸ With intramuscular use The BP directs that when vitamin B_{12} injection is prescribed or demanded, hydroxocobalamin injection shall be dispensed or supplied.
Poisoning by cyanides
▸ With intravenous use *Cyanokit*® is the only preparation of hydroxocobalamin that is suitable for use in victims of smoke inhalation who show signs of significant cyanide poisoning.

● **NATIONAL FUNDING/ACCESS DECISIONS**
NHS restrictions *Cobalin-H*® is not prescribable under National Health Service (NHS).
Neo-Cytamen® is not prescribable under National Health Service (NHS).

● **MEDICINAL FORMS**
There can be variation in the licensing of different medicines containing the same drug. Forms available from special-order manufacturers include: oral suspension, oral solution
Solution for injection
▸ Hydroxocobalamin (Non-proprietary)
  Hydroxocobalamin 1 mg per 1 ml Hydroxocobalamin 1mg/1ml solution for injection ampoules | 5 ampoule PoM £12.49 DT price = £7.12
  Hydroxocobalamin 2.5 mg per 1 ml Hepavit 5mg/2ml solution for injection ampoules | 2 ampoule PoM no price available
  Hydroxocobalamin 5 mg per 1 ml Megamilbedoce 10mg/2ml solution for injection ampoules | 10 ampoule PoM no price available
▸ Cobalin (AMCo)
  Hydroxocobalamin 1 mg per 1 ml Cobalin-H 1mg/1ml solution for injection ampoules | 5 ampoule PoM £9.50 DT price = £7.12
▸ Neo-Cytamen (Focus Pharmaceuticals Ltd)
  Hydroxocobalamin 1 mg per 1 ml Neo-Cytamen 1000micrograms/1ml solution for injection ampoules | 5 ampoule PoM £12.49 DT price = £7.12
Powder for solution for infusion
▸ Cyanokit (Swedish Orphan Biovitrum Ltd)
  Hydroxocobalamin 5 gram Cyanokit 5g powder for solution for infusion vials | 1 vial PoM no price available

2 Iron overload

Iron overload

Overview

Severe tissue iron overload can occur in aplastic and other refractory anaemias, mainly as the result of repeated blood transfusions. It is a particular problem in refractory anaemias with hyperplastic bone marrow, especially *thalassaemia major*, where excessive iron absorption from the gut and inappropriate iron therapy can add to the tissue siderosis.

Iron overload associated with haemochromatosis can be treated with repeated venesection. Venesection may also be used for patients who have received multiple transfusions and whose bone marrow has recovered. Where venesection is contra-indicated, and in thalassaemia, the long-term administration of the iron chelating compound desferrioxamine mesilate p. 550 is useful. Desferrioxamine mesilate (up to 2 g per unit of blood) may also be given at the time of blood transfusion, provided that the desferrioxamine mesilate is **not** added to the blood and is **not** given through the same line as the blood (but the two may be given through the same cannula).

Iron excretion induced by desferrioxamine mesilate is enhanced by ascorbic acid (vitamin C) p. 602 daily by mouth; it should be given separately from food since it also enhances iron absorption. Ascorbic acid should not be given to children with cardiac dysfunction; in children with normal cardiac function ascorbic acid should be introduced 1 month after starting desferrioxamine mesilate.

Desferrioxamine mesilate infusion can be used to treat *aluminium overload* in dialysis patients; theoretically 100 mg of desferrioxamine binds with 4.1 mg of aluminium.

ANTIDOTES AND CHELATORS ⟩ IRON CHELATORS

Deferasirox

14-Jun-2017

● **DRUG ACTION** Deferasirox, is an oral iron chelator.

● **INDICATIONS AND DOSE**
Transfusion-related chronic iron overload when desferrioxamine is contra-indicated or inadequate in patients with beta thalassaemia major who receive frequent blood transfusions (7 mL/kg/month or more of packed red blood cells) (specialist use only)
▸ BY MOUTH USING DISPERSIBLE TABLETS
▸ Child 2–5 years: Initially 10–30 mg/kg once daily, dose adjusted according to serum-ferritin concentration and amount of transfused blood—consult product literature, then adjusted in steps of 5–10 mg/kg every 3–6 months, maintenance dose adjusted according to serum-ferritin concentration; maximum 40 mg/kg per day; Usual maximum 30 mg/kg

Transfusion-related chronic iron overload in patients with beta thalassaemia major who receive frequent blood transfusions (7 mL/kg/month or more of packed red blood cells) (specialist use only)
▸ BY MOUTH USING DISPERSIBLE TABLETS
▸ Child 6–17 years: Initially 10–30 mg/kg once daily, dose adjusted according to serum-ferritin concentration and amount of transfused blood—consult product literature, then adjusted in steps of 5–10 mg/kg every 3–6 months, maintenance dose adjusted according to serum-ferritin concentration; maximum 40 mg/kg per day; Usual maximum 30 mg/kg

**Transfusion-related chronic iron overload when desferrioxamine is contra-indicated or inadequate in patients with beta thalassaemia major who receive infrequent blood transfusions (less than 7 mL/kg/month of packed red blood cells) (specialist use only) |
Transfusion-related chronic iron overload when desferrioxamine is contra-indicated or inadequate in patients with other anaemias (specialist use only)**
▸ BY MOUTH USING DISPERSIBLE TABLETS
▸ Child 2–17 years: Initially 10–30 mg/kg once daily, dose adjusted according to serum-ferritin concentration and amount of transfused blood—consult product literature, then adjusted in steps of 5–10 mg/kg every 3–6 months, maintenance dose adjusted according to serum-ferritin concentration maximum 40 mg/kg per day; Usual maximum 30 mg/kg

Chronic iron overload when desferrioxamine is contra-indicated or inadequate in non-transfusion-dependent thalassaemia syndromes (specialist use only)
▸ BY MOUTH USING DISPERSIBLE TABLETS
▸ Child 10–17 years: Initially 10 mg/kg once daily, maintenance dose adjusted according to serum-ferritin concentration and liver-iron concentration (consult product literature); maximum 10 mg/kg per day

Transfusion-related chronic iron overload when desferrioxamine is contra-indicated or inadequate in patients with beta thalassaemia major who receive frequent blood transfusions (7 mL/kg/month or more of packed red blood cells) (specialist use only)
▸ BY MOUTH USING FILM-COATED TABLETS
▸ Child 2–5 years: Initially 7–21 mg/kg once daily, dose adjusted according to serum-ferritin concentration and amount of transfused blood—consult product literature, then adjusted in steps of 3.5–7 mg/kg every 3–6 months, maintenance dose adjusted according to

serum-ferritin concentration; maximum 28 mg/kg per day; Usual maximum 21 mg/kg

Transfusion-related chronic iron overload in patients with beta thalassaemia major who receive frequent blood transfusions (7 mL/kg/month or more of packed red blood cells) (specialist use only)
▶ BY MOUTH USING FILM-COATED TABLETS
▶ Child 6-17 years: Initially 7–21 mg/kg once daily, dose adjusted according to serum-ferritin concentration and amount of transfused blood—consult product literature, then adjusted in steps of 3.5–7 mg/kg every 3–6 months, maintenance dose adjusted according to serum-ferritin concentration; maximum 28 mg/kg per day; Usual maximum 21 mg/kg

**Transfusion-related chronic iron overload when desferrioxamine is contra-indicated or inadequate in patients with beta thalassaemia major who receive infrequent blood transfusions (less than 7 mL/kg/month of packed red blood cells) (specialist use only) |
Transfusion-related chronic iron overload when desferrioxamine is contra-indicated or inadequate in patients with other anaemias (specialist use only)**
▶ BY MOUTH USING FILM-COATED TABLETS
▶ Child 2-17 years: Initially 7–21 mg/kg once daily, dose adjusted according to serum-ferritin concentration and amount of transfused blood—consult product literature, then adjusted in steps of 3.5–7 mg/kg every 3–6 months, maintenance dose adjusted according to serum-ferritin concentration; maximum 28 mg/kg per day; Usual maximum 21 mg/kg

Chronic iron overload when desferrioxamine is contra-indicated or inadequate in non-transfusion-dependent thalassaemia syndromes (specialist use only)
▶ BY MOUTH USING FILM-COATED TABLETS
▶ Child 10-17 years: Initially 7 mg/kg once daily, maintenance dose adjusted according to serum-ferritin concentration and liver-iron concentration (consult product literature); maximum 7 mg/kg per day

DOSE EQUIVALENCE AND CONVERSION
▶ The bioavailability of dispersible tablets is lower than that of film-coated tablets; dispersible tablets are not interchangeable with film-coated tablets on a milligram-for-milligram basis—consult product literature for information on switching between formulations.

● **CAUTIONS** History of liver cirrhosis · not recommended in conditions which may reduce life expectancy (e.g. high-risk myelodysplastic syndromes) · platelet count less than 50×10^9/litre · risk of gastro-intestinal ulceration and haemorrhage · unexplained cytopenia—consider treatment interruption

● **INTERACTIONS** → Appendix 1: deferasirox

● **SIDE-EFFECTS**
▶ **Common or very common** Abdominal distension · abdominal pain · constipation · diarrhoea · dyspepsia · gastro-intestinal haemorrhage (including fatal cases) · gastro-intestinal ulceration · headache · nausea · proteinuria · pruritus · raised serum creatinine · raised transaminases · rash · vomiting
▶ **Uncommon** Anxiety · cataract · cholelithiasis · disturbances of hearing and vision · dizziness · fatigue · gastritis · glucosuria · hepatitis · laryngeal pain · maculopathy · oedema · pyrexia · renal tubulopathy · skin pigmentation · sleep disorder
▶ **Rare** Oesophagitis · optic neuritis
▶ **Frequency not known** Acute pancreatitis · acute renal failure · alopecia · anaphylaxis · angioedema · blood disorders · erythema multiforme · hepatic failure · hypersensitivity reactions · hypersensitivity vasculitis · metabolic acidosis · nephrolithiasis · Stevens-Johnson

syndrome · toxic epidermal necrolysis · tubulointerstitial nephritis · urticaria

● **PREGNANCY** Manufacturer advises avoid unless essential— toxicity in *animal* studies.

● **BREAST FEEDING** Manufacturer advises avoid—present in milk in *animal* studies.

● **HEPATIC IMPAIRMENT** Use with caution in moderate impairment, reduce dose considerably then gradually increase to max. 50% of normal dose. Avoid in severe impairment.

● **RENAL IMPAIRMENT** Manufacturer advises reduce dose if serum-creatinine increased above age-appropriate limits or creatinine clearance less than 90 mL/minute on 2 consecutive occasions—consult product literature. Manufacturer advises avoid if estimated creatinine clearance less than 60 mL/minute.

● **MONITORING REQUIREMENTS**
▶ Manufacturer advises monitoring of the following patient parameters: baseline serum creatinine twice and creatinine clearance once before initiation of treatment, weekly in the first month after treatment initiation or modification, then monthly thereafter; proteinuria before treatment initiation then monthly thereafter, and other markers of renal tubular function as needed; liver function before treatment initiation, every 2 weeks during the first month of treatment, then monthly thereafter; eye and ear examinations before treatment and annually during treatment; serum-ferritin concentration monthly.
▶ Manufacturer advises monitor liver-iron concentration every three months in children with non-transfusion-dependent thalassaemia syndromes when serum ferritin is ≤800 micrograms/litre.
▶ Manufacturer advises monitor body-weight, height, and sexual development before treatment and then annually thereafter.

● **DIRECTIONS FOR ADMINISTRATION** For *dispersible tablets*, manufacturer advises tablets should be dispersed in 100–200 mL of water, orange juice, or apple juice; if necessary any residue should be resuspended in a small volume of water or juice then administered; do not chew or swallow whole. For *film-coated tablets*, manufacturer advises tablets may be crushed and sprinkled on to soft food (yoghurt or apple sauce), then administered immediately.

● **PATIENT AND CARER ADVICE**
Patient or carers should be given advice on how to administer deferasirox dispersible tablets.
Medicines for Children leaflet: Deferasirox for removing excess iron www.medicinesforchildren.org.uk/deferasirox-for-removing-excess-iron

● **NATIONAL FUNDING/ACCESS DECISIONS**
Scottish Medicines Consortium (SMC) Decisions
The *Scottish Medicines Consortium* has advised (January 2007) that deferasirox is accepted for restricted use within NHS Scotland for the treatment of chronic iron overload associated with the treatment of rare acquired or inherited anaemias requiring recurrent blood transfusions. It is not recommended for patients with myelodysplastic syndromes.

The *Scottish Medicines Consortium* has advised (January 2017) that deferasirox (*Exjade*®) is accepted for restricted use within NHS Scotland for the treatment of chronic iron overload due to blood transfusions when deferoxamine treatment is contra-indicated or inadequate, in adult and paediatric patients aged 2 years and older with rare acquired or inherited anaemias. This advice relates only for use in patients with myelodysplastic syndrome with an International Prognostic Scoring System score of low or intermediate -1 risk.

9

Blood and nutrition

- **MEDICINAL FORMS**
  There can be variation in the licensing of different medicines containing the same drug.

  Dispersible tablet
  CAUTIONARY AND ADVISORY LABELS 13, 22
  - ▸ **Exjade** (Novartis Pharmaceuticals UK Ltd) ▼
    Deferasirox 125 mg Exjade 125mg dispersible tablets sugar-free | 28 tablet PoM £117.60
    Deferasirox 250 mg Exjade 250mg dispersible tablets sugar-free | 28 tablet PoM £235.20
    Deferasirox 500 mg Exjade 500mg dispersible tablets sugar-free | 28 tablet PoM £470.40

  Tablet
  CAUTIONARY AND ADVISORY LABELS 25
  - ▸ **Exjade** (Novartis Pharmaceuticals UK Ltd) ▼
    Deferasirox 90 mg Exjade 90mg tablets | 30 tablet PoM £126.00
    Deferasirox 180 mg Exjade 180mg tablets | 30 tablet PoM £252.00
    Deferasirox 360 mg Exjade 360mgtablets | 30 tablet PoM £504.00

Deferiprone

- **DRUG ACTION** Deferiprone, is an oral iron chelator.

- **INDICATIONS AND DOSE**

  Treatment of iron overload in patients with thalassaemia major in whom desferrioxamine is contra-indicated or is inadequate
  - ▸ BY MOUTH
    - ▸ Child 6–17 years: 25 mg/kg 3 times a day; maximum 100 mg/kg per day

- **UNLICENSED USE** Not licensed for use in children under 6 years.

- **CONTRA-INDICATIONS** History of agranulocytosis or recurrent neutropenia

- **INTERACTIONS** → Appendix 1: deferiprone

- **SIDE-EFFECTS** Agranulocytosis · arthropathy · blood dyscrasias · gastro-intestinal disturbances (reducing dose and increasing gradually may improve tolerance) · headache · increased appetite · neutropenia · red-brown urine discoloration · zinc deficiency

- **CONCEPTION AND CONTRACEPTION** Manufacturer advises avoid before intended conception—teratogenic and embryotoxic in *animal* studies. Contraception advised in females of child-bearing potential.

- **PREGNANCY** Manufacturer advises avoid during pregnancy—teratogenic and embryotoxic in *animal* studies.

- **BREAST FEEDING** Manufacturer advises avoid—no information available.

- **HEPATIC IMPAIRMENT** Manufacturer advises monitor liver function—interrupt treatment if persistent elevation in serum alanine aminotransferase.

- **RENAL IMPAIRMENT** Manufacturer advises caution—no information available.

- **MONITORING REQUIREMENTS** Monitor neutrophil count weekly and discontinue treatment if neutropenia develops.

- **PATIENT AND CARER ADVICE**
  Blood disorders Patients or their carers should be told how to recognise signs of neutropenia and advised to seek immediate medical attention if symptoms such as fever or sore throat develop.

- **MEDICINAL FORMS**
  There can be variation in the licensing of different medicines containing the same drug. Forms available from special-order manufacturers include: capsule, oral suspension, oral solution

  Oral solution
  CAUTIONARY AND ADVISORY LABELS 14
  - ▸ **Ferriprox** (Swedish Orphan Biovitrum Ltd)
    Deferiprone 100 mg per 1 ml Ferriprox 100mg/ml oral solution sugar-free | 500 ml PoM £152.39 DT price = £152.39

Tablet
CAUTIONARY AND ADVISORY LABELS 14
- ▸ **Ferriprox** (Swedish Orphan Biovitrum Ltd)
  Deferiprone 500 mg Ferriprox 500mg tablets | 100 tablet PoM £152.39 DT price = £152.39
  Deferiprone 1 gram Ferriprox 1000mg tablets | 50 tablet PoM £175.25 DT price = £175.25

Desferrioxamine mesilate

(Deferoxamine Mesilate)

- **INDICATIONS AND DOSE**

  Iron poisoning
  - ▸ BY CONTINUOUS INTRAVENOUS INFUSION
    - ▸ Neonate: Initially up to 15 mg/kg/hour, max. 80 mg/kg in 24 hours, dose to be reduced after 4–6 hours, in severe cases, higher doses may be given on advice from the National Poisons Information Service.
    - ▸ Child: Initially up to 15 mg/kg/hour, max. 80 mg/kg in 24 hours, dose to be reduced after 4–6 hours, in severe cases, higher doses may be given on advice from the National Poisons Information Service.

  Aluminium overload in dialysis patients
  - ▸ BY INTRAVENOUS INFUSION
    - ▸ Child: 5 mg/kg once weekly

  Chronic iron overload (low iron overload)
  - ▸ BY SUBCUTANEOUS INFUSION
    - ▸ Child: Initially up to 30 mg/kg 3–7 times a week, to be given over 8–12 hours, the dose should reflect the degree of iron overload

  Chronic iron overload (established overload)
  - ▸ BY SUBCUTANEOUS INFUSION
    - ▸ Child: 20–50 mg/kg daily

- **UNLICENSED USE**
  - ▸ When used for Iron poisoning Licensed for use in children (age range not specified by manufacturer).

- **CAUTIONS** Aluminium-related encephalopathy (may exacerbate neurological dysfunction)

- **INTERACTIONS** → Appendix 1: desferrioxamine

- **SIDE-EFFECTS**
  - ▸ **Common or very common** Abdominal pain · arthralgia · bone disorders · growth retardation · headache · hearing disturbances · injection-site reactions · myalgia · nausea · pyrexia · vomiting
  - ▸ **Rare** Anaphylaxis · blood dyscrasias · bone pain · diarrhoea · hepatic impairment · hypotension (especially when given too rapidly by intravenous injection) · leg cramps · lens opacity · leucopenia · rash · retinopathy · thrombocytopenia · visual disturbances · Yersinia and mucormycosis infections
  - ▸ **Very rare** Acute respiratory distress · convulsions · dizziness · neurological disturbances · neuropathy · paraesthesia · renal impairment
  - ▸ **Frequency not known** Muscle spasms

- **PREGNANCY** Teratogenic in *animal* studies. Manufacturer advises use only if potential benefit outweighs risk.

- **BREAST FEEDING** Manufacturer advises use only if potential benefit outweighs risk—no information available.

- **RENAL IMPAIRMENT** Use with caution.

- **MONITORING REQUIREMENTS**
  - ▸ Eye and ear examinations before treatment and at 3-month intervals during treatment.
  - ▸ Monitor body-weight and height in children at 3-month intervals—risk of growth retardation with excessive doses.

9

Blood and nutrition

Reduction in the duration of neutropenia and associated complications following treatment with cytotoxic chemotherapy associated with a significant incidence of febrile neutropenia (specialist use only)
▸ BY SUBCUTANEOUS INJECTION
▸ Child 2–17 years: 150 micrograms/m^2 daily until neutrophil count stable in acceptable range (max. 28 days), to be started on the day after completion of chemotherapy

Mobilisation of peripheral blood progenitor cells for harvesting and subsequent infusion, used alone (specialist use only)
▸ BY SUBCUTANEOUS INJECTION
▸ Child 2–17 years: 10 micrograms/kg daily for 4–6 days (5–6 days in healthy donors)

Mobilisation of peripheral blood progenitor cells, used following adjunctive myelosuppressive chemotherapy (to improve yield) (specialist use only)
▸ BY SUBCUTANEOUS INJECTION
▸ Child 2–17 years: 150 micrograms/m^2 daily until neutrophil count stable in acceptable range, to be started 1–5 days after completion of chemotherapy, for timing of leucopheresis, consult product literature

● UNLICENSED USE Not licensed for use in children for cytotoxic-induced neutropenia, mobilisation of peripheral blood progenitor cells (monotherapy or adjunctive therapy), or following peripheral stem cells transplantation.

● SIDE-EFFECTS Mucositis · splenic rupture · toxic epidermal necrolysis

● DIRECTIONS FOR ADMINISTRATION For *intravenous infusion*, dilute reconstituted solution to a concentration of not less than 2 micrograms/mL (*Granocyte*-13) or 2.5 micrograms/mL (*Granocyte*-34) with Sodium Chloride 0.9%.

● PRESCRIBING AND DISPENSING INFORMATION *Granocyte*® solution for injection contains 105 micrograms of lenograstim per 13.4 mega unit vial and 263 micrograms lenograstim per 33.6 mega unit vial.

● MEDICINAL FORMS
There can be variation in the licensing of different medicines containing the same drug.
Powder and solvent for solution for injection
EXCIPIENTS: May contain Phenylalanine
▸ Granocyte (Chugai Pharma UK Ltd)
Lenograstim 13.4 mega u Granocyte-13 powder and solvent for solution for injection vials | 1 vial [PoM] £40.11 | 5 vial [PoM] £200.55
Lenograstim 33.6 mega u Granocyte-34 powder and solvent for solution for injection vials | 1 vial [PoM] £62.54 | 5 vial [PoM] £312.69

4 Platelet disorders

Platelet disorders

Idiopathic thrombocytopenic purpura
Acute idiopathic thrombocytopenic purpura is usually self-limiting in children. A corticosteroid, such as prednisolone p. 421, is sometimes used if idiopathic thrombocytopenic purpura does not resolve spontaneously or if it is associated with severe cutaneous symptoms or mucous membrane bleeding; corticosteroid treatment should not be continued longer than 14 days regardless of the response.

Immunoglobulin preparations may be used in idiopathic thrombocytopenic purpura or where a temporary rapid rise in platelets is needed, as in pregnancy or pre-operatively;

they are often used in preference to a corticosteroid. Anti-D (Rh$_0$) immunoglobulin p. 741 is licensed for the management of idiopathic thrombocytopenic purpura.

Other therapy that has been tried under specialist supervision in refractory idiopathic thrombocytopenic purpura includes azathioprine p. 495, cyclophosphamide p. 509, vincristine sulfate p. 523, and ciclosporin p. 496. Rituximab p. 505 is also used in specialist centres but experience of its use in children is limited. For patients with chronic severe thrombocytopenia refractory to other therapy, tranexamic acid p. 80 may be given to reduce the severity of haemorrhage.

Splenectomy is considered in chronic thrombocytopenic purpura if a satisfactory platelet count is not achieved with regular immunoglobulin infusions, if there is a relapse on withdrawing or reducing the dose of corticosteroid, and if other therapies are considered inappropriate.

Essential thrombocythaemia
Anagrelide below reduces platelets in essential thrombocythaemia in patients at risk of thrombo-haemorrhagic events who have not responded adequately to other drugs or who cannot tolerate other drugs.

4.1 Essential thrombocythaemia

ANTITHROMBOTIC DRUGS ❯ CYCLIC AMP PHOSPHODIESTERASE III INHIBITORS

Anagrelide

● INDICATIONS AND DOSE
Essential thrombocythaemia in patients at risk of thrombo-haemorrhagic events who have not responded adequately to other drugs or who cannot tolerate other drugs (initiated under specialist supervision)
▸ BY MOUTH
▸ Child 7–17 years: Initially 500 micrograms daily, dose to be adjusted at weekly intervals according to response, increased in steps of 500 micrograms daily; usual dose 1–3 mg daily in divided doses (max. per dose 2.5 mg); maximum 10 mg per day

● UNLICENSED USE Not licensed for use in children.

● CAUTIONS Cardiovascular disease—assess cardiac function before and regularly during treatment · concomitant use of drugs that prolong QT-interval—assess cardiac function before and regularly during treatment · risk factors for QT-interval prolongation—assess cardiac function before and regularly during treatment

● INTERACTIONS → Appendix 1: anagrelide

● SIDE-EFFECTS
▸ **Common or very common** Anaemia · dizziness · fatigue · fluid retention · gastro-intestinal disturbances · headache · palpitation · rash · tachycardia
▸ **Uncommon** Alopecia · amnesia · anorexia · arrhythmias · arthralgia · back pain · blood disorders · chest pain · confusion · congestive heart failure · depression · dry mouth · dyspnoea · ecchymosis · epistaxis · fever · gastro-intestinal haemorrhage · haemorrhage · hypertension · hypoaesthesia · impotence · malaise · myalgia · nervousness · oedema · pancreatitis · paraesthesia · pneumonia pleural effusion · pruritus · skin discoloration · sleep disturbances · syncope · weight changes
▸ **Rare** Angina · asthenia · cardiomegaly · cardiomyopathy · colitis · dry skin · dysarthria · gastritis · gingival bleeding · impaired coordination · migraine · myocardial infarction · nocturia · pericardial effusion · postural hypotension · pulmonary hypertension · pulmonary infiltrates · renal

9

Blood and nutrition

failure · somnolence · tinnitus · vasodilatation · visual disturbances

- **Frequency not known** Hepatitis · interstitial lung disease · Torsade de pointes · tubulointerstitial nephritis

- **CONCEPTION AND CONTRACEPTION** Effective contraception required during treatment.

- **PREGNANCY** Manufacturer advises avoid (toxicity in *animal* studies).

- **BREAST FEEDING** Manufacturer advises avoid—present in milk in *animal* studies.

- **HEPATIC IMPAIRMENT** Manufacturer advises caution in mild impairment. Avoid in moderate to severe impairment.

- **RENAL IMPAIRMENT** Manufacturer advises avoid if estimated glomerular filtration rate less than 50 mL/minute/1.73 m^2

- **MONITORING REQUIREMENTS**
- Monitor full blood count (monitor platelet count every 2 days for 1 week, then weekly until maintenance dose established).
- Monitor liver function.
- Monitor serum creatinine.
- Monitor urea.
- Monitor electrolytes (including potassium, magnesium and calcium) before and during treatment.
- Monitor closely for further signs of disease progression such as malignant transformation.

- **PRESCRIBING AND DISPENSING INFORMATION** Initiate only when signs of disease progression or patient suffers from thrombosis. Consider stopping treatment after 3 months if inadequate response.

- **PATIENT AND CARER ADVICE**
  Driving and skilled tasks
  Dizziness may affect performance of skilled tasks (e.g. cycling, driving).

- **MEDICINAL FORMS**
  There can be variation in the licensing of different medicines containing the same drug.
  Capsule
  - Xagrid (Shire Pharmaceuticals Ltd) ▼
  Anagrelide (as Anagrelide hydrochloride) 500 microgram Xagrid 500microgram capsules | 100 capsule [PoM] £404.57

4.2 Idiopathic thrombocytopenic purpura

ANTIHAEMORRHAGICS › THROMBOPOIETIN RECEPTOR AGONISTS

▎ Eltrombopag

09-Jun-2017

- **INDICATIONS AND DOSE**
  Chronic immune (idiopathic) thrombocytopenic purpura in patients refractory to other treatments (such as corticosteroids or immunoglobulins) (under expert supervision)
  - BY MOUTH
  - Child 1–5 years: Initially 25 mg once daily, dose to be adjusted to achieve a platelet count of 50x10^9/litre or more—consult product literature for dose adjustments, discontinue if inadequate response after 4 weeks treatment at maximum dose; maximum 75 mg per day
  - Child 6–17 years: Initially 50 mg once daily, dose to be adjusted to achieve a platelet count of 50x10^9/litre or more—consult product literature for dose adjustments, discontinue if inadequate response after 4 weeks treatment at maximum dose; maximum 75 mg per day

- Child 6–17 years (patients of East Asian origin): Initially 25 mg once daily, dose to be adjusted to achieve a platelet count of 50x10^9/litre or more—consult product literature for dose adjustments, discontinue if inadequate response after 4 weeks treatment at maximum dose; maximum 75 mg per day.

- **CAUTIONS** Patients of East Asian origin · risk factors for thromboembolism

- **INTERACTIONS** → Appendix 1: eltrombopag

- **SIDE-EFFECTS**
- **Common or very common** Abdominal pain · alopecia · anaemia · asthenia · blood disorder · bone pain · cataract · changes in appetite · changes in weight · chest pain · cough · depression · diarrhoea · dry eye · dry mouth · erythema · eye disorders · faeces discoloured · flatulence · headache · hepatobiliary disorders · hepatotoxicity including drug-induced liver injury · hyperhidrosis · influenza · irritability · malaise · menorrhagia · mood disturbances · mouth ulceration · muscle spasms · musculoskeletal pain · myalgia · nasopharyngitis · nausea · oral herpes · oropharyngeal pain · paraesthesia · pharyngitis · pruritus · pyrexia · rash · respiratory tract infection · rhinorrhoea · sleep disorders · toothache · urinary tract infections · vertigo · visual disturbances · vomiting

- **Uncommon** Acute myocardial infarction · anorexia · balance disorder · blood uric acid increased · cardiovascular disorders · cholestasis · cyanosis · dysaesthesia · ear pain · electrolyte disturbances · flushing · frequent bowel movements · gingivitis · glossodynia · gout · haematemesis · haematoma · hemiparesis · hepatic lesions · hepatitis · hypoaesthesia · lupus nephritis · migraine · muscular weakness · nasal discomfort · nocturia · oral discomfort · oropharyngeal blistering · peripheral neuropathy · QT-interval prolongation · rectosigmoid cancer · renal failure · sinus disorder · skin discolouration · skin infection · speech disorder · tachycardia · thromboembolic events · toxic neuropathy · tremor

- **Frequency not known** Increased bone marrow reticulin—discontinue

- **CONCEPTION AND CONTRACEPTION** Ensure effective contraception during treatment.

- **PREGNANCY** Avoid—toxicity in *animal* studies.

- **BREAST FEEDING** Manufacturer advises avoid.

- **HEPATIC IMPAIRMENT** For *idiopathic thrombocytopenic purpura*, manufacturer advises avoid unless potential benefit outweighs risk—reduce initial dose to 25 mg once daily and wait at least 3 weeks before upwards titration of dose.

- **RENAL IMPAIRMENT** Use with caution.

- **MONITORING REQUIREMENTS**
- Manufacturer advises monitor liver function before treatment, every two weeks when adjusting the dose, and monthly thereafter.
- Manufacturer advises regular ophthalmological examinations for cataract formation.
- Manufacturer advises peripheral blood smear prior to initiation to establish baseline level of cellular morphologic abnormalities; once stabilised, full blood count with white blood cell count differential should be performed monthly.
- For *idiopathic thrombocytopenic purpura*, manufacturer advises monitor full blood count including platelet count and peripheral blood smears every week during treatment until a stable platelet count is reached (50x10^9/litre or more for at least 4 weeks), then monthly thereafter; monitor platelet count weekly for 4 weeks following treatment discontinuation.

- **DIRECTIONS FOR ADMINISTRATION** Each dose must be taken at least 4 hours before or after any dairy products (or foods containing calcium), indigestion remedies, or intravenous infusion of a weaker solution (usually 1.26%)

Renal hyperkalaemia
▶ BY SLOW INTRAVENOUS INJECTION
▶ **Neonate:** 1 mmol/kg daily.

▶ **Child:** 1 mmol/kg daily

Persistent cyanotic spell in a child with congenital heart disease despite optimal use of 100% oxygen and propranolol
▶ BY INTRAVENOUS INFUSION
▶ **Child:** 1 mmol/kg, dose given to correct acidosis (or dose calculated according to arterial blood gas results), sodium bicarbonate 4.2% intravenous infusion is appropriate for a child under 1 year and sodium bicarbonate 8.4% intravenous infusion in children over 1 year

● CONTRA-INDICATIONS
▶ With oral use Salt restricted diet
● CAUTIONS Respiratory acidosis
● INTERACTIONS → Appendix 1: sodium bicarbonate
● SIDE-EFFECTS
▶ When used for chronic acidotic states such as uraemic acidosis or renal tubular acidosis Fluid retention (in those at risk) · hypokalaemia may be exacerbated · increase blood pressure · pulmonary oedema (in those at risk)
● MONITORING REQUIREMENTS
▶ With intravenous use Plasma-pH and electrolytes should be monitored.
● DIRECTIONS FOR ADMINISTRATION
▶ With intravenous use For *peripheral infusion* dilute 8.4% solution at least 1 in 10. For *central line infusion* dilute 1 in 5 with Glucose 5% or 10% *or* Sodium Chloride 0.9%. Extravasation can cause severe tissue damage.
▶ With oral use Sodium bicarbonate may affect the stability or absorption of other drugs if administered at the same time. If possible, allow 1–2 hours before administering other drugs orally.
● PRESCRIBING AND DISPENSING INFORMATION
▶ With oral use *Sodium bicarbonate* 500*mg* capsules contain approximately 6 mmol each of Na$^+$ and HCO$_3^-$; *Sodium bicarbonate* 600*mg* capsules contain approximately 7 mmol each of Na$^+$ and HCO$_3^-$. Oral solutions of sodium bicarbonate are required occasionally; these are available from 'special-order' manufacturers or specialist importing companies; the strength of sodium bicarbonate should be stated on the prescription.
▶ With intravenous use Usual strength Sodium bicarbonate 1.26% (12.6 g, 150 mmol each of Na$^+$ and HCO$_3^-$/litre), various other strengths available.
● PATIENT AND CARER ADVICE
Patients or carers should be given advice on the administration of sodium bicarbonate oral medicines. Medicines for Children leaflet: Sodium bicarbonate for acidosis www.medicinesforchildren.org.uk/sodium-bicarbonate-for-acidosis

● MEDICINAL FORMS
There can be variation in the licensing of different medicines containing the same drug. Forms available from special-order manufacturers include: capsule, oral suspension, oral solution, solution for injection.

Tablet
▶ Sodium bicarbonate (Non-proprietary)
  Sodium bicarbonate 600 mg Sodium bicarbonate 600mg tablets | 100 tablet GSL £29.75 DT price = £26.52 | 100 tablet £125.50 DT price = £26.52

Solution for injection
▶ Sodium bicarbonate (Non-proprietary)
  Sodium bicarbonate 84 mg per 1 ml Sodium bicarbonate 8.4% (1mmol/ml) solution for injection 10ml ampoules | 10 ampoule PoM £81.27
  Sodium bicarbonate 8.4% (1mmol/ml) solution for injection 250ml bottles | 10 bottle PoM £65.34
  Sodium bicarbonate 8.4% (1mmol/ml) solution for injection 100ml bottles | 10 bottle PoM £62.04

Oral solution
▶ Sodium bicarbonate (Non-proprietary)
  Sodium bicarbonate 84 mg per 1 ml S-Bicarb SF 420mg/5ml (1mmol/ml) oral solution sugar-free | 100 ml £26.25 DT price = £39.80 S-Bicarb 420mg/5ml (1mmol/ml) oral solution | 100 ml no price available
  SodiBic 420mg/5ml (1mmol/ml) oral solution sugar-free | 100 ml £17.71 DT price = £39.80
▶ Thamicarb (Thame Laboratories Ltd)
  Sodium bicarbonate 84 mg per 1 ml Thamicarb 84mg/1ml oral solution sugar-free | 100 ml P £39.80 DT price = £39.80 sugar-free | 500 ml P £199.20 DT price = £199.20

Capsule
▶ Sodium bicarbonate (Non-proprietary)
  Sodium bicarbonate 500 mg Sodium bicarbonate 500mg capsules | 56 capsule P £17.56 DT price = £2.01 | 100 capsule PoM no price available

Infusion
▶ Sodium bicarbonate (Non-proprietary)
  Sodium bicarbonate 12.6 mg per 1 ml Polyfusor BC sodium bicarbonate 1.26% infusion 500ml bottles | 1 bottle PoM £9.86
  Sodium bicarbonate 14 mg per 1 ml Polyfusor BD sodium bicarbonate 1.4% infusion 500ml bottles | 1 bottle PoM £9.86
  Sodium bicarbonate 27.4 mg per 1 ml Polyfusor V sodium bicarbonate 2.74% infusion 500ml bottles | 1 bottle PoM £9.86
  Sodium bicarbonate 42 mg per 1 ml Polyfusor BE sodium bicarbonate 4.2% infusion 500ml bottles | 1 bottle PoM £9.86
  Sodium bicarbonate 84 mg per 1 ml Polyfusor B sodium bicarbonate 8.4% infusion 200ml bottles | 1 bottle PoM £9.86

ELECTROLYTES AND MINERALS ⟩ POTASSIUM

Potassium chloride with calcium chloride and sodium chloride and sodium lactate

(Sodium Lactate Intravenous Infusion, Compound; Compound, Hartmann's Solution for Injection; Ringer-Lactate Solution for Injection)

The properties listed below are those particular to the combination only. For the properties of the components please consider, potassium chloride p. 575, sodium chloride p. 561, calcium chloride p. 567.

● INDICATIONS AND DOSE
For prophylaxis, and replacement therapy, requiring the use of sodium chloride and lactate, with minimal amounts of calcium and potassium
▶ BY INTRAVENOUS INFUSION
▶ **Child:** (consult product literature)

● INTERACTIONS → Appendix 1: calcium salts, potassium chloride
● PRESCRIBING AND DISPENSING INFORMATION Compound sodium lactate intravenous infusion contains Na$^+$ 131 mmol, K$^+$ 5 mmol, Ca^{2+} 2 mmol, HCO$_3^-$ (as lactate) 29 mmol, Cl$^-$ 111 mmol/litre.

● MEDICINAL FORMS
There can be variation in the licensing of different medicines containing the same drug.

Infusion
▶ Potassium chloride with calcium chloride and sodium chloride and sodium lactate (Non-proprietary)
  Calcium chloride 270 microgram per 1 ml, Potassium chloride 400 microgram per 1 ml, Sodium lactate 3.17 mg per 1 ml,

9

Blood and nutrition

Sodium chloride 6 mg per 1 ml Sodium lactate compound infusion 1litre Macoflex N bags | 1 bag [PoM] no price available | 10 bag [PoM] no price available
Sodium lactate compound infusion 1litre Viaflex bags | 1 bag [PoM] no price available | 10 bag [PoM] no price available
Sodium lactate compound infusion 1litre Macoflex bags | 1 bag [PoM] no price available | 12 bag [PoM] no price available
Sodium lactate compound infusion 1litre Viaflo bags | 1 bag [PoM] no price available | 10 bag [PoM] no price available
Ringer lactate infusion 1litre Viaflo bags | 1 bag [PoM] no price available | 10 bag [PoM] no price available

Potassium chloride with calcium chloride dihydrate and sodium chloride

(Ringer's solution)

The properties listed below are those particular to the combination only. For the properties of the components please consider, potassium chloride p. 575, sodium chloride p. 561.

- **INDICATIONS AND DOSE**
Electrolyte imbalance
  - BY INTRAVENOUS INFUSION
  - Child: Dosed according to the deficit or daily maintenance requirements (consult product literature)

- **INTERACTIONS** → Appendix 1: potassium chloride

- **PRESCRIBING AND DISPENSING INFORMATION** Ringer's solution for injection provides the following ions (in mmol/litre), Ca^{2+} 2.2, K^+ 4, Na^+ 147, Cl^- 156.

- **MEDICINAL FORMS**
There can be variation in the licensing of different medicines containing the same drug.
Infusion
  - Potassium chloride with calcium chloride dihydrate and sodium chloride (Non-proprietary)
  Potassium chloride 300 microgram per 1 ml, Calcium chloride 320 microgram per 1 ml, Sodium chloride 8.6 mg per 1 ml Polyfusor C ringers infusion 500ml bottles | 1 bottle [PoM] £2.95
  Steriflex No.9 ringers infusion 1litre bags | 1 bag [PoM] £2.22
  Steriflex No.9 ringers infusion 500ml bags | 1 bag [PoM] £1.96

Potassium chloride with glucose

The properties listed below are those particular to the combination only. For the properties of the components please consider, potassium chloride p. 575, glucose p. 564.

- **INDICATIONS AND DOSE**
Electrolyte imbalance
  - BY INTRAVENOUS INFUSION
  - Child: Dosed according to the deficit or daily maintenance requirements

- **INTERACTIONS** → Appendix 1: glucose, potassium chloride

- **PRESCRIBING AND DISPENSING INFORMATION** Potassium chloride 0.3% contains 40 mmol each of K^+ and Cl^-/litre or 0.15% contains 20 mmol each of K^+ and Cl^-/litre with 5% of anhydrous glucose.

- **MEDICINAL FORMS**
There can be variation in the licensing of different medicines containing the same drug. Forms available from special-order manufacturers include: infusion, solution for infusion
Infusion
  - Potassium chloride with glucose (Non-proprietary)
  Potassium chloride 3 mg per 1 ml, Glucose anhydrous 50 mg per 1 ml Potassium chloride 0.3% (potassium 40mmol/1litre) / Glucose 5% infusion 1litre Macoflex bags | 1 bag [PoM] no price available
  Steriflex No.16 Potassium chloride 0.3% (potassium 20mmol/500ml) / glucose 5% infusion 500ml bags | 1 bag [PoM] £1.67

Potassium chloride 0.3% (potassium 20mmol/500ml) / glucose 5% infusion 500ml Macoflex bags | 1 bag [PoM] no price available
Potassium chloride 0.3% (potassium 40mmol/1litre) / Glucose 5% infusion 1litre bags | 1 bag [PoM] £2.82
Steriflex No.16 potassium chloride 0.3% (potassium 40mmol/1litre) / glucose 5% infusion 1litre bags | 1 bag [PoM] £2.20
Potassium chloride 0.3% (potassium 20mmol/500ml) / Glucose 5% infusion 500ml Viaflo bags | 1 bag [PoM] no price available
Potassium chloride 0.3% (potassium 40mmol/1litre) / Glucose 5% infusion 1litre Viaflo bags | 1 bag [PoM] no price available
Potassium chloride 2 mg per 1 ml, Glucose anhydrous 50 mg per 1 ml Steriflex No.29 potassium chloride 0.2% (potassium 27mmol/1litre) / glucose 5% infusion 1litre bags | 1 bag [PoM] £2.20
Steriflex No.29 potassium chloride 0.2% (potassium 13.3mmol/500ml) / glucose 5% infusion 500ml bags | 1 bag [PoM] £1.67
Potassium chloride 1.5 mg per 1 ml, Glucose anhydrous 50 mg per 1 ml Steriflex No.13 potassium chloride 0.15% (potassium 10mmol/500ml) / glucose 5% infusion 500ml bags | 1 bag [PoM] £1.67 | 15 bag [PoM] no price available
Steriflex No.13 potassium chloride 0.15% (potassium 20mmol/1litre) / glucose 5% infusion 1litre bags | 1 bag [PoM] £2.20 | 10 bag [PoM] no price available
Potassium chloride 0.15% (potassium 20mmol/1litre) / Glucose 5% infusion 1litre Macoflex bags | 1 bag [PoM] no price available
Potassium chloride 0.15% (potassium 10mmol/500ml) / Glucose 5% infusion 500ml bags | 10 bag [PoM] £0.67
Potassium chloride 0.15% (potassium 10mmol/500ml) / Glucose 5% infusion 500ml Macoflex bags | 1 bag [PoM] no price available
Potassium chloride 0.15% (potassium 20mmol/1litre) / Glucose 5% infusion 1litre Viaflo bags | 1 bag [PoM] no price available
Potassium chloride 0.15% (potassium 20mmol/1litre) / Glucose 5% infusion 1litre Viaflex bags | 1 bag [PoM] no price available

Potassium chloride with glucose and sodium chloride

The properties listed below are those particular to the combination only. For the properties of the components please consider, potassium chloride p. 575, glucose p. 564, sodium chloride p. 561.

- **INDICATIONS AND DOSE**
Electrolyte imbalance
  - BY INTRAVENOUS INFUSION
  - Child: Dosed according to the deficit or daily maintenance requirements

- **INTERACTIONS** → Appendix 1: glucose, potassium chloride

- **PRESCRIBING AND DISPENSING INFORMATION** Concentration of potassium chloride to be specified by the prescriber (usually K^+ 10–40 mmol/litre).

- **MEDICINAL FORMS**
There can be variation in the licensing of different medicines containing the same drug. Forms available from special-order manufacturers include: infusion, solution for infusion
Infusion
  - Potassium chloride with glucose and sodium chloride (Non-proprietary)
  Sodium chloride 1.8 mg per 1 ml, Potassium chloride 3 mg per 1 ml, Glucose anhydrous 40 mg per 1 ml Steriflex No.17 potassium chloride 0.3% (potassium 40mmol/1litre) / glucose 4% / sodium chloride 0.18% infusion 1litre bags | 1 bag [PoM] £2.20
  Steriflex No.17 potassium chloride 0.3% (potassium 20mmol/500ml) / glucose 4% / sodium chloride 0.18% infusion 500ml bags | 1 bag [PoM] £1.67 | 15 bag [PoM] no price available
  Potassium chloride 0.3% (potassium 20mmol/500ml) / Glucose 4% / Sodium chloride 0.18% infusion 500ml Macoflex bags | 1 bag [PoM] no price available | 20 bag [PoM] no price available
  Potassium chloride 0.3% (potassium 40mmol/1litre) / Glucose 4% / Sodium chloride 0.18% infusion 1litre Macoflex bags | 1 bag [PoM] no price available | 12 bag [PoM] no price available
  Potassium chloride 0.3% (potassium 40mmol/1litre) / Glucose 4% / Sodium chloride 0.18% infusion 1litre Viaflo bags | 1 bag [PoM] no price available | 10 bag [PoM] no price available
  Potassium chloride 1.5 mg per 1 ml, Sodium chloride 1.8 mg per 1 ml, Glucose anhydrous 40 mg per 1 ml Potassium chloride 0.15% (potassium 20mmol/1litre) / Glucose 4% / Sodium chloride 0.18% infusion 1litre Viaflo bags | 1 bag [PoM] no price available

Glucose 5% infusion 500ml Macoflex N bags | 1 bag [PoM] no price available | 18 bag [PoM] no price available

Glucose 5% infusion 100ml bags | 1 bag [PoM] £2.00

Glucose 5% infusion 1litre Easyflex N bags | 1 bag [PoM] no price available | 10 bag [PoM] no price available

Glucose 5% infusion 100ml Easyflex N bags | 1 bag [PoM] no price available | 60 bag [PoM] no price available

Glucose 5% infusion 500ml Viaflo bags | 1 bag [PoM] no price available | 20 bag [PoM] no price available

Glucose 5% infusion 100ml Macoflex N bags | 1 bag [PoM] no price available | 60 bag [PoM] no price available

Glucose 5% infusion 500ml Viaflex bags | 1 bag [PoM] no price available | 20 bag [PoM] no price available

Glucose 5% infusion 250ml Macoflex N bags | 1 bag [PoM] no price available | 30 bag [PoM] no price available

Glucose 5% infusion 500ml Macoflex bags | 1 bag [PoM] no price available | 20 bag [PoM] no price available

Polyfusor D glucose 5% infusion 1litre bottles | 1 bottle [PoM] £3.02

Glucose 5% infusion 500ml Easyflex N bags | 1 bag [PoM] no price available | 18 bag [PoM] no price available

Glucose 5% infusion 1litre Viaflex bags | 1 bag [PoM] no price available | 10 bag [PoM] no price available

Glucose 5% infusion 50ml Viaflo bags | 1 bag [PoM] no price available | 50 bag [PoM] no price available

Glucose 5% infusion 250ml Easyflex N bags | 1 bag [PoM] no price available | 30 bag [PoM] no price available

Glucose 5% infusion 1litre bags | 10 bag [PoM] £11.11

Glucose 5% infusion 100ml Macoflex N bags | 1 bag [PoM] no price available | 60 bag [PoM] no price available

Glucose 5% infusion 50ml Easyflex N bags | 1 bag [PoM] no price available | 70 bag [PoM] no price available

Glucose 5% infusion 50ml Macoflex N bags | 1 bag [PoM] no price available | 70 bag [PoM] no price available

Glucose 5% infusion 250ml Viaflex bags | 1 bag [PoM] no price available | 30 bag [PoM] no price available

Polyfusor D glucose 5% infusion 500ml bottles | 1 bottle [PoM] £2.25

Glucose 5% infusion 50ml Viaflex bags | 1 bag [PoM] no price available | 50 bag [PoM] no price available

Glucose 5% infusion 100ml Viaflex bags | 1 bag [PoM] no price available | 50 bag [PoM] no price available

Glucose 5% infusion 100ml Viaflo bags | 1 bag [PoM] no price available | 50 bag [PoM] no price available

Glucose 5% infusion 1litre Macoflex N bags | 1 bag [PoM] no price available | 10 bag [PoM] no price available

Glucose 5% infusion 250ml Macoflex bags | 1 bag [PoM] no price available | 30 bag [PoM] no price available

Glucose 5% infusion 50ml Macoflex bags | 1 bag [PoM] no price available | 70 bag [PoM] no price available

Glucose 5% infusion 250ml Viaflo bags | 1 bag [PoM] no price available | 30 bag [PoM] no price available

Glucose anhydrous 100 mg per 1 ml Steriflex No.7 glucose 10% infusion 1litre bags | 1 bag [PoM] £2.54

Glucose 10% infusion 1litre Viaflo bags | 1 bag [PoM] no price available | 10 bag [PoM] no price available

Glucose 10% infusion 500ml Macoflex bags | 1 bag [PoM] no price available | 20 bag [PoM] no price available

Glucose 10% infusion 500ml Viaflo bags | 1 bag [PoM] no price available | 20 bag [PoM] no price available

Glucose 10% infusion 1litre Macoflex bags | 1 bag [PoM] no price available | 12 bag [PoM] no price available

Steriflex No.7 glucose 10% infusion 500ml bags | 1 bag [PoM] £1.85

Glucose anhydrous 200 mg per 1 ml Steriflex No.31 glucose 20% infusion 500ml bags | 1 bag [PoM] £2.64 | 15 bag [PoM] no price available

Glucose 20% infusion 500ml bags | 1 bag [PoM] £3.47

Glucose (as Glucose monohydrate) 300 mg per 1 ml Glucose 30% infusion 500ml polyethylene bottles | 10 bottle [PoM] no price available

Glucose anhydrous 400 mg per 1 ml Steriflex No.33 glucose 40% infusion 500ml bags | 1 bag [PoM] £2.81 | 15 bag [PoM] no price available

Glucose anhydrous 500 mg per 1 ml Steriflex No.34 glucose 50% infusion 500ml bags | 1 bag [PoM] £3.11 | 15 bag [PoM] no price available

Glucose 50% infusion 500ml polyethylene bottles | 1 bottle [PoM] £4.64

Glucose anhydrous 700 mg per 1 ml Glucose 70% concentrate for solution for infusion 500ml Viaflex bags | 1 bag [PoM] no price available

Combinations available: *Potassium chloride with glucose,* p. 560 · *Potassium chloride with glucose and sodium chloride,* p. 560 · *Sodium chloride with glucose,* p. 563

ORAL REHYDRATION SALTS

Disodium hydrogen citrate with glucose, potassium chloride and sodium chloride

(Formulated as oral rehydration salts)

● **INDICATIONS AND DOSE**

Fluid and electrolyte loss in diarrhoea

▸ BY MOUTH

▸ Child 1–11 months: 1–1½ times usual feed volume to be given

▸ Child 1–11 years: 200 mL, to be given after every loose motion

▸ Child 12–17 years: 200–400 mL, to be given after every loose motion, dose according to fluid loss

● **DIRECTIONS FOR ADMINISTRATION** Reconstitute 1 sachet with 200mL of water (freshly boiled and cooled for infants); 5 sachets reconstituted with 1 litre of water provide Na^+ 60 mmol, K^+ 20 mmol, Cl^- 60 mmol, citrate 10 mmol, and glucose 90 mmol.

● **PRESCRIBING AND DISPENSING INFORMATION** Flavours of oral powder formulations may include black currant, citrus, or natural.

● **PATIENT AND CARER ADVICE**

After reconstitution any unused solution should be discarded no later than 1 hour after preparation unless stored in a refrigerator when it may be kept for up to 24 hours.

Medicines for Children leaflet: Oral rehydration salts www.medicinesforchildren.org.uk/oral-rehydration-salts

● **MEDICINAL FORMS**

There can be variation in the licensing of different medicines containing the same drug.

Powder

▸ Dioralyte (Sanofi)

Potassium chloride 300 mg, Sodium chloride 470 mg, Disodium hydrogen citrate 530 mg, Glucose 3.56 gram Dioralyte oral powder sachets citrus | 20 sachet [P] £6.72

Dioralyte oral powder sachets plain | 20 sachet [P] £6.72

Dioralyte oral powder sachets blackcurrant | 20 sachet [P] £6.72

Glucose with potassium chloride, sodium bicarbonate and sodium chloride

(Formulated as oral rehydration salts)

● **INDICATIONS AND DOSE**

Fluid and electrolyte loss in diarrhoea

▸ BY MOUTH

▸ Child 1–11 months: 1–1½ times usual feed volume to be given

▸ Child 1–11 years: 200 mL, to be given after every loose motion

▸ Child 12–17 years: 200–400 mL, to be given after every loose motion, dose according to fluid loss

● **DIRECTIONS FOR ADMINISTRATION** Reconstitute 1 sachet with 200 mL of water (freshly boiled and cooled for infants); 5 sachets when reconstituted with 1 litre of water provide Na^+ 50 mmol, K^+ 20 mmol, Cl^- 40 mmol, HCO_3^- 30 mmol, and glucose 111 mmol.

● **PRESCRIBING AND DISPENSING INFORMATION** Flavours of oral powder formulations may include banana, orange, black current, lemon and lime, plain, or multiflavoured.

9

Blood and nutrition

- **PATIENT AND CARER ADVICE** Patients and carers should be advised how to reconstitute *Electrolade®* oral powder. After reconstitution any unused solution should be discarded no later than 1 hour after preparation unless stored in a refrigerator when it may be kept for up to 24 hours.

- **MEDICINAL FORMS**
There can be variation in the licensing of different medicines containing the same drug.
No licensed medicines listed.

Potassium chloride with rice powder, sodium chloride and sodium citrate

(Formulated as oral rehydation salts)

- **INDICATIONS AND DOSE**

Fluid and electrolyte loss in diarrhoea
▸ BY MOUTH
▸ Child 1–11 months: 1–1½ times usual feed volume to be given
▸ Child 1–11 years: 200 mL, to be given after every loose motion
▸ Child 12–17 years: 200–400 mL, to be given after every loose motion, dose according to fluid loss

- **UNLICENSED USE** *Dioralyte Relief®* not licensed for use in children under 3 months.

- **DIRECTIONS FOR ADMINISTRATION** Reconstitute 1 sachet with 200 mL of water (freshly boiled and cooled for infants); 5 sachets when reconstituted with 1 litre of water provide Na^+ 60 mmol, K^+ 20 mmol, Cl^- 50 mmol and citrate 10 mmol.

- **PRESCRIBING AND DISPENSING INFORMATION** Flavours of oral powder formulations may include apricot, black currant, or raspberry.

- **PATIENT AND CARER ADVICE**
Patients and carers should be advised how to reconstitute *Dioralyte®* Relief oral powder.
After reconstitution any unused solution should be discarded no later than 1 hour after preparation unless stored in a refrigerator when it may be kept for up to 24 hours.
Medicines for Children leaflet: Oral rehydration salts www.medicinesforchildren.org.uk/oral-rehydration-salts

- **MEDICINAL FORMS**
There can be variation in the licensing of different medicines containing the same drug.
Powder
EXCIPIENTS: May contain Aspartame
▸ **Dioralyte Relief** (Sanofi)
Potassium chloride 300 mg, Sodium chloride 350 mg, Sodium citrate 580 mg, Rice powder pre-cooked 6 gram Dioralyte Relief oral powder sachets raspberry sugar-free | 6 sachet GSL £2.50
Dioralyte Relief oral powder sachets blackcurrant sugar-free | 20 sachet P £7.13

2.1 Calcium imbalance

Calcium

Calcium supplements

Calcium supplements are usually only required where dietary calcium intake is deficient. This dietary requirement varies with age and is relatively greater in childhood, pregnancy, and lactation, due to an increased demand. Hypocalcaemia may be caused by vitamin D deficiency (see Vitamin D under Vitamins p. 596), impaired metabolism, a failure of secretion (hypoparathyroidism), or resistance to parathyroid hormone (pseudohypoparathyroidism).

Mild asymptomatic hypocalcaemia may be managed with oral calcium supplements. *Severe symptomatic hypocalcaemia* requires an intravenous infusion of calcium gluconate 10% p. 568 over 5 to 10 minutes, repeating the dose if symptoms persist; in exceptional cases it may be necessary to maintain a continuous calcium infusion over a day or more. Calcium chloride injection p. 567 is also available, but is more irritant; care should be taken to prevent extravasation.

See the role of calcium gluconate in temporarily reducing the toxic effects of *hyperkalaemia*.

Persistent hypocalcaemia requires oral calcium supplements and either a vitamin D analogue (alfacalcidol p. 603 or calcitriol p. 603) for hypoparathyroidism and pseudohypoparathyroidism or natural vitamin D (calciferol) if due to vitamin D deficiency. It is important to monitor plasma and urinary calcium during long-term maintenance therapy.

Severe hypercalcaemia

Severe hypercalcaemia calls for urgent treatment before detailed investigation of the cause. Rehydration should be corrected first with intravenous infusion of sodium chloride 0.9% p. 561. Drugs (such as thiazide and vitamin D compounds) which promote hypercalcaemia, should be discontinued and dietary calcium should be restricted.

If *severe hypercalcaemia persists* drugs which inhibit mobilisation of calcium from the skeleton may be required. The **bisphosphonates** are useful and pamidronate disodium p. 448 is probably the most effective.

Corticosteroids are widely given, but may only be useful where hypercalcaemia is due to sarcoidosis or vitamin D intoxication; they often take several days to achieve the desired effect.

Calcitonin (salmon) p. 450 can be used by specialists for the treatment of hypercalcaemia associated with malignancy; it is rarely effective where bisphosphonates have failed to reduce serum calcium adequately.

After treatment of severe hypercalcaemia the underlying cause must be established. *Further treatment* is governed by the same principles as for initial therapy. Salt and water depletion and drugs promoting hypercalcaemia should be avoided; oral administration of a bisphosphonate may be useful. Parathyroidectomy may be indicated for hyperparathyroidism.

Hypercalciuria

Hypercalciuria should be investigated for an underlying cause, which should be treated. Reducing dietary calcium intake may be beneficial but severe restriction of calcium intake has not proved beneficial and may even be harmful.

Neonates

Hypocalcaemia is common in the first few days of life, particularly following birth asphyxia or respiratory distress. Late onset at 4–10 days after birth may be secondary to vitamin D deficiency, hypoparathyroidism or hypomagnesaemia and may be associated with seizures.

2.1a Hypocalcaemia

ELECTROLYTES AND MINERALS › CALCIUM

Calcium salts

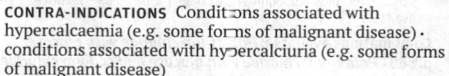

- **CONTRA-INDICATIONS** Conditions associated with hypercalcaemia (e.g. some forms of malignant disease) · conditions associated with hypercalciuria (e.g. some forms of malignant disease)

- **CAUTIONS** History of nephrolithiasis · sarcoidosis

Magnesium glycerophosphate

02-Jun-2016

- **INDICATIONS AND DOSE**

Hypomagnesaemia

▶ BY MOUTH

▶ Child 1 month–11 years: Initially 0.2 mmol/kg 3 times a day, dose to be adjusted as necessary, dose expressed as Mg^{2+}

▶ Child 12–17 years: Initially 4–8 mmol 3 times a day, dose to be adjusted as necessary, dose expressed as Mg^{2+}

DOSE EQUIVALENCE AND CONVERSION

▶ Magnesium glycerophosphate 1 g is approximately equivalent to Mg^{2+} 4 mmol or magnesium 97 mg.

- **UNLICENSED USE** Not licensed for use.
- **INTERACTIONS** → Appendix 1: magnesium
- **SIDE-EFFECTS** Arrhythmias · colic · coma · confusion · diarrhoea · drowsiness · flushing of skin · hypermagnesaemia associated side-effects · hypotension · loss of tendon reflexes · muscle weakness · nausea · respiratory depression · thirst · vomiting
- **RENAL IMPAIRMENT** Avoid or reduce dose. Increased risk of toxicity.
- **MONITORING REQUIREMENTS** Monitor blood pressure, respiratory rate, urinary output and for signs of overdosage (loss of patellar reflexes, weakness, nausea, sensation of warmth, flushing, drowsiness, double vision, and slurred speech).
- **DIRECTIONS FOR ADMINISTRATION** Tablets may be dispersed in water.

- **MEDICINAL FORMS**
There can be variation in the licensing of different medicines containing the same drug. Forms available from special-order manufacturers include: tablet, chewable tablet, capsule, oral suspension, oral solution, powder

Tablet

▶ Magnesium glycerophosphate (Non-proprietary)
Magnesium (as Magnesium glycerophosphate) 97.2 mg Mag-4 (magnesium 97.2mg (4mmol)) tablets | 30 tablet £84.50

Oral solution

▶ LiquaMag GP (Fontus Health Ltd)
Magnesium (as Magnesium glycerophosphate) 24.25 mg per 1 ml LiquaMag GP (magnesium 121.25mg/5ml (5mmol/5ml)) oral solution sugar-free | 200 ml £49.99 sugar-free | 250 ml £55.00

Chewable tablet

▶ Magnesium glycerophosphate (Non-proprietary)
Magnesium (as Magnesium glycerophosphate) 97.2 mg YourMAG (magnesium 97.2mg (4mmol)) chewable tablets | 50 tablet £20.00
Mag-4 (magnesium 97.2mg (4mmol)) chewable tablets sugar-free | 30 tablet £84.50
MagnaPhos 97.2mg (4mmol) chewable tablets sugar-free | 50 tablet £17.89
Neomag (magnesium 97mg (4mmol)) chewable tablets sugar-free | 50 tablet £48.50

▶ MagnaPhate (Arjun Products Ltd)
Magnesium (as Magnesium glycerophosphate) 97.2 mg MagnaPhate (magnesium 97.2mg (4mmol)) chewable tablets sugar-free | 50 tablet £22.64

Capsule

▶ Magnesium glycerophosphate (Non-proprietary)
Magnesium (as Magnesium glycerophosphate) 48.6 mg Mag-4 (magnesium 48.6mg (2mmol)) capsules | 30 capsule £85.70
MagnaPhos 48.6mg (2mmol) capsules | 50 capsule £35.87
Magnesium (as Magnesium glycerophosphate) 97.2 mg Mag-4 (magnesium 97.2mg (4mmol)) capsules | 30 capsule £89.30
MagnaPhos 97.2mg (4mmol) capsules | 50 capsule £37.87

Magnesium sulfate

- **INDICATIONS AND DOSE**

Severe acute asthma | Continuing respiratory deterioration in anaphylaxis

▶ BY INTRAVENOUS INFUSION

▶ Child 2–17 years: 40 mg/kg (max. per dose 2 g), to be given over 20 minutes

Persistent pulmonary hypertension of the newborn

▶ INITIALLY BY INTRAVENOUS INFUSION

▶ Neonate: Initially 200 mg/kg, to be given over 20–30 minutes, then (by continuous intravenous infusion) 20–75 mg/kg/hour for up to 5 days if response occurs after initial dose (to maintain plasma magnesium concentration between 3.5–5.5 mmol/litre).

Hypomagnesaemia

▶ BY INTRAVENOUS INJECTION

▶ Neonate: 100 mg/kg every 6–12 hours as required, to be given over at least 10 minutes.

▶ Child 1 month–11 years: 50 mg/kg every 12 hours as required, to be given over at least 10 minutes

▶ Child 12–17 years: 1 g every 12 hours as required, to be given over at least 10 minutes

Hypomagnesaemia maintenance (e.g. in intravenous nutrition)

▶ BY INTRAVENOUS INFUSION, OR BY INTRAMUSCULAR INJECTION

▶ Child: 50–100 mg/kg daily; maximum 5 g per day

Neonatal hypocalaemia

▶ BY DEEP INTRAMUSCULAR INJECTION, OR BY INTRAVENOUS INFUSION

▶ Neonate: 100 mg/kg every 12 hours for 2–3 doses.

Torsade de pointes

▶ BY INTRAVENOUS INJECTION

▶ Child: 25–50 mg/kg (max. per dose 2 g), to be given over 10–15 minutes, dose may be repeated once if necessary (consult local protocol)

DOSE EQUIVALENCE AND CONVERSION

▶ Magnesium sulfate heptahydrate 1 g equivalent to Mg^{2+} approx. 4 mmol.

- **UNLICENSED USE** Unlicensed indication in severe acute asthma. Continuing respiratory deterioration in anaphylaxis.
- **INTERACTIONS** → Appendix 1: magnesium
- **SIDE-EFFECTS** Arrhythmias · coma · confusion · drowsiness · flushing of skin · hypermagnesaemia associated side-effects · hypotension · loss of tendon reflexes · muscle weakness · nausea · respiratory depression · thirst · vomiting
- **PREGNANCY** Sufficient amount may cross the placenta in mothers treated with high doses e.g. in pre-eclampsia, causing hypotonia and respiratory depression in newborns.
- **HEPATIC IMPAIRMENT** Avoid in hepatic coma if risk of renal failure.
- **RENAL IMPAIRMENT** Avoid or reduce dose. Increased risk of toxicity.
- **MONITORING REQUIREMENTS** Monitor blood pressure, respiratory rate, urinary output and for signs of overdosage (loss of patellar reflexes, weakness, nausea, sensation of warmth, flushing, drowsiness, double vision, and slurred speech).
- **DIRECTIONS FOR ADMINISTRATION**

▶ With intravenous use In severe hypomagnesaemia administer initially via controlled infusion device (preferably syringe pump).

9

Blood and nutrition

‣ With intravenous use For *intravenous infusion*, in persistent pulmonary hypertension of the newborn, dilute to a max. concentration of 100 mg/mL (10%) (0.4 mmol/mL Mg^{2+}) magnesium sulfate heptahydrate (200 mg/mL (0.8 mmol/mL Mg^{2+}) if fluid restricted) with Glucose 5% *or* Sodium Chloride 0.9%.

‣ With intravenous use For neonatal hypocalcaemia, hypomagnaesemia, and torsade de pointes, dilute to 10% (100 mg magnesium sulfate heptahydrate (0.4 mmol Mg^{2+}) in 1 mL) with Glucose 5% *or* 10%, Sodium Chloride 0.45% *or* 0.9% *or* Glucose and Sodium Chloride combinations. Up to 20% solution may be given in fluid restriction. Rate of administration should not exceed 10 mg/kg/minute (0.04 mmol/kg/minute Mg^{2+}) of magnesium sulfate heptahydrate.

● PRESCRIBING AND DISPENSING INFORMATION
The BP directs that the label states the strength as the % w/v of magnesium sulfate heptahydrate and as the approximate concentration of magnesium ions (Mg^{2+}) in mmol/mL. Magnesium Sulfate Injection BP is a sterile solution of Magnesium Sulfate Heptahydrate.

● MEDICINAL FORMS
There can be variation in the licensing of different medicines containing the same drug. Forms available from special-order manufacturers include: solution for injection, infusion, solution for infusion

Solution for injection
‣ **Magnesium sulfate (Non-proprietary)**
Magnesium sulfate heptahydrate 500 mg per 1 ml Magnesium sulfate 50% (magnesium 2mmol/ml) solution for injection 10ml ampoules | 10 ampoule [PoM] £11.85–£35.25
Magnesium sulfate 50% (magnesium 2mmol/ml) solution for injection 20ml vials | 10 vial [PoM] £46.40
Magnesium sulfate 50% (magnesium 2mmol/ml) solution for injection 5ml ampoules | 10 ampoule [PoM] £21.80–£61.26
Magnesium sulfate 50% (magnesium 2mmol/ml) solution for injection 2ml ampoules | 10 ampoule [PoM] £11.72–£17.90 DT price = £11.85

Solution for infusion
‣ **Magnesium sulfate (Non-proprietary)**
Magnesium sulfate heptahydrate 100 mg per 1 ml Magnesium sulfate 10% (magnesium 0.4mmol/ml) solution for injection 10ml ampoules | 10 ampoule [PoM] £59.98–£60.50
Magnesium sulfate heptahydrate 500 mg per 1 ml Magnesium sulfate 50% (magnesium 2mmol/ml) solution for infusion 50ml vials | 10 vial [PoM] £63.70

2.4 Phosphate imbalance

Phosphorus

Phosphate supplements
Oral phosphate supplements p. 573 may be required in addition to vitamin D in children with hypophosphataemic vitamin D-resistant rickets, see also Vitamin D, under Vitamins p. 596.

Phosphate infusion is occasionally needed in phosphate deficiency arising from use of parenteral nutrition deficient in phosphate supplements; phosphate depletion also occurs in severe diabetic ketoacidosis. It is difficult to provide detailed guidelines for the treatment of *severe hypophosphatemia* because the extent of total body deficits and response to therapy are difficult to predict. High doses of phosphate may result in a transient serum elevation followed by redistribution into intracellular compartments or bone tissue. It is recommended that severe hypophosphataemia be treated intravenously as large doses of oral phosphate may cause diarrhoea; intestinal absorption may be unreliable and dose adjustment may be necessary.

Phosphate is not the first choice for the treatment of hypercalcaemia because of the risk of precipitation of calcium phosphate in the kidney and other tissues. If used,

the child should be well hydrated and electrolytes monitored.

Neonates
Phosphate deficiency may occur in very low-birthweight infants and may compromise bone growth if not corrected. Parenterally fed infants may be at risk of phosphate deficiency due to the limited solubility of phosphate. Some units routinely supplement expressed breast milk with phosphate, although the effect on the osmolality of the milk should be considered.

Phosphate-binding agents
Calcium-containing preparations are used as phosphate-binding agents in the management of hyperphosphataemia complicating renal failure. Aluminium- containing preparations are rarely used as phosphate- binding agents and can cause aluminium accumulation.

Sevelamer hydrochloride is licensed for the treatment of hyperphosphataemia in adults on haemodialysis or peritoneal dialysis. Although experience is limited in children sevelamer hydrochloride may be useful when hypercalcaemia prevents the use of calcium carbonate p. 567.

2.4a Hyperphosphataemia

ELECTROLYTES AND MINERALS › ALUMINIUM

Aluminium hydroxide

● INDICATIONS AND DOSE
Hyperphosphataemia in renal failure
‣ BY MOUTH USING CAPSULES
‣ Child 5–11 years: 1–2 capsules 3–4 times a day, dose adjusted as necessary
‣ Child 12–17 years: 1–5 capsules 3–4 times a day, dose adjusted as necessary

● CONTRA-INDICATIONS Hypophosphataemia · infants · neonates
CONTRA-INDICATIONS, FURTHER INFORMATION
‣ Neonates and infants Aluminium-containing antacids should not be used because accumulation may lead to increased plasma-aluminium concentrations.

● INTERACTIONS → Appendix 1: antacids

● SIDE-EFFECTS Constipation · hyperaluminaemia

● HEPATIC IMPAIRMENT Avoid; can cause constipation which can precipitate coma.

● RENAL IMPAIRMENT There is a risk of accumulation and aluminium toxicity with antacids containing aluminium salts. Absorption of aluminium from aluminium salts is increased by citrates, which are contained in many effervescent preparations (such as effervescent analgesics).

● MEDICINAL FORMS
There can be variation in the licensing of different medicines containing the same drug.
Capsule
‣ **Alu-Cap** (Meda Pharmaceuticals Ltd)
Aluminium hydroxide 475 mg Alu-Cap 475mg capsules | 120 capsule [P] £13.71 DT price = £13.71

ELECTROLYTES AND MINERALS ⟩
CALCIUM

⟨ 566

Calcium acetate

- **INDICATIONS AND DOSE**

PHOSEX® TABLETS

Phosphate binding in renal failure and hyperphosphataemia
▸ BY MOUTH
▸ Child: Dose to be adjusted according to requirements of patient, dose to be taken with meals (consult product literature)

- **INTERACTIONS** → Appendix 1: calcium salts
- **DIRECTIONS FOR ADMINISTRATION**
PHOSEX® TABLETS *Phosex*® tablets are taken with meals. Tablets can be broken to aid swallowing, but not chewed (bitter taste).
- **PRESCRIBING AND DISPENSING INFORMATION** *Phosex*® tablets contain calcium acetate 1 g (equivalent to calcium 250 mg or Ca^{2+} 6.2 mmol).
- **PATIENT AND CARER ADVICE**
Medicines for Children leaflet: Calcium salts for kidney disease www.medicinesforchildren.org.uk/calcium-salts-kidney-disease-0
PHOSEX® TABLETS Patients or carers should be given advice on how to administer *Phosex*® tablets.

- **MEDICINAL FORMS**
There can be variation in the licensing of different medicines containing the same drug.
Tablet
CAUTIONARY AND ADVISORY LABELS 25
▸ Phosex (Pharmacosmos UK Ltd)
Calcium acetate 1 gram Phosex 1g tablets | 180 tablet [PoM] £19.79
DT price = £19.79

PHOSPHATE BINDERS

Sevelamer

31-Oct-2016

- **INDICATIONS AND DOSE**

RENAGEL®

Hyperphosphataemia in patients on haemodialysis or peritoneal dialysis
▸ BY MOUTH
▸ Child 12-17 years: Initially 0.8-1.6 g 3 times a day, dose to be given with meals and adjusted according to serum-phosphate concentration

- **UNLICENSED USE** Not licensed for use in children under 18 years.
- **CONTRA-INDICATIONS** Bowel obstruction
- **CAUTIONS** Gastro-intestinal disorders
- **SIDE-EFFECTS**
▸ **Common or very common** Abdominal pain · constipation · diarrhoea · dyspepsia · flatulence · nausea · vomiting
▸ **Frequency not known** Diverticulitis · ileus · intestinal obstruction (higher incidence with sevelamer hydrochloride salt) · intestinal perforation · pruritus · rash
- **PREGNANCY** Manufacturer advises use only if potential benefit outweighs risk.
- **BREAST FEEDING** Manufacturer advises use only if potential benefit outweighs risk.
- **PATIENT AND CARER ADVICE**
Medicines for Children leaflet: Sevelamer in dialysis www.medicinesforchildren.org.uk/sevelamer-in-dialysis

- **MEDICINAL FORMS**
There can be variation in the licensing of different medicines containing the same drug.
Tablet
CAUTIONARY AND ADVISORY LABELS 25
EXCIPIENTS: May contain Propylene glycol
▸ Renagel (Sanofi)
Sevelamer 800 mg Renagel 800mg tablets | 180 tablet [PoM] £167.04 DT price = £48.87

2.4b Hypophosphataemia

ELECTROLYTES AND MINERALS ⟩ PHOSPHATES

Phosphate

- **INDICATIONS AND DOSE**

Hypophosphataemia | Hypophosphataemic rickets | Osteomalacia
▸ BY MOUTH USING EFFERVESCENT TABLETS
▸ Neonate: 1 mmol/kg daily in 1-2 divided doses, dose can be taken as a supplement in breast milk—caution advised as solubility in breast milk is limited to 1.2 mmol in 100 mL if calcium also added, contact pharmacy department for details.
▸ Child 1 month-4 years: 2-3 mmol/kg daily in 2-4 divided doses, dose to be adjusted as necessary, dose can be taken as a supplement in breast milk—caution advised as solubility in breast milk is limited to 1.2 mmol in 100 mL if calcium also added, contact pharmacy department for details; maximum 48 mmol per day
▸ Child 5-17 years: 2-3 mmol/kg daily in 2-4 divided doses, dose to be adjusted as necessary; maximum 97 mmol per day
▸ BY INTRAVENOUS INFUSION
▸ Neonate: 1 mmol/kg daily, dose to be adjusted as necessary.
▸ Child 1 month-1 year: 0.7 mmol/kg daily, dose to be adjusted as necessary
▸ Child 2-17 years: 0.4 mmol/kg daily, dose to be adjusted as necessary

> **IMPORTANT SAFETY INFORMATION**
> Some phosphate injection preparations also contain potassium. For peripheral intravenous administration the *concentration* of potassium should not usually exceed 40 mmol/litre. The infusion solution should be **thoroughly mixed**. Local policies on avoiding inadvertent use of potassium concentrate should be followed. The potassium content of some phosphate preparations may also limit the *rate* at which they may be administered.

- **CAUTIONS**
GENERAL CAUTIONS
Cardiac disease · dehydration · diabetes mellitus · sodium and potassium concentrations of preparations
SPECIFIC CAUTIONS
▸ With intravenous use Avoid extravasation · severe tissue necrosis
- **SIDE-EFFECTS**
▸ **Common or very common** Diarrhoea
▸ **Frequency not known** Acute renal failure · hypocalcaemia · hypotension · metastatic calcification · nausea · oedema · phlebitis · tissue necrosis on extravasation
SIDE-EFFECTS, FURTHER INFORMATION
Diarrhoea is a common side-effect and should prompt a reduction in dosage.

9

Blooc and nutrition

- **RENAL IMPAIRMENT** Reduce dose. Monitor closely in renal impairment.
- **MONITORING REQUIREMENTS** It is essential to monitor closely plasma concentrations of calcium, phosphate, potassium, and other electrolytes—excessive doses of phosphates may cause hypocalcaemia and metastatic calcification.
- **DIRECTIONS FOR ADMINISTRATION**
  ▸ With intravenous use Dilute injection with Sodium Chloride 0.9% or 0.45% or Glucose 5% or 10%. Administration rate of phosphate should not exceed 0.05 mmol/kg/hour. In emergencies in intensive care faster rates may be used—seek specialist advice.
- **PRESCRIBING AND DISPENSING INFORMATION** *Phosphate Sandoz®* contains sodium dihydrogen phosphate anhydrous (anhydrous sodium acid phosphate) 1.936 g, sodium bicarbonate 350 mg, potassium bicarbonate 315 mg, equivalent to phosphorus 500 mg (phosphate 16.1 mmol), sodium 468.8 mg (Na$^+$ 20.4 mmol), potassium 123 mg (K$^+$ 3.1 mmol); *Polyfusor NA®* contains Na$^+$ 162 mmol/litre, K$^+$ 19 mmol/litre, PO$_4$$^{3-}$ 100 mmol/litre; non-proprietary *potassium dihydrogen phosphate injection* (potassium acid phosphate)13.6% may contain 1 mmol/mL phosphate, 1 mmol/mL potassium.
- **PATIENT AND CARER ADVICE**
  Medicines for Children leaflet: Phosphate supplements for low phosphate levels www.medicinesforchildren.org.uk/phosphate-supplements-low-phosphate-levels

- **MEDICINAL FORMS**
  There can be variation in the licensing of different medicines containing the same drug. Forms available from special-order manufacturers include: infusion, solution for infusion

  Effervescent tablet
  CAUTIONARY AND ADVISORY LABELS 13
  ▸ Phosphate Sandoz (HK Pharma Ltd)
  Sodium dihydrogen phosphate anhydrous 1.936 gram Phosphate Sandoz effervescent tablets | 100 tablet P £16.43

  Solution for infusion
  ▸ Phosphate (Non-proprietary)
  Potassium dihydrogen phosphate 136 mg per 1 ml Potassium dihydrogen phosphate 13.6% (potassium 10mmol/10ml) solution for infusion 10ml ampoules | 10 ampoule PoM £80.25–£85.00 DT price = £84.63

  Infusion
  ▸ Phosphate (Non-proprietary)
  Potassium dihydrogen phosphate 1.295 gram per 1 litre, Disodium hydrogen phosphate anhydrous 5.75 gram per 1 litre Polyfusor NA phosphates infusion 500ml bottles | 1 bottle PoM £5.15

2.5 Potassium imbalance

2.5a Hyperkalaemia

Other drugs used for Hyperkalaemia Calcium gluconate, p. 568 · Insulin, p. 436 · Salbutamol, p. 150

Calcium polystyrene sulfonate

- **INDICATIONS AND DOSE**

  Hyperkalaemia associated with anuria or severe oliguria, and in dialysis patients
  ▸ BY MOUTH
  ▸ Child: 0.5–1 g/kg daily in divided doses; maximum 60 g per day
  ▸ BY RECTUM
  ▸ Neonate: 0.5–1 g/kg daily, irrigate colon to remove resin after 8–12 hours.

  ▸ Child: 0.5–1 g/kg daily, irrigate colon to remove resin after 8–12 hours; maximum 30 g per day

  SORBISTERIT® POWDER

  Hyperkalaemia associated with anuria or severe oliguria, and in dialysis patients
  ▸ BY MOUTH
  ▸ Child: 0.5–1 g/kg daily, to be given in at least 3 divided doses; maximum 60 g per day
  ▸ BY RECTUM
  ▸ Neonate: 0.5–1 g/kg daily, retained for 6 hours followed by irrigation to remove resin from colon.

  ▸ Child: 0.5–1 g/kg daily, retained for 6 hours followed by irrigation to remove resin from colon; maximum 40 g per day

- **CONTRA-INDICATIONS** Hyperparathyroidism · metastatic carcinoma · multiple myeloma · obstructive bowel disease · reduced gut motility (in neonates) · sarcoidosis
- **CAUTIONS** Impaction of resin with excessive dosage or inadequate dilution
- **INTERACTIONS** → Appendix 1: polystyrene sulfonate
- **SIDE-EFFECTS**

  GENERAL SIDE-EFFECTS
  Anorexia · constipation (discontinue treatment—avoid magnesium-containing laxatives) · diarrhoea · gastric irritation · gastro-intestinal obstruction · hypercalcaemia (including in dialysed patients and occasionally in those with renal impairment) · hypomagnesaemia · intestinal necrosis (reported with concomitant sorbitol) · ischaemic colitis · nausea · necrosis · ulceration · vomiting

  SPECIFIC SIDE-EFFECTS
  ▸ With oral use Gastro-intestinal concretions
  ▸ With rectal use Faecal impaction

- **PREGNANCY** Manufacturers advise use only if potential benefit outweighs risk—no information available.
- **BREAST FEEDING** Manufacturers advise use only if potential benefit outweighs risk—no information available.
- **MONITORING REQUIREMENTS** Monitor for electrolyte disturbances (stop if plasma-potassium concentration below 5 mmol/litre).
- **DIRECTIONS FOR ADMINISTRATION**
  ▸ With rectal use Mix each 1 g of resin with 5 mL of water or 10% glucose.

  SORBISTERIT® POWDER *By mouth*, administer in a small amount of water or soft drink—do not give with fruit juice or squash, which have a high potassium content.

  By rectum, mix each 1 g of resin with 4 mL of 5% glucose.

- **MEDICINAL FORMS**
There can be variation in the licensing of different medicines containing the same drug. Forms available from special-order manufacturers include: enema
Powder
CAUTIONARY AND ADVISORY LABELS 13, 21 (Sorbisterit ® powder only)
EXCIPIENTS: May contain Sucrose
▸ **Calcium Resonium** (Sanofi)
Calcium polystyrene sulfonate 999.34 mg per 1 gram Calcium Resonium powder sugar-free | 300 gram | P | £82.16

Sodium polystyrene sulfonate

- **INDICATIONS AND DOSE**

Hyperkalaemia associated with anuria or severe oliguria, and in dialysis patients
▸ BY MOUTH
▸ Child: 0.5–1 g/kg daily in divided doses; maximum 60 g per day
▸ BY RECTUM
▸ Neonate: 0.5–1 g/kg daily, irrigate colon to remove resin after 8–12 hours.
▸ Child: 0.5–1 g/kg daily, irrigate colon to remove resin after 8–12 hours; maximum 30 g per day

- **CONTRA-INDICATIONS** Obstructive bowel disease · reduced gut motility (in neonates)
- **CAUTIONS** Congestive heart failure · hypertension · impaction of resin with excessive dosage or inadequate dilution · oedema
- **INTERACTIONS** → Appendix 1: polystyrene sulfonate
- **SIDE-EFFECTS**
GENERAL SIDE-EFFECTS
Anorexia · constipation (discontinue treatment—avoid magnesium-containing laxatives) · diarrhoea · gastric irritation · gastro-intestinal obstruction · hypocalcaemia · hypomagnesaemia · intestinal necrosis (reported with concomitant use of sorbitol) · ischaemic colitis · nausea · necrosis · sodium retention · ulceration · vomiting
SPECIFIC SIDE-EFFECTS
▸ With oral use Gastro-intestinal concretions
▸ With rectal use Faecal impaction
- **PREGNANCY** Manufacturers advise use only if potential benefit outweighs risk—no information available.
- **BREAST FEEDING** Manufacturers advise use only if potential benefit outweighs risk—no information available.
- **RENAL IMPAIRMENT** Use with caution.
- **MONITORING REQUIREMENTS** Monitor for electrolyte disturbances (stop if plasma-potassium concentration below 5 mmol/litre).
- **DIRECTIONS FOR ADMINISTRATION**
▸ With rectal use Mix each 1 g of resin with 5 mL of water or 10% glucose.
▸ With oral use Administer dose (powder) in a small amount of water or honey—do not give with fruit juice or squash, which have a high potassium content.
- **MEDICINAL FORMS**
There can be variation in the licensing of different medicines containing the same drug. Forms available from special-order manufacturers include: oral suspension
Powder
CAUTIONARY AND ADVISORY LABELS 13
▸ **Resonium A** (Sanofi)
Sodium polystyrene sulfonate 999.34 mg per 1 gram Resonium A powder sugar-free | 454 gram | P | £81.11

2.5b Hypokalaemia

ELECTROLYTES AND MINERALS ⟩ POTASSIUM

Potassium bicarbonate with potassium acid tartrate

- **INDICATIONS AND DOSE**

Hyperchloraemic acidosis associated with potassium deficiency (as in some renal tubular and gastro-intestinal disorders)
▸ BY MOUTH
▸ Child: (consult product literature)

- **CONTRA-INDICATIONS** Hypochloraemia · plasma-potassium concentration above 5 mmol/litre
- **CAUTIONS** Cardiac disease
- **SIDE-EFFECTS** Abdominal pain · diarrhoea · flatulence · nausea · vomiting
- **RENAL IMPAIRMENT** Avoid in severe impairment. Close monitoring required in renal impairment—high risk of hyperkalaemia.
- **DIRECTIONS FOR ADMINISTRATION** To be dissolved in water before administration.
- **PRESCRIBING AND DISPENSING INFORMATION** These tablets do not contain chloride.

- **MEDICINAL FORMS**
There can be variation in the licensing of different medicines containing the same drug.
Effervescent tablet
CAUTIONARY AND ADVISORY LABELS 13, 21
▸ Potassium bicarbonate with potassium acid tartrate (Non-proprietary)
Potassium acid tartrate 300 mg, Potassium bicarbonate 500 mg Potassium (potassium 6.5mmol) effervescent tablets BPC 1968 | 56 tablet | GSL | £77.77–£99.15 DT price = £92.02

Potassium chloride

- **INDICATIONS AND DOSE**

Prevention of hypokalaemia (patients with normal diet)
▸ BY MOUTH
▸ Child: 1–2 mmol/kg daily; Usual maximum 50 mmol
Electrolyte imbalance
▸ BY INTRAVENOUS INFUSION
▸ Neonate: 1–2 mmol/kg daily, dose dependent on deficit or the daily maintenance requirements.
▸ Child: 1–2 mmol/kg daily, dose dependent on deficit or the daily maintenance requirements
Potassium depletion
▸ BY MOUTH
▸ Neonate: 0.5–1 mmol/kg twice daily, total daily dose may alternatively be given in 3 divided doses, dose to be adjusted according to plasma-potassium concentration.
▸ Child: 0.5–1 mmol/kg twice daily, total daily dose may alternatively be given in 3 divided doses, dose to be adjusted according to plasma-potassium concentration

IMPORTANT SAFETY INFORMATION
SAFE PRACTICE
Potassium overdose can be fatal. Ready-mixed infusion solutions containing potassium should be used. Exceptionally, if potassium chloride concentrate is used for preparing an infusion, the infusion solution should be **thoroughly mixed**. Local policies on avoiding

9

Blood and nutrition

9

Blood and nutrition

inadvertent use of potassium chloride concentrate should be followed.

- **CONTRA-INDICATIONS** Plasma-potassium concentration above 5 mmol/litre
- **CAUTIONS**
  ‣ With intravenous use Seek specialist advice in very severe potassium depletion or difficult cases
  ‣ With oral use Cardiac disease · hiatus hernia (*with modified-release preparations*) · history of peptic ulcer (*with modified-release preparations*) · intestinal stricture (*with modified-release preparations*)
- **INTERACTIONS** → Appendix 1: potassium chloride
- **SIDE-EFFECTS**
  ‣ Common or very common
  ‣ With oral use Abdominal pain · diarrhoea · flatulence · nausea · vomiting
  ‣ Frequency not known
  ‣ With intravenous use Heart toxicity (with rapid infusion)
  ‣ With oral use Bleeding (*with modified-release preparations*) · gastro-intestinal obstruction (*with modified-release preparations*) · ulceration (*with modified-release preparations*)
- **RENAL IMPAIRMENT** Smaller doses must be used in the prevention of hypokalaemia, to reduce the risk of hyperkalaemia. Avoid in severe impairment. Close monitoring required in renal impairment—high risk of hyperkalaemia.
- **MONITORING REQUIREMENTS**
  ‣ Regular monitoring of plasma-potassium concentration is essential in those taking potassium supplements.
  ‣ With intravenous use ECG monitoring should be performed in difficult cases.
- **DIRECTIONS FOR ADMINISTRATION**
  ‣ With oral use in neonates Potassium chloride solutions suitable for use by mouth in neonates are available from 'special order' manufacturers or specialist importing companies; they should be used with care because they are hypertonic and can damage the gastric mucosa.
  ‣ With oral use Potassium salts are preferably given as a liquid (or effervescent) preparation, rather than modified-release tablets; they should be given as the chloride (the use of effervescent potassium tablets BPC 1968 should be restricted to *hyperchloraemic* states).
  ‣ With intravenous use Potassium chloride concentrate must be diluted with **not less** than 50 times its volume of sodium chloride intravenous infusion 0.9% or other suitable diluent and **mixed well**.
  ‣ With intravenous use Ready-mixed infusion solutions should be used when possible. For *peripheral intravenous infusion*, the concentration of potassium should not usually exceed 40 mmol/L. Potassium infusions should be given slowly over at least 2–3 hours and at a rate not exceeding 0.2 mmol/kg/hour with specialist advice and ECG monitoring in difficult cases. Higher concentrations of potassium chloride or faster infusion rates may be given in very severe depletion, but require specialist advice.
- **PRESCRIBING AND DISPENSING INFORMATION** Kay-Cee-L® contains 1 mmol/mL each of K⁺ and Cl⁻.
  Potassium Tablets
  Do not confuse Effervescent Potassium Tablets BPC 1968 with effervescent potassium chloride tablets. Effervescent Potassium Tablets BPC 1968 do not contain chloride ions and their use should be restricted to hyperchloraemic states.
- **PATIENT AND CARER ADVICE** Patient or carers should be given advice on how to administer potassium chloride modified-release tablets.
  Salt substitutes A number of salt substitutes which contain significant amounts of potassium chloride are readily available as health food products (e.g. *LoSalt®* and

Ruthmol®). These should not be used by patients with renal failure as potassium intoxication may result.

- **LESS SUITABLE FOR PRESCRIBING** Modified-release tablets are less suitable for prescribing. Modified-release preparations should be avoided unless effervescent tablets or liquid preparations inappropriate.

- **MEDICINAL FORMS**
  There can be variation in the licensing of different medicines containing the same drug. Forms available from special-order manufacturers include: modified-release tablet, oral solution, infusion, solution for infusion

  Modified-release tablet
  CAUTIONARY AND ADVISORY LABELS 25, 27
  ‣ **Potassium chloride (Non-proprietary)**
  Potassium chloride 600 mg Kaleorid LP 600mg tablets | 30 tablet [PoM] no price available
  Duro-K 600mg tablets | 100 tablet [PoM] no price available

  Solution for infusion
  ‣ **Potassium chloride (Non-proprietary)**
  Potassium chloride 150 mg per 1 ml Potassium chloride 15% (potassium 20mmol/10ml) solution for infusion 10ml ampoules | 10 ampoule [PoM] £6.50 | 20 ampoule [PoM] £6.50
  Potassium chloride 15% (potassium 20mmol/10ml) solution for infusion 10ml Mini-Plasco ampoules | 20 ampoule [PoM] £10.70
  Potassium chloride 200 mg per 1 ml Potassium chloride 20% (potassium 13.3mmol/5ml) solution for infusion 5ml ampoules | 10 ampoule [PoM] £3.84-£4.00
  Potassium chloride 20% (potassium 27mmol/10ml) solution for infusion 10ml ampoules | 10 ampoule [PoM] £121.25

  Oral solution
  CAUTIONARY AND ADVISORY LABELS 21
  ‣ **Kay-Cee-L** (Geistlich Sons Ltd)
  Potassium chloride 75 mg per 1 ml Kay-Cee-L syrup sugar-free | 500 ml [P] £7.95

3 Metabolic disorders

Metabolic disorders

Use of medicines in metabolic disorders

Metabolic disorders should be managed under the guidance of a specialist. As many preparations are unlicensed and may be difficult to obtain, arrangements for continued prescribing and supply should be made in primary care.

General advice on the use of medicines in metabolic disorders can be obtained from:
Alder Hey Children's Hospital, Medicines Information Centre
(0151) 252 5381
and
Great Ormond Street Hospital for Children, pharmacy
(020) 7405 9200

Urea cycle disorders

Sodium benzoate p. 587 and sodium phenylbutyrate p. 588 are used in the management of urea cycle disorders. Both, either singly or in combination, are indicated as adjunctive therapy in all patients with neonatal-onset disease and in those with late-onset disease who have a history of hyperammonaemic encephalopathy. Sodium benzoate is also used in non-ketotic hyperglycinaemia.

The long-term management of urea cycle disorders includes oral maintenance treatment with sodium benzoate and sodium phenylbutyrate combined with a low protein diet and other drugs such as arginine p. 586 or citrulline p. 587, depending on the specific disorder.

Emergency management

For further information on the emergency management of urea cycle disorders consult the British Inherited Metabolic Disease Group (BIMDG) website at: www.bimdg.org.uk.

3.1 Acute porphyrias

Acute porphyrias

Overview

The acute porphyrias (acute intermittent porphyria, variegate porphyria, hereditary coproporphyria, and 5-aminolaevulinic acid dehydratase deficiency porphyria) are hereditary disorders of haem biosynthesis; they have a prevalence of about 1 in 10 000 of the population.

Great care must be taken when prescribing for patients with acute porphyria, since certain drugs can induce acute porphyric crises. Since acute porphyrias are hereditary, relatives of affected individuals should be screened and advised about the potential danger of certain drugs. Acute attacks of porphyria are exceptionally rare before puberty. When acute porphyria is suspected in a child, support from an expert porphyria service should be sought.

Treatment of serious or life-threatening conditions should not be withheld from patients with acute porphyria. When there is no safe alternative, treatment should be started and urinary porphobilinogen excretion should be measured regularly; if it increases or symptoms occur, the drug can be withdrawn and the acute attack treated. If an acute attack of porphyria occurs during pregnancy, contact an expert porphyria service for further advice.

Haem arginate p. 578 is administered by short intravenous infusion as haem replacement in moderate, severe, or unremitting acute porphyria crises.

In the United Kingdom the National Acute Porphyria Service (NAPS) provides clinical support and treatment with haem arginate from three centres (University Hospital of Wales, Addenbrooke's Hospital, and King's College Hospital). To access the service telephone (029) 2074 7747 and ask for the Acute Porphyria Service.

Drugs unsafe for use in acute porphyrias

The following list contains drugs on the UK market that have been classified as 'unsafe' in porphyria because they have been shown to be porphyrinogenic in animals or in vitro, or have been associated with acute attacks in patients. Absence of a drug from the following lists does not necessarily imply that the drug is safe. For many drugs no information about porphyria is available.

An up-to-date list of drugs considered **safe** in acute porphyrias is available at www.wmic.wales.nhs.uk/specialist-services/drugs-in-porphyria/. Further information may be obtained from: www.porphyria-europe.org and also from:

Welsh Medicines Information Centre
University Hospital of Wales
CF14 4XW
Cardiff
(029) 2074 2979/3877

Quite modest changes in chemical structure can lead to changes in porphyrinogenicity but where possible general statements have been made about groups of drugs; these should be checked first.

Unsafe Drug Groups (check first)

- Alkylating drugs (contact Welsh Medicines Information Centre for further advice)
- Anabolic steroids
- Antidepressants (includes tricyclic (and related) antidepressants and MAOIs; fluoxetine, duloxetine, venlafaxine, and trazodone thought to be safe)
- Antihistamines (alimemazine, chlorphenamine, desloratadine, fexofenadine, ketotifen, loratadine, and promethazine thought to be safe)
- Barbiturates (includes primidone and thiopental)
- Calcium channel blockers (amlodipine, felodipine, and nifedipine thought to be safe)
- Contraceptives, hormonal (progestogens are more porphyrinogenic than oestrogens; oestrogens may be safe at least in replacement doses. Progestogens should be avoided whenever possible by all women susceptible to acute porphyria; however, when non-hormonal contraception is inappropriate, progestogens may be used with extreme caution if the potential benefit outweighs risk. The risk of an acute attack is greatest in young women who have had a previous attack. Long-acting progestogen preparations should **never** be used in those at risk of acute porphyria.)
- Ergot derivatives (includes ergometrine (oxytocin probably safe) and pergolide)
- Imidazole antifungals (applies to oral and intravenous use; topical antifungals are thought to be safe due to low systemic exposure)
- Non-nucleoside reverse transcriptase inhibitors (contact Welsh Medicines Information Centre for further advice)
- Progestogens (progestogens are more porphyrinogenic than oestrogens; oestrogens may be safe at least in replacement doses. Progestogens should be avoided whenever possible by all women susceptible to acute porphyria; however, when non-hormonal contraception is inappropriate, progestogens may be used with extreme caution if the potential benefit outweighs risk. The risk of an acute attack is greatest in young women who have had a previous attack. Long-acting progestogen preparations should **never** be used in those at risk of acute porphyria.)
- Protease inhibitors (contact Welsh Medicines Information Centre for further advice)
- Sulfonamides (includes co-trimoxazole and sulfasalazine)
- Sulfonylureas (glipizide is thought to be safe)
- Taxanes (contact Welsh Medicines Information Centre for further advice)
- Thiazolidinediones (contact Welsh Medicines Information Centre for further advice)
- Triazole antifungals (applies to oral and intravenous use; topical antifungals are thought to be safe due to low systemic exposure)

Unsafe drugs (check groups above first)

- Aceclofenac
- Alcohol
- Amiodarone
- Aprepitant (contact Welsh Medicines Information Centre for further advice)
- Artemether with lumefantrine
- Bexarotene
- Bosentan
- Bromocriptine
- Buspirone
- Cabergoline
- Carbamazepine
- Chloral hydrate (although evidence of hazard is uncertain, manufacturer advises avoid)
- Chloramphenicol
- Chloroform (small amounts in medicines probably safe)
- Clindamycin
- Cocaine
- Colistimethate sodium
- Danazol
- Dapsone
- Dexfenfluramine
- Disopyramide
- Disulfiram
- Erythromycin

- Etamsylate
- Ethosuximide
- Etomidate
- Fenfluramine
- Flupentixol
- Flutamide
- Fosaprepitant (contact Welsh Medicines Information Centre for further advice)
- Fosphenytoin
- Griseofulvin
- Hydralazine
- Indapamide
- Isometheptene mucate
- Isoniazid (safety uncertain, contact Welsh Medicines Information Centre for further advice)
- Ketamine
- Mefenamic acid (may be used with caution if safer alternative not available)
- Meprobamate
- Methyldopa
- Metolazone
- Metyrapone
- Mifepristone
- Minoxidil (may be used with caution if safer alternative not available)
- Mitotane
- Nalidixic acid
- Nitrazepam
- Nitrofurantoin
- Orphenadrine
- Oxcarbazepine
- Oxybutynin
- Pentazocine (buprenorphine, codeine, diamorphine, dihydrocodeine, fentanyl, methadone, morphine, oxycodone, pethidine, and tramadol are thought to be safe)
- Pentoxifylline
- Phenoxybenzamine
- Phenytoin
- Pivmecillinam
- Porfimer
- Potassium canrenoate (evidence of hazard uncertain—contact Welsh Medicines Information Centre for further advice)
- Raloxifene
- Rifabutin (safety uncertain, contact Welsh Medicines Information Centre for further advice)
- Rifampicin
- Riluzole
- Risperidone
- Selegiline
- Spironolactone
- Sulfinpyrazone
- Tamoxifen
- Telithromycin
- Temoporfin
- Tiagabine
- Tibolone
- Tinidazole
- Topiramate
- Toremifene
- Trimethoprim
- Valproate
- Xipamide
- Zidovudine (contact Welsh Medicines Information Centre for further advice)
- Zuclopenthixol

BLOOD AND RELATED PRODUCTS ⟩ HAEM DERIVATIVES

Haem arginate

(Human hemin)

- **INDICATIONS AND DOSE**

Acute porphyrias | Acute intermittent porphyria | Porphyria variegata | Hereditary coproporphyria
▸ BY INTRAVENOUS INFUSION
  ▸ Child: Initially 3 mg/kg once daily for 4 days, if response inadequate, repeat 4-day course with close biochemical monitoring; maximum 250 mg per day

- **SIDE-EFFECTS**
▸ **Common or very common** Pain at injection site · thrombophlebitis at injection site
▸ **Rare** Fever · hypersensitivity reactions
▸ **Frequency not known** Headache

- **PREGNANCY** Manufacturer advises avoid unless essential.
- **BREAST FEEDING** Manufacturer advises avoid unless essential—no information available.
- **DIRECTIONS FOR ADMINISTRATION** Administer over at least 30 minutes through a filter via large antebrachial or central vein; dilute requisite dose in 100 mL Sodium Chloride 0.9% in glass bottle; administer within 1 hour after dilution; max. concentration 2.5 mg/mL.

- **MEDICINAL FORMS**
There can be variation in the licensing of different medicines containing the same drug.
Solution for infusion
▸ **Normosang** (Orphan Europe (UK) Ltd)
  Haem arginate 25 mg per 1 ml Normosang 250mg/10ml solution for infusion ampoules | 4 ampoule [PoM] £1,737.00

3.2 Carnitine deficiency

AMINO ACIDS AND DERIVATIVES

Levocarnitine

(Carnitine)

- **INDICATIONS AND DOSE**

Primary carnitine deficiency due to inborn errors of metabolism
▸ BY MOUTH
  ▸ Neonate: Up to 200 mg/kg daily in 2–4 divided doses.

  ▸ Child: Up to 200 mg/kg daily in 2–4 divided doses; maximum 3 g per day
  ▸ INITIALLY BY INTRAVENOUS INFUSION

  ▸ Neonate: Initially 100 mg/kg, to be administered over 30 minutes, followed by (by continuous intravenous infusion) 4 mg/kg/hour.

  ▸ Child: Initially 100 mg/kg, to be administered over 30 minutes, followed by (by continuous intravenous infusion) 4 mg/kg/hour
  ▸ BY SLOW INTRAVENOUS INJECTION

  ▸ Neonate: Up to 100 mg/kg daily in 2–4 divided doses, to be administered over 2–3 minutes.

  ▸ Child: Up to 100 mg/kg daily in 2–4 divided doses, to be administered over 2–3 minutes

Secondary carnitine deficiency in haemodialysis patients
▸ INITIALLY BY SLOW INTRAVENOUS INJECTION
▸ **Child:** 20 mg/kg, to be administered over 2–3 minutes, after each dialysis session, dosage adjusted according to plasma-carnitine concentration, then (by mouth) maintenance 1 g daily, administered if benefit is gained from first intravenous course

Organic acidaemias
▸ BY MOUTH
▸ **Neonate:** Up to 200 mg/kg daily in 2–4 divided doses.

▸ **Child:** Up to 200 mg/kg daily in 2–4 divided doses; maximum 3 g per day
▸ INITIALLY BY INTRAVENOUS INFUSION
▸ **Neonate:** Initially 100 mg/kg, to be administered over 30 minutes, followed by (by continuous intravenous infusion) 4 mg/kg/hour.

▸ **Child:** Initially 100 mg/kg, to be administered over 30 minutes, followed by (by continuous intravenous infusion) 4 mg/kg/hour
▸ BY SLOW INTRAVENOUS INJECTION
▸ **Neonate:** Up to 100 mg/kg daily in 2–4 divided doses, to be administered over 2–3 minutes.

▸ **Child:** Up to 100 mg/kg daily in 2–4 divided doses, to be administered over 2–3 minutes

● **UNLICENSED USE** Not licensed for use in organic acidaemias. Not licensed for use by intravenous infusion. Tablets, chewable tablets, and oral liquid (10%) not licensed in children under 12 years. Paediatric oral solution (30%) not licensed in children over 12 years.

● **CAUTIONS** Diabetes mellitus

● **SIDE-EFFECTS** Abdominal pain · body odour · diarrhoea · nausea · vomiting

SIDE-EFFECTS, FURTHER INFORMATION
Side-effects may be dose-related—monitor tolerance during first week and after any dose increase.

● **PREGNANCY** Appropriate to use; no evidence of teratogenicity in *animal* studies.

● **RENAL IMPAIRMENT** Accumulation of metabolites may occur with chronic oral administration in severe impairment.

● **MONITORING REQUIREMENTS**
▸ Monitoring of free and acyl carnitine in blood and urine recommended.

● **DIRECTIONS FOR ADMINISTRATION**
▸ With intravenous use For *intravenous infusion*, dilute injection with Sodium Chloride 0.9% or Glucose 5% or 10%.

● **PRESCRIBING AND DISPENSING INFORMATION**
▸ When used for Organic acidaemias Levocarnitine is used in the treatment of some organic acidaemias; however, use in fatty acid oxidation is controversial.

● **PATIENT AND CARER ADVICE**
Medicines for Children leaflet: Carnitine for metabolic disorders www.medicinesforchildren.org.uk/carnitine-metabolic-disorders-0

● **MEDICINAL FORMS**
There can be variation in the licensing of different medicines containing the same drug. Forms available from special-order manufacturers include: capsule

Solution for injection
▸ Carnitor (Logixx Pharma Solutions Ltd)
L-Carnitine 200 mg per 1 ml Carnitor 1g/5ml solution for injection ampoules | 5 ampoule PoM £59.50

Oral solution
▸ Levocarnitine (Non-proprietary)
L-Carnitine 300 mg per 1 ml Levocarnitine 1.5g/5ml (30%) oral solution paediatric | 20 ml PoM £71.40 DT price = £71.40
▸ Carnitor (Logixx Pharma Solutions Ltd)
L-Carnitine 100 mg per 1 ml Carnitor oral single dose 1g solution sugar-free | 10 unit dose PoM £35.00

Chewable tablet
▸ Carnitor (Logixx Pharma Solutions Ltd)
L-Carnitine 1 gram Carnitor 1g chewable tablets | 10 tablet PoM £35.00

Capsule
▸ Levocarnitine (Non-proprietary)
L-Carnitine 250 mg Carnitine 250mg capsules | 125 capsule £11.06
L-Carnitine 500 mg L-Carnitine 500mg capsules | 60 capsule £11.14

3.3 Fabry's disease

ENZYMES

Agalsidase alfa

● **DRUG ACTION** Agalsidase alfa, an enzyme produced by recombinant DNA technology are licensed for long-term enzyme replacement therapy in Fabry's disease (a lysosomal storage disorder caused by deficiency of alpha-galactosidase A).

● **INDICATIONS AND DOSE**
Fabry's disease (specialist use only)
▸ BY INTRAVENOUS INFUSION
▸ **Child 7-17 years:** 200 micrograms/kg every 2 weeks

● **INTERACTIONS** → Appendix 1: agalsidase

● **SIDE-EFFECTS**
▸ **Common or very common** Acne · angioedema · arthralgia · asthenia · bradycardia · chest pain · cough · dizziness · dyspnoea · eye irritation · fatigue · flushing · gastro-intestinal disturbances · headache · hypersensitivity reactions · hypertension · hypotension · influenza- like symptoms · muscle spasms · myalgia · nasopharyngitis · neuropathic pain · oedema · palpitation · paraesthesia · pruritus · rash · rhinorrhoea · sleep disturbances · syncope · tachycardia · taste disturbances · tinnitus · tremor · urticaria
▸ **Uncommon** Cold extremities · ear pain · ear swelling · injection-site reactions · parosmia · skin discoloration

SIDE-EFFECTS, FURTHER INFORMATION
▸ Infusion-related reactions Infusion-related reactions very common; manage by slowing the infusion rate or interrupting the infusion, or minimise by pre-treatment with an antihistamine, antipyretic, or corticosteroid—consult product literature.

● **PREGNANCY** Use with caution.

● **BREAST FEEDING** Use with caution—no information available.

● **DIRECTIONS FOR ADMINISTRATION** Administration for *intravenous infusion*, dilute requisite dose with 100 mL Sodium Chloride 0.9% and give over 40 minutes using an in-line filter; use within 3 hours of dilution.

● **MEDICINAL FORMS**
There can be variation in the licensing of different medicines containing the same drug.
Solution for infusion
▸ Replagal (Shire Pharmaceuticals Ltd)
Agalsidase alfa 1 mg per 1 ml Replagal 3.5mg/3.5ml solution for infusion vials | 1 vial PoM £1,068.64

9

Blood and nutrition

Agalsidase beta

- **DRUG ACTION** Agalsidase beta, an enzyme produced by recombinant DNA technology are licensed for long-term enzyme replacement therapy in Fabry's disease (a lysosomal storage disorder caused by deficiency of alpha-galactosidase A).

- **INDICATIONS AND DOSE**

Fabry's disease (specialist use only)
  ▶ BY INTRAVENOUS INFUSION
  ▸ Child 8-17 years: 1 mg/kg every 2 weeks

- **INTERACTIONS** → Appendix 1: agalsidase

- **SIDE-EFFECTS**
  ▸ **Common or very common** Acne · angioedema · arthralgia · asthenia · bradycardia · chest pain · cough · dizziness · dyspnoea · eye irritation · fatigue · flushing · gastro-intestinal disturbances · headache · hypersensitivity reactions · hypertension · hypotension · influenza- like symptoms · muscle spasms · myalgia · nasopharyngitis · neuropathic pain · oedema · palpitation · paraesthesia · pruritus · rash · rhinorrhoea · sleep disturbances · syncope · tachycardia · taste disturbances · tinnitus · tremor · urticaria
  ▸ **Uncommon** Cold extremities · ear pain · ear swelling · injection-site reactions · parosmia · skin discoloration

  SIDE-EFFECTS, FURTHER INFORMATION
  ▸ Infusion-related reactions Infusion-related reactions very common; manage by slowing the infusion rate or interrupting the infusion, or minimise by pre-treatment with an antihistamine, antipyretic, or corticosteroid—consult product literature.

- **PREGNANCY** Use with caution.

- **BREAST FEEDING** Use with caution—no information available.

- **DIRECTIONS FOR ADMINISTRATION** For *intravenous infusion*, given intermittently in Sodium chloride 0.9%, reconstitute initially with Water for Injections (5 mg in 1.1 mL, 35 mg in 7.2 mL) to produce a solution containing 5 mg/mL. Dilute with Sodium Chloride 0.9% (for doses less than 35 mg dilute with at least 50 mL; doses 35–70 mg dilute with at least 100 mL; doses 70–100 mg dilute with at least 250 mL; doses greater than 100 mg dilute with 500 mL) and give through an in-line low protein-binding 0.2 micron filter at an initial rate of no more than 15 mg/hour; for subsequent infusions, infusion rate may be increased gradually once tolerance has been established.

- **MEDICINAL FORMS**
  There can be variation in the licensing of different medicines containing the same drug.
  Powder for solution for infusion
  ▸ Fabrazyme (Genzyme Therapeutics Ltd)
  Agalsidase beta 5 mg Fabrazyme 5mg powder for solution for infusion vials | 1 vial PoM £315.08
  Agalsidase beta 35 mg Fabrazyme 35mg powder for solution for infusion vials | 1 vial PoM £2,196.59

3.4 Gaucher's disease

ENZYMES

Imiglucerase

- **DRUG ACTION** Imiglucerase is an enzyme produced by recombinant DNA technology that is administered as enzyme replacement therapy for non-neurological manifestations of type I or type III Gaucher's disease, a familial disorder affecting principally the liver, spleen, bone marrow, and lymph nodes.

- **INDICATIONS AND DOSE**

Gaucher's disease type I (specialist use only)
  ▶ BY INTRAVENOUS INFUSION
  ▸ Neonate: Initially 60 units/kg every 2 weeks, adjusted according to response, doses as low as 30 units/kg once every 2 weeks may be appropriate.
  ▸ Child: Initially 60 units/kg every 2 weeks, adjusted according to response, doses as low as 30 units/kg once every 2 weeks may be appropriate

Gaucher's disease type III (specialist use only)
  ▶ BY INTRAVENOUS INFUSION
  ▸ Neonate: Initially 60–120 units/kg every 2 weeks, adjusted according to response.
  ▸ Child: Initially 60–120 units/kg every 2 weeks, adjusted according to response

- **SIDE-EFFECTS**
  ▸ **Common or very common** Angioedema · backache · cyanosis · flushing · hypersensitivity reactions · hypotension · paraesthesia · tachycardia · urticaria
  ▸ **Uncommon** Abdominal cramps · arthralgia · diarrhoea · dizziness · fatigue · fever · headache · injection-site reactions · nausea · vomiting

- **PREGNANCY** Manufacturer advises use with caution—limited information available.

- **BREAST FEEDING** No information available.

- **MONITORING REQUIREMENTS**
  ▸ Monitor for immunoglobulin G (IgG) antibodies to imiglucerase.
  ▸ When stabilised, monitor all parameters and response to treatment at intervals of 6–12 months.

- **DIRECTIONS FOR ADMINISTRATION** For *intravenous infusion* (*Cerezyme®*), give intermittently in Sodium chloride 0.9%; initially reconstitute with water for injections (200 units in 5.1 mL, 400 units in 10.2 mL) to give 40 units/mL solution; dilute requisite dose with infusion fluid to a final volume of 100–200 mL and give initial dose at a rate not exceeding 0.5 units/kg/minute, subsequent doses to be given at a rate not exceeding 1 unit/kg/minute; administer within 3 hours after reconstitution.

- **MEDICINAL FORMS**
  There can be variation in the licensing of different medicines containing the same drug.
  Powder for solution for infusion
  ELECTROLYTES: May contain Sodium
  ▸ Cerezyme (Genzyme Therapeutics Ltd)
  Imiglucerase 400 unit Cerezyme 400unit powder for solution for infusion vials | 1 vial PoM £1,071.29

Velaglucerase alfa

- **DRUG ACTION** Velaglucerase alfa is an enzyme produced by recombinant DNA technology that is administered as enzyme replacement therapy for the treatment of type I Gaucher's disease.

- **INDICATIONS AND DOSE**

Type I Gaucher's disease (specialist use only)
- ▸ BY INTRAVENOUS INFUSION
- ▸ Child 4–17 years: Initially 60 units/kg every 2 weeks; adjusted according to response to 15–60 units/kg every 2 weeks

- **SIDE-EFFECTS** Abdominal pain · arthralgia · back pain · bone pain · dizziness · flushing · headache · hypersensitivity reactions · hypertension · hypotension · malaise · nausea · pyrexia · rash · tachycardia · urticaria

SIDE-EFFECTS, FURTHER INFORMATION
- ▸ Infusion-related reactions Infusion-related reactions very common; manage by slowing the infusion rate, or interrupting the infusion, or minimise by pre-treatment with an antihistamine, antipyretic, or corticosteroid—consult product literature.

- **PREGNANCY** Manufacturer advises use with caution—limited information available.

- **BREAST FEEDING** Manufacturer advises use with caution—no information available.

- **MONITORING REQUIREMENTS** Monitor immunoglobulin G (IgG) antibody concentration in severe infusion-related reactions or if there is a lack or loss of effect with velaglucerase alfa.

- **DIRECTIONS FOR ADMINISTRATION** For *intravenous infusion*, reconstitute each 400-unit vial with 4.3 mL water for injections; dilute requisite dose in 100 mL Sodium Chloride 0.9% and give over 60 minutes through a 0.22 micron filter; start infusion within 24 hours of reconstitution.

- **MEDICINAL FORMS**
There can be variation in the licensing of different medicines containing the same drug.
Powder for solution for infusion
ELECTROLYTES: May contain Sodium
- ▸ VPRIV (Shire Pharmaceuticals Ltd)
Velaglucerase alfa 400 unit VPRIV 400units powder for solution for infusion vials | 1 vial [PoM] £1,410.20

3.5 Homocystinuria

METHYL DONORS

Betaine

- **INDICATIONS AND DOSE**

Adjunctive treatment of homocystinuria involving deficiencies or defects in cystathionine beta-synthase, 5,10-methylene-tetrahydrofolate reductase, or cobalamin cofactor metabolism (specialist use only)
- ▸ BY MOUTH
- ▸ Neonate: Initially 50 mg/kg twice daily (max. per dose 75 mg/kg), adjusted according to response; maximum 150 mg/kg per day.
- ▸ Child 1 month–9 years: Initially 50 mg/kg twice daily (max. per dose 75 mg/kg), adjusted according to response; maximum 150 mg/kg per day
- ▸ Child 10–17 years: 3 g twice daily (max. per dose 10 g), adjusted according to response; maximum 20 g per day

- **SIDE-EFFECTS**
- ▸ **Uncommon** Agitation · alopecia · anorexia · depression · gastro-intestinal disorders · personality disorder · reversible cerebral oedema · sleep disturbances · urinary incontinence · urticaria

- **PREGNANCY** Manufacturer advises avoid unless essential—limited information available.

- **BREAST FEEDING** Manufacturer advises caution—no information available.

- **MONITORING REQUIREMENTS** Monitor plasma-methionine concentration before and during treatment—interrupt treatment if symptoms of cerebral oedema occur.

- **DIRECTIONS FOR ADMINISTRATION** Powder should be mixed with water, juice, milk, formula, or food until completely dissolved and taken immediately; measuring spoons are provided to measure 1 g, 150 mg, and 100 mg of *Cystadane*® powder.

- **PRESCRIBING AND DISPENSING INFORMATION** Betaine should be used in conjunction with dietary restrictions and may be given with supplements of Vitamin B_{12}, pyridoxine, and folate under specialist advice.

- **NATIONAL FUNDING/ACCESS DECISIONS**

Scottish Medicines Consortium (SMC) Decisions
The *Scottish Medicines Consortium* has advised (July 2010) that betaine anhydrous (Cystadane®) is accepted for restricted use within NHS Scotland for the adjunctive treatment of homocystinuria involving deficiencies or defects in cystathionine beta-synthase, 5,10-methylene-tetrahydrofolate reductase, or cobalamin cofactor metabolism in patients who are not responsive to pyridoxine treatment.

- **MEDICINAL FORMS**
There can be variation in the licensing of different medicines containing the same drug. Forms available from special-order manufacturers include: tablet, oral solution
Powder
- ▸ Cystadane (Orphan Europe (UK) Ltd)
Betaine 1 gram per 1 gram Cystadane oral powder | 180 gram [PoM] £347.00

3.6 Mitochondrial disorders

CO-ENZYMES

Ubidecarenone

(Ubiquinone; Co-enzyme Q10)

- **INDICATIONS AND DOSE**

Mitochondrial disorders
- ▸ BY MOUTH
- ▸ Neonate: Initially 5 mg 1–2 times a day, adjusted according to response, dose too be taken with food, increased if necessary up to 200 mg daily.
- ▸ Child: Initially 5 mg 1–2 times a day, adjusted according to response, dose to be taken with food, increased if necessary up to 300 mg daily

- **UNLICENSED USE** Not licensed.

- **CAUTIONS** May reduce insulin requirement in diabetes mellitus

- **SIDE-EFFECTS**
- ▸ **Common or very common** Diarrhoea · heartburn · nausea
- ▸ **Rare** Agitation · dizziness · headache · irritability

- **HEPATIC IMPAIRMENT** Reduce dose in moderate and severe impairment.

9

Blood and nutrition

- **PATIENT AND CARER ADVICE**
  Medicines for Children leaflet: Ubidecarenone for mitochondrial disease www.medicinesforchildren.org.uk/ubidecarenone-for-mitochondrial-disease

- **MEDICINAL FORMS**
  There can be variation in the licensing of different medicines containing the same drug. Forms available from special-order manufacturers include: oral solution, oral drops

Tablet
  ▸ **Ubidecarenone** (Non-proprietary)
    Ubidecarenone 30 mg Co-enzyme Q10 30mg tablets | 30 tablet £6.90 | 90 tablet £19.21

Oral drops
  ▸ **Ubidecarenone** (Non-proprietary)
    Ubidecarenone 5 mg per 1 ml Ubicor 5mg/ml oral drops | 10 ml [PoM] no price available

Chewable tablet
  ▸ **Ubidecarenone** (Non-proprietary)
    Ubidecarenone 25 mg Coenzyme Q10 25mg chewable tablets sugar-free | 250 tablet [PoM] no price available

Capsule
  ▸ **Ubidecarenone** (Non-proprietary)
    Ubidecarenone 30 mg Co-Enzyme Q10 30mg capsules | 60 capsule £8.51 | 180 capsule £17.64
    Co-Enzyme Q10 30mg capsules | 30 capsule £6.96 | 60 capsule £12.17 | 120 capsule £21.78
    Ubidecarenone 60 mg Solgar CoQ-10 60mg capsules | 30 capsule no price available
    Ubidecarenone 100 mg BioActive Q10 Uniquinol 100mg capsules | 60 capsule £26.57 | 150 capsule £53.14
    G & G CoQ10 100mg capsules | 60 capsule £9.00
    Natures Aid Co-Q-10 100mg capsules | 30 capsule £9.42 | 90 capsule £22.69
    Co-Enzyme Q10 100mg capsules | 60 capsule £16.50
    Bio-Quinone Q10 GOLD 100mg capsules | 20 capsule £8.12 | 60 capsule £21.03 | 150 capsule £42.09
    Ubidecarenone 120 mg HealthAid Mega CO-Q-10 120mg capsules | 30 capsule £15.07
    Ubidecarenone 200 mg Co-Enzyme Q10 200mg capsules | 60 capsule £20.07
    Ubidecarenone 300 mg Natures Aid Co-Q-10 300mg capsules | 60 capsule £22.21
  ▸ **Super Bio-Quinone** (Pharma Nord (UK) Ltd)
    Ubidecarenone 30 mg Super Bio-Quinone Q10 30mg capsules | 30 capsule £4.96 | 60 capsule £8.84 | 150 capsule £15.77

3.7 Mucopolysaccharidosis

ENZYMES

Elosulfase alfa

01-Sep-2016

- **DRUG ACTION** Elosulfase alfa is an enzyme produced by recombinant DNA technology that provides replacement therapy in conditions caused by N-acetylgalactosamine-6-sulfatase (GALNS) deficiency.

- **INDICATIONS AND DOSE**
  Mucopolysaccharidosis IVA (specialist use only)
  ▸ BY INTRAVENOUS INFUSION

  ▸ Neonate: 2 mg/kg once weekly.

  ▸ Child: 2 mg/kg once weekly

- **CAUTIONS** Infusion-related reactions
  CAUTIONS, FURTHER INFORMATION
  ▸ Infusion-related reactions Infusion-related reactions can occur; manufacturer advises these may be minimised by pre-treatment with an antihistamine and antipyretic, given 30-60 minutes before treatment. If reaction is severe, stop infusion and start appropriate treatment. Caution and close monitoring is advised during re-administration following a severe reaction.

- **SIDE-EFFECTS**
  ▸ Common or very common Abdominal pain · chills · diarrhoea · dizziness · dyspnoea · headache · hypersensitivity · infusion-related reactions · myalgia · nausea · oropharyngeal pain · pyrexia · vomiting
  ▸ Uncommon Anaphylaxis

- **PREGNANCY** Manufacturer advises avoid unless essential—limited information available.

- **BREAST FEEDING** Manufacturer advises use only if potential benefit outweighs risk—present in milk in *animal* studies.

- **DIRECTIONS FOR ADMINISTRATION** For *intravenous infusion* (*Vimizim*®), give intermittently *in* Sodium chloride 0.9%; body-weight under 25 kg, dilute requisite dose to final volume of 100 mL infusion fluid and mix gently, give over 4 hours through in-line filter (0.2 micron) initially at a rate of 3 mL/hour, then increase to a rate of 6 mL/hour after 15 minutes, then increase gradually if tolerated every 15 minutes by 6 mL/hour to max. 36 mL/hour; body-weight 25 kg or over, dilute requisite dose to final volume of 250 mL and mix gently, give over 4 hours through in-line filter (0.2 micron) initially at a rate of 6 mL/hour, then increase to a rate of 12 mL/hour after 15 minutes, then increase gradually if tolerated every 15 minutes by 12 mL/hour to max. 72 mL/hour.

- **HANDLING AND STORAGE** Manufacturer advises store in a refrigerator at 2–8°C. After dilution use immediately or, if necessary, store at 2-8°C for max. 24 hours, followed by up to 24 hours at 23–27°C.

- **PATIENT AND CARER ADVICE**
  Driving and skilled tasks
  Manufacturer advises patients and carers should be counselled about the effects on driving and performance of skilled tasks—increased risk of dizziness.

- **MEDICINAL FORMS**
  There can be variation in the licensing of different medicines containing the same drug.
  Solution for infusion
  EXCIPIENTS: May contain Polysorbates, sorbitol
  ELECTROLYTES: May contain Sodium
  ▸ **Vimizim** (BioMarin Europe Ltd) ▼
    Elosulfase alfa 1 mg per 1 ml Vimizim 5mg/5ml concentrate for solution for infusion vials | 1 vial [PoM] £750.00

Galsulfase

- **DRUG ACTION** Galsulfase is a recombinant form of human N-acetylgalactosamine-4-sulfatase.

- **INDICATIONS AND DOSE**
  Mucopolysaccharidosis VI (specialist use only)
  ▸ BY INTRAVENOUS INFUSION
  ▸ Child 5-17 years: 1 mg/kg once weekly

- **CAUTIONS** Acute febrile illness (consider delaying treatment) · acute respiratory illness (consider delaying treatment) · infusion-related reactions can occur · respiratory disease

- **SIDE-EFFECTS** Abdominal pain · apnoea · areflexia · chest pain · conjunctivitis · corneal opacity · dyspnoea · ear pain · facial oedema · gastroenteritis · hypertension · infusion-related reactions · malaise · nasal congestion · pharyngitis · rigors · umbilical hernia

  SIDE-EFFECTS, FURTHER INFORMATION
  ▸ Infusion-related reactions Infusion-related reactions often occur, they can be managed by slowing the infusion rate or interrupting the infusion, and can be minimised by pre-treatment with an antihistamine and an antipyretic. Recurrent infusion-related reactions may require

pre-treatment with a corticosteroid—consult product literature for details.
- **PREGNANCY** Manufacturer advises avoid unless essential.
- **BREAST FEEDING** Manufacturer advises avoid—no information available.
- **DIRECTIONS FOR ADMINISTRATION** For *intravenous infusion*, dilute requisite dose with Sodium Chloride 0.9% to a final volume of 250 mL and mix gently; infuse through a 0.2 micron in-line filter; give approx. 2.5% of the total volume over 1 hour, then infuse remaining volume over next 3 hours; if body-weight under 20 kg and at risk of fluid overload, dilute requisite dose in 100 mL Sodium Chloride 0.9% and give over at least 4 hours.

- **MEDICINAL FORMS** There can be variation in the licensing of different medicines containing the same drug.

  Solution for infusion
  - Naglazyme (BioMarin Europe Ltd) ▼
    Galsulfase 1 mg per 1 ml Naglazyme 5mg/5ml solution for infusion vials | 1 vial PoM £982.00

Idursulfase

- **DRUG ACTION** Idursulfase is an enzyme produced by recombinant DNA technology licensed for long-term replacement therapy in mucopolysaccharidosis II (Hunter syndrome), a lysosomal storage disorder caused by deficiency of iduronate-2-sulfatase.

- **INDICATIONS AND DOSE**
  Mucopolysaccharidosis II (specialist use only)
  - BY INTRAVENOUS INFUSION
  - Child 5-17 years: 500 micrograms/kg once weekly

- **CAUTIONS** Acute febrile respiratory illness (consider delaying treatment) · infusion-related reactions can occur · severe respiratory disease

- **SIDE-EFFECTS**
  - **Common or very common** Arrhythmia · arthralgia · bronchospasm · chest pain · cough · cyanosis · dizziness · dyspnoea · erythema · facial oedema · flushing · gastro-intestinal disturbances · headache · hypertension · hypotension · hypoxia · infusion-site swelling · peripheral oedema · pruritus · pyrexia · rash · swollen tongue · tachycardia · tachypnoea · tremor · urticaria · wheezing
  - **Frequency not known** Anaphylaxis · infusion-related reactions · pulmonary embolism

  SIDE-EFFECTS, FURTHER INFORMATION
  - Infusion-related reactions Infusion-related reactions often occur, they can be managed by slowing the infusion rate or interrupting the infusion, and can be minimised by pre-treatment with an antihistamine and an antipyretic. Recurrent infusion-related reactions may require pre-treatment with a corticosteroid—consult product literature for details.

- **CONCEPTION AND CONTRACEPTION** Contra-indicated in women of child-bearing potential.
- **PREGNANCY** Manufacturer advises avoid.
- **BREAST FEEDING** Manufacturer advises avoid—present in milk in *animal* studies.
- **DIRECTIONS FOR ADMINISTRATION** For *intravenous infusion*, dilute requisite dose in 100 mL Sodium Chloride 0.9% and mix gently (do not shake); give over 3 hours (gradually reduced to 1 hour if no infusion-related reactions).

- **MEDICINAL FORMS** There can be variation in the licensing of different medicines containing the same drug.

  Solution for infusion
  - Elaprase (Shire Pharmaceuticals Ltd) ▼
    Idursulfase 2 mg per 1 ml Elaprase 6mg/3ml concentrate for solution for infusion vials | 1 vial PoM £1,985.00

Laronidase

- **DRUG ACTION** Laronidase is an enzyme produced by recombinant DNA technology licensed for long-term replacement therapy in the treatment of non-neurological manifestations of mucopolysaccharidosis I, a lysosomal storage disorder caused by deficiency of alpha-L-iduronidase.

- **INDICATIONS AND DOSE**
  Non-neurological manifestations of mucopolysaccharidosis I (specialist use only)
  - BY INTRAVENOUS INFUSION
  - Child: 100 units/kg once weekly

- **CAUTIONS** Infusion-related reactions can occur
- **INTERACTIONS** → Appendix 1: laronidase
- **SIDE-EFFECTS**
  - **Common or very common** Abdominal pain · alopecia · anaphylaxis · angioedema · blood pressure changes · cold extremities · cough · diarrhoea · dizziness · dyspnoea · fatigue · flushing · headache · influenza-like symptoms · infusion-site reactions · musculoskeletal pain · nausea · pain in extremities · pallor · paraesthesia · pruritus · rash · restlessness · tachycardia · urticaria · vomiting
  - **Frequency not known** Bronchospasm · infusion-related reactions · respiratory arrest

  SIDE-EFFECTS, FURTHER INFORMATION
  - Infusion-related reactions Infusion-related reactions often occur, they can be managed by slowing the infusion rate or interrupting the infusion, and can be minimised by pre-treatment with an antihistamine and an antipyretic. Recurrent infusion-related reactions may require pre-treatment with a corticosteroid—consult product literature for details.

- **PREGNANCY** Manufacturer advises avoid unless essential—no information available.
- **BREAST FEEDING** Manufacturer advises avoid—no information available.
- **MONITORING REQUIREMENTS** Monitor immunoglobulin G (IgG) antibody concentration.
- **DIRECTIONS FOR ADMINISTRATION** For *intravenous infusion*, dilute with Sodium Chloride 0.9%; body-weight under 20 kg, dilute to 100 mL, body-weight over 20 kg dilute to 250 mL; give through an in-line filter (0.22 micron) initially at a rate of 2 units/kg/hour then increase gradually every 15 minutes to max. 43 units/kg/hour.

- **MEDICINAL FORMS** There can be variation in the licensing of different medicines containing the same drug.

  Solution for infusion
  ELECTROLYTES: May contain Sodium
  - Aldurazyme (Genzyme Therapeutics Ltd)
    Laronidase 100 unit per 1 ml Aldurazyme 500units/5ml solution for infusion vials | 1 vial PoM £444.70

9

Blood and nutrition

3.8 Nephropathic cystinosis

AMINO ACIDS AND DERIVATIVES

Mercaptamine

(Cysteamine)

- **INDICATIONS AND DOSE**

Nephropathic cystinosis (specialist use only)
▶ BY MOUTH

▸ **Neonate:** Initially one-sixth to one-quarter of the expected maintenance dose, increased gradually over 4–6 weeks to avoid intolerance, maintenance 1.3 g/m² daily in 4 divided doses.

▸ **Child 1 month-11 years (body-weight up to 50 kg):** Initially one-sixth to one-quarter of the expected maintenance dose, increased gradually over 4–6 weeks to avoid intolerance, maintenance 1.3 g/m² daily in 4 divided doses

▸ **Child 12-17 years (body-weight up to 50 kg):** Initially one-sixth to one-quarter of the expected maintenance dose, increased gradually over 4–6 weeks to avoid intolerance, maintenance 1.3 g/m² daily in 4 divided doses

▸ **Child 12-17 years (body-weight 50 kg and above):** Initially one-sixth to one-quarter of the expected maintenance dose, increased gradually over 4–6 weeks to avoid intolerance, maintenance 2 g daily in 4 divided doses

DOSE EQUIVALENCE AND CONVERSION
▸ 1.3 g/m² is approximately equivalent to 50 mg/kg.

- **UNLICENSED USE** Mercaptamine eye drops for the management of ocular symptoms arising from the deposition of cystine crystals in the eye are not licensed.

> **IMPORTANT SAFETY INFORMATION**
> SAFE PRACTICE
> Mercaptamine has been confused with mercaptopurine; care must be taken to ensure the correct drug is prescribed and dispensed.

- **CAUTIONS** Dose of phosphate supplement may need to be adjusted if transferring from phosphocysteamine to mercaptamine
- **SIDE-EFFECTS**
▶ **Common or very common** Abdominal pain · anorexia · breath and body odour · diarrhoea · dyspepsia · encephalopathy · fever · gastroenteritis · headache · malaise · nausea · rash · vomiting
▶ **Uncommon** Drowsiness · gastro-intestinal ulcer · hallucinations · leucopenia · nephrotic syndrome · nervousness · seizures
- **ALLERGY AND CROSS-SENSITIVITY** Contra-indicated if history of hypersensitivity to penicillamine.
- **PREGNANCY** Avoid—teratogenic and toxic in *animal* studies.
- **BREAST FEEDING** Avoid.
- **MONITORING REQUIREMENTS** Leucocyte-cystine concentration and haematological monitoring required—consult product literature.
▶ All patients receiving mercaptamine should be registered (contact local specialist centre for details).
- **DIRECTIONS FOR ADMINISTRATION** For children under 6 years at risk of aspiration, capsules can be opened and contents sprinkled on food (at a temperature suitable for eating); avoid adding to acidic drinks (e.g. orange juice).

- **PRESCRIBING AND DISPENSING INFORMATION** Mercaptamine has a very unpleasant taste and smell, which can affect compliance.

- **PATIENT AND CARER ADVICE** Medicines for Children leaflet: Mercaptamine eye drops for ocular symptoms of cystinosis www.medicinesforchildren.org.uk/ nercaptamine-eye-drops-for-cystinosis

- **MEDICINAL FORMS** There can be variation in the licensing of different medicines containing the same drug.

Gastro-resistant capsule
▶ Procysbi (Horizon Pharma Europe B.V.)
Mercaptamine (as Mercaptamine bitartrate) **25 mg** Procysbi 25mg gastro-resistant capsules | 60 capsule PoM £335.97
Mercaptamine (as Mercaptamine bitartrate) **75 mg** Procysbi 75mg gastro-resistant capsules | 250 capsule PoM £4,199.65

Capsule
CAUTIONARY AND ADVISORY LABELS 21
▶ Cystagon (Orphan Europe (UK) Ltd)
Mercaptamine (as Mercaptamine bitartrate) **50 mg** Cystagon 50mg capsules | 100 capsule PoM £70.00
Mercaptamine (as Mercaptamine bitartrate) **150 mg** Cystagon 150mg capsules | 100 capsule PoM £190.00

3.9 Niemann-Pick type C disease

ENZYME INHIBITORS ⟩ GLUCOSYLCERAMIDE SYNTHASE INHIBITORS

Miglustat

- **DRUG ACTION** Miglustat is an inhibitor of glucosylceramide synthase.

- **INDICATIONS AND DOSE**

Treatment of progressive neurological manifestations of Niemann-Pick type C disease (under expert supervision)
▶ BY MOUTH

▸ **Child 4-11 years (body surface area up to 0.48 m²):** 100 mg once daily

▸ **Child 4-11 years (body surface area 0.48-0.73 m²):** 100 mg twice daily

▸ **Child 4-11 years (body surface area 0.74-0.88 m²):** 100 mg 3 times a day

▸ **Child 4-11 years (body surface area 0.89-1.25 m²):** 200 mg twice daily

▸ **Child 4-11 years (body surface area 1.26 m² and above):** 200 mg 3 times a day

▸ **Child 12-17 years:** 200 mg 3 times a day

- **SIDE-EFFECTS** Abdominal pain · amnesia · anorexia · ataxia · chills · constipation · decreased libido · depression · diarrhoea · dizziness · dyspepsia · flatulence · headache · hypoaesthesia · insomnia · malaise · muscle spasm · muscle weakness · nausea · paraesthesia · peripheral neuropathy · thrombocytopenia · tremor · vomiting · weight changes

- **CONCEPTION AND CONTRACEPTION** Effective contraception must be used during treatment. Men should avoid fathering a child during and for 3 months after treatment.

- **PREGNANCY** Manufacturer advises avoid—toxicity in *animal* studies.

- **BREAST FEEDING** Manufacturer advises avoid—no information available.

- **HEPATIC IMPAIRMENT** No information available—manufacturer advises caution.

- **RENAL IMPAIRMENT** Child 12–17 years, initially 200 mg twice daily if estimated glomerular filtration rate 50–70 mL/minute/1.73 m². Child 12–17 years, initially 100 mg twice daily if estimated glomerular filtration rate

30–50 mL/minute/1.73 m^2. Avoid if estimated glomerular filtration less than 30 mL/minute/1.73 m^2.

Child under 12 years—consult product literature.

- **MONITORING REQUIREMENTS**
- ▸ Monitor cognitive and neurological function.
- ▸ Monitor growth and platelet count in Niemann-Pick type C disease.

- **MEDICINAL FORMS**
There can be variation in the licensing of different medicines containing the same drug.

Capsule
- ▸ Zavesca (Actelion Pharmaceuticals UK Ltd)
Miglustat 100 mg Zavesca 100mg capsules | 84 capsule [PoM] £3,934.17 (Hospital only)

3.10 Pompe disease

ENZYMES

Alglucosidase alfa

- **DRUG ACTION** Alglucosidase alfa is an enzyme produced by recombinant DNA technology licensed for long-term replacement therapy in Pompe disease, a lysosomal storage disorder caused by deficiency of acid alpha-glucosidase.

- **INDICATIONS AND DOSE**
Pompe disease (specialist use only)
- ▸ BY INTRAVENOUS INFUSION
- ▸ Neonate: 20 mg/kg every 2 weeks.
- ▸ Child: 20 mg/kg every 2 weeks

- **CAUTIONS** Cardiac dysfunction · infusion-related reactions—consult product literature · respiratory dysfunction
- **SIDE-EFFECTS**
- ▸ **Common or very common** Agitation · anaphylaxis · antibody formation · blood pressure changes · bronchospasm · chest discomfort · cold extremities · cough · cyanosis · diarrhoea · dizziness · facial oedema · fatigue · flushing · headache · hypersensitivity reactions · injection-site reactions · irritability · muscle spasm · myalgia · nausea · paraesthesia · pruritus · pyrexia · rash · restlessness · sweating · tachycardia · tachypnoea · tremor · urticaria · vomiting
- ▸ **Frequency not known** Infusion-related reactions · necrotising skin lesions · severe skin reactions · ulcerative skin lesions

SIDE-EFFECTS, FURTHER INFORMATION
- ▸ Infusion-related reactions Infusion-related reactions very common, calling for use of antihistamine, antipyretic, or corticosteroid; consult product literature for details.

- **PREGNANCY** Toxicity in *animal* studies, but treatment should not be withheld.
- **BREAST FEEDING** Manufacturer advises avoid—no information available.
- **MONITORING REQUIREMENTS**
- ▸ Monitor closely if cardiac dysfunction.
- ▸ Monitor closely if respiratory dysfunction.
- ▸ Monitor immunoglobulin G (IgG) antibody concentration.
- **DIRECTIONS FOR ADMINISTRATION** For *intravenous infusion*, reconstitute 50 mg with 10.3 mL water for injections to produce 5 mg/mL solution; gently rotate vial without shaking; dilute requisite dose with Sodium Chloride 0.9% to give a final concentration of 0.5–4 mg/mL; give through a low protein-binding in-line filter (0.2 micron) at an initial rate of 1 mg/kg/hour increased by 2 mg/kg/hour every 30 minutes to max. 7mg/kg/hour.

- **MEDICINAL FORMS**
There can be variation in the licensing of different medicines containing the same drug.
Powder for solution for infusion
- ▸ Myozyme (Genzyme Therapeutics Ltd)
Alglucosidase alfa 50 mg Myozyme 50mg powder for concentrate for solution for infusion vials | 1 vial [PoM] £356.06 (Hospital only)

3.11 Tyrosinaemia type I

ENZYME INHIBITORS ›
4-HYDROXYPHENYLPYRUVATE DIOXYGENASE INHIBITORS

Nitisinone
(NTBC)

- **INDICATIONS AND DOSE**
Hereditary tyrosinaemia type I (in combination with dietary restriction of tyrosine and phenylalanine) (specialist use only)
- ▸ BY MOUTH
- ▸ Neonate: Initially 500 micrograms/kg twice daily, adjusted according to response; maximum 2 mg/kg per day.
- ▸ Child: Initially 500 micrograms/kg twice daily, adjusted according to response; maximum 2 mg/kg per day

- **INTERACTIONS** → Appendix 1: nitisinone
- **SIDE-EFFECTS**
- ▸ **Common or very common** Conjunctivitis · corneal opacity · eye pain · granulocytopenia · keratitis · leucopenia · photophobia · thrombocytopenia
- ▸ **Uncommon** Blepharitis · erythematous rash · exfoliative dermatitis · leucocytosis · pruritus
- **PREGNANCY** Manufacturer advises avoid unless potential benefit outweighs risk—toxicity in *animal* studies.
- **BREAST FEEDING** Manufacturer advises avoid—adverse effects in *animal* studies.
- **PRE-TREATMENT SCREENING** Slit-lamp examination of eyes recommended before treatment.
- **MONITORING REQUIREMENTS**
- ▸ Monitor liver function regularly.
- ▸ Monitor platelet and white blood cell count every 6 months.
- **DIRECTIONS FOR ADMINISTRATION** Capsules can be opened and the contents suspended in a small amount of water or formula diet and taken immediately.

- **MEDICINAL FORMS**
There can be variation in the licensing of different medicines containing the same drug.
Oral suspension
- ▸ Orfadin (Swedish Orphan Biovitrum Ltd)
Nitisinone 4 mg per 1 ml Orfadin 4mg/1ml oral suspension sugar-free | 90 ml [PoM] £1,692.00
Capsule
- ▸ Orfadin (Swedish Orphan Biovitrum Ltd)
Nitisinone 2 mg Orfadin 2mg capsules | 60 capsule [PoM] £564.00
Nitisinone 5 mg Orfadin 5mg capsules | 60 capsule [PoM] £1,127.00
Nitisinone 10 mg Orfadin 10mg capsules | 60 capsule [PoM] £2,062.00
Nitisinone 20 mg Orfadin 20mg capsules | 60 capsule [PoM] £4,512.00

9

Blood and nutrition

3.12 Urea cycle disorders

AMINO ACIDS AND DERIVATIVES

Arginine

- **INDICATIONS AND DOSE**

Acute hyperammonaemia in carbamylphosphate synthetase deficiency (specialist use only) | Acute hyperammonaemia in ornithine transcarbamylase deficiency (specialist use only)
▸ BY INTRAVENOUS INFUSION

▸ Neonate: 6 mg/kg/hour.

▸ Child (body-weight up to 40 kg): 6 mg/kg/hour
▸ Child (body-weight 40 kg and above): 4 mg/kg/hour

Maintenance treatment of hyperammonaemia in carbamylphosphate synthetase deficiency (specialist use only) | Maintenance treatment of hyperammonaemia in ornithine transcarbamylase deficiency (specialist use only)
▸ BY MOUTH

▸ Neonate: 100–200 mg/kg daily in 3–4 divided doses, dose to be taken with feeds.

▸ Child (body-weight up to 20 kg): 100–200 mg/kg daily in 3–4 divided doses, dose to be given with feeds or meals
▸ Child (body-weight 20 kg and above): 2.5–6 g/m^2 daily in 3–4 divided doses, dose to be taken with meals; maximum 6 g per day

Acute hyperammonaemia in citrullinaemia (specialist use only) | Acute hyperammonaemia in arginosuccinic aciduria (specialist use only)
▸ BY INTRAVENOUS INFUSION

▸ Neonate: Initially 300 mg/kg, to be administered over 90 minutes, followed by 12.5 mg/kg/hour, to be administered over 24 hours (maximum 25 mg/kg/hour thereafter).

▸ Child (body-weight up to 40 kg): Initially 300 mg/kg, to be administered over 90 minutes, followed by 12.5 mg/kg/hour, to be administered over 24 hours (maximum 25 mg/kg/hour thereafter)
▸ Child (body-weight 40 kg and above): 21 mg/kg/hour

Maintenance treatment of hyperammonaemia in citrullinaemia (specialist use only) | Maintenance treatment of hyperammonaemia in arginosuccinic aciduria (specialist use only)
▸ BY MOUTH

▸ Neonate: 100–300 mg/kg daily in 3–4 divided doses, dose to be taken with feeds.

▸ Child (body-weight up to 20 kg): 100–300 mg/kg daily in 3–4 divided doses, dose to be taken with feed or meals
▸ Child (body-weight 20 kg and above): 2.5–6 g/m^2 daily in 3–4 divided doses, doses to be taken with meals; maximum 6 g per day

- **UNLICENSED USE** Injection not licensed in children. Tablets not licensed in children. Powder licensed for urea cycle disorders in children.

- **CONTRA-INDICATIONS** Not to be used in the treatment of arginase deficiency

- **SIDE-EFFECTS**
▸ With intravenous use Flushing · headache · hyperchloraemic metabolic acidosis · hypotension · irritation at injection-site · nausea · numbness · vomiting

- **PREGNANCY** No information available.

- **BREAST FEEDING** No information available.

- **MONITORING REQUIREMENTS** Monitor plasma pH and chloride.

- **DIRECTIONS FOR ADMINISTRATION**
▸ With intravenous use For *intravenous infusion*, dilute to a max. concentration of 50 mg/mL with glucose 10%.

- **PRESCRIBING AND DISPENSING INFORMATION**
▸ With oral use Powder to be prescribed as a borderline substance (ACBS). For use as a supplement in urea cycle disorders other than arginase deficiency, such as hyperammonaemia types I and II, citrullinaemia, arginosuccinic aciduria, and deficiency of N-acetyl glutamate synthetase.

- **PATIENT AND CARER ADVICE**
Medicines for Children leaflet: Arginine for urea cycle disorders www.medicinesforchildren.org.uk/arginine-urea-cycle-disorders-0

- **MEDICINAL FORMS**
There can be variation in the licensing of different medicines containing the same drug. Forms available from special-order manufacturers include: tablet, capsule, oral solution, solution for infusion

Tablet
▸ Arginine (Non-proprietary)
L-Arginine 500 mg L-Arginine 500mg tablets | 60 tablet £5.30
L-Arginine 1 gram Arginine 1g tablets | 90 tablet £11.14

Solution for infusion
▸ Arginine (Non-proprietary)
L-Arginine monohydrochloride 210.7 mg per 1 ml L-Arginin-Hydrochlorid 21% concentrate for solution for infusion 20ml ampoules | 5 ampoule [PoM] no price available

Capsule
▸ Arginine (Non-proprietary)
L-Arginine 500 mg L-Arginine 500mg capsules | 30 capsule £3.35 | 60 capsule £6.50

Powder
▸ Arginine (Non-proprietary)
L-Arginine 1 gram per 1 gram L-Arginine powder | 100 gram £42.69

Carglumic acid

- **INDICATIONS AND DOSE**

Hyperammonaemia due to N-acetylglutamate synthase deficiency (under expert supervision)
▸ BY MOUTH

▸ Neonate: Initially 50–125 mg/kg twice daily, to be taken immediately before feeds, dose adjusted according to plasma–ammonia concentration; maintenance 5–50 mg/kg twice daily, the total daily dose may alternatively be given in 3–4 divided doses.

▸ Child: Initially 50–125 mg/kg twice daily, to be taken immediately before food, dose adjusted according to plasma–ammonia concentration; maintenance 5–50 mg/kg twice daily, the total daily dose may alternatively be given in 3–4 divided doses

Hyperammonaemia due to organic acidaemia (under expert supervision)
▸ BY MOUTH

▸ Neonate: Initially 50–125 mg/kg twice daily, to be taken immediately before feeds, dose adjusted according to plasma-ammonia concentration, the total daily dose may alternatively be given in 3–4 divided doses.

▸ Child: Initially 50–125 mg/kg twice daily, to be taken immediately before food, dose adjusted according to plasma-ammonia concentration, the total daily dose may alternatively be given in 3–4 divided doses

---

IMPORTANT SAFETY INFORMATION

EMERGENCY MANAGEMENT OF UREA CYCLE DISORDERS
For further information on the emergency management of urea cycle disorders consult the British Inherited Metabolic Disease Group (BIMDG) website at www.bimdg.org.uk.

- **SIDE-EFFECTS**
- ▶ Common or very common Sweating
- ▶ Uncommon Bradycardia · diarrhoea · pyrexia · vomiting
- **PREGNANCY** Manufacturer advises avoid unless essential—no information available.
- **BREAST FEEDING** Manufacturer advises avoid—present in milk in *animal* studies.
- **DIRECTIONS FOR ADMINISTRATION** Dispersible tablets must be dispersed in at least 5–10 mL of water and taken orally immediately, or administered via a nasogastric tube.

- **MEDICINAL FORMS**
There can be variation in the licensing of different medicines containing the same drug.
Dispersible tablet
CAUTIONARY AND ADVISORY LABELS 13
- ▶ Carbaglu (Orphan Europe (UK) Ltd)
Carglumic acid 200 mg Carbaglu 200mg dispersible tablets sugar-free | 5 tablet [PoM] £299.00 sugar-free | 60 tablet [PoM] £3,499.00

Citrulline

- **INDICATIONS AND DOSE**
Carbamyl phosphate synthase deficiency | Ornithine carbamyl transferase deficiency
- ▶ BY MOUTH
- ▶ Neonate: 150 mg/kg daily in 3–4 divided doses, adjusted according to response.
- ▶ Child: 150 mg/kg daily in 3–4 divided doses, adjusted according to response

- **PREGNANCY** No information available.
- **BREAST FEEDING** No information available.
- **DIRECTIONS FOR ADMINISTRATION** Powder may be mixed with drinks or taken as a paste.

- **MEDICINAL FORMS**
There can be variation in the licensing of different medicines containing the same drug. Forms available from special-order manufacturers include: tablet, oral solution, powder
Powder
- ▶ Citrulline (Non-proprietary)
L-citrulline 1 mg per 1 mg L-Citrulline powder | 100 gram £225.70

BENZOATES

Sodium benzoate

- **INDICATIONS AND DOSE**
Acute hyperammonaemia due to urea cycle disorder (specialist use only)
- ▶ BY INTRAVENOUS INFUSION
- ▶ Neonate: Initially 250 mg/kg, to be administered over 90 minutes, followed by 10 mg/kg/hour, adjusted according to response.
- ▶ Child: Initially 250 mg/kg, to be administered over 90 minutes, followed by 10 mg/kg/hour, adjusted according to response

Maintenance treatment of hyperammonaemia due to urea cycle disorders (specialist use only) | Non-ketotic hyperglycinaemia (specialist use only)
- ▶ BY MOUTH
- ▶ Neonate: Up to 250 mg/kg daily in 3–4 divided doses, dose to be taken with feeds.
- ▶ Child: Up to 250 mg/kg daily in 3–4 divided doses, dose to be taken with feeds or meals; maximum 12 g per day

- **UNLICENSED USE** Not licensed for use in children.
- **CAUTIONS** Conditions involving sodium retention or oedema (preparations contain significant amounts of sodium) · congestive heart failure (preparations contain significant amounts of sodium) · neonates (risk of kernicterus and increased side-effects)
- **SIDE-EFFECTS** Anorexia · coma · irritability · lethargy · nausea · vomiting
SIDE-EFFECTS, FURTHER INFORMATION
Gastro-intestinal side-effects may be reduced by giving smaller doses more frequently.
- **PREGNANCY** No information available.
- **BREAST FEEDING** No information available.
- **RENAL IMPAIRMENT** Caution in renal insufficiency—preparations contain significant amounts of sodium.
- **DIRECTIONS FOR ADMINISTRATION**
- ▶ With oral use For administration *by mouth*, oral solution or powder may be administered in fruit drinks; less soluble in acidic drinks.
- ▶ With intravenous use For *intravenous infusion*, dilute to a max. concentration of 50 mg/mL with Glucose 10%.
- **PATIENT AND CARER ADVICE**
Medicines for Children leaflet: Sodium benzoate for urea cycle disorders www.medicinesforchildren.org.uk/sodium-benzoate-for-urea-cycle-disorders

- **MEDICINAL FORMS**
There can be variation in the licensing of different medicines containing the same drug. Forms available from special-order manufacturers include: tablet, capsule, oral solution, solution for infusion

DRUGS FOR METABOLIC DISORDERS ›
ACETIC ACIDS

Sodium dichloroacetate

- **INDICATIONS AND DOSE**
Pyruvate dehydrogenase defects
- ▶ BY MOUTH
- ▶ Neonate: Initially 12.5 mg/kg 4 times a day, adjusted according to response, increased if necessary up to 200 mg/kg daily.
- ▶ Child: Initially 12.5 mg/kg 4 times a day, adjusted according to response, increased if necessary up to 200 mg/kg daily

- **SIDE-EFFECTS** Abnormal oxalate metabolism · metabolic acidosis · polyneuropathy on prolonged use
- **PREGNANCY** No information available.
- **BREAST FEEDING** No information available.

- **MEDICINAL FORMS**
There can be variation in the licensing of different medicines containing the same drug.
No licensed medicines listed.

DRUGS FOR METABOLIC DISORDERS ›
AMMONIA LOWERING DRUGS

Sodium phenylbutyrate

- **INDICATIONS AND DOSE**

Acute hyperammonaemia due to urea cycle disorders (specialist use only)
▸ BY INTRAVENOUS INFUSION

- Neonate: Initially 250 mg/kg, to be administered over 90 minutes, followed by 10 mg/kg/hour, adjusted according to response.

- Child: Initially 250 mg/kg, to be administered over 90 minutes, followed by 10 mg/kg/hour, adjusted according to response

Maintenance treatment of hyperammonaemia due to urea cycle disorders (specialist use only)
▸ BY MOUTH

- Neonate: Up to 250 mg/kg daily in 3–4 divided doses, with feeds.

- Child (body-weight up to 20 kg): Up to 250 mg/kg daily in 3–4 divided doses, with feeds or meals
- Child (body-weight 20 kg and above): 5 g/m^2 daily in 3–4 divided doses, with meals; maximum 12 g per day

- **UNLICENSED USE** Injection not licensed for use in children.

> **IMPORTANT SAFETY INFORMATION**
> EMERGENCY MANAGEMENT OF UREA CYCLE DISORDERS
> For further information on the emergency management of urea cycle disorders consult the British Inherited Metabolic Disease Group (BIMDG) website at www.bimdg.org.uk.

- **CAUTIONS** Conditions involving sodium retention with oedema (preparations contain significant amounts of sodium) · congestive heart failure (preparations contain significant amounts of sodium)
- **INTERACTIONS** → Appendix 1: sodium phenylbutyrate
- **SIDE-EFFECTS**
- **Common or very common** Amenorrhoea · body odour · decreased appetite · depression · gastro-intestinal disturbances · headache · irregular menstrual cycles · oedema · rash · renal tubular acidosis · syncope · taste disturbance · weight gain
- **Uncommon** Abdominal pain · aplastic anaemia · arrhythmias · ecchymoses · nausea · oedema · pancreatitis · peptic ulcer · rectal bleeding · vomiting
  SIDE-EFFECTS, FURTHER INFORMATION
  Gastro-intestinal side-effects may be reduced by giving smaller doses more frequently.
- **CONCEPTION AND CONTRACEPTION** Manufacturer advises adequate contraception during administration in women of child-bearing potential.
- **PREGNANCY** Avoid—toxicity in *animal* studies.
- **BREAST FEEDING** Manufacturer advises avoid—no information available.
- **HEPATIC IMPAIRMENT** Manufacturer advises use with caution.
- **RENAL IMPAIRMENT** Manufacturer advises use with caution (preparations contain significant amounts of sodium).
- **DIRECTIONS FOR ADMINISTRATION**
- With oral use Oral dose may be mixed with fruit drinks, milk, or feeds. Granules should be mixed with food before taking. *Pheburane*® granules must not be administered by nasogastric or gastrostomy tubes.

- With intravenous use For *intravenous infusion*, dilute to a maximum concentration of 50 mg/mL with Glucose 10%.

- **PATIENT AND CARER ADVICE**
  Medicines for Children leaflet: Sodium phenylbutyrate for urea cycle disorders www.medicinesforchildren.org.uk/sodium-phenylbutyrate-for-urea-cycle-disorders

- **MEDICINAL FORMS**
  There can be variation in the licensing of different medicines containing the same drug. Forms available from special-order manufacturers include: capsule, oral suspension, oral solution, solution for infusion

  Granules
  ▸ Ammonaps (Swedish Orphan Biovitrum Ltd)
  Sodium phenylbutyrate 940 mg per 1 gram Ammonaps 940mg/g granules sugar-free | 266 gram [PoM] £860.00
  ▸ Pheburane (Lucane Pharma Ltd)
  Sodium phenylbutyrate 483 mg per 1 gram Pheburane 483mg/g granules | 174 gram [PoM] £331.00

  Tablet
  ▸ Ammonaps (Swedish Orphan Biovitrum Ltd)
  Sodium phenylbutyrate 500 mg Ammonaps 500mg tablets | 250 tablet [PoM] £493.00

3.13 Wilson's disease

ANTIDOTES AND CHELATORS › COPPER ABSORPTION INHIBITORS

Zinc acetate

- **DRUG ACTION** Zinc prevents the absorption of copper in Wilson's disease.

- **INDICATIONS AND DOSE**

Wilson's disease (initiated under specialist supervision)
▸ BY MOUTH

- Child 1–5 years: 25 mg twice daily
- Child 6–15 years (body-weight up to 57 kg): 25 mg 3 times a day
- Child 6–15 years (body-weight 57 kg and above): 50 mg 3 times a day
- Child 16–17 years: 50 mg 3 times a day

DOSE EQUIVALENCE AND CONVERSION
- Doses expressed as elemental zinc.

PHARMACOKINETICS
Symptomatic Wilson's disease patients should be treated initially with a chelating agent because zinc has a slow onset of action. When transferring from chelating treatment to zinc maintenance therapy, chelating treatment should be co-administered for 2–3 weeks until zinc produces its maximal effect.

- **CAUTIONS** Portal hypertension (risk of hepatic decompensation when switching from chelating agent)
- **INTERACTIONS** → Appendix 1: zinc
- **SIDE-EFFECTS**
- **Common or very common** Gastric irritation (usually transient)
- **Uncommon** Leucopenia · sideroblastic anaemia
  SIDE-EFFECTS, FURTHER INFORMATION
  Transient gastric irritation may be reduced if first dose is taken mid-morning or with a little protein.
- **PREGNANCY** Usual dose 25 mg 3 times daily adjusted according to plasma-copper concentration and urinary copper excretion.
- **BREAST FEEDING** Manufacturer advises avoid; present in milk—may cause zinc-induced copper deficiency in infant.
- **MONITORING REQUIREMENTS** Monitor full blood count and serum cholesterol.

- **DIRECTIONS FOR ADMINISTRATION** Capsules may be opened and the contents mixed with water.

- **MEDICINAL FORMS**
There can be variation in the licensing of different medicines containing the same drug.
  Capsule
  CAUTIONARY AND ADVISORY LABELS 23
  ▸ Wilzin (Orphan Europe (UK) Ltd)
  Zinc (as Zinc acetate) 25 mg Wilzin 25mg capsules |
  250 capsule [PoM] £132.00
  Zinc (as Zinc acetate) 50 mg Wilzin 50mg capsules |
  250 capsule [PoM] £242.00

ANTIDOTES AND CHELATORS 〉 COPPER CHELATORS

Penicillamine

- **DRUG ACTION** Penicillamine aids the elimination of copper ions in Wilson's disease (hepatolenticular degeneration).

- **INDICATIONS AND DOSE**
Wilson's disease
  ▸ BY MOUTH
  ▸ Child 1 month-11 years: 20 mg/kg daily in 2-3 divided doses, to be taken 1 hour before food; maximum 2 g per day
  ▸ Child 12-17 years: Initially 20 mg/kg daily in 2-3 divided doses. maintenance 0.75-1 g daily, to be taken 1 hour before food; maximum 2 g per day

Cystinuria
  ▸ BY MOUTH
  ▸ Child: 20-30 mg/kg daily in 2-3 divided doses, lower doses may be used initially and increased gradually, doses to be adjusted to maintain 24-hour urinary cystine below 1 mmol/litre, maintain adequate fluid intake, to be taken 1 hour before food; maximum 3 g per day

- **CONTRA-INDICATIONS** Lupus erythematosus
- **CAUTIONS** Neurological involvement in Wilson's disease
- **INTERACTIONS** → Appendix 1: penicillamine
- **SIDE-EFFECTS**
  ▸ **Common or very common** Anorexia · fever · nausea · proteinuria · rash · thrombocytopenia
  ▸ **Rare** Alopecia · breast enlargement (male and female) · elastosis perforans · haematuria (withdraw immediately if cause unknown) · mouth ulceration · pseudoxanthoma elasticum · skin laxity · stomatitis
  ▸ **Frequency not known** Agranulocytosis · aplastic anaemia · blood disorders · bronchiolitis · cholestatic jaundice · dermatomyositis · glomerulonephritis · Goodpasture's syndrome · haemolytic anaemia · haemolytic leucopenia · late rashes (consider dose reduction) · lupus erythematosus · myasthenia gravis · nephrotic syndrome · neuropathy (especially if neurological involvement in Wilson's disease—prophylactic pyridoxine recommended) · neutropenia · pancreatitis · pemphigus · pneumonitis · polymyositis · pulmonary haemorrhage · rheumatoid arthritis · Stevens-Johnson syndrome · taste loss (mineral supplements not recommended) · urticaria · vomiting

- **ALLERGY AND CROSS-SENSITIVITY** Patients who are hypersensitive to penicillin may react rarely to penicillamine.

- **PREGNANCY** Fetal abnormalities reported rarely; avoid if possible.

- **BREAST FEEDING** Manufacturer advises avoid unless potential benefit outweighs risk—no information available.

- **RENAL IMPAIRMENT** Reduce dose and monitor renal function or avoid (consult product literature).

- **MONITORING REQUIREMENTS**
  ▸ Consider withdrawal if platelet count falls below 120 000/mm³ or white blood cells below 2500/mm³ or if 3 successive falls within reference range (can restart at reduced dose when counts return to within reference range but permanent withdrawal necessary if recurrence of leucopenia or thrombocytopenia).
  ▸ Monitor urine for proteinuria.
  ▸ Monitor blood and platelet count regularly.

- **PATIENT AND CARER ADVICE** Counselling on the symptoms of blood disorders is advised. Warn patient and carers to tell doctor immediately if sore throat, fever, infection, non-specific illness, unexplained bleeding and bruising, purpura, mouth ulcers, or rashes develop.

- **MEDICINAL FORMS**
There can be variation in the licensing of different medicines containing the same drug. Forms available from special-order manufacturers include: oral solution
  Tablet
  CAUTIONARY AND ADVISORY LABELS 6, 22
  ▸ Penicillamine (Non-proprietary)
  Penicillamine 125 mg Penicillamine 125mg tablets | 56 tablet [PoM] £45.00 DT price = £45.00
  Penicillamine 250 mg Penicillamine 250mg tablets | 56 tablet [PoM] £88.78 DT price = £88.75
  ▸ Distamine (Alliance Pharmaceuticals Ltd)
  Penicillamine 125 mg Distamine 125mg tablets | 100 tablet [PoM] £10.34
  Penicillamine 250 mg Distamine 250mg tablets | 100 tablet [PoM] £17.78

Trientine dihydrochloride

- **INDICATIONS AND DOSE**
Wilson's disease in patients intolerant of penicillamine
  ▸ BY MOUTH
  ▸ Child 2-11 years: Initially 0.6-1.5 g daily in 2-4 divided doses, adjusted according to response, to be taken before food
  ▸ Child 12-17 years: 1.2-2.4 g daily in 2-4 divided doses, adjusted according to response, to be taken before food

- **INTERACTIONS** → Appendix 1: trientine
- **SIDE-EFFECTS**
  ▸ **Common or very common** Nausea · rash
  ▸ **Very rare** Anaemia
  ▸ **Frequency not known** Colitis · duodenitis

- **PREGNANCY** Teratogenic in *animal* studies—use only if benefit outweighs risk. Monitor maternal and neonatal serum-copper concentrations.

- **PRESCRIBING AND DISPENSING INFORMATION** Trientine is **not** an alternative to penicillamine for rheumatoid arthritis or cystinuria. Penicillamine-induced systemic lupus erythematosus may not resolve on transfer to trientine.

- **MEDICINAL FORMS**
There can be variation in the licensing of different medicines containing the same drug.
  Capsule
  CAUTIONARY AND ADVISORY LABELS 6, 22
  ▸ Trientine dihydrochloride (Non-proprietary)
  Trientine dihydrochloride 300 mg Trientine dihydrochloride 300mg capsules | 100 capsule [PoM] £3,090.00 DT price = £3,090.00

9

Blood and nutrition

4 Mineral and trace elements deficiencies

4.1 Zinc deficiency

Zinc

Zinc supplements should not be given unless there is good evidence of deficiency (hypoproteinaemia spuriously lowers plasma-zinc concentration) or in zinc-losing conditions. Zinc deficiency can occur as a result of inadequate diet or malabsorption; excessive loss of zinc can occur in trauma, burns, and protein-losing conditions. A zinc supplement is given until clinical improvement occurs, but it may need to be continued in severe malabsorption, metabolic disease, or in zinc-losing states.

Zinc is used in the treatment of Wilson's disease and acrodermatitis enteropathica, a rare inherited abnormality of zinc absorption.

Parenteral nutrition regimens usually include trace amounts of zinc, see also Intravenous nutrition below. If necessary, further zinc can be added to intravenous feeding regimens.

ELECTROLYTES AND MINERALS ❭ ZINC

Zinc sulfate

● **INDICATIONS AND DOSE**

Zinc deficiency or supplementation in zinc-losing conditions

▸ BY MOUTH USING EFFERVESCENT TABLETS

▸ **Neonate:** 1 mg/kg daily, dose expressed as elemental zinc, to be dissolved in water and taken after food.

▸ **Child (body-weight up to 10 kg):** 22.5 mg daily, dose to be adjusted as necessary, to be dissolved in water and taken after food, dose expressed as elemental zinc
▸ **Child (body-weight 10–30 kg):** 22.5 mg 1–3 times a day, dose to be adjusted as necessary, to be dissolved in water and taken after food, dose expressed as elemental zinc
▸ **Child (body-weight 31 kg and above):** 45 mg 1–3 times a day, dose to be adjusted as necessary, to be dissolved in water and taken after food, dose expressed as elemental zinc

Acrodermatitis enteropathica

▸ BY MOUTH USING EFFERVESCENT TABLETS

▸ **Neonate:** 0.5–1 mg/kg twice daily, dose to be adjusted as necessary, total daily dose may alternatively be given in 3 divided doses, dose expressed as elemental zinc.

▸ **Child:** 0.5–1 mg/kg twice daily, dose to be adjusted as necessary, total daily dose may alternatively be given in 3 divided doses, dose expressed as elemental zinc

● **UNLICENSED USE** *Solvazinc®* is not licensed for use in acrodermatitis enteropathica.

● **INTERACTIONS** → Appendix 1: zinc

● **SIDE-EFFECTS** Abdominal pain · diarrhoea · dyspepsia · gastric irritation · gastritis · headache · irritability · lethargy · nausea · vomiting

● **PREGNANCY** Crosses placenta; risk theoretically minimal, but no information available.

● **BREAST FEEDING** Present in milk; risk theoretically minimal, but no information available.

● **RENAL IMPAIRMENT** Accumulation may occur in acute renal failure.

● **PRESCRIBING AND DISPENSING INFORMATION** Each *Solvazinc®* tablet contains zinc sulfate monohydrate 125 mg (45 mg zinc).

● **MEDICINAL FORMS** There can be variation in the licensing of different medicines containing the same drug.

Effervescent tablet

CAUTIONARY AND ADVISORY LABELS 13, 21

▸ Solvazinc (Galen Ltd)
Zinc sulfate monohydrate 125 mg Solvazinc 125mg effervescent tablets sugar-free | 90 tablet Ⓟ £16.45 DT price = £16.45

5 Nutrition (intravenous)

Intravenous nutrition

Overview

When adequate feeding through the alimentary tract is not possible, nutrients may be given by intravenous infusion. This may be in addition to oral or enteral tube feeding—**supplemental parenteral nutrition**, or may be the sole source of nutrition—**total parenteral nutrition** (TPN). Complete enteral starvation is undesirable and total parenteral nutrition is a last resort.

Indications for parenteral nutrition include prematurity; severe or prolonged disorders of the gastro-intestinal tract; preparation of undernourished patients for surgery, chemotherapy, or radiation therapy; major surgery, trauma, or burns; prolonged coma or inability to eat; and some patients with renal or hepatic failure. The composition of proprietary preparations used in children is given under Proprietary Infusion Fluids for Parenteral Feeding p. 591.

Parenteral nutrition requires the use of a solution containing amino acids, glucose, lipids, electrolytes, trace elements, and vitamins. This is now commonly provided by the pharmacy in the form of an amino-acid, glucose, electrolyte bag, and a separate lipid infusion or, in older children a single 'all-in-one' bag. If the patient is able to take small amounts by mouth, vitamins may be given orally.

The nutrition solution is infused through a central venous catheter inserted under full surgical precautions. Alternatively, infusion through a peripheral vein may be used for supplementary as well as total parenteral nutrition, depending on the availability of peripheral veins; factors prolonging cannula life and preventing thrombophlebitis include the use of soft polyurethane paediatric cannulas and use of nutritional solutions of low osmolality and neutral pH. Nutritional fluids should be given by a dedicated intravenous line; if not possible, compatibility with any drugs or fluids should be checked as precipitation of components may occur. Extravasation of parenteral nutrition solution can cause severe tissue damage and injury; the infusion site should be regularly monitored.

Before starting intravenous nutrition the patient should be clinically stable and renal function and acid-base status should be assessed. Appropriate biochemical tests should have been carried out beforehand and serious deficits corrected. Nutritional and electrolyte status must be monitored throughout treatment. The nutritional components of parenteral nutrition regimens are usually increased gradually over a number of days to prevent metabolic complications and to allow metabolic adaptation to the infused nutrients. The solutions are usually infused over 24 hours but this may be gradually reduced if long-term nutrition is required. Home parenteral nutrition is usually infused over 12 hours overnight.

Complications of long-term parenteral nutrition include gall bladder sludging, gall stones, cholestasis and abnormal liver function tests. For details of the prevention and

Proprietary Infusion Fluids for Parenteral Feeding

Preparation	Nitrogen g/litre	[1,2]Energy kJ/litre	Electrolytes					Other components/litre
			K^+	Mg^{2+}	Na^+	Acet⁻	Cl⁻	
ClinOleic 20% (Baxter Healthcare Ltd) Net price 100 ml: no price available; Net price 250 ml: no price available; Net price 500 ml: no price available	–	8360	–	–	–	–	–	purified olive and soya oil 200 g, glycerol 22.5 g, egg phosphatides 12 g
Intralipid 10% (Fresenius Kabi Ltd) Net price 100 ml = £4.12; Net price 500 ml = £9.01	–	4600	–	–	–	–	–	soya oil 100 g, glycerol 22 g, purified egg phospholipids 12 g, phosphate 15 mmol
Intralipid 20% (Fresenius Kabi Ltd) Net price 100 ml = £6.21; Net price 250 ml = £10.16; Net price 500 ml = £13.52	–	8400	–	–	–	–	–	soya oil 200 g, glycerol 22 g, purified egg phospholipids 12 g, phosphate 15 mmol
Intralipid 30% (Fresenius Kabi Ltd) Net price 333 ml = £17.80	–	12600	–	–	–	–	–	soya oil 300 g, glycerol 16.7 g, purified egg phospholipids 12 g, phosphate 15 mmol
Lipofundin MCT/LCT 10% (B.Braun Medical Ltd) Net price 100 ml: no price available; Net price 500 ml = £13.70	–	4430	–	–	–	–	–	soya oil 50 g, medium-chain triglycerides 50 g
Lipofundin MCT/LCT 20% (B.Braun Medical Ltd) Net price 100 ml = £13.28; Net price 250 ml: no price available; Net price 500 ml = £20.36	–	8000	–	–	–	–	–	soya oil 100 g, medium-chain triglycerides 100 g
Primene 10% (Baxter Healthcare Ltd) Net price 100 ml: no price available; Net price 250 ml: no price available	15.0	–	–	–	–	–	19.0	
Synthamin 9 (Baxter Healthcare Ltd) Net price 500 ml: no price available; Net price 1 litre: no price available	9.1	–	60.0	5.0	70.0	100.0	70.0	acid phosphate 30 mmol
Synthamin 9 EF (electrolyte-free) (Baxter Healthcare Ltd) Net price 500 ml: no price available; Net price 1 litre: no price available	9.1	–	–	–	–	44.0	22.0	
Vamin 9 Glucose (Fresenius Kabi Ltd) Net price 100 ml = £3.90; Net price 500 ml = £7.95; Net price 1 litre = £13.80	9.4	1700	20.0	1.5	50.0	–	50.0	CA^{2+} 2.5 mmol, anhydrous glucose 100 g
Vaminolact (Fresenius Kabi Ltd) Net price 100 ml = £3.70; Net price 500 ml = £8.50	9.3	–	–	–	–	–	–	

1　1000 kcal = 4200kJ; 1000 kJ = 238.8 kcal. All entries are Prescription-only medicines.

2　Excludes protein- or amino acid-derived energy

management of parenteral nutrition complications, specialist literature should be consulted.

Protein (nitrogen) is given as mixtures of essential and non-essential synthetic L-amino acids. Ideally, all essential amino acids should be included with a wide variety of non-essential ones to provide sufficient nitrogen together with electrolytes. Solutions vary in their composition of amino acids; they often contain an energy source (usually glucose) and electrolytes. Solutions for use in neonates and children under 1 year of age are based on the amino acid profile of umbilical cord blood (*Primene*®) or breast milk (*Vaminolact*®) and contain amino acids that are essential in this age group; these amino acids may not be present in sufficient quantities in preparations designed for older children and adults.

Energy requirements must be met if amino acids are to be utilised for tissue maintenance. An appropriate energy to protein ratio is essential and requirements will vary depending on the child's age and condition. A mixture of carbohydrate and fat energy sources (usually 30–50% as fat) gives better utilisation of amino acids than glucose alone.

Glucose p. 564 is the preferred source of carbohydrate, but frequent monitoring of blood glucose is required particularly during initiation and build-up of the regimen; insulin may be necessary. Glucose above a concentration of 12.5% must be infused through a central venous catheter to avoid thrombosis; the maximum concentration of glucose that should normally be infused in fluid restricted children is 20–25%.

In parenteral nutrition regimens, it is necessary to provide adequate **phosphate** in order to allow phosphorylation of glucose and to prevent hypophosphataemia. Neonates, particularly preterm neonates, and young children also require phosphorus and calcium to ensure adequate bone mineralisation. The compatibility and solubility of calcium and phosphorus salts is complex and unpredictable; precipitation is a risk and specialist pharmacy advice should be sought.

Fat (lipid) emulsions have the advantages of a high energy to fluid volume ratio, neutral pH, and iso-osmolarity with plasma, and provide essential fatty acids. Several days of adaptation may be required to attain maximal utilisation.

Reactions include occasional febrile episodes (usually only with 20% emulsions) and rare anaphylactic responses. Interference with biochemical measurements such as those for blood gases and calcium may occur if samples are taken before fat has been cleared. Regular monitoring of plasma cholesterol and triglyceride is necessary to ensure clearance from the plasma, particularly in conditions where fat metabolism may be disturbed e.g. infection. Emulsions containing 20% or 30% fat should be used in neonates as they are cleared more efficiently. **Additives should not be mixed with fat emulsions unless compatibility is known.**

Electrolytes are usually provided as the chloride salts of potassium and sodium. Acetate salts can be used to reduce the amount of chloride infused; hyperchloraemic acidosis or hypochloraemic alkalosis can occur in preterm neonates or children with renal impairment.

Adminstration
Because of the complex requirements relating to parenteral nutrition full details relating to administration have been omitted. In all cases *specialist pharmacy advice, product literature and other specialist literature should be consulted.*

NUTRIENTS > PARENTERAL NUTRITION

Parenteral nutrition supplements

- **INDICATIONS AND DOSE**

DIPEPTIVEN 20G/100ML CONCENTRATE FOR SOLUTION FOR INFUSION BOTTLES

Amino acid supplement for hypercatabolic or hypermetabolic states

▶ BY INTRAVENOUS INFUSION

▶ Child: 300–400 mg/kg daily, dose not to exceed 20% of total amino acid intake

- **CAUTIONS**

PEDITRACE SOLUTION FOR INFUSION 10ML VIALS Reduced biliary excretion · reduced biliary excretion in cholestatic liver disease · reduced biliary excretion in markedly reduced urinary excretion (careful biochemical monitoring required) · total parenteral nutrition exceeding one month

CAUTIONS, FURTHER INFORMATION

▶ Total parenteral nutrition exceeding one month Measure serum manganese concentration and check liver function before commencing treatment and regularly during treatment— discontinue if manganese concentration raised or if cholestasis develops.

- **DIRECTIONS FOR ADMINISTRATION** Because of the complex requirements relating to parenteral nutrition, full details relating to administration have been omitted. In all cases *specialist pharmacy advice, product literature, and other specialist literature should be consulted.* Compatibility with the infusion solution must be ascertained before adding supplementary preparations. **Additives should not be mixed with fat emulsions unless compatibility is known.**

CERNEVIT SOLUTION FOR INJECTION VIALS AND DILUENT Dissolve in 5 mL water for injections.

PEDITRACE SOLUTION FOR INFUSION 10ML VIALS For addition to *Vaminolact®*, *Vamin®* 14 *Electrolyte-Free* solutions, and glucose intravenous infusions.

DECAN CONCENTRATE FOR SOLUTION FOR INFUSION 40ML BOTTLES For addition to infusion solutions.

ADDIPHOS® VIALS For addition to *Vamin®* solutions and glucose intravenous infusions.

DIPEPTIVEN 20G/100ML CONCENTRATE FOR SOLUTION FOR INFUSION BOTTLES For addition to infusion solutions containing amino acids.

ADDITRACE SOLUTION FOR INFUSION 10ML AMPOULES For adddition to *Vamin®* solutions and glucose intravenous infusions.

GLYCOPHOS® VIALS For addition to *Vamin®* and *Vaminolact®* solutions, and glucose intravenous infusions.

SOLIVITO N POWDER FOR SOLUTION FOR INFUSION VIALS Dissolve in water for injections or glucose intravenous infusion for adding to glucose intravenous infusion or *Intralipid®*; dissolve in *Vitlipid N®* or *Intralipid®* for adding to *Intralipid®* only.

VITLIPID N INFANT EMULSION FOR INJECTION 10ML AMPOULES For addition to *Intralipid®*.

VITLIPID N ADULT EMULSION FOR INJECTION 10ML AMPOULES For addition to *Intralipid®*.

- **PRESCRIBING AND DISPENSING INFORMATION**

CERNEVIT SOLUTION FOR INJECTION VIALS AND DILUENT *Cernevit®* solution contains *dl*-alpha tocopherol 11.2 units, ascorbic acid 125 mg, biotin 69 micrograms, colecalciferol 220 units, cyanocobalamin 6 micrograms, folic acid 414 micrograms, glycine 250 mg, nicotinamide 46 mg, pantothenic acid (as dexpanthenol) 17.25 mg, pyridoxine hydrochloride 5.5 mg, retinol (as palmitate) 3500 units, riboflavin (as dihydrated sodium phosphate) 4.14 mg, thiamine (as cocarboxylase tetrahydrate) 3.51 mg.

PEDITRACE SOLUTION FOR INFUSION 10ML VIALS For use in neonates (when kidney function established, usually second day of life), infants, and children.

Peditrace® solution contains traces of Zn^{2+}, Cu^{2+}, Mn^{2+}, Se^{4+}, F^-, I^-.

DECAN CONCENTRATE FOR SOLUTION FOR INFUSION 40ML BOTTLES For patients over 40 kg.

Decan® solution contains trace elements Fe^{2+}, Zn^{2+}, Cu^{2+}, Mn^{2+}, F^-, Co^{2+}, I^-, Se^{4+}, Mo^{6+}, Cr^{3+}.

ADDIPHOS® VIALS *Addiphos®* sterile solution contains phosphate 40 mmol, K^+ 30 mmol, Na^+ 30 mmol/20 mL.

DIPEPTIVEN 20G/100ML CONCENTRATE FOR SOLUTION FOR INFUSION BOTTLES *Dipeptiven®* solution contains N(2)-L-alanyl-L-glutamine 200 mg/mL (providing L-alanine 82 mg, L-glutamine 134.6 mg).

ADDITRACE SOLUTION FOR INFUSION 10ML AMPOULES For patients over 40 kg.

Additrace® solution contains traces of Fe^{3+}, Zn^{2+}, Mn^{2+}, Cu^{2+}, Cr^{3+}, Se^{4+}, Mo^{6+}, F^-, I^-.

GLYCOPHOS® VIALS *Glycophos®* Sterile Concentrate solution contains phosphate 20 mmol, Na^+ 40 mmol/20 mL.

SOLIVITO N POWDER FOR SOLUTION FOR INFUSION VIALS *Solivito N®* powder for reconstitution contains biotin 60 micrograms, cyanocobalamin 5 micrograms, folic acid 400 micrograms, glycine 300 mg, nicotinamide 40 mg, pyridoxine hydrochloride 4.9 mg, riboflavin sodium phosphate 4.9 mg, sodium ascorbate 113 mg, sodium pantothenate 16.5 mg, thiamine mononitrate 3.1 mg.

VITLIPID N INFANT EMULSION FOR INJECTION 10ML AMPOULES *Vitlipid N®* infant emulsion contains vitamin A 230 units, ergocalciferol 40 units, *dl*-alpha tocopherol 0.7 unit, phytomenadione 20 micrograms/mL.

VITLIPID N ADULT EMULSION FOR INJECTION 10ML AMPOULES *Vitlipid N®* adult emulsion contains vitamin A 330 units, ergocalciferol 20 units, *dl*-alpha tocopherol 1 unit, phytomenadione 15 micrograms/mL.

For adults and children over 11 years.

● **MEDICINAL FORMS**
There can be variation in the licensing of different medicines
containing the same drug. Forms available from special-order
manufacturers include: solution for infusion

Solution for injection

▸ Cernevit (Baxter Healthcare Ltd)
 Cyanocobalamin 6 microgram, Biotin 69 microgram, Folic acid
 414 microgram, Thiamine 3.51 mg, Riboflavin (as Riboflavin
 sodium phosphate) 4.14 mg, Pyridoxine (as Pyridoxine
 hydrochloride) 4.53 mg, Pantothenic acid (as Dexpanthenol)
 17.25 mg, Nicotinamide 46 mg, Ascorbic acid 125 mg, Alpha
 tocopherol 11.2 unit, Colecalciferol 220 unit, Retinol
 3500 unit Cernevit solution for injection vials and diluent |
 10 vial PoM no price available

Solution for infusion

▸ Parenteral nutrition supplements (Non-proprietary)
 Sodium glycerophosphate 216 mg per 1 ml Sodium
 glycerophosphate 4.32g/20ml concentrate for solution for infusion
 vials | 1 vial PoM £5.07 | 10 vial PoM no price available

▸ Additrace (Fresenius Kabi Ltd)
 Sodium molybdate 4.85 microgram per 1 ml, Chromic chloride
 5.33 microgram per 1 ml, Sodium selenite 10.5 microgram per
 1 ml, Potassium iodide 16.6 microgram per 1 ml, Manganese
 chloride 99 microgram per 1 ml, Sodium fluoride 210 microgram
 per 1 ml, Copper chloride 340 microgram per 1 ml, Ferric chloride
 544 microgram per 1 ml, Zinc chloride 1.36 mg per 1 ml Additrace
 solution for infusion 10ml ampoules | 1 ampoule PoM £1.96 |
 20 ampoule PoM no price available

▸ Dipeptiven (Fresenius Kabi Ltd)
 N(2)-L-alanyl-L-glutamine 200 mg per 1 ml Dipeptiven 20g/100ml
 concentrate for solution for infusion bottles | 1 bottle PoM £25.93 |
 10 bottle PoM no price available
 Dipeptiven 10g/50ml concentrate for solution for infusion bottles |
 1 bottle PoM £13.94 | 10 bottle PoM no price available

▸ Peditrace (Fresenius Kabi Ltd)
 Manganese (as Manganese chloride) 1 microgram per 1 ml, Iodine
 (as Potassium iodide) 1 microgram per 1 ml, Selenium (as Sodium
 selenite) 2 microgram per 1 ml, Copper (as Copper chloride)
 20 microgram per 1 ml, Fluoride (as Sodium fluoride)
 57 microgram per 1 ml, Zinc (as Zinc chloride) 250 microgram per
 1 ml Peditrace solution for infusion 10ml vials | 1 vial PoM £3.55 |
 10 vial PoM no price available

▸ Tracutil (B.Braun Melsungen AG)
 Sodium molybdate dihydrate 2.42 microgram per 1 ml, Chromic
 chloride 5.3 microgram per 1 ml, Sodium selenite pentahydrate
 7.89 microgram per 1 ml, Potassium iodide 16.6 microgram per
 1 ml, Sodium fluoride 126 microgram per 1 ml, Manganese
 chloride 197.9 microgram per 1 ml, Copper chloride
 204.6 microgram per 1 ml, Zinc chloride 681.5 microgram per
 1 ml, Ferrous chloride 695.8 microgram per 1 ml Tracutil
 concentrate for solution for infusion 10ml ampoules |
 5 ampoule PoM £7.96

Powder for solution for infusion

▸ Solivito N (Fresenius Kabi Ltd)
 Cyanocobalamin 5 microgram, Biotin 60 microgram, Folic acid
 400 microgram, Thiamine nitrate 3.1 mg, Pyridoxine
 hydrochloride 4.9 mg, Riboflavin sodium phosphate 4.9 mg,
 Sodium pantothenate 16.5 mg, Nicotinamide 40 mg, Sodium
 ascorbate 113 mg Solivito N powder for solution for infusion vials |
 1 vial PoM £1.97 | 10 vial PoM no price available

Emulsion for injection

▸ Vitlipid N Adult (Fresenius Kabi Ltd)
 Ergocalciferol 500 nanogram per 1 ml, Phytomenadione
 15 microgram per 1 ml, Retinol palmitate 99 microgram per 1 ml,
 Alpha tocopherol 910 microgram per 1 ml Vitlipid N Adult
 emulsion for injection 10ml ampoules | 1 ampoule PoM £1.97 |
 10 ampoule PoM no price available

▸ Vitlipid N Infant (Fresenius Kabi Ltd)
 Ergocalciferol 1 microgram per 1 ml, Phytomenadione
 20 microgram per 1 ml, Retinol palmitate 69 microgram per 1 ml,
 Alpha tocopherol 640 microgram per 1 ml Vitlipid N Infant
 emulsion for injection 10ml ampoules | 1 ampoule PoM £1.97 |
 10 ampoule PoM no price available

6   Nutrition (oral)

Enteral nutrition

Overview

Children have higher nutrient requirements per kg
bodyweight, different metabolic rates, and physiological
responses compared to adults. They have low nutritional
stores and are particularly vulnerable to growth and
nutritional problems during critical periods of development.
Major illness, operations, or trauma impose increased
metabolic demands and can rapidly exhaust nutritional
reserves.

Every effort should be made to optimise oral food intake
before beginning enteral tube feeding; this may include
change of posture, special seating, feeding equipment, oral
desensitisation, food texture changes, thickening of liquids,
increasing energy density of food, treatment of reflux or
oesophagitis, as well as using age-specific nutritional
supplements.

Enteral tube feeding has a role in both short-term
rehabilitation and long-term nutritional management in
paediatrics. It can be used as supportive therapy, in which
the enteral feed supplies a proportion of the required
nutrients, or as primary therapy, in which the enteral feed
delivers all the necessary nutrients. Most children receiving
tube feeds should also be encouraged to take oral food and
drink. Tube feeding should be considered in the following
situations:

● unsafe swallowing and risk of aspiration
● inability to consume at least 60% of energy needs by
 mouth
● total feeding time of more than 4 hours per day
● weight loss or no weight gain for a period of 3 months (less
 for younger children and infants)
● weight for height (or length) less than 2nd percentile for
 age and sex

Most feeds for enteral use contain protein derived from
cows' milk or soya. Elemental feeds containing protein
hydrolysates or free amino acids can be used for children
who have diminished ability to break down protein, for
example in inflammatory bowel disease or pancreatic
insufficiency.

Even when nutritionally complete feeds are given, water
and electrolyte balance should be monitored.
Haematological and biochemical parameters should also be
monitored, particularly in the clinically unstable child. Extra
minerals (e.g. magnesium and zinc) may be needed in
patients where gastro-intestinal secretions are being lost.
Additional vitamins may also be needed..

Choosing the best formula for children depends on several
factors including: nutritional requirements, gastro-intestinal
function, underlying disease, nutrient restrictions, age, and
feed characteristics (nutritional composition, viscosity,
osmolality, availability and cost). Children have specific
dietary requirements and in many situations liquid feeds
prepared for adults are totally unsuitable and should not be
given. Expert advice from a dietician should be sought before
prescribing enteral feeds for a child.

Infant formula feeds

Child 0–12 months. Term infants with normal gastro-
intestinal function are given either breast milk or normal
infant formula during the first year of life. The average
intake is between 150 mL and 200 mL/kg/day. Infant milk
formulas are based on whey- or casein-dominant protein,
lactose with or without maltodextrin, amylose, vegetable oil
and milk fat. The composition of all normal and soya infant
formulas have to meet The Infant Formula and Follow-on
Formula Regulations (England and Wales) 2007, which enact

9

Blood and nutrition

the European Community Regulations 2006/141/EC; the composition of other enteral and specialist feeds has to meet the Commission Directive (1999/21/EC) on Dietary Foods for Special Medical Purposes.

A high-energy feed, which contains 9–11% of energy derived from protein can be used for infants who fail to grow adequately. Alternatively, energy supplements may be added to normal infant formula to achieve a higher energy content (but this will reduce the protein to energy ratio) or the normal infant formula concentration may be increased slightly. Care should be taken not to present an osmotic load of more than 500 milliosmols/kg water to the normal functioning gut, otherwise osmotic diarrhoea will result. Concentrating or supplementing feeds should not be attempted without the advice of a paediatric dietician.

Enteral feeds

Child 1–6 years (body-weight 8–20 kg). Ready-to-use feeds based on caseinates, maltodextrin and vegetable oils (with or without added medium chain triglyceride (MCT) oil or fibre) are well tolerated and effective in improving nutritional status in this age group. Although originally designed for children 1–6 years (body-weight 8–20 kg), some products have ACBS approval for use in children weighing up to 30 kg (approx. 10 years of age). Enteral feeds formulated for children 1–6 years are low in sodium and potassium; electrolyte intake and biochemical status should be monitored. Older children in this age range taking small feed volumes may need to be given additional micronutrients. Fibre-enriched feeds may be helpful for children with chronic constipation or diarrhoea.

Child 7–12 years (body-weight 21–45 kg). Depending on age, weight, clinical condition and nutritional requirements, ready-to-use feeds formulated for 7–12 year olds may be given at appropriate rates.

Child over 12 years (body-weight over 45 kg). As there are no standard enteral feeds formulated for this age group, adult formulations are used. The intake of protein, electrolytes, vitamins, and trace minerals should be carefully assessed and monitored. Note: Adult feeds containing more than 6 g/100 mL protein or 2 g/100 mL fibre should be used with caution and expert advice.

Specialised formula

It is essential that any infant who is intolerant of breast milk or normal infant formula, or whose condition requires nutrient-specific adaptation, is prescribed an adequate volume of a nutritionally complete replacement formula. In the first 4 months of life, a volume of 150–200 mL/kg/day is recommended. After 6 months, should the formula still be required, a volume of 600 mL/day should be maintained, in addition to solid food.

Products for cow's milk protein intolerance or lactose intolerance. There are a number of infant formulas formulated for cow's milk protein intolerance or lactose intolerance; these feeds may contain a residual amount of lactose (less than 1 g/100 mL formula)—sometimes described as clinically lactose-free or 'lactose-free' by manufacturers. If the total daily intake of these formulas is low, it may be necessary to supplement with calcium, and a vitamin and mineral supplement.

Soya-based infant formulas have a high phytoestrogen content and this may be a long-term reproductive health risk. The Chief Medical Officer has advised that soya-based infant formulas should not be used as the first choice for the management of infants with proven cow's milk sensitivity, lactose intolerance, galactokinase deficiency and galactosaemia. Most UK paediatricians with expertise in inherited metabolic disease still advocate soya-based formulations for infants with galactosaemia as there are concerns about the residual lactose content of low lactose formulas and protein hydrolysates based on cow's milk protein.

Low lactose infant formulations, based on whole cow's milk protein, are unsuitable for children with cow's milk protein intolerance. Liquid soya milks purchased from supermarkets and health food stores are not nutritionally complete and should never be used for infants under 1 year of age.

Protein hydrolysate formulas. Non-milk, peptide-based feeds containing hydrolysates of casein, whey, meat and soya protein, are suitable for infants with disaccharide or whole protein intolerance. The total daily intake of electrolytes, vitamins and minerals should be carefully assessed and modified to meet the child's nutritional requirements; these feeds have a high osmolality when given at recommended dilution and need gradual and careful introduction.

Elemental (amino acid based formula). Specially formulated elemental feeds containing essential and nonessential amino acids are available for use in infants and children under 6 years with proven whole protein intolerance. Adult elemental formula may be used for children over 6 years; the intake of electrolytes, vitamins and minerals should be carefully assessed and modified to meet nutritional requirements. These feeds have a high osmolality when given at the recommended concentration and therefore need gradual and careful introduction.

Modular feeds. Modular feeds (see Specialised Formulas for Specific Clinical Conditions) are based on individual protein, fat, carbohydrate, vitamin and mineral components or modules which can be combined to meet the specific needs of a child. Modular feeds are used when nutritionally complete specialised formula are not tolerated, or if the fluid and nutrient requirements change e.g. in gastro-intestinal, renal or liver disease. The main advantage of modular feeds is their flexibility; disadvantages include their complexity and preparation difficulties. Modular feeds should not be used without the supervision of a paediatric dietician.

Specialised formula. Highly specialised formulas are designed to meet the specific requirements in various clinical conditions such as renal and liver diseases. When using these formulas, both the biochemical status of the child and their growth parameters need to be monitored.

Feed thickeners

Carob based thickeners may be used to thicken feeds for infants under 1 year with significant gastro-oesophageal reflux. Breast-fed infants can be given the thickener mixed to a paste with water or breast-milk prior to feeds.

Pre-thickened formula Milk-protein- or casein-dominant infant formula, which contains small quantities of pre-gelatinised starch, is recommended primarily for infants with mild gastro-oesophageal reflux. Pre-thickened formula is prepared in the same way as normal infant formula and flows through a standard teat. The feeds do not thicken on standing but thicken in the stomach when exposed to acid pH.

Starched based thickeners can be used to thicken liquids and feeds for children over 1 year of age with dysphagia.

Dietary supplements for oral use

Three types of prescribable fortified dietary supplements are available: fortified milk and non-milk tasting (juice-style) drinks, and fortified milk-based semi-solid preparations. The recommended daily quantity is age-dependent. The following is a useful guide: 1–2 years, 200 kcal (840 kJ); 3–5 years, 400 kcal (1680 kJ); 6–11 years, 600 kcal (2520 kJ); and over 12 years, 800 kcal (3360 kJ). Supplements containing 1.5 kcal/mL are high in protein and should not be used for children under 3 years of age. Many supplements are high in sugar or maltodextrin; care should be taken to prevent prolonged contact with teeth. Ideally supplements should be administered after meals or at bedtime so as not to affect appetite.

Products for metabolic diseases

There is a large range of disease-specific infant formulas and amino acid-based supplements available for use in children with metabolic diseases (see under specific metabolic diseases. Some of these formulas are nutritionally incomplete and supplementation with vitamins and other nutrients may be necessary. Many of the product names are similar; to prevent metabolic complications in children who cannot tolerate specific amino acids it is important to ensure the correct supplement is supplied.

Enteral feeding tubes

Care is required in choosing an appropriate formulation of a drug for administration through a nasogastric narrow-bore feeding tube or through a percutaneous endoscopic gastrostomy (PEG) or jejunostomy tube. Liquid preparations (or soluble tablets) are preferred; injection solutions may also be suitable for administration through an enteral tube.

If a solid formulation of a medicine needs to be given, it should be given as a suspension of particles fine enough to pass through the tube. It is possible to crush many immediate-release tablets but enteric-coated or modified-release preparations should **not** be crushed.

Enteral feeds may affect the absorption of drugs and it is therefore important to consider the timing of drug administration in relation to feeds. If more than one drug needs to be given, they should be given separately and the tube should be flushed with water after each drug has been given.

Clearing blockages

Carbonated (sugar-free) drinks may be marginally more effective than water in unblocking feeding tubes, but mildly acidic liquids (such as pineapple juice or cola-based drinks) can coagulate protein in feeds, causing further blockage. If these measures fail to clear the enteral feeding tube, an alkaline solution containing pancreatic enzymes may be introduced into the tube (followed after at least 5 minutes by water). Specific products designed to break up blockages caused by formula feeds are also available.

6.1 Special diets

Nutrition in special diets

Overview

These are preparations that have been modified to eliminate a particular constituent from a food or that are nutrient mixtures formulated as food substitutes for children who either cannot tolerate or cannot metabolise certain common constituents of food.

Coeliac disease

Coeliac disease is caused by an abnormal immune response to gluten. For management and further information, see Coeliac disease p. 33.

Phenylketonuria

Phenylketonuria (hyperphenylalaninaemia, PKU), which results from the inability to metabolise **phenylalanine**, is managed by restricting dietary intake of **phenylalanine** to a small amount sufficient for tissue building and repair.

Aspartame (used as a sweetener in some foods and medicines) contributes to the **phenylalanine** intake and may affect control of *phenylketonuria*. If alternatives are unavailable, children with phenylketonuria should not be denied access to appropriate medication; the amount of **aspartame** consumed can be taken in to account in the management of the condition. Where the presence of **aspartame** in a preparation is specified in the product literature, **aspartame** is listed as an excipient in the relevant

product entry in *BNF for Children*; the child or carer should be informed of this.

Some rare forms *of phenylketonuria* are caused by a deficiency of **tetrahydrobiopterin**. Treatment involves oral supplementation of tetrahydrobiopterin p. 596; in some severe cases, the addition of the neurotransmitter precursors, levodopa and 5-hydroxytryptophan, is also necessary.

Sapropterin dihydrochloride below, a synthetic form of tetrahydrobiopterin, is licensed as an adjunct to dietary restriction of **phenylalanine** in the management of patients with *phenylketonuria* and *tetrahydrobiopterin deficiency*.

Products for metabolic diseases

There is a large range of disease-specific infant formulas and amino acid-based supplements available for use in children with metabolic diseases (see under specific metabolic diseases. Some of these formulas are nutritionally incomplete and supplementation with vitamins and other nutrients may be necessary. Many of the product names are similar; to prevent metabolic complications in children who cannot tolerate specific amino acids it is important to ensure the correct supplement is supplied.

6.1a Phenylketonuria

DRUGS FOR METABOLIC DISORDERS 〉
TETRAHYDROBIOPTERIN AND DERIVATIVES

▍ Sapropterin dihydrochloride

● **INDICATIONS AND DOSE**

Phenylketonuria (adjunct to dietary restriction of phenylalanine) (specialist use only)

▸ BY MOUTH

▸ Child 4–17 years: Initially 10 mg/kg once daily, adjusted according to response; usual dose 5–20 mg/kg once daily, dose to be taken preferably in the morning

Tetrahydrobiopterin deficiency (adjunct to dietary restriction of phenylalanine) (specialist use only)

▸ BY MOUTH

▸ Neonate: Initially 2–5 mg/kg once daily, adjusted according to response, dose to be taken preferably in the morning, the total daily dose may alternatively be given in 2–3 divided doses; maximum 20 mg/kg per day.

▸ Child: Initially 2–5 mg/kg once daily, adjusted according to response, dose to be taken preferably in the morning, the total daily dose may alternatively be given in 2–3 divided doses; maximum 20 mg/kg per day

● **CAUTIONS** History of convulsions

● **INTERACTIONS** → Appendix 1: sapropterin

● **SIDE-EFFECTS**

▸ **Common or very common** Abdominal pain · cough · diarrhoea · headache · nasal congestion · pharyngolaryngeal pain · vomiting

▸ **Frequency not known** Hypersensitivity reactions

● **PREGNANCY** Manufacturer advises caution—consider only if strict dietary management inadequate.

● **BREAST FEEDING** Manufacturer advises avoid—no information available.

● **HEPATIC IMPAIRMENT** Manufacturer advises caution—no information available.

● **RENAL IMPAIRMENT** Manufacturer advises caution—no information available.

● **MONITORING REQUIREMENTS**

▸ Monitor blood-phenylalanine concentration before and after first week of treatment—if unsatisfactory response

9

Blood and nutrition

increase dose at weekly intervals to max. dose and monitor blood-phenylalanine concentration weekly; discontinue treatment if unsatisfactory response after 1 month.
▸ Monitor blood-phenylalanine and tyrosine concentrations 1–2 weeks after dose adjustment and during treatment.
● DIRECTIONS FOR ADMINISTRATION Tablets should be dissolved in water and taken within 20 minutes.
● PRESCRIBING AND DISPENSING INFORMATION Sapropterin is a synthetic form of tetrahydrobiopterin.
● PATIENT AND CARER ADVICE Patient or carers should be given advice on how to administer sapropterin dihydrochloride dispersible tablets.

● MEDICINAL FORMS
There can be variation in the licensing of different medicines containing the same drug.
Soluble tablet
CAUTIONARY AND ADVISORY LABELS 13, 21
▸ Kuvan (BioMarin Europe Ltd)
Sapropterin dihydrochloride 100 mg   Kuvan 100mg soluble tablets sugar-free | 30 tablet [PoM] £597.22

Tetrahydrobiopterin

● INDICATIONS AND DOSE
Monotherapy in tetrahydrobiopterin-sensitive phenylketonuria (specialist use only)
▸ BY MOUTH
▸ Child: 10 mg/kg twice daily, adjusted according to response, total daily dose may alternatively be given in 3 divided doses

In combination with neurotransmitter precursors for tetrahydrobiopterin-sensitive phenylketonuria (specialist use only)
▸ BY MOUTH
▸ Child 1 month–1 year: Initially 250–750 micrograms/kg 4 times a day, adjusted according to response, total daily dose may alternatively be given in 3 divided doses; maximum 7 mg/kg per day
▸ Child 2–17 years: Initially 250–750 micrograms/kg 4 times a day, adjusted according to response, total daily dose may alternatively be given in 3 divided doses; maximum 10 mg/kg per day

● UNLICENSED USE Not licensed.
● SIDE-EFFECTS Diarrhoea · disturbed sleep · urinary frequency
● PREGNANCY Crosses the placenta; use only if benefit outweighs risk.
● BREAST FEEDING Present in milk, effects unknown.
● RENAL IMPAIRMENT Use with caution—accumulation of metabolites.

● MEDICINAL FORMS
There can be variation in the licensing of different medicines containing the same drug.
No licensed medicines listed.

7   Vitamin deficiency

Vitamins

Overview

Vitamins are used for the prevention and treatment of specific deficiency states or where the diet is known to be inadequate; they may be prescribed in the NHS to prevent or treat deficiency but not as dietary supplements. Except for iron-deficiency anaemia, a primary vitamin or mineral

deficiency due to simple dietary inadequacy is rare in the developed world. Some children may be at risk of developing deficiencies because of an inadequate intake, impaired vitamin synthesis or malabsorption in disease states such as cystic fibrosis and Crohn's disease.

The use of vitamins as general 'pick-me-ups' is of unproven value and, the 'fad' for mega-vitamin therapy with water-soluble vitamins, such as ascorbic acid p. 602 and pyridoxine hydrochloride p. 600, is unscientific and can be harmful. Many vitamin supplements are described as 'multivitamin' but few contain the whole range of essential vitamins and many contain relatively high amounts of vitamins A and D. Care should be taken to ensure the correct dose is not exceeded.

Dietary reference values for vitamins are available in the Department of Health publication:

Dietary Reference Values for Food Energy and Nutrients for the United Kingdom: Report of the Panel on Dietary Reference Values of the Committee on Medical Aspects of Food Policy. Report on Health and Social Subjects 41. London: HMSO, 1991.

Dental patients

It is unjustifiable to treat stomatitis or glossitis with mixtures of vitamin preparations; this delays diagnosis and correct treatment.

Most patients who develop a nutritional deficiency despite an adequate intake of vitamins have malabsorption and if this is suspected the patient should be referred to a medical practitioner.

Vitamin A

Deficiency of vitamin A (retinol) p. 599 is associated with ocular defects (particularly xerophthalmia) and an increased susceptibility to infections, but deficiency is rare in the UK (even in disorders of fat absorption).

Vitamin A supplementation may be required in children with liver disease, particularly cholestatic liver disease, due to the malabsorption of fat soluble vitamins. In those with complete biliary obstruction an intramuscular dose once a month may be appropriate.

Preterm neonates have low plasma concentrations of vitamin A and are usually given vitamin A supplements, often as part of an oral multivitamin preparation once enteral feeding has been established.

Vitamin B group

Deficiency of the B vitamins, other than vitamin B_{12}, is rare in the UK and is usually treated by preparations containing thiamine (B_1) p. 601, and riboflavin (B_2). Other members (or substances traditionally classified as members) of the vitamin B complex such as aminobenzoic acid, biotin, choline, inositol nicotinate, and pantothenic acid or panthenol may be included in vitamin B preparations, but there is no evidence of their value as supplements; however, they can be used in the management of certain metabolic disorders. Anaphylaxis has been reported with parenteral B vitamins.

As with other vitamins of the B group, pyridoxine hydrochloride (B_6) deficiency is rare, but it may occur during isoniazid p. 352 therapy or penicillamine p. 589 treatment in Wilson's disease and is characterised by peripheral neuritis. High doses of pyridoxine hydrochloride are given in some metabolic disorders, such as hyperoxaluria, cystathioninuria and homocystinuria; folic acid p. 546 supplementation may also be beneficial in these disorders. Pyridoxine hydrochloride is also used in sideroblastic anaemia. Rarely, seizures in the neonatal period or during infancy respond to pyridoxine hydrochloride treatment; pyridoxine hydrochloride should be tried in all cases of early-onset intractable seizures and status epilepticus. Pyridoxine hydrochloride has been tried for a wide variety of other disorders, but there is little sound evidence to support the claims of efficacy.

A number of mitochondrial disorders may respond to treatment with certain B vitamins but these disorders require specialist management. Thiamine is used in the treatment of maple syrup urine disease, mitochondrial respiratory chain defects and, together with riboflavin, in the treatment of congenital lactic acidosis; riboflavin is also used in glutaric acidaemias and cytochrome oxidase deficiencies; biotin is used in carboxylase defects.

Folic acid and vitamin B_{12} are used in the treatment of megaloblastic anaemia. Folinic acid p. 528 (available as calcium folinate) is used in association with cytotoxic therapy.

Vitamin C

Vitamin C (ascorbic acid) therapy is essential in scurvy, but less florid manifestations of vitamin C deficiency have been reported. Vitamin C is used to enhance the excretion of iron one month after starting desferrioxamine mesilate p. 550 therapy; it is given separately from food as it also enhances iron absorption. Vitamin C is also used in the treatment of some inherited metabolic disorders, particularly mitochondrial disorders; specialist management of these conditions is required.

Severe scurvy causes gingival swelling and bleeding margins as well as petechiae on the skin. This is, however, exceedingly rare and a child with these signs is more likely to have leukaemia. Investigation should not be delayed by a trial period of vitamin treatment.

Claims that vitamin C ameliorates colds or promotes wound healing have not been proved.

Vitamin D

The term Vitamin D is used for a range of compounds including ergocalciferol (calciferol, vitamin D_2) p. 607, colecalciferol (vitamin D_3) p. 604, dihydrotachysterol, alfacalcidol (1α-hydroxycholecalciferol) p. 603, and calcitriol (1,25- dihydroxycholecalciferol) p. 603.

Asymptomatic vitamin D deficiency is common in the United Kingdom; symptomatic deficiency may occur in certain ethnic groups, particularly as rickets or hypocalcaemia, and rarely in association with malabsorption. The amount of vitamin D required in infancy is related to the stores built up *in-utero* and subsequent exposure to sunlight. The amount of vitamin D in breast milk varies and some breast-fed babies, particularly if preterm or born to vitamin D deficient mothers, may become deficient. Most formula milk and supplement feeds contain adequate vitamin D to prevent deficiency.

Simple, nutritional vitamin D deficiency can be prevented by oral supplementation of ergocalciferol (calciferol, vitamin D_2) or colecalciferol (vitamin D_3) daily, using multi-vitamin drops, preparations of vitamins A and D, manufactured 'special' solutions, or as calcium and ergocalciferol tablets (although the calcium and other vitamins in supplements are unnecessary); excessive supplementation may cause hypercalcaemia.

Inadequate bone mineralisation can be caused by a deficiency, or a lack of action of vitamin D or its active metabolite. In childhood this causes bowing and distortion of bones (rickets). In nutritional vitamin D deficiency rickets, initial high doses of ergocalciferol or colecalciferol should be reduced to supplemental doses after 8–12 weeks, as there is a significant risk of hypercalcaemia. However, calcium supplements are recommended if there is hypocalcaemia or evidence of a poor dietary calcium intake. A single large dose of ergocalciferol or colecalciferol can also be effective for the treatment of nutritional vitamin D deficiency rickets.

Poor bone mineralisation in neonates and young children may also be due to inadequate intake of phosphate or calcium particularly during long-term parenteral nutrition—supplementation with phosphate or calcium may be required.

Hypophosphataemic rickets occurs due to abnormal phosphate excretion; treatment with high doses of oral phosphate, and hydroxylated (activated) forms of vitamin D allow bone mineralisation and optimise growth.

Nutritional deficiency of vitamin D is best treated with colecalciferol or ergocalciferol. Preparations containing calcium and colecalciferol are also occasionally used in children where there is evidence of combined calcium and vitamin D deficiency. Vitamin D deficiency caused by *intestinal malabsorption* or *chronic liver disease* usually requires vitamin D in pharmacological doses; the hypocalcaemia of *hypoparathyroidism* often requires higher doses in order to achieve normocalcaemia and alfacalcidol is generally preferred.

Vitamin D supplementation is often given in combination with calcium supplements for persistent hypocalcaemia in neonates, and in chronic renal disease

Vitamin D requires hydroxylation, by the kidney and liver, to its active form therefore the hydroxylated derivatives alfacalcidol or calcitriol should be prescribed if patients with *severe liver or renal impairment* require vitamin D therapy. Alfacalcidol is generally preferred in children as there is more experience of its use and appropriate formulations are available. Calcitriol is unlicensed for use in children and is generally reserved for those with severe liver disease.

Vitamin E

The daily requirement of vitamin E (tocopherol) has not been well defined. Vitamin E supplements are given to children with fat malabsorption such as in cystic fibrosis and cholestatic liver disease. In children with abetalipoproteinaemia abnormally low vitamin E concentrations may occur in association with neuromuscular problems; this usually responds to high doses of vitamin E. Some neonatal units still administer a single intramuscular dose of vitamin E at birth to preterm neonates to reduce the risk of complications; no trials of long-term outcome have been carried out. The intramuscular route should also be considered in children with severe liver disease when response to oral therapy is inadequate.

Vitamin E has been tried for various other conditions but there is little scientific evidence of its value.

Vitamin K

Vitamin K is necessary for the production of blood clotting factors and proteins necessary for the normal calcification of bone.

Because vitamin K is fat soluble, children with fat malabsorption, especially in biliary obstruction or hepatic disease, may become deficient. For oral administration to prevent vitamin K deficiency in malabsorption syndromes, a water-soluble synthetic vitamin K derivative, menadiol sodium phosphate p. 609 can be used if supplementation with phytomenadione p. 609 by mouth has been insufficient. Oral coumarin anticoagulants act by interfering with vitamin K metabolism in the hepatic cells and their effects can be antagonised by giving vitamin K; see advice on the use of vitamin K in haemorrhage.

Multivitamins

Multivitamin supplements are used in children with vitamin deficiencies and also in malabsorption conditions such as cystic fibrosis or liver disease. Supplementation is not required if nutrient enriched feeds are used; consult a dietician for further advice.

Neonates

Vitamin K deficiency bleeding

Neonates are relatively deficient in vitamin K and those who do not receive supplements of vitamin K are at risk of serious bleeding including intracranial bleeding. The Chief Medical Officer and the Chief Nursing Officer have recommended that all newborn babies should receive vitamin K to prevent vitamin K deficiency bleeding (previously termed haemorrhagic disease of the newborn). An appropriate regimen should be selected after discussion with parents in the antenatal period.

Vitamin K (as phytomenadione) may be given by a single intramuscular injection at birth; this prevents vitamin K deficiency bleeding in virtually all babies.

Alternatively, in healthy babies who are not at particular risk of bleeding disorders, vitamin K may be given by mouth, and arrangements must be in place to ensure the appropriate regimen is followed. Two doses of a colloidal (mixed micelle) preparation of phytomenadione should be given by mouth in the first week, the first dose being given at birth and the second dose at 4–7 days. For exclusively breast-fed babies, a third dose of colloidal phytomenadione is given by mouth at 1 month of age; the third dose is omitted in formula-fed babies because formula foods contain adequate vitamin K. An alternative regimen is to give one dose of phytomenadione by mouth at birth (using the contents of a phytomenadione capsule) to protect from the risk of vitamin K deficiency bleeding in the first week; for exclusively breast-fed babies, further doses of phytomenadione are given by mouth (using the contents of a phytomenadione capsule) at weekly intervals for 12 weeks.

VITAMINS AND TRACE ELEMENTS ⟩
MULTIVITAMINS

Vitamins A and D

● **INDICATIONS AND DOSE**

Prevention of vitamin A and D deficiency
▸ BY MOUTH
  ▸ Child: 1 capsule daily, 1 capsule contains 4000 units vitamin A and 400 units (10 micrograms) vitamin D

● **UNLICENSED USE** Not licensed in children under 6 months of age.

● **SIDE-EFFECTS**

Overdose
Excessive ingestion Prolonged excessive ingestion of vitamins A and D can lead to hypervitaminosis.

● **PRESCRIBING AND DISPENSING INFORMATION** This drug contains vitamin D; consult individual vitamin D monographs.

● **MEDICINAL FORMS**
There can be variation in the licensing of different medicines containing the same drug.

Capsule
▸ Vitamins a and d (Non-proprietary)
  Vitamin D 400 unit, Vitamin A 4000 unit Vitamins A and D capsules BPC 1973 | 28 capsule £2.81 | 28 capsule GSL £2.81 | 84 capsule £6.75–£8.42 DT price = £8.42

Vitamins A, B group, C and D

● **INDICATIONS AND DOSE**

Prevention of deficiency
▸ BY MOUTH USING CAPSULES
  ▸ Child 1–11 years: 1 capsule daily
  ▸ Child 12–17 years: 2 capsules daily

Cystic Fibrosis: prevention of deficiency
▸ BY MOUTH USING CAPSULES
  ▸ Child 1–17 years: 2–3 capsules daily

ABIDEC MULTIVITAMIN DROPS®
Prevention of deficiency
▸ BY MOUTH USING ORAL DROPS
  ▸ Preterm neonate: 0.6 mL daily.

  ▸ Neonate: 0.3 mL daily.

  ▸ Child 1–11 months: 0.3 mL daily
  ▸ Child 1–17 years: 0.6 mL daily
Cystic Fibrosis: prevention of deficiency
▸ BY MOUTH USING ORAL DROPS
  ▸ Child 1–11 months: 0.6 mL daily
  ▸ Child 1–17 years: 1.2 mL daily

DALIVIT ORAL DROPS®
Prevention of deficiency
▸ BY MOUTH USING ORAL DROPS
  ▸ Preterm neonate: 0.3 mL daily.

  ▸ Neonate: 0.3 mL daily.

  ▸ Child 1–11 months: 0.3 mL daily
  ▸ Child 1–17 years: 0.6 mL daily
Cystic Fibrosis: prevention of deficiency
▸ BY MOUTH USING ORAL DROPS
  ▸ Child 1–11 months: 0.6 mL daily
  ▸ Child 1–17 years: 1 mL daily

● **UNLICENSED USE** *Dalavit®* not licensed for use in children under 6 weeks.

● **PRESCRIBING AND DISPENSING INFORMATION** This drug contains vitamin D; consult individual vitamin D monographs.
  To avoid potential toxicity, the content of all vitamin preparations, particularly vitamin A, should be considered when used together with other supplements.
  Vitamin A concentration of preparations varies.
ABIDEC MULTIVITAMIN DROPS® *Abidec®* contains 1333 units of vitamin A (as palmitate) per 0.6 mL dose.
DALIVIT ORAL DROPS® *Dalavit®* contains 5000 units of vitamin A (as palmitate) per 0.6 mL dose.

● **MEDICINAL FORMS**
There can be variation in the licensing of different medicines containing the same drug.
Oral drops
EXCIPIENTS: May contain Arachis (peanut) oil, sucrose
▸ Abidec Multivitamin (Omega Pharma Ltd)
  Nicotinamide 1333 microgram per 1 ml, Pyridoxine hydrochloride 1333 microgram per 1 ml, Riboflavin 1333 microgram per 1 ml, Thiamine hydrochloride 1.67 mg per 1 ml, Ascorbic acid 66.7 mg per 1 ml, Ergocalciferol 667 iu per 1 ml, Retinol (as Vitamin A palmitate) 2222 iu per 1 ml Abidec Multivitamin drops | 25 ml GSL £3.33
▸ Dalivit (Boston Healthcare Ltd)
  Riboflavin 667 microgram per 1 ml, Pyridoxine 833 microgram per 1 ml, Thiamine 1667 microgram per 1 ml, Nicotinamide 8.3 mg per 1 ml, Ascorbic acid 83 mg per 1 ml, Ergocalciferol 667 iu per 1 ml, Vitamin A 8333 iu per 1 ml Dalivit oral drops | 25 ml GSL £6.19 | 50 ml GSL £10.82

Capsule
▸ Vitamins a, b group, c and d (Non-proprietary)
  Riboflavin 500 microgram, Thiamine hydrochloride 1 mg, Nicotinamide 7.5 mg, Ascorbic acid 15 mg, Vitamin D 300 unit, Vitamin A 2500 unit Vitamins capsules | 84 capsule no price available | 1000 capsule £48.20 DT price = £15.48

Vitamins A, C and D

The properties listed below are those particular to the combination only. For the properties of the components please consider, vitamin A below, ascorbic acid p. 602.

- **INDICATIONS AND DOSE**

Prevention of vitamin deficiency
▸ BY MOUTH
 ‣ Child 1 month-4 years: 5 drops daily, 5 drops contain vitamin A approx. 700 units, vitamin D approx. 300 units (7.5 micrograms), ascorbic acid approx. 20 mg

- **INTERACTIONS** → Appendix 1: ascorbic acid, vitamin A
- **PRESCRIBING AND DISPENSING INFORMATION** This drug contains vitamin D; consult individual vitamin D monographs.

 Available free of charge to children under 4 years in families on the Healthy Start Scheme, or alternatively may be available direct to the public—further information for healthcare professionals can be accessed at www.healthystart.nhs.uk. Beneficiaries can contact their midwife or health visitor for further information on where to obtain supplies.

 Healthy Start Vitamins for women (containing ascorbic acid, vitamin D, and folic acid) are also available free of charge to women on the Healthy Start Scheme during pregnancy and until their baby is one year old, or alternatively may be available direct to the public—further information for healthcare professionals can be accessed at www.healthystart.nhs.uk. Beneficiaries can contact their midwife or health visitor for further information on where to obtain supplies.

- **MEDICINAL FORMS**
 There can be variation in the licensing of different medicines containing the same drug.
 Oral drops
 ▸ Healthy Start Children's Vitamin (Secretary of State for Health) Vitamin A and D3 concentrate.55 mg per 1 ml, Sodium ascorbate 18.58 mg per 1 ml, Ascorbic acid 150 mg per 1 ml, Vitamin D 2000 iu per 1 ml, Vitamin A 5000 iu per 1 ml Healthy Start Children's Vitamin drops | 10 ml no price available

VITAMINS AND TRACE ELEMENTS ⟩ VITAMIN A

Vitamin A

(Retinol)

- **INDICATIONS AND DOSE**

Vitamin A deficiency
▸ BY MOUTH
 ‣ Neonate: 5000 units daily, higher doses may be used initially for treatment of severe deficiency.
 ‣ Child 1-11 months: 5000 units daily, to be taken with or after food, higher doses may be used initially for treatment of severe deficiency
 ‣ Child 1-17 years: 10 000 units daily, to be taken with or after food, higher doses may be used initially for treatment of severe deficiency

Prevention of deficiency in complete biliary obstruction
▸ BY INTRAMUSCULAR INJECTION
 ‣ Neonate: 50 000 units once a month.
 ‣ Child 1-11 months: 50 000 units once a month

- **UNLICENSED USE** Preparations containing only vitamin A are not licensed.
- **INTERACTIONS** → Appendix 1: vitamin A

- **SIDE-EFFECTS**
 Overdose
 Massive overdose can cause rough skin, dry hair, an enlarged liver, and a raised erythrocyte sedimentation rate and raised serum calcium and serum alkaline phosphatase concentrations.
- **PREGNANCY** Excessive doses may be teratogenic. In view of evidence suggesting that high levels of vitamin A may cause birth defects, women who are (or may become) pregnant are advised not to take vitamin A supplements (including tablets and fish liver oil drops), except on the advice of a doctor or an antenatal clinic; nor should they eat liver or products such as liver paté or liver sausage.
- **BREAST FEEDING** Theoretical risk of toxicity in infants of mothers taking large doses.
- **MONITORING REQUIREMENTS** Treatment is sometimes initiated with very high doses of vitamin A and the child should be monitored closely; very high doses are associated with acute toxicity.

- **MEDICINAL FORMS**
 There can be variation in the licensing of different medicines containing the same drug. Forms available from special-order manufacturers include: drops, solution for injection
 Solution for injection
 ▸ Vitamin A (Non-proprietary)
  Retinol (as Vitamin A palmitate) 50000 unit per 1 ml Vitamin A 100,000units/2ml solution for injection ampoules | 6 ampoule PoM no price available
 Drops
 ▸ Vitamin A (Non-proprietary)
  Vitamin A 150000 unit per 1 ml Arovit 150,000units/ml drops | 7.5 ml PoM no price available

 Combinations available: *Vitamins A, C and D,* above

VITAMINS AND TRACE ELEMENTS ⟩ VITAMIN B GROUP

Biotin

(Vitamin H)

- **INDICATIONS AND DOSE**

Isolated carboxylase defects
▸ BY MOUTH, OR BY SLOW INTRAVENOUS INJECTION
 ‣ Neonate: 5 mg once daily, adjusted according to response, maintenance 10–50 mg daily, higher doses may be required.
 ‣ Child: 10 mg once daily, adjusted according to response; maintenance 10–50 mg daily, increased if necessary up to 100 mg daily

Defects of biotin metabolism
▸ BY MOUTH, OR BY SLOW INTRAVENOUS INJECTION
 ‣ Neonate: Initially 10 mg once daily, adjusted according to response; maintenance 5–20 mg daily, higher doses may be required.
 ‣ Child: Initially 10 mg once daily, adjusted according to response; maintenance 5–20 mg daily, higher doses may be required

- **PREGNANCY** No information available.
- **BREAST FEEDING** No information available.
- **DIRECTIONS FOR ADMINISTRATION** For administration *by mouth*, tablets may be crushed and mixed with food or drink.
- **PATIENT AND CARER ADVICE**
 Medicines for Children leaflet: Biotin for metabolic disorders www.medicinesforchildren.org.uk/biotin-metabolic-disorders-0

9

Blood and nutrition

● MEDICINAL FORMS
There can be variation in the licensing of different medicines containing the same drug. Forms available from special-order manufacturers include: tablet, oral suspension, oral solution

Solution for injection
▸ Biotin (Non-proprietary)
Biotin 5 mg per 1 ml Biodermatin 5mg/1ml solution for injection vials | 10 vial [PoM] no price available

Tablet
▸ Biotin (Non-proprietary)
Biotin 5 mg Biotin 5 tablets | 30 tablet [PoM] no price available
Biotin 10 mg Biotin 10mg tablets | 30 tablet no price available
▸ OroB7 (Rhodes Pharma Ltd)
Biotin 5 mg OroB7 5mg tablets | 30 tablet £33.99

Pyridoxine hydrochloride

(Vitamin B₆)

● INDICATIONS AND DOSE
Isoniazid-induced neuropathy (prophylaxis)
▸ BY MOUTH

▸ Neonate: 5 mg daily.

▸ Child 1 month–11 years: 5–10 mg daily
▸ Child 12–17 years: 10 mg daily

Isoniazid-induced neuropathy (treatment)
▸ BY MOUTH

▸ Neonate: 5–10 mg daily.

▸ Child 1 month–11 years: 10–20 mg 2–3 times a day
▸ Child 12–17 years: 30–50 mg 2–3 times a day

Prevention of penicillamine-induced neuropathy in Wilson's disease
▸ BY MOUTH

▸ Child 1–11 years: 5–10 mg daily
▸ Child 12–17 years: 10 mg daily

Metabolic diseases | Cystathioninuria | Homocystinuria
▸ BY MOUTH

▸ Neonate: 50–100 mg 1–2 times a day.

▸ Child: 50–250 mg 1–2 times a day

Pyridoxine-dependent seizures
▸ INITIALLY BY INTRAVENOUS INJECTION

▸ Neonate: Test dose 50–100 mg, repeated if necessary, if responsive, followed by an oral maintenance dose; (by mouth) maintenance 50–100 mg once daily, dose to be adjusted as necessary.

▸ Child 1 month–11 years: Test dose 50–100 mg daily, if responsive, followed by an oral maintenance dose, (by mouth) maintenance 20–50 mg 1–2 times a day, dose to be adjusted as necessary, (by mouth) increased if necessary up to 30 mg/kg daily, alternatively (by mouth) increased if necessary up to 1 g daily

● UNLICENSED USE Not licensed for prophylaxis of penicillamine-induced neuropathy in Wilson's disease. Not licensed for use in children.

● CAUTIONS
▸ With intravenous use Risk of cardiovascular collapse (with intravenous injection—resuscitation facilities must be available and monitor closely)

● INTERACTIONS → Appendix 1: pyridoxine

● SIDE-EFFECTS Sensory neuropathy (with high doses when given for extended periods)

Overdose
Overdosage induces toxic effects.

● MEDICINAL FORMS
There can be variation in the licensing of different medicines containing the same drug. Forms available from special-order manufacturers include: capsule, oral suspension, oral solution, solution for injection

Tablet
▸ Pyridoxine hydrochloride (Non-proprietary)
Pyridoxine hydrochloride 10 mg Pyridoxine 10mg tablets | 28 tablet £12.95–£14.50 DT price = £12.95 | 28 tablet [GSL] no price available DT price = £12.95 | 30 tablet [GSL] no price available | 60 tablet [GSL] no price available | 500 tablet [GSL] no price available
Pyridoxine (as Pyridoxine hydrochloride) 20 mg Pyridoxine 20mg tablets | 500 tablet [GSL] no price available
Pyridoxine hydrochloride 50 mg Pyridoxine 50mg tablets | 28 tablet [P] no price available DT price = £8.74 | 500 tablet [P] no price available
Pyridoxine (as Pyridoxine hydrochloride) 100 mg Vitamin B6 100mg tablets | 90 tablet £5.02
▸ Pyrid (Ennogen Healthcare Ltd)
Pyridoxine hydrochloride 10 mg Pyrid-10 tablets | 30 tablet £12.95
Pyridoxine (as Pyridoxine hydrochloride) 20 mg Pyrid-20 tablets | 30 tablet £89.80

Solution for injection
▸ Pyridoxine hydrochloride (Non-proprietary)
Pyridoxine hydrochloride 25 mg per 1 ml Sicovit B6 50mg/2ml solution for injection vials | 5 vial [PoM] no price available
Pyridoxine hydrochloride 50 mg per 1 ml Vitamin B6 100mg/2ml solution for injection ampoules | 10 ampoule [PoM] no price available

Capsule
▸ Pyridoxine hydrochloride (Non-proprietary)
Pyridoxine (as Pyridoxine hydrochloride) 100 mg Vitamin B6 100mg capsules | 120 capsule £6.00

Riboflavin

(Riboflavine; Vitamin B₂)

● INDICATIONS AND DOSE
Metabolic diseases
▸ BY MOUTH

▸ Neonate: 50 mg 1–2 times a day, adjusted according to response.

▸ Child: 50–100 mg 1–2 times a day, adjusted according to response to up to 400 mg daily

● UNLICENSED USE Not licensed in children.

● SIDE-EFFECTS Bright yellow urine

● PREGNANCY Crosses the placenta but no adverse effects reported, information at high doses limited.

● BREAST FEEDING Present in breast milk but no adverse effects reported, information at high doses limited.

● MEDICINAL FORMS
There can be variation in the licensing of different medicines containing the same drug. Forms available from special-order manufacturers include: tablet, modified-release tablet, capsule, oral suspension, oral solution

Modified-release tablet
▸ Riboflavin (Non-proprietary)
Riboflavin 100 mg Vitamin B2 100mg modified-release tablets | 60 tablet £4.18

Tablet
▸ Riboflavin (Non-proprietary)
Riboflavin 10 mg 10mg tablets | 20 tablet no price available
Riboflavin 100 mg Vitamin B2 100mg tablets | 100 tablet no price available

Capsule
▸ Riboflavin (Non-proprietary)
Riboflavin 50 mg Riboflavin 50mg capsules | 30 capsule £3.02 | 100 capsule £5.00
Riboflavin 100 mg Vitamin B2 100mg capsules | 100 capsule no price available

▸ **B-2-50** (Bio-Tech Pharmacal Inc)
Riboflavin 50 mg B-2-50 capsules | 100 capsule no price available
▸ **E-B2** (Ennogen Healthcare Ltd)
Riboflavin 50 mg E-B2 50mg capsules | 30 capsule £84.70
Riboflavin 100 mg E-B2 100mg capsules | 30 capsule £89.20

Thiamine

(Vitamin B₁)

- **INDICATIONS AND DOSE**

Maple syrup urine disease
▸ BY MOUTH

▸ **Neonate:** 5 mg/kg daily, dose to be adjusted as necessary.

▸ **Child:** 5 mg/kg daily, dose to be adjusted as necessary

Metabolic disorders | Congenital lactic acidosis
▸ BY MOUTH, OR BY INTRAVENOUS INFUSION

▸ **Neonate:** 50–200 mg once daily, dose to be adjusted as
necessary, the total dose may alternatively be given in
2–3 divided doses, administer intravenous infusion over
30 minutes.

▸ **Child:** 100–300 mg once daily, dose to be adjusted as
necessary, the total dose may alternatively be given in
2–3 divided doses, administer intravenous infusion
over 30 minutes, increased if necessary up to 2 g daily

- **UNLICENSED USE** Not licensed in children.

> **IMPORTANT SAFETY INFORMATION**
> MHRA/CHM ADVICE (SEPTEMBER 2007)
> Although potentially serious allergic adverse reactions
> may rarely occur during, or shortly after, parenteral
> administration, the CHM has recommended that:
>
> - This should not preclude the use of parenteral
>   thiamine in patients where this route of
>   administration is required, particularly in patients at
>   risk of Wernicke-Korsakoff syndrome where treatment
>   with thiamine is essential;
> - Intravenous administration should be by infusion over
>   30 minutes;
> - Facilities for treating anaphylaxis (including
>   resuscitation facilities) should be available when
>   parenteral thiamine is administered.

- **CAUTIONS** Anaphylaxis may occasionally follow injection
- **SIDE-EFFECTS**
▸ With intravenous use Hypersensitivity reactions
- **BREAST FEEDING** Severely thiamine-deficient mothers
  should avoid breast-feeding as toxic methyl-glyoxal
  present in milk.
- **PRESCRIBING AND DISPENSING INFORMATION**
▸ With intravenous use Some preparations may contain phenol
  as a preservative.
- **MEDICINAL FORMS**
  There can be variation in the licensing of different medicines
  containing the same drug. Forms available from special-order
  manufacturers include: oral suspension, oral solution
  Modified-release tablet
▸ Thiamine (Non-proprietary)
  Thiamine hydrochloride 100 mg Vitamin B1 100mg modified-
  release tablets | 90 tablet £4.18
  Tablet
▸ Thiamine (Non-proprietary)
  Thiamine hydrochloride 25 mg Vitamin B1 25mg tablets |
  100 tablet P no price available
  Thiamine hydrochloride 50 mg Thiamine 50mg tablets |
  28 tablet P £1.80–£2.00 | 100 tablet P £7.14 DT price = £7.14
  Thiamine hydrochloride 100 mg Thiamine 100mg tablets |
  28 tablet P £2.50–£2.80 | 100 tablet P £10.00 DT price = £10.00

▸ **Benerva** (Teofarma)
  Thiamine hydrochloride 50 mg Benerva 50mg tablets |
  100 tablet P £4.00 DT price = £7.14
  Thiamine hydrochloride 100 mg Benerva 100mg tablets |
  100 tablet P £6.29 DT price = £10.00
▸ **Tyvera** (Auden McKenzie (Pharma Division) Ltd)
  Thiamine hydrochloride 50 mg Tyvera 50mg tablets |
  100 tablet P £4.99 DT price = £7.14
  Thiamine hydrochloride 100 mg Tyvera 100mg tablets |
  100 tablet P £6.99 DT price = £10.00
  Solution for injection
▸ Thiamine (Non-proprietary)
  Thiamine hydrochloride 50 mg per 1 ml Bevitine 100mg/2ml
  solution for injection ampoules | 5 ampoule PoM no price available
  Thiamine hydrochloride 100 mg per 1 ml Vitamin B1 Streuli
  100mg/1ml solution for injection ampoules | 10 ampoule PoM no
  price available

Vitamin B complex

- **INDICATIONS AND DOSE**

VIGRANON B® SYRUP

Treatment of deficiency
▸ BY MOUTH

▸ Child 1–11 months: 5 mL 3 times a day
▸ Child 1–11 years: 10 mL 3 times a day
▸ Child 12–17 years: 10–15 mL 3 times a day

Prophylaxis of deficiency
▸ BY MOUTH

▸ Child 1–11 months: 5 mL once daily
▸ Child 1–11 years: 5 mL twice daily
▸ Child 12–17 years: 5 mL 3 times a day

- **NATIONAL FUNDING/ACCESS DECISIONS**
  NHS restrictions Vigranon B® syrup is not prescribable
  under the National Health Service (NHS).
- **LESS SUITABLE FOR PRESCRIBING** Vigranon B® syrup is
  less suitable for prescribing.

- **MEDICINAL FORMS**
  There can be variation in the licensing of different medicines
  containing the same drug.
  Oral solution
▸ Vigranon-B (Wallace Manufacturing Chemists Ltd)
  **Pyridoxine hydrochloride 400 microgram per 1 ml, Riboflavin
  sodium phosphate 548 microgram per 1 ml, Dexpanthenol
  600 microgram per 1 ml, Thiamine hydrochloride 1 mg per 1 ml,
  Nicotinamide 4 mg per 1 ml** Vigranon-B syrup sugar-free |
  150 ml P £26.00

Vitamins with minerals and trace elements

- **INDICATIONS AND DOSE**

FORCEVAL® CAPSULES

**Vitamin and mineral deficiency and as adjunct in
synthetic diets**
▸ BY MOUTH

▸ Child 12–17 years: 1 capsule daily, one hour after a meal

KETOVITE® LIQUID

**Prevention of vitamin deficiency in disorders of
carbohydrate or amino-acid metabolism | Adjunct in
restricted, specialised, or synthetic diets**
▸ BY MOUTH

▸ Child: 5 mL daily, dose adjusted according to condition,
  diet, or age, use with Ketovite® Tablets for complete
  vitamin supplementation. continued →

9

Blood and nutrition

KETOVITE® TABLETS

Prevention of vitamin deficiency in disorders of carbohydrate or amino-acid metabolism | Adjunct in restricted, specialised, or synthetic diets

▶ BY MOUTH

▶ Child: 1 tablet 3 times a day, dose adjusted according to condition, diet, or age, use with *Ketovite® Liquid* for complete vitamin supplementation.

● PRESCRIBING AND DISPENSING INFORMATION To avoid potential toxicity, the content of all vitamin preparations, particularly vitamin A, should be considered when used together with other supplements.

● PATIENT AND CARER ADVICE
Medicines for Children leaflet: Multivitamin preparations for vitamin deficiency www.medicinesforchildren.org.uk/multivitamin-preparations-vitamin-deficiency
KETOVITE® LIQUID *Ketovite®* liquid may be mixed with milk, cereal, or fruit juice.
KETOVITE® TABLETS Tablets may be crushed immediately before use.

● MEDICINAL FORMS
There can be variation in the licensing of different medicines containing the same drug.
Oral emulsion
▶ Vitamins with minerals and trace elements (Non-proprietary)
Cyanocobalamin 2.5 microgram per 1 ml, Choline chloride 30 mg per 1 ml, Ergocalciferol 80 unit per 1 ml, Vitamin A 500 unit per 1 ml Ketovite liquid sugar-free | 150 ml [P] £19.10
Tablet
▶ Ketovite (Essential Pharmaceuticals Ltd)
Biotin 170 microgram, Folic acid 250 microgram, Pyridoxine hydrochloride 330 microgram, Acetomenaphthone 500 microgram, Riboflavin 1 mg, Thiamine hydrochloride 1 mg, Calcium pantothenate 1.16 mg, Nicotinamide 3.3 mg, Alpha tocopheryl acetate 5 mg, Ascorbic acid 16.6 mg, Inositol 50 mg Ketovite tablets | 100 tablet [PoM] £9.21
Capsule
▶ Forceval (Alliance Pharmaceuticals Ltd)
Cyanocobalamin 3 microgram, Selenium 50 microgram, Biotin 100 microgram, Iodine 140 microgram, Chromium 200 microgram, Molybdenum 250 microgram, Folic acid 400 microgram, Thiamine 1.2 mg, Riboflavin 1.6 mg, Copper 2 mg, Pyridoxine 2 mg, Manganese 3 mg, Pantothenic acid 4 mg, Potassium 4 mg, Tocopheryl acetate 10 mg, Iron 12 mg, Zinc 15 mg, Nicotinamide 18 mg, Magnesium 30 mg, Ascorbic acid 60 mg, Phosphorus 77 mg, Calcium 100 mg, Ergocalciferol 400 unit, Vitamin A 2500 unit Forceval capsules | 15 capsule [P] £4.86 | 30 capsule [P] £8.48 | 90 capsule [P] £25.44

VITAMINS AND TRACE ELEMENTS > VITAMIN C

Ascorbic acid
(Vitamin C)

● INDICATIONS AND DOSE
Treatment of scurvy
▶ BY MOUTH
▶ Child 1 month-3 years: 125–250 mg daily in 1–2 divided doses
▶ Child 4-11 years: 250–500 mg daily in 1–2 divided doses
▶ Child 12-17 years: 0.5–1 g daily in 1–2 divided doses
Adjunct to desferrioxamine (to enhance the excretion of iron 1 month after treatment)
▶ BY MOUTH
▶ Child: 100–200 mg daily, to be taken 1 hour before food

Metabolic disorders | Tyrosinaemia type III | Transient tyrosinaemia of the newborn | Glutathione synthase deficiency | Hawkinsinuria
▶ BY MOUTH
▶ Neonate: 50–200 mg daily, dose to be adjusted as necessary.
▶ Child: 200–400 mg daily in 1–2 divided doses, dose to be adjusted as necessary, increased if necessary up to 1 g daily

● UNLICENSED USE Not licensed for metabolic disorders.
● CONTRA-INDICATIONS Hyperoxaluria
● CAUTIONS
CAUTIONS, FURTHER INFORMATION
▶ Iron overload Ascorbic acid should not be given to patients with cardiac dysfunction.
In patients with normal cardiac function ascorbic acid should be introduced 1 month after starting desferrioxamine.
● INTERACTIONS → Appendix 1: ascorbic acid
● SIDE-EFFECTS Diarrhoea · fatigue · headache · hyperoxaluria · nausea
● PRESCRIBING AND DISPENSING INFORMATION It is rarely necessary to prescribe more than 100 mg daily except early in the treatment of scurvy.

● MEDICINAL FORMS
There can be variation in the licensing of different medicines containing the same drug. Forms available from special-order manufacturers include: oral suspension, oral solution, solution for infusion
Tablet
EXCIPIENTS: May contain Aspartame
▶ Ascorbic acid (Non-proprietary)
Ascorbic acid 50 mg Ascorbic acid 50mg tablets | 28 tablet [GSL] £15.05 DT price = £15.05 | 500 tablet [GSL] no price available
Ascorbic acid 100 mg Ascorbic acid 100mg tablets | 28 tablet [GSL] £14.30 DT price = £14.30
Ascorbic acid 200 mg Ascorbic acid 200mg tablets | 28 tablet [GSL] £19.86 DT price = £19.86 | 100 tablet [GSL] no price available
Ascorbic acid 250 mg Ascorbic acid 250mg tablets | 1000 tablet [PoM] no price available
Ascorbic acid 500 mg Ascorbic acid 500mg tablets | 28 tablet [GSL] £26.87 DT price = £26.87 | 100 tablet [GSL] no price available
Chewable tablet
CAUTIONARY AND ADVISORY LABELS 24
EXCIPIENTS: May contain Aspartame
▶ Ascorbic acid (Non-proprietary)
Ascorbic acid 60 mg Vitamin C 60mg chewable tablets | 60 tablet no price available | 180 tablet no price available
Ascorbic acid 500 mg Vitamin C 500mg chewable tablets | 25 tablet £0.90 | 60 tablet £3.90 | 100 tablet £5.58
Ascorbic acid (as Sodium ascorbate) 500 mg Vitamin C 500mg chewable tablets sugar-free | 60 tablet no price available
Ascorbic acid 1 gram Vitamin C 1000mg chewable tablets | 30 tablet £2.35 | 60 tablet £4.29 | 100 tablet £9.49
▶ Ascur (Ennogen Healthcare Ltd)
Ascorbic acid 100 mg Ascur 100mg chewable tablets | 30 tablet £3.95
Ascorbic acid (as Sodium ascorbate) 500 mg Ascur 500mg chewable tablets sugar-free | 30 tablet £2.99
Capsule
▶ Ascorbic acid (Non-proprietary)
Ascorbic acid 500 mg Vitamin C 500mg capsules | 100 capsule no price available
Ascorbic acid 1 gram Vitamin C 1000mg capsules | 100 capsule no price available | 250 capsule no price available

Combinations available: *Vitamins A, C and D,* p. 599

Vitamin D and analogues (systemic)

- **CONTRA-INDICATIONS** Hypercalcaemia · metastatic calcification
- **SIDE-EFFECTS**

Overdose
Symptoms of overdosage include anorexia, lassitude, nausea and vomiting, diarrhoea, constipation, weight loss, polyuria, sweating, headache, thirst, vertigo, and raised concentrations of calcium and phosphate in plasma and urine.

- **PREGNANCY** High doses teratogenic in *animals* but therapeutic doses unlikely to be harmful.
- **BREAST FEEDING** Caution with high doses; may cause hypercalcaemia in infant—monitor serum-calcium concentration.
- **MONITORING REQUIREMENTS Important:** All patients receiving pharmacological doses of vitamin D should have their plasma-calcium concentration checked at intervals (initially once or twice weekly) and whenever nausea or vomiting occur.

☞ above

Alfacalcidol

(1α-Hydroxycholecalciferol)

- **INDICATIONS AND DOSE**

Hypophosphataemic rickets | Persistent hypocalcaemia due to hypoparathyroidism or pseudohypoparathyroidism
▸ BY MOUTH, OR BY INTRAVENOUS INJECTION
‣ Child 1 month–11 years: 25–50 nanograms/kg once daily, dose to be adjusted as necessary; maximum 1 microgram per day
‣ Child 12–17 years: 1 microgram once daily, dose to be adjusted as necessary

Persistent neonatal hypocalcaemia
▸ BY MOUTH, OR BY INTRAVENOUS INJECTION
‣ Neonate: 50–100 nanograms/kg once daily, dose to be adjusted as necessary, in resistant cases higher doses may be needed; increased if necessary up to 2 micrograms/kg daily.

Prevention of vitamin D deficiency in renal or cholestatic liver disease
▸ BY MOUTH, OR BY INTRAVENOUS INJECTION
‣ Neonate: 20 nanograms/kg once daily, dose to be adjusted as necessary.
‣ Child 1 month–11 years (body-weight up to 20 kg): 15–30 nanograms/kg once daily (max. per dose 500 nanograms)
‣ Child 1 month–11 years (body-weight 20 kg and above): 250–500 nanograms once daily, dose to be adjusted as necessary
‣ Child 12–17 years: 250–500 nanograms once daily, dose to be adjusted as necessary

DOSE EQUIVALENCE AND CONVERSION
▸ One drop of alfacalcidol 2 microgram/mL oral drops contains approximately 100 nanograms alfacalcidol.

- **CAUTIONS** Nephrolithiasis · take care to ensure correct dose in infants
- **INTERACTIONS** → Appendix 1: vitamin D substances

- **SIDE-EFFECTS**
▸ **Rare** Nephrocalcinosis · pruritus · rash · urticaria
- **RENAL IMPAIRMENT** Monitor plasma-calcium concentration in renal impairment.
- **MONITORING REQUIREMENTS** Monitor plasma-calcium concentration in patients receiving high doses.
- **DIRECTIONS FOR ADMINISTRATION**
▸ With intravenous use For injection, shake ampoule for at least 5 seconds before use, and give over 30 seconds.
- **MEDICINAL FORMS**
There can be variation in the licensing of different medicines containing the same drug. Forms available from special-order manufacturers include: oral suspension, oral solution

Solution for injection
EXCIPIENTS: May contain Alcohol, propylene glycol
▸ One-Alpha (LEO Pharma)
Alfacalcidol 2 microgram per 1 ml One-Alpha 2micrograms/1ml solution for injection ampoules | 10 ampoule PoM £41.13
One-Alpha 1micrograms/0.5ml solution for injection ampoules | 10 ampoule PoM £21.57

Oral drops
EXCIPIENTS: May contain Alcohol
▸ One-Alpha (LEO Pharma)
Alfacalcidol 2 microgram per 1 ml One-Alpha 2micrograms/ml oral drops sugar-free | 10 ml PoM £21.30 DT price = £21.30

Capsule
EXCIPIENTS: May contain Sesame oil
▸ Alfacalcidol (Non-proprietary)
Alfacalcidol 250 nanogram Alfacalcidol 250nanogram capsules | 30 capsule PoM £5.20 DT price = £3.64
Alfacalcidol 500 nanogram Alfacalcidol 500nanogram capsules | 30 capsule PoM £10.00 DT price = £7.62
Alfacalcidol 1 microgram Alfacalcidol 1microgram capsules | 30 capsule PoM £14.03 DT price = £10.23 | 30 capsule no price available DT price = £10.23
▸ One-Alpha (LEO Pharma)
Alfacalcidol 250 nanogram One-Alpha 250nanogram capsules | 30 capsule PoM £3.37 DT price = £3.64
Alfacalcidol 500 nanogram One-Alpha 0.5microgram capsules | 30 capsule PoM £6.27 DT price = £7.62
Alfacalcidol 1 microgram One-Alpha 1microgram capsules | 30 capsule PoM £8.75 DT price = £10.23

☞ above

Calcitriol

(1,25-Dihydroxycholecalciferol)

- **INDICATIONS AND DOSE**

Vitamin D dependent rickets | Hypophosphataemic rickets | Persistent hypocalcaemia due to hypoparathyroidism | Pseudo-hypoparathyroidism (limited experience)
▸ BY MOUTH
‣ Child 1 month–11 years: Initially 15 nanograms/kg once daily (max. per dose 250 nanograms), increased in steps of 5 nanograms/kg daily (max. per dose 250 nanograms) if required, dose to be increased every 2–4 weeks
‣ Child 12–17 years: Initially 250 nanograms once daily, increased in steps of 5 nanograms/kg daily (max. per dose 250 nanograms) if required, dose to be increased every 2–4 weeks; usual dose 0.5–1 microgram daily

- **UNLICENSED USE** Not licensed for use in children.
- **CAUTIONS** Take care to ensure correct dose in infants
- **INTERACTIONS** → Appendix 1: vitamin D substances
- **HEPATIC IMPAIRMENT** Manufacturer advises avoid—no information available.
- **RENAL IMPAIRMENT** Manufacturer advises avoid—no information available. Monitor plasma-calcium concentration in renal impairment.

9

Blood and nutrition

9

Blooe and nutrition

- MONITORING REQUIREMENTS
- Monitor plasma calcium, phosphate, and creatinine during dosage titration.
- Monitor plasma-calcium concentration in patients receiving high doses.
- DIRECTIONS FOR ADMINISTRATION Contents of capsule may be administered by oral syringe.
- MEDICINAL FORMS
  There can be variation in the licensing of different medicines containing the same drug. Forms available from special-order manufacturers include: oral suspension, oral solution

Oral solution
- Calcitriol (Non-proprietary)
  Calcitriol 1 microgram per 1 ml Rocaltrol 1micrograms/ml oral solution sugar-free | 10 ml [PoM] no price available

Capsule
- Calcitriol (Non-proprietary)
  Calcitriol 250 nanogram Calcitriol 250nanogram capsules | 30 capsule [PoM] £18.04 | 100 capsule [PoM] no price available DT price £10.01
  Calcitriol 500 nanogram Calcitriol 500nanogram capsules | 30 capsule [PoM] £32.25 | 100 capsule [PoM] no price available DT price = £32.25
- Rocaltrol (Roche Products Ltd)
  Calcitriol 250 nanogram Rocaltrol 250nanogram capsules | 100 capsule [PoM] £18.04 DT price = £18.04
  Calcitriol 500 nanogram Rocaltrol 500nanogram capsules | 100 capsule [PoM] £32.25 DT price = £32.25

F 603

Colecalciferol

(Cholecalciferol; Vitamin D₃)

- INDICATIONS AND DOSE

Prevention of vitamin D deficiency
- BY MOUTH
- Child: 400 units daily

- UNLICENSED USE *Adcal-D3*®, *Calceos*®, and *Fultium-D₃*® 800 units and *Fultium-D₃*® 20000 units are not licensed for use in children under 12 years. *Cacit*® D3, *Calcichew-D₃*® *Forte*, *Calcichew-D₃*® 500 mg/400 unit, and *Kalcipos-D*® not licensed for use in children (age range not specified by manufacturers). *Accrete D3*®, *Calfovit D3*®, and *Natecal D3*® not licensed for use in children under 18 years.
- CAUTIONS Take care to ensure correct dose in infants
- INTERACTIONS → Appendix 1: vitamin D substances
- RENAL IMPAIRMENT Monitor plasma-calcium concentration in renal impairment.
- MONITORING REQUIREMENTS Monitor plasma-calcium concentration in patients receiving high doses.
- DIRECTIONS FOR ADMINISTRATION
  INVITA D3® 25,000UNITS/1ML ORAL SOLUTION
  May be mixed with a small amount of milk or cold or lukewarm food immediately before administration.

- MEDICINAL FORMS
  There can be variation in the licensing of different medicines containing the same drug. Forms available from special-order manufacturers include: tablet, capsule, oral suspension, oral solution, oral drops

Tablet
- Colecalciferol (Non-proprietary)
  Colecalciferol 400 unit Colecalciferol 400unit tablets | 30 tablet no price available | 60 tablet £15.50
  Colecalciferol 800 unit Colecalciferol 800unit tablets | 30 tablet [PoM] £3.60–£4.32 DT price = £3.60
  Colecalciferol 1000 unit Colecalciferol 1,000unit tablets | 28 tablet £2.85–£2.95 DT price = £2.95 | 30 tablet no price available | 90 tablet £34.50 | 180 tablet no price available
  Colecalciferol 5000 unit Vitamin D3 5,000unit tablets | 100 tablet £3.50

Colecalciferol 10000 unit Colecalciferol 10,000unit tablets | 30 tablet £36.00
Colecalciferol 20000 unit Colecalciferol 20,000unit tablets | 20 tablet £36.00 | 30 tablet no price available
Colecalciferol 50000 unit Vitamin D3 50,000unit tablets | 30 tablet £16.74
- Aciferol D3 (Rhodes Pharma Ltd)
  Colecalciferol 400 unit Aciferol D3 400unit tablets | 90 tablet £9.99
  Colecalciferol 1000 unit Aciferol D3 1,000unit tablets | 90 tablet £14.99
  Colecalciferol 2200 unit Aciferol D3 2,200unit tablets | 90 tablet £25.99
  Colecalciferol 3000 unit Aciferol D3 3,000unit tablets | 60 tablet £14.99
  Colecalciferol 5000 unit Aciferol D3 5,000unit tablets | 60 tablet £19.99
  Colecalciferol 10000 unit Aciferol D3 10,000unit tablets | 30 tablet £13.99
  Colecalciferol 20000 unit Aciferol D3 20,000unit tablets | 30 tablet £18.99
- Cubicole D3 (Cubic Pharmaceuticals Ltd)
  Colecalciferol 400 unit Cubicole D3 400unit tablets | 30 tablet £5.95
  Colecalciferol 2200 unit Cubicole D3 2,200unit tablets | 30 tablet £12.95
  Colecalciferol 10000 unit Cubicole D3 10,000unit tablets | 30 tablet £14.95
- Desunin (Meda Pharmaceuticals Ltd)
  Colecalciferol 800 unit Desunin 800unit tablets | 30 tablet [PoM] £3.60 DT price = £3.60 | 90 tablet [PoM] £10.17
  Colecalciferol 4000 unit Desunin 4,000unit tablets | 70 tablet [PoM] £15.90 DT price = £15.90
- E-D3 (Ennogen Healthcare Ltd)
  Colecalciferol 400 unit E-D3 400unit tablets | 30 tablet £78.50
  Colecalciferol 1000 unit E-D3 1,000unit tablets | 30 tablet £2.95
  Colecalciferol 10000 unit E-D3 10,000unit tablets | 30 tablet £95.00
  Colecalciferol 20000 unit E-D3 20,000unit tablets | 30 tablet £95.90
- Iso D3 (Nutri Advanced Ltd)
  Colecalciferol 2000 unit Iso D3 2,000unit tablets | 90 tablet £14.37
- Stexerol-D3 (Kyowa Kirin Ltd)
  Colecalciferol 1000 unit Stexerol-D3 1,000unit tablets | 28 tablet [PoM] £2.95 DT price = £2.95
  Colecalciferol 25000 unit Stexerol-D3 25,000unit tablets | 12 tablet [PoM] £17.00 DT price = £17.00
- SunVit D3 (SunVit-D3 Ltd)
  Colecalciferol 400 unit SunVit-D3 400unit tablets | 28 tablet £2.55
  Colecalciferol 1000 unit SunVit-D3 1,000unit tablets | 28 tablet £3.56 DT price = £2.95
  Colecalciferol 2000 unit SunVit-D3 2,000unit tablets | 28 tablet £3.99
  Colecalciferol 3000 unit SunVit-D3 3,000unit tablets | 28 tablet £5.49
  Colecalciferol 5000 unit SunVit-D3 5,000unit tablets | 28 tablet £4.99
  Colecalciferol 10000 unit SunVit-D3 10,000unit tablets | 28 tablet £6.99
  Colecalciferol 20000 unit SunVit-D3 20,000unit tablets | 28 tablet £4.40
  Colecalciferol 50000 unit SunVit-D3 50,000unit tablets | 15 tablet £19.99

Oral drops
- Colecalciferol (Non-proprietary)
  Colecalciferol 200 unit per 1 drop Vitamin D3 200units/drop for infants and children oral drops sugar-free | 50 ml £3.86 | 15 ml £4.46
  Colecalciferol 2500 unit per 1 drop Vitamin D3 2,500units/drop oral drops sugar-free | 50 ml £6.64
- E-D3 (Ennogen Healthcare Ltd)
  Colecalciferol 2000 unit per 1 ml E-D3 2,000units/ml oral drops sugar-free | 20 ml no price available
- Fultium daily D3 (Internis Pharmaceuticals Ltd)
  Colecalciferol 2740 unit per 1 ml Fultium daily D3 2,740units/ml drops sugar-free | 15 ml £5.16
- Fultium-D3 (Internis Pharmaceuticals Ltd)
  Colecalciferol 2740 unit per 1 ml Fultium-D3 2,740units/ml oral drops sugar-free | 25 ml [PoM] £10.70 DT price = £10.70
- InVita D3 (Consilient Health Ltd)
  Colecalciferol 2400 unit per 1 ml InVita D3 2,400units/ml oral drops sugar-free | 10 ml [PoM] £3.60

- **Pro D3** (Synergy Biologics Ltd)
  Colecalciferol 2000 unit per 1 ml Pro D3 2,000units/ml liquid drops sugar-free | 20 ml £9.80
- **SunVit D3** (SunVit-D3 Ltd)
  Colecalciferol 2000 unit per 1 ml SunVit-D3 2,000units/ml oral drops sugar-free | 20 ml £6.20
- **Thorens** (Galen Ltd)
  Colecalciferol 10000 unit per 1 ml Thorens 10,000units/ml oral drops sugar-free | 10 ml [PoM] £5.85 DT price = £5.85

Oral solution
CAUTIONARY AND ADVISORY LABELS 21
- **Colecalciferol** (Non-proprietary)
  Colecalciferol 3000 unit per 1 ml Colecalciferol 3,000units/ml oral solution | 100 ml [PoM] £144.00 DT price = £144.00
  Colecalciferol 10000 unit per 1 ml Colecalciferol 10,000units/ml oral solution | 10 ml no price available
- **Aciferol D3** (Rhodes Pharma Ltd)
  Colecalciferol 2000 unit per 1 ml Aciferol D3 2,000units/ml liquid | 100 ml £18.00
- **Baby D** (KoRa Healthcare)
  Colecalciferol 1000 unit per 1 ml Baby D 1,000units/ml oral solution | 30 ml £4.50
- **E-D3** (Ennogen Healthcare Ltd)
  Colecalciferol 1000 unit per 1 ml E-D3 1,000units/ml oral solution | 15 ml no price available
- **InVita D3** (Consilient Health Ltd)
  Colecalciferol 25000 unit per 1 ml InVita D3 25,000units/1ml oral solution sugar-free | 3 ampoule [PoM] £4.45 DT price = £4.45
  Colecalciferol 50000 unit per 1 ml InVita D3 50,000units/1ml oral solution sugar-free | 3 ampoule [PoM] £6.25 DT price = £6.25
- **Pro D3** (Synergy Biologics Ltd)
  Colecalciferol 2000 unit per 1 ml Pro D3 2,000units/ml liquid | 50 ml £16.80 | 100 ml £22.50
- **SunVit D3** (SunVit-D3 Ltd)
  Colecalciferol 2000 unit per 1 ml SunVit-D3 2,000units/ml oral solution | 50 ml £8.90
- **Thorens** (Galen Ltd)
  Colecalciferol 10000 unit per 1 ml Thorens 25,000units/2.5ml oral solution sugar-free | 2.5 ml [PoM] £1.55 DT price = £1.55 sugar-free | 10 ml [PoM] £5.85 DT price = £5.85

Chewable tablet
- **Colecalciferol** (Non-proprietary)
  Colecalciferol 1000 unit Vitamin D3 1,000unit chewable tablets | 100 tablet no price available

Capsule
CAUTIONARY AND ADVISORY LABELS 25
- **Colecalciferol** (Non-proprietary)
  Colecalciferol 500 unit Vitamin D3 500IU capsules | 90 capsule [GSL] £3.50
  Colecalciferol 600 unit Vitamin D3 600unit capsules | 60 capsule no price available | 120 capsule no price available
  Colecalciferol 2200 unit Colecalciferol 2,200unit capsules | 30 capsule no price available
  Colecalciferol 2500 unit Colecalciferol 2,500unit capsules | 30 capsule no price available
  Colecalciferol 3000 unit Colecalciferol 3,000unit capsules | 30 capsule no price available
  Colecalciferol 4000 unit Vitamin D3 4,000unit capsules | 60 capsule no price available | 120 capsule no price available
  Colecalciferol 5000 unit Colecalciferol 5,000unit capsules | 30 capsule no price available | 40 capsule no price available | 100 capsule [PoM] no price available
  Colecalciferol 5600 unit InVita D3 5,600unit capsules | 4 capsule [PoM] £2.50
  Colecalciferol 10000 unit Vitamin D3 10,000unit capsules | 30 capsule £5.58
  Colecalciferol 20000 unit Colecalciferol 20,000unit capsules | 30 capsule [PoM] £29.00 DT price = £29.00
  Colecalciferol 30000 unit Colecalciferol 30,000unit capsules | 10 capsule no price available
  Colecalciferol 50000 unit Colecalciferol 50,000unit capsules | 10 capsule £36.00 | 100 capsule [PoM] no price available
- **Aciferol D3** (Rhodes Pharma Ltd)
  Colecalciferol 30000 unit Aciferol D3 30,000unit capsules | 10 capsule £19.99

- **Aviticol** (Colonis Pharma Ltd)
  Colecalciferol 800 unit Aviticol 800unit capsules | 30 capsule [PoM] £2.22 DT price = £3.60
  Colecalciferol 1000 unit Aviticol 1,000unit capsules | 30 capsule [PoM] £2.34 DT price = £2.34
  Colecalciferol 20000 unit Aviticol 20,000unit capsules | 30 capsule [PoM] £20.25 DT price = £29.00
- **ColeKal-D3** (Essential-Healthcare Ltd)
  Colecalciferol 3200 unit ColeKal-D3 3,200unit capsules | 30 capsule £5.97 DT price = £13.32
- **Cubicole D3** (Cubic Pharmaceuticals Ltd)
  Colecalciferol 600 unit Cubicole D3 600unit capsules | 30 capsule £6.95
  Colecalciferol 2200 unit Cubicole D3 2,200unit capsules | 30 capsule £9.95
  Colecalciferol 3000 unit Cubicole D3 3,000unit capsules | 30 capsule £11.95
  Colecalciferol 10000 unit Cubicole D3 10,000unit capsules | 30 capsule £12.95
- **E-D3** (Ennogen Healthcare Ltd)
  Colecalciferol 600 unit E-D3 600unit capsules | 30 capsule £82.10
  Colecalciferol 2200 unit E-D3 2,200unit capsules | 30 capsule £86.20
  Colecalciferol 2500 unit E-D3 2,500unit capsules | 30 capsule £86.20
  Colecalciferol 3000 unit E-D3 3,000unit capsules | 30 capsule £88.60
  Colecalciferol 30000 unit E-D3 30,000unit capsules | 10 capsule £94.40
- **Fultium daily D3** (Internis Pharmaceuticals Ltd)
  Colecalciferol 400 unit Fultium daily D3 400unit capsules | 30 capsule £2.58 | 60 capsule £4.84 | 90 capsule £7.09
- **Fultium-D3** (Internis Pharmaceuticals Ltd)
  Colecalciferol 800 unit Fultium-D3 800unit capsules | 30 capsule [PoM] £3.60 DT price = £3.60 | 90 capsule [PoM] £8.85
  Colecalciferol 3200 unit Fultium-D3 3,200unit capsules | 30 capsule [PoM] £13.32 DT price = £13.32 | 90 capsule [PoM] £39.96
  Colecalciferol 20000 unit Fultium-D3 20,000unit capsules | 15 capsule [PoM] £17.04 DT price = £17.04 | 30 capsule [PoM] £29.00 DT price = £29.00
- **InVita D3** (Consilient Health Ltd)
  Colecalciferol 400 unit Invita D3 400unit capsules | 28 capsule [PoM] £1.85
  Colecalciferol 800 unit InVita D3 800unit capsules | 28 capsule [PoM] £2.50
  Colecalciferol 25000 unit Invita D3 25,000unit capsules | 3 capsule [PoM] £3.95
- **Plenachol** (Auden McKenzie (Pharma Division) Ltd)
  Colecalciferol 20000 unit Plenachol 20,000unit capsules | 10 capsule [PoM] £9.00
  Colecalciferol 40000 unit Plenachol 40,000unit capsules | 10 capsule [PoM] £15.00 DT price = £15.00
- **Pro D3** (Synergy Biologics Ltd)
  Colecalciferol 2500 unit Pro D3 2,500unit capsules | 30 capsule £9.99
  Colecalciferol 30000 unit Pro D3 30,000unit capsules | 10 capsule £24.99
- **Strivit-D3** (Strides Arcolab International Ltd)
  Colecalciferol 800 unit Strivit-D3 800unit capsules | 30 capsule [PoM] £2.34 DT price = £3.60

Orodispersible tablet
- **Colecalciferol** (Non-proprietary)
  Colecalciferol 2000 unit D3 Lemon Melts 2,000unit tablets sugar-free | 120 tablet £4.88

Colecalciferol with calcium carbonate

The properties listed below are those particular to the combination only. For the properties of the components please consider, colecalciferol p. 604, calcium carbonate p. 567.

● **INDICATIONS AND DOSE**
Prevention and treatment of vitamin D and calcium deficiency
- BY MOUTH
- Child: Dosed according to the deficit or daily maintenance requirements (consult product literature)

9

Blood and nutrition

- **UNLICENSED USE** *Adcal-D3*® and *Calceos*® are not licensed for use in children under 12 years. *Cacit*® *D3*, *Calcichew D3*® *Forte*, *Calcichew-D₃*® and *Kalcipos-D*® not licensed for use in children (age range not specified by manufacturers). *Accrete D3*® and *Natecal D3*® not licensed for use in children under 18 years.
- **INTERACTIONS** → Appendix 1: calcium salts, vitamin D substances
- **PRESCRIBING AND DISPENSING INFORMATION** *Accrete D3*® contains calcium carbonate 1.5 g (calcium 600 mg or Ca²⁺ 15 mmol), colecalciferol 10 micrograms (400 units); *Adcal-D3*® tablets contain calcium carbonate 1.5 g (calcium 600 mg or Ca²⁺ 15 mmol), colecalciferol 10 micrograms (400 units); *Cacit*® *D3* contains calcium carbonate 1.25 g (calcium 500 mg or Ca²⁺ 12.5 mmol), colecalciferol 11 micrograms (440 units)/sachet; *Calceos*® contains calcium carbonate 1.25 g (calcium 500 mg or Ca²⁺ 12.5 mmol), colecalciferol 10 micrograms (400 units); *Calcichew-D3*® tablets contain calcium carbonate 1.25 g (calcium 500 mg or Ca²⁺ 12.5 mmol), colecalciferol 10 micrograms (400 units); *Calcichew-D3*® 500 mg/400 unit caplets contain calcium carbonate (calcium 500 mg or Ca²⁺ 12.5 mmol), colecalciferol 10 micrograms (400 units); *Kalcipos-D*® contains calcium carbonate (calcium 500 mg or Ca²⁺ 12.5 mmol), colecalciferol 20 micrograms (800 units); *Natecal D3*® contains calcium carbonate 1.5 g (calcium 600 mg or Ca²⁺ 15 mmol), colecalciferol 10 micrograms (400 units); consult product literature for details of other available products.

Flavours of chewable and soluble forms may include orange, lemon, aniseed, peppermint, molasses, or tutti-frutti.

- **MEDICINAL FORMS**
There can be variation in the licensing of different medicines containing the same drug.
Effervescent granules
CAUTIONARY AND ADVISORY LABELS 13
  ‣ **Colecalciferol with calcium carbonate (Non-proprietary)**
  Calcium carbonate 2.5 gram, Colecalciferol 880 unit Colecalciferol 880unit / Calcium carbonate 2.5g effervescent granules sachets | 24 sachet [PoM] no price available
  ‣ **Cacit D3** (Teva UK Ltd)
  Calcium carbonate 1.25 gram, Colecalciferol 440 unit Cacit D3 effervescent granules sachets | 30 sachet [P] £4.06 DT price = £4.06

Effervescent tablet
CAUTIONARY AND ADVISORY LABELS 13
  ‣ **Adcal-D3** (Kyowa Kirin Ltd)
  Calcium carbonate 1.5 gram, Colecalciferol 400 unit Adcal-D3 Dissolve 1500mg/400unit effervescent tablets | 56 tablet [P] £5.99 DT price = £5.99

Tablet
EXCIPIENTS: May contain Propylene glycol
  ‣ **Colecalciferol with calcium carbonate (Non-proprietary)**
  Calcium carbonate 400 mg, Colecalciferol 100 unit Calcium & Vitamin D tablets | 30 tablet no price available | 60 tablet no price available
  ‣ **Accrete D3** (Internis Pharmaceuticals Ltd)
  Calcium carbonate 1.5 gram, Colecalciferol 400 unit Accrete D3 tablets | 60 tablet [P] £2.95 DT price = £2.95
  ‣ **Adcal-D3** (Kyowa Kirin Ltd)
  Calcium carbonate 750 mg, Colecalciferol 200 unit Adcal-D3 750mg/200unit caplets | 112 tablet [P] £2.95 DT price = £2.95
  ‣ **Calcichew D3** (Forum Health Products Ltd)
  Calcium carbonate 1.25 gram, Colecalciferol 400 unit Calcichew D3 500mg/400unit caplets | 100 tablet [P] £7.43 DT price = £7.43
  ‣ **Kalcipos-D** (Meda Pharmaceuticals Ltd)
  Calcium carbonate 1.25 gram, Colecalciferol 800 unit Kalcipos-D 500mg/800unit tablets | 30 tablet [PoM] £4.21 DT price = £4.21

Chewable tablet
CAUTIONARY AND ADVISORY LABELS 24
EXCIPIENTS: May contain Aspartame
  ‣ **Colecalciferol with calcium carbonate (Non-proprietary)**
  Calcium carbonate 1.25 gram, Colecalciferol 400 unit Colecalciferol 400unit / Calcium carbonate 1.25g chewable tablets | 100 tablet £14.75
  Calcium carbonate 1.5 gram, Colecalciferol 400 unit Colecalciferol 400unit / Calcium carbonate 1.5g chewable tablets | 56 tablet [P] £3.65 DT price = £3.65 | 60 tablet [P] £4.38
  ‣ **Adcal-D3** (Kyowa Kirin Ltd)
  Calcium carbonate 1.5 gram, Colecalciferol 400 unit Adcal-D3 Lemon chewable tablets | 56 tablet [P] £3.65 DT price = £3.65 | 112 tablet [P] £7.49
  Adcal-D3 chewable tablets tutti frutti | 56 tablet [P] £3.65 DT price = £3.65 | 112 tablet [P] £7.49
  ‣ **Calceos** (Galen Ltd)
  Calcium carbonate 1.25 gram, Colecalciferol 400 unit Calceos 500mg/400unit chewable tablets | 60 tablet [P] £3.88 DT price = £4.24
  ‣ **Calci-D** (Consilient Health Ltd)
  Calcium carbonate 2.5 gram, Colecalciferol 1000 iu Calci-D 1000mg/1,000unit chewable tablets | 28 tablet [PoM] £2.25 DT price = £2.25
  ‣ **Calcichew D3** (Forum Health Products Ltd)
  Calcium carbonate 2.5 gram, Colecalciferol 800 iu Calcichew D3 1000mg/800unit Once Daily chewable tablets | 30 tablet [P] £6.75 DT price = £6.75
  Calcium carbonate 1.25 gram, Colecalciferol 200 unit Calcichew D3 chewable tablets | 100 tablet [P] £7.68 DT price = £7.68
  ‣ **Calcichew D3 Forte** (Forum Health Products Ltd)
  Calcium carbonate 1.25 gram, Colecalciferol 400 unit Calcichew D3 Forte chewable tablets | 60 tablet [P] £4.24 DT price = £4.24 | 100 tablet [P] £7.08
  ‣ **Evacal D3** (Teva UK Ltd)
  Calcium carbonate 1.5 gram, Colecalciferol 400 unit Evacal D3 1500mg/400unit chewable tablets | 56 tablet [P] £2.75 DT price = £3.65 | 112 tablet [P] £5.50
  ‣ **Kalcipos-D** (Meda Pharmaceuticals Ltd)
  Calcium carbonate 1.25 gram, Colecalciferol 800 unit Kalcipos-D 500mg/800unit chewable tablets | 30 tablet [PoM] £4.21 DT price = £4.21
  ‣ **Natecal** (Chiesi Ltd)
  Calcium carbonate 1.5 gram, Colecalciferol 400 unit Natecal D3 600mg/400unit chewable tablets | 60 tablet [P] £3.63
  ‣ **TheiCal-D3** (Stirling Anglian Pharmaceuticals Ltd)
  Calcium carbonate 2.5 gram, Colecalciferol 880 unit TheiCal-D3 1000mg/880unit chewable tablets | 30 tablet [P] £2.95 DT price = £2.95

Colecalciferol with calcium phosphate

The properties listed below are those particular to the combination only. For the properties of the components please consider, colecalciferol p. 604, calcium phosphate p. 568.

- **INDICATIONS AND DOSE**
Calcium and vitamin D deficiency
  ‣ BY MOUTH
  ‣ Child: (consult product literature)

- **INTERACTIONS** → Appendix 1: calcium salts, vitamin D substances

- **MEDICINAL FORMS**
There can be variation in the licensing of different medicines containing the same drug.
Powder
CAUTIONARY AND ADVISORY LABELS 13, 21
  ‣ **Calfovit D3** (A. Menarini Farmaceutica Internazionale SRL)
  Calcium phosphate 3.1 gram, Colecalciferol 800 unit Calfovit D3 oral powder sachets | 30 sachet [P] £4.32 DT price = £4.32

Ergocalciferol

(Calciferol; Vitamin D₂)

F 603

- ● **INDICATIONS AND DOSE**
  Nutritional vitamin-D deficiency rickets
  - ▸ BY MOUTH
  - ▸ Child 1-5 months: 3000 units daily, dose to be adjusted as necessary
  - ▸ Child 6 months-11 years: 6000 units daily, dose to be adjusted as necessary
  - ▸ Child 12-17 years: 10 000 units daily, dose to be adjusted as necessary

  Nutritional or physiological supplement | Prevention of rickets
  - ▸ BY MOUTH
  - ▸ Neonate: 400 units daily.

  - ▸ Child: 400–600 units daily

  Vitamin D deficiency in intestinal malabsorption or in chronic liver disease
  - ▸ BY MOUTH, OR BY INTRAMUSCULAR INJECTION
  - ▸ Child 1-11 years: 10 000–25 000 units daily, dose to be adjusted as necessary
  - ▸ Child 12-17 years: 10 000–40 000 units daily, dose to be adjusted as necessary

- ● **CAUTIONS** Take care to ensure correct dose in infants
- ● **INTERACTIONS** → Appendix 1: vitamin D substances
- ● **RENAL IMPAIRMENT** Monitor plasma-calcium concentration in renal impairment.
- ● **MONITORING REQUIREMENTS** Monitor plasma-calcium concentration in patients receiving high doses.
- ● **PRESCRIBING AND DISPENSING INFORMATION** The BP directs that when calciferol is prescribed or demanded, colecalciferol or ergocalciferol should be dispensed or supplied.
  When the strength of the tablets ordered or prescribed is not clear, the intention of the prescriber with respect to the strength (expressed in micrograms or milligrams per tablet) should be ascertained.

- ● **MEDICINAL FORMS**
  There can be variation in the licensing of different medicines containing the same drug. Forms available from special-order manufacturers include: tablet, oral suspension, oral solution, solution for injection

  Tablet
  - ▸ Ergocalciferol (Non-proprietary)
    Ergocalciferol 12.5 microgram Ergocalciferol 12.5microgram tablets | 30 tablet no price available | 60 tablet £3.74
  - ▸ Ergoral (Cubic Pharmaceuticals Ltd)
    Ergocalciferol 125 microgram Ergoral D2 5,000unit tablets | 30 tablet £19.95
    Ergocalciferol 250 microgram Ergoral D2 10,000unit tablets | 30 tablet £23.95

  Solution for injection
  - ▸ Ergocalciferol (Non-proprietary)
    Ergocalciferol 300000 unit per 1 ml Ergocalciferol 300,000units/1ml solution for injection ampoules | 10 ampoule PoM £93.50 DT price = £93.50
    Ergocalciferol 400000 unit per 1 ml Sterogyl 15H 600,000units/1.5ml solution for injection ampoules | 1 ampoule PoM no price available

  Oral solution
  - ▸ Ergocalciferol (Non-proprietary)
    Ergocalciferol 1500 unit per 1 ml Uvesterol D 1,500units/ml oral solution sugar-free | 20 ml PoM no price available
    Ergocalciferol 20000 unit per 1 ml Sterogyl 100,000units/5ml oral solution | 20 ml PoM no price available DT price = £72.68
  - ▸ Eciferol (Rhodes Pharma Ltd)
    Ergocalciferol 3000 unit per 1 ml Eciferol D2 3,000units/ml liquid | 60 ml £55.00 DT price = £102.44

Capsule
- ▸ Ergocalciferol (Non-proprietary)
  Ergocalciferol 1.25 mg Ergocalciferol 1.25mg capsules | 30 capsule PoM no price available | 50 capsule PoM £230.00
- ▸ Eciferol (Rhodes Pharma Ltd)
  Ergocalciferol 1.25 mg Eciferol D2 50,000unit capsules | 10 capsule £29.99
- ▸ Ergoral (Cubic Pharmaceuticals Ltd)
  Ergocalciferol 1.25 mg Ergoral D2 50,000unit capsules | 10 capsule £19.95

Ergocalciferol with calcium lactate and calcium phosphate

(Calcium and vitamin D)

The properties listed below are those particular to the combination only. For the properties of the components please consider, ergocalciferol above, calcium lactate p. 568.

- ● **INDICATIONS AND DOSE**
  Prevention of calcium and vitamin D deficiency | Treatment of calcium and vitamin D deficiency
  - ▸ BY MOUTH
  - ▸ Child: (consult product literature)

- ● **UNLICENSED USE** Calcium and Ergocalciferol tablets not licensed for use in children under 6 years.
- ● **INTERACTIONS** → Appendix 1: calcium salts, vitamin D substances
- ● **DIRECTIONS FOR ADMINISTRATION** Tablets may be crushed before administration, or may be chewed.
- ● **PRESCRIBING AND DISPENSING INFORMATION** Each tablet contains calcium lactate 300 mg, calcium phosphate 150 mg (calcium 97 mg or Ca^{2+} 2.4 mmol), ergocalciferol 10 micrograms (400 units).
- ● **PATIENT AND CARER ADVICE** Patient or carers should be given advice on how to administer calcium and ergocalciferol tablets.

- ● **MEDICINAL FORMS**
  There can be variation in the licensing of different medicines containing the same drug.
  Tablet
  - ▸ Ergocalciferol with calcium lactate and calcium phosphate (Non-proprietary)
    Ergocalciferol 10 microgram, Calcium phosphate 150 mg, Calcium lactate 300 mg Calcium and Ergocalciferol tablets | 28 tablet P £18.50 DT price = £18.26 | 500 tablet P no price available

VITAMINS AND TRACE ELEMENTS > VITAMIN E

Alpha tocopherol

(Tocopherol)

- ● **INDICATIONS AND DOSE**
  Vitamin E deficiency because of malabsorption in congenital or hereditary chronic cholestasis
  - ▸ BY MOUTH USING ORAL SOLUTION
  - ▸ Neonate: 17 mg/kg daily, dose to be adjusted as necessary.

  - ▸ Child: 17 mg/kg daily, dose to be adjusted as necessary

- ● **CONTRA-INDICATIONS** Preterm neonates
- ● **CAUTIONS** Predisposition to thrombosis
- ● **INTERACTIONS** → Appendix 1: vitamin E substances
- ● **SIDE-EFFECTS**
  - ▸ Common or very common Diarrhoea

9

Blood and nutrition

▸ **Uncommon** Alopecia · asthenia · disturbances in serum-potassium concentration · disturbances in serum-sodium concentration · headache · pruritus · rash

● **PREGNANCY** Manufacturer advises caution, no evidence of harm in *animal* studies.

● **BREAST FEEDING** Manufacturer advises use only if potential benefit outweighs risk—no information available.

● **HEPATIC IMPAIRMENT** Manufacturer advises caution—no information available. Manufacturer advises monitor closely in hepatic impairment.

● **RENAL IMPAIRMENT** Manufacturer advises caution. Risk of renal toxicity due to polyethylene glycol content. Manufacturer advises monitor closely in renal impairment.

● **PRESCRIBING AND DISPENSING INFORMATION** Tocofersolan is a water-soluble form of D-alpha tocopherol.

● **MEDICINAL FORMS** There can be variation in the licensing of different medicines containing the same drug.

Oral solution
▸ Vedrop (Orphan Europe (UK) Ltd) ▼
D-alpha tocopherol (as Tocofersolan) 50 mg per 1 ml Vedrop 50mg/ml oral solution sugar-free | 20 ml [PoM] £54.55 sugar-free | 60 ml [PoM] £163.65

Alpha tocopheryl acetate

(Tocopherol)

● **INDICATIONS AND DOSE**

Vitamin E deficiency
▸ BY MOUTH

▸ Neonate: 10 mg/kg once daily.

▸ Child: 2–10 mg/kg daily, increased if necessary up to 20 mg/kg daily

Malabsorption in cystic fibrosis
▸ BY MOUTH

▸ Child 1–11 months: 50 mg once daily, dose to be adjusted as necessary, to be taken with food and pancreatic enzymes
▸ Child 1–11 years: 100 mg once daily, dose to be adjusted as necessary, to be taken with food and pancreatic enzymes
▸ Child 12–17 years: 100–200 mg once daily, dose to be adjusted as necessary, to be taken with food and pancreatic enzymes

Vitamin E deficiency in cholestasis and severe liver disease
▸ BY MOUTH

▸ Neonate: 10 mg/kg daily.

▸ Child 1 month–11 years: Initially 100 mg daily, adjusted according to response, increased if necessary up to 200 mg/kg daily
▸ Child 12–17 years: Initially 200 mg daily, adjusted according to response, increased if necessary up to 200 mg/kg daily
▸ BY INTRAMUSCULAR INJECTION

▸ Neonate: 10 mg/kg once a month.

▸ Child: 10 mg/kg once a month (max. per dose 100 mg)

Malabsorption in abetalipoproteinaemia
▸ BY MOUTH

▸ Neonate: 100 mg/kg once daily.

▸ Child: 50–100 mg/kg once daily

● **CAUTIONS** Increased risk of necrotising enterocolitis in neonate weighing less than 1.5 kg or in a preterm neonate · predisposition to thrombosis

● **INTERACTIONS** → Appendix 1: vitamin E substances

● **SIDE-EFFECTS** Abdominal pain (particularly with high doses) · diarrhoea (particularly with high doses)

● **PREGNANCY** No evidence of safety of high doses.

● **BREAST FEEDING** Excreted in milk; minimal risk, although caution with large doses.

● **MONITORING REQUIREMENTS** Increased bleeding tendency in vitamin-K deficient patients or those taking anticoagulants (prothrombin time and INR should be monitored).

● **DIRECTIONS FOR ADMINISTRATION**
▸ In neonates Consider dilution of oral suspension for use in neonates due to high osmolality.

● **MEDICINAL FORMS** There can be variation in the licensing of different medicines containing the same drug. Forms available from special-order manufacturers include: chewable tablet, solution for injection

Solution for injection
▸ Alpha tocopheryl acetate (Non-proprietary)
Alpha tocopheryl acetate 50 mg per 1 ml E-Vicotrat 100mg/2ml solution for injection ampoules | 10 ampoule [PoM] no price available

Oral suspension
EXCIPIENTS: May contain Sucrose
▸ Alpha tocopheryl acetate (Non-proprietary)
Alpha tocopheryl acetate 100 mg per 1 ml Alpha tocopheryl acetate 500mg/5ml oral suspension | 100 ml [GSL] £58.85 DT price = £58.85

Chewable tablet
▸ Alpha tocopheryl acetate (Non-proprietary)
Alpha tocopheryl acetate 100 mg Alpha tocopheryl acetate 100mg chewable tablets | 30 tablet no price available
▸ E-Tabs (Ennogen Healthcare Ltd)
Alpha tocopheryl acetate 100 mg E-Tabs 100mg chewable tablets | 30 tablet £87.30
▸ Ephynal (Imported (Italy))
Alpha tocopheryl acetate 100 mg Ephynal 100mg chewable tablets | 30 tablet no price available

Capsule
▸ Alpha tocopheryl acetate (Non-proprietary)
Alpha tocopherol 100 unit Vitamin E 100unit capsules | 30 capsule £0.77
Alpha tocopherol 200 unit Vitamin E 200unit capsules | 60 capsule £5.58 | 100 capsule £8.09
Alpha tocopherol 250 unit Vitamin E 250unit capsules | 100 capsule £7.23
Alpha tocopherol 400 unit Vitamin E 400unit capsules | 30 capsule £6.69 | 60 capsule £11.72
Alpha tocopherol 600 unit Vitamin E 600unit capsules | 30 capsule £8.37 | 60 capsule £13.95
Alpha tocopherol 1000 unit Vitamin E 1,000unit capsules | 30 capsule £6.64
▸ E-Caps (Ennogen Healthcare Ltd)
Alpha tocopherol 75 unit E-Caps 75unit capsules | 100 capsule £109.50
Alpha tocopherol 100 unit E-Caps 100unit capsules | 30 capsule £84.40
Alpha tocopherol 200 unit E-Caps 200unit capsules | 30 capsule £89.50
Alpha tocopherol 400 unit E-Caps 400unit capsules | 30 capsule £128.50
Alpha tocopherol 1000 unit E-Caps 1,000unit capsules | 30 capsule £130.20
▸ Vita-E (Typharm Ltd)
Alpha tocopherol 75 unit Vita-E 75unit capsules | 100 capsule £4.35
Alpha tocopherol 200 unit Vita-E 200unit capsules | 30 capsule £3.35 | 100 capsule £10.34
Alpha tocopherol 400 unit Vita-E 400unit capsules | 30 capsule £5.04 | 100 capsule £16.44

VITAMINS AND TRACE ELEMENTS > VITAMIN K

Menadiol sodium phosphate

- ● **INDICATIONS AND DOSE**
Supplementation in vitamin K malabsorption
  - ▶ BY MOUTH
  - ▶ Child 1–11 years: 5–10 mg daily, dose to be adjusted as necessary
  - ▶ Child 12–17 years: 10–20 mg daily, dose to be adjusted as necessary

- ● **CONTRA-INDICATIONS** Infants · neonates
- ● **CAUTIONS** G6PD deficiency (risk of haemolysis) · vitamin E deficiency (risk of haemolysis)
- ● **PREGNANCY** Avoid in late pregnancy and labour unless benefit outweighs risk of neonatal haemolytic anaemia, hyperbilirubinaemia, and kernicterus in neonate.

- ● **MEDICINAL FORMS**
There can be variation in the licensing of different medicines containing the same drug. Forms available from special-order manufacturers include: oral suspension, oral solution
  Tablet
  - ▶ Menadiol sodium phosphate (Non-proprietary)
  Menadiol phosphate (as Menadiol sodium phosphate)
  10 mg Menadiol 10mg tablets | 100 tablet P £185.90 DT price = £185.90

Phytomenadione

(Vitamin K₁)

- ● **INDICATIONS AND DOSE**
Neonatal prophylaxis of vitamin-K deficiency bleeding
  - ▶ BY INTRAMUSCULAR INJECTION
  - ▶ Preterm neonate: 400 micrograms/kg (max. per dose 1 mg) for 1 dose, to be given at birth, the intravenous route may be used in preterm neonates with very low birth-weight if intramuscular injection is not possible, however, it may not provide the prolonged protection of the intramuscular injection, any neonate receiving intravenous vitamin K should be given subsequent oral doses.
  - ▶ Neonate: 1 mg for 1 dose, to be given at birth.

Neonatal prophylaxis of vitamin-K deficiency bleeding in healthy babies who are not at particular risk of bleeding disorders
  - ▶ BY MOUTH USING CAPSULES
  - ▶ Neonate: 1 mg for 1 dose at birth (to protect from the risk of vitamin K deficiency bleeding in the first week).

Neonatal prophylaxis of vitamin-K deficiency bleeding in healthy babies who are not at particular risk of bleeding disorders (exclusively breast-fed babies)
  - ▶ BY MOUTH USING CAPSULES
  - ▶ Neonate: Initially 1 mg for 1 dose at birth, then 1 mg every week for 12 weeks.

Neonatal hypoprothrombinaemia | Vitamin-K deficiency bleeding
  - ▶ BY INTRAVENOUS INJECTION
  - ▶ Neonate: 1 mg every 8 hours if required.

Neonatal biliary atresia and liver disease
  - ▶ BY MOUTH
  - ▶ Neonate: 1 mg daily.

Reversal of coumarin anticoagulation when continued anticoagulation required or if no significant bleeding—seek specialist advice
  - ▶ BY INTRAVENOUS INJECTION
  - ▶ Child: 15–30 micrograms/kg (max. per dose 1 mg) for 1 dose, dose may be repeated as necessary

Reversal of coumarin anticoagulation when anticoagulation not required or if significant bleeding—seek specialist advice | Treatment of haemorrhage associated with vitamin-K deficiency—seek specialist advice
  - ▶ BY INTRAVENOUS INJECTION
  - ▶ Child: 250–300 micrograms/kg (max. per dose 10 mg) for 1 dose

KONAKION® MM PAEDIATRIC
Neonatal prophylaxis of vitamin-K deficiency bleeding in healthy babies who are not at risk of bleeding disorders
  - ▶ BY MOUTH
  - ▶ Neonate: Initially 2 mg for 1 dose at birth, then 2 mg after 4–7 days.

Neonatal prophylaxis of vitamin-K deficiency bleeding in healthy babies who are not at risk of bleeding disorders (exclusively breast fed babies)
  - ▶ BY MOUTH
  - ▶ Neonate: Initially 2 mg for 1 dose at birth, then 2 mg after 4–7 days for a further 1 dose, then 2 mg for a further 1 dose 1 month after birth.

- ● **CAUTIONS** Intravenous injections should be given very slowly—risk of vascular collapse
KONAKION® MM PAEDIATRIC
Parenteral administration in premature infant or neonate of less than 2.5 kg (increased risk of kernicterus)
- ● **SIDE-EFFECTS**
KONAKION® MM Anaphylactoid reactions
- ● **PREGNANCY** Use if potential benefit outweighs risk.
- ● **BREAST FEEDING** Present in milk.
- ● **HEPATIC IMPAIRMENT**
KONAKION® MM Caution—glycocholic acid may displace bilirubin.
- ● **DIRECTIONS FOR ADMINISTRATION**
  - ▶ With oral use in neonates The contents of one capsule should be administered by cutting the narrow tubular tip off and squeezing the liquid contents into the mouth; if the baby spits out the dose or is sick within three hours of administration a replacement dose should be given.
  KONAKION® MM PAEDIATRIC *Konakion® MM Paediatric* may be administered *by mouth* or *by intramuscular injection* or *by intravenous injection.*
      For *intravenous injection*, may be diluted with Glucose 5% if necessary.
  KONAKION® MM *Konakion® MM* may be administered by slow intravenous injection or by intravenous infusion in glucose 5%; **not** for intramuscular injection.

- ● **MEDICINAL FORMS**
There can be variation in the licensing of different medicines containing the same drug. Forms available from special-order manufacturers include: tablet, capsule, oral suspension, oral solution, drops
  Tablet
  - ▶ Phytomenadione (Non-proprietary)
  Phytomenadione 100 microgram Vitamin K1 100microgram tablets | 30 tablet no price available
  Solution for injection
  EXCIPIENTS: May contain Glycocholic acid, lecithin
  - ▶ Konakion MM (Roche Products Ltd)
  Phytomenadione 10 mg per 1 ml Konakion MM Paediatric 2mg/0.2ml solution for injection ampoules | 5 ampoule PoM £4.71

9

Blood and nutrition

Konakion MM 10mg/1ml solution for injection ampoules |
10 ampoule PoM £3.78 DT price = £3.78

Drops

▶ **Phytomenadione (Non-proprietary)**
Phytomenadione 20 mg per 1 ml Kanavit 20mg/ml oral drops sugar
free sugar-free | 5 ml PoM no price available

▶ **Neokay** (Neoceuticals Ltd)
Phytomenadione 200 microgram per 1 ml NeoKay
200micrograms/ml oral drops sugar-free | 25 ml £3.95

Capsule

▶ **Neokay** (Neoceuticals Ltd)
Phytomenadione 1 mg NeoKay 1mg capsules | 12 capsule PoM
£3.95 DT price = £3.95 | 100 capsule PoM £34.00

7.1 Neural tube defects (prevention in pregnancy)

Neural tube defects (prevention in pregnancy)

Prevention in pregnancy

Folic acid supplements p. 546 taken before and during
pregnancy can reduce the occurrence of neural tube defects.
The risk of a neural tube defect occurring in a child should be
assessed and folic acid given as follows:

- Women at a low risk of conceiving a child with a neural
  tube defect should be advised to take folic acid as a
  medicinal or food supplement daily (at low-risk group
  dose) before conception and until week 12 of pregnancy.
  Women who have not been taking folic acid and who
  suspect they are pregnant should start at once and
  continue until week 12 of pregnancy.
- Couples are at a high risk of conceiving a child with a
  neural tube defect if either partner has a neural tube defect
  (or either partner has a family history of neural tube
  defects), if they have had a previous pregnancy affected by
  a neural tube defect, or if the woman has *coeliac disease* (or
  other malabsorption state), diabetes mellitus, sickle-cell
  anaemia, or is taking **antiepileptic medicines**.
- Women in the high-risk group who wish to become
  pregnant (or who are at risk of becoming pregnant) should
  be advised to take folic acid daily (at high-risk group dose)
  and continue until week 12 of pregnancy (women with
  sickle-cell disease should continue taking their normal
  dose of folic acid (or to increase the dose to high-risk
  group daily dose) and continue this throughout
  pregnancy).

There is no justification for prescribing multiple-ingredient
vitamin preparations containing vitamin B_{12} or folic acid.

Chapter 10
Musculoskeletal system

10

Musculoskeletal system

1   Arthritis

Juvenile idiopathic arthritis

Management

Rheumatic diseases require symptomatic treatment to relieve pain, swelling, and stiffness, together with treatment to control and suppress disease activity. Treatment of juvenile idiopathic arthritis may involve Non-steroidal anti-inflammatory drugs (NSAIDs) p. 621, a disease modifying anti-rheumatic drug (DMARD) such as methotrexate p. 517 or a cytokine modulator, and intra-articular, intravenous, or oral corticosteroids.

Rheumatic disease, suppressing drugs

Overview

Certain drugs, such as methotrexate p. 517, cytokine modulators, and sulfasalazine p. 30, are used to suppress the disease process in *juvenile idiopathic arthritis* (juvenile chronic arthritis); these drugs are known as disease-modifying antirheumatic drugs (DMARDs). In children, disease modifying antirheumatic drugs should be used under specialist supervision.

Some children with juvenile idiopathic arthritis do not require disease-modifying antirheumatic drugs. Methotrexate is effective in juvenile idiopathic arthritis; sulfasalazine is an alternative but should be avoided in *systemic-onset juvenile idiopathic arthritis*. Gold and penicillamine p. 589 are no longer used. Cytokine modulators have a role in *polyarticular juvenile idiopathic arthritis*.

Unlike NSAIDs, disease-modifying antirheumatic drugs can affect the progression of disease but they may require 3–6 months of treatment for a full therapeutic response. Response to a disease-modifying antirheumatic drug may allow the dose of the NSAID to be reduced.

Disease-modifying antirheumatic drugs can improve not only the symptoms of inflammatory joint disease but also extra-articular manifestations. They reduce the erythrocyte sedimentation rate and C-reactive protein.

Antimalarials

The antimalarial hydroxychloroquine sulfate p. 612 is rarely used to treat juvenile idiopathic arthritis.
Hydroxychloroquine sulfate can also be useful for systemic or discoid lupus erythematosus, particularly involving the skin and joints, and in sarcoidosis.

Retinopathy rarely occurs provided that the recommended doses are not exceeded.

Mepacrine hydrochloride is used on rare occasions to treat discoid lupus erythematosus [unlicensed].

Drugs affecting the immune response

Methotrexate, given as a once weekly dose, is the disease-modifying antirheumatic drug of choice in the treatment of juvenile idiopathic arthritis and also has a role in juvenile dermatomyositis, vasculitis, uveitis, systemic lupus erythematosus, localised scleroderma, and sarcoidosis; for these indications it is given by the subcutaneous, oral, or rarely, the intramuscular route. Absorption from intramuscular or subcutaneous routes may be more predictable than from the oral route; if the oral route is ineffective subcutaneous administration is generally preferred. Folic acid may reduce mucosal or gastro-intestinal side-effects of methotrexate. The dosage regimen for folic acid p. 546 has not been established—in children over 2 years a weekly dose [unlicensed indication], may be given on a different day from the methotrexate.

Azathioprine p. 495 may be used in children for vasculitis which has failed to respond to other treatments, for the management of severe cases of *systemic lupus erythematosus* and other connective tissue disorders, in conjunction with corticosteroids for patients with severe or progressive renal disease, and in cases of *polymyositis* which are resistant to corticosteroids. Azathioprine has a corticosteroid-sparing effect in patients whose corticosteroid requirements are excessive.

Ciclosporin is rarely used in juvenile idiopathic arthritis, connective tissue diseases, vasculitis, and uveitis; it may be considered if the condition has failed to respond to other treatments.

Cytokine modulators

Cytokine modulators should be used under specialist supervision.

Adalimumab p. 614, etanercept p. 616, and infliximab p. 31 inhibit the activity of tumour necrosis factor alpha (TNF-α). Adalimumab can be used for the management of active polyarticular juvenile idiopathic arthritis and enthesitis-related arthritis. Etanercept is licensed for the treatment of the following subtypes of juvenile idiopathic arthritis: polyarticular juvenile idiopathic arthritis in children who have had an inadequate response to methotrexate or who cannot tolerate it, oligoarthritis in children who have had an inadequate response to methotrexate or who cannot tolerate it, psoriatic arthritis in children over 12 years who have had an inadequate response to methotrexate or cannot tolerate it, and enthesitis-related arthritis in children over 12 years who have had an inadequate response to conventional therapy or cannot tolerate it. Infliximab has been used in refractory polyarticular juvenile idiopathic arthritis [unlicensed indication] when other treatments, such as etanercept, have failed.

Abatacept p. 614 prevents the full activation of T-lymphocytes; it can be used for the management of active polyarticular juvenile idiopathic arthritis. Abatacept is not recommended for use in combination with TNF inhibitors.

Canakinumab p. 502 inhibits the activity of interleukin-1 beta (IL-1β) and is licensed for the treatment of active systemic juvenile idiopathic arthritis in children over 2 years, when there has been an inadequate response to NSAIDs and systemic corticosteroids.

Tocilizumab p. 613 antagonises the actions of interleukin-6; it can be used for the management of active systemic juvenile idiopathic arthritis when there has been an inadequate response to NSAIDs and systemic corticosteroids and polyarticular juvenile idiopathic arthritis when there has been an inadequate response to methotrexate. Tocilizumab can be used in combination with methotrexate, or as monotherapy if methotrexate is not tolerated or is contra-indicated. Tocilizumab is not recommended for use with other cytokine modulators.

Sulfasalazine

Sulfasalazine has a beneficial effect in suppressing the inflammatory activity associated with some forms of juvenile idiopathic arthritis; it is generally not used in systemic-onset disease.

Other drugs used for Arthritis Diclofenac potassium, p. 622 · Diclofenac sodium, p. 623 · Etoricoxib, p. 624 · Flurbiprofen, p. 625 · Ibuprofen, p. 625 · Indometacin, p. 628 · Ketoprofen, p. 629 · Meloxicam, p. 630 · Naproxen, p. 631 · Piroxicam, p. 632

DISEASE-MODIFYING ANTI-RHEUMATIC DRUGS

Hydroxychloroquine sulfate

● **INDICATIONS AND DOSE**

Active rheumatoid arthritis (including juvenile idiopathic arthritis) (administered on expert advice) | Systemic and discoid lupus erythematosus (administered on expert advice) | Dermatological conditions caused or aggravated by sunlight (administered on expert advice)
▶ BY MOUTH
▶ Child: 5–6.5 mg/kg once daily (max. per dose 400 mg), dose given based on ideal body-weight

● **UNLICENSED USE** *Plaquenil®* not licensed for use in children for dermatological conditions caused or aggravated by sunlight.

● **CAUTIONS** Acute porphyrias p. 577 · diabetes (may lower blood glucose) · G6PD deficiency · may aggravate myasthenia gravis · may exacerbate psoriasis · neurological disorders (especially in those with a history of epilepsy) · severe gastro-intestinal disorders

CAUTIONS, FURTHER INFORMATION
▶ Screening for ocular toxicity Hydroxychloroquine is rarely associated with ocular toxicity. The British Society for Paediatric and Adolescent Rheumatology recommends that children should have their vision tested before long-term treatment with hydroxychloroquine and have an annual review of visual acuity. Children should be referred to an ophthalmologist if there is visual impairment, changes in visual acuity, or blurred vision. The Royal College of Ophthalmologists has recommended that a locally agreed protocol between the prescribing doctor and ophthalmologist be established to monitor the vision of

these children. A review group convened by the Royal College of Ophthalmologists has updated guidelines for screening to prevent ocular toxicity on long-term treatment with hydroxychloroquine (*Hydroxychloroquine and Ocular Toxicity: Recommendations on Screening* 2009); this includes the recommendation that a child treated for juvenile idiopathic arthritis should receive slit-lamp examination routinely to check for uveitis.

● **INTERACTIONS** → Appendix 1: hydroxychloroquine

● **SIDE-EFFECTS**
▶ **Common or very common** Gastro-intestinal disturbances · headache · pruritus · rashes · skin reactions
▶ **Uncommon** Convulsions · discoloration of skin, nails, and mucous membranes · ECG changes · hair depigmentation · hair loss · keratopathy · ototoxicity · retinal damage · visual changes
▶ **Rare** Acute generalised exanthematous pustulosis · agranulocytosis · aplastic anaemia · blood disorders · cardiomyopathy · emotional disturbances · exfoliative dermatitis · hepatic damage · mental changes · myopathy · neuromyopathy · photosensitivity · psychosis · Stevens-Johnson syndrome · thrombocytopenia
▶ **Frequency not known** Angioedema · bronchospasm

Overdose
Hydroxychloroquine is very toxic in overdosage; overdosage is extremely hazardous and difficult to treat. Urgent advice from the National Poisons Information Service is essential. Life-threatening features include arrhythmias (which can have a very rapid onset) and convulsions (which can be intractable).

● **PREGNANCY** It is not necessary to withdraw an antimalarial drug during pregnancy if the rheumatic disease is well controlled; however, the manufacturer of hydroxychloroquine advises avoiding use.

● **BREAST FEEDING** Avoid—risk of toxicity in infant.

● **HEPATIC IMPAIRMENT** Caution in moderate to severe hepatic impairment.

● **RENAL IMPAIRMENT** Manufacturer advises caution. Monitor plasma-hydroxychloroquine concentration in severe renal impairment.

● **PRESCRIBING AND DISPENSING INFORMATION** To avoid excessive dosage in obese patients, the dose of hydroxychloroquine should be calculated on the basis of ideal body-weight.

● **PATIENT AND CARER ADVICE** Do not take antacids for at least 4 hours before or after hydroxychloroquine to reduce possible interference with hydroxychloroquine absorption.

● **MEDICINAL FORMS**
There can be variation in the licensing of different medicines containing the same drug. Forms available from special-order manufacturers include: oral suspension, oral solution

Tablet
CAUTIONARY AND ADVISORY LABELS 21
▶ **Hydroxychloroquine sulfate** (Non-proprietary)
Hydroxychloroquine sulfate 200 mg Hydroxychloroquine 200mg tablets | 60 tablet [PoM] £5.15 DT price = £3.64
▶ **Plaquenil** (Sanofi)
Hydroxychloroquine sulfate 200 mg Plaquenil 200mg tablets | 60 tablet [PoM] £5.15 DT price = £3.64
▶ **Quinoric** (Bristol Laboratories Ltd)
Hydroxychloroquine sulfate 200 mg Quinoric 200mg tablets | 60 tablet [PoM] £4.75 DT price = £3.64

IMMUNOSUPPRESSANTS > INTERLEUKIN INHIBITORS

Tocilizumab

31-May-2016

- **INDICATIONS AND DOSE**

Active systemic juvenile idiopathic arthritis (in combination with methotrexate or alone if methotrexate inappropriate) in children who have had an inadequate response to NSAIDs and systemic corticosteroids
- ▸ BY INTRAVENOUS INFUSION
- ▸ Child 2-17 years (body-weight up to 30 kg): 12 mg/kg every 2 weeks, review treatment if no improvement within 6 weeks
- ▸ Child 2-17 years (body-weight 30 kg and above): 8 mg/kg every 2 weeks, review treatment if no improvement within 6 weeks

Polyarticular juvenile idiopathic arthritis (in combination with methotrexate or alone if methotrexate inappropriate) in children who have had an inadequate response to methotrexate
- ▸ BY INTRAVENOUS INFUSION
- ▸ Child 2-17 years (body-weight up to 30 kg): 10 mg/kg every 4 weeks, review treatment if no improvement within 12 weeks
- ▸ Child 2-17 years (body-weight 30 kg and above): 8 mg/kg every 4 weeks, review treatment if no improvement within 12 weeks

- **CONTRA-INDICATIONS** Do not initiate if absolute neutrophil count less than 2×10^9/litre · severe active infection
- **CAUTIONS** History of diverticulitis · history of intestinal ulceration · history of recurrent or chronic infection (interrupt treatment if serious infection occurs) · low absolute neutrophil count · low platelet count · predisposition to infection (interrupt treatment if serious infection occurs)

  CAUTIONS, FURTHER INFORMATION
- ▸ Tuberculosis Patients with latent tuberculosis should be treated with standard therapy before starting tocilizumab.
- **INTERACTIONS** → Appendix 1: monoclonal antibodies
- **SIDE-EFFECTS**
- ▸ **Common or very common** Headache · hypercholesterolaemia · infection · neutropenia · raised hepatic transaminases · upper respiratory-tract infection
- ▸ **Frequency not known** Antibody formation · diarrhoea · infusion related reactions · nausea · thrombocytopenia

  SIDE-EFFECTS, FURTHER INFORMATION
- ▸ Neutrophil and platelet counts Discontinue if absolute neutrophil count less than 0.5×10^9/litre or platelet count less than 50×10^3/microlitre.
- **CONCEPTION AND CONTRACEPTION** Effective contraception required during and for 3 months after treatment.
- **PREGNANCY** Manufacturer advises avoid unless essential—toxicity in *animal* studies.
- **BREAST FEEDING** Manufacturer advises use only if potential benefit outweighs risk—no information available.
- **HEPATIC IMPAIRMENT** Manufacturer advises caution—consult product literature.
- **RENAL IMPAIRMENT** Manufacturer advises monitor renal function closely in moderate or severe impairment.
- **PRE-TREATMENT SCREENING**
  Tuberculosis Patients should be evaluated for tuberculosis before treatment.

- **MONITORING REQUIREMENTS**
- ▸ Monitor lipid profile 4–8 weeks after starting treatment and then as indicated.
- ▸ Monitor for demyelinating disorders.
- ▸ Monitor hepatic transaminases.
- ▸ Monitor neutrophil and platelet counts.

- **DIRECTIONS FOR ADMINISTRATION** For *intravenous infusion*; body-weight less than 30 kg, dilute requisite dose to a volume of 50 mL with Sodium chloride 0.9% and give over 1 hour; body-weight over 30 kg, dilute requisite dose to a volume of 100 mL with Sodium chloride 0.9% and give over 1 hour.

- **PATIENT AND CARER ADVICE** An alert card should be provided.

  Patients and their carers should be advised to seek immediate medical attention if symptoms of infection occur, or if symptoms of diverticular perforation such as abdominal pain, haemorrhage, or fever accompanying change in bowel habits occur.

- **NATIONAL FUNDING/ACCESS DECISIONS**

  NICE technology appraisals (TAs)
- ▸ **Tocilizumab for the treatment of systemic juvenile idiopathic arthritis (December 2011)** NICE TA238
  Tocilizumab is recommended for the treatment of systemic juvenile idiopathic arthritis in children aged over 2 years who have not responded adequately to NSAIDs, systemic corticosteroids and methotrexate, if the manufacturer makes tocilizumab available with the discount agreed as part of the patient access scheme.

  Tocilizumab is not recommended for the treatment of systemic juvenile idiopathic arthritis in children whose disease continues to respond to methotrexate or who have not been treated with methotrexate.

  Children currently receiving tocilizumab for systemic juvenile idiopathic arthritis who do not meet these criteria should have the option to continue treatment until it is considered appropriate to stop.
  www.nice.org.uk/TA238
- ▸ **Abatacept, adalimumab, etanercept and tocilizumab for treating juvenile idiopathic arthritis (December 2015)** NICE TA373
  Tocilizumab is recommended as an option for treatment of polyarticular juvenile idiopathic arthritis (JIA), including polyarticular-onset, polyarticular-course and extended oligoarticular JIA in children 2 years and older whose disease has responded inadequately to previous therapy with methotrexate and if the manufacturer provides tocilizumab with the discounts agreed in the patient access schemes.
  www.nice.org.uk/TA373

- **MEDICINAL FORMS**
  There can be variation in the licensing of different medicines containing the same drug.
  Solution for infusion
- ▸ RoActemra (Roche Products Ltd)
  Tocilizumab 20 mg per 1 ml RoActemra 400mg/20ml concentrate for solution for infusion vials | 1 vial [PoM] £512.00 (Hospital only)
  RoActemra 200mg/10ml concentrate for solution for infusion vials | 1 vial [PoM] £256.00 (Hospital only)
  RoActemra 80mg/4ml concentrate for solution for infusion vials | 1 vial [PoM] £102.40 (Hospital only)

10

Musculoskeletal system

10

Musculoskeletal system

IMMUNOSUPPRESSANTS > T-CELL ACTIVATION INHIBITORS

Abatacept

31-May-2016

- **INDICATIONS AND DOSE**

  Moderate to severe active polyarticular juvenile idiopathic arthritis (in combination with methotrexate) in children who have not responded adequately to other disease-modifying antirheumatic drugs (including at least one tumour necrosis factor (TNF) inhibitor)
  - BY INTRAVENOUS INFUSION
  - Child 6–17 years (body-weight up to 75 kg): 10 mg/kg every 2 weeks for 3 doses, then 10 mg/kg every 4 weeks, review treatment if no response within 6 months
  - Child 6–17 years (body-weight 75–100 kg): 750 mg every 2 weeks for 3 doses, then 750 mg every 4 weeks, review treatment if no response within 6 months
  - Child 6–17 years (body-weight 101 kg and above): 1 g every 2 weeks for 3 doses, then 1 g every 4 weeks, review treatment if no response within 6 months

- **CONTRA-INDICATIONS** Severe infection
- **CAUTIONS** Children should be brought up to date with current immunisation schedule before initiating therapy · do not initiate until active infections are controlled · predisposition to infection (screen for latent tuberculosis and viral hepatitis) · progressive multifocal leucoencephalopathy (discontinue treatment if neurological symptoms present)
- **INTERACTIONS** → Appendix 1: abatacept
- **SIDE-EFFECTS**
  - **Common or very common** Abdominal pain · conjunctivitis · cough · diarrhoea · dizziness · dyspepsia · fatigue · flushing · headache · hypertension · infection · leucopenia · nausea · pain in extremities · paraesthesia · stomatitis · vomiting
  - **Uncommon** Psoriasis · alopecia · anxiety · arthralgia · basal and squamous cell carcinoma · bradycardia · bronchospasm · bruising · depression · dry eye · dry skin · dyspnoea · gastritis · hyperhidrosis · hypotension · menstrual disturbances · palpitation · skin papilloma · sleep disorder · tachycardia · thrombocytopenia · visual disturbance · weight gain
  - **Frequency not known** Lung cancer · lymphoma
- **CONCEPTION AND CONTRACEPTION** Effective contraception required during treatment and for 14 weeks after last dose.
- **PREGNANCY** Manufacturer advises avoid unless essential.
- **BREAST FEEDING** Present in milk in *animal* studies—manufacturer advises avoid breast-feeding during treatment and for 14 weeks after last dose.
- **DIRECTIONS FOR ADMINISTRATION** For *intravenous infusion*, given intermittently *in* Sodium chloride 0.9%; reconstitute each vial with 10 mL water for injections using the silicone-free syringe provided; dilute requisite dose in Sodium Chloride 0.9% to 100 mL (using the same silicone-free syringe); give over 30 minutes through a low protein-binding filter (pore size 0.2–1.2 micron).
- **NATIONAL FUNDING/ACCESS DECISIONS**

  NICE technology appraisals (TAs)
  - Abatacept, adalimumab, etanercept and tocilizumab for treating juvenile idiopathic arthritis (December 2015) NICE TA373

  Abatacept is recommended as options for treating polyarticular juvenile idiopathic arthritis (JIA), including polyarticular-onset, polyarticular-course and extended oligoarticular JIA in patients 6 years and older whose disease has responded inadequately to other disease-modifying anti-rheumatic drugs (DMARDs) including at least 1 tumour necrosis factor (TNF) inhibitor,

only if the manufacturer provides abatacept with the discounts agreed in the patient access schemes. www.nice.org.uk/TA373

- **MEDICINAL FORMS**
  There can be variation in the licensing of different medicines containing the same drug.

  Powder for solution for infusion
  ELECTROLYTES: May contain Sodium
  - **Orencia** (Bristol-Myers Squibb Pharmaceuticals Ltd)
    Abatacept 250 mg Orencia 250mg powder for concentrate for solution for infusion vials | 1 vial [PoM] £302.40 (Hospital only)

IMMUNOSUPPRESSANTS > TUMOR NECROSIS FACTOR ALPHA (TNF-α) INHIBITORS

Adalimumab

27-Apr-2017

- **INDICATIONS AND DOSE**

  Severe chronic plaque psoriasis in children who have had an inadequate response to, or are inappropriate for topical therapy and phototherapies
  - BY SUBCUTANEOUS INJECTION
  - Child 4–17 years: Initially 0.8 mg/kg every week (max. per dose 40 mg) for 2 doses, then 0.8 mg/kg every 2 weeks (max. per dose 40 mg), review treatment if no response within 16 weeks; for further information on dose banding, consult product literature

  Active polyarticular juvenile idiopathic arthritis (in combination with methotrexate or alone if methotrexate inappropriate) in children who have not responded adequately to one or more disease-modifying antirheumatic drug
  - BY SUBCUTANEOUS INJECTION
  - Child 2–3 years: 24 mg/m² every 2 weeks (max. per dose 20 mg), review treatment if no response within 12 weeks; for further information on dose banding, consult product literature
  - Child 4–12 years: 24 mg/m² every 2 weeks (max. per dose 40 mg), review treatment if no response within 12 weeks; for further information on dose banding, consult product literature
  - Child 13–17 years: 40 mg every 2 weeks, review treatment if no response within 12 weeks; for further information on dose banding, consult product literature

  Active enthesitis-related arthritis in children who have had an inadequate response to, or who are intolerant of, conventional therapy
  - BY SUBCUTANEOUS INJECTION
  - Child 6–17 years: 24 mg/m² every 2 weeks (max. per dose 40 mg), for further information on dose banding, consult product literature

  Severe active Crohn's disease
  - BY SUBCUTANEOUS INJECTION
  - Child 6–17 years (body-weight up to 40 kg): Initially 40 mg, then 20 mg after 2 weeks; maintenance 20 mg every 2 weeks, increased if necessary to 20 mg once weekly, review treatment if no response within 12 weeks of initial dose
  - Child 6–17 years (body-weight 40 kg and above): Initially 80 mg, then 40 mg after 2 weeks; maintenance 40 mg every 2 weeks, increased if necessary to 40 mg once weekly, maximum 40 mg administered at a single site, review treatment if no response within 12 weeks of initial dose

  Severe active Crohn's disease (accelerated regimen)
  - BY SUBCUTANEOUS INJECTION
  - Child 6–17 years (body-weight up to 40 kg): Initially 80 mg, then 40 mg after 2 weeks; maintenance 20 mg every 2 weeks, increased if necessary to 20 mg once

weekly, maximum 40 mg administered at a single site, review treatment if no response within 12 weeks of initial dose
▸ **Child 6-17 years (body-weight 40 kg and above):** Initially 160 mg, dose can alternatively be given as divided injections over 2 days, then 80 mg after 2 weeks; maintenance 40 mg every 2 weeks, then increased if necessary to 40 mg once weekly, maximum 40 mg administered at a single site, review treatment if no response within 12 weeks of initial dose

Active moderate to severe hidradenitis suppurativa (acne inversa) in patients with an inadequate response to conventional systemic therapy
▸ BY SUBCUTANEOUS INJECTION
▸ **Child 12-17 years (body-weight 30 kg and above):** Initially 80 mg, given as two 40 mg injections in one day, followed by 40 mg after 1 week, then maintenance 40 mg every 2 weeks; increased if necessary to 40 mg once weekly, review treatment if no response within 12 weeks; if treatment interrupted—consult product literature

● CONTRA-INDICATIONS Moderate or severe heart failure · severe infection
● CAUTIONS Children should be brought up to date with current immunisation schedule before initiating therapy · demyelinating disorders (risk of exacerbation) · development of malignancy · do not initiate until active infections are controlled (discontinue if new serious infection develops) · hepatitis B virus—monitor for active infection · history of malignancy · mild heart failure (discontinue if symptoms develop or worsen) · predisposition to infection
CAUTIONS, FURTHER INFORMATION
▸ Tuberculosis Active tuberculosis should be treated with standard treatment for at least 2 months before starting adalimumab. Patients who have previously received adequate treatment for tuberculosis can start adalimumab but should be monitored every 3 months for possible recurrence. In patients without active tuberculosis but who were previously not treated adequately, chemoprophylaxis should ideally be completed before starting adalimumab. In patients at high risk of tuberculosis who cannot be assessed by tuberculin skin test, chemoprophylaxis can be given concurrently with adalimumab.
● INTERACTIONS → Appendix 1: monoclonal antibodies
● SIDE-EFFECTS
▸ **Common or very common** Anxiety · benign tumours · chest pain · cough · dehydration · dermatitis · dizziness · dyspepsia · dyspnoea · electrolyte disturbances · eye disorders · flushing · gastrointestinal haemorrhage · haematuria · hyperlipidaemia · hypertension · hyperuricaemia · impaired healing · mood changes · musculoskeletal pain · oedema · onycholysis · paraesthesia · rash · renal impairment · skin cancer · sleep disturbances · tachycardia · vomiting
▸ **Uncommon** Aortic aneurysm · arrhythmias · cholecystitis · cholelithiasis · dysphagia · erectile dysfunction · hearing loss · hepatic steatosis · interstitial lung disease · leukaemia · lymphoma · malignancy · neuropathy · nocturia · pancreatitis · pneumonitis · rhabdomyolysis · solid tumours · tinnitus · tremor · vascular occlusion
▸ **Rare** Autoimmune hepatitis · demyelinating disorders · myocardial infarction
▸ **Frequency not known** Abdominal pain · anaemia · antibody formation · aplastic anaemia · blood disorders · cutaneous vasculitis · depression · fever · headache · hypersensitivity reactions · injection-site reactions · leucopenia · lupus erythematosus-like syndrome · nausea · new onset psoriasis · pancytopenia · pleural effusion · pruritus ·

pulmonary embolism · sarcoidosis · Stevens-Johnson syndrome · thrombocytopenia · worsening heart failure · worsening of symptoms of dermatomyositis · worsening psoriasis
SIDE-EFFECTS, FURTHER INFORMATION
Associated with infections, sometimes severe, including tuberculosis, septicaemia, and hepatitis B reactivation.
● CONCEPTION AND CONTRACEPTION Manufacturer advises effective contraception required during treatment and for at least 5 months after last dose.
● PREGNANCY Avoid.
● BREAST FEEDING Avoid; manufacturer advises avoid for at least 5 months after last dose.
● PRE-TREATMENT SCREENING Tuberculosis Patients should be evaluated for tuberculosis before treatment.
● MONITORING REQUIREMENTS
▸ Manufacturer advises monitor for infection before, during, and for 4 months after treatment.
▸ Manufacturer advises monitor for non-melanoma skin cancer before and during treatment, especially in patients with a history of PUVA treatment for psoriasis or extensive immunosuppressant therapy.
▸ For uveitis, manufacturer advises patients should be assessed for pre-existing or developing central demyelinating disorders before and at regular intervals during treatment.
● PATIENT AND CARER ADVICE An alert card should be provided.
   When used to treat *hidradenitis suppurativa*, patients and their carers should be advised to use a daily topical antiseptic wash on lesions during treatment with adalimumab.
Tuberculosis patients and their carers should be advised to seek medical attention if symptoms suggestive of tuberculosis (e.g. persistent cough, weight loss, or, and fever) develop.
Blood disorders Patients and their carers should be advised to seek medical attention if symptoms suggestive of blood disorders (such as fever, sore throat, bruising, or bleeding) develop.
● NATIONAL FUNDING/ACCESS DECISIONS
NICE technology appraisals (TAs)
▸ **Abatacept, adalimumab, etanercept and tocilizumab for treating juvenile idiopathic arthritis (December 2015)**
NICE TA373
Adalimumab is recommended as an option for treating polyarticular juvenile idiopathic arthritis (JIA), including polyarticular-onset, polyarticular-course and extended oligoarticular JIA in patients 2 years and older whose disease has responded inadequately to 1 or more disease-modifying antirheumatic drugs (DMARDs) and for treating enthesitis-related JIA in patients 6 years and older whose disease has responded inadequately to, or who are intolerant of, conventional therapy.
www.nice.org.uk/TA373
Scottish Medicines Consortium (SMC) Decisions
The *Scottish Medicines Consortium* has advised (April 2015) that adalimumab (*Humira®*) is accepted for restricted use within NHS Scotland for the treatment of active enthesitis-related arthritis in children over 6 years of age who have had an inadequate response to, or who are intolerant of, conventional therapy, and is used within specialist rheumatology services (including those working within the network for paediatric rheumatology).
   The *Scottish Medicines Consortium* has advised (June 2015) that adalimumab (*Humira®*) is accepted for restricted use within NHS Scotland for the treatment of severe chronic plaque psoriasis in children over 4 years who have had an inadequate response to, or are

10

Musculoskeletal system

inappropriate for, topical therapy and phototherapies, and have severe disease as defined by a total Psoriasis Area Severity Index (PASI) score of ≥10 and a Dermatology Life Quality Index (DLQI) of >10.

All Wales Medicines Strategy Group (AWMSG) Decisions
The *All Wales Medicines Strategy Group* has advised (January 2017) that adalimumab (*Humira*®) is recommended as an option for use within NHS Wales for the treatment of moderately to severely active Crohn's disease in children 6 years and over, who have had an inadequate response to conventional therapy including primary nutrition therapy and a corticosteroid and/or an immunomodulator, or who are intolerant to or have contra-indications for such therapies.

● MEDICINAL FORMS
There can be variation in the licensing of different medicines containing the same drug.

Solution for injection
CAUTIONARY AND ADVISORY LABELS 10
▸ Humira (AbbVie Ltd)
Adalimumab 50 mg per 1 ml Humira 40mg/0.8ml solution for injection pre-filled syringes | 2 pre-filled disposable injection PoM £704.28
Humira 40mg/0.8ml solution for injection pre-filled pen | 2 pre-filled disposable injection PoM £704.28
Humira 40mg/0.8ml solution for injection vials | 2 vial PoM £704.28
Adalimumab 100 mg per 1 ml Humira 40mg/0.4ml solution for injection pre-filled pen | 2 pre-filled disposable injection PoM £704.28
Humira 40mg/0.4ml solution for injection pre-filled syringes | 2 pre-filled disposable injection PoM £704.28

Etanercept
07-Jun-2017

● INDICATIONS AND DOSE

BENEPALI® SOLUTION FOR INJECTION

Polyarthritis in children who have had an inadequate response to methotrexate or who cannot tolerate it | Extended oligoarthritis in children who have had an inadequate response to methotrexate or who cannot tolerate it
▸ BY SUBCUTANEOUS INJECTION
▸ Child 2–17 years: 800 micrograms/kg once weekly (max. per dose 50 mg), consider discontinuation if no response after 4 months

Psoriatic arthritis in adolescents who have had an inadequate response to methotrexate or who cannot tolerate it | Enthesitis-related arthritis in adolescents who have had an inadequate response to conventional therapy or who cannot tolerate it
▸ BY SUBCUTANEOUS INJECTION
▸ Child 12–17 years: 800 micrograms/kg once weekly (max. per dose 50 mg), consider discontinuation if no response after 4 months

Chronic, severe plaque psoriasis in children who have had an inadequate response to other systemic therapies or phototherapies or who cannot tolerate them
▸ BY SUBCUTANEOUS INJECTION
▸ Child 6–17 years: 800 micrograms/kg once weekly (max. per dose 50 mg) for up to 24 weeks, discontinue if no response after 12 weeks

ENBREL® POWDER AND SOLVENT FOR SOLUTION FOR INJECTION

Polyarthritis in children who have had an inadequate response to methotrexate or who cannot tolerate it | Extended oligoarthritis in children who have had an inadequate response to methotrexate or who cannot tolerate it
▸ BY SUBCUTANEOUS INJECTION
▸ Child 2–17 years: 400 micrograms/kg twice weekly (max. per dose 25 mg), to be given at an interval of 3–4 days between doses, alternatively 800 micrograms/kg once weekly (max. per dose 50 mg), consider discontinuation if no response after 4 months

Psoriatic arthritis in adolescents who have had an inadequate response to methotrexate or who cannot tolerate it | Enthesitis-related arthritis in adolescents who have had an inadequate response to conventional therapy or who cannot tolerate it
▸ BY SUBCUTANEOUS INJECTION
▸ Child 12–17 years: 400 micrograms/kg twice weekly (max. per dose 25 mg), to be given at an interval of 3–4 days between doses, alternatively 800 micrograms/kg once weekly (max. per dose 50 mg), consider discontinuation if no response after 4 months

Chronic, severe plaque psoriasis in children who have had an inadequate response to other systemic therapies or phototherapies or who cannot tolerate them
▸ BY SUBCUTANEOUS INJECTION
▸ Child 6–17 years: 800 micrograms/kg once weekly (max. per dose 50 mg) for up to 24 weeks, discontinue if no response after 12 weeks

ENBREL® SOLUTION FOR INJECTION

Polyarthritis in children who have had an inadequate response to methotrexate or who cannot tolerate it | Extended oligoarthritis in children who have had an inadequate response to methotrexate or who cannot tolerate it
▸ BY SUBCUTANEOUS INJECTION
▸ Child 2–17 years: 400 micrograms/kg twice weekly (max. per dose 25 mg), to be given at an interval of 3–4 days between doses, alternatively 800 micrograms/kg once weekly (max. per dose 50 mg), consider discontinuation if no response after 4 months

Psoriatic arthritis in adolescents who have had an inadequate response to methotrexate or who cannot tolerate it | Enthesitis-related arthritis in adolescents who have had an inadequate response to conventional therapy or who cannot tolerate it
▸ BY SUBCUTANEOUS INJECTION
▸ Child 12–17 years: 400 micrograms/kg twice weekly (max. per dose 25 mg), to be given at an interval of 3–4 days between doses, alternatively 800 micrograms/kg once weekly (max. per dose 50 mg), consider discontinuation if no response after 4 months

Chronic, severe plaque psoriasis in children who have had an inadequate response to other systemic therapies or phototherapies or who cannot tolerate them
▸ BY SUBCUTANEOUS INJECTION
▸ Child 6–17 years: 800 micrograms/kg once weekly (max. per dose 50 mg) for up to 24 weeks, discontinue if no response after 12 weeks

● CONTRA-INDICATIONS Active infection · avoid injections containing benzyl alcohol in neonates
● CAUTIONS Children should be brought up to date with current immunisation schedule before initiating therapy · development of malignancy · diabetes mellitus · heart failure (risk of exacerbation) · hepatitis B virus—monitor for active infection · hepatitis C infection (monitor for worsening infection) · history of blood disorders · history of malignancy · history or increased risk of demyelinating

disorders · predisposition to infection (avoid if predisposition to septicaemia) · significant exposure to herpes zoster virus—interrupt treatment and consider varicella–zoster immunoglobulin

CAUTIONS, FURTHER INFORMATION

▸ **Tuberculosis** Active tuberculosis should be treated with standard treatment for at least 2 months before starting etanercept. Patients who have previously received adequate treatment for tuberculosis can start etanercept but should be monitored every 3 months for possible recurrence. In patients without active tuberculosis but who were previously not treated adequately, chemoprophylaxis should ideally be completed before starting etanercept. In patients at high risk of tuberculosis who cannot be assessed by tuberculin skin test, chemoprophylaxis can be given concurrently with etanercept.

● INTERACTIONS → Appendix 1: etanercept

● SIDE-EFFECTS

▸ **Uncommon** Interstitial lung disease · new onset or worsening psoriasis · rash · skin cancer · uveitis

▸ **Rare** Demyelinating disorders · lymphoma · seizures · Stevens-Johnson syndrome · vasculitis

▸ **Very rare** Toxic epidermal necrolysis

▸ **Frequency not known** Abdominal pain · anaemia · antibody formation · aplastic anaemia · appendicitis · blood disorders · cutaneous ulcer · depression · diabetes mellitus · fever · gastritis · headache · hypersensitivity reactions · inflammatory bowel disease · injection-site reactions · leucopenia · leukaemia · lupus erythematosus-like syndrome · macrophage activation syndrome · malignancy · nausea · oesophagitis · pancytopenia · pruritus · solid tumours · thrombocytopenia · vomiting · worsening heart failure

SIDE-EFFECTS, FURTHER INFORMATION
Associated with infections, sometimes severe, including tuberculosis, septicaemia, and hepatitis B reactivation.

● **CONCEPTION AND CONTRACEPTION** Manufacturer advises effective contraception required during treatment and for 3 weeks after last dose.

● **PREGNANCY** Avoid—limited information available.

● **BREAST FEEDING** Manufacturer advises avoid—present in milk in *animal* studies.

● **HEPATIC IMPAIRMENT** Use with caution in moderate to severe alcoholic hepatitis.

● **PRE-TREATMENT SCREENING**
Tuberculosis Patients should be evaluated for tuberculosis before treatment.

● **MONITORING REQUIREMENTS** Monitor for skin cancer before and during treatment, particularly in those at risk (including patients with psoriasis or a history of PUVA treatment).

● **PRESCRIBING AND DISPENSING INFORMATION** Etanercept is a biological medicine. Biological medicines must be prescribed and dispensed by brand name, see *Biological medicines* and *Biosimilar medicines*, under Guidance on prescribing p. 1.

BENEPALI® SOLUTION FOR INJECTION Manufacturer advises patients requiring less than the full 50 mg dose should **not** receive *Benepali*®—if an alternate dose is required, other etanercept formulations providing this option should be used.

● **PATIENT AND CARER ADVICE** An alert card should be provided.
Blood disorders Patients and their carers should be advised to seek medical attention if symptoms suggestive of blood disorders (such as fever, sore throat, bruising, or bleeding) develop.
Tuberculosis Patients and their carers should be advised to seek medical attention if symptoms suggestive of

tuberculosis (e.g. persistent cough, weight loss, and fever) develop.

● NATIONAL FUNDING/ACCESS DECISIONS

NICE technology appraisals (TAs)

▸ **Abatacept, adalimumab, etanercept and tocilizumab for treating juvenile idiopathic arthritis (December 2015)**
NICE TA373
Etanercept is recommended as an option for treating:

● polyarticular juvenile idiopathic arthritis (JIA), including polyarticular-onset, polyarticular-course and extended oligoarticular JIA, in patients 2 years and over whose disease has responded inadequately to, or who are intolerant of, methotrexate;

● enthesitis-related JIA in patients 12 years and over whose disease has responded inadequately to, or who are intolerant of, conventional therapy;

● psoriatic JIA in patients 12 years and over whose disease has responded inadequately to, or who are intolerant of, methotrexate.
www.nice.org.uk/TA373

Scottish Medicines Consortium (SMC) Decisions
The *Scottish Medicines Consortium* issued similar advice to NICE TA103 on the use of etanercept for severe plaque psoriasis in adults (August 2009) and children over 6 years old (April 2012).

The *Scottish Medicines Consortium* has advised (January 2013) that etanercept (*Enbrel*®) is accepted for restricted use within NHS Scotland for the treatment of polyarthritis (rheumatoid factor positive or negative) and extended oligoarthritis in children and adolescents from the age of 2 years who have had an inadequate response to or are intolerant of methotrexate, psoriatic arthritis in adolescents from the age of 12 years who have had an inadequate response to or are intolerant of methotrexate, and enthesitis-related arthritis in adolescents from the age of 12 years who have had an inadequate response to or are intolerant of conventional therapy. It is further restricted to use within specialist rheumatology services (including those working within the network for paediatric rheumatology).

● MEDICINAL FORMS
There can be variation in the licensing of different medicines containing the same drug.

Solution for injection
CAUTIONARY AND ADVISORY LABELS 10

▸ **Benepali** (Biogen Idec Ltd) ▼
Etanercept 50 mg per 1 ml Benepali 50mg/1ml solution for injection pre-filled syringes | 4 pre-filled disposable injection PoM £656.00
Benepali 50mg/1ml solution for injection pre-filled pen | 4 pre-filled disposable injection PoM £656.00

▸ **Enbrel** (Pfizer Ltd)
Etanercept 50 mg per 1 ml Enbrel 50mg/1ml solution for injection pre-filled syringes | 4 pre-filled disposable injection PoM £715.00
Enbrel 25mg/0.5ml solution for injection pre-filled syringes | 4 pre-filled disposable injection PoM £357.50

▸ **Enbrel MyClic** (Pfizer Ltd)
Etanercept 50 mg per 1 ml Enbrel 50mg/1ml solution for injection pre-filled MyClic pen | 4 pre-filled disposable injection PoM £715.00

Powder and solvent for solution for injection
CAUTIONARY AND ADVISORY LABELS 10
EXCIPIENTS: May contain Benzyl alcohol

▸ **Enbrel** (Pfizer Ltd)
Etanercept 10 mg Enbrel Paediatric 10mg powder and solvent for solution for injection vials | 1 vial PoM £143.00
Etanercept 25 mg Enbrel 25mg powder and solvent for solution for injection vials | 4 vial PoM £357.50

2 Neuromuscular disorders

Neuromuscular disorders

Drugs that enhance neuromuscular transmission

Anticholinesterases are used as first-line treatment in *ocular myasthenia gravis* and as an adjunct to immunosuppressant therapy for *generalised myasthenia gravis*.

Corticosteroids are used when anticholinesterases do not control symptoms completely. A second-line immunosuppressant such as azathioprine p. 495 is frequently used to reduce the dose of corticosteroid.

Plasmapheresis or infusion of intravenous immunoglobulin [unlicensed indication] may induce temporary remission in severe relapses, particularly where bulbar or respiratory function is compromised or before thymectomy.

Anticholinesterases

Anticholinesterase drugs enhance neuromuscular transmission in voluntary and involuntary muscle in myasthenia gravis. Excessive dosage of these drugs can impair neuromuscular transmission and precipitate cholinergic crises by causing a depolarising block. This may be difficult to distinguish from a worsening myasthenic state.

Muscarinic side-effects of anticholinesterases include increased sweating, increased salivary and gastric secretions, increased gastro-intestinal and uterine motility, and bradycardia. These parasympathomimetic effects are antagonised by atropine sulfate p. 779.

Neostigmine p. 619 produces a therapeutic effect for up to 4 hours. Its pronounced muscarinic action is a disadvantage, and simultaneous administration of an antimuscarinic drug such as atropine sulfate or propantheline bromide p. 61 may be required to prevent colic, excessive salivation, or diarrhoea. In severe disease neostigmine can be given every 2 hours. In infants, neostigmine by either subcutaneous or intramuscular injection is preferred for the short-term management of myasthenia.

Pyridostigmine bromide p. 620 is less powerful and slower in action than neostigmine but it has a longer duration of action. It is preferable to neostigmine because of its smoother action and the need for less frequent dosage. It is particularly preferred in patients whose muscles are weak on waking. It has a comparatively mild gastrointestinal effect but an antimuscarinic drug may still be required. It is inadvisable to use excessive doses because acetylcholine receptor down regulation may occur. Immunosuppressant therapy may be considered if high doses of pyridostigmine bromide are needed.

Neostigmine and pyridostigmine bromide should be given to neonates 30 minutes before feeds to improve suckling.

Neostigmine is also used to reverse the actions of the non-depolarising neuromuscular blocking drugs.

Immunosuppressant therapy

A course of **corticosteroids** is an established treatment in severe cases of myasthenia gravis and may be particularly useful when antibodies to the acetylcholine receptor are present in high titre. Short courses of high-dose ('pulsed') methylprednisolone p. 421 followed by maintenance therapy with oral corticosteroids may also be useful.

Corticosteroid treatment is usually initiated under specialist supervision. Transient but very serious worsening of symptoms can occur in the first 2–3 weeks, especially if the corticosteroid is started at a high dose. Once remission has occurred (usually after 2–6 months), the dose of prednisolone p. 421 should be reduced slowly to the minimum effective dose.

Skeletal muscle relaxants

The drugs described are used for the relief of chronic muscle spasm or spasticity associated with neurological damage; they are not indicated for spasm associated with minor injuries. They act principally on the central nervous system with the exception of dantrolene, which has a peripheral site of action. They differ in action from the muscle relaxants used in anaesthesia, which block transmission at the neuromuscular junction.

The underlying cause of spasticity should be treated and any aggravating factors (e.g. pressure sores, infection) remedied. Skeletal muscle relaxants are effective in most forms of spasticity except the rare alpha variety. The major disadvantage of treatment with these drugs is that reduction in muscle tone can cause a loss of splinting action of the spastic leg and trunk muscles and sometimes lead to an increase in disability.

Dantrolene sodium p. 791 acts directly on skeletal muscle and produces fewer central adverse effects. It is generally used in resistant cases. The dose should be increased slowly.

Baclofen p. 620 inhibits transmission at spinal level and also depresses the central nervous system. The dose should be increased slowly to avoid the major side-effects of sedation and muscular hypotonia (other adverse events are uncommon).

Diazepam p. 212 has undoubted efficacy in some children. Sedation and occasionally extensor hypotonus are disadvantages. Other benzodiazepines also have muscle-relaxant properties.

2.1 Muscular dystrophy

DRUGS FOR NEUROMUSCULAR DISORDERS

Ataluren

24-May-2017

- **DRUG ACTION** Ataluren restores the synthesis of dystrophin by allowing ribosomes to read through premature stop codons that cause incomplete dystrophin synthesis in nonsense mutation Duchenne muscular dystrophy.

- **INDICATIONS AND DOSE**

  Duchenne muscular dystrophy resulting from a nonsense mutation in the dystrophin gene, in ambulatory patients (initiated by a specialist)
  - BY MOUTH
    - Child 5–17 years: (consult product literature)

- **INTERACTIONS** → Appendix 1: ataluren

- **SIDE-EFFECTS**
- **Common or very common** Abdominal discomfort · constipation · cough · decreased appetite · diarrhoea · enuresis · epistaxis · flatulence · haematuria · headache · hypertension · hypertriglyceridaemia · musculoskeletal chest pain · nausea · pain in extremity · pyrexia · rash · upper abdominal pain · vomiting · weight loss
- **Frequency not known** Changes in renal function tests · raised cholesterol

- **PREGNANCY** Manufacturer advises avoid—toxicity in *animal* studies.

- **BREAST FEEDING** Manufacturer advises discontinue breastfeeding—present in milk in *animal* studies.

- **HEPATIC IMPAIRMENT** Manufacturer advises close monitoring—safety and efficacy not established.

- **RENAL IMPAIRMENT** Manufacturer advises close monitoring—safety and efficacy not established.

- **MONITORING REQUIREMENTS** Manufacturer advises monitor renal function at least every 6–12 months, and cholesterol and triglyceride concentrations at least annually.

- **DIRECTIONS FOR ADMINISTRATION** Manufacturer advises the contents of each sachet should be mixed with at least 30 mL of liquid (water, milk, fruit juice), or 3 tablespoons of semi-solid food (yoghurt or apple sauce).
- **PATIENT AND CARER ADVICE**
Manufacturer advises patients should maintain adequate hydration during treatment.

  Missed doses
  Manufacturer advises if a morning or midday dose is more than 3 hours late, or an evening dose is more than 6 hours late, the missed dose should not be taken and the next dose should be taken at the normal time.
- **NATIONAL FUNDING/ACCESS DECISIONS**

  Scottish Medicines Consortium (SMC) Decisions
  The *Scottish Medicines Consortium* has advised (April 2016) that ataluren (*Translarna*®) is not recommended for use within NHS Scotland for the treatment of Duchenne muscular dystrophy resulting from a nonsense mutation in the dystrophin gene, in ambulatory patients aged 5 years and older as the economic case was not demonstrated.
- **MEDICINAL FORMS**
There can be variation in the licensing of different medicines containing the same drug.

  Granules
  ▸ **Translarna** (PTC Therapeutics Ltd) ▼
  Ataluren 125 mg Translarna 125mg granules for oral suspension sachets | 30 sachet PoM no price available
  Ataluren 250 mg Translarna 250mg granules for oral suspension sachets | 30 sachet PoM no price available
  Ataluren 1 gram Translarna 1,000mg granules for oral suspension sachets | 30 sachet PoM no price available

2.2 Myasthenia gravis

ANTICHOLINESTERASES

Anticholinesterases

- **DRUG ACTION** They prolong the action of acetylcholine by inhibiting the action of the enzyme acetylcholinesterase.
- **CONTRA-INDICATIONS** Intestinal obstruction · urinary obstruction
- **CAUTIONS** Arrhythmias · asthma (extreme caution) · atropine or other antidote to muscarinic effects may be necessary (particularly when neostigmine is given by injection) but not given routinely because it may mask signs of overdosage · bradycardia · epilepsy · hyperthyroidism · hypotension · parkinsonism · peptic ulceration · recent myocardial infarction · vagotonia
- **SIDE-EFFECTS** Abdominal cramps (more marked with higher doses) · diarrhoea · increased salivation · nausea · vomiting

  Overdose
  Signs of overdosage include bronchoconstriction, increased bronchial secretions, lacrimation, excessive sweating, involuntary defaecation, involuntary micturition, miosis, nystagmus, bradycardia, heart block, arrhythmias, hypotension, agitation, excessive dreaming, and weakness eventually leading to fasciculation and paralysis.
- **PREGNANCY** Manufacturer advises use only if potential benefit outweighs risk.
- **BREAST FEEDING** Amount probably too small to be harmful.

▯ above

Neostigmine
(Neostigmine methylsulfate)

- **INDICATIONS AND DOSE**

  Treatment of myasthenia gravis
  ▸ BY MOUTH

  ▸ Neonate: Initially 1–2 mg, then 1–5 mg every 4 hours, given 30 minutes before feeds.

  ▸ Child 1 month–5 years: Initially 7.5 mg, dose repeated at suitable intervals throughout the day, total daily dose 15–90 mg

  ▸ Child 6–11 years: Initially 15 mg, dose repeated at suitable intervals throughout the day, total daily dose 15–90 mg

  ▸ Child 12–17 years: Initially 15–30 mg, dose repeated at suitable intervals throughout the day, total daily dose 75–300 mg, the maximum that most patients can tolerate is 180 mg daily

  ▸ BY SUBCUTANEOUS INJECTION, OR BY INTRAMUSCULAR INJECTION

  ▸ Neonate: 150 micrograms/kg every 6–8 hours, to be given 30 minutes before feeds, then increased if necessary up to 300 micrograms/kg every 4 hours.

  ▸ Child 1 month–11 years: 200–500 micrograms, dose repeated at suitable intervals throughout the day

  ▸ Child 12–17 years: 1–2.5 mg, dose repeated at suitable intervals throughout the day

  Reversal of non-depolarising (competitive) neuromuscular blockade
  ▸ BY INTRAVENOUS INJECTION

  ▸ Neonate: 50 micrograms/kg, to be given over 1 minute after or with glycopyrronium or atropine, followed by 25 micrograms/kg if required.

  ▸ Child 1 month–11 years: 50 micrograms/kg (max. per dose 2.5 mg), to be given over 1 minute after or with glycopyrronium or atropine, then 25 micrograms/kg if required

  ▸ Child 12–17 years: 50 micrograms/kg (max. per dose 2.5 mg), to be given over 1 minute after or with glycopyrronium or atropine, then 25 micrograms/kg (max. per dose 2.5 mg) if required

- **UNLICENSED USE**
  ▸ In neonates Dose for treatment of myasthenia gravis by subcutaneous or intramuscular injection is unlicensed.
- **CAUTIONS**
  ▸ With intravenous use Glycopyrronium or atropine should also be given when reversing neuromuscular blockade
- **INTERACTIONS** → Appendix 1: neostigmine
- **RENAL IMPAIRMENT** May need dose reduction.
- **DIRECTIONS FOR ADMINISTRATION** For *intravenous injection*, give undiluted or dilute with Glucose 5% or Sodium Chloride 0.9%.
- **MEDICINAL FORMS**
There can be variation in the licensing of different medicines containing the same drug. Forms available from special-order manufacturers include: oral solution

  Solution for injection
  ▸ **Neostigmine** (Non-proprietary)
  Neostigmine metilsulfate 2.5 mg per 1 ml Neostigmine 2.5mg/1ml solution for injection ampoules | 10 ampoule PoM £5.06–£5.45

  Tablet
  ▸ **Neostigmine** (Non-proprietary)
  Neostigmine bromide 15 mg Neostigmine 15mg tablets | 140 tablet PoM £99.60 DT price = £99.60

☞ 619

Pyridostigmine bromide

- **DRUG ACTION** Pyridostigmine bromide has weaker muscarinic action than neostigmine.

- **INDICATIONS AND DOSE**

Myasthenia gravis
▸ INITIALLY BY MOUTH

▸ **Neonate:** Initially 1–1.5 mg/kg, dose repeated throughout the day, then (by mouth using immediate-release medicines) increased if necessary to 10 mg, to be increased gradually and given 30-60 minutes before feeds.

▸ **Child 1 month-11 years:** Initially 1–1.5 mg/kg daily, then (by mouth using immediate-release medicines) increased to 7 mg/kg daily in 6 divided doses, to be increased gradually; (by mouth using immediate-release medicines) usual dose 30–360 mg daily in divided doses

▸ **Child 12-17 years:** 30–120 mg, dose repeated throughout the day; (by mouth using immediate-release medicines) usual dose 300–600 mg daily in divided doses, consider immunosuppressant therapy if total daily dose exceeds 360 mg, down-regulation of acetylcholine receptors possible if total daily dose exceeds 450 mg

- **INTERACTIONS** → Appendix 1: pyridostigmine

- **RENAL IMPAIRMENT** Reduce dose; excreted by kidney.

- **MEDICINAL FORMS**
There can be variation in the licensing of different medicines containing the same drug. Forms available from special-order manufacturers include: oral suspension, oral solution

Tablet
▸ **Pyridostigmine bromide (Non-proprietary)**
Pyridostigmine bromide 60 mg Pyridostigmine bromide 60mg tablets | 200 tablet [PoM] £45.54 DT price = £45.54
▸ **Mestinon** (Meda Pharmaceuticals Ltd)
Pyridostigmine bromide 60 mg Mestinon 60mg tablets | 200 tablet [PoM] £45.57 DT price = £45.54

2.3 Spasticity

MUSCLE RELAXANTS ⟩ CENTRALLY ACTING

Baclofen

- **INDICATIONS AND DOSE**

Chronic severe spasticity of voluntary muscle
▸ BY MOUTH

▸ **Child 1 month-7 years:** Initially 300 micrograms/kg daily in 4 divided doses, increased gradually at weekly intervals until satisfactory response; maintenance 0.75–2 mg/kg daily in divided doses, review treatment if no benefit within 6 weeks of achieving maximum dose; maximum 40 mg per day

▸ **Child 8-17 years:** Initially 300 micrograms/kg daily in 4 divided doses, increased gradually at weekly intervals until satisfactory response; maintenance 0.75–2 mg/kg daily in divided doses, review treatment if no benefit within 6 weeks of achieving maximum dose; maximum 60 mg per day

Severe chronic spasticity of cerebral or spinal origin unresponsive to oral antispastic drugs (or oral therapy not tolerated) (specialist use only)
▸ BY INTRATHECAL INJECTION

▸ **Child 4-17 years:** Test dose 25–50 micrograms, to be given over at least 1 minute via catheter or lumbar puncture, then increased in steps of 25 micrograms (maximum per dose 100 micrograms), not more often than every 24 hours to determine initial maintenance dose; maintenance 25–200 micrograms daily, adjusted according to response, dose-titration phase, most often using infusion pump (implanted into chest wall or abdominal wall tissues) to establish maintenance dose retaining some spasticity to avoid sensation of paralysis

> **IMPORTANT SAFETY INFORMATION**
> Consult product literature for details on test dose and titration—important to monitor patients closely in appropriately equipped and staffed environment during screening and immediately after pump implantation. Resuscitation equipment must be available for immediate use. Treatment with continuous pump-administered intrathecal baclofen should be initiated within 3 months of a satisfactory response to intrathecal baclofen testing.

- **CONTRA-INDICATIONS**
▸ With intrathecal use Local infection · systemic infection
▸ With oral use Avoid oral route in active peptic ulceration

- **CAUTIONS**
GENERAL CAUTIONS
Diabetes · epilepsy · history of peptic ulcer · hypertonic bladder sphincter · psychiatric illness · respiratory impairment

SPECIFIC CAUTIONS
▸ With intrathecal use Coagulation disorders · malnutrition (increased risk of post-surgical complications) · previous spinal fusion procedure

- **INTERACTIONS** → Appendix 1: baclofen

- **SIDE-EFFECTS**
▸ **Common or very common** Agitation · anxiety · ataxia · cardiovascular depression · confusion · depression · dizziness · drowsiness · dry mouth · euphoria · gastro-intestinal disturbances · hallucinations · headache · hyperhidrosis · hypotension · insomnia · myalgia · nightmares · rash · respiratory depression · sedation · seizure · tremor · urinary disturbances · visual disorders
▸ **Rare** Abdominal pain · changes in hepatic function · dysarthria · erectile dysfunction · paraesthesia · taste disturbances
▸ **Very rare** Hypothermia

- **PREGNANCY** Manufacturer advises use only if potential benefit outweighs risk (toxicity in *animal* studies).

- **BREAST FEEDING** Present in milk—amount probably too small to be harmful.

- **HEPATIC IMPAIRMENT**
▸ With oral use Manufacturer advises use with caution.

- **RENAL IMPAIRMENT**
▸ With oral use Risk of toxicity—use smaller oral doses and if necessary increase dosage interval; if estimated glomerular filtration rate less than 15 mL/minute/1.73 m^2 use by mouth only if potential benefit outweighs risk. Excreted by the kidney.

- **TREATMENT CESSATION** Avoid abrupt withdrawal (risk of hyperactive state, may exacerbate spasticity, and precipitate autonomic dysfunction including hyperthermia, psychiatric reactions and convulsions; to minimise risk, discontinue by gradual dose reduction over at least 1–2 weeks (longer if symptoms occur).

- **PRESCRIBING AND DISPENSING INFORMATION** Flavours of oral liquid formulations may include raspberry.

- **PATIENT AND CARER ADVICE**

Driving and skilled tasks
Drowsiness may affect performance of skilled tasks (e.g. driving); effects of alcohol enhanced.

Medicines for Children leaflet: Baclofen for muscle spasm www.medicinesforchildren.org.uk/baclofen-muscle-spasm

- **MEDICINAL FORMS**
There can be variation in the licensing of different medicines containing the same drug. Forms available from special-order manufacturers include: oral suspension, oral solution

Tablet
CAUTIONARY AND ADVISORY LABELS 2, 8, 21
EXCIPIENTS: May contain Gluten
▸ **Baclofen** (Non-proprietary)
Baclofen 10 mg Baclofen 10mg tablets | 84 tablet PoM £9.99 DT price = £2.69
▸ **Lioresal** (Novartis Pharmaceuticals UK Ltd)
Baclofen 10 mg Lioresal 10mg tablets | 100 tablet PoM £14.86

Oral solution
CAUTIONARY AND ADVISORY LABELS 2, 8, 21
▸ **Baclofen** (Non-proprietary)
Baclofen 1 mg per 1 ml Baclofen 5mg/5ml oral solution sugar free sugar-free | 300 ml PoM £22.45 DT price = £3.43
▸ **Lioresal** (Novartis Pharmaceuticals UK Ltd)
Baclofen 1 mg per 1 ml Lioresal 5mg/5ml liquid sugar-free | 300 ml PoM £10.31 DT price = £3.43
▸ **Lyflex** (Chemidex Pharma Ltd)
Baclofen 1 mg per 1 ml Lyflex 5mg/5ml oral solution sugar-free | 300 ml PoM £7.95 DT price = £3.43

Solution for injection
▸ **Baclofen** (Non-proprietary)
Baclofen 50 microgram per 1 ml Baclofen 50micrograms/1ml solution for injection ampoules | 5 ampoule PoM £10.95 | 10 ampoule PoM £25.00-£27.60
▸ **Lioresal** (Novartis Pharmaceuticals UK Ltd)
Baclofen 50 microgram per 1 ml Lioresal Intrathecal 50micrograms/1ml solution for injection ampoules | 1 ampoule PoM £3.16

Solution for infusion
▸ **Baclofen** (Non-proprietary)
Baclofen 500 microgram per 1 ml Baclofen 10mg/20ml solution for infusion ampoules | 1 ampoule PoM £48.62-£57.00
Baclofen 2 mg per 1 ml Baclofen 40mg/20ml solution for infusion ampoules | 1 ampoule PoM £228.00-£250.00
Baclofen 10mg/5ml solution for infusion ampoules | 5 ampoule £243.10 | 10 ampoule PoM £500.00-£570.00
▸ **Lioresal** (Novartis Pharmaceuticals UK Ltd)
Baclofen 500 microgram per 1 ml Lioresal Intrathecal 10mg/20ml solution for infusion ampoules | 1 ampoule PoM £70.01
Baclofen 2 mg per 1 ml Lioresal Intrathecal 10mg/5ml solution for infusion ampoules | 1 ampoule PoM £70.01

3 Pain and inflammation in musculoskeletal disorders

Non-steroidal anti-inflammatory drugs

Therapeutic effects
In *single doses* non-steroidal anti-inflammatory drugs (NSAIDs) have analgesic activity comparable to that of paracetamol p. 260 but paracetamol is preferred.

In regular *full dosage* NSAIDs have both a lasting analgesic and an anti-inflammatory effect which makes them particularly useful for the treatment of continuous or regular pain associated with inflammation.

Choice
Differences in anti-inflammatory activity between NSAIDs are small, but there is considerable variation in individual response and tolerance of these drugs. A large proportion of

children will respond to any NSAID; of the others, those who do not respond to one may well respond to another. Pain relief starts soon after taking the first dose and a full analgesic effect should normally be obtained within a week, whereas an anti-inflammatory effect may not be achieved (or may not be clinically assessable) for up to 3 weeks. However, in juvenile idiopathic arthritis NSAIDs may take 4–12 weeks to be effective. If appropriate responses are not obtained within these times, another NSAID should be tried. The availability of appropriate formulations needs to be considered when prescribing NSAIDs for children.

NSAIDs reduce the production of prostaglandins by inhibiting the enzyme cyclo-oxygenase. They vary in their selectivity for inhibiting different types of cyclo-oxygenase; selective inhibition of cyclo-oxygenase-2 is associated with less gastro-intestinal intolerance. However, in children gastro-intestinal symptoms are rare in those taking NSAIDs for short periods. The role of selective inhibitors of cyclo-oxygenase-2 is undetermined in children.

Ibuprofen p. 625 and naproxen p. 631 are propionic acid derivatives used in children.

Ibuprofen combines anti-inflammatory, analgesic, and antipyretic properties. It has fewer side-effects than other NSAIDs but its anti-inflammatory properties are weaker.

Naproxen combines good efficacy with a low incidence of side-effects.

Diclofenac sodium p. 623, diclofenac potassium p. 622, indometacin p. 628, mefenamic acid p. 629, and piroxicam p. 632 have properties similar to those of propionic acid derivatives:

Diclofenac sodium and diclofenac potassium are similar in efficacy to naproxen.

Indometacin has an action equal to or superior to that of naproxen, but with a high incidence of side-effects including headache, dizziness, and gastro-intestinal disturbances. It is rarely used in children and should be reserved for when other NSAIDs have been unsuccessful.

Mefenamic acid has minor anti-inflammatory properties. It has occasionally been associated with diarrhoea and haemolytic anaemia which require discontinuation of treatment.

Piroxicam is as effective as naproxen and has a long duration of action which permits once-daily administration. However, it has more gastro-intestinal side-effects than most other NSAIDs, and is associated with more frequent serious skin reactions.

Meloxicam p. 630 is a selective inhibitor of cyclo-oxygenase-2. Its use may be considered in adolescents intolerant to other NSAIDs.

Ketorolac trometamol p. 787 can be used for the short-term management of postoperative pain.

Etoricoxib p. 624, a selective inhibitor of cyclo-oxygenase-2, is licensed for the relief of pain in osteoarthritis, rheumatoid arthritis, ankylosing spondylitis, and acute gout in children aged 16 years and over.

Dental and orofacial pain
Most mild to moderate dental pain and inflammation is effectively relieved by ibuprofen, diclofenac potassium or diclofenac sodium.

NSAIDs and cardiovascular events
The risk of cardiovascular events secondary to NSAID use is undetermined in children. In adults, all NSAID use (including cyclo-oxygenase-2 selective inhibitors) can, to varying degrees, be associated with a small increased risk of thrombotic events (e.g. myocardial infarction and stroke) independent of baseline cardiovascular risk factors or duration of NSAID use; however, the greatest risk may be in those patients receiving high doses long term. A small increased thrombotic risk cannot be excluded in children.

In adults, cyclo-oxygenase-2 selective inhibitors, diclofenac (150 mg daily) and ibuprofen (2.4 g daily) are

10

Musculoskeletal system

associated with an increased risk of thrombotic events. The increased risk for diclofenac is similar to that of etoricoxib. Naproxen (in adults, 1 g daily) is associated with a lower thrombotic risk, and lower doses of ibuprofen (in adults, 1.2 g daily or less) have not been associated with an increased risk of myocardial infarction.

The lowest effective dose of NSAID should be prescribed for the shortest period of time to control symptoms, and the need for long-term treatment should be reviewed periodically.

NSAIDs and gastro-intestinal events

All NSAIDs are associated with gastro-intestinal toxicity. In adults, evidence on the relative safety of NSAIDs indicates differences in the risks of serious upper gastro-intestinal side-effects—piroxicam and ketorolac trometamol are associated with the highest risk; indometacin, diclofenac, and naproxen are associated with intermediate risk, and ibuprofen with the lowest risk (although high doses of ibuprofen have been associated with intermediate risk). Selective inhibitors of cyclo-oxygenase-2 are associated with a *lower risk* of serious upper gastro-intestinal side-effects than non-selective NSAIDs.

Children appear to tolerate NSAIDs better than adults and gastro-intestinal side-effects are less common although they do still occur and can be significant; use of gastro-protective drugs may be necessary.

Asthma

All NSAIDs have the potential to worsen asthma, either acutely or as a gradual worsening of symptoms; consider both prescribed NSAIDs and those that are purchased over the counter.

ANALGESICS › NON-STEROIDAL ANTI-INFLAMMATORY DRUGS

Diclofenac potassium

- ● **INDICATIONS AND DOSE**

Pain and inflammation in rheumatic disease and other musculoskeletal disorders
- ▶ BY MOUTH
- ▶ Child 14–17 years: 75–100 mg daily in 2–3 divided doses

Postoperative pain
- ▶ BY MOUTH
- ▶ Child 9–13 years (body-weight 35 kg and above): Up to 2 mg/kg daily in 3 divided doses; maximum 100 mg per day
- ▶ Child 14–17 years: 75–100 mg daily in 2–3 divided doses

Fever in ear, nose, or throat infection
- ▶ BY MOUTH
- ▶ Child 9–17 years (body-weight 35 kg and above): Up to 2 mg/kg daily in 3 divided doses; maximum 100 mg per day

- ● **UNLICENSED USE** *Voltarol® Rapid* not licensed for use in children under 14 years or in fever.

- ● **CONTRA-INDICATIONS** Active gastro-intestinal bleeding · active gastro-intestinal ulceration · cerebrovascular disease · history of gastro-intestinal bleeding related to previous NSAID therapy · history of gastro-intestinal perforation related to previous NSAID therapy · history of recurrent gastro-intestinal haemorrhage (two or more distinct episodes) · history of recurrent gastro-intestinal ulceration (two or more distinct episodes) · ischaemic heart disease · mild to severe heart failure · peripheral arterial disease

- ● **CAUTIONS** Allergic disorders · cardiac impairment (NSAIDs may impair renal function) · coagulation defects · connective-tissue disorders · Crohn's disease (may be

exacerbated) · history of cardiac failure · hypertension · left ventricular dysfunction · oedema · risk factors for cardiovascular events · ulcerative colitis (may be exacerbated)

- ● **INTERACTIONS** → Appendix 1: NSAIDs

- ● **SIDE-EFFECTS**
- ▶ **Rare** Alveolitis · aseptic meningitis (patients with connective-tissue disorders such as systemic lupus erythematosus may be especially susceptible) · hepatic damage · interstitial fibrosis associated with NSAIDs can lead to renal failure · pancreatitis · papillary necrosis associated with NSAIDs can lead to renal failure · pulmonary eosinophilia · Stevens-Johnson syndrome · toxic epidermal necrolysis · visual disturbances
- ▶ **Frequency not known** Angioedema · blood disorders · bronchospasm · colitis (induction of or exacerbation of) · Crohn's disease (induction of or exacerbation of) · depression · diarrhoea · dizziness · drowsiness · fluid retention (rarely precipitating congestive heart failure) · gastro-intestinal bleeding · gastro-intestinal discomfort · gastro-intestinal disturbances · gastro-intestinal ulceration · haematuria · headache · hearing disturbances · hypersensitivity reactions · insomnia · nausea · nervousness · photosensitivity · raised blood pressure · rashes · renal failure (especially in patients with pre-existing renal impairment) · tinnitus · vertigo

- ● **ALLERGY AND CROSS-SENSITIVITY** Contra-indicated in patients with a history of hypersensitivity to aspirin or any other NSAID—which includes those in whom attacks of asthma, angioedema, urticaria or rhinitis have been precipitated by aspirin or any other NSAID.

- ● **PREGNANCY** Avoid unless the potential benefit outweighs the risk. Avoid during the third trimester (risk of closure of fetal ductus arteriosus *in utero* and possibly persistent pulmonary hypertension of the newborn); onset of labour may be delayed and duration may be increased.

- ● **BREAST FEEDING** Use with caution during breast-feeding. Amount in milk too small to be harmful.

- ● **HEPATIC IMPAIRMENT** Use with caution; there is an increased risk of gastro-intestinal bleeding and fluid retention. Avoid in severe liver disease.

- ● **RENAL IMPAIRMENT** The lowest effective dose should be used for the shortest possible duration. Avoid if possible or use with caution. Avoid in severe impairment. In renal impairment monitor renal function; sodium and water retention may occur and renal function may deteriorate, possibly leading to renal failure.

- ● **PATIENT AND CARER ADVICE**
Medicines for Children leaflet: Diclofenac for pain and inflammation www.medicinesforchildren.org.uk/diclofenac-for-pain-and-inflammation

- ● **MEDICINAL FORMS**
There can be variation in the licensing of different medicines containing the same drug.

Tablet
CAUTIONARY AND ADVISORY LABELS 21
- ▶ **Diclofenac potassium** (Non-proprietary)
  Diclofenac potassium 25 mg Diclofenac potassium 25mg tablets | 28 tablet PoM £3.87 DT price = £3.87
  Diclofenac potassium 50 mg Diclofenac potassium 50mg tablets | 28 tablet PoM £7.41
- ▶ **Voltarol Rapid** (Novartis Pharmaceuticals UK Ltd)
  Diclofenac potassium 50 mg Voltarol Rapid 50mg tablets | 30 tablet PoM £7.94 DT price = £7.94

Diclofenac sodium

- **INDICATIONS AND DOSE**

Pain and inflammation in rheumatic disease including juvenile idiopathic arthritis
▸ BY MOUTH USING IMMEDIATE-RELEASE MEDICINES
▸ Child 6 months-17 years: 1.5–2.5 mg/kg twice daily, total daily dose may alternatively be given in 3 divided doses; maximum 150 mg per day

Postoperative pain
▸ BY RECTUM
▸ Child 6 months-17 years (body-weight 8–11 kg): 12.5 mg twice daily for maximum 4 days
▸ Child 6 months-17 years (body-weight 12 kg and above): 1 mg/kg 3 times a day (max. per dose 50 mg) for maximum 4 days

Inflammation | Mild to moderate pain
▸ BY MOUTH USING IMMEDIATE-RELEASE MEDICINES, OR BY RECTUM
▸ Child 6 months-17 years: 0.3–1 mg/kg 3 times a day (max. per dose 50 mg)

DICLOMAX RETARD®

Pain and inflammation
▸ BY MOUTH
▸ Child 12-17 years: 1 capsule once daily

DICLOMAX SR®

Pain and inflammation
▸ BY MOUTH
▸ Child 12-17 years: 1 capsule 1–2 times a day

MOTIFENE®

Pain and inflammation
▸ BY MOUTH
▸ Child 12-17 years: 1 capsule 1–2 times a day

VOLTAROL® 75MG SR TABLETS

Pain and inflammation
▸ BY MOUTH
▸ Child 12-17 years: 1 tablet 1–2 times a day

VOLTAROL® RETARD

Pain and inflammation
▸ BY MOUTH
▸ Child 12-17 years: 1 tablet once daily

VOLTAROL® SOLUTION FOR INJECTION

Postoperative pain
▸ BY INTRAVENOUS INFUSION, OR BY DEEP INTRAMUSCULAR INJECTION
▸ Child 2-17 years: 0.3–1 mg/kg 1–2 times a day for maximum 2 days, for intramuscular injection, to be injected into the gluteal muscle; maximum 150 mg per day

- **UNLICENSED USE** Not licensed for use in children under 1 year. *Suppositories* not licensed for use in children under 6 years except for use in children over 1 year for juvenile idiopathic arthritis. Solid dose forms containing more than 25 mg not licensed for use in children. *Injection* not licensed for use in children.
- **CONTRA-INDICATIONS** Active gastro-intestinal bleeding · active gastro-intestinal ulceration · avoid injections containing benzyl alcohol in neonates · avoid suppositories in proctitis · cerebrovascular disease · history of gastro-intestinal bleeding related to previous NSAID therapy · history of gastro-intestinal perforation related to previous NSAID therapy · history of recurrent gastro-intestinal haemorrhage (two or more distinct episodes) · history of recurrent gastro-intestinal ulceration (two or more distinct episodes) · ischaemic heart disease · mild to severe heart failure · peripheral arterial disease

▸ With intravenous use Dehydration · history of asthma · history of confirmed or suspected cerebrovascular bleeding · history of haemorrhagic diathesis · hypovolaemia · operations with high risk of haemorrhage

- **CAUTIONS** Allergic disorders · cardiac impairment (NSAIDs may impair renal function) · coagulation defects · connective-tissue disorders · Crohn's disease (may be exacerbated) · history of cardiac failure · hypertension · left ventricular dysfunction · oedema · risk factors for cardiovascular events · ulcerative colitis (may be exacerbated)
- **INTERACTIONS** → Appendix 1: NSAIDs
- **SIDE-EFFECTS**
▸ **Rare** Alveolitis · aseptic meningitis (patients with connective-tissue disorders such as systemic lupus erythematosus may be especially susceptible) · hepatic damage · interstitial fibrosis associated with NSAIDs can lead to renal failure · pancreatitis · papillary necrosis associated with NSAIDs can lead to renal failure · pulmonary eosinophilia · Stevens-Johnson syndrome · toxic epidermal necrolysis · visual disturbances
▸ **Frequency not known** Angioedema · blood disorders · bronchospasm · colitis (induction of or exacerbation of) · Crohn's disease (induction of or exacerbation of) · depression · diarrhoea · dizziness · drowsiness · fluid retention (rarely precipitating congestive heart failure) · gastro-intestinal bleeding · gastro-intestinal discomfort · gastro-intestinal disturbances · gastro-intestinal ulceration · haematuria · headache · hearing disturbances · hypersensitivity reactions · insomnia · nausea · nervousness · photosensitivity · raised blood pressure · rashes · renal failure (especially in patients with pre-existing renal impairment) · tinnitus · vertigo
▸ With intramuscular use or intravenous use Injection site reactions
▸ With rectal use Suppositories may cause rectal irritation
  SIDE-EFFECTS, FURTHER INFORMATION
▸ Serious side-effects For information about cardiovascular and gastro-intestinal side-effects, and a possible exacerbation of symptoms in asthma, see Non-steroidal anti-inflammatory drugs p. 621.
- **ALLERGY AND CROSS-SENSITIVITY** Contra-indicated in patients with a history of hypersensitivity to aspirin or any other NSAID—which includes those in whom attacks of asthma, angioedema, urticaria or rhinitis have been precipitated by aspirin or any other NSAID.
- **PREGNANCY** Avoid unless the potential benefit outweighs the risk. Avoid during the third trimester (risk of closure of fetal ductus arteriosus *in utero* and possibly persistent pulmonary hypertension of the newborn); onset of labour may be delayed and duration may be increased.
- **BREAST FEEDING** Use with caution during breast-feeding. Amount in milk too small to be harmful.
- **HEPATIC IMPAIRMENT** Use with caution; there is an increased risk of gastro-intestinal bleeding and fluid retention. Avoid in severe liver disease.
- **RENAL IMPAIRMENT** The lowest effective dose should be used for the shortest possible duration. Avoid in severe impairment. Monitor renal function; sodium and water retention may occur and renal function may deteriorate, possibly leading to renal failure.
▸ With intravenous use Contra-indicated in moderate or severe renal impairment.
- **DIRECTIONS FOR ADMINISTRATION**
For *intravenous infusion*, dilute 75 mg with 100–500 mL Glucose 5% *or* Sodium Chloride 0.9% (previously buffered with 0.5 mL Sodium Bicarbonate 8.4% solution *or* with 1 mL Sodium Bicarbonate 4.2% solution); give over 30–120 minutes.

10

Musculoskeletal system

Musculoskeletal system

10

● PATIENT AND CARER ADVICE

Medicines for Children leaflet: Diclofenac for pain and inflammation www.medicinesforchildren.org.uk/diclofenac-for-pain-and-inflammation

● MEDICINAL FORMS

There can be variation in the licensing of different medicines containing the same drug. Forms available from special-order manufacturers include: dispersible tablet, oral suspension, oral solution

Gastro-resistant tablet

CAUTIONARY AND ADVISORY LABELS 5, 25
▸ Diclofenac sodium (Non-proprietary)
   Diclofenac sodium 25 mg Diclofenac sodium 25mg gastro-resistant tablets | 28 tablet PoM £2.49-£8.99 DT price = £2.52 | 84 tablet PoM £26.97
   Diclofenac sodium 50 mg Diclofenac sodium 50mg gastro-resistant tablets | 28 tablet PoM £4.97 DT price = £2.86 | 84 tablet PoM £15.00 | 100 tablet PoM no price available
▸ Dicloflex (Dexcel-Pharma Ltd)
   Diclofenac sodium 25 mg Dicloflex 25mg gastro-resistant tablets | 84 tablet PoM £4.42
   Diclofenac sodium 50 mg Dicloflex 50mg gastro-resistant tablets | 28 tablet PoM £2.75 DT price = £2.86 (Hospital only) | 84 tablet PoM £8.05
▸ Fenactol (Discovery Pharmaceuticals)
   Diclofenac sodium 50 mg Fenactol 50mg gastro-resistant tablets | 100 tablet PoM £3.50
▸ Voltarol (Novartis Pharmaceuticals UK Ltd)
   Diclofenac sodium 25 mg Voltarol 25mg gastro-resistant tablets | 84 tablet PoM £2.94

Suppository

▸ Diclofenac sodium (Non-proprietary)
   Diclofenac sodium 100 mg Diclofenac 100mg suppositories | 10 suppository PoM £4.05 DT price = £3.64
▸ Econac (AMCo)
   Diclofenac sodium 100 mg Econac 100mg suppositories | 10 suppository PoM £3.04 DT price = £3.64
▸ Voltarol (Novartis Pharmaceuticals UK Ltd)
   Diclofenac sodium 12.5 mg Voltarol 12.5mg suppositories | 10 suppository PoM £0.70 DT price = £0.70
   Diclofenac sodium 25 mg Voltarol 25mg suppositories | 10 suppository PoM £1.24 DT price = £1.24
   Diclofenac sodium 50 mg Voltarol 50mg suppositories | 10 suppository PoM £2.04 DT price = £2.04
   Diclofenac sodium 100 mg Voltarol 100mg suppositories | 10 suppository PoM £3.64 DT price = £3.64

Solution for injection

EXCIPIENTS: May contain Benzyl alcohol, propylene glycol
▸ Voltarol (Novartis Pharmaceuticals UK Ltd)
   Diclofenac sodium 25 mg per 1 ml Voltarol 75mg/3ml solution for injection ampoules | 10 ampoule PoM £9.91 DT price = £9.91

Modified-release capsule

CAUTIONARY AND ADVISORY LABELS 21(does not apply to Motifene® 75 mg), 25
EXCIPIENTS: May contain Propylene glycol
▸ Diclomax Retard (Galen Ltd)
   Diclofenac sodium 100 mg Diclomax Retard 100mg capsules | 28 capsule PoM £6.97 DT price = £6.97
▸ Diclomax SR (Galen Ltd)
   Diclofenac sodium 75 mg Diclomax SR 75mg capsules | 56 capsule PoM £9.69 DT price = £9.69
▸ Motifene (Daiichi Sankyo UK Ltd)
   Diclofenac sodium 75 mg Motifene 75mg modified-release capsules | 56 capsule PoM £8.00 DT price = £8.00

Etoricoxib

23-Nov-2016

● INDICATIONS AND DOSE

Pain and inflammation in osteoarthritis

▸ BY MOUTH
▸ Child 16-17 years: 30 mg once daily, increased if necessary to 60 mg once daily

Pain and inflammation in rheumatoid arthritis | Ankylosing spondylitis

▸ BY MOUTH
▸ Child 16-17 years: 60 mg once daily, increased if necessary to 90 mg once daily

Acute gout

▸ BY MOUTH
▸ Child 16-17 years: 120 mg once daily for maximum 8 days

● CONTRA-INDICATIONS Active gastro-intestinal bleeding · active gastro-intestinal ulceration · cerebrovascular disease · inflammatory bowel disease · ischaemic heart disease · mild to severe heart failure · peripheral arterial disease · uncontrolled hypertension (persistently above 140/90 mmHg)

● CAUTIONS Allergic disorders · cardiac impairment (NSAIDs may impair renal function) · coagulation defects · connective-tissue disorders · Crohn's disease (may be exacerbated) · dehydration · history of cardiac failure · hypertension · left ventricular dysfunction · oedema · risk factors for cardiovascular events · ulcerative colitis (may be exacerbated)

● INTERACTIONS → Appendix 1: NSAIDs

● SIDE-EFFECTS

▸ **Common or very common** Ecchymosis · fatigue · influenza-like symptoms · palpitation
▸ **Uncommon** Anxiety · appetite change · arthralgia · atrial fibrillation · chest pain · cough · dry mouth · dyspnoea · electrolyte disturbance · epistaxis · flushing · mental acuity impaired · mouth ulcer · myalgia · paraesthesia · taste disturbance · transient ischaemic attack · weight change
▸ **Rare** Alveolitis · aseptic meningitis (patients with connective-tissue disorders such as systemic lupus erythematosus may be especially susceptible) · hepatic damage · interstitial fibrosis associated with NSAIDs can lead to renal failure · pancreatitis · papillary necrosis associated with NSAIDs can lead to renal failure · pulmonary eosinophilia · Stevens-Johnson syndrome · toxic epidermal necrolysis · visual disturbances
▸ **Very rare** Confusion · hallucinations
▸ **Frequency not known** Angioedema · blood disorders · bronchospasm · colitis (induction of or exacerbation of) · Crohn's disease (induction of or exacerbation of) · depression · diarrhoea · dizziness · drowsiness · fluid retention (rarely precipitating congestive heart failure) · gastro-intestinal bleeding · gastro-intestinal discomfort · gastro-intestinal disturbances · gastro-intestinal ulceration · haematuria · headache · hearing disturbances · hypersensitivity reactions · insomnia · nausea · nervousness · photosensitivity · raised blood pressure · rashes · renal failure (especially in patients with pre-existing renal impairment) · tinnitus · vertigo

SIDE-EFFECTS, FURTHER INFORMATION
▸ Serious side-effects For information about cardiovascular and gastro-intestinal side-effects, and a possible exacerbation of symptoms in asthma, see Non-steroidal anti-inflammatory drugs p. 621.

● ALLERGY AND CROSS-SENSITIVITY Contra-indicated in patients with a history of hypersensitivity to aspirin or any other NSAID—which includes those in whom attacks of asthma, angioedema, urticaria or rhinitis have been precipitated by aspirin or any other NSAID.

● CONCEPTION AND CONTRACEPTION Caution—long-term use of some NSAIDs is associated with reduced female fertility, which is reversible on stopping treatment.

● PREGNANCY Manufacturer advises avoid (teratogenic in *animal* studies). Avoid during the third trimester (risk of closure of fetal ductus arteriosus *in utero* and possibly persistent pulmonary hypertension of the newborn); onset of labour may be delayed and duration may be increased.

- **BREAST FEEDING** Use with caution during breast-feeding. Manufacturer advises avoid—present in milk in *animal* studies.
- **HEPATIC IMPAIRMENT** Max. 60 mg daily in mild impairment. Max. 60 mg on alternate days or 30 mg once daily in moderate impairment. Use with caution; there is an increased risk of gastro-intestinal bleeding and fluid retention. Avoid in severe liver disease.
- **RENAL IMPAIRMENT** The lowest effective dose should be used for the shortest possible duration. Avoid if possible or use with caution.

  Avoid if estimated glomerular filtration rate less than 30 mL/minute/1.73 m². In renal impairment monitor renal function; sodium and water retention may occur and renal function may deteriorate, possibly leading to renal failure.
- **MONITORING REQUIREMENTS** Monitor blood pressure before treatment, 2 weeks after initiation and periodically during treatment.

- **MEDICINAL FORMS**
There can be variation in the licensing of different medicines containing the same drug.

Tablet
▸ Arcoxia (Grunenthal Ltd)
  Etoricoxib 30 mg Arcoxia 30mg tablets | 28 tablet PoM £13.99 DT price = £13.99
  Etoricoxib 60 mg Arcoxia 60mg tablets | 28 tablet PoM £20.11 DT price = £20.11
  Etoricoxib 90 mg Arcoxia 90mg tablets | 5 tablet PoM £4.10 | 28 tablet PoM £22.96 DT price = £22.96
  Etoricoxib 120 mg Arcoxia 120mg tablets | 7 tablet PoM £6.03 | 28 tablet PoM £24.11 DT price = £24.11

Flurbiprofen

- **INDICATIONS AND DOSE**

Pain and inflammation in rheumatic disease and other musculoskeletal disorders | Migraine | Postoperative analgesia | Mild to moderate pain
▸ BY MOUTH
▸ **Child 12–17 years:** 150–200 mg daily in 2–4 divided doses, then increased to 300 mg daily, dose to be increased only in acute conditions

Dysmenorrhoea
▸ BY MOUTH
▸ **Child 12–17 years:** Initially 100 mg, then 50–100 mg every 4–6 hours; maximum 300 mg per day

- **CONTRA-INDICATIONS** Active gastro-intestinal bleeding · active gastro-intestinal ulceration · history of gastro-intestinal bleeding related to previous NSAID therapy · history of gastro-intestinal perforation related to previous NSAID therapy · history of recurrent gastro-intestinal haemorrhage (two or more distinct episodes) · history of recurrent gastro-intestinal ulceration (two or more distinct episodes) · severe heart failure
- **CAUTIONS** Allergic disorders · cardiac impairment (NSAIDs may impair renal function) · cerebrovascular disease · coagulation defects · connective-tissue disorders · Crohn's disease (may be exacerbated) · heart failure · ischaemic heart disease · peripheral arterial disease · risk factors for cardiovascular events · ulcerative colitis (may be exacerbated) · uncontrolled hypertension
- **INTERACTIONS** → Appendix 1: NSAIDs
- **SIDE-EFFECTS**
▸ **Common or very common** Stomatitis
▸ **Uncommon** Confusion · fatigue · hallucinations · paraesthesia
▸ **Rare** Alveolitis · aseptic meningitis (patients with connective-tissue disorders such as systemic lupus erythematosus may be especially susceptible) · hepatic

damage · interstitial fibrosis associated with NSAIDs can lead to renal failure · pancreatitis · papillary necrosis associated with NSAIDs can lead to renal failure · pulmonary eosinophilia · Stevens-Johnson syndrome · toxic epidermal necrolysis · visual disturbances
▸ **Frequency not known** Angioedema · blood disorders · bronchospasm · colitis (induction of or exacerbation of) · Crohn's disease (induction of or exacerbation of) · depression · diarrhoea · dizziness · drowsiness · fluid retention (rarely precipitating congestive heart failure) · gastro-intestinal bleeding · gastro-intestinal discomfort · gastro-intestinal disturbances · gastro-intestinal ulceration · haematuria · headache · hearing disturbances · hypersensitivity reactions · insomnia · nausea · nervousness · photosensitivity · raised blood pressure · rashes · renal failure (especially in patients with pre-existing renal impairment) · tinnitus · vertigo

SIDE-EFFECTS, FURTHER INFORMATION
▸ **Serious side-effects** For information about cardiovascular and gastro-intestinal side-effects, and a possible exacerbation of symptoms in asthma, see Non-steroidal anti-inflammatory drugs p. 621.

- **ALLERGY AND CROSS-SENSITIVITY** Contra-indicated in patients with a history of hypersensitivity to aspirin or any other NSAID—which includes those in whom attacks of asthma, angioedema, urticaria or rhinitis have been precipitated by aspirin or any other NSAID.
- **PREGNANCY** Avoid unless the potential benefit outweighs the risk. Avoid during the third trimester (risk of closure of fetal ductus arteriosus *in utero* and possibly persistent pulmonary hypertension of the newborn); onset of labour may be delayed and duration may be increased.
- **BREAST FEEDING** Use with caution during breast-feeding. Small amount present in milk—manufacturer advises avoid.
- **HEPATIC IMPAIRMENT** Use with caution; there is an increased risk of gastro-intestinal bleeding and fluid retention. Avoid in severe liver disease.
- **RENAL IMPAIRMENT** The lowest effective dose should be used for the shortest possible duration. Avoid if possible or use with caution.

  Deterioration in renal function has also been reported after topical use.

  Avoid in severe impairment. In renal impairment monitor renal function; sodium and water retention may occur and renal function may deteriorate, possibly leading to renal failure.

- **MEDICINAL FORMS**
There can be variation in the licensing of different medicines containing the same drug.

Tablet
CAUTIONARY AND ADVISORY LABELS 21
▸ Flurbiprofen (Non-proprietary)
  Flurbiprofen 50 mg Flurbiprofen 50mg tablets | 100 tablet PoM £21.30–£35.97 DT price = £35.96
  Flurbiprofen 100 mg Flurbiprofen 100mg tablets | 100 tablet PoM £64.34 DT price = £64.33

Ibuprofen

- **INDICATIONS AND DOSE**

Closure of ductus arteriosus
▸ BY SLOW INTRAVENOUS INJECTION
▸ **Neonate:** Initially 10 mg/kg for 1 dose, followed by 5 mg/kg every 24 hours for 2 doses, the course may be repeated after 48 hours if necessary.

continued →

10

Musculoskeletal system

Mild to moderate pain | Pain and inflammation of soft-tissue injuries | Pyrexia with discomfort

▸ BY MOUTH USING IMMEDIATE-RELEASE MEDICINES
▸ Child 1–2 months: 5 mg/kg 3–4 times a day
▸ Child 3–5 months: 50 mg 3 times a day, maximum daily dose to be given in 3–4 divided doses; maximum 30 mg/kg per day
▸ Child 6–11 months: 50 mg 3–4 times a day, maximum daily dose to be given in 3–4 divided doses; maximum 30 mg/kg per day
▸ Child 1–3 years: 100 mg 3 times a day, maximum daily dose to be given in 3–4 divided doses; maximum 30 mg/kg per day
▸ Child 4–6 years: 150 mg 3 times a day, maximum daily dose to be given in 3–4 divided doses; maximum 30 mg/kg per day
▸ Child 7–9 years: 200 mg 3 times a day, maximum daily dose to be given in 3–4 divided doses; maximum 30 mg/kg per day; maximum 2.4 g per day
▸ Child 10–11 years: 300 mg 3 times a day, maximum daily dose to be given in 3–4 divided doses; maximum 30 mg/kg per day; maximum 2.4 g per day
▸ Child 12–17 years: Initially 300–400 mg 3–4 times a day; increased if necessary up to 600 mg 4 times a day; maintenance 200–400 mg 3 times a day, may be adequate

Pain and inflammation

▸ BY MOUTH USING MODIFIED-RELEASE MEDICINES
▸ Child 12–17 years: 1.6 g once daily, dose preferably taken in the early evening, increased to 2.4 g daily in 2 divided doses, dose to be increased only in severe cases

Pain and inflammation in rheumatic disease including juvenile idiopathic arthritis

▸ BY MOUTH USING IMMEDIATE-RELEASE MEDICINES
▸ Child 3 months–17 years: 30–40 mg/kg daily in 3–4 divided doses; maximum 2.4 g per day

Pain and inflammation in systemic juvenile idiopathic arthritis

▸ BY MOUTH USING IMMEDIATE-RELEASE MEDICINES
▸ Child 3 months–17 years: Up to 60 mg/kg daily in 4–6 divided doses; maximum 2.4 g per day

Post-immunisation pyrexia in infants (on doctor's advice only)

▸ BY MOUTH USING IMMEDIATE-RELEASE MEDICINES
▸ Child 2–3 months: 50 mg for 1 dose, followed by 50 mg after 6 hours if required

● UNLICENSED USE
▸ With intravenous use Orphan licence for the injection for closure of ductus arteriosus in premature neonates less than 34 weeks corrected gestational age.
▸ With oral use Not licensed for use in children under 3 months or body-weight under 5 kg. Maximum dose for systemic juvenile idiopathic arthritis is unlicensed.

● CONTRA-INDICATIONS Active gastro-intestinal bleeding · active gastro-intestinal ulceration · history of gastro-intestinal bleeding related to previous NSAID therapy · history of gastro-intestinal perforation related to previous NSAID therapy · history of recurrent gastro-intestinal haemorrhage (two or more distinct episodes) · history of recurrent gastro-intestinal ulceration (two or more distinct episodes) · severe heart failure
▸ With intravenous use Active bleeding (especially intracranial or gastro-intestinal) · coagulation defects · known or suspected necrotising enterocolitis · life-threatening infection · marked unconjugated hyperbilirubinaemia · pulmonary hypertension · thrombocytopenia

● CAUTIONS Cardiac impairment (NSAIDs may impair renal function) · cerebrovascular disease · coagulation defects · connective-tissue disorders · Crohn's disease (may be

exacerbated) · heart failure · ischaemic heart disease · peripheral arterial disease · risk factors for cardiovascular events · risk factors for cardiovascular events · ulcerative colitis (may be exacerbated) · uncontrolled hypertension
▸ With intravenous use May mask symptoms of infection

CAUTIONS, FURTHER INFORMATION
▸ High-dose ibuprofen A small increase in cardiovascular risk, similar to the risk associated with cyclo-oxygenase-2 inhibitors and diclofenac, has been reported with high-dose ibuprofen (≥ 2.4 g daily); use should be avoided in patients with established ischaemic heart disease, peripheral arterial disease, cerebrovascular disease, congestive heart failure (New York Heart Association classification II-III), and uncontrolled hypertension.

● INTERACTIONS → Appendix 1: NSAIDs

● SIDE-EFFECTS
▸ Common or very common
▸ With intravenous use Bronchopulmonary dysplasia · fluid retention · haematuria · hyponatraemia · intestinal perforation · intraventricular haemorrhage · ischaemic brain injury · neutropenia · oliguria · pulmonary haemorrhage · thrombocytopenia
▸ Uncommon
▸ With intravenous use Gastrointestinal haemorrhage
▸ Rare Alveolitis · aseptic meningitis (patients with connective-tissue disorders such as systemic lupus erythematosus may be especially susceptible) · hepatic damage · interstitial fibrosis associated with NSAIDs can lead to renal failure · pancreatitis · papillary necrosis associated with NSAIDs can lead to renal failure · pulmonary eosinophilia · Stevens-Johnson syndrome · toxic epidermal necrolysis · visual disturbances
▸ Frequency not known Angioedema · blood disorders · bronchospasm · colitis (induction of or exacerbation of) · Crohn's disease (induction of or exacerbation of) · depression · diarrhoea · dizziness · drowsiness · fluid retention (rarely precipitating congestive heart failure) · gastro-intestinal bleeding · gastro-intestinal discomfort · gastro-intestinal disturbances · gastro-intestinal ulceration · haematuria · headache · hearing disturbances · hypersensitivity reactions · insomnia · nausea · nervousness · photosensitivity · raised blood pressure · rashes · renal failure (especially in patients with pre-existing renal impairment) · tinnitus · vertigo
▸ With intravenous use Hypoxaemia

SIDE-EFFECTS, FURTHER INFORMATION
▸ Serious side-effects For information about cardiovascular and gastro-intestinal side-effects, and a possible exacerbation of symptoms in asthma, see Non-steroidal anti-inflammatory drugs p. 621.

Overdose
Overdosage with ibuprofen may cause nausea, vomiting, epigastric pain, and tinnitus, but more serious toxicity is very uncommon. Charcoal, activated p. 810 followed by symptomatic measures are indicated if more than 100 mg/kg has been ingested within the preceding hour.

For details on the management of poisoning, see Emergency treatment of poisoning p. 803.

● ALLERGY AND CROSS-SENSITIVITY Contra-indicated in patients with a history of hypersensitivity to aspirin or any other NSAID—which includes those in whom attacks of asthma, angioedema, urticaria or rhinitis have been precipitated by aspirin or any other NSAID.

● PREGNANCY Avoid unless the potential benefit outweighs the risk. Avoid during the third trimester (risk of closure of fetal ductus arteriosus *in utero* and possibly persistent pulmonary hypertension of the newborn); onset of labour may be delayed and duration may be increased.

● BREAST FEEDING Use with caution during breast-feeding. Amount too small to be harmful but some manufacturers advise avoid.

- **HEPATIC IMPAIRMENT**
▸ With intravenous use Increased risk of gastro-intestinal bleeding and fluid retention. Avoid in severe liver disease.
▸ With oral use Use with caution; there is an increased risk of gastro-intestinal bleeding and fluid retention. Avoid in severe liver disease.

- **RENAL IMPAIRMENT** Monitor renal function; sodium and water retention may occur and renal function may deteriorate, possibly leading to renal failure.
▸ With intravenous use Use lowest effective dose. Avoid if possible in severe impairment.
▸ With oral use The lowest effective dose should be used for the shortest possible duration. Avoid if possible or use with caution. Avoid in severe impairment.

- **MONITORING REQUIREMENTS**
▸ With intravenous use Monitor for bleeding. Monitor gastro-intestinal function.

- **DIRECTIONS FOR ADMINISTRATION** For *slow intravenous injection*, give over 15 minutes, preferably undiluted. May be diluted with Glucose 5% *or* Sodium Chloride 0.9%.

- **PRESCRIBING AND DISPENSING INFORMATION** Flavours of syrup may include orange.

- **PATIENT AND CARER ADVICE**
Medicines for Children leaflet: Ibuprofen for pain and inflammation www.medicinesforchildren.org.uk/ibuprofen-for-pain-and-inflammation

- **PROFESSION SPECIFIC INFORMATION**
Dental practitioners' formulary
Ibuprofen Oral Suspension Sugar-free may be prescribed. Ibuprofen Tablets may be prescribed.

- **EXCEPTIONS TO LEGAL CATEGORY** Oral preparations can be sold to the public in certain circumstances.

- **MEDICINAL FORMS**
There can be variation in the licensing of different medicines containing the same drug. Forms available from special-order manufacturers include: oral suspension

Effervescent granules
CAUTIONARY AND ADVISORY LABELS 13, 21
ELECTROLYTES: May contain Sodium
▸ Brufen (Mylan Ltd)
Ibuprofen 600 mg Brufen 600mg effervescent granules sachets | 20 sachet [PoM] £6.80 DT price = £6.80

Modified-release tablet
CAUTIONARY AND ADVISORY LABELS 25, 27
▸ Brufen Retard (Mylan Ltd)
Ibuprofen 800 mg Brufen Retard 800mg tablets | 56 tablet [PoM] £7.74 DT price = £7.74

Tablet
CAUTIONARY AND ADVISORY LABELS 21
▸ Ibuprofen (Non-proprietary)
Ibuprofen 200 mg Ibuprofen 200mg tablets | 16 tablet [P] £0.20 | 24 tablet [P] £0.92 DT price = £0.92 | 48 tablet [P] £1.84 | 84 tablet [P] £3.29 DT price = £3.22 | 96 tablet [P] £1.69
Ibuprofen 200mg tablets film coated | 84 tablet [P] £1.38 DT price = £3.22
Ibuprofen 200mg caplets | 16 tablet [P] £0.20 | 24 tablet [P] no price available DT price = £0.92 | 48 tablet [P] no price available | 96 tablet [P] no price available | 100 tablet [P] no price available
Ibuprofen 400 mg Ibuprofen 400mg tablets film coated | 24 tablet [P] £0.89 DT price = £0.86 | 84 tablet [P] £1.52 DT price = £3.01
Ibuprofen 400mg caplets | 12 tablet [P] no price available | 24 tablet [P] no price available DT price = £0.86 | 48 tablet [P] no price available | 96 tablet [P] no price available
Ibuprofen 400mg tablets | 24 tablet [P] £1.39 DT price = £0.86 | 48 tablet [P] £2.56 | 84 tablet [P] £6.84 DT price = £3.01 | 96 tablet [P] £2.46 | 250 tablet [PoM] £8.96
Ibuprofen 600 mg Ibuprofen 600mg tablets | 84 tablet [PoM] £6.95 DT price = £4.07
Ibuprofen 600mg tablets film coated | 84 tablet [PoM] £4.07 DT price = £4.07
▸ Brufen (Mylan Ltd)
Ibuprofen 400 mg Brufen 400mg tablets | 60 tablet [PoM] £4.90
Ibuprofen 600 mg Brufen 600mg tablets | 60 tablet [PoM] £7.34

▸ Cuprofen (SSL International Plc)
Ibuprofen 400 mg Cuprofen Maximum Strength 400mg tablets | 12 tablet [P] £1.03 | 24 tablet [P] £1.61 DT price = £0.86 | 48 tablet [P] £2.91 | 96 tablet [P] £5.04
▸ Ibucalm (Aspar Pharmaceuticals Ltd)
Ibuprofen 200 mg Ibucalm 200mg tablets | 24 tablet [P] £0.77 DT price = £0.92 | 48 tablet [P] £1.43 | 96 tablet [P] £2.43
Ibuprofen 400 mg Ibucalm 400mg tablets | 16 tablet [P] £0.88 | 24 tablet [P] £1.36 DT price = £0.86 | 48 tablet [P] £2.44 | 96 tablet [P] £4.19
▸ Nurofen (Reckitt Benckiser Healthcare (UK) Ltd)
Ibuprofen 200 mg Nurofen 200mg caplets | 24 tablet [P] £2.48 DT price = £0.92
Nurofen 200mg tablets | 24 tablet [P] £2.37 DT price = £0.92 | 48 tablet [P] £4.36 | 96 tablet [P] £7.20
Ibuprofen (as Ibuprofen lysine) 400 mg Nurofen Maximum Strength Migraine Pain 684mg caplets | 12 tablet [P] £3.49
▸ Nurofen Express (Reckitt Benckiser Healthcare (UK) Ltd)
Ibuprofen (as Ibuprofen lysine) 400 mg Nurofen Express 684mg caplets | 24 tablet [P] £6.14

Oral suspension
CAUTIONARY AND ADVISORY LABELS 21
▸ Ibuprofen (Non-proprietary)
Ibuprofen 20 mg per 1 ml Ibuprofen 100mg/5ml oral suspension sugar free sugar-free | 100 ml [P] £1.32 DT price = £1.25 sugar-free | 150 ml [P] no price available sugar-free | 500 ml [PoM] £6.25 sugar-free | 500 ml [P] no price available
Junior Ibuprofen 100mg/5ml oral suspension sugar-free | 100 ml [P] £0.90 DT price = £1.25
▸ Brufen (Mylan Ltd)
Ibuprofen 20 mg per 1 ml Brufen 100mg/5ml syrup | 500 ml [PoM] £8.88 DT price = £8.88
▸ Calprofen (McNeil Products Ltd)
Ibuprofen 20 mg per 1 ml Calprofen 100mg/5ml oral suspension sugar-free | 200 ml [P] £3.42
Nurofen for Children 100mg/5ml oral suspension orange sugar-free | 200 ml [P] £4.20
Nurofen for Children 100mg/5ml oral suspension strawberry sugar-free | 200 ml [P] £4.20
▸ Orbifen (Orbis Consumer Products Ltd)
Ibuprofen 20 mg per 1 ml Orbifen For Children 100mg/5ml oral suspension sugar-free | 100 ml [P] £1.67 DT price = £1.25 sugar-free | 150 ml [P] £2.71

Modified-release capsule
▸ Ibuprofen (Non-proprietary)
Ibuprofen 200 mg Ibuprofen Long Lasting 200mg capsules | 16 capsule [GSL] no price available

Solution for infusion
▸ Ibuprofen (Non-proprietary)
Ibuprofen (as Ibuprofen lysine) 10 mg per 1 ml NeoProfen 20mg/2ml solution for infusion vials | 3 vial [PoM] no price available
▸ Pedea (Orphan Europe (UK) Ltd)
Ibuprofen 5 mg per 1 ml Pedea 10mg/2ml solution for infusion ampoules | 4 ampoule [PoM] £288.00 (Hospital only)

Chewable capsule
▸ Nurofen (Reckitt Benckiser Healthcare (UK) Ltd)
Ibuprofen 100 mg Nurofen for Children 100mg chewable capsules | 12 capsule [P] £3.23

Capsule
▸ Ibuprofen (Non-proprietary)
Ibuprofen 200 mg Ibuprofen 200mg capsules | 30 capsule [P] no price available DT price = £4.40 | 32 capsule [P] £0.79
Ibuprofen 400 mg Ibuprofen 400mg capsules | 10 capsule [P] no price available | 20 capsule [P] no price available DT price = £5.82

Orodispersible tablet
▸ Ibuprofen (Non-proprietary)
Ibuprofen 200 mg Ibuprofen 200mg orodispersible tablets sugar free sugar-free | 12 tablet [GSL] no price available DT price = £2.19
▸ Brands may include Nurofen Meltlets

10

Musculoskeletal system

Indometacin

(Indomethacin)

- ● **INDICATIONS AND DOSE**

Symptomatic ductus arteriosus
- ▸ BY INTRAVENOUS INFUSION
- ▸ Neonate: Initially 100–200 micrograms/kg for 1 dose, followed by 100 micrograms/kg after 24 hours for 2 doses, at 24-hour intervals, doses to be given over 20–30 minutes, if residual patency present, 100 micrograms/kg to be given for a further 3 doses at 24-hour intervals.

Relief of pain and inflammation in rheumatic diseases including juvenile idiopathic arthritis
- ▸ BY MOUTH USING IMMEDIATE-RELEASE MEDICINES
- ▸ Child: 0.5–1 mg/kg twice daily, higher doses may be used under specialist supervision

- ● **UNLICENSED USE**
- ▸ With oral use Not licensed for use in children.

- ● **CONTRA-INDICATIONS**
- ▸ With intravenous use Bleeding (especially with active intracranial haemorrhage or gastro-intestinal bleeding) · coagulation defects · necrotising enterocolitis · thrombocytopenia · untreated infection
- ▸ With oral use Active gastro-intestinal bleeding · active gastro-intestinal ulceration · history of gastro-intestinal bleeding related to previous NSAID therapy · history of gastro-intestinal perforation related to previous NSAID therapy · history of recurrent gastro-intestinal haemorrhage (two or more distinct episodes) · history of recurrent gastro-intestinal ulceration (two or more distinct episodes) · severe heart failure

- ● **CAUTIONS**
  GENERAL CAUTIONS
  Heart failure
  SPECIFIC CAUTIONS
- ▸ With intravenous use Inhibition of platelet aggregation (monitor for bleeding) · may induce hyponatraemia · may mask symptoms of infection · may reduce urine output by 50% or more and precipitate renal impairment especially if extracellular volume depleted · sepsis
- ▸ With oral use Allergic disorders · cardiac impairment (NSAIDs may impair renal function) · cerebrovascular disease · coagulation defects · connective-tissue disorders · Crohn's disease (may be exacerbated) · epilepsy · ischaemic heart disease · peripheral arterial disease · psychiatric disturbances · risk factors for cardiovascular events · ulcerative colitis (may be exacerbated) · uncontrolled hypertension

- ● **INTERACTIONS** → Appendix 1: NSAIDs

- ● **SIDE-EFFECTS**
- ▸ Rare
- ▸ With oral use Alveolitis · aseptic meningitis (patients with connective-tissue disorders such as systemic lupus erythematosus may be especially susceptible) · blood disorders · confusion · convulsions · hepatic damage · hyperglycaemia · interstitial fibrosis associated with NSAIDs can lead to renal failure · intestinal strictures · pancreatitis · papillary necrosis associated with NSAIDs can lead to renal failure · peripheral neuropathy · psychiatric disturbances · pulmonary eosinophilia · Stevens-Johnson syndrome · syncope · thrombocytopenia · toxic epidermal necrolysis · visual disturbances
- ▸ Frequency not known
- ▸ With intravenous use Coagulation disorders · exacerbation of infection · fluid retention · gastro-intestinal disorders · haemorrhagic disorders · intracranial bleeding · metabolic disorders · pulmonary hypertension · renal disorders

- ▸ With oral use Angioedema · blood disorders · bronchospasm · colitis (induction of or exacerbation of) · Crohn's disease (induction of or exacerbation of) · depression · diarrhoea · dizziness · drowsiness · fluid retention (rarely precipitating congestive heart failure) · gastro-intestinal bleeding · gastro-intestinal discomfort · gastro-intestinal disturbances · gastro-intestinal ulceration · haematuria · headache · hearing disturbances · hyperkalaemia · hypersensitivity reactions · insomnia · nausea · nervousness · photosensitivity · raised blood pressure · rashes · renal failure (especially in patients with pre-existing renal impairment) · tinnitus · vertigo
  SIDE-EFFECTS, FURTHER INFORMATION
- ▸ Serious side-effects For information about cardiovascular and gastro-intestinal side-effects, and a possible exacerbation of symptoms in asthma, see Non-steroidal anti-inflammatory drugs p. 621.

- ● **ALLERGY AND CROSS-SENSITIVITY** Contra-indicated in patients with a history of hypersensitivity to aspirin or any other NSAID—which includes those in whom attacks of asthma, angioedema, urticaria or rhinitis have been precipitated by aspirin or any other NSAID.

- ● **PREGNANCY**
- ▸ With oral use Avoid unless the potential benefit outweighs the risk. Avoid during the third trimester (risk of closure of fetal ductus arteriosus *in utero* and possibly persistent pulmonary hypertension of the newborn); onset of labour may be delayed and duration may be increased.

- ● **BREAST FEEDING**
- ▸ With oral use Amount probably too small to be harmful—manufacturers advise avoid. Use with caution during breast-feeding.

- ● **HEPATIC IMPAIRMENT**
- ▸ With intravenous use Increased risk of gastro-intestinal bleeding and fluid retention. Avoid in severe impairment.
- ▸ With oral use or rectal use Use with caution; there is an increased risk of gastro-intestinal bleeding and fluid retention. Avoid in severe liver disease.

- ● **RENAL IMPAIRMENT**
- ▸ With intravenous use Use lowest effective dose. Avoid if possible in severe impairment If anuria or marked oliguria (urinary output less than 0.6 mL/kg/hour), delay further doses until renal function returns to normal.
- ▸ With oral use The lowest effective dose should be used for the shortest possible duration. Avoid if possible or use with caution. Avoid in severe impairment. Monitor renal function; sodium and water retention may occur and renal function may deteriorate, possibly leading to renal failure.

- ● **MONITORING REQUIREMENTS**
- ▸ With oral use During prolonged therapy ophthalmic and blood examinations particularly advisable.

- ● **DIRECTIONS FOR ADMINISTRATION** For *intravenous infusion*, dilute each vial with 1–2 mL Sodium Chloride 0.9% *or* Water for Injections.

- ● **PATIENT AND CARER ADVICE**

Driving and skilled tasks
Dizziness may affect performance of skilled tasks (e.g. driving).

- ● **MEDICINAL FORMS**
  There can be variation in the licensing of different medicines containing the same drug. Forms available from special-order manufacturers include: oral suspension, oral solution

Capsule
CAUTIONARY AND ADVISORY LABELS 21
- ▸ **Indometacin (Non-proprietary)**
  Indometacin 25 mg Indometacin 25mg capsules I 28 capsule [PoM]
  £5.00 DT price = £1.22
  Indometacin 50 mg Indometacin 50mg capsules I 28 capsule [PoM]
  £7.50 DT price = £1.36

Ketoprofen

- **INDICATIONS AND DOSE**

For use as a component of Ketoprofen with omeprazole, below
- ▸ BY MOUTH
- ▸ Child 15-17 years: (consult product literature)

- **CONTRA-INDICATIONS** Active gastro-intestinal bleeding · active gastro-intestinal ulceration · history of gastro-intestinal bleeding · history of gastro-intestinal perforation · history of gastro-intestinal ulceration · severe heart failure
- **CAUTIONS** Allergic disorders · cardiac impairment (NSAIDs may impair renal function) · cerebrovascular disease · coagulation defects · connective-tissue disorders · Crohn's disease (may be exacerbated) · heart failure · ischaemic heart disease · peripheral arterial disease · risk factors for cardiovascular events · ulcerative colitis (may be exacerbated) · uncontrolled hypertension
- **SIDE-EFFECTS**
- ▸ **Rare** Alveolitis · aseptic meningitis (patients with connective-tissue disorders such as systemic lupus erythematosus may be especially susceptible) · hepatic damage · interstitial fibrosis associated with NSAIDs can lead to renal failure · pancreatitis · papillary necrosis associated with NSAIDs can lead to renal failure · pulmonary eosinophilia · Stevens-Johnson syndrome · toxic epidermal necrolysis · visual disturbances
- ▸ **Frequency not known** Angioedema · blood disorders · bronchospasm · colitis (induction of or exacerbation of) · Crohn's disease (induction of or exacerbation of) · depression · diarrhoea · dizziness · drowsiness · fluid retention (rarely precipitating congestive heart failure) · gastro-intestinal bleeding · gastro-intestinal discomfort · gastro-intestinal disturbances · gastro-intestinal ulceration · haematuria · headache · hearing disturbances · hypersensitivity reactions · insomnia · nausea · nervousness · photosensitivity · raised blood pressure · rashes · renal failure (especially in patients with pre-existing renal impairment) · tinnitus · vertigo
  SIDE-EFFECTS, FURTHER INFORMATION
- ▸ Serious side-effects For information about cardiovascular and gastro-intestinal side-effects, and a possible exacerbation of symptoms in asthma, see Non-steroidal anti-inflammatory drugs p. 621.
- **ALLERGY AND CROSS-SENSITIVITY** Contra-indicated in patients with a history of hypersensitivity to aspirin or any other NSAID—which includes those in whom attacks of asthma, angioedema, urticaria or rhinitis have been precipitated by aspirin or any other NSAID.
- **CONCEPTION AND CONTRACEPTION** Caution—long-term use of some NSAIDs is associated with reduced female fertility, which is reversible on stopping treatment.
- **PREGNANCY** Avoid unless the potential benefit outweighs the risk. Avoid during the third trimester (risk of closure of fetal ductus arteriosus *in utero* and possibly persistent pulmonary hypertension of the newborn); onset of labour may be delayed and duration may be increased.
- **BREAST FEEDING** Use with caution during breast-feeding. Amount probably too small to be harmful but manufacturers advise avoid.
- **HEPATIC IMPAIRMENT** Use with caution; there is an increased risk of gastro-intestinal bleeding and fluid retention. Should be avoided in severe liver disease.
- **RENAL IMPAIRMENT** The lowest effective dose should be used for the shortest possible duration.
  Avoid if possible or use with caution. Avoid in severe impairment. Monitor renal function; sodium and water

retention may occur and renal function may deteriorate, possibly leading to renal failure.
- **PRESCRIBING AND DISPENSING INFORMATION** Flavours of oral liquid formulations may include strawberry.

- **MEDICINAL FORMS**
  There can be variation in the licensing of different medicines containing the same drug.

Ketoprofen with omeprazole

The properties listed below are those particular to the combination only. For the properties of the components please consider, ketoprofen above, omeprazole p. 57.

- **INDICATIONS AND DOSE**

Patients requiring ketoprofen for osteoarthritis, rheumatoid arthritis, and ankylosing spondylitis, who are at risk of NSAID associated duodenal or gastric ulcer or gastroduodenal erosions
- ▸ BY MOUTH USING MODIFIED-RELEASE MEDICINES
- ▸ Child 15-17 years: Initially 100/20 mg daily, increased if necessary to 200/20 mg daily, depending on severity of symptoms, dose expressed as *x*/*y* mg ketoprofen/omeprazole

- **INTERACTIONS** → Appendix 1: NSAIDs, proton pump inhibitors
- **PRESCRIBING AND DISPENSING INFORMATION** Capsules enclose microgranules containing modified-release ketoprofen and gastro-resistant omperazole.

- **MEDICINAL FORMS**
  There can be variation in the licensing of different medicines containing the same drug.
  No licensed medicines listed.

Mefenamic acid

- **INDICATIONS AND DOSE**

Acute pain including dysmenorrhoea | Menorrhagia
- ▸ BY MOUTH
- ▸ Child 12-17 years: 500 mg 3 times a day

- **CONTRA-INDICATIONS** Active gastro-intestinal bleeding · active gastro-intestinal ulceration · history of gastro-intestinal bleeding related to previous NSAID therapy · history of gastro-intestinal perforation related to previous NSAID therapy · history of recurrent gastro-intestinal haemorrhage (two or more distinct episodes) · history of recurrent gastro-intestinal ulceration (two or more distinct episodes) · inflammatory bowel disease · severe heart failure
- **CAUTIONS** Acute porphyrias p. 577 · allergic disorders · cardiac impairment (NSAIDs may impair renal function) · cerebrovascular disease · coagulation defects · connective-tissue disorders · Crohn's disease (may be exacerbated) · epilepsy · heart failure · ischaemic heart disease · peripheral arterial disease · risk factors for cardiovascular events · ulcerative colitis (may be exacerbated) · uncontrolled hypertension
- **INTERACTIONS** → Appendix 1: NSAIDs
- **SIDE-EFFECTS**
- ▸ **Common or very common** Diarrhoea (withdraw treatment) · rashes (withdraw treatment) · stomatitis
- ▸ **Uncommon** Fatigue · paraesthesia
- ▸ **Rare** Alveolitis · aplastic anaemia · aseptic meningitis (patients with connective-tissue disorders such as systemic lupus erythematosus may be especially susceptible) · glucose intolerance · haemolytic anaemia (positive Coombs' test) · hepatic damage · hypotension ·

10

Musculoskeletal system

interstitial fibrosis associated with NSAIDs can lead to renal failure · palpitation · pancreatitis · papillary necrosis associated with NSAIDs can lead to renal failure · pulmonary eosinophilia · Stevens-Johnson syndrome · thrombocytopenia · toxic epidermal necrolysis · visual disturbances

▶ **Frequency not known** Angioedema · blood disorders · bronchospasm · colitis (induction of or exacerbation of) · Crohn's disease (induction of or exacerbation of) · depression · dizziness · drowsiness · fluid retention (rarely precipitating congestive heart failure) · gastro-intestinal bleeding · gastro-intestinal discomfort · gastro-intestinal disturbances · gastro-intestinal ulceration · haematuria · headache · hearing disturbances · hypersensitivity reactions · insomnia · nausea · nervousness · photosensitivity · raised blood pressure · renal failure (especially in patients with pre-existing renal impairment) · tinnitus · vertigo

SIDE-EFFECTS, FURTHER INFORMATION

▶ Serious side-effects For information about cardiovascular and gastro-intestinal side-effects, and a possible exacerbation of symptoms in asthma, see Non-steroidal anti-inflammatory drugs p. 621.

Overdose
Mefenamic acid has important consequences in overdosage because it can cause convulsions, which if prolonged or recurrent, require treatment.

For details on the management of poisoning, see Emergency treatment of poisoning p. 803, in particular, Convulsions.

● **ALLERGY AND CROSS-SENSITIVITY** Contra-indicated in patients with a history of hypersensitivity to aspirin or any other NSAID—which includes those in whom attacks of asthma, angioedema, urticaria or rhinitis have been precipitated by aspirin or any other NSAID.

● **PREGNANCY** Avoid unless the potential benefit outweighs the risk. Avoid during the third trimester (risk of closure of fetal ductus arteriosus *in utero* and possibly persistent pulmonary hypertension of the newborn); onset of labour may be delayed and duration may be increased.

● **BREAST FEEDING** Use with caution during breast-feeding. Amount too small to be harmful but manufacturer advises avoid.

● **HEPATIC IMPAIRMENT** Use with caution; there is an increased risk of gastro-intestinal bleeding and fluid retention. Avoid in severe liver disease.

● **RENAL IMPAIRMENT** The lowest effective dose should be used for the shortest possible duration. Avoid if possible or use with caution. Avoid in severe impairment. In renal impairment monitor renal function; sodium and water retention may occur and renal function may deteriorate, possibly leading to renal failure.

● **MEDICINAL FORMS**
There can be variation in the licensing of different medicines containing the same drug. Forms available from special-order manufacturers include: oral suspension

Oral suspension
CAUTIONARY AND ADVISORY LABELS 21
EXCIPIENTS: May contain Ethanol
▶ Mefenamic acid (Non-proprietary)
  Mefenamic acid 10 mg per 1 ml Mefenamic acid 50mg/5ml oral suspension ┃ 125 ml 〔PoM〕 £179.00 DT price = £179.00

Tablet
CAUTIONARY AND ADVISORY LABELS 21
▶ Mefenamic acid (Non-proprietary)
  Mefenamic acid 500 mg Mefenamic acid 500mg tablets ┃ 28 tablet 〔PoM〕 £50.20 DT price = £6.15 ┃ 84 tablet 〔PoM〕 £44.99
▶ Ponstan (Chemidex Pharma Ltd)
  Mefenamic acid 500 mg Ponstan Forte 500mg tablets ┃ 100 tablet 〔PoM〕 £15.72

Capsule
CAUTIONARY AND ADVISORY LABELS 21
▶ Mefenamic acid (Non-proprietary)
  Mefenamic acid 250 mg Mefenamic acid 250mg capsules ┃ 100 capsule 〔PoM〕 £60.10 DT price = £9.54
▶ Ponstan (Chemidex Pharma Ltd)
  Mefenamic acid 250 mg Ponstan 250mg capsules ┃ 100 capsule 〔PoM〕 £8.17 DT price = £9.54

Meloxicam

● **INDICATIONS AND DOSE**

Exacerbation of osteoarthritis (short-term)
▶ BY MOUTH
  ▶ Child 16-17 years: 7.5 mg once daily, then increased if necessary up to 15 mg once daily

Pain and inflammation in rheumatic disease | Ankylosing spondylitis
▶ BY MOUTH
  ▶ Child 16-17 years: 15 mg once daily, then reduced to 7.5 mg once daily if required

Relief of pain and inflammation in juvenile idiopathic arthritis and other musculoskeletal disorders in children intolerant to other NSAIDs
▶ BY MOUTH
  ▶ Child 12-17 years (body-weight up to 50 kg): 7.5 mg once daily
  ▶ Child 12-17 years (body-weight 50 kg and above): 15 mg once daily

● **UNLICENSED USE** Not licensed for use in children under 16 years.

● **CONTRA-INDICATIONS** Active gastro-intestinal bleeding · active gastro-intestinal ulceration · history of gastro-intestinal bleeding related to previous NSAID therapy · history of gastro-intestinal perforation related to previous NSAID therapy · history of recurrent gastro-intestinal haemorrhage (two or more distinct episodes) · history of recurrent gastro-intestinal ulceration (two or more distinct episodes) · severe heart failure

● **CAUTIONS** Allergic disorders · cardiac impairment (NSAIDs may impair renal function) · cerebrovascular disease · coagulation defects · connective-tissue disorders · Crohn's disease (may be exacerbated) · heart failure · ischaemic heart disease · peripheral arterial disease · risk factors for cardiovascular events · ulcerative colitis (may be exacerbated) · uncontrolled hypertension

● **INTERACTIONS** → Appendix 1: NSAIDs

● **SIDE-EFFECTS**

▶ **Rare** Alveolitis · aseptic meningitis (patients with connective-tissue disorders such as systemic lupus erythematosus may be especially susceptible) · hepatic damage · interstitial fibrosis associated with NSAIDs can lead to renal failure · pancreatitis · papillary necrosis associated with NSAIDs can lead to renal failure · pulmonary eosinophilia · Stevens-Johnson syndrome · toxic epidermal necrolysis · visual disturbances

▶ **Frequency not known** Angioedema · blood disorders · bronchospasm · colitis (induction of or exacerbation of) · Crohn's disease (induction of or exacerbation of) · depression · diarrhoea · dizziness · drowsiness · fluid retention (rarely precipitating congestive heart failure) · gastro-intestinal bleeding · gastro-intestinal discomfort · gastro-intestinal disturbances · gastro-intestinal ulceration · haematuria · headache · hearing disturbances · hypersensitivity reactions · insomnia · nausea · nervousness · photosensitivity · raised blood pressure · rashes · renal failure (especially in patients with pre-existing renal impairment) · tinnitus · vertigo

SIDE-EFFECTS, FURTHER INFORMATION

▸ Serious side-effects For information about cardiovascular and gastro-intestinal side-effects, and a possible exacerbation of symptoms in asthma, see Non-steroidal anti-inflammatory drugs p. 621.

● **ALLERGY AND CROSS-SENSITIVITY** Contra-indicated in patients with a history of hypersensitivity to aspirin or any other NSAID—which includes those in whom attacks of asthma, angioedema, urticaria or rhinitis have been precipitated by aspirin or any other NSAID.

● **PREGNANCY** Avoid unless the potential benefit outweighs the risk. Avoid during the third trimester (risk of closure of fetal ductus arteriosus *in utero* and possibly persistent pulmonary hypertension of the newborn); onset of labour may be delayed and duration may be increased.

● **BREAST FEEDING** Use with caution during breast-feeding. Present in milk in *animal* studies—manufacturer advises avoid.

● **HEPATIC IMPAIRMENT** Use with caution; there is an increased risk of gastro-intestinal bleeding and fluid retention. Avoid in severe liver disease.

● **RENAL IMPAIRMENT** The lowest effective dose should be used for the shortest possible duration. Avoid if possible or use with caution.

  Avoid if estimated glomerular filtration rate less than 25 mL/minute/1.73 m². In renal impairment monitor renal function; sodium and water retention may occur and renal function may deteriorate, possibly leading to renal failure.

● **MEDICINAL FORMS**
There can be variation in the licensing of different medicines containing the same drug. Forms available from special-order manufacturers include: oral suspension

Orodispersible tablet
▸ Meloxicam (Non-proprietary)

  Meloxicam 7.5 mg Meloxicam 7.5mg orodispersible tablets sugar free sugar-free I 30 tablet [PoM] £15.50
  Meloxicam 15 mg Meloxicam 15mg orodispersible tablets sugar free sugar-free I 30 tablet [PoM] £15.50

Tablet
CAUTIONARY AND ADVISORY LABELS 21
▸ Meloxicam (Non-proprietary)

  Meloxicam 7.5 mg Meloxicam 7.5mg tablets I 30 tablet [PoM] £4.00 DT price = £0.94
  Meloxicam 15 mg Meloxicam 15mg tablets I 30 tablet [PoM] £4.00 DT price = £1.06

Naproxen

● **INDICATIONS AND DOSE**

Pain and inflammation in musculoskeletal disorders | Dysmenorrhoea
▸ BY MOUTH
▸ Child: 5 mg/kg twice daily; maximum 1 g per day

Pain and inflammation in juvenile idiopathic arthritis
▸ BY MOUTH
▸ Child 2–17 years: 5–7.5 mg/kg twice daily; maximum 1 g per day

● **UNLICENSED USE** Not licensed for use in children under 5 years for juvenile idiopathic arthritis. Not licensed for use in children under 16 years for musculoskeletal disorders or dysmenorrhoea.

● **CONTRA-INDICATIONS** Active gastro-intestinal bleeding · active gastro-intestinal ulceration · history of gastro-intestinal bleeding related to previous NSAID therapy · history of gastro-intestinal perforation related to previous NSAID therapy · history of recurrent gastro-intestinal haemorrhage (two or more distinct episodes) · history of recurrent gastro-intestinal ulceration (two or more distinct episodes) · severe heart failure

● **CAUTIONS** Allergic disorders · cardiac impairment (NSAIDs may impair renal function) · cerebrovascular disease · coagulation defects · connective-tissue disorders · Crohn's disease (may be exacerbated) · heart failure · ischaemic heart disease · peripheral arterial disease · risk factors for cardiovascular events · ulcerative colitis (may be exacerbated) · uncontrolled hypertension

● **INTERACTIONS** → Appendix 1: NSAIDs

● **SIDE-EFFECTS**

▸ **Rare** Alveolitis · aseptic meningitis (patients with connective-tissue disorders such as systemic lupus erythematosus may be especially susceptible) · hepatic damage · interstitial fibrosis associated with NSAIDs can lead to renal failure · pancreatitis · papillary necrosis associated with NSAIDs can lead to renal failure · pulmonary eosinophilia · Stevens-Johnson syndrome · toxic epidermal necrolysis · visual disturbances

▸ **Frequency not known** Angioedema · blood disorders · bronchospasm · colitis (induction of or exacerbation of) · Crohn's disease (induction of or exacerbation of) · depression · diarrhoea · dizziness · drowsiness · fluid retention (rarely precipitating congestive heart failure) · gastro-intestinal bleeding · gastro-intestinal discomfort · gastro-intestinal disturbances · gastro-intestinal ulceration · haematuria · headache · hearing disturbances · hypersensitivity reactions · insomnia · nausea · nervousness · photosensitivity · raised blood pressure · rashes · renal failure (especially in patients with pre-existing renal impairment) · tinnitus · vertigo

SIDE-EFFECTS, FURTHER INFORMATION
▸ Serious side-effects For information about cardiovascular and gastro-intestinal side-effects, and a possible exacerbation of symptoms in asthma, see Non-steroidal anti-inflammatory drugs p. 621.

● **ALLERGY AND CROSS-SENSITIVITY** Contra-indicated in patients with a history of hypersensitivity to aspirin or any other NSAID—which includes those in whom attacks of asthma, angioedema, urticaria or rhinitis have been precipitated by aspirin or any other NSAID.

● **PREGNANCY** Avoid unless the potential benefit outweighs the risk. Avoid during the third trimester (risk of closure of fetal ductus arteriosus *in utero* and possibly persistent pulmonary hypertension of the newborn); onset of labour may be delayed and duration may be increased.

● **BREAST FEEDING** Use with caution during breast-feeding. Amount too small to be harmful but manufacturer advises avoid.

● **HEPATIC IMPAIRMENT** Use with caution; there is an increased risk of gastro-intestinal bleeding and fluid retention. Avoid in severe liver disease.

● **RENAL IMPAIRMENT** The lowest effective dose should be used for the shortest possible duration. Avoid if possible or use with caution.

  Avoid if estimated glomerular filtration rate less than 30 mL/minute/1.73 m². In renal impairment monitor renal function; sodium and water retention may occur and renal function may deteriorate, possibly leading to renal failure.

● **EXCEPTIONS TO LEGAL CATEGORY** Can be sold to the public for the treatment of primary dysmenorrhoea in women aged 15–50 years subject to max. single dose of 500 mg, max. daily dose of 750 mg for max. 3 days, and a max. pack size of 9 × 250 mg tablets.

● **MEDICINAL FORMS**
There can be variation in the licensing of different medicines containing the same drug. Forms available from special-order manufacturers include: oral suspension

Oral suspension
▸ Naproxen (Non-proprietary)

  Naproxen 25 mg per 1 ml Naproxen 25mg/ml oral suspension sugar free sugar-free I 100 ml [PoM] £110.00 DT price = £110.00

10

Musculoskeletal system

Naproxen 125mg/5ml oral suspension sugar free sugar-free |
100 ml [PoM] £110.00 £120.00 DT price = £110.00

Naproxen 50 mg per 1 ml Naproxen 50mg/ml oral suspension |
100 ml [PoM] £75.00

Gastro-resistant tablet

CAUTIONARY AND ADVISORY LABELS 5, 25

▸ **Naproxen (Non-proprietary)**
Naproxen 250 mg Naproxen 250mg gastro-resistant tablets |
56 tablet [PoM] £7.00 DT price = £2.97
Naproxen 375 mg Naproxen 375mg gastro-resistant tablets |
56 tablet [PoM] £26.82 DT price = £26.82
Naproxen 500 mg Naproxen 500mg gastro-resistant tablets |
56 tablet [PoM] £17.03 DT price = £7.01

▸ **Naprosyn EC** (Atnahs Pharma UK Ltd)
Naproxen 250 mg Naprosyn EC 250mg tablets | 56 tablet [PoM]
£4.29 DT price = £2.97
Naproxen 375 mg Naprosyn EC 375mg tablets | 56 tablet [PoM]
£6.42 DT price = £26.82
Naproxen 500 mg Naprosyn EC 500mg tablets | 56 tablet [PoM]
£8.56 DT price = £7.01

Effervescent tablet

▸ **Stirlescent** (Stirling Anglian Pharmaceuticals Ltd)
Naproxen 250 mg Stirlescent 250mg effervescent tablets sugar-free
| 20 tablet [PoM] £7.90 DT price = £7.90

Tablet

CAUTIONARY AND ADVISORY LABELS 21

▸ **Naproxen (Non-proprietary)**
Naproxen 250 mg Naproxen 250mg tablets | 28 tablet [PoM] £2.10
DT price = £0.93 | 56 tablet [PoM] £2.33
Naproxen 500 mg Naproxen 500mg tablets | 28 tablet [PoM] £4.27
DT price = £1.42 | 56 tablet [PoM] £3.99

▸ **Naprosyn** (Atnahs Pharma UK Ltd)
Naproxen 250 mg Naprosyn 250mg tablets | 56 tablet [PoM] £4.29
Naproxen 500 mg Naprosyn 500mg tablets | 56 tablet [PoM] £8.56

Piroxicam

● **INDICATIONS AND DOSE**

**Relief of pain and inflammation in juvenile idiopathic
arthritis**

▸ BY MOUTH

▸ Child 6–17 years (body-weight up to 15 kg): 5 mg daily
▸ Child 6–17 years (body-weight 15–25 kg): 10 mg daily
▸ Child 6–17 years (body-weight 26–45 kg): 15 mg daily
▸ Child 6–17 years (body-weight 46 kg and above): 20 mg
daily

● **UNLICENSED USE** Not licensed for use in children.

IMPORTANT SAFETY INFORMATION
The CHMP has recommended restrictions on the use of
piroxicam because of the increased risk of gastro-
intestinal side effects and serious skin reactions. The
CHMP has advised that:
● piroxicam should be initiated only by physicians
experienced in treating inflammatory or degenerative
rheumatic diseases
● piroxicam should not be used as first-line treatment
● in adults, use of piroxicam should be limited to the
symptomatic relief of osteoarthritis, rheumatoid
arthritis, and ankylosing spondylitis
● piroxicam dose should not exceed 20 mg daily
● piroxicam should no longer be used for the treatment
of acute painful and inflammatory conditions
● treatment should be reviewed 2 weeks after initiating
piroxicam, and periodically thereafter
● concomitant administration of a gastro-protective
agent should be considered.
Topical preparations containing piroxicam are not
affected by these restrictions.

● **CONTRA-INDICATIONS** Active gastro-intestinal bleeding ·
active gastro-intestinal ulceration · history of gastro-
intestinal bleeding · history of gastro-intestinal

perforation · history of gastro-intestinal ulceration ·
inflammatory bowel disease · severe heart failure

● **CAUTIONS** Allergic disorders · cardiac impairment (NSAIDs
may impair renal function) · cerebrovascular disease ·
coagulation defects · connective-tissue disorders · Crohn's
disease (may be exacerbated) · heart failure · ischaemic
heart disease · peripheral arterial disease · risk factors for
cardiovascular events · ulcerative colitis (may be
exacerbated) · uncontrolled hypertension

● **INTERACTIONS** → Appendix 1: NSAIDs

● **SIDE-EFFECTS**

▸ **Rare** Alveolitis · aseptic meningitis (patients with
connective-tissue disorders such as systemic lupus
erythematosus may be especially susceptible) · hepatic
damage · interstitial fibrosis associated with NSAIDs can
lead to renal failure · pancreatitis · papillary necrosis
associated with NSAIDs can lead to renal failure ·
pulmonary eosinophilia · Stevens-Johnson syndrome ·
toxic epidermal necrolysis · visual disturbances

▸ **Frequency not known** Angioedema · blood disorders ·
bronchospasm · colitis (induction of or exacerbation of) ·
Crohn's disease (induction of or exacerbation of) ·
depression · diarrhoea · dizziness · drowsiness · fluid
retention (rarely precipitating congestive heart failure) ·
gastro-intestinal bleeding · gastro-intestinal discomfort ·
gastro-intestinal disturbances · gastro-intestinal
ulceration · haematuria · headache · hearing disturbances ·
hypersensitivity reactions · insomnia · nausea ·
nervousness · photosensitivity · raised blood pressure ·
rashes · renal failure (especially in patients with pre-
existing renal impairment) · tinnitus · vertigo

SIDE-EFFECTS, FURTHER INFORMATION

▸ **Serious side-effects** For information about cardiovascular
and gastro-intestinal side-effects, and a possible
exacerbation of symptoms in asthma, see Non-steroidal
anti-inflammatory drugs p. 621.

● **ALLERGY AND CROSS-SENSITIVITY** Contra-indicated in
patients with a history of hypersensitivity to aspirin or any
other NSAID—which includes those in whom attacks of
asthma, angioedema, urticaria or rhinitis have been
precipitated by aspirin or any other NSAID.

● **PREGNANCY** Avoid unless the potential benefit outweighs
the risk. Avoid during the third trimester (risk of closure of
fetal ductus arteriosus *in utero* and possibly persistent
pulmonary hypertension of the newborn); onset of labour
may be delayed and duration may be increased.

● **BREAST FEEDING** Use with caution during breast-feeding.
Amount too small to be harmful.

● **HEPATIC IMPAIRMENT** Use with caution; there is an
increased risk of gastro-intestinal bleeding and fluid
retention. Avoid in severe liver disease.

● **RENAL IMPAIRMENT** The lowest effective dose should be
used for the shortest possible duration. Avoid if possible or
use with caution. Monitor renal function; sodium and
water retention may occur and renal function may
deteriorate, possibly leading to renal failure.

● **DIRECTIONS FOR ADMINISTRATION** Piroxicam
orodispersible tablets can be taken by placing on the
tongue and allowing to dissolve or by swallowing.
    Piroxicam orodispersible tablets may be halved to give
10 mg dose.

● **LESS SUITABLE FOR PRESCRIBING**
Piroxicam is less suitable for prescribing.

- **MEDICINAL FORMS**
There can be variation in the licensing of different medicines containing the same drug.

Orodispersible tablet
CAUTIONARY AND ADVISORY LABELS 10, 21
EXCIPIENTS: May contain Aspartame

▸ **Feldene Melt** (Pfizer Ltd)
Piroxicam 20 mg Feldene Melt 20mg tablets sugar-free | 30 tablet [PoM] £10.53 DT price = £10.53

Capsule
CAUTIONARY AND ADVISORY LABELS 21

▸ **Piroxicam** (Non-proprietary)
Piroxicam 10 mg Piroxicam 10mg capsules | 56 capsule [PoM] £16.82 DT price = £4.18
Piroxicam 20 mg Piroxicam 20mg capsules | 28 capsule [PoM] £17.60 DT price = £3.61

▸ **Feldene** (Pfizer Ltd)
Piroxicam 10 mg Feldene 10mg capsules | 30 capsule [PoM] £3.86
Piroxicam 20 mg Feldene 20 capsules | 30 capsule [PoM] £7.71

4 Soft tissue and joint disorders

4.1 Local inflammation of joints and soft tissue

CORTICOSTEROIDS

Corticosteroids, inflammatory disorders

Systemic corticosteroids

In children with rheumatic diseases corticosteroids should be reserved for specific indications (e.g. when other therapies are unsuccessful or while waiting for DMARDs to take effect) and should be used only under the supervision of a specialist.

Systemic corticosteroids may be considered for the management of juvenile idiopathic arthritis in systemic disease or when several joints are affected. Systemic corticosteroids may also be considered in severe, possibly life-threatening conditions such as systemic lupus erythematosus, systemic vasculitis, juvenile dermatomyositis, Behçet's disease, and polyarticular joint disease.

In severe conditions, short courses ('pulses') of high dose intravenous methylprednisolone p. 421 or a pulsed oral corticosteroid may be particularly effective for providing rapid relief, and has fewer long-term adverse effects than continuous treatment.

Corticosteroid doses should be reduced with care because of the possibility of relapse if the reduction is too rapid. If complete discontinuation of corticosteroids is not possible, consideration should be given to alternate-day (or alternate high-dose, low-dose) administration; on days when no corticosteroid is given, or a lower dose is given, an additional dose of a NSAID may be helpful. In some conditions, alternative treatment using an antimalarial or concomitant use of an immunosuppressant drug, such as azathioprine p. 495, methotrexate p. 517 or cyclophosphamide p. 509 may prove useful; in less severe conditions treatment with a NSAID alone may be adequate.

Administration of corticosteroids may result in suppression of growth and may affect the development of puberty. The risk of corticosteroid-induced osteoporosis should be considered for those on long-term corticosteroid treatment; corticosteroids may also increase the risk of osteopenia in those unable to exercise. See the disadvantages of corticosteroid treatment.

Local corticosteroid injections

Corticosteroids are injected locally for an anti-inflammatory effect. In inflammatory conditions of the joints, including juvenile idiopathic arthritis, they are given by *intra-articular injection* as monotherapy, or as an adjunct to long-term therapy to reduce swelling and deformity in one or a few joints. Aseptic precautions (e.g. a no-touch technique) are essential, as is a clinician skilled in the technique; infected areas should be avoided and general anaesthesia, or local anaesthesia, or conscious sedation should be used. Occasionally an acute inflammatory reaction develops after an intra-articular or soft-tissue injection of a corticosteroid. This may be a reaction to the microcrystalline suspension of the corticosteroid used, but must be distinguished from sepsis introduced into the injection site.

Triamcinolone hexacetonide p. 634 [unlicensed] is preferred for intra-articular injection because it is almost insoluble and has a long-acting (depot) effect. Triamcinolone acetonide p. 634 and methylprednisolone may also be considered for intra-articular injection into larger joints, whilst hydrocortisone below acetate should be reserved for smaller joints or for soft-tissue injections. Intra-articular corticosteroid injections can cause flushing and, in adults, may affect the hyaline cartilage. Each joint should usually be treated no more than 3–4 times in one year.

A smaller amount of corticosteroid may also be injected directly into soft tissues for the relief of inflammation in conditions such as *tennis* or *golfer's elbow* or *compression neuropathies*, which occur rarely in children. In *tendinitis*, injections should be made into the tendon sheath and not directly into the tendon (due to the absence of a true tendon sheath and a high risk of rupture, the Achilles tendon should not be injected).

Corticosteroid injections are also injected into soft tissues for the treatment of skin lesions.

☞ 416

Hydrocortisone

18-May-2017

- **INDICATIONS AND DOSE**

HYDROCORTISTAB®

Local inflammation of joints and soft-tissues
▸ BY INTRA-ARTICULAR INJECTION
▸ Child 1 month–11 years: 5–30 mg, select dose according to size of child and joint; where appropriate dose may be repeated at intervals of 21 days. Not more than 3 joints should be treated on any one day, for details consult product literature
▸ Child 12–17 years: 5–50 mg, select dose according to size of patient and joint; where appropriate dose may be repeated at intervals of 21 days. Not more than 3 joints should be treated on any one day, for details consult product literature

- **INTERACTIONS** → Appendix 1: corticosteroids

- **MEDICINAL FORMS**
There can be variation in the licensing of different medicines containing the same drug.
Suspension for injection
▸ Hydrocortisone (AMCo)
Hydrocortisone acetate 25 mg per 1 ml Hydrocortistab 25mg/1ml suspension for injection ampoules | 10 ampoule [PoM] £68.72 DT price = £68.72

☞ 416

Methylprednisolone

10-Aug-2016

- **INDICATIONS AND DOSE**

DEPO-MEDRONE®

Local inflammation of joints and soft tissues
▸ BY INTRA-ARTICULAR INJECTION
▸ Child: (consult product literature)

10

Musculoskeletal system

- INTERACTIONS → Appendix 1: corticosteroids
- PATIENT AND CARER ADVICE Patient counselling is advised for methylprednisolone injections (steroid card).

- MEDICINAL FORMS
There can be variation in the licensing of different medicines containing the same drug.
Suspension for injection
CAUTIONARY AND ADVISORY LABELS 10
  - Depo-Medrone (Pfizer Ltd)
  Methylprednisolone acetate 40 mg per 1 ml Depo-Medrone 40mg/1ml suspension for injection vials | 1 vial [PoM] £3.44 DT price = £3.44 | 10 vial [PoM] £34.04
  Depo-Medrone 80mg/2ml suspension for injection vials | 1 vial [PoM] £6.18 DT price = £6.18 | 10 vial [PoM] £61.39
  Depo-Medrone 120mg/3ml suspension for injection vials | 1 vial [PoM] £8.96 DT price = £8.96 | 10 vial [PoM] £88.81

F 416

Triamcinolone acetonide

- INDICATIONS AND DOSE

ADCORTYL® INTRA-ARTICULAR/INTRADERMAL

Local inflammation of joints and soft tissues
  - BY INTRA-ARTICULAR INJECTION
  - Child 1-17 years: 2 mg/kg (max. per dose 15 mg), for details consult product literature, dose applies for larger joints. For doses above 15 mg use *Kenalog® Intra-articular/Intramuscular*. If appropriate repeat treatment for relapse.

KENALOG® VIALS

Local inflammation of joints and soft tissues
  - BY INTRA-ARTICULAR INJECTION
  - Child 1-17 years: 2 mg/kg, for details consult product literature, if appropriate repeat treatment for relapse, higher doses than usual maximum have been used; Usual maximum 40 mg

- UNLICENSED USE Not licensed for use in children under 6 years.
- INTERACTIONS → Appendix 1: corticosteroids
- PATIENT AND CARER ADVICE Patient counselling is advised for triamcinolone acetonide injection (steroid card).

- MEDICINAL FORMS
There can be variation in the licensing of different medicines containing the same drug.
Suspension for injection
CAUTIONARY AND ADVISORY LABELS 10
EXCIPIENTS: May contain Benzyl alcohol
  - Adcortyl Intra-articular / Intradermal (Bristol-Myers Squibb Pharmaceuticals Ltd)
  Triamcinolone acetonide 10 mg per 1 ml Adcortyl Intra-articular / Intradermal 50mg/5ml suspension for injection vials | 1 vial [PoM] £3.63
  Adcortyl Intra-articular / Intradermal 10mg/1ml suspension for injection ampoules | 5 ampoule [PoM] £4.47 DT price = £4.47
  - Kenalog (Bristol-Myers Squibb Pharmaceuticals Ltd)
  Triamcinolone acetonide 40 mg per 1 ml Kenalog Intra-articular / Intramuscular 40mg/1ml suspension for injection vials | 5 vial [PoM] £7.45 DT price = £7.45

F 416

Triamcinolone hexacetonide

- INDICATIONS AND DOSE

Symptomatic treatment of subacute and chronic inflammatory joint diseases (for details, consult product literature)
  - BY INTRA-ARTICULAR INJECTION
  - Child 12-17 years: 2-20 mg, according to size of the joint; if appropriate repeat treatment at intervals of 3-4 weeks, no more than 2 joints should be treated on any one day

  - BY PERI-ARTICULAR INJECTION
  - Child 12-17 years: 10-20 mg, according to size of the joint, no more than 2 joints should be treated on any one day

Juvenile idiopathic arthritis
  - BY INTRA-ARTICULAR INJECTION
  - Child 3-11 years: (consult product literature)

- CONTRA-INDICATIONS Consult product literature
- CAUTIONS Consult product literature
- INTERACTIONS → Appendix 1: corticosteroids
- SIDE-EFFECTS Consult product literature
- PRESCRIBING AND DISPENSING INFORMATION Various strengths available from 'special order' manufacturers or specialist importing companies.

- MEDICINAL FORMS
There can be variation in the licensing of different medicines containing the same drug.
Suspension for injection
EXCIPIENTS: May contain Benzyl alcohol
  - Triamcinolone hexacetonide (Non-proprietary)
  Triamcinolone hexacetonide 20 mg per 1 ml Triamcinolone hexacetonide 20mg/1ml suspension for injection ampoules | 10 ampoule [PoM] £120.00

4.2 Soft tissue disorders

Soft-tissue disorders

Soft-tissue and musculoskeletal disorders

The management of children with soft-tissue injuries and strains, and musculoskeletal disorders, may include temporary rest together with the local application of heat or cold, local massage and physiotherapy. For pain relief, paracetamol p. 260 is often adequate and should be used first. Alternatively, the lowest effective dose of a NSAID (e.g. ibuprofen p. 625) can be used. If pain relief with either drug is inadequate, both paracetamol (in a full dose appropriate for the child) and a low dose of a NSAID may be required.

Extravasation

Local guidelines for the management of extravasation should be followed where they exist or specialist advice sought.

Extravasation injury follows leakage of drugs or intravenous fluids from the veins or inadvertent administration into the subcutaneous or subdermal tissue. It must be dealt with **promptly** to prevent tissue necrosis.

Acidic or alkaline preparations and those with an osmolarity greater than that of plasma can cause extravasation injury; excipients including alcohol and polyethylene glycol have also been implicated. Cytotoxic drugs commonly cause extravasation injury. Very young children are at increased risk. Those receiving anticoagulants are more likely to lose blood into surrounding tissues if extravasation occurs, while those receiving sedatives or analgesics may not notice the early signs or symptoms of extravasation.

Prevention of extravasation
Precautions should be taken to avoid extravasation; ideally, drugs likely to cause extravasation injury should be given through a central line and children receiving repeated doses of hazardous drugs peripherally should have the cannula resited at regular intervals. Attention should be paid to the manufacturers' recommendations for administration. Placing a glyceryl trinitrate patch or using glyceryl trinitrate ointment distal to the cannula may improve the patency of the vessel in children with small veins or in those whose

veins are prone to collapse. Children or their carers should be asked to report any pain or burning at the site of injection immediately.

Management of extravasation
If extravasation is suspected the infusion should be stopped immediately but the cannula should not be removed until after an attempt has been made to aspirate the area (through the cannula) in order to remove as much of the drug as possible. Aspiration is sometimes possible if the extravasation presents with a raised bleb or blister at the injection site and is surrounded by hardened tissue, but it is often unsuccessful if the tissue is soft or soggy.
Corticosteroids are usually given to treat inflammation, although there is little evidence to support their use in extravasation. Hydrocortisone p. 633 or dexamethasone p. 419 can be given either locally by subcutaneous injection or intravenously at a site distant from the injury. Antihistamines and analgesics may be required for symptom relief.

  The management of extravasation beyond these measures is not well standardised and calls for specialist advice. Treatment depends on the nature of the offending substance; one approach is to localise and neutralise the substance whereas another is to spread and dilute it. The first method may be appropriate following extravasation of vesicant drugs and involves administration of an antidote (if available) and the application of cold compresses 3–4 times a day (consult specialist literature for details of specific antidotes). Spreading and diluting the offending substance involves infiltrating the area with physiological saline, applying warm compresses, elevating the affected limb, and administering hyaluronidase below. A saline flush-out technique (involving flushing the subcutaneous tissue with physiological saline) may be effective but requires specialist advice. Hyaluronidase should **not** be administered following extravasation of vesicant drugs (unless it is either specifically indicated or used in the saline flush-out technique).

Enzymes
Hyaluronidase is used for the management of extravasation.

ENZYMES

Hyaluronidase

● INDICATIONS AND DOSE
Extravasation
▸ BY LOCAL INFILTRATION
▸ **Child:** (consult product literature)

● **UNLICENSED USE** Licensed for use in children, but age range not specified by the manufacturer.

● **CONTRA-INDICATIONS** Avoid sites where infection is present · avoid sites where malignancy is present · do not apply direct to cornea · not for anaesthesia in unexplained premature labour · not for intravenous administration · not to be used to enhance the absorption and dispersion of dopamine and/or alpha-adrenoceptor agonists · not to be used to reduce swelling of bites · not to be used to reduce swelling of stings

● **CAUTIONS** Infants (control speed and total volume and avoid overhydration especially in renal impairment)

● **SIDE-EFFECTS**
▸ **Common or very common** Oedema
▸ **Rare** Bleeding · bruising · infection · local irritation
▸ **Frequency not known** Anaphylaxis · severe allergy

● MEDICINAL FORMS
There can be variation in the licensing of different medicines containing the same drug.
Powder for solution for injection
▸ Hyaluronidase (Non-proprietary)
  Hyaluronidase 1500 unit Hyaluronidase 1,500unit powder for solution for injection ampoules | 10 ampoule [PoM] £136.55

Chapter 11
Eye

CONTENTS

Eye

Administration of drugs to the eye

Drugs are most commonly administered to the eye by topical application as eye drops or eye ointments. When a higher drug concentration is required within the eye, a local injection may be necessary.

Eye-drop dispenser devices are available to aid the instillation of eye drops from plastic bottles and some are prescribable on the NHS (consult Drug Tariff—see Appliances and Reagents). Product-specific devices may be supplied by manufacturers—contact individual manufacturers for further information. They are particularly useful for children in whom normal application is difficult, for the visually impaired, or otherwise physically limited patients.

Eye drops and eye ointments

Eye drops are generally instilled into the pocket formed by gently pulling down the lower eyelid and keeping the eye closed for as long as possible after application; in neonates and infants it may be more appropriate to administer the drop in the inner angle of the open eye. One drop is all that is needed; instillation of more than one drop at a time should be discouraged because it may increase systemic side-effects. A small amount of eye ointment is applied similarly; the ointment melts rapidly and blinking helps to spread it.

When two different eye-drop preparations are used at the same time of day, dilution and overflow can occur when one immediately follows the other. The carer or child should therefore leave an interval of at least 5 minutes between the two; the interval should be extended when eye drops with a prolonged contact time, such as gels and suspensions, are used. Eye ointment should be applied after drops. Both drops and ointment can cause transient blurred vision; children should be warned, where appropriate, not to perform skilled tasks (e.g. cycling or driving) until vision is clear.

Systemic effects may arise from absorption of drugs into the general circulation from conjunctival vessels or from the nasal mucosa after the excess preparation has drained down through the tear ducts. The extent of systemic absorption following ocular administration is highly variable; nasal drainage of drugs is associated with eye drops much more often than with eye ointments. Pressure on the lacrimal punctum for at least a minute after applying eye drops reduces nasolacrimal drainage and therefore decreases systemic absorption from the nasal mucosa.

Also see warnings relating to eye drops and contact lenses.

Eye lotions

These are solutions for the irrigation of the conjunctival sac. They act mechanically to flush out irritants or foreign bodies as a first-aid treatment. Sterile sodium chloride 0.9% p. 645 solution is usually used. Clean water will suffice in an emergency.

Other preparations administered to the eye

Subconjunctival injection may be used to administer anti-infective drugs, mydriatics, or corticosteroids for conditions not responding to topical therapy; intracameral and intravitreal routes can also be used to administer certain drugs, for example antibacterials. These injections should only be used under specialist supervision.

Drugs such as antimicrobials and corticosteroids may be administered systemically to treat susceptible eye conditions.

Ophthalmic Specials

The Royal College of Ophthalmologists and the UK Ophthalmic Pharmacy Group have produced the Ophthalmic Specials Guidance to help prescribers and pharmacists manage and restrict the use of unlicensed eye preparations. 'Specials' should only be prescribed in situations where a licensed product will not be suitable for a child's needs. The Ophthalmic Specials Guidance can be accessed on the Royal College of Ophthalmologists website (www.rcophth.ac.uk). The guidance will be reviewed every six months to ensure the most accurate and up-to-date information is available.

Preservatives and sensitisers

Information on preservatives and substances identified as skin sensitisers is provided under Excipients statements in preparation entries. Very rarely, cases of corneal calcification have been reported with the use of phosphate-containing eye drops in patients with significantly damaged corneas—consult product literature for further information.

Control of microbial contamination

Preparations for the eye should be sterile when issued. Care should be taken to avoid contamination of the contents during use.

Eye drops in multiple-application containers for *domiciliary use* should not be used for more than 4 weeks after first opening (unless otherwise stated by the manufacturer).

Multiple application eye drops for use in *hospital wards* are normally discarded 1 week after first opening—local practice may vary. Individual containers should be provided for each patient. A separate container should be supplied for each eye only if there are special concerns about contamination. Containers used before an eye operation should be discarded at the time of the operation and fresh containers supplied postoperatively. A fresh supply should also be provided upon discharge from hospital; in specialist ophthalmology units, it may be acceptable to issue containers that have been dispensed to the patient on the day of discharge.

In *out-patient departments* single-application containers should be used; if multiple-application containers are used, they should be discarded after single patient use within one clinical session.

In *eye surgery* single-application containers should be used if possible; if a multiple-application container is used, it should be discarded after single use. Preparations used during intra-ocular procedures and others that may penetrate into the anterior chamber must be isotonic and without preservatives and buffered if necessary to a neutral pH. Specially formulated fluids should be used for intra-ocular surgery; intravenous infusion preparations are not usually suitable for this purpose (Hartmann's solution may be used in some ocular surgery). For all surgical procedures, a previously unopened container is used for each patient.

Contact lenses

For cosmetic reasons many people prefer to wear contact lenses rather than spectacles; contact lenses are also sometimes required for medical indications. Visual defects are corrected by either rigid ('hard' or gas permeable) lenses or soft (hydrogel or silicone hydrogel—in adults only) lenses; soft lenses are the most popular type, because they are initially the most comfortable, but they may not give the best vision. Lenses should usually be worn for a specified number of hours each day and removed for sleeping. The risk of infectious and non-infectious keratitis is increased by extended continuous contact lens wear, which is not recommended, except when medically indicated.

Contact lenses require meticulous care. Poor compliance with directions for use, and with daily cleaning and disinfection, can result in complications including ulcerative keratitis or conjunctivitis. One-day disposable lenses, which are worn only once and therefore require no disinfection or cleaning, are becoming increasingly popular.

Acanthamoeba keratitis, a painful and sight-threatening condition, is associated with ineffective lens cleaning and disinfection, the use of contaminated lens cases, or tap water coming into contact with the lenses. The condition is especially associated with the use of soft lenses (including frequently replaced lenses) and should be treated by specialists.

Contact lenses and drug treatment

Special care is required in prescribing eye preparations for contact lens users. Some drugs and preservatives in eye preparations can accumulate in hydrogel lenses and may induce toxic and adverse reactions. Therefore, unless medically indicated, the lenses should be removed before instillation of the eye preparation and not worn during the period of treatment. Alternatively, unpreserved drops can be used. Eye drops may, however, be instilled while patients are wearing rigid corneal contact lenses. Ointment preparations should never be used in conjunction with contact lens wear; oily eye drops should also be avoided.

Many drugs given systemically can also have adverse effects on contact lens wear. These include oral contraceptives (particularly those with a higher oestrogen content), drugs which reduce blink rate (e.g. anxiolytics, hypnotics, antihistamines, and muscle relaxants), drugs which reduce lacrimation (e.g. antihistamines, antimuscarinics, phenothiazines and related drugs, some beta-blockers, diuretics, and tricyclic antidepressants), and drugs which increase lacrimation (including ephedrine hydrochloride p. 120 and hydralazine hydrochloride p. 113). Other drugs that may affect contact lens wear are isotretinoin p. 727 (can cause conjunctival inflammation),

aspirin p. 89 (salicylic acid appears in tears and can be absorbed by contact lenses—leading to irritation), and rifampicin p. 349 and sulfasalazine p. 30 (can discolour lenses).

1 Allergic and inflammatory eye conditions

Eye, allergy and inflammation

Corticosteroids

Corticosteroids administered locally to the eye or given by mouth are effective for treating anterior segment inflammation, including that which results from surgery.

Topical corticosteroids should normally only be used under expert supervision; three main dangers are associated with their use:

- a 'red eye', when the diagnosis is unconfirmed, may be due to herpes simplex virus, and a corticosteroid may aggravate the condition, leading to corneal ulceration, with possible damage to vision and even loss of the eye. Bacterial, fungal, and amoebic infections pose a similar hazard;
- 'steroid glaucoma' can follow the use of corticosteroid eye preparations in susceptible individuals;
- a 'steroid cataract' can follow prolonged use.

Products combining a corticosteroid with an antimicrobial are used after ocular surgery to reduce inflammation and prevent infection: use of combination products is otherwise rarely justified.

Systemic corticosteroids may be useful for ocular conditions. The risk of producing a 'steroid cataract' increases with the dose and duration of corticosteroid use.

Other anti-inflammatory preparations

Eye drops containing **antihistamines**, such as **antazoline** (with xylometazoline hydrochloride p. 637 as *Otrivine-Antistin®*), azelastine hydrochloride p. 638, epinastine hydrochloride p. 638, ketotifen p. 638, and olopatadine p. 638, can be used for allergic conjunctivitis.

Sodium cromoglicate p. 639 and nedocromil sodium p. 639 eye drops may be useful for vernal keratoconjunctivitis and other allergic forms of conjunctivitis.

Lodoxamide eye drops p. 639 are used for allergic conjunctival conditions including seasonal allergic conjunctivitis.

Emedastine eye drops p. 638 are licensed for seasonal allergic conjunctivitis.

1.1 Allergic conjunctivitis

ANTIHISTAMINES

Antazoline with xylometazoline

- **INDICATIONS AND DOSE**
Allergic conjunctivitis
  ▸ TO THE EYE
  ▸ Child 12–17 years: Apply 2–3 times a day for maximum 7 days

- **CAUTIONS** Angle-closure glaucoma · cardiovascular disease · diabetes mellitus · hypertension · hyperthyroidism · phaeochromocytoma · urinary retention
- **INTERACTIONS** → Appendix 1: sympathomimetics, vasoconstrictor

11

Eye

- **SIDE-EFFECTS**
- ▶ **Common or very common** Transient stinging
- ▶ **Frequency not known** Blurred vision · eye irritation · mydriasis

SIDE-EFFECTS, FURTHER INFORMATION
Absorption of antazoline and xylometazoline may result in systemic side-effects.

- **MEDICINAL FORMS**
There can be variation in the licensing of different medicines containing the same drug.
Eye drops
EXCIPIENTS: May contain Benzalkonium chloride, disodium edetate
- ▶ **Otrivine Antistin** (Thea Pharmaceuticals Ltd)
Xylometazoline hydrochloride 500 microgram per 1 ml, Antazoline sulfate 5 mg per 1 ml Otrivine Antistin 0.5%/0.05% eye drops | 10 ml Ⓟ £3.35 DT price = £3.35

Azelastine hydrochloride

- **INDICATIONS AND DOSE**
Seasonal allergic conjunctivitis
- ▶ TO THE EYE
- ▶ Child 4-17 years: Apply twice daily, increased if necessary to 4 times a day
Perennial conjunctivitis
- ▶ TO THE EYE
- ▶ Child 12-17 years: Apply twice daily; increased if necessary to 4 times a day, maximum duration of treatment 6 weeks

- **INTERACTIONS** → Appendix 1: antihistamines (non-sedating)
- **SIDE-EFFECTS**
- ▶ Frequency not known Bitter taste · mild transient irritation

- **MEDICINAL FORMS**
There can be variation in the licensing of different medicines containing the same drug.
Eye drops
EXCIPIENTS: May contain Benzalkonium chloride, disodium edetate
- ▶ **Optilast** (Meda Pharmaceuticals Ltd)
Azelastine hydrochloride 500 microgram per 1 ml Optilast 0.05% eye drops | 8 ml PoM £6.40 DT price = £6.40

Emedastine

- **INDICATIONS AND DOSE**
Seasonal allergic conjunctivitis
- ▶ TO THE EYE
- ▶ Child 3-17 years: Apply twice daily

- **SIDE-EFFECTS** Blurred vision · corneal infiltrates (discontinue) · corneal staining · dry eye · headache · irritation · keratitis · lacrimation · local oedema · photophobia · rhinitis · transient burning · transient stinging

- **MEDICINAL FORMS**
There can be variation in the licensing of different medicines containing the same drug.
No licensed medicines listed.

Epinastine hydrochloride

- **INDICATIONS AND DOSE**
Seasonal allergic conjunctivitis
- ▶ TO THE EYE
- ▶ Child 12-17 years: Apply twice daily for maximum 8 weeks

- **SIDE-EFFECTS**
- ▶ **Common or very common** Burning
- ▶ **Uncommon** Conjunctival hyperaemia · dry eye · eye pain · eye pruritus · headache · increased lacrimation · nasal irritation · rhinitis · taste disturbance · visual disturbance

- **MEDICINAL FORMS**
There can be variation in the licensing of different medicines containing the same drug.
Eye drops
EXCIPIENTS: May contain Benzalkonium chloride, disodium edetate
- ▶ **Relestat** (Allergan Ltd)
Epinastine hydrochloride 500 microgram per 1 ml Relestat 500micrograms/ml eye drops | 5 ml PoM £9.90 DT price = £9.90

Ketotifen

- **INDICATIONS AND DOSE**
Seasonal allergic conjunctivitis
- ▶ TO THE EYE
- ▶ Child 3-17 years: Apply twice daily

- **INTERACTIONS** → Appendix 1: antihistamines (sedating)
- **SIDE-EFFECTS**
- ▶ **Common or very common** Punctate corneal epithelial erosion · transient burning · transient stinging
- ▶ **Uncommon** Dry eye · photophobia · subconjunctival haemorrhage
- ▶ **Frequency not known** Drowsiness · dry mouth · headache · skin reactions

- **MEDICINAL FORMS**
There can be variation in the licensing of different medicines containing the same drug.
Eye drops
EXCIPIENTS: May contain Benzalkonium chloride
- ▶ **Zaditen** (Thea Pharmaceuticals Ltd)
Ketotifen (as Ketotifen fumarate) 250 microgram per 1 ml Zaditen 250micrograms/ml eye drops | 5 ml PoM £7.80 DT price = £7.80

Olopatadine

- **INDICATIONS AND DOSE**
Seasonal allergic conjunctivitis
- ▶ TO THE EYE
- ▶ Child 3-17 years: Apply twice daily for maximum 4 months

- **SIDE-EFFECTS**
- ▶ **Common or very common** Local irritation
- ▶ **Uncommon** Asthenia · dizziness · dry eye · headache · keratitis · local oedema · photophobia
- ▶ **Frequency not known** Dry nose

- **MEDICINAL FORMS**
There can be variation in the licensing of different medicines containing the same drug.
Eye drops
EXCIPIENTS: May contain Benzalkonium chloride
- ▶ **Opatanol** (Alcon Laboratories (UK) Ltd)
Olopatadine (as Olopatadine hydrochloride) 1 mg per 1 ml Opatanol 1mg/ml eye drops | 5 ml PoM £4.68 DT price = £4.68

MAST-CELL STABILISERS

Lodoxamide

• INDICATIONS AND DOSE

Allergic conjunctivitis
▸ TO THE EYE
▸ Child 4-17 years: Apply 4 times a day, improvement of symptoms may sometimes require treatment for up to 4 weeks

• SIDE-EFFECTS
▸ **Common or very common** Blurred vision · burning · itching · ocular discomfort · stinging · tear production disturbance
▸ **Uncommon** Blepharitis · dizziness · drowsiness · flushing · headache · keratitis · nasal dryness
● **EXCEPTIONS TO LEGAL CATEGORY** Lodoxamide 0.1% eye drops can be sold to the public for treatment of allergic conjunctivitis in children over 4 years.

• MEDICINAL FORMS
There can be variation in the licensing of different medicines containing the same drug.

Eye drops
EXCIPIENTS: May contain Benzalkonium chloride, disodium edetate
▸ **Alomide** (Alcon Laboratories (UK) Ltd)
Lodoxamide (as Lodoxamide trometamol) 1 mg per 1 ml Alomide 0.1% eye drops | 10 ml PoM £5.21 DT price = £5.21
Alomide Allergy 0.1% eye drops | 5 ml P £3.12

Nedocromil sodium

• INDICATIONS AND DOSE

Seasonal and perennial conjunctivitis
▸ TO THE EYE
▸ Child 6-17 years: Apply twice daily, increased if necessary to 4 times a day, max.12 weeks duration of treatment for seasonal allergic conjunctivitis

Seasonal keratoconjunctivitis
▸ TO THE EYE
▸ Child 6-17 years: Apply 4 times a day

● **SIDE-EFFECTS** Distinctive taste · transient burning · transient stinging

• MEDICINAL FORMS
There can be variation in the licensing of different medicines containing the same drug.

Eye drops
EXCIPIENTS: May contain Benzalkonium chloride, disodium edetate
▸ **Rapitil** (Sanofi)
Nedocromil sodium 20 mg per 1 ml Rapitil 2% eye drops | 5 ml PoM £2.86 DT price = £2.86

Sodium cromoglicate

(Sodium cromoglycate)

• INDICATIONS AND DOSE

Allergic conjunctivitis | Seasonal keratoconjunctivitis
▸ TO THE EYE
▸ Child: Apply 4 times a day

● **SIDE-EFFECTS** Transient burning · transient stinging
● **PREGNANCY** Not known to be harmful. Inhaled drugs can be taken as normal during pregnancy.
● **EXCEPTIONS TO LEGAL CATEGORY** Sodium cromoglicate 2% eye drops can be sold to the public (in max. pack size of 10 mL) for treatment of acute seasonal and perennial allergic conjunctivitis.

• MEDICINAL FORMS
There can be variation in the licensing of different medicines containing the same drug. Forms available from special-order manufacturers include: eye drops

Eye drops
▸ **Sodium cromoglicate** (Non-proprietary)
Sodium cromoglicate 20 mg per 1 ml Sodium cromoglicate 2% eye drops | 13.5 ml PoM £8.03 DT price = £2.35
▸ **Cromolux** (Tubilux Pharma Ltd)
Sodium cromoglicate 20 mg per 1 ml Cromolux 2% eye drops | 13.5 ml PoM £3.20 DT price = £2.35
▸ **Opticrom** (Sanofi)
Sodium cromoglicate 20 mg per 1 ml Opticrom Aqueous 2% eye drops | 13.5 ml PoM £8.03 DT price = £2.35
▸ **Vividrin** (Bausch & Lomb UK Ltd)
Sodium cromoglicate 20 mg per 1 ml Vividrin 2% eye drops | 13.5 ml PoM £10.95 DT price = £2.35

1.2 Inflammatory eye conditions

CORTICOSTEROIDS

Betamethasone

• INDICATIONS AND DOSE

Local treatment of inflammation (short-term)
▸ TO THE EYE USING EYE DROP
▸ Child: Apply every 1–2 hours until controlled then reduce frequency
▸ TO THE EYE USING EYE OINTMENT
▸ Child: Apply 2–4 times a day, alternatively apply at night when used in combination with eye drops

● **INTERACTIONS** → Appendix 1: corticosteroids
● **SIDE-EFFECTS** Adrenal suppression following prolonged use in neonates · corneal thinning · scleral thinning

• MEDICINAL FORMS
There can be variation in the licensing of different medicines containing the same drug.

Ear/eye/nose drops solution
EXCIPIENTS: May contain Benzalkonium chloride, disodium edetate
▸ **Betamethasone** (Non-proprietary)
Betamethasone sodium phosphate 1 mg per 1 ml Betamethasone 0.1% ear/eye/nose drops | 5 ml PoM no price available
▸ **Betnesol** (Focus Pharmaceuticals Ltd)
Betamethasone sodium phosphate 1 mg per 1 ml Betnesol 0.1% eye/ear/nose drops | 10 ml PoM £2.32 DT price = £2.32
▸ **Vistamethasone** (Martindale Pharmaceuticals Ltd)
Betamethasone sodium phosphate 1 mg per 1 ml Vistamethasone 0.1% ear/eye/nose drops | 5 ml PoM £0.87 | 10 ml PoM £0.99 DT price = £2.32

Eye ointment
▸ **Betnesol** (Focus Pharmaceuticals Ltd)
Betamethasone sodium phosphate 1 mg per 1 gram Betnesol 0.1% eye ointment | 3 gram PoM £1.41 DT price = £1.41

Combinations available: *Betamethasone with neomycin*, p. 640

Dexamethasone

06-Jun-2016

• INDICATIONS AND DOSE

Local treatment of inflammation (short-term)
▸ TO THE EYE USING EYE DROP
▸ Child: Apply 4–6 times a day

Short term local treatment of inflammation (severe conditions)
▸ TO THE EYE USING EYE DROP
▸ Child: Apply every 30–60 minutes until controlled, reduce frequency when control achieved

11

Eye

● UNLICENSED USE *Maxidex*® not licensed for use in children under 2 years. *Dropodex*® not licensed for use in children.

● INTERACTIONS → Appendix 1: corticosteroids

● SIDE-EFFECTS Adrenal suppression following prolonged use in neonates · corneal thinning · scleral thinning

● PREGNANCY Dexamethasone readily crosses the placenta.

● PRESCRIBING AND DISPENSING INFORMATION Although multi-dose Dexamethasone eye drops commonly contain preservatives, preservative-free unit dose vials may be available.

● MEDICINAL FORMS
There can be variation in the licensing of different medicines containing the same drug. Forms available from special-order manufacturers include: eye drops
Eye drops
EXCIPIENTS: May contain Benzalkonium chloride, disodium edetate, polysorbates
▸ **Dexamethasone (Non-proprietary)**
Dexamethasone sodium phosphate 1 mg per 1 ml Dexamethasone 0.1% eye drops 0.4ml unit dose preservative free | 20 unit dose PoM £9.75 DT price = £9.75
Minims dexamethasone 0.1% eye drops 0.5ml unit dose | 20 unit dose PoM £11.46 DT price = £11.46
▸ **Dexafree** (Thea Pharmaceuticals Ltd)
Dexamethasone sodium phosphate 1 mg per 1 ml Dexafree 1mg/1ml eye drops 0.4ml unit dose | 30 unit dose PoM £9.70
▸ **Dropodex** (Rayner Pharmaceuticals Ltd)
Dexamethasone sodium phosphate 1 mg per 1 ml Dropodex 0.1% eye drops 0.4ml unit dose | 20 unit dose PoM £9.75 DT price = £9.75
▸ **Maxidex** (Alcon Laboratories (UK) Ltd)
Dexamethasone 1 mg per 1 ml Maxidex 0.1% eye drops | 5 ml PoM £1.42 DT price = £1.42 | 10 ml PoM £2.80 DT price = £2.80

Combinations available: *Dexamethasone with framycetin sulfate and gramicidin*, below · *Dexamethasone with hypromellose, neomycin and polymyxin B sulfate*, p. 641

Fluorometholone

● INDICATIONS AND DOSE
Local treatment of inflammation (short term)
▸ TO THE EYE
  ▸ Child 2-17 years: Apply every 1 hour for 24–48 hours, then reduced to 2–4 times a day

● UNLICENSED USE Not licensed for use in children under 2 years.

● SIDE-EFFECTS Adrenal suppression following prolonged use in neonates · corneal thinning · scleral thinning

● MEDICINAL FORMS
There can be variation in the licensing of different medicines containing the same drug.
Eye drops
EXCIPIENTS: May contain Benzalkonium chloride, disodium edetate, polysorbates
▸ **FML Liquifilm** (Allergan Ltd)
Fluorometholone 1 mg per 1 ml FML Liquifilm 0.1% ophthalmic suspension | 5 ml PoM £1.71 DT price = £1.71 | 10 ml PoM £2.95 DT price = £2.95

Prednisolone

● INDICATIONS AND DOSE
Local treatment of inflammation (short-term)
▸ TO THE EYE
  ▸ Child: Apply every 1–2 hours until controlled then reduce frequency

● UNLICENSED USE *Pred Forte*® not licensed for use in children (age range not specified by manufacturer).

● INTERACTIONS → Appendix 1: corticosteroids

● SIDE-EFFECTS Adrenal suppression following prolonged use in neonates · corneal thinning · scleral thinning

● PRESCRIBING AND DISPENSING INFORMATION Although multi-dose prednisolone eye drops commonly contain preservatives, preservative-free unit dose vials may be available.

● MEDICINAL FORMS
There can be variation in the licensing of different medicines containing the same drug. Forms available from special-order manufacturers eye drops
Eye drops
EXCIPIENTS: May contain Benzalkonium chloride, disodium edetate, polysorbates
▸ **Prednisolone (Non-proprietary)**
Prednisolone sodium phosphate 5 mg per 1 ml Minims prednisolone sodium phosphate 0.5% eye drops 0.5ml unit dose | 20 unit dose PoM £11.78 DT price = £11.78
▸ **Pred Forte** (Allergan Ltd)
Prednisolone acetate 10 mg per 1 ml Pred Forte 1% eye drops | 5 ml PoM £1.82 DT price = £1.82 | 10 ml PoM £3.66 DT price = £3.66
Ear/eye drops solution
EXCIPIENTS: May contain Benzalkonium chloride, disodium edetate
▸ **Predsol** (Focus Pharmaceuticals Ltd)
Prednisolone sodium phosphate 5 mg per 1 ml Predsol 0.5% ear/eye drops | 10 ml PoM £2.00 DT price = £2.00

CORTICOSTEROIDS 〉 CORTICOSTEROID COMBINATIONS WITH ANTI-INFECTIVES

Betamethasone with neomycin

The properties listed below are those particular to the combination only. For the properties of the components please consider, betamethasone p. 639, neomycin sulfate p. 662.

● INDICATIONS AND DOSE
Local treatment of eye inflammation and bacterial infection (short-term)
▸ TO THE EYE USING EYE DROP
▸ Child: (consult product literature)

● LESS SUITABLE FOR PRESCRIBING Betamethasone with neomycin eye-drops are less suitable for prescribing.

● MEDICINAL FORMS
There can be variation in the licensing of different medicines containing the same drug.
Ear/eye/nose drops solution
EXCIPIENTS: May contain Benzalkonium chloride, disodium edetate
▸ **Betnesol-N** (Focus Pharmaceuticals Ltd)
Betamethasone (as Betamethasone sodium phosphate) 1 mg per 1 ml, Neomycin sulfate 5 mg per 1 ml Betnesol-N ear/eye/nose drops | 10 ml PoM £2.39 DT price = £2.39

Dexamethasone with framycetin sulfate and gramicidin

The properties listed below are those particular to the combination only. For the properties of the components please consider, dexamethasone p. 639, framycetin sulfate p. 661.

● INDICATIONS AND DOSE
Local treatment of inflammation (short-term)
▸ TO THE EYE
▸ Child: Apply 4–6 times a day, may be administered every 30–60 minutes in severe conditions until controlled, then reduce frequency

- **LESS SUITABLE FOR PRESCRIBING** *Sofradex*® is less suitable for prescribing.

- **MEDICINAL FORMS**
There can be variation in the licensing of different medicines containing the same drug.
  Ear/eye drops solution
  EXCIPIENTS: May contain Polysorbates
  ▸ Sofradex (Sanofi)
  Gramicidin 50 microgram per 1 ml, Dexamethasone (as Dexamethasone sodium metasulfobenzoate) 500 microgram per 1 ml, Framycetin sulfate 5 mg per 1 ml Sofradex ear/eye drops | 10 ml PoM £7.50

Dexamethasone with hypromellose, neomycin and polymyxin B sulfate

The properties listed below are those particular to the combination only. For the properties of the components please consider, dexamethasone p. 639, neomycin sulfate p. 662.

- **INDICATIONS AND DOSE**
  Local treatment of inflammation (short-term)
  ▸ TO THE EYE USING EYE DROP
  ▸ Child: Apply every 30–60 minutes until controlled, then reduced to 4–6 times a day
  Local treatment of inflammation (short-term)
  ▸ TO THE EYE USING EYE OINTMENT
  ▸ Child: Apply 3–4 times a day, alternatively, apply at night when used with eye drops

- **LESS SUITABLE FOR PRESCRIBING** Dexamethasone with neomycin and polymyxin B sulfate is less suitable for prescribing.

- **MEDICINAL FORMS**
There can be variation in the licensing of different medicines containing the same drug.
  Eye ointment
  EXCIPIENTS: May contain Hydroxybenzoates (parabens), wool fat and related substances including lanolin
  ▸ Maxitrol (Alcon Laboratories (UK) Ltd)
  Dexamethasone 1 mg per 1 gram, Neomycin (as Neomycin sulfate) 3500 unit per 1 gram, Polymyxin B sulfate 6000 unit per 1 gram Maxitrol eye ointment | 3.5 gram PoM £1.44
  Eye drops
  EXCIPIENTS: May contain Benzalkonium chloride, polysorbates
  ▸ Maxitrol (Alcon Laboratories (UK) Ltd)
  Dexamethasone 1 mg per 1 ml, Hypromellose 5 mg per 1 ml, Neomycin (as Neomycin sulfate) 3500 unit per 1 ml, Polymyxin B sulfate 6000 unit per 1 ml Maxitrol eye drops | 5 ml PoM £1.68

1.2a Anterior uveitis

ANTIMUSCARINICS

Antimuscarinics (eye)

- **CAUTIONS** Children under 3 months owing to the possible association between cycloplegia and the development of amblyopia · darkly pigmented iris is more resistant to pupillary dilatation and caution should be exercised to avoid overdosage · mydriasis can precipitate acute angle-closure glaucoma (usually in those who are predisposed to the condition because of a shallow anterior chamber) · neonates at increased risk of systemic toxicity

- **SIDE-EFFECTS** Conjunctivitis (on prolonged administration) · contact dermatitis · eye oedema (on prolonged administration) · hyperaemia (on prolonged administration) · local irritation (on prolonged administration) · raised intraocular pressure · transient stinging

- **PATIENT AND CARER ADVICE** Patients may not be able to undertake skilled tasks until vision clears after mydriasis.

Atropine sulfate

- **INDICATIONS AND DOSE**
  Cycloplegia
  ▸ TO THE EYE USING EYE DROP
  ▸ Child 3 months–17 years: Apply twice daily for 3 days, before procedure
  Anterior uveitis
  ▸ TO THE EYE USING EYE DROP
  ▸ Child 2–17 years: Apply 1 drop up to 4 times a day

- **UNLICENSED USE** Not licensed for use in children for uveitis.

- **INTERACTIONS** → Appendix 1: atropine

- **SIDE-EFFECTS**
  SIDE-EFFECTS, FURTHER INFORMATION Toxic systemic reactions can occur. Systemic side-effects can occur.

- **PRESCRIBING AND DISPENSING INFORMATION** Although multi-dose atropine sulphate eye drops commonly contain preservatives, preservative-free unit dose vials may be available.

- **MEDICINAL FORMS**
There can be variation in the licensing of different medicines containing the same drug. Forms available from special-order manufacturers include: eye drops
  Eye drops
  ▸ Atropine sulfate (Non-proprietary)
  Atropine sulfate 10 mg per 1 ml Atropine 1% eye drops | 10 ml PoM £108.47 DT price = £89.80
  ▸ Atropine sulfate (Bausch & Lomb UK Ltd)
  Atropine sulfate 10 mg per 1 ml Minims atropine sulfate 1% eye drops 0.5ml unit dose | 20 unit dose PoM £15.10 DT price = £15.10

Cyclopentolate hydrochloride

- **INDICATIONS AND DOSE**
  Cycloplegia
  ▸ TO THE EYE
  ▸ Child 3 months–11 years: Apply 1 drop, 30–60 minutes before examination, using 1% eye drops
  ▸ Child 12–17 years: Apply 1 drop, 30–60 minutes before examination, using 0.5% eye drops
  Uveitis
  ▸ TO THE EYE
  ▸ Child 3 months–17 years: Apply 1 drop 2–4 times a day, using 0.5% eye drops (1% for deeply pigmented eyes)

- **INTERACTIONS** → Appendix 1: cyclopentolate

- **SIDE-EFFECTS**
  SIDE-EFFECTS, FURTHER INFORMATION
  Toxic systemic reactions can occur. Systemic side-effects can occur.

- **PRESCRIBING AND DISPENSING INFORMATION** Although multi-dose cyclopentolate eye drops commonly contain preservatives, preservative-free unit dose vials may be available.

11

Eye

- **MEDICINAL FORMS**
There can be variation in the licensing of different medicines containing the same drug.
Eye drops
EXCIPIENTS: May contain Benzalkonium chloride
▸ **Cyclopentolate hydrochloride** (Bausch & Lomb UK Ltd)
Cyclopentolate hydrochloride 5 mg per 1 ml Minims cyclopentolate hydrochloride 0.5% eye drops 0.5ml unit dose | 20 unit dose [PoM] £10.97 DT price = £10.97
Cyclopentolate hydrochloride 10 mg per 1 ml Minims cyclopentolate hydrochloride 1% eye drops 0.5ml unit dose | 20 unit dose [PoM] £11.23 DT price = £11.23
▸ **Mydrilate** (Intrapharm Laboratories Ltd)
Cyclopentolate hydrochloride 5 mg per 1 ml Mydrilate 0.5% solution | 5 ml [PoM] £6.73 DT price = £6.73
Cyclopentolate hydrochloride 10 mg per 1 ml Mydrilate 1% solution | 5 ml [PoM] £6.73 DT price = £6.73

▶ 641

Homatropine hydrobromide

- **INDICATIONS AND DOSE**
Anterior uveitis
▸ TO THE EYE
▸ Child 3 months–1 year: Apply 1 drop daily, alternatively apply 1 drop once daily on alternate days, adjusted according to response, only 0.5% eye drops to be used
▸ Child 2–17 years: Apply 1 drop twice daily, adjusted according to response

- **INTERACTIONS** → Appendix 1: homatropine

- **MEDICINAL FORMS**
There can be variation in the licensing of different medicines containing the same drug. Forms available from special-order manufacturers include: eye drops

2 Dry eye conditions

Dry eye

Tear deficiency, ocular lubricants, and astringents

Chronic soreness of the eyes associated with reduced or abnormal tear secretion often responds to tear replacement therapy. The severity of the condition and child's preference will often guide the choice of preparation.

Hypromellose p. 643 is the traditional choice of treatment for tear deficiency. It may need to be instilled frequently (e.g. hourly) for adequate relief. Ocular surface mucin is often abnormal in tear deficiency and the combination of hypromellose with a mucolytic such as acetylcysteine below can be helpful.

The ability of **carbomers** to cling to the eye surface may help reduce frequency of application to 4 times daily.

Polyvinyl alcohol p. 644 increases the persistence of the tear film and is useful when the ocular surface mucin is reduced.

Sodium hyaluronate eye drops p. 645 are also used in the management of tear deficiency.

Sodium chloride 0.9% drops p. 645 are sometimes useful in tear deficiency, and can be used as 'comfort drops' by contact lens wearers, and to facilitate lens removal. Special presentations of sodium chloride 0.9% and other irrigation solutions are used routinely for intra-ocular surgery and in first aid for removal of harmful substances.

Eye ointments containing a paraffin can be used to lubricate the eye surface, especially in cases of recurrent corneal epithelial erosion. They may cause temporary visual disturbance and are best suited for application before sleep. Ointments should not be used during contact lens wear.

OCULAR LUBRICANTS

Acetylcysteine

07-Feb-2017

- **INDICATIONS AND DOSE**
Tear deficiency | Impaired or abnormal mucus production
▸ TO THE EYE
▸ Child: Apply 3–4 times a day

- **MEDICINAL FORMS**
There can be variation in the licensing of different medicines containing the same drug. Forms available from special-order manufacturers include: eye drops
Eye drops
EXCIPIENTS: May contain Benzalkonium chloride, disodium edetate
▸ **Ilube** (Rayner Pharmaceuticals Ltd)
Acetylcysteine 50 mg per 1 ml Ilube 5% eye drops | 10 ml [PoM] £14.93 DT price = £14.93

Carbomers

(Polyacrylic acid)

- **INDICATIONS AND DOSE**
Dry eyes including keratoconjunctivitis sicca, unstable tear film
▸ TO THE EYE
▸ Child: Apply 3–4 times a day or when required

- **UNLICENSED USE** Some preparations not licensed for use in children.

- **PRESCRIBING AND DISPENSING INFORMATION** Synthetic high molecular weight polymers of acrylic acid cross-linked with either allyl ethers of sucrose or allyl ethers of pentaerithrityl.

- **MEDICINAL FORMS**
There can be variation in the licensing of different medicines containing the same drug.
Eye gel
EXCIPIENTS: May contain Benzalkonium chloride, cetrimide, disodium edetate
▸ **Blephagel** (Thea Pharmaceuticals Ltd)
Carbomer 3.5 mg per 1 gram Blephagel 0.35% eye gel | 40 gram £6.66
Carbomer 3.6 mg per 1 gram Blephagel 0.36% eye gel preservative free | 30 gram £7.53
▸ **Liquivisc** (Thea Pharmaceuticals Ltd)
Carbomer 974P 2.5 mg per 1 gram Liquivisc 0.25% eye gel | 10 gram [P] £4.50 DT price = £4.50
Eye drops
▸ **Carbomers** (Non-proprietary)
Carbomer 980 2 mg per 1 gram EyeGel 0.2% eye gel | 10 gram £2.80 DT price = £2.80
Carbomer '980' 0.2% eye drops | 10 gram [P] £2.80 DT price = £2.80
Carbomer 0.2% eye gel | 10 gram £2.80 DT price = £2.80
▸ **Artelac Nighttime** (Bausch & Lomb UK Ltd)
Carbomer 980 2 mg per 1 gram Artelac Nighttime 0.2% eye gel | 10 gram £2.96 DT price = £2.80
▸ **Clinitas Carbomer** (Altacor Ltd)
Carbomer 980 2 mg per 1 gram Clinitas Carbomer 0.2% eye gel | 10 gram £1.49 DT price = £2.80
▸ **GelTears** (Bausch & Lomb UK Ltd)
Carbomer 980 2 mg per 1 gram GelTears 0.2% gel | 10 gram [P] £2.80 DT price = £2.80
▸ **Lumecare Long Lasting** (Medicom Healthcare Ltd)
Carbomer 980 2 mg per 1 gram Lumecare Carbomer 0.2% eye gel | 10 gram £1.51 DT price = £2.80
▸ **Viscotears** (Bausch & Lomb UK Ltd)
Carbomer 980 2 mg per 1 gram Viscotears 2mg/g liquid gel | 10 gram [P] £1.59 DT price = £2.80
Viscotears 2mg/g eye gel 0.6ml unit dose | 30 unit dose [P] £5.42 DT price = £5.42

▸ **Xailin** (Nicox Pharma)
Carbomer 980 2 mg per 1 gram Xailin 0.2% eye gel | 10 gram
£3.25 DT price = £2.80

Carmellose sodium

● **INDICATIONS AND DOSE**
Dry eye conditions
▸ TO THE EYE
▸ **Child:** Apply as required

● **PRESCRIBING AND DISPENSING INFORMATION** Some
preparations are contained units which are resealable and
may be used for up to 12 hours.

● **MEDICINAL FORMS**
There can be variation in the licensing of different medicines
containing the same drug.
Eye drops
▸ Carmellose sodium (Non-proprietary)
Carmellose sodium 5 mg per 1 ml Carmellose 0.5% eye drops 0.4ml
unit dose preservative free | 30 unit dose Ⓟ no price available DT
price = £4.80 | 30 unit dose £5.75 DT price = £4.80 | 90 unit dose Ⓟ
no price available
Carmellose 0.5% eye drops | 10 ml £7.49
Carmellose 1% eye drops 0.4ml unit dose preservative free | 30 unit
dose PoM no price available DT price = £3.00 | 30 unit dose £3.00 DT
price = £3.00 | 30 unit dose Ⓟ no price available DT price = £3.00 |
60 unit dose Ⓟ no price available
▸ Carmeleze (Martindale Pharmaceuticals Ltd)
Carmellose sodium 5 mg per 1 ml Melophthal 0.5% eye drops 0.4ml
unit dose | 30 unit dose £5.75 DT price = £4.80
Melophthal 1% eye drops 0.4ml unit dose | 30 unit dose £3.00 DT price
= £3.00
▸ Carmellose (Moorfields Pharmaceuticals, Medicom Healthcare Ltd)
PF Drops Carmellose 0.5% eye drops preservative free | 10 ml £7.49
PF Drops Carmellose 1% eye drops preservative free | 10 ml £7.49
Lumecare Advance Carmellose 0.5% eye drops | 10 ml £5.99
▸ Carmize (Aspire Pharma Ltd)
Carmellose sodium 5 mg per 1 ml Carmize 0.5% eye drops 0.4ml
unit dose preservative free | 30 unit dose £5.75 DT price = £4.80 |
90 unit dose £15.53
Carmize 1% eye drops | 10 ml £8.49
Carmize 1% eye drops 0.4ml unit dose preservative free | 30 unit dose
£3.00 DT price = £3.00 | 60 unit dose £6.00
Carmize 0.5% eye drops | 10 ml £7.49
▸ Cellusan (Farmigea S.p.A.)
Carmellose sodium 5 mg per 1 ml Cellusan Light 0.5% eye drops
0.4ml unit dose preservative free | 30 unit dose £5.75 DT price = £4.80
Cellusan 1% eye drops preservative free | 10 ml £4.80
Cellusan 1% eye drops 0.4ml unit dose preservative free | 30 unit
dose £3.00 DT price = £3.00
Cellusan Light 0.5% eye drops preservative free | 10 ml £4.80
▸ Celluvisc (Allergan Ltd)
Carmellose sodium 5 mg per 1 ml Celluvisc 0.5% eye drops 0.4ml
unit dose | 30 unit dose Ⓟ £4.80 DT price = £4.80 | 90 unit dose Ⓟ
£15.53
Celluvisc 1% eye drops 0.4ml unit dose | 30 unit dose Ⓟ £3.00 DT
price = £3.00 | 60 unit dose Ⓟ £10.99
▸ Lumecare (Carmellose) (Medicom Healthcare Ltd)
Carmellose sodium 5 mg per 1 ml Lumecare Singles Carmellose
0.5% eye drops 0.4ml unit dose | 30 unit dose £4.60 DT price = £4.80
▸ Optho-Lique (Essential-Healthcare Ltd)
Optho-Lique 0.5% eye drops | 10 ml £3.73
Optho-Lique Forte 1% eye drops | 10 ml £5.47
▸ Optive (Allergan Ltd)
Optive 0.5% eye drops | 10 ml £7.49
▸ Optive Plus (Allergan Ltd)
Optive Plus 0.5% eye drops | 10 ml £7.49
▸ Xailin Fresh (Nicox Pharma)
Carmellose sodium 5 mg per 1 ml Xailin Fresh 0.5% eye drops 0.4ml
unit dose | 30 unit dose £3.84 DT price = £4.80

Hydroxyethylcellulose

● **INDICATIONS AND DOSE**
Tear deficiency
▸ TO THE EYE
▸ **Child:** Apply as required

● **PRESCRIBING AND DISPENSING INFORMATION** Although
multi-dose hydroxyethylcellulose eye drops commonly
contain preservatives, preservative-free unit dose vials
may be available.

● **MEDICINAL FORMS**
There can be variation in the licensing of different medicines
containing the same drug.
Eye drops
▸ Artificial tears (Bausch & Lomb UK Ltd)
Hydroxyethylcellulose 4.4 mg per 1 ml Minims artificial tears
0.44% eye drops 0.5ml unit dose | 20 unit dose Ⓟ £8.97

Hydroxypropyl guar with polyethylene glycol and propylene glycol
(Formulated as an ocular lubricant)

● **INDICATIONS AND DOSE**
Dry eye conditions
▸ TO THE EYE
▸ **Child:** Apply as required

● **MEDICINAL FORMS**
There can be variation in the licensing of different medicines
containing the same drug.
Eye drops
▸ Systane (Novartis Pharmaceuticals UK Ltd)
Systane Gel eye drops | 10 ml Ⓟ £7.49

Hypromellose

● **INDICATIONS AND DOSE**
Tear deficiency
▸ TO THE EYE
▸ **Child:** Apply as required

● **PRESCRIBING AND DISPENSING INFORMATION** The Royal
Pharmaceutical Society has stated that where it is not
possible to ascertain the strength of hypromellose prescribed,
the prescriber should be contacted to clarify
the strength intended.
Although multi-dose hypromellose eye drops commonly
contain preservatives, preservative-free unit dose vials
may be available.

● **MEDICINAL FORMS**
There can be variation in the licensing of different medicines
containing the same drug. Forms available from special-order
manufacturers include: eye drops
Eye drops
EXCIPIENTS: May contain Benzalkonium chloride, cetrimide, disodium
edetate
▸ Hypromellose (Non-proprietary)
Hypromellose 3 mg per 1 ml Hypromellose 0.3% eye drops
preservative free | 10 ml £5.75
Hypromellose 0.3% eye drops | 10 ml £0.99–£1.50 DT price = £1.42 |
10 ml Ⓟ £1.42 DT price = £1.42
▸ Artelac (Bausch & Lomb UK Ltd)
Hypromellose 3.2 mg per 1 ml Artelac Single Dose Unit 0.32% eye
drops 0.5ml unit dose | 30 unit dose Ⓟ £16.95 | 60 unit dose Ⓟ
£32.85
Artelac 0.32% eye drops | 10 ml Ⓟ £4.99
▸ Hydromoor (Moorfields Pharmaceuticals)
Hydromoor 0.3% eye drops 0.4ml unit dose preservative free | 30 unit
dose £5.75

11

Eye

‣ **Hypromellose** (Moorfields Pharmaceuticals)
  Hypromellose 3 mg per 1 ml PF Drops Hypromellose 0.3% eye drops preservative free │ 10 ml £5.75
‣ **Hypromol** (Ennogen Healthcare Ltd)
  Hypromellose 3 mg per 1 ml Hypromol 0.3% eye drops preservative free │ 10 ml £4.55
‣ **Isopto Alkaline** (Alcon Laboratories (UK) Ltd)
  Hypromellose 10 mg per 1 ml Isopto Alkaline 1% eye drops │ 10 ml ℗ £0.94 DT price = £0.94
‣ **Isopto Plain** (Alcon Laboratories (UK) Ltd)
  Hypromellose 5 mg per 1 ml Isopto Plain 0.5% eye drops │ 10 ml ℗ £0.81 DT price = £0.81
‣ **Lumecare (Hypromellose)** (Medicom Healthcare Ltd)
  Hypromellose 3 mg per 1 ml Lumecare Hypromellose 0.3% eye drops │ 10 ml £1.67 DT price = £1.42
‣ **Lumecare Tear Drops** (Medicom Healthcare Ltd)
  Hypromellose 3 mg per 1 ml Lumecare Tear Drops 0.3% eye drops │ 10 ml £0.79 DT price = £1.42
‣ **Mandanol (Hydroxypropyl methylcellulose)** (M & A Pharmachem Ltd)
  Hypromellose 3 mg per 1 ml Mandanol eye drops │ 10 ml £1.33 DT price £1.12
‣ **Ocu-Lube** (Sai-Meds Ltd)
  Hypromellose 3 mg per 1 ml Ocu-Lube 0.3% eye drops preservative free │ 10 ml £5.75
‣ **SoftDrops** (Farmigea S.p.A.)
  Hypromellose 3 mg per 1 ml SoftDrops 0.3% eye drops │ 10 ml £1.67 DT price = £1.42
‣ **Tear-Lac** (Scope Ophthalmics Ltd)
  Hypromellose 3 mg per 1 ml Tear-Lac Hypromellose 0.3% eye drops preservative free │ 10 ml £5.75
‣ **Vizulize Hypromellose** (East Midlands Pharma Ltd)
  Hypromellose 3 mg per 1 ml Vizulize Hypromellose 0.3% eye drops │ 10 ml £1.25 DT price = £1.42
‣ **Xailin Hydrate** (Nicox Pharma)
  Hypromellose 3 mg per 1 ml Xailin Hydrate 0.3% eye drops preservative free │ 10 ml £4.60

Hypromellose with dextran 70

The properties listed below are those particular to the combination only. For the properties of the components please consider, hypromellose p. 643.

● **INDICATIONS AND DOSE**

Tear deficiency
▸ TO THE EYE
‣ **Child:** Apply as required

● **MEDICINAL FORMS**
There can be variation in the licensing of different medicines containing the same drug.

Eye drops
EXCIPIENTS: May contain Benzalkonium chloride, disodium edetate
‣ **Tears Naturale** (Alcon Laboratories (UK) Ltd)
  Dextran 70 1 mg per 1 ml, Hypromellose 3 mg per 1 ml Tears Naturale eye drops │ 15 ml ℗ £1.89
  Tears Naturale eye drops 0.4ml unit dose │ 28 unit dose ℗ £13.26

Liquid paraffin with white soft paraffin and wool alcohols

● **INDICATIONS AND DOSE**

Dry eye conditions
▸ TO THE EYE
‣ **Child:** Apply as required, best suited for application before sleep

● **PATIENT AND CARER ADVICE** May cause temporary visual disturbance. Should not be used during contact lens wear.

● **MEDICINAL FORMS**
There can be variation in the licensing of different medicines containing the same drug.

Eye ointment
‣ **Lacri-Lube** (Allergan Ltd)
  Wool alcohols 2 mg per 1 gram, Liquid paraffin 425 mg per 1 gram, White soft paraffin 573 mg per 1 gram Lacri-lube eye ointment │ 3.5 gram ℗ £2.94 │ 5 gram ℗ £3.88

Paraffin, yellow, soft

● **INDICATIONS AND DOSE**

Eye surface lubrication
▸ TO THE EYE
‣ **Child:** Apply every 2 hours as required

● **PATIENT AND CARER ADVICE** Ophthalmic preparations may cause temporary visual disturbance. Should not be used during contact lens wear.

● **MEDICINAL FORMS**
There can be variation in the licensing of different medicines containing the same drug.

Eye ointment
‣ **Paraffin, yellow, soft** (Non-proprietary)
  Liquid paraffin 100 mg per 1 gram, Wool fat 100 mg per 1 gram, Yellow soft paraffin 800 mg per 1 gram Simple eye ointment │ 4 gram ℗ £17.45 DT price = £14.12

Polyvinyl alcohol

● **INDICATIONS AND DOSE**

Tear deficiency
▸ TO THE EYE
‣ **Child:** Apply as required

● **PRESCRIBING AND DISPENSING INFORMATION** Although multi-dose polyvinyl alcohol eye drops commonly contain preservatives, preservative-free unit dose vials may be available.

● **MEDICINAL FORMS**
There can be variation in the licensing of different medicines containing the same drug. Forms available from special-order manufacturers include: eye drops

Eye drops
EXCIPIENTS: May contain Benzalkonium chloride, disodium edetate
‣ **Liquifilm Tears** (Allergan Ltd)
  Polyvinyl alcohol 14 mg per 1 ml Liquifilm Tears 1.4% eye drops │ 15 ml £1.93
  Liquifilm Tears 1.4% eye drops 0.4ml unit dose preservative free │ 30 unit dose £5.35
‣ **PVA** (Tubilux Pharma Ltd)
  Polyvinyl alcohol 14 mg per 1 ml PVA 1.4% eye drops │ 15 ml £1.63
‣ **Refresh Ophthalmic** (Allergan Ltd)
  Polyvinyl alcohol 14 mg per 1 ml Refresh Ophthalmic 1.4% eye drops 0.4ml unit dose │ 30 unit dose £2.25
‣ **Sno Tears** (Bausch & Lomb UK Ltd)
  Polyvinyl alcohol 14 mg per 1 ml Sno Tears 1.4% eye drops │ 10 ml £1.06

Retinol palmitate with white soft paraffin and light liquid paraffin and liquid paraffin and wool fat

(Formulated as an ocular lubricant)

● **INDICATIONS AND DOSE**

Dry eye conditions
▸ TO THE EYE
‣ **Child:** Apply as required

- **MEDICINAL FORMS**
There can be variation in the licensing of different medicines containing the same drug.
Eye ointment
  ▸ **VitA-POS** (Scope Ophthalmics Ltd)
  VitA-POS eye ointment preservative free | 5 gram £2.75

Sodium chloride

- **INDICATIONS AND DOSE**

Tear deficiency | Ocular lubricants and astringents | Irrigation, including first-aid removal of harmful substances | Intra-ocular or topical irrigation during surgical procedures
  ▸ TO THE EYE
  ▸ **Child:** Apply as required, use 0.9% eye preparations

- **PRESCRIBING AND DISPENSING INFORMATION** Although multi-dose sodium chloride eye drops commonly contain preservatives, preservative-free unit dose vials may be available.

- **MEDICINAL FORMS**
There can be variation in the licensing of different medicines containing the same drug. Forms available from special-order manufacturers include: eye drops, eye ointment
Eye drops
  ▸ **Sodium chloride (Non-proprietary)**
  Sodium chloride 50 mg per 1 ml Sodium chloride 5% eye drops | 10 ml £25.25
  ▸ **Hypersal** (Ennogen Healthcare Ltd)
  Sodium chloride 50 mg per 1 ml Hypersal 5% eye drops | 10 ml £25.25
  ▸ **ODM5** (Kestrel Ophthalmics Ltd)
  Sodium chloride 50 mg per 1 ml ODM5 5% eye drops preservative free | 10 ml £24.00 DT price = £0.00
  ▸ **Saline** (Bausch & Lomb UK Ltd)
  Sodium chloride 9 mg per 1 ml Minims saline 0.9% eye drops 0.5ml unit dose | 20 unit dose Ⓟ £7.14 DT price = £7.14
  ▸ **Sodium chloride** (Essential Pharmaceuticals Ltd, Moorfields Pharmaceuticals)
  Sodium chloride 50 mg per 1 ml NaCl 5% eye drops 0.45ml unit dose preservative free | 20 unit dose £19.70
  PF Drops Sodium Chloride 5% eye drops preservative free | 10 ml £25.20 DT price = £0.00
Eye ointment
  ▸ **Sodium chloride (Non-proprietary)**
  Sodium chloride 50 mg per 1 gram Muro 128 5% eye ointment | 3.5 gram [PoM] no price available
  Sodium chloride 50 mg per 1 ml Sodium chloride 5% eye ointment preservative free | 5 gram £22.50

Sodium hyaluronate

- **INDICATIONS AND DOSE**
Dry eye conditions
  ▸ TO THE EYE
  ▸ **Child:** Apply as required

- **PRESCRIBING AND DISPENSING INFORMATION** Some preparations are contained in units which are resealable and may be used for up to 12 hours.
  Although multi-dose sodium hyaluronate eye drops commonly contain preservatives, preservative-free unit dose vials may be available.

- **MEDICINAL FORMS**
There can be variation in the licensing of different medicines containing the same drug.
Eye drops
  ▸ **Artelac Rebalance** (Bausch & Lomb UK Ltd)
  Artelac Rebalance 0.15% eye drops | 10 ml £4.00

  ▸ **Artelac Splash** (Bausch & Lomb UK Ltd)
  Artelac Splash 0.2% eye drops 0.5ml unit dose | 30 unit dose £7.00 | 60 unit dose £11.20
  ▸ **Blink Intensive** (AMO UK Ltd)
  Blink Intensive Tears 0.2% eye drops 0.4ml unit dose | 20 unit dose £2.97
  Blink Intensive Tears 0.2% eye drops | 10 ml £2.97
  ▸ **Clinitas** (Altacor Ltd)
  Clinitas Multi 0.4% eye drops preservative free | 10 ml £6.99
  Clinitas 0.4% eye drops 0.5ml unit dose | 30 unit dose £5.70
  ▸ **Evolve HA** (Medicom Healthcare Ltd)
  Evolve HA 0.2% eye drops preservative free | 10 ml £5.99
  ▸ **Hy-Opti** (Alissa Healthcare Research Ltd)
  Hy-Opti 0.1% eye drops preservative free | 10 ml £8.50
  Hy-Opti 0.2% eye drops preservative free | 10 ml £9.50
  ▸ **Hyabak** (Thea Pharmaceuticals Ltd)
  Hyabak 0.15% eye drops preservative free | 10 ml £7.99
  Hyabak UD 0.15% eye drops 0.4ml unit dose preservative free | 30 unit dose £4.99
  ▸ **Hycosan** (Scope Ophthalmics Ltd)
  Hycosan Extra 0.2% eye drops | 7.5 ml no price available
  Hycosan 0.1% eye drops | 7.5 ml no price available
  ▸ **HydraMed** (Farmigea S.p.A.)
  HydraMed 0.2% eye drops preservative free | 10 ml £5.60
  HydraMed 0.2% eye drops 0.5ml unit dose preservative free | 30 unit dose £5.60
  ▸ **Hylo-Comod** (Scope Ophthalmics Ltd)
  Hylo-Tear 0.1% eye drops preservative free | 10 ml £8.50
  Hylo-Forte 0.2% eye drops preservative free | 10 ml £9.50
  ▸ **Hylo-fresh** (Scope Ophthalmics Ltd)
  Hylo-Fresh 0.03% eye drops preservative free | 10 ml £4.95
  ▸ **Lubristil** (Moorfields Pharmaceuticals)
  Lubristil 0.15% eye drops 0.3ml unit dose preservative free | 20 unit dose £4.99
  ▸ **Ocusan** (Agepha Pharma s.r.o.)
  Ocusan 0.2% eye drops 0.5ml unit dose | 20 unit dose £5.37
  ▸ **Optive Fusion** (Allergan Ltd)
  Optive Fusion 0.1% eye drops | 10 ml £7.49
  ▸ **Oxyal** (Bausch & Lomb UK Ltd)
  Oxyal 0.15% eye drops | 10 ml £4.15
  ▸ **Vismed** (TRB Chemidica (UK) Ltd)
  Vismed Gel Multi 0.3% eye drops preservative free | 10 ml £7.95
  Vismed Multi 0.18% eye drops preservative free | 10 ml £6.81
  Vismed 0.18% eye drops 0.3ml unit dose preservative free | 20 unit dose £5.10
  ▸ **Vizulize** (East Midlands Pharma Ltd)
  Vizulize 0.1% eye drops | 10 ml £1.71
  ▸ **Xailin HA** (Nicox Pharma)
  Xailin HA 0.2% eye drops preservative free | 10 ml £7.13
Eye gel
  ▸ **Lubristil** (Moorfields Pharmaceuticals)
  Lubristil 0.15% eye gel 0.4ml unit dose preservative free | 20 unit dose £6.49
  ▸ **Vismed** (TRB Chemidica (UK) Ltd)
  Vismed Gel 0.3% eye gel 0.45ml unit dose preservative free | 20 unit dose £5.98

Soybean oil

- **INDICATIONS AND DOSE**
Dry eye conditions
  ▸ TO THE EYE
  ▸ **Child:** Apply up to 4 times a day

- **MEDICINAL FORMS**
There can be variation in the licensing of different medicines containing the same drug.
Eye drops
  ▸ **Emustil** (Moorfields Pharmaceuticals)
  Emustil eye drops 0.3ml unit dose preservative free | 20 unit dose £6.22

3 Eye infections

Eye infections

Most acute superficial eye infections can be treated topically. Blepharitis and conjunctivitis are often caused by staphylococci; keratitis and endophthalmitis may be bacterial, viral, or fungal.

Bacterial *blepharitis* is treated by lid hygiene and application of antibacterial eye drops to the conjunctival sac or to the lid margins. Systemic treatment may be required and may be necessary for 3 months or longer.

Most cases of acute bacterial conjunctivitis are self-limiting; where treatment is appropriate, antibacterial eye drops or an eye ointment are used. A poor response might indicate viral or allergic conjunctivitis or antibiotic resistance.

Corneal *ulcer* and *keratitis* require specialist treatment, usually under inpatient care, and may call for intensive topical, subconjunctival, or systemic administration of antimicrobials.

Endophthalmitis is a medical emergency which also calls for specialist management and requires intravitreal administration of antimicrobials; concomitant systemic treatment is required in some cases. Surgical intervention, such as vitrectomy, is sometimes indicated.

See reference to the treatment of *crab lice of the eyelashes*.

Antibacterials

Bacterial eye infections are generally treated topically with eye drops and eye ointments. Systemic administration is sometimes appropriate in blepharitis.

Chloramphenicol p. 648 has a broad spectrum of activity and is the drug of choice for *superficial eye infections*. Chloramphenicol eye drops are well tolerated and the recommendation that chloramphenicol eye drops should be avoided because of an increased risk of aplastic anaemia is not well founded.

Other antibacterials with a broad spectrum of activity include the quinolones, ciprofloxacin p. 647, levofloxacin p. 648, moxifloxacin p. 648, and ofloxacin p. 648; the aminoglycosides, gentamicin p. 647 and tobramycin p. 647 are also active against a wide variety of bacteria. Gentamicin, tobramycin, quinolones (except moxifloxacin), and polymyxin B are effective for infections caused by *Pseudomonas aeruginosa*.

Ciprofloxacin eye drops are licensed for corneal ulcers; intensive application (especially in the first 2 days) is required throughout the day and night.

Azithromycin eye drops p. 647 are licensed for trachomatous conjunctivitis caused by *Chlamydia trachomatis* and for purulent bacterial conjunctivitis. *Trachoma* which results from chronic infection with *Chlamydia trachomatis* can be treated with azithromycin by mouth [unlicensed indication].

Fusidic acid is useful for staphylococcal infections. Propamidine isetionate p. 649 is of little value in bacterial infections but is used by specialists to treat the rare, but potentially sight-threatening, condition of *acanthamoeba keratitis* [unlicensed indication].

Other antibacterial eye drops may be prepared aseptically in a specialist manufacturing unit from material supplied for injection.

With corticosteroids

Many antibacterial preparations also incorporate a corticosteroid but such mixtures should **not** be used unless a patient is under close specialist supervision. In particular they should not be prescribed for undiagnosed 'red eye' which is sometimes caused by the herpes simplex virus and may be difficult to diagnose.

Administration

Frequency of application depends on the severity of the infection and the potential for irreversible ocular damage; antibacterial eye preparations are usually administered as follows:

- *Eye drops*, apply 1 drop at least every 2 hours in severe infection then reduce frequency as infection is controlled and continue for 48 hours after healing. For less severe infection 3-4 times daily is generally sufficient.
- *Eye ointment*, apply *either* at night (if eye drops used during the day) *or* 3-4 times daily (if eye ointment used alone).

Antifungals

Fungal infections of the cornea are rare. Orbital mycosis is rarer, and when it occurs it is usually because of direct spread of infection from the paranasal sinuses. Debility or immunosuppression can encourage fungal proliferation. The spread of infection through blood occasionally produces metastatic endophthalmitis.

Many different fungi are capable of producing ocular infection; they can be identified by appropriate laboratory procedures.

Antifungal preparations for the eye are not generally available. Treatment will normally be carried out at specialist centres, but requests for information about supplies of preparations not available commercially should be addressed to the Strategic Health Authority (or equivalent in Scotland or Northern Ireland), or to the nearest hospital ophthalmology unit, or to Moorfields Eye Hospital, 162 City Road, London EC1V 2PD (tel. (020) 7253 3411) or www.moorfields.nhs.uk .

Antivirals

Herpes simplex infections producing, for example, dendritic corneal ulcers can be treated with aciclovir p. 649. Aciclovir eye ointment is used in combination with systemic treatment for ophthalmic zoster.

Also see systemic treatment of CMV retinitis.

Antibacterials in neonates

Antibacterial eye drops are used to treat acute bacterial conjunctivitis in neonates (ophthalmia neonatorum); where possible the causative microorganism should be identified. Chloramphenicol eye drops are used to treat mild conjunctivitis; more serious infections also require a systemic antibacterial. Failure to respond to initial treatment requires further investigation; chlamydial infection is one of the most frequent causes of neonatal conjunctivitis and should be considered. Azithromycin eye drops are licensed to treat trachomatous conjunctivitis caused by *Chlamydia trachomatis* and purulent bacterial conjunctivitis in neonates. However, as there is a risk of simultaneous infection at other sites in neonates and children under 3 months presenting with conjunctivitis caused by *Chlamydia trachomatis*, systemic treatment with oral erythromycin p. 316 is required. *Gonococcal eye infections* are treated with a single-dose of parenteral cefotaxime p. 307 or ceftriaxone p. 308. Gentamicin eye drops together with appropriate systemic antibacterials are used in the treatment of *pseudomonal eye infections*; high-strength gentamicin eye drops (1.5%) [unlicensed] are available for severe infections.

3.1 Bacterial eye infection

ANTIBACTERIALS > AMINOGLYCOSIDES

Gentamicin

- **INDICATIONS AND DOSE**

Bacterial eye infections
- ▶ TO THE EYE
- ▶ Child: Apply 1 drop at least every 2 hours in severe infection, reduce frequency as infection is controlled and continue for 48 hours after healing, frequency of eye drops depends on the severity of the infection and the potential for irreversible ocular damage; for less severe infection 3–4 times daily is generally sufficient

- **INTERACTIONS** → Appendix 1: aminoglycosides
- **PRESCRIBING AND DISPENSING INFORMATION** Eye drops may be sourced as a manufactured special or from specialist importing companies.

- **MEDICINAL FORMS**
There can be variation in the licensing of different medicines containing the same drug. Forms available from special-order manufacturers include: eye drops

Ear/eye drops solution
EXCIPIENTS: May contain Benzalkonium chloride
- ▶ Gentamicin (Non-proprietary)
  Gentamicin (as Gentamicin sulfate) 3 mg per 1 ml Gentamicin 0.3% ear/eye drops⏐ 10 ml PoM £2.14 DT price = £2.15

Tobramycin
30-Nov-2016

- **INDICATIONS AND DOSE**

Local treatment of infections
- ▶ TO THE EYE
- ▶ Child 1-17 years: Apply twice daily for 6–8 days

Local treatment of infections (severe infection)
- ▶ TO THE EYE
- ▶ Child 1-17 years: Apply 4 times a day for first day, then apply twice daily for 5–7 days

- **INTERACTIONS** → Appendix 1: aminoglycosides

- **MEDICINAL FORMS**
There can be variation in the licensing of different medicines containing the same drug.

Eye drops
EXCIPIENTS: May contain Benzododecinium bromide
- ▶ Tobravisc (Alcon Laboratories (UK) Ltd)
  Tobramycin 3 mg per 1 ml Tobravisc 3mg/ml eye drops⏐ 15 ml PoM £4.74

ANTIBACTERIALS > MACROLIDES

Azithromycin

- **INDICATIONS AND DOSE**

Trachomatous conjunctivitis caused by *Chlamydia trachomatis*⏐Purulent bacterial conjunctivitis
- ▶ TO THE EYE
- ▶ Child: Apply twice daily for 3 days, review if no improvement after 3 days of treatment

- **INTERACTIONS** → Appendix 1: macrolides
- **SIDE-EFFECTS**
- ▶ **Common or very common** Blurred vision · ocular burning · ocular discomfort · ocular pruritus
- ▶ **Uncommon** Conjunctival hyperaemia · eyelid eczema · eyelid erythema · eyelid oedema · keratitis

- **MEDICINAL FORMS**
There can be variation in the licensing of different medicines containing the same drug.

Eye drops
- ▶ Azyter (Thea Pharmaceuticals Ltd)
  Azithromycin dihydrate 15 mg per 1 gram Azyter 15mg/g eye drops 0.25g unit dose⏐ 6 unit dose PoM £6.99 DT price = £6.99

ANTIBACTERIALS > QUINOLONES

Ciprofloxacin

- **INDICATIONS AND DOSE**

Superficial bacterial eye infection
- ▶ TO THE EYE USING EYE DROP
- ▶ Child: Apply 4 times a day for maximum duration of treatment 21 days
- ▶ TO THE EYE USING EYE OINTMENT
- ▶ Child 1-17 years: Apply 1.25 centimetres 3 times a day for 2 days, then apply 1.25 centimetres twice daily for 5 days

Superficial bacterial eye infection (severe infection)
- ▶ TO THE EYE USING EYE DROP
- ▶ Child: Apply every 2 hours during waking hours for 2 days, then apply 4 times a day for maximum duration of treatment 21 days

Corneal ulcer
- ▶ TO THE EYE USING EYE DROP
- ▶ Child: Apply every 15 minutes for 6 hours, then apply every 30 minutes for the remainder of day 1, then apply every 1 hour on day 2, then apply every 4 hours on days 3–14, maximum duration of treatment 21 days, to be administered throughout the day and night
- ▶ TO THE EYE USING EYE OINTMENT
- ▶ Child 1-17 years: Apply 1.25 centimetres every 1–2 hours for 2 days, then apply 1.25 centimetres every 4 hours for the next 12 days, to be administered throughout the day and night

- **UNLICENSED USE** Eye ointment not licensed for use in children under 1 year.
- **INTERACTIONS** → Appendix 1: quinolones
- **SIDE-EFFECTS**
- ▶ **Common or very common** Corneal deposits (reversible after completion of treatment) · ocular discomfort · ocular hyperaemia · taste disturbance
- ▶ **Uncommon** Increased lacrimation · blurred vision · conjunctival hyperaemia · corneal infiltrates · corneal staining · eye dryness · eye irritation · eye pain · eye pruritus · eye swelling · eyelid disorders · eyelid erythema · eyelid exfoliation · eyelid oedema · headache · keratopathy · nausea · photophobia
- ▶ **Rare** Abdominal pain · asthenopia · corneal disorders · corneal epithelium defect · dermatitis · diarrhoea · diplopia · dizziness · ear pain · eye hypoaesthesia · keratitis · paranasal sinus hypersecretion · rhinitis
- **PREGNANCY** Manufacturer advises use only if potential benefit outweighs risk.
- **BREAST FEEDING** Manufacturer advises caution.

- **MEDICINAL FORMS**
There can be variation in the licensing of different medicines containing the same drug. Forms available from special-order manufacturers include: eye drops

Eye drops
EXCIPIENTS: May contain Benzalkonium chloride
- ▶ Ciloxan (Alcon Laboratories (UK) Ltd)
  Ciprofloxacin (as Ciprofloxacin hydrochloride) 3 mg per 1 ml Ciloxan 0.3% eye drops⏐ 5 ml PoM £4.70 DT price = £4.70

11

Eye

Eye ointment
- Ciloxan (Alcon Laboratories (UK) Ltd)
 Ciprofloxacin (as Ciprofloxacin hydrochloride) 3 mg per
 1 gram Ciloxan 3mg/g eye ointment | 3.5 gram PoM £5.22

Levofloxacin

● **INDICATIONS AND DOSE**
Local treatment of eye infections
▸ TO THE EYE
▸ Child 1–17 years: Apply every 2 hours for first 2 days, to
 be applied maximum 8 times a day, then apply 4 times
 a day for 3 days

● **INTERACTIONS** → Appendix 1: quinolones
● **SIDE-EFFECTS**
▸ **Common or very common** Ocular burning · visual
 disturbances
▸ **Uncommon** Conjunctival follicles · headache · lid erythema
 · lid oedema · ocular discomfort · ocular dryness · ocular
 itching · ocular pain · photophobia · rhinitis
● **PREGNANCY** Manufacturer advises use only if potential
 benefit outweighs risk.
● **BREAST FEEDING** Manufacturer advises use only if
 potential benefit outweighs risk.
● **PRESCRIBING AND DISPENSING INFORMATION** Although
 multi-dose levofloxacin eye drops commonly contain
 preservatives, preservative-free unit dose vials may be
 available.

● **MEDICINAL FORMS**
There can be variation in the licensing of different medicines
containing the same drug.
Eye drops
EXCIPIENTS: May contain Benzalkonium chloride
▸ Levofloxacin (Non-proprietary)
 Levofloxacin (as Levofloxacin hemihydrate) 5 mg per
 1 ml Levofloxacin 5mg/ml eye drops | 5 ml PoM £6.25
▸ Oftaquix (Santen UK Ltd)
 Levofloxacin (as Levofloxacin hemihydrate) 5 mg per
 1 ml Oftaquix 5mg/ml eye drops 0.3ml unit dose | 30 unit dose PoM
 £17.95
 Oftaquix 5mg/ml eye drops | 5 ml PoM £6.95

Moxifloxacin

● **INDICATIONS AND DOSE**
Local treatment of infections
▸ TO THE EYE
▸ Child: Apply 3 times a day continue treatment for
 2–3 days after infection improves; review if no
 improvement within 5 days

● **CAUTIONS** Not recommended for neonates
● **INTERACTIONS** → Appendix 1: quinolones
● **SIDE-EFFECTS**
▸ **Common or very common** Hyperaemia · ocular discomfort ·
 ocular dryness · ocular irritation · ocular pain · taste
 disturbances
▸ **Uncommon** Conjunctival haemorrhage · corneal disorders ·
 corneal erosion · corneal keratitis · corneal staining · eyelid
 erythema · headache · nasal discomfort · paraesthesia ·
 pharyngolaryngeal pain · visual disturbances · vomiting
▸ **Frequency not known** Dizziness · dyspnoea · nausea ·
 palpitation · photophobia · pruritus · raised intra-ocular
 pressure · rash

● **MEDICINAL FORMS**
There can be variation in the licensing of different medicines
containing the same drug.
Eye drops
▸ Moxivig (Alcon Laboratories (UK) Ltd)
 Moxifloxacin (as Moxifloxacin hydrochloride) 5 mg per
 1 ml Moxivig 0.5% eye drops | 5 ml PoM £9.80

Ofloxacin

● **INDICATIONS AND DOSE**
Local treatment of infections
▸ TO THE EYE
▸ Child 1–17 years: Apply every 2–4 hours for the first
 2 days, then reduced to 4 times a day for maximum
 10 days treatment

● **CAUTIONS** Corneal ulcer (risk of corneal perforation) ·
 epithelial defect (risk of corneal perforation)
● **INTERACTIONS** → Appendix 1: quinolones
● **SIDE-EFFECTS**
▸ **Common or very common** Ocular discomfort
▸ **Frequency not known** Dry eyes · facial oedema · increased
 lacrimation · keratitis · ocular hyperaemia · ocular oedema ·
 photophobia · visual disturbances
● **PREGNANCY** Manufacturer advises use only if benefit
 outweighs risk (systemic quinolones have caused
 arthropathy in *animal* studies).
● **BREAST FEEDING** Manufacturer advises avoid.

● **MEDICINAL FORMS**
There can be variation in the licensing of different medicines
containing the same drug.
Eye drops
EXCIPIENTS: May contain Benzalkonium chloride
▸ Exocin (Allergan Ltd)
 Ofloxacin 3 mg per 1 ml Exocin 0.3% eye drops | 5 ml PoM £2.17
 DT price = £2.17

ANTIBACTERIALS ❭ OTHER

Chloramphenicol

● **DRUG ACTION** Chloramphenicol is a potent broad-
spectrum antibiotic.

● **INDICATIONS AND DOSE**
Superficial eye infections
▸ TO THE EYE USING EYE DROP
▸ Child: Apply 1 drop every 2 hours then reduce
 frequency as infection is controlled and continue for
 48 hours after healing, frequency dependent on the
 severity of the infection. For less severe infection
 3–4 times daily is generally sufficient
▸ TO THE EYE USING EYE OINTMENT
▸ Child: Apply daily, to be applied at night (if eye drops
 used during the day), alternatively apply 3–4 times a
 day, if ointment used alone

● **INTERACTIONS** → Appendix 1: chloramphenicol
● **SIDE-EFFECTS** Transient stinging
● **PREGNANCY** Avoid unless essential—no information on
 topical use but risk of 'neonatal grey-baby syndrome' with
 oral use in third trimester.
● **BREAST FEEDING** Avoid unless essential—*theoretical* risk
 of bone-marrow toxicity.
● **PRESCRIBING AND DISPENSING INFORMATION** Although
 multi-dose chloramphenicol eye drops commonly contain
 preservatives, preservative-free unit dose vials may be
 available.

- **PATIENT AND CARER ADVICE**
  Medicines for Children leaflet: Chloramphenicol for eye infections
  www.medicinesforchildren.org.uk/chloramphenicol-eye-infections-0
- **EXCEPTIONS TO LEGAL CATEGORY** Chloramphenicol 0.5% eye drops (in max. pack size 10 mL) and 1% ointment (in max. pack size 4 g) can be sold to the public for treatment of acute bacterial conjunctivitis in adults and children over 2 years; max. duration of treatment 5 days.

- **MEDICINAL FORMS**
  There can be variation in the licensing of different medicines containing the same drug. Forms available from special-order manufacturers include: eye drops
  Eye drops
  EXCIPIENTS: May contain Phenylmercuric acetate
  ▸ Chloramphenicol (Non-proprietary)
  Chloramphenicol 5 mg per 1 ml Minims chloramphenicol 0.5% eye drops 0.5ml unit dose| 20 unit dose [PoM] £10.99 DT price = £10.99
  Chloramphenicol Antibiotic 0.5% eye drops| 10 ml [P] £1.70 DT price = £1.52
  Chloramphenicol 0.5% eye drops| 10 ml [PoM] £2.20 DT price = £1.52
  ▸ Chloromycetin (AMCo)
  Chloromycetin 5 mg per 1 ml Chloromycetin Redidrops 0.5%| 10 ml [PoM] £0.90 DT price = £1.52
  Eye ointment
  ▸ Chloramphenicol (Non-proprietary)
  Chloramphenicol 10 mg per 1 gram Chloramphenicol 1% eye ointment| 4 gram [PoM] £2.27 DT price = £2.27
  ▸ Chloromycetin (AMCo)
  Chloromycetin 10 mg per 1 gram Chloromycetin 1% eye ointment| 4 gram [PoM] £1.08 DT price = £2.27
  ▸ Klorafect (Blumont Pharma Ltd)
  Chloramphenicol 10 mg per 1 gram Klorafect 1% eye ointment| 4 gram [PoM] £1.81 DT price = £2.27

Fusidic acid

16-Jun-2017

- **DRUG ACTION** Fusidic acid and its salts are narrow-spectrum antibiotics used for staphylococcal infections.

- **INDICATIONS AND DOSE**
  Staphylococcal eye infections
  ▸ TO THE EYE
  ▸ Child: Apply twice daily

- **INTERACTIONS** → Appendix 1: fusidic acid

- **MEDICINAL FORMS**
  There can be variation in the licensing of different medicines containing the same drug.
  Modified-release drops
  EXCIPIENTS: May contain Benzalkonium chloride, disodium edetate
  ▸ Fusidic acid (Non-proprietary)
  Fusidic acid 10 mg per 1 gram Fusidic acid 1% modified-release eye drops| 5 gram [PoM] £29.06 DT price = £29.06

ANTIPROTOZOALS

Propamidine isetionate

- **INDICATIONS AND DOSE**
  Acanthamoeba keratitis infections (specialist use only) |
  Local treatment of eye infections
  ▸ TO THE EYE USING EYE OINTMENT
  ▸ Child: Apply 1–2 times a day
  ▸ TO THE EYE USING EYE DROP
  ▸ Child: Apply up to 4 times a day

- **UNLICENSED USE** Not licensed for _acanthamoeba keratitis_ infections.
- **SIDE-EFFECTS** Eye irritation · eye pain
- **PREGNANCY** Manufacturer advises avoid unless essential—no information available.

- **BREAST FEEDING** Manufacturer advises avoid unless essential—no information available.

- **MEDICINAL FORMS**
  There can be variation in the licensing of different medicines containing the same drug.
  Eye ointment
  ▸ Brolene (dibrompropamidine) (Sanofi)
  Dibrompropamidine isetionate 1.5 mg per 1 gram Brolene 0.15% eye ointment| 5 gram [P] £2.92 DT price = £3.49
  ▸ Golden Eye (dibrompropamidine) (Cambridge Healthcare Supplies Ltd)
  Dibrompropamidine isetionate 1.5 mg per 1 gram Golden Eye 0.15% ointment| 5 gram [P] £3.49 DT price = £3.49
  Eye drops
  EXCIPIENTS: May contain Benzalkonium chloride
  ▸ Brolene (Propamidine) (Sanofi)
  Propamidine isetionate 1 mg per 1 ml Brolene 0.1% eye drops| 10 ml [P] £2.80
  ▸ Golden Eye (propamidine) (Cambridge Healthcare Supplies Ltd)
  Propamidine isetionate 1 mg per 1 ml Golden Eye 0.1% drops| 10 ml [P] £3.26

3.2 Viral eye infection
3.2a Ophthalmic herpes simplex

ANTIVIRALS 〉 NUCLEOSIDE ANALOGUES

Aciclovir
(Acyclovir)

- **INDICATIONS AND DOSE**
  Herpes simplex infection (local treatment)
  ▸ TO THE EYE USING EYE OINTMENT
  ▸ Child: Apply 1 centimetre 5 times a day continue for at least 3 days after complete healing

- **INTERACTIONS** → Appendix 1: aciclovir
- **SIDE-EFFECTS**
  ▸ Common or very common Local inflammation · local irritation · superficial punctate keratopathy
  ▸ Rare Blepharitis
  ▸ Very rare Angioedema · hypersensitivity reactions
- **PATIENT AND CARER ADVICE**
  Medicines for Children leaflet: Aciclovir eye ointment for herpes simplex infections www.medicinesforchildren.org.uk/aciclovir-eye-ointment-for-herpes-simplex-infection

- **MEDICINAL FORMS**
  There can be variation in the licensing of different medicines containing the same drug.
  Eye ointment
  ▸ Zovirax (GlaxoSmithKline UK Ltd)
  Aciclovir 30 mg per 1 gram Zovirax 3% ophthalmic ointment| 4.5 gram [PoM] £9.34 DT price = £9.34

4 Eye procedures

Mydriatics and cycloplegics

Overview

Antimuscarinics dilate the pupil and paralyse the ciliary muscle; they vary in potency and duration of action.
Short-acting, relatively weak mydriatics, such as tropicamide 0.5% p. 650 (action lasts for 4–6 hours), facilitate the examination of the fundus of the eye. Cyclopentolate hydrochloride 1% p. 641 (action up to 24 hours) or atropine sulfate p. 641 (action up to 7 days) are

11

Eye

preferable for producing cycloplegia for refraction in young children; tropicamide may be preferred in neonates.

Phenylephrine hydrochloride p. 651 is used for mydriasis in diagnostic or therapeutic procedures; mydriasis occurs within 60–90 minutes and lasts up to 5–7 hours.

Mydriatics and cycloplegics are used in the treatment of anterior uveitis, usually as an adjunct to corticosteroids. Atropine sulfate is used in anterior uveitis mainly to prevent posterior synechiae and to relieve ciliary spasm; cyclopentolate hydrochloride or homatropine hydrobromide p. 642 (action up to 3 days) can also be used and may be preferred because they have a shorter duration of action.

ANTIMUSCARINICS

F 641

Tropicamide

- **INDICATIONS AND DOSE**

Funduscopy
- ▸ TO THE EYE

- ▸ Neonate: 0.5% eye drops to be applied 20 minutes before examination.

- ▸ Child: 0.5% eye drops to be applied 20 minutes before examination

- **INTERACTIONS** → Appendix 1: tropicamide
- **PRESCRIBING AND DISPENSING INFORMATION** Although multi-dose tropicamide eye drops commonly contain preservatives, preservative-free unit dose vials may be available.

- **MEDICINAL FORMS**
There can be variation in the licensing of different medicines containing the same drug.
Eye drops
EXCIPIENTS: May contain Benzalkonium chloride, edetic acid (edta)
- ▸ Mydriacyl (Alcon Laboratories (UK) Ltd)
Tropicamide 5 mg per 1 ml Mydriacyl 0.5% eye drops | 5 ml [PoM] £1.29
Tropicamide 10 mg per 1 ml Mydriacyl 1% eye drops | 5 ml [PoM] £1.60
- ▸ Tropicamide (Bausch & Lomb UK Ltd)
Tropicamide 5 mg per 1 ml Minims tropicamide 0.5% eye drops 0.5ml unit dose | 20 unit dose [PoM] £10.75
Tropicamide 10 mg per 1 ml Minims tropicamide 1% eye drops 0.5ml unit dose | 20 unit dose [PoM] £10.77

ANTISEPTICS AND DISINFECTANTS ﹥ IODINE PRODUCTS

Povidone-iodine

- **INDICATIONS AND DOSE**

Cutaneous peri-ocular and conjunctival antisepsis before ocular surgery
- ▸ TO THE EYE

- ▸ Neonate: Apply, leave for 2 minutes, then irrigate thoroughly with sodium chloride 0.9%.

- ▸ Child: Apply, leave for 2 minutes, then irrigate thoroughly with sodium chloride 0.9%

- **CONTRA-INDICATIONS** Concomitant use of ocular antimicrobial drugs · concomitant use of ocular formulations containing mercury-based preservatives · preterm neonates
- **SIDE-EFFECTS**
- ▸ **Rare** Conjunctival hyperaemia · superficial punctuate keratitis
- ▸ **Frequency not known** Cytotoxicity on deep tissue · cytotoxicity on mucous membranes · hypothyroidism in neonates · residual yellow coloration of the conjunctiva

- **PRESCRIBING AND DISPENSING INFORMATION** Although multi-dose povidone iodine eye drops commonly contain preservatives, preservative-free unit dose vials may be available.

- **MEDICINAL FORMS**
There can be variation in the licensing of different medicines containing the same drug. Forms available from special-order manufacturers include: eye drops
Eye drops
- ▸ Povidone iodine (Bausch & Lomb UK Ltd)
Povidone-Iodine 50 mg per 1 ml Minims povidone iodine 5% eye drops 0.4ml unit dose | 20 unit dose [PoM] £16.00

DIAGNOSTIC AGENTS ﹥ DYES

Fluorescein sodium

- **INDICATIONS AND DOSE**

Detection of lesions and foreign bodies
- ▸ TO THE EYE USING EYE DROP
- ▸ Child: Use sufficient amount to stain damaged areas

- **PRESCRIBING AND DISPENSING INFORMATION** Although multi-dose fluorescein eye drops commonly contain preservatives, preservative-free unit dose vials may be available.

- **MEDICINAL FORMS**
There can be variation in the licensing of different medicines containing the same drug.
Eye drops
- ▸ Fluorescein sodium (Bausch & Lomb UK Ltd)
Fluorescein sodium 10 mg per 1 ml Minims fluorescein sodium 1% eye drops 0.5ml unit dose | 20 unit dose [P] £8.89
Fluorescein sodium 20 mg per 1 ml Minims fluorescein sodium 2% eye drops 0.5ml unit dose | 20 unit dose [P] £8.89

MIOTICS ﹥ PARASYMPATHOMIMETICS

Acetylcholine chloride

- **INDICATIONS AND DOSE**

Cataract surgery | Penetrating keratoplasty | Iridectomy | Anterior segment surgery requiring rapid complete miosis
- ▸ TO THE EYE
- ▸ Child: (consult product literature)

- **UNLICENSED USE** Not licensed for use in children.
- **CAUTIONS** Asthma · gastro-intestinal spasm · heart failure · hyperthyroidism · peptic ulcer · urinary-tract obstruction
- **INTERACTIONS** → Appendix 1: acetylcholine
- **PREGNANCY** Avoid unless potential benefit outweighs risk—no information available.
- **BREAST FEEDING** Avoid unless potential benefit outweighs risk—no information available.

- **MEDICINAL FORMS**
There can be variation in the licensing of different medicines containing the same drug.
Irrigation
- ▸ Miochol-E (Bausch & Lomb UK Ltd)
Acetylcholine chloride 20 mg Miochol-E 20mg powder and solvent for solution for intraocular irrigation vials | 1 vial [PoM] £7.28
- ▸ Miphtel (Alan Pharmaceuticals)
Acetylcholine chloride 20 mg Miphtel 20mg powder and solvent for solution for intraocular irrigation ampoules | 6 ampoule [PoM] £43.68 (Hospital only)

SYMPATHOMIMETICS > VASOCONSTRICTOR

Phenylephrine hydrochloride

- **INDICATIONS AND DOSE**
Mydriasis
▶ TO THE EYE
- Child: Apply 1 drop, to be administered before procedure, a drop of proxymetacaine topical anaesthetic may be applied to the eye a few minutes before using phenylephrine to prevent stinging

- **CONTRA-INDICATIONS** 10% strength eye drops in children · 10% strength eye drops in neonates · aneurysms · cardiovascular disease · hypertension · thyrotoxicosis

- **CAUTIONS** Asthma · corneal epithelial damage · darkly pigmented iris is more resistant to pupillary dilatation and caution should be exercised to avoid overdosage. · diabetes (avoid eye drops in long standing diabetes) · mydriasis can precipitate acute angle-closure glaucoma in the very few children who are predisposed to the condition because of a shallow anterior chamber · neonates are at an increased risk of systemic toxicity · ocular hyperaemia · susceptibility to angle-closure glaucoma

- **INTERACTIONS** → Appendix 1: sympathomimetics, vasoconstrictor

- **SIDE-EFFECTS** Arrhythmias · blurred vision · conjunctivitis on prolonged administration · coronary artery spasm · extrasystoles · hyperaemia on prolonged administration · hypertension · local irritation on prolonged administration · myocardial infarction (usually after use of 10% strength in patients with pre-existing cardiovascular disease) · oedema on prolonged administration · palpitation · photophobia · raised intraocular pressure · tachycardia · transient stinging

- **PREGNANCY** Use only if potential benefit outweighs risk.

- **BREAST FEEDING** Use only if potential benefit outweighs risk—no information available.

- **PRESCRIBING AND DISPENSING INFORMATION** Although multi-dose phenylephrine eye drops commonly contain preservatives, preservative-free unit dose vials may be available.

- **PATIENT AND CARER ADVICE**
Driving and skilled tasks
Patients should be warned not to undertake skilled tasks (e.g. driving) until vision clears after mydriasis.

- **MEDICINAL FORMS**
There can be variation in the licensing of different medicines containing the same drug. Forms available from special-order manufacturers include: eye drops
Eye drops
EXCIPIENTS: May contain Disodium edetate, sodium metabisulfite
▶ **Phenylephrine hydrochloride** (Bausch & Lomb UK Ltd)
Phenylephrine hydrochloride 25 mg per 1 ml Minims phenylephrine hydrochloride 2.5% eye drops 0.5ml unit dose | 20 unit dose Ⓟ £11.41

4.1 Post-operative pain and inflammation

Eye, surgical and peri-operative drug use

Ocular peri-operative drugs

Drugs used to prepare the eye for surgery and drugs that are injected into the anterior chamber at the time of surgery are included here.

Sodium hyaluronate p. 645 is used during surgical procedures on the eye.

Apraclonidine p. 658, an alpha₂-adrenoceptor agonist, reduces intra-ocular pressure possibly by reducing the production of aqueous humour. It is used for short-term treatment only.

Balanced Salt Solution is used routinely in intra-ocular surgery.

Povidone-iodine p. 650 is used for peri-ocular and conjunctival antisepsis before ocular surgery to support postoperative infection control.

Local anaesthetics

Oxybuprocaine hydrochloride below and tetracaine p. 652 are widely used topical local anaesthetics. Proxymetacaine hydrochloride p. 652 causes less initial stinging and is useful for children. Oxybuprocaine hydrochloride or a combined preparation of lidocaine hydrochloride p. 796 and fluorescein sodium p. 650 is used for tonometry. Tetracaine produces a more profound anaesthesia and is suitable for use before minor surgical procedures, such as the removal of corneal sutures. It has a temporary disruptive effect on the corneal epithelium. Lidocaine hydrochloride, with or without adrenaline/epinephrine p. 132, is injected into the eyelids for minor surgery. Local anaesthetics should never be used for the management of ocular symptoms.

Local anaesthetic eye drops should be avoided in preterm neonates because of the immaturity of the metabolising enzyme system.

ANAESTHETICS, LOCAL

Fluorescein with lidocaine

- **INDICATIONS AND DOSE**
Local anaesthesia
▶ TO THE EYE
- Child: Apply as required

- **CONTRA-INDICATIONS** Avoid in pre-term neonate (immature metabolising enzyme system)

- **PRESCRIBING AND DISPENSING INFORMATION** Although multi-dose lidocaine and fluorescein eye drops commonly contain preservatives, preservative-free unit dose vials may be available.

- **MEDICINAL FORMS**
There can be variation in the licensing of different medicines containing the same drug.
Eye drops
▶ **Lidocaine and Fluorescein** (Bausch & Lomb UK Ltd)
Fluorescein sodium 2.5 mg per 1 ml, Lidocaine hydrochloride 40 mg per 1 ml Minims lidocaine and fluorescein eye drops 0.5ml unit dose | 20 unit dose PoM £11.24

Oxybuprocaine hydrochloride
(Benoxinate hydrochloride)

- **INDICATIONS AND DOSE**
Local anaesthetic
▶ TO THE EYE
- Child: Apply as required

- **CONTRA-INDICATIONS** Avoid in preterm neonates
- **INTERACTIONS** → Appendix 1: anaesthetics, local
- **PRESCRIBING AND DISPENSING INFORMATION** Although multi-dose oxybuprocaine eye drops commonly contain preservatives, preservative-free unit dose vials may be available.

- **MEDICINAL FORMS**
  There can be variation in the licensing of different medicines containing the same drug.
  Eye drops
  ‣ Oxybuprocaine hydrochloride (Bausch & Lomb UK Ltd)
    Oxybuprocaine hydrochloride 4 mg per 1 ml Minims oxybuprocaine hydrochloride 0.4% eye drops 0.5ml unit dose| 20 unit dose PoM| £10.15

Proxymetacaine hydrochloride

- **INDICATIONS AND DOSE**
  Local anaesthetic
  ‣ TO THE EYE
  ‣ Child: Apply as required

- **CONTRA-INDICATIONS** Avoid in preterm neonates
- **INTERACTIONS** → Appendix 1: anaesthetics, local
- **PRESCRIBING AND DISPENSING INFORMATION** Although multi-dose proxymetacaine eye drops commonly contain preservatives, preservative-free unit dose vials may be available.

- **MEDICINAL FORMS**
  There can be variation in the licensing of different medicines containing the same drug.
  Eye drops
  ‣ Proxymetacaine (Bausch & Lomb UK Ltd)
    Proxymetacaine hydrochloride 5 mg per 1 ml Minims proxymetacaine 0.5% eye drops 0.5ml unit dose| 20 unit dose PoM| £11.54

Tetracaine

(Amethocaine)

- **INDICATIONS AND DOSE**
  Local anaesthetic
  ‣ TO THE EYE
  ‣ Child: Apply as required

- **UNLICENSED USE** Not licensed for use in neonates.
- **CONTRA-INDICATIONS** Avoid in preterm neonates
- **INTERACTIONS** → Appendix 1: anaesthetics, local
- **SIDE-EFFECTS** Local skin reactions
  SIDE-EFFECTS, FURTHER INFORMATION
  The systemic toxicity of local anaesthetics mainly involves the central nervous and cardiovascular systems; systemic side effects unlikely as minimal absorption following topical application.
- **ALLERGY AND CROSS-SENSITIVITY** Hypersensitivity reactions occur mainly with the ester-type local anaesthetics, such as tetracaine and chloroprocaine; reactions are less frequent with the amide types, such as articaine, bupivacaine, levobupivacaine, lidocaine, mepivacaine, prilocaine, and ropivacaine. Cross-sensitivity reactions may be avoided by using the alternative chemical type.
- **PRESCRIBING AND DISPENSING INFORMATION** Although multi-dose tetracaine eye drops commonly contain preservatives, preservative-free unit dose vials may be available.

- **MEDICINAL FORMS**
  There can be variation in the licensing of different medicines containing the same drug.
  Eye drops
  ‣ Tetracaine (Non-proprietary)
    Tetracaine hydrochloride 5 mg per 1 ml Minims tetracaine hydrochloride 0.5% eye drops 0.5ml unit dose| 20 unit dose PoM| £10.16

Tetracaine hydrochloride 10 mg per 1 ml Minims tetracaine hydrochloride 1% eye drops 0.5ml unit dose| 20 unit dose PoM| £10.16

ANALGESICS ⟩ NON-STEROIDAL ANTI-INFLAMMATORY DRUGS

Diclofenac sodium

- **INDICATIONS AND DOSE**
  Inhibition of intra-operative miosis during cataract surgery (but does not possess intrinsic mydriatic properties) | Postoperative inflammation in cataract surgery, strabismus surgery, argon laser trabeculoplasty
  ‣ TO THE EYE
  ‣ Child: (consult product literature)

- **UNLICENSED USE** Not licensed for use in children.
- **INTERACTIONS** → Appendix 1: NSAIDs
- **ALLERGY AND CROSS-SENSITIVITY** Contra-indicated in patients with a history of hypersensitivity to aspirin or any other NSAID—which includes those in whom attacks of asthma, angioedema, urticaria or rhinitis have been precipitated by aspirin or any other NSAID.
- **PRESCRIBING AND DISPENSING INFORMATION** Although multi-dose diclofenac sodium eye drops commonly contain preservatives, preservative-free unit dose vials may be available.

- **MEDICINAL FORMS**
  There can be variation in the licensing of different medicines containing the same drug.
  Eye drops
  EXCIPIENTS: May contain Benzalkonium chloride, disodium edetate, propylene glycol
  ‣ Voltarol Ophtha (Thea Pharmaceuticals Ltd)
    Diclofenac sodium 1 mg per 1 ml Voltarol Ophtha 0.1% eye drops 0.3ml unit dose| 5 unit dose PoM| £4.00| 40 unit dose PoM| £32.00
  ‣ Voltarol Ophtha Multidose (Thea Pharmaceuticals Ltd)
    Diclofenac sodium 1 mg per 1 ml Voltarol Ophtha Multidose 0.1% eye drops| 5 ml PoM| £6.68

Flurbiprofen

- **INDICATIONS AND DOSE**
  Inhibition of intra-operative miosis (but does not possess intrinsic mydriatic properties) | Control of anterior segment inflammation following postoperative and post-laser trabeculoplasty when corticosteroids contra-indicated
  ‣ TO THE EYE
  ‣ Child: (consult product literature)

- **UNLICENSED USE** Not licensed for use in children.
- **INTERACTIONS** → Appendix 1: NSAIDs
- **ALLERGY AND CROSS-SENSITIVITY** Contra-indicated in patients with a history of hypersensitivity to aspirin or any other NSAID—which includes those in whom attacks of asthma, angioedema, urticaria or rhinitis have been precipitated by aspirin or any other NSAID.

- **MEDICINAL FORMS**
  There can be variation in the licensing of different medicines containing the same drug.
  Eye drops
  ‣ Ocufen (Allergan Ltd)
    Flurbiprofen sodium 300 microgram per 1 ml Ocufen 0.03% eye drops 0.4ml unit dose| 40 unit dose PoM| £37.15

Ketorolac trometamol

- **INDICATIONS AND DOSE**

Prophylaxis and reduction of inflammation and associated symptoms following ocular surgery
▸ TO THE EYE
▸ Child: (consult product literature)

- **UNLICENSED USE** Not licensed for use in children.
- **INTERACTIONS** → Appendix 1: NSAIDs
- **ALLERGY AND CROSS-SENSITIVITY** Contra-indicated in patients with a history of hypersensitivity to aspirin or any other NSAID—which includes those in whom attacks of asthma, angioedema, urticaria or rhinitis have been precipitated by aspirin or any other NSAID.

- **MEDICINAL FORMS**
There can be variation in the licensing of different medicines containing the same drug.

Eye drops
EXCIPIENTS: May contain Benzalkonium chloride, disodium edetate
▸ **Acular** (Allergan Ltd)
Ketorolac trometamol 5 mg per 1 ml Acular 0.5% eye drops |
5 ml [PoM] £3.00 DT price = £3.00

5   Glaucoma and ocular hypertension

Glaucoma

Overview

Glaucoma describes a group of disorders characterised by a loss of visual field associated with cupping of the optic disc and optic nerve damage and is generally associated with raised intra-ocular pressure.

Glaucoma is rare in children and should always be managed by a specialist. *Primary congenital glaucoma* is the most common form of glaucoma in children, followed by *secondary glaucomas*, such as following hereditary anterior segment malformations; *juvenile open-angle glaucoma* is less common and usually occurs in older children.

Treatment of glaucoma is determined by the pathophysiology and usually involves controlling raised intra-ocular pressure with surgery. Drug therapy is generally supportive, and can be used temporarily, pre- or post-operatively, or both, to reduce intra-ocular pressure. In secondary glaucomas, drug therapy is often used first-line, and long-term treatment may be required. Drugs that reduce intra-ocular pressure by different mechanisms are available for managing glaucoma. A topical beta-blocker or a prostaglandin analogue can be used. It may be necessary to combine these drugs or add others, such as carbonic anhydrase inhibitors, or miotics to control intra-ocular pressure.

Children with an acute form of glaucoma (usually presenting with pain in older children, a cloudy cornea, and may be associated with a previous history of controlled glaucoma or recent intra-ocular surgery) need immediate referral for specialist ophthalmology assessment and treatment.

Beta-blockers

Topical application of a beta-blocker to the eye reduces intra-ocular pressure effectively in primary and secondary glaucomas, probably by reducing the rate of production of aqueous humour.

Prostaglandin analogues

The prostaglandin analogues latanoprost p. 657, and travoprost, and the synthetic prostamide, bimatoprost, increase uveoscleral outflow and subsequently reduce intra-ocular pressure. They are used to reduce intra-ocular pressure. Only latanoprost (*Xalatan*®) and certain non-proprietary preparations of latanoprost) is licensed for use in children. Children receiving prostaglandin analogues should be managed by a specialist.

Sympathomimetics

Apraclonidine p. 658 is an alpha$_2$-adrenoceptor agonist that lowers intra-ocular pressure by reducing aqueous humour formation. Eye drops containing apraclonidine 0.5% are used for a short period to delay laser treatment or surgery for glaucoma in patients not adequately controlled by another drug; eye drops containing 1% are used for control of intra-ocular pressure after anterior segment laser surgery.

Brimonidine tartrate, an alpha$_2$-adrenoceptor agonist, is thought to lower intra-ocular pressure by reducing aqueous humour formation and increasing uveoscleral outflow.

Carbonic anhydrase inhibitors and systemic drugs

The **carbonic anhydrase inhibitors**, acetazolamide p. 655, brinzolamide p. 656, and dorzolamide p. 656, reduce intra-ocular pressure by reducing aqueous humour production. Systemic use of acetazolamide also produces weak diuresis.

Acetazolamide is given by mouth or, rarely in children, by intravenous injection (intramuscular injections are painful because of the alkaline pH of the solution). It is used as an adjunct to other treatment for reducing intra-ocular pressure. Acetazolamide is not generally recommended for long-term use.

Dorzolamide and brinzolamide are topical carbonic anhydrase inhibitors. They are unlicensed in children but are used in those resistant to beta-blockers or those in whom beta-blockers are contra-indicated. They are used alone or as an adjunct to a topical beta-blocker. Brinzolamide can also be used as an adjunct to a prostaglandin analogue. Systemic absorption can rarely cause sulfonamide-like side-effects and may require discontinuation if severe.

Metabolic acidosis can occur in children using topical carbonic anhydrase inhibitors; symptoms may include poor feeding and lack of weight gain.

Miotics

Miotics act by opening up the inefficient drainage channels in the trabecular meshwork. Pilocarpine p. 657 is a miotic used pre- and post-operatively in goniotomy and trabeculotomy; it is used occasionally for aphakic glaucoma.

BETA-ADRENOCEPTOR BLOCKERS

Betaxolol

- **INDICATIONS AND DOSE**

Primary and secondary glaucomas
▸ TO THE EYE
▸ Child: Apply twice daily

- **UNLICENSED USE** Not licensed for use in children.
- **CONTRA-INDICATIONS** Also consider contra-indications listed for systemically administered beta blockers ·
bradycardia · heart block
- **CAUTIONS** Patients with corneal disease
CAUTIONS, FURTHER INFORMATION
Systemic absorption can follow topical application to the eyes; consider cautions listed for systemically administered beta blockers.
- **INTERACTIONS** → Appendix 1: beta blockers (selective)

11

Eye

- SIDE-EFFECTS Anaphylaxis · blepharoconjunctivitis · burning · corneal disorders · cough, rather than wheeze, may occur · dry eyes · erythema · itching · ocular stinging · pain

  SIDE-EFFECTS, FURTHER INFORMATION
  Systemic absorption can follow topical application to the eyes; consider side effects listed for systemically administered beta blockers.

- PRESCRIBING AND DISPENSING INFORMATION Although multi-dose bextaxolol eye drops commonly contain preservatives, preservative-free unit dose vials may be available.

- MEDICINAL FORMS
  There can be variation in the licensing of different medicines containing the same drug.
  Eye drops
  EXCIPIENTS: May contain Benzalkonium chloride, disodium edetate
  ▸ Betaxolol (Non-proprietary)
  Betaxolol (as Betaxolol hydrochloride) 2.5 mg per 1 ml Betaxolol 0.25% eye drops 0.25ml unit dose preservative free | 50 unit dose PoM no price available
  Betaxolol (as Betaxolol hydrochloride) 5 mg per 1 ml Betaxolol 0.5% eye drops | 5 ml PoM £1.90 DT price = £1.90
  ▸ Betoptic (Alcon Laboratories (UK) Ltd)
  Betaxolol (as Betaxolol hydrochloride) 2.5 mg per 1 ml Betoptic 0.25% suspension eye drops | 5 ml PoM £2.66 DT price = £2.66
  Betoptic 0.25% eye drops suspension 0.25ml unit dose | 50 unit dose PoM £13.77
  Betaxolol (as Betaxolol hydrochloride) 5 mg per 1 ml Betoptic 0.5% eye drops | 5 ml PoM £1.90 DT price = £1.90

Carteolol hydrochloride

- INDICATIONS AND DOSE
  Primary and secondary glaucomas
  ▸ TO THE EYE
  ▸ Child: Apply twice daily

- UNLICENSED USE Not licensed for use in children.

- CONTRA-INDICATIONS Also consider contra-indications listed for systemically administered beta blockers · bradycardia · heart block

- CAUTIONS Patients with corneal disease
  CAUTIONS, FURTHER INFORMATION
  Systemic absorption can follow topical application to the eyes; consider cautions listed for systemically administered beta blockers.

- INTERACTIONS → Appendix 1: beta blockers (non-selective)

- SIDE-EFFECTS Anaphylaxis · blepharoconjunctivitis · burning · corneal disorders · cough, rather than wheeze, may occur · dry eyes · erythema · itching · ocular stinging · pain

  SIDE-EFFECTS, FURTHER INFORMATION
  Systemic absorption can follow topical application to the eyes; consider side effects listed for systemically administered beta blockers.

- MEDICINAL FORMS
  There can be variation in the licensing of different medicines containing the same drug.
  Eye drops
  EXCIPIENTS: May contain Benzalkonium chloride
  ▸ Teoptic (Thea Pharmaceuticals Ltd)
  Carteolol hydrochloride 10 mg per 1 ml Teoptic 1% eye drops | 5 ml PoM £7.60 DT price = £7.60
  Carteolol hydrochloride 20 mg per 1 ml Teoptic 2% eye drops | 5 ml PoM £8.40 DT price = £8.40

Levobunolol hydrochloride

- INDICATIONS AND DOSE
  Primary and secondary glaucomas
  ▸ TO THE EYE
  ▸ Child: Apply 1–2 times a day

- UNLICENSED USE Not licensed for use in children.

- CONTRA-INDICATIONS Also consider contra-indications listed for systemically administered beta blockers · bradycardia · heart block

- CAUTIONS Patients with corneal disease
  CAUTIONS, FURTHER INFORMATION
  Systemic absorption can follow topical application to the eyes; consider cautions listed for systemically administered beta blockers.

- INTERACTIONS → Appendix 1: beta blockers (non-selective)

- SIDE-EFFECTS Anaphylaxis · anterior uveitis · blepharoconjunctivitis · burning · corneal disorders · cough, rather than wheeze, may occur · dry eyes · erythema · itching · ocular stinging · pain

  SIDE-EFFECTS, FURTHER INFORMATION
  Systemic absorption can follow topical application to the eyes; consider side effects listed for systemically administered beta blockers.

- PRESCRIBING AND DISPENSING INFORMATION Although multi-dose (Levobunolol) eye drops commonly contain preservatives, preservative-free unit dose vials may be available.

- MEDICINAL FORMS
  There can be variation in the licensing of different medicines containing the same drug.
  Eye drops
  EXCIPIENTS: May contain Benzalkonium chloride, disodium edetate, sodium metabisulfite
  ▸ Betagan (Allergan Ltd)
  Levobunolol hydrochloride 5 mg per 1 ml Betagan 0.5% eye drops | 5 ml PoM £1.85 DT price = £1.85
  Betagan Unit Dose 0.5% eye drops 0.4ml unit dose | 30 unit dose PoM £9.98

Timolol maleate

- INDICATIONS AND DOSE
  Primary congenital and primary juvenile glaucoma, for a transitional period, before surgery or following failed surgery
  ▸ TO THE EYE
  ▸ Child: (consult product literature)
  TIMOPTOL-LA®

  Reduction of intra-ocular pressure in primary and secondary glaucoma
  ▸ TO THE EYE
  ▸ Child: Apply once daily
  TIOPEX®

  Reduction of intra-ocular pressure primary and secondary glaucomas
  ▸ TO THE EYE
  ▸ Child: Apply once daily, to be applied in the morning

- UNLICENSED USE Not licensed for use in children.

- CONTRA-INDICATIONS Also consider contra-indications listed for systemically administered beta blockers · bradycardia · heart block

- CAUTIONS Consider also cautions listed for systemically administered beta blockers · patients with corneal disease

- **INTERACTIONS** → Appendix 1: beta blockers (non-selective)
- **SIDE-EFFECTS** Anaphylaxis · blepharoconjunctivitis · burning · corneal disorders · cough, rather than wheeze, may occur · dry eyes · erythema · itching · ocular stinging · pain

SIDE-EFFECTS, FURTHER INFORMATION

Systemic absorption can follow topical application to the eyes; consider side effects listed for systemically administered beta blockers.

- **BREAST FEEDING** Manufacturer advises avoidance.
- **NATIONAL FUNDING/ACCESS DECISIONS**

TIOPEX®

Scottish Medicines Consortium (SMC) Decisions
The *Scottish Medicines Consortium* has advised (February 2014) that timolol gel eye drops (*Tiopex®*) are accepted for restricted use within NHS Scotland for the reduction of elevated intraocular pressure in patients with ocular hypertension or chronic open angle glaucoma who have proven sensitivity to preservatives.

- **MEDICINAL FORMS**
There can be variation in the licensing of different medicines containing the same drug. Forms available from special-order manufacturers include: eye drops

Eye gel
EXCIPIENTS: May contain Benzododecinium bromide
▸ Timoptol-LA (Santen UK Ltd)
   Timolol (as Timolol maleate) 2.5 mg per 1 ml Timoptol-LA 0.25% ophthalmic gel-forming solution | 2.5 ml [PoM] £3.12 DT price = £3.12
   Timolol (as Timolol maleate) 5 mg per 1 ml Timoptol-LA 0.5% ophthalmic gel-forming solution | 2.5 ml [PoM] £3.12 DT price = £3.12

Eye drops
EXCIPIENTS: May contain Benzalkonium chloride
▸ Timolol maleate (Non-proprietary)
   Timolol (as Timolol maleate) 2.5 mg per 1 ml Timolol 0.25% eye drops | 5 ml [PoM] £1.76 DT price = £1.43
   Timolol (as Timolol maleate) 5 mg per 1 ml Timolol 0.5% eye drops | 5 ml [PoM] £1.95 DT price = £1.25
▸ Timoptol (Santen UK Ltd)
   Timolol (as Timolol maleate) 2.5 mg per 1 ml Timoptol 0.25% eye drops | 5 ml [PoM] £3.12 DT price = £1.43
   Timoptol Unit Dose 0.25% ophthalmic solution 0.2ml unit dose | 30 unit dose [PoM] £8.45 DT price = £8.45
   Timolol (as Timolol maleate) 5 mg per 1 ml Timoptol 0.5% eye drops | 5 ml [PoM] £3.12 DT price = £1.25
   Timoptol Unit Dose 0.5% ophthalmic solution 0.2ml unit dose | 30 unit dose [PoM] £9.65 DT price = £9.65
▸ Tiopex (Thea Pharmaceuticals Ltd)
   Timolol (as Timolol maleate) 1 mg per 1 gram Tiopex 1mg/g eye gel 0.4g unit dose | 30 unit dose [PoM] £7.49 DT price = £7.49

Combinations available: *Dorzolamide with timolol,* p. 657

CARBONIC ANHYDRASE INHIBITORS

Acetazolamide

- **INDICATIONS AND DOSE**

Glaucoma
▸ BY MOUTH USING MODIFIED-RELEASE MEDICINES
▸ Child 12–17 years: 250–500 mg daily

Epilepsy
▸ BY MOUTH USING IMMEDIATE-RELEASE MEDICINES, OR BY SLOW INTRAVENOUS INJECTION

▸ Neonate: Initially 2.5 mg/kg 2–3 times a day, followed by maintenance 5–7 mg/kg 2–3 times a day.

▸ Child 1 month–11 years: Initially 2.5 mg/kg 2–3 times a day, followed by maintenance 5–7 mg/kg 2–3 times a day; maximum 750 mg per day
▸ Child 12–17 years: 250 mg 2–4 times a day

Reduction of intra-ocular pressure in primary and secondary glaucoma (specialist use only)
▸ BY MOUTH USING IMMEDIATE-RELEASE MEDICINES, OR BY INTRAVENOUS INJECTION
▸ Child 1 month–11 years: 5 mg/kg 2–4 times a day, adjusted according to response; maximum 750 mg per day
▸ Child 12–17 years: 250 mg 2–4 times a day

Raised intracranial pressure
▸ BY MOUTH USING IMMEDIATE-RELEASE MEDICINES, OR BY SLOW INTRAVENOUS INJECTION
▸ Child 1 month–11 years: Initially 8 mg/kg 3 times a day, then increased if necessary up to 100 mg/kg daily

- **UNLICENSED USE** Not licensed for the treatment of glaucoma.
- **CONTRA-INDICATIONS** Adrenocortical insufficiency · hyperchloraemic acidosis · hypokalaemia · hyponatraemia · long-term administration in chronic angle-closure glaucoma
- **CAUTIONS** Avoid extravasation at injection site (risk of necrosis) · diabetes mellitus · impaired alveolar ventilation (risk of acidosis) · not generally recommended for long-term use · pulmonary obstruction (risk of acidosis) · renal calculi
- **INTERACTIONS** → Appendix 1: acetazolamide
- **SIDE-EFFECTS**
▸ **Common or very common** Ataxia · depression · diarrhoea · dizziness · excitement · fatigue · flushing · headache · irritability · loss of appetite · nausea · paraesthesia · polyuria · taste disturbance · thirst · vomiting
▸ **Uncommon** Blood disorders · bone marrow suppression · confusion · crystalluria · drowsiness · electrolyte disturbances on long-term therapy · fever · glycosuria · haematuria · hearing disturbances · melaena · metabolic acidosis · rash · renal calculi · renal colic · renal failure · renal lesions · Stevens-Johnson syndrome · toxic epidermal necrosis · ureteric colic
▸ **Rare** Cholestatic jaundice · convulsions · flaccid paralysis · fulminant hepatic necrosis · hepatitis · photosensitivity
▸ **Frequency not known** Transient myopia
SIDE-EFFECTS, FURTHER INFORMATION

Acetazolamide is a sulfonamide derivative; blood disorders, rashes, and other sulfonamide-related side-effects occur occasionally—patients should be told to report any unusual skin rash.

If electrolyte disturbances and metabolic acidosis occur, these can be corrected by administering potassium bicarbonate (as effervescent potassium tablets).

- **ALLERGY AND CROSS-SENSITIVITY** Contra-indicated if history of sulfonamide hypersensitivity.
- **PREGNANCY** Manufacturer advises avoid, especially in first trimester (toxicity in *animal* studies).
- **BREAST FEEDING** Amount too small to be harmful.
- **HEPATIC IMPAIRMENT** Manufacturer advises avoid.
- **RENAL IMPAIRMENT** Avoid—risk of metabolic acidosis.
- **MONITORING REQUIREMENTS** Monitor blood count and plasma electrolyte concentrations with prolonged use.

- **MEDICINAL FORMS**
There can be variation in the licensing of different medicines containing the same drug.

Tablet
CAUTIONARY AND ADVISORY LABELS 3
▸ Acetazolamide (Non-proprietary)
   Acetazolamide 250 mg Acetazolamide 250mg tablets | 112 tablet [PoM] £75.36 DT price = £28.20
Powder for solution for injection
▸ Diamox (AMCo)
   Acetazolamide 500 mg Diamox Sodium Parenteral 500mg powder for solution for injection vials | 1 vial [PoM] £14.76

Modified-release capsule
CAUTIONARY AND ADVISORY LABELS 3, 25
▸ Diamox SR (AMCo)
Acetazolamide 250 mg Diamox SR 250mg capsules |
30 capsule PoM £16.66 DT price = £16.66
▸ Eytazox (Teva UK Ltd)
Acetazolamide 250 mg Eytazox 250mg modified-release capsules |
30 capsule PoM £16.60 DT price = £16.66

Brinzolamide

● INDICATIONS AND DOSE
Reduction of intra-ocular pressure in primary and secondary glaucoma either as adjunct to beta-blockers or prostaglandin analogues or used alone if unresponsive to beta-blockers or if beta-blockers contra-indicated
▸ TO THE EYE
▸ Child: Apply twice daily, then increased if necessary up to 3 times a day

● UNLICENSED USE Not licensed for use in children.
● CONTRA-INDICATIONS Hyperchloraemic acidosis
● CAUTIONS Renal tubular immaturity or abnormality—risk of metabolic acidosis · systemic absorption follows topical application
● INTERACTIONS → Appendix 1: brinzolamide
● SIDE-EFFECTS
▸ **Common or very common** Corneal erosion · corneal oedema · dry mouth · headache · ocular disturbances · photophobia · reduced visual acuity · taste disturbances
▸ **Uncommon** Alopecia · amnesia · bradycardia · chest pain · cough · decreased libido · depression · diarrhoea · dizziness · drowsiness · dyspepsia · dyspnoea · epistaxis · erectile dysfunction · flatulence · malaise · nasal dryness · nausea · nervousness · oesophagitis · oral hypoaesthesia and paraesthesia · palpitation · paraesthesia · pharyngitis · renal pain · sinusitis · sleep disturbances · throat irritation · tinnitus · upper respiratory tract congestion · vomiting
▸ **Frequency not known** Arrhythmia · asthma · dermatitis · erythema · hypertension · peripheral oedema · pollakiuria · rhinitis · tachycardia · tremor · vertigo

SIDE-EFFECTS, FURTHER INFORMATION
Systemic absorption can rarely cause sulfonamide-like side-effects and may require discontinuation if severe.

● ALLERGY AND CROSS-SENSITIVITY Contra-indicated if history of sulfonamide hypersensitivity.
● PREGNANCY Avoid—toxicity in *animal* studies.
● BREAST FEEDING Use only if benefit outweighs risk.
● HEPATIC IMPAIRMENT Manufacturer advises avoid.
● RENAL IMPAIRMENT Avoid if estimated glomerular filtration rate less than 30 mL/minute/1.73 m^2.

● MEDICINAL FORMS
There can be variation in the licensing of different medicines containing the same drug.
Eye drops
EXCIPIENTS: May contain Benzalkonium chloride, disodium edetate
▸ Brinzolamide (Non-proprietary)
Brinzolamide 10 mg per 1 ml Brinzolamide 10mg/ml eye drops |
5 ml PoM £6.92 DT price = £2.11
▸ Azopt (Alcon Laboratories (UK) Ltd)
Brinzolamide 10 mg per 1 ml Azopt 10mg/ml eye drops |
5 ml PoM £6.92 DT price = £2.11

Dorzolamide

● INDICATIONS AND DOSE
Raised intra-ocular pressure in primary and secondary glaucoma used alone in patients unresponsive to beta-blockers or if beta-blockers contra-indicated
▸ TO THE EYE
▸ Child: Apply 3 times a day

Raised intra-ocular pressure in primary and secondary glaucoma as adjunct to a beta-blocker
▸ TO THE EYE
▸ Child: Apply twice daily

● UNLICENSED USE Not licensed for use in children.
● CONTRA-INDICATIONS Hyperchloraemic acidosis
● CAUTIONS Chronic corneal defects · history of intra-ocular surgery · history of renal calculi · immature renal tubules (neonates and infants)—risk of metabolic acidosis · low endothelial cell count · systemic absorption follows topical application
● INTERACTIONS → Appendix 1: dorzolamide
● SIDE-EFFECTS
▸ **Common or very common** Asthenia · bitter taste · blurred vision · conjunctivitis · eyelid inflammation · headache · lacrimation · nausea · ocular irritation · superficial punctate keratitis
▸ **Uncommon** Iridocyclitis
▸ **Rare** Contact dermatitis · corneal oedema · dizziness · dry mouth · epistaxis · eyelid crusting · paraesthesia · Stevens-Johnson syndrome · throat irritation · toxic epidermal necrolysis · transient myopia · urolithiasis
▸ **Frequency not known** Metabolic acidosis

SIDE-EFFECTS, FURTHER INFORMATION
Systemic absorption can rarely cause sulfonamide-like side-effects and may require discontinuation if severe.

● ALLERGY AND CROSS-SENSITIVITY Contra-indicated if history of sulfonamide hypersensitivity.
● PREGNANCY Manufacturer advises avoid—toxicity in *animal* studies.
● BREAST FEEDING Manufacturer advises avoid—no information available.
● HEPATIC IMPAIRMENT Manufacturer advises caution— no information available.
● RENAL IMPAIRMENT Avoid if estimated glomerular filtration rate less than 30 mL/minute/1.73 m^2.
● PRESCRIBING AND DISPENSING INFORMATION Although multi-dose dorzolamide eye drops commonly contain preservatives, preservative-free unit dose vials may be available.

● MEDICINAL FORMS
There can be variation in the licensing of different medicines containing the same drug.
Eye drops
EXCIPIENTS: May contain Benzalkonium chloride
▸ Dorzolamide (Non-proprietary)
Dorzolamide (as Dorzolamide hydrochloride) 20 mg per 1 ml Dorzolamide 2% eye drops | 5 ml PoM £6.33 DT price = £1.90
▸ Trusopt (Santen UK Ltd)
Dorzolamide (as Dorzolamide hydrochloride) 20 mg per 1 ml Trusopt 2% eye drops | 5 ml PoM £6.33 DT price = £1.90
Trusopt 2% eye drops 0.2ml unit dose preservative free | 60 unit dose PoM £24.18 DT price = £24.18

Dorzolamide with timolol

The properties listed below are those particular to the combination only. For the properties of the components please consider, dorzolamide p. 656, timolol maleate p. 654.

- **INDICATIONS AND DOSE**
  Raised intra-ocular pressure in open-angle glaucoma when beta-blockers alone not adequate | Raised intra-ocular pressure in pseudo-exfoliative glaucoma when beta-blockers alone not adequate
  ▸ TO THE EYE
  ▸ Child: Apply twice daily

- **PRESCRIBING AND DISPENSING INFORMATION** Although multi-dose dorzolamide with timolol eye drops commonly contain preservatives, preservative-free unit dose vials may be available.

- **MEDICINAL FORMS**
  There can be variation in the licensing of different medicines containing the same drug.
  Eye drops
  EXCIPIENTS: May contain Benzalkonium chloride
  ▸ **Dorzolamide with timolol** (Non-proprietary)
  Timolol (as Timolol maleate) 5 mg per 1 ml, **Dorzolamide** (as Dorzolamide hydrochloride) 20 mg per 1 ml Dorzolamide 2% / Timolol 0.5% eye drops | 5 ml [PoM] £27.16 DT price = £1.81
  Dorzolamide 2% / Timolol 0.5% eye drops 0.2ml unit dose preservative free | 60 unit dose [PoM] £28.59 DT price = £28.59
  ▸ **Cosopt** (Santen UK Ltd)
  Timolol (as Timolol maleate) 5 mg per 1 ml, **Dorzolamide** (as Dorzolamide hydrochloride) 20 mg per 1 ml Cosopt eye drops 0.2ml unit dose preservative free | 60 unit dose [PoM] £28.59 DT price = £28.59
  Cosopt eye drops | 5 ml [PoM] £10.05 DT price = £1.81

MIOTICS > PARASYMPATHOMIMETICS

Pilocarpine

- **DRUG ACTION** Pilocarpine acts by opening the inefficient drainage channels in the trabecular meshwork.

- **INDICATIONS AND DOSE**
  Raised intra-ocular pressure
  ▸ TO THE EYE
  ▸ Child 1 month-1 year: Apply 1 drop 3 times a day, doses are for 0.5% or 1% solution
  ▸ Child 2-17 years: Apply 1 drop 4 times a day
  Pre- and postoperatively in goniotomy and trabeculotomy
  ▸ TO THE EYE
  ▸ Child: Apply once daily, 1% or 2% solution to be applied

- **UNLICENSED USE** Not licensed for use in children.

- **CONTRA-INDICATIONS** Acute inflammatory disease of the anterior segment · acute iritis · anterior uveitis · conditions where pupillary constriction is undesirable · some forms of secondary glaucoma (where pupillary constriction is undesirable)

- **CAUTIONS** A darkly pigmented iris may require a higher concentration of the miotic or more frequent administration and care should be taken to avoid overdosage · asthma · cardiac disease · care in conjunctival damage · care in corneal damage · epilepsy · gastro-intestinal spasm · hypertension · hyperthyroidism · hypotension · peptic ulceration · retinal detachment has occurred in susceptible individuals and those with retinal disease · urinary-tract obstruction

- **INTERACTIONS** → Appendix 1: pilocarpine

- **SIDE-EFFECTS**
  ▸ **Rare** Parasympathomimetics systemic side effects

- **Frequency not known** Blurred vision · ciliary spasm (leads to headache and browache which may be more severe in the initial 2-4 weeks of treatment—a particular disadvantage in patients under 40 years of age) · conjunctival vascular congestion · lens changes (with chronic use) · myopia · ocular burning · ocular itching · pupillary block · smarting · vitreous haemorrhage

- **PREGNANCY** Avoid unless the potential benefit outweighs risk—limited information available.

- **BREAST FEEDING** Avoid unless the potential benefit outweighs risk—no information available.

- **PRE-TREATMENT SCREENING** Fundus examination is advised before starting treatment with a miotic (retinal detachment has occurred).

- **MONITORING REQUIREMENTS** Intra-ocular pressure and visual fields should be monitored in those with chronic simple glaucoma and those receiving long-term treatment with a miotic.

- **PRESCRIBING AND DISPENSING INFORMATION** Although multi-dose pilocarpine eye drops commonly contain preservatives, preservative-free unit dose vials may be available.

- **PATIENT AND CARER ADVICE**
  Driving and skilled tasks
  Blurred vision may affect performance of skilled tasks (e.g. driving) particularly at night or in reduced lighting.

- **MEDICINAL FORMS**
  There can be variation in the licensing of different medicines containing the same drug. Forms available from special-order manufacturers include: eye drops
  Eye drops
  EXCIPIENTS: May contain Benzalkonium chloride
  ▸ **Pilocarpine** (Non-proprietary)
  Pilocarpine hydrochloride 10 mg per 1 ml Pilocarpine hydrochloride 1% eye drops | 10 ml [PoM] £16.10 DT price = £13.44
  Pilocarpine hydrochloride 20 mg per 1 ml Pilocarpine hydrochloride 2% eye drops | 10 ml [PoM] £19.71 DT price = £16.48
  Pilocarpine hydrochloride 40 mg per 1 ml Pilocarpine hydrochloride 4% eye drops | 10 ml [PoM] £21.99 DT price = £18.35
  ▸ **Pilocarpine nitrate** (Bausch & Lomb UK Ltd)
  Pilocarpine nitrate 20 mg per 1 ml Minims pilocarpine nitrate 2% eye drops 0.5ml unit dose | 20 unit dose [PoM] £11.99

PROSTAGLANDIN ANALOGUES AND PROSTAMIDES

Latanoprost

- **INDICATIONS AND DOSE**
  Reduction of intra-ocular pressure in raised intra-ocular pressure and glaucoma
  ▸ TO THE EYE
  ▸ Child: Apply once daily, to be administered preferably in the evening

---

IMPORTANT SAFETY INFORMATION

MHRA/CHM ADVICE: LATANOPROST (*XALATAN*®): INCREASED REPORTING OF EYE IRRITATION SINCE REFORMULATION (JULY 2015)

Following reformulation of *Xalatan*®, to allow for long-term storage at room temperature, there has been an increase in the number of reports of eye irritation from across the EU. Patients should be advised to tell their health professional promptly (within a week) if they experience eye irritation (e.g. excessive watering) severe enough to make them consider stopping treatment. Review treatment and prescribe a different formulation if necessary.

11

Eye

- CONTRA-INDICATIONS Active herpes simplex keratitis · history of recurrent herpetic keratitis associated with prostaglandin analogues
- CAUTIONS Aphakia · asthma · children less than 1 year—limited information available · history of herpetic keratitis · history of significant ocular viral infections · peri-operative period of cataract surgery · preterm neonates less than 36 weeks gestational age—no information available · pseudophakia with torn posterior lens capsule or anterior chamber lenses · risk factors for cystoid macular oedema · risk factors for iritis · risk factors for uveitis
- SIDE-EFFECTS
  - **Common or very common** Blepharitis · conjunctival hyperaemia · eye irritation · eye pain · eyelash and vellus hair changes · increased iris pigmentation · transient punctate epithelial erosion
  - **Uncommon** Blurred vision · conjunctivitis · dry eye · eyelid oedema · keratitis · skin rash
  - **Rare** Corneal erosion · corneal oedema · distichiasis · iritis · macular oedema · misdirected eyelashes · periorbital oedema · photophobia · uveitis
  - **Very rare** Chest pain · darkening of palpebral skin of the eyelids · localised skin reaction on the eyelids · periorbital changes resulting in deepening of the eyelid sulcus
  - **Frequency not known** Arthralgia · asthma · dizziness · dyspnoea · exacerbation of asthma · headache · herpetic keratitis · iris cyst · myalgia · nasopharyngitis · palpitation · pyrexia
- PREGNANCY Manufacturer advises avoid.
- BREAST FEEDING May be present in milk—manufacturer advises avoid.
- MONITORING REQUIREMENTS Monitor for changes to eye coloration.
- PRESCRIBING AND DISPENSING INFORMATION Although multi-dose latanoprost eye drops commonly contain preservatives, preservative-free unit dose vials may be available.
- PATIENT AND CARER ADVICE
  Changes in eye colour Before initiating treatment, patients should be warned of a possible change in eye colour as an increase in the brown pigment in the iris can occur, which may be permanent; particular care is required in those with mixed coloured irides and those receiving treatment to one eye only. Changes in eyelashes and vellus hair can also occur, and patients should also be advised to avoid repeated contact of the eye drop solution with skin as this can lead to hair growth or skin pigmentation.
- NATIONAL FUNDING/ACCESS DECISIONS
  MONOPOST®
  Scottish Medicines Consortium (SMC) Decisions
  The *Scottish Medicines Consortium* has advised (June 2013) that *Monopost®* is accepted for restricted use within NHS Scotland for the reduction of elevated intra-ocular pressure in patients with open-angle glaucoma and ocular hypertension who have proven sensitivity to benzalkonium chloride.

- MEDICINAL FORMS
  There can be variation in the licensing of different medicines containing the same drug.
  Eye drops
  EXCIPIENTS: May contain Benzalkonium chloride
  - Latanoprost (Non-proprietary)
    Latanoprost 50 microgram per 1 ml Latanoprost 50micrograms/ml eye drops | 2.5 ml [PoM] £12.48 DT price = £1.40
  - Monopost (Thea Pharmaceuticals Ltd)
    Latanoprost 50 microgram per 1 ml Monopost 50micrograms/ml eye drops 0.2ml unit dose | 30 unit dose [PoM] £8.49 DT price = £8.49 | 90 unit dose [PoM] £25.47 DT price = £25.47
  - Xalatan (Pfizer Ltd)
    Latanoprost 50 microgram per 1 ml Xalatan 50micrograms/ml eye drops | 2.5 ml [PoM] £12.48 DT price = £1.40

SYMPATHOMIMETICS > ALPHA$_2$-ADRENOCEPTOR AGONISTS

Apraclonidine

- DRUG ACTION Apraclonidine is an alpha$_2$-adrenoceptor agonist that lowers intra-ocular pressure by reducing aqueous humour formation. It is a derivative of clonidine.

- INDICATIONS AND DOSE

Control or prevention of postoperative elevation of intra-ocular pressure after anterior segment laser surgery
  - ▶ TO THE EYE
  - ▶ Child: Apply 1 drop, 1 hour before laser procedure, then 1 drop, immediately after completion of procedure, 1% eye drops to be administered

Short-term adjunctive treatment of chronic glaucoma in patients not adequately controlled by another drug
  - ▶ TO THE EYE
  - ▶ Child 12–17 years: Apply 1 drop 3 times a day usually for maximum 1 month, 0.5% eye drops to be administered, may not provide additional benefit if patient already using two drugs that suppress the production of aqueous humour

- UNLICENSED USE 0.5% drops are not licensed for use in children under 12 years. 1% drops are not licensed for use in children.
- CONTRA-INDICATIONS History of severe or unstable and uncontrolled cardiovascular disease
- CAUTIONS Cerebrovascular disease · depression · heart failure · history of angina · hypertension · loss of effect may occur over time · Raynaud's syndrome · recent myocardial infarction · reduction in vision in end-stage glaucoma (suspend treatment) · severe coronary insufficiency · thromboangiitis obliterans · vasovagal attack
- INTERACTIONS → Appendix 1: apraclonidine
- SIDE-EFFECTS
  - **Common or very common** Conjunctivitis · dry eye · ocular intolerance · rhinitis · taste disturbance
  - **Uncommon** Asthma · blepharitis · blepharospasm · chest pain · conjunctival vascular disorders · corneal erosion and infiltrates · dyspnoea · eyelid ptosis or retraction · impaired co-ordination · irritability · keratitis · keratopathy · myalgia · mydriasis · nervousness · parosmia · photophobia · rhinorrhoea · throat irritation · visual impairment
  SIDE-EFFECTS, FURTHER INFORMATION
  - ▶ Ocular intolerance Withdraw if eye pruritus, ocular hyperaemia, increased lacrimation, or oedema of the eyelids and conjunctiva occur.
  - ▶ Systemic effects Since absorption may follow topical application, see clonidine hydrochloride p. 99.
- PREGNANCY Manufacturer advises avoid—no information available.
- BREAST FEEDING Manufacturer advises avoid—no information available.
- HEPATIC IMPAIRMENT Manufacturer advises caution.
- RENAL IMPAIRMENT Use with caution in chronic renal failure.
- MONITORING REQUIREMENTS
  - ▶ Monitor intra-ocular pressure and visual fields.
  - ▶ Monitor for excessive reduction in intra-ocular pressure following peri-operative use.
- PATIENT AND CARER ADVICE
  Driving and skilled tasks
  Drowsiness may affect performance of skilled tasks (e.g. driving).

● **MEDICINAL FORMS**
There can be variation in the licensing of different medicines containing the same drug.

Eye drops
EXCIPIENTS: May contain Benzalkonium chloride
▸ **Iopidine** (Alcon Laboratories (UK) Ltd)
Apraclonidine (as Apraclonidine hydrochloride) 5 mg per 1 ml Iopidine 5mg/ml eye drops | 5 ml [PoM] £10.88 DT price = £10.88
Apraclonidine (as Apraclonidine hydrochloride) 10 mg per 1 ml Iopidine 1% eye drops 0.25ml unit dose | 24 unit dose [PoM] £77.85 DT price = £77.85

6 Retinal disorders

6.1 Optic neuropathy

DRUGS FOR METABOLIC DISORDERS ›
ANTIOXIDANTS

Idebenone   31-May-2017

● **DRUG ACTION** Idebenone is a nootropic and antioxidant that is thought to act by restoring cellular ATP generation, thereby reactivating retinal ganglion cells.

● **INDICATIONS AND DOSE**
Leber's Hereditary Optic Neuropathy (initiated by a specialist)
▸ **BY MOUTH**
▸ Child 12–17 years: 300 mg 3 times a day

● **SIDE-EFFECTS**
▸ **Common or very common** Back pain · cough · diarrhoea · nasopharyngitis
▸ **Frequency not known** Anorexia · azotaemia · blood disorders · bronchitis · chromaturia · dyspepsia · hepatitis · malaise · nausea · nervous system disorders · pain in extremity · pruritus · raised lipids · raised liver enzymes · rash · vomiting

SIDE-EFFECTS, FURTHER INFORMATION
▸ **Chromaturia** The metabolites of idebenone may cause red-brown discolouration of the urine. This effect is harmless, but the manufacturer advises caution as this may mask colour changes due to other causes (e.g. renal or blood disorders).

● **PREGNANCY** Manufacturer advises avoid unless potential benefit outweighs risk—no information available.

● **BREAST FEEDING** Manufacturer advises avoid—present in milk in *animal* studies.

● **HEPATIC IMPAIRMENT** Manufacturer advises use with caution—no information available.

● **RENAL IMPAIRMENT** Manufacturer advises use with caution—no information available.

● **NATIONAL FUNDING/ACCESS DECISIONS**
Scottish Medicines Consortium (SMC) Decisions
The *Scottish Medicines Consortium* has advised (May 2017) that idebenone (*Raxone*®) is accepted for restricted use within NHS Scotland for the treatment of visual impairment in patients with Leber's Hereditary Optic Neuropathy (LHON) who are not yet blind i.e. they do not meet the UK criteria to be registered as severely sight impaired. This advice is contingent upon the continuing availability of the Patient Access Scheme in NHS Scotland or a list price that is equivalent or lower.

● **MEDICINAL FORMS**
There can be variation in the licensing of different medicines containing the same drug. Forms available from special-order manufacturers include: tablet

Tablet
CAUTIONARY AND ADVISORY LABELS 14, 21
▸ **Raxone** (Santhera (UK) Ltd) ▼
Idebenone 150 mg Raxone 150mg tablets | 180 tablet [PoM] £6,364.00

11
Eye

Chapter 12
Ear, nose and oropharynx

CONTENTS

Ear

Ear

Otitis externa

Otitis externa is an inflammatory reaction of the lining of the ear canal usually associated with an underlying seborrhoeic dermatitis or eczema; it is important to exclude an underlying chronic otitis media before treatment is commenced. Many cases recover after thorough cleansing of the external ear canal by suction or dry mopping.

A frequent problem in resistant cases is the difficulty in applying lotions and ointments satisfactorily to the relatively inaccessible affected skin. The most effective method is to introduce a ribbon gauze dressing or sponge wick soaked with **corticosteroid** ear drops or with an astringent such as aluminium acetate solution p. 664. When this is not practical, the ear should be gently cleansed with a probe covered in cotton wool and the patient encouraged to lie with the affected ear uppermost for ten minutes after the canal has been filled with a liberal quantity of the appropriate solution.

Secondary infection in otitis externa may be of bacterial, fungal, or viral origin. If infection is present, a topical anti-infective which is not used systemically (such as neomycin sulfate p. 662 or **clioquinol**) may be used, but for only about a week because excessive use may result in fungal infections that are difficult to treat. Sensitivity to the anti-infective or solvent may occur and resistance to antibacterials is a possibility with prolonged use. Aluminium acetate ear drops are also effective against bacterial infection and inflammation of the ear. Chloramphenicol p. 662 may be used, but the ear drops contain propylene glycol and cause hypersensitivity reactions in about 10% of patients. Solutions containing an anti-infective and a corticosteroid are used for treating children when infection is present with inflammation and eczema. Clotrimazole 1% solution p. 662 is used topically to treat fungal infection in otitis externa.

In view of reports of ototoxicity, manufacturers contra-indicate treatment with topical **aminoglycosides** or **polymyxins** in children with a perforated tympanic membrane (eardrum) or patent grommet. However, some specialists do use these drops cautiously in the presence of a perforation or patent grommet in children with chronic suppurative otitis media and when other measures have failed for otitis externa; treatment should be considered only by **specialists** in the following circumstances:

- drops should only be used in the presence of obvious infection;
- treatment should be for no longer than 2 weeks;
- the carer and child should be counselled on the risk of ototoxicity and given justification for the use of these topical antibiotics;
- baseline audiometry should be performed, if possible, before treatment is commenced.

Clinical expertise and judgement should be used to assess the risk of treatment versus the benefit to the patient in such circumstances.

A solution of **acetic acid** 2% acts as an antifungal and antibacterial in the external ear canal. It may be used to treat mild otitis externa but in severe cases an anti-inflammatory preparation with or without an anti-infective drug is required. A proprietary preparation containing acetic acid 2% (*EarCalm®* spray) is on sale to the public for children over 12 years.

For severe pain associated with otitis externa, a simple analgesic, such as paracetamol p. 260 or ibuprofen p. 625, can be used. A systemic antibacterial can be used if there is spreading cellulitis or if the patient is systemically unwell. When a resistant staphylococcal infection (a boil) is present in the external auditory meatus, flucloxacillin p. 330 is the drug of choice; oral ciprofloxacin p. 333 or a systemic aminoglycoside may be needed for pseudomonal infections, particularly in children with diabetes or compromised immunity.

The skin of the pinna adjacent to the ear canal is often affected by eczema. Topical corticosteroid creams and ointments are then required, but prolonged use should be avoided.

Otitis media

Acute otitis media

Acute otitis media is the commonest cause of severe aural pain in young children and may occur with even minor upper respiratory tract infections. Children diagnosed with acute otitis media should not be prescribed antibacterials routinely as many infections, especially those accompanying coryza, are caused by viruses. Most uncomplicated cases resolve without antibacterial treatment and a **simple analgesic**, such as paracetamol, may be sufficient. In children without systemic features, a **systemic antibacterial** may be started after 72 hours if there is no improvement, or earlier if there is deterioration, if the child is systemically unwell, if the child is at high risk of serious complications (e.g. in immunosuppression, cystic fibrosis), if mastoiditis is present, or in children under 2 years of age with bilateral otitis media. Perforation of the tympanic membrane in children with *acute otitis media* usually heals spontaneously without treatment; if there is no improvement, e.g. pain or discharge persists, a systemic antibacterial can be given. Topical antibacterial treatment of acute otitis media is ineffective and there is no place for ear drops containing a local anaesthetic.

Otitis media with effusion

Otitis media with effusion (glue ear) occurs in about 10% of children and in 90% of children with cleft palates. Antimicrobials, corticosteroids, decongestants, and antihistamines have little place in the routine management of otitis media with effusion. If glue ear persists for more than a month or two, the child should be referred for assessment and follow up because of the risk of long-term hearing impairment which can delay language development. Untreated or resistant glue ear may be responsible for some types of *chronic otitis media*.

Chronic otitis media

Opportunistic organisms are often present in the debris, keratin, and necrotic bone of the middle ear and mastoid in children with chronic otitis media. The mainstay of treatment is thorough cleansing with aural microsuction, which may completely resolve long-standing infection. Cleansing may be followed by topical treatment as for otitis externa; this is particularly beneficial for discharging ears or infections of the mastoid cavity. Acute exacerbations of chronic infection may require treatment with an oral antibacterial; a swab should be taken to identify infecting organisms and antibacterial sensitivity.

In view of reports of ototoxicity, manufacturers contraindicate topical treatment with ototoxic antibacterials in the presence of a tympanic perforation or patent grommet. Ciprofloxacin p. 647 or ofloxacin eye drops p. 648 used in the ear [unlicensed use] or ear drops [both unlicensed; available from 'special-order' manufacturers or specialist importing companies] are an effective alternative to such ototoxic ear drops for chronic otitis media in patients with perforation of the tympanic membrane.

However, some specialists do use ear drops containing **aminoglycosides** or **polymyxins** [unlicensed indications] cautiously in children with chronic suppurative otitis media and perforation of the tympanic membrane, if the otitis media has failed to settle with systemic antibacterials; treatment should be considered only **by specialists** in the following circumstances:

- drops should only be used in the presence of obvious infection;
- treatment should be for no longer than 2 weeks;
- the carer and child should be counselled on the risk of ototoxicity and given justification for the use of these topical antibiotics;
- baseline audiometry should be performed, if possible, before treatment is commenced.

Clinical expertise and judgement should be used to assess the risk of treatment versus the benefit to the patient in such circumstances. It is considered that the pus in the middle ear associated with otitis media also carries a risk of ototoxicity.

Removal of ear wax

Ear wax (cerumen) is a normal bodily secretion which provides a protective film on the meatal skin and need only be removed if it causes hearing loss or interferes with a proper view of the ear drum.

Ear wax causing discomfort or impaired hearing may be softened using simple remedies such as **olive oil** ear drops or **almond oil** ear drops; sodium bicarbonate ear drops p. 664 are also effective, but may cause dryness of the ear canal. If the wax is hard and impacted, the drops can be used twice daily for several days and this may reduce the need for mechanical removal of the wax. The child should lie with the affected ear uppermost for 5 to 10 minutes after a generous amount of the softening remedy has been introduced into the ear. Proprietary preparations containing organic solvents can irritate the meatal skin, and in most cases the simple remedies indicated above are just as effective and less likely to cause irritation. Docusate sodium p. 664 or urea hydrogen peroxide p. 665 are ingredients in a number of proprietary preparations for softening ear wax.

If necessary, wax may be removed by irrigation with water (warmed to body temperature). Ear irrigation is generally best avoided in young children, in children unable to co-operate with the procedure, in children who have had otitis media in the last six weeks, in otitis externa, in children with cleft palate, a history of ear drum perforation, or previous ear surgery. A child who has hearing in one ear only should not have that ear irrigated because even a very slight risk of damage is unacceptable in this situation.

Administration

To administer ear drops, lay the child down with the head turned to one side; for an infant pull the earlobe back and down, for an older child pull the earlobe back and up.

1   Otitis externa

ANTIBACTERIALS 〉 AMINOGLYCOSIDES

Framycetin sulfate

- **INDICATIONS AND DOSE**
Bacterial infection in otitis externa
  ▸ TO THE EAR
  ▸ Child: (consult product literature)

- **CONTRA-INDICATIONS** Perforated tympanic membrane
- **CAUTIONS** Avoid prolonged use
- **SIDE-EFFECTS** Local sensitivity

- **MEDICINAL FORMS**
There can be variation in the licensing of different medicines containing the same drug.
No licensed medicines listed.

  Combinations available: *Dexamethasone with framycetin sulfate and gramicidin*, p. 663

Gentamicin

- **INDICATIONS AND DOSE**
Bacterial infection in otitis externa
  ▸ TO THE EAR
  ▸ Child: Apply 2–3 drops 4–5 times a day, (including a dose at bedtime)

- **CONTRA-INDICATIONS** Patent grommet (although may be used by specialists, see Ear p. 660) · perforated tympanic membrane (although may be used by specialists, see Ear p. 660)
- **CAUTIONS** Avoid prolonged use
- **SIDE-EFFECTS** Local sensitivity

12

Ear, nose and oropharynx

Ear, nose and oropharynx

12

- **MEDICINAL FORMS**
There can be variation in the licensing of different medicines containing the same drug.
Ear/eye drops solution
EXCIPIENTS: May contain Benzalkonium chloride
  ‣ Gentamicin (Non-proprietary)
  Gentamicin (as Gentamicin sulfate) 3 mg per 1 ml Gentamicin 0.3% ear/eye drops | 10 ml PoM £2.14 DT price = £2.15

Gentamicin with hydrocortisone

- **INDICATIONS AND DOSE**
Eczematous inflammation in otitis externa
  ‣ TO THE EAR
  ‣ Child: Apply 2–4 drops 4–5 times a day, (including a dose at bedtime)

- **CONTRA-INDICATIONS** Patent grommet (although may be used by specialists, see Ear p. 660) · perforated tympanic membrane (although may be used by specialists, see Ear p. 660)
- **CAUTIONS** Avoid prolonged use
- **SIDE-EFFECTS** Local sensitivity reactions
- **PATIENT AND CARER ADVICE**
Medicines for Children leaflet: Gentamicin and hydrocortisone ear drops for inflammatory ear infections
www.medicinesforchildren.org.uk/gentamicin-and-hydrocortisone-ear-drops-inflammatory-ear-infections

- **MEDICINAL FORMS**
There can be variation in the licensing of different medicines containing the same drug.
Ear drops
EXCIPIENTS: May contain Benzalkonium chloride, disodium edetate
  ‣ Gentamicin with hydrocortisone (Non-proprietary)
  Gentamicin (as Gentamicin sulfate) 3 mg per 1 ml, Hydrocortisone acetate 10 mg per 1 ml Gentamicin 0.3% / Hydrocortisone acetate 1% ear drops | 10 ml PoM £23.92 DT price = £23.92

Neomycin sulfate

- **INDICATIONS AND DOSE**
Bacterial infection in otitis externa
  ‣ TO THE EAR
  ‣ Child: (consult product literature)

- **CONTRA-INDICATIONS** Patent grommet (although may be used by specialists, see Ear p. 660) · perforated tympanic membrane (although may be used by specialists, see Ear p. 660)
- **SIDE-EFFECTS** Local sensitivity
- **MEDICINAL FORMS**
There can be variation in the licensing of different medicines containing the same drug. No licensed medicines listed.

Combinations available: *Betamethasone with neomycin*, p. 663 · *Dexamethasone with glacial acetic acid and neomycin sulfate*, p. 664

ANTIBACTERIALS › OTHER

Chloramphenicol

- **DRUG ACTION** Chloramphenicol is a potent broad-spectrum antibiotic.

- **INDICATIONS AND DOSE**
Bacterial infection in otitis externa
  ‣ TO THE EAR
  ‣ Child: Apply 2–3 drops 2–3 times a day

- **CAUTIONS** Avoid prolonged use
- **SIDE-EFFECTS**
  ‣ **Common or very common** High incidence of sensitivity reactions to vehicle
- **PATIENT AND CARER ADVICE**
Medicines for Children leaflet: Chloramphenicol ear drops for ear infections (otitis externa) www.medicinesforchildren.org.uk/chloramphenicol-ear-drops-ear-infections-otitis-externa-0
- **LESS SUITABLE FOR PRESCRIBING** Chloramphenicol ear drops are less suitable for prescribing.

- **MEDICINAL FORMS**
There can be variation in the licensing of different medicines containing the same drug.
Ear drops
EXCIPIENTS: May contain Propylene glycol
  ‣ Chloramphenicol (Non-proprietary)
  Chloramphenicol 50 mg per 1 ml Chloramphenicol 5% ear drops | 10 ml PoM £78.17 DT price = £57.90
  Chloramphenicol 100 mg per 1 ml Chloramphenicol 10% ear drops | 10 ml PoM £48.21 DT price = £38.95

ANTIFUNGALS › IMIDAZOLE ANTIFUNGALS

Clotrimazole

- **INDICATIONS AND DOSE**
Fungal infection in otitis externa
  ‣ TO THE EAR
  ‣ Child: Apply 2–3 times a day continue for at least 14 days after disappearance of infection

- **SIDE-EFFECTS** Local irritation · local sensitivity

- **MEDICINAL FORMS**
There can be variation in the licensing of different medicines containing the same drug.
Liquid
  ‣ Canesten (clotrimazole) (Bayer Plc)
  Clotrimazole 10 mg per 1 ml Canesten 1% solution | 20 ml P £2.30 DT price = £2.30

CORTICOSTEROIDS

Betamethasone

- **INDICATIONS AND DOSE**
BETNESOL®
Eczematous inflammation in otitis externa
  ‣ TO THE EAR
  ‣ Child: Apply 2–3 drops every 2–3 hours, reduce frequency when relief obtained
VISTAMETHASONE®
Eczematous inflammation in otitis externa
  ‣ TO THE EAR
  ‣ Child: Apply 2–3 drops every 3–4 hours, reduce frequency when relief obtained

- **CONTRA-INDICATIONS** Avoid alone in the presence of untreated infection (combine with suitable anti-infective)
- **CAUTIONS** Avoid prolonged use
- **SIDE-EFFECTS** Local sensitivity reactions

- **MEDICINAL FORMS**
There can be variation in the licensing of different medicines containing the same drug.
Ear/eye/nose drops solution
EXCIPIENTS: May contain Benzalkonium chloride, disodium edetate
  ‣ Betnesol (Focus Pharmaceuticals Ltd)
  Betamethasone sodium phosphate 1 mg per 1 ml Betnesol 0.1% eye/ear/nose drops | 10 ml PoM £2.32 DT price = £2.32

▸ **Vistamethasone** (Martindale Pharmaceuticals Ltd)
Betamethasone sodium phosphate 1 mg per 1 ml Vistamethasone
0.1% ear/eye/nose drops | 5 ml [PoM] £0.87 | 10 ml [PoM] £0.99 DT
price = £2.32

Combinations available: *Betamethasone with neomycin,* below

Clioquinol with flumetasone pivalate

- **INDICATIONS AND DOSE**

**Eczematous inflammation in otitis externa | Mild bacterial
or fungal infections in otitis externa**
▸ TO THE EAR
▸ Child 2-17 years: 2–3 drops twice daily for 7–10 days, to
be instilled into the ear

- **CONTRA-INDICATIONS** Iodine sensitivity
- **CAUTIONS** Avoid prolonged use · manufacturer advises
avoid in perforated tympanic membrane (but used by
specialists for short periods)
- **SIDE-EFFECTS** Local sensitivity
- **PATIENT AND CARER ADVICE** Clioquinol stains skin and
clothing

- **MEDICINAL FORMS**
There can be variation in the licensing of different medicines
containing the same drug.
Ear drops
▸ Clioquinol with flumetasone pivalate (Non-proprietary)
Flumetasone pivalate 200 microgram per 1 ml, Clioquinol 10 mg
per 1 ml Flumetasone 0.02% / Clioquinol 1% ear drops |
7.5 ml [PoM] £10.37 DT price = £10.37 | 10 ml [PoM] £13.82 DT price =
£13.82

Prednisolone

- **INDICATIONS AND DOSE**

Eczematous inflammation in otitis externa
▸ TO THE EAR
▸ Child: Apply 2–3 drops every 2–3 hours, frequency to
be reduced when relief obtained

- **CONTRA-INDICATIONS** Avoid alone in the presence of
untreated infection (combine with suitable anti-infective)
- **CAUTIONS** Avoid prolonged use
- **SIDE-EFFECTS** Local sensitivity reactions

- **MEDICINAL FORMS**
There can be variation in the licensing of different medicines
containing the same drug. Forms available from special-order
manufacturers include: ear drops
Ear/eye drops solution
EXCIPIENTS: May contain Benzalkonium chloride, disodium edetate
▸ Predsol (Focus Pharmaceuticals Ltd)
Prednisolone sodium phosphate 5 mg per 1 ml Predsol 0.5%
ear/eye drops | 10 ml [PoM] £2.00 DT price = £2.00

CORTICOSTEROIDS › CORTICOSTEROID
COMBINATIONS WITH ANTI-INFECTIVES

Betamethasone with neomycin

The properties listed below are those particular to the
combination only. For the properties of the components
please consider, betamethasone p. 662, neomycin sulfate
p. 662.

- **INDICATIONS AND DOSE**

Eczematous inflammation in otitis externa
▸ TO THE EAR USING EAR DROPS
▸ Child: Apply 2–3 drops 3–4 times a day

- **CONTRA-INDICATIONS** Patent grommet (although may be
used by specialists, see Ear p. 660) · perforated tympanic
membrane (although may be used by specialists, see Ear
p. 660)
- **CAUTIONS** Avoid prolonged use
- **SIDE-EFFECTS** Local sensitivity

- **MEDICINAL FORMS**
There can be variation in the licensing of different medicines
containing the same drug.
Ear/eye/nose drops solution
EXCIPIENTS: May contain Benzalkonium chloride, disodium edetate
▸ Betnesol-N (Focus Pharmaceuticals Ltd)
Betamethasone (as Betamethasone sodium phosphate) 1 mg per
1 ml, Neomycin sulfate 5 mg per 1 ml Betnesol-N ear/eye/nose
drops | 10 ml [PoM] £2.39 DT price = £2.39

Dexamethasone with ciprofloxacin

09-Mar-2017

- **INDICATIONS AND DOSE**

Acute otitis media in patients with tympanostomy tubes
▸ TO THE EAR
▸ Child 6 months-17 years: Apply 4 drops twice daily for
7 days

Acute otitis externa
▸ TO THE EAR
▸ Child 1-17 years: Apply 4 drops twice daily for 7 days

- **CONTRA-INDICATIONS** Fungal ear infections · viral ear
infections
- **CAUTIONS** Avoid prolonged use
- **SIDE-EFFECTS**
▸ **Common or very common** Ear pain
▸ **Uncommon** Ear congestion · flushing · fungal ear infections
· irritability · malaise · otorrhoea · paraesthesia of the ear ·
skin exfoliation · taste disturbances · vomiting
▸ **Rare** Dizziness · erythematous rash · headache · hearing
loss · tinnitus
SIDE-EFFECTS, FURTHER INFORMATION
▸ Otorrhoea Manufacturer advises further evaluation of
underlying conditions if otorrhoea persists after a full
course, or if at least two episodes of otorrhoea occur within
6 months.
- **PREGNANCY** Manufacturer advises use only if potential
benefit outweighs risk—no information available.
- **BREAST FEEDING** Manufacturer advises caution—no
information available.
- **PATIENT AND CARER ADVICE** Manufacturer advises
counselling on administration.

- **MEDICINAL FORMS**
There can be variation in the licensing of different medicines
containing the same drug.
Ear drops
EXCIPIENTS: May contain Benzalkonium chloride, disodium edetate
▸ Cilodex (Alcon Laboratories (UK) Ltd)
Dexamethasone 1 mg per 1 ml, Ciprofloxacin (as Ciprofloxacin
hydrochloride) 3 mg per 1 ml Cilodex ear drops | 5 ml [PoM] £6.12
DT price = £6.12

Dexamethasone with framycetin sulfate and gramicidin

- **INDICATIONS AND DOSE**

Eczematous inflammation in otitis externa
▸ TO THE EAR
▸ Child: 2–3 drops 3–4 times a day

12

Ear, nose and oropharynx

- **LESS SUITABLE FOR PRESCRIBING** *Sofradex*® is less suitable for prescribing.

- **MEDICINAL FORMS**
There can be variation in the licensing of different medicines containing the same drug.
Ear/eye drops solution
EXCIPIENTS: May contain polysorbates
  ‣ Sofradex (Sanofi)
    Gramicidin 50 microgram per 1ml, Dexamethasone (as Dexamethasone sodium metasolfobenzoate) 500 microgram per 1 ml, Framycetin sulfate 5mg per 1 ml Sofradex ear/eye drops | 10 ml PoM £7.50

Dexamethasone with glacial acetic acid and neomycin sulfate

The properties listed below are those particular to the combination only. For the properties of the components please consider neomycin sulfate p. 662

- **INDICATIONS AND DOSE**
Eczematous inflammation in otitis externa
  ▸ TO THE EAR
  ▸ Child 2–17 years: Apply 1 spray 3 times a day

- **CONTRA-INDICATIONS** Patent grommet (although may be used by specialists, see Ear p. 660) · perforated tympanic membrane (although may be used by specialists, see Ear p. 660)
- **CAUTIONS** Avoid prolonged use
- **SIDE-EFFECTS** Local sensitivity

- **MEDICINAL FORMS**
There can be variation in the licensing of different medicines containing the same drug.
Spray
EXCIPIENTS: May contain Hydroxybenzoates (parabens)
  ‣ Otomize (Teva UK Ltd)
    Dexamethasone 1 mg per 1 gram, Neomycin sulfate 5 mg per 1 gram, Acetic acid glacial 20 mg per 1 gram Otomize ear spray | 5 ml PoM £3.27

ASTRINGENTS

Aluminium acetate

- **INDICATIONS AND DOSE**
Inflammation in otitis externa
  ▸ TO THE EAR
  ▸ Child: To be inserted into meatus or apply on a ribbon gauze dressing or sponge wick which should be kept saturated with the ear drops

- **UNLICENSED USE** Not licensed for use in children.
- **DIRECTIONS FOR ADMINISTRATION**
For ear drops 8%—dilute 8 parts aluminium acetate ear drops (13%) with 5 parts purified water. Must be freshly prepared.

- **MEDICINAL FORMS**
There can be variation in the licensing of different medicines containing the same drug. Forms available from special-order manufacturers include: ear drops

2   Removal of earwax

BICARBONATE

Sodium bicarbonate

- **INDICATIONS AND DOSE**
Removal of earwax (with 5% ear drop solution)
  ▸ TO THE EAR
  ▸ Child: (consult product literature)

- **SIDE-EFFECTS** Dryness of the ear canal

- **MEDICINAL FORMS**
There can be variation in the licensing of different medicines containing the same drug.
Ear drops
  ‣ Sodium bicarbonate (Non-proprietary)
    Sodium bicarbonate 50 mg per 1 ml Sodium bicarbonate 5% ear drops | 10 ml £1.23–£1.25

SOFTENING DRUGS

Almond oil

- **INDICATIONS AND DOSE**
Removal of earwax
  ▸ TO THE EAR
  ▸ Child: Allow drops to warm to room temperature before use (consult product literature)

- **DIRECTIONS FOR ADMINISTRATION** The patient should lie with the affected ear uppermost for 5 to 10 minutes after a generous amount of the softening remedy has been introduced into the ear.

- **MEDICINAL FORMS**
There can be variation in the licensing of different medicines containing the same drug.
Liquid
  ‣ Almond oil (Non-proprietary)
    Almond oil 1 ml per 1 ml Almond oil liquid | 50 ml £0.91 DT price = £0.91 | 70 ml £0.73–£0.82 | 200 ml £2.54 | 500 ml £11.90

Arachis oil with chlorobutanol

- **INDICATIONS AND DOSE**
Removal of earwax
  ▸ TO THE EAR
  ▸ Child 1–17 years: (consult product literature)

- **LESS SUITABLE FOR PRESCRIBING** Arachis (peanut) oil with chlorobutanol ear drops are less suitable for prescribing.

- **MEDICINAL FORMS**
There can be variation in the licensing of different medicines containing the same drug.
Ear drops
  ‣ Cerumol (Thornton & Ross Ltd)
    Chlorobutanol 50 mg per 1 ml, Arachis oil 573 mg per 1 ml Cerumol ear drops | 11 ml P £2.05

Docusate sodium
(Dioctyl sodium sulphosuccinate)

20-Apr-2016

- **INDICATIONS AND DOSE**
Removal of ear wax
  ▸ TO THE EAR
  ▸ Child 1–17 years: (consult product literature)

12

Ear, nose and oropharynx

- **LESS SUITABLE FOR PRESCRIBING** Ear drops less suitable for prescribing.

- **MEDICINAL FORMS**
There can be variation in the licensing of different medicines containing the same drug.

Ear drops
EXCIPIENTS: May contain Propylene glycol

▸ Molcer (Wallace Manufacturing Chemists Ltd)
Docusate sodium 50 mg per 1 ml Molcer ear drops | 15 ml Ⓟ £8.08

▸ Waxsol (Meda Pharmaceuticals Ltd)
Docusate sodium 5 mg per 1 ml Waxsol ear drops | 10 ml Ⓟ £1.95
DT price = £1.95

Olive oil

- **INDICATIONS AND DOSE**

Removal of earwax
▸ TO THE EAR
▸ **Child:** Apply twice daily for several days (if wax is hard and impacted)

- **DIRECTIONS FOR ADMINISTRATION** The patient should lie with the affected ear uppermost for 5 to 10 minutes after a generous amount of the softening remedy has been introduced into the ear. Allow ear drops to warm to room temperature before use.

- **MEDICINAL FORMS**
There can be variation in the licensing of different medicines containing the same drug.

Ear drops
▸ Olive oil (Non-proprietary)
Olive oil ear drops | 10 ml £1.35-£1.42 | 15 ml £0.92 | 20 ml £2.70
▸ Arjun (Arjun Products Ltd)
Arjun ear drops | 10 ml £1.26
▸ Cerumol (olive oil) (Thornton & Ross Ltd)
Cerumol olive oil ear drops | 10 ml no price available
▸ Oleax (JR Biomedical Ltd)
Oleax ear drops | 15 ml £1.40
▸ Olive oil (Thornton & Ross Ltd)
Care olive oil ear drops | 10 ml £1.42

Spray
▸ Earol (HL Healthcare Ltd)
Earol olive oil ear spray | 10 ml no price available

Urea hydrogen peroxide

- **INDICATIONS AND DOSE**

Softening and removal of earwax
▸ TO THE EAR
▸ **Child:** (consult product literature)

- **PATIENT AND CARER ADVICE** The patient should lie with the affected ear uppermost for 5 to 10 minutes after a generous amount of the softening remedy has been introduced into the ear.

- **LESS SUITABLE FOR PRESCRIBING** Urea-hydrogen peroxide ear drops are less suitable for prescribing.

- **MEDICINAL FORMS**
There can be variation in the licensing of different medicines containing the same drug.

Ear drops
▸ Exterol (Dermal Laboratories Ltd)
Urea hydrogen peroxide 50 mg per 1 gram Exterol 5% ear drops | 8 ml Ⓟ £1.75 DT price = £2.89
▸ Otex (Dendron Ltd)
Urea hydrogen peroxide 50 mg per 1 gram Otex 5% ear drops | 8 ml Ⓟ £2.89 DT price = £2.89

Nose

Nose

Rhinitis and bacterial sinusitis

Rhinitis is often self-limiting but bacterial sinusitis may require treatment with antibacterials. Many nasal preparations contain sympathomimetic drugs which can give rise to rebound congestion (*rhinitis medicamentosa*) and may damage the nasal cilia. Sodium chloride 0.9% solution p. 561 may be used as a douche or 'sniff' following endonasal surgery.

Administration
To administer nasal drops, lay the child face-upward with the neck extended, instil the drops, then sit the child up and tilt the head forward.

Drugs used in nasal allergy

Mild allergic rhinitis is controlled by **antihistamines** (see under Antihistamines, allergen immunotherapy and allergic emergencies p. 165) or topical **nasal corticosteroids**; systemic nasal decongestants are not recommended for use in children. Topical nasal decongestants can be used for a short period to relieve congestion and allow penetration of a topical nasal corticosteroid.

More persistent symptoms can be relieved by topical nasal **corticosteroids**; sodium cromoglicate p. 671 is an alternative, but may be less effective. The topical antihistamine, azelastine hydrochloride p. 638, is useful for controlling breakthrough symptoms in allergic rhinitis. Azelastine hydrochloride is less effective than nasal corticosteroids, but probably more effective than sodium cromoglicate. In seasonal allergic rhinitis (e.g. hay fever), treatment should begin 2 to 3 weeks before the season commences and may have to be continued for several months; continuous long-term treatment may be required in perennial rhinitis.

Montelukast p. 159 is less effective than topical nasal corticosteroids; it can be used in children with seasonal allergic rhinitis (unresponsive to other treatments) and concomitant asthma.

Children with disabling symptoms of seasonal rhinitis (e.g. students taking important examinations), may be treated with oral **corticosteroids** for short periods. Oral corticosteroids may also be used at the beginning of a course of treatment with a corticosteroid spray to relieve severe mucosal oedema and allow the spray to penetrate the nasal mucosa.

Sometimes allergic rhinitis is accompanied by vasomotor rhinitis. In this situation, the addition of topical nasal ipratropium bromide p. 668 can reduce watery rhinorrhoea.

Corticosteroids

Corticosteroid nasal preparations should be avoided in the presence of untreated nasal infections, after nasal surgery (until healing has occurred), and in pulmonary tuberculosis. Systemic absorption may follow nasal administration particularly if high doses are used or if treatment is prolonged; for cautions and side-effects of systemic corticosteroids. The risk of systemic effects may be greater with nasal drops than with nasal sprays; drops are administered incorrectly more often than sprays. The height of children receiving prolonged treatment with nasal corticosteroids should be monitored; if growth is slowed, referral to a paediatrician should be considered.

Nasal polyps

Short-term use of corticosteroid nasal drops helps to shrink nasal polyps; to be effective, the drops must be administered with the child in the 'head down' position. A short course of a systemic corticosteroid may be required initially to shrink

12

Ear, nose and oropharynx

Ear, nose and oropharynx

12

large polyps. A corticosteroid nasal spray can be used to maintain the reduction in swelling and also for the initial treatment of small polyps.

Pregnancy
If a pregnant woman cannot tolerate the symptoms of allergic rhinitis, treatment with nasal beclometasone dipropionate p. 669, budesonide p. 669, fluticasone p. 670, or sodium cromoglicate may be considered.

Topical nasal decongestants

Sodium chloride 0.9% given as nasal drops or spray may relieve nasal congestion by helping to liquefy mucous secretions in children with rhinitis. In infants, 1–2 drops of sodium chloride 0.9% solution in each nostril before feeds will help relieve congestion and allow more effective suckling.

Inhalation of **warm moist air** is useful in the treatment of symptoms of acute nasal congestion in infants and children, but the use of boiling water for steam inhalation is dangerous for children and should not be recommended. Volatile substances such as menthol and eucalyptus may encourage inhalation of warm moist air (see also Aromatic inhalations, cough preparations and systemic nasal decongestants p. 180).

Topical nasal decongestants containing sympathomimetics can cause rebound congestion (*rhinitis medicamentosa*) following prolonged use (more than 7 days), and are therefore of limited value in the treatment of nasal congestion.

Ephedrine hydrochloride nasal drops below is the least likely of the sympathomimetic nasal decongestants to cause rebound congestion and can provide relief for several hours. The more potent sympathomimetic drugs **oxymetazoline** and xylometazoline hydrochloride p. 667 are more likely to cause a rebound effect.

Non-allergic watery rhinorrhoea often responds well to treatment with the antimuscarinic ipratropium bromide.

Recurrent, persistent bleeding may respond to the use of a sympathomimetic nasal spray; if infection is present, chlorhexidine and neomycin (*Naseptin*®) cream may be effective.

Sinusitis and oral pain
Sinusitis affecting the maxillary antrum can cause pain in the upper jaw. Where this is associated with blockage of the opening from the sinus into the nasal cavity, it may be helpful to relieve the congestion with inhalation of warm moist air or with ephedrine hydrochloride nasal drops.

Systemic antibacterials may sometimes be required for sinusitis (see under Nose infections, bacterial p. 295).

Nasal preparations for infection

There is **no** evidence that topical anti-infective nasal preparations have any therapeutic value in rhinitis or sinusitis; see elimination of nasal staphylococci. In children, acute complications such as periorbital cellulitis require hospital treatment.

Nasal staphylococci
Elimination of organisms such as staphylococci from the nasal vestibule can be achieved by the use of a cream containing **chlorhexidine** and **neomycin** (*Naseptin*®), but re-colonisation frequently occurs. Coagulase-positive staphylococci are present in the noses of 40% of the population.

A nasal ointment containing mupirocin p. 668 is also available; it should probably be held in reserve for resistant infections. In hospitals or in care establishments, mupirocin nasal ointment should be reserved for the eradication (in both patients and staff) of nasal carriage of meticillin-resistant *Staphylococcus aureus* (MRSA). A sample should be taken 2 days after treatment to confirm eradication. The course may be repeated if the sample is positive (and the

throat is not colonised). To avoid the development of resistance, the treatment course should not exceed 7 days and the course should not be repeated on more than one occasion. If the MRSA strain is mupirocin-resistant or does not respond after 2 courses, consider alternative products such as chlorhexidine and neomycin cream.

For eradication of MRSA also consult local infection control policy. See also MRSA p. 345.

1   Nasal congestion

SYMPATHOMIMETICS ＞ VASOCONSTRICTOR

Ephedrine hydrochloride

● **INDICATIONS AND DOSE**

Nasal congestion | Sinusitis affecting the maxillary antrum
▸ BY INTRANASAL ADMINISTRATION
  ▸ Child 12–17 years: Apply 1–2 drops up to 4 times a day as required for a maximum of 7 days, to be instilled into each nostril, administer ephedrine 0.5% nasal drops

---

IMPORTANT SAFETY INFORMATION

CHM/MHRA ADVICE
The CHM/MHRA has stated that non-prescription cough and cold medicines containing ephedrine can be considered for up to 5 days' treatment in children aged 6–12 years after basic principles of best care have been tried; these medicines should not be used in children under 6 years of age.

● **CAUTIONS** Avoid excessive or prolonged use · cardiovascular disease · diabetes mellitus · hypertension · hyperthyroidism

● **INTERACTIONS** → Appendix 1: sympathomimetics, vasoconstrictor

● **SIDE-EFFECTS**
  ▸ Common or very common Headache · nausea
  ▸ Frequency not known After excessive use tolerance with diminished effect · cardiovascular effect · local irritation · rebound congestion

● **PREGNANCY** Manufacturer advises avoid.

● **BREAST FEEDING** Present in milk; manufacturer advises avoid—irritability and disturbed sleep reported.

● **PRESCRIBING AND DISPENSING INFORMATION** For nasal drops, the BP directs that if no strength is specified 0.5% drops should be supplied.

● **PROFESSION SPECIFIC INFORMATION**
  Dental practitioners' formulary
  Ephedrine nasal drops may be prescribed.

● **EXCEPTIONS TO LEGAL CATEGORY** Ephedrine nasal drops can be sold to the public provided no more than 180 mg of ephedrine base (or salts) are supplied at one time, and pseudoephedrine salts are not supplied at the same time; for conditions that apply to supplies made at the request of a patient, see *Medicines, Ethics and Practice*, London, Pharmaceutical Press (always consult latest edition).

● **MEDICINAL FORMS**
There can be variation in the licensing of different medicines containing the same drug. Forms available from special-order manufacturers include: nasal drops

Nasal drops
  ▸ Ephedrine hydrochloride (Non-proprietary)
    Ephedrine hydrochloride 5 mg per 1 ml Ephedrine 0.5% nasal drops | 10 ml Ⓟ £1.87–£1.90 DT price = £1.87
    Ephedrine hydrochloride 10 mg per 1 ml Ephedrine 1% nasal drops | 10 ml Ⓟ £1.91–£1.94 DT price = £1.91

Pseudoephedrine hydrochloride

- **INDICATIONS AND DOSE**

Congestion of mucous membranes of upper respiratory tract

▶ BY MOUTH

- Child 6–11 years: 30 mg 3–4 times a day
- Child 12–17 years: 60 mg 3–4 times a day

IMPORTANT SAFETY INFORMATION

MHRA/CHM ADVICE (MARCH 2008 AND FEBRUARY 2009): OVER-THE-COUNTER COUGH AND COLD MEDICINES FOR CHILDREN
Children under 6 years should not be given over-the-counter cough and cold medicines containing pseudoephedrine.

- **CAUTIONS** Diabetes · heart disease · hypertension · hyperthyroidism · raised intra-ocular pressure
- **INTERACTIONS** → Appendix 1: sympathomimetics, vasoconstrictor
- **SIDE-EFFECTS**
  ▶ **Common or very common** Anxiety · headache · hypertension · insomnia · nausea · restlessness · tachycardia · vomiting
  ▶ **Rare** Hallucinations · rash
  ▶ **Very rare** Angle-closure glaucoma
  ▶ **Frequency not known** Urinary retention
- **PREGNANCY** Defective closure of the abdominal wall (gastroschisis) reported very rarely in newborns after first trimester exposure.
- **BREAST FEEDING** May suppress lactation; avoid if lactation not well established or if milk production insufficient.
- **HEPATIC IMPAIRMENT** Manufacturer advises use with caution in severe impairment.
- **RENAL IMPAIRMENT** Use with caution in mild to moderate renal impairment. Manufacturer advises avoid in severe renal impairment.
- **LESS SUITABLE FOR PRESCRIBING** Pseudoephedrine hydrochloride is less suitable for prescribing.
- **EXCEPTIONS TO LEGAL CATEGORY** *Galpseud* ® and *Sudafed* ® can be sold to the public provided no more than 720 mg of pseudoephedrine salts are supplied, and ephedrine base (or salts) are not supplied at the same time; for details see *Medicines, Ethics and Practice*, London, Pharmaceutical Press (always consult latest edition).

- **MEDICINAL FORMS**
  There can be variation in the licensing of different medicines containing the same drug.
  Oral solution
  EXCIPIENTS: May contain Alcohol
  ▶ Galpseud (Thornton & Ross Ltd)
  Pseudoephedrine hydrochloride 6 mg per 1 ml Galpseud 30mg/5ml linctus sugar-free | 2000 ml PoM £14.00
  ▶ Sudafed Non-Drowsy Decongestant (pseudoephedrine) (McNeil Products Ltd)
  Pseudoephedrine hydrochloride 6 mg per 1 ml Sudafed Decongestant 30mg/5ml liquid | 100 ml P £1.92
  Tablet
  ▶ Galpseud (Thornton & Ross Ltd)
  Pseudoephedrine hydrochloride 60 mg Galpseud 60mg tablets | 24 tablet PoM £2.25 | 100 tablet PoM £5.42 DT price = £5.42
  ▶ Sudafed Non-Drowsy Decongestant (pseudoephedrine) (McNeil Products Ltd)
  Pseudoephedrine hydrochloride 60 mg Sudafed Decongestant 60mg tablets | 12 tablet P £2.04

Xylometazoline hydrochloride

- **DRUG ACTION** Xylometazoline is a sympathomimetic.

- **INDICATIONS AND DOSE**

Nasal congestion

▶ BY INTRANASAL ADMINISTRATION USING NASAL DROPS

- Child 6–11 years: 1–2 drops 1–2 times a day as required for maximum duration of 5 days, 0.05% solution to be administered into each nostril
- Child 12–17 years: 2–3 drops 2–3 times a day as required for maximum duration of 7 days, 0.1% solution to be administered into each nostril

▶ BY INTRANASAL ADMINISTRATION USING NASAL SPRAY

- Child 12–17 years: 1 spray 1–3 times a day as required for maximum duration of 7 days, to be administered into each nostril

---

IMPORTANT SAFETY INFORMATION

The CHM/MHRA has stated that non-prescription cough and cold medicines containing oxymetazoline or xylometazoline can be considered for up to 5 days' treatment in children aged 6–12 years after basic principles of best care have been tried; these medicines should not be used in children under 6 years of age.

- **CAUTIONS** Angle-closure glaucoma · avoid excessive or prolonged use · cardiovascular disease · diabetes mellitus · hypertension · hyperthyroidism · rebound congestion
  CAUTIONS, FURTHER INFORMATION
  ▶ **Rebound congestion** Sympathomimetic drugs are of limited value in the treatment of nasal congestion because they can, following prolonged use (more than 7 days), give rise to a rebound congestion (rhinitis medicamentosa) on withdrawal, due to a secondary vasodilatation with a subsequent temporary increase in nasal congestion. This in turn tempts the further use of the decongestant, leading to a vicious cycle of events.
- **INTERACTIONS** → Appendix 1: sympathomimetics, vasoconstrictor
- **SIDE-EFFECTS** Cardiovascular effects · hallucinations in small children · headache · local irritation · nausea · rebound congestion · restlessness in small children · sleep disturbances in small children · tolerance with diminished effect (after excessive use) · transient visual disturbances
  SIDE-EFFECTS, FURTHER INFORMATION
  ▶ **Hallucinations (in small children)** Discontinue treatment if the hallucinations occur.
- **PREGNANCY** Manufacturer advises avoid.
- **BREAST FEEDING** Manufacturer advises caution—no information available.

- **MEDICINAL FORMS**
  There can be variation in the licensing of different medicines containing the same drug.
  Spray
  ▶ Otrivine (GlaxoSmithKline Consumer Healthcare)
  Xylometazoline hydrochloride 1 mg per 1 ml Otrivine Congestion Relief 0.1% nasal spray | 10 ml GSL £3.05 DT price = £2.18
  Otrivine Adult Measured Dose Sinusitis spray | 10 ml GSL £2.62 DT price = £2.18
  Otrivine Allergy Relief 0.1% nasal spray | 10 ml GSL £2.62 DT price = £2.18
  Otrivine Adult nasal spray | 10 ml GSL £2.18 DT price = £2.18
  Otrivine Adult Metered Dose 0.1% nasal spray | 10 ml GSL £2.62 DT price = £2.18
  ▶ Sudafed Congestion Relief (McNeil Products Ltd)
  Xylometazoline hydrochloride 1 mg per 1 ml Sudafed Congestion Relief 0.1% nasal spray | 10 ml GSL £3.25 DT price = £2.18
  ▶ Sudafed Mucus Relief (McNeil Products Ltd)
  Xylometazoline hydrochloride 1 mg per 1 ml Sudafed Mucus Relief 0.1% nasal spray | 15 ml GSL £2.37

12

Ear, nose and oropharynx

Ear, nose and oropharynx

12

▸ Sudafed Non-Drowsy Decongestant (xylometazoline) (McNeil Products Ltd)
Xylometazoline hydrochloride 1 mg per 1 ml Sudafed Blocked Nose 0.1% spray | 15 ml GSL £2.38

Nasal drops
▸ Otrivine (GlaxoSmithKline Consumer Healthcare)
Xylometazoline hydrochloride 500 microgram per 1 ml Otrivine Child nasal drops | 10 ml P £1.91 DT price = £1.91
Xylometazoline hydrochloride 1 mg per 1 ml Otrivine Adult 0.1% nasal drops | 10 ml GSL £2.18 DT price = £2.18

2   Nasal infection

ANTIBACTERIALS ⟩ AMINOGLYCOSIDES

Chlorhexidine with neomycin

● INDICATIONS AND DOSE
Eradication of nasal carriage of staphylococci
▸ BY INTRANASAL ADMINISTRATION
▸ Child: Apply 4 times a day for 10 days
Preventing nasal carriage of staphylococci
▸ BY INTRANASAL ADMINISTRATION
▸ Child: Apply twice daily

● MEDICINAL FORMS
There can be variation in the licensing of different medicines containing the same drug.
Cream
EXCIPIENTS: May contain Arachis (peanut) oil, cetostearyl alcohol (including cetyl and stearyl alcohol)
▸ Naseptin (Alliance Pharmaceuticals Ltd)
Chlorhexidine hydrochloride 1 mg per 1 gram, Neomycin sulfate 5 mg per 1 gram Naseptin nasal cream | 15 gram PoM £2.24 DT price = £2.24

ANTIBACTERIALS ⟩ OTHER

Mupirocin

● INDICATIONS AND DOSE
BACTROBAN NASAL®
For eradication of nasal carriage of staphylococci, including meticillin-resistant *Staphylococcus aureus* (MRSA)
▸ BY INTRANASAL ADMINISTRATION
▸ Child: Apply 2–3 times a day for 5 days; a sample should be taken 2 days after treatment to confirm eradication. Course may be repeated once if sample positive (and throat not colonised), dose to be applied to the inner surface of each nostril

● PREGNANCY Manufacturer advises avoid unless potential benefit outweighs risk—no information available.
● BREAST FEEDING No information available.
● RENAL IMPAIRMENT Manufacturer advises caution when mupirocin ointment used in moderate or severe impairment because it contains macrogols (polyethylene glycol).

● MEDICINAL FORMS
There can be variation in the licensing of different medicines containing the same drug.
Nasal ointment
▸ Bactroban (GlaxoSmithKline UK Ltd)
Mupirocin (as Mupirocin calcium) 20 mg per 1 gram Bactroban 2% nasal ointment | 3 gram PoM £4.24 DT price = £4.24

CORTICOSTEROIDS ⟩ CORTICOSTEROID COMBINATIONS WITH ANTI-INFECTIVES

Betamethasone with neomycin

The properties listed below are those particular to the combination only. For the properties of the components please consider, betamethasone p. 662, neomycin sulfate p. 662.

● INDICATIONS AND DOSE
Nasal infection
▸ BY INTRANASAL ADMINISTRATION USING NASAL DROPS
▸ Child: Apply 2–3 drops 2–3 times a day, to be applied into each nostril

● LESS SUITABLE FOR PRESCRIBING Betamethasone with neomycin nasal-drops are less suitable for prescribing; there is no evidence that topical anti-infective nasal preparations have any therapeutic value in rhinitis or sinusitis.

● MEDICINAL FORMS
There can be variation in the licensing of different medicines containing the same drug.
Ear/eye/nose drops solution
EXCIPIENTS: May contain Benzalkonium chloride, disodium edetate
▸ Betnesol-N (Focus Pharmaceuticals Ltd)
Betamethasone (as Betamethasone sodium phosphate) 1 mg per 1 ml, Neomycin sulfate 5 mg per 1 ml Betnesol-N ear/eye/nose drops | 10 ml PoM £2.39 DT price = £2.39

3   Nasal inflammation, nasal polyps and rhinitis

Other drugs used for Nasal inflammation, nasal polyps and rhinitis Desloratadine, p. 168 · Fexofenadine hydrochloride, p. 169 · Ketotifen, p. 174

ANTIMUSCARINICS

F 147

Ipratropium bromide

24-Feb-2016

● INDICATIONS AND DOSE
Rhinorrhoea associated with allergic and non-allergic rhinitis
▸ BY INTRANASAL ADMINISTRATION
▸ Child 12–17 years: 2 sprays 2–3 times a day, dose to be sprayed into each nostril
DOSE EQUIVALENCE AND CONVERSION
▸ 1 metered spray of nasal spray = 21 micrograms.

● CAUTIONS Avoid spraying near eyes · bladder outflow obstruction · cystic fibrosis · susceptibility to angle-closure glaucoma
● INTERACTIONS → Appendix 1: ipratropium
● SIDE-EFFECTS
▸ Common or very common Epistaxis · nasal dryness · nasal irritation
▸ Uncommon Headache · nausea
▸ Very rare Gastro-intestinal motility disturbances · palpitations · urinary retention
● PREGNANCY Manufacturer advises only use if potential benefit outweighs the risk.
● BREAST FEEDING No information available—manufacturer advises only use if potential benefit outweighs risk.

- **MEDICINAL FORMS**
There can be variation in the licensing of different medicines containing the same drug.

Spray
EXCIPIENTS: May contain Benzalkonium chloride, disodium edetate
- **Rinatec** (Boehringer Ingelheim Ltd)
Ipratropium bromide 21 microgram per 1 dose Rinatec 21micrograms/dose nasal spray | 180 dose [PoM] £6.54 DT price = £6.54

CORTICOSTEROIDS

Corticosteroids (intranasal)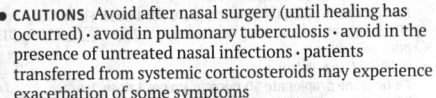

- **CAUTIONS** Avoid after nasal surgery (until healing has occurred) · avoid in pulmonary tuberculosis · avoid in the presence of untreated nasal infections · patients transferred from systemic corticosteroids may experience exacerbation of some symptoms

CAUTIONS, FURTHER INFORMATION
- Systemic absorption Systemic absorption may follow nasal administration particularly if high doses are used or if treatment is prolonged; therefore also consider the cautions and side-effects of systemic corticosteroids. The risk of systemic effects may be greater with nasal drops than with nasal sprays; drops are administered incorrectly more often than sprays.

- **SIDE-EFFECTS**
- **Rare** Glaucoma · raised intra-ocular pressure
- **Very rare** Nasal septal perforation (usually following nasal surgery)
- **Frequency not known** Aggression (particularly in children) · anxiety (particularly in children) · bronchospasm · depression (particularly in children) · dryness · epistaxis · headache · hyperactivity (particularly in children) · hypersensitivity reactions · nasal irritation · nasal ulceration · sleep disturbances (particularly in children) · smell disturbances · taste disturbances · throat irritation

SIDE-EFFECTS, FURTHER INFORMATION
- Systemic absorption Systemic absorption may follow nasal administration particularly if high doses are used or if treatment is prolonged. Therefore also consider the side-effects of systemic corticosteroids. The risk of systemic effects may be greater with nasal drops than with nasal sprays; drops are administered incorrectly more often than sprays.

- **MONITORING REQUIREMENTS** The height of children receiving prolonged treatment with nasal corticosteroids should be monitored; if growth is slowed, referral to a paediatrician should be considered.

🏳 above

Beclometasone dipropionate
(Beclomethasone dipropionate)

- **INDICATIONS AND DOSE**
Prophylaxis and treatment of allergic and vasomotor rhinitis
- BY INTRANASAL ADMINISTRATION
- Child 6-17 years: 100 micrograms twice daily, dose to be administered into each nostril, reduced to 50 micrograms twice daily, dose to be administered into each nostril, dose to be reduced when symptoms controlled; maximum 400 micrograms per day

- **INTERACTIONS** → Appendix 1: corticosteroids

- **MEDICINAL FORMS**
There can be variation in the licensing of different medicines containing the same drug

Spray
EXCIPIENTS: May contain Benzalkonium chloride, polysorbates
- **Beclometasone dipropionate (Non-proprietary)**
Beclometasone dipropionate 50 microgram per 1 dose
Beclometasone 50micrograms/dose nasal spray | 200 dose [P] £2.52 DT price = £2.10
- **Beconase** (GlaxoSmithKline UK Ltd, Omega Pharma Ltd)
Beclometasone dipropionate 50 microgram per 1 dose Beconase Aqueous 50micrograms/dose nasal spray | 200 dose [PoM] £2.63 DT price = £2.10
- **Nasobec** (Teva UK Ltd)
Beclometasone dipropionate 50 microgram per 1 dose Nasobec Aqueous 50micrograms/dose nasal spray | 200 dose [PoM] £3.06 DT price = £2.10

🏳 above

Betamethasone

- **INDICATIONS AND DOSE**
BETNESOL®
Non-infected inflammatory conditions of nose
- BY INTRANASAL ADMINISTRATION
- Child: Apply 2–3 drops 2–3 times a day, dose to be applied into each nostril

VISTAMETHASONE®
Non-infected inflammatory conditions of nose
- BY INTRANASAL ADMINISTRATION
- Child: Apply 2–3 drops twice daily, dose to be applied into each nostril

- **INTERACTIONS** → Appendix 1: corticosteroids

- **MEDICINAL FORMS**
There can be variation in the licensing of different medicines containing the same drug.

Ear/eye/nose drops solution
EXCIPIENTS: May contain Benzalkonium chloride, disodium edetate
- **Betnesol** (Focus Pharmaceuticals Ltd)
Betamethasone sodium phosphate 1 mg per 1 ml Betnesol 0.1% eye/ear/nose drops | 10 ml [PoM] £2.32 DT price = £2.32
- **Vistamethasone** (Martindale Pharmaceuticals Ltd)
Betamethasone sodium phosphate 1 mg per 1 ml Vistamethasone 0.1% ear/eye/nose drops | 5 ml [PoM] £0.87 | 10 ml [PoM] £0.99 DT price = £2.32

🏳 above

Budesonide   20-Nov-2016

- **INDICATIONS AND DOSE**
Prophylaxis and treatment of allergic and vasomotor rhinitis
- BY INTRANASAL ADMINISTRATION
- Child 12-17 years: Initially 200 micrograms once daily, dose to be administered into each nostril in the morning, alternatively initially 100 micrograms twice daily, dose to be administered to each nostril; reduced to 100 micrograms once daily, dose to be administered into each nostril, dose can be reduced when control achieved

Nasal polyps
- BY INTRANASAL ADMINISTRATION
- Child 12-17 years: 100 micrograms twice daily for up to 3 months, dose to be administered into each nostril

RHINOCORT AQUA®
Rhinitis
- BY INTRANASAL ADMINISTRATION
- Child 12-17 years: 128 micrograms once daily, dose to be administered into each nostril in the morning, alternatively 64 micrograms twice daily, dose to be administered into each nostril; reduced to continued →

12

Ear, nose and oropharynx

64 micrograms once daily when control achieved. Use for maximum 3 months, doses to be administered into each nostril

Nasal polyps
▸ BY INTRANASAL ADMINISTRATION
• Child 12-17 years: 64 micrograms twice daily for up to 3 months, dose to be administered into each nostril

• INTERACTIONS → Appendix 1: corticosteroids

• MEDICINAL FORMS
There can be variation in the licensing of different medicines containing the same drug.

Spray
EXCIPIENTS: May contain Disodium edetate, polysorbates, potassium sorbate
▸ Budesonide (Non-proprietary)

Budesonide 64 microgram per 1 dose Budesonide 64micrograms/dose nasal spray | 120 dose [PoM] £4.77 DT price = £4.77

Budesonide 100 microgram per 1 dose Budeflam Aquanase 100micrograms/dose nasal spray | 150 dose [PoM] no price available Aircort 100micrograms/dose nasal spray | 200 dose [PoM] no price available
▸ Rhinocort (AstraZeneca UK Ltd)

Budesonide 64 microgram per 1 dose Rhinocort Aqua 64 nasal spray | 120 dose [PoM] £3.49 DT price = £4.77

F 669

Fluticasone

04-Jan-2016

• INDICATIONS AND DOSE

Prophylaxis and treatment of allergic rhinitis and perennial rhinitis
▸ BY INTRANASAL ADMINISTRATION USING NASAL SPRAY
• Child 4-11 years: 50 micrograms once daily, to be administered into each nostril preferably in the morning, increased if necessary to 50 micrograms twice daily
• Child 12-17 years: 100 micrograms once daily, to be administered into each nostril preferably in the morning, increased if necessary to 100 micrograms twice daily; reduced to 50 micrograms once daily, dose to be administered into each nostril, dose to be reduced when control achieved

Nasal polyps
▸ BY INTRANASAL ADMINISTRATION USING NASAL DROPS
• Child 16-17 years: 200 micrograms 1–2 times a day, to be administered into each nostril, alternative treatment should be considered if no improvement after 4–6 weeks, (200 micrograms is equivalent to approximately 6 drops)

AVAMYS® SPRAY

Prophylaxis and treatment of allergic rhinitis
▸ BY INTRANASAL ADMINISTRATION
• Child 6-11 years: 27.5 micrograms once daily, dose to be sprayed into each nostril, then increased if necessary to 55 micrograms once daily, dose to be sprayed into each nostril, reduced to 27.5 micrograms once daily, to be sprayed into each nostril, dose to be reduced once control achieved; use minimum effective dose
• Child 12-17 years: 55 micrograms once daily, dose to be sprayed into each nostril, reduced to 27.5 micrograms once daily, to be sprayed into each nostril, dose to be reduced once control achieved; use minimum effective dose

DOSE EQUIVALENCE AND CONVERSION
▸ For Avamys® spray: 1 spray equivalent to 27.5 micrograms.

• INTERACTIONS → Appendix 1: corticosteroids

• SIDE-EFFECTS Nasal ulceration occurs commonly with nasal preparations containing fluticasone furoate.

• MEDICINAL FORMS
There can be variation in the licensing of different medicines containing the same drug.

Spray
EXCIPIENTS: May contain Benzalkonium chloride, disodium edetate, polysorbates
▸ Fluticasone (Non-proprietary)

Fluticasone propionate 50 microgram per 1 dose Fluticasone propionate 50micrograms/dose nasal spray | 60 dose [PoM] no price available | 150 dose [PoM] no price available DT price = £11.01
▸ Avamys (GlaxoSmithKline UK Ltd)

Fluticasone furoate 27.5 microgram per 1 dose Avamys 27.5micrograms/dose nasal spray | 120 dose [PoM] £6.44 DT price = £6.44
▸ Flixonase (GlaxoSmithKline UK Ltd)

Fluticasone propionate 50 microgram per 1 dose Flixonase 50micrograms/dose aqueous nasal spray | 150 dose [PoM] £11.01 DT price = £11.01
▸ Nasofan (Teva UK Ltd)

Fluticasone propionate 50 microgram per 1 dose Nasofan 50micrograms/dose aqueous nasal spray | 150 dose [PoM] £8.04 DT price = £11.01

Nasal drops
EXCIPIENTS: May contain Polysorbates
▸ Flixonase (GlaxoSmithKline UK Ltd)

Fluticasone propionate 400 microgram Flixonase Nasule 400microgram/unit dose nasal drops | 28 unit dose [PoM] £12.99 DT price = £12.99

Fluticasone with azelastine

The properties listed below are those particular to the combination only. For the properties of the components please consider fluticasone above.

• INDICATIONS AND DOSE

Moderate to severe seasonal and perennial allergic rhinitis, if monotherapy with antihistamine or corticosteroid is inadequate
▸ BY INTRANASAL ADMINISTRATION
• Child 12-17 years: 1 spray twice daily, dose to be administered into each nostril

• MEDICINAL FORMS
There can be variation in the licensing of different medicines containing the same drug.

Spray
EXCIPIENTS: May contain Benzalkonium chloride, polysorbates
▸ Fluticasone with azelastine (Non-proprietary)

Fluticasone propionate 50 microgram per 1 actuation, Azelastine hydrochloride 137 microgram per 1 actuation Fluticasone propionate 50micrograms/dose / Azelastine 137micrograms/dose nasal spray | 120 dose [PoM] no price available DT price = £14.80
▸ Dymista (Meda Pharmaceuticals Ltd)

Fluticasone propionate 50 microgram per 1 actuation, Azelastine hydrochloride 137 microgram per 1 actuation Dymista 137micrograms/dose / 50micrograms/dose nasal spray | 120 dose [PoM] £14.80 DT price = £14.80

F 669

Mometasone furoate

• INDICATIONS AND DOSE

Prophylaxis and treatment of allergic rhinitis
▸ BY INTRANASAL ADMINISTRATION
• Child 6-11 years: 50 micrograms daily, dose to be sprayed into each nostril
• Child 12-17 years: 100 micrograms daily, increased if necessary up to 200 micrograms daily, dose to be sprayed into each nostril; reduced to 50 micrograms daily, dose to be reduced when control achieved, dose to be sprayed into each nostril

• INTERACTIONS → Appendix 1: corticosteroids

- **SIDE-EFFECTS**

SIDE-EFFECTS, FURTHER INFORMATION Nasal ulceration occurs commonly with preparations containing mometasone furoate.

- **MEDICINAL FORMS**

There can be variation in the licensing of different medicines containing the same drug.

Spray
EXCIPIENTS: May contain Benzalkonium chloride, polysorbates
▸ **Mometasone furoate** (Non-proprietary)
   Mometasone furoate 50 microgram per 1 dose Mometasone 50micrograms/dose nasal spray ⎮ 140 dose PoM £7.30 DT price = £2.12
▸ **Nasonex** (Merck Sharp & Dohme Ltd)
   Mometasone furoate 50 microgram per 1 dose Nasonex 50micrograms/dose nasal spray ⎮ 140 dose PoM £7.68 DT price = £2.12

▸ 669

Triamcinolone acetonide

- **INDICATIONS AND DOSE**

Prophylaxis and treatment of allergic rhinitis
▸ BY INTRANASAL ADMINISTRATION
▸ Child 2-5 years: 55 micrograms once daily for maximum 3 months, dose to be sprayed into each nostril
▸ Child 6-11 years: 55 micrograms once daily, dose to be sprayed into each nostril, increased if necessary to 110 micrograms once daily, dose to be sprayed into each nostril; reduced to 55 micrograms once daily, dose to be sprayed into each nostril, reduce dose when control achieved; maximum duration of treatment 3 months
▸ Child 12-17 years: 110 micrograms once daily, dose to be sprayed into each nostril, reduced to 55 micrograms once daily, dose to be sprayed into each nostril, reduce dose when control achieved

- **UNLICENSED USE** Not licensed for use in children under 6 years.
- **INTERACTIONS** → Appendix 1: corticosteroids

- **MEDICINAL FORMS**

There can be variation in the licensing of different medicines containing the same drug.

Spray
EXCIPIENTS: May contain Benzalkonium chloride, disodium edetate, polysorbates
▸ **Nasacort** (Sanofi)
   Triamcinolone acetonide 55 microgram per 1 dose Nasacort 55micrograms/dose nasal spray ⎮ 120 dose PoM £7.39 DT price = £7.39

MAST-CELL STABILISERS

Sodium cromoglicate

(Sodium cromoglycate)

- **INDICATIONS AND DOSE**

Prophylaxis of allergic rhinitis
▸ BY INTRANASAL ADMINISTRATION
▸ Child: 1 spray 2–4 times a day, to be administered into each nostril

- **UNLICENSED USE** Licensed for use in children (age range not specified by manufacturers).
- **SIDE-EFFECTS**
▸ **Rare** Transient bronchospasm
▸ **Frequency not known** Local irritation

- **MEDICINAL FORMS**

There can be variation in the licensing of different medicines containing the same drug. No licensed medicines listed.

Oropharynx

1 Dry mouth

Treatment of dry mouth

Overview

Dry mouth (xerostomia) may be caused by drugs with antimuscarinic (anticholinergic) side-effects (e.g. antispasmodics and sedating antihistamines), by irradiation of the head and neck region or by damage to or disease of the salivary glands. Children with a persistently dry mouth may develop a burning or scalded sensation and have poor oral hygiene; they may develop dental caries, periodontal disease, and oral infections (particularly candidiasis). Dry mouth may be relieved in many patients by simple measures such as frequent sips of cool drinks or sucking pieces of ice or sugar-free fruit pastilles. Sugar-free chewing gum stimulates salivation in patients with residual salivary function.

Artificial saliva can provide useful relief of dry mouth. A properly balanced artificial saliva should be of a neutral pH and contain electrolytes (including fluoride) to correspond approximately to the composition of saliva. The acidic pH of some artificial saliva products may be inappropriate.

Artificial saliva products

- **ARTIFICIAL SALIVA PRODUCTS**

AS SALIVA ORTHANA® LOZENGES

Mucin 65 mg, xylitol 59 mg, in a sorbitol basis, pH neutral

- **INDICATIONS AND DOSE**

Dry mouth as a result of having (or having undergone) radiotherapy (ACBS) | Dry mouth as a result of sicca syndrome (ACBS)
▸ BY MOUTH
▸ Child: 1 lozenge as required, allow to dissolve slowly in the mouth

- **PRESCRIBING AND DISPENSING INFORMATION** AS Saliva Orthana® lozenges do not contain fluoride.
▸ **AS Saliva Orthana lozenges** (A S Pharma Ltd)
   30 lozenge(ACBS) · NHS indicative price = £3.50

AS SALIVA ORTHANA® SPRAY

Gastric mucin (porcine) 3.5%, xylitol 2%, sodium fluoride 4.2 mg/litre, with preservatives and flavouring agents, pH neutral.

- **INDICATIONS AND DOSE**

Symptomatic treatment of dry mouth
▸ BY MOUTH
▸ Child: Apply 2–3 sprays as required, spray onto oral and pharyngeal mucosa

- **PROFESSION SPECIFIC INFORMATION**

Dental practitioners' formulary
AS Saliva Orthana® Oral Spray may be prescribed.

12

Ear, nose and oropharynx

BIOXTRA® GEL

Lactoperoxidase, lactoferrin, lysozyme, whey colostrum, xylitol and other ingredients.

● INDICATIONS AND DOSE

Dry mouth as a result of having (or having undergone) radiotherapy (ACBS) | Dry mouth as a result of sicca syndrome (ACBS)
▸ BY MOUTH
▸ Child: Apply as required, apply to oral mucosa

● PROFESSION SPECIFIC INFORMATION

Dental practitioners' formulary
BioXtra® Gel may be prescribed.
▸ BioXtra Dry Mouth oral gel (R.I.S. Products Ltd)
  40 ml · NHS indicative price = £3.94 · Drug Tariff (Part IXa)

BIOTENE ORALBALANCE®

Lactoperoxidase, lactoferrin, lysozyme, glucose oxidase, xylitol in a gel basis

● INDICATIONS AND DOSE

Symptomatic treatment of dry mouth
▸ BY MOUTH
▸ Child: Apply as required, apply to gums and tongue

● PATIENT AND CARER ADVICE Avoid use with toothpastes containing detergents (including foaming agents).

● PROFESSION SPECIFIC INFORMATION

Dental practitioners' formulary
Biotene Oralbalance® Saliva Replacement Gel may be prescribed as Artificial Saliva Gel.
▸ Biotene Oralbalance dry mouth saliva replacement gel
  (GlaxoSmithKline Consumer Healthcare) Glucose oxidase 12000 unit,
  Lactoferrin 12 mg, Lactoperoxidase 12000 unit, Muramidase
  12 mg 50 gram · NHS indicative price = £4.46 · Drug Tariff (Part IXa)

GLANDOSANE®

Carmellose sodium 500 mg, sorbitol 1.5 g, potassium chloride 60 mg, sodium chloride 42.2 mg, magnesium chloride 2.6 mg, calcium chloride 7.3 mg, and dipotassium hydrogen phosphate 17.1 mg/50 g, pH 5.75.

● INDICATIONS AND DOSE

Dry mouth as a result of having (or having undergone) radiotherapy (ACBS) | Dry mouth as a result of sicca syndrome (ACBS)
▸ BY MOUTH
▸ Child: Apply as required, spray onto oral and pharyngeal mucosa

● PROFESSION SPECIFIC INFORMATION

Dental practitioners' formulary
Glandosane® Aerosol Spray may be prescribed.
▸ Glandosane synthetic saliva spray lemon (Fresenius Kabi Ltd)
  50 ml · NHS indicative price = £5.68
▸ Glandosane synthetic saliva spray natural (Fresenius Kabi Ltd)
  50 ml · NHS indicative price = £5.68
▸ Glandosane synthetic saliva spray peppermint (Fresenius Kabi Ltd)
  50 ml · NHS indicative price = £5.68

ORALIEVE GEL

● INDICATIONS AND DOSE

Symptomatic treatment of dry mouth
▸ BY MOUTH
▸ Child: Apply as required, particularly at night, to oral mucosa

● PRESCRIBING AND DISPENSING INFORMATION Contains traces of milk protein and egg white protein.

SST®

Sugar-free, citric acid, malic acid and other ingredients in a sorbitol base.

● INDICATIONS AND DOSE

Symptomatic treatment of dry mouth in patients with impaired salivary gland function and patent salivary ducts
▸ BY MOUTH
▸ Child: 1 tablet as required, allow tablet to dissolve slowly in the mouth

● PROFESSION SPECIFIC INFORMATION

Dental practitioners' formulary
May be prescribed as Saliva Stimulating Tablets.
▸ SST saliva stimulating tablets (Sinclair IS Pharma Plc)
  100 tablet · NHS indicative price = £4.86 · Drug Tariff (Part IXa)

SALIVEZE®

Carmellose sodium (sodium carboxymethylcellulose), calcium chloride, magnesium chloride, potassium chloride, sodium chloride, and dibasic sodium phosphate, pH neutral

● INDICATIONS AND DOSE

Dry mouth as a result of having (or having undergone) radiotherapy (ACBS) | Dry mouth as a result of sicca syndrome (ACBS)
▸ BY MOUTH
▸ Child: Apply 1 spray as required, spray onto oral mucosa

● PROFESSION SPECIFIC INFORMATION

Dental practitioners' formulary
Saliveze® Oral Spray may be prescribed.
▸ Saliveze mouth spray (Wyvern Medical Ltd)
  50 ml(ACBS) · NHS indicative price = £3.50

SALIVIX®

Sugar-free, reddish-amber, acacia, malic acid and other ingredients.

● INDICATIONS AND DOSE

Symptomatic treatment of dry mouth
▸ BY MOUTH USING PASTILLES
▸ Child: 1 unit as required, suck pastille

● PROFESSION SPECIFIC INFORMATION

Dental practitioners' formulary
Salivix® Pastilles may be prescribed as Artificial Saliva Pastilles.
▸ Salivix pastilles (Galen Ltd)
  50 pastille · NHS indicative price = £3.55 · Drug Tariff (Part IXa)

XEROTIN®

Sugar-free, water, sorbitol, carmellose (carboxymethylcellulose), potassium chloride, sodium chloride, potassium phosphate, magnesium chloride, calcium chloride and other ingredients, pH neutral.

● INDICATIONS AND DOSE

Symptomatic treatment of dry mouth
▸ BY MOUTH
▸ Child: 1 spray as required

● PROFESSION SPECIFIC INFORMATION

Dental practitioners' formulary
Xerotin® Oral Spray may be prescribed as Artificial Saliva Oral Spray.
▸ Xerotin spray (SpePharm UK Ltd)
  100 ml · NHS indicative price = £6.86 · Drug Tariff (Part IXa)

2 Oral hygiene

Mouthwashes and other preparations for oropharyngeal use

Lozenges and sprays

There is no convincing evidence that antiseptic lozenges and sprays have a beneficial action and they sometimes irritate and cause sore tongue and sore lips. Some of these preparations also contain local anaesthetics which relieve pain but may cause sensitisation.

Mouthwashes and gargles

Superficial infections of the mouth are often helped by warm mouthwashes which have a mechanical cleansing effect and cause some local hyperaemia. However, to be effective, they must be used frequently and vigorously. Mouthwashes may not be suitable for children under 7 years (risk of the solution being swallowed); the mouthwash or dental gel may be applied using a cotton bud.

A warm saline mouthwash is ideal and can be prepared either by dissolving half a teaspoonful of salt in a glassful of warm water or by diluting compound sodium chloride mouthwash p. 674 with an equal volume of warm water.

Mouthwashes containing an oxidising agent, such as hydrogen peroxide p. 674, may be useful in the treatment of acute ulcerative gingivitis (Vincent's infection) since the organisms involved are anaerobes. It also has a mechanical cleansing effect arising from frothing when in contact with oral debris. Concentrations greater than 1.5% in children may cause ulceration and tissue damage.

Chlorhexidine below is an effective antiseptic which has the advantage of inhibiting plaque formation on the teeth. It does not, however, completely control plaque deposition and is not a substitute for effective toothbrushing. Moreover, chlorhexidine preparations do not penetrate significantly into stagnation areas and are therefore of little value in the control of dental caries or of periodontal disease once pocketing has developed. Chlorhexidine preparations are of little value in the control of acute necrotising ulcerative gingivitis. With prolonged use, chlorhexidine causes reversible brown staining of teeth and tongue. Chlorhexidine may be incompatible with some ingredients in toothpaste, causing an unpleasant taste in the mouth; rinse the mouth thoroughly with water between using toothpaste and chlorhexidine-containing products.

Chlorhexidine can be used as a mouthwash, spray or gel for secondary infection in mucosal ulceration and for controlling gingivitis, as an adjunct to other oral hygiene measures. These preparations may also be used instead of toothbrushing where there is a painful periodontal condition (e.g. primary herpetic stomatitis) or if the patient has a haemorrhagic disorder, or is disabled. Chlorhexidine mouthwash is used in the prevention of oral candidiasis in immunocompromised patients. Chlorhexidine mouthwash reduces the incidence of alveolar osteitis following tooth extraction. Chlorhexidine mouthwash should not be used for the prevention of endocarditis in children undergoing dental procedures.

ANTISEPTICS AND DISINFECTANTS

Chlorhexidine

- **INDICATIONS AND DOSE**

Oral hygiene and plaque inhibition | Oral candidiasis | Gingivitis | Management of aphthous ulcers
▸ BY MOUTH USING MOUTHWASH
▸ Child: Rinse or gargle 10 mL twice daily (rinse or gargle for about 1 minute)

Oral hygiene and plaque inhibition and gingivitis
▸ BY MOUTH USING DENTAL GEL
▸ Child: Apply 1–2 times a day, to be brushed on the teeth

Oral candidiasis | Management of aphthous ulcers
▸ BY MOUTH USING DENTAL GEL
▸ Child: Apply 1–2 times a day, to affected areas

Oral hygiene and plaque inhibition | Oral candidiasis | Gingivitis | Management of aphthous ulcers
▸ BY MOUTH USING OROMUCOSAL SPRAY
▸ Child: Apply up to 12 sprays twice daily as required, to be applied tooth, gingival, or ulcer surfaces

Bladder irrigation and catheter patency solutions
▸ BY INTRAVESICAL INSTILLATION
▸ Child: (consult product literature)

- **UNLICENSED USE** *Corsodyl*® not licensed for use in children under 12 years (unless on the advice of a healthcare professional).

- **SIDE-EFFECTS** Anaphylaxis · hypersensitivity · mucosal irritation · parotid gland swelling · reversible brown staining of composite restorations · reversible brown staining of silicate compositions · reversible brown staining of teeth · taste disturbance · tongue discolouration
  SIDE-EFFECTS, FURTHER INFORMATION If desquamation occurs with mucosal irritation, discontinue treatment or dilute mouthwash with an equal volume of water.

- **PATIENT AND CARER ADVICE** Chlorhexidine gluconate may be incompatible with some ingredients in toothpaste; rinse the mouth thoroughly with water between using toothpaste and chlorhexidine-containing product.

- **PROFESSION SPECIFIC INFORMATION**

Dental practitioners' formulary
Corsodyl® dental gel may be prescribed as Chlorhexidine Gluconate Gel; *Corsodyl*® mouthwash may be prescribed as Chlorhexidine Mouthwash; *Corsodyl*® oral spray may be prescribed as Chlorhexidine Oral Spray.

- **MEDICINAL FORMS**
There can be variation in the licensing of different medicines containing the same drug.

Dental gel
▸ Corsodyl (GlaxoSmithKline Consumer Healthcare)
  Chlorhexidine gluconate 10 mg per 1 gram Corsodyl 1% dental gel sugar-free | 50 gram Ⓟ £1.26 DT price = £1.26

Irrigation
▸ Chlorhexidine (Non-proprietary)
  Chlorhexidine acetate 200 microgram per 1 ml Chlorhexidine acetate 0.02% catheter maintenance solution | 100 ml Ⓟ no price available
▸ Uro-Tainer (chlorhexidine) (B.Braun Medical Ltd)
  Chlorhexidine acetate 200 microgram per 1 ml Uro-Tainer chlorhexidine 1:5000 catheter maintenance solution | 100 ml Ⓟ £2.70

Mouthwash
▸ Chlorhexidine (Non-proprietary)
  Chlorhexidine gluconate 2 mg per 1 ml Chlorhexidine gluconate 0.2% mouthwash aniseed | 300 ml GSL £1.99 DT price = £3.82
  Chlorhexidine gluconate 0.2% mouthwash natural | 300 ml GSL £4.02 DT price = £3.82
  Chlorhexidine gluconate 0.2% mouthwash | 300 ml GSL £2.09 DT price = £3.82

12

Ear, nose and oropharynx

Chlorhexidine gluconate 0.2% mouthwash plain | 300 ml [GSL] £3.77 DT price = £3.82

Chlorhexidine gluconate 0.2% mouthwash peppermint | 300 ml [GSL] £4.02 DT price = £3.82

Colgate Pro Gum Health 0.2% antiseptic mouthwash | 300 ml [GSL] £3.06 DT price = £3.82

Chlorhexidine gluconate 0.2% mouthwash original | 300 ml [GSL] £4.02 DT price = £3.82

Chlorhexidine gluconate 0.2% mouthwash alcohol free | 300 ml [GSL] no price available DT price = £3.82 | 500 ml [GSL] no price available

▸ **Corsodyl** (GlaxoSmithKline Consumer Healthcare)

Chlorhexidine gluconate 2 mg per 1 ml Corsodyl Mint 0.2% mouthwash | 300 ml [GSL] £2.44 DT price = £3.82 | 600 ml [GSL] £4.76

Corsodyl 0.2% mouthwash aniseed | 300 ml [GSL] £2.44 DT price = £3.82

Corsodyl 0.2% mouthwash alcohol free | 300 ml [GSL] £3.06 DT price = £3.82

▸ **Curasept** (Curaprox (UK) Ltd)

Chlorhexidine gluconate 2 mg per 1 ml Curasept 0.2% oral rinse | 200 ml no price available

Chlorhexidine with chlorobutanol

The properties listed below are those particular to the combination only. For the properties of the components please consider, chlorhexidine p. 673.

- **INDICATIONS AND DOSE**

Oral hygiene and plaque inhibition

▸ BY MOUTH USING MOUTHWASH

▸ Child 6–17 years: Rinse or gargle 10–15 mL 2–3 times a day, to be diluted with lukewarm water in measuring cup provided

- **PRESCRIBING AND DISPENSING INFORMATION** Flavours of mouthwash may include mint.

- **MEDICINAL FORMS**
There can be variation in the licensing of different medicines containing the same drug.
No licensed medicines listed.

Hexetidine

- **INDICATIONS AND DOSE**

Oral hygiene

▸ BY MOUTH USING MOUTHWASH

▸ Child 6–17 years: Rinse or gargle 15 mL 2–3 times a day, to be used undiluted

- **SIDE-EFFECTS**
▸ **Very rare** Taste disturbance · transient anaesthesia
▸ **Frequency not known** Local irritation

- **MEDICINAL FORMS**
There can be variation in the licensing of different medicines containing the same drug.
No licensed medicines listed.

Hydrogen peroxide

- **DRUG ACTION** Hydrogen peroxide is an oxidising agent.

- **INDICATIONS AND DOSE**

Oral hygiene (with hydrogen peroxide 6%)

▸ BY MOUTH USING MOUTHWASH

▸ Child: Rinse or gargle 15 mL 2–3 times a day for 2–3 minutes, to be diluted in half a tumblerful of warm water

PEROXYL®

Oral hygiene

▸ BY MOUTH USING MOUTHWASH

▸ Child 6–17 years: Rinse or gargle 10 mL 3 times a day for about 1 minute, for maximum 7 days, to be used after meals and at bedtime

- **SIDE-EFFECTS** Hypertrophy of papillae of tongue on prolonged used

- **PRESCRIBING AND DISPENSING INFORMATION** When prepared extemporaneously, the BP states Hydrogen Peroxide Mouthwash, BP consists of hydrogen peroxide 6% solution (= approx. 20 volume) BP.

- **HANDLING AND STORAGE** Hydrogen peroxide bleaches fabric.

- **PROFESSION SPECIFIC INFORMATION**

Dental practitioners' formulary
Hydrogen Peroxide Mouthwash may be prescribed.

- **MEDICINAL FORMS**
There can be variation in the licensing of different medicines containing the same drug.

Mouthwash

▸ **Peroxyl** (Colgate-Palmolive (UK) Ltd)

Hydrogen peroxide 15 mg per 1 ml Peroxyl 1.5% mouthwash sugar-free | 300 ml [GSL] £2.94

Sodium bicarbonate with sodium chloride

- **INDICATIONS AND DOSE**

Oral hygiene

▸ BY MOUTH USING MOUTHWASH

▸ Child: (consult product literature)

- **DIRECTIONS FOR ADMINISTRATION** For mouthwash, extemporaneous preparations should be prepared according to the following formula: sodium chloride 1.5 g, sodium bicarbonate 1 g, concentrated peppermint emulsion 2.5 mL, double-strength chloroform water 50 mL, water to 100 mL. To be diluted with an equal volume of warm water prior to administration.

- **PRESCRIBING AND DISPENSING INFORMATION** Flavours of mouthwash may include peppermint.

- **PROFESSION SPECIFIC INFORMATION**

Dental practitioners' formulary
Compound sodium chloride mouthwash may be prescribed.

- **MEDICINAL FORMS**
There can be variation in the licensing of different medicines containing the same drug. Forms available from special-order manufacturers include: mouthwash

Sodium chloride

- **INDICATIONS AND DOSE**

Oral hygiene

▸ BY MOUTH USING MOUTHWASH

▸ Child: Rinse or gargle as required

- **DIRECTIONS FOR ADMINISTRATION** Extemporaneous mouthwash preparations should be prepared according to the following formula: sodium chloride 1.5 g, sodium bicarbonate 1 g, concentrated peppermint emulsion 2.5 mL, double-strength chloroform water 50 mL, water to 100 mL. To be diluted with an equal volume of warm water.

- **PRESCRIBING AND DISPENSING INFORMATION** No mouthwash preparations available—when prepared extemporaneously, the BP states Sodium Chloride

Mouthwash, Compound, BP consists of sodium bicarbonate 1%, sodium chloride 1.5% in a suitable vehicle with peppermint flavour.

- **PROFESSION SPECIFIC INFORMATION**
Dental practitioners' formulary
Compound Sodium Chloride Mouthwash may be prescribed.

- **MEDICINAL FORMS**
There can be variation in the licensing of different medicines containing the same drug.
No licensed preparations listed

2.1 Dental caries

Fluoride

Availability of adequate fluoride confers significant resistance to dental caries. It is now considered that the topical action of fluoride on enamel and plaque is more important than the systemic effect.

When the fluoride content of drinking water is less than 700 micrograms per litre (0.7 parts per million), daily administration of fluoride tablets or drops provides suitable supplementation. Systemic fluoride supplements should not be prescribed without reference to the fluoride content of the local water supply. Infants need not receive fluoride supplements until the age of 6 months.

Dentifrices which incorporate sodium fluoride or monofluorophosphate are also a convenient source of fluoride.

Individuals who are either particularly caries prone or medically compromised may be given additional protection by use of fluoride rinses or by application of fluoride gels. Rinses may be used daily or weekly; daily use of a less concentrated rinse is more effective than weekly use of a more concentrated one. High-strength gels must be applied regularly under professional supervision; extreme caution is necessary to prevent children from swallowing any excess. Less concentrated gels are available for home use. Varnishes are also available and are particularly valuable for young or disabled children since they adhere to the teeth and set in the presence of moisture.

VITAMINS AND TRACE ELEMENTS

Sodium fluoride

- **INDICATIONS AND DOSE**
Prophylaxis of dental caries for water content less than 300micrograms/litre (0.3 parts per million) of fluoride ion
 ▸ BY MOUTH USING TABLETS
 ▸ Child 6 months–2 years: 250 micrograms daily, doses expressed as fluoride ion (F⁻)
 ▸ Child 3–5 years: 500 micrograms daily, doses expressed as fluoride ion (F⁻)
 ▸ Child 6–17 years: 1 mg daily, doses expressed as fluoride ion (F⁻)

Prophylaxis of dental caries for water content between 300 and 700micrograms/litre (0.3–0.7 parts per million) of fluoride ion
 ▸ BY MOUTH USING TABLETS
 ▸ Child 3–5 years: 250 micrograms daily, doses expressed as fluoride ion (F⁻)
 ▸ Child 6–17 years: 500 micrograms daily, doses expressed as fluoride ion (F⁻)

Prophylaxis of dental caries for water content above 700micrograms/litre (0.7 parts per million) of fluoride ion
 ▸ Child 6 months–17 years: Supplements not advised

Prophylaxis of dental caries for individuals who are caries prone or medically compromised
 ▸ BY MOUTH USING MOUTHWASH
 ▸ Child 6–17 years: Rinse or gargle 10 mL daily

COLGATE DURAPHAT® 2800PPM FLUORIDE TOOTHPASTE
Prophylaxis of dental caries
 ▸ BY MOUTH USING PASTE
 ▸ Child 10–17 years: Apply 1 centimetre twice daily, to be applied using a toothbrush

COLGATE DURAPHAT® 5000PPM FLUORIDE TOOTHPASTE
Prophylaxis of dental caries
 ▸ BY MOUTH USING PASTE
 ▸ Child 16–17 years: Apply 2 centimetres 3 times a day, to be applied after meals using a toothbrush

EN-DE-KAY® FLUORINSE
Prophylaxis of dental carries for individuals who are caries prone or medically compromised
 ▸ BY MOUTH USING MOUTHWASH
 ▸ Child 8–17 years: 5 drops daily, dilute 5 drops to 10 mL of water, alternatively 20 drops once weekly, dilute 20 drops to 10 mL

DOSE EQUIVALENCE AND CONVERSION
 ▸ Sodium fluoride 2.2 mg provides approx. 1 mg fluoride ion.
 ▸ These doses reflect the recommendations of the British Dental Association, the British Society of Paediatric Dentistry and the British Association for the Study of Community Dentistry (*Br Dent J* 1997; **182**: 6–7).

- **CONTRA-INDICATIONS** Not for areas where drinking water is fluoridated
- **SIDE-EFFECTS**
 ▸ **Uncommon** Occasional white flecks on teeth with recommended doses
 ▸ **Rare** Yellowish-brown discoloration if recommended doses are exceeded
- **DIRECTIONS FOR ADMINISTRATION** Tablets should be sucked or dissolved in the mouth and taken preferably in the evening. For mouthwash, rinse mouth for 1 minute and then spit out.
COLGATE DURAPHAT® 2800PPM FLUORIDE TOOTHPASTE Brush teeth for 1 minute before spitting out.
COLGATE DURAPHAT® 5000PPM FLUORIDE TOOTHPASTE Brush teeth for 3 minutes before spitting out.
- **PRESCRIBING AND DISPENSING INFORMATION** Flavours of oral tablet formulations may include orange.
- **PATIENT AND CARER ADVICE**
Mouthwash Avoid eating, drinking, or rinsing mouth for 15 minutes after use.
COLGATE DURAPHAT® 2800PPM FLUORIDE TOOTHPASTE Patients or carers should be given advice on how to administer sodium fluoride toothpaste. Avoid drinking or rinsing mouth for 30 minutes after use.
COLGATE DURAPHAT® 5000PPM FLUORIDE TOOTHPASTE Patients or carers should be given advice on how to administer Sodium fluoride toothpaste.
- **PROFESSION SPECIFIC INFORMATION**
Dental practitioners' formulary
Tablets may be prescribed as Sodium Fluoride Tablets. Oral drops may be prescribed as Sodium Fluoride Oral Drops.
Mouthwashes may be prescribed as Sodium Fluoride Mouthwash 0.05% or Sodium Fluoride Mouthwash 2%.

12

Ear, nose and oropharynx

COLGATE DURAPHAT® 2800PPM FLUORIDE TOOTHPASTE
May be prescribed as Sodium Fluoride Toothpaste 0.619%.

COLGATE DURAPHAT® 5000PPM FLUORIDE TOOTHPASTE
May be prescribed as Sodium Fluoride Toothpaste 1.1%.

Dental information
Fluoride mouthwash, oral drops, tablets and toothpaste
are prescribable on form FP10D (GP14 in Scotland, WP10D
in Wales).

There are also arrangements for health authorities to
supply fluoride tablets in the course of pre-school dental
schemes, and they may also be supplied in school dental
schemes.

Fluoride gels are not prescribable on form FP10D (GP14
in Scotland, WP10D in Wales).

● MEDICINAL FORMS
There can be variation in the licensing of different medicines
containing the same drug. Forms available from special-order
manufacturers include: capsule, oral solution

Tablet
▸ Endekay (Manx Healthcare Ltd)
Sodium fluoride 1.1 mg Endekay Fluotabs 3-6 Years 1.1mg tablets |
200 tablet P £2.38 DT price = £2.38
Sodium fluoride 2.2 mg Endekay Fluotabs 6+ Years 2.2mg tablets |
200 tablet P £2.38 DT price = £2.38

Paste
▸ Colgate Duraphat (Colgate-Palmolive (UK) Ltd)
Fluoride (as Sodium fluoride) 2.8 mg per 1 gram Colgate Duraphat
2800ppm fluoride toothpaste sugar-free | 75 ml PoM £3.26 DT price
= £3.26
Fluoride (as Sodium fluoride) 5 mg per 1 gram Colgate Duraphat
5000ppm fluoride toothpaste sugar-free | 51 gram PoM £6.50 DT
price = £6.50

Oral drops
▸ Endekay (Manx Healthcare Ltd)
Sodium fluoride 3.7 mg per 1 ml Endekay Fluodrops 0.37% drops
paediatric sugar-free | 60 ml P £2.38 DT price = £2.38

Chewable tablet
▸ Fluor-a-day (Dental Health Products Ltd)
Sodium fluoride 1.1 mg Fluor-a-day 1.1mg chewable tablets sugar-
free | 200 tablet P £3.38 DT price = £2.79
Sodium fluoride 2.2 mg Fluor-a-day 2.2mg chewable tablets sugar-
free | 200 tablet P £3.38 DT price = £2.79

Mouthwash
▸ Sodium fluoride (Non-proprietary)
Sodium fluoride 500 microgram per 1 ml Sodium fluoride 0.05%
mouthwash sugar free sugar-free | 250 ml GSL no price available DT
price = £1.51 sugar-free | 400 ml GSL no price available sugar-free
| 500 ml GSL no price available
▸ Colgate FluoriGard (Colgate-Palmolive (UK) Ltd)
Sodium fluoride 500 microgram per 1 ml Colgate FluoriGard 0.05%
daily dental rinse alcohol free sugar-free | 400 ml £2.99
Colgate FluoriGard 0.05% daily dental rinse sugar-free | 400 ml GSL
£2.99
▸ Endekay (Manx Healthcare Ltd)
Sodium fluoride 500 microgram per 1 ml Endekay 0.05% daily
fluoride mouthrinse sugar-free | 250 ml GSL £1.51 DT price = £1.51
sugar-free | 500 ml GSL £2.45
Sodium fluoride 20 mg per 1 ml Endekay Fluorinse 2% mouthwash
sugar-free | 100 ml PoM £4.97

3   Oral ulceration and inflammation

Oral ulceration and inflammation

Ulceration and inflammation

Ulceration of the oral mucosa may be caused by trauma
(physical or chemical), recurrent aphthae, infections,
carcinoma, dermatological disorders, nutritional
deficiencies, gastro-intestinal disease, haematopoietic
disorders, and drug therapy. It is important to establish the
diagnosis in each case as the majority of these lesions
require specific management in addition to local treatment.
Local treatment aims to protect the ulcerated area, to relieve
pain, to reduce inflammation, or to control secondary
infection. Children with an unexplained mouth ulcer of more
than 3 weeks' duration require urgent referral to hospital to
exclude oral cancer in adults or secondary causes such as
leukaemia.

Simple mouthwashes
A **saline** mouthwash may relieve the pain of traumatic
ulceration. The mouthwash is made up with warm water and
used at frequent intervals until the discomfort and swelling
subsides.

Antiseptic mouthwashes
Secondary bacterial infection may be a feature of any
mucosal ulceration; it can increase discomfort and delay
healing. Use of chlorhexidine mouthwash p. 673 is often
beneficial and may accelerate healing of recurrent aphthae.

Corticosteroids
Topical corticosteroid therapy may be used for some forms of
oral ulceration. In the case of aphthous ulcers it is most
effective if applied in the 'prodromal' phase. Thrush or other
types of candidiasis are recognised complications of
corticosteroid treatment.

Hydrocortisone **oromucosal tablets** p. 678 are allowed to
dissolve next to an ulcer and are useful in recurrent aphthae
and erosive lichenoid lesions.

Beclometasone dipropionate inhaler p. 154 sprayed on the
oral mucosa is used to manage oral ulceration [unlicensed
indication]. Alternatively, betamethasone soluble tablets
p. 662 dissolved in water can be used as a mouthwash to
treat oral ulceration [unlicensed indication].

Systemic corticosteroid therapy (see under
Corticosteroids, inflammatory disorders p. 633) is reserved
for severe conditions such as pemphigus vulgaris.

Local analgesics
Local analgesics have a limited role in the management of
oral ulceration. When applied topically their action is of a
relatively short duration so that analgesia cannot be
maintained continuously throughout the day. When local
anaesthetics are used in the mouth, care must be taken not
to produce anaesthesia of the pharynx before meals as this
might lead to choking.

Benzydamine hydrochloride p. 677 and flurbiprofen p. 678
are non-steroidal anti-inflammatory drugs (NSAIDs).
Benzydamine hydrochloride mouthwash or spray may be
useful in reducing the discomfort associated with a variety of
ulcerative conditions. It has also been found to be effective
in reducing the discomfort of tonsillectomy and post-
irradiation mucositis. Some patients find the full-strength
mouthwash causes some stinging and, for them, it should be
diluted with an equal volume of water. Flurbiprofen lozenges
are licensed for the relief of sore throat in adolescents.

Choline salicylate p. 678 is a derivative of salicylic acid and
has some analgesic action. The dental gel may provide relief
for recurrent aphthae, but excessive application or
confinement under a denture irritates the mucosa and can
itself cause ulceration in adults and children over 16 years of
age.

Other preparations
Doxycycline p. 679 rinsed in the mouth may be of value for
recurrent aphthous ulceration.

Periodontitis
Low-dose doxycycline (*Periostat®*) is licensed as an adjunct
to scaling and root planing for the treatment of
periodontitis; a low dose of doxycycline reduces collagenase
activity without inhibiting bacteria associated with
periodontitis.

For anti-infectives used in the treatment of destructive
(refractory) forms of periodontal disease, see under

Ear, nose and oropharynx

12

Oropharyngeal bacterial infections p. 679. See also Mouthwashes and other preparations for oropharyngeal use p. 673 for mouthwashes used for oral hygiene and plaque inhibition.

ANAESTHETICS, LOCAL

Lidocaine hydrochloride
(Lignocaine hydrochloride)

- **INDICATIONS AND DOSE**

Dental practice
▶ BY BUCCAL ADMINISTRATION USING OINTMENT
▶ Child: Rub gently into dry gum

LARYNGOJET®

Anaesthesia of mucous membranes of oropharynx, trachea, or respiratory tract
▶ TO MUCOUS MEMBRANES
▶ Child: Up to 3 mg/kg (max. per dose 200 mg), to be given as a single dose sprayed, instilled (if a cavity) or applied with a swab; reduce dose according to size, age, and condition of child

XYLOCAINE®

Bronchoscopy | Laryngoscopy | Oesophagoscopy | Endotracheal intubation
▶ TO MUCOUS MEMBRANES
▶ Child: Up to 3 mg/kg

- **CAUTIONS** Can damage plastic cuffs of endotracheal tubes
- **INTERACTIONS** → Appendix 1: antiarrhythmics
- **SIDE-EFFECTS**
  SIDE-EFFECTS, FURTHER INFORMATION A single application of a topical lidocaine preparation does not generally cause systemic side-effects.
- **ALLERGY AND CROSS-SENSITIVITY** Hypersensitivity reactions occur mainly with the ester-type local anaesthetics, such as tetracaine and chloroprocaine; reactions are less frequent with the amide types, such as articaine, bupivacaine, levobupivacaine, lidocaine, mepivacaine, prilocaine, and ropivacaine. Cross-sensitivity reactions may be avoided by using the alternative chemical type.
- **PREGNANCY** Crosses the placenta but not known to be harmful in *animal* studies—use if benefit outweighs risk. When used as a local anaesthetic, large doses can cause fetal bradycardia; if given during delivery can also cause neonatal respiratory depression, hypotonia, or bradycardia after paracervical or epidural block.
- **BREAST FEEDING** Present in milk but amount too small to be harmful.
- **HEPATIC IMPAIRMENT** Caution—increased risk of side-effects.
- **RENAL IMPAIRMENT** Possible accumulation of lidocaine and active metabolite; caution in severe impairment.
- **PROFESSION SPECIFIC INFORMATION**
  Dental practitioners' formulary
  Lidocaine ointment 5% may be prescribed.
  Spray may be prescribed as Lidocaine Spray 10%
  XYLOCAINE®
  May be prescribed as lidocaine spray 10%.

- **MEDICINAL FORMS**
  There can be variation in the licensing of different medicines containing the same drug
  Spray
  ▶ Xylocaine (Aspen Pharma Trading Ltd)
  Lidocaine 10 mg per 1 actuation Xylocaine 10mg/dose spray sugar-free | 50 ml P £6.29

Ointment
▶ Lidocaine hydrochloride (Non-proprietary)
Lidocaine hydrochloride 50 mg per 1 gram Lidocaine 5% ointment | 15 gram P £6.50 DT price = £6.18
Liquid
▶ LaryngoJet (UCB Pharma Ltd)
Lidocaine hydrochloride 40 mg per 1 ml Lidocaine 4% oromucosal solution LaryngoJet pre-filled syringes | 1 pre-filled disposable injection PoM £5.10

ANALGESICS ❭ NON-STEROIDAL ANTI-INFLAMMATORY DRUGS

Benzydamine hydrochloride

- **INDICATIONS AND DOSE**

Painful inflammatory conditions of oropharynx
▶ TO THE LESION USING MOUTHWASH
▶ Child 13-17 years: Rinse or gargle 15 mL every 1.5–3 hours as required usually for not more than 7 days, dilute with an equal volume of water if stinging occurs
▶ TO THE LESION USING OROMUCOSAL SPRAY
▶ Child 1 month-5 years (body-weight 4–7 kg): 1 spray every 1.5–3 hours, to be administered onto the affected area
▶ Child 1 month-5 years (body-weight 8–11 kg): 2 sprays every 1.5–3 hours, to be administered onto the affected area
▶ Child 1 month-5 years (body-weight 12–15 kg): 3 sprays every 1.5–3 hours, to be administered onto the affected area
▶ Child 1 month-5 years (body-weight 16 kg and above): 4 sprays every 1.5–3 hours, to be administered onto the affected area
▶ Child 6-11 years: 4 sprays every 1.5–3 hours, to be administered onto affected area
▶ Child 12-17 years: 4–8 sprays every 1.5–3 hours, to be administered onto affected area

- **INTERACTIONS** → Appendix 1: NSAIDs
- **SIDE-EFFECTS**
▶ Rare Hypersensitivity reactions
▶ Frequency not known Occasional numbness or stinging
- **PROFESSION SPECIFIC INFORMATION**
  Dental practitioners' formulary
  Benzydamine Oromucosal Spray 0.15% may be prescribed. Benzydamine mouthwash may be prescribed as Benzydamine Mouthwash 0.15%.

- **MEDICINAL FORMS**
  There can be variation in the licensing of different medicines containing the same drug.
  Spray
  ▶ Benzydamine hydrochloride (Non-proprietary)
  Benzydamine hydrochloride 1.5 mg per 1 ml Benzydamine 0.15% oromucosal spray sugar free sugar-free | 30 ml P £4.53 DT price = £4.10
  ▶ Difflam (Meda Pharmaceuticals Ltd)
  Benzydamine hydrochloride 1.5 mg per 1 ml Difflam 0.15% spray sugar-free | 30 ml P £4.24 DT price = £4.10
  Mouthwash
  ▶ Benzydamine hydrochloride (Non-proprietary)
  Benzydamine hydrochloride 1.5 mg per 1 ml Benzydamine 0.15% mouthwash sugar free sugar-free | 300 ml P £7.14 DT price = £6.21
  ▶ Difflam (Meda Pharmaceuticals Ltd)
  Benzydamine hydrochloride 1.5 mg per 1 ml Difflam Oral Rinse 0.15% solution sugar-free | 300 ml P £6.50 DT price = £6.21
  Difflam 0.15% Sore Throat Rinse sugar-free | 200 ml P £4.64

12

Ear, nose and oropharynx

Flurbiprofen

- **INDICATIONS AND DOSE**

Relief of sore throat
▸ BY MOUTH USING LOZENGES
▸ Child 12-17 years: 1 lozenge every 3–6 hours for maximum 3 days, allow lozenge to dissolve slowly in the mouth; maximum 5 lozenges per day

- **INTERACTIONS** → Appendix 1: NSAIDs
- **SIDE-EFFECTS** Mouth ulcers (move lozenge around mouth) · taste disturbance
- **ALLERGY AND CROSS-SENSITIVITY** Contra-indicated in patients with a history of hypersensitivity to aspirin or any other NSAID—which includes those in whom attacks of asthma, angioedema, urticaria or rhinitis have been precipitated by aspirin or any other NSAID.
- **MEDICINAL FORMS** There can be variation in the licensing of different medicines containing the same drug.

Lozenge
▸ **Strefen** (Reckitt Benckiser Healthcare (UK) Ltd)
Flurbiprofen 8.75 mg Strefen 8.75mg lozenges | 16 lozenge ℗ £2.58 DT price = £2.58

CORTICOSTEROIDS

Betamethasone

- **INDICATIONS AND DOSE**

Oral ulceration
▸ TO THE LESION USING SOLUBLE TABLETS
▸ Child 12-17 years: 500 micrograms 4 times a day, to be dissolved in 20 mL water and rinsed around the mouth; not to be swallowed

- **UNLICENSED USE** Betamethasone soluble tablets not licensed for use as mouthwash or in oral ulceration.
- **CONTRA-INDICATIONS** Untreated local infection
- **INTERACTIONS** → Appendix 1: corticosteroids
- **SIDE-EFFECTS** Candidal infection · exacerbation of local infection
- **PATIENT AND CARER ADVICE** Patient counselling is advised for betamethasone soluble tablets (administration).
- **PROFESSION SPECIFIC INFORMATION**

Dental practitioners' formulary
Betamethasone Soluble Tablets 500 micrograms may be prescribed for oral ulceration.

- **MEDICINAL FORMS** There can be variation in the licensing of different medicines containing the same drug.

Soluble tablet
CAUTIONARY AND ADVISORY LABELS 10, 13, 21 (not for use as mouthwash for oral ulceration)
▸ **Betamethasone** (Non-proprietary)
Betamethasone (as Betamethasone sodium phosphate)
500 microgram Betamethasone 500microgram soluble tablets sugar free sugar-free | 100 tablet PoM £42.60 DT price = £42.60

Hydrocortisone

18-May-2017

- **INDICATIONS AND DOSE**

Oral and perioral lesions
▸ TO THE LESION USING BUCCAL TABLET
▸ Child 1 month–11 years: Only on medical advice
▸ Child 12-17 years: 1 lozenge 4 times a day, allowed to dissolve slowly in the mouth in contact with the ulcer

- **UNLICENSED USE** Hydrocortisone mucoadhesive buccal tablets licensed for use in children (under 12 years—on medical advice only).
- **CONTRA-INDICATIONS** Untreated local infection
- **INTERACTIONS** → Appendix 1: corticosteroids
- **SIDE-EFFECTS** Candidal infection · exacerbation of local infection
- **PROFESSION SPECIFIC INFORMATION**

Dental practitioners' formulary
Mucoadhesive buccal tablets may be prescribed as Hydrocortisone Oromucosal Tablets.

- **MEDICINAL FORMS** There can be variation in the licensing of different medicines containing the same drug.

Muco-adhesive buccal tablet
▸ Hydrocortisone (Non-proprietary)
Hydrocortisone (as Hydrocortisone sodium succinate)
2.5 mg Hydrocortisone 2.5mg muco-adhesive buccal tablets sugar free sugar-free | 20 tablet ℗ £8.30 DT price = £7.30

SALICYLIC ACID AND DERIVATIVES

Choline salicylate

- **INDICATIONS AND DOSE**

Mild oral and perioral lesions
▸ TO THE LESION
▸ Child 16-17 years: Apply 0.5 inch, apply with gentle massage, not more often than every 3 hours

- **CONTRA-INDICATIONS** Children under 16 years
CONTRA-INDICATIONS, FURTHER INFORMATION
▸ Reye's syndrome The CHM has advised that topical oral pain relief products containing salicylate salts should not be used in children under 16 years, as a cautionary measure due to the theoretical risk of Reye's syndrome.
- **CAUTIONS** Frequent application, especially in children, may give rise to salicylate poisoning
- **INTERACTIONS** → Appendix 1: choline salicylate
- **SIDE-EFFECTS** Transient local burning sensation
- **PRESCRIBING AND DISPENSING INFORMATION** When prepared extemporaneously, the BP states Choline Salicylate Dental Gel, BP consists of choline salicylate 8.7% in a flavoured gel basis.
- **PROFESSION SPECIFIC INFORMATION**

Dental practitioners' formulary
Choline Salicylate Dental Gel may be prescribed.

- **MEDICINAL FORMS** There can be variation in the licensing of different medicines containing the same drug.

Oromucosal gel
▸ **Bonjela** (Reckitt Benckiser Healthcare (UK) Ltd)
Choline salicylate 87 mg per 1 gram Bonjela Cool Mint gel sugar-free | 15 gram GSL £3.55 DT price = £2.58
Bonjela Original gel sugar-free | 15 gram GSL £2.58 DT price = £2.58

Salicylic acid with rhubarb extract

- **INDICATIONS AND DOSE**

Mild oral and perioral lesions
▸ TO THE LESION
▸ Child 16-17 years: Apply 3–4 times a day maximum duration 7 days

- **CONTRA-INDICATIONS** Children under 16 years
CONTRA-INDICATIONS, FURTHER INFORMATION
▸ Reye's syndrome The CHM has advised that topical oral pain relief products containing salicylate salts should not be

used in children under 16 years, as a cautionary measure due to the theoretical risk of Reye's syndrome.

- **CAUTIONS** Frequent application, especially in children, may give rise to salicylate poisoning
- **SIDE-EFFECTS** Temporary discolouration of oral mucosa · temporary discolouration of teeth · transient local burning sensation
- **PATIENT AND CARER ADVICE** May cause temporary discolouration of teeth and oral mucosa.

- **MEDICINAL FORMS**
  There can be variation in the licensing of different medicines containing the same drug.
  Paint
  EXCIPIENTS: May contain Ethanol
  ‣ **Pyralvex** (Meda Pharmaceuticals Ltd)
  Salicylic acid 10 mg per 1 ml, Rhubarb extract 50 mg per 1 ml Pyralvex solution | 10 ml [P] £3.25

4   Oropharyngeal bacterial infections

Oropharyngeal bacterial infections

Antibacterial therapy for pericoronitis

Antibacterial required only in presence of systemic features of infection, or of trismus, or persistent swelling despite local treatment.

- Metronidazole p. 319, or *alternatively*, amoxicillin p. 325
- ‣ *Suggested duration of treatment* 3 days or until symptoms resolve.

Antibacterial therapy for gingivitis: acute necrotising ulcerative

Antibacterial required only if systemic features of infection.

- Metronidazole, or *alternatively*, amoxicillin
- ‣ *Suggested duration of treatment* 3 days or until symptoms resolve.

Antibacterial therapy for periapical or periodontal abscess

Antibacterial required only in severe disease with cellulitis or if systemic features of infection.

- Amoxicillin, or *alternatively*, metronidazole
- ‣ *Suggested duration of treatment* 5 days.

Antibacterial therapy for periodontitis

Antibacterial used as an adjunct to debridement in severe disease or disease unresponsive to local treatment alone.

- Metronidazole, or *alternatively in adults and children over 12 years*, doxycycline below

Antibacterial therapy for throat infections

Most throat infections are caused by viruses and many do not require antibacterial therapy. Consider antibacterial, if history of valvular heart disease, if marked systemic upset, if peritonsillar cellulitis or abscess, or if at increased risk from acute infection (e.g. in immunosuppression, cystic fibrosis); prescribe antibacterial for beta-haemolytic streptococcal pharyngitis.

- Phenoxymethylpenicillin p. 324
- ‣ In severe infection, initial parenteral therapy with benzylpenicillin sodium p. 323, then oral therapy with phenoxymethylpenicillin *or* amoxicillin (*or* ampicillin p. 326). **Avoid** amoxicillin if possibility of glandular fever.
- ‣ *Suggested duration of treatment* 10 days.

- If *penicillin-allergic*, clarithromycin p. 315 (*or* azithromycin p. 314 *or* erythromycin p. 316)
- ‣ *Suggested duration of treatment* 10 days

ANTIBACTERIALS ⟩ TETRACYCLINES AND RELATED DRUGS

▌ Doxycycline

- **INDICATIONS AND DOSE**
  Treatment of recurrent aphthous ulceration
  ‣ BY MOUTH USING SOLUBLE TABLETS
  ‣ Child 12–17 years: 100 mg 4 times a day usually for 3 days, dispersible tablet can be stirred into a small amount of water then rinsed around the mouth for 2–3 minutes, it should preferably not be swallowed

- **UNLICENSED USE** Not licensed for use in children under 12 years.
- **CAUTIONS** Alcohol dependence
- **INTERACTIONS** → Appendix 1: tetracyclines
- **SIDE-EFFECTS** Anorexia · anxiety · dry mouth · flushing · fungal superinfection (when used for periodontitis) · tinnitus
- **RENAL IMPAIRMENT** Use with caution (avoid excessive doses).
- **PATIENT AND CARER ADVICE** Counselling on administration advised.
  Photosensitivity Patients should be advised to avoid exposure to sunlight or sun lamps.
- **PROFESSION SPECIFIC INFORMATION**
  Dental practitioners' formulary
  Dispersible tablets may be prescribed as Dispersible Doxycycline Tablets.

- **MEDICINAL FORMS**
  There can be variation in the licensing of different medicines containing the same drug.
  Dispersible tablet
  CAUTIONARY AND ADVISORY LABELS 6, 9, 11, 13
  ‣ **Vibramycin-D** (Pfizer Ltd)
  Doxycycline (as Doxycycline monohydrate) 100 mg Vibramycin-D 100mg dispersible tablets sugar-free | 8 tablet [PoM] £4.91 DT price = £4.91

5   Oropharyngeal fungal infections

Oropharyngeal fungal infections

Overview

Fungal infections of the mouth are usually caused by *Candida* spp. (candidiasis or candidosis). Different types of oropharyngeal candidiasis are managed as follows:

Thrush

Acute pseudomembranous candidiasis (thrush), is usually an acute infection but it may persist for months in patients receiving inhaled corticosteroids, cytotoxics, or broad-spectrum antibacterials. Thrush also occurs in patients with serious systemic disease associated with reduced immunity such as leukaemia, other malignancies, and HIV infection. Any predisposing condition should be managed appropriately. When thrush is associated with corticosteroid inhalers, rinsing the mouth with water (or cleaning a child's teeth) immediately after using the inhaler may avoid the problem. Treatment with nystatin p. 680 or miconazole p. 680 may be needed. Fluconazole p. 358 is effective for

12

Ear, nose and oropharynx

unresponsive infections or if a topical antifungal drug cannot be used. Topical therapy may not be adequate in immunocompromised children and an oral triazole antifungal is preferred.

Acute erythematous candidiasis

Acute erythematous (atrophic) candidiasis is a relatively uncommon condition associated with corticosteroid and broad-spectrum antibacterial use and with HIV disease. It is usually treated with fluconazole.

Angular cheilitis

Angular cheilitis (angular stomatitis) is characterised by soreness, erythema and fissuring at the angles of the mouth. It may represent a nutritional deficiency or it may be related to orofacial granulomatosis or HIV infection. Both yeasts (*Candida* spp.) and bacteria (*Staphylococcus aureus* and beta-haemolytic streptococci) are commonly involved as interacting, infective factors. While the underlying cause is being identified and treated, it is often helpful to apply miconazole cream or fusidic acid ointment p. 342; if the angular cheilitis is unresponsive to treatment, hydrocortisone with miconazole cream or ointment p. 714 can be used.

Immunocompromised patients

See advice on prevention of fungal infections under *Immunocompromised children* in Antifungals, systemic use p. 355.

Antiseptic mouthwashes can have a role in the prevention of oral candidiasis in immunocompromised children.

Drugs used in oropharyngeal candidiasis

Nystatin is not absorbed from the gastro-intestinal tract and is applied locally (as a suspension) to the mouth for treating local fungal infections. Miconazole is used by local application (as an oral gel) in the mouth but it is also absorbed to the extent that potential interactions need to be considered. Miconazole also has some activity against Gram-positive bacteria including streptococci and staphylococci. In neonates, nystatin oral suspension or miconazole oral gel is used for the treatment of oropharyngeal candidiasis; to prevent re-infection it is important to ensure that the mother's breast nipples and the teats of feeding bottles are cleaned adequately.

Fluconazole given by mouth is reliably absorbed; it is used for infections that do not respond to topical therapy or when topical therapy cannot be used. Itraconazole p. 360 can be used for fluconazole-resistant infections.

If candidal infection fails to respond after 1 to 2 weeks of treatment with antifungal drugs the child should be sent for investigation to eliminate the possibility of underlying disease. Persistent infection may also be caused by re-infection from the genito-urinary or gastro-intestinal tract.

ANTIFUNGALS > IMIDAZOLE ANTIFUNGALS

Miconazole

- **INDICATIONS AND DOSE**

  Prevention and treatment of oral candidiasis
  ▸ BY MOUTH USING ORAL GEL

  ▸ Neonate: 1 mL 2–4 times a day treatment should be continued for at least 7 days after lesions have healed or symptoms have cleared, to be smeared around the inside of the mouth after feeds

  ▸ Child 1 month–1 year: 1.25 mL 4 times a day treatment should be continued for at least 7 days after lesions have healed or symptoms have cleared, to be smeared around the inside of the mouth after feeds

  ▸ Child 2–17 years: 2.5 mL 4 times a day treatment should be continued for at least 7 days after lesions have healed or symptoms have cleared, to be administered

after meals, retain near oral lesions before swallowing (dental prostheses and orthodontic appliances should be removed at night and brushed with gel)

  Prevention and treatment of intestinal candidiasis
  ▸ BY MOUTH USING ORAL GEL

  ▸ Child 4 months–17 years: 5 mg/kg 4 times a day (max. per dose 250 mg 4 times a day) treatment should be continued for at least 7 days after lesions have healed or symptoms have cleared

- **UNLICENSED USE** Not licensed for use in children under 4 months of age or during first 5–6 months of life of an infant born pre-term.

- **CONTRA-INDICATIONS** Infants with impaired swallowing reflex

- **CAUTIONS** Avoid in acute porphyrias p. 577

- **INTERACTIONS** → Appendix 1: antifungals, azoles

- **SIDE-EFFECTS**
  ▸ **Common or very common** Nausea · rash · vomiting
  ▸ **Very rare** Diarrhoea (usually on long term treatment) · hepatitis · rash · Stevens-Johnson syndrome · toxic epidermal necrolysis

- **PREGNANCY** Manufacturer advises avoid if possible—toxicity at high doses in *animal* studies.

- **BREAST FEEDING** Manufacturer advises caution—no information available.

- **HEPATIC IMPAIRMENT** Avoid.

- **DIRECTIONS FOR ADMINISTRATION** Oral gel should be held in mouth, after food.

- **PRESCRIBING AND DISPENSING INFORMATION** Flavours of oral gel may include orange.

- **PATIENT AND CARER ADVICE** Patients or carers should be given advice on how to administer miconazole oromucosal gel.

- **PROFESSION SPECIFIC INFORMATION**

  Dental practitioners' formulary
  Miconazole Oromucosal Gel may be prescribed.

- **EXCEPTIONS TO LEGAL CATEGORY** 15-g tube of oral gel can be sold to the public.

- **MEDICINAL FORMS**
  There can be variation in the licensing of different medicines containing the same drug.

  Oromucosal gel
  CAUTIONARY AND ADVISORY LABELS 9
  ▸ Daktarin (McNeil Products Ltd, Janssen-Cilag Ltd)
  Miconazole 20 mg per 1 gram Daktarin 20mg/g oromucosal gel sugar-free | 15 gram Ⓟ £3.23 DT price = £3.23 sugar-free | 80 gram PoM £4.38 DT price = £4.38

ANTIFUNGALS > POLYENE ANTIFUNGALS

Nystatin

08-Feb-2017

- **INDICATIONS AND DOSE**

  Oral candidiasis
  ▸ BY MOUTH

  ▸ Neonate: 100 000 units 4 times a day usually for 7 days, and continued for 48 hours after lesions have resolved, to be given after feeds.

  ▸ Child: 100 000 units 4 times a day usually for 7 days, and continued for 48 hours after lesions have resolved

- **UNLICENSED USE** EvGr Not licensed for use in neonates. ⟨E⟩

- **CAUTIONS** Contact with eyes and mucous membranes should be avoided

- **SIDE-EFFECTS** Burning sensation · erythema · hypersensitivity reactions · itching · local irritation · local sensitisation · nausea

  SIDE-EFFECTS, FURTHER INFORMATION
  Treatment should be discontinued if symptoms are severe.

- **PATIENT AND CARER ADVICE** Counselling advised with oral suspension (use of pipette, hold in mouth, after food).
  Medicines for Children leaflet: Nystatin for Candida infection
  www.medicinesforchildren.org.uk/nystatin-for-candida-infection

- **PROFESSION SPECIFIC INFORMATION**

  Dental practitioners' formulary
  Nystatin Oral Suspension may be prescribed.

- **MEDICINAL FORMS**
  There can be variation in the licensing of different medicines containing the same drug. Forms available from special-order manufacturers include: tablet, capsule, oral suspension

  Oral suspension
  CAUTIONARY AND ADVISORY LABELS 9
  EXCIPIENTS: May contain Ethanol
  ▸ **Nystatin (Non-proprietary)**
    Nystatin 100000 unit per 1 ml Nystatin 100,000units/ml oral suspension | 30 ml PoM £2.33 DT price = £2.09
  ▸ **Nystan (Bristol-Myers Squibb Pharmaceuticals Ltd)**
    Nystatin 100000 unit per 1 ml Nystan 100,000units/ml oral suspension (ready mixed) | 30 ml PoM £1.80 DT price = £2.09

6   Oropharyngeal viral infections

Oropharyngeal viral infections

Management

Viral infections are the most common cause of a sore throat. It is usually a self-limiting condition which does not benefit from anti-infective treatment. Adequate analgesia may be all that is required.

Children with varicella–zoster infection often develop painful lesions in the mouth and throat. Benzydamine hydrochloride p. 677 may be used to provide local analgesia. Chlorhexidine mouthwash or gel p. 673 will control plaque accumulation if toothbrushing is painful and will also help to control secondary infection in general.

In severe herpetic stomatitis systemic aciclovir p. 387 or valaciclovir p. 389 may be used for oral lesions associated with herpes zoster. Aciclovir and valaciclovir are also used to prevent frequently recurring herpes simplex lesions of the mouth particularly when associated with the initiation of erythema multiforme. See the treatment of labial herpes simplex infections.

12

Ear, nose and oropharynx

Chapter 13
Skin

CONTENTS

Skin conditions, management

Topical preparations

When prescribing topical preparations for the treatment of skin conditions in children, the site of application, the condition being treated, and the child's (and carer's) preference for a particular vehicle all need to be taken into consideration.

Vehicles

The British Association of Dermatologists list of preferred unlicensed dermatological preparations (specials) is available at www.bad.org.uk.

The vehicle in topical preparations for the skin affects the degree of hydration, has a mild anti-inflammatory effect, and aids the penetration of the active drug. Therefore, the vehicle, as well as the active drug, should be chosen on the basis of their suitability for the child's skin condition.

Applications are usually viscous solutions, emulsions, or suspensions for application to the skin (including the scalp) or nails.

Collodions are painted on the skin and allowed to dry to leave a flexible film over the site of application.

Creams are emulsions of oil and water and are generally well absorbed into the skin. They may contain an antimicrobial preservative unless the active ingredient or basis is intrinsically bactericidal and fungicidal. Generally, creams are cosmetically more acceptable than ointments because they are less greasy and easier to apply.

Gels consist of active ingredients in suitable hydrophilic or hydrophobic bases; they generally have a high water content. Gels are particularly suitable for application to the face and scalp.

Lotions have a cooling effect and may be preferred to ointments or creams for application over a hairy area. Lotions in alcoholic basis can sting if used on broken skin. *Shake lotions* (such as calamine lotion) contain insoluble powders which leave a deposit on the skin surface.

Ointments are greasy preparations which are normally anhydrous and insoluble in water, and are more occlusive than creams. They are particularly suitable for chronic, dry lesions. The most commonly used ointment bases consist of soft paraffin or a combination of soft, liquid, and hard paraffin. Some ointment bases have both *hydrophilic and lipophilic* properties; they may have occlusive properties on the skin surface, encourage hydration, and also be miscible with water;

they often have a mild anti-inflammatory effect. *Water-soluble ointments* contain macrogols which are freely soluble in water and are therefore readily washed off; they have a limited but useful role where ready removal is desirable.

Pastes are stiff preparations containing a high proportion of finely powdered solids such as zinc oxide and starch suspended in an ointment. They are used for circumscribed lesions such as those which occur in lichen simplex, chronic eczema, or psoriasis. They are less occlusive than ointments and can be used to protect inflamed, lichenified, or excoriated skin.

Dusting powders are used only rarely. They reduce friction between opposing skin surfaces. Dusting powders should not be applied to moist areas because they can cake and abrade the skin. Talc is a lubricant but it does not absorb moisture; it can cause respiratory irritation. Starch is less lubricant but absorbs water.

Dilution

The BP directs that creams and ointments should **not** normally be diluted but that should dilution be necessary care should be taken, in particular, to prevent microbial contamination. The appropriate diluent should be used and heating should be avoided during mixing; excessive dilution may affect the stability of some creams. Diluted creams should normally be used within 2 weeks of preparation.

Suitable quantities for prescribing

Suitable quantities of dermatological preparations to be prescribed for specific areas of the body		
Area of body	Creams and Ointments	Lotions
Face	15-30 g	100 ml
Both hands	25-50 g	200 ml
Scalp	50-100 g	200 ml
Both arms or both legs	100-200 g	200 ml
Trunk	400 g	500 ml
Groins and genitalia	15-25 g	100 ml

These amounts are usually suitable for children 12-18 years for twice daily application for 1 week; smaller quantities will be required for children under 12 years. These recommendations do **not** apply to corticosteroid preparations.

Excipients and sensitisation

Excipients in topical products rarely cause problems. If a patch test indicates allergy to an excipient, products containing the substance should be avoided (see also Anaphylaxis). The following excipients in topical preparations are associated, rarely, with sensitisation; the presence of these excipients is indicated in the entries for topical products. See also Excipients, under General Guidance.

- Beeswax
- Benzyl alcohol
- Butylated hydroxyanisole
- Butylated hydroxytoluene
- Cetostearyl alcohol (including cetyl and stearyl alcohol)
- Chlorocresol
- Edetic acid (EDTA)
- Ethylenediamine
- Fragrances
- Hydroxybenzoates (parabens)
- Imidurea
- Isopropyl palmitate
- N-(3-Chloroallyl)hexaminium chloride (quaternium 15)
- Polysorbates
- Propylene glycol
- Sodium metabisulfite
- Sorbic acid
- Wool fat and related substances including lanolin (purified versions of wool fat have reduced the problem)

Neonates

Caution is required when prescribing topical preparations for neonates—their large body surface area in relation to body mass increases susceptibility to toxicity from systemic absorption of substances applied to the skin. Topical preparations containing potentially sensitising substances such as corticosteroids, aminoglycosides, iodine, and parasiticidal drugs should be avoided. Preparations containing alcohol should be avoided because they can dehydrate the skin, cause pain if applied to raw areas, and the alcohol can cause necrosis. In *preterm neonates*, the skin is more fragile and offers a poor barrier, especially in the first fortnight after birth. Preterm infants, especially if below 32 weeks corrected gestational age, may also require special measures to maintain skin hydration.

1 Dry and scaling skin disorders

Emollient and barrier preparations

Borderline substances

The preparations marked 'ACBS' are regarded as drugs when prescribed in accordance with the advice of the Advisory Committee on Borderline Substances for the clinical conditions listed. Prescriptions issued in accordance with this advice and endorsed 'ACBS' will normally not be investigated.

Emollients

Emollients hydrate the skin, soften the skin, act as barrier to water and external irritants, and are indicated for all dry or scaling disorders. Their effects are short-lived and they should be applied frequently even after improvement occurs. They are useful in dry and eczematous disorders, and to a lesser extent in psoriasis; they should be applied immediately after washing or bathing to maximise the effect of skin hydration. The choice of an appropriate emollient will depend on the severity of the condition, the child's (or

carer's) preference, and the site of application. Ointments may exacerbate acne and folliculitis. Some ingredients rarely cause sensitisation and this should be suspected if an eczematous reaction occurs. The use of aqueous cream as a leave-on emollient may increase the risk of skin reactions, particularly in eczema.

Preparations such as **aqueous cream** and **emulsifying ointment** can be used as soap substitutes for handwashing and in the bath; the preparation is rubbed on the skin before rinsing off completely. The addition of a bath oil may also be helpful.

Urea is occasionally used with other topical agents such as corticosteroids to enhance penetration of the skin.

Emollient bath and shower preparations

In dry skin conditions soap should be avoided.

The quantities of bath additives recommended for older children are suitable for an adult-size bath. Proportionately less should be used for a child-size bath or a washbasin; recommended bath additive quantities for younger children reflect this.

MHRA/CHM update (April 2016): Fire risk with paraffin-based skin emollients on dressings and clothing

When patients are being treated with a paraffin-based emollient product that is covered by a dressing or clothing, there is a danger that smoking or using a naked flame could cause dressings or clothing to catch fire.

Patients should be advised not to smoke, use naked flames (or be near people who are smoking or using naked flames), or go near anything that may cause a fire while emollients are in contact with their medical dressings or clothing. Patients' clothing and bedding should be changed regularly—preferably daily—because emollients soak into fabric and can become a fire hazard.

Barrier preparations

Barrier preparations often contain water-repellent substances such as dimeticone p. 698, natural oils, and paraffins, to help protect the skin from abrasion and irritation; they are used to protect intact skin around stomas and pressure sores, and as a barrier against nappy rash. In neonates, barrier preparations which do not contain potentially sensitising excipients are preferred. Where the skin has broken down, barrier preparations have a limited role in protecting adjacent skin. Barrier preparations with zinc oxide or titanium salts are used to aid healing of uninfected, excoriated skin.

Nappy rash (Dermatitis)

The first line of treatment is to ensure that nappies are changed frequently and that tightly fitting water-proof pants are avoided. The rash may clear when left exposed to the air and a barrier preparation, applied with each nappy change, can be helpful. A mild corticosteroid such as hydrocortisone 0.5% or 1% p. 709 can be used if inflammation is causing discomfort, but it should be avoided in neonates. The barrier preparation should be applied after the corticosteroid preparation to prevent further damage. Preparations containing hydrocortisone should be applied for no more than a week; the hydrocortisone should be discontinued as soon as the inflammation subsides. The occlusive effect of nappies and waterproof pants may increase absorption of corticosteroids (see cautions). If the rash is associated with candidal infection, a topical antifungal such as clotrimazole cream p. 694 can be used. Topical antibacterial preparations can be used if bacterial infection is present; treatment with an oral antibacterial may occasionally be required in severe or recurrent infection. Hydrocortisone may be used in combination with antimicrobial preparations if there is considerable inflammation, erosion, and infection.

13

Skin

Emollients

In the *neonate*, a preservative-free paraffin-based emollient hydrates the skin without affecting the normal skin flora; substances such as olive oil are also used. The development of blisters (epidermolysis bullosa) or ichthyosis may be alleviated by applying liquid and white soft paraffin ointment while awaiting dermatological investigation.

DERMATOLOGICAL DRUGS > BARRIER PREPARATIONS

Barrier creams and ointments

- **INDICATIONS AND DOSE**

For use as a barrier preparation
- ▸ TO THE SKIN
- ▸ Child: (consult product literature)

- **MEDICINAL FORMS**
There can be variation in the licensing of different medicines containing the same drug.

Ointment
EXCIPIENTS: May contain Wool fat and related substances including lanolin
- ▸ Barrier creams and ointments (Non-proprietary)
Cetostearyl alcohol 20 mg per 1 gram, Zinc oxide 75 mg per 1 gram, Beeswax white 100 mg per 1 gram, Arachis oil 305 mg per 1 gram, Castor oil 500 mg per 1 gram Zinc and Castor oil ointment | 100 gram GSL £1.45 | 500 gram GSL £4.99–£5.37 DT price = £5.37
Zinc and Castor oil cream | 100 gram GSL £1.45
- ▸ Brands may include Metanium

Spray
CAUTIONARY AND ADVISORY LABELS 15
EXCIPIENTS: May contain Cetostearyl alcohol (including cetyl and stearyl alcohol), hydroxybenzoates (parabens), wool fat and related substances including lanolin
- ▸ Sprilon (J M Loveridge Ltd)
Dimeticone 10.4 mg per 1 gram, Zinc oxide 125 mg per 1 gram Sprilon aerosol spray | 115 gram GSL £8.90 DT price = £8.90

Cream
EXCIPIENTS: May contain Beeswax, butylated hydroxyanisole, butylated hydroxytoluene, cetostearyl alcohol (including cetyl and stearyl alcohol), chlorocresol, fragrances, hydroxybenzoates (parabens), propylene glycol, wool fat and related substances including lanolin
- ▸ Conotrane (LEO Pharma)
Benzalkonium chloride 1 mg per 1 gram, Dimeticone 220 mg per 1 gram Conotrane cream | 100 gram GSL £0.88 DT price = £0.88 | 500 gram GSL £3.51
- ▸ Drapolene (Omega Pharma Ltd)
Benzalkonium chloride 100 microgram per 1 gram, Cetrimide 2 mg per 1 gram Drapolene cream | 100 gram GSL £1.76 | 200 gram GSL £2.86 | 350 gram GSL £4.28
- ▸ Siopel (Derma UK Ltd)
Cetrimide 3 mg per 1 gram, Dimeticone 1000 100 mg per 1 gram Siopel cream | 50 gram GSL £4.65
- ▸ Sudocrem (Teva UK Ltd)
Benzyl cinnamate 1.5 mg per 1 gram, Benzyl alcohol 3.9 mg per 1 gram, Benzyl benzoate 10.1 mg per 1 gram, Wool fat hydrous 40 mg per 1 gram, Zinc oxide 152.5 mg per 1 gram Sudocrem antiseptic healing cream | 60 gram GSL £1.45 | 125 gram GSL £2.15 | 250 gram GSL £3.67 | 400 gram GSL £5.25

DERMATOLOGICAL DRUGS > EMOLLIENTS

Emollient bath and shower products, antimicrobial-containing

31-Aug-2016

- **INDICATIONS AND DOSE**

DERMOL® 200 SHOWER EMOLLIENT
Dry and pruritic skin conditions including eczema and dermatitis
- ▸ TO THE SKIN
- ▸ Child: To be applied to the skin or used as a soap substitute

DERMOL® 600® BATH EMOLLIENT
Dry and pruritic skin conditions including eczema and dermatitis
- ▸ TO THE SKIN
- ▸ Child 1-23 months: 5–15 mL/bath, not to be used undiluted
- ▸ Child 2-17 years: 15–30 mL/bath, not to be used undiluted

DERMOL® WASH EMULSION
Dry and pruritic skin conditions including eczema and dermatitis
- ▸ TO THE SKIN
- ▸ Child: To be applied to the skin or used as a soap substitute

EMULSIDERM®
Dry skin conditions including eczema and ichthyosis
- ▸ TO THE SKIN
- ▸ Child 1-23 months: 5–10 mL/bath, alternatively, to be rubbed into dry skin until absorbed
- ▸ Child 2-17 years: 7–30 mL/bath, alternatively, to be rubbed into dry skin until absorbed

OILATUM® PLUS
Topical treatment of eczema, including eczema at risk from infection
- ▸ TO THE SKIN
- ▸ Child 6-11 months: 1 mL/bath, not to be used undiluted
- ▸ Child 1-17 years: 1–2 capfuls/bath, not to be used undiluted

---

IMPORTANT SAFETY INFORMATION
These preparations make skin and surfaces slippery—particular care is needed when bathing.

MHRA/CHM UPDATE (APRIL 2016): FIRE RISK WITH PARAFFIN-BASED SKIN EMOLLIENTS ON DRESSINGS OR CLOTHING
See Emollient and barrier preparations p. 683.

- **DIRECTIONS FOR ADMINISTRATION** Emollient bath additives should be added to bath water; hydration can be improved by soaking in the bath for 10–20 minutes. Some bath emollients can be applied to wet skin undiluted and rinsed off. Emollient preparations contained in tubs should be removed with a clean spoon or spatula to reduce bacterial contamination of the emollient. Emollients should be applied in the direction of hair growth to reduce the risk of folliculitis.

- **PRESCRIBING AND DISPENSING INFORMATION**
Preparations containing an antibacterial should be avoided unless infection is present or is a frequent complication.

- **MEDICINAL FORMS**
There can be variation in the licensing of different medicines containing the same drug.
Bath additive
CAUTIONARY AND ADVISORY LABELS 15
EXCIPIENTS: May contain Acetylated lanolin alcohols, isopropyl palmitate, polysorbates

13

Skin

▸ Dermol 600 (Dermal Laboratories Ltd)
Benzalkonium chloride 5 mg per 1 gram, Isopropyl myristate 250 mg per 1 gram, Liquid paraffin 250 mg per 1 gram Dermol 600 bath emollient | 600 ml P £7.55

▸ Emulsiderm (Dermal Laboratories Ltd)
Benzalkonium chloride 5 mg per 1 gram, Isopropyl myristate 250 mg per 1 gram, Liquid paraffin 250 mg per 1 gram Emulsiderm emollient | 300 ml P £3.85 | 1000 ml P £12.00

▸ Oilatum Plus (GlaxoSmithKline Consumer Healthcare)
Triclosan 20 mg per 1 gram, Benzalkonium chloride 60 mg per 1 gram, Liquid paraffin light 525 mg per 1 gram Oilatum Plus bath additive | 500 ml GSL £7.22

Liquid

CAUTIONARY AND ADVISORY LABELS 15
EXCIPIENTS: May contain Cetostearyl alcohol (including cetyl and stearyl alcohol)

▸ Dermol 200 (Dermal Laboratories Ltd)
Benzalkonium chloride 1 mg per 1 gram, Chlorhexidine hydrochloride 1 mg per 1 gram, Isopropyl myristate 25 mg per 1 gram, Liquid paraffin 25 mg per 1 gram Dermol 200 shower emollient | 200 ml P £3.55

▸ Dermol Wash (Dermal Laboratories Ltd)
Benzalkonium chloride 1 mg per 1 gram, Chlorhexidine hydrochloride 1 mg per 1 gram, Isopropyl myristate 25 mg per 1 gram, Liquid paraffin 25 mg per 1 gram Dermol Wash cutaneous emulsion | 200 ml P £3.55

Emollient bath and shower products, colloidal oatmeal-containing

● **INDICATIONS AND DOSE**

Endogenous and exogenous eczema | Xeroderma | Ichthyosis
▸ TO THE SKIN
▸ Child 2–17 years: 20–30 mL/bath, alternatively apply to wet skin and rinse

> **IMPORTANT SAFETY INFORMATION**
> These preparations make skin and surfaces slippery—particular care is needed when bathing.

● **DIRECTIONS FOR ADMINISTRATION** Emollient bath additives should be added to bath water; hydration can be improved by soaking in the bath for 10–20 minutes. Some bath emollients can be applied to wet skin undiluted and rinsed off. Emollient preparations contained in tubs should be removed with a clean spoon or spatula to reduce bacterial contamination of the emollient. Emollients should be applied in the direction of hair growth to reduce the risk of folliculitis.

● **MEDICINAL FORMS**
There can be variation in the licensing of different medicines containing the same drug.
No licensed medicines listed.

Emollient bath and shower products, paraffin-containing

15-Aug-2016

● **INDICATIONS AND DOSE**

AQUAMAX® WASH
Dry skin conditions
▸ TO THE SKIN
▸ Child: To be applied to wet or dry skin and rinse

CETRABEN® BATH
Dry skin conditions, including eczema
▸ TO THE SKIN
▸ Neonate: 0.5 capful/bath, alternatively, to be applied to wet skin and rinse.

▸ Child 1 month–11 years: 0.5–1 capful/bath, alternatively, to be applied to wet skin and rinse
▸ Child 12–17 years: 1–2 capfuls/bath, alternatively, to be applied to wet skin and rinse

DERMALO®
Dermatitis | Dry skin conditions, including ichthyosis
▸ TO THE SKIN
▸ Neonate: 5 mL/bath, alternatively, to be applied to wet skin and rinse.

▸ Child 1 month–11 years: 5–10 mL/bath, alternatively, to be applied to wet skin and rinse
▸ Child 12–17 years: 15–20 mL/bath, alternatively, to be applied to wet skin and rinse

DOUBLEBASE® EMOLLIENT BATH ADDITIVE
Dry skin conditions including dermatitis and ichthyosis
▸ TO THE SKIN
▸ Neonate: 5–10 mL/bath.

▸ Child 1 month–11 years: 5–10 mL/bath
▸ Child 12–17 years: 15–20 mL/bath

DOUBLEBASE® EMOLLIENT SHOWER GEL
Dry, chapped, or itchy skin conditions
▸ TO THE SKIN
▸ Child: To be applied to wet or dry skin and rinse, or apply to dry skin after showering

E45® BATH OIL
Endogenous and exogenous eczema, xeroderma, and ichthyosis
▸ TO THE SKIN
▸ Neonate: 5 mL/bath, alternatively, to be applied to wet skin and rinse.

▸ Child 1 month–11 years: 5–10 mL/bath, alternatively, to be applied to wet skin and rinse
▸ Child 12–17 years: 15 mL/bath, alternatively, to be applied to wet skin and rinse

E45® WASH CREAM
Endogenous and exogenous eczema, xeroderma, and ichthyosis
▸ TO THE SKIN
▸ Child: To be used as a soap substitute

HYDROMOL® BATH AND SHOWER EMOLLIENT
Dry skin conditions | Eczema | Ichthyosis
▸ TO THE SKIN
▸ Neonate: 0.5 capful/bath, alternatively apply to wet skin and rinse.

▸ Child 1 month–11 years: 0.5–2 capfuls/bath, alternatively apply to wet skin and rinse
▸ Child 12–17 years: 1–3 capfuls/bath, alternatively apply to wet skin and rinse

LPL 63.4®
Dry skin conditions
▸ TO THE SKIN
▸ Neonate: 0.5 capful/bath, alternatively, to be applied to wet skin and rinse.

▸ Child 1 month–11 years: 0.5–2 capfuls/bath, alternatively, to be applied to wet skin and rinse
▸ Child 12–17 years: 1–3 capfuls/bath, alternatively, to be applied to wet skin and rinse continued →

13

Skin

OILATUM® EMOLLIENT BATH ADDITIVE

Dry skin conditions including dermatitis and ichthyosis
▸ TO THE SKIN

▸ **Neonate:** 0.5 capful/bath, alternatively, to be applied to wet skin and rinse.

▸ **Child 1 month-11 years:** Apply 0.5-2 capfuls/bath, alternatively, to be applied to wet skin and rinse
▸ **Child 12-17 years:** 1-3 capfuls/bath, alternatively, to be applied to wet skin and rinse

OILATUM® JUNIOR BATH ADDITIVE

Dry skin conditions including dermatitis and ichthyosis
▸ TO THE SKIN

▸ **Neonate:** 0.5 capful/bath, alternatively, apply to wet skin and rinse.

▸ **Child 1 month-11 years:** 0.5-2 capfuls/bath, alternatively, apply to wet skin and rinse
▸ **Child 12-17 years:** 1-3 capfuls/bath, alternatively, apply to wet skin and rinse

QV® BATH OIL

Dry skin conditions including eczema, psoriasis, ichthyosis, and pruritus
▸ TO THE SKIN

▸ **Neonate:** 5 mL/bath, alternatively, to be applied to wet skin and rinse.

▸ **Child 1-11 months:** 5 mL/bath, alternatively, to be applied to wet skin and rinse
▸ **Child 1-17 years:** 10 mL/bath, alternatively, to be applied to wet skin and rinse

QV® GENTLE WASH

Dry skin conditions including eczema, psoriasis, ichthyosis, and pruritus
▸ TO THE SKIN
▸ **Child:** To be used as a soap substitute

ZEROLATUM®

Dry skin conditions | Dermatitis | Ichthyosis
▸ TO THE SKIN

▸ **Child 1 month-11 years:** 5-10 mL/bath
▸ **Child 12-17 years:** 15-20 mL/bath

IMPORTANT SAFETY INFORMATION
These preparations make the skin and surfaces slippery—particular care is needed when bathing.

MHRA/CHM UPDATE (APRIL 2016): FIRE RISK WITH PARAFFIN-BASED SKIN EMOLLIENTS ON DRESSINGS OR CLOTHING
See Emollient and barrier preparations p. 683.

● **DIRECTIONS FOR ADMINISTRATION** Emollient bath additives should be added to bath water; hydration can be improved by soaking in the bath for 10-20 minutes. Some bath emollients can be applied to wet skin undiluted and rinsed off. Emollient preparations contained in tubs should be removed with a clean spoon or spatula to reduce bacterial contamination of the emollient. Emollients should be applied in the direction of hair growth to reduce the risk of folliculitis.

● **MEDICINAL FORMS**
There can be variation in the licensing of different medicines containing the same drug.
Bath additive
CAUTIONARY AND ADVISORY LABELS 15
EXCIPIENTS: May contain Acetylated lanolin alcohols, cetostearyl alcohol (including cetyl and stearyl alcohol), fragrances, isopropyl palmitate
▸ **Cetraben** (Genus Pharmaceuticals Ltd)
Liquid paraffin light 828 mg per 1 gram Cetraben emollient 82.8% bath additive | 500 ml GSL £5.75

▸ **Dermalo** (Dermal Laboratories Ltd)
Acetylated wool alcohols 50 mg per 1 gram, Liquid paraffin 650 mg per 1 gram Dermalo bath emollient | 500 ml GSL £3.44
▸ **Doublebase emollient bath** (Dermal Laboratories Ltd)
Liquid paraffin 650 mg per 1 gram Doublebase emollient bath additive | 500 ml GSL £5.45
▸ **E45 emollient bath** (Forum Health Products Ltd)
E45 emollient bath oil | 250 ml(ACBS) £3.30 | 500 ml(ACBS) £5.29
▸ **Hydromol** (Alliance Pharmaceuticals Ltd)
Isopropyl myristate 130 mg per 1 ml, Liquid paraffin light 378 mg per 1 ml Hydromol Bath & Shower emollient | 350 ml GSL £3.88 | 500 ml GSL £4.42 | 1000 ml GSL £8.80
▸ **LPL** (Huxley Europe Ltd)
Liquid paraffin light 634 mg per 1 ml LPL 63.4 bath additive and emollient | 500 ml £3.10 DT price = £4.57
▸ **Oilatum** (GlaxoSmithKline Consumer Healthcare)
Liquid paraffin light 634 mg per 1 ml Oilatum Bath Formula | 150 ml GSL £2.95 DT price = £2.84 | 300 ml GSL £5.02 DT price = £4.88
Oilatum Emollient | 250 ml GSL £2.75 DT price = £2.75 | 500 ml GSL £5.27 DT price = £4.57
▸ **Oilatum junior** (GlaxoSmithKline Consumer Healthcare)
Liquid paraffin light 634 mg per 1 ml Oilatum Junior bath additive | 150 ml GSL £2.95 DT price = £2.84 | 250 ml GSL £4.44 DT price = £2.75 | 300 ml GSL £5.02 DT price = £4.88 | 600 ml GSL £6.67 DT price = £5.89
▸ **QV** (Crawford Healthcare Ltd)
Liquid paraffin light 850.9 mg per 1 gram QV 85.09% bath oil | 250 ml £2.91 | 500 ml £4.76
▸ **Zerolatum** (Thornton & Ross Ltd)
Acetylated wool alcohols 50 mg per 1 gram, Liquid paraffin 650 mg per 1 gram Zerolatum Emollient bath additive | 500 ml £4.79

Gel
CAUTIONARY AND ADVISORY LABELS 15
EXCIPIENTS: May contain Cetostearyl alcohol (including cetyl and stearyl alcohol)
▸ **Doublebase** (Dermal Laboratories Ltd)
Isopropyl myristate 150 mg per 1 gram, Liquid paraffin 150 mg per 1 gram Doublebase emollient shower gel | 200 gram P £5.21

Wash
CAUTIONARY AND ADVISORY LABELS 15
EXCIPIENTS: May contain Cetostearyl alcohol (including cetyl and stearyl alcohol), polysorbates
▸ **Aquamax** (Intrapharm Laboratories Ltd)
Aquamax wash | 250 gram £2.99
▸ **E45 emollient wash** (Forum Health Products Ltd)
E45 emollient wash cream | 250 ml(ACBS) £3.30
▸ **QV Gentle** (Crawford Healthcare Ltd)
QV Gentle wash | 250 ml £3.17 | 500 ml £5.29

Emollient bath and shower products, soya-bean oil-containing

● **INDICATIONS AND DOSE**

BALNEUM® BATH OIL

Dry skin conditions including those associated with dermatitis and eczema
▸ TO THE SKIN

▸ **Neonate:** 5-15 mL/bath, not to be used undiluted.

▸ **Child 1-23 months:** 5-15 mL/bath, not to be used undiluted
▸ **Child 2-17 years:** 20-60 mL/bath, not to be used undiluted

BALNEUM® PLUS BATH OIL

Dry skin conditions including those associated with dermatitis and eczema where pruritus also experienced
▸ TO THE SKIN

▸ **Neonate:** 5 mL/bath, alternatively, to be applied to wet skin and rinse.

▸ **Child 1-23 months:** 5 mL/bath, alternatively, to be applied to wet skin and rinse

▸ Child 2–17 years: 10–20 mL/bath, alternatively, to be applied to wet skin and rinse

ZERONEUM®

Dry skin conditions including eczema

▸ TO THE SKIN

▸ Child 1 month–11 years: 5 mL/bath

▸ Child 12–17 years: 20 mL/bath

IMPORTANT SAFETY INFORMATION

These preparations make skin and surfaces slippery—particular care is needed when bathing.

● **DIRECTIONS FOR ADMINISTRATION** Emollient bath additives should be added to bath water; hydration can be improved by soaking in the bath for 10–20 minutes. Some bath emollients can be applied to wet skin undiluted and rinsed off. Emollient preparations contained in tubs should be removed with a clean spoon or spatula to reduce bacterial contamination of the emollient. Emollients should be applied in the direction of hair growth to reduce the risk of folliculitis.

● **MEDICINAL FORMS**

There can be variation in the licensing of different medicines containing the same drug.

Bath additive

EXCIPIENTS: May contain Butylated hydroxytoluene, fragrances, propylene glycol

▸ **Balneum** (Almirall Ltd)

Lauromacrogols 150 mg per 1 gram, Soya oil 829.5 mg per 1 gram Balneum Plus bath oil | 500 ml [GSL] £6.66

Soya oil 847.5 mg per 1 gram Balneum 84.75% bath oil | 200 ml [GSL] £2.48 | 500 ml [GSL] £5.38 | 1000 ml [GSL] £10.39

▸ **Zeroneum** (Thornton & Ross Ltd)

Soya oil 833.5 mg per 1 gram Zeroneum 83.35% bath additive | 500 ml £4.48

Emollient bath and shower products, tar-containing

17-Aug-2016

● **INDICATIONS AND DOSE**

POLYTAR EMOLLIENT®

Psoriasis, eczema, atopic and pruritic dermatoses

▸ TO THE SKIN

▸ Child: 2–4 capfuls/bath, add 15–30 mL to an adult-size bath and proportionally less for a child's bath; soak for 20 minutes

PSORIDERM® EMULSION

Psoriasis

▸ TO THE SKIN

▸ Child: Up to 30 mL/bath, use 30mL in adult-size bath, and proportionally less for a child's bath, soak for 5 minutes

---

IMPORTANT SAFETY INFORMATION

These preparations make skin and surfaces slippery—particular care is needed when bathing.

● **DIRECTIONS FOR ADMINISTRATION** Emollient bath additives should be added to bath water; hydration can be improved by soaking in the bath for 10–20 minutes. Some bath emollients can be applied to wet skin undiluted and rinsed off. Emollient preparations contained in tubs should be removed with a clean spoon or spatula to reduce bacterial contamination of the emollient. Emollients should be applied in the direction of hair growth to reduce the risk of folliculitis.

● **MEDICINAL FORMS**

There can be variation in the licensing of different medicines containing the same drug.

Bath additive

EXCIPIENTS: May contain Isopropyl palmitate, polysorbates

▸ **Psoriderm** (Dermal Laboratories Ltd)

Coal tar distilled 400 mg per 1 ml Psoriderm Emulsion 40% bath additive | 200 ml [P] £2.74

Emollient creams and ointments, antimicrobial-containing

17-Aug-2016

● **INDICATIONS AND DOSE**

Dry and pruritic skin conditions including eczema and dermatitis

▸ TO THE SKIN

▸ Child: To be applied to the skin or used as a soap substitute

---

IMPORTANT SAFETY INFORMATION

These preparations make skin and surfaces slippery—particular care is needed when bathing.

MHRA/CHM UPDATE (APRIL 2016): FIRE RISK WITH PARAFFIN-BASED SKIN EMOLLIENTS ON DRESSINGS OR CLOTHING

See Emollient and barrier preparations p. 683.

● **DIRECTIONS FOR ADMINISTRATION** Emollients should be applied immediately after washing or bathing to maximise the effect of skin hydration. Emollient preparations contained in tubs should be removed with a clean spoon or spatula to reduce bacterial contamination of the emollient. Emollients should be applied in the direction of hair growth to reduce the risk of folliculitis.

● **PRESCRIBING AND DISPENSING INFORMATION** Preparations containing an antibacterial should be avoided unless infection is present or is a frequent complication.

● **MEDICINAL FORMS**

There can be variation in the licensing of different medicines containing the same drug.

Cream

CAUTIONARY AND ADVISORY LABELS 15

EXCIPIENTS: May contain Cetostearyl alcohol (including cetyl and stearyl alcohol)

▸ **Dermol** (Dermal Laboratories Ltd)

Benzalkonium chloride 1 mg per 1 gram, Chlorhexidine hydrochloride 1 mg per 1 gram, Isopropyl myristate 100 mg per 1 gram, Liquid paraffin 100 mg per 1 gram Dermol cream | 100 gram [P] £2.86 | 500 gram [P] £6.63

▸ **Eczmol** (Genus Pharmaceuticals Ltd)

Chlorhexidine gluconate 10 mg per 1 gram Eczmol 1% cream | 250 ml [GSL] £3.70

▸ **Hibitane** (Derma UK Ltd)

Chlorhexidine gluconate 10 mg per 1 gram Hibitane Obstetric 1% cream | 250 ml [GSL] £16.95

Liquid

CAUTIONARY AND ADVISORY LABELS 15

EXCIPIENTS: May contain Cetostearyl alcohol (including cetyl and stearyl alcohol)

▸ **Dermol 500** (Dermal Laboratories Ltd)

Benzalkonium chloride 1 mg per 1 gram, Chlorhexidine hydrochloride 1 mg per 1 gram, Isopropyl myristate 25 mg per 1 gram, Liquid paraffin 25 mg per 1 gram Dermol 500 lotion | 500 ml [P] £6.04

13

Skin

13

Skin

Emollient creams and ointments, colloidal oatmeal-containing

● INDICATIONS AND DOSE

Endogenous and exogenous eczema | Xeroderma | Ichthyosis

▸ TO THE SKIN
▸ Child: (consult product literature)

● DIRECTIONS FOR ADMINISTRATION Emollients should be applied immediately after washing or bathing to maximise the effect of skin hydration. Emollient preparations contained in tubs should be removed with a clean spoon or spatula to reduce bacterial contamination of the emollient. Emollients should be applied in the direction of hair growth to reduce the risk of folliculitis.

● MEDICINAL FORMS
There can be variation in the licensing of different medicines containing the same drug.

Cream/Lotion
EXCIPIENTS: May contain Benzyl alcohol, cetostearyl alcohol (including cetyl and stearyl alcohol), isopropyl palmitate
▸ Aveeno (Johnson & Johnson Ltd)
Aveeno lotion | 500 ml(ACBS) £6.66
Aveeno cream | 100 ml(ACBS) £3.97 | 300 ml(ACBS) £6.80 | 500 ml (ACBS) £7.19

Emollient creams and ointments, paraffin-containing

31-Aug-2016

● INDICATIONS AND DOSE

Dry skin conditions | Eczema | Psoriasis | Ichthyosis | Pruritus

▸ TO THE SKIN
▸ Child: (consult product literature)

IMPORTANT SAFETY INFORMATION
MHRA/CHM UPDATE (APRIL 2016): FIRE RISK WITH PARAFFIN-BASED SKIN EMOLLIENTS ON DRESSINGS OR CLOTHING
See Emollient and barrier preparations p. 683.

● DIRECTIONS FOR ADMINISTRATION Emollients should be applied immediately after washing or bathing to maximise the effect of skin hydration. Emollient preparations contained in tubs should be removed with a clean spoon or spatula to reduce bacterial contamination of the emollient. Emollients should be applied in the direction of hair growth to reduce the risk of folliculitis.

● MEDICINAL FORMS
There can be variation in the licensing of different medicines containing the same drug.

Spray
CAUTIONARY AND ADVISORY LABELS 15
▸ Dermamist (Alliance Pharmaceuticals Ltd)
White soft paraffin 100 mg per 1 gram Dermamist 10% spray | 250 ml [P] £5.97
▸ Emollin (C D Medical Ltd)
Emollin aerosol spray | 150 ml £4.00 | 240 ml £6.39

Cream
CAUTIONARY AND ADVISORY LABELS 15
EXCIPIENTS: May contain Benzyl alcohol, cetostearyl alcohol (including cetyl and stearyl alcohol), chlorocresol, disodium edetate, fragrances, hydroxybenzoates (parabens), polysorbates, propylene glycol, sorbic acid, lanolin
▸ Aquamax (Intrapharm Laboratories Ltd)
Aquamax cream | 100 gram £1.89 | 500 gram £3.99
▸ Aquamol (Thornton & Ross Ltd)
Aquamol cream | 50 gram £1.22 | 500 gram £6.40

▸ Cetraben (Thornton & Ross Ltd)
Liquid paraffin light 105 mg per 1 gram, White soft paraffin 132 mg per 1 gram Cetraben cream | 50 gram £1.40 | 150 gram £3.98 | 500 gram £5.99 | 1050 gram £11.62
▸ Diprobase (Bayer Plc)
Diprobase cream | 50 gram [GSL] £1.28 | 500 gram [GSL] £6.32
▸ E45 (Forum Health Products Ltd)
Wool fat 10 mg per 1 gram, Liquid paraffin light 126 mg per 1 gram, White soft paraffin 145 mg per 1 gram E45 cream | 50 gram [GSL] £1.61 | 125 gram [GSL] £2.90 | 350 gram [GSL] £5.49 | 500 gram [GSL] £5.99
▸ Enopen (Ennogen Healthcare Ltd)
Liquid paraffin light 105 mg per 1 gram, White soft paraffin 132 mg per 1 gram Enopen cream | 50 gram £1.40 | 150 gram £3.98 | 500 gram £5.99 | 1050 gram £11.62
▸ Epaderm (Molnlycke Health Care Ltd)
Epaderm cream | 50 gram £1.70 | 500 gram £6.95
▸ Hydromol (Alliance Pharmaceuticals Ltd)
Sodium lactate 10 mg per 1 gram, Sodium pidolate 25 mg per 1 gram, Isopropyl myristate 50 mg per 1 gram, Liquid paraffin 100 mg per 1 gram Hydromol 2.5% cream | 50 gram £2.19 | 100 gram £4.09 | 500 gram £11.92
▸ Lipobase (LEO Pharma)
Lipobase cream | 50 gram [P] £1.46
▸ Oilatum (GlaxoSmithKline Consumer Healthcare)
Liquid paraffin light 60 mg per 1 gram, White soft paraffin 150 mg per 1 gram Oilatum cream | 50 gram [GSL] £1.67 DT price = £1.67 | 150 gram [GSL] £3.06 DT price = £3.06 | 500 ml [GSL] £5.28 DT price = £5.28 | 1050 ml [GSL] £9.98 DT price = £9.98
▸ Oilatum junior (GlaxoSmithKline Consumer Healthcare)
Liquid paraffin light 60 mg per 1 gram, White soft paraffin 150 mg per 1 gram Oilatum Junior cream | 150 gram [GSL] £3.06 DT price = £3.06 | 350 ml [GSL] £4.65 DT price = £4.65 | 500 ml [GSL] £5.28 DT price = £5.28
▸ QV (Crawford Healthcare Ltd)
White soft paraffin 50 mg per 1 gram, Glycerol 100 mg per 1 gram, Liquid paraffin light 100 mg per 1 gram QV cream | 100 gram £2.06 | 500 gram £5.92 | 1050 gram £12.05
▸ Soffen (Vitame Ltd)
Liquid paraffin light 105 mg per 1 gram, White soft paraffin 132 mg per 1 gram Soffen cream | 500 gram £4.79
▸ Unguentum M (Almirall Ltd)
Unguentum M cream | 50 gram [GSL] £1.41 | 60 gram [GSL] no price available | 100 gram [GSL] £2.78 | 200 ml [GSL] £5.50 | 500 gram [GSL] £8.48
▸ ZeroAQS (Thornton & Ross Ltd)
ZeroAQS emollient cream | 500 gram £3.29
▸ Zerobase (Thornton & Ross Ltd)
Liquid paraffin 110 mg per 1 gram Zerobase 11% cream | 50 gram £1.04 | 500 gram £5.26
▸ Zerocream (Thornton & Ross Ltd)
Liquid paraffin 126 mg per 1 gram, White soft paraffin 145 mg per 1 gram Zerocream | 50 gram £1.17 | 500 gram £4.08
▸ Zeroguent (Thornton & Ross Ltd)
White soft paraffin 40 mg per 1 gram, Soya oil 50 mg per 1 gram, Liquid paraffin light 80 mg per 1 gram Zeroguent cream | 100 gram £2.33 | 500 gram £6.99

Ointment
CAUTIONARY AND ADVISORY LABELS 15
EXCIPIENTS: May contain Cetostearyl alcohol (including cetyl and stearyl alcohol), polysorbates
▸ Emollient creams and ointments, paraffin-containing (Non-proprietary)
Liquid paraffin 200 mg per 1 gram, Emulsifying wax 300 mg per 1 gram, White soft paraffin 500 mg per 1 gram Emulsifying ointment | 100 gram [GSL] no price available | 500 gram [PoM] no price available DT price = £2.92 | 500 gram [GSL] £3.43 DT price = £2.92
Liquid paraffin 500 mg per 1 gram, White soft paraffin 500 mg per 1 gram White soft paraffin 50% / Liquid paraffin 50% ointment | 250 gram £1.87 | 500 gram £4.19 DT price = £4.57 | 500 gram [P] £4.57 DT price = £4.57
Magnesium sulfate dried 5 mg per 1 gram, Phenoxyethanol 10 mg per 1 gram, Wool alcohols ointment 500 mg per 1 gram Hydrous ointment | 500 gram [GSL] £4.89 DT price = £4.89
White soft paraffin 1 mg per 1 mg White soft paraffin solid | 500 gram [GSL] £4.33 DT price = £3.23 | 4500 gram [GSL] £19.17-£29.07

Yellow soft paraffin 1 mg per 1 mg   Yellow soft paraffin solid |
15 gram GSL £1.16 | 500 gram GSL £15.44 DT price = £15.44 |
4500 gram GSL £19.02
▸ **Diprobase** (Bayer Plc)
**Liquid paraffin 50 mg per 1 gram, White soft paraffin 950 mg per
1 gram**   Diprobase ointment | 50 gram GSL £1.28 DT price = £1.28
| 500 gram GSL £5.99 DT price = £5.99
▸ **Emelpin** (Vitame Ltd)
**Emulsifying wax 300 mg per 1 gram, Yellow soft paraffin 300 mg
per 1 gram**   Emelpin ointment | 125 gram £3.08 | 500 gram £5.22
▸ **Epaderm** (Molnlycke Health Care Ltd)
**Emulsifying wax 300 mg per 1 gram, Yellow soft paraffin 300 mg
per 1 gram**   Epaderm ointment | 125 gram £3.85 | 500 gram £6.53 |
1000 gram £12.02
▸ **Fifty:50** (Ennogen Healthcare Ltd)
**Liquid paraffin 500 mg per 1 gram, White soft paraffin 500 mg
per 1 gram**   Fifty:50 ointment | 250 gram £1.83 | 500 gram £3.66 DT
price = £4.57
▸ **Hydromol** (Alliance Pharmaceuticals Ltd)
**Emulsifying wax 300 mg per 1 gram, Yellow soft paraffin 300 mg
per 1 gram**   Hydromol ointment | 125 gram £2.88 | 500 gram £4.89
| 1000 gram £9.09
▸ **Thirty:30** (Ennogen Healthcare Ltd)
**Emulsifying wax 300 mg per 1 gram, Yellow soft paraffin 300 mg
per 1 gram**   Thirty:30 ointment | 125 gram £3.81 | 250 gram £4.29 |
500 gram £6.47
▸ **Vaseline** (Unilever UK Home & Personal Care)
White soft paraffin 1 mg per 1 mg   Vaseline Pure Petroleum jelly |
50 ml GSL no price available | 100 ml GSL no price available |
250 ml GSL no price available

Liquid
CAUTIONARY AND ADVISORY LABELS 15
EXCIPIENTS: May contain Benzyl alcohol, cetostearyl alcohol (including
cetyl and stearyl alcohol), hydroxybenzoates (parabens), isopropyl
palmitate
▸ **E45** (Forum Health Products Ltd)
E45 lotion | 200 ml £2.45 | 500 ml £4.59
▸ **QV** (Crawford Healthcare Ltd)
White soft paraffin 50 mg per 1 gram   QV 5% skin lotion | 250 ml
£3.17 | 500 ml £5.29

Emollients, urea-containing

- **DRUG ACTION** Urea is a keratin softener and hydrating
agent used in the treatment of dry, scaling conditions
(including ichthyosis) and may be useful in elderly
patients.

- **INDICATIONS AND DOSE**

AQUADRATE®

Dry, scaling, and itching skin
▸ TO THE SKIN
▸ Child: Apply twice daily, to be applied thinly

BALNEUM® CREAM

Dry skin conditions
▸ TO THE SKIN
▸ Child: Apply twice daily

BALNEUM® PLUS CREAM

Dry, scaling, and itching skin
▸ TO THE SKIN
▸ Child: Apply twice daily

CALMURID®

Dry, scaling, and itching skin
▸ TO THE SKIN
▸ Child: Apply twice daily, apply a thick layer for
3–5 minutes, massage into area, and remove excess.
Can be diluted with aqueous cream (life of diluted
cream is 14 days). Half-strength cream can be used for
1 week if stinging occurs

DERMATONICS ONCE HEEL BALM®

Dry skin on soles of feet
▸ TO THE SKIN
▸ Child 12–17 years: Apply once daily

E45® ITCH RELIEF CREAM

Dry, scaling, and itching skin
▸ TO THE SKIN
▸ Child: Apply twice daily

EUCERIN® INTENSIVE CREAM

**Dry skin conditions including eczema, ichthyosis,
xeroderma, and hyperkeratosis**
▸ TO THE SKIN
▸ Child: Apply twice daily, to be applied thinly and
rubbed into area

EUCERIN® INTENSIVE LOTION

**Dry skin conditions including eczema, ichthyosis,
xeroderma, and hyperkeratosis**
▸ TO THE SKIN
▸ Child: Apply twice daily, to be applied sparingly and
rubbed into area

FLEXITOL®

Dry skin on soles of feet and heels
▸ TO THE SKIN
▸ Child 12–17 years: Apply 1–2 times a day

HYDROMOL® INTENSIVE

Dry, scaling, and itching skin
▸ TO THE SKIN
▸ Child: Apply twice daily, to be applied thinly

IMUDERM® EMOLLIENT

**Dry skin conditions including eczema, psoriasis or
dermatitis**
▸ TO THE SKIN
▸ Child: Apply to skin or use as a soap substitute

NUTRAPLUS®

Dry, scaling, and itching skin
▸ TO THE SKIN
▸ Child: Apply 2–3 times a day

- **DIRECTIONS FOR ADMINISTRATION** Emollients should be
applied immediately after washing or bathing to maximise
the effect of skin hydration. Emollient preparations
contained in tubs should be removed with a clean spoon or
spatula to reduce bacterial contamination of the emollient.
Emollients should be applied in the direction of hair
growth to reduce the risk of folliculitis.

- **MEDICINAL FORMS**
There can be variation in the licensing of different medicines
containing the same drug.
Cream
EXCIPIENTS: May contain Benzyl alcohol, cetostearyl alcohol (including
cetyl and stearyl alcohol), hydroxybenzoates (parabens), isopropyl
palmitate, polysorbates, propylene glycol, wool fat and related
substances including lanolin
▸ **Aquadrate** (Alliance Pharmaceuticals Ltd)
Urea 100 mg per 1 gram   Aquadrate 10% cream | 100 gram P
£4.37
▸ **Balneum** (Almirall Ltd)
Balneum cream | 50 gram £2.85 | 500 gram £9.97
▸ **Balneum Plus** (Almirall Ltd)
**Lauromacrogols 30 mg per 1 gram, Urea 50 mg per
1 gram**   Balneum Plus cream | 100 gram GSL £3.29 |
500 gram GSL £14.99
▸ **Calmurid** (Galderma (UK) Ltd)
Lactic acid 50 mg per 1 gram, Urea 100 mg per 1 gram   Calmurid
cream | 100 gram P £5.75 DT price = £5.75 | 500 gram P £33.40
DT price = £33.40
▸ **E45 Itch Relief** (Forum Health Products Ltd)
Lauromacrogols 30 mg per 1 gram, Urea 50 mg per 1 gram   E45
Itch Relief cream | 50 gram GSL £2.81 | 100 gram GSL £4.28 |
500 gram GSL £14.99

13

Skin

▸ **Eucerin** (Beiersdorf UK Ltd)
Urea 100 mg per 1 gram Eucerin Intensive 10% cream |
100 ml GSL £7.59
▸ **Hydromol Intensive** (Alliance Pharmaceuticals Ltd)
Urea 100 mg per 1 gram Hydromol Intensive 10% cream |
30 gram P £1.64 | 100 gram P £4.37
▸ **Nutraplus** (Galderma (UK) Ltd)
Urea 100 mg per 1 gram Nutraplus 10% cream | 100 gram P
£4.37

Liquid
EXCIPIENTS: May contain Benzyl alcohol, isopropyl palmitate
▸ **Eucerin** (Beiersdorf UK Ltd)
Urea 100 mg per 1 gram Eucerin Intensive 10% lotion |
250 ml GSL £7.93 DT price = £7.93

Balms
EXCIPIENTS: May contain Beeswax, benzyl alcohol, cetostearyl alcohol
(including cetyl and stearyl alcohol), fragrances, lanolin
▸ **Emollients, urea-containing (Non-proprietary)**
imuDERM emollient | 500 gram £6.50
▸ **Dermatonics Once** (Dermatonics Ltd)
Dermatonics Once Heel Balm | 75 ml £3.60 | 200 ml £8.50
▸ **Flexitol** (Thornton & Ross Ltd)
Flexitol Heel Balm | 40 gram £2.75 | 56 gram no price available |
75 gram £3.80 | 112 gram no price available | 200 gram £9.40 |
500 gram £14.75

2   Infections of the skin

Skin infections

Antibacterial preparations

Topical antibacterial preparations are used to treat localised
bacterial skin infections caused by Gram-positive organisms
(particularly by staphylococci or streptococci). Systemic
antibacterial treatment is more appropriate for deep-seated
skin infections.

Problems associated with the use of topical antibacterials
include bacterial resistance, contact sensitisation, and
superinfection. In order to minimise the development of
resistance, antibacterials used systemically (e.g. fusidic acid
p. 342) should not generally be chosen for topical use.
Resistant organisms are more common in hospitals, and
whenever possible swabs should be taken for bacteriological
examination before beginning treatment.

Neomycin sulfate p. 692 applied topically may cause
sensitisation and cross-sensitivity with other
aminoglycoside antibacterials such as gentamicin p. 299 may
occur. Topical antibacterials applied over large areas can
cause systemic toxicity; ototoxicity with neomycin sulfate
and with polymyxins p. 693 is a particular risk for neonates
and children with renal impairment.

Superficial bacterial infection of the skin may be treated
with a topical antiseptic such as povidone-iodine p. 731
which also softens crusts, or hydrogen peroxide 1% cream
p. 733.

Bacterial infections such as *impetigo* and *folliculitis* can be
treated with a short course of topical fusidic acid; mupirocin
p. 694 should be used only to treat meticillin-resistant
Staphylococcus aureus.

For extensive or long-standing impetigo, an oral
antibacterial such as flucloxacillin p. 330 (or clarithromycin
p. 315 in children with penicillin-allergy), should be used. A
mild antiseptic may help to soften crusts. Mild antiseptics
may be useful in reducing the spread of infection, but there
is little evidence to support the use of topical antiseptics
alone in the treatment of impetigo.

Cellulitis, a rapidly spreading deeply seated inflammation
of the skin and subcutaneous tissue, requires systemic
antibacterial treatment. Lower leg infections or infections
spreading around wounds are almost always cellulitis.

Erysipelas, a superficial infection with clearly defined edges

(and often affecting the face), is also treated with a systemic
antibacterial.

Staphylococcal scalded-skin syndrome requires urgent
treatment with a systemic antibacterial, such as
flucloxacillin.

Mupirocin is not related to any other antibacterial in use;
it is effective for skin infections, particularly those due to
Gram-positive organisms but it is not indicated for
pseudomonal infection. Although *Staphylococcus aureus*
strains with low-level resistance to mupirocin are emerging,
it is generally useful in infections resistant to other
antibacterials. To avoid the development of resistance,
mupirocin or fusidic acid should not be used for longer than
10 days and local microbiology advice should be sought
before using it in hospital. In the presence of mupirocin-
resistant MRSA infection, a topical antiseptic, such as
povidone-iodine, chlorhexidine p. 732, or alcohol, can be
used; their use should be discussed with the local
microbiologist.

Mupirocin ointment contains macrogols, extensive
absorption of macrogols through the mucous membranes or
through application to thin or damaged skin may result in
renal toxicity, especially in neonates. Mupirocin nasal
ointment is formulated in a paraffin base and may be more
suitable for the treatment of MRSA-infected open wound in
neonates.

Metronidazole gel p. 692 is used topically in children to
reduce the odour associated with anaerobic infections and
for the treatment of periorificial rosacea; oral metronidazole
is used to treat wounds infected with anaerobic bacteria.

Retapamulin p. 694 can be used for impetigo and other
superficial bacterial skin infections caused by *Staphylococcus
aureus* and *Streptococcus pyogenes* that are resistant to first-
line topical antibacterials. However, it is not effective against
MRSA.

Silver sulfadiazine p. 693 is licensed for the prevention and
treatment of infection in burns but the use of appropriate
dressings may be more effective. Systemic effects may occur
following extensive application of silver sulfadiazine; its use
is not recommended in neonates.

Antibacterial preparations also used systemically

Fusidic acid is a narrow-spectrum antibacterial used for
staphylococcal infections. Fusidic acid has a role in the
treatment of impetigo.

An ointment containing fusidic acid is used in the fissures
of angular cheilitis when associated with staphylococcal
infection. See Oropharyngeal fungal infections p. 679 for
further information on angular cheilitis.

Metronidazole is used topically to treat rosacea and to
reduce the odour associated with anaerobic infections; oral
metronidazole is used to treat wounds infected with
anaerobic bacteria.

Antifungal preparations

Most localised fungal infections are treated with topical
preparations. To prevent relapse, local antifungal treatment
should be continued for 1–2 weeks after the disappearance
of all signs of infection. Systemic therapy is necessary for
scalp infection or if the skin infection is widespread,
disseminated or intractable; although topical therapy may be
used to treat some nail infections, systemic therapy is more
effective. Specimens of scale, nail or hair should be sent for
mycological examination before starting treatment, unless
the diagnosis is certain.

Dermatophytoses

Ringworm infection can affect the scalp (tinea capitis), body
(tinea corporis), groin (tinea cruris), hand (tinea manuum),
foot (tinea pedis, athlete's foot), or nail (tinea unguium,
onychomycosis). Tinea capitis is a common childhood
infection that requires systemic treatment with an oral
antifungal; additional application of a topical antifungal,
during the early stages of treatment, may reduce the risk of

transmission. A topical antifungal can also be used to treat asymptomatic carriers of scalp ringworm.

Tinea corporis and tinea pedis infections in children respond to treatment with a topical **imidazole** (clotrimazole p. 694, econazole nitrate p. 695, or miconazole p. 695) or terbinafine cream p. 696. Nystatin p. 680 is less effective against tinea.

Compound benzoic acid ointment (Whitfield's ointment) has been used for ringworm infections but it is cosmetically less acceptable than proprietary preparations. Antifungal dusting powders are of little therapeutic value in the treatment of fungal skin infections and may cause skin irritation; they may have some role in preventing re-infection.

Antifungal treatment may not be necessary in asymptomatic children with tinea infection of the nails. If treatment is necessary, a systemic antifungal is more effective than topical therapy. However, topical application of tioconazole p. 696 may be useful for treating early onychomycosis when involvement is limited to mild distal disease, or for superficial white onychomycosis, or where there are contra-indications to systemic therapy. Chronic paronychia on the fingers (usually due to a candidal infection) should be treated with topical clotrimazole or nystatin, but these preparations should be used with caution in children who suck their fingers. Chronic paronychia of the toes (usually due to dermatophyte infection) can be treated with topical terbinafine.

Pityriasis versicolor

Pityriasis (tinea) versicolor can be treated with ketoconazole shampoo p. 695 or **selenium sulfide** shampoo. Topical imidazole antifungals such as clotrimazole, econazole nitrate and miconazole or topical terbinafine are alternatives, but large quantities may be required.

If topical therapy fails, or if the infection is widespread, pityriasis versicolor is treated systemically with an azole antifungal. Relapse is common, especially in the immunocompromised.

Candidiasis

Candidal skin infections can be treated with topical imidazole antifungals clotrimazole p. 694, econazole nitrate p. 695, or miconazole p. 695; topical terbinafine p. 696 is an alternative. Topical application of nystatin p. 680 is also effective for candidiasis but it is ineffective against dermatophytosis. Refractory candidiasis requires systemic treatment generally with a triazole such as fluconazole p. 358; systemic treatment with griseofulvin p. 363 or terbinafine is **not appropriate** for refractory candidiasis. See the treatment of oral candiasis and for the management of nappy rash.

Angular cheilitis

Miconazole cream is used in the fissures of angular cheilitis when associated with *Candida*.

Compound topical preparations

Combination of an imidazole and a mild corticosteroid (such as hydrocortisone 1% p. 709) may be of value in the treatment of eczematous intertrigo and, in the first few days only, of a severely inflamed patch of ringworm. Combination of a mild corticosteroid with either an imidazole or nystatin may be of use in the treatment of *intertriginous eczema* associated with candida.

Antiviral preparations

Aciclovir cream p. 699 is used for the treatment of initial and recurrent labial, cutaneous, and genital *herpes simplex infections* in children; treatment should begin as early as possible. Systemic treatment is necessary for buccal or vaginal infections or if cold sores recur frequently.

Herpes labialis

Aciclovir cream can be used for the treatment of initial and recurrent labial herpes simplex infections (cold sores). It is best applied at the earliest possible stage, usually when prodromal changes of sensation are felt in the lip and before vesicles appear.

Penciclovir cream is also licensed for the treatment of herpes labialis; it needs to be applied more frequently than aciclovir cream.

Parasiticidal preparations

Suitable quantities of parasiticidal preparations

Area of body	Skin creams	Lotions	Cream rinses
Scalp (head lice)		50-100 mL	50-100 mL
Body (scabies)	30-60 g	100 mL	
Body (crab lice)	30-60 g	100 mL	

These amounts are usually suitable for a child 12–17 years for single application.

Scabies

Permethrin p. 699 is used for the treatment of *scabies* (*Sarcoptes scabiei*); malathion p. 699 can be used if permethrin is inappropriate.

Benzyl benzoate is an irritant and should be avoided in children; it is less effective than malathion and permethrin.

Ivermectin p. 367 (available from 'special-order' manufacturers or specialist importing companies) by mouth has been used, in combination with topical drugs, for the treatment of hyperkeratotic (crusted or 'Norwegian') scabies that does not respond to topical treatment alone.

Application

Although acaricides have traditionally been applied after a hot bath, this is **not** necessary and there is even evidence that a hot bath may increase absorption into the blood, removing them from their site of action on the skin.

All members of the affected household should be treated simultaneously. Treatment should be applied to the whole body including the scalp, neck, face, and ears. Particular attention should be paid to the webs of the fingers and toes and lotion brushed under the ends of nails. It is now recommended that malathion and permethrin should be applied twice, one week apart; in the case of benzyl benzoate in adults, up to 3 applications on consecutive days may be needed. It is important to warn users to reapply treatment to the hands if they are washed. Patients with hyperkeratotic scabies may require 2 or 3 applications of acaricide on consecutive days to ensure that enough penetrates the skin crusts to kill all the mites.

Itching

The *itch* and *eczema* of scabies persists for some weeks after the infestation has been eliminated and treatment for pruritus and eczema may be required. Application of crotamiton p. 723 can be used to control itching after treatment with more effective acaricides. A topical corticosteroid may help to reduce itch and inflammation after scabies has been treated successfully; however, persistent symptoms suggest that scabies eradication was not successful. Oral administration of a **sedating antihistamine** at night may also be useful.

Head lice

Dimeticone p. 698 is effective against head lice (*Pediculus humanus capitis*) and acts on the surface of the organism. Malathion, an organophosphorus insecticide, is an alternative, but resistance has been reported. Benzyl benzoate is licensed for the treatment of head lice but it is not recommended for use in children.

Head lice infestation (pediculosis) should be treated using lotion or liquid formulations only if live lice are present.

13

Skin

Shampoos are diluted too much in use to be effective. A contact time of 8–12 hours or overnight treatment is recommended for lotions and liquids; a 2-hour treatment is not sufficient to kill eggs.

In general, a course of treatment for head lice should be 2 applications of product 7 days apart to kill lice emerging from any eggs that survive the first application. All affected household members should be treated at the same time.

Wet combing methods

Head lice can be mechanically removed by combing wet hair meticulously with a plastic detection comb (probably for at least 30 minutes each time) over the whole scalp at 4-day intervals for a minimum of 2 weeks, and continued until no lice are found on 3 consecutive sessions; hair conditioner or vegetable oil can be used to facilitate the process.

Several devices for the removal of head lice such as combs and topical solutions, are available and some are prescribable on the NHS.

The Drug Tariffs can be accessed online at:

- National Health Service Drug Tariff for England and Wales: www.ppa.org.uk/ppa/edt_intro.htm
- Health and Personal Social Services for Northern Ireland Drug Tariff: www.dhsspsni.gov.uk/pas-tariff
- Scottish Drug Tariff: www.isdscotland.org/Health-topics/Prescribing-and-Medicines/Scottish-Drug-Tariff/

Crab lice

Permethrin and malathion are used to eliminate *crab lice* (*Pthirus pubis*); permethrin is not licensed for treatment of crab lice in children under 18 years. An aqueous preparation should be applied, allowed to dry naturally and washed off after 12 hours; a second treatment is needed after 7 days to kill lice emerging from surviving eggs. All surfaces of the body should be treated, including the scalp, neck, and face (paying particular attention to the eyebrows and other facial hair). A different insecticide should be used if a course of treatment fails.

Parasiticidal preparations

Dimeticone coats head lice and interferes with water balance in lice by preventing the excretion of water; it is less active against eggs and treatment should be repeated after 7 days.

Malathion is recommended for *scabies, head lice* and *crab lice*. The risk of systemic effects associated with 1–2 applications of malathion p. 699 is considered to be very low; however, except in the treatment of hyperkeratotic scabies in children, applications of malathion liquid repeated at intervals of less than 1 week or application for more than 3 consecutive weeks should be **avoided** since the likelihood of eradication of lice is not increased.

Permethrin p. 699 is effective for *scabies*. It is also active against *head lice* but the formulation and licensed methods of application of the current products make them unsuitable for the treatment of head lice. Permethrin is also effective against *crab lice* but it is not licensed for this purpose in children under 18 years.

2.1 Bacterial skin infections

ANTIBACTERIALS ⟩ AMINOGLYCOSIDES

Neomycin sulfate

- **INDICATIONS AND DOSE**

Bacterial skin infections
▸ TO THE SKIN
▸ Child: Apply up to 3 times a day, for short-term use only

- **UNLICENSED USE** *Neomycin Cream BPC*—no information available.

- **CONTRA-INDICATIONS** Neonates
- **CAUTIONS**

CAUTIONS, FURTHER INFORMATION
▸ Large areas If large areas of skin are being treated ototoxicity may be a hazard in children, particularly in those with renal impairment.

- **INTERACTIONS** → Appendix 1: neomycin
- **SIDE-EFFECTS** Sensitisation (cross sensitivity with other aminoglycosides may occur)
- **RENAL IMPAIRMENT** Ototoxicity may be a hazard if large areas of skin are treated.
- **LESS SUITABLE FOR PRESCRIBING** Neomycin sulfate cream is less suitable for prescribing.

- **MEDICINAL FORMS**

There can be variation in the licensing of different medicines containing the same drug. Forms available from special-order manufacturers include: cream

ANTIBACTERIALS ⟩ NITROIMIDAZOLE DERIVATIVES

Metronidazole

- **DRUG ACTION** Metronidazole is an antimicrobial drug with high activity against anaerobic bacteria and protozoa.

- **INDICATIONS AND DOSE**

ACEA®

Acute inflammatory exacerbation of rosacea
▸ TO THE SKIN
▸ Child 1-17 years: Apply twice daily, to be applied thinly

ANABACT®

Malodorous fungating tumours and malodorous gravitational and decubitus ulcers
▸ TO THE SKIN
▸ Child: Apply 1–2 times a day, to be applied to clean wound and covered with non-adherent dressing

METROGEL®

Acute inflammatory exacerbation of rosacea
▸ TO THE SKIN
▸ Child 1-17 years: Apply twice daily, to be applied thinly

Malodorous fungating tumours
▸ TO THE SKIN
▸ Child: Apply 1–2 times a day, to be applied to clean wound and covered with non-adherent dressing

METROSA®

Acute exacerbation of rosacea
▸ TO THE SKIN
▸ Child 1-17 years: Apply twice daily, to be applied thinly

ROSICED®

Inflammatory papules and pustules of rosacea
▸ TO THE SKIN
▸ Child 1-17 years: Apply twice daily for 6 weeks (longer if necessary)

ROZEX® CREAM

Inflammatory papules, pustules and erythema of rosacea
▸ TO THE SKIN
▸ Child 1-17 years: Apply twice daily

ROZEX® GEL

Inflammatory papules, pustules and erythema of rosacea
▸ TO THE SKIN
▸ Child 1-17 years: Apply twice daily

ZYOMET®

Acute inflammatory exacerbation of rosacea
▸ TO THE SKIN
▸ Child 1-17 years: Apply twice daily, to be applied thinly

13

Skin

- **UNLICENSED USE**
  METROGEL®. METROSA®, ROSICED®, ROZEX® CREAM,
  ROZEX® GEL, ZYOMET® Not licensed for use in children.
  ANABACT®, ACEA® Not licensed for use in children under
  12 years.
- **CAUTIONS** Avoid exposure to strong sunlight or UV light
- **INTERACTIONS** → Appendix 1: metronidazole
- **SIDE-EFFECTS** Skin irritation
- **PATIENT AND CARER ADVICE**
  Medicines for Children leaflet: Metronidazole for bacterial
  infections www.medicinesforchildren.org.uk/
  metronidazole-bacterial-infections

- **MEDICINAL FORMS**
  There can be variation in the licensing of different medicines
  containing the same drug. Forms available from special-order
  manufacturers include: cream, gel
  Gel
  EXCIPIENTS: May contain Benzyl alcohol, disodium edetate,
  hydroxybenzoates (parabens), propylene glycol
  ‣ **Acea** (Ferndale Pharmaceuticals Ltd)
    Metronidazole 7.5 mg per 1 gram Acea 0.75% gel | 40 gram PoM
    £9.95 DT price = £22.63
  ‣ **Anabact** (Cambridge Healthcare Supplies Ltd)
    Metronidazole 7.5 mg per 1 gram Anabact 0.75% gel |
    15 gram PoM £4.47 DT price = £4.47 | 30 gram PoM £7.89
  ‣ **Metrogel** (Galderma (UK) Ltd)
    Metronidazole 7.5 mg per 1 gram Metrogel 0.75% gel |
    40 gram PoM £22.63 DT price = £22.63
  ‣ **Metrosa** (M & A Pharmachem Ltd)
    Metronidazole 7.5 mg per 1 gram Metrosa 0.75% gel |
    30 gram PoM £12.00 | 40 gram PoM £19.90 DT price = £22.63
  ‣ **Rozex** (Galderma (UK) Ltd)
    Metronidazole 7.5 mg per 1 gram Rozex 0.75% gel | 30 gram PoM
    £6.60 | 40 gram PoM £9.88 DT price = £22.63
  ‣ **Zyomet** (AMCo)
    Metronidazole 7.5 mg per 1 gram Zyomet 0.75% gel |
    30 gram PoM £12.00
  Cream
  EXCIPIENTS: May contain Benzyl alcohol, isopropyl palmitate, propylene
  glycol
  ‣ **Rosiced** (Pierre Fabre Dermo-Cosmetique)
    Metronidazole 7.5 mg per 1 gram Rosiced 0.75% cream |
    30 gram PoM £7.50 DT price = £6.60
  ‣ **Rozex** (Galderma (UK) Ltd)
    Metronidazole 7.5 mg per 1 gram Rozex 0.75% cream |
    30 gram PoM £6.60 DT price = £6.60 | 40 gram PoM £9.88 DT price
    = £9.88

ANTIBACTERIALS > POLYMYXINS

Polymyxins

- **INDICATIONS AND DOSE**
  Bacterial skin infections
  ‣ TO THE SKIN
  ‣ **Child:** Apply twice daily, may be applied more
    frequently if required

- **UNLICENSED USE** Licensed for use in children (age range
  not specified by manufacturer).
- **CAUTIONS**

  CAUTIONS, FURTHER INFORMATION
  ‣ Large areas If large areas of skin are being treated
    nephrotoxicity and neurotoxicity may be a hazard,
    particularly in children with renal impairment.
- **INTERACTIONS** → Appendix 1: polymyxins
- **SIDE-EFFECTS** Sensitisation

- **MEDICINAL FORMS**
  There can be variation in the licensing of different medicines
  containing the same drug.
  No licensed medicines listed.

  Combinations available: *Bacitracin with polymyxin B*, p. 694

ANTIBACTERIALS > SULFONAMIDES

Silver sulfadiazine

- **INDICATIONS AND DOSE**
  Prophylaxis and treatment of infection in burn wounds
  ‣ TO THE SKIN
  ‣ **Child:** Apply daily, may be applied more frequently if
    very exudative
  For conservative management of finger-tip injuries
  ‣ TO THE SKIN
  ‣ **Child:** Apply every 2–3 days, consult product literature
    for details
  **Adjunct to prophylaxis of infection in skin graft donor
  sites and extensive abrasions**
  ‣ TO THE SKIN
  ‣ **Child:** (consult product literature)
  **Adjunct to short-term treatment of infection in pressure
  sores**
  ‣ TO THE SKIN
  ‣ **Child:** (consult product literature)

- **UNLICENSED USE** No age range specified by manufacturer.
- **CONTRA-INDICATIONS** Not recommended for neonates
- **CAUTIONS** G6PD deficiency

  CAUTIONS, FURTHER INFORMATION
  ‣ Large areas Plasma-sulfadiazine concentrations may
    approach therapeutic levels with *side-effects* and
    interactions as for sulfonamides if large areas of skin are
    treated.
- **INTERACTIONS** → Appendix 1: silver sulfadiazine
- **SIDE-EFFECTS** Allergic reactions · argyria (following
  treatment of large areas of skin or prolonged use) · burning
  · itching · leucopenia · rashes

  SIDE-EFFECTS, FURTHER INFORMATION
  ‣ Severe blood and skin disorders Owing to the association of
    sulfonamides with severe blood and skin disorders,
    treatment should be stopped immediately if blood
    disorders or rashes develop.

    Leucopenia developing 2–3 days after starting treatment
    of burns patients is reported usually to be self-limiting and
    silver sulfadiazine need not usually be discontinued
    provided blood counts are monitored carefully to ensure
    return to normality within a few days.
- **ALLERGY AND CROSS-SENSITIVITY** Contra-indicated in
  patients with sensitivity to sulfonamides.
- **PREGNANCY** Risk of neonatal haemolysis and
  methaemoglobinaemia in third trimester.
- **BREAST FEEDING** Small risk of kernicterus in jaundiced
  infants and of haemolysis in G6PD-deficient infants.
- **HEPATIC IMPAIRMENT** Manufacturer advises caution if
  significant impairment.
- **RENAL IMPAIRMENT** Manufacturer advises caution if
  significant impairment.
- **MONITORING REQUIREMENTS** Monitor for leucopenia.
- **DIRECTIONS FOR ADMINISTRATION** Apply with sterile
  applicator.

- **MEDICINAL FORMS**
  There can be variation in the licensing of different medicines
  containing the same drug.
  Cream
  EXCIPIENTS: May contain Cetostearyl alcohol (including cetyl and
  stearyl alcohol), polysorbates, propylene glycol
  ‣ **Flamazine** (Smith & Nephew Healthcare Ltd)
    Sulfadiazine silver 10 mg per 1 gram Flamazine 1% cream |
    20 gram PoM £2.91 | 50 gram PoM £3.85 DT price = £3.85 |
    250 gram PoM £10.32 DT price = £10.32 | 500 gram PoM £18.27 DT
    price = £18.27

13

Skin

ANTIBACTERIALS ⟩ OTHER

Bacitracin with polymyxin B

- **INDICATIONS AND DOSE**

Bacterial skin infections

▸ TO THE SKIN
  ▸ Child: Apply twice daily, can be applied more frequently if required

- **UNLICENSED USE** Licensed for use in children (age range not specified by manufacturer).
- **CAUTIONS** Nephrotoxicity · neurotoxicity

CAUTIONS, FURTHER INFORMATION
If large areas of skin are being treated nephrotoxicity and neurotoxicity may be a hazard, particularly in children with renal impairment.

- **INTERACTIONS** → Appendix 1: bacitracin, polymyxins
- **SIDE-EFFECTS** Contact sensitisation
- **RENAL IMPAIRMENT** Renal impairment increases the risk of nephrotoxicity and neurotoxicity.

- **MEDICINAL FORMS**
There can be variation in the licensing of different medicines containing the same drug.

Ointment
▸ Polyfax (Teva UK Ltd)
  Bacitracin zinc 500 unit per 1 gram, Polymyxin B sulfate 10000 unit per 1 gram Polyfax ointment | 4 gram [PoM] £3.26 | 20 gram [PoM] £4.62 DT price = £4.62

Mupirocin

- **INDICATIONS AND DOSE**

Bacterial skin infections, particularly those caused by Gram-positive organisms (except pseudomonal infection)

▸ TO THE SKIN
  ▸ Child: Apply up to 3 times a day for up to 10 days

- **UNLICENSED USE** Mupirocin ointment licensed for use in children (age range not specified by manufacturer). *Bactroban* ® cream not recommended for use in children under 1 year.
- **SIDE-EFFECTS** Burning sensation · local reactions · pruritus · rash · urticaria
- **PREGNANCY** Manufacturer advises avoid unless potential benefit outweighs risk—no information available.
- **BREAST FEEDING** No information available.
- **RENAL IMPAIRMENT** Manufacturer advises caution when mupirocin ointment used in moderate or severe impairment because it contains macrogols (polyethylene glycol).

- **MEDICINAL FORMS**
There can be variation in the licensing of different medicines containing the same drug.

Ointment
▸ Mupirocin (Non-proprietary)
  Mupirocin 20 mg per 1 gram Mupirocin 2% ointment | 15 gram [PoM] £12.50 DT price = £5.26
▸ Bactroban (GlaxoSmithKline UK Ltd)
  Mupirocin 20 mg per 1 gram Bactroban 2% ointment | 15 gram [PoM] £5.26 DT price = £5.26

Cream
EXCIPIENTS: May contain Benzyl alcohol, cetostearyl alcohol (including cetyl and stearyl alcohol)
▸ Bactroban (GlaxoSmithKline UK Ltd)
  Mupirocin (as Mupirocin calcium) 20 mg per 1 gram Bactroban 2% cream | 15 gram [PoM] £5.26 DT price = £5.26

Retapamulin

- **INDICATIONS AND DOSE**

Superficial bacterial skin infection caused by *Staphylococcus aureus* and *Streptococcus pyogenes* (if resistant to first line topical antibacterials)

▸ TO THE SKIN
  ▸ Child 9 months-17 years: Apply twice daily for 5 days, to be applied thinly, maximum area of skin treated 2% of body surface area, review treatment if no response within 2–3 days

- **CONTRA-INDICATIONS** Contact with eyes · contact with mucous membranes
- **SIDE-EFFECTS** Contact dermatitis · localised erythema · localised irritation · localised pain · pruritus
- **NATIONAL FUNDING/ACCESS DECISIONS**

Scottish Medicines Consortium (SMC) Decisions
The Scottish Medicines Consortium has advised (March 2008) that retapamulin (*Altargo* ®) is **not** recommended for use within NHS Scotland for the treatment of superficial skin infections.

- **MEDICINAL FORMS**
There can be variation in the licensing of different medicines containing the same drug.

Ointment
CAUTIONARY AND ADVISORY LABELS 28
EXCIPIENTS: May contain Butylated hydroxytoluene
▸ Altargo (GlaxoSmithKline UK Ltd)
  Retapamulin 10 mg per 1 gram Altargo 10mg/g ointment | 5 gram [PoM] £7.89

2.2 Fungal skin infections

Other drugs used for **Fungal skin infections** Griseofulvin, p. 363

ANTIFUNGALS ⟩ IMIDAZOLE ANTIFUNGALS

Clotrimazole

- **INDICATIONS AND DOSE**

Fungal skin infections

▸ TO THE SKIN
  ▸ Child: Apply 2–3 times a day

- **CAUTIONS** Contact with eyes and mucous membranes should be avoided
- **INTERACTIONS** → Appendix 1: antifungals, azoles
- **SIDE-EFFECTS** Local irritation · erythema · hypersensitivity reactions · itching · mild burning sensation

SIDE-EFFECTS, FURTHER INFORMATION
Treatment should be discontinued if side-effects are severe.

- **PREGNANCY** Minimal absorption from skin; not known to be harmful.
- **PRESCRIBING AND DISPENSING INFORMATION** Spray may be useful for application of clotrimazole to large or hairy areas of the skin.

- **MEDICINAL FORMS**
There can be variation in the licensing of different medicines containing the same drug. Forms available from special-order manufacturers include: powder

Cream
EXCIPIENTS: May contain Benzyl alcohol, cetostearyl alcohol (including cetyl and stearyl alcohol), polysorbates

‣ Clotrimazole (Non-proprietary)
Clotrimazole 10 mg per 1 gram Clotrimazole 1% cream |
20 gram Ⓟ £2.06 DT price = £1.12 | 50 gram Ⓟ £5.45 DT price =
£2.80
‣ Canesten (clotrimazole) (Bayer Plc)
Clotrimazole 10 mg per 1 gram Canesten 1% cream | 20 gram Ⓟ
£2.14 DT price = £1.12 | 50 gram Ⓟ £3.50 DT price = £2.80
Canesten Antifungal 1% cream | 20 gram Ⓟ £1.85 DT price = £1.12
Clotrimazole 20 mg per 1 gram Canesten 2% thrush cream |
10 gram Ⓟ no price available | 20 gram Ⓟ £4.46 DT price = £4.46
Clotrimazole 100 mg per 1 gram Canesten Internal 10% cream |
5 gram Ⓟ £6.23 DT price = £6.23
Canesten 10% VC cream | 5 gram PoM £4.50 DT price = £6.23

Liquid
‣ Canesten (clotrimazole) (Bayer Plc)
Clotrimazole 10 mg per 1 ml Canesten 1% solution | 20 ml Ⓟ
£2.30 DT price = £2.30

**Combinations available: *Hydrocortisone with clotrimazole,*
p. 714**

Econazole nitrate

● **INDICATIONS AND DOSE**
Fungal skin infections
▶ TO THE SKIN
▶ Child: Apply twice daily
Fungal nail infections
▶ BY TRANSUNGUAL APPLICATION
▶ Child: Apply once daily, applied under occlusive
dressing

● CAUTIONS Avoid contact with eyes and mucous
membranes
● SIDE-EFFECTS Burning sensation · erythema ·
hypersensitivity reactions · itching · occasional local
irritation
SIDE-EFFECTS, FURTHER INFORMATION
Treatment should be discontinued if side-effects are
severe.
● PREGNANCY Minimal absorption from skin; not known to
be harmful.

● MEDICINAL FORMS
There can be variation in the licensing of different medicines
containing the same drug.
Cream
EXCIPIENTS: May contain Butylated hydroxyanisole, fragrances
‣ Gyno-Pevaryl (Janssen-Cilag Ltd)
Econazole nitrate 10 mg per 1 gram Gyno-Pevaryl 1% cream |
15 gram PoM £2.11 | 30 gram PoM £3.78
‣ Pevaryl (Janssen-Cilag Ltd)
Econazole nitrate 10 mg per 1 gram Pevaryl 1% cream |
30 gram Ⓟ £3.71

Ketoconazole

16-Jun-2017

● **INDICATIONS AND DOSE**
Treatment of seborrhoeic dermatitis and dandruff
▶ TO THE SKIN USING SHAMPOO
▶ Child 12–17 years: Apply twice weekly for 2–4 weeks,
leave preparation on for 3–5 minutes before rinsing
Prophylaxis of seborrhoeic dermatitis and dandruff
▶ TO THE SKIN USING SHAMPOO
▶ Child 12–17 years: Apply every 1–2 weeks, leave
preparation on for 3–5 minutes before rinsing
Treatment of pityriasis versicolor
▶ TO THE SKIN USING SHAMPOO
▶ Child 12–17 years: Apply once daily for maximum 5 days,
leave preparation on for 3–5 minutes before rinsing

Prophylaxis of pityriasis versicolor
▶ TO THE SKIN USING SHAMPOO
▶ Child 12–17 years: Apply once daily for up to 3 days
before sun exposure, leave preparation on for
3–5 minutes before rinsing

● CAUTIONS Avoid contact with eyes · avoid contact with
mucous membranes
● INTERACTIONS → Appendix 1: antifungals, azoles
● SIDE-EFFECTS Erythema · hypersensitivity reactions ·
itching · mild burning sensation · occasional local irritation
SIDE-EFFECTS, FURTHER INFORMATION Treatment should
be discontinued if side-effects are severe.
● EXCEPTIONS TO LEGAL CATEGORY Can be sold to the
public for the prevention and treatment of dandruff and
seborrhoeic dermatitis of the scalp as a shampoo
formulation containing ketoconazole maximum 2%, in a
pack containing maximum 120 mL and labelled to show a
maximum frequency of application of once every 3 days.

● MEDICINAL FORMS
There can be variation in the licensing of different medicines
containing the same drug.
Shampoo
EXCIPIENTS: May contain Imidurea
‣ Ketoconazole (Non-proprietary)
Ketoconazole 20 mg per 1 gram Ketoconazole 2% shampoo |
120 ml PoM £2.77 DT price = £2.77
‣ Dandrazol (Transdermal Ltd)
Ketoconazole 20 mg per 1 gram Dandrazol 2% shampoo |
120 ml PoM £5.20 DT price = £2.77
‣ Nizoral (Janssen-Cilag Ltd, McNeil Products Ltd)
Ketoconazole 20 mg per 1 gram Nizoral 2% shampoo |
120 ml PoM £3.59 DT price = £2.77

Miconazole

● **INDICATIONS AND DOSE**
Fungal skin infections
▶ TO THE SKIN
▶ Neonate: Apply twice daily continuing for 10 days after
lesions have healed.

▶ Child: Apply twice daily continuing for 10 days after
lesions have healed
Fungal nail infections
▶ TO THE SKIN
▶ Child: Apply 1–2 times a day

● UNLICENSED USE Licensed for use in children (age range
not specified by manufacturer).
● CAUTIONS Avoid in acute porphyrias p. 577 · contact with
eyes and mucous membranes should be avoided
● INTERACTIONS → Appendix 1: antifungals, azoles
● SIDE-EFFECTS
▶ Common or very common Nausea · rash · vomiting
▶ Frequency not known Burning sensation · erythema ·
hypersensitivity reactions · itching · occasional local
irritation
SIDE-EFFECTS, FURTHER INFORMATION
Treatment should be discontinued if side effects are
severe.
● PREGNANCY Absorbed from the skin in small amounts;
manufacturer advises caution.
● BREAST FEEDING Manufacturer advises caution—no
information available.
● PROFESSION SPECIFIC INFORMATION
Dental practitioners' formulary
Miconazole cream may be prescribed.

13

Skin

13

Skin

● MEDICINAL FORMS
There can be variation in the licensing of different medicines containing the same drug.

Cream
EXCIPIENTS: May contain Butylated hydroxyanisole
▸ Daktarin (McNeil Products Ltd, Janssen-Cilag Ltd)
Miconazole nitrate 20 mg per 1 gram Daktarin 2% cream |
15 gram [P] £2.14 | 30 gram [P] £1.82 DT price = £1.82
▸ Gyno-Daktarin (Janssen-Cilag Ltd)
Miconazole nitrate 20 mg per 1 gram Gyno-Daktarin 2% vaginal cream | 78 gram [PoM] £4.33

Powder
▸ Daktarin (McNeil Products Ltd)
Miconazole nitrate 20 mg per 1 gram Daktarin 2% powder |
20 gram [P] £2.58 DT price = £2.58

Tioconazole

● INDICATIONS AND DOSE

Fungal nail infection
▸ BY TRANSUNGUAL APPLICATION
▸ Child: Apply twice daily usually for up to 6 months (may be extended to 12 months), apply to nails and surrounding skin

● UNLICENSED USE Licensed for use in children (age range not specified by manufacturer).

● CAUTIONS Contact with eyes and mucous membranes should be avoided · use with caution if child likely to suck affected digits

● SIDE-EFFECTS Burning sensation · dry skin · erythema · exfoliation · hypersensitivity reactions · itching · local oedema · nail discoloration · nail pain · occasional local irritation · periungual inflammation · rash

SIDE-EFFECTS, FURTHER INFORMATION
Treatment should be discontinued if side-effects are severe.

● PREGNANCY Manufacturer advises avoid.

● MEDICINAL FORMS
There can be variation in the licensing of different medicines containing the same drug.

Paint
▸ Tioconazole (Non-proprietary)
Tioconazole 283 mg per 1 ml Tioconazole 283mg/ml medicated nail lacquer | 12 ml [PoM] £27.38–£28.74 DT price = £28.74
▸ Trosyl (Pfizer Ltd)
Tioconazole 283 mg per 1 ml Trosyl 283mg/ml nail solution |
12 ml [PoM] £27.38 DT price = £28.74

ANTIFUNGALS › OTHER

Amorolfine

● INDICATIONS AND DOSE

Fungal nail infections
▸ BY TRANSUNGUAL APPLICATION
▸ Child 1 month-11 years: Apply 1–2 times a week for 6 months to treat finger nails and for toe nails 9–12 months (review at intervals of 3 months), apply to infected nails after filing and cleansing, allow to dry for approximately 3 minutes
▸ Child 12-17 years: Apply 1–2 times a week for 6 months to treat finger nails and for toe nails 9–12 months (review at intervals of 3 months), apply to infected nails after filing and cleansing, allow to dry for approximately 3 minutes

● UNLICENSED USE Not licensed for use in children under 12 years.

● CAUTIONS Avoid contact with ears · avoid contact with eyes and mucous membranes · use with caution in child likely to suck affected digits

● SIDE-EFFECTS Burning sensation · erythema · hypersensitivity reactions · itching · occasional local irritation

SIDE-EFFECTS, FURTHER INFORMATION
Treatment should be discontinued if side-effects are severe.

● PATIENT AND CARER ADVICE Avoid nail varnish or artificial nails during treatment.

● MEDICINAL FORMS
There can be variation in the licensing of different medicines containing the same drug.
Medicated nail lacquer
CAUTIONARY AND ADVISORY LABELS 10
▸ Amorolfine (Non-proprietary)
Amorolfine (as Amorolfine hydrochloride) 50 mg per
1 ml Amorolfine 5% medicated nail lacquer | 3 ml [PoM] no price available | 5 ml [PoM] £16.21 DT price = £6.99
▸ Loceryl (Galderma (UK) Ltd)
Amorolfine (as Amorolfine hydrochloride) 50 mg per 1 ml Loceryl 5% medicated nail lacquer | 2.5 ml [PoM] £7.26 | 5 ml [PoM] £9.08 DT price = £6.99
▸ Omicur (Morningside Healthcare Ltd)
Amorolfine (as Amorolfine hydrochloride) 50 mg per 1 ml Omicur 5% medicated nail lacquer | 2.5 ml [PoM] £9.09 | 5 ml [PoM] £9.09 DT price = £6.99

Terbinafine

● INDICATIONS AND DOSE

Tinea pedis
▸ TO THE SKIN USING CREAM
▸ Child: Apply 1–2 times a day for up to 1 week, to be applied thinly
▸ BY MOUTH USING TABLETS
▸ Child 1-17 years (body-weight 10-19 kg): 62.5 mg once daily for 2-6 weeks
▸ Child 1-17 years (body-weight 20-39 kg): 125 mg once daily for 2-6 weeks
▸ Child 1-17 years (body-weight 40 kg and above): 250 mg once daily for 2-6 weeks

Tinea corporis
▸ TO THE SKIN USING CREAM
▸ Child: Apply 1–2 times a day for up to 1–2 weeks, to be applied thinly, review treatment after 2 weeks
▸ BY MOUTH USING TABLETS
▸ Child 1-17 years (body-weight 10-19 kg): 62.5 mg once daily for 4 weeks
▸ Child 1-17 years (body-weight 20-39 kg): 125 mg once daily for 4 weeks
▸ Child 1-17 years (body-weight 40 kg and above): 250 mg once daily for 4 weeks

Tinea cruris
▸ TO THE SKIN USING CREAM
▸ Child: Apply 1–2 times a day for up to 1–2 weeks, to be applied thinly, review treatment after 2 weeks
▸ BY MOUTH USING TABLETS
▸ Child 1-17 years (body-weight 10-19 kg): 62.5 mg once daily for 2-4 weeks
▸ Child 1-17 years (body-weight 20-39 kg): 125 mg once daily for 2-4 weeks
▸ Child 1-17 years (body-weight 40 kg and above): 250 mg once daily for 2-4 weeks

Tinea capitis
▸ BY MOUTH USING TABLETS
▸ Child 1-17 years (body-weight 10-19 kg): 62.5 mg once daily for 4 weeks

- Child 1-17 years (body-weight 20-39 kg): 125 mg once daily for 4 weeks
- Child 1-17 years (body-weight 40 kg and above): 250 mg once daily for 4 weeks

Dermatophyte infections of the nails
▶ BY MOUTH USING TABLETS
- Child 1-17 years (body-weight 10-19 kg): 62.5 mg once daily for 6 weeks-3 months (occasionally longer in toenail infections)
- Child 1-17 years (body-weight 20-39 kg): 125 mg once daily for 6 weeks-3 months (occasionally longer in toenail infections)
- Child 1-17 years (body-weight 40 kg and above): 250 mg once daily for 6 weeks-3 months (occasionally longer in toenail infections)

Cutaneous candidiasis | Pityriasis versicolor
▶ TO THE SKIN USING CREAM
- Child: Apply 1-2 times a day for 2 weeks, to be applied thinly, review treatment after 2 weeks

● UNLICENSED USE Not licensed for use in children.
● CAUTIONS
▶ With oral use Autoimmune disease (risk of lupus-erythematosus-like effect) · psoriasis (risk of exacerbation)
▶ With topical use Contact with eyes and mucous membranes should be avoided
● INTERACTIONS → Appendix 1: terbinafine
● SIDE-EFFECTS
▶ Common or very common
▶ With oral use Abdominal discomfort · anorexia · arthralgia · diarrhoea · dyspepsia · headache · myalgia · nausea · rash · urticaria
▶ Uncommon
▶ With oral use Taste disturbance
▶ Rare
▶ With oral use Cholestasis · dizziness · hepatitis · hypoaesthesia · jaundice · liver toxicity · malaise · paraesthesia
▶ Very rare
▶ With oral use Alopecia · blood disorders · lupus erythematosus-like effect · neutropenia · photosensitivity · serious skin reactions · Stevens-Johnson syndrome · thrombocytopenia · toxic epidermal necrolysis
▶ Frequency not known
▶ With oral use Disturbances in smell · exacerbation of psoriasis · hearing disturbances · influenza-like symptoms · pancreatitis · rhabdomyolysis · vasculitis
▶ With topical use Erythema · hypersensitivity reactions · itching · mild burning sensation · occasional local irritation
SIDE-EFFECTS, FURTHER INFORMATION
▶ Liver toxicity
▶ With oral use Discontinue treatment if liver toxicity develops (including jaundice, cholestasis and hepatitis).
▶ Serious skin reactions
▶ With oral use Discontinue treatment in progressive skin rash (including Stevens-Johnson syndrome and toxic epidermal necrolysis).
▶ Topical application Treatment should be discontinued if side effects are severe.
● PREGNANCY
▶ With topical use Manufacturer advises use only if potential benefit outweighs risk—*animal* studies suggest no adverse effects.
▶ With oral use Manufacturer advises use only if potential benefit outweighs risk—no information available.
● BREAST FEEDING
▶ With topical use Manufacturer advises avoid—present in milk. Less than 5% of the dose is absorbed after topical application of terbinafine; avoid application to mother's chest.
▶ With oral use Avoid—present in milk.

● HEPATIC IMPAIRMENT
▶ With oral use Manufacturer advises avoid—elimination reduced.
● RENAL IMPAIRMENT
▶ With oral use Use half normal dose if estimated glomerular filtration rate less than 50 mL/minute/1.73 m^2 and no suitable alternative available.
● MONITORING REQUIREMENTS
▶ With oral use Monitor hepatic function before treatment and then every 4–6 weeks during treatment—discontinue if abnormalities in liver function tests.
● EXCEPTIONS TO LEGAL CATEGORY
Preparations of terbinafine hydrochloride (maximum 1%) can be sold to the public for use in those over 16 years for external use for the treatment of tinea pedis as a cream in a pack containing maximum 15 g, or for the treatment of tinea pedis and cruris as a cream in a pack containing maximum 15 g, or for the treatment of tinea pedis, cruris, and corporis as a spray in a pack containing maximum 30 mL spray or as a gel in a pack containing maximum 30 g gel.

● MEDICINAL FORMS
There can be variation in the licensing of different medicines containing the same drug.
Tablet
CAUTIONARY AND ADVISORY LABELS 9
▶ Terbinafine (Non-proprietary)
  Terbinafine (as Terbinafine hydrochloride) 250 mg Terbinafine 250mg tablets | 14 tablet [PoM] £18.11 DT price = £1.21 | 28 tablet [PoM] £34.93
▶ Lamisil (Novartis Pharmaceuticals UK Ltd)
  Terbinafine (as Terbinafine hydrochloride) 250 mg Lamisil 250mg tablets | 14 tablet [PoM] £21.30 DT price = £1.21 | 28 tablet [PoM] £41.09
Cream
EXCIPIENTS: May contain Benzyl alcohol, cetostearyl alcohol (including cetyl and stearyl alcohol), polysorbates
▶ Terbinafine (Non-proprietary)
  Terbinafine hydrochloride 10 mg per 1 gram Terbinafine 1% cream | 7.5 gram [PoM] £1.06 | 15 gram [PoM] £3.17 DT price = £1.29 | 30 gram [PoM] £6.33 DT price = £2.58
▶ Lamisil (GlaxoSmithKline Consumer Healthcare)
  Terbinafine hydrochloride 10 mg per 1 gram Lamisil 1% cream | 30 gram [PoM] £7.45 DT price = £2.58
  Lamisil AT 1% cream | 7.5 gram [GSL] £2.39 | 15 gram [GSL] £3.60 DT price = £1.29

ANTISEPTICS AND DISINFECTANTS ›
UNDECENOATES

Undecenoic acid with zinc undecenoate

● INDICATIONS AND DOSE
Treatment of athletes foot
▶ TO THE SKIN
- Child: Apply twice daily, continue use for 7 days after lesions have healed

Prevention of athletes foot
▶ TO THE SKIN
- Child: Apply once daily

● UNLICENSED USE *Mycota*® licensed for use in children (age range not specified by manufacturer).
● CAUTIONS Avoid broken skin · contact with eyes should be avoided · contact with mucous membranes should be avoided
● SIDE-EFFECTS Erythema · hypersensitivity reactions · itching · local irritation · mild burning sensation

13

Skin

SIDE-EFFECTS, FURTHER INFORMATION
Treatment should be discontinued if side effects are severe.

● **MEDICINAL FORMS**
There can be variation in the licensing of different medicines containing the same drug.
Cream
EXCIPIENTS: May contain Cetostearyl alcohol (including cetyl and stearyl alcohol), fragrances
▸ Mycota (zinc undecenoate / undecenoic acid) (Thornton & Ross Ltd)
Undecenoic acid 50 mg per 1 gram, Zinc undecenoate 200 mg per 1 gram Mycota cream | 25 gram GSL £2.01
Powder
EXCIPIENTS: May contain Fragrances
▸ Mycota (zinc undecenoate / undecenoic acid) (Thornton & Ross Ltd)
Undecenoic acid 20 mg per 1 gram, Zinc undecenoate 200 mg per 1 gram Mycota powder | 70 gram GSL £2.94

ANTISEPTICS AND DISINFECTANTS ▸ OTHER

Chlorhexidine with nystatin

● **INDICATIONS AND DOSE**
Skin infections due to Candida spp.
▸ TO THE SKIN
▸ Child: Apply 2–3 times a day, continuing for 7 days after lesions have healed

● **UNLICENSED USE** Licensed for use in children (age range not specified by manufacturer).
● **CAUTIONS** Avoid contact with eyes and mucous membranes
● **SIDE-EFFECTS** Burning sensation · erythema · hypersensitivity reactions · itching · occasional local irritation
SIDE-EFFECTS, FURTHER INFORMATION
Treatment should be discontinued if side-effects are severe.

● **MEDICINAL FORMS**
There can be variation in the licensing of different medicines containing the same drug.
Cream
EXCIPIENTS: May contain Benzyl alcohol, cetostearyl alcohol (including cetyl and stearyl alcohol), polysorbates
▸ Chlorhexidine with nystatin (Non-proprietary)
Chlorhexidine hydrochloride 10 mg per 1 gram, Nystatin 100000 unit per 1 gram Nystatin 100,000units/g / Chlorhexidine hydrochloride 1% cream | 30 gram PoM £4.99 DT price = £2.62
▸ Nystaform (Typharm Ltd)
Chlorhexidine hydrochloride 10 mg per 1 gram, Nystatin 100000 unit per 1 gram Nystaform cream | 30 gram PoM £2.62 DT price = £2.62

BENZOATES

Benzoic acid with salicylic acid

● **INDICATIONS AND DOSE**
Ringworm (tinea)
▸ TO THE SKIN
▸ Child: Apply twice daily

● **UNLICENSED USE** Licensed for use in children (age range not specified by manufacturer).
● **CAUTIONS** Avoid broken or inflamed skin · avoid contact with eyes · avoid contact with mucous membranes
CAUTIONS, FURTHER INFORMATION
▸ Salicylate toxicity Salicylate toxicity may occur particularly if applied on large areas of skin.

● **SIDE-EFFECTS** Erythema · hypersensitivity reactions · itching · mild burning sensation · occasional local irritation
SIDE-EFFECTS, FURTHER INFORMATION
Treatment should be discontinued if side effects are severe.

● **PRESCRIBING AND DISPENSING INFORMATION** Benzoic Acid Ointment, Compound, BP has also been referred to as Whitfield's ointment.

● **MEDICINAL FORMS**
There can be variation in the licensing of different medicines containing the same drug. Forms available from special-order manufacturers include: cream, ointment

SALICYLIC ACID AND DERIVATIVES

Boric acid with salicylic acid and tannic acid

● **INDICATIONS AND DOSE**
Fungal nail infection, particularly tinea
▸ BY TRANSUNGUAL APPLICATION
▸ Child 5–17 years: Apply twice daily, and after washing

● **CAUTIONS** Avoid broken or inflamed skin · contact with eyes and mucous membranes should be avoided · use with caution in children likely to suck affected digits
CAUTIONS, FURTHER INFORMATION
▸ Salicylate toxicity Salicylate toxicity can occur particularly if applied on large areas of skin.
● **SIDE-EFFECTS** Burning sensation · erythema · hypersensitivity reactions · itching · occasional local irritation
SIDE-EFFECTS, FURTHER INFORMATION
Treatment should be discontinued if side-effects are severe.
● **PREGNANCY** Avoid.
● **LESS SUITABLE FOR PRESCRIBING** *Phytex*® is less suitable for prescribing.

● **MEDICINAL FORMS**
There can be variation in the licensing of different medicines containing the same drug.
No licensed medicines listed.

2.3 Parasitic skin infections

Other drugs used for Parasitic skin infections Ivermectin, p. 367

PARASITICIDES

Dimeticone

● **INDICATIONS AND DOSE**
Head lice
▸ TO THE SKIN
▸ Child: Apply once weekly for 2 doses, rub into dry hair and scalp, allow to dry naturally, shampoo after minimum 8 hours (or overnight)

● **UNLICENSED USE** Not licensed for use in children under 6 months except under medical supervision.
● **CAUTIONS** Avoid contact with eyes · children under 6 months, medical supervision required
● **SIDE-EFFECTS** Skin irritation
● **PATIENT AND CARER ADVICE** Patients should be told to keep hair away from fire and flames during treatment.

Skin 13

- **MEDICINAL FORMS**
There can be variation in the licensing of different medicines containing the same drug.

Liquid
▸ **Hedrin** (Thornton & Ross Ltd)
Dimeticone 40 mg per 1 gram Hedrin 4% lotion | 50 ml P £3.06 DT price = £3.06 | 150 ml P £7.13 DT price = £7.13
▸ **Lyclear (dimeticone)** (Omega Pharma Ltd)
Dimeticone 40 mg per 1 gram Lyclear lotion | 100 ml no price available

Cutaneous spray solution
▸ **Hedrin** (Thornton & Ross Ltd)
Dimeticone 40 mg per 1 gram Hedrin 4% spray | 120 ml GSL £7.33

Malathion

- **INDICATIONS AND DOSE**

Head lice
▸ TO THE SKIN
▸ Child: Apply once weekly for 2 doses, rub preparation into dry hair and scalp, allow to dry naturally, remove by washing after 12 hours

Crab lice
▸ TO THE SKIN
▸ Child: Apply once weekly for 2 doses, apply preparation over whole body, allow to dry naturally, wash off after 12 hours or overnight

Scabies
▸ TO THE SKIN
▸ Child: Apply once weekly for 2 doses, apply preparation over whole body, and wash off after 24 hours, if hands are washed with soap within 24 hours, they should be retreated

- **UNLICENSED USE** Not licensed for use in children under 6 months except under medical supervision.
- **CAUTIONS** Alcoholic lotions **not** recommended for head lice in children with severe eczema or asthma, or for scabies or crab lice · avoid contact with eyes · children under 6 months, medical supervision required · do not use lotion more than once a week for 3 consecutive weeks · do not use on broken or secondarily infected skin
- **SIDE-EFFECTS** Chemical burns · hypersensitivity reactions · skin irritation
- **PRESCRIBING AND DISPENSING INFORMATION** For scabies, manufacturer recommends application to the body but not necessarily to the head and neck. However, application should be extended to the scalp, neck, face, and ears.
- **MEDICINAL FORMS**
There can be variation in the licensing of different medicines containing the same drug.

Liquid
EXCIPIENTS: May contain Cetostearyl alcohol (including cetyl and stearyl alcohol), fragrances, hydroxybenzoates (parabens)
▸ **Derbac-M** (G.R. Lane Health Products Ltd)
Malathion 5 mg per 1 gram Derbac-M 0.5% liquid | 50 ml P £3.89 DT price = £3.57 | 200 ml P £9.09 DT price = £8.44

Permethrin

- **INDICATIONS AND DOSE**

Scabies
▸ TO THE SKIN
▸ Child: Apply once weekly for 2 doses, apply 5% preparation over whole body including face, neck, scalp and ears then wash off after 8–12 hours. If hands are washed with soap within 8 hours of application, they should be treated again with cream

- **UNLICENSED USE** *Dermal Cream* (scabies), not licensed for use in children under 2 months; not licensed for treatment of crab lice in children under 18 years. *Creme Rinse* (head lice) not licensed for use in children under 6 months except under medical supervision.
- **CAUTIONS** Avoid contact with eyes · children aged 2 months–2 years, medical supervision required for dermal cream (scabies) · children under 6 months, medical supervision required for cream rinse (head lice) · do not use on broken or secondarily infected skin
- **SIDE-EFFECTS**
▸ **Rare** Oedema · rashes
▸ **Frequency not known** Erythema · pruritus · stinging
- **PRESCRIBING AND DISPENSING INFORMATION** Manufacturer recommends application to the body but to exclude head and neck. However, application should be extended to the scalp, neck, face, and ears.
Larger patients may require up to two 30-g packs for adequate treatment.
- **LESS SUITABLE FOR PRESCRIBING** Lyclear® Creme Rinse is less suitable for prescribing.
- **MEDICINAL FORMS**
There can be variation in the licensing of different medicines containing the same drug.

Cream
CAUTIONARY AND ADVISORY LABELS 10 (Dermal cream only)
EXCIPIENTS: May contain Butylated hydroxytoluene, wool fat and related substances including lanolin
▸ **Permethrin (Non-proprietary)**
Permethrin 50 mg per 1 gram Permethrin 5% cream | 30 gram P £7.46 DT price = £7.46
▸ **Lyclear** (Omega Pharma Ltd)
Permethrin 50 mg per 1 gram Lyclear 5% dermal cream | 30 gram P £5.71 DT price = £7.46

Liquid
EXCIPIENTS: May contain Cetostearyl alcohol (including cetyl and stearyl alcohol)
▸ **Lyclear** (Omega Pharma Ltd)
Permethrin 10 mg per 1 gram Lyclear 1% creme rinse | 59 ml P £3.55 DT price = £3.55 | 118 ml P £6.46 DT price = £6.46

2.4 Viral skin infections

ANTIVIRALS ⟩ NUCLEOSIDE ANALOGUES

Aciclovir

(Acyclovir)

- **INDICATIONS AND DOSE**

Herpes simplex infection (local treatment)
▸ TO THE SKIN
▸ Child: Apply 5 times a day for 5–10 days, to be applied to lesions approximately every 4 hours, starting at first sign of attack

- **UNLICENSED USE** Cream licensed for use in children (age range not specified by manufacturer).
- **CAUTIONS** Avoid cream coming in to contact with eyes and mucous membranes
- **INTERACTIONS** → Appendix 1: aciclovir
- **SIDE-EFFECTS** Drying of the skin · erythema · itching of the skin · transient burning · transient stinging
- **PREGNANCY** Limited absorption from topical aciclovir preparations.
- **PATIENT AND CARER ADVICE**
Medicines for Children leaflet: Aciclovir cream for herpes www.medicinesforchildren.org.uk/aciclovir-cream-for-herpes

13

Skin

● **PROFESSION SPECIFIC INFORMATION**

Dental practitioners' formulary
Aciclovir Cream may be prescribed.

● **EXCEPTIONS TO LEGAL CATEGORY** A 2-g tube and a pump pack are on sale to the public for the treatment of cold sores.

● **MEDICINAL FORMS**
There can be variation in the licensing of different medicines containing the same drug.

Cream
EXCIPIENTS: May contain Cetostearyl alcohol (including cetyl and stearyl alcohol), propylene glycol

▸ **Aciclovir (Non-proprietary)**
Aciclovir 50 mg per 1 gram Aciclovir 5% cream | 2 gram PoM
£1.31 DT price = £1.10 | 10 gram PoM £6.00 DT price = £5.50

▸ **Zovirax** (GlaxoSmithKline Consumer Healthcare, GlaxoSmithKline UK Ltd)
Aciclovir 50 mg per 1 gram Zovirax 5% cream | 2 gram PoM £4.63
DT price = £1.10 | 10 gram PoM £13.96 DT price = £5.50

3 Inflammatory skin conditions

3.1 Eczema and psoriasis

Eczema

Types and management
The main types of eczema (dermatitis) in children are atopic, irritant and allergic contact; different types may co-exist. *Atopic eczema* is the most common type and it usually involves dry skin as well as infection and lichenification caused by scratching and rubbing. *Seborrhoeic dermatitis* is also common in infants.

Management of eczema involves the removal or treatment of contributory factors; known or suspected irritants and contact allergens should be avoided. Rarely, ingredients in topical medicinal products may sensitise the skin; *BNF for Children* lists active ingredients together with excipients that have been associated with skin sensitisation.

Skin dryness and the consequent irritant eczema requires **emollients** applied regularly (at least twice daily) and liberally to the affected area; this can be supplemented with bath or shower emollients. The use of emollients should continue even if the eczema improves or if other treatment is being used.

Topical corticosteroids are also required in the management of eczema; the potency of the corticosteroid should be appropriate to the severity and site of the condition, and the age of the child. Mild corticosteroids are generally used on the face and on flexures; the more potent corticosteroids are generally required for use on lichenified areas of eczema or for severe eczema on the scalp, limbs, and trunk. Treatment should be reviewed regularly, especially if a potent corticosteroid is required. In children with frequent flares (2–3 per month), a topical corticosteroid can be applied on 2 consecutive days each week to prevent further flares.

Bandages (including those containing ichthammol with zinc oxide p. 715) are sometimes applied over topical corticosteroids or emollients to treat eczema of the limbs. Dry-wrap dressings can be used to provide a physical barrier to help prevent scratching and improve retention of emollients. Wet elasticated viscose stockinette is used for 'wet-wrap' bandaging over topical corticosteroids or emollients to cool the skin and relieve itching, but there is an increased risk of infection and excessive absorption of the corticosteroid; 'wet-wrap' bandaging should be used under specialist supervision.

See *Wound management products and elasticated garments* for details of elasticated viscose stockinette tubular bandages and garments, and silk clothing.

See Eczema and psoriasis, drugs affecting the immune response p. 701 for the role of topical pimecrolimus p. 718 and tacrolimus p. 718 in atopic eczema.

Infection
Bacterial infection (commonly with *Staphylococcus aureus* and occasionally with *Streptococcus pyogenes*) can exacerbate eczema. A topical antibacterial may be used for small areas of mild infection; treatment should be limited to a short course (typically 1 week) to reduce the risk of drug resistance or skin sensitisation. Associated eczema is treated simultaneously with a topical corticosteroid which can be combined with a topical antimicrobial.

Eczema involving moderate to severe, widespread, or recurrent infection requires the use of a systemic antibacterial that is active against the infecting organism. Preparations that combine an antiseptic with an emollient application and with a bath emollient can also be used; antiseptic shampoos can be used on the scalp.

Intertriginous eczema commonly involves candida and bacteria; it is best treated with a mild or moderately potent topical corticosteroid combined with a suitable antimicrobial drug.

Widespread *herpes simplex infection* may complicate atopic eczema (eczema herpeticum) and treatment under specialist supervision with a systemic antiviral drug is indicated. Secondary bacterial infection often exacerbates eczema herpeticum.

Management of other features of eczema
Lichenification, which results from repeated scratching, is treated initially with a potent corticosteroid. Bandages containing ichthammol p. 715 (to reduce pruritus) and other substances such as **zinc oxide** can be applied over the corticosteroid or emollient. **Coal tar** and ichthammol can be useful in some cases of chronic eczema. *Discoid eczema*, with thickened plaques in chronic atopic eczema, is usually treated with a topical antiseptic preparation, a potent topical corticosteroid, and paste bandages containing ichthammol with zinc oxide.

A *non-sedating* antihistamine may be of some value in relieving severe itching or urticaria associated with eczema. A *sedating* antihistamine can be used at night if itching causes sleep disturbance, but a large dose may be needed and drowsiness may persist on the following day.

Exudative ('weeping') eczema requires a potent corticosteroid initially; infection may also be present and require specific treatment. Potassium permanganate solution (1 in 10,000) p. 731 can be used as a soak in exudating eczema for its antiseptic and astringent effects; treatment should be stopped when exudation stops.

Severe refractory eczema is best managed under specialist supervision; it may require phototherapy or drugs that act on the immune system.

Seborrhoeic dermatitis
Seborrhoeic dermatitis (seborrhoeic eczema) is associated with species of the yeast *Malassezia*. *Infantile seborrhoeic dermatitis* affects particularly the body folds, nappy area and scalp; it is treated with emollients and mild topical corticosteroids with suitable antimicrobials. Infantile seborrhoeic dermatitis affecting the scalp (*cradle cap*) is treated by hydrating the scalp using natural oils and the use of mild shampoo.

In older children, seborrhoeic dermatitis affects the scalp, paranasal areas, and eyebrows. Shampoos active against the yeast (including those containing ketoconazole p. 695 and coal tar) and combinations of mild topical corticosteroids with suitable antimicrobials are used to treat older children.

Medicated bandages

Zinc paste bandages (see *Wound management products and elasticated garments*) are used with **coal tar** or ichthammol in chronic lichenified skin conditions such as chronic eczema (ichthammol often being preferred since its action is considered to be milder). They are also used with calamine in milder eczematous skin conditions.

Eczema and psoriasis, drugs affecting the immune response

Overview

Drugs affecting the immune response are used for eczema or psoriasis. Pimecrolimus p. 718 by topical application is licensed for *mild to moderate atopic eczema*. Tacrolimus p. 718 is licensed for topical use in *moderate to severe atopic eczema*. Both are drugs whose long-term safety is still being evaluated and they should not usually be considered first-line treatment unless there is a specific reason to avoid or reduce the use of topical corticosteroids. Treatment with topical pimecrolimus or topical tacrolimus should be initiated only by prescribers experienced in treating atopic eczema.

Topical corticosteroids have a role in eczema and a limited role in psoriasis. A systemic corticosteroid such as prednisolone p. 421 may be used in severe refractory eczema.

Systemic drugs acting on the immune system are generally used by **specialists** in a hospital setting.

Ciclosporin p. 496 by mouth can be used for *severe psoriasis* and for *severe eczema*. Azathioprine p. 495 or mycophenolate mofetil p. 503 are also used for severe refractory eczema in children.

Methotrexate p. 517 can be used for *severe resistant* psoriasis; the dose is given **once weekly** and adjusted according to severity of the condition and haematological and biochemical measurements. Folic acid p. 546 should be given to reduce the possibility of methotrexate toxicity [unlicensed indication]. Folic acid can be given once weekly on a different day to the methotrexate; alternative regimens may be used in some settings.

Etanercept p. 616 (a cytokine modulator) is licensed in children over 6 years of age for the treatment of *severe plaque psoriasis* that is inadequately controlled by other systemic treatments and photochemotherapy, or when these other treatments cannot be used because of intolerance or contra-indications.

Adalimumab p. 614 (a cytokine modulator) is licensed in children over 4 years for the treatment of *severe chronic plaque psoriasis* that is inadequately controlled by other topical treatments and phototherapies, or when these treatments are inappropriate.

Psoriasis

Management

Psoriasis is characterised by epidermal thickening and scaling. It commonly affects extensor surfaces and the scalp. For mild psoriasis, reassurance and treatment with an emollient may be all that is necessary. *Guttate psoriasis* is a distinctive form of psoriasis that characteristically occurs in children and young adults, often following a streptococcal throat infection or tonsillitis.

Occasionally psoriasis is provoked or exacerbated by drugs such as lithium, chloroquine and hydroxychloroquine, beta-blockers, non-steroidal anti-inflammatory drugs, and ACE inhibitors. Psoriasis may not occur until the drug has been taken for weeks or months.

Emollients, in addition to their effects on dryness, scaling and cracking, may have an antiproliferative effect in psoriasis. They are particularly useful in *inflammatory psoriasis* and in *chronic stable plaque psoriasis*.

For *chronic stable plaque psoriasis* on extensor surfaces of trunk and limbs preparations containing **coal tar** are moderately effective, but the smell is unacceptable to some children. **Vitamin D** and its analogues are effective and cosmetically acceptable alternatives to preparations containing coal tar or dithranol p. 715. Dithranol is an effective topical antipsoriatic agent but it irritates and stains the skin and it should be used only under specialist supervision. Adverse effects of dithranol are minimised by using a 'short-contact technique' and by starting with low concentration preparations. Tazarotene, a topical retinoid for the treatment of mild to moderate plaque psoriasis, is not recommended for use in children under 18 years. These medications can irritate the skin particularly in the flexures and they are not suitable for the more inflammatory forms of psoriasis; their use should be suspended during an inflammatory phase of psoriasis. The efficacy and the irritancy of each substance varies between patients. If a substance irritates significantly, it should be stopped or the concentration reduced; if it is tolerated, its effects should be assessed after 4 to 6 weeks and treatment continued if it is effective.

Widespread *unstable psoriasis* of erythrodermic or generalised pustular type requires urgent specialist assessment. Initial topical treatment should be limited to using emollients frequently and generously. More localised acute or subacute *inflammatory psoriasis* with hot, spreading or itchy lesions, should be treated topically with emollients or with a corticosteroid of moderate potency.

Scalp psoriasis is usually scaly, and the scale may be thick and adherent. This requires softening with an emollient ointment, cream, or oil and usually combined with salicylic acid as a keratolytic.

Some preparations for psoriasis affecting the scalp combine salicylic acid with coal tar or **sulfur**. The preparation should be applied generously and left on for at least an hour, often more conveniently overnight, before washing it off. If a corticosteroid lotion or gel is required (e.g. for itch), it can be used in the morning.

Flexural psoriasis can be managed with short-term use of a mild potency topical corticosteroid. Calcitriol p. 720 or tacalcitol p. 721 can be used in the longer term; calcipotriol p. 720 is more likely to cause irritation in flexures and should be avoided. Low-strength tar preparations can also be used.

Facial psoriasis can be treated with short-term use of a mild topical corticosteroid; if this is ineffective, calcitriol, tacalcitol, or a low-strength tar preparation can be used.

Calcipotriol and tacalcitol are analogues of vitamin D that affect cell division and differentiation. Calcitriol is an active form of vitamin D. Vitamin D and its analogues are used as first-line treatment for plaque psoriasis; they do not smell or stain and they may be more acceptable than tar or dithranol products. Of the vitamin D analogues, tacalcitol and calcitriol are less likely to irritate.

Coal tar p. 716 has anti-inflammatory properties that are useful in chronic plaque psoriasis; it also has antiscaling properties. Contact of coal tar products with normal skin is not normally harmful and preparations containing coal tar can be used for widespread small lesions; however, irritation, contact allergy, and sterile folliculitis can occur. Leave-on preparations that remain in contact with the skin, such as creams or ointments, containing up to 6% coal tar may be used on children 1 month to 2 years; leave-on preparations containing coal tar 10% may be used on children over 2 years with more severe psoriasis. Tar baths and tar shampoos may also be helpful.

Dithranol is effective for chronic plaque psoriasis. Its major disadvantages are irritation (for which individual

13

Skin

susceptibility varies) and staining of skin and of clothing. Dithranol is not generally suitable for widespread small lesions nor should it be used in the flexures or on the face. Proprietary preparations are more suitable for home use; they are usually washed off after 20–30 minutes ('short contact' technique). Specialist nurses may apply intensive treatment with dithranol paste which is covered by stockinette dressings and usually retained overnight. Dithranol should be discontinued if even a low concentration causes acute inflammation; continued use can result in the psoriasis becoming unstable.

A topical **corticosteroid** is not generally suitable for long-term use or as the sole treatment of extensive chronic plaque psoriasis; any early improvement is not usually maintained and there is a risk of the condition deteriorating or of precipitating an unstable form of psoriasis e.g. erythrodermic psoriasis or generalised pustular psoriasis on withdrawal. Topical use of potent corticosteroids on widespread psoriasis can also lead to systemic as well as local side-effects. However, topical corticosteroids used short term may be appropriate to treat psoriasis in specific sites such as the face or flexures with a mild corticosteroid, and psoriasis of the scalp, palms, and soles with a potent corticosteroid. Very potent topical corticosteroids should only be used under specialist supervision.

Combining the use of a corticosteroid with another specific topical treatment may be beneficial in chronic plaque psoriasis; the drugs may be used separately at different times of the day or used together in a single formulation. *Eczema* co-existing with psoriasis may be treated with a corticosteroid, or coal tar, or both.

Phototherapy

Phototherapy is available in specialist centres under the supervision of a dermatologist. Narrow band ultraviolet B (UVB) radiation is usually effective for *chronic stable psoriasis* and for *guttate psoriasis*. It can be considered for children with moderately severe psoriasis in whom topical treatment has failed, but it may irritate inflammatory psoriasis. The use of phototherapy and photochemotherapy in children is limited by concerns over carcinogenicity and premature ageing.

Photochemotherapy combining long-wave ultraviolet A radiation with a psoralen (PUVA) is available in specialist centres under the supervision of a dermatologist. The psoralen, which enhances the effect of irradiation, is administered either by mouth or topically. PUVA is effective in most forms of psoriasis, including the *localised palmoplantar pustular psoriasis*. Early adverse effects include phototoxicity and pruritus. Higher cumulative doses exaggerate skin ageing, increase the risk of dysplastic and neoplastic skin lesions especially squamous cancer, and pose a theoretical risk of cataracts.

Phototherapy combined with coal tar, dithranol, topical vitamin D or vitamin D analogues, or oral acitretin, allows reduction of the cumulative dose of phototherapy required to treat psoriasis.

Systemic treatment

Systemic treatment is required for severe, resistant, unstable or complicated forms of psoriasis, and it should be initiated only under specialist supervision. Systemic drugs for psoriasis include acitretin and drugs that affect the immune response (see Eczema and psoriasis, drugs affecting the immune response p. 701).

Acitretin p. 719, a metabolite of etretinate, is a retinoid (vitamin A derivative); it is prescribed by specialists. The main indication of acitretin is severe psoriasis resistant to other forms of therapy. It is also used in disorders of keratinisation such as severe *Darier's disease* (keratosis follicularis), and some forms of *ichthyosis*. Although a minority of cases of psoriasis respond well to acitretin alone, it is only moderately effective in many cases; adverse effects

are a limiting factor. A therapeutic effect occurs after 2 to 4 weeks and the maximum benefit after 4 months. Consideration should be given to stopping acitretin if the response is inadequate after 4 months at the optimum dose. Continuous treatment for longer than 6 months is not usually necessary in psoriasis. However, some patients, particularly those with severe ichthyosis, may benefit from longer treatment, provided that the lowest effective dose is used, patients are monitored carefully for adverse effects, and the need for treatment is reviewed regularly. Topical preparations containing keratolytics should normally be stopped before administration of acitretin. Liberal use of emollients should be encouraged and topical corticosteroids can be continued if necessary.

Acitretin is teratogenic; in females of child-bearing age, the possibility of pregnancy must be excluded before treatment and effective contraception must be used during treatment and for at least 3 years afterwards (oral progestogen-only contraceptives not considered effective).

Topical treatment

The vitamin D and analogues, calcipotriol p. 720, calcitriol p. 720, and tacalcitol p. 721 are used for the management of plaque psoriasis. They should be avoided by those with calcium metabolism disorders, and used with caution in generalised pustular or erythrodermic exfoliative psoriasis (enhanced risk of hypercalcaemia).

CORTICOSTEROIDS

Topical corticosteroids

Overview

Topical corticosteroids are used for the treatment of inflammatory conditions of the skin (other than those arising from an infection), particularly eczema, contact dermatitis, insect stings, and eczema of scabies. Corticosteroids suppress the inflammatory reaction during use; they are not curative and on discontinuation a rebound exacerbation of the condition may occur. They are generally used to relieve symptoms and suppress signs of the disorder when other measures such as emollients are ineffective.

Children, especially infants, are particularly susceptible to side-effects. However, concern about the safety of topical corticosteroids in children should not result in the child being undertreated. The aim is to control the condition as well as possible; inadequate treatment will perpetuate the condition. Carers of young children should be advised that treatment should **not** necessarily be reserved to 'treat only the worst areas' and they may need to be advised that patient information leaflets may contain inappropriate advice for the child's condition.

In an acute flare-up of atopic eczema, it may be appropriate to use more potent formulations of topical corticosteroids for a short period to regain control of the condition.

Topical corticosteroids are not recommended in the routine treatment of urticaria; treatment should only be initiated and supervised by a specialist. Topical corticosteroids may worsen ulcerated or secondarily infected lesions. They should not be used indiscriminately in pruritus (where they will only benefit if inflammation is causing the itch) and are **not** recommended for acne vulgaris.

Systemic or very potent topical corticosteroids should be avoided or given only under specialist supervision in psoriasis because, although they may suppress the psoriasis in the short term, relapse or vigorous rebound occurs on withdrawal (sometimes precipitating severe pustular psoriasis). Topical use of potent corticosteroids on widespread psoriasis can lead to systemic as well as to local side-effects. It is reasonable, however, to prescribe a mild topical corticosteroid for a short period (2–4 weeks) for *flexural* and *facial psoriasis*, and to use a more potent corticosteroid such as betamethasone p. 705 or fluocinonide p. 708 for *psoriasis* of the *scalp*, *palms*, or *soles*.

In general, the most potent topical corticosteroids should be reserved for recalcitrant dermatoses such as *chronic discoid lichen erythematosus*, *lichen simplex chronicus*, *hypertrophic lichen planus*, and *palmoplantar pustulosis*. Potent corticosteroids should generally be avoided on the face and skin flexures, but specialists occasionally prescribe them for use on these areas in certain circumstances.

When topical treatment has failed, intralesional corticosteroid injections may be used. These are more effective than the very potent topical corticosteroid preparations and should be reserved for severe cases where there are localised lesions such as *keloid scars*, *hypertrophic lichen planus*, or *localised alopecia areata*.

Perioral lesions

Hydrocortisone cream 1% p. 709 can be used for up to 7 days to treat uninfected inflammatory lesions on the lips. Hydrocortisone with miconazole cream or ointment p. 714 is useful where infection by susceptible organisms and inflammation co-exist, particularly for initial treatment (up to 7 days) e.g. in angular cheilitis. Organisms susceptible to miconazole include *Candida* spp. and many Gram-positive bacteria including streptococci and staphylococci.

Choice

Water-miscible corticosteroid creams are suitable for moist or weeping lesions whereas ointments are generally chosen for dry, lichenified or scaly lesions or where a more occlusive effect is required. Lotions may be useful when minimal application to a large or hair-bearing area is required or for the treatment of exudative lesions. *Occlusive polythene* or *hydrocolloid dressings* increase absorption, but also increase the risk of side-effects; they are therefore used only under supervision on a short-term basis for areas of very thick skin (such as the palms and soles). Disposable nappies and tight fitting pants also increase the risk of side-effects by increasing absorption of the corticosteroid. The inclusion of urea or salicylic acid also increases the penetration of the corticosteroid.

In the *BNF for Children*, topical corticosteroids for the skin are categorised as 'mild', 'moderately potent', 'potent' or 'very potent'; the least potent preparation which is effective should be chosen but dilution should be avoided whenever possible.

Topical hydrocortisone is usually used in children under 1 year of age. Moderately potent and potent corticosteroids should be used with great care in children and for short periods (1–2 weeks) only. A very potent corticosteroid should be initiated under the supervision of a specialist.

Appropriate topical corticosteroids for specific conditions are:

- *insect bites and stings*—mild corticosteroid such as hydrocortisone 1% cream;
- *inflamed nappy rash causing discomfort* in infant over 1 month—mild corticosteroid such as hydrocortisone 0.5% or 1% for up to 7 days (combined with antimicrobial if infected);
- *mild to moderate eczema, flexural and facial eczema or psoriasis*—mild corticosteroid such as hydrocortisone 1%;
- *severe eczema of the face and neck*—moderately potent corticosteroid for 3–5 days only, if not controlled by a mild corticosteroid;
- *severe eczema on the trunk and limbs*—moderately potent or potent corticosteroid for 1–2 weeks only, switching to a less potent preparation as the condition improves;
- *eczema affecting area with thickened skin (e.g. soles of feet)*—potent topical corticosteroid in combination with urea or salicylic acid (to increase penetration of corticosteroid).

Absorption through the skin

Mild and *moderately potent* topical corticosteroids are associated with few side-effects but particular care is required when treating neonates and infants, and in the use of *potent* and *very potent* corticosteroids. Absorption through the skin can rarely cause adrenal suppression and even Cushing's syndrome, depending on the area of the body being treated and the duration of treatment. Absorption of corticosteroid is greatest from severely inflamed skin, thin skin (especially on the face and genital area), from flexural sites (e.g. axillae, groin), and in infants where skin surface area is higher in relation to body-weight; absorption is increased by occlusion.

Compound preparations

The advantages of including other substances (such as antibacterials or antifungals) with corticosteroids in topical preparations are uncertain, but such combinations may have a place where inflammatory skin conditions are associated with bacterial or fungal infection, such as infected eczema. In these cases the antimicrobial drug should be chosen according to the sensitivity of the infecting organism and used regularly for a short period (typically twice daily for 1 week). Longer use increases the likelihood of resistance and of sensitisation.

The keratolytic effect of salicylic acid facilitates the absorption of topical corticosteroids; however, excessive and prolonged use of topical preparations containing salicylic acid may cause salicylism.

Topical corticosteroid preparation potencies

Potency of a topical corticosteroid preparation is a result of the formulation as well as the corticosteroid. Therefore, proprietary names are shown.

Mild
- Hydrocortisone 0.1–2.5%
- Dioderm
- Mildison
- Synalar 1 in 10 dilution

Mild with antimicrobials
- Canesten HC
- Daktacort
- Econacort
- Fucidin H
- Nystaform-HC
- Terra-Cortril
- Timodine

Moderate
- Betnovate-RD
- Eumovate
- Haelan
- Modrasone
- Synalar 1 in 4 Dilution
- Ultralanum Plain

Moderate with antimicrobials
- Trimovate

Moderate with urea:
- Alphaderm

Potent
- Beclometasone dipropionate 0.025%
- Betamethasone valerate 0.1%
- Betacap
- Betesil
- Bettamousse
- Betnovate
- Cutivate
- Diprosone
- Elocon
- Hydrocortisone butyrate
- Locoid

- Locoid Crelo
- Metosyn
- Mometasone furoate 0.1%
- Nerisone
- Synalar

Potent with antimicrobials

- Aureocort
- Betamethasone and clioquinol
- Betamethasone and neomycin
- Fucibet
- Lotriderm
- Synalar C
- Synalar N

Potent with salicylic acid

- Diprosalic

Very potent

- Dermovate
- Nerisone Forte

Very potent with antimicrobials

- Clobetasol propionate 0.05% with neomycin and nystatin

Corticosteroids (topical)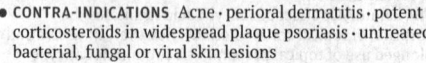

- **CONTRA-INDICATIONS** Acne · perioral dermatitis · potent corticosteroids in widespread plaque psoriasis · untreated bacterial, fungal or viral skin lesions
- **CAUTIONS** Avoid prolonged use (particularly on the face) · cautions applicable to systemic corticosteroids may also apply if absorption occurs following topical and local use · dermatoses of infancy, including nappy rash (extreme caution required—treatment should be limited to 5–7 days) · infection · keep away from eyes · use potent or very potent topical corticosteroids under specialist supervision
- **SIDE-EFFECTS**
  ‣ **Rare** Adrenal suppression · Cushing's syndrome
  ‣ **Frequency not known** Acne · contact dermatitis · hypertrichosis · irreversible striae atrophicae · irreversible telangiectasia · mild depigmentation (may be reversible) · perioral dermatitis · side-effects applicable to systemic corticosteroids may also apply if absorption occurs following topical and local use · spread and worsening of untreated infection · thinning of the skin (may be restored over a period after stopping treatment but the original structure may never return) · worsening of acne · worsening of rosacea

  SIDE-EFFECTS, FURTHER INFORMATION
  In order to minimise the side-effects of a topical corticosteroid, it is important to apply it **thinly** to affected areas **only**, no more frequently than **twice daily**, and to use the least potent formulation which is fully effective.

- **DIRECTIONS FOR ADMINISTRATION** Topical corticosteroid preparations should be applied no more frequently than twice daily; once daily is often sufficient. Topical corticosteroids should be spread thinly on the skin but in sufficient quantity to cover the affected areas. The length of cream or ointment expelled from a tube may be used to specify the quantity to be applied to a given area of skin. This length can be measured in terms of a *fingertip unit* (the distance from the tip of the adult index finger to the first crease). One fingertip unit (approximately 500 mg from a tube with a standard 5 mm diameter nozzle) is sufficient to cover an area that is twice that of the flat adult handprint (palm and fingers). Mixing topical preparations on the skin should be avoided where possible; several minutes should elapse between application of different preparations.

  'Wet-wrap bandaging' increases absorption into the skin, but should be initiated only by a dermatologist and application supervised by a healthcare professional trained in the technique.

- **PRESCRIBING AND DISPENSING INFORMATION** The potency of each topical corticosteroid should be included on the label with the directions for use. The label should be attached to the container (for example, the tube) rather than the outer packaging.
- **PATIENT AND CARER ADVICE** Patients or carers should be given advice on how to administer corticosteroid creams and ointments. If a patient is using topical corticosteroids of different potencies, the patient should be told when to use each corticosteroid. Patients and their carers should be reassured that side effects such as skin thinning and systemic effects rarely occur when topical corticosteroids are used appropriately.

☛ above

Alclometasone dipropionate

- **INDICATIONS AND DOSE**

  Inflammatory skin disorders such as eczemas
  ‣ TO THE SKIN
  ‣ Child: Apply 1–2 times a day, to be applied thinly

  POTENCY
  Alclometasone dipropionate cream 0.05%: moderate

- **UNLICENSED USE** Licensed for use in children (age range not specified by manufacturer).
- **PATIENT AND CARER ADVICE** Patients or carers should be counselled on the application of alclometasone dipropionate cream.

- **MEDICINAL FORMS**
  There can be variation in the licensing of different medicines containing the same drug.
  Cream
  CAUTIONARY AND ADVISORY LABELS 28
  EXCIPIENTS: May contain Cetostearyl alcohol (including cetyl and stearyl alcohol), chlorocresol, propylene glycol
  ‣ Alclometasone dipropionate (Non-proprietary)
  Alclometasone dipropionate 500 microgram per 1 gram Boots Derma Care Eczema & Dermatitis Flare-Up 0.05% cream | 15 gram Ⓟ no price available

☛ above

Beclometasone dipropionate

(Beclomethasone dipropionate)

- **INDICATIONS AND DOSE**

  Severe inflammatory skin disorders such as eczemas unresponsive to less potent corticosteroids | Psoriasis
  ‣ TO THE SKIN
  ‣ Child: Apply 1–2 times a day, thin layer to be applied

  POTENCY
  Beclometasone dipropionate cream and ointment 0.025%: potent.

- **UNLICENSED USE** Not licensed for use in children under 1 year.
- **INTERACTIONS** → Appendix 1: corticosteroids

- **MEDICINAL FORMS**
  There can be variation in the licensing of different medicines containing the same drug. Forms available from special-order manufacturers include: cream, ointment
  Cream
  CAUTIONARY AND ADVISORY LABELS 28
  ‣ Beclometasone dipropionate (Non-proprietary)
  Beclometasone dipropionate 250 microgram per 1 gram Beclometasone 0.025% cream | 30 gram PoM £68.00 DT price = £68.00

Ointment
CAUTIONARY AND ADVISORY LABELS 28
▶ Beclometasone dipropionate (Non-proprietary)
Beclometasone dipropionate 250 microgram per
1 gram Beclometasone 0.025% ointment ┃ 30 gram PoM £68.00 DT
price = £68.00

⏴ 704

Betamethasone

● **INDICATIONS AND DOSE**

Severe inflammatory skin disorders such as eczemas
unresponsive to less potent corticosteroids ┃ Psoriasis
▶ TO THE SKIN
› Child: Apply 1–2 times a day, to be applied thinly

POTENCY
Betamethasone valerate 0.025% cream and ointment:
moderate. Betamethasone valerate 0.1% cream, lotion,
ointment, and scalp application: potent. Betamethasone
valerate 0.12% foam: potent. Betamethasone
dipropionate 0.05% cream, lotion, and ointment: potent.

● **UNLICENSED USE** *Betacap*®, *Betnovate*® and *Betnovate-*
RD® are not licensed for use in children under 1 year.
Bettamousse® is not licensed for use in children under
6 years.

● **CAUTIONS** Use of more than 100 g per week of 0.1%
preparation likely to cause adrenal suppression

● **INTERACTIONS** → Appendix 1: corticosteroids

● **PATIENT AND CARER ADVICE** Patient counselling is advised
for betamethasone cream, ointment, scalp application and
foam (application).

● **MEDICINAL FORMS**
There can be variation in the licensing of different medicines
containing the same drug. Forms available from special-order
manufacturers include: cream, ointment

Foam
CAUTIONARY AND ADVISORY LABELS 28, 15
EXCIPIENTS: May contain Cetostearyl alcohol (including cetyl and
stearyl alcohol), polysorbates, propylene glycol
▶ Bettamousse (Focus Pharmaceuticals Ltd)
Betamethasone (as Betamethasone valerate) 1 mg per
1 gram Bettamousse 0.1% cutaneous foam ┃ 100 gram PoM £9.75
DT price = £9.75

Cream
CAUTIONARY AND ADVISORY LABELS 28
EXCIPIENTS: May contain Cetostearyl alcohol (including cetyl and
stearyl alcohol), chlorocresol
▶ Betamethasone (Non-proprietary)
Betamethasone (as Betamethasone valerate) 1 mg per
1 gram Betamethasone valerate 0.1% cream ┃ 15 gram PoM £3.00
┃ 30 gram PoM £5.99 DT price = £2.87 ┃ 100 gram PoM £11.99 DT
price = £9.57
▶ Audavate (Auden McKenzie (Pharma Division) Ltd)
Betamethasone (as Betamethasone valerate) 250 microgram per
1 gram Audavate RD 0.025% cream ┃ 100 gram PoM £2.52 DT price
= £3.15
▶ Betnovate (GlaxoSmithKline UK Ltd)
Betamethasone (as Betamethasone valerate) 250 microgram per
1 gram Betnovate RD 0.025% cream ┃ 100 gram PoM £3.15 DT
price = £3.15
Betamethasone (as Betamethasone valerate) 1 mg per
1 gram Betnovate 0.1% cream ┃ 30 gram PoM £1.43 DT price =
£2.87 ┃ 100 gram PoM £4.05 DT price = £9.57
▶ Diprosone (Merck Sharp & Dohme Ltd)
Betamethasone (as Betamethasone dipropionate)
500 microgram per 1 gram Diprosone 0.05% cream ┃
30 gram PoM £2.16 DT price = £2.16 ┃ 100 gram PoM £6.12 DT
price = £6.12

Ointment
CAUTIONARY AND ADVISORY LABELS 28
▶ Betamethasone (Non-proprietary)
Betamethasone (as Betamethasone valerate) 1 mg per
1 gram Betamethasone valerate 0.1% ointment ┃ 30 gram PoM
£5.55 DT price = £2.20 ┃ 100 gram PoM £14.99 DT price = £7.33

▶ Audavate (Auden McKenzie (Pharma Division) Ltd)
Betamethasone (as Betamethasone valerate) 250 microgram per
1 gram Audavate RD 0.025% ointment ┃ 100 gram PoM £2.52 DT
price = £3.15
Betamethasone (as Betamethasone valerate) 1 mg per
1 gram Audavate 0.1% ointment ┃ 30 gram PoM £1.14 DT price =
£2.20 ┃ 100 gram PoM £3.24 DT price = £7.33
▶ Betnovate (GlaxoSmithKline UK Ltd)
Betamethasone (as Betamethasone valerate) 250 microgram per
1 gram Betnovate RD 0.025% ointment ┃ 100 gram PoM £3.15 DT
price = £3.15
Betamethasone (as Betamethasone valerate) 1 mg per
1 gram Betnovate 0.1% ointment ┃ 30 gram PoM £1.43 DT price =
£2.20 ┃ 100 gram PoM £4.05 DT price = £7.33
▶ Diprosone (Merck Sharp & Dohme Ltd)
Betamethasone (as Betamethasone dipropionate)
500 microgram per 1 gram Diprosone 0.05% ointment ┃
30 gram PoM £2.16 DT price = £2.16 ┃ 100 gram PoM £6.12 DT
price = £6.12

Liquid
CAUTIONARY AND ADVISORY LABELS 15(scalp lotion only), 28
EXCIPIENTS: May contain Cetostearyl alcohol (including cetyl and
stearyl alcohol), hydroxybenzoates (parabens)
▶ Betacap (Dermal Laboratories Ltd)
Betamethasone (as Betamethasone valerate) 1 mg per
1 gram Betacap 0.1% scalp application ┃ 100 ml PoM £3.19 DT price
= £3.19
▶ Betnovate (GlaxoSmithKline UK Ltd)
Betamethasone (as Betamethasone valerate) 1 mg per
1 gram Betnovate 0.1% scalp application ┃ 100 ml PoM £4.99 DT
price = £3.19
Betnovate 0.1% lotion ┃ 100 ml PoM £4.58 DT price = £4.58
▶ Diprosone (Merck Sharp & Dohme Ltd)
Betamethasone (as Betamethasone dipropionate)
500 microgram per 1 ml Diprosone 0.05% lotion ┃ 30 ml PoM
£2.73 DT price = £2.73 ┃ 100 ml PoM £7.80 DT price = £7.80

Combinations available: *Betamethasone with clioquinol,*
p. 710 · *Betamethasone with clotrimazole,* p. 710 ·
Betamethasone with fusidic acid, p. 711 · *Betamethasone with*
neomycin, p. 711 · *Betamethasone with salicylic acid,* p. 711

Calcipotriol with betamethasone
30-May-2017

The properties listed below are those particular to the
combination only. For the properties of the components
please consider, calcipotriol p. 720, betamethasone above.

● **INDICATIONS AND DOSE**

DOVOBET® GEL

Scalp psoriasis
▶ TO THE SKIN
› Child 12–17 years (specialist use only): Apply 1–4 g once
daily usual duration of therapy 4 weeks; if necessary,
treatment may be continued beyond 4 weeks or
repeated, on the advice of a specialist, shampoo off
after leaving on scalp overnight or during day, when
different preparations containing calcipotriol used
together, maximum total calcipiotriol 3.75 mg in any
one week

Mild to moderate plaque psoriasis
▶ TO THE SKIN
› Child 12–17 years (specialist use only): Apply once daily
usual duration for up to 4 weeks; if necessary
treatment should be continued beyond 4 weeks, or
repeated, only on the advice of a specialist, apply to
maximum 30% of body surface, when different
preparations containing calcipotriol used together,
max. total calcipotriol 3.75 mg in any one week;
maximum 75 g per week   continued →

13

Skin

DOVOBET® OINTMENT

Stable plaque psoriasis

▶ TO THE SKIN

▶ Child 12–17 years (specialist use only): Apply once daily for up to 4 weeks; if necessary, treatment may be continued beyond 4 weeks or repeated, on the advice of a specialist, apply to a maximum 30% of body surface, when different preparations containing calcipotriol used together, max. total calcipotriol 3.75 mg in any one week; maximum 75 g per week

● UNLICENSED USE *Dovobet®* not licensed for use in children.

● MEDICINAL FORMS
There can be variation in the licensing of different medicines containing the same drug.

Ointment
CAUTIONARY AND ADVISORY LABELS 28
EXCIPIENTS: May contain Butylated hydroxytoluene
▶ Dovobet (LEO Pharma)
Calcipotriol (as Calcipotriol hydrate) 50 microgram per 1 gram, Betamethasone (as Betamethasone dipropionate) 500 microgram per 1 gram Dovobet ointment | 30 gram PoM £19.84 DT price = £19.84 | 60 gram PoM £39.68 | 120 gram PoM £73.86

Gel
CAUTIONARY AND ADVISORY LABELS 28
EXCIPIENTS: May contain Butylated hydroxytoluene
▶ Dovobet (LEO Pharma)
Calcipotriol (as Calcipotriol monohydrate) 50 microgram per 1 gram, Betamethasone (as Betamethasone dipropionate) 500 microgram per 1 gram Dovobet gel Applicator | 60 gram PoM £37.21 DT price = £37.21
Dovobet gel | 60 gram PoM £37.21 DT price = £37.21 | 120 gram PoM £69.11

F 704

Clobetasol propionate

● INDICATIONS AND DOSE

Short-term treatment only of severe resistant inflammatory skin disorders such as recalcitrant eczemas unresponsive to less potent corticosteroids | Psoriasis

▶ TO THE SKIN

▶ Child: Apply 1–2 times a day for up to 4 weeks, to be applied thinly

POTENCY
Clobetasol propionate 0.05% cream, foam, ointment, scalp application, and shampoo: very potent.

● UNLICENSED USE *Dermovate®* not licensed for use in children under 1 year.

● PATIENT AND CARER ADVICE Patients or carers should be given advice on how to administer clobetasol propionate foam, liquid (scalp application), cream, ointment and shampoo.
Scalp application Patients or carers should be advised to apply foam directly to scalp lesions (foam begins to subside immediately on contact with skin).

● MEDICINAL FORMS
There can be variation in the licensing of different medicines containing the same drug. Forms available from special-order manufacturers include: cream, ointment, paste

Foam
CAUTIONARY AND ADVISORY LABELS 15, 28
EXCIPIENTS: May contain Cetostearyl alcohol (including cetyl and stearyl alcohol), polysorbates, propylene glycol
▶ Clarelux (Pierre Fabre Dermo-Cosmetique)
Clobetasol propionate 500 microgram per 1 gram Clarelux 500micrograms/g foam | 100 gram PoM £11.06

Shampoo
CAUTIONARY AND ADVISORY LABELS 28
▶ Etrivex (Galderma (UK) Ltd)
Clobetasol propionate 500 microgram per 1 gram Etrivex 500micrograms/g shampoo | 125 ml PoM £9.15 DT price = £9.15

Cream
CAUTIONARY AND ADVISORY LABELS 28
EXCIPIENTS: May contain Beeswax, cetostearyl alcohol (including cetyl and stearyl alcohol), chlorocresol, propylene glycol
▶ Clobetasol propionate (Non-proprietary)
Clobetasol propionate 500 microgram per 1 gram Clobetasol 0.05% cream | 30 gram PoM no price available DT price = £2.69 | 100 gram PoM no price available DT price = £7.90
▶ ClobaDerm (Auden McKenzie (Pharma Division) Ltd)
Clobetasol propionate 500 microgram per 1 gram ClobaDerm 0.05% cream | 30 gram PoM £2.15 DT price = £2.69 | 100 gram PoM £6.32 DT price = £7.90
▶ Dermovate (GlaxoSmithKline UK Ltd)
Clobetasol propionate 500 microgram per 1 gram Dermovate 0.05% cream | 30 gram PoM £2.69 DT price = £2.69 | 100 gram PoM £7.90 DT price = £7.90

Ointment
CAUTIONARY AND ADVISORY LABELS 28
EXCIPIENTS: May contain Propylene glycol
▶ Clobetasol propionate (Non-proprietary)
Clobetasol propionate 500 microgram per 1 gram Clobetasol 0.05% ointment | 30 gram PoM no price available DT price = £2.69 | 100 gram PoM no price available DT price = £7.90
▶ ClobaDerm (Auden McKenzie (Pharma Division) Ltd)
Clobetasol propionate 500 microgram per 1 gram ClobaDerm 0.05% ointment | 30 gram PoM £2.15 DT price = £2.69 | 100 gram PoM £6.32 DT price = £7.90
▶ Dermovate (GlaxoSmithKline UK Ltd)
Clobetasol propionate 500 microgram per 1 gram Dermovate 0.05% ointment | 30 gram PoM £2.69 DT price = £2.69 | 100 gram PoM £7.90 DT price = £7.90

Liquid
CAUTIONARY AND ADVISORY LABELS 15, 28
▶ Dermovate (GlaxoSmithKline UK Ltd)
Clobetasol propionate 500 microgram per 1 gram Dermovate 0.05% scalp application | 30 ml PoM £3.07 DT price = £3.07 | 100 ml PoM £10.42 DT price = £10.42

Combinations available: *Clobetasol propionate with neomycin sulfate and nystatin*, p. 712

F 704

Clobetasone butyrate

● INDICATIONS AND DOSE

Eczemas and dermatitis of all types | Maintenance between courses of more potent corticosteroids

▶ TO THE SKIN

▶ Child: Apply 1–2 times a day, to be applied thinly

POTENCY
Clobetasone butyrate 0.05% cream and ointment: moderate.

● UNLICENSED USE Licensed for use in children (age range not specified by manufacturer).

● PATIENT AND CARER ADVICE Patients or carers should be advised on the application of clobetasone butyrate containing preparations.

● EXCEPTIONS TO LEGAL CATEGORY Cream can be sold to the public for short-term symptomatic treatment and control of patches of eczema and dermatitis (but not seborrhoeic dermatitis) in adults and children over 12 years provided pack does not contain more than 15 g.

- **MEDICINAL FORMS**
There can be variation in the licensing of different medicines containing the same drug. Forms available from special-order manufacturers include: cream, ointment

Ointment
CAUTIONARY AND ADVISORY LABELS 28
▸ Clobavate (Teva UK Ltd)
  Clobetasone butyrate 500 microgram per 1 gram Clobavate 0.05% ointment | 30 gram PoM £1.49 DT price = £1.86 | 100 gram PoM £4.35 DT price = £5.44
▸ Eumovate (GlaxoSmithKline UK Ltd)
  Clobetasone butyrate 500 microgram per 1 gram Eumovate 0.05% ointment | 30 gram PoM £1.86 DT price = £1.86 | 100 gram PoM £5.44 DT price = £5.44

Cream
CAUTIONARY AND ADVISORY LABELS 28
EXCIPIENTS: May contain Cetostearyl alcohol (including cetyl and stearyl alcohol), chlorocresol
▸ Eumovate (GlaxoSmithKline Consumer Healthcare, GlaxoSmithKline UK Ltd)
  Clobetasone butyrate 500 microgram per 1 gram Eumovate Eczema and Dermatitis 0.05% cream | 15 gram P £3.73 DT price = £3.57
  Eumovate 0.05% cream | 30 gram PoM £1.86 DT price = £1.86 | 100 gram PoM £5.44 DT price = £5.44

Combinations available: *Clobetasone butyrate with nystatin and oxytetracycline*, p. 712

F 704

Diflucortolone valerate

- **INDICATIONS AND DOSE**
Severe inflammatory skin disorders such as eczemas unresponsive to less potent corticosteroids (using 0.3% diflucortolone valerate) | Short-term treatment of severe exacerbations (using 0.3% diflucortolone valerate) | Psoriasis (using 0.3% diflucortolone valerate)
▸ TO THE SKIN
▸ Child 1 month-3 years: Apply 1–2 times a day for up to 2 weeks, reducing strength as condition responds, to be applied thinly
▸ Child 4-17 years: Apply 1–2 times a day for up to 2 weeks, reducing strength as condition responds, to be applied thinly; maximum 60 g per week

Severe inflammatory skin disorders such as eczemas unresponsive to less potent corticosteroids (using 0.1% diflucortolone valerate) | Psoriasis (using 0.1% diflucortolone valerate)
▸ TO THE SKIN
▸ Child: Apply 1–2 times a day for up to 4 weeks, to be applied thinly

POTENCY
Diflucortolone valerate 0.1% cream and ointment: potent.
Diflucortolone valerate 0.3% cream and ointment: very potent.

- **UNLICENSED USE** *Nerisone* ® licensed for use in children (age range not specified by manufacturer); *Nerisone Forte* ® not licensed for use in children under 4 years.

- **PRESCRIBING AND DISPENSING INFORMATION** Patients or carers should be advised on application of diflucortolone valerate containing preparations.

- **MEDICINAL FORMS**
There can be variation in the licensing of different medicines containing the same drug.

Ointment
CAUTIONARY AND ADVISORY LABELS 28
▸ Nerisone (Meadow Laboratories Ltd)
  Diflucortolone valerate 1 mg per 1 gram Nerisone 0.1% ointment | 30 gram PoM £3.98
  Diflucortolone valerate 3 mg per 1 gram Nerisone Forte 0.3% ointment | 15 gram PoM £4.70

Cream
CAUTIONARY AND ADVISORY LABELS 28
EXCIPIENTS: May contain Beeswax, cetostearyl alcohol (including cetyl and stearyl alcohol), disodium edetate, hydroxybenzoates (parabens)
▸ Nerisone (Meadow Laboratories Ltd)
  Diflucortolone valerate 1 mg per 1 gram Nerisone 0.1% cream | 30 gram PoM £3.98
  Nerisone 0.1% oily cream | 30 gram PoM £4.95 DT price = £4.95
  Diflucortolone valerate 3 mg per 1 gram Nerisone Forte 0.3% oily cream | 15 gram PoM £4.70 DT price = £4.70

F 704

Fludroxycortide

(Flurandrenolone)

- **INDICATIONS AND DOSE**
Inflammatory skin disorders such as eczemas
▸ TO THE SKIN
▸ Child: Apply 1–2 times a day, to be applied thinly

HAELAN® TAPE
Chronic localised recalcitrant dermatoses (but not acute or weeping)
▸ TO THE SKIN
▸ Child: Cut tape to fit lesion, apply to clean, dry skin shorn of hair, usually for 12 hours daily

POTENCY
Fludroxycortide 0.0125% cream and ointment: moderate

- **UNLICENSED USE** Licensed for use in children (age range not specified by manufacturer).

- **PATIENT AND CARER ADVICE** Patients or carers should be counselled on application of fludroxycortide cream and ointment.

- **MEDICINAL FORMS**
There can be variation in the licensing of different medicines containing the same drug.

Ointment
CAUTIONARY AND ADVISORY LABELS 28
EXCIPIENTS: May contain Beeswax, cetostearyl alcohol (including cetyl and stearyl alcohol), polysorbates
▸ Fludroxycortide (Non-proprietary)
  Fludroxycortide 125 microgram per 1 gram Fludroxycortide 0.0125% ointment | 60 gram PoM £5.99
▸ Haelan (Typharm Ltd)
  Fludroxycortide 125 microgram per 1 gram Haelan 0.0125% ointment | 60 gram PoM £3.26

Cream
CAUTIONARY AND ADVISORY LABELS 28
EXCIPIENTS: May contain Cetostearyl alcohol (including cetyl and stearyl alcohol), propylene glycol
▸ Fludroxycortide (Non-proprietary)
  Fludroxycortide 125 microgram per 1 gram Fludroxycortide 0.0125% cream | 60 gram PoM £5.99
▸ Haelan (Typharm Ltd)
  Fludroxycortide 125 microgram per 1 gram Haelan 0.0125% cream | 60 gram PoM £3.26

Impregnated dressing
▸ Fludroxycortide (Non-proprietary)
  Fludroxycortide 4 microgram per 1 square cm Fludroxycortide 4micrograms/square cm tape 7.5cm | 20 cm PoM £12.49 DT price = £12.49 | 40 cm PoM £19.99 | 80 cm PoM £28.66

F 704

Fluocinolone acetonide

- **INDICATIONS AND DOSE**
Severe inflammatory skin disorders such as eczemas | Psoriasis
▸ TO THE SKIN
▸ Child 1-17 years: Apply 1–2 times a day, to be applied thinly, reduce strength as condition responds

continued →

13

Skin

POTENCY

Fluocinolone acetonide 0.025% cream, gel, and ointment: potent.
Fluocinolone acetonide 0.00625% cream and ointment: moderate.
Fluocinolone acetonide 0.0025% cream: mild.

- **UNLICENSED USE** Not licensed for use in children under 1 year.
- **PRESCRIBING AND DISPENSING INFORMATION** Gel is useful for application to the scalp and other hairy areas.
- **PATIENT AND CARER ADVICE** Patient counselling is advised for fluocinolone acetonide cream, gel and ointment (application).

- **MEDICINAL FORMS**
There can be variation in the licensing of different medicines containing the same drug.
Ointment
CAUTIONARY AND ADVISORY LABELS 28
EXCIPIENTS: May contain Propylene glycol, wool fat and related substances including lanolin
▸ **Synalar** (Reig Jofre UK Ltd)
Fluocinolone acetonide 62.5 microgram per 1 gram Synalar 1 in 4 Dilution 0.00625% ointment | 50 gram [PoM] £4.84 DT price = £4.84
Fluocinolone acetonide 250 microgram per 1 gram Synalar 0.025% ointment | 30 gram [PoM] £4.14 DT price = £4.14 | 100 gram [PoM] £11.75 DT price = £11.75
Cream
CAUTIONARY AND ADVISORY LABELS 28
EXCIPIENTS: May contain Benzyl alcohol, cetostearyl alcohol (including cetyl and stearyl alcohol), polysorbates, propylene glycol
▸ **Synalar** (Reig Jofre UK Ltd)
Fluocinolone acetonide 25 microgram per 1 gram Synalar 1 in 10 Dilution 0.0025% cream | 50 gram [PoM] £4.58 DT price = £4.58
Fluocinolone acetonide 62.5 microgram per 1 gram Synalar 1 in 4 Dilution 0.00625% cream | 50 gram [PoM] £4.84 DT price = £4.84
Fluocinolone acetonide 250 microgram per 1 gram Synalar 0.025% cream | 30 gram [PoM] £4.14 DT price = £4.14 | 100 gram [PoM] £11.75 DT price = £11.75
Gel
CAUTIONARY AND ADVISORY LABELS 28
EXCIPIENTS: May contain Hydroxybenzoates (parabens), propylene glycol
▸ **Synalar** (Reig Jofre UK Ltd)
Fluocinolone acetonide 250 microgram per 1 gram Synalar 0.025% gel | 30 gram [PoM] £5.56 DT price = £5.56 | 60 gram [PoM] £10.02 DT price = £10.02

Combinations available: *Fluocinolone acetonide with clioquinol*, p. 712 · *Fluocinolone acetonide with neomycin*, p. 713

F 704

Fluocinonide

- **INDICATIONS AND DOSE**
Severe inflammatory skin disorders such as eczemas unresponsive to less potent corticosteroids | Psoriasis
▸ TO THE SKIN
▸ **Child:** Apply 1–2 times a day, to be applied thinly
POTENCY
Fluocinonide 0.05% cream and ointment: potent.

- **UNLICENSED USE** Not licensed for use in children under 1 year.
- **PATIENT AND CARER ADVICE** Patients or carers should be advised on the application of fluocinonide preparations.

- **MEDICINAL FORMS**
There can be variation in the licensing of different medicines containing the same drug. Forms available from special-order manufacturers include: ointment
Ointment
CAUTIONARY AND ADVISORY LABELS 28
EXCIPIENTS: May contain Propylene glycol, wool fat and related substances including lanolin
▸ **Metosyn** (Reig Jofre UK Ltd)
Fluocinonide 500 microgram per 1 gram Metosyn 0.05% ointment | 25 gram [PoM] £3.50 DT price = £3.50 | 100 gram [PoM] £13.15 DT price = £13.15
Cream
CAUTIONARY AND ADVISORY LABELS 28
EXCIPIENTS: May contain Propylene glycol
▸ **Metosyn FAPG** (Reig Jofre UK Ltd)
Fluocinonide 500 microgram per 1 gram Metosyn FAPG 0.05% cream | 25 gram [PoM] £3.96 DT price = £3.96 | 100 gram [PoM] £13.34 DT price = £13.34

F 704

Fluocortolone

- **INDICATIONS AND DOSE**
Severe inflammatory skin disorders such as eczemas unresponsive to less potent corticosteroides | Psoriasis
▸ TO THE SKIN
▸ **Child:** Apply 1–2 times a day, to be applied thinly
POTENCY
Fluocortolone hexanoate 0.25% cream and ointment; fluocortolone pivalate 0.25% cream and fluocortolone 0.25% ointment: moderate.

- **UNLICENSED USE** Licensed for use in children (age range not specified by manufacturer).
- **PRESCRIBING AND DISPENSING INFORMATION** Patients or carers should be counselled on the application of fluocortolone preparations.

- **MEDICINAL FORMS**
There can be variation in the licensing of different medicines containing the same drug.
No licensed medicines listed.

F 704

Fluticasone

04-Jan-2016

- **INDICATIONS AND DOSE**
Severe inflammatory skin disorders such as dermatitis and eczemas unresponsive to less potent corticosteroids | Psoriasis
▸ TO THE SKIN
▸ **Child 1-2 months:** Apply 1–2 times a day, to be applied thinly
▸ **Child 3 months-17 years:** Apply 1–2 times a day, to be applied thinly
POTENCY
Fluticasone cream 0.05%: potent.
Fluticasone ointment 0.005%: potent.

- **UNLICENSED USE** Not licensed for use in children under 3 months.
- **INTERACTIONS** → Appendix 1: corticosteroids
- **PATIENT AND CARER ADVICE** Patients or carers should be given advice on application of fluticasone creams and ointments.

- **MEDICINAL FORMS**
There can be variation in the licensing of different medicines containing the same drug.
Cream
CAUTIONARY AND ADVISORY LABELS 28
EXCIPIENTS: May contain Cetostearyl alcohol (including cetyl and stearyl alcohol), imidurea, propylene glycol

▸ **Cutivate** (GlaxoSmithKline UK Ltd)
Fluticasone propionate 500 microgram per 1 gram Cutivate
0.05% cream | 15 gram [PoM] £2.27 DT price = £2.27 |
30 gram [PoM] £4.24 DT price = £4.24

Ointment
CAUTIONARY AND ADVISORY LABELS 28
EXCIPIENTS: May contain Propylene glycol
▸ **Cutivate** (GlaxoSmithKline UK Ltd)
Fluticasone propionate 50 microgram per 1 gram Cutivate 0.005%
ointment | 15 gram [PoM] £2.27 DT price = £2.27 | 30 gram [PoM]
£4.24 DT price = £4.24

[F 704]

Hydrocortisone
18-May-2017

● **INDICATIONS AND DOSE**

Mild inflammatory skin disorders such as eczemas
▸ TO THE SKIN
▸ **Child:** Apply 1–2 times a day, to be applied thinly

Nappy rash
▸ TO THE SKIN
▸ **Child:** Apply 1–2 times a day for no longer than 1 week,
discontinued as soon as the inflammation subsides

POTENCY
Hydrocortisone cream and ointment 0.5 to 2.5%: mild

● **INTERACTIONS** → Appendix 1: corticosteroids

● **PRESCRIBING AND DISPENSING INFORMATION** When
hydrocortisone cream or ointment is prescribed and no
strength is stated, the 1% strength should be supplied.
Although *Dioderm®* contains only 0.1% hydrocortisone,
the formulation is designed to provide a clinical activity
comparable to that of Hydrocortisone Cream 1% BP.

● **PATIENT AND CARER ADVICE** Patient counselling is advised
for hydrocortisone cream and ointment (application).

● **PROFESSION SPECIFIC INFORMATION**

Dental practitioners' formulary
Hydrocortisone Cream 1% 15 g may be prescribed.

● **EXCEPTIONS TO LEGAL CATEGORY** Skin creams and
ointments containing hydrocortisone (alone or with other
ingredients) can be sold to the public for the treatment of
allergic contact dermatitis, irritant dermatitis, insect bite
reactions and mild to moderate eczema in patients over
10 years, to be applied sparingly over the affected area
1–2 times daily for max. 1 week. Over-the-counter
hydrocortisone preparations should not be sold without
medical advice for children under 10 years or for pregnant
women; they should **not** be sold for application to the
face, anogenital region, broken or infected skin (including
cold sores, acne, and athlete's foot).

● **MEDICINAL FORMS**
There can be variation in the licensing of different medicines
containing the same drug. Forms available from special-order
manufacturers include: liquid, cream, ointment

Cream
CAUTIONARY AND ADVISORY LABELS 28
EXCIPIENTS: May contain Benzyl alcohol, cetostearyl alcohol (including
cetyl and stearyl alcohol), hydroxybenzoates (parabens), propylene glycol
▸ **Hydrocortisone** (Non-proprietary)
Hydrocortisone 5 mg per 1 gram Hydrocortisone 0.5% cream |
15 gram [PoM] £3.00 DT price = £1.13 | 30 gram [PoM] £2.69–£4.90
Hydrocortisone 10 mg per 1 gram Hydrocortisone 1% cream |
15 gram [PoM] £10.50 DT price = £0.90 | 15 gram [P] £1.64 DT price =
£0.90 | 30 gram [PoM] £23.83 DT price = £1.80 | 50 gram [PoM]
£36.12 DT price = £3.00
Hydrocortisone 25 mg per 1 gram Hydrocortisone 2.5% cream |
15 gram [PoM] £44.00 DT price = £4.95 | 30 gram [PoM] £88.00
▸ **Derma Care Hydrocortisone** (The Boots Company Plc)
Hydrocortisone 10 mg per 1 gram Derma Care Hydrocortisone 1%
cream | 15 gram [P] no price available DT price = £0.90
▸ **Dermacort** (Marlborough Pharmaceuticals Ltd)
Hydrocortisone 1 mg per 1 gram Dermacort hydrocortisone 0.1%
cream | 15 gram [P] £2.83 DT price = £2.83

▸ **Dioderm** (Dermal Laboratories Ltd)
Hydrocortisone 1 mg per 1 gram Dioderm 0.1% cream |
30 gram [PoM] £2.03 DT price = £2.03
▸ **Hc45** (Reckitt Benckiser Healthcare (UK) Ltd)
Hydrocortisone acetate 10 mg per 1 gram Hc45 Hydrocortisone 1%
cream | 15 gram [P] £2.58
▸ **Mildison Lipocream** (LEO Pharma)
Hydrocortisone 10 mg per 1 gram Mildison Lipocream 1% cream |
30 gram [PoM] £1.71 DT price = £1.80
▸ **Zenoxone** (Teva UK Ltd)
Hydrocortisone 10 mg per 1 gram Zenoxone 1% cream |
15 gram [P] £1.25 DT price = £0.90

Ointment
CAUTIONARY AND ADVISORY LABELS 28
▸ **Hydrocortisone** (Non-proprietary)
Hydrocortisone 5 mg per 1 gram Hydrocortisone 0.5% ointment |
15 gram [PoM] £5.55 DT price = £5.55 | 30 gram [PoM] £11.10–£12.00
Hydrocortisone 10 mg per 1 gram Hydrocortisone 1% ointment |
15 gram [PoM] £10.50 DT price = £0.99 | 30 gram [P] £3.31 DT price =
£1.98 | 30 gram [PoM] £23.83 DT price = £1.98 | 50 gram [PoM]
£36.12 DT price = £3.30
Hydrocortisone 25 mg per 1 gram Hydrocortisone 2.5% ointment |
15 gram [PoM] £44.00 DT price = £24.43 | 30 gram [PoM] £88.00

Combinations available: *Hydrocortisone with benzalkonium
chloride, dimeticone and nystatin*, p. 713 · *Hydrocortisone with
chlorhexidine hydrochloride and nystatin*, p. 713 ·
Hydrocortisone with clotrimazole, p. 714 · *Hydrocortisone with
fusidic acid*, p. 714 · *Hydrocortisone with miconazole*, p. 714 ·
Hydrocortisone with oxytetracycline, p. 714

[F 704]

Hydrocortisone butyrate

● **INDICATIONS AND DOSE**

**Severe inflammatory skin disorders such as eczemas
unresponsive to less potent corticosteroids | Psoriasis**
▸ TO THE SKIN
▸ **Child 1–17 years:** Apply 1–2 times a day, to be applied
thinly

POTENCY
Hydrocortisone butyrate 0.1% cream, liquid, and
ointment: potent

● **PATIENT AND CARER ADVICE** Patients or carers should be
given advice on how to administer hydrocortisone butyrate
lotion, cream, ointment and scalp lotion.
Medicines for Children leaflet: Hydrocortisone (topical) for eczema
www.medicinesforchildren.org.uk/hydrocortisone-topical-for-
eczema

● **MEDICINAL FORMS**
There can be variation in the licensing of different medicines
containing the same drug. Forms available from special-order
manufacturers include: ointment

Ointment
CAUTIONARY AND ADVISORY LABELS 28
▸ **Locoid** (LEO Pharma)
Hydrocortisone butyrate 1 mg per 1 gram Locoid 0.1% ointment |
30 gram [PoM] £1.60 DT price = £1.60 | 100 gram [PoM] £4.93 DT
price = £4.93

Cream
CAUTIONARY AND ADVISORY LABELS 28
EXCIPIENTS: May contain Benzyl alcohol, cetostearyl alcohol (including
cetyl and stearyl alcohol), hydroxybenzoates (parabens)
▸ **Locoid** (LEO Pharma)
Hydrocortisone butyrate 1 mg per 1 gram Locoid 0.1% cream |
30 gram [PoM] £1.60 DT price = £1.60 | 100 gram [PoM] £4.93 DT
price = £4.93
▸ **Locoid Lipocream** (LEO Pharma)
Hydrocortisone butyrate 1 mg per 1 gram Locoid 0.1% Lipocream
| 30 gram [PoM] £1.69 DT price = £1.60 | 100 gram [PoM] £5.17 DT
price = £4.93

13

Skin

Liquid

CAUTIONARY AND ADVISORY LABELS 15(excluding Locoid Crelo topical emulsion), 28

EXCIPIENTS: May contain Butylated hydroxytoluene, cetostearyl alcohol (including cetyl and stearyl alcohol), hydroxybenzoates (parabens), propylene glycol

‣ Locoid (LEO Pharma)
  Hydrocortisone butyrate 1 mg per 1 ml Locoid 0.1% scalp lotion | 100 ml PoM £6.83 DT price = £6.83

‣ Locoid Crelo (LEO Pharma)
  Hydrocortisone butyrate 1 mg per 1 gram Locoid Crelo 0.1% topical emulsion | 100 gram PoM £5.91

Hydrocortisone with urea

The properties listed below are those particular to the combination only. For the properties of the components please consider, hydrocortisone p. 709.

● **INDICATIONS AND DOSE**

Mild inflammatory skin disorders such as eczemas
‣ TO THE SKIN
‣ Child: To be applied thinly (consult product literature)

POTENCY
Hydrocortisone 1% with urea cream: moderate

● **PATIENT AND CARER ADVICE** Patients or carers should be advised on application of hydrocortisone with urea cream.

● **MEDICINAL FORMS**
There can be variation in the licensing of different medicines containing the same drug.
Cream
CAUTIONARY AND ADVISORY LABELS 28
‣ Alphaderm (Alliance Pharmaceuticals Ltd)
  Hydrocortisone 10 mg per 1 gram, Urea 100 mg per 1 gram Alphaderm 1%/10% cream | 30 gram PoM £2.38 DT price = £2.38 | 100 gram PoM £7.03 DT price = £7.03

☞ 704

Mometasone furoate

● **INDICATIONS AND DOSE**

Severe inflammatory skin disorders such as eczemas unresponsive to less potent corticosteroids | Psoriasis
‣ TO THE SKIN
‣ Child 1 month-1 year: Apply once daily, to be applied thinly (to scalp in case of lotion)
‣ Child 2-17 years: Apply once daily, to be applied thinly (to scalp in case of lotion)

POTENCY
Mometasone furoate 0.1% cream, ointment, and scalp lotion: potent.

● **UNLICENSED USE** Not licensed for use in children under 2 years.

● **INTERACTIONS** → Appendix 1: corticosteroids

● **PATIENT AND CARER ADVICE** Patients and carers should be advised on the application of topical mometasone.

● **MEDICINAL FORMS**
There can be variation in the licensing of different medicines containing the same drug. Forms available from special-order manufacturers include: ointment
Cream
CAUTIONARY AND ADVISORY LABELS 28
EXCIPIENTS: May contain Beeswax
‣ Mometasone furoate (Non-proprietary)
  Mometasone furoate 1 mg per 1 gram Mometasone 0.1% cream | 30 gram PoM £4.36 DT price = £1.81 | 100 gram PoM £12.58 DT price = £6.03
‣ Elocon (Merck Sharp & Dohme Ltd)
  Mometasone furoate 1 mg per 1 gram Elocon 0.1% cream | 30 gram PoM £4.80 DT price = £1.81 | 100 gram PoM £15.10 DT price = £6.03

Ointment

CAUTIONARY AND ADVISORY LABELS 28
EXCIPIENTS: May contain Beeswax, propylene glycol
‣ Mometasone furoate (Non-proprietary)
  Mometasone furoate 1 mg per 1 gram Mometasone 0.1% ointment | 15 gram PoM £4.32 | 30 gram PoM £4.45 DT price = £1.86 | 50 gram PoM £12.44 | 100 gram PoM £12.82 DT price = £6.20
‣ Elocon (Merck Sharp & Dohme Ltd)
  Mometasone furoate 1 mg per 1 gram Elocon 0.1% ointment | 30 gram PoM £4.32 DT price = £1.86 | 100 gram PoM £12.44 DT price = £6.20

Liquid
CAUTIONARY AND ADVISORY LABELS 28
EXCIPIENTS: May contain Propylene glycol
‣ Elocon (Merck Sharp & Dohme Ltd)
  Mometasone furoate 1 mg per 1 gram Elocon 0.1% scalp lotion | 30 ml PoM £4.36 DT price = £4.36

CORTICOSTEROIDS › CORTICOSTEROID COMBINATIONS WITH ANTI-INFECTIVES

Betamethasone with clioquinol   18-Nov-2015

The properties listed below are those particular to the combination only. For the properties of the components please consider, betamethasone p. 705.

● **INDICATIONS AND DOSE**

Severe inflammatory skin disorders such as eczemas unresponsive to less potent corticosteroids | Psoriasis
‣ TO THE SKIN
‣ Child: (consult product literature)

POTENCY
Betamethasone (as valerate) 0.1% with clioquinol cream and ointment: potent.

● **UNLICENSED USE** Betamethasone and clioquinol preparations is not licensed for use in children under 1 year.

● **PATIENT AND CARER ADVICE** Stains clothing. Patients or carers should be counselled on application of betamethasone with clioquinol preparations.

● **MEDICINAL FORMS**
There can be variation in the licensing of different medicines containing the same drug.
Ointment
CAUTIONARY AND ADVISORY LABELS 28
‣ Betamethasone with clioquinol (Non-proprietary)
  Betamethasone (as Betamethasone valerate) 1 mg per 1 gram, Clioquinol 30 mg per 1 gram Betamethasone valerate 0.1% / Clioquinol 3% ointment | 30 gram PoM £38.88 DT price = £38.88
Cream
CAUTIONARY AND ADVISORY LABELS 28
EXCIPIENTS: May contain Cetostearyl alcohol (including cetyl and stearyl alcohol), chlorocresol
‣ Betamethasone with clioquinol (Non-proprietary)
  Betamethasone (as Betamethasone valerate) 1 mg per 1 gram, Clioquinol 30 mg per 1 gram Betamethasone valerate 0.1% / Clioquinol 3% cream | 30 gram PoM £38.88 DT price = £38.88

Betamethasone with clotrimazole

The properties listed below are those particular to the combination only. For the properties of the components please consider, betamethasone p. 705, clotrimazole p. 694.

● **INDICATIONS AND DOSE**

Severe inflammatory skin disorders such as eczemas unresponsive to less potent corticosteroids | Psoriasis
‣ TO THE SKIN
‣ Child: (consult product literature)

POTENCY
Betamethasone dipropionate 0.064% (=betamethasone 0.5%) with clotrimazole cream: potent.

13

Skin

- UNLICENSED USE *Lotriderm*® not licensed for use in children under 12 years.
- PATIENT AND CARER ADVICE Patients or carers should be given advice on how to administer betamethasone with clotrimazole cream.

- MEDICINAL FORMS
There can be variation in the licensing of different medicines containing the same drug.
Cream
CAUTIONARY AND ADVISORY LABELS 28
EXCIPIENTS: May contain Benzyl alcohol, cetostearyl alcohol (including cetyl and stearyl alcohol), propylene glycol
  ▸ Lotriderm (Merck Sharp & Dohme Ltd)
    Betamethasone dipropionate 640 microgram per 1 gram, Clotrimazole 10 mg per 1 gram Lotriderm cream | 30 gram PoM £6.34 DT price = £6.34

Betamethasone with fusidic acid

The properties listed below are those particular to the combination only. For the properties of the components please consider, betamethasone p. 705, fusidic acid p. 342.

- INDICATIONS AND DOSE
Severe inflammatory skin disorders such as eczemas unresponsive to less potent corticosteroids | Psoriasis
  ▸ TO THE SKIN
  ▸ Child: (consult product literature)
POTENCY
Betamethasone (as valerate) 0.1% with fusidic acid cream: potent.

- UNLICENSED USE *Fucibet*® *Lipid Cream* is not licensed for use in children under 6 years.
- PATIENT AND CARER ADVICE Patients or carers should be counselled on application of betamethasone with fusidic acid preparations.

- MEDICINAL FORMS
There can be variation in the licensing of different medicines containing the same drug.
Cream
CAUTIONARY AND ADVISORY LABELS 28
EXCIPIENTS: May contain Cetostearyl alcohol (including cetyl and stearyl alcohol), chlorocresol, hydroxybenzoates (parabens)
  ▸ Betamethasone with fusidic acid (Non-proprietary)
    Betamethasone (as Betamethasone valerate) 1 mg per 1 gram, Fusidic acid 20 mg per 1 gram Betamethasone valerate 0.1% / Fusidic acid 2% cream | 30 gram PoM £7.71 DT price = £6.38 | 60 gram PoM £15.42 DT price = £12.76
  ▸ Fucibet (LEO Pharma)
    Betamethasone (as Betamethasone valerate) 1 mg per 1 gram, Fusidic acid 20 mg per 1 gram Fucibet cream | 30 gram PoM £6.38 DT price = £6.38 | 60 gram PoM £12.76 DT price = £12.76
    Fucibet Lipid cream | 30 gram PoM £6.74 DT price = £6.38
  ▸ Xemacort (Mylan Ltd)
    Betamethasone (as Betamethasone valerate) 1 mg per 1 gram, Fusidic acid 20 mg per 1 gram Xemacort cream | 30 gram PoM £6.05 DT price = £6.38 | 60 gram PoM £12.45 DT price = £12.76

Betamethasone with neomycin

The properties listed below are those particular to the combination only. For the properties of the components please consider, betamethasone p. 705, neomycin sulfate p. 662.

- INDICATIONS AND DOSE
Severe inflammatory skin disorders such as eczemas unresponsive to less potent corticosteroids | Psoriasis
  ▸ TO THE SKIN USING OINTMENT, OR TO THE SKIN USING CREAM
  ▸ Child 1-23 months: Apply 1–2 times a day, to be applied thinly
  ▸ Child 2-17 years: Apply 1–2 times a day, to be applied thinly
POTENCY
Betamethasone (as valerate) 0.1% with neomycin cream and ointment: potent.

- UNLICENSED USE Betamethasone and neomycin preparations not licensed for use in children under 2 years.
- PATIENT AND CARER ADVICE Patient counselling is advised for betamethasone with neomycin cream and ointment (application).

- MEDICINAL FORMS
There can be variation in the licensing of different medicines containing the same drug.
Ointment
CAUTIONARY AND ADVISORY LABELS 28
  ▸ Betamethasone with neomycin (Non-proprietary)
    Betamethasone (as Betamethasone valerate) 1 mg per 1 gram, Neomycin sulfate 5 mg per 1 gram Betamethasone valerate 0.1% / Neomycin 0.5% ointment | 30 gram PoM £38.88 DT price = £31.36 | 100 gram PoM £97.00 DT price = £104.52
Cream
CAUTIONARY AND ADVISORY LABELS 28
EXCIPIENTS: May contain Cetostearyl alcohol (including cetyl and stearyl alcohol), chlorocresol
  ▸ Betamethasone with neomycin (Non-proprietary)
    Betamethasone (as Betamethasone valerate) 1 mg per 1 gram, Neomycin sulfate 5 mg per 1 gram Betamethasone valerate 0.1% / Neomycin 0.5% cream | 30 gram PoM £38.88 DT price = £31.36 | 100 gram PoM £97.00 DT price = £104.52

Betamethasone with salicylic acid

The properties listed below are those particular to the combination only. For the properties of the components please consider, betamethasone p. 705.

- INDICATIONS AND DOSE
DIPROSALIC® OINTMENT
Severe inflammatory skin disorders such as eczemas unresponsive to less potent corticosteroids | Psoriasis
  ▸ TO THE SKIN
  ▸ Child: Apply 1–2 times a day, max. 60 g per week
POTENCY
For *Diprosalic*® ointment: Betamethasone (as dipropionate) 0.05% with salicylic acid 3%: potent.

DIPROSALIC® SCALP APPLICATION
Severe inflammatory skin disorders such as eczemas unresponsive to less potent corticosteroids | Psoriasis
  ▸ TO THE SKIN
  ▸ Child: Apply 1–2 times a day, apply a few drops
POTENCY
For *Diprosalic*® scalp application: Betamethasone (as dipropionate) 0.05% with salicylic acid 2%: potent.

13

Skin

● PATIENT AND CARER ADVICE

DIPROSALIC® OINTMENT Patients or carers should be counselled on application of betamethasone and salicylic acid preparations.

DIPROSALIC® SCALP APPLICATION Patients or carers should be counselled on application of betamethasone and salicylic acid scalp application.

● MEDICINAL FORMS
There can be variation in the licensing of different medicines containing the same drug.

Ointment
CAUTIONARY AND ADVISORY LABELS 28
▸ Diprosalic (Merck Sharp & Dohme Ltd)
Betamethasone (as Betamethasone dipropionate) 500 microgram per 1 gram, Salicylic acid 30 mg per 1 gram Diprosalic 0.05%/3% ointment | 30 gram [PoM] £3.18 DT price = £3.18 | 100 gram [PoM] £9.14 DT price = £9.14

Liquid
CAUTIONARY AND ADVISORY LABELS 28
EXCIPIENTS: May contain Disodium edetate
▸ Diprosalic (Merck Sharp & Dohme Ltd)
Betamethasone (as Betamethasone dipropionate) 500 microgram per 1 ml, Salicylic acid 20 mg per 1 ml Diprosalic 0.05%/2% scalp application | 100 ml [PoM] £10.10 DT price = £10.10

Chlortetracycline with triamcinolone

● INDICATIONS AND DOSE

Severe inflammatory skin disorders such as eczemas unresponsive to less potent corticosteroids (associated with infection) | Psoriasis (associated with infection)
▸ TO THE SKIN
▸ Child 1 month-7 years: To be applied thinly (consult product literature)
▸ Child 8-17 years: To be applied thinly (consult product literature)

POTENCY
Triamcinolone acetonide 0.1%, chlortetracycline hydrochloride 3% ointment: potent.

● UNLICENSED USE Not licensed for use in children under 8 years.
● PATIENT AND CARER ADVICE Stains clothing. Patients or carers should be counselled on the application of chlortetracycline with triamcinolone products.

● MEDICINAL FORMS
There can be variation in the licensing of different medicines containing the same drug.
No licensed medicines listed.

Clobetasol propionate with neomycin sulfate and nystatin

The properties listed below are those particular to the combination only. For the properties of the components please consider, clobetasol propionate p. 706, neomycin sulfate p. 662.

● INDICATIONS AND DOSE

Short-term treatment only of severe resistant inflammatory skin disorders such as recalcitrant eczemas associated with infection and unresponsive to less potent corticosteroids | Psoriasis associated with infection
▸ TO THE SKIN
▸ Child: (consult product literature)

POTENCY
Clobetasol propionate 0.05% with neomycin sulfate and nystatin cream and ointment: very potent.

● UNLICENSED USE Clobetasol with neomycin and nystatin preparations not licensed for use in children under 2 years.
● PATIENT AND CARER ADVICE Patients or carers should be advised on application of clobetasol propionate, neomycin sulfate and nystatin containing preparations.

● MEDICINAL FORMS
There can be variation in the licensing of different medicines containing the same drug.

Ointment
CAUTIONARY AND ADVISORY LABELS 28
▸ Clobetasol propionate with neomycin sulfate and nystatin (Non-proprietary)
Clobetasol propionate 500 microgram per 1 gram, Neomycin sulfate 5 mg per 1 gram, Nystatin 100000 unit per 1 gram Clobetasol 500microgram / Neomycin 5mg / Nystatin 100,000units/g ointment | 30 gram [PoM] £87.00 DT price = £87.00

Cream
CAUTIONARY AND ADVISORY LABELS 28
▸ Clobetasol propionate with neomycin sulfate and nystatin (Non-proprietary)
Clobetasol propionate 500 microgram per 1 gram, Neomycin sulfate 5 mg per 1 gram, Nystatin 100000 unit per 1 gram Clobetasol 500microgram / Neomycin 5mg / Nystatin 100,000units/g cream | 30 gram [PoM] £87.00 DT price = £87.00

Clobetasone butyrate with nystatin and oxytetracycline

The properties listed below are those particular to the combination only. For the properties of the components please consider, clobetasone butyrate p. 706, oxytetracycline p. 339.

● INDICATIONS AND DOSE

Steroid-responsive dermatoses where candidal or bacterial infection is present
▸ TO THE SKIN
▸ Child: (consult product literature)

POTENCY
Clobetasone butyrate 0.05% with nystatin and oxytetracyline cream: moderate.

● PATIENT AND CARER ADVICE Stains clothing.

● MEDICINAL FORMS
There can be variation in the licensing of different medicines containing the same drug.
Cream
CAUTIONARY AND ADVISORY LABELS 28
EXCIPIENTS: May contain Cetostearyl alcohol (including cetyl and stearyl alcohol), chlorocresol, sodium metabisulfite
▸ Trimovate (GlaxoSmithKline UK Ltd)
Clobetasone butyrate 500 microgram per 1 gram, Oxytetracycline (as Oxytetracycline calcium) 30 mg per 1 gram, Nystatin 100000 unit per 1 gram Trimovate cream | 30 gram [PoM] £3.29

Fluocinolone acetonide with clioquinol

The properties listed below are those particular to the combination only. For the properties of the components please consider, fluocinolone acetonide p. 707.

● INDICATIONS AND DOSE

Inflammatory skin disorders such as eczemas associated with infection | Psoriasis associated with infection
▸ TO THE SKIN
▸ Child: Apply 1–2 times a day, to be applied thinly, reducing strength as condition responds

POTENCY
Clioquinol 3% with fluocinolone acetonide 0.025% cream and ointment: potent

- **PATIENT AND CARER ADVICE** Patient counselling is advised for clioquinol with fluocinolone acetonide cream and ointment (application). Ointment stains clothing.

- **MEDICINAL FORMS**
  There can be variation in the licensing of different medicines containing the same drug.
  Ointment
  CAUTIONARY AND ADVISORY LABELS 28
  EXCIPIENTS: May contain Propylene glycol, wool fat and related substances including lanolin
  ‣ Synalar C (Reig Jofre UK Ltd)
  Fluocinolone acetonide 250 microgram per 1 gram, Clioquinol 30 mg per 1 gram Synalar C ointment | 15 gram PoM £2.66
  Cream
  CAUTIONARY AND ADVISORY LABELS 28
  EXCIPIENTS: May contain Cetostearyl alcohol (including cetyl and stearyl alcohol), disodium edetate, hydroxybenzoates (parabens), polysorbates, propylene glycol
  ‣ Synalar C (Reig Jofre UK Ltd)
  Fluocinolone acetonide 250 microgram per 1 gram, Clioquinol 30 mg per 1 gram Synalar C cream | 15 gram PoM £2.66

Fluocinolone acetonide with neomycin

The properties listed below are those particular to the combination only. For the properties of the components please consider, fluocinolone acetonide p. 707, neomycin sulfate p. 692.

- **INDICATIONS AND DOSE**
  Inflammatory skin disorders such as eczemas associated with infection | Psoriasis associated with infection
  ‣ TO THE SKIN
  ‣ Child 1-11 months: Apply 1–2 times a day, to be applied thinly, reducing strength as condition responds
  ‣ Child 1-17 years: Apply 1–2 times a day, to be applied thinly, reducing strength as condition responds
  POTENCY
  Fluocinolone acetonide 0.025% with neomycin 0.5% cream and ointment: potent.

- **PATIENT AND CARER ADVICE** Patients or carers should be counselled on the application of fluocinolone acetonide with neomycin preparations.

- **MEDICINAL FORMS**
  There can be variation in the licensing of different medicines containing the same drug.
  Ointment
  CAUTIONARY AND ADVISORY LABELS 28
  EXCIPIENTS: May contain Propylene glycol, wool fat and related substances including lanolin
  ‣ Synalar N (Reig Jofre UK Ltd)
  Fluocinolone acetonide 250 microgram per 1 gram, Neomycin sulfate 5 mg per 1 gram Synalar N ointment | 30 gram PoM £4.36
  Cream
  CAUTIONARY AND ADVISORY LABELS 28
  EXCIPIENTS: May contain Cetostearyl alcohol (including cetyl and stearyl alcohol), hydroxybenzoates (parabens), polysorbates, propylene glycol
  ‣ Synalar N (Reig Jofre UK Ltd)
  Fluocinolone acetonide 250 microgram per 1 gram, Neomycin sulfate 5 mg per 1 gram Synalar N cream | 30 gram PoM £4.36

Hydrocortisone with benzalkonium chloride, dimeticone and nystatin

15-Mar-2016

The properties listed below are those particular to the combination only. For the properties of the components please consider, hydrocortisone p. 709, dimeticone p. 698.

- **INDICATIONS AND DOSE**
  Mild inflammatory skin disorders such as eczemas associated with infection
  ‣ TO THE SKIN
  ‣ Child: Apply 3 times a day until lesion has healed, to be applied thinly
  POTENCY
  Benzalkonium with dimeticone, hydrocortisone acetate 0.5%, and nystatin cream: mild.

- **PATIENT AND CARER ADVICE** Patients or carers should be advised on application of benzalkonium with dimeticone and hydrocortisone and nystatin preparations.

- **MEDICINAL FORMS**
  There can be variation in the licensing of different medicines containing the same drug.
  Cream
  CAUTIONARY AND ADVISORY LABELS 28
  EXCIPIENTS: May contain Butylated hydroxyanisole, cetostearyl alcohol (including cetyl and stearyl alcohol), hydroxybenzoates (parabens), sodium metabisulfite, sorbic acid
  ‣ Timodine (Alliance Pharmaceuticals Ltd)
  Benzalkonium chloride 1 mg per 1 gram, Hydrocortisone 5 mg per 1 gram, Dimeticone 350 100 mg per 1 gram, Nystatin 100000 unit per 1 gram Timodine cream | 30 gram PoM £3.37

Hydrocortisone with chlorhexidine hydrochloride and nystatin

The properties listed below are those particular to the combination only. For the properties of the components please consider, hydrocortisone p. 709, chlorhexidine p. 673.

- **INDICATIONS AND DOSE**
  Mild inflammatory skin disorders such as eczemas
  ‣ TO THE SKIN
  ‣ Child: To be applied thinly (consult product literature)
  POTENCY
  Hydrocortisone 0.5% with chlorhexidine hydrochloride 1% and nystatin cream: mild
  Hydrocortisone 1% with chlorhexidine hydrochloride 1% and nystatin ointment: mild

- **PATIENT AND CARER ADVICE** Patients or carers should be given advice on application of chlorhexidine hydrochloride with hydrocortisone and nystatin preparations.

- **MEDICINAL FORMS**
  There can be variation in the licensing of different medicines containing the same drug.
  Ointment
  CAUTIONARY AND ADVISORY LABELS 28
  ‣ Hydrocortisone with chlorhexidine hydrochloride and nystatin (Non-proprietary)
  Chlorhexidine acetate 10 mg per 1 gram, Hydrocortisone 10 mg per 1 gram, Nystatin 100000 unit per 1 gram Nystatin 100,000units/g / Chlorhexidine acetate 1% / Hydrocortisone 1% ointment | 30 gram PoM £5.29
  ‣ Nystaform HC (Typharm Ltd)
  Chlorhexidine acetate 10 mg per 1 gram, Hydrocortisone 10 mg per 1 gram, Nystatin 100000 unit per 1 gram Nystaform HC ointment | 30 gram PoM £2.66

13

Skin

Cream

CAUTIONARY AND ADVISORY LABELS 28

EXCIPIENTS: May contain Benzyl alcohol, cetostearyl alcohol (including cetyl and stearyl alcohol), polysorbates

▸ Hydrocortisone with chlorhexidine hydrochloride and nystatin (Non-proprietary)

Hydrocortisone 5 mg per 1 gram, Chlorhexidine hydrochloride 10 mg per 1 gram, Nystatin 100000 unit per 1 gram Nystatin 100,000units/g / Chlorhexidine hydrochloride 1% / Hydrocortisone 0.5% cream | 30 gram PoM £5.29

▸ Nystaform HC (Typharm Ltd)

Hydrocortisone 5 mg per 1 gram, Chlorhexidine hydrochloride 10 mg per 1 gram, Nystatin 100000 unit per 1 gram Nystaform HC cream | 30 gram PoM £2.66

Hydrocortisone with clotrimazole

The properties listed below are those particular to the combination only. For the properties of the components please consider, hydrocortisone p. 709, clotrimazole p. 694.

● **INDICATIONS AND DOSE**

Mild inflammatory skin disorders such as eczemas (associated with fungal infection)

▸ TO THE SKIN

▸ Child: (consult product literature)

POTENCY

Clotrimazole with hydrocortisone 1% cream: mild

● **PATIENT AND CARER ADVICE** Patients or carers should be given advice on how to administer clotrimazole with hydrocortisone cream.

● **EXCEPTIONS TO LEGAL CATEGORY** A 15-g tube is on sale to the public for the treatment of athlete's foot and fungal infection of skin folds with associated inflammation in patients 10 years and over.

● **MEDICINAL FORMS**

There can be variation in the licensing of different medicines containing the same drug.

Cream

CAUTIONARY AND ADVISORY LABELS 28

EXCIPIENTS: May contain Benzyl alcohol, cetostearyl alcohol (including cetyl and stearyl alcohol)

▸ Canesten HC (Bayer Plc)

Clotrimazole 10 mg per 1 gram, Hydrocortisone 10 mg per 1 gram Canesten HC cream | 30 gram PoM £2.42 DT price = £2.42

▸ Canesten Hydrocortisone (Bayer Plc)

Clotrimazole 10 mg per 1 gram, Hydrocortisone 10 mg per 1 gram Canesten Hydrocortisone cream | 15 gram P £3.11 DT price = £3.11

Hydrocortisone with fusidic acid

The properties listed below are those particular to the combination only. For the properties of the components please consider, hydrocortisone p. 709, fusidic acid p. 342.

● **INDICATIONS AND DOSE**

Mild inflammatory skin disorders such as eczemas

▸ TO THE SKIN

▸ Child: To be applied thinly (consult product literature)

POTENCY

Hydrocortisone with fusidic acid cream: mild

● **PATIENT AND CARER ADVICE** Patients or carers should be advised on application of hydrocortisone with fusidic acid preparations.

● **MEDICINAL FORMS**

There can be variation in the licensing of different medicines containing the same drug.

Cream

CAUTIONARY AND ADVISORY LABELS 28

EXCIPIENTS: May contain Butylated hydroxyanisole, cetostearyl alcohol (including cetyl and stearyl alcohol), polysorbates, potassium sorbate

▸ Fucidin H (Fusidic acid / Hydrocortisone) (LEO Pharma)

Hydrocortisone acetate 10 mg per 1 gram, Fusidic acid 20 mg per 1 gram Fucidin H cream | 30 gram PoM £6.02 DT price = £6.02 | 60 gram PoM £12.05 DT price = £12.05

Hydrocortisone with miconazole

The properties listed below are those particular to the combination only. For the properties of the components please consider, hydrocortisone p. 709, miconazole p. 695.

● **INDICATIONS AND DOSE**

Mild inflammatory skin disorders such as eczemas associated with infections

▸ TO THE SKIN

▸ Child: (consult product literature)

POTENCY

Hydrocortisone 1% with miconazole cream and ointment: mild

● **PATIENT AND CARER ADVICE** Patients or carers should be advised on application of hydrocortisone with miconazole preparations.

● **PROFESSION SPECIFIC INFORMATION**

Dental practitioners' formulary

May be prescribed as Miconazole and Hydrocortisone Cream or Ointment for max. 7 days.

● **EXCEPTIONS TO LEGAL CATEGORY** A 15-g tube of hydrocortisone with miconazole cream is on sale to the public for the treatment of athlete's foot and candidal intertrigo in children over 10 years.

● **MEDICINAL FORMS**

There can be variation in the licensing of different medicines containing the same drug.

Ointment

CAUTIONARY AND ADVISORY LABELS 28

▸ Daktacort (Janssen-Cilag Ltd)

Hydrocortisone 10 mg per 1 gram, Miconazole nitrate 20 mg per 1 gram Daktacort ointment | 30 gram PoM £2.50 DT price = £2.50

Cream

CAUTIONARY AND ADVISORY LABELS 28

EXCIPIENTS: May contain Butylated hydroxyanisole, disodium edetate

▸ Daktacort (McNeil Products Ltd, Janssen-Cilag Ltd)

Hydrocortisone 10 mg per 1 gram, Miconazole nitrate 20 mg per 1 gram Daktacort Hydrocortisone cream | 15 gram P £3.17 DT price = £3.17

Daktacort 2%/1% cream | 30 gram PoM £2.49 DT price = £2.49

Hydrocortisone with oxytetracycline

The properties listed below are those particular to the combination only. For the properties of the components please consider, hydrocortisone p. 709, oxytetracycline p. 339.

● **INDICATIONS AND DOSE**

Mild inflammatory skin disorders such as eczemas

▸ TO THE SKIN

▸ Child 12–17 years: (consult product literature)

POTENCY

Hydrocortisone 1% with oxytetracycline ointment: mild.

● **CONTRA-INDICATIONS** Children under 12 years

- **PREGNANCY** Tetracyclines should not be given to pregnant women. Effects on skeletal development have been documented when tetracyclines have been used in the first trimester in animal studies. Administration during the second or third trimester may cause discoloration of the child's teeth.

- **BREAST FEEDING** Tetracyclines should not be given to women who are breast-feeding (although absorption and therefore discoloration of teeth in the infant is probably usually prevented by chelation with calcium in milk).

- **PATIENT AND CARER ADVICE** Patients should be given advice on the application of hydrocortisone with oxytetracycline ointment.

- **MEDICINAL FORMS**
There can be variation in the licensing of different medicines containing the same drug.
Ointment
CAUTIONARY AND ADVISORY LABELS 28
  ▸ Terra-Cortril (Intrapharm Laboratories Ltd)
  Hydrocortisone 10 mg per 1 gram, Oxytetracycline (as Oxytetracycline hydrochloride) 30 mg per 1 gram Terra-Cortril ointment | 30 gram PoM £5.01 DT price = £5.01

DERMATOLOGICAL DRUGS > ANTI-INFECTIVES

Ichthammol

- **INDICATIONS AND DOSE**
Chronic lichenified eczema
  ▸ TO THE SKIN
  ▸ Child 1-17 years: Apply 1–3 times a day

- **UNLICENSED USE** No information available.
- **SIDE-EFFECTS** Skin irritation

- **MEDICINAL FORMS**
There can be variation in the licensing of different medicines containing the same drug. Forms available from special-order manufacturers include: ointment, paste
Liquid
  ▸ Ichthammol (Non-proprietary)
  Ichthammol 1 mg per 1 mg Ichthammol liquid | 100 gram GSL £11.42 DT price = £11.42 | 500 gram GSL £34.27

Ichthammol with zinc oxide

The properties listed below are those particular to the combination only. For the properties of the components please consider, ichthammol above.

- **INDICATIONS AND DOSE**
Chronic lichenified eczema
  ▸ TO THE SKIN
  ▸ Child: (consult product literature)

- **MEDICINAL FORMS**
There can be variation in the licensing of different medicines containing the same drug. Forms available from special-order manufacturers include: cream, ointment
Impregnated dressing
  ▸ Ichthopaste (Smith & Nephew Healthcare Ltd)
  Ichthopaste bandage 7.5cm × 6m | 1 bandage £3.72

DERMATOLOGICAL DRUGS > ANTRACEN DERIVATIVES

Dithranol

(Anthralin)

- **INDICATIONS AND DOSE**
Subacute and chronic psoriasis
  ▸ TO THE SKIN
  ▸ Child: (consult product literature)
DITHROCREAM®
Subacute and chronic psoriasis
  ▸ TO THE SKIN
  ▸ Child: For application to skin or scalp, 0.1–0.5% cream suitable for overnight treatment, 1–2% cream for maximum 1 hour (consult product literature)
MICANOL®
Subacute and chronic psoriasis
  ▸ TO THE SKIN
  ▸ Child: Apply once daily, for application to skin or scalp, to be applied for up to 30 minutes, apply 1% cream, if necessary 3% cream can be used under medical supervision

- **UNLICENSED USE**
DITHROCREAM® *Dithrocream®* is licensed for use in children (age range not specified by manufacturer).
MICANOL® *Micanol®* licensed for use in children, but not recommended for infants or young children (age range not specified by manufacturer).

- **CONTRA-INDICATIONS** Acute and pustular psoriasis · hypersensitivity

- **CAUTIONS** Avoid sensitive areas of skin · avoid use near eyes

- **SIDE-EFFECTS** Local burning sensation · local irritation · stains hair · stains skin

- **PREGNANCY** No adverse effects reported.

- **BREAST FEEDING** No adverse effects reported.

- **DIRECTIONS FOR ADMINISTRATION** When applying dithranol, hands should be protected by gloves or they should be washed thoroughly afterwards. Dithranol should be applied to chronic extensor plaques only, carefully avoiding normal skin.
MICANOL® At the end of contact time, use plenty of lukewarm (not hot) water to rinse off cream; soap may be used after the cream has been rinsed off; use shampoo before applying cream to scalp and if necessary after cream has been rinsed off.

- **PRESCRIBING AND DISPENSING INFORMATION** Treatment should be started with a low concentration such as dithranol 0.1%, and the strength increased gradually every few days up to 3%, according to tolerance.

- **PATIENT AND CARER ADVICE** Dithranol can stain the skin, hair and fabrics.

- **EXCEPTIONS TO LEGAL CATEGORY** Prescription only medicine if dithranol content more than 1%, otherwise may be sold to the public.

- **MEDICINAL FORMS**
There can be variation in the licensing of different medicines containing the same drug. Forms available from special-order manufacturers include: ointment
Cream
CAUTIONARY AND ADVISORY LABELS 28
EXCIPIENTS: May contain Cetostearyl alcohol (including cetyl and stearyl alcohol), chlorocresol
  ▸ Dithrocream (Dermal Laboratories Ltd)
  Dithranol 1 mg per 1 gram Dithrocream 0.1% cream | 50 gram P £3.77

13

Skin

Dithranol 2.5 mg per 1 gram Dithrocream 0.25% cream |
50 gram P £4.04
Dithranol 5 mg per 1 gram Dithrocream 0.5% cream | 50 gram P
£4.66
Dithranol 10 mg per 1 gram Dithrocream HP 1% cream |
50 gram P £5.42
Dithranol 20 mg per 1 gram Dithrocream 2% cream |
50 gram PoM £5.77

▸ Micanol (Reig Jofre UK Ltd)
Dithranol 10 mg per 1 gram Micanol 1% cream | 50 gram P
£16.18
Dithranol 30 mg per 1 gram Micanol 3% cream | 50 gram PoM
£20.15

Combinations available: *Coal tar with dithranol and salicylic acid*, p. 717

Dithranol with salicylic acid and zinc oxide

The properties listed below are those particular to the combination only. For the properties of the components please consider, dithranol p. 715.

● **INDICATIONS AND DOSE**

Subacute and chronic psoriasis
▸ TO THE SKIN
▸ Child: (consult local protocol)

● **MEDICINAL FORMS**
There can be variation in the licensing of different medicines containing the same drug. Forms available from special-order manufacturers include: ointment, paste

DERMATOLOGICAL DRUGS ❭ TARS

Coal tar

● **INDICATIONS AND DOSE**

Psoriasis | Chronic atopic eczema
▸ TO THE SKIN USING PASTE
▸ Child: Apply 1–3 times a day, start application with low-strength preparations
▸ TO THE SKIN
▸ Child: 100 mL/bath, to be added to an adult sized bath; add proportionally less for a child's bath. Use Coal Tar Solution BP

ALPHOSYL 2 IN 1® SHAMPOO

Psoriasis | Seborrhoeic dermatitis | Scaling | Itching
▸ TO THE SKIN
▸ Child: Apply every 2–3 days

Dandruff
▸ TO THE SKIN
▸ Child: Apply 1–2 times a week as required

EXOREX® LOTION

Psoriasis
▸ TO THE SKIN
▸ Child: Apply 2–3 times a day, to be applied to skin or scalp; can be diluted with a few drops of water before applying

● **CONTRA-INDICATIONS** Avoid broken or inflamed skin · avoid eye area · avoid genital area · avoid mucosal areas · avoid rectal area · infection · sore, acute, or pustular psoriasis

● **CAUTIONS** Application to face · application to skin flexures

● **SIDE-EFFECTS** Acne-like eruptions · photosensitivity · skin irritation

● **PRESCRIBING AND DISPENSING INFORMATION** Coal Tar Solution BP contains coal tar 20%, Strong Coal Tar Solution BP contains coal tar 40%.

● **HANDLING AND STORAGE** Use suitable chemical protection gloves for extemporaneous preparation. May stain skin, hair and fabric.

● **PATIENT AND CARER ADVICE** May stain skin, hair and fabric.

● **MEDICINAL FORMS**
There can be variation in the licensing of different medicines containing the same drug. Forms available from special-order manufacturers include: cream, ointment, paste

Bath additive
▸ Psoriderm (Dermal Laboratories Ltd)
Coal tar distilled 400 mg per 1 ml Psoriderm Emulsion 40% bath additive | 200 ml P £2.74

Cutaneous emulsion
EXCIPIENTS: May contain Hydroxybenzoates (parabens)
▸ Exorex (Teva UK Ltd)
Coal tar solution 50 mg per 1 gram Exorex lotion | 100 ml GSL
£8.11 DT price = £8.11 | 250 ml GSL £16.24 DT price = £16.24

Shampoo
EXCIPIENTS: May contain Fragrances, hydroxybenzoates (parabens)
▸ Coal tar (Non-proprietary)
Coal tar extract 20 mg per 1 gram Coal tar extract 2% shampoo |
125 ml GSL no price available DT price = £3.61 | 250 ml GSL no price available DT price = £5.38
▸ Brands may include Alphosyl 2 in 1, Neutrogena T/Gel Therapeutic, Polytar Scalp

Coal tar with arachis oil extract of coal tar, cade oil, light liquid paraffin and tar

The properties listed below are those particular to the combination only. For the properties of the components please consider, coal tar above.

● **INDICATIONS AND DOSE**

Psoriasis | Eczema | Atopic dermatoses | Pruritic dermatoses
▸ TO THE SKIN
▸ Child: 2–4 capfuls/bath, alternatively 15–30 mL, to be added in an adult-size bath and soak for 20 minutes (proportionally less for a child's bath)

● **MEDICINAL FORMS**
There can be variation in the licensing of different medicines containing the same drug.
No licensed medicines listed.

Coal tar with coconut oil and salicylic acid

The properties listed below are those particular to the combination only. For the properties of the components please consider, coal tar above.

● **INDICATIONS AND DOSE**

Scaly scalp disorders | Psoriasis | Seborrhoeic dermatitis | Dandruff | Cradle cap
▸ TO THE SKIN USING SHAMPOO
▸ Child: Apply daily as required

● **MEDICINAL FORMS**
There can be variation in the licensing of different medicines containing the same drug.

Shampoo
▸ Capasal (Dermal Laboratories Ltd)
Salicylic acid 5 mg per 1 gram, Coal tar distilled 10 mg per 1 gram, Coconut oil 10 mg per 1 gram Capasal Therapeutic shampoo |
250 ml P £4.69

Coal tar with dithranol and salicylic acid

The properties listed below are those particular to the combination only. For the properties of the components please consider, coal tar p. 716, dithranol p. 715.

- ● **INDICATIONS AND DOSE**
  Subacute and chronic psoriasis
  ▸ TO THE SKIN
  ▸ Child: Apply up to twice daily

- ● UNLICENSED USE *Psorin* ® is licensed for use in children (age range not specified by manufacturer).

- ● **MEDICINAL FORMS**
  There can be variation in the licensing of different medicines containing the same drug. Forms available from special-order manufacturers include: ointment

Coal tar with lecithin

The properties listed below are those particular to the combination only. For the properties of the components please consider, coal tar p. 716.

- ● **INDICATIONS AND DOSE**
  PSORIDERM® CREAM
  Psoriasis
  ▸ TO THE SKIN
  ▸ Child: Apply 1–2 times a day, cream to be applied to the skin or scalp
  PSORIDERM® SCALP LOTION
  Scalp psoriasis
  ▸ TO THE SKIN
  ▸ Child: Apply as required

- ● **MEDICINAL FORMS**
  There can be variation in the licensing of different medicines containing the same drug.
  Cream
  EXCIPIENTS: May contain Isopropyl palmitate, propylene glycol
  ▸ Psoriderm (Dermal Laboratories Ltd)
  Lecithin 4 mg per 1 gram, Coal tar distilled 60 mg per 1 gram Psoriderm cream | 225 ml P £9.42
  Shampoo
  EXCIPIENTS: May contain Disodium edetate
  ▸ Psoriderm (Dermal Laboratories Ltd)
  Lecithin 3 mg per 1 ml, Coal tar distilled 25 mg per 1 ml Psoriderm scalp lotion | 250 ml P £4.74

Coal tar with salicylic acid and precipitated sulfur

The properties listed below are those particular to the combination only. For the properties of the components please consider, coal tar p. 716.

- ● **INDICATIONS AND DOSE**
  COCOIS® OINTMENT
  Scaly scalp disorders including psoriasis, eczema, seborrhoeic dermatitis and dandruff
  ▸ INITIALLY TO THE SKIN USING SCALP OINTMENT
  ▸ Child 6–11 years: Medical supervision required
  ▸ Child 12–17 years: Apply once weekly as required, alternatively (to the skin) apply daily for the first 3–7 days (if severe), shampoo off after 1 hour

SEBCO® OINTMENT
Scaly scalp disorders including psoriasis, eczema, seborrhoeic dermatitis
▸ TO THE SKIN USING SCALP OINTMENT
▸ Child 6–11 years: Medical supervision required
▸ Child 12–17 years: Apply as required, alternatively apply daily for the first 3–7 days (if severe), shampoo off after 1 hour

- ● **MEDICINAL FORMS**
  There can be variation in the licensing of different medicines containing the same drug.
  Ointment
  EXCIPIENTS: May contain Cetostearyl alcohol (including cetyl and stearyl alcohol)
  ▸ Cocois (Focus Pharmaceuticals Ltd)
  Salicylic acid 20 mg per 1 gram, Sulfur precipitated 40 mg per 1 gram, Coal tar solution 120 mg per 1 gram Cocois ointment | 40 gram GSL £6.22 | 100 gram GSL £11.69
  ▸ Sebco (Derma UK Ltd)
  Salicylic acid 20 mg per 1 gram, Sulfur precipitated 40 mg per 1 gram, Coal tar solution 120 mg per 1 gram Sebco ointment | 40 gram GSL £5.91 | 100 gram GSL £11.11

Coal tar with zinc oxide
26-Aug-2016

The properties listed below are those particular to the combination only. For the properties of the components please consider, coal tar p. 716.

- ● **INDICATIONS AND DOSE**
  Psoriasis | Chronic atopic eczema
  ▸ TO THE SKIN
  ▸ Child: Apply 1–2 times a day

IMPORTANT SAFETY INFORMATION
MHRA/CHM UPDATE (APRIL 2016): FIRE RISK WITH PARAFFIN-BASED SKIN EMOLLIENTS ON DRESSINGS OR CLOTHING
See Emollient and barrier preparations p. 683.

- ● **PRESCRIBING AND DISPENSING INFORMATION** No preparations available—when prepared extemporaneously, the BP states Zinc and Coal Tar Paste, BP consists of zinc oxide 6%, coal tar 6%, emulsifying wax 5%, starch 38%, yellow soft paraffin 45%.

- ● **MEDICINAL FORMS**
  There can be variation in the licensing of different medicines containing the same drug. Forms available from special-order manufacturers include: ointment, paste

Extract of coal tar with arachis oil

The properties listed below are those particular to the combination only. For the properties of the components please consider, coal tar p. 716.

- ● **INDICATIONS AND DOSE**
  Scalp disorders | Psoriasis | Seborrhoea | Eczema | Pruritus | Dandruff
  ▸ TO THE SKIN
  ▸ Child: Apply 1–2 times a week, to the scalp

- ● **MEDICINAL FORMS**
  There can be variation in the licensing of different medicines containing the same drug.
  No licensed medicines listed.

13

Skin

IMMUNOSUPPRESSANTS > CALCINEURIN INHIBITORS AND RELATED DRUGS

Pimecrolimus

- **INDICATIONS AND DOSE**

Short-term treatment of mild to moderate atopic eczema (including flares) when topical corticosteroids cannot be used (initiated by a specialist)

▶ TO THE SKIN

▸ Child 2–17 years: Apply twice daily until symptoms resolve (stop treatment if eczema worsens or no response after 6 weeks)

- **CONTRA-INDICATIONS** Application to malignant or potentially malignant skin lesions · application under occlusion · congenital epidermal barrier defects · contact with eyes · contact with mucous membranes · generalised erythroderma · immunodeficiency · infection at treatment site

- **CAUTIONS** Alcohol consumption (risk of facial flushing and skin irritation) · avoid other topical treatments except emollients at treatment site · UV light (avoid excessive exposure to sunlight and sunlamps)

- **INTERACTIONS** → Appendix 1: pimecrolimus

- **SIDE-EFFECTS**
- ▸ **Common or very common** Burning sensation · erythema · folliculitis · pruritus · skin infections
- ▸ **Uncommon** Herpes simplex · herpes zoster · impetigo · molluscum contagiosum
- ▸ **Rare** Dryness · local reactions including pain · oedema · papilloma · paraesthesia · peeling · skin discolouration · worsening of eczema
- ▸ **Frequency not known** Skin malignancy

- **PREGNANCY** Manufacturer advises avoid; toxicity in *animal* studies following systemic administration.

- **BREAST FEEDING** Manufacturer advises caution; ensure infant does not come in contact with treated areas.

- **NATIONAL FUNDING/ACCESS DECISIONS**

NICE technology appraisals (TAs)
- ▸ Tacrolimus and pimecrolimus for atopic eczema (August 2004) NICE TA82

Topical pimecrolimus is an option for atopic eczema not controlled by maximal topical corticosteroid treatment or if there is a risk of important corticosteroid side-effects (particularly skin atrophy).

Topical pimecrolimus is recommended for moderate atopic eczema on the face and neck of children aged 2–16 years. Pimecrolimus should be used within its licensed indications.
www.nice.org.uk/TA82

- **MEDICINAL FORMS**
There can be variation in the licensing of different medicines containing the same drug.

Cream
CAUTIONARY AND ADVISORY LABELS 4, 11, 28
EXCIPIENTS: May contain Benzyl alcohol, cetostearyl alcohol (including cetyl and stearyl alcohol), propylene glycol
- ▸ **Elidel** (Meda Pharmaceuticals Ltd)
Pimecrolimus 10 mg per 1 gram Elidel 1% cream | 30 gram [PoM] £19.69 DT price = £19.69 | 60 gram [PoM] £37.41 DT price = £37.41 | 100 gram [PoM] £59.07 DT price = £59.07

Tacrolimus

- **DRUG ACTION** Tacrolimus is a calcineurin inhibitor.

- **INDICATIONS AND DOSE**

Short-term treatment of moderate to severe atopic eczema (including flares) in patients unresponsive to, or intolerant of conventional therapy (initiated by a specialist)

▶ TO THE SKIN

▸ Child 2–15 years: Apply twice daily for up to 3 weeks (consider other treatment if eczema worsens or if no improvement after 2 weeks), 0.03% ointment to be applied thinly, then reduced to once daily until lesion clears

▸ Child 16–17 years: Apply twice daily until lesion clears (consider other treatment if eczema worsens or no improvement after 2 weeks), initially 0.1% ointment to be applied thinly, reduce frequency to once daily or strength of ointment to 0.03% if condition allows

Prevention of flares in patients with moderate to severe atopic eczema and 4 or more flares a year who have responded to initial treatment with topical tacrolimus (initiated by a specialist)

▶ TO THE SKIN

▸ Child 2–15 years: Apply twice weekly, 0.03% ointment to be applied thinly, with an interval of 2–3 days between applications, use short-term treatment regimen during an acute flare; review need for preventative therapy after 1 year

▸ Child 16–17 years: Apply twice weekly, 0.1% ointment to be applied thinly, with an interval of 2–3 days between applications, use short-term treatment regimen during an acute flare; review need for preventative therapy after 1 year

- **CONTRA-INDICATIONS** Application to malignant or potentially malignant skin lesions · application under occlusion · avoid contact with eyes · avoid contact with mucous membranes · congenital epidermal barrier defects · generalised erythroderma · immunodeficiency · infection at treatment site

- **CAUTIONS** UV light (avoid excessive exposure to sunlight and sunlamps)

- **INTERACTIONS** → Appendix 1: tacrolimus

- **SIDE-EFFECTS**
- ▸ **Common or very common** Application-site infections · application-site reactions · herpes simplex infection · irritation (at application-site) · Kaposi's varicelliform eruption · pain at application-site · rash
- ▸ **Uncommon** Acne
- ▸ **Frequency not known** Cutaneous lymphoma · malignancies · other types of lymphomas · rosacea · skin malignancy

- **ALLERGY AND CROSS-SENSITIVITY** Contra-indicated if history of hypersensitivity to macrolides.

- **PREGNANCY** Manufacturer advises avoid unless essential; toxicity in *animal* studies following systemic administration.

- **BREAST FEEDING** Avoid—present in breast milk (following systemic administration).

- **PATIENT AND CARER ADVICE** Avoid excessive exposure to UV light including sunlight.

- **NATIONAL FUNDING/ACCESS DECISIONS**

NICE technology appraisals (TAs)
- ▸ Tacrolimus and pimecrolimus for atopic eczema (August 2004) NICE TA82

Topical tacrolimus is an option for atopic eczema not controlled by maximal topical corticosteroid treatment or if there is a risk of important corticosteroid side-effects (particularly skin atrophy).

Topical tacrolimus is recommended for moderate to severe atopic eczema in children over 2 years. Tacrolimus should be used within its licensed indications. www.nice.org.uk/TA82

Scottish Medicines Consortium (SMC) Decisions
The *Scottish Medicines Consortium* has advised (March 2010) that tacrolimus ointment (*Protopic*®) is accepted for restricted use within NHS Scotland for the prevention of flares in patients aged over 2 years with moderate to severe atopic eczema in accordance with the licensed indications; initiation of treatment is restricted to doctors (including general practitioners) with a specialist interest and experience in treating atopic eczema with immunomodulatory therapy.

● **MEDICINAL FORMS**
There can be variation in the licensing of different medicines containing the same drug.
Ointment
CAUTIONARY AND ADVISORY LABELS 4, 11, 28
EXCIPIENTS: May contain Beeswax
▸ Protopic (LEO Pharma)
  Tacrolimus (as Tacrolimus monohydrate) 300 microgram per 1 gram Protopic 0.03% ointment | 30 gram [PoM] £23.33 DT price = £23.33 | 60 gram [PoM] £42.55 DT price = £42.55
  Tacrolimus (as Tacrolimus monohydrate) 1 mg per 1 gram Protopic 0.1% ointment | 30 gram [PoM] £25.92 DT price = £25.92 | 60 gram [PoM] £47.28 DT price = £47.28

RETINOID AND RELATED DRUGS

Acitretin

● **DRUG ACTION** Acitretin is a metabolite of etretinate.

● **INDICATIONS AND DOSE**
Severe extensive psoriasis resistant to other forms of therapy (under expert supervision) | Palmoplantar pustular psoriasis (under expert supervision) | Severe congenital ichthyosis (under expert supervision)
▸ BY MOUTH
▸ **Child 1 month–11 years:** 0.5 mg/kg once daily; increased if necessary to 1 mg/kg once daily, to be taken with food or milk, careful monitoring of musculoskeletal development required; maximum 35 mg per day
▸ **Child 12–17 years:** Initially 25–30 mg daily for 2–4 weeks, then adjusted according to response to 25–50 mg daily, increased to up to 75 mg daily, dose only increased to 75 mg daily for short periods in psoriasis

Severe Darier's disease (keratosis follicularis) (under expert supervision)
▸ BY MOUTH
▸ **Child 1 month–11 years:** 0.5 mg/kg once daily; increased if necessary to 1 mg/kg once daily, to be taken with food or milk, careful monitoring of musculoskeletal development required; maximum 35 mg per day
▸ **Child 12–17 years:** Initially 10 mg daily for 2–4 weeks, then adjusted according to response to 25–50 mg daily

Harlequin ichthyosis (under expert supervision)
▸ BY MOUTH
▸ **Neonate:** 0.5 mg/kg once daily; increased if necessary to 1 mg/kg once daily, to be taken with food or milk, careful monitoring of musculoskeletal development required.

● **CONTRA-INDICATIONS** Hyperlipidaemia
● **CAUTIONS** Avoid excessive exposure to sunlight and unsupervised use of sunlamps · diabetes (can alter glucose tolerance—initial frequent blood glucose checks) · do not donate blood during and for 2 years after stopping therapy (teratogenic risk) · in children use only in exceptional

circumstances and monitor growth parameters and bone development (premature epiphyseal closure reported) · investigate atypical musculoskeletal symptoms

● **INTERACTIONS** → Appendix 1: retinoids
● **SIDE-EFFECTS**
▸ **Common or very common** Abdominal pain · abnormal hair texture · alopecia (reversible on withdrawal) · arthralgia · brittle nails · dermatitis · diarrhoea · dryness and inflammation of mucous membranes · dryness of conjunctiva (causing conjunctivitis and decreased tolerance to contact lenses) · epidermal fragility · erythema · headache · myalgia · nausea · paronychia · peripheral oedema · pruritus · reversible increase in serum-cholesterol (with high doses) · reversible increase in serum-triglyceride concentrations (with high doses) · skin exfoliation · sticky skin · vomiting
▸ **Uncommon** Dizziness · hepatitis · photosensitivity · visual disturbances
▸ **Rare** Peripheral neuropathy
▸ **Very rare** Benign intracranial hypertension · bone pain · exostosis · night blindness · ulcerative keratitis
▸ **Frequency not known** Drowsiness · dry skin · flushing · granulomatous lesions · impaired hearing · initial worsening of psoriasis · malaise · rectal haemorrhage · sweating · taste disturbance · tinnitus

SIDE-EFFECTS, FURTHER INFORMATION
▸ Exostosis Skeletal hyperostosis and extra-osseous calcification reported following long-term treatment with etretinate (of which Acitretin is a metabolite) and premature epiphyseal closure in children.
▸ Benign intracranial hypertension Discontinue if severe headache, nausea, vomiting, or visual disturbances occur.

● **CONCEPTION AND CONTRACEPTION** Effective contraception must be used.
Pregnancy prevention In females of child-bearing potential (including those with a history of infertility), exclude pregnancy up to 3 days before treatment, every month during treatment, and every 1–3 months for 3 years after stopping treatment. Treatment should be started on day 2 or 3 of menstrual cycle. Females of child-bearing age must practise effective contraception for at least 1 month before starting treatment, during treatment, and for at least 3 years after stopping treatment. Females should be advised to use at least 1 method of contraception, but ideally they should use 2 methods of contraception. Oral progestogen-only contraceptives are not considered effective. Barrier methods should not be used alone but can be used in conjunction with other contraceptive methods. Females should be advised to seek medical attention immediately if they become pregnant during treatment or within 3 years of stopping treatment. They should also be advised to avoid alcohol during treatment and for 2 months after stopping treatment.

● **PREGNANCY** Avoid—teratogenic.
● **BREAST FEEDING** Avoid.
● **HEPATIC IMPAIRMENT** Avoid in severe impairment—risk of further impairment.
● **RENAL IMPAIRMENT** Avoid in severe impairment; increased risk of toxicity.
● **MONITORING REQUIREMENTS**
▸ Monitor serum-triglyceride and serum-cholesterol concentrations before treatment, 1 month after starting, then every 3 months.
▸ Check liver function at start, at least every 4 weeks for first 2 months and then every 3 months.
● **PRESCRIBING AND DISPENSING INFORMATION**
Prescribing for women of child-bearing potential Each prescription for acitretin should be limited to a supply of up to 30 days' treatment and dispensed within 7 days of the date stated on the prescription.

- **PATIENT AND CARER ADVICE** A patient information leaflet should be provided.
  Females of child-bearing potential must be advised on pregnancy prevention.

- **MEDICINAL FORMS**
  There can be variation in the licensing of different medicines containing the same drug. Forms available from special-order manufacturers include: oral suspension, oral solution

  Capsule
  CAUTIONARY AND ADVISORY LABELS 10, 11, 21
  ▸ Acitretin (Non-proprietary)
    Acitretin 10 mg Acitretin 10mg capsules | 60 capsule PoM £23.80 DT price = £23.80
    Acitretin 25 mg Acitretin 25mg capsules | 60 capsule PoM £55.24 DT price = £55.24
  ▸ Neotigason (Teva UK Ltd)
    Acitretin 10 mg Neotigason 10mg capsules | 60 capsule PoM £17.30 DT price = £23.80 (Hospital only)
    Acitretin 25 mg Neotigason 25mg capsules | 60 capsule PoM £43.00 DT price = £55.24 (Hospital only)

SALICYLIC ACID AND DERIVATIVES

Salicylic acid with zinc oxide

- **INDICATIONS AND DOSE**

  Hyperkeratotic skin disorders
  ▸ TO THE SKIN
  ▸ Child: Apply twice daily

- **CAUTIONS** Avoid broken skin · avoid inflamed skin
  CAUTIONS, FURTHER INFORMATION
  ▸ Salicylate toxicity Salicylate toxicity may occur particularly if applied on large areas of skin or neonatal skin.

- **SIDE-EFFECTS** Excessive drying · irritation · sensitivity · systemic effects (after widespread use)

- **PRESCRIBING AND DISPENSING INFORMATION** Zinc and Salicylic Acid Paste BP is also referred to as Lassar's Paste. When prepared extemporaneously, the BP states Zinc and Salicylic Acid Paste, BP (Lassar's Paste) consists of zinc oxide 24%, salicylic acid 2%, starch 24%, white soft paraffin 50%.

- **MEDICINAL FORMS**
  There can be variation in the licensing of different medicines containing the same drug. Forms available from special-order manufacturers include: paste

VITAMINS AND TRACE ELEMENTS › VITAMIN D AND ANALOGUES

Calcipotriol

- **INDICATIONS AND DOSE**

  Plaque psoriasis
  ▸ TO THE SKIN USING OINTMENT
  ▸ Child 6–11 years: Apply twice daily, when preparations used together maximum total calcipotriol 2.5 mg in any one week (e.g. scalp solution 20 mL with ointment 30 g); maximum 50 g per week
  ▸ Child 12–17 years: Apply twice daily, when preparations used together maximum total calcipotriol 3.75 mg in any one week (e.g. scalp solution 30 mL with ointment 45 g); maximum 75 g per week

  Scalp psoriasis
  ▸ TO THE SKIN USING SCALP LOTION
  ▸ Child 6–11 years (specialist use only): Apply twice daily, when preparations used together max. total calcipotriol 2.5 mg in any one week (e.g. scalp solution 20 mL with ointment 30 g); maximum 30 mL per week

  ▸ Child 12–17 years (specialist use only): Apply twice daily, when preparations used together maximum total calcipotriol 3.75 mg in any one week (e.g. scalp solution 30 mL with ointment 45 g); maximum 45 mL per week

- **UNLICENSED USE** Calcipotriol ointment and scalp solution not licensed for use in children.

- **CONTRA-INDICATIONS** Calcium metabolism disorders

- **CAUTIONS** Avoid excessive exposure to sunlight and sunlamps · avoid use on face · erythrodermic exfoliative psoriasis (enhanced risk of hypercalcaemia) · generalised pustular psoriasis (enhanced risk of hypercalcaemia)

- **INTERACTIONS** → Appendix 1: vitamin D substances

- **SIDE-EFFECTS**
- **Common or very common** Burning · dermatitis · erythema · itching · local skin reactions · paraesthesia
- **Rare** Facial dermatitis · perioral dermatitis
- **Frequency not known** Aggravation of psoriasis · dry skin · photosensitivity

- **PREGNANCY** Manufacturers advise avoid unless essential.

- **BREAST FEEDING** No information available.

- **HEPATIC IMPAIRMENT** Manufacturers advise avoid in severe impairment.

- **RENAL IMPAIRMENT** Manufacturers advise avoid in severe impairment.

- **PATIENT AND CARER ADVICE**
  Advice on application Patient information leaflet for *Dovonex®* ointment advises liberal application. However, patients should be advised of maximum recommended weekly dose.
  Hands should be washed thoroughly after application to avoid inadvertent transfer to other body areas.

- **MEDICINAL FORMS**
  There can be variation in the licensing of different medicines containing the same drug. Forms available from special-order manufacturers include: ointment

  Ointment
  EXCIPIENTS: May contain Disodium edetate, propylene glycol
  ▸ Calcipotriol (Non-proprietary)
    Calcipotriol 50 microgram per 1 gram Calcipotriol 50micrograms/g ointment | 30 gram PoM £7.37 DT price = £5.78 | 60 gram PoM £11.56–£13.86 | 120 gram PoM £23.12–£27.75
  ▸ Dovonex (LEO Pharma)
    Calcipotriol 50 microgram per 1 gram Dovonex 50micrograms/g ointment | 30 gram PoM £5.78 DT price = £5.78 | 60 gram PoM £11.56

  Liquid
  ▸ Calcipotriol (Non-proprietary)
    Calcipotriol (as Calcipotriol hydrate) 50 microgram per 1 ml Calcipotriol 50micrograms/ml scalp solution | 60 ml PoM £56.94 DT price = £56.94 | 120 ml PoM £113.88 DT price = £113.88

  Combinations available: *Calcipotriol with betamethasone*, p. 705

Calcitriol

(1,25-Dihydroxycholecalciferol)

- **INDICATIONS AND DOSE**

  Mild to moderate plaque psoriasis
  ▸ TO THE SKIN
  ▸ Child 12–17 years: Apply twice daily, not more than 35% of body surface to be treated daily; maximum 30 g per day

- **CONTRA-INDICATIONS** Do not apply under occlusion · patients with calcium metabolism disorders

- **CAUTIONS** Erythrodermic exfoliative psoriasis (enhanced risk of hypercalcaemia) · generalised pustular psoriasis (enhanced risk of hypercalcaemia)
- **INTERACTIONS** → Appendix 1: vitamin D substances
- **SIDE-EFFECTS**
  - **Common or very common** Burning · dermatitis · erythema · itching · local skin reactions · paraesthesia
  - **Frequency not known** Aggravation of psoriasis
- **PREGNANCY** Manufacturer advises use in restricted amounts only if clearly necessary.
  Monitor urine- and serum-calcium concentration in pregnancy.
- **BREAST FEEDING** Manufacturer advises avoid.
- **HEPATIC IMPAIRMENT** Manufacturer advises avoid—no information available.
- **RENAL IMPAIRMENT** Manufacturer advises avoid—no information available.
- **HANDLING AND STORAGE** Hands should be washed thoroughly after application to avoid inadvertent transfer to other body areas.

- **MEDICINAL FORMS**
  There can be variation in the licensing of different medicines containing the same drug.
  Ointment
  - ▸ Silkis (Galderma (UK) Ltd)
    Calcitriol 3 microgram per 1 gram Silkis ointment |
    100 gram PoM £18.06 DT price = £18.06

Tacalcitol

- **INDICATIONS AND DOSE**
  Plaque psoriasis
  - ▸ TO THE SKIN
  - ▸ Child 12–17 years: Apply once daily, preferably at bedtime, maximum 10 g ointment or 10 mL lotion daily, when lotion and ointment used together, maximum total tacalcitol 280 micrograms in any one week (e.g. lotion 30 mL with ointment 40 g)

- **CONTRA-INDICATIONS** Calcium metabolism disorders
- **CAUTIONS** Avoid eyes · erythrodermic exfoliative psoriasis (enhanced risk of hypercalcaemia) · generalised pustular psoriasis (enhanced risk of hypercalcaemia) · if used in conjunction with UV treatment
  CAUTIONS, FURTHER INFORMATION
  - ▸ UV treatment If tacalcitol is used in conjunction with UV treatment, UV radiation should be given in the morning and tacalcitol applied at bedtime.
- **INTERACTIONS** → Appendix 1: vitamin D substances
- **SIDE-EFFECTS**
  - **Common or very common** Burning · dermatitis · erythema · itching · local skin reactions · paraesthesia
  - **Frequency not known** Aggravation of psoriasis
- **PREGNANCY** Manufacturer advises avoid unless no safer alternative—no information available.
- **BREAST FEEDING** Manufacturer advises avoid application to breast area; no information available on presence in milk.
- **RENAL IMPAIRMENT** Monitor serum calcium concentration.
- **MONITORING REQUIREMENTS** Monitor serum calcium if risk of hypercalcaemia.
- **PATIENT AND CARER ADVICE** Hands should be washed thoroughly after application to avoid inadvertent transfer to other body areas.

- **MEDICINAL FORMS**
  There can be variation in the licensing of different medicines containing the same drug.
  Ointment
  - ▸ Curatoderm (Almirall Ltd)
    Tacalcitol (as Tacalcitol monohydrate) 4 microgram per 1 gram Curatoderm 4micrograms/g ointment | 30 gram PoM £13.40 DT price = £13.40 | 60 gram PoM £23.14 DT price = £23.14 | 100 gram PoM £30.86 DT price = £30.86
  Liquid
  EXCIPIENTS: May contain Disodium edetate, propylene glycol
  - ▸ Curatoderm (Almirall Ltd)
    Tacalcitol (as Tacalcitol monohydrate) 4 microgram per 1 gram Curatoderm 4micrograms/g lotion | 30 ml PoM £12.73

4 Perspiration
4.1 Hyperhidrosis

Hyperhidrosis

Overview

Aluminium chloride hexahydrate p. 722 is a potent antiperspirant used in the treatment of axillary, palmar, and plantar hyperhidrosis. Aluminium salts are also incorporated in preparations used for minor fungal skin infections associated with hyperhidrosis.

In more severe cases specialists use tap water or glycopyrronium bromide below (as a 0.05% solution) in the iontophoretic treatment of hyperhidrosis of palms and soles.

Botox® contains botulinum toxin type A complex p. 248 and is available for use intradermally for severe hyperhidrosis of the axillae unresponsive to topical antiperspirant or other antihidrotic treatment; intradermal treatment is unlikely to be tolerated by most children and should be administered under hospital specialist supervision.

ANTIMUSCARINICS

Glycopyrronium bromide
17-Oct-2016

(Glycopyrrolate)

- **INDICATIONS AND DOSE**
  Iontophoretic treatment of hyperhidrosis
  - ▸ TO THE SKIN
  - ▸ Child: Only 1 site to be treated at a time, maximum 2 sites treated in any 24 hours, treatment not to be repeated within 7 days (consult product literature)

- **UNLICENSED USE** Licensed for use in children (age range not specified by manufacturer).
- **CONTRA-INDICATIONS** Infections affecting the treatment site
  CONTRA-INDICATIONS, FURTHER INFORMATION
  Contra-indications applicable to systemic use should be considered; however, glycopyrronium is poorly absorbed and systemic effects unlikely with topical use.
- **CAUTIONS**
  CAUTIONS, FURTHER INFORMATION
  Cautions applicable to systemic use should be considered; however, glycopyrronium is poorly absorbed and systemic effects unlikely with topical use.
- **INTERACTIONS** → Appendix 1: glycopyrronium

13

Skin

- **SIDE-EFFECTS** Tingling at administration site

SIDE-EFFECTS, FURTHER INFORMATION
The possibility of systemic side-effects should be considered; however, glycopyrronium is poorly absorbed and systemic effects unlikely with topical use.

- **MEDICINAL FORMS**
There can be variation in the licensing of different medicines containing the same drug.

Powder for solution for iontophoresis
▸ Glycopyrronium bromide (Non-proprietary)
  Glycopyrronium bromide 1 mg per 1 mg Glycopyrronium bromide powder for solution for iontophoresis | 3 gram [PoM] £327.00

DERMATOLOGICAL DRUGS 〉 ASTRINGENTS

Aluminium chloride hexahydrate

- **INDICATIONS AND DOSE**

Hyperhidrosis affecting axillae, hands or feet
▸ TO THE SKIN
▸ Child: Apply once daily, apply liquid formulation at night to dry skin, wash off the following morning, reduce frequency as condition improves—do not bathe immediately before use

Hyperhidrosis | Bromidrosis | Intertrigo | Prevention of tinea pedis and related conditions
▸ TO THE SKIN
▸ Child: Apply powder to dry skin

- **UNLICENSED USE** Licensed for use in children (age range not specified by manufacturer).
- **CAUTIONS** Avoid contact with eyes · avoid contact with mucous membranes · avoid use on broken or irritated skin · do not shave axillae or use depilatories within 12 hours of application
- **SIDE-EFFECTS** Skin irritation
- **PATIENT AND CARER ADVICE** Avoid contact with clothing.
- **EXCEPTIONS TO LEGAL CATEGORY** A 30 mL pack of aluminium chloride hexahydrate 20% is on sale to the public.

- **MEDICINAL FORMS**
There can be variation in the licensing of different medicines containing the same drug.

Liquid
CAUTIONARY AND ADVISORY LABELS 15
▸ Aluminium chloride hexahydrate (Non-proprietary)
  Aluminium chloride 200 mg per 1 ml Aluminium chloride 20% solution | 60 ml [P] no price available DT price = £2.51
▸ Anhydrol (Dermal Laboratories Ltd)
  Aluminium chloride 200 mg per 1 ml Anhydrol Forte 20% solution | 60 ml [P] £2.51 DT price = £2.51
▸ Driclor (GlaxoSmithKline Consumer Healthcare)
  Aluminium chloride 200 mg per 1 ml Driclor 20% solution | 75 ml [P] £3.01 DT price = £3.01

5   Pruritus

Topical local antipruritics

Overview

Pruritus may be caused by systemic disease (such as obstructive jaundice, endocrine disease, chronic renal disease, iron deficiency, and certain malignant diseases), skin disease (such as eczema, psoriasis, urticaria, and scabies), drug hypersensitivity, or as a side-effect of opioid analgesics. Where possible, the underlying cause should be treated. Local antipruritics have a role in the treatment of

pruritus in palliative care. Pruritus caused by cholestasis generally requires a bile acid sequestrant.

An **emollient** may be of value where the pruritus is associated with dry skin. Preparations containing calamine or crotamiton p. 723 are sometimes used but are of uncertain value.

A topical preparation containing doxepin 5% p. 723 is licensed for the relief of pruritus in eczema in children over 12 years; it can cause drowsiness and there may be a risk of sensitisation.

Topical antihistamines and local anaesthetics are only marginally effective and occasionally cause sensitisation. For *insect stings* and *insect bites*, a short course of a topical corticosteroid is appropriate. Short-term treatment with a **sedating antihistamine** may help in insect stings and in intractable pruritus where sedation is desirable. Calamine preparations are of little value for the treatment of insect stings or bites.

In *pruritus ani*, the underlying cause such as faecal soiling, eczema, psoriasis, or helminth infection should be treated.

> **Other drugs used for Pruritus** Alimemazine tartrate, p. 171 · Cetirizine hydrochloride, p. 168 · Chlorphenamine maleate, p. 172 · Hydroxyzine hydrochloride, p. 173 · Levocetirizine hydrochloride, p. 169

ANTIPRURITICS

Calamine with zinc oxide   31-Aug-2016

- **INDICATIONS AND DOSE**

Pruritus
▸ TO THE SKIN
▸ Child: (consult product literature)

IMPORTANT SAFETY INFORMATION

MHRA/CHM UPDATE (APRIL 2016): FIRE RISK WITH PARAFFIN-BASED SKIN EMOLLIENTS ON DRESSINGS OR CLOTHING
See Emollient and barrier preparations p. 683.

- **CONTRA-INDICATIONS** Avoid application of preparations containing zinc oxide prior to x-ray (zinc oxide may affect outcome of x-ray)
- **LESS SUITABLE FOR PRESCRIBING** Less suitable for prescribing.

- **MEDICINAL FORMS**
There can be variation in the licensing of different medicines containing the same drug.

Cream
CAUTIONARY AND ADVISORY LABELS 15
▸ Calamine with zinc oxide (Non-proprietary)
  Phenoxyethanol 5 mg per 1 gram, Zinc oxide 30 mg per 1 gram, Calamine 40 mg per 1 gram, Cetomacrogol emulsifying wax 50 mg per 1 gram, Self-emulsifying glyceryl monostearate 50 mg per 1 gram, Liquid paraffin 200 mg per 1 gram Aqueous calamine cream | 100 gram [GSL] £1.38 DT price = £1.38
▸ Cala Soothe (Ennogen Healthcare Ltd)
  Phenoxyethanol 5 mg per 1 gram, Zinc oxide 30 mg per 1 gram, Calamine 40 mg per 1 gram, Cetomacrogol emulsifying wax 50 mg per 1 gram, Self-emulsifying glyceryl monostearate 50 mg per 1 gram, Liquid paraffin 200 mg per 1 gram Cala Soothe cream | 100 ml £18.80

Liquid
▸ Calamine with zinc oxide (Non-proprietary)
  Phenol liquefied 5 mg per 1 ml, Sodium citrate 5 mg per 1 ml, Bentonite 30 mg per 1 ml, Glycerol 50 mg per 1 ml, Zinc oxide 50 mg per 1 ml, Calamine 150 mg per 1 ml Calamine lotion | 200 ml [GSL] £0.74–£1.04 DT price = £1.04
▸ Cala Soothe (Ennogen Healthcare Ltd)
  Phenol liquefied 5 mg per 1 ml, Sodium citrate 5 mg per 1 ml, Bentonite 30 mg per 1 ml, Glycerol 50 mg per 1 ml, Zinc oxide

13

Skin

50 mg per 1 ml, Calamine 150 mg per 1 ml Cala Soothe lotion |
200 ml £19.50 DT price = £1.04

Crotamiton

- **INDICATIONS AND DOSE**
Pruritus (including pruritus after scabies)
▸ TO THE SKIN
▸ Child 1 month–2 years (on doctor's advice only): Apply
  once daily
▸ Child 3–17 years: Apply 2–3 times a day

- **CONTRA-INDICATIONS** Acute exudative dermatoses

- **CAUTIONS** Avoid use in buccal mucosa · avoid use near
eyes · avoid use on broken skin · avoid use on very inflamed
skin · use on doctor's advice for children under 3 years

- **PREGNANCY** Manufacturer advises avoid, especially during
the first trimester—no information available.

- **BREAST FEEDING** No information available; avoid
application to nipple area.

- **MEDICINAL FORMS**
There can be variation in the licensing of different medicines
containing the same drug.
Cream
EXCIPIENTS: May contain Beeswax, cetostearyl alcohol (including cetyl
and stearyl alcohol), fragrances, hydroxybenzoates (parabens)
▸ Crotamiton (Non-proprietary)
  Crotamiton 100 mg per 1 gram Itch Relief cream | 30 gram GSL
  no price available DT price = £2.50
▸ Brands may include Eurax

Doxepin

- **INDICATIONS AND DOSE**
Pruritus in eczema
▸ TO THE SKIN
▸ Child 12–17 years: Apply up to 3 g 3–4 times a day, apply
  thinly; coverage should be less than 10% of body
  surface area; maximum 12 g per day

- **CAUTIONS** Avoid application to large areas · cardiac
arrhythmias · mania · severe heart disease · susceptibility
to angle-closure glaucoma · urinary retention

- **INTERACTIONS** → Appendix 1: tricyclic antidepressants

- **SIDE-EFFECTS**
▸ **Common or very common** Dizziness · drowsiness
▸ **Frequency not known** Antimuscarinic effects · fever ·
gastro-intestinal disturbances · headache · irritation · local
burning · rash · stinging · tingling

- **PREGNANCY** Manufacturer advises use only if potential
benefit outweighs risk.

- **BREAST FEEDING** Manufacturer advises use only if
potential benefit outweighs risk.

- **HEPATIC IMPAIRMENT** Manufacturer advises caution in
severe liver disease.

- **PATIENT AND CARER ADVICE**
A patient information leaflet should be provided.
Driving and skilled tasks
Drowsiness may affect performance of skilled tasks (e.g.
driving). Effects of alcohol enhanced.

- **MEDICINAL FORMS**
There can be variation in the licensing of different medicines
containing the same drug.
Cream
CAUTIONARY AND ADVISORY LABELS 2, 10
EXCIPIENTS: May contain Benzyl alcohol
▸ Xepin (Cambridge Healthcare Supplies Ltd)
  Doxepin hydrochloride 50 mg per 1 gram Xepin 5% cream |
  30 gram PoM £11.70

6   Rosacea and acne

Rosacea and Acne

Acne vulgaris in children
Acne vulgaris commonly affects children around puberty and
occasionally affects infants. Treatment of acne should be
commenced early to prevent scarring; lesions may worsen
before improving. The choice of treatment depends on age,
severity, and whether the acne is predominantly
inflammatory or comedonal.

Mild to moderate acne is generally treated with topical
preparations, such as benzoyl peroxide p. 726, azelaic acid
p. 726, and retinoids.

For *moderate to severe inflammatory acne* or where topical
preparations are not tolerated or are ineffective or where
application to the site is difficult, systemic treatment with
oral antibacterials may be effective. Co-cyprindiol
(cyproterone acetate with ethinylestradiol) p. 725 has anti-
androgenic properties and may be useful in young women
with acne refractory to other treatments.

Severe acne, acne unresponsive to prolonged courses of
oral antibacterials, acne with scarring, or acne associated
with psychological problems calls for early referral to a
consultant dermatologist who may prescribe oral
isotretinoin p. 727.

Neonatal and infantile acne
Inflammatory papules, pustules, and occasionally
comedones may develop at birth or within the first month;
most neonates with acne do not require treatment. Acne
developing at 3–6 months of age may be more severe and
persistent; lesions are usually confined to the face. Topical
preparations containing benzoyl peroxide (at the lowest
strength possible to avoid irritation), adapalene p. 727, or
tretinoin p. 729 may be used if treatment for infantile acne is
necessary. In infants with inflammatory acne, oral
erythromycin p. 316 is used because topical preparations for
acne are not well tolerated. In cases of erythromycin-
resistant acne, oral isotretinoin can be given on the advice of
a consultant dermatologist.

Topical preparations for acne
In mild to moderate acne, comedones and inflamed lesions
respond well to benzoyl peroxide or topical retinoids.
Alternatively, topical application of an antibacterial such as
erythromycin or clindamycin p. 725 may be effective for
inflammatory acne. However, topical antibacterials are
probably no more effective than benzoyl peroxide and may
promote the emergence of resistant organisms. If topical
preparations prove inadequate, oral preparations may be
needed. The choice of product and formulation (gel,
solution, lotion, or cream) is largely determined by skin type,
patient preference, and previous usage of acne products.

Benzoyl peroxide and azelaic acid
Benzoyl peroxide is effective in mild to moderate acne. Both
comedones and inflamed lesions respond well to benzoyl
peroxide. The lower concentrations seem to be as effective as
higher concentrations in reducing inflammation. It is usual
to start with a lower strength and to increase the
concentration of benzoyl peroxide gradually. The usefulness
of benzoyl peroxide washes is limited by the short time the
products are in contact with the skin. Adverse effects include
local skin irritation, particularly when therapy is initiated,
but the scaling and redness often subside with a reduction in
benzoyl peroxide concentration, frequency, and area of
application. If the acne does not respond after 2 months then
use of a topical antibacterial should be considered.

13

Skin

Azelaic acid has antimicrobial and anticomedonal properties. It may be used as an alternative to benzoyl peroxide or to a topical retinoid for treating mild to moderate comedonal acne, particularly of the face; azelaic acid is less likely to cause local irritation than benzoyl peroxide.

Topical antibacterials for acne

In the treatment of mild to moderate inflammatory acne, topical antibacterials may be no more effective than topical benzoyl peroxide or tretinoin. Topical antibacterials are probably best reserved for children who wish to avoid oral antibacterials or who cannot tolerate them.

Topical preparations of erythromycin and clindamycin may be used to treat *inflamed lesions* in mild to moderate acne when topical benzoyl peroxide or tretinoin is ineffective or poorly tolerated. Topical benzoyl peroxide, azelaic acid, or retinoids used in combination with an antibacterial (topical or systemic) may be more effective than an antibacterial used alone. Topical antibacterials can produce mild irritation of the skin, and on rare occasions cause sensitisation; gastro-intestinal disturbances have been reported with topical clindamycin.

Antibacterial resistance of *Propionibacterium acnes* is increasing; there is cross-resistance between erythromycin and clindamycin. To avoid development of resistance:

- when possible use non-antibiotic antimicrobials (such as benzoyl peroxide or azelaic acid);
- avoid concomitant treatment with different oral and topical antibacterials;
- if a particular antibacterial is effective, use it for repeat courses if needed (short intervening courses of benzoyl peroxide or azelaic acid may eliminate any resistant propionibacteria);
- do not continue treatment for longer than necessary (but treatment with a topical preparation should be continued for at least 6 months).

Topical retinoids and related preparations for acne

Topical tretinoin, its isomer isotretinoin, and adapalene (a retinoid-like drug), are useful for treating comedones and inflammatory lesions in mild to moderate acne. Patients should be warned that some redness and skin peeling can occur initially but settles with time. If undue irritation occurs, the frequency of application should be reduced or treatment suspended until the reaction subsides; if irritation persists, discontinue treatment. Several months of treatment may be needed to achieve an optimal response and the treatment should be continued until no new lesions develop.

Tretinoin can be used under specialist supervision to treat infantile acne; adapalene can also be used.

Other topical preparations for acne

A topical preparation of nicotinamide p. 730 is available for inflammatory acne.

Oral preparations for acne

Oral antibacterials for acne

Oral antibacterials may be used in *moderate to severe inflammatory acne* when topical treatment is not adequately effective or is inappropriate. Concomitant anticomedonal treatment with topical benzoyl peroxide or azelaic acid may also be required.

Tetracyclines should not be given to children under 12 years. In children over 12 years, either oxytetracycline p. 339 or tetracycline p. 339 is usually given for acne. If there is no improvement after the first 3 months another oral antibacterial should be used. Maximum improvement usually occurs after 4 to 6 months but in more severe cases treatment may need to be continued for 2 years or longer. Doxycycline p. 338 and lymecycline p. 338 are alternatives to tetracycline in children over 12 years.

Although minocycline p. 339 is as effective as other tetracyclines for acne, it is associated with a greater risk of lupus erythematosus-like syndrome. Minocycline sometimes causes irreversible pigmentation.

Erythromycin is an alternative for the management of moderate to severe acne with inflamed lesions, but propionibacteria strains resistant to erythromycin are becoming widespread and this may explain poor response. In cases of erythromycin-resistant *P. acnes* in infants, oral isotretinoin may be used on the advice of a consultant dermatologist.

Concomitant use of different topical and systemic antibacterials is undesirable owing to the increased likelihood of the development of bacterial resistance.

Hormone treatment for acne

Co-cyprindiol (cyproterone acetate with ethinylestradiol) p. 725 contains an anti-androgen. It is no more effective than an oral broad-spectrum antibacterial but is useful in females of childbearing age who also wish to receive oral contraception.

Improvement of acne with co-cyprindiol probably occurs because of decreased sebum secretion which is under androgen control. Some females with moderately severe hirsutism may also benefit because hair growth is also androgen-dependent.

Oral retinoid for acne

The retinoid isotretinoin p. 727 reduces sebum secretion. It is used for the systemic treatment of nodulo-cystic and conglobate acne, severe acne, acne with scarring, or for acne which has not responded to an adequate course of a systemic antibacterial. Isotretinoin is used for the treatment of severe infantile acne resistant to erythromycin p. 316.

Isotretinoin is a toxic drug that should be prescribed **only** by, or under the supervision of, a consultant dermatologist. It is given for at least 16 weeks; repeat courses are not normally required. The drug is **teratogenic** and must **not** be given to females of child-bearing age unless they practise effective contraception (oral progestogen-only contraceptives not considered effective) and then only after detailed assessment and explanation by the physician. They must also be registered with a pregnancy prevention programme.

Although a causal link between isotretinoin use and psychiatric changes (including suicidal ideation) has not been established, the possibility should be considered before initiating treatment; if psychiatric changes occur during treatment, isotretinoin should be stopped, the prescriber informed, and specialist psychiatric advice should be sought.

Rosacea

The adult form of rosacea rarely occurs in children. Persistent or repeated use of potent topical corticosteroids may cause periorificial rosacea (steroid acne). The pustules and papules of rosacea may be treated for at least 6 weeks with a topical metronidazole preparation p. 692, or a systemic antibacterial such as erythromycin, or for a child over 12 years, oxytetracycline p. 339. Tetracyclines are **contra-indicated** in children under 12 years of age.

6.1 Acne

ANTI-ANDROGENS

Co-cyprindiol

● **INDICATIONS AND DOSE**

Moderate to severe acne in females of child-bearing age refractory to topical therapy or oral antibacterials | Moderately severe hirsutism

▸ BY MOUTH

▸ Females of childbearing potential: 1 tablet daily for 21 days, to be started on day 1 of menstrual cycle; subsequent courses repeated after a 7-day interval (during which withdrawal bleeding occurs), time to symptom remission, at least 3 months; review need for treatment regularly

● **CONTRA-INDICATIONS** Acute porphyria p. 577 · gallstones · heart disease associated with pulmonary hypertension or risk of embolus · history during pregnancy of cholestatic jaundice · history during pregnancy of chorea · history during pregnancy of pemphigoid gestationis · history during pregnancy of pruritus · history of breast cancer but can be used after 5 years if no evidence of disease and non-hormonal methods unacceptable · history of haemolytic uraemic syndrome · migraine with aura · personal history of venous or arterial thrombosis · sclerosing treatment for varicose veins · severe or multiple risk factors for arterial disease or for venous thromboembolism · systemic lupus erythematosus with (or unknown) antiphospholipid antibodies · transient cerebral ischaemic attacks without headaches · undiagnosed vaginal bleeding

● **CAUTIONS** Active trophoblastic disease (until return to normal of urine- and plasma-gonadotrophin concentration)—seek specialist advice · arterial disease · gene mutations associated with breast cancer (e.g. BRCA 1) · history of severe depression especially if induced by hormonal contraceptive · hyperprolactinaemia—seek specialist advice · inflammatory bowel disease including Crohn's disease · migraine · personal or family history of hypertriglyceridaemia (increased risk of pancreatitis) · risk factors for venous thromboembolism · sickle-cell disease · undiagnosed breast mass

CAUTIONS, FURTHER INFORMATION

▸ **Venous thromboembolism** There is an increased risk of venous thromboembolism in women taking co-cyprindiol, particularly during the first year of use. The incidence of venous thromboembolism is 1.5–2 times higher in women using co-cyprindiol than in women using combined oral contraceptives containing levonorgestrel, but the risk may be similar to that associated with use of combined oral contraceptives containing third generation progestogens (desogestrel and gestodene) or drospirenone. Women requiring co-cyprindiol may have an inherently increased risk of cardiovascular disease.

● **INTERACTIONS** → Appendix 1: combined hormonal contraceptives

● **SIDE-EFFECTS**

▸ **Rare** Rarely gallstones · systemic lupus erythematosus

▸ **Very rare** Photosensitivity

▸ **Frequency not known** Abdominal cramps · absence of withdrawal bleeding · amenorrhoea after discontinuation · breast enlargement · breast secretion · breast tenderness · cervical erosion · changes in libido · changes in lipid metabolism · changes in vaginal discharge · chloasma · chorea · contact lenses may irritate · depression · fluid retention · headache · hepatic tumours · hypertension · irritability · leg cramps · liver impairment · nausea · nervousness · reduced menstrual loss · skin reactions ·

thrombosis (more common when factor V Leiden present or in blood groups A, B, and AB · visual disturbances · vomiting · 'spotting' in early cycles

● **PREGNANCY** Avoid—risk of feminisation of male fetus with cyproterone.

● **BREAST FEEDING** Manufacturer advises avoid; possibility of anti-androgen effects in neonate with cyproterone.

● **HEPATIC IMPAIRMENT** Avoid in active liver disease including disorders of hepatic excretion (e.g. Dubin-Johnson or Rotor syndromes), infective hepatitis (until liver function returns to normal), and liver tumours.

● **PRESCRIBING AND DISPENSING INFORMATION** A mixture of cyproterone acetate and ethinylestradiol in the mass proportions 2000 parts to 35 parts, respectively.

● **MEDICINAL FORMS**
There can be variation in the licensing of different medicines containing the same drug.

Tablet

▸ Co-cyprindiol (Non-proprietary)
Ethinylestradiol 35 microgram, Cyproterone acetate 2 mg Co-cyprindiol 2000microgram/35microgram tablets | 63 tablet [PoM] £5.70 DT price = £5.70

▸ Clairette (Stragen UK Ltd)
Ethinylestradiol 35 microgram, Cyproterone acetate 2 mg Clairette 2000/35 tablets | 63 tablet [PoM] £5.90 DT price = £5.70

▸ Dianette (Bayer Plc)
Ethinylestradiol 35 microgram, Cyproterone acetate 2 mg Dianette tablets | 63 tablet [PoM] £7.71 DT price = £5.70

▸ Teragezza (Morningside Healthcare Ltd)
Ethinylestradiol 35 microgram, Cyproterone acetate 2 mg Teragezza 2000microgram/35microgram tablets | 63 tablet [PoM] £11.10 DT price = £5.70

ANTIBACTERIALS ⟩ LINCOSAMIDES

Clindamycin

● **INDICATIONS AND DOSE**

DALACIN T ® LOTION

Acne vulgaris

▸ TO THE SKIN

▸ Child: Apply twice daily, to be applied thinly

DALACIN T ® SOLUTION

Acne vulgaris

▸ TO THE SKIN

▸ Child: Apply twice daily, to be applied thinly

ZINDACLIN ® GEL

Acne vulgaris

▸ TO THE SKIN

▸ Child 12–17 years: Apply once daily, to be applied thinly

● **INTERACTIONS** → Appendix 1: clindamycin

● **MEDICINAL FORMS**
There can be variation in the licensing of different medicines containing the same drug.

Gel
EXCIPIENTS: May contain Propylene glycol

▸ Zindaclin (Crawford Healthcare Ltd)
Clindamycin (as Clindamycin phosphate) 10 mg per
1 gram Zindaclin 1% gel | 30 gram [PoM] £8.66 DT price = £8.66

Cream
EXCIPIENTS: May contain Benzyl alcohol, cetostearyl alcohol (including cetyl and stearyl alcohol), polysorbates, propylene glycol

▸ Dalacin (Pfizer Ltd)
Clindamycin (as Clindamycin phosphate) 20 mg per
1 gram Dalacin 2% cream | 40 gram [PoM] £10.86 DT price = £10.86

Liquid
EXCIPIENTS: May contain Cetostearyl alcohol (including cetyl and stearyl alcohol), hydroxybenzoates (parabens), propylene glycol

13

Skin

▸ **Dalacin T** (Pfizer Ltd)
Clindamycin (as Clindamycin phosphate) 10 mg per 1 ml Dalacin T
1% topical lotion | 30 ml [PoM] £5.08 DT price = £5.08 | 60 ml [PoM]
£10.16
Dalacin T 1% topical solution | 30 ml [PoM] £4.34 DT price = £4.34 |
50 ml [PoM] £7.23

Combinations available: *Benzoyl peroxide with clindamycin*,
below · *Tretinoin with clindamycin*, p. 729

ANTIBACTERIALS > MACROLIDES

Erythromycin with zinc acetate

● **INDICATIONS AND DOSE**

Acne vulgaris

▸ TO THE SKIN

▸ **Child:** Apply twice daily

● **CAUTIONS** Some manufacturers advise preparations
containing alcohol are not suitable for use with benzoyl
peroxide

● **MEDICINAL FORMS**
There can be variation in the licensing of different medicines
containing the same drug.
Liquid
▸ **Zineryt** (LEO Pharma)
Zinc acetate 12 mg per 1 ml, Erythromycin 40 mg per 1 ml Zineryt
lotion | 30 ml [PoM] £9.25 DT price = £9.25 | 90 ml [PoM] £20.02 DT
price = £20.02

ANTISEPTICS AND DISINFECTANTS > PEROXIDES

Benzoyl peroxide

● **INDICATIONS AND DOSE**

Acne vulgaris

▸ TO THE SKIN

▸ **Child 12–17 years:** Apply 1–2 times a day, preferably
apply after washing with soap and water, start
treatment with lower-strength preparations

Infantile acne

▸ TO THE SKIN

▸ **Child 1 month-1 year:** Apply 1–2 times a day, start
treatment with lower-strength preparations

● **UNLICENSED USE** Not licensed for use in treatment of
infantile acne.

● **CAUTIONS** Avoid contact with broken skin · avoid contact
with eyes · avoid contact with mouth · avoid contact with
mucous membranes · avoid excessive exposure to sunlight

● **SIDE-EFFECTS** Skin irritation

SIDE-EFFECTS, FURTHER INFORMATION
▸ Skin irritation Reduce frequency or suspend use until
irritation subsides and re-introduce at reduced frequency.

● **PATIENT AND CARER ADVICE** May bleach fabrics and hair.

● **MEDICINAL FORMS**
There can be variation in the licensing of different medicines
containing the same drug.
Cream
EXCIPIENTS: May contain Cetostearyl alcohol (including cetyl and
stearyl alcohol), fragrances, isopropyl palmitate, propylene glycol
▸ **Brevoxyl** (GlaxoSmithKline Consumer Healthcare)
Benzoyl peroxide 40 mg per 1 gram Brevoxyl 4% cream |
50 gram [P] £4.13 DT price = £4.13
Gel
EXCIPIENTS: May contain Fragrances, propylene glycol
▸ **Acnecide** (Galderma (UK) Ltd)
Benzoyl peroxide 50 mg per 1 gram Acnecide 5% gel | 30 gram [P]
£5.44 DT price = £5.44 | 60 gram [P] £10.68 DT price = £10.68
Acnecide Wash 5% gel | 50 gram [P] £5.44 DT price = £5.44

Combinations available: *Adapalene with benzoyl peroxide*,
p. 727

Benzoyl peroxide with clindamycin

The properties listed below are those particular to the
combination only. For the properties of the components
please consider, benzoyl peroxide above, clindamycin p. 725.

● **INDICATIONS AND DOSE**

Acne vulgaris

▸ TO THE SKIN

▸ **Child 12–17 years:** Apply once daily, dose to be applied in
the evening

● **MEDICINAL FORMS**
There can be variation in the licensing of different medicines
containing the same drug.
Gel
EXCIPIENTS: May contain Disodium edetate
▸ **Duac** (Stiefel Laboratories (UK) Ltd)
Clindamycin (as Clindamycin phosphate) 10 mg per 1 gram,
Benzoyl peroxide 30 mg per 1 gram Duac Once Daily gel (3% and
1%) | 30 gram [PoM] £13.14 DT price = £13.14 | 60 gram [PoM]
£26.28
Clindamycin (as Clindamycin phosphate) 10 mg per 1 gram,
Benzoyl peroxide 50 mg per 1 gram Duac Once Daily gel (5% and
1%) | 30 gram [PoM] £13.14 DT price = £13.14 | 60 gram [PoM]
£26.28 DT price = £26.28

DERMATOLOGICAL DRUGS > ANTICOMEDONALS

Azelaic acid

● **INDICATIONS AND DOSE**

FINACEA®

Facial acne vulgaris

▸ TO THE SKIN

▸ **Child 12–17 years:** Apply twice daily, discontinue if no
improvement after 1 month

SKINOREN®

Acne vulgaris

▸ TO THE SKIN

▸ **Child 12–17 years:** Apply twice daily

Acne vulgaris in patients with sensitive skin

▸ TO THE SKIN

▸ **Child 12–17 years:** Apply once daily for 1 week, then
apply twice daily

● **CAUTIONS** Avoid contact with eyes · avoid contact with
mouth · avoid contact with mucous membranes

● **SIDE-EFFECTS**
▸ **Common or very common** Local irritation (reduce frequency
or discontinue temporarily)
▸ **Uncommon** Skin discoloration
▸ **Frequency not known** Worsening of asthma

● **MEDICINAL FORMS**
There can be variation in the licensing of different medicines
containing the same drug.
Cream
EXCIPIENTS: May contain Propylene glycol
▸ **Skinoren** (Bayer Plc)
Azelaic acid 200 mg per 1 gram Skinoren 20% cream |
30 gram [PoM] £3.74 DT price = £3.74
Gel
EXCIPIENTS: May contain Disodium edetate, polysorbates, propylene
glycol
▸ **Finacea** (Bayer Plc)
Azelaic acid 150 mg per 1 gram Finacea 15% gel | 30 gram [PoM]
£7.48 DT price = £7.48

RETINOID AND RELATED DRUGS

❙ Adapalene

- ● **INDICATIONS AND DOSE**

Mild to moderate acne vulgaris
▸ TO THE SKIN
▸ Child 12–17 years: Apply once daily, apply thinly in the evening

Infantile acne
▸ TO THE SKIN
▸ Child 1 month–1 year: Apply once daily, apply thinly in the evening

- ● **UNLICENSED USE** Not licensed for use in infantile acne.
- ● **CAUTIONS** Avoid accumulation in angles of the nose · avoid contact with eyes, nostrils, mouth and mucous membranes, eczematous, broken or sunburned skin · avoid exposure to UV light (including sunlight, solariums) · avoid in severe acne involving large areas · caution in sensitive areas such as the neck
- ● **INTERACTIONS** → Appendix 1: retinoids
- ● **CONCEPTION AND CONTRACEPTION** Females of child-bearing age must use effective contraception (oral progestogen-only contraceptives not considered effective).
- ● **PREGNANCY** Avoid.
- ● **BREAST FEEDING** Amount of drug in milk probably too small to be harmful; ensure infant does not come in contact with treated areas.
- ● **PATIENT AND CARER ADVICE** If sun exposure is unavoidable, an appropriate sunscreen or protective clothing should be used.
- ● **MEDICINAL FORMS**
There can be variation in the licensing of different medicines containing the same drug.

Cream
CAUTIONARY AND ADVISORY LABELS 11
EXCIPIENTS: May contain Disodium edetate, hydroxybenzoates (parabens)
▸ **Adapalene** (Non-proprietary)
Adapalene 1 mg per 1 gram   Adapalene 0.1% cream |
45 gram [PoM] £19.73 DT price = £16.43
▸ **Differin** (Galderma (UK) Ltd)
Adapalene 1 mg per 1 gram   Differin 0.1% cream | 45 gram [PoM]
£16.43 DT price = £16.43

Gel
CAUTIONARY AND ADVISORY LABELS 11
EXCIPIENTS: May contain Disodium edetate, hydroxybenzoates (parabens), propylene glycol
▸ **Adapalene** (Non-proprietary)
Adapalene 1 mg per 1 gram   Adapalene 0.1% gel | 45 gram [PoM]
£19.73 DT price = £16.43
▸ **Differin** (Galderma (UK) Ltd)
Adapalene 1 mg per 1 gram   Differin 0.1% gel | 45 gram [PoM]
£16.43 DT price = £16.43

❙ Adapalene with benzoyl peroxide

The properties listed below are those particular to the combination only. For the properties of the components please consider, adapalene above, benzoyl peroxide p. 726.

- ● **INDICATIONS AND DOSE**

Acne vulgaris
▸ TO THE SKIN
▸ Child 9–17 years: Apply once daily, to be applied thinly in the evening

- ● **INTERACTIONS** → Appendix 1: retinoids

- ● **CONCEPTION AND CONTRACEPTION** Females of child-bearing age must use effective contraception (oral progestogen-only contraceptives not considered effective).
- ● **PATIENT AND CARER ADVICE** Gel may bleach clothing and hair.
- ● **NATIONAL FUNDING/ACCESS DECISIONS**
Scottish Medicines Consortium (SMC) Decisions
The *Scottish Medicines Consortium* has advised (March 2014) that *Epiduo*® should be restricted for use in mild to moderate facial acne when monotherapy with benzoyl peroxide or adapalene is inappropriate.

- ● **MEDICINAL FORMS**
There can be variation in the licensing of different medicines containing the same drug.

Gel
CAUTIONARY AND ADVISORY LABELS 11
EXCIPIENTS: May contain Disodium edetate, polysorbates, propylene glycol
▸ **Adapalene with benzoyl peroxide** (Non-proprietary)
Adapalene 1 mg per 1 gram, Benzoyl peroxide 25 mg per
1 gram   Adapalene 0.1% / Benzoyl peroxide 2.5% gel |
45 gram [PoM] no price available DT price = £19.53
▸ **Epiduo** (Galderma (UK) Ltd)
Adapalene 1 mg per 1 gram, Benzoyl peroxide 25 mg per
1 gram   Epiduo 0.1%/2.5% gel | 45 gram [PoM] £19.53 DT price =
£19.53

❙ Isotretinoin

- ● **INDICATIONS AND DOSE**

Topical treatment of mild to moderate acne
▸ TO THE SKIN
▸ Child: Apply 1–2 times a day, to be applied thinly

Severe acne (under expert supervision) | Acne which is associated with psychological problems (under expert supervision) | Acne which has not responded to an adequate course of a systemic antibacterial (under expert supervision) | Acne with scarring (under expert supervision) | Systemic treatment of nodulo-cystic and conglobate acne (under expert supervision)
▸ BY MOUTH
▸ Child 12–17 years: Initially 500 micrograms/kg daily in 1–2 divided doses, increased if necessary to 1 mg/kg daily for 16–24 weeks, repeat treatment course after a period of at least 8 weeks if relapse after first course; maximum 150 mg/kg per course

Severe infantile acne (under expert supervision)
▸ BY MOUTH
▸ Child 1 month–1 year: Initially 200 micrograms/kg daily in 1–2 divided doses, increased if necessary to 1 mg/kg daily for 16–24 weeks; maximum 150 mg/kg per course

- ● **UNLICENSED USE** Not licensed for use in infantile acne.
- ● **CONTRA-INDICATIONS**
▸ With oral use Hyperlipidaemia · hypervitaminosis A
▸ With topical use Perioral dermatitis · rosacea
- ● **CAUTIONS**
▸ With oral use Avoid blood donation during treatment and for at least 1 month after treatment · diabetes · dry eye syndrome (associated with risk of keratitis) · history of depression · monitor for depression
▸ With topical use Allow peeling (resulting from other irritant treatments) to subside before using a topical retinoid · alternating a preparation that causes peeling with a topical retinoid may give rise to contact dermatitis (reduce frequency of retinoid application) · avoid accumulation in angles of the nose · avoid contact with eyes, nostrils, mouth and mucous membranes, eczematous, broken or sunburned skin · avoid exposure to UV light (including

13

Skin

sunlight, solariums) · avoid in severe acne involving large areas · avoid use of topical retinoids with abrasive cleaners, comedogenic or astringent cosmetics · caution in sensitive areas such as the neck · personal or familial history of non-melanoma skin cancer

- **INTERACTIONS** → Appendix 1: retinoids
- **SIDE-EFFECTS**
- ▸ **Common or very common**
- ▸ With oral use Anaemia · arthralgia · dryness of eyes (with blepharitis and conjunctivitis) · dryness of lips (sometimes cheilitis) · dryness of nasal mucosa (with epistaxis) · dryness of pharyngeal mucosa (with hoarseness) · dryness of skin (with dermatitis, scaling, thinning, erythema, pruritus) · epidermal fragility (trauma may cause blistering) · haematuria · headache · myalgia · neutropenia · proteinuria · raised blood-glucose concentration · raised plasma-triglyceride concentration · raised serum-cholesterol concentration (with reduced high-density lipoprotein concentration) · raised serum-transaminase concentration · thrombocytopenia · thrombocytosis
- ▸ **Rare**
- ▸ With oral use Aggressive behaviour · alopecia · anxiety · depression · mood changes · skin reactions
- ▸ **Very rare**
- ▸ With oral use Acne fulminans · allergic vasculitis · arthritis · benign intracranial hypertension · blurred vision · bone changes following long-term administration · calcification of tendons and ligaments following long-term administration · cataracts · colour blindness · convulsions · corneal opacities · decreased night vision · decreased tolerance to contact lenses · diabetes mellitus · dizziness · drowsiness · early epiphyseal closure following long-term administration · exacerbation of acne · gastrointestinal haemorrhage · glomerulonephritis · Gram-positive infections of skin and mucous membranes · granulomatous lesions · haemorrhagic diarrhoea · hepatitis · hirsutism · hyperuricaemia · impaired hearing · increased sweating · inflammatory bowel disease · keratitis · lymphadenopathy · malaise · nail dystrophy · nausea · papilloedema · paronychia · photophobia · photosensitivity · psychosis · raised serum-creatine kinase concentration · reduced bone density following long-term administration · skeletal hyperostosis following long-term administration · skin hyperpigmentation · suicidal ideation · tendinitis · visual disturbances
- ▸ **Frequency not known**
- ▸ With oral use Stevens-Johnson syndrome · toxic epidermal necrolysis
- ▸ With topical use Blistering of skin · burning · crusting of skin · dry or peeling skin · erythema · eye irritation · increased sensitivity to UVB light or sunlight · oedema · pruritus · stinging

SIDE-EFFECTS, FURTHER INFORMATION
- ▸ Management of side-effects Risk of pancreatitis if triglycerides above 9 mmol/litre—discontinue if uncontrolled hypertriglyceridaemia or pancreatitis. Psychiatric side-effects require expert referral. Discontinue treatment if skin peeling severe or haemorrhagic diarrhoea develops. Visual disturbances require expert referral and possible withdrawal.

- **CONCEPTION AND CONTRACEPTION**
Pregnancy prevention
- ▸ With oral use Effective contraception must be used. In women of child-bearing potential, exclude pregnancy up to 3 days before treatment (start treatment on day 2 or 3 of menstrual cycle), every month during treatment (unless there are compelling reasons to indicate that there is no risk of pregnancy), and 5 weeks after stopping treatment—perform pregnancy test in the first 3 days of the menstrual cycle. Women must practise effective contraception for at least 1 month before starting treatment, during treatment,

and for at least 1 month after stopping treatment. Women should be advised to use at least 1 method of contraception, but ideally they should use 2 methods of contraception. Oral progestogen-only contraceptives are not considered effective. Barrier methods should not be used alone, but can be used in conjunction with other contraceptive methods. Each prescription for isotretinoin should be limited to a supply of up to 30 days' treatment and dispensed within 7 days of the date stated on the prescription; repeat prescriptions or faxed prescriptions are not acceptable. Women should be advised to discontinue treatment and to seek prompt medical attention if they become pregnant during treatment or within 1 month of stopping treatment.
- ▸ With topical use Females of child-bearing age must use effective contraception (oral progestogen-only contraceptives not considered effective).

- **PREGNANCY** Contra-indicated in pregnancy (teratogenic).
- **BREAST FEEDING** Avoid.
- **HEPATIC IMPAIRMENT**
- ▸ With oral use Avoid—further impairment may occur.
- **RENAL IMPAIRMENT**
- ▸ With oral use In severe impairment, reduce initial dose and increase gradually, if necessary, up to 1 mg/kg daily as tolerated.

- **MONITORING REQUIREMENTS**
- ▸ With oral use Measure hepatic function and serum lipids before treatment, 1 month after starting and then every 3 months (reduce dose or discontinue if transaminase or serum lipids persistently raised).

- **PRESCRIBING AND DISPENSING INFORMATION** Isotretinoin is an isomer of tretinoin.

- **PATIENT AND CARER ADVICE**
- ▸ With oral use Warn patient to avoid wax epilation (risk of epidermal stripping), dermabrasion, and laser skin treatments (risk of scarring) during treatment and for at least 6 months after stopping; patient should avoid exposure to UV light (including sunlight) and use sunscreen and emollient (including lip balm) preparations from the start of treatment.

  Patients and carers should be told how to recognise signs and symptoms of psychiatric disorders such as depression, anxiety, and rarely suicidal thoughts.
- ▸ With topical use Patients should be warned that some redness and skin peeling can occur initially but settles with time. If undue irritation occurs, the frequency of application should be reduced or treatment suspended until the reaction subsides; if irritation persists, discontinue treatment. Several months of treatment may be needed to achieve an optimal response and the treatment should be continued until no new lesions develop. If sun exposure is unavoidable, an appropriate sunscreen or protective clothing should be used.

- **MEDICINAL FORMS**
There can be variation in the licensing of different medicines containing the same drug.

Capsule
CAUTIONARY AND ADVISORY LABELS 10, 11, 21
- ▸ **Isotretinoin (Non-proprietary)**
  Isotretinoin 5 mg Isotretinoin 5mg capsules | 30 capsule PoM £10.15 | 56 capsule PoM £14.78 DT price = £14.78
  Isotretinoin 10 mg Isotretinoin 10mg capsules | 30 capsule PoM £14.54 DT price = £14.54
  Isotretinoin 20 mg Isotretinoin 20mg capsules | 30 capsule PoM £20.00 DT price = £16.46 | 56 capsule PoM £37.85
  Isotretinoin 40 mg Isotretinoin 40mg capsules | 30 capsule PoM £38.98 DT price = £38.98
- ▸ **Roaccutane** (Roche Products Ltd)
  Isotretinoin 10 mg Roaccutane 10mg capsules | 30 capsule PoM £14.54 DT price = £14.54
  Isotretinoin 20 mg Roaccutane 20mg capsules | 30 capsule PoM £20.02 DT price = £16.46

Isotretinoin with erythromycin

The properties listed below are those particular to the combination only. For the properties of the components please consider, isotretinoin p. 727, erythromycin p. 316.

● **INDICATIONS AND DOSE**

Topical treatment of mild to moderate acne

▸ TO THE SKIN

▸ Child: (consult product literature)

● **INTERACTIONS** → Appendix 1: macrolides, retinoids

● **MEDICINAL FORMS**
There can be variation in the licensing of different medicines containing the same drug.
Gel
CAUTIONARY AND ADVISORY LABELS 11
EXCIPIENTS: May contain Butylated hydroxytoluene
▸ Isotrexin (Stiefel Laboratories (UK) Ltd)
  Isotretinoin 500 microgram per 1 gram, Erythromycin 20 mg per 1 gram Isotrexin gel | 30 gram [PoM] £7.47 DT price = £7.47

Tretinoin with clindamycin

The properties listed below are those particular to the combination only. For the properties of the components please consider, tretinoin p. 527, clindamycin p. 725.

● **INDICATIONS AND DOSE**

Facial acne

▸ TO THE SKIN

▸ Child 12–17 years: Apply daily, (to be applied thinly at bedtime)

● **CONTRA-INDICATIONS** Perioral dermatitis · personal or familial history of non-melanoma skin cancer · rosacea

● **CAUTIONS** Allow peeling (resulting from other irritant treatments) to subside before using a topical retinoid · alternating a preparation that causes peeling with a topical retinoid may give rise to contact dermatitis (reduce frequency of retinoid application) · avoid accumulation in angles of the nose · avoid contact with eyes, nostrils, mouth and mucous membranes, eczematous, broken or sunburned skin · avoid exposure to UV light (including sunlight, solariums) · avoid in severe acne involving large areas · avoid use of topical retinoids with abrasive cleaners, comedogenic or astringent cosmetics · caution in sensitive areas such as the neck

● **INTERACTIONS** → Appendix 1: clindamycin, retinoids

● **SIDE-EFFECTS** Blistering of skin · burning · crusting of skin · dry or peeling skin (discontinue if severe) · erythema · eye irritation · increased sensitivity to UVB light or sunlight · oedema · pruritus · stinging · temporary changes of skin pigmentation

● **CONCEPTION AND CONTRACEPTION** Females of child-bearing age must use effective contraception (oral progestogen-only contraceptives not considered effective).

● **PREGNANCY** Contra-indicated in pregnancy.

● **BREAST FEEDING** Amount of drug in milk after topical application probably too small to be harmful; ensure infant does not come in contact with treated areas.

● **PATIENT AND CARER ADVICE** If sun exposure is unavoidable, an appropriate sunscreen or protective clothing should be used.
  Patients and carers should be warned that some redness and skin peeling can occur initially but settles with time. If undue irritation occurs, the frequency of application should be reduced or treatment suspended until the reaction subsides; if irritation persists, discontinue treatment. Several months of treatment may be needed to

achieve an optimal response and the treatment should be continued until no new lesions develop.

● **MEDICINAL FORMS**
There can be variation in the licensing of different medicines containing the same drug.
Gel
CAUTIONARY AND ADVISORY LABELS 11
EXCIPIENTS: May contain Butylated hydroxytoluene, hydroxybenzoates (parabens), polysorbates
▸ Treclin (Meda Pharmaceuticals Ltd)
  Tretinoin 250 microgram per 1 gram, Clindamycin (as Clindamycin phosphate) 10 mg per 1 gram Treclin 1%/0.025% gel | 30 gram [PoM] £11.94

Tretinoin with erythromycin

The properties listed below are those particular to the combination only. For the properties of the components please consider, tretinoin p. 527, erythromycin p. 316.

● **INDICATIONS AND DOSE**

Acne

▸ TO THE SKIN

▸ Child: Apply 1–2 times a day, apply thinly

● **CONTRA-INDICATIONS** Perioral dermatitis · personal or familial history of non-melanoma skin cancer · rosacea

● **CAUTIONS** Allow peeling (resulting from other irritant treatments) to subside before using a topical retinoid · alternating a preparation that causes peeling with a topical retinoid may give rise to contact dermatitis (reduce frequency of retinoid application) · avoid accumulation in angles of the nose · avoid contact with eyes, nostrils, mouth and mucous membranes, eczematous, broken or sunburned skin · avoid exposure to UV light (including sunlight, solariums) · avoid in severe acne involving large areas · avoid use of topical retinoids with abrasive cleaners, comedogenic or astringent cosmetics · caution in sensitive areas such as the neck

● **INTERACTIONS** → Appendix 1: macrolides, retinoids

● **SIDE-EFFECTS** Blistering of skin · burning · crusting of skin · dry or peeling skin (discontinue if severe) · erythema · eye irritation · increased sensitivity to UVB light or sunlight · oedema · pruritus · stinging · temporary changes of skin pigmentation

● **CONCEPTION AND CONTRACEPTION** Females of child-bearing age must use effective contraception (oral progestogen-only contraceptives not considered effective).

● **PREGNANCY** Contra-indicated in pregnancy.

● **BREAST FEEDING** Amount of drug in milk after topical application probably too small to be harmful; ensure infant does not come in contact with treated areas.

● **PATIENT AND CARER ADVICE** Patients and carers should be warned that some redness and skin peeling can occur initially but settles with time. If undue irritation occurs, the frequency of application should be reduced or treatment suspended until the reaction subsides; if irritation persists, discontinue treatment. Several months of treatment may be needed to achieve an optimal response and the treatment should be continued until no new lesions develop. If sun exposure is unavoidable, an appropriate sunscreen or protective clothing should be used.

13

Skin

- **MEDICINAL FORMS**
  There can be variation in the licensing of different medicines containing the same drug.
  Liquid
  CAUTIONARY AND ADVISORY LABELS 11
  ‣ Aknemycin Plus (Almirall Ltd)
  Tretinoin 250 microgram per 1 gram, Erythromycin 40 mg per 1 gram Aknemycin Plus solution | 25 ml PoM £7.05 DT price = £7.05

VITAMINS AND TRACE ELEMENTS > VITAMIN B GROUP

Nicotinamide

- **INDICATIONS AND DOSE**
  Inflammatory acne vulgaris
  ‣ TO THE SKIN
  ‣ Child: Apply twice daily, reduced to once daily or on alternate days, dose reduced if irritation occurs

- **UNLICENSED USE** Licensed for use in children (age range not specified by manufacturer).
- **CAUTIONS** Avoid contact with eyes · avoid contact with mucous membranes (including nose and mouth) · reduce frequency of application if excessive dryness, irritation or peeling
- **SIDE-EFFECTS** Burning · dry skin · erythema · irritation · pruritus

- **MEDICINAL FORMS**
  There can be variation in the licensing of different medicines containing the same drug.
  Gel
  ‣ Freederm (Dendron Ltd)
  Nicotinamide 40 mg per 1 gram Freederm 4% gel | 10 gram GSL £3.10 | 25 gram P £5.56
  ‣ Nicam (Dermal Laboratories Ltd)
  Nicotinamide 40 mg per 1 gram Nicam 4% gel | 60 gram P £7.10

7 Scalp and hair conditions

Scalp and hair conditions

Overview

The detergent action of shampoo removes grease (sebum) from hair. Prepubertal children produce very little grease and require shampoo less frequently than adults. Shampoos can be used as vehicles for medicinal products, but their usefulness is limited by the short time the product is in contact with the scalp and by their irritant nature.

Oils and ointments are very useful for scaly, dry scalp conditions; if a greasy appearance is cosmetically unacceptable, the preparation may be applied at night and washed out in the morning. Alcohol-based lotions are rarely used in children; alcohol causes painful stinging on broken skin and the fumes may exacerbate asthma.

Itchy, inflammatory, eczematous scalp conditions may be relieved by a simple emollient oil such as **olive oil** or **coconut oil** (arachis oil (ground nut oil, peanut oil) is best avoided in children under 5 years). In more severe cases a topical **corticosteroid** may be required. Preparations containing **coal tar** are used for the common scaly scalp conditions of childhood including seborrhoeic dermatitis, dandruff (a mild form of seborrhoeic dermatitis), and psoriasis; salicylic acid is used as a keratolytic in some scalp preparations.

Shampoos containing antimicrobials such as selenium below or ketoconazole p. 695 are used for seborrhoeic dermatitis and dandruff in which yeast infection has been implicated, and for tinea capitis (ringworm of the scalp).

Bacterial infection affecting the scalp (usually secondary to eczema, head lice, or ringworm) may be treated with shampoos containing antimicrobials such as **pyrithione zinc**, cetrimide, or povidone-iodine p. 731.

In neonates and infants, *cradle cap* (which is also a form of seborrhoeic eczema) can be treated by massaging **coconut oil** or **olive oil** into the scalp; a bland emollient such as **emulsifying ointment** can be rubbed onto the affected area once or twice daily before bathing and a mild shampoo used.

ANTISEPTICS AND DISINFECTANTS > UNDECENOATES

Cetrimide with undecenoic acid

- **INDICATIONS AND DOSE**
  Scalp psoriasis | Seborrhoeic dermatitis | Dandruff
  ‣ TO THE SKIN
  ‣ Child: Apply 3 times a week for 1 week, then apply twice weekly

- **MEDICINAL FORMS**
  There can be variation in the licensing of different medicines containing the same drug.
  Shampoo
  ‣ Ceanel (Alliance Pharmaceuticals Ltd)
  Undecenoic acid 10 mg per 1 ml, Phenylethyl alcohol 75 mg per 1 ml, Cetrimide 100 mg per 1 ml Ceanel Concentrate shampoo | 150 ml P £3.40 | 500 ml P £9.80

ANTISEPTICS AND DISINFECTANTS > OTHER

Benzalkonium chloride

- **INDICATIONS AND DOSE**
  Seborrhoeic scalp conditions associated with dandruff and scaling
  ‣ TO THE SKIN
  ‣ Child: Apply as required

- **MEDICINAL FORMS**
  There can be variation in the licensing of different medicines containing the same drug.
  Shampoo
  ‣ Dermax (Dermal Laboratories Ltd)
  Benzalkonium chloride 5 mg per 1 ml Dermax Therapeutic 0.5% shampoo | 250 ml P £5.69

VITAMINS AND TRACE ELEMENTS

Selenium

- **INDICATIONS AND DOSE**
  Seborrhoeic dermatitis | Dandruff
  ‣ TO THE SKIN USING SHAMPOO
  ‣ Child 5-17 years: Apply twice weekly for 2 weeks, then apply once weekly for 2 weeks, then apply as required
  Pityriasis versicolor
  ‣ TO THE SKIN USING SHAMPOO
  ‣ Child 5-17 years: Apply once daily for 7 days, apply to the affected area and leave on for 10 minutes before rinsing off. The course may be repeated if necessary. Diluting with a small amount of water prior to application can reduce irritation

- **UNLICENSED USE** The use of selenium sulfide shampoo as a lotion for the treatment of pityriasis (tinea) versicolor is an unlicensed indication.
- **INTERACTIONS** → Appendix 1: selenium

- **PATIENT AND CARER ADVICE** Avoid using 48 hours before or after applying hair colouring, straightening or waving preparations.

- **MEDICINAL FORMS**
There can be variation in the licensing of different medicines containing the same drug.
Shampoo
EXCIPIENTS: May contain Fragrances
▸ **Selsun** (Chattem (U.K.) Ltd)
   Selenium sulfide 25 mg per 1 ml Selsun 2.5% shampoo | 50 ml P
   £1.61 DT price = £1.61 | 100 ml P £2.15 DT price = £2.15 |
   150 ml P £3.06 DT price = £3.06

8 Skin cleansers, antiseptics and desloughing agents

Skin cleansers, antiseptics and desloughing agents

Skin cleansers and antiseptics

Soap or detergent is used with water to cleanse intact skin but they can irritate infantile skin; emollient preparations such as aqueous cream or emulsifying ointment can be used in place of soap or detergent for cleansing dry or irritated skin.

An antiseptic is used for skin that is infected or that is susceptible to recurrent infection. Detergent preparations containing chlorhexidine p. 732 or povidone-iodine below, which should be thoroughly rinsed off, are used. Emollients may also contain antiseptics.

Antiseptics such as chlorhexidine or povidone-iodine are used on intact skin before surgical procedures; their antiseptic effect is enhanced by an alcoholic solvent. Antiseptic solutions containing cetrimide can be used if a detergent effect is also required.

Preparations containing alcohol, and regular use of povidone-iodine, should be avoided on neonatal skin.

Hydrogen peroxide p. 733, an oxidising agent, is available as a cream and can be used for superficial bacterial skin infections.

For irrigating ulcers or wounds, lukewarm sterile sodium chloride 0.9% solution p. 561 is used but tap water is often appropriate.

Potassium permanganate below solution 1 in 10 000, a mild antiseptic with astringent properties, can be used as a soak for exudative eczematous areas; treatment should be stopped when the skin becomes dry.

Desloughing agents

Alginate, hydrogel, and hydrocolloid dressings are effective in wound debridement. Sterile larvae (maggots) (available from BioMonde) are also used for managing sloughing wounds and are prescribable on the NHS.

Desloughing solutions and creams are of little clinical value. Substances applied to an open area are easily absorbed and perilesional skin is easily sensitised.

ANTISEPTICS AND DISINFECTANTS

Potassium permanganate

- **INDICATIONS AND DOSE**
Cleansing and deodorising suppurating eczematous reactions and wounds
▸ TO THE SKIN
▸ Child: For wet dressings or baths, use approximately 0.01% (1 in 10 000) solution

- **CAUTIONS** Irritant to mucous membranes
- **DIRECTIONS FOR ADMINISTRATION** Potassium permanganate 0.1% solution to be diluted 1 in 10 to provide a 0.01% (1 in 10 000) solution. With potassium permanganate tablets for solution, 1 tablet dissolved in 4 litres of water provides a 0.01% (1 in 10 000) solution.

- **PATIENT AND CARER ADVICE** Can stain clothing, skin and nails (especially with prolonged use).

- **MEDICINAL FORMS**
There can be variation in the licensing of different medicines containing the same drug. Forms available from special-order manufacturers include: liquid
Tablet for cutaneous solution
▸ Potassium permanganate (Non-proprietary)
   Potassium permanganate 400 mg Potassium permanganate 400mg tablets for cutaneous solution | 30 tablet no price available DT price = £17.50
▸ Permitabs (Alliance Pharmaceuticals Ltd)
   Potassium permanganate 400 mg Permitabs 400mg tablets for cutaneous solution | 30 tablet £17.50 DT price = £17.50

ANTISEPTICS AND DISINFECTANTS ⟩ ALCOHOL DISINFECTANTS

Alcohol
(Industrial methylated spirit)

- **INDICATIONS AND DOSE**
Skin preparation before injection
▸ TO THE SKIN
▸ Child: Apply as required

- **CONTRA-INDICATIONS** Neonates
- **CAUTIONS** Avoid broken skin · flammable · patients have suffered severe burns when diathermy has been preceded by application of alcoholic skin disinfectants

- **SIDE-EFFECTS**
Overdose
Features of acute alcohol intoxication include ataxia, dysarthria, nystagmus, and drowsiness, which may progress to coma, with hypotension and acidosis.
For details on the management of poisoning, see Alcohol, under Emergency treatment of poisoning p. 803.

- **PRESCRIBING AND DISPENSING INFORMATION** Industrial methylated spirits defined by the BP as a mixture of 19 volumes of ethyl alcohol of an appropriate strength with 1 volume of approved wood naphtha.

- **MEDICINAL FORMS**
There can be variation in the licensing of different medicines containing the same drug.
Liquid
▸ Alcohol (Non-proprietary)
   Industrial methylated spirit 70% | 600 ml £6.30
   Wood naphtha 50 ml per 1 litre, Ethanol 950 ml per 1 litre Industrial methylated spirit 95% | 600 ml £5.04 | 1000 ml £4.46-£12.45

ANTISEPTICS AND DISINFECTANTS ⟩ IODINE PRODUCTS

Povidone-iodine

- **INDICATIONS AND DOSE**
Skin disinfection
▸ TO THE SKIN
▸ Child: (consult product literature)   continued →

13

Skin

BETADINE® DRY POWDER SPRAY

Skin disinfection, particularly minor wounds and infections

▸ TO THE SKIN
▸ Child 2-17 years: Not for use in serous cavities (consult product literature)

SAVLON® DRY

Skin disinfection of minor wounds

▸ TO THE SKIN
▸ Child: (consult product literature)

VIDENE® SOLUTION

Skin disinfection

▸ TO THE SKIN
▸ Child: Apply undiluted in pre-operative skin disinfection and general antisepsis

VIDENE® SURGICAL SCRUB®

Skin disinfection

▸ TO THE SKIN
▸ Child: Use as a pre-operative scrub for hand and skin disinfection

VIDENE® TINCTURE

Skin disinfection

▸ TO THE SKIN
▸ Child: Apply undiluted in pre-operative skin disinfection

- **CONTRA-INDICATIONS** Concomitant use of lithium · corrected gestational age under 32 weeks · infants body-weight under 1.5 kg · regular use in neonates
  VIDENE® TINCTURE Neonates
- **CAUTIONS** Broken skin · large open wounds
  CAUTIONS, FURTHER INFORMATION
  ▸ Large open wounds The application of povidone–iodine to large wounds or severe burns may produce systemic adverse effects such as metabolic acidosis, hypernatraemia and impairment of renal function.
  VIDENE® TINCTURE Procedures involving hot wire cautery and diathermy
- **SIDE-EFFECTS**
  ▸ Rare Sensitivity
- **PREGNANCY** Sufficient iodine may be absorbed to affect the fetal thyroid in the second and third trimester.
- **BREAST FEEDING** Avoid regular or excessive use.
- **RENAL IMPAIRMENT** Avoid regular application to inflamed or broken skin or mucosa.
- **EFFECT ON LABORATORY TESTS** May interfere with thyroid function tests.

- **MEDICINAL FORMS**
  There can be variation in the licensing of different medicines containing the same drug. Forms available from special-order manufacturers include: liquid

Spray
▸ Betadine (Aspire Pharma Ltd)
  Povidone-Iodine 25 mg per 1 gram Betadine 2.5% dry powder spray | 100 ml GSL £9.95 DT price = £9.95

Liquid
CAUTIONARY AND ADVISORY LABELS 15 (Only for use with alcoholic solutions)
▸ Videne (Ecolab Healthcare Division)
  Povidone-Iodine 75 mg per 1 ml Videne 7.5% surgical scrub solution | 500 ml P £7.67
  Povidone-Iodine 100 mg per 1 ml Videne 10% antiseptic solution | 500 ml P £7.67
  Videne 10% alcoholic tinrure | 500 ml P £7.68

ANTISEPTICS AND DISINFECTANTS ⟩ OTHER

Chlorhexidine

- **INDICATIONS AND DOSE**
  CX ANTISEPTIC DUSTING POWDER
  For skin disinfection
  ▸ TO THE SKIN
  ▸ Child: (consult product literature)
  CEPTON® LOTION
  For skin disinfection in acne
  ▸ TO THE SKIN
  ▸ Child: (consult product literature)
  CEPTON® SKIN WASH
  For use as skin wash in acne
  ▸ TO THE SKIN
  ▸ Child: (consult product literature)
  HIBITANE® PLUS 5% CONCENTRATE SOLUTION
  General and pre-operative skin disinfection
  ▸ TO THE SKIN
  ▸ Child: (consult product literature)
  HIBISCRUB®
  Pre-operative hand and skin disinfection | General hand and skin disinfection
  ▸ TO THE SKIN
  ▸ Child: Use as alternative to soap (consult product literature)
  HIBITANE OBSTETRIC®
  For use in obstetrics and gynaecology as an antiseptic and lubricant
  ▸ TO THE SKIN
  ▸ Child: To be applied to skin around vulva and perineum and to hands of midwife or doctor
  HIBI® LIQUID HAND RUB+
  Hand and skin disinfection
  ▸ TO THE SKIN
  ▸ Child: To be used undiluted (consult product literature)
  HYDREX® SOLUTION
  For pre-operative skin disinfection
  ▸ TO THE SKIN
  ▸ Child: (consult product literature)
  HYDREX® SURGICAL SCRUB
  For pre-operative hand and skin disinfection | General hand disinfection
  ▸ TO THE SKIN
  ▸ Child: (consult product literature)
  UNISEPT®
  For cleansing and disinfecting wounds and burns and swabbing in obstetrics
  ▸ TO THE SKIN
  ▸ Child: (consult product literature)

> **IMPORTANT SAFETY INFORMATION**
> In preterm neonates, use sparingly, monitor for skin reactions, and do not allow solution to pool—risk of severe chemical burns.

- **CONTRA-INDICATIONS** Alcoholic solutions not suitable before diathermy · alcoholic solutions not suitable for use on neonatal skin · not for use in body cavities
- **CAUTIONS** Avoid contact with brain · avoid contact with eyes · avoid contact with meninges · avoid contact with middle ear
- **SIDE-EFFECTS** Chemical burns in preterm neonates · sensitivity

● **DIRECTIONS FOR ADMINISTRATION**

HIBITANE ® PLUS 5% CONCENTRATE SOLUTION
For pre-operative skin preparation, dilute 1 in 10 (0.5%) with alcohol 70%. For general skin disinfection, dilute 1 in 100 (0.05%) with water. Alcoholic solutions not suitable for use before diathermy or on neonatal skin.

● **MEDICINAL FORMS**
There can be variation in the licensing of different medicines containing the same drug.

Cream
▸ Chlorhexidine (Non-proprietary)
  Chlorhexidine hydrochloride 5 mg per 1 gram cream | 30 gram GSL £2.07
▸ Brands may include Acriflex, Eczmol, Hibitane

Powder
▸ CX (Ecolab Healthcare Division)
  Chlorhexidine acetate 10 mg per 1 gram CX 1% powder | 15 gram GSL £5.47

Liquid
CAUTIONARY AND ADVISORY LABELS 15 (For ethanolic solutions e.g. ChloraPrep ® and Hydrex ® only)
EXCIPIENTS: May contain Fragrances
▸ Cepton (Boston Healthcare Ltd)
  Chlorhexidine gluconate 10 mg per 1 ml Cepton 1% medicated skin wash | 150 ml GSL £31.45
▸ HiBiTane Plus (Molnlycke Health Care Ltd)
  Chlorhexidine gluconate 50 mg per 1 ml HiBiTane Plus 5% concentrate solution | 5000 ml GSL £14.50
▸ Hibi (Molnlycke Health Care Ltd)
  Chlorhexidine gluconate 5 mg per 1 ml HiBi Liquid Hand Rub+ 0.5% solution | 500 ml GSL £5.25
▸ Hibiscrub (Molnlycke Health Care Ltd)
  Chlorhexidine gluconate 40 mg per 1 ml Hibiscrub 4% solution | 250 ml GSL £4.25 | 500 ml GSL £5.25 | 5000 ml GSL £24.00
▸ Hydrex (Ecolab Healthcare Division)
  Chlorhexidine gluconate 5 mg per 1 ml Hydrex pink chlorhexidine gluconate 0.5% solution | 600 ml GSL £4.72
  Hydrex clear chlorhexidine gluconate 0.5% solution | 600 ml GSL £4.72
  Chlorhexidine gluconate 40 mg per 1 ml Hydrex 4% Surgical Scrub | 250 ml GSL £4.30 | 500 ml GSL £4.77 | 5000 ml GSL £39.75

Chlorhexidine gluconate with isopropyl alcohol

The properties listed below are those particular to the combination only. For the properties of the components please consider, chlorhexidine p. 732.

● **INDICATIONS AND DOSE**

Skin disinfection before invasive procedures
▸ TO THE SKIN
▸ Child 2 months-17 years: (consult product literature)

● **MEDICINAL FORMS**
There can be variation in the licensing of different medicines containing the same drug. Forms available from special-order manufacturers include: liquid

Liquid
CAUTIONARY AND ADVISORY LABELS 15
▸ ChloraPrep (CareFusion U.K. Ltd)
  Chlorhexidine gluconate 20 mg per 1 ml, Isopropyl alcohol 700 ml per 1 litre ChloraPrep with Tint solution 10.5ml applicators | 25 applicator GSL £76.65
  ChloraPrep with Tint solution 26ml applicators | 25 applicator £170.75
  ChloraPrep solution 3ml applicators | 25 applicator GSL £21.25
  ChloraPrep solution 1.5ml applicators | 20 applicator GSL £11.00
  ChloraPrep with Tint solution 3ml applicator | 25 applicator GSL £22.31
  ChloraPrep solution 0.67ml applicators | 200 applicator GSL £60.00
  ChloraPrep solution 10.5ml applicators | 25 applicator GSL £73.00
  ChloraPrep solution 26ml applicators | 25 applicator GSL £162.50

Chlorhexidine with cetrimide

The properties listed below are those particular to the combination only. For the properties of the components please consider, chlorhexidine p. 732.

● **INDICATIONS AND DOSE**

Skin disinfection such as wound cleansing and obstetrics
▸ TO THE SKIN
▸ Child: To be used undiluted

● **MEDICINAL FORMS**
There can be variation in the licensing of different medicines containing the same drug.

Cream
▸ Chlorhexidine with cetrimide (Non-proprietary)
  Chlorhexidine gluconate 1 mg per 1 gram, Cetrimide 5 mg per 1 gram Savlon antiseptic cream | 15 gram GSL £0.90 | 30 gram GSL £1.19 | 60 gram GSL £1.91 | 100 gram GSL £2.78

Irrigation solution
▸ Chlorhexidine with cetrimide (Non-proprietary)
  Chlorhexidine acetate 150 microgram per 1 ml, Cetrimide 1.5 mg per 1 ml Chlorhexidine acetate 0.015% / Cetrimide 0.15% irrigation solution 1litre bottles | 1 bottle P no price available

Liquid
▸ Savlon disinfectant (GlaxoSmithKline Consumer Healthcare)
  Chlorhexidine gluconate 3 mg per 1 ml, Cetrimide 30 mg per 1 ml Savlon disinfectant liquid | 500 ml £1.32
▸ Sterets Tisept (Molnlycke Health Care Ltd)
  Chlorhexidine gluconate 150 microgram per 1 ml, Cetrimide 1.5 mg per 1 ml Sterets Tisept solution 25ml sachets | 25 sachet P £5.33
  Sterets Tisept solution 100ml sachets | 10 sachet P £6.85

Diethyl phthalate with methyl salicylate

● **INDICATIONS AND DOSE**

Skin preparation before injection
▸ TO THE SKIN
▸ Child: Apply to the area to be disinfected

● **MEDICINAL FORMS**
There can be variation in the licensing of different medicines containing the same drug.

Liquid
CAUTIONARY AND ADVISORY LABELS 15
▸ Diethyl phthalate with methyl salicylate (Non-proprietary)
  Methyl salicylate 5 ml per 1 litre, Diethyl phthalate 20 ml per 1 litre, Castor oil 25 ml per 1 litre, Industrial methylated spirit 950 ml per 1 litre Surgical spirit | 200 ml GSL £1.15 DT price = £1.15 | 1000 ml GSL £3.62

Hydrogen peroxide

● **DRUG ACTION** Hydrogen peroxide is an oxidising agent.

● **INDICATIONS AND DOSE**

CRYSTACIDE®

Superficial bacterial skin infection
▸ TO THE SKIN
▸ Child: Apply 2–3 times a day for up to 3 weeks

● **UNLICENSED USE** Licensed for use in children (age range not specified by manufacturer).

● **CAUTIONS** Avoid on eyes · avoid on healthy skin · incompatible with products containing iodine or potassium permanganate

● **PRESCRIBING AND DISPENSING INFORMATION** The BP directs that when hydrogen peroxide is prescribed,

13

Skin

hydrogen peroxide solution 6% (20 vols) should be dispensed.

Strong solutions of hydrogen peroxide which contain 27% (90 vols) and 30% (100 vols) are only for the preparation of weaker solutions.

- **HANDLING AND STORAGE** Hydrogen peroxide bleaches fabric.

- **MEDICINAL FORMS**
There can be variation in the licensing of different medicines containing the same drug.
Cream
EXCIPIENTS: May contain Edetic acid (edta), propylene glycol
▸ Crystacide (Reig Jofre UK Ltd)
Hydrogen peroxide 10 mg per 1 gram Crystacide 1% cream | 25 gram P £8.07 DT price = £8.07 | 40 gram P £11.62

Proflavine

The properties listed below are those particular to the combination only. For the properties of the components please consider, liquid paraffin.

- **INDICATIONS AND DOSE**
Infected wounds | Infected burns
▸ TO THE SKIN
▸ Child: (consult product literature)

- **PATIENT AND CARER ADVICE** Stains clothing.

- **MEDICINAL FORMS**
There can be variation in the licensing of different medicines containing the same drug. Forms available from special-order manufacturers include: liquid

Irrigation solutions

- **IRRIGATION SOLUTIONS**

Flowfusor sodium chloride 0.9% irrigation solution 120ml bottles (Fresenius Kabi Ltd) Sodium chloride 9 mg per 1 ml 1 bottle · NHS indicative price = £1.71 · Drug Tariff (Part IXa)

Irriclens sodium chloride 0.9% irrigation solution aerosol spray (ConvaTec Ltd) Sodium chloride 9 mg per 1 ml 240 ml · NHS indicative price = £3.54 · Drug Tariff (Part IXa)

Normasol sodium chloride 0.9% irrigation solution 100ml sachets (Molnlycke Health Care Ltd) Sodium chloride 9 mg per 1 ml 10 unit dose · NHS indicative price = £7.92 · Drug Tariff (Part IXa)

Normasol sodium chloride 0.9% irrigation solution 25ml sachets (Molnlycke Health Care Ltd) Sodium chloride 9 mg per 1 ml 25 unit dose · NHS indicative price = £6.42 · Drug Tariff (Part IXa)

Sodium chloride 0.9% irrigation solution 20ml Clinipod unit dose (Mayors Healthcare Ltd) Sodium chloride 9 mg per 1 ml 25 unit dose · NHS indicative price = £4.80 · Drug Tariff (Part IXa)

Sodium chloride 0.9% irrigation solution 20ml ISO-POD unit dose (St Georges Medical Ltd) Sodium chloride 9 mg per 1 ml 25 unit dose · NHS indicative price = £4.95 · Drug Tariff (Part IXa)

Sodium chloride 0.9% irrigation solution 20ml Irripod unit dose (C D Medical Ltd) Sodium chloride 9 mg per 1 ml 25 unit dose · NHS indicative price = £5.84 · Drug Tariff (Part IXa)

Sodium chloride 0.9% irrigation solution 20ml Sal-e Pods unit dose (Ennogen Healthcare Ltd) Sodium chloride 9 mg per 1 ml 25 unit dose · NHS indicative price = £4.80 · Drug Tariff (Part IXa)

Sodium chloride 0.9% irrigation solution 20ml Salipod unit dose (Sai-Meds Ltd) Sodium chloride 9 mg per 1 ml 25 unit dose · NHS indicative price = £4.99 · Drug Tariff (Part IXa)

Sodium chloride 0.9% irrigation solution 20ml Steripod unit dose (Molnlycke Health Care Ltd) Sodium chloride 9 mg per 1 ml 25 unit dose · NHS indicative price = £7.90 · Drug Tariff (Part IXa)

Sodium chloride 0.9% irrigation solution 20ml Sterowash unit dose (Steroplast Healthcare Ltd) Sodium chloride 9 mg per 1 ml 25 unit dose · NHS indicative price = £5.40 · Drug Tariff (Part IXa)

Sodium chloride 0.9% irrigation solution 20ml unit dose (Alissa Healthcare Research Ltd) Sodium chloride 9 mg per 1 ml 25 unit dose · NHS indicative price = £7.36 · Drug Tariff (Part IXa)

Sodium chloride 0.9% irrigation solution 20ml unit dose (Crest Medical Ltd) Sodium chloride 9 mg per 1 ml 25 unit dose · NHS indicative price = £4.99 · Drug Tariff (Part IXa)

Sodium chloride 0.9% irrigation solution 20ml unit dose (Mylan Ltd) Sodium chloride 9 mg per 1 ml 25 unit dose · NHS indicative price = £5.50 · Drug Tariff (Part IXa)

Stericlens sodium chloride 0.9% irrigation solution aerosol spray (C D Medical Ltd) Sodium chloride 9 mg per 1 ml 100 ml · NHS indicative price = £2.07 · Drug Tariff (Part IXa) 240 ml · NHS indicative price = £3.15 · Drug Tariff (Part IXa)

8.1 Minor cuts and abrasions

Minor cuts and abrasions

Management

Many preparations traditionally used to manage minor burns, and abrasions have fallen out of favour. Preparations containing camphor and sulfonamides should be avoided. Preparations such as magnesium sulfate paste are now rarely used to treat carbuncles and boils as these are best treated with antibiotics.

Cetrimide is used to treat minor cuts and abrasions and proflavine above may be used to treat infected wounds or burns, but its use has now been largely superseded by other antisepics or suitable antibacterials. The effervescent effect of hydrogen peroxide p. 733 is used to clean minor cuts and abrasions.

Flexible collodion (see castor oil with collodion and colophony below) may be used to seal minor cuts and wounds that have partially healed; skin tissue adhesives are used similarly, and also for additional suture support.

DERMATOLOGICAL DRUGS › COLLODIONS

Castor oil with collodion and colophony

- **INDICATIONS AND DOSE**
Used to seal minor cuts and wounds that have partially healed
▸ TO THE SKIN
▸ Child: (consult product literature)

- **ALLERGY AND CROSS-SENSITIVITY** Contra-indicated if patient has an allergy to colophony in elastic adhesive plasters and tape.

- **MEDICINAL FORMS**
There can be variation in the licensing of different medicines containing the same drug.
Liquid
▸ Castor oil with collodion and colophony (Non-proprietary)
Castor oil 25 mg per 1 ml, Colophony 25 mg per 1 ml, Collodion methylated 950 microlitre per 1 ml Flexible collodion methylated | 100 ml £13.54 | 500 ml £27.79

Skin adhesives

- **SKIN ADHESIVES**

Derma+Flex skin adhesive (Chemence Ltd)
.5 ml · NHS indicative price = £5.36 · Drug Tariff (Part IXa)

Dermabond ProPen skin adhesive (Ethicon Ltd)
.5 ml · NHS indicative price = £19.46 · Drug Tariff (Part IXa)

Histoacryl L skin adhesive (B.Braun Medical Ltd)
.5 ml · NHS indicative price = £6.72 · Drug Tariff (Part IXa)

Histoacryl skin adhesive (B.Braun Medical Ltd)
.5 ml · NHS indicative price = £6.50 · Drug Tariff (Part IXa)

Indermil skin adhesive (Covidien (UK) Commercial Ltd)
.5 gram · NHS indicative price = £6.50 · Drug Tariff (Part IXa)

LiquiBand flow control tissue adhesive (MedLogic Global Ltd)
.5 gram · NHS indicative price = £5.50 · Drug Tariff (Part IXa)

LiquiBand tissue adhesive (MedLogic Global Ltd)
.5 gram · NHS indicative price = £5.50 · Drug Tariff (Part IXa)

9 Skin disfigurement

Camouflagers

Overview

Disfigurement of the skin can be very distressing to patients and may have a marked psychological effect. In skilled hands, or with experience, camouflage cosmetics can be very effective in concealing scars and birthmarks. The depigmented patches in vitiligo are also very disfiguring and camouflage creams are of great cosmetic value.

Opaque cover foundation or cream is used to mask skin pigment abnormalities; careful application using a combination of dark- and light-coloured cover creams set with powder helps to minimise the appearance of skin deformities.

Borderline substances

The preparations marked 'ACBS' can be prescribed on the NHS for postoperative scars and other deformities and as adjunctive therapy in the relief of emotional disturbances due to disfiguring skin disease, such as vitiligo.

Camouflages

● CAMOUFLAGES

Covermark classic foundation (Derma UK Ltd)
15 ml(ACBS) · NHS indicative price = £11.86

Covermark finishing powder (Derma UK Ltd)
25 gram(ACBS) · NHS indicative price = £11.86

Dermablend Dermasmooth Corrective Foundation (Vichy)
30 ml · No NHS indicative price available

Dermacolor body camouflage (Kryolan UK Ltd)
50 ml · NHS indicative price = £8.94

Dermacolor camouflage creme (Kryolan UK Ltd)
30 gram · NHS indicative price = £11.00

Dermacolor fixing powder (Kryolan UK Ltd)
60 gram(ACBS) · NHS indicative price = £9.85

Keromask finishing powder (Bellava Ltd)
20 gram(ACBS) · NHS indicative price = £5.80

Keromask masking cream (Bellava Ltd)
15 ml(ACBS) · NHS indicative price = £5.90

Veil cover cream (Thomas Blake Cosmetic Creams Ltd)
19 gram(ACBS) · NHS indicative price = £22.42 44 gram(ACBS) · NHS indicative price = £33.35 70 gram(ACBS) · NHS indicative price = £42.10

Veil finishing powder (Thomas Blake Cosmetic Creams Ltd)
35 gram(ACBS) · NHS indicative price = £24.58

10 Sun protection and photodamage

Photodamage

Overview

Actinic keratoses occur very rarely in healthy children; actinic cheilitis may occur on the lips of adolescents following excessive sun exposure.

Diclofenac gel (Solaraze®) and topical preparations of fluorouracil are licensed for the treatment of actinic keratoses but they are not licensed for use in children.

In children with photosensitivity disorders, such as erythropoietic protoporphyria, specialists may use betacarotene p. 736, mepacrine, chloroquine or hydroxychloroquine to reduce skin reactions.

Sunscreen

Sunscreen preparations

Solar ultraviolet irradiation can be harmful to the skin. It is responsible for disorders such as *polymorphic light eruption, solar urticaria,* and it provokes the various *cutaneous porphyrias.* It also provokes (or at least aggravates) skin lesions of *lupus erythematosus* and may aggravate some other *dermatoses.* Certain drugs, such as demeclocycline, phenothiazines, or amiodarone, can cause photosensitivity. All these conditions (as well as *sunburn*) may occur after relatively short periods of exposure to the sun. Solar ultraviolet irradiation may provoke attacks of recurrent herpes labialis (but it is not known whether the effect of sunlight exposure is local or systemic).

The effects of exposure over longer periods include *ageing changes* and more importantly the initiation of *skin cancer.*

Solar ultraviolet radiation is approximately 200–400 m in wavelength. The medium wavelengths (290–320 nm, known as UVB) cause sunburn. The long wavelengths (320–400 nm, known as UVA) are responsible for many *photosensitivity reactions* and *photodermatoses.* Both UVA and UVB contribute to long-term *photodamage* and to the changes responsible for *skin cancer* and ageing.

Sunscreen preparations contain substances that protect the skin against UVA and UVB radiation, but they are no substitute for covering the skin and avoiding sunlight. Protective clothing and sun avoidance (rather than the use of sunscreen preparations) are recommended for children under 6 months of age.

The sun protection factor (SPF, usually indicated in the preparation title) provides guidance on the degree of protection offered against UVB; it indicates the multiples of protection provided against burning, compared with unprotected skin; for example, an SPF of 8 should enable a child to remain 8 times longer in the sun without burning. However, in practice users do not apply sufficient sunscreen product and the protection is lower than that found in experimental studies. Some manufacturers use a star rating system to indicate the protection against UVA relative to protection against UVB for sunscreen products. However, the usefulness of the star rating system remains controversial. The EU Commission (September 2006) has recommended that the UVA protection factor for a sunscreen should be at least one-third of the sun protection factor (SPF); products that achieve this requirement will be labelled with a UVA logo alongside the SPF classification. Preparations that also contain reflective substances, such as titanium dioxide, provide the most effective protection against UVA.

13

Skin

Sunscreen preparations may rarely cause allergic reactions.

For optimum photoprotection, sunscreen preparations should be applied **thickly** and **frequently** (approximately 2 hourly). In photodermatoses, they should be used from spring to autumn. As maximum protection from sunlight is desirable, preparations with the highest SPF should be prescribed.

Ingredient nomenclature in sunscreen preparations

rINN	INCI
amiloxate	isoamyl *p*-methoxycinnamate
avobenzone	butyl methoxydibenzoylmethane
bemotrizinol	bis-ethylhexyloxyphenol methoxyphenyl triazine
bisoctrizole	methylene bis-benzotriazolyl tetramethylbutylphenol
ecamsule	terephthalylidene dicamphor sulfonic acid
ensulizole	phenylbenzimidazole sulfonic acid
enzacamene	4-methylbenzylidene camphor
octinoxate	octyl (*or* ethylhexyl) methoxycinnamate
octocrilene	octocrylene
oxybenzone	benzophenone-3

The European Commission Cosmetic Products Regulation (EC) 1223/2009 requires the use of INCI (International Nomenclature of Cosmetic Ingredients) for cosmetics and sunscreens. This table includes the rINN and the INCI synonym for the active ingredients of sunscreen preparations in the BNFC

Borderline substances

Anthelios® XL SPF 50+ Melt-in cream; *Sunsense*® Ultra; *Uvistat*® Lipscreen SPF 50; and *Uvistat*® Suncream SPF 30 and 50 (see *Borderline substances*) cannot be prescribed on the NHS except for skin protection against ultraviolet radiation in abnormal cutaneous photosensitivity resulting from genetic disorders or photodermatoses, including vitiligo and those resulting from radiotherapy; chronic or recurrent herpes simplex labialis. Preparations with SPF less than 30 should not normally be prescribed.

VITAMINS AND TRACE ELEMENTS › VITAMIN A

Betacarotene

● **DRUG ACTION** Betacarotene is a precursor to vitamin A.

● **INDICATIONS AND DOSE**

Management of photosensitivity reactions in erythropoietic protoporphyria (specialist use only)
▶ BY MOUTH
▸ Child 1-4 years: 60–90 mg daily, to be given as a single dose or in divided doses
▸ Child 5-8 years: 90–120 mg daily, to be given as a single dose or in divided doses
▸ Child 9-11 years: 120–150 mg daily, to be given as a single dose or in divided doses
▸ Child 12-15 years: 150–180 mg daily, to be given as a single dose or in divided doses
▸ Child 16-17 years: 180–300 mg daily, to be given as a single dose or in divided doses

● **UNLICENSED USE** Not licensed.

● **CAUTIONS** Monitor vitamin A intake

● **CAUTIONS, FURTHER INFORMATION**
Protection not total avoid strong sunlight and use sunscreen preparations; generally 2–6 weeks of treatment (resulting in yellow coloration of palms and soles) necessary before increasing exposure to sunlight; dose should be adjusted according to level of exposure to sunlight.

● **SIDE-EFFECTS**
▸ **Rare** Arthralgia · bruising
▸ **Frequency not known** Loose stools · yellow discoloration of skin

● **PREGNANCY** Partially converted to vitamin A, but does not give rise to abnormally high serum concentration; manufacturer advises use only if potential benefit outweighs risk.

● **BREAST FEEDING** Use with caution—present in milk.

● **HEPATIC IMPAIRMENT** Avoid.

● **RENAL IMPAIRMENT** Use with caution.

● **MEDICINAL FORMS**
There can be variation in the licensing of different medicines containing the same drug. Forms available from special-order manufacturers include: tablet, capsule

Capsule
CAUTIONARY AND ADVISORY LABELS 21
▸ **Betacarotene** (Non-proprietary)
Betacarotene 15 mg Betacarotene 15mg capsules | 90 capsule £6.11
G & G Natural Betacarotene 15mg capsules | 120 capsule £13.50
Betacarotene 25 mg Carotaben 25mg capsules | 100 capsule P no price available
Betacarotene 30 mg Lumitene 30mg capsules | 100 capsule PoM no price available
▸ **Bio-Carotene** (Pharma Nord (UK) Ltd)
Betacarotene 9 mg Bio-Carotene 9mg capsules | 150 capsule no price available
▸ **Super Betavit** (Health+Plus Ltd)
Betacarotene 15 mg Super Betavit 15mg capsules | 30 capsule £3.59

11 Superficial soft-tissue injuries and superficial thrombophlebitis

Topical circulatory preparations

Overview

These preparations are used to improve circulation in conditions such as bruising and superficial thrombophlebitis but are of little value. First aid measures such as rest, ice, compression, and elevation should be used. Chilblains are best managed by avoidance of exposure to cold; neither systemic nor topical vasodilator therapy is established as being effective.

HEPARINOIDS

Heparinoid

● **INDICATIONS AND DOSE**

Superficial thrombophlebitis | Bruising | Haematoma
▶ TO THE SKIN
▸ Child 5-17 years: Apply up to 4 times a day

● **CONTRA-INDICATIONS** Should not be used on large areas of skin, broken or sensitive skin, or mucous membranes

● **LESS SUITABLE FOR PRESCRIBING** Hirudoid® is less suitable for prescribing.

- **MEDICINAL FORMS**
There can be variation in the licensing of different medicines containing the same drug.

Cream
EXCIPIENTS: May contain Cetostearyl alcohol (including cetyl and stearyl alcohol), hydroxybenzoates (parabens)
- Hirudoid (Genus Pharmaceuticals Ltd)
  Heparinoid 3 mg per 1 gram Hirudoid 0.3% cream | 50 gram P
  £3.99 DT price = £3.99

Gel
EXCIPIENTS: May contain Fragrances, propylene glycol
- Hirudoid (Genus Pharmaceuticals Ltd)
  Heparinoid 3 mg per 1 gram Hirudoid 0.3% gel | 50 gram P £3.99
  DT price = £3.99

12 Warts and calluses

Warts and calluses

Overview

Warts (verruca vulgaris) are common, benign, self-limiting, and usually asymptomatic. They are caused by a human papillomavirus, which most frequently affects the hands, feet (plantar warts), and the anogenital region; treatment usually relies on local tissue destruction and is required only if the warts are painful, unsightly, persistent, or cause distress. In immunocompromised children, warts may be more difficult to eradicate.

Preparations of salicylic acid p. 739, formaldehyde below, glutaraldehyde p. 738 or silver nitrate p. 738 are used for the removal of warts on hands and feet. Salicylic acid is a useful keratolytic which may be considered first-line in the treatment of warts; it is also suitable for the removal of *corns and calluses*. Preparations of salicylic acid in a collodion basis are available but some patients may develop an allergy to colophony in the formulation; collodion should be avoided in children allergic to elastic adhesive plaster. Cryotherapy causes pain, swelling, and blistering, and may be no more effective than topical salicylic acid in the treatment of warts.

Anogenital warts

Anogenital warts (condylomata acuminata) in children are often asymptomatic and require only a simple barrier preparation. If treatment is required it should be supervised by a hospital specialist. Persistent warts on genital skin may require treatment with cryotherapy or other forms of physical ablation under general anaesthesia.

Podophyllotoxin below (the major active ingredient of podophyllum), or imiquimod p. 738 are used to treat external anogenital warts; these preparations can cause considerable irritation of the treated area and are therefore suitable only for children who are able to co-operate with the treatment.

ANTINEOPLASTIC DRUGS > PLANT ALKALOIDS

Podophyllotoxin

- **INDICATIONS AND DOSE**

CONDYLINE®

Condylomata acuminata affecting the penis or the female external genitalia
- TO THE LESION
- Child 2–17 years (initiated under specialist supervision):
  Apply twice daily for 3 consecutive days, treatment may be repeated at weekly intervals if necessary for a total of five 3-day treatment courses, direct medical supervision for lesions in the female and for lesions greater than 4 cm^2 in the male, maximum 50 single applications ('loops') per session (consult product literature)

WARTICON® CREAM

Condylomata acuminata affecting the penis or the female external genitalia
- TO THE LESION
- Child 2–17 years (initiated under specialist supervision):
  Apply twice daily for 3 consecutive days, treatment may be repeated at weekly intervals if necessary for a total of four 3-day treatment courses, direct medical supervision for lesions greater than 4 cm^2

WARTICON® LIQUID

Condylomata acuminata affecting the penis or the female external genitalia
- TO THE LESION
- Child 2–17 years (initiated under specialist supervision):
  Apply twice daily for 3 consecutive days, treatment may be repeated at weekly intervals if necessary for a total of four 3-day treatment courses, direct medical supervision for lesions greater than 4 cm^2, maximum 50 single applications ('loops') per session (consult product literature)

- **UNLICENSED USE** Not licensed for use in children.
- **CAUTIONS** Avoid normal skin · avoid open wounds · keep away from face · very irritant to eyes
- **SIDE-EFFECTS** Local irritation
- **PREGNANCY** Avoid.
- **BREAST FEEDING** Avoid.

- **MEDICINAL FORMS**
There can be variation in the licensing of different medicines containing the same drug.

Cream
EXCIPIENTS: May contain Butylated hydroxyanisole, cetostearyl alcohol (including cetyl and stearyl alcohol), hydroxybenzoates (parabens), sorbic acid
- Warticon (Stiefel Laboratories (UK) Ltd)
  Podophyllotoxin 1.5 mg per 1 gram Warticon 0.15% cream |
  5 gram PoM £17.83 DT price = £17.83

Liquid
CAUTIONARY AND ADVISORY LABELS 15
- Condyline (Takeda UK Ltd)
  Podophyllotoxin 5 mg per 1 ml Condyline 0.5% solution |
  3.5 ml PoM £14.49 DT price = £14.49
- Warticon (Stiefel Laboratories (UK) Ltd)
  Podophyllotoxin 5 mg per 1 ml Warticon 0.5% solution | 3 ml PoM
  £14.86 DT price = £14.86

ANTISEPTICS AND DISINFECTANTS >
ALDEHYDES AND DERIVATIVES

Formaldehyde

- **INDICATIONS AND DOSE**

Warts, particularly plantar warts
- TO THE LESION
- Child: Apply twice daily

- **UNLICENSED USE** Licensed for use in children (age range not specified by manufacturer).
- **CAUTIONS** Impaired peripheral circulation · not suitable for application to anogenital region · not suitable for application to face · not suitable for application to large areas · patients with diabetes at risk of neuropathic ulcers · protect surrounding skin and avoid broken skin · significant peripheral neuropathy
- **SIDE-EFFECTS** Skin irritation · skin ulceration (with high concentrations)

13

Skin

● **MEDICINAL FORMS**
There can be variation in the licensing of different medicines containing the same drug. Forms available from special-order manufacturers include: liquid

Gel
▸ Veracur (Typharm Ltd)
Formaldehyde 7.5 mg per 1 gram Veracur 0.75% gel | 15 gram GSL £2.41

Liquid
▸ Formaldehyde (Non-proprietary)
Formaldehyde 40 mg per 1 ml Formaldehyde (Buffered) 4% solution | 1000 ml £3.90
Formaldehyde 350 mg per 1 gram Formaldehyde solution | 500 ml £5.90 DT price = £5.90 | 2000 ml £16.98

Glutaraldehyde

● **INDICATIONS AND DOSE**

Warts, particularly plantar warts
▸ TO THE LESION
▸ Child: Apply twice daily

● **UNLICENSED USE** Licensed for use in children (age range not specified by manufacturer).

● **CAUTIONS** Not for application to anogenital areas · not for application to face · not for application to mucosa · protect surrounding skin

● **SIDE-EFFECTS** Rashes · skin irritation (discontinue if severe) · stains skin brown

● **MEDICINAL FORMS**
There can be variation in the licensing of different medicines containing the same drug.

Paint
▸ Glutarol (Dermal Laboratories Ltd)
Glutaraldehyde 100 mg per 1 ml Glutarol 10% cutaneous solution | 10 ml P £2.07 DT price = £2.07

ANTISEPTICS AND DISINFECTANTS 〉 OTHER

Silver nitrate

● **INDICATIONS AND DOSE**

Common warts
▸ TO THE LESION
▸ Child: Apply every 24 hours for up to 3 applications, apply moistened caustic pencil tip for 1–2 minutes. Instructions in proprietary packs generally incorporate advice to remove dead skin before use by gentle filing and to cover with adhesive dressing after application

Verrucas
▸ TO THE LESION
▸ Child: Apply every 24 hours for up to 6 applications, apply moistened caustic pencil tip for 1–2 minutes. Instructions in proprietary packs generally incorporate advice to remove dead skin before use by gentle filing and to cover with adhesive dressing after application

Umbilical granulomas
▸ TO THE SKIN
▸ Child: Apply moistened caustic pencil tip (usually containing silver nitrate 40%) for 1–2 minutes, protect surrounding skin with soft paraffin

● **UNLICENSED USE** No age range specified by manufacturer.

● **CAUTIONS** Avoid broken skin · not suitable for application to ano-genital region · not suitable for application to face · not suitable for application to large areas · protect surrounding skin

● **SIDE-EFFECTS** Chemical burns on surrounding skin · stains skin

● **PATIENT AND CARER ADVICE** Patients should be advised that silver nitrate may stain fabric.

● **MEDICINAL FORMS**
There can be variation in the licensing of different medicines containing the same drug.

Stick
▸ Silver nitrate (Non-proprietary)
Silver nitrate 400 mg per 1 gram Silver nitrate 40% caustic pencils | 1 applicator P no price available
▸ Avoca (Bray Group Ltd)
Silver nitrate 400 mg per 1 gram Avoca 40% silver nitrate pencils | 1 applicator P £1.03
Silver nitrate 750 mg per 1 gram Avoca 75% silver nitrate applicators | 100 applicator P £44.48
Avoca 75% silver nitrate applicators with thick handles | 50 applicator P £43.41
Silver nitrate 950 mg per 1 gram Avoca 95% silver nitrate applicators | 100 applicator P £44.52
Avoca 95% silver nitrate pencils | 1 applicator P £1.99 DT price = £2.44
Avoca wart and verruca treatment set | 1 applicator P £2.44 DT price = £2.44

ANTIVIRALS 〉 IMMUNE RESPONSE MODIFIERS

Imiquimod

● **INDICATIONS AND DOSE**

ALDARA®

Warts (external genital and perianal)
▸ TO THE LESION
▸ Child (initiated under specialist supervision): Apply 3 times a week until lesions resolve (maximum 16 weeks), to be applied thinly at night

● **UNLICENSED USE**
ALDARA® Not licensed for use in children.

● **CAUTIONS** Autoimmune disease · avoid broken skin · avoid normal skin · avoid open wounds · immunosuppressed patients · not suitable for internal genital warts · uncircumcised males (risk of phimosis or stricture of foreskin)

● **SIDE-EFFECTS**
▸ Common or very common Burning sensation · erosion · erythema · excoriation · headache · influenza-like symptoms · itching · local reactions · myalgia · oedema · scabbing
▸ Uncommon Alopecia · local ulceration
▸ Rare Cutaneous lupus erythematosus-like effect · Stevens-Johnson syndrome
▸ Very rare Dysuria
▸ Frequency not known Permanent hyperpigmentation · permanent hypopigmentation

● **CONCEPTION AND CONTRACEPTION** May damage latex condoms and diaphragms.

● **PREGNANCY** No evidence of teratogenicity or toxicity in *animal* studies; manufacturer advises caution.

● **BREAST FEEDING** No information available.

● **DIRECTIONS FOR ADMINISTRATION**
ALDARA®
▸ Important Should be rubbed in and allowed to stay on the treated area for 6–10 hours then washed off with mild soap and water (uncircumcised males treating warts under foreskin should wash the area daily). The cream should be washed off before sexual contact.

● **PATIENT AND CARER ADVICE** A patient information leaflet should be provided.

- **MEDICINAL FORMS**
  There can be variation in the licensing of different medicines containing the same drug.
  Cream
  CAUTIONARY AND ADVISORY LABELS 10
  EXCIPIENTS: May contain Benzyl alcohol, cetostearyl alcohol (including cetyl and stearyl alcohol), hydroxybenzoates (parabens), polysorbates
  ▸ Aldara (Meda Pharmaceuticals Ltd)
    Imiquimod 50 mg per 1 gram Aldara 5% cream 250mg sachets | 12 sachet [PoM] £48.60 DT price = £48.60

SALICYLIC ACID AND DERIVATIVES

Salicylic acid

- **INDICATIONS AND DOSE**

OCCLUSAL®

Common and plantar warts
▸ TO THE LESION
▸ **Child:** Apply daily, treatment may need to be continued for up to 3 months

VERRUGON®

For plantar warts
▸ TO THE LESION
▸ **Child:** Apply daily, treatment may need to be continued for up to 3 months

- **UNLICENSED USE** Not licensed for use in children under 2 years.
- **CAUTIONS** Avoid broken skin · impaired peripheral circulation · not suitable for application to anogenital region · not suitable for application to face · not suitable for application to large areas · patients with diabetes at risk of neuropathic ulcers · significant peripheral neuropathy
- **SIDE-EFFECTS** Skin irritation · skin ulceration (with high concentrations)
- **PATIENT AND CARER ADVICE** Advise patient to apply carefully to wart and to protect surrounding skin (e.g. with soft paraffin or specially designed plaster); rub wart surface gently with file or pumice stone once weekly.

- **MEDICINAL FORMS**
  There can be variation in the licensing of different medicines containing the same drug.
  Ointment
  ▸ Verrugon (Optima Consumer Health Ltd)
    Salicylic acid 500 mg per 1 gram Verrugon complete 50% ointment | 6 gram [P] £3.61 DT price = £3.61
  Liquid
  CAUTIONARY AND ADVISORY LABELS 15
  ▸ Occlusal (Alliance Pharmaceuticals Ltd)
    Salicylic acid 260 mg per 1 ml Occlusal 26% solution | 10 ml [P] £3.56 DT price = £3.56

Salicylic acid with lactic acid

The properties listed below are those particular to the combination only. For the properties of the components please consider, salicylic acid, above.

- **INDICATIONS AND DOSE**

CUPLEX®

Plantar and mosaic warts | Corns | Calluses
▸ TO THE LESION
▸ **Child:** Apply twice daily, treatment may need to be continued for up to 3 months

DUOFILM®

Plantar and mosaic warts
▸ TO THE LESION
▸ **Child:** Apply daily, treatment may need to be continued for up to 3 months

SALACTOL®

Warts, particularly plantar warts | Verrucas | Corns | Calluses
▸ TO THE LESION
▸ **Child:** Apply daily, treatment may need to be continued for up to 3 months

SALATAC®

Warts | Verrucas | Corns | Calluses
▸ TO THE LESION
▸ **Child:** Apply daily, treatment may need to be continued for up to 3 months

- **PRESCRIBING AND DISPENSING INFORMATION**
  Preparations of salicylic acid in a collodion basis (Cuplex® and Salactol®) are available but some patients may develop an allergy to colophony in the formulation.

- **MEDICINAL FORMS**
  There can be variation in the licensing of different medicines containing the same drug.
  Paint
  CAUTIONARY AND ADVISORY LABELS 15
  ▸ Duofilm (GlaxoSmithKline UK Ltd)
    Lactic acid 150 mg per 1 gram, Salicylic acid 167 mg per 1 gram Duofilm paint | 15 ml [P] £2.25
  ▸ Salactol (Dermal Laboratories Ltd)
    Lactic acid 167 mg per 1 gram, Salicylic acid 167 mg per 1 gram Salactol paint | 10 ml [P] £1.71 DT price = £1.71
  Gel
  CAUTIONARY AND ADVISORY LABELS 15
  ▸ Cuplex (Crawford Healthcare Ltd)
    Lactic acid 40 mg per 1 gram, Salicylic acid 110 mg per 1 gram Cuplex Verruca gel | 5 gram [GSL] £2.88 DT price = £2.88
  ▸ Salatac (Dermal Laboratories Ltd)
    Lactic acid 40 mg per 1 gram, Salicylic acid 120 mg per 1 gram Salatac gel | 8 gram [P] £2.98 DT price = £2.98

13

Skin

Chapter 14
Vaccines

CONTENTS

1 Immunoglobulin therapy

IMMUNE SERA AND IMMUNOGLOBULINS ⟩
IMMUNOGLOBULINS

Immunoglobulins

Passive immunity

Immunity with immediate protection against certain infective organisms can be obtained by injecting preparations made from the plasma of immune individuals with adequate levels of antibody to the disease for which protection is sought. The duration of this passive immunity varies according to the dose and the type of immunoglobulin. Passive immunity may last only a few weeks; when necessary, passive immunisation can be repeated. Antibodies of human origin are usually termed immunoglobulins. The term antiserum is applied to material prepared in animals. Because of serum sickness and other allergic-type reactions that may follow injections of antisera, this therapy has been replaced wherever possible by the use of immunoglobulins. Reactions are theoretically possible after injection of human immunoglobulins but reports of such reactions are very rare.

Two types of human immunoglobulin preparation are available, normal immunoglobulin p. 743 and **disease-specific immunoglobulins**.

Human immunoglobulin is a sterile preparation of concentrated antibodies (immune globulins) recovered from pooled human plasma or serum obtained from outside the UK, tested and found non-reactive for hepatitis B surface antigen and for antibodies against hepatitis C virus and human immunodeficiency virus (types 1 and 2). A global shortage of human immunoglobulin and the rapidly increasing range of clinical indications for treatment with immunoglobulins has resulted in the need for a Demand Management programme in the UK, for further information consult www.ivig.nhs.uk and *Clinical Guidelines for Immunoglobulin Use*, www.gov.uk/dh.

Further information on the use of immunoglobulins is included in Public Health England's *Immunoglobulin Handbook* www.gov.uk/phe, and in the Department of Health's publication, *Immunisation against Infectious Disease*, www.gov.uk/dh.

Availability

Normal immunoglobulin for intramuscular administration is available from some regional Public Health laboratories for protection of contacts and the control of outbreaks of hepatitis A, measles, and rubella only. For other indications, subcutaneous or intravenous normal immunoglobulin should be purchased from the manufacturer.

Disease-specific immunoglobulins are available from some regional Public Health laboratories, with the exception of tetanus immunoglobulin p. 745 which is available from BPL,

hospital pharmacies, or blood transfusion departments. Rabies immunoglobulin p. 745 is available from the Specialist and Reference Microbiology Division, Public Health England, Colindale. Hepatitis B immunoglobulin p. 743 required by transplant centres should be obtained commercially.

In Scotland all immunoglobulins are available from the *Scottish National Blood Transfusion Service* (SNBTS).

In Wales all immunoglobulins are available from the *Welsh Blood Service* (WBS).

In Northern Ireland all immunoglobulins are available from the *Northern Ireland Blood Transfusion Service* (NIBTS).

Normal immunoglobulin

Human normal immunoglobulin ('HNIG') is prepared from pools of at least 1000 donations of human plasma; it contains immunoglobulin G (IgG) and antibodies to hepatitis A, measles, mumps, rubella, varicella, and other viruses that are currently prevalent in the general population.

Uses

Normal immunoglobulin (containing 10–18% protein) is administered by *intramuscular injection* for the protection of susceptible contacts against **hepatitis A** virus (infectious hepatitis), **measles** and, to a lesser extent, **rubella**. Injection of immunoglobulin produces immediate protection lasting for several weeks.

Normal immunoglobulin (containing 3–12% protein) for *intravenous administration* is used as *replacement therapy* for children with congenital agammaglobulinaemia and hypogammaglobulinaemia, and for the short-term treatment of idiopathic thrombocytopenic purpura and Kawasaki disease; it is also used for the prophylaxis of infection following bone-marrow transplantation and in children with symptomatic HIV infection who have recurrent bacterial infections. Normal immunoglobulin for replacement therapy may also be given intramuscularly or subcutaneously, but intravenous formulations are normally preferred. Intravenous immunoglobulin is also used in the treatment of Guillain-Barré syndrome as an alternative to plasma exchange.

The dose of normal immunoglobulin used as replacement therapy in patients with immunodeficiencies is **not the same** as the dose required for treatment of acute conditions. For Kawasaki disease a single dose by intravenous infusion should be given with concomitant aspirin p. 89 within 10 days of onset of symptoms (but children with a delayed diagnosis may also benefit).

For guidance on the use of intravenous normal immunoglobulin and alternative therapies for other conditions, consult *Clinical Guidelines for Immunoglobulin Use* (www.gov.uk/dh).

Hepatitis A

Hepatitis A vaccine p. 764 is preferred for individuals at risk of infection including those visiting areas where the disease is highly endemic (all countries excluding Northern and Western Europe, North America, Japan, Australia, and New

Zealand). In unimmunised individuals, transmission of hepatitis A is reduced by good hygiene. Intramuscular normal immunoglobulin is no longer recommended for routine prophylaxis in travellers, but it may be indicated for immunocompromised patients if their antibody response to the vaccine is unlikely to be adequate.

Intramuscular normal immunoglobulin is recommended for prevention of infection in close contacts (of confirmed cases of hepatitis A) who have chronic liver disease or HIV infection, or who are immunosuppressed; normal immunoglobulin should be given as soon as possible, preferably within 14 days of exposure to the primary case. However, normal immunoglobulin can still be given to contacts at risk of severe disease up to 28 days after exposure to the primary case. Hepatitis A vaccine can be given at the same time, but it should be given at a separate injection site.

Measles
Intravenous or subcutaneous normal immunoglobulin may be given to prevent or attenuate an attack of measles in individuals who do not have adequate immunity. Children with compromised immunity who have come into contact with measles should receive intravenous or subcutaneous normal immunoglobulin as soon as possible after exposure. It is most effective if given within 72 hours but can be effective if given within 6 days.

Subcutaneous or intramuscular normal immunoglobulin should also be considered for the following individuals if they have been in contact with a confirmed case of measles or with a person associated with a local outbreak:

- non-immune pregnant women
- infants under 9 months

Further advice should be sought from the Centre for Infections, Public Health England (tel. (020) 8200 6868).

Individuals with normal immunity who are not in the above categories and who have not been fully immunised against measles, can be given measles, mumps and rubella vaccine, live p. 769 for prophylaxis following exposure to measles.

Rubella
Intramuscular immunoglobulin after exposure to rubella does **not** prevent infection in non-immune contacts and is **not** recommended for protection of pregnant women exposed to rubella. It may, however, reduce the likelihood of a clinical attack which may possibly reduce the risk to the fetus. Risk of intra-uterine transmission is greatest in the first 11 weeks of pregnancy, between 16 and 20 weeks there is minimal risk of deafness only, after 20 weeks there is no increased risk. Intramuscular normal immunoglobulin p. 743 should be used only if termination of pregnancy would be unacceptable to the pregnant woman—it should be given as soon as possible after exposure. Serological follow-up of recipients is essential to determine if the woman has become infected despite receiving immunoglobulin.

For routine prophylaxis against Rubella, see measles, mumps and rubella vaccine, live p. 769.

Disease-specific immunoglobulins
Specific immunoglobulins are prepared by pooling the plasma of selected human donors with high levels of the specific antibody required. For further information, see *Immunoglobulin Handbook* (www.gov.uk/phe).

There are no specific immunoglobulins for hepatitis A, measles, or rubella—normal immunoglobulin is used in certain circumstances. There is no specific immunoglobulin for mumps; neither normal immunoglobulin nor measles, mumps and rubella vaccine, live is effective as postexposure prophylaxis.

Hepatitis B immunoglobulin
Disease-specific hepatitis B immunoglobulin ('HBIG') p. 743 is available for use in association with hepatitis B vaccine p. 765 for the prevention of infection in infants born to

mothers who have become infected with this virus in pregnancy or who are high-risk carriers (see hepatitis B vaccine). Hepatitis B immunoglobulin will not inhibit the antibody response when given at the same time as hepatitis B vaccine but should be given at different sites.

An intravenous and preparation of hepatitis B immunoglobulin is licensed for the prevention of hepatitis B recurrence in HBV-DNA negative patients who have undergone liver transplantation for liver failure caused by the virus.

Rabies immunoglobulin
Following exposure of an unimmunised individual to an animal in or from a country where the risk of rabies is high the site of the bite should be washed with soapy water and specific rabies immunoglobulin p. 745 of human origin administered. All of the dose should be injected around the site of the wound; if this is difficult or the wound has completely healed it can be given in the anterolateral thigh (remote from the site used for vaccination).

Rabies vaccine p. 770 should also be given intramuscularly at a different site (for details see rabies vaccine). If there is delay in giving the rabies immunoglobulin, it should be given within 7 days of starting the course of rabies vaccine.

Tetanus immunoglobulin
For the management of tetanus-prone wounds, tetanus immunoglobulin p. 745 should be used in addition to wound cleansing and, where appropriate, antibacterial prophylaxis and a tetanus-containing vaccine. Tetanus immunoglobulin, together with metronidazole p. 319 and wound cleansing, should also be used for the treatment of established cases of tetanus.

Varicella-zoster immunoglobulin
Varicella-zoster immunoglobulin (VZIG) p. 746 is recommended for individuals who are at increased risk of severe varicella *and* who have no antibodies to varicella–zoster virus *and* who have significant exposure to chickenpox or herpes zoster. Those at increased risk include:

- neonates whose mothers develop chickenpox in the period 7 days before to 7 days after delivery;
- susceptible neonates exposed in the first 7 days of life;
- susceptible neonates or infants exposed whilst requiring intensive or prolonged special care nursing;
- susceptible women exposed at any stage of pregnancy (but when supplies of VZIG are short, may only be issued to those exposed in the first 20 weeks' gestation or to those near term) providing VZIG is given within 10 days of contact;
- immunocompromised individuals including those who have received corticosteroids in the previous 3 months at the following dose equivalents of prednisolone; *children* 2 mg/kg daily (or more than 40 mg) for at least 1 week or 1 mg/kg daily for 1 month.

Important: for full details consult *Immunisation against Infectious Disease*. Varicella-zoster vaccine p. 771 is available.

Anti-D (Rh₀) immunoglobulin

- **INDICATIONS AND DOSE**

To rhesus-negative woman for prevention of Rh₀(D) sensitisation, following birth of rhesus-positive infant
▶ BY DEEP INTRAMUSCULAR INJECTION
▸ Females of childbearing potential: 500 units, dose to be administered immediately or within 72 hours; for transplacental bleed of over 4 mL fetal red cells, extra 100–125 units per mL fetal red cells, subcutaneous route used for patients with bleeding disorders

continued →

To rhesus-negative woman for prevention of Rh$_0$(D) sensitisation, following any potentially sensitising episode (e.g. stillbirth, abortion, amniocentesis) up to 20 weeks' gestation
‣ BY DEEP INTRAMUSCULAR INJECTION
‣ Females of childbearing potential: 250 units per episode, dose to be administered immediately or within 72 hours, subcutaneous route used for patients with bleeding disorders

To rhesus-negative woman for prevention of Rh$_0$(D) sensitisation, following any potentially sensitising episode (e.g. stillbirth, abortion, amniocentesis) after 20 weeks' gestation
‣ BY DEEP INTRAMUSCULAR INJECTION
‣ Females of childbearing potential: 500 units per episode, dose to be administered immediately or within 72 hours, subcutaneous route used for patients with bleeding disorders

To rhesus-negative woman for prevention of Rh$_0$(D) sensitisation, antenatal prophylaxis
‣ BY DEEP INTRAMUSCULAR INJECTION
‣ Females of childbearing potential: 500 units, dose to be given at weeks 28 and 34 of pregnancy, if infant rhesus-positive, a further dose is still needed immediately or within 72 hours of delivery, subcutaneous route used for patients with bleeding disorders

To rhesus-negative woman for prevention of Rh$_0$(D) sensitisation, antenatal prophylaxis (alternative NICE recommendation)
‣ BY DEEP INTRAMUSCULAR INJECTION
‣ Females of childbearing potential: 1000–1650 units, dose to be given at weeks 28 and 34 of pregnancy, alternatively 1500 units for 1 dose, dose to be given between 28 and 30 weeks gestation

To rhesus-negative woman for prevention of Rh$_0$(D) sensitisation, following Rh$_0$(D) incompatible blood transfusion
‣ BY DEEP INTRAMUSCULAR INJECTION
‣ Females of childbearing potential: 100–125 units per mL of transfused rhesus-positive red cells, subcutaneous route used for patients with bleeding disorders

RHOPHYLAC®

To rhesus-negative woman for prevention of Rh$_0$(D) sensitisation, following birth of rhesus-positive infant
‣ BY INTRAMUSCULAR INJECTION, OR BY INTRAVENOUS INJECTION
‣ Females of childbearing potential: 1000–1500 units, dose to be administered immediately or within 72 hours; for large transplacental bleed, extra 100 units per mL fetal red cells (preferably by intravenous injection), intravenous route recommended for patients with bleeding disorders

To rhesus-negative woman for prevention of Rh$_0$(D) sensitisation, following any potentially sensitising episode (e.g. abortion, amniocentesis, chorionic villous sampling) up to 12 weeks' gestation
‣ BY INTRAMUSCULAR INJECTION, OR BY INTRAVENOUS INJECTION
‣ Females of childbearing potential: 1000 units per episode, dose to be administered immediately or within 72 hours, intravenous route recommended for patients with bleeding disorders, higher doses may be required after 12 weeks gestation

To rhesus-negative woman for prevention of Rh$_0$(D) sensitisation, antenatal prophylaxis
‣ BY INTRAMUSCULAR INJECTION, OR BY INTRAVENOUS INJECTION
‣ Females of childbearing potential: 1500 units, dose to be given between weeks 28–30 of pregnancy; if infant rhesus-positive, a further dose is still needed

immediately or within 72 hours of delivery, intravenous route recommended for patients with bleeding disorders

To rhesus-negative woman for prevention of Rh$_0$(D) sensitisation, following Rh$_0$(D) incompatible blood transfusion
‣ BY INTRAVENOUS INJECTION
‣ Females of childbearing potential: 50 units per mL of transfused rhesus-positive blood, alternatively 100 units per of mL of erythrocyte concentrate, intravenous route recommended for patients with bleeding disorders

● CONTRA-INDICATIONS Treatment of idiopathic thrombocytopenia purpura in rhesus negative patients · treatment of idiopathic thrombocytopenia purpura in splenectomised patients
● CAUTIONS Immunoglobulin A deficiency · possible interference with live virus vaccines
CAUTIONS, FURTHER INFORMATION
‣ MMR vaccine MMR vaccine may be given in the postpartum period with anti-D (Rh$_0$) immunoglobulin injection provided that separate syringes are used and the products are administered into different limbs. If blood is transfused, the antibody response to the vaccine may be inhibited—measure rubella antibodies after 6–8 weeks and revaccinate if necessary.
● SIDE-EFFECTS
GENERAL SIDE-EFFECTS
‣ **Rare** Anaphylaxis · dyspnoea · hypotension · tachycardia · urticaria
‣ **Frequency not known** Abdominal pain · arthralgia · asthenia · back pain · diarrhoea · dizziness · drowsiness · fever · headache · hypertension · hypotension · injection site pain · malaise · myalgia · nausea · pruritus · rash · sweating · vomiting
SPECIFIC SIDE-EFFECTS
‣ With intravenous use Abdominal distension · blood pressure fluctuations · deep vein thrombosis · haemolytic anaemia · injection site reactions · myocardial infarction · pulmonary embolism · stroke · thromboembolic events
● HANDLING AND STORAGE Care must be taken to store all immunological products under the conditions recommended in the product literature, otherwise the preparation may become ineffective. **Refrigerated storage** is usually necessary; many immunoglobulins need to be stored at 2–8°C and not allowed to freeze. Immunoglobulins should be protected from light. Opened multidose vials must be used within the period recommended in the product literature.
● NATIONAL FUNDING/ACCESS DECISIONS
NICE technology appraisals (TAs)
‣ **Routine antenatal anti-D prophylaxis for rhesus-negative women (August 2008)** NICE TA156
Routine antenatal anti-D prophylaxis should be offered to all non-sensitised pregnant women who are rhesus negative.
www.nice.org.uk/TA156

● MEDICINAL FORMS
There can be variation in the licensing of different medicines containing the same drug.
Solution for injection
‣ **D-Gam** (Bio Products Laboratory Ltd)
Anti-D (RHO) immunoglobulin 500 unit D-Gam Anti-D immunoglobulin 500unit solution for injection vials | 1 vial PoM £33.75
Anti-D (RHO) immunoglobulin 1500 unit D-Gam Anti-D immunoglobulin 1,500unit solution for injection vials | 1 vial PoM £58.00

▸ **Rhophylac** (CSL Behring UK Ltd)
Anti-D (RHO) immunoglobulin 750 unit per 1 ml Rhophylac
1,500units/2ml solution for injection pre-filled syringes | 1 pre-filled
disposable injection [PoM] £39.52

Hepatitis B immunoglobulin

● **INDICATIONS AND DOSE**
Prophylaxis against hepatitis B infection
▸ BY INTRAMUSCULAR INJECTION

▸ Neonate: 200 units, dose to be administered as soon as
possible after exposure; ideally within 12–48 hours, but
no later than 7 days after exposure.

▸ Child 1 month-4 years: 200 units, dose to be
administered as soon as possible after exposure; ideally
within 12–48 hours, but no later than 7 days after
exposure
▸ Child 5-9 years: 300 units, dose to be administered as
soon as possible after exposure; ideally within
12–48 hours, but no later than 7 days after exposure
▸ Child 10-17 years: 500 units, dose to be administered as
soon as possible after exposure; ideally within
12–48 hours, but no later than 7 days after exposure
Prevention of transmitted infection at birth
▸ BY INTRAMUSCULAR INJECTION

▸ Neonate: 200 units, dose to be administered as soon as
possible after birth; for full details consult
Immunisation against Infectious Disease
(www.dh.gov.uk).

▸ BY INTRAVENOUS INFUSION
▸ Neonate: (consult product literature).

**Prophylaxis against hepatitis B infection, after exposure
to hepatitis B virus-contaminated material**
▸ BY INTRAVENOUS INFUSION
▸ Child: Dose to be administered as soon as possible after
exposure, but no later than 72 hours (consult product
literature)
Prophylaxis against re-infection of transplanted liver
▸ BY INTRAVENOUS INFUSION
▸ Child: (consult product literature)

● **CAUTIONS** IgA deficiency · interference with live virus
vaccines
● **SIDE-EFFECTS**
GENERAL SIDE-EFFECTS
▸ **Rare** Anaphylaxis · chest tightness · dyspnoea
▸ **Frequency not known** Arthralgia · buccal ulceration ·
dizziness · facial oedema · glossitis · pain at injection site ·
swelling at injection site · tremor
SPECIFIC SIDE-EFFECTS
▸ With intravenous use Abdominal distension · abdominal pain
· blood pressure fluctuations · deep vein thrombosis ·
haemolytic anaemia · injection site reactions · myocardial
infarction · pulmonary embolism · stroke · thromboembolic
events
● **PRESCRIBING AND DISPENSING INFORMATION** Vials
containing 200 units or 500 units (for intramuscular
injection), available from selected Public Health England
and NHS laboratories (except for Transplant Centres), also
available from BPL.
● **HANDLING AND STORAGE** Care must be taken to store all
immunological products under the conditions
recommended in the product literature, otherwise the
preparation may become ineffective. **Refrigerated
storage** is usually necessary; many immunoglobulins need
to be stored at 2–8°C and not allowed to freeze.
Immunoglobulins should be protected from light. Opened

multidose vials must be used within the period
recommended in the product literature.
● **MEDICINAL FORMS**
There can be variation in the licensing of different medicines
containing the same drug.
Solution for injection
▸ Hepatitis B immunoglobulin (Non-proprietary)
Hepatitis B immunoglobulin human 200 unit Hepatitis B
immunoglobulin human 200unit solution for injection vials |
1 vial [PoM] £150.00
Hepatitis B immunoglobulin human 500 unit Hepatitis B
immunoglobulin human 500unit solution for injection vials |
1 vial [PoM] £300.00
▸ Zutectra (Biotest (UK) Ltd)
Zutectra 500units/1ml solution for injection pre-filled syringes |
5 syringe [PoM] £1,275.00
Solution for infusion
▸ Hepatect CP (Biotest (UK) Ltd)
Hepatitis B immunoglobulin human 50 unit per 1 ml Hepatect CP
100units/2ml solution for infusion vials | 1 vial [PoM] £51.00
Hepatect CP 2000units/40ml solution for infusion vials | 1 vial [PoM]
£935.00
Hepatect CP 500units/10ml solution for infusion vials | 1 vial [PoM]
£255.00
Hepatect CP 5000units/100ml solution for infusion vials | 1 vial [PoM]
£2,337.50
▸ Omri-Hep-B (Imported (Israel))
Hepatitis B immunoglobulin human 50 unit per 1 ml Omri-Hep-B
5000units/100ml solution for infusion vials | 1 vial [PoM] no price
available

Normal immunoglobulin

● **INDICATIONS AND DOSE**
To control outbreaks of hepatitis A
▸ BY DEEP INTRAMUSCULAR INJECTION
▸ Child 1 month-9 years: 250 mg
▸ Child 10-17 years: 500 mg
Rubella in pregnancy, prevention of clinical attack
▸ BY DEEP INTRAMUSCULAR INJECTION
▸ Females of childbearing potential: 750 mg
Antibody deficiency syndromes
▸ BY SUBCUTANEOUS INFUSION
▸ Child: (consult product literature)
Kawasaki disease (with concomitant aspirin)
▸ BY INTRAVENOUS INFUSION
▸ Child: 2 g/kg daily for 1 dose, treatment should be given
within 10 days of onset of symptom (but children with
a delayed diagnosis may also benefit)
SUBGAM®
Hepatitis A prophylaxis in outbreaks
▸ BY INTRAMUSCULAR INJECTION
▸ Child 1 month-9 years: 500 mg
▸ Child 10-17 years: 750 mg

● **UNLICENSED USE**
SUBGAM® *Subgam*® is not licensed for prophylactic use,
but due to difficulty in obtaining suitable immunoglobulin
products, Public Health England recommends
intramuscular use for prophylaxis against Hepatitis A or
rubella.
● **CONTRA-INDICATIONS** Patients with selective IgA
deficiency who have known antibody against IgA
HIZENTRA® Hyperprolinaemia (contains -proline)
FLEBOGAMMA® DIF Hereditary fructose intolerance
(contains sorbitol)
PRIVIGEN® Hyperprolinaemia (contains -proline)
GAMMAPLEX® Hereditary fructose intolerance (contains
sorbitol)

14

Vaccines

● **CAUTIONS**

GENERAL CAUTIONS

Agammaglobulinaemia with or without IgA deficiency · hypogammaglobulinaemia with or without IgA deficiency · interference with live virus vaccines

SPECIFIC CAUTIONS

▶ With intravenous use Ensure adequate hydration · obesity · renal insufficiency · risk factors for arterial or venous thromboembolic events · thrombophilic disorders

CAUTIONS, FURTHER INFORMATION

▶ Interference with live virus vaccines Normal immunoglobulin may **interfere with the immune response to live virus vaccines** which should therefore only be given **at least 3 weeks before or 3 months after** an injection of normal immunoglobulin (this does not apply to yellow fever vaccine since normal immunoglobulin does not contain antibody to this virus).

OCTAGAM® Falsely elevated results with blood glucose testing systems (contains maltose)

● **SIDE-EFFECTS**

GENERAL SIDE-EFFECTS

▶ Rare Acute renal failure · anaphylaxis · aseptic meningitis · cutaneous skin reactions · hypotension

▶ **Frequency not known** Arthralgia · chills · diarrhoea · dizziness · fever · headache · low back pain · muscle spasms · myalgia · nausea

SPECIFIC SIDE-EFFECTS

▶ With intravenous use Abdominal distension · abdominal pain · blood pressure fluctuations · deep vein thrombosis · haemolytic anaemia · injection site reactions · myocardial infarction · pulmonary embolism · stroke · thromboembolic events

SIDE-EFFECTS, FURTHER INFORMATION

Adverse reactions are more likely to occur in patients receiving normal immunoglobulin for the first time, or following a prolonged period between treatments, or when a different brand of normal immunoglobulin is administered.

● **MONITORING REQUIREMENTS** Monitor for acute renal failure; consider discontinuation if renal function deteriorates. Intravenous preparations with added sucrose have been associated with cases of renal dysfunction and acute renal failure.

● **DIRECTIONS FOR ADMINISTRATION**

Preparations for subcutaneous use May be administered by intramuscular injection if subcutaneous route not possible; intramuscular route **not** for patients with thrombocytopenia or other bleeding disorders.

GAMUNEX® Use Glucose 5% intravenous infusion if dilution prior to infusion is required.

KIOVIG® Use Glucose 5% intravenous infusion if dilution prior to infusion is required.

● **PRESCRIBING AND DISPENSING INFORMATION** Antibody titres can vary widely between normal immunoglobulin preparations from different manufacturers—formulations are **not interchangeable**; patients should be maintained on the same formulation throughout long-term treatment to avoid adverse effects.

▶ With intramuscular use Available from the Centre for Infections and other regional Public Health England offices (for contacts and control of outbreaks only).

● **HANDLING AND STORAGE** Care must be taken to store all immunological products under the conditions recommended in the product literature, otherwise the preparation may become ineffective. **Refrigerated storage** is usually necessary; many immunoglobulins need to be stored at 2–8°C and not allowed to freeze. Immunoglobulins should be protected from light. Opened multidose vials must be used within the period recommended in the product literature.

● **MEDICINAL FORMS**

There can be variation in the licensing of different medicines containing the same drug.

Solution for injection

ELECTROLYTES: May contain Sodium

▶ **Gammanorm** (Octapharma Ltd)

Normal immunoglobulin human 165 mg per 1 ml Gammanorm 8g/48ml solution for injection vials | 1 vial PoM £469.20

Gammanorm 2g/12ml solution for injection vials | 1 vial PoM £117.30

Gammanorm 4g/24ml solution for injection vials | 1 vial PoM £234.60

Gammanorm 1.65g/10ml solution for injection vials | 1 vial PoM £96.77 | 10 vial PoM no price available (Hospital only)

Gammanorm 3.3g/20ml solution for injection vials | 1 vial PoM £193.55 | 10 vial PoM no price available (Hospital only)

Gammanorm 1g/6ml solution for injection vials | 1 vial PoM £58.65

▶ **Subcuvia** (Baxalta UK Ltd)

Normal immunoglobulin human 160 mg per 1 ml Subcuvia 800mg/5ml solution for injection vials | 1 vial PoM no price available

Subcuvia 1.6g/10ml solution for injection vials | 1 vial PoM no price available

▶ **Subgam** (Bio Products Laboratory Ltd)

Normal immunoglobulin human 150 mg per 1 ml Subgam 750mg/5ml solution for injection vials | 1 vial PoM £37.50

Subgam 1.5g/10ml solution for injection vials | 1 vial PoM £75.00

Solution for infusion

EXCIPIENTS: May contain Glucose, maltose, sorbitol, sucrose

▶ **Normal immunoglobulin (Non-proprietary)**

Normal immunoglobulin human 100 mg per 1 ml Normal immunoglobulin human 5g/50ml solution for infusion vials | 1 vial PoM no price available

Normal immunoglobulin human 2.5g/25ml solution for infusion vials | 1 vial PoM no price available

Normal immunoglobulin human 20g/200ml solution for infusion vials | 1 vial PoM no price available

Normal immunoglobulin human 10g/100ml solution for infusion vials | 1 vial PoM no price available

Normal immunoglobulin human 30g/300ml solution for infusion vials | 1 vial PoM no price available

▶ **Aragam** (Oxbridge Pharma Ltd)

Normal immunoglobulin human 50 mg per 1 ml Aragam 5g/100ml solution for infusion vials | 1 vial PoM no price available

Aragam 2.5g/50ml solution for infusion vials | 1 vial PoM no price available

▶ **Flebogamma DIF** (Grifols UK Ltd)

Normal immunoglobulin human 50 mg per 1 ml Flebogamma DIF 10g/200ml solution for infusion vials | 1 vial PoM £510.00

Flebogamma DIF 2.5g/50ml solution for infusion vials | 1 vial PoM £127.50

Flebogamma DIF 5g/100ml solution for infusion vials | 1 vial PoM £255.00

Flebogamma DIF 500mg/10ml solution for infusion vials | 1 vial PoM £30.00

Flebogamma DIF 20g/400ml solution for infusion vials | 1 vial PoM £1,020.00

Normal immunoglobulin human 100 mg per 1 ml Flebogamma DIF 20g/200ml solution for infusion vials | 1 vial PoM £1,020.00

Flebogamma DIF 10g/100ml solution for infusion vials | 1 vial PoM £510.00

Flebogamma DIF 5g/50ml solution for infusion vials | 1 vial PoM £255.00

▶ **Gammaplex** (Bio Products Laboratory Ltd)

Normal immunoglobulin human 50 mg per 1 ml Gammaplex 10g/200ml solution for infusion vials | 1 vial PoM £418.00 (Hospital only)

Gammaplex 5g/100ml solution for infusion vials | 1 vial PoM £209.00 (Hospital only)

Gammaplex 20g/400ml solution for infusion vials | 1 vial PoM £836.00 (Hospital only)

▶ **Gamunex** (Grifols UK Ltd)

Normal immunoglobulin human 100 mg per 1 ml Gamunex 10% 1g/10ml solution for infusion vials | 1 vial PoM £42.50

Gamunex 10% 10g/100ml solution for infusion vials | 1 vial PoM £425.00

Gamunex 10% 20g/200ml solution for infusion vials | 1 vial PoM £850.00

Gamunex 10% 5g/50ml solution for infusion vials | 1 vial PoM £212.50

▸ **Hizentra** (CSL Behring UK Ltd)
Normal immunoglobulin human 200 mg per 1 ml Hizentra
2g/10ml solution for infusion vials | 1 vial PoM £91.80
Hizentra 1g/5ml solution for infusion vials | 1 vial PoM £45.90
Hizentra 4g/20ml solution for infusion vials | 1 vial PoM £183.60

▸ **Intratect** (Biotest (UK) Ltd)
Normal immunoglobulin human 50 mg per 1 ml Intratect
5g/100ml solution for infusion vials | 1 vial PoM £191.25
Intratect 1g/20ml solution for infusion vials | 1 vial PoM £38.25
Intratect 2.5g/50ml solution for infusion vials | 1 vial PoM £95.63
Intratect 10g/200ml solution for infusion vials | 1 vial PoM £382.50
Normal immunoglobulin human 100 mg per 1 ml Intratect
10g/100ml solution for infusion vials | 1 vial PoM £382.50
Intratect 20g/200ml solution for infusion vials | 1 vial PoM £765.00
Intratect 5g/50ml solution for infusion vials | 1 vial PoM £191.25
Intratect 1g/10ml solution for infusion vials | 1 vial PoM £38.25

▸ **Kiovig** (Baxalta UK Ltd)
Normal immunoglobulin human 100 mg per 1 ml Kiovig 5g/50ml
solution for infusion vials | 1 vial PoM no price available
Kiovig 20g/200ml solution for infusion vials | 1 vial PoM no price
available
Kiovig 10g/100ml solution for infusion vials | 1 vial PoM no price
available
Kiovig 30g/300ml solution for infusion vials | 1 vial PoM £1,470.00
Kiovig 2.5g/25ml solution for infusion vials | 1 vial PoM no price
available
Kiovig 1g/10ml solution for infusion vials | 1 vial PoM no price
available

▸ **Octagam** (Octapharma Ltd)
Normal immunoglobulin human 50 mg per 1 ml Octagam 5%
10g/200ml solution for infusion bottles | 1 bottle PoM £408.00
(Hospital only)
Octagam 5% 5g/100ml solution for infusion bottles | 1 bottle PoM
£204.00 (Hospital only)
Octagam 5% 2.5g/50ml solution for infusion bottles | 1 bottle PoM
£102.00 (Hospital only)
Normal immunoglobulin human 100 mg per 1 ml Octagam 10%
5g/50ml solution for infusion bottles | 1 bottle PoM £293.25
(Hospital only)
Octagam 10% 10g/100ml solution for infusion bottles | 1 bottle PoM
£586.50 (Hospital only)
Octagam 10% 20g/200ml solution for infusion bottles | 1 bottle PoM
£1,173.00 (Hospital only)
Octagam 10% 2g/20ml solution for infusion vials | 1 vial PoM
£117.30 (Hospital only)

▸ **Privigen** (CSL Behring UK Ltd)
Normal immunoglobulin human 100 mg per 1 ml Privigen
5g/50ml solution for infusion vials | 1 vial PoM £229.50
Privigen 20g/200ml solution for infusion vials | 1 vial PoM £918.00
Privigen 10g/100ml solution for infusion vials | 1 vial PoM £459.00
Privigen 2.5g/25ml solution for infusion vials | 1 vial PoM £114.75

▸ **Vigam** (Bio Products Laboratory Ltd)
Normal immunoglobulin human 50 mg per 1 ml Vigam Liquid
5g/100ml solution for infusion vials | 1 vial PoM £209.00
Vigam Liquid 10g/200ml solution for infusion vials | 1 vial PoM
£418.00

Powder and solvent for solution for injection
▸ **Gammagard S/D** (Baxalta UK Ltd)
Normal immunoglobulin human 5 gram Gammagard S/D 5g
powder and solvent for solution for injection bottles | 1 bottle PoM
no price available
Normal immunoglobulin human 10 gram Gammagard S/D 10g
powder and solvent for solution for injection bottles | 1 bottle PoM
no price available

Rabies immunoglobulin

● **INDICATIONS AND DOSE**
Post-exposure prophylaxis against rabies infection
▸ BY LOCAL INFILTRATION, OR BY INTRAMUSCULAR INJECTION
▸ Child: 20 units/kg, dose administered by infiltration in
and around the cleansed wound; if the wound not
visible or healed or if infiltration of whole volume not
possible, give remainder by intramuscular injection
into anterolateral thigh (remote from vaccination site)

● CAUTIONS IgA deficiency · interference with live virus
vaccines

● SIDE-EFFECTS
▸ **Rare** Anaphylaxis · arthralgia · buccal ulceration · chest
tightness · dizziness · dyspnoea · glossitis · tremor
▸ **Frequency not known** Facial oedema · injection site pain ·
injection site swelling

● PRESCRIBING AND DISPENSING INFORMATION The potency
of individual batches of rabies immunoglobulin from the
manufacturer may vary; potency may also be described
differently by different manufacturers. It is therefore
critical to know the potency of the batch to be used and
the weight of the patient in order to calculate the specific
volume required to provide the necessary dose.
Available from Specialist and Reference Microbiology
Division, Public Health England (also from BPL).

● HANDLING AND STORAGE Care must be taken to store all
immunological products under the conditions
recommended in the product literature, otherwise the
preparation may become ineffective. **Refrigerated
storage** is usually necessary; many immunoglobulins need
to be stored at 2-8°C and not allowed to freeze.
Immunoglobulins should be protected from light. Opened
multidose vials must be used within the period
recommended in the product literature.

● MEDICINAL FORMS
There can be variation in the licensing of different medicines
containing the same drug.
Solution for injection
▸ Rabies immunoglobulin (Non-proprietary)
Rabies immunoglobulin human 500 unit Rabies immunoglobulin
human 500unit solution for injection vials | 1 vial PoM £600.00

Tetanus immunoglobulin

● **INDICATIONS AND DOSE**
Post-exposure prophylaxis
▸ BY INTRAMUSCULAR INJECTION
▸ Child: Initially 250 units, then increased to 500 units,
dose is only increased if more than 24 hours have
elapsed or there is risk of heavy contamination or
following burns
Treatment of tetanus infection
▸ BY INTRAMUSCULAR INJECTION
▸ Child: 150 units/kg, dose may be given over multiple
sites

● CAUTIONS IgA deficiency · interference with live virus
vaccines

● SIDE-EFFECTS
▸ **Rare** Anaphylaxis · arthralgia · buccal ulceration · chest
tightness · dizziness · dyspnoea · glossitis · tremor
▸ **Frequency not known** Facial oedema · injection site
swelling · pain at injection site

● HANDLING AND STORAGE Care must be taken to store all
immunological products under the conditions
recommended in the product literature, otherwise the
preparation may become ineffective. **Refrigerated
storage** is usually necessary; many immunoglobulins need
to be stored at 2-8°C and not allowed to freeze.
Immunoglobulins should be protected from light. Opened
multidose vials must be used within the period
recommended in the product literature.

● MEDICINAL FORMS
There can be variation in the licensing of different medicines
containing the same drug.
Solution for injection
▸ Tetanus immunoglobulin (Non-proprietary)
Tetanus immunoglobulin human 250 unit Tetanus immunoglobulin
human 250unit solution for injection vials | 1 vial PoM £125.00

14

Vaccines

Varicella-zoster immunoglobulin

(Antivaricella-zoster Immunoglobulin)

- **INDICATIONS AND DOSE**

Prophylaxis against varicella infection
▸ BY DEEP INTRAMUSCULAR INJECTION

▸ Neonate: 250 mg, to be administered as soon as possible—not later than 10 days after exposure, second dose to be given if further exposure occurs more than 3 weeks after first dose, no evidence that effective in severe disease.

▸ Child 1 month–5 years: 250 mg, to be administered as soon as possible—not later than 10 days after exposure, second dose to be given if further exposure occurs more than 3 weeks after first dose, no evidence that effective in severe disease

▸ Child 6–10 years: 500 mg, to be administered as soon as possible—not later than 10 days after exposure, second dose to be given if further exposure occurs more than 3 weeks after first dose, no evidence that effective in severe disease

▸ Child 11–14 years: 750 mg, to be administered as soon as possible—not later than 10 days after exposure, second dose to be given if further exposure occurs more than 3 weeks after first dose, no evidence that effective in severe disease

▸ Child 15–17 years: 1 g, to be administered as soon as possible—not later than 10 days after exposure, second dose to be given if further exposure occurs more than 3 weeks after first dose, no evidence that effective in severe disease

- **CAUTIONS** IgA deficiency · interference with live virus vaccines
- **SIDE-EFFECTS**
▸ **Rare** Anaphylaxis
▸ **Frequency not known** Injection site pain · injection site swelling
- **DIRECTIONS FOR ADMINISTRATION** Normal immunoglobulin for intravenous use may be used in those unable to receive intramuscular injections.
- **PRESCRIBING AND DISPENSING INFORMATION** Available from selected Public Health England and NHS laboratories (also from BPL).
- **HANDLING AND STORAGE** Care must be taken to store all immunological products under the conditions recommended in the product literature, otherwise the preparation may become ineffective. **Refrigerated storage** is usually necessary; many immunoglobulins need to be stored at 2–8°C and not allowed to freeze. Immunoglobulins should be protected from light. Opened multidose vials must be used within the period recommended in the product literature.
- **MEDICINAL FORMS**
There can be variation in the licensing of different medicines containing the same drug.
Solution for injection
▸ Varicella-Zoster (Bio Products Laboratory Ltd)
Varicella-Zoster immunoglobulin human 250 mg Varicella-Zoster immunoglobulin human 250mg solution for injection vials |
1 vial [PoM] £450.00

2   Post-exposure prophylaxis

IMMUNE SERA AND IMMUNOGLOBULINS >
ANTITOXINS

Botulism antitoxin

- **DRUG ACTION** A preparation containing the specific antitoxic globulins that have the power of neutralising the toxins formed by types A, B, and E of *Clostridium botulinum*.

- **INDICATIONS AND DOSE**

Post exposure prophylaxis of botulism
▸ BY INTRAMUSCULAR INJECTION
▸ Child: (consult product literature)

- **SIDE-EFFECTS** Hypersensitivity reactions
SIDE-EFFECTS, FURTHER INFORMATION
▸ **Hypersensitivity reactions** It is essential to read the contra-indications, warnings, and details of sensitivity tests on the package insert. Prior to treatment checks should be made regarding previous administration of any antitoxin and history of any allergic condition, e.g. asthma, hay fever, etc.
- **PRE-TREATMENT SCREENING** All patients should be tested for sensitivity (diluting the antitoxin if history of allergy).
- **PRESCRIBING AND DISPENSING INFORMATION** Available from local designated centres, for details see TOXBASE (requires registration) www.toxbase.org. For supplies outside working hours apply to other designated centres or to the Public Health England Colindale duty doctor (Tel (020) 8200 6868). For major incidents, obtain supplies from the local blood bank.
The BP title Botulinum Antitoxin is not used because the preparation currently in use may have a different specification.

- **MEDICINAL FORMS**
There can be variation in the licensing of different medicines containing the same drug.
No licensed medicines listed.

Diphtheria antitoxin

(Dip/Ser)

- **INDICATIONS AND DOSE**

Passive immunisation in suspected cases of diphtheria
▸ BY INTRAVENOUS INFUSION
▸ Child: Dose should be given without waiting for bacteriological confirmation (consult product literature)

- **CAUTIONS**
CAUTIONS, FURTHER INFORMATION
▸ **Hypersensitivity** Hypersensitivity is common after administration; resuscitation facilities should be available.
Diphtheria antitoxin is no longer used for prophylaxis because of the risk of hypersensitivity; unimmunised contacts should be promptly investigated and given antibacterial prophylaxis and vaccine.
- **SIDE-EFFECTS**
▸ **Common or very common** Hypersensitivity reactions
- **PRE-TREATMENT SCREENING** Diphtheria antitoxin is derived from horse serum and reactions are common; tests for hypersensitivity should be carried out before use.
- **PRESCRIBING AND DISPENSING INFORMATION** Available from Centre for Infections (Tel (020) 8200 6868) or in

Northern Ireland from Public Health Laboratory, Belfast City Hospital (Tel (028) 9032 9241).

● MEDICINAL FORMS
There can be variation in the licensing of different medicines containing the same drug.
Solution for injection
▸ Diphtheria antitoxin (Non-proprietary)
   Diphtheria antitoxin 1000 unit per 1 ml Antidiphtheria serum 10,000units/10ml solution for injection ampoules | 1 ampoule PoM no price available

3 Tuberculosis diagnostic test

DIAGNOSTIC AGENTS

Tuberculin purified protein derivative
(Tuberculin PPD)

● INDICATIONS AND DOSE
Mantoux test
▸ BY INTRADERMAL INJECTION
▸ Child: 2 units for one dose
Mantoux test (if first test is negative and a further test is considered appropriate)
▸ BY INTRADERMAL INJECTION
▸ Child: 10 units for 1 dose
DOSE EQUIVALENCE AND CONVERSION
▸ 2 units is equivalent to 0.1 mL of 20 units/mL strength.
▸ 10 units is equivalent to 0.1 mL of 100 units/mL strength.

● CAUTIONS
CAUTIONS, FURTHER INFORMATION
▸ Mantoux test Response to tuberculin may be suppressed by viral infection, sarcoidosis, corticosteroid therapy, or immunosuppression due to disease or treatment and the MMR vaccine. If a tuberculin skin test has already been initiated, then the MMR should be delayed until the skin test has been read unless protection against measles is required urgently. If a child has had a recent MMR, and requires a tuberculin test, then a 4 week interval should be observed. Apart from tuberculin and MMR, all other live vaccines can be administered at any time before or after tuberculin.

● PRESCRIBING AND DISPENSING INFORMATION Available from ImmForm (SSI brand).
   The strength of tuberculin PPD in currently available products may be different to the strengths of products used previously for the Mantoux test; care is required to select the correct strength.

● MEDICINAL FORMS
There can be variation in the licensing of different medicines containing the same drug. Forms available from special-order manufacturers include: solution for injection
Solution for injection
▸ Tuberculin purified protein derivative (Non-proprietary)
   Tuberculin purified protein derivative 20 tuberculin unit per 1 ml Tuberculin PPD RT23 SSI 20 tuberculin units/ml solution for injection 1.5ml vials | 1 vial no price available
   Tuberculin purified protein derivative 100 tuberculin unit per 1 ml Tuberculin PPD RT23 SSI 100 tuberculin units/ml solution for injection 1.5ml vials | 1 vial no price available

4 Vaccination

Vaccines
14-Jun-2017

Active immunity

Active immunity can be acquired by natural disease or by vaccination. **Vaccines** stimulate production of antibodies and other components of the immune mechanism; they consist of either:

● a *live attenuated* form of a virus (e.g. measles, mumps and rubella vaccine) or bacteria (e.g. BCG vaccine), or
● *inactivated* preparations of the virus (e.g. influenza vaccine) or bacteria, or
● *detoxified exotoxins* produced by a micro-organism (e.g. tetanus vaccine), or
● *extracts of* a micro-organism, which may be derived from the organism (e.g. pneumococcal vaccine) or produced by recombinant DNA technology (e.g. hepatitis B vaccine).

Live attenuated vaccines usually produce a durable immunity, but not always as long-lasting as that resulting from natural infection.
   Inactivated vaccines may require a primary series of injections of vaccine to produce an adequate antibody response, and in most cases booster (reinforcing) injections are required; the duration of immunity varies from months to many years. Some inactivated vaccines are adsorbed onto an adjuvant (such as aluminium hydroxide) to enhance the antibody response.
   Advice reflects that in the handbook *Immunisation against Infectious Disease* (2013), which in turn reflects the guidance of the Joint Committee on Vaccination and Immunisation (JCVI).
   Chapters from the handbook (including updates since 2013) are available at www.gov.uk/government/collections/immunisation-against-infectious-disease-the-green-book.
   The advice also incorporates changes announced by the Chief Medical Officer and Health Department Updates.

Children with unknown or incomplete immunisation history

For children born in the UK who present with an inadequate or unknown immunisation history, investigation into immunisations received should be carried out. Outstanding doses should be administered where the routine childhood immunisation schedule has not been completed.
   For advice on the immunisation of children coming to the UK, consult the handbook *Immunisation against Infectious Disease* (2006) (available at www.dh.gov.uk**).**

Immunisation schedule

Vaccines for the childhood immunisation schedule should be obtained from **local health organisations** or from ImmForm (www.immform.dh.gov.uk)—not to be prescribed on FP10 (HS21 in Northern Ireland; GP10 in Scotland; WP10 in Wales).
   For the most up to date immunisation schedule consult 'The complete routine immunisation schedule', available at www.gov.uk.

Preterm birth

Babies born preterm should receive all routine immunisations based on their actual date of birth. The risk of apnoea following vaccination is increased in preterm babies, particularly in those born at or before 28 weeks postmenstrual age. If babies at risk of apnoea are in hospital at the time of their first immunisation, they should be monitored for 48–72 hours after immunisation. If a baby develops apnoea, bradycardia, or desaturation after the first immunisation, the second immunisation should also be given in hospital with similar monitoring. Seroconversion

14

Vaccines

Routine immunisation schedule

When to immunise (for preterm infants-see note below)	Vaccine given and dose schedule (for details of dose, see under individual vaccines)
Neonates at risk only (see BCG vaccine and Hepatitis B vaccine, below)	▸ Bacillus Calmette-Guérin vaccine p. 760 ▸ Hepatitis B vaccine p. 765
2 months	▸ Diphtheria with haemophilus influenzae type b vaccine, pertussis, poliomyelitis and tetanus p. 759 First dose ▸ Meningococcal group B vaccine (rDNA, component, adsorbed) p. 762 First dose ▸ Pneumococcal polysaccharide conjugate vaccine (adsorbed) p. 763 First dose ▸ Rotavirus vaccine p. 770 First dose
3 months	▸ Diphtheria with haemophilus influenzae type b vaccine, pertussis, poliomyelitis and tetanus p. 759 Second dose ▸ Rotavirus vaccine p. 770 Second dose
4 months	▸ Diphtheria with haemophilus influenzae type b vaccine, pertussis, poliomyelitis and tetanus p. 759 Third dose ▸ Meningococcal group B vaccine (rDNA, component, adsorbed) p. 762 Second dose ▸ Pneumococcal polysaccharide conjugate vaccine (adsorbed) p. 763 Second dose
12-13 months	▸ Measles, mumps and rubella vaccine, live p. 769 First dose ▸ Meningococcal group B vaccine (rDNA, component, adsorbed) p. 762 Single booster dose ▸ Pneumococcal polysaccharide conjugate vaccine (adsorbed) p. 763 Single booster dose ▸ Haemophilus influenzae type B with meningococcal group C vaccine p. 761 Single booster dose
2-8 years (including children in school years 1, 2, 3 and 4)	▸ Influenza vaccine p. 767 Each year from September. **Note:** Flu nasal spray is recommended (*Fluenz Tetra*®). If contra-indicated and child is in clinical risk group, use inactivated flu vaccine
Between 3 years and 4 months, and 5 years	▸ Diphtheria with pertussis, poliomyelitis vaccine and tetanus p. 759 Single booster dose. **Note:** Preferably allow interval of at least 3 years after completing primary course ▸ Measles, mumps and rubella vaccine, live p. 769 Second dose
11-14 years (females only). First dose of HPV vaccine will be offered to females aged 12-13 years of age in England, Wales, and Northern Ireland, and 11-13 years of age in Scotland.	▸ Human papillomavirus vaccines p. 767 Two doses; second dose 6-24 months after first dose. If a 3-dose course of HPV vaccine has been started under the 2013/2014 programme, where possible, the course should be completed (2 doses less than 6 months apart does not provide long-term protection). The two human papillomavirus vaccines are not interchangeable and, ideally, one vaccine product should be used for the entire course. However, since 2012, only *Gardasil*® is offered as part of the national immunisation programme; for those females who started the schedule with *Cervarix*® under the national immunisation programme, but did not complete the vaccination course, the course can be completed with *Gardasil*®.
13-15 years	▸ Meningococcal groups A with C and W135 and Y vaccine p. 762 Single booster dose
13-18 years	▸ Diphtheria with poliomyelitis and tetanus vaccine p. 760 Single booster dose. **Note:** Can be given at the same time as the booster dose of meningococcal group A with C and W135 and Y vaccine at 13-15 years of age
During adult life, women of child-bearing age susceptible to rubella	▸ Measles, mumps and rubella vaccine, live p. 769 Women of child-bearing age who have not received 2 doses of a rubella-containing vaccine or who do not have a positive antibody test for rubella should be offered rubella immunisation (using the MMR vaccine)—exclude pregnancy before immunisation.
Pregnant females	▸ Acellular pertussis-containing vaccine administered as diphtheria with pertussis, poliomyelitis vaccine and tetanus p. 759 (*Boostrix-IPV*®) 1 dose from the 16th week of pregnancy, preferably after the foetal anomaly scan (weeks 18-20) ▸ Influenza vaccine p. 767 (inactivated), Single dose administered from September, regardless of the stage of pregnancy

may be unreliable in babies born earlier than 28 weeks' gestation or in babies treated with corticosteroids for chronic lung disease; consideration should be given to testing for antibodies against Haemophilus influenzae type b, meningococcal C, and hepatitis B after primary immunisation.

Vaccines and HIV infection
HIV-positive children with or without symptoms can receive the following live vaccines:

• MMR (but avoid if immunity significantly impaired), varicella-zoster vaccine against chickenpox (but avoid if immunity significantly impaired—consult product literature; use of normal immunoglobulin should be considered after exposure to measles and varicella–zoster immunoglobulin considered after exposure to chickenpox or herpes zoster), rotavirus;

and the following inactivated vaccines:

• anthrax, cholera (oral), diphtheria, haemophilus influenzae type b, hepatitis A, hepatitis B, human papillomavirus, influenza (injection), meningococcal, pertussis, pneumococcal, poliomyelitis (inactivated poliomyelitis vaccine is now used instead of oral poliomyelitis vaccine for routine immunisation of children), rabies, tetanus, tick-borne encephalitis, typhoid (injection).

HIV-positive children should **not** receive:

• BCG, influenza nasal spray (unless stable HIV infection and receiving antiretroviral therapy), typhoid (oral), yellow fever (if yellow fever risk is unavoidable, specialist advice should be sought).

The above advice differs from that for other immunocompromised patients; *Immunisation of HIV infected*

Children issued by *Children's HIV Association* (CHIVA) are available at www.chiva.org.uk.

Vaccines and asplenia

The following vaccines are recommended for asplenic patients, those with splenic dysfunction or complement disorders, depending on the age at which their condition is diagnosed:

- Haemophilus influenzae type b with meningococcal group C vaccine p. 761;
- Influenza vaccine p. 767;
- Meningococcal groups A with C and W135 and Y vaccine p. 762 and meningococcal group B vaccine (rDNA, component, adsorbed) p. 762;
- pneumococcal polysaccharide vaccine.

Children first diagnosed under 1 *year of age* should be vaccinated according to the Immunisation Schedule. Additionally, one dose of meningococcal groups A with C and W135 and Y vaccine should be given during infancy followed by a second dose at least one month apart. Two months following the routine 12 month booster vaccines, give a dose of meningococcal groups A with C and W135 and Y vaccine and an additional dose of 13-valent pneumococcal polysaccharide vaccine. An additional dose of haemophilus influenzae type B with meningococcal group C vaccine and 23-valent pneumococcal polysaccharide vaccine should be given after the second birthday. The influenza vaccine should be administered annually in children aged 6 months or older.

Children first diagnosed between 1 *and* 2 *years of age* should be vaccinated according to the Immunisation Schedule, including the 12 month boosters. Two months after the routine 12 month booster vaccines, give a dose of meningococcal groups A with C and W135 and Y vaccine and an additional dose of 13-valent pneumococcal polysaccharide vaccine. An additional dose of haemophilus influenzae type B with meningococcal group C vaccine and 23-valent pneumococcal polysaccharide vaccine should be given after the second birthday. The influenza vaccine should be administered annually.

Children first diagnosed over 2 *years of age* should be vaccinated according to the Immunisation schedule, including the 12 month boosters. The child should receive one additional booster dose of haemophilus influenzae type B with meningococcal group C vaccine along with the 23-valent pneumococcal polysaccharide vaccine, followed by one dose of meningococcal groups A with C and W135 and Y vaccine after 2 months. The influenza vaccine should be administered annually.

Passive immunity

Immunity with immediate protection against certain infective organisms can be obtained by injecting preparations made from the plasma of immune individuals with adequate levels of antibody to the disease for which protection is sought (see under Immunoglobulins). The duration of this passive immunity varies according to the dose and the type of immunoglobulin. Passive immunity may last only a few weeks; when necessary, passive immunisation can be repeated.

Antibodies of human origin are usually termed *immunoglobulins*. The term *antiserum* is applied to material prepared in animals. Because of serum sickness and other allergic-type reactions that may follow injections of antisera, this therapy has been replaced whenever possible by the use of immunoglobulins. Reactions are theoretically possible after injection of human immunoglobulins, but reports of such reactions are very rare.

Vaccines and antisera availability

Anthrax vaccine and yellow fever vaccine, live p. 771, botulism antitoxin p. 746, diphtheria antitoxin p. 746, and snake and spider venom antitoxins are available from local designated holding centres.

For antivenom, see Emergency Treatment of Poisoning.

Enquiries for vaccines not available commercially can also be made to:

Vaccines and Countermeasures Response Department
Public Health England
Wellington House
133–155 Waterloo Road
London
SE1 8UG
vaccinesupply@phe.gov.uk

In Scotland information about availability of vaccines can be obtained from a Specialist in Pharmaceutical Public Health.

In Wales enquiries for vaccines not available commercially should be directed to:

Welsh Medicines Information Centre
University Hospital of Wales
Cardiff
CF14 4XW
(029) 2074 2979

In Northern Ireland:

Pharmacy and Medicines Management Centre
Northern Health and Social Care Trust
Beech House
Antrim Hospital Site
Bush Road
Antrim
BT41 2RL
rphps.admin@northerntrust.hscni.net

For further details of availability, see under individual vaccines.

Anthrax vaccine

Anthrax vaccine is rarely required for children.

BCG vaccine

BCG (Bacillus Calmette-Guérin vaccine p. 760) is a live attenuated strain derived from *Mycobacterium bovis* which stimulates the development of hypersensitivity to *M. tuberculosis*. Bacillus Calmette-Guérin vaccine should be given intradermally by operators skilled in the technique.

The expected reaction to successful Bacillus Calmette-Guérin vaccine is induration at the site of injection followed by a local lesion which starts as a papule 2 or more weeks after vaccination; the lesion may ulcerate then subside over several weeks or months, leaving a small flat scar. A dry dressing may be used if the ulcer discharges, but air should **not** be excluded.

All children of 6 years and over being considered for Bacillus Calmette-Guérin vaccine must first be given a skin test for hypersensitivity to tuberculoprotein (see under Diagnostic agents). A skin test is not necessary for a child under 6 years, provided that the child has not stayed for longer than 3 months in a country with an incidence of tuberculosis greater than 40 per 100 000 (a list of countries or primary care trusts where the incidence of tuberculosis is greater than 40 cases per 100 000 is available at www.gov.uk/phe), the child has not had contact with a person with tuberculosis, and there is no family history of tuberculosis within the last 5 years.

Bacillus Calmette-Guérin vaccine is recommended for the following groups of children if BCG immunisation has not previously been carried out and they are negative for tuberculoprotein hypersensitivity:

- neonates with a family history of tuberculosis in the last 5 years;
- all neonates and infants (0–12 months) born in areas where the incidence of tuberculosis is greater than 40 per 100 000;

14

Vaccines

- neonates, infants, and children under 16 years with a parent or grandparent born in a country with an incidence of tuberculosis greater than 40 per 100 000;
- new immigrants aged under 16 years who were born in, or lived for more than 3 months in a country with an incidence of tuberculosis greater than 40 per 100 000;
- new immigrants aged 16–18 years from Sub-Saharan Africa or a country with an incidence of tuberculosis greater than 500 per 100 000;
- contacts of those with active respiratory tuberculosis;
- children under 16 years intending to live with local people for more than 3 months in a country with an incidence of tuberculosis greater than 40 per 100 000.

Bacillus Calmette-Guérin vaccine can be given simultaneously with another live vaccine, but if they are not given at the same time, an interval of 4 weeks should normally be allowed between them. When Bacillus Calmette-Guérin vaccine is given to infants, there is no need to delay routine primary immunisations. No further vaccination should be given in the arm used for BCG vaccination for at least 3 months because of the risk of regional lymphadenitis.

For advice on chemoprophylaxis against tuberculosis; for treatment of infection following vaccination, seek expert advice.

Tuberculosis Diagnostic Agents

The *Mantoux test* is recommended for tuberculin skin testing, but no licensed preparation is currently available. Guidance for healthcare professionals is available at www.dh.gov.uk/immunisation.

In the Mantoux test, the diagnostic dose is administered by intradermal injection of Tuberculin Purified Protein Derivative (PPD).

The *Heaf test* (involving the use of multiple-puncture apparatus) is no longer available.

Two interferon gamma release assay (IGRA) tests are also available as an aid in the diagnosis of tuberculosis infection: *QuantiFERON® TB Gold* and *T-SPOT®.TB*. Both tests measure T-cell mediated immune response to synthetic antigens. For further information on the use of interferon gamma release assay tests for tuberculosis, see www.gov.uk/phe.

Botulism antitoxin

A polyvalent botulism antitoxin p. 746 is available for the post-exposure prophylaxis of botulism and for the treatment of persons thought to be suffering from botulism. It specifically neutralises the toxins produced by *Clostridium botulinum* types A, B, and E. It is not effective against infantile botulism as the toxin (type A) is seldom, if ever, found in the blood in this type of infection.

Hypersensitivity reactions are a problem. It is essential to read the contra-indications, warnings, and details of sensitivity tests on the package insert. Prior to treatment checks should be made regarding previous administration of any antitoxin and history of any allergic condition, e.g. asthma, hay fever, etc. All patients should be tested for sensitivity (diluting the antitoxin if history of allergy).

Cholera vaccine

Cholera vaccine p. 761 (oral) contains inactivated Inaba (including El-Tor biotype) and Ogawa strains of *Vibrio cholerae*, serotype O1 together with recombinant B-subunit of the cholera toxin produced in Inaba strains of *V.cholerae*, serotype O1.

Oral cholera vaccine is licensed for travellers to endemic or epidemic areas on the basis of current recommendations. Immunisation should be completed at least 1 week before potential exposure. However, there is no requirement for cholera vaccination for international travel.

Immunisation with cholera vaccine does not provide complete protection and all travellers to a country where cholera exists should be warned that scrupulous attention to food, water, and personal hygiene is **essential**.

Injectable cholera vaccine provides unreliable protection and is no longer available in the UK.

Diphtheria vaccine

Diphtheria vaccines are prepared from the toxin of *Corynebacterium diphtheriae* and adsorption on aluminium hydroxide or aluminium phosphate improves antigenicity. The vaccine stimulates the production of the protective antitoxin. The quantity of diphtheria toxoid in a preparation determines whether the vaccine is defined as 'high dose' or 'low dose'. Vaccines containing the higher dose of diphtheria toxoid are used for primary immunisation of children under 10 years of age. Vaccines containing the lower dose of diphtheria toxoid are used for primary immunisation in adults and children over 10 years. Single-antigen diphtheria vaccine is not available and adsorbed diphtheria vaccine is given as a combination product containing other vaccines.

For primary immunisation *of children aged between 2 months and 10 years* vaccination is recommended usually in the form of 3 doses (separated by 1-month intervals) of **diphtheria, tetanus, pertussis (acellular, component), poliomyelitis (inactivated) and haemophilus type b conjugate vaccine (adsorbed)** (see Immunisation schedule). In unimmunised individuals aged *over 10 years* the primary course comprises of 3 doses of **adsorbed diphtheria** [low dose], **tetanus and poliomyelitis (inactivated) vaccine**.

A booster dose should be given 3 years after the primary course (this interval can be reduced to a minimum of 1 year if the primary course was delayed). Children *under 10 years* should receive *either* **adsorbed diphtheria, tetanus, pertussis (acellular, component) and poliomyelitis (inactivated) vaccine** *or* **adsorbed diphtheria** [low dose], **tetanus, pertussis (acellular, component) and poliomyelitis (inactivated) vaccine**. Individuals aged *over 10 years* should receive **adsorbed diphtheria** [low dose], **tetanus, and poliomyelitis (inactivated) vaccine**.

A second booster dose, of adsorbed diphtheria [low dose], tetanus and poliomyelitis (inactivated) vaccine, should be given 10 years after the previous booster dose (this interval can be reduced to a minimum of 5 years if previous doses were delayed). For children who have been vaccinated following a tetanus-prone wound, see tetanus vaccines.

Travel

Those intending to travel to areas with a risk of diphtheria infection should be fully immunised according to the UK schedule. If more than 10 years have lapsed since completion of the UK schedule, a dose of **adsorbed diphtheria** [low dose], **tetanus and poliomyelitis (inactivated) vaccine** should be administered.

Contacts

Advice on the management of cases of diphtheria, carriers, contacts and outbreaks must be sought from health protection units. The immunisation history of infected children and their contacts should be determined; those who have been incompletely immunised should complete their immunisation and fully immunised individuals should receive a reinforcing dose. Also see advice on antibacterial treatment to prevent a secondary case of diphtheria in a non-immune child.

Haemophilus influenzae type b conjugate vaccine

Haemophilus influenzae type b (Hib) vaccine is made from capsular polysaccharide; it is conjugated with a protein such as tetanus toxoid to increase immunogenicity, especially in young children. Haemophilus influenzae type b vaccine immunisation is given in combination with diphtheria, tetanus, pertussis (acellular, component) and poliomyelitis (inactivated) vaccine, as a component of the primary course of childhood immunisation (see

Immunisation schedule) (see under Diphtheria-containing Vaccines). For infants under 1 year, the course consists of 3 doses of a vaccine containing *Haemophilus influenzae* type b component with an interval of 1 month between doses. A booster dose of haemophilus influenzae type b vaccine (combined with meningococcal group C conjugate vaccine) should be given at 12–13 months of age.

Children 1–10 years who have not been immunised against *Haemophilus influenzae* type b need to receive only 1 dose of Haemophilus influenzae type b vaccine (combined with meningococcal group C conjugate vaccine). However, if a primary course of immunisation has not been completed, these children should be given 3 doses of diphtheria with haemophilus influenzae type b vaccine, pertussis, poliomyelitis and tetanus p. 759. The risk of infection falls sharply in older children and the vaccine is not normally required for children over 10 years.

Haemophilus influenzae type b vaccine may be given to those over 10 years who are considered to be at increased risk of invasive *H. influenzae* type b disease (such as those with sickle-cell disease or complement deficiency, or those receiving treatment for malignancy).

Invasive *Haemophilus influenzae* type b disease

After recovery from infection, unimmunised and partially immunised index cases under 10 years of age should complete their age-specific course of immunisation. Previously vaccinated cases under 10 years of age should be given an additional dose of haemophilus influenzae type b vaccine (combined with meningococcal group C conjugate vaccine) if Hib antibody concentrations are low or if it is not possible to measure antibody concentrations. Index cases of any age with asplenia or splenic dysfunction should complete their immunisation according to the recommendations below; fully vaccinated cases with asplenia or splenic dysfunction should be given an additional dose of haemophilus influenzae type b vaccine (combined with meningococcal group C conjugate vaccine) if they received their previous dose over 1 year ago.

Also see use of rifampicin p. 349 in the prevention of secondary cases of *Haemophilus influenzae* type b disease.

Hepatitis A vaccine

Hepatitis A vaccine p. 764 is prepared from formaldehyde-inactivated hepatitis A virus grown in human diploid cells. Immunisation is recommended for:

- residents of homes for those with severe learning difficulties;
- children with haemophilia or other conditions treated with plasma-derived clotting factors;
- children with severe liver disease;
- children travelling to high-risk areas;
- adolescents who are at risk due to their sexual behaviour;
- parenteral drug abusers.

Immunisation should be considered for:

- children with chronic liver disease including chronic hepatitis B or chronic hepatitis C;
- prevention of secondary cases in close contacts of confirmed cases of hepatitis A, within 14 days of exposure to the primary case (within 8 weeks of exposure to the primary case where there is more than 1 contact in the household).

A booster dose of hepatitis A vaccine is usually given 6–12 months after the initial dose. A second booster dose can be given 20 years after the previous booster dose to those who continue to be at risk. Specialist advice should be sought on re-immunisation of immunocompromised individuals.

In children under 16 years, a single dose of the combined vaccine *Ambirix*® can be used to provide rapid protection against hepatitis A. Intramuscular normal immunoglobulin p. 743 is recommended for use in addition to hepatitis A vaccine for close contacts (of confirmed cases of hepatitis A)

who have chronic liver disease or HIV infection, or who are immunosuppressed.

Post-exposure prophylaxis is not required for healthy children under 1 year of age, so long as all those involved in nappy changing are vaccinated against hepatitis A. However, children 2–12 months of age can be given a dose of hepatitis A vaccine if it is not possible to vaccinate their carers, or if the child becomes a source of infection to others [unlicensed use]; in these cases, if the child goes on to require long-term protection against hepatitis A after the first birthday, the full course of 2 doses should be given.

Hepatitis B vaccine

Hepatitis B vaccine p. 765 contains inactivated hepatitis B virus surface antigen (HBsAg) adsorbed on to aluminium hydroxide adjuvant. It is made biosynthetically using recombinant DNA technology. The vaccine is used in individuals at high risk of contracting hepatitis B. In the UK, high-risk groups include:

- parenteral drug misusers, their sexual partners, and household contacts; other drug misusers who are likely to 'progress' to injecting;
- adolescents who are at risk from their sexual behaviour;
- close family contacts of an individual with chronic hepatitis B infection;
- babies whose mothers have had acute hepatitis B during pregnancy or are positive for hepatitis B surface antigen (regardless of e-antigen markers); hepatitis B vaccination is started immediately on delivery and *hepatitis B immunoglobulin* given at the same time (but at a different site). Babies whose mothers are positive for hepatitis B surface antigen and for e-antigen antibody should receive the vaccine only (but babies weighing 1.5 kg or less should also receive the immunoglobulin regardless of the mother's e-antigen antibody status);
- children with haemophilia, those receiving regular blood transfusions or blood products, and carers responsible for the administration of such products;
- children with chronic renal failure including those on haemodialysis. Children receiving haemodialysis should be monitored for antibodies annually and re-immunised if necessary. Home carers (of dialysis patients) should be vaccinated;
- children with chronic liver disease
- patients of day-care or residential accommodation for those with severe learning difficulties;
- children in custodial institutions;
- children travelling to areas of high or intermediate prevalence who are at increased risk or who plan to remain there for lengthy periods;
- families adopting children from countries with a high or intermediate prevalence of hepatitis B;
- foster carers and their families.

Different immunisation schedules for hepatitis B vaccine are recommended for specific circumstances; an 'accelerated schedule' is recommended for pre-exposure prophylaxis in high–risk groups where rapid protection is required, and for post-exposure prophylaxis. Generally, three or four doses are required for primary immunisation. Immunisation may take up to 6 months to confer adequate protection; the duration of immunity is not known precisely, but a single booster 5 years after the primary course may be sufficient to maintain immunity for those who continue to be at risk.

Immunisation does not eliminate the need for commonsense precautions for avoiding the risk of infection from known carriers by the routes of infection which have been clearly established, consult *Guidance for Clinical Health Care Workers: Protection against Infection with Blood-borne Viruses* (available at www.dh.gov.uk). Accidental inoculation of hepatitis B virus-infected blood into a wound, incision, needle-prick, or abrasion may lead to infection, whereas it is unlikely that indirect exposure to a carrier will do so.

14

Vaccines

Following significant exposure to hepatits B, an accelerated schedule, with the second dose given 1 month, and the third dose 2 months after the initial dose, is recommended. For those at continued risk, a fourth dose should be given 12 months after the first dose. More detailed guidance is given in the *Immunisation against Infectious Disease* handbook.

Specific hepatitis B immunoglobulin ('HBIG') p. 743 is available for use with the vaccine in those accidentally inoculated and in neonates at special risk of infection.

A combined hepatitis A and B vaccine p. 764 is also available.

Human papillomavirus vaccine

Human papillomavirus vaccine is available as a bivalent vaccine (*Cervarix*®) or a quadrivalent vaccine (*Gardasil*®). Since 2012, only *Gardasil*® is offered as part of the national immunisation programme. *Cervarix*® is licensed for use in females for the prevention of cervical cancer and other pre-cancerous lesions caused by human papillomavirus types 16 and 18. *Gardasil*® is licensed for use in females for the prevention of cervical and anal cancers, genital warts and pre-cancerous genital (cervical, vulvar, and vaginal) and anal lesions caused by human papillomavirus types 6, 11, 16, and 18. The vaccines may also provide limited protection against disease caused by other types of human papillomavirus. The two vaccines are not interchangeable and one vaccine product should be used for an entire course.

Human papillomavirus vaccine will be most effective if given before sexual activity starts. From September 2014, a 2-dose schedule is recommended, as long as the first dose is received before the age of 15 years. The first dose is given to females aged 11 to 14 years, and the second dose is given 6-24 months after the first dose (for the purposes of planning the national immunisation programme, it is appropriate to give the second dose 12 months after the first—see Immunisation schedule). If the course is interrupted, it should be resumed (using the same vaccine) but not repeated, even if more than 24 months have elapsed since the first dose or if the girl is then aged 15 years or more.

Females aged 15 years or older require a 3-dose schedule (see *Cervarix*® and *Gardasil*®), with the second and third doses given 1 and 4–6 months after the first dose; all 3 doses should be given within a 12-month period. If the course is interrupted, it should be resumed (using the same vaccine) but not repeated, allowing the appropriate interval between the remaining doses.

If a 3-dose course of vaccination had been started before September 2014 in a female aged under 15 years, then where possible this should be completed; the interrupted course should be resumed (using the same vaccine) but not repeated, allowing the appropriate interval between the remaining doses.

Under the national programme in England, females remain eligible to receive the vaccine up to the age of 18 years if they did not receive the vaccine when scheduled. Where appropriate, immunisation with human papillomavirus vaccine should be offered to females coming into the UK as they may not have been offered protection in their country of origin. The duration of protection has not been established, but current studies suggest that protection is maintained for at least 6 years after completion of the primary course.

Influenza vaccine

While most viruses are antigenically stable, the influenza viruses A and B (especially A) are constantly altering their antigenic structure as indicated by changes in the haemagglutinins (H) and neuraminidases (N) on the surface of the viruses. It is essential that influenza vaccine p. 767 in use contain the H and N components of the prevalent strain or strains recommended each year by the World Health Organization.

The inactivated influenza vaccine is recommended for children aged 6 months–2 years in an at risk group (see below), those aged 18 years and over, in pregnancy and in children with a contra-indication to the live influenza vaccine.

Unless contra-indicated, the live influenza vaccine, administered as a nasal spray (*Fluenz Tetra*®), is preferred in children aged 2–17 years because it provides a higher level of protection than the inactivated *influenza vaccine*.

Immunisation is recommended *for persons at high risk*, and to reduce transmission of infection. Annual immunisation is strongly recommended for children (including infants that were preterm or low birth-weight) aged over 6 months with the following conditions:

- chronic respiratory disease (includes asthma treated with continuous or repeated use of inhaled or systemic corticosteroids or asthma with previous exacerbations requiring hospital admission);
- chronic heart disease;
- chronic liver disease;
- chronic renal disease at stage 3, 4 or 5;
- chronic neurological disease;
- complement disorders;
- diabetes mellitus;
- immunosuppression because of disease (including asplenia or splenic dysfunction) or treatment (including prolonged systemic corticosteroid treatment [for over 1 month at dose equivalents of prednisolone: *child under* 20 *kg*, 1 mg/kg or more daily; *child over* 20 *kg*, 20 mg or more daily] and chemotherapy);
- HIV infection (regardless of immune status);
- morbid obesity.

Seasonal influenza vaccine is also recommended for all pregnant women, for children living in long-stay facilities, and for carers of children whose welfare may be at risk if the carer falls ill. Influenza immunisation should also be considered for household contacts of immunocompromised individuals.

In the 2017/2018 national influenza immunisation programme, seasonal influenza vaccine will also be offered to all children who were aged 2–8 years on 31 August 2017 (including those in school years 1, 2, 3 and 4), and all primary school-aged children in former primary school pilot areas.

Further information on pandemic influenza, avian influenza, and swine influenza may be found at www.gov.uk/pandemic-flu and at www.gov.uk/phe.

Japanese encephalitis vaccine

Japanese encephalitis vaccine p. 768 is indicated for travellers to areas in Asia and the Far East where infection is endemic and for laboratory staff at risk of exposure to the virus. The primary immunisation course of 2 doses should be completed at least one week before potential exposure to Japanese encephalitis virus.

Up-to-date information on the risk of Japanese encephalitis in specific countries can be obtained from the National Travel Health Network and Centre (www.nathnac.org).

Management of Measles, Mumps and Rubella

Measles vaccine has been replaced by a combined measles, mumps and rubella vaccine, live (MMR vaccine) p. 769.

A combined measles, mumps and rubella vaccine, live (MMR vaccine) aims to eliminate measles, mumps, and rubella (German measles) and congenital rubella syndrome. Every child should receive two doses of measles, mumps and rubella vaccine, live by entry to primary school, unless there is a valid contra-indication. Measles, mumps and rubella vaccine, live should be given irrespective of previous measles, mumps, or rubella infection or vaccination.

The first dose of measles, mumps and rubella vaccine, live is given to children aged 12–13 months. A second dose is given before starting school at 3 years and 4 months–5 years of age (see Immunisation Schedule).

Children presenting for pre-school booster who have not received the first dose of measles, mumps and rubella vaccine, live should be given a dose of measles, mumps and rubella vaccine, live followed 3 months later by a second dose.

At school-leaving age or at entry into further education, MMR immunisation should be offered to individuals of both sexes who have not received 2 doses during childhood. In those who have received only a single dose of MMR in childhood, a second dose is recommended to achieve full protection. If 2 doses of measles, mumps and rubella vaccine, live p. 769 are required, the second dose should be given one month after the initial dose.

Measles, mumps and rubella vaccine, live should be used to protect against rubella in *seronegative women of child-bearing age* (see Immunisation Schedule); unimmunised healthcare workers who might put pregnant women and other vulnerable groups at risk of rubella or measles should be vaccinated. Measles, mumps and rubella vaccine, live may also be offered to previously *unimmunised and seronegative post-partum women* (see measles, mumps and rubella vaccine, live)—vaccination a few days after delivery is important because about 60% of congenital abnormalities from rubella infection occur in babies of women who have borne more than one child. Immigrants arriving after the age of school immunisation are particularly likely to require immunisation.

Contacts

Measles, mumps and rubella vaccine, live may also be used in the control of outbreaks of measles and should be offered to susceptible children aged over 6 months who are contacts of a case, within 3 days of exposure to infection. Children immunised before 12 months of age should still receive two doses of measles, mumps and rubella vaccine, live at the recommended ages. If one dose of measles, mumps and rubella vaccine, live has already been given to a child, then the second dose may be brought forward to at least one month after the first, to ensure complete protection. If the child is under 18 months of age and the second dose is given within 3 months of the first, then the routine dose before starting school at 3 years and 4 months–5 years should still be given. Children aged under 9 months for whom avoidance of measles infection is particularly important (such as those with history of recent severe illness) can be given normal immunoglobulin p. 743 after exposure to measles; routine MMR immunisation should then be given after at least 3 months at the appropriate age.

Measles, mumps and rubella vaccine, live is **not suitable** for prophylaxis following exposure to mumps or rubella since the antibody response to the mumps and rubella components is too slow for effective prophylaxis.

Children with impaired immune response should not receive live vaccines (for advice on HIV). If they have been exposed to measles infection they should be given normal immunoglobulin.

Travel

Unimmunised travellers, including children over 6 months, to areas where measles is endemic or epidemic should receive measles, mumps and rubella vaccine, live. Children immunised before 12 months of age should still receive two doses of measles, mumps and rubella vaccine, live at the recommended ages. If one dose of measles, mumps and rubella vaccine, live has already been given to a child, then the second dose should be brought forward to at least one month after the first, to ensure complete protection. If the child is under 18 months of age and the second dose is given within 3 months of the first, then the routine dose before starting school at 3 years and 4 months–5 years should still be given.

Meningococcal vaccine

Almost all childhood meningococcal disease in the UK is caused by *Neisseria meningitidis* serogroups B and C. **Meningococcal group C conjugate vaccine** protects only against infection by serogroup C and **meningococcal group B vaccine** protects only against infection by serogroup B. The risk of meningococcal disease declines with age— immunisation is not generally recommended after the age of 25 years.

Tetravalent meningococcal vaccines that cover serogroups A, C, W135, and Y are available. Although the duration of protection has not been established, the **meningococcal groups A, C, W135, and Y conjugate vaccine** is likely to provide longer-lasting protection than the unconjugated meningococcal polysaccharide vaccine. The antibody response to serogroup C in unconjugated meningococcal polysaccharide vaccines in young children may be suboptimal [not currently available in the UK].

A meningococcal group B vaccine (rDNA, component, adsorbed) p. 762, *Bexsero*®, is licensed in the UK against infection caused by *Neisseria meningitidis* serogroup B and is recommended in the Immunisation Schedule. *Bexsero*® contains 3 recombinant *Neisseria meningitidis* serogroup B proteins and the outer membrane vesicles from the NZ 98/254 strain, in order to achieve broad protection against *Neisseria meningitidis* serogroup B; the proteins are adsorbed onto an aluminium compound to stimulate an enhanced immune response.

Childhood immunisation

Meningococcal group C conjugate vaccine provides long-term protection against infection by serogroup C of *Neisseria meningitidis*. Immunisation consists of 1 dose given at 12 months of age (as the haemophilus influenzae type B with meningococcal group C vaccine p. 761) and a second dose given at 13–15 years of age (as the meningococcal groups A with C and W135 and Y vaccine p. 762) (see Immunisation Schedule).

Meningococcal group B vaccine provides protection against infection by serogroup B of *Neisseria meningitidis*. Immunisation consists of 1 dose given at 2 months of age, a second dose at 4 months of age, and a booster dose at 12 months of age (see *Immunisation Schedule* above).

Unimmunised children aged under 12 months should be given 1 dose of meningococcal group B vaccine (rDNA, component, adsorbed) followed by a second dose two months later. They should then be vaccinated according to the Immunisation Schedule (ensuring at least a two month interval between doses of meningococcal group B vaccines). Unimmunised children aged 12–23 months should be given 2 doses of meningococcal group B vaccine (rDNA, component, adsorbed) separated by an interval of two months if they have received less than 2 doses in the first year of life. Unimmunised children aged 2–9 years should be given a single dose of meningococcal group C vaccine (as the haemophilus influenzae type B with meningococcal group C vaccine), followed by a booster dose of meningococcal groups A with C and W135 and Y vaccine at 13–15 years of age.

From 2015, unimmunised individuals aged 10–25 years, including those aged under 25 years who are attending university for the first time, should be given a single dose of meningococcal groups A with C and W135 and Y vaccine; a booster dose is not required.

Children with confirmed serogroup C disease, who have previously been immunised with meningococcal group C vaccine, should be offered meningococcal group C conjugate vaccine before discharge from hospital.

14

Vaccines

Travel

Individuals travelling to countries of risk should be immunised with meningococcal groups A, C, W135, and Y conjugate vaccine, even if they have previously received meningococcal group C conjugate vaccine. If an individual has recently received meningococcal group C conjugate vaccine, an interval of at least 4 weeks should be allowed before administration of the tetravalent (meningococcal groups A, C, W135, and Y) vaccine.

Vaccination is particularly important for those living or working with local people or visiting an area of risk during outbreaks.

Immunisation recommendations and requirements for visa entry for individual countries should be checked before travelling, particularly to countries in Sub-Saharan Africa, Asia, and the Indian sub-continent where epidemics of meningococcal outbreaks and infection are reported. Country-by-country information is available from the National Travel Health Network and Centre (www.nathnac.org).

Proof of vaccination with the tetravalent (meningococcal groups A, C, W135, and Y) vaccine is required for those travelling to Saudi Arabia during the Hajj and Umrah pilgrimages (where outbreaks of the W135 strain have occurred).

Contacts

For advice on the immunisation of *laboratory workers and close contacts* of cases of meningococcal disease in the UK and on the role of the vaccine in the control of *local outbreaks*, consult Guidelines for Public Health Management of Meningococcal Disease in the UK at www.gov.uk/phe. Also see antibacterial prophylaxis for prevention of secondary cases of meningococcal meningitis.

Pertussis vaccine

Pertussis vaccine is given as a combination preparation containing other vaccines. Acellular vaccines are derived from highly purified components of *Bordetella pertussis*. Primary immunisation against pertussis (whooping cough) requires 3 doses of an acellular pertussis-containing vaccine (see Immunisation schedule), given at intervals of 1 month from the age of 2 months.

All children up to the age of 10 years should receive primary immunisation with diphtheria, tetanus, pertussis (acellular, component), poliomyelitis (inactivated) and haemophilus type b conjugate vaccine (adsorbed).

A booster dose of an acellular pertussis-containing vaccine should ideally be given 3 years after the primary course, although, the interval can be reduced to 1 year if the primary course was delayed.

Children aged 1-10 years who have not received a *pertussis-containing* vaccine as part of their primary immunisation should be offered 1 dose of a suitable pertussis-containing vaccine; after an interval of at least 1 year, a booster dose of a suitable pertussis-containing vaccine should be given. Immunisation against pertussis is not routinely recommended in individuals over 10 years of age.

Vaccination of pregnant women against pertussis

In response to the pertussis outbreak, the UK health departments introduced a temporary programme (October 2012) to vaccinate pregnant women against pertussis, and this programme will continue until further notice. The aim of the programme is to boost the levels of pertussis-specific antibodies that are transferred, through the placenta, from the mother to the fetus, so that the newborn is protected before routine immunisation begins at 2 months of age.

Pregnant women should be offered a single dose of acellular pertussis-containing vaccine (as adsorbed diphtheria [low dose], tetanus, pertussis (acellular, component) and poliomyelitis (inactivated) vaccine; *Boostrix-IPV®*) between 16 and 32 weeks of pregnancy.

Public Health England has advised (2016) that the vaccine is probably best offered on or after the foetal anomaly scan at around 18-20 weeks. Pregnant women should be offered a single dose of acellular pertussis-containing vaccine up to the onset of labour if they missed the opportunity for vaccination at 16-32 weeks of pregnancy. A single dose of acellular pertussis-containing vaccine may also be offered to new mothers, who have never previously been vaccinated against pertussis, until the child receives the first vaccination.

While this programme is in place, women who become pregnant again should be offered vaccination during each pregnancy to maximise transplacental transfer of antibody.

Contacts

Vaccination against pertussis should be considered for close contacts of cases with pertussis who have been offered antibacterial prophylaxis. Unimmunised or partially immunised contacts under 10 years of age should complete their vaccination against pertussis. A booster dose of an acellular pertussis-containing vaccine is recommended for contacts aged over 10 years who have not received a pertussis-containing vaccine in the last 5 years and who have not received adsorbed diphtheria [low dose], tetanus, and poliomyelitis (inactivated) vaccine in the last month.

Side-effects

Local reactions do not contra-indicate further doses.

The vaccine should not be withheld from children with a history to a preceding dose of:

- fever, irrespective of severity;
- persistent crying or screaming for more than 3 hours;
- severe local reaction, irrespective of extent.

Pneumococcal vaccine

Pneumococcal polysaccharide conjugate vaccine (adsorbed) p. 763 protect against infection with *Streptococcus pneumoniae* (pneumococcus); the vaccines contain polysaccharide from capsular pneumococci, **Pneumococcal polysaccharide vaccine** contains purified polysaccharide from 23 capsular types of pneumococcus, whereas **pneumococcal polysaccharide conjugate vaccine** (adsorbed) contains polysaccharide from either 10 capsular types (*Synflorix®*) or 13 capsular types (*Prevenar 13®*) with the polysaccharide being conjugated to protein.

The 13-valent conjugate vaccine is used for childhood immunisation. The recommended schedule consists of 3 doses, the first at 2 months of age, the second at 4 months, and the third at 12-13 months (see Immunisation Schedule).

Pneumococcal vaccination is recommended for individuals at increased risk of pneumococcal infection as follows:

- child under 5 years with a history of invasive pneumococcal disease;
- asplenia or splenic dysfunction (including homozygous sickle cell disease and coeliac disease which could lead to splenic dysfunction);
- chronic respiratory disease (includes asthma treated with continuous or frequent use of a systemic corticosteroid);
- chronic heart disease;
- chronic renal disease;
- chronic liver disease;
- chronic neurological conditions;
- complement disorders;
- diabetes mellitus;
- immune deficiency because of disease (e.g. HIV infection) or treatment (including prolonged systemic corticosteroid treatment for over 1 month at dose equivalents of prednisolone: *child under 20 kg*, 1 mg/kg or more daily; *child over 20 kg*, 20 mg or more daily);
- presence of cochlear implant;
- conditions where leakage of cerebrospinal fluid could occur.

Where possible, the vaccine should be given at least 2 weeks before splenectomy, cochlear implant surgery, chemotherapy, or radiotherapy; children and carers should be given advice about increased risk of pneumococcal infection. If it is not practical to vaccinate at least 2 weeks before splenectomy, chemotherapy, or radiotherapy, the vaccine should be given at least 2 weeks after the splenectomy or, where possible, at least 3 months after completion of chemotherapy or radiotherapy. Prophylactic antibacterial therapy against pneumococcal infection should not be stopped after immunisation. A patient card and information leaflet for patients with asplenia are available from the Department of Health or in Scotland from the Scottish Government, Health Protection Division (Tel (0131) 244 2879).

Choice of vaccine

Children under 2 years at increased risk of pneumococcal infection (see list above) should receive the 13-valent pneumococcal polysaccharide conjugate vaccine (adsorbed) at the recommended ages, followed by a single dose of the 23-valent pneumococcal polysaccharide vaccine after their second birthday. Children at increased risk of pneumococcal infection presenting late for vaccination should receive 2 doses (separated by at least 1 month) of the 13-valent pneumococcal polysaccharide conjugate vaccine (adsorbed) before the age of 12 months, and a third dose at 12–13 months. Children over 12 months and under 5 years (who have not been vaccinated or not completed the primary course) should receive a single dose of 13-valent pneumococcal polysaccharide conjugate vaccine (adsorbed) (2 doses separated by an interval of 2 months in the immunocompromised or those with asplenia or splenic dysfunction). All children under 5 years at increased risk of pneumococcal infection should receive a single dose of the 23-valent pneumococcal polysaccharide vaccine after their second birthday and at least 2 months after the final dose of the 13- valent pneumococcal polysaccharide conjugate vaccine (adsorbed).

Children over 5 years who are at increased risk of pneumococcal disease should receive a single dose of the 23-valent unconjugated pneumococcal polysaccharide vaccine.

Revaccination

In individuals with higher concentrations of antibodies to pneumococcal polysaccharides, revaccination with the 23-valent pneumococcal polysaccharide vaccine more commonly produces adverse reactions. Revaccination is therefore not recommended, except every 5 years in individuals in whom the antibody concentration is likely to decline rapidly (e.g. asplenia, splenic dysfunction and nephrotic syndrome). If there is doubt, the need for revaccination should be discussed with a haematologist, immunologist, or microbiologist.

Poliomyelitis vaccine

Two types of poliomyelitis vaccines (containing strains of poliovirus types 1, 2, and 3) are available, inactivated poliomyelitis vaccines (for injection) and live (oral) poliomyelitis vaccines. **Inactivated** poliomyelitis vaccines, only available in combined preparation, is recommended for routine immunisation; it is given by injection and contains inactivated strains of human poliovirus types 1, 2 and 3.

A course of primary immunisation consists of 3 doses of a combined preparation containing inactivated poliomyelitis vaccines starting at 2 months of age with intervals of 1 month between doses (see Immunisation schedule). A course of 3 doses should also be given to all unimmunised children; no child should remain unimmunised against poliomyelitis.

Two booster doses of a preparation containing inactivated poliomyelitis vaccines are recommended, the first before school entry and the second before leaving school (see Immunisation schedule). Further booster doses should be given every 10 years only to individuals at special risk.

Live (oral) poliomyelitis vaccines is no longer available for routine use; its use may be considered during large outbreaks, but advice should be sought from Public Health England. The live (oral) vaccine poses a very rare risk of vaccine-associated paralytic polio because the attenuated strain of the virus can revert to a virulent form. For this reason the live (oral) vaccine must **not** be used for immunosuppressed individuals or their household contacts. The use of inactivated poliomyelitis vaccines removes the risk of vaccine-associated paralytic polio altogether.

Travel

Unimmunised travellers to areas with a high incidence of poliomyelitis should receive a full 3–dose course of a preparation containing inactivated poliomyelitis vaccines. Those who have not been vaccinated in the last 10 years should receive a booster dose of **adsorbed diphtheria [low dose], tetanus and poliomyelitis (inactivated) vaccine**. Information about countries with a high incidence of poliomyelitis can be obtained from www.travax.nhs.uk or from the National Travel Health Network and Centre, (www.nathnac.org).

Rabies vaccine

Rabies vaccine p. 770 contains inactivated rabies virus cultivated in either human diploid cells or purified chick embryo cells; vaccines are used for pre- and postexposure prophylaxis.

Pre-exposure prophylaxis

Immunisation should be offered to children at high risk of exposure to rabies—where there is limited access to prompt medical care for those living in areas where rabies is enzootic, for those travelling to such areas for longer than 1 month, and for those on shorter visits who may be exposed to unusual risk. Transmission of rabies by humans has not been recorded but it is advised that those caring for children with the disease should be vaccinated.

Up-to-date country-by-country information on the incidence of rabies can be obtained from the National Travel Health Network and Centre (www.nathnac.org) and, in Scotland, from Health Protection Scotland (www.hps.scot.nhs.uk).

Immunisation against rabies requires 3 doses of rabies vaccine, with further booster doses for those who remain at frequent risk.

Post-exposure management

Following potential exposure to rabies, the wound or site of exposure (e.g. mucous membrane) should be cleansed under running water and washed for several minutes with soapy water as soon as possible after exposure. Disinfectant and a simple dressing can be applied, but suturing should be delayed because it may increase the risk of introducing rabies virus into the nerves.

Post-exposure prophylaxis against rabies depends on the level of risk in the country, the nature of exposure, and the individual's immunity. In each case, expert risk assessment and advice on appropriate management should be obtained from the local Public Health England Centre or Public Health England's Virus Reference Department, Colindale (tel. (020) 8200 4400) or the PHE Colindale Duty Doctor (tel. (020) 8200 6868), in Wales from the Public Health Wales local Health Protection Team or Public Health Wales Virus Reference Laboratory (tel. (029) 2074 7747), in Scotland from the local on-call infectious diseases consultant, and in Northern Ireland from the Public Health Agency Duty Room (tel (028) 9055 3997/(028) 9063 2662) or the Regional Virology Service (tel. (028) 9024 0503).

There are no specific contra-indications to the use of rabies vaccine for post-exposure prophylaxis and its use should be considered whenever a child has been attacked by

14

Vaccines

an animal in a country where rabies is enzootic, even if there is no direct evidence of rabies in the attacking animal. Because of the potential consequences of untreated rabies exposure and because rabies vaccination has not been associated with fetal abnormalities, pregnancy is not considered a contra-indication to post-exposure prophylaxis.

For post-exposure prophylaxis of *fully immunised* individuals (who have previously received pre-exposure or post-exposure prophylaxis with cell-derived rabies vaccine), 2 doses of cell-derived vaccine are likely to be sufficient; the first dose is given on day 0 and the second dose is given between day 3–7. Rabies immunoglobulin p. 745 is not necessary in such cases.

Post-exposure treatment for *unimmunised individuals* (or those whose prophylaxis is possibly incomplete) comprises 5 doses of rabies vaccine given over 1 month (on days 0, 3, 7, 14, and the fifth dose is given between day 28–30); also, depending on the level of risk (determined by factors such as the nature of the bite and the country where it was sustained), rabies immunoglobulin is given to unimmunised individuals on day 0 or within 7 days of starting the course of rabies vaccine. The immunisation course can be discontinued if it is proved that the child was not at risk.

Rotavirus vaccine

Rotavirus vaccine p. 770 is a live, oral vaccine that protects young children against gastro-enteritis caused by rotavirus infection. The recommended schedule consists of 2 doses, the first at 2 months of age, and the second at 3 months of age (see Immunisation schedule). The first dose of rotavirus vaccine p. 770 must be given between 6–15 weeks of age and the second dose should be given after an interval of at least 4 weeks; the vaccine should not be started in children 15 weeks of age or older. Ideally, the full course should be completed before 16 weeks of age to provide protection before the main burden of disease, and to avoid a temporal association between vaccination and intussusception; the course must be completed before 24 weeks of age.

The rotavirus vaccine virus is excreted in the stool and may be transmitted to close contacts; however, vaccination of those with *immunosuppressed* close contacts may protect the contacts from wild-type rotavirus disease and outweigh any risk from transmission of vaccine virus. Carers of a recently vaccinated baby should be advised of the need to wash their hands after changing the baby's nappies.

Smallpox vaccine

Limited supplies of **smallpox vaccine** are held at the Specialist and Reference Microbiology Division, Public Health England Colindale (Tel. (020) 8200 4400) for the exclusive use of workers in laboratories where pox viruses (such as vaccinia) are handled.

If a wider use of the vaccine is being considered, *Guidelines for smallpox response and management in the post-eradication era* should be consulted at www.gov.uk/phe.

Tetanus vaccine

Tetanus vaccine contains a cell-free purified toxin of *Clostridium tetani* adsorbed on aluminium hydroxide or aluminium phosphate to improve antigenicity.

Primary immunisation for children under 10 years consists of 3 doses of a combined preparation containing adsorbed tetanus vaccine, with an interval of 1 month between doses. Following routine childhood vaccination, 2 booster doses of a preparation containing adsorbed tetanus vaccine are recommended, the first before school entry and the second before leaving school (see Immunisation schedule).

The recommended schedule of tetanus vaccination not only gives protection against tetanus in childhood but also gives the basic immunity for subsequent booster doses. In most circumstances, a total of 5 doses of tetanus vaccine is considered sufficient for long term protection.

For primary immunisation of adults and children over 10 years previously unimmunised against tetanus, 3 doses of **adsorbed diphtheria [low dose], tetanus and poliomyelitis (inactivated) vaccine** are given with an interval of 1 month between doses.

When an individual presents for a booster dose but has been vaccinated following a tetanus-prone wound, the vaccine preparation administered at the time of injury should be determined. If this is not possible, the booster should still be given to ensure adequate protection against all antigens in the booster vaccine.

Very rarely, tetanus has developed after abdominal surgery; patients awaiting elective surgery should be asked about tetanus immunisation and immunised if necessary.

Parenteral drug abuse is also associated with tetanus; those abusing drugs by injection should be vaccinated if unimmunised—booster doses should be given if there is any doubt about their immunisation status.

All laboratory staff should be offered a primary course if unimmunised.

Wounds

Wounds are considered to be tetanus-prone if they are sustained more than 6 hours before surgical treatment or at any interval after injury and are puncture-type (particularly if contaminated with soil or manure) *or* show much devitalised tissue *or* are septic or are compound fractures *or* contain foreign bodies. All wounds should receive thorough cleansing.

- For *clean wounds*: fully immunised individuals (those who have received a total of 5 doses of a tetanus-containing vaccine at appropriate intervals) and those whose primary immunisation is complete (with boosters up to date), do not require tetanus vaccine; individuals whose primary immunisation is incomplete or whose boosters are not up to date require a reinforcing dose of a tetanus-containing vaccine (followed by further doses as required to complete the schedule); non-immunised individuals (or those whose immunisation status is not known or who have been fully immunised but are now immunocompromised) should be given a dose of the appropriate tetanus-containing vaccine immediately (followed by completion of the full course of the vaccine if records confirm the need)
- For *tetanus-prone wounds*: management is as for clean wounds with the addition of a dose of tetanus immunoglobulin given at a different site; in fully immunised individuals and those whose primary immunisation is complete (with boosters up to date) the immunoglobulin is needed only if the risk of infection is especially high (e.g. contamination with manure). Antibacterial prophylaxis (with benzylpenicillin, co-amoxiclav, or metronidazole) may also be required for tetanus-prone wounds.

Tick-borne encephalitis vaccine

Tick-borne encephalitis vaccine, inactivated p. 770 contains inactivated tick-borne encephalitis virus cultivated in chick embryo cells. It is recommended for immunisation of those working in, or visiting, high-risk areas (see International Travel). Those working, walking or camping in warm forested areas of Central and Eastern Europe, Scandinavia, Northern and Eastern China, and some parts of Japan, particularly from April to November when ticks are most prevalent, are at greatest risk of tick-borne encephalitis. For full protection, 3 doses of the vaccine are required; booster doses are required every 3–5 years for those still at risk. Ideally, immunisation should be completed at least one month before travel.

Typhoid vaccine

Typhoid vaccine p. 763 is available as Vi capsular polysaccharide (from *Salmonella typhi*) vaccine for injection and as live attenuated *Salmonella typhi* vaccine for oral use. Typhoid immunisation is advised for children travelling to:

- areas where typhoid is endemic, especially if staying with or visiting local people;
- endemic areas where frequent or prolonged exposure to poor sanitation and poor food hygiene is likely;

Typhoid vaccination is not a substitute for scrupulous personal hygiene.

Capsular **polysaccharide typhoid vaccine** is usually given by *intramuscular* injection. Children under 2 years may respond suboptimally to the vaccine, but children aged between 1–2 years should be immunised if the risk of typhoid fever is considered high (immunisation is not recommended for infants under 12 months). Revaccination is needed every 3 years on continued exposure.

Oral typhoid vaccine is a **live attenuated** vaccine contained in an enteric-coated capsule. One capsule taken on alternate days for a total of 3 doses provides protection 7–10 days after the last dose. Protection may persist for up to 3 years in those constantly (or repeatedly) exposed to *Salmonella typhi*, but those who only occasionally travel to endemic areas require further courses at intervals of 1 year.

Varicella-zoster vaccine

Varicella-zoster vaccine (live) p. 771 is licensed for immunisation against varicella (chickenpox) in seronegative individuals. It is not recommended for routine use in children but can be given to seronegative healthy children over 1 year who come into close contact with individuals at high risk of severe varicella infections.

Rarely, the varicella-zoster vaccine virus has been transmitted from the vaccinated individual to close contacts. Therefore, contact with the following should be avoided if a vaccine-related cutaneous rash develops within 4–6 weeks of the first or second dose:

- varicella-susceptible pregnant females;
- individuals at high risk of severe varicella, including those with immunodeficiency or those receiving immunosuppressive therapy.

Varicella-zoster immunoglobulin p. 746 is used to protect susceptible children at increased risk of varicella infection.

Yellow fever vaccine

Live yellow fever vaccine, live p. 771 is indicated for those travelling to or living in areas where infection is endemic. Infants under 6 months of age should not be vaccinated because there is a small risk of encephalitis; infants aged 6–9 months should be vaccinated only if the risk of yellow fever is high and unavoidable (seek expert advice). The immunity which probably lasts for life is officially accepted for 10 years starting from 10 days after primary immunisation and for a further 10 years immediately after revaccination.

Very rarely vaccine-associated adverse effects have been reported, such as viscerotropic disease (yellow fever vaccine, live-associated viscerotropic disease, YEL–AVD), a syndrome which may include metabolic acidosis, muscle and liver cytolysis, and multi-organ failure. Neurological disorders (yellow fever vaccine, live-associated neurotropic disease, YEL-AND) such as encephalitis have also been reported. These *very rare* adverse effects have usually occurred after the first dose of yellow fever vaccine, live in those with no previous immunity.

Vaccines for travel

Immunisation

See advice on Malaria, treatment p. 371.

No special immunisation is required for travellers to the United States, Europe, Australia, or New Zealand, although all travellers should have immunity to tetanus and poliomyelitis (and childhood immunisations should be up to date); Tick-borne encephalitis vaccine is recommended for immunisation of those working in, or visiting, high-risk areas. Certain special precautions are required in non-European areas surrounding the Mediterranean, in Africa, the Middle East, Asia, and South America.

Travellers to areas that have a high incidence of **poliomyelitis** or **tuberculosis** should be immunised with the appropriate vaccine; in the case of poliomyelitis previously immunised travellers may be given a booster dose of a preparation containing inactivated poliomyelitis vaccine. BCG immunisation is recommended for travellers aged under 16 years proposing to stay for longer than 3 months (or in close contact with the local population) in countries with an incidence of tuberculosis greater than 40 per 100 000 (list of countries where the incidence of tuberculosis is greater than 40 cases per 100 000 is available from www.gov.uk/phe); it should preferably be given 3 months or more before departure.

Yellow fever immunisation is recommended for travel to the endemic zones of Africa and South America. Many countries require an International Certificate of Vaccination from individuals arriving from, or who have been travelling through, endemic areas; other countries require a certificate from all entering travellers (consult the Department of Health handbook, *Health Information for Overseas Travel*, www.dh.gov.uk).

Immunisation against **meningococcal meningitis** is recommended for a number of areas of the world.

Protection against **hepatitis A** is recommended for travellers to high-risk areas outside Northern and Western Europe, North America, Japan, Australia and New Zealand. Hepatitis A vaccine is preferred and it is likely to be effective even if given shortly before departure; normal immunoglobulin is no longer given routinely but may be indicated in the immunocompromised. Special care must also be taken with food hygiene.

Hepatitis B vaccine is recommended for those travelling to areas of high or intermediate prevalence who intend to seek employment as healthcare workers or who plan to remain there for lengthy periods and who may therefore be at increased risk of acquiring infection as the result of medical or dental procedures carried out in those countries. Short-term tourists or business travellers are not generally at increased risk of infection but may put themselves at risk by their sexual behaviour when abroad.

Prophylactic immunisation against **rabies** is recommended for travellers to enzootic areas on long journeys or to areas out of reach of immediate medical attention.

Travellers who have not had a **tetanus** booster in the last 10 years and are visiting areas where medical attention may not be accessible should receive a booster dose of adsorbed diphtheria [low dose], tetanus and poliomyelitis (inactivated) vaccine, even if they have received 5 doses of a tetanus-containing vaccine previously.

Typhoid vaccine is indicated for travellers to countries where typhoid is endemic, but the vaccine is no substitute for personal precautions.

There is no requirement for cholera vaccination as a condition for entry into any country, but **oral cholera vaccine** should be considered for backpackers and those travelling to situations where the risk is greatest (e.g. refugee camps). Regardless of vaccination, travellers to areas where

14

Vaccines

cholera is endemic should take special care with food hygiene.

Advice on **diphtheria**, on **Japanese encephalitis**, and on **tick-borne encephalitis** is included in *Health Information for Overseas Travel*.

Food hygiene

In areas where sanitation is poor, good food hygiene is important to help prevent hepatitis A, typhoid, cholera, and other diarrhoeal diseases (including travellers' diarrhoea). Food should be freshly prepared and hot, and uncooked vegetables (including green salads) should be avoided; only fruits which can be peeled should be eaten. Only suitable bottled water, or tap water that has been boiled or treated with sterilising tablets, should be used for drinking.

Information on health advice for travellers

Health professionals and travellers can find the latest information on immunisation requirements and precautions for avoiding illness while travelling from: www.nathnac.org.

The handbook, *Health Information for Overseas Travel* (2010), which draws together essential information *for healthcare professionals* regarding health advice for travellers, can also be obtained from this website.

Immunisation requirements change from time to time, and information on the current requirements for any particular country may be obtained from the embassy or legation of the appropriate country or from:

National Travel Health Network and Centre
UCLH NHS Foundation Trust
3rd Floor Central,
250 Euston Road,
London, NW1 2PG
Tel: 0845 602 6712
(8:30–11:45 a.m, 1–3:15 p.m. weekdays for healthcare professionals only) www.nathnac.org

Travel Medicine Team
Health Protection Scotland
Meridian Court,
5 Cadogan Street,
Glasgow, G2 6QE
Tel: (0141) 300 1130
(2–4 p.m. Monday to Wednesday, 9:30–11:30 a.m. Friday; for registered TRAVAX users only) www.travax.nhs.uk
(TRAVAX is free for NHS Scotland users (registration required); subscription fee may be payable for users outside NHS Scotland)

Welsh Assembly Government
Tel (029) 2082 5397
(9 a.m.–5:30 p.m. weekdays)

Department of Health, Social Services and Public Safety
Castle Buildings,
Stormont,
Belfast, BT4 3SQ
Tel: (028) 9052 2118
(9 a.m.–5 p.m. weekdays) www.dhsspsni.gov.uk

VACCINES

Vaccines

IMPORTANT SAFETY INFORMATION
MHRA/CHM ADVICE (APRIL 2016)
Following reports of death in neonates who received a live attenuated vaccine after exposure to a tumor necrosis factor alpha (TNF-a) inhibitor in utero, the MHRA has issued the following advice:
- any infant who has been exposed to immunosuppressive treatment from the mother either in utero during pregnancy or via breastfeeding should have any live attenuated vaccination deferred for as long as a postnatal influence on the immune status of the infant remains possible;
- in the case of infants who have been exposed to TNF-a inhibitors and other biological medicines in utero, any live attenuated vaccination should be deferred until the infant is age 6 months, after which time vaccination should be considered.

- **CONTRA-INDICATIONS**
CONTRA-INDICATIONS, FURTHER INFORMATION
▸ Impaired immune response Severely immunosuppressed patients should not be given live vaccines (including those with severe primary immunodeficiency).

- **CAUTIONS** Acute illness · minor illnesses
CAUTIONS, FURTHER INFORMATION
Vaccination may be postponed if the individual is suffering from an acute illness; however, it is not necessary to postpone immunisation in patients with minor illnesses without fever or systemic upset.
▸ Impaired immune response and drugs affecting immune response Immune response to vaccines may be reduced in immunosuppressed patients and there is also a risk of generalised infection with live vaccines.

Specialist advice should be sought for those being treated with high doses of corticosteroids (dose equivalents of prednisolone: **adults**, at least 40 mg daily for more than 1 week; **children**, 2 mg/kg (or more than 40 mg) daily for at least 1 week or 1 mg/kg daily for 1 month), or other immunosuppressive drugs, and those being treated for malignant conditions with chemotherapy or generalised radiotherapy. Live vaccines should be postponed until at least 3 months after stopping high-dose systemic corticosteroids and at least 6 months after stopping other immunosuppressive drugs or generalised radiotherapy (at least 12 months after discontinuing immunosuppressants following bone-marrow transplantation).

The Royal College of Paediatrics and Child Health has produced a statement, *Immunisation of the Immunocompromised Child* (2002) (available at www.rcpch.ac.uk).
▸ Predisposition to neurological problems When there is a personal or family history of *febrile* convulsions, there is an increased risk of these occurring during fever from any cause including immunisation, but this is not a contra-indication to immunisation. In children who have had a seizure associated with fever without neurological deterioration, immunisation is *recommended*; advice on the *management of fever* (see Post-immunisation Pyrexia in Infants) should be given before immunisation. When a child has had a convulsion not associated with fever, and the neurological condition is not deteriorating, immunisation is *recommended*.

Children with stable neurological disorders (e.g. spina bifida, congenital brain abnormality, and peri-natal hypoxic-ischaemic encephalopathy) should be immunised according to the recommended schedule.

When there is a *still evolving neurological problem*, including poorly controlled epilepsy, immunisation should be deferred and the child referred to a specialist. Immunisation is recommended if a cause for the neurological disorder is identified. If a cause is not identified, immunisation should be deferred until the condition is stable.

- **SIDE-EFFECTS**
GENERAL SIDE-EFFECTS
▸ **Common or very common** Fatigue · fever · gastro-intestinal disturbances · headache · irritability · loss of appetite · lymphangitis · malaise · myalgia

▸ **Very rare** Anaphylaxis (can be fatal) · angioedema (can be fatal) · bronchospasm (can be fatal) · hypersensitivity reactions (can be fatal) · urticaria (can be fatal)

▸ **Frequency not known** Arthralgia · asthenia · dizziness · drowsiness · influenza-like symptoms · lymphadenopathy · paraesthesia · rash

SPECIFIC SIDE-EFFECTS

▸ **Common or very common**

▸ With intradermal use or intramuscular use or subcutaneous use Induration may develop at the injection site · inflammation · local reactions · pain · redness · sterile abscess may develop at the injection site

SIDE-EFFECTS, FURTHER INFORMATION
Occasionally serious adverse reactions can occur—these should always be reported to the CHM.

▸ Post-immunisation pyrexia in infants The parent should be advised that if pyrexia develops after childhood immunisation, and the infant seems distressed, paracetamol can be given. Ibuprofen can be used if paracetamol is unsuitable. The parent should be warned to seek medical advice if the pyrexia persists.

● **ALLERGY AND CROSS-SENSITIVITY** Contra-indicated in patients with a confirmed anaphylactic reaction to a preceding dose of a vaccine containing the same antigens or vaccine component (such as antibacterials in viral vaccines).

● **PREGNANCY** Live vaccines should not be administered routinely to pregnant women because of the theoretical risk of fetal infection but where there is a significant risk of exposure to disease, the need for vaccination usually outweighs any possible risk to the fetus. Termination of pregnancy following inadvertent immunisation is not recommended. There is no evidence of risk from vaccinating pregnant women with inactivated viral or bacterial vaccines or toxoids.

● **BREAST FEEDING** Although there is a theoretical risk of live vaccine being present in breast milk, vaccination is not contra-indicated for women who are breast-feeding when there is significant risk of exposure to disease. There is no evidence of risk from vaccinating women who are breast-feeding, with inactivated viral or bacterial vaccines or toxoids.

● **DIRECTIONS FOR ADMINISTRATION** If alcohol or disinfectant is used for cleansing the skin it should be allowed to evaporate before vaccination to prevent possible inactivation of live vaccines.

When 2 or more live vaccines are required (and are not available as a combined preparation), they can be administered at any time before or after each other at different sites, preferably in a different limb; if more than one injection is to be given in the same limb, they should be administered at least 2.5 cm apart. See also Bacillus Calmette-Guérin vaccine p. 760.

Vaccines should not be given intravenously. Most vaccines are given by the intramuscular route, although some are given by either the intradermal, deep subcutaneous, or oral route. The intramuscular route should not be used in patients with **bleeding disorders** such as haemophilia or thrombocytopenia, vaccines usually given by the intramuscular route should be given by deep subcutaneous injection instead.

The Department of Health has advised *against the use of jet guns* for vaccination owing to the risk of transmitting blood borne infections, such as HIV.

Particular attention must be paid to instructions on the use of diluents. Vaccines which are liquid suspensions or are reconstituted before use should be adequately mixed to ensure uniformity of the material to be injected.

● **HANDLING AND STORAGE** Care must be taken to store all vaccines under the conditions recommended in the product literature, otherwise the preparation may become ineffective. **Refrigerated storage** is usually necessary; many vaccines need to be stored at 2–8°C and not allowed to freeze. Vaccines should be protected from light. Reconstituted vaccines and opened multidose vials must be used within the period recommended in the product literature. Unused vaccines should be disposed of by incineration at a registered disposal contractor.

VACCINES ⟩ BACTERIAL AND VIRAL VACCINES, COMBINED

[F 758]

Diphtheria with haemophilus influenzae type b vaccine, pertussis, poliomyelitis and tetanus

● **INDICATIONS AND DOSE**

Primary immunisation

▸ BY INTRAMUSCULAR INJECTION

▸ Child 2 months-10 years: 0.5 mL every month for 3 doses

● **UNLICENSED USE** *Infanrix-IPV + Hib*® not licensed for use in children over 36 months; *Pediacel*® not licensed in children over 4 years. However, the Department of Health recommends that these be used for children up to 10 years.

● **SIDE-EFFECTS** Atopic dermatitis · hypotonia · restlessness · sleep disturbances · unusual crying in infants

SIDE-EFFECTS, FURTHER INFORMATION

▸ Side effects of vaccines containing pertussis The incidence of local and systemic effects is generally lower with vaccines containing acellular pertussis components than with the whole-cell pertussis vaccine used previously. However, compared with primary vaccination, booster doses with vaccines containing acellular pertussis are reported to increase the risk of injection-site reactions (some of which affect the entire limb); local reactions do not contra-indicate further doses.

The vaccine should not be withheld from children with a history to a preceding dose of:

● fever, irrespective of severity;
● persistent crying or screaming for more than 3 hours;
● severe local reaction, irrespective of extent.

● **PRESCRIBING AND DISPENSING INFORMATION** Available as part of childhood schedule from health organisations or ImmForm.

● **MEDICINAL FORMS**
There can be variation in the licensing of different medicines containing the same drug.

Powder and suspension for suspension for injection

▸ **Infanrix-IPV + Hib** (GlaxoSmithKline UK Ltd)
Infanrix-IPV + Hib vaccine powder and suspension for suspension for injection 0.5ml pre-filled syringes | 1 pre-filled disposable injection [PoM] £27.86

Suspension for injection
EXCIPIENTS: May contain Neomycin, polymyxin b, streptomycin

▸ **Pediacel** (sanofi pasteur MSD Ltd)
Pediacel vaccine suspension for injection 0.5ml vials | 1 vial [PoM] £32.00

[F 758]

Diphtheria with pertussis, poliomyelitis vaccine and tetanus

● **INDICATIONS AND DOSE**

First booster dose

▸ BY INTRAMUSCULAR INJECTION

▸ Child 3-9 years: 0.5 mL, to be given 3 years after primary immunisation   continued →

14

Vaccines

Vaccination of pregnant women against pertussis (using low dose vaccines)
▶ BY INTRAMUSCULAR INJECTION
▶ Females of childbearing potential: 0.5 mL for 1 dose

● SIDE-EFFECTS Restlessness · sleep disturbances · unusual crying in infants

SIDE-EFFECTS, FURTHER INFORMATION
▶ Side effects of vaccines containing pertussis The incidence of local and systemic effects is generally lower with vaccines containing acellular pertussis components than with the whole-cell pertussis vaccine used previously. However, compared with primary vaccination, booster doses with vaccines containing acellular pertussis are reported to increase the risk of injection-site reactions (some of which affect the entire limb); local reactions do not contra-indicate further doses.
    The vaccine should not be withheld from children with a history to a preceding dose of:
    ● fever, irrespective of severity;
    ● persistent crying or screaming for more than 3 hours;
    ● severe local reaction, irrespective of extent.
● PREGNANCY Contra-indicated in pregnant women with a history of encephalopathy of unknown origin within 7 days of previous immunisation with a pertussis-containing vaccine. Contra-indicated in pregnant women with a history of transient thrombocytopenia or neurological complications following previous immunisation against diphtheria or tetanus.
● PRESCRIBING AND DISPENSING INFORMATION Pregnant women should be vaccinated using low dose vaccines (brands may include *Boostrix-IPV*® or *Repevax*®).
    Available as part of childhood immunisation schedule from health organisations or ImmForm.
    Available for vaccination of pregnant women from ImmForm.

● MEDICINAL FORMS
There can be variation in the licensing of different medicines containing the same drug.
Suspension for injection
EXCIPIENTS: May contain Neomycin, polymyxin b, streptomycin
▶ Boostrix-IPV (GlaxoSmithKline UK Ltd)
    Boostrix-IPV suspension for injection 0.5ml pre-filled syringes | 1 pre-filled disposable injection [PoM] £22.74
▶ Infanrix-IPV (GlaxoSmithKline UK Ltd)
    Infanrix-IPV vaccine suspension for injection 0.5ml pre-filled syringes | 1 pre-filled disposable injection [PoM] £17.56
▶ Repevax (sanofi pasteur MSD Ltd)
    Repevax vaccine suspension for injection 0.5ml pre-filled syringes | 1 pre-filled disposable injection [PoM] £20.00

F 758

Diphtheria with poliomyelitis and tetanus vaccine

● INDICATIONS AND DOSE
Primary immunisation
▶ BY INTRAMUSCULAR INJECTION
▶ Child 10-17 years: 0.5 mL every month for 3 doses
Booster doses
▶ BY INTRAMUSCULAR INJECTION
▶ Child 10-17 years: 0.5 mL for 1 dose, first booster dose—should be given 3 years after primary course (this interval can be reduced to a minimum of 1 year if the primary course was delayed), then 0.5 mL for 1 dose, second booster dose—should be given 10 years after first booster dose (this interval can be reduced to a minimum of 5 years if previous doses were delayed), second booster dose may also be used as first booster dose in those over 10 years who have received only 3 previous doses of a diphtheria-containing vaccine

● SIDE-EFFECTS Restlessness · sleep disturbances · unusual crying in infants
● PRESCRIBING AND DISPENSING INFORMATION Available as part of childhood schedule from health organisations or ImmForm.

● MEDICINAL FORMS
There can be variation in the licensing of different medicines containing the same drug.
Suspension for injection
EXCIPIENTS: May contain Neomycin, polymyxin b, streptomycin
▶ Revaxis (sanofi pasteur MSD Ltd)
    Revaxis vaccine suspension for injection 0.5ml pre-filled syringes | 1 pre-filled disposable injection [PoM] £6.50

VACCINES > BACTERIAL VACCINES

F 758

Bacillus Calmette-Guérin vaccine
(BCG Vaccine)

● DRUG ACTION BCG (Bacillus Calmette-Guérin) is a live attenuated strain derived from *Mycobacterium bovis* which stimulates the development of immunity to *M. tuberculosis*.

● INDICATIONS AND DOSE
Immunisation against tuberculosis
▶ BY INTRADERMAL INJECTION
▶ Neonate: 0.05 mL, to be injected at insertion of deltoid muscle onto humerus (keloid formation more likely with sites higher on arm); tip of shoulder should be **avoided**.
▶ Child 1-11 months: 0.05 mL, to be injected at insertion of deltoid muscle onto humerus (keloid formation more likely with sites higher on arm); tip of shoulder should be **avoided**
▶ Child 1-17 years: 0.1 mL, to be injected at insertion of deltoid muscle onto humerus (keloid formation more likely with sites higher on arm); tip of shoulder should be **avoided**

● CONTRA-INDICATIONS Generalised septic skin conditions · neonate in household contact with known or suspected case of active tuberculosis
CONTRA-INDICATIONS, FURTHER INFORMATION
A lesion-free site should be used to administer BCG vaccine to patients with eczema.
● CAUTIONS
CAUTIONS, FURTHER INFORMATION
BCG vaccine can be given simultaneously with another live vaccine, but if they are not given at the same time an interval of 4 weeks should normally be allowed. When BCG is given to infants, there is no need to delay routine primary immunisations. No further vaccination should be given in the arm used for BCG vaccination for at least 3 months because of the risk of regional lymphadenitis.
● INTERACTIONS → Appendix 1: live vaccines
● SIDE-EFFECTS
▶ Rare Disseminated complications · osteitis · osteomyelitis
▶ Frequency not known Prolonged ulceration at the injection site · subcutaneous abscess at the injection site
● PRE-TREATMENT SCREENING Apart from children under 6 years, any person being considered for BCG immunisation must first be given a skin test for hypersensitivity to tuberculoprotein (see tuberculin purified protein derivative p. 747). A skin test is not necessary for a child under 6 years provided that the child has not stayed for longer than 3 months in a country with an incidence of tuberculosis greater than 40 per 100 000, the child has not had contact with a person with

tuberculosis, and there is no family history of tuberculosis within the last 5 years.

● **DIRECTIONS FOR ADMINISTRATION**
Intradermal injection technique Skin is stretched between thumb and forefinger and needle (size 25G or 26G) inserted (bevel upwards) for about 3 mm into superficial layers of dermis (almost parallel with surface). Needle should be short with short bevel (can usually be seen through epidermis during insertion). Tense raised blanched bleb showing tips of hair follicles is sign of correct injection; 7 mm bleb ≡ 0.1 mL injection, 3 mm bleb ≡ 0.05 mL injection; if considerable resistance not felt, needle too deep and should be removed and reinserted before giving more vaccine.

● **PRESCRIBING AND DISPENSING INFORMATION** Available from health organisations or direct from ImmForm www.immform.dh.gov.uk (SSI brand, multidose vial with diluent).

● **MEDICINAL FORMS**
There can be variation in the licensing of different medicines containing the same drug.
Powder and solvent for suspension for injection
▸ Bacillus calmette-guérin vaccine (Non-proprietary)
  Bacillus Calmette-Guerin vaccine powder and solvent for suspension for injection vials | 10 vial [PoM] no price available

☞ 758

Cholera vaccine

● **INDICATIONS AND DOSE**
Immunisation against cholera (for travellers to endemic or epidemic areas on the basis of current recommendations)
▸ BY MOUTH
▸ Child 2–5 years: 1 dose every 1–6 weeks for 3 doses, if more than 6 weeks have elapsed between doses, the primary course should be restarted, immunisation should be completed at least one week before potential exposure
▸ Child 6–17 years: 1 dose every 1–6 weeks for 2 doses, if more than 6 weeks have elapsed between doses, the primary course should be restarted, immunisation should be completed at least one week before potential exposure

Booster
▸ BY MOUTH
▸ Child 2–5 years: A single booster dose can be given within 6 months after primary course, if more than 6 months have elapsed since the last vaccination, the primary course should be repeated
▸ Child 6–17 years: A single booster dose can be given within 2 years after primary course, if more than 2 years have elapsed since the last vaccination, the primary course should be repeated

● **CONTRA-INDICATIONS** Acute gastro-intestinal illness
● **INTERACTIONS** → Appendix 1: cholera vaccine
● **SIDE-EFFECTS**
▸ **Rare** Cough · respiratory symptoms · rhinitis
▸ **Very rare** Insomnia · sore throat
▸ **Frequency not known** Abdominal pain and cramps · diarrhoea · nausea · vomiting
● **DIRECTIONS FOR ADMINISTRATION** Dissolve effervescent sodium bicarbonate granules in a glassful of water *or* chlorinated water (approximately 150 mL). For children over 6 years, add vaccine suspension to make one dose. For child 2–5 years, discard half (approximately 75 mL) of the solution, then add vaccine suspension to make one dose. Drink within 2 hours. Food, drink, and other oral medicines should be avoided for 1 hour before and after vaccination.

● **PATIENT AND CARER ADVICE** Counselling on administration advised. Immunisation with cholera vaccine does not provide complete protection and all travellers to a country where cholera exists should be warned that scrupulous attention to food, water, and personal hygiene is **essential**.

● **MEDICINAL FORMS**
There can be variation in the licensing of different medicines containing the same drug.
Oral suspension
▸ Dukoral (Valneva UK Ltd)
  Dukoral cholera vaccine oral suspension | 2 dose [PoM] £23.42

☞ 758

Haemophilus influenzae type B with meningococcal group C vaccine

● **INDICATIONS AND DOSE**
Booster dose (for infants who have received primary immunisation with a vaccine containing *Haemophilus influenzae* type b component) and primary immunisation against *Neisseria meningitidis*
▸ BY INTRAMUSCULAR INJECTION
▸ Child 12–13 months: 0.5 mL for 1 dose
Immunisation against *Neisseria meningitidis* in an unimmunised patient
▸ BY INTRAMUSCULAR INJECTION
▸ Child 1–9 years: 0.5 mL for 1 dose
Booster dose (for children who have not been immunised against *Haemophilus influenza* type b) | Booster dose after recovery from *Haemophilus influenzae* type b disease (for index cases previously vaccinated, with low Hib antibody concentration or if it is not possible to measure antibody concentration)
▸ BY INTRAMUSCULAR INJECTION
▸ Child 1–9 years: 0.5 mL for 1 dose
Booster dose after recovery from *Haemophilus influenzae* type b disease (for fully vaccinated index cases with asplenia or splenic dysfunction, if previous dose received over 1 year ago)
▸ BY INTRAMUSCULAR INJECTION
▸ Child 1–17 years: 0.5 mL for 1 dose
Booster dose (for patients diagnosed with asplenia, splenic dysfunction or complement deficiency at under 2 years of age)
▸ BY INTRAMUSCULAR INJECTION
▸ Child 2–17 years: 0.5 mL for 1 dose, this booster dose should be given after the second birthday, this is the second dose of haemophilus influenzae type B vaccine combined with meningococcal group C conjugate vaccine (the first dose is given during the routine immunisation schedule)
Booster dose (for patients diagnosed with asplenia, splenic dysfunction or complement deficiency at over 2 years of age)
▸ BY INTRAMUSCULAR INJECTION
▸ Child 2–17 years: 0.5 mL for 1 dose, this booster dose should be followed 2 months later by one dose of meningococcal A, C, W135, and Y conjugate vaccine (in patients from 11 years of age, this interval can be reduced to one month)

● **UNLICENSED USE** Not licensed for use in patients over 2 years.
● **SIDE-EFFECTS**
▸ **Rare** Symptoms of meningitis reported (but no evidence that the vaccine causes meningococcal C meningitis)
▸ **Frequency not known** Atopic dermatitis · hypotonia

14

Vaccines

- **PRESCRIBING AND DISPENSING INFORMATION** Available as part of the childhood immunisation schedule from ImmForm.

- **MEDICINAL FORMS**
There can be variation in the licensing of different medicines containing the same drug.
Powder and solvent for solution for injection
  - Menitorix (GlaxoSmithKline UK Ltd)
    Menitorix vaccine powder and solvent for solution for injection 0.5ml vials | 1 vial [PoM] £37.76

F 758

Meningococcal group B vaccine (rDNA, component, adsorbed)

- **INDICATIONS AND DOSE**
Immunisation against _Neisseria meningitidis_, primary immunisation
  ▸ BY DEEP INTRAMUSCULAR INJECTION
  - Child 2 months: 0.5 mL for 1 dose, injected preferably into deltoid region (or anterolateral thigh in infants), for information about the use of paracetamol for prophylaxis of post-immunisation pyrexia, see p. 260.
  - Child 4 months: 0.5 mL for 1 dose, injected preferably into deltoid region (or anterolateral thigh in infants), for information about the use of paracetamol for prophylaxis of post-immunisation pyrexia, see p. 260.

Immunisation against _Neisseria meningitidis_, primary immunisation booster dose
  ▸ BY DEEP INTRAMUSCULAR INJECTION
  - Child 12–23 months: 0.5 mL for 1 dose, injected preferably into deltoid region (or anterolateral thigh in infants)

Immunisation against _Neisseria meningitidis_, primary immunisation (in unimmunised patients)
  ▸ BY DEEP INTRAMUSCULAR INJECTION
  - Child 6–11 months: 0.5 mL for 2 doses, separated by an interval of at least 2 months; booster dose of 0.5 mL given between 1–2 years of age and at least 2 months after completion of primary immunisation, injected preferably into deltoid region (or anterolateral thigh in infants)
  - Child 12–23 months: 0.5 mL for 2 doses, separated by an interval of at least 2 months; booster dose of 0.5 mL given 12–24 months after completion of primary immunisation, injected preferably into deltoid region (or anterolateral thigh in infants)
  - Child 2–10 years: 0.5 mL for 2 doses, separated by an interval of at least 2 months. Injected preferably into deltoid region (or anterolateral thigh in infants)
  - Child 11–17 years: 0.5 mL for 2 doses, separated by an interval of at least 1 month. Injected preferably into deltoid region

- **SIDE-EFFECTS**
  ▸ Rare Kawasaki disease · symptoms of meningitis reported (but no evidence that the vaccine causes meningococcal C meningitis)
  ▸ Frequency not known Unusual crying

- **MEDICINAL FORMS**
There can be variation in the licensing of different medicines containing the same drug.
Suspension for injection
  EXCIPIENTS: May contain Kanamycin
  ▸ Bexsero (GlaxoSmithKline UK Ltd) ▼
    Bexsero vaccine suspension for injection 0.5ml pre-filled syringes | 1 pre-filled disposable injection [PoM] £75.00

F 758

Meningococcal group C vaccine

- **INDICATIONS AND DOSE**
Patients with confirmed serogroup C disease (who have previously been immunised)
  ▸ BY INTRAMUSCULAR INJECTION
  - Child 1–17 years: 0.5 mL for 1 dose, dose to be given before discharge from hospital

- **SIDE-EFFECTS**
  ▸ Rare Symptoms of meningitis (but no evidence that vaccine causes meningococcal C meningitis)

- **DIRECTIONS FOR ADMINISTRATION** _Menjugate Kit®_ may be used via subcutaneous route in children with bleeding disorders.

- **PRESCRIBING AND DISPENSING INFORMATION** Available as part of childhood immunisation schedule from www.immform.dh.gov.uk.

- **MEDICINAL FORMS**
There can be variation in the licensing of different medicines containing the same drug.
Suspension for injection
  ▸ NeisVac-C (Pfizer Ltd)
    NeisVac-C vaccine suspension for injection 0.5ml pre-filled syringes | 10 pre-filled disposable injection [PoM] £187.50

F 758

Meningococcal groups A with C and W135 and Y vaccine

- **INDICATIONS AND DOSE**
MENVEO®
Primary immunisation against _Neisseria meningitidis_
  ▸ BY INTRAMUSCULAR INJECTION
  - Child 13–15 years: 0.5 mL for 1 dose, dose preferably injected into deltoid region

Immunisation against _Neisseria meningitidis_ in an unimmunised patient
  ▸ BY INTRAMUSCULAR INJECTION
  - Child 10–17 years: 0.5 mL for 1 dose, booster dose is not required

Immunisation against _Neisseria meningitidis_ in those at risk of exposure to prevent invasive disease
  ▸ BY INTRAMUSCULAR INJECTION
  - Child 3–11 months: 0.5 mL every month for 2 doses, dose preferably injected into deltoid region
  - Child 1–17 years: 0.5 mL for 1 dose, dose preferably injected into deltoid region

Patients attending university for the first time (who have not received the routine meningococcal A, C, W135, and Y conjugate vaccine over the age of 10 years)
  ▸ BY INTRAMUSCULAR INJECTION
  - Child 16–17 years: 0.5 mL for 1 dose

NIMENRIX®
Primary immunisation against _Neisseria meningitidis_
  ▸ BY INTRAMUSCULAR INJECTION
  - Child 13–15 years: 0.5 mL for 1 dose, to be injected preferably into deltoid region

Immunisation against _Neisseria meningitidis_ in an unimmunised patient
  ▸ BY INTRAMUSCULAR INJECTION
  - Child 10–17 years: 0.5 mL for 1 dose, booster dose is not required

Immunisation against *Neisseria meningitidis* in those at risk of exposure

▸ BY INTRAMUSCULAR INJECTION

▸ Child 1-17 years: 0.5 mL for 1 dose, to be injected preferably into deltoid region (or anterolateral thigh in child 12–23 months), then 0.5 mL after 1 year if required for 1 dose, second dose should be considered in those who continue to be at risk of *Neisseria meningitidis* serogroup A infection

Patients attending university for the first time (who have not received the routine meningococcal A, C, W135, and Y conjugate vaccine over the age of 10 years)

▸ BY INTRAMUSCULAR INJECTION

▸ Child 16-17 years: 0.5 mL for 1 dose

● UNLICENSED USE

MENVEO® *Menveo*® is not licensed for use in children under 2 years.

● SIDE-EFFECTS

▸ **Rare** Symptoms of meningitis reported (but no evidence that the vaccine causes meningococcal C meningitis)

● MEDICINAL FORMS

There can be variation in the licensing of different medicines containing the same drug.

Powder and solvent for solution for injection

▸ Menveo (GlaxoSmithKline UK Ltd)
Menveo vaccine powder and solvent for solution for injection 0.5ml vials | 1 vial PoM £30.00

▸ Nimenrix (Pfizer Ltd) ▼
Nimenrix vaccine powder and solvent for solution for injection 0.5ml pre-filled syringes | 1 pre-filled disposable injection PoM £30.00

F 758

Pneumococcal polysaccharide conjugate vaccine (adsorbed)

● INDICATIONS AND DOSE

PREVENAR 13®

Primary immunisation against pneumococcal infection (first dose)

▸ BY INTRAMUSCULAR INJECTION

▸ Child 2 months: 0.5 mL for 1 dose, anterolateral thigh is preferred site of injection in infants

Primary immunisation against pneumococcal infection (second dose)

▸ BY INTRAMUSCULAR INJECTION

▸ Child 4 months: 0.5 mL for 1 dose, anterolateral thigh is preferred site of injection in infants

Primary immunisation against pneumococcal infection (booster dose)

▸ BY INTRAMUSCULAR INJECTION

▸ Child 12-13 months: 0.5 mL for 1 dose, anterolateral thigh is preferred site of injection in infants

Immunisation against pneumococcal infection (in patients who have not been vaccinated or not completed the primary course)

▸ BY INTRAMUSCULAR INJECTION

▸ Child 12 months-4 years: 0.5 mL for 1 dose, deltoid muscle is preferred site of injection in young children; anterolateral thigh is preferred site in infants

Immunisation against pneumococcal infection, in immunocompromised or asplenic patients or patients with splenic dysfunction (who have not been vaccinated or not completed the primary course)

▸ BY INTRAMUSCULAR INJECTION

▸ Child 12 months-4 years: 0.5 mL every 2 months for 2 doses, deltoid muscle is preferred site of injection in young children; anterolateral thigh is preferred site in infants

SYNFLORIX®

Immunisation against pneumococcal infection

▸ BY INTRAMUSCULAR INJECTION

▸ Child 6 weeks-4 years: Deltoid muscle is preferred site of injection in young children; anterolateral thigh is preferred site of injection in infants (consult product literature)

● UNLICENSED USE

PREVENAR 13® The dose in BNF publications may differ from that in product literature.

● PRESCRIBING AND DISPENSING INFORMATION

PREVENAR 13® Available as part of childhood immunisation schedule from ImmForm www.immform.dh.gov.uk.

● MEDICINAL FORMS

There can be variation in the licensing of different medicines containing the same drug.

Suspension for injection

▸ Prevenar (Pfizer Ltd)
Prevenar 13 vaccine suspension for injection 0.5ml pre-filled syringes | 1 pre-filled disposable injection PoM £49.10 | 10 pre-filled disposable injection PoM £491.00

▸ Synflorix (GlaxoSmithKline UK Ltd)
Synflorix vaccine suspension for injection 0.5ml pre-filled syringes | 1 pre-filled disposable injection PoM £27.60

F 758

Pneumococcal polysaccharide vaccine

● INDICATIONS AND DOSE

Immunisation against pneumococcal infection

▸ BY INTRAMUSCULAR INJECTION, OR BY SUBCUTANEOUS INJECTION

▸ Child 2-17 years: 0.5 mL for 1 dose

Immunisation in patients at increased risk of pneumococcal disease

▸ BY INTRAMUSCULAR INJECTION, OR BY SUBCUTANEOUS INJECTION

▸ Child 2-4 years: 0.5 mL for 1 dose, dose should be administered after the second birthday or at least 2 months after the final dose of the 13-valent pneumococcal polysaccharide conjugate vaccine (adsorbed)

▸ Child 5-17 years: 0.5 mL for 1 dose

● MEDICINAL FORMS

There can be variation in the licensing of different medicines containing the same drug.

Solution for injection

▸ Pneumococcal polysaccharide vaccine (Non-proprietary)
Pneumococcal polysaccharide vaccine solution for injection 0.5ml vials | 1 vial PoM £8.32

F 758

Typhoid vaccine

● INDICATIONS AND DOSE

Immunisation against typhoid fever in children at high risk of typhoid fever

▸ BY INTRAMUSCULAR INJECTION

▸ Child 12-23 months: 0.5 mL for 1 dose, dose should be given at least 2 weeks before potential exposure to typhoid infection, response may be suboptimal

Immunisation against typhoid fever

▸ BY INTRAMUSCULAR INJECTION

▸ Child 2-17 years: 0.5 mL for 1 dose, dose should be given at least 2 weeks before potential exposure to typhoid infection

▸ BY MOUTH

▸ Child 6-17 years: 1 capsule every 2 days for 3 doses (on days 1, 3, and 5)

14

Vaccines

14

Vaccines

- **UNLICENSED USE**
  ‣ With intramuscular use Not licensed for use in children under 2 years.
- **CONTRA-INDICATIONS**
  ‣ With oral use Acute gastro-intestinal illness
- **INTERACTIONS** → Appendix 1: live vaccines
- **SIDE-EFFECTS**
  ‣ With oral use Abdominal cramps · abdominal pain · diarrhoea · nausea · vomiting
- **DIRECTIONS FOR ADMINISTRATION** Capsule should be taken one hour before a meal. Swallow as soon as possible after placing in mouth with a cold or lukewarm drink.
- **HANDLING AND STORAGE** It is important to store capsules in a refrigerator.
- **PATIENT AND CARER ADVICE** Patients or carers should be given advice on how to administer and store typhoid vaccine capsules.

▪ MEDICINAL FORMS
There can be variation in the licensing of different medicines containing the same drug.

Solution for injection
‣ Typherix (GlaxoSmithKline UK Ltd)
  Salmonella typhi Vi capsular polysaccharide 50 microgram per 1 ml Typherix 25micrograms/0.5ml vaccine solution for injection pre-filled syringes | 1 pre-filled disposable injection PoM £9.93 | 10 pre-filled disposable injection PoM £99.32
‣ Typhim Vi (sanofi pasteur MSD Ltd)
  Salmonella typhi Vi capsular polysaccharide 50 microgram per 1 ml Typhim Vi 25micrograms/0.5ml vaccine solution for injection pre-filled syringes | 1 pre-filled disposable injection PoM £9.30 | 10 pre-filled disposable injection PoM £93.00

Gastro-resistant capsule
CAUTIONARY AND ADVISORY LABELS 25
‣ Vivotif (PaxVax Ltd)
  Vivotif vaccine gastro-resistant capsules | 3 capsule PoM £14.77

Combinations available: *Hepatitis A with typhoid vaccine,* p. 765

VACCINES › VIRAL VACCINES

Hepatitis A and B vaccine

The properties listed below are those particular to the combination only. For the properties of the components please consider, hepatitis A vaccine below, hepatitis B vaccine p. 765.

- **INDICATIONS AND DOSE**

AMBIRIX®

Immunisation against hepatitis A and hepatitis B infection (primary course)
  ‣ BY INTRAMUSCULAR INJECTION
  ‣ Child 1–15 years: Initially 1 mL for 1 dose, then 1 mL after 6–12 months for 1 dose, the deltoid region is the preferred site of injection in older children; anterolateral thigh is the preferred site in infants; not to be injected into the buttock (vaccine efficacy reduced), subcutaneous route used for patients with bleeding disorders (but immune response may be reduced)

TWINRIX® ADULT

Immunisation against hepatitis A and hepatitis B infection (primary course)
  ‣ BY INTRAMUSCULAR INJECTION
  ‣ Child 16–17 years: Initially 1 mL every month for 2 doses, then 1 mL after 5 months for 1 dose, the deltoid region is the preferred site of injection; not to be injected into the buttock (vaccine efficacy reduced), subcutaneous route used for patients with bleeding disorders (but immune response may be reduced)

Immunisation against hepatitis A and hepatitis B infection—accelerated schedule for travellers departing within 1 month
  ‣ BY INTRAMUSCULAR INJECTION
  ‣ Child 16–17 years: Initially 1 mL for 1 dose, then 1 mL after 7 days for 1 dose, then 1 mL after 14 days for 1 dose, then 1 mL for 1 dose given 12 months after the first dose, the deltoid region is the preferred site of injection; not to be injected into the buttock (vaccine efficacy reduced), subcutaneous route used for patients with bleeding disorders (but immune response may be reduced)

TWINRIX® PAEDIATRIC

Immunisation against hepatitis A and hepatitis B infection (primary course)
  ‣ BY INTRAMUSCULAR INJECTION
  ‣ Child 1–15 years: Initially 0.5 mL every month for 2 doses, then 0.5 mL after 5 months for 1 dose, the deltoid region is the preferred site of injection in older children; anterolateral thigh is the preferred site in infants; not to be injected into the buttock (vaccine efficacy reduced), subcutaneous route used for patients with bleeding disorders (but immune response may be reduced)

> **IMPORTANT SAFETY INFORMATION**
> *Ambirix*® and *Twinrix*® are not recommended for post-exposure prophylaxis following percutaneous (needle-stick), ocular, or mucous membrane exposure to hepatitis B virus.

- **PRESCRIBING AND DISPENSING INFORMATION**
  TWINRIX® PAEDIATRIC Primary course should be completed with *Twinrix*® (single component vaccines given at appropriate intervals may be used for booster dose).
  AMBIRIX® Primary course should be completed with *Ambirix*® (single component vaccines given at appropriate intervals may be used for booster dose).
  TWINRIX® ADULT Primary course should be completed with *Twinrix*® (single component vaccines given at appropriate intervals may be used for booster dose).

- **MEDICINAL FORMS**
  There can be variation in the licensing of different medicines containing the same drug.

Suspension for injection
EXCIPIENTS: May contain Neomycin
  ‣ Ambirix (GlaxoSmithKline UK Ltd)
    Ambirix vaccine suspension for injection 1ml pre-filled syringes | 1 pre-filled disposable injection PoM £31.18
  ‣ Twinrix (GlaxoSmithKline UK Ltd)
    Twinrix Paediatric vaccine suspension for injection 0.5ml pre-filled syringes | 1 pre-filled disposable injection PoM £20.79
    Twinrix Adult vaccine suspension for injection 1ml pre-filled syringes | 1 pre-filled disposable injection PoM £33.31 | 10 pre-filled disposable injection PoM £333.13

⚑ 758

Hepatitis A vaccine

- **INDICATIONS AND DOSE**

AVAXIM®

Immunisation against hepatitis A infection
  ‣ BY INTRAMUSCULAR INJECTION
  ‣ Child 16–17 years: Initially 0.5 mL for 1 dose, then 0.5 mL after 6–12 months, dose given as booster; booster dose may be delayed by up to 3 years if not given after recommended interval following primary dose, the deltoid region is the preferred site of injection. The subcutaneous route may be used for patients with bleeding disorders; not to be injected into the buttock (vaccine efficacy reduced)

HAVRIX MONODOSE®

Immunisation against hepatitis A infection

▸ BY INTRAMUSCULAR INJECTION

▸ **Child 1–15 years:** Initially 0.5 mL for 1 dose, then 0.5 mL after 6–12 months, dose given as booster; booster dose may be delayed by up to 3 years if not given after recommended interval following primary dose, the deltoid region is the preferred site of injection. The subcutaneous route may be used for patients with bleeding disorders

▸ **Child 16–17 years:** Initially 1 mL for 1 dose, then 1 mL after 6–12 months, dose given as booster; booster dose may be delayed by up to 3 years if not given after recommended interval following primary dose, the deltoid region is the preferred site of injection. The subcutaneous route may be used for patients with bleeding disorders

VAQTA® PAEDIATRIC

Immunisation against hepatitis A infection

▸ BY INTRAMUSCULAR INJECTION

▸ **Child 1–17 years:** Initially 0.5 mL for 1 dose, then 0.5 mL after 6–18 months, dose given as booster, the deltoid region is the preferred site of injection. The subcutaneous route may be used for patients with bleeding disorders (but immune response may be reduced)

● MEDICINAL FORMS
There can be variation in the licensing of different medicines containing the same drug.
Suspension for injection
EXCIPIENTS: May contain Neomycin

▸ **Avaxim** (sanofi pasteur MSD Ltd)
Avaxim vaccine suspension for injection 0.5ml pre-filled syringes | 1 pre-filled disposable injection [PoM] £18.10 | 10 pre-filled disposable injection [PoM] £181.00

▸ **Havrix** (GlaxoSmithKline UK Ltd)
Havrix Monodose vaccine suspension for injection 1ml pre-filled syringes | 1 pre-filled disposable injection [PoM] £22.14 | 10 pre-filled disposable injection [PoM] £221.43
Havrix Junior Monodose vaccine suspension for injection 0.5ml pre-filled syringes | 1 pre-filled disposable injection [PoM] £16.77 | 10 pre-filled disposable injection [PoM] £167.68
Havrix Junior Monodose vaccine suspension for injection 0.5ml vials | 1 vial [PoM] £16.77
Havrix Monodose vaccine suspension for injection 1ml vials | 1 vial [PoM] £22.14

▸ **VAQTA** (Merck Sharp & Dohme Ltd)
VAQTA Paediatric vaccine suspension for injection 0.5ml pre-filled syringes | 1 pre-filled disposable injection [PoM] £14.74

Hepatitis A with typhoid vaccine

The properties listed below are those particular to the combination only. For the properties of the components please consider, hepatitis A vaccine p. 764, typhoid vaccine p. 763.

● INDICATIONS AND DOSE

HEPATYRIX®

Immunisation against hepatitis A and typhoid infection (primary course)

▸ BY INTRAMUSCULAR INJECTION

▸ **Child 15–17 years:** 1 mL for 1 dose, the deltoid region is the preferred site of injection; not to be injected into the buttock (vaccine efficacy reduced). The subcutaneous route may be used for patients with bleeding disorders, booster dose given using single component vaccines

VIATIM®

Immunisation against hepatitis A and typhoid infection (primary course)

▸ BY INTRAMUSCULAR INJECTION

▸ **Child 16–17 years:** 1 mL for 1 dose, the deltoid region is the preferred site of injection; not to be injected into the buttock (vaccine efficacy reduced). The subcutaneous route may be used for patients with bleeding disorders, booster dose given using single component vaccines

● INTERACTIONS → Appendix 1: live vaccines

● MEDICINAL FORMS
There can be variation in the licensing of different medicines containing the same drug.
Suspension for injection
EXCIPIENTS: May contain Neomycin

▸ **Hepatyrix** (GlaxoSmithKline UK Ltd)
Hepatyrix vaccine suspension for injection 1ml pre-filled syringes | 1 pre-filled disposable injection [PoM] £37.21 | 10 pre-filled disposable injection [PoM] £372.10

▸ **ViATIM** (sanofi pasteur MSD Ltd)
ViATIM vaccine suspension for injection 1ml pre-filled syringes | 1 pre-filled disposable injection [PoM] £29.80

⚑ 758

Hepatitis B vaccine

● INDICATIONS AND DOSE

ENGERIX B®

Immunisation against hepatitis B infection

▸ BY INTRAMUSCULAR INJECTION

▸ **Neonate:** 10 micrograms for 1 dose, then 10 micrograms after 1 month for 1 dose, followed by 10 micrograms after 5 months for 1 dose, anterolateral thigh is preferred site in neonates; not to be injected into the buttock (vaccine efficacy reduced), this dose should not be given to neonates born to hepatitis B surface antigen positive mother.

▸ **Child 1 month–15 years:** 10 micrograms for 1 dose, then 10 micrograms after 1 month for 1 dose, followed by 10 micrograms after 5 months for 1 dose, deltoid muscle is preferred site of injection in older children; anterolateral thigh is preferred site in infants and young children; not to be injected into the buttock (vaccine efficacy reduced)

▸ **Child 16–17 years:** 20 micrograms for 1 dose, then 20 micrograms after 1 month for 1 dose, followed by 20 micrograms after 5 months for 1 dose, deltoid muscle is preferred site of injection; not to be injected into the buttock (vaccine efficacy reduced)

Immunisation against hepatitis B infection (accelerated schedule)

▸ BY INTRAMUSCULAR INJECTION

▸ **Neonate:** 10 micrograms every month for 3 doses, followed by 10 micrograms after 10 months for 1 dose, anterolateral thigh is preferred site in neonates; not to be injected into the buttock (vaccine efficacy reduced), this dose should not be given to neonates born to hepatitis B surface antigen positive mother.

▸ **Child 1 month–15 years:** 10 micrograms every month for 3 doses, followed by 10 micrograms after 10 months for 1 dose, deltoid muscle is preferred site of injection in older children; anterolateral thigh is preferred site in infants and young children; not to be injected into the buttock (vaccine efficacy reduced)

▸ **Child 16–17 years:** 20 micrograms every month for 3 doses, followed by 20 micrograms after 10 months for 1 dose, deltoid muscle is preferred site of injection; not to be injected into the buttock (vaccine efficacy reduced)   continued →

14

Vaccines

Immunisation against hepatitis B infection, alternative accelerated schedule

▸ BY INTRAMUSCULAR INJECTION

▸ Child 11–15 years: 20 micrograms for 1 dose, followed by 20 micrograms after 6 months, this schedule is not suitable if high risk of infection between doses or if compliance with second dose uncertain, deltoid muscle is preferred site of injection; not to be injected into the buttock (vaccine efficacy reduced)

Immunisation against hepatitis B infection (for neonates born to hepatitis B surface antigen positive mother)

▸ BY INTRAMUSCULAR INJECTION

▸ Neonate: 10 micrograms once a month for 3 doses, first dose to be given at birth with hepatitis B immunoglobulin injection (separate site), followed by 10 micrograms after 10 months for 1 dose, anterolateral thigh is preferred site in neonates; not to be injected into the buttock (vaccine efficacy reduced).

Immunisation against hepatitis B infection (in renal insufficiency, including haemodialysis patients)

▸ BY INTRAMUSCULAR INJECTION

▸ Neonate: 10 micrograms every month for 2 doses, followed by 10 micrograms after 5 months for 1 dose, immunisation schedule and booster doses may need to be adjusted in those with low antibody concentration, anterolateral thigh is preferred site in neonates; not to be injected into the buttock (vaccine efficacy reduced), this dose should not be given to neonates born to hepatitis B surface antigen positive mother.

▸ Child 1 month–15 years: 10 micrograms every month for 2 doses, followed by 10 micrograms after 5 months for 1 dose, immunisation schedule and booster doses may need to be adjusted in those with low antibody concentration, deltoid muscle is preferred site of injection in older children; anterolateral thigh is preferred site in infants and young children; not to be injected into the buttock (vaccine efficacy reduced)

▸ Child 16–17 years: 40 micrograms every month for 3 doses, followed by 40 micrograms after 4 months for 1 dose, immunisation schedule and booster doses may need to be adjusted in those with low antibody concentration, deltoid muscle is preferred site of injection; not to be injected into the buttock (vaccine efficacy reduced)

Immunisation against hepatitis B infection (in renal insufficiency, including haemodialysis patients (accelerated schedule))

▸ BY INTRAMUSCULAR INJECTION

▸ Neonate: 10 micrograms every month for 3 doses, followed by 10 micrograms after 10 months for 1 dose, immunisation schedule and booster doses may need to be adjusted in those with low antibody concentration, anterolateral thigh is preferred site in neonates; not to be injected into the buttock (vaccine efficacy reduced), this dose should not be given to neonates born to hepatitis B surface antigen positive mother.

▸ Child 1 month–15 years: 10 micrograms every month for 3 doses, followed by 10 micrograms after 10 months for 1 dose, immunisation schedule and booster doses may need to be adjusted in those with low antibody concentration, deltoid muscle is preferred site of injection in older children; anterolateral thigh is preferred site in infants and young children; not to be injected into the buttock (vaccine efficacy reduced)

FENDRIX®

Immunisation against hepatitis B infection in renal insufficiency (including pre-haemodialysis and haemodialysis patients)

▸ BY INTRAMUSCULAR INJECTION

▸ Child 15–17 years: 20 micrograms every month for 3 doses, followed by 20 micrograms after 4 months for 1 dose, immunisation schedule and booster doses may need to be adjusted in those with low antibody concentration, deltoid muscle is preferred site of injection; not to be injected into the buttock (vaccine efficacy reduced)

HBVAXPRO®

Immunisation against hepatitis B infection

▸ BY INTRAMUSCULAR INJECTION

▸ Neonate: 5 micrograms for 1 dose, followed by 5 micrograms after 1 month for 1 dose, then 5 micrograms after 5 months for 1 dose, booster doses may be required in immunocompromised patients with low antibody concentration, anterolateral thigh is preferred site in neonates; not to be injected into the buttock (vaccine efficacy reduced), dose not to be used for neonate born to hepatitis B surface antigen positive mother.

▸ Child 1 month–15 years: 5 micrograms for 1 dose, followed by 5 micrograms after 1 month for 1 dose, then 5 micrograms after 5 months for 1 dose, booster doses may be required in immunocompromised patients with low antibody concentration, deltoid muscle is preferred site of injection in adults and older children; anterolateral thigh is preferred site in infants; not to be injected into the buttock (vaccine efficacy reduced)

▸ Child 16–17 years: 10 micrograms for 1 dose, followed by 10 micrograms after 1 month for 1 dose, followed by 10 micrograms after 5 months for 1 dose, booster doses may be required in immunocompromised patients with low antibody concentration, deltoid muscle is preferred site of injection in adults and older children; not to be injected into the buttock (vaccine efficacy reduced)

Immunisation against hepatitis B infection (accelerated schedule)

▸ BY INTRAMUSCULAR INJECTION

▸ Neonate: 5 micrograms every month for 3 doses, followed by 5 micrograms after 10 months for 1 dose, booster doses may be required in immunocompromised patients with low antibody concentration, anterolateral thigh is preferred site in neonates; not to be injected into the buttock (vaccine efficacy reduced), dose not to be used for neonate born to hepatitis B surface antigen positive mother.

▸ Child 1 month–15 years: 5 micrograms every month for 3 doses, followed by 5 micrograms after 10 months for 1 dose, booster doses may be required in immunocompromised patients with low antibody concentration, deltoid muscle is preferred site of injection in older children; anterolateral thigh is preferred site in infants; not to be injected into the buttock (vaccine efficacy reduced)

▸ Child 16–17 years: 10 micrograms every month for 3 doses, followed by 10 micrograms after 10 months for 1 dose, booster doses may be required in immunocompromised patients with low antibody concentration, deltoid muscle is preferred site of injection in older children; not to be injected into the buttock (vaccine efficacy reduced)

Neonate born to hepatitis B surface antigen-positive mother

▶ BY INTRAMUSCULAR INJECTION

▸ **Neonate:** 5 micrograms every month for 3 doses, first dose given at birth with hepatitis B immunoglobulin injection (separate site), followed by 5 micrograms after 10 months for 1 dose, anterolateral thigh is preferred site in neonates; not to be injected into the buttock (vaccine efficacy reduced).

Chronic haemodialysis patients

▶ BY INTRAMUSCULAR INJECTION

▸ **Child 16–17 years:** 40 micrograms every month for 2 doses, followed by 40 micrograms after 5 months for 1 dose, booster doses may be required in those with low antibody concentration, deltoid muscle is preferred site of injection in older children; not to be injected into the buttock (vaccine efficacy reduced)

● **MEDICINAL FORMS**
There can be variation in the licensing of different medicines containing the same drug.

Suspension for injection
EXCIPIENTS: May contain Thiomersal

▸ **Engerix B** (GlaxoSmithKline UK Ltd)
Hepatitis B virus surface antigen 20 microgram per 1 ml Engerix B 20micrograms/1ml vaccine suspension for injection vials | 1 vial PoM £12.34 | 10 vial PoM £123.41
Engerix B 10micrograms/0.5ml vaccine suspension for injection pre-filled syringes | 1 pre-filled disposable injection PoM £9.67
Engerix B 20micrograms/1ml vaccine suspension for injection pre-filled syringes | 1 pre-filled disposable injection PoM £12.99 | 10 pre-filled disposable injection PoM £129.92

▸ **Fendrix** (GlaxoSmithKline UK Ltd)
Hepatitis B virus surface antigen 40 microgram per 1 ml Fendrix 20micrograms/0.5ml vaccine suspension for injection pre-filled syringes | 1 pre-filled disposable injection PoM £38.10

▸ **HBVAXPRO** (Merck Sharp & Dohme Ltd)
Hepatitis B virus surface antigen 10 microgram per 1 ml HBVAXPRO 10micrograms/1ml vaccine suspension for injection pre-filled syringes | 1 pre-filled disposable injection PoM £12.20
HBVAXPRO 5micrograms/0.5ml vaccine suspension for injection pre-filled syringes | 1 pre-filled disposable injection PoM £8.95
Hepatitis B virus surface antigen 40 microgram per 1 ml HBvaxPRO 40micrograms/1ml vaccine suspension for injection vials | 1 vial PoM £27.60

F 758

Human papillomavirus vaccines

02-Mar-2017

● **INDICATIONS AND DOSE**

CERVARIX®

Prevention of premalignant genital lesions and cervical cancer

▶ BY INTRAMUSCULAR INJECTION

▸ **Child 9–14 years (female):** 0.5 mL for 1 dose, followed by 0.5 mL after 5–7 months for 1 dose, if second dose administered earlier than 5 months after the first, a third dose should be administered, dose to be administered into deltoid region, if the course is interrupted, it should be resumed (using the same vaccine) but not repeated, even if more than 24 months have elapsed since the first dose or if the girl is then aged 15 years or more.

▸ **Child 15–17 years (female):** 0.5 mL for 1 dose, followed by 0.5 mL after 1–2.5 months for 1 dose, then 0.5 mL after 5–12 months from the first dose for 1 dose, dose to be administered into deltoid region, if the course is interrupted, it should be resumed (using the same vaccine) but not repeated, allowing the appropriate interval between the remaining doses.

GARDASIL®

Prevention of premalignant genital (cervical, vulvar and vaginal) and anal lesions, cervical and anal cancers, and genital warts

▶ BY INTRAMUSCULAR INJECTION

▸ **Child 9–14 years (female):** 0.5 mL for 1 dose, followed by 0.5 mL after 6 months for 1 dose, if the second dose is administered earlier than 6 months after the first dose, a third dose should be administered, dose to be administered preferably into deltoid region or higher anterolateral thigh, if the course is interrupted, it should be resumed (using the same vaccine) but not repeated, even if more than 24 months have elapsed since the first dose or if the girl is then aged 15 years or more.

▸ **Child 15–17 years (female):** 0.5 mL for 1 dose, followed by 0.5 mL for 1 dose, second dose to be given at least 1 month after the first dose, then 0.5 mL for 1 dose, third dose to be given at least 3 months after the second dose, schedule should be completed within 12 months of the first dose, dose to be administered preferably into deltoid region or higher anterolateral thigh, if the course is interrupted, it should be resumed (using the same vaccine) but not repeated, allowing the appropriate interval between the remaining doses.

Prevention of premalignant genital (cervical, vulvar, and vaginal) and anal lesions, cervical and anal cancers, and genital warts (alternative schedule)

▶ BY INTRAMUSCULAR INJECTION

▸ **Child 9–14 years (female):** 0.5 mL for 1 dose, followed by 0.5 mL for 1 dose, second dose to be given at least 1 month after the first dose, then 0.5 mL for 1 dose, third dose to be given at least 3 months after the second dose, schedule should be completed within 12 months of the first dose, dose to be administered preferably into deltoid region or higher anterolateral thigh, if the course is interrupted, it should be resumed (using the same vaccine) but not repeated, allowing the appropriate interval between the remaining doses.

● **UNLICENSED USE**
GARDASIL® Two dose schedule not licensed for use in girls aged 14 years.

● **PREGNANCY** Not known to be harmful, but vaccination should be postponed until completion of pregnancy.

● **PRESCRIBING AND DISPENSING INFORMATION** To avoid confusion, prescribers should specify the brand to be dispensed.

● **MEDICINAL FORMS**
There can be variation in the licensing of different medicines containing the same drug.

Suspension for injection

▸ **Cervarix** (GlaxoSmithKline UK Ltd)
Cervarix vaccine suspension for injection 0.5ml pre-filled syringes | 1 pre-filled disposable injection PoM £80.50

▸ **Gardasil** (Merck Sharp & Dohme Ltd)
Gardasil vaccine suspension for injection 0.5ml pre-filled syringes | 1 pre-filled disposable injection PoM £86.50

F 758

Influenza vaccine

● **INDICATIONS AND DOSE**

Annual immunisation against seasonal influenza

▶ BY INTRAMUSCULAR INJECTION

▸ **Child 6 months–17 years:** 0.5 mL for 1 dose

▶ BY INTRANASAL ADMINISTRATION

▸ **Child 2–17 years:** 0.1 mL for 1 dose, dose to be administered into each nostril

continued →

14

Vaccines

Annual immunisation against seasonal influenza (for children who have not received seasonal influenza vaccine previously)
▶ BY INTRAMUSCULAR INJECTION
  ▸ Child 6 months–9 years: 0.5 mL for 1 dose, followed by 0.5 mL for 1 dose, after at least 4 weeks
▶ BY INTRANASAL ADMINISTRATION
  ▸ Child 2–9 years: 0.1 mL for 1 dose, followed by 0.1 mL for 1 dose, after at least 4 weeks. 0.1 mL dose to be administered to each nostril

● UNLICENSED USE Some products containing inactivated influenza vaccine (surface antigen) are not licensed for use in children under 4 years—check product literature.
  FLUVIRIN® Not licensed for use in children under 4 years.
  FLUARIX TETRA® Not licensed for use in children under 3 years of age.
  OPTAFLU® Not licensed for use in children and adolescents under 18 years.

● CONTRA-INDICATIONS Preparations marketed by Pfizer, or CSL Biotherapies in child under 5 years— increased risk of febrile convulsions
  FLUENZ TETRA® Active wheezing · concomitant use with antiviral therapy for influenza · concomitant use with salicylates · severe asthma
  CONTRA-INDICATIONS, FURTHER INFORMATION
  ▸ Concomitant use with antivirals Avoid antivirals for at least 2 weeks after immunisation; avoid immunisation for at least 48 hours after stopping the antiviral.
  ENZIRA® Child under 5 years—increased risk of febrile convulsions

● CAUTIONS Increased risk of fever in child 5–9 years with preparations marketed by Pfizer or CSL Biotherapies—use alternative influenza vaccine if available
  ENZIRA® Child 5–9 years (increased risk of fever)—use alternative influenza vaccine if available

● INTERACTIONS → Appendix 1: live vaccines

● SIDE-EFFECTS
  GENERAL SIDE-EFFECTS
  ▸ Uncommon Epistaxis
  ▸ Frequency not known Febrile convulsions · transient thrombocytopenia
  SPECIFIC SIDE-EFFECTS
  ▸ With intranasal use Rhinorrhoea

● ALLERGY AND CROSS-SENSITIVITY Individuals with a history of egg allergy can be immunised with either an egg free influenza vaccine, if available, or an influenza vaccine with an ovalbumin content less than 120 nanograms/mL (facilities should be available to treat anaphylaxis). Vaccines with an ovalbumin content more than 120 nanograms/mL or where content is not stated should not be used in individuals with egg allergy. If an influenza vaccine containing ovalbumin is being considered in those with a history of anaphylaxis to egg or egg allergy with uncontrolled asthma, these individuals should be referred to a specialist in hospital.

● PREGNANCY Inactivated vaccines not known to be harmful.
  FLUENZ TETRA® Avoid in pregnancy.

● BREAST FEEDING Inactivated vaccines not known to be harmful.
  FLUENZ TETRA® Avoid in breast-feeding.

● PRESCRIBING AND DISPENSING INFORMATION
  FLUARIX TETRA® Ovalbumin content less than 100 nanograms/mL.

● PATIENT AND CARER ADVICE
  FLUENZ TETRA® Avoid close contact with severely immunocompromised patients for 1–2 weeks after vaccination.

● MEDICINAL FORMS
There can be variation in the licensing of different medicines containing the same drug.
Spray
EXCIPIENTS: May contain Gelatin, gentamicin
▸ FluMist Quadrivalent (AstraZeneca UK Ltd)
  FluMist Quadrivalent vaccine nasal suspension 0.2ml unit dose | 10 unit dose PoM £180.00
▸ Fluenz Tetra (AstraZeneca UK Ltd) ▼
  Fluenz Tetra vaccine nasal suspension 0.2ml unit dose | 10 unit dose PoM £180.00

Suspension for injection
EXCIPIENTS: May contain Gentamicin, kanamycin, neomycin penicillins, polymyxin b, thiomersal
▸ Influenza vaccine (Non-proprietary)
  Influenza vaccine (split virion, inactivated) suspension for injection 0.5ml pre-filled syringes | 1 pre-filled disposable injection PoM £5.00–£6.59 | 10 pre-filled disposable injection PoM £65.90
▸ Agrippal (Seqirus Ltd)
  Agrippal vaccine suspension for injection 0.5ml pre-filled syringes | 10 pre-filled disposable injection PoM £58.50
▸ Enzira (Pfizer Ltd)
  Enzira vaccine suspension for injection 0.5ml pre-filled syringes | 1 pre-filled disposable injection PoM £5.25 | 10 pre-filled disposable injection PoM £52.50
▸ Fluarix Tetra (GlaxoSmithKline UK Ltd) ▼
  Fluarix Tetra vaccine suspension for injection 0.5ml pre-filled syringes | 1 pre-filled disposable injection PoM £9.94 | 10 pre-filled disposable injection PoM £99.40
▸ Imuvac (BGP Products Ltd)
  Imuvac vaccine suspension for injection 0.5ml pre-filled syringes | 1 pre-filled disposable injection PoM £6.59 | 10 pre-filled disposable injection PoM £65.90
▸ Influvac Sub-unit (BGP Products Ltd)
  Influvac Sub-unit vaccine suspension for injection 0.5ml pre-filled syringes | 1 pre-filled disposable injection PoM £5.22 | 10 pre-filled disposable injection PoM £52.20
▸ Intanza (sanofi pasteur MSD Ltd)
  Intanza 15microgram strain vaccine suspension for injection 0.1ml pre-filled syringes | 1 pre-filled disposable injection PoM £9.05 | 10 pre-filled disposable injection PoM £90.50

F 758

Japanese encephalitis vaccine

● INDICATIONS AND DOSE
Immunisation against Japanese encephalitis
▶ BY INTRAMUSCULAR INJECTION
  ▸ Child 2 months–2 years: 0.25 mL every 28 days for 2 doses, anterolateral thigh is preferred site of injection in infants, the subcutaneous route may be used for patients with bleeding disorders
  ▸ Child 3–17 years: 0.5 mL every 28 days for 2 doses, deltoid muscle is preferred site in older children; anterolateral thigh is preferred in infants, the subcutaneous route may be used for patients with bleeding disorders

● SIDE-EFFECTS
▸ Uncommon Cough

● PREGNANCY Although manufacturer advises avoid because of limited information, miscarriage has been associated with Japanese encephalitis virus infection acquired during the first 2 trimesters of pregnancy.

● MEDICINAL FORMS
There can be variation in the licensing of different medicines containing the same drug.
Solution for injection
▸ Japanese encephalitis vaccine (Non-proprietary)
  Japanese encephalitis GCVC vaccine solution for injection 1ml vials | 1 vial no price available

Japanese encephalitis GCVC vaccine solution for injection 20ml vials |
1 vial no price available
Japanese encephalitis GCVC vaccine solution for injection 10ml vials |
1 vial no price available

Suspension for injection
▸ Ixiaro (Valneva UK Ltd)
Ixiaro vaccine suspension for injection 0.5ml pre-filled syringes |
1 pre-filled disposable injection PoM £59.50

⌖ 758

Measles, mumps and rubella vaccine, live

● **INDICATIONS AND DOSE**
Primary immunisation against measles, mumps, and rubella (first dose)
▸ BY INTRAMUSCULAR INJECTION, OR BY DEEP SUBCUTANEOUS INJECTION
▸ Child 12-13 months: 0.5 mL for 1 dose
Primary immunisation against measles, mumps, and rubella (second dose)
▸ BY INTRAMUSCULAR INJECTION, OR BY DEEP SUBCUTANEOUS INJECTION
▸ Child 40 months-5 years: 0.5 mL for 1 dose
Rubella immunisation (in seronegative women, susceptible to rubella and in unimmunised, seronegative women, post-partum)
▸ BY INTRAMUSCULAR INJECTION, OR BY DEEP SUBCUTANEOUS INJECTION
▸ Females of childbearing potential: (consult product literature or local protocols)
Children presenting for pre-school booster, who have not received the primary immunisation (first dose) | Immunisation for patients at school-leaving age or at entry into further education, who have not completed the primary immunisation course | Control of measles outbreak | Immunisation for patients travelling to areas where measles is endemic or epidemic, who have not completed the primary immunisation
▸ BY INTRAMUSCULAR INJECTION, OR BY DEEP SUBCUTANEOUS INJECTION
▸ Child 6 months-17 years: (consult product literature or local protocols)

● **UNLICENSED USE** Not licensed for use in children under 9 months.

IMPORTANT SAFETY INFORMATION
MMR VACCINATION AND BOWEL DISEASE OR AUTISM
Reviews undertaken on behalf of the CSM, the Medical Research Council, and the Cochrane Collaboration, have not found any evidence of a link between MMR vaccination and bowel disease or autism. The Chief Medical Officers have advised that the MMR vaccine is the safest and best way to protect children against measles, mumps, and rubella. Information (including fact sheets and a list of references) may be obtained from www.dh.gov.uk/immunisation.

● **CAUTIONS** Antibody response to measles component may be reduced after immunoglobulin administration or blood transfusion—leave an interval of at least 3 months before MMR immunisation
CAUTIONS, FURTHER INFORMATION
▸ Administration with other vaccines MMR vaccine should not be administered on the same day as yellow fever vaccine; there should be a 4-week minimum interval between the vaccines. When protection is rapidly required, the vaccines can be given at any interval and an additional dose of MMR may be considered.
MMR and varicella-zoster vaccine can be given on the same day or separated by a 4-week minimum interval.

When protection is rapidly required, the vaccines can be given at any interval and an additional dose of the vaccine given second may be considered.
● **INTERACTIONS** → Appendix 1: live vaccines
● **SIDE-EFFECTS**
▸ **Uncommon** Parotid swelling (usually in the third week) · sleep disturbances · unusual crying in infants
▸ **Rare** Arthropathy (2 to 3 weeks after immunisation) · idiopathic thrombocytopenic purpura
▸ **Frequency not known** Optic neuritis · peripheral neuritis
SIDE-EFFECTS, FURTHER INFORMATION
Malaise, fever, or a rash can occur after the first dose of MMR vaccine—most commonly about a week after vaccination and lasting about 2 to 3 days. Leaflets are available for parents on advice for reducing fever (including the use of paracetamol).
▸ Febrile seizures—occur rarely 6 to 11 days after MMR vaccination (the incidence is lower than that following measles infection)
▸ Idiopathic thrombocytopenic purpura Idiopathic thrombocytopenic purpura has occurred rarely following MMR vaccination, usually within 6 weeks of the first dose. The risk of idiopathic thrombocytopenic purpura after MMR vaccine is much less than the risk after infection with wild measles or rubella virus. Children who develop idiopathic thrombocytopenic purpura within 6 weeks of the first dose of MMR should undergo serological testing before the second dose is due; if the results suggest incomplete immunity against measles, mumps or rubella then a second dose of MMR is recommended. The Specialist and Reference Microbiology Division, Health Protection Agency offers free serological testing for children who develop idiopathic thrombocytopenic purpura *within 6 weeks* of the first dose of MMR.
▸ Aseptic meningitis Post-vaccination aseptic meningitis was reported (rarely and with complete recovery) following vaccination with MMR vaccine containing Urabe mumps vaccine, which has now been discontinued; no cases have been confirmed in association with the currently used Jeryl Lynn mumps vaccine. Children with post-vaccination symptoms are not infectious.
▸ Frequency of side effects Adverse reactions are considerably less frequent after the second dose of MMR vaccine than after the first.
● **ALLERGY AND CROSS-SENSITIVITY** MMR vaccine can be given safely even when the child has had an anaphylactic reaction to food containing egg. Dislike of eggs, refusal to eat egg, or confirmed anaphylactic reactions to egg-containing food is not a contra-indication to MMR vaccination. Children with a confirmed anaphylactic reaction to the MMR vaccine should be assessed by a specialist.
● **CONCEPTION AND CONTRACEPTION** Exclude pregnancy before immunisation. Avoid pregnancy for at least 1 month after vaccination.
● **PRESCRIBING AND DISPENSING INFORMATION** Available as part of childhood immunisation schedule from health organisations or ImmForm www.immform.dh.gov.uk.

● **MEDICINAL FORMS**
There can be variation in the licensing of different medicines containing the same drug.
Powder and solvent for suspension for injection
EXCIPIENTS: May contain Gelatin, neomycin
▸ M-M-RVAXPRO (Merck Sharp & Dohme Ltd)
M-M-RVAXPRO vaccine powder and solvent for suspension for injection 0.5ml pre-filled syringes | 1 pre-filled disposable injection PoM £11.00
Powder and solvent for solution for injection
EXCIPIENTS: May contain Neomycin
▸ Priorix (GlaxoSmithKline UK Ltd)
Priorix vaccine powder and solvent for solution for injection 0.5ml vials | 1 vial PoM £7.64

14

Vaccines

Rabies vaccine

☞ 758

- **INDICATIONS AND DOSE**

Pre-exposure prophylaxis
- ▸ BY INTRAMUSCULAR INJECTION
  - ▸ **Child:** 1 mL for 2 doses (on days 0 and 7), followed by 1 mL for 1 dose (on day 28), to be administered in deltoid region or anterolateral thigh in infants, for those at continuous risk, measure plasma-concentration of antirabies antibodies every 6 months and give a booster dose if the titre is less than 0.5 units/mL, final dose may be given from day 21, if insufficient time before travel

Pre-exposure prophylaxis booster dose (for patients at frequent risk of exposure)
- ▸ BY INTRAMUSCULAR INJECTION
  - ▸ **Child:** 1 mL after 1 year for 1 dose, to be given 1 year after primary course is completed, then 1 mL every 3–5 years, to be administered in deltoid region or anterolateral thigh in infants, the frequency of booster doses may alternatively be determined according to plasma-concentration of antirabies antibodies

Pre-exposure prophylaxis booster dose (for patients at infrequent risk of exposure)
- ▸ BY INTRAMUSCULAR INJECTION
  - ▸ **Child:** 1 mL for 1 dose, to be given 10 years after primary course is completed, administered in deltoid region or anterolateral thigh in infants

Post-exposure prophylaxis of fully immunised individuals (who have previously received pre-exposure or post-exposure prophylaxis with cell-derived rabies vaccine)
- ▸ BY INTRAMUSCULAR INJECTION
  - ▸ **Child** (administered on expert advice): 1 mL for 1 dose, followed by 1 mL after 3–7 days for 1 dose, to be administered in deltoid region or anterolateral thigh in infants, rabies immunoglobulin is not necessary

Post-exposure treatment for unimmunised individuals (or those whose prophylaxis is possibly incomplete)
- ▸ BY INTRAMUSCULAR INJECTION
  - ▸ **Child** (administered on expert advice): 1 mL 5 times a month for 1 month, doses should be given on days 0, 3, 7, 14, and the fifth dose is given between day 28–30, to be administered in deltoid region or anterolateral thigh in infants, depending on the level of risk (determined by factors such as the nature of the bite and the country where it was sustained), rabies immunoglobulin is given to unimmunised individuals on day 0 or within 7 days of starting the course of rabies vaccine, the immunisation course can be discontinued if it is proved that the individual was not at risk

- **INTERACTIONS** → Appendix 1: rabies vaccine
- **SIDE-EFFECTS** Paresis
- **PREGNANCY** Because of the potential consequences of untreated rabies exposure and because rabies vaccination has not been associated with fetal abnormalities, pregnancy is not considered a contra-indication to post-exposure prophylaxis. Immunisation against rabies is indicated during pregnancy if there is substantial risk of exposure to rabies and rapid access to post-exposure prophylaxis is likely to be limited.

- **MEDICINAL FORMS**
There can be variation in the licensing of different medicines containing the same drug.

Powder and solvent for suspension for injection
EXCIPIENTS: May contain Neomycin
- ▸ **Rabies vaccine (Non-proprietary)**
  Verorab powder and solvent for suspension for injection 0.5ml vials | 1 vial PoM no price available

Rabies vaccine powder and solvent for suspension for injection 1ml vials | 1 vial PoM £40.84

Powder and solvent for solution for injection
EXCIPIENTS: May contain Neomycin
- ▸ **Rabipur** (GlaxoSmithKline UK Ltd)
  Rabipur vaccine powder and solvent for solution for injection 1ml vials | 1 vial PoM £34.56
  Rabipur vaccine powder and solvent for solution for injection 1ml pre-filled syringes | 1 pre-filled disposable injection PoM £34.56

Rotavirus vaccine

☞ 758

- **DRUG ACTION** Rotavirus vaccine is a live, oral vaccine that protects young children against gastro-enteritis caused by rotavirus infection.

- **INDICATIONS AND DOSE**

Immunisation against gastro-enteritis caused by rotavirus
- ▸ BY MOUTH
  - ▸ **Child 6-23 weeks:** 1.5 mL for 2 doses separated by an interval of at least 4 weeks, first dose must be given between 6–14 weeks of age; course should be completed before 24 weeks of age (preferably before 16 weeks)

- **CONTRA-INDICATIONS** History of intussusception · predisposition to intussusception · severe combined immunosuppression

  CONTRA-INDICATIONS, FURTHER INFORMATION
- ▸ Immunosuppresion With the exception of severe combined immunodeficiency, rotavirus vaccine is not contra-indicated in immunosuppressed patients—benefit from vaccination is likely to outweigh the risk, if there is any doubt, seek specialist advice.

- **CAUTIONS** Diarrhoea (postpone vaccination) · immunosuppressed close contacts · vomiting (postpone vaccination)

  CAUTIONS, FURTHER INFORMATION
  The rotavirus vaccine virus is excreted in the stool and may be transmitted to close contacts; however, vaccination of those with immunosuppressed close contacts may protect the contacts from wild-type rotavirus disease and outweigh any risk from transmission of vaccine virus.

- **INTERACTIONS** → Appendix 1: live vaccines
- **SIDE-EFFECTS** Abdominal cramps · abdominal pain · diarrhoea · nausea · vomiting
- **PATIENT AND CARER ADVICE** The rotavirus vaccine virus is excreted in the stool and may be transmitted to close contacts; carers of a recently vaccinated baby should be advised of the need to wash their hands after changing the baby's nappies.

- **MEDICINAL FORMS**
There can be variation in the licensing of different medicines containing the same drug.

Oral suspension
- ▸ **Rotarix** (GlaxoSmithKline UK Ltd)
  Rotarix vaccine live oral suspension 1.5ml pre-filled syringes | 1 unit dose PoM £34.76

Tick-borne encephalitis vaccine, inactivated

☞ 758

- **INDICATIONS AND DOSE**

Initial immunisation against tick-borne encephalitis
- ▸ BY INTRAMUSCULAR INJECTION
  - ▸ **Child 1-15 years:** 0.25 mL for 1 dose, followed by 0.25 mL after 1–3 months for 1 dose, then 0.25 mL after further 5–12 months for 1 dose, to achieve more rapid

protection, second dose may be given 14 days after first dose, dose to be administered in deltoid region or anterolateral thigh in infants, in immunocompromised patients (including those receiving immunosuppressants), antibody concentration may be measured 4 weeks after second dose and dose repeated if protective levels not achieved

▸ Child 16-17 years: 0.5 mL for 1 dose, followed by 0.5 mL after 1-3 months for 1 dose, then 0.5 mL after further 5-12 months for 1 dose, to achieve more rapid protection, second dose may be given 14 days after first dose, dose to be administered in deltoid region, in immunocompromised patients (including those receiving immunosuppressants), antibody concentration may be measured 4 weeks after second dose and dose repeated if protective levels not achieved

Immunisation against tick-borne encephalitis, booster doses

▸ BY INTRAMUSCULAR INJECTION

▸ Child 1-17 years: First dose to be given within 3 years after initial course completed and then every 3-5 years, dose to be administered in deltoid region or anterolateral thigh in infants (consult product literature)

● **ALLERGY AND CROSS-SENSITIVITY** Individuals with evidence of previous anaphylactic reaction to egg should not be given tick-borne encephalitis vaccine.

● **MEDICINAL FORMS**
There can be variation in the licensing of different medicines containing the same drug.
Suspension for injection
EXCIPIENTS: May contain Gentamicin, neomycin

▸ TicoVac (Masta Ltd)
TicoVac Junior vaccine suspension for injection 0.25ml pre-filled syringes | 1 pre-filled disposable injection PoM £28.00
TicoVac vaccine suspension for injection 0.5ml pre-filled syringes | 1 pre-filled disposable injection PoM £32.00

F 758

Varicella-zoster vaccine

● **INDICATIONS AND DOSE**

VARILRIX®

Prevention of varicella infection (chickenpox)

▸ BY SUBCUTANEOUS INJECTION

▸ Child 1-17 years: 0.5 mL every 4-6 weeks for 2 doses, to be administered into the deltoid region or anterolateral thigh

VARIVAX®

Prevention of varicella infection (chickenpox)

▸ BY SUBCUTANEOUS INJECTION, OR BY INTRAMUSCULAR INJECTION

▸ Child 1-12 years: 0.5 mL for 2 doses, interval of at least 4 weeks between each dose, to be administered into the deltoid region (or higher anterolateral thigh in young children)

▸ Child 13-17 years: 0.5 mL every 4-8 weeks for 2 doses, to be administered preferably into the deltoid region

Prevention of varicella infection (chickenpox) in children with asymptomatic HIV infection

▸ BY SUBCUTANEOUS INJECTION, OR BY INTRAMUSCULAR INJECTION

▸ Child 1-12 years: 0.5 mL every 12 weeks for 2 doses, to be administered into the deltoid region (or higher anterolateral thigh in young children)

● **CAUTIONS** Post-vaccination close contact with susceptible individuals

● CAUTIONS, FURTHER INFORMATION
Rarely, the varicella-zoster vaccine virus has been transmitted from the vaccinated individual to close contacts. Therefore, contact with the following should be avoided if a vaccine-related cutaneous rash develops within 4-6 weeks of the first or second dose:
● varicella-susceptible pregnant women;
● individuals at high risk of severe varicella, including those with immunodeficiency or those receiving immunosuppressive therapy.
Healthcare workers who develop a generalised papular or vesicular rash on vaccination should avoid contact with patients until the lesions have crusted. Those who develop a localised rash after vaccination should cover the lesions and be allowed to continue working unless in contact with patients at high risk of severe varicella.

▸ Administration with MMR vaccine Varicella-zoster and MMR vaccines can be given on the same day or separated by a 4-week minimum interval. When protection is rapidly required, the vaccines can be given at any interval and an additional dose of the vaccine given second may be considered.

● **INTERACTIONS** → Appendix 1: live vaccines

● **SIDE-EFFECTS**

▸ **Rare** Thrombocytopenia

▸ **Frequency not known** Conjunctivitis · varicella-like rash

● **CONCEPTION AND CONTRACEPTION** Avoid pregnancy for 3 months after vaccination.

● **PRESCRIBING AND DISPENSING INFORMATION**
ZOSTAVAX® Advice in BNF Publications may differ from that in product literature.

● **MEDICINAL FORMS**
There can be variation in the licensing of different medicines containing the same drug.
Powder and solvent for suspension for injection
EXCIPIENTS: May contain Gelatin, neomycin

▸ Varivax (Merck Sharp & Dohme Ltd)
Varivax vaccine powder and solvent for suspension for injection 0.5ml vials | 1 vial PoM £30.28

Powder and solvent for solution for injection
EXCIPIENTS: May contain Neomycin

▸ Varilrix (GlaxoSmithKline UK Ltd)
Varilrix vaccine powder and solvent for solution for injection 0.5ml vials | 1 vial PoM £27.31

F 758

Yellow fever vaccine, live

● **INDICATIONS AND DOSE**

Immunisation against yellow fever

▸ BY DEEP SUBCUTANEOUS INJECTION

▸ Child 6-8 months (administered on expert advice): Infants under 9 months should be vaccinated only if the risk of yellow fever is high and unavoidable (consult product literature or local protocols)

▸ Child 9 months-17 years: 0.5 mL for 1 dose

● **CONTRA-INDICATIONS** Children under 6 months · history of thymus dysfunction

● **CAUTIONS**

CAUTIONS, FURTHER INFORMATION

▸ Administration with MMR vaccine Yellow fever and MMR vaccines should not be administered on the same day; there should be a 4-week minimum interval between the vaccines. When protection is rapidly required, the vaccines can be given at any interval and an additional dose of MMR may be considered.

● **INTERACTIONS** → Appendix 1: live vaccines

● **SIDE-EFFECTS** Neurotropic disease · viscerotropic disease

14

Vaccines

SIDE-EFFECTS, FURTHER INFORMATION

▸ Vaccine-associated adverse effects *Very rare* adverse effects, such as viscerotropic disease (yellow-fever vaccine-associated viscerotropic disease, YEL-AVD), a syndrome which may include metabolic acidosis, muscle and liver cirrhosis, and multi-organ failure. Neurological disorders (yellow fever vaccine-associated neurotropic disease, YEL-AND) such as encephalitis have also been reported. These *very rare* adverse effects usually occur after the first dose of yellow fever vaccine in those with no previous immunity.

● **ALLERGY AND CROSS-SENSITIVITY** Yellow fever vaccine should only be considered under the guidance of a specialist in individuals with evidence of previous anaphylactic reaction to egg.

● **PREGNANCY** Live yellow fever vaccine should not be given during pregnancy because there is a theoretical risk of fetal infection. Pregnant women should be advised not to travel to areas at high risk of yellow fever. If exposure cannot be avoided during pregnancy, then the vaccine should be given if the risk from disease in the mother outweighs the risk to the fetus from vaccination.

● **BREAST FEEDING** Avoid; seek specialist advice if exposure to virus cannot be avoided.

● **MEDICINAL FORMS**
There can be variation in the licensing of different medicines containing the same drug.

Powder and solvent for suspension for injection
▸ **Stamaril** (sanofi pasteur MSD Ltd)
Stamaril vaccine powder and solvent for suspension for injection 0.5ml vials | 1 vial [PoM] £33.10

Chapter 15
Anaesthesia

CONTENTS

General anaesthesia

General anaesthesia

Overview

Several different types of drug are given together during general anaesthesia. Anaesthesia is induced with either a volatile drug given by inhalation or with an intravenously administered drug; anaesthesia is maintained with an intravenous or inhalational anaesthetic. Analgesics, usually short-acting opioids, are also used. The use of neuromuscular blocking drugs necessitates intermittent positive-pressure ventilation. Following surgery, anticholinesterases can be given to reverse the effects of neuromuscular blocking drugs; specific antagonists can be used to reverse central and respiratory depression caused by some drugs used in surgery. A local topical anaesthetic can be used to reduce pain at the injection site.

Individual requirements vary considerably and the recommended doses are only a guide. Smaller doses are indicated in ill, shocked, or debilitated children and in significant hepatic impairment, while robust individuals may require larger doses. The required dose of induction agent may be less if the patient has been premedicated with a sedative agent or if an opioid analgesic has been used.

Intravenous anaesthetics

Intravenous anaesthetics may be used either to induce anaesthesia or for maintenance of anaesthesia throughout surgery. Intravenous anaesthetics nearly all produce their effect in one arm-brain circulation time. Extreme care is required in surgery of the mouth, pharynx, or larynx where the airway may be difficult to maintain (e.g. in the presence of a tumour in the pharynx or larynx).

To facilitate tracheal intubation, induction is usually followed by a neuromuscular blocking drug or a short-acting opioid.

The doses of all intravenous anaesthetic drugs should be titrated to effect (except when using 'rapid sequence induction').

Total intravenous anaesthesia

This is a technique in which major surgery is carried out with all drugs given intravenously. Respiration can be spontaneous, or controlled with oxygen-enriched air. Neuromuscular blocking drugs can be used to provide relaxation and prevent reflex muscle movements. The main problem to be overcome is the assessment of depth of anaesthesia. Target Controlled Infusion (TCI) systems can be used to titrate intravenous anaesthetic infusions to predicted plasma-drug concentrations; specific models with paediatric pharmacokinetic data should be used for children.

Drugs used for intravenous anaesthesia

Propofol p. 775, the most widely used intravenous anaesthetic, can be used for induction or maintenance of anaesthesia in children, but it is not commonly used in neonates. Propofol is associated with rapid recovery and less hangover effect than other intravenous anaesthetics. Propofol can also be used for sedation during diagnostic procedures.

Thiopental sodium p. 214 is a barbiturate that is used for induction of anaesthesia, but has no analgesic properties. Induction is generally smooth and rapid, but dose-related cardiovascular and respiratory depression can occur. Awakening from a moderate dose of thiopental sodium is rapid because the drug redistributes into other tissues, particularly fat. However, metabolism is slow and sedative effects can persist for 24 hours. Repeated doses have a cumulative effect particularly in neonates and recovery is much slower.

Etomidate p. 774 is an intravenous agent associated with rapid recovery without a hangover effect. Etomidate causes less hypotension than thiopental sodium and propofol during induction. It produces a high incidence of extraneous muscle movements, which can be minimised by an opioid analgesic or a short-acting benzodiazepine given just before induction.

Ketamine p. 790 causes less hypotension than thiopental sodium and propofol during induction. It is sometimes used in children requiring repeat anaesthesia (such as for serial burns dressings), however recovery is relatively slow and there is a high incidence of extraneous muscle movements. Ketamine can cause hallucinations, nightmares, and other transient psychotic effects; these can be reduced by a benzodiazepine such as diazepam p. 212 or midazolam p. 215.

Inhalational anaesthetics

Inhalational anaesthetics include gases and volatile liquids. *Gaseous anaesthetics* require suitable equipment for storage and administration. *Volatile liquid anaesthetics* are administered using calibrated vaporisers, using air, oxygen, or nitrous oxide-oxygen mixtures as the carrier gas. To prevent hypoxia, the inspired gas mixture should contain a minimum of 25% oxygen at all times. Higher concentrations of oxygen (greater than 30%) are usually required during inhalational anaesthesia when nitrous oxide p. 777 is being administered.

Volatile liquid anaesthetics

Volatile liquid anaesthetics can be used for induction and maintenance of anaesthesia, and following induction with an intravenous anaesthetic.

Isoflurane p. 777 is a volatile liquid anaesthetic. Heart rhythm is generally stable during isoflurane anaesthesia, but heart-rate can rise. Systemic arterial pressure and cardiac

15

Anaesthesia

output can fall, owing to a decrease in systemic vascular resistance. Muscle relaxation occurs and the effects of muscle relaxant drugs are potentiated. Isoflurane is not recommended for induction of anaesthesia in infants and children of all ages because of the occurrence of cough, breath-holding, desaturation, increased secretions, and laryngospasm. Isoflurane is the preferred inhalational anaesthetic for use in obstetrics.

Desflurane p. 777 is a rapid acting volatile liquid anaesthetic; it is reported to have about one-fifth the potency of isoflurane. Emergence and recovery from anaesthesia are particularly rapid because of its low solubility. Desflurane is not recommended for induction of anaesthesia as it is irritant to the upper respiratory tract.

Sevoflurane p. 778 is a rapid acting volatile liquid anaesthetic and is more potent than desflurane. Emergence and recovery are particularly rapid, but slower than desflurane. Sevoflurane is non-irritant and is therefore often used for inhalational induction of anaesthesia.

Nitrous oxide

Nitrous oxide is used for maintenance of anaesthesia and, in sub-anaesthetic concentrations, for analgesia. For *anaesthesia*, it is commonly used in a concentration of 50 to 66% in oxygen as part of a balanced technique in association with other inhalational or intravenous agents. Nitrous oxide is unsatisfactory as a sole anaesthetic owing to lack of potency, but is useful as part of a combination of drugs since it allows a significant reduction in dosage.

For analgesia (without loss of consciousness), a mixture of nitrous oxide and oxygen containing 50% of each gas (Entonox®, Equanox®) is used. Self-administration using a demand valve may be used in children who are able to self-regulate their intake (usually over 5 years of age) for painful dressing changes, as an aid to postoperative physiotherapy, for wound debridement and in emergency ambulances.

Nitrous oxide may have a deleterious effect if used in children with an air-containing closed space since nitrous oxide diffuses into such a space with a resulting increase in pressure. This effect may be dangerous in conditions such as pneumothorax, which may enlarge to compromise respiration, or in the presence of intracranial air after head injury, entrapped air following recent underwater dive, or recent intra-ocular gas injection.

Malignant hyperthermia

Malignant hyperthermia is a rare but potentially lethal complication of anaesthesia. It is characterised by a rapid rise in temperature, increased muscle rigidity, tachycardia, and acidosis. The most common triggers of malignant hyperthermia are the volatile anaesthetics. Suxamethonium chloride p. 782 has also been implicated, but malignant hyperthermia is more likely if it is given following a volatile anaesthetic. Volatile anaesthetics and suxamethonium chloride should be avoided during anaesthesia in children at high risk of malignant hyperthermia.

Dantrolene sodium p. 791 is used in the treatment of malignant hyperthermia.

Sedation, anaesthesia, and resuscitation in dental practice

Overview

Sedation for dental procedures should be limited to conscious sedation whenever possible. Nitrous oxide p. 777 alone and midazolam p. 215 are effective for many children.

For details of anaesthesia, sedation, and resuscitation in dental practice see *A Conscious Decision: A review of the use of general anaesthesia and conscious sedation in primary dental care*; report by a group chaired by the Chief Medical Officer and Chief Dental Officer, July 2000 and associated

documents. Further details can also be found in *Standards for Conscious Sedation in the Provision of Dental Care*; report of an Intercollegiate Advisory Committee for Sedation in Dentistry, 2015 www.rcseng.ac.uk/-/media/files/rcs/library-and-publications/non-journal-publications/dental-sedation-report.pdf.

Surgery and long-term medication

Overview

The risk of losing disease control on stopping long-term medication before surgery is often greater than the risk posed by continuing it during surgery. It is vital that the anaesthetist knows about **all** drugs that a patient is (or has been) taking.

Patients with adrenal atrophy resulting from long-term corticosteroid use may suffer a precipitous fall in blood pressure unless corticosteroid cover is provided during anaesthesia and in the immediate postoperative period. Anaesthetists must therefore know whether **a patient is**, or has been, receiving corticosteroids (including high-dose inhaled corticosteroids).

Other drugs that should normally not be stopped before surgery include drugs for epilepsy, asthma, immunosuppression, and metabolic, endocrine and cardiovascular disorders (but see potassium sparing diuretics). Expert advice is required for children receiving antivirals for HIV infection. See general advice on surgery in children with diabetes in Diabetes, surgery and medical illness p. 429.

Children taking antiplatelet medication or an oral anticoagulant present an increased risk for surgery. In these circumstances, the anaesthetist and surgeon should assess the relative risks and decide jointly whether the antiplatelet or the anticoagulant drug should be stopped or replaced with heparin (unfractionated) p. 92 or low molecular weight heparin therapy.

Drugs that should be stopped before surgery include combined oral contraceptives, see Contraceptives, hormonal p. 472. If antidepressants need to be stopped, they should be withdrawn gradually to avoid withdrawal symptoms. Tricyclic antidepressants need not be stopped, but there may be an increased risk of arrhythmias and hypotension (and dangerous interactions with vasopressor drugs); therefore, the anaesthetist should be informed if they are not stopped. Lithium should be stopped 24 hours before major surgery but the normal dose can be continued for minor surgery (with careful monitoring of fluids and electrolytes). Potassium-sparing diuretics may need to be withheld on the morning of surgery because hyperkalaemia may develop if renal perfusion is impaired or if there is tissue damage. Herbal medicines may be associated with adverse effects when given with anaesthetic drugs and consideration should be given to stopping them before surgery.

ANAESTHETICS, GENERAL › INTRAVENOUS ANAESTHETICS

| Etomidate

- **INDICATIONS AND DOSE**
  Induction of anaesthesia
  ▶ BY SLOW INTRAVENOUS INJECTION
  ▶ Child 1 month–14 years: 150–300 micrograms/kg (max. per dose 60 mg), to be administered over 30-60 seconds (60 seconds for children in whom hypotension might be hazardous), increased if necessary to 400 micrograms/kg
  ▶ Child 15–17 years: 150–300 micrograms/kg (max. per dose 60 mg), to be administered over 30–60 seconds (60 seconds for children in whom hypotension might be hazardous)

- **UNLICENSED USE** *Hypnomidate* ® licensed for use in children (age range not specified by manufacturer). *Etomidate-Lipuro* ® not licensed for children under 6 months except for imperative indications during inpatient treatment. Doses in *BNF for Children* may differ from those in the product literature.

IMPORTANT SAFETY INFORMATION

Etomidate should only be administered by, or under the direct supervision of, personnel experienced in its use, with adequate training in anaesthesia and airway management, and when resuscitation equipment is available.

- **CAUTIONS** Acute circulatory failure (shock) · acute porphyrias p. 577 (avoid) · adrenal insufficiency · cardiovascular disease · fixed cardiac output · hypovolaemia

  CAUTIONS, FURTHER INFORMATION
  ‣ Adrenal insufficiency Etomidate suppresses adrenocortical function, particularly during continuous administration, and it should not be used for maintenance of anaesthesia. It should be used with caution in patients with underlying adrenal insufficiency, for example, those with sepsis.

- **INTERACTIONS** → Appendix 1: etomidate

- **SIDE-EFFECTS**
  ‣ **Common or very common** Apnoea · hyperventilation · hypotension · nausea · rash · stridor · vomiting
  ‣ **Uncommon** Arrhythmias · bradycardia · cough · hiccups · hypersalivation · hypertension · phlebitis
  ‣ **Frequency not known** AV block · cardiac arrest · extraneous muscle movement (high incidence) · pain on injection · respiratory depression · seizures · shivering · Stevens-Johnson syndrome

  SIDE-EFFECTS, FURTHER INFORMATION
  ‣ Pain on injection Can be reduced by injecting into a larger vein or by giving an opioid analgesic just before induction.
  ‣ Extraneous muscle movement Extraneous muscle movements can be minimised by an opioid analgesic or a short-acting benzodiazepine given just before induction.

- **PREGNANCY** May depress neonatal respiration if used during delivery.

- **BREAST FEEDING** Breast-feeding can be resumed as soon as mother has recovered sufficiently from anaesthesia.

- **HEPATIC IMPAIRMENT** Reduce dose in liver cirrhosis.

- **DIRECTIONS FOR ADMINISTRATION** To be administered over 30–60 seconds (60 seconds in patients in whom hypotension might be hazardous).

- **PATIENT AND CARER ADVICE**
  Driving and skilled tasks
  Patients given sedatives and analgesics during minor outpatient procedures should be very carefully warned about the risk of driving or undertaking skilled tasks afterwards. For a short general anaesthetic the risk extends to **at least 24 hours** after administration. Responsible persons should be available to take patients home. The dangers of taking **alcohol** should also be emphasised.

- **MEDICINAL FORMS**
  There can be variation in the licensing of different medicines containing the same drug.
  Solution for injection
  EXCIPIENTS: May contain Propylene glycol
  ‣ Hypnomidate (Janssen-Cilag Ltd)
    Etomidate 2 mg per 1 ml Hypnomidate 20mg/10ml solution for injection ampoules | 5 ampoule [PoM] £6.90
  Emulsion for injection
  ‣ Etomidate-Lipuro (B.Braun Medical Ltd)
    Etomidate 2 mg per 1 ml Etomidate-Lipuro 20mg/10ml emulsion for injection ampoules | 10 ampoule [PoM] £15.62

Propofol

- **INDICATIONS AND DOSE**

  Induction of anaesthesia using 0.5% or 1% injection
  ▸ BY SLOW INTRAVENOUS INJECTION, OR BY INTRAVENOUS INFUSION
  ‣ Child 1 month–16 years: Usual dose 2.5–4 mg/kg, dose adjusted according to age, body-weight and response
  ‣ Child 17 years: Usual dose 1.5–2.5 mg/kg, to be administered at a rate of 20–40 mg every 10 seconds until response

  Induction of anaesthesia using 2% injection
  ▸ BY INTRAVENOUS INFUSION
  ‣ Child 3–16 years: Usual dose 2.5–4 mg/kg, dose adjusted according to age, body-weight and response
  ‣ Child 17 years: Usual dose 1.5–2.5 mg/kg, to be administered at a rate of 20–40 mg every 10 seconds until response

  Maintenance of anaesthesia using 1% injection
  ▸ BY CONTINUOUS INTRAVENOUS INFUSION
  ‣ Child 1 month–16 years: Usual dose 9–15 mg/kg/hour, dose adjusted according to age, body-weight and response
  ‣ Child 17 years: Usual dose 4–12 mg/kg/hour, adjusted according to response

  Maintenance of anaesthesia using 2% injection
  ▸ BY CONTINUOUS INTRAVENOUS INFUSION
  ‣ Child 3–16 years: Usual dose 9–15 mg/kg/hour, dose adjusted according to age, body-weight and response
  ‣ Child 17 years: Usual dose 4–12 mg/kg/hour, adjusted according to response

  Sedation of ventilated patients in intensive care using 1% or 2% injection
  ▸ BY CONTINUOUS INTRAVENOUS INFUSION
  ‣ Child 16–17 years: Usual dose 0.3–4 mg/kg/hour, adjusted according to response

  Induction of sedation for surgical and diagnostic procedures using 0.5% or 1% injection
  ▸ BY SLOW INTRAVENOUS INJECTION
  ‣ Child 1 month–16 years: Initially 1–2 mg/kg, dose and rate of administration adjusted according to desired level of sedation and response
  ‣ Child 17 years: Initially 0.5–1 mg/kg, to be administered over 1–5 minutes, dose and rate of administration adjusted according to desired level of sedation and response

  Maintenance of sedation for surgical and diagnostic procedures using 0.5% injection
  ▸ INITIALLY BY INTRAVENOUS INFUSION
  ‣ Child 17 years: Initially 1.5–4.5 mg/kg/hour, dose and rate of administration adjusted according to desired level of sedation and response, followed by (by slow intravenous injection) 10–20 mg, (if rapid increase in sedation required)

  Maintenance of sedation for surgical and diagnostic procedures using 1% injection
  ▸ INITIALLY BY INTRAVENOUS INFUSION
  ‣ Child 1 month–16 years: Usual dose 1.5–9 mg/kg/hour, dose and rate of administration adjusted according to desired level of sedation and response, followed by (by slow intravenous injection) up to 1 mg/kg, (if rapid increase in sedation required)
  ‣ Child 17 years: Initially 1.5–4.5 mg/kg/hour, dose and rate of administration adjusted according to desired level of sedation and response, followed by (by slow intravenous injection) 10–20 mg, (if rapid increase in sedation required)   continued →

15

Anaesthesia

Maintenance of sedation for surgical and diagnostic procedures using 2% injection

▶ INITIALLY BY INTRAVENOUS INFUSION

▶ **Child 3–16 years:** Usual dose 1.5–9 mg/kg/hour, dose and rate of administration adjusted according to desired level of sedation and response

▶ **Child 17 years:** Initially 1.5–4.5 mg/kg/hour, dose and rate of administration adjusted according to desired level of sedation and response, followed by (by slow intravenous injection) 10–20 mg, using 0.5% or 1% injection (if rapid increase in sedation required)

IMPORTANT SAFETY INFORMATION

Propofol should only be administered by, or under the direct supervision of, personnel experienced in its use, with adequate training in anaesthesia and airway management, and when resuscitation equipment is available.

● **CONTRA-INDICATIONS** Children under 16 years receiving intensive care

CONTRA-INDICATIONS, FURTHER INFORMATION Use in intensive care associated with a risk of propofol infusion syndrome (potentially fatal effects, including metabolic acidosis, arrhythmias, cardiac failure, rhabdomyolysis, hyperlipidaemia, hyperkalaemia, hepatomegaly, and renal failure).

● **CAUTIONS** Acute circulatory failure (shock) · cardiac impairment · cardiovascular disease · epilepsy · fixed cardiac output · hypotension · hypovolaemia · raised intracranial pressure · respiratory impairment

● **INTERACTIONS** → Appendix 1: propofol

● **SIDE-EFFECTS**

▶ **Common or very common** Headache · hypotension · tachycardia · transient apnoea

▶ **Uncommon** Phlebitis · thrombosis

▶ **Rare** Anaphylaxis · arrhythmia · convulsions (onset can be delayed) · delayed recovery from anaesthesia · euphoria

▶ **Very rare** Discoloration of urine · pancreatitis · pulmonary oedema · sexual disinhibition

▶ **Frequency not known** Bradycardia · pain on intravenous injection · propofol infusion syndrome · significant extraneous muscle movements

SIDE-EFFECTS, FURTHER INFORMATION

▶ **Bradycardia** Bardycardia may be profound and may be treated with intravenous administration of an antimuscarinic drug.

▶ **Extraneous muscle movement** Extraneous muscle movements can be minimised by an opioid analgesic or a short-acting benzodiazepine given just before induction.

▶ **Pain on injection** Can be reduced by intravenous lidocaine.

▶ **Propofol infusion syndrome** Prolonged infusion of propofol doses exceeding 4 mg/kg/hour may result in potentially fatal effects, including metabolic acidosis, arrhythmias, cardiac failure, rhabdomyolysis, hyperlipidaemia, hyperkalaemia, hepatomegaly, and renal failure.

● **PREGNANCY** Max. dose for maintenance of anaesthesia 6 mg/kg/hour. May depress neonatal respiration if used during delivery.

● **BREAST FEEDING** Breast-feeding can be resumed as soon as mother has recovered sufficiently from anaesthesia.

● **HEPATIC IMPAIRMENT** Use with caution.

● **RENAL IMPAIRMENT** Use with caution.

● **MONITORING REQUIREMENTS** Monitor blood-lipid concentration if risk of fat overload or if sedation longer than 3 days.

● **DIRECTIONS FOR ADMINISTRATION** Shake before use; microbiological filter not recommended; may be administered via a Y-piece close to injection site

co-administered with Glucose 5% *or* Sodium chloride 0.9%. 0.5% **emulsion** for injection or intermittent infusion; may be administered undiluted, or diluted with Glucose 5% *or* Sodium chloride 0.9%; dilute to a concentration not less than 1 mg/mL. 1% **emulsion** for injection or infusion; may be administered undiluted, or diluted with Glucose 5% (*Diprivan*®) or (*Propofol-Lipuro*®) *or* Sodium chloride 0.9% (*Propofol-Lipuro*® only); dilute to a concentration not less than 2 mg/mL; use within 6 hours of preparation. 2% **emulsion** for infusion; do not dilute.

● **PATIENT AND CARER ADVICE**

Driving and skilled tasks

Patients given sedatives and analgesics during minor outpatient procedures should be very carefully warned about the risk of driving or undertaking skilled tasks afterwards. For a short general anaesthetic the risk extends to **at least 24 hours** after administration. Responsible persons should be available to take patients home. The dangers of taking **alcohol** should also be emphasised.

● **MEDICINAL FORMS**

There can be variation in the licensing of different medicines containing the same drug.

Emulsion for infusion

▶ **Diprivan** (Aspen Pharma Trading Ltd)

Propofol 10 mg per 1 ml Diprivan 1% emulsion for infusion 50ml pre-filled syringes | 1 pre-filled disposable injection PoM £10.68

Propofol 20 mg per 1 ml Diprivan 2% emulsion for infusion 50ml pre-filled syringes | 1 pre-filled disposable injection PoM £15.16

Emulsion for injection

▶ **Diprivan** (Aspen Pharma Trading Ltd)

Propofol 10 mg per 1 ml Diprivan 1% emulsion for injection 20ml ampoules | 5 ampoule PoM £15.36 (Hospital only)

▶ **Propofol-Lipuro** (B.Braun Melsungen AG)

Propofol 5 mg per 1 ml Propofol-Lipuro 0.5% emulsion for injection 20ml ampoules | 5 ampoule £14.71

ANAESTHETICS, GENERAL > VOLATILE LIQUID ANAESTHETICS

Volatile halogenated anaesthetics

IMPORTANT SAFETY INFORMATION

Should only be administered by, or under the direct supervision of, personnel experienced in their use, with adequate training in anaesthesia and airway management, and when resuscitation equipment is available.

● **CONTRA-INDICATIONS** Susceptibility to malignant hyperthermia

● **CAUTIONS** Can trigger malignant hyperthermia · neuromuscular disease (inhalational anaesthetics are very rarely associated with hyperkalaemia, resulting in cardiac arrhythmias and death) · raised intracranial pressure (can increase cerebrospinal pressure)

● **SIDE-EFFECTS**

▶ **Common or very common** Arrhythmias · cardiorespiratory depression · hypotension

▶ **Frequency not known** Convulsions · mood changes (that can last several days)

● **ALLERGY AND CROSS-SENSITIVITY** Can cause hepatotoxicity in those sensitised to halogenated anaesthetics.

● **DIRECTIONS FOR ADMINISTRATION** Volatile liquid anaesthetics are administered using calibrated vaporisers, using air, oxygen, or nitrous oxide-oxygen mixtures as the carrier gas. To prevent hypoxia, the inspired gas mixture should contain a minimum of 25% oxygen at all times.

- **PATIENT AND CARER ADVICE**
  Driving and skilled tasks
  Patients given sedatives and analgesics during minor outpatient procedures should be very carefully warned about the risks of driving or undertaking skilled tasks afterwards. For a short general anaesthetic, the risk extends **to at least 24 hours** after administration. Responsible persons should be available to take patients home. The dangers of taking **alcohol** should also be emphasised.

⟩ 776

Desflurane

- **INDICATIONS AND DOSE**
  Induction of anaesthesia (but not recommended)
  ▸ BY INHALATION
  ▹ Child 12-17 years: 4-11 %, to be inhaled through specifically calibrated vaporiser

  Maintenance of anaesthesia (in nitrous oxide-oxygen)
  ▸ BY INHALATION
  ▹ Neonate: 2-6 %, to be inhaled through a specifically calibrated vaporiser.
  ▹ Child: 2-6 %, to be inhaled through a specifically calibrated vaporiser

  Maintenance of anaesthesia (in oxygen or oxygen-enriched air)
  ▸ BY INHALATION
  ▹ Neonate: 2.5-8.5 %, to be inhaled through a specifically calibrated vaporiser.
  ▹ Child: 2.5-8.5 %, to be inhaled through a specifically calibrated vaporiser

- **INTERACTIONS** → Appendix 1: volatile halogenated anaesthetics
- **SIDE-EFFECTS** Apnoea · breath-holding · cough · increased secretions · laryngospasm
- **PREGNANCY** May depress neonatal respiration if used during delivery.
- **BREAST FEEDING** Breast-feeding can be resumed as soon as mother has recovered sufficiently from anaesthesia.

- **MEDICINAL FORMS**
  There can be variation in the licensing of different medicines containing the same drug.
  Inhalation vapour
  ▸ Desflurane (Non-proprietary)
  Desflurane 1 ml per 1 ml Desflurane volatile liquid | 240 ml [PoM] no price available (Hospital only)

⟩ 776

Isoflurane

- **INDICATIONS AND DOSE**
  Induction of anaesthesia (in oxygen or nitrous oxide-oxygen) (but indication not recommended in infants and children of all ages)
  ▸ BY INHALATION
  ▹ Neonate: Initially 0.5 %, increased to 3 %, adjusted according to response, administered using specifically calibrated vaporiser.
  ▹ Child: Initially 0.5 %, increased to 3 %, adjusted according to response, administered using specifically calibrated vaporiser

Maintenance of anaesthesia (in nitrous oxide-oxygen)
▸ BY INHALATION
▹ Neonate: 1-2.5 %, to be administered using specifically calibrated vaporiser; an additional 0.5-1% may be required when given with oxygen alone.
▹ Child: 1-2.5 %, to be administered using specifically calibrated vaporiser; an additional 0.5-1% may be required when given with oxygen alone

Maintenance of anaesthesia in caesarean section (in nitrous oxide-oxygen)
▸ BY INHALATION
▹ Child: 0.5-0.75 %, to be administered using specifically calibrated vaporiser

IMPORTANT SAFETY INFORMATION
Isoflurane is not recommended for induction of anaesthesia in infants and children of all ages because of the occurence of cough, breath-holding, desaturation, increased secretions, and laryngospasm.

- **CAUTIONS** Children under 2 years—limited experience
- **INTERACTIONS** → Appendix 1: volatile halogenated anaesthetics
- **SIDE-EFFECTS** Breath-holding · cough · irritate mucous membrane · laryngospasm
- **PREGNANCY** May depress neonatal respiration if used during delivery.
- **BREAST FEEDING** Breast-feeding can be resumed as soon as mother has recovered sufficiently from anaesthesia.
- **MEDICINAL FORMS**
  There can be variation in the licensing of different medicines containing the same drug.
  Inhalation vapour
  ▸ Isoflurane (Non-proprietary)
  Isoflurane 1 ml per 1 ml Isoflurane inhalation vapour | 250 ml [PoM] £35.29 (Hospital only)
  Isoflurane volatile liquid | 250 ml [P] £47.50 (Hospital only)
  ▸ AErrane (Baxter Healthcare Ltd)
  Isoflurane 1 ml per 1 ml AErrane volatile liquid | 250 ml [P] no price available (Hospital only)

Nitrous oxide

- **INDICATIONS AND DOSE**
  Maintenance of anaesthesia in conjunction with other anaesthetic agents
  ▸ BY INHALATION
  ▹ Neonate: 50-66 %, to be administered using suitable anaesthetic apparatus in oxygen.
  ▹ Child: 50-66 %, to be administered using suitable anaesthetic apparatus in oxygen

  Analgesia
  ▸ BY INHALATION
  ▹ Neonate: Up to 50 %, to be administered using suitable anaesthetic apparatus in oxygen, adjusted according to the patient's needs.
  ▹ Child: Up to 50 %, to be administered using suitable anaesthetic apparatus in oxygen, adjusted according to the patient's needs

IMPORTANT SAFETY INFORMATION
Nitrous oxide should only be administered by, or under the direct supervision of, personnel experienced in its use, with adequate training in anaesthesia and airway

15

Anaesthesia

management, and when resuscitation equipment is available.

- **CAUTIONS** Entrapped air following recent underwater dive · pneumothorax · presence of intracranial air after head injury · recent intra-ocular gas injection

CAUTIONS, FURTHER INFORMATION
Nitrous oxide may have a deleterious effect if used in patients with an air-containing closed space since nitrous oxide diffuses into such a space with a resulting increase in pressure. This effect may be dangerous in conditions such as pneumothorax, which may enlarge to compromise respiration, or in the presence of intracranial air after head injury, entrapped air following recent underwater dive, or recent intra-ocular gas injection.

- **INTERACTIONS** → Appendix 1: nitrous oxide
- **SIDE-EFFECTS** Depression of white cell formation · hypoxia · megaloblastic anaemia · neurological toxic effects

SIDE-EFFECTS, FURTHER INFORMATION
- Hypoxia Hypoxia can occur immediately following the administration of nitrous oxide; additional oxygen should always be given for several minutes after stopping the flow of nitrous oxide.
- Prolonged exposure Exposure of patients to nitrous oxide for prolonged periods, either by continuous or by intermittent administration, may result in megaloblastic anaemia owing to interference with the action of vitamin B_{12}; neurological toxic effects can occur without preceding overt haematological changes. Depression of white cell formation may also occur.

- **PREGNANCY** May depress neonatal respiration if used during delivery.
- **BREAST FEEDING** Breast-feeding can be resumed as soon as mother has recovered sufficiently from anaesthesia.
- **MONITORING REQUIREMENTS**
- Assessment of plasma-vitamin B_{12} concentration should be considered in those at risk of deficiency, including those who have a poor vegetarian, or vegan diet, and those with a history of anaemia.
- Nitrous oxide should **not** be given continuously for longer than 24 hours or more frequently than every 4 days without close supervision and haematological monitoring.
- **DIRECTIONS FOR ADMINISTRATION** For analgesia (without loss of consciousness), a mixture of nitrous oxide and oxygen containing 50% of each gas (Entonox®, Equanox®) is used.
- **HANDLING AND STORAGE** Exposure of theatre staff to nitrous oxide should be minimised (risk of serious side-effects).
- **PATIENT AND CARER ADVICE**
Medicines for Children leaflet: Nitrous oxide for pain www.medicinesforchildren.org.uk/nitrous-oxide-for-pain
- **MEDICINAL FORMS**
There can be variation in the licensing of different medicines containing the same drug.
Inhalation gas
- Nitrous oxide (Non-proprietary)
Nitrous oxide 1 ml per 1 ml Nitrous oxide cylinders size E | 1800 litre P no price available
Medical Nitrous Oxide cylinders size D | 900 litre P no price available
Medical Nitrous Oxide cylinders size G | 9000 litre P no price available
Nitrous oxide cylinders size F | 3600 litre P no price available
Nitrous oxide cylinders size J | 18000 litre P no price available
Nitrous oxide cylinders size G | 9000 litre P no price available
Nitrous oxide cylinders size C | 450 litre P no price available
Medical Nitrous Oxide cylinders size F | 3600 litre P no price available
Nitrous oxide cylinders size D | 900 litre P no price available
Medical Nitrous Oxide cylinders size E | 1800 litre P no price available

---

F 776

Sevoflurane

- **INDICATIONS AND DOSE**
Induction of anaesthesia (in oxygen or nitrous oxide–oxygen)
▸ BY INHALATION
- Neonate: Up to 4 %, adjusted according to response, to be administered using specifically calibrated vaporiser.
- Child: Initially 0.5–1 %, then increased to up to 8 %, increased gradually, according to response, to be administered using specifically calibrated vaporiser
Maintenance of anaesthesia (in oxygen or nitrous oxide–oxygen)
▸ BY INHALATION
- Neonate: 0.5–2 %, adjusted according to response, to be administered using specifically calibrated vaporiser.
- Child: 0.5–3 %, adjusted according to response, to be administered using specifically calibrated vaporiser

- **CAUTIONS** Susceptibility to QT-interval prolongation
- **INTERACTIONS** → Appendix 1: volatile halogenated anaesthetics
- **SIDE-EFFECTS** Agitation · cardiac arrest · dystonia · leucopenia · torsade de pointes · urinary retention
- **PREGNANCY** May depress neonatal respiration if used during delivery.
- **BREAST FEEDING** Breast-feeding can be resumed as soon as mother has recovered sufficiently from anaesthesia.
- **RENAL IMPAIRMENT** Use with caution.

- **MEDICINAL FORMS**
There can be variation in the licensing of different medicines containing the same drug.
Inhalation vapour
- Sevoflurane (Non-proprietary)
Sevoflurane 1 ml per 1 ml Sevoflurane volatile liquid | 250 ml PoM £123.00 (Hospital only)

---

1 Anaesthesia adjuvants

Pre-medication and peri-operative drugs

Drugs that affect gastric pH

Regurgitation and aspiration of gastric contents (Mendelson's syndrome) can be a complication of general anaesthesia, particularly in obstetrics and in gastro-oesophageal reflux disease; prophylaxis against acid aspiration is not routinely used in children but may be required in high-risk cases.

An **H_2-receptor antagonist** can be used before surgery to increase the pH and reduce the volume of gastric fluid. It does not affect the pH of fluid already in the stomach and this limits its value in emergency procedures; an oral H_2-receptor antagonist can be given 1–2 hours before the procedure.

Antimuscarinic drugs

Antimuscarinic drugs are used (less commonly nowadays) as premedicants to dry bronchial and salivary secretions which are increased by intubation, upper airway surgery, or some inhalational anaesthetics. They are also used before or with neostigmine p. 619 to prevent bradycardia, excessive salivation, and other muscarinic actions of neostigmine. They also prevent bradycardia and hypotension associated with drugs such as propofol p. 775 and suxamethonium chloride p. 782.

Atropine sulfate p. 779 is now rarely used for premedication but still has an emergency role in the treatment of vagotonic side-effects. Atropine sulfate may have a role in cardiopulmonary resuscitation.

Hyoscine hydrobromide p. 256 reduces secretions and also provides a degree of amnesia, sedation, and anti-emesis. Unlike atropine sulfate it may produce bradycardia rather than tachycardia.

Glycopyrronium bromide p. 780 reduces salivary secretions. When given intravenously it produces less tachycardia than atropine sulfate. It is widely used with neostigmine for reversal of non-depolarising muscle relaxants.

Glycopyrronium bromide or hyoscine hydrobromide are also used to control excessive secretions in upper airways or hypersalivation in palliative care and in children unable to control posture or with abnormal swallowing reflex; effective dose varies and tolerance may develop. The intramuscular route should be avoided if possible. Hyoscine hydrobromide transdermal patches may also be used.

Sedative drugs

Premedication

Fear and anxiety before a procedure (including the night before) can be minimised by using a sedative drug, usually a **benzodiazepine**. Premedication may also augment the action of anaesthetics and provide some degree of pre-operative amnesia. The choice of drug depends on the individual, the nature of the procedure, the anaesthetic to be used, and other prevailing circumstances such as outpatients, obstetrics, and availability of recovery facilities. The choice also varies between elective and emergency procedures. Oral administration is preferred if possible; the rectal route should only be used in exceptional circumstances.

Premedicants can be given the night before major surgery; a further, smaller dose may be required before surgery. Alternatively, the first dose may be given on the day of the procedure.

Oral midazolam p. 215 is the most common premedicant for children; temazepam p. 790 may be used in older children. The antihistamine alimemazine tartrate p. 171 is occasionally used orally, but when given alone it may cause postoperative restlessness in the presence of pain.

Benzodiazepines

Benzodiazepines possess useful properties for premedication including relief of anxiety, sedation, and amnesia; short-acting benzodiazepines taken by mouth are the most common premedicants. Benzodiazepines are also used for sedation prior to clinical procedures and for sedation in intensive care.

Benzodiazepines may occasionally cause marked respiratory depression and facilities for its treatment are essential; flumazenil p. 811 is used to antagonise the effects of benzodiazepines.

Midazolam, a water-soluble benzodiazepine, is the preferred benzodiazepine for premedication and for sedation for clinical procedures in children. It has a fast onset of action, and recovery is faster than for other benzodiazepines. Recovery may be longer in children with a low cardiac output, or after repeated dosing.

Midazolam can be given by mouth [unlicensed], but its bitter acidic taste may need to be disguised. It can also be given buccally [unlicensed indication] or intranasally [unlicensed]. Midazolam is associated with profound sedation when high doses are given or when it is used with certain other drugs. It can cause severe disinhibition and restlessness in some children. Midazolam is not recommended for prolonged sedation in neonates; drug accumulation is likely to occur.

Temazepam is given by mouth for premedication in older children and has a short duration of action. Anxiolytic and sedative effects last about 90 minutes, although there may be residual drowsiness. Temazepam is rarely used for dental procedures in children.

Lorazepam p. 214 produces more prolonged sedation than temazepam and it has marked amnesic effects.

Peri-operative use of diazepam p. 212 is not recommended in children; onset and magnitude of response are unreliable, and paradoxical effects may occur. Diazepam is not used for dental procedures in children.

Antagonists for central and respiratory depression

Respiratory depression is a major concern with opioid analgesics and it may be treated by artificial ventilation or be reversed by an opioid antagonist. Naloxone hydrochloride p. 813 given intravenously immediately reverses opioid-induced respiratory depression but the dose may have to be repeated because of its **short duration of action**. Intramuscular injection of naloxone hydrochloride produces a more gradual and prolonged effect but absorption may be erratic. Care is required in children requiring pain relief because naloxone hydrochloride also antagonises the analgesic effect of opioids.

Flumazenil is a benzodiazepine antagonist for the reversal of the central sedative effects of benzodiazepines after anaesthetic and similar procedures. Flumazenil has a shorter half-life and duration of action than diazepam or midazolam so patients may become resedated.

Neonates

Naloxone hydrochloride is used in newborn infants to reverse respiratory depression and sedation resulting from the use of opioids by the mother, usually for pain during labour. In neonates the effects of opioids may persist for up to 48 hours and in such cases naloxone hydrochloride is often given by intramuscular injection for its prolonged effect. In severe respiratory depression after birth, breathing should first be established (using artificial means if necessary) and naloxone hydrochloride administered only if use of opioids by the mother is thought to cause the respiratory depression; the infant should be monitored closely and further doses of naloxone hydrochloride administered as necessary.

ANTIMUSCARINICS
F 468

Atropine sulfate

● INDICATIONS AND DOSE

Bradycardia due to acute massive overdosage of beta-blockers

▶ BY INTRAVENOUS INJECTION
▶ Child: 40 micrograms/kg (max. per dose 3 mg)

Treatment of poisoning by organophosphorus insecticide or nerve agent (in combination with pralidoxime chloride)

▶ BY INTRAVENOUS INJECTION
▶ Child: 20 micrograms/kg every 5–10 minutes (max. per dose 2 mg) until the skin becomes flushed and dry, the pupils dilate, and bradycardia is abolished, frequency of administration dependent on the severity of poisoning

Premedication

▶ BY INTRAVENOUS INJECTION
▶ Neonate: 10 micrograms/kg, to be administered immediately before induction of anaesthesia.

▶ Child 1 month-11 years: 20 micrograms/kg, to be administered immediately before induction of anaesthesia (minimum 100 micrograms, max. 600 micrograms)

continued →

- Child 12-17 years: 300–600 micrograms, to be administered immediately before induction of anaesthesia
▸ BY SUBCUTANEOUS INJECTION, OR BY INTRAMUSCULAR INJECTION
- Neonate: 10 micrograms/kg, to be administered 30–60 minutes before induction of anaesthesia.

- Child 1 month-11 years: 10–30 micrograms/kg, to be administered 30–60 minutes before induction of anaesthesia (minimum 100 micrograms, max. 600 micrograms)
- Child 12-17 years: 300–600 micrograms, to be administered 30–60 minutes before induction of anaesthesia
▸ BY MOUTH
- Neonate: 20–40 micrograms/kg, to be administered 1–2 hours before induction of anaesthesia.

- Child: 20–40 micrograms/kg (max. per dose 900 micrograms), to be administered 1–2 hours before induction of anaesthesia

Intra-operative bradycardia
▸ BY INTRAVENOUS INJECTION
- Neonate: 10–20 micrograms/kg.

- Child 1 month-11 years: 10–20 micrograms/kg
- Child 12-17 years: 300–600 micrograms, larger doses may be used in emergencies

Control of muscarinic side-effects of neostigmine in reversal of competitive neuromuscular block
▸ BY INTRAVENOUS INJECTION
- Neonate: 20 micrograms/kg.

- Child 1 month-11 years: 20 micrograms/kg (max. per dose 1.2 mg)
- Child 12-17 years: 0.6–1.2 mg

● UNLICENSED USE Not licensed for use in children under 12 years for intra-operative bradycardia or by intravenous route for premedication. Not licensed for use by oral route.

IMPORTANT SAFETY INFORMATION
Antimuscarinic drugs used for premedication to general anaesthesia should only be administered by, or under the direct supervision of, personnel experienced in their use.

● INTERACTIONS → Appendix 1: atropine

● PREGNANCY Not known to be harmful; manufacturer advises caution.

● BREAST FEEDING May suppress lactation; small amount present in milk—manufacturer advises caution.

● MONITORING REQUIREMENTS
▸ Control of muscarinic side-effects of neostigmine in reversal of competitive neuromuscular block Since atropine has a shorter duration of action than neostigmine, late unopposed bradycardia may result; close monitoring of the patient is necessary.

● DIRECTIONS FOR ADMINISTRATION For administration *by mouth*, injection solution may be given orally.

● EXCEPTIONS TO LEGAL CATEGORY
▸ With intramuscular use or intravenous use or subcutaneous use Prescription only medicine restriction does not apply where administration is for saving life in emergency.

● MEDICINAL FORMS
There can be variation in the licensing of different medicines containing the same drug. Forms available from special-order manufacturers include: oral suspension, oral solution, solution for injection, solution for infusion

Tablet
▸ Atropine sulfate (Non-proprietary)
  Atropine sulfate 600 microgram Atropine 600microgram tablets | 28 tablet [PoM] £52.92 DT price = £49.53

Solution for injection
▸ Atropine sulfate (Non-proprietary)
  Atropine sulfate 100 microgram per 1 ml Atropine 500micrograms/5ml solution for injection pre-filled syringes | 1 pre-filled disposable injection [PoM] £7.40–£13.00 | 10 pre-filled disposable injection [PoM] £69.00–£130.00
  Atropine sulfate 200 microgram per 1 ml Atropine 1mg/5ml solution for injection pre-filled syringes | 1 pre-filled disposable injection [PoM] £7.08–£13.00 | 10 pre-filled disposable injection [PoM] £130.00
  Atropine sulfate 300 microgram per 1 ml Atropine 3mg/10ml solution for injection pre-filled syringes | 1 pre-filled disposable injection [PoM] £7.08–£13.00 DT price = £7.19 | 10 pre-filled disposable injection [PoM] £130.00
  Atropine sulfate 400 microgram per 1 ml Atropine 400micrograms/1ml solution for injection ampoules | 10 ampoule [PoM] £80.48–£82.32 DT price = £79.11
  Atropine sulfate 600 microgram per 1 ml Atropine 600micrograms/1ml solution for injection ampoules | 10 ampoule [PoM] £11.71 DT price = £11.70
  Atropine 600micrograms/1ml solution for injection pre-filled syringes | 1 pre-filled disposable injection [PoM] £7.08
  Atropine sulfate 1 mg per 1 ml Atropine 1mg/1ml solution for injection ampoules | 10 ampoule [PoM] £74.29–£75.98 DT price = £73.03

F 468

Glycopyrronium bromide

13-Jun-2017

(Glycopyrrolate)

● INDICATIONS AND DOSE
Premedication at induction
▸ BY INTRAMUSCULAR INJECTION, OR BY INTRAVENOUS INJECTION
- Neonate: 5 micrograms/kg.

- Child 1 month-11 years: 4–8 micrograms/kg (max. per dose 200 micrograms)
- Child 12-17 years: 200–400 micrograms, alternatively 4–5 micrograms/kg (max. per dose 400 micrograms)

Intra-operative bradycardia
▸ BY INTRAVENOUS INJECTION
- Neonate: 10 micrograms/kg, repeated if necessary.

- Child: 4–8 micrograms/kg (max. per dose 200 micrograms), repeated if necessary

Control of muscarinic side-effects of neostigmine in reversal of non-depolarising neuromuscular block
▸ BY INTRAVENOUS INJECTION
- Neonate: 10 micrograms/kg.

- Child 1 month-11 years: 10 micrograms/kg (max. per dose 500 micrograms)
- Child 12-17 years: 10–15 micrograms/kg, alternatively, 200 micrograms per 1 mg of neostigmine to be administered

Control of upper airways secretion | Hypersalivation
▸ BY MOUTH
- Child: 40–100 micrograms/kg 3–4 times a day (max. per dose 2 mg), adjusted according to response, dose to be administered using tablets or injection solution, see *Directions for administration*
▸ BY SUBCUTANEOUS INFUSION
- Child 1 month-11 years: 12–40 micrograms/kg (max. per dose 1.2 mg) over 24 hours

- Child 12–17 years: 0.6–1.2 mg/24 hours
- ▶ BY SUBCUTANEOUS INJECTION, OR BY INTRAMUSCULAR INJECTION, OR BY INTRAVENOUS INJECTION
- Child 1 month–11 years: 4–10 micrograms/kg 4 times a day (max. per dose 200 micrograms) as required
- Child 12–17 years: 200 micrograms every 4 hours as required

SIALANAR® ORAL SOLUTION

Severe sialorrhoea (chronic pathological drooling)
- ▶ BY MOUTH
- Child 3–17 years: (consult product literature)

- **UNLICENSED USE** Not licensed for use in control of upper airways secretion and hypersalivation.

> **IMPORTANT SAFETY INFORMATION**
> Antimuscarinic drugs used for premedication to general anaesthesia should only be administered by, or under the direct supervision of, personnel experienced in their use.

- **CAUTIONS**
  SIALANAR® ORAL SOLUTION Compromised blood-brain barrier—monitor for behavioural changes
- **INTERACTIONS** → Appendix 1: glycopyrronium
- **PREGNANCY**
  SIALANAR® ORAL SOLUTION Manufacturer advises avoid—no information available.
- **BREAST FEEDING**
  SIALANAR® ORAL SOLUTION Manufacturer advises avoid—no information available.
- **RENAL IMPAIRMENT**
  SIALANAR® ORAL SOLUTION Manufacturer advises reduce dose by 30% if estimated glomerular filtration rate is 30–89 mL/minute/1.73 m²—consult product literature. Manufacturer advises avoid if estimated glomerular filtration rate is less than 30 mL/minute/1.73 m².
- **DIRECTIONS FOR ADMINISTRATION**
  ▶ With oral use for Control of upper airways secretion or Hypersalivation For administration *by mouth*, injection solution may be given or crushed tablets suspended in water.
  SIALANAR® ORAL SOLUTION Doses should be given at least 1 hour before or 2 hours after food, or at consistent times with respect to food if co-administration with food is required—high-fat food should be avoided; for administration by a nasogastric or feeding tube, flush with 10 mL of water immediately after dosing.
- **PRESCRIBING AND DISPENSING INFORMATION**
  Tablets may be available on a named-patient basis from specialist importing companies.
- **PATIENT AND CARER ADVICE**
  SIALANAR® ORAL SOLUTION Manufacturer advises patients and their carers should be informed to stop treatment and seek medical advice if constipation, urinary retention, pneumonia, allergic reaction, pyrexia, or changes in behaviour occur; treatment should also be stopped and medical advice sought in very hot weather.

- **MEDICINAL FORMS**
  There can be variation in the licensing of different medicines containing the same drug. Forms available from special-order manufacturers include: oral solution

  Tablet
  ▶ Glycopyrronium bromide (Non-proprietary)
  Glycopyrronium bromide 1 mg Glycopyrronium bromide 1mg tablets | 30 tablet [PoM] £180.00–£216.00 DT price = £215.97
  Glycopyrronium bromide 2 mg Glycopyrronium bromide 2mg tablets | 30 tablet [PoM] £198.00–£237.60 DT price = £237.57

Solution for injection
▶ Glycopyrronium bromide (Non-proprietary)
  Glycopyrronium bromide 200 microgram per 1 ml Glycopyrronium bromide 200micrograms/1ml solution for injection ampoules | 10 ampoule [PoM] £14.00 DT price = £12.40
  Glycopyrronium bromide 600micrograms/3ml solution for injection ampoules | 3 ampoule [PoM] £8.00–£9.75 | 10 ampoule [PoM] £11.50

Oral solution
▶ Glycopyrronium bromide (Non-proprietary)
  Glycopyrronium bromide 200 microgram per 1 ml Glycopyrronium bromide 1mg/5ml oral solution sugar free sugar-free | 150 ml [PoM] £91.00 DT price = £91.00
▶ Sialanar (Proveca Ltd)
  Glycopyrronium bromide 400 microgram per 1 ml Sialanar 320micrograms/ml oral solution sugar-free | 250 ml [PoM] £320.00 DT price = £320.00

1.1 Neuromuscular blockade

Neuromuscular blockade

Neuromuscular blocking drugs

Neuromuscular blocking drugs used in anaesthesia are also known as **muscle relaxants**. By specific blockade of the neuromuscular junction they enable light anaesthesia to be used with adequate relaxation of the muscles of the abdomen and diaphragm. They also relax the vocal cords and allow the passage of a tracheal tube. Their action differs from the muscle relaxants used in musculoskeletal disorders that act on the spinal cord or brain.

Children who have received a neuromuscular blocking drug should **always** have their respiration assisted or controlled until the drug has been inactivated or antagonised. They should also receive sufficient concomitant inhalational or intravenous anaesthetic or sedative drugs to prevent awareness.

Non-depolarising neuromuscular blocking drugs

Non-depolarising neuromuscular blocking drugs (also known as competitive muscle relaxants) compete with acetylcholine for receptor sites at the neuromuscular junction and their action can be reversed with anticholinesterases such as neostigmine p. 619. Non-depolarising neuromuscular blocking drugs can be divided into the **aminosteroid** group, comprising pancuronium bromide p. 785, rocuronium bromide p. 785, and vecuronium bromide p. 785, and the **benzylisoquinolinium** group, comprising atracurium besilate p. 783, cisatracurium p. 784, and mivacurium p. 784.

Non-depolarising neuromuscular blocking drugs have a slower onset of action than suxamethonium chloride p. 782. These drugs can be classified by their duration of action as short-acting (15–30 minutes), intermediate-acting (30–40 minutes), and long-acting (60–120 minutes), although duration of action is dose-dependent. Drugs with a shorter or intermediate duration of action, such as atracurium besilate and vecuronium bromide, are more widely used than those with a longer duration of action, such as pancuronium bromide.

Non-depolarising neuromuscular blocking drugs have no sedative or analgesic effects and are not considered to trigger malignant hyperthermia.

For patients receiving intensive care and who require tracheal intubation and mechanical ventilation, a non-depolarising neuromuscular blocking drug is chosen according to its onset of effect, duration of action, and side-effects. Rocuronium bromide, with a rapid onset of effect, may facilitate intubation. Atracurium besilate or cisatracurium may be suitable for long-term neuromuscular blockade since their duration of action is not dependent on elimination by the liver or the kidneys.

15

Anaesthesia

Atracurium besilate, a mixture of 10 isomers, is a benzylisoquinolinium neuromuscular blocking drug with an intermediate duration of action. It undergoes non-enzymatic metabolism which is independent of liver and kidney function, thus allowing its use in children with hepatic or renal impairment. Cardiovascular effects are associated with significant histamine release; histamine release can be minimised by administering slowly or in divided doses over at least 1 minute. Neonates may be more sensitive to the effects of atracurium besilate and lower doses may be required.

Cisatracurium is a single isomer of atracurium besilate. It is more potent and has a slightly longer duration of action than atracurium besilate and provides greater cardiovascular stability because cisatracurium lacks histamine-releasing effects. In children aged 1 month to 12 years, cisatracurium has a shorter duration of action and produces faster spontaneous recovery.

Mivacurium, a benzylisoquinolinium neuromuscular blocking drug, has a short duration of action. It is metabolised by plasma cholinesterase and muscle paralysis is prolonged in individuals deficient in this enzyme. It is not associated with vagolytic activity or ganglionic blockade although histamine release can occur, particularly with rapid injection. In children under 12 years mivacurium has a faster onset, shorter duration of action, and produces more rapid spontaneous recovery.

Pancuronium bromide, an aminosteroid neuromuscular blocking drug, has a long duration of action and is often used in children receiving long-term mechanical ventilation in intensive care units. It lacks a histamine-releasing effect, but vagolytic and sympathomimetic effects can cause tachycardia and hypertension. The half-life of pancuronium bromide is prolonged in neonates; neonates should receive postoperative intermittent positive pressure ventilation.

Rocuronium bromide exerts an effect within 2 minutes and has the most rapid onset of any of the non-depolarising neuromuscular blocking drugs. It is an aminosteroid neuromuscular blocking drug with an intermediate duration of action. It is reported to have minimal cardiovascular effects; high doses produce mild vagolytic activity. In most children, the duration of action of rocuronium bromide may be shorter than in adults; however, in neonates and children under 2 years, usual doses may produce a more prolonged action.

Vecuronium bromide, an aminosteroid neuromuscular blocking drug, has an intermediate duration of action. It does not generally produce histamine release and lacks cardiovascular effects. In most children, the duration of action of vecuronium bromide may be shorter than in adults; however, in neonates and children under 2 years, usual doses may produce a more prolonged action.

Depolarising neuromuscular blocking drugs
Suxamethonium chloride has the most rapid onset of action of any of the neuromuscular blocking drugs and is ideal if fast onset and brief duration of action are required e.g. with tracheal intubation. Neonates and young children are less sensitive to suxamethonium chloride and a higher dose may be required. Unlike the non-depolarising neuromuscular blocking drugs, its action cannot be reversed and recovery is spontaneous; anticholinesterases such as neostigmine potentiate the neuromuscular block.

Suxamethonium chloride should be given after anaesthetic induction because paralysis is usually preceded by painful muscle fasciculations. Bradycardia may occur; premedication with atropine sulfate p. 779 reduces bradycardia as well as the excessive salivation associated with suxamethonium chloride use.

Prolonged paralysis may occur in dual block, which occurs with high or repeated doses of suxamethonium chloride and is caused by the development of a non-depolarising block following the initial depolarising block. Children with myasthenia gravis are resistant to suxamethonium chloride but can develop dual block resulting in delayed recovery. Prolonged paralysis may also occur in those with low or atypical plasma cholinesterase. Assisted ventilation should be continued until muscle function is restored.

NEUROMUSCULAR BLOCKING DRUGS >
DEPOLARISING

Suxamethonium chloride

(Succinylcholine chloride)

- **DRUG ACTION** Suxamethonium acts by mimicking acetylcholine at the neuromuscular junction but hydrolysis is much slower than for acetylcholine; depolarisation is therefore prolonged, resulting in neuromuscular blockade.

- **INDICATIONS AND DOSE**
  Neuromuscular blockade (short duration) during surgery
  ▸ BY INTRAVENOUS INJECTION
  ▸ Neonate: 2 mg/kg, produces 5–10 minutes neuromuscular blockade.

  ▸ Child 1-11 months: 2 mg/kg
  ▸ Child 1-17 years: 1 mg/kg
  ▸ BY INTRAMUSCULAR INJECTION
  ▸ Neonate: Up to 4 mg/kg, produces 10–30 minutes neuromuscular blockade.

  ▸ Child 1-11 months: Up to 5 mg/kg
  ▸ Child 1-11 years: Up to 4 mg/kg (max. per dose 150 mg)
  PHARMACOKINETICS
  Intramuscular injection has a duration of onset of 2–3 minutes.

  IMPORTANT SAFETY INFORMATION
  Should only be administered by, or under the direct supervision of, personnel experienced in its use.

- **CONTRA-INDICATIONS** Duchenne muscular dystrophy · family history of malignant hyperthermia · hyperkalaemia · low plasma-cholinesterase activity (including severe liver disease) · major trauma · neurological disease involving acute wasting of major muscle · personal or family history of congenital myotonic disease · prolonged immobilisation (risk of hyperkalaemia) · severe burns

- **CAUTIONS** Cardiac disease · neuromuscular disease · raised intra-ocular pressure (avoid in penetrating eye injury) · respiratory disease · severe sepsis (risk of hyperkalaemia)

- **INTERACTIONS** → Appendix 1: suxamethonium

- **SIDE-EFFECTS**
  ▸ **Common or very common** Flushing · hyperkalaemia · increased gastric pressure · increased intra-ocular pressure · myoglobinaemia · myoglobinuria · postoperative muscle pain · rash
  ▸ **Rare** Apnoea · arrhythmias · bronchospasm · cardiac arrest · limited jaw mobility · prolonged respiratory depression
  ▸ **Very rare** Anaphylactic reactions · malignant hyperthermia
  ▸ **Frequency not known** Bradycardia (may occur with the first dose) · hypertension · hypotension · rhabdomyolysis · tachycardia (occurs with single use)

  SIDE-EFFECTS, FURTHER INFORMATION
  ▸ Bradycardia Premedication with atropine reduces bradycardia as well as the excessive salivation associated with suxamethonium use.

- **ALLERGY AND CROSS-SENSITIVITY** Allergic cross-reactivity between neuromuscular blocking drugs has been reported; caution is advised in cases of hypersensitivity to these drugs.

- PREGNANCY Mildly prolonged maternal neuromuscular blockade may occur.

- BREAST FEEDING Unlikely to be present in breast milk in significant amounts (ionised at physiological pH). Breast-feeding may be resumed once the mother recovered from neuromuscular block.

- HEPATIC IMPAIRMENT Prolonged apnoea may occur in severe liver disease because of reduced hepatic synthesis of pseudocholinesterase.

- DIRECTIONS FOR ADMINISTRATION For *intravenous injection*, give undiluted or dilute with Glucose 5% or Sodium Chloride 0.9%.

- MEDICINAL FORMS
  There can be variation in the licensing of different medicines containing the same drug. Forms available from special-order manufacturers include: solution for injection

  Solution for injection
  ▸ Suxamethonium chloride (Non-proprietary)
    Suxamethonium chloride 50 mg per 1 ml Suxamethonium chloride 100mg/2ml solution for injection ampoules | 10 ampoule [PoM] £28.80–£50.00
  ▸ Anectine (GlaxoSmithKline UK Ltd)
    Suxamethonium chloride 50 mg per 1 ml Anectine 100mg/2ml solution for injection ampoules | 5 ampoule [PoM] £3.57

NEUROMUSCULAR BLOCKING DRUGS ›
NON-DEPOLARISING

Non-depolarising neuromuscular blocking drugs

> IMPORTANT SAFETY INFORMATION
> Non-depolarising neuromuscular blocking drugs should only be administered by, or under direct supervision of, personnel experienced in their use, with adequate training in anaesthesia and airway management.

- CAUTIONS Burns (resistance can develop, increased doses may be required) · cardiovascular disease (reduce rate of administration) · electrolyte disturbances (response unpredictable) · fluid disturbances (response unpredictable) · hypothermia (activity prolonged, lower doses required) · myasthenia gravis (activity prolonged, lower doses required) · neuromuscular disorders (response unpredictable)

- ALLERGY AND CROSS-SENSITIVITY Allergic cross-reactivity between neuromuscular blocking drugs has been reported; caution is advised in cases of hypersensitivity to these drugs.

- PREGNANCY Non-depolarising neuromuscular blocking drugs are highly ionised at physiological pH and are therefore unlikely to cross the placenta in significant amounts.

- BREAST FEEDING Non-depolarising neuromuscular blocking drugs are ionised at physiological pH and are unlikely to be present in milk in significant amounts. Breast-feeding may be resumed once the mother has recovered from neuromuscular block.

[☞ above]

Atracurium besilate
(Atracurium besylate)

- INDICATIONS AND DOSE
  Neuromuscular blockade (short to intermediate duration) for surgery
  ▸ INITIALLY BY INTRAVENOUS INJECTION

  ▸ Neonate: Initially 300–500 micrograms/kg, followed by (by intravenous injection) 100–200 micrograms/kg, repeated if necessary, alternatively (by intravenous infusion) 300–400 micrograms/kg/hour, adjusted according to response.

  ▸ Child: Initially 300–600 micrograms/kg, then (by intravenous injection) 100–200 micrograms/kg, repeated if necessary, alternatively (by intravenous injection) initially 300–600 micrograms/kg, followed by (by intravenous infusion) 300–600 micrograms/kg/hour, adjusted according to response

  Neuromuscular blockade during intensive care
  ▸ INITIALLY BY INTRAVENOUS INJECTION

  ▸ Neonate: Initially 300–500 micrograms/kg, followed by (by intravenous injection) 100–200 micrograms/kg, repeated if necessary, alternatively (by intravenous infusion) 300–400 micrograms/kg/hour, adjusted according to response, higher doses may be necessary.

  ▸ Child: Initially 300–600 micrograms/kg, initial dose is optional, then (by intravenous infusion) 270–1770 micrograms/kg/hour; (by intravenous infusion) usual dose 650–780 micrograms/kg/hour

  DOSES AT EXTREMES OF BODY-WEIGHT
  To avoid excessive dosage in obese patients, dose should be calculated on the basis of ideal body-weight.

- UNLICENSED USE Not licensed for use in neonates.

- INTERACTIONS → Appendix 1: neuromuscular blocking drugs, non-depolarising

- SIDE-EFFECTS
  ▸ **Very rare** Anaphylactoid reactions
  ▸ **Frequency not known** Acute myopathy (after prolonged use in intensive care) · bronchospasm · hypotension · seizures · skin flushing · tachycardia

  SIDE-EFFECTS, FURTHER INFORMATION
  ▸ Cardiovascular effects Cardiovascular effects are associated with significant histamine release; histamine release can be minimised by administering slowly or in divided doses over at least 1 minute. Neonates may be more sensitive to the effects of atracurium and lower doses may be required.

- DIRECTIONS FOR ADMINISTRATION For *continuous intravenous infusion*, dilute to a concentration of 0.5–5 mg/mL with Glucose 5% or Sodium Chloride 0.9%; stability varies with diluent.
  Neonatal intensive care, dilute 60 mg/kg body-weight to a final volume of 50 mL with Glucose 5% or Sodium Chloride 0.9%; minimum concentration of 500 micrograms/mL, maximum concentration of 5 mg/mL; an intravenous infusion rate of 0.1 mL/hour provides a dose of 120 micrograms/kg/hour.

15

Anaesthesia

● MEDICINAL FORMS
There can be variation in the licensing of different medicines containing the same drug.

Solution for injection
▸ Atracurium besilate (Non-proprietary)
Atracurium besilate 10 mg per 1 ml Atracurium besilate 250mg/25ml solution for injection vials | 1 vial PoM £16.50
Atracurium besilate 25mg/2.5ml solution for injection ampoules | 5 ampoule PoM £9.25
Atracurium besilate 50mg/5ml solution for injection ampoules | 5 ampoule PoM £17.50 | 10 ampoule PoM £35.00
▸ Tracrium (GlaxoSmithKline UK Ltd)
Atracurium besilate 10 mg per 1 ml Tracrium 250mg/25ml solution for injection vials | 2 vial PoM £25.81
Tracrium 25mg/2.5ml solution for injection ampoules | 5 ampoule PoM £8.28
Tracrium 50mg/5ml solution for injection ampoules | 5 ampoule PoM £15.02

F 783

Cisatracurium

● INDICATIONS AND DOSE

Neuromuscular blockade (intermediate duration) during surgery
▸ INITIALLY BY INTRAVENOUS INJECTION
▸ Child 1 month-1 year: Initially 150 micrograms/kg, then (by intravenous injection) 30 micrograms/kg every 20 minutes as required
▸ Child 2-11 years: Initially 150 micrograms/kg, 80–100 micrograms/kg if not for intubation, then (by intravenous injection) 20 micrograms/kg every 10 minutes as required, alternatively (by intravenous injection) initially 150 micrograms/kg, followed by (by intravenous infusion) 180 micrograms/kg/hour, (by intravenous infusion) reduced to 60–120 micrograms/kg/hour, adjusted according to response
▸ Child 12-17 years: Initially 150 micrograms/kg, then (by intravenous injection) 30 micrograms/kg every 20 minutes as required, alternatively (by intravenous injection) initially 150 micrograms/kg, followed by (by intravenous infusion) 180 micrograms/kg/hour, (by intravenous infusion) reduced to 60–120 micrograms/kg/hour, adjusted according to response

DOSES AT EXTREMES OF BODY-WEIGHT
To avoid excessive dosage in obese patients, dose should be calculated on the basis of ideal body-weight.

● INTERACTIONS → Appendix 1: neuromuscular blocking drugs, non-depolarising
● SIDE-EFFECTS Acute myopathy (after prolonged use in intensive care) · bradycardia
● DIRECTIONS FOR ADMINISTRATION For *continuous intravenous infusion*, dilute to a concentration of 0.1–2 mg/mL with Glucose 5% or Sodium Chloride 0.9%; solutions of 2 mg/mL and 5 mg/mL may be infused undiluted.

● MEDICINAL FORMS
There can be variation in the licensing of different medicines containing the same drug.

Solution for injection
▸ Cisatracurium (Non-proprietary)
Cisatracurium (as Cisatracurium besilate) 2 mg per 1 ml Cisatracurium besilate 20mg/10ml solution for injection ampoules | 5 ampoule PoM £32.09
Cisatracurium besilate 20mg/10ml solution for injection vials | 5 vial PoM £37.75 (Hospital only)
Cisatracurium (as Cisatracurium besilate) 5 mg per 1 ml Cisatracurium besilate 150mg/30ml solution for injection vials | 1 vial PoM £45.00 (Hospital only) | 1 vial PoM £26.43

▸ Nimbex (GlaxoSmithKline UK Ltd)
Cisatracurium (as Cisatracurium besilate) 2 mg per 1 ml Nimbex 20mg/10ml solution for injection ampoules | 5 ampoule PoM £37.75
Cisatracurium (as Cisatracurium besilate) 5 mg per 1 ml Nimbex Forte 150mg/30ml solution for injection vials | 1 vial PoM £31.09

F 783

Mivacurium

● INDICATIONS AND DOSE

Neuromuscular blockade (short duration) during surgery
▸ INITIALLY BY INTRAVENOUS INJECTION
▸ Child 2-5 months: Initially 150 micrograms/kg, then (by intravenous injection) 100 micrograms/kg every 6–9 minutes as required, alternatively (by intravenous infusion) 8–10 micrograms/kg/minute, (by intravenous infusion) adjusted in steps of 1 microgram/kg/minute every 3 minutes if required; (by intravenous infusion) usual dose 11–14 micrograms/kg/minute
▸ Child 6 months-11 years: Initially 200 micrograms/kg, then (by intravenous injection) 100 micrograms/kg every 6–9 minutes as required, alternatively (by intravenous infusion) 8–10 micrograms/kg/minute, (by intravenous infusion) adjusted in steps of 1 microgram/kg/minute every 3 minutes if required; (by intravenous infusion) usual dose 11–14 micrograms/kg/minute
▸ Child 12-17 years: Initially 70–250 micrograms/kg, then (by intravenous injection) 100 micrograms/kg every 15 minutes as required, alternatively (by intravenous infusion) 8–10 micrograms/kg/minute, (by intravenous infusion) adjusted in steps of 1 microgram/kg/minute every 3 minutes if required; (by intravenous infusion) usual dose 6–7 micrograms/kg/minute

DOSES AT EXTREMES OF BODY-WEIGHT
To avoid excessive dosage in obese patients, dose should be calculated on the basis of ideal bodyweight.

● CAUTIONS Burns (low plasma cholinesterase activity; dose titration required)
● INTERACTIONS → Appendix 1: neuromuscular blocking drugs, non-depolarising
● SIDE-EFFECTS
▸ Very rare Anaphylactoid reactions
▸ Frequency not known Bronchospasm · hypotension · skin flushing · tachycardia
● HEPATIC IMPAIRMENT Reduce dose in severe impairment.
● RENAL IMPAIRMENT Clinical effect prolonged in renal failure—reduce dose according to response.
● DIRECTIONS FOR ADMINISTRATION For *intravenous injection*, give undiluted or dilute in Glucose 5% or Sodium Chloride 0.9%. Doses up to 150 micrograms/kg may be given over 5–15 seconds, higher doses should be given over 30 seconds. In asthma, cardiovascular disease or in those sensitive to reduced arterial blood pressure, give over 60 seconds.

● MEDICINAL FORMS
There can be variation in the licensing of different medicines containing the same drug.

Solution for injection
▸ Mivacron (GlaxoSmithKline UK Ltd)
Mivacurium (as Mivacurium chloride) 2 mg per 1 ml Mivacron 10mg/5ml solution for injection ampoules | 5 ampoule PoM £13.95
Mivacron 20mg/10ml solution for injection ampoules | 5 ampoule PoM £22.57

Pancuronium bromide

F 783

● **INDICATIONS AND DOSE**

Neuromuscular blockade (long duration) during surgery
▸ BY INTRAVENOUS INJECTION

▸ **Neonate:** Initially 100 micrograms/kg, then 50 micrograms/kg, repeated if necessary.

▸ **Child:** Initially 100 micrograms/kg, then 20 micrograms/kg, repeated if necessary

DOSES AT EXTREMES OF BODY-WEIGHT
To avoid excessive dosage in obese patients, dose should be calculated on the basis of ideal bodyweight.

● **INTERACTIONS** → Appendix 1: neuromuscular blocking drugs, non-depolarising

● **SIDE-EFFECTS** Acute myopathy (after prolonged use in intensive care) · hypertension · tachycardia

SIDE-EFFECTS, FURTHER INFORMATION
Pancuronium lacks histamine-releasing effect, but vagolytic and sympathomimetic effects can cause tachycardia and hypertension.

● **HEPATIC IMPAIRMENT** Possibly slower onset, higher dose requirement, and prolonged recovery time.

● **RENAL IMPAIRMENT** Use with caution; prolonged duration of block.

● **DIRECTIONS FOR ADMINISTRATION** For *intravenous injection*, give undiluted or dilute in Glucose 5% or Sodium Chloride 0.9%.

● **MEDICINAL FORMS**
There can be variation in the licensing of different medicines containing the same drug.
Solution for injection
▸ Pancuronium bromide (Non-proprietary)
Pancuronium bromide 2 mg per 1 ml Pancuronium bromide 4mg/2ml solution for injection ampoules | 10 ampoule PoM £50.00

Rocuronium bromide

F 783

● **INDICATIONS AND DOSE**

Neuromuscular blockade (intermediate duration) during surgery
▸ INITIALLY BY INTRAVENOUS INJECTION

▸ **Neonate:** Initially 600 micrograms/kg, then (by intravenous injection) 150 micrograms/kg, repeated if necessary, alternatively (by intravenous infusion) 300–600 micrograms/kg/hour, adjusted according to response.

▸ **Child:** Initially 600 micrograms/kg, then (by intravenous injection) 150 micrograms/kg, repeated if necessary, alternatively (by intravenous infusion) 300–600 micrograms/kg/hour, adjusted according to response

Assisted ventilation in intensive care
▸ INITIALLY BY INTRAVENOUS INJECTION

▸ **Child:** Initially 600 micrograms/kg, initial dose is optional, then (by intravenous infusion) 300–600 micrograms/kg/hour for first hour, then (by intravenous infusion), adjusted according to response

DOSES AT EXTREMES OF BODY-WEIGHT
To avoid excessive dosage in obese patients, dose should be calculated on the basis of ideal bodyweight.

● **UNLICENSED USE** Not licensed for use in children for assisted ventilation in intensive care.

● **INTERACTIONS** → Appendix 1: neuromuscular blocking drugs, non-depolarising

● **SIDE-EFFECTS**
▸ **Very rare** Anaphylactoid reactions
▸ **Frequency not known** Acute myopathy (after prolonged use in intensive care) · bronchospasm · hypotension · skin flushing · tachycardia

● **HEPATIC IMPAIRMENT** Reduce dose.

● **RENAL IMPAIRMENT** Reduce maintenance dose; prolonged paralysis.

● **DIRECTIONS FOR ADMINISTRATION** For *continuous intravenous infusion* or via drip tubing, may be diluted with Glucose 5% or Sodium Chloride 0.9%.

● **MEDICINAL FORMS**
There can be variation in the licensing of different medicines containing the same drug.
Solution for injection
▸ Rocuronium bromide (Non-proprietary)
Rocuronium bromide 10 mg per 1 ml Rocuronium bromide 50mg/5ml solution for injection ampoules | 10 ampoule PoM £24.00
Rocuronium bromide 50mg/5ml solution for injection vials | 10 vial PoM £28.00–£30.00
Rocuronium bromide 100mg/10ml solution for injection vials | 10 vial PoM £57.00–£57.90
▸ Esmeron (Merck Sharp & Dohme Ltd)
Rocuronium bromide 10 mg per 1 ml Esmeron 50mg/5ml solution for injection vials | 10 vial PoM £28.92 (Hospital only)
Esmeron 100mg/10ml solution for injection vials | 10 vial PoM £57.85 (Hospital only)

F 783

Vecuronium bromide

● **INDICATIONS AND DOSE**

Neuromuscular blockade (intermediate duration) during surgery
▸ INITIALLY BY INTRAVENOUS INJECTION

▸ **Neonate:** Initially 80 micrograms/kg, then (by intravenous injection) 30–50 micrograms/kg, adjusted according to response.

▸ **Child:** Initially 80–100 micrograms/kg, then (by intravenous injection) 20–30 micrograms/kg, repeated if necessary, alternatively (by intravenous infusion) 0.8–1.4 micrograms/kg/minute, adjusted according to response

Assisted ventilation in intensive care
▸ INITIALLY BY INTRAVENOUS INJECTION

▸ **Neonate:** Initially 80 micrograms/kg, then (by intravenous injection) 30–50 micrograms/kg, adjusted according to response, alternatively (by intravenous injection) initially 80 micrograms/kg, then (by intravenous infusion) 0.8–1.4 micrograms/kg/minute, adjusted according to response, risk of accumulation—consider interruption of infusion.

▸ **Child:** Initially 80–100 micrograms/kg, initial dose is optional, then (by intravenous infusion) 0.8–1.4 micrograms/kg/minute, adjusted according to response, (by intravenous infusion) increased if necessary up to 3 micrograms/kg/minute

DOSES AT EXTREMES OF BODY-WEIGHT
To avoid excessive dosage in obese patients, dose should be calculated on the basis of ideal bodyweight.

● **UNLICENSED USE** Not licensed for assisted ventilation in intensive care.

● **INTERACTIONS** → Appendix 1: neuromuscular blocking drugs, non-depolarising

● **SIDE-EFFECTS**
▸ **Very rare** Anaphylactoid reactions
▸ **Frequency not known** Acute myopathy (after prolonged use in intensive care) · bronchospasm · hypotension · skin flushing · tachycardia

15

Anaesthesia

15

Anaesthesia

- **HEPATIC IMPAIRMENT** Use with caution in significant impairment.
- **RENAL IMPAIRMENT** Use with caution.
- **DIRECTIONS FOR ADMINISTRATION** Reconstitute each vial with 5 mL Water for Injections to give 2 mg/mL solution; *alternatively* reconstitute with up to 10 mL Glucose 5% *or* Sodium Chloride 0.9% *or* Water for Injections—unsuitable for further dilution if not reconstituted with Water for Injections. For *continuous intravenous infusion*, dilute reconstituted solution to a concentration up to 40 micrograms/mL with Glucose 5% or Sodium Chloride 0.9%; reconstituted solution can also be given via drip tubing.
  Neonatal intensive care, reconstitute each vial with 5 mL Water for Injections to give a 2 mg/mL solution. Dilute 5 mg/kg body-weight to a final volume of 50 mL with Glucose 5% or Sodium Chloride 0.9%; an intravenous infusion rate of 0.5 mL/hour provides a dose of 50 micrograms/kg/hour; minimum concentration of 40 micrograms/mL.
- **MEDICINAL FORMS** There can be variation in the licensing of different medicines containing the same drug. No licensed medicines listed.

1.2 Neuromuscular blockade reversal

Drugs for reversal of neuromuscular blockade

Anticholinesterases

Anticholinesterases reverse the effects of the non-depolarising (competitive) neuromuscular blocking drugs such as pancuronium bromide but they prolong the action of the depolarising neuromuscular blocking drug suxamethonium chloride.

Neostigmine is used specifically for reversal of non-depolarising (competitive) blockade. It acts within one minute of intravenous injection and its effects last for 20 to 30 minutes; a second dose may then be necessary. Glycopyrronium bromide p. 780 or alternatively atropine sulfate, given before or with neostigmine, prevent bradycardia, excessive salivation, and other muscarinic effects of neostigmine.

Other drugs for reversal of neuromuscular blockade

Sugammadex p. 786 is a modified gamma cyclodextrin that can be used in children for the routine reversal of neuromuscular blockade induced by rocuronium bromide.

ANTICHOLINESTERASES

Neostigmine with glycopyrronium bromide

The properties listed below are those particular to the combination only. For the properties of the components please consider, neostigmine p. 619, glycopyrronium bromide p. 780.

- **INDICATIONS AND DOSE**
  Reversal of non-depolarising neuromuscular blockade
  ▶ BY INTRAVENOUS INJECTION
  ▶ Child: 0.02 mL/kilogram, repeated if necessary, alternatively dilute to 1 in 10 solution and give 0.2 mL/kg; maximum 2 mL per course
- **INTERACTIONS** → Appendix 1: glycopyrronium, neostigmine
- **DIRECTIONS FOR ADMINISTRATION** For *intravenous injection*, may be diluted with Sodium Chloride 0.9%, give over 10–30 seconds
- **MEDICINAL FORMS** There can be variation in the licensing of different medicines containing the same drug.
  Solution for injection
  ▶ Neostigmine with glycopyrronium bromide (Non-proprietary)
  Glycopyrronium bromide 500 microgram per 1 ml, Neostigmine metilsulfate 2.5 mg per 1 ml Neostigmine 2.5mg/1ml / Glycopyrronium bromide 500micrograms/1ml solution for injection ampoules | 10 ampoule [PoM] £11.50

ANTIDOTES AND CHELATORS

Sugammadex

- **INDICATIONS AND DOSE**
  Routine reversal of neuromuscular blockade induced by rocuronium
  ▶ BY INTRAVENOUS INJECTION
  ▶ Child 2-17 years: 2 mg/kg (consult product literature)

> **IMPORTANT SAFETY INFORMATION**
> Should only be administered by, or under the direct supervision of, personnel experienced in its use.

- **CAUTIONS** Cardiovascular disease (recovery may be delayed) · pre-existing coagulation disorders · recurrence of neuromuscular blockade— monitor respiratory function until fully recovered · use of anticoagulants (unrelated to surgery) · wait 24 hours before re-administering rocuronium
- **INTERACTIONS** → Appendix 1: sugammadex
- **SIDE-EFFECTS** Bradycardia · bronchospasm · cardiac arrest · hypersensitivity reactions
- **PREGNANCY** Use with caution—no information available.
- **RENAL IMPAIRMENT** Avoid if estimated glomerular filtration rate less than 30 mL/minute/1.73 m^2.
- **DIRECTIONS FOR ADMINISTRATION** For *intravenous injection* dose may be diluted to a concentration of 10 mg/mL with Sodium Chloride 0.9%.
- **NATIONAL FUNDING/ACCESS DECISIONS**
  Scottish Medicines Consortium (SMC) Decisions
  The *Scottish Medicines Consortium*, has advised (February 2013) that sugammadex (*Bridion* ®) is accepted for restricted use within NHS Scotland for the routine reversal of neuromuscular blockade in high-risk patients only, or where prompt reversal of neuromuscular block is required.

- **MEDICINAL FORMS**
There can be variation in the licensing of different medicines
containing the same drug.
 Solution for injection
 ELECTROLYTES: May contain Sodium
 ▸ **Bridion** (Merck Sharp & Dohme Ltd)
 Sugammadex (as Sugammadex sodium) 100 mg per 1 ml Bridion
 500mg/5ml solution for injection vials | 10 vial PoM £1,491.00
 (Hospital only)
 Bridion 200mg/2ml solution for injection vials | 10 vial PoM £596.40
 (Hospital only)

1.3 Peri-operative analgesia

Peri-operative analgesia

Non-opioid analgesics

Since non-steroidal anti-inflammatory drugs (NSAIDs) do
not depress respiration, do not impair gastro-intestinal
motility, and do not cause dependence, they may be useful
alternatives or adjuncts to opioids for the relief of
postoperative pain. NSAIDs may be inadequate for the relief
of severe pain.
 Diclofenac sodium p. 623, diclofenac potassium p. 622,
ibuprofen p. 625, paracetamol p. 260, and ketorolac
trometamol p. 787 are used to relieve postoperative pain in
children; diclofenac sodium and paracetamol can be given
parenterally and rectally as well as by mouth. Ketorolac
trometamol is given by intravenous injection.

Opioid analgesics

Opioid analgesics are now rarely used as premedicants; they
are more likely to be administered at induction. Pre-
operative use of opioid analgesics is generally limited to
children who require control of existing pain. The main side-
effects of opioid analgesics are respiratory depression,
cardiovascular depression, nausea, and vomiting; see
general notes on opioid analgesics and their use in
postoperative pain.
 See the management of opioid-induced respiratory
depression in Pre-medication and peri-operative drugs
p. 778.

Intra-operative analgesia

Opioid analgesics given in small doses before or with
induction reduce the dose requirement of some drugs used
during anaesthesia.
 Alfentanil p. 788, fentanyl p. 268, and remifentanil p. 789
are particularly useful because they act within 1-2 minutes
and have short durations of action. The initial doses of
alfentanil or fentanyl are followed either by successive
intravenous injections or by an intravenous infusion;
prolonged infusions increase the duration of effect.
 In contrast to other opioids which are metabolised in the
liver, remifentanil undergoes rapid metabolism by
nonspecific blood and tissue esterases; its short duration of
action allows prolonged administration at high dosage,
without accumulation, and with little risk of residual
postoperative respiratory depression. Remifentanil should
not be given by intravenous injection intraoperatively, but it
is well suited to continuous infusion; a supplementary
analgesic is given before stopping the infusion of
remifentanil.

ANALGESICS › NON-STEROIDAL ANTI-INFLAMMATORY DRUGS

Ketorolac trometamol

- **INDICATIONS AND DOSE**

**Short-term management of moderate to severe acute
postoperative pain only**
▸ BY INTRAMUSCULAR INJECTION, OR BY INTRAVENOUS
 INJECTION
 ▸ Child 16-17 years (body-weight up to 50 kg): Initially
 10 mg, then 10-30 mg every 4-6 hours as required for
 maximum duration of treatment 2 days, frequency may
 be increased to up to every 2 hours during initial
 postoperative period; maximum 60 mg per day
 ▸ Child 16-17 years (body-weight 50 kg and above): Initially
 10 mg, then 10-30 mg every 4-6 hours as required for
 maximum duration of treatment 2 days, frequency may
 be increased to up to every 2 hours during initial
 postoperative period; maximum 90 mg per day
▸ BY INTRAVENOUS INJECTION
 ▸ Child 6 months-15 years: Initially 0.5-1 mg/kg (max. per
 dose 15 mg), then 500 micrograms/kg every 6 hours
 (max. per dose 15 mg) as required for maximum
 duration of treatment 2 days; maximum 60 mg per day

- **UNLICENSED USE** Not licensed for use in children under
 16 years.
- **CONTRA-INDICATIONS** Active or history of gastro-
 intestinal bleeding · active or history of gastro-intestinal
 ulceration · coagulation disorders · complete or partial
 syndrome of nasal polyps · confirmed or suspected
 cerebrovascular bleeding · dehydration · following
 operations with high risk of haemorrhage or incomplete
 haemostasis · haemorrhagic diatheses · history of gastro-
 intestinal perforation · hypovolaemia · severe heart failure
- **CAUTIONS** Allergic disorders · cardiac impairment (NSAIDs
 may impair renal function) · cerebrovascular disease ·
 coagulation defects · connective-tissue disorders · Crohn's
 disease (may be exacerbated) · heart failure · ischaemic
 heart disease · peripheral arterial disease · risk factors for
 cardiovascular events · ulcerative colitis (may be
 exacerbated) · uncontrolled hypertension
- **INTERACTIONS** → Appendix 1: NSAIDs
- **SIDE-EFFECTS**
▸ **Rare** Alveolitis · aseptic meningitis (patients with
 connective-tissue disorders such as systemic lupus
 erythematosus may be especially susceptible) · hepatic
 damage · interstitial fibrosis associated with NSAIDs can
 lead to renal failure · pancreatitis · papillary necrosis
 associated with NSAIDs can lead to renal failure ·
 pulmonary eosinophilia · Stevens-Johnson syndrome ·
 toxic epidermal necrolysis
▸ **Frequency not known** Abnormal dreams · angioedema ·
 asthma · blood disorders · bradycardia · bronchospasm ·
 chest pain · colitis (induction of or exacerbation of) ·
 confusion · convulsions · Crohn's disease (induction of or
 exacerbation of) · depression · diarrhoea · dizziness ·
 drowsiness · dry mouth · dyspnoea · euphoria · fluid
 retention (rarely precipitating congestive heart failure) ·
 flushing · gastro-intestinal bleeding · gastro-intestinal
 discomfort · gastro-intestinal disturbances · gastro-
 intestinal ulceration · haematuria · hallucinations ·
 headache · hearing disturbances · hyperkalaemia ·
 hyperkinesia · hypersensitivity reactions · hypertension ·
 hyponatraemia · insomnia · malaise · myalgia · nausea ·
 nervousness · optic neuritis · pain at injection site · pallor ·
 palpitation · paraesthesia · photosensitivity · psychosis ·
 purpura · raised blood pressure · rashes · renal failure
 (especially in patients with pre-existing renal

impairment) · sweating · taste disturbances · thirst · tinnitus · urinary frequency · vertigo · visual disturbances

SIDE-EFFECTS, FURTHER INFORMATION

▸ **Serious side-effects** For information about cardiovascular and gastro-intestinal side-effects, and a possible exacerbation of symptoms in asthma, see Non-steroidal anti-inflammatory drugs p. 621.

● **ALLERGY AND CROSS-SENSITIVITY** Contra-indicated in patients with a history of hypersensitivity to aspirin or any other NSAID—which includes those in whom attacks of asthma, angioedema, urticaria or rhinitis have been precipitated by aspirin or any other NSAID.

● **PREGNANCY** Avoid unless the potential benefit outweighs the risk. Avoid during the third trimester (risk of closure of fetal ductus arteriosus *in utero* and possibly persistent pulmonary hypertension of the newborn); onset of labour may be delayed and duration may be increased.

● **BREAST FEEDING** Amount too small to be harmful.

● **HEPATIC IMPAIRMENT** Use with caution; there is an increased risk of gastro-intestinal bleeding and fluid retention. Avoid in severe liver disease.

● **RENAL IMPAIRMENT** Avoid if possible or use with caution. Avoid if serum creatinine greater than 160 micromol/litre. The lowest effective dose should be used for the shortest possible duration. Max. 60 mg daily by intramuscular injection or intravenous injection. Monitor renal function; sodium and water retention may occur and renal function may deteriorate, possibly leading to renal failure.

● **DIRECTIONS FOR ADMINISTRATION** For *intravenous injection*, give over at least 15 seconds.

● **MEDICINAL FORMS**
There can be variation in the licensing of different medicines containing the same drug.
Solution for injection
▸ Ketorolac trometamol (Non-proprietary)
Ketorolac trometamol 30 mg per 1 ml Ketorolac 30mg/1ml solution for injection ampoules | 5 ampoule PoM £5.47 (Hospital only) | 6 ampoule PoM £6.56
▸ Toradol (Atnahs Pharma UK Ltd)
Ketorolac trometamol 30 mg per 1 ml Toradol 30mg/1ml solution for injection ampoules | 5 ampoule PoM £5.36

ANALGESICS ⟩ OPIOIDS

⬛ **F 262**

▍Alfentanil

● **INDICATIONS AND DOSE**

Assisted ventilation: analgesia and enhancement of anaesthesia for short procedures
▸ BY INTRAVENOUS INJECTION

▸ **Neonate:** Initially 5–20 micrograms/kg, dose to be administered over 30 seconds; supplemental doses up to 10 micrograms/kg.

▸ **Child:** Initially 10–20 micrograms/kg, dose to be administered over 30 seconds; supplemental doses up to 10 micrograms/kg

Assisted ventilation: analgesia and enhancement of anaesthesia during maintenance of anaesthesia for longer procedures
▸ BY INTRAVENOUS INFUSION

▸ **Neonate:** Initially 10–50 micrograms/kg, dose to be administered over 10 minutes, followed by 30–60 micrograms/kg/hour.

▸ **Child:** Initially 50–100 micrograms/kg, dose to be administered over 10 minutes, followed by 30–120 micrograms/kg/hour, usual dose with intravenous anaesthetic, 60 micrograms/kg/hour

DOSES AT EXTREMES OF BODY-WEIGHT
To avoid excessive dosage in obese patients, dose should be calculated on the basis of ideal body-weight.

PHARMACOKINETICS
Half-life is prolonged in neonates and accumulation is likely with prolonged use. Clearance may be increased in children 1 month–12 years and higher infusion doses might be needed.

● **CAUTIONS**

CAUTIONS, FURTHER INFORMATION

▸ **Repeated intra-operative doses** Repeated intra-operative doses of alfentanil should be given with care since the resulting respiratory depression can persist postoperatively and occasionally it may become apparent for the first time postoperatively when monitoring of the patient might be less intensive.

● **INTERACTIONS** → Appendix 1: opioids

● **SIDE-EFFECTS**

▸ **Common or very common** Hypertension · myoclonic movements

▸ **Uncommon** Arrhythmias · hiccup · laryngospasm

▸ **Rare** Epistaxis

▸ **Frequency not known** Cardiac arrest · convulsions · cough · muscle rigidity · pyrexia

SIDE-EFFECTS, FURTHER INFORMATION

▸ **Muscle rigidity** Alfentanil can cause muscle rigidity, particularly of the chest wall or jaw; this can be managed by the use of neuromuscular blocking drugs.

● **BREAST FEEDING** Present in milk—withhold breast-feeding for 24 hours.

● **RENAL IMPAIRMENT** Avoid use or reduce dose; opioid effects increased and prolonged and increased cerebral sensitivity occurs.

● **DIRECTIONS FOR ADMINISTRATION** 5 mg/mL injection to be diluted before use. For *continuous or intermittent intravenous infusion* dilute in Glucose 5% *or* Sodium Chloride 0.9%.

● **MEDICINAL FORMS**
There can be variation in the licensing of different medicines containing the same drug. Forms available from special-order manufacturers include: solution for injection
Solution for injection
▸ Alfentanil (Non-proprietary)
Alfentanil (as Alfentanil hydrochloride) 500 microgram per 1 ml Alfentanil 1mg/2ml solution for injection ampoules | 10 ampoule PoM £5.95 CD2
Alfentanil 5mg/10ml solution for injection ampoules | 5 ampoule PoM £13.90 CD2
Alfentanil (as Alfentanil hydrochloride) 5 mg per 1 ml Alfentanil 5mg/1ml solution for injection ampoules | 10 ampoule PoM £21.95 CD2
▸ Rapifen (Janssen-Cilag Ltd)
Alfentanil (as Alfentanil hydrochloride) 500 microgram per 1 ml Rapifen 5mg/10ml solution for injection ampoules | 5 ampoule PoM £14.50 CD2
Rapifen 1mg/2ml solution for injection ampoules | 10 ampoule PoM £6.34 CD2
Alfentanil (as Alfentanil hydrochloride) 5 mg per 1 ml Rapifen Intensive Care 5mg/1ml solution for injection ampoules | 10 ampoule PoM £23.19 (Hospital only) CD2

⟟ 262

Remifentanil

- **INDICATIONS AND DOSE**

Analgesia and enhancement of anaesthesia at induction (initial bolus injection)
▸ BY INTRAVENOUS INJECTION
▸ Child 12-17 years: Initially 0.25–1 microgram/kg, dose to be administered over at least 30 seconds, if child is to be intubated more than 8 minutes after start of intravenous infusion, initial bolus intravenous injection dose is not necessary

Analgesia and enhancement of anaesthesia at induction with or without initial bolus dose
▸ BY INTRAVENOUS INFUSION
▸ Child 12-17 years: 30–60 micrograms/kg/hour, if child is to be intubated more than 8 minutes after start of intravenous infusion, initial bolus intravenous injection dose is not necessary

Assisted ventilation: analgesia and enhancement of anaesthesia during maintenance of anaesthesia (initial bolus injection)
▸ BY INTRAVENOUS INJECTION
▸ Child 1 month-11 years: Initially 0.1–1 microgram/kg, dose to be administered over at least 30 seconds (omitted if not required)
▸ Child 12-17 years: Initially 0.1–1 microgram/kg, dose to be administered over at least 30 seconds (omitted if not required)

Assisted ventilation: analgesia and enhancement of anaesthesia during maintenance of anaesthesia with or without initial bolus dose
▸ BY INTRAVENOUS INFUSION
▸ Neonate: 24–60 micrograms/kg/hour, additional doses of 1 microgram/kg can be given *by intravenous injection* during the intravenous infusion
▸ Child 1 month-11 years: 3–78 micrograms/kg/hour, dose to be administered according to anaesthetic technique and adjusted according to response, additional doses can be given *by intravenous injection* during the intravenous infusion
▸ Child 12-17 years: 3–120 micrograms/kg/hour, dose to be administered according to anaesthetic technique and adjusted according to response, additional doses can be given *by intravenous injection* during the intravenous infusion

Spontaneous respiration: analgesia and enhancement of anaesthesia during maintenance of anaesthesia
▸ BY INTRAVENOUS INFUSION
▸ Child 12-17 years: Initially 2.4 micrograms/kg/hour, adjusted according to response; usual dose 1.5–6 micrograms/kg/hour

DOSES AT EXTREMES OF BODY-WEIGHT
To avoid excessive dosage in obese patients, dose should be calculated on the basis of ideal body-weight.

- **UNLICENSED USE** Not licensed for use in children under 1 year.
- **CONTRA-INDICATIONS** Analgesia in conscious patients
- **INTERACTIONS** → Appendix 1: opioids
- **SIDE-EFFECTS**
▸ **Common or very common** Hypertension
▸ **Uncommon** Hypoxia
▸ **Rare** Asystole
▸ **Frequency not known** AV block · convulsions
   SIDE-EFFECTS, FURTHER INFORMATION
▸ Muscle rigidity Alfentanil can cause muscle rigidity, particularly of the chest wall or jaw; this can be managed by the use of neuromuscular blocking drugs.

▸ Respiratory depression In contrast to other opioids which are metabolised in the liver, remifentanil undergoes rapid metabolism by non-specific blood and tissue esterases; its short duration of action allows prolonged administration at high dosage, without accumulation, and with little risk of residual postoperative respiratory depression.
- **PREGNANCY** No information available.
- **BREAST FEEDING** Avoid breast-feeding for 24 hours after administration—present in milk in *animal* studies.
- **RENAL IMPAIRMENT** No dose adjustment necessary in renal impairment.
- **DIRECTIONS FOR ADMINISTRATION** For *intravenous injection*, reconstitute to a concentration of 1 mg/mL; for *continuous intravenous infusion*, dilute further with Glucose 5% or Sodium Chloride 0.9% to a concentration of 20–25 micrograms/mL for child 1–12 years or 20–250 micrograms/mL (usually 50 micrograms/mL) for child 12–18 years.
- **PRESCRIBING AND DISPENSING INFORMATION** Remifentanil should not be given by intravenous injection intra-operatively, but it is well suited to continuous infusion; a supplementary analgesic is given before stopping the infusion of remifentanil.

- **MEDICINAL FORMS**
There can be variation in the licensing of different medicines containing the same drug.
Powder for solution for injection
▸ Remifentanil (Non-proprietary)
   Remifentanil (as Remifentanyl hydrochloride) 1 mg Remifentanil 1mg powder for concentrate for solution for injection vials | 5 vial PoM £25.58–£25.60 (Hospital only) CD2
   Remifentanil (as Remifentanyl hydrochloride) 2 mg Remifentanil 2mg powder for concentrate for solution for injection vials | 5 vial PoM £51.13–£51.15 (Hospital only) CD2
   Remifentanil (as Remifentanyl hydrochloride) 5 mg Remifentanil 5mg powder for concentrate for solution for injection vials | 5 vial PoM £127.88–£127.90 (Hospital only) CD2
▸ Ultiva (GlaxoSmithKline UK Ltd)
   Remifentanil (as Remifentanyl hydrochloride) 1 mg Ultiva 1mg powder for solution for injection vials | 5 vial PoM £25.58 (Hospital only) CD2
   Remifentanil (as Remifentanyl hydrochloride) 2 mg Ultiva 2mg powder for solution for injection vials | 5 vial PoM £51.15 (Hospital only) CD2
   Remifentanil (as Remifentanyl hydrochloride) 5 mg Ultiva 5mg powder for solution for injection vials | 5 vial PoM £127.88 (Hospital only) CD2

1.4 Peri-operative sedation

Conscious sedation for clinical procedures

Overview

Sedation of children during diagnostic and therapeutic procedures is used to reduce fear and anxiety, to control pain, and to minimise excessive movement. The choice of sedative drug will depend upon the intended procedure and whether the child is cooperative; some procedures are safer and more successful under anaesthesia.

Midazolam p. 215 and chloral hydrate p. 282 are suitable for sedating children for painless procedures, such as imaging. For painful procedures, alternative choices include nitrous oxide p. 777, local anaesthesia, ketamine p. 790, or concomitant use of sedation with **opioid** or **non-opioid analgesia**.

15

Anaesthesia

ANAESTHETICS, GENERAL > NMDA RECEPTOR ANTAGONISTS

Ketamine

● **INDICATIONS AND DOSE**

Induction and maintenance of anaesthesia for short procedures

▶ BY INTRAMUSCULAR INJECTION

▶ Neonate: 4 mg/kg, adjusted according to response, a dose of 4 mg/kg usually produces 15 minutes of surgical anaesthesia.

▶ Child: 4–13 mg/kg, adjusted according to response, a dose of 4 mg/kg sufficient for some diagnostic procedures, a dose of 10 mg/kg usually produces 12–25 minutes of surgical anaesthesia

▶ BY INTRAVENOUS INJECTION

▶ Neonate: 1–2 mg/kg, adjusted according to response, to be given over at least 60 seconds, a dose of 1–2 mg/kg produces 5–10 minutes of surgical anaesthesia.

▶ Child 1 month–11 years: 1–2 mg/kg, adjusted according to response, to be given over at least 60 seconds, a dose of 1–2 mg/kg produces 5–10 minutes of surgical anaesthesia

▶ Child 12–17 years: 1–4.5 mg/kg, adjusted according to response, to be given over at least 60 seconds, a dose of 2 mg/kg usually produces 5–10 minutes of surgical anaesthesia

Induction and maintenance of anaesthesia for long procedures

▶ INITIALLY BY INTRAVENOUS INJECTION

▶ Neonate: Initially 0.5–2 mg/kg, followed by (by continuous intravenous infusion) 8 micrograms/kg/minute, adjusted according to response, doses up to 30 micrograms/kg/minute may be used to produce deep anaesthesia.

▶ Child: Initially 0.5–2 mg/kg, followed by (by continuous intravenous infusion) 10–45 micrograms/kg/minute, adjusted according to response

Sedation prior to invasive or painful procedures

▶ BY INTRAVENOUS INJECTION

▶ Child: 1–2 mg/kg for 1 dose

IMPORTANT SAFETY INFORMATION

Ketamine should only be administered by, or under the direct supervision of, personnel experienced in its use, with adequate training in anaesthesia and airway management, and when resuscitation equipment is available.

● **CONTRA-INDICATIONS** Acute porphyrias p. 577 · eclampsia · head trauma · hypertension · pre-eclampsia · raised intracranial pressure · severe cardiac disease · stroke

● **CAUTIONS** Acute circulatory failure (shock) · cardiovascular disease · dehydration · fixed cardiac output · hallucinations · head injury · hypertension · hypovolaemia · increased cerebrospinal fluid pressure · intracranial mass lesions · nightmares · predisposition to seizures · psychotic disorders · raised intra-ocular pressure · respiratory tract infection · thyroid dysfunction

● **INTERACTIONS** → Appendix 1: ketamine

● **SIDE-EFFECTS**

▶ **Common or very common** Diplopia · hallucinations · hypertension · nausea · nightmares · nystagmus · rash · tachycardia · transient psychotic effects · vomiting

▶ **Uncommon** Arrhythmias · bradycardia · hypotension · laryngospasm · respiratory depression

▶ **Rare** Apnoea · cystitis · cystitis · haemorrhagic cystitis · hypersalivation · insomnia

▶ **Frequency not known** Raised intra-ocular pressure

SIDE-EFFECTS, FURTHER INFORMATION

▶ Transient psychotic effects Incidence of hallucinations, nightmares, and other transient psychotic effects can be reduced by a benzodiazepine such as diazepam or midazolam.

● **PREGNANCY** May depress neonatal respiration if used during delivery.

● **BREAST FEEDING** Avoid for at least 12 hours after last dose.

● **HEPATIC IMPAIRMENT** Consider dose reduction.

● **DIRECTIONS FOR ADMINISTRATION** For *intravenous injection*, dilute 100 mg/mL strength to a concentration of not more than 50 mg/mL with Glucose 5% *or* Sodium Chloride 0.9%. For *continuous intravenous infusion*, dilute to a concentration of 1 mg/mL with Glucose 5% *or* Sodium Chloride 0.9%; use microdrip infusion for maintenance of anaesthesia.

● **PATIENT AND CARER ADVICE**

Driving and skilled tasks

Patients given sedatives and analgesics during minor outpatient procedures should be very carefully warned about the risk of driving or undertaking skilled tasks afterwards. For a short general anaesthetic the risk extends to **at least 24 hours** after administration. Responsible persons should be available to take patients home. The dangers of taking **alcohol** should also be emphasised.

For information on 2015 legislation regarding driving whilst taking certain controlled drugs, including ketamine, see *Drugs and driving* under Guidance on prescribing p. 1.

● **MEDICINAL FORMS**

There can be variation in the licensing of different medicines containing the same drug. Forms available from special-order manufacturers include: solution for injection

Solution for injection

▶ **Ketamine (Non-proprietary)**

Ketamine (as Ketamine hydrochloride) 10 mg per 1 ml Ketamin 10 Curamed 50mg/5ml solution for injection ampoules | 10 ampoule PoM no price available CD2

Ketamine (as Ketamine hydrochloride) 50 mg per 1 ml Ketamine 500mg/10ml solution for injection vials | 10 vial PoM £70.00 CD2

Ketamin 100mg/2ml solution for injection ampoules | 10 ampoule PoM no price available CD2

▶ **Ketalar** (Pfizer Ltd)

Ketamine (as Ketamine hydrochloride) 10 mg per 1 ml Ketalar 200mg/20ml solution for injection vials | 1 vial PoM £5.06 (Hospital only) CD2

Ketamine (as Ketamine hydrochloride) 50 mg per 1 ml Ketalar 500mg/10ml solution for injection vials | 1 vial PoM £8.77 (Hospital only) CD2

HYPNOTICS, SEDATIVES AND ANXIOLYTICS > BENZODIAZEPINES

F 210

Temazepam

● **INDICATIONS AND DOSE**

Premedication before surgery or investigatory procedures

▶ BY MOUTH

▶ Child 12–17 years: 10–20 mg, to be taken 1 hour before procedure

● **UNLICENSED USE** Tablets not licensed for use in children.

● **CONTRA-INDICATIONS** CNS depression · compromised airway · hyperkinesis · obsessional state · phobic states · respiratory depression

● **CAUTIONS** Hypoalbuminaemia · muscle weakness · organic brain changes · personality disorder (within the fearful group—dependent, avoidant, obsessive-compulsive)—may increase risk of dependence

CAUTIONS, FURTHER INFORMATION
▶ Paradoxical effects A paradoxical increase in hostility and aggression may be reported by patients taking benzodiazepines. The effects range from talkativeness and excitement to aggressive and antisocial acts. Adjustment of the dose (up or down) sometimes attenuates the impulses. Increased anxiety and perceptual disorders are other paradoxical effects.

● INTERACTIONS → Appendix 1: temazepam

● SIDE-EFFECTS
▶ Common or very common Amnesia · ataxia · confusion · dependence · drowsiness the next day · lightheadedness the next day · muscle weakness · paradoxical increase in aggression
▶ Uncommon Dizziness · dysarthria · gastro-intestinal disturbances · gynaecomastia · incontinence · salivation changes · tremor · visual disturbances
▶ Rare Apnoea · blood disorders · changes in libido · headache · hypotension · jaundice · skin reactions · urinary retention · vertigo
▶ Frequency not known Delusions · excitement · hallucinations · irritability · psychosis · respiratory depression (may be marked when used for sedation; facilities for its treatment are essential) · restlessness

● BREAST FEEDING Benzodiazepines are present in milk, and should be avoided if possible during breast-feeding.

● HEPATIC IMPAIRMENT Start with smaller initial doses or reduce dose. Can precipitate coma. Avoid in severe impairment.

● RENAL IMPAIRMENT Start with small doses in severe impairment.

● PATIENT AND CARER ADVICE
Driving and skilled tasks
May impair judgement and increase reaction time, and so affect ability to drive or operate machinery; they increase the effects of alcohol. Moreover the hangover effects of a night dose may impair driving on the following day.
  Patients given sedatives and analgesics during minor outpatient procedures should be very carefully warned about the risks of undertaking skilled tasks (e.g. driving) afterwards. Responsible persons should be available to take patients home afterwards. The dangers of taking **alcohol** should be emphasised.

● PROFESSION SPECIFIC INFORMATION
Dental practitioners' formulary
Temazepam Tablets and Oral Solution may be prescribed.

● MEDICINAL FORMS
There can be variation in the licensing of different medicines containing the same drug. Forms available from special-order manufacturers include: oral suspension, oral solution

Oral solution
CAUTIONARY AND ADVISORY LABELS 19
▶ Temazepam (Non-proprietary)
Temazepam 2 mg per 1 ml Temazepam 10mg/5ml oral solution sugar free sugar-free | 300 ml PoM £121.08 DT price = £121.08 CD3

Tablet
CAUTIONARY AND ADVISORY LABELS 19
▶ Temazepam (Non-proprietary)
Temazepam 10 mg Temazepam 10mg tablets | 28 tablet PoM £35.00 DT price = £1.89 CD3 | 500 tablet PoM £624.82 CD3
Temazepam 20 mg Temazepam 20mg tablets | 28 tablet PoM £35.00 DT price = £1.91 CD3 | 250 tablet PoM £307.94 CD3

2   Malignant hyperthermia

MUSCLE RELAXANTS ⟩ DIRECTLY ACTING

Dantrolene sodium

● DRUG ACTION Acts on skeletal muscle cells by interfering with calcium efflux, thereby stopping the contractile process.

● INDICATIONS AND DOSE
Malignant hyperthermia
▶ BY RAPID INTRAVENOUS INJECTION
▶ Child: Initially 2–3 mg/kg, then 1 mg/kg, repeated if necessary; maximum 10 mg/kg per course
Chronic severe spasticity of voluntary muscle
▶ BY MOUTH
▶ Child 5-11 years: Initially 500 micrograms/kg once daily for 7 days, then increased to 500 micrograms/kg/dose 3 times a day, then increased in steps of 500 micrograms/kg/dose every 7 days (max. per dose 2 mg/kg 3–4 times a day) until satisfactory response; maximum 400 mg per day
▶ Child 12-17 years: Initially 25 mg once daily for 7 days, then increased to 25 mg 3 times a day, then increased in steps of 500 micrograms/kg/dose every 7 days (max. per dose 2 mg/kg 3–4 times a day) until satisfactory response; maximum 400 mg per day

● UNLICENSED USE Not licensed for use in children.

IMPORTANT SAFETY INFORMATION
Should only be administered by, or under the direct supervision of, personnel experienced in the use of dantrolene when used for malignant hyperthermia.

● CONTRA-INDICATIONS
▶ With oral use Acute muscle spasm · avoid when spasticity is useful, for example, locomotion

● CAUTIONS
▶ With intravenous use Avoid extravasation (risk of tissue necrosis)
▶ With oral use Females (hepatotoxicity) · history of liver disorders (hepatotoxicity) · if doses greater than 400 mg daily (hepatotoxicity) · impaired cardiac function · impaired pulmonary function · therapeutic effect may take a few weeks to develop— discontinue if no response within 6–8 weeks

● INTERACTIONS → Appendix 1: dantrolene

● SIDE-EFFECTS
▶ Common or very common
▶ With oral use Abdominal pain · anorexia · asthenia · chills · diarrhoea (withdraw if severe, discontinue treatment if recurs on re-introduction) · dizziness · drowsiness · fatigue · fever · headache · hepatotoxicity · nausea · pericarditis · pleural effusion · rash · respiratory depression · seizures · speech disturbances · visual disturbances · vomiting
▶ Uncommon
▶ With oral use Confusion · constipation · crystalluria · depression · dysphagia · dyspnoea · erratic blood pressure · exacerbation of cardiac insufficiency · haematuria · increased sweating · increased urinary frequency · insomnia · nervousness · tachycardia · urinary incontinence · urinary retention
▶ Frequency not known
▶ With intravenous use Dizziness · erythema · hepatotoxicity · injection-site reactions · pulmonary oedema · rash · swelling · thrombophlebitis · weakness

15

Anaesthesia

SIDE-EFFECTS, FURTHER INFORMATION
▸ Hepatotoxicity Potentially life-threatening hepatotoxicity reported—discontinue if abnormal liver function tests or symptoms of liver disorder; re-introduce only if complete reversal of hepatotoxicity.

● PREGNANCY
▸ With intravenous use Use only if potential benefit outweighs risk.
▸ With oral use Avoid use in chronic spasticity—embryotoxic in *animal* studies.

● BREAST FEEDING
▸ With intravenous use Present in milk—use only if potential benefit outweighs risk.
▸ With oral use Present in milk—manufacturer advises avoid use in chronic spasticity.

● HEPATIC IMPAIRMENT Avoid—may cause severe liver damage (injection may be used in an emergency for malignant hyperthermia).

● MONITORING REQUIREMENTS
▸ With oral use Test liver function before and at intervals during therapy.

● PATIENT AND CARER ADVICE
Hepatotoxicity
▸ With oral use Patients should be told how to recognise signs of liver disorder and advised to seek prompt medical attention if symptoms such as anorexia, nausea, vomiting, fatigue, abdominal pain, dark urine, or pruritus develop.
Driving and skilled tasks
▸ With oral use Drowsiness may affect performance of skilled tasks (e.g. driving); effects of alcohol enhanced.

● MEDICINAL FORMS
There can be variation in the licensing of different medicines containing the same drug. Forms available from special-order manufacturers include: oral suspension, oral solution

Powder for solution for injection
▸ Dantrium (Norgine Pharmaceuticals Ltd)
Dantrolene sodium 20 mg Dantrium Intravenous 20mg powder for solution for injection vials | 12 vial PoM £612.00 (Hospital only) | 36 vial PoM £1,836.00 (Hospital only)

Capsule
CAUTIONARY AND ADVISORY LABELS 2
▸ Dantrium (Norgine Pharmaceuticals Ltd)
Dantrolene sodium 25 mg Dantrium 25mg capsules | 100 capsule PoM £16.87 DT price = £16.87
Dantrolene sodium 100 mg Dantrium 100mg capsules | 100 capsule PoM £43.07 DT price = £43.07

Local anaesthesia

Local anaesthesia

Local anaesthetic drugs

The use of local anaesthetics by injection or by application to mucous membranes to produce local analgesia is discussed in this section.

Local anaesthetic drugs act by causing a reversible block to conduction along nerve fibres. They vary widely in their potency, toxicity, duration of action, stability, solubility in water, and ability to penetrate mucous membranes. These factors determine their application, e.g. topical (surface), infiltration, peripheral nerve block, intravenous regional anaesthesia (Bier's block), plexus, epidural (extradural), or spinal (intrathecal or subarachnoid) block. Local anaesthetics may also be used for postoperative pain relief, thereby reducing the need for analgesics such as opioids.

Bupivacaine hydrochloride p. 794 has a longer duration of action than other local anaesthetics. It has a slow onset of action, taking up to 30 minutes for full effect. It is often used in lumbar epidural blockade and is particularly suitable for continuous epidural analgesia in labour, or for postoperative pain relief. It is the principal drug used for spinal anaesthesia. Hyperbaric solutions containing glucose may be used for spinal block.

Levobupivacaine p. 795, an isomer of bupivacaine hydrochloride, has anaesthetic and analgesic properties similar to bupivacaine hydrochloride, but is thought to have fewer adverse effects.

Lidocaine hydrochloride p. 796 is effectively absorbed from mucous membranes and is a useful surface anaesthetic in concentrations up to 10%. Except for surface anaesthesia and dental anaesthesia, solutions should **not** usually exceed 1% in strength. The duration of the block (with adrenaline/epinephrine p. 132) is about 90 minutes.

Application of a mixture of lidocaine and prilocaine (*EMLA®*) under an occlusive dressing provides surface anaesthesia for 1–2 hours. *EMLA®* does not appear to be effective in providing local anaesthesia for heel lancing in neonates.

Prilocaine hydrochloride p. 800 is a local anaesthetic of low toxicity which is similar to lidocaine hydrochloride.

Ropivacaine hydrochloride p. 800 is an amide-type local anaesthetic agent similar to bupivacaine hydrochloride. It is less cardiotoxic than bupivacaine hydrochloride, but also less potent.

Tetracaine p. 801, a para-aminobenzoic acid ester, is an effective local anaesthetic for topical application; a 4% gel is indicated for anaesthesia before venepuncture or venous cannulation. Tetracaine is effective for 4–6 hours after a single application in most children. It is not recommended prior to neonatal heel lancing.

Tetracaine is rapidly absorbed from mucous membranes and should never be applied to inflamed, traumatised, or highly vascular surfaces. It should never be used to provide anaesthesia for bronchoscopy or cystoscopy because lidocaine hydrochloride is a safer alternative.

Administration by injection

The dose of local anaesthetic depends on the injection site and the procedure used. In determining the safe dosage, it is important to take account of the rate of absorption and excretion, and of the potency. The child's age, weight, physique, and clinical condition, and the vascularity of the administration site and the duration of administration, must also be considered.

Uptake of local anaesthetics into the systemic circulation determines their duration of action and produces toxicity.

NHS Improvement has advised (September 2016) that, prior to administration, all injectable medicines must be drawn directly from their original ampoule or container into a syringe and should **never** be decanted into gallipots or open containers. This is to avoid the risk of medicines being confused with other substances, e.g. skin disinfectants, and to reduce the risk of contamination.

Great care must be taken to avoid accidental intravascular injection; local anaesthetic injections should be given slowly in order to detect inadvertent intravascular administration. When prolonged analgesia is required, a long-acting local anaesthetic is preferred to minimise the likelihood of cumulative systemic toxicity. Local anaesthesia around the oral cavity may impair swallowing and therefore increases the risk of aspiration.

Epidural anaesthesia is combined with general anaesthesia for certain surgical procedures in children.

Use of vasoconstrictors

Local anaesthetics cause dilatation of blood vessels. The addition of a vasoconstrictor such as adrenaline/epinephrine to the local anaesthetic preparation diminishes local blood flow, slowing the rate of absorption and thereby prolonging the anaesthetic effect. Great care should be taken to avoid inadvertent intravenous administration of a preparation containing adrenaline/epinephrine, and it is not advisable to give adrenaline/epinephrine with a local anaesthetic injection in digits or appendages because of the risk of ischaemic necrosis.

Adrenaline/epinephrine must be used in a low concentration when administered with a local anaesthetic. Care must also be taken to calculate a safe maximum dose of local anaesthetic when using combination products.

In children with severe hypertension or unstable cardiac rhythm, the use of adrenaline/epinephrine with a local anaesthetic may be hazardous. For these children an anaesthetic without adrenaline/epinephrine should be used.

Dental anaesthesia

Lidocaine hydrochloride is widely used in dental procedures; it is most often used in combination with adrenaline/epinephrine. Lidocaine hydrochloride 2% combined with adrenaline/epinephrine 1 in 80 000 (12.5 micrograms/mL) is a safe and effective preparation; there is no justification for using higher concentrations of adrenaline/epinephrine. The amide-type local anaesthetics articaine and mepivacaine hydrochloride p. 799 are also used in dentistry; they are available in cartridges suitable for dental use. Mepivacaine hydrochloride is available with or without adrenaline/epinephrine, and articaine is available with adrenaline/epinephrine. In children with severe hypertension or unstable cardiac rhythm, mepivacaine hydrochloride without adrenaline/epinephrine may be used. Alternatively, prilocaine hydrochloride with or without felypressin can be used but there is no evidence that it is any safer. Felypressin can cause coronary vasoconstriction when used at high doses; limit dose in children with coronary artery disease.

Toxicity

For management of toxicity see Severe local anaesthetic-induced cardiovascular toxicity below.

Severe local anaesthetic-induced cardiovascular toxicity

Overview

After injection of a bolus of local anaesthetic, toxicity may develop at any time in the following hour. In the event of signs of toxicity during injection, the administration of the local anaesthetic must be stopped immediately.

Cardiovascular status must be assessed and cardiopulmonary resuscitation procedures must be followed.

In the event of local anaesthetic-induced cardiac arrest, standard cardiopulmonary resuscitation should be initiated immediately. Lidocaine must not be used as anti-arrhythmic therapy.

If the patient does not respond rapidly to standard procedures, 20% lipid emulsion such as *Intralipid*® [unlicensed indication] should be given intravenously at an initial bolus dose of 1.5 mL/kg over 1 minute, followed by an infusion of 15 mL/kg/hour. After 5 minutes, if cardiovascular stability has not been restored or circulation deteriorates, give a maximum of two further bolus doses of 1.5 mL/kg over 1 minute, 5 minutes apart, and increase the infusion rate to 30 mL/kg/hour. Continue infusion until cardiovascular stability and adequate circulation are restored or maximum cumulative dose of 12 mL/kg is given.

Standard cardiopulmonary resuscitation must be maintained throughout lipid emulsion treatment.

Propofol is not a suitable alternative to lipid emulsion.

Further advice on ongoing treatment should be obtained from the National Poisons Information Service.

Detailed treatment algorithms and accompanying notes are available at www.toxbase.org *or* can be found in the

Association of Anaesthetists of Great Britain and Ireland safety guideline, Management of Severe Local Anaesthetic Toxicity and Management of Severe Local Anaesthetic Toxicity – Accompanying notes.

ANAESTHETICS, LOCAL

Adrenaline with articaine hydrochloride

(Carticaine hydrochloride with epinephrine)

● **INDICATIONS AND DOSE**

Infiltration anaesthesia in dentistry

▶ BY REGIONAL ADMINISTRATION

▸ Child 4-17 years: Consult expert dental sources

DOSES AT EXTREMES OF BODY-WEIGHT

To avoid excessive dosage in obese patients, dose should be calculated on the basis of ideal body-weight.

> IMPORTANT SAFETY INFORMATION
>
> Should only be administered by, or under the direct supervision of, personnel experienced in their use, with adequate training in anaesthesia and airway management, and should not be administered parenterally unless adequate resuscitation equipment is available.
>
> Adrenaline/epinephrine must be used in a low concentration when administered with a local anaesthetic. The total dose of adrenaline should not exceed 5 micrograms/kg (1 mL/kg of a 1 in 200 000 solution) and it is essential not to exceed a concentration of 1 in 200 000 (5 micrograms/mL) if more than 50 mL of the mixture is to be injected.

● **CONTRA-INDICATIONS** Application to damaged skin · application to the middle ear (may cause ototoxicity) · complete heart block · injection into infected tissues · injection into inflamed tissues · preparations containing preservatives should not be used for caudal, epidural, or spinal block, or for intravenous regional anaesthesia (Bier's block)

CONTRA-INDICATIONS, FURTHER INFORMATION

▸ Injection site Local anaesthetics should not be injected into inflamed or infected tissues nor should they be applied to damaged skin. Increased absorption into the blood increases the possibility of systemic side-effects, and the local anaesthetic effect may also be reduced by altered local pH.

● **CAUTIONS** Arrhythmias · cardiovascular disease · cerebrovascular disease · children (consider dose reduction) · cor pulmonale · debilitated patients (consider dose reduction) · diabetes mellitus · epilepsy · hypercalcaemia · hyperreflexia · hypertension · hyperthyroidism · hypokalaemia · hypovolaemia · impaired cardiac conduction · impaired respiratory function · ischaemic heart disease · myasthenia gravis · obstructive cardiomyopathy · occlusive vascular disease · organic brain damage · phaeochromocytoma · prostate disorders · psychoneurosis · severe angina · shock · susceptibility to angle-closure glaucoma

CAUTIONS, FURTHER INFORMATION

▸ Use of vasoconstrictors In patients with severe hypertension or unstable cardiac rhythm, the use of adrenaline with a local anaesthetic may be hazardous. For these patients an anaesthetic without adrenaline should be used.

● **INTERACTIONS** → Appendix 1: articaine, sympathomimetics, vasoconstrictor

● **SIDE-EFFECTS** Angina · angle-closure glaucoma · anorexia · anxiety · arrhythmias · blurred vision · cardiac arrest · cold

15

Anaesthesia

extremities · confusion · convulsions · difficulty in micturition · dizziness · drowsiness · dry mouth · dyspnoea · feeling of inebriation · headache · hyperglycaemia · hypersalavation · hypertension (risk of cerebral haemorrhage) · hypokalaemia · insomnia · lightheadedness · metabolic acidosis · methaemoglobinaemia · muscle twitching · mydriasis · myocardial depression (resulting in hypotension and bradycardia) · myocardial infarction · nausea · numbness of the tongue and perioral region · pallor · palpitation · paraesthesia (including sensations of hot and cold) · peripheral vasodilatation (resulting in hypotension and bradycardia) · psychosis · pulmonary oedema (on excessive dosage or extreme sensitivity) · restlessness · sweating · tachycardia · tinnitus · tissue necrosis at injection site and of extremities, bowel, liver and kidneys · transient excitation (followed by depression with drowsiness, respiratory failure, unconsciousness, and coma) · tremor · urinary retention · vomiting · weakness
SIDE-EFFECTS, FURTHER INFORMATION
▸ Toxic effects Toxic effects after administration of local anaesthetics are a result of excessively high plasma concentrations; severe toxicity usually results from inadvertent intravascular injection or too rapid injection.

Following most regional anaesthetic procedures, maximum arterial plasma concentration of anaesthetic develops within about 10 to 25 minutes, so careful surveillance for toxic effects is necessary during the first 30 minutes after injection.

The systemic toxicity of local anaesthetics mainly involves the central nervous and cardiovascular systems.

● **ALLERGY AND CROSS-SENSITIVITY**
Hypersensitivity reactions occur mainly with the ester-type local anaesthetics, such as tetracaine and chloroprocaine; reactions are less frequent with the amide types, such as articaine, bupivacaine, levobupivacaine, lidocaine, mepivacaine, prilocaine, and ropivacaine. Cross-sensitivity reactions may be avoided by using the alternative chemical type.

● **PREGNANCY** Use only if potential benefit outweighs risk—no information available.

● **BREAST FEEDING** Avoid breast-feeding for 48 hours after administration.

● **HEPATIC IMPAIRMENT** Use with caution; increased risk of side-effects in severe impairment.

● **RENAL IMPAIRMENT** Manufacturers advise use with caution in severe impairment.

● **MONITORING REQUIREMENTS** Consider monitoring blood pressure and ECG (advised with systemic adrenaline/epinephrine).

● **MEDICINAL FORMS**
There can be variation in the licensing of different medicines containing the same drug.

Solution for injection
EXCIPIENTS: May contain Sulfites
▸ Septanest (Septodont Ltd)
Adrenaline (as Adrenaline acid tartrate) 10 microgram per 1 ml, Articaine hydrochloride 40 mg per 1 ml Septanest 1 in 100,000 solution for injection cartridges | 50 cartridge PoM no price available
Adrenaline (as Adrenaline acid tartrate) 5 microgram per 1 ml, Articaine hydrochloride 40 mg per 1 ml Septanest 1 in 200,000 solution for injection cartridges | 50 cartridge PoM no price available

Bupivacaine hydrochloride

● **INDICATIONS AND DOSE**
Surgical anaesthesia | Acute pain
▸ BY REGIONAL ADMINISTRATION
▸ Child: Doses adjusted according to child's physical status and nature of procedure, seek expert advice (consult product literature or local protocols)

DOSES AT EXTREMES OF BODY-WEIGHT
To avoid excessive dosage in obese patients, dose should be calculated on the basis of ideal body-weight.

IMPORTANT SAFETY INFORMATION
The licensed doses stated may not be appropriate in some settings and expert advice should be sought.

Should only be administered by, or under the direct supervision of, personnel experienced in their use, with adequate training in anaesthesia and airway management, and should not be administered parenterally unless adequate resuscitation equipment is available.

● **CONTRA-INDICATIONS** Application to the middle ear (can cause ototoxicity) · avoid injection into infected tissues · avoid injection into inflamed tissues · complete heart block · preparations containing preservatives should not be used for caudal, epidural, or spinal block, or for intravenous regional anaesthesia (Bier's block) · should not be applied to damaged skin

CONTRA-INDICATIONS, FURTHER INFORMATION
▸ Injection site Local anaesthetics should not be injected into inflamed or infected tissues nor should they be applied to damaged skin. Increased absorption into the blood increases the possibility of systemic side-effects, and the local anaesthetic effect may also be reduced by altered local pH.

● **CAUTIONS** Cardiovascular disease · cerebral atheroma · children (consider dose reduction) · debilitated patients (consider dose reduction) · epilepsy · hypertension · hypotension · hypovolaemia · impaired cardiac conduction · impaired respiratory function · myasthenia gravis · myocardial depression may be more severe and more resistant to treatment · shock

● **INTERACTIONS** → Appendix 1: anaesthetics, local

● **SIDE-EFFECTS** Arrhythmias · blurred vision · cardiac arrest · convulsions · dizziness · drowsiness · feeling of inebriation · headache · lightheadedness · muscle twitching · myocardial depression (resulting in hypotension and bradycardia) · nausea · numbness of the tongue and perioral region · paraesthesia (including sensations of hot and cold) · peripheral vasodilatation (resulting in hypotension and bradycardia) · restlessness · tinnitus · transient excitation (followed by depression with drowsiness, respiratory failure, unconsciousness, and coma) · tremors · vomiting
SIDE-EFFECTS, FURTHER INFORMATION
▸ Toxic effects Toxic effects after administration of local anaesthetics are a result of excessively high plasma concentrations; severe toxicity usually results from inadvertent intravascular injection or too rapid injection.

Following most regional anaesthetic procedures, maximum arterial plasma concentration of anaesthetic develops within about 10 to 25 minutes, so careful surveillance for toxic effects is necessary during the first 30 minutes after injection.

The systemic toxicity of local anaesthetics mainly involves the central nervous and cardiovascular systems.

● **ALLERGY AND CROSS-SENSITIVITY**
Hypersensitivity reactions occur mainly with the ester-type local anaesthetics, such as tetracaine and

chloroprocaine; reactions are less frequent with the amide types, such as articaine, bupivacaine, levobupivacaine, lidocaine, mepivacaine, prilocaine, and ropivacaine. Cross-sensitivity reactions may be avoided by using the alternative chemical type.

- **PREGNANCY** Use lower doses for intrathecal use during late pregnancy. Large doses during delivery can cause neonatal respiratory depression, hypotonia, and bradycardia after epidural block.
- **BREAST FEEDING** Amount too small to be harmful.
- **HEPATIC IMPAIRMENT** Use with caution in severe impairment.
- **RENAL IMPAIRMENT** Use with caution in severe impairment.

- **MEDICINAL FORMS**
There can be variation in the licensing of different medicines containing the same drug. Forms available from special-order manufacturers include: solution for injection, infusion, solution for infusion

Solution for injection
▸ Bupivacaine hydrochloride (Non-proprietary)
Bupivacaine hydrochloride 2.5 mg per 1 ml Bupivacaine 0.25% solution for injection 10ml Sure-Amp ampoules | 20 ampoule PoM £17.50
Bupivacaine hydrochloride 5 mg per 1 ml Bupivacaine 0.5% solution for injection 10ml Sure-Amp ampoules | 20 ampoule PoM £18.30
Bupivacaine 50mg/10ml (0.5%) solution for injection ampoules | 10 ampoule PoM no price available
▸ Marcain (Aspen Pharma Trading Ltd)
Bupivacaine hydrochloride 2.5 mg per 1 ml Marcain 0.25% solution for injection 10ml Polyamp Steripack ampoules | 5 ampoule PoM £7.92
Bupivacaine hydrochloride 5 mg per 1 ml Marcain 0.5% solution for injection 10ml Polyamp Steripack ampoules | 5 ampoule PoM £9.25

Infusion
▸ Bupivacaine hydrochloride (Non-proprietary)
Bupivacaine hydrochloride 1 mg per 1 ml Bupivacaine 100mg/100ml (0.1%) infusion bags | 20 bag PoM no price available
Bupivacaine 250mg/250ml (0.1%) infusion bags | 20 bag PoM no price available
Bupivacaine hydrochloride 1.25 mg per 1 ml Bupivacaine 312.5mg/250ml (0.125%) infusion bags | 20 bag PoM no price available

Bupivacaine with adrenaline

The properties listed below are those particular to the combination only. For the properties of the components please consider, bupivacaine hydrochloride p. 794, adrenaline/epinephrine p. 132.

- **INDICATIONS AND DOSE**
Surgical anaesthesia
▸ BY LUMBAR EPIDURAL, OR BY LOCAL INFILTRATION, OR BY CAUDAL EPIDURAL
▸ Child 12-17 years: (consult product literature)

Acute pain management
▸ BY LUMBAR EPIDURAL, OR BY LOCAL INFILTRATION
▸ Child 1-17 years: (consult product literature)

IMPORTANT SAFETY INFORMATION
Adrenaline/epinephrine must be used in a low concentration when administered with a local anaesthetic. The total dose of adrenaline should not exceed 5 micrograms/kg (1 mL/kg of a 1 in 200 000 solution) and it is essential not to exceed a concentration of 1 in 200 000 (5 micrograms/mL) if more than 50 mL of the mixture is to be injected.

- **CAUTIONS**
CAUTIONS, FURTHER INFORMATION
In patients with severe hypertension or unstable cardiac rhythm, the use of adrenaline with a local anaesthetic may be hazardous. For these patients an anaesthetic without adrenaline should be used.
- **INTERACTIONS** → Appendix 1: anaesthetics, local, sympathomimetics, vasoconstrictor

- **MEDICINAL FORMS**
There can be variation in the licensing of different medicines containing the same drug.
Solution for injection
▸ Bupivacaine with adrenaline (Non-proprietary)
Adrenaline (as Adrenaline acid tartrate) 5 microgram per 1 ml, Bupivacaine hydrochloride 2.5 mg per 1 ml Bupivacaine 25mg/10ml (0.25%) / Adrenaline (base) 50micrograms/10ml (1 in 200,000) solution for injection ampoules | 10 ampoule PoM £40.00
Adrenaline (as Adrenaline acid tartrate) 5 microgram per 1 ml, Bupivacaine hydrochloride anhydrous 2.5 mg per 1 ml Carbostesin-adrenaline 0.25% / 100micrograms/20ml (1 in 200,000) solution for injection ampoules | 1 ampoule PoM no price available
Carbostesin-adrenaline 0.25% / 25micrograms/5ml (1 in 200,000) solution for injection ampoules | 1 ampoule PoM no price available
Adrenaline (as Adrenaline acid tartrate) 5 microgram per 1 ml, Bupivacaine hydrochloride 5 mg per 1 ml Bupivacaine 50mg/10ml (0.5%) / Adrenaline (base) 50micrograms/10ml (1 in 200,000) solution for injection ampoules | 10 ampoule PoM £45.00
Adrenaline (as Adrenaline acid tartrate) 5 microgram per 1 ml, Bupivacaine hydrochloride anhydrous 5 mg per 1 ml Carbostesin-adrenaline 0.5% / 25micrograms/5ml (1 in 200,000) solution for injection ampoules | 1 ampoule PoM no price available
Carbostesin-adrenaline 0.5% / 100micrograms/20ml (1 in 200,000) solution for injection ampoules | 1 ampoule PoM no price available

Levobupivacaine

- **INDICATIONS AND DOSE**
Surgical anaesthesia | Acute pain
▸ BY REGIONAL ADMINISTRATION
▸ Child: Doses adjusted according to child's physical status and nature of procedure, seek expert advice (consult product literature or local protocols)

DOSES AT EXTREMES OF BODY-WEIGHT
To avoid excessive dosage in obese patients, dose should be calculated on the basis of ideal body-weight.

- **UNLICENSED USE** Not licensed for use in children except for analgesia by ilioinguinal or iliohypogastric block.

IMPORTANT SAFETY INFORMATION
The licensed doses stated may not be appropriate in some settings and expert advice should be sought.
    Should only be administered by, or under the direct supervision of, personnel experienced in their use, with adequate training in anaesthesia and airway management, and should not be administered parenterally unless adequate resuscitation equipment is available.

- **CONTRA-INDICATIONS** Application to the middle ear (can cause ototoxicity) · avoid injection into infected tissues · avoid injection into inflamed tissues · complete heart block · preparations containing preservatives should not be used for caudal, epidural, or spinal block, or for intravenous regional anaesthesia (Bier's block) · should not be applied to damaged skin
CONTRA-INDICATIONS, FURTHER INFORMATION
▸ Injection site Local anaesthetics should not be injected into inflamed or infected tissues nor should they be applied to damaged skin. Increased absorption into the blood increases the possibility of systemic side-effects, and the

15

Anaesthesia

local anaesthetic effect may also be reduced by altered local pH.

- **CAUTIONS** Cardiovascular disease · children (consider dose reduction) · debilitated patients (consider dose reduction) · epilepsy · hypovolaemia · impaired cardiac conduction · impaired respiratory function · myasthenia gravis · shock
- **INTERACTIONS** → Appendix 1: anaesthetics, local
- **SIDE-EFFECTS** Anaemia · arrhythmias · blurred vision · cardiac arrest · convulsions · dizziness · drowsiness · feeling of inebriation · headache · lightheadedness · muscle twitching · myocardial depression (resulting in hypotension and bradycardia) · nausea · numbness of the tongue and perioral region · paraesthesia (including sensations of hot and cold) · peripheral vasodilatation (resulting in hypotension and bradycardia) · pyrexia · restlessness · sweating · tinnitus · transient excitation (followed by depression with drowsiness, respiratory failure, unconsciousness, and coma) · tremors · vomiting
  SIDE-EFFECTS, FURTHER INFORMATION
  ‣ Toxic effects Toxic effects after administration of local anaesthetics are a result of excessively high plasma concentrations; severe toxicity usually results from inadvertent intravascular injection or too rapid injection.
  Following most regional anaesthetic procedures, maximum arterial plasma concentration of anaesthetic develops within about 10 to 25 minutes, so careful surveillance for toxic effects is necessary during the first 30 minutes after injection.
  The systemic toxicity of local anaesthetics mainly involves the central nervous and cardiovascular systems.
- **ALLERGY AND CROSS-SENSITIVITY**
  Hypersensitivity reactions occur mainly with the ester-type local anaesthetics, such as tetracaine and chloroprocaine; reactions are less frequent with the amide types, such as articaine, bupivacaine, levobupivacaine, lidocaine, mepivacaine, prilocaine, and ropivacaine. Cross-sensitivity reactions may be avoided by using the alternative chemical type.
- **PREGNANCY** Large doses during delivery can cause neonatal respiratory depression, hypotonia, and bradycardia after epidural block. Avoid if possible in the first trimester—toxicity in *animal* studies. May cause fetal distress syndrome. Do not use for paracervical block in obstetrics. Do not use 7.5 mg/mL strength in obstetrics.
- **BREAST FEEDING** Amount too small to be harmful.
- **HEPATIC IMPAIRMENT** Use with caution.
- **DIRECTIONS FOR ADMINISTRATION** For 1.25 mg/mL concentration dilute standard solutions with sodium chloride 0.9%.
- **PRESCRIBING AND DISPENSING INFORMATION**
  Levobupivacaine is an isomer of bupivacaine.

- **MEDICINAL FORMS**
  There can be variation in the licensing of different medicines containing the same drug.
  Solution for injection
  ‣ Chirocaine (AbbVie Ltd)
  Levobupivacaine (as Levobupivacaine hydrochloride) 2.5 mg per 1 ml Chirocaine 25mg/10ml solution for injection ampoules | 10 ampoule [PoM] £14.11 (Hospital only)
  Levobupivacaine (as Levobupivacaine hydrochloride) 5 mg per 1 ml Chirocaine 50mg/10ml solution for injection ampoules | 10 ampoule [PoM] £16.15 (Hospital only)
  Levobupivacaine (as Levobupivacaine hydrochloride) 7.5 mg per 1 ml Chirocaine 75mg/10ml solution for injection ampoules | 10 ampoule [PoM] £24.23 (Hospital only)
  Infusion
  ‣ Chirocaine (AbbVie Ltd)
  Levobupivacaine (as Levobupivacaine hydrochloride) 1.25 mg per 1 ml Chirocaine 125mg/100ml infusion bags | 24 bag [PoM] £174.22 Chirocaine 250mg/200ml infusion bags | 12 bag [PoM] no price available

Lidocaine hydrochloride
(Lignocaine hydrochloride)

- **INDICATIONS AND DOSE**
  Infiltration anaesthesia
  ▸ BY LOCAL INFILTRATION

  ‣ Neonate: Up to 3 mg/kg, dose to be given according to patient's weight and nature of procedure, dose may be repeated not more often than every 4 hours, 3 mg/kg equivalent to 0.3 mL/kg of 1% solution.

  ‣ Child 1 month–11 years: Up to 3 mg/kg, dose to be given according to patient's weight and nature of procedure, dose may be repeated not more often than every 4 hours, 3 mg/kg equivalent to 0.3 mL/kg of 1% solution
  ‣ Child 12–17 years: (max. per dose 200 mg), dose to be given according to child's weight and nature of procedure, dose may be repeated not more often than every 4 hours

  DOSES AT EXTREMES OF BODY-WEIGHT
  ‣ When used by local infiltration To avoid excessive dosage in obese patients, weight-based doses for non-emergency indications may need to be calculated on the basis of ideal body-weight.
  Intravenous regional anaesthesia and nerve block
  ▸ BY REGIONAL ADMINISTRATION
  ‣ Child: Seek expert advice
  Dental anaesthesia
  ▸ BY REGIONAL ADMINISTRATION
  ‣ Child: Seek expert advice
  Pain relief (in anal fissures, haemorrhoids, pruritus ani, pruritus vulvae, herpes zoster, or herpes labialis) | **Lubricant in cystoscopy** | **Lubricant in proctoscopy**
  ▸ TO THE SKIN USING OINTMENT
  ‣ Child: Apply 1–2 mL as required, avoid long-term use
  LMX 4®
  Anaesthesia before venous cannulation or venepuncture
  ▸ TO THE SKIN
  ‣ Child 1–2 months: Apply up to 1 g, apply thick layer to small area (2.5 cm × 2.5 cm) of non-irritated skin at least 30 minutes before procedure; may be applied under an occlusive dressing; max. application time 60 minutes, remove cream with gauze and perform procedure after approximately 5 minutes
  ‣ Child 3–11 months: Apply up to 1 g, apply thick layer to small area (2.5 cm × 2.5 cm) of non-irritated skin at least 30 minutes before procedure; may be applied under an occlusive dressing; max. application time 4 hours, remove cream with gauze and perform procedure after approximately 5 minutes
  ‣ Child 1–17 years: Apply 1–2.5 g, apply thick layer to small area (2.5 cm × 2.5 cm) of non-irritated skin at least 30 minutes before procedure; may be applied under an occlusive dressing; max. application time 5 hours, remove cream with gauze and perform procedure after approximately 5 minutes

IMPORTANT SAFETY INFORMATION
▸ When used by local infiltration
The licensed doses stated may not be appropriate in some settings and expert advice should be sought. Should only be administered by, or under the direct supervision of, personnel experienced in their use, with adequate training in anaesthesia and airway management, and should not be administered parenterally unless adequate resuscitation equipment is available.

- **CONTRA-INDICATIONS**
▸ When used by regional administration Application to the middle ear (can cause ototoxicity) · avoid injection into infected tissues · avoid injection into inflamed tissues · preparations containing preservatives should not be used for caudal, epidural, or spinal block, or for intravenous regional anaesthesia (Bier's block) · should not be applied to damaged skin

  CONTRA-INDICATIONS, FURTHER INFORMATION
▸ When used by regional administration Local anaesthetics should not be injected into inflamed or infected tissues nor should they be applied to damaged skin. Increased absorption into the blood increases the possibility of systemic side-effects, and the local anaesthetic effect may also be reduced by altered local pH.

- **CAUTIONS**
▸ When used by regional administration Children (consider dose reduction) · debilitated patients (consider dose reduction) · epilepsy · hypovolaemia · impaired cardiac conduction · impaired respiratory function · myasthenia gravis · shock

- **INTERACTIONS** → Appendix 1: antiarrhythmics

- **SIDE-EFFECTS**
▸ Frequency not known
▸ When used by regional administration Transient excitation (followed by depression with drowsiness, respiratory failure, unconsciousness, and coma) · arrhythmias · blurred vision · cardiac arrest · feeling of inebriation · headache · hypoglycaemia (following intrathecal or extradural administration) · methaemoglobinaemia · muscle twitching · myocardial depression (resulting in hypotension and bradycardia) · nausea · numbness of the tongue and perioral region · nystagmus · peripheral vasodilatation (resulting in hypotension and bradycardia) · rash · restlessness · tinnitus · tremors · vomiting

  SIDE-EFFECTS, FURTHER INFORMATION
▸ Topical application A single application of a topical lidocaine preparation does not generally cause systemic side-effects.
▸ Toxic effects
▸ When used by regional administration Toxic effects after administration of local anaesthetics are a result of excessively high plasma concentrations; severe toxicity usually results from inadvertent intravascular injection or too rapid injection. Following most regional anaesthetic procedures, maximum arterial plasma concentration of anaesthetic develops within about 10 to 25 minutes, so careful surveillance for toxic effects is necessary during the first 30 minutes after injection. The systemic toxicity of local anaesthetics mainly involves the central nervous and cardiovascular systems.
▸ Methaemoglobinaemia
▸ When used by regional administration Methaemoglobinaemia can be treated with an intravenous injection of methylthioninium chloride; neonates and infants under 6 months are particularly susceptible to methaemoglobinaemia.

- **ALLERGY AND CROSS-SENSITIVITY**
Hypersensitivity reactions occur mainly with the ester-type local anaesthetics, such as tetracaine and chloroprocaine; reactions are less frequent with the amide types, such as articaine, bupivacaine, levobupivacaine, lidocaine, mepivacaine, prilocaine, and ropivacaine. Cross-sensitivity reactions may be avoided by using the alternative chemical type.

- **PREGNANCY** Crosses the placenta but not known to be harmful in *animal* studies—use if benefit outweighs risk. When used as a local anaesthetic, large doses can cause fetal bradycardia; if given during delivery can also cause neonatal respiratory depression, hypotonia, or bradycardia after paracervical or epidural block.

- **BREAST FEEDING** Present in milk but amount too small to be harmful.

- **HEPATIC IMPAIRMENT** Caution—increased risk of side-effects.

- **RENAL IMPAIRMENT** Possible accumulation of lidocaine and active metabolite; caution in severe impairment.

- **MONITORING REQUIREMENTS**
▸ With systemic use Monitor ECG and have resuscitation facilities available.

- **MEDICINAL FORMS**
There can be variation in the licensing of different medicines containing the same drug. Forms available from special-order manufacturers include: solution for injection

Solution for injection
▸ **Lidocaine hydrochloride (Non-proprietary)**
  Lidocaine hydrochloride 5 mg per 1 ml Lidocaine 50mg/10ml (0.5%) solution for injection ampoules | 10 ampoule [PoM] £7.00
  Lidocaine hydrochloride 10 mg per 1 ml Lidocaine 100mg/10ml (1%) solution for injection Mini-Plasco ampoules | 20 ampoule [PoM] £10.89
  Lidocaine 100mg/10ml (1%) solution for injection ampoules | 10 ampoule [PoM] £4.40 DT price = £4.36
  Lidocaine 100mg/10ml (1%) solution for injection Sure-Amp ampoules | 20 ampoule [PoM] £8.80
  Lidocaine 200mg/10ml (1%) solution for injection vials | 10 vial [PoM] £19.00
  Lidocaine 200mg/20ml (1%) solution for injection ampoules | 10 ampoule [PoM] £7.00–£9.63 DT price = £9.63
  Lidocaine 50mg/5ml (1%) solution for injection ampoules | 10 ampoule [PoM] £2.57–£3.10 DT price = £2.57
  Lidocaine 20mg/2ml (1%) solution for injection ampoules | 10 ampoule [PoM] £3.50 DT price = £2.18
  Lidocaine 50mg/5ml (1%) solution for injection Sure-Amp ampoules | 20 ampoule [PoM] £6.00
  Lidocaine hydrochloride 20 mg per 1 ml Lidocaine 100mg/5ml (2%) solution for injection ampoules | 10 ampoule [PoM] £2.67–£3.80 DT price = £2.67
  Lidocaine 400mg/20ml (2%) solution for injection vials | 10 vial [PoM] £19.50
  Lidocaine 200mg/10ml (2%) solution for injection Mini-Plasco ampoules | 20 ampoule [PoM] £14.52
  Lidocaine 40mg/2ml (2%) solution for injection ampoules | 10 ampoule [PoM] £4.00 DT price = £2.34
  Lidocaine 100mg/5ml (2%) solution for injection Sure-Amp ampoules | 20 ampoule [PoM] £6.00
  Lidocaine 400mg/20ml (2%) solution for injection ampoules | 10 ampoule [PoM] £8.00–£9.90 DT price = £9.90

Cream
EXCIPIENTS: May contain Benzyl alcohol, propylene glycol
▸ **LMX 4** (Ferndale Pharmaceuticals Ltd)
  Lidocaine 40 mg per 1 gram LMX 4 cream | 5 gram [P] £2.98 DT price = £2.98 | 30 gram [P] £14.90 DT price = £14.90

Ointment
▸ **Lidocaine hydrochloride (Non-proprietary)**
  Lidocaine hydrochloride 50 mg per 1 gram Lidocaine 5% ointment | 15 gram [P] £6.50 DT price = £6.18

Lidocaine with adrenaline

The properties listed below are those particular to the combination only. For the properties of the components please consider, lidocaine hydrochloride p. 796, adrenaline/epinephrine p. 132.

- **INDICATIONS AND DOSE**
Local anaesthesia
▸ BY LOCAL INFILTRATION
▸ Child 12-17 years: Dosed according to the type of nerve block required (consult product literature)

IMPORTANT SAFETY INFORMATION
Adrenaline/epinephrine must be used in a low concentration when administered with a local anaesthetic. The total dose of adrenaline should not exceed 5 micrograms/kg (1 mL/kg of a 1 in 200 000 solution) and it is essential not to exceed a

15

Anaesthesia

concentration of 1 in 200 000 (5 micrograms/mL) if more than 50 mL of the mixture is to be injected.

- **INTERACTIONS** → Appendix 1: antiarrhythmics, sympathomimetics, vasoconstrictor
- **PROFESSION SPECIFIC INFORMATION**

Dental information
A variety of lidocaine injections with adrenaline is available in dental cartridges.
Consult expert dental sources for specific advice in relation to dose of lidocaine for dental anaesthesia.

- **MEDICINAL FORMS**
There can be variation in the licensing of different medicines containing the same drug. Forms available from special-order manufacturers include: solution for injection

Solution for injection
EXCIPIENTS: May contain Sulfites
- Lignospan Special (Kent Pharmaceuticals Ltd)
Adrenaline (as Adrenaline acid tartrate) 12.5 microgram per 1 ml, Lidocaine hydrochloride 20 mg per 1 ml Lignospan Special 2% injection 2.2ml cartridges | 50 cartridge [PoM] £19.95
- Rexocaine (Henry Schein Ltd)
Adrenaline (as Adrenaline acid tartrate) 12.5 microgram per 1 ml, Lidocaine hydrochloride 20 mg per 1 ml Rexocaine 2% injection 2.2ml cartridges | 50 cartridge [PoM] no price available
- Xylocaine with Adrenaline (Aspen Pharma Trading Ltd)
Adrenaline (as Adrenaline acid tartrate) 5 microgram per 1 ml, Lidocaine hydrochloride 10 mg per 1 ml Xylocaine 1% with Adrenaline 100micrograms/20ml (1 in 200,000) solution for injection vials | 5 vial [PoM] £9.66 DT price = £9.66
Adrenaline (as Adrenaline acid tartrate) 5 microgram per 1 ml, Lidocaine hydrochloride 20 mg per 1 ml Xylocaine 2% with Adrenaline 100micrograms/20ml (1 in 200,000) solution for injection vials | 5 vial [PoM] £8.85 DT price = £8.85

Lidocaine with phenylephrine

The properties listed below are those particular to the combination only. For the properties of the components please consider, lidocaine hydrochloride p. 796, phenylephrine hydrochloride p. 121.

- **INDICATIONS AND DOSE**

Anaesthesia before nasal surgery, endoscopy, laryngoscopy, or removal of foreign bodies from the nose
▸ BY INTRANASAL ADMINISTRATION
‣ Child 12-17 years: Up to 8 sprays

- **INTERACTIONS** → Appendix 1: antiarrhythmics, sympathomimetics, vasoconstrictor

- **MEDICINAL FORMS**
There can be variation in the licensing of different medicines containing the same drug.

Spray
▸ Lidocaine with phenylephrine (Non-proprietary)
Phenylephrine hydrochloride 5 mg per 1 ml, Lidocaine hydrochloride 50 mg per 1 ml Lidocaine 5% / Phenylephrine 0.5% nasal spray | 2.5 ml [PoM] £12.99 DT price = £12.27

Lidocaine with prilocaine

14-Jun-2017

The properties listed below are those particular to the combination only. For the properties of the components please consider, lidocaine hydrochloride p. 796, prilocaine hydrochloride p. 800.

- **INDICATIONS AND DOSE**

Anaesthesia before minor skin procedures including venepuncture
▸ TO THE SKIN

‣ Neonate: Apply up to 1 g for maximum 1 hour before procedure, to be applied under occlusive dressing, shorter application time of 15–30 minutes is recommended for children with atopic dermatitis (30 minutes before removal of mollusca); maximum 1 dose per day.

‣ Child 1-2 months: Apply up to 1 g for maximum 1 hour before procedure, to be applied under occlusive dressing, shorter application time of 15–30 minutes is recommended for children with atopic dermatitis (30 minutes before removal of mollusca); maximum 1 dose per day

‣ Child 3-11 months: Apply up to 2 g for maximum 1 hour before procedure, to be applied under occlusive dressing, shorter application time of 15–30 minutes is recommended for children with atopic dermatitis (30 minutes before removal of mollusca); maximum 2 doses per day

‣ Child 1-11 years: Apply 1–5 hours before procedure, a thick layer should be applied under occlusive dressing, shorter application time of 15–30 minutes is recommended for children with atopic dermatitis (30 minutes before removal of mollusca); maximum 2 doses per day

‣ Child 12-17 years: Apply 1–5 hours before procedure (2–5 hours before procedures on large areas e.g. split skin grafting), a thick layer should be applied under occlusive dressing, shorter application time of 15–30 minutes is recommended for children with atopic dermatitis (30 minutes before removal of mollusca)

Anaesthesia on genital skin before injection of local anaesthetics
▸ TO THE SKIN
‣ Child 12-17 years: Apply under occlusive dressing for 15 minutes (males) or 60 minutes (females) before procedure

Anaesthesia before surgical treatment of lesions on genital mucosa
▸ TO THE SKIN
‣ Child 12-17 years: Apply up to 10 g, to be applied 5–10 minutes before procedure, maximum dose should be proportionally reduced in adolescents with body-weight less than 20 kg

Anaesthesia before cervical curettage
▸ TO THE SKIN
‣ Child 12-17 years: Apply 10 g in lateral vaginal fornices for 10 minutes

- **CONTRA-INDICATIONS** Use in child less than 37 weeks corrected gestational age
- **INTERACTIONS** → Appendix 1: anaesthetics, local, antiarrhythmics
- **PATIENT AND CARER ADVICE**
Medicines for Children leaflet: EMLA cream for local anaesthesia www.medicinesforchildren.org.uk/emla-cream-for-local-anaesthesia

- **MEDICINAL FORMS**
  There can be variation in the licensing of different medicines containing the same drug.
  Cream
  - Lidocaine with prilocaine (Non-proprietary)
    Lidocaine 25 mg per 1 gram, Prilocaine 25 mg per 1 gram Lidocaine 2.5% / Prilocaine 2.5% cream | 5 gram P no price available
  - Denela (Teva UK Ltd)
    Lidocaine 25 mg per 1 gram, Prilocaine 25 mg per 1 gram Denela 5% cream | 5 gram P £2.84–£3.29 | 25 gram P £12.99 | 30 gram P £14.75 DT price = £12.30
  - Emla (Aspen Pharma Trading Ltd)
    Lidocaine 25 mg per 1 gram, Prilocaine 25 mg per 1 gram Emla 5% cream | 5 gram P £2.25–£2.99 | 25 gram P £11.70 | 30 gram P £12.30 DT price = £12.30

Mepivacaine hydrochloride

- **INDICATIONS AND DOSE**
  Infiltration anaesthesia and nerve block in dentistry
  - Child 3-17 years: Consult expert dental sources
  DOSES AT EXTREMES OF BODY-WEIGHT
  To avoid excessive dosage in obese patients, dose should be calculated on the basis of ideal body-weight.

  IMPORTANT SAFETY INFORMATION
  Should only be administered by, or under the direct supervision of, personnel experienced in their use, with adequate training in anaesthesia and airway management, and should not be administered parenterally unless adequate resuscitation equipment is available.

- **CONTRA-INDICATIONS** Application to the middle ear (can cause ototoxicity) · avoid injection into infected tissues · avoid injection into inflamed tissues · complete heart block · preparations containing preservatives should not be used for caudal, epidural, or spinal block, or for intravenous regional anaesthesia (Bier's block) · should not be applied to damaged skin
  CONTRA-INDICATIONS, FURTHER INFORMATION
  - Injection site Local anaesthetics should not be injected into inflamed or infected tissues nor should they be applied to damaged skin. Increased absorption into the blood increases the possibility of systemic side-effects, and the local anaesthetic effect may also be reduced by altered local pH.
- **CAUTIONS** Cardiovascular disease · children (consider dose reduction) · debilitated patients (consider dose reduction) · epilepsy · hypovolaemia · impaired cardiac conduction · impaired respiratory function · myasthenia gravis · shock
- **INTERACTIONS** → Appendix 1: anaesthetics, local
- **SIDE-EFFECTS** Arrhythmias · blurred vision · cardiac arrest · convulsions · dizziness · drowsiness · feeling of inebriation · headache · lightheadedness · muscle twitching · myocardial depression (resulting in hypotension and bradycardia) · nausea · numbness of the tongue and perioral region · paraesthesia (including sensations of hot and cold) · peripheral vasodilatation (resulting in hypotension and bradycardia) · restlessness · tinnitus · transient excitation (followed by depression with drowsiness, respiratory failure, unconsciousness, and coma) · tremors · vomiting
  SIDE-EFFECTS, FURTHER INFORMATION
  - Toxic effects Toxic effects after administration of local anaesthetics are a result of excessively high plasma concentrations; severe toxicity usually results from inadvertent intravascular injection or too rapid injection.
    Following most regional anaesthetic procedures, maximum arterial plasma concentration of anaesthetic

develops within about 10 to 25 minutes, so careful surveillance for toxic effects is necessary during the first 30 minutes after injection.
  The systemic toxicity of local anaesthetics mainly involves the central nervous and cardiovascular systems.

- **ALLERGY AND CROSS-SENSITIVITY**
  Hypersensitivity reactions occur mainly with the ester-type local anaesthetics, such as tetracaine and chloroprocaine; reactions are less frequent with the amide types, such as articaine, bupivacaine, levobupivacaine, lidocaine, mepivacaine, prilocaine, and ropivacaine. Cross-sensitivity reactions may be avoided by using the alternative chemical type.
- **PREGNANCY** Use with caution in early pregnancy.
- **BREAST FEEDING** Use with caution.
- **HEPATIC IMPAIRMENT** Use with caution; increased risk of side-effects in severe impairment.
- **RENAL IMPAIRMENT** Use with caution; increased risk of side-effects.
- **MEDICINAL FORMS**
  There can be variation in the licensing of different medicines containing the same drug.
  Solution for injection
  - Scandonest plain (Deproco UK Ltd)
    Mepivacaine hydrochloride 30 mg per 1 ml Scandonest plain 3% solution for injection 2.2ml cartridges | 50 cartridge PoM no price available

Mepivacaine with adrenaline

The properties listed below are those particular to the combination only. For the properties of the components please consider, mepivacaine hydrochloride above, adrenaline/epinephrine p. 132.

- **INDICATIONS AND DOSE**
  Infiltration anaesthesia and nerve block in dentistry
  - BY LOCAL INFILTRATION
  - Child: (consult product literature)

  IMPORTANT SAFETY INFORMATION
  Adrenaline/epinephrine must be used in a low concentration when administered with a local anaesthetic. The total dose of adrenaline should not exceed 5 micrograms/kg (1 mL/kg of a 1 in 200 000 solution) and it is essential not to exceed a concentration of 1 in 200 000 (5 micrograms/mL) if more than 50 mL of the mixture is to be injected.

- **INTERACTIONS** → Appendix 1: anaesthetics, local, sympathomimetics, vasoconstrictor

- **MEDICINAL FORMS**
  There can be variation in the licensing of different medicines containing the same drug.
  Solution for injection
  EXCIPIENTS: May contain Sulfites
  - Scandonest special (Deproco UK Ltd)
    Adrenaline 10 microgram per 1 ml, Mepivacaine hydrochloride 20 mg per 1 ml Scandonest special 2% solution for injection 2.2ml cartridges | 50 cartridge PoM no price available

15

Anaesthesia

Prilocaine hydrochloride

● **INDICATIONS AND DOSE**

CITANEST 1%®

Infiltration anaesthesia | Nerve block
▶ BY REGIONAL ADMINISTRATION
▶ Child 6 months–11 years: Up to 5 mg/kg, dose adjusted according to site of administration and response; maximum 400 mg per course
▶ Child 12–17 years: 100–200 mg/minute, alternatively, may be given in incremental doses; dose adjusted according to site of administration and response; maximum 400 mg per course

DOSES AT EXTREMES OF BODY-WEIGHT
To avoid excessive dosage in obese patients, dose should be calculated on the basis of ideal body-weight.

IMPORTANT SAFETY INFORMATION
Should only be administered by, or under the direct supervision of, personnel experienced in their use, with adequate training in anaesthesia and airway management, and should not be administered parenterally unless adequate resuscitation equipment is available.

● **CONTRA-INDICATIONS** Acquired methaemoglobinaemia · anaemia · application to the middle ear (can cause ototoxicity) · avoid injection into infected tissues · avoid injection into inflamed tissues · complete heart block · congenital methaemoglobinaemia · preparations containing preservatives should not be used for caudal, epidural, or spinal block, or for intravenous regional anaesthesia (Bier's block) · should not be applied to damaged skin

CONTRA-INDICATIONS, FURTHER INFORMATION
▶ Injection site Local anaesthetics should not be injected into inflamed or infected tissues or should they be applied to damaged skin. Increased absorption into the blood increases the possibility of systemic side-effects, and the local anaesthetic effect may also be reduced by altered local pH.

● **CAUTIONS** Acute porphyrias p. 577 · cardiovascular disease · children (consider dose reduction) · debilitated patients (consider dose reduction) · epilepsy · hypovolaemia · impaired cardiac conduction · impaired respiratory function · myasthenia gravis · neonates and infants under 6 months are particularly susceptible to methaemoglobinaemia · severe or untreated hypertension · shock

● **INTERACTIONS** → Appendix 1: anaesthetics, local

● **SIDE-EFFECTS** Arrhythmias · blurred vision · cardiac arrest · convulsions · dizziness · drowsiness · feeling of inebriation · headache · hypertension · lightheadedness · methaemoglobinaemia (with high doses) · muscle twitching · myocardial depression (resulting in hypotension and bradycardia) · nausea · numbness of the tongue and perioral region · paraesthesia (including sensations of hot and cold) · peripheral vasodilatation (resulting in hypotension and bradycardia) · restlessness · tinnitus · transient excitation (followed by depression with drowsiness, respiratory failure, unconsciousness, and coma) · tremors · vomiting

SIDE-EFFECTS, FURTHER INFORMATION
▶ Toxic effects Toxic effects after administration of local anaesthetics are a result of excessively high plasma concentrations; severe toxicity usually results from inadvertent intravascular injection or too rapid injection.
  Following most regional anaesthetic procedures, maximum arterial plasma concentration of anaesthetic develops within about 10 to 25 minutes, so careful

surveillance for toxic effects is necessary during the first 30 minutes after injection.
  The systemic toxicity of local anaesthetics mainly involves the central nervous and cardiovascular systems.

▶ Methaemoglobinaemia Methaemoglobinaemia can be treated with an intravenous injection of **methylthioninium chloride**.

● **ALLERGY AND CROSS-SENSITIVITY**
Hypersensitivity reactions occur mainly with the ester-type local anaesthetics, such as tetracaine and chloroprocaine; reactions are less frequent with the amide types, such as articaine, bupivacaine, levobupivacaine, lidocaine, mepivacaine, prilocaine, and ropivacaine. Cross-sensitivity reactions may be avoided by using the alternative chemical type.

● **PREGNANCY** Use lower doses for intrathecal use during late pregnancy. Large doses during delivery can cause neonatal respiratory depression, hypotonia, and bradycardia after epidural block. Avoid paracervical or pudendal block in obstetrics (neonatal methaemoglobinaemia reported).

● **BREAST FEEDING** Present in milk but not known to be harmful.

● **HEPATIC IMPAIRMENT** Lower doses may be required for intrathecal anaesthesia. Use with caution.

● **RENAL IMPAIRMENT** Lower doses may be required for intrathecal anaesthesia. Use with caution.

● **MEDICINAL FORMS**
There can be variation in the licensing of different medicines containing the same drug. Forms available from special-order manufacturers include: solution for injection
Solution for injection
▶ Citanest (Aspen Pharma Trading Ltd)
  Prilocaine hydrochloride 10 mg per 1 ml Citanest 1% solution for injection 50ml vials | 1 vial [PoM] £5.06

Prilocaine with felypressin

The properties listed below are those particular to the combination only. For the properties of the components please consider, prilocaine hydrochloride above.

● **INDICATIONS AND DOSE**

Dental anaesthesia
▶ BY REGIONAL ADMINISTRATION
▶ Child: Consult expert dental sources for specific advice

● **INTERACTIONS** → Appendix 1: anaesthetics, local

● **MEDICINAL FORMS**
There can be variation in the licensing of different medicines containing the same drug.
Solution for injection
▶ Citanest with Octapressin (Dentsply Ltd)
  Prilocaine hydrochloride 30 mg per 1 ml, Felypressin.03 unit per 1 ml Citanest 3% with Octapressin Dental 0.054units/1.8ml solution for injection self aspirating cartridges | 100 cartridge [PoM] no price available
  Citanest 3% with Octapressin Dental 0.066units/2.2ml solution for injection self aspirating cartridges | 100 cartridge [PoM] no price available

Ropivacaine hydrochloride

● **INDICATIONS AND DOSE**

Acute pain | Surgical anaesthesia
▶ BY REGIONAL ADMINISTRATION
▶ Child: Adjust according to child's physical status and nature of procedure, seek expert advice

DOSES AT EXTREMES OF BODY-WEIGHT
To avoid excessive dosage in obese patients, dose may need to be calculated on the basis of ideal bodyweight.

● **UNLICENSED USE** 2 mg/mL strength not licensed for use in children under 12 years except for acute pain management by caudal epidural block and continuous epidural infusion. 7.5 mg/mL and 10 mg/mL strengths not licensed for use in children under 12 years.

IMPORTANT SAFETY INFORMATION
Should only be administered by, or under the direct supervision of, personnel experienced in their use, with adequate training in anaesthesia and airway management, and should not be administered parenterally unless adequate resuscitation equipment is available.

● **CONTRA-INDICATIONS** Application to the middle ear (can cause ototoxicity) · avoid injection into infected tissues · avoid injection into inflamed tissues · complete heart block · preparations containing preservatives should not be used for caudal, epidural, or spinal block, or for intravenous regional anaesthesia (Bier's block) · should not be applied to damaged skin

CONTRA-INDICATIONS, FURTHER INFORMATION
▶ Injection site Local anaesthetics should not be injected into inflamed or infected tissues nor should they be applied to damaged skin. Increased absorption into the blood increases the possibility of systemic side-effects, and the local anaesthetic effect may also be reduced by altered local pH.

● **CAUTIONS** Acute porphyrias p. 577 · cardiovascular disease · children (consider dose reduction) · debilitated patients (consider dose reduction) · epilepsy · hypovolaemia · impaired cardiac conduction · impaired respiratory function · myasthenia gravis · shock

● **INTERACTIONS** → Appendix 1: anaesthetics, local

● **SIDE-EFFECTS**
▶ **Common or very common** Hypertension · pyrexia
▶ **Uncommon** Hypothermia · syncope
▶ **Frequency not known** Arrhythmias · blurred vision · cardiac arrest · convulsions · dizziness · drowsiness · feeling of inebriation · headache · lightheadedness · muscle twitching · myocardial depression (resulting in hypotension and bradycardia) · nausea · numbness of the tongue and perioral region · paraesthesia (including sensations of hot and cold) · peripheral vasodilatation (resulting in hypotension and bradycardia) · restlessness · tinnitus · transient excitation (followed by depression with drowsiness, respiratory failure, unconsciousness, and coma) · tremors · vomiting

SIDE-EFFECTS, FURTHER INFORMATION
▶ Toxic effects Toxic effects after administration of local anaesthetics are a result of excessively high plasma concentrations; severe toxicity usually results from inadvertent intravascular injection or too rapid injection.
    Following most regional anaesthetic procedures, maximum arterial plasma concentration of anaesthetic develops within about 10 to 25 minutes, so careful surveillance for toxic effects is necessary during the first 30 minutes after injection.
    The systemic toxicity of local anaesthetics mainly involves the central nervous and cardiovascular systems.

● **ALLERGY AND CROSS-SENSITIVITY**
Hypersensitivity reactions occur mainly with the ester-type local anaesthetics, such as tetracaine and chloroprocaine; reactions are less frequent with the amide types, such as articaine, bupivacaine, levobupivacaine, lidocaine, mepivacaine, prilocaine, and ropivacaine. Cross-sensitivity reactions may be avoided by using the alternative chemical type.

● **PREGNANCY** Not known to be harmful. Do not use for paracervical block in obstetrics.

● **BREAST FEEDING** Not known to be harmful.

● **HEPATIC IMPAIRMENT** Use with caution in severe impairment.

● **RENAL IMPAIRMENT** Caution in severe impairment. Increased risk of systemic toxicity in chronic renal failure.

● **MEDICINAL FORMS**
There can be variation in the licensing of different medicines containing the same drug.

Solution for injection
ELECTROLYTES: May contain Sodium
▶ **Ropivacaine hydrochloride (Non-proprietary)**
Ropivacaine hydrochloride 2 mg per 1 ml Ropivacaine 20mg/10ml solution for injection ampoules | 10 ampoule [PoM] £16.50 (Hospital only)
Ropivacaine hydrochloride 7.5 mg per 1 ml Ropivacaine 75mg/10ml solution for injection ampoules | 10 ampoule [PoM] £25.00 (Hospital only)
Ropivacaine hydrochloride 10 mg per 1 ml Ropivacaine 100mg/10ml solution for injection ampoules | 10 ampoule [PoM] £30.00 (Hospital only)
▶ **Naropin** (Aspen Pharma Trading Ltd)
Ropivacaine hydrochloride 2 mg per 1 ml Naropin 20mg/10ml solution for injection ampoules | 5 ampoule [PoM] £12.79
Ropivacaine hydrochloride 7.5 mg per 1 ml Naropin 75mg/10ml solution for injection ampoules | 5 ampoule [PoM] £15.90
Ropivacaine hydrochloride 10 mg per 1 ml Naropin 100mg/10ml solution for injection ampoules | 5 ampoule [PoM] £19.22

Infusion
ELECTROLYTES: May contain Sodium
▶ **Ropivacaine hydrochloride (Non-proprietary)**
Ropivacaine hydrochloride 2 mg per 1 ml Ropivacaine 400mg/200ml infusion bags | 5 bag [PoM] £72.25 | 10 bag [PoM] £137.00 (Hospital only)
▶ **Naropin** (AstraZeneca UK Ltd)
Ropivacaine hydrochloride 2 mg per 1 ml Naropin 400mg/200ml infusion Polybags | 5 bag [PoM] £86.70

Tetracaine

(Amethocaine)

● **INDICATIONS AND DOSE**
Anaesthesia before venepuncture or venous cannulation
▶ TO THE SKIN

▶ **Neonate:** Apply contents of tube (or appropriate proportion) to site of venepuncture or venous cannulation and cover with occlusive dressing; remove gel and dressing after 30 minutes for venepuncture and after 45 minutes for venous cannulation.

▶ **Child 1 month–4 years:** Apply contents of up to 1 tube (applied at separate sites at a single time or appropriate proportion) to site of venepuncture or venous cannulation and cover with occlusive dressing; remove gel and dressing after 30 minutes for venepuncture and after 45 minutes for venous cannulation

▶ **Child 5–17 years:** Apply contents of up to 5 tubes (applied at separate sites at a single time or appropriate proportion) to site of venepuncture or venous cannulation and cover with occlusive dressing; remove gel and dressing after 30 minutes for venepuncture and after 45 minutes for venous cannulation

● **UNLICENSED USE** Not licensed for use in neonates.

● **CONTRA-INDICATIONS** Should not be applied to damaged skin

● **INTERACTIONS** → Appendix 1: anaesthetics, local

● **SIDE-EFFECTS** Local skin reactions

15

Anaesthesia

SIDE-EFFECTS, FURTHER INFORMATION
The systemic toxicity of local anaesthetics mainly involves the central nervous and cardiovascular systems; systemic side effects unlikely as minimal absorption following topical application.

- **ALLERGY AND CROSS-SENSITIVITY**
Hypersensitivity reactions occur mainly with the ester-type local anaesthetics, such as tetracaine and chloroprocaine; reactions are less frequent with the amide types, such as articaine, bupivacaine, levobupivacaine, lidocaine, mepivacaine, prilocaine, and ropivacaine. Cross-sensitivity reactions may be avoided by using the alternative chemical type.

- **BREAST FEEDING** Not known to be harmful.

- **PATIENT AND CARER ADVICE**
Medicines for Children leaflet: Tetracaine gel for local anaesthesia www.medicinesforchildren.org.uk/tetracaine-gel-for-local-anaesthesia

- **MEDICINAL FORMS**
There can be variation in the licensing of different medicines containing the same drug.

Gel
EXCIPIENTS: May contain Hydroxybenzoates (parabens)
▸ **Ametop** (Smith & Nephew Healthcare Ltd)
 Tetracaine 40 mg per 1 gram Ametop 4% gel | 1.5 gram Ⓟ £1.08
 | 18 gram Ⓟ no price available

severity of poisoning is less below a plasma-salicylate concentration of 500 mg/litre (3.6 mmol/litre), unless there is evidence of metabolic acidosis. Activated charcoal can be given within 1 hour of ingesting more than 125 mg/kg of aspirin. Fluid losses should be replaced and intravenous sodium bicarbonate may be given (ensuring plasma-potassium concentration is within the reference range) to enhance urinary salicylate excretion (optimum urinary pH 7.5–8.5).

Plasma-potassium concentration should be corrected before giving sodium bicarbonate as hypokalaemia may complicate alkalinisation of the urine.

Haemodialysis is the treatment of choice for severe salicylate poisoning and should be considered when the plasma-salicylate concentration exceeds 700 mg/litre (5.1 mmol/litre) or in the presence of severe metabolic acidosis, convulsions, respiratory failure, pulmonary oedema or persistently high plasma-salicylate concentrations unresponsive to urinary alkalinisation.

Opioids

Opioids (narcotic analgesics) cause varying degrees of coma, respiratory depression, and pinpoint pupils. The specific antidote naloxone hydrochloride p. 813 is indicated if there is coma or bradypnoea. Since naloxone has a shorter duration of action than many opioids, close monitoring and repeated injections are necessary according to the respiratory rate and depth of coma. When repeated administration of naloxone is required, it can be given by continuous intravenous infusion instead and the rate of infusion adjusted according to vital signs. All children should be observed for at least 6 hours after the last dose of naloxone. The effects of some opioids, such as buprenorphine, are only partially reversed by naloxone. Dextropropoxyphene and methadone have very long durations of action; patients may need to be monitored for long periods following large overdoses.

Naloxone reverses the opioid effects of dextropropoxyphene. The long duration of action of dextropropoxyphene calls for prolonged monitoring and further doses of naloxone may be required.

Norpropoxyphene, a metabolite of dextropropoxyphene, also has cardiotoxic effects which may require treatment with sodium bicarbonate p. 558 or magnesium sulfate p. 571, or both. Arrhythmias may occur for up to 12 hours.

Paracetamol

In cases of **intravenous** paracetamol poisoning contact the National Poisons Information Service for advice on risk assessment and management.

Toxic doses of paracetamol may cause severe hepatocellular necrosis and, much less frequently, renal tubular necrosis. Nausea and vomiting, the only early features of poisoning, usually settle within 24 hours. Persistence beyond this time, often associated with the onset of right subcostal pain and tenderness, usually indicates development of hepatic necrosis. Liver damage is maximal 3–4 days after paracetamol overdose and may lead to encephalopathy, haemorrhage, hypoglycaemia, cerebral oedema, and death. Therefore, despite a lack of significant early symptoms, children who have taken an overdose of paracetamol should be transferred to hospital urgently.

To avoid underestimating the potentially toxic paracetamol dose ingested by obese children who weigh more than 110 kg, use a body-weight of 110 kg (rather than their actual body-weight) when calculating the total dose of paracetamol ingested (in mg/kg).

Acetylcysteine p. 814 protects the liver if infused up to, and possibly beyond, 24 hours of ingesting paracetamol. It is most effective if given within 8 hours of ingestion, after which effectiveness declines. Very rarely, giving acetylcysteine by mouth [unlicensed route] is an alternative

if intravenous access is not possible—contact the National Poisons Information Service for advice.

Neonates less than 45 weeks corrected gestational age may be more susceptible to paracetamol-induced liver toxicity, therefore, treatment with acetylcysteine should be considered in all paracetamol overdoses, and advice should be sought from the National Poisons Information Service.

Acute overdose

Hepatotoxicity may occur after a single ingestion of more than 150 mg/kg paracetamol taken in less than 1 hour. Rarely, hepatotoxicity may develop with single ingestions as low as 75 mg/kg of paracetamol taken in less than 1 hour.

Children who have ingested 75 mg/kg or more of paracetamol in less than 1 hour should be referred to hospital. Administration of charcoal, activated p. 810 should be considered if paracetamol in excess of 150 mg/kg is thought to have been ingested within the previous hour.

Children at risk of liver damage and, therefore, requiring acetylcysteine, can be identified from a single measurement of the plasma-paracetamol concentration, related to the time from ingestion, provided this time interval is not less than 4 hours; earlier samples may be misleading. The concentration is plotted on a paracetamol treatment graph, with a reference line ('treatment line') joining plots of 100 mg/litre (0.66 mmol/litre) at 4 hours and 3.13 mg/litre (0.02 mmol/litre) at 24 hours. Acetylcysteine treatment should commence immediately in children:

- whose plasma-paracetamol concentration falls on or above the *treatment line* on the paracetamol treatment graph;
- who present 8–24 hours after taking an acute overdose of more than 150 mg/kg of paracetamol, even if the plasma-paracetamol concentration is not yet available; acetylcysteine can be discontinued if the plasma-paracetamol concentration is later reported to be below the *treatment line* on the paracetamol treatment graph, provided that the child is asymptomatic and liver function tests, serum creatinine and INR are normal.

The prognostic accuracy of a plasma-paracetamol concentration taken after 15 hours is uncertain, but a concentration on or above the *treatment line* on the paracetamol treatment graph should be regarded as carrying a serious risk of liver damage. If more than 15 hours have elapsed since ingestion, or there is doubt about appropriate management, advice should be sought from the National Poisons Information Service.

'Staggered' overdose, uncertain time of overdose, or therapeutic excess

A 'staggered' overdose involves ingestion of a potentially toxic dose of paracetamol over more than one hour, with the possible intention of causing self-harm. Therapeutic excess is the inadvertent ingestion of a potentially toxic dose of paracetamol during its clinical use. The paracetamol treatment graph is unreliable if a 'staggered' overdose is taken, if there is uncertainty about the time of the overdose, or if there is therapeutic excess. In these cases, children who have taken more than 150 mg/kg of paracetamol in any 24-hour period are at risk of toxicity and should be commenced on acetylcysteine immediately, unless it is more than 24 hours since the last ingestion, the patient is asymptomatic, the plasma-paracetamol concentration is undetectable, and liver function tests, serum creatinine and INR are normal.

Rarely, toxicity can occur with paracetamol doses between 75–150 mg/kg in any 24-hour period; for some children this may be within the licensed dose, but ingestion of a licensed dose of paracetamol is not considered an overdose. Clinical judgement of the individual case is necessary to determine whether to treat those who have ingested this amount of paracetamol.

Although there is some evidence suggesting that factors such as the use of liver enzyme-inducing drugs (e.g.

16

Emergency treatment of poisoning

Paracetamol overdose treatment graph

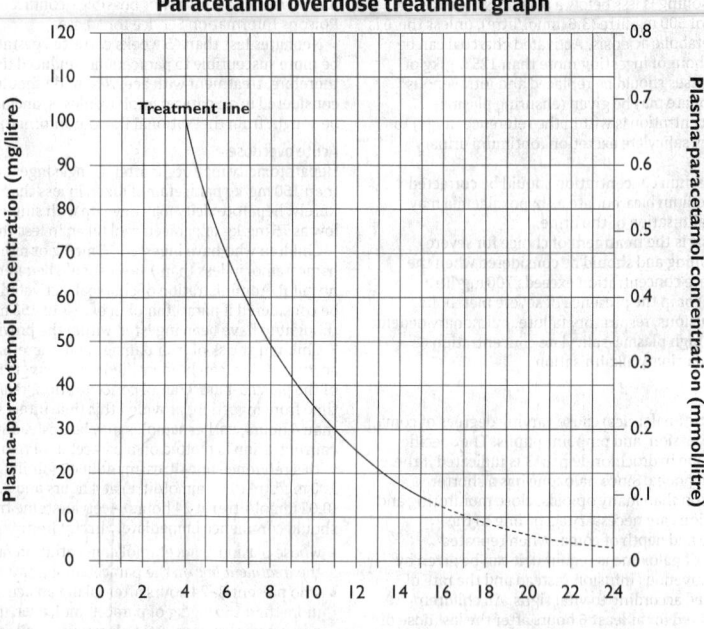

Patients whose plasma-paracetamol concentrations are on or above the **treatment line** should be treated with acetylcysteine by intravenous infusion.

The prognostic accuracy after 15 hours is uncertain, but a plasma-paracetamol concentration on or above the treatment line should be regarded as carrying a serious risk of liver damage.

Graph reproduced courtesy of Medicines and Healthcare products Regulatory Agency

carbamazepine p. 189, efavirenz p. 394, nevirapine p. 395, phenobarbital p. 208, phenytoin p. 198, primidone p. 209, rifabutin p. 348, rifampicin p. 349, St John's wort), chronic alcoholism, and starvation may increase the risk of hepatotoxicity, the CHM has advised that these should no longer be used in the assessment of paracetamol toxicity.

Significant toxicity is unlikely if, 24 hours or longer after the last paracetamol ingestion, the patient is asymptomatic, the plasma-paracetamol concentration is undetectable, and liver function tests, serum creatinine and INR are normal. Children with clinical features of hepatic injury such as jaundice or hepatic tenderness should be treated urgently with acetylcysteine. If there is uncertainty about a patient's risk of toxicity after paracetamol overdose, treatment with acetylcysteine should be commenced. Advice should be sought from the National Poisons Information Service whenever necessary.

Antidepressants

Tricyclic and related antidepressants

Tricyclic and related antidepressants cause dry mouth, coma of varying degree, hypotension, hypothermia, hyperreflexia, extensor plantar responses, convulsions, respiratory failure, cardiac conduction defects, and arrhythmias. Dilated pupils and urinary retention also occur. Metabolic acidosis may complicate severe poisoning; delirium with confusion, agitation, and visual and auditory hallucinations are common during recovery.

Assessment in hospital is strongly advised in case of poisoning by tricyclic and related antidepressants but symptomatic treatment can be given before transfer.

Supportive measures to ensure a clear airway and adequate ventilation during transfer are mandatory. Intravenous lorazepam or intravenous diazepam (preferably in emulsion form) may be required to treat convulsions. Activated charcoal given within 1 hour of the overdose reduces absorption of the drug. Although arrhythmias are worrying, some will respond to correction of hypoxia and acidosis. The use of anti-arrhythmic drugs is best avoided, but intravenous infusion of sodium bicarbonate can arrest arrhythmias or prevent them in those with an extended QRS duration. Diazepam p. 212 given by mouth is usually adequate to sedate delirious patients but large doses may be required.

Selective serotonin re-uptake inhibitors (SSRIs)

Symptoms of poisoning by selective serotonin re-uptake inhibitors include nausea, vomiting, agitation, tremor, nystagmus, drowsiness, and sinus tachycardia; convulsions may occur. Rarely, severe poisoning results in the serotonin syndrome, with marked neuropsychiatric effects, neuromuscular hyperactivity, and autonomic instability; hyperthermia, rhabdomyolysis, renal failure, and coagulopathies may develop.

Management of SSRI poisoning is supportive. Activated charcoal given within 1 hour of the overdose reduces absorption of the drug. Convulsions can be treated with lorazepam p. 214, diazepam p. 212, or buccal midazolam p. 215 (see *Convulsions*). Contact the National Poisons Information Service for the management of hyperthermia or the serotonin syndrome.

Antimalarials

Overdosage with quinine, chloroquine, or hydroxychloroquine is extremely hazardous and difficult to treat. Urgent advice from the National Poisons Information Service is essential. Life-threatening features include arrhythmias (which can have a very rapid onset) and convulsions (which can be intractable).

Antipsychotics

Phenothiazines and related drugs

Phenothiazines cause less depression of consciousness and respiration than other sedatives. Hypotension, hypothermia, sinus tachycardia, and arrhythmias may complicate poisoning. Dystonic reactions can occur with therapeutic doses (particularly with prochlorperazine and trifluoperazine), and convulsions may occur in severe cases. Arrhythmias may respond to correction of hypoxia, acidosis, and other biochemical abnormalities, but specialist advice should be sought if arrhythmias result from a prolonged QT interval; the use of some anti-arrhythmic drugs can worsen such arrhythmias. Dystonic reactions are rapidly abolished by injection of drugs such as procyclidine hydrochloride p. 246 or diazepam (emulsion preferred).

Second-generation antipsychotic drugs

Features of poisoning by second-generation antipsychotic drugs include drowsiness, convulsions, extrapyramidal symptoms, hypotension, and ECG abnormalities (including prolongation of the QT interval). Management is supportive. Charcoal, activated p. 810 can be given within 1 hour of ingesting a significant quantity of a second-generation antipsychotic drug.

Benzodiazepines

Benzodiazepines taken alone cause drowsiness, ataxia, dysarthria, nystagmus, and occasionally respiratory depression, and coma. Charcoal, activated can be given within 1 hour of ingesting a significant quantity of benzodiazepine, provided the patient is awake and the airway is protected. Benzodiazepines potentiate the effects of other central nervous system depressants taken concomitantly. Use of the benzodiazepine antagonist flumazenil p. 811 [unlicensed indication] can be hazardous, particularly in mixed overdoses involving tricyclic antidepressants or in benzodiazepine-dependent patients. Flumazenil may prevent the need for ventilation, particularly in patients with severe respiratory disorders; it should be used on expert advice only and not as a diagnostic test in children with a reduced level of consciousness.

Beta blockers

Therapeutic overdosages with beta-blockers may cause lightheadedness, dizziness, and possibly syncope as a result of bradycardia and hypotension; heart failure may be precipitated or exacerbated. These complications are most likely in children with conduction system disorders or impaired myocardial function. Bradycardia is the most common arrhythmia caused by beta-blockers, but sotalol may induce ventricular tachyarrhythmias (sometimes of the torsade de pointes type). The effects of massive overdosage can vary from one beta-blocker to another; propranolol overdosage in particular may cause coma and convulsions.

Acute massive overdosage must be managed in hospital and expert advice should be obtained. Maintenance of a clear airway and adequate ventilation is mandatory. An intravenous injection of atropine sulfate p. 779 is required to treat bradycardia. Cardiogenic shock unresponsive to atropine sulfate is probably best treated with an intravenous injection of glucagon p. 444 [unlicensed] in glucose 5% (with precautions to protect the airway in case of vomiting) followed by an intravenous infusion. If glucagon is not available, intravenous isoprenaline (available from 'special-

order' manufacturers or specialist importing companies) is an alternative. A cardiac pacemaker can be used to increase the heart rate.

Calcium-channel blockers

Features of calcium-channel blocker poisoning include nausea, vomiting, dizziness, agitation, confusion, and coma in severe poisoning. Metabolic acidosis and hyperglycaemia may occur. Verapamil and diltiazem have a profound cardiac depressant effect causing hypotension and arrhythmias, including complete heart block and asystole. The dihydropyridine calcium-channel blockers cause severe hypotension secondary to profound peripheral vasodilatation.

Charcoal, activated should be considered if the patient presents within 1 hour of overdosage with a calcium-channel blocker; repeated doses of activated charcoal are considered if a modified-release preparation is involved. In patients with significant features of poisoning, calcium chloride p. 567 or calcium gluconate p. 568 is given by injection; atropine sulfate is given to correct symptomatic bradycardia. In severe cases, an insulin and glucose infusion may be required in the management of hypotension and myocardial failure. For the management of hypotension, the choice of inotropic sympathomimetic depends on whether hypotension is secondary to vasodilatation or to myocardial depression—advice should be sought from the National Poisons Information Service.

Iron salts

Iron poisoning in childhood is usually accidental. The symptoms are nausea, vomiting, abdominal pain, diarrhoea, haematemesis, and rectal bleeding. Hypotension and hepatocellular necrosis can occur later. Coma, shock, and metabolic acidosis indicate severe poisoning.

Advice should be sought from the National Poisons Information Service if a significant quantity of iron has been ingested within the previous hour.

Mortality is reduced by intensive and specific therapy with desferrioxamine mesilate p. 550, which chelates iron. The serum-iron concentration is measured as an emergency and intravenous desferrioxamine mesilate given to chelate absorbed iron in excess of the expected iron binding capacity. In severe toxicity intravenous desferrioxamine mesilate should be given immediately without waiting for the result of the serum-iron measurement.

Lithium

Most cases of lithium intoxication occur as a complication of long-term therapy and are caused by reduced excretion of the drug because of a variety of factors including dehydration, deterioration of renal function, infections, and co-administration of diuretics or NSAIDs (or other drugs that interact). Acute deliberate overdoses may also occur with delayed onset of symptoms (12 hours or more) owing to slow entry of lithium into the tissues and continuing absorption from modified-release formulations.

The early clinical features are non-specific and may include apathy and restlessness which could be confused with mental changes arising from the child's depressive illness. Vomiting, diarrhoea, ataxia, weakness, dysarthria, muscle twitching, and tremor may follow. Severe poisoning is associated with convulsions, coma, renal failure, electrolyte imbalance, dehydration, and hypotension.

Therapeutic serum-lithium concentrations are within the range of 0.4–1 mmol/litre; concentrations in excess of 2 mmol/litre are usually associated with serious toxicity and such cases may need treatment with haemodialysis if neurological symptoms or renal failure are present. In acute overdosage much higher serum-lithium concentrations may be present without features of toxicity and all that is usually necessary is to take measures to increase urine output (e.g.

16

Emergency treatment of poisoning

by increasing fluid intake but avoiding diuretics). Otherwise, treatment is supportive with special regard to electrolyte balance, renal function, and control of convulsions. Whole-bowel irrigation should be considered for significant ingestion, but advice should be sought from the National Poisons Information Service.

Stimulants

Amfetamines

Amfetamines cause wakefulness, excessive activity, paranoia, hallucinations, and hypertension followed by exhaustion, convulsions, hyperthermia, and coma. The early stages can be controlled by diazepam p. 212 or lorazepam p. 214; advice should be sought from the National Poisons Information Service on the management of hypertension. Later, tepid sponging, anticonvulsants, and artificial respiration may be needed.

Cocaine

Cocaine stimulates the central nervous system, causing agitation, dilated pupils, tachycardia, hypertension, hallucinations, hyperthermia, hypertonia, and hyperreflexia; cardiac effects include chest pain, myocardial infarction, and arrhythmias.

Initial treatment of cocaine poisoning involves cooling measures for hyperthermia (see *Body temperature*); agitation, hypertension and cardiac effects require specific treatment and expert advice should be sought.

Ecstasy

Ecstasy (methylenedioxymethamfetamine, MDMA) may cause severe reactions, even at doses that were previously tolerated. The most serious effects are delirium, coma, convulsions, ventricular arrhythmias, hyperthermia, rhabdomyolysis, acute renal failure, acute hepatitis, disseminated intravascular coagulation, adult respiratory distress syndrome, hyperreflexia, hypotension and intracerebral haemorrhage; hyponatraemia has also been associated with ecstasy use and syndrome of inappropriate antidiuretic hormone secretion (SIADH) can occur.

Treatment of methylenedioxymethamfetamine poisoning is supportive, with diazepam to control persistent convulsions and close monitoring including ECG. For the management of agitation, seek specialist advice. Self-induced water intoxication should be considered in patients with ecstasy poisoning.

'Liquid ecstasy' is a term used for sodium oxybate (gamma-hydroxybutyrate, GHB), which is a sedative.

Theophylline

Theophylline and related drugs are often prescribed as modified-release formulations and toxicity can therefore be delayed. They cause vomiting (which may be severe and intractable), agitation, restlessness, dilated pupils, sinus tachycardia, and hyperglycaemia. More serious effects are haematemesis, convulsions, and supraventricular and ventricular arrhythmias. Severe hypokalaemia may develop rapidly.

Repeated doses of charcoal, activated p. 810 can be used to eliminate theophylline even if more than 1 hour has elapsed after ingestion and especially if a modified-release preparation has been taken (see also under Active Elimination Techniques). Ondansetron p. 253 may be effective for severe vomiting that is resistant to other antiemetics. Hypokalaemia is corrected by intravenous infusion of potassium chloride p. 575 and may be so severe as to require high doses under ECG monitoring. Convulsions should be controlled by intravenous administration of lorazepam or diazepam (see Convulsions). For the management of agitation associated with theophylline overdosage, seek specialist advice.

Provided the child does **not** suffer from asthma, a short-acting beta-blocker can be administered intravenously to

reverse severe tachycardia, hypokalaemia, and hyperglycaemia.

Other poisons

Consult either the National Poisons Information Service day and night or TOXBASE, see under the National Poisons Information Service.

Cyanides

Oxygen should be administered to children with cyanide poisoning. The choice of antidote depends on the severity of poisoning, certainty of diagnosis, and the cause. Dicobalt edetate p. 810 is the antidote of choice when there is a strong clinical suspicion of severe cyanide poisoning, but it should **not** be used as a precautionary measure. Dicobalt edetate itself is toxic, associated with anaphylactoid reactions, and is potentially fatal if administered in the absence of cyanide poisoning. A regimen of sodium nitrite p. 810 followed by sodium thiosulfate p. 810 is an alternative if dicobalt edetate is not available.

Hydroxocobalamin p. 541 (Cyanokit® or other preparation of hydroxocobalamin is suitable) can be considered for use in victims of smoke inhalation who show signs of significant cyanide poisoning.

Ethylene glycol and methanol

Fomepizole (available from 'special-order' manufacturers or specialist importing companies) is the treatment of choice for ethylene glycol and methanol (methyl alcohol) poisoning. If necessary, **ethanol** (by mouth or by intravenous infusion) can be used, but with caution. Advice on the treatment of ethylene glycol and methanol poisoning should be obtained from the National Poisons Information Service. It is important to start antidote treatment promptly in cases of suspected poisoning with these agents.

Heavy metals

Heavy metal antidotes include succimer (DMSA) [unlicensed], unithiol (DMPS) [unlicensed], sodium calcium edetate [unlicensed], and dimercaprol. Dimercaprol in the management of heavy metal poisoning has been superseded by other chelating agents. In all cases of heavy metal poisoning, the advice of the National Poisons Information Service should be sought.

Noxious gases

Carbon monoxide

Carbon monoxide poisoning is usually due to inhalation of smoke, car exhaust, or fumes caused by blocked flues or incomplete combustion of fuel gases in confined spaces.

Immediate treatment of carbon monoxide poisoning is essential. The patient should be moved to fresh air, the airway cleared, and high-flow **oxygen** 100% administered as soon as available. Artificial respiration should be given as necessary and continued until adequate spontaneous breathing starts, or stopped only after persistent and efficient treatment of cardiac arrest has failed. The child should be admitted to hospital because complications may arise after a delay of hours or days. Cerebral oedema may occur in severe poisoning and is treated with an intravenous infusion of mannitol p. 137. Referral for hyperbaric oxygen treatment should be discussed with the National Poisons Information Service if the patient is pregnant or in cases of severe poisoning such as if the patient is or has been unconscious, or has psychiatric or neurological features other than a headache or has myocardial ischaemia or an arrhythmia, or has a blood carboxyhaemoglobin concentration of more than 20%.

Sulfur dioxide, chlorine, phosgene, ammonia

All of these gases can cause upper respiratory tract and conjunctival irritation. Pulmonary oedema, with severe breathlessness and cyanosis may develop suddenly up to

36 hours after exposure. Death may occur. Patients are kept under observation and those who develop pulmonary oedema are given oxygen. Assisted ventilation may be necessary in the most serious cases.

CS spray

CS spray, which is used for riot control, irritates the eyes (hence 'tear gas') and the respiratory tract; symptoms normally settle spontaneously within 15 minutes. If symptoms persist, the patient should be removed to a well-ventilated area, and the exposed skin washed with soap and water after removal of contaminated clothing. Contact lenses should be removed and rigid ones washed (soft ones should be discarded). Eye symptoms should be treated by irrigating the eyes with physiological saline (or water if saline is not available) and advice sought from an ophthalmologist. Patients with features of severe poisoning, particularly respiratory complications, should be admitted to hospital for symptomatic treatment.

Nerve agents

Treatment of nerve agent poisoning is similar to organophosphorus insecticide poisoning, but advice must be sought from the National Poisons Information Service. The risk of cross-contamination is significant; adequate decontamination and protective clothing for healthcare personnel are essential. In emergencies involving the release of **nerve agents**, kits ('NAAS pods') containing **pralidoxime chloride** p. 811 can be obtained through the Ambulance Service from the National Blood Service (or the Welsh Blood Service in South Wales or designated hospital pharmacies in Northern Ireland and Scotland—see TOXBASE for list of designated centres).

Pesticides

Organophosphorus insecticides

Organophosphorus insecticides are usually supplied as powders or dissolved in organic solvents. All are absorbed through the bronchi and intact skin as well as through the gut and inhibit cholinesterase activity, thereby prolonging and intensifying the effects of acetylcholine. Toxicity between different compounds varies considerably, and onset may be delayed after skin exposure.

Anxiety, restlessness, dizziness, headache, miosis, nausea, hypersalivation, vomiting, abdominal colic, diarrhoea, bradycardia, and sweating are common features of organophosphorus poisoning. Muscle weakness and fasciculation may develop and progress to generalised flaccid paralysis, including the ocular and respiratory muscles. Convulsions, coma, pulmonary oedema with copious bronchial secretions, hypoxia, and arrhythmias occur in severe cases. Hyperglycaemia and glycosuria without ketonuria may also be present.

Further absorption of the organophosphorus insecticide should be prevented by moving the child to fresh air, removing soiled clothing, and washing contaminated skin. In severe poisoning it is vital to ensure a clear airway, frequent removal of bronchial secretions, and adequate ventilation and oxygenation; gastric lavage may be considered provided that the airway is protected. Atropine sulfate p. 779 will reverse the muscarinic effects of acetylcholine and is given by intravenous injection until the skin becomes flushed and dry, the pupils dilate, and bradycardia is abolished.

Pralidoxime chloride, a cholinesterase reactivator, is used as an adjunct to atropine sulfate in moderate or severe poisoning. It improves muscle tone within 30 minutes of administration. Pralidoxime chloride is continued until the patient has not required atropine sulfate for 12 hours. Pralidoxime chloride can be obtained from designated centres, the names of which are held by the National Poisons Information Service.

Snake bites and animal stings

Snake bites

Envenoming from snake bite is uncommon in the UK. Many exotic snakes are kept, some illegally, but the only indigenous venomous snake is the adder (*Vipera berus*). The bite may cause local and systemic effects. Local effects include pain, swelling, bruising, and tender enlargement of regional lymph nodes. Systemic effects include early anaphylactic symptoms (transient hypotension with syncope, angioedema, urticaria, abdominal colic, diarrhoea, and vomiting), with later persistent or recurrent hypotension, ECG abnormalities, spontaneous systemic bleeding, coagulopathy, adult respiratory distress syndrome, and acute renal failure. Fatal envenoming is rare but the potential for severe envenoming must not be underestimated.

Early anaphylactic symptoms should be treated with adrenaline/epinephrine p. 132. Indications for european viper snake venom antiserum treatment p. 815 include *systemic envenoming*, especially hypotension, ECG abnormalities, vomiting, haemostatic abnormalities, and marked local envenoming such that after bites on the hand or foot, swelling extends beyond the wrist or ankle within 4 hours of the bite. For those children who present with clinical features of *severe envenoming* (e.g. shock, ECG abnormalities, or local swelling that has advanced from the foot to above the knee or from the hand to above the elbow within 2 hours of the bite), a higher initial dose of the european viper snake venom antiserum is recommended; if symptoms of *systemic envenoming* persist contact the National Poisons Information Service.

Adrenaline/epinephrine injection must be immediately to hand for treatment of anaphylactic reactions to the european viper snake venom antiserum.

European viper snake venom antiserum is available for bites by certain foreign snakes and spiders, stings by scorpions and fish. For information on identification, management, and for supply in an emergency, telephone the National Poisons Information Service. Whenever possible the TOXBASE entry should be read, and relevant information collected, before telephoning the National Poisons Information Service.

Insect stings

Stings from ants, wasps, hornets, and bees cause local pain and swelling but seldom cause severe direct toxicity unless many stings are inflicted at the same time. If the sting is in the mouth or on the tongue local swelling may threaten the upper airway. The stings from these insects are usually treated by cleaning the area with a topical antiseptic. Bee stings should be removed as quickly as possible. Anaphylactic reactions require immediate treatment with intramuscular **adrenaline/epinephrine**; self-administered (or administered by a carer) intramuscular adrenaline/epinephrine (e.g. *EpiPen*®) is the best first-aid treatment for patients with severe hypersensitivity. An inhaled bronchodilator should be used for asthmatic reactions, see also the management of anaphylaxis. A short course of an **oral antihistamine** or a **topical corticosteroid** may help to reduce inflammation and relieve itching. A vaccine containing extracts of bee and wasp venom can be used to reduce the risk of anaphylaxis and systemic reactions in patients with systemic hypersensitivity to bee or wasp stings.

Marine stings

The severe pain of weeverfish (*Trachinus vipera*) and Portuguese man-o'-war stings can be relieved by immersing the stung area immediately in uncomfortably hot, but not scalding, water (not more than 45°C). People stung by jellyfish and Portuguese man-o'-war around the UK coast should be removed from the sea as soon as possible. Adherent tentacles should be lifted off carefully (wearing gloves or using tweezers) or washed off with seawater. Alcoholic solutions, including suntan lotions, should **not** be applied because they can cause further discharge of stinging hairs. Ice packs can be used to reduce pain.

Other poisons

Consult either the National Poisons Information Service day and night or TOXBASE.

The **National Poisons Information Service** (Tel: 0344 892 0111) will provide specialist advice on all aspects of poisoning day and night.

1 Active elimination from the gastro-intestinal tract

ANTIDOTES AND CHELATORS ⟩ INTESTINAL ADSORBENTS

Charcoal, activated

● **INDICATIONS AND DOSE**
Reduction of absorption of poisons in the gastro-intestinal system
▸ BY MOUTH

▸ Neonate: 1 g/kg.

▸ Child 1 month–11 years: 1 g/kg (max. per dose 50 g)
▸ Child 12–17 years: 50 g
Active elimination of poisons
▸ BY MOUTH

▸ Neonate: 1 g/kg every 4 hours, dose may be reduced and the frequency increased if not tolerated, reduced dose may compromise efficacy.

▸ Child 1 month–11 years: 1 g/kg every 4 hours (max. per dose 50 g), dose may be reduced and the frequency increased if not tolerated, reduced dose may compromise efficacy

▸ Child 12–17 years: Initially 50 g, then 50 g every 4 hours, reduced if not tolerated to 25 g every 2 hours, alternatively 12.5 g every 1 hour, reduced dose may compromise efficacy

● **CAUTIONS** Comatose patient (risk of aspiration—ensure airway is protected) · drowsy patient (risk of aspiration—ensure airway protected) · reduced gastrointestinal motility (risk of obstruction)

● **SIDE-EFFECTS** Black stools

● **DIRECTIONS FOR ADMINISTRATION** Suspension or reconstituted powder may be mixed with soft drinks (e.g. caffeine-free diet cola) or fruit juices to mask the taste.

● **MEDICINAL FORMS**
There can be variation in the licensing of different medicines containing the same drug.
Oral suspension
▸ Actidose-Aqua Advance (Alliance Pharmaceuticals Ltd)
Activated charcoal 208 mg per 1 ml Actidose-Aqua Advance 1.04g/5ml oral suspension | 240 ml Ⓟ £12.89
▸ Charcodote (Teva UK Ltd)
Activated charcoal 200 mg per 1 ml Charcodote 200mg/ml oral suspension sugar-free | 250 ml Ⓟ £11.88
Granules
▸ Carbomix (Beacon Pharmaceuticals Ltd)
Activated charcoal 813 mg per 1 gram Carbomix 81.3% granules sugar-free | 50 gram Ⓟ £11.90

2 Chemical toxicity

2.1 Cyanide toxicity

ANTIDOTES AND CHELATORS

Dicobalt edetate

● **INDICATIONS AND DOSE**
Severe poisoning with cyanides
▸ BY INTRAVENOUS INJECTION
▸ Child: Consult the National Poisons Information Service

● **CAUTIONS** Owing to toxicity to be used only for definite cyanide poisoning when patient tending to lose, or has lost, consciousness

● **SIDE-EFFECTS** Anaphylactoid reactions · cardiac abnormalities · facial oedema · hypotension · laryngeal oedema · tachycardia · vomiting

● **EXCEPTIONS TO LEGAL CATEGORY** Prescription only medicine restriction does not apply where administration is for saving life in emergency.

● **MEDICINAL FORMS**
There can be variation in the licensing of different medicines containing the same drug.
Solution for injection
▸ Dicobalt edetate (Non-proprietary)
Dicobalt edetate 15 mg per 1 ml Dicobalt edetate 300mg/20ml solution for injection ampoules | 6 ampoule PoM £117.20

Sodium nitrite

● **INDICATIONS AND DOSE**
Poisoning with cyanides (used in conjunction with sodium thiosulfate)
▸ BY INTRAVENOUS INJECTION
▸ Child: 4–10 mg/kg (max. per dose 300 mg), to be given over 5–20 minutes followed by sodium thiosulphate injection

DOSE EQUIVALENCE AND CONVERSION
▸ 4–10 mg/kg equates to 0.13–0.33 mL/kg of a 3% solution.
▸ Dose max. of 300 mg equates to 10 mL of a 3% solution.

● **SIDE-EFFECTS** Flushing (due to vasodilatation) · headache (due to vasodilatation)

● **EXCEPTIONS TO LEGAL CATEGORY** Prescription only medicine restriction does not apply where administration is for saving life in emergency.

● **MEDICINAL FORMS**
There can be variation in the licensing of different medicines containing the same drug. Forms available from special-order manufacturers include: solution for injection

Sodium thiosulfate

● **INDICATIONS AND DOSE**
Poisoning with cyanides (used in conjunction with sodium nitrite)
▸ BY INTRAVENOUS INJECTION
▸ Child: 400 mg/kg (max. per dose 12.5 g), to be given over 10 minutes, dose may be repeated in severe cyanide poisoning if dicobalt edetate not available

DOSE EQUIVALENCE AND CONVERSION
▸ 400 mg/kg equates to 0.8 mL/kg of a 50% solution.
▸ 12.5 g equates to 25 mL of a 50% solution.

- **EXCEPTIONS TO LEGAL CATEGORY** Prescription only medicine restriction does not apply where administration is for saving life in emergency.

- **MEDICINAL FORMS** There can be variation in the licensing of different medicines containing the same drug. Forms available from special-order manufacturers include: solution for injection, solution for infusion

2.2 Organophosphorus toxicity

Other drugs used for Organophosphorus toxicity Atropine sulfate, p. 779

ANTIDOTES AND CHELATORS

Pralidoxime chloride

- **INDICATIONS AND DOSE**

  Adjunct to atropine in the treatment of poisoning by organophosphorus insecticide or nerve agent
  - ▸ BY INTRAVENOUS INFUSION
  - ▸ Child: Initially 30 mg/kg, to be given over 20 minutes, followed by 8 mg/kg/hour; maximum 12 g per day

- **UNLICENSED USE** Pralidoxime chloride doses may differ from those in product literature. Licensed for use in children (age range not specified by manufacturer).

- **CONTRA-INDICATIONS** Poisoning with carbamates · poisoning with organophosphorus compounds without anticholinesterase activity

- **CAUTIONS** Myasthenia gravis

- **SIDE-EFFECTS** Disturbances of vision · dizziness · drowsiness · headache · hyperventilation · muscular weakness · nausea · tachycardia

- **RENAL IMPAIRMENT** Use with caution.

- **DIRECTIONS FOR ADMINISTRATION** The loading dose may be administered by intravenous injection (diluted to a concentration of 50 mg/mL with water for injections) over at least 5 minutes if pulmonary oedema is present or if it is not practical to administer an intravenous infusion.
     For *intravenous infusion*, reconstitute each vial with 20 mL Water for Injections, then dilute to a concentration of 10–20 mg/mL with Sodium Chloride 0.9%.

- **PRESCRIBING AND DISPENSING INFORMATION** Available from designated centres for organophosphorus insecticide poisoning or from the National Blood Service (or Welsh Ambulance Services for Mid West and South East Wales)—see TOXBASE for list of designated centres).

- **EXCEPTIONS TO LEGAL CATEGORY** Prescription only medicine restriction does not apply where administration is for saving life in emergency.

- **MEDICINAL FORMS** There can be variation in the licensing of different medicines containing the same drug.
  Powder for solution for injection
  - ▸ Pralidoxime chloride (Non-proprietary)
    Pralidoxime chloride 1 gram Protopam Chloride 1g powder for solution for injection vials | 6 vial [PoM] no price available

3   Drug toxicity

3.1   Benzodiazepine toxicity

ANTIDOTES AND CHELATORS ⟩
BENZODIAZEPINE ANTAGONISTS

Flumazenil

- **INDICATIONS AND DOSE**

  Reversal of sedative effects of benzodiazepines
  - ▸ BY INTRAVENOUS INJECTION
  - ▸ Neonate: 10 micrograms/kg every 1 minute if required, dose to be administered over 15 seconds.
  - ▸ Child: 10 micrograms/kg every 1 minute (max. per dose 200 micrograms) if required, dose to be administered over 15 seconds; maximum 1 mg per course; maximum 50 micrograms/kg per course

  Reversal of sedative effects of benzodiazepines (if drowsiness recurs after injection)
  - ▸ BY INTRAVENOUS INFUSION
  - ▸ Neonate: 2–10 micrograms/kg/hour, adjusted according to response.
  - ▸ Child: 2–10 micrograms/kg/hour (max. per dose 400 micrograms/hour), adjusted according to response

  Reversal of sedative effects of benzodiazepines in intensive care
  - ▸ BY INTRAVENOUS INJECTION
  - ▸ Child: 10 micrograms/kg every 1 minute (max. per dose 200 micrograms) if required, dose to be administered over 15 seconds; maximum 2 mg per course; maximum 50 micrograms/kg per course

- **UNLICENSED USE** Not licensed for use in children under 1 year. Not licensed for use by intravenous infusion in children. Not licensed for use in children in intensive care.

> **IMPORTANT SAFETY INFORMATION**
> Flumazenil should only be administered by, or under the direct supervision of, personnel experienced in its use.

- **CONTRA-INDICATIONS** Life-threatening condition (e.g. raised intracranial pressure, status epilepticus) controlled by benzodiazepines

- **CAUTIONS** Avoid rapid injection following major surgery · avoid rapid injection in high-risk or anxious patients · benzodiazepine dependence (may precipitate withdrawal symptoms) · children · ensure neuromuscular blockade cleared before giving · head injury (rapid reversal of benzodiazepine sedation may cause convulsions) · history of panic disorders (risk of recurrence) · prolonged benzodiazepine therapy for epilepsy (risk of convulsions) · short-acting (repeat doses may be necessary—benzodiazepine effects may persist for at least 24 hours)

- **SIDE-EFFECTS**
  - ▸ **Common or very common** Nausea · vomiting
  - ▸ **Uncommon** Anxiety · fear · palpitation
  - ▸ **Frequency not known** Agitation · chills · convulsions (particularly in those with epilepsy) · dizziness · flushing · sensory disturbance · sweating · tachycardia · transient hypertension

- **PREGNANCY** Not known to be harmful.

- **BREAST FEEDING** Avoid breast-feeding for 24 hours.

- **HEPATIC IMPAIRMENT** Carefully titrate dose.

- **DIRECTIONS FOR ADMINISTRATION** For *continuous intravenous infusion*, dilute with Glucose 5% or Sodium Chloride 0.9%.

16

Emergency treatment of poisoning

● MEDICINAL FORMS
There can be variation in the licensing of different medicines containing the same drug.
Solution for injection
▸ Flumazenil (Non-proprietary)
Flumazenil 100 microgram per 1 ml Flumazenil 500micrograms/5ml solution for injection ampoules | 5 ampoule [PoM] £65.50–£72.46

3.2 Digoxin toxicity

ANTIDOTES AND CHELATORS > ANTIBODIES

Digoxin-specific antibody

● INDICATIONS AND DOSE
Treatment of known or strongly suspected life-threatening digoxin toxicity associated with ventricular arrhythmias or bradyarrhythmias unresponsive to atropine and when measures beyond the withdrawal of digoxin and correction of any electrolyte abnormalities are considered necessary
▸ BY INTRAVENOUS INFUSION
▸ Child: Serious cases of digoxin toxicity should be discussed with the National Poisons Information Service (consult product literature)

● MEDICINAL FORMS
There can be variation in the licensing of different medicines containing the same drug.
Powder for solution for infusion
▸ DigiFab (BTG International Ltd)
Digoxin-specific antibody fragments 40 mg DigiFab 40mg powder for solution for infusion vials | 1 vial [PoM] £750.00 (Hospital only)

3.3 Heparin toxicity

ANTIDOTES AND CHELATORS

Protamine sulfate

● INDICATIONS AND DOSE
Overdosage with intravenous injection or intravenous infusion of unfractionated heparin (less than 30 minutes lapsed since overdose)
▸ BY INTRAVENOUS INJECTION
▸ Child: 1 mg (max. per dose 50 mg), to be administered at a rate not exceeding 5 mg/minute, to neutralise each 100 units of unfractionated heparin
Overdosage with intravenous injection or intravenous infusion of unfractionated heparin (if 30–60 minutes lapsed since overdose)
▸ BY INTRAVENOUS INJECTION
▸ Child: 500–750 micrograms (max. per dose 50 mg), to be administered at a rate not exceeding 5 mg/minute, to neutralise each 100 units of unfractionated heparin
Overdosage with intravenous injection or intravenous infusion of unfractionated heparin (if 60–120 minutes lapsed since overdose)
▸ BY INTRAVENOUS INJECTION
▸ Child: 375–500 micrograms (max. per dose 50 mg), to be administered at a rate not exceeding 5 mg/minute, to neutralise each 100 units of unfractionated heparin

Overdosage with intravenous injection or intravenous infusion of unfractionated heparin (if over 120 minutes lapsed since overdose)
▸ BY INTRAVENOUS INJECTION
▸ Child: 250–375 micrograms (max. per dose 50 mg), to be administered at a rate not exceeding 5 mg/minute, to neutralise each 100 units of unfractionated heparin
Overdosage with subcutaneous injection of unfractionated heparin
▸ BY INTRAVENOUS INJECTION, OR BY INTRAVENOUS INFUSION
▸ Child: (max. per dose 50 mg), 50–100% of the total dose to be given by intravenous injection (rate not exceeding 5 mg/minute), then give any remainder of dose by intravenous infusion over 8–16 hours, 1 mg neutralises approx. 100 units of unfractionated heparin
Overdosage with subcutaneous injection of low molecular weight heparin
▸ BY INTRAVENOUS INJECTION, OR BY CONTINUOUS INTRAVENOUS INFUSION
▸ Child: (max. per dose 50 mg), to be administered by intermittent intravenous injection at a rate not exceeding 5 mg/minute or by continuous intravenous infusion, 1 mg neutralises approx. 100 units of low molecular weight heparin, consult product literature of low molecular weight heparin for details

● CAUTIONS Excessive doses can have an anticoagulant effect

● SIDE-EFFECTS Anaphylaxis · angioedema · back pain · bradycardia · dyspnoea · flushing · hypersensitivity reactions · hypertension · hypotension · lassitude · nausea · pulmonary oedema · rebound bleeding · vomiting

● ALLERGY AND CROSS-SENSITIVITY Caution if increased risk of allergic reaction to protamine (includes previous treatment with protamine or protamine insulin, allergy to fish, men who are infertile or who have had a vasectomy and who may have antibodies to protamine).

● MONITORING REQUIREMENTS Monitor activated partial thromboplastin time or other appropriate blood clotting parameters.

● DIRECTIONS FOR ADMINISTRATION May be diluted if necessary with Sodium Chloride 0.9%.

● PRESCRIBING AND DISPENSING INFORMATION The long half-life of low molecular weight heparins should be taken into consideration when determining the dose of protamine sulfate; the effects of low molecular weight heparins can persist for up to 24 hours after administration.

● MEDICINAL FORMS
There can be variation in the licensing of different medicines containing the same drug.
Solution for injection
▸ Protamine sulfate (Non-proprietary)
Protamine sulfate 10 mg per 1 ml Protamine sulfate 100mg/10ml solution for injection ampoules [PoM] no price available
Protamine sulfate 50mg/5ml solution for injection ampoules | 10 ampoule [PoM] £49.55

3.4 Opioid toxicity

OPIOID RECEPTOR ANTAGONISTS

Naloxone hydrochloride

- **INDICATIONS AND DOSE**

Overdosage with opioids
▸ BY INTRAVENOUS INJECTION, OR BY SUBCUTANEOUS
INJECTION, OR BY INTRAMUSCULAR INJECTION

▸ Neonate: Initially 100 micrograms/kg, if no response, repeat at intervals of 1 minute to a total max. 2 mg, then review diagnosis; further doses may be required if respiratory function deteriorates.

▸ Child 1 month–11 years: Initially 100 micrograms/kg, if no response, repeat at intervals of 1 minute to a total max. 2 mg, then review diagnosis; further doses may be required if respiratory function deteriorates

▸ Child 12–17 years: Initially 400 micrograms, then 800 micrograms for up to 2 doses at 1 minute intervals if no response to preceding dose, then increased to 2 mg for 1 dose if still no response (4 mg dose may be required in seriously poisoned patients), then review diagnosis; further doses may be required if respiratory function deteriorates

▸ BY CONTINUOUS INTRAVENOUS INFUSION

▸ Neonate: Using an infusion pump, adjust rate according to response (initially, rate may be set at 60% of the initial resuscitative intravenous injection dose per hour). The initial resuscitative *intravenous injection* dose is that which maintained satisfactory ventilation for at least 15 minutes.

▸ Child: Using an infusion pump, adjust rate according to response (initially, rate may be set at 60% of the initial resuscitative intravenous injection dose per hour). The initial resuscitative *intravenous injection* dose is that which maintained satisfactory ventilation for at least 15 minutes

Reversal of postoperative respiratory depression
▸ INITIALLY BY INTRAVENOUS INJECTION

▸ Neonate: 1 microgram/kg, repeated every 2–3 minutes if required.

▸ Child 1 month–11 years: 1 microgram/kg, repeated every 2–3 minutes if required

▸ Child 12–17 years: Initially 100–200 micrograms, alternatively (by intravenous injection) initially 1.5–3 micrograms/kg, if response inadequate, give subsequent doses, (by intravenous injection) 100 micrograms every 2 minutes, alternatively (by intramuscular injection) 100 micrograms every 1–2 hours

Reversal of respiratory and CNS depression resulting from opioid administration to mother during labour
▸ BY INTRAMUSCULAR INJECTION

▸ Neonate: 200 micrograms, alternatively 60 micrograms/kg, to be given as a single dose at birth.

▸ BY INTRAVENOUS INJECTION, OR BY SUBCUTANEOUS INJECTION

▸ Neonate: 10 micrograms/kg, repeated every 2–3 minutes if required.

PHARMACOKINETICS
Naloxone has a short duration of action; repeated doses or infusion may be necessary to reverse effects of opioids with longer duration of action.
Important: Only give by subcutaneous or intramuscular routes if intravenous route is not feasible; intravenous administration has more rapid onset of action.

- **UNLICENSED USE** Naloxone doses in BNF may differ from those in product literature.

IMPORTANT SAFETY INFORMATION
SAFE PRACTICE
Doses used in acute opioid overdosage may not be appropriate for the management of opioid-induced respiratory depression and sedation in those receiving palliative care and in chronic opioid use.

- **CAUTIONS** Cardiovascular disease or those receiving cardiotoxic drugs (serious adverse cardiovascular effects reported) · maternal physical dependence on opioids (may precipitate withdrawal in newborn) · pain · physical dependence on opioids (precipitates withdrawal)
CAUTIONS, FURTHER INFORMATION
▸ Titration of dose In postoperative use, the dose should be titrated for each patient in order to obtain sufficient respiratory response; however, naloxone antagonises analgesia.

- **INTERACTIONS** → Appendix 1: naloxone
- **SIDE-EFFECTS**
▸ **Common or very common** Cardiac arrest · dizziness · dyspnoea · headache · hypertension · hyperventilation · hypotension · nausea · pulmonary oedema · tachycardia · ventricular fibrillation · vomiting
▸ **Uncommon** Agitation · diarrhoea · dry mouth · excitement · paraesthesia · sweating · tremor
▸ **Very rare** Erythema multiforme · seizures
- **PREGNANCY** Use only if potential benefit outweighs risk.
- **BREAST FEEDING** Not orally bioavailable.
- **DIRECTIONS FOR ADMINISTRATION** For *continuous intravenous infusion*, dilute to a concentration of up to 200 micrograms/mL with Glucose 5% or Sodium Chloride 0.9%.

- **MEDICINAL FORMS**
There can be variation in the licensing of different medicines containing the same drug.
Solution for injection
▸ Naloxone hydrochloride (Non-proprietary)
Naloxone hydrochloride 20 microgram per 1 ml Naloxone 40micrograms/2ml solution for injection ampoules |
10 ampoule [PoM] £55.00
Naloxone hydrochloride 400 microgram per 1 ml Naloxone 400micrograms/1ml solution for injection ampoules |
3 ampoule [PoM] £17.70 | 10 ampoule [PoM] £41.00–£53.70
Naloxone hydrochloride 1 mg per 1 ml Naloxone 2mg/2ml solution for injection pre-filled syringes | 1 pre-filled disposable injection [PoM] £16.80
▸ Prenoxad (Martindale Pharmaceuticals Ltd)
Naloxone hydrochloride 1 mg per 1 ml Prenoxad 2mg/2ml solution for injection pre-filled syringes | 1 pre-filled disposable injection [PoM] £15.30

16

Emergency treatment of poisoning

3.5 Paracetamol toxicity

ANTIDOTES AND CHELATORS

Acetylcysteine

07-Feb-2017

● **INDICATIONS AND DOSE**

Paracetamol overdosage
▶ BY INTRAVENOUS INFUSION

▶ **Neonate:** Initially 150 mg/kg over 1 hour, dose to be administered in 3 mL/kg glucose 5%, followed by 50 mg/kg over 4 hours, dose to be administered in 7 mL/kg glucose 5%, then 100 mg/kg over 16 hours, dose to be administered in 14 mL/kg glucose 5%.

▶ **Child (body-weight up to 20 kg):** Initially 150 mg/kg over 1 hour, dose to be administered in 3 mL/kg glucose 5%, followed by 50 mg/kg over 4 hours, dose to be administered in 7 mL/kg glucose 5%, then 100 mg/kg over 16 hours, dose to be administered in 14 mL/kg glucose 5%

▶ **Child (body-weight 20-39 kg):** Initially 150 mg/kg over 1 hour, dose to be administered in 100 mL glucose 5%, followed by 50 mg/kg over 4 hours, dose to be administered in 250 mL glucose 5%, then 100 mg/kg over 16 hours, dose to be administered in 500 mL glucose 5%

▶ **Child (body-weight 40 kg and above):** 150 mg/kg over 1 hour, dose to be administered in 200 mL Glucose Intravenous Infusion 5%, then 50 mg/kg over 4 hours, to be started immediately after completion of first infusion, dose to be administered in 500 mL Glucose Intravenous Infusion 5%, then 100 mg/kg over 16 hours, to be started immediately after completion of second infusion, dose to be administered in 1 litre Glucose Intravenous Infusion 5%

Meconium ileus
▶ BY MOUTH

▶ **Neonate:** 200–400 mg up to 3 times a day if required.

Treatment of distal intestinal obstructive syndrome
▶ BY MOUTH

▶ Child 1 month-1 year: 0.4–3 g as a single dose
▶ Child 2-6 years: 2–3 g as a single dose
▶ Child 7-17 years: 4–6 g as a single dose

Prevention of distal intestinal obstruction syndrome
▶ BY MOUTH

▶ Child 1 month-1 year: 100–200 mg 3 times a day
▶ Child 2-11 years: 200 mg 3 times a day
▶ Child 12-17 years: 200–400 mg 3 times a day

DOSES AT EXTREMES OF BODY-WEIGHT
To avoid excessive dosage in obese patients, a ceiling weight of 110 kg should be used when calculating the dose for paracetamol overdosage.

● **UNLICENSED USE** Not licensed for use in meconium ileus or for distal intestinal obstructive syndrome in children with cystic fibrosis.

IMPORTANT SAFETY INFORMATION
MHRA/CHM ADVICE: INTRAVENOUS ACETYLCYSTEINE FOR PARACETAMOL OVERDOSE: REMINDER OF AUTHORISED DOSE REGIMEN; POSSIBLE NEED FOR CONTINUED TREATMENT (JANUARY 2017)
The authorised dose regimen for acetylcysteine in paracetamol overdose is 3 consecutive intravenous infusions given over a total of 21 hours.
Continued treatment (given at the dose and rate as used in the third infusion) may be necessary depending on the clinical evaluation of the individual patient.

● **CAUTIONS**
▶ With intravenous use Asthma (see Side-effects for management of asthma but do not delay acetylcysteine treatment) · atopy · may slightly increase INR · may slightly increase prothrombin time
▶ With oral use Asthma · history of peptic ulceration

● **SIDE-EFFECTS**
▶ With intravenous use Hypersensitivity-like reactions · rashes · slight increase in INR and prothrombin time
▶ With oral use Anaphylaxis · Hypersensitivity-like reactions · rashes

SIDE-EFFECTS, FURTHER INFORMATION
▶ Hypersensitivity-like reactions
▶ With intravenous use Hypersensitivity-like reactions managed by reducing infusion rate or suspending until reaction settled (rash also managed by giving antihistamine; acute asthma managed by giving nebulised short-acting beta$_2$ agonist)—contact the National Poisons Information Service if reaction severe.

● **DIRECTIONS FOR ADMINISTRATION**
▶ With oral use For *oral* administration, use oral granules, or dilute injection solution (200 mg/mL) to a concentration of 50 mg/mL; orange or blackcurrant juice or cola drink may be used as a diluent to mask the bitter taste.
▶ With intravenous use Glucose 5% is preferred fluid; Sodium Chloride 0.9% is an alternative if Glucose 5% unsuitable.

● **MEDICINAL FORMS**
There can be variation in the licensing of different medicines containing the same drug.

Granules
CAUTIONARY AND ADVISORY LABELS 13
▶ Acetylcysteine (Non-proprietary)
Acetylcysteine 100 mg Fluimucil N 100mg granules sachets | 20 sachet [PoM] no price available | 50 sachet [PoM] no price available
Acetylcysteine 200 mg Fluimucil N 200mg granules sachets | 20 sachet [PoM] no price available | 50 sachet [PoM] no price available | 100 sachet [PoM] no price available
▶ A-CYS (Ennogen Healthcare Ltd)
Acetylcysteine 200 mg A-CYS 200mg granules sachets | 20 sachet £75.00

Solution for infusion
ELECTROLYTES: May contain Sodium
▶ Acetylcysteine (Non-proprietary)
Acetylcysteine 200 mg per 1 ml Acetylcysteine 2g/10ml solution for infusion ampoules | 10 ampoule [PoM] £21.26-£24.99
▶ Parvolex (Phoenix Labs Ltd)
Acetylcysteine 200 mg per 1 ml Parvolex 2g/10ml concentrate for solution for infusion ampoules | 10 ampoule [PoM] £22.50

4 Methaemoglobinaemia

ANTIDOTES AND CHELATORS

Methylthioninium chloride
(Methylene blue)

● **INDICATIONS AND DOSE**

Drug- or chemical-induced methaemoglobinaemia
▶ BY SLOW INTRAVENOUS INJECTION

▶ **Neonate:** Seek advice from National Poisons Information Service.

▶ Child 1-2 months: Seek advice from National Poisons Information Service
▶ Child 3 months-17 years: Initially 1–2 mg/kg, then 1–2 mg/kg after 30–60 minutes if required, to be given over 5 minutes, seek advice from National Poisons Information Service if further repeat doses are required; maximum 7 mg/kg per course

Aniline- or dapsone-induced methaemoglobinaemia
▸ BY SLOW INTRAVENOUS INJECTION
▸ Child 3 months–17 years: Initially 1–2 mg/kg, then
1–2 mg/kg after 30–60 minutes if required, to be given
over 5 minutes, seek advice from National Poisons
Information Service if further repeat doses are
required; maximum 4 mg/kg per course

● CAUTIONS Children under 3 months (more susceptible to
methaemoglobinaemia from high doses of
methylthioninium) · chlorate poisoning (reduces efficacy
of methylthioninium) · G6PD deficiency (seek advice from
National Poisons Information Service) ·
methaemoglobinaemia due to treatment of cyanide
poisoning with sodium nitrite (seek advice from National
Poisons Information Service) · pulse oximetry may give
false estimation of oxygen saturation

● INTERACTIONS → Appendix 1: methylthioninium chloride

● SIDE-EFFECTS Abdominal pain · agitation · anxiety ·
arrhythmia · blue-green discoloration of faeces · blue-
green discoloration of skin · blue-green discoloration of
urine · chest pain · confusion · dizziness · dyspnoea · fever ·
haemolytic anaemia · headache · hyperbilirubinaemia (in
infants) · hypertension · hypotension ·
methaemoglobinaemia · mydriasis · nausea · sweating ·
tachypnoea · tremor · vomiting

● PREGNANCY No information available, but risk to fetus of
untreated methaemoglobinaemia likely to be significantly
higher than risk of treatment.

● BREAST FEEDING Manufacturer advises avoid
breastfeeding for up to 6 days after administration—no
information available.

● RENAL IMPAIRMENT Use with caution in severe
impairment; dose reduction may be required.

● DIRECTIONS FOR ADMINISTRATION For *intravenous
injection*, may be diluted with Glucose 5% to minimise
injection-site pain; not compatible with Sodium Chloride
0.9%.

● MEDICINAL FORMS
There can be variation in the licensing of different medicines
containing the same drug. Forms available from special-order
manufacturers include: solution for injection
Solution for injection
▸ **Methylthioninium chloride (Non-proprietary)**
  Methylthioninium chloride 5 mg per 1 ml Methylthioninium
  chloride Proveblue 50mg/10ml solution for injection ampoules |
  5 ampoule PoM £167.36

5 Snake bites

IMMUNE SERA AND IMMUNOGLOBULINS ›
ANTITOXINS

European viper snake venom antiserum

● INDICATIONS AND DOSE
**Systemic envenoming from snake bites | Marked local
envenoming**
▸ BY INTRAVENOUS INJECTION, OR BY INTRAVENOUS INFUSION
▸ Child: Initially 10 mL for 1 dose, then 10 mL after
1–2 hours if required, the second dose should only be
given if symptoms of systemic envenoming persist
after the first dose, if symptoms of systemic
envenoming persist contact the National Poisons
Information Service

**Severe systemic envenoming from snake bites in patients
presenting with clinical features**
▸ BY INTRAVENOUS INJECTION, OR BY INTRAVENOUS INFUSION
▸ Child: Initially 20 mL for 1 dose, if symptoms of
systemic envenoming persist contact the National
Poisons Information Service

● DIRECTIONS FOR ADMINISTRATION By *intravenous injection*
given over 10–15 minutes or by *intravenous infusion* over
30 minutes after diluting in sodium chloride 0.9% (use
5 mL diluent/kg body-weight).

● PRESCRIBING AND DISPENSING INFORMATION To order,
email immform@dh.gsi.gov.uk.

● MEDICINAL FORMS
There can be variation in the licensing of different medicines
containing the same drug.
Solution for injection
▸ **European viper snake venom antiserum (Non-proprietary)**
  European viper snake venom antiserum 100 mg per 1 ml Viper
  venom antiserum, European (equine) 1g/10ml solution for injection
  vials | 1 vial PoM no price available

16

Emergency treatment of poisoning

Appendix 1
Interactions

Changes have been made to Appendix 1. For more information, see www.bnf.org.

Two or more drugs given at the same time can exert their effects independently or they can interact. Interactions may be beneficial and exploited therapeutically; this type of interaction is not within the scope of this appendix. Many interactions are harmless, and even those that are potentially harmful can often be managed, allowing the drugs to be used safely together. Nevertheless, adverse drug interactions should be reported to the Medicines and Healthcare products Regulatory Agency (MHRA), through the Yellow Card Scheme (see Adverse Reactions to Drugs, p. 12), as for other adverse drug reactions.

Potentially harmful drug interactions may occur in only a small number of patients, but the true incidence is often hard to establish. Furthermore the severity of a harmful interaction is likely to vary from one patient to another. Patients at increased risk from drug interactions include the elderly and those with impaired renal or hepatic function.

Interactions can result in the potentiation or antagonism of one drug by another, or result in another effect, such as renal impairment. Drug interactions may develop either through pharmacokinetic or pharmacodynamic mechanisms.

Pharmacodynamic interactions

These are interactions between drugs that have similar or antagonistic pharmacological effects or side-effects. They might be due to competition at receptor sites, or occur between drugs acting on the same physiological system. They are usually predictable from a knowledge of the pharmacology of the interacting drugs; in general, those demonstrated with one drug are likely to occur with related drugs.

Pharmacokinetic interactions

These occur when one drug alters the absorption, distribution, metabolism, or excretion of another, thus increasing or decreasing the amount of drug available to produce its pharmacological effects. Pharmacokinetic interactions occurring with one drug do not necessarily occur uniformly across a group of related drugs.

Affecting absorption

The rate of absorption and the total amount absorbed can both be altered by drug interactions. Delayed absorption is rarely of clinical importance unless a rapid effect is required (e.g. when giving an analgesic). Reduction in the total amount absorbed, however, can result in ineffective therapy.

Affecting distribution

Due to changes in protein binding

To a variable extent most drugs are loosely bound to plasma proteins. Protein-binding sites are non-specific and one drug can displace another thereby increasing the proportion free to diffuse from the plasma to its site of action. This only produces a detectable increase in effect if it is an extensively bound drug (more than 90%) that is not widely distributed throughout the body. Even so displacement rarely produces

more than transient potentiation because this increased concentration of free drug will usually be eliminated.

Displacement from protein binding does play a part in the potentiation of warfarin by sulfonamides but these interactions become clinically relevant mainly because warfarin metabolism is also inhibited.

Induction or inhibition of drug transporter proteins

Drug transporter proteins, such as P-glycoprotein, actively transport drugs across biological membranes. Transporters can be induced or inhibited, resulting in changes in the concentrations of drugs that are substrates for the transporter. For example, rifampicin induces P-glycoprotein, particularly in the gut wall, resulting in decreased plasma concentrations of digoxin, a P-glycoprotein substrate.

Affecting metabolism

Many drugs are metabolised in the liver. Drugs are either metabolised by phase I reactions (oxidation, reduction, or hydrolysis) or by phase II reactions (e.g. glucuronidation).

Phase I reactions are mainly carried out by the cytochrome P450 family of isoenzymes, of which CYP3A4 is the most important isoenzyme involved in the metabolism of drugs. Induction of cytochrome P450 isoenzymes by one drug can increase the rate of metabolism of another, resulting in lower plasma concentrations and a reduced effect. On withdrawal of the inducing drug, plasma concentrations increase and toxicity can occur.

Conversely when one drug inhibits cytochrome P450 isoenzymes, it can decrease the metabolism of another, leading to higher plasma concentrations, resulting in an increased effect with a risk of toxicity.

Isoenzymes of the hepatic cytochrome P450 system interact with a wide range of drugs. With knowledge of which isoenzymes are involved in a drug's metabolism, it is possible to predict whether certain pharmacokinetic interactions will occur. For example, carbamazepine is a potent inducer, ketoconazole is a potent inhibitor, and midazolam is a substrate of CYP3A4. Carbamazepine reduces midazolam concentrations, and it is therefore likely that other drugs that are potent inducers of CYP3A4 will interact similarly with midazolam. Ketoconazole, however, increases midazolam concentrations, and it can be predicted that other drugs that are potent inhibitors of CYP3A4 will interact similarly.

Less is known about the enzymes involved in phase II reactions. These might include UDP-glucuronyltransferases which, for example, might be induced by rifampicin, resulting in decreased metabolism of mycophenolate (a substrate for this enzyme) to its active form, mycophenolic acid.

Affecting renal excretion

Drugs are eliminated through the kidney both by glomerular filtration and by active tubular secretion. Competition occurs between those which share active transport mechanisms in the proximal tubule. For example, salicylates and some other NSAIDs delay the excretion of methotrexate; serious methotrexate toxicity is possible. Changes in urinary pH can also affect the reabsorption of a small number of drugs, including methenamine.

Relative importance of interactions

Severity of interactions

Most interactions have been assigned a severity; this describes the likely effect of an unmanaged interaction on the patient.

Severe – the result may be a life-threatening event or have a permanent detrimental effect.

Moderate – the result could cause considerable distress or partially incapacitate a patient; they are unlikely to be life-threatening or result in long-term effects.

Mild – the result is unlikely to cause concern or incapacitate the majority of patients.

Unknown – used for those interactions that are predicted, but there is insufficient evidence to hazard a guess at the outcome.

Evidence for interactions

Most interactions have been assigned a rating to indicate the weight of evidence behind the interaction.

Study – for interactions where the information is based on formal study including those for other drugs with the same mechanism (e.g. known inducers, inhibitors, or substrates of cytochrome P450 isoenzymes or P-glycoprotein).

Anecdotal – interactions based on either a single case report or a limited number of case reports.

Theoretical – interactions that are predicted based on sound theoretical considerations. The information may have been derived from *in vitro* studies or based on the way other members in the same class act.

Appendix 1 structure

❶ Drugs

Drugs are listed alphabetically. If a drug is a member of a drug class, all interactions for that drug will be listed under the drug class entry; in this case the drug entry provides direction to the relevant drug class where its interactions can be found.

    Within a drug or drug class entry, interactions are listed alphabetically by the interacting drug or drug class. The interactions describe the effect that occurs, and the action to be taken, either based on manufacturer's advice from the relevant Summary of Product Characteristics or advice from a relevant authority (e.g. MHRA). An action message is only included where the combination is to be avoided, where a dose adjustment is required, or where specific administration requirements (e.g. timing of doses) are recommended. If two drugs have a pharmacodynamic effect in addition to a pharmacokinetic interaction, a cross-reference to the relevant pharmacodynamic effect table is included at the end of the pharmacokinetic message.

❷ Drug classes

The drugs that are members of a drug class are listed underneath the drug class entry in a blue box. Interactions for the class are then listed alphabetically by the interacting drug or drug class. If the interaction only applies to certain drugs in the class, these drugs will be shown in brackets after the drug class name.

❸ Supplementary information

If a drug has additional important information to be considered, this is shown in a blue box underneath the drug or drug class entry. This information might be food and lifestyle advice (including smoking and alcohol consumption), relate to the pharmacology of the drug or applicability of interactions to certain routes of administration, or it might be advice about separating administration times.

---

❶ Drug entry
- ▸ Details of interaction between **drug entry** and another **drug** or **drug class**. Action statement. Severity Evidence
- ▸ Details of interaction between **drug entry** and another **drug** or **drug class**. Action statement. Severity Evidence
  → Also see **TABLE 1**

Drug entry → see Drug class entry

❷ Drug class entry

    Drug A · Drug B · Drug C · Drug D

- ▸ Details of interaction between **drug class entry** and another **drug** or **drug class**. Action statement. Severity Evidence

❸ Drug entry or Drug class entry

    Supplementary information

❹ Drug entry or Drug class entry → see **TABLE 1**

TABLE 1		
Name of pharmacodynamic effect		
Explanation of the effect		
Drug	Drug	Drug
Drug	Drug	Drug

---

❹ Pharmacodynamic effects

Tables at the beginning of Appendix 1 cover pharmacodynamic effects. If a drug is included in one or more of these tables, this will be indicated at the top of the list of interactions for the drug or drug class. In addition to the list of interactions for a drug or drug class, these tables should always be consulted.

    Each table describes the relevant pharmacodynamic effect and lists those drugs that are commonly associated with the effect. Concurrent use of two or more drugs from the same table is expected to increase the risk of the pharmacodynamic effect occurring. Please note these tables are not exhaustive.

    Other than for QT interval prolongation, actions for pharmacodynamic effects are not included in the BNF, as these will depend on individual patient circumstances.

TABLE 1
Drugs that cause hepatotoxicity

The following is a list of some drugs that cause hepatotoxicity (note that this list is not exhaustive). Concurrent use of two or more drugs from the list might increase this risk.

alcohol (beverage)	demeclocycline	leflunomide	minocycline	sulfasalazine
asparaginase	didanosine	lenalidomide	oxytetracycline	tetracycline
atorvastatin	doxycycline	lomitapide	paracetamol	tigecycline
carbamazepine	fluconazole	lymecycline	pegaspargase	trabectedin
crisantaspase	fluvastatin	mercaptopurine	pravastatin	valproate
dactinomycin	isoniazid	methotrexate	rosuvastatin	vincristine
dantrolene	itraconazole	micafungin	simvastatin	

TABLE 2
Drugs that cause nephrotoxicity

The following is a list of some drugs that cause nephrotoxicity (note that this list is not exhaustive). Concurrent use of two or more drugs from the list might increase this risk.

aceclofenac	ceftaroline	etoricoxib	nabumetone	tenofovir
acemetacin	ceftazidime	fenoprofen	naproxen	tenoxicam
aciclovir	ceftobiprole	flurbiprofen	neomycin	tiaprofenic acid
amikacin	ceftolozane	foscarnet	oxaliplatin	tobramycin
amphotericin	ceftriaxone	ganciclovir	parecoxib	tolfenamic acid
bacitracin	cefuroxime	gentamicin	pemetrexed	trimethoprim
capreomycin	celecoxib	ibuprofen	penicillamine	valaciclovir
carboplatin	ciclosporin	ifosfamide	pentamidine	valganciclovir
cefaclor	cisplatin	indometacin	piroxicam	vancomycin
cefadroxil	colistimethate	ketoprofen	polymyxins	zidovudine
cefalexin	dexibuprofen	ketorolac	streptomycin	zoledronic acid
cefixime	dexketoprofen	mefenamic acid	sulindac	
cefotaxime	diclofenac	meloxicam	tacrolimus	
cefradine	etodolac	methotrexate	telavancin	

TABLE 3
Drugs with anticoagulant effects

The following is a list of drugs that have anticoagulant effects. Concurrent use of two or more drugs from this list might increase the risk of bleeding; concurrent use of drugs with antiplatelet effects (see table of drugs with antiplatelet effects) might also increase this risk.

acenocoumarol	dabigatran	fondaparinux	phenindione	tinzaparin
alteplase	dalteparin	glucose	reteplase-to be deleted	urokinase
apixaban	danaparoid	heparin (unfractionated)	rivaroxaban	warfarin
argatroban	edoxaban	nicotinic acid	streptokinase	
bivalirudin	enoxaparin	omega-3-acid ethyl esters	tenecteplase	

TABLE 4
Drugs with antiplatelet effects

The following is a list of drugs that have antiplatelet effects (note that this list is not exhaustive). Concurrent use of two or more drugs from this list might increase the risk of bleeding; concurrent use of drugs with anticoagulant effects (see table of drugs with anticoagulant effects) might also increase this risk.

abciximab	dapoxetine	etoricoxib	mefenamic acid	sulindac
aceclofenac	dasatinib	fenoprofen	meloxicam	tenoxicam
acemetacin	dexibuprofen	fluoxetine	nabumetone	tiaprofenic acid
anagrelide	dexketoprofen	flurbiprofen	naproxen	ticagrelor
aspirin	diclofenac	fluvoxamine	parecoxib	tirofiban
bevacizumab	dipyridamole	ibrutinib	paroxetine	tolfenamic acid
cangrelor	duloxetine	ibuprofen	piroxicam	trastuzumab
celecoxib	epoprostenol	iloprost	prasugrel	trastuzumab emtansine
cilostazol	eptifibatide	indometacin	regorafenib	venlafaxine
citalopram	escitalopram	ketoprofen	sertraline	vortioxetine
clopidogrel	etodolac	ketorolac	sulfinpyrazone	

TABLE 5
Drugs that cause thromboembolism

The following is a list of some drugs that cause thromboembolism (note that this list is not exhaustive). Concurrent use of two or more drugs from the list might increase this risk.

bleomycin	epoetin zeta	pentostatin	tibolone	vindesine
cyclophosphamide	fluorouracil	pomalidomide	toremifene	vinflunine
darbepoetin alfa	fulvestrant	raloxifene	tranexamic acid	vinorelbine
doxorubicin	lenalidomide	strontium ranelate	tretinoin	
epoetin alfa	methotrexate	tamoxifen	vinblastine	
epoetin beta	mitomycin	thalidomide	vincristine	

TABLE 6

Drugs that cause bradycardia

The following is a list of drugs that cause bradycardia (note that this list is not exhaustive). Concurrent use of two or more drugs from the list might increase this risk.

acebutolol	carvedilol	fentanyl	nadolol	rivastigmine
alfentanil	celiprolol	fingolimod	nebivolol	selegiline
amiodarone	cisatracurium	flecainide	neostigmine	sotalol
apraclonidine	clonidine	galantamine	oxprenolol	sufentanil
atenolol	crizotinib	ivabradine	pasireotide	thalidomide
betaxolol	digoxin	labetalol	pindolol	timolol
bisoprolol	diltiazem	levobunolol	propranolol	tizanidine
brimonidine	donepezil	methadone	pyridostigmine	verapamil
carteolol	esmolol	metoprolol	remifentanil	

TABLE 7

Drugs that cause first dose hypotension

The following is a list of some drugs that can cause first-dose hypotension (note that this list is not exhaustive). Concurrent use of two or more drugs from the list might increase this risk.

alfuzosin	eprosartan	isosorbide dinitrate	perindopril	terazosin
azilsartan	fosinopril	isosorbide mononitrate	prazosin	trandolapril
candesartan	glyceryl trinitrate	lisinopril	quinapril	valsartan
captopril	imidapril	losartan	ramipril	
doxazosin	indoramin	moexipril	tamsulosin	
enalapril	irbesartan	olmesartan	telmisartan	

TABLE 8

Drugs that cause hypotension

The following is a list of some drugs that cause hypotension (note that this list is not exhaustive). Concurrent use of two or more drugs from the list might increase this risk.

acebutolol	chlorpromazine	haloperidol	moxisylyte	riociguat
alcohol (beverage)	chlortalidone	histamine	moxonidine	risperidone
alfuzosin	clevidipine	hydralazine	nadolol	ropinirole
aliskiren	clomipramine	hydrochlorothiazide	nebivolol	rotigotine
alprostadil	clonidine	imidapril	nicardipine	sacubitril
amantadine	clopamide	imipramine	nicorandil	sapropterin
amitriptyline	clozapine	indapamide	nifedipine	selegiline
amlodipine	cyclopenthiazide	indoramin	nimodipine	sevoflurane
apomorphine	dapagliflozin	irbesartan	nitrous oxide	sildenafil
apraclonidine	desflurane	isocarboxazid	nortriptyline	sodium nitroprusside
aripiprazole	diazoxide	isoflurane	olanzapine	sodium oxybate
asenapine	diltiazem	isosorbide dinitrate	olmesartan	sotalol
atenolol	dipyridamole	isosorbide mononitrate	oxprenolol	spironolactone
avanafil	dosulepin	isradipine	paliperidone	sulpiride
azilsartan	doxazosin	ketamine	pergolide	tadalafil
baclofen	doxepin	labetalol	pericyazine	tamsulosin
bendroflumethiazide	droperidol	lercanidipine	perindopril	telmisartan
benperidol	empagliflozin	levobunolol	perphenazine	terazosin
betaxolol	enalapril	levodopa	phenelzine	thiopental
bisoprolol	eplerenone	levomepromazine	phenoxybenzamine	timolol
bortezomib	eprosartan	lisinopril	pimozide	tizanidine
brimonidine	esmolol	lofepramine	pindolol	torasemide
bromocriptine	etomidate	lofexidine	pramipexole	trandolapril
bumetanide	felodipine	losartan	prazosin	tranylcypromine
cabergoline	flupentixol	loxapine	prochlorperazine	trifluoperazine
canagliflozin	fluphenazine	lurasidone	promazine	trimipramine
candesartan	fosinopril	methyldopa	propofol	valsartan
captopril	furosemide	metolazone	propranolol	vardenafil
carteolol	glyceryl trinitrate	metoprolol	quetiapine	verapamil
carvedilol	guanethidine	minoxidil	quinagolide	xipamide
celiprolol	guanfacine	moexipril	quinapril	zuclopenthixol
			ramipril	

TABLE 9
Drugs that prolong the QT interval

The following is a list of some drugs that prolong the QT-interval (note that this list is not exhaustive). In general, manufacturers advise that the use of two or more drugs that are associated with QT prolongation should be avoided. Increasing age, female sex, cardiac disease, and some metabolic disturbances (notably hypokalaemia) predispose to QT prolongation—concurrent use of drugs that reduce serum potassium might further increase this risk (see table of drugs that reduce serum potassium).

Drugs that are not known to prolong the QT interval but are predicted (by the manufacturer) to increase the risk of QT prolongation include: domperidone, erythromycin, fingolimod, granisetron, ivabradine, mefloquine, mizolastine, palonosetron, and pentamidine. Most manufacturers advise avoiding concurrent use with drugs that prolong the QT interval.

amifampridine	clarithromycin	hydroxyzine	pazopanib	tizanidine
amiodarone	clomipramine	lapatinib	pimozide	tolterodine
amisulpride	crizotinib	levomepromazine	quinine	toremifene
apomorphine	dasatinib	lithium	ranolazine	vandetanib
arsenic trioxide	delamanid	lofexidine	risperidone	vardenafil
artemether	disopyramide	methadone	saquinavir	vemurafenib
artenimol	dronedarone	moxifloxacin	sildenafil	venlafaxine
bedaquiline	droperidol	nilotinib	sorafenib	vinflunine
bosutinib	eribulin	ondansetron	sotalol	voriconazole
cabozantinib	escitalopram	osimertinib	sulpiride	zuclopenthixol
ceritinib	flecainide	paliperidone	sunitinib	
chlorpromazine	fluphenazine	panobinostat	telavancin	
citalopram	haloperidol	pasireotide	tetrabenazine	

TABLE 10
Drugs with antimuscarinic effects

The following is a list of some drugs that have antimuscarinic effects (note that this list is not exhaustive). Concurrent use of two or more drugs from this list might increase the risk of these effects occurring.

aclidinium	cyclopentolate	haloperidol	orphenadrine	tiotropium
amantadine	cyproheptadine	homatropine	oxybutynin	tolterodine
amitriptyline	darifenacin	hydroxyzine	perphenazine	trifluoperazine
atropine	dicycloverine	hyoscine	pimozide	trihexyphenidyl
baclofen	dimenhydrinate	imipramine	prochlorperazine	trimipramine
chlorphenamine	disopyramide	ipratropium	procyclidine	tropicamide
chlorpromazine	dosulepin	levomepromazine	promethazine	trospium
clemastine	doxepin	lofepramine	propafenone	umeclidinium
clomipramine	fesoterodine	loxapine	propantheline	
clozapine	flavoxate	nefopam	propiverine	
cyclizine	glycopyrronium	nortriptyline	solifenacin	

TABLE 11
Drugs with CNS depressant effects

The following is a list of some drugs with CNS depressant effects (note that this list is not exhaustive). Concurrent use of two or more drugs from this list might increase the risk of CNS depressant effects, such as drowsiness, which might affect the ability to perform skilled tasks (see Drugs and Driving p. 3).

agomelatine	clomethiazole	isoflurane	nabilone	remifentanil
alcohol (beverage)	clonazepam	ketamine	nitrazepam	risperidone
alfentanil	clonidine	ketotifen	nitrous oxide	ropivacaine
alimemazine	clozapine	lamotrigine	olanzapine	sevoflurane
alprazolam	codeine	levetiracetam	oxazepam	sodium oxybate
amisulpride	cyclizine	levomepromazine	oxycodone	sufentanil
apraclonidine	cyproheptadine	lidocaine	paliperidone	sulpiride
aripiprazole	desflurane	loprazolam	papaveretum	tapentadol
articaine	dexmedetomidine	lorazepam	pentazocine	temazepam
asenapine	diamorphine	lormetazepam	perampanel	tetracaine
baclofen	diazepam	loxapine	pericyazine	thalidomide
benperidol	dihydrocodeine	lurasidone	perphenazine	thiopental
brimonidine	dipipanone	melatonin	pethidine	tizanidine
buclizine	droperidol	mepivacaine	phenobarbital	tramadol
bupivacaine	etomidate	meprobamate	pimozide	trazodone
buprenorphine	fentanyl	meptazinol	pizotifen	trifluoperazine
cannabis extract	flupentixol	methadone	pregabalin	venlafaxine
chloral hydrate	fluphenazine	methocarbamol	prilocaine	zaleplon
chlordiazepoxide	flurazepam	mianserin	primidone	zolpidem
chloroprocaine	gabapentin	midazolam	prochlorperazine	zopiclone
chlorphenamine	guanfacine	mirtazapine	promazine	zuclopenthixol
chlorpromazine	haloperidol	morphine	promethazine	
cinnarizine	hydromorphone	moxonidine	propofol	
clemastine	hydroxyzine		quetiapine	

TABLE 12
Drugs that cause peripheral neuropathy

The following is a list of some drugs that cause peripheral neuropathy (note that this list is not exhaustive). Concurrent use of two or more drugs from the list might increase this risk.

amiodarone	didanosine	isoniazid	stavudine	vinflunine
bortezomib	disulfiram	lamivudine	thalidomide	vinorelbine
brentuximab vedotin	docetaxel	metronidazole	vinblastine	
cabazitaxel	eribulin	paclitaxel	vincristine	
cisplatin	fosphenytoin	phenytoin	vindesine	

TABLE 13
Drugs that cause serotonin syndrome

The following is a list of some drugs that cause serotonin syndrome (note that this list is not exhaustive). See Antidepressant drugs p. 226 for more information and specific advice on avoiding monoamine-oxidase inhibitors during and after administration of other serotonergic drugs.

almotriptan	fentanyl	methadone	pethidine	tapentadol
bupropion	fluoxetine	methylthioninium chloride	phenelzine	tedizolid
buspirone	fluvoxamine	mianserin	procarbazine	tramadol
citalopram	frovatriptan	mirtazapine	rasagiline	tranylcypromine
clomipramine	granisetron	moclobemide	rizatriptan	trazodone
dapoxetine	imipramine	naratriptan	safinamide	venlafaxine
dexamfetamine	isocarboxazid	ondansetron	selegiline	vortioxetine
duloxetine	linezolid	palonosetron	sertraline	zolmitriptan
eletriptan	lisdexamfetamine	paroxetine	St John's Wort	
escitalopram	lithium	pentazocine	sumatriptan	

TABLE 14
Antidiabetic drugs

The following is a list of antidiabetic drugs (note that this list is not exhaustive). Concurrent use of two or more drugs from the list might increase the risk of hypoglycaemia.

acarbose	dulaglutide	insulin aspart	linagliptin	saxagliptin
albiglutide	empagliflozin	insulin degludec	liraglutide	sitagliptin
alogliptin	exenatide	insulin detemir	lixisenatide	tolbutamide
biphasic insulin aspart	glibenclamide	insulin glargine	metformin	vildagliptin
biphasic insulin lispro	gliclazide	insulin glulisine	nateglinide	
biphasic isophane insulin	glimepiride	insulin lispro	pioglitazone	
canagliflozin	glipizide	insulin zinc suspension	protamine zinc insulin	
dapagliflozin	insulin	isophane insulin	repaglinide	

TABLE 15
Drugs that cause myelosuppression

The following is a list of some drugs that cause myelosuppression (note that this list is not exhaustive). Concurrent use of two or more drugs from the list might increase this risk.

afatinib	carmustine	everolimus	nilotinib	rituximab
aflibercept	ceritinib	fludarabine	nivolumab	ruxolitinib
alemtuzumab	cetuximab	fluorouracil	obinutuzumab	siltuximab
amsacrine	chlorambucil	ganciclovir	ofatumumab	sorafenib
anakinra	cisplatin	gefitinib	olanzapine	sulfadiazine
arsenic trioxide	cladribine	gemcitabine	olaparib	sulfasalazine
asparaginase	clofarabine	hydroxycarbamide	olsalazine	sunitinib
axitinib	clozapine	ibrutinib	oxaliplatin	temozolomide
azacitidine	co-trimoxazole	idarubicin	paclitaxel	temsirolimus
azathioprine	crisantaspase	idelalisib	panitumumab	thalidomide
balsalazide	crizotinib	ifosfamide	panobinostat	thiotepa
belimumab	cyclophosphamide	imatinib	pazopanib	tioguanine
bendamustine	cytarabine	interferon alfa	pegaspargase	topotecan
bevacizumab	dabrafenib	interferon beta	peginterferon alfa	trabectedin
blinatumomab	dacarbazine	irinotecan	peginterferon beta-1a	trastuzumab emtansine
bortezomib	dactinomycin	leflunomide	pemetrexed	treosulfan
bosutinib	dasatinib	lenalidomide	pentamidine	valganciclovir
brentuximab vedotin	daunorubicin	linezolid	pentostatin	vinblastine
busulfan	decitabine	lomustine	pixantrone	vincristine
cabazitaxel	deferiprone	melphalan	pomalidomide	vindesine
cabozantinib	docetaxel	mercaptopurine	primaquine	vinflunine
canakinumab	doxorubicin	methotrexate	procarbazine	vinorelbine
capecitabine	epirubicin	mitomycin	propylthiouracil	vismodegib
carbimazole	eribulin	mitotane	pyrimethamine	zidovudine
carboplatin	estramustine	mitoxantrone	raltitrexed	
carfilzomib	ethosuximide	mycophenolate	ramucirumab	
	etoposide	nelarabine	regorafenib	

TABLE 16
Drugs that increase serum potassium

The following is a list of some drugs that increase serum potassium concentrations (note that this list is not exhaustive). Concurrent use of two or more drugs from this list might increase the risk of hyperkalaemia (hyperkalaemia is particularly notable when ACE inhibitors or angiotensin-II receptor antagonists are given with spironolactone or eplerenone).

aceclofenac	dexibuprofen	felbinac	meloxicam	spironolactone
acemetacin	dexketoprofen	fenoprofen	moexipril	sulindac
aliskiren	diclofenac	flurbiprofen	nabumetone	tacrolimus
amiloride	drospirenone	heparin (unfractionated)	naproxen	telmisartan
azilsartan	enalapril	ibuprofen	nepafenac	tenoxicam
benzydamine	enoxaparin	imidapril	olmesartan	tiaprofenic acid
bromfenac	eplerenone	indometacin	parecoxib	tinzaparin
candesartan	epoetin alfa	irbesartan	perindopril	tolfenamic acid
captopril	epoetin beta	ketoprofen	piroxicam	tolvaptan
celecoxib	epoetin zeta	ketorolac	potassium canrenoate	trandolapril
ciclosporin	eprosartan	lisinopril	potassium chloride	triamterene
dalteparin	etodolac	losartan	quinapril	trimethoprim
darbepoetin alfa	etoricoxib	mefenamic acid	ramipril	valsartan

TABLE 17
Drugs that reduce serum potassium

The following is a list of some drugs that reduce serum potassium concentrations (note that this list is not exhaustive). Concurrent use of two or more drugs from this list might increase the risk of hypokalaemia. Hypokalaemia can increase the risk of torsade de pointes, which might be additive with the effects of drugs that prolong the QT interval (see table of drugs that prolong the QT interval).

aminophylline	bumetanide	fludrocortisone	indapamide	senna
amphotericin	chlortalidone	formoterol	methylprednisolone	sodium picosulfate
bambuterol	clopamide	furosemide	metolazone	terbutaline
beclometasone	cyclopenthiazide	glycerol	olodaterol	theophylline
bendroflumethiazide	dantron	hydrochlorothiazide	prednisolone	torasemide
betamethasone	deflazacort	hydrocortisone	prednisone	triamcinolone
bisacodyl	dexamethasone	hydroflumethiazide	salbutamol	vilanterol
budesonide	docusate sodium	indacaterol	salmeterol	xipamide

TABLE 18
Drugs that cause hyponatraemia

The following is a list of some drugs that reduce sodium concentrations (note that this list is not exhaustive). Concurrent use of two or more drugs from this list might increase the risk of hyponatraemia.

aceclofenac	cyclopenthiazide	etoricoxib	ketorolac	spironolactone
acemetacin	dapoxetine	fenoprofen	mefenamic acid	sulindac
amiloride	desmopressin	fluoxetine	meloxicam	tenoxicam
amitriptyline	dexibuprofen	flurbiprofen	metolazone	tiaprofenic acid
bendroflumethiazide	dexketoprofen	fluvoxamine	nabumetone	tolfenamic acid
bumetanide	diclofenac	furosemide	naproxen	torasemide
carbamazepine	dosulepin	hydrochlorothiazide	nortriptyline	triamterene
celecoxib	doxepin	ibuprofen	parecoxib	trimethoprim
chlortalidone	duloxetine	imipramine	paroxetine	trimipramine
citalopram	eplerenone	indapamide	piroxicam	xipamide
clomipramine	escitalopram	indometacin	sertraline	
clopamide	etodolac	ketoprofen	sodium picosulfate	

TABLE 19
Drugs that cause ototoxicity

The following is a list of some drugs that cause ototoxicity (note that this list is not exhaustive). Concurrent use of two or more drugs from the list might increase this risk.

amikacin	cisplatin	oxaliplatin	torasemide	vindesine
bumetanide	furosemide	streptomycin	vancomycin	vinflunine
capreomycin	gentamicin	telavancin	vinblastine	vinorelbine
carboplatin	neomycin	tobramycin	vincristine	

TABLE 20
Drugs with neuromuscular blocking effects

The following is a list of some drugs with neuromuscular blocking effects (note that this list is not exhaustive). Concurrent use of two or more drugs from the list might increase this risk.

amikacin	cisatracurium	neomycin	pyridostigmine	tobramycin
atracurium	colistimethate	neostigmine	rocuronium	vecuronium
botulinum toxin type A	gentamicin	pancuronium	streptomycin	
botulinum toxin type B	mivacurium	polymyxins	suxamethonium	

List of drug interactions

The following is an alphabetical list of drugs and their interactions; to avoid excessive cross-referencing each drug or group is listed twice: in the alphabetical list and also against the drug or group with which it interacts.

Abacavir
- Antiepileptics (carbamazepine, fosphenytoin, phenobarbital, phenytoin, primidone) are predicted to decrease the exposure to abacavir. Moderate Theoretical
- Enzalutamide is predicted to decrease the exposure to abacavir. Moderate Theoretical
- HIV-protease inhibitors (tipranavir) slightly decrease the exposure to abacavir. Avoid. Severe Study
- Rifampicin is predicted to decrease the exposure to abacavir. Moderate Theoretical

Abatacept
- Live vaccines are predicted to increase the risk of generalised infection (possibly life-threatening) when given with abatacept. Public Health England advises avoid. Severe Theoretical

Abciximab → see TABLE 4 p. 818 (antiplatelet effects)

Abiraterone

GENERAL INFORMATION Caution with concurrent chemotherapy—safety and efficacy not established.

- Abiraterone is predicted to increase the exposure to antiarrhythmics (flecainide). Severe Theoretical
- Antiepileptics (carbamazepine, fosphenytoin, phenobarbital, phenytoin, primidone) are predicted to decrease the exposure to abiraterone. Avoid. Severe Theoretical
- Antifungals, azoles (itraconazole, ketoconazole, voriconazole) are predicted to increase the exposure to abiraterone. Severe Theoretical
- Abiraterone is predicted to increase the exposure to beta blockers, non-selective (carvedilol, timolol). Moderate Theoretical
- Abiraterone is predicted to increase the exposure to beta blockers, selective (metoprolol, nebivolol). Moderate Study
- Cobicistat is predicted to increase the exposure to abiraterone. Severe Theoretical
- Enzalutamide is predicted to decrease the exposure to abiraterone. Avoid. Severe Theoretical
- HIV-protease inhibitors (atazanavir, darunavir, fosamprenavir, lopinavir, ritonavir, saquinavir, tipranavir) are predicted to increase the exposure to abiraterone. Severe Theoretical
- Idelalisib is predicted to increase the exposure to abiraterone. Severe Theoretical
- Macrolides (clarithromycin) are predicted to increase the exposure to abiraterone. Severe Theoretical
- Abiraterone is predicted to decrease the efficacy of opioids (tramadol). Moderate Study
- Abiraterone is predicted to increase the exposure to pitolisant. Use with caution and adjust dose. Moderate Study
- Rifampicin is predicted to decrease the exposure to abiraterone. Avoid. Severe Theoretical
- Abiraterone potentially increases the exposure to venlafaxine. Severe Theoretical

Acarbose → see TABLE 14 p. 821 (antidiabetic drugs)
- Acarbose decreases the concentration of digoxin. Moderate Study
- Pancreatin is predicted to decrease the effects of acarbose. Avoid. Moderate Theoretical

ACE inhibitors → see TABLE 7 p. 819 (first-dose hypotension), TABLE 8 p. 819 (hypotension), TABLE 16 p. 822 (increased serum potassium)

captopril · enalapril · fosinopril · imidapril · lisinopril · moexipril · perindopril · quinapril · ramipril · trandolapril

- ACE inhibitors increase the risk of renal impairment when given with aliskiren. Use with caution or avoid aliskiren in selected patients. Severe Study → Also see TABLE 8 p. 819 → Also see TABLE 16 p. 822
- ACE inhibitors are predicted to increase the risk of hypersensitivity and haematological reactions when given with allopurinol. Severe Anecdotal
- ACE inhibitors are predicted to increase the risk of anaemia and/or leucopenia when given with azathioprine. Severe Anecdotal
- ACE inhibitors increase the risk of hypersensitivity when given with bee venom extract. Avoid. Severe Study
- ACE inhibitors are predicted to decrease the efficacy of icatibant and icatibant is predicted to decrease the efficacy of ACE inhibitors. Avoid. Moderate Theoretical
- ACE inhibitors are predicted to increase the concentration of lithium. Monitor and adjust dose. Severe Anecdotal
- ACE inhibitors are predicted to increase the risk of hypersensitivity when given with sodium aurothiomalate. Severe Anecdotal
- Quinapril (tablet) decreases the absorption of oral tetracyclines (tetracycline). Avoid. Moderate Study
- ACE inhibitors increase the risk of hypersensitivity when given with wasp venom extract. Avoid. Severe Study

Acebutolol → see beta blockers, selective
Aceclofenac → see NSAIDs
Acemetacin → see NSAIDs
Acenocoumarol → see coumarins

Acetazolamide
- Acetazolamide potentially increases the risk of overheating and dehydration when given with antiepileptics (zonisamide). Avoid in children. Severe Theoretical
- Acetazolamide increases the risk of severe toxic reaction when given with aspirin (high-dose). Severe Study
- Acetazolamide alters the concentration of lithium. Severe Anecdotal
- Acetazolamide is predicted to decrease the efficacy of methenamine. Avoid. Moderate Theoretical
- Acetazolamide increases the urinary excretion of methotrexate. Moderate Study

Aciclovir → see TABLE 2 p. 818 (nephrotoxicity)

ROUTE-SPECIFIC INFORMATION Since systemic absorption can follow topical application, the possibility of interactions should be borne in mind.

- Aciclovir increases the exposure to aminophylline. Monitor theophylline concentration and adjust dose. Severe Anecdotal
- Mycophenolate is predicted to increase the risk of haematological toxicity when given with aciclovir. Moderate Theoretical
- Aciclovir is predicted to increase the exposure to theophylline. Monitor theophylline concentration and adjust dose. Severe Theoretical

Acitretin → see retinoids
Aclidinium → see TABLE 10 p. 820 (antimuscarinics)
Acrivastine → see antihistamines, non-sedating
Adalimumab → see monoclonal antibodies
Adapalene → see retinoids

Adefovir
- Ataluren increases the exposure to adefovir. Moderate Study

Adenosine → see antiarrhythmics
Adrenaline/epinephrine → see sympathomimetics, vasoconstrictor
Afatinib → see TABLE 15 p. 821 (myelosuppression)
- Antiarrhythmics (amiodarone, dronedarone) are predicted to increase the exposure to afatinib. Separate administration by 12 hours. Moderate Study
- Antiepileptics (carbamazepine) are predicted to decrease the exposure to afatinib. Moderate Study
- Antifungals, azoles (itraconazole, ketoconazole) are predicted to increase the exposure to afatinib. Separate administration by 12 hours. Moderate Study
- Calcium channel blockers (verapamil) are predicted to increase the exposure to afatinib. Separate administration by 12 hours. Moderate Study
- Ciclosporin is predicted to increase the exposure to afatinib. Separate administration by 12 hours. Moderate Study
- HIV-protease inhibitors (lopinavir, ritonavir, saquinavir) are predicted to increase the exposure to afatinib. Separate administration by 12 hours. Moderate Study
- Lapatinib is predicted to increase the exposure to afatinib. Separate administration by 12 hours. Moderate Study
- Macrolides are predicted to increase the exposure to afatinib. Separate administration by 12 hours. Moderate Study

A1

Interactions | **Appendix 1**

Afatinib (continued)
- Ranolazine is predicted to increase the exposure to afatinib. Separate administration by 12 hours. Moderate Study
- Rifampicin is predicted to decrease the exposure to afatinib. Moderate Study
- St John's Wort is predicted to decrease the exposure to afatinib. Moderate Study
- Vemurafenib is predicted to increase the exposure to afatinib. Separate administration by 12 hours. Moderate Study

Aflibercept → see TABLE 15 p. 821 (myelosuppression)

Agalsidase
- Aminoglycosides are predicted to decrease the effects of agalsidase. Avoid. Moderate Theoretical
- Antiarrhythmics (amiodarone) are predicted to decrease the effects of agalsidase. Avoid. Moderate Theoretical
- Antimalarials (chloroquine) are predicted to decrease the effects of agalsidase. Avoid. Moderate Theoretical
- Hydroxychloroquine is predicted to decrease the effects of agalsidase. Moderate Theoretical

Agomelatine → see TABLE 11 p. 820 (CNS depressant effects)

> - Dose adjustment might be necessary if smoking started or stopped during treatment.
> - Caution with concomitant use of drugs associated with hepatic injury.

- Antiepileptics (fosphenytoin, phenytoin) are predicted to decrease the exposure to agomelatine. Moderate Theoretical
- Combined hormonal contraceptives are predicted to increase the exposure to agomelatine. Moderate Study
- HIV-protease inhibitors (ritonavir) are predicted to decrease the exposure to agomelatine. Moderate Theoretical
- Quinolones (ciprofloxacin) are predicted to increase the exposure to agomelatine. Moderate Study
- Rifampicin is predicted to decrease the exposure to agomelatine. Moderate Theoretical
- SSRIs (fluvoxamine) very markedly increase the exposure to agomelatine. Avoid. Severe Study

Albendazole
- Antiepileptics (carbamazepine, fosphenytoin, phenobarbital, phenytoin, primidone) decrease the concentration of albendazole. Moderate Study
- H₂ receptor antagonists (cimetidine) decrease the clearance of albendazole. Moderate Study
- HIV-protease inhibitors (ritonavir) decrease the exposure to albendazole. Moderate Study
- Albendazole slightly decreases the exposure to levamisole and levamisole moderately decreases the exposure to albendazole. Moderate Study

Albiglutide → see TABLE 14 p. 821 (antidiabetic drugs)

Alcohol (beverage) → see TABLE 1 p. 818 (hepatotoxicity), TABLE 8 p. 819 (hypotension), TABLE 11 p. 820 (CNS depressant effects)

Aldosterone antagonists → see TABLE 18 p. 822 (hyponatraemia), TABLE 8 p. 819 (hypotension), TABLE 16 p. 822 (increased serum potassium)

eplerenone · spironolactone

- Antiarrhythmics (amiodarone) are predicted to increase the exposure to eplerenone. Adjust eplerenone dose. Severe Theoretical
- Antiarrhythmics (dronedarone) are predicted to increase the exposure to eplerenone. Adjust eplerenone dose. Severe Study
- Antiepileptics (carbamazepine, fosphenytoin, phenobarbital, phenytoin, primidone) are predicted to decrease the exposure to eplerenone. Avoid. Moderate Theoretical → Also see TABLE 18 p. 822
- Antifungals, azoles (fluconazole, isavuconazole, posaconazole) are predicted to increase the exposure to eplerenone. Adjust eplerenone dose. Severe Study
- Antifungals, azoles (itraconazole, ketoconazole, voriconazole) are predicted to markedly increase the exposure to eplerenone. Avoid. Severe Study
- Aprepitant is predicted to increase the exposure to eplerenone. Adjust eplerenone dose. Severe Study
- Calcium channel blockers (diltiazem, verapamil) are predicted to increase the exposure to eplerenone. Adjust eplerenone dose. Severe Study → Also see TABLE 8 p. 819

- Cobicistat is predicted to markedly increase the exposure to eplerenone. Avoid. Severe Study
- Crizotinib is predicted to increase the exposure to eplerenone. Adjust eplerenone dose. Severe Study
- Eplerenone very slightly increases the exposure to digoxin. Mild Study
- Spironolactone increases the concentration of digoxin. Monitor and adjust dose. Moderate Study
- Enzalutamide is predicted to decrease the exposure to eplerenone. Avoid. Moderate Theoretical
- HIV-protease inhibitors (atazanavir, darunavir, fosamprenavir, lopinavir, ritonavir, saquinavir, tipranavir) are predicted to markedly increase the exposure to eplerenone. Avoid. Severe Study
- HIV-protease inhibitors (indinavir) are predicted to increase the exposure to eplerenone. Adjust eplerenone dose. Severe Study
- Idelalisib is predicted to markedly increase the exposure to eplerenone. Avoid. Severe Study
- Imatinib is predicted to increase the exposure to eplerenone. Adjust eplerenone dose. Severe Study
- Eplerenone is predicted to increase the concentration of lithium. Avoid. Moderate Theoretical
- Spironolactone potentially increases the concentration of lithium. Avoid. Moderate Study
- Macrolides (clarithromycin) are predicted to markedly increase the exposure to eplerenone. Avoid. Severe Study
- Macrolides (erythromycin) are predicted to increase the exposure to eplerenone. Adjust eplerenone dose. Severe Study
- Spironolactone is predicted to decrease the effects of mitotane. Avoid. Severe Anecdotal
- Netupitant is predicted to increase the exposure to eplerenone. Adjust eplerenone dose. Severe Study
- Nilotinib is predicted to increase the exposure to eplerenone. Adjust eplerenone dose. Severe Study
- Rifampicin is predicted to decrease the exposure to eplerenone. Avoid. Moderate Theoretical
- St John's Wort is predicted to slightly decrease the exposure to eplerenone. Avoid. Moderate Study

Alemtuzumab → see monoclonal antibodies
Alendronic acid → see bisphosphonates
Alfacalcidol → see vitamin D substances
Alfentanil → see opioids
Alfuzosin → see alpha blockers
Alimemazine → see antihistamines, sedating
Alirocumab → see monoclonal antibodies
Aliskiren → see TABLE 8 p. 819 (hypotension), TABLE 16 p. 822 (increased serum potassium)

FOOD AND LIFESTYLE Avoid apple juice and orange juice as they greatly decrease aliskiren concentrations and plasma renin activity.

- ACE inhibitors increase the risk of renal impairment when given with aliskiren. Use with caution or avoid aliskiren in selected patients. Severe Study → Also see TABLE 8 p. 819 → Also see TABLE 16 p. 822
- Angiotensin-II receptor antagonists increase the risk of renal impairment when given with aliskiren. Use with caution or avoid aliskiren in selected patients. Severe Study → Also see TABLE 8 p. 819 (hypotension) → Also see TABLE 16 p. 822
- Antiarrhythmics (amiodarone, dronedarone) are predicted to increase the exposure to aliskiren. Severe Study
- Antiepileptics (carbamazepine) decrease the exposure to aliskiren. Moderate Study
- Antifungals, azoles (itraconazole) markedly increase the exposure to aliskiren. Avoid. Severe Study
- Antifungals, azoles (ketoconazole) moderately increase the exposure to aliskiren. Moderate Study
- Calcium channel blockers (verapamil) moderately increase the exposure to aliskiren. Moderate Study → Also see TABLE 8 p. 819
- Ceritinib is predicted to increase the exposure to aliskiren. Moderate Theoretical
- Ciclosporin markedly increases the exposure to aliskiren. Avoid. Severe Study → Also see TABLE 16 p. 822
- Grapefruit juice moderately decreases the exposure to aliskiren. Avoid. Moderate Study

- HIV-protease inhibitors **(ritonavir, saquinavir)** are predicted to increase the exposure to **aliskiren**. [Moderate] Theoretical
- **Lapatinib** is predicted to increase the exposure to **aliskiren**. [Moderate] Theoretical
- **Aliskiren** slightly decreases the exposure to loop diuretics **(furosemide)**. [Moderate] Study → Also see **TABLE 8** p. 819
- **Lumacaftor** is predicted to affect the exposure to **aliskiren**. [Moderate] Theoretical
- Macrolides **(azithromycin)** are predicted to increase the exposure to **aliskiren**. [Moderate] Theoretical
- Macrolides **(clarithromycin, erythromycin)** are predicted to increase the exposure to **aliskiren**. [Moderate] Study
- **Mirabegron** is predicted to increase the exposure to **aliskiren**. [Mild] Theoretical
- **Ranolazine** is predicted to increase the exposure to **aliskiren**. [Moderate] Theoretical
- **Rifampicin** decreases the exposure to **aliskiren**. [Moderate] Study
- **St John's Wort** decreases the exposure to **aliskiren**. [Moderate] Study
- Statins **(atorvastatin)** slightly to moderately increase the exposure to **aliskiren**. [Moderate] Study
- **Velpatasvir** is predicted to increase the exposure to **aliskiren**. [Severe] Theoretical
- **Vemurafenib** is predicted to increase the exposure to **aliskiren**. Use with caution and adjust dose. [Moderate] Theoretical

Alitretinoin → see retinoids

Alkylating agents → see **TABLE 15** p. 821 (myelosuppression), **TABLE 2** p. 818 (nephrotoxicity), **TABLE 5** p. 818 (thromboembolism)

bendamustine · busulfan · carmustine · chlorambucil · cyclophosphamide · dacarbazine · estramustine · ifosfamide · lomustine · melphalan · temozolomide · thiotepa · treosulfan

- **Antacids** are predicted to decrease the absorption of **estramustine**. Avoid. [Moderate] Study
- Antifungals, azoles **(itraconazole)** increase the risk of **busulfan** toxicity when given with **busulfan**. Monitor and adjust dose. [Moderate] Study
- Antifungals, azoles **(miconazole)** are predicted to increase the concentration of **busulfan**. Use with caution and adjust dose. [Moderate] Theoretical
- Oral **calcium salts** decrease the absorption of **estramustine**. [Severe] Study
- **Live vaccines** are predicted to increase the risk of generalised infection (possibly life-threatening) when given with **alkylating agents**. Public Health England advises avoid. [Severe] Theoretical
- **Metronidazole** increases the risk of toxicity when given with **busulfan**. [Severe] Study
- **Paracetamol** is predicted to decrease the clearance of **busulfan**. [Moderate] Theoretical
- **Cyclophosphamide** (high-dose) increases the risk of toxicity when given with **pentostatin**. Avoid. [Severe] Anecdotal → Also see **TABLE 15** p. 821 → Also see **TABLE 5** p. 818
- **Cyclophosphamide** increases the risk of prolonged neuromuscular blockade when given with **suxamethonium**. [Moderate] Study

Allopurinol

- **ACE inhibitors** are predicted to increase the risk of hypersensitivity and haematological reactions when given with **allopurinol**. [Severe] Anecdotal
- **Allopurinol** potentially increases the risk of haematological toxicity when given with **azathioprine**. Adjust **azathioprine** dose, p. 495. [Severe] Study
- **Allopurinol** is predicted to decrease the effects of **capecitabine**. Avoid. [Severe] Study
- **Allopurinol** moderately increases the exposure to **didanosine**. Avoid. [Severe] Study
- **Allopurinol** potentially increases the risk of haematological toxicity when given with **mercaptopurine**. Adjust **mercaptopurine** dose, p. 516. [Severe] Study
- **Allopurinol** increases the risk of skin rash when given with penicillins **(amoxicillin, ampicillin)**. [Moderate] Study
- **Allopurinol** is predicted to increase the risk of hyperuricaemia when given with **pyrazinamide**. [Moderate] Theoretical

- **Thiazide diuretics** are predicted to increase the risk of hypersensitivity reactions when given with **allopurinol**. [Severe] Theoretical

Almotriptan → see **TABLE 13** p. 821 (serotonin syndrome)

- Antifungals, azoles **(itraconazole, ketoconazole, voriconazole)** increase the exposure to **almotriptan**. [Mild] Study
- **Cobicistat** increases the exposure to **almotriptan**. [Mild] Study
- **Almotriptan** is predicted to increase the risk of vasoconstriction when given with **ergotamine**. Ergotamine should be taken at least 24 hours before or 6 hours after **almotriptan**. [Severe] Theoretical
- HIV-protease inhibitors **(atazanavir, darunavir, fosamprenavir, lopinavir, ritonavir, saquinavir, tipranavir)** increase the exposure to **almotriptan**. [Mild] Study
- **Idelalisib** increases the exposure to **almotriptan**. [Mild] Study
- Macrolides **(clarithromycin)** increase the exposure to **almotriptan**. [Mild] Study

Alogliptin → see **TABLE 14** p. 821 (antidiabetic drugs)

Alpha blockers → see **TABLE 7** p. 819 (first-dose hypotension), **TABLE 8** p. 819 (hypotension)

alfuzosin · doxazosin · indoramin · prazosin · tamsulosin · terazosin

- Antiarrhythmics **(dronedarone)** are predicted to increase the exposure to **tamsulosin**. [Moderate] Theoretical
- Antifungals, azoles **(fluconazole, isavuconazole, posaconazole)** are predicted to increase the exposure to **tamsulosin**. [Moderate] Theoretical
- Antifungals, azoles **(itraconazole, ketoconazole, voriconazole)** are predicted to increase the exposure to **doxazosin**. [Moderate] Study
- Antifungals, azoles **(itraconazole, ketoconazole, voriconazole)** are predicted to moderately increase the exposure to alpha blockers **(alfuzosin, tamsulosin)**. Use with caution or avoid. [Moderate] Study
- **Aprepitant** is predicted to increase the exposure to **tamsulosin**. [Moderate] Theoretical
- Calcium channel blockers **(diltiazem, verapamil)** are predicted to increase the exposure to **tamsulosin**. [Moderate] Theoretical → Also see **TABLE 8** p. 819
- **Cobicistat** is predicted to moderately increase the exposure to alpha blockers **(alfuzosin, tamsulosin)**. Use with caution or avoid. [Moderate] Study
- **Cobicistat** is predicted to increase the exposure to **doxazosin**. [Moderate] Study
- **Crizotinib** is predicted to increase the exposure to **tamsulosin**. [Moderate] Theoretical
- HIV-protease inhibitors **(atazanavir, darunavir, fosamprenavir, lopinavir, ritonavir, saquinavir, tipranavir)** are predicted to increase the exposure to **doxazosin**. [Moderate] Study
- HIV-protease inhibitors **(indinavir)** are predicted to increase the exposure to **tamsulosin**. [Moderate] Theoretical
- HIV-protease inhibitors **(atazanavir, darunavir, fosamprenavir, lopinavir, ritonavir, saquinavir, tipranavir)** are predicted to moderately increase the exposure to alpha blockers **(alfuzosin, tamsulosin)**. Use with caution or avoid. [Moderate] Study
- **Idelalisib** is predicted to moderately increase the exposure to alpha blockers **(alfuzosin, tamsulosin)**. Use with caution or avoid. [Moderate] Study
- **Idelalisib** is predicted to increase the exposure to **doxazosin**. [Moderate] Study
- **Imatinib** is predicted to increase the exposure to **tamsulosin**. [Moderate] Theoretical
- Macrolides **(clarithromycin)** are predicted to increase the exposure to **doxazosin**. [Moderate] Study
- Macrolides **(erythromycin)** are predicted to increase the exposure to **tamsulosin**. [Moderate] Theoretical
- Macrolides **(clarithromycin)** are predicted to moderately increase the exposure to alpha blockers **(alfuzosin, tamsulosin)**. Use with caution or avoid. [Moderate] Study
- **Monoamine-oxidase A and B inhibitors, irreversible** are predicted to increase the effects of **indoramin**. Avoid. [Severe] Theoretical → Also see **TABLE 8** p. 819
- **Netupitant** is predicted to increase the exposure to **tamsulosin**. [Moderate] Theoretical
- **Nilotinib** is predicted to increase the exposure to **tamsulosin**. [Moderate] Theoretical

Alpha blockers (continued)

▸ **Alpha blockers** cause significant hypotensive effects when given with **phosphodiesterase type-5 inhibitors**. Patient should be stabilised on first drug then second drug should be added at the lowest recommended dose. Severe Study → Also see **TABLE 8** p. 819

Alpha tocopherol → see vitamin E substances
Alpha tocopheryl acetate → see vitamin E substances
Alprazolam → see **TABLE 11** p. 820 (CNS depressant effects)

▸ Antiarrhythmics (**dronedarone**) are predicted to increase the exposure to **alprazolam**. Severe Study
▸ Antiepileptics (**carbamazepine, fosphenytoin, phenobarbital, phenytoin, primidone**) are predicted to decrease the exposure to **alprazolam** dose. Moderate Theoretical → Also see **TABLE 11** p. 820
▸ Antifungals, azoles (**fluconazole, isavuconazole, posaconazole**) are predicted to increase the exposure to **alprazolam**. Severe Study
▸ Antifungals, azoles (**itraconazole, ketoconazole, voriconazole**) moderately increase the exposure to **alprazolam**. Avoid. Moderate Study
▸ Antifungals, azoles (**miconazole**) are predicted to increase the exposure to **alprazolam**. Use with caution and adjust dose. Moderate Theoretical
▸ **Aprepitant** is predicted to increase the exposure to **alprazolam**. Severe Study
▸ Calcium channel blockers (**diltiazem, verapamil**) are predicted to increase the exposure to **alprazolam**. Severe Study
▸ **Cobicistat** moderately increases the exposure to **alprazolam**. Avoid. Moderate Study
▸ **Crizotinib** is predicted to increase the exposure to **alprazolam**. Severe Study
▸ **Enzalutamide** is predicted to decrease the exposure to **alprazolam**. Adjust **alprazolam** dose. Moderate Theoretical
▸ HIV-protease inhibitors (**atazanavir, darunavir, fosamprenavir, lopinavir, ritonavir, saquinavir, tipranavir**) moderately increase the exposure to **alprazolam**. Avoid. Moderate Study
▸ HIV-protease inhibitors (**indinavir**) are predicted to increase the exposure to **alprazolam**. Severe Study
▸ **Idelalisib** moderately increases the exposure to **alprazolam**. Avoid. Moderate Study
▸ **Imatinib** is predicted to increase the exposure to **alprazolam**. Severe Study
▸ **Alprazolam** is predicted to increase the exposure to **lomitapide**. Separate administration by 12 hours. Theoretical
▸ Macrolides (**clarithromycin**) moderately increase the exposure to **alprazolam**. Avoid. Moderate Study
▸ Macrolides (**erythromycin**) are predicted to increase the exposure to **alprazolam**. Severe Study
▸ **Netupitant** is predicted to increase the exposure to **alprazolam**. Severe Study
▸ **Nilotinib** is predicted to increase the exposure to **alprazolam**. Severe Study
▸ **Rifampicin** is predicted to decrease the exposure to **alprazolam**. Adjust **alprazolam** dose. Moderate Theoretical
▸ SSRIs (**fluvoxamine**) moderately increase the exposure to **alprazolam**. Adjust dose. Moderate Study
▸ **St John's Wort** moderately decreases the exposure to **alprazolam**. Moderate Study

Alprostadil → see **TABLE 8** p. 819 (hypotension)
Alteplase → see **TABLE 3** p. 818 (anticoagulant effects)
Aluminium hydroxide → see antacids
Amantadine → see dopamine receptor agonists
Ambrisentan

▸ **Ciclosporin** moderately increases the exposure to **ambrisentan**. Adjust **ambrisentan** dose. Moderate Study
▸ **Rifampicin** transiently increases the exposure to **ambrisentan**. Moderate Study

Amfetamines → see **TABLE 13** p. 821 (serotonin syndrome)

dexamfetamine · lisdexamfetamine

▸ **Amfetamines** are predicted to decrease the effects of **apraclonidine**. Avoid. Severe Theoretical
▸ **Amfetamines** are predicted to increase the risk of side-effects when given with **atomoxetine**. Severe Theoretical

▸ **Dexamfetamine** decreases the effects of **guanethidine**. Severe Study
▸ HIV-protease inhibitors (**ritonavir, tipranavir**) are predicted to increase the exposure to **amfetamines**. Severe Theoretical
▸ **Moclobemide** is predicted to increase the risk of a hypertensive crisis when given with **dexamfetamine**. Avoid. Severe Theoretical → Also see **TABLE 13** p. 821
▸ **Moclobemide** is predicted to increase the risk of a hypertensive crisis when given with **lisdexamfetamine**. Avoid. Severe Anecdotal → Also see **TABLE 13** p. 821
▸ Monoamine-oxidase A and B inhibitors, irreversible are predicted to increase the risk of a hypertensive crisis when given with **amfetamines**. Avoid and for 14 days after stopping the MAOI. Severe Anecdotal → Also see **TABLE 13** p. 821
▸ Monoamine-oxidase B inhibitors (**rasagiline, selegiline**) are predicted to increase the risk of severe hypertension when given with **amfetamines**. Avoid. Severe Theoretical → Also see **TABLE 13** p. 821
▸ Monoamine-oxidase B inhibitors (**safinamide**) are predicted to increase the risk of severe hypertension when given with **amfetamines**. Severe Theoretical → Also see **TABLE 13** p. 821
▸ **Nabilone** is predicted to increase the risk of cardiovascular side-effects when given with **amfetamines**. Severe Theoretical
▸ **Phenothiazines** are predicted to decrease the effects of **amfetamines**. Moderate Study
▸ **Amfetamines** are predicted to decrease the effects of phenothiazines (**chlorpromazine**). Moderate Study
▸ SSRIs (**fluoxetine, paroxetine**) are predicted to increase the exposure to **amfetamines**. Severe Theoretical → Also see **TABLE 13** p. 821

Amifampridine → see **TABLE 9** p. 820 (QT-interval prolongation)
Amikacin → see aminoglycosides
Amiloride → see potassium-sparing diuretics
Aminoglycosides → see **TABLE 2** p. 818 (nephrotoxicity), **TABLE 19** p. 822 (ototoxicity), **TABLE 20** p. 822 (neuromuscular blocking effects)

amikacin · gentamicin · streptomycin · tobramycin

▸ **Aminoglycosides** are predicted to decrease the effects of **agalsidase**. Avoid. Moderate Theoretical
▸ Antifungals, azoles (**miconazole**) potentially decrease the exposure to **tobramycin**. Moderate Anecdotal
▸ **Ataluren** is predicted to increase the risk of nephrotoxicity when given with intravenous **aminoglycosides**. Avoid. Severe Study
▸ **Aminoglycosides** increase the risk of hypocalcaemia when given with **bisphosphonates**. Moderate Anecdotal → Also see **TABLE 2** p. 818
▸ **Aminoglycosides** potentially increase the concentration of **digoxin**. Monitor and adjust dose. Mild Study
▸ **Loop diuretics** increase the risk of nephrotoxicity and ototoxicity when given with **aminoglycosides**. Avoid. Moderate Study → Also see **TABLE 19** p. 822
▸ **Aminoglycosides** are predicted to decrease the effects of **neostigmine**. Moderate Theoretical → Also see **TABLE 20** p. 822
▸ **Aminoglycosides** are predicted to increase the risk of prolonged neuromuscular blockade when given with **neuromuscular blocking drugs, non-depolarising**. Severe Theoretical → Also see **TABLE 20** p. 822
▸ **Aminoglycosides** are predicted to decrease the effects of **pyridostigmine**. Moderate Theoretical → Also see **TABLE 20** p. 822
▸ **Aminoglycosides** are predicted to increase the risk of prolonged neuromuscular blockade when given with **suxamethonium**. Severe Theoretical → Also see **TABLE 20** p. 822
▸ **Telavancin** is predicted to increase the risk of ototoxicity when given with **aminoglycosides**. Moderate Theoretical → Also see **TABLE 2** p. 818 → Also see **TABLE 19** p. 822
▸ **Vancomycin** increases the risk of nephrotoxicity when given with **aminoglycosides**. Avoid. Moderate Study → Also see **TABLE 2** p. 818 → Also see **TABLE 19** p. 822

Aminophylline → see **TABLE 17** p. 822 (reduced serum potassium)

FOOD AND LIFESTYLE Smoking can increase aminophylline clearance and increased doses of aminophylline are therefore required; dose adjustments are likely to be necessary if smoking started or stopped during treatment.

- Aciclovir increases the exposure to **aminophylline**. Monitor theophylline concentration and adjust dose. [Severe] Anecdotal
- **Aminophylline** is predicted to decrease the efficacy of antiarrhythmics **(adenosine)**. Separate administration by 24 hours. [Mild] Theoretical
- Antiepileptics **(fosphenytoin)** are predicted to decrease the exposure to **aminophylline**. Adjust dose. [Moderate] Study
- Antiepileptics **(phenobarbital)** are predicted to decrease the exposure to **aminophylline**. Adjust dose. [Moderate] Theoretical
- Antiepileptics **(phenytoin)** decrease the exposure to **aminophylline**. Adjust dose. [Moderate] Study
- Antiepileptics **(primidone)** are predicted to increase the clearance of **aminophylline**. Adjust dose. [Moderate] Theoretical
- Beta blockers, non-selective are predicted to increase the risk of bronchospasm when given with **aminophylline**. Avoid. [Severe] Theoretical
- Beta blockers, selective are predicted to increase the risk of bronchospasm when given with **aminophylline**. Avoid. [Severe] Theoretical
- **Combined hormonal contraceptives** are predicted to increase the exposure to **aminophylline**. Adjust dose. [Moderate] Theoretical
- **Aminophylline** increases the risk of agitation when given with doxapram. [Moderate] Study
- H$_2$ receptor antagonists **(cimetidine)** increase the concentration of **aminophylline**. Adjust dose. [Severe] Study
- HIV-protease inhibitors **(ritonavir)** decrease the exposure to **aminophylline**. Adjust dose. [Moderate] Study
- Interferons are predicted to slightly increase the exposure to **aminophylline**. Adjust dose. [Moderate] Theoretical
- Iron chelators **(deferasirox)** are predicted to increase the exposure to **aminophylline**. Avoid. [Moderate] Theoretical
- Isoniazid is predicted to affect the clearance of **aminophylline**. [Severe] Theoretical
- **Aminophylline** is predicted to decrease the concentration of lithium. [Moderate] Theoretical
- Macrolides **(azithromycin)** are predicted to increase the exposure to **aminophylline**. [Moderate] Theoretical
- Macrolides **(clarithromycin)** are predicted to increase the exposure to **aminophylline**. Adjust **aminophylline** dose. [Moderate] Theoretical
- **Aminophylline** is predicted to decrease the exposure to macrolides **(erythromycin)**. Adjust dose. [Severe] Study
- Methotrexate is predicted to decrease the clearance of **aminophylline**. [Moderate] Theoretical
- Monoclonal antibodies **(blinatumomab)** are predicted to transiently increase the exposure to **aminophylline**. Monitor and adjust dose. [Moderate] Theoretical
- Pentoxifylline is predicted to increase the concentration of **aminophylline**. Use with caution or avoid. [Severe] Theoretical
- Quinolones **(ciprofloxacin, norfloxacin)** are predicted to increase the exposure to **aminophylline**. Adjust dose. [Moderate] Theoretical
- Rifampicin decreases the exposure to **aminophylline**. Adjust dose. [Moderate] Study
- **Aminophylline** is predicted to slightly increase the exposure to roflumilast. Avoid. [Moderate] Theoretical
- SSRIs **(fluvoxamine)** moderately to markedly increase the exposure to **aminophylline**. Avoid. [Severe] Study
- St John's Wort is predicted to decrease the concentration of **aminophylline**. [Severe] Theoretical
- Sympathomimetics, vasoconstrictor **(ephedrine)** increase the risk of side-effects when given with **aminophylline**. Avoid in children. [Moderate] Study
- Valaciclovir is predicted to increase the exposure to **aminophylline**. [Severe] Anecdotal

Aminosalicylic acid
- **Aminosalicylic acid** is predicted to increase the risk of methaemoglobinaemia when given with topical anaesthetics, local **(prilocaine)**. Use with caution or avoid. [Severe] Theoretical
- **Aminosalicylic acid** is predicted to increase the risk of methaemoglobinaemia when given with dapsone. [Severe] Theoretical

Amiodarone → see antiarrhythmics

Amisulpride → see TABLE 9 p. 820 (QT-interval prolongation), TABLE 11 p. 820 (CNS depressant effects)
- **Amisulpride** is predicted to decrease the effects of dopamine receptor agonists. Avoid. [Moderate] Theoretical → Also see TABLE 9 p. 820
- **Amisulpride** is predicted to decrease the effects of levodopa. Avoid. [Severe] Theoretical

Amitriptyline → see tricyclic antidepressants

Amlodipine → see calcium channel blockers

Amoxicillin → see penicillins

Amphotericin → see TABLE 2 p. 818 (nephrotoxicity), TABLE 17 p. 822 (reduced serum potassium)
- **Amphotericin** increases the risk of toxicity when given with flucytosine. [Severe] Study
- Micafungin slightly increases the exposure to **amphotericin**. Avoid or monitor toxicity. [Moderate] Study
- Sodium stibogluconate increases the risk of cardiovascular side-effects when given with **amphotericin**. Separate administration by 14 days. [Severe] Study

Ampicillin → see penicillins

Amsacrine → see TABLE 15 p. 821 (myelosuppression)
- Live vaccines are predicted to increase the risk of generalised infection (possibly life-threatening) when given with **amsacrine**. Public Health England advises avoid. [Severe] Theoretical

Anaesthetics, local → see TABLE 11 p. 820 (CNS depressant effects)

bupivacaine · levobupivacaine · mepivacaine · oxybuprocaine · prilocaine · proxymetacaine · ropivacaine · tetracaine

- **Aminosalicylic acid** is predicted to increase the risk of methaemoglobinaemia when given with topical **prilocaine**. Use with caution or avoid. [Severe] Theoretical
- **Anaesthetics, local** are predicted to increase the risk of cardiodepression when given with antiarrhythmics. [Severe] Theoretical → Also see TABLE 11 p. 820
- Antiepileptics **(fosphenytoin, phenobarbital, phenytoin, primidone)** are predicted to increase the risk of methaemoglobinaemia when given with topical **prilocaine**. Use with caution or avoid. [Severe] Theoretical → Also see TABLE 11 p. 820
- Antimalarials **(chloroquine, primaquine)** are predicted to increase the risk of methaemoglobinaemia when given with topical **prilocaine**. Use with caution or avoid. [Severe] Theoretical
- Dapsone is predicted to increase the risk of methaemoglobinaemia when given with topical **prilocaine**. Use with caution or avoid. [Severe] Theoretical
- Metoclopramide is predicted to increase the risk of methaemoglobinaemia when given with topical **prilocaine**. Avoid. [Severe] Theoretical
- Nitrates are predicted to increase the risk of methaemoglobinaemia when given with topical **prilocaine**. Avoid. [Severe] Theoretical
- Nitrofurantoin is predicted to increase the risk of methaemoglobinaemia when given with topical **prilocaine**. Use with caution or avoid. [Severe] Theoretical
- Paracetamol is predicted to increase the risk of methaemoglobinaemia when given with topical **prilocaine**. Use with caution or avoid. [Severe] Theoretical
- Sodium nitroprusside is predicted to increase the risk of methaemoglobinaemia when given with topical **prilocaine**. Use with caution or avoid. [Severe] Theoretical
- SSRIs **(fluvoxamine)** decrease the clearance of **ropivacaine**. Avoid prolonged use. [Moderate] Study
- Sulfonamides potentially increase the risk of methaemoglobinaemia when given with topical **prilocaine**. Use with caution or avoid. [Severe] Anecdotal

Anagrelide → see TABLE 4 p. 818 (antiplatelet effects)
- Combined hormonal contraceptives are predicted to increase the exposure to **anagrelide**. [Moderate] Theoretical
- Quinolones **(ciprofloxacin)** are predicted to increase the exposure to **anagrelide**. [Moderate] Theoretical
- SSRIs **(fluvoxamine)** are predicted to increase the exposure to **anagrelide**. [Moderate] Theoretical → Also see TABLE 4 p. 818

Anakinra → see TABLE 15 p. 821 (myelosuppression)
- Live vaccines are predicted to increase the risk of generalised infection (possibly life-threatening) when given with

Anakinra (continued)

anakinra. Public Health England advises avoid. Severe Theoretical

Angiotensin-II receptor antagonists → see TABLE 7 p. 819 (first-dose hypotension), TABLE 8 p. 819 (hypotension), TABLE 16 p. 822 (increased serum potassium)

azilsartan · candesartan · eprosartan · irbesartan · losartan · olmesartan · telmisartan · valsartan

▸ **Angiotensin-II receptor antagonists** increase the risk of renal impairment when given with **aliskiren**. Use with caution or avoid **aliskiren** in selected patients. Severe Study → Also see TABLE 8 p. 819 → Also see TABLE 16 p. 822

▸ **Angiotensin-II receptor antagonists** potentially increase the concentration of **lithium**. Monitor concentration and adjust dose. Severe Anecdotal

Antacids

aluminium hydroxide · magnesium carbonate · magnesium trisilicate

SEPARATION OF ADMINISTRATION Antacids should preferably not be taken at the same time as other drugs since they might impair absorption. Antacids might damage enteric coatings designed to prevent dissolution in the stomach.

▸ **Antacids** are predicted to decrease the absorption of alkylating agents (**estramustine**). Avoid. Moderate Study

▸ **Antacids** decrease the absorption of antiepileptics (**gabapentin**). Gabapentin should be taken 2 hours after **antacids**. Moderate Study

▸ **Antacids** decrease the absorption of antifungals, azoles (**itraconazole**). Antacids should be taken 1 hour before or 2 hours after **itraconazole**. Moderate Study

▸ **Antacids** decrease the absorption of antifungals, azoles (**ketoconazole**). Separate administration by at least 2 hours. Moderate Study

▸ **Antacids** decrease the absorption of antihistamines, non-sedating (**fexofenadine**). Separate administration by 2 hours. Moderate Study

▸ **Antacids** decrease the absorption of antimalarials (**chloroquine**). Separate administration by at least 4 hours. Moderate Study

▸ **Antacids** are predicted to decrease the absorption of antimalarials (**proguanil**). Separate administration by at least 2 hours. Moderate Study

▸ **Antacids** decrease the absorption of **aspirin** (high-dose). Moderate Study

▸ **Antacids** decrease the absorption of bisphosphonates (**alendronic acid**). Alendronic acid should be taken at least 30 minutes before **antacids**. Moderate Study

▸ **Antacids** are predicted to decrease the absorption of bisphosphonates (**ibandronic acid**). Avoid **antacids** for at least 6 hours before or 1 hour after ibandronic acid. Moderate Theoretical

▸ **Antacids** decrease the absorption of bisphosphonates (**risedronate**). Separate administration by at least 2 hours. Moderate Study

▸ **Antacids** decrease the absorption of bisphosphonates (**sodium clodronate**). Avoid **antacids** for 2 hours before or 1 hour after sodium clodronate. Moderate Study

▸ **Antacids** are predicted to decrease the absorption of bosutinib. Bosutinib should be taken at least 12 hours before **antacids**. Moderate Theoretical

▸ **Antacids** are predicted to decrease the absorption of ceritinib. Separate administration by 2 hours. Moderate Theoretical

▸ **Antacids** are predicted to decrease the absorption of **chenodeoxycholic acid**. Mild Theoretical

▸ **Antacids** are predicted to decrease the absorption of **cholic acid**. Separate administration by 5 hours. Mild Theoretical

▸ **Antacids** are predicted to decrease the absorption of corticosteroids (**deflazacort**). Separate administration by 2 hours. Moderate Theoretical

▸ **Antacids** decrease the absorption of corticosteroids (**dexamethasone**). Moderate Study

▸ **Antacids** are predicted to decrease the absorption of **dabrafenib**. Avoid. Severe Theoretical

▸ **Antacids** decrease the absorption of **dasatinib**. Separate administration by at least 2 hours. Moderate Study

▸ **Aluminium hydroxide** is predicted to decrease the absorption of **deferiprone**. Avoid. Moderate Theoretical

▸ **Antacids** decrease the absorption of **digoxin**. Separate administration by 2 hours. Mild Study

▸ **Antacids** are predicted to decrease the absorption of **dipyridamole** (immediate release tablets). Moderate Theoretical

▸ **Antacids** moderately decrease the exposure to **dolutegravir**. Dolutegravir should be taken 2 hours before or 6 hours after antacids. Moderate Study

▸ **Antacids** decrease the absorption of **eltrombopag**. Eltrombopag should be taken 2 hours before or 4 hours after **antacids**. Severe Study

▸ **Antacids** moderately decrease the exposure to **elvitegravir**. Separate administration by at least 4 hours. Moderate Study

▸ **Aluminium hydroxide** increases the risk of blocked enteral or nasogastric tubes when given with **enteral feeds**. Moderate Study

▸ **Antacids** are predicted to decrease the absorption of **erlotinib**. Antacids should be taken 4 hours before or 2 hours after erlotinib. Moderate Theoretical

▸ **Antacids** slightly to moderately decrease the exposure to fibrates (**gemfibrozil**). Moderate Study

▸ **Antacids** are predicted to slightly decrease the exposure to **gefitinib**. Moderate Theoretical

▸ **Antacids** are predicted to decrease the absorption of HIV-protease inhibitors (**atazanavir**). Atazanavir should be taken 2 hours before or 1 hour after **antacids**. Severe Theoretical

▸ **Antacids** are predicted to decrease the absorption of HIV-protease inhibitors (**tipranavir**). Separate administration by 2 hours. Moderate Study

▸ **Antacids** decrease the absorption of **hydroxychloroquine**. Separate administration by at least 4 hours. Moderate Study

▸ **Antacids** decrease the absorption of **iron (oral)**. Iron (oral) should be taken 1 hour before or 2 hours after **antacids**. Moderate Study

▸ **Aluminium hydroxide** is predicted to decrease the exposure to iron chelators (**deferasirox**). Avoid. Moderate Theoretical

▸ **Antacids** are predicted to decrease the absorption of **lapatinib**. Avoid. Moderate Theoretical

▸ **Antacids** are predicted to decrease the exposure to **ledipasvir**. Separate administration by 4 hours. Moderate Theoretical

▸ **Antacids** are predicted to decrease the absorption of **levothyroxine**. Separate administration by at least 4 hours. Moderate Anecdotal

▸ **Antacids** decrease the exposure to **mycophenolate**. Moderate Study

▸ **Antacids** are predicted to decrease the absorption of **nilotinib**. Separate administration by at least 2 hours. Moderate Theoretical

▸ **Magnesium trisilicate** decreases the absorption of **nitrofurantoin**. Moderate Study

▸ **Antacids** are predicted to decrease the absorption of **pazopanib**. Pazopanib should be taken 1 hour before or 2 hours after **antacids**. Moderate Theoretical

▸ **Antacids** decrease the absorption of **penicillamine**. Separate administration by 2 hours. Mild Study

▸ **Antacids** are predicted to decrease the absorption of **phenothiazines**. Moderate Anecdotal

▸ **Antacids** increase the risk of metabolic alkalosis when given with **polystyrene sulfonate**. Severe Anecdotal

▸ **Antacids** decrease the absorption of **quinolones**. Quinolones should be taken 2 hours before or 4 hours after **antacids**. Moderate Study

▸ **Antacids** slightly decrease the exposure to **raltegravir**. Avoid. Moderate Study

▸ **Antacids** decrease the absorption of **rifampicin**. Rifampicin should be taken 1 hour before **antacids**. Moderate Study

▸ **Antacids** are predicted to decrease the absorption of **rilpivirine**. Antacids should be taken 2 hours before or 4 hours after **rilpivirine**. Theoretical

▸ **Antacids** slightly decrease the exposure to **riociguat**. Antacids should be taken 2 hours before or 1 hour after **riociguat**. Mild Study

- **Antacids** moderately decrease the absorption of statins (rosuvastatin). Separate administration by 2 hours. Moderate Study
- **Antacids** decrease the absorption of **strontium ranelate**. Separate administration by 2 hours. Moderate Study
- **Antacids** decrease the absorption of **tetracyclines**. Separate administration by 2 to 3 hours. Moderate Study
- **Antacids** are predicted to decrease the absorption of **ursodeoxycholic acid**. Separate administration by 2 hours. Moderate Theoretical
- **Antacids** are predicted to decrease the concentration of **velpatasvir**. Separate administration by 4 hours. Moderate Theoretical

Anthracyclines → see TABLE 15 p. 821 (myelosuppression), TABLE 5 p. 818 (thromboembolism)

daunorubicin · doxorubicin · epirubicin · idarubicin · mitoxantrone · pixantrone

GENERAL INFORMATION　Caution is necessary with concurrent use of cardiotoxic drugs, or drugs that reduce cardiac contractility.

- Calcium channel blockers **(verapamil)** moderately increase the exposure to **doxorubicin**. Moderate Study
- **Ciclosporin** increases the concentration of anthracyclines **(daunorubicin, doxorubicin, epirubicin, idarubicin, mitoxantrone)**. Severe Study
- H₂ receptor antagonists **(cimetidine)** slightly increase the exposure to **epirubicin**. Avoid. Moderate Study
- **Live vaccines** are predicted to increase the risk of generalised infection (possibly life-threatening) when given with **anthracyclines**. Public Health England advises avoid. Severe Theoretical
- **Anthracyclines** are predicted to increase the risk of cardiotoxicity when given with monoclonal antibodies **(trastuzumab, trastuzumab emtansine)**. Avoid. Severe Theoretical → Also see TABLE 15 p. 821

Antiarrhythmics → see TABLE 6 p. 819 (bradycardia), TABLE 12 p. 821 (peripheral neuropathy), TABLE 9 p. 820 (QT-interval prolongation), TABLE 11 p. 820 (CNS depressant effects), TABLE 10 p. 820 (antimuscarinics)

adenosine · amiodarone · disopyramide · dronedarone · flecainide · lidocaine · propafenone

- Amiodarone has a long half-life; there is potential for drug interactions to occur for several weeks (or even months) after treatment with it has been stopped.
- Since systemic absorption can follow topical application of **lidocaine** the possibility of interactions should be borne in mind.

- **Abiraterone** is predicted to increase the exposure to **flecainide**. Severe Theoretical
- Antiarrhythmics **(amiodarone, dronedarone)** are predicted to increase the exposure to **afatinib**. Separate administration by 12 hours. Moderate Study
- **Amiodarone** is predicted to decrease the effects of **agalsidase**. Avoid. Moderate Theoretical
- **Amiodarone** is predicted to increase the exposure to aldosterone antagonists **(eplerenone)**. Adjust **eplerenone** dose. Severe Theoretical
- **Dronedarone** is predicted to increase the exposure to aldosterone antagonists **(eplerenone)**. Adjust **eplerenone** dose. Severe Study
- Antiarrhythmics **(amiodarone, dronedarone)** are predicted to increase the exposure to **aliskiren**. Severe Study
- **Dronedarone** is predicted to increase the exposure to alpha blockers **(tamsulosin)**. Moderate Theoretical
- **Dronedarone** is predicted to increase the exposure to **alprazolam**. Severe Study
- **Aminophylline** is predicted to decrease the efficacy of **adenosine**. Separate administration by 24 hours. Mild Theoretical
- **Anaesthetics, local** are predicted to increase the risk of cardiodepression when given with **antiarrhythmics**. Severe Theoretical → Also see TABLE 11 p. 820

- Antiarrhythmics **(propafenone)** are predicted to increase the risk of cardiodepression when given with antiarrhythmics **(amiodarone)**. Monitor and adjust dose. Severe Theoretical
- Antiarrhythmics **(amiodarone)** increase the concentration of antiarrhythmics **(flecainide)**. Adjust **flecainide** dose and monitor side effects. Severe Study → Also see TABLE 6 p. 819 → Also see TABLE 9 p. 820
- Antiarrhythmics **(propafenone)** are predicted to increase the exposure to antiarrhythmics **(flecainide)**. Severe Theoretical
- Antiarrhythmics **(propafenone)** are predicted to increase the risk of cardiodepression when given with antiarrhythmics **(lidocaine)**. Moderate Study
- Antiarrhythmics **(dronedarone)** are predicted to increase the exposure to antiarrhythmics **(propafenone)**. Monitor and adjust dose. Moderate Study
- **Amiodarone** increases the risk of bradycardia when given with **anticholinesterases, centrally acting**. Moderate Anecdotal → Also see TABLE 6 p. 819
- **Antiepileptics (carbamazepine, fosphenytoin, phenobarbital, phenytoin, primidone)** are predicted to decrease the efficacy of **propafenone**. Moderate Study
- **Antiepileptics (fosphenytoin, phenytoin)** are predicted to decrease the exposure to **lidocaine**. Severe Anecdotal
- **Antiepileptics (carbamazepine, fosphenytoin, phenobarbital, phenytoin, primidone)** are predicted to decrease the exposure to antiarrhythmics **(disopyramide, dronedarone)**. Avoid. Severe Study
- **Amiodarone** is predicted to slightly increase the concentration of antiepileptics **(fosphenytoin, phenytoin)**. Monitor and adjust dose. Severe Study → Also see TABLE 12 p. 821
- Antifungals, azoles **(fluconazole)** are predicted to increase the exposure to **dronedarone**. Severe Theoretical
- Antifungals, azoles **(fluconazole, isavuconazole, posaconazole)** are predicted to increase the exposure to **propafenone**. Monitor and adjust dose. Moderate Study
- Antifungals, azoles **(itraconazole, ketoconazole, voriconazole)** are predicted to increase the exposure to **disopyramide**. Avoid. Severe Theoretical → Also see TABLE 9 p. 820
- Antifungals, azoles **(itraconazole, ketoconazole, voriconazole)** very markedly increase the exposure to **dronedarone**. Avoid. Severe Study → Also see TABLE 9 p. 820
- Antifungals, azoles **(itraconazole, ketoconazole, voriconazole)** are predicted to increase the exposure to **propafenone**. Monitor and adjust dose. Severe Study
- Antifungals, azoles **(miconazole)** are predicted to increase the exposure to **disopyramide**. Use with caution and adjust dose. Severe Theoretical
- Antifungals, azoles **(posaconazole)** are predicted to increase the exposure to antiarrhythmics **(disopyramide, dronedarone)**. Avoid. Severe Theoretical
- **Dronedarone** is predicted to increase the exposure to antifungals, azoles **(isavuconazole)**. Severe Theoretical
- **Dronedarone** is predicted to increase the exposure to antihistamines, non-sedating **(fexofenadine, mizolastine)**. Severe Theoretical
- **Dronedarone** is predicted to increase the concentration of antimalarials **(piperaquine)**. Severe Theoretical
- **Dronedarone** is predicted to increase the exposure to **apixaban**. Moderate Theoretical
- **Aprepitant** increases the exposure to **dronedarone**. Severe Theoretical
- **Aprepitant** is predicted to increase the exposure to **propafenone**. Monitor and adjust dose. Moderate Study
- **Dronedarone** is predicted to increase the exposure to **axitinib**. Moderate Theoretical
- **Dronedarone** is predicted to increase the exposure to **bedaquiline**. Avoid prolonged use. Mild Theoretical → Also see TABLE 9 p. 820
- Antiarrhythmics **(amiodarone, disopyramide, dronedarone, flecainide, lidocaine)** are predicted to increase the risk of cardiovascular side-effects when given with beta blockers, non-selective. Use with caution or avoid. Severe Study → Also see TABLE 6 p. 819 → Also see TABLE 9 p. 820
- **Propafenone** is predicted to increase the risk of cardiovascular

A1

Interactions | Appendix 1

Antiarrhythmics (continued)

side-effects when given with beta blockers, non-selective (carteolol, labetalol, levobunolol, nadolol, oxprenolol, pindolol, sotalol). Use with caution or avoid. Severe Study

▸ **Propafenone** is predicted to increase the exposure to beta blockers, non-selective (**carvedilol**). Moderate Theoretical

▸ **Propafenone** increases the risk of cardiovascular side-effects when given with beta blockers, non-selective (**propranolol**). Use with caution or avoid. Severe Study

▸ **Propafenone** is predicted to increase the exposure to beta blockers, non-selective (**timolol**) and beta blockers, non-selective (**timolol**) are predicted to increase the risk of cardiodepression when given with **propafenone**. Severe Anecdotal

▸ Antiarrhythmics (**amiodarone, disopyramide, dronedarone, flecainide, lidocaine**) are predicted to increase the risk of cardiovascular side-effects when given with beta blockers, selective. Use with caution or avoid. Severe Study → Also see TABLE 6 p. 819 → Also see TABLE 9 p. 820

▸ **Propafenone** is predicted to increase the risk of cardiovascular side-effects when given with beta blockers, selective (**acebutolol, atenolol, betaxolol, bisoprolol, celiprolol, esmolol**). Use with caution or avoid. Severe Study

▸ **Propafenone** is predicted to increase the exposure to beta blockers, selective (**metoprolol**). Moderate Study

▸ **Propafenone** is predicted to increase the exposure to beta blockers, selective (**nebivolol**) and beta blockers, selective (**nebivolol**) are predicted to increase the risk of cardiodepression when given with **propafenone**. Avoid. Severe Theoretical

▸ **Bosentan** is predicted to decrease the exposure to dronedarone. Severe Theoretical

▸ **Dronedarone** is predicted to increase the exposure to bosutinib. Avoid or adjust bosutinib dose. Severe Theoretical → Also see TABLE 9 p. 820

▸ **Bupropion** is predicted to increase the exposure to flecainide. Severe Theoretical

▸ **Bupropion** is predicted to increase the exposure to propafenone. Monitor and adjust dose. Moderate Study

▸ **Dronedarone** is predicted to increase the exposure to buspirone. Use with caution and adjust dose. Moderate Study

▸ **Dronedarone** is predicted to increase the exposure to cabozantinib. Moderate Theoretical → Also see TABLE 9 p. 820

▸ **Caffeine citrate** decreases the efficacy of **adenosine**. Separate administration by 24 hours. Mild Study

▸ Calcium channel blockers (**diltiazem, verapamil**) increase the exposure to **dronedarone** and **dronedarone** increases the exposure to calcium channel blockers (**diltiazem, verapamil**). Moderate Study

▸ Calcium channel blockers (**diltiazem, verapamil**) are predicted to increase the exposure to **propafenone**. Monitor and adjust dose. Moderate Study

▸ Calcium channel blockers (**verapamil**) increase the risk of cardiodepression when given with **flecainide**. Severe Anecdotal → Also see TABLE 6 p. 819

▸ **Dronedarone** is predicted to increase the exposure to calcium channel blockers (**amlodipine, felodipine, isradipine, lacidipine, lercanidipine, nicardipine, nifedipine, nimodipine**). Monitor and adjust dose. Moderate Study

▸ **Amiodarone** is predicted to increase the risk of cardiodepression when given with calcium channel blockers (**diltiazem, verapamil**). Avoid. Severe Theoretical → Also see TABLE 6 p. 819

▸ **Disopyramide** is predicted to increase the risk of cardiodepression when given with calcium channel blockers (**verapamil**). Severe Theoretical

▸ Antiarrhythmics (**amiodarone, dronedarone**) are predicted to increase the exposure to ceritinib. Moderate Theoretical → Also see TABLE 9 p. 820

▸ **Amiodarone** increases the concentration of ciclosporin. Monitor ciclosporin concentration and adjust dose. Severe Study

▸ **Dronedarone** increases the concentration of ciclosporin. Severe Study

▸ **Ciclosporin** increases the exposure to dronedarone. Avoid. Severe Theoretical

▸ **Cinacalcet** is predicted to increase the exposure to flecainide. Severe Theoretical

▸ **Cinacalcet** is predicted to increase the exposure to propafenone. Monitor and adjust dose. Moderate Study

▸ **Cobicistat** very markedly increases the exposure to dronedarone. Avoid. Severe Study

▸ **Cobicistat** is predicted to increase the exposure to propafenone. Monitor and adjust dose. Severe Study

▸ **Dronedarone** is predicted to increase the exposure to cobimetinib. Severe Theoretical

▸ **Dronedarone** is predicted to increase the exposure to colchicine. Adjust colchicine dose. Severe Study

▸ **Dronedarone** is predicted to increase the exposure to corticosteroids (**methylprednisolone**). Monitor and adjust dose. Moderate Study

▸ **Amiodarone** increases the anticoagulant effect of coumarins. Severe Study

▸ **Propafenone** increases the anticoagulant effect of coumarins. Monitor INR and adjust dose. Moderate Study

▸ **Dronedarone** is predicted to increase the exposure to crizotinib. Moderate Theoretical → Also see TABLE 9 p. 820

▸ **Crizotinib** is predicted to increase the exposure to propafenone. Monitor and adjust dose. Moderate Study

▸ **Amiodarone** increases the exposure to dabigatran. Adjust dabigatran dose. Moderate Study

▸ **Dronedarone** slightly increases the exposure to dabigatran. Avoid. Severe Study

▸ **Daclatasvir** is predicted to increase the risk of severe bradycardia or heart block when given with amiodarone. Refer to specialist literature. Severe Anecdotal

▸ **Dronedarone** is predicted to slightly increase the exposure to darifenacin. Moderate Study

▸ **Darifenacin** is predicted to increase the concentration of flecainide. Moderate Theoretical

▸ **Dronedarone** is predicted to increase the exposure to dasatinib. Severe Study → Also see TABLE 9 p. 820

▸ Antiarrhythmics (**amiodarone, dronedarone**) are predicted to moderately increase the exposure to digoxin. Monitor and adjust digoxin dose, p. 79. Severe Study → Also see TABLE 6 p. 819

▸ **Propafenone** increases the concentration of digoxin. Monitor and adjust dose. Severe Study

▸ **Dipyridamole** increases the exposure to adenosine. Avoid or adjust dose. Severe Study

▸ **Dronedarone** increases the risk of QT-prolongation when given with domperidone. Avoid. Severe Study

▸ **Dronedarone** is predicted to increase the exposure to dopamine receptor agonists (**bromocriptine, cabergoline**). Severe Theoretical

▸ **Duloxetine** is predicted to increase the exposure to flecainide. Severe Theoretical

▸ **Dronedarone** is predicted to moderately increase the exposure to dutasteride. Mild Study

▸ **Amiodarone** slightly increases the exposure to edoxaban. Severe Study

▸ **Dronedarone** slightly increases the exposure to edoxaban. Adjust edoxaban dose. Severe Study

▸ **Efavirenz** is predicted to decrease the exposure to dronedarone. Severe Theoretical

▸ **Enzalutamide** is predicted to decrease the exposure to antiarrhythmics (**disopyramide, dronedarone**). Avoid. Severe Study

▸ **Enzalutamide** is predicted to decrease the efficacy of propafenone. Moderate Study

▸ **Dronedarone** is predicted to increase the risk of ergotism when given with ergometrine. Severe Theoretical

▸ **Dronedarone** is predicted to increase the risk of ergotism when given with ergotamine. Severe Theoretical

▸ Antiarrhythmics (**amiodarone, dronedarone**) are predicted to increase the exposure to erlotinib. Moderate Theoretical

▸ **Dronedarone** is predicted to increase the concentration of everolimus. Avoid or adjust dose. Moderate Study

▸ **Dronedarone** is predicted to increase the concentration of fesoterodine. Adjust fesoterodine dose in hepatic and renal impairment. Mild Study

▸ Antiarrhythmics (**amiodarone, dronedarone**) are predicted to increase the exposure to fidaxomicin. Avoid. Moderate Study

- ▸ **Dronedarone** is predicted to increase the exposure to **gefitinib**. Moderate Theoretical
- ▸ **Grapefruit juice** increases the exposure to **amiodarone**. Avoid. Moderate Study
- ▸ **Grapefruit juice** moderately increases the exposure to **dronedarone**. Avoid. Severe Study
- ▸ **Grapefruit juice** increases the exposure to **propafenone**. Monitor and adjust dose. Moderate Study
- ▸ **Dronedarone** is predicted to increase the concentration of **guanfacine**. Adjust **guanfacine** dose, p. 222. Moderate Theoretical
- ▸ H₂ receptor antagonists (**cimetidine**) increase the exposure to **amiodarone**. Moderate Study
- ▸ H₂ receptor antagonists (**cimetidine**) slightly increase the exposure to **flecainide**. Monitor and adjust dose. Mild Study
- ▸ H₂ receptor antagonists (**cimetidine**) increase the exposure to **lidocaine**. Monitor and adjust dose. Moderate Study
- ▸ H₂ receptor antagonists (**cimetidine**) are predicted to increase the exposure to **propafenone**. Monitor and adjust dose. Moderate Theoretical
- ▸ **HIV-protease inhibitors** are predicted to increase the exposure to **amiodarone**. Avoid. Severe Theoretical → Also see TABLE 9 p. 820
- ▸ **HIV-protease inhibitors** are predicted to increase the exposure to **disopyramide**. Severe Theoretical → Also see TABLE 9 p. 820
- ▸ **HIV-protease inhibitors** (**atazanavir, darunavir, fosamprenavir, lopinavir, ritonavir, saquinavir, tipranavir**) very markedly increase the exposure to **dronedarone**. Avoid. Severe Study → Also see TABLE 9 p. 820
- ▸ **HIV-protease inhibitors** are predicted to increase the exposure to **lidocaine**. Avoid. Severe Study
- ▸ **HIV-protease inhibitors** (**atazanavir, darunavir, fosamprenavir, lopinavir, ritonavir, saquinavir, tipranavir**) are predicted to increase the exposure to **propafenone**. Monitor and adjust dose. Severe Study
- ▸ **HIV-protease inhibitors** (**indinavir**) are predicted to increase the exposure to **propafenone**. Monitor and adjust dose. Moderate Study
- ▸ **HIV-protease inhibitors** (**ritonavir**) are predicted to increase the exposure to **flecainide**. Severe Theoretical
- ▸ **Dronedarone** is predicted to increase the exposure to **ibrutinib**. Avoid or adjust **ibrutinib** dose. Severe Theoretical
- ▸ **Idelalisib** very markedly increases the exposure to **dronedarone**. Avoid. Severe Study
- ▸ **Idelalisib** is predicted to increase the exposure to **propafenone**. Monitor and adjust dose. Severe Study
- ▸ **Imatinib** is predicted to increase the exposure to **dronedarone**. Severe Theoretical
- ▸ **Imatinib** is predicted to increase the exposure to **propafenone**. Monitor and adjust dose. Moderate Study
- ▸ **Dronedarone** is predicted to increase the exposure to **ivabradine**. Adjust **ivabradine** dose. Severe Theoretical
- ▸ **Dronedarone** is predicted to increase the exposure to **ivacaftor**. Adjust **ivacaftor** dose, p. 179. Severe Study
- ▸ **Dronedarone** is predicted to increase the exposure to **lapatinib**. Moderate Study → Also see TABLE 9 p. 820
- ▸ **Ledipasvir** increases the risk of severe bradycardia or heart block when given with **amiodarone**. Refer to specialist literature. Severe Anecdotal
- ▸ **Amiodarone** increases the risk of thyroid dysfunction when given with **levothyroxine**. Avoid. Moderate Study
- ▸ **Amiodarone** is predicted to increase the risk of thyroid dysfunction when given with **liothyronine**. Avoid. Moderate Theoretical
- ▸ **Amiodarone** is predicted to increase the exposure to **lomitapide**. Separate administration by 12 hours. Moderate Theoretical
- ▸ **Dronedarone** is predicted to increase the exposure to **lomitapide**. Avoid. Moderate Theoretical
- ▸ **Dronedarone** is predicted to increase the exposure to **loperamide**. Severe Theoretical
- ▸ **Dronedarone** is predicted to increase the exposure to **lurasidone**. Moderate Study
- ▸ **Macrolides** (**clarithromycin**) very markedly increase the exposure to **dronedarone**. Avoid. Severe Study → Also see TABLE 9 p. 820

- ▸ **Macrolides** (**clarithromycin**) are predicted to increase the exposure to **propafenone**. Monitor and adjust dose. Severe Study
- ▸ **Macrolides** (**clarithromycin, erythromycin**) are predicted to increase the exposure to **lidocaine**. Moderate Theoretical
- ▸ **Macrolides** (**erythromycin**) are predicted to moderately increase the exposure to **dronedarone**. Avoid. Severe Theoretical
- ▸ **Macrolides** (**erythromycin**) are predicted to increase the exposure to **propafenone**. Monitor and adjust dose. Moderate Study
- ▸ **Dronedarone** is predicted to increase the exposure to **midazolam**. Monitor side effects and adjust dose. Severe Study
- ▸ **Mirabegron** is predicted to increase the exposure to **flecainide**. Severe Theoretical
- ▸ **Dronedarone** increases the risk of neutropenia when given with monoclonal antibodies (**brentuximab vedotin**). Monitor and adjust dose. Severe Theoretical
- ▸ **Dronedarone** is predicted to increase the exposure to **naloxegol**. Adjust **naloxegol** dose and monitor side effects. Moderate Study
- ▸ **Netupitant** is predicted to increase the exposure to **propafenone**. Monitor and adjust dose. Moderate Study
- ▸ **Nevirapine** is predicted to decrease the exposure to **dronedarone**. Severe Theoretical
- ▸ **Dronedarone** is predicted to increase the exposure to **nilotinib**. Moderate Theoretical → Also see TABLE 9 p. 820
- ▸ **Nilotinib** is predicted to increase the exposure to **propafenone**. Monitor and adjust dose. Moderate Study
- ▸ Antiarrhythmics (**amiodarone, dronedarone**) are predicted to increase the exposure to **nintedanib**. Moderate Study
- ▸ NSAIDs (**celecoxib**) are predicted to increase the exposure to antiarrhythmics (**flecainide, propafenone**). Monitor and adjust dose. Moderate Theoretical
- ▸ **Dronedarone** is predicted to increase the exposure to **olaparib**. Avoid or adjust **olaparib** dose. Moderate Theoretical
- ▸ **Dronedarone** is predicted to increase the exposure to opioids (**alfentanil, buprenorphine, fentanyl, oxycodone**). Monitor and adjust dose. Moderate Study
- ▸ **Amiodarone** is predicted to increase the concentration of opioids (**fentanyl**). Moderate Theoretical → Also see TABLE 6 p. 819
- ▸ **Dronedarone** is predicted to increase the exposure to opioids (**methadone, sufentanil**). Moderate Theoretical → Also see TABLE 9 p. 820
- ▸ **Propafenone** is predicted to decrease the efficacy of opioids (**tramadol**). Moderate Study
- ▸ **Dronedarone** is predicted to increase the exposure to **oxybutynin**. Mild Theoretical
- ▸ **Dronedarone** is predicted to increase the exposure to **pazopanib**. Moderate Theoretical → Also see TABLE 9 p. 820
- ▸ **Propafenone** is predicted to increase the anticoagulant effect of **phenindione**. Monitor and adjust dose. Moderate Theoretical
- ▸ **Dronedarone** is predicted to increase the exposure to phosphodiesterase type-5 inhibitors (**avanafil**). Adjust **avanafil** dose. Moderate Theoretical
- ▸ **Dronedarone** is predicted to increase the exposure to phosphodiesterase type-5 inhibitors (**sildenafil**). Monitor and adjust **sildenafil** dose, p. 117. Moderate Study → Also see TABLE 9 p. 820
- ▸ **Dronedarone** is predicted to increase the exposure to phosphodiesterase type-5 inhibitors (**tadalafil**). Severe Theoretical
- ▸ **Dronedarone** is predicted to increase the exposure to phosphodiesterase type-5 inhibitors (**vardenafil**). Adjust dose. Severe Theoretical → Also see TABLE 9 p. 820
- ▸ **Dronedarone** is predicted to increase the exposure to **pimozide**. Avoid. Severe Theoretical → Also see TABLE 9 p. 820
- ▸ **Propafenone** is predicted to increase the exposure to **pitolisant**. Use with caution and adjust dose. Moderate Study
- ▸ **Dronedarone** is predicted to increase the exposure to **quetiapine**. Avoid. Moderate Study
- ▸ Quinolones (**ciprofloxacin**) slightly increase the exposure to **lidocaine**. Mild Study
- ▸ **Dronedarone** is predicted to increase the exposure to **ranolazine**. Severe Study → Also see TABLE 9 p. 820
- ▸ **Amiodarone** is predicted to increase the exposure to retinoids (**alitretinoin**). Adjust **alitretinoin** dose. Moderate Theoretical

Antiarrhythmics (continued)

▸ Rifampicin is predicted to decrease the exposure to antiarrhythmics (disopyramide, dronedarone). Avoid. Severe Study

▸ Rifampicin is predicted to decrease the efficacy of propafenone. Moderate Study

▸ Dronedarone is predicted to increase the exposure to rivaroxaban. Avoid. Moderate Theoretical

▸ Dronedarone is predicted to increase the exposure to ruxolitinib. Moderate Theoretical

▸ Dronedarone is predicted to increase the exposure to saxagliptin. Mild Study

▸ Simeprevir is predicted to increase the concentration of amiodarone. Refer to specialist literature. Severe Anecdotal

▸ Dronedarone is predicted to increase the exposure to simeprevir. Avoid. Severe Study

▸ Amiodarone is predicted to increase the concentration of sirolimus. Severe Anecdotal

▸ Dronedarone increases the concentration of sirolimus. Monitor and adjust dose. Moderate Study

▸ Sofosbuvir is predicted to increase the risk of severe bradycardia or heart block when given with amiodarone. Refer to specialist literature. Severe Anecdotal

▸ SSRIs (fluoxetine, fluvoxamine, paroxetine) are predicted to increase the exposure to propafenone. Monitor and adjust dose. Moderate Study

▸ SSRIs (fluoxetine, paroxetine) are predicted to increase the exposure to flecainide. Severe Theoretical

▸ Dronedarone is predicted to increase the exposure to SSRIs (citalopram, escitalopram, fluoxetine, fluvoxamine, paroxetine, sertraline). Severe Theoretical → Also see TABLE 9 p. 820

▸ Dronedarone is predicted to increase the exposure to SSRIs (dapoxetine). Adjust dapoxetine dose. Moderate Theoretical

▸ St John's Wort is predicted to decrease the exposure to dronedarone. Avoid. Severe Theoretical

▸ Amiodarone is predicted to increase the risk of rhabdomyolysis when given with statins (atorvastatin). Monitor and adjust dose. Moderate Theoretical

▸ Dronedarone is predicted to increase the exposure to statins (atorvastatin). Monitor and adjust dose. Severe Theoretical

▸ Amiodarone is predicted to increase the exposure to statins (fluvastatin). Severe Theoretical

▸ Dronedarone slightly increases the exposure to statins (rosuvastatin). Adjust dose. Severe Study

▸ Amiodarone increases the risk of rhabdomyolysis when given with statins (simvastatin). Adjust simvastatin dose, p. 130. Severe Study

▸ Dronedarone is predicted to increase the exposure to statins (simvastatin). Use with caution and adjust simvastatin dose, p. 130. Severe Study

▸ Amiodarone is predicted to increase the exposure to sulfonylureas. Use with caution and adjust dose. Moderate Study

▸ Dronedarone is predicted to increase the exposure to sunitinib. Moderate Theoretical → Also see TABLE 9 p. 820

▸ Lidocaine is predicted to increase the effects of suxamethonium. Moderate Study

▸ Amiodarone is predicted to increase the concentration of tacrolimus. Severe Anecdotal

▸ Dronedarone is predicted to increase the concentration of tacrolimus. Severe Study

▸ Dronedarone is predicted to increase the exposure to taxanes (cabazitaxel). Moderate Theoretical

▸ Dronedarone is predicted to increase the exposure to taxanes (paclitaxel). Severe Theoretical

▸ Dronedarone is predicted to increase the concentration of temsirolimus. Moderate Theoretical

▸ Terbinafine is predicted to increase the exposure to flecainide. Severe Theoretical

▸ Terbinafine is predicted to increase the exposure to propafenone. Monitor and adjust dose. Moderate Study

▸ Theophylline decreases the efficacy of adenosine. Separate administration by 24 hours. Mild Study

▸ Amiodarone is predicted to increase the exposure to ticagrelor. Use with caution or avoid. Severe Study

▸ Dronedarone is predicted to increase the exposure to tolterodine. Mild Theoretical → Also see TABLE 9 p. 820

▸ Dronedarone is predicted to increase the exposure to tolvaptan. Adjust dose. Moderate Theoretical

▸ Antiarrhythmics (amiodarone, dronedarone) are predicted to increase the exposure to topotecan. Severe Study

▸ Antiarrhythmics (amiodarone, dronedarone) are predicted to increase the concentration of trametinib. Moderate Theoretical

▸ Dronedarone is predicted to increase the exposure to trazodone. Moderate Theoretical

▸ Dronedarone is predicted to increase the risk of torsade de pointes when given with tricyclic antidepressants. Avoid. Severe Theoretical → Also see TABLE 9 p. 820

▸ Propafenone is predicted to increase the concentration of tricyclic antidepressants. Moderate Theoretical → Also see TABLE 10 p. 820

▸ Dronedarone is predicted to increase the exposure to ulipristal. Avoid if used for uterine fibroids. Moderate Study

▸ Amiodarone is predicted to increase the concentration of velpatasvir. Avoid or monitor. Moderate Theoretical

▸ Amiodarone is predicted to increase the exposure to venetoclax. Avoid or monitor for toxicity. Severe Theoretical

▸ Dronedarone is predicted to increase the exposure to venetoclax. Avoid or adjust venetoclax dose. Severe Study

▸ Dronedarone is predicted to increase the exposure to vinca alkaloids. Severe Theoretical → Also see TABLE 9 p. 820

▸ Dronedarone is predicted to increase the exposure to zopiclone. Adjust dose. Moderate Study

Anticholinesterases, centrally acting → see TABLE 6 p. 819
(bradycardia)

donepezil · galantamine · rivastigmine

▸ Antiarrhythmics (amiodarone) increase the risk of bradycardia when given with anticholinesterases, centrally acting. Moderate Anecdotal → Also see TABLE 6 p. 819

▸ Antiepileptics (carbamazepine, fosphenytoin, phenobarbital, phenytoin, primidone) are predicted to decrease the exposure to donepezil. Mild Study

▸ Antifungals, azoles (itraconazole, ketoconazole, voriconazole) are predicted to increase the exposure to galantamine. Monitor and adjust dose. Moderate Study

▸ Anticholinesterases, centrally acting are predicted to increase the risk of bradycardia when given with beta blockers, non-selective. Moderate Anecdotal → Also see TABLE 6 p. 819

▸ Anticholinesterases, centrally acting are predicted to increase the risk of bradycardia when given with beta blockers, selective. Moderate Anecdotal → Also see TABLE 6 p. 819

▸ Bupropion is predicted to increase the exposure to donepezil. Moderate Theoretical

▸ Bupropion is predicted to increase the exposure to galantamine. Monitor and adjust dose. Moderate Study

▸ Calcium channel blockers (diltiazem, verapamil) increase the risk of bradycardia when given with anticholinesterases, centrally acting. Moderate Anecdotal → Also see TABLE 6 p. 819

▸ Cinacalcet is predicted to increase the exposure to donepezil. Moderate Theoretical

▸ Cinacalcet is predicted to increase the exposure to galantamine. Monitor and adjust dose. Moderate Study

▸ Cobicistat is predicted to increase the exposure to galantamine. Monitor and adjust dose. Moderate Study

▸ Enzalutamide is predicted to decrease the exposure to donepezil. Mild Study

▸ HIV-protease inhibitors (atazanavir, darunavir, fosamprenavir, lopinavir, ritonavir, saquinavir, tipranavir) are predicted to increase the exposure to galantamine. Monitor and adjust dose. Moderate Study

▸ Idelalisib is predicted to increase the exposure to galantamine. Monitor and adjust dose. Moderate Study

▸ Macrolides (clarithromycin) are predicted to increase the exposure to galantamine. Monitor and adjust dose. Moderate Study

▸ Anticholinesterases, centrally acting are predicted to decrease the effects of neuromuscular blocking drugs, non-depolarising. Moderate Theoretical → Also see TABLE 6 p. 819

▸ Rifampicin is predicted to decrease the exposure to donepezil. Mild Study

- SSRIs **(fluoxetine, paroxetine)** are predicted to increase the exposure to **donepezil.** Moderate Theoretical
- SSRIs **(fluoxetine, paroxetine)** are predicted to increase the exposure to **galantamine.** Monitor and adjust dose. Moderate Study
- **Anticholinesterases, centrally acting** increase the effects of **suxamethonium.** Moderate Theoretical
- **Terbinafine** is predicted to increase the exposure to **donepezil.** Moderate Theoretical
- **Terbinafine** is predicted to increase the exposure to **galantamine.** Monitor and adjust dose. Moderate Study

Antiepileptics → see TABLE 1 p. 818 (hepatotoxicity), TABLE 18 p. 822 (hyponatraemia), TABLE 15 p. 821 (myelosuppression), TABLE 12 p. 821 (peripheral neuropathy), TABLE 11 p. 820 (CNS depressant effects)

brivaracetam · carbamazepine · eslicarbazepine · ethosuximide · fosphenytoin · gabapentin · lacosamide · lamotrigine · levetiracetam · oxcarbazepine · paraldehyde · perampanel · phenobarbital · phenytoin · pregabalin · primidone · retigabine · rufinamide · stiripentol · tiagabine · topiramate · valproate · vigabatrin · zonisamide

FOOD AND LIFESTYLE   Increased risk of blurred vision when retigabine taken with alcohol.

- Antiepileptics **(carbamazepine, fosphenytoin, phenobarbital, phenytoin, primidone)** are predicted to decrease the exposure to **abacavir.** Moderate Theoretical
- Antiepileptics **(carbamazepine, fosphenytoin, phenobarbital, phenytoin, primidone)** are predicted to decrease the exposure to **abiraterone.** Avoid. Severe Theoretical
- **Acetazolamide** potentially increases the risk of overheating and dehydration when given with **zonisamide.** Avoid in children. Severe Theoretical
- **Carbamazepine** is predicted to decrease the exposure to **afatinib.** Moderate Study
- Antiepileptics **(fosphenytoin, phenytoin)** are predicted to decrease the exposure to **agomelatine.** Moderate Theoretical
- Antiepileptics **(carbamazepine, fosphenytoin, phenobarbital, phenytoin, primidone)** decrease the concentration of **albendazole.** Moderate Study
- Antiepileptics **(carbamazepine, fosphenytoin, phenobarbital, phenytoin, primidone)** are predicted to decrease the exposure to aldosterone antagonists **(eplerenone).** Avoid. Moderate Theoretical → Also see TABLE 18 p. 822
- **Carbamazepine** decreases the exposure to **aliskiren.** Moderate Study
- Antiepileptics **(carbamazepine, fosphenytoin, phenobarbital, phenytoin, primidone)** are predicted to decrease the exposure to **alprazolam.** Adjust **alprazolam** dose. Moderate Theoretical → Also see TABLE 11 p. 820
- **Fosphenytoin** is predicted to decrease the exposure to **aminophylline.** Adjust dose. Moderate Study
- **Phenobarbital** is predicted to decrease the exposure to **aminophylline.** Adjust dose. Moderate Theoretical
- **Phenytoin** decreases the exposure to **aminophylline.** Adjust dose. Moderate Study
- **Primidone** is predicted to increase the clearance of **aminophylline.** Adjust dose. Moderate Theoretical
- Antiepileptics **(fosphenytoin, phenobarbital, phenytoin, primidone)** are predicted to increase the risk of methaemoglobinaemia when given with topical anaesthetics, local **(prilocaine).** Use with caution or avoid. Severe Theoretical → Also see TABLE 11 p. 820
- **Antacids** decrease the absorption of **gabapentin.** Gabapentin should be taken 2 hours after **antacids.** Moderate Study
- Antiepileptics **(carbamazepine, fosphenytoin, phenobarbital, phenytoin, primidone)** are predicted to decrease the exposure to antiarrhythmics **(disopyramide, dronedarone).** Avoid. Severe Study
- Antiarrhythmics **(amiodarone)** are predicted to slightly increase the concentration of antiepileptics **(fosphenytoin, phenytoin).** Monitor and adjust dose. Severe Study → Also see TABLE 12 p. 821
- Antiepileptics **(fosphenytoin, phenytoin)** are predicted to decrease the exposure to antiarrhythmics **(lidocaine).** Severe Anecdotal

- Antiepileptics **(carbamazepine, fosphenytoin, phenobarbital, phenytoin, primidone)** are predicted to decrease the efficacy of antiarrhythmics **(propafenone).** Moderate Study
- Antiepileptics **(carbamazepine, fosphenytoin, phenobarbital, phenytoin, primidone)** are predicted to decrease the exposure to anticholinesterases, centrally acting **(donepezil).** Mild Study
- Antiepileptics **(carbamazepine)** decrease the concentration of antiepileptics **(brivaracetam).** Moderate Study
- Antiepileptics **(fosphenytoin, phenytoin)** decrease the concentration of antiepileptics **(brivaracetam).** Moderate Study
- Antiepileptics **(lamotrigine)** potentially increase the concentration of antiepileptics **(carbamazepine)** and antiepileptics **(carbamazepine)** decrease the concentration of antiepileptics **(lamotrigine).** Adjust **lamotrigine** dose and monitor **carbamazepine** concentration, p. 194. Moderate Study
- Antiepileptics **(phenobarbital)** affect the concentration of antiepileptics **(carbamazepine)** and antiepileptics **(carbamazepine)** increase the concentration of antiepileptics **(phenobarbital).** Adjust dose. Moderate Study
- Antiepileptics **(stiripentol)** increase the concentration of antiepileptics **(carbamazepine).** Severe Study
- Antiepileptics **(topiramate)** increase the risk of carbamazepine toxicity when given with antiepileptics **(carbamazepine).** Moderate Study
- Antiepileptics **(carbamazepine)** slightly decrease the exposure to antiepileptics **(eslicarbazepine, oxcarbazepine).** Monitor and adjust dose. Moderate Study
- Antiepileptics **(oxcarbazepine)** are predicted to increase the concentration of antiepileptics **(fosphenytoin).** Monitor concentration and adjust dose. Moderate Study
- Antiepileptics **(carbamazepine)** affect the concentration of antiepileptics **(fosphenytoin, phenytoin)** and antiepileptics **(fosphenytoin, phenytoin)** decrease the concentration of antiepileptics **(carbamazepine).** Monitor and adjust dose. Severe Study
- Antiepileptics **(eslicarbazepine)** increase the exposure to antiepileptics **(fosphenytoin, phenytoin)** and antiepileptics **(fosphenytoin, phenytoin)** decrease the exposure to antiepileptics **(eslicarbazepine).** Monitor and adjust dose. Moderate Study
- Antiepileptics **(stiripentol)** are predicted to increase the concentration of antiepileptics **(fosphenytoin, phenytoin).** Severe Study
- Antiepileptics **(valproate)** affect the concentration of antiepileptics **(fosphenytoin, phenytoin)** and antiepileptics **(fosphenytoin, phenytoin)** decrease the concentration of antiepileptics **(valproate).** Severe Study
- Antiepileptics **(vigabatrin)** decrease the concentration of antiepileptics **(fosphenytoin, phenytoin).** Mild Study
- Antiepileptics **(fosphenytoin)** decrease the concentration of antiepileptics **(lamotrigine).** Monitor and adjust **lamotrigine** dose, p. 194. Moderate Study
- Antiepileptics **(phenobarbital, phenytoin, primidone)** decrease the concentration of antiepileptics **(lamotrigine).** Monitor and adjust **lamotrigine** dose, p. 194. Moderate Study → Also see TABLE 11 p. 820
- Antiepileptics **(valproate)** increase the exposure to antiepileptics **(lamotrigine).** Adjust **lamotrigine** dose and monitor rash, p. 194. Severe Study
- Antiepileptics **(lamotrigine)** are predicted to increase the concentration of antiepileptics **(oxcarbazepine)** and antiepileptics **(oxcarbazepine)** are predicted to decrease the concentration of antiepileptics **(lamotrigine).** Monitor side effects and adjust dose. Moderate Study
- Antiepileptics **(carbamazepine, fosphenytoin)** are predicted to decrease the exposure to antiepileptics **(perampanel).** Monitor and adjust dose. Moderate Study
- Antiepileptics **(oxcarbazepine)** decrease the concentration of antiepileptics **(perampanel)** and antiepileptics **(perampanel)** increase the concentration of antiepileptics **(oxcarbazepine).** Monitor and adjust dose. Moderate Study
- Antiepileptics **(phenobarbital, phenytoin, primidone)** are predicted to decrease the exposure to antiepileptics **(perampanel).** Monitor and adjust dose. Moderate Study → Also see TABLE 11 p. 820

A1

Interactions | Appendix 1

Antiepileptics (continued)

▸ Antiepileptics **(phenytoin)** increase the concentration of antiepileptics **(phenobarbital)** and antiepileptics **(phenobarbital)** affect the concentration of antiepileptics **(phenytoin)**. Moderate Study

▸ Antiepileptics **(fosphenytoin)** increase the concentration of antiepileptics **(phenobarbital, primidone)** and antiepileptics **(phenobarbital, primidone)** affect the concentration of antiepileptics **(fosphenytoin)**. Moderate Study

▸ Antiepileptics **(stiripentol)** are predicted to increase the concentration of antiepileptics **(phenobarbital, primidone)**. Severe Theoretical

▸ Antiepileptics **(oxcarbazepine)** are predicted to increase the concentration of antiepileptics **(phenytoin)**. Monitor concentration and adjust dose. Moderate Study

▸ Antiepileptics **(carbamazepine)** potentially decrease the concentration of antiepileptics **(primidone)** and antiepileptics **(primidone)** potentially decrease the concentration of antiepileptics **(carbamazepine)**. Adjust dose. Moderate Anecdotal

▸ Antiepileptics **(phenytoin)** increase the concentration of antiepileptics **(primidone)** and antiepileptics **(primidone)** affect the concentration of antiepileptics **(phenytoin)**. Moderate Study

▸ Antiepileptics **(valproate)** affect the concentration of antiepileptics **(primidone)**. Monitor and adjust dose. Severe Study

▸ Antiepileptics **(carbamazepine, fosphenytoin, phenytoin)** decrease the exposure to antiepileptics **(retigabine)**. Moderate Study

▸ Antiepileptics **(valproate)** increase the exposure to antiepileptics **(rufinamide)**. Adjust rufinamide dose, p. 200. Moderate Study

▸ Antiepileptics **(carbamazepine, fosphenytoin, phenobarbital, phenytoin, primidone)** decrease the exposure to antiepileptics **(tiagabine)**. Monitor and adjust tiagabine dose, p. 203. Moderate Study

▸ Antiepileptics **(fosphenytoin, phenytoin)** decrease the concentration of antiepileptics **(topiramate)** and antiepileptics **(topiramate)** increase the concentration of antiepileptics **(fosphenytoin, phenytoin)**. Monitor and adjust dose. Moderate Study

▸ Antiepileptics **(phenobarbital, primidone)** are predicted to decrease the concentration of antiepileptics **(topiramate)**. Mild Study

▸ Antiepileptics **(phenobarbital)** decrease the concentration of antiepileptics **(valproate)** and antiepileptics **(valproate)** increase the concentration of antiepileptics **(phenobarbital)**. Monitor and adjust dose. Moderate Study

▸ Antiepileptics **(topiramate)** increase the risk of toxicity when given with antiepileptics **(valproate)**. Severe Study

▸ Antiepileptics **(carbamazepine)** slightly to moderately decrease the concentration of antiepileptics **(zonisamide)** and antiepileptics **(zonisamide)** affect the concentration of antiepileptics **(carbamazepine)**. Monitor and adjust dose. Moderate Study

▸ Antiepileptics **(fosphenytoin, phenytoin)** slightly to moderately decrease the concentration of antiepileptics **(zonisamide)**. Monitor and adjust dose. Moderate Study

▸ Antiepileptics **(phenobarbital, primidone)** are predicted to decrease the concentration of antiepileptics **(zonisamide)**. Monitor and adjust dose. Moderate Study

▸ Antiepileptics **(topiramate)** potentially increase the risk of overheating and dehydration when given with antiepileptics **(zonisamide)**. Avoid in children. Severe Theoretical

▸ Antifungals, azoles **(itraconazole, ketoconazole, voriconazole)** are predicted to slightly increase the exposure to perampanel. Mild Study

▸ Antifungals, azoles **(miconazole)** increase the risk of **carbamazepine** toxicity when given with **carbamazepine**. Monitor and adjust dose. Severe Anecdotal

▸ Antifungals, azoles **(miconazole)** increase the risk of phenytoin toxicity when given with **fosphenytoin**. Monitor and adjust dose. Severe Anecdotal

▸ Antifungals, azoles **(miconazole)** increase the risk of **phenytoin** toxicity when given with **phenytoin**. Monitor and adjust dose. Severe Anecdotal

▸ **Carbamazepine** is predicted to decrease the efficacy of antifungals, azoles **(fluconazole)** and antifungals, azoles **(fluconazole)** increase the concentration of **carbamazepine**. Avoid or monitor **carbamazepine** concentration and adjust dose accordingly. Severe Theoretical → Also see TABLE 1 p. 818

▸ Antifungals, azoles **(fluconazole)** increase the concentration of antiepileptics **(fosphenytoin, phenytoin)**. Monitor concentration and adjust dose. Moderate Study

▸ Antiepileptics **(carbamazepine, fosphenytoin, phenobarbital, phenytoin, primidone)** are predicted to decrease the exposure to antifungals, azoles **(isavuconazole)**. Avoid. Severe Study

▸ **Fosphenytoin** very markedly decreases the exposure to antifungals, azoles **(itraconazole)**. Avoid **fosphenytoin** for 14 days before and during treatment with itraconazole. Moderate Study

▸ **Phenobarbital** decreases the concentration of antifungals, azoles **(itraconazole)**. Avoid **phenobarbital** for 14 days before and during treatment with itraconazole. Moderate Study

▸ **Phenytoin** very markedly decreases the exposure to antifungals, azoles **(itraconazole)**. Avoid **phenytoin** for 14 days before and during treatment with itraconazole. Moderate Study

▸ **Primidone** is predicted to decrease the concentration of antifungals, azoles **(itraconazole)**. Moderate Theoretical

▸ **Carbamazepine** is predicted to decrease the efficacy of antifungals, azoles **(itraconazole, voriconazole)** and antifungals, azoles **(itraconazole, voriconazole)** increase the concentration of **carbamazepine**. Avoid or adjust dose. Moderate Theoretical → Also see TABLE 1 p. 818

▸ **Carbamazepine** is predicted to decrease the efficacy of antifungals, azoles **(ketoconazole)** and antifungals, azoles **(ketoconazole)** slightly increase the concentration of **carbamazepine**. Avoid or monitor **carbamazepine** concentration and adjust dose accordingly. Moderate Study

▸ **Phenobarbital** is predicted to decrease the concentration of antifungals, azoles **(ketoconazole)**. Avoid. Moderate Study

▸ Antiepileptics **(fosphenytoin, phenytoin)** decrease the exposure to antifungals, azoles **(ketoconazole)**. Avoid. Moderate Study

▸ **Primidone** is predicted to decrease the concentration of antifungals, azoles **(ketoconazole, posaconazole)**. Avoid. Moderate Study

▸ **Carbamazepine** is predicted to decrease the efficacy of antifungals, azoles **(posaconazole)** and antifungals, azoles **(posaconazole)** increase the concentration of **carbamazepine**. Avoid. Moderate Theoretical

▸ **Phenobarbital** is predicted to decrease the concentration of antifungals, azoles **(posaconazole)**. Avoid. Moderate Study

▸ Antiepileptics **(fosphenytoin, phenytoin)** are predicted to decrease the exposure to antifungals, azoles **(posaconazole)**. Avoid. Moderate Study

▸ **Fosphenytoin** decreases the exposure to antifungals, azoles **(voriconazole)** and antifungals, azoles **(voriconazole)** increase the exposure to **fosphenytoin**. Avoid or adjust **voriconazole** dose and monitor phenytoin concentration, p. 361. Moderate Study

▸ **Phenytoin** decreases the exposure to antifungals, azoles **(voriconazole)** and antifungals, azoles **(voriconazole)** increase the exposure to **phenytoin**. Avoid or adjust **voriconazole** dose and monitor phenytoin concentration, p. 361. Moderate Study

▸ Antiepileptics **(phenobarbital, primidone)** are predicted to decrease the concentration of antifungals, azoles **(voriconazole)**. Avoid. Moderate Theoretical

▸ Antihistamines, sedating **(hydroxyzine)** potentially increase the risk of overheating and dehydration when given with **zonisamide**. Avoid in children. Severe Theoretical

▸ Antiepileptics **(carbamazepine, fosphenytoin, phenobarbital, phenytoin, primidone)** are predicted to decrease the exposure to antimalarials **(artemether)** (with lumefantrine). Avoid. Severe Study

▸ Antimalarials **(pyrimethamine)** increase the risk of haematological toxicity when given with antiepileptics **(fosphenytoin, phenytoin)**. Severe Study

▸ Antimalarials **(pyrimethamine)** are predicted to increase the risk of haematological toxicity when given with antiepileptics **(phenobarbital, primidone)**. Severe Theoretical

- Antiepileptics **(carbamazepine, fosphenytoin, phenobarbital, phenytoin, primidone)** are predicted to decrease the concentration of antimalarials **(piperaquine)**. Avoid. Moderate Theoretical
- Antiepileptics **(carbamazepine, fosphenytoin, phenobarbital, phenytoin, primidone)** are predicted to moderately decrease the exposure to apixaban. Use with caution or avoid. Severe Study
- Antiepileptics **(carbamazepine, fosphenytoin, phenobarbital, phenytoin, primidone)** moderately decrease the exposure to apremilast. Avoid. Severe Study
- Antiepileptics **(carbamazepine, fosphenytoin, phenobarbital, phenytoin, primidone)** are predicted to markedly decrease the exposure to aprepitant. Avoid. Moderate Study
- Antiepileptics **(carbamazepine, fosphenytoin, phenobarbital, phenytoin, primidone)** are predicted to moderately decrease the exposure to aripiprazole. Adjust aripiprazole dose, p. 240. Moderate Study → Also see TABLE 11 p. 820
- Antiepileptics **(carbamazepine, fosphenytoin, phenobarbital, phenytoin, primidone)** are predicted to decrease the exposure to axitinib. Avoid or adjust dose. Moderate Study
- Antiepileptics **(carbamazepine, fosphenytoin, phenobarbital, phenytoin, primidone)** are predicted to decrease the exposure to bazedoxifene. Moderate Theoretical
- Antiepileptics **(carbamazepine, fosphenytoin, phenobarbital, phenytoin, primidone)** decrease the exposure to bedaquiline. Avoid. Severe Study
- Antiepileptics **(phenobarbital, primidone)** are predicted to decrease the exposure to beta blockers, non-selective **(carvedilol, labetalol)**. Moderate Theoretical
- Antiepileptics **(phenobarbital, primidone)** are predicted to decrease the exposure to beta blockers, non-selective **(propranolol)**. Moderate Study
- Antiepileptics **(phenobarbital, primidone)** are predicted to decrease the exposure to beta blockers, selective **(acebutolol, bisoprolol, metoprolol, nebivolol)**. Moderate Study
- Antiepileptics **(carbamazepine, fosphenytoin, phenobarbital, phenytoin, primidone)** slightly decrease the exposure to bortezomib. Avoid. Severe Study → Also see TABLE 12 p. 821
- Antiepileptics **(carbamazepine, fosphenytoin, phenobarbital, phenytoin, primidone)** affect the exposure to bosentan. Avoid. Severe Study
- Antiepileptics **(carbamazepine, fosphenytoin, phenobarbital, phenytoin, primidone)** are predicted to very markedly decrease the exposure to bosutinib. Avoid. Severe Study
- Antiepileptics **(carbamazepine, fosphenytoin, phenobarbital, phenytoin, primidone)** are predicted to markedly decrease the exposure to bupropion. Severe Study
- **Valproate** increases the exposure to bupropion. Severe Study
- Antiepileptics **(carbamazepine, fosphenytoin, phenobarbital, phenytoin, primidone)** are predicted to decrease the exposure to buspirone. Use with caution and adjust dose. Severe Study
- Antiepileptics **(carbamazepine, fosphenytoin, phenobarbital, phenytoin, primidone)** moderately decrease the exposure to cabozantinib. Moderate Study
- Antiepileptics **(fosphenytoin, phenytoin)** are predicted to moderately increase the clearance of caffeine citrate. Monitor and adjust dose. Moderate Study
- Calcium channel blockers **(diltiazem, verapamil)** increase the concentration of carbamazepine. Severe Anecdotal
- Antiepileptics **(carbamazepine, fosphenytoin, phenobarbital, phenytoin, primidone)** are predicted to decrease the exposure to calcium channel blockers **(amlodipine, felodipine, lacidipine, lercanidipine, nicardipine, nifedipine, nimodipine)**. Monitor and adjust dose. Moderate Study
- Antiepileptics **(carbamazepine, fosphenytoin, phenobarbital, phenytoin, primidone)** decrease the exposure to calcium channel blockers **(diltiazem)**. Severe Study
- Antiepileptics **(carbamazepine, fosphenytoin, phenobarbital, phenytoin, primidone)** decrease the exposure to calcium channel blockers **(isradipine)**. Avoid. Moderate Study
- Antiepileptics **(carbamazepine, fosphenytoin, phenobarbital, phenytoin, primidone)** are predicted to decrease the exposure to calcium channel blockers **(verapamil)**. Severe Study

- Antiepileptics **(carbamazepine, fosphenytoin, phenobarbital, phenytoin, primidone)** are predicted to decrease the exposure to cannabis extract. Avoid. Severe Theoretical → Also see TABLE 11 p. 820
- **Capecitabine** increases the concentration of antiepileptics **(fosphenytoin, phenytoin)**. Severe Anecdotal
- **Carbapenems** decrease the concentration of valproate. Avoid. Severe Anecdotal
- Antiepileptics **(carbamazepine, fosphenytoin, phenytoin)** are predicted to decrease the concentration of caspofungin. Adjust caspofungin dose, p. 356. Moderate Theoretical
- Antiepileptics **(carbamazepine, fosphenytoin, phenobarbital, phenytoin, primidone)** are predicted to decrease the exposure to ceritinib. Avoid. Severe Study
- Antiepileptics **(phenobarbital, primidone)** decrease the concentration of chloramphenicol. Moderate Study
- Intravenous **chloramphenicol** increases the concentration of antiepileptics **(fosphenytoin, phenytoin)** and antiepileptics **(fosphenytoin, phenytoin)** affect the concentration of intravenous chloramphenicol. Monitor concentration and adjust dose. Severe Study
- **Chlordiazepoxide** affects the concentration of antiepileptics **(fosphenytoin, phenytoin)**. Severe Study
- **Phenobarbital** decreases the effects of cholic acid. Avoid. Moderate Study
- Antiepileptics **(carbamazepine, fosphenytoin, phenobarbital, phenytoin, primidone)** decrease the concentration of ciclosporin. Severe Study
- **Oxcarbazepine** decreases the concentration of ciclosporin. Severe Anecdotal
- Antiepileptics **(carbamazepine, fosphenytoin, phenobarbital, phenytoin, primidone)** are predicted to alter the effects of cilostazol. Moderate Theoretical
- **Clobazam** potentially affects the concentration of antiepileptics **(fosphenytoin, phenytoin)**. Severe Anecdotal
- **Stiripentol** increases the concentration of clobazam. Severe Study
- Antiepileptics **(carbamazepine, fosphenytoin, phenobarbital, phenytoin, primidone)** decrease the exposure to clomethiazole. Monitor and adjust dose. Moderate Study → Also see TABLE 11 p. 820
- **Clonazepam** potentially affects the concentration of antiepileptics **(fosphenytoin, phenytoin)**. Severe Anecdotal
- Antiepileptics **(fosphenytoin, phenytoin)** are predicted to decrease the exposure to clozapine. Moderate Anecdotal
- Antiepileptics **(phenobarbital, primidone)** decrease the exposure to clozapine. Moderate Anecdotal → Also see TABLE 11 p. 820
- Antiepileptics **(carbamazepine, fosphenytoin, phenobarbital, phenytoin, primidone)** are predicted to decrease the exposure to cobicistat. Avoid. Severe Theoretical
- **Oxcarbazepine** is predicted to decrease the concentration of cobicistat. Severe Theoretical
- **Cobicistat** is predicted to slightly increase the exposure to perampanel. Mild Study
- Antiepileptics **(carbamazepine, fosphenytoin, phenobarbital, phenytoin, primidone)** are predicted to decrease the exposure to cobimetinib. Avoid. Severe Theoretical
- Antiepileptics **(carbamazepine, eslicarbazepine, fosphenytoin, oxcarbazepine, perampanel, phenobarbital, phenytoin, primidone, rufinamide, topiramate)** are predicted to decrease the efficacy of combined hormonal contraceptives. For FSRH guidance, see Contraceptives, interactions p. 474. Severe Study
- **Combined hormonal contraceptives** alter the exposure to lamotrigine. Adjust lamotrigine dose, p. 194. Moderate Study
- Antiepileptics **(carbamazepine, fosphenytoin, phenobarbital, phenytoin, primidone)** are predicted to decrease the exposure to corticosteroids **(budesonide, dexamethasone, methylprednisolone, prednisolone)**. Monitor and adjust dose. Moderate Study
- Antiepileptics **(carbamazepine, fosphenytoin, phenobarbital, phenytoin, primidone)** are predicted to decrease the exposure to corticosteroids **(fluticasone)**. Unknown Theoretical
- Antiepileptics **(carbamazepine, fosphenytoin, phenobarbital, phenytoin, primidone)** are predicted to decrease the exposure to corticosteroids **(prednisone)**. Mild Study

Antiepileptics (continued)

▸ Antiepileptics (fosphenytoin, phenytoin) are predicted to alter the anticoagulant effect of coumarins. Moderate Anecdotal

▸ Antiepileptics (phenobarbital, primidone) decrease the anticoagulant effect of coumarins. Monitor INR and adjust dose. Moderate Study

▸ Carbamazepine decreases the effects of coumarins. Monitor and adjust dose. Severe Study

▸ Antiepileptics (carbamazepine, fosphenytoin, phenobarbital, phenytoin, primidone) are predicted to markedly decrease the exposure to crizotinib. Avoid. Severe Study

▸ Carbamazepine is predicted to decrease the exposure to dabigatran. Avoid. Severe Study

▸ Antiepileptics (carbamazepine, fosphenytoin, phenobarbital, phenytoin, primidone) are predicted to decrease the exposure to dabrafenib. Avoid. Moderate Theoretical

▸ Antiepileptics (carbamazepine, fosphenytoin, phenobarbital, phenytoin, primidone) are predicted to moderately decrease the exposure to daclatasvir. Avoid. Severe Study

▸ Oxcarbazepine is predicted to decrease the exposure to daclatasvir. Avoid. Severe Theoretical

▸ Danazol moderately increases the concentration of carbamazepine. Monitor carbamazepine concentration and adjust dose. Severe Study

▸ Antiepileptics (fosphenytoin, phenobarbital, phenytoin, primidone) are predicted to increase the risk of methaemoglobinaemia when given with dapsone. Severe Theoretical

▸ Antiepileptics (carbamazepine, fosphenytoin, phenobarbital, phenytoin, primidone) are predicted to decrease the exposure to darifenacin. Moderate Theoretical

▸ Antiepileptics (carbamazepine, fosphenytoin, phenobarbital, phenytoin, primidone) are predicted to decrease the exposure to dasabuvir. Avoid. Severe Theoretical

▸ Antiepileptics (carbamazepine, fosphenytoin, phenobarbital, phenytoin, primidone) are predicted to markedly decrease the exposure to dasatinib. Avoid. Severe Study

▸ Antiepileptics (carbamazepine, fosphenytoin, phenobarbital, phenytoin, primidone) are predicted to slightly decrease the exposure to delamanid. Avoid. Moderate Study

▸ Lamotrigine is predicted to increase the risk of hyponatraemia when given with desmopressin. Severe Theoretical

▸ Antiepileptics (carbamazepine, eslicarbazepine, fosphenytoin, oxcarbazepine, perampanel, phenobarbital, phenytoin, primidone, rufinamide, topiramate) are predicted to decrease the efficacy of desogestrel. For FSRH guidance, see Contraceptives, interactions p. 474. Severe Theoretical

▸ Desogestrel is predicted to increase the exposure to lamotrigine. Moderate Study

▸ Diazepam potentially affects the concentration of antiepileptics (fosphenytoin, phenytoin). Monitor concentration and adjust dose. Severe Study

▸ Diazoxide decreases the concentration of antiepileptics (fosphenytoin, phenytoin) and antiepileptics (fosphenytoin, phenytoin) are predicted to decrease the effects of diazoxide. Monitor concentration and adjust dose. Moderate Anecdotal

▸ Antiepileptics (fosphenytoin, phenytoin) are predicted to decrease the concentration of digoxin. Moderate Anecdotal

▸ Disulfiram increases the concentration of antiepileptics (fosphenytoin, phenytoin). Monitor concentration and adjust dose. Severe Study → Also see TABLE 12 p. 821

▸ Antiepileptics (carbamazepine, fosphenytoin, phenobarbital, phenytoin, primidone) decrease the exposure to dolutegravir. Adjust dose. Severe Study

▸ Oxcarbazepine is predicted to decrease the exposure to dolutegravir. Adjust dose. Severe Theoretical

▸ Carbamazepine is predicted to decrease the exposure to edoxaban. Moderate Study

▸ Antiepileptics (fosphenytoin, phenytoin) slightly decrease the exposure to efavirenz and efavirenz affects the concentration of antiepileptics (fosphenytoin, phenytoin). Severe Theoretical

▸ Carbamazepine slightly decreases the exposure to efavirenz and efavirenz slightly decreases the exposure to carbamazepine. Severe Study

▸ Phenobarbital is predicted to decrease the exposure to efavirenz and efavirenz affects the concentration of phenobarbital. Severe Theoretical

▸ Efavirenz is predicted to affect the efficacy of primidone and primidone is predicted to slightly decrease the exposure to efavirenz. Severe Theoretical

▸ Antiepileptics (carbamazepine, fosphenytoin, phenobarbital, phenytoin, primidone) are predicted to decrease the exposure to elbasvir. Avoid. Severe Study

▸ Antiepileptics (carbamazepine, fosphenytoin, phenobarbital, phenytoin, primidone) are predicted to decrease the concentration of elvitegravir. Avoid. Severe Theoretical

▸ Enteral feeds decreases the absorption of phenytoin. Severe Study

▸ Enzalutamide is predicted to slightly decrease the exposure to brivaracetam. Moderate Theoretical

▸ Enzalutamide is predicted to decrease the exposure to perampanel. Monitor and adjust dose. Moderate Study

▸ Antiepileptics (carbamazepine, fosphenytoin, phenobarbital, phenytoin, primidone) are predicted to decrease the effects of ergotamine. Moderate Theoretical

▸ Antiepileptics (carbamazepine, fosphenytoin, phenobarbital, phenytoin, primidone) are predicted to decrease the exposure to erlotinib. Avoid or adjust erlotinib dose. Severe Study

▸ Antiepileptics (carbamazepine, eslicarbazepine, fosphenytoin, oxcarbazepine, perampanel, phenobarbital, phenytoin, primidone, rufinamide, topiramate) are predicted to decrease the efficacy of etonogestrel. For FSRH guidance, see Contraceptives, interactions p. 474. Severe Theoretical

▸ Antiepileptics (carbamazepine, fosphenytoin, phenobarbital, phenytoin, primidone) are predicted to decrease the efficacy of etoposide. Moderate Study

▸ Antiepileptics (carbamazepine, fosphenytoin, phenobarbital, phenytoin, primidone) are predicted to decrease the exposure to etravirine. Avoid. Severe Theoretical

▸ Antiepileptics (carbamazepine, fosphenytoin, phenobarbital, phenytoin, primidone) are predicted to decrease the concentration of everolimus. Avoid or adjust dose. Severe Study

▸ Antiepileptics (carbamazepine, fosphenytoin, phenobarbital, phenytoin, primidone) moderately decrease the exposure to exemestane. Moderate Study

▸ Antiepileptics (carbamazepine, fosphenytoin, phenobarbital, phenytoin, primidone) are predicted to decrease the exposure to fesoterodine. Avoid. Moderate Study

▸ Antiepileptics (carbamazepine, fosphenytoin, phenobarbital, phenytoin, primidone) are predicted to decrease the exposure to fingolimod. Moderate Study

▸ Fluorouracil increases the concentration of antiepileptics (fosphenytoin, phenytoin). Monitor concentration and adjust dose. Severe Anecdotal

▸ Folates (folic acid) decrease the concentration of antiepileptics (fosphenytoin, phenobarbital, phenytoin, primidone). Monitor concentration and adjust dose. Severe Study

▸ Folates (folinic acid) are predicted to decrease the concentration of antiepileptics (fosphenytoin, phenobarbital, phenytoin, primidone). Severe Theoretical

▸ Antiepileptics (carbamazepine, fosphenytoin, phenobarbital, phenytoin, primidone) are predicted to decrease the exposure to fosaprepitant. Avoid. Moderate Theoretical

▸ Antiepileptics (carbamazepine, fosphenytoin, phenobarbital, phenytoin, primidone) are predicted to decrease the exposure to gefitinib. Avoid. Severe Study

▸ Grapefruit juice slightly increases the exposure to carbamazepine. Monitor carbamazepine concentration and adjust dose. Moderate Study

▸ Antiepileptics (carbamazepine, fosphenytoin, phenobarbital, phenytoin, primidone) are predicted to decrease the exposure to grazoprevir. Avoid. Severe Study

▸ Antiepileptics (phenobarbital, primidone) decrease the effects of griseofulvin. Moderate Study

▸ Antiepileptics (carbamazepine, fosphenytoin, phenobarbital, phenytoin, primidone) are predicted to decrease the concentration of guanfacine. Adjust guanfacine dose, p. 222. Moderate Study → Also see TABLE 11 p. 820

▸ **Oxcarbazepine** is predicted to decrease the concentration of guanfacine. Monitor and adjust **guanfacine** dose, p. 222. Moderate Theoretical

▸ **Guanfacine** increases the concentration of **valproate**. Monitor and adjust dose. Moderate Study

▸ H₂ receptor antagonists **(cimetidine)** transiently increase the concentration of **carbamazepine**. Moderate Study

▸ H₂ receptor antagonists **(cimetidine)** increase the concentration of **fosphenytoin**. Monitor phenytoin concentration and adjust dose. Severe Study

▸ H₂ receptor antagonists **(cimetidine)** increase the concentration of **phenytoin**. Monitor **phenytoin** concentration and adjust dose. Severe Study

▸ **Antiepileptics (carbamazepine, fosphenytoin, phenobarbital, phenytoin, primidone)** decrease the concentration of **haloperidol**. Adjust dose. Moderate Study → Also see TABLE 11 p. 820

▸ **Haloperidol** potentially increases the risk of overheating and dehydration when given with **zonisamide**. Avoid in children. Severe Theoretical

▸ **HIV-protease inhibitors (ritonavir)** are predicted to decrease the concentration of **valproate**. Severe Anecdotal

▸ **HIV-protease inhibitors** are predicted to affect the exposure to antiepileptics **(fosphenytoin, phenytoin)** and antiepileptics **(fosphenytoin, phenytoin)** decrease the concentration of **HIV-protease inhibitors**. Severe Theoretical

▸ **HIV-protease inhibitors** are predicted to affect the concentration of antiepileptics **(phenobarbital, primidone)** and antiepileptics **(phenobarbital, primidone)** are predicted to decrease the concentration of **HIV-protease inhibitors**. Severe Theoretical

▸ **HIV-protease inhibitors** are predicted to increase the exposure to **carbamazepine** and **carbamazepine** is predicted to decrease the exposure to **HIV-protease inhibitors**. Monitor and adjust dose. Severe Theoretical

▸ **HIV-protease inhibitors (atazanavir, darunavir, fosamprenavir, lopinavir, ritonavir, saquinavir, tipranavir)** are predicted to slightly increase the exposure to **perampanel**. Mild Study

▸ **HIV-protease inhibitors (ritonavir)** slightly decrease the exposure to **lamotrigine**. Severe Study

▸ **Antiepileptics (carbamazepine, eslicarbazepine, fosphenytoin, oxcarbazepine, perampanel, phenobarbital, phenytoin, primidone, rufinamide, topiramate)** are predicted to decrease the effects of **Hormone replacement therapy**. Moderate Anecdotal

▸ **Hormone replacement therapy** is predicted to alter the exposure to **lamotrigine**. Moderate Theoretical

▸ **Antiepileptics (carbamazepine, fosphenytoin, phenobarbital, phenytoin, primidone)** are predicted to decrease the exposure to **ibrutinib**. Avoid. Severe Study

▸ **Antiepileptics (carbamazepine, fosphenytoin, phenobarbital, phenytoin, primidone)** are predicted to decrease the exposure to **idelalisib**. Avoid. Severe Study

▸ **Idelalisib** is predicted to slightly increase the exposure to **perampanel**. Mild Study

▸ **Antiepileptics (carbamazepine, fosphenytoin, phenobarbital, phenytoin, primidone)** are predicted to decrease the exposure to **imatinib**. Avoid. Moderate Study

▸ **Oxcarbazepine** decreases the exposure to **imatinib**. Avoid. Moderate Study

▸ **Antiepileptics (carbamazepine, fosphenytoin, phenobarbital, phenytoin, primidone)** are predicted to decrease the exposure to **irinotecan**. Avoid. Severe Study

▸ **Antiepileptics (carbamazepine, fosphenytoin, phenobarbital, phenytoin, primidone)** are predicted to decrease the exposure to **iron chelators (deferasirox)**. Monitor serum ferritin and adjust dose. Moderate Theoretical

▸ **Isoniazid** increases the concentration of antiepileptics **(fosphenytoin, phenytoin)**. Moderate Study → Also see TABLE 12 p. 821

▸ **Isoniazid** markedly increases the concentration of **carbamazepine** and **carbamazepine** increases the risk of hepatotoxicity when given with **isoniazid**. Monitor **carbamazepine** concentration and adjust dose. Severe Study → Also see TABLE 1 p. 818

▸ **Antiepileptics (carbamazepine, fosphenytoin, phenobarbital, phenytoin, primidone)** are predicted to decrease the exposure to **ivabradine**. Adjust dose. Moderate Theoretical

▸ **Antiepileptics (carbamazepine, fosphenytoin, phenobarbital, phenytoin, primidone)** markedly decrease the exposure to **ivacaftor**. Avoid. Severe Study

▸ **Antiepileptics (carbamazepine, fosphenytoin, phenobarbital, phenytoin, primidone)** are predicted to decrease the exposure to **ixazomib**. Avoid. Severe Study

▸ **Antiepileptics (carbamazepine, fosphenytoin, phenobarbital, phenytoin, primidone)** are predicted to decrease the exposure to **lapatinib**. Avoid. Severe Study

▸ **Carbamazepine** is predicted to decrease the exposure to **ledipasvir**. Avoid. Severe Theoretical

▸ **Antiepileptics (fosphenytoin, phenytoin)** decrease the effects of **levodopa**. Moderate Study

▸ **Antiepileptics (carbamazepine, eslicarbazepine, fosphenytoin, oxcarbazepine, perampanel, phenobarbital, phenytoin, primidone, rufinamide, topiramate)** are predicted to decrease the efficacy of **levonorgestrel**. For FSRH guidance, see Contraceptives, interactions p. 474. Severe Theoretical

▸ **Antiepileptics (fosphenytoin, phenytoin)** increase the risk of hypothyroidism when given with **levothyroxine**. Moderate Study

▸ **Antiepileptics (phenobarbital, primidone)** are predicted to decrease the effects of **levothyroxine**. Moderate Theoretical

▸ **Carbamazepine** increases the risk of hypothyroidism when given with **levothyroxine**. Monitor and adjust dose. Moderate Study

▸ **Antiepileptics (carbamazepine, fosphenytoin, phenobarbital, phenytoin, primidone)** are predicted to decrease the exposure to **linagliptin**. Moderate Study

▸ **Antiepileptics (fosphenytoin, phenytoin)** are predicted to increase the risk of hypothyroidism when given with **liothyronine**. Moderate Theoretical

▸ **Antiepileptics (phenobarbital, primidone)** are predicted to decrease the effects of **liothyronine**. Moderate Theoretical

▸ **Carbamazepine** increases the risk of neurotoxicity when given with **lithium**. Severe Anecdotal

▸ **Oxcarbazepine** is predicted to increase the risk of neurotoxicity when given with **lithium**. Severe Theoretical

▸ **Antiepileptics (carbamazepine, fosphenytoin, phenobarbital, phenytoin, primidone)** are predicted to decrease the exposure to **lomitapide**. Monitor and adjust dose. Moderate Theoretical → Also see TABLE 1 p. 818

▸ **Antiepileptics (fosphenytoin, phenytoin)** decrease the effects of loop diuretics **(furosemide)**. Moderate Study

▸ **Lumacaftor** is predicted to decrease the exposure to antiepileptics **(carbamazepine, fosphenytoin, phenobarbital, phenytoin, primidone)**. Avoid. Severe Theoretical

▸ **Antiepileptics (carbamazepine, fosphenytoin, phenobarbital, phenytoin, primidone)** are predicted to decrease the exposure to **lurasidone**. Avoid. Moderate Study → Also see TABLE 11 p. 820

▸ **Antiepileptics (carbamazepine, fosphenytoin, phenobarbital, phenytoin, primidone)** are predicted to decrease the exposure to **macitentan**. Avoid. Severe Study

▸ **Macrolides (clarithromycin)** slightly increase the concentration of **carbamazepine**. Monitor **carbamazepine** concentration and adjust dose. Severe Study

▸ **Macrolides (clarithromycin)** are predicted to slightly increase the exposure to **perampanel**. Mild Study

▸ **Macrolides (erythromycin)** markedly increase the concentration of **carbamazepine**. Monitor **carbamazepine** concentration and adjust dose. Severe Study

▸ **Antiepileptics (carbamazepine, fosphenytoin, phenobarbital, phenytoin, primidone)** are predicted to decrease the exposure to **maraviroc**. Adjust dose. Severe Study

▸ **Levetiracetam** decreases the clearance of **methotrexate**. Severe Anecdotal

▸ **Antiepileptics (phenobarbital, primidone)** are predicted to decrease the exposure to **metronidazole**. Moderate Study

▸ **Antiepileptics (fosphenytoin, phenobarbital, phenytoin, primidone)** decrease the effects of **metyrapone**. Avoid. Moderate Study

Antiepileptics (continued)

▶ Antiepileptics **(phenobarbital, primidone)** are predicted to decrease the exposure to **mianserin**. Moderate Study → Also see **TABLE 11** p. 820

▶ **Carbamazepine** markedly decreases the exposure to **mianserin**. Adjust dose. Moderate Study

▶ Antiepileptics **(carbamazepine, fosphenytoin, phenobarbital, phenytoin, primidone)** are predicted to decrease the exposure to **midazolam**. Monitor and adjust dose. Moderate Study → Also see **TABLE 11** p. 820

▶ Antiepileptics **(carbamazepine, fosphenytoin, phenobarbital, phenytoin, primidone)** are predicted to decrease the exposure to **mirtazapine**. Adjust dose. Moderate Study → Also see **TABLE 11** p. 820

▶ Antiepileptics **(carbamazepine, phenobarbital, primidone)** are predicted to decrease the exposure to **modafinil**. Mild Theoretical

▶ Antiepileptics **(fosphenytoin, phenytoin)** are predicted to decrease the exposure to **modafinil** and **modafinil** is predicted to increase the concentration of antiepileptics **(fosphenytoin, phenytoin)**. Monitor concentration and adjust dose. Moderate Theoretical

▶ Antiepileptics **(phenobarbital, primidone)** are predicted to increase the effects of **monoamine-oxidase A and B inhibitors, irreversible**. Severe Theoretical

▶ **Carbamazepine** is predicted to decrease the effects of monoclonal antibodies **(brentuximab vedotin)**. Severe Theoretical

▶ Antiepileptics **(carbamazepine, fosphenytoin, phenobarbital, phenytoin, primidone)** are predicted to decrease the exposure to monoclonal antibodies **(trastuzumab emtansine)**. Severe Theoretical

▶ Antiepileptics **(carbamazepine, fosphenytoin, phenobarbital, phenytoin, primidone)** are predicted to decrease the exposure to **montelukast**. Mild Study

▶ Antiepileptics **(carbamazepine, fosphenytoin, phenobarbital, phenytoin, primidone)** are predicted to markedly decrease the exposure to **naloxegol**. Avoid. Moderate Study

▶ Antiepileptics **(carbamazepine, fosphenytoin, phenobarbital, phenytoin, primidone)** are predicted to slightly decrease the exposure to **nateglinide**. Mild Study

▶ Antiepileptics **(carbamazepine, fosphenytoin, phenobarbital, phenytoin, primidone)** are predicted to decrease the exposure to **netupitant**. Avoid. Moderate Study

▶ Antiepileptics **(fosphenytoin, phenytoin)** decrease the effects of (but acute use increases the effects of) neuromuscular blocking drugs, non-depolarising **(atracurium, cisatracurium, pancuronium, rocuronium, vecuronium)**. Moderate Study

▶ **Carbamazepine** is predicted to decrease the effects of (but acute use increases the effects of) neuromuscular blocking drugs, non-depolarising. Monitor and adjust dose. Moderate Study

▶ **Nevirapine** is predicted to decrease the concentration of antiepileptics **(carbamazepine, fosphenytoin, phenobarbital, phenytoin, primidone)** and antiepileptics **(carbamazepine, fosphenytoin, phenobarbital, phenytoin, primidone)** are predicted to decrease the concentration of **nevirapine**. Severe Theoretical

▶ Antiepileptics **(carbamazepine, fosphenytoin, phenobarbital, phenytoin, primidone)** are predicted to moderately decrease the exposure to **nilotinib**. Avoid. Severe Study

▶ **Carbamazepine** is predicted to decrease the exposure to **nintedanib**. Moderate Study

▶ Antiepileptics **(carbamazepine, fosphenytoin, phenobarbital, phenytoin, primidone)** are predicted to decrease the exposure to **nitisinone**. Adjust **nitisinone** dose. Moderate Theoretical

▶ Antiepileptics **(carbamazepine, eslicarbazepine, fosphenytoin, oxcarbazepine, perampanel, phenobarbital, phenytoin, primidone, rufinamide, topiramate)** are predicted to decrease the efficacy of **norethisterone**. For FSRH guidance, see Contraceptives, interactions, p. 474. Severe Anecdotal

▶ **Carbamazepine** potentially decreases the exposure to **olanzapine**. Monitor and adjust dose. Moderate Study

▶ Antiepileptics **(carbamazepine, fosphenytoin, phenobarbital, phenytoin, primidone)** are predicted to decrease the exposure to **olaparib**. Avoid. Moderate Theoretical

▶ **Carbamazepine** is predicted to decrease the exposure to **ombitasvir**. Avoid. Severe Theoretical

▶ Antiepileptics **(carbamazepine, fosphenytoin, phenobarbital, phenytoin, primidone)** are predicted to decrease the exposure to **ondansetron**. Moderate Study

▶ Antiepileptics **(carbamazepine, fosphenytoin, phenobarbital, phenytoin, primidone)** are predicted to decrease the exposure to opioids **(alfentanil, fentanyl)**. Moderate Study → Also see **TABLE 11** p. 820

▶ Antiepileptics **(carbamazepine, fosphenytoin, phenobarbital, phenytoin, primidone)** are predicted to decrease the exposure to opioids **(buprenorphine)**. Monitor and adjust dose. Moderate Theoretical → Also see **TABLE 11** p. 820

▶ Antiepileptics **(carbamazepine, fosphenytoin, phenobarbital, phenytoin, primidone)** decrease the exposure to opioids **(methadone)**. Monitor and adjust dose. Severe Study → Also see **TABLE 11** p. 820

▶ Antiepileptics **(carbamazepine, fosphenytoin, phenobarbital, phenytoin, primidone)** are predicted to decrease the exposure to opioids **(oxycodone)**. Monitor and adjust dose. Moderate Study → Also see **TABLE 11** p. 820

▶ **Carbamazepine** decreases the concentration of opioids **(tramadol)**. Adjust dose. Severe Study

▶ Antiepileptics **(carbamazepine, fosphenytoin, phenobarbital, phenytoin, primidone)** are predicted to moderately decrease the exposure to **osimertinib**. Avoid. Moderate Study

▶ **Oxybutynin** potentially increases the risk of overheating and dehydration when given with **zonisamide**. Avoid in children. Severe Theoretical

▶ Antiepileptics **(carbamazepine, fosphenytoin, phenobarbital, phenytoin, primidone)** are predicted to decrease the exposure to **palbociclib**. Avoid. Severe Study

▶ **Carbamazepine** decreases the concentration of **paliperidone**. Adjust dose. Moderate Study

▶ Antiepileptics **(carbamazepine, fosphenytoin, phenobarbital, phenytoin, primidone)** are predicted to decrease the exposure to **panobinostat**. Avoid. Moderate Theoretical

▶ Antiepileptics **(carbamazepine, fosphenytoin, phenobarbital, phenytoin, primidone)** are predicted to decrease the exposure to **paracetamol**. Moderate Study → Also see **TABLE 1** p. 818

▶ Antiepileptics **(carbamazepine, fosphenytoin, phenobarbital, phenytoin, primidone)** are predicted to decrease the exposure to **paritaprevir** (with ritonavir and ombitasvir). Avoid. Severe Study

▶ Antiepileptics **(carbamazepine, fosphenytoin, phenobarbital, phenytoin, primidone)** are predicted to decrease the exposure to **pazopanib**. Avoid. Severe Theoretical

▶ Phenothiazines **(chlorpromazine)** decrease the concentration of antiepileptics **(phenobarbital, primidone)** and antiepileptics **(phenobarbital, primidone)** decrease the concentration of phenothiazines **(chlorpromazine)**. Moderate Study → Also see **TABLE 11** p. 820

▶ Antiepileptics **(carbamazepine, fosphenytoin, phenobarbital, phenytoin, primidone)** are predicted to decrease the exposure to phosphodiesterase type-5 inhibitors **(avanafil, tadalafil)**. Avoid. Severe Study

▶ Antiepileptics **(carbamazepine, fosphenytoin, phenobarbital, phenytoin, primidone)** are predicted to decrease the exposure to phosphodiesterase type-5 inhibitors **(sildenafil, vardenafil)**. Moderate Theoretical

▶ Antiepileptics **(fosphenytoin, phenytoin)** are predicted to decrease the exposure to **pirfenidone**. Avoid. Moderate Theoretical

▶ Antiepileptics **(carbamazepine, fosphenytoin, phenobarbital, phenytoin, primidone)** are predicted to moderately decrease the exposure to **pitolisant**. Moderate Study

▶ Antiepileptics **(carbamazepine, fosphenytoin, phenobarbital, phenytoin, primidone)** are predicted to decrease the exposure to **ponatinib**. Avoid. Moderate Theoretical

▶ Antiepileptics **(carbamazepine, fosphenytoin, phenobarbital, phenytoin, primidone)** are predicted to markedly decrease the exposure to **praziquantel**. Avoid. Moderate Study

▶ Antiepileptics **(carbamazepine, fosphenytoin, phenobarbital, phenytoin, primidone)** are predicted to increase the risk of hypersensitivity reactions when given with procarbazine. Severe Anecdotal

▸ Antiepileptics **(carbamazepine, fosphenytoin, phenobarbital, phenytoin, primidone)** are predicted to decrease the exposure to quetiapine. Moderate Study → Also see TABLE 11 p. 820

▸ Quinolones **(ciprofloxacin)** affect the concentration of antiepileptics **(fosphenytoin, phenytoin)**. Monitor concentration and adjust dose. Severe Study

▸ Antiepileptics **(carbamazepine, fosphenytoin, phenobarbital, phenytoin, primidone)** are predicted to decrease the exposure to ranolazine. Avoid. Severe Study

▸ Antiepileptics **(carbamazepine, fosphenytoin, phenobarbital, phenytoin, primidone)** are predicted to decrease the exposure to reboxetine. Moderate Anecdotal

▸ Antiepileptics **(carbamazepine, fosphenytoin, phenobarbital, phenytoin, primidone)** are predicted to decrease the exposure to regorafenib. Avoid. Moderate Study

▸ Antiepileptics **(carbamazepine, fosphenytoin, phenobarbital, phenytoin, primidone)** are predicted to decrease the exposure to repaglinide. Monitor blood glucose and adjust dose. Moderate Study

▸ Antiepileptics **(phenobarbital, primidone)** are predicted to decrease the exposure to rifampicin and rifampicin is predicted to decrease the exposure to antiepileptics **(phenobarbital, primidone)**. Use with caution and adjust dose. Moderate Study

▸ Rifampicin decreases the concentration of antiepileptics **(fosphenytoin, phenytoin)**. Use with caution and adjust dose. Moderate Study

▸ Rifampicin slightly decreases the exposure to **brivaracetam**. Adjust dose. Moderate Study

▸ Rifampicin markedly increases the clearance of **lamotrigine**. Adjust **lamotrigine** dose, p. 194. Moderate Study

▸ Rifampicin is predicted to decrease the exposure to **perampanel**. Monitor and adjust dose. Moderate Study

▸ Antiepileptics **(carbamazepine, fosphenytoin, phenobarbital, phenytoin, primidone)** markedly decrease the exposure to rilpivirine. Avoid. Severe Study

▸ Oxcarbazepine is predicted to decrease the concentration of rilpivirine. Avoid. Severe Theoretical

▸ Antiepileptics **(carbamazepine, fosphenytoin, phenobarbital, phenytoin, primidone)** are predicted to decrease the exposure to risperidone. Adjust **risperidone** dose. Moderate Study → Also see TABLE 11 p. 820

▸ Antiepileptics **(carbamazepine, fosphenytoin, phenobarbital, phenytoin, primidone)** are predicted to moderately decrease the exposure to rivaroxaban. Avoid unless patient can be monitored for signs of thrombosis. Severe Study

▸ Antiepileptics **(carbamazepine, fosphenytoin, phenobarbital, phenytoin, primidone)** are predicted to decrease the exposure to roflumilast. Avoid. Moderate Study

▸ Antiepileptics **(carbamazepine, fosphenytoin, phenobarbital, phenytoin, primidone)** are predicted to decrease the exposure to ruxolitinib. Monitor and adjust dose. Moderate Study

▸ Antiepileptics **(carbamazepine, fosphenytoin, phenobarbital, phenytoin, primidone)** are predicted to moderately decrease the exposure to saxagliptin. Moderate Study

▸ Valproate is predicted to increase the exposure to selexipag. Unknown Theoretical

▸ Antiepileptics **(carbamazepine, fosphenytoin, phenobarbital, phenytoin, primidone)** are predicted to decrease the exposure to simeprevir. Avoid. Severe Study

▸ Oxcarbazepine is predicted to decrease the exposure to simeprevir. Avoid. Severe Theoretical

▸ Antiepileptics **(carbamazepine, fosphenytoin, phenobarbital, phenytoin, primidone)** are predicted to decrease the concentration of sirolimus. Avoid. Severe Study

▸ Valproate increases the exposure to sodium oxybate. Adjust **sodium oxybate** dose. Moderate Study

▸ Valproate potentially decreases the effects of sodium phenylbutyrate. Moderate Anecdotal

▸ Antiepileptics **(carbamazepine, fosphenytoin, oxcarbazepine, phenobarbital, phenytoin, primidone)** are predicted to decrease the exposure to sofosbuvir. Avoid. Severe Study

▸ Antiepileptics **(carbamazepine, fosphenytoin, phenobarbital, phenytoin, primidone)** are predicted to decrease the exposure to solifenacin. Moderate Theoretical

▸ Antiepileptics **(carbamazepine, fosphenytoin, phenobarbital, phenytoin, primidone)** are predicted to decrease the exposure to sorafenib. Moderate Theoretical

▸ SSRIs **(fluoxetine, fluvoxamine)** are predicted to increase the concentration of antiepileptics **(fosphenytoin, phenytoin)**. Monitor and adjust dose. Severe Anecdotal

▸ SSRIs **(sertraline)** potentially increase the risk of toxicity when given with antiepileptics **(fosphenytoin, phenytoin)**. Monitor concentration and adjust dose. Severe Anecdotal

▸ Antiepileptics **(fosphenytoin, phenytoin)** decrease the concentration of SSRIs **(paroxetine)**. Moderate Study

▸ St John's Wort is predicted to decrease the concentration of antiepileptics **(fosphenytoin, phenobarbital, phenytoin, primidone)**. Avoid. Moderate Theoretical

▸ St John's Wort is predicted to decrease the exposure to **brivaracetam**. Moderate Theoretical

▸ St John's Wort is predicted to decrease the concentration of carbamazepine. Monitor and adjust dose. Moderate Theoretical

▸ St John's Wort is predicted to decrease the exposure to **perampanel**. Monitor and adjust dose. Moderate Theoretical

▸ Antiepileptics **(carbamazepine, eslicarbazepine)** are predicted to decrease the exposure to statins **(atorvastatin)**. Monitor and adjust dose. Moderate Theoretical → Also see TABLE 1 p. 818

▸ Antiepileptics **(fosphenytoin, phenytoin)** potentially decrease the exposure to statins **(atorvastatin, simvastatin)**. Moderate Anecdotal

▸ Carbamazepine moderately decreases the exposure to statins **(simvastatin)**. Monitor and adjust dose. Severe Study → Also see TABLE 1 p. 818

▸ Eslicarbazepine moderately decreases the exposure to statins **(simvastatin)**. Monitor and adjust dose. Moderate Study

▸ Sulfinpyrazone increases the concentration of antiepileptics **(fosphenytoin, phenytoin)**. Moderate Study

▸ Sulfonamides **(sulfadiazine)** are predicted to increase the concentration of fosphenytoin. Monitor and adjust dose. Moderate Study

▸ Sulfonamides **(sulfadiazine)** increase the concentration of phenytoin. Monitor and adjust dose. Moderate Study

▸ Antiepileptics **(carbamazepine, fosphenytoin, phenobarbital, phenytoin, primidone)** are predicted to decrease the exposure to sunitinib. Avoid or adjust **sunitinib** dose. Moderate Study

▸ Antiepileptics **(fosphenytoin, phenytoin)** increase the effects of suxamethonium. Moderate Study

▸ Carbamazepine increases the risk of prolonged neuromuscular blockade when given with suxamethonium. Moderate Study

▸ Antiepileptics **(carbamazepine, fosphenytoin, phenobarbital, phenytoin, primidone)** decrease the concentration of tacrolimus. Monitor and adjust dose. Severe Study

▸ Antiepileptics **(carbamazepine, fosphenytoin, phenobarbital, phenytoin, primidone)** are predicted to decrease the exposure to taxanes **(cabazitaxel, paclitaxel)**. Avoid. Severe Study → Also see TABLE 12 p. 821

▸ Antiepileptics **(carbamazepine, fosphenytoin, phenobarbital, phenytoin, primidone)** are predicted to decrease the exposure to taxanes **(docetaxel)**. Severe Theoretical → Also see TABLE 12 p. 821

▸ Tegafur potentially increases the concentration of antiepileptics **(fosphenytoin, phenytoin)**. Monitor concentration and adjust dose. Severe Anecdotal

▸ Antiepileptics **(carbamazepine, fosphenytoin, phenobarbital, phenytoin, primidone)** are predicted to decrease the concentration of temsirolimus. Avoid. Severe Study

▸ Antiepileptics **(carbamazepine, fosphenytoin, phenobarbital, phenytoin, primidone)** decrease the exposure to tetracyclines **(doxycycline)**. Monitor and adjust dose. Moderate Study → Also see TABLE 1 p. 818

▸ Antiepileptics **(phenobarbital, primidone)** are predicted to increase the clearance of theophylline. Adjust dose. Moderate Theoretical

▸ Carbamazepine potentially increases the clearance of theophylline and theophylline decreases the exposure to carbamazepine. Adjust dose. Moderate Anecdotal

Antiepileptics (continued)

‣ **Fosphenytoin** is predicted to increase the clearance of theophylline. Adjust dose. Moderate Study

‣ **Phenytoin** is predicted to decrease the exposure to theophylline. Adjust dose. Moderate Study

‣ Antiepileptics **(carbamazepine, fosphenytoin, phenobarbital, phenytoin, primidone)** are predicted to markedly decrease the exposure to **ticagrelor**. Avoid. Severe Study

‣ Antiepileptics **(fosphenytoin, phenytoin)** moderately decrease the exposure to **tizanidine**. Mild Study

‣ Antiepileptics **(carbamazepine, fosphenytoin, phenobarbital, phenytoin, primidone)** are predicted to decrease the exposure to **tolvaptan**. Avoid. Severe Study

‣ Antiepileptics **(fosphenytoin, phenytoin)** increase the clearance of **topotecan**. Moderate Study

‣ Antiepileptics **(carbamazepine, fosphenytoin, phenobarbital, phenytoin, primidone)** are predicted to decrease the exposure to **toremifene**. Adjust dose. Moderate Study

‣ Antiepileptics **(carbamazepine, fosphenytoin, phenobarbital, phenytoin, primidone)** are predicted to decrease the exposure to **trabectedin**. Avoid. Severe Theoretical → Also see **TABLE 1** p. 818

‣ **Carbamazepine** decreases the concentration of **trazodone**. Adjust dose. Moderate Anecdotal

‣ Antiepileptics **(phenobarbital, primidone)** are predicted to decrease the exposure to **tricyclic antidepressants**. Moderate Study

‣ **Carbamazepine** decreases the exposure to **tricyclic antidepressants**. Adjust dose. Moderate Study → Also see **TABLE 18** p. 822

‣ Tricyclic antidepressants **(clomipramine, imipramine)** potentially increase the risk of overheating and dehydration when given with **zonisamide**. Avoid in children. Severe Theoretical

‣ **Trimethoprim** increases the concentration of antiepileptics **(fosphenytoin, phenytoin)**. Moderate Study

‣ Antiepileptics **(carbamazepine, eslicarbazepine, fosphenytoin, oxcarbazepine, perampanel, phenobarbital, phenytoin, primidone, rufinamide, topiramate)** decrease the efficacy of ulipristal. For FSRH guidance, see Contraceptives, interactions p. 474. Severe Anecdotal

‣ Antiepileptics **(carbamazepine, fosphenytoin, phenobarbital, phenytoin, primidone)** are predicted to decrease the exposure to **vandetanib**. Avoid. Moderate Study

‣ Antiepileptics **(carbamazepine, fosphenytoin, phenobarbital, phenytoin, primidone)** are predicted to moderately decrease the exposure to **velpatasvir**. Avoid. Severe Study

‣ **Oxcarbazepine** is predicted to decrease the exposure to **velpatasvir**. Avoid. Severe Theoretical

‣ Antiepileptics **(carbamazepine, fosphenytoin, phenobarbital, phenytoin, primidone)** are predicted to decrease the exposure to **vemurafenib**. Avoid. Severe Theoretical

‣ Antiepileptics **(carbamazepine, fosphenytoin, phenobarbital, phenytoin, primidone)** are predicted to decrease the exposure to **venetoclax**. Avoid. Severe Study

‣ Antiepileptics **(carbamazepine, fosphenytoin, phenobarbital, phenytoin, primidone)** are predicted to decrease the exposure to vinca alkaloids **(vinblastine, vincristine, vindesine)**. Severe Theoretical → Also see **TABLE 1** p. 818 → Also see **TABLE 12** p. 821

‣ Antiepileptics **(carbamazepine, fosphenytoin, phenobarbital, phenytoin, primidone)** are predicted to decrease the exposure to vinca alkaloids **(vinflunine)**. Avoid. Severe Theoretical → Also see **TABLE 12** p. 821

‣ Antiepileptics **(carbamazepine, fosphenytoin, phenobarbital, phenytoin, primidone)** are predicted to decrease the exposure to vinca alkaloids **(vinorelbine)**. Use with caution or avoid. Severe Theoretical → Also see **TABLE 12** p. 821

‣ Antiepileptics **(carbamazepine, fosphenytoin, phenobarbital, phenytoin, primidone)** are predicted to decrease the exposure to **vismodegib**. Avoid. Moderate Theoretical

‣ Antiepileptics **(fosphenytoin, phenytoin)** decrease the effects of **vitamin D substances**. Moderate Study

‣ Antiepileptics **(phenobarbital, primidone)** are predicted to decrease the effects of **vitamin D substances**. Moderate Theoretical

‣ **Carbamazepine** is predicted to decrease the effects of **vitamin D substances**. Moderate Study

‣ Antiepileptics **(carbamazepine, fosphenytoin, phenobarbital, phenytoin, primidone)** are predicted to decrease the exposure to **vortioxetine**. Monitor and adjust dose. Moderate Study

‣ **Valproate** slightly increases the exposure to **zidovudine**. Moderate Study

‣ **Carbamazepine** moderately decreases the exposure to **zolpidem**. Moderate Study

‣ Antiepileptics **(carbamazepine, fosphenytoin, phenobarbital, phenytoin, primidone)** are predicted to decrease the exposure to **zopiclone**. Adjust dose. Moderate Study → Also see **TABLE 11** p. 820

Antifungals, azoles → see **TABLE 1** p. 818 (hepatotoxicity), **TABLE 9** p. 820 (QT-interval prolongation)

clotrimazole · fluconazole · isavuconazole · itraconazole · ketoconazole · miconazole · posaconazole · voriconazole

‣ In general, **fluconazole** interactions relate to multiple-dose treatment.

‣ The use of carbonated drinks, such as cola, improves **itraconazole, ketoconazole,** and **posaconazole** bioavailability.

‣ Disulfiram-like reaction might occur with **ketoconazole** on consumption of alcohol.

‣ Since systemic absorption can follow topical application, the possibility of interactions with topical **ketoconazole** should be borne in mind.

‣ Interactions of **miconazole** apply to the oral gel formulation, as a sufficient quantity can be absorbed to cause systemic effects. Systemic absorption from intravaginal and topical formulations might also occur.

‣ Antifungals, azoles **(itraconazole, ketoconazole, voriconazole)** are predicted to increase the exposure to **abiraterone**. Severe Theoretical

‣ Antifungals, azoles **(itraconazole, ketoconazole)** are predicted to increase the exposure to **afatinib**. Separate administration by 12 hours. Moderate Study

‣ Antifungals, azoles **(fluconazole, isavuconazole, posaconazole)** are predicted to increase the exposure to aldosterone antagonists **(eplerenone)**. Adjust eplerenone dose. Severe Study

‣ Antifungals, azoles **(itraconazole, ketoconazole, voriconazole)** are predicted to markedly increase the exposure to aldosterone antagonists **(eplerenone)**. Avoid. Severe Study

‣ **Itraconazole** markedly increases the exposure to **aliskiren**. Avoid. Severe Study

‣ **Ketoconazole** moderately increases the exposure to **aliskiren**. Moderate Study

‣ **Itraconazole** increases the risk of busulfan toxicity when given with alkylating agents **(busulfan)**. Monitor and adjust dose. Moderate Study

‣ **Miconazole** is predicted to increase the concentration of alkylating agents **(busulfan)**. Use with caution and adjust dose. Moderate Theoretical

‣ Antifungals, azoles **(itraconazole, ketoconazole, voriconazole)** increase the exposure to **almotriptan**. Mild Study

‣ Antifungals, azoles **(itraconazole, ketoconazole, voriconazole)** are predicted to moderately increase the exposure to alpha blockers **(alfuzosin, tamsulosin)**. Use with caution or avoid. Moderate Study

‣ Antifungals, azoles **(itraconazole, ketoconazole, voriconazole)** are predicted to increase the exposure to alpha blockers **(doxazosin)**. Moderate Study

‣ Antifungals, azoles **(fluconazole, isavuconazole, posaconazole)** are predicted to increase the exposure to alpha blockers **(tamsulosin)**. Moderate Theoretical

‣ Antifungals, azoles **(fluconazole, isavuconazole, posaconazole)** are predicted to increase the exposure to **alprazolam**. Severe Study

‣ Antifungals, azoles **(itraconazole, ketoconazole, voriconazole)** moderately increase the exposure to **alprazolam**. Avoid. Moderate Study

‣ **Miconazole** is predicted to increase the exposure to **alprazolam**. Use with caution and adjust dose. Moderate Theoretical

▶ **Miconazole** potentially decreases the exposure to aminoglycosides **(tobramycin)**. Moderate Anecdotal

▶ **Antacids** decrease the absorption of **itraconazole**. **Antacids** should be taken 1 hour before or 2 hours after **itraconazole**. Moderate Study

▶ **Antacids** decrease the absorption of **ketoconazole**. Separate administration by at least 2 hours. Moderate Study

▶ **Antiarrhythmics (dronedarone)** are predicted to increase the exposure to **isavuconazole**. Severe Theoretical

▶ **Miconazole** is predicted to increase the exposure to antiarrhythmics **(disopyramide)**. Use with caution and adjust dose. Severe Theoretical

▶ **Antifungals, azoles (itraconazole, ketoconazole, voriconazole)** are predicted to increase the exposure to antiarrhythmics **(disopyramide)**. Avoid. Severe Theoretical → Also see TABLE 9 p. 820

▶ **Posaconazole** is predicted to increase the exposure to antiarrhythmics **(disopyramide, dronedarone)**. Avoid. Severe Theoretical

▶ **Fluconazole** is predicted to increase the exposure to antiarrhythmics **(dronedarone)**. Severe Theoretical

▶ **Antifungals, azoles (itraconazole, ketoconazole, voriconazole)** very markedly increase the exposure to antiarrhythmics **(dronedarone)**. Avoid. Severe Study → Also see TABLE 9 p. 820

▶ **Antifungals, azoles (fluconazole, isavuconazole, posaconazole)** are predicted to increase the exposure to antiarrhythmics **(propafenone)**. Monitor and adjust dose. Moderate Study

▶ **Antifungals, azoles (itraconazole, ketoconazole, voriconazole)** are predicted to increase the exposure to antiarrhythmics **(propafenone)**. Monitor and adjust dose. Severe Study

▶ **Antifungals, azoles (itraconazole, ketoconazole, voriconazole)** are predicted to increase the exposure to anticholinesterases, centrally acting **(galantamine)**. Monitor and adjust dose. Moderate Study

▶ **Antiepileptics (carbamazepine)** are predicted to decrease the efficacy of **fluconazole** and **fluconazole** increases the concentration of antiepileptics **(carbamazepine)**. Avoid or monitor **carbamazepine** concentration and adjust dose accordingly. Severe Theoretical → Also see TABLE 1 p. 818

▶ **Antiepileptics (carbamazepine)** are predicted to decrease the efficacy of **ketoconazole** and **ketoconazole** slightly increases the concentration of antiepileptics **(carbamazepine)**. Avoid or monitor **carbamazepine** concentration and adjust dose accordingly. Moderate Study

▶ **Antiepileptics (carbamazepine)** are predicted to decrease the efficacy of **posaconazole** and **posaconazole** increases the concentration of antiepileptics **(carbamazepine)**. Avoid. Moderate Theoretical

▶ **Antiepileptics (carbamazepine, fosphenytoin, phenobarbital, phenytoin, primidone)** are predicted to decrease the exposure to **isavuconazole**. Avoid. Severe Study

▶ **Antiepileptics (fosphenytoin)** very markedly decrease the exposure to **itraconazole**. Avoid **fosphenytoin** for 14 days before and during treatment with **itraconazole**. Moderate Study

▶ **Antiepileptics (fosphenytoin)** decrease the exposure to **voriconazole** and **voriconazole** increases the exposure to antiepileptics **(fosphenytoin)**. Avoid or adjust **voriconazole** dose and monitor phenytoin concentration, p. 361. Moderate Study

▶ **Antiepileptics (fosphenytoin, phenytoin)** decrease the exposure to **ketoconazole**. Avoid. Moderate Study

▶ **Antiepileptics (fosphenytoin, phenytoin)** are predicted to decrease the exposure to **posaconazole**. Avoid. Moderate Study

▶ **Antiepileptics (phenobarbital)** decrease the concentration of **itraconazole**. Avoid **phenobarbital** for 14 days before and during treatment with **itraconazole**. Moderate Study

▶ **Antiepileptics (phenobarbital)** are predicted to decrease the concentration of **ketoconazole**. Avoid. Moderate Study

▶ **Antiepileptics (phenobarbital)** are predicted to decrease the concentration of **posaconazole**. Avoid. Moderate Study

▶ **Antiepileptics (phenobarbital, primidone)** are predicted to decrease the concentration of **voriconazole**. Avoid. Moderate Theoretical

▶ **Antiepileptics (phenytoin)** very markedly decrease the exposure to **itraconazole**. Avoid **phenytoin** for 14 days before and during treatment with **itraconazole**. Moderate Study

▶ **Antiepileptics (phenytoin)** decrease the exposure to **voriconazole** and **voriconazole** increases the exposure to antiepileptics **(phenytoin)**. Avoid or adjust **voriconazole** dose and monitor phenytoin concentration, p. 361. Moderate Study

▶ **Antiepileptics (primidone)** are predicted to decrease the concentration of **itraconazole**. Moderate Theoretical

▶ **Miconazole** increases the risk of **carbamazepine** toxicity when given with antiepileptics **(carbamazepine)**. Monitor and adjust dose. Severe Anecdotal

▶ **Miconazole** increases the risk of phenytoin toxicity when given with antiepileptics **(fosphenytoin)**. Monitor and adjust dose. Severe Anecdotal

▶ **Fluconazole** increases the concentration of antiepileptics **(fosphenytoin, phenytoin)**. Monitor concentration and adjust dose. Moderate Study

▶ **Antiepileptics (carbamazepine)** are predicted to decrease the efficacy of antifungals, azoles **(itraconazole, voriconazole)** and antifungals, azoles **(itraconazole, voriconazole)** increase the concentration of antiepileptics **(carbamazepine)**. Avoid or adjust dose. Moderate Theoretical → Also see TABLE 1 p. 818

▶ **Antiepileptics (primidone)** are predicted to decrease the concentration of antifungals, azoles **(ketoconazole, posaconazole)**. Avoid. Moderate Study

▶ **Antifungals, azoles (itraconazole, ketoconazole, voriconazole)** are predicted to slightly increase the exposure to antiepileptics **(perampanel)**. Mild Study

▶ **Miconazole** increases the risk of phenytoin toxicity when given with antiepileptics **(phenytoin)**. Monitor and adjust dose. Severe Anecdotal

▶ **Antifungals, azoles (fluconazole)** are predicted to increase the exposure to antifungals, azoles **(isavuconazole)**. Severe Theoretical

▶ **Antifungals, azoles (itraconazole, ketoconazole, voriconazole)** are predicted to increase the exposure to antifungals, azoles **(isavuconazole)**. Avoid or monitor side effects. Severe Study

▶ **Antifungals, azoles (posaconazole)** are predicted to increase the exposure to antifungals, azoles **(isavuconazole)**. Moderate Theoretical

▶ **Miconazole** is predicted to increase the exposure to antihistamines, non-sedating **(mizolastine)**. Avoid. Moderate Theoretical

▶ **Antifungals, azoles (fluconazole, isavuconazole, posaconazole)** are predicted to increase the exposure to antihistamines, non-sedating **(mizolastine)**. Severe Theoretical

▶ **Antifungals, azoles (itraconazole, ketoconazole, voriconazole)** are predicted to increase the exposure to antihistamines, non-sedating **(mizolastine)**. Avoid. Severe Study

▶ **Antifungals, azoles (itraconazole, ketoconazole, voriconazole)** are predicted to increase the exposure to antimalarials **(artemether)** (with lumefantrine). Moderate Study → Also see TABLE 9 p. 820

▶ **Ketoconazole** increases the exposure to antimalarials **(mefloquine)**. Moderate Study

▶ **Antifungals, azoles (fluconazole, itraconazole, posaconazole, voriconazole)** are predicted to increase the exposure to antimalarials **(mefloquine)**. Moderate Theoretical

▶ **Antifungals, azoles (fluconazole, isavuconazole, itraconazole, ketoconazole, posaconazole, voriconazole)** are predicted to increase the concentration of antimalarials **(piperaquine)**. Severe Theoretical

▶ **Itraconazole** is predicted to increase the exposure to apixaban. Avoid. Severe Theoretical

▶ **Ketoconazole** slightly to moderately increases the exposure to apixaban. Avoid. Severe Study

▶ **Antifungals, azoles (itraconazole, ketoconazole, voriconazole)** are predicted to markedly increase the exposure to aprepitant. Moderate Study

▶ **Aprepitant** is predicted to increase the exposure to **isavuconazole**. Moderate Theoretical

▶ **Antifungals, azoles (itraconazole, ketoconazole, voriconazole)** are predicted to slightly increase the exposure to aripiprazole. Adjust **aripiprazole** dose, p. 240. Moderate Study

▶ **Antifungals, azoles (fluconazole, isavuconazole, posaconazole)** are predicted to increase the exposure to axitinib. Moderate Theoretical

A1

Interactions | **Appendix 1**

Antifungals, azoles (continued)

▶ Antifungals, azoles **(itraconazole, ketoconazole, voriconazole)** are predicted to increase the exposure to **axitinib**. Avoid or adjust dose. Moderate Study

▶ Antifungals, azoles **(fluconazole, isavuconazole, posaconazole)** are predicted to increase the exposure to **bedaquiline**. Avoid prolonged use. Mild Theoretical

▶ Antifungals, azoles **(itraconazole, ketoconazole, voriconazole)** are predicted to increase the exposure to **bedaquiline**. Avoid prolonged use. Mild Study → Also see TABLE 9 p. 820

▶ Antifungals, azoles **(itraconazole, ketoconazole)** are predicted to increase the exposure to beta blockers, non-selective **(nadolol)**. Moderate Study

▶ Antifungals, azoles **(itraconazole, ketoconazole, voriconazole)** are predicted to increase the exposure to beta₂ agonists **(salmeterol)**. Avoid. Severe Study

▶ Antifungals, azoles **(itraconazole, ketoconazole, voriconazole)** slightly increase the exposure to **bortezomib**. Moderate Study

▶ **Fluconazole** is predicted to increase the exposure to **bosentan**. Avoid. Severe Study

▶ **Bosentan** is predicted to decrease the exposure to **isavuconazole**. Avoid. Severe Theoretical

▶ **Itraconazole** is predicted to increase the exposure to **bosentan**. Moderate Theoretical

▶ **Ketoconazole** moderately increases the exposure to **bosentan**. Moderate Study

▶ **Voriconazole** is predicted to increase the exposure to **bosentan**. Avoid. Severe Theoretical

▶ Antifungals, azoles **(fluconazole, isavuconazole, posaconazole)** are predicted to increase the exposure to **bosutinib**. Avoid or adjust **bosutinib** dose. Severe Theoretical

▶ Antifungals, azoles **(itraconazole, ketoconazole, voriconazole)** are predicted to markedly increase the exposure to **bosutinib**. Avoid or adjust **bosutinib** dose. Severe Study → Also see TABLE 9 p. 820

▶ Antifungals, azoles **(fluconazole, isavuconazole, posaconazole)** are predicted to increase the exposure to **buspirone**. Use with caution and adjust dose. Moderate Study

▶ Antifungals, azoles **(itraconazole, ketoconazole, voriconazole)** are predicted to increase the exposure to **buspirone**. Adjust **buspirone** dose. Severe Study

▶ **Miconazole** is predicted to increase the concentration of **buspirone**. Use with caution and adjust dose. Moderate Theoretical

▶ Antifungals, azoles **(fluconazole, isavuconazole, posaconazole)** are predicted to increase the exposure to **cabozantinib**. Moderate Theoretical

▶ Antifungals, azoles **(itraconazole, ketoconazole, voriconazole)** slightly increase the exposure to **cabozantinib**. Moderate Study → Also see TABLE 9 p. 820

▶ Calcium channel blockers **(diltiazem, verapamil)** are predicted to increase the exposure to **isavuconazole**. Moderate Theoretical

▶ **Miconazole** is predicted to increase the exposure to calcium channel blockers **(amlodipine, clevidipine, felodipine, isradipine, lacidipine, lercanidipine, nicardipine, nifedipine, nimodipine, verapamil)**. Use with caution and adjust dose. Moderate Theoretical

▶ Antifungals, azoles **(fluconazole, isavuconazole, itraconazole, ketoconazole, posaconazole, voriconazole)** are predicted to increase the exposure to calcium channel blockers **(amlodipine, felodipine, isradipine, lacidipine, nicardipine, nifedipine, nimodipine)**. Monitor and adjust dose. Moderate Study

▶ **Fluconazole** (high-dose) is predicted to increase the exposure to calcium channel blockers **(diltiazem, verapamil)**. Moderate Theoretical

▶ **Posaconazole** is predicted to increase the exposure to calcium channel blockers **(diltiazem, verapamil)**. Moderate Theoretical

▶ Antifungals, azoles **(itraconazole, ketoconazole, voriconazole)** are predicted to increase the exposure to calcium channel blockers **(diltiazem, verapamil)**. Severe Study

▶ Antifungals, azoles **(itraconazole, ketoconazole, voriconazole)** are predicted to markedly increase the exposure to calcium channel blockers **(lercanidipine)**. Avoid. Severe Study

▶ Antifungals, azoles **(itraconazole, ketoconazole, voriconazole)** are predicted to increase the exposure to **cannabis extract**. Use with caution and adjust dose. Moderate Theoretical

▶ Antifungals, azoles **(fluconazole, isavuconazole, posaconazole)** are predicted to increase the exposure to **ceritinib**. Moderate Theoretical

▶ Antifungals, azoles **(itraconazole, ketoconazole, voriconazole)** are predicted to increase the exposure to **ceritinib**. Avoid or adjust **ceritinib** dose. Severe Study → Also see TABLE 9 p. 820

▶ Antifungals, azoles **(fluconazole, isavuconazole, itraconazole, ketoconazole, posaconazole, voriconazole)** increase the concentration of **ciclosporin**. Severe Study

▶ **Miconazole** increases the concentration of **ciclosporin**. Monitor and adjust dose. Severe Anecdotal

▶ Antifungals, azoles **(itraconazole, ketoconazole, voriconazole)** are predicted to moderately increase the exposure to **cilostazol**. Adjust **cilostazol** dose. Moderate Study

▶ **Fluconazole** is predicted to increase the exposure to **cilostazol**. Adjust **cilostazol** dose. Moderate Theoretical

▶ **Miconazole** is predicted to increase the exposure to **cilostazol**. Use with caution and adjust dose. Moderate Theoretical

▶ Antifungals, azoles **(itraconazole, ketoconazole, voriconazole)** are predicted to moderately increase the exposure to **cinacalcet**. Adjust dose. Moderate Study

▶ **Fluconazole** is predicted to decrease the efficacy of **clopidogrel**. Avoid. Severe Theoretical

▶ **Voriconazole** is predicted to decrease the efficacy of **clopidogrel**. Avoid. Moderate Study

▶ **Cobicistat** is predicted to increase the exposure to antifungals, azoles **(fluconazole, posaconazole)**. Moderate Theoretical

▶ **Cobicistat** is predicted to increase the exposure to **isavuconazole**. Avoid or monitor side effects. Severe Study

▶ **Cobicistat** is predicted to increase the exposure to **itraconazole**. Adjust **itraconazole** dose. Moderate Theoretical

▶ **Cobicistat** is predicted to increase the exposure to **ketoconazole**. Adjust **ketoconazole** dose. Moderate Theoretical

▶ **Cobicistat** is predicted to affect the exposure to **voriconazole**. Avoid. Moderate Theoretical

▶ Antifungals, azoles **(fluconazole, isavuconazole, miconazole, posaconazole)** are predicted to increase the exposure to **cobimetinib**. Severe Theoretical

▶ Antifungals, azoles **(itraconazole, ketoconazole, voriconazole)** are predicted to markedly increase the exposure to **cobimetinib**. Avoid or monitor for toxicity. Severe Study

▶ Antifungals, azoles **(fluconazole, isavuconazole, posaconazole)** are predicted to increase the exposure to **colchicine**. Adjust **colchicine** dose. Severe Study

▶ Antifungals, azoles **(itraconazole, ketoconazole, voriconazole)** are predicted to increase the exposure to **colchicine**. Avoid or adjust **colchicine** dose. Severe Study

▶ Antifungals, azoles **(itraconazole, ketoconazole, voriconazole)** are predicted to increase the exposure to corticosteroids **(budesonide)**. Avoid. Severe Study

▶ Antifungals, azoles **(itraconazole, ketoconazole, voriconazole)** are predicted to increase the exposure to corticosteroids **(ciclesonide)**. Avoid. Moderate Theoretical

▶ Antifungals, azoles **(itraconazole, ketoconazole, voriconazole)** are predicted to increase the exposure to corticosteroids **(dexamethasone, methylprednisolone)**. Monitor and adjust dose. Moderate Study

▶ Antifungals, azoles **(itraconazole, ketoconazole, voriconazole)** are predicted to increase the exposure to inhaled corticosteroids **(fluticasone)**. Severe Study

▶ **Miconazole** is predicted to increase the concentration of corticosteroids **(methylprednisolone)**. Monitor and adjust dose. Moderate Theoretical

▶ Antifungals, azoles **(fluconazole, isavuconazole, posaconazole)** are predicted to increase the exposure to corticosteroids **(methylprednisolone)**. Monitor and adjust dose. Moderate Study

▶ Antifungals, azoles **(itraconazole, ketoconazole, voriconazole)** are predicted to increase the exposure to corticosteroids **(mometasone)**. Moderate Theoretical

▶ Antifungals, azoles **(itraconazole, ketoconazole, voriconazole)** are predicted to increase the risk of side-effects when given with corticosteroids **(triamcinolone)**. Severe Theoretical

▶ **Fluconazole** increases the anticoagulant effect of **coumarins**. Monitor INR and adjust dose. Severe Study

▶ **Itraconazole** potentially increases the anticoagulant effect of **coumarins**. Severe Anecdotal

▶ **Ketoconazole** potentially increases the anticoagulant effect of coumarins **(warfarin)**. Monitor INR and adjust dose. Severe Anecdotal

▶ **Miconazole** greatly increases the anticoagulant effect of **coumarins**. Severe Study

▶ **Voriconazole** increases the anticoagulant effect of **coumarins**. Monitor INR and adjust dose. Moderate Study

▶ Antifungals, azoles **(fluconazole, posaconazole)** are predicted to increase the exposure to **crizotinib**. Moderate Theoretical

▶ Antifungals, azoles **(itraconazole, ketoconazole, voriconazole)** are predicted to moderately increase the exposure to **crizotinib**. Avoid. Moderate Study → Also see **TABLE 9** p. 820

▶ **Crizotinib** is predicted to increase the exposure to **isavuconazole**. Moderate Theoretical

▶ Antifungals, azoles **(itraconazole, ketoconazole)** are predicted to increase the exposure to **dabigatran**. Avoid. Severe Study

▶ Antifungals, azoles **(itraconazole, ketoconazole, voriconazole)** are predicted to increase the exposure to **dabrafenib**. Use with caution or avoid. Moderate Study

▶ Antifungals, azoles **(itraconazole, ketoconazole, voriconazole)** are predicted to moderately increase the exposure to **daclatasvir**. Adjust **daclatasvir** dose. Moderate Study

▶ Antifungals, azoles **(fluconazole, isavuconazole, posaconazole)** are predicted to slightly increase the exposure to **darifenacin**. Moderate Study

▶ Antifungals, azoles **(itraconazole, ketoconazole, voriconazole)** are predicted markedly to very markedly increase the exposure to **darifenacin**. Avoid. Severe Study

▶ Antifungals, azoles **(fluconazole, isavuconazole, posaconazole)** are predicted to increase the exposure to **dasatinib**. Severe Study

▶ Antifungals, azoles **(itraconazole, ketoconazole, voriconazole)** are predicted to markedly increase the exposure to **dasatinib**. Avoid. Severe Study → Also see **TABLE 9** p. 820

▶ Antifungals, azoles **(itraconazole, ketoconazole, voriconazole)** very slightly increase the exposure to **delamanid**. Severe Study → Also see **TABLE 9** p. 820

▶ Antifungals, azoles **(fluconazole, voriconazole)** moderately increase the exposure to **diazepam**. Monitor and adjust dose. Moderate Study

▶ **Didanosine** (buffered) decreases the exposure to antifungals, azoles **(itraconazole, ketoconazole)**. Separate administration by 2 hours. Severe Study → Also see **TABLE 1** p. 818

▶ **Itraconazole** markedly increases the concentration of **digoxin**. Monitor and adjust dose. Severe Study

▶ **Ketoconazole** is predicted to markedly increase the concentration of **digoxin**. Severe Theoretical

▶ **Posaconazole** is predicted to increase the concentration of **digoxin**. Severe Theoretical

▶ Antifungals, azoles **(fluconazole, isavuconazole, itraconazole, ketoconazole, posaconazole, voriconazole)** increase the risk of QT-prolongation when given with **domperidone**. Avoid. Severe Study

▶ Antifungals, azoles **(fluconazole, isavuconazole, posaconazole)** are predicted to increase the exposure to dopamine receptor agonists **(bromocriptine, cabergoline)**. Severe Theoretical

▶ Antifungals, azoles **(itraconazole, ketoconazole, voriconazole)** increase the exposure to dopamine receptor agonists **(bromocriptine, cabergoline)**. Severe Study

▶ **Ketoconazole** moderately increases the exposure to **drospirenone**. Severe Study

▶ Antifungals, azoles **(fluconazole, isavuconazole, posaconazole)** are predicted to moderately increase the exposure to **dutasteride**. Mild Study

▶ Antifungals, azoles **(itraconazole, ketoconazole, voriconazole)** are predicted to increase the exposure to **dutasteride**. Monitor side effects and adjust dose. Moderate Theoretical

▶ **Itraconazole** is predicted to slightly increase the exposure to **edoxaban**. Severe Theoretical

▶ **Ketoconazole** slightly increases the exposure to **edoxaban**. Adjust **edoxaban** dose. Severe Study

▶ **Efavirenz** is predicted to decrease the exposure to **isavuconazole**. Avoid. Severe Theoretical

▶ **Efavirenz** slightly decreases the exposure to **itraconazole**. Avoid **efavirenz** for 14 days before and during treatment with **itraconazole**. Moderate Study

▶ **Efavirenz** moderately decreases the exposure to **ketoconazole**. Severe Study

▶ **Efavirenz** slightly decreases the exposure to **posaconazole**. Avoid. Moderate Study

▶ **Efavirenz** moderately decreases the exposure to **voriconazole** and **voriconazole** slightly increases the exposure to **efavirenz**. Adjust dose. Severe Study

▶ Antifungals, azoles **(itraconazole, ketoconazole, voriconazole)** slightly to moderately increase the exposure to **elbasvir**. Avoid. Moderate Study

▶ Antifungals, azoles **(itraconazole, ketoconazole, voriconazole)** are predicted to markedly increase the exposure to **eletriptan**. Avoid. Severe Study

▶ **Enzalutamide** is predicted to decrease the exposure to **isavuconazole**. Avoid. Severe Study

▶ Antifungals, azoles **(fluconazole, isavuconazole, posaconazole)** are predicted to increase the risk of ergotism when given with **ergometrine**. Severe Theoretical

▶ Antifungals, azoles **(itraconazole, ketoconazole, voriconazole)** are predicted to increase the risk of ergotism when given with **ergometrine**. Avoid. Severe Study

▶ **Miconazole** is predicted to increase the exposure to **ergometrine**. Avoid. Moderate Theoretical

▶ Antifungals, azoles **(fluconazole, isavuconazole, posaconazole)** are predicted to increase the risk of ergotism when given with **ergotamine**. Severe Theoretical

▶ Antifungals, azoles **(itraconazole, ketoconazole, voriconazole)** are predicted to increase the risk of ergotism when given with **ergotamine**. Avoid. Severe Theoretical

▶ **Miconazole** is predicted to increase the exposure to **ergotamine**. Avoid. Moderate Theoretical

▶ Antifungals, azoles **(fluconazole, isavuconazole, posaconazole)** are predicted to increase the exposure to **erlotinib**. Moderate Theoretical

▶ Antifungals, azoles **(itraconazole, ketoconazole, voriconazole)** are predicted to slightly increase the exposure to **erlotinib**. Use with caution and adjust dose. Moderate Study

▶ Antifungals, azoles **(fluconazole, isavuconazole, posaconazole)** are predicted to increase the concentration of **everolimus**. Avoid or adjust dose. Moderate Study

▶ Antifungals, azoles **(itraconazole, ketoconazole, voriconazole)** are predicted to increase the concentration of **everolimus**. Avoid. Severe Study

▶ Antifungals, azoles **(fluconazole, isavuconazole, posaconazole)** are predicted to increase the exposure to **fesoterodine**. Adjust **fesoterodine** dose in hepatic and renal impairment. Mild Study

▶ Antifungals, azoles **(itraconazole, ketoconazole, voriconazole)** are predicted to moderately increase the exposure to **fesoterodine**. Adjust **fesoterodine** dose; avoid in hepatic and renal impairment. Severe Study

▶ Antifungals, azoles **(itraconazole, ketoconazole)** are predicted to increase the exposure to **fidaxomicin**. Avoid. Moderate Study

▶ Antifungals, azoles **(itraconazole, ketoconazole, voriconazole)** are predicted to increase the exposure to **fosaprepitant**. Moderate Theoretical

▶ Antifungals, azoles **(fluconazole, isavuconazole, posaconazole)** are predicted to increase the exposure to **gefitinib**. Moderate Theoretical

▶ Antifungals, azoles **(itraconazole, ketoconazole, voriconazole)** are predicted to increase the exposure to **gefitinib**. Moderate Study

▶ Antifungals, azoles **(itraconazole, ketoconazole, voriconazole)** are predicted to moderately to markedly increase the exposure to **grazoprevir**. Avoid. Severe Study

▶ Antifungals, azoles **(fluconazole, isavuconazole, posaconazole)** are predicted to increase the concentration of **guanfacine**. Adjust **guanfacine** dose, p. 222. Moderate Theoretical

▶ Antifungals, azoles **(itraconazole, ketoconazole, voriconazole)** are predicted to increase the exposure to **guanfacine**. Adjust **guanfacine** dose, p. 222. Moderate Study

Antifungals, azoles (continued)

▶ H₂ **receptor antagonists** are predicted to decrease the absorption of **itraconazole**. Administer **itraconazole** capsules with an acidic beverage. Moderate Study

▶ H₂ **receptor antagonists** are predicted to decrease the absorption of **ketoconazole**. Administer **ketoconazole** with an acidic beverage. Moderate Study

▶ H₂ **receptor antagonists** are predicted to slightly decrease the exposure to **posaconazole**. Avoid use of posaconazole oral suspension. Moderate Study

▶ **Itraconazole** increases the concentration of **haloperidol**. Moderate Study

▶ **HIV-protease inhibitors (atazanavir, darunavir, fosamprenavir, lopinavir, ritonavir, saquinavir, tipranavir)** are predicted to increase the exposure to **isavuconazole**. Avoid or monitor side effects. Severe Study

▶ **Fluconazole** slightly increases the exposure to **HIV-protease inhibitors (tipranavir)**. Avoid or adjust dose. Moderate Study

▶ **HIV-protease inhibitors** are predicted to increase the exposure to **itraconazole**. Use with caution and adjust dose. Severe Study

▶ **HIV-protease inhibitors** are predicted to increase the exposure to **ketoconazole**. Use with caution and adjust dose. Moderate Study

▶ **Miconazole** is predicted to increase the concentration of **HIV-protease inhibitors**. Use with caution and adjust dose. Moderate Theoretical

▶ **Posaconazole** is predicted to increase the exposure to **HIV-protease inhibitors**. Moderate Study

▶ **HIV-protease inhibitors** are predicted to affect the exposure to **voriconazole** and **voriconazole** potentially affects the exposure to **HIV-protease inhibitors**. Severe Study → Also see **TABLE 9** p. 820

▶ Antifungals, azoles **(fluconazole, isavuconazole, posaconazole)** are predicted to increase the exposure to **ibrutinib**. Avoid or adjust **ibrutinib** dose. Severe Theoretical

▶ Antifungals, azoles **(itraconazole, ketoconazole, voriconazole)** are predicted to very markedly increase the exposure to **ibrutinib**. Avoid or adjust **ibrutinib** dose. Severe Study

▶ **Idelalisib** is predicted to increase the exposure to **isavuconazole**. Avoid or monitor side effects. Severe Study

▶ Antifungals, azoles **(fluconazole, posaconazole)** are predicted to increase the exposure to **imatinib**. Moderate Theoretical

▶ Antifungals, azoles **(itraconazole, ketoconazole, voriconazole)** are predicted to increase the exposure to **imatinib**. Moderate Study

▶ **Imatinib** is predicted to decrease the exposure to **isavuconazole**. Moderate Theoretical

▶ Antifungals, azoles **(itraconazole, ketoconazole, voriconazole)** are predicted to increase the risk of toxicity when given with **irinotecan**. Avoid. Moderate Study

▶ Antifungals, azoles **(fluconazole, isavuconazole, posaconazole)** are predicted to increase the exposure to **ivabradine**. Adjust **ivabradine** dose. Severe Theoretical

▶ Antifungals, azoles **(itraconazole, ketoconazole, voriconazole)** are predicted to increase the exposure to **ivabradine**. Avoid. Severe Study

▶ Antifungals, azoles **(fluconazole, isavuconazole, posaconazole)** are predicted to increase the exposure to **ivacaftor**. Adjust **ivacaftor** dose, p. 179. Severe Study

▶ Antifungals, azoles **(itraconazole, ketoconazole, voriconazole)** are predicted to increase the exposure to **ivacaftor**. Adjust **ivacaftor** or lumacaftor with ivacaftor dose, p. 179. Severe Study

▶ **Lanthanum** is predicted to decrease the absorption of **ketoconazole**. Separate administration by at least 2 hours. Moderate Theoretical

▶ Antifungals, azoles **(fluconazole, isavuconazole, posaconazole)** are predicted to increase the exposure to **lapatinib**. Moderate Study

▶ Antifungals, azoles **(itraconazole, ketoconazole, voriconazole)** are predicted to increase the exposure to **lapatinib**. Avoid. Moderate Study → Also see **TABLE 9** p. 820

▶ Antifungals, azoles **(fluconazole, isavuconazole, posaconazole)** are predicted to increase the exposure to **lomitapide**. Avoid. Moderate Theoretical → Also see **TABLE 1** p. 818

▶ Antifungals, azoles **(itraconazole, ketoconazole, voriconazole)** are predicted to markedly increase the exposure to **lomitapide**. Avoid. Severe Study → Also see **TABLE 1** p. 818

▶ **Clotrimazole** is predicted to increase the exposure to **lomitapide**. Separate administration by 12 hours. Moderate Theoretical

▶ **Lumacaftor** is predicted to decrease the exposure to antifungals, azoles **(itraconazole, ketoconazole, voriconazole)**. Moderate Theoretical

▶ **Lumacaftor** is predicted to decrease the exposure to **fluconazole**. Adjust dose. Mild Theoretical

▶ **Lumacaftor** is predicted to decrease the exposure to **posaconazole**. Avoid. Moderate Theoretical

▶ Antifungals, azoles **(fluconazole, isavuconazole, posaconazole)** are predicted to increase the exposure to **lurasidone**. Moderate Study

▶ Antifungals, azoles **(itraconazole, ketoconazole, voriconazole)** are predicted to increase the exposure to **lurasidone**. Avoid. Severe Study

▶ Antifungals, azoles **(itraconazole, ketoconazole, voriconazole)** are predicted to increase the exposure to **macitentan**. Moderate Study

▶ **Macrolides (clarithromycin)** are predicted to increase the exposure to **isavuconazole**. Avoid or monitor side effects. Severe Study

▶ **Macrolides (erythromycin)** are predicted to increase the exposure to **isavuconazole**. Moderate Theoretical

▶ Antifungals, azoles **(itraconazole, ketoconazole, voriconazole)** markedly increase the exposure to **maraviroc**. Adjust dose. Severe Study

▶ Antifungals, azoles **(fluconazole, isavuconazole, posaconazole)** are predicted to increase the exposure to **midazolam**. Monitor side effects and adjust dose. Severe Study

▶ Antifungals, azoles **(itraconazole, ketoconazole, voriconazole)** are predicted to markedly to very markedly increase the exposure to **midazolam**. Avoid or adjust **midazolam** dose. Severe Study

▶ **Miconazole** is predicted to increase the exposure to intravenous **midazolam**. Use with caution and adjust dose. Moderate Theoretical

▶ **Miconazole** is predicted to increase the exposure to oral **midazolam**. Avoid. Moderate Theoretical

▶ Antifungals, azoles **(itraconazole, ketoconazole, voriconazole)** are predicted to increase the exposure to **mirabegron**. Adjust **mirabegron** dose in hepatic and renal impairment. Moderate Study

▶ Antifungals, azoles **(itraconazole, ketoconazole, voriconazole)** are predicted to increase the exposure to **mirtazapine**. Moderate Study

▶ Antifungals, azoles **(itraconazole, ketoconazole, voriconazole)** are predicted to increase the exposure to **modafinil**. Mild Theoretical

▶ Antifungals, azoles **(itraconazole, ketoconazole, voriconazole)** increase the risk of neutropenia when given with **monoclonal antibodies (brentuximab vedotin)**. Monitor and adjust dose. Severe Study

▶ Antifungals, azoles **(itraconazole, ketoconazole, voriconazole)** are predicted to increase the exposure to **monoclonal antibodies (trastuzumab emtansine)**. Avoid. Severe Theoretical

▶ Antifungals, azoles **(fluconazole, isavuconazole, posaconazole)** are predicted to increase the exposure to **naloxegol**. Adjust **naloxegol** dose and monitor side effects. Moderate Study

▶ Antifungals, azoles **(itraconazole, ketoconazole, voriconazole)** are predicted to markedly increase the exposure to **naloxegol**. Avoid. Severe Study

▶ Antifungals, azoles **(itraconazole, ketoconazole, voriconazole)** are predicted to increase the exposure to **netupitant**. Mild Study

▶ **Netupitant** is predicted to decrease the exposure to **isavuconazole**. Moderate Theoretical

▶ **Fluconazole** slightly to moderately increases the exposure to **nevirapine**. Moderate Study

▶ **Nevirapine** is predicted to decrease the exposure to **isavuconazole**. Avoid. Severe Theoretical

▶ **Nevirapine** moderately decreases the exposure to **itraconazole**. Avoid **nevirapine** for 14 days before and during treatment with **itraconazole**. Moderate Study

▶ **Nevirapine** moderately decreases the exposure to **ketoconazole**. Avoid. Severe Study

▶ **Nevirapine** is predicted to decrease the exposure to **voriconazole** and **voriconazole** increases the exposure to **nevirapine**. Monitor and adjust dose. Severe Theoretical

▸ Antifungals, azoles **(fluconazole, posaconazole)** are predicted to increase the exposure to nilotinib. Moderate Theoretical

▸ Antifungals, azoles **(itraconazole, ketoconazole, voriconazole)** are predicted to moderately increase the exposure to nilotinib. Avoid. Severe Study → Also see TABLE 9 p. 820

▸ **Nilotinib** is predicted to increase the exposure to isavuconazole. Moderate Theoretical

▸ Antifungals, azoles **(itraconazole, ketoconazole)** are predicted to increase the exposure to nintedanib. Moderate Study

▸ Antifungals, azoles **(itraconazole, ketoconazole, voriconazole)** are predicted to increase the exposure to nitisinone. Adjust nitisinone dose. Moderate Theoretical

▸ **Fluconazole** moderately increases the exposure to NSAIDs **(celecoxib)**. Adjust celecoxib dose. Moderate Study

▸ **Voriconazole** slightly increases the exposure to NSAIDs **(diclofenac)**. Monitor and adjust dose. Moderate Study

▸ **Voriconazole** moderately increases the exposure to NSAIDs **(ibuprofen)**. Adjust dose. Moderate Study

▸ **Fluconazole** increases the exposure to NSAIDs **(parecoxib)**. Monitor and adjust dose. Moderate Study

▸ Antifungals, azoles **(fluconazole, isavuconazole, posaconazole)** are predicted to increase the exposure to olaparib. Avoid or adjust olaparib dose. Moderate Theoretical

▸ Antifungals, azoles **(itraconazole, ketoconazole, voriconazole)** are predicted to increase the exposure to olaparib. Avoid or adjust olaparib dose. Moderate Study

▸ **Miconazole** is predicted to increase the exposure to opioids **(alfentanil)**. Use with caution and adjust dose. Moderate Theoretical

▸ Antifungals, azoles **(fluconazole, isavuconazole, posaconazole)** are predicted to increase the exposure to opioids **(alfentanil, buprenorphine, fentanyl, oxycodone)**. Monitor and adjust dose. Moderate Study

▸ Antifungals, azoles **(itraconazole, ketoconazole, voriconazole)** are predicted to increase the exposure to opioids **(alfentanil, buprenorphine, fentanyl, oxycodone, sufentanil)**. Monitor and adjust dose. Severe Study

▸ Antifungals, azoles **(itraconazole, ketoconazole, voriconazole)** are predicted to increase the exposure to opioids **(methadone)**. Moderate Theoretical → Also see TABLE 9 p. 820

▸ Antifungals, azoles **(fluconazole, isavuconazole, posaconazole)** are predicted to increase the exposure to opioids **(methadone, sufentanil)**. Moderate Theoretical

▸ Antifungals, azoles **(fluconazole, isavuconazole, posaconazole)** are predicted to increase the exposure to oxybutynin. Mild Theoretical

▸ Antifungals, azoles **(itraconazole, ketoconazole, voriconazole)** are predicted to increase the exposure to oxybutynin. Mild Study

▸ Antifungals, azoles **(itraconazole, ketoconazole, voriconazole)** are predicted to increase the exposure to palbociclib. Avoid or adjust palbociclib dose. Severe Study

▸ Antifungals, azoles **(itraconazole, ketoconazole, voriconazole)** are predicted to increase the exposure to panobinostat. Adjust panobinostat dose; in hepatic impairment avoid. Moderate Study → Also see TABLE 9 p. 820

▸ Antifungals, azoles **(itraconazole, ketoconazole, voriconazole)** are predicted to increase the exposure to paritaprevir (with ritonavir and ombitasvir). Avoid. Severe Theoretical

▸ **Posaconazole** is predicted to increase the exposure to paritaprevir (with ritonavir and ombitasvir) and **paritaprevir** (with ritonavir and ombitasvir) is predicted to increase the exposure to posaconazole. Avoid. Severe Theoretical

▸ Antifungals, azoles **(fluconazole, isavuconazole, posaconazole)** are predicted to increase the exposure to pazopanib. Moderate Theoretical

▸ Antifungals, azoles **(itraconazole, ketoconazole, voriconazole)** are predicted to increase the exposure to pazopanib. Avoid or adjust pazopanib dose. Moderate Study → Also see TABLE 9 p. 820

▸ **Miconazole** greatly increases the anticoagulant effect of phenindione. Severe Theoretical

▸ Antifungals, azoles **(fluconazole, isavuconazole, posaconazole)** are predicted to increase the exposure to phosphodiesterase type-5 inhibitors **(avanafil)**. Adjust avanafil dose. Moderate Theoretical

▸ Antifungals, azoles **(itraconazole, ketoconazole, voriconazole)** are predicted to increase the exposure to phosphodiesterase type-5 inhibitors **(avanafil, vardenafil)**. Avoid. Severe Study → Also see TABLE 9 p. 820

▸ **Miconazole** is predicted to increase the exposure to phosphodiesterase type-5 inhibitors **(sildenafil)**. Use with caution and adjust dose. Severe Theoretical

▸ Antifungals, azoles **(fluconazole, isavuconazole, posaconazole)** are predicted to increase the exposure to phosphodiesterase type-5 inhibitors **(sildenafil)**. Monitor and adjust sildenafil dose, p. 117. Moderate Study

▸ Antifungals, azoles **(itraconazole, ketoconazole, voriconazole)** are predicted to increase the exposure to phosphodiesterase type-5 inhibitors **(sildenafil)**. Avoid or adjust sildenafil dose, p. 117. Severe Study → Also see TABLE 9 p. 820

▸ Antifungals, azoles **(fluconazole, isavuconazole, posaconazole)** are predicted to increase the exposure to phosphodiesterase type-5 inhibitors **(tadalafil)**. Severe Theoretical

▸ Antifungals, azoles **(itraconazole, ketoconazole, voriconazole)** are predicted to increase the exposure to phosphodiesterase type-5 inhibitors **(tadalafil)**. Use with caution or avoid. Severe Study

▸ Antifungals, azoles **(fluconazole, isavuconazole, posaconazole)** are predicted to increase the exposure to phosphodiesterase type-5 inhibitors **(vardenafil)**. Adjust dose. Severe Theoretical

▸ Antifungals, azoles **(fluconazole, isavuconazole, posaconazole)** are predicted to increase the exposure to pimozide. Avoid. Severe Theoretical

▸ Antifungals, azoles **(itraconazole, ketoconazole, voriconazole)** are predicted to increase the exposure to pimozide. Avoid. Severe Study → Also see TABLE 9 p. 820

▸ **Miconazole** is predicted to increase the exposure to pimozide. Avoid. Moderate Theoretical

▸ Antifungals, azoles **(itraconazole, ketoconazole, voriconazole)** are predicted to slightly increase the exposure to ponatinib. Monitor and adjust ponatinib dose. Moderate Study

▸ Antifungals, azoles **(itraconazole, ketoconazole, voriconazole)** are predicted to moderately increase the exposure to praziquantel. Mild Study

▸ **Fluconazole** is predicted to increase the exposure to proton pump inhibitors. Mild Study

▸ **Proton pump inhibitors** decrease the absorption of itraconazole. Administer **itraconazole** capsules with an acidic beverage. Moderate Study

▸ **Proton pump inhibitors** decrease the absorption of ketoconazole. Administer **ketoconazole** with an acidic beverage. Moderate Study

▸ **Proton pump inhibitors** decrease the absorption of posaconazole (oral suspension). Avoid. Moderate Study

▸ **Voriconazole** increases the exposure to proton pump inhibitors **(esomeprazole, omeprazole)**. Adjust dose. Moderate Study

▸ Antifungals, azoles **(fluconazole, isavuconazole, posaconazole)** are predicted to increase the exposure to quetiapine. Avoid. Moderate Study

▸ Antifungals, azoles **(itraconazole, ketoconazole, voriconazole)** are predicted to increase the exposure to quetiapine. Avoid. Severe Study

▸ Antifungals, azoles **(fluconazole, isavuconazole, posaconazole)** are predicted to increase the exposure to ranolazine. Severe Study

▸ Antifungals, azoles **(itraconazole, ketoconazole, voriconazole)** are predicted to increase the exposure to ranolazine. Avoid. Severe Study → Also see TABLE 9 p. 820

▸ Antifungals, azoles **(itraconazole, ketoconazole, voriconazole)** are predicted to increase the exposure to reboxetine. Avoid. Moderate Study

▸ **Miconazole** is predicted to increase the concentration of reboxetine. Use with caution and adjust dose. Moderate Theoretical

▸ Antifungals, azoles **(itraconazole, ketoconazole, voriconazole)** are predicted to increase the exposure to regorafenib. Avoid. Moderate Study

▸ Antifungals, azoles **(itraconazole, ketoconazole, voriconazole)** are predicted to increase the exposure to repaglinide. Moderate Study

A1

Interactions | Appendix 1

Antifungals, azoles (continued)

▸ Antifungals, azoles **(fluconazole, itraconazole, ketoconazole, miconazole, voriconazole)** are predicted to increase the exposure to retinoids **(alitretinoin)**. Adjust **alitretinoin** dose. Moderate Theoretical

▸ Antifungals, azoles **(fluconazole, ketoconazole, voriconazole)** are predicted to increase the risk of **tretinoin** toxicity when given with retinoids **(tretinoin)**. Moderate Study

▸ Antifungals, azoles **(itraconazole, posaconazole)** increase the concentration of rifabutin and rifabutin decreases the concentration of antifungals, azoles **(itraconazole, posaconazole)**. Avoid. Severe Study

▸ **Fluconazole** increases the risk of uveitis when given with rifabutin. Adjust dose. Severe Study

▸ Rifabutin is predicted to decrease the exposure to **isavuconazole**. Avoid. Severe Theoretical

▸ **Ketoconazole** is predicted to increase the concentration of rifabutin and rifabutin is predicted to decrease the concentration of **ketoconazole**. Avoid. Severe Theoretical

▸ **Miconazole** is predicted to increase the concentration of rifabutin. Use with caution and adjust dose. Moderate Theoretical

▸ Rifabutin decreases the concentration of **voriconazole** and **voriconazole** increases the concentration of rifabutin. Avoid or adjust **voriconazole** dose, p. 361. Severe Study

▸ Rifampicin slightly decreases the exposure to **fluconazole**. Adjust dose. Moderate Study

▸ Rifampicin is predicted to decrease the exposure to **isavuconazole**. Avoid. Severe Study

▸ Rifampicin markedly decreases the exposure to **itraconazole**. Avoid **rifampicin** for 14 days before and during treatment with **itraconazole**. Moderate Study

▸ Rifampicin markedly decreases the exposure to **ketoconazole** and **ketoconazole** potentially decreases the exposure to rifampicin. Avoid. Moderate Study

▸ Rifampicin is predicted to decrease the exposure to **posaconazole**. Avoid. Moderate Anecdotal

▸ Rifampicin very markedly decreases the exposure to **voriconazole**. Avoid. Moderate Study

▸ **Itraconazole** is predicted to increase the exposure to **riociguat**. Avoid. Moderate Study

▸ **Ketoconazole** moderately increases the exposure to **riociguat**. Avoid. Moderate Study

▸ Antifungals, azoles **(itraconazole, ketoconazole, voriconazole)** are predicted to increase the exposure to **risperidone**. Adjust dose. Moderate Study → Also see **TABLE 9** p. 820

▸ Antifungals, azoles **(itraconazole, ketoconazole)** increase the exposure to **rivaroxaban**. Avoid. Severe Study

▸ Antifungals, azoles **(fluconazole, isavuconazole, posaconazole)** are predicted to increase the exposure to **ruxolitinib**. Moderate Theoretical

▸ Antifungals, azoles **(itraconazole, ketoconazole, voriconazole)** are predicted to increase the exposure to **ruxolitinib**. Adjust dose and monitor side effects. Moderate Study

▸ Antifungals, azoles **(fluconazole, isavuconazole, posaconazole)** are predicted to increase the exposure to **saxagliptin**. Mild Study

▸ Antifungals, azoles **(itraconazole, ketoconazole, voriconazole)** are predicted to increase the exposure to **saxagliptin**. Moderate Study

▸ **Fluconazole** is predicted to increase the exposure to **selexipag**. Unknown Theoretical

▸ Antifungals, azoles **(fluconazole, isavuconazole, itraconazole, ketoconazole, posaconazole, voriconazole)** are predicted to increase the exposure to **simeprevir**. Avoid. Severe Study

▸ Antifungals, azoles **(fluconazole, isavuconazole, posaconazole)** increase the concentration of **sirolimus**. Monitor and adjust dose. Moderate Study

▸ Antifungals, azoles **(itraconazole, ketoconazole, voriconazole)** are predicted to increase the concentration of **sirolimus**. Avoid. Severe Study

▸ **Miconazole** is predicted to increase the concentration of **sirolimus**. Monitor and adjust dose. Moderate Study

▸ Antifungals, azoles **(itraconazole, ketoconazole, voriconazole)** are predicted to increase the exposure to **solifenacin**. Adjust solifenacin or tamsulosin with solifenacin dose; avoid in hepatic and renal impairment. Severe Study

▸ **Voriconazole** is predicted to increase the exposure to SSRIs **(citalopram)**. Severe Theoretical → Also see **TABLE 9** p. 820

▸ Antifungals, azoles **(fluconazole, isavuconazole, posaconazole)** are predicted to increase the exposure to SSRIs **(dapoxetine)**. Adjust **dapoxetine** dose. Moderate Theoretical

▸ Antifungals, azoles **(itraconazole, ketoconazole, voriconazole)** are predicted to moderately increase the exposure to SSRIs **(dapoxetine)**. Avoid or adjust **dapoxetine** dose. Severe Study

▸ St John's Wort is predicted to decrease the exposure to **isavuconazole**. Avoid. Severe Theoretical

▸ St John's Wort moderately decreases the exposure to **voriconazole**. Avoid. Moderate Study

▸ **Miconazole** potentially increases the exposure to statins **(atorvastatin)**. Severe Anecdotal

▸ Antifungals, azoles **(fluconazole, isavuconazole, posaconazole)** are predicted to increase the exposure to statins **(atorvastatin)**. Monitor and adjust dose. Severe Theoretical → Also see **TABLE 1** p. 818

▸ Antifungals, azoles **(itraconazole, ketoconazole, voriconazole)** are predicted to increase the exposure to statins **(atorvastatin)**. Avoid or adjust dose and monitor rhabdomyolysis. Severe Study → Also see **TABLE 1** p. 818

▸ Antifungals, azoles **(fluconazole, miconazole)** are predicted to increase the exposure to statins **(fluvastatin)**. Severe Theoretical → Also see **TABLE 1** p. 818

▸ **Miconazole** is predicted to increase the exposure to statins **(simvastatin)**. Avoid. Severe Theoretical

▸ Antifungals, azoles **(fluconazole, isavuconazole, posaconazole)** are predicted to increase the exposure to statins **(simvastatin)**. Use with caution and adjust **simvastatin** dose, p. 130. Severe Study → Also see **TABLE 1** p. 818

▸ Antifungals, azoles **(itraconazole, ketoconazole, voriconazole)** are predicted to increase the exposure to statins **(simvastatin)**. Avoid. Severe Study → Also see **TABLE 1** p. 818

▸ Antifungals, azoles **(fluconazole, miconazole, voriconazole)** are predicted to increase the exposure to **sulfonylureas**. Use with caution and adjust dose. Moderate Study

▸ Antifungals, azoles **(fluconazole, isavuconazole, posaconazole)** are predicted to increase the exposure to **sunitinib**. Moderate Theoretical

▸ Antifungals, azoles **(itraconazole, ketoconazole, voriconazole)** are predicted to slightly increase the exposure to **sunitinib**. Avoid or adjust **sunitinib** dose. Moderate Study → Also see **TABLE 9** p. 820

▸ Antifungals, azoles **(fluconazole, isavuconazole, posaconazole)** are predicted to increase the concentration of **tacrolimus**. Severe Study

▸ Antifungals, azoles **(itraconazole, ketoconazole, voriconazole)** are predicted to increase the concentration of **tacrolimus**. Monitor and adjust dose. Severe Study

▸ **Miconazole** is predicted to increase the concentration of **tacrolimus**. Monitor and adjust dose. Severe Theoretical

▸ Antifungals, azoles **(fluconazole, isavuconazole, posaconazole)** are predicted to increase the exposure to taxanes **(cabazitaxel)**. Moderate Theoretical

▸ Antifungals, azoles **(itraconazole, ketoconazole, voriconazole)** are predicted to increase the exposure to taxanes **(cabazitaxel)**. Avoid. Severe Study

▸ **Miconazole** is predicted to increase the concentration of taxanes **(docetaxel)**. Use with caution and adjust dose. Moderate Theoretical

▸ Antifungals, azoles **(itraconazole, ketoconazole, voriconazole)** are predicted to moderately increase the exposure to taxanes **(docetaxel)**. Avoid or adjust dose. Severe Study

▸ Antifungals, azoles **(itraconazole, ketoconazole, voriconazole)** are predicted to increase the exposure to taxanes **(paclitaxel)**. Severe Theoretical

▸ Antifungals, azoles **(fluconazole, isavuconazole, posaconazole)** are predicted to increase the concentration of **temsirolimus**. Moderate Theoretical

▸ Antifungals, azoles **(itraconazole, ketoconazole, voriconazole)** are predicted to increase the concentration of **temsirolimus**. Avoid. Severe Theoretical

▸ Antifungals, azoles **(itraconazole, ketoconazole, voriconazole)** are predicted to markedly increase the exposure to ticagrelor. Avoid. [Severe] Study

▸ Antifungals, azoles **(fluconazole, isavuconazole, posaconazole)** are predicted to increase the exposure to tolterodine. [Mild] Theoretical

▸ Antifungals, azoles **(itraconazole, ketoconazole, voriconazole)** are predicted to increase the exposure to tolterodine. Avoid. [Severe] Study → Also see TABLE 9 p. 820

▸ Antifungals, azoles **(fluconazole, isavuconazole, posaconazole)** are predicted to increase the exposure to tolvaptan. Adjust dose. [Moderate] Theoretical

▸ Antifungals, azoles **(itraconazole, ketoconazole, voriconazole)** are predicted to increase the exposure to tolvaptan. Adjust dose. [Severe] Study

▸ Antifungals, azoles **(itraconazole, ketoconazole)** are predicted to increase the exposure to topotecan. [Severe] Study

▸ Antifungals, azoles **(itraconazole, ketoconazole, voriconazole)** are predicted to increase the exposure to toremifene. [Moderate] Theoretical → Also see TABLE 9 p. 820

▸ Antifungals, azoles **(itraconazole, ketoconazole, voriconazole)** are predicted to increase the exposure to trabectedin. Avoid or adjust dose. [Severe] Theoretical → Also see TABLE 1 p. 818

▸ Antifungals, azoles **(itraconazole, ketoconazole)** are predicted to increase the concentration of trametinib. [Moderate] Theoretical

▸ Antifungals, azoles **(fluconazole, isavuconazole, posaconazole)** are predicted to increase the exposure to trazodone. [Moderate] Theoretical

▸ Antifungals, azoles **(itraconazole, ketoconazole, voriconazole)** are predicted to moderately increase the exposure to trazodone. Avoid or adjust dose. [Moderate] Study

▸ Antifungals, azoles **(fluconazole, isavuconazole, posaconazole)** are predicted to increase the exposure to ulipristal. Avoid if used for uterine fibroids. [Moderate] Study

▸ Antifungals, azoles **(itraconazole, ketoconazole, voriconazole)** are predicted to increase the exposure to ulipristal. Avoid if used for uterine fibroids. [Severe] Study

▸ Antifungals, azoles **(itraconazole, ketoconazole, voriconazole)** are predicted to increase the exposure to vemurafenib. [Severe] Theoretical → Also see TABLE 9 p. 820

▸ Antifungals, azoles **(fluconazole, isavuconazole, itraconazole, ketoconazole, posaconazole, voriconazole)** are predicted to increase the exposure to venetoclax. Avoid or adjust venetoclax dose. [Severe] Study

▸ Antifungals, azoles **(itraconazole, ketoconazole, voriconazole)** are predicted to increase the exposure to venlafaxine. [Moderate] Study → Also see TABLE 9 p. 820

▸ Antifungals, azoles **(fluconazole, isavuconazole, itraconazole, ketoconazole, posaconazole, voriconazole)** are predicted to increase the exposure to vinca alkaloids. [Severe] Theoretical → Also see TABLE 1 p. 818 → Also see TABLE 9 p. 820

▸ **Miconazole** is predicted to increase the concentration of vinca alkaloids. Use with caution and adjust dose. [Moderate] Theoretical

▸ Antifungals, azoles **(clotrimazole, ketoconazole)** are predicted to decrease the exposure to vitamin D substances **(colecalciferol)**. [Moderate] Theoretical

▸ Antifungals, azoles **(itraconazole, ketoconazole, voriconazole)** are predicted to increase the exposure to vitamin D substances **(paricalcitol)**. [Moderate] Study

▸ Antifungals, azoles **(fluconazole, isavuconazole, posaconazole)** are predicted to increase the exposure to zopiclone. Adjust dose. [Moderate] Study

▸ Antifungals, azoles **(itraconazole, ketoconazole, voriconazole)** are predicted to increase the exposure to zopiclone. Adjust dose. [Moderate] Theoretical

Antihistamines, non-sedating → see TABLE 9 p. 820 (QT-interval prolongation)

acrivastine · azelastine · bilastine · cetirizine · desloratadine · fexofenadine · levocetirizine · loratadine · mizolastine

FOOD AND LIFESTYLE Apple juice and orange juice decrease the exposure to fexofenadine.

▸ **Antacids** decrease the absorption of **fexofenadine**. Separate administration by 2 hours. [Mild] Study

▸ **Antiarrhythmics (dronedarone)** are predicted to increase the exposure to antihistamines, non-sedating **(fexofenadine, mizolastine)**. [Severe] Theoretical

▸ Antifungals, azoles **(fluconazole, isavuconazole, posaconazole)** are predicted to increase the exposure to **mizolastine**. [Severe] Theoretical

▸ Antifungals, azoles **(itraconazole, ketoconazole, voriconazole)** are predicted to increase the exposure to **mizolastine**. Avoid. [Severe] Study

▸ Antifungals, azoles **(miconazole)** are predicted to increase the exposure to **mizolastine**. Avoid. [Moderate] Theoretical

▸ **Aprepitant** is predicted to increase the exposure to **mizolastine**. [Severe] Theoretical

▸ **Antihistamines, non-sedating** are predicted to decrease the effects of betahistine. [Moderate] Theoretical

▸ **Calcium channel blockers (diltiazem, verapamil)** are predicted to increase the exposure to **mizolastine**. [Severe] Theoretical

▸ **Ceritinib** is predicted to increase the exposure to **fexofenadine**. [Moderate] Theoretical

▸ **Cobicistat** is predicted to increase the exposure to **mizolastine**. Avoid. [Severe] Study

▸ **Crizotinib** is predicted to increase the exposure to **mizolastine**. [Severe] Theoretical

▸ **Grapefruit juice** slightly decreases the exposure to **bilastine**. Bilastine should be taken 1 hour before or 2 hours after grapefruit juice. [Moderate] Study

▸ **Antihistamines, non-sedating** are predicted to decrease the effects of histamine. Avoid. [Severe] Theoretical

▸ **HIV-protease inhibitors (atazanavir, darunavir, fosamprenavir, lopinavir, ritonavir, saquinavir, tipranavir)** are predicted to increase the exposure to **mizolastine**. Avoid. [Severe] Study

▸ **HIV-protease inhibitors (indinavir)** are predicted to increase the exposure to **mizolastine**. [Severe] Theoretical

▸ **Idelalisib** is predicted to increase the exposure to **mizolastine**. Avoid. [Severe] Study

▸ **Imatinib** is predicted to increase the exposure to **mizolastine**. [Severe] Theoretical

▸ **Lapatinib** is predicted to increase the exposure to **fexofenadine**. [Moderate] Theoretical

▸ **Lumacaftor** is predicted to affect the exposure to **fexofenadine**. Monitor and adjust dose. [Moderate] Theoretical

▸ **Macrolides (clarithromycin)** are predicted to increase the exposure to **mizolastine**. Avoid. [Severe] Study

▸ **Macrolides (erythromycin)** are predicted to increase the exposure to **mizolastine**. [Severe] Theoretical

▸ **Mirabegron** is predicted to increase the exposure to **fexofenadine**. [Mild] Theoretical

▸ **Monoamine-oxidase A and B inhibitors, irreversible** are predicted to increase the risk of antimuscarinic side-effects when given with **antihistamines, non-sedating**. Avoid. [Severe] Theoretical

▸ **Netupitant** is predicted to increase the exposure to **mizolastine**. [Severe] Theoretical

▸ **Nilotinib** is predicted to increase the exposure to **mizolastine**. [Severe] Theoretical

▸ **Rifampicin** is predicted to decrease the exposure to **bilastine**. [Moderate] Theoretical

▸ **Rifampicin** increases the clearance of **fexofenadine**. [Moderate] Study

▸ **Velpatasvir** is predicted to increase the exposure to **fexofenadine**. [Severe] Theoretical

Antihistamines, sedating → see TABLE 9 p. 820 (QT-interval prolongation), TABLE 11 p. 820 (CNS depressant effects), TABLE 10 p. 820 (antimuscarinics)

alimemazine · buclizine · chlorphenamine · cinnarizine · clemastine · cyclizine · cyproheptadine · hydroxyzine · ketotifen · pizotifen · promethazine

ROUTE-SPECIFIC INFORMATION Since systemic absorption can follow topical application of **ketotifen**, the possibility of interactions should be borne in mind.

▸ **Hydroxyzine** potentially increases the risk of overheating and dehydration when given with antiepileptics **(zonisamide)**. Avoid in children. [Severe] Theoretical

Antihistamines, sedating (continued)

▸ **Antihistamines, sedating** are predicted to decrease the effects of **betahistine**. [Moderate] Theoretical

▸ **Antihistamines, sedating** are predicted to decrease the effects of **histamine**. Avoid. [Severe] Theoretical

▸ **Cyproheptadine** decreases the effects of **metyrapone**. Avoid. [Moderate] Study

▸ **Monoamine-oxidase A and B inhibitors, irreversible** are predicted to increase the risk of antimuscarinic side-effects when given with **antihistamines, sedating**. Avoid. [Severe] Theoretical

▸ **Antihistamines, sedating** are predicted to decrease the efficacy of **pitolisant**. [Unknown] Theoretical

▸ **Cyproheptadine** potentially decreases the effects of **SSRIs**. [Moderate] Anecdotal

Antimalarials → see TABLE 15 p. 821 (myelosuppression), TABLE 9 p. 820 (QT-interval prolongation)

artemether · artenimol · atovaquone · chloroquine · lumefantrine · mefloquine · piperaquine · primaquine · proguanil · pyrimethamine · quinine

PHARMACOLOGY Piperaquine has a long half-life; there is a potential for drug interactions to occur for up to 3 months after treatment has been stopped.

▸ **Chloroquine** is predicted to decrease the effects of **agalsidase**. Avoid. [Moderate] Theoretical

▸ **Antimalarials (chloroquine, primaquine)** are predicted to increase the risk of methaemoglobinaemia when given with topical **anaesthetics, local (prilocaine)**. Use with caution or avoid. [Severe] Theoretical

▸ **Antacids** decrease the absorption of **chloroquine**. Separate administration by at least 4 hours. [Moderate] Study

▸ **Antacids** are predicted to decrease the absorption of **proguanil**. Separate administration by at least 2 hours. [Moderate] Study

▸ **Antiarrhythmics (dronedarone)** are predicted to increase the concentration of **piperaquine**. [Severe] Theoretical

▸ **Antiepileptics (carbamazepine, fosphenytoin, phenobarbital, phenytoin, primidone)** are predicted to decrease the exposure to **artemether** (with lumefantrine). Avoid. [Severe] Study

▸ **Antiepileptics (carbamazepine, fosphenytoin, phenobarbital, phenytoin, primidone)** are predicted to decrease the concentration of **piperaquine**. Avoid. [Moderate] Theoretical

▸ **Pyrimethamine** increases the risk of haematological toxicity when given with antiepileptics **(fosphenytoin, phenytoin)**. [Severe] Study

▸ **Pyrimethamine** is predicted to increase the risk of haematological toxicity when given with antiepileptics **(phenobarbital, primidone)**. [Severe] Theoretical

▸ **Antifungals, azoles (fluconazole, isavuconazole, itraconazole, ketoconazole, posaconazole, voriconazole)** are predicted to increase the concentration of **piperaquine**. [Severe] Theoretical

▸ **Antifungals, azoles (fluconazole, itraconazole, posaconazole, voriconazole)** are predicted to increase the exposure to **mefloquine**. [Moderate] Theoretical

▸ **Antifungals, azoles (itraconazole, ketoconazole, voriconazole)** are predicted to increase the exposure to **artemether** (with lumefantrine). [Moderate] Study → Also see TABLE 9 p. 820

▸ **Antifungals, azoles (ketoconazole)** increase the exposure to **mefloquine**. [Moderate] Study

▸ **Antimalarials (proguanil)** are predicted to increase the risk of side-effects when given with antimalarials **(pyrimethamine)**. [Severe] Theoretical

▸ **Aprepitant** is predicted to increase the concentration of **piperaquine**. [Severe] Theoretical

▸ **Mefloquine** is predicted to increase the risk of bradycardia when given with **beta blockers, non-selective**. [Severe] Theoretical

▸ **Mefloquine** is predicted to increase the risk of bradycardia when given with **beta blockers, selective**. [Severe] Theoretical

▸ **Mefloquine** is predicted to increase the risk of bradycardia when given with **calcium channel blockers**. [Severe] Theoretical

▸ **Calcium channel blockers (diltiazem, verapamil)** are predicted to increase the concentration of **piperaquine**. [Severe] Theoretical

▸ **Calcium salts (calcium carbonate)** decrease the absorption of **chloroquine**. Separate administration by at least 4 hours. [Moderate] Study

▸ **Calcium salts (calcium carbonate)** are predicted to decrease the absorption of **proguanil**. Separate administration by at least 2 hours. [Moderate] Study

▸ **Chloroquine** decreases the efficacy of oral **cholera vaccine**. [Moderate] Study

▸ **Cobicistat** is predicted to increase the exposure to **artemether** (with lumefantrine). [Moderate] Study

▸ **Cobicistat** is predicted to increase the concentration of **piperaquine**. [Severe] Theoretical

▸ **Crizotinib** is predicted to increase the concentration of **piperaquine**. [Severe] Theoretical

▸ **Antimalarials (chloroquine, primaquine)** are predicted to increase the risk of methaemoglobinaemia when given with **dapsone**. [Severe] Theoretical

▸ **Mefloquine** is predicted to increase the risk of bradycardia when given with **digoxin**. [Severe] Theoretical

▸ **Quinine** increases the concentration of **digoxin**. Monitor and adjust **digoxin** dose, p. 79. [Severe] Anecdotal

▸ **Efavirenz** decreases the concentration of **artemether**. [Severe] Study

▸ **Efavirenz** moderately decreases the exposure to **atovaquone**. Avoid. [Moderate] Study

▸ **Efavirenz** affects the exposure to **proguanil**. Avoid. [Moderate] Study

▸ **Enzalutamide** is predicted to decrease the exposure to **artemether** (with lumefantrine). Avoid. [Severe] Study

▸ **Enzalutamide** is predicted to decrease the concentration of **piperaquine**. Avoid. [Moderate] Theoretical

▸ **Etravirine** decreases the exposure to **artemether**. [Moderate] Study

▸ **Grapefruit juice** increases the exposure to **artemether**. [Unknown] Study

▸ **Grapefruit juice** is predicted to increase the concentration of **piperaquine**. Avoid. [Severe] Theoretical

▸ **H₂ receptor antagonists (cimetidine)** decrease the clearance of **chloroquine**. [Moderate] Study

▸ **H₂ receptor antagonists (cimetidine)** slightly increase the exposure to **quinine**. [Moderate] Study

▸ **Antimalarials (artemether, atovaquone, chloroquine, mefloquine, primaquine, proguanil, pyrimethamine, quinine)** are predicted to affect the exposure to **histamine**. Avoid. [Severe] Theoretical

▸ **HIV-protease inhibitors (atazanavir, darunavir, fosamprenavir, lopinavir, ritonavir, saquinavir, tipranavir)** are predicted to increase the exposure to **artemether** (with lumefantrine). [Moderate] Study → Also see TABLE 9 p. 820

▸ **HIV-protease inhibitors** decrease the exposure to **atovaquone**. Avoid if boosted with ritonavir. [Moderate] Study

▸ **HIV-protease inhibitors** are predicted to increase the concentration of **piperaquine**. [Severe] Theoretical

▸ **HIV-protease inhibitors** are predicted to decrease the exposure to **proguanil**. Avoid. [Moderate] Study

▸ **HIV-protease inhibitors** are predicted to affect the exposure to **quinine**. [Severe] Study → Also see TABLE 9 p. 820

▸ **Idelalisib** is predicted to increase the exposure to **artemether** (with lumefantrine). [Moderate] Study

▸ **Idelalisib** is predicted to increase the concentration of **piperaquine**. [Severe] Theoretical

▸ **Imatinib** is predicted to increase the concentration of **piperaquine**. [Severe] Theoretical

▸ **Lanthanum** is predicted to decrease the absorption of **chloroquine**. Separate administration by at least 2 hours. [Moderate] Theoretical

▸ **Chloroquine** is predicted to decrease the exposure to **laronidase**. Avoid simultaneous administration. [Severe] Theoretical

▸ **Macrolides (clarithromycin)** are predicted to increase the exposure to **artemether** (with lumefantrine). [Moderate] Study → Also see TABLE 9 p. 820

▸ **Macrolides (clarithromycin, erythromycin)** are predicted to increase the concentration of **piperaquine**. [Severe] Theoretical

▸ **Mepacrine** is predicted to increase the concentration of **primaquine**. Avoid. [Moderate] Theoretical

▸ **Pyrimethamine** is predicted to increase the risk of side-effects when given with **methotrexate**. [Severe] Theoretical → Also see TABLE 15 p. 821

▸ Metoclopramide decreases the concentration of **atovaquone**. Avoid. Moderate Study
▸ Netupitant is predicted to increase the concentration of **piperaquine**. Severe Theoretical
▸ Nilotinib is predicted to increase the concentration of **piperaquine**. Severe Theoretical
▸ Pyrimethamine is predicted to increase the risk of side-effects when given with **pemetrexed**. Severe Theoretical → Also see **TABLE 15** p. 821
▸ Chloroquine is predicted to increase the risk of haematological toxicity when given with **penicillamine**. Avoid. Severe Theoretical
▸ Chloroquine moderately decreases the exposure to **praziquantel**. Use with caution and adjust dose. Moderate Study
▸ Chloroquine decreases the efficacy of **rabies vaccine**. Avoid. Moderate Study
▸ Rifabutin slightly decreases the exposure to **atovaquone**. Avoid. Moderate Study
▸ Rifampicin is predicted to decrease the exposure to **artemether** (with lumafantrine). Avoid. Severe Study
▸ Rifampicin moderately decreases the exposure to **atovaquone** and **atovaquone** slightly increases the exposure to **rifampicin**. Avoid. Moderate Study
▸ Rifampicin moderately decreases the exposure to **mefloquine**. Severe Study
▸ Rifampicin is predicted to decrease the concentration of **piperaquine**. Avoid. Moderate Theoretical
▸ Rifampicin decreases the exposure to **quinine**. Severe Study
▸ St John's Wort is predicted to decrease the concentration of **piperaquine**. Avoid. Moderate Theoretical
▸ Pyrimethamine increases the risk of side-effects when given with **sulfonamides**. Severe Study → Also see **TABLE 15** p. 821
▸ Tetracyclines (tetracycline) decrease the concentration of **atovaquone**. Moderate Study
▸ Pyrimethamine increases the risk of side-effects when given with **trimethoprim**. Severe Study
▸ Pyrimethamine is predicted to increase the risk of side-effects when given with **zidovudine**. Severe Theoretical → Also see **TABLE 15** p. 821

Apixaban → see **TABLE 3** p. 818 (anticoagulant effects)
▸ Antiarrhythmics (dronedarone) are predicted to increase the exposure to **apixaban**. Moderate Theoretical
▸ Antiepileptics (carbamazepine, fosphenytoin, phenobarbital, phenytoin, primidone) are predicted to moderately decrease the exposure to **apixaban**. Use with caution or avoid. Severe Study
▸ Antifungals, azoles (itraconazole) are predicted to increase the exposure to **apixaban**. Avoid. Severe Theoretical
▸ Antifungals, azoles (ketoconazole) slightly to moderately increase the exposure to **apixaban**. Avoid. Severe Study
▸ Calcium channel blockers (verapamil) are predicted to increase the exposure to **apixaban**. Moderate Theoretical
▸ Enzalutamide is predicted to moderately decrease the exposure to **apixaban**. Use with caution or avoid. Severe Study
▸ HIV-protease inhibitors (ritonavir) are predicted to increase the exposure to **apixaban**. Severe Theoretical
▸ Macrolides (clarithromycin) are predicted to increase the exposure to **apixaban**. Severe Theoretical
▸ Macrolides (erythromycin) are predicted to increase the exposure to **apixaban**. Moderate Theoretical
▸ Rifampicin is predicted to moderately decrease the exposure to **apixaban**. Use with caution or avoid. Severe Study
▸ St John's Wort is predicted to decrease the exposure to **apixaban**. Use with caution or avoid. Moderate Theoretical

Apomorphine → see dopamine receptor agonists
Apraclonidine → see **TABLE 6** p. 819 (bradycardia), **TABLE 8** p. 819 (hypotension), **TABLE 11** p. 820 (CNS depressant effects)
▸ Amfetamines are predicted to decrease the effects of **apraclonidine**. Avoid. Severe Theoretical
▸ Methylphenidate is predicted to decrease the effects of **apraclonidine**. Avoid. Severe Theoretical
▸ Sympathomimetics, inotropic are predicted to decrease the effects of **apraclonidine**. Avoid. Severe Theoretical
▸ Sympathomimetics, vasoconstrictor are predicted to decrease the effects of **apraclonidine**. Avoid. Severe Theoretical

Apremilast
▸ Antiepileptics (carbamazepine, fosphenytoin, phenobarbital, phenytoin, primidone) moderately decrease the exposure to **apremilast**. Avoid. Severe Study
▸ Enzalutamide moderately decreases the exposure to **apremilast**. Avoid. Severe Study
▸ Rifampicin moderately decreases the exposure to **apremilast**. Avoid. Severe Study
▸ St John's Wort is predicted to decrease the exposure to **apremilast**. Avoid. Severe Theoretical

Aprepitant
▸ **Aprepitant** is predicted to increase the exposure to aldosterone antagonists (eplerenone). Adjust eplerenone dose. Severe Study
▸ **Aprepitant** is predicted to increase the exposure to alpha blockers (tamsulosin). Moderate Theoretical
▸ **Aprepitant** is predicted to increase the exposure to alprazolam. Severe Study
▸ **Aprepitant** increases the exposure to antiarrhythmics (dronedarone). Severe Theoretical
▸ **Aprepitant** is predicted to increase the exposure to antiarrhythmics (propafenone). Monitor and adjust dose. Moderate Study
▸ Antiepileptics (carbamazepine, fosphenytoin, phenobarbital, phenytoin, primidone) are predicted to markedly decrease the exposure to **aprepitant**. Avoid. Moderate Study
▸ Antifungals, azoles (itraconazole, ketoconazole, voriconazole) are predicted to markedly increase the exposure to **aprepitant**. Moderate Study
▸ **Aprepitant** is predicted to increase the exposure to antifungals, azoles (isavuconazole). Moderate Theoretical
▸ **Aprepitant** is predicted to increase the exposure to antihistamines, non-sedating (mizolastine). Severe Theoretical
▸ **Aprepitant** is predicted to increase the concentration of antimalarials (piperaquine). Severe Theoretical
▸ **Aprepitant** is predicted to increase the exposure to axitinib. Moderate Theoretical
▸ **Aprepitant** is predicted to increase the exposure to bedaquiline. Avoid prolonged use. Mild Theoretical
▸ **Aprepitant** is predicted to increase the exposure to bosutinib. Avoid or adjust bosutinib dose. Severe Theoretical
▸ **Aprepitant** is predicted to increase the exposure to buspirone. Use with caution and adjust dose. Moderate Study
▸ **Aprepitant** is predicted to increase the exposure to cabozantinib. Moderate Theoretical
▸ Calcium channel blockers (diltiazem) increase the exposure to **aprepitant** and **aprepitant** increases the exposure to calcium channel blockers (diltiazem). Moderate Study
▸ Calcium channel blockers (verapamil) are predicted to increase the exposure to **aprepitant** and **aprepitant** is predicted to increase the exposure to calcium channel blockers (verapamil). Moderate Theoretical
▸ **Aprepitant** is predicted to increase the exposure to calcium channel blockers (amlodipine, felodipine, isradipine, lacidipine, lercanidipine, nicardipine, nifedipine, nimodipine). Monitor and adjust dose. Moderate Study
▸ **Aprepitant** is predicted to increase the exposure to ceritinib. Moderate Theoretical
▸ **Aprepitant** increases the concentration of ciclosporin. Severe Study
▸ Cobicistat is predicted to markedly increase the exposure to **aprepitant**. Moderate Study
▸ **Aprepitant** is predicted to increase the exposure to cobimetinib. Severe Theoretical
▸ **Aprepitant** is predicted to increase the exposure to colchicine. Adjust colchicine dose. Severe Study
▸ **Aprepitant** is predicted to decrease the efficacy of combined hormonal contraceptives. For FSRH guidance, see Contraceptives, interactions p. 474. Severe Study
▸ **Aprepitant** moderately increases the exposure to corticosteroids (dexamethasone). Monitor and adjust dose. Moderate Study
▸ **Aprepitant** is predicted to increase the exposure to corticosteroids (methylprednisolone). Monitor and adjust dose. Moderate Study
▸ **Aprepitant** decreases the anticoagulant effect of coumarins. Moderate Study

Aprepitant (continued)

▶ **Aprepitant** is predicted to increase the exposure to **crizotinib**. Moderate Theoretical

▶ **Aprepitant** is predicted to slightly increase the exposure to **darifenacin**. Moderate Study

▶ **Aprepitant** is predicted to increase the exposure to **dasatinib**. Severe Study

▶ **Aprepitant** is predicted to decrease the efficacy of **desogestrel**. For FSRH guidance, see Contraceptives, interactions p. 474. Severe Theoretical

▶ **Aprepitant** increases the risk of QT-prolongation when given with **domperidone**. Avoid. Severe Study

▶ **Aprepitant** is predicted to increase the exposure to dopamine receptor agonists (**bromocriptine, cabergoline**). Severe Theoretical

▶ **Aprepitant** is predicted to moderately increase the exposure to **dutasteride**. Mild Study

▶ **Enzalutamide** is predicted to markedly decrease the exposure to **aprepitant**. Avoid. Moderate Study

▶ **Aprepitant** is predicted to increase the risk of ergotism when given with **ergometrine**. Severe Theoretical

▶ **Aprepitant** is predicted to increase the risk of ergotism when given with **ergotamine**. Severe Theoretical

▶ **Aprepitant** is predicted to increase the exposure to **erlotinib**. Moderate Theoretical

▶ **Aprepitant** is predicted to decrease the efficacy of **etonogestrel**. For FSRH guidance, see Contraceptives, interactions p. 474. Severe Theoretical

▶ **Aprepitant** is predicted to increase the concentration of **everolimus**. Avoid or adjust dose. Moderate Study

▶ **Aprepitant** is predicted to increase the exposure to **fesoterodine**. Adjust **fesoterodine** dose in hepatic and renal impairment. Mild Study

▶ **Aprepitant** is predicted to increase the exposure to **gefitinib**. Moderate Theoretical

▶ **Aprepitant** is predicted to increase the concentration of **guanfacine**. Adjust **guanfacine** dose, p. 222. Moderate Theoretical

▶ HIV-protease inhibitors (**atazanavir, darunavir, fosamprenavir, lopinavir, ritonavir, saquinavir, tipranavir**) are predicted to markedly increase the exposure to **aprepitant**. Moderate Study

▶ **Aprepitant** is predicted to decrease the effects of Hormone replacement therapy. Moderate Anecdotal

▶ **Aprepitant** is predicted to increase the exposure to **ibrutinib**. Avoid or adjust **ibrutinib** dose. Severe Theoretical

▶ **Idelalisib** is predicted to markedly increase the exposure to **aprepitant**. Moderate Study

▶ **Aprepitant** is predicted to increase the exposure to **imatinib**. Moderate Theoretical

▶ **Aprepitant** is predicted to increase the exposure to **ivabradine**. Adjust **ivabradine** dose. Severe Theoretical

▶ **Aprepitant** is predicted to increase the exposure to **ivacaftor**. Adjust **ivacaftor** dose, p. 179. Severe Study

▶ **Aprepitant** is predicted to increase the exposure to **lapatinib**. Moderate Study

▶ **Aprepitant** is predicted to decrease the efficacy of **levonorgestrel**. For FSRH guidance, see Contraceptives, interactions p. 474. Severe Theoretical

▶ **Aprepitant** is predicted to increase the exposure to **lomitapide**. Avoid. Moderate Theoretical

▶ **Aprepitant** is predicted to increase the exposure to **lurasidone**. Moderate Study

▶ Macrolides (**clarithromycin**) are predicted to markedly increase the exposure to **aprepitant**. Moderate Study

▶ **Aprepitant** is predicted to increase the exposure to **midazolam**. Monitor side effects and adjust dose. Severe Study

▶ **Aprepitant** is predicted to increase the exposure to **naloxegol**. Adjust **naloxegol** dose and monitor side effects. Moderate Study

▶ **Aprepitant** is predicted to increase the exposure to **nilotinib**. Moderate Theoretical

▶ **Aprepitant** is predicted to decrease the efficacy of **norethisterone**. For FSRH guidance, see Contraceptives, interactions p. 474. Severe Anecdotal

▶ **Aprepitant** is predicted to increase the exposure to **olaparib**. Avoid or adjust **olaparib** dose. Moderate Theoretical

▶ **Aprepitant** is predicted to increase the exposure to opioids (**alfentanil, buprenorphine, fentanyl, oxycodone**). Monitor and adjust dose. Moderate Study

▶ **Aprepitant** is predicted to increase the exposure to opioids (**methadone, sufentanil**). Moderate Theoretical

▶ **Aprepitant** is predicted to increase the exposure to **oxybutynin**. Mild Theoretical

▶ **Aprepitant** is predicted to increase the exposure to **pazopanib**. Moderate Theoretical

▶ **Aprepitant** is predicted to increase the exposure to phosphodiesterase type-5 inhibitors (**avanafil**). Adjust **avanafil** dose. Moderate Theoretical

▶ **Aprepitant** is predicted to increase the exposure to phosphodiesterase type-5 inhibitors (**sildenafil**). Monitor and adjust **sildenafil** dose, p. 117. Moderate Study

▶ **Aprepitant** is predicted to increase the exposure to phosphodiesterase type-5 inhibitors (**tadalafil**). Severe Theoretical

▶ **Aprepitant** is predicted to increase the exposure to phosphodiesterase type-5 inhibitors (**vardenafil**). Adjust dose. Severe Theoretical

▶ **Aprepitant** is predicted to increase the exposure to **pimozide**. Avoid. Severe Theoretical

▶ **Aprepitant** is predicted to increase the exposure to **quetiapine**. Avoid. Moderate Study

▶ **Aprepitant** is predicted to increase the exposure to **ranolazine**. Severe Study

▶ **Rifampicin** is predicted to markedly decrease the exposure to **aprepitant**. Avoid. Moderate Study

▶ **Aprepitant** is predicted to increase the exposure to **ruxolitinib**. Moderate Theoretical

▶ **Aprepitant** is predicted to increase the exposure to **saxagliptin**. Mild Study

▶ **Aprepitant** is predicted to increase the exposure to **simeprevir**. Avoid. Severe Study

▶ **Aprepitant** increases the concentration of **sirolimus**. Monitor and adjust dose. Moderate Study

▶ **Aprepitant** is predicted to increase the exposure to SSRIs (**dapoxetine**). Adjust **dapoxetine** dose. Moderate Theoretical

▶ **St John's Wort** is predicted to decrease the exposure to **aprepitant**. Avoid. Moderate Theoretical

▶ **Aprepitant** is predicted to increase the exposure to statins (**atorvastatin**). Monitor and adjust dose. Severe Theoretical

▶ **Aprepitant** is predicted to increase the exposure to statins (**simvastatin**). Use with caution and adjust **simvastatin** dose, p. 130. Severe Study

▶ **Aprepitant** is predicted to increase the exposure to **sunitinib**. Moderate Theoretical

▶ **Aprepitant** is predicted to increase the concentration of **tacrolimus**. Severe Study

▶ **Aprepitant** is predicted to increase the exposure to taxanes (**cabazitaxel**). Moderate Theoretical

▶ **Aprepitant** is predicted to increase the concentration of **temsirolimus**. Moderate Theoretical

▶ **Aprepitant** is predicted to increase the exposure to **tolterodine**. Mild Theoretical

▶ **Aprepitant** is predicted to increase the exposure to **tolvaptan**. Adjust dose. Moderate Theoretical

▶ **Aprepitant** is predicted to increase the exposure to **trazodone**. Moderate Theoretical

▶ **Aprepitant** decreases the efficacy of **ulipristal**. For FSRH guidance, see Contraceptives, interactions p. 474. Severe Anecdotal

▶ **Aprepitant** is predicted to increase the exposure to **venetoclax**. Avoid or adjust **venetoclax** dose. Severe Study

▶ **Aprepitant** is predicted to increase the exposure to vinca alkaloids. Severe Theoretical

▶ **Aprepitant** is predicted to increase the exposure to **zopiclone**. Adjust dose. Moderate Study

Argatroban → see TABLE 3 p. 818 (anticoagulant effects)

▶ **Ranibizumab** is predicted to increase the risk of bleeding events when given with **argatroban**. Severe Theoretical

Aripiprazole → see TABLE 8 p. 819 (hypotension), TABLE 11 p. 820 (CNS depressant effects)

▶ Antiepileptics (**carbamazepine, fosphenytoin, phenobarbital, phenytoin, primidone**) are predicted to moderately decrease the exposure to **aripiprazole**. Adjust **aripiprazole** dose, p. 240. Moderate Study → Also see TABLE 11 p. 820

▸ Antifungals, azoles (itraconazole, ketoconazole, voriconazole) are predicted to slightly increase the exposure to **aripiprazole**. Adjust **aripiprazole** dose, p. 240. Moderate Study

▸ **Bupropion** is predicted to moderately increase the exposure to **aripiprazole**. Adjust **aripiprazole** dose, p. 240. Moderate Study

▸ **Cinacalcet** is predicted to moderately increase the exposure to **aripiprazole**. Adjust **aripiprazole** dose, p. 240. Moderate Study

▸ **Cobicistat** is predicted to slightly increase the exposure to **aripiprazole**. Adjust **aripiprazole** dose, p. 240. Moderate Study

▸ **Aripiprazole** is predicted to decrease the effects of **dopamine receptor agonists**. Moderate Theoretical → Also see TABLE 8 p. 819

▸ **Enzalutamide** is predicted to moderately decrease the exposure to **aripiprazole**. Adjust **aripiprazole** dose, p. 240. Moderate Study

▸ HIV-protease inhibitors (atazanavir, darunavir, fosamprenavir, lopinavir, ritonavir, saquinavir, tipranavir) are predicted to slightly increase the exposure to **aripiprazole**. Adjust **aripiprazole** dose, p. 240. Moderate Study

▸ **Idelalisib** is predicted to slightly increase the exposure to **aripiprazole**. Adjust **aripiprazole** dose, p. 240. Moderate Study

▸ **Aripiprazole** is predicted to decrease the effects of **levodopa**. Severe Theoretical → Also see TABLE 8 p. 819

▸ Macrolides (clarithromycin) are predicted to slightly increase the exposure to **aripiprazole**. Adjust **aripiprazole** dose, p. 240. Moderate Study

▸ **Rifampicin** is predicted to moderately decrease the exposure to **aripiprazole**. Adjust **aripiprazole** dose, p. 240. Moderate Study

▸ SSRIs (fluoxetine, paroxetine) are predicted to moderately increase the exposure to **aripiprazole**. Adjust **aripiprazole** dose, p. 240. Moderate Study

▸ **Terbinafine** is predicted to moderately increase the exposure to **aripiprazole**. Adjust **aripiprazole** dose, p. 240. Moderate Study

Arsenic trioxide → see TABLE 15 p. 821 (myelosuppression), TABLE 9 p. 820 (QT-interval prolongation)

Artemether → see antimalarials

Artenimol → see antimalarials

Articaine → see TABLE 11 p. 820 (CNS depressant effects)

Ascorbic acid

▸ **Ascorbic acid** is predicted to increase the risk of cardiovascular side-effects when given with **deferiprone**. Severe Theoretical

▸ **Ascorbic acid** is predicted to increase the risk of cardiovascular side-effects when given with iron chelators (desferrioxamine). Severe Theoretical

Asenapine → see TABLE 8 p. 819 (hypotension), TABLE 11 p. 820 (CNS depressant effects)

▸ **Asenapine** is predicted to decrease the effects of **dopamine receptor agonists**. Adjust dose. Moderate Theoretical → Also see TABLE 8 p. 819

▸ **Asenapine** is predicted to decrease the effects of **levodopa**. Adjust dose. Severe Theoretical → Also see TABLE 8 p. 819

▸ SSRIs (fluvoxamine) increase the exposure to **asenapine**. Moderate Study

▸ SSRIs (paroxetine) moderately increase the exposure to **asenapine**. Moderate Study

Asparaginase → see TABLE 1 p. 818 (hepatotoxicity), TABLE 15 p. 821 (myelosuppression)

▸ **Asparaginase** is predicted to increase the risk of hepatotoxicity when given with **imatinib**. Severe Theoretical → Also see TABLE 15 p. 821

▸ **Asparaginase** affects the efficacy of **methotrexate**. Severe Anecdotal → Also see TABLE 1 p. 818 → Also see TABLE 15 p. 821

▸ **Asparaginase** potentially increases the risk of neurotoxicity when given with vinca alkaloids (vincristine). Vincristine should be taken 3 to 24 hours before **asparaginase**. Severe Anecdotal → Also see TABLE 1 p. 818 → Also see TABLE 15 p. 821

Aspirin → see TABLE 4 p. 818 (antiplatelet effects)

▸ **Acetazolamide** increases the risk of severe toxic reaction when given with **aspirin** (high-dose). Severe Study

▸ **Antacids** decrease the absorption of **aspirin** (high-dose). Moderate Study

▸ **Aspirin** (high-dose) is predicted to increase the risk of gastrointestinal irritation when given with bisphosphonates (alendronic acid, ibandronic acid). Moderate Study

▸ **Aspirin** (high-dose) is predicted to increase the risk of renal impairment when given with bisphosphonates (sodium clodronate). Severe Theoretical

▸ **Corticosteroids** are predicted to decrease the concentration of **aspirin** (high-dose) and **aspirin** (high-dose) increases the risk of gastrointestinal bleeding when given with **corticosteroids**. Moderate Study

▸ **Aspirin** (high-dose) increases the risk of renal impairment when given with **daptomycin**. Moderate Theoretical

▸ **Erlotinib** is predicted to increase the risk of gastrointestinal perforation when given with **aspirin** (high-dose). Severe Theoretical

▸ **Aspirin** (high-dose) is predicted to increase the risk of gastrointestinal bleeds when given with iron chelators (deferasirox). Severe Theoretical

▸ **Aspirin** (high-dose) is predicted to increase the risk of toxicity when given with **methotrexate**. Severe Theoretical

▸ **Aspirin** is predicted to increase the risk of gastrointestinal perforation when given with **nicorandil**. Severe Theoretical

▸ **Aspirin** (high-dose) potentially increases the exposure to **pemetrexed**. Use with caution or avoid. Severe Theoretical

▸ **Aspirin** (high-dose) potentially increases the risk of seizures when given with **quinolones**. Severe Theoretical

▸ **Aspirin** decreases the effects of **sulfinpyrazone**. Moderate Study → Also see TABLE 4 p. 818

▸ **Aspirin** (high-dose) increases the risk of acute renal failure when given with **thiazide diuretics**. Severe Theoretical

▸ **Zidovudine** increases the risk of haematological toxicity when given with **aspirin** (high-dose). Severe Study

Ataluren

▸ **Ataluren** increases the exposure to **adefovir**. Moderate Study

▸ **Ataluren** is predicted to increase the risk of nephrotoxicity when given with intravenous **aminoglycosides**. Avoid. Severe Study

▸ **Rifampicin** decreases the exposure to **ataluren**. Moderate Study

Atazanavir → see HIV-protease inhibitors

Atenolol → see beta blockers, selective

Atomoxetine

▸ **Amfetamines** are predicted to increase the risk of side-effects when given with **atomoxetine**. Severe Theoretical

▸ **Atomoxetine** is predicted to increase the risk of cardiovascular side-effects when given with beta₂ agonists (high-dose). Moderate Study

▸ **Bupropion** is predicted to markedly increase the exposure to **atomoxetine**. Adjust dose. Severe Study

▸ **Cinacalcet** is predicted to markedly increase the exposure to **atomoxetine**. Adjust dose. Severe Study

▸ Monoamine-oxidase A and B inhibitors, irreversible are predicted to increase the risk of side-effects when given with **atomoxetine**. Avoid and for 2 weeks after stopping the MAOI. Severe Theoretical

▸ **Panobinostat** is predicted to increase the exposure to **atomoxetine**. Monitor and adjust dose. Severe Theoretical

▸ SSRIs (fluoxetine, paroxetine) are predicted to markedly increase the exposure to **atomoxetine**. Adjust dose. Severe Study

▸ **Terbinafine** is predicted to markedly increase the exposure to **atomoxetine**. Adjust dose. Severe Study

Atorvastatin → see statins

Atovaquone → see antimalarials

Atracurium → see neuromuscular blocking drugs, non-depolarising

Atropine → see TABLE 10 p. 820 (antimuscarinics)

▸ **Atropine** increases the risk of severe hypertension when given with sympathomimetics, vasoconstrictor (phenylephrine). Severe Study

Avanafil → see phosphodiesterase type-5 inhibitors

Axitinib → see TABLE 15 p. 821 (myelosuppression)

▸ Antiarrhythmics (dronedarone) are predicted to increase the exposure to **axitinib**. Moderate Theoretical

▸ Antiepileptics (carbamazepine, fosphenytoin, phenobarbital, phenytoin, primidone) are predicted to decrease the exposure to **axitinib**. Avoid or adjust dose. Moderate Study

▸ Antifungals, azoles (fluconazole, isavuconazole, posaconazole) are predicted to increase the exposure to **axitinib**. Moderate Theoretical

Axitinib (continued)

▸ Antifungals, azoles (itraconazole, ketoconazole, voriconazole) are predicted to increase the exposure to **axitinib**. Avoid or adjust dose. Moderate Study

▸ Aprepitant is predicted to increase the exposure to **axitinib**. Moderate Theoretical

▸ Bosentan is predicted to decrease the exposure to **axitinib**. Moderate Theoretical

▸ Calcium channel blockers (diltiazem, verapamil) are predicted to increase the exposure to **axitinib**. Moderate Theoretical

▸ Cobicistat is predicted to increase the exposure to **axitinib**. Avoid or adjust dose. Moderate Study

▸ **Axitinib** is predicted to increase the risk of bleeding events when given with coumarins. Severe Theoretical

▸ Crizotinib is predicted to increase the exposure to **axitinib**. Moderate Theoretical → Also see TABLE 15 p. 821

▸ Efavirenz is predicted to decrease the exposure to **axitinib**. Moderate Theoretical

▸ Enzalutamide is predicted to decrease the exposure to **axitinib**. Avoid or adjust dose. Moderate Study

▸ Grapefruit juice is predicted to increase the exposure to **axitinib**. Moderate Theoretical

▸ HIV-protease inhibitors (atazanavir, darunavir, fosamprenavir, lopinavir, ritonavir, saquinavir, tipranavir) are predicted to increase the exposure to **axitinib**. Avoid or adjust dose. Moderate Study

▸ HIV-protease inhibitors (indinavir) are predicted to increase the exposure to **axitinib**. Moderate Theoretical

▸ Idelalisib is predicted to increase the exposure to **axitinib**. Avoid or adjust dose. Moderate Study → Also see TABLE 15 p. 821

▸ Imatinib is predicted to increase the exposure to **axitinib**. Moderate Theoretical → Also see TABLE 15 p. 821

▸ Macrolides (clarithromycin) are predicted to increase the exposure to **axitinib**. Avoid or adjust dose. Moderate Study

▸ Macrolides (erythromycin) are predicted to increase the exposure to **axitinib**. Moderate Theoretical

▸ Netupitant is predicted to increase the exposure to **axitinib**. Moderate Theoretical

▸ Nevirapine is predicted to decrease the exposure to **axitinib**. Moderate Theoretical

▸ Nilotinib is predicted to increase the exposure to **axitinib**. Moderate Theoretical → Also see TABLE 15 p. 821

▸ **Axitinib** is predicted to increase the risk of bleeding events when given with phenindione. Severe Theoretical

▸ Rifampicin is predicted to decrease the exposure to **axitinib**. Avoid or adjust dose. Moderate Study

▸ St John's Wort is predicted to decrease the exposure to **axitinib**. Moderate Theoretical

Azacitidine → see TABLE 15 p. 821 (myelosuppression)

Azathioprine → see TABLE 15 p. 821 (myelosuppression)

▸ ACE inhibitors are predicted to increase the risk of anaemia and/or leucopenia when given with **azathioprine**. Severe Anecdotal

▸ Allopurinol potentially increases the risk of haematological toxicity when given with **azathioprine**. Adjust **azathioprine** dose, p. 495. Severe Study

▸ **Azathioprine** decreases the anticoagulant effect of coumarins. Moderate Study

▸ Febuxostat is predicted to increase the exposure to **azathioprine**. Avoid. Severe Theoretical

▸ Live vaccines are predicted to increase the risk of generalised infection (possibly life-threatening) when given with **azathioprine**. Public Health England advises avoid. Severe Theoretical

Azelastine → see antihistamines, non-sedating

Azilsartan → see angiotensin-II receptor antagonists

Azithromycin → see macrolides

Bacillus Calmette-Guérin vaccine → see live vaccines

Bacitracin → see TABLE 2 p. 818 (nephrotoxicity)

Baclofen → see TABLE 8 p. 819 (hypotension), TABLE 11 p. 820 (CNS depressant effects), TABLE 10 p. 820 (antimuscarinics)

▸ Baclofen is predicted to increase the risk of side-effects when given with levodopa. Severe Anecdotal → Also see TABLE 8 p. 819

Balsalazide → see TABLE 15 p. 821 (myelosuppression)

▸ Balsalazide is predicted to decrease the concentration of digoxin. Moderate Theoretical

Bambuterol → see beta₂ agonists

Basiliximab → see monoclonal antibodies

Bazedoxifene

▸ Antiepileptics (carbamazepine, fosphenytoin, phenobarbital, phenytoin, primidone) are predicted to decrease the exposure to **bazedoxifene**. Moderate Theoretical

▸ Rifampicin is predicted to decrease the exposure to **bazedoxifene**. Moderate Theoretical

Beclometasone → see corticosteroids

Bedaquiline → see TABLE 9 p. 820 (QT-interval prolongation)

▸ Antiarrhythmics (dronedarone) are predicted to increase the exposure to **bedaquiline**. Avoid prolonged use. Mild Theoretical → Also see TABLE 9 p. 820

▸ Antiepileptics (carbamazepine, fosphenytoin, phenobarbital, phenytoin, primidone) decrease the exposure to **bedaquiline**. Avoid. Severe Study

▸ Antifungals, azoles (fluconazole, isavuconazole, posaconazole) are predicted to increase the exposure to **bedaquiline**. Avoid prolonged use. Mild Theoretical

▸ Antifungals, azoles (itraconazole, ketoconazole, voriconazole) are predicted to increase the exposure to **bedaquiline**. Avoid prolonged use. Mild Study → Also see TABLE 9 p. 820

▸ Aprepitant is predicted to increase the exposure to **bedaquiline**. Avoid prolonged use. Mild Theoretical

▸ Bosentan is predicted to decrease the exposure to **bedaquiline**. Avoid. Severe Study

▸ Calcium channel blockers (diltiazem, verapamil) are predicted to increase the exposure to **bedaquiline**. Avoid prolonged use. Mild Theoretical

▸ Clofazimine potentially increases the risk of QT-prolongation when given with **bedaquiline**. Severe Study

▸ Cobicistat is predicted to increase the exposure to **bedaquiline**. Avoid prolonged use. Mild Study

▸ Crizotinib is predicted to increase the exposure to **bedaquiline**. Avoid prolonged use. Mild Theoretical → Also see TABLE 9 p. 820

▸ Efavirenz is predicted to decrease the exposure to **bedaquiline**. Avoid. Severe Study

▸ Enzalutamide decreases the exposure to **bedaquiline**. Avoid. Severe Study

▸ Etravirine is predicted to decrease the exposure to **bedaquiline**. Avoid. Severe Theoretical

▸ HIV-protease inhibitors (atazanavir, darunavir, fosamprenavir, lopinavir, ritonavir, saquinavir, tipranavir) are predicted to increase the exposure to **bedaquiline**. Avoid prolonged use. Mild Study → Also see TABLE 9 p. 820

▸ HIV-protease inhibitors (indinavir) are predicted to increase the exposure to **bedaquiline**. Avoid prolonged use. Mild Theoretical

▸ Idelalisib is predicted to increase the exposure to **bedaquiline**. Avoid prolonged use. Mild Study

▸ Imatinib is predicted to increase the exposure to **bedaquiline**. Avoid prolonged use. Mild Theoretical

▸ Macrolides (clarithromycin) are predicted to increase the exposure to **bedaquiline**. Avoid prolonged use. Mild Study → Also see TABLE 9 p. 820

▸ Macrolides (erythromycin) are predicted to increase the exposure to **bedaquiline**. Avoid prolonged use. Mild Theoretical

▸ Netupitant is predicted to increase the exposure to **bedaquiline**. Avoid prolonged use. Mild Theoretical

▸ Nevirapine is predicted to decrease the exposure to **bedaquiline**. Avoid. Severe Study

▸ Nilotinib is predicted to increase the exposure to **bedaquiline**. Avoid prolonged use. Mild Theoretical → Also see TABLE 9 p. 820

▸ Rifampicin decreases the exposure to **bedaquiline**. Avoid. Severe Study

▸ St John's Wort is predicted to decrease the exposure to **bedaquiline**. Avoid. Severe Study

Bee venom extract

GENERAL INFORMATION Desensitising vaccines should be avoided in patients taking beta-blockers (adrenaline might be ineffective in case of a hypersensitivity reaction) or ACE inhibitors (risk of severe anaphylactoid reactions).

▸ ACE inhibitors increase the risk of hypersensitivity when given with **bee venom extract**. Avoid. Severe Study

Belatacept
▸ Live vaccines are predicted to increase the risk of generalised infection (possibly life-threatening) when given with **belatacept**. Public Health England advises avoid. Severe
Theoretical

Belimumab → see monoclonal antibodies
Bendamustine → see alkylating agents
Bendroflumethiazide → see thiazide diuretics
Benperidol → see **TABLE 8** p. 819 (hypotension), **TABLE 11** p. 820 (CNS depressant effects)
▸ **Benperidol** is predicted to decrease the effects of **dopamine receptor agonists**. Avoid. Moderate Theoretical → Also see **TABLE 8** p. 819
▸ **Benperidol** is predicted to decrease the effects of **guanethidine**. Moderate Theoretical → Also see **TABLE 8** p. 819
▸ **Benperidol** is predicted to decrease the effects of **levodopa**. Severe Study → Also see **TABLE 8** p. 819

Benzydamine → see NSAIDs
Benzylpenicillin → see penicillins
Beta blockers, non-selective → see **TABLE 6** p. 819 (bradycardia), **TABLE 8** p. 819 (hypotension), **TABLE 9** p. 820 (QT-interval prolongation)

carteolol · carvedilol · labetalol · levobunolol · nadolol · oxprenolol · pindolol · propranolol · sotalol · timolol

ROUTE-SPECIFIC INFORMATION Since systemic absorption can follow topical application of **carteolol, levobunolol,** and **timolol** the possibility of interactions should be borne in mind.

▸ **Abiraterone** is predicted to increase the exposure to beta blockers, non-selective (**carvedilol, timolol**). Moderate Theoretical
▸ **Beta blockers, non-selective** are predicted to increase the risk of bronchospasm when given with **aminophylline**. Avoid. Severe Theoretical
▸ **Antiarrhythmics (amiodarone, disopyramide, dronedarone, flecainid, lidocaine)** are predicted to increase the risk of cardiovascular side-effects when given with **beta blockers, non-selective**. Use with caution or avoid. Severe Study → Also see **TABLE 6** p. 819 → Also see **TABLE 9** p. 820
▸ **Antiarrhythmics (propafenone)** are predicted to increase the exposure to **carvedilol**. Moderate Theoretical
▸ **Antiarrhythmics (propafenone)** increase the risk of cardiovascular side-effects when given with **propranolol**. Use with caution or avoid. Severe Study
▸ **Antiarrhythmics (propafenone)** are predicted to increase the exposure to **timolol** and **timolol** is predicted to increase the risk of cardiodepression when given with antiarrhythmics (**propafenone**). Severe Anecdotal
▸ **Antiarrhythmics (propafenone)** are predicted to increase the risk of cardiovascular side-effects when given with beta blockers, non-selective (**carteolol, labetalol, levobunolol, nadolol, oxprenolol, pindolol, sotalol**). Use with caution or avoid. Severe Study
▸ **Anticholinesterases, centrally acting** are predicted to increase the risk of bradycardia when given with **beta blockers, non-selective**. Moderate Anecdotal → Also see **TABLE 6** p. 819
▸ **Antiepileptics (phenobarbital, primidone)** are predicted to decrease the exposure to **propranolol**. Moderate Study
▸ **Antiepileptics (phenobarbital, primidone)** are predicted to decrease the exposure to beta blockers, non-selective (**carvedilol, labetalol**). Moderate Theoretical
▸ **Antifungals, azoles (itraconazole, ketoconazole)** are predicted to increase the exposure to **nadolol**. Moderate Study
▸ **Antimalarials (mefloquine)** are predicted to increase the risk of bradycardia when given with **beta blockers, non-selective**. Severe Theoretical
▸ **Bupropion** is predicted to increase the exposure to beta blockers, non-selective (**carvedilol, timolol**). Moderate Study
▸ Calcium channel blockers (**diltiazem**) are predicted to increase the risk of cardiodepression when given with **beta blockers, non-selective**. Severe Study → Also see **TABLE 6** p. 819 → Also see **TABLE 8** p. 819
▸ Intravenous calcium channel blockers (**verapamil**) increase the risk of cardiovascular side-effects when given with **beta blockers, non-selective**. Avoid. Severe Study → Also see **TABLE 6** p. 819 → Also see **TABLE 8** p. 819

▸ Oral calcium channel blockers (**verapamil**) increase the risk of cardiovascular side-effects when given with **beta blockers, non-selective**. Severe Study → Also see **TABLE 6** p. 819 → Also see **TABLE 8** p. 819
▸ **Ciclosporin** is predicted to increase the exposure to **nadolol**. Moderate Study
▸ **Cinacalcet** is predicted to increase the exposure to beta blockers, non-selective (**carvedilol, timolol**). Moderate Study
▸ **Duloxetine** is predicted to increase the exposure to beta blockers, non-selective (**carvedilol, timolol**). Moderate Theoretical
▸ **Beta blockers, non-selective** are predicted to increase the risk of peripheral vasoconstriction when given with **ergometrine**. Severe Theoretical
▸ **Beta blockers, non-selective** are predicted to increase the risk of peripheral vasoconstriction when given with **ergotamine**. Severe Study
▸ **HIV-protease inhibitors (lopinavir, ritonavir, saquinavir)** are predicted to increase the exposure to **nadolol**. Moderate Study
▸ **HIV-protease inhibitors (ritonavir)** are predicted to increase the exposure to **carvedilol**. Moderate Theoretical
▸ **HIV-protease inhibitors (ritonavir)** (high-dose) are predicted to increase the exposure to **timolol**. Moderate Theoretical
▸ **Beta blockers, non-selective** are predicted to increase the risk of bradycardia when given with **lanreotide**. Moderate Theoretical
▸ **Lapatinib** is predicted to increase the exposure to **nadolol**. Moderate Study
▸ **Macrolides** are predicted to increase the exposure to **nadolol**. Moderate Study
▸ **Mirabegron** is predicted to increase the exposure to beta blockers, non-selective (**carvedilol, timolol**). Moderate Theoretical
▸ **Ranolazine** is predicted to increase the exposure to **nadolol**. Moderate Study
▸ **Rifampicin** moderately decreases the exposure to **carvedilol**. Moderate Study
▸ **Rifampicin** decreases the exposure to **propranolol**. Monitor and adjust **propranolol** dose, p. 101. Moderate Study
▸ **Propranolol** slightly to moderately increases the exposure to rizatriptan. Adjust **rizatriptan** dose and separate administration by at least 2 hours. Moderate Study
▸ **SSRIs (fluvoxamine)** moderately increase the concentration of **propranolol**. Moderate Study
▸ **SSRIs (fluoxetine, paroxetine)** are predicted to increase the exposure to beta blockers, non-selective (**carvedilol, timolol**). Moderate Study
▸ **Beta blockers, non-selective** increase the risk of hypertension and bradycardia when given with sympathomimetics, inotropic (**dobutamine**). Severe Theoretical
▸ **Beta blockers, non-selective** are predicted to increase the risk of hypertension and bradycardia when given with sympathomimetics, vasoconstrictor (**adrenaline/epinephrine, noradrenaline/norepinephrine**). Severe Study
▸ **Terbinafine** is predicted to increase the exposure to beta blockers, non-selective (**carvedilol, timolol**). Moderate Study
▸ **Beta blockers, non-selective** are predicted to increase the risk of bronchospasm when given with **theophylline**. Avoid. Severe Theoretical
▸ **Vemurafenib** is predicted to increase the exposure to **nadolol**. Moderate Study

Beta blockers, selective → see **TABLE 6** p. 819 (bradycardia), **TABLE 8** p. 819 (hypotension)

acebutolol · atenolol · betaxolol · bisoprolol · celiprolol · esmolol · metoprolol · nebivolol

▸ Since systemic absorption can follow topical application of **betaxolol**, the possibility of interactions should be borne in mind.
▸ Orange juice greatly decreases the exposure to **celiprolol**.

▸ **Abiraterone** is predicted to increase the exposure to beta blockers, selective (**metoprolol, nebivolol**). Moderate Study
▸ **Beta blockers, selective** are predicted to increase the risk of bronchospasm when given with **aminophylline**. Avoid. Severe Theoretical
▸ **Antiarrhythmics (amiodarone, disopyramide, dronedarone, flecainide, lidocaine)** are predicted to increase the risk of cardiovascular side-effects when given with **beta blockers,**

A1

Interactions | **Appendix 1**

Beta blockers, selective (continued)

selective. Use with caution or avoid. Severe Study → Also see TABLE 6 p. 819

▶ Antiarrhythmics (propafenone) are predicted to increase the exposure to metoprolol. Moderate Study

▶ Antiarrhythmics (propafenone) are predicted to increase the exposure to nebivolol and nebivolol is predicted to increase the risk of cardiodepression when given with antiarrhythmics (propafenone). Avoid. Severe Theoretical

▶ Antiarrhythmics (propafenone) are predicted to increase the risk of cardiovascular side-effects when given with beta blockers, selective (acebutolol, atenolol, betaxolol, bisoprolol, celiprolol, esmolol). Use with caution or avoid. Severe Study

▶ Anticholinesterases, centrally acting are predicted to increase the risk of bradycardia when given with beta blockers, selective. Moderate Anecdotal → Also see TABLE 6 p. 819

▶ Antiepileptics (phenobarbital, primidone) are predicted to decrease the exposure to beta blockers, selective (acebutolol, bisoprolol, metoprolol, nebivolol). Moderate Study

▶ Antimalarials (mefloquine) are predicted to increase the risk of bradycardia when given with beta blockers, selective. Severe Theoretical

▶ Bupropion is predicted to increase the exposure to beta blockers, selective (metoprolol, nebivolol). Moderate Study

▶ Calcium channel blockers (diltiazem) are predicted to increase the risk of cardiodepression when given with beta blockers, selective. Severe Study → Also see TABLE 6 p. 819 → Also see TABLE 8 p. 819

▶ Intravenous calcium channel blockers (verapamil) increase the risk of cardiovascular side-effects when given with beta blockers, selective. Avoid. Severe Study → Also see TABLE 6 p. 819 → Also see TABLE 8 p. 819

▶ Oral calcium channel blockers (verapamil) increase the risk of cardiovascular side-effects when given with beta blockers, selective. Severe Study → Also see TABLE 6 p. 819 → Also see TABLE 8 p. 819

▶ Cinacalcet is predicted to increase the exposure to beta blockers, selective (metoprolol, nebivolol). Moderate Study

▶ Duloxetine is predicted to increase the exposure to beta blockers, selective (metoprolol, nebivolol). Moderate Study

▶ Beta blockers, selective are predicted to increase the risk of peripheral vasoconstriction when given with ergometrine. Severe Theoretical

▶ Beta blockers, selective are predicted to increase the risk of peripheral vasoconstriction when given with ergotamine. Severe Study

▶ Grapefruit juice greatly decreases the exposure to celiprolol. Moderate Study

▶ HIV-protease inhibitors (ritonavir) are predicted to increase the exposure to beta blockers, selective (metoprolol, nebivolol). Moderate Study

▶ Beta blockers, selective are predicted to increase the risk of bradycardia when given with lanreotide. Moderate Theoretical

▶ Mirabegron is predicted to increase the exposure to beta blockers, selective (metoprolol, nebivolol). Moderate Study

▶ Panobinostat is predicted to increase the exposure to metoprolol. Monitor and adjust dose. Moderate Theoretical

▶ Rifampicin slightly decreases the exposure to beta blockers, selective (bisoprolol, metoprolol). Mild Study

▶ Rifampicin moderately decreases the exposure to celiprolol. Moderate Study

▶ SSRIs (fluoxetine, paroxetine) are predicted to increase the exposure to beta blockers, selective (metoprolol, nebivolol). Moderate Study

▶ Beta blockers, selective increase the risk of hypertension and bradycardia when given with sympathomimetics, inotropic (dobutamine). Moderate Theoretical

▶ Beta blockers, selective are predicted to increase the risk of hypertension and bradycardia when given with sympathomimetics, vasoconstrictor (adrenaline/epinephrine, noradrenaline/norepinephrine). Severe Study

▶ Terbinafine is predicted to increase the exposure to beta blockers, selective (metoprolol, nebivolol). Moderate Study

▶ Beta blockers, selective are predicted to increase the risk of bronchospasm when given with theophylline. Avoid. Severe Theoretical

Beta₂ agonists → see TABLE 17 p. 822 (reduced serum potassium)

bambuterol · formoterol · indacaterol · olodaterol · salbutamol · salmeterol · terbutaline · vilanterol

▶ Antifungals, azoles (itraconazole, ketoconazole, voriconazole) are predicted to increase the exposure to salmeterol. Avoid. Severe Study

▶ Atomoxetine is predicted to increase the risk of cardiovascular side-effects when given with beta₂ agonists (high-dose). Moderate Study

▶ Cobicistat is predicted to increase the exposure to salmeterol. Avoid. Severe Study

▶ HIV-protease inhibitors (atazanavir, darunavir, fosamprenavir, lopinavir, ritonavir, saquinavir, tipranavir) are predicted to increase the exposure to salmeterol. Avoid. Severe Study

▶ Idelalisib is predicted to increase the exposure to salmeterol. Avoid. Severe Study

▶ Beta₂ agonists are predicted to increase the risk of glaucoma when given with ipratropium. Moderate Anecdotal

▶ Beta₂ agonists are predicted to increase the risk of elevated blood pressure when given with linezolid. Avoid. Severe Theoretical

▶ Macrolides (clarithromycin) are predicted to increase the exposure to salmeterol. Avoid. Severe Study

▶ Monoamine-oxidase A and B inhibitors, irreversible are predicted to increase the risk of cardiovascular side-effects when given with beta₂ agonists. Moderate Anecdotal

▶ Monoamine-oxidase B inhibitors (rasagiline, selegiline) are predicted to increase the risk of severe hypertension when given with beta₂ agonists. Avoid. Severe Theoretical

▶ Monoamine-oxidase B inhibitors (safinamide) are predicted to increase the risk of severe hypertension when given with beta₂ agonists. Severe Theoretical

Betahistine

▶ Antihistamines, non-sedating are predicted to decrease the effects of betahistine. Moderate Theoretical

▶ Antihistamines, sedating are predicted to decrease the effects of betahistine. Moderate Theoretical

Betamethasone → see corticosteroids

Betaxolol → see beta blockers, selective

Bevacizumab → see monoclonal antibodies

Bexarotene → see retinoids

Bezafibrate → see fibrates

Bicalutamide

▶ Bicalutamide is predicted to increase the exposure to lomitapide. Separate administration by 12 hours. Moderate Theoretical

Bilastine → see antihistamines, non-sedating

Biphasic insulin aspart → see insulins

Biphasic insulin lispro → see insulins

Biphasic isophane insulin → see insulins

Bisacodyl → see TABLE 17 p. 822 (reduced serum potassium)

Bisoprolol → see beta blockers, selective

Bisphosphonates → see TABLE 2 p. 818 (nephrotoxicity)

alendronic acid · ibandronic acid · pamidronate · risedronate · sodium clodronate · zoledronic acid

▶ Aminoglycosides increase the risk of hypocalcaemia when given with bisphosphonates. Moderate Anecdotal → Also see TABLE 2 p. 818

▶ Antacids decrease the absorption of alendronic acid. Alendronic acid should be taken at least 30 minutes before antacids. Moderate Study

▶ Antacids are predicted to decrease the absorption of ibandronic acid. Avoid antacids for at least 6 hours before or 1 hour after ibandronic acid. Moderate Theoretical

▶ Antacids decrease the absorption of risedronate. Separate administration by at least 2 hours. Moderate Study

▶ Antacids decrease the absorption of sodium clodronate. Avoid antacids for 2 hours before or 1 hour after sodium clodronate. Moderate Study

‣ **Aspirin** (high-dose) is predicted to increase the risk of gastrointestinal irritation when given with bisphosphonates **(alendronic acid, ibandronic acid)**. Moderate Study

‣ **Aspirin** (high-dose) is predicted to increase the risk of renal impairment when given with **sodium clodronate**. Severe Theoretical

‣ Oral **calcium salts** decrease the absorption of **alendronic acid**. **Alendronic acid** should be taken at least 30 minutes before **calcium salts**. Moderate Study

‣ Oral **calcium salts** are predicted to decrease the absorption of oral **ibandronic acid**. Avoid **calcium salts** for at least 6 hours before or 1 hour after **ibandronic acid**. Moderate Theoretical

‣ Oral **calcium salts** decrease the absorption of **risedronate**. Separate administration by at least 2 hours. Moderate Study

‣ Oral **calcium salts** decrease the absorption of **sodium clodronate**. Avoid **calcium salts** for 2 hours before or 1 hour after **sodium clodronate**. Moderate Study

‣ **Iron (oral)** is predicted to decrease the absorption of oral **ibandronic acid**. Avoid **iron (oral)** for at least 6 hours before or 1 hour after **ibandronic acid**. Moderate Theoretical

‣ **Iron (oral)** decreases the absorption of **risedronate**. Separate administration by at least 2 hours. Moderate Study

‣ **Iron (oral)** decreases the absorption of **sodium clodronate**. Avoid **iron (oral)** for 2 hours before or 1 hour after **sodium clodronate**. Moderate Study

‣ **Bisphosphonates** are predicted to increase the risk of gastrointestinal bleeding when given with iron chelators **(deferasirox)**. Severe Theoretical

‣ Oral **magnesium** decreases the absorption of **alendronic acid**. **Alendronic acid** should be taken at least 30 minutes before **magnesium**. Moderate Study

‣ Oral **magnesium** is predicted to decrease the absorption of oral **ibandronic acid**. Avoid **magnesium** for at least 6 hours before or 1 hour after **ibandronic acid**. Moderate Theoretical

‣ Oral **magnesium** decreases the absorption of **risedronate**. Separate administration by at least 2 hours. Moderate Study

‣ Oral **magnesium** decreases the absorption of **sodium clodronate**. Avoid **magnesium** for 2 hours before or 1 hour after **sodium clodronate**. Moderate Study

‣ **NSAIDs** are predicted to increase the risk of gastrointestinal irritation when given with bisphosphonates **(alendronic acid, ibandronic acid)**. Moderate Study

‣ **NSAIDs** are predicted to increase the risk of renal impairment when given with **sodium clodronate**. Severe Theoretical

‣ Oral **zinc** decreases the absorption of oral **alendronic acid**. **Zinc** should be taken at least 30 minutes before **alendronic acid**. Moderate Study

‣ Oral **zinc** is predicted to decrease the absorption of oral **ibandronic acid**. Avoid **zinc** for at least 6 hours before or 1 hour after **ibandronic acid**. Moderate Theoretical

‣ Oral **zinc** decreases the absorption of oral **risedronate**. Separate administration by at least 2 hours. Moderate Study

‣ Oral **zinc** decreases the absorption of oral **sodium clodronate**. Avoid **zinc** for 2 hours before or 1 hour after **sodium clodronate**. Moderate Study

Bivalirudin → see TABLE 3 p. 818 (anticoagulant effects)

‣ **Ranibizumab** is predicted to increase the risk of bleeding events when given with **bivalirudin**. Moderate Theoretical

Bleomycin → see TABLE 15 p. 821 (myelosuppression), TABLE 5 p. 818 (thromboembolism)

‣ **Live vaccines** are predicted to increase the risk of generalised infection (possibly life-threatening) when given with **bleomycin**. Public Health England advises avoid. Severe Theoretical

‣ Monoclonal antibodies **(brentuximab vedotin)** increase the risk of pulmonary toxicity when given with **bleomycin**. Avoid. Severe Study → Also see TABLE 15 p. 821

‣ Platinum compounds **(cisplatin)** increase the risk of pulmonary toxicity when given with **bleomycin**. Severe Study → Also see TABLE 15 p. 821

Blinatumomab → see monoclonal antibodies

Bortezomib → see TABLE 8 p. 819 (hypotension), TABLE 15 p. 821 (myelosuppression), TABLE 12 p. 821 (peripheral neuropathy)

‣ Antiepileptics **(carbamazepine, fosphenytoin, phenobarbital, phenytoin, primidone)** slightly decrease the exposure to bortezomib. Avoid. Severe Study → Also see TABLE 12 p. 821

‣ Antifungals, azoles **(itraconazole, ketoconazole, voriconazole)** slightly increase the exposure to **bortezomib**. Moderate Study

‣ **Cobicistat** slightly increases the exposure to **bortezomib**. Moderate Study

‣ **Enzalutamide** slightly decreases the exposure to **bortezomib**. Avoid. Severe Study

‣ HIV-protease inhibitors **(atazanavir, darunavir, fosamprenavir, lopinavir, ritonavir, saquinavir, tipranavir)** slightly increase the exposure to **bortezomib**. Moderate Study

‣ **Idelalisib** slightly increases the exposure to **bortezomib**. Moderate Study → Also see TABLE 15 p. 821

‣ Macrolides **(clarithromycin)** slightly increase the exposure to **bortezomib**. Moderate Study

‣ **Rifampicin** slightly decreases the exposure to **bortezomib**. Avoid. Severe Study

Bosentan

‣ **Bosentan** is predicted to decrease the exposure to antiarrhythmics **(dronedarone)**. Severe Theoretical

‣ Antiepileptics **(carbamazepine, fosphenytoin, phenobarbital, phenytoin, primidone)** affect the exposure to **bosentan**. Avoid. Severe Study

‣ Antifungals, azoles **(fluconazole)** are predicted to increase the exposure to **bosentan**. Avoid. Severe Study

‣ Antifungals, azoles **(itraconazole)** are predicted to increase the exposure to **bosentan**. Moderate Theoretical

‣ Antifungals, azoles **(ketoconazole)** moderately increase the exposure to **bosentan**. Moderate Study

‣ Antifungals, azoles **(voriconazole)** are predicted to increase the exposure to **bosentan**. Avoid. Severe Theoretical

‣ **Bosentan** is predicted to decrease the exposure to antifungals, azoles **(isavuconazole)**. Avoid. Severe Theoretical

‣ **Bosentan** is predicted to decrease the exposure to **axitinib**. Moderate Theoretical

‣ **Bosentan** is predicted to decrease the exposure to **bedaquiline**. Avoid. Severe Study

‣ **Bosentan** is predicted to decrease the exposure to **bosutinib**. Avoid. Severe Theoretical

‣ **Bosentan** is predicted to decrease the exposure to **cabozantinib**. Moderate Theoretical

‣ **Bosentan** is predicted to decrease the exposure to calcium channel blockers **(amlodipine, felodipine, isradipine, lacidipine, lercanidipine, nicardipine, nifedipine, nimodipine)**. Monitor and adjust dose. Moderate Theoretical

‣ **Bosentan** is predicted to decrease the exposure to calcium channel blockers **(diltiazem, verapamil)**. Moderate Theoretical

‣ Cephalosporins **(ceftobiprole)** are predicted to increase the exposure to **bosentan**. Moderate Theoretical

‣ **Bosentan** moderately decreases the exposure to ciclosporin and ciclosporin moderately increases the exposure to **bosentan**. Avoid. Severe Study

‣ **Bosentan** is predicted to decrease the exposure to **cobicistat**. Avoid. Severe Theoretical

‣ **Bosentan** is predicted to decrease the exposure to **cobimetinib**. Avoid. Severe Theoretical

‣ **Bosentan** is predicted to decrease the efficacy of combined hormonal contraceptives. For FSRH guidance, see Contraceptives, interactions p. 474. Severe Study

‣ **Bosentan** decreases the anticoagulant effect of **coumarins**. Moderate Study

‣ **Bosentan** is predicted to decrease the exposure to **crizotinib**. Avoid. Severe Theoretical

‣ **Bosentan** is predicted to decrease the exposure to **daclatasvir**. Adjust **daclatasvir** dose. Moderate Theoretical

‣ **Bosentan** is predicted to decrease the exposure to **dasatinib**. Severe Study

‣ **Bosentan** is predicted to decrease the efficacy of **desogestrel**. For FSRH guidance, see Contraceptives, interactions p. 474. Severe Theoretical

‣ **Bosentan** decreases the exposure to **dolutegravir**. Adjust dose. Severe Study

‣ **Bosentan** is predicted to moderately decrease the exposure to **elbasvir**. Avoid. Severe Study

Bosentan (continued)

▸ **Bosentan** is predicted to decrease the concentration of elvitegravir. Avoid. Severe Theoretical

▸ Enzalutamide affects the exposure to **bosentan**. Avoid. Severe Study

▸ **Bosentan** is predicted to decrease the effects of ergotamine. Moderate Theoretical

▸ **Bosentan** is predicted to decrease the exposure to erlotinib. Severe Theoretical

▸ **Bosentan** is predicted to decrease the efficacy of etonogestrel. For FSRH guidance, see Contraceptives, interactions p. 474. Severe Theoretical

▸ **Bosentan** is predicted to decrease the exposure to etravirine. Avoid. Severe Study

▸ **Bosentan** is predicted to decrease the concentration of everolimus. Avoid or adjust dose. Severe Study

▸ **Bosentan** is predicted to decrease the exposure to gefitinib. Avoid. Severe Theoretical

▸ **Bosentan** is predicted to markedly decrease the exposure to grazoprevir. Avoid. Severe Study

▸ **Bosentan** is predicted to decrease the concentration of guanfacine. Adjust dose. Moderate Theoretical

▸ HIV-protease inhibitors are predicted to increase the exposure to **bosentan**. Severe Study

▸ **Bosentan** is predicted to decrease the effects of Hormone replacement therapy. Moderate Anecdotal

▸ **Bosentan** is predicted to decrease the exposure to imatinib. Moderate Study

▸ **Bosentan** is predicted to decrease the exposure to lapatinib. Avoid. Severe Study

▸ **Bosentan** is predicted to decrease the efficacy of levonorgestrel. For FSRH guidance, see Contraceptives, interactions p. 474. Severe Theoretical

▸ **Bosentan** is predicted to decrease the exposure to lurasidone. Monitor and adjust dose. Moderate Theoretical

▸ Macrolides (clarithromycin) are predicted to increase the exposure to **bosentan**. Moderate Theoretical

▸ **Bosentan** is predicted to decrease the exposure to maraviroc. Avoid. Moderate Theoretical

▸ **Bosentan** is predicted to decrease the concentration of midazolam. Monitor and adjust dose. Moderate Theoretical

▸ **Bosentan** is predicted to decrease the exposure to nilotinib. Avoid. Severe Theoretical

▸ **Bosentan** is predicted to decrease the efficacy of norethisterone. For FSRH guidance, see Contraceptives, interactions p. 474. Severe Anecdotal

▸ **Bosentan** is predicted to decrease the exposure to olaparib. Avoid. Moderate Theoretical

▸ **Bosentan** decreases the exposure to opioids (methadone). Monitor and adjust dose. Severe Study

▸ **Bosentan** is predicted to decrease the exposure to osimertinib. Moderate Theoretical

▸ **Bosentan** is predicted to decrease the exposure to paritaprevir (with ritonavir and ombitasvir). Avoid. Severe Study

▸ **Bosentan** decreases the exposure to phosphodiesterase type-5 inhibitors. Moderate Study

▸ Rifampicin affects the exposure to **bosentan**. Avoid. Severe Study

▸ **Bosentan** is predicted to decrease the exposure to rilpivirine. Avoid. Severe Theoretical

▸ **Bosentan** is predicted to decrease the exposure to ruxolitinib. Monitor and adjust dose. Moderate Theoretical

▸ **Bosentan** is predicted to decrease the exposure to simeprevir. Avoid. Severe Study

▸ **Bosentan** is predicted to decrease the concentration of sirolimus and sirolimus potentially increases the concentration of **bosentan**. Avoid. Severe Theoretical

▸ St John's Wort is predicted to decrease the exposure to **bosentan**. Avoid. Moderate Theoretical

▸ **Bosentan** slightly decreases the exposure to statins (atorvastatin). Mild Study

▸ **Bosentan** moderately decreases the exposure to statins (simvastatin). Moderate Study

▸ **Bosentan** increases the risk of hepatotoxicity when given with sulfonylureas (glibenclamide). Avoid. Severe Study

▸ **Bosentan** is predicted to decrease the concentration of tacrolimus and tacrolimus potentially increases the concentration of **bosentan**. Avoid. Severe Theoretical

▸ **Bosentan** is predicted to decrease the exposure to taxanes (cabazitaxel). Avoid. Severe Study

▸ **Bosentan** is predicted to decrease the concentration of temsirolimus. Avoid. Severe Theoretical

▸ **Bosentan** is predicted to decrease the exposure to ticagrelor. Moderate Theoretical

▸ **Bosentan** is predicted to decrease the exposure to tolvaptan. Moderate Theoretical

▸ **Bosentan** decreases the efficacy of ulipristal. For FSRH guidance, see Contraceptives, interactions p. 474. Severe Anecdotal

▸ **Bosentan** is predicted to decrease the exposure to velpatasvir. Avoid. Moderate Theoretical

Bosutinib → see TABLE 15 p. 821 (myelosuppression), TABLE 9 p. 820 (QT-interval prolongation)

▸ Antacids are predicted to decrease the absorption of **bosutinib**. **Bosutinib** should be taken at least 12 hours before antacids. Moderate Theoretical

▸ Antiarrhythmics (dronedarone) are predicted to increase the exposure to **bosutinib**. Avoid or adjust **bosutinib** dose. Severe Theoretical → Also see TABLE 9 p. 820

▸ Antiepileptics (carbamazepine, fosphenytoin, phenobarbital, phenytoin, primidone) are predicted to very markedly decrease the exposure to **bosutinib**. Avoid. Severe Study

▸ Antifungals, azoles (fluconazole, isavuconazole, posaconazole) are predicted to increase the exposure to **bosutinib**. Avoid or adjust **bosutinib** dose. Severe Theoretical

▸ Antifungals, azoles (itraconazole, ketoconazole, voriconazole) are predicted to markedly increase the exposure to **bosutinib**. Avoid or adjust **bosutinib** dose. Severe Study → Also see TABLE 9 p. 820

▸ Aprepitant is predicted to increase the exposure to **bosutinib**. Avoid or adjust **bosutinib** dose. Severe Theoretical

▸ **Bosentan** is predicted to decrease the exposure to **bosutinib**. Avoid. Severe Theoretical

▸ Calcium channel blockers (diltiazem, verapamil) are predicted to increase the exposure to **bosutinib**. Avoid or adjust **bosutinib** dose. Severe Theoretical

▸ Cobicistat is predicted to markedly increase the exposure to **bosutinib**. Avoid or adjust **bosutinib** dose. Severe Study

▸ **Bosutinib** is predicted to increase the risk of bleeding events when given with coumarins. Severe Theoretical

▸ Crizotinib is predicted to increase the exposure to **bosutinib**. Avoid or adjust **bosutinib** dose. Severe Theoretical → Also see TABLE 15 p. 821 → Also see TABLE 9 p. 820

▸ Efavirenz is predicted to decrease the exposure to **bosutinib**. Avoid. Severe Theoretical

▸ Enzalutamide is predicted to very markedly decrease the exposure to **bosutinib**. Avoid. Severe Study

▸ Etravirine is predicted to decrease the exposure to **bosutinib**. Avoid. Severe Theoretical

▸ Fosaprepitant is predicted to increase the exposure to **bosutinib**. Severe Theoretical

▸ Grapefruit juice is predicted to increase the exposure to **bosutinib**. Avoid. Moderate Theoretical

▸ H_2 receptor antagonists are predicted to decrease the absorption of **bosutinib**. Moderate Theoretical

▸ HIV-protease inhibitors (atazanavir, darunavir, fosamprenavir, lopinavir, ritonavir, saquinavir, tipranavir) are predicted to markedly increase the exposure to **bosutinib**. Avoid or adjust **bosutinib** dose. Severe Study → Also see TABLE 9 p. 820

▸ HIV-protease inhibitors (indinavir) are predicted to increase the exposure to **bosutinib**. Avoid or adjust **bosutinib** dose. Severe Theoretical

▸ Idelalisib is predicted to markedly increase the exposure to **bosutinib**. Avoid or adjust **bosutinib** dose. Severe Study → Also see TABLE 15 p. 821

▸ Imatinib is predicted to increase the exposure to **bosutinib**. Avoid or adjust **bosutinib** dose. Severe Theoretical → Also see TABLE 15 p. 821

▸ Macrolides (**clarithromycin**) are predicted to markedly increase the exposure to **bosutinib**. Avoid or adjust **bosutinib** dose. Severe Study → Also see TABLE 9 p. 820

▸ Macrolides (**erythromycin**) are predicted to increase the exposure to **bosutinib**. Avoid or adjust **bosutinib** dose. Severe Theoretical

▸ **Modafinil** is predicted to decrease the exposure to **bosutinib**. Avoid. Severe Theoretical

▸ **Netupitant** is predicted to increase the exposure to **bosutinib**. Avoid or adjust **bosutinib** dose. Severe Theoretical

▸ **Nevirapine** is predicted to decrease the exposure to **bosutinib**. Avoid. Severe Theoretical

▸ **Nilotinib** is predicted to increase the exposure to **bosutinib**. Avoid or adjust **bosutinib** dose. Severe Theoretical → Also see TABLE 15 p. 821 → Also see TABLE 9 p. 820

▸ **Bosutinib** is predicted to increase the risk of bleeding events when given with **phenindione**. Severe Theoretical

▸ **Pitolisant** is predicted to decrease the exposure to **bosutinib**. Avoid. Severe Theoretical

▸ **Proton pump inhibitors** are predicted to decrease the absorption of **bosutinib**. Moderate Study

▸ **Rifampicin** is predicted to very markedly decrease the exposure to **bosutinib**. Avoid. Severe Study

▸ **St John's Wort** is predicted to decrease the exposure to **bosutinib**. Avoid. Severe Theoretical

Botulinum toxin type A → see TABLE 20 p. 822 (neuromuscular blocking effects)

Botulinum toxin type B → see TABLE 20 p. 822 (neuromuscular blocking effects)

Bowel cleansing preparations

SEPARATION OF ADMINISTRATION   Other oral drugs should not be taken 1 hour before, or after, administration of bowel cleansing preparations because absorption may be imparred. Consider withholding ACE inhibitors, angiotensin-II receptor antagonists, and NSAIDs on the day that bowel cleaning preparations are given and for up to 72 hours after the procedure. Also consider witholding diuretics on the day that bowel cleaning preparations are given.

Brentuximab vedotin → see monoclonal antibodies

Brimonidine → see TABLE 6 p. 819 (bradycardia), TABLE 8 p. 819 (hypotension), TABLE 11 p. 820 (CNS depressant effects)

Brinzolamide

ROUTE-SPECIFIC INFORMATION   Since systemic absorption can follow topical application, the possibility of interactions should be borne in mind.

Brivaracetam → see antiepileptics

Bromfenac → see NSAIDs

Bromocriptine → see dopamine receptor agonists

Buclizine → see antihistamines, sedating

Budesonide → see corticosteroids

Bumetanide → see loop diuretics

Bupivacaine → see anaesthetics, local

Buprenorphine → see opioids

Bupropion → see TABLE 13 p. 821 (serotonin syndrome)

▸ **Bupropion** is predicted to increase the exposure to antiarrhythmics (**flecainide**). Severe Theoretical

▸ **Bupropion** is predicted to increase the exposure to antiarrhythmics (**propafenone**). Monitor and adjust dose. Moderate Study

▸ **Bupropion** is predicted to increase the exposure to anticholinesterases, centrally acting (**donepezil**). Moderate Theoretical

▸ **Bupropion** is predicted to increase the exposure to anticholinesterases, centrally acting (**galantamine**). Monitor and adjust dose. Moderate Study

▸ Antiepileptics (**carbamazepine, fosphenytoin, phenobarbital, phenytoin, primidone**) are predicted to markedly decrease the exposure to **bupropion**. Severe Study

▸ Antiepileptics (**valproate**) increase the exposure to **bupropion**. Severe Study

▸ **Bupropion** is predicted to moderately increase the exposure to aripiprazole. Adjust **aripiprazole** dose, p. 240. Moderate Study

▸ **Bupropion** is predicted to markedly increase the exposure to atomoxetine. Adjust dose. Severe Study

▸ **Bupropion** is predicted to increase the exposure to beta blockers, non-selective (**carvedilol, timolol**). Moderate Study

▸ **Bupropion** is predicted to increase the exposure to beta blockers, selective (**metoprolol, nebivolol**). Moderate Study

▸ **Bupropion** is predicted to slightly increase the exposure to darifenacin. Mild Study

▸ **Bupropion** increases the risk of side-effects when given with dopamine receptor agonists (**amantadine**). Moderate Study

▸ **Efavirenz** moderately decreases the exposure to **bupropion**. Moderate Study

▸ **Enzalutamide** is predicted to markedly decrease the exposure to **bupropion**. Severe Study

▸ HIV-protease inhibitors (**ritonavir**) slightly to moderately decrease the exposure to **bupropion**. Moderate Study

▸ **Bupropion** increases the risk of side-effects when given with levodopa. Moderate Study

▸ **Bupropion** is predicted to increase the risk of intraoperative hypertension when given with **linezolid**. Severe Anecdotal → Also see TABLE 13 p. 821

▸ **Lumacaftor** is predicted to decrease the exposure to **bupropion**. Adjust dose. Moderate Theoretical

▸ **Methylthioninium chloride** is predicted to increase the risk of severe hypertension when given with **bupropion**. Avoid. Severe Theoretical → Also see TABLE 13 p. 821

▸ **Moclobemide** is predicted to increase the risk of severe hypertension when given with **bupropion**. Avoid. Severe Theoretical → Also see TABLE 13 p. 821

▸ **Monoamine-oxidase A and B inhibitors, irreversible** are predicted to increase the risk of severe hypertension when given with **bupropion**. Avoid and for 14 days after stopping the MAOI. Severe Theoretical → Also see TABLE 13 p. 821

▸ **Monoamine-oxidase B inhibitors** are predicted to increase the risk of severe hypertension when given with **bupropion**. Avoid. Moderate Theoretical → Also see TABLE 13 p. 821

▸ **Bupropion** is predicted to decrease the efficacy of opioids (**codeine**). Moderate Theoretical

▸ **Bupropion** is predicted to decrease the efficacy of opioids (**tramadol**). Severe Study → Also see TABLE 13 p. 821

▸ **Bupropion** is predicted to moderately increase the exposure to pitolisant. Use with caution and adjust dose. Moderate Study

▸ **Rifampicin** is predicted to markedly decrease the exposure to **bupropion**. Severe Study

▸ **Bupropion** is predicted to increase the exposure to risperidone. Adjust dose. Moderate Study

▸ **Bupropion** is predicted to increase the exposure to SSRIs (**dapoxetine**). Moderate Theoretical → Also see TABLE 13 p. 821

▸ **Bupropion** is predicted to decrease the efficacy of tamoxifen. Avoid. Severe Study

▸ **Bupropion** is predicted to increase the exposure to tricyclic antidepressants. Monitor for toxicity and adjust dose. Severe Study → Also see TABLE 13 p. 821

▸ **Bupropion** is predicted to increase the exposure to vortioxetine. Monitor and adjust dose. Moderate Study → Also see TABLE 13 p. 821

Buspirone → see TABLE 13 p. 821 (serotonin syndrome)

▸ Antiarrhythmics (**dronedarone**) are predicted to increase the exposure to **buspirone**. Use with caution and adjust dose. Moderate Study

▸ Antiepileptics (**carbamazepine, fosphenytoin, phenobarbital, phenytoin, primidone**) are predicted to decrease the exposure to **buspirone**. Use with caution and adjust dose. Severe Study

▸ Antifungals, azoles (**fluconazole, isavuconazole, posaconazole**) are predicted to increase the exposure to **buspirone**. Use with caution and adjust dose. Moderate Study

▸ Antifungals, azoles (**itraconazole, ketoconazole, voriconazole**) are predicted to increase the exposure to **buspirone**. Adjust **buspirone** dose. Severe Study

▸ Antifungals, azoles (**miconazole**) are predicted to increase the concentration of **buspirone**. Use with caution and adjust dose. Moderate Theoretical

▸ **Aprepitant** is predicted to increase the exposure to **buspirone**. Use with caution and adjust dose. Moderate Study

▸ Calcium channel blockers (**diltiazem, verapamil**) are predicted to increase the exposure to **buspirone**. Use with caution and adjust dose. Moderate Study

Buspirone (continued)

▸ Cobicistat is predicted to increase the exposure to buspirone. Adjust buspirone dose. Severe Study

▸ Crizotinib is predicted to increase the exposure to buspirone. Use with caution and adjust dose. Moderate Study

▸ Enzalutamide is predicted to decrease the exposure to buspirone. Use with caution and adjust dose. Severe Study

▸ Grapefruit juice increases the exposure to buspirone. Avoid. Mild Study

▸ HIV-protease inhibitors (atazanavir, darunavir, fosamprenavir, lopinavir, ritonavir, saquinavir, tipranavir) are predicted to increase the exposure to buspirone. Adjust buspirone dose. Severe Study

▸ HIV-protease inhibitors (indinavir) are predicted to increase the exposure to buspirone. Use with caution and adjust dose. Moderate Study

▸ Idelalisib is predicted to increase the exposure to buspirone. Adjust buspirone dose. Severe Study

▸ Imatinib is predicted to increase the exposure to buspirone. Use with caution and adjust dose. Moderate Study

▸ Buspirone is predicted to increase the risk of elevated blood pressure when given with linezolid. Avoid. Severe Theoretical → Also see TABLE 13 p. 821

▸ Macrolides (clarithromycin) are predicted to increase the exposure to buspirone. Adjust buspirone dose. Severe Study

▸ Macrolides (erythromycin) are predicted to increase the exposure to buspirone. Use with caution and adjust dose. Moderate Study

▸ Buspirone is predicted to increase the risk of elevated blood pressure when given with monoamine-oxidase A and B inhibitors, irreversible. Avoid. Severe Anecdotal → Also see TABLE 13 p. 821

▸ Netupitant is predicted to increase the exposure to buspirone. Use with caution and adjust dose. Moderate Study

▸ Nilotinib is predicted to increase the exposure to buspirone. Use with caution and adjust dose. Moderate Study

▸ Rifampicin is predicted to decrease the exposure to buspirone. Use with caution and adjust dose. Severe Study

Busulfan → see alkylating agents
Cabazitaxel → see taxanes
Cabergoline → see dopamine receptor agonists
Cabozantinib → see TABLE 15 p. 821 (myelosuppression), TABLE 9 p. 820 (QT-interval prolongation)

▸ Antiarrhythmics (dronedarone) are predicted to increase the exposure to cabozantinib. Moderate Theoretical → Also see TABLE 9 p. 820

▸ Antiepileptics (carbamazepine, fosphenytoin, phenobarbital, phenytoin, primidone) moderately decrease the exposure to cabozantinib. Avoid. Moderate Study

▸ Antifungals, azoles (fluconazole, isavuconazole, posaconazole) are predicted to increase the exposure to cabozantinib. Moderate Theoretical

▸ Antifungals, azoles (itraconazole, ketoconazole, voriconazole) slightly increase the exposure to cabozantinib. Moderate Study → Also see TABLE 9 p. 820

▸ Aprepitant is predicted to increase the exposure to cabozantinib. Moderate Theoretical

▸ Bosentan is predicted to decrease the exposure to cabozantinib. Moderate Theoretical

▸ Calcium channel blockers (diltiazem, verapamil) are predicted to increase the exposure to cabozantinib. Moderate Theoretical

▸ Cobicistat slightly increases the exposure to cabozantinib. Moderate Study

▸ Cabozantinib is predicted to increase the risk of bleeding events when given with coumarins. Severe Theoretical

▸ Crizotinib is predicted to increase the exposure to cabozantinib. Moderate Theoretical → Also see TABLE 15 p. 821 → Also see TABLE 9 p. 820

▸ Efavirenz is predicted to decrease the exposure to cabozantinib. Moderate Theoretical

▸ Enzalutamide moderately decreases the exposure to cabozantinib. Avoid. Moderate Study

▸ Grapefruit juice is predicted to increase the exposure to cabozantinib. Moderate Theoretical

▸ HIV-protease inhibitors (atazanavir, darunavir, fosamprenavir, lopinavir, ritonavir, saquinavir, tipranavir) slightly increase the exposure to cabozantinib. Moderate Study → Also see TABLE 9 p. 820

▸ HIV-protease inhibitors (indinavir) are predicted to increase the exposure to cabozantinib. Moderate Theoretical

▸ Idelalisib slightly increases the exposure to cabozantinib. Moderate Study → Also see TABLE 15 p. 821

▸ Imatinib is predicted to increase the exposure to cabozantinib. Moderate Theoretical → Also see TABLE 15 p. 821

▸ Macrolides (clarithromycin) slightly increase the exposure to cabozantinib. Moderate Study → Also see TABLE 9 p. 820

▸ Macrolides (erythromycin) are predicted to increase the exposure to cabozantinib. Moderate Theoretical

▸ Netupitant is predicted to increase the exposure to cabozantinib. Moderate Theoretical

▸ Nevirapine is predicted to decrease the exposure to cabozantinib. Moderate Theoretical

▸ Nilotinib is predicted to increase the exposure to cabozantinib. Moderate Theoretical → Also see TABLE 15 p. 821 → Also see TABLE 9 p. 820

▸ Cabozantinib is predicted to increase the risk of bleeding events when given with phenindione. Severe Theoretical

▸ Rifampicin moderately decreases the exposure to cabozantinib. Avoid. Moderate Study

▸ St John's Wort is predicted to decrease the exposure to cabozantinib. Moderate Theoretical

Caffeine citrate

▸ Caffeine citrate decreases the efficacy of antiarrhythmics (adenosine). Separate administration by 24 hours. Mild Study

▸ Antiepileptics (fosphenytoin, phenytoin) are predicted to moderately increase the clearance of caffeine citrate. Monitor and adjust dose. Moderate Study

▸ HIV-protease inhibitors (ritonavir) are predicted to moderately increase the clearance of caffeine citrate. Monitor and adjust dose. Moderate Study

▸ Rifampicin is predicted to moderately increase the clearance of caffeine citrate. Monitor and adjust dose. Moderate Study

▸ SSRIs (fluvoxamine) markedly decrease the clearance of caffeine citrate. Monitor and adjust dose. Severe Study

▸ Caffeine citrate decreases the clearance of theophylline. Moderate Study

Calcipotriol → see vitamin D substances
Calcitonin (salmon)

▸ Calcitonin (salmon) decreases the concentration of lithium. Monitor lithium concentration and adjust dose. Moderate Study

Calcitriol → see vitamin D substances
Calcium acetate → see calcium salts
Calcium carbonate → see calcium salts
Calcium channel blockers → see TABLE 6 p. 819 (bradycardia), TABLE 8 p. 819 (hypotension)

amlodipine · clevidipine · diltiazem · felodipine · isradipine · lacidipine · lercanidipine · nicardipine · nifedipine · nimodipine · verapamil

▸ Verapamil is predicted to increase the exposure to afatinib. Separate administration by 12 hours. Moderate Study

▸ Calcium channel blockers (diltiazem, verapamil) are predicted to increase the exposure to aldosterone antagonists (eplerenone). Adjust eplerenone dose. Severe Study → Also see TABLE 8 p. 819

▸ Verapamil moderately increases the exposure to aliskiren. Moderate Study → Also see TABLE 8 p. 819

▸ Calcium channel blockers (diltiazem, verapamil) are predicted to increase the exposure to alpha blockers (tamsulosin). Moderate Theoretical → Also see TABLE 8 p. 819

▸ Calcium channel blockers (diltiazem, verapamil) are predicted to increase the exposure to alprazolam. Severe Study

▸ Verapamil moderately increases the exposure to anthracyclines (doxorubicin). Moderate Study

▸ Antiarrhythmics (disopyramide) are predicted to increase the risk of cardiodepression when given with verapamil. Severe Theoretical

▸ Antiarrhythmics (dronedarone) are predicted to increase the exposure to calcium channel blockers (amlodipine, felodipine, isradipine, lacidipine, lercanidipine, nicardipine, nifedipine, nimodipine). Monitor and adjust dose. Moderate Study

▶ Antiarrhythmics **(amiodarone)** are predicted to increase the risk of cardiodepression when given with calcium channel blockers **(diltiazem, verapamil)**. Avoid. Severe Theoretical → Also see **TABLE 6** p. 819

▶ Calcium channel blockers **(diltiazem, verapamil)** increase the exposure to antiarrhythmics **(dronedarone)** and antiarrhythmics **(dronedarone)** increase the exposure to calcium channel blockers **(diltiazem, verapamil)**. Moderate

▶ Verapamil increases the risk of cardiodepression when given with antiarrhythmics **(flecainide)**. Severe Anecdotal → Also see **TABLE 6** p. 819

▶ Calcium channel blockers **(diltiazem, verapamil)** are predicted to increase the exposure to antiarrhythmics **(propafenone)**. Monitor and adjust dose. Moderate Study

▶ Calcium channel blockers **(diltiazem, verapamil)** increase the risk of bradycardia when given with anticholinesterases, centrally acting. Moderate Anecdotal → Also see **TABLE 6** p. 819

▶ Antiepileptics **(carbamazepine, fosphenytoin, phenobarbital, phenytoin, primidone)** decrease the exposure to diltiazem. Severe Study

▶ Antiepileptics **(carbamazepine, fosphenytoin, phenobarbital, phenytoin, primidone)** decrease the exposure to isradipine. Avoid. Moderate Study

▶ Antiepileptics **(carbamazepine, fosphenytoin, phenobarbital, phenytoin, primidone)** are predicted to decrease the exposure to verapamil. Severe Study

▶ Antiepileptics **(carbamazepine, fosphenytoin, phenobarbital, phenytoin, primidone)** are predicted to decrease the exposure to calcium channel blockers **(amlodipine, felodipine, lacidipine, lercanidipine, nicardipine, nifedipine, nimodipine)**. Monitor and adjust dose. Moderate Study

▶ Calcium channel blockers **(diltiazem, verapamil)** increase the concentration of antiepileptics **(carbamazepine)**. Severe Anecdotal

▶ Antifungals, azoles **(itraconazole, ketoconazole, voriconazole)** are predicted to markedly increase the exposure to lercanidipine. Avoid. Severe Study

▶ Antifungals, azoles **(miconazole)** are predicted to increase the exposure to calcium channel blockers **(amlodipine, clevidipine, felodipine, isradipine, lacidipine, lercanidipine, nicardipine, nifedipine, nimodipine, verapamil)**. Use with caution and adjust dose. Moderate Theoretical

▶ Antifungals, azoles **(fluconazole, isavuconazole, itraconazole, ketoconazole, posaconazole, voriconazole)** are predicted to increase the exposure to calcium channel blockers **(amlodipine, felodipine, isradipine, lacidipine, nicardipine, nifedipine, nimodipine)**. Monitor and adjust dose. Moderate Study

▶ Antifungals, azoles **(fluconazole)** (high-dose) are predicted to increase the exposure to calcium channel blockers **(diltiazem, verapamil)**. Moderate Theoretical

▶ Antifungals, azoles **(itraconazole, ketoconazole, voriconazole)** are predicted to increase the exposure to calcium channel blockers **(diltiazem, verapamil)**. Severe Study

▶ Antifungals, azoles **(posaconazole)** are predicted to increase the exposure to calcium channel blockers **(diltiazem, verapamil)**. Moderate Theoretical

▶ Calcium channel blockers **(diltiazem, verapamil)** are predicted to increase the exposure to antifungals, azoles **(isavuconazole)**. Moderate Theoretical

▶ Calcium channel blockers **(diltiazem, verapamil)** are predicted to increase the exposure to antihistamines, non-sedating **(mizolastine)**. Severe Theoretical

▶ Antimalarials **(mefloquine)** are predicted to increase the risk of bradycardia when given with calcium channel blockers. Severe Theoretical

▶ Calcium channel blockers **(diltiazem, verapamil)** are predicted to increase the concentration of antimalarials **(piperaquine)**. Severe Theoretical

▶ Verapamil is predicted to increase the exposure to apixaban. Moderate Theoretical

▶ Aprepitant is predicted to increase the exposure to calcium channel blockers **(amlodipine, felodipine, isradipine, lacidipine, lercanidipine, nicardipine, nifedipine, nimodipine)**. Monitor and adjust dose. Moderate Study

▶ Diltiazem increases the exposure to aprepitant and aprepitant increases the exposure to diltiazem. Moderate Study

▶ Verapamil is predicted to increase the exposure to aprepitant and aprepitant is predicted to increase the exposure to verapamil. Moderate Theoretical

▶ Calcium channel blockers **(diltiazem, verapamil)** are predicted to increase the exposure to axitinib. Moderate Theoretical

▶ Calcium channel blockers **(diltiazem, verapamil)** are predicted to increase the exposure to bedaquiline. Avoid prolonged use. Mild Theoretical

▶ Diltiazem is predicted to increase the risk of cardiodepression when given with beta blockers, non-selective. Severe Study → Also see **TABLE 6** p. 819 → Also see **TABLE 8** p. 819

▶ Intravenous verapamil increases the risk of cardiovascular side-effects when given with beta blockers, non-selective. Avoid. Severe Study → Also see **TABLE 6** p. 819 → Also see **TABLE 8** p. 819

▶ Oral verapamil increases the risk of cardiovascular side-effects when given with beta blockers, non-selective. Severe Study → Also see **TABLE 6** p. 819 → Also see **TABLE 8** p. 819

▶ Diltiazem is predicted to increase the risk of cardiodepression when given with beta blockers, selective. Severe Study → Also see **TABLE 6** p. 819 → Also see **TABLE 8** p. 819

▶ Intravenous verapamil increases the risk of cardiovascular side-effects when given with beta blockers, selective. Avoid. Severe Study → Also see **TABLE 6** p. 819 → Also see **TABLE 8** p. 819

▶ Oral verapamil increases the risk of cardiovascular side-effects when given with beta blockers, selective. Severe Study → Also see **TABLE 6** p. 819 → Also see **TABLE 8** p. 819

▶ Bosentan is predicted to decrease the exposure to calcium channel blockers **(amlodipine, felodipine, isradipine, lacidipine, lercanidipine, nicardipine, nifedipine, nimodipine)**. Monitor and adjust dose. Moderate Theoretical

▶ Bosentan is predicted to decrease the exposure to calcium channel blockers **(diltiazem, verapamil)**. Moderate Theoretical

▶ Calcium channel blockers **(diltiazem, verapamil)** are predicted to increase the exposure to bosutinib. Avoid or adjust bosutinib dose. Severe Theoretical

▶ Calcium channel blockers **(diltiazem, verapamil)** are predicted to increase the exposure to buspirone. Use with caution and adjust dose. Moderate Study

▶ Calcium channel blockers **(diltiazem, verapamil)** are predicted to increase the exposure to cabozantinib. Moderate Theoretical

▶ Calcium channel blockers **(diltiazem)** are predicted to increase the exposure to calcium channel blockers **(amlodipine)**. Monitor and adjust dose. Moderate Study → Also see **TABLE 8** p. 819

▶ Calcium channel blockers **(verapamil)** are predicted to increase the exposure to calcium channel blockers **(amlodipine, felodipine, isradipine, lacidipine, lercanidipine, nicardipine, nifedipine, nimodipine)**. Monitor and adjust dose. Moderate Study → Also see **TABLE 8** p. 819

▶ Calcium channel blockers **(diltiazem)** are predicted to increase the exposure to calcium channel blockers **(felodipine, isradipine, lacidipine, lercanidipine, nicardipine, nifedipine, nimodipine)**. Monitor and adjust dose. Moderate Study → Also see **TABLE 8** p. 819

▶ Calcium channel blockers **(diltiazem, verapamil)** are predicted to increase the exposure to ceritinib. Moderate Theoretical

▶ Calcium channel blockers **(diltiazem, nicardipine, verapamil)** increase the concentration of ciclosporin. Severe Study

▶ Ciclosporin moderately increases the exposure to lercanidipine. Use with caution or avoid. Severe Study

▶ Cobicistat is predicted to increase the exposure to calcium channel blockers **(amlodipine, felodipine, isradipine, lacidipine, nicardipine, nifedipine, nimodipine)**. Monitor and adjust dose. Moderate Study

▶ Cobicistat is predicted to increase the exposure to calcium channel blockers **(diltiazem, verapamil)**. Severe Study

▶ Cobicistat is predicted to markedly increase the exposure to lercanidipine. Avoid. Severe Study

▶ Calcium channel blockers **(diltiazem, verapamil)** are predicted to increase the exposure to cobimetinib. Severe Theoretical

▶ Calcium channel blockers **(diltiazem, verapamil)** are predicted to increase the exposure to colchicine. Adjust colchicine dose. Severe Study

Calcium channel blockers (continued)

▶ Calcium channel blockers **(diltiazem, verapamil)** are predicted to increase the exposure to corticosteroids **(methylprednisolone)**. Monitor and adjust dose. Moderate Study

▶ Calcium channel blockers **(diltiazem, verapamil)** are predicted to increase the exposure to **crizotinib**. Moderate Theoretical → Also see **TABLE 6** p. 819

▶ Crizotinib is predicted to increase the exposure to calcium channel blockers **(amlodipine, felodipine, isradipine, lacidipine, lercanidipine, nicardipine, nifedipine, nimodipine)**. Monitor and adjust dose. Moderate Study

▶ Verapamil increases the exposure to **dabigatran**. Adjust **dabigatran** dose. Severe Study

▶ Intravenous **dantrolene** potentially increases the risk of acute hyperkalaemia and cardiovascular collapse when given with calcium channel blockers **(diltiazem, verapamil)**. Avoid. Severe Anecdotal

▶ Calcium channel blockers **(diltiazem, verapamil)** are predicted to slightly increase the exposure to **darifenacin**. Moderate Study

▶ Calcium channel blockers **(diltiazem, verapamil)** are predicted to increase the exposure to **dasatinib**. Severe Study

▶ Calcium channel blockers **(diltiazem, verapamil)** increase the concentration of **digoxin**. Monitor and adjust dose. Severe Study → Also see **TABLE 6** p. 819

▶ Calcium channel blockers **(diltiazem, verapamil)** increase the risk of QT-prolongation when given with **domperidone**. Avoid. Severe Study

▶ Calcium channel blockers **(diltiazem, verapamil)** are predicted to increase the exposure to dopamine receptor agonists **(bromocriptine, cabergoline)**. Severe Theoretical → Also see **TABLE 8** p. 819

▶ Calcium channel blockers **(diltiazem, verapamil)** are predicted to moderately increase the exposure to **dutasteride**. Mild Study

▶ Verapamil is predicted to slightly increase the exposure to **edoxaban**. Severe Theoretical

▶ Efavirenz is predicted to decrease the exposure to calcium channel blockers **(amlodipine, felodipine, isradipine, lacidipine, lercanidipine, nicardipine, nifedipine, nimodipine)**. Monitor and adjust dose. Moderate Theoretical

▶ Efavirenz is predicted to decrease the exposure to calcium channel blockers **(diltiazem, verapamil)**. Moderate Theoretical

▶ Enzalutamide is predicted to decrease the exposure to calcium channel blockers **(amlodipine, felodipine, lacidipine, lercanidipine, nicardipine, nifedipine, nimodipine)**. Monitor and adjust dose. Moderate Study

▶ Enzalutamide decreases the exposure to **diltiazem**. Severe Study

▶ Enzalutamide decreases the exposure to **isradipine**. Avoid. Moderate Study

▶ Enzalutamide is predicted to decrease the exposure to **verapamil**. Severe Study

▶ Calcium channel blockers **(diltiazem, verapamil)** are predicted to increase the risk of ergotism when given with **ergometrine**. Severe Theoretical

▶ Calcium channel blockers **(diltiazem, verapamil)** are predicted to increase the risk of ergotism when given with **ergotamine**. Severe Theoretical

▶ Calcium channel blockers **(diltiazem, verapamil)** are predicted to increase the exposure to **erlotinib**. Moderate Theoretical

▶ Calcium channel blockers **(diltiazem, verapamil)** are predicted to increase the concentration of **everolimus**. Avoid or adjust dose. Moderate Study

▶ Calcium channel blockers **(diltiazem, verapamil)** are predicted to increase the exposure to **fesoterodine**. Adjust **fesoterodine** dose in hepatic and renal impairment. Mild Study

▶ Verapamil is predicted to increase the exposure to **fidaxomicin**. Avoid. Moderate Study

▶ Calcium channel blockers **(diltiazem, verapamil)** are predicted to increase the exposure to **fingolimod**. Avoid. Moderate Theoretical → Also see **TABLE 6** p. 819

▶ Calcium channel blockers **(diltiazem, verapamil)** are predicted to increase the exposure to **gefitinib**. Moderate Theoretical

▶ Grapefruit juice very slightly increases the exposure to **amlodipine**. Avoid. Mild Study

▶ Grapefruit juice increases the exposure to calcium channel blockers **(nifedipine, verapamil)**. Avoid. Mild Study

▶ Grapefruit juice increases the exposure to **felodipine**. Avoid. Moderate Study

▶ Grapefruit juice is predicted to increase the exposure to **lercanidipine**. Avoid. Moderate Theoretical

▶ Grapefruit juice increases the exposure to **nicardipine**. Mild Study

▶ Calcium channel blockers **(diltiazem, verapamil)** are predicted to increase the concentration of **guanfacine**. Adjust **guanfacine** dose, p. 222. Moderate Theoretical → Also see **TABLE 8** p. 819

▶ H₂ receptor antagonists **(cimetidine)** (high-dose) are predicted to increase the exposure to **lercanidipine**. Moderate Theoretical

▶ H₂ receptor antagonists **(cimetidine)** moderately increase the exposure to **nifedipine**. Monitor and adjust dose. Severe Study

▶ H₂ receptor antagonists **(cimetidine)** increase the exposure to **verapamil**. Moderate Study

▶ H₂ receptor antagonists **(cimetidine)** slightly increase the exposure to calcium channel blockers **(diltiazem, isradipine, nimodipine)**. Monitor and adjust dose. Moderate Study

▶ HIV-protease inhibitors **(atazanavir, darunavir, fosamprenavir, lopinavir, ritonavir, saquinavir, tipranavir)** are predicted to markedly increase the exposure to **lercanidipine**. Avoid. Severe Study

▶ HIV-protease inhibitors are predicted to increase the exposure to calcium channel blockers **(amlodipine, felodipine, isradipine, lacidipine, nicardipine, nifedipine, nimodipine)**. Monitor and adjust dose. Moderate Study

▶ HIV-protease inhibitors **(atazanavir, darunavir, fosamprenavir, lopinavir, ritonavir, saquinavir, tipranavir)** are predicted to increase the exposure to calcium channel blockers **(diltiazem, verapamil)**. Severe Study

▶ Calcium channel blockers **(diltiazem, verapamil)** are predicted to increase the exposure to **ibrutinib**. Avoid or adjust **ibrutinib** dose. Severe Theoretical

▶ Idelalisib is predicted to increase the exposure to calcium channel blockers **(amlodipine, felodipine, isradipine, lacidipine, nicardipine, nifedipine, nimodipine)**. Monitor and adjust dose. Moderate Study

▶ Idelalisib is predicted to increase the exposure to calcium channel blockers **(diltiazem, verapamil)**. Severe Study

▶ Idelalisib is predicted to markedly increase the exposure to **lercanidipine**. Avoid. Severe Study

▶ Calcium channel blockers **(diltiazem, verapamil)** are predicted to increase the exposure to **imatinib**. Moderate Theoretical

▶ Imatinib is predicted to increase the exposure to calcium channel blockers **(amlodipine, felodipine, isradipine, lacidipine, lercanidipine, nicardipine, nifedipine, nimodipine)**. Monitor and adjust dose. Moderate Study

▶ Calcium channel blockers **(diltiazem, verapamil)** are predicted to increase the exposure to **ivabradine**. Avoid. Moderate Study → Also see **TABLE 6** p. 819

▶ Calcium channel blockers **(diltiazem, verapamil)** are predicted to increase the exposure to **ivacaftor**. Adjust **ivacaftor** dose, p. 179. Severe Study

▶ Calcium channel blockers **(diltiazem, verapamil)** are predicted to increase the exposure to **lapatinib**. Moderate Study

▶ Calcium channel blockers **(diltiazem, verapamil)** are predicted to increase the risk of neurotoxicity when given with **lithium**. Severe Anecdotal

▶ Calcium channel blockers **(amlodipine, lacidipine)** are predicted to increase the exposure to **lomitapide**. Separate administration by 12 hours. Moderate Theoretical

▶ Calcium channel blockers **(diltiazem, verapamil)** are predicted to increase the exposure to **lomitapide**. Avoid. Moderate Theoretical

▶ Calcium channel blockers **(diltiazem, verapamil)** are predicted to increase the exposure to **lurasidone**. Moderate Study → Also see **TABLE 8** p. 819

▶ Macrolides **(clarithromycin)** are predicted to markedly increase the exposure to **lercanidipine**. Avoid. Severe Study

▶ Macrolides **(erythromycin)** are predicted to increase the exposure to **diltiazem**. Severe Theoretical

▶ Macrolides **(erythromycin)** are predicted to increase the exposure to **verapamil**. Severe Study

▶ Macrolides **(clarithromycin, erythromycin)** are predicted to increase the exposure to calcium channel blockers **(amlodipine, felodipine, isradipine, lacidipine, lercanidipine, nicardipine,** nifedipine, nimodipine). Monitor and adjust dose. Moderate Study

▸ Macrolides (clarithromycin) are predicted to increase the exposure to calcium channel blockers (diltiazem, verapamil). Severe Study

▸ Intravenous magnesium potentially increases the risk of hypotension when given with calcium channel blockers (amlodipine, clevidipine, felodipine, isradipine, lacidipine, lercanidipine, nicardipine, nifedipine, nimodipine, verapamil) in pregnant women. Severe Anecdotal

▸ Calcium channel blockers (diltiazem, verapamil) are predicted to increase the exposure to midazolam. Monitor side effects and adjust dose. Severe Study

▸ Calcium channel blockers (diltiazem, verapamil) are predicted to increase the exposure to naloxegol. Adjust naloxegol dose and monitor side effects. Moderate Study

▸ Netupitant is predicted to increase the exposure to calcium channel blockers (amlodipine, felodipine, isradipine, lacidipine, lercanidipine, nicardipine, nifedipine, nimodipine). Monitor and adjust dose. Moderate Study

▸ Nevirapine is predicted to decrease the exposure to calcium channel blockers (amlodipine, felodipine, isradipine, lacidipine, lercanidipine, nicardipine, nifedipine, nimodipine). Monitor and adjust dose. Moderate Theoretical

▸ Nevirapine is predicted to decrease the exposure to calcium channel blockers (diltiazem, verapamil). Moderate Theoretical

▸ Calcium channel blockers (diltiazem, verapamil) are predicted to increase the exposure to nilotinib. Moderate Theoretical

▸ Nilotinib is predicted to increase the exposure to calcium channel blockers (amlodipine, felodipine, isradipine, lacidipine, lercanidipine, nicardipine, nifedipine, nimodipine). Monitor and adjust dose. Moderate Study

▸ Verapamil is predicted to increase the exposure to nintedanib. Moderate Study

▸ Calcium channel blockers (diltiazem, verapamil) are predicted to increase the exposure to olaparib. Avoid or adjust olaparib dose. Moderate Theoretical

▸ Calcium channel blockers (diltiazem, verapamil) are predicted to increase the exposure to opioids (alfentanil, buprenorphine, fentanyl, oxycodone). Monitor and adjust dose. Moderate Study → Also see TABLE 6 p. 819

▸ Calcium channel blockers (diltiazem, verapamil) are predicted to increase the exposure to opioids (methadone, sufentanil). Moderate Theoretical → Also see TABLE 6 p. 819

▸ Calcium channel blockers (diltiazem, verapamil) are predicted to increase the exposure to oxybutynin. Mild Theoretical

▸ Calcium channel blockers (diltiazem, verapamil) are predicted to increase the exposure to pazopanib. Moderate Theoretical

▸ Calcium channel blockers (diltiazem, verapamil) are predicted to increase the exposure to phosphodiesterase type-5 inhibitors (avanafil). Adjust avanafil dose. Moderate Theoretical → Also see TABLE 8 p. 819

▸ Calcium channel blockers (diltiazem, verapamil) are predicted to increase the exposure to phosphodiesterase type-5 inhibitors (sildenafil). Monitor and adjust sildenafil dose, p. 117. Moderate Study → Also see TABLE 8 p. 819

▸ Calcium channel blockers (diltiazem, verapamil) are predicted to increase the exposure to phosphodiesterase type-5 inhibitors (tadalafil). Severe Theoretical → Also see TABLE 8 p. 819

▸ Calcium channel blockers (diltiazem, verapamil) are predicted to increase the exposure to phosphodiesterase type-5 inhibitors (vardenafil). Adjust dose. Severe Theoretical → Also see TABLE 8 p. 819

▸ Calcium channel blockers (diltiazem, verapamil) are predicted to increase the exposure to pimozide. Avoid. Severe Theoretical → Also see TABLE 8 p. 819

▸ Calcium channel blockers (diltiazem, verapamil) are predicted to increase the exposure to quetiapine. Avoid. Moderate Study → Also see TABLE 8 p. 819

▸ Calcium channel blockers (diltiazem, verapamil) are predicted to increase the exposure to ranolazine. Severe Study

▸ Rifampicin is predicted to decrease the exposure to calcium channel blockers (amlodipine, felodipine, lacidipine, lercanidipine, nicardipine, nimodipine). Monitor and adjust dose. Moderate Study

▸ Rifampicin decreases the exposure to diltiazem. Severe Study

▸ Rifampicin decreases the exposure to isradipine. Avoid. Moderate Study

▸ Rifampicin moderately decreases the exposure to nifedipine. Avoid. Severe Study

▸ Rifampicin is predicted to decrease the exposure to verapamil. Severe Study

▸ Calcium channel blockers (diltiazem, verapamil) are predicted to increase the exposure to ruxolitinib. Moderate Theoretical

▸ Calcium channel blockers (diltiazem, verapamil) are predicted to increase the exposure to saxagliptin. Mild Study

▸ Calcium channel blockers (diltiazem, verapamil) are predicted to increase the exposure to simeprevir. Avoid. Severe Study

▸ Calcium channel blockers (diltiazem, verapamil) increase the concentration of sirolimus. Monitor and adjust dose. Moderate Study

▸ Calcium channel blockers (diltiazem, verapamil) are predicted to increase the exposure to SSRIs (dapoxetine). Adjust dapoxetine dose. Moderate Theoretical

▸ St John's Wort is predicted to decrease the exposure to calcium channel blockers (amlodipine, felodipine, isradipine, lacidipine, lercanidipine, nicardipine, nifedipine, nimodipine). Monitor and adjust dose. Moderate Theoretical

▸ St John's Wort is predicted to decrease the exposure to calcium channel blockers (diltiazem, verapamil). Moderate Theoretical

▸ Calcium channel blockers (diltiazem, verapamil) are predicted to increase the exposure to statins (atorvastatin). Monitor and adjust dose. Severe Theoretical

▸ Amlodipine slightly increases the exposure to statins (simvastatin). Adjust simvastatin dose, p. 130. Mild Study

▸ Calcium channel blockers (diltiazem, verapamil) are predicted to increase the exposure to statins (simvastatin). Use with caution and adjust simvastatin dose, p. 130. Severe Study

▸ Sulfinpyrazone decreases the exposure to verapamil. Moderate Study

▸ Calcium channel blockers (diltiazem, verapamil) are predicted to increase the exposure to sunitinib. Moderate Theoretical

▸ Calcium channel blockers (diltiazem, verapamil) are predicted to increase the concentration of tacrolimus. Severe Study

▸ Nicardipine potentially increases the concentration of tacrolimus. Monitor concentration and adjust dose. Severe Anecdotal

▸ Calcium channel blockers (diltiazem, verapamil) are predicted to increase the exposure to taxanes (cabazitaxel). Moderate Theoretical

▸ Calcium channel blockers (diltiazem, verapamil) are predicted to increase the concentration of temsirolimus. Moderate Theoretical

▸ Calcium channel blockers (diltiazem, verapamil) are predicted to increase the exposure to tolterodine. Mild Theoretical

▸ Calcium channel blockers (diltiazem, verapamil) are predicted to increase the exposure to tolvaptan. Adjust dose. Moderate Theoretical

▸ Verapamil is predicted to increase the exposure to topotecan. Severe Study

▸ Verapamil is predicted to increase the concentration of trametinib. Moderate Theoretical

▸ Calcium channel blockers (diltiazem, verapamil) are predicted to increase the exposure to trazodone. Moderate Theoretical

▸ Calcium channel blockers (diltiazem, verapamil) are predicted to increase the exposure to ulipristal. Avoid if used for uterine fibroids. Moderate Study

▸ Calcium channel blockers (diltiazem, verapamil) are predicted to increase the exposure to venetoclax. Avoid or adjust venetoclax dose. Severe Study

▸ Calcium channel blockers (diltiazem, verapamil) are predicted to increase the exposure to vinca alkaloids. Severe Theoretical

▸ Calcium channel blockers (diltiazem, verapamil) are predicted to increase the exposure to zopiclone. Adjust dose. Moderate Study

Calcium chloride → see calcium salts

Calcium gluconate → see calcium salts

Calcium lactate → see calcium salts

Calcium phosphate → see calcium salts

Calcium salts

calcium acetate · calcium carbonate · calcium chloride · calcium gluconate · calcium lactate · calcium phosphate

SEPARATION OF ADMINISTRATION Calcium carbonate-containing antacids should preferably not be taken at the same time as other drugs since they might impair absorption. Antacids might damage enteric coatings designed to prevent dissolution in the stomach.

▸ Oral **calcium salts** decrease the absorption of alkylating agents (estramustine). Severe Study
▸ **Calcium carbonate** decreases the absorption of antimalarials (chloroquine). Separate administration by at least 4 hours. Moderate Study
▸ **Calcium carbonate** is predicted to decrease the absorption of antimalarials (proguanil). Separate administration by at least 2 hours. Moderate Study
▸ Oral **calcium salts** decrease the absorption of bisphosphonates (alendronic acid). **Alendronic acid** should be taken at least 30 minutes before **calcium salts**. Moderate Study
▸ Oral **calcium salts** are predicted to decrease the absorption of oral bisphosphonates (ibandronic acid). Avoid **calcium salts** for at least 6 hours before or 1 hour after **ibandronic acid**. Moderate Theoretical
▸ Oral **calcium salts** decrease the absorption of bisphosphonates (risedronate). Separate administration by at least 2 hours. Moderate Study
▸ Oral **calcium salts** decrease the absorption of bisphosphonates (sodium clodronate). Avoid **calcium salts** for 2 hours before or 1 hour after **sodium clodronate**. Moderate Study
▸ Cephalosporins (ceftriaxone) increase the risk of cardio-respiratory arrest when given with **calcium chloride**. Avoid. Severe Anecdotal
▸ Cephalosporins (ceftriaxone) increase the risk of cardio-respiratory arrest when given with intravenous **calcium gluconate**. Avoid. Severe Anecdotal
▸ Intravenous **calcium salts** increase the concentration of digoxin. Avoid. Moderate Anecdotal
▸ Oral **calcium salts** decrease the absorption of dolutegravir. **Dolutegravir** should be taken 2 hours before or 6 hours after **calcium salts**. Moderate Study
▸ Oral **calcium salts** decrease the absorption of eltrombopag. **Eltrombopag** should be taken 2 hours before or 4 hours after **calcium salts**. Severe Study
▸ **Calcium carbonate** decreases the absorption of hydroxychloroquine. Separate administration by at least 4 hours. Moderate Study
▸ **Calcium carbonate** decreases the absorption of iron (oral). **Calcium carbonate** should be taken 1 hour before or 2 hours after iron (oral). Moderate Study
▸ **Calcium carbonate** is predicted to decrease the exposure to ledipasvir. Separate administration by 4 hours. Moderate Theoretical
▸ Oral **calcium salts** are predicted to decrease the absorption of levothyroxine. Separate administration by at least 4 hours. Moderate Anecdotal
▸ **Calcium carbonate** decreases the absorption of quinolones (ciprofloxacin, nalidixic acid). Separate administration by 2 hours. Moderate Study
▸ **Calcium carbonate** decreases the absorption of quinolones (norfloxacin). **Norfloxacin** should be taken 2 hours before or 4 hours after **calcium carbonate**. Moderate Study
▸ **Calcium carbonate** is predicted to slightly decrease the exposure to rilpivirine. **Calcium carbonate** should be taken 2 hours before or 4 hours after **rilpivirine**. Severe Theoretical
▸ Oral **calcium salts** decrease the absorption of strontium ranelate. Separate administration by 2 hours. Moderate Study
▸ **Calcium carbonate** is predicted to decrease the absorption of tetracyclines. Separate administration by 2 to 3 hours. Moderate Theoretical
▸ Thiazide diuretics increase the risk of hypercalcaemia when given with **calcium salts**. Severe Anecdotal
▸ **Calcium carbonate** is predicted to decrease the concentration of velpatasvir. Separate administration by 4 hours. Moderate Anecdotal

▸ Oral **calcium salts** decrease the absorption of zinc. Moderate Study

Canagliflozin → see TABLE 14 p. 821 (antidiabetic drugs), TABLE 8 p. 819 (hypotension)
▸ Rifampicin moderately decreases the exposure to **canagliflozin**. Adjust **canagliflozin** dose. Moderate Study
Canakinumab → see monoclonal antibodies
Candesartan → see angiotensin-II receptor antagonists
Cangrelor → see TABLE 4 p. 818 (antiplatelet effects)
Cannabis extract → see TABLE 11 p. 820 (CNS depressant effects)
▸ Antiepileptics (carbamazepine, fosphenytoin, phenobarbital, phenytoin, primidone) are predicted to decrease the exposure to **cannabis extract**. Avoid. Severe Theoretical → Also see TABLE 11 p. 820
▸ Antifungals, azoles (itraconazole, ketoconazole, voriconazole) are predicted to increase the exposure to **cannabis extract**. Use with caution and adjust dose. Moderate Theoretical
▸ Cobicistat is predicted to increase the exposure to **cannabis extract**. Use with caution and adjust dose. Moderate Theoretical
▸ Enzalutamide is predicted to decrease the exposure to **cannabis extract**. Avoid. Severe Theoretical
▸ HIV-protease inhibitors (atazanavir, darunavir, fosamprenavir, lopinavir, ritonavir, saquinavir, tipranavir) are predicted to increase the exposure to **cannabis extract**. Use with caution and adjust dose. Moderate Theoretical
▸ Idelalisib is predicted to increase the exposure to **cannabis extract**. Use with caution and adjust dose. Moderate Theoretical
▸ Macrolides (clarithromycin) are predicted to increase the exposure to **cannabis extract**. Use with caution and adjust dose. Moderate Theoretical
▸ Rifampicin is predicted to decrease the exposure to **cannabis extract**. Avoid. Severe Theoretical
Capecitabine → see TABLE 15 p. 821 (myelosuppression)
▸ Allopurinol is predicted to decrease the effects of **capecitabine**. Avoid. Severe Study
▸ **Capecitabine** increases the concentration of antiepileptics (fosphenytoin, phenytoin). Severe Anecdotal
▸ **Capecitabine** increases the effects of coumarins. Monitor INR and adjust dose. Moderate Anecdotal
▸ Folates (folic acid) are predicted to increase the risk of toxicity when given with **capecitabine**. Severe Anecdotal
▸ Folates (folinic acid) increase the risk of toxicity when given with **capecitabine**. Severe Study
▸ H_2 receptor antagonists (cimetidine) are predicted to slightly increase the exposure to **capecitabine**. Severe Theoretical
▸ Live vaccines are predicted to increase the risk of generalised infection (possibly life-threatening) when given with **capecitabine**. Public Health England advises avoid. Severe Theoretical
▸ Metronidazole is predicted to increase the risk of **capecitabine** toxicity when given with **capecitabine**. Severe Theoretical
Capreomycin → see TABLE 2 p. 818 (nephrotoxicity), TABLE 19 p. 822 (ototoxicity)
Captopril → see ACE inhibitors
Carbamazepine → see antiepileptics
Carbapenems

ertapenem · imipenem · meropenem

▸ **Carbapenems** decrease the concentration of antiepileptics (valproate). Avoid. Severe Anecdotal
▸ Ganciclovir is predicted to increase the risk of seizures when given with **imipenem**. Avoid. Severe Anecdotal
▸ Valganciclovir is predicted to increase the risk of seizures when given with **imipenem**. Avoid. Severe Anecdotal
Carbidopa
▸ Iron (oral) is predicted to decrease the exposure to **carbidopa**. Moderate Theoretical
Carbimazole → see TABLE 15 p. 821 (myelosuppression)
▸ **Carbimazole** affects the concentration of digoxin. Monitor and adjust dose. Moderate Theoretical
▸ **Carbimazole** decreases the effects of metyrapone. Avoid. Moderate Theoretical
Carboplatin → see platinum compounds
Carfilzomib → see TABLE 15 p. 821 (myelosuppression)
Carmustine → see alkylating agents
Carteolol → see beta blockers, non-selective

Carvedilol → see beta blockers, non-selective

Caspofungin

▸ **Antiepileptics (carbamazepine, fosphenytoin, phenytoin)** are predicted to decrease the concentration of **caspofungin**. Adjust caspofungin dose, p. 356. Moderate Theoretical
▸ **Ciclosporin** slightly increases the exposure to **caspofungin**. Severe Study
▸ **Corticosteroids (dexamethasone)** are predicted to decrease the concentration of **caspofungin**. Adjust **caspofungin** dose, p. 356. Moderate Theoretical
▸ **Efavirenz** is predicted to decrease the concentration of caspofungin. Adjust dose. Moderate Study
▸ **Nevirapine** is predicted to decrease the concentration of caspofungin. Adjust dose. Moderate Theoretical
▸ **Rifampicin** decreases the concentration of **caspofungin**. Adjust caspofungin dose, p. 356. Moderate Study

Catumaxomab → see monoclonal antibodies

Cefaclor → see cephalosporins

Cefadroxil → see cephalosporins

Cefalexin → see cephalosporins

Cefixime → see cephalosporins

Cefotaxime → see cephalosporins

Cefradine → see cephalosporins

Ceftaroline → see cephalosporins

Ceftazidime → see cephalosporins

Ceftobiprole → see cephalosporins

Ceftolozane → see cephalosporins

Ceftriaxone → see cephalosporins

Cefuroxime → see cephalosporins

Celecoxib → see NSAIDs

Celiprolol → see beta blockers, selective

Cephalosporins → see TABLE 2 p. 818 (nephrotoxicity)

cefaclor · cefadroxil · cefalexin · cefixime · cefotaxime · cefradine · ceftaroline · ceftazidime · ceftobiprole · ceftolozane · ceftriaxone · cefuroxime

▸ **Ceftobiprole** is predicted to increase the exposure to **bosentan**. Moderate Theoretical
▸ **Ceftriaxone** increases the risk of cardio-respiratory arrest when given with calcium salts **(calcium chloride)**. Avoid. Severe Anecdotal
▸ **Ceftriaxone** increases the risk of cardio-respiratory arrest when given with intravenous calcium salts **(calcium gluconate)**. Avoid. Severe Anecdotal
▸ **Ceftriaxone** potentially increases the risk of bleeding events when given with coumarins. Severe Anecdotal
▸ **Ceftriaxone** potentially increases the risk of bleeding events when given with phenindione. Severe Anecdotal
▸ **Ceftobiprole** is predicted to increase the concentration of statins. Moderate Theoretical
▸ **Ceftobiprole** is predicted to increase the concentration of sulfonylureas **(glibenclamide)**. Moderate Theoretical

Ceritinib → see TABLE 15 p. 821 (myelosuppression), TABLE 9 p. 820 (QT-interval prolongation)

▸ **Ceritinib** is predicted to increase the exposure to **aliskiren**. Moderate Theoretical
▸ **Antacids** are predicted to decrease the absorption of **ceritinib**. Separate administration by 2 hours. Moderate Theoretical
▸ **Antiarrhythmics (amiodarone, dronedarone)** are predicted to increase the exposure to **ceritinib**. Moderate Theoretical → Also see TABLE 9 p. 820
▸ **Antiepileptics (carbamazepine, fosphenytoin, phenobarbital, phenytoin, primidone)** are predicted to decrease the exposure to **ceritinib**. Avoid. Severe Study
▸ **Antifungals, azoles (fluconazole, isavuconazole, posaconazole)** are predicted to increase the exposure to **ceritinib**. Moderate Theoretical
▸ **Antifungals, azoles (itraconazole, ketoconazole, voriconazole)** are predicted to increase the exposure to **ceritinib**. Avoid or adjust **ceritinib** dose. Severe Study → Also see TABLE 9 p. 820
▸ **Ceritinib** is predicted to increase the exposure to antihistamines, non-sedating **(fexofenadine)**. Moderate Theoretical
▸ **Aprepitant** is predicted to increase the exposure to **ceritinib**. Moderate Theoretical
▸ Calcium channel blockers **(diltiazem, verapamil)** are predicted to increase the exposure to **ceritinib**. Moderate Theoretical

▸ **Ceritinib** is predicted to increase the exposure to ciclosporin. Avoid. Severe Theoretical
▸ **Cobicistat** is predicted to increase the exposure to **ceritinib**. Avoid or adjust **ceritinib** dose. Severe Study
▸ **Ceritinib** is predicted to increase the exposure to colchicine. Moderate Theoretical
▸ **Ceritinib** is predicted to increase the exposure to coumarins **(warfarin)**. Avoid. Severe Theoretical
▸ **Crizotinib** is predicted to increase the exposure to **ceritinib**. Moderate Theoretical → Also see TABLE 15 p. 821 → Also see TABLE 9 p. 820
▸ **Ceritinib** is predicted to increase the exposure to dabigatran. Moderate Theoretical
▸ **Ceritinib** is predicted to increase the risk of bradycardia when given with digoxin. Avoid. Severe Theoretical
▸ **Ceritinib** is predicted to increase the exposure to edoxaban. Moderate Theoretical
▸ **Enzalutamide** is predicted to decrease the exposure to ceritinib. Avoid. Severe Study
▸ **Ceritinib** is predicted to increase the exposure to ergotamine. Avoid. Severe Theoretical
▸ **Ceritinib** is predicted to increase the exposure to everolimus. Moderate Theoretical → Also see TABLE 15 p. 821
▸ **Grapefruit juice** is predicted to increase the exposure to ceritinib. Avoid. Severe Theoretical
▸ **H₂ receptor antagonists** are predicted to decrease the absorption of **ceritinib**. Moderate Theoretical
▸ HIV-protease inhibitors **(atazanavir, darunavir, fosamprenavir, lopinavir, ritonavir, saquinavir, tipranavir)** are predicted to increase the exposure to **ceritinib**. Avoid or adjust ceritinib dose. Severe Study → Also see TABLE 9 p. 820
▸ HIV-protease inhibitors **(indinavir)** are predicted to increase the exposure to **ceritinib**. Moderate Theoretical
▸ **Idelalisib** is predicted to increase the exposure to **ceritinib**. Avoid or adjust **ceritinib** dose. Severe Study → Also see TABLE 15 p. 821
▸ **Imatinib** is predicted to increase the exposure to **ceritinib**. Moderate Theoretical → Also see TABLE 15 p. 821
▸ **Lapatinib** is predicted to increase the exposure to **ceritinib**. Moderate Theoretical → Also see TABLE 9 p. 820
▸ **Ceritinib** is predicted to increase the exposure to loperamide. Moderate Theoretical
▸ Macrolides **(azithromycin, erythromycin)** are predicted to increase the exposure to **ceritinib**. Moderate Theoretical
▸ Macrolides **(clarithromycin)** are predicted to increase the exposure to **ceritinib**. Avoid or adjust **ceritinib** dose. Severe Study → Also see TABLE 9 p. 820
▸ **Netupitant** is predicted to increase the exposure to **ceritinib**. Moderate Theoretical
▸ **Nilotinib** is predicted to increase the exposure to **ceritinib**. Moderate Theoretical → Also see TABLE 15 p. 821 → Also see TABLE 9 p. 820
▸ **Ceritinib** is predicted to increase the exposure to NSAIDs **(celecoxib, diclofenac)**. Adjust dose. Moderate Theoretical
▸ **Ceritinib** is predicted to increase the exposure to opioids **(alfentanil, fentanyl)**. Avoid. Severe Theoretical
▸ **Ceritinib** is predicted to increase the exposure to pimozide. Avoid. Severe Theoretical → Also see TABLE 9 p. 820
▸ **Proton pump inhibitors** are predicted to decrease the absorption of **ceritinib**. Moderate Theoretical
▸ **Ranolazine** is predicted to increase the exposure to **ceritinib**. Moderate Theoretical → Also see TABLE 9 p. 820
▸ **Rifampicin** is predicted to decrease the exposure to **ceritinib**. Avoid. Severe Study
▸ **Ceritinib** is predicted to increase the exposure to sirolimus. Avoid. Severe Theoretical
▸ **St John's Wort** is predicted to decrease the exposure to ceritinib. Avoid. Severe Theoretical
▸ **Ceritinib** is predicted to increase the exposure to sulfonylureas **(glimepiride)**. Adjust dose. Moderate Theoretical
▸ **Ceritinib** is predicted to increase the exposure to tacrolimus. Avoid. Severe Theoretical
▸ **Ceritinib** is predicted to increase the exposure to taxanes **(paclitaxel)**. Moderate Theoretical → Also see TABLE 15 p. 821

Ceritinib (continued)

‣ **Ceritinib** is predicted to increase the exposure to **topotecan**. Moderate Theoretical → Also see TABLE 15 p. 821

Certolizumab pegol → see monoclonal antibodies

Cetirizine → see antihistamines, non-sedating

Cetuximab → see monoclonal antibodies

Chenodeoxycholic acid

‣ **Antacids** are predicted to decrease the absorption of chenodeoxycholic acid. Mild Theoretical

Chloral hydrate → see TABLE 11 p. 820 (CNS depressant effects)

‣ Intravenous loop diuretics (**furosemide**) potentially increase the risk of sweating, variable blood pressure, and tachycardia when given after **chloral hydrate**. Moderate Anecdotal

Chlorambucil → see alkylating agents

Chloramphenicol

ROUTE-SPECIFIC INFORMATION Since systemic absorption can follow topical application, the possibility of interactions should be borne in mind.

‣ Antiepileptics (**phenobarbital, primidone**) decrease the concentration of **chloramphenicol**. Moderate Study

‣ Intravenous **chloramphenicol** increases the concentration of antiepileptics (**fosphenytoin, phenytoin**) and antiepileptics (**fosphenytoin, phenytoin**) affect the concentration of intravenous **chloramphenicol**. Monitor concentration and adjust dose. Severe Study

‣ **Chloramphenicol** potentially increases the anticoagulant effect of **coumarins**. Moderate Anecdotal

‣ **Chloramphenicol** decreases the efficacy of intravenous **iron** (injectable). Moderate Anecdotal

‣ **Chloramphenicol** decreases the efficacy of oral **iron** (oral). Moderate Theoretical

‣ **Rifampicin** decreases the concentration of **chloramphenicol**. Moderate Study

‣ **Chloramphenicol** is predicted to increase the exposure to **sulfonylureas**. Severe Study

‣ **Chloramphenicol** increases the concentration of **tacrolimus**. Severe Study

Chlordiazepoxide → see TABLE 11 p. 820 (CNS depressant effects)

‣ **Chlordiazepoxide** affects the concentration of antiepileptics (**fosphenytoin, phenytoin**). Severe Study

‣ **Rifampicin** is predicted to decrease the exposure to **chlordiazepoxide**. Moderate Theoretical

Chloroprocaine → see TABLE 11 p. 820 (CNS depressant effects)

Chloroquine → see antimalarials

Chlorphenamine → see antihistamines, sedating

Chlorpromazine → see phenothiazines

Chlortalidone → see thiazide diuretics

Cholera vaccine

‣ Antimalarials (**chloroquine**) decrease the efficacy of oral **cholera vaccine**. Moderate Study

‣ **Hydroxychloroquine** is predicted to decrease the efficacy of oral **cholera vaccine**. Moderate Theoretical

Cholic acid

‣ **Antacids** are predicted to decrease the absorption of **cholic acid**. Separate administration by 5 hours. Mild Theoretical

‣ Antiepileptics (**phenobarbital**) decrease the effects of **cholic acid**. Avoid. Moderate Study

‣ **Ciclosporin** affects the concentration of **cholic acid**. Avoid. Moderate Study

Choline salicylate

‣ **Corticosteroids** are predicted to decrease the concentration of **choline salicylate**. Moderate Study

Ciclesonide → see corticosteroids

Ciclosporin → see TABLE 2 p. 818 (nephrotoxicity), TABLE 16 p. 822 (increased serum potassium)

‣ Pomelo juice is predicted to increase ciclosporin exposure, and purple grape juice is predicted to decrease ciclosporin exposure.

‣ Since systemic absorption can follow topical application, the possibility of interactions should be borne in mind.

‣ **Ciclosporin** is predicted to increase the exposure to **afatinib**. Separate administration by 12 hours. Moderate Study

‣ **Ciclosporin** markedly increases the exposure to **aliskiren**. Avoid. Severe Study → Also see TABLE 16 p. 822

‣ **Ciclosporin** moderately increases the exposure to **ambrisentan**. Adjust **ambrisentan** dose. Moderate Study

‣ **Ciclosporin** increases the concentration of anthracyclines (**daunorubicin, doxorubicin, epirubicin, idarubicin, mitoxantrone**). Severe Study

‣ Antiarrhythmics (**amiodarone**) increase the concentration of **ciclosporin**. Monitor **ciclosporin** concentration and adjust dose. Severe Study

‣ Antiarrhythmics (**dronedarone**) increase the concentration of **ciclosporin**. Severe Study

‣ **Ciclosporin** increases the exposure to antiarrhythmics (**dronedarone**). Avoid. Severe Theoretical

‣ Antiepileptics (**carbamazepine, fosphenytoin, phenobarbital, phenytoin, primidone**) decrease the concentration of **ciclosporin**. Severe Study

‣ Antiepileptics (**oxcarbazepine**) decrease the concentration of **ciclosporin**. Severe Anecdotal

‣ Antifungals, azoles (**fluconazole, isavuconazole, itraconazole, ketoconazole, posaconazole, voriconazole**) increase the concentration of **ciclosporin**. Severe Study

‣ Antifungals, azoles (**miconazole**) increase the concentration of **ciclosporin**. Monitor and adjust dose. Severe Anecdotal

‣ **Aprepitant** increases the concentration of **ciclosporin**. Severe Study

‣ **Ciclosporin** is predicted to increase the exposure to beta blockers, non-selective (**nadolol**). Moderate Study

‣ **Bosentan** moderately decreases the exposure to **ciclosporin** and **ciclosporin** moderately increases the exposure to **bosentan**. Avoid. Severe Study

‣ Calcium channel blockers (**diltiazem, nicardipine, verapamil**) increase the concentration of **ciclosporin**. Severe Study

‣ **Ciclosporin** moderately increases the exposure to calcium channel blockers (**lercanidipine**). Use with caution or avoid. Severe Study

‣ **Ciclosporin** slightly increases the exposure to **caspofungin**. Severe Study

‣ **Ceritinib** is predicted to increase the exposure to **ciclosporin**. Avoid. Severe Theoretical

‣ **Ciclosporin** affects the concentration of **cholic acid**. Avoid. Moderate Study

‣ **Cobicistat** increases the concentration of **ciclosporin**. Severe Study

‣ **Ciclosporin** increases the exposure to **colchicine**. Avoid or adjust **colchicine** dose. Severe Study

‣ **Crizotinib** increases the concentration of **ciclosporin**. Severe Study

‣ **Ciclosporin** is predicted to increase the exposure to **dabigatran**. Avoid. Severe Theoretical

‣ **Danazol** increases the concentration of **ciclosporin**. Severe Study

‣ **Ciclosporin** is predicted to increase the risk of rhabdomyolysis when given with **daptomycin**. Severe Theoretical

‣ **Ciclosporin** is predicted to increase the exposure to **darifenacin**. Avoid. Moderate Theoretical

‣ **Ciclosporin** increases the concentration of **digoxin**. Monitor and adjust dose. Severe Theoretical

‣ **Ciclosporin** slightly increases the exposure to **edoxaban**. Adjust **edoxaban** dose. Severe Study

‣ **Efavirenz** decreases the concentration of **ciclosporin**. Monitor **ciclosporin** concentration and adjust dose. Moderate Study

‣ **Enzalutamide** decreases the concentration of **ciclosporin**. Severe Study

‣ **Ciclosporin** is predicted to increase the exposure to **erlotinib**. Moderate Theoretical

‣ **Ciclosporin** increases the exposure to **etoposide**. Monitor and adjust dose. Severe Study

‣ **Ciclosporin** moderately increases the exposure to **everolimus**. Avoid or adjust dose. Severe Study

‣ **Ciclosporin** moderately increases the exposure to **ezetimibe** and **ezetimibe** slightly increases the exposure to **ciclosporin**. Moderate Study

‣ Fibrates (**bezafibrate**) are predicted to increase the risk of nephrotoxicity when given with **ciclosporin**. Severe Theoretical

‣ Fibrates (**fenofibrate**) increase the risk of nephrotoxicity when given with **ciclosporin**. Severe Study

▶ **Ciclosporin** is predicted to increase the exposure to fidaxomicin. Avoid. Moderate Study

▶ Grapefruit juice increases the concentration of **ciclosporin**. Avoid. Severe Study

▶ **Ciclosporin** greatly increases the exposure to grazoprevir. Avoid. Severe Study

▶ H₂ receptor antagonists (cimetidine) increase the concentration of **ciclosporin**. Mild Study

▶ HIV-protease inhibitors increase the concentration of **ciclosporin**. Severe Study

▶ Idelalisib increases the concentration of **ciclosporin**. Severe Study

▶ Imatinib increases the concentration of **ciclosporin**. Severe Study

▶ Lanreotide is predicted to decrease the absorption of oral **ciclosporin**. Adjust dose. Severe Theoretical

▶ Live vaccines are predicted to increase the risk of generalised infection (possibly life-threatening) when given with **ciclosporin**. Public Health England advises avoid. Severe Theoretical

▶ **Ciclosporin** is predicted to increase the exposure to lomitapide. Separate administration by 12 hours. Moderate Theoretical

▶ Lumacaftor is predicted to decrease the exposure to **ciclosporin**. Avoid. Severe Theoretical

▶ Macrolides (clarithromycin, erythromycin) increase the concentration of **ciclosporin**. Severe Study

▶ **Ciclosporin** is predicted to decrease the efficacy of mifamurtide. Avoid. Severe Theoretical

▶ Monoclonal antibodies (blinatumomab) are predicted to transiently increase the exposure to **ciclosporin**. Monitor and adjust dose. Moderate Theoretical

▶ Netupitant increases the concentration of **ciclosporin**. Severe Study

▶ Nevirapine is predicted to decrease the concentration of **ciclosporin**. Moderate Study

▶ Nilotinib increases the concentration of **ciclosporin**. Severe Study

▶ **Ciclosporin** is predicted to increase the exposure to nintedanib. Moderate Study

▶ **Ciclosporin** increases the concentration of NSAIDs (diclofenac). Severe Study → Also see **TABLE 2** p. 818 → Also see **TABLE 16** p. 822

▶ Octreotide decreases the absorption of oral **ciclosporin**. Adjust **ciclosporin** dose, p. 496. Severe Anecdotal

▶ Palbociclib is predicted to increase the exposure to **ciclosporin**. Adjust dose. Moderate Theoretical

▶ Pasireotide is predicted to decrease the absorption of oral **ciclosporin**. Adjust dose. Severe Theoretical

▶ Pitolisant is predicted to decrease the exposure to **ciclosporin**. Avoid. Severe Theoretical

▶ **Ciclosporin** is predicted to increase the concentration of ranolazine and ranolazine is predicted to increase the concentration of **ciclosporin**. Moderate Theoretical

▶ **Ciclosporin** moderately increases the exposure to repaglinide. Moderate Study

▶ Rifampicin decreases the concentration of **ciclosporin**. Severe Study

▶ **Ciclosporin** very markedly increases the exposure to rifaximin. Severe Study

▶ **Ciclosporin** is predicted to increase the exposure to riociguat. Moderate Theoretical

▶ **Ciclosporin** is predicted to increase the exposure to sacubitril. Moderate Theoretical

▶ **Ciclosporin** moderately increases the exposure to sirolimus. Separate administration by 4 hours. Severe Study

▶ St John's Wort decreases the concentration of **ciclosporin**. Avoid. Moderate Study

▶ **Ciclosporin** very markedly increases the exposure to statins (atorvastatin). Avoid or adjust **atorvastatin** dose, p. 128. Severe Study

▶ **Ciclosporin** moderately increases the exposure to statins (fluvastatin). Severe Study

▶ **Ciclosporin** markedly to very markedly increases the exposure to statins (pravastatin). Adjust **pravastatin** dose. Severe Study

▶ **Ciclosporin** markedly increases the exposure to statins (rosuvastatin, simvastatin). Avoid. Severe Study

▶ Sulfinpyrazone decreases the concentration of **ciclosporin**. Severe Study

▶ **Ciclosporin** increases the concentration of tacrolimus. Avoid. Severe Study → Also see **TABLE 2** p. 818 → Also see **TABLE 16** p. 822

▶ **Ciclosporin** is predicted to increase the exposure to ticagrelor. Use with caution or avoid. Severe Study

▶ **Ciclosporin** is predicted to increase the exposure to topotecan. Severe Study

▶ **Ciclosporin** is predicted to increase the concentration of trametinib. Moderate Theoretical

▶ Ursodeoxycholic acid affects the concentration of **ciclosporin**. Use with caution and adjust dose. Severe Anecdotal

▶ **Ciclosporin** is predicted to increase the exposure to venetoclax. Avoid or monitor for toxicity. Severe Theoretical

▶ Vitamin E substances affect the exposure to **ciclosporin**. Moderate Study

Cilostazol → see **TABLE 4** p. 818 (antiplatelet effects)

GENERAL INFORMATION Concurrent use with 2 or more antiplatelets or anticoagulants is contra-indicated.

▶ Antiepileptics (carbamazepine, fosphenytoin, phenobarbital, phenytoin, primidone) are predicted to alter the effects of **cilostazol**. Moderate Theoretical

▶ Antifungals, azoles (fluconazole) are predicted to increase the exposure to **cilostazol**. Adjust **cilostazol** dose. Moderate Theoretical

▶ Antifungals, azoles (itraconazole, ketoconazole, voriconazole) are predicted to moderately increase the exposure to **cilostazol**. Adjust **cilostazol** dose. Moderate Study

▶ Antifungals, azoles (miconazole) are predicted to increase the exposure to **cilostazol**. Use with caution and adjust dose. Moderate Theoretical

▶ Cobicistat is predicted to moderately increase the exposure to **cilostazol**. Adjust **cilostazol** dose. Moderate Study

▶ Enzalutamide is predicted to alter the effects of **cilostazol**. Moderate Theoretical

▶ HIV-protease inhibitors (atazanavir, darunavir, fosamprenavir, lopinavir, ritonavir, saquinavir, tipranavir) are predicted to moderately increase the exposure to **cilostazol**. Adjust **cilostazol** dose. Moderate Study

▶ Idelalisib is predicted to moderately increase the exposure to **cilostazol**. Adjust **cilostazol** dose. Moderate Study

▶ **Cilostazol** is predicted to increase the exposure to lomitapide. Separate administration by 12 hours. Moderate Theoretical

▶ Macrolides (clarithromycin) are predicted to moderately increase the exposure to **cilostazol**. Adjust **cilostazol** dose. Moderate Study

▶ Macrolides (erythromycin) slightly increase the exposure to **cilostazol**. Adjust **cilostazol** dose. Moderate Study

▶ Moclobemide is predicted to increase the exposure to **cilostazol**. Moderate Theoretical

▶ Proton pump inhibitors (esomeprazole) are predicted to increase the exposure to **cilostazol**. Moderate Theoretical

▶ Proton pump inhibitors (omeprazole) are predicted to increase the exposure to **cilostazol**. Adjust **cilostazol** dose. Moderate Study

▶ Rifampicin is predicted to alter the effects of **cilostazol**. Moderate Theoretical

▶ SSRIs (fluvoxamine) are predicted to increase the exposure to **cilostazol**. Adjust **cilostazol** dose. Moderate Theoretical → Also see **TABLE 4** p. 818

▶ St John's Wort is predicted to alter the effects of **cilostazol**. Moderate Theoretical

Cimetidine → see H₂ receptor antagonists

Cinacalcet

FOOD AND LIFESTYLE Dose adjustment might be necessary if smoking started or stopped during treatment.

▶ **Cinacalcet** is predicted to increase the exposure to antiarrhythmics (flecainide). Severe Theoretical

▶ **Cinacalcet** is predicted to increase the exposure to antiarrhythmics (propafenone). Monitor and adjust dose. Moderate Study

▶ **Cinacalcet** is predicted to increase the exposure to anticholinesterases, centrally acting (donepezil). Moderate Theoretical

A1

Interactions | **Appendix 1**

Cinacalcet (continued)

▶ **Cinacalcet** is predicted to increase the exposure to anticholinesterases, centrally acting (**galantamine**). Monitor and adjust dose. Moderate Study

▶ **Antifungals, azoles** (**itraconazole, ketoconazole, voriconazole**) are predicted to moderately increase the exposure to **cinacalcet**. Adjust dose. Moderate Study

▶ **Cinacalcet** is predicted to moderately increase the exposure to **aripiprazole**. Adjust **aripiprazole** dose, p. 240. Moderate Study

▶ **Cinacalcet** is predicted to markedly increase the exposure to **atomoxetine**. Adjust dose. Severe Study

▶ **Cinacalcet** is predicted to increase the exposure to beta blockers, non-selective (**carvedilol, timolol**). Moderate Study

▶ **Cinacalcet** is predicted to increase the exposure to beta blockers, selective (**metoprolol, nebivolol**). Moderate Study

▶ **Cobicistat** is predicted to moderately increase the exposure to **cinacalcet**. Adjust dose. Moderate Study

▶ **Cinacalcet** is predicted to slightly increase the exposure to **darifenacin**. Mild Study

▶ **HIV-protease inhibitors** (**atazanavir, darunavir, fosamprenavir, lopinavir, ritonavir, saquinavir, tipranavir**) are predicted to moderately increase the exposure to **cinacalcet**. Adjust dose. Moderate Study

▶ **Idelalisib** is predicted to moderately increase the exposure to **cinacalcet**. Adjust dose. Moderate Study

▶ **Macrolides** (**clarithromycin**) are predicted to moderately increase the exposure to **cinacalcet**. Adjust dose. Moderate Study

▶ **Cinacalcet** is predicted to decrease the efficacy of **opioids** (**codeine**). Moderate Theoretical

▶ **Cinacalcet** is predicted to decrease the efficacy of **opioids** (**tramadol**). Severe Study

▶ **Cinacalcet** is predicted to moderately increase the exposure to **pitolisant**. Use with caution and adjust dose. Moderate Study

▶ **Cinacalcet** is predicted to increase the exposure to **risperidone**. Adjust dose. Moderate Study

▶ **SSRIs** (**fluvoxamine**) are predicted to increase the exposure to **cinacalcet**. Adjust dose. Moderate Theoretical

▶ **Cinacalcet** is predicted to increase the exposure to **SSRIs** (**dapoxetine**). Moderate Theoretical

▶ **Cinacalcet** is predicted to decrease the efficacy of **tamoxifen**. Avoid. Severe Study

▶ **Cinacalcet** is predicted to increase the exposure to **tricyclic antidepressants**. Monitor for toxicity and adjust dose. Severe Study

▶ **Cinacalcet** is predicted to increase the exposure to **vortioxetine**. Monitor and adjust dose. Moderate Study

Cinnarizine → see antihistamines, sedating

Ciprofibrate → see fibrates

Ciprofloxacin → see quinolones

Cisatracurium → see neuromuscular blocking drugs, non-depolarising

Cisplatin → see platinum compounds

Citalopram → see SSRIs

Cladribine → see TABLE 15 p. 821 (myelosuppression)

▶ **Live vaccines** are predicted to increase the risk of generalised infection (possibly life-threatening) when given with **cladribine**. Public Health England advises avoid. Severe Theoretical

Clarithromycin → see macrolides

Clemastine → see antihistamines, sedating

Clevidipine → see calcium channel blockers

Clindamycin

ROUTE-SPECIFIC INFORMATION Since systemic absorption can follow topical application, the possibility of interactions should be borne in mind.

▶ **Clindamycin** increases the effects of **neuromuscular blocking drugs, non-depolarising**. Severe Anecdotal

▶ **Clindamycin** increases the effects of **suxamethonium**. Severe Anecdotal

Clobazam

▶ **Antiepileptics** (**stiripentol**) increase the concentration of **clobazam**. Severe Study

▶ **Clobazam** potentially affects the concentration of antiepileptics (**fosphenytoin, phenytoin**). Severe Anecdotal

Clofarabine → see TABLE 15 p. 821 (myelosuppression)

▶ **Live vaccines** are predicted to increase the risk of generalised infection (possibly life-threatening) when given with **clofarabine**. Public Health England advises avoid. Severe Theoretical

Clofazimine

▶ **Clofazimine** potentially increases the risk of QT-prolongation when given with **bedaquiline**. Severe Study

Clomethiazole → see TABLE 11 p. 820 (CNS depressant effects)

FOOD AND LIFESTYLE Alcohol consumption can cause serious, potentially fatal, CNS depression with clomethiazole.

▶ **Antiepileptics** (**carbamazepine, fosphenytoin, phenobarbital, phenytoin, primidone**) decrease the exposure to **clomethiazole**. Monitor and adjust dose. Moderate Study → Also see TABLE 11 p. 820

▶ **Enzalutamide** decreases the exposure to **clomethiazole**. Monitor and adjust dose. Moderate Study

▶ **Rifampicin** decreases the exposure to **clomethiazole**. Monitor and adjust dose. Moderate Study

Clomipramine → see tricyclic antidepressants

Clonazepam → see TABLE 11 p. 820 (CNS depressant effects)

▶ **Clonazepam** potentially affects the concentration of antiepileptics (**fosphenytoin, phenytoin**). Severe Anecdotal

Clonidine → see TABLE 6 p. 819 (bradycardia), TABLE 8 p. 819 (hypotension), TABLE 11 p. 820 (CNS depressant effects)

▶ **Clonidine** is predicted to decrease the effects of **histamine**. Avoid. Severe Theoretical → Also see TABLE 8 p. 819

▶ **Tricyclic antidepressants** decrease the antihypertensive effects of **clonidine**. Monitor and adjust dose. Moderate Anecdotal → Also see TABLE 8 p. 819

Clopamide → see thiazide diuretics

Clopidogrel → see TABLE 4 p. 818 (antiplatelet effects)

▶ **Antifungals, azoles** (**fluconazole**) are predicted to decrease the efficacy of **clopidogrel**. Avoid. Severe Theoretical

▶ **Antifungals, azoles** (**voriconazole**) are predicted to decrease the efficacy of **clopidogrel**. Avoid. Moderate Study

▶ **Grapefruit juice** markedly decreases the exposure to **clopidogrel**. Severe Study

▶ **Clopidogrel** is predicted to increase the exposure to **loperamide**. Severe Theoretical

▶ **Moclobemide** is predicted to decrease the efficacy of **clopidogrel**. Avoid. Moderate Study

▶ **Clopidogrel** is predicted to increase the exposure to **pioglitazone**. Severe Theoretical

▶ **Proton pump inhibitors** (**esomeprazole, omeprazole**) are predicted to decrease the efficacy of **clopidogrel**. Avoid. Moderate Study

▶ **Clopidogrel** increases the exposure to **repaglinide**. Severe Study

▶ **SSRIs** (**fluvoxamine**) are predicted to decrease the efficacy of **clopidogrel**. Avoid. Severe Theoretical → Also see TABLE 4 p. 818

▶ **Clopidogrel** increases the exposure to statins (**rosuvastatin**). Adjust **rosuvastatin** dose, p. 130. Moderate Study

Clotrimazole → see antifungals, azoles

Clozapine → see TABLE 8 p. 819 (hypotension), TABLE 15 p. 821 (myelosuppression), TABLE 11 p. 820 (CNS depressant effects), TABLE 10 p. 820 (antimuscarinics)

▶ Dose adjustment might be necessary if smoking started or stopped during treatment.

▶ Avoid concomitant use of clozapine with drugs that have a substantial potential for causing agranulocytosis.

▶ **Antiepileptics** (**fosphenytoin, phenytoin**) are predicted to decrease the exposure to **clozapine**. Moderate Anecdotal

▶ **Antiepileptics** (**phenobarbital, primidone**) decrease the exposure to **clozapine**. Moderate Anecdotal → Also see TABLE 11 p. 820

▶ **Combined hormonal contraceptives** increase the concentration of **clozapine**. Monitor side effects and adjust dose. Severe Study

▶ **Clozapine** is predicted to decrease the effects of **dopamine receptor agonists**. Moderate Theoretical → Also see TABLE 8 p. 819 → Also see TABLE 10 p. 820

▶ **Clozapine** is predicted to decrease the effects of **histamine**. Avoid. Severe Theoretical → Also see TABLE 8 p. 819

▶ **HIV-protease inhibitors** (**ritonavir**) are predicted to increase the exposure to **clozapine**. Avoid. Severe Theoretical

▶ **Iron chelators** (**deferasirox**) are predicted to increase the exposure to **clozapine**. Avoid. Moderate Theoretical

▸ **Clozapine** is predicted to decrease the effects of **levodopa**. Severe Theoretical → Also see TABLE 8 p. 819

▸ Quinolones **(ciprofloxacin)** increase the concentration of **clozapine**. Monitor side effects and adjust dose. Severe Study

▸ **Rifampicin** decreases the exposure to **clozapine**. Severe Anecdotal

▸ SSRIs **(fluvoxamine)** increase the concentration of **clozapine**. Monitor side effects and adjust dose. Severe Study

Co-trimoxazole → see sulfonamides

Cobicistat

▸ **Cobicistat** is predicted to increase the exposure to **abiraterone**. Severe Theoretical

▸ **Cobicistat** is predicted to markedly increase the exposure to aldosterone antagonists **(eplerenone)**. Avoid. Severe Study

▸ **Cobicistat** increases the exposure to **almotriptan**. Mild Study

▸ **Cobicistat** is predicted to moderately increase the exposure to alpha blockers **(alfuzosin, tamsulosin)**. Use with caution or avoid. Moderate Study

▸ **Cobicistat** is predicted to increase the exposure to alpha blockers **(doxazosin)**. Moderate Study

▸ **Cobicistat** moderately increases the exposure to **alprazolam**. Avoid. Moderate Study

▸ **Cobicistat** very markedly increases the exposure to antiarrhythmics **(dronedarone)**. Avoid. Severe Study

▸ **Cobicistat** is predicted to increase the exposure to antiarrhythmics **(propafenone)**. Monitor and adjust dose. Severe Study

▸ **Cobicistat** is predicted to increase the exposure to anticholinesterases, centrally acting **(galantamine)**. Monitor and adjust dose. Moderate Study

▸ Antiepileptics **(carbamazepine, fosphenytoin, phenobarbital, phenytoin, primidone)** are predicted to decrease the exposure to **cobicistat**. Avoid. Severe Theoretical

▸ Antiepileptics **(oxcarbazepine)** are predicted to decrease the concentration of **cobicistat**. Severe Theoretical

▸ **Cobicistat** is predicted to slightly increase the exposure to antiepileptics **(perampanel)**. Mild Study

▸ **Cobicistat** is predicted to increase the exposure to antifungals, azoles **(fluconazole, posaconazole)**. Moderate Theoretical

▸ **Cobicistat** is predicted to increase the exposure to antifungals, azoles **(isavuconazole)**. Avoid or monitor side effects. Severe Study

▸ **Cobicistat** is predicted to increase the exposure to antifungals, azoles **(itraconazole)**. Adjust **itraconazole** dose. Moderate Theoretical

▸ **Cobicistat** is predicted to increase the exposure to antifungals, azoles **(ketoconazole)**. Adjust **ketoconazole** dose. Moderate Theoretical

▸ **Cobicistat** is predicted to affect the exposure to antifungals, azoles **(voriconazole)**. Avoid. Moderate Theoretical

▸ **Cobicistat** is predicted to increase the exposure to antihistamines, non-sedating **(mizolastine)**. Avoid. Severe Study

▸ **Cobicistat** is predicted to increase the exposure to antimalarials **(artemether) (with lumafantrine)**. Moderate Study

▸ **Cobicistat** is predicted to increase the concentration of antimalarials **(piperaquine)**. Severe Theoretical

▸ **Cobicistat** is predicted to markedly increase the exposure to **aprepitant**. Moderate Study

▸ **Cobicistat** is predicted to slightly increase the exposure to **aripiprazole**. Adjust **aripiprazole** dose, p. 240. Moderate Study

▸ **Cobicistat** is predicted to increase the exposure to **axitinib**. Avoid or adjust dose. Moderate Study

▸ **Cobicistat** is predicted to increase the exposure to **bedaquiline**. Avoid prolonged use. Mild Study

▸ **Cobicistat** is predicted to increase the exposure to beta₂ agonists **(salmeterol)**. Avoid. Severe Study

▸ **Cobicistat** slightly increases the exposure to **bortezomib**. Moderate Study

▸ **Bosentan** is predicted to decrease the exposure to **cobicistat**. Avoid. Severe Theoretical

▸ **Cobicistat** is predicted to markedly increase the exposure to **bosutinib**. Avoid or adjust **bosutinib** dose. Severe Study

▸ **Cobicistat** is predicted to increase the exposure to **buspirone**. Adjust **buspirone** dose. Severe Study

▸ **Cobicistat** slightly increases the exposure to **cabozantinib**. Moderate Study

▸ **Cobicistat** is predicted to increase the exposure to calcium channel blockers **(amlodipine, felodipine, isradipine, lacidipine, nicardipine, nifedipine, nimodipine)**. Monitor and adjust dose. Moderate Study

▸ **Cobicistat** is predicted to increase the exposure to calcium channel blockers **(diltiazem, verapamil)**. Severe Study

▸ **Cobicistat** is predicted to markedly increase the exposure to calcium channel blockers **(lercanidipine)**. Avoid. Severe Study

▸ **Cobicistat** is predicted to increase the exposure to cannabis extract. Use with caution and adjust dose. Moderate Theoretical

▸ **Cobicistat** is predicted to increase the exposure to **ceritinib**. Avoid or adjust **ceritinib** dose. Severe Study

▸ **Cobicistat** increases the concentration of **ciclosporin**. Severe Study

▸ **Cobicistat** is predicted to moderately increase the exposure to **cilostazol**. Adjust **cilostazol** dose. Moderate Study

▸ **Cobicistat** is predicted to moderately increase the exposure to **cinacalcet**. Adjust dose. Moderate Study

▸ **Cobicistat** is predicted to markedly increase the exposure to **cobimetinib**. Avoid or monitor for toxicity. Severe Study

▸ **Cobicistat** is predicted to increase the exposure to **colchicine**. Avoid or adjust **colchicine** dose. Severe Study

▸ **Cobicistat** is predicted to decrease the efficacy of combined hormonal contraceptives. Avoid. Severe Study

▸ **Cobicistat** is predicted to increase the concentration of corticosteroids **(beclometasone)** (risk with beclometasone is likely to be lower than with other corticosteroids). MHRA advises avoid or monitor for **beclometasone** side effects. Moderate Theoretical

▸ **Cobicistat** is predicted to increase the concentration of corticosteroids **(betamethasone)**. MHRA advises avoid or monitor side effects and consider beclomethasone as an alternative. Severe Theoretical

▸ **Cobicistat** is predicted to increase the concentration of corticosteroids **(budesonide)**. MHRA advises avoid or monitor side effects and consider beclomethasone as an alternative. Severe Theoretical

▸ **Cobicistat** is predicted to increase the concentration of corticosteroids **(ciclesonide)**. Avoid. Moderate Theoretical

▸ **Cobicistat** is predicted to increase the concentration of corticosteroids **(deflazacort)**. MHRA advises avoid or monitor side effects and consider beclomethasone as an alternative. Severe Theoretical

▸ **Cobicistat** is predicted to increase the concentration of corticosteroids **(dexamethasone)**. MHRA advises avoid or monitor side effects and consider beclomethasone as an alternative. Severe Theoretical

▸ **Cobicistat** is predicted to increase the exposure to inhaled corticosteroids **(fluticasone)**. Severe Study

▸ **Cobicistat** is predicted to increase the concentration of corticosteroids **(hydrocortisone)**. MHRA advises avoid or monitor side effects and consider beclomethasone as an alternative. Severe Theoretical

▸ **Cobicistat** potentially increases the concentration of corticosteroids **(methylprednisolone)**. MHRA advises avoid or monitor side effects and consider beclomethasone as an alternative. Severe Theoretical

▸ **Cobicistat** is predicted to increase the exposure to corticosteroids **(mometasone)**. Moderate Theoretical

▸ **Cobicistat** is predicted to increase the concentration of corticosteroids **(prednisolone)**. MHRA advises avoid or monitor side effects and consider beclomethasone as an alternative. Severe Theoretical

▸ **Cobicistat** is predicted to increase the concentration of corticosteroids **(prednisone)**. MHRA advises avoid or monitor side effects and consider beclomethasone as an alternative. Severe Theoretical

▸ **Cobicistat** is predicted to increase the concentration of corticosteroids **(triamcinolone)**. MHRA advises avoid or monitor side effects and consider beclomethasone as an alternative. Severe Theoretical

▸ **Cobicistat** is predicted to moderately increase the exposure to **crizotinib**. Avoid. Moderate Study

Interactions | Appendix 1

Cobicistat (continued)

▸ **Cobicistat** is predicted to increase the exposure to **dabrafenib**. Use with caution or avoid. Moderate Study

▸ **Cobicistat** is predicted to moderately increase the exposure to daclatasvir. Adjust **daclatasvir** dose. Moderate Study

▸ **Cobicistat** is predicted to markedly to very markedly increase the exposure to **darifenacin**. Avoid. Severe Study

▸ **Cobicistat** is predicted to markedly increase the exposure to dasatinib. Avoid. Severe Study

▸ **Cobicistat** very slightly increases the exposure to delamanid. Severe Study

▸ **Cobicistat** increases the risk of QT-prolongation when given with domperidone. Avoid. Severe Study

▸ **Cobicistat** increases the exposure to dopamine receptor agonists (bromocriptine, cabergoline). Severe Study

▸ **Cobicistat** is predicted to increase the exposure to dutasteride. Monitor side effects and adjust dose. Moderate Theoretical

▸ **Efavirenz** is predicted to decrease the exposure to **cobicistat**. Avoid. Severe Theoretical

▸ **Cobicistat** slightly to moderately increases the exposure to elbasvir. Avoid. Moderate Study

▸ **Cobicistat** is predicted to markedly increase the exposure to eletriptan. Avoid. Severe Study

▸ **Enzalutamide** is predicted to decrease the exposure to **cobicistat**. Avoid. Severe Theoretical

▸ **Cobicistat** is predicted to increase the risk of ergotism when given with ergometrine. Avoid. Severe Theoretical

▸ **Cobicistat** is predicted to increase the risk of ergotism when given with ergotamine. Avoid. Severe Theoretical

▸ **Cobicistat** is predicted to slightly increase the exposure to erlotinib. Use with caution and adjust dose. Moderate Study

▸ **Cobicistat** is predicted to increase the concentration of everolimus. Avoid. Severe Study

▸ **Cobicistat** is predicted to moderately increase the exposure to fesoterodine. Adjust **fesoterodine** dose; avoid in hepatic and renal impairment. Severe Study

▸ **Cobicistat** is predicted to increase the exposure to fosaprepitant. Moderate Theoretical

▸ **Cobicistat** is predicted to increase the exposure to gefitinib. Moderate Study

▸ **Cobicistat** is predicted to moderately to markedly increase the exposure to grazoprevir. Avoid. Severe Study

▸ **Cobicistat** is predicted to increase the exposure to guanfacine. Adjust **guanfacine** dose, p. 222. Moderate Study

▸ **Cobicistat** is predicted to very markedly increase the exposure to ibrutinib. Avoid or adjust **ibrutinib** dose. Severe Study

▸ **Cobicistat** is predicted to increase the exposure to imatinib. Moderate Study

▸ **Cobicistat** is predicted to increase the risk of toxicity when given with irinotecan. Avoid. Moderate Study

▸ **Cobicistat** is predicted to increase the exposure to ivabradine. Avoid. Severe Study

▸ **Cobicistat** is predicted to increase the exposure to ivacaftor. Adjust **ivacaftor** or lumacaftor with ivacaftor dose, p. 179. Severe Study

▸ **Cobicistat** is predicted to increase the exposure to lapatinib. Avoid. Moderate Study

▸ **Cobicistat** is predicted to markedly increase the exposure to lomitapide. Avoid. Severe Study

▸ **Cobicistat** is predicted to increase the exposure to lurasidone. Avoid. Severe Study

▸ **Cobicistat** is predicted to increase the exposure to macitentan. Moderate Study

▸ **Cobicistat** markedly increases the exposure to maraviroc. Refer to specialist literature. Severe Study

▸ **Cobicistat** is predicted to markedly to very markedly increase the exposure to midazolam. Avoid or adjust **midazolam** dose. Severe Study

▸ **Cobicistat** is predicted to increase the exposure to mirabegron. Adjust **mirabegron** dose in hepatic and renal impairment. Moderate Study

▸ **Cobicistat** is predicted to increase the exposure to mirtazapine. Moderate Study

▸ **Cobicistat** is predicted to increase the exposure to modafinil. Mild Theoretical

▸ **Cobicistat** is predicted to increase the exposure to monoclonal antibodies (trastuzumab emtansine). Avoid. Severe Theoretical

▸ **Cobicistat** is predicted to markedly increase the exposure to naloxegol. Avoid. Severe Study

▸ **Cobicistat** is predicted to increase the exposure to netupitant. Mild Study

▸ **Nevirapine** is predicted to decrease the exposure to **cobicistat**. Avoid. Severe Theoretical

▸ **Cobicistat** is predicted to moderately increase the exposure to nilotinib. Avoid. Severe Study

▸ **Cobicistat** is predicted to increase the exposure to nitisinone. Adjust **nitisinone** dose. Moderate Theoretical

▸ **Cobicistat** is predicted to increase the exposure to olaparib. Avoid or adjust **olaparib** dose. Moderate Study

▸ **Cobicistat** is predicted to increase the exposure to opioids (alfentanil, buprenorphine, fentanyl, oxycodone, sufentanil). Monitor and adjust dose. Severe Study

▸ **Cobicistat** is predicted to increase the exposure to opioids (methadone). Moderate Theoretical

▸ **Cobicistat** is predicted to increase the exposure to oxybutynin. Mild Study

▸ **Cobicistat** is predicted to increase the exposure to palbociclib. Avoid or adjust **palbociclib** dose. Severe Study

▸ **Cobicistat** is predicted to increase the exposure to panobinostat. Adjust **panobinostat** dose; in hepatic impairment avoid. Moderate Study

▸ **Cobicistat** is predicted to increase the exposure to paritaprevir (with ritonavir and ombitasvir). Avoid. Severe Theoretical

▸ **Cobicistat** is predicted to increase the exposure to pazopanib. Avoid or adjust **pazopanib** dose. Moderate Study

▸ **Cobicistat** is predicted to increase the exposure to phosphodiesterase type-5 inhibitors (avanafil, vardenafil). Avoid. Severe Study

▸ **Cobicistat** is predicted to increase the exposure to phosphodiesterase type-5 inhibitors (sildenafil). Avoid or adjust **sildenafil** dose, p. 117. Severe Study

▸ **Cobicistat** is predicted to increase the exposure to phosphodiesterase type-5 inhibitors (tadalafil). Use with caution or avoid. Severe Study

▸ **Cobicistat** is predicted to increase the exposure to pimozide. Avoid. Severe Study

▸ **Cobicistat** is predicted to slightly increase the exposure to ponatinib. Monitor and adjust **ponatinib** dose. Moderate Study

▸ **Cobicistat** is predicted to moderately increase the exposure to praziquantel. Mild Study

▸ **Cobicistat** is predicted to increase the exposure to quetiapine. Avoid. Severe Study

▸ **Cobicistat** is predicted to increase the exposure to ranolazine. Avoid. Severe Study

▸ **Cobicistat** is predicted to increase the exposure to reboxetine. Avoid. Moderate Study

▸ **Cobicistat** is predicted to increase the exposure to regorafenib. Avoid. Moderate Study

▸ **Cobicistat** is predicted to increase the exposure to repaglinide. Moderate Study

▸ **Cobicistat** is predicted to increase the exposure to retinoids (alitretinoin). Adjust **alitretinoin** dose. Moderate Theoretical

▸ **Rifabutin** decreases the concentration of **cobicistat** and cobicistat increases the exposure to rifabutin. Avoid or adjust dose. Severe Study

▸ **Rifampicin** is predicted to decrease the exposure to **cobicistat**. Avoid. Severe Theoretical

▸ **Cobicistat** is predicted to increase the exposure to risperidone. Adjust dose. Moderate Study

▸ **Cobicistat** is predicted to increase the exposure to ruxolitinib. Adjust dose and monitor side effects. Moderate Study

▸ **Cobicistat** is predicted to increase the exposure to saxagliptin. Moderate Study

▸ **Cobicistat** is predicted to increase the exposure to simeprevir. Avoid. Severe Study

▸ **Cobicistat** is predicted to increase the concentration of sirolimus. Avoid. Severe Study

▸ **Cobicistat** is predicted to increase the exposure to solifenacin. Adjust **solifenacin** or tamsulosin with solifenacin dose; avoid in hepatic and renal impairment. Severe Study

▶ **Cobicistat** is predicted to moderately increase the exposure to SSRIs (**dapoxetine**). Avoid or adjust **dapoxetine** dose. Severe Study

▶ **St John's Wort** is predicted to decrease the exposure to **cobicistat**. Avoid. Severe Theoretical

▶ **Cobicistat** is predicted to increase the exposure to statins (**atorvastatin**). Avoid or adjust dose and monitor rhabdomyolysis. Severe Study

▶ **Cobicistat** is predicted to increase the exposure to statins (**simvastatin**). Avoid. Severe Study

▶ **Cobicistat** is predicted to slightly increase the exposure to **sunitinib**. Avoid or adjust **sunitinib** dose. Moderate Study

▶ **Cobicistat** is predicted to increase the concentration of **tacrolimus**. Monitor and adjust dose. Severe Study

▶ **Cobicistat** is predicted to increase the exposure to taxanes (**cabazitaxel**). Avoid. Severe Study

▶ **Cobicistat** is predicted to moderately increase the exposure to taxanes (**docetaxel**). Avoid or adjust dose. Severe Study

▶ **Cobicistat** is predicted to increase the exposure to taxanes (**paclitaxel**). Severe Theoretical

▶ **Cobicistat** is predicted to increase the concentration of **temsirolimus**. Avoid. Severe Theoretical

▶ **Cobicistat** is predicted to markedly increase the exposure to **ticagrelor**. Avoid. Severe Study

▶ **Cobicistat** is predicted to increase the exposure to **tolterodine**. Avoid. Severe Study

▶ **Cobicistat** is predicted to increase the exposure to **tolvaptan**. Adjust dose. Severe Study

▶ **Cobicistat** is predicted to increase the exposure to **toremifene**. Moderate Theoretical

▶ **Cobicistat** is predicted to increase the exposure to **trabectedin**. Avoid or adjust dose. Severe Theoretical

▶ **Cobicistat** is predicted to moderately increase the exposure to **trazodone**. Avoid or adjust dose. Moderate Study

▶ **Cobicistat** is predicted to slightly increase the exposure to tricyclic antidepressants. Mild Study

▶ **Cobicistat** is predicted to increase the exposure to **ulipristal**. Avoid if used for uterine fibroids. Severe Study

▶ **Cobicistat** is predicted to increase the exposure to **vemurafenib**. Severe Theoretical

▶ **Cobicistat** is predicted to increase the exposure to **venetoclax**. Avoid or adjust **venetoclax** dose. Severe Study

▶ **Cobicistat** is predicted to increase the exposure to **venlafaxine**. Moderate Study

▶ **Cobicistat** is predicted to increase the exposure to vinca alkaloids. Severe Theoretical

▶ **Cobicistat** is predicted to increase the exposure to vitamin D substances (**paricalcitol**). Moderate Study

▶ **Cobicistat** is predicted to increase the exposure to **zopiclone**. Adjust dose. Moderate Theoretical

Cobimetinib

▶ Antiarrhythmics (**dronedarone**) are predicted to increase the exposure to **cobimetinib**. Severe Theoretical

▶ Antiepileptics (**carbamazepine, fosphenytoin, phenobarbital, phenytoin, primidone**) are predicted to decrease the exposure to **cobimetinib**. Avoid. Severe Theoretical

▶ Antifungals, azoles (**fluconazole, isavuconazole, miconazole, posaconazole**) are predicted to increase the exposure to **cobimetinib**. Severe Theoretical

▶ Antifungals, azoles (**itraconazole, ketoconazole, voriconazole**) are predicted to markedly increase the exposure to **cobimetinib**. Avoid or monitor for toxicity. Severe Study

▶ **Aprepitant** is predicted to increase the exposure to **cobimetinib**. Severe Theoretical

▶ **Bosentan** is predicted to decrease the exposure to **cobimetinib**. Avoid. Severe Theoretical

▶ Calcium channel blockers (**diltiazem, verapamil**) are predicted to increase the exposure to **cobimetinib**. Severe Theoretical

▶ **Cobicistat** is predicted to markedly increase the exposure to **cobimetinib**. Avoid or monitor for toxicity. Severe Study

▶ **Crizotinib** is predicted to increase the exposure to **cobimetinib**. Severe Theoretical

▶ **Efavirenz** is predicted to decrease the exposure to **cobimetinib**. Avoid. Severe Theoretical

▶ **Enzalutamide** is predicted to decrease the exposure to **cobimetinib**. Avoid. Severe Theoretical

▶ **Grapefruit juice** is predicted to increase the exposure to **cobimetinib**. Avoid. Severe Theoretical

▶ HIV-protease inhibitors (**atazanavir, darunavir, fosamprenavir, lopinavir, ritonavir, saquinavir, tipranavir**) are predicted to markedly increase the exposure to **cobimetinib**. Avoid or monitor for toxicity. Severe Study

▶ HIV-protease inhibitors (**indinavir**) are predicted to increase the exposure to **cobimetinib**. Severe Theoretical

▶ **Idelalisib** is predicted to markedly increase the exposure to **cobimetinib**. Avoid or monitor for toxicity. Severe Study

▶ **Imatinib** is predicted to increase the exposure to **cobimetinib**. Severe Theoretical

▶ Macrolides (**clarithromycin**) are predicted to markedly increase the exposure to **cobimetinib**. Avoid or monitor for toxicity. Severe Study

▶ Macrolides (**erythromycin**) are predicted to increase the exposure to **cobimetinib**. Severe Theoretical

▶ **Netupitant** is predicted to increase the exposure to **cobimetinib**. Severe Theoretical

▶ **Nevirapine** is predicted to decrease the exposure to **cobimetinib**. Avoid. Severe Theoretical

▶ **Nilotinib** is predicted to increase the exposure to **cobimetinib**. Severe Theoretical

▶ **Rifampicin** is predicted to decrease the exposure to **cobimetinib**. Avoid. Severe Theoretical

▶ **St John's Wort** is predicted to decrease the exposure to **cobimetinib**. Avoid. Severe Theoretical

Codeine → see opioids

Colchicine

▶ Antiarrhythmics (**dronedarone**) are predicted to increase the exposure to **colchicine**. Adjust **colchicine** dose. Severe Study

▶ Antifungals, azoles (**fluconazole, isavuconazole, posaconazole**) are predicted to increase the exposure to **colchicine**. Adjust **colchicine** dose. Severe Study

▶ Antifungals, azoles (**itraconazole, ketoconazole, voriconazole**) are predicted to increase the exposure to **colchicine**. Avoid or adjust **colchicine** dose. Severe Study

▶ **Aprepitant** is predicted to increase the exposure to **colchicine**. Adjust **colchicine** dose. Severe Study

▶ Calcium channel blockers (**diltiazem, verapamil**) are predicted to increase the exposure to **colchicine**. Adjust **colchicine** dose. Severe Study

▶ **Ceritinib** is predicted to increase the exposure to **colchicine**. Moderate Theoretical

▶ **Ciclosporin** increases the exposure to **colchicine**. Avoid or adjust **colchicine** dose. Severe Study

▶ **Cobicistat** is predicted to increase the exposure to **colchicine**. Avoid or adjust **colchicine** dose. Severe Study

▶ **Crizotinib** is predicted to increase the exposure to **colchicine**. Adjust **colchicine** dose. Severe Study

▶ **Colchicine** increases the risk of rhabdomyolysis when given with **fibrates**. Severe Anecdotal

▶ HIV-protease inhibitors (**atazanavir, darunavir, fosamprenavir, lopinavir, ritonavir, saquinavir, tipranavir**) are predicted to increase the exposure to **colchicine**. Avoid or adjust **colchicine** dose. Severe Study

▶ HIV-protease inhibitors (**indinavir**) are predicted to increase the exposure to **colchicine**. Adjust **colchicine** dose. Severe Study

▶ **Idelalisib** is predicted to increase the exposure to **colchicine**. Avoid or adjust **colchicine** dose. Severe Study

▶ **Imatinib** is predicted to increase the exposure to **colchicine**. Adjust **colchicine** dose. Severe Study

▶ **Lapatinib** is predicted to increase the exposure to **colchicine**. Avoid or adjust **colchicine** dose. Moderate Theoretical

▶ **Lumacaftor** is predicted to affect the exposure to **colchicine**. Moderate Theoretical

▶ Macrolides (**azithromycin**) are predicted to increase the exposure to **colchicine**. Avoid or adjust **colchicine** dose. Severe Theoretical

▶ Macrolides (**clarithromycin**) are predicted to increase the exposure to **colchicine**. Avoid or adjust **colchicine** dose. Severe Study

Interactions | Appendix 1

A1

Colchicine (continued)

▸ Macrolides (**erythromycin**) are predicted to increase the exposure to **colchicine**. Adjust **colchicine** dose. [Severe] Study
▸ **Mirabegron** is predicted to increase the exposure to **colchicine**. [Mild] Theoretical
▸ **Netupitant** is predicted to increase the exposure to **colchicine**. Adjust **colchicine** dose. [Severe] Study
▸ **Nilotinib** is predicted to increase the exposure to **colchicine**. Adjust **colchicine** dose. [Severe] Study
▸ **Ranolazine** is predicted to increase the exposure to **colchicine**. Avoid or adjust **colchicine** dose. [Severe] Theoretical
▸ **Colchicine** increases the risk of rhabdomyolysis when given with **statins**. [Severe] Anecdotal
▸ **Velpatasvir** is predicted to increase the exposure to **colchicine**. [Severe] Theoretical
▸ **Vemurafenib** is predicted to increase the exposure to **colchicine**. Avoid or adjust **colchicine** dose. [Severe] Theoretical

Colecalciferol → see vitamin D substances

Colesevelam

SEPARATION OF ADMINISTRATION Manufacturer advises take 4 hours before, or after, other drugs.

Colestipol

SEPARATION OF ADMINISTRATION Manufacturer advises take other drugs at least 1 hour before, or 4 hours after, colestipol.

Colestyramine

SEPARATION OF ADMINISTRATION Manufacturer advises take other drugs at least 1 hour before, or 4-6 hours after, colestyramine.

Colistimethate → see TABLE 2 p. 818 (nephrotoxicity), TABLE 20 p. 822 (neuromuscular blocking effects)

▸ **Colistimethate** increases the effects of **neuromuscular blocking drugs, non-depolarising**. Monitor and adjust dose. [Moderate] Study → Also see TABLE 20 p. 822 (neuromuscular blocking effects)
▸ **Colistimethate** increases the effects of **suxamethonium**. Monitor and adjust dose. [Moderate] Study → Also see TABLE 20 p. 822

Combined hormonal contraceptives

▸ **Combined hormonal contraceptives** are predicted to increase the exposure to **agomelatine**. [Moderate] Study
▸ **Combined hormonal contraceptives** are predicted to increase the exposure to **aminophylline**. Adjust dose. [Moderate] Theoretical
▸ **Combined hormonal contraceptives** are predicted to increase the exposure to **anagrelide**. [Moderate] Theoretical
▸ **Antiepileptics** (**carbamazepine, eslicarbazepine, fosphenytoin, oxcarbazepine, perampanel, phenobarbital, phenytoin, primidone, rufinamide, topiramate**) are predicted to decrease the efficacy of **combined hormonal contraceptives**. For FSRH guidance, see Contraceptives, interactions p. 474. [Severe] Study
▸ **Combined hormonal contraceptives** alter the exposure to antiepileptics (**lamotrigine**). Adjust **lamotrigine** dose. [Moderate] Study
▸ **Aprepitant** is predicted to decrease the efficacy of **combined hormonal contraceptives**. For FSRH guidance, see Contraceptives, interactions p. 474. [Severe] Study
▸ **Bosentan** is predicted to decrease the efficacy of **combined hormonal contraceptives**. For FSRH guidance, see Contraceptives, interactions p. 474. [Severe] Study
▸ **Combined hormonal contraceptives** increase the concentration of **clozapine**. Monitor side effects and adjust dose. [Severe] Study
▸ **Cobicistat** is predicted to decrease the efficacy of **combined hormonal contraceptives**. Avoid. [Severe] Study
▸ **Combined hormonal contraceptives** increase the risk of raised liver function tests when given with **dasabuvir**. Avoid. [Severe] Study
▸ **Combined hormonal contraceptives** are predicted to increase the exposure to dopamine receptor agonists (**ropinirole**). Adjust dose. [Moderate] Study
▸ **Efavirenz** is predicted to decrease the efficacy of **combined hormonal contraceptives**. For FSRH guidance, see Contraceptives, interactions p. 474. [Severe] Study

▸ **Combined hormonal contraceptives** slightly increase the exposure to eriotinib. Monitor side effects and adjust dose. [Moderate] Study
▸ **Fosaprepitant** is predicted to decrease the efficacy of **combined hormonal contraceptives**. For FSRH guidance, see Contraceptives, interactions p. 474. [Severe] Study
▸ **Griseofulvin** potentially decreases the efficacy of **combined hormonal contraceptives**. For FSRH guidance, see Contraceptives, interactions p. 474. [Severe] Anecdotal
▸ HIV-protease inhibitors (**atazanavir**) (unboosted) increase the exposure to **combined hormonal contraceptives**. Adjust dose. [Severe] Study
▸ HIV-protease inhibitors (**ritonavir**) are predicted to decrease the efficacy of **combined hormonal contraceptives**. For FSRH guidance, see Contraceptives, interactions p. 474. [Severe] Study
▸ **Combined hormonal contraceptives** are predicted to increase the risk of venous thromboembolism when given with **lenalidomide**. Avoid. [Severe] Study
▸ Oral **combined hormonal contraceptives** slightly increase the exposure to **lomitapide**. Separate administration by 12 hours. [Moderate] Theoretical
▸ **Combined hormonal contraceptives** are predicted to increase the exposure to **loxapine**. Avoid. [Unknown] Theoretical
▸ **Lumacaftor** is predicted to decrease the efficacy of **combined hormonal contraceptives**. Use additional contraceptive precautions. [Severe] Theoretical
▸ **Combined hormonal contraceptives** are predicted to increase the exposure to **melatonin**. [Moderate] Theoretical
▸ **Combined hormonal contraceptives** decrease the effects of **metyrapone**. Avoid. [Moderate] Theoretical
▸ **Modafinil** is predicted to decrease the efficacy of **combined hormonal contraceptives**. For FSRH guidance, see Contraceptives, interactions p. 474. [Severe] Study
▸ **Combined hormonal contraceptives** slightly increase the exposure to monoamine-oxidase B inhibitors (**rasagiline**). [Moderate] Study
▸ **Combined hormonal contraceptives** increase the exposure to monoamine-oxidase B inhibitors (**selegiline**). Avoid. [Severe] Study
▸ **Nevirapine** is predicted to decrease the efficacy of **combined hormonal contraceptives**. For FSRH guidance, see Contraceptives, interactions p. 474. [Severe] Study
▸ NSAIDs (**etoricoxib**) slightly increase the exposure to **combined hormonal contraceptives**. [Moderate] Study
▸ **Paritaprevir** (with ritonavir and ombitasvir) increases the risk of raised liver function tests when given with **combined hormonal contraceptives**. Avoid. [Severe] Study
▸ **Combined hormonal contraceptives** are predicted to increase the exposure to **pirfenidone**. Use with caution and adjust dose. [Moderate] Study
▸ **Pitolisant** is predicted to decrease the efficacy of **combined hormonal contraceptives**. Avoid. [Severe] Theoretical
▸ **Combined hormonal contraceptives** are predicted to increase the risk of venous thromboembolism when given with **pomalidomide**. Avoid. [Severe] Theoretical
▸ **Rifabutin** is predicted to decrease the efficacy of **combined hormonal contraceptives**. For FSRH guidance, see Contraceptives, interactions p. 474. [Severe] Study
▸ **Rifampicin** is predicted to decrease the efficacy of **combined hormonal contraceptives**. For FSRH guidance, see Contraceptives, interactions p. 474. [Severe] Study
▸ **Combined hormonal contraceptives** are predicted to increase the exposure to **roflumilast**. [Moderate] Theoretical
▸ **St John's Wort** decreases the efficacy of **combined hormonal contraceptives**. MHRA advises avoid. For FSRH guidance, see Contraceptives, interactions p. 474. [Severe] Anecdotal
▸ **Sugammadex** is predicted to decrease the exposure to oral **combined hormonal contraceptives**. Refer to patient information leaflet for missed pill advice. [Severe] Theoretical
▸ **Combined hormonal contraceptives** are predicted to increase the risk of venous thromboembolism when given with **thalidomide**. Avoid. [Severe] Study
▸ **Combined hormonal contraceptives** are predicted to increase the exposure to **theophylline**. Monitor and adjust dose. [Moderate] Theoretical

▸ **Combined hormonal contraceptives** increase the exposure to tizanidine. Avoid. Moderate Study

▸ **Ulipristal** is predicted to decrease the efficacy of **combined hormonal contraceptives**. Avoid. Severe Theoretical

▸ **Combined hormonal contraceptives** are predicted to increase the exposure to zolmitriptan. Adjust **zolmitriptan** dose, p. 280. Moderate Theoretical

Corticosteroids → see TABLE 17 p. 822 (reduced serum potassium)

beclometasone · betamethasone · budesonide · ciclesonide · deflazacort · dexamethasone · fluticasone · hydrocortisone · methylprednisolone · mometasone · prednisolone · prednisone · triamcinolone

ROUTE-SPECIFIC INFORMATION Interactions do not generally apply to corticosteroids used for topical action (including inhalation) unless specified.

▸ **Antacids** are predicted to decrease the absorption of **deflazacort**. Separate administration by 2 hours. Moderate Theoretical

▸ **Antacids** decrease the absorption of **dexamethasone**. Moderate Study

▸ **Antiarrhythmics (dronedarone)** are predicted to increase the exposure to **methylprednisolone**. Monitor and adjust dose. Moderate Study

▸ **Antiepileptics (carbamazepine, fosphenytoin, phenobarbital, phenytoin, primidone)** are predicted to decrease the exposure to **fluticasone**. Unknown Theoretical

▸ **Antiepileptics (carbamazepine, fosphenytoin, phenobarbital, phenytoin, primidone)** are predicted to decrease the exposure to **prednisone**. Mild Study

▸ **Antiepileptics (carbamazepine, fosphenytoin, phenobarbital, phenytoin, primidone)** are predicted to decrease the exposure to corticosteroids **(budesonide, dexamethasone, methylprednisolone, prednisolone)**. Monitor and adjust dose. Moderate Study

▸ **Antifungals, azoles (fluconazole, isavuconazole, posaconazole)** are predicted to increase the exposure to **methylprednisolone**. Monitor and adjust dose. Moderate Study

▸ **Antifungals, azoles (itraconazole, ketoconazole, voriconazole)** are predicted to increase the exposure to **budesonide**. Avoid. Severe Study

▸ **Antifungals, azoles (itraconazole, ketoconazole, voriconazole)** are predicted to increase the exposure to **ciclesonide**. Avoid. Moderate Theoretical

▸ **Antifungals, azoles (itraconazole, ketoconazole, voriconazole)** are predicted to increase the exposure to inhaled **fluticasone**. Severe Study

▸ **Antifungals, azoles (itraconazole, ketoconazole, voriconazole)** are predicted to increase the exposure to **mometasone**. Moderate Theoretical

▸ **Antifungals, azoles (itraconazole, ketoconazole, voriconazole)** are predicted to increase the risk of side-effects when given with **triamcinolone**. Severe Theoretical

▸ **Antifungals, azoles (miconazole)** are predicted to increase the concentration of **methylprednisolone**. Monitor and adjust dose. Moderate Theoretical

▸ **Antifungals, azoles (itraconazole, ketoconazole, voriconazole)** are predicted to increase the exposure to corticosteroids **(dexamethasone, methylprednisolone)**. Monitor and adjust dose. Moderate Study

▸ **Aprepitant** moderately increases the exposure to **dexamethasone**. Monitor and adjust dose. Moderate Study

▸ **Aprepitant** is predicted to increase the exposure to **methylprednisolone**. Monitor and adjust dose. Moderate Study

▸ **Corticosteroids** are predicted to decrease the concentration of **aspirin** (high-dose) and **aspirin** (high-dose) increases the risk of gastrointestinal bleeding when given with **corticosteroids**. Moderate Study

▸ **Calcium channel blockers (diltiazem, verapamil)** are predicted to increase the exposure to **methylprednisolone**. Monitor and adjust dose. Moderate Study

▸ **Dexamethasone** is predicted to decrease the concentration of **caspofungin**. Adjust **caspofungin** dose, p. 356. Moderate Theoretical

▸ **Corticosteroids** are predicted to decrease the concentration of **choline salicylate**. Moderate Study

▸ **Cobicistat** is predicted to increase the concentration of **beclometasone** (risk with beclometasone is likely to be lower than with other corticosteroids). MHRA advises avoid or monitor for **beclometasone** side effects. Moderate Theoretical

▸ **Cobicistat** is predicted to increase the concentration of **betamethasone**. MHRA advises avoid or monitor side effects and consider beclometasone as an alternative. Severe Theoretical

▸ **Cobicistat** is predicted to increase the concentration of **budesonide**. MHRA advises avoid or monitor side effects and consider beclometasone as an alternative. Severe Theoretical

▸ **Cobicistat** is predicted to increase the exposure to **ciclesonide**. Avoid. Moderate Theoretical

▸ **Cobicistat** is predicted to increase the concentration of **deflazacort**. MHRA advises avoid or monitor side effects and consider beclometasone as an alternative. Severe Theoretical

▸ **Cobicistat** is predicted to increase the concentration of **dexamethasone**. MHRA advises avoid or monitor side effects and consider beclometasone as an alternative. Severe Theoretical

▸ **Cobicistat** is predicted to increase the exposure to inhaled **fluticasone**. Severe Study

▸ **Cobicistat** is predicted to increase the concentration of **hydrocortisone**. MHRA advises avoid or monitor side effects and consider beclometasone as an alternative. Severe Theoretical

▸ **Cobicistat** potentially increases the concentration of **methylprednisolone**. MHRA advises avoid or monitor side effects and consider beclometasone as an alternative. Severe Theoretical

▸ **Cobicistat** is predicted to increase the exposure to **mometasone**. Moderate Theoretical

▸ **Cobicistat** is predicted to increase the concentration of **prednisolone**. MHRA advises avoid or monitor side effects and consider beclometasone as an alternative. Severe Theoretical

▸ **Cobicistat** is predicted to increase the concentration of **prednisone**. MHRA advises avoid or monitor side effects and consider beclometasone as an alternative. Severe Theoretical

▸ **Cobicistat** is predicted to increase the concentration of **triamcinolone**. MHRA advises avoid or monitor side effects and consider beclometasone as an alternative. Severe Theoretical

▸ **Corticosteroids** are predicted to increase the effects of **coumarins**. Moderate Study

▸ **Crizotinib** is predicted to increase the exposure to **methylprednisolone**. Monitor and adjust dose. Moderate Study

▸ **Enzalutamide** is predicted to decrease the exposure to corticosteroids **(budesonide, dexamethasone, methylprednisolone, prednisolone)**. Monitor and adjust dose. Moderate Study

▸ **Enzalutamide** is predicted to decrease the exposure to **fluticasone**. Unknown Theoretical

▸ **Enzalutamide** is predicted to decrease the exposure to **prednisone**. Mild Study

▸ **Corticosteroids** increase the risk of gastrointestinal perforation when given with **erlotinib**. Severe Theoretical

▸ **Fosaprepitant** is predicted to increase the exposure to corticosteroids **(dexamethasone, methylprednisolone)**. Monitor and adjust dose. Moderate Theoretical

▸ **Grapefruit juice** moderately increases the exposure to oral **budesonide**. Avoid. Moderate Study

▸ **Corticosteroids** are predicted to decrease the effects of **histamine**. Avoid. Severe Theoretical

▸ HIV-protease inhibitors **(atazanavir, darunavir, fosamprenavir, lopinavir, ritonavir, saquinavir, tipranavir)** are predicted to increase the exposure to **ciclesonide**. Avoid. Moderate Theoretical

▸ HIV-protease inhibitors **(atazanavir, darunavir, fosamprenavir, lopinavir, ritonavir, saquinavir, tipranavir)** are predicted to increase the exposure to inhaled **fluticasone**. Severe Study

▸ HIV-protease inhibitors **(atazanavir, darunavir, fosamprenavir, lopinavir, ritonavir, saquinavir, tipranavir)** are predicted to increase the exposure to **mometasone**. Moderate Theoretical

Corticosteroids (continued)

▸ HIV-protease inhibitors (atazanavir, darunavir, fosamprenavir, lopinavir, saquinavir, tipranavir) are predicted to increase the exposure to budesonide. Avoid. Severe Study

▸ HIV-protease inhibitors (atazanavir, darunavir, fosamprenavir, lopinavir, saquinavir, tipranavir) are predicted to increase the risk of side-effects when given with triamcinolone. Severe Theoretical

▸ HIV-protease inhibitors (indinavir) are predicted to increase the exposure to methylprednisolone. Monitor and adjust dose. Moderate Study

▸ HIV-protease inhibitors (ritonavir) are predicted to increase the concentration of beclometasone (risk with beclometasone is likely to be lower than with other corticosteroids). MHRA advises avoid or monitor for beclometasone side-effects. Moderate Theoretical

▸ HIV-protease inhibitors (ritonavir) are predicted to increase the concentration of corticosteroids (betamethasone, budesonide, deflazacort, dexamethasone, hydrocortisone, methylprednisolone, prednisolone, prednisone, triamcinolone). MHRA advises avoid or monitor side effects and consider beclometasone as an alternative. Severe Theoretical

▸ HIV-protease inhibitors (atazanavir, darunavir, fosamprenavir, lopinavir, saquinavir, tipranavir) are predicted to increase the exposure to corticosteroids (dexamethasone, methylprednisolone). Monitor and adjust dose. Moderate Study

▸ Idelalisib is predicted to increase the exposure to budesonide. Avoid. Severe Study

▸ Idelalisib is predicted to increase the exposure to ciclesonide. Avoid. Moderate Theoretical

▸ Idelalisib is predicted to increase the exposure to corticosteroids (dexamethasone, methylprednisolone). Monitor and adjust dose. Moderate Study

▸ Idelalisib is predicted to increase the exposure to inhaled fluticasone. Severe Study

▸ Idelalisib is predicted to increase the exposure to mometasone. Moderate Theoretical

▸ Idelalisib is predicted to increase the risk of side-effects when given with triamcinolone. Severe Theoretical

▸ Imatinib is predicted to increase the exposure to methylprednisolone. Monitor and adjust dose. Moderate Study

▸ Corticosteroids are predicted to increase the risk of gastrointestinal bleeding when given with iron chelators (deferasirox). Severe Theoretical

▸ Live vaccines are predicted to increase the risk of generalised infection (possibly life-threatening) when given with corticosteroids (high-dose). Public Health England advises avoid. Severe Theoretical

▸ Lumacaftor is predicted to decrease the exposure to corticosteroids (methylprednisolone, prednisone). Adjust dose. Severe Theoretical

▸ Macrolides (clarithromycin) are predicted to increase the exposure to budesonide. Avoid. Severe Study

▸ Macrolides (clarithromycin) are predicted to increase the exposure to ciclesonide. Moderate Theoretical

▸ Macrolides (clarithromycin) are predicted to increase the exposure to inhaled fluticasone. Severe Study

▸ Macrolides (clarithromycin) are predicted to increase the exposure to mometasone. Moderate Theoretical

▸ Macrolides (clarithromycin) are predicted to increase the risk of side-effects when given with triamcinolone. Severe Theoretical

▸ Macrolides (erythromycin) are predicted to increase the exposure to methylprednisolone. Monitor and adjust dose. Moderate Study

▸ Macrolides (clarithromycin) are predicted to increase the exposure to corticosteroids (dexamethasone, methylprednisolone). Moderate Study

▸ Corticosteroids are predicted to decrease the efficacy of mifamurtide. Avoid. Severe Theoretical

▸ Mifepristone is predicted to decrease the efficacy of corticosteroids. Use with caution and adjust dose. Moderate Theoretical

▸ Netupitant increases the exposure to dexamethasone. Adjust dose. Moderate Study

▸ Netupitant is predicted to increase the exposure to methylprednisolone. Monitor and adjust dose. Moderate Study

▸ Corticosteroids are predicted to decrease the effects of neuromuscular blocking drugs, non-depolarising. Severe Anecdotal

▸ Corticosteroids increase the risk of gastrointestinal perforation when given with nicorandil. Severe Anecdotal

▸ Nilotinib is predicted to increase the exposure to methylprednisolone. Monitor and adjust dose. Moderate Study

▸ NSAIDs increase the risk of gastrointestinal bleeding when given with corticosteroids. Severe Study

▸ Corticosteroids are predicted to increase the effects of phenindione. Moderate Anecdotal

▸ Dexamethasone decreases the exposure to praziquantel. Moderate Study

▸ Rifampicin is predicted to decrease the exposure to corticosteroids (budesonide, dexamethasone, methylprednisolone, prednisolone). Monitor and adjust dose. Moderate Study

▸ Rifampicin is predicted to decrease the exposure to fluticasone. Unknown Theoretical

▸ Rifampicin is predicted to decrease the exposure to prednisone. Mild Study

▸ Corticosteroids potentially decrease the effects of sodium phenylbutyrate. Moderate Anecdotal

▸ Corticosteroids are predicted to decrease the effects of somatropin. Moderate Theoretical

▸ Corticosteroids are predicted to decrease the effects of suxamethonium. Severe Anecdotal

Coumarins → see TABLE 3 p. 818 (anticoagulant effects)

acenocoumarol · warfarin

FOOD AND LIFESTYLE The effects of coumarins can be reduced or abolished by vitamin K, including that found in health foods, food supplements, enteral feeds, or large amounts of some green vegetables or green tea. Major changes in diet (especially involving salads and vegetables) and in alcohol consumption can affect anticoagulant control. Pomegranate is predicted to increase the INR in response to acenocoumarol and warfarin.

▸ Antiarrhythmics (amiodarone) increase the anticoagulant effect of coumarins. Severe Study

▸ Antiarrhythmics (propafenone) increase the anticoagulant effect of coumarins. Monitor INR and adjust dose. Moderate Study

▸ Antiepileptics (carbamazepine) decrease the effects of coumarins. Monitor and adjust dose. Severe Study

▸ Antiepileptics (fosphenytoin, phenytoin) are predicted to alter the anticoagulant effect of coumarins. Moderate Anecdotal

▸ Antiepileptics (phenobarbital, primidone) decrease the anticoagulant effect of coumarins. Monitor INR and adjust dose. Moderate Study

▸ Antifungals, azoles (fluconazole) increase the anticoagulant effect of coumarins. Monitor INR and adjust dose. Severe Study

▸ Antifungals, azoles (itraconazole) potentially increase the anticoagulant effect of coumarins. Severe Anecdotal

▸ Antifungals, azoles (ketoconazole) potentially increase the anticoagulant effect of warfarin. Monitor INR and adjust dose. Severe Anecdotal

▸ Antifungals, azoles (miconazole) greatly increase the anticoagulant effect of coumarins. Severe Study

▸ Antifungals, azoles (voriconazole) increase the anticoagulant effect of coumarins. Monitor INR and adjust dose. Moderate Study

▸ Aprepitant decreases the anticoagulant effect of coumarins. Moderate Study

▸ Axitinib is predicted to increase the risk of bleeding events when given with coumarins. Severe Theoretical

▸ Azathioprine decreases the anticoagulant effect of coumarins. Moderate Study

▸ Bosentan decreases the anticoagulant effect of coumarins. Moderate Study

▸ Bosutinib is predicted to increase the risk of bleeding events when given with coumarins. Severe Theoretical

‣ **Cabozantinib** is predicted to increase the risk of bleeding events when given with **coumarins**. Severe Theoretical

‣ **Capecitabine** increases the effects of **coumarins**. Monitor INR and adjust dose. Moderate Anecdotal

‣ **Cephalosporins** (**ceftriaxone**) potentially increase the risk of bleeding events when given with **coumarins**. Severe Anecdotal

‣ **Ceritinib** is predicted to increase the exposure to **warfarin**. Avoid. Severe Theoretical

‣ **Chloramphenicol** potentially increases the anticoagulant effect of **coumarins**. Moderate Anecdotal

‣ **Corticosteroids** are predicted to increase the effects of **coumarins**. Moderate Study

‣ **Cranberry juice** potentially increases the anticoagulant effect of **warfarin**. Avoid. Severe Anecdotal

‣ **Crizotinib** is predicted to increase the risk of bleeding events when given with **coumarins**. Severe Theoretical

‣ **Dabrafenib** is predicted to decrease the anticoagulant effect of **coumarins**. Severe Theoretical

‣ **Danazol** potentially increases the anticoagulant effect of **coumarins**. Severe Anecdotal

‣ **Dasatinib** is predicted to increase the risk of bleeding events when given with **coumarins**. Severe Theoretical

‣ **Disulfiram** increases the anticoagulant effect of **coumarins**. Monitor and adjust dose. Severe Study

‣ **Efavirenz** is predicted to affect the concentration of **coumarins**. Adjust dose. Moderate Theoretical

‣ **Elvitegravir** is predicted to decrease the anticoagulant effect of **coumarins**. Moderate Theoretical

‣ **Enteral feeds** (vitamin-K containing) potentially decreases the anticoagulant effect of **coumarins**. Severe Anecdotal

‣ **Enzalutamide** potentially decreases the exposure to **coumarins**. Avoid or adjust dose and monitor INR. Severe Study

‣ **Erlotinib** increases the anticoagulant effect of **coumarins**. Severe Anecdotal

‣ **Etravirine** increases the anticoagulant effect of **coumarins**. Moderate Theoretical

‣ **Fibrates** are predicted to increase the anticoagulant effect of **coumarins**. Monitor INR and adjust dose. Severe Study

‣ **Fluorouracil** increases the anticoagulant effect of **coumarins**. Severe Anecdotal

‣ **Fosaprepitant** is predicted to decrease the anticoagulant effect of **coumarins**. Moderate Theoretical

‣ **Gefitinib** is predicted to increase the anticoagulant effect of **coumarins**. Severe Anecdotal

‣ **Glucagon** increases the anticoagulant effect of **warfarin**. Severe Study

‣ **Glucosamine** increases the anticoagulant effect of **warfarin**. Avoid. Moderate Anecdotal

‣ **Griseofulvin** potentially decreases the anticoagulant effect of **coumarins**. Moderate Anecdotal

‣ **H₂ receptor antagonists** (**cimetidine**) increase the anticoagulant effect of **coumarins**. Severe Study

‣ **HIV-protease inhibitors** are predicted to affect the anticoagulant effect of **coumarins**. Moderate Study

‣ **Imatinib** is predicted to increase the risk of bleeding events when given with **coumarins**. Severe Theoretical

‣ **Ivacaftor** is predicted to increase the anticoagulant effect of **warfarin**. Severe Theoretical

‣ **Ivermectin** potentially increases the anticoagulant effect of **coumarins**. Severe Anecdotal

‣ **Lapatinib** is predicted to increase the risk of bleeding events when given with **coumarins**. Severe Theoretical

‣ **Leflunomide** increases the anticoagulant effect of **coumarins**. Severe Anecdotal

‣ **Live vaccines** (influenza vaccine) potentially increase the risk of bleeding events when given with **coumarins**. Severe Anecdotal

‣ **Lomitapide** increases the exposure to **warfarin**. Monitor INR and adjust **warfarin** dose. Severe Study

‣ **Lumacaftor** is predicted to affect the exposure to **warfarin**. Severe Theoretical

‣ **Macrolides** (**clarithromycin**, **erythromycin**) increase the anticoagulant effect of **coumarins**. Monitor INR and adjust dose. Severe Anecdotal

‣ **Mercaptopurine** decreases the anticoagulant effect of **coumarins**. Moderate Anecdotal

‣ **Metronidazole** increases the anticoagulant effect of **coumarins**. Monitor INR and adjust dose. Severe Study

‣ **Monoclonal antibodies** (**blinatumomab**) are predicted to transiently increase the exposure to **warfarin**. Monitor and adjust dose. Moderate Theoretical

‣ **Nandrolone** is predicted to increase the anticoagulant effect of **coumarins**. Monitor and adjust dose. Severe Theoretical

‣ **Nevirapine** potentially alters the anticoagulant effect of **coumarins**. Severe Anecdotal

‣ **Nilotinib** is predicted to increase the risk of bleeding events when given with **coumarins**. Severe Theoretical

‣ **Oxymetholone** increases the anticoagulant effect of **coumarins**. Severe Anecdotal

‣ **Paracetamol** increases the anticoagulant effect of **coumarins**. Severe Study

‣ **Pazopanib** is predicted to increase the risk of bleeding events when given with **coumarins**. Severe Theoretical

‣ **Penicillins** potentially alter the anticoagulant effect of **coumarins**. Monitor INR and adjust dose. Severe Anecdotal

‣ **Pitolisant** is predicted to decrease the exposure to **warfarin**. Unknown Theoretical

‣ **Ponatinib** is predicted to increase the risk of bleeding events when given with **coumarins**. Severe Theoretical

‣ **Quinolones** increase the anticoagulant effect of **coumarins**. Severe Anecdotal

‣ **Ranibizumab** increases the risk of bleeding events when given with **coumarins**. Severe Anecdotal

‣ **Regorafenib** is predicted to increase the risk of bleeding events when given with **coumarins**. Severe Study

‣ **Rifampicin** decreases the anticoagulant effect of **coumarins**. Severe Study

‣ **Ruxolitinib** is predicted to increase the risk of bleeding events when given with **coumarins**. Severe Theoretical

‣ **Sorafenib** increases the anticoagulant effect of **coumarins**. Severe Anecdotal

‣ **St John's Wort** decreases the anticoagulant effect of **coumarins**. Avoid. Severe Anecdotal

‣ **Statins** (**fluvastatin**, **rosuvastatin**) increase the anticoagulant effect of **coumarins**. Monitor INR and adjust dose. Severe Study

‣ **Sucralfate** potentially decreases the effects of **warfarin**. Separate administration by 2 hours. Moderate Anecdotal

‣ **Sulfamethoxazole** increases the anticoagulant effect of **coumarins**. Severe Study

‣ **Sulfinpyrazone** increases the anticoagulant effect of **coumarins**. Avoid. Severe Study

‣ **Sulfonamides** (**sulfadiazine**) are predicted to increase the anticoagulant effect of **coumarins**. Severe Theoretical

‣ **Sunitinib** is predicted to increase the risk of bleeding events when given with **coumarins**. Severe Theoretical

‣ **Tamoxifen** increases the anticoagulant effect of **coumarins**. Severe Study

‣ **Tegafur** increases the anticoagulant effect of **coumarins**. Moderate Theoretical

‣ **Teriflunomide** affects the anticoagulant effect of **coumarins**. Severe Study

‣ **Tetracyclines** increase the risk of bleeding events when given with **coumarins**. Moderate Anecdotal

‣ **Tinidazole** is predicted to increase the anticoagulant effect of **coumarins**. Monitor INR and adjust dose. Severe Theoretical

‣ **Toremifene** is predicted to increase the anticoagulant effect of **coumarins**. Severe Theoretical

‣ **Trimethoprim** is predicted to increase the anticoagulant effect of **coumarins**. Severe Study

‣ **Vandetanib** is predicted to increase the risk of bleeding events when given with **coumarins**. Severe Theoretical

‣ **Venetoclax** slightly increases the exposure to **warfarin**. Moderate Study

Cranberry juice

‣ **Cranberry juice** potentially increases the anticoagulant effect of coumarins (**warfarin**). Avoid. Severe Anecdotal

Crisantaspase → see TABLE 1 p. 818 (hepatotoxicity), TABLE 15 p. 821 (myelosuppression)

‣ **Crisantaspase** is predicted to increase the risk of hepatotoxicity when given with **imatinib**. Severe Theoretical
→ Also see TABLE 15 p. 821

Crisantaspase (continued)

▸ Crisantaspase affects the efficacy of methotrexate. [Severe] Anecdotal → Also see TABLE 1 p. 818 → Also see TABLE 15 p. 821

▸ Crisantaspase potentially increases the risk of neurotoxicity when given with vinca alkaloids (vincristine). Vincristine should be taken 3 to 24 hours before crisantaspase. [Severe] Anecdotal → Also see TABLE 1 p. 818 → Also see TABLE 15 p. 821

Crizotinib → see TABLE 6 p. 819 (bradycardia), TABLE 15 p. 821 (myelosuppression), TABLE 9 p. 820 (QT-interval prolongation)

> **GENERAL INFORMATION** Caution with concurrent use of drugs that cause gastrointestinal perforation—discontinue treatment if gastrointestinal perforation occurs.

▸ Crizotinib is predicted to increase the exposure to aldosterone antagonists (eplerenone). Adjust eplerenone dose. [Severe] Study

▸ Crizotinib is predicted to increase the exposure to alpha blockers (tamsulosin). [Moderate] Theoretical

▸ Crizotinib is predicted to increase the exposure to alprazolam. [Severe] Study

▸ Antiarrhythmics (dronedarone) are predicted to increase the exposure to crizotinib. [Moderate] Theoretical → Also see TABLE 9 p. 820

▸ Crizotinib is predicted to increase the exposure to antiarrhythmics (propafenone). Monitor and adjust dose. [Moderate] Study

▸ Antiepileptics (carbamazepine, fosphenytoin, phenobarbital, phenytoin, primidone) are predicted to markedly decrease the exposure to crizotinib. Avoid. [Severe] Study

▸ Antifungals, azoles (fluconazole, posaconazole) are predicted to increase the exposure to crizotinib. [Moderate] Theoretical

▸ Antifungals, azoles (itraconazole, ketoconazole, voriconazole) are predicted to moderately increase the exposure to crizotinib. Avoid. [Moderate] Study → Also see TABLE 9 p. 820

▸ Crizotinib is predicted to increase the exposure to antifungals, azoles (isavuconazole). [Moderate] Theoretical

▸ Crizotinib is predicted to increase the exposure to antihistamines, non-sedating (mizolastine). [Severe] Theoretical

▸ Crizotinib is predicted to increase the concentration of antimalarials (piperaquine). [Severe] Theoretical

▸ Aprepitant is predicted to increase the exposure to crizotinib. [Moderate] Theoretical

▸ Crizotinib is predicted to increase the exposure to axitinib. [Moderate] Theoretical → Also see TABLE 15 p. 821

▸ Crizotinib is predicted to increase the exposure to bedaquiline. Avoid prolonged use. [Mild] Theoretical → Also see TABLE 9 p. 820

▸ Bosentan is predicted to decrease the exposure to crizotinib. Avoid. [Severe] Theoretical

▸ Crizotinib is predicted to increase the exposure to bosutinib. Avoid or adjust bosutinib dose. [Severe] Theoretical → Also see TABLE 15 p. 821 → Also see TABLE 9 p. 820

▸ Crizotinib is predicted to increase the exposure to buspirone. Use with caution and adjust dose. [Moderate] Study

▸ Crizotinib is predicted to increase the exposure to cabozantinib. [Moderate] Theoretical → Also see TABLE 15 p. 821 → Also see TABLE 9 p. 820

▸ Calcium channel blockers (diltiazem, verapamil) are predicted to increase the exposure to crizotinib. [Moderate] Theoretical → Also see TABLE 6 p. 819

▸ Crizotinib is predicted to increase the exposure to calcium channel blockers (amlodipine, felodipine, isradipine, lacidipine, lercanidipine, nicardipine, nifedipine, nimodipine). Monitor and adjust dose. [Moderate] Study

▸ Crizotinib is predicted to increase the exposure to ceritinib. [Moderate] Theoretical → Also see TABLE 15 p. 821 → Also see TABLE 9 p. 820

▸ Crizotinib increases the concentration of ciclosporin. [Severe] Study

▸ Cobicistat is predicted to moderately increase the exposure to crizotinib. Avoid. [Moderate] Study

▸ Crizotinib is predicted to increase the exposure to cobimetinib. [Severe] Theoretical

▸ Crizotinib is predicted to increase the exposure to colchicine. Adjust colchicine dose. [Severe] Study

▸ Crizotinib is predicted to increase the exposure to corticosteroids (methylprednisolone). Monitor and adjust dose. [Moderate] Study

▸ Crizotinib is predicted to increase the risk of bleeding events when given with coumarins. [Severe] Theoretical

▸ Crizotinib is predicted to slightly increase the exposure to darifenacin. [Moderate] Study

▸ Crizotinib is predicted to increase the exposure to dasatinib. [Severe] Study → Also see TABLE 15 p. 821 → Also see TABLE 9 p. 820

▸ Crizotinib increases the risk of QT-prolongation when given with domperidone. Avoid. [Severe] Study

▸ Crizotinib is predicted to increase the exposure to dopamine receptor agonists (bromocriptine, cabergoline). [Severe] Theoretical

▸ Crizotinib is predicted to moderately increase the exposure to dutasteride. [Mild] Study

▸ Efavirenz is predicted to decrease the exposure to crizotinib. Avoid. [Severe] Theoretical

▸ Enzalutamide is predicted to markedly decrease the exposure to crizotinib. Avoid. [Severe] Study

▸ Crizotinib is predicted to increase the risk of ergotism when given with ergometrine. [Severe] Theoretical

▸ Crizotinib is predicted to increase the risk of ergotism when given with ergotamine. [Severe] Theoretical

▸ Crizotinib is predicted to increase the exposure to erlotinib. [Moderate] Theoretical

▸ Crizotinib is predicted to increase the concentration of everolimus. Avoid or adjust dose. [Moderate] Study → Also see TABLE 15 p. 821

▸ Crizotinib is predicted to increase the exposure to fesoterodine. Adjust fesoterodine dose in hepatic and renal impairment. [Mild] Study

▸ Crizotinib is predicted to increase the exposure to gefitinib. [Moderate] Theoretical → Also see TABLE 15 p. 821

▸ Grapefruit juice is predicted to increase the exposure to crizotinib. Avoid. [Moderate] Theoretical

▸ Crizotinib is predicted to increase the concentration of guanfacine. Adjust guanfacine dose, p. 222. [Moderate] Theoretical

▸ HIV-protease inhibitors (atazanavir, darunavir, fosamprenavir, lopinavir, ritonavir, saquinavir, tipranavir) are predicted to moderately increase the exposure to crizotinib. Avoid. [Moderate] Study → Also see TABLE 9 p. 820

▸ HIV-protease inhibitors (indinavir) are predicted to increase the exposure to crizotinib. [Moderate] Theoretical

▸ Crizotinib is predicted to increase the exposure to ibrutinib. Avoid or adjust ibrutinib dose. [Severe] Theoretical → Also see TABLE 15 p. 821

▸ Idelalisib is predicted to moderately increase the exposure to crizotinib. Avoid. [Moderate] Study → Also see TABLE 15 p. 821

▸ Crizotinib is predicted to increase the exposure to ivabradine. Adjust ivabradine dose. [Severe] Theoretical → Also see TABLE 6 p. 819

▸ Crizotinib is predicted to increase the exposure to ivacaftor. Adjust ivacaftor dose, p. 179. [Severe] Study

▸ Crizotinib is predicted to increase the exposure to lapatinib. [Moderate] Study → Also see TABLE 9 p. 820

▸ Crizotinib is predicted to increase the exposure to lomitapide. Avoid. [Moderate] Theoretical

▸ Crizotinib is predicted to increase the exposure to lurasidone. [Moderate] Study

▸ Macrolides (clarithromycin) are predicted to moderately increase the exposure to crizotinib. Avoid. [Moderate] Study → Also see TABLE 9 p. 820

▸ Macrolides (erythromycin) are predicted to increase the exposure to crizotinib. [Moderate] Theoretical

▸ Crizotinib is predicted to increase the exposure to midazolam. Monitor side effects and adjust dose. [Severe] Study

▸ Crizotinib is predicted to increase the exposure to naloxegol. Adjust naloxegol dose and monitor side effects. [Moderate] Study

▸ Netupitant is predicted to increase the exposure to crizotinib. [Severe] Theoretical

▸ Nevirapine is predicted to decrease the exposure to crizotinib. Avoid. [Severe] Theoretical

▸ Crizotinib is predicted to increase the exposure to olaparib. Avoid or adjust olaparib dose. [Moderate] Theoretical → Also see TABLE 15 p. 821

▸ Crizotinib is predicted to increase the exposure to opioids (alfentanil, buprenorphine, fentanyl, oxycodone). Monitor and adjust dose. [Moderate] Study → Also see TABLE 6 p. 819

- **Darifenacin** is predicted to increase the concentration of antiarrhythmics (**flecainide**). [Moderate] Theoretical
- Antiepileptics (**carbamazepine, fosphenytoin, phenobarbital, phenytoin, primidone**) are predicted to decrease the exposure to **darifenacin**. [Moderate] Theoretical
- Antifungals, azoles (**fluconazole, isavuconazole, posaconazole**) are predicted to slightly increase the exposure to **darifenacin**. [Moderate] Study
- Antifungals, azoles (**itraconazole, ketoconazole, voriconazole**) are predicted to markedly to very markedly increase the exposure to **darifenacin**. Avoid. [Severe] Study
- **Aprepitant** is predicted to slightly increase the exposure to **darifenacin**. [Moderate] Study
- **Bupropion** is predicted to slightly increase the exposure to **darifenacin**. [Mild] Study
- Calcium channel blockers (**diltiazem, verapamil**) are predicted to slightly increase the exposure to **darifenacin**. [Moderate] Study
- **Ciclosporin** is predicted to increase the exposure to **darifenacin**. Avoid. [Moderate] Theoretical
- **Cinacalcet** is predicted to slightly increase the exposure to **darifenacin**. [Mild] Study
- **Cobicistat** is predicted to markedly to very markedly increase the exposure to **darifenacin**. Avoid. [Severe] Study
- **Crizotinib** is predicted to slightly increase the exposure to **darifenacin**. [Moderate] Study
- **Enzalutamide** is predicted to decrease the exposure to **darifenacin**. [Moderate] Theoretical
- **Grapefruit juice** is predicted to increase the exposure to **darifenacin**. [Moderate] Study
- HIV-protease inhibitors (**atazanavir, darunavir, fosamprenavir, lopinavir, ritonavir, saquinavir, tipranavir**) are predicted to markedly to very markedly increase the exposure to **darifenacin**. Avoid. [Severe] Study
- HIV-protease inhibitors (**indinavir**) are predicted to slightly increase the exposure to **darifenacin**. [Moderate] Study
- **Idelalisib** is predicted to markedly to very markedly increase the exposure to **darifenacin**. Avoid. [Severe] Study
- **Imatinib** is predicted to slightly increase the exposure to **darifenacin**. [Moderate] Study
- Macrolides (**clarithromycin**) are predicted to markedly to very markedly increase the exposure to **darifenacin**. Avoid. [Severe] Study
- Macrolides (**erythromycin**) are predicted to slightly increase the exposure to **darifenacin**. [Moderate] Study
- **Netupitant** is predicted to slightly increase the exposure to **darifenacin**. [Moderate] Study
- **Nilotinib** is predicted to slightly increase the exposure to **darifenacin**. [Moderate] Study
- **Rifampicin** is predicted to decrease the exposure to **darifenacin**. [Moderate] Theoretical
- SSRIs (**fluoxetine, paroxetine**) are predicted to slightly increase the exposure to **darifenacin**. [Mild] Study
- **St John's Wort** is predicted to decrease the exposure to **darifenacin**. [Moderate] Theoretical
- **Terbinafine** is predicted to slightly increase the exposure to **darifenacin**. [Mild] Study
- **Darifenacin** is predicted to increase the exposure to tricyclic antidepressants. [Moderate] Theoretical → Also see TABLE 10 p. 820

Darunavir → see HIV-protease inhibitors

Dasabuvir
- Antiepileptics (**carbamazepine, fosphenytoin, phenobarbital, phenytoin, primidone**) are predicted to decrease the exposure to **dasabuvir**. Avoid. [Severe] Theoretical
- **Combined hormonal contraceptives** increase the risk of raised liver function tests when given with **dasabuvir**. Avoid. [Severe] Study
- **Enzalutamide** is predicted to decrease the exposure to **dasabuvir**. Avoid. [Severe] Theoretical
- Fibrates (**gemfibrozil**) very markedly increase the exposure to **dasabuvir**. Avoid. [Severe] Study
- **Dasabuvir** (with ombitasvir, paritaprevir and ritonavir) increases the concentration of loop diuretics (**furosemide**). Adjust dose. [Moderate] Study
- **Rifampicin** is predicted to decrease the exposure to **dasabuvir**. Avoid. [Severe] Theoretical

- **St John's Wort** is predicted to decrease the exposure to **dasabuvir**. Avoid. [Severe] Theoretical
- **Dasabuvir** increases the exposure to statins (**rosuvastatin**). Adjust **rosuvastatin** dose, p. 130. [Moderate] Study

Dasatinib → see TABLE 15 p. 821 (myelosuppression), TABLE 9 p. 820 (QT-interval prolongation), TABLE 4 p. 818 (antiplatelet effects)
- **Antacids** decrease the absorption of **dasatinib**. Separate administration by at least 2 hours. [Moderate] Study
- Antiarrhythmics (**dronedarone**) are predicted to increase the exposure to **dasatinib**. [Severe] Study → Also see TABLE 9 p. 820
- Antiepileptics (**carbamazepine, fosphenytoin, phenobarbital, phenytoin, primidone**) are predicted to markedly decrease the exposure to **dasatinib**. Avoid. [Severe] Study
- Antifungals, azoles (**fluconazole, isavuconazole, posaconazole**) are predicted to increase the exposure to **dasatinib**. [Severe] Study
- Antifungals, azoles (**itraconazole, ketoconazole, voriconazole**) are predicted to markedly increase the exposure to **dasatinib**. Avoid. [Severe] Study → Also see TABLE 9 p. 820
- **Aprepitant** is predicted to increase the exposure to **dasatinib**. [Severe] Study
- **Bosentan** is predicted to decrease the exposure to **dasatinib**. [Severe] Study
- Calcium channel blockers (**diltiazem, verapamil**) are predicted to increase the exposure to **dasatinib**. [Severe] Study
- **Cobicistat** is predicted to markedly increase the exposure to **dasatinib**. Avoid. [Severe] Study
- **Dasatinib** is predicted to increase the risk of bleeding events when given with **coumarins**. [Severe] Theoretical
- **Crizotinib** is predicted to increase the exposure to **dasatinib**. [Severe] Study → Also see TABLE 15 p. 821 → Also see TABLE 9 p. 820
- **Efavirenz** is predicted to decrease the exposure to **dasatinib**. [Severe] Study
- **Enzalutamide** is predicted to markedly decrease the exposure to **dasatinib**. Avoid. [Severe] Study
- **Grapefruit juice** is predicted to increase the exposure to **dasatinib**. Avoid. [Moderate] Theoretical
- H₂ receptor antagonists are predicted to decrease the exposure to **dasatinib**. Avoid. [Moderate] Study
- HIV-protease inhibitors (**atazanavir, darunavir, fosamprenavir, lopinavir, ritonavir, saquinavir, tipranavir**) are predicted to markedly increase the exposure to **dasatinib**. Avoid. [Severe] Study → Also see TABLE 9 p. 820
- HIV-protease inhibitors (**indinavir**) are predicted to increase the exposure to **dasatinib**. [Severe] Study
- **Idelalisib** is predicted to markedly increase the exposure to **dasatinib**. Avoid. [Severe] Study → Also see TABLE 15 p. 821
- **Imatinib** is predicted to increase the exposure to **dasatinib**. [Severe] Study → Also see TABLE 15 p. 821
- Macrolides (**clarithromycin**) are predicted to markedly increase the exposure to **dasatinib**. Avoid. [Severe] Study → Also see TABLE 9 p. 820
- Macrolides (**erythromycin**) are predicted to increase the exposure to **dasatinib**. [Severe] Study
- **Netupitant** is predicted to increase the exposure to **dasatinib**. [Severe] Study
- **Nevirapine** is predicted to decrease the exposure to **dasatinib**. [Severe] Study
- **Nilotinib** is predicted to increase the exposure to **dasatinib**. [Severe] Study → Also see TABLE 15 p. 821 → Also see TABLE 9 p. 820
- **Dasatinib** is predicted to increase the risk of bleeding events when given with **phenindione**. [Severe] Theoretical
- **Pitolisant** is predicted to decrease the exposure to **dasatinib**. Avoid. [Severe] Theoretical
- **Proton pump inhibitors** are predicted to slightly to moderately decrease the exposure to **dasatinib**. Avoid. [Severe] Study
- **Rifampicin** is predicted to markedly decrease the exposure to **dasatinib**. Avoid. [Severe] Study
- **St John's Wort** is predicted to decrease the exposure to **dasatinib**. [Severe] Study
- **Dasatinib** is predicted to increase the exposure to statins (**simvastatin**). [Moderate] Theoretical

Daunorubicin → see anthracyclines

Decitabine → see TABLE 15 p. 821 (myelosuppression)

Deferasirox → see iron chelators

Interactions | Appendix 1

Deferiprone → see TABLE 15 p. 821 (myelosuppression)
▸ Antacids (aluminium hydroxide) are predicted to decrease the absorption of **deferiprone**. Avoid. Moderate Theoretical
▸ Ascorbic acid is predicted to increase the risk of cardiovascular side-effects when given with **deferiprone**. Severe Theoretical

Deflazacort → see corticosteroids

Delamanid → see TABLE 9 p. 820 (QT-interval prolongation)
▸ Antiepileptics (carbamazepine, fosphenytoin, phenobarbital, phenytoin, primidone) are predicted to slightly decrease the exposure to **delamanid**. Avoid. Moderate Study
▸ Antifungals, azoles (itraconazole, ketoconazole, voriconazole) very slightly increase the exposure to **delamanid**. Severe Study → Also see TABLE 9 p. 820
▸ Cobicistat very slightly increases the exposure to **delamanid**. Severe Study
▸ Enzalutamide is predicted to slightly decrease the exposure to **delamanid**. Avoid. Moderate Study
▸ HIV-protease inhibitors (atazanavir, darunavir, fosamprenavir, lopinavir, ritonavir, saquinavir, tipranavir) very slightly increase the exposure to **delamanid**. Severe Study → Also see TABLE 9 p. 820
▸ Idelalisib very slightly increases the exposure to **delamanid**. Severe Study
▸ Macrolides (clarithromycin) very slightly increase the exposure to **delamanid**. Severe Study → Also see TABLE 9. 820
▸ Rifampicin is predicted to slightly decrease the exposure to **delamanid**. Avoid. Moderate Study

Demeclocycline → see tetracyclines
Denosumab → see monoclonal antibodies
Desferrioxamine → see iron chelators
Desflurane → see volatile halogenated anaesthetics
Desloratadine → see antihistamines, non-sedating
Desmopressin → see TABLE 18 p. 822 (hyponatraemia)
▸ Antiepileptics (lamotrigine) are predicted to increase the risk of hyponatraemia when given with **desmopressin**. Severe Theoretical
▸ Loperamide greatly increases the absorption of oral **desmopressin** (and possibly sublingual). Moderate Study
▸ Phenothiazines (chlorpromazine) are predicted to increase the risk of hyponatraemia when given with **desmopressin**. Severe Theoretical

Desogestrel
▸ Antiepileptics (carbamazepine, eslicarbazepine, fosphenytoin, oxcarbazepine, perampanel, phenobarbital, phenytoin, primidone, rufinamide, topiramate) are predicted to decrease the efficacy of **desogestrel**. For FSRH guidance, see Contraceptives, interactions p. 474. Severe Theoretical
▸ Desogestrel is predicted to increase the exposure to antiepileptics (lamotrigine). Moderate Study
▸ Aprepitant is predicted to decrease the efficacy of **desogestrel**. For FSRH guidance, see Contraceptives, interactions p. 474. Severe Theoretical
▸ Bosentan is predicted to decrease the efficacy of **desogestrel**. For FSRH guidance, see Contraceptives, interactions p. 474. Severe Theoretical
▸ Efavirenz is predicted to decrease the efficacy of **desogestrel**. For FSRH guidance, see Contraceptives, interactions p. 474. Severe Theoretical
▸ Fosaprepitant is predicted to decrease the efficacy of **desogestrel**. For FSRH guidance, see Contraceptives, interactions p. 474. Severe Theoretical
▸ Griseofulvin potentially decreases the efficacy of **desogestrel**. For FSRH guidance, see Contraceptives, interactions p. 474. Severe Anecdotal
▸ HIV-protease inhibitors (ritonavir) are predicted to decrease the efficacy of **desogestrel**. For FSRH guidance, see Contraceptives, interactions p. 474. Severe Theoretical
▸ Modafinil is predicted to decrease the efficacy of **desogestrel**. For FSRH guidance, see Contraceptives, interactions p. 474. Severe Theoretical
▸ Nevirapine is predicted to decrease the efficacy of **desogestrel**. For FSRH guidance, see Contraceptives, interactions p. 474. Severe Theoretical

▸ Rifabutin is predicted to decrease the efficacy of **desogestrel**. For FSRH guidance, see Contraceptives, interactions p. 474. Severe Theoretical
▸ Rifampicin is predicted to decrease the efficacy of **desogestrel**. For FSRH guidance, see Contraceptives, interactions p. 474. Severe Theoretical
▸ St John's Wort is predicted to decrease the efficacy of **desogestrel**. MHRA advises avoid. For FSRH guidance, see Contraceptives, interactions p. 474. Severe Theoretical
▸ Sugammadex is predicted to decrease the exposure to **desogestrel**. Refer to patient information leaflet for missed pill advice. Severe Theoretical
▸ Ulipristal is predicted to decrease the efficacy of **desogestrel**. Avoid. Severe Theoretical

Dexamethasone → see corticosteroids
Dexamfetamine → see amfetamines
Dexibuprofen → see NSAIDs
Dexketoprofen → see NSAIDs
Dexmedetomidine → see TABLE 11 p. 820 (CNS depressant effects)
Dexrazoxane → see iron chelators
Diamorphine → see opioids
Diazepam → see TABLE 11 p. 820 (CNS depressant effects)
▸ Diazepam potentially affects the concentration of antiepileptics (fosphenytoin, phenytoin). Monitor concentration and adjust dose. Severe Study
▸ Antifungals, azoles (fluconazole, voriconazole) moderately increase the exposure to **diazepam**. Monitor and adjust dose. Moderate Study
▸ HIV-protease inhibitors (ritonavir) are predicted to increase the exposure to **diazepam**. Avoid. Moderate Theoretical
▸ Rifampicin moderately decreases the exposure to **diazepam**. Avoid. Moderate Study
▸ SSRIs (fluvoxamine) moderately increase the exposure to **diazepam**. Moderate Study

Diazoxide → see TABLE 8 p. 819 (hypotension)
▸ Diazoxide decreases the concentration of antiepileptics (fosphenytoin, phenytoin) and antiepileptics (fosphenytoin, phenytoin) are predicted to decrease the effects of **diazoxide**. Monitor concentration and adjust dose. Moderate Anecdotal
▸ Diazoxide increases the risk of severe hypotension when given with hydralazine. Severe Study → Also see TABLE 8 p. 819

Diclofenac → see NSAIDs
Dicycloverine → see TABLE 10 p. 820 (antimuscarinics)
Didanosine → see TABLE 1 p. 818 (hepatotoxicity), TABLE 12 p. 821 (peripheral neuropathy)

ROUTE-SPECIFIC INFORMATION Antacids in tablet formulation might affect absorption of other drugs—give at least 2 hours apart.

▸ Allopurinol moderately increases the exposure to **didanosine**. Avoid. Severe Study
▸ Didanosine (buffered) decreases the exposure to antifungals, azoles (itraconazole, ketoconazole). Separate administration by 2 hours. Severe Study → Also see TABLE 1 p. 818
▸ Febuxostat is predicted to increase the exposure to **didanosine**. Severe Theoretical
▸ Ganciclovir is predicted to increase the exposure to **didanosine**. Moderate Study
▸ HIV-protease inhibitors (tipranavir) decrease the exposure to **didanosine**. Separate administration by 2 hours. Moderate Study
▸ Didanosine (buffered) decreases the exposure to HIV-protease inhibitors (atazanavir). Didanosine should be taken 2 hours after atazanavir. Severe Study
▸ Didanosine (buffered) is predicted to decrease the exposure to HIV-protease inhibitors (darunavir) boosted with ritonavir. Didanosine should be taken 1 hour before or 2 hours after darunavir. Moderate Theoretical
▸ Didanosine (buffered) decreases the exposure to HIV-protease inhibitors (indinavir). Separate administration by 1 hour. Severe Study
▸ Hydroxycarbamide increases the risk of toxicity when given with **didanosine**. Avoid. Severe Study
▸ Isoniazid is predicted to increase the risk of peripheral neuropathy when given with **didanosine**. Severe Theoretical → Also see TABLE 1 p. 818 → Also see TABLE 12 p. 821

▸ **Didanosine** is predicted to increase the risk of pancreatitis when given with **pentamidine**. Avoid. [Severe] Study

▸ **Didanosine** (buffered) is predicted to greatly decrease the exposure to oral **quinolones**. **Didanosine** should be taken 2 hours after quinolones. [Moderate] Study

▸ **Ribavirin** is predicted to increase the exposure to **didanosine**. Avoid. [Severe] Study

▸ **Didanosine** increases the risk of toxicity when given with **stavudine**. Avoid. [Severe] Study → Also see **TABLE 12** p. 821

▸ **Tenofovir** increases the risk of toxicity when given with **didanosine**. Avoid. [Severe] Study

▸ **Valganciclovir** is predicted to increase the exposure to **didanosine**. [Moderate] Study

Digoxin → see **TABLE 6** p. 819 (bradycardia)

GENERAL INFORMATION   Drugs that reduce serum potassium are predicted to increase the risk of digoxin toxicity, see **TABLE 17** p. 822.

▸ **Acarbose** decreases the concentration of **digoxin**. [Moderate] Study

▸ **Aldosterone antagonists (eplerenone)** very slightly increase the exposure to **digoxin**. [Mild] Study

▸ **Aldosterone antagonists (spironolactone)** increase the concentration of **digoxin**. Monitor and adjust dose. [Moderate] Study

▸ **Aminoglycosides** potentially increase the concentration of **digoxin**. Monitor and adjust dose. [Mild] Study

▸ **Antacids** decrease the absorption of **digoxin**. Separate administration by 2 hours. [Mild] Study

▸ **Antiarrhythmics (amiodarone, dronedarone)** are predicted to moderately increase the exposure to **digoxin**. Monitor and adjust **digoxin** dose, p. 79. [Severe] Study → Also see **TABLE 6** p. 819

▸ **Antiarrhythmics (propafenone)** increase the concentration of **digoxin**. Monitor and adjust dose. [Severe] Study

▸ **Antiepileptics (fosphenytoin, phenytoin)** are predicted to decrease the concentration of **digoxin**. [Moderate] Anecdotal

▸ **Antifungals, azoles (itraconazole)** markedly increase the concentration of **digoxin**. Monitor and adjust dose. [Severe] Study

▸ **Antifungals, azoles (ketoconazole)** are predicted to markedly increase the concentration of **digoxin**. [Severe] Theoretical

▸ **Antifungals, azoles (posaconazole)** are predicted to increase the concentration of **digoxin**. [Severe] Theoretical

▸ **Antimalarials (mefloquine)** are predicted to increase the risk of bradycardia when given with **digoxin**. [Severe] Theoretical

▸ **Antimalarials (quinine)** increase the concentration of **digoxin**. Monitor and adjust **digoxin** dose, p. 79. [Severe] Anecdotal

▸ **Balsalazide** is predicted to decrease the concentration of **digoxin**. [Moderate] Theoretical

▸ **Calcium channel blockers (diltiazem, verapamil)** increase the concentration of **digoxin**. Monitor and adjust dose. [Severe] Study → Also see **TABLE 6** p. 819

▸ **Intravenous calcium salts** increase the concentration of **digoxin**. Avoid. [Moderate] Anecdotal

▸ **Carbimazole** affects the concentration of **digoxin**. Monitor and adjust dose. [Moderate] Theoretical

▸ **Ceritinib** is predicted to increase the risk of bradycardia when given with **digoxin**. Avoid. [Severe] Theoretical

▸ **Ciclosporin** increases the concentration of **digoxin**. Monitor and adjust dose. [Severe] Theoretical

▸ **Daclatasvir** slightly increases the concentration of **digoxin**. [Severe] Study

▸ **HIV-protease inhibitors (ritonavir)** increase the concentration of **digoxin**. Adjust dose and monitor concentration. [Severe] Study

▸ **Lapatinib** is predicted to increase the exposure to **digoxin**. [Moderate] Theoretical

▸ **Levothyroxine** is predicted to affect the concentration of **digoxin**. Monitor and adjust dose. [Moderate] Theoretical

▸ **Liothyronine** is predicted to affect the concentration of **digoxin**. Monitor and adjust dose. [Moderate] Theoretical

▸ **Lumacaftor** is predicted to affect the exposure to **digoxin**. Monitor and adjust dose. [Moderate] Theoretical

▸ **Macrolides** increase the concentration of **digoxin**. [Severe] Anecdotal

▸ **Mirabegron** slightly increases the exposure to **digoxin**. Monitor **digoxin** concentration and adjust dose, p. 79. [Severe] Study

▸ **Neomycin** decreases the absorption of **digoxin**. [Moderate] Study

▸ **Neuromuscular blocking drugs, non-depolarising (pancuronium)** are predicted to increase the risk of cardiovascular side-effects when given with **digoxin**. [Severe] Anecdotal

▸ **NSAIDs (indometacin)** increase the concentration of **digoxin**. [Severe] Study

▸ **Penicillamine** potentially decreases the concentration of **digoxin**. Separate administration by 2 hours. [Severe] Anecdotal

▸ **Pitolisant** is predicted to decrease the exposure to **digoxin**. [Unknown] Theoretical

▸ **Ranolazine** increases the concentration of **digoxin**. [Moderate] Study

▸ **Rifampicin** decreases the concentration of **digoxin**. [Moderate] Study

▸ **St John's Wort** decreases the concentration of **digoxin**. Avoid. [Severe] Anecdotal

▸ **Sucralfate** decreases the absorption of **digoxin**. Separate administration by 2 hours. [Severe] Anecdotal

▸ **Sulfasalazine** decreases the concentration of **digoxin**. [Moderate] Study

▸ **Suxamethonium** is predicted to increase the risk of cardiovascular side-effects when given with **digoxin**. [Severe] Anecdotal

▸ **Ticagrelor** increases the concentration of **digoxin**. [Moderate] Study

▸ **Tolvaptan** increases the concentration of **digoxin**. [Mild] Study

▸ **Trimethoprim** increases the concentration of **digoxin**. [Moderate] Study

▸ **Vandetanib** slightly increases the exposure to **digoxin**. Monitor ECG and adjust dose. [Moderate] Study

▸ **Velpatasvir** is predicted to increase the exposure to **digoxin**. [Severe] Study

▸ **Vitamin D substances** are predicted to increase the risk of toxicity when given with **digoxin**. [Severe] Theoretical

Dihydrocodeine → see opioids

Dihydrotachysterol → see vitamin D substances

Diltiazem → see calcium channel blockers

Dimenhydrinate → see **TABLE 10** p. 820 (antimuscarinics)

Dimethyl fumarate

▸ **Live vaccines** are predicted to increase the risk of generalised infection (possibly life-threatening) when given with **dimethyl fumarate**. Public Health England advises avoid. [Severe] Theoretical

Dimethyl sulfoxide

▸ Topical **dimethyl sulfoxide** potentially increases the risk of peripheral neuropathy when given with **NSAIDs (sulindac)**. Avoid. [Severe] Anecdotal

Diphenoxylate → see opioids

Dipipanone → see opioids

Dipyridamole → see **TABLE 8** p. 819 (hypotension), **TABLE 4** p. 818 (antiplatelet effects)

▸ **Antacids** are predicted to decrease the absorption of **dipyridamole** (immediate release tablets). [Moderate] Theoretical

▸ **Dipyridamole** increases the exposure to antiarrhythmics **(adenosine)**. Avoid or adjust dose. [Severe] Study

▸ **H_2 receptor antagonists** are predicted to decrease the absorption of **dipyridamole** (immediate release tablets). [Moderate] Theoretical

▸ **Proton pump inhibitors** are predicted to decrease the absorption of **dipyridamole** (immediate release tablets). [Moderate] Theoretical

Disopyramide → see antiarrhythmics

Disulfiram → see **TABLE 12** p. 821 (peripheral neuropathy)

FOOD AND LIFESTYLE   Disulfiram gives rise to an extremely unpleasant systemic reaction after the ingestion of even a small amount of alcohol. Ensure that alcohol is not consumed for at least 24 hours before initiating treatment and should be avoided for at least 1 week after stopping treatment.

▸ **Disulfiram** increases the concentration of antiepileptics **(fosphenytoin, phenytoin)**. Monitor concentration and adjust dose. [Severe] Study → Also see **TABLE 12** p. 821

▸ **Disulfiram** increases the anticoagulant effect of **coumarins**. Monitor and adjust dose. [Severe] Study

▸ **Disulfiram** increases the risk of acute psychoses when given with **metronidazole**. [Severe] Study → Also see **TABLE 12** p. 821

A1

Interactions | Appendix 1

Disulfiram (continued)
▸ **Disulfiram** is predicted to increase the anticoagulant effect of phenindione. Severe Theoretical

Dobutamine → see sympathomimetics, inotropic

Docetaxel → see taxanes

Docusate sodium → see TABLE 17 p. 822 (reduced serum potassium)

Dolutegravir
▸ **Antacids** moderately decrease the exposure to **dolutegravir**. Dolutegravir should be taken 2 hours before or 6 hours after antacids. Moderate Study
▸ **Antiepileptics (carbamazepine, fosphenytoin, phenobarbital, phenytoin, primidone)** decrease the exposure to **dolutegravir**. Adjust dose. Severe Study
▸ **Antiepileptics (oxcarbazepine)** are predicted to decrease the exposure to **dolutegravir**. Adjust dose. Severe Theoretical
▸ **Bosentan** decreases the exposure to **dolutegravir**. Adjust dose. Severe Study
▸ **Oral calcium salts** decrease the absorption of **dolutegravir**. Dolutegravir should be taken 2 hours before or 6 hours after calcium salts. Moderate Study
▸ **Efavirenz** decreases the exposure to **dolutegravir**. Adjust dose. Severe Study
▸ **Enzalutamide** decreases the exposure to **dolutegravir**. Adjust dose. Severe Study
▸ **Etravirine** moderately decreases the exposure to **dolutegravir**. Avoid unless given with atazanavir, darunavir, or lopinavir (all boosted with ritonavir). Severe Study
▸ **HIV-protease inhibitors (fosamprenavir)** boosted with ritonavir slightly decrease the exposure to **dolutegravir**. Avoid if resistant to HIV-integrase inhibitors. Severe Study
▸ **HIV-protease inhibitors (tipranavir)** moderately decrease the exposure to **dolutegravir**. Refer to specialist literature. Severe Study
▸ **Iron (oral)** decreases the absorption of **dolutegravir**. Iron (oral) should be taken 2 hours before or 6 hours after **dolutegravir**. Moderate Study
▸ **Dolutegravir** slightly to moderately increases the exposure to metformin. Use with caution and adjust dose. Severe Study
▸ **Nevirapine** decreases the exposure to **dolutegravir**. Adjust dose. Severe Study
▸ **Rifampicin** decreases the exposure to **dolutegravir**. Adjust dose. Severe Study
▸ **St John's Wort** decreases the exposure to **dolutegravir**. Adjust dose. Severe Study
▸ **Sucralfate** decreases the absorption of **dolutegravir**. Moderate Study

Domperidone → see TABLE 9 p. 820 (QT-interval prolongation)
▸ **Antiarrhythmics (dronedarone)** increase the risk of QT-prolongation when given with **domperidone**. Avoid. Severe Study
▸ **Antifungals, azoles (fluconazole, isavuconazole, itraconazole, ketoconazole, posaconazole, voriconazole)** increase the risk of QT-prolongation when given with **domperidone**. Avoid. Severe Study
▸ **Aprepitant** increases the risk of QT-prolongation when given with **domperidone**. Avoid. Severe Study
▸ **Calcium channel blockers (diltiazem, verapamil)** increase the risk of QT-prolongation when given with **domperidone**. Avoid. Severe Study
▸ **Cobicistat** increases the risk of QT-prolongation when given with **domperidone**. Avoid. Severe Study
▸ **Crizotinib** increases the risk of QT-prolongation when given with **domperidone**. Avoid. Severe Study
▸ **Domperidone** is predicted to decrease the prolactin-lowering effect of dopamine receptor agonists (**bromocriptine, cabergoline**). Moderate Theoretical
▸ **HIV-protease inhibitors** increase the risk of QT-prolongation when given with **domperidone**. Avoid. Severe Study
▸ **Idelalisib** increases the risk of QT-prolongation when given with **domperidone**. Avoid. Severe Study
▸ **Imatinib** increases the risk of QT-prolongation when given with **domperidone**. Avoid. Severe Study
▸ **Macrolides (clarithromycin, erythromycin)** increase the risk of QT-prolongation when given with **domperidone**. Avoid. Severe Study

▸ **Netupitant** increases the risk of QT-prolongation when given with **domperidone**. Avoid. Severe Study
▸ **Nilotinib** increases the risk of QT-prolongation when given with **domperidone**. Avoid. Severe Study

Donepezil → see anticholinesterases, centrally acting

Dopamine → see sympathomimetics, inotropic

Dopamine receptor agonists → see TABLE 8 p. 819 (hypotension), TABLE 9 p. 820 (QT-interval prolongation), TABLE 10 p. 820 (antimuscarinics)

amantadine · apomorphine · bromocriptine · cabergoline · pergolide · pramipexole · quinagolide · ropinirole · rotigotine

FOOD AND LIFESTYLE Dose adjustment might be necessary if smoking started or stopped during treatment with **ropinirole**.

▸ **Amisulpride** is predicted to decrease the effects of **dopamine receptor agonists**. Avoid. Moderate Theoretical → Also see TABLE 9 p. 820
▸ **Antiarrhythmics (dronedarone)** are predicted to increase the exposure to dopamine receptor agonists (**bromocriptine, cabergoline**). Severe Theoretical
▸ **Antifungals, azoles (fluconazole, isavuconazole, posaconazole)** are predicted to increase the exposure to dopamine receptor agonists (**bromocriptine, cabergoline**). Severe Theoretical
▸ **Antifungals, azoles (itraconazole, ketoconazole, voriconazole)** increase the exposure to dopamine receptor agonists (**bromocriptine, cabergoline**). Severe Study
▸ **Aprepitant** is predicted to increase the exposure to dopamine receptor agonists (**bromocriptine, cabergoline**). Severe Theoretical
▸ **Aripiprazole** is predicted to decrease the effects of **dopamine receptor agonists**. Moderate Theoretical → Also see TABLE 8 p. 819
▸ **Asenapine** is predicted to decrease the effects of **dopamine receptor agonists**. Adjust dose. Moderate Theoretical → Also see TABLE 8 p. 819
▸ **Benperidol** is predicted to decrease the effects of **dopamine receptor agonists**. Avoid. Moderate Theoretical → Also see TABLE 8 p. 819
▸ **Bupropion** increases the risk of side-effects when given with amantadine. Moderate Study
▸ **Calcium channel blockers (diltiazem, verapamil)** are predicted to increase the exposure to dopamine receptor agonists (**bromocriptine, cabergoline**). Severe Theoretical → Also see TABLE 8 p. 819
▸ **Clozapine** is predicted to decrease the effects of **dopamine receptor agonists**. Moderate Theoretical → Also see TABLE 8 p. 819 → Also see TABLE 10 p. 820
▸ **Cobicistat** increases the exposure to dopamine receptor agonists (**bromocriptine, cabergoline**). Severe Study
▸ **Combined hormonal contraceptives** are predicted to increase the exposure to **ropinirole**. Adjust dose. Moderate Study
▸ **Crizotinib** is predicted to increase the exposure to dopamine receptor agonists (**bromocriptine, cabergoline**). Severe Theoretical
▸ **Domperidone** is predicted to decrease the prolactin-lowering effect of dopamine receptor agonists (**bromocriptine, cabergoline**). Moderate Theoretical
▸ Dopamine receptor agonists (**cabergoline**) are predicted to increase the risk of ergotism when given with dopamine receptor agonists (**bromocriptine**). Moderate Theoretical → Also see TABLE 8 p. 819
▸ Dopamine receptor agonists (**bromocriptine, cabergoline**) are predicted to increase the risk of ergotism with dopamine receptor agonists (**pergolide**). Avoid. Moderate Theoretical → Also see TABLE 8 p. 819
▸ Dopamine receptor agonists (**amantadine**) are predicted to increase the exposure to dopamine receptor agonists (**pramipexole**). Adjust pramipexole dose. Moderate Theoretical → Also see TABLE 8 p. 819
▸ **Droperidol** is predicted to decrease the effects of **dopamine receptor agonists**. Avoid. Moderate Theoretical → Also see TABLE 8 p. 819 → Also see TABLE 9 p. 820
▸ **Ergometrine** is predicted to increase the risk of ergotism when given with dopamine receptor agonists (**cabergoline, pergolide**). Avoid. Moderate Theoretical
▸ **Ergotamine** is predicted to increase the risk of ergotism when given with dopamine receptor agonists (**bromocriptine, cabergoline**). Avoid. Moderate Theoretical

- Ergotamine is predicted to increase the risk of ergotism when given with **pergolide**. Moderate Theoretical
- Flupentixol is predicted to decrease side effects of **dopamine receptor agonists**. Avoid. Moderate Theoretical → Also see TABLE 8 p. 819
- Apomorphine is predicted to increase the risk of severe hypotension when given with granisetron. Severe Theoretical
- H₂ receptor antagonists (cimetidine) slightly increase the exposure to **pramipexole**. Adjust dose. Moderate Study
- Haloperidol is predicted to decrease the effects of **dopamine receptor agonists**. Avoid. Moderate Theoretical → Also see TABLE 9 p. 820 → Also see TABLE 10 p. 820
- HIV-protease inhibitors (atazanavir, darunavir, fosamprenavir, lopinavir, ritonavir, saquinavir, tipranavir) increase the exposure to dopamine receptor agonists (**bromocriptine, cabergoline**). Severe Study
- HIV-protease inhibitors (indinavir) are predicted to increase the exposure to dopamine receptor agonists (**bromocriptine, cabergoline**). Severe Theoretical
- Hormone replacement therapy decreases the clearance of **ropinirole**. Monitor and adjust dose. Moderate Study
- Idelalisib increases the exposure to dopamine receptor agonists (**bromocriptine, cabergoline**). Severe Study
- Imatinib is predicted to increase the exposure to dopamine receptor agonists (**bromocriptine, cabergoline**). Severe Theoretical
- Loxapine is predicted to decrease the effects of **dopamine receptor agonists**. Moderate Theoretical → Also see TABLE 8 p. 819 → Also see TABLE 9 p. 820
- Macrolides (clarithromycin) increase the exposure to dopamine receptor agonists (**bromocriptine, cabergoline**). Severe Study
- Macrolides (erythromycin) are predicted to increase the exposure to dopamine receptor agonists (**bromocriptine, cabergoline**). Severe Theoretical
- Amantadine increases the risk of CNS toxicity when given with memantine. Use with caution or avoid. Severe Theoretical
- Memantine is predicted to increase the effects of dopamine receptor agonists (**apomorphine, bromocriptine, cabergoline, pergolide, pramipexole, quinagolide, ropinirole, rotigotine**). Moderate Theoretical
- Metoclopramide is predicted to decrease the effects of dopamine receptor agonists, (**apomorphine, bromocriptine, cabergoline, pergolide, pramipexole, quinagolide, ropinirole, rotigotine**). Avoid. Moderate Study
- Netupitant is predicted to increase the exposure to dopamine receptor agonists (**bromocriptine, cabergoline**). Severe Theoretical
- Nilotinib is predicted to increase the exposure to dopamine receptor agonists (**bromocriptine, cabergoline**). Severe Theoretical
- Olanzapine is predicted to decrease the effects of **dopamine receptor agonists**. Avoid. Moderate Theoretical → Also see TABLE 8 p. 819
- Apomorphine increases the risk of severe hypotension when given with ondansetron. Avoid. Severe Study → Also see TABLE 9 p. 820
- Paliperidone is predicted to decrease the effects of **dopamine receptor agonists**. Avoid. Moderate Theoretical → Also see TABLE 8 p. 819 → Also see TABLE 9 p. 820
- Apomorphine is predicted to increase the risk of severe hypotension when given with palonosetron. Severe Theoretical
- Phenothiazines are predicted to decrease the effects of dopamine receptor agonists. Avoid. Moderate Study → Also see TABLE 8 p. 819 → Also see TABLE 9 p. 820 → Also see TABLE 10 p. 820
- Pimozide is predicted to decrease the effects of **dopamine receptor agonists**. Avoid. Moderate Theoretical → Also see TABLE 8 p. 819 → Also see TABLE 9 p. 820 → Also see TABLE 10 p. 820
- Quetiapine is predicted to decrease the effects of **dopamine receptor agonists**. Avoid. Moderate Theoretical→ Also see TABLE 8 p. 819
- Quinolones (ciprofloxacin) are predicted to increase the exposure to **ropinirole**. Adjust dose. Moderate Study
- Risperidone is predicted to decrease the effects of **dopamine receptor agonists**. Avoid. Moderate Theoretical → Also see TABLE 8 p. 819 → Also see TABLE 10 p. 820
- SSRIs (fluvoxamine) are predicted to increase the exposure to **ropinirole**. Adjust dose. Moderate Study

- Sulpiride is predicted to decrease the effects of **dopamine receptor agonists**. Avoid. Moderate Theoretical → Also see TABLE 8 p. 819 → Also see TABLE 9 p. 820
- Zuclopenthixol is predicted to decrease the effects of **dopamine receptor agonists**. Avoid. Moderate Theoretical → Also see TABLE 8 p. 819 → Also see TABLE 9 p. 820

Dopexamine → see sympathomimetics, inotropic

Dorzolamide

> **ROUTE-SPECIFIC INFORMATION** Since systemic absorption can follow topical application, the possibility of interactions should be borne in mind.

Dosulepin → see tricyclic antidepressants

Doxapram
- Aminophylline increases the risk of agitation when given with doxapram. Moderate Study
- Monoamine-oxidase A and B inhibitors, irreversible are predicted to increase the effects of doxapram. Moderate Theoretical
- Theophylline increases the risk of agitation when given with doxapram. Moderate Study

Doxazosin → see alpha blockers
Doxepin → see tricyclic antidepressants
Doxorubicin → see anthracyclines
Doxycycline → see tetracyclines
Dronedarone → see antiarrhythmics
Droperidol → see TABLE 8 p. 819 (hypotension), TABLE 9 p. 820 (QT-interval prolongation), TABLE 11 p. 820 (CNS depressant effects)
- Droperidol is predicted to decrease the effects of **dopamine receptor agonists**. Avoid. Moderate Theoretical → Also see TABLE 8 p. 819 → Also see TABLE 9 p. 820
- Droperidol is predicted to decrease the effects of **guanethidine**. Monitor and adjust dose. Moderate Theoretical → Also see TABLE 8 p. 819
- Droperidol decreases the effects of **levodopa**. Severe Study → Also see TABLE 8 p. 819

Drospirenone → see TABLE 16 p. 822 (increased serum potassium)
- Antifungals, azoles (ketoconazole) moderately increase the exposure to **drospirenone**. Severe Study

Dulaglutide → see TABLE 14 p. 821 (antidiabetic drugs)
Duloxetine → see TABLE 18 p. 822 (hyponatraemia), TABLE 13 p. 821 (serotonin syndrome), TABLE 4 p. 818 (antiplatelet effects)
- Duloxetine is predicted to increase the exposure to antiarrhythmics (flecainide). Severe Theoretical
- Duloxetine is predicted to increase the exposure to beta blockers, non-selective (carvedilol, timolol). Moderate Theoretical
- Duloxetine is predicted to increase the exposure to beta blockers, selective (metoprolol, nebivolol). Moderate Study
- Duloxetine is predicted to decrease the efficacy of opioids (tramadol). Moderate Study → Also see TABLE 13 p. 821
- Duloxetine is predicted to increase the exposure to pitolisant. Use with caution and adjust dose. Moderate Study
- Quinolones (ciprofloxacin) are predicted to increase the exposure to duloxetine. Avoid. Moderate Theoretical
- SSRIs (fluvoxamine) markedly increase the exposure to duloxetine. Avoid. Severe Study → Also see TABLE 18 p. 822 → Also see TABLE 13 p. 821 → Also see TABLE 4 p. 818

Dutasteride
- Antiarrhythmics (dronedarone) are predicted to moderately increase the exposure to dutasteride. Mild Study
- Antifungals, azoles (fluconazole, isavuconazole, posaconazole) are predicted to moderately increase the exposure to dutasteride. Mild Study
- Antifungals, azoles (itraconazole, ketoconazole, voriconazole) are predicted to increase the exposure to dutasteride. Monitor side effects and adjust dose. Moderate Theoretical
- Aprepitant is predicted to moderately increase the exposure to dutasteride. Mild Study
- Calcium channel blockers (diltiazem, verapamil) are predicted to moderately increase the exposure to dutasteride. Mild Study
- Cobicistat is predicted to increase the exposure to dutasteride. Monitor side effects and adjust dose. Moderate Theoretical
- Crizotinib is predicted to moderately increase the exposure to dutasteride. Mild Study
- HIV-protease inhibitors (atazanavir, darunavir, fosamprenavir, lopinavir, ritonavir, saquinavir, tipranavir) are predicted to

A1

Interactions | Appendix 1

Dutasteride (continued)
increase the exposure to **dutasteride**. Monitor side effects and adjust dose. Moderate Theoretical

▶ HIV-protease inhibitors (**indinavir**) are predicted to moderately increase the exposure to **dutasteride**. Mild Study

▶ Idelalisib is predicted to increase the exposure to **dutasteride**. Monitor side effects and adjust dose. Moderate Theoretical

▶ Imatinib is predicted to moderately increase the exposure to **dutasteride**. Mild Study

▶ Macrolides (**clarithromycin**) are predicted to increase the exposure to **dutasteride**. Monitor side effects and adjust dose. Moderate Theoretical

▶ Macrolides (**erythromycin**) are predicted to moderately increase the exposure to **dutasteride**. Mild Study

▶ Netupitant is predicted to moderately increase the exposure to **dutasteride**. Mild Study

▶ Nilotinib is predicted to moderately increase the exposure to **dutasteride**. Mild Study

Eculizumab → see monoclonal antibodies
Edoxaban → see TABLE 3 p. 818 (anticoagulant effects)

▶ Antiarrhythmics (**amiodarone**) slightly increase the exposure to **edoxaban**. Severe Study

▶ Antiarrhythmics (**dronedarone**) slightly increase the exposure to **edoxaban**. Adjust **edoxaban** dose. Severe Study

▶ Antiepileptics (**carbamazepine**) are predicted to decrease the exposure to **edoxaban**. Moderate Study

▶ Antifungals, azoles (**itraconazole**) are predicted to slightly increase the exposure to **edoxaban**. Severe Theoretical

▶ Antifungals, azoles (**ketoconazole**) slightly increase the exposure to **edoxaban**. Adjust **edoxaban** dose. Severe Study

▶ Calcium channel blockers (**verapamil**) are predicted to slightly increase the exposure to **edoxaban**. Severe Theoretical

▶ Ceritinib is predicted to increase the exposure to **edoxaban**. Moderate Theoretical

▶ Ciclosporin slightly increases the exposure to **edoxaban**. Adjust **edoxaban** dose. Severe Study

▶ HIV-protease inhibitors (**lopinavir, ritonavir, saquinavir**) are predicted to slightly increase the exposure to **edoxaban**. Severe Theoretical

▶ Lapatinib is predicted to slightly increase the exposure to **edoxaban**. Severe Theoretical

▶ Lumacaftor is predicted to affect the exposure to **edoxaban**. Moderate Theoretical

▶ Macrolides (**azithromycin, clarithromycin**) are predicted to slightly increase the exposure to **edoxaban**. Severe Theoretical

▶ Macrolides (**erythromycin**) slightly increase the exposure to **edoxaban**. Adjust **edoxaban** dose. Severe Study

▶ Mirabegron is predicted to increase the exposure to **edoxaban**. Mild Theoretical

▶ Ranolazine is predicted to slightly increase the exposure to **edoxaban**. Severe Theoretical

▶ Rifampicin is predicted to decrease the exposure to **edoxaban**. Moderate Study

▶ St John's Wort is predicted to decrease the exposure to **edoxaban**. Moderate Study

▶ Velpatasvir is predicted to increase the exposure to **edoxaban**. Severe Theoretical

▶ Vemurafenib is predicted to slightly increase the exposure to **edoxaban**. Severe Theoretical

Efavirenz

▶ **Efavirenz** is predicted to decrease the exposure to antiarrhythmics (**dronedarone**). Severe Theoretical

▶ Antiepileptics (**carbamazepine**) slightly decrease the exposure to **efavirenz** and **efavirenz** slightly decreases the exposure to antiepileptics (**carbamazepine**). Severe Study

▶ Antiepileptics (**fosphenytoin, phenytoin**) slightly decrease the exposure to **efavirenz** and **efavirenz** affects the concentration of antiepileptics (**fosphenytoin, phenytoin**). Severe Theoretical

▶ Antiepileptics (**phenobarbital**) are predicted to decrease the exposure to **efavirenz** and **efavirenz** affects the concentration of antiepileptics (**phenobarbital**). Severe Theoretical

▶ **Efavirenz** is predicted to affect the efficacy of antiepileptics (**primidone**) and antiepileptics (**primidone**) are predicted to slightly decrease the exposure to **efavirenz**. Severe Theoretical

▶ **Efavirenz** is predicted to decrease the exposure to antifungals, azoles (**isavuconazole**). Avoid. Severe Theoretical

▶ **Efavirenz** slightly decreases the exposure to antifungals, azoles (**itraconazole**). Avoid **efavirenz** for 14 days before and during treatment with **itraconazole**. Moderate Study

▶ **Efavirenz** moderately decreases the exposure to antifungals, azoles (**ketoconazole**). Severe Study

▶ **Efavirenz** slightly decreases the exposure to antifungals, azoles (**posaconazole**). Avoid. Moderate Study

▶ **Efavirenz** moderately decreases the exposure to antifungals, azoles (**voriconazole**) and antifungals, azoles (**voriconazole**) slightly increase the exposure to **efavirenz**. Adjust dose. Severe Study

▶ **Efavirenz** decreases the concentration of antimalarials (**artemether**). Severe Study

▶ **Efavirenz** moderately decreases the exposure to antimalarials (**atovaquone**). Avoid. Moderate Study

▶ **Efavirenz** affects the exposure to antimalarials (**proguanil**). Avoid. Moderate Study

▶ **Efavirenz** is predicted to decrease the exposure to axitinib. Moderate Theoretical

▶ **Efavirenz** is predicted to decrease the exposure to bedaquiline. Avoid. Severe Study

▶ **Efavirenz** is predicted to decrease the exposure to bosutinib. Avoid. Severe Theoretical

▶ **Efavirenz** moderately decreases the exposure to bupropion. Moderate Study

▶ **Efavirenz** is predicted to decrease the exposure to cabozantinib. Moderate Theoretical

▶ **Efavirenz** is predicted to decrease the exposure to calcium channel blockers (**amlodipine, felodipine, isradipine, lacidipine, lercanidipine, nicardipine, nifedipine, nimodipine**). Monitor and adjust dose. Moderate Theoretical

▶ **Efavirenz** is predicted to decrease the exposure to calcium channel blockers (**diltiazem, verapamil**). Moderate Theoretical

▶ **Efavirenz** is predicted to decrease the concentration of caspofungin. Adjust dose. Moderate Study

▶ **Efavirenz** decreases the concentration of ciclosporin. Monitor ciclosporin concentration and adjust dose. Moderate Study

▶ **Efavirenz** is predicted to decrease the exposure to cobicistat. Avoid. Severe Theoretical

▶ **Efavirenz** is predicted to decrease the exposure to cobimetinib. Avoid. Severe Study

▶ **Efavirenz** is predicted to decrease the efficacy of combined hormonal contraceptives. For FSRH guidance, see Contraceptives, interactions p. 474. Severe Study

▶ **Efavirenz** is predicted to affect the concentration of coumarins. Adjust dose. Moderate Theoretical

▶ **Efavirenz** is predicted to decrease the exposure to crizotinib. Avoid. Severe Study

▶ **Efavirenz** is predicted to decrease the exposure to daclatasvir. Adjust dose. Severe Study

▶ **Efavirenz** is predicted to decrease the exposure to dasatinib. Severe Study

▶ **Efavirenz** is predicted to decrease the efficacy of desogestrel. For FSRH guidance, see Contraceptives, interactions p. 474. Severe Theoretical

▶ **Efavirenz** decreases the exposure to dolutegravir. Adjust dose. Severe Study

▶ **Efavirenz** is predicted to moderately decrease the exposure to elbasvir. Avoid. Severe Study

▶ **Efavirenz** is predicted to decrease the concentration of elvitegravir. Avoid. Severe Theoretical

▶ **Efavirenz** is predicted to decrease the effects of ergotamine. Moderate Theoretical

▶ **Efavirenz** is predicted to decrease the exposure to erlotinib. Severe Theoretical

▶ **Efavirenz** is predicted to decrease the efficacy of etonogestrel. For FSRH guidance, see Contraceptives, interactions p. 474. Severe Theoretical

▶ **Efavirenz** is predicted to decrease the exposure to etravirine. Avoid. Severe Study

▶ **Efavirenz** is predicted to decrease the concentration of everolimus. Avoid or adjust dose. Severe Study

▸ **Efavirenz** is predicted to decrease the exposure to gefitinib. Avoid. Severe Theoretical

▸ **Efavirenz** is predicted to markedly decrease the exposure to grazoprevir. Avoid. Severe Study

▸ **Efavirenz** is predicted to decrease the concentration of guanfacine. Adjust dose. Moderate Theoretical

▸ **Efavirenz** decreases the exposure to HIV-protease inhibitors. Refer to specialist literature. Severe Study

▸ **Efavirenz** is predicted to decrease the effects of Hormone replacement therapy. Moderate Anecdotal

▸ **Efavirenz** is predicted to decrease the exposure to imatinib. Moderate Study

▸ **Efavirenz** is predicted to decrease the exposure to lapatinib. Avoid. Severe Study

▸ **Efavirenz** is predicted to decrease the efficacy of levonorgestrel. For FSRH guidance, see Contraceptives, interactions p. 474. Severe Theoretical

▸ **Efavirenz** is predicted to decrease the exposure to lurasidone. Monitor and adjust dose. Moderate Theoretical

▸ **Efavirenz** decreases the exposure to macrolides (clarithromycin). Moderate Study

▸ **Efavirenz** decreases the exposure to maraviroc. Refer to specialist literature. Severe Theoretical

▸ **Efavirenz** is predicted to alter the effects of midazolam. Avoid. Moderate Theoretical

▸ Nevirapine decreases the concentration of **efavirenz**. Avoid. Severe Study

▸ **Efavirenz** is predicted to decrease the exposure to nilotinib. Avoid. Severe Theoretical

▸ **Efavirenz** is predicted to decrease the efficacy of norethisterone. For FSRH guidance, see Contraceptives, interactions p. 474. Severe Anecdotal

▸ **Efavirenz** is predicted to decrease the exposure to olaparib. Avoid. Moderate Theoretical

▸ **Efavirenz** decreases the exposure to opioids (methadone). Monitor and adjust dose. Severe Study

▸ **Efavirenz** is predicted to decrease the exposure to osimertinib. Moderate Theoretical

▸ **Efavirenz** is predicted to decrease the exposure to paritaprevir with ritonavir and ombitasvir. Avoid. Severe Study

▸ **Efavirenz** is predicted to decrease the exposure to phosphodiesterase type-5 inhibitors. Moderate Theoretical

▸ Pitolisant is predicted to decrease the exposure to **efavirenz**. Unknown Theoretical

▸ **Efavirenz** slightly decreases the exposure to rifabutin. Adjust dose. Severe Study

▸ Rifampicin slightly decreases the exposure to **efavirenz**. Adjust dose. Severe Study

▸ **Efavirenz** is predicted to decrease the exposure to rilpivirine. Avoid. Severe Theoretical

▸ **Efavirenz** is predicted to decrease the exposure to ruxolitinib. Monitor and adjust dose. Moderate Theoretical

▸ **Efavirenz** is predicted to decrease the exposure to simeprevir. Avoid. Severe Study

▸ **Efavirenz** is predicted to decrease the concentration of sirolimus. Monitor and adjust dose. Moderate Theoretical

▸ St John's Wort is predicted to decrease the concentration of **efavirenz**. Avoid. Severe Theoretical

▸ **Efavirenz** slightly decreases the exposure to statins (atorvastatin). Mild Study

▸ **Efavirenz** moderately decreases the exposure to statins (simvastatin). Moderate Study

▸ **Efavirenz** is predicted to decrease the concentration of tacrolimus. Monitor and adjust dose. Moderate Theoretical

▸ **Efavirenz** is predicted to decrease the exposure to taxanes (cabazitaxel). Avoid. Severe Study

▸ **Efavirenz** is predicted to decrease the concentration of temsirolimus. Avoid. Severe Theoretical

▸ **Efavirenz** is predicted to decrease the exposure to ticagrelor. Moderate Theoretical

▸ **Efavirenz** is predicted to decrease the exposure to tolvaptan. Moderate Theoretical

▸ **Efavirenz** decreases the efficacy of ulipristal. For FSRH guidance, see Contraceptives, interactions p. 474. Severe Anecdotal

▸ **Efavirenz** is predicted to decrease the exposure to velpatasvir. Avoid. Moderate Theoretical

Elbasvir

▸ Antiepileptics (carbamazepine, fosphenytoin, phenobarbital, phenytoin, primidone) are predicted to decrease the exposure to **elbasvir**. Avoid. Severe Study

▸ Antifungals, azoles (itraconazole, ketoconazole, voriconazole) slightly to moderately increase the exposure to **elbasvir**. Avoid. Moderate Study

▸ Bosentan is predicted to moderately decrease the exposure to **elbasvir**. Avoid. Severe Study

▸ Cobicistat slightly to moderately increases the exposure to **elbasvir**. Avoid. Moderate Study

▸ **Elbasvir** is predicted to increase the concentration of dabigatran. Moderate Theoretical

▸ Efavirenz is predicted to moderately decrease the exposure to **elbasvir**. Avoid. Severe Study

▸ Enzalutamide is predicted to decrease the exposure to **elbasvir**. Avoid. Severe Study

▸ Etravirine is predicted to decrease the exposure to **elbasvir**. Avoid. Unknown Theoretical

▸ HIV-protease inhibitors (atazanavir, darunavir, fosamprenavir, lopinavir, ritonavir, saquinavir, tipranavir) slightly to moderately increase the exposure to **elbasvir**. Avoid. Moderate Study

▸ Idelalisib slightly to moderately increases the exposure to **elbasvir**. Avoid. Moderate Study

▸ Macrolides (clarithromycin) slightly to moderately increase the exposure to **elbasvir**. Avoid. Moderate Study

▸ Modafinil is predicted to decrease the exposure to **elbasvir**. Avoid. Unknown Theoretical

▸ Nevirapine is predicted to moderately decrease the exposure to **elbasvir**. Avoid. Severe Study

▸ Rifampicin is predicted to decrease the exposure to **elbasvir**. Avoid. Severe Study

▸ St John's Wort is predicted to moderately decrease the exposure to **elbasvir**. Avoid. Severe Study

▸ **Elbasvir** potentially increases the exposure to statins (atorvastatin). Adjust atorvastatin dose, p. 128. Moderate Study

▸ **Elbasvir** is predicted to increase the exposure to statins (fluvastatin). Adjust fluvastatin dose, p. 129. Unknown Theoretical

▸ **Elbasvir** increases the exposure to statins (rosuvastatin). Adjust rosuvastatin dose, p. 130. Moderate Study

▸ **Elbasvir** is predicted to increase the exposure to statins (simvastatin). Adjust simvastatin dose, p. 130. Unknown Theoretical

Eletriptan → see TABLE 13 p. 821 (serotonin syndrome)

▸ Antifungals, azoles (itraconazole, ketoconazole, voriconazole) are predicted to markedly increase the exposure to **eletriptan**. Avoid. Severe Study

▸ Cobicistat is predicted to markedly increase the exposure to **eletriptan**. Avoid. Severe Study

▸ **Eletriptan** increases the risk of vasoconstriction when given with ergotamine. Separate administration by 24 hours. Severe Study

▸ HIV-protease inhibitors (atazanavir, darunavir, fosamprenavir, lopinavir, ritonavir, saquinavir, tipranavir) are predicted to markedly increase the exposure to **eletriptan**. Avoid. Severe Study

▸ Idelalisib is predicted to markedly increase the exposure to **eletriptan**. Avoid. Severe Study

▸ Macrolides (clarithromycin) are predicted to markedly increase the exposure to **eletriptan**. Avoid. Severe Study

▸ Macrolides (erythromycin) moderately increase the exposure to **eletriptan**. Avoid. Moderate Study

Elotuzumab → see monoclonal antibodies

Eltrombopag

▸ Antacids decrease the absorption of **eltrombopag**. **Eltrombopag** should be taken 2 hours before or 4 hours after antacids. Severe Study

▸ Oral calcium salts decrease the absorption of **eltrombopag**. **Eltrombopag** should be taken 2 hours before or 4 hours after calcium salts. Severe Study

A1

Interactions | Appendix 1

Eltrombopag (continued)

▸ **Dairy products** are predicted to decrease the absorption of **eltrombopag**. **Eltrombopag** should be taken 2 hours before or 4 hours after **dairy products**. Severe Theoretical

▸ **Iron (oral)** is predicted to decrease the absorption of **eltrombopag**. **Eltrombopag** should be taken 2 hours before or 4 hours after **iron (oral)**. Severe Theoretical

▸ **Selenium** is predicted to decrease the absorption of **eltrombopag**. **Eltrombopag** should be taken 2 hours before or 4 hours after **selenium**. Severe Theoretical

▸ **Eltrombopag** is predicted to increase the exposure to **statins**. Monitor and adjust dose. Moderate Study

▸ **Zinc** is predicted to decrease the absorption of **eltrombopag**. **Eltrombopag** should be taken 2 hours before or 4 hours after **zinc**. Severe Theoretical

Elvitegravir

▸ **Antacids** moderately decrease the exposure to **elvitegravir**. Separate administration by at least 4 hours. Moderate Study

▸ **Antiepileptics (carbamazepine, fosphenytoin, phenobarbital, phenytoin, primidone)** are predicted to decrease the concentration of **elvitegravir**. Avoid. Severe Theoretical

▸ **Bosentan** is predicted to decrease the concentration of **elvitegravir**. Avoid. Severe Theoretical

▸ **Elvitegravir** is predicted to decrease the anticoagulant effect of **coumarins**. Moderate Theoretical

▸ **Efavirenz** is predicted to decrease the concentration of **elvitegravir**. Avoid. Severe Theoretical

▸ **Enzalutamide** is predicted to decrease the concentration of **elvitegravir**. Avoid. Severe Theoretical

▸ **HIV-protease inhibitors (atazanavir, lopinavir)** increase the concentration of **elvitegravir**. Refer to specialist literature. Moderate Study

▸ **Nevirapine** is predicted to decrease the concentration of **elvitegravir**. Severe Theoretical

▸ **Rifampicin** is predicted to decrease the concentration of **elvitegravir**. Avoid. Severe Theoretical

▸ **St John's Wort** is predicted to decrease the concentration of **elvitegravir**. Avoid. Severe Theoretical

Empagliflozin → see TABLE 14 p. 821 (antidiabetic drugs), TABLE 8 p. 819 (hypotension)

Enalapril → see ACE inhibitors

Enoxaparin → see low molecular-weight heparins

Entacapone

▸ **Iron (oral)** is predicted to decrease the absorption of **entacapone**. Separate administration by at least 2 hours. Moderate Theoretical

▸ **Entacapone** increases the exposure to **levodopa**. Monitor side effects and adjust dose. Moderate Study

▸ **Entacapone** is predicted to increase the exposure to **methyldopa**. Moderate Theoretical

▸ **Entacapone** is predicted to increase the risk of elevated blood pressure when given with **monoamine-oxidase A and B inhibitors, irreversible**. Avoid. Severe Theoretical

▸ **Entacapone** is predicted to increase the risk of cardiovascular side-effects when given with **sympathomimetics, inotropic (dobutamine, dopamine)**. Moderate Theoretical

▸ **Entacapone** is predicted to increase the risk of cardiovascular side-effects when given with **sympathomimetics, vasoconstrictor (adrenaline/epinephrine, noradrenaline/norepinephrine)**. Moderate Study

Enteral feeds

▸ **Antacids (aluminium hydroxide)** increase the risk of blocked enteral or nasogastric tubes when given with **enteral feeds**. Moderate Study

▸ **Enteral feeds** decrease the absorption of **antiepileptics (phenytoin)**. Severe Study

▸ **Enteral feeds (vitamin-K containing)** potentially decrease the anticoagulant effect of **coumarins**. Severe Anecdotal

▸ **Enteral feeds (vitamin-K containing)** potentially decrease the effects of **phenindione**. Severe Theoretical

▸ **Enteral feeds** decrease the exposure to quinolones **(ciprofloxacin)**. Moderate Study

▸ **Sucralfate** increases the risk of blocked enteral or nasogastric tubes when given with **enteral feeds**. Separate administration by 1 hour. Moderate Study

▸ **Enteral feeds** decrease the exposure to **theophylline**. Moderate Study

Enzalutamide

GENERAL INFORMATION Caution with concurrent chemotherapy—safety and efficacy not established.

▸ **Enzalutamide** is predicted to decrease the exposure to **abacavir**. Moderate Theoretical

▸ **Enzalutamide** is predicted to decrease the exposure to **abiraterone**. Avoid. Severe Theoretical

▸ **Enzalutamide** is predicted to decrease the exposure to aldosterone antagonists **(eplerenone)**. Avoid. Moderate Theoretical

▸ **Enzalutamide** is predicted to decrease the exposure to **alprazolam**. Adjust **alprazolam** dose. Moderate Theoretical

▸ **Enzalutamide** is predicted to decrease the exposure to antiarrhythmics **(disopyramide, dronedarone)**. Avoid. Severe Study

▸ **Enzalutamide** is predicted to decrease the efficacy of antiarrhythmics **(propafenone)**. Moderate Study

▸ **Enzalutamide** is predicted to decrease the exposure to anticholinesterases, centrally acting **(donepezil)**. Mild Study

▸ **Enzalutamide** is predicted to slightly decrease the exposure to antiepileptics **(brivaracetam)**. Moderate Theoretical

▸ **Enzalutamide** is predicted to decrease the exposure to antiepileptics **(perampanel)**. Monitor and adjust dose. Moderate Study

▸ **Enzalutamide** is predicted to decrease the exposure to antifungals, azoles **(isavuconazole)**. Avoid. Severe Study

▸ **Enzalutamide** is predicted to decrease the exposure to antimalarials **(artemether)** with lumefantrine. Avoid. Severe Study

▸ **Enzalutamide** is predicted to decrease the concentration of antimalarials **(piperaquine)**. Avoid. Moderate Study

▸ **Enzalutamide** is predicted to moderately decrease the exposure to **apixaban**. Use with caution or avoid. Severe Study

▸ **Enzalutamide** moderately decreases the exposure to **apremilast**. Avoid. Severe Study

▸ **Enzalutamide** is predicted to markedly decrease the exposure to **aprepitant**. Avoid. Moderate Study

▸ **Enzalutamide** is predicted to moderately decrease the exposure to **aripiprazole**. Adjust **aripiprazole** dose, p. 240. Moderate Study

▸ **Enzalutamide** is predicted to decrease the exposure to **axitinib**. Avoid or adjust dose. Moderate Study

▸ **Enzalutamide** decreases the exposure to **bedaquiline**. Avoid. Severe Study

▸ **Enzalutamide** slightly decreases the exposure to **bortezomib**. Avoid. Severe Study

▸ **Enzalutamide** affects the exposure to **bosentan**. Avoid. Severe Study

▸ **Enzalutamide** is predicted to very markedly decrease the exposure to **bosutinib**. Avoid. Severe Study

▸ **Enzalutamide** is predicted to markedly decrease the exposure to **bupropion**. Severe Study

▸ **Enzalutamide** is predicted to decrease the exposure to **buspirone**. Use with caution and adjust dose. Severe Study

▸ **Enzalutamide** moderately decreases the exposure to **cabozantinib**. Avoid. Moderate Study

▸ **Enzalutamide** is predicted to decrease the exposure to calcium channel blockers **(amlodipine, felodipine, lacidipine, lercanidipine, nicardipine, nifedipine, nimodipine)**. Monitor and adjust dose. Moderate Study

▸ **Enzalutamide** decreases the exposure to calcium channel blockers **(diltiazem)**. Severe Study

▸ **Enzalutamide** decreases the exposure to calcium channel blockers **(isradipine)**. Avoid. Moderate Study

▸ **Enzalutamide** is predicted to decrease the exposure to calcium channel blockers **(verapamil)**. Severe Study

▸ **Enzalutamide** is predicted to decrease the exposure to cannabis extract. Avoid. Severe Theoretical

▸ **Enzalutamide** is predicted to decrease the exposure to **ceritinib**. Avoid. Severe Study

▸ **Enzalutamide** decreases the concentration of **ciclosporin**. Severe Study

▸ **Enzalutamide** is predicted to alter the effects of **cilostazol**. Moderate Theoretical

▸ **Enzalutamide** decreases the exposure to **clomethiazole**. Monitor and adjust dose. [Moderate] Study

▸ **Enzalutamide** is predicted to decrease the exposure to **cobicistat**. Avoid. [Severe] Theoretical

▸ **Enzalutamide** is predicted to decrease the exposure to **cobimetinib**. Avoid. [Severe] Theoretical

▸ **Enzalutamide** is predicted to decrease the exposure to corticosteroids (**budesonide, dexamethasone, methylprednisolone, prednisolone**). Monitor and adjust dose. [Moderate] Study

▸ **Enzalutamide** is predicted to decrease the exposure to corticosteroids (**fluticasone**). [Unknown] Theoretical

▸ **Enzalutamide** is predicted to decrease the exposure to corticosteroids (**prednisone**). [Mild] Study

▸ **Enzalutamide** potentially decreases the exposure to **coumarins**. Avoid or adjust dose and monitor INR. [Severe] Study

▸ **Enzalutamide** is predicted to markedly decrease the exposure to **crizotinib**. Avoid. [Severe] Study

▸ **Enzalutamide** is predicted to decrease the exposure to **dabrafenib**. Avoid. [Moderate] Theoretical

▸ **Enzalutamide** is predicted to moderately decrease the exposure to **daclatasvir**. Avoid. [Severe] Study

▸ **Enzalutamide** is predicted to decrease the exposure to **darifenacin**. [Moderate] Theoretical

▸ **Enzalutamide** is predicted to decrease the exposure to **dasabuvir**. Avoid. [Severe] Theoretical

▸ **Enzalutamide** is predicted to markedly decrease the exposure to **dasatinib**. Avoid. [Severe] Study

▸ **Enzalutamide** is predicted to slightly decrease the exposure to **delamanid**. Avoid. [Moderate] Study

▸ **Enzalutamide** decreases the exposure to **dolutegravir**. Adjust dose. [Severe] Study

▸ **Enzalutamide** is predicted to decrease the exposure to **elbasvir**. Avoid. [Severe] Study

▸ **Enzalutamide** is predicted to decrease the concentration of **elvitegravir**. Avoid. [Severe] Theoretical

▸ **Enzalutamide** is predicted to decrease the effects of **ergotamine**. [Moderate] Theoretical

▸ **Enzalutamide** is predicted to decrease the exposure to **erlotinib**. Avoid or adjust **erlotinib** dose. [Severe] Study

▸ **Enzalutamide** is predicted to decrease the exposure to **etravirine**. Avoid. [Severe] Theoretical

▸ **Enzalutamide** is predicted to decrease the concentration of **everolimus**. Avoid or adjust dose. [Severe] Study

▸ **Enzalutamide** moderately decreases the exposure to **exemestane**. [Moderate] Study

▸ **Enzalutamide** is predicted to decrease the exposure to **fesoterodine**. Avoid. [Moderate] Study

▸ Fibrates (**gemfibrozil**) moderately increase the exposure to **enzalutamide**. Avoid or adjust **enzalutamide** dose. [Severe] Study

▸ **Enzalutamide** is predicted to decrease the exposure to **fingolimod**. [Moderate] Study

▸ **Enzalutamide** is predicted to decrease the exposure to **fosaprepitant**. Avoid. [Moderate] Theoretical

▸ **Enzalutamide** is predicted to decrease the exposure to **gefitinib**. Avoid. [Severe] Study

▸ **Enzalutamide** is predicted to decrease the exposure to **grazoprevir**. Avoid. [Severe] Study

▸ **Enzalutamide** is predicted to decrease the concentration of **guanfacine**. Adjust **guanfacine** dose, p. 222. [Moderate] Study

▸ **Enzalutamide** decreases the concentration of **haloperidol**. Adjust dose. [Moderate] Study

▸ **Enzalutamide** is predicted to decrease the exposure to **ibrutinib**. Avoid. [Severe] Study

▸ **Enzalutamide** is predicted to decrease the exposure to **idelalisib**. Avoid. [Severe] Study

▸ **Enzalutamide** is predicted to decrease the exposure to **imatinib**. Avoid. [Moderate] Study

▸ **Enzalutamide** is predicted to decrease the exposure to **irinotecan**. Avoid. [Severe] Study

▸ **Enzalutamide** is predicted to decrease the exposure to **ivabradine**. Adjust dose. [Moderate] Theoretical

▸ **Enzalutamide** markedly decreases the exposure to **ivacaftor**. Avoid. [Severe] Study

▸ **Enzalutamide** is predicted to decrease the exposure to **ixazomib**. Avoid. [Severe] Study

▸ **Enzalutamide** is predicted to decrease the exposure to **lapatinib**. Avoid. [Severe] Study

▸ **Enzalutamide** is predicted to decrease the exposure to **linagliptin**. [Moderate] Study

▸ **Enzalutamide** is predicted to decrease the exposure to **lomitapide**. Monitor and adjust dose. [Moderate] Theoretical

▸ **Enzalutamide** is predicted to decrease the exposure to **lurasidone**. Avoid. [Moderate] Study

▸ **Enzalutamide** is predicted to decrease the exposure to **macitentan**. Avoid. [Severe] Study

▸ **Enzalutamide** is predicted to decrease the exposure to **maraviroc**. Adjust dose. [Severe] Study

▸ **Enzalutamide** is predicted to decrease the exposure to **midazolam**. Monitor and adjust dose. [Moderate] Study

▸ **Enzalutamide** is predicted to decrease the exposure to **mirtazapine**. Adjust dose. [Moderate] Study

▸ **Enzalutamide** is predicted to decrease the exposure to monoclonal antibodies (**trastuzumab emtansine**). [Severe] Theoretical

▸ **Enzalutamide** is predicted to decrease the exposure to **montelukast**. [Mild] Study

▸ **Enzalutamide** is predicted to markedly decrease the exposure to **naloxegol**. Avoid. [Moderate] Study

▸ **Enzalutamide** is predicted to slightly decrease the exposure to **nateglinide**. [Mild] Study

▸ **Enzalutamide** is predicted to decrease the exposure to **netupitant**. Avoid. [Moderate] Study

▸ **Enzalutamide** is predicted to moderately decrease the exposure to **nilotinib**. Avoid. [Severe] Study

▸ **Enzalutamide** is predicted to decrease the exposure to **nitisinone**. Adjust **nitisinone** dose. [Moderate] Theoretical

▸ **Enzalutamide** is predicted to decrease the exposure to **olaparib**. Avoid. [Moderate] Theoretical

▸ **Enzalutamide** is predicted to decrease the exposure to **ondansetron**. [Moderate] Study

▸ **Enzalutamide** is predicted to decrease the exposure to opioids (**alfentanil, fentanyl**). [Moderate] Study

▸ **Enzalutamide** is predicted to decrease the exposure to opioids (**buprenorphine**). Monitor and adjust dose. [Moderate] Study

▸ **Enzalutamide** decreases the exposure to opioids (**methadone**). Monitor and adjust dose. [Severe] Study

▸ **Enzalutamide** is predicted to decrease the exposure to opioids (**oxycodone**). Monitor and adjust dose. [Moderate] Study

▸ **Enzalutamide** is predicted to moderately decrease the exposure to **osimertinib**. Avoid. [Moderate] Study

▸ **Enzalutamide** is predicted to decrease the exposure to **palbociclib**. Avoid. [Severe] Study

▸ **Enzalutamide** is predicted to decrease the exposure to **panobinostat**. Avoid. [Moderate] Theoretical

▸ **Enzalutamide** is predicted to decrease the exposure to **paracetamol**. [Moderate] Study

▸ **Enzalutamide** is predicted to decrease the exposure to **paritaprevir with ritonavir and ombitasvir**. Avoid. [Severe] Study

▸ **Enzalutamide** is predicted to decrease the exposure to **pazopanib**. Avoid. [Severe] Theoretical

▸ **Enzalutamide** is predicted to decrease the exposure to phosphodiesterase type-5 inhibitors (**avanafil, tadalafil**). Avoid. [Severe] Study

▸ **Enzalutamide** is predicted to decrease the exposure to phosphodiesterase type-5 inhibitors (**sildenafil, vardenafil**). [Moderate] Theoretical

▸ **Enzalutamide** is predicted to moderately decrease the exposure to **pitolisant**. [Moderate] Study

▸ **Enzalutamide** is predicted to decrease the exposure to **ponatinib**. Avoid. [Moderate] Theoretical

▸ **Enzalutamide** is predicted to markedly decrease the exposure to **praziquantel**. Avoid. [Moderate] Study

▸ **Enzalutamide** is predicted to moderately decrease the exposure to proton pump inhibitors (**omeprazole**). [Moderate] Study

▸ **Enzalutamide** is predicted to decrease the exposure to **quetiapine**. [Moderate] Study

▸ **Enzalutamide** is predicted to decrease the exposure to **ranolazine**. Avoid. [Severe] Study

Enzalutamide (continued)

▶ **Enzalutamide** is predicted to decrease the exposure to reboxetine. Moderate Anecdotal

▶ **Enzalutamide** is predicted to decrease the exposure to regorafenib. Avoid. Moderate Study

▶ **Enzalutamide** is predicted to decrease the exposure to repaglinide. Monitor blood glucose and adjust dose. Moderate Study

▶ **Enzalutamide** markedly decreases the exposure to rilpivirine. Avoid. Severe Study

▶ **Enzalutamide** is predicted to decrease the exposure to risperidone. Adjust risperidone dose. Moderate Study

▶ **Enzalutamide** is predicted to moderately decrease the exposure to rivaroxaban. Avoid unless patient can be monitored for signs of thrombosis. Severe Study

▶ **Enzalutamide** is predicted to decrease the exposure to roflumilast. Avoid. Moderate Study

▶ **Enzalutamide** is predicted to decrease the exposure to ruxolitinib. Monitor and adjust dose. Moderate Study

▶ **Enzalutamide** is predicted to moderately decrease the exposure to saxagliptin. Moderate Study

▶ **Enzalutamide** is predicted to decrease the exposure to simeprevir. Avoid. Severe Study

▶ **Enzalutamide** is predicted to decrease the concentration of sirolimus. Avoid. Severe Study

▶ **Enzalutamide** is predicted to decrease the exposure to solifenacin. Moderate Theoretical

▶ **Enzalutamide** is predicted to decrease the exposure to sorafenib. Moderate Theoretical

▶ **Enzalutamide** is predicted to decrease the exposure to sunitinib. Avoid or adjust sunitinib dose. Moderate Study

▶ **Enzalutamide** decreases the concentration of tacrolimus. Monitor and adjust dose. Severe Study

▶ **Enzalutamide** is predicted to decrease the exposure to taxanes (cabazitaxel, paclitaxel). Avoid. Severe Study

▶ **Enzalutamide** is predicted to decrease the exposure to taxanes (docetaxel). Severe Theoretical

▶ **Enzalutamide** is predicted to decrease the concentration of temsirolimus. Avoid. Severe Study

▶ **Enzalutamide** decreases the exposure to tetracyclines (doxycycline). Monitor and adjust dose. Moderate Study

▶ **Enzalutamide** is predicted to markedly decrease the exposure to ticagrelor. Avoid. Severe Study

▶ **Enzalutamide** is predicted to decrease the exposure to tolvaptan. Avoid. Severe Study

▶ **Enzalutamide** is predicted to decrease the exposure to toremifene. Adjust dose. Moderate Study

▶ **Enzalutamide** is predicted to decrease the exposure to trabectedin. Avoid. Severe Theoretical

▶ **Enzalutamide** is predicted to markedly decrease the exposure to ulipristal. Avoid and for 4 weeks after stopping ulipristal. Severe Theoretical

▶ **Enzalutamide** is predicted to decrease the exposure to vandetanib. Avoid. Moderate Study

▶ **Enzalutamide** is predicted to moderately decrease the exposure to velpatasvir. Avoid. Severe Study

▶ **Enzalutamide** is predicted to decrease the exposure to vemurafenib. Avoid. Severe Theoretical

▶ **Enzalutamide** is predicted to decrease the exposure to venetoclax. Avoid. Severe Study

▶ **Enzalutamide** is predicted to decrease the exposure to vinca alkaloids (vinblastine, vincristine, vindesine). Severe Theoretical

▶ **Enzalutamide** is predicted to decrease the exposure to vinca alkaloids (vinflunine). Avoid. Severe Theoretical

▶ **Enzalutamide** is predicted to decrease the exposure to vinca alkaloids (vinorelbine). Use with caution or avoid. Severe Theoretical

▶ **Enzalutamide** is predicted to decrease the exposure to vismodegib. Avoid. Moderate Theoretical

▶ **Enzalutamide** is predicted to decrease the exposure to vortioxetine. Monitor and adjust dose. Moderate Study

▶ **Enzalutamide** is predicted to decrease the exposure to zopiclone. Adjust dose. Moderate Study

Ephedrine → see sympathomimetics, vasoconstrictor

Epirubicin → see anthracyclines

Eplerenone → see aldosterone antagonists

Epoetin alfa → see **TABLE 5** p. 818 (thromboembolism), **TABLE 16** p. 822 (increased serum potassium)

Epoetin beta → see **TABLE 5** p. 818 (thromboembolism), **TABLE 16** p. 822 (increased serum potassium)

Epoetin zeta → see **TABLE 5** p. 818 (thromboembolism), **TABLE 16** p. 822 (increased serum potassium)

Epoprostenol → see **TABLE 4** p. 818 (antiplatelet effects)

Eprosartan → see angiotensin-II receptor antagonists

Eptifibatide → see **TABLE 4** p. 818 (antiplatelet effects)

Ergocalciferol → see vitamin D substances

Ergometrine

▶ Antiarrhythmics (dronedarone) are predicted to increase the risk of ergotism when given with **ergometrine**. Severe Theoretical

▶ Antifungals, azoles (fluconazole, isavuconazole, posaconazole) are predicted to increase the risk of ergotism when given with **ergometrine**. Severe Theoretical

▶ Antifungals, azoles (itraconazole, ketoconazole, voriconazole) are predicted to increase the risk of ergotism when given with **ergometrine**. Avoid. Severe Theoretical

▶ Antifungals, azoles (miconazole) are predicted to increase the exposure to **ergometrine**. Avoid. Moderate Theoretical

▶ Aprepitant is predicted to increase the risk of ergotism when given with **ergometrine**. Severe Theoretical

▶ Beta blockers, non-selective are predicted to increase the risk of peripheral vasoconstriction when given with **ergometrine**. Severe Theoretical

▶ Beta blockers, selective are predicted to increase the risk of peripheral vasoconstriction when given with **ergometrine**. Severe Theoretical

▶ Calcium channel blockers (diltiazem, verapamil) are predicted to increase the risk of ergotism when given with **ergometrine**. Severe Theoretical

▶ Cobicistat is predicted to increase the risk of ergotism when given with **ergometrine**. Avoid. Severe Theoretical

▶ Crizotinib is predicted to increase the risk of ergotism when given with **ergometrine**. Severe Theoretical

▶ **Ergometrine** is predicted to increase the risk of ergotism when given with dopamine receptor agonists (cabergoline, pergolide). Avoid. Moderate Theoretical

▶ Grapefruit juice is predicted to increase the risk of ergotism when given with **ergometrine**. Severe Theoretical

▶ HIV-protease inhibitors (atazanavir, darunavir, fosamprenavir, lopinavir, ritonavir, saquinavir, tipranavir) are predicted to increase the risk of ergotism when given with **ergometrine**. Avoid. Severe Theoretical

▶ HIV-protease inhibitors (indinavir) are predicted to increase the risk of ergotism when given with **ergometrine**. Severe Theoretical

▶ Idelalisib is predicted to increase the risk of ergotism when given with **ergometrine**. Avoid. Severe Theoretical

▶ Imatinib is predicted to increase the risk of ergotism when given with **ergometrine**. Severe Theoretical

▶ Macrolides (clarithromycin) are predicted to increase the risk of ergotism when given with **ergometrine**. Avoid. Severe Theoretical

▶ Macrolides (erythromycin) are predicted to increase the risk of ergotism when given with **ergometrine**. Severe Theoretical

▶ Netupitant is predicted to increase the risk of ergotism when given with **ergometrine**. Severe Theoretical

▶ Nilotinib is predicted to increase the risk of ergotism when given with **ergometrine**. Severe Theoretical

▶ **Ergometrine** potentially increases the risk of peripheral vasoconstriction when given with sympathomimetics, inotropic (dopamine). Avoid. Severe Anecdotal

▶ **Ergometrine** is predicted to increase the risk of peripheral vasoconstriction when given with sympathomimetics, vasoconstrictor (noradrenaline/norepinephrine). Severe Anecdotal

Ergotamine

▶ Almotriptan is predicted to increase the risk of vasoconstriction when given with **ergotamine**. **Ergotamine** should be taken at least 24 hours before or 6 hours after almotriptan. Severe Theoretical

▸ Antiarrhythmics **(dronedarone)** are predicted to increase the risk of ergotism when given with **ergotamine**. [Severe] Theoretical

▸ Antiepileptics **(carbamazepine, fosphenytoin, phenobarbital, phenytoin, primidone)** are predicted to decrease the effects of **ergotamine**. [Moderate] Theoretical

▸ Antifungals, azoles **(fluconazole, isavuconazole, posaconazole)** are predicted to increase the risk of ergotism when given with **ergotamine**. [Severe] Theoretical

▸ Antifungals, azoles **(itraconazole, ketoconazole, voriconazole)** are predicted to increase the risk of ergotism when given with **ergotamine**. Avoid. [Severe] Theoretical

▸ Antifungals, azoles **(miconazole)** are predicted to increase the exposure to **ergotamine**. Avoid. [Moderate] Theoretical

▸ Aprepitant is predicted to increase the risk of ergotism when given with **ergotamine**. [Severe] Theoretical

▸ Beta blockers, non-selective are predicted to increase the risk of peripheral vasoconstriction when given with **ergotamine**. [Severe] Study

▸ Beta blockers, selective are predicted to increase the risk of peripheral vasoconstriction when given with **ergotamine**. [Severe] Study

▸ Bosentan is predicted to decrease the effects of **ergotamine**. [Moderate] Theoretical

▸ Calcium channel blockers **(diltiazem, verapamil)** are predicted to increase the risk of ergotism when given with **ergotamine**. [Severe] Theoretical

▸ Ceritinib is predicted to increase the exposure to **ergotamine**. Avoid. [Severe] Theoretical

▸ Cobicistat is predicted to increase the risk of ergotism when given with **ergotamine**. Avoid. [Severe] Theoretical

▸ Crizotinib is predicted to increase the risk of ergotism when given with **ergotamine**. [Severe] Theoretical

▸ Ergotamine is predicted to increase the risk of ergotism when given with dopamine receptor agonists **(bromocriptine, cabergoline)**. Avoid. [Moderate] Theoretical

▸ Ergotamine is predicted to increase the risk of ergotism when given with dopamine receptor agonists **(pergolide)**. [Moderate] Theoretical

▸ Efavirenz is predicted to decrease the effects of **ergotamine**. [Moderate] Theoretical

▸ Eletriptan increases the risk of vasoconstriction when given with **ergotamine**. Separate administration by 24 hours. [Severe] Study

▸ Enzalutamide is predicted to decrease the effects of **ergotamine**. [Moderate] Theoretical

▸ Grapefruit juice is predicted to increase the exposure to **ergotamine**. [Severe] Theoretical

▸ HIV-protease inhibitors **(atazanavir, darunavir, fosamprenavir, lopinavir, ritonavir, saquinavir, tipranavir)** are predicted to increase the risk of ergotism when given with **ergotamine**. Avoid. [Severe] Theoretical

▸ HIV-protease inhibitors **(indinavir)** are predicted to increase the risk of ergotism when given with **ergotamine**. [Severe] Theoretical

▸ Idelalisib is predicted to increase the risk of ergotism when given with **ergotamine**. Avoid. [Severe] Theoretical

▸ Imatinib is predicted to increase the risk of ergotism when given with **ergotamine**. [Severe] Theoretical

▸ Macrolides **(clarithromycin)** are predicted to increase the risk of ergotism when given with **ergotamine**. Avoid. [Severe] Theoretical

▸ Macrolides **(erythromycin)** are predicted to increase the risk of ergotism when given with **ergotamine**. [Severe] Theoretical

▸ Naratriptan is predicted to increase the risk of vasoconstriction when given with **ergotamine**. Separate administration by 24 hours. [Severe] Theoretical

▸ Netupitant is predicted to increase the risk of ergotism when given with **ergotamine**. [Severe] Theoretical

▸ Nevirapine is predicted to decrease the effects of **ergotamine**. [Moderate] Theoretical

▸ Nilotinib is predicted to increase the risk of ergotism when given with **ergotamine**. [Severe] Theoretical

▸ Palbociclib is predicted to increase the exposure to **ergotamine**. Adjust dose. [Moderate] Theoretical

▸ Rifampicin is predicted to decrease the effects of **ergotamine**. [Moderate] Theoretical

▸ Rizatriptan is predicted to increase the risk of vasoconstriction when given with **ergotamine**. **Ergotamine** should be taken at least 24 hours before or 6 hours after **rizatriptan**. [Severe] Theoretical

▸ St John's Wort is predicted to decrease the effects of **ergotamine**. [Moderate] Theoretical

▸ Sumatriptan increases the risk of vasoconstriction when given with **ergotamine**. **Ergotamine** should be taken at least 24 hours before or 6 hours after **sumatriptan**. [Severe] Study

Eribulin → see TABLE 15 p. 821 (myelosuppression), TABLE 12 p. 821 (peripheral neuropathy), TABLE 9 p. 820 (QT-interval prolongation)

Erlotinib

> **FOOD AND LIFESTYLE** Dose adjustment may be necessary if smoking started or stopped during treatment.

▸ Antacids are predicted to decrease the absorption of **erlotinib**. Antacids should be taken 4 hours before or 2 hours after **erlotinib**. [Moderate] Theoretical

▸ Antiarrhythmics **(amiodarone, dronedarone)** are predicted to increase the exposure to **erlotinib**. [Moderate] Theoretical

▸ Antiepileptics **(carbamazepine, fosphenytoin, phenobarbital, phenytoin, primidone)** are predicted to decrease the exposure to **erlotinib**. Avoid or adjust **erlotinib** dose. [Severe] Study

▸ Antifungals, azoles **(fluconazole, isavuconazole, posaconazole)** are predicted to increase the exposure to **erlotinib**. [Moderate] Theoretical

▸ Antifungals, azoles **(itraconazole, ketoconazole, voriconazole)** are predicted to slightly increase the exposure to **erlotinib**. Use with caution and adjust dose. [Moderate] Study

▸ Aprepitant is predicted to increase the exposure to **erlotinib**. [Moderate] Theoretical

▸ Erlotinib is predicted to increase the risk of gastrointestinal perforation when given with aspirin (high-dose). [Severe] Theoretical

▸ Bosentan is predicted to decrease the exposure to **erlotinib**. [Severe] Theoretical

▸ Calcium channel blockers **(diltiazem, verapamil)** are predicted to increase the exposure to **erlotinib**. [Moderate] Theoretical

▸ Ciclosporin is predicted to increase the exposure to **erlotinib**. [Moderate] Theoretical

▸ Cobicistat is predicted to slightly increase the exposure to **erlotinib**. Use with caution and adjust dose. [Moderate] Study

▸ Combined hormonal contraceptives slightly increase the exposure to **erlotinib**. Monitor side effects and adjust dose. [Moderate] Study

▸ Corticosteroids increase the risk of gastrointestinal perforation when given with **erlotinib**. [Severe] Theoretical

▸ Erlotinib increases the anticoagulant effect of coumarins. [Severe] Anecdotal

▸ Crizotinib is predicted to increase the exposure to **erlotinib**. [Moderate] Theoretical

▸ Efavirenz is predicted to decrease the exposure to **erlotinib**. [Severe] Theoretical

▸ Enzalutamide is predicted to decrease the exposure to **erlotinib**. Avoid or adjust **erlotinib** dose. [Severe] Study

▸ Grapefruit juice is predicted to increase the exposure to **erlotinib**. [Moderate] Theoretical

▸ H$_2$ receptor antagonists are predicted to decrease the exposure to **erlotinib**. **Erlotinib** should be taken 2 hours before or 10 hours after H$_2$ receptor antagonists. [Moderate] Study

▸ HIV-protease inhibitors **(atazanavir, darunavir, fosamprenavir, lopinavir, ritonavir, saquinavir, tipranavir)** are predicted to slightly increase the exposure to **erlotinib**. Use with caution and adjust dose. [Moderate] Study

▸ HIV-protease inhibitors **(indinavir)** are predicted to increase the exposure to **erlotinib**. [Moderate] Theoretical

▸ Idelalisib is predicted to slightly increase the exposure to **erlotinib**. Use with caution and adjust dose. [Moderate] Study

▸ Imatinib is predicted to increase the exposure to **erlotinib**. [Moderate] Theoretical

▸ Lapatinib is predicted to increase the exposure to **erlotinib**. [Moderate] Theoretical

▸ Macrolides **(azithromycin, erythromycin)** are predicted to increase the exposure to **erlotinib**. [Moderate] Theoretical

A1

Interactions | Appendix 1

Erlotinib (continued)

▶ Macrolides **(clarithromycin)** are predicted to slightly increase the exposure to **erlotinib**. Use with caution and adjust dose. Moderate Study

▶ **Netupitant** is predicted to increase the exposure to **erlotinib**. Moderate Theoretical

▶ **Nevirapine** is predicted to decrease the exposure to **erlotinib**. Severe Theoretical

▶ **Nilotinib** is predicted to increase the exposure to **erlotinib**. Moderate Theoretical

▶ **Erlotinib** is predicted to increase the risk of gastrointestinal perforation when given with **NSAIDs**. Severe Theoretical

▶ **Erlotinib** is predicted to increase the risk of bleeding events when given with **phenindione**. Severe Theoretical

▶ **Proton pump inhibitors** are predicted to slightly decrease the exposure to **erlotinib**. Avoid. Moderate Study

▶ Quinolones **(ciprofloxacin)** slightly increase the exposure to **erlotinib**. Monitor side effects and adjust dose. Moderate Study

▶ **Ranolazine** is predicted to increase the exposure to **erlotinib**. Moderate Theoretical

▶ **Rifampicin** is predicted to decrease the exposure to **erlotinib**. Avoid or adjust **erlotinib** dose. Severe Study

▶ SSRIs **(fluvoxamine)** are predicted to increase the exposure to **erlotinib**. Monitor side effects and adjust dose. Moderate Theoretical

▶ **St John's Wort** is predicted to decrease the exposure to **erlotinib**. Severe Theoretical

▶ **Vemurafenib** is predicted to increase the exposure to **erlotinib**. Moderate Theoretical

Ertapenem → see carbapenems
Erythromycin → see macrolides
Escitalopram → see SSRIs
Eslicarbazepine → see antiepileptics
Esmolol → see beta blockers, selective
Esomeprazole → see proton pump inhibitors
Estramustine → see alkylating agents
Etanercept

▶ **Live vaccines** are predicted to increase the risk of generalised infection (possibly life-threatening) when given with **etanercept**. Public Health England advises avoid. Severe Theoretical

Ethambutol

▶ **Isoniazid** increases the risk of optic neuropathy when given with **ethambutol**. Severe Anecdotal

Ethosuximide → see antiepileptics
Etodolac → see NSAIDs
Etomidate → see TABLE 8 p. 819 (hypotension), TABLE 11 p. 820 (CNS depressant effects)

Etonogestrel

▶ **Antiepileptics (carbamazepine, eslicarbazepine, fosphenytoin, oxcarbazepine, perampanel, phenobarbital, phenytoin, primidone, rufinamide, topiramate)** are predicted to decrease the efficacy of **etonogestrel**. For FSRH guidance, see Contraceptives, interactions p. 474. Severe Theoretical

▶ **Aprepitant** is predicted to decrease the efficacy of **etonogestrel**. For FSRH guidance, see Contraceptives, interactions p. 474. Severe Theoretical

▶ **Bosentan** is predicted to decrease the efficacy of **etonogestrel**. For FSRH guidance, see Contraceptives, interactions p. 474. Severe Theoretical

▶ **Efavirenz** is predicted to decrease the efficacy of **etonogestrel**. For FSRH guidance, see Contraceptives, interactions p. 474. Severe Theoretical

▶ **Fosaprepitant** is predicted to decrease the efficacy of **etonogestrel**. For FSRH guidance, see Contraceptives, interactions p. 474. Severe Theoretical

▶ **Griseofulvin** decreases the efficacy of **etonogestrel**. For FSRH guidance, see Contraceptives, interactions p. 474. Severe Anecdotal

▶ **HIV-protease inhibitors (ritonavir)** are predicted to decrease the efficacy of **etonogestrel**. For FSRH guidance, see Contraceptives, interactions p. 474. Severe Theoretical

▶ **Modafinil** is predicted to decrease the efficacy of **etonogestrel**. For FSRH guidance, see Contraceptives, interactions p. 474. Severe Theoretical

▶ **Nevirapine** is predicted to decrease the efficacy of **etonogestrel**. For FSRH guidance, see Contraceptives, interactions p. 474. Severe Theoretical

▶ **Rifabutin** is predicted to decrease the efficacy of **etonogestrel**. For FSRH guidance, see Contraceptives, interactions p. 474. Severe Theoretical

▶ **Rifampicin** is predicted to decrease the efficacy of **etonogestrel**. For FSRH guidance, see Contraceptives, interactions p. 474. Severe Theoretical

▶ **St John's Wort** is predicted to decrease the efficacy of **etonogestrel**. MHRA advises avoid. For FSRH guidance, see Contraceptives, interactions p. 474. Severe Theoretical

▶ **Sugammadex** is predicted to decrease the efficacy of **etonogestrel**. Use additional contraceptive precautions. Severe Theoretical

▶ **Ulipristal** is predicted to decrease the efficacy of **etonogestrel**. Avoid. Severe Theoretical

Etoposide → see TABLE 15 p. 821 (myelosuppression)

▶ **Antiepileptics (carbamazepine, fosphenytoin, phenobarbital, phenytoin, primidone)** are predicted to decrease the efficacy of **etoposide**. Moderate Theoretical

▶ **Ciclosporin** increases the exposure to **etoposide**. Monitor and adjust dose. Severe Study

▶ **Live vaccines** are predicted to increase the risk of generalised infection (possibly life-threatening) when given with **etoposide**. Public Health England advises avoid. Severe Theoretical

Etoricoxib → see NSAIDs

Etravirine

▶ **Antiepileptics (carbamazepine, fosphenytoin, phenobarbital, phenytoin, primidone)** are predicted to decrease the exposure to **etravirine**. Avoid. Severe Theoretical

▶ **Etravirine** decreases the exposure to antimalarials **(artemether)**. Moderate Study

▶ **Etravirine** is predicted to decrease the exposure to **bedaquiline**. Avoid. Severe Theoretical

▶ **Bosentan** is predicted to decrease the exposure to **etravirine**. Avoid. Severe Study

▶ **Etravirine** is predicted to decrease the exposure to **bosutinib**. Avoid. Severe Theoretical

▶ **Etravirine** increases the anticoagulant effect of **coumarins**. Moderate Theoretical

▶ **Etravirine** is predicted to decrease the exposure to **daclatasvir**. Avoid. Moderate Theoretical

▶ **Etravirine** moderately decreases the exposure to **dolutegravir**. Avoid unless given with atazanavir, darunavir, or lopinavir (all boosted with ritonavir). Severe Study

▶ **Efavirenz** is predicted to decrease the exposure to **etravirine**. Avoid. Severe Study

▶ **Etravirine** is predicted to decrease the exposure to **elbasvir**. Avoid. Unknown Theoretical

▶ **Enzalutamide** is predicted to decrease the exposure to **etravirine**. Avoid. Severe Theoretical

▶ **Etravirine** is predicted to decrease the exposure to **grazoprevir**. Avoid. Mild Theoretical

▶ **HIV-protease inhibitors (tipranavir)** decrease the exposure to **etravirine**. Avoid. Severe Study

▶ **Etravirine** increases the exposure to HIV-protease inhibitors **(fosamprenavir)** boosted with ritonavir. Refer to specialist literature. Moderate Study

▶ **Etravirine** is predicted to decrease the exposure to HIV-protease inhibitors **(indinavir)**. Avoid. Severe Study

▶ **Etravirine** decreases the exposure to macrolides **(clarithromycin)**. Severe Study

▶ **Etravirine** (with a boosted protease inhibitor) increases the exposure to **maraviroc**. Avoid or adjust dose. Moderate Study

▶ **Nevirapine** is predicted to decrease the exposure to **etravirine**. Avoid. Severe Study

▶ **Etravirine** moderately decreases the exposure to **phosphodiesterase type-5 inhibitors**. Adjust dose. Moderate Study

▶ **Rifabutin** decreases the exposure to **etravirine**. Moderate Study

▶ **Rifampicin** is predicted to decrease the exposure to **etravirine**. Avoid. Severe Theoretical

‣ **Etravirine** is predicted to decrease the exposure to rilpivirine. Avoid. [Severe] Theoretical

‣ **Etravirine** is predicted to decrease the exposure to simeprevir. Avoid. [Moderate] Study

▸ **St John's Wort** is predicted to decrease the exposure to etravirine. Avoid. [Severe] Study

Everolimus → see TABLE 15 p. 821 (myelosuppression)

▸ **Antiarrhythmics (dronedarone)** are predicted to increase the concentration of **everolimus**. Avoid or adjust dose. [Moderate] Study

▸ **Antiepileptics (carbamazepine, fosphenytoin, phenobarbital, phenytoin, primidone)** are predicted to decrease the concentration of **everolimus**. Avoid or adjust dose. [Severe] Study

▸ **Antifungals, azoles (fluconazole, isavuconazole, posaconazole)** are predicted to increase the concentration of **everolimus**. Avoid or adjust dose. [Moderate] Study

▸ **Antifungals, azoles (itraconazole, ketoconazole, voriconazole)** are predicted to increase the concentration of **everolimus**. Avoid. [Severe] Study

▸ **Aprepitant** is predicted to increase the concentration of **everolimus**. Avoid or adjust dose. [Moderate] Study

▸ **Bosentan** is predicted to decrease the concentration of **everolimus**. Avoid or adjust dose. [Severe] Study

▸ **Calcium channel blockers (diltiazem, verapamil)** are predicted to increase the concentration of **everolimus**. Avoid or adjust dose. [Moderate] Study

▸ **Ceritinib** is predicted to increase the exposure to **everolimus**. [Moderate] Theoretical → Also see TABLE 15 p. 821

▸ **Ciclosporin** moderately increases the exposure to **everolimus**. Avoid or adjust dose. [Severe] Study

▸ **Cobicistat** is predicted to increase the concentration of **everolimus**. Avoid. [Severe] Study

▸ **Crizotinib** is predicted to increase the concentration of **everolimus**. Avoid or adjust dose. [Moderate] Study → Also see TABLE 15 p. 821

▸ **Efavirenz** is predicted to decrease the concentration of **everolimus**. Avoid or adjust dose. [Severe] Study

▸ **Enzalutamide** is predicted to decrease the concentration of **everolimus**. Avoid or adjust dose. [Severe] Study

▸ **Grapefruit juice** is predicted to increase the exposure to **everolimus**. Avoid. [Severe] Theoretical

▸ **HIV-protease inhibitors (atazanavir, darunavir, fosamprenavir, lopinavir, ritonavir, saquinavir, tipranavir)** are predicted to increase the concentration of **everolimus**. Avoid. [Severe] Study

▸ **HIV-protease inhibitors (indinavir)** are predicted to increase the concentration of **everolimus**. Avoid or adjust dose. [Moderate] Study

▸ **Idelalisib** is predicted to increase the concentration of **everolimus**. Avoid. [Severe] Study → Also see TABLE 15 p. 821

▸ **Imatinib** is predicted to increase the concentration of **everolimus**. Avoid or adjust dose. [Moderate] Study → Also see TABLE 15 p. 821

▸ **Lapatinib** is predicted to increase the exposure to **everolimus**. [Moderate] Theoretical

▸ **Live vaccines** are predicted to increase the risk of generalised infection (possibly life-threatening) when given with **everolimus**. Public Health England advises avoid. [Severe] Theoretical

▸ **Everolimus** is predicted to increase the exposure to lomitapide. Separate administration by 12 hours. [Moderate] Theoretical

▸ **Lumacaftor** is predicted to decrease the exposure to **everolimus**. Avoid. [Severe] Theoretical

▸ **Macrolides (clarithromycin)** are predicted to increase the concentration of **everolimus**. Avoid. [Severe] Study

▸ **Macrolides (erythromycin)** are predicted to increase the concentration of **everolimus**. Avoid or adjust dose. [Moderate] Study

▸ **Mirabegron** is predicted to increase the exposure to **everolimus**. [Mild] Theoretical

▸ **Netupitant** is predicted to increase the concentration of **everolimus**. Avoid or adjust dose. [Moderate] Study

▸ **Nevirapine** is predicted to decrease the concentration of **everolimus**. Avoid or adjust dose. [Severe] Study

▸ **Nilotinib** is predicted to increase the concentration of **everolimus**. Avoid or adjust dose. [Moderate] Study → Also see TABLE 15 p. 821

▸ **Palbociclib** is predicted to increase the exposure to **everolimus**. Adjust dose. [Moderate] Theoretical

▸ **Pitolisant** is predicted to decrease the exposure to **everolimus**. Avoid. [Severe] Theoretical

▸ **Rifampicin** is predicted to decrease the concentration of **everolimus**. Avoid or adjust dose. [Severe] Study

▸ **St John's Wort** is predicted to decrease the concentration of **everolimus**. Avoid or adjust dose. [Severe] Study

▸ **Velpatasvir** is predicted to increase the exposure to **everolimus**. [Severe] Theoretical

Evolocumab → see monoclonal antibodies

Exemestane

▸ **Antiepileptics (carbamazepine, fosphenytoin, phenobarbital, phenytoin, primidone)** moderately decrease the exposure to **exemestane**. [Moderate] Study

▸ **Enzalutamide** moderately decreases the exposure to **exemestane**. [Moderate] Study

▸ **Rifampicin** moderately decreases the exposure to **exemestane**. [Moderate] Study

▸ **St John's Wort** is predicted to decrease the exposure to **exemestane**. [Moderate] Theoretical

Exenatide → see TABLE 14 p. 821 (antidiabetic drugs)

SEPARATION OF ADMINISTRATION With standard-release exenatide: some orally administered drugs should be taken at least 1 hour before, or 4 hours after, exenatide injection.

Ezetimibe

▸ **Ciclosporin** moderately increases the exposure to **ezetimibe** and **ezetimibe** slightly increases the exposure to ciclosporin. [Moderate] Study

▸ **Fibrates** are predicted to increase the risk of gallstones when given with **ezetimibe**. [Severe] Theoretical

▸ **Ezetimibe** potentially increases the risk of rhabdomyolysis when given with statins. [Severe] Anecdotal

Famotidine → see H₂ receptor antagonists

Fampridine

▸ **H₂ receptor antagonists (cimetidine)** increase the concentration of **fampridine**. Avoid. [Severe] Theoretical

Febuxostat

▸ **Febuxostat** is predicted to increase the exposure to azathioprine. Avoid. [Severe] Theoretical

▸ **Febuxostat** is predicted to increase the exposure to didanosine. [Severe] Theoretical

▸ **Febuxostat** is predicted to increase the exposure to mercaptopurine. Avoid. [Severe] Theoretical

Felbinac → see NSAIDs

Felodipine → see calcium channel blockers

Fenofibrate → see fibrates

Fenoprofen → see NSAIDs

Fentanyl → see opioids

Ferric carboxymaltose → see iron (injectable)

Ferric maltol → see iron (oral)

Ferrous fumarate → see iron (oral)

Ferrous gluconate → see iron (oral)

Ferrous sulfate → see iron (oral)

Fesoterodine → see TABLE 10 p. 820 (antimuscarinics)

▸ **Antiarrhythmics (dronedarone)** are predicted to increase the exposure to **fesoterodine**. Adjust **fesoterodine** dose in hepatic and renal impairment. [Mild] Study

▸ **Antiepileptics (carbamazepine, fosphenytoin, phenobarbital, phenytoin, primidone)** are predicted to decrease the exposure to **fesoterodine**. [Moderate] Study

▸ **Antifungals, azoles (fluconazole, isavuconazole, posaconazole)** are predicted to increase the exposure to **fesoterodine**. Adjust **fesoterodine** dose in hepatic and renal impairment. [Mild] Study

▸ **Antifungals, azoles (itraconazole, ketoconazole, voriconazole)** are predicted to moderately increase the exposure to **fesoterodine**. Adjust **fesoterodine** dose; avoid in hepatic and renal impairment. [Severe] Study

▸ **Aprepitant** is predicted to increase the exposure to **fesoterodine**. Adjust **fesoterodine** dose in hepatic and renal impairment. [Mild] Study

A1

Interactions | Appendix 1

Fesoterodine (continued)
- Calcium channel blockers (diltiazem, verapamil) are predicted to increase the exposure to **fesoterodine**. Adjust **fesoterodine** dose in hepatic and renal impairment. Mild Study
- Cobicistat is predicted to moderately increase the exposure to **fesoterodine**. Adjust **fesoterodine** dose; avoid in hepatic and renal impairment. Severe Study
- Crizotinib is predicted to increase the exposure to **fesoterodine**. Adjust **fesoterodine** dose in hepatic and renal impairment. Mild Study
- Enzalutamide is predicted to decrease the exposure to **fesoterodine**. Avoid. Moderate Study
- HIV-protease inhibitors (atazanavir, darunavir, fosamprenavir, lopinavir, ritonavir, saquinavir, tipranavir) are predicted to moderately increase the exposure to **fesoterodine**. Adjust **fesoterodine** dose; avoid in hepatic and renal impairment. Severe Study
- HIV-protease inhibitors (indinavir) are predicted to increase the exposure to **fesoterodine**. Adjust **fesoterodine** dose in hepatic and renal impairment. Mild Study
- Idelalisib is predicted to moderately increase the exposure to **fesoterodine**. Adjust **fesoterodine** dose; avoid in hepatic and renal impairment. Severe Study
- Imatinib is predicted to increase the exposure to **fesoterodine**. Adjust **fesoterodine** dose in hepatic and renal impairment. Mild Study
- Macrolides (clarithromycin) are predicted to moderately increase the exposure to **fesoterodine**. Adjust **fesoterodine** dose; avoid in hepatic and renal impairment. Severe Study
- Macrolides (erythromycin) are predicted to increase the exposure to **fesoterodine**. Adjust **fesoterodine** dose in hepatic and renal impairment. Mild Study
- Netupitant is predicted to increase the exposure to **fesoterodine**. Adjust **fesoterodine** dose in hepatic and renal impairment. Mild Study
- Nilotinib is predicted to increase the exposure to **fesoterodine**. Adjust **fesoterodine** dose in hepatic and renal impairment. Mild Study
- Rifampicin is predicted to decrease the exposure to **fesoterodine**. Avoid. Moderate Study
- St John's Wort is predicted to decrease the exposure to **fesoterodine**. Avoid. Severe Theoretical

Fexofenadine → see antihistamines, non-sedating

Fibrates

bezafibrate · ciprofibrate · fenofibrate · gemfibrozil

- Antacids slightly to moderately decrease the exposure to gemfibrozil. Moderate Study
- Bezafibrate is predicted to increase the risk of nephrotoxicity when given with ciclosporin. Severe Theoretical
- Fenofibrate increases the risk of nephrotoxicity when given with ciclosporin. Severe Study
- Colchicine increases the risk of rhabdomyolysis when given with fibrates. Severe Anecdotal
- Fibrates are predicted to increase the anticoagulant effect of coumarins. Monitor INR and adjust dose. Severe Study
- Gemfibrozil is predicted to increase the exposure to dabrafenib. Moderate Theoretical
- Fibrates are predicted to increase the risk of rhabdomyolysis when given with daptomycin. Severe Theoretical
- Gemfibrozil very markedly increases the exposure to dasabuvir. Avoid. Severe Study
- Gemfibrozil moderately increases the exposure to enzalutamide. Avoid or adjust enzalutamide dose. Severe Study
- Fibrates are predicted to increase the risk of gallstones when given with ezetimibe. Severe Theoretical
- Fibrates are predicted to increase the risk of hypoglycaemia when given with insulins. Moderate Theoretical
- Gemfibrozil is predicted to moderately increase the exposure to montelukast. Moderate Study
- Fibrates are predicted to increase the anticoagulant effect of phenindione. Monitor INR and adjust dose. Severe Study
- Gemfibrozil markedly increases the exposure to pioglitazone. Monitor blood glucose and adjust dose. Severe Study
- Gemfibrozil markedly increases the exposure to repaglinide. Avoid. Severe Study

- Gemfibrozil is predicted to increase the exposure to retinoids (alitretinoin). Adjust alitretinoin dose. Moderate Theoretical
- Gemfibrozil increases the concentration of retinoids (bexarotene). Avoid. Severe Study
- Gemfibrozil is predicted to increase the exposure to selexipag. Avoid. Severe Theoretical
- Ciprofibrate increases the risk of rhabdomyolysis when given with statins (atorvastatin). Avoid or adjust dose. Severe Study
- Bezafibrate increases the risk of rhabdomyolysis when given with statins (atorvastatin, fluvastatin). Severe Study
- Fenofibrate increases the risk of rhabdomyolysis when given with statins (atorvastatin, simvastatin). Adjust fenofibrate dose, p. 127. Severe Anecdotal
- Ciprofibrate increases the risk of rhabdomyolysis when given with statins (fluvastatin). Severe Study
- Fenofibrate is predicted to increase the risk of rhabdomyolysis when given with statins (fluvastatin). Adjust fenofibrate dose, p. 127. Severe Theoretical
- Fenofibrate is predicted to increase the risk of rhabdomyolysis when given with statins (pravastatin). Avoid. Severe Theoretical
- Fibrates (bezafibrate, ciprofibrate) increase the risk of rhabdomyolysis when given with statins (pravastatin). Avoid. Severe Study
- Fenofibrate increases the risk of rhabdomyolysis when given with statins (rosuvastatin). Adjust fenofibrate and rosuvastatin doses, p. 127, p. 130. Severe Anecdotal
- Fibrates (bezafibrate, ciprofibrate) increase the risk of rhabdomyolysis when given with statins (rosuvastatin). Adjust rosuvastatin dose, p. 130. Severe Study
- Fibrates (bezafibrate, ciprofibrate) increase the risk of rhabdomyolysis when given with statins (simvastatin). Adjust simvastatin dose, p. 130. Severe Study
- Gemfibrozil increases the risk of rhabdomyolysis when given with statins. Severe Anecdotal
- Fibrates are predicted to increase the risk of hypoglycaemia when given with sulfonylureas. Moderate Theoretical
- Fibrates are predicted to decrease the efficacy of ursodeoxycholic acid. Avoid. Severe Theoretical

Fidaxomicin
- Antiarrhythmics (amiodarone, dronedarone) are predicted to increase the exposure to **fidaxomicin**. Avoid. Moderate Study
- Antifungals, azoles (itraconazole, ketoconazole) are predicted to increase the exposure to **fidaxomicin**. Avoid. Moderate Study
- Calcium channel blockers (verapamil) are predicted to increase the exposure to **fidaxomicin**. Avoid. Moderate Study
- Ciclosporin is predicted to increase the exposure to **fidaxomicin**. Avoid. Moderate Study
- HIV-protease inhibitors (lopinavir, ritonavir, saquinavir) are predicted to increase the exposure to **fidaxomicin**. Avoid. Moderate Study
- Lapatinib is predicted to increase the exposure to **fidaxomicin**. Avoid. Moderate Study
- Macrolides are predicted to increase the exposure to **fidaxomicin**. Avoid. Moderate Study
- Ranolazine is predicted to increase the exposure to **fidaxomicin**. Avoid. Moderate Study
- Vemurafenib is predicted to increase the exposure to **fidaxomicin**. Avoid. Moderate Study

Fingolimod → see TABLE 6 p. 819 (bradycardia), TABLE 9 p. 820 (QT-interval prolongation)
- Antiepileptics (carbamazepine, fosphenytoin, phenobarbital, phenytoin, primidone) are predicted to decrease the exposure to **fingolimod**. Moderate Study
- Calcium channel blockers (diltiazem, verapamil) are predicted to increase the exposure to **fingolimod**. Avoid. Moderate Theoretical → Also see TABLE 6 p. 819
- Enzalutamide is predicted to decrease the exposure to **fingolimod**. Moderate Study
- Live vaccines are predicted to increase the risk of generalised infection (possibly life-threatening) when given with **fingolimod**. Public Health England advises avoid. Severe Theoretical
- Rifampicin is predicted to decrease the exposure to **fingolimod**. Moderate Study

- St John's Wort is predicted to decrease the exposure to fingolimod. Avoid. Moderate Theoretical
Flavoxate → see TABLE 10 p. 820 (antimuscarinics)
Flecainide → see antiarrhythmics
Flucloxacillin → see penicillins
Fluconazole → see antifungals, azoles
Flucytosine
- Amphotericin increases the risk of toxicity when given with flucytosine. Severe Study
- Cytarabine decreases the concentration of flucytosine. Avoid. Severe Study
Fludarabine → see TABLE 15 p. 821 (myelosuppression)
- Live vaccines are predicted to increase the risk of generalised infection (possibly life-threatening) when given with fludarabine. Public Health England advises avoid. Severe Theoretical
- Fludarabine increases the risk of pulmonary toxicity when given with pentostatin. Avoid. Severe Study → Also see TABLE 15 p. 821
Fludrocortisone → see TABLE 17 p. 822 (reduced serum potassium)
Fluocinolone

ROUTE-SPECIFIC INFORMATION With intravitreal use in adults: caution with concurrent administration of anticoagulant or antiplatelet drugs (higher incidence of conjunctival haemorrhage).

Fluorouracil → see TABLE 15 p. 821 (myelosuppression), TABLE 5 p. 818 (thromboembolism)

ROUTE-SPECIFIC INFORMATION Since systemic absorption can follow topical application, the possibility of interactions should be borne in mind.

- Fluorouracil increases the concentration of antiepileptics (fosphenytoin, phenytoin). Monitor concentration and adjust dose. Severe Anecdotal
- Fluorouracil increases the anticoagulant effect of coumarins. Severe Anecdotal
- Folates (folic acid) are predicted to increase the risk of toxicity when given with fluorouracil. Avoid. Severe Theoretical
- Folates (folinic acid) are predicted to increase the risk of toxicity when given with fluorouracil. Severe Theoretical
- H₂ receptor antagonists (cimetidine) slightly increase the exposure to fluorouracil. Severe Study
- Live vaccines are predicted to increase the risk of generalised infection (possibly life-threatening) when given with fluorouracil. Public Health England advises avoid. Severe Theoretical
- Metronidazole increases the risk of toxicity when given with fluorouracil. Severe Study
Fluoxetine → see SSRIs
Flupentixol → see TABLE 8 p. 819 (hypotension), TABLE 11 p. 820 (CNS depressant effects)
- Flupentixol is predicted to decrease side effects dopamine receptor agonists. Avoid. Moderate Theoretical → Also see TABLE 8 p. 819
- Flupentixol decreases the effects of levodopa. Avoid or monitor worsening parkinsonian symptoms. Severe Theoretical → Also see TABLE 8 p. 819
Fluphenazine → see phenothiazines
Flurazepam → see TABLE 11 p. 820 (CNS depressant effects)
- HIV-protease inhibitors (ritonavir) are predicted to increase the exposure to flurazepam. Avoid. Moderate Theoretical
Flurbiprofen → see NSAIDs
Fluticasone → see corticosteroids
Fluvastatin → see statins
Fluvoxamine → see SSRIs
Folates

folic acid · folinic acid · levofolinic acid

- Folic acid decreases the concentration of antiepileptics (fosphenytoin, phenobarbital, phenytoin, primidone). Monitor concentration and adjust dose. Severe Study
- Folinic acid is predicted to decrease the concentration of antiepileptics (fosphenytoin, phenobarbital, phenytoin, primidone). Severe Theoretical

- Folic acid is predicted to increase the risk of toxicity when given with capecitabine. Severe Anecdotal
- Folinic acid increases the risk of toxicity when given with capecitabine. Severe Study
- Folic acid is predicted to increase the risk of toxicity when given with fluorouracil. Avoid. Severe Theoretical
- Folinic acid is predicted to increase the risk of toxicity when given with fluorouracil. Severe Theoretical
- Folic acid is predicted to alter the effects of raltitrexed. Avoid. Moderate Theoretical
- Folinic acid alters the effects of raltitrexed. Avoid. Moderate Study
- Sulfasalazine decreases the absorption of folic acid. Moderate Study
- Sulfasalazine is predicted to decrease the absorption of folinic acid. Moderate Theoretical
- Folic acid is predicted to increase the risk of tegafur toxicity when given with tegafur. Severe Theoretical
- Folinic acid is predicted to increase the risk of toxicity when given with tegafur. Severe Theoretical
Folic acid → see folates
Folinic acid → see folates
Fondaparinux → see TABLE 3 p. 818 (anticoagulant effects)
Formoterol → see beta₂ agonists
Fosamprenavir → see HIV-protease inhibitors
Fosaprepitant
- Antiepileptics (carbamazepine, fosphenytoin, phenobarbital, phenytoin, primidone) are predicted to decrease the exposure to fosaprepitant. Avoid. Moderate Theoretical
- Antifungals, azoles (itraconazole, ketoconazole, voriconazole) are predicted to increase the exposure to fosaprepitant. Moderate Theoretical
- Fosaprepitant is predicted to increase the exposure to bosutinib. Severe Theoretical
- Cobicistat is predicted to increase the exposure to fosaprepitant. Moderate Theoretical
- Fosaprepitant is predicted to decrease the efficacy of combined hormonal contraceptives. For FSRH guidance, see Contraceptives, interactions p. 474. Severe Study
- Fosaprepitant is predicted to increase the exposure to corticosteroids (dexamethasone, methylprednisolone). Monitor and adjust dose. Moderate Theoretical
- Fosaprepitant is predicted to decrease the anticoagulant effect of coumarins. Moderate Theoretical
- Fosaprepitant is predicted to decrease the efficacy of desogestrel. For FSRH guidance, see Contraceptives, interactions p. 474. Severe Theoretical
- Enzalutamide is predicted to decrease the exposure to fosaprepitant. Avoid. Moderate Theoretical
- Fosaprepitant is predicted to decrease the efficacy of etonogestrel. For FSRH guidance, see Contraceptives, interactions p. 474. Severe Theoretical
- Fosaprepitant is predicted to increase the concentration of guanfacine. Moderate Theoretical
- HIV-protease inhibitors (atazanavir, darunavir, fosamprenavir, lopinavir, ritonavir, saquinavir, tipranavir) are predicted to increase the exposure to fosaprepitant. Moderate Theoretical
- Fosaprepitant is predicted to decrease the effects of Hormone replacement therapy. Moderate Anecdotal
- Fosaprepitant is predicted to slightly increase the exposure to ibrutinib. Moderate Theoretical
- Idelalisib is predicted to increase the exposure to fosaprepitant. Moderate Theoretical
- Fosaprepitant is predicted to decrease the efficacy of levonorgestrel. For FSRH guidance, see Contraceptives, interactions p. 474. Severe Theoretical
- Fosaprepitant is predicted to increase the exposure to lomitapide. Separate administration by 12 hours. Moderate Theoretical
- Macrolides (clarithromycin) are predicted to increase the exposure to fosaprepitant. Moderate Theoretical
- Fosaprepitant slightly increases the exposure to midazolam. Moderate Study

A1

Interactions | Appendix 1

Fosaprepitant (continued)
- **Fosaprepitant** is predicted to decrease the efficacy of norethisterone. For FSRH guidance, see Contraceptives, interactions p. 474. Severe Anecdotal
- **Fosaprepitant** is predicted to increase the exposure to pimozide. Avoid. Severe Theoretical
- **Rifampicin** is predicted to decrease the exposure to fosaprepitant. Avoid. Moderate Theoretical
- **St John's Wort** is predicted to decrease the exposure to fosaprepitant. Avoid. Moderate Theoretical
- **Fosaprepitant** decreases the efficacy of ulipristal. For FSRH guidance, see Contraceptives, interactions p. 474. Severe Anecdotal

Foscarnet → see TABLE 2 p. 818 (nephrotoxicity)
- **Foscarnet** increases the risk of hypocalcaemia when given with pentamidine. Severe Anecdotal → Also see TABLE 2 p. 818

Fosinopril → see ACE inhibitors

Fosphenytoin → see antiepileptics

Frovatriptan → see TABLE 13 p. 821 (serotonin syndrome)
- **SSRIs** (fluvoxamine) increase the concentration of frovatriptan. Severe Study → Also see TABLE 13 p. 821

Fulvestrant → see TABLE 5 p. 818 (thromboembolism)

Furosemide → see loop diuretics

Fusidic acid
- **Fusidic acid** increases the risk of rhabdomyolysis when given with statins. Avoid. Severe Anecdotal

Gabapentin → see antiepileptics

Galantamine → see anticholinesterases, centrally acting

Ganciclovir → see TABLE 15 p. 821 (myelosuppression), TABLE 2 p. 818 (nephrotoxicity)

ROUTE-SPECIFIC INFORMATION Since systemic absorption can follow topical application, the possibility of interactions should be borne in mind.

- **Ganciclovir** is predicted to increase the risk of seizures when given with carbapenems (imipenem). Avoid. Severe Anecdotal
- **Ganciclovir** is predicted to increase the exposure to didanosine. Moderate Study
- **Mycophenolate** is predicted to increase the risk of haematological toxicity when given with ganciclovir. Moderate Theoretical → Also see TABLE 15 p. 821

Gefitinib → see TABLE 15 p. 821 (myelosuppression)
- **Antacids** are predicted to slightly decrease the exposure to gefitinib. Moderate Theoretical
- **Antiarrhythmics** (dronedarone) are predicted to increase the exposure to gefitinib. Moderate Theoretical
- **Antiepileptics** (carbamazepine, fosphenytoin, phenobarbital, phenytoin, primidone) are predicted to decrease the exposure to gefitinib. Avoid. Severe Study
- **Antifungals, azoles** (fluconazole, isavuconazole, posaconazole) are predicted to increase the exposure to gefitinib. Moderate Theoretical
- **Antifungals, azoles** (itraconazole, ketoconazole, voriconazole) are predicted to increase the exposure to gefitinib. Moderate Study
- **Aprepitant** is predicted to increase the exposure to gefitinib. Moderate Theoretical
- **Bosentan** is predicted to decrease the exposure to gefitinib. Avoid. Severe Theoretical
- **Calcium channel blockers** (diltiazem, verapamil) are predicted to increase the exposure to gefitinib. Moderate Theoretical
- **Cobicistat** is predicted to increase the exposure to gefitinib. Moderate Study
- **Gefitinib** is predicted to increase the anticoagulant effect of coumarins. Severe Anecdotal
- **Crizotinib** is predicted to increase the exposure to gefitinib. Moderate Theoretical → Also see TABLE 15 p. 821
- **Efavirenz** is predicted to decrease the exposure to gefitinib. Avoid. Severe Theoretical
- **Enzalutamide** is predicted to decrease the exposure to gefitinib. Avoid. Severe Study
- **H₂ receptor antagonists** are predicted to slightly to moderately decrease the exposure to gefitinib. Moderate Study
- **HIV-protease inhibitors** (atazanavir, darunavir, fosamprenavir, lopinavir, ritonavir, saquinavir, tipranavir) are predicted to increase the exposure to gefitinib. Moderate Study

- **HIV-protease inhibitors** (indinavir) are predicted to increase the exposure to gefitinib. Moderate Theoretical
- **Idelalisib** is predicted to increase the exposure to gefitinib. Moderate Study → Also see TABLE 15 p. 821
- **Imatinib** is predicted to increase the exposure to gefitinib. Moderate Theoretical → Also see TABLE 15 p. 821
- **Macrolides** (clarithromycin) are predicted to increase the exposure to gefitinib. Moderate Study
- **Macrolides** (erythromycin) are predicted to increase the exposure to gefitinib. Moderate Theoretical
- **Netupitant** is predicted to increase the exposure to gefitinib. Moderate Theoretical
- **Nevirapine** is predicted to decrease the exposure to gefitinib. Avoid. Severe Theoretical
- **Nilotinib** is predicted to increase the exposure to gefitinib. Moderate Theoretical → Also see TABLE 15 p. 821
- **Gefitinib** is predicted to increase the risk of bleeding events when given with phenindione. Severe Theoretical
- **Proton pump inhibitors** are predicted to decrease the exposure to gefitinib. Severe Theoretical
- **Rifampicin** is predicted to decrease the exposure to gefitinib. Avoid. Severe Study
- **St John's Wort** is predicted to decrease the exposure to gefitinib. Avoid. Severe Theoretical

Gemcitabine → see TABLE 15 p. 821 (myelosuppression)
- **Live vaccines** are predicted to increase the risk of generalised infection (possibly life-threatening) when given with gemcitabine. Public Health England advises avoid. Severe Theoretical

Gemfibrozil → see fibrates

Gentamicin → see aminoglycosides

Glibenclamide → see sulfonylureas

Gliclazide → see sulfonylureas

Glimepiride → see sulfonylureas

Glipizide → see sulfonylureas

Glucagon
- **Glucagon** increases the anticoagulant effect of coumarins (warfarin). Severe Study

Glucosamine
- **Glucosamine** increases the anticoagulant effect of coumarins (warfarin). Avoid. Moderate Anecdotal

Glucose → see TABLE 3 p. 818 (anticoagulant effects)

Glycerol → see TABLE 17 p. 822 (reduced serum potassium)

Glyceryl trinitrate → see nitrates

Glycopyrronium → see TABLE 10 p. 820 (antimuscarinics)

Golimumab → see monoclonal antibodies

Granisetron → see TABLE 9 p. 820 (QT-interval prolongation), TABLE 13 p. 821 (serotonin syndrome)
- **Dopamine receptor agonists** (apomorphine) are predicted to increase the risk of severe hypotension when given with granisetron. Severe Theoretical

Grapefruit juice
- **Grapefruit juice** moderately decreases the exposure to aliskiren. Avoid. Severe Study
- **Grapefruit juice** increases the exposure to antiarrhythmics (amiodarone). Avoid. Moderate Study
- **Grapefruit juice** moderately increases the exposure to antiarrhythmics (dronedarone). Avoid. Severe Study
- **Grapefruit juice** increases the exposure to antiarrhythmics (propafenone). Monitor and adjust dose. Moderate Study
- **Grapefruit juice** slightly increases the exposure to antiepileptics (carbamazepine). Monitor carbamazepine concentration and adjust dose. Moderate Study
- **Grapefruit juice** slightly decreases the exposure to antihistamines, non-sedating (bilastine). Bilastine should be taken 1 hour before or 2 hours after grapefruit juice. Moderate Study
- **Grapefruit juice** increases the exposure to antimalarials (artemether). Unknown Study
- **Grapefruit juice** is predicted to increase the concentration of antimalarials (piperaquine). Avoid. Severe Theoretical
- **Grapefruit juice** is predicted to increase the exposure to axitinib. Moderate Theoretical
- **Grapefruit juice** greatly decreases the exposure to beta blockers, selective (celiprolol). Moderate Study

- **Grapefruit juice** is predicted to increase the exposure to bosutinib. Avoid. Moderate Theoretical
- **Grapefruit juice** increases the exposure to **buspirone**. Avoid. Mild Study
- **Grapefruit juice** is predicted to increase the exposure to cabozantinib. Moderate Theoretical
- **Grapefruit juice** very slightly increases the exposure to calcium channel blockers **(amlodipine)**. Avoid. Mild Study
- **Grapefruit juice** increases the exposure to calcium channel blockers **(felodipine)**. Avoid. Moderate Study
- **Grapefruit juice** is predicted to increase the exposure to calcium channel blockers **(lercanidipine)**. Avoid. Moderate Theoretical
- **Grapefruit juice** increases the exposure to calcium channel blockers **(nicardipine)**. Mild Study
- **Grapefruit juice** increases the exposure to calcium channel blockers **(nifedipine, verapamil)**. Avoid. Mild Study
- **Grapefruit juice** is predicted to increase the exposure to ceritinib. Severe Theoretical
- **Grapefruit juice** increases the concentration of **ciclosporin**. Avoid. Severe Study
- **Grapefruit juice** markedly decreases the exposure to clopidogrel. Severe Study
- **Grapefruit juice** is predicted to increase the exposure to cobimetinib. Avoid. Severe Theoretical
- **Grapefruit juice** moderately increases the exposure to oral corticosteroids **(budesonide)**. Avoid. Moderate Study
- **Grapefruit juice** is predicted to increase the exposure to crizotinib. Avoid. Moderate Theoretical
- **Grapefruit juice** is predicted to increase the exposure to darifenacin. Moderate Study
- **Grapefruit juice** is predicted to increase the exposure to dasatinib. Avoid. Moderate Theoretical
- **Grapefruit juice** is predicted to increase the risk of ergotism when given with **ergometrine**. Severe Theoretical
- **Grapefruit juice** is predicted to increase the exposure to ergotamine. Severe Theoretical
- **Grapefruit juice** is predicted to increase the exposure to erlotinib. Moderate Theoretical
- **Grapefruit juice** is predicted to increase the exposure to everolimus. Avoid. Severe Theoretical
- **Grapefruit juice** is predicted to increase the exposure to ibrutinib. Avoid. Moderate Theoretical
- **Grapefruit juice** is predicted to increase the exposure to imatinib. Moderate Theoretical
- **Grapefruit juice** is predicted to increase the exposure to ivabradine. Avoid. Moderate Study
- **Grapefruit juice** is predicted to increase the exposure to ivacaftor. Avoid. Moderate Theoretical
- **Grapefruit juice** is predicted to increase the exposure to lapatinib. Avoid. Moderate Theoretical
- **Grapefruit juice** is predicted to increase the exposure to lomitapide. Separate administration by 12 hours. Moderate Theoretical
- **Grapefruit juice** is predicted to increase the exposure to lurasidone. Avoid. Severe Theoretical
- **Grapefruit juice** is predicted to increase the exposure to naloxegol. Avoid. Moderate Theoretical
- **Grapefruit juice** is predicted to increase the exposure to nilotinib. Avoid. Severe Theoretical
- **Grapefruit juice** is predicted to increase the exposure to olaparib. Avoid. Moderate Theoretical
- **Grapefruit juice** is predicted to increase the exposure to palbociclib. Avoid. Severe Theoretical
- **Grapefruit juice** is predicted to increase the exposure to pazopanib. Avoid. Severe Theoretical
- **Grapefruit juice** is predicted to increase the exposure to phosphodiesterase type-5 inhibitors. Use with caution or avoid. Moderate Study
- **Grapefruit juice** increases the exposure to **pimozide**. Avoid. Severe Theoretical
- **Grapefruit juice** is predicted to increase the exposure to ponatinib. Moderate Theoretical
- **Grapefruit juice** is predicted to increase the exposure to praziquantel. Moderate Study

- **Grapefruit juice** is predicted to increase the exposure to quetiapine. Avoid. Severe Theoretical
- **Grapefruit juice** is predicted to increase the concentration of ranolazine. Avoid. Severe Theoretical
- **Grapefruit juice** is predicted to increase the exposure to regorafenib. Avoid. Moderate Theoretical
- **Grapefruit juice** is predicted to increase the exposure to ruxolitinib. Severe Theoretical
- **Grapefruit juice** is predicted to increase the exposure to saxagliptin. Mild Theoretical
- **Grapefruit juice** increases the concentration of **sirolimus**. Avoid. Moderate Study
- **Grapefruit juice** moderately increases the exposure to SSRIs **(sertraline)**. Avoid. Moderate Study
- **Grapefruit juice** increases the exposure to statins **(atorvastatin)**. Mild Study
- **Grapefruit juice** increases the exposure to statins **(simvastatin)**. Avoid. Severe Study
- **Grapefruit juice** is predicted to increase the exposure to sunitinib. Avoid. Moderate Theoretical
- **Grapefruit juice** increases the concentration of **tacrolimus**. Avoid. Severe Study
- **Grapefruit juice** is predicted to increase the concentration of temsirolimus. Use with caution or avoid. Moderate Theoretical
- **Grapefruit juice** moderately increases the exposure to ticagrelor. Moderate Study
- **Grapefruit juice** increases the exposure to **tolvaptan**. Avoid. Moderate Study
- **Grapefruit juice** is predicted to increase the exposure to ulipristal. Avoid if used for uterine fibroids. Moderate Theoretical
- **Grapefruit juice** is predicted to increase the exposure to venetoclax. Avoid. Severe Theoretical

Grass pollen extract

> **GENERAL INFORMATION** Desensitising vaccines should be avoided in patients taking beta-blockers (adrenaline might be ineffective in case of a hypersensitivity reaction) or ACE inhibitors (risk of severe anaphylactoid reactions).

Grazoprevir

- Antiepileptics **(carbamazepine, fosphenytoin, phenobarbital, phenytoin, primidone)** are predicted to decrease the exposure to **grazoprevir**. Avoid. Severe Study
- Antifungals, azoles **(itraconazole, ketoconazole, voriconazole)** are predicted to moderately to markedly increase the exposure to **grazoprevir**. Avoid. Severe Study
- Bosentan is predicted to markedly decrease the exposure to **grazoprevir**. Avoid. Severe Study
- Ciclosporin greatly increases the exposure to **grazoprevir**. Avoid. Severe Study
- Cobicistat is predicted to moderately to markedly increase the exposure to **grazoprevir**. Avoid. Severe Study
- Efavirenz is predicted to markedly decrease the exposure to **grazoprevir**. Avoid. Severe Study
- Enzalutamide is predicted to decrease the exposure to **grazoprevir**. Avoid. Severe Study
- Etravirine is predicted to decrease the exposure to **grazoprevir**. Avoid. Mild Theoretical
- HIV-protease inhibitors **(atazanavir, darunavir, fosamprenavir, lopinavir, ritonavir, saquinavir, tipranavir)** are predicted to moderately to markedly increase the exposure to **grazoprevir**. Avoid. Severe Study
- Idelalisib is predicted to moderately to markedly increase the exposure to **grazoprevir**. Avoid. Severe Study
- Macrolides **(clarithromycin)** are predicted to moderately to markedly increase the exposure to **grazoprevir**. Avoid. Severe Study
- Modafinil is predicted to decrease the exposure to **grazoprevir**. Avoid. Unknown Theoretical
- Nevirapine is predicted to markedly decrease the exposure to **grazoprevir**. Avoid. Severe Study
- Rifampicin is predicted to decrease the exposure to **grazoprevir**. Avoid. Severe Study
- St John's Wort is predicted to markedly decrease the exposure to **grazoprevir**. Avoid. Severe Study
- **Grazoprevir** increases the exposure to statins **(atorvastatin)**. Adjust **atorvastatin** dose, p. 128. Moderate Study

Grazoprevir (continued)

▸ **Grazoprevir** is predicted to increase the exposure to statins (**fluvastatin**). Adjust **fluvastatin** dose, p. 129. [Unknown] Theoretical

▸ **Grazoprevir** increases the exposure to statins (**rosuvastatin**). Adjust **rosuvastatin** dose, p. 130. [Moderate] Study

▸ **Grazoprevir** is predicted to increase the exposure to statins (**simvastatin**). Adjust **simvastatin** dose, p. 130. [Unknown] Theoretical

▸ **Grazoprevir** increases the exposure to **tacrolimus**. [Moderate] Study

Griseofulvin

> **FOOD AND LIFESTYLE** Disulfiram-like reaction might occur on consumption of alcohol.

▸ Antiepileptics (**phenobarbital, primidone**) decrease the effects of griseofulvin. [Moderate] Study

▸ **Griseofulvin** potentially decreases the efficacy of combined hormonal contraceptives. For FSRH guidance, see Contraceptives, interactions p. 474. [Severe] Anecdotal

▸ **Griseofulvin** potentially decreases the anticoagulant effect of coumarins. [Moderate] Anecdotal

▸ **Griseofulvin** potentially decreases the efficacy of **desogestrel**. For FSRH guidance, see Contraceptives, interactions p. 474. [Severe] Anecdotal

▸ **Griseofulvin** decreases the efficacy of **etonogestrel**. For FSRH guidance, see Contraceptives, interactions p. 474. [Severe] Anecdotal

▸ **Griseofulvin** potentially decreases the efficacy of oral **levonorgestrel**. For FSRH guidance, see Contraceptives, interactions p. 474. [Severe] Anecdotal

▸ **Griseofulvin** potentially decreases the efficacy of **norethisterone**. For FSRH guidance, see Contraceptives, interactions p. 474. [Severe] Anecdotal

▸ **Griseofulvin** potentially decreases the efficacy of **ulipristal**. For FSRH guidance, see Contraceptives, interactions p. 474. [Severe] Anecdotal

Guanethidine → see TABLE 8 p. 819 (hypotension)

▸ Amfetamines (**dexamfetamine**) decrease the effects of guanethidine. [Severe] Study

▸ **Benperidol** is predicted to decrease the effects of guanethidine. [Moderate] Theoretical → Also see TABLE 8 p. 819

▸ **Droperidol** is predicted to decrease the effects of guanethidine. Monitor and adjust dose. [Moderate] Theoretical → Also see TABLE 8 p. 819

▸ **Haloperidol** is predicted to decrease the antihypertensive effects of **guanethidine**. Monitor and adjust dose. [Moderate] Theoretical → Also see TABLE 8 p. 819

▸ Monoamine-oxidase A and B inhibitors, irreversible are predicted to decrease the antihypertensive effects of **guanethidine**. Avoid and for 14 days after stopping the MAOI. [Severe] Theoretical → Also see TABLE 8 p. 819

▸ **Phenothiazines** are predicted to decrease the antihypertensive effects of **guanethidine**. [Moderate] Theoretical → Also see TABLE 8 p. 819

▸ **Guanethidine** is predicted to increase the effects of sympathomimetics, inotropic (**dopamine**). [Severe] Theoretical

▸ **Guanethidine** is predicted to increase the effects of sympathomimetics, vasoconstrictor (**adrenaline/epinephrine, noradrenaline/norepinephrine**). [Moderate] Study

▸ **Guanethidine** increases the effects of sympathomimetics, vasoconstrictor (**metaraminol**). [Severe] Anecdotal

▸ **Guanethidine** increases the effects of sympathomimetics, vasoconstrictor (**phenylephrine**). [Severe] Study

▸ Tricyclic antidepressants are predicted to decrease the antihypertensive effects of **guanethidine**. [Moderate] Study → Also see TABLE 8 p. 819

Guanfacine → see TABLE 8 p. 819 (hypotension), TABLE 11 p. 820 (CNS depressant effects)

▸ Antiarrhythmics (**dronedarone**) are predicted to increase the concentration of **guanfacine**. Adjust **guanfacine** dose, p. 222. [Moderate] Theoretical

▸ Antiepileptics (**carbamazepine, fosphenytoin, phenobarbital, phenytoin, primidone**) are predicted to decrease the concentration of **guanfacine**. Adjust **guanfacine** dose, p. 222. [Moderate] Study → Also see TABLE 11 p. 820

▸ Antiepileptics (**oxcarbazepine**) are predicted to decrease the concentration of **guanfacine**. Monitor and adjust **guanfacine** dose, p. 222. [Moderate] Theoretical

▸ **Guanfacine** increases the concentration of antiepileptics (**valproate**). Monitor and adjust dose. [Moderate] Study

▸ Antifungals, azoles (**fluconazole, isavuconazole, posaconazole**) are predicted to increase the concentration of **guanfacine**. Adjust **guanfacine** dose, p. 222. [Moderate] Theoretical

▸ Antifungals, azoles (**itraconazole, ketoconazole, voriconazole**) are predicted to increase the exposure to **guanfacine**. Adjust **guanfacine** dose, p. 222. [Moderate] Study

▸ **Aprepitant** is predicted to increase the concentration of **guanfacine**. Adjust **guanfacine** dose, p. 222. [Moderate] Theoretical

▸ **Bosentan** is predicted to decrease the concentration of **guanfacine**. Adjust **guanfacine** dose. [Moderate] Theoretical

▸ Calcium channel blockers (**diltiazem, verapamil**) are predicted to increase the concentration of **guanfacine**. Adjust **guanfacine** dose, p. 222. [Moderate] Theoretical → Also see TABLE 8 p. 819

▸ **Cobicistat** is predicted to increase the exposure to **guanfacine**. Adjust **guanfacine** dose, p. 222. [Moderate] Study

▸ **Crizotinib** is predicted to increase the concentration of **guanfacine**. Adjust **guanfacine** dose, p. 222. [Moderate] Theoretical

▸ **Efavirenz** is predicted to decrease the concentration of **guanfacine**. Adjust dose. [Moderate] Theoretical

▸ **Enzalutamide** is predicted to decrease the concentration of **guanfacine**. Adjust **guanfacine** dose, p. 222. [Moderate] Study

▸ **Fosaprepitant** is predicted to increase the concentration of **guanfacine**. [Moderate] Theoretical

▸ HIV-protease inhibitors (**atazanavir, darunavir, fosamprenavir, lopinavir, ritonavir, saquinavir, tipranavir**) are predicted to increase the exposure to **guanfacine**. Adjust **guanfacine** dose, p. 222. [Moderate] Study

▸ HIV-protease inhibitors (**indinavir**) are predicted to increase the concentration of **guanfacine**. Adjust **guanfacine** dose, p. 222. [Moderate] Theoretical

▸ **Idelalisib** is predicted to increase the exposure to **guanfacine**. Adjust **guanfacine** dose, p. 222. [Moderate] Study

▸ **Imatinib** is predicted to increase the concentration of **guanfacine**. Adjust **guanfacine** dose, p. 222. [Moderate] Theoretical

▸ Macrolides (**clarithromycin**) are predicted to increase the exposure to **guanfacine**. Adjust **guanfacine** dose, p. 222. [Moderate] Study

▸ Macrolides (**erythromycin**) are predicted to increase the concentration of **guanfacine**. Adjust **guanfacine** dose, p. 222. [Moderate] Theoretical

▸ **Netupitant** is predicted to increase the concentration of **guanfacine**. Adjust **guanfacine** dose, p. 222. [Moderate] Theoretical

▸ **Nevirapine** is predicted to decrease the concentration of **guanfacine**. Adjust dose. [Moderate] Theoretical

▸ **Nilotinib** is predicted to increase the concentration of **guanfacine**. Adjust **guanfacine** dose, p. 222. [Moderate] Theoretical

▸ **Rifampicin** is predicted to decrease the concentration of **guanfacine**. Adjust **guanfacine** dose, p. 222. [Moderate] Study

▸ **St John's Wort** is predicted to decrease the concentration of **guanfacine**. Adjust dose. [Moderate] Theoretical

H₂ receptor antagonists

cimetidine · famotidine · nizatidine · ranitidine

▸ **Cimetidine** decreases the clearance of **albendazole**. [Moderate] Study

▸ **Cimetidine** increases the concentration of **aminophylline**. Adjust dose. [Severe] Study

▸ **Cimetidine** slightly increases the exposure to anthracyclines (**epirubicin**). Avoid. [Moderate] Study

▸ **Cimetidine** increases the exposure to antiarrhythmics (**amiodarone**). [Moderate] Study

▸ **Cimetidine** slightly increases the exposure to antiarrhythmics (**flecainide**). Monitor and adjust dose. [Mild] Study

▸ **Cimetidine** increases the exposure to antiarrhythmics (**lidocaine**). Monitor and adjust dose. [Moderate] Study

▸ **Cimetidine** is predicted to increase the exposure to antiarrhythmics (**propafenone**). Monitor and adjust dose. [Moderate] Theoretical

▸ **Cimetidine** transiently increases the concentration of antiepileptics (**carbamazepine**). [Moderate] Study

- **Cimetidine** increases the concentration of antiepileptics (**fosphenytoin**). Monitor phenytoin concentration and adjust dose. Severe Study
- **Cimetidine** increases the concentration of antiepileptics (**phenytoin**). Monitor **phenytoin** concentration and adjust dose. Severe Study
- **H₂ receptor antagonists** are predicted to decrease the absorption of antifungals, azoles (**itraconazole**). Administer itraconazole capsules with an acidic beverage. Moderate Study
- **H₂ receptor antagonists** are predicted to decrease the absorption of antifungals, azoles (**ketoconazole**). Administer ketoconazole with an acidic beverage. Severe Study
- **H₂ receptor antagonists** are predicted to slightly decrease the exposure to antifungals, azoles (**posaconazole**). Avoid use of posaconazole oral suspension. Moderate Study
- **Cimetidine** decreases the clearance of antimalarials (**chloroquine**). Moderate Study
- **Cimetidine** slightly increases the exposure to antimalarials (**quinine**). Moderate Study
- **H₂ receptor antagonists** are predicted to decrease the absorption of **bosutinib**. Moderate Theoretical
- **Cimetidine** slightly increases the exposure to calcium channel blockers (**diltiazem, isradipine, nimodipine**). Monitor and adjust dose. Moderate Study
- **Cimetidine** (high-dose) is predicted to increase the exposure to calcium channel blockers (**lercanidipine**). Moderate Theoretical
- **Cimetidine** moderately increases the exposure to calcium channel blockers (**nifedipine**). Monitor and adjust dose. Severe Study
- **Cimetidine** increases the exposure to calcium channel blockers (**verapamil**). Moderate Study
- **Cimetidine** is predicted to slightly increase the exposure to **capecitabine**. Severe Theoretical
- **H₂ receptor antagonists** are predicted to decrease the absorption of **ceritinib**. Moderate Theoretical
- **Cimetidine** increases the concentration of **ciclosporin**. Mild Study
- **Cimetidine** increases the anticoagulant effect of **coumarins**. Severe Study
- **H₂ receptor antagonists** are predicted to decrease the exposure to **dabrafenib**. Avoid. Severe Theoretical
- **H₂ receptor antagonists** are predicted to decrease the exposure to **dasatinib**. Avoid. Moderate Study
- **H₂ receptor antagonists** are predicted to decrease the absorption of **dipyridamole** (immediate release tablets). Moderate Theoretical
- **Cimetidine** slightly increases the exposure to dopamine receptor agonists (**pramipexole**). Adjust dose. Moderate Study
- **H₂ receptor antagonists** are predicted to decrease the exposure to **erlotinib**. Erlotinib should be taken 2 hours before or 10 hours after **H₂ receptor antagonists**. Moderate Study
- **Cimetidine** increases the concentration of **fampridine**. Avoid. Severe Theoretical
- **Cimetidine** slightly increases the exposure to **fluorouracil**. Severe Study
- **H₂ receptor antagonists** are predicted to slightly to moderately decrease the exposure to **gefitinib**. Moderate Study
- **H₂ receptor antagonists** are predicted to decrease the effects of **histamine**. Avoid. Severe Theoretical
- **H₂ receptor antagonists** decrease the exposure to HIV-protease inhibitors (**atazanavir**). Monitor and adjust dose. Moderate Study
- **Cimetidine** is predicted to decrease the clearance of **hydroxychloroquine**. Moderate Theoretical
- **H₂ receptor antagonists** are predicted to decrease the absorption of **lapatinib**. Avoid. Moderate Theoretical
- **H₂ receptor antagonists** are predicted to decrease the exposure to **ledipasvir**. Adjust dose, see sofosbuvir with ledipasvir. Moderate Study
- **H₂ receptor antagonists** (**cimetidine, ranitidine**) are predicted to increase the exposure to **lomitapide**. Separate administration by 12 hours. Moderate Theoretical
- **Lumacaftor** is predicted to affect the exposure to **ranitidine**. Monitor and adjust dose. Moderate Theoretical
- **Cimetidine** slightly increases the exposure to macrolides (**erythromycin**). Moderate Study

- **Cimetidine** increases the concentration of **mebendazole**. Moderate Study
- **Cimetidine** slightly increases the exposure to **metformin**. Monitor and adjust dose. Moderate Study
- **Cimetidine** slightly increases the exposure to **mirtazapine**. Use with caution and adjust dose. Moderate Study
- **Cimetidine** increases the exposure to **moclobemide**. Adjust **moclobemide** dose. Mild Study
- **H₂ receptor antagonists** are predicted to decrease the absorption of **nilotinib**. **H₂ receptor antagonists** should be taken 10 hours before or 2 hours after **nilotinib**. Mild Theoretical
- **Cimetidine** increases the concentration of opioids (**alfentanil**). Use with caution and adjust dose. Severe Study
- **Cimetidine** increases the exposure to opioids (**fentanyl**). Moderate Study
- **H₂ receptor antagonists** are predicted to decrease the exposure to **pazopanib**. **H₂ receptor antagonists** should be taken 10 hours before or 2 hours after **pazopanib**. Moderate Theoretical
- **Cimetidine** increases the exposure to **phenindione**. Severe Anecdotal
- **Cimetidine** moderately increases the exposure to **praziquantel**. Moderate Study
- **H₂ receptor antagonists** are predicted to decrease the exposure to **rilpivirine**. **H₂ receptor antagonists** should be taken 12 hours before or 4 hours after **rilpivirine**. Severe Study
- **Cimetidine** slightly increases the exposure to **roflumilast**. Moderate Study
- **H₂ receptor antagonists** potentially decrease the exposure to **sofosbuvir**. Adjust dose, see sofosbuvir with ledipasvir and sofosbuvir with velpatasvir. Moderate Study
- **Cimetidine** slightly increases the exposure to SSRIs (**citalopram, escitalopram**). Adjust dose. Moderate Study
- **Cimetidine** slightly increases the exposure to SSRIs (**paroxetine, sertraline**). Moderate Study
- **Cimetidine** is predicted to increase the risk of toxicity when given with **tegafur**. Severe Theoretical
- **Cimetidine** increases the concentration of **theophylline**. Adjust dose. Severe Study
- **Cimetidine** increases the exposure to tricyclic antidepressants. Moderate Study
- **H₂ receptor antagonists** are predicted to decrease the concentration of **velpatasvir**. Adjust dose, see sofosbuvir with velpatasvir. Moderate Study
- **Cimetidine** slightly increases the exposure to **venlafaxine**. Mild Study
- **Cimetidine** slightly increases the exposure to **zolmitriptan**. Adjust **zolmitriptan** dose, p. 280. Moderate Study

Haloperidol → see TABLE 8 p. 819 (hypotension), TABLE 9 p. 820 (QT-interval prolongation), TABLE 11 p. 820 (CNS depressant effects), TABLE 10 p. 820 (antimuscarinics)

FOOD AND LIFESTYLE Dose adjustment might be necessary if smoking started or stopped during treatment.

- Antiepileptics (**carbamazepine, fosphenytoin, phenobarbital, phenytoin, primidone**) decrease the concentration of **haloperidol**. Adjust dose. Moderate Study → Also see TABLE 11 p. 820
- **Haloperidol** potentially increases the risk of overheating and dehydration when given with antiepileptics (**zonisamide**). Avoid in children. Severe Theoretical
- Antifungals, azoles (**itraconazole**) increase the concentration of **haloperidol**. Moderate Study
- **Haloperidol** is predicted to decrease the effects of dopamine receptor agonists. Avoid. Moderate Theoretical → Also see TABLE 8 p. 819 → Also see TABLE 9 p. 820 → Also see TABLE 10 p. 820
- **Enzalutamide** decreases the concentration of **haloperidol**. Adjust dose. Moderate Study
- **Haloperidol** is predicted to decrease the antihypertensive effects of **guanethidine**. Monitor and adjust dose. Moderate Theoretical → Also see TABLE 8 p. 819
- HIV-protease inhibitors (**ritonavir**) are predicted to increase the exposure to **haloperidol**. Severe Theoretical
- **Haloperidol** decreases the effects of **levodopa**. Severe Study → Also see TABLE 8 p. 819
- **Rifampicin** decreases the concentration of **haloperidol**. Adjust dose. Moderate Study

A1

Interactions | Appendix 1

Haloperidol (continued)
▸ **Haloperidol** potentially decreases the effects of **sodium phenylbutyrate**. Moderate Anecdotal
▸ SSRIs **(fluoxetine)** increase the concentration of **haloperidol**. Adjust dose. Moderate Anecdotal
▸ SSRIs **(fluvoxamine)** increase the concentration of **haloperidol**. Adjust dose. Moderate Study
▸ **Venlafaxine** slightly increases the exposure to **haloperidol**. Severe Study → Also see **TABLE 9** p. 820 → Also see **TABLE 11** p. 820

Heparin (unfractionated) → see **TABLE 16** p. 822 (increased serum potassium), **TABLE 3** p. 818 (anticoagulant effects)
▸ **Ranibizumab** increases the risk of bleeding events when given with **heparin (unfractionated)**. Severe Theoretical

Histamine → see **TABLE 8** p. 819 (hypotension)
▸ **Antihistamines, non-sedating** are predicted to decrease the effects of **histamine**. Avoid. Severe Theoretical
▸ **Antihistamines, sedating** are predicted to decrease the effects of **histamine**. Avoid. Severe Theoretical
▸ **Antimalarials (artemether, atovaquone, chloroquine, mefloquine, primaquine, proguanil, pyrimethamine, quinine)** are predicted to affect the exposure to **histamine**. Avoid. Severe Theoretical
▸ **Clonidine** is predicted to decrease the effects of **histamine**. Avoid. Severe Theoretical → Also see **TABLE 8** p. 819
▸ **Clozapine** is predicted to decrease the effects of **histamine**. Avoid. Severe Theoretical → Also see **TABLE 8** p. 819
▸ **Corticosteroids** are predicted to decrease the effects of **histamine**. Avoid. Severe Theoretical
▸ **H₂ receptor antagonists** are predicted to decrease the effects of **histamine**. Avoid. Severe Theoretical
▸ **Monoamine-oxidase A and B inhibitors, irreversible** are predicted to affect the exposure to **histamine**. Avoid. Severe Theoretical → Also see **TABLE 8** p. 819
▸ **Olanzapine** is predicted to decrease the effects of **histamine**. Avoid. Severe Theoretical → Also see **TABLE 8** p. 819
▸ **Phenothiazines** are predicted to decrease the effects of **histamine**. Avoid. Severe Theoretical → Also see **TABLE 8** p. 819
▸ **Quetiapine** is predicted to decrease the effects of **histamine**. Avoid. Severe Theoretical → Also see **TABLE 8** p. 819
▸ **Risperidone** is predicted to decrease the effects of **histamine**. Avoid. Severe Theoretical → Also see **TABLE 8** p. 819
▸ **Tricyclic antidepressants** are predicted to decrease the effects of **histamine**. Avoid. Severe Theoretical → Also see **TABLE 8** p. 819
▸ **Zuclopenthixol** is predicted to decrease the effects of **histamine**. Avoid. Severe Theoretical → Also see **TABLE 8** p. 819

HIV-protease inhibitors → see **TABLE 9** p. 820 (QT-interval prolongation)

atazanavir · darunavir · fosamprenavir · indinavir · lopinavir · ritonavir · saquinavir · tipranavir

▸ Caution on concurrent use of **atazanavir, lopinavir** with **ritonavir**, or **ritonavir** with drugs that prolong the PR interval.
▸ Concurrent use of **saquinavir** with drugs that prolong the PR interval is contra-indicated.
▸ Caution with concurrent use of **tipranavir** with drugs that increase risk of bleeding.

▸ **Tipranavir** slightly decreases the exposure to **abacavir**. Avoid. Severe Study
▸ **HIV-protease inhibitors (atazanavir, darunavir, fosamprenavir, lopinavir, ritonavir, saquinavir, tipranavir)** are predicted to increase the exposure to **abiraterone**. Severe Theoretical
▸ **HIV-protease inhibitors (lopinavir, ritonavir, saquinavir)** are predicted to increase the exposure to **afatinib**. Separate administration by 12 hours. Moderate Study
▸ **Ritonavir** is predicted to decrease the exposure to **agomelatine**. Moderate Theoretical
▸ **Ritonavir** decreases the exposure to **albendazole**. Moderate Study
▸ **Indinavir** is predicted to increase the exposure to **aldosterone antagonists (eplerenone)**. Adjust **eplerenone** dose. Severe Study
▸ **HIV-protease inhibitors (atazanavir, darunavir, fosamprenavir, lopinavir, ritonavir, saquinavir, tipranavir)** are predicted to markedly increase the exposure to aldosterone antagonists **(eplerenone)**. Avoid. Severe Study

▸ **HIV-protease inhibitors (ritonavir, saquinavir)** are predicted to increase the exposure to **aliskiren**. Moderate Theoretical
▸ **HIV-protease inhibitors (atazanavir, darunavir, fosamprenavir, lopinavir, ritonavir, saquinavir, tipranavir)** increase the exposure to **almotriptan**. Mild Study
▸ **HIV-protease inhibitors (atazanavir, darunavir, fosamprenavir, lopinavir, ritonavir, saquinavir, tipranavir)** are predicted to moderately increase the exposure to alpha blockers **(alfuzosin, tamsulosin)**. Use with caution or avoid. Moderate Study
▸ **HIV-protease inhibitors (atazanavir, darunavir, fosamprenavir, lopinavir, ritonavir, saquinavir, tipranavir)** are predicted to increase the exposure to alpha blockers **(doxazosin)**. Moderate Study
▸ **Indinavir** is predicted to increase the exposure to alpha blockers **(tamsulosin)**. Moderate Theoretical
▸ **HIV-protease inhibitors (atazanavir, darunavir, fosamprenavir, lopinavir, ritonavir, saquinavir, tipranavir)** moderately increase the exposure to **alprazolam**. Avoid. Moderate Study
▸ **Indinavir** is predicted to increase the exposure to **alprazolam**. Severe Study
▸ **HIV-protease inhibitors (ritonavir, tipranavir)** are predicted to increase the exposure to **antihistamines**. Severe Theoretical
▸ **Ritonavir** decreases the exposure to **aminophylline**. Adjust dose. Moderate Study
▸ **Antacids** are predicted to decrease the absorption of **atazanavir**. Atazanavir should be taken 2 hours before or 1 hour after **antacids**. Severe Theoretical
▸ **Antacids** are predicted to decrease the absorption of **tipranavir**. Separate administration by 2 hours. Moderate Study
▸ **HIV-protease inhibitors** are predicted to increase the exposure to antiarrhythmics **(amiodarone)**. Avoid. Severe Theoretical → Also see **TABLE 9** p. 820
▸ **HIV-protease inhibitors** are predicted to increase the exposure to antiarrhythmics **(disopyramide)**. Severe Theoretical → Also see **TABLE 9** p. 820
▸ **HIV-protease inhibitors (atazanavir, darunavir, fosamprenavir, lopinavir, ritonavir, saquinavir, tipranavir)** very markedly increase the exposure to antiarrhythmics **(dronedarone)**. Avoid. Severe Study → Also see **TABLE 9** p. 820
▸ **Ritonavir** is predicted to increase the exposure to antiarrhythmics **(flecainide)**. Severe Theoretical
▸ **HIV-protease inhibitors** are predicted to increase the exposure to antiarrhythmics **(lidocaine)**. Avoid. Severe Study
▸ **Indinavir** is predicted to increase the exposure to antiarrhythmics **(propafenone)**. Monitor and adjust dose. Moderate Study
▸ **HIV-protease inhibitors (atazanavir, darunavir, fosamprenavir, lopinavir, ritonavir, saquinavir, tipranavir)** are predicted to increase the exposure to antiarrhythmics **(propafenone)**. Monitor and adjust dose. Severe Study
▸ **HIV-protease inhibitors (atazanavir, darunavir, fosamprenavir, lopinavir, ritonavir, saquinavir, tipranavir)** are predicted to increase the exposure to anticholinesterases, centrally acting **(galantamine)**. Monitor and adjust dose. Moderate Study
▸ **HIV-protease inhibitors** are predicted to increase the exposure to antiepileptics **(carbamazepine)** and antiepileptics **(carbamazepine)** are predicted to decrease the exposure to **HIV-protease inhibitors**. Monitor and adjust dose. Severe Theoretical
▸ **HIV-protease inhibitors** are predicted to affect the exposure to antiepileptics **(fosphenytoin, phenytoin)** and antiepileptics **(fosphenytoin, phenytoin)** decrease the concentration of **HIV-protease inhibitors**. Severe Theoretical
▸ **Ritonavir** slightly decreases the exposure to antiepileptics **(lamotrigine)**. Severe Study
▸ **HIV-protease inhibitors (atazanavir, darunavir, fosamprenavir, lopinavir, ritonavir, saquinavir, tipranavir)** are predicted to slightly increase the exposure to antiepileptics **(perampanel)**. Mild Study
▸ **HIV-protease inhibitors** are predicted to affect the concentration of antiepileptics **(phenobarbital, primidone)** and antiepileptics **(phenobarbital, primidone)** are predicted to decrease the concentration of **HIV-protease inhibitors**. Severe Theoretical

▸ **Ritonavir** is predicted to decrease the concentration of antiepileptics (**valproate**). Severe Anecdotal

▸ Antifungals, azoles (**fluconazole**) slightly increase the exposure to **tipranavir**. Avoid or adjust dose. Moderate Study

▸ Antifungals, azoles (**miconazole**) are predicted to increase the concentration of **HIV-protease inhibitors**. Use with caution and adjust dose. Moderate Theoretical

▸ Antifungals, azoles (**posaconazole**) are predicted to increase the exposure to **HIV-protease inhibitors**. Moderate Study

▸ **HIV-protease inhibitors** (**atazanavir, darunavir, fosamprenavir, lopinavir, ritonavir, saquinavir, tipranavir**) are predicted to increase the exposure to antifungals, azoles (**isavuconazole**). Avoid or monitor side effects. Severe Study

▸ **HIV-protease inhibitors** are predicted to increase the exposure to antifungals, azoles (**itraconazole**). Use with caution and adjust dose. Severe Study

▸ **HIV-protease inhibitors** are predicted to increase the exposure to antifungals, azoles (**ketoconazole**). Use with caution and adjust dose. Moderate Study

▸ **HIV-protease inhibitors** are predicted to affect the exposure to antifungals, azoles (**voriconazole**) and antifungals, azoles (**voriconazole**) potentially affect the exposure to **HIV-protease inhibitors**. Severe Study → Also see TABLE 9 p. 820

▸ **Indinavir** is predicted to increase the exposure to antihistamines, non-sedating (**mizolastine**). Severe Theoretical

▸ **HIV-protease inhibitors** (**atazanavir, darunavir, fosamprenavir, lopinavir, ritonavir, saquinavir, tipranavir**) are predicted to increase the exposure to antihistamines, non-sedating (**mizolastine**). Avoid. Severe Study

▸ **HIV-protease inhibitors** (**atazanavir, darunavir, fosamprenavir, lopinavir, ritonavir, saquinavir, tipranavir**) are predicted to increase the exposure to antimalarials (**artemether**) with lumafantrine. Moderate Study → Also see TABLE 9 p. 820

▸ **HIV-protease inhibitors** decrease the exposure to antimalarials (**atovaquone**). Avoid if boosted with ritonavir. Moderate Study

▸ **HIV-protease inhibitors** are predicted to increase the concentration of antimalarials (**piperaquine**). Severe Theoretical

▸ **HIV-protease inhibitors** are predicted to decrease the exposure to antimalarials (**proguanil**). Avoid. Moderate Study

▸ **HIV-protease inhibitors** are predicted to affect the exposure to antimalarials (**quinine**). Severe Study → Also see TABLE 9 p. 820

▸ **Ritonavir** is predicted to increase the exposure to apixaban. Avoid. Severe Theoretical

▸ **HIV-protease inhibitors** (**atazanavir, darunavir, fosamprenavir, lopinavir, ritonavir, saquinavir, tipranavir**) are predicted to markedly increase the exposure to aprepitant. Moderate Study

▸ **HIV-protease inhibitors** (**atazanavir, darunavir, fosamprenavir, lopinavir, ritonavir, saquinavir, tipranavir**) are predicted to slightly increase the exposure to aripiprazole. Adjust **aripiprazole** dose, p. 240. Moderate Study

▸ **HIV-protease inhibitors** (**atazanavir, darunavir, fosamprenavir, lopinavir, ritonavir, saquinavir, tipranavir**) are predicted to increase the exposure to axitinib. Avoid or adjust dose. Moderate Study

▸ **Indinavir** is predicted to increase the exposure to axitinib. Moderate Theoretical

▸ **HIV-protease inhibitors** (**atazanavir, darunavir, fosamprenavir, lopinavir, ritonavir, saquinavir, tipranavir**) are predicted to increase the exposure to bedaquiline. Avoid prolonged use. Mild Study → Also see TABLE 9 p. 820

▸ **Indinavir** is predicted to increase the exposure to bedaquiline. Avoid prolonged use. Mild Theoretical

▸ **Ritonavir** is predicted to increase the exposure to beta blockers, non-selective (**carvedilol**). Moderate Theoretical

▸ **HIV-protease inhibitors** (**lopinavir, ritonavir, saquinavir**) are predicted to increase the exposure to beta blockers, non-selective (**nadolol**). Moderate Study

▸ **Ritonavir** (high-dose) is predicted to increase the exposure to beta blockers, non-selective (**timolol**). Moderate Theoretical

▸ **Ritonavir** is predicted to increase the exposure to beta blockers, selective (**metoprolol, nebivolol**). Moderate Study

▸ **HIV-protease inhibitors** (**atazanavir, darunavir, fosamprenavir, lopinavir, ritonavir, saquinavir, tipranavir**) are predicted to increase the exposure to beta₂ agonists (**salmeterol**). Avoid. Severe Study

▸ HIV-protease inhibitors (**atazanavir, darunavir, fosamprenavir, lopinavir, ritonavir, saquinavir, tipranavir**) slightly increase the exposure to bortezomib. Moderate Study

▸ **HIV-protease inhibitors** are predicted to increase the exposure to bosentan. Severe Study

▸ HIV-protease inhibitors (**atazanavir, darunavir, fosamprenavir, lopinavir, ritonavir, saquinavir, tipranavir**) are predicted to markedly increase the exposure to bosutinib. Avoid or adjust **bosutinib** dose. Severe Study → Also see TABLE 9 p. 820

▸ **Indinavir** is predicted to increase the exposure to bosutinib. Avoid or adjust **bosutinib** dose. Severe Theoretical

▸ **Ritonavir** slightly to moderately decreases the exposure to **bupropion**. Moderate Study

▸ HIV-protease inhibitors (**atazanavir, darunavir, fosamprenavir, lopinavir, ritonavir, saquinavir, tipranavir**) are predicted to increase the exposure to buspirone. Adjust **buspirone** dose. Severe Study

▸ **Indinavir** is predicted to increase the exposure to buspirone. Use with caution and adjust dose. Moderate Study

▸ HIV-protease inhibitors (**atazanavir, darunavir, fosamprenavir, lopinavir, ritonavir, saquinavir, tipranavir**) slightly increase the exposure to cabozantinib. Moderate Study → Also see TABLE 9 p. 820

▸ **Indinavir** is predicted to increase the exposure to cabozantinib. Moderate Theoretical

▸ **Ritonavir** is predicted to moderately increase the clearance of caffeine citrate. Monitor and adjust dose. Moderate Study

▸ **HIV-protease inhibitors** are predicted to increase the exposure to calcium channel blockers (**amlodipine, felodipine, isradipine, lacidipine, nicardipine, nifedipine, nimodipine**). Monitor and adjust dose. Moderate Study

▸ HIV-protease inhibitors (**atazanavir, darunavir, fosamprenavir, lopinavir, ritonavir, saquinavir, tipranavir**) are predicted to increase the exposure to calcium channel blockers (**diltiazem, verapamil**). Severe Study

▸ HIV-protease inhibitors (**atazanavir, darunavir, fosamprenavir, lopinavir, ritonavir, saquinavir, tipranavir**) are predicted to markedly increase the exposure to calcium channel blockers (**lercanidipine**). Avoid. Severe Study

▸ HIV-protease inhibitors (**atazanavir, darunavir, fosamprenavir, lopinavir, ritonavir, saquinavir, tipranavir**) are predicted to increase the exposure to cannabis extract. Use with caution and adjust dose. Moderate Theoretical

▸ HIV-protease inhibitors (**atazanavir, darunavir, fosamprenavir, lopinavir, ritonavir, saquinavir, tipranavir**) are predicted to increase the exposure to ceritinib. Avoid or adjust **ceritinib** dose. Severe Study → Also see TABLE 9 p. 820

▸ **Indinavir** is predicted to increase the exposure to ceritinib. Moderate Theoretical

▸ **HIV-protease inhibitors** increase the concentration of ciclosporin. Severe Study

▸ HIV-protease inhibitors (**atazanavir, darunavir, fosamprenavir, lopinavir, ritonavir, saquinavir, tipranavir**) are predicted to moderately increase the exposure to cilostazol. Adjust **cilostazol** dose. Moderate Study

▸ HIV-protease inhibitors (**atazanavir, darunavir, fosamprenavir, lopinavir, ritonavir, saquinavir, tipranavir**) are predicted to moderately increase the exposure to cinacalcet. Adjust dose. Moderate Study

▸ **Ritonavir** is predicted to increase the exposure to clozapine. Avoid. Severe Theoretical

▸ HIV-protease inhibitors (**atazanavir, darunavir, fosamprenavir, lopinavir, ritonavir, saquinavir, tipranavir**) are predicted to markedly increase the exposure to cobimetinib. Avoid or monitor for toxicity. Severe Study

▸ **Indinavir** is predicted to increase the exposure to cobimetinib. Severe Theoretical

▸ HIV-protease inhibitors (**atazanavir, darunavir, fosamprenavir, lopinavir, ritonavir, saquinavir, tipranavir**) are predicted to increase the exposure to colchicine. Avoid or adjust **colchicine** dose. Severe Study

▸ **Indinavir** is predicted to increase the exposure to colchicine. Adjust **colchicine** dose. Severe Study

▸ **Atazanavir** (unboosted) increases the exposure to combined hormonal contraceptives. Adjust dose. Severe Study

Interactions | Appendix 1

A1

HIV-protease inhibitors (continued)

▸ **Ritonavir** is predicted to decrease the efficacy of **combined hormonal contraceptives.** For FSRH guidance, see Contraceptives, interactions p. 474. Severe Study

▸ **Ritonavir** is predicted to increase the concentration of corticosteroids (**beclometasone**) (risk with beclometasone is likely to be lower than with other corticosteroids). MHRA advises avoid or monitor for **beclometasone** side effects. Moderate Theoretical

▸ **Ritonavir** is predicted to increase the concentration of corticosteroids (**betamethasone, budesonide, dexamethasone, deflazacort, hydrocortisone, methylprednisolone, prednisolone, prednisone, triamcinolone**). MHRA advises avoid or monitor side effects and consider beclomethasone as an alternative. Severe Theoretical

▸ **HIV-protease inhibitors (atazanavir, darunavir, fosamprenavir, lopinavir, saquinavir, tipranavir)** are predicted to increase the exposure to corticosteroids (**budesonide**). Avoid. Severe Study

▸ **HIV-protease inhibitors (atazanavir, darunavir, fosamprenavir, lopinavir, ritonavir, saquinavir, tipranavir)** are predicted to increase the exposure to corticosteroids (**ciclesonide**). Avoid. Moderate Theoretical

▸ **HIV-protease inhibitors (atazanavir, darunavir, fosamprenavir, lopinavir, saquinavir, tipranavir)** are predicted to increase the exposure to corticosteroids (**dexamethasone, methylprednisolone**). Monitor and adjust dose. Moderate Study

▸ **HIV-protease inhibitors (atazanavir, darunavir, fosamprenavir, lopinavir, ritonavir, saquinavir, tipranavir)** are predicted to increase the exposure to inhaled corticosteroids (**fluticasone**). Severe Study

▸ **Indinavir** is predicted to increase the exposure to corticosteroids (**methylprednisolone**). Monitor and adjust dose. Moderate Study

▸ **HIV-protease inhibitors (atazanavir, darunavir, fosamprenavir, lopinavir, ritonavir, saquinavir, tipranavir)** are predicted to increase the exposure to corticosteroids (**mometasone**). Moderate Theoretical

▸ **HIV-protease inhibitors (atazanavir, darunavir, fosamprenavir, lopinavir, saquinavir, tipranavir)** are predicted to increase the risk of side-effects when given with corticosteroids (**triamcinolone**). Severe Theoretical

▸ **HIV-protease inhibitors** are predicted to affect the anticoagulant effect of **coumarins.** Moderate Study

▸ **HIV-protease inhibitors (atazanavir, darunavir, fosamprenavir, lopinavir, ritonavir, saquinavir, tipranavir)** are predicted to moderately increase the exposure to **crizotinib.** Avoid. Moderate Study → Also see **TABLE 9** p. 820

▸ **Indinavir** is predicted to increase the exposure to **crizotinib.** Moderate Theoretical

▸ **HIV-protease inhibitors (lopinavir, ritonavir, saquinavir)** are predicted to increase the exposure to **dabigatran.** Avoid. Severe Theoretical

▸ **HIV-protease inhibitors (atazanavir, darunavir, fosamprenavir, lopinavir, ritonavir, saquinavir, tipranavir)** are predicted to increase the exposure to **dabrafenib.** Use with caution or avoid. Moderate Study

▸ **HIV-protease inhibitors (atazanavir, darunavir, fosamprenavir, lopinavir, ritonavir, saquinavir, tipranavir)** are predicted to moderately increase the exposure to **daclatasvir.** Adjust **daclatasvir** dose. Moderate Study

▸ **HIV-protease inhibitors (atazanavir, darunavir, fosamprenavir, lopinavir, ritonavir, saquinavir, tipranavir)** are predicted to markedly to very markedly increase the exposure to **darifenacin.** Avoid. Severe Study

▸ **Indinavir** is predicted to slightly increase the exposure to **darifenacin.** Moderate Study

▸ **HIV-protease inhibitors (atazanavir, darunavir, fosamprenavir, lopinavir, ritonavir, saquinavir, tipranavir)** are predicted to markedly increase the exposure to **dasatinib.** Avoid. Severe Study → Also see **TABLE 9** p. 820

▸ **Indinavir** is predicted to increase the exposure to **dasatinib.** Severe Study

▸ **HIV-protease inhibitors (atazanavir, darunavir, fosamprenavir, lopinavir, ritonavir, saquinavir, tipranavir)** very slightly increase

the exposure to **delamanid.** Severe Study → Also see **TABLE 9** p. 820

▸ **Ritonavir** is predicted to decrease the efficacy of **desogestrel.** For FSRH guidance, see Contraceptives, interactions p. 474. Severe Theoretical

▸ **Ritonavir** is predicted to increase the exposure to **diazepam.** Avoid. Moderate Theoretical

▸ **Didanosine** (buffered) decreases the exposure to **atazanavir. Didanosine** should be taken 2 hours after **atazanavir.** Severe Study

▸ **Didanosine** (buffered) is predicted to decrease the exposure to **darunavir** (boosted with ritonavir). **Didanosine** should be taken 1 hour before or 2 hours after **darunavir.** Moderate Theoretical

▸ **Didanosine** (buffered) decreases the exposure to **indinavir.** Separate administration by 1 hour. Severe Study

▸ **Tipranavir** decreases the exposure to didanosine. Separate administration by 2 hours. Moderate Study

▸ **Ritonavir** increases the concentration of digoxin. Adjust dose and monitor concentration. Severe Study

▸ **Fosamprenavir** (boosted with ritonavir) slightly decreases the exposure to **dolutegravir.** Avoid if resistant to HIV-integrase inhibitors. Severe Study

▸ **Tipranavir** moderately decreases the exposure to **dolutegravir.** Refer to specialist literature. Severe Study

▸ **HIV-protease inhibitors** increase the risk of QT-prolongation when given with **domperidone.** Avoid. Severe Study

▸ **Indinavir** is predicted to increase the exposure to dopamine receptor agonists (**bromocriptine, cabergoline**). Severe Theoretical

▸ **HIV-protease inhibitors (atazanavir, darunavir, fosamprenavir, lopinavir, ritonavir, saquinavir, tipranavir)** increase the exposure to dopamine receptor agonists (**bromocriptine, cabergoline**). Severe Study

▸ **HIV-protease inhibitors (atazanavir, darunavir, fosamprenavir, lopinavir, ritonavir, saquinavir, tipranavir)** are predicted to increase the exposure to **dutasteride.** Monitor side effects and adjust dose. Moderate Theoretical

▸ **Indinavir** is predicted to moderately increase the exposure to **dutasteride.** Mild Study

▸ **HIV-protease inhibitors (lopinavir, ritonavir, saquinavir)** are predicted to slightly increase the exposure to **edoxaban.** Severe Theoretical

▸ **Efavirenz** decreases the exposure to **HIV-protease inhibitors.** Refer to specialist literature. Severe Study

▸ **HIV-protease inhibitors (atazanavir, darunavir, fosamprenavir, lopinavir, ritonavir, saquinavir, tipranavir)** slightly to moderately increase the exposure to **elbasvir.** Avoid. Moderate Study

▸ **HIV-protease inhibitors (atazanavir, darunavir, fosamprenavir, lopinavir, ritonavir, saquinavir, tipranavir)** are predicted to markedly increase the exposure to **eletriptan.** Avoid. Severe Study

▸ **Atazanavir** increases the concentration of **elvitegravir.** Refer to specialist literature. Moderate Study

▸ **Lopinavir** increases the concentration of **elvitegravir.** Refer to specialist literature. Moderate Study

▸ **HIV-protease inhibitors (atazanavir, darunavir, fosamprenavir, lopinavir, ritonavir, saquinavir, tipranavir)** are predicted to increase the risk of ergotism when given with **ergometrine.** Avoid. Severe Theoretical

▸ **Indinavir** is predicted to increase the risk of ergotism when given with **ergometrine.** Severe Theoretical

▸ **HIV-protease inhibitors (atazanavir, darunavir, fosamprenavir, lopinavir, ritonavir, saquinavir, tipranavir)** are predicted to increase the risk of ergotism when given with **ergotamine.** Avoid. Severe Theoretical

▸ **Indinavir** is predicted to increase the risk of ergotism when given with **ergotamine.** Severe Theoretical

▸ **HIV-protease inhibitors (atazanavir, darunavir, fosamprenavir, lopinavir, ritonavir, saquinavir, tipranavir)** are predicted to slightly increase the exposure to **erlotinib.** Use with caution and adjust dose. Moderate Study

▸ **Indinavir** is predicted to increase the exposure to **erlotinib.** Moderate Theoretical

- Ritonavir is predicted to decrease the efficacy of etonogestrel. For FSRH guidance, see Contraceptives, interactions p. 474. Severe Theoretical
- Etravirine increases the exposure to fosamprenavir (boosted with ritonavir). Refer to specialist literature. Moderate Study
- Etravirine is predicted to decrease the exposure to indinavir. Avoid. Severe Theoretical
- Tipranavir decreases the exposure to etravirine. Avoid. Severe Study
- HIV-protease inhibitors (atazanavir, darunavir, fosamprenavir, lopinavir, ritonavir, saquinavir, tipranavir) are predicted to increase the concentration of everolimus. Avoid. Severe Study
- Indinavir is predicted to increase the concentration of everolimus. Avoid or adjust dose. Moderate Study
- HIV-protease inhibitors (atazanavir, darunavir, fosamprenavir, lopinavir, ritonavir, saquinavir, tipranavir) are predicted to moderately increase the exposure to fesoterodine. Adjust fesoterodine dose; avoid in hepatic and renal impairment. Severe Study
- Indinavir is predicted to increase the exposure to fesoterodine. Adjust fesoterodine dose in hepatic and renal impairment. Mild Study
- HIV-protease inhibitors (lopinavir, ritonavir, saquinavir) are predicted to increase the exposure to fidaxomicin. Avoid. Moderate Study
- Ritonavir is predicted to increase the exposure to flurazepam. Avoid. Moderate Theoretical
- HIV-protease inhibitors (atazanavir, darunavir, fosamprenavir, lopinavir, ritonavir, saquinavir, tipranavir) are predicted to increase the exposure to fosaprepitant. Moderate Theoretical
- HIV-protease inhibitors (atazanavir, darunavir, fosamprenavir, lopinavir, ritonavir, saquinavir, tipranavir) are predicted to increase the exposure to gefitinib. Moderate Study
- Indinavir is predicted to increase the exposure to gefitinib. Moderate Theoretical
- HIV-protease inhibitors (atazanavir, darunavir, fosamprenavir, lopinavir, ritonavir, saquinavir, tipranavir) are predicted to moderately to markedly increase the exposure to grazoprevir. Avoid. Severe Study
- HIV-protease inhibitors (atazanavir, darunavir, fosamprenavir, lopinavir, ritonavir, saquinavir, tipranavir) are predicted to increase the exposure to guanfacine. Adjust guanfacine dose, p. 222. Moderate Study
- Indinavir is predicted to increase the concentration of guanfacine. Adjust guanfacine dose, p. 222. Moderate Theoretical
- H$_2$ receptor antagonists decrease the exposure to atazanavir. Monitor and adjust dose. Moderate Study
- Ritonavir is predicted to increase the exposure to haloperidol. Severe Theoretical
- Ritonavir is predicted to decrease the effects of Hormone replacement therapy. Moderate Anecdotal
- HIV-protease inhibitors (atazanavir, darunavir, fosamprenavir, lopinavir, ritonavir, saquinavir, tipranavir) are predicted to very markedly increase the exposure to ibrutinib. Avoid or adjust ibrutinib dose. Severe Study
- Indinavir is predicted to increase the exposure to ibrutinib. Avoid or adjust ibrutinib dose. Severe Theoretical
- HIV-protease inhibitors (atazanavir, darunavir, fosamprenavir, lopinavir, ritonavir, saquinavir, tipranavir) are predicted to increase the exposure to imatinib. Moderate Study
- HIV-protease inhibitors (atazanavir, darunavir, fosamprenavir, lopinavir, ritonavir, saquinavir, tipranavir) are predicted to increase the risk of toxicity when given with irinotecan. Avoid. Moderate Study
- Ritonavir is predicted to decrease the exposure to iron chelators (deferasirox). Monitor serum ferritin and adjust dose. Moderate Theoretical
- HIV-protease inhibitors (atazanavir, darunavir, fosamprenavir, lopinavir, ritonavir, saquinavir, tipranavir) are predicted to increase the exposure to ivabradine. Avoid. Severe Study
- Indinavir increases the exposure to ivabradine. Adjust dose. Severe Theoretical
- HIV-protease inhibitors (atazanavir, darunavir, fosamprenavir, lopinavir, ritonavir, saquinavir, tipranavir) are predicted to

increase the exposure to ivacaftor. Adjust ivacaftor or lumacaftor with ivacaftor dose, p. 179. Severe Study
- Indinavir is predicted to increase the exposure to ivacaftor. Adjust ivacaftor dose, p. 179. Severe Study
- HIV-protease inhibitors (atazanavir, darunavir, fosamprenavir, lopinavir, ritonavir, saquinavir, tipranavir) are predicted to increase the exposure to lapatinib. Avoid. Moderate Study → Also see **TABLE 9** p. 820
- Indinavir is predicted to increase the exposure to lapatinib. Moderate Study
- Ritonavir is predicted to decrease the efficacy of levonorgestrel. For FSRH guidance, see Contraceptives, interactions p. 474. Severe Theoretical
- HIV-protease inhibitors (atazanavir, darunavir, fosamprenavir, lopinavir, ritonavir, saquinavir, tipranavir) are predicted to markedly increase the exposure to lomitapide. Avoid. Severe Study
- Indinavir is predicted to increase the exposure to lomitapide. Avoid. Moderate Theoretical
- HIV-protease inhibitors (atazanavir, darunavir, fosamprenavir, lopinavir, ritonavir, saquinavir, tipranavir) are predicted to increase the exposure to lurasidone. Avoid. Severe Study
- Indinavir is predicted to increase the exposure to lurasidone. Moderate Study
- HIV-protease inhibitors (atazanavir, darunavir, fosamprenavir, lopinavir, ritonavir, saquinavir, tipranavir) are predicted to increase the exposure to macitentan. Moderate Study
- Macrolides (clarithromycin) increase the exposure to saquinavir and saquinavir increases the exposure to macrolides (clarithromycin). Avoid. Severe Study → Also see **TABLE 9** p. 820
- Macrolides (erythromycin) are predicted to increase the exposure to saquinavir. Avoid. Severe Theoretical
- HIV-protease inhibitors (atazanavir, darunavir, fosamprenavir, indinavir, lopinavir, ritonavir) are predicted to increase the exposure to macrolides (clarithromycin). Monitor renal function and adjust dose. Severe Study
- HIV-protease inhibitors (atazanavir, darunavir, fosamprenavir, indinavir, lopinavir, ritonavir, tipranavir) are predicted to increase the exposure to macrolides (erythromycin). Severe Theoretical
- Maraviroc potentially decreases the exposure to fosamprenavir and fosamprenavir potentially decreases the exposure to maraviroc. Avoid. Severe Study
- HIV-protease inhibitors (atazanavir, darunavir, lopinavir, ritonavir, saquinavir) increase the exposure to maraviroc. Refer to specialist literature. Severe Study
- HIV-protease inhibitors (atazanavir, darunavir, fosamprenavir, lopinavir, ritonavir, saquinavir, tipranavir) are predicted to markedly to very markedly increase the exposure to midazolam. Avoid or adjust midazolam dose. Severe Study
- Indinavir is predicted to increase the exposure to midazolam. Monitor side effects and adjust dose. Severe Study
- HIV-protease inhibitors (atazanavir, darunavir, fosamprenavir, lopinavir, ritonavir, saquinavir, tipranavir) are predicted to increase the exposure to mirabegron. Adjust mirabegron dose in hepatic and renal impairment. Moderate Study
- HIV-protease inhibitors (atazanavir, darunavir, fosamprenavir, lopinavir, ritonavir, saquinavir, tipranavir) are predicted to increase the exposure to mirtazapine. Moderate Study
- HIV-protease inhibitors (atazanavir, darunavir, fosamprenavir, lopinavir, ritonavir, saquinavir, tipranavir) are predicted to increase the exposure to modafinil. Mild Theoretical
- HIV-protease inhibitors (lopinavir, ritonavir, saquinavir) are predicted to increase the risk of neutropenia when given with monoclonal antibodies (brentuximab vedotin). Monitor and adjust dose. Severe Study
- HIV-protease inhibitors (atazanavir, darunavir, fosamprenavir, lopinavir, ritonavir, saquinavir, tipranavir) are predicted to increase the exposure to monoclonal antibodies (trastuzumab emtansine). Avoid. Severe Theoretical
- HIV-protease inhibitors (atazanavir, darunavir, fosamprenavir, lopinavir, ritonavir, saquinavir, tipranavir) are predicted to markedly increase the exposure to naloxegol. Avoid. Severe Study

HIV-protease inhibitors (continued)

▸ **Indinavir** is predicted to increase the exposure to **naloxegol**. Adjust **naloxegol** dose and monitor side effects. Moderate Study

▸ HIV-protease inhibitors **(atazanavir, darunavir, fosamprenavir, lopinavir, ritonavir, saquinavir, tipranavir)** are predicted to increase the exposure to **netupitant**. Mild Study

▸ **Nevirapine** decreases the exposure to **HIV-protease inhibitors**. Refer to specialist literature. Moderate Study

▸ HIV-protease inhibitors **(atazanavir, darunavir, fosamprenavir, lopinavir, ritonavir, saquinavir, tipranavir)** are predicted to moderately increase the exposure to **nilotinib**. Avoid. Severe Study → Also see TABLE 9 p. 820

▸ HIV-protease inhibitors **(lopinavir, ritonavir, saquinavir)** are predicted to increase the exposure to **nintedanib**. Moderate Study

▸ HIV-protease inhibitors **(atazanavir, darunavir, fosamprenavir, lopinavir, ritonavir, saquinavir, tipranavir)** are predicted to increase the exposure to **nitisinone**. Adjust **nitisinone** dose. Moderate Theoretical

▸ **Ritonavir** is predicted to decrease the efficacy of **norethisterone**. For FSRH guidance, see Contraceptives, interactions p. 474. Anecdotal

▸ **Ritonavir** moderately decreases the exposure to **olanzapine**. Moderate Study

▸ HIV-protease inhibitors **(atazanavir, darunavir, fosamprenavir, lopinavir, ritonavir, saquinavir, tipranavir)** are predicted to increase the exposure to **olaparib**. Avoid or adjust **olaparib** dose. Moderate Study

▸ **Indinavir** is predicted to increase the exposure to **olaparib**. Avoid or adjust **olaparib** dose. Moderate Theoretical

▸ **Indinavir** is predicted to increase the exposure to opioids **(alfentanil, buprenorphine, fentanyl, oxycodone)**. Monitor and adjust dose. Moderate Study

▸ HIV-protease inhibitors **(atazanavir, darunavir, fosamprenavir, lopinavir, ritonavir, saquinavir, tipranavir)** are predicted to increase the exposure to opioids **(alfentanil, buprenorphine, fentanyl, oxycodone, sufentanil)**. Monitor and adjust dose. Severe Study

▸ HIV-protease inhibitors **(atazanavir, darunavir, fosamprenavir, lopinavir, ritonavir, saquinavir, tipranavir)** are predicted to increase the exposure to opioids **(methadone)**. Moderate Theoretical → Also see TABLE 9 p. 820

▸ **Indinavir** is predicted to increase the exposure to opioids **(methadone, sufentanil)**. Moderate Theoretical

▸ **Ritonavir** is predicted to decrease the concentration of opioids **(morphine)**. Moderate Theoretical

▸ **Ritonavir** increases the risk of CNS toxicity when given with opioids **(pethidine)**. Avoid. Severe Study

▸ **Ritonavir** is predicted to decrease the efficacy of opioids **(tramadol)**. Moderate Study

▸ HIV-protease inhibitors **(atazanavir, darunavir, fosamprenavir, lopinavir, ritonavir, saquinavir, tipranavir)** are predicted to increase the exposure to **oxybutynin**. Mild Study

▸ **Indinavir** is predicted to increase the exposure to **oxybutynin**. Mild Theoretical

▸ HIV-protease inhibitors **(atazanavir, darunavir, fosamprenavir, lopinavir, ritonavir, saquinavir, tipranavir)** are predicted to increase the exposure to **palbociclib**. Avoid or adjust **palbociclib** dose. Severe Study

▸ HIV-protease inhibitors **(atazanavir, darunavir, fosamprenavir, lopinavir, ritonavir, saquinavir, tipranavir)** are predicted to increase the exposure to **panobinostat**. Adjust **panobinostat** dose; in hepatic impairment avoid. Moderate Study → Also see TABLE 9 p. 820

▸ HIV-protease inhibitors **(atazanavir, darunavir, fosamprenavir, lopinavir, ritonavir, saquinavir, tipranavir)** are predicted to increase the exposure to **paritaprevir** (with ritonavir and ombitasvir). Avoid. Severe Theoretical

▸ **Indinavir** potentially increases the exposure to **paritaprevir**. Avoid. Severe Theoretical

▸ HIV-protease inhibitors **(atazanavir, darunavir, fosamprenavir, lopinavir, ritonavir, saquinavir, tipranavir)** are predicted to increase the exposure to **pazopanib**. Avoid or adjust **pazopanib** dose. Moderate Study → Also see TABLE 9 p. 820

▸ **Indinavir** is predicted to increase the exposure to **pazopanib**. Moderate Theoretical

▸ **Indinavir** is predicted to increase the exposure to phosphodiesterase type-5 inhibitors **(avanafil)**. Adjust **avanafil** dose. Moderate Theoretical

▸ HIV-protease inhibitors **(atazanavir, darunavir, fosamprenavir, lopinavir, ritonavir, saquinavir, tipranavir)** are predicted to increase the exposure to phosphodiesterase type-5 inhibitors **(avanafil, vardenafil)**. Avoid. Severe Study → Also see TABLE 9 p. 820

▸ **Indinavir** is predicted to increase the exposure to phosphodiesterase type-5 inhibitors **(sildenafil)**. Monitor and adjust **sildenafil** dose, p. 117. Moderate Study

▸ HIV-protease inhibitors **(atazanavir, darunavir, fosamprenavir, lopinavir, ritonavir, saquinavir, tipranavir)** are predicted to increase the exposure to phosphodiesterase type-5 inhibitors **(sildenafil)**. Avoid or adjust **sildenafil** dose, p. 117. Severe Study → Also see TABLE 9 p. 820

▸ **Indinavir** is predicted to increase the exposure to phosphodiesterase type-5 inhibitors **(tadalafil)**. Severe Theoretical

▸ HIV-protease inhibitors **(atazanavir, darunavir, fosamprenavir, lopinavir, ritonavir, saquinavir, tipranavir)** are predicted to increase the exposure to phosphodiesterase type-5 inhibitors **(tadalafil)**. Use with caution or avoid. Severe Study

▸ **Indinavir** is predicted to increase the exposure to phosphodiesterase type-5 inhibitors **(vardenafil)**. Adjust dose. Severe Theoretical

▸ HIV-protease inhibitors **(atazanavir, darunavir, fosamprenavir, lopinavir, ritonavir, saquinavir, tipranavir)** are predicted to increase the exposure to **pimozide**. Avoid. Severe Study → Also see TABLE 9 p. 820

▸ **Indinavir** is predicted to increase the exposure to **pimozide**. Avoid. Severe Theoretical

▸ **Ritonavir** is predicted to decrease the exposure to **pirfenidone**. Avoid. Moderate Theoretical

▸ **Ritonavir** is predicted to increase the exposure to **pitolisant**. Use with caution and adjust dose. Moderate Study

▸ HIV-protease inhibitors **(atazanavir, darunavir, fosamprenavir, lopinavir, ritonavir, saquinavir, tipranavir)** are predicted to slightly increase the exposure to **ponatinib**. Monitor and adjust **ponatinib** dose. Moderate Study

▸ HIV-protease inhibitors **(atazanavir, darunavir, fosamprenavir, lopinavir, ritonavir, saquinavir, tipranavir)** are predicted to moderately increase the exposure to **praziquantel**. Mild Study

▸ **Proton pump inhibitors** decrease the exposure to **atazanavir**. Avoid or adjust dose. Severe Study

▸ **Proton pump inhibitors** increase the exposure to **saquinavir**. Avoid. Severe Study

▸ **Proton pump inhibitors** decrease the exposure to **tipranavir**. Avoid. Severe Study

▸ HIV-protease inhibitors **(atazanavir, darunavir, fosamprenavir, lopinavir, ritonavir, saquinavir, tipranavir)** are predicted to increase the exposure to **quetiapine**. Avoid. Severe Study

▸ **Indinavir** is predicted to increase the exposure to **quetiapine**. Avoid. Moderate Study

▸ **Darunavir** increases the risk of rash when given with **raltegravir**. Moderate Study

▸ **Fosamprenavir** (boosted with ritonavir) decreases the exposure to **raltegravir** and **raltegravir** decreases the exposure to **fosamprenavir** (boosted with ritonavir). Avoid. Severe Study

▸ HIV-protease inhibitors **(atazanavir, darunavir, fosamprenavir, lopinavir, ritonavir, saquinavir, tipranavir)** are predicted to increase the exposure to **ranolazine**. Avoid. Severe Study → Also see TABLE 9 p. 820

▸ **Indinavir** is predicted to increase the exposure to **ranolazine**. Severe Study

▸ HIV-protease inhibitors **(atazanavir, darunavir, fosamprenavir, lopinavir, ritonavir, saquinavir, tipranavir)** are predicted to increase the exposure to **reboxetine**. Avoid. Moderate Study

▸ HIV-protease inhibitors **(atazanavir, darunavir, fosamprenavir, lopinavir, ritonavir, saquinavir, tipranavir)** are predicted to increase the exposure to **regorafenib**. Avoid. Moderate Study

▸ HIV-protease inhibitors **(atazanavir, darunavir, fosamprenavir, lopinavir, ritonavir, saquinavir, tipranavir)** are predicted to increase the exposure to **repaglinide**. Moderate Study

- HIV-protease inhibitors (atazanavir, darunavir, fosamprenavir, lopinavir, ritonavir, saquinavir, tipranavir) are predicted to increase the exposure to retinoids (alitretinoin). Adjust alitretinoin dose. Moderate Theoretical
- HIV-protease inhibitors (atazanavir, darunavir, fosamprenavir, lopinavir, saquinavir, tipranavir) increase the exposure to rifabutin. Monitor and adjust dose. Severe Study
- Indinavir increases the exposure to rifabutin and rifabutin decreases the exposure to indinavir. Avoid. Severe Study
- Ritonavir markedly increases the exposure to rifabutin. Avoid or adjust dose. Severe Study
- Rifampicin is predicted to moderately to markedly decrease the exposure to HIV-protease inhibitors (atazanavir, darunavir, fosamprenavir, indinavir, lopinavir, saquinavir, tipranavir). Avoid. Severe Study
- Rifampicin slightly decreases the exposure to ritonavir. Severe Study
- Ritonavir is predicted to increase the exposure to riociguat. Avoid. Moderate Theoretical
- HIV-protease inhibitors (atazanavir, darunavir, fosamprenavir, lopinavir, ritonavir, saquinavir, tipranavir) are predicted to increase the exposure to risperidone. Adjust dose. Moderate Study → Also see TABLE 9 p. 820
- Ritonavir moderately increases the exposure to rivaroxaban. Avoid. Severe Study
- HIV-protease inhibitors (atazanavir, darunavir, fosamprenavir, lopinavir, ritonavir, saquinavir, tipranavir) are predicted to increase the exposure to ruxolitinib. Adjust dose and monitor side effects. Moderate Study
- Indinavir is predicted to increase the exposure to ruxolitinib. Moderate Theoretical
- HIV-protease inhibitors (atazanavir, darunavir, fosamprenavir, lopinavir, ritonavir, saquinavir, tipranavir) are predicted to increase the exposure to saxagliptin. Moderate Study
- Indinavir is predicted to increase the exposure to saxagliptin. Mild Study
- HIV-protease inhibitors are predicted to increase the exposure to simeprevir. Avoid. Severe Study
- HIV-protease inhibitors (atazanavir, darunavir, fosamprenavir, lopinavir, ritonavir, saquinavir, tipranavir) are predicted to increase the concentration of sirolimus. Avoid. Severe Study
- Indinavir increases the concentration of sirolimus. Monitor and adjust dose. Moderate Study
- Tipranavir is predicted to decrease the exposure to sofosbuvir. Avoid. Severe Theoretical
- HIV-protease inhibitors (atazanavir, darunavir, fosamprenavir, lopinavir, ritonavir, saquinavir, tipranavir) are predicted to increase the exposure to solifenacin. Adjust solifenacin or tamsulosin with solifenacin dose; avoid in hepatic and renal impairment. Severe Study
- Indinavir is predicted to increase the exposure to SSRIs (dapoxetine). Adjust dapoxetine dose. Moderate Theoretical
- HIV-protease inhibitors (atazanavir, darunavir, fosamprenavir, lopinavir, ritonavir, saquinavir, tipranavir) are predicted to moderately increase the exposure to SSRIs (dapoxetine). Avoid, or adjust dapoxetine dose. Severe Study
- St John's Wort is predicted to decrease the exposure to HIV-protease inhibitors. Avoid. Severe Study
- Indinavir is predicted to increase the exposure to statins (atorvastatin). Monitor and adjust dose. Severe Theoretical
- HIV-protease inhibitors (atazanavir, darunavir, fosamprenavir, lopinavir, ritonavir, saquinavir, tipranavir) are predicted to increase the exposure to statins (atorvastatin). Avoid or adjust dose and monitor rhabdomyolysis. Severe Study
- HIV-protease inhibitors slightly to moderately increase the exposure to statins (rosuvastatin). Avoid or adjust dose. Severe Study
- Indinavir is predicted to increase the exposure to statins (simvastatin). Use with caution and adjust simvastatin dose, p. 130. Severe Study
- HIV-protease inhibitors (atazanavir, darunavir, fosamprenavir, lopinavir, ritonavir, saquinavir, tipranavir) are predicted to increase the exposure to statins (simvastatin). Avoid. Severe Study

- HIV-protease inhibitors (atazanavir, darunavir, fosamprenavir, lopinavir, ritonavir, saquinavir, tipranavir) are predicted to slightly increase the exposure to sunitinib. Avoid or adjust sunitinib dose. Moderate Study → Also see TABLE 9 p. 820
- Indinavir is predicted to increase the exposure to sunitinib. Moderate Theoretical
- HIV-protease inhibitors (atazanavir, darunavir, fosamprenavir, lopinavir, ritonavir, saquinavir, tipranavir) are predicted to increase the concentration of tacrolimus. Monitor and adjust dose. Severe Study
- Indinavir is predicted to increase the concentration of tacrolimus. Severe Study
- Indinavir is predicted to increase the exposure to taxanes (cabazitaxel). Moderate Theoretical
- HIV-protease inhibitors (atazanavir, darunavir, fosamprenavir, lopinavir, ritonavir, saquinavir, tipranavir) are predicted to increase the exposure to taxanes (cabazitaxel). Avoid. Severe Study
- HIV-protease inhibitors (atazanavir, darunavir, fosamprenavir, lopinavir, ritonavir, saquinavir, tipranavir) are predicted to moderately increase the exposure to taxanes (docetaxel). Avoid or adjust dose. Severe Study
- HIV-protease inhibitors (atazanavir, darunavir, fosamprenavir, lopinavir, ritonavir, saquinavir, tipranavir) are predicted to increase the exposure to taxanes (paclitaxel). Severe Theoretical
- HIV-protease inhibitors (atazanavir, darunavir, fosamprenavir, lopinavir, ritonavir, saquinavir, tipranavir) are predicted to increase the concentration of temsirolimus. Avoid. Severe Theoretical
- Indinavir is predicted to increase the concentration of temsirolimus. Moderate Theoretical
- Ritonavir is predicted to decrease the exposure to theophylline. Adjust dose. Moderate Study
- HIV-protease inhibitors (atazanavir, darunavir, fosamprenavir, lopinavir, ritonavir, saquinavir, tipranavir) are predicted to markedly increase the exposure to ticagrelor. Avoid. Severe Study
- Ritonavir moderately decreases the exposure to tizanidine. Mild Study
- HIV-protease inhibitors (atazanavir, darunavir, fosamprenavir, lopinavir, ritonavir, saquinavir, tipranavir) are predicted to increase the exposure to tolterodine. Avoid. Severe Study → Also see TABLE 9 p. 820
- Indinavir is predicted to increase the exposure to tolterodine. Mild Theoretical
- HIV-protease inhibitors (atazanavir, darunavir, fosamprenavir, lopinavir, ritonavir, saquinavir, tipranavir) are predicted to increase the exposure to tolvaptan. Adjust dose. Severe Study
- Indinavir is predicted to increase the exposure to tolvaptan. Adjust dose. Moderate Theoretical
- HIV-protease inhibitors (lopinavir, ritonavir, saquinavir) are predicted to increase the exposure to topotecan. Severe Study
- HIV-protease inhibitors (atazanavir, darunavir, fosamprenavir, lopinavir, ritonavir, saquinavir, tipranavir) are predicted to increase the exposure to toremifene. Moderate Theoretical → Also see TABLE 9 p. 820
- HIV-protease inhibitors (atazanavir, darunavir, fosamprenavir, lopinavir, ritonavir, saquinavir, tipranavir) are predicted to increase the exposure to trabectedin. Avoid or adjust dose. Severe Theoretical
- HIV-protease inhibitors (lopinavir, ritonavir, saquinavir) are predicted to increase the concentration of trametinib. Moderate Theoretical
- HIV-protease inhibitors (atazanavir, darunavir, fosamprenavir, lopinavir, ritonavir, saquinavir, tipranavir) are predicted to moderately increase the exposure to trazodone. Avoid or adjust dose. Moderate Study
- Indinavir is predicted to increase the exposure to trazodone. Moderate Theoretical
- HIV-protease inhibitors (ritonavir, tipranavir) are predicted to increase the exposure to tricyclic antidepressants. Moderate Theoretical
- HIV-protease inhibitors (atazanavir, darunavir, fosamprenavir, lopinavir, saquinavir, tipranavir) are predicted to increase the

HIV-protease inhibitors (continued)
exposure to **uliprital**. Avoid if used for uterine fibroids. [Severe] Study

▸ **Indinavir** is predicted to increase the exposure to **uliprital**. Avoid if used for uterine fibroids. [Moderate] Study

▸ **Ritonavir** decreases the efficacy of **uliprital**. For FSRH guidance, see Contraceptives, interactions p. 474. [Severe] Anecdotal

▸ **HIV-protease inhibitors (atazanavir, darunavir, fosamprenavir, lopinavir, ritonavir, saquinavir, tipranavir)** are predicted to increase the exposure to **vemurafenib**. [Severe] Theoretical → Also see TABLE 9 p. 820

▸ **HIV-protease inhibitors** are predicted to increase the exposure to **venetoclax**. Avoid or adjust **venetoclax** dose. [Severe] Study

▸ **HIV-protease inhibitors (atazanavir, darunavir, fosamprenavir, lopinavir, ritonavir, saquinavir, tipranavir)** are predicted to increase the exposure to **venlafaxine**. [Moderate] Study → Also see TABLE 9 p. 820

▸ **HIV-protease inhibitors** are predicted to increase the exposure to **vinca alkaloids**. [Severe] Theoretical → Also see TABLE 9 p. 820

▸ **HIV-protease inhibitors (atazanavir, darunavir, fosamprenavir, lopinavir, ritonavir, saquinavir, tipranavir)** are predicted to increase the exposure to vitamin D substances **(paricalcitol)**. [Moderate] Study

▸ **Tipranavir** slightly decreases the exposure to **zidovudine**. Avoid. [Moderate] Study

▸ **HIV-protease inhibitors (atazanavir, darunavir, fosamprenavir, lopinavir, ritonavir, saquinavir, tipranavir)** are predicted to increase the exposure to **zopiclone**. Adjust dose. [Moderate] Theoretical

▸ **Indinavir** is predicted to increase the exposure to **zopiclone**. Adjust dose. [Moderate] Study

Homatropine → see TABLE 10 p. 820 (antimuscarinics)
Hormone replacement therapy

▸ **Antiepileptics (carbamazepine, eslicarbazepine, fosphenytoin, oxcarbazepine, perampanel, phenobarbital, phenytoin, primidone, rufinamide, topiramate)** are predicted to decrease the effects of **Hormone replacement therapy**. [Moderate] Anecdotal

▸ **Hormone replacement therapy** is predicted to alter the exposure to antiepileptics **(lamotrigine)**. [Moderate] Theoretical

▸ **Aprepitant** is predicted to decrease the effects of **Hormone replacement therapy**. [Moderate] Anecdotal

▸ **Bosentan** is predicted to decrease the effects of **Hormone replacement therapy**. [Moderate] Anecdotal

▸ **Hormone replacement therapy** decreases the clearance of dopamine receptor agonists **(ropinirole)**. Monitor and adjust dose. [Moderate] Study

▸ **Efavirenz** is predicted to decrease the effects of **Hormone replacement therapy**. [Moderate] Anecdotal

▸ **Fosaprepitant** is predicted to decrease the effects of **Hormone replacement therapy**. [Moderate] Anecdotal

▸ **HIV-protease inhibitors (ritonavir)** are predicted to decrease the effects of **Hormone replacement therapy**. [Moderate] Anecdotal

▸ **Hormone replacement therapy** is predicted to increase the risk of venous thromboembolism when given with **lenalidomide**. [Severe] Theoretical

▸ Oral **Hormone replacement therapy** is predicted to decrease the effects of **levothyroxine**. [Moderate] Theoretical

▸ Oral **Hormone replacement therapy** is predicted to decrease the effects of **liothyronine**. [Moderate] Theoretical

▸ **Modafinil** is predicted to decrease the effects of **Hormone replacement therapy**. [Moderate] Anecdotal

▸ **Hormone replacement therapy** is predicted to increase the exposure to monoamine-oxidase B inhibitors **(selegiline)**. Avoid. [Moderate] Study

▸ **Nevirapine** is predicted to decrease the effects of **Hormone replacement therapy**. [Moderate] Anecdotal

▸ **NSAIDs (etoricoxib)** slightly increase the exposure to **Hormone replacement therapy**. [Moderate] Study

▸ **Hormone replacement therapy** is predicted to increase the risk of venous thromboembolism when given with **pomalidomide**. [Severe] Theoretical

▸ **Rifabutin** is predicted to decrease the effects of **Hormone replacement therapy**. [Moderate] Anecdotal

▸ **Rifampicin** is predicted to decrease the effects of **Hormone replacement therapy**. [Moderate] Anecdotal

▸ **St John's Wort** is predicted to decrease the efficacy of **Hormone replacement therapy**. [Moderate] Theoretical

▸ **Hormone replacement therapy** is predicted to increase the risk of venous thromboembolism when given with **thalidomide**. [Severe] Theoretical

Hydralazine → see TABLE 8 p. 819 (hypotension)

▸ **Diazoxide** increases the risk of severe hypotension when given with **hydralazine**. [Severe] Study → Also see TABLE 8 p. 819

Hydrochlorothiazide → see thiazide diuretics
Hydrocortisone → see corticosteroids
Hydroflumethiazide → see thiazide diuretics
Hydromorphone → see opioids
Hydroxycarbamide → see TABLE 15 p. 821 (myelosuppression)

▸ **Hydroxycarbamide** increases the risk of toxicity when given with **didanosine**. Avoid. [Severe] Study

▸ **Live vaccines** are predicted to increase the risk of generalised infection (possibly life-threatening) when given with **hydroxycarbamide**. Public Health England advises avoid. [Severe] Theoretical

▸ **Hydroxycarbamide** increases the risk of toxicity when given with **stavudine**. Avoid. [Severe] Study

Hydroxychloroquine

▸ **Hydroxychloroquine** is predicted to decrease the effects of **agalsidase**. [Moderate] Theoretical

▸ **Antacids** decrease the absorption of **hydroxychloroquine**. Separate administration by at least 4 hours. [Moderate] Study

▸ **Calcium salts (calcium carbonate)** decrease the absorption of **hydroxychloroquine**. Separate administration by at least 4 hours. [Moderate] Study

▸ **Hydroxychloroquine** is predicted to decrease the efficacy of oral **cholera vaccine**. [Moderate] Theoretical

▸ H₂ receptor antagonists **(cimetidine)** are predicted to decrease the clearance of **hydroxychloroquine**. [Moderate] Theoretical

▸ **Lanthanum** is predicted to decrease the absorption of **hydroxychloroquine**. Separate administration by at least 2 hours. [Moderate] Theoretical

▸ **Hydroxychloroquine** is predicted to decrease the exposure to **laronidase**. Avoid simultaneous administration. [Severe] Theoretical

▸ **Hydroxychloroquine** is predicted to increase the risk of haematological toxicity when given with **penicillamine**. Avoid. [Severe] Theoretical

▸ **Hydroxychloroquine** is predicted to decrease efficacy **rabies vaccine**. [Moderate] Theoretical

Hydroxyzine → see antihistamines, sedating
Hyoscine → see TABLE 10 p. 820 (antimuscarinics)
Ibandronic acid → see bisphosphonates
Ibrutinib → see TABLE 15 p. 821 (myelosuppression), TABLE 4 p. 818 (antiplatelet effects)

> **FOOD AND LIFESTYLE** Avoid food or drink containing bitter (Seville) oranges as they are predicted to increase the exposure to ibrutinib.

▸ **Antiarrhythmics (dronedarone)** are predicted to increase the exposure to **ibrutinib**. Avoid or adjust **ibrutinib** dose. [Severe] Theoretical

▸ **Antiepileptics (carbamazepine, fosphenytoin, phenobarbital, phenytoin, primidone)** are predicted to decrease the exposure to **ibrutinib**. Avoid. [Severe] Study

▸ **Antifungals, azoles (fluconazole, isavuconazole, posaconazole)** are predicted to increase the exposure to **ibrutinib**. Avoid or adjust **ibrutinib** dose. [Severe] Theoretical

▸ **Antifungals, azoles (itraconazole, ketoconazole, voriconazole)** are predicted to very markedly increase the exposure to **ibrutinib**. Avoid or adjust **ibrutinib** dose. [Severe] Study

▸ **Aprepitant** is predicted to increase the exposure to **ibrutinib**. Avoid or adjust **ibrutinib** dose. [Severe] Theoretical

▸ **Calcium channel blockers (diltiazem, verapamil)** are predicted to increase the exposure to **ibrutinib**. Avoid or adjust **ibrutinib** dose. [Severe] Theoretical

▸ **Cobicistat** is predicted to very markedly increase the exposure to **ibrutinib**. Avoid or adjust **ibrutinib** dose. [Severe] Study

- Crizotinib is predicted to increase the exposure to **ibrutinib**. Avoid or adjust **ibrutinib** dose. Severe Theoretical → Also see TABLE 15 p. 821
- Enzalutamide is predicted to decrease the exposure to **ibrutinib**. Avoid. Severe Study
- Fosaprepitant is predicted to slightly increase the exposure to **ibrutinib**. Moderate Theoretical
- Grapefruit juice is predicted to increase the exposure to **ibrutinib**. Avoid. Moderate Theoretical
- HIV-protease inhibitors (atazanavir, darunavir, fosamprenavir, lopinavir, ritonavir, saquinavir, tipranavir) are predicted to very markedly increase the exposure to **ibrutinib**. Avoid or adjust **ibrutinib** dose. Severe Study
- HIV-protease inhibitors (indinavir) are predicted to increase the exposure to **ibrutinib**. Avoid or adjust **ibrutinib** dose. Severe Theoretical
- Idelalisib is predicted to very markedly increase the exposure to **ibrutinib**. Avoid or adjust **ibrutinib** dose. Severe Study → Also see TABLE 15 p. 821
- Imatinib is predicted to increase the exposure to **ibrutinib**. Avoid or adjust **ibrutinib** dose. Severe Theoretical → Also see TABLE 15 p. 821
- Macrolides (clarithromycin) are predicted to very markedly increase the exposure to **ibrutinib**. Avoid or adjust **ibrutinib** dose. Severe Study
- Macrolides (erythromycin) are predicted to increase the exposure to **ibrutinib**. Avoid or adjust **ibrutinib** dose. Severe Theoretical
- Netupitant is predicted to increase the exposure to **ibrutinib**. Avoid or adjust **ibrutinib** dose. Severe Theoretical
- Nilotinib is predicted to increase the exposure to **ibrutinib**. Avoid or adjust **ibrutinib** dose. Severe Theoretical → Also see TABLE 15 p. 821
- Quinolones (ciprofloxacin) are predicted to increase the exposure to **ibrutinib**. Avoid or adjust **ibrutinib** dose. Severe Theoretical
- Rifampicin is predicted to decrease the exposure to **ibrutinib**. Avoid. Severe Study
- St John's Wort is predicted to decrease the exposure to **ibrutinib**. Avoid. Severe Theoretical

Ibuprofen → see NSAIDs
Icatibant
- ACE inhibitors are predicted to decrease the efficacy of **icatibant** and **icatibant** is predicted to decrease the efficacy of ACE inhibitors. Avoid. Moderate Theoretical

Idarubicin → see anthracyclines
Idarucizumab → see monoclonal antibodies
Idelalisib → see TABLE 15 p. 821 (myelosuppression)
- Idelalisib is predicted to increase the exposure to abiraterone. Severe Theoretical
- Idelalisib is predicted to markedly increase the exposure to aldosterone antagonists (eplerenone). Avoid. Severe Study
- Idelalisib increases the exposure to almotriptan. Mild Study
- Idelalisib is predicted to moderately increase the exposure to alpha blockers (alfuzosin, tamsulosin). Use with caution or avoid. Moderate Study
- Idelalisib is predicted to increase the exposure to alpha blockers (doxazosin). Moderate Study
- Idelalisib moderately increases the exposure to alprazolam. Avoid. Moderate Study
- Idelalisib very markedly increases the exposure to antiarrhythmics (dronedarone). Avoid. Severe Study
- Idelalisib is predicted to increase the exposure to antiarrhythmics (propafenone). Monitor and adjust dose. Severe Study
- Idelalisib is predicted to increase the exposure to anticholinesterases, centrally acting (galantamine). Monitor and adjust dose. Moderate Study
- Antiepileptics (carbamazepine, fosphenytoin, phenobarbital, phenytoin, primidone) are predicted to decrease the exposure to **idelalisib**. Avoid. Severe Study
- Idelalisib is predicted to slightly increase the exposure to antiepileptics (perampanel). Mild Study

- Idelalisib is predicted to increase the exposure to antifungals, azoles (isavuconazole). Avoid or monitor side effects. Severe Study
- Idelalisib is predicted to increase the exposure to antihistamines, non-sedating (mizolastine). Avoid. Severe Study
- Idelalisib is predicted to increase the exposure to antimalarials (artemether) with lumefantrine. Moderate Study
- Idelalisib is predicted to increase the concentration of antimalarials (piperaquine). Severe Theoretical
- Idelalisib is predicted to markedly increase the exposure to aprepitant. Moderate Study
- Idelalisib is predicted to slightly increase the exposure to aripiprazole. Adjust **aripiprazole** dose, p. 240. Moderate Study
- Idelalisib is predicted to increase the exposure to axitinib. Avoid or adjust dose. Moderate Study → Also see TABLE 15 p. 821
- Idelalisib is predicted to increase the exposure to bedaquiline. Avoid prolonged use. Mild Study
- Idelalisib is predicted to increase the exposure to beta$_2$ agonists (salmeterol). Avoid. Severe Study
- Idelalisib slightly increases the exposure to bortezomib. Moderate Study → Also see TABLE 15 p. 821
- Idelalisib is predicted to markedly increase the exposure to bosutinib. Avoid or adjust **bosutinib** dose. Severe Study → Also see TABLE 15 p. 821
- Idelalisib is predicted to increase the exposure to buspirone. Adjust **buspirone** dose. Severe Study
- Idelalisib slightly increases the exposure to cabozantinib. Moderate Study → Also see TABLE 15 p. 821
- Idelalisib is predicted to increase the exposure to calcium channel blockers (amlodipine, felodipine, isradipine, lacidipine, nicardipine, nifedipine, nimodipine). Monitor and adjust dose. Moderate Study
- Idelalisib is predicted to increase the exposure to calcium channel blockers (diltiazem, verapamil). Severe Study
- Idelalisib is predicted to markedly increase the exposure to calcium channel blockers (lercanidipine). Avoid. Severe Study
- Idelalisib is predicted to increase the exposure to cannabis extract. Use with caution and adjust dose. Moderate Theoretical
- Idelalisib is predicted to increase the exposure to ceritinib. Avoid or adjust **ceritinib** dose. Severe Study → Also see TABLE 15 p. 821
- Idelalisib increases the concentration of ciclosporin. Severe Study
- Idelalisib is predicted to moderately increase the exposure to cilostazol. Adjust **cilostazol** dose. Moderate Study
- Idelalisib is predicted to moderately increase the exposure to cinacalcet. Adjust dose. Moderate Study
- Idelalisib is predicted to markedly increase the exposure to cobimetinib. Avoid or monitor for toxicity. Severe Study
- Idelalisib is predicted to increase the exposure to colchicine. Avoid or adjust **colchicine** dose. Severe Study
- Idelalisib is predicted to increase the exposure to corticosteroids (budesonide). Avoid. Severe Study
- Idelalisib is predicted to increase the exposure to corticosteroids (ciclesonide). Avoid. Moderate Theoretical
- Idelalisib is predicted to increase the exposure to corticosteroids (dexamethasone, methylprednisolone). Monitor and adjust dose. Moderate Study
- Idelalisib is predicted to increase the exposure to inhaled corticosteroids (fluticasone). Severe Study
- Idelalisib is predicted to increase the exposure to corticosteroids (mometasone). Moderate Theoretical
- Idelalisib is predicted to increase the risk of side-effects when given with corticosteroids (triamcinolone). Severe Theoretical
- Idelalisib is predicted to moderately increase the exposure to crizotinib. Avoid. Moderate Study → Also see TABLE 15 p. 821
- Idelalisib is predicted to increase the exposure to dabrafenib. Use with caution or avoid. Moderate Study → Also see TABLE 15 p. 821
- Idelalisib is predicted to moderately increase the exposure to daclatasvir. Adjust **daclatasvir** dose. Moderate Study
- Idelalisib is predicted to markedly to very markedly increase the exposure to darifenacin. Avoid. Severe Study
- Idelalisib is predicted to markedly increase the exposure to dasatinib. Avoid. Severe Study → Also see TABLE 15 p. 821

Idelalisib (continued)
- **Idelalisib** very slightly increases the exposure to **delamanid**. Severe Study
- **Idelalisib** increases the risk of QT-prolongation when given with **domperidone**. Avoid. Severe Study
- **Idelalisib** increases the exposure to dopamine receptor agonists (**bromocriptine, cabergoline**). Severe Study
- **Idelalisib** is predicted to increase the exposure to **dutasteride**. Monitor side effects and adjust dose. Moderate Theoretical
- **Idelalisib** slightly to moderately increases the exposure to **elbasvir**. Avoid. Moderate Study
- **Idelalisib** is predicted to markedly increase the exposure to **eletriptan**. Avoid. Severe Study
- **Enzalutamide** is predicted to decrease the exposure to **idelalisib**. Avoid. Severe Study
- **Idelalisib** is predicted to increase the risk of ergotism when given with **ergometrine**. Avoid. Severe Theoretical
- **Idelalisib** is predicted to increase the risk of ergotism when given with **ergotamine**. Avoid. Severe Theoretical
- **Idelalisib** is predicted to slightly increase the exposure to **erlotinib**. Use with caution and adjust dose. Moderate Study
- **Idelalisib** is predicted to increase the concentration of **everolimus**. Avoid. Severe Study → Also see TABLE 15 p. 821
- **Idelalisib** is predicted to moderately increase the exposure to **fesoterodine**. Adjust **fesoterodine** dose; avoid in hepatic and renal impairment. Severe Study
- **Idelalisib** is predicted to increase the exposure to **fosaprepitant**. Moderate Theoretical
- **Idelalisib** is predicted to increase the exposure to **gefitinib**. Moderate Study → Also see TABLE 15 p. 821
- **Idelalisib** is predicted to moderately to markedly increase the exposure to **grazoprevir**. Avoid. Severe Study
- **Idelalisib** is predicted to increase the exposure to **guanfacine**. Adjust **guanfacine** dose, p. 222. Moderate Study
- **Idelalisib** is predicted to very markedly increase the exposure to **ibrutinib**. Avoid or adjust **ibrutinib** dose. Severe Study → Also see TABLE 15 p. 821
- **Idelalisib** is predicted to increase the exposure to **imatinib**. Moderate Study → Also see TABLE 15 p. 821
- **Idelalisib** is predicted to increase the risk of toxicity when given with **irinotecan**. Avoid. Moderate Study → Also see TABLE 15 p. 821
- **Idelalisib** is predicted to increase the exposure to **ivabradine**. Avoid. Severe Study
- **Idelalisib** is predicted to increase the exposure to **ivacaftor**. Adjust **ivacaftor** or lumacaftor with ivacaftor dose, p. 179 . Severe Study
- **Idelalisib** is predicted to increase the exposure to **lapatinib**. Avoid. Moderate Study
- **Idelalisib** is predicted to markedly increase the exposure to **lomitapide**. Avoid. Severe Study
- **Idelalisib** is predicted to increase the exposure to **lurasidone**. Avoid. Severe Study
- **Idelalisib** is predicted to increase the exposure to **macitentan**. Moderate Study
- **Idelalisib** markedly increases the exposure to **maraviroc**. Adjust dose. Severe Theoretical
- **Idelalisib** is predicted to markedly to very markedly increase the exposure to **midazolam**. Avoid or adjust **midazolam** dose. Severe Study
- **Idelalisib** is predicted to increase the exposure to **mirabegron**. Adjust **mirabegron** dose in hepatic and renal impairment. Moderate Study
- **Idelalisib** is predicted to increase the exposure to **mirtazapine**. Moderate Study
- **Idelalisib** is predicted to increase the exposure to **modafinil**. Mild Theoretical
- **Idelalisib** is predicted to increase the exposure to monoclonal antibodies (**trastuzumab emtansine**). Avoid. Severe Theoretical → Also see TABLE 15 p. 821
- **Idelalisib** is predicted to markedly increase the exposure to **naloxegol**. Avoid. Severe Study
- **Idelalisib** is predicted to increase the exposure to **netupitant**. Mild Study

- **Idelalisib** is predicted to moderately increase the exposure to **nilotinib**. Avoid. Severe Study → Also see TABLE 15 p. 821
- **Idelalisib** is predicted to increase the exposure to **nitisinone**. Adjust **nitisinone** dose, p. 585. Moderate Theoretical
- **Idelalisib** is predicted to increase the exposure to **olaparib**. Avoid or adjust **olaparib** dose. Moderate Study → Also see TABLE 15 p. 821
- **Idelalisib** is predicted to increase the exposure to opioids (**alfentanil, buprenorphine, fentanyl, oxycodone, sufentanil**). Monitor and adjust dose. Severe Study
- **Idelalisib** is predicted to increase the exposure to opioids (**methadone**). Moderate Theoretical
- **Idelalisib** is predicted to increase the exposure to **oxybutynin**. Mild Study
- **Idelalisib** is predicted to increase the exposure to **palbociclib**. Avoid or adjust **palbociclib** dose. Severe Study
- **Idelalisib** is predicted to increase the exposure to **panobinostat**. Adjust **panobinostat** dose; in hepatic impairment avoid. Moderate Study → Also see TABLE 15 p. 821
- **Idelalisib** is predicted to increase the exposure to **paritaprevir** (with **ritonavir and ombitasvir**). Avoid. Severe Theoretical
- **Idelalisib** is predicted to increase the exposure to **pazopanib**. Avoid or adjust **pazopanib** dose. Moderate Study → Also see TABLE 15 p. 821
- **Idelalisib** is predicted to increase the exposure to phosphodiesterase type-5 inhibitors (**avanafil, vardenafil**). Avoid. Severe Study
- **Idelalisib** is predicted to increase the exposure to phosphodiesterase type-5 inhibitors (**sildenafil**). Avoid or adjust **sildenafil** dose, p. 117. Severe Study
- **Idelalisib** is predicted to increase the exposure to phosphodiesterase type-5 inhibitors (**tadalafil**). Use with caution or avoid. Severe Study
- **Idelalisib** is predicted to increase the exposure to **pimozide**. Avoid. Severe Study
- **Idelalisib** is predicted to slightly increase the exposure to **ponatinib**. Monitor and adjust **ponatinib** dose. Moderate Study
- **Idelalisib** is predicted to moderately increase the exposure to **praziquantel**. Mild Study
- **Idelalisib** is predicted to increase the exposure to **quetiapine**. Avoid. Severe Study
- **Idelalisib** is predicted to increase the exposure to **ranolazine**. Avoid. Severe Study
- **Idelalisib** is predicted to increase the exposure to **reboxetine**. Avoid. Moderate Study
- **Idelalisib** is predicted to increase the exposure to **regorafenib**. Avoid. Moderate Study → Also see TABLE 15 p. 821
- **Idelalisib** is predicted to increase the exposure to **repaglinide**. Moderate Study
- **Idelalisib** is predicted to increase the exposure to retinoids (**alitretinoin**). Adjust **alitretinoin** dose. Moderate Theoretical
- **Rifampicin** is predicted to decrease the exposure to **idelalisib**. Avoid. Severe Study
- **Idelalisib** is predicted to increase the exposure to **risperidone**. Adjust dose. Moderate Study
- **Idelalisib** is predicted to increase the exposure to **ruxolitinib**. Adjust dose and monitor side effects. Moderate Study → Also see TABLE 15 p. 821
- **Idelalisib** is predicted to increase the exposure to **saxagliptin**. Moderate Study
- **Idelalisib** is predicted to increase the exposure to **simeprevir**. Avoid. Severe Study
- **Idelalisib** is predicted to increase the concentration of **sirolimus**. Avoid. Severe Study
- **Idelalisib** is predicted to increase the exposure to **solifenacin**. Adjust **solifenacin** or tamsulosin with solifenacin dose; avoid in hepatic and renal impairment. Severe Study
- **Idelalisib** is predicted to moderately increase the exposure to SSRIs (**dapoxetine**). Avoid, or adjust **dapoxetine** dose. Severe Study
- **St John's Wort** is predicted to decrease the exposure to **idelalisib**. Severe Theoretical
- **Idelalisib** is predicted to increase the exposure to statins (**atorvastatin**). Avoid or adjust dose and monitor rhabdomyolysis. Severe Study

- **Idelalisib** is predicted to increase the exposure to statins (simvastatin). Avoid. Severe Study
- **Idelalisib** is predicted to slightly increase the exposure to sunitinib. Avoid or adjust **sunitinib** dose. Moderate Study → Also see TABLE 15 p. 821
- **Idelalisib** is predicted to increase the concentration of tacrolimus. Monitor and adjust dose. Severe Study
- **Idelalisib** is predicted to increase the exposure to taxanes (cabazitaxel). Avoid. Severe Study → Also see TABLE 15 p. 821
- **Idelalisib** is predicted to moderately increase the exposure to taxanes (docetaxel). Avoid or adjust dose. Severe Study → Also see TABLE 15 p. 821
- **Idelalisib** is predicted to increase the exposure to taxanes (paclitaxel). Severe Theoretical → Also see TABLE 15 p. 821
- **Idelalisib** is predicted to increase the concentration of temsirolimus. Avoid. Severe Theoretical → Also see TABLE 15 p. 821
- **Idelalisib** is predicted to markedly increase the exposure to ticagrelor. Avoid. Severe Study
- **Idelalisib** is predicted to increase the exposure to tolterodine. Avoid. Severe Study
- **Idelalisib** is predicted to increase the exposure to tolvaptan. Adjust dose. Severe Study
- **Idelalisib** is predicted to increase the exposure to toremifene. Moderate Theoretical
- **Idelalisib** is predicted to increase the exposure to trabectedin. Avoid or adjust dose. Severe Theoretical → Also see TABLE 15 p. 821
- **Idelalisib** is predicted to moderately increase the exposure to trazodone. Avoid or adjust dose. Moderate Study
- **Idelalisib** is predicted to increase the exposure to ulipristal. Avoid if used for uterine fibroids. Severe Study
- **Idelalisib** is predicted to increase the exposure to vemurafenib. Severe Theoretical
- **Idelalisib** is predicted to increase the exposure to venetoclax. Avoid or adjust **venetoclax** dose. Severe Study
- **Idelalisib** is predicted to increase the exposure to venlafaxine. Moderate Study
- **Idelalisib** is predicted to increase the exposure to vinca alkaloids. Severe Theoretical → Also see TABLE 15 p. 821
- **Idelalisib** is predicted to increase the exposure to vitamin D substances (paricalcitol). Moderate Study
- **Idelalisib** is predicted to increase the exposure to zopiclone. Adjust dose. Moderate Theoretical

Ifosfamide → see alkylating agents

Iloprost → see TABLE 4 p. 818 (antiplatelet effects)

Imatinib → see TABLE 15 p. 821 (myelosuppression)

- **Imatinib** is predicted to increase the exposure to aldosterone antagonists (eplerenone). Adjust **eplerenone** dose. Severe Study
- **Imatinib** is predicted to increase the exposure to alpha blockers (tamsulosin). Moderate Theoretical
- **Imatinib** is predicted to increase the exposure to alprazolam. Severe Study
- **Imatinib** is predicted to increase the exposure to antiarrhythmics (dronedarone). Severe Theoretical
- **Imatinib** is predicted to increase the exposure to antiarrhythmics (propafenone). Monitor and adjust dose. Moderate Study
- Antiepileptics (carbamazepine, fosphenytoin, phenobarbital, phenytoin, primidone) are predicted to decrease the exposure to **imatinib**. Avoid. Moderate Study
- Antiepileptics (oxcarbazepine) decrease the exposure to **imatinib**. Avoid. Moderate Study
- Antifungals, azoles (fluconazole, posaconazole) are predicted to increase the exposure to **imatinib**. Moderate Theoretical
- Antifungals, azoles (itraconazole, ketoconazole, voriconazole) are predicted to increase the exposure to **imatinib**. Moderate Study
- **Imatinib** is predicted to decrease the exposure to antifungals, azoles (isavuconazole). Moderate Theoretical
- **Imatinib** is predicted to increase the exposure to antihistamines, non-sedating (mizolastine). Severe Theoretical
- **Imatinib** is predicted to increase the concentration of antimalarials (piperaquine). Severe Theoretical
- **Aprepitant** is predicted to increase the exposure to **imatinib**. Moderate Theoretical

- **Asparaginase** is predicted to increase the risk of hepatotoxicity when given with **imatinib**. Severe Theoretical → Also see TABLE 15 p. 821
- **Imatinib** is predicted to increase the exposure to axitinib. Moderate Theoretical → Also see TABLE 15 p. 821
- **Imatinib** is predicted to increase the exposure to bedaquiline. Avoid prolonged use. Mild Theoretical
- **Bosentan** is predicted to decrease the exposure to **imatinib**. Moderate Study
- **Imatinib** is predicted to increase the exposure to bosutinib. Avoid or adjust **bosutinib** dose. Severe Theoretical → Also see TABLE 15 p. 821
- **Imatinib** is predicted to increase the exposure to buspirone. Use with caution and adjust dose. Moderate Study
- **Imatinib** is predicted to increase the exposure to cabozantinib. Moderate Theoretical → Also see TABLE 15 p. 821
- Calcium channel blockers (diltiazem, verapamil) are predicted to increase the exposure to **imatinib**. Moderate Theoretical
- **Imatinib** is predicted to increase the exposure to calcium channel blockers (amlodipine, felodipine, isradipine, lacidipine, lercanidipine, nicardipine, nifedipine, nimodipine). Monitor and adjust dose. Moderate Study
- **Imatinib** is predicted to increase the exposure to ceritinib. Moderate Theoretical → Also see TABLE 15 p. 821
- **Imatinib** increases the concentration of ciclosporin. Severe Study
- **Cobicistat** is predicted to increase the exposure to **imatinib**. Moderate Study
- **Imatinib** is predicted to increase the exposure to cobimetinib. Severe Theoretical
- **Imatinib** is predicted to increase the exposure to colchicine. Adjust **colchicine** dose. Severe Study
- **Imatinib** is predicted to increase the exposure to corticosteroids (methylprednisolone). Monitor and adjust dose. Moderate Study
- **Imatinib** is predicted to increase the risk of bleeding events when given with coumarins. Severe Theoretical
- **Crisantaspase** is predicted to increase the risk of hepatotoxicity when given with **imatinib**. Severe Theoretical → Also see TABLE 15 p. 821
- **Imatinib** is predicted to slightly increase the exposure to darifenacin. Moderate Study
- **Imatinib** is predicted to increase the exposure to dasatinib. Severe Study → Also see TABLE 15 p. 821
- **Imatinib** increases the risk of QT-prolongation when given with domperidone. Avoid. Severe Study
- **Imatinib** is predicted to increase the exposure to dopamine receptor agonists (bromocriptine, cabergoline). Severe Theoretical
- **Imatinib** is predicted to moderately increase the exposure to dutasteride. Mild Study
- **Efavirenz** is predicted to decrease the exposure to **imatinib**. Moderate Study
- **Enzalutamide** is predicted to decrease the exposure to **imatinib**. Avoid. Moderate Study
- **Imatinib** is predicted to increase the risk of ergotism when given with ergometrine. Severe Theoretical
- **Imatinib** is predicted to increase the risk of ergotism when given with ergotamine. Severe Theoretical
- **Imatinib** is predicted to increase the exposure to erlotinib. Moderate Theoretical
- **Imatinib** is predicted to increase the concentration of everolimus. Avoid or adjust dose. Moderate Study → Also see TABLE 15 p. 821
- **Imatinib** is predicted to increase the exposure to fesoterodine. Adjust **fesoterodine** dose in hepatic and renal impairment. Mild Study
- **Imatinib** is predicted to increase the exposure to gefitinib. Moderate Theoretical → Also see TABLE 15 p. 821
- **Grapefruit juice** is predicted to increase the exposure to **imatinib**. Moderate Theoretical
- **Imatinib** is predicted to increase the concentration of guanfacine. Adjust **guanfacine** dose, p. 222. Moderate Theoretical
- HIV-protease inhibitors (atazanavir, darunavir, fosamprenavir, lopinavir, ritonavir, saquinavir, tipranavir) are predicted to increase the exposure to **imatinib**. Moderate Study

Imatinib (continued)

▶ **Imatinib** is predicted to increase the exposure to **ibrutinib**. Avoid or adjust **ibrutinib** dose. Severe Theoretical → Also see TABLE 15 p. 821

▶ **Idelalisib** is predicted to increase the exposure to **imatinib**. Moderate Study → Also see TABLE 15 p. 821

▶ **Imatinib** is predicted to increase the exposure to **ivabradine**. Adjust **ivabradine** dose. Severe Theoretical

▶ **Imatinib** is predicted to increase the exposure to **ivacaftor**. Adjust **ivacaftor** dose, p. 179. Severe Study

▶ **Imatinib** is predicted to increase the exposure to **lapatinib**. Moderate Study

▶ **Imatinib** is predicted to increase the exposure to **lomitapide**. Avoid. Moderate Theoretical

▶ **Imatinib** is predicted to increase the exposure to **lurasidone**. Moderate Study

▶ Macrolides **(clarithromycin)** are predicted to increase the exposure to **imatinib**. Moderate Study

▶ Macrolides **(erythromycin)** are predicted to increase the exposure to **imatinib**. Moderate Theoretical

▶ **Imatinib** is predicted to increase the exposure to **midazolam**. Monitor side effects and adjust dose. Severe Study

▶ **Imatinib** is predicted to increase the exposure to **naloxegol**. Adjust **naloxegol** dose and monitor side effects. Moderate Study

▶ **Netupitant** is predicted to increase the exposure to **imatinib**. Moderate Theoretical

▶ **Nevirapine** is predicted to decrease the exposure to **imatinib**. Moderate Study

▶ **Imatinib** is predicted to increase the exposure to **olaparib**. Avoid or adjust **olaparib** dose. Moderate Theoretical → Also see TABLE 15 p. 821

▶ **Imatinib** is predicted to increase the exposure to opioids **(alfentanil, buprenorphine, fentanyl, oxycodone)**. Monitor and adjust dose. Moderate Study

▶ **Imatinib** is predicted to increase the exposure to opioids **(methadone, sufentanil)**. Moderate Theoretical

▶ **Imatinib** is predicted to increase the exposure to **oxybutynin**. Mild Theoretical

▶ **Imatinib** increases the risk of hepatotoxicity when given with **paracetamol**. Severe Anecdotal

▶ **Imatinib** is predicted to increase the exposure to **pazopanib**. Moderate Theoretical → Also see TABLE 15 p. 821

▶ **Pegaspargase** is predicted to increase the risk of hepatotoxicity when given with **imatinib**. Severe Theoretical → Also see TABLE 15 p. 821

▶ **Imatinib** is predicted to increase the risk of bleeding events when given with **phenindione**. Severe Theoretical

▶ **Imatinib** is predicted to increase the exposure to phosphodiesterase type-5 inhibitors **(avanafil)**. Adjust **avanafil** dose. Moderate Theoretical

▶ **Imatinib** is predicted to increase the exposure to phosphodiesterase type-5 inhibitors **(sildenafil)**. Monitor and adjust **sildenafil** dose, p. 117. Moderate Study

▶ **Imatinib** is predicted to increase the exposure to phosphodiesterase type-5 inhibitors **(tadalafil)**. Severe Theoretical

▶ **Imatinib** is predicted to increase the exposure to phosphodiesterase type-5 inhibitors **(vardenafil)**. Adjust dose. Severe Theoretical

▶ **Imatinib** is predicted to increase the exposure to **pimozide**. Avoid. Severe Theoretical

▶ **Imatinib** is predicted to increase the exposure to **quetiapine**. Avoid. Moderate Study

▶ **Imatinib** is predicted to increase the exposure to **ranolazine**. Severe Study

▶ **Rifampicin** is predicted to decrease the exposure to **imatinib**. Avoid. Moderate Study

▶ **Imatinib** is predicted to increase the exposure to **ruxolitinib**. Moderate Theoretical → Also see TABLE 15 p. 821

▶ **Imatinib** is predicted to increase the exposure to **saxagliptin**. Mild Study

▶ **Imatinib** is predicted to increase the exposure to **simeprevir**. Avoid. Severe Study

▶ **Imatinib** increases the concentration of **sirolimus**. Monitor and adjust dose. Moderate Study

▶ **Imatinib** is predicted to increase the exposure to SSRIs **(dapoxetine)**. Adjust **dapoxetine** dose. Moderate Theoretical

▶ **St John's Wort** is predicted to decrease the exposure to **imatinib**. Moderate Study

▶ **Imatinib** is predicted to increase the exposure to statins **(atorvastatin)**. Monitor and adjust dose. Severe Theoretical

▶ **Imatinib** is predicted to increase the exposure to statins **(simvastatin)**. Use with caution and adjust **simvastatin** dose, p. 130. Severe Study

▶ **Imatinib** is predicted to increase the exposure to **sunitinib**. Moderate Theoretical → Also see TABLE 15 p. 821

▶ **Imatinib** is predicted to increase the concentration of **tacrolimus**. Severe Study

▶ **Imatinib** is predicted to increase the exposure to taxanes **(cabazitaxel)**. Moderate Theoretical → Also see TABLE 15 p. 821

▶ **Tedizolid** is predicted to increase the exposure to **imatinib**. Avoid. Moderate Theoretical

▶ **Imatinib** is predicted to increase the concentration of **temsirolimus**. Moderate Theoretical → Also see TABLE 15 p. 821

▶ **Imatinib** is predicted to increase the exposure to **tolterodine**. Mild Theoretical

▶ **Imatinib** is predicted to increase the exposure to **tolvaptan**. Adjust dose. Moderate Theoretical

▶ **Imatinib** is predicted to increase the exposure to **trazodone**. Moderate Theoretical

▶ **Imatinib** is predicted to increase the exposure to **ulipristal**. Avoid if used for uterine fibroids. Moderate Study

▶ **Imatinib** is predicted to increase the exposure to **venetoclax**. Avoid or adjust **venetoclax** dose. Severe Study

▶ **Imatinib** is predicted to increase the exposure to vinca alkaloids. Severe Theoretical → Also see TABLE 15 p. 821

▶ **Imatinib** is predicted to increase the exposure to **zopiclone**. Adjust dose. Moderate Study

Imidapril → see ACE inhibitors

Imipenem → see carbapenems

Imipramine → see tricyclic antidepressants

Indacaterol → see beta$_2$ agonists

Indapamide → see thiazide diuretics

Indinavir → see HIV-protease inhibitors

Indometacin → see NSAIDs

Indoramin → see alpha blockers

Infliximab → see monoclonal antibodies

Influenza vaccine → see live vaccines

Insulin → see insulins

Insulin aspart → see insulins

Insulin degludec → see insulins

Insulin detemir → see insulins

Insulin glargine → see insulins

Insulin glulisine → see insulins

Insulin lispro → see insulins

Insulin zinc suspension → see insulins

Insulins → see TABLE 14 p. 821 (antidiabetic drugs)

biphasic insulin aspart · biphasic insulin lispro · biphasic isophane insulin · insulin · insulin aspart · insulin degludec · insulin detemir · insulin glargine · insulin glulisine · insulin lispro · insulin zinc suspension · isophane insulin · protamine zinc insulin

▶ **Fibrates** are predicted to increase the risk of hypoglycaemia when given with **insulins**. Moderate Theoretical

Interferon alfa → see interferons

Interferon beta → see interferons

Interferons → see TABLE 15 p. 821 (myelosuppression)

interferon alfa · interferon beta · peginterferon alfa

▶ **Interferons** are predicted to slightly increase the exposure to **aminophylline**. Adjust dose. Moderate Theoretical

▶ **Interferon alfa** is predicted to increase the risk of peripheral neuropathy when given with **telbivudine**. Avoid. Severe Theoretical

▶ **Peginterferon alfa** increases the risk of peripheral neuropathy when given with **telbivudine**. Avoid. Severe Study

▶ **Interferons** slightly increase the exposure to **theophylline**. Adjust dose. Moderate Study

Ipilimumab → see monoclonal antibodies

Ipratropium → see TABLE 10 p. 820 (antimuscarinics)

▸ Beta$_2$ agonists are predicted to increase the risk of glaucoma when given with **ipratropium**. Moderate Anecdotal

Irbesartan → see angiotensin-II receptor antagonists

Irinotecan → see TABLE 15 p. 821 (myelosuppression)

▸ Antiepileptics (carbamazepine, fosphenytoin, phenobarbital, phenytoin, primidone) are predicted to decrease the exposure to **irinotecan**. Avoid. Severe Study

▸ Antifungals, azoles (itraconazole, ketoconazole, voriconazole) are predicted to increase the risk of toxicity when given with **irinotecan**. Avoid. Moderate Study

▸ Cobicistat is predicted to increase the risk of toxicity when given with **irinotecan**. Avoid. Moderate Study

▸ Enzalutamide is predicted to decrease the exposure to **irinotecan**. Avoid. Severe Study

▸ HIV-protease inhibitors (atazanavir, darunavir, fosamprenavir, lopinavir, ritonavir, saquinavir, tipranavir) are predicted to increase the risk of toxicity when given with **irinotecan**. Avoid. Moderate Study

▸ Idelalisib is predicted to increase the risk of toxicity when given with **irinotecan**. Avoid. Moderate Study → Also see TABLE 15 p. 821

▸ Live vaccines are predicted to increase the risk of generalised infection (possibly life-threatening) when given with **irinotecan**. Public Health England advises avoid. Severe Theoretical

▸ Macrolides (clarithromycin) are predicted to increase the risk of toxicity when given with **irinotecan**. Avoid. Moderate Study

▸ **Irinotecan** is predicted to decrease the effects of neuromuscular blocking drugs, non-depolarising. Moderate Theoretical

▸ Pitolisant is predicted to decrease the exposure to **irinotecan**. Unknown Theoretical

▸ Rifampicin is predicted to decrease the exposure to **irinotecan**. Avoid. Moderate Study

▸ St John's Wort slightly decreases the exposure to **irinotecan**. Avoid. Severe Study

▸ **Irinotecan** is predicted to increase the risk of prolonged neuromuscular blockade when given with suxamethonium. Moderate Theoretical

Iron (injectable)

ferric carboxymaltose · iron dextran · iron isomaltoside 1000 · iron sucrose

▸ Chloramphenicol decreases the efficacy of intravenous **iron (injectable)**. Moderate Anecdotal

Iron (oral)

ferric maltol · ferrous fumarate · ferrous gluconate · ferrous sulfate · polysaccharide-iron complex · sodium feredetate

▸ Antacids decrease the absorption of **iron (oral)**. **Iron (oral)** should be taken 1 hour before or 2 hours after **antacids**. Moderate Study

▸ **Iron (oral)** is predicted to decrease the absorption of oral bisphosphonates (ibandronic acid). Avoid **iron (oral)** for at least 6 hours before or 1 hour after **ibandronic acid**. Moderate Theoretical

▸ **Iron (oral)** decreases the absorption of bisphosphonates (risedronate). Separate administration by at least 2 hours. Moderate Study

▸ **Iron (oral)** decreases the absorption of bisphosphonates (sodium clodronate). Avoid **iron (oral)** for 2 hours before or 1 hour after **sodium clodronate**. Moderate Study

▸ Calcium salts (calcium carbonate) decrease the absorption of **iron (oral)**. **Calcium carbonate** should be taken 1 hour before or 2 hours after **iron (oral)**. Moderate Study

▸ **Iron (oral)** is predicted to decrease the exposure to carbidopa. Moderate Theoretical

▸ Chloramphenicol decreases the efficacy of oral **iron (oral)**. Moderate Theoretical

▸ **Iron (oral)** decreases the absorption of dolutegravir. **Iron (oral)** should be taken 2 hours before or 6 hours after **dolutegravir**. Moderate Study

▸ **Iron (oral)** is predicted to decrease the absorption of eltrombopag. **Eltrombopag** should be taken 2 hours before or 4 hours after **iron (oral)**. Severe Theoretical

▸ **Iron (oral)** is predicted to decrease the absorption of entacapone. Separate administration by at least 2 hours. Moderate Theoretical

▸ **Iron (oral)** decreases the absorption of levodopa. Moderate Study

▸ **Iron (oral)** decreases the absorption of levothyroxine. Separate administration by at least 4 hours. Moderate Study

▸ **Iron (oral)** decreases the effects of methyldopa. Moderate Study

▸ **Iron (oral)** is predicted to decrease the absorption of penicillamine. Separate administration by at least 2 hours. Mild Study

▸ **Iron (oral)** decreases the exposure to quinolones. Separate administration by at least 2 hours. Moderate Study

▸ **Iron (oral)** decreases the absorption of tetracyclines. Tetracyclines should be taken 2 to 3 hours after **iron (oral)**. Moderate Study

▸ Trientine potentially decreases the absorption of **iron (oral)**. Moderate Theoretical

▸ Zinc is predicted to decrease the efficacy of **iron (oral)** and **iron (oral)** is predicted to decrease the efficacy of zinc. Moderate Study

Iron chelators

deferasirox · desferrioxamine · dexrazoxane

▸ **Deferasirox** is predicted to increase the exposure to aminophylline. Avoid. Moderate Theoretical

▸ Antacids (aluminium hydroxide) are predicted to decrease the exposure to **deferasirox**. Avoid. Moderate Theoretical

▸ Antiepileptics (carbamazepine, fosphenytoin, phenobarbital, phenytoin, primidone) are predicted to decrease the exposure to **deferasirox**. Monitor serum ferritin and adjust dose. Moderate Theoretical

▸ Ascorbic acid is predicted to increase the risk of cardiovascular side-effects when given with **desferrioxamine**. Severe Theoretical

▸ Aspirin (high-dose) is predicted to increase the risk of gastrointestinal bleeds when given with **deferasirox**. Severe Theoretical

▸ Bisphosphonates are predicted to increase the risk of gastrointestinal bleeding when given with **deferasirox**. Severe Theoretical

▸ **Deferasirox** is predicted to increase the exposure to clozapine. Avoid. Moderate Theoretical

▸ Corticosteroids are predicted to increase the risk of gastrointestinal bleeding when given with **deferasirox**. Severe Theoretical

▸ HIV-protease inhibitors (ritonavir) are predicted to decrease the exposure to **deferasirox**. Monitor serum ferritin and adjust dose. Moderate Theoretical

▸ Live vaccines are predicted to increase the risk of generalised infection (possibly life-threatening) when given with **dexrazoxane**. Avoid. Severe Theoretical

▸ NSAIDs are predicted to increase the risk of gastrointestinal bleeding when given with **deferasirox**. Severe Theoretical

▸ **Deferasirox** moderately increases the exposure to repaglinide. Avoid. Moderate Study

▸ Rifampicin is predicted to decrease the exposure to **deferasirox**. Monitor serum ferritin and adjust dose. Moderate Study

▸ **Deferasirox** increases the exposure to theophylline. Avoid. Moderate Study

▸ **Deferasirox** is predicted to increase the exposure to tizanidine. Avoid. Moderate Theoretical

Iron dextran → see iron (injectable)

Iron isomaltoside 1000 → see iron (injectable)

Iron sucrose → see iron (injectable)

Isavuconazole → see antifungals, azoles

Isocarboxazid → see monoamine-oxidase A and B inhibitors, irreversible

Isoflurane → see volatile halogenated anaesthetics

Isomethepene → see sympathomimetics, vasoconstrictor

Isoniazid → see TABLE 1 p. 818 (hepatotoxicity), TABLE 12 p. 821 (peripheral neuropathy)

FOOD AND LIFESTYLE Avoid tyramine or histamine rich foods, as tachycardia, palpitation, hypotension, flushing, headache, dizziness, and sweating reported.

Interactions | Appendix 1

A1

Isoniazid (continued)

▶ Isoniazid is predicted to affect the clearance of aminophylline. Severe Theoretical

▶ Isoniazid markedly increases the concentration of antiepileptics (carbamazepine) and antiepileptics (carbamazepine) increase the risk of hepatotoxicity when given with isoniazid. Monitor carbamazepine concentration and adjust dose. Severe Study → Also see TABLE 1 p. 818

▶ Isoniazid increases the concentration of antiepileptics (fosphenytoin, phenytoin). Moderate Study → Also see TABLE 12 p. 821

▶ Cycloserine increases the risk of CNS toxicity when given with isoniazid. Monitor and adjust dose. Moderate Study

▶ Isoniazid is predicted to increase the risk of peripheral neuropathy when given with didanosine. Severe Theoretical → Also see TABLE 1 p. 818 → Also see TABLE 12 p. 821

▶ Isoniazid increases the risk of optic neuropathy when given with ethambutol. Severe Study

▶ Isoniazid decreases the effects of levodopa. Moderate Study

▶ Isoniazid is predicted to increase the exposure to lomitapide. Separate administration by 12 hours. Unknown Theoretical → Also see TABLE 1 p. 818

▶ Isoniazid is predicted to increase the risk of peripheral neuropathy when given with stavudine. Severe Theoretical → Also see TABLE 12 p. 821

▶ Isoniazid is predicted to affect the clearance of theophylline. Severe Anecdotal

Isophane insulin → see insulins

Isosorbide dinitrate → see nitrates

Isosorbide mononitrate → see nitrates

Isotretinoin → see retinoids

Isradipine → see calcium channel blockers

Itraconazole → see antifungals, azoles

Ivabradine → see TABLE 6 p. 819 (bradycardia), TABLE 9 p. 820 (QT-interval prolongation)

▶ Antiarrhythmics (dronedarone) are predicted to increase the exposure to ivabradine. Adjust ivabradine dose. Severe Theoretical

▶ Antiepileptics (carbamazepine, fosphenytoin, phenobarbital, phenytoin, primidone) are predicted to decrease the exposure to ivabradine. Adjust dose. Moderate Theoretical

▶ Antifungals, azoles (fluconazole, isavuconazole, posaconazole) are predicted to increase the exposure to ivabradine. Adjust ivabradine dose. Severe Theoretical

▶ Antifungals, azoles (itraconazole, ketoconazole, voriconazole) are predicted to increase the exposure to ivabradine. Avoid. Severe Study

▶ Aprepitant is predicted to increase the exposure to ivabradine. Adjust ivabradine dose. Severe Theoretical

▶ Calcium channel blockers (diltiazem, verapamil) are predicted to increase the exposure to ivabradine. Avoid. Moderate Study → Also see TABLE 6 p. 819

▶ Cobicistat is predicted to increase the exposure to ivabradine. Avoid. Severe Study

▶ Crizotinib is predicted to increase the exposure to ivabradine. Adjust ivabradine dose. Severe Theoretical → Also see TABLE 6 p. 819

▶ Enzalutamide is predicted to decrease the exposure to ivabradine. Adjust dose. Moderate Theoretical

▶ Grapefruit juice is predicted to increase the exposure to ivabradine. Avoid. Moderate Study

▶ HIV-protease inhibitors (atazanavir, darunavir, fosamprenavir, lopinavir, ritonavir, saquinavir, tipranavir) are predicted to increase the exposure to ivabradine. Avoid. Severe Study

▶ HIV-protease inhibitors (indinavir) increase the exposure to ivabradine. Adjust dose. Severe Theoretical

▶ Idelalisib is predicted to increase the exposure to ivabradine. Avoid. Severe Study

▶ Imatinib is predicted to increase the exposure to ivabradine. Adjust ivabradine dose. Severe Theoretical

▶ Macrolides (clarithromycin) are predicted to increase the exposure to ivabradine. Severe Study

▶ Macrolides (erythromycin) are predicted to increase the exposure to ivabradine. Avoid. Severe Theoretical

▶ Netupitant is predicted to increase the exposure to ivabradine. Adjust ivabradine dose. Severe Theoretical

▶ Nilotinib is predicted to increase the exposure to ivabradine. Adjust ivabradine dose. Severe Theoretical

▶ Rifampicin is predicted to decrease the exposure to ivabradine. Adjust dose. Moderate Study

▶ St John's Wort decreases the exposure to ivabradine. Avoid. Moderate Study

Ivacaftor

FOOD AND LIFESTYLE Avoid bitter (Seville) oranges as they are predicted to increase the exposure to ivacaftor.

▶ Antiarrhythmics (dronedarone) are predicted to increase the exposure to ivacaftor. Adjust ivacaftor dose, p. 179. Severe Study

▶ Antiepileptics (carbamazepine, fosphenytoin, phenobarbital, phenytoin, primidone) markedly decrease the exposure to ivacaftor. Avoid. Severe Study

▶ Antifungals, azoles (fluconazole, isavuconazole, posaconazole) are predicted to increase the exposure to ivacaftor. Adjust ivacaftor dose, p. 179. Severe Study

▶ Antifungals, azoles (itraconazole, ketoconazole, voriconazole) are predicted to increase the exposure to ivacaftor. Adjust ivacaftor or lumacaftor with ivacaftor dose, p. 179. Severe Study

▶ Aprepitant is predicted to increase the exposure to ivacaftor. Adjust ivacaftor dose, p. 179. Severe Study

▶ Calcium channel blockers (diltiazem, verapamil) are predicted to increase the exposure to ivacaftor. Adjust ivacaftor dose, p. 179. Severe Study

▶ Cobicistat is predicted to increase the exposure to ivacaftor. Adjust ivacaftor or lumacaftor with ivacaftor dose, p. 179. Severe Study

▶ Ivacaftor is predicted to increase the anticoagulant effect of coumarins (warfarin). Severe Theoretical

▶ Crizotinib is predicted to increase the exposure to ivacaftor. Adjust ivacaftor dose, p. 179. Severe Study

▶ Enzalutamide markedly decreases the exposure to ivacaftor. Avoid. Severe Study

▶ Grapefruit juice is predicted to increase the exposure to ivacaftor. Avoid. Moderate Theoretical

▶ HIV-protease inhibitors (atazanavir, darunavir, fosamprenavir, lopinavir, ritonavir, saquinavir, tipranavir) are predicted to increase the exposure to ivacaftor. Adjust ivacaftor or lumacaftor with ivacaftor dose, p. 179. Severe Study

▶ HIV-protease inhibitors (indinavir) are predicted to increase the exposure to ivacaftor. Adjust ivacaftor dose, p. 179. Severe Study

▶ Idelalisib is predicted to increase the exposure to ivacaftor. Adjust ivacaftor or lumacaftor with ivacaftor dose, p. 179. Severe Study

▶ Imatinib is predicted to increase the exposure to ivacaftor. Adjust ivacaftor dose, p. 179. Severe Study

▶ Ivacaftor is predicted to increase the exposure to lomitapide. Separate administration by 12 hours. Moderate Theoretical

▶ Macrolides (clarithromycin) are predicted to increase the exposure to ivacaftor. Adjust ivacaftor or lumacaftor with ivacaftor dose, p. 179. Severe Study

▶ Macrolides (erythromycin) are predicted to increase the exposure to ivacaftor. Adjust ivacaftor dose, p. 179. Severe Study

▶ Netupitant is predicted to increase the exposure to ivacaftor. Adjust ivacaftor dose, p. 179. Severe Study

▶ Nilotinib is predicted to increase the exposure to ivacaftor. Adjust ivacaftor dose, p. 179. Severe Study

▶ Rifampicin markedly decreases the exposure to ivacaftor. Avoid. Severe Study

▶ St John's Wort is predicted to decrease the exposure to ivacaftor. Avoid. Severe Theoretical

Ivermectin

▶ Ivermectin potentially increases the anticoagulant effect of coumarins. Severe Anecdotal

▶ Levamisole increases the exposure to ivermectin. Moderate Study

Ixazomib

▶ Antiepileptics (carbamazepine, fosphenytoin, phenobarbital, phenytoin, primidone) are predicted to decrease the exposure to ixazomib. Avoid. Severe Study

▶ Enzalutamide is predicted to decrease the exposure to ixazomib. Avoid. Severe Study

- **Rifampicin** is predicted to decrease the exposure to **ixazomib**. Avoid. [Severe] Study
- **St John's Wort** is predicted to decrease the exposure to **ixazomib**. Avoid. [Severe] Theoretical

Ixekizumab → see monoclonal antibodies

Kaolin

- **Kaolin** is predicted to decrease the absorption of **tetracyclines**. [Moderate] Theoretical

Ketamine → see TABLE 8 p. 819 (hypotension), TABLE 11 p. 820 (CNS depressant effects)

- **Memantine** is predicted to increase the risk of CNS side-effects when given with **ketamine**. Avoid. [Severe] Theoretical

Ketoconazole → see antifungals, azoles

Ketoprofen → see NSAIDs

Ketorolac → see NSAIDs

Ketotifen → see antihistamines, sedating

Labetalol → see beta blockers, non-selective

Lacidipine → see calcium channel blockers

Lacosamide → see antiepileptics

Lamivudine → see TABLE 12 p. 821 (peripheral neuropathy)

- **Trimethoprim** slightly increases the exposure to **lamivudine**. [Moderate] Study

Lamotrigine → see antiepileptics

Lanreotide

- **Beta blockers, non-selective** are predicted to increase the risk of bradycardia when given with **lanreotide**. [Moderate] Theoretical
- **Beta blockers, selective** are predicted to increase the risk of bradycardia when given with **lanreotide**. [Moderate] Theoretical
- **Lanreotide** is predicted to decrease the absorption of oral **ciclosporin**. Adjust dose. [Severe] Theoretical

Lansoprazole → see proton pump inhibitors

Lanthanum

- **Lanthanum** is predicted to decrease the absorption of antifungals, azoles (**ketoconazole**). Separate administration by at least 2 hours. [Moderate] Theoretical
- **Lanthanum** is predicted to decrease the absorption of antimalarials (**chloroquine**). Separate administration by at least 2 hours. [Moderate] Theoretical
- **Lanthanum** is predicted to decrease the absorption of **hydroxychloroquine**. Separate administration by at least 2 hours. [Moderate] Theoretical
- **Lanthanum** decreases the absorption of **levothyroxine**. Separate administration by 2 hours. [Moderate] Study
- **Lanthanum** decreases the absorption of **liothyronine**. Separate administration by 2 hours. [Moderate] Study
- **Lanthanum** moderately decreases the exposure to **quinolones**. Quinolones should be taken 2 hours before or 4 hours after **lanthanum**. [Moderate] Study
- **Lanthanum** is predicted to decrease the absorption of **tetracyclines**. Separate administration by 2 hours. [Moderate] Theoretical

Lapatinib → see TABLE 9 p. 820 (QT-interval prolongation)

- **Lapatinib** is predicted to increase the exposure to **afatinib**. Separate administration by 12 hours. [Moderate] Study
- **Lapatinib** is predicted to increase the exposure to **aliskiren**. [Moderate] Theoretical
- **Antacids** are predicted to decrease the absorption of **lapatinib**. Avoid. [Moderate] Theoretical
- **Antiarrhythmics (dronedarone)** are predicted to increase the exposure to **lapatinib**. [Moderate] Study → Also see TABLE 9 p. 820
- **Antiepileptics (carbamazepine, fosphenytoin, phenobarbital, phenytoin, primidone)** are predicted to decrease the exposure to **lapatinib**. Avoid. [Severe] Study
- **Antifungals, azoles (fluconazole, isavuconazole, posaconazole)** are predicted to increase the exposure to **lapatinib**. [Moderate] Study
- **Antifungals, azoles (itraconazole, ketoconazole, voriconazole)** are predicted to increase the exposure to **lapatinib**. Avoid. [Moderate] Study → Also see TABLE 9 p. 820
- **Lapatinib** is predicted to increase the exposure to antihistamines, non-sedating (**fexofenadine**). [Moderate] Theoretical
- **Aprepitant** is predicted to increase the exposure to **lapatinib**. [Moderate] Study
- **Lapatinib** is predicted to increase the exposure to beta blockers, non-selective (**nadolol**). [Moderate] Study

- **Bosentan** is predicted to decrease the exposure to **lapatinib**. Avoid. [Severe] Study
- **Calcium channel blockers (diltiazem, verapamil)** are predicted to increase the exposure to **lapatinib**. [Moderate] Study
- **Lapatinib** is predicted to increase the exposure to **ceritinib**. [Moderate] Theoretical → Also see TABLE 9 p. 820
- **Cobicistat** is predicted to increase the exposure to **lapatinib**. Avoid. [Moderate] Study
- **Lapatinib** is predicted to increase the exposure to **colchicine**. Avoid or adjust colchicine dose. [Moderate] Theoretical
- **Lapatinib** is predicted to increase the risk of bleeding events when given with **coumarins**. Avoid. [Severe] Theoretical
- **Crizotinib** is predicted to increase the exposure to **lapatinib**. [Moderate] Study → Also see TABLE 9 p. 820
- **Lapatinib** is predicted to increase the exposure to **dabigatran**. [Severe] Theoretical
- **Lapatinib** is predicted to increase the exposure to **digoxin**. [Moderate] Theoretical
- **Lapatinib** is predicted to slightly increase the exposure to **edoxaban**. [Severe] Theoretical
- **Efavirenz** is predicted to decrease the exposure to **lapatinib**. Avoid. [Severe] Study
- **Enzalutamide** is predicted to decrease the exposure to **lapatinib**. Avoid. [Severe] Study
- **Lapatinib** is predicted to increase the exposure to **erlotinib**. [Moderate] Theoretical
- **Lapatinib** is predicted to increase the exposure to **everolimus**. [Moderate] Theoretical
- **Lapatinib** is predicted to increase the exposure to **fidaxomicin**. Avoid. [Moderate] Study
- **Grapefruit juice** is predicted to increase the exposure to **lapatinib**. Avoid. [Moderate] Theoretical
- **H₂ receptor antagonists** are predicted to decrease the absorption of **lapatinib**. [Moderate] Theoretical
- **HIV-protease inhibitors (atazanavir, darunavir, fosamprenavir, lopinavir, ritonavir, saquinavir, tipranavir)** are predicted to increase the exposure to **lapatinib**. Avoid. [Moderate] Study → Also see TABLE 9 p. 820
- **HIV-protease inhibitors (indinavir)** are predicted to increase the exposure to **lapatinib**. [Moderate] Study
- **Idelalisib** is predicted to increase the exposure to **lapatinib**. Avoid. [Moderate] Study
- **Imatinib** is predicted to increase the exposure to **lapatinib**. [Moderate] Study
- **Lapatinib** is predicted to increase the exposure to **lomitapide**. Separate administration by 12 hours. [Moderate] Theoretical
- **Lapatinib** is predicted to increase the exposure to **loperamide**. [Moderate] Theoretical
- **Macrolides (clarithromycin)** are predicted to increase the exposure to **lapatinib**. Avoid. [Moderate] Study → Also see TABLE 9 p. 820
- **Macrolides (erythromycin)** are predicted to increase the exposure to **lapatinib**. [Moderate] Theoretical
- **Netupitant** is predicted to increase the exposure to **lapatinib**. [Moderate] Study
- **Nevirapine** is predicted to decrease the exposure to **lapatinib**. Avoid. [Severe] Study
- **Nilotinib** is predicted to increase the exposure to **lapatinib**. [Moderate] Study → Also see TABLE 9 p. 820
- **Lapatinib** is predicted to increase the exposure to **nintedanib**. [Moderate] Theoretical
- **Lapatinib** is predicted to increase the risk of bleeding events when given with **phenindione**. [Severe] Theoretical
- **Rifampicin** is predicted to decrease the exposure to **lapatinib**. Avoid. [Severe] Study
- **Lapatinib** is predicted to increase the exposure to **sirolimus**. [Moderate] Theoretical
- **St John's Wort** is predicted to decrease the exposure to **lapatinib**. Avoid. [Severe] Study
- **Lapatinib** slightly increases the exposure to taxanes (**paclitaxel**). [Severe] Study
- **Tedizolid** is predicted to increase the exposure to **lapatinib**. Avoid. [Moderate] Theoretical
- **Lapatinib** is predicted to increase the exposure to **topotecan**. [Severe] Study

A1

Interactions | Appendix 1

Lapatinib (continued)

▸ Lapatinib is predicted to increase the concentration of trametinib. Moderate Theoretical

▸ Lapatinib is predicted to increase the exposure to venetoclax. Avoid or monitor for toxicity. Severe Theoretical

Laronidase

▸ Antimalarials **(chloroquine)** are predicted to decrease the exposure to **laronidase**. Avoid simultaneous administration. Severe Theoretical

▸ Hydroxychloroquine is predicted to decrease the exposure to **laronidase**. Avoid simultaneous administration. Severe Theoretical

Ledipasvir

▸ Antacids are predicted to decrease the exposure to **ledipasvir**. Separate administration by 4 hours. Severe Theoretical

▸ Ledipasvir increases the risk of severe bradycardia or heart block when given with antiarrhythmics **(amiodarone)**. Refer to specialist literature. Severe Anecdotal

▸ Antiepileptics **(carbamazepine)** are predicted to decrease the exposure to **ledipasvir**. Avoid Severe Theoretical

▸ Calcium salts **(calcium carbonate)** are predicted to decrease the exposure to **ledipasvir**. Separate administration by 4 hours. Moderate Theoretical

▸ H₂ receptor antagonists are predicted to decrease the exposure to **ledipasvir**. Adjust dose, see sofosbuvir with ledipasvir. Moderate Study

▸ Proton pump inhibitors are predicted to decrease the exposure to **ledipasvir**. Adjust dose, see sofosbuvir with ledipasvir. Moderate Theoretical

▸ Rifampicin is predicted to decrease the exposure to **ledipasvir**. Avoid. Severe Theoretical

▸ Ledipasvir moderately increases the exposure to simeprevir and simeprevir slightly increases the exposure to **ledipasvir**. Avoid. Severe Study

▸ St John's Wort is predicted to decrease the exposure to **ledipasvir**. Avoid. Severe Theoretical

▸ Ledipasvir is predicted to increase the exposure to statins **(atorvastatin, simvastatin)**. Monitor and adjust dose. Moderate Theoretical

▸ Ledipasvir (with sofosbuvir) is predicted to increase the exposure to statins **(fluvastatin, pravastatin)**. Monitor and adjust dose. Moderate Theoretical

▸ Ledipasvir is predicted to increase the exposure to statins **(rosuvastatin)**. Avoid. Severe Theoretical

▸ Ledipasvir (with sofosbuvir) slightly increases the exposure to tenofovir. Moderate Study

Leflunomide → see TABLE 1 p. 818 (hepatotoxicity), TABLE 15 p. 821 (myelosuppression)

> **PHARMACOLOGY** Leflunomide has a long half-life; washout procedure recommended before switching to other DMARDs (consult product literature).

▸ Leflunomide increases the anticoagulant effect of coumarins. Severe Anecdotal

▸ Live vaccines are predicted to increase the risk of generalised infection (possibly life-threatening) when given with **leflunomide**. Public Health England advises avoid. Severe Theoretical

Lenalidomide → see TABLE 1 p. 818 (hepatotoxicity), TABLE 15 p. 821 (myelosuppression), TABLE 5 p. 818 (thromboembolism)

▸ Combined hormonal contraceptives are predicted to increase the risk of venous thromboembolism when given with **lenalidomide**. Avoid. Severe Theoretical

▸ Hormone replacement therapy is predicted to increase the risk of venous thromboembolism when given with **lenalidomide**. Severe Theoretical

Lercanidipine → see calcium channel blockers

Levamisole

> **FOOD AND LIFESTYLE** Disulfiram-like reaction might occur on consumption of alcohol.

▸ Albendazole slightly decreases the exposure to **levamisole** and **levamisole** moderately decreases the exposure to albendazole. Moderate Study

▸ Levamisole increases the exposure to ivermectin. Moderate Study

Levetiracetam → see antiepileptics

Levobunolol → see beta blockers, non-selective

Levobupivacaine → see anaesthetics, local

Levocetirizine → see antihistamines, non-sedating

Levodopa → see TABLE 8 p. 819 (hypotension)

> **GENERAL INFORMATION** Drugs with antimuscarinic effects might reduce the absorption of levodopa.

▸ Amisulpride is predicted to decrease the effects of **levodopa**. Avoid. Severe Theoretical

▸ Antiepileptics **(fosphenytoin, phenytoin)** decrease the effects of **levodopa**. Moderate Study

▸ Aripiprazole is predicted to decrease the effects of **levodopa**. Severe Theoretical → Also see TABLE 8 p. 819

▸ Asenapine is predicted to decrease the effects of **levodopa**. Adjust dose. Severe Theoretical → Also see TABLE 8 p. 819

▸ Baclofen is predicted to increase the risk of side-effects when given with **levodopa**. Severe Anecdotal → Also see TABLE 8 p. 819

▸ Benperidol is predicted to decrease the effects of **levodopa**. Severe Study → Also see TABLE 8 p. 819

▸ Bupropion increases the risk of side-effects when given with **levodopa**. Moderate Study

▸ Clozapine is predicted to decrease the effects of **levodopa**. Severe Theoretical → Also see TABLE 8 p. 819

▸ Droperidol decreases the effects of **levodopa**. Severe Study → Also see TABLE 8 p. 819

▸ Entacapone increases the exposure to **levodopa**. Monitor side effects and adjust dose. Moderate Study

▸ Flupentixol decreases the effects of **levodopa**. Avoid or monitor worsening parkinsonian symptoms. Severe Theoretical → Also see TABLE 8 p. 819

▸ Haloperidol decreases the effects of **levodopa**. Severe Study → Also see TABLE 8 p. 819

▸ Iron (oral) decreases the absorption of **levodopa**. Moderate Study

▸ Isoniazid decreases the effects of **levodopa**. Moderate Study

▸ Levodopa is predicted to increase the risk of elevated blood pressure when given with linezolid. Avoid. Severe Theoretical

▸ Loxapine is predicted to decrease the effects of **levodopa**. Severe Theoretical → Also see TABLE 8 p. 819

▸ Lurasidone is predicted to decrease the effects of **levodopa**. Severe Theoretical → Also see TABLE 8 p. 819

▸ Memantine is predicted to increase the effects of **levodopa**. Moderate Theoretical

▸ Metoclopramide decreases the effects of **levodopa**. Avoid. Moderate Study

▸ Levodopa increases the risk of side-effects when given with moclobemide. Moderate Study

▸ Levodopa increases the risk of a hypertensive crisis when given with monoamine-oxidase A and B inhibitors, irreversible. Avoid and for 14 days after stopping the MAOI. Severe Study → Also see TABLE 8 p. 819

▸ Monoamine-oxidase B inhibitors are predicted to increase the effects of **levodopa**. Adjust dose. Mild Study → Also see TABLE 8 p. 819

▸ Olanzapine decreases the effects of **levodopa**. Avoid or monitor worsening parkinsonian symptoms. Severe Anecdotal → Also see TABLE 8 p. 819

▸ Opicapone increases the exposure to **levodopa**. Adjust **levodopa** dose. Moderate Study

▸ Paliperidone is predicted to decrease the effects of **levodopa**. Severe Theoretical → Also see TABLE 8 p. 819

▸ Phenothiazines decrease the effects of **levodopa**. Avoid or monitor worsening parkinsonian symptoms. Severe Study → Also see TABLE 8 p. 819

▸ Pimozide decreases the effects of **levodopa**. Severe Theoretical → Also see TABLE 8 p. 819

▸ Quetiapine decreases the effects of **levodopa**. Severe Anecdotal → Also see TABLE 8 p. 819

▸ Risperidone is predicted to decrease the effects of **levodopa**. Avoid or adjust dose. Severe Anecdotal → Also see TABLE 8 p. 819

▸ Sulpiride is predicted to decrease the effects of **levodopa**. Avoid. Severe Theoretical → Also see TABLE 8 p. 819

▸ Tetrabenazine is predicted to decrease the effects of **levodopa**. Use with caution or avoid. Moderate Theoretical

▶ Tolcapone increases the exposure to **levodopa**. Monitor and adjust dose. [Moderate] Study

▶ Zuclopenthixol is predicted to decrease the effects of **levodopa**. Avoid or monitor worsening parkinsonian symptoms. [Severe] Theoretical → Also see TABLE 8 p. 819

Levofloxacin → see quinolones

Levofolinic acid → see folates

Levomepromazine → see phenothiazines

Levonorgestrel

▶ Antiepileptics (carbamazepine, eslicarbazepine, fosphenytoin, oxcarbazepine, perampanel, phenobarbital, phenytoin, primidone, rufinamide, topiramate) are predicted to decrease the efficacy of **levonorgestrel**. For FSRH guidance, see Contraceptives, interactions p. 474. [Severe] Theoretical

▶ Aprepitant is predicted to decrease the efficacy of **levonorgestrel**. For FSRH guidance, see Contraceptives, interactions p. 474. [Severe] Theoretical

▶ Bosentan is predicted to decrease the efficacy of **levonorgestrel**. For FSRH guidance, see Contraceptives, interactions p. 474. [Severe] Theoretical

▶ Efavirenz is predicted to decrease the efficacy of **levonorgestrel**. For FSRH guidance, see Contraceptives, interactions p. 474. [Severe] Theoretical

▶ Fosaprepitant is predicted to decrease the efficacy of **levonorgestrel**. For FSRH guidance, see Contraceptives, interactions p. 474. [Severe] Theoretical

▶ Griseofulvin potentially decreases the efficacy of oral **levonorgestrel**. For FSRH guidance, see Contraceptives, interactions p. 474. [Severe] Anecdotal

▶ HIV-protease inhibitors (ritonavir) are predicted to decrease the efficacy of **levonorgestrel**. For FSRH guidance, see Contraceptives, interactions p. 474. [Severe] Theoretical

▶ Modafinil is predicted to decrease the efficacy of **levonorgestrel**. For FSRH guidance, see Contraceptives, interactions p. 474. [Severe] Theoretical

▶ Nevirapine is predicted to decrease the efficacy of **levonorgestrel**. For FSRH guidance, see Contraceptives, interactions p. 474. [Severe] Theoretical

▶ Rifabutin is predicted to decrease the efficacy of **levonorgestrel**. For FSRH guidance, see Contraceptives, interactions p. 474. [Severe] Theoretical

▶ Rifampicin is predicted to decrease the efficacy of **levonorgestrel**. For FSRH guidance, see Contraceptives, interactions p. 474. [Severe] Theoretical

▶ St John's Wort is predicted to decrease the efficacy of **levonorgestrel**. MHRA advises avoid. For FSRH guidance, see Contraceptives, interactions p. 474. [Severe] Theoretical

▶ Sugammadex is predicted to decrease the exposure to **levonorgestrel**. Use additional contraceptive precautions. [Severe] Theoretical

▶ Ulipristal is predicted to decrease the efficacy of **levonorgestrel**. Avoid. [Severe] Theoretical

Levothyroxine

▶ Antacids are predicted to decrease the absorption of **levothyroxine**. Separate administration by at least 4 hours. [Moderate] Anecdotal

▶ Antiarrhythmics (amiodarone) increase the risk of thyroid dysfunction when given with **levothyroxine**. Avoid. [Moderate] Study

▶ Antiepileptics (carbamazepine) increase the risk of hypothyroidism when given with **levothyroxine**. Monitor and adjust dose. [Moderate] Study

▶ Antiepileptics (fosphenytoin, phenytoin) increase the risk of hypothyroidism when given with **levothyroxine**. [Moderate] Study

▶ Antiepileptics (phenobarbital, primidone) are predicted to decrease the effects of **levothyroxine**. [Moderate] Theoretical

▶ Oral calcium salts are predicted to decrease the absorption of **levothyroxine**. Separate administration by at least 4 hours. [Moderate] Anecdotal

▶ Levothyroxine is predicted to affect the concentration of digoxin. Monitor and adjust dose. [Moderate] Theoretical

▶ Oral Hormone replacement therapy is predicted to decrease the effects of **levothyroxine**. [Moderate] Theoretical

▶ Iron (oral) decreases the absorption of **levothyroxine**. Separate administration by at least 4 hours. [Moderate] Study

▶ Lanthanum decreases the absorption of **levothyroxine**. Separate administration by 2 hours. [Moderate] Study

▶ Polystyrene sulfonate is predicted to decrease the absorption of **levothyroxine**. Separate administration by at least 4 hours. [Moderate] Study

▶ Sucralfate decreases the absorption of **levothyroxine**. Separate administration by at least 4 hours. [Moderate] Study

Lidocaine → see antiarrhythmics

Linagliptin → see TABLE 14 p. 821 (antidiabetic drugs)

▶ Antiepileptics (carbamazepine, fosphenytoin, phenobarbital, phenytoin, primidone) are predicted to decrease the exposure to **linagliptin**. [Moderate] Study

▶ Enzalutamide is predicted to decrease the exposure to **linagliptin**. [Moderate] Study

▶ Linagliptin is predicted to increase the exposure to lomitapide. Separate administration by 12 hours. [Moderate] Theoretical

▶ Rifampicin is predicted to decrease the exposure to **linagliptin**. [Moderate] Study

Linezolid → see TABLE 15 p. 821 (myelosuppression), TABLE 13 p. 821 (serotonin syndrome)

FOOD AND LIFESTYLE Patients taking linezolid should avoid consuming large amounts of tyramine-rich foods (such as mature cheese, salami, pickled herring, Bovril®, Oxo®, Marmite® or any similar meat or yeast extract or fermented soya bean extract, and some beers, lagers or wines).

▶ Beta$_2$ agonists are predicted to increase the risk of elevated blood pressure when given with **linezolid**. Avoid. [Severe] Theoretical

▶ Bupropion is predicted to increase the risk of intraoperative hypertension when given with **linezolid**. [Severe] Anecdotal → Also see TABLE 13 p. 821

▶ Buspirone is predicted to increase the risk of elevated blood pressure when given with **linezolid**. Avoid. [Severe] Theoretical → Also see TABLE 13 p. 821

▶ Levodopa is predicted to increase the risk of elevated blood pressure when given with **linezolid**. Avoid. [Severe] Theoretical

▶ Methylphenidate is predicted to increase the risk of elevated blood pressure when given with **linezolid**. Avoid. [Severe] Theoretical

▶ Moclobemide is predicted to increase the risk of side-effects when given with **linezolid**. Avoid and for 14 days after stopping moclobemide. [Severe] Theoretical → Also see TABLE 13 p. 821

▶ Monoamine-oxidase A and B inhibitors, irreversible are predicted to increase the risk of side-effects when given with **linezolid**. Avoid and for 14 days after stopping the MAOI. [Severe] Theoretical → Also see TABLE 13 p. 821

▶ Monoamine-oxidase B inhibitors (rasagiline, selegiline) are predicted to increase the risk of side-effects when given with **linezolid**. Avoid and for 14 days after stopping the MAOI. [Severe] Theoretical → Also see TABLE 13 p. 821

▶ Monoamine-oxidase B inhibitors (safinamide) are predicted to increase the risk of side-effects when given with **linezolid**. Avoid and for 1 week after stopping safinamide. [Severe] Theoretical → Also see TABLE 13 p. 821

▶ Reboxetine is predicted to increase the risk of a hypertensive crisis when given with **linezolid**. Avoid. [Severe] Theoretical

▶ Rifampicin slightly decreases the exposure to **linezolid**. [Moderate] Study

▶ Sympathomimetics, inotropic (dobutamine, dopamine) are predicted to increase the risk of elevated blood pressure when given with **linezolid**. Avoid. [Severe] Theoretical

▶ Sympathomimetics, vasoconstrictor (adrenaline/epinephrine, ephedrine, isometheptene, noradrenaline/norepinephrine, phenylephrine) are predicted to increase the risk of elevated blood pressure when given with **linezolid**. Avoid. [Severe] Theoretical

▶ Sympathomimetics, vasoconstrictor (pseudoephedrine) increase the risk of elevated blood pressure when given with **linezolid**. Avoid. [Severe] Study

Liothyronine

▶ Antiarrhythmics (amiodarone) are predicted to increase the risk of thyroid dysfunction when given with **liothyronine**. Avoid. [Moderate] Theoretical

A1

Interactions | Appendix 1

Liothyronine (continued)

▶ Antiepileptics **(fosphenytoin, phenytoin)** are predicted to increase the risk of hypothyroidism when given with **liothyronine**. Moderate Theoretical

▶ Antiepileptics **(phenobarbital, primidone)** are predicted to decrease the effects of **liothyronine**. Moderate Theoretical

▶ **Liothyronine** is predicted to affect the concentration of digoxin. Monitor and adjust dose. Moderate Theoretical

▶ Oral **Hormone replacement therapy** is predicted to decrease the effects of **liothyronine**. Moderate Theoretical

▶ **Lanthanum** decreases the absorption of **liothyronine**. Separate administration by 2 hours. Moderate Study

Liraglutide → see TABLE 14 p. 821 (antidiabetic drugs)

Lisdexamfetamine → see amfetamines

Lisinopril → see ACE inhibitors

Lithium → see TABLE 13 p. 821 (serotonin syndrome), TABLE 9 p. 820 (QT-interval prolongation)

▶ **ACE inhibitors** are predicted to increase the concentration of **lithium**. Monitor and adjust dose. Severe Anecdotal

▶ **Acetazolamide** alters the concentration of **lithium**. Severe Anecdotal

▶ **Aldosterone antagonists (eplerenone)** are predicted to increase the concentration of **lithium**. Avoid. Moderate Theoretical

▶ **Aldosterone antagonists (spironolactone)** potentially increase the concentration of **lithium**. Moderate Study

▶ **Aminophylline** is predicted to decrease the concentration of **lithium**. Moderate Theoretical

▶ **Angiotensin-II receptor antagonists** potentially increase the concentration of **lithium**. Monitor concentration and adjust dose. Severe Anecdotal

▶ Antiepileptics **(carbamazepine)** increase the risk of neurotoxicity when given with **lithium**. Severe Anecdotal

▶ Antiepileptics **(oxcarbazepine)** are predicted to increase the risk of neurotoxicity when given with **lithium**. Severe Theoretical

▶ **Calcitonin (salmon)** decreases the concentration of **lithium**. Monitor **lithium** (lithium carbonate, lithium citrate) concentration and adjust dose. Moderate Study

▶ **Calcium channel blockers (diltiazem, verapamil)** are predicted to increase the risk of neurotoxicity when given with **lithium**. Severe Anecdotal

▶ **Loop diuretics** increase the concentration of **lithium**. Monitor and adjust dose. Severe Study

▶ **Methyldopa** increases the risk of neurotoxicity when given with **lithium**. Severe Anecdotal

▶ **NSAIDs** increase the concentration of **lithium**. Monitor and adjust **lithium** (lithium carbonate, lithium citrate) dose. Severe Study

▶ **Phenothiazines** potentially increase the risk of neurotoxicity when given with **lithium**. Severe Anecdotal → Also see TABLE 9 p. 820

▶ **Potassium-sparing diuretics (triamterene)** potentially increase the clearance of **lithium**. Moderate Study

▶ **Quetiapine** potentially increases the risk of neurotoxicity when given with **lithium**. Severe Anecdotal

▶ **Risperidone** potentially increases the risk of neurotoxicity when given with **lithium**. Severe Anecdotal → Also see TABLE 9 p. 820

▶ **Sodium bicarbonate** decreases the concentration of **lithium**. Severe Anecdotal

▶ **Sulpiride** potentially increases the risk of neurotoxicity when given with **lithium**. Severe Anecdotal → Also see TABLE 9 p. 820

▶ **Theophylline** is predicted to decrease the concentration of **lithium**. Moderate Anecdotal

▶ **Thiazide diuretics** increase the concentration of **lithium**. Avoid or adjust **lithium** (lithium carbonate, lithium citrate) dose and monitor **lithium** (lithium carbonate, lithium citrate) concentration. Severe Study

▶ **Tricyclic antidepressants** potentially increase the risk of neurotoxicity when given with **lithium**. Severe Anecdotal → Also see TABLE 9 p. 820 → Also see TABLE 13 p. 821

▶ **Zuclopenthixol** potentially increases the risk of neurotoxicity when given with **lithium**. Severe Anecdotal → Also see TABLE 9 p. 820

Live vaccines

Bacillus Calmette-Guérin vaccine · influenza vaccine · measles, mumps and rubella vaccine, live · rotavirus vaccine · typhoid vaccine · varicella-zoster vaccine · yellow fever vaccine, live

ROUTE-SPECIFIC INFORMATION **Oral typhoid vaccine** is inactivated by concurrent administration of antibacterials or antimalarials: antibacterials should be avoided for 3 days before and after oral typhoid vaccination; mefloquine should be avoided for at least 12 hours before or after oral typhoid vaccination; for other antimalarials oral typhoid vaccine vaccination should be completed at least 3 days before the first dose of the antimalarial (except proguanil hydrochloride with atovaquone, which can be given concurrently).

▶ **Live vaccines** are predicted to increase the risk of generalised infection (possibly life-threatening) when given with **abatacept**. Public Health England advises avoid. Severe Theoretical

▶ **Live vaccines** are predicted to increase the risk of generalised infection (possibly life-threatening) when given with **alkylating agents**. Public Health England advises avoid. Severe Theoretical

▶ **Live vaccines** are predicted to increase the risk of generalised infection (possibly life-threatening) when given with **amsacrine**. Public Health England advises avoid. Severe Theoretical

▶ **Live vaccines** are predicted to increase the risk of generalised infection (possibly life-threatening) when given with **anakinra**. Public Health England advises avoid. Severe Theoretical

▶ **Live vaccines** are predicted to increase the risk of generalised infection (possibly life-threatening) when given with **anthracyclines**. Public Health England advises avoid. Severe Theoretical

▶ **Live vaccines** are predicted to increase the risk of generalised infection (possibly life-threatening) when given with **azathioprine**. Public Health England advises avoid. Severe Theoretical

▶ **Live vaccines** are predicted to increase the risk of generalised infection (possibly life-threatening) when given with **belatacept**. Public Health England advises avoid. Severe Theoretical

▶ **Live vaccines** are predicted to increase the risk of generalised infection (possibly life-threatening) when given with **bleomycin**. Public Health England advises avoid. Severe Theoretical

▶ **Live vaccines** are predicted to increase the risk of generalised infection (possibly life-threatening) when given with **capecitabine**. Public Health England advises avoid. Severe Theoretical

▶ **Live vaccines** are predicted to increase the risk of generalised infection (possibly life-threatening) when given with **ciclosporin**. Public Health England advises avoid. Severe Theoretical

▶ **Live vaccines** are predicted to increase the risk of generalised infection (possibly life-threatening) when given with **cladribine**. Public Health England advises avoid. Severe Theoretical

▶ **Live vaccines** are predicted to increase the risk of generalised infection (possibly life-threatening) when given with **clofarabine**. Public Health England advises avoid. Severe Theoretical

▶ **Live vaccines** are predicted to increase the risk of generalised infection (possibly life-threatening) when given with **corticosteroids** (high-dose). Public Health England advises avoid. Severe Theoretical

▶ **Influenza vaccine** potentially increases the risk of bleeding events when given with **coumarins**. Severe Anecdotal

▶ **Live vaccines** are predicted to increase the risk of generalised infection (possibly life-threatening) when given with **cytarabine**. Public Health England advises avoid. Severe Theoretical

▶ **Live vaccines** are predicted to increase the risk of generalised infection (possibly life-threatening) when given with dactinomycin. Public Health England advises avoid. Severe Theoretical

▸ **Live vaccines** are predicted to increase the risk of generalised infection (possibly life-threatening) when given with dimethyl fumarate. Public Health England advises avoid. Severe Theoretical

▸ **Live vaccines** are predicted to increase the risk of generalised infection (possibly life-threatening) when given with etanercept. Public Health England advises avoid. Severe Theoretical

▸ **Live vaccines** are predicted to increase the risk of generalised infection (possibly life-threatening) when given with etoposide. Public Health England advises avoid. Severe Theoretical

▸ **Live vaccines** are predicted to increase the risk of generalised infection (possibly life-threatening) when given with everolimus. Public Health England advises avoid. Severe Theoretical

▸ **Live vaccines** are predicted to increase the risk of generalised infection (possibly life-threatening) when given with fingolimod. Public Health England advises avoid. Severe Theoretical

▸ **Live vaccines** are predicted to increase the risk of generalised infection (possibly life-threatening) when given with fludarabine. Public Health England advises avoid. Severe Theoretical

▸ **Live vaccines** are predicted to increase the risk of generalised infection (possibly life-threatening) when given with fluorouracil. Public Health England advises avoid. Severe Theoretical

▸ **Live vaccines** are predicted to increase the risk of generalised infection (possibly life-threatening) when given with gemcitabine. Public Health England advises avoid. Severe Theoretical

▸ **Live vaccines** are predicted to increase the risk of generalised infection (possibly life-threatening) when given with hydroxycarbamide. Public Health England advises avoid. Severe Theoretical

▸ **Live vaccines** are predicted to increase the risk of generalised infection (possibly life-threatening) when given with irinotecan. Public Health England advises avoid. Severe Theoretical

▸ **Live vaccines** are predicted to increase the risk of generalised infection (possibly life-threatening) when given with iron chelators (dexrazoxane). Avoid. Severe Theoretical

▸ **Live vaccines** are predicted to increase the risk of generalised infection (possibly life-threatening) when given with leflunomide. Public Health England advises avoid. Severe Theoretical

▸ **Live vaccines** are predicted to increase the risk of generalised infection (possibly life-threatening) when given with mercaptopurine. Public Health England advises avoid. Severe Theoretical

▸ **Live vaccines** are predicted to increase the risk of generalised infection (possibly life-threatening) when given with methotrexate. Public Health England advises avoid. Severe Theoretical

▸ **Live vaccines** are predicted to increase the risk of generalised infection (possibly life-threatening) when given with mitomycin. Public Health England advises avoid. Severe Theoretical

▸ **Live vaccines** are predicted to increase the risk of generalised infection (possibly life-threatening) when given with monoclonal antibodies. Public Health England advises avoid. Severe Theoretical

▸ **Live vaccines** are predicted to increase the risk of generalised infection (possibly life-threatening) when given with mycophenolate. Public Health England advises avoid. Severe Theoretical

▸ **Live vaccines** are predicted to increase the risk of generalised infection (possibly life-threatening) when given with pemetrexed. Public Health England advises avoid. Severe Theoretical

▸ **Live vaccines** are predicted to increase the risk of generalised infection (possibly life-threatening) when given with platinum

compounds. Public Health England advises avoid. Severe Theoretical

▸ **Live vaccines** are predicted to increase the risk of generalised infection (possibly life-threatening) when given with procarbazine. Public Health England advises avoid. Severe Theoretical

▸ **Live vaccines** are predicted to increase the risk of generalised infection (possibly life-threatening) when given with raltitrexed. Public Health England advises avoid. Severe Theoretical

▸ **Live vaccines** are predicted to increase the risk of generalised infection (possibly life-threatening) when given with sirolimus. Public Health England advises avoid. Severe Theoretical

▸ **Live vaccines** are predicted to increase the risk of generalised infection (possibly life-threatening) when given with tacrolimus. Public Health England advises avoid. Severe Theoretical

▸ **Live vaccines** are predicted to increase the risk of generalised infection (possibly life-threatening) when given with taxanes (docetaxel, paclitaxel). Public Health England advises avoid. Severe Theoretical

▸ **Live vaccines** are predicted to increase the risk of generalised infection (possibly life-threatening) when given with tegafur. Public Health England advises avoid. Severe Theoretical

▸ **Live vaccines** are predicted to increase the risk of generalised infection (possibly life-threatening) when given with temsirolimus. Public Health England advises avoid. Severe Theoretical

▸ **Live vaccines** are predicted to increase the risk of generalised infection (possibly life-threatening) when given with teriflunomide. Public Health England advises avoid. Severe Theoretical

▸ **Live vaccines** are predicted to increase the risk of generalised infection (possibly life-threatening) when given with tioguanine. Public Health England advises avoid. Severe Theoretical

▸ **Live vaccines** are predicted to increase the risk of generalised infection (possibly life-threatening) when given with topotecan. Public Health England advises avoid. Severe Theoretical

▸ **Live vaccines** are predicted to increase the risk of generalised infection (possibly life-threatening) when given with trabectedin. Public Health England advises avoid. Severe Theoretical

▸ Venetoclax potentially decreases the efficacy of **live vaccines**. Avoid. Severe Theoretical

▸ **Live vaccines** are predicted to increase the risk of generalised infection (possibly life-threatening) when given with vinca alkaloids. Public Health England advises avoid. Severe Theoretical

Lixisenatide → see TABLE 14 p. 821 (antidiabetic drugs)

SEPARATION OF ADMINISTRATION Some orally administered drugs should be taken at least 1 hour before, or 4 hours after, lixisenatide injection.

Lofepramine → see tricyclic antidepressants

Lofexidine → see TABLE 8 p. 819 (hypotension), TABLE 9 p. 820 (QT-interval prolongation), TABLE 11 p. 820 (CNS depressant effects)

Lomitapide → see TABLE 1 p. 818 (hepatotoxicity)

FOOD AND LIFESTYLE Bitter (Seville) orange is predicted to increase the exposure to lomitapide; separate administration by 12 hours.

▸ Alprazolam is predicted to increase the exposure to **lomitapide**. Separate administration by 12 hours. Moderate Theoretical

▸ Antiarrhythmics (amiodarone) are predicted to increase the exposure to **lomitapide**. Separate administration by 12 hours. Moderate Theoretical

▸ Antiarrhythmics (dronedarone) are predicted to increase the exposure to **lomitapide**. Avoid. Moderate Theoretical

▸ Antiepileptics (carbamazepine, fosphenytoin, phenobarbital, phenytoin, primidone) are predicted to decrease the exposure to **lomitapide**. Monitor and adjust dose. Moderate Theoretical
→ Also see TABLE 1 p. 818

A1

Interactions | **Appendix 1**

Lomitapide (continued)

▶ Antifungals, azoles **(clotrimazole)** are predicted to increase the exposure to **lomitapide**. Separate administration by 12 hours. Moderate Theoretical

▶ Antifungals, azoles **(fluconazole, isavuconazole, posaconazole)** are predicted to increase the exposure to **lomitapide**. Avoid. Moderate Theoretical → Also see TABLE 1 p. 818

▶ Antifungals, azoles **(itraconazole, ketoconazole, voriconazole)** are predicted to markedly increase the exposure to **lomitapide**. Avoid. Severe Study → Also see TABLE 1 p. 818

▶ **Aprepitant** is predicted to increase the exposure to **lomitapide**. Avoid. Moderate Theoretical

▶ **Bicalutamide** is predicted to increase the exposure to **lomitapide**. Separate administration by 12 hours. Moderate Theoretical

▶ Calcium channel blockers **(amlodipine, lacidipine)** are predicted to increase the exposure to **lomitapide**. Separate administration by 12 hours. Moderate Theoretical

▶ Calcium channel blockers **(diltiazem, verapamil)** are predicted to increase the exposure to **lomitapide**. Avoid. Moderate Theoretical

▶ **Ciclosporin** is predicted to increase the exposure to **lomitapide**. Separate administration by 12 hours. Moderate Theoretical

▶ **Cilostazol** is predicted to increase the exposure to **lomitapide**. Separate administration by 12 hours. Moderate Theoretical

▶ **Cobicistat** is predicted to markedly increase the exposure to **lomitapide**. Avoid. Severe Study

▶ Oral **combined hormonal contraceptives** slightly increase the exposure to **lomitapide**. Separate administration by 12 hours. Moderate Theoretical

▶ **Lomitapide** increases the exposure to coumarins **(warfarin)**. Monitor INR and adjust **warfarin** dose. Severe Study

▶ **Crizotinib** is predicted to increase the exposure to **lomitapide**. Avoid. Moderate Theoretical

▶ **Enzalutamide** is predicted to decrease the exposure to **lomitapide**. Monitor and adjust dose. Moderate Theoretical

▶ **Everolimus** is predicted to increase the exposure to **lomitapide**. Separate administration by 12 hours. Moderate Theoretical

▶ **Fosaprepitant** is predicted to increase the exposure to **lomitapide**. Separate administration by 12 hours. Moderate Theoretical

▶ **Grapefruit juice** is predicted to increase the exposure to **lomitapide**. Separate administration by 12 hours. Moderate Theoretical

▶ H_2 receptor antagonists **(cimetidine, ranitidine)** are predicted to increase the exposure to **lomitapide**. Separate administration by 12 hours. Moderate Theoretical

▶ HIV-protease inhibitors **(atazanavir, darunavir, fosamprenavir, lopinavir, ritonavir, saquinavir, tipranavir)** are predicted to markedly increase the exposure to **lomitapide**. Avoid. Severe Study

▶ HIV-protease inhibitors **(indinavir)** are predicted to increase the exposure to **lomitapide**. Avoid. Moderate Theoretical

▶ **Idelalisib** is predicted to markedly increase the exposure to **lomitapide**. Avoid. Severe Study

▶ **Imatinib** is predicted to increase the exposure to **lomitapide**. Avoid. Moderate Theoretical

▶ **Isoniazid** is predicted to increase the exposure to **lomitapide**. Separate administration by 12 hours. Unknown Theoretical → Also see TABLE 1 p. 818

▶ **Ivacaftor** is predicted to increase the exposure to **lomitapide**. Separate administration by 12 hours. Moderate Theoretical

▶ **Lapatinib** is predicted to increase the exposure to **lomitapide**. Separate administration by 12 hours. Moderate Theoretical

▶ **Linagliptin** is predicted to increase the exposure to **lomitapide**. Separate administration by 12 hours. Moderate Theoretical

▶ Macrolides **(azithromycin)** are predicted to increase the exposure to **lomitapide**. Separate administration by 12 hours. Moderate Theoretical

▶ Macrolides **(clarithromycin)** are predicted to markedly increase the exposure to **lomitapide**. Avoid. Severe Study

▶ Macrolides **(erythromycin)** are predicted to increase the exposure to **lomitapide**. Avoid. Moderate Theoretical

▶ **Netupitant** is predicted to increase the exposure to **lomitapide**. Avoid. Moderate Theoretical

▶ **Nilotinib** is predicted to increase the exposure to **lomitapide**. Avoid. Moderate Theoretical

▶ **Pazopanib** is predicted to increase the exposure to **lomitapide**. Separate administration by 12 hours. Moderate Theoretical

▶ **Peppermint oil** is predicted to increase the exposure to **lomitapide**. Separate administration by 12 hours. Moderate Theoretical

▶ **Propiverine** is predicted to increase the exposure to **lomitapide**. Separate administration by 12 hours. Moderate Theoretical

▶ **Ranolazine** is predicted to increase the exposure to **lomitapide**. Separate administration by 12 hours. Moderate Theoretical

▶ **Rifampicin** is predicted to decrease the exposure to **lomitapide**. Monitor and adjust dose. Moderate Theoretical

▶ SSRIs **(fluoxetine)** are predicted to increase the exposure to **lomitapide**. Separate administration by 12 hours. Unknown Theoretical

▶ SSRIs **(fluvoxamine)** are predicted to increase the exposure to **lomitapide**. Separate administration by 12 hours. Moderate Theoretical

▶ **Lomitapide** increases the exposure to statins **(atorvastatin)**. Adjust **lomitapide** dose or separate administration by 12 hours. Mild Study → Also see TABLE 1 p. 818

▶ **Lomitapide** increases the exposure to statins **(simvastatin)**. Monitor and adjust **simvastatin** dose, p. 130. Moderate Study → Also see TABLE 1 p. 818

▶ **Tacrolimus** is predicted to increase the exposure to **lomitapide**. Separate administration by 12 hours. Moderate Theoretical

▶ **Ticagrelor** is predicted to increase the exposure to **lomitapide**. Separate administration by 12 hours. Moderate Theoretical

▶ **Tolvaptan** is predicted to increase the exposure to **lomitapide**. Separate administration by 12 hours. Moderate Theoretical

Lomustine → see alkylating agents

Loop diuretics → see TABLE 18 p. 822 (hyponatraemia), TABLE 8 p. 819 (hypotension), TABLE 19 p. 822 (ototoxicity), TABLE 17 p. 822 (reduced serum potassium)

bumetanide · furosemide · torasemide

▶ **Aliskiren** slightly decreases the exposure to **furosemide**. Moderate Study → Also see TABLE 8 p. 819

▶ **Loop diuretics** increase the risk of nephrotoxicity and ototoxicity when given with **aminoglycosides**. Avoid. Moderate Study → Also see TABLE 19 p. 822

▶ Antiepileptics **(fosphenytoin, phenytoin)** decrease the effects of **furosemide**. Moderate Study

▶ Intravenous **furosemide** potentially increases the risk of sweating, variable blood pressure, and tachycardia when given after **chloral hydrate**. Moderate Anecdotal

▶ **Dasabuvir** (with ombitasvir, paritaprevir and ritonavir) increases the concentration of **furosemide**. Adjust dose. Moderate Study

▶ **Loop diuretics** increase the concentration of **lithium**. Monitor and adjust dose. Severe Study

▶ **Paritaprevir** (with ritonavir and ombitasvir) is predicted to increase the exposure to **furosemide**. Adjust **furosemide** dose, p. 136. Moderate Theoretical

▶ **Reboxetine** is predicted to increase the risk of hypokalaemia when given with **loop diuretics**. Moderate Theoretical

Loperamide

▶ Antiarrhythmics **(dronedarone)** are predicted to increase the exposure to **loperamide**. Severe Theoretical

▶ **Ceritinib** is predicted to increase the exposure to **loperamide**. Moderate Theoretical

▶ **Clopidogrel** is predicted to increase the exposure to **loperamide**. Severe Theoretical

▶ **Loperamide** greatly increases the absorption of oral **desmopressin** (and possibly sublingual). Moderate Study

▶ **Lapatinib** is predicted to increase the exposure to **loperamide**. Moderate Theoretical

▶ **Lumacaftor** is predicted to affect the exposure to **loperamide**. Moderate Theoretical

▶ **Mirabegron** is predicted to increase the exposure to **loperamide**. Mild Theoretical

▶ **Velpatasvir** is predicted to increase the exposure to **loperamide**. Severe Theoretical

Lopinavir → see HIV-protease inhibitors

Loprazolam → see TABLE 11 p. 820 (CNS depressant effects)

Loratadine → see antihistamines, non-sedating

Lorazepam → see TABLE 11 p. 820 (CNS depressant effects)

▸ **Rifampicin** increases the clearance of **lorazepam**. Moderate Study

Lormetazepam → see TABLE 11 p. 820 (CNS depressant effects)

Losartan → see angiotensin-II receptor antagonists

Low molecular-weight heparins → see TABLE 16 p. 822 (increased serum potassium), TABLE 3 p. 818 (anticoagulant effects)

dalteparin · enoxaparin · tinzaparin

▸ **Ranibizumab** increases the risk of bleeding events when given with **low molecular-weight heparins**. Severe Theoretical

Loxapine → see TABLE 8 p. 819 (hypotension), TABLE 11 p. 820 (CNS depressant effects), TABLE 10 p. 820 (antimuscarinics)

▸ **Combined hormonal contraceptives** are predicted to increase the exposure to **loxapine**. Avoid. Unknown Theoretical

▸ **Loxapine** is predicted to decrease the effects of **dopamine receptor agonists**. Moderate Theoretical → Also see TABLE 8 p. 819 → Also see TABLE 10 p. 820

▸ **Loxapine** is predicted to decrease the effects of **levodopa**. Severe Theoretical → Also see TABLE 8 p. 819

▸ **Quinolones (ciprofloxacin)** are predicted to increase the exposure to **loxapine**. Unknown Theoretical

▸ **SSRIs (fluvoxamine)** are predicted to increase the exposure to **loxapine**. Avoid. Unknown Theoretical

Lumacaftor

▸ **Lumacaftor** is predicted to affect the exposure to **aliskiren**. Moderate Theoretical

▸ **Lumacaftor** is predicted to decrease the exposure to **antiepileptics (carbamazepine, fosphenytoin, phenobarbital, phenytoin, primidone)**. Avoid. Severe Theoretical

▸ **Lumacaftor** is predicted to decrease the exposure to **antifungals, azoles (fluconazole)**. Adjust dose. Mild Theoretical

▸ **Lumacaftor** is predicted to decrease the exposure to **antifungals, azoles (itraconazole, ketoconazole, voriconazole)**. Moderate Theoretical

▸ **Lumacaftor** is predicted to decrease the exposure to **antifungals, azoles (posaconazole)**. Avoid. Moderate Theoretical

▸ **Lumacaftor** is predicted to affect the exposure to **antihistamines, non-sedating (fexofenadine)**. Monitor and adjust dose. Moderate Theoretical

▸ **Lumacaftor** is predicted to decrease the exposure to **bupropion**. Adjust dose. Moderate Theoretical

▸ **Lumacaftor** is predicted to decrease the exposure to **ciclosporin**. Avoid. Severe Theoretical

▸ **Lumacaftor** is predicted to affect the exposure to **colchicine**. Moderate Theoretical

▸ **Lumacaftor** is predicted to decrease the efficacy of **combined hormonal contraceptives**. Use additional contraceptive precautions. Severe Theoretical

▸ **Lumacaftor** is predicted to decrease the exposure to **corticosteroids (methylprednisolone, prednisone)**. Adjust dose. Severe Theoretical

▸ **Lumacaftor** is predicted to affect the exposure to **coumarins (warfarin)**. Severe Theoretical

▸ **Lumacaftor** is predicted to affect the exposure to **dabigatran**. Monitor and adjust dose. Moderate Theoretical

▸ **Lumacaftor** is predicted to affect the exposure to **digoxin**. Monitor and adjust dose. Moderate Theoretical

▸ **Lumacaftor** is predicted to affect the exposure to **edoxaban**. Moderate Theoretical

▸ **Lumacaftor** is predicted to decrease the exposure to **everolimus**. Avoid. Severe Theoretical

▸ **Lumacaftor** is predicted to decrease the exposure to **H₂ receptor antagonists (ranitidine)**. Monitor and adjust dose. Moderate Theoretical

▸ **Lumacaftor** is predicted to affect the exposure to **loperamide**. Moderate Theoretical

▸ **Lumacaftor** is predicted to decrease the exposure to **macrolides (clarithromycin, erythromycin)**. Moderate Theoretical

▸ **Lumacaftor** is predicted to decrease the exposure to **midazolam**. Avoid. Severe Theoretical

▸ **Lumacaftor** is predicted to decrease the exposure to **montelukast**. Moderate Theoretical

▸ **Lumacaftor** is predicted to decrease the exposure to **NSAIDs (ibuprofen)**. Adjust dose. Moderate Theoretical

▸ **Lumacaftor** is predicted to decrease the exposure to **proton pump inhibitors (esomeprazole, lansoprazole, omeprazole)**. Adjust dose. Moderate Theoretical

▸ **Lumacaftor** is predicted to decrease the exposure to **repaglinide**. Adjust dose. Moderate Theoretical

▸ **Lumacaftor** is predicted to decrease the exposure to **rifabutin**. Adjust dose. Moderate Theoretical

▸ **Lumacaftor** is predicted to decrease the exposure to **sirolimus**. Avoid. Severe Theoretical

▸ **Lumacaftor** is predicted to decrease the exposure to **SSRIs (citalopram, escitalopram, sertraline)**. Adjust dose. Moderate Theoretical

▸ **Lumacaftor** is predicted to decrease the exposure to **tacrolimus**. Avoid. Severe Theoretical

▸ **Lumacaftor** is predicted to affect the exposure to **taxanes (paclitaxel)**. Moderate Theoretical

▸ **Lumacaftor** is predicted to decrease the exposure to **temsirolimus**. Severe Theoretical

▸ **Lumacaftor** is predicted to affect the exposure to **topotecan**. Moderate Theoretical

Lumefantrine → see antimalarials

Lurasidone → see TABLE 8 p. 819 (hypotension), TABLE 11 p. 820 (CNS depressant effects)

▸ **Antiarrhythmics (dronedarone)** are predicted to increase the exposure to **lurasidone**. Moderate Theoretical

▸ **Antiepileptics (carbamazepine, fosphenytoin, phenobarbital, phenytoin, primidone)** are predicted to decrease the exposure to **lurasidone**. Avoid. Moderate Study → Also see TABLE 11 p. 820

▸ **Antifungals, azoles (fluconazole, isavuconazole, posaconazole)** are predicted to increase the exposure to **lurasidone**. Moderate Study

▸ **Antifungals, azoles (itraconazole, ketoconazole, voriconazole)** are predicted to increase the exposure to **lurasidone**. Avoid. Severe Study

▸ **Aprepitant** is predicted to increase the exposure to **lurasidone**. Moderate Study

▸ **Bosentan** is predicted to decrease the exposure to **lurasidone**. Monitor and adjust dose. Moderate Theoretical

▸ **Calcium channel blockers (diltiazem, verapamil)** are predicted to increase the exposure to **lurasidone**. Moderate Study → Also see TABLE 8 p. 819

▸ **Cobicistat** is predicted to increase the exposure to **lurasidone**. Avoid. Severe Study

▸ **Crizotinib** is predicted to increase the exposure to **lurasidone**. Moderate Study

▸ **Efavirenz** is predicted to decrease the exposure to **lurasidone**. Monitor and adjust dose. Moderate Theoretical

▸ **Enzalutamide** is predicted to decrease the exposure to **lurasidone**. Avoid. Moderate Study

▸ **Grapefruit juice** is predicted to increase the exposure to **lurasidone**. Avoid. Severe Theoretical

▸ **HIV-protease inhibitors (atazanavir, darunavir, fosamprenavir, lopinavir, ritonavir, saquinavir, tipranavir)** are predicted to increase the exposure to **lurasidone**. Avoid. Severe Study

▸ **HIV-protease inhibitors (indinavir)** are predicted to increase the exposure to **lurasidone**. Moderate Study

▸ **Idelalisib** is predicted to increase the exposure to **lurasidone**. Avoid. Severe Study

▸ **Imatinib** is predicted to increase the exposure to **lurasidone**. Moderate Study

▸ **Lurasidone** is predicted to decrease the effects of **levodopa**. Severe Theoretical → Also see TABLE 8 p. 819

▸ **Macrolides (clarithromycin)** are predicted to increase the exposure to **lurasidone**. Avoid. Severe Study

▸ **Macrolides (erythromycin)** are predicted to increase the exposure to **lurasidone**. Moderate Study

▸ **Netupitant** is predicted to increase the exposure to **lurasidone**. Moderate Study

▸ **Nevirapine** is predicted to decrease the exposure to **lurasidone**. Monitor and adjust dose. Moderate Theoretical

▸ **Nilotinib** is predicted to increase the exposure to **lurasidone**. Moderate Study

Lurasidone (continued)
- Rifampicin is predicted to decrease the exposure to **lurasidone**. Avoid. Moderate Study
- St John's Wort is predicted to decrease the exposure to **lurasidone**. Monitor and adjust dose. Moderate Theoretical

Lymecycline → see tetracyclines

Macitentan
- Antiepileptics (**carbamazepine, fosphenytoin, phenobarbital, phenytoin, primidone**) are predicted to decrease the exposure to **macitentan**. Avoid. Severe Study
- Antifungals, azoles (**itraconazole, ketoconazole, voriconazole**) are predicted to increase the exposure to **macitentan**. Moderate Study
- Cobicistat is predicted to increase the exposure to **macitentan**. Moderate Study
- Enzalutamide is predicted to decrease the exposure to **macitentan**. Avoid. Severe Study
- HIV-protease inhibitors (**atazanavir, darunavir, fosamprenavir, lopinavir, ritonavir, saquinavir, tipranavir**) are predicted to increase the exposure to **macitentan**. Moderate Study
- Idelalisib is predicted to increase the exposure to **macitentan**. Moderate Study
- Macrolides (**clarithromycin**) are predicted to increase the exposure to **macitentan**. Moderate Study
- Rifampicin is predicted to decrease the exposure to **macitentan**. Avoid. Severe Study
- St John's Wort is predicted to decrease the exposure to **macitentan**. Avoid. Severe Theoretical

Macrolides → see TABLE 9 p. 820 (QT-interval prolongation)

azithromycin · clarithromycin · erythromycin

ROUTE-SPECIFIC INFORMATION Since systemic absorption can follow topical application, the possibility of interactions should be borne in mind.

- **Clarithromycin** is predicted to increase the exposure to **abiraterone**. Severe Theoretical
- **Macrolides** are predicted to increase the exposure to **afatinib**. Separate administration by 12 hours. Moderate Study
- **Clarithromycin** is predicted to markedly increase the exposure to aldosterone antagonists (**eplerenone**). Avoid. Severe Study
- **Erythromycin** is predicted to increase the exposure to aldosterone antagonists (**eplerenone**). Adjust **eplerenone** dose. Severe Study
- Azithromycin is predicted to increase the exposure to **aliskiren**. Moderate Theoretical
- Macrolides (**clarithromycin, erythromycin**) are predicted to increase the exposure to **aliskiren**. Moderate Study
- **Clarithromycin** increases the exposure to **almotriptan**. Mild Study
- **Clarithromycin** is predicted to moderately increase the exposure to alpha blockers (**alfuzosin, tamsulosin**). Use with caution or avoid. Moderate Study
- **Clarithromycin** is predicted to increase the exposure to alpha blockers (**doxazosin**). Moderate Study
- **Erythromycin** is predicted to increase the exposure to alpha blockers (**tamsulosin**). Moderate Theoretical
- **Clarithromycin** moderately increases the exposure to **alprazolam**. Avoid. Moderate Study
- **Erythromycin** is predicted to increase the exposure to **alprazolam**. Severe Study
- Azithromycin is predicted to increase the exposure to **aminophylline**. Moderate Theoretical
- **Clarithromycin** is predicted to increase the exposure to **aminophylline**. Adjust **aminophylline** dose, p. 161. Moderate Theoretical
- Aminophylline is predicted to decrease the exposure to **erythromycin**. Adjust dose. Severe Study
- **Clarithromycin** very markedly increases the exposure to antiarrhythmics (**dronedarone**). Avoid. Severe Study → Also see TABLE 9 p. 820
- **Erythromycin** is predicted to moderately increase the exposure to antiarrhythmics (**dronedarone**). Avoid. Severe Theoretical
- Macrolides (**clarithromycin, erythromycin**) are predicted to increase the exposure to antiarrhythmics (**lidocaine**). Moderate Theoretical

- Clarithromycin is predicted to increase the exposure to antiarrhythmics (**propafenone**). Monitor and adjust dose. Severe Study
- **Erythromycin** is predicted to increase the exposure to antiarrhythmics (**propafenone**). Monitor and adjust dose. Moderate Study
- Clarithromycin is predicted to increase the exposure to anticholinesterases, centrally acting (**galantamine**). Monitor and adjust dose. Moderate Study
- Clarithromycin slightly increases the concentration of antiepileptics (**carbamazepine**). Monitor **carbamazepine** concentration and adjust dose. Severe Study
- **Erythromycin** markedly increases the concentration of antiepileptics (**carbamazepine**). Monitor **carbamazepine** concentration and adjust dose. Severe Study
- Clarithromycin is predicted to slightly increase the exposure to antiepileptics (**perampanel**). Mild Study
- Clarithromycin is predicted to increase the exposure to antifungals, azoles (**isavuconazole**). Avoid or monitor side effects. Severe Study
- Erythromycin is predicted to increase the exposure to antifungals, azoles (**isavuconazole**). Moderate Theoretical
- Clarithromycin is predicted to increase the exposure to antihistamines, non-sedating (**mizolastine**). Avoid. Severe Study
- **Erythromycin** is predicted to increase the exposure to antihistamines, non-sedating (**mizolastine**). Severe Theoretical
- Clarithromycin is predicted to increase the exposure to antimalarials (**artemether**) with lumefantrine. Moderate Study → Also see TABLE 9 p. 820
- Macrolides (**clarithromycin, erythromycin**) are predicted to increase the concentration of antimalarials (**piperaquine**). Severe Theoretical
- Clarithromycin is predicted to increase the exposure to **apixaban**. Avoid. Severe Theoretical
- **Erythromycin** is predicted to increase the exposure to **apixaban**. Moderate Theoretical
- Clarithromycin is predicted to markedly increase the exposure to **aprepitant**. Moderate Study
- Clarithromycin is predicted to slightly increase the exposure to **aripiprazole**. Adjust **aripiprazole** dose, p. 240. Moderate Study
- Clarithromycin is predicted to increase the exposure to **axitinib**. Avoid or adjust dose. Moderate Study
- **Erythromycin** is predicted to increase the exposure to **axitinib**. Moderate Theoretical
- Clarithromycin is predicted to increase the exposure to **bedaquiline**. Avoid prolonged use. Mild Study → Also see TABLE 9 p. 820
- **Erythromycin** is predicted to increase the exposure to **bedaquiline**. Avoid prolonged use. Mild Theoretical
- **Macrolides** are predicted to increase the exposure to beta blockers, non-selective (**nadolol**). Moderate Study
- Clarithromycin is predicted to increase the exposure to beta₂ agonists (**salmeterol**). Avoid. Severe Study
- Clarithromycin slightly increases the exposure to **bortezomib**. Moderate Study
- Clarithromycin is predicted to increase the exposure to **bosentan**. Moderate Theoretical
- Clarithromycin is predicted to markedly increase the exposure to **bosutinib**. Avoid or adjust **bosutinib** dose. Severe Study → Also see TABLE 9 p. 820
- **Erythromycin** is predicted to increase the exposure to **bosutinib**. Avoid or adjust **bosutinib** dose. Severe Theoretical
- Clarithromycin is predicted to increase the exposure to **buspirone**. Adjust **buspirone** dose. Severe Study
- **Erythromycin** is predicted to increase the exposure to **buspirone**. Use with caution and adjust dose. Moderate Study
- Clarithromycin slightly increases the exposure to **cabozantinib**. Moderate Study → Also see TABLE 9 p. 820
- **Erythromycin** is predicted to increase the exposure to **cabozantinib**. Moderate Theoretical
- Macrolides (**clarithromycin, erythromycin**) are predicted to increase the exposure to calcium channel blockers (**amlodipine, felodipine, isradipine, lacidipine, lercanidipine, nicardipine, nifedipine, nimodipine**). Monitor and adjust dose. Moderate Study

- Erythromycin is predicted to increase the exposure to calcium channel blockers (diltiazem). [Severe] Theoretical
- Clarithromycin is predicted to increase the exposure to calcium channel blockers (diltiazem, verapamil). [Severe] Study
- Clarithromycin is predicted to markedly increase the exposure to calcium channel blockers (lercanidipine). Avoid. [Severe] Study
- Erythromycin is predicted to increase the exposure to calcium channel blockers (verapamil). [Severe] Study
- Clarithromycin is predicted to increase the exposure to cannabis extract. Use with caution and adjust dose. [Moderate] Theoretical
- Clarithromycin is predicted to increase the exposure to ceritinib. Avoid or adjust ceritinib dose. [Severe] Study → Also see **TABLE 9** p. 820
- Macrolides (azithromycin, erythromycin) are predicted to increase the exposure to ceritinib. [Moderate] Theoretical
- Macrolides (clarithromycin, erythromycin) increase the concentration of ciclosporin. [Severe] Study
- Clarithromycin is predicted to moderately increase the exposure to cilostazol. Adjust cilostazol dose. [Moderate] Study
- Erythromycin slightly increases the exposure to cilostazol. Adjust cilostazol dose. [Moderate] Study
- Clarithromycin is predicted to moderately increase the exposure to cinacalcet. Adjust dose. [Moderate] Study
- Clarithromycin is predicted to markedly increase the exposure to cobimetinib. Avoid or monitor for toxicity. [Severe] Study
- Erythromycin is predicted to increase the exposure to cobimetinib. [Severe] Theoretical
- Azithromycin is predicted to increase the exposure to colchicine. Avoid or adjust colchicine dose. [Severe] Theoretical
- Clarithromycin is predicted to increase the exposure to colchicine. Avoid or adjust colchicine dose. [Severe] Study
- Erythromycin is predicted to increase the exposure to colchicine. Adjust colchicine dose. [Severe] Study
- Clarithromycin is predicted to increase the exposure to corticosteroids (budesonide). Avoid. [Severe] Study
- Clarithromycin is predicted to increase the exposure to corticosteroids (ciclesonide). Avoid. [Moderate] Theoretical
- Clarithromycin is predicted to increase the exposure to corticosteroids (dexamethasone, methylprednisolone). Monitor and adjust dose. [Moderate] Study
- Clarithromycin is predicted to increase the exposure to inhaled corticosteroids (fluticasone). [Severe] Study
- Erythromycin is predicted to increase the exposure to corticosteroids (methylprednisolone). Monitor and adjust dose. [Moderate] Study
- Clarithromycin is predicted to increase the exposure to corticosteroids (mometasone). [Moderate] Theoretical
- Clarithromycin is predicted to increase the risk of side-effects when given with corticosteroids (triamcinolone). [Severe] Theoretical
- Macrolides (clarithromycin, erythromycin) increase the anticoagulant effect of coumarins. Monitor INR and adjust dose. [Severe] Anecdotal
- Clarithromycin is predicted to moderately increase the exposure to crizotinib. Avoid. [Moderate] Study → Also see **TABLE 9** p. 820
- Erythromycin is predicted to increase the exposure to crizotinib. [Moderate] Theoretical
- Macrolides (azithromycin, clarithromycin, erythromycin) are predicted to increase the exposure to dabigatran. [Moderate] Theoretical
- Clarithromycin is predicted to increase the exposure to dabrafenib. Use with caution or avoid. [Moderate] Study
- Clarithromycin is predicted to moderately increase the exposure to daclatasvir. Adjust daclatasvir dose. [Moderate] Study
- Clarithromycin is predicted to markedly to very markedly increase the exposure to darifenacin. Avoid. [Severe] Study
- Erythromycin is predicted to slightly increase the exposure to darifenacin. [Moderate] Study
- Clarithromycin is predicted to markedly increase the exposure to dasatinib. Avoid. [Severe] Study → Also see **TABLE 9** p. 820
- Erythromycin is predicted to increase the exposure to dasatinib. [Severe] Study

- Clarithromycin very slightly increases the exposure to delamanid. [Severe] Study → Also see **TABLE 9** p. 820
- Macrolides increase the concentration of digoxin. [Severe] Anecdotal
- Macrolides (clarithromycin, erythromycin) increase the risk of QT-prolongation when given with domperidone. Avoid. [Severe] Study
- Clarithromycin increases the exposure to dopamine receptor agonists (bromocriptine, cabergoline). [Severe] Study
- Erythromycin is predicted to increase the exposure to dopamine receptor agonists (bromocriptine, cabergoline). [Severe] Theoretical
- Clarithromycin is predicted to increase the exposure to dutasteride. Monitor side effects and adjust dose. [Moderate] Theoretical
- Erythromycin is predicted to moderately increase the exposure to dutasteride. [Mild] Study
- Erythromycin slightly increases the exposure to edoxaban. Adjust edoxaban dose. [Severe] Study
- Macrolides (azithromycin, clarithromycin) are predicted to slightly increase the exposure to edoxaban. [Severe] Theoretical
- Efavirenz decreases the exposure to clarithromycin. [Moderate] Study
- Clarithromycin slightly to moderately increases the exposure to elbasvir. Avoid. [Moderate] Study
- Clarithromycin is predicted to markedly increase the exposure to eletriptan. Avoid. [Severe] Study
- Erythromycin moderately increases the exposure to eletriptan. Avoid. [Moderate] Study
- Clarithromycin is predicted to increase the risk of ergotism when given with ergometrine. Avoid. [Severe] Theoretical
- Erythromycin is predicted to increase the risk of ergotism when given with ergometrine. [Severe] Theoretical
- Clarithromycin is predicted to increase the risk of ergotism when given with ergotamine. Avoid. [Severe] Theoretical
- Erythromycin is predicted to increase the risk of ergotism when given with ergotamine. [Severe] Theoretical
- Clarithromycin is predicted to slightly increase the exposure to erlotinib. Use with caution and adjust dose. [Moderate] Study
- Macrolides (azithromycin, clarithromycin) are predicted to increase the exposure to erlotinib. [Moderate] Theoretical
- Etravirine decreases the exposure to clarithromycin. [Severe] Study
- Clarithromycin is predicted to increase the concentration of everolimus. Avoid. [Severe] Study
- Erythromycin is predicted to increase the concentration of everolimus. Avoid or adjust dose. [Moderate] Study
- Clarithromycin is predicted to moderately increase the exposure to fesoterodine. Adjust fesoterodine dose; avoid in hepatic and renal impairment. [Severe] Study
- Erythromycin is predicted to increase the exposure to fesoterodine. Adjust fesoterodine dose in hepatic and renal impairment. [Mild] Study
- Macrolides are predicted to increase the exposure to fidaxomicin. Avoid. [Moderate] Study
- Clarithromycin is predicted to increase the exposure to fosaprepitant. [Moderate] Theoretical
- Clarithromycin is predicted to increase the exposure to gefitinib. [Moderate] Study
- Erythromycin is predicted to increase the exposure to gefitinib. [Moderate] Theoretical
- Clarithromycin is predicted to moderately to markedly increase the exposure to grazoprevir. Avoid. [Severe] Study
- Clarithromycin is predicted to increase the exposure to guanfacine. Adjust guanfacine dose, p. 222. [Moderate] Study
- Erythromycin is predicted to increase the concentration of guanfacine. Adjust guanfacine dose, p. 222. [Moderate] Theoretical
- H₂ receptor antagonists (cimetidine) slightly increase the exposure to erythromycin. [Moderate] Study
- HIV-protease inhibitors (atazanavir, darunavir, fosamprenavir, indinavir, lopinavir, ritonavir) slightly to moderately increase the exposure to clarithromycin. Adjust dose in renal impairment. [Severe] Study

A1

Interactions | Appendix 1

Macrolides (continued)

▶ HIV-protease inhibitors (atazanavir, darunavir, fosamprenavir, indinavir, lopinavir, ritonavir, tipranavir) are predicted to increase the exposure to erythromycin. [Severe] Theoretical

▶ Clarithromycin increases the exposure to HIV-protease inhibitors (saquinavir) and HIV-protease inhibitors (saquinavir) increase the exposure to clarithromycin. Avoid. [Severe] Study → Also see TABLE 9 p. 820

▶ Erythromycin is predicted to increase the exposure to HIV-protease inhibitors (saquinavir). Avoid. [Severe] Theoretical

▶ Clarithromycin is predicted to very markedly increase the exposure to ibrutinib. Avoid or adjust ibrutinib dose. [Severe] Study

▶ Erythromycin is predicted to increase the exposure to ibrutinib. Avoid or adjust ibrutinib dose. [Severe] Theoretical

▶ Clarithromycin is predicted to increase the exposure to imatinib. [Moderate] Study

▶ Erythromycin is predicted to increase the exposure to imatinib. [Moderate] Theoretical

▶ Clarithromycin is predicted to increase the risk of toxicity when given with irinotecan. Avoid. [Moderate] Study

▶ Clarithromycin is predicted to increase the exposure to ivabradine. Avoid. [Severe] Study

▶ Erythromycin is predicted to increase the exposure to ivabradine. Avoid. [Severe] Theoretical

▶ Clarithromycin is predicted to increase the exposure to ivacaftor. Adjust ivacaftor or lumacaftor with ivacaftor dose, p. 179. [Severe] Study

▶ Erythromycin is predicted to increase the exposure to ivacaftor. Adjust ivacaftor dose, p. 179. [Severe] Study

▶ Clarithromycin is predicted to increase the exposure to lapatinib. Avoid. [Moderate] Study → Also see TABLE 9 p. 820

▶ Erythromycin is predicted to increase the exposure to lapatinib. [Moderate] Study

▶ Azithromycin is predicted to increase the exposure to lomitapide. Separate administration by 12 hours. [Moderate] Theoretical

▶ Clarithromycin is predicted to markedly increase the exposure to lomitapide. Avoid. [Severe] Study

▶ Erythromycin is predicted to increase the exposure to lomitapide. Avoid. [Moderate] Theoretical

▶ Lumacaftor is predicted to decrease the exposure to macrolides (clarithromycin, erythromycin). [Moderate] Theoretical

▶ Clarithromycin is predicted to increase the exposure to lurasidone. Avoid. [Severe] Study

▶ Erythromycin is predicted to increase the exposure to lurasidone. [Moderate] Study

▶ Clarithromycin is predicted to increase the exposure to macitentan. [Moderate] Study

▶ Clarithromycin is predicted to markedly increase the exposure to maraviroc. Adjust dose. [Severe] Study

▶ Clarithromycin is predicted to markedly to very markedly increase the exposure to midazolam. Avoid or adjust midazolam dose. [Severe] Study

▶ Erythromycin is predicted to increase the exposure to midazolam. Monitor side effects and adjust dose. [Severe] Study

▶ Clarithromycin is predicted to increase the exposure to mirabegron. Adjust mirabegron dose in hepatic and renal impairment. [Moderate] Study

▶ Clarithromycin is predicted to increase the exposure to mirtazapine. [Moderate] Study

▶ Clarithromycin is predicted to markedly to increase the exposure to modafinil. [Mild] Theoretical

▶ Clarithromycin increases the risk of neutropenia when given with monoclonal antibodies (brentuximab vedotin). Monitor and adjust dose. [Severe] Theoretical

▶ Clarithromycin is predicted to increase the exposure to monoclonal antibodies (trastuzumab emtansine). Avoid. [Severe] Theoretical

▶ Clarithromycin is predicted to markedly increase the exposure to naloxegol. Avoid. [Severe] Study

▶ Erythromycin is predicted to increase the exposure to naloxegol. Adjust naloxegol dose and monitor side effects. [Moderate] Study

▶ Clarithromycin is predicted to increase the exposure to netupitant. [Mild] Study

▶ Nevirapine decreases the exposure to clarithromycin. [Moderate] Study

▶ Clarithromycin is predicted to moderately increase the exposure to nilotinib. Avoid. [Severe] Study → Also see TABLE 9 p. 820

▶ Erythromycin is predicted to increase the exposure to nilotinib. [Moderate] Theoretical

▶ Macrolides are predicted to increase the exposure to nintedanib. [Moderate] Study

▶ Clarithromycin is predicted to increase the exposure to nitisinone. Adjust nitisinone dose. [Moderate] Theoretical

▶ Clarithromycin is predicted to increase the exposure to olaparib. Avoid or adjust olaparib dose. [Moderate] Study

▶ Erythromycin is predicted to increase the exposure to olaparib. Avoid or adjust olaparib dose. [Moderate] Theoretical

▶ Erythromycin is predicted to increase the exposure to opioids (alfentanil, buprenorphine, fentanyl, oxycodone). Monitor and adjust dose. [Moderate] Study

▶ Clarithromycin is predicted to increase the exposure to opioids (alfentanil, buprenorphine, fentanyl, oxycodone, sufentanil). Monitor and adjust dose. [Severe] Study

▶ Clarithromycin is predicted to increase the exposure to opioids (methadone). [Moderate] Theoretical → Also see TABLE 9 p. 820

▶ Erythromycin is predicted to increase the exposure to opioids (methadone, sufentanil). [Moderate] Theoretical

▶ Clarithromycin is predicted to increase the exposure to oxybutynin. [Mild] Study

▶ Erythromycin is predicted to increase the exposure to oxybutynin. [Mild] Theoretical

▶ Clarithromycin is predicted to increase the exposure to palbociclib. Avoid or adjust palbociclib dose. [Severe] Study

▶ Clarithromycin is predicted to increase the exposure to panobinostat. Adjust panobinostat dose; in hepatic impairment avoid. [Moderate] Study → Also see TABLE 9 p. 820

▶ Clarithromycin is predicted to increase the exposure to paritaprevir (with ritonavir and ombitasvir). Avoid. [Severe] Theoretical

▶ Clarithromycin is predicted to increase the exposure to pazopanib. Avoid or adjust pazopanib dose. [Moderate] Study → Also see TABLE 9 p. 820

▶ Erythromycin is predicted to increase the exposure to pazopanib. [Moderate] Theoretical

▶ Erythromycin is predicted to increase the exposure to phosphodiesterase type-5 inhibitors (avanafil). Adjust avanafil dose. [Moderate] Theoretical

▶ Clarithromycin is predicted to increase the exposure to phosphodiesterase type-5 inhibitors (avanafil, vardenafil). Avoid. [Severe] Study → Also see TABLE 9 p. 820

▶ Clarithromycin is predicted to increase the exposure to phosphodiesterase type-5 inhibitors (sildenafil). Avoid or adjust sildenafil dose, p. 117. [Severe] Study → Also see TABLE 9 p. 820

▶ Erythromycin is predicted to increase the exposure to phosphodiesterase type-5 inhibitors (sildenafil). Monitor and adjust sildenafil dose, p. 117. [Moderate] Study

▶ Clarithromycin is predicted to increase the exposure to phosphodiesterase type-5 inhibitors (tadalafil). Use with caution or avoid. [Severe] Study

▶ Erythromycin is predicted to increase the exposure to phosphodiesterase type-5 inhibitors (tadalafil). [Severe] Theoretical

▶ Erythromycin is predicted to increase the exposure to phosphodiesterase type-5 inhibitors (vardenafil). Adjust dose. [Severe] Theoretical

▶ Clarithromycin is predicted to increase the exposure to pimozide. Avoid. [Severe] Study → Also see TABLE 9 p. 820

▶ Erythromycin is predicted to increase the exposure to pimozide. Avoid. [Severe] Theoretical

▶ Clarithromycin is predicted to slightly increase the exposure to ponatinib. Monitor and adjust ponatinib dose. [Moderate] Study

▶ Clarithromycin is predicted to moderately increase the exposure to praziquantel. [Mild] Study

▶ Clarithromycin is predicted to increase the exposure to quetiapine. Avoid. [Severe] Study

- **Erythromycin** is predicted to increase the exposure to quetiapine. Avoid. [Moderate] Study
- **Clarithromycin** is predicted to increase the exposure to ranolazine. Avoid. [Severe] Study → Also see **TABLE 9** p. 820
- **Erythromycin** is predicted to increase the exposure to ranolazine. [Severe] Study
- **Clarithromycin** is predicted to increase the exposure to reboxetine. Avoid. [Moderate] Study
- **Clarithromycin** is predicted to increase the exposure to regorafenib. Avoid. [Moderate] Study
- **Clarithromycin** is predicted to increase the exposure to repaglinide. [Moderate] Study
- **Clarithromycin** is predicted to increase the exposure to retinoids (**alitretinoin**). Adjust **alitretinoin** dose. [Moderate] Theoretical
- **Azithromycin** increases the risk of neutropenia when given with rifabutin. [Severe] Study
- **Clarithromycin** increases the risk of uveitis when given with rifabutin. Adjust dose. [Severe] Study
- **Rifampicin** decreases the concentration of **clarithromycin**. [Severe] Study
- **Clarithromycin** is predicted to increase the exposure to risperidone. Adjust dose. [Moderate] Study → Also see **TABLE 9** p. 820
- **Clarithromycin** is predicted to increase the exposure to ruxolitinib. Adjust dose and monitor side effects. [Moderate] Study
- **Erythromycin** is predicted to increase the exposure to ruxolitinib. [Moderate] Theoretical
- **Clarithromycin** is predicted to increase the exposure to saxagliptin. [Moderate] Study
- **Erythromycin** is predicted to increase the exposure to saxagliptin. [Mild] Study
- **Macrolides (clarithromycin, erythromycin)** are predicted to increase the exposure to simeprevir. Avoid. [Severe] Study
- **Clarithromycin** is predicted to increase the concentration of sirolimus. Avoid. [Severe] Study
- **Erythromycin** increases the concentration of sirolimus. Monitor and adjust dose. [Moderate] Study
- **Clarithromycin** is predicted to increase the exposure to solifenacin. Adjust **solifenacin** or tamsulosin with solifenacin dose; avoid in hepatic and renal impairment. [Severe] Study
- **Clarithromycin** is predicted to moderately increase the exposure to SSRIs (**dapoxetine**). Avoid or adjust **dapoxetine** dose. [Severe] Study
- **Erythromycin** is predicted to increase the exposure to SSRIs (**dapoxetine**). Adjust **dapoxetine** dose. [Moderate] Theoretical
- **Clarithromycin** is predicted to increase the exposure to statins (**atorvastatin**). Avoid or adjust dose and monitor rhabdomyolysis. [Severe] Study
- **Erythromycin** is predicted to increase the exposure to statins (**atorvastatin**). Monitor and adjust dose. [Severe] Theoretical
- **Clarithromycin** moderately increases the exposure to statins (**pravastatin**). [Severe] Study
- **Erythromycin** is predicted to increase the exposure to statins (**pravastatin**). [Severe] Study
- **Clarithromycin** is predicted to increase the exposure to statins (**simvastatin**). Avoid. [Severe] Study
- **Erythromycin** is predicted to increase the exposure to statins (**simvastatin**). Use with caution and adjust **simvastatin** dose, p. 130. [Severe] Study
- **Clarithromycin** is predicted to slightly increase the exposure to sulfonylureas. [Moderate] Theoretical
- **Clarithromycin** is predicted to slightly increase the exposure to sunitinib. Avoid or adjust **sunitinib** dose. [Moderate] Study → Also see **TABLE 9** p. 820
- **Erythromycin** is predicted to increase the exposure to sunitinib. [Moderate] Theoretical
- **Clarithromycin** is predicted to increase the concentration of tacrolimus. Monitor and adjust dose. [Severe] Study
- **Erythromycin** is predicted to increase the concentration of tacrolimus. [Severe] Study
- **Clarithromycin** is predicted to increase the exposure to taxanes (**cabazitaxel**). Avoid. [Severe] Study

- **Erythromycin** is predicted to increase the exposure to taxanes (**cabazitaxel**). [Moderate] Theoretical
- **Clarithromycin** is predicted to moderately increase the exposure to taxanes (**docetaxel**). Avoid or adjust dose. [Severe] Study
- **Clarithromycin** is predicted to increase the exposure to taxanes (**paclitaxel**). [Severe] Theoretical
- **Clarithromycin** is predicted to increase the concentration of temsirolimus. Avoid. [Severe] Theoretical
- **Erythromycin** is predicted to increase the concentration of temsirolimus. [Moderate] Theoretical
- **Erythromycin** decreases the clearance of **theophylline** and theophylline potentially decreases the clearance of erythromycin. Adjust dose. [Severe] Study
- **Macrolides (azithromycin, clarithromycin)** are predicted to increase the exposure to theophylline. Adjust dose. [Moderate] Anecdotal
- **Azithromycin** is predicted to increase the exposure to ticagrelor. Use with caution or avoid. [Severe] Study
- **Clarithromycin** is predicted to markedly increase the exposure to ticagrelor. Avoid. [Severe] Study
- **Clarithromycin** is predicted to increase the exposure to tolterodine. Avoid. [Severe] Study → Also see **TABLE 9** p. 820
- **Erythromycin** is predicted to increase the exposure to tolterodine. [Mild] Theoretical
- **Clarithromycin** is predicted to increase the exposure to tolvaptan. Adjust dose. [Severe] Study
- **Erythromycin** is predicted to increase the exposure to tolvaptan. Adjust dose. [Moderate] Theoretical
- **Macrolides** are predicted to increase the exposure to topotecan. [Severe] Study
- **Clarithromycin** is predicted to increase the exposure to toremifene. [Moderate] Theoretical → Also see **TABLE 9** p. 820
- **Clarithromycin** is predicted to increase the exposure to trabectedin. Avoid or adjust dose. [Severe] Theoretical
- **Macrolides** are predicted to increase the concentration of trametinib. [Moderate] Theoretical
- **Clarithromycin** is predicted to moderately increase the exposure to trazodone. Avoid or adjust dose. [Moderate] Study
- **Erythromycin** is predicted to increase the exposure to trazodone. [Moderate] Theoretical
- **Clarithromycin** is predicted to increase the exposure to ulipristal. Avoid if used for uterine fibroids. [Severe] Study
- **Erythromycin** is predicted to increase the exposure to ulipristal. Avoid if used for uterine fibroids. [Moderate] Study
- **Clarithromycin** is predicted to increase the exposure to vemurafenib. [Severe] Theoretical → Also see **TABLE 9** p. 820
- **Azithromycin** is predicted to increase the exposure to venetoclax. Avoid or monitor for toxicity. [Severe] Theoretical
- **Macrolides (clarithromycin, erythromycin)** are predicted to increase the exposure to **venetoclax**. Avoid or adjust **venetoclax** dose. [Severe] Study
- **Clarithromycin** is predicted to increase the exposure to venlafaxine. [Moderate] Study → Also see **TABLE 9** p. 820
- **Macrolides (clarithromycin, erythromycin)** are predicted to increase the exposure to **vinca alkaloids**. [Severe] Theoretical → Also see **TABLE 9** p. 820
- **Clarithromycin** is predicted to increase the exposure to vitamin D substances (**paricalcitol**). [Moderate] Study
- **Clarithromycin** decreases the absorption of zidovudine. Separate administration by at least 2 hours. [Moderate] Study
- **Clarithromycin** is predicted to increase the exposure to zopiclone. Adjust dose. [Moderate] Theoretical
- **Erythromycin** is predicted to increase the exposure to zopiclone. Adjust dose. [Moderate] Study

Magnesium

- Oral **magnesium** decreases the absorption of bisphosphonates (**alendronic acid**). Alendronic acid should be taken at least 30 minutes before **magnesium**. [Moderate] Study
- Oral **magnesium** is predicted to decrease the absorption of oral bisphosphonates (**ibandronic acid**). Avoid **magnesium** for at least 6 hours before or 1 hour after **ibandronic acid**. [Moderate] Theoretical

Magnesium (continued)
- Oral **magnesium** decreases the absorption of bisphosphonates (**risedronate**). Separate administration by at least 2 hours. Moderate Study
- Oral **magnesium** decreases the absorption of bisphosphonates (**sodium clodronate**). Avoid **magnesium** for 2 hours before or 1 hour after **sodium clodronate**. Moderate Study
- Intravenous **magnesium** potentially increases the risk of hypotension when given with calcium channel blockers (**amlodipine, clevidipine, felodipine, isradipine, lacidipine, lercanidipine, nicardipine, nifedipine, nimodipine, verapamil**) in pregnant women. Severe Anecdotal
- Intravenous **magnesium** increases the effects of neuromuscular blocking drugs, non-depolarising. Moderate Study
- Intravenous **magnesium** is predicted to increase the effects of **suxamethonium**. Moderate Study

Magnesium carbonate → see antacids
Magnesium trisilicate → see antacids
Maraviroc
- Antiepileptics (carbamazepine, fosphenytoin, phenobarbital, phenytoin, primidone) are predicted to decrease the exposure to **maraviroc**. Adjust dose. Severe Study
- Antifungals, azoles (**itraconazole, ketoconazole, voriconazole**) markedly increase the exposure to **maraviroc**. Adjust dose. Severe Study
- **Bosentan** is predicted to decrease the exposure to **maraviroc**. Avoid. Moderate Theoretical
- **Cobicistat** markedly increases the exposure to **maraviroc**. Refer to specialist literature. Severe Study
- **Efavirenz** decreases the exposure to **maraviroc**. Refer to specialist literature. Severe Theoretical
- **Enzalutamide** is predicted to decrease the exposure to **maraviroc**. Adjust dose. Severe Study
- **Etravirine** (with a boosted protease inhibitor) increases the exposure to **maraviroc**. Avoid or adjust dose. Moderate Study
- HIV-protease inhibitors (**atazanavir, darunavir, lopinavir, ritonavir, saquinavir**) increase the exposure to **maraviroc**. Refer to specialist literature. Severe Study
- **Maraviroc** potentially decreases the exposure to HIV-protease inhibitors (**fosamprenavir**) and HIV-protease inhibitors (**fosamprenavir**) potentially decrease the exposure to **maraviroc**. Avoid. Severe Study
- **Idelalisib** markedly increases the exposure to **maraviroc**. Adjust dose. Severe Theoretical
- Macrolides (**clarithromycin**) are predicted to markedly increase the exposure to **maraviroc**. Adjust dose. Severe Study
- **Rifampicin** is predicted to decrease the exposure to **maraviroc**. Adjust dose. Severe Study
- **St John's Wort** is predicted to decrease the exposure to **maraviroc**. Avoid. Severe Theoretical

Measles, mumps and rubella vaccine, live → see live vaccines
Mebendazole
- H₂ receptor antagonists (**cimetidine**) increase the concentration of **mebendazole**. Moderate Study
Medroxyprogesterone
- **Sugammadex** is predicted to decrease the exposure to **medroxyprogesterone**. Use additional contraceptive precautions. Severe Theoretical
Mefenamic acid → see NSAIDs
Mefloquine → see antimalarials
Melatonin → see TABLE 11 p. 820 (CNS depressant effects)
- Combined hormonal contraceptives are predicted to increase the exposure to **melatonin**. Moderate Theoretical
- Quinolones (**ciprofloxacin**) are predicted to increase the exposure to **melatonin**. Moderate Theoretical
- SSRIs (**fluvoxamine**) very markedly increase the exposure to **melatonin**. Avoid. Severe Study
Meloxicam → see NSAIDs
Melphalan → see alkylating agents
Memantine
- Dopamine receptor agonists (**amantadine**) increase the risk of CNS toxicity when given with **memantine**. Use with caution or avoid. Severe Theoretical
- **Memantine** is predicted to increase the effects of dopamine receptor agonists (**apomorphine, bromocriptine, cabergoline,**

pergolide, pramipexole, quinagolide, ropinirole, rotigotine). Moderate Theoretical
- **Memantine** is predicted to increase the risk of CNS side-effects when given with **ketamine**. Avoid. Severe Theoretical
- **Memantine** is predicted to increase the effects of **levodopa**. Moderate Theoretical
Mepacrine
- **Mepacrine** is predicted to increase the concentration of antimalarials (**primaquine**). Avoid. Moderate Theoretical
Mepivacaine → see anaesthetics, local
Mepolizumab → see monoclonal antibodies
Meprobamate → see TABLE 11 p. 820 (CNS depressant effects)
Meptazinol → see opioids
Mercaptopurine → see TABLE 1 p. 818 (hepatotoxicity), TABLE 15 p. 821 (myelosuppression)
- **Allopurinol** potentially increases the risk of haematological toxicity when given with **mercaptopurine**. Adjust mercaptopurine dose, p. 516. Severe Study
- **Mercaptopurine** decreases the anticoagulant effect of coumarins. Moderate Anecdotal
- **Febuxostat** is predicted to increase the exposure to **mercaptopurine**. Avoid. Severe Study
- Live vaccines are predicted to increase the risk of generalised infection (possibly life-threatening) when given with **mercaptopurine**. Public Health England advises avoid. Severe Theoretical
Meropenem → see carbapenems
Mesalazine

ROUTE-SPECIFIC INFORMATION The manufacturers of some mesalazine gastro-resistant and modified-release medicines (Asacol MR tablets, Ipocol, Salofalk granules) suggest that preparations that lower stool pH (e.g. lactulose) might prevent the release of mesalazine.

Metaraminol → see sympathomimetics, vasoconstrictor
Metformin → see TABLE 14 p. 821 (antidiabetic drugs)

FOOD AND LIFESTYLE Excessive alcohol consumption might increase the risk of lactic acidosis with metformin.

- **Dolutegravir** slightly to moderately increases the exposure to **metformin**. Use with caution and adjust dose. Severe Study
- H₂ receptor antagonists (**cimetidine**) slightly increase the exposure to **metformin**. Monitor and adjust dose. Moderate Study
- **Pitolisant** is predicted to increase the exposure to **metformin**. Unknown Theoretical
- **Vandetanib** slightly increases the exposure to **metformin**. Monitor and adjust dose. Moderate Study
Methadone → see opioids
Methenamine
- **Acetazolamide** is predicted to decrease the efficacy of **methenamine**. Avoid. Moderate Theoretical
- **Potassium citrate** is predicted to decrease the efficacy of **methenamine**. Avoid. Moderate Theoretical
- **Sodium bicarbonate** is predicted to decrease the efficacy of **methenamine**. Avoid. Moderate Theoretical
- **Sodium citrate** is predicted to decrease the efficacy of **methenamine**. Avoid. Moderate Theoretical
Methocarbamol → see TABLE 11 p. 820 (CNS depressant effects)
Methotrexate → see TABLE 1 p. 818 (hepatotoxicity), TABLE 15 p. 821 (myelosuppression), TABLE 2 p. 818 (nephrotoxicity), TABLE 5 p. 818 (thromboembolism)
- **Acetazolamide** increases the urinary excretion of **methotrexate**. Moderate Study
- **Methotrexate** is predicted to decrease the clearance of **aminophylline**. Moderate Theoretical
- Antiepileptics (**levetiracetam**) decrease the clearance of **methotrexate**. Severe Anecdotal
- Antimalarials (**pyrimethamine**) are predicted to increase the risk of side-effects when given with **methotrexate**. Severe Theoretical → Also see TABLE 15 p. 821
- **Asparaginase** affects the efficacy of **methotrexate**. Severe Anecdotal → Also see TABLE 1 p. 818 → Also see TABLE 15 p. 821
- **Aspirin** (high-dose) is predicted to increase the risk of toxicity when given with **methotrexate**. Severe Theoretical

- Crisantaspase affects the efficacy of **methotrexate**. Severe
Anecdotal → Also see TABLE 1 p. 818 → Also see TABLE 15 p. 821
- Live vaccines are predicted to increase the risk of generalised infection (possibly life-threatening) when given with **methotrexate**. Public Health England advises avoid. Severe Theoretical
- NSAIDs are predicted to increase the risk of toxicity when given with **methotrexate**. Monitor and adjust dose. Severe Study → Also see TABLE 2 p. 818
- Pegaspargase affects the efficacy of **methotrexate**. Severe Anecdotal → Also see TABLE 1 p. 818 → Also see TABLE 15 p. 821
- Penicillins are predicted to increase the risk of toxicity when given with **methotrexate**. Severe Theoretical
- Proton pump inhibitors decrease the clearance of **methotrexate**. Use with caution or avoid. Severe Study
- Quinolones (ciprofloxacin) potentially increase the risk of toxicity when given with **methotrexate**. Avoid. Severe Anecdotal
- Regorafenib is predicted to increase the exposure to **methotrexate**. Severe Theoretical → Also see TABLE 15 p. 821
- Retinoids (acitretin) are predicted to increase the concentration of **methotrexate**. Avoid. Moderate Anecdotal
- **Methotrexate** is predicted to decrease the efficacy of sapropterin. Moderate Theoretical
- Sulfonamides are predicted to increase the exposure to **methotrexate**. Use with caution or avoid. Severe Theoretical → Also see TABLE 15 p. 821
- Tedizolid is predicted to increase the exposure to **methotrexate**. Avoid. Moderate Theoretical
- **Methotrexate** is predicted to increase the risk of toxicity when given with tegafur. Severe Theoretical
- **Methotrexate** decreases the clearance of theophylline. Moderate Study
- Trimethoprim is predicted to increase the risk of side-effects when given with **methotrexate**. Avoid. Severe Theoretical → Also see TABLE 2 p. 818

Methyldopa → see TABLE 8 p. 819 (hypotension)
- Entacapone is predicted to increase the exposure to **methyldopa**. Moderate Theoretical
- Iron (oral) decreases the effects of **methyldopa**. Moderate Study
- **Methyldopa** increases the risk of neurotoxicity when given with lithium. Severe Anecdotal
- Monoamine-oxidase A and B inhibitors, irreversible are predicted to alter the antihypertensive effects of **methyldopa**. Avoid. Severe Theoretical → Also see TABLE 8 p. 819

Methylphenidate
- **Methylphenidate** is predicted to decrease the effects of apraclonidine. Severe Theoretical
- **Methylphenidate** is predicted to increase the risk of elevated blood pressure when given with linezolid. Avoid. Severe Theoretical
- **Methylphenidate** is predicted to increase the risk of a hypertensive crisis when given with moclobemide. Severe Theoretical
- **Methylphenidate** is predicted to increase the risk of a hypertensive crisis when given with monoamine-oxidase A and B inhibitors, irreversible. Avoid and for 14 days after stopping the MAOI. Severe Theoretical
- Monoamine-oxidase B inhibitors (rasagiline, selegiline) are predicted to increase the risk of a hypertensive crisis when given with **methylphenidate**. Avoid. Severe Theoretical

Methylprednisolone → see corticosteroids
Methylthioninium chloride → see TABLE 13 p. 821 (serotonin syndrome)
- **Methylthioninium chloride** is predicted to increase the risk of severe hypertension when given with bupropion. Avoid. Severe Theoretical → Also see TABLE 13 p. 821

Metoclopramide
- **Metoclopramide** is predicted to increase the risk of methaemoglobinaemia when given with topical anaesthetics, local (prilocaine). Avoid. Severe Theoretical
- **Metoclopramide** decreases the concentration of antimalarials (atovaquone). Avoid. Moderate Study
- **Metoclopramide** is predicted to decrease the effects of dopamine receptor agonists (apomorphine, bromocriptine,

cabergoline ,pergolide, pramipexole, quinagolide, ropinirole, rotigotine). Avoid. Moderate Study
- **Metoclopramide** decreases the effects of levodopa. Avoid. Moderate Study
- **Metoclopramide** is predicted to increase the effects of neuromuscular blocking drugs, non-depolarising. Moderate Theoretical
- **Metoclopramide** increases the effects of suxamethonium. Moderate Study

Metolazone → see thiazide diuretics
Metoprolol → see beta blockers, selective
Metronidazole → see TABLE 12 p. 821 (peripheral neuropathy)

- Disulfiram-like reaction can occur on the ingestion of alcohol. Ensure that alcohol is not consumed for at least 48 hours after stopping metronidazole.
- Since systemic absorption can follow topical application, the possibility of interactions should be borne in mind.

- **Metronidazole** increases the risk of toxicity when given with alkylating agents (busulfan). Severe Study
- Antiepileptics (phenobarbital, primidone) are predicted to decrease the exposure to **metronidazole**. Moderate Study
- **Metronidazole** is predicted to increase the risk of capecitabine toxicity when given with capecitabine. Severe Theoretical
- **Metronidazole** increases the anticoagulant effect of coumarins. Monitor INR and adjust dose. Severe Study
- Disulfiram increases the risk of acute psychoses when given with **metronidazole**. Severe Study → Also see TABLE 12 p. 821
- **Metronidazole** increases the risk of toxicity when given with fluorouracil. Severe Study

Metyrapone
- Antiepileptics (fosphenytoin, phenobarbital, phenytoin, primidone) decrease the effects of **metyrapone**. Avoid. Moderate Study
- Antihistamines, sedating (cyproheptadine) decrease the effects of **metyrapone**. Avoid. Moderate Study
- Carbimazole decreases the effects of **metyrapone**. Avoid. Moderate Theoretical
- Combined hormonal contraceptives decrease the effects of **metyrapone**. Avoid. Moderate Theoretical
- Phenothiazines (chlorpromazine) decrease the effects of **metyrapone**. Avoid. Moderate Theoretical
- Progesterone is predicted to decrease the effects of **metyrapone**. Avoid. Moderate Theoretical
- Propylthiouracil is predicted to decrease the effects of **metyrapone**. Avoid. Moderate Theoretical
- Tricyclic antidepressants (amitriptyline) decrease the effects of **metyrapone**. Avoid. Moderate Theoretical

Mianserin → see TABLE 13 p. 821 (serotonin syndrome), TABLE 11 p. 820 (CNS depressant effects)
- Antiepileptics (carbamazepine) markedly decrease the exposure to **mianserin**. Adjust dose. Moderate Study
- Antiepileptics (phenobarbital, primidone) are predicted to decrease the exposure to **mianserin**. Moderate Study → Also see TABLE 11 p. 820
- **Mianserin** is predicted to increase the risk of toxicity when given with moclobemide. Avoid and for 1 week after stopping **mianserin**. Severe Theoretical → Also see TABLE 13 p. 821
- **Mianserin** is predicted to increase the risk of toxicity when given with monoamine-oxidase A and B inhibitors, irreversible. Avoid and for 14 days after stopping the MAOI. Severe Theoretical → Also see TABLE 13 p. 821
- **Mianserin** is predicted to decrease the efficacy of pitolisant. Unknown Theoretical
- **Mianserin** decreases the effects of sympathomimetics, vasoconstrictor (ephedrine). Severe Anecdotal

Micafungin → see TABLE 1 p. 818 (hepatotoxicity)
- **Micafungin** slightly increases the exposure to amphotericin. Avoid or monitor toxicity. Moderate Study

Miconazole → see antifungals, azoles
Midazolam → see TABLE 11 p. 820 (CNS depressant effects)
- Antiarrhythmics (dronedarone) are predicted to increase the exposure to **midazolam**. Monitor side effects and adjust dose. Severe Study

A1

Interactions | Appendix 1

Midazolam (continued)

▸ Antiepileptics **(carbamazepine, fosphenytoin, phenobarbital, phenytoin, primidone)** are predicted to decrease the exposure to **midazolam**. Monitor and adjust dose. [Moderate] Study → Also see **TABLE 11** p. 820

▸ Antifungals, azoles **(fluconazole, isavuconazole, posaconazole)** are predicted to increase the exposure to **midazolam**. Monitor side effects and adjust dose. [Severe] Study

▸ Antifungals, azoles **(itraconazole, ketoconazole, voriconazole)** are predicted to markedly to very markedly increase the exposure to **midazolam**. Avoid or adjust **midazolam** dose. [Severe] Study

▸ Antifungals, azoles **(miconazole)** are predicted to increase the exposure to intravenous **midazolam**. Use with caution and adjust dose. [Moderate] Theoretical

▸ Antifungals, azoles **(miconazole)** are predicted to increase the exposure to oral **midazolam**. Avoid. [Moderate] Theoretical

▸ Aprepitant is predicted to increase the exposure to **midazolam**. Monitor side effects and adjust dose. [Severe] Study

▸ Bosentan is predicted to decrease the concentration of **midazolam**. Monitor and adjust dose. [Moderate] Theoretical

▸ Calcium channel blockers **(diltiazem, verapamil)** are predicted to increase the exposure to **midazolam**. Monitor side effects and adjust dose. [Severe] Study

▸ Cobicistat is predicted to markedly to very markedly increase the exposure to **midazolam**. Avoid or adjust **midazolam** dose. [Severe] Study

▸ Crizotinib is predicted to increase the exposure to **midazolam**. Monitor side effects and adjust dose. [Severe] Study

▸ Dabrafenib decreases the exposure to **midazolam**. Monitor and adjust dose. [Moderate] Study

▸ Efavirenz is predicted to alter the effects of **midazolam**. Avoid. [Moderate] Theoretical

▸ Enzalutamide is predicted to decrease the exposure to **midazolam**. Monitor and adjust dose. [Moderate] Study

▸ Fosaprepitant slightly increases the exposure to **midazolam**. [Moderate] Study

▸ HIV-protease inhibitors **(atazanavir, darunavir, fosamprenavir, lopinavir, ritonavir, saquinavir, tipranavir)** are predicted to markedly to very markedly increase the exposure to **midazolam**. Avoid or adjust **midazolam** dose. [Severe] Study

▸ HIV-protease inhibitors **(indinavir)** are predicted to increase the exposure to **midazolam**. Monitor side effects and adjust dose. [Severe] Study

▸ Idelalisib is predicted to markedly to very markedly increase the exposure to **midazolam**. Avoid or adjust **midazolam** dose. [Severe] Study

▸ Imatinib is predicted to increase the exposure to **midazolam**. Monitor side effects and adjust dose. [Severe] Study

▸ Lumacaftor is predicted to decrease the exposure to **midazolam**. Avoid. [Severe] Theoretical

▸ Macrolides **(clarithromycin)** are predicted to markedly to very markedly increase the exposure to **midazolam**. Avoid or adjust **midazolam** dose. [Severe] Study

▸ Macrolides **(erythromycin)** are predicted to increase the exposure to **midazolam**. Monitor side effects and adjust dose. [Severe] Study

▸ Netupitant is predicted to increase the exposure to **midazolam**. Monitor side effects and adjust dose. [Severe] Study

▸ Nevirapine decreases the concentration of **midazolam**. Monitor and adjust dose. [Moderate] Study

▸ Nilotinib is predicted to increase the exposure to **midazolam**. Monitor side effects and adjust dose. [Severe] Study

▸ Palbociclib increases the exposure to **midazolam**. [Moderate] Study

▸ Rifampicin is predicted to decrease the exposure to **midazolam**. Monitor and adjust dose. [Moderate] Study

▸ St John's Wort moderately decreases the exposure to **midazolam**. Monitor and adjust dose. [Moderate] Study

Midodrine → see sympathomimetics, vasoconstrictor

Mifamurtide

▸ Ciclosporin is predicted to decrease the efficacy of **mifamurtide**. Avoid. [Severe] Theoretical

▸ Corticosteroids are predicted to decrease the efficacy of **mifamurtide**. Avoid. [Severe] Theoretical

▸ NSAIDs (high-dose) are predicted to decrease the efficacy of **mifamurtide**. Avoid. [Severe] Theoretical

▸ Pimecrolimus is predicted to decrease the efficacy of **mifamurtide**. Avoid. [Severe] Theoretical

▸ Sirolimus is predicted to decrease the efficacy of **mifamurtide**. Avoid. [Severe] Theoretical

▸ Tacrolimus is predicted to affect the efficacy of **mifamurtide**. Avoid. [Severe] Theoretical

Mifepristone

▸ Mifepristone is predicted to decrease the efficacy of corticosteroids. Use with caution and adjust dose. [Moderate] Theoretical

Minocycline → see tetracyclines

Minoxidil → see **TABLE 8** p. 819 (hypotension)

Mirabegron

▸ Mirabegron is predicted to increase the exposure to aliskiren. [Mild] Theoretical

▸ Mirabegron is predicted to increase the exposure to antiarrhythmics **(flecainide)**. [Severe] Theoretical

▸ Antifungals, azoles **(itraconazole, ketoconazole, voriconazole)** are predicted to increase the exposure to **mirabegron**. Adjust **mirabegron** dose in hepatic and renal impairment. [Moderate] Study

▸ Mirabegron is predicted to increase the exposure to antihistamines, non-sedating **(fexofenadine)**. [Mild] Theoretical

▸ Mirabegron is predicted to increase the exposure to beta blockers, non-selective **(carvedilol, timolol)**. [Moderate] Theoretical

▸ Mirabegron is predicted to increase the exposure to beta blockers, selective **(metoprolol, nebivolol)**. [Moderate] Study

▸ Cobicistat is predicted to increase the exposure to **mirabegron**. Adjust **mirabegron** dose in hepatic and renal impairment. [Moderate] Study

▸ Mirabegron is predicted to increase the exposure to colchicine. [Mild] Theoretical

▸ Mirabegron is predicted to increase the exposure to dabigatran. [Severe] Theoretical

▸ Mirabegron slightly increases the exposure to digoxin. Monitor digoxin concentration and adjust dose, p. 79. [Severe] Study

▸ Mirabegron is predicted to increase the exposure to edoxaban. [Mild] Theoretical

▸ Mirabegron is predicted to increase the exposure to everolimus. [Mild] Theoretical

▸ HIV-protease inhibitors **(atazanavir, darunavir, fosamprenavir, lopinavir, ritonavir, saquinavir, tipranavir)** are predicted to increase the exposure to **mirabegron**. Adjust **mirabegron** dose in hepatic and renal impairment. [Moderate] Study

▸ Idelalisib is predicted to increase the exposure to **mirabegron**. Adjust **mirabegron** dose in hepatic and renal impairment. [Moderate] Study

▸ Mirabegron is predicted to increase the exposure to loperamide. [Mild] Theoretical

▸ Macrolides **(clarithromycin)** are predicted to increase the exposure to **mirabegron**. Adjust **mirabegron** dose in hepatic and renal impairment. [Moderate] Study

▸ Mirabegron is predicted to decrease the efficacy of opioids **(tramadol)**. [Moderate] Study

▸ Mirabegron is predicted to increase the exposure to pitolisant. Use with caution and adjust dose. [Moderate] Study

▸ Mirabegron is predicted to increase the exposure to sirolimus. [Mild] Theoretical

▸ Mirabegron is predicted to increase the exposure to taxanes **(paclitaxel)**. [Mild] Theoretical

▸ Mirabegron is predicted to increase the exposure to topotecan. [Mild] Theoretical

Mirtazapine → see **TABLE 13** p. 821 (serotonin syndrome), **TABLE 11** p. 820 (CNS depressant effects)

▸ Antiepileptics **(carbamazepine, fosphenytoin, phenobarbital, phenytoin, primidone)** are predicted to decrease the exposure to **mirtazapine**. Adjust dose. [Moderate] Study → Also see **TABLE 11** p. 820

▸ Antifungals, azoles **(itraconazole, ketoconazole, voriconazole)** are predicted to increase the exposure to **mirtazapine**. [Moderate] Study

▸ Cobicistat is predicted to increase the exposure to **mirtazapine**. [Moderate] Study

- **Enzalutamide** is predicted to decrease the exposure to mirtazapine. Adjust dose. Moderate Study
- **H$_2$ receptor antagonists (cimetidine)** slightly increase the exposure to **mirtazapine**. Use with caution and adjust dose. Moderate Theoretical
- **HIV-protease inhibitors (atazanavir, darunavir, fosamprenavir, lopinavir, ritonavir, saquinavir, tipranavir)** are predicted to increase the exposure to **mirtazapine**. Moderate Study
- **Idelalisib** is predicted to increase the exposure to **mirtazapine**. Moderate Study
- **Macrolides (clarithromycin)** are predicted to increase the exposure to **mirtazapine**. Moderate Study
- **Mirtazapine** is predicted to decrease the efficacy of **pitolisant**. Unknown Theoretical
- **Rifampicin** is predicted to decrease the exposure to **mirtazapine**. Adjust dose. Moderate Study

Mitomycin → see TABLE 15 p. 821 (myelosuppression), TABLE 5 p. 818 (thromboembolism)

- **Live vaccines** are predicted to increase the risk of generalised infection (possibly life-threatening) when given with **mitomycin**. Public Health England advises avoid. Severe Theoretical

Mitotane → see TABLE 15 p. 821 (myelosuppression)

- **Aldosterone antagonists (spironolactone)** are predicted to decrease the effects of **mitotane**. Avoid. Severe Anecdotal

Mitoxantrone → see anthracyclines

Mivacurium → see neuromuscular blocking drugs, non-depolarising

Mizolastine → see antihistamines, non-sedating

Moclobemide → see TABLE 13 p. 821 (serotonin syndrome)

> **FOOD AND LIFESTYLE** Moclobemide is claimed to cause less potentiation of the pressor effect of tyramine than the traditional (irreversible) MAOIs, but patients should avoid consuming large amounts of tyramine-rich foods (such as mature cheese, salami, pickled herring, Bovril®, Oxo®, Marmite® or any similar meat or yeast extract or fermented soya bean extract, and some beers, lagers or wines).

- **Moclobemide** is predicted to increase the risk of a hypertensive crisis when given with amfetamines **(dexamfetamine)**. Avoid. Severe Theoretical → Also see TABLE 13 p. 821
- **Moclobemide** is predicted to increase the risk of a hypertensive crisis when given with amfetamines **(lisdexamfetamine)**. Avoid. Severe Anecdotal → Also see TABLE 13 p. 821
- **Moclobemide** is predicted to increase the risk of severe hypertension when given with **bupropion**. Avoid. Severe Theoretical → Also see TABLE 13 p. 821
- **Moclobemide** is predicted to increase the exposure to **cilostazol**. Moderate Theoretical
- **Moclobemide** is predicted to decrease the efficacy of **clopidogrel**. Avoid. Moderate Study
- **H$_2$ receptor antagonists (cimetidine)** increase the exposure to **moclobemide**. Adjust **moclobemide** dose. Mild Study
- **Levodopa** increases the risk of side-effects when given with **moclobemide**. Moderate Study
- **Moclobemide** is predicted to increase the risk of side-effects when given with **linezolid**. Avoid and for 14 days after stopping **moclobemide**. Severe Theoretical → Also see TABLE 13 p. 821
- **Methylphenidate** is predicted to increase the risk of a hypertensive crisis when given with **moclobemide**. Severe Theoretical
- **Mianserin** is predicted to increase the risk of toxicity when given with **moclobemide**. Avoid and for 1 week after stopping mianserin. Severe Theoretical → Also see TABLE 13 p. 821
- **Moclobemide** is predicted to increase the effects of monoamine-oxidase B inhibitors **(rasagiline, selegiline)**. Avoid. Severe Theoretical → Also see TABLE 13 p. 821
- **Moclobemide** is predicted to increase the risk of side-effects when given with monoamine-oxidase B inhibitors **(safinamide)**. Avoid and for 1 week after stopping **safinamide**. Severe Theoretical → Also see TABLE 13 p. 821
- **Opicapone** is predicted to increase the risk of elevated blood pressure when given with **moclobemide**. Avoid. Severe Theoretical
- **Moclobemide** increases the risk of side-effects when given with phenothiazines **(levomepromazine)**. Moderate Study

- **Reboxetine** is predicted to increase the risk of a hypertensive crisis when given with **moclobemide**. Avoid. Severe Theoretical
- **Moclobemide** moderately increases the exposure to **rizatriptan**. Avoid. Moderate Study → Also see TABLE 13 p. 821
- **Moclobemide** moderately increases the exposure to **sumatriptan**. Avoid. Moderate Study → Also see TABLE 13 p. 821
- **Moclobemide** is predicted to increase the risk of a hypertensive crisis when given with sympathomimetics, vasoconstrictor **(ephedrine, isometheptene, phenylephrine, pseudoephedrine)**. Avoid. Severe Study
- **Moclobemide** is predicted to increase the risk of side-effects when given with **tedizolid**. Severe Theoretical → Also see TABLE 13 p. 821
- **Tricyclic antidepressants** are predicted to increase the effects of **moclobemide**. Avoid. Severe Theoretical → Also see TABLE 13 p. 821
- **Moclobemide** slightly increases the exposure to **zolmitriptan**. Adjust **zolmitriptan** dose, p. 280. Moderate Study → Also see TABLE 13 p. 821

Modafinil

- **Antiepileptics (carbamazepine, phenobarbital, primidone)** are predicted to decrease the exposure to **modafinil**. Mild Theoretical
- **Antiepileptics (fosphenytoin, phenytoin)** are predicted to decrease the exposure to **modafinil** and **modafinil** is predicted to increase the concentration of antiepileptics **(fosphenytoin, phenytoin)**. Monitor concentration and adjust dose. Moderate Theoretical
- **Antifungals, azoles (itraconazole, ketoconazole, voriconazole)** are predicted to increase the exposure to **modafinil**. Mild Theoretical
- **Modafinil** is predicted to decrease the exposure to **bosutinib**. Avoid. Severe Theoretical
- **Cobicistat** is predicted to increase the exposure to **modafinil**. Mild Theoretical
- **Modafinil** is predicted to decrease the efficacy of **combined hormonal contraceptives**. For FSRH guidance, see Contraceptives, interactions p. 474. Severe Study
- **Modafinil** is predicted to decrease the efficacy of **desogestrel**. For FSRH guidance, see Contraceptives, interactions p. 474. Severe Theoretical
- **Modafinil** is predicted to decrease the exposure to **elbasvir**. Avoid. Unknown Theoretical
- **Modafinil** is predicted to decrease the efficacy of **etonogestrel**. For FSRH guidance, see Contraceptives, interactions p. 474. Severe Theoretical
- **Modafinil** is predicted to decrease the exposure to **grazoprevir**. Avoid. Unknown Theoretical
- **HIV-protease inhibitors (atazanavir, darunavir, fosamprenavir, lopinavir, ritonavir, saquinavir, tipranavir)** are predicted to increase the exposure to **modafinil**. Mild Theoretical
- **Modafinil** is predicted to decrease the effects of **Hormone replacement therapy**. Moderate Anecdotal
- **Idelalisib** is predicted to increase the exposure to **modafinil**. Mild Theoretical
- **Modafinil** is predicted to decrease the efficacy of **levonorgestrel**. For FSRH guidance, see Contraceptives, interactions p. 474. Severe Theoretical
- **Macrolides (clarithromycin)** are predicted to increase the exposure to **modafinil**. Mild Theoretical
- **Modafinil** is predicted to decrease the efficacy of **norethisterone**. For FSRH guidance, see Contraceptives, interactions p. 474. Severe Anecdotal
- **Rifampicin** is predicted to decrease the exposure to **modafinil**. Moderate Theoretical
- **Modafinil** decreases the efficacy of **ulipristal**. For FSRH guidance, see Contraceptives, interactions p. 474. Severe Anecdotal

Moexipril → see ACE inhibitors

Mometasone → see corticosteroids

Monoamine-oxidase A and B inhibitors, irreversible → see TABLE 8 p. 819 (hypotension), TABLE 13 p. 821 (serotonin syndrome)

> isocarboxazid · phenelzine · tranylcypromine

> **FOOD AND LIFESTYLE** Potentially life-threatening hypertensive crisis can develop in those taking MAOIs who eat tyramine-

Interactions | **Appendix 1**

Monoamine-oxidase A and B inhibitors, irreversible (continued)

rich food (such as mature cheese, salami, pickled herring, Bovril®, Oxo®, Marmite® or any similar meat or yeast extract or fermented soya bean extract, and some beers, lagers or wines) or foods containing dopa (such as broad bean pods). Avoid tyramine-rich or dopa-rich food or drinks with, or for 2 to 3 weeks after stopping, the MAOI.

- **Monoamine-oxidase A and B inhibitors, irreversible** are predicted to increase the effects of alpha blockers (**indoramin**). Avoid. Severe Theoretical → Also see TABLE 8 p. 819
- **Monoamine-oxidase A and B inhibitors, irreversible** are predicted to increase the risk of a hypertensive crisis when given with **amfetamines**. Avoid and for 14 days after stopping the MAOI. Severe Anecdotal → Also see TABLE 13 p. 821
- Antiepileptics (**phenobarbital, primidone**) are predicted to increase the effects of **monoamine-oxidase A and B inhibitors, irreversible**. Severe Theoretical
- **Monoamine-oxidase A and B inhibitors, irreversible** are predicted to increase the risk of antimuscarinic side-effects when given with **antihistamines, non-sedating**. Avoid. Severe Theoretical
- **Monoamine-oxidase A and B inhibitors, irreversible** are predicted to increase the risk of antimuscarinic side-effects when given with **antihistamines, sedating**. Avoid. Severe Theoretical
- **Monoamine-oxidase A and B inhibitors, irreversible** are predicted to increase the risk of side-effects when given with **atomoxetine**. Avoid and for 2 weeks after stopping the MAOI. Severe Theoretical
- **Monoamine-oxidase A and B inhibitors, irreversible** are predicted to increase the risk of cardiovascular side-effects when given with **beta$_2$ agonists**. Moderate Anecdotal
- **Monoamine-oxidase A and B inhibitors, irreversible** are predicted to increase the risk of severe hypertension when given with **bupropion**. Avoid and for 14 days after stopping the MAOI. Severe Theoretical → Also see TABLE 13 p. 821
- **Buspirone** is predicted to increase the risk of elevated blood pressure when given with **monoamine-oxidase A and B inhibitors, irreversible**. Avoid. Severe Anecdotal → Also see TABLE 13 p. 821
- **Monoamine-oxidase A and B inhibitors, irreversible** are predicted to increase the effects of **doxapram**. Moderate Theoretical
- **Entacapone** is predicted to increase the risk of elevated blood pressure when given with **monoamine-oxidase A and B inhibitors, irreversible**. Avoid. Severe Theoretical
- **Monoamine-oxidase A and B inhibitors, irreversible** are predicted to decrease the antihypertensive effects of **guanethidine**. Avoid and for 14 days after stopping the MAOI. Severe Theoretical → Also see TABLE 8 p. 819
- **Monoamine-oxidase A and B inhibitors, irreversible** are predicted to affect the exposure to **histamine**. Avoid. Severe Theoretical → Also see TABLE 8 p. 819
- **Levodopa** increases the risk of a hypertensive crisis when given with **monoamine-oxidase A and B inhibitors, irreversible**. Avoid and for 14 days after stopping the MAOI. Severe Study → Also see TABLE 8 p. 819
- **Monoamine-oxidase A and B inhibitors, irreversible** are predicted to increase the risk of side-effects when given with **linezolid**. Avoid and for 14 days after stopping the MAOI. Severe Theoretical → Also see TABLE 13 p. 821
- **Monoamine-oxidase A and B inhibitors, irreversible** are predicted to alter the antihypertensive effects of **methyldopa**. Avoid. Severe Theoretical → Also see TABLE 8 p. 819
- **Methylphenidate** is predicted to increase the risk of a hypertensive crisis when given with **monoamine-oxidase A and B inhibitors, irreversible**. Avoid and for 14 days after stopping the MAOI. Severe Theoretical
- **Mianserin** is predicted to increase the risk of toxicity when given with **monoamine-oxidase A and B inhibitors, irreversible**. Avoid and for 14 days after stopping the MAOI. Severe Theoretical → Also see TABLE 13 p. 821
- Monoamine-oxidase B inhibitors (**rasagiline, selegiline**) are predicted to increase the risk of side-effects when given with **monoamine-oxidase A and B inhibitors, irreversible**. Avoid and for 14 days after stopping the MAOI. Severe Theoretical → Also see TABLE 13 p. 821
- Monoamine-oxidase B inhibitors (**safinamide**) are predicted to increase the risk of side-effects when given with **monoamine-oxidase A and B inhibitors, irreversible**. Avoid and for 1 week after stopping **safinamide**. Severe Theoretical → Also see TABLE 13 p. 821
- **Nefopam** is predicted to increase the risk of serious elevations in blood pressure when given with **monoamine-oxidase A and B inhibitors, irreversible**. Avoid. Severe Theoretical
- **Opicapone** is predicted to increase the risk of elevated blood pressure when given with **monoamine-oxidase A and B inhibitors, irreversible**. Avoid. Severe Theoretical
- **Opioids** are predicted to increase the risk of CNS excitation or depression when given with **monoamine-oxidase A and B inhibitors, irreversible**. Avoid. Severe Study → Also see TABLE 13 p. 821
- **Monoamine-oxidase A and B inhibitors, irreversible** are predicted to increase the risk of neuroleptic malignant syndrome when given with **phenothiazines**. Severe Theoretical → Also see TABLE 8 p. 819
- **Pholcodine** is predicted to increase the risk of CNS excitation or depression when given with **monoamine-oxidase A and B inhibitors, irreversible**. Avoid and for 14 days after stopping the MAOI. Severe Theoretical
- **Reboxetine** is predicted to increase the risk of a hypertensive crisis when given with **monoamine-oxidase A and B inhibitors, irreversible**. Avoid. Severe Theoretical
- **Monoamine-oxidase A and B inhibitors, irreversible** are predicted to increase the exposure to **rizatriptan**. Avoid and for 14 days after stopping the MAOI. Severe Theoretical → Also see TABLE 13 p. 821
- **Monoamine-oxidase A and B inhibitors, irreversible** are predicted to increase the exposure to **sumatriptan**. Avoid and for 14 days after stopping the MAOI. Severe Theoretical → Also see TABLE 13 p. 821
- **Monoamine-oxidase A and B inhibitors, irreversible** are predicted to increase the risk of a hypertensive crisis when given with **sympathomimetics, inotropic**. Avoid and for 14 days after stopping the MAOI. Severe Theoretical
- **Monoamine-oxidase A and B inhibitors, irreversible** are predicted to increase the risk of a hypertensive crisis when given with **sympathomimetics, vasoconstrictor**. Avoid and for 14 days after stopping the MAOI. Severe Study
- **Monoamine-oxidase A and B inhibitors, irreversible** are predicted to increase the risk of side-effects when given with **tedizolid**. Severe Theoretical → Also see TABLE 13 p. 821
- **Tetrabenazine** is predicted to increase the risk of CNS toxicity when given with **monoamine-oxidase A and B inhibitors, irreversible**. Avoid and for 14 days after stopping the MAOI. Severe Theoretical
- **Tolcapone** is predicted to increase the effects of **monoamine-oxidase A and B inhibitors, irreversible**. Avoid. Severe Theoretical
- **Tricyclic antidepressants** are predicted to increase the effects of **monoamine-oxidase A and B inhibitors, irreversible**. Avoid. Severe Theoretical → Also see TABLE 8 p. 819 → Also see TABLE 13 p. 821
- **Monoamine-oxidase A and B inhibitors, irreversible** are predicted to increase the exposure to **zolmitriptan**. Severe Theoretical → Also see TABLE 13 p. 821

Monoamine-oxidase B inhibitors → see TABLE 6 p. 819 (bradycardia), TABLE 8 p. 819 (hypotension), TABLE 13 p. 821 (serotonin syndrome)

rasagiline · safinamide · selegiline

FOOD AND LIFESTYLE Hypertension is predicted to occur when high-dose **selegiline** is taken with tyramine-rich foods (such as mature cheese, salami, pickled herring, Bovril®, Oxo®, Marmite® or any similar meat or yeast extract or fermented soya bean extract, and some beers, lagers or wines).

- Monoamine-oxidase B inhibitors (**rasagiline, selegiline**) are predicted to increase the risk of severe hypertension when given with **amfetamines**. Avoid. Severe Theoretical → Also see TABLE 13 p. 821

▸ **Safinamide** is predicted to increase the risk of severe hypertension when given with **amfetamines**. [Severe] Theoretical → Also see **TABLE 13** p. 821

▸ Monoamine-oxidase B inhibitors **(rasagiline, selegiline)** are predicted to increase the risk of severe hypertension when given with **beta₂ agonists**. Avoid. [Severe] Theoretical

▸ **Safinamide** is predicted to increase the risk of severe hypertension when given with **beta₂ agonists**. [Severe] Theoretical

▸ **Monoamine-oxidase B inhibitors** are predicted to increase the risk of severe hypertension when given with **bupropion**. Avoid. [Moderate] Theoretical → Also see **TABLE 13** p. 821

▸ **Combined hormonal contraceptives** slightly increases the exposure to **rasagiline**. [Moderate] Study

▸ **Combined hormonal contraceptives** increase the exposure to **selegiline**. Avoid. [Severe] Study

▸ **Hormone replacement therapy** is predicted to increase the exposure to **selegiline**. Avoid. [Moderate] Study

▸ **Monoamine-oxidase B inhibitors** are predicted to increase the effects of **levodopa**. Adjust dose. [Mild] Study → Also see **TABLE 8** p. 819

▸ Monoamine-oxidase B inhibitors **(rasagiline, selegiline)** are predicted to increase the risk of side-effects when given with **linezolid**. Avoid and for 14 days after stopping the MAOI. [Severe] Theoretical → Also see **TABLE 13** p. 821

▸ **Safinamide** is predicted to increase the risk of side-effects when given with **linezolid**. Avoid and for 1 week after stopping **safinamide**. [Severe] Theoretical → Also see **TABLE 13** p. 821

▸ Monoamine-oxidase B inhibitors **(rasagiline, selegiline)** are predicted to increase the risk of a hypertensive crisis when given with **methylphenidate**. Avoid. [Severe] Theoretical

▸ **Moclobemide** is predicted to increase the effects of monoamine-oxidase B inhibitors **(rasagiline, selegiline)**. Avoid. [Severe] Theoretical → Also see **TABLE 13** p. 821

▸ **Moclobemide** is predicted to increase the risk of side-effects when given with **safinamide**. Avoid and for 1 week after stopping **safinamide**. [Severe] Theoretical → Also see **TABLE 13** p. 821

▸ Monoamine-oxidase B inhibitors **(rasagiline, selegiline)** are predicted to increase the risk of side-effects when given with **monoamine-oxidase A and B inhibitors, irreversible**. Avoid and for 14 days after stopping the MAOI. [Severe] Theoretical → Also see **TABLE 8** p. 819 → Also see **TABLE 13** p. 821

▸ **Safinamide** is predicted to increase the risk of side-effects when given with **monoamine-oxidase A and B inhibitors, irreversible**. Avoid and for 1 week after stopping **safinamide**. [Severe] Theoretical → Also see **TABLE 13** p. 821

▸ **Opicapone** is predicted to increase the risk of elevated blood pressure when given with monoamine-oxidase B inhibitors **(rasagiline, selegiline)**. [Severe] Theoretical

▸ **Rasagiline** is predicted to increase the risk of side-effects when given with opioids **(pethidine)**. Avoid and for 14 days after stopping **rasagiline**. [Severe] Theoretical → Also see **TABLE 13** p. 821

▸ **Safinamide** is predicted to increase the risk of side-effects when given with opioids **(pethidine)**. Avoid and for 1 week after stopping **safinamide**. [Severe] Theoretical → Also see **TABLE 13** p. 821

▸ **Selegiline** increases the risk of side-effects when given with opioids **(pethidine)**. Avoid. [Severe] Anecdotal → Also see **TABLE 13** p. 821

▸ Quinolones **(ciprofloxacin)** slightly increase the exposure to **rasagiline**. [Moderate] Study

▸ **Reboxetine** is predicted to increase the risk of a hypertensive crisis when given with monoamine-oxidase B inhibitors **(rasagiline, selegiline)**. Avoid. [Severe] Theoretical

▸ **Monoamine-oxidase B inhibitors** are predicted to increase the risk of a hypertensive crisis when given with sympathomimetics, inotropic. Avoid. [Severe] Anecdotal

▸ **Monoamine-oxidase B inhibitors** are predicted to increase the risk of a hypertensive crisis when given with sympathomimetics, vasoconstrictor. Avoid. [Severe] Anecdotal

▸ Monoamine-oxidase B inhibitors **(rasagiline, selegiline)** are predicted to increase the risk of side-effects when given with **tedizolid**. [Severe] Theoretical → Also see **TABLE 13** p. 821

▸ **Safinamide** is predicted to increase the risk of side-effects when given with **tedizolid**. Avoid and for 1 week after stopping **safinamide**. [Severe] Theoretical → Also see **TABLE 13** p. 821

Monoclonal antibodies → see **TABLE 15** p. 821 (myelosuppression), **TABLE 12** p. 821 (peripheral neuropathy), **TABLE 4** p. 818 (antiplatelet effects)

adalimumab · alemtuzumab · alirocumab · basiliximab · belimumab · bevacizumab · blinatumomab · brentuximab vedotin · canakinumab · catumaxomab · certolizumab pegol · cetuximab · daclizumab · daratumumab · denosumab · eculizumab · elotuzumab · evolocumab · golimumab · idarucizumab · infliximab · ipilimumab · ixekizumab · mepolizumab · natalizumab · necitumumab · nivolumab · obinutuzumab · ofatumumab · omalizumab · panitumumab · pembrolizumab · pertuzumab · ramucirumab · reslizumab · rituximab · secukinumab · siltuximab · tocilizumab · trastuzumab · trastuzumab emtansine · ustekinumab · vedolizumab

▸ **Blinatumomab** is predicted to transiently increase the exposure to **aminophylline**. Monitor and adjust dose. [Moderate] Theoretical

▸ **Anthracyclines** are predicted to increase the risk of cardiotoxicity when given with monoclonal antibodies **(trastuzumab, trastuzumab emtansine)**. Avoid. [Severe] Theoretical → Also see **TABLE 15** p. 821

▸ **Antiarrhythmics (dronedarone)** increase the risk of neutropenia when given with **brentuximab vedotin**. Monitor and adjust dose. [Severe] Theoretical

▸ **Antiepileptics (carbamazepine)** are predicted to decrease the effects of **brentuximab vedotin**. [Severe] Theoretical

▸ **Antiepileptics (carbamazepine, fosphenytoin, phenobarbital, phenytoin, primidone)** are predicted to decrease the exposure to **trastuzumab emtansine**. [Severe] Theoretical

▸ **Antifungals, azoles (itraconazole, ketoconazole)** increase the risk of neutropenia when given with **brentuximab vedotin**. Monitor and adjust dose. [Severe] Study

▸ **Antifungals, azoles (itraconazole, ketoconazole, voriconazole)** are predicted to increase the exposure to **trastuzumab emtansine**. Avoid. [Severe] Theoretical

▸ **Brentuximab vedotin** increases the risk of pulmonary toxicity when given with **bleomycin**. Avoid. [Severe] Study → Also see **TABLE 15** p. 821

▸ **Blinatumomab** is predicted to transiently increase the exposure to **ciclosporin**. Monitor and adjust dose. [Moderate] Theoretical

▸ **Cobicistat** is predicted to increase the exposure to **trastuzumab emtansine**. Avoid. [Severe] Theoretical

▸ **Blinatumomab** is predicted to transiently increase the exposure to coumarins **(warfarin)**. Monitor and adjust dose. [Moderate] Theoretical

▸ **Enzalutamide** is predicted to decrease the exposure to **trastuzumab emtansine**. [Severe] Theoretical

▸ **HIV-protease inhibitors (atazanavir, darunavir, fosamprenavir, lopinavir, ritonavir, saquinavir, tipranavir)** are predicted to increase the exposure to **trastuzumab emtansine**. Avoid. [Severe] Theoretical

▸ **HIV-protease inhibitors (lopinavir, ritonavir, saquinavir)** are predicted to increase the risk of neutropenia when given with **brentuximab vedotin**. Monitor and adjust dose. [Severe] Study

▸ **Idelalisib** is predicted to increase the exposure to **trastuzumab emtansine**. Avoid. [Severe] Theoretical → Also see **TABLE 15** p. 821

▸ **Live vaccines** are predicted to increase the risk of generalised infection (possibly life-threatening) when given with **monoclonal antibodies**. Public Health England advises avoid. [Severe] Theoretical

▸ **Macrolides (clarithromycin)** increase the risk of neutropenia when given with **brentuximab vedotin**. Monitor and adjust dose. [Severe] Theoretical

▸ **Macrolides (clarithromycin)** are predicted to increase the exposure to **trastuzumab emtansine**. Avoid. [Severe] Theoretical

▸ **Rifampicin** decreases the effects of **brentuximab vedotin**. [Severe] Study

▸ **Rifampicin** is predicted to decrease the exposure to **trastuzumab emtansine**. [Severe] Theoretical

▸ **Tocilizumab** is predicted to decrease the exposure to statins **(atorvastatin)**. Monitor and adjust dose. [Moderate] Theoretical

▸ **Tocilizumab** moderately decreases the exposure to statins **(simvastatin)**. Monitor and adjust dose. [Moderate] Study

A1

Interactions | Appendix 1

Monoclonal antibodies (continued)

▸ Blinatumomab is predicted to transiently increase the exposure to theophylline. Monitor and adjust dose. [Moderate] Theoretical

Montelukast

▸ Antiepileptics (carbamazepine, fosphenytoin, phenobarbital, phenytoin, primidone) are predicted to decrease the exposure to montelukast. [Mild] Study
▸ Enzalutamide is predicted to decrease the exposure to montelukast. [Mild] Study
▸ Fibrates (gemfibrozil) are predicted to moderately increase the exposure to montelukast. [Moderate] Study
▸ Lumacaftor is predicted to decrease the exposure to montelukast. [Moderate] Theoretical
▸ Rifampicin is predicted to decrease the exposure to montelukast. [Mild] Study

Morphine → see opioids

Moxifloxacin → see quinolones

Moxisylyte → see TABLE 8 p. 819 (hypotension)

Moxonidine → see TABLE 8 p. 819 (hypotension), TABLE 11 p. 820 (CNS depressant effects)

▸ Tricyclic antidepressants are predicted to decrease the effects of moxonidine. Avoid. [Moderate] Theoretical → Also see TABLE 8 p. 819

Mycophenolate → see TABLE 15 p. 821 (myelosuppression)

▸ Mycophenolate is predicted to increase the risk of haematological toxicity when given with aciclovir. [Moderate] Theoretical
▸ Antacids decrease the exposure to mycophenolate. [Moderate] Study
▸ Mycophenolate is predicted to increase the risk of haematological toxicity when given with ganciclovir. [Moderate] Theoretical → Also see TABLE 15 p. 821
▸ Live vaccines are predicted to increase the risk of generalised infection (possibly life-threatening) when given with mycophenolate. Public Health England advises avoid. [Severe] Theoretical
▸ Rifampicin decreases the concentration of mycophenolate. Monitor and adjust dose. [Severe] Study
▸ Mycophenolate is predicted to increase the risk of haematological toxicity when given with valaciclovir. [Moderate] Theoretical
▸ Mycophenolate is predicted to increase the risk of haematological toxicity when given with valganciclovir. [Moderate] Theoretical → Also see TABLE 15 p. 821

Nabilone → see TABLE 11 p. 820 (CNS depressant effects)

▸ Nabilone is predicted to increase the risk of cardiovascular side-effects when given with amfetamines. [Severe] Theoretical

Nabumetone → see NSAIDs

Nadolol → see beta blockers, non-selective

Nalidixic acid → see quinolones

Nalmefene

GENERAL INFORMATION Discontinue treatment 1 week before anticipated use of opioids; if emergency analgesia is required during treatment, an increased dose of opioid analgesic might be necessary (monitor for opioid intoxication).

▸ Nalmefene is predicted to decrease the efficacy of opioids. Avoid. [Severe] Theoretical

Naloxegol

▸ Antiarrhythmics (dronedarone) are predicted to increase the exposure to naloxegol. Adjust naloxegol dose and monitor side effects. [Moderate] Study
▸ Antiepileptics (carbamazepine, fosphenytoin, phenobarbital, phenytoin, primidone) are predicted to markedly decrease the exposure to naloxegol. Avoid. [Moderate] Study
▸ Antifungals, azoles (fluconazole, isavuconazole, posaconazole) are predicted to increase the exposure to naloxegol. Adjust naloxegol dose and monitor side effects. [Moderate] Study
▸ Antifungals, azoles (itraconazole, ketoconazole, voriconazole) are predicted to markedly increase the exposure to naloxegol. Avoid. [Severe] Study
▸ Aprepitant is predicted to increase the exposure to naloxegol. Adjust naloxegol dose and monitor side effects. [Moderate] Study

▸ Calcium channel blockers (diltiazem, verapamil) are predicted to increase the exposure to naloxegol. Adjust naloxegol dose and monitor side effects. [Moderate] Study
▸ Cobicistat is predicted to markedly increase the exposure to naloxegol. [Severe] Study
▸ Crizotinib is predicted to increase the exposure to naloxegol. Adjust naloxegol dose and monitor side effects. [Moderate] Study
▸ Enzalutamide is predicted to markedly decrease the exposure to naloxegol. Avoid. [Moderate] Study
▸ Grapefruit juice is predicted to increase the exposure to naloxegol. Avoid. [Moderate] Study
▸ HIV-protease inhibitors (atazanavir, darunavir, fosamprenavir, lopinavir, ritonavir, saquinavir, tipranavir) are predicted to markedly increase the exposure to naloxegol. Avoid. [Severe] Study
▸ HIV-protease inhibitors (indinavir) are predicted to increase the exposure to naloxegol. Adjust naloxegol dose and monitor side effects. [Moderate] Study
▸ Idelalisib is predicted to markedly increase the exposure to naloxegol. Avoid. [Severe] Study
▸ Imatinib is predicted to increase the exposure to naloxegol. Adjust naloxegol dose and monitor side effects. [Moderate] Study
▸ Macrolides (clarithromycin) are predicted to markedly increase the exposure to naloxegol. Avoid. [Severe] Study
▸ Macrolides (erythromycin) are predicted to increase the exposure to naloxegol. Adjust naloxegol dose and monitor side effects. [Moderate] Study
▸ Netupitant is predicted to increase the exposure to naloxegol. Adjust naloxegol dose and monitor side effects. [Moderate] Study
▸ Nilotinib is predicted to increase the exposure to naloxegol. Adjust naloxegol dose and monitor side effects. [Moderate] Study
▸ Rifampicin is predicted to markedly decrease the exposure to naloxegol. Avoid. [Moderate] Study
▸ St John's Wort is predicted to decrease the exposure to naloxegol. Avoid. [Moderate] Theoretical

Naltrexone

GENERAL INFORMATION Avoid concurrent use of opioids.

Nandrolone

▸ Nandrolone is predicted to increase the anticoagulant effect of coumarins. Monitor and adjust dose. [Severe] Theoretical
▸ Nandrolone is predicted to increase the anticoagulant effect of phenindione. Monitor and adjust dose. [Severe] Theoretical

Naproxen → see NSAIDs

Naratriptan → see TABLE 13 p. 821 (serotonin syndrome)

▸ Naratriptan is predicted to increase the risk of vasoconstriction when given with ergotamine. Separate administration by 24 hours. [Severe] Theoretical

Natalizumab → see monoclonal antibodies

Nateglinide → see TABLE 14 p. 821 (antidiabetic drugs)

▸ Antiepileptics (carbamazepine, fosphenytoin, phenobarbital, phenytoin, primidone) are predicted to slightly decrease the exposure to nateglinide. [Mild] Study
▸ Enzalutamide is predicted to slightly decrease the exposure to nateglinide. [Mild] Study
▸ Rifampicin is predicted to slightly decrease the exposure to nateglinide. [Mild] Study
▸ Sulfinpyrazone slightly increases the exposure to nateglinide. [Mild] Study

Nebivolol → see beta blockers, selective

Necitumumab → see monoclonal antibodies

Nefopam → see TABLE 10 p. 820 (antimuscarinics)

▸ Nefopam is predicted to increase the risk of serious elevations in blood pressure when given with monoamine-oxidase A and B inhibitors, irreversible. Avoid. [Severe] Theoretical

Nelarabine → see TABLE 15 p. 821 (myelosuppression)

Neomycin → see TABLE 2 p. 818 (nephrotoxicity), TABLE 19 p. 822 (ototoxicity), TABLE 20 p. 822 (neuromuscular blocking effects)

▸ Neomycin decreases the absorption of digoxin. [Moderate] Study
▸ Neomycin moderately decreases the exposure to sorafenib. [Moderate] Study

Neostigmine → see TABLE 6 p. 819 (bradycardia), TABLE 20 p. 822 (neuromuscular blocking effects)

▸ Aminoglycosides are predicted to decrease the effects of neostigmine. [Moderate] Theoretical → Also see TABLE 20 p. 822

Nepafenac → see NSAIDs

Netupitant

- **Netupitant** is predicted to increase the exposure to aldosterone antagonists (**eplerenone**). Adjust **eplerenone** dose. [Severe] Study
- **Netupitant** is predicted to increase the exposure to alpha blockers (**tamsulosin**). [Moderate] Theoretical
- **Netupitant** is predicted to increase the exposure to alprazolam. [Severe] Study
- **Netupitant** is predicted to increase the exposure to antiarrhythmics (**propafenone**). Monitor and adjust dose. [Moderate] Study
- Antiepileptics (**carbamazepine, fosphenytoin, phenobarbital, phenytoin, primidone**) are predicted to decrease the exposure to **netupitant**. Avoid. [Moderate] Study
- Antifungals, azoles (**itraconazole, ketoconazole, voriconazole**) are predicted to increase the exposure to **netupitant**. [Mild] Study
- **Netupitant** is predicted to decrease the exposure to antifungals, azoles (**isavuconazole**). [Moderate] Theoretical
- **Netupitant** is predicted to increase the exposure to antihistamines, non-sedating (**mizolastine**). [Severe] Theoretical
- **Netupitant** is predicted to increase the concentration of antimalarials (**piperaquine**). [Severe] Theoretical
- **Netupitant** is predicted to increase the exposure to axitinib. [Moderate] Theoretical
- **Netupitant** is predicted to increase the exposure to bedaquiline. Avoid prolonged use. [Mild] Theoretical
- **Netupitant** is predicted to increase the exposure to bosutinib. Avoid or adjust **bosutinib** dose. [Severe] Theoretical
- **Netupitant** is predicted to increase the exposure to buspirone. Use with caution and adjust dose. [Moderate] Study
- **Netupitant** is predicted to increase the exposure to cabozantinib. [Moderate] Theoretical
- **Netupitant** is predicted to increase the exposure to calcium channel blockers (**amlodipine, felodipine, isradipine, lacidipine, lercanidipine, nicardipine, nifedipine, nimodipine**). Monitor and adjust dose. [Moderate] Study
- **Netupitant** is predicted to increase the exposure to ceritinib. [Moderate] Theoretical
- **Netupitant** increases the concentration of ciclosporin. [Severe] Study
- Cobicistat is predicted to increase the exposure to **netupitant**. [Mild] Study
- **Netupitant** is predicted to increase the exposure to cobimetinib. [Severe] Theoretical
- **Netupitant** is predicted to increase the exposure to colchicine. Adjust **colchicine** dose. [Severe] Study
- **Netupitant** is predicted to increase the exposure to corticosteroids (**dexamethasone, methylprednisolone**). Monitor and adjust dose. [Moderate] Study
- **Netupitant** is predicted to increase the exposure to crizotinib. [Severe] Theoretical
- **Netupitant** is predicted to slightly increase the exposure to darifenacin. [Moderate] Study
- **Netupitant** is predicted to increase the exposure to dasatinib. [Severe] Study
- **Netupitant** increases the risk of QT-prolongation when given with domperidone. Avoid. [Severe] Study
- **Netupitant** is predicted to increase the exposure to dopamine receptor agonists (**bromocriptine, cabergoline**). [Severe] Theoretical
- **Netupitant** is predicted to moderately increase the exposure to dutasteride. [Mild] Study
- Enzalutamide is predicted to decrease the exposure to **netupitant**. Avoid. [Moderate] Study
- **Netupitant** is predicted to increase the risk of ergotism when given with ergometrine. [Severe] Theoretical
- **Netupitant** is predicted to increase the risk of ergotism when given with ergotamine. [Severe] Theoretical
- **Netupitant** is predicted to increase the exposure to erlotinib. [Moderate] Theoretical
- **Netupitant** is predicted to increase the concentration of everolimus. Avoid or adjust dose. [Moderate] Study
- **Netupitant** is predicted to increase the exposure to fesoterodine. Adjust **fesoterodine** dose in hepatic and renal impairment. [Mild] Study
- **Netupitant** is predicted to increase the exposure to gefitinib. [Moderate] Theoretical

- **Netupitant** is predicted to increase the concentration of guanfacine. Adjust **guanfacine** dose, p. 222. [Moderate] Theoretical
- HIV-protease inhibitors (**atazanavir, darunavir, fosamprenavir, lopinavir, ritonavir, saquinavir, tipranavir**) are predicted to increase the exposure to **netupitant**. [Mild] Study
- **Netupitant** is predicted to increase the exposure to ibrutinib. Avoid or adjust **ibrutinib** dose. [Severe] Theoretical
- Idelalisib is predicted to increase the exposure to **netupitant**. [Mild] Study
- **Netupitant** is predicted to increase the exposure to imatinib. [Moderate] Theoretical
- **Netupitant** is predicted to increase the exposure to ivabradine. Adjust **ivabradine** dose. [Severe] Theoretical
- **Netupitant** is predicted to increase the exposure to ivacaftor. Adjust **ivacaftor** dose, p. 179. [Severe] Study
- **Netupitant** is predicted to increase the exposure to lapatinib. [Moderate] Study
- **Netupitant** is predicted to increase the exposure to lomitapide. Avoid. [Moderate] Theoretical
- **Netupitant** is predicted to increase the exposure to lurasidone. [Moderate] Study
- Macrolides (**clarithromycin**) are predicted to increase the exposure to **netupitant**. [Mild] Study
- **Netupitant** is predicted to increase the exposure to midazolam. Monitor side effects and adjust dose. [Severe] Study
- **Netupitant** is predicted to increase the exposure to naloxegol. Adjust **naloxegol** dose and monitor side effects. [Moderate] Study
- **Netupitant** is predicted to increase the exposure to nilotinib. [Moderate] Theoretical
- **Netupitant** is predicted to increase the exposure to olaparib. Avoid or adjust **olaparib** dose. [Moderate] Theoretical
- **Netupitant** is predicted to increase the exposure to opioids (**alfentanil, buprenorphine, fentanyl, oxycodone**). Monitor and adjust dose. [Moderate] Study
- **Netupitant** is predicted to increase the exposure to opioids (**methadone, sufentanil**). [Moderate] Theoretical
- **Netupitant** is predicted to increase the exposure to oxybutynin. [Mild] Theoretical
- **Netupitant** is predicted to increase the exposure to pazopanib. [Moderate] Theoretical
- **Netupitant** is predicted to increase the exposure to phosphodiesterase type-5 inhibitors (**avanafil**). Adjust **avanafil** dose. [Moderate] Theoretical
- **Netupitant** is predicted to increase the exposure to phosphodiesterase type-5 inhibitors (**sildenafil**). Monitor and adjust **sildenafil** dose, p. 117. [Moderate] Study
- **Netupitant** is predicted to increase the exposure to phosphodiesterase type-5 inhibitors (**tadalafil**). [Severe] Theoretical
- **Netupitant** is predicted to increase the exposure to phosphodiesterase type-5 inhibitors (**vardenafil**). Adjust dose. [Severe] Theoretical
- **Netupitant** is predicted to increase the exposure to pimozide. Avoid. [Severe] Theoretical
- **Netupitant** is predicted to increase the exposure to quetiapine. Avoid. [Moderate] Study
- **Netupitant** is predicted to increase the exposure to ranolazine. [Severe] Study
- Rifampicin is predicted to decrease the exposure to **netupitant**. Avoid. [Moderate] Study
- **Netupitant** is predicted to increase the exposure to ruxolitinib. [Moderate] Theoretical
- **Netupitant** is predicted to increase the exposure to saxagliptin. [Mild] Study
- **Netupitant** is predicted to increase the exposure to simeprevir. Avoid. [Severe] Study
- **Netupitant** increases the concentration of sirolimus. Monitor and adjust dose. [Moderate] Study
- **Netupitant** is predicted to increase the exposure to SSRIs (**dapoxetine**). Adjust **dapoxetine** dose. [Moderate] Theoretical
- **Netupitant** is predicted to increase the exposure to statins (**atorvastatin**). Monitor and adjust dose. [Severe] Theoretical
- **Netupitant** is predicted to increase the exposure to statins (**simvastatin**). Use with caution and adjust **simvastatin** dose, p. 130. [Severe] Study

Netupitant (continued)
▶ **Netupitant** is predicted to increase the exposure to **sunitinib**. Moderate Theoretical
▶ **Netupitant** is predicted to increase the concentration of **tacrolimus**. Severe Study
▶ **Netupitant** is predicted to increase the exposure to **taxanes (cabazitaxel)**. Moderate Theoretical
▶ **Netupitant** is predicted to increase the concentration of **temsirolimus**. Moderate Theoretical
▶ **Netupitant** is predicted to increase the exposure to **tolterodine**. Mild Theoretical
▶ **Netupitant** is predicted to increase the exposure to **tolvaptan**. Adjust dose. Moderate Theoretical
▶ **Netupitant** is predicted to increase the exposure to **trazodone**. Moderate Theoretical
▶ **Netupitant** is predicted to increase the exposure to **ulipristal**. Avoid if used for uterine fibroids. Moderate Study
▶ **Netupitant** is predicted to increase the exposure to **venetoclax**. Avoid or adjust **venetoclax** dose. Severe Study
▶ **Netupitant** is predicted to increase the exposure to **vinca alkaloids**. Severe Theoretical
▶ **Netupitant** is predicted to increase the exposure to **zopiclone**. Adjust dose. Moderate Study

Neuromuscular blocking drugs, non-depolarising → see TABLE 6 p. 819 (bradycardia), TABLE 20 p. 822 (neuromuscular blocking effects)

atracurium · cisatracurium · mivacurium · pancuronium · rocuronium · vecuronium

▶ **Aminoglycosides** are predicted to increase the risk of prolonged neuromuscular blockade when given with **neuromuscular blocking drugs, non-depolarising**. Severe Theoretical → Also see TABLE 20 p. 822
▶ **Anticholinesterases, centrally acting** are predicted to decrease the effects of **neuromuscular blocking drugs, non-depolarising**. Moderate Theoretical → Also see TABLE 6 p. 819
▶ **Antiepileptics (carbamazepine)** are predicted to decrease the effects of (but acute use increases the effects of) **neuromuscular blocking drugs, non-depolarising**. Monitor and adjust dose. Moderate Study
▶ **Antiepileptics (fosphenytoin, phenytoin)** decrease the effects of (but acute use increases the effects of) neuromuscular blocking drugs, non-depolarising (atracurium, cisatracurium, pancuronium, rocuronium, vecuronium). Moderate Study
▶ **Clindamycin** increases the effects of **neuromuscular blocking drugs, non-depolarising**. Severe Anecdotal
▶ **Colistimethate** increases the effects of **neuromuscular blocking drugs, non-depolarising**. Monitor and adjust dose. Moderate Study → Also see TABLE 20 p. 822
▶ **Corticosteroids** are predicted to decrease the effects of **neuromuscular blocking drugs, non-depolarising**. Severe Anecdotal
▶ **Pancuronium** is predicted to increase the risk of cardiovascular side-effects when given with **digoxin**. Severe Anecdotal
▶ **Irinotecan** is predicted to decrease the effects of **neuromuscular blocking drugs, non-depolarising**. Moderate Theoretical
▶ Intravenous **magnesium** increases the effects of **neuromuscular blocking drugs, non-depolarising**. Moderate Study
▶ **Metoclopramide** is predicted to increase the effects of **neuromuscular blocking drugs, non-depolarising**. Moderate Theoretical
▶ **Penicillins (piperacillin)** increase the effects of **neuromuscular blocking drugs, non-depolarising**. Moderate Study
▶ **SSRIs** potentially increase the risk of prolonged neuromuscular blockade when given with **mivacurium**. Unknown Theoretical

Nevirapine
▶ **Nevirapine** is predicted to decrease the exposure to antiarrhythmics **(dronedarone)**. Severe Theoretical
▶ **Nevirapine** is predicted to decrease the concentration of antiepileptics **(carbamazepine, fosphenytoin, phenobarbital, phenytoin, primidone)** and antiepileptics **(carbamazepine, fosphenytoin, phenobarbital, phenytoin, primidone)** are predicted to decrease the concentration of **nevirapine**. Severe Study

▶ Antifungals, azoles **(fluconazole)** slightly to moderately increase the exposure to **nevirapine**. Moderate Study
▶ **Nevirapine** is predicted to decrease the exposure to antifungals, azoles **(isavuconazole)**. Avoid. Severe Theoretical
▶ **Nevirapine** moderately decreases the exposure to antifungals, azoles **(itraconazole)**. Avoid **nevirapine** for 14 days before and during treatment with **itraconazole**. Moderate Study
▶ **Nevirapine** moderately decreases the exposure to antifungals, azoles **(ketoconazole)**. Avoid. Severe Study
▶ **Nevirapine** is predicted to decrease the exposure to antifungals, azoles **(voriconazole)** and antifungals, azoles **(voriconazole)** increase the exposure to **nevirapine**. Monitor and adjust dose. Severe Theoretical
▶ **Nevirapine** is predicted to decrease the exposure to **axitinib**. Moderate Theoretical
▶ **Nevirapine** is predicted to decrease the exposure to **bedaquiline**. Avoid. Severe Study
▶ **Nevirapine** is predicted to decrease the exposure to **bosutinib**. Avoid. Severe Theoretical
▶ **Nevirapine** is predicted to decrease the exposure to **cabozantinib**. Moderate Theoretical
▶ **Nevirapine** is predicted to decrease the exposure to calcium channel blockers **(amlodipine, felodipine, isradipine, lacidipine, lercanidipine, nicardipine, nifedipine, nimodipine)**. Monitor and adjust dose. Moderate Theoretical
▶ **Nevirapine** is predicted to decrease the exposure to calcium channel blockers **(diltiazem, verapamil)**. Moderate Theoretical
▶ **Nevirapine** is predicted to decrease the concentration of **caspofungin**. Adjust dose. Moderate Theoretical
▶ **Nevirapine** is predicted to decrease the concentration of **ciclosporin**. Moderate Study
▶ **Nevirapine** is predicted to decrease the exposure to **cobicistat**. Avoid. Severe Theoretical
▶ **Nevirapine** is predicted to decrease the exposure to **cobimetinib**. Avoid. Severe Theoretical
▶ **Nevirapine** is predicted to decrease the efficacy of **combined hormonal contraceptives**. For FSRH guidance, see Contraceptives, interactions p. 474. Severe Study
▶ **Nevirapine** potentially alters the anticoagulant effect of **coumarins**. Severe Anecdotal
▶ **Nevirapine** is predicted to decrease the exposure to **crizotinib**. Avoid. Severe Theoretical
▶ **Nevirapine** is predicted to decrease the exposure to **daclatasvir**. Avoid. Severe Theoretical
▶ **Nevirapine** is predicted to decrease the exposure to **dasatinib**. Severe Study
▶ **Nevirapine** is predicted to decrease the efficacy of **desogestrel**. For FSRH guidance, see Contraceptives, interactions p. 474. Severe Theoretical
▶ **Nevirapine** decreases the exposure to **dolutegravir**. Adjust dose. Severe Study
▶ **Nevirapine** decreases the concentration of **efavirenz**. Avoid. Severe Study
▶ **Nevirapine** is predicted to moderately decrease the exposure to **elbasvir**. Avoid. Severe Study
▶ **Nevirapine** is predicted to decrease the concentration of **elvitegravir**. Avoid. Severe Theoretical
▶ **Nevirapine** is predicted to decrease the effects of **ergotamine**. Moderate Theoretical
▶ **Nevirapine** is predicted to decrease the exposure to **erlotinib**. Severe Theoretical
▶ **Nevirapine** is predicted to decrease the efficacy of **etonogestrel**. For FSRH guidance, see Contraceptives, interactions p. 474. Severe Theoretical
▶ **Nevirapine** is predicted to decrease the exposure to **etravirine**. Avoid. Severe Study
▶ **Nevirapine** is predicted to decrease the concentration of **everolimus**. Avoid or adjust dose. Severe Study
▶ **Nevirapine** is predicted to decrease the exposure to **gefitinib**. Avoid. Severe Theoretical
▶ **Nevirapine** is predicted to markedly decrease the exposure to **grazoprevir**. Avoid. Severe Study
▶ **Nevirapine** is predicted to decrease the concentration of **guanfacine**. Adjust dose. Moderate Theoretical

▸ **Nevirapine** decreases the exposure to **HIV-protease inhibitors**. Refer to specialist literature. Moderate Study
▸ **Nevirapine** is predicted to decrease the effects of **Hormone replacement therapy**. Moderate Anecdotal
▸ **Nevirapine** is predicted to decrease the exposure to **imatinib**. Moderate Study
▸ **Nevirapine** is predicted to decrease the exposure to **lapatinib**. Avoid. Severe Study
▸ **Nevirapine** is predicted to decrease the efficacy of **levonorgestrel**. For FSRH guidance, see Contraceptives, interactions p. 474. Severe Theoretical
▸ **Nevirapine** is predicted to decrease the exposure to **lurasidone**. Monitor and adjust dose. Moderate Theoretical
▸ **Nevirapine** decreases the exposure to macrolides **(clarithromycin)**. Moderate Study
▸ **Nevirapine** decreases the concentration of **midazolam**. Monitor and adjust dose. Moderate Study
▸ **Nevirapine** is predicted to decrease the exposure to **nilotinib**. Avoid. Severe Theoretical
▸ **Nevirapine** is predicted to decrease the efficacy of **norethisterone**. For FSRH guidance, see Contraceptives, interactions p. 474. Severe Anecdotal
▸ **Nevirapine** is predicted to decrease the exposure to **olaparib**. Avoid. Moderate Theoretical
▸ **Nevirapine** decreases the exposure to opioids **(methadone)**. Monitor and adjust dose. Severe Study
▸ **Nevirapine** is predicted to decrease the exposure to **osimertinib**. Severe Theoretical
▸ **Nevirapine** is predicted to decrease the exposure to **paritaprevir** (with ritonavir and ombitasvir). Avoid. Severe Study
▸ **Nevirapine** is predicted to decrease the exposure to **phosphodiesterase type-5 inhibitors**. Moderate Theoretical
▸ **Rifampicin** decreases the concentration of **nevirapine**. Avoid. Severe Study
▸ **Nevirapine** is predicted to decrease the exposure to **rilpivirine**. Avoid. Severe Theoretical
▸ **Nevirapine** is predicted to decrease the exposure to **ruxolitinib**. Monitor and adjust dose. Moderate Theoretical
▸ **Nevirapine** is predicted to decrease the exposure to **simeprevir**. Avoid. Severe Study
▸ **Nevirapine** is predicted to decrease the concentration of **sirolimus**. Monitor and adjust dose. Moderate Theoretical
▸ **St John's Wort** is predicted to decrease the concentration of **nevirapine**. Avoid. Severe Theoretical
▸ **Nevirapine** slightly decreases the exposure to statins **(atorvastatin)**. Mild Study
▸ **Nevirapine** moderately decreases the exposure to statins **(simvastatin)**. Moderate Study
▸ **Nevirapine** is predicted to decrease the concentration of **tacrolimus**. Monitor and adjust dose. Moderate Theoretical
▸ **Nevirapine** is predicted to decrease the exposure to taxanes **(cabazitaxel)**. Avoid. Severe Study
▸ **Nevirapine** is predicted to decrease the concentration of **temsirolimus**. Avoid. Severe Theoretical
▸ **Nevirapine** is predicted to decrease the exposure to **ticagrelor**. Moderate Theoretical
▸ **Nevirapine** is predicted to decrease the exposure to **tolvaptan**. Moderate Theoretical
▸ **Nevirapine** decreases the efficacy of **uliprista**l. For FSRH guidance, see Contraceptives, interactions p. 474. Severe Anecdotal
▸ **Nevirapine** is predicted to decrease the exposure to **velpatasvir**. Avoid. Moderate Theoretical
▸ **Nevirapine** is predicted to decrease the concentration of **zidovudine**. Refer to specialist literature. Severe Theoretical
Nicardipine → see calcium channel blockers
Nicorandil → see TABLE 8 p. 819 (hypotension)
▸ **Aspirin** is predicted to increase the risk of gastrointestinal perforation when given with **nicorandil**. Severe Theoretical
▸ **Corticosteroids** increase the risk of gastrointestinal perforation when given with **nicorandil**. Severe Anecdotal
▸ **Nicorandil** is predicted to increase the risk of gastrointestinal perforation when given with **NSAIDs**. Severe Theoretical

▸ **Nicorandil** is predicted to increase the risk of hypotension when given with **phosphodiesterase type-5 inhibitors**. Avoid. Severe Theoretical → Also see TABLE 8 p. 819
Nicotinic acid → see TABLE 3 p. 818 (anticoagulant effects)
▸ **Nicotinic acid** is predicted to increase the risk of rhabdomyolysis when given with **statins**. Severe Theoretical
Nifedipine → see calcium channel blockers
Nilotinib → see TABLE 15 p. 821 (myelosuppression), TABLE 9 p. 820 (QT-interval prolongation)
▸ **Nilotinib** is predicted to increase the exposure to aldosterone antagonists **(eplerenone)**. Adjust eplerenone dose. Severe Study
▸ **Nilotinib** is predicted to increase the exposure to alpha blockers **(tamsulosin)**. Moderate Theoretical
▸ **Nilotinib** is predicted to increase the exposure to **alprazolam**. Severe Study
▸ **Antacids** are predicted to decrease the absorption of **nilotinib**. Separate administration by at least 2 hours. Moderate Theoretical
▸ **Antiarrhythmics (dronedarone)** are predicted to increase the exposure to **nilotinib**. Moderate Theoretical → Also see TABLE 9 p. 820
▸ **Nilotinib** is predicted to increase the exposure to antiarrhythmics **(propafenone)**. Monitor and adjust dose. Moderate Study
▸ **Antiepileptics (carbamazepine, fosphenytoin, phenobarbital, phenytoin, primidone)** are predicted to moderately decrease the exposure to **nilotinib**. Avoid. Severe Study
▸ **Antifungals, azoles (fluconazole, posaconazole)** are predicted to increase the exposure to **nilotinib**. Moderate Theoretical
▸ **Antifungals, azoles (itraconazole, ketoconazole, voriconazole)** are predicted to moderately increase the exposure to **nilotinib**. Avoid. Severe Study → Also see TABLE 9 p. 820
▸ **Nilotinib** is predicted to increase the exposure to antifungals, azoles **(isavuconazole)**. Moderate Theoretical
▸ **Nilotinib** is predicted to increase the exposure to antihistamines, non-sedating **(mizolastine)**. Severe Theoretical
▸ **Nilotinib** is predicted to increase the concentration of antimalarials **(piperaquine)**. Severe Theoretical
▸ **Aprepitant** is predicted to increase the exposure to **nilotinib**. Moderate Theoretical
▸ **Nilotinib** is predicted to increase the exposure to **axitinib**. Moderate Theoretical → Also see TABLE 15 p. 821
▸ **Nilotinib** is predicted to increase the exposure to **bedaquiline**. Avoid prolonged use. Mild Theoretical → Also see TABLE 9 p. 820
▸ **Bosentan** is predicted to decrease the exposure to **nilotinib**. Avoid. Severe Theoretical
▸ **Nilotinib** is predicted to increase the exposure to **bosutinib**. Avoid or adjust bosutinib dose. Severe Theoretical → Also see TABLE 15 p. 821 → Also see TABLE 9 p. 820
▸ **Nilotinib** is predicted to increase the exposure to **buspirone**. Use with caution and adjust dose. Moderate Study
▸ **Nilotinib** is predicted to increase the exposure to **cabozantinib**. Moderate Theoretical → Also see TABLE 15 p. 821 → Also see TABLE 9 p. 820
▸ **Calcium channel blockers (diltiazem, verapamil)** are predicted to increase the exposure to **nilotinib**. Moderate Theoretical
▸ **Nilotinib** is predicted to increase the exposure to calcium channel blockers **(amlodipine, felodipine, isradipine, lacidipine, lercanidipine, nicardipine, nifedipine, nimodipine)**. Monitor and adjust dose. Moderate Study
▸ **Nilotinib** is predicted to increase the exposure to **ceritinib**. Moderate Theoretical → Also see TABLE 15 p. 821 → Also see TABLE 9 p. 820
▸ **Nilotinib** increases the concentration of **ciclosporin**. Severe Study
▸ **Cobicistat** is predicted to moderately increase the exposure to **nilotinib**. Avoid. Severe Study
▸ **Nilotinib** is predicted to increase the exposure to **cobimetinib**. Severe Theoretical
▸ **Nilotinib** is predicted to increase the exposure to **colchicine**. Adjust colchicine dose. Severe Study
▸ **Nilotinib** is predicted to increase the exposure to corticosteroids **(methylprednisolone)**. Monitor and adjust dose. Moderate Study
▸ **Nilotinib** is predicted to increase the risk of bleeding events when given with **coumarins**. Severe

Interactions | Appendix 1

A1

Nilotinib (continued)

‣ **Nilotinib** is predicted to slightly increase the exposure to **darifenacin**. Moderate Study

‣ **Nilotinib** is predicted to increase the exposure to **dasatinib**. Severe Study → Also see TABLE 15 p. 821 → Also see TABLE 9 p. 820

‣ **Nilotinib** increases the risk of QT-prolongation when given with **domperidone**. Avoid. Severe Study

‣ **Nilotinib** is predicted to increase the exposure to dopamine receptor agonists (**bromocriptine, cabergoline**). Severe Theoretical

‣ **Nilotinib** is predicted to moderately increase the exposure to **dutasteride**. Mild Study

‣ **Efavirenz** is predicted to decrease the exposure to **nilotinib**. Avoid. Severe Theoretical

‣ **Enzalutamide** is predicted to moderately decrease the exposure to **nilotinib**. Avoid. Severe Study

‣ **Nilotinib** is predicted to increase the risk of ergotism when given with **ergometrine**. Severe Theoretical

‣ **Nilotinib** is predicted to increase the risk of ergotism when given with **ergotamine**. Severe Theoretical

‣ **Nilotinib** is predicted to increase the exposure to **erlotinib**. Moderate Theoretical

‣ **Nilotinib** is predicted to increase the concentration of **everolimus**. Avoid or adjust dose. Moderate Study → Also see TABLE 15 p. 821

‣ **Nilotinib** is predicted to increase the exposure to **fesoterodine**. Adjust **fesoterodine** dose in hepatic and renal impairment. Mild Study

‣ **Nilotinib** is predicted to increase the exposure to **gefitinib**. Moderate Theoretical → Also see TABLE 15 p. 821

‣ **Grapefruit juice** is predicted to increase the exposure to **nilotinib**. Avoid. Severe Theoretical

‣ **Nilotinib** is predicted to increase the concentration of **guanfacine**. Adjust **guanfacine** dose, p. 222. Moderate Theoretical

‣ **H₂ receptor antagonists** are predicted to decrease the absorption of **nilotinib**. **H₂ receptor antagonists** should be taken 10 hours before or 2 hours after **nilotinib**. Mild Theoretical

‣ **HIV-protease inhibitors** (**atazanavir, darunavir, fosamprenavir, lopinavir, ritonavir, saquinavir, tipranavir**) are predicted to moderately increase the exposure to **nilotinib**. Avoid. Severe Study → Also see TABLE 9 p. 820

‣ **Nilotinib** is predicted to increase the exposure to **ibrutinib**. Avoid or adjust **ibrutinib** dose. Severe Theoretical → Also see TABLE 15 p. 821

‣ **Idelalisib** is predicted to moderately increase the exposure to **nilotinib**. Avoid. Severe Study → Also see TABLE 15 p. 821

‣ **Nilotinib** is predicted to increase the exposure to **ivabradine**. Adjust **ivabradine** dose. Severe Theoretical

‣ **Nilotinib** is predicted to increase the exposure to **ivacaftor**. Adjust **ivacaftor** dose, p. 179. Severe Study

‣ **Nilotinib** is predicted to increase the exposure to **lapatinib**. Moderate Study → Also see TABLE 9 p. 820

‣ **Nilotinib** is predicted to increase the exposure to **lomitapide**. Avoid. Moderate Theoretical

‣ **Nilotinib** is predicted to increase the exposure to **lurasidone**. Moderate Study

‣ **Macrolides** (**clarithromycin**) are predicted to moderately increase the exposure to **nilotinib**. Avoid. Severe Study → Also see TABLE 9 p. 820

‣ **Macrolides** (**erythromycin**) are predicted to increase the exposure to **nilotinib**. Moderate Theoretical

‣ **Nilotinib** is predicted to increase the exposure to **midazolam**. Monitor side effects and adjust dose. Severe Study

‣ **Nilotinib** is predicted to increase the exposure to **naloxegol**. Adjust **naloxegol** dose and monitor side effects. Moderate Study

‣ **Netupitant** is predicted to increase the exposure to **nilotinib**. Moderate Theoretical

‣ **Nevirapine** is predicted to decrease the exposure to **nilotinib**. Avoid. Severe Theoretical

‣ **Nilotinib** is predicted to increase the exposure to **olaparib**. Avoid or adjust **olaparib** dose. Moderate Theoretical → Also see TABLE 15 p. 821

‣ **Nilotinib** is predicted to increase the exposure to opioids (**alfentanil, buprenorphine, fentanyl, oxycodone**). Monitor and adjust dose. Moderate Study

‣ **Nilotinib** is predicted to increase the exposure to opioids (**methadone, sufentanil**). Moderate Theoretical → Also see TABLE 9 p. 820

‣ **Nilotinib** is predicted to increase the exposure to **oxybutynin**. Mild Theoretical

‣ **Nilotinib** is predicted to increase the exposure to **pazopanib**. Moderate Theoretical → Also see TABLE 15 p. 821 → Also see TABLE 9 p. 820

‣ **Nilotinib** is predicted to increase the risk of bleeding events when given with **phenindione**. Severe Theoretical

‣ **Nilotinib** is predicted to increase the exposure to phosphodiesterase type-5 inhibitors (**avanafil**). Adjust avanafil dose. Moderate Theoretical

‣ **Nilotinib** is predicted to increase the exposure to phosphodiesterase type-5 inhibitors (**sildenafil**). Monitor and adjust sildenafil dose, p. 117. Moderate Study → Also see TABLE 9 p. 820

‣ **Nilotinib** is predicted to increase the exposure to phosphodiesterase type-5 inhibitors (**tadalafil**). Severe Theoretical

‣ **Nilotinib** is predicted to increase the exposure to phosphodiesterase type-5 inhibitors (**vardenafil**). Adjust dose. Severe Theoretical → Also see TABLE 9 p. 820

‣ **Nilotinib** is predicted to increase the exposure to **pimozide**. Avoid. Severe Theoretical → Also see TABLE 9 p. 820

‣ **Nilotinib** is predicted to increase the exposure to **quetiapine**. Avoid. Moderate Study

‣ **Nilotinib** is predicted to increase the exposure to **ranolazine**. Severe Study → Also see TABLE 9 p. 820

‣ **Rifampicin** is predicted to moderately decrease the exposure to **nilotinib**. Avoid. Severe Study

‣ **Nilotinib** is predicted to increase the exposure to **ruxolitinib**. Moderate Theoretical → Also see TABLE 15 p. 821

‣ **Nilotinib** is predicted to increase the exposure to **saxagliptin**. Mild Study

‣ **Nilotinib** is predicted to increase the exposure to **simeprevir**. Avoid. Severe Study

‣ **Nilotinib** increases the concentration of **sirolimus**. Monitor and adjust dose. Moderate Study

‣ **Nilotinib** is predicted to increase the exposure to SSRIs (**dapoxetine**). Adjust **dapoxetine** dose. Moderate Theoretical

‣ **St John's Wort** is predicted to decrease the exposure to **nilotinib**. Avoid. Severe Theoretical

‣ **Nilotinib** is predicted to increase the exposure to statins (**atorvastatin**). Monitor and adjust dose. Severe Theoretical

‣ **Nilotinib** is predicted to increase the exposure to statins (**simvastatin**). Use with caution and adjust **simvastatin** dose, p. 130. Severe Study

‣ **Nilotinib** is predicted to increase the exposure to **sunitinib**. Moderate Theoretical → Also see TABLE 15 p. 821 → Also see TABLE 9 p. 820

‣ **Nilotinib** is predicted to increase the concentration of **tacrolimus**. Severe Study

‣ **Nilotinib** is predicted to increase the exposure to taxanes (**cabazitaxel**). Moderate Theoretical → Also see TABLE 15 p. 821

‣ **Nilotinib** is predicted to increase the concentration of **temsirolimus**. Moderate Theoretical → Also see TABLE 15 p. 821

‣ **Nilotinib** is predicted to increase the exposure to **tolterodine**. Mild Theoretical → Also see TABLE 9 p. 820

‣ **Nilotinib** is predicted to increase the exposure to **tolvaptan**. Adjust dose. Moderate Theoretical

‣ **Nilotinib** is predicted to increase the exposure to **trazodone**. Moderate Theoretical

‣ **Nilotinib** is predicted to increase the exposure to **ulipristal**. Avoid if used for uterine fibroids. Moderate Study

‣ **Nilotinib** is predicted to increase the exposure to **venetoclax**. Avoid or adjust **venetoclax** dose. Severe Study

‣ **Nilotinib** is predicted to increase the exposure to vinca alkaloids. Severe Theoretical → Also see TABLE 9 p. 820 → Also see TABLE 15 p. 821

‣ **Nilotinib** is predicted to increase the exposure to **zopiclone**. Adjust dose. Moderate Study

Nimodipine → see calcium channel blockers

Nintedanib
‣ **Antiarrhythmics** (**amiodarone, dronedarone**) are predicted to increase the exposure to **nintedanib**. Moderate Study

▸ Antiepileptics (**carbamazepine**) are predicted to decrease the exposure to **nintedanib**. Moderate Study

▸ Antifungals, azoles (**itraconazole, ketoconazole**) are predicted to increase the exposure to **nintedanib**. Moderate Study

▸ Calcium channel blockers (**verapamil**) are predicted to increase the exposure to **nintedanib**. Moderate Study

▸ Ciclosporin is predicted to increase the exposure to **nintedanib**. Moderate Study

▸ HIV-protease inhibitors (**lopinavir, ritonavir, saquinavir**) are predicted to increase the exposure to **nintedanib**. Moderate Study

▸ Lapatinib is predicted to increase the exposure to **nintedanib**. Moderate Study

▸ Macrolides are predicted to increase the exposure to **nintedanib**. Moderate Study

▸ Ranolazine is predicted to increase the exposure to **nintedanib**. Moderate Study

▸ Rifampicin is predicted to decrease the exposure to **nintedanib**. Moderate Study

▸ St John's Wort is predicted to decrease the exposure to **nintedanib**. Moderate Study

▸ Vemurafenib is predicted to increase the exposure to **nintedanib**. Moderate Study

Nitisinone

▸ Antiepileptics (**carbamazepine, fosphenytoin, phenobarbital, phenytoin, primidone**) are predicted to decrease the exposure to **nitisinone**. Adjust **nitisinone** dose. Moderate Study

▸ Antifungals, azoles (**itraconazole, ketoconazole, voriconazole**) are predicted to increase the exposure to **nitisinone**. Adjust **nitisinone** dose. Moderate Theoretical

▸ Cobicistat is predicted to increase the exposure to **nitisinone**. Adjust **nitisinone** dose. Moderate Theoretical

▸ Enzalutamide is predicted to decrease the exposure to **nitisinone**. Adjust **nitisinone** dose. Moderate Theoretical

▸ HIV-protease inhibitors (**atazanavir, darunavir, fosamprenavir, lopinavir, ritonavir, saquinavir, tipranavir**) are predicted to increase the exposure to **nitisinone**. Adjust **nitisinone** dose. Moderate Theoretical

▸ Idelalisib is predicted to increase the exposure to **nitisinone**. Adjust **nitisinone** dose. Moderate Theoretical

▸ Macrolides (**clarithromycin**) are predicted to increase the exposure to **nitisinone**. Adjust **nitisinone** dose. Moderate Theoretical

▸ Rifampicin is predicted to decrease the exposure to **nitisinone**. Adjust **nitisinone** dose. Moderate Theoretical

Nitrates → see TABLE 7 p. 819 (first-dose hypotension), TABLE 8 p. 819 (hypotension)

glyceryl trinitrate · isosorbide dinitrate · isosorbide mononitrate

PHARMACOLOGY Drugs with antimuscarinic effects can cause dry mouth, which can reduce the effectiveness of sublingual glyceryl trinitrate tablets.

▸ Nitrates are predicted to increase the risk of methaemoglobinaemia when given with topical anaesthetics, local (**prilocaine**). Avoid. Severe Theoretical

▸ Nitrates are predicted to increase the risk of methaemoglobinaemia when given with **dapsone**. Severe Theoretical

▸ Nitrates potentially increase the risk of hypotension when given with **phosphodiesterase type-5 inhibitors**. Avoid. Severe Study → Also see TABLE 8 p. 819

Nitrazepam → see TABLE 11 p. 820 (CNS depressant effects)

▸ Rifampicin increases the clearance of **nitrazepam**. Moderate Study

Nitrofurantoin

▸ Nitrofurantoin is predicted to increase the risk of methaemoglobinaemia when given with topical anaesthetics, local (**prilocaine**). Use with caution or avoid. Severe Theoretical

▸ Antacids (**magnesium trisilicate**) decrease the absorption of nitrofurantoin. Moderate Study

▸ Nitrofurantoin is predicted to increase the risk of methaemoglobinaemia when given with **dapsone**. Severe Theoretical

Nitrous oxide → see TABLE 8 p. 819 (hypotension), TABLE 11 p. 820 (CNS depressant effects)

Nivolumab → see monoclonal antibodies

Nizatidine → see H$_2$ receptor antagonists

Noradrenaline/norepinephrine → see sympathomimetics, vasoconstrictor

Norethisterone

▸ Antiepileptics (**carbamazepine, eslicarbazepine, fosphenytoin, oxcarbazepine, perampanel, phenobarbital, phenytoin, primidone, rufinamide, topiramate**) are predicted to decrease the efficacy of **norethisterone**. For FSRH guidance, see Contraceptives, interactions p. 474. Severe Anecdotal

▸ Aprepitant is predicted to decrease the efficacy of **norethisterone**. For FSRH guidance, see Contraceptives, interactions p. 474. Severe Anecdotal

▸ Bosentan is predicted to decrease the efficacy of **norethisterone**. For FSRH guidance, see Contraceptives, interactions p. 474. Severe Anecdotal

▸ Efavirenz is predicted to decrease the efficacy of **norethisterone**. For FSRH guidance, see Contraceptives, interactions p. 474. Severe Anecdotal

▸ Fosaprepitant is predicted to decrease the efficacy of **norethisterone**. For FSRH guidance, see Contraceptives, interactions p. 474. Severe Anecdotal

▸ Griseofulvin potentially decreases the efficacy of **norethisterone**. For FSRH guidance, see Contraceptives, interactions p. 474. Severe Anecdotal

▸ HIV-protease inhibitors (**ritonavir**) are predicted to decrease the efficacy of **norethisterone**. For FSRH guidance, see Contraceptives, interactions p. 474. Severe Anecdotal

▸ Modafinil is predicted to decrease the efficacy of **norethisterone**. For FSRH guidance, see Contraceptives, interactions p. 474. Severe Anecdotal

▸ Nevirapine is predicted to decrease the efficacy of **norethisterone**. For FSRH guidance, see Contraceptives, interactions p. 474. Severe Anecdotal

▸ Rifabutin is predicted to decrease the efficacy of **norethisterone**. For FSRH guidance, see Contraceptives, interactions p. 474. Severe Anecdotal

▸ Rifampicin is predicted to decrease the efficacy of **norethisterone**. For FSRH guidance, see Contraceptives, interactions p. 474. Severe Anecdotal

▸ St John's Wort is predicted to decrease the efficacy of **norethisterone**. MHRA advises avoid. For FSRH guidance, see Contraceptives, interactions p. 474. Severe Anecdotal

▸ Sugammadex is predicted to decrease the exposure to **norethisterone**. Use additional contraceptive precautions. Severe Theoretical

▸ Ulipristal is predicted to decrease the efficacy of **norethisterone**. Avoid. Severe Theoretical

Norfloxacin → see quinolones

Nortriptyline → see tricyclic antidepressants

NSAIDs → see TABLE 18 p. 822 (hyponatraemia), TABLE 2 p. 818 (nephrotoxicity), TABLE 16 p. 822 (increased serum potassium), TABLE 4 p. 818 (antiplatelet effects)

aceclofenac · acemetacin · benzydamine · bromfenac · celecoxib · dexibuprofen · dexketoprofen · diclofenac · etodolac · etoricoxib · felbinac · fenoprofen · flurbiprofen · ibuprofen · indometacin · ketoprofen · ketorolac · mefenamic acid · meloxicam · nabumetone · naproxen · nepafenac · parecoxib · piroxicam · sulindac · tenoxicam · tiaprofenic acid · tolfenamic acid

ROUTE-SPECIFIC INFORMATION Since systemic absorption can follow topical application, the possibility of interactions should be borne in mind.

▸ Celecoxib is predicted to increase the exposure to antiarrhythmics (**flecainide, propafenone**). Monitor and adjust dose. Moderate Theoretical

▸ Antifungals, azoles (**fluconazole**) moderately increase the exposure to **celecoxib**. Adjust **celecoxib** dose. Moderate Study

▸ Antifungals, azoles (**fluconazole**) increase the exposure to **parecoxib**. Monitor and adjust dose. Moderate Study

▸ Antifungals, azoles (**voriconazole**) slightly increase the exposure to **diclofenac**. Monitor and adjust dose. Moderate Study

▸ Antifungals, azoles (**voriconazole**) moderately increase the exposure to **ibuprofen**. Adjust dose. Moderate Study

A1

Interactions | Appendix 1

NSAIDs (continued)

▶ **NSAIDs** are predicted to increase the risk of gastrointestinal irritation when given with bisphosphonates (alendronic acid, ibandronic acid). [Moderate] Study

▶ **NSAIDs** are predicted to increase the risk of renal impairment when given with bisphosphonates (sodium clodronate). [Severe] Theoretical

▶ **Ceritinib** is predicted to increase the exposure to NSAIDs (celecoxib, diclofenac). Adjust dose. [Moderate] Theoretical

▶ **Ciclosporin** increases the concentration of diclofenac. [Severe] Study → Also see TABLE 2 p. 818 → Also see TABLE 16 p. 822

▶ **Etoricoxib** slightly increases the exposure to combined hormonal contraceptives. [Moderate] Study

▶ **NSAIDs** increase the risk of gastrointestinal bleeding when given with corticosteroids. [Severe] Study

▶ **NSAIDs** increase the risk of renal impairment when given with daptomycin. [Moderate] Theoretical

▶ **Indometacin** increases the concentration of digoxin. [Severe] Study

▶ **Topical dimethyl sulfoxide** potentially increases the risk of peripheral neuropathy when given with sulindac. Avoid. [Severe] Anecdotal

▶ **Erlotinib** is predicted to increase the risk of gastrointestinal perforation when given with NSAIDs. [Severe] Theoretical

▶ **Etoricoxib** slightly increases the exposure to Hormone replacement therapy. [Moderate] Study

▶ **NSAIDs** are predicted to increase the risk of gastrointestinal bleeding when given with iron chelators (deferasirox). [Severe] Theoretical

▶ **NSAIDs** increase the concentration of lithium. Monitor and adjust lithium (lithium carbonate, lithium citrate) dose. [Severe] Study

▶ **Lumacaftor** is predicted to decrease the exposure to ibuprofen. Adjust dose. [Moderate] Theoretical

▶ **NSAIDs** are predicted to increase the risk of toxicity when given with methotrexate. Monitor and adjust dose. [Severe] Study → Also see TABLE 2 p. 818

▶ **NSAIDs** (high-dose) are predicted to decrease the efficacy of mifamurtide. Avoid. [Severe] Theoretical

▶ **Nicorandil** is predicted to increase the risk of gastrointestinal perforation when given with NSAIDs. [Severe] Theoretical

▶ **NSAIDs** are predicted to increase the exposure to pemetrexed. Use with caution or avoid. [Severe] Theoretical → Also see TABLE 2 p. 818

▶ **NSAIDs** potentially increase the risk of seizures when given with quinolones. [Severe] Theoretical

▶ **Regorafenib** is predicted to increase the exposure to mefenamic acid. Avoid. [Moderate] Theoretical → Also see TABLE 4 p. 818

▶ **Rifampicin** moderately decreases the exposure to NSAIDs (celecoxib, diclofenac, etoricoxib). [Moderate] Study

▶ **NSAIDs** increase the risk of acute renal failure when given with thiazide diuretics. [Severe] Theoretical → Also see TABLE 18 p. 822

▶ **Zidovudine** increases the risk of haematological toxicity when given with NSAIDs. [Severe] Study → Also see TABLE 2 p. 818

Obinutuzumab → see monoclonal antibodies

Octreotide

▶ **Octreotide** decreases the absorption of oral ciclosporin. Adjust ciclosporin dose, p. 496. [Severe] Anecdotal

Ofatumumab → see monoclonal antibodies

Ofloxacin → see quinolones

Olanzapine → see TABLE 8 p. 819 (hypotension), TABLE 15 p. 821 (myelosuppression), TABLE 11 p. 820 (CNS depressant effects)

FOOD AND LIFESTYLE   Dose adjustment might be necessary if smoking started or stopped during treatment.

▶ **Antiepileptics** (carbamazepine) potentially decrease the exposure to olanzapine. Monitor and adjust dose. [Moderate] Study

▶ **Olanzapine** is predicted to decrease the effects of dopamine receptor agonists. Avoid. [Moderate] Theoretical → Also see TABLE 8 p. 819

▶ **Olanzapine** is predicted to decrease the effects of histamine. Avoid. [Severe] Theoretical → Also see TABLE 8 p. 819

▶ **HIV-protease inhibitors** (ritonavir) moderately decrease the exposure to olanzapine. [Moderate] Study

▶ **Olanzapine** decreases the effects of levodopa. Avoid or monitor worsening parkinsonian symptoms. [Severe] Anecdotal → Also see TABLE 8 p. 819

▶ **SSRIs** (fluvoxamine) moderately increase the exposure to olanzapine. Adjust dose. [Severe] Anecdotal

Olaparib → see TABLE 15 p. 821 (myelosuppression)

FOOD AND LIFESTYLE   Bitter (Seville) orange is predicted to increase the exposure to olaparib.

▶ **Antiarrhythmics** (dronedarone) are predicted to increase the exposure to olaparib. Avoid or adjust olaparib dose. [Moderate] Theoretical

▶ **Antiepileptics** (carbamazepine, fosphenytoin, phenobarbital, phenytoin, primidone) are predicted to decrease the exposure to olaparib. Avoid. [Moderate] Theoretical

▶ **Antifungals, azoles** (fluconazole, isavuconazole, posaconazole) are predicted to increase the exposure to olaparib. Avoid or adjust olaparib dose. [Moderate] Theoretical

▶ **Antifungals, azoles** (itraconazole, ketoconazole, voriconazole) are predicted to increase the exposure to olaparib. Avoid or adjust olaparib dose. [Moderate] Study

▶ **Aprepitant** is predicted to increase the exposure to olaparib. Avoid or adjust olaparib dose. [Moderate] Theoretical

▶ **Bosentan** is predicted to decrease the exposure to olaparib. Avoid. [Moderate] Theoretical

▶ **Calcium channel blockers** (diltiazem, verapamil) are predicted to increase the exposure to olaparib. Avoid or adjust olaparib dose. [Moderate] Theoretical

▶ **Cobicistat** is predicted to increase the exposure to olaparib. Avoid or adjust olaparib dose. [Moderate] Study

▶ **Crizotinib** is predicted to increase the exposure to olaparib. Avoid or adjust olaparib dose. [Moderate] Theoretical → Also see TABLE 15 p. 821

▶ **Efavirenz** is predicted to decrease the exposure to olaparib. Avoid. [Moderate] Theoretical

▶ **Enzalutamide** is predicted to decrease the exposure to olaparib. Avoid. [Moderate] Theoretical

▶ **Grapefruit juice** is predicted to increase the exposure to olaparib. Avoid. [Moderate] Theoretical

▶ **HIV-protease inhibitors** (atazanavir, darunavir, fosamprenavir, lopinavir, ritonavir, saquinavir, tipranavir) are predicted to increase the exposure to olaparib. Avoid or adjust olaparib dose. [Moderate] Study

▶ **HIV-protease inhibitors** (indinavir) are predicted to increase the exposure to olaparib. Avoid or adjust olaparib dose. [Moderate] Theoretical

▶ **Idelalisib** is predicted to increase the exposure to olaparib. Avoid or adjust olaparib dose. [Moderate] Study → Also see TABLE 15 p. 821

▶ **Imatinib** is predicted to increase the exposure to olaparib. Avoid or adjust olaparib dose. [Moderate] Theoretical → Also see TABLE 15 p. 821

▶ **Macrolides** (clarithromycin) are predicted to increase the exposure to olaparib. Avoid or adjust olaparib dose. [Moderate] Study

▶ **Macrolides** (erythromycin) are predicted to increase the exposure to olaparib. Avoid or adjust olaparib dose. [Moderate] Theoretical

▶ **Netupitant** is predicted to increase the exposure to olaparib. Avoid or adjust olaparib dose. [Moderate] Theoretical

▶ **Nevirapine** is predicted to decrease the exposure to olaparib. Avoid. [Moderate] Theoretical

▶ **Nilotinib** is predicted to increase the exposure to olaparib. Avoid or adjust olaparib dose. [Moderate] Theoretical → Also see TABLE 15 p. 821

▶ **Rifampicin** is predicted to decrease the exposure to olaparib. Avoid. [Moderate] Theoretical

▶ **St John's Wort** is predicted to decrease the exposure to olaparib. Avoid. [Moderate] Theoretical

Olmesartan → see angiotensin-II receptor antagonists

Olodaterol → see beta₂ agonists

Olsalazine → see TABLE 15 p. 821 (myelosuppression)

Omalizumab → see monoclonal antibodies

Ombitasvir

▶ **Antiepileptics** (carbamazepine) are predicted to decrease the exposure to ombitasvir. Avoid. [Severe] Theoretical

► **Rifampicin** is predicted to decrease the exposure to **ombitasvir**. Avoid. Severe Theoretical

► **St John's Wort** is predicted to decrease the exposure to **ombitasvir**. Avoid. Severe Theoretical

Omega-3-acid ethyl esters → see TABLE 3 p. 818 (anticoagulant effects)

Omeprazole → see proton pump inhibitors

Ondansetron → see TABLE 13 p. 821 (serotonin syndrome), TABLE 9 p. 820 (QT-interval prolongation)

► **Antiepileptics (carbamazepine, fosphenytoin, phenobarbital, phenytoin, primidone)** are predicted to decrease the exposure to **ondansetron**. Moderate Study

► **Dopamine receptor agonists (apomorphine)** increase the risk of severe hypotension when given with **ondansetron**. Avoid. Severe Study → Also see TABLE 9 p. 820

► **Enzalutamide** is predicted to decrease the exposure to **ondansetron**. Moderate Study

► **Rifampicin** is predicted to decrease the exposure to **ondansetron**. Moderate Study

Opicapone

► **Opicapone** increases the exposure to **levodopa**. Adjust **levodopa** dose. Moderate Study

► **Opicapone** is predicted to increase the risk of elevated blood pressure when given with **moclobemide**. Avoid. Severe Theoretical

► **Opicapone** is predicted to increase the risk of elevated blood pressure when given with **monoamine-oxidase A and B inhibitors, irreversible**. Avoid. Severe Theoretical

► **Opicapone** is predicted to increase the risk of elevated blood pressure when given with monoamine-oxidase B inhibitors **(rasagiline, selegiline)**. Severe Theoretical

► **Opicapone** is predicted to increase the risk of cardiovascular side-effects when given with sympathomimetics, inotropic **(dobutamine, dopamine)**. Severe Theoretical

► **Opicapone** is predicted to increase the risk of cardiovascular side-effects when given with sympathomimetics, vasoconstrictor **(adrenaline/epinephrine, noradrenaline/norepinephrine)**. Severe Theoretical

Opioids → see TABLE 6 p. 819 (bradycardia), TABLE 13 p. 821 (serotonin syndrome), TABLE 9 p. 820 (QT-interval prolongation), TABLE 11 p. 820 (CNS depressant effects)

alfentanil · buprenorphine · codeine · diamorphine · dihydrocodeine · diphenoxylate · dipipanone · fentanyl · hydromorphone · meptazinol · methadone · morphine · oxycodone · papaveretum · pentazocine · pethidine · remifentanil · sufentanil · tapentadol · tramadol

FOOD AND LIFESTYLE Alcohol has been associated with rapid release of **hydromorphone** and **morphine** from extended-release preparations. Avoid alcohol consumption with extended-release preparations.

► **Abiraterone** is predicted to decrease the efficacy of **tramadol**. Moderate Study

► **Antiarrhythmics (amiodarone)** are predicted to increase the concentration of **fentanyl**. Moderate Theoretical → Also see TABLE 6 p. 819

► **Antiarrhythmics (propafenone)** are predicted to decrease the efficacy of **tramadol**. Moderate Study

► **Antiarrhythmics (dronedarone)** are predicted to increase the exposure to opioids **(alfentanil, buprenorphine, fentanyl, oxycodone)**. Monitor and adjust dose. Moderate Study

► **Antiarrhythmics (dronedarone)** are predicted to increase the exposure to opioids **(methadone, sufentanil)**. Moderate Theoretical → Also see TABLE 9 p. 820

► **Antiepileptics (carbamazepine)** decrease the concentration of **tramadol**. Adjust dose. Severe Study

► **Antiepileptics (carbamazepine, fosphenytoin, phenobarbital, phenytoin, primidone)** are predicted to decrease the exposure to **buprenorphine**. Monitor and adjust dose. Moderate Theoretical → Also see TABLE 11 p. 820

► **Antiepileptics (carbamazepine, fosphenytoin, phenobarbital, phenytoin, primidone)** decrease the exposure to **methadone**. Monitor and adjust dose. Severe Study → Also see TABLE 11 p. 820

► **Antiepileptics (carbamazepine, fosphenytoin, phenobarbital, phenytoin, primidone)** are predicted to decrease the exposure

to **oxycodone**. Monitor and adjust dose. Moderate Study → Also see TABLE 11 p. 820

► **Antiepileptics (carbamazepine, fosphenytoin, phenobarbital, phenytoin, primidone)** are predicted to decrease the exposure to opioids **(alfentanil, fentanyl)**. Moderate Study → Also see TABLE 11 p. 820

► **Antifungals, azoles (itraconazole, ketoconazole, voriconazole)** are predicted to increase the exposure to **methadone**. Moderate Theoretical → Also see TABLE 9 p. 820

► **Antifungals, azoles (miconazole)** are predicted to increase the exposure to **alfentanil**. Use with caution and adjust dose. Moderate Theoretical

► **Antifungals, azoles (fluconazole, isavuconazole, posaconazole)** are predicted to increase the exposure to opioids **(alfentanil, buprenorphine, fentanyl, oxycodone)**. Monitor and adjust dose. Moderate Study

► **Antifungals, azoles (itraconazole, ketoconazole, voriconazole)** are predicted to increase the exposure to opioids **(alfentanil, buprenorphine, fentanyl, oxycodone, sufentanil)**. Monitor and adjust dose. Severe Study

► **Antifungals, azoles (fluconazole, isavuconazole, posaconazole)** are predicted to increase the exposure to opioids **(methadone, sufentanil)**. Moderate Theoretical

► **Aprepitant** is predicted to increase the exposure to opioids **(alfentanil, buprenorphine, fentanyl, oxycodone)**. Monitor and adjust dose. Moderate Study

► **Aprepitant** is predicted to increase the exposure to opioids **(methadone, sufentanil)**. Moderate Theoretical

► **Bosentan** decreases the exposure to **methadone**. Monitor and adjust dose. Severe Study

► **Bupropion** is predicted to decrease the efficacy of **codeine**. Moderate Theoretical

► **Bupropion** is predicted to decrease the efficacy of **tramadol**. Severe Study → Also see TABLE 13 p. 821

► **Calcium channel blockers (diltiazem, verapamil)** are predicted to increase the exposure to opioids **(alfentanil, buprenorphine, fentanyl, oxycodone)**. Monitor and adjust dose. Moderate Study → Also see TABLE 6 p. 819

► **Calcium channel blockers (diltiazem, verapamil)** are predicted to increase the exposure to opioids **(methadone, sufentanil)**. Moderate Theoretical → Also see TABLE 6 p. 819

► **Ceritinib** is predicted to increase the exposure to opioids **(alfentanil, fentanyl)**. Avoid. Severe Theoretical

► **Cinacalcet** is predicted to decrease the efficacy of **codeine**. Moderate Theoretical

► **Cinacalcet** is predicted to decrease the efficacy of **tramadol**. Severe Study

► **Cobicistat** is predicted to increase the exposure to **methadone**. Moderate Theoretical

► **Cobicistat** is predicted to increase the exposure to opioids **(alfentanil, buprenorphine, fentanyl, oxycodone, sufentanil)**. Monitor and adjust dose. Severe Study

► **Crizotinib** is predicted to increase the exposure to opioids **(alfentanil, buprenorphine, fentanyl, oxycodone)**. Monitor and adjust dose. Moderate Study → Also see TABLE 6 p. 819

► **Crizotinib** is predicted to increase the exposure to opioids **(methadone, sufentanil)**. Moderate Theoretical → Also see TABLE 6 p. 819 → Also see TABLE 9 p. 820

► **Duloxetine** is predicted to decrease the efficacy of **tramadol**. Moderate Study → Also see TABLE 13 p. 821

► **Efavirenz** decreases the exposure to **methadone**. Monitor and adjust dose. Severe Study

► **Enzalutamide** is predicted to decrease the exposure to **buprenorphine**. Monitor and adjust dose. Moderate Theoretical

► **Enzalutamide** decreases the exposure to **methadone**. Monitor and adjust dose. Severe Study

► **Enzalutamide** is predicted to decrease the exposure to opioids **(alfentanil, fentanyl)**. Moderate Study

► **Enzalutamide** is predicted to decrease the exposure to **oxycodone**. Monitor and adjust dose. Moderate Study

► **H₂ receptor antagonists (cimetidine)** increase the concentration of **alfentanil**. Use with caution and adjust dose. Severe Study

► **H₂ receptor antagonists (cimetidine)** increase the exposure to **fentanyl**. Moderate Study

Opioids (continued)

▸ HIV-protease inhibitors **(atazanavir, darunavir, fosamprenavir, lopinavir, ritonavir, saquinavir, tipranavir)** are predicted to increase the exposure to **methadone**. Moderate Theoretical → Also see TABLE 9 p. 820

▸ HIV-protease inhibitors **(ritonavir)** are predicted to decrease the concentration of **morphine**. Moderate Theoretical

▸ HIV-protease inhibitors **(ritonavir)** increase the risk of CNS toxicity when given with **pethidine**. Avoid. Severe Study

▸ HIV-protease inhibitors **(ritonavir)** are predicted to decrease the efficacy of **tramadol**. Moderate Study

▸ HIV-protease inhibitors **(indinavir)** are predicted to increase the exposure to opioids **(alfentanil, buprenorphine, fentanyl, oxycodone)**. Monitor and adjust dose. Moderate Study

▸ HIV-protease inhibitors **(atazanavir, darunavir, fosamprenavir, lopinavir, ritonavir, saquinavir, tipranavir)** are predicted to increase the exposure to opioids **(alfentanil, buprenorphine, fentanyl, oxycodone, sufentanil)**. Monitor and adjust dose. Severe Study

▸ HIV-protease inhibitors **(indinavir)** are predicted to increase the exposure to opioids **(methadone, sufentanil)**. Moderate Theoretical

▸ Idelalisib is predicted to increase the exposure to **methadone**. Moderate Theoretical

▸ Idelalisib is predicted to increase the exposure to opioids **(alfentanil, buprenorphine, fentanyl, oxycodone, sufentanil)**. Monitor and adjust dose. Severe Study

▸ Imatinib is predicted to increase the exposure to opioids **(alfentanil, buprenorphine, fentanyl, oxycodone)**. Monitor and adjust dose. Moderate Study

▸ Imatinib is predicted to increase the exposure to opioids **(methadone, sufentanil)**. Moderate Theoretical

▸ Macrolides **(clarithromycin)** are predicted to increase the exposure to **methadone**. Moderate Theoretical → Also see TABLE 9 p. 820

▸ Macrolides **(erythromycin)** are predicted to increase the exposure to opioids **(alfentanil, buprenorphine, fentanyl, oxycodone)**. Monitor and adjust dose. Moderate Study

▸ Macrolides **(clarithromycin)** are predicted to increase the exposure to opioids **(alfentanil, buprenorphine, fentanyl, oxycodone, sufentanil)**. Monitor and adjust dose. Severe Study

▸ Macrolides **(erythromycin)** are predicted to increase the exposure to opioids **(methadone, sufentanil)**. Moderate Theoretical

▸ **Mirabegron** is predicted to decrease the efficacy of **tramadol**. Moderate Study

▸ **Opioids** are predicted to increase the risk of CNS excitation or depression when given with **monoamine-oxidase A and B inhibitors, irreversible**. Avoid. Severe Study → Also see TABLE 13 p. 821

▸ Monoamine-oxidase B inhibitors **(rasagiline)** are predicted to increase the risk of side-effects when given with **pethidine**. Avoid and for 14 days after stopping **rasagiline**. Severe Theoretical → Also see TABLE 13 p. 821

▸ Monoamine-oxidase B inhibitors **(safinamide)** are predicted to increase the risk of side-effects when given with **pethidine**. Avoid and for 1 week after stopping **safinamide**. Severe Theoretical → Also see TABLE 13 p. 821

▸ Monoamine-oxidase B inhibitors **(selegiline)** increase the risk of side-effects when given with **pethidine**. Avoid. Severe Anecdotal → Also see TABLE 13 p. 821

▸ **Nalmefene** is predicted to decrease the efficacy of **opioids**. Avoid. Severe Theoretical

▸ **Netupitant** is predicted to increase the exposure to opioids **(alfentanil, buprenorphine, fentanyl, oxycodone)**. Monitor and adjust dose. Moderate Study

▸ **Netupitant** is predicted to increase the exposure to opioids **(methadone, sufentanil)**. Moderate Theoretical

▸ **Nevirapine** decreases the exposure to **methadone**. Monitor and adjust dose. Severe Study

▸ **Nilotinib** is predicted to increase the exposure to opioids **(alfentanil, buprenorphine, fentanyl, oxycodone)**. Monitor and adjust dose. Moderate Study

▸ **Nilotinib** is predicted to increase the exposure to opioids **(methadone, sufentanil)**. Moderate Theoretical → Also see TABLE 9 p. 820

▸ Opioids **(buprenorphine)** are predicted to increase the risk of opiate withdrawal when given with opioids **(alfentanil)**. Severe Theoretical → Also see TABLE 11 p. 820

▸ Opioids **(pentazocine)** are predicted to increase the risk of opiate withdrawal when given with opioids **(alfentanil, codeine, diamorphine, dihydrocodeine, dipipanone, fentanyl, hydromorphone, meptazinol, methadone, morphine, oxycodone, papaveretum)**. Severe Theoretical → Also see TABLE 13 p. 821 → Also see TABLE 11 p. 820

▸ Opioids **(buprenorphine, pentazocine)** are predicted to increase the risk of opiate withdrawal when given with opioids **(pethidine, remifentanil, tapentadol, tramadol)**. Severe Theoretical → Also see TABLE 11 p. 820 → Also see TABLE 13 p. 821

▸ Opioids **(pentazocine)** are predicted to increase the risk of opiate withdrawal when given with opioids **(sufentanil)**. Severe Anecdotal → Also see TABLE 11 p. 820

▸ **Palbociclib** is predicted to increase the exposure to opioids **(alfentanil, fentanyl)**. Adjust dose. Moderate Theoretical

▸ **Pitolisant** is predicted to decrease the exposure to **morphine**. Unknown Theoretical

▸ **Rifampicin** is predicted to decrease the exposure to **buprenorphine**. Monitor and adjust dose. Moderate Theoretical

▸ **Rifampicin** decreases the exposure to **methadone**. Monitor and adjust dose. Severe Study

▸ **Rifampicin** is predicted to decrease the exposure to opioids **(alfentanil, fentanyl)**. Moderate Study

▸ **Rifampicin** decreases the exposure to opioids **(codeine, morphine)**. Moderate Study

▸ **Rifampicin** is predicted to decrease the exposure to **oxycodone**. Monitor and adjust dose. Moderate Study

▸ SSRIs **(fluoxetine, paroxetine)** are predicted to decrease the efficacy of **codeine**. Moderate Theoretical

▸ SSRIs **(fluoxetine, paroxetine)** are predicted to decrease the efficacy of **tramadol**. Severe Study → Also see TABLE 13 p. 821

▸ **St John's Wort** decreases the exposure to **methadone**. Monitor and adjust dose. Severe Study → Also see TABLE 13 p. 821

▸ **St John's Wort** moderately decreases the exposure to **oxycodone**. Adjust dose. Moderate Study

▸ **Terbinafine** is predicted to decrease the efficacy of **codeine**. Moderate Theoretical

▸ **Terbinafine** is predicted to decrease the efficacy of **tramadol**. Severe Study

Orlistat

SEPARATION OF ADMINISTRATION Orlistat might affect the absorption of concurrently administered drugs—consider separating administration. Particular care should be taken with antiepileptics, antiretrovirals, and drugs that have a narrow therapeutic index.

Orphenadrine → see TABLE 10 p. 820 (antimuscarinics)

Osimertinib → see TABLE 9 p. 820 (QT-interval prolongation)

▸ Antiepileptics **(carbamazepine, fosphenytoin, phenobarbital, phenytoin, primidone)** are predicted to moderately decrease the exposure to **osimertinib**. Avoid. Moderate Study

▸ **Bosentan** is predicted to decrease the exposure to **osimertinib**. Moderate Theoretical

▸ **Efavirenz** is predicted to decrease the exposure to **osimertinib**. Moderate Theoretical

▸ **Enzalutamide** is predicted to moderately decrease the exposure to **osimertinib**. Avoid. Moderate Study

▸ **Nevirapine** is predicted to decrease the exposure to **osimertinib**. Severe Theoretical

▸ **Rifampicin** is predicted to moderately decrease the exposure to **osimertinib**. Avoid. Moderate Study

▸ **St John's Wort** is predicted to decrease the exposure to **osimertinib**. Avoid. Moderate Theoretical

▸ **Osimertinib** slightly increases the exposure to statins **(rosuvastatin)**. Moderate Study

Oxaliplatin → see platinum compounds

Oxazepam → see TABLE 11 p. 820 (CNS depressant effects)

Oxcarbazepine → see antiepileptics

Oxprenolol → see beta blockers, non-selective

Oxybuprocaine → see anaesthetics, local

Oxybutynin → see TABLE 10 p. 820 (antimuscarinics)
▶ Antiarrhythmics **(dronedarone)** are predicted to increase the exposure to **oxybutynin**. Mild Theoretical
▶ **Oxybutynin** potentially increases the risk of overheating and dehydration when given with antiepileptics **(zonisamide)**. Avoid in children. Severe Theoretical
▶ Antifungals, azoles **(fluconazole, isavuconazole, posaconazole)** are predicted to increase the exposure to **oxybutynin**. Mild Theoretical
▶ Antifungals, azoles **(itraconazole, ketoconazole, voriconazole)** are predicted to increase the exposure to **oxybutynin**. Mild Study
▶ **Aprepitant** is predicted to increase the exposure to **oxybutynin**. Mild Theoretical
▶ Calcium channel blockers **(diltiazem, verapamil)** are predicted to increase the exposure to **oxybutynin**. Mild Theoretical
▶ **Cobicistat** is predicted to increase the exposure to **oxybutynin**. Mild Study
▶ **Crizotinib** is predicted to increase the exposure to **oxybutynin**. Mild Theoretical
▶ HIV-protease inhibitors **(atazanavir, darunavir, fosamprenavir, lopinavir, ritonavir, saquinavir, tipranavir)** are predicted to increase the exposure to **oxybutynin**. Mild Study
▶ HIV-protease inhibitors **(indinavir)** are predicted to increase the exposure to **oxybutynin**. Mild Theoretical
▶ **Idelalisib** is predicted to increase the exposure to **oxybutynin**. Mild Study
▶ **Imatinib** is predicted to increase the exposure to **oxybutynin**. Mild Theoretical
▶ Macrolides **(clarithromycin)** are predicted to increase the exposure to **oxybutynin**. Mild Study
▶ Macrolides **(erythromycin)** are predicted to increase the exposure to **oxybutynin**. Mild Theoretical
▶ **Netupitant** is predicted to increase the exposure to **oxybutynin**. Mild Theoretical
▶ **Nilotinib** is predicted to increase the exposure to **oxybutynin**. Mild Theoretical

Oxycodone → see opioids

Oxymetholone
▶ **Oxymetholone** increases the anticoagulant effect of **coumarins**. Severe Anecdotal
▶ **Oxymetholone** increases the anticoagulant effect of **phenindione**. Severe Anecdotal

Oxytetracycline → see tetracyclines

Paclitaxel → see taxanes

Palbociclib
▶ Antiepileptics **(carbamazepine, fosphenytoin, phenobarbital, phenytoin, primidone)** are predicted to decrease the exposure to **palbociclib**. Avoid. Severe Study
▶ Antifungals, azoles **(itraconazole, ketoconazole, voriconazole)** are predicted to increase the exposure to **palbociclib**. Avoid or adjust **palbociclib** dose. Severe Study
▶ **Palbociclib** is predicted to increase the exposure to **ciclosporin**. Adjust dose. Moderate Theoretical
▶ **Cobicistat** is predicted to increase the exposure to **palbociclib**. Avoid or adjust **palbociclib** dose. Severe Study
▶ **Enzalutamide** is predicted to decrease the exposure to **palbociclib**. Avoid. Severe Study
▶ **Palbociclib** is predicted to increase the exposure to **ergotamine**. Adjust dose. Moderate Theoretical
▶ **Palbociclib** is predicted to increase the exposure to **everolimus**. Adjust dose. Moderate Theoretical
▶ **Grapefruit juice** is predicted to increase the exposure to **palbociclib**. Avoid. Severe Theoretical
▶ HIV-protease inhibitors **(atazanavir, darunavir, fosamprenavir, lopinavir, ritonavir, saquinavir, tipranavir)** are predicted to increase the exposure to **palbociclib**. Avoid or adjust **palbociclib** dose. Severe Study
▶ **Idelalisib** is predicted to increase the exposure to **palbociclib**. Avoid or adjust **palbociclib** dose. Severe Study
▶ Macrolides **(clarithromycin)** are predicted to increase the exposure to **palbociclib**. Avoid or adjust **palbociclib** dose. Severe Study
▶ **Palbociclib** increases the exposure to **midazolam**. Moderate Study
▶ **Palbociclib** is predicted to increase the exposure to opioids **(alfentanil, fentanyl)**. Adjust dose. Moderate Theoretical
▶ **Palbociclib** is predicted to increase the exposure to **pimozide**. Adjust dose. Moderate Theoretical
▶ **Rifampicin** is predicted to decrease the exposure to **palbociclib**. Avoid. Severe Study
▶ **Palbociclib** is predicted to increase the exposure to **sirolimus**. Adjust dose. Moderate Theoretical
▶ **St John's Wort** is predicted to decrease the exposure to **palbociclib**. Avoid. Severe Theoretical
▶ **Palbociclib** is predicted to increase the exposure to **tacrolimus**. Adjust dose. Moderate Theoretical

Paliperidone → see TABLE 8 p. 819 (hypotension), TABLE 9 p. 820 (QT-interval prolongation), TABLE 11 p. 820 (CNS depressant effects)
▶ Antiepileptics **(carbamazepine)** decrease the concentration of **paliperidone**. Adjust dose. Moderate Study
▶ **Paliperidone** is predicted to decrease the effects of **dopamine receptor agonists**. Avoid. Moderate Study → Also see TABLE 8 p. 819 → Also see TABLE 9 p. 820
▶ **Paliperidone** is predicted to decrease the effects of **levodopa**. Severe Theoretical → Also see TABLE 8 p. 819
▶ **Rifampicin** is predicted to decrease the exposure to **paliperidone**. Monitor and adjust **paliperidone** dose. Moderate Theoretical

Palonosetron → see TABLE 9 p. 820 (QT-interval prolongation), TABLE 13 p. 821 (serotonin syndrome)
▶ Dopamine receptor agonists **(apomorphine)** are predicted to increase the risk of severe hypotension when given with **palonosetron**. Severe Theoretical

Pamidronate → see bisphosphonates

Pancreatin
▶ **Pancreatin** is predicted to decrease the effects of **acarbose**. Avoid. Moderate Theoretical

Pancuronium → see neuromuscular blocking drugs, non-depolarising

Panitumumab → see monoclonal antibodies

Panobinostat → see TABLE 9 p. 820 (QT-interval prolongation), TABLE 15 p. 821 (myelosuppression)

FOOD AND LIFESTYLE Avoid pomegranate, pomegranate juice, and star fruit as they are predicted to increase panobinostat exposure.

▶ Antiepileptics **(carbamazepine, fosphenytoin, phenobarbital, phenytoin, primidone)** are predicted to decrease the exposure to **panobinostat**. Avoid. Moderate Theoretical
▶ Antifungals, azoles **(itraconazole, ketoconazole, voriconazole)** are predicted to increase the exposure to **panobinostat**. Adjust **panobinostat** dose; in hepatic impairment avoid. Moderate Study → Also see TABLE 9 p. 820
▶ **Panobinostat** is predicted to increase the exposure to **atomoxetine**. Monitor and adjust dose. Severe Theoretical
▶ **Panobinostat** is predicted to increase the exposure to beta blockers, selective **(metoprolol)**. Monitor and adjust dose. Moderate Theoretical
▶ **Cobicistat** is predicted to increase the exposure to **panobinostat**. Adjust **panobinostat** dose; in hepatic impairment avoid. Moderate Study
▶ **Enzalutamide** is predicted to decrease the exposure to **panobinostat**. Avoid. Moderate Theoretical
▶ HIV-protease inhibitors **(atazanavir, darunavir, fosamprenavir, lopinavir, ritonavir, saquinavir, tipranavir)** are predicted to increase the exposure to **panobinostat**. Adjust **panobinostat** dose; in hepatic impairment avoid. Moderate Study → Also see TABLE 9 p. 820
▶ **Idelalisib** is predicted to increase the exposure to **panobinostat**. Adjust **panobinostat** dose; in hepatic impairment avoid. Moderate Study → Also see TABLE 15 p. 821
▶ Macrolides **(clarithromycin)** are predicted to increase the exposure to **panobinostat**. Adjust **panobinostat** dose; in hepatic impairment avoid. Moderate Study → Also see TABLE 9 p. 820
▶ **Panobinostat** is predicted to increase the exposure to phenothiazines **(perphenazine)**. Monitor and adjust dose. Severe Theoretical
▶ **Panobinostat** is predicted to increase the exposure to **pimozide**. Avoid. Severe Theoretical → Also see TABLE 9 p. 820

Panobinostat (continued)
▸ **Rifampicin** is predicted to decrease the exposure to panobinostat. Avoid. Moderate Theoretical
▸ **St John's Wort** is predicted to decrease the exposure to panobinostat. Avoid. Moderate Theoretical
▸ **Panobinostat** is predicted to increase the exposure to tolterodine. Moderate Theoretical → Also see **TABLE 9** p. 820

Pantoprazole → see proton pump inhibitors

Papaveretum → see opioids

Paracetamol → see **TABLE 1** p. 818 (hepatotoxicity)

> **FOOD AND LIFESTYLE** Severe liver damage can occur with chronic alcohol consumption in some alcoholics and persistent heavy drinkers who take only moderate doses of paracetamol.

▸ **Paracetamol** is predicted to decrease the clearance of alkylating agents (busulfan). Moderate Theoretical
▸ **Paracetamol** is predicted to increase the risk of methaemoglobinaemia when given with topical anaesthetics, local (prilocaine). Use with caution or avoid. Severe Theoretical
▸ **Antiepileptics (carbamazepine, fosphenytoin, phenobarbital, phenytoin, primidone)** are predicted to decrease the exposure to paracetamol. Moderate Study → Also see **TABLE 1** p. 818
▸ **Paracetamol** increases the anticoagulant effect of **coumarins**. Severe Study
▸ **Paracetamol** is predicted to increase the risk of methaemoglobinaemia when given with **dapsone**. Severe Theoretical
▸ **Enzalutamide** is predicted to decrease the exposure to paracetamol. Moderate Study
▸ **Imatinib** increases the risk of hepatotoxicity when given with paracetamol. Severe Anecdotal
▸ **Paracetamol** is predicted to increase the anticoagulant effect of **phenindione**. Severe Theoretical
▸ **Pitolisant** is predicted to decrease the exposure to paracetamol. Unknown Theoretical
▸ **Rifampicin** is predicted to decrease the exposure to paracetamol. Moderate Study

Paraldehyde → see antiepileptics

Parecoxib → see NSAIDs

Paricalcitol → see vitamin D substances

Paritaprevir
▸ **Antiepileptics (carbamazepine, fosphenytoin, phenobarbital, phenytoin, primidone)** are predicted to decrease the exposure to paritaprevir (with ritonavir and ombitasvir). Avoid. Severe Study
▸ **Antifungals, azoles (itraconazole, ketoconazole, voriconazole)** are predicted to increase the exposure to **paritaprevir** (with ritonavir and ombitasvir). Avoid. Severe Theoretical
▸ **Antifungals, azoles (posaconazole)** are predicted to increase the exposure to **paritaprevir** (with ritonavir and ombitasvir) and **paritaprevir** (with ritonavir and ombitasvir) is predicted to increase the exposure to antifungals, azoles (posaconazole). Avoid. Severe Theoretical
▸ **Bosentan** is predicted to decrease the exposure to **paritaprevir** (with ritonavir and ombitasvir). Avoid. Severe Study
▸ **Cobicistat** is predicted to increase the exposure to **paritaprevir** (with ritonavir and ombitasvir). Avoid. Severe Theoretical
▸ **Paritaprevir** (with ritonavir and ombitasvir) increases the risk of raised liver function tests when given with **combined hormonal contraceptives**. Avoid. Severe Study
▸ **Efavirenz** is predicted to decrease the exposure to **paritaprevir** (with ritonavir and ombitasvir). Avoid. Severe Study
▸ **Enzalutamide** is predicted to decrease the exposure to **paritaprevir** (with ritonavir and ombitasvir). Avoid. Severe Study
▸ **HIV-protease inhibitors (atazanavir, darunavir, fosamprenavir, lopinavir, ritonavir, saquinavir, tipranavir)** are predicted to increase the exposure to **paritaprevir** (with ritonavir and ombitasvir). Avoid. Severe Theoretical
▸ **HIV-protease inhibitors (indinavir)** potentially increase the exposure to **paritaprevir**. Avoid. Severe Theoretical
▸ **Idelalisib** is predicted to increase the exposure to **paritaprevir** (with ritonavir and ombitasvir). Avoid. Severe Theoretical

▸ **Paritaprevir** (with ritonavir and ombitasvir) is predicted to increase the exposure to loop diuretics (furosemide). Adjust **furosemide** dose, p. 136. Moderate Theoretical
▸ **Macrolides (clarithromycin)** are predicted to increase the exposure to **paritaprevir** (with ritonavir and ombitasvir). Avoid. Severe Theoretical
▸ **Nevirapine** is predicted to decrease the exposure to **paritaprevir** (with ritonavir and ombitasvir). Avoid. Severe Study
▸ **Rifampicin** is predicted to decrease the exposure to **paritaprevir** (with ritonavir and ombitasvir). Avoid. Severe Study
▸ **St John's Wort** is predicted to decrease the exposure to **paritaprevir** (with ritonavir and ombitasvir). Avoid. Severe Study
▸ **Paritaprevir** (with ritonavir and ombitasvir) is predicted to increase the exposure to statins (fluvastatin). Avoid. Moderate Theoretical
▸ **Paritaprevir** (with ritonavir and ombitasvir) increases the exposure to statins (pravastatin). Adjust **pravastatin** dose Moderate Study
▸ **Paritaprevir** (with ritonavir and ombitasvir) increases the exposure to statins (rosuvastatin). Adjust **rosuvastatin** dose, p. 130. Moderate Study

Paroxetine → see SSRIs

Pasireotide → see **TABLE 6** p. 819 (bradycardia), **TABLE 9** p. 820 (QT-interval prolongation)
▸ **Pasireotide** is predicted to decrease the absorption of oral ciclosporin. Adjust dose. Severe Theoretical

Pazopanib → see **TABLE 9** p. 820 (QT-interval prolongation), **TABLE 15** p. 821 (myelosuppression)
▸ **Antacids** are predicted to decrease the absorption of pazopanib. **Pazopanib** should be taken 1 hour before or 2 hours after **antacids**. Moderate Theoretical
▸ **Antiarrhythmics (dronedarone)** are predicted to increase the exposure to **pazopanib**. Moderate Theoretical → Also see **TABLE 9** p. 820
▸ **Antiepileptics (carbamazepine, fosphenytoin, phenobarbital, phenytoin, primidone)** are predicted to decrease the exposure to **pazopanib**. Avoid. Severe Theoretical
▸ **Antifungals, azoles (fluconazole, isavuconazole, posaconazole)** are predicted to increase the exposure to **pazopanib**. Moderate Theoretical
▸ **Antifungals, azoles (itraconazole, ketoconazole, voriconazole)** are predicted to increase the exposure to **pazopanib**. Avoid or adjust **pazopanib** dose. Moderate Study → Also see **TABLE 9** p. 820
▸ **Aprepitant** is predicted to increase the exposure to **pazopanib**. Moderate Theoretical
▸ **Calcium channel blockers (diltiazem, verapamil)** are predicted to increase the exposure to **pazopanib**. Moderate Theoretical
▸ **Cobicistat** is predicted to increase the exposure to **pazopanib**. Avoid or adjust **pazopanib** dose. Moderate Study
▸ **Pazopanib** is predicted to increase the risk of bleeding events when given with **coumarins**. Severe Theoretical
▸ **Crizotinib** is predicted to increase the exposure to **pazopanib**. Moderate Theoretical → Also see **TABLE 9** p. 820→ Also see **TABLE 15** p. 821
▸ **Enzalutamide** is predicted to decrease the exposure to **pazopanib**. Avoid. Severe Theoretical
▸ **Grapefruit juice** is predicted to increase the exposure to **pazopanib**. Avoid. Severe Theoretical
▸ **H₂ receptor antagonists** are predicted to decrease the exposure to **pazopanib**. **H₂ receptor antagonists** should be taken 10 hours before or 2 hours after **pazopanib**. Moderate Theoretical
▸ **HIV-protease inhibitors (atazanavir, darunavir, fosamprenavir, lopinavir, ritonavir, saquinavir, tipranavir)** are predicted to increase the exposure to **pazopanib**. Avoid or adjust **pazopanib** dose. Moderate Study → Also see **TABLE 9** p. 820
▸ **HIV-protease inhibitors (indinavir)** are predicted to increase the exposure to **pazopanib**. Moderate Theoretical
▸ **Idelalisib** is predicted to increase the exposure to **pazopanib**. Avoid or adjust **pazopanib** dose. Moderate Study → Also see **TABLE 15** p. 821
▸ **Imatinib** is predicted to increase the exposure to **pazopanib**. Moderate Theoretical → Also see **TABLE 15** p. 821

‣ **Pazopanib** is predicted to increase the exposure to lomitapide. Separate administration by 12 hours. [Moderate] Theoretical
‣ Macrolides (clarithromycin) are predicted to increase the exposure to **pazopanib**. Avoid or adjust **pazopanib** dose. [Moderate] Study → Also see TABLE 9 p. 820
‣ Macrolides (erythromycin) are predicted to increase the exposure to **pazopanib**. [Moderate] Theoretical
‣ Netupitant is predicted to increase the exposure to **pazopanib**. [Moderate] Theoretical
‣ Nilotinib is predicted to increase the exposure to **pazopanib**. [Moderate] Theoretical → Also see TABLE 15 p. 821 → Also see TABLE 9 p. 820
‣ **Pazopanib** is predicted to increase the risk of bleeding events when given with phenindione. [Severe] Theoretical
‣ Proton pump inhibitors are predicted to decrease the exposure to **pazopanib**. Avoid or administer concurrently without food. [Moderate] Study
‣ Rifampicin is predicted to decrease the exposure to **pazopanib**. Avoid. [Severe] Theoretical

Pegaspargase → see TABLE 1 p. 818 (hepatotoxicity), TABLE 15 p. 821 (myelosuppression)
‣ **Pegaspargase** is predicted to increase the risk of hepatotoxicity when given with imatinib. [Severe] Theoretical → Also see TABLE 15 p. 821
‣ **Pegaspargase** affects the efficacy of methotrexate. [Severe] Anecdotal → Also see TABLE 1 p. 818 → Also see TABLE 15 p. 821
‣ **Pegaspargase** potentially increases the risk of neurotoxicity when given with vinca alkaloids (vincristine). Vincristine should be taken 3 to 24 hours before **pegaspargase**. [Severe] Anecdotal → Also see TABLE 1 p. 818 → Also see TABLE 15 p. 821

Peginterferon alfa → see interferons
Peginterferon beta-1a → see TABLE 15 p. 821 (myelosuppression)
Pembrolizumab → see monoclonal antibodies
Pemetrexed → see TABLE 15 p. 821 (myelosuppression), TABLE 2 p. 818 (nephrotoxicity)
‣ Antimalarials (pyrimethamine) are predicted to increase the risk of side-effects when given with **pemetrexed**. [Severe] Theoretical → Also see TABLE 15 p. 821
‣ Aspirin (high-dose) potentially increases the exposure to **pemetrexed**. Use with caution or avoid. [Severe] Theoretical
‣ Live vaccines are predicted to increase the risk of generalised infection (possibly life-threatening) when given with **pemetrexed**. Public Health England advises avoid. [Severe] Theoretical
‣ NSAIDs are predicted to increase the exposure to **pemetrexed**. Use with caution or avoid. [Severe] Theoretical → Also see TABLE 2 p. 818

Penicillamine → see TABLE 2 p. 818 (nephrotoxicity)
‣ Antacids decrease the absorption of **penicillamine**. Separate administration by 2 hours. [Mild] Study
‣ Antimalarials (chloroquine) are predicted to increase the risk of haematological toxicity when given with **penicillamine**. Avoid. [Severe] Theoretical
‣ **Penicillamine** potentially decreases the concentration of digoxin. Separate administration by 2 hours. [Severe] Anecdotal
‣ Hydroxychloroquine is predicted to increase the risk of haematological toxicity when given with **penicillamine**. Avoid. [Severe] Theoretical
‣ Iron (oral) is predicted to decrease the absorption of **penicillamine**. Separate administration by at least 2 hours. [Mild] Study
‣ Sodium aurothiomalate potentially increases the risk of side-effects when given with **penicillamine** (in those who have had previous adverse reactions to gold). Avoid. [Severe] Study
‣ Zinc is predicted to decrease the absorption of **penicillamine**. [Mild] Theoretical

Penicillins

amoxicillin · ampicillin · benzylpenicillin · flucloxacillin · phenoxymethylpenicillin · piperacillin · pivmecillinam · temocillin · ticarcillin

‣ Allopurinol increases the risk of skin rash when given with penicillins (amoxicillin, ampicillin). [Moderate] Study
‣ **Penicillins** potentially alter the anticoagulant effect of coumarins. Monitor INR and adjust dose. [Severe] Anecdotal

‣ **Penicillins** are predicted to increase the risk of toxicity when given with methotrexate. [Severe] Theoretical
‣ Piperacillin increases the effects of neuromuscular blocking drugs, non-depolarising. [Moderate] Study
‣ **Penicillins** are predicted to increase the risk of bleeding events when given with phenindione. [Severe] Theoretical
‣ Piperacillin increases the effects of suxamethonium. [Moderate] Study

Pentamidine → see TABLE 2 p. 818 (nephrotoxicity), TABLE 9 p. 820 (QT-interval prolongation), TABLE 15 p. 821 (myelosuppression)
‣ Didanosine is predicted to increase the risk of pancreatitis when given with **pentamidine**. Avoid. [Severe] Study
‣ Foscarnet increases the risk of hypocalcaemia when given with **pentamidine**. [Severe] Anecdotal → Also see TABLE 2 p. 818

Pentazocine → see opioids
Pentostatin → see TABLE 15 p. 821 (myelosuppression), TABLE 5 p. 818 (thromboembolism)
‣ Alkylating agents (cyclophosphamide) (high-dose) increase the risk of toxicity when given with **pentostatin**. Avoid. [Severe] Anecdotal → Also see TABLE 15 p. 821 → Also see TABLE 5 p. 818
‣ Fludarabine increases the risk of pulmonary toxicity when given with **pentostatin**. Avoid. [Severe] Study → Also see TABLE 15 p. 821

Pentoxifylline
‣ **Pentoxifylline** is predicted to increase the concentration of aminophylline. Use with caution or avoid. [Severe] Theoretical
‣ Quinolones (ciprofloxacin) very slightly increase the exposure to **pentoxifylline**. [Moderate] Study
‣ SSRIs (fluvoxamine) are predicted to increase the exposure to **pentoxifylline**. [Moderate] Theoretical
‣ **Pentoxifylline** increases the concentration of theophylline. Monitor and adjust dose. [Severe] Study

Peppermint oil
‣ Peppermint oil is predicted to increase the exposure to lomitapide. Separate administration by 12 hours. [Moderate] Theoretical

Perampanel → see antiepileptics
Pergolide → see dopamine receptor agonists
Pericyazine → see phenothiazines
Perindopril → see ACE inhibitors
Perphenazine → see phenothiazines
Pertuzumab → see monoclonal antibodies
Pethidine → see opioids
Phenelzine → see monoamine-oxidase A and B inhibitors, irreversible
Phenindione → see TABLE 3 p. 818 (anticoagulant effects)

FOOD AND LIFESTYLE The effects of phenindione can be reduced or abolished by vitamin K, including that found in health foods, food supplements, enteral feeds, or large amounts of some green vegetables or green tea. Major changes in diet (especially involving salads and vegetables) and in alcohol consumption can affect anticoagulant control.

‣ Antiarrhythmics (propafenone) are predicted to increase the anticoagulant effect of **phenindione**. Monitor and adjust dose. [Moderate] Theoretical
‣ Antifungals, azoles (miconazole) greatly increase the anticoagulant effect of **phenindione**. [Severe] Theoretical
‣ Axitinib is predicted to increase the risk of bleeding events when given with **phenindione**. [Severe] Theoretical
‣ Bosutinib is predicted to increase the risk of bleeding events when given with **phenindione**. [Severe] Theoretical
‣ Cabozantinib is predicted to increase the risk of bleeding events when given with **phenindione**. [Severe] Theoretical
‣ Cephalosporins (ceftriaxone) potentially increase the risk of bleeding events when given with **phenindione**. [Severe] Anecdotal
‣ Corticosteroids are predicted to increase the effects of **phenindione**. [Moderate] Anecdotal
‣ Crizotinib is predicted to increase the risk of bleeding events when given with **phenindione**. [Severe] Theoretical
‣ Dasatinib is predicted to increase the risk of bleeding events when given with **phenindione**. [Severe] Theoretical
‣ Disulfiram is predicted to increase the anticoagulant effect of **phenindione**. [Severe] Theoretical
‣ Enteral feeds (vitamin-K containing) potentially decreases the effects of **phenindione**. [Severe] Theoretical

A1

Interactions | Appendix 1

Phenindione (continued)

▸ Erlotinib is predicted to increase the risk of bleeding events when given with **phenindione**. Severe Theoretical

▸ Fibrates are predicted to increase the anticoagulant effect of **phenindione**. Monitor INR and adjust dose. Severe Study

▸ Gefitinib is predicted to increase the risk of bleeding events when given with **phenindione**. Severe Theoretical

▸ H₂ receptor antagonists (cimetidine) increase the exposure to **phenindione**. Severe Anecdotal

▸ Imatinib is predicted to increase the risk of bleeding events when given with **phenindione**. Severe Theoretical

▸ Lapatinib is predicted to increase the risk of bleeding events when given with **phenindione**. Severe Theoretical

▸ Nandrolone is predicted to increase the anticoagulant effect of **phenindione**. Monitor and adjust dose. Severe Theoretical

▸ Nilotinib is predicted to increase the risk of bleeding events when given with **phenindione**. Severe Theoretical

▸ Oxymetholone increases the anticoagulant effect of **phenindione**. Severe Anecdotal

▸ Paracetamol is predicted to increase the anticoagulant effect of **phenindione**. Severe Theoretical

▸ Pazopanib is predicted to increase the risk of bleeding events when given with **phenindione**. Severe Theoretical

▸ Penicillins are predicted to increase the risk of bleeding events when given with **phenindione**. Severe Theoretical

▸ Ponatinib is predicted to increase the risk of bleeding events when given with **phenindione**. Severe Theoretical

▸ Ranibizumab is predicted to increase the risk of bleeding events when given with **phenindione**. Severe Theoretical

▸ Regorafenib is predicted to increase the risk of bleeding events when given with **phenindione**. Severe Theoretical

▸ Ruxolitinib is predicted to increase the risk of bleeding events when given with **phenindione**. Severe Theoretical

▸ Sorafenib is predicted to increase the risk of bleeding events when given with **phenindione**. Severe Theoretical

▸ Statins (rosuvastatin) are predicted to increase the anticoagulant effect of **phenindione**. Monitor INR and adjust dose. Severe Theoretical

▸ Sunitinib is predicted to increase the risk of bleeding events when given with **phenindione**. Severe Theoretical

▸ Vandetanib is predicted to increase the risk of bleeding events when given with **phenindione**. Severe Theoretical

Phenobarbital → see antiepileptics

Phenothiazines → see TABLE 8 p. 819 (hypotension), TABLE 9 p. 820 (QT-interval prolongation), TABLE 11 p. 820 (CNS depressant effects), TABLE 10 p. 820 (antimuscarinics)

chlorpromazine · fluphenazine · levomepromazine · pericyazine · perphenazine · prochlorperazine · promazine · trifluoperazine

FOOD AND LIFESTYLE Dose adjustment of **chlorpromazine** and **fluphenazine** might be necessary if smoking started or stopped during treatment.

▸ Amfetamines are predicted to decrease the effects of **chlorpromazine**. Moderate Study

▸ Phenothiazines are predicted to decrease the effects of amfetamines. Moderate Study

▸ Antacids decrease the absorption of **phenothiazines**. Moderate Anecdotal

▸ Chlorpromazine decreases the concentration of antiepileptics (phenobarbital, primidone) and antiepileptics (phenobarbital, primidone) decrease the concentration of **chlorpromazine**. Moderate Study → Also see TABLE 11 p. 820

▸ Chlorpromazine is predicted to increase the risk of hyponatraemia when given with desmopressin. Severe Theoretical

▸ Phenothiazines are predicted to decrease the effects of dopamine receptor agonists. Avoid. Moderate Study → Also see TABLE 8 p. 819 → Also see TABLE 9 p. 820 → Also see TABLE 10 p. 820

▸ Phenothiazines are predicted to decrease the antihypertensive effects of guanethidine. Moderate Theoretical → Also see TABLE 8 p. 819

▸ Phenothiazines are predicted to decrease the effects of histamine. Avoid. Severe Theoretical → Also see TABLE 8 p. 819

▸ Phenothiazines decrease the effects of levodopa. Avoid or monitor worsening parkinsonian symptoms. Severe Study → Also see TABLE 8 p. 819

▸ Phenothiazines potentially increase the risk of neurotoxicity when given with lithium. Severe Anecdotal → Also see TABLE 9 p. 820

▸ Chlorpromazine decreases the effects of metyrapone. Avoid. Moderate Theoretical

▸ Moclobemide increases the risk of side-effects when given with levomepromazine. Moderate Study

▸ Monoamine-oxidase A and B inhibitors, irreversible are predicted to increase the risk of neuroleptic malignant syndrome when given with **phenothiazines**. Severe Theoretical → Also see TABLE 8 p. 819

▸ Panobinostat is predicted to increase the exposure to **perphenazine**. Monitor and adjust dose. Severe Theoretical

▸ SSRIs (paroxetine) markedly increase the exposure to **perphenazine**. Severe Study

Phenoxymethylpenicillin → see penicillins

Phenylephrine → see sympathomimetics, vasoconstrictor

Phenytoin → see antiepileptics

Pholcodine

▸ Pholcodine is predicted to increase the risk of CNS excitation or depression when given with monoamine-oxidase A and B inhibitors, irreversible. Avoid and for 14 days after stopping the MAOI. Severe Theoretical

Phosphodiesterase type-5 inhibitors → see TABLE 8 p. 819 (hypotension), TABLE 9 p. 820 (QT-interval prolongation)

avanafil · sildenafil · tadalafil · vardenafil

▸ Alpha blockers cause significant hypotensive effects when given with **phosphodiesterase type-5 inhibitors**. Patient should be stabilised on first drug then second drug should be added at the lowest recommended dose. Severe Study → Also see TABLE 8 p. 819

▸ Antiarrhythmics (dronedarone) are predicted to increase the exposure to **avanafil**. Adjust avanafil dose. Moderate Theoretical

▸ Antiarrhythmics (dronedarone) are predicted to increase the exposure to **sildenafil**. Monitor and adjust sildenafil dose, p. 117. Moderate Study → Also see TABLE 9 p. 820

▸ Antiarrhythmics (dronedarone) are predicted to increase the exposure to **tadalafil**. Severe Theoretical

▸ Antiarrhythmics (dronedarone) are predicted to increase the exposure to **vardenafil**. Adjust dose. Severe Theoretical → Also see TABLE 9 p. 820

▸ Antiepileptics (carbamazepine, fosphenytoin, phenobarbital, phenytoin, primidone) are predicted to decrease the exposure to phosphodiesterase type-5 inhibitors (**avanafil, tadalafil**). Avoid. Severe Study

▸ Antiepileptics (carbamazepine, fosphenytoin, phenobarbital, phenytoin, primidone) are predicted to decrease the exposure to phosphodiesterase type-5 inhibitors (**sildenafil, vardenafil**). Moderate Theoretical

▸ Antifungals, azoles (fluconazole, isavuconazole, posaconazole) are predicted to increase the exposure to **avanafil**. Adjust avanafil dose. Moderate Theoretical

▸ Antifungals, azoles (fluconazole, isavuconazole, posaconazole) are predicted to increase the exposure to **sildenafil**. Monitor and adjust sildenafil dose, p. 117. Moderate Study

▸ Antifungals, azoles (fluconazole, isavuconazole, posaconazole) are predicted to increase the exposure to **tadalafil**. Severe Theoretical

▸ Antifungals, azoles (fluconazole, isavuconazole, posaconazole) are predicted to increase the exposure to **vardenafil**. Adjust dose. Severe Theoretical

▸ Antifungals, azoles (itraconazole, ketoconazole, voriconazole) are predicted to increase the exposure to **sildenafil**. Avoid or adjust sildenafil dose, p. 117. Severe Study → Also see TABLE 9 p. 820

▸ Antifungals, azoles (itraconazole, ketoconazole, voriconazole) are predicted to increase the exposure to **tadalafil**. Use with caution or avoid. Severe Study

▸ Antifungals, azoles (miconazole) are predicted to increase the exposure to **sildenafil**. Use with caution and adjust dose. Severe Theoretical

▸ Antifungals, azoles (itraconazole, ketoconazole, voriconazole) are predicted to increase the exposure to phosphodiesterase type-5 inhibitors **(avanafil, vardenafil)**. Avoid. ⟨Severe⟩ Study → Also see TABLE 9 p. 820

▸ **Aprepitant** is predicted to increase the exposure to **avanafil**. Adjust **avanafil** dose. ⟨Moderate⟩ Theoretical

▸ **Aprepitant** is predicted to increase the exposure to **sildenafil**. Monitor and adjust **sildenafil** dose, p. 117. ⟨Moderate⟩ Study

▸ **Aprepitant** is predicted to increase the exposure to **tadalafil**. ⟨Severe⟩ Theoretical

▸ **Aprepitant** is predicted to increase the exposure to **vardenafil**. Adjust dose. ⟨Severe⟩ Theoretical

▸ **Bosentan** decreases the exposure to **phosphodiesterase type-5 inhibitors**. ⟨Moderate⟩ Study

▸ **Calcium channel blockers (diltiazem, verapamil)** are predicted to increase the exposure to **avanafil**. Adjust **avanafil** dose. ⟨Moderate⟩ Theoretical → Also see TABLE 8 p. 819

▸ **Calcium channel blockers (diltiazem, verapamil)** are predicted to increase the exposure to **sildenafil**. Monitor and adjust **sildenafil** dose, p. 117. ⟨Moderate⟩ Study → Also see TABLE 8 p. 819

▸ **Calcium channel blockers (diltiazem, verapamil)** are predicted to increase the exposure to **tadalafil**. ⟨Severe⟩ Theoretical → Also see TABLE 8 p. 819

▸ **Calcium channel blockers (diltiazem, verapamil)** are predicted to increase the exposure to **vardenafil**. Adjust dose. ⟨Severe⟩ Theoretical → Also see TABLE 8 p. 819

▸ **Cobicistat** is predicted to increase the exposure to **phosphodiesterase type-5 inhibitors (avanafil, vardenafil)**. Avoid. ⟨Severe⟩ Study

▸ **Cobicistat** is predicted to increase the exposure to **sildenafil**. Avoid or adjust **sildenafil** dose, p. 117. ⟨Severe⟩ Study

▸ **Cobicistat** is predicted to increase the exposure to **tadalafil**. Use with caution or avoid. ⟨Severe⟩ Study

▸ **Crizotinib** is predicted to increase the exposure to **avanafil**. Adjust **avanafil** dose. ⟨Moderate⟩ Theoretical

▸ **Crizotinib** is predicted to increase the exposure to **sildenafil**. Monitor and adjust **sildenafil** dose, p. 117. ⟨Moderate⟩ Study → Also see TABLE 9 p. 820

▸ **Crizotinib** is predicted to increase the exposure to **tadalafil**. ⟨Severe⟩ Theoretical

▸ **Crizotinib** is predicted to increase the exposure to **vardenafil**. Adjust dose. ⟨Severe⟩ Theoretical → Also see TABLE 9 p. 820

▸ **Efavirenz** is predicted to decrease the exposure to **phosphodiesterase type-5 inhibitors**. ⟨Moderate⟩ Theoretical

▸ **Enzalutamide** is predicted to decrease the exposure to **phosphodiesterase type-5 inhibitors (avanafil, tadalafil)**. Avoid. ⟨Severe⟩ Study

▸ **Enzalutamide** is predicted to decrease the exposure to **phosphodiesterase type-5 inhibitors (sildenafil, vardenafil)**. ⟨Moderate⟩ Theoretical

▸ **Etravirine** moderately decreases the exposure to **phosphodiesterase type-5 inhibitors**. Adjust dose. ⟨Moderate⟩ Study

▸ **Grapefruit juice** is predicted to increase the exposure to **phosphodiesterase type-5 inhibitors**. Use with caution or avoid. ⟨Moderate⟩ Study

▸ **HIV-protease inhibitors (atazanavir, darunavir, fosamprenavir, lopinavir, ritonavir, saquinavir, tipranavir)** are predicted to increase the exposure to phosphodiesterase type-5 inhibitors **(avanafil, vardenafil)**. Avoid. ⟨Severe⟩ Study → Also see TABLE 9 p. 820

▸ **HIV-protease inhibitors (atazanavir, darunavir, fosamprenavir, lopinavir, ritonavir, saquinavir, tipranavir)** are predicted to increase the exposure to **sildenafil**. Avoid or adjust **sildenafil** dose, p. 117. ⟨Severe⟩ Study → Also see TABLE 9 p. 820

▸ **HIV-protease inhibitors (atazanavir, darunavir, fosamprenavir, lopinavir, ritonavir, saquinavir, tipranavir)** are predicted to increase the exposure to **tadalafil**. Use with caution or avoid. ⟨Severe⟩ Study

▸ **HIV-protease inhibitors (indinavir)** are predicted to increase the exposure to **avanafil**. Adjust **avanafil** dose. ⟨Moderate⟩ Theoretical

▸ **HIV-protease inhibitors (indinavir)** are predicted to increase the exposure to **sildenafil**. Monitor and adjust **sildenafil** dose, p. 117. ⟨Moderate⟩ Study

▸ **HIV-protease inhibitors (indinavir)** are predicted to increase the exposure to **tadalafil**. ⟨Severe⟩ Theoretical

▸ **HIV-protease inhibitors (indinavir)** are predicted to increase the exposure to **vardenafil**. Adjust dose. ⟨Severe⟩ Theoretical

▸ **Idelalisib** is predicted to increase the exposure to phosphodiesterase type-5 inhibitors **(avanafil, vardenafil)**. Avoid. ⟨Severe⟩ Study

▸ **Idelalisib** is predicted to increase the exposure to **sildenafil**. Avoid or adjust **sildenafil** dose, p. 117. ⟨Severe⟩ Study

▸ **Idelalisib** is predicted to increase the exposure to **tadalafil**. Use with caution or avoid. ⟨Severe⟩ Study

▸ **Imatinib** is predicted to increase the exposure to **avanafil**. Adjust **avanafil** dose. ⟨Moderate⟩ Theoretical

▸ **Imatinib** is predicted to increase the exposure to **sildenafil**. Monitor and adjust **sildenafil** dose, p. 117. ⟨Moderate⟩ Study

▸ **Imatinib** is predicted to increase the exposure to **tadalafil**. ⟨Severe⟩ Theoretical

▸ **Imatinib** is predicted to increase the exposure to **vardenafil**. Adjust dose. ⟨Severe⟩ Theoretical

▸ **Macrolides (clarithromycin)** are predicted to increase the exposure to **sildenafil**. Avoid or adjust **sildenafil** dose, p. 117. ⟨Severe⟩ Study → Also see TABLE 9 p. 820

▸ **Macrolides (clarithromycin)** are predicted to increase the exposure to **tadalafil**. Use with caution or avoid. ⟨Severe⟩ Study

▸ **Macrolides (erythromycin)** are predicted to increase the exposure to **avanafil**. Adjust **avanafil** dose. ⟨Moderate⟩ Theoretical

▸ **Macrolides (erythromycin)** are predicted to increase the exposure to **sildenafil**. Monitor and adjust **sildenafil** dose, p. 117. ⟨Moderate⟩ Study

▸ **Macrolides (erythromycin)** are predicted to increase the exposure to **tadalafil**. ⟨Severe⟩ Theoretical

▸ **Macrolides (erythromycin)** are predicted to increase the exposure to **vardenafil**. Adjust dose. ⟨Severe⟩ Theoretical

▸ **Macrolides (clarithromycin)** are predicted to increase the exposure to phosphodiesterase type-5 inhibitors **(avanafil, vardenafil)**. Avoid. ⟨Severe⟩ Study → Also see TABLE 9 p. 820

▸ **Netupitant** is predicted to increase the exposure to **avanafil**. Adjust **avanafil** dose. ⟨Moderate⟩ Theoretical

▸ **Netupitant** is predicted to increase the exposure to **sildenafil**. Monitor and adjust **sildenafil** dose, p. 117. ⟨Moderate⟩ Study

▸ **Netupitant** is predicted to increase the exposure to **tadalafil**. ⟨Severe⟩ Theoretical

▸ **Netupitant** is predicted to increase the exposure to **vardenafil**. Adjust dose. ⟨Severe⟩ Theoretical

▸ **Nevirapine** is predicted to decrease the exposure to **phosphodiesterase type-5 inhibitors**. ⟨Moderate⟩ Theoretical

▸ **Nicorandil** is predicted to increase the risk of hypotension when given with **phosphodiesterase type-5 inhibitors**. Avoid. ⟨Severe⟩ Theoretical → Also see TABLE 8 p. 819

▸ **Nilotinib** is predicted to increase the exposure to **avanafil**. Adjust **avanafil** dose. ⟨Moderate⟩ Theoretical

▸ **Nilotinib** is predicted to increase the exposure to **sildenafil**. Monitor and adjust **sildenafil** dose, p. 117. ⟨Moderate⟩ Study → Also see TABLE 9 p. 820

▸ **Nilotinib** is predicted to increase the exposure to **tadalafil**. ⟨Severe⟩ Theoretical

▸ **Nilotinib** is predicted to increase the exposure to **vardenafil**. Adjust dose. ⟨Severe⟩ Theoretical → Also see TABLE 9 p. 820

▸ **Nitrates** potentially increase the risk of hypotension when given with **phosphodiesterase type-5 inhibitors**. Avoid. ⟨Severe⟩ Study → Also see TABLE 8 p. 819

▸ **Rifampicin** is predicted to decrease the exposure to phosphodiesterase type-5 inhibitors **(avanafil, tadalafil)**. Avoid. ⟨Severe⟩ Study

▸ **Rifampicin** is predicted to decrease the exposure to phosphodiesterase type-5 inhibitors **(sildenafil, vardenafil)**. ⟨Moderate⟩ Theoretical

▸ **Riociguat** is predicted to increase the risk of hypotension when given with **phosphodiesterase type-5 inhibitors**. Avoid. ⟨Severe⟩ Theoretical → Also see TABLE 8 p. 819

▸ **Phosphodiesterase type-5 inhibitors** are predicted to increase the risk of hypotension when given with **sapropterin**. ⟨Moderate⟩ Theoretical → Also see TABLE 8 p. 819

▸ **St John's Wort** is predicted to decrease the exposure to **phosphodiesterase type-5 inhibitors**. ⟨Moderate⟩ Theoretical

Interactions | Appendix 1

A1

Pilocarpine

ROUTE-SPECIFIC INFORMATION Since systemic absorption can follow topical application, the possibility of interactions should be borne in mind.

Pimecrolimus

FOOD AND LIFESTYLE Risk of facial flushing and skin irritation with alcohol consumption.

‣ **Pimecrolimus** is predicted to decrease the efficacy of mifamurtide. Avoid. Severe Theoretical

Pimozide → see TABLE 8 p. 819 (hypotension), TABLE 9 p. 820 (QT-interval prolongation), TABLE 11 p. 820 (CNS depressant effects), TABLE 10 p. 820 (antimuscarinics)

‣ Antiarrhythmics **(dronedarone)** are predicted to increase the exposure to **pimozide**. Avoid. Severe Theoretical → Also see TABLE 9 p. 820

‣ Antifungals, azoles **(fluconazole, isavuconazole, posaconazole)** are predicted to increase the exposure to **pimozide**. Avoid. Severe Theoretical

‣ Antifungals, azoles **(itraconazole, ketoconazole, voriconazole)** are predicted to increase the exposure to **pimozide**. Avoid. Severe Study → Also see TABLE 9 p. 820

‣ Antifungals, azoles **(miconazole)** are predicted to increase the exposure to **pimozide**. Avoid. Moderate Theoretical

‣ **Aprepitant** is predicted to increase the exposure to **pimozide**. Avoid. Severe Theoretical

‣ Calcium channel blockers **(diltiazem, verapamil)** are predicted to increase the exposure to **pimozide**. Avoid. Severe Theoretical → Also see TABLE 8 p. 819

‣ **Ceritinib** is predicted to increase the exposure to **pimozide**. Avoid. Severe Theoretical → Also see TABLE 9 p. 820

‣ **Cobicistat** is predicted to increase the exposure to **pimozide**. Avoid. Severe Study

‣ **Crizotinib** is predicted to increase the exposure to **pimozide**. Avoid. Severe Theoretical → Also see TABLE 9 p. 820

‣ **Pimozide** is predicted to decrease the effects of dopamine receptor agonists. Avoid. Moderate Theoretical → Also see TABLE 8 p. 819 → Also see TABLE 9 p. 820 → Also see TABLE 10 p. 820

‣ **Fosaprepitant** is predicted to increase the exposure to **pimozide**. Avoid. Severe Theoretical

‣ **Grapefruit juice** increases the exposure to **pimozide**. Avoid. Severe Theoretical

‣ HIV-protease inhibitors **(atazanavir, darunavir, fosamprenavir, lopinavir, ritonavir, saquinavir, tipranavir)** are predicted to increase the exposure to **pimozide**. Avoid. Severe Study → Also see TABLE 9 p. 820

‣ HIV-protease inhibitors **(indinavir)** are predicted to increase the exposure to **pimozide**. Avoid. Severe Theoretical

‣ **Idelalisib** is predicted to increase the exposure to **pimozide**. Avoid. Severe Study

‣ **Imatinib** is predicted to increase the exposure to **pimozide**. Avoid. Severe Theoretical

‣ **Pimozide** decreases the effects of levodopa. Severe Theoretical → Also see TABLE 8 p. 819

‣ Macrolides **(clarithromycin)** are predicted to increase the exposure to **pimozide**. Avoid. Severe Study → Also see TABLE 9 p. 820

‣ Macrolides **(erythromycin)** are predicted to increase the exposure to **pimozide**. Avoid. Severe Theoretical

‣ **Netupitant** is predicted to increase the exposure to **pimozide**. Avoid. Severe Theoretical

‣ **Nilotinib** is predicted to increase the exposure to **pimozide**. Avoid. Severe Theoretical → Also see TABLE 9 p. 820

‣ **Palbociclib** is predicted to increase the exposure to **pimozide**. Adjust dose. Moderate Theoretical

‣ **Panobinostat** is predicted to increase the exposure to **pimozide**. Avoid. Severe Theoretical → Also see TABLE 9 p. 820

‣ **Pitolisant** is predicted to decrease the exposure to **pimozide**. Avoid. Severe Theoretical

Pindolol → see beta blockers, non-selective

Pioglitazone → see TABLE 14 p. 821 (antidiabetic drugs)

‣ **Clopidogrel** is predicted to increase the exposure to pioglitazone. Severe Theoretical

‣ Fibrates **(gemfibrozil)** markedly increase the exposure to pioglitazone. Monitor blood glucose and adjust dose. Severe Study

‣ **Rifampicin** moderately decreases the exposure to **pioglitazone**. Monitor and adjust **pioglitazone** dose. Moderate Study

‣ **St John's Wort** slightly decreases the exposure to **pioglitazone**. Mild Study

Piperacillin → see penicillins

Piperaquine → see antimalarials

Pirfenidone

FOOD AND LIFESTYLE Smoking increases pirfenidone clearance; patients should be encouraged to stop smoking before and during treatment with pirfenidone.

‣ Antiepileptics **(fosphenytoin, phenytoin)** are predicted to decrease the exposure to **pirfenidone**. Avoid. Moderate Theoretical

‣ **Combined hormonal contraceptives** are predicted to increase the exposure to **pirfenidone**. Use with caution and adjust dose. Moderate Study

‣ HIV-protease inhibitors **(ritonavir)** are predicted to decrease the exposure to **pirfenidone**. Avoid. Moderate Theoretical

‣ Quinolones **(ciprofloxacin)** are predicted to increase the exposure to **pirfenidone**. Use with caution and adjust dose. Moderate Study

‣ **Rifampicin** is predicted to decrease the exposure to pirfenidone. Moderate Theoretical

‣ SSRIs **(fluvoxamine)** are predicted to moderately increase the exposure to **pirfenidone**. Avoid. Moderate Study

Piroxicam → see NSAIDs

Pitolisant

‣ **Abiraterone** is predicted to increase the exposure to **pitolisant**. Use with caution and adjust dose. Moderate Study

‣ Antiarrhythmics **(propafenone)** are predicted to increase the exposure to **pitolisant**. Use with caution and adjust dose. Moderate Study

‣ Antiepileptics **(carbamazepine, fosphenytoin, phenobarbital, phenytoin, primidone)** are predicted to moderately decrease the exposure to **pitolisant**. Moderate Study

‣ Antihistamines, sedating are predicted to decrease the efficacy of **pitolisant**. Unknown Theoretical

‣ **Pitolisant** is predicted to decrease the exposure to bosutinib. Avoid. Severe Theoretical

‣ **Bupropion** is predicted to moderately increase the exposure to **pitolisant**. Use with caution and adjust dose. Moderate Study

‣ **Pitolisant** is predicted to decrease the exposure to ciclosporin. Avoid. Severe Theoretical

‣ **Cinacalcet** is predicted to moderately increase the exposure to **pitolisant**. Use with caution and adjust dose. Moderate Study

‣ **Pitolisant** is predicted to decrease the efficacy of combined hormonal contraceptives. Avoid. Severe Theoretical

‣ **Pitolisant** is predicted to decrease the exposure to coumarins **(warfarin)**. Unknown Theoretical

‣ **Pitolisant** is predicted to decrease the exposure to crizotinib. Avoid. Severe Theoretical

‣ **Pitolisant** is predicted to decrease the exposure to dabigatran. Unknown Theoretical

‣ **Pitolisant** is predicted to decrease the exposure to dasatinib. Avoid. Severe Theoretical

‣ **Pitolisant** is predicted to decrease the exposure to digoxin. Unknown Theoretical

‣ **Duloxetine** is predicted to increase the exposure to **pitolisant**. Use with caution and adjust dose. Moderate Study

‣ **Pitolisant** is predicted to decrease the exposure to efavirenz. Unknown Theoretical

‣ **Enzalutamide** is predicted to moderately decrease the exposure to **pitolisant**. Moderate Study

‣ **Pitolisant** is predicted to decrease the exposure to everolimus. Avoid. Severe Theoretical

‣ HIV-protease inhibitors **(ritonavir)** are predicted to increase the exposure to **pitolisant**. Use with caution and adjust dose. Moderate Study

‣ **Pitolisant** is predicted to decrease the exposure to irinotecan. Unknown Theoretical

‣ **Pitolisant** is predicted to increase the exposure to metformin. Unknown Theoretical

- Mianserin is predicted to decrease the efficacy of **pitolisant**. Unknown Theoretical
- Mirabegron is predicted to increase the exposure to **pitolisant**. Use with caution and adjust dose. Moderate Study
- Mirtazapine is predicted to decrease the efficacy of **pitolisant**. Unknown Theoretical
- **Pitolisant** is predicted to decrease the exposure to opioids (morphine). Unknown Theoretical
- **Pitolisant** is predicted to decrease the exposure to paracetamol. Unknown Theoretical
- **Pitolisant** is predicted to decrease the exposure to pimozide. Avoid. Severe Theoretical
- **Pitolisant** is predicted to decrease the exposure to repaglinide. Unknown Theoretical
- Rifampicin is predicted to moderately decrease the exposure to **pitolisant**. Moderate Study
- **Pitolisant** is predicted to decrease the exposure to sirolimus. Avoid. Severe Theoretical
- SSRIs (fluoxetine, paroxetine) are predicted to moderately increase the exposure to **pitolisant**. Use with caution and adjust dose. Moderate Study
- St John's Wort is predicted to decrease the exposure to **pitolisant**. Monitor and adjust dose. Moderate Theoretical
- **Pitolisant** is predicted to decrease the exposure to tacrolimus. Avoid. Severe Theoretical
- **Pitolisant** is predicted to decrease the exposure to taxanes (docetaxel). Avoid. Severe Theoretical
- **Pitolisant** is predicted to decrease the exposure to temsirolimus. Avoid. Severe Theoretical
- Terbinafine is predicted to moderately increase the exposure to **pitolisant**. Use with caution and adjust dose. Moderate Study
- Tricyclic antidepressants are predicted to decrease the efficacy of **pitolisant**. Mild Theoretical

Pivmecillinam → see penicillins
Pixantrone → see anthracyclines
Pizotifen → see antihistamines, sedating
Platinum compounds → see TABLE 15 p. 821 (myelosuppression), TABLE 2 p. 818 (nephrotoxicity), TABLE 19 p. 822 (ototoxicity), TABLE 12 p. 821 (peripheral neuropathy)

carboplatin · cisplatin · oxaliplatin

- Cisplatin increases the risk of pulmonary toxicity when given with bleomycin. Severe Study → Also see TABLE 15 p. 821
- Live vaccines are predicted to increase the risk of generalised infection (possibly life-threatening) when given with **platinum compounds**. Public Health England advises avoid. Severe Theoretical

Polymyxins → see TABLE 2 p. 818 (nephrotoxicity), TABLE 20 p. 822 (neuromuscular blocking effects)
Polysaccharide-iron complex → see iron (oral)
Polystyrene sulfonate

- Antacids increase the risk of metabolic alkalosis when given with polystyrene sulfonate. Severe Anecdotal
- **Polystyrene sulfonate** is predicted to decrease the absorption of levothyroxine. Separate administration by at least 4 hours. Moderate Theoretical

Pomalidomide → see TABLE 15 p. 821 (myelosuppression), TABLE 5 p. 818 (thromboembolism)

- Combined hormonal contraceptives are predicted to increase the risk of venous thromboembolism when given with **pomalidomide**. Avoid. Severe Theoretical
- Hormone replacement therapy is predicted to increase the risk of venous thromboembolism when given with **pomalidomide**. Severe Theoretical
- Quinolones (ciprofloxacin) are predicted to increase the exposure to **pomalidomide**. Adjust **pomalidomide** dose. Moderate Theoretical
- SSRIs (fluvoxamine) moderately increase the exposure to **pomalidomide**. Adjust **pomalidomide** dose. Moderate Study

Ponatinib

- Antiepileptics (carbamazepine, fosphenytoin, phenobarbital, phenytoin, primidone) are predicted to decrease the exposure to **ponatinib**. Avoid. Moderate Theoretical
- Antifungals, azoles (itraconazole, ketoconazole, voriconazole) are predicted to slightly increase the exposure to **ponatinib**. Monitor and adjust **ponatinib** dose. Moderate Study

- Cobicistat is predicted to slightly increase the exposure to **ponatinib**. Monitor and adjust **ponatinib** dose. Moderate Study
- **Ponatinib** is predicted to increase the risk of bleeding events when given with coumarins. Severe Theoretical
- Enzalutamide is predicted to decrease the exposure to **ponatinib**. Avoid. Moderate Theoretical
- Grapefruit juice is predicted to increase the exposure to **ponatinib**. Moderate Theoretical
- HIV-protease inhibitors (atazanavir, darunavir, fosamprenavir, lopinavir, ritonavir, saquinavir, tipranavir) are predicted to slightly increase the exposure to **ponatinib**. Monitor and adjust **ponatinib** dose. Moderate Study
- Idelalisib is predicted to slightly increase the exposure to **ponatinib**. Monitor and adjust **ponatinib** dose. Moderate Study
- Macrolides (clarithromycin) are predicted to slightly increase the exposure to **ponatinib**. Monitor and adjust **ponatinib** dose. Moderate Study
- **Ponatinib** is predicted to increase the risk of bleeding events when given with phenindione. Severe Theoretical
- Rifampicin is predicted to decrease the exposure to **ponatinib**. Avoid. Moderate Theoretical
- St John's Wort is predicted to decrease the exposure to **ponatinib**. Avoid. Severe Theoretical

Posaconazole → see antifungals, azoles
Potassium canrenoate → see TABLE 16 p. 822 (increased serum potassium)
Potassium chloride → see TABLE 16 p. 822 (increased serum potassium)
Potassium citrate

- **Potassium citrate** is predicted to decrease the efficacy of methenamine. Avoid. Moderate Theoretical
- Potassium citrate increases the risk of side-effects when given with sucralfate. Avoid. Moderate Theoretical

Potassium-sparing diuretics → see TABLE 18 p. 822 (hyponatraemia), TABLE 16 p. 822 (increased serum potassium)

amiloride · triamterene

- Triamterene potentially increases the clearance of lithium. Moderate Study

Pramipexole → see dopamine receptor agonists
Prasugrel → see TABLE 4 p. 818 (antiplatelet effects)
Pravastatin → see statins
Praziquantel

- Antiepileptics (carbamazepine, fosphenytoin, phenobarbital, phenytoin, primidone) are predicted to markedly decrease the exposure to **praziquantel**. Avoid. Moderate Study
- Antifungals, azoles (itraconazole, ketoconazole, voriconazole) are predicted to moderately increase the exposure to **praziquantel**. Mild Study
- Antimalarials (chloroquine) moderately decrease the exposure to **praziquantel**. Use with caution and adjust dose. Moderate Study
- Cobicistat is predicted to moderately increase the exposure to **praziquantel**. Mild Study
- Corticosteroids (dexamethasone) decrease the exposure to **praziquantel**. Moderate Study
- Enzalutamide is predicted to markedly decrease the exposure to **praziquantel**. Avoid. Moderate Study
- Grapefruit juice is predicted to increase the exposure to **praziquantel**. Moderate Study
- H$_2$ receptor antagonists (cimetidine) moderately increase the exposure to **praziquantel**. Moderate Study
- HIV-protease inhibitors (atazanavir, darunavir, fosamprenavir, lopinavir, ritonavir, saquinavir, tipranavir) are predicted to moderately increase the exposure to **praziquantel**. Mild Study
- Idelalisib is predicted to moderately increase the exposure to **praziquantel**. Mild Study
- Macrolides (clarithromycin) are predicted to moderately increase the exposure to **praziquantel**. Mild Study
- Rifampicin is predicted to markedly decrease the exposure to **praziquantel**. Avoid. Moderate Study

Prazosin → see alpha blockers
Prednisolone → see corticosteroids
Prednisone → see corticosteroids
Pregabalin → see antiepileptics
Prilocaine → see anaesthetics, local
Primaquine → see antimalarials

Primidone → see antiepileptics

Procarbazine → see TABLE 15 p. 821 (myelosuppression), TABLE 13 p. 821 (serotonin syndrome)

FOOD AND LIFESTYLE Procarbazine is a mild monoamine-oxidase inhibitor and might rarely interact with tyramine-rich foods (such as mature cheese, salami, pickled herring, Bovril®, Oxo®, Marmite® or any similar meat or yeast extract or fermented soya bean extract, and some beers, lagers or wines). Alcohol consumption can cause a disulfiram-like reaction.

▸ Antiepileptics **(carbamazepine, fosphenytoin, phenobarbital, phenytoin, primidone)** potentially increase the risk of hypersensitivity reactions when given with **procarbazine**. Severe Anecdotal

▸ Live vaccines are predicted to increase the risk of generalised infection (possibly life-threatening) when given with **procarbazine**. Public Health England advises avoid. Severe Theoretical

Prochlorperazine → see phenothiazines

Procyclidine → see TABLE 10 p. 820 (antimuscarinics)

▸ SSRIs **(paroxetine)** slightly increase the exposure to **procyclidine**. Monitor and adjust **procyclidine** dose. Moderate Study

Proguanil → see antimalarials

Promazine → see phenothiazines

Promethazine → see antihistamines, sedating

Propafenone → see antiarrhythmics

Propantheline → see TABLE 10 p. 820 (antimuscarinics)

Propiverine → see TABLE 10 p. 820 (antimuscarinics)

▸ **Propiverine** is predicted to increase the exposure to **lomitapide**. Separate administration by 12 hours. Moderate Theoretical

Propofol → see TABLE 8 p. 819 (hypotension), TABLE 11 p. 820 (CNS depressant effects)

Propranolol → see beta blockers, non-selective

Propylthiouracil → see TABLE 15 p. 821 (myelosuppression)

▸ **Propylthiouracil** is predicted to decrease the effects of **metyrapone**. Avoid. Moderate Theoretical

Protamine zinc insulin → see insulins

Proton pump inhibitors

esomeprazole · lansoprazole · omeprazole · pantoprazole · rabeprazole

▸ Antifungals, azoles **(fluconazole)** are predicted to increase the exposure to **proton pump inhibitors**. Mild Study

▸ Antifungals, azoles **(voriconazole)** increase the exposure to proton pump inhibitors **(esomeprazole, omeprazole)**. Adjust dose. Moderate Study

▸ **Proton pump inhibitors** decrease the absorption of antifungals, azoles **(itraconazole)**. Administer **itraconazole** capsules with an acidic beverage. Moderate Study

▸ **Proton pump inhibitors** decrease the absorption of antifungals, azoles **(ketoconazole)**. Administer **ketoconazole** with an acidic beverage. Moderate Study

▸ **Proton pump inhibitors** decrease the absorption of antifungals, azoles **(posaconazole)** (oral suspension). Avoid. Moderate Study

▸ **Proton pump inhibitors** are predicted to decrease the absorption of **bosutinib**. Moderate Study

▸ **Proton pump inhibitors** are predicted to decrease the absorption of **ceritinib**. Moderate Theoretical

▸ **Esomeprazole** is predicted to increase the exposure to **cilostazol**. Moderate Theoretical

▸ **Omeprazole** is predicted to increase the exposure to **cilostazol**. Adjust **cilostazol** dose. Moderate Study

▸ Proton pump inhibitors **(esomeprazole, omeprazole)** are predicted to decrease the efficacy of **clopidogrel**. Avoid. Moderate Study

▸ **Proton pump inhibitors** are predicted to decrease the exposure to **dabrafenib**. Avoid. Severe Theoretical

▸ **Proton pump inhibitors** are predicted to slightly to moderately decrease the exposure to **dasatinib**. Avoid. Severe Study

▸ **Proton pump inhibitors** are predicted to decrease the absorption of **dipyridamole** (immediate release tablets). Moderate Theoretical

▸ **Enzalutamide** is predicted to moderately decrease the exposure to **omeprazole**. Moderate Study

▸ **Proton pump inhibitors** are predicted to slightly decrease the exposure to **erlotinib**. Avoid. Moderate Study

▸ **Proton pump inhibitors** are predicted to decrease the exposure to **gefitinib**. Severe Theoretical

▸ **Proton pump inhibitors** decrease the exposure to HIV-protease inhibitors **(atazanavir)**. Avoid or adjust dose. Severe Study

▸ **Proton pump inhibitors** increase the exposure to HIV-protease inhibitors **(saquinavir)**. Avoid. Severe Study

▸ HIV-protease inhibitors **(tipranavir)** decrease the exposure to **proton pump inhibitors**. Avoid. Severe Study

▸ **Proton pump inhibitors** are predicted to decrease the exposure to **ledipasvir**. Adjust dose, see sofosbuvir with ledipasvir. Moderate Theoretical

▸ **Lumacaftor** is predicted to decrease the exposure to proton pump inhibitors **(esomeprazole, lansoprazole, omeprazole)**. Adjust dose. Moderate Theoretical

▸ **Proton pump inhibitors** decrease the clearance of **methotrexate**. Use with caution or avoid. Severe Study

▸ **Proton pump inhibitors** are predicted to decrease the exposure to **pazopanib**. Avoid or administer concurrently without food. Moderate Study

▸ **Rifampicin** is predicted to moderately decrease the exposure to **omeprazole**. Moderate Study

▸ **Proton pump inhibitors** are predicted to decrease the exposure to **rilpivirine**. Severe Study

▸ **Proton pump inhibitors** potentially decrease the exposure to **sofosbuvir**. Adjust dose, see sofosbuvir with ledipasvir and sofosbuvir with velpatasvir. Moderate Study

▸ SSRIs **(fluvoxamine)** are predicted to increase the exposure to **proton pump inhibitors**. Mild Study

▸ **Esomeprazole** is predicted to slightly to moderately increase the exposure to SSRIs **(citalopram, escitalopram)**. Monitor and adjust dose. Severe Theoretical

▸ **Omeprazole** slightly to moderately increases the exposure to SSRIs **(citalopram, escitalopram)**. Monitor and adjust dose. Severe Study

▸ **Proton pump inhibitors** are predicted to decrease the concentration of **velpatasvir**. Adjust dose, see sofosbuvir with velpatasvir. Moderate Study

Proxymetacaine → see anaesthetics, local

Pseudoephedrine → see sympathomimetics, vasoconstrictor

Pyrazinamide

▸ **Allopurinol** is predicted to increase the risk of hyperuricaemia when given with **pyrazinamide**. Moderate Theoretical

▸ **Pyrazinamide** is predicted to decrease the effects of **sulfinpyrazone**. Moderate Theoretical

Pyridostigmine → see TABLE 6 p. 819 (bradycardia), TABLE 20 p. 822 (neuromuscular blocking effects)

▸ **Aminoglycosides** are predicted to decrease the effects of **pyridostigmine**. Moderate Theoretical → Also see TABLE 20 p. 822

Pyrimethamine → see antimalarials

Quetiapine → see TABLE 8 p. 819 (hypotension), TABLE 11 p. 820 (CNS depressant effects)

▸ Antiarrhythmics **(dronedarone)** are predicted to increase the exposure to **quetiapine**. Avoid. Moderate Study

▸ Antiepileptics **(carbamazepine, fosphenytoin, phenobarbital, phenytoin, primidone)** are predicted to decrease the exposure to **quetiapine**. Moderate Study → Also see TABLE 11 p. 820

▸ Antifungals, azoles **(fluconazole, isavuconazole, posaconazole)** are predicted to increase the exposure to **quetiapine**. Avoid. Moderate Study

▸ Antifungals, azoles **(itraconazole, ketoconazole, voriconazole)** are predicted to increase the exposure to **quetiapine**. Avoid. Severe Study

▸ **Aprepitant** is predicted to increase the exposure to **quetiapine**. Avoid. Moderate Study

▸ Calcium channel blockers **(diltiazem, verapamil)** are predicted to increase the exposure to **quetiapine**. Avoid. Moderate Study → Also see TABLE 8 p. 819

▸ **Cobicistat** is predicted to increase the exposure to **quetiapine**. Avoid. Severe Study

▸ **Crizotinib** is predicted to increase the exposure to **quetiapine**. Avoid. Moderate Study

- **Quetiapine** is predicted to decrease the effects of **dopamine receptor agonists**. Avoid. Moderate Theoretical → Also see **TABLE 8** p. 819
- **Enzalutamide** is predicted to decrease the exposure to **quetiapine**. Moderate Study
- **Grapefruit juice** is predicted to increase the exposure to **quetiapine**. Avoid. Severe Theoretical
- **Quetiapine** is predicted to decrease the effects of **histamine**. Avoid. Severe Theoretical → Also see **TABLE 8** p. 819
- **HIV-protease inhibitors (atazanavir, darunavir, fosamprenavir, lopinavir, ritonavir, saquinavir, tipranavir)** are predicted to increase the exposure to **quetiapine**. Avoid. Severe Study
- **HIV-protease inhibitors (indinavir)** are predicted to increase the exposure to **quetiapine**. Avoid. Moderate Study
- **Idelalisib** is predicted to increase the exposure to **quetiapine**. Avoid. Severe Study
- **Imatinib** is predicted to increase the exposure to **quetiapine**. Avoid. Moderate Study
- **Quetiapine** decreases the effects of **levodopa**. Severe Anecdotal → Also see **TABLE 8** p. 819
- **Quetiapine** potentially increases the risk of neurotoxicity when given with **lithium**. Severe Anecdotal
- **Macrolides (clarithromycin)** are predicted to increase the exposure to **quetiapine**. Avoid. Severe Study
- **Macrolides (erythromycin)** are predicted to increase the exposure to **quetiapine**. Avoid. Moderate Study
- **Netupitant** is predicted to increase the exposure to **quetiapine**. Avoid. Moderate Study
- **Nilotinib** is predicted to increase the exposure to **quetiapine**. Avoid. Moderate Study
- **Rifampicin** is predicted to decrease the exposure to **quetiapine**. Moderate Study

Quinagolide → see dopamine receptor agonists
Quinapril → see ACE inhibitors
Quinine → see antimalarials
Quinolones → see **TABLE 9** p. 820 (QT-interval prolongation)

ciprofloxacin · levofloxacin · moxifloxacin · nalidixic acid · norfloxacin · ofloxacin

ROUTE-SPECIFIC INFORMATION Since systemic absorption can follow topical application, the possibility of interactions should be borne in mind.

- **Ciprofloxacin** is predicted to increase the exposure to **agomelatine**. Moderate Study
- **Quinolones (ciprofloxacin, norfloxacin)** are predicted to increase the exposure to **aminophylline**. Adjust dose. Moderate Theoretical
- **Ciprofloxacin** is predicted to increase the exposure to **anagrelide**. Moderate Theoretical
- **Antacids** decrease the absorption of **quinolones**. Quinolones should be taken 2 hours before or 4 hours after **antacids**. Moderate Study
- **Ciprofloxacin** slightly increases the exposure to antiarrhythmics (lidocaine). Mild Study
- **Ciprofloxacin** affects the concentration of antiepileptics (fosphenytoin, phenytoin). Monitor concentration and adjust dose. Severe Study
- **Aspirin** (high-dose) potentially increases the risk of seizures when given with **quinolones**. Severe Theoretical
- Calcium salts (**calcium carbonate**) decrease the absorption of **norfloxacin**. Norfloxacin should be taken 2 hours before or 4 hours after **calcium carbonate**. Moderate Study
- Calcium salts (**calcium carbonate**) decrease the absorption of quinolones (**ciprofloxacin, nalidixic acid**). Separate administration by 2 hours. Moderate Study
- **Ciprofloxacin** increases the concentration of **clozapine**. Monitor side effects and adjust dose. Severe Study
- **Quinolones** increase the anticoagulant effect of **coumarins**. Severe Anecdotal
- **Didanosine** (buffered) is predicted to greatly decrease the exposure to oral **quinolones**. Didanosine should be taken 2 hours after quinolones. Moderate Study
- **Ciprofloxacin** is predicted to increase the exposure to dopamine receptor agonists (**ropinirole**). Adjust dose. Moderate Study

- **Ciprofloxacin** is predicted to increase the exposure to **duloxetine**. Avoid. Moderate Theoretical
- **Enteral feeds** decreases the exposure to **ciprofloxacin**. Moderate Study
- **Ciprofloxacin** slightly increases the exposure to **erlotinib**. Monitor side effects and adjust dose. Moderate Study
- **Ciprofloxacin** is predicted to increase the exposure to **ibrutinib**. Avoid or adjust **ibrutinib** dose. Severe Study
- **Iron (oral)** decreases the exposure to **quinolones**. Separate administration by at least 2 hours. Moderate Study
- **Lanthanum** moderately decreases the exposure to **quinolones**. Quinolones should be taken 2 hours before or 4 hours after **lanthanum**. Moderate Study
- **Ciprofloxacin** is predicted to increase the exposure to **loxapine**. Avoid. Unknown Theoretical
- **Ciprofloxacin** is predicted to increase the exposure to **melatonin**. Moderate Theoretical
- **Ciprofloxacin** potentially increases the risk of toxicity when given with **methotrexate**. Avoid. Severe Anecdotal
- **Ciprofloxacin** slightly increases the exposure to monoamine-oxidase B inhibitors (**rasagiline**). Moderate Study
- **NSAIDs** potentially increase the risk of seizures when given with **quinolones**. Severe Theoretical
- **Ciprofloxacin** very slightly increases the exposure to **pentoxifylline**. Moderate Study
- **Ciprofloxacin** is predicted to increase the exposure to **pirfenidone**. Use with caution and adjust dose. Moderate Study
- **Ciprofloxacin** is predicted to increase the exposure to **pomalidomide**. Adjust **pomalidomide** dose. Moderate Theoretical
- **Ciprofloxacin** is predicted to increase the exposure to **roflumilast**. Moderate Theoretical
- **Strontium ranelate** is predicted to decrease the absorption of **quinolones**. Moderate Theoretical
- **Sucralfate** decreases the exposure to **quinolones**. Separate administration by 2 hours. Moderate Study
- **Ciprofloxacin** is predicted to increase the exposure to **theophylline**. Monitor and adjust dose. Moderate Theoretical
- **Norfloxacin** is predicted to increase the exposure to **theophylline**. Adjust dose. Moderate Anecdotal
- **Ciprofloxacin** increases the exposure to **tizanidine**. Avoid. Moderate Study
- **Zinc** is predicted to decrease the exposure to **quinolones**. Separate administration by 2 hours. Moderate Study
- **Ciprofloxacin** is predicted to increase the exposure to **zolmitriptan**. Adjust **zolmitriptan** dose, p. 280. Moderate Theoretical

Rabeprazole → see proton pump inhibitors
Rabies vaccine
- **Antimalarials (chloroquine)** decrease the efficacy of **rabies vaccine**. Avoid. Moderate Study
- **Hydroxychloroquine** is predicted to decrease efficacy **rabies vaccine**. Moderate Theoretical
Raloxifene → see **TABLE 5** p. 818 (thromboembolism)
Raltegravir
- **Antacids** slightly decrease the exposure to **raltegravir**. Avoid. Moderate Study
- **HIV-protease inhibitors (darunavir)** increase the risk of rash when given with **raltegravir**. Moderate Study
- **HIV-protease inhibitors (fosamprenavir)** boosted with ritonavir decrease the exposure to **raltegravir** and raltegravir decreases the exposure to HIV-protease inhibitors (**fosamprenavir**) boosted with ritonavir. Avoid. Severe Study
- **Rifampicin** slightly decreases the exposure to **raltegravir**. Avoid or adjust dose. Moderate Study
Raltitrexed → see **TABLE 15** p. 821 (myelosuppression)
- **Folates (folic acid)** are predicted to alter the effects of **raltitrexed**. Avoid. Moderate Theoretical
- **Folates (folinic acid)** alter the effects of **raltitrexed**. Avoid. Moderate Study
- **Live vaccines** are predicted to increase the risk of generalised infection (possibly life-threatening) when given with **raltitrexed**. Public Health England advises avoid. Severe Theoretical
Ramipril → see ACE inhibitors
Ramucirumab → see monoclonal antibodies

Interactions | Appendix 1　A1

Ranibizumab

▶ **Ranibizumab** is predicted to increase the risk of bleeding events when given with **argatroban**. Severe Theoretical
▶ **Ranibizumab** is predicted to increase the risk of bleeding events when given with **bivalirudin**. Moderate Theoretical
▶ **Ranibizumab** increases the risk of bleeding events when given with **coumarins**. Severe Theoretical
▶ **Ranibizumab** is predicted to increase the risk of bleeding events when given with **danaparoid**. Severe Theoretical
▶ **Ranibizumab** increases the risk of bleeding events when given with **heparin (unfractionated)**. Severe Theoretical
▶ **Ranibizumab** increases the risk of bleeding events when given with **low molecular-weight heparins**. Severe Theoretical
▶ **Ranibizumab** is predicted to increase the risk of bleeding events when given with **phenindione**. Severe Theoretical

Ranitidine → see H₂ receptor antagonists

Ranolazine → see TABLE 9 p. 820 (QT-interval prolongation)
▶ **Ranolazine** is predicted to increase the exposure to **afatinib**. Separate administration by 12 hours. Moderate Study
▶ **Ranolazine** is predicted to increase the exposure to **aliskiren**. Moderate Theoretical
▶ Antiarrhythmics (**dronedarone**) are predicted to increase the exposure to **ranolazine**. Severe Study → Also see TABLE 9 p. 820
▶ Antiepileptics (**carbamazepine, fosphenytoin, phenobarbital, phenytoin, primidone**) are predicted to decrease the exposure to **ranolazine**. Severe Study
▶ Antifungals, azoles (**fluconazole, isavuconazole, posaconazole**) are predicted to increase the exposure to **ranolazine**. Severe Study
▶ Antifungals, azoles (**itraconazole, ketoconazole, voriconazole**) are predicted to increase the exposure to **ranolazine**. Avoid. Severe Study → Also see TABLE 9 p. 820
▶ **Aprepitant** is predicted to increase the exposure to **ranolazine**. Severe Study
▶ **Ranolazine** is predicted to increase the exposure to beta blockers, non-selective (**nadolol**). Moderate Study
▶ Calcium channel blockers (**diltiazem, verapamil**) are predicted to increase the exposure to **ranolazine**. Severe Study
▶ **Ranolazine** is predicted to increase the exposure to **ceritinib**. Moderate Theoretical → Also see TABLE 9 p. 820
▶ **Ciclosporin** is predicted to increase the concentration of **ranolazine** and **ranolazine** is predicted to increase the concentration of **ciclosporin**. Moderate Theoretical
▶ **Cobicistat** is predicted to increase the exposure to **ranolazine**. Avoid. Severe Study
▶ **Ranolazine** is predicted to increase the exposure to **colchicine**. Avoid or adjust **colchicine** dose. Severe Theoretical
▶ **Crizotinib** is predicted to increase the exposure to **ranolazine**. Severe Study → Also see TABLE 9 p. 820
▶ **Ranolazine** is predicted to increase the exposure to **dabigatran**. Severe Theoretical
▶ **Ranolazine** increases the concentration of **digoxin**. Moderate Study
▶ **Ranolazine** is predicted to slightly increase the exposure to **edoxaban**. Severe Theoretical
▶ **Enzalutamide** is predicted to decrease the exposure to **ranolazine**. Avoid. Severe Study
▶ **Ranolazine** is predicted to increase the exposure to **erlotinib**. Moderate Theoretical
▶ **Ranolazine** is predicted to increase the exposure to **fidaxomicin**. Avoid. Moderate Study
▶ **Grapefruit juice** is predicted to increase the concentration of **ranolazine**. Avoid. Severe Theoretical
▶ HIV-protease inhibitors (**atazanavir, darunavir, fosamprenavir, lopinavir, ritonavir, saquinavir, tipranavir**) are predicted to increase the exposure to **ranolazine**. Avoid. Severe Study → Also see TABLE 9 p. 820
▶ HIV-protease inhibitors (**indinavir**) are predicted to increase the exposure to **ranolazine**. Severe Study
▶ **Idelalisib** is predicted to increase the exposure to **ranolazine**. Avoid. Severe Study
▶ **Imatinib** is predicted to increase the exposure to **ranolazine**. Severe Study
▶ **Ranolazine** is predicted to increase the exposure to **lomitapide**. Separate administration by 12 hours. Moderate Theoretical

▶ Macrolides (**clarithromycin**) are predicted to increase the exposure to **ranolazine**. Avoid. Severe Study → Also see TABLE 9 p. 820
▶ Macrolides (**erythromycin**) are predicted to increase the exposure to **ranolazine**. Severe Study
▶ **Netupitant** is predicted to increase the exposure to **ranolazine**. Severe Study
▶ **Nilotinib** is predicted to increase the exposure to **ranolazine**. Severe Study → Also see TABLE 9 p. 820
▶ **Ranolazine** is predicted to increase the exposure to **nintedanib**. Moderate Study
▶ **Rifampicin** is predicted to decrease the exposure to **ranolazine**. Avoid. Severe Study
▶ **St John's Wort** is predicted to decrease the exposure to **ranolazine**. Avoid. Severe Study
▶ **Ranolazine** is predicted to increase the exposure to statins (**atorvastatin**). Moderate Theoretical
▶ **Ranolazine** slightly increases the exposure to statins (**simvastatin**). Adjust **simvastatin** dose, p. 130. Moderate Study
▶ **Ranolazine** increases the concentration of **tacrolimus**. Adjust dose. Severe Anecdotal
▶ **Ranolazine** is predicted to increase the exposure to **ticagrelor**. Use with caution or avoid. Severe Study
▶ **Ranolazine** is predicted to increase the exposure to **topotecan**. Severe Study
▶ **Ranolazine** is predicted to increase the concentration of **trametinib**. Moderate Theoretical
▶ **Ranolazine** is predicted to increase the exposure to **venetoclax**. Avoid or monitor for toxicity. Severe Theoretical

Rasagiline → see monoamine-oxidase B inhibitors

Reboxetine

▶ Antiepileptics (**carbamazepine, fosphenytoin, phenobarbital, phenytoin, primidone**) are predicted to decrease the exposure to **reboxetine**. Moderate Anecdotal
▶ Antifungals, azoles (**itraconazole, ketoconazole, voriconazole**) are predicted to increase the exposure to **reboxetine**. Avoid. Moderate Study
▶ Antifungals, azoles (**miconazole**) are predicted to increase the concentration of **reboxetine**. Use with caution and adjust dose. Moderate Theoretical
▶ **Cobicistat** is predicted to increase the exposure to **reboxetine**. Avoid. Moderate Study
▶ **Enzalutamide** is predicted to decrease the exposure to **reboxetine**. Moderate Anecdotal
▶ HIV-protease inhibitors (**atazanavir, darunavir, fosamprenavir, lopinavir, ritonavir, saquinavir, tipranavir**) are predicted to increase the exposure to **reboxetine**. Avoid. Moderate Study
▶ **Idelalisib** is predicted to increase the exposure to **reboxetine**. Avoid. Moderate Study
▶ **Reboxetine** is predicted to increase the risk of a hypertensive crisis when given with **linezolid**. Avoid. Severe Theoretical
▶ **Reboxetine** is predicted to increase the risk of hypokalaemia when given with **loop diuretics**. Moderate Theoretical
▶ Macrolides (**clarithromycin**) are predicted to increase the exposure to **reboxetine**. Avoid. Moderate Study
▶ **Reboxetine** is predicted to increase the risk of a hypertensive crisis when given with **moclobemide**. Avoid. Severe Theoretical
▶ **Reboxetine** is predicted to increase the risk of a hypertensive crisis when given with **monoamine-oxidase A and B inhibitors, irreversible**. Avoid. Severe Theoretical
▶ **Reboxetine** is predicted to increase the risk of a hypertensive crisis when given with monoamine-oxidase B inhibitors (**rasagiline, selegiline**). Avoid. Severe Theoretical
▶ **Rifampicin** is predicted to decrease the exposure to **reboxetine**. Moderate Anecdotal
▶ **Reboxetine** is predicted to increase the risk of hypokalaemia when given with **thiazide diuretics**. Moderate Anecdotal

Regorafenib → see TABLE 15 p. 821 (myelosuppression), TABLE 4 p. 818 (antiplatelet effects)
▶ Antiepileptics (**carbamazepine, fosphenytoin, phenobarbital, phenytoin, primidone**) are predicted to decrease the exposure to **regorafenib**. Avoid. Moderate Study
▶ Antifungals, azoles (**itraconazole, ketoconazole, voriconazole**) are predicted to increase the exposure to **regorafenib**. Avoid. Moderate Study

▸ **Cobicistat** is predicted to increase the exposure to **regorafenib**. Avoid. Moderate Study
▸ **Regorafenib** is predicted to increase the risk of bleeding events when given with **coumarins**. Severe Study
▸ **Enzalutamide** is predicted to decrease the exposure to **regorafenib**. Avoid. Moderate Study
▸ **Grapefruit juice** is predicted to increase the exposure to **regorafenib**. Avoid. Moderate Theoretical
▸ **HIV-protease inhibitors (atazanavir, darunavir, fosamprenavir, lopinavir, ritonavir, saquinavir, tipranavir)** are predicted to increase the exposure to **regorafenib**. Avoid. Moderate Study
▸ **Idelalisib** is predicted to increase the exposure to **regorafenib**. Avoid. Moderate Study → Also see **TABLE 15** p. 821
▸ **Macrolides (clarithromycin)** are predicted to increase the exposure to **regorafenib**. Avoid. Moderate Study
▸ **Regorafenib** is predicted to increase the exposure to **methotrexate**. Severe Theoretical → Also see **TABLE 15** p. 821
▸ **Regorafenib** is predicted to increase the exposure to NSAIDs **(mefenamic acid)**. Avoid. Moderate Theoretical → Also see **TABLE 4** p. 818
▸ **Regorafenib** is predicted to increase the risk of bleeding events when given with **phenindione**. Severe Theoretical
▸ **Rifampicin** is predicted to decrease the exposure to **regorafenib**. Avoid. Moderate Study
▸ **Regorafenib** is predicted to increase the exposure to statins **(atorvastatin, fluvastatin, rosuvastatin)**. Severe Theoretical

Remifentanil → see opioids

Repaglinide → see **TABLE 14** p. 821 (antidiabetic drugs)
▸ **Antiepileptics (carbamazepine, fosphenytoin, phenobarbital, phenytoin, primidone)** are predicted to decrease the exposure to **repaglinide**. Monitor blood glucose and adjust dose. Moderate Study
▸ **Antifungals, azoles (itraconazole, ketoconazole, voriconazole)** are predicted to increase the exposure to **repaglinide**. Moderate Study
▸ **Ciclosporin** moderately increases the exposure to **repaglinide**. Moderate Study
▸ **Clopidogrel** increases the exposure to **repaglinide**. Severe Study
▸ **Cobicistat** is predicted to increase the exposure to **repaglinide**. Moderate Study
▸ **Enzalutamide** is predicted to decrease the exposure to **repaglinide**. Monitor blood glucose and adjust dose. Moderate Study
▸ **Fibrates (gemfibrozil)** markedly increase the exposure to **repaglinide**. Avoid. Severe Study
▸ **HIV-protease inhibitors (atazanavir, darunavir, fosamprenavir, lopinavir, ritonavir, saquinavir, tipranavir)** are predicted to increase the exposure to **repaglinide**. Moderate Study
▸ **Idelalisib** is predicted to increase the exposure to **repaglinide**. Moderate Study
▸ **Iron chelators (deferasirox)** moderately increase the exposure to **repaglinide**. Avoid. Moderate Study
▸ **Lumacaftor** is predicted to decrease the exposure to **repaglinide**. Adjust dose. Moderate Theoretical
▸ **Macrolides (clarithromycin)** are predicted to increase the exposure to **repaglinide**. Moderate Study
▸ **Pitolisant** is predicted to decrease the exposure to **repaglinide**. Unknown Theoretical
▸ **Rifampicin** is predicted to decrease the exposure to **repaglinide**. Monitor blood glucose and adjust dose. Moderate Study
▸ **Teriflunomide** increases the exposure to **repaglinide**. Moderate Study
▸ **Trimethoprim** slightly increases the exposure to **repaglinide**. Avoid or monitor blood glucose. Moderate Study

Reslizumab → see monoclonal antibodies

Reteplase → see **TABLE 3** p. 818 (anticoagulant effects)

Retigabine → see antiepileptics

Retinoids → see **TABLE 5** p. 818 (thromboembolism)

acitretin · adapalene · alitretinoin · bexarotene · isotretinoin · tazarotene · tretinoin

▸ Consumption of alcohol might increase the serum concentration of etretinate in patients taking **acitretin**.

▸ Avoid concomitant use of keratolytics in patients taking **acitretin** and **isotretinoin**.
▸ Since systemic absorption can follow topical application, the possibility of interactions should be borne in mind.

▸ **Antiarrhythmics (amiodarone)** are predicted to increase the exposure to **alitretinoin**. Adjust **alitretinoin** dose. Moderate Theoretical
▸ **Antifungals, azoles (fluconazole, itraconazole, ketoconazole, miconazole, voriconazole)** are predicted to increase the exposure to **alitretinoin**. Adjust **alitretinoin** dose. Moderate Theoretical
▸ **Antifungals, azoles (fluconazole, ketoconazole, voriconazole)** are predicted to increase the risk of tretinoin toxicity when given with **tretinoin**. Moderate Study
▸ **Cobicistat** is predicted to increase the exposure to **alitretinoin**. Adjust **alitretinoin** dose. Moderate Theoretical
▸ **Fibrates (gemfibrozil)** are predicted to increase the exposure to **alitretinoin**. Adjust **alitretinoin** dose. Moderate Theoretical
▸ **Fibrates (gemfibrozil)** increase the concentration of **bexarotene**. Avoid. Severe Study
▸ **HIV-protease inhibitors (atazanavir, darunavir, fosamprenavir, lopinavir, ritonavir, saquinavir, tipranavir)** are predicted to increase the exposure to **alitretinoin**. Adjust **alitretinoin** dose. Moderate Theoretical
▸ **Idelalisib** is predicted to increase the exposure to **alitretinoin**. Adjust **alitretinoin** dose. Moderate Theoretical
▸ **Macrolides (clarithromycin)** are predicted to increase the exposure to **alitretinoin**. Adjust **alitretinoin** dose. Moderate Theoretical
▸ **Acitretin** is predicted to increase the concentration of **methotrexate**. Avoid. Moderate Anecdotal
▸ **Sulfinpyrazone** is predicted to increase the exposure to **alitretinoin**. Adjust **alitretinoin** dose. Moderate Theoretical
▸ **Retinoids (acitretin, alitretinoin, isotretinoin, tretinoin)** increase the risk of benign intracranial hypertension when given with **tetracyclines**. Avoid. Severe Anecdotal
▸ **Bexarotene** is predicted to increase the risk of toxicity when given with **vitamin A**. Adjust dose. Moderate Theoretical
▸ **Retinoids (acitretin, alitretinoin, isotretinoin)** are predicted to increase the risk of vitamin A toxicity when given with **vitamin A**. Avoid. Severe Theoretical
▸ **Tretinoin** is predicted to increase the risk of vitamin A toxicity when given with **vitamin A**. Avoid. Severe Study

Ribavirin
▸ **Ribavirin** is predicted to increase the exposure to **didanosine**. Avoid. Severe Study
▸ **Ribavirin** increases the risk of toxicity when given with **stavudine**. Avoid. Severe Study
▸ **Ribavirin** increases the risk of anaemia and/or leucopenia when given with **zidovudine**. Avoid. Severe Study

Rifabutin

GENERAL INFORMATION Although some manufacturers class rifabutin as a potent inducer of CYP3A4, clinical data suggests it is potentially a weak inducer, and therefore the BNF does not extrapolate the interactions of potent CYP3A4 inducers to rifabutin. For those who wish to err on the side of caution, see the interactions of rifampicin but bear in mind other mechanisms might be involved.

▸ **Antifungals, azoles (fluconazole)** increase the risk of uveitis when given with **rifabutin**. Adjust dose. Severe Study
▸ **Antifungals, azoles (itraconazole, posaconazole)** increase the concentration of **rifabutin** and **rifabutin** decreases the concentration of antifungals, azoles **(itraconazole, posaconazole)**. Severe Study
▸ **Antifungals, azoles (ketoconazole)** are predicted to increase the concentration of **rifabutin** and **rifabutin** is predicted to decrease the concentration of antifungals, azoles **(ketoconazole)**. Avoid. Severe Study
▸ **Antifungals, azoles (miconazole)** are predicted to increase the concentration of **rifabutin**. Use with caution and adjust dose. Moderate Theoretical
▸ **Rifabutin** is predicted to decrease the exposure to antifungals, azoles **(isavuconazole)**. Avoid. Severe Theoretical

Interactions | Appendix 1

A1

Rifabutin (continued)

▶ Rifabutin decreases the concentration of antifungals, azoles (voriconazole) and antifungals, azoles (voriconazole) increase the concentration of **rifabutin**. Avoid or adjust **voriconazole** dose, p. 361. Severe Study

▶ Rifabutin slightly decreases the exposure to antimalarials (atovaquone). Avoid. Moderate Study

▶ Rifabutin decreases the concentration of cobicistat and cobicistat increases the exposure to **rifabutin**. Avoid or adjust dose. Severe Study

▶ Rifabutin is predicted to decrease the efficacy of combined hormonal contraceptives. For FSRH guidance, see Contraceptives, interactions p. 474. Severe Study

▶ Rifabutin increases the clearance of dapsone. Moderate Study

▶ Rifabutin is predicted to decrease the efficacy of desogestrel. For FSRH guidance, see Contraceptives, interactions p. 474. Severe Theoretical

▶ Efavirenz slightly decreases the exposure to **rifabutin**. Adjust dose. Severe Study

▶ Rifabutin is predicted to decrease the efficacy of etonogestrel. For FSRH guidance, see Contraceptives, interactions p. 474. Severe Theoretical

▶ Rifabutin decreases the exposure to etravirine. Moderate Study

▶ HIV-protease inhibitors (atazanavir, darunavir, fosamprenavir, lopinavir, saquinavir, tipranavir) increase the exposure to **rifabutin**. Monitor and adjust dose. Severe Study

▶ HIV-protease inhibitors (indinavir) increase the exposure to **rifabutin** and **rifabutin** decreases the exposure to HIV-protease inhibitors (indinavir). Avoid. Severe Study

▶ HIV-protease inhibitors (ritonavir) markedly increase the exposure to **rifabutin**. Avoid or adjust dose. Severe Study

▶ Rifabutin is predicted to decrease the effects of Hormone replacement therapy. Moderate Anecdotal

▶ Rifabutin is predicted to decrease the efficacy of levonorgestrel. For FSRH guidance, see Contraceptives, interactions p. 474. Severe Theoretical

▶ Lumacaftor is predicted to decrease the exposure to **rifabutin**. Adjust dose. Moderate Theoretical

▶ Macrolides (azithromycin) increase the risk of neutropenia when given with **rifabutin**. Severe Study

▶ Macrolides (clarithromycin) increase the risk of uveitis when given with **rifabutin**. Adjust dose. Severe Study

▶ Rifabutin is predicted to decrease the efficacy of norethisterone. For FSRH guidance, see Contraceptives, interactions p. 474. Severe Anecdotal

▶ Rifabutin slightly decreases the exposure to rilpivirine. Adjust dose. Severe Study

▶ Rifabutin is predicted to decrease the exposure to simeprevir. Avoid. Moderate Theoretical

▶ Rifabutin decreases the efficacy of ulipristal. For FSRH guidance, see Contraceptives, interactions p. 474. Severe Anecdotal

Rifampicin

▶ **Rifampicin** is predicted to decrease the exposure to abacavir. Moderate Theoretical

▶ Rifampicin is predicted to decrease the exposure to abiraterone. Avoid. Severe Theoretical

▶ Rifampicin is predicted to decrease the exposure to afatinib. Moderate Study

▶ Rifampicin is predicted to decrease the exposure to agomelatine. Moderate Theoretical

▶ Rifampicin is predicted to decrease the exposure to aldosterone antagonists (eplerenone). Avoid. Moderate Theoretical

▶ Rifampicin decreases the exposure to aliskiren. Moderate Study

▶ Rifampicin is predicted to decrease the exposure to alprazolam. Adjust **alprazolam** dose. Moderate Theoretical

▶ Rifampicin transiently increases the exposure to ambrisentan. Moderate Study

▶ Rifampicin decreases the exposure to aminophylline. Adjust dose. Moderate Study

▶ Antacids decrease the absorption of **rifampicin**. **Rifampicin** should be taken 1 hour before antacids. Moderate Study

▶ Rifampicin is predicted to decrease the exposure to antiarrhythmics (disopyramide, dronedarone). Avoid. Severe Study

▶ Rifampicin is predicted to decrease the efficacy of antiarrhythmics (propafenone). Moderate Study

▶ Rifampicin is predicted to decrease the exposure to anticholinesterases, centrally acting (donepezil). Mild Study

▶ Antiepileptics (phenobarbital, primidone) are predicted to decrease the exposure to **rifampicin** and **rifampicin** is predicted to decrease the exposure to antiepileptics (phenobarbital, primidone). Use with caution and adjust dose. Moderate Study

▶ Rifampicin slightly decreases the exposure to antiepileptics (brivaracetam). Adjust dose. Moderate Study

▶ Rifampicin decreases the concentration of antiepileptics (fosphenytoin, phenytoin). Use with caution and adjust dose. Moderate Study

▶ Rifampicin markedly increases the clearance of antiepileptics (lamotrigine). Adjust **lamotrigine** dose, p. 194. Moderate Study

▶ Rifampicin is predicted to decrease the exposure to antiepileptics (perampanel). Monitor and adjust dose. Moderate Study

▶ Rifampicin slightly decreases the exposure to antifungals, azoles (fluconazole). Adjust dose. Moderate Study

▶ Rifampicin is predicted to decrease the exposure to antifungals, azoles (isavuconazole). Avoid. Severe Study

▶ Rifampicin markedly decreases the exposure to antifungals, azoles (itraconazole). Avoid **rifampicin** for 14 days before and during treatment with **itraconazole**. Moderate Study

▶ Rifampicin markedly decreases the exposure to antifungals, azoles (ketoconazole) and antifungals, azoles (ketoconazole) potentially decrease the exposure to **rifampicin**. Avoid. Moderate Study

▶ Rifampicin is predicted to decrease the exposure to antifungals, azoles (posaconazole). Avoid. Moderate Anecdotal

▶ Rifampicin very markedly decreases the exposure to antifungals, azoles (voriconazole). Avoid. Moderate Study

▶ Rifampicin is predicted to decrease the efficacy of antihistamines, non-sedating (bilastine). Moderate Theoretical

▶ Rifampicin increases the clearance of antihistamines, non-sedating (fexofenadine). Moderate Study

▶ Rifampicin is predicted to decrease the exposure to antimalarials (artemether) with lumafantrine. Avoid. Severe Study

▶ Rifampicin moderately decreases the exposure to antimalarials (atovaquone) and antimalarials (atovaquone) slightly increase the exposure to **rifampicin**. Avoid. Moderate Study

▶ Rifampicin moderately decreases the exposure to antimalarials (mefloquine). Severe Study

▶ Rifampicin is predicted to decrease the concentration of antimalarials (piperaquine). Avoid. Moderate Theoretical

▶ Rifampicin decreases the exposure to antimalarials (quinine). Severe Study

▶ Rifampicin is predicted to moderately decrease the exposure to apixaban. Use with caution or avoid. Severe Study

▶ Rifampicin moderately decreases the exposure to apremilast. Avoid. Severe Study

▶ Rifampicin is predicted to markedly decrease the exposure to aprepitant. Avoid. Moderate Study

▶ Rifampicin is predicted to moderately decrease the exposure to aripiprazole. Adjust **aripiprazole** dose, p. 240. Moderate Study

▶ Rifampicin decreases the exposure to ataluren. Moderate Study

▶ Rifampicin is predicted to decrease the exposure to axitinib. Avoid or adjust dose. Moderate Study

▶ Rifampicin is predicted to decrease the exposure to bazedoxifene. Moderate Theoretical

▶ Rifampicin decreases the exposure to bedaquiline. Avoid. Severe Study

▶ Rifampicin moderately decreases the exposure to beta blockers, non-selective (carvedilol). Moderate Study

▶ Rifampicin decreases the exposure to beta blockers, non-selective (propranolol). Monitor and adjust **propranolol** dose. Moderate Study

▶ Rifampicin slightly decreases the exposure to beta blockers, selective (bisoprolol, metoprolol). Mild Study

▶ Rifampicin moderately decreases the exposure to beta blockers, selective (celiprolol). Moderate Study

▶ Rifampicin slightly decreases the exposure to bortezomib. Avoid. Severe Study

▶ **Rifampicin** affects the exposure to **bosentan**. Avoid. Severe Study

▶ **Rifampicin** is predicted to very markedly decrease the exposure to **bosutinib**. Avoid. Severe Study

▶ **Rifampicin** is predicted to markedly decrease the exposure to **bupropion**. Severe Study

▶ **Rifampicin** is predicted to decrease the exposure to **buspirone**. Use with caution and adjust dose. Severe Study

▶ **Rifampicin** moderately decreases the exposure to **cabozantinib**. Avoid. Moderate Study

▶ **Rifampicin** is predicted to moderately increase the clearance of **caffeine citrate**. Monitor and adjust dose. Moderate Study

▶ **Rifampicin** is predicted to decrease the exposure to calcium channel blockers (**amlodipine, felodipine, lacidipine, lercanidipine, nicardipine, nimodipine**). Monitor and adjust dose. Moderate Study

▶ **Rifampicin** decreases the exposure to calcium channel blockers (**diltiazem**). Severe Study

▶ **Rifampicin** decreases the exposure to calcium channel blockers (**isradipine**). Avoid. Moderate Study

▶ **Rifampicin** moderately decreases the exposure to calcium channel blockers (**nifedipine**). Avoid. Severe Study

▶ **Rifampicin** is predicted to decrease the exposure to calcium channel blockers (**verapamil**). Severe Study

▶ **Rifampicin** moderately decreases the exposure to **canagliflozin**. Adjust **canagliflozin** dose. Moderate Study

▶ **Rifampicin** is predicted to decrease the exposure to **cannabis extract**. Avoid. Severe Theoretical

▶ **Rifampicin** decreases the concentration of **caspofungin**. Adjust **caspofungin** dose, p. 356. Moderate Study

▶ **Rifampicin** is predicted to decrease the exposure to **ceritinib**. Avoid. Severe Study

▶ **Rifampicin** decreases the concentration of **chloramphenicol**. Moderate Study

▶ **Rifampicin** is predicted to decrease the exposure to **chlordiazepoxide**. Moderate Theoretical

▶ **Rifampicin** decreases the concentration of **ciclosporin**. Severe Study

▶ **Rifampicin** is predicted to alter the effects of **cilostazol**. Moderate Theoretical

▶ **Rifampicin** decreases the exposure to **clomethiazole**. Monitor and adjust dose. Moderate Study

▶ **Rifampicin** decreases the exposure to **clozapine**. Severe Anecdotal

▶ **Rifampicin** is predicted to decrease the exposure to **cobicistat**. Avoid. Severe Theoretical

▶ **Rifampicin** is predicted to decrease the exposure to **cobimetinib**. Avoid. Severe Theoretical

▶ **Rifampicin** is predicted to decrease the efficacy of **combined hormonal contraceptives**. For FSRH guidance, see Contraceptives, interactions p. 474. Severe Study

▶ **Rifampicin** is predicted to decrease the exposure to corticosteroids (**budesonide, dexamethasone, methylprednisolone, prednisolone**). Monitor and adjust dose. Moderate Study

▶ **Rifampicin** is predicted to decrease the exposure to corticosteroids (**fluticasone**). Unknown Theoretical

▶ **Rifampicin** is predicted to decrease the exposure to corticosteroids (**prednisone**). Mild Study

▶ **Rifampicin** decreases the anticoagulant effect of **coumarins**. Severe Study

▶ **Rifampicin** is predicted to markedly decrease the exposure to **crizotinib**. Avoid. Severe Study

▶ **Rifampicin** is predicted to decrease the exposure to **dabigatran**. Avoid. Severe Study

▶ **Rifampicin** is predicted to decrease the exposure to **dabrafenib**. Avoid. Moderate Theoretical

▶ **Rifampicin** is predicted to moderately decrease the exposure to **daclatasvir**. Avoid. Severe Study

▶ **Rifampicin** moderately decreases the exposure to **dapsone**. Moderate Study

▶ **Rifampicin** is predicted to decrease the exposure to **darifenacin**. Moderate Theoretical

▶ **Rifampicin** is predicted to decrease the exposure to **dasabuvir**. Avoid. Severe Theoretical

▶ **Rifampicin** is predicted to markedly decrease the exposure to **dasatinib**. Avoid. Severe Study

▶ **Rifampicin** is predicted to slightly decrease the exposure to **delamanid**. Avoid. Moderate Study

▶ **Rifampicin** is predicted to decrease the efficacy of **desogestrel**. For FSRH guidance, see Contraceptives, interactions p. 474. Severe Theoretical

▶ **Rifampicin** moderately decreases the exposure to **diazepam**. Avoid. Moderate Study

▶ **Rifampicin** decreases the concentration of **digoxin**. Moderate Study

▶ **Rifampicin** decreases the exposure to **dolutegravir**. Adjust dose. Severe Study

▶ **Rifampicin** is predicted to decrease the exposure to **edoxaban**. Moderate Study

▶ **Rifampicin** slightly decreases the exposure to **efavirenz**. Adjust dose. Severe Study

▶ **Rifampicin** is predicted to decrease the exposure to **elbasvir**. Avoid. Severe Study

▶ **Rifampicin** is predicted to decrease the concentration of **elvitegravir**. Avoid. Severe Theoretical

▶ **Rifampicin** is predicted to decrease the effects of **ergotamine**. Moderate Theoretical

▶ **Rifampicin** is predicted to decrease the exposure to **erlotinib**. Avoid or adjust **erlotinib** dose. Severe Study

▶ **Rifampicin** is predicted to decrease the efficacy of **etonogestrel**. For FSRH guidance, see Contraceptives, interactions p. 474. Severe Theoretical

▶ **Rifampicin** is predicted to decrease the exposure to **etravirine**. Avoid. Severe Theoretical

▶ **Rifampicin** is predicted to decrease the concentration of **everolimus**. Avoid or adjust dose. Severe Study

▶ **Rifampicin** moderately decreases the exposure to **exemestane**. Moderate Study

▶ **Rifampicin** is predicted to decrease the exposure to **fesoterodine**. Avoid. Moderate Study

▶ **Rifampicin** is predicted to decrease the exposure to **fingolimod**. Moderate Study

▶ **Rifampicin** is predicted to decrease the exposure to **fosaprepitant**. Avoid. Moderate Theoretical

▶ **Rifampicin** is predicted to decrease the exposure to **gefitinib**. Avoid. Severe Study

▶ **Rifampicin** is predicted to decrease the exposure to **grazoprevir**. Avoid. Severe Study

▶ **Rifampicin** is predicted to decrease the concentration of **guanfacine**. Adjust **guanfacine** dose, p. 222. Moderate Study

▶ **Rifampicin** decreases the concentration of **haloperidol**. Adjust dose. Moderate Study

▶ **Rifampicin** is predicted to moderately to markedly decrease the exposure to HIV-protease inhibitors (**atazanavir, darunavir, fosamprenavir, indinavir, lopinavir, saquinavir, tipranavir**). Avoid. Severe Study

▶ **Rifampicin** slightly decreases the exposure to HIV-protease inhibitors (**ritonavir**). Severe Study

▶ **Rifampicin** is predicted to decrease the effects of Hormone replacement therapy. Moderate Anecdotal

▶ **Rifampicin** is predicted to decrease the exposure to **ibrutinib**. Avoid. Severe Study

▶ **Rifampicin** is predicted to decrease the exposure to **idelalisib**. Avoid. Severe Study

▶ **Rifampicin** is predicted to decrease the exposure to **imatinib**. Avoid. Moderate Study

▶ **Rifampicin** is predicted to decrease the exposure to **irinotecan**. Avoid. Severe Study

▶ **Rifampicin** is predicted to decrease the exposure to iron chelators (**deferasirox**). Monitor serum ferritin and adjust dose. Moderate Study

▶ **Rifampicin** is predicted to decrease the exposure to **ivabradine**. Adjust dose. Moderate Theoretical

▶ **Rifampicin** markedly decreases the exposure to **ivacaftor**. Avoid. Severe Study

▶ **Rifampicin** is predicted to decrease the exposure to **ixazomib**. Avoid. Severe Study

▶ **Rifampicin** is predicted to decrease the exposure to **lapatinib**. Avoid. Severe Study

Rifampicin (continued)

▶ **Rifampicin** is predicted to decrease the exposure to ledipasvir. Avoid. Severe Theoretical

▶ **Rifampicin** is predicted to decrease the efficacy of levonorgestrel. For FSRH guidance, see Contraceptives, interactions p. 474. Severe Theoretical

▶ **Rifampicin** is predicted to decrease the exposure to linagliptin. Moderate Study

▶ **Rifampicin** slightly decreases the exposure to linezolid. Moderate Study

▶ **Rifampicin** is predicted to decrease the exposure to lomitapide. Monitor and adjust dose. Moderate Theoretical

▶ **Rifampicin** increases the clearance of lorazepam. Moderate Study

▶ **Rifampicin** is predicted to decrease the exposure to lurasidone. Avoid. Moderate Study

▶ **Rifampicin** is predicted to decrease the exposure to macitentan. Avoid. Severe Study

▶ **Rifampicin** decreases the concentration of macrolides (clarithromycin). Severe Study

▶ **Rifampicin** is predicted to decrease the exposure to maraviroc. Adjust dose. Severe Study

▶ **Rifampicin** is predicted to decrease the exposure to midazolam. Monitor and adjust dose. Moderate Study

▶ **Rifampicin** is predicted to decrease the exposure to mirtazapine. Adjust dose. Moderate Study

▶ **Rifampicin** is predicted to decrease the exposure to modafinil. Moderate Theoretical

▶ **Rifampicin** decreases the effects of monoclonal antibodies (brentuximab vedotin). Severe Study

▶ **Rifampicin** is predicted to decrease the exposure to monoclonal antibodies (trastuzumab emtansine). Severe Theoretical

▶ **Rifampicin** is predicted to decrease the exposure to montelukast. Mild Study

▶ **Rifampicin** decreases the concentration of mycophenolate. Monitor and adjust dose. Severe Study

▶ **Rifampicin** is predicted to markedly decrease the exposure to naloxegol. Avoid. Moderate Study

▶ **Rifampicin** is predicted to slightly decrease the exposure to nateglinide. Mild Study

▶ **Rifampicin** is predicted to decrease the exposure to netupitant. Avoid. Moderate Study

▶ **Rifampicin** decreases the concentration of nevirapine. Avoid. Severe Study

▶ **Rifampicin** is predicted to moderately decrease the exposure to nilotinib. Avoid. Severe Study

▶ **Rifampicin** is predicted to decrease the exposure to nintedanib. Moderate Study

▶ **Rifampicin** is predicted to decrease the exposure to nitisinone. Adjust nitisinone dose. Moderate Theoretical

▶ **Rifampicin** increases the clearance of nitrazepam. Moderate Study

▶ **Rifampicin** is predicted to decrease the efficacy of norethisterone. For FSRH guidance, see Contraceptives, interactions p. 474. Severe Anecdotal

▶ **Rifampicin** moderately decreases the exposure to NSAIDs (celecoxib, diclofenac, etoricoxib). Moderate Study

▶ **Rifampicin** is predicted to decrease the exposure to olaparib. Avoid. Moderate Theoretical

▶ **Rifampicin** is predicted to decrease the exposure to ombitasvir. Avoid. Severe Theoretical

▶ **Rifampicin** is predicted to decrease the exposure to ondansetron. Moderate Study

▶ **Rifampicin** is predicted to decrease the exposure to opioids (alfentanil, fentanyl). Moderate Study

▶ **Rifampicin** is predicted to decrease the exposure to opioids (buprenorphine). Monitor and adjust dose. Moderate Theoretical

▶ **Rifampicin** decreases the exposure to opioids (codeine, morphine). Moderate Study

▶ **Rifampicin** decreases the exposure to opioids (methadone). Monitor and adjust dose. Severe Study

▶ **Rifampicin** is predicted to decrease the exposure to opioids (oxycodone). Monitor and adjust dose. Moderate Study

▶ **Rifampicin** is predicted to moderately decrease the exposure to osimertinib. Avoid. Moderate Study

▶ **Rifampicin** is predicted to decrease the exposure to palbociclib. Avoid. Severe Study

▶ **Rifampicin** is predicted to decrease the exposure to paliperidone. Monitor and adjust paliperidone dose. Moderate Theoretical

▶ **Rifampicin** is predicted to decrease the exposure to panobinostat. Avoid. Moderate Theoretical

▶ **Rifampicin** is predicted to decrease the exposure to paracetamol. Moderate Study

▶ **Rifampicin** is predicted to decrease the exposure to paritaprevir (with ritonavir and ombitasvir). Avoid. Severe Study

▶ **Rifampicin** is predicted to decrease the exposure to pazopanib. Avoid. Severe Theoretical

▶ **Rifampicin** is predicted to decrease the exposure to phosphodiesterase type-5 inhibitors (avanafil, tadalafil). Avoid. Severe Study

▶ **Rifampicin** is predicted to decrease the exposure to phosphodiesterase type-5 inhibitors (sildenafil, vardenafil). Moderate Theoretical

▶ **Rifampicin** moderately decreases the exposure to pioglitazone. Monitor and adjust pioglitazone dose. Moderate Study

▶ **Rifampicin** is predicted to decrease the exposure to pirfenidone. Avoid. Moderate Theoretical

▶ **Rifampicin** is predicted to moderately decrease the exposure to pitolisant. Moderate Study

▶ **Rifampicin** is predicted to decrease the exposure to ponatinib. Avoid. Moderate Theoretical

▶ **Rifampicin** is predicted to markedly decrease the exposure to praziquantel. Avoid. Moderate Study

▶ **Rifampicin** is predicted to moderately decrease the exposure to proton pump inhibitors (omeprazole). Moderate Study

▶ **Rifampicin** is predicted to decrease the exposure to quetiapine. Moderate Study

▶ **Rifampicin** slightly decreases the exposure to raltegravir. Avoid or adjust dose. Moderate Study

▶ **Rifampicin** is predicted to decrease the exposure to ranolazine. Avoid. Severe Study

▶ **Rifampicin** is predicted to decrease the exposure to reboxetine. Moderate Anecdotal

▶ **Rifampicin** is predicted to decrease the exposure to regorafenib. Avoid. Moderate Study

▶ **Rifampicin** is predicted to decrease the exposure to repaglinide. Monitor blood glucose and adjust dose. Moderate Study

▶ **Rifampicin** markedly decreases the exposure to rilpivirine. Avoid. Severe Study

▶ **Rifampicin** is predicted to decrease the exposure to risperidone. Adjust risperidone dose. Moderate Study

▶ **Rifampicin** is predicted to moderately decrease the exposure to rivaroxaban. Avoid unless patient can be monitored for signs of thrombosis. Severe Study

▶ **Rifampicin** is predicted to decrease the exposure to roflumilast. Avoid. Moderate Study

▶ **Rifampicin** is predicted to decrease the exposure to ruxolitinib. Monitor and adjust dose. Moderate Study

▶ **Rifampicin** is predicted to increase the exposure to sacubitril. Moderate Theoretical

▶ **Rifampicin** is predicted to moderately decrease the exposure to saxagliptin. Moderate Study

▶ **Rifampicin** is predicted to decrease the exposure to selexipag. Unknown Theoretical

▶ **Rifampicin** is predicted to decrease the exposure to simeprevir. Avoid. Severe Study

▶ **Rifampicin** is predicted to decrease the concentration of sirolimus. Avoid. Severe Study

▶ **Rifampicin** is predicted to decrease the exposure to sofosbuvir. Avoid. Severe Study

▶ **Rifampicin** is predicted to decrease the exposure to solifenacin. Moderate Theoretical

▶ **Rifampicin** is predicted to decrease the exposure to sorafenib. Moderate Theoretical

▶ **Rifampicin** markedly decreases the exposure to statins (atorvastatin). Atorvastatin should be taken at the same time as **rifampicin**. Moderate Study

- ▸ **Rifampicin** moderately decreases the exposure to statins (**fluvastatin**). Monitor and adjust dose. Moderate Study
- ▸ **Rifampicin** very markedly decreases the exposure to statins (**simvastatin**). Moderate Study
- ▸ **Rifampicin** is predicted to decrease the exposure to sulfonylureas. Moderate Study
- ▸ **Rifampicin** is predicted to decrease the exposure to sunitinib. Avoid or adjust **sunitinib** dose. Moderate Study
- ▸ **Rifampicin** decreases the concentration of **tacrolimus**. Monitor and adjust dose. Severe Study
- ▸ **Rifampicin** markedly decreases the exposure to **tamoxifen**. Unknown Study
- ▸ **Rifampicin** is predicted to decrease the exposure to taxanes (**cabazitaxel, paclitaxel**). Avoid. Severe Study
- ▸ **Rifampicin** is predicted to decrease the exposure to taxanes (**docetaxel**). Severe Theoretical
- ▸ **Rifampicin** is predicted to decrease the concentration of **temsirolimus**. Avoid. Severe Study
- ▸ **Rifampicin** decreases the exposure to **terbinafine**. Adjust dose. Moderate Study
- ▸ **Rifampicin** decreases the exposure to tetracyclines (**doxycycline**). Monitor and adjust dose. Moderate Study
- ▸ **Rifampicin** is predicted to decrease the exposure to theophylline. Adjust dose. Moderate Study
- ▸ **Rifampicin** is predicted to markedly decrease the exposure to **ticagrelor**. Avoid. Severe Study
- ▸ **Rifampicin** moderately decreases the exposure to **tizanidine**. Mild Study
- ▸ **Rifampicin** is predicted to decrease the exposure to **tolvaptan**. Avoid. Severe Study
- ▸ **Rifampicin** is predicted to decrease the exposure to **toremifene**. Adjust dose. Moderate Study
- ▸ **Rifampicin** is predicted to decrease the exposure to **trabectedin**. Avoid. Severe Theoretical
- ▸ **Rifampicin** decreases the exposure to **trimethoprim**. Moderate Study
- ▸ **Rifampicin** decreases the efficacy of **ulipristal**. For FSRH guidance, see Contraceptives, interactions p. 474. Severe Anecdotal
- ▸ **Rifampicin** is predicted to decrease the exposure to **vandetanib**. Avoid. Moderate Study
- ▸ **Rifampicin** is predicted to moderately decrease the exposure to **velpatasvir**. Avoid. Severe Study
- ▸ **Rifampicin** is predicted to decrease the exposure to **vemurafenib**. Avoid. Severe Theoretical
- ▸ **Rifampicin** is predicted to decrease the exposure to **venetoclax**. Avoid. Severe Study
- ▸ **Rifampicin** is predicted to decrease the exposure to vinca alkaloids (**vinblastine, vincristine, vindesine**). Severe Theoretical
- ▸ **Rifampicin** is predicted to decrease the exposure to vinca alkaloids (**vinflunine**). Avoid. Severe Theoretical
- ▸ **Rifampicin** is predicted to decrease the exposure to vinca alkaloids (**vinorelbine**). Use with caution or avoid. Severe Theoretical
- ▸ **Rifampicin** is predicted to decrease the exposure to **vismodegib**. Avoid. Moderate Theoretical
- ▸ **Rifampicin** is predicted to decrease the exposure to **vortioxetine**. Monitor and adjust dose. Moderate Study
- ▸ **Rifampicin** markedly decreases the exposure to **zaleplon**. Moderate Study
- ▸ **Rifampicin** moderately decreases the exposure to **zolpidem**. Moderate Study
- ▸ **Rifampicin** is predicted to decrease the exposure to **zopiclone**. Adjust dose. Moderate Study

Rifaximin
- ▸ **Ciclosporin** very markedly increases the exposure to **rifaximin**. Severe Study

Rilpivirine
- ▸ **Antacids** are predicted to decrease the exposure to **rilpivirine**. **Antacids** should be taken 2 hours before or 4 hours after **rilpivirine**. Severe Theoretical
- ▸ Antiepileptics (**carbamazepine, fosphenytoin, phenobarbital, phenytoin, primidone**) markedly decrease the exposure to **rilpivirine**. Avoid. Severe Study

- ▸ Antiepileptics (**oxcarbazepine**) are predicted to decrease the concentration of **rilpivirine**. Avoid. Severe Theoretical
- ▸ **Bosentan** is predicted to decrease the exposure to **rilpivirine**. Avoid. Severe Theoretical
- ▸ Calcium salts (**calcium carbonate**) are predicted to slightly decrease the exposure to **rilpivirine**. **Calcium carbonate** should be taken 2 hours before or 4 hours after **rilpivirine**. Severe Theoretical
- ▸ **Efavirenz** is predicted to decrease the exposure to **rilpivirine**. Avoid. Severe Theoretical
- ▸ **Enzalutamide** markedly decreases the exposure to **rilpivirine**. Avoid. Severe Study
- ▸ **Etravirine** is predicted to decrease the exposure to **rilpivirine**. Avoid. Severe Theoretical
- ▸ H_2 receptor antagonists are predicted to decrease the exposure to **rilpivirine**. H_2 receptor antagonists should be taken 12 hours before or 4 hours after **rilpivirine**. Severe Study
- ▸ **Nevirapine** is predicted to decrease the exposure to **rilpivirine**. Avoid. Severe Theoretical
- ▸ Proton pump inhibitors are predicted to decrease the exposure to **rilpivirine**. Avoid. Severe Study
- ▸ **Rifabutin** slightly decreases the exposure to **rilpivirine**. Adjust dose. Severe Study
- ▸ **Rifampicin** markedly decreases the exposure to **rilpivirine**. Avoid. Severe Study
- ▸ **St John's Wort** is predicted to decrease the exposure to **rilpivirine**. Avoid. Severe Theoretical

Riluzole

> **FOOD AND LIFESTYLE** Charcoal-grilled foods are predicted to decrease the exposure to riluzole.

- ▸ SSRIs (**fluvoxamine**) are predicted to increase the exposure to **riluzole**. Moderate Theoretical

Riociguat → see TABLE 8 p. 819 (hypotension)
- ▸ **Antacids** slightly decrease the exposure to **riociguat**. **Antacids** should be taken 2 hours before or 1 hour after **riociguat**. Mild Study
- ▸ Antifungals, azoles (**itraconazole**) are predicted to increase the exposure to **riociguat**. Avoid. Moderate Study
- ▸ Antifungals, azoles (**ketoconazole**) moderately increase the exposure to **riociguat**. Avoid. Moderate Study
- ▸ **Ciclosporin** is predicted to increase the exposure to **riociguat**. Moderate Theoretical
- ▸ HIV-protease inhibitors (**ritonavir**) are predicted to increase the exposure to **riociguat**. Moderate Theoretical
- ▸ **Riociguat** is predicted to increase the risk of hypotension when given with phosphodiesterase type-5 inhibitors. Avoid. Severe Theoretical → Also see TABLE 8 p. 819

Risedronate → see bisphosphonates

Risperidone → see TABLE 8 p. 819 (hypotension), TABLE 9 p. 820 (QT-interval prolongation), TABLE 11 p. 820 (CNS depressant effects)
- ▸ Antiepileptics (**carbamazepine, fosphenytoin, phenobarbital, phenytoin, primidone**) are predicted to decrease the exposure to **risperidone**. Adjust **risperidone** dose. Moderate Study → Also see TABLE 11 p. 820
- ▸ Antifungals, azoles (**itraconazole, ketoconazole, voriconazole**) are predicted to increase the exposure to **risperidone**. Adjust dose. Moderate Study → Also see TABLE 9 p. 820
- ▸ **Bupropion** is predicted to increase the exposure to **risperidone**. Adjust dose. Moderate Study
- ▸ **Cinacalcet** is predicted to increase the exposure to **risperidone**. Adjust dose. Moderate Study
- ▸ **Cobicistat** is predicted to increase the exposure to **risperidone**. Adjust dose. Moderate Study
- ▸ **Risperidone** is predicted to decrease the effects of dopamine receptor agonists. Avoid. Moderate Theoretical → Also see TABLE 8 p. 819 → Also see TABLE 9 p. 820
- ▸ **Enzalutamide** is predicted to decrease the exposure to **risperidone**. Adjust **risperidone** dose. Moderate Study
- ▸ **Risperidone** is predicted to decrease the effects of histamine. Avoid. Severe Theoretical → Also see TABLE 8 p. 819
- ▸ HIV-protease inhibitors (**atazanavir, darunavir, fosamprenavir, lopinavir, ritonavir, saquinavir, tipranavir**) are predicted to increase the exposure to **risperidone**. Adjust dose. Moderate Study → Also see TABLE 9 p. 820

Risperidone (continued)
- Idelalisib is predicted to increase the exposure to **risperidone**. Adjust dose. Moderate Study
- **Risperidone** is predicted to decrease the effects of levodopa. Avoid or adjust dose. Severe Anecdotal → Also see **TABLE 8** p. 819
- **Risperidone** potentially increases the risk of neurotoxicity when given with lithium. Severe Anecdotal → Also see **TABLE 9** p. 820
- Macrolides **(clarithromycin)** are predicted to increase the exposure to **risperidone**. Adjust dose. Moderate Study → Also see **TABLE 9** p. 820
- Rifampicin is predicted to decrease the exposure to **risperidone**. Adjust **risperidone** dose. Moderate Study
- SSRIs **(fluoxetine, paroxetine)** are predicted to increase the exposure to **risperidone**. Adjust dose. Moderate Study
- Terbinafine is predicted to increase the exposure to **risperidone**. Adjust dose. Moderate Study

Ritonavir → see HIV-protease inhibitors
Rituximab → see monoclonal antibodies
Rivaroxaban → see **TABLE 3** p. 818 (anticoagulant effects)
- Antiarrhythmics **(dronedarone)** are predicted to increase the exposure to **rivaroxaban**. Avoid. Moderate Theoretical
- Antiepileptics **(carbamazepine, fosphenytoin, phenobarbital, phenytoin, primidone)** are predicted to moderately decrease the exposure to **rivaroxaban**. Avoid unless patient can be monitored for signs of thrombosis. Severe Study
- Antifungals, azoles **(itraconazole, ketoconazole)** are predicted to increase the exposure to **rivaroxaban**. Avoid. Severe Study
- Enzalutamide is predicted to moderately decrease the exposure to **rivaroxaban**. Avoid unless patient can be monitored for signs of thrombosis. Severe Study
- HIV-protease inhibitors **(ritonavir)** moderately increase the exposure to **rivaroxaban**. Avoid. Severe Study
- Rifampicin is predicted to moderately decrease the exposure to **rivaroxaban**. Avoid unless patient can be monitored for signs of thrombosis. Severe Study

Rivastigmine → see anticholinesterases, centrally acting
Rizatriptan → see **TABLE 13** p. 821 (serotonin syndrome)
- Beta blockers, non-selective **(propranolol)** slightly to moderately increase the exposure to **rizatriptan**. Adjust **rizatriptan** dose and separate administration by at least 2 hours. Moderate Study
- **Rizatriptan** is predicted to increase the risk of vasoconstriction when given with ergotamine. Ergotamine should be taken at least 24 hours before or 6 hours after **rizatriptan**. Severe Theoretical
- Moclobemide moderately increases the exposure to **rizatriptan**. Avoid. Moderate Study → Also see **TABLE 13** p. 821
- Monoamine-oxidase A and B inhibitors, irreversible are predicted to increase the exposure to **rizatriptan**. Avoid and for 14 days after stopping the MAOI. Severe Theoretical → Also see **TABLE 13** p. 821

Rocuronium → see neuromuscular blocking drugs, non-depolarising
Roflumilast
- Aminophylline is predicted to slightly increase the exposure to **roflumilast**. Avoid. Moderate Theoretical
- Antiepileptics **(carbamazepine, fosphenytoin, phenobarbital, phenytoin, primidone)** are predicted to decrease the exposure to **roflumilast**. Avoid. Moderate Study
- Combined hormonal contraceptives are predicted to increase the exposure to **roflumilast**. Moderate Theoretical
- Enzalutamide is predicted to decrease the exposure to **roflumilast**. Moderate Study
- H₂ receptor antagonists **(cimetidine)** slightly increase the exposure to **roflumilast**. Moderate Study
- Quinolones **(ciprofloxacin)** are predicted to increase the exposure to **roflumilast**. Moderate Theoretical
- Rifampicin is predicted to decrease the exposure to **roflumilast**. Avoid. Moderate Study
- SSRIs **(fluvoxamine)** are predicted to increase the exposure to **roflumilast**. Moderate Study
- Theophylline is predicted to slightly increase the exposure to **roflumilast**. Avoid. Moderate Theoretical

Ropinirole → see dopamine receptor agonists
Ropivacaine → see anaesthetics, local
Rosuvastatin → see statins

Rotavirus vaccine → see live vaccines
Rotigotine → see dopamine receptor agonists
Rufinamide → see antiepileptics
Ruxolitinib → see **TABLE 15** p. 821 (myelosuppression)
- Antiarrhythmics **(dronedarone)** are predicted to increase the exposure to **ruxolitinib**. Moderate Theoretical
- Antiepileptics **(carbamazepine, fosphenytoin, phenobarbital, phenytoin, primidone)** are predicted to decrease the exposure to **ruxolitinib**. Monitor and adjust dose. Moderate Study
- Antifungals, azoles **(fluconazole, isavuconazole, posaconazole)** are predicted to increase the exposure to **ruxolitinib**. Moderate Theoretical
- Antifungals, azoles **(itraconazole, ketoconazole, voriconazole)** are predicted to increase the exposure to **ruxolitinib**. Adjust dose and monitor side effects. Moderate Study
- Aprepitant is predicted to increase the exposure to **ruxolitinib**. Moderate Theoretical
- Bosentan is predicted to decrease the exposure to **ruxolitinib**. Monitor and adjust dose. Moderate Theoretical
- Calcium channel blockers **(diltiazem, verapamil)** are predicted to increase the exposure to **ruxolitinib**. Moderate Theoretical
- Cobicistat is predicted to increase the exposure to **ruxolitinib**. Adjust dose and monitor side effects. Moderate Study
- **Ruxolitinib** is predicted to increase the risk of bleeding events when given with coumarins. Severe Theoretical
- Crizotinib is predicted to increase the exposure to **ruxolitinib**. Moderate Theoretical → Also see **TABLE 15** p. 821
- Efavirenz is predicted to decrease the exposure to **ruxolitinib**. Monitor and adjust dose. Moderate Theoretical
- Enzalutamide is predicted to decrease the exposure to **ruxolitinib**. Monitor and adjust dose. Moderate Study
- Grapefruit juice is predicted to increase the exposure to **ruxolitinib**. Severe Theoretical
- HIV-protease inhibitors **(atazanavir, darunavir, fosamprenavir, lopinavir, ritonavir, saquinavir, tipranavir)** are predicted to increase the exposure to **ruxolitinib**. Adjust dose and monitor side effects. Moderate Study
- HIV-protease inhibitors **(indinavir)** are predicted to increase the exposure to **ruxolitinib**. Moderate Theoretical
- Idelalisib is predicted to increase the exposure to **ruxolitinib**. Adjust dose and monitor side effects. Moderate Study → Also see **TABLE 15** p. 821
- Imatinib is predicted to increase the exposure to **ruxolitinib**. Moderate Theoretical → Also see **TABLE 15** p. 821
- Macrolides **(clarithromycin)** are predicted to increase the exposure to **ruxolitinib**. Adjust dose and monitor side effects. Moderate Study
- Macrolides **(erythromycin)** are predicted to increase the exposure to **ruxolitinib**. Moderate Theoretical
- Netupitant is predicted to increase the exposure to **ruxolitinib**. Moderate Theoretical
- Nevirapine is predicted to decrease the exposure to **ruxolitinib**. Monitor and adjust dose. Moderate Theoretical
- Nilotinib is predicted to increase the exposure to **ruxolitinib**. Moderate Theoretical → Also see **TABLE 15** p. 821
- **Ruxolitinib** is predicted to increase the risk of bleeding events when given with phenindione. Severe Theoretical
- Rifampicin is predicted to decrease the exposure to **ruxolitinib**. Monitor and adjust dose. Moderate Study
- St John's Wort is predicted to decrease the exposure to **ruxolitinib**. Monitor and adjust dose. Moderate Theoretical

Sacubitril → see **TABLE 8** p. 819 (hypotension)
- Ciclosporin is predicted to increase the exposure to **sacubitril**. Moderate Theoretical
- Rifampicin is predicted to increase the exposure to **sacubitril**. Moderate Theoretical
- **Sacubitril** is predicted to increase the exposure to statins. Severe Study
- Tenofovir is predicted to increase the exposure to **sacubitril**. Moderate Theoretical

Safinamide → see monoamine-oxidase B inhibitors
Salbutamol → see beta₂ agonists
Salmeterol → see beta₂ agonists
Sapropterin → see **TABLE 8** p. 819 (hypotension)

- Methotrexate is predicted to decrease the efficacy of sapropterin. Moderate Theoretical
- Phosphodiesterase type-5 inhibitors are predicted to increase the risk of hypotension when given with sapropterin. Moderate Theoretical → Also see TABLE 8 p. 819
- Trimethoprim is predicted to decrease the efficacy of sapropterin. Moderate Theoretical

Saquinavir → see HIV-protease inhibitors

Saxagliptin → see TABLE 14 p. 821 (antidiabetic drugs)
- Antiarrhythmics (dronedarone) are predicted to increase the exposure to saxagliptin. Mild Study
- Antiepileptics (carbamazepine, fosphenytoin, phenobarbital, phenytoin, primidone) are predicted to moderately decrease the exposure to saxagliptin. Moderate Study
- Antifungals, azoles (fluconazole, isavuconazole, posaconazole) are predicted to increase the exposure to saxagliptin. Mild Study
- Antifungals, azoles (itraconazole, ketoconazole, voriconazole) are predicted to increase the exposure to saxagliptin. Moderate Study
- Aprepitant is predicted to increase the exposure to saxagliptin. Mild Study
- Calcium channel blockers (diltiazem, verapamil) are predicted to increase the exposure to saxagliptin. Mild Study
- Cobicistat is predicted to increase the exposure to saxagliptin. Moderate Study
- Crizotinib is predicted to increase the exposure to saxagliptin. Mild Study
- Enzalutamide is predicted to moderately decrease the exposure to saxagliptin. Moderate Study
- Grapefruit juice is predicted to increase the exposure to saxagliptin. Mild Theoretical
- HIV-protease inhibitors (atazanavir, darunavir, fosamprenavir, lopinavir, ritonavir, saquinavir, tipranavir) are predicted to increase the exposure to saxagliptin. Moderate Study
- HIV-protease inhibitors (indinavir) are predicted to increase the exposure to saxagliptin. Mild Study
- Idelalisib is predicted to increase the exposure to saxagliptin. Moderate Study
- Imatinib is predicted to increase the exposure to saxagliptin. Mild Study
- Macrolides (clarithromycin) are predicted to increase the exposure to saxagliptin. Moderate Study
- Macrolides (erythromycin) are predicted to increase the exposure to saxagliptin. Mild Study
- Netupitant is predicted to increase the exposure to saxagliptin. Mild Study
- Nilotinib is predicted to increase the exposure to saxagliptin. Mild Study
- Rifampicin is predicted to moderately decrease the exposure to saxagliptin. Moderate Study

Secukinumab → see monoclonal antibodies

Selegiline → see monoamine-oxidase B inhibitors

Selenium
- Selenium is predicted to decrease the absorption of eltrombopag. Eltrombopag should be taken 2 hours before or 4 hours after selenium. Severe Theoretical

Selexipag
- Antiepileptics (valproate) are predicted to increase the exposure to selexipag. Unknown Theoretical
- Antifungals, azoles (fluconazole) are predicted to increase the exposure to selexipag. Unknown Theoretical
- Fibrates (gemfibrozil) are predicted to increase the exposure to selexipag. Avoid. Severe Theoretical
- Rifampicin is predicted to decrease the exposure to selexipag. Unknown Theoretical

Senna → see TABLE 17 p. 822 (reduced serum potassium)

Sertraline → see SSRIs

Sevoflurane → see volatile halogenated anaesthetics

Sildenafil → see phosphodiesterase type-5 inhibitors

Siltuximab → see monoclonal antibodies

Silver sulfadiazine

PHARMACOLOGY Silver might inactivate enzymatic debriding agents—concurrent use might not be appropriate.

Simeprevir
- Antiarrhythmics (dronedarone) are predicted to increase the exposure to simeprevir. Avoid. Severe Study
- Simeprevir is predicted to increase the concentration of antiarrhythmics (amiodarone). Refer to specialist literature. Severe Anecdotal
- Antiepileptics (carbamazepine, fosphenytoin, phenobarbital, phenytoin, primidone) are predicted to decrease the exposure to simeprevir. Avoid. Severe Study
- Antiepileptics (oxcarbazepine) are predicted to decrease the exposure to simeprevir. Avoid. Severe Theoretical
- Antifungals, azoles (fluconazole, isavuconazole, itraconazole, ketoconazole, posaconazole, voriconazole) are predicted to increase the exposure to simeprevir. Avoid. Severe Study
- Aprepitant is predicted to increase the exposure to simeprevir. Avoid. Severe Study
- Bosentan is predicted to decrease the exposure to simeprevir. Avoid. Severe Study
- Calcium channel blockers (diltiazem, verapamil) are predicted to increase the exposure to simeprevir. Avoid. Severe Study
- Cobicistat is predicted to increase the exposure to simeprevir. Avoid. Severe Study
- Crizotinib is predicted to increase the exposure to simeprevir. Avoid. Severe Study
- Efavirenz is predicted to decrease the exposure to simeprevir. Avoid. Severe Study
- Enzalutamide is predicted to decrease the exposure to simeprevir. Avoid. Severe Study
- Etravirine is predicted to decrease the exposure to simeprevir. Avoid. Moderate Study
- HIV-protease inhibitors are predicted to increase the exposure to simeprevir. Avoid. Severe Study
- Idelalisib is predicted to increase the exposure to simeprevir. Avoid. Severe Study
- Imatinib is predicted to increase the exposure to simeprevir. Avoid. Severe Study
- Ledipasvir moderately increases the exposure to simeprevir and simeprevir slightly increases the exposure to ledipasvir. Avoid. Severe Study
- Macrolides (clarithromycin, erythromycin) are predicted to increase the exposure to simeprevir. Avoid. Severe Study
- Netupitant is predicted to increase the exposure to simeprevir. Avoid. Severe Study
- Nevirapine is predicted to decrease the exposure to simeprevir. Avoid. Severe Study
- Nilotinib is predicted to increase the exposure to simeprevir. Avoid. Severe Study
- Rifabutin is predicted to decrease the exposure to simeprevir. Avoid. Moderate Theoretical
- Rifampicin is predicted to decrease the exposure to simeprevir. Avoid. Severe Study
- St John's Wort is predicted to decrease the exposure to simeprevir. Avoid. Severe Study
- Simeprevir moderately increases the exposure to statins (atorvastatin). Monitor and adjust dose. Moderate Study
- Simeprevir is predicted to increase the exposure to statins (pravastatin). Monitor and adjust dose. Severe Theoretical
- Simeprevir moderately increases the exposure to statins (rosuvastatin). Adjust rosuvastatin dose, p. 130. Moderate Study
- Simeprevir slightly increases the exposure to statins (simvastatin). Monitor and adjust dose. Moderate Study

Simvastatin → see statins

Sirolimus
- Antiarrhythmics (amiodarone) are predicted to increase the concentration of sirolimus. Severe Anecdotal
- Antiarrhythmics (dronedarone) increase the concentration of sirolimus. Monitor and adjust dose. Moderate Study
- Antiepileptics (carbamazepine, fosphenytoin, phenobarbital, phenytoin, primidone) are predicted to decrease the concentration of sirolimus. Avoid. Severe Study
- Antifungals, azoles (fluconazole, isavuconazole, posaconazole) increase the concentration of sirolimus. Monitor and adjust dose. Moderate Study

A1

Interactions | Appendix 1

Sirolimus (continued)

▶ Antifungals, azoles **(itraconazole, ketoconazole, voriconazole)** are predicted to increase the concentration of **sirolimus**. Avoid. Severe Study

▶ Antifungals, azoles **(miconazole)** are predicted to increase the concentration of **sirolimus**. Monitor and adjust dose. Moderate Study

▶ Aprepitant increases the concentration of **sirolimus**. Monitor and adjust dose. Moderate Study

▶ Bosentan is predicted to decrease the concentration of **sirolimus** and **sirolimus** potentially increases the concentration of **bosentan**. Avoid. Severe Theoretical

▷ Calcium channel blockers **(diltiazem, verapamil)** increase the concentration of **sirolimus**. Monitor and adjust dose. Moderate Study

▶ Ceritinib is predicted to increase the exposure to **sirolimus**. Avoid. Severe Theoretical

▷ Ciclosporin moderately increases the exposure to **sirolimus**. Separate administration by 4 hours. Severe Study

▶ Cobicistat is predicted to increase the concentration of **sirolimus**. Avoid. Severe Study

▶ Crizotinib increases the concentration of **sirolimus**. Monitor and adjust dose. Moderate Study

▶ Efavirenz is predicted to decrease the concentration of **sirolimus**. Monitor and adjust dose. Moderate Theoretical

▶ Enzalutamide is predicted to decrease the concentration of **sirolimus**. Avoid. Severe Study

▶ Grapefruit juice increases the concentration of **sirolimus**. Avoid. Moderate Study

▶ HIV-protease inhibitors **(atazanavir, darunavir, fosamprenavir, lopinavir, ritonavir, saquinavir, tipranavir)** are predicted to increase the concentration of **sirolimus**. Avoid. Severe Study

▶ HIV-protease inhibitors **(indinavir)** increase the concentration of **sirolimus**. Monitor and adjust dose. Moderate Study

▶ Idelalisib is predicted to increase the concentration of **sirolimus**. Avoid. Severe Study

▶ Imatinib increases the concentration of **sirolimus**. Monitor and adjust dose. Moderate Study

▶ Lapatinib is predicted to increase the exposure to **sirolimus**. Moderate Theoretical

▶ Live vaccines are predicted to increase the risk of generalised infection (possibly life-threatening) when given with **sirolimus**. Public Health England advises avoid. Severe Theoretical

▶ Lumacaftor is predicted to decrease the exposure to **sirolimus**. Avoid. Severe Study

▷ Macrolides **(clarithromycin)** are predicted to increase the concentration of **sirolimus**. Avoid. Severe Study

▶ Macrolides **(erythromycin)** increase the concentration of **sirolimus**. Monitor and adjust dose. Moderate Study

▶ Sirolimus is predicted to decrease the efficacy of **mifamurtide**. Avoid. Severe Theoretical

▶ Mirabegron is predicted to increase the exposure to **sirolimus**. Mild Theoretical

▶ Netupitant increases the concentration of **sirolimus**. Monitor and adjust dose. Moderate Study

▶ Nevirapine is predicted to decrease the concentration of **sirolimus**. Monitor and adjust dose. Moderate Theoretical

▶ Nilotinib increases the concentration of **sirolimus**. Monitor and adjust dose. Moderate Study

▶ Palbociclib is predicted to increase the exposure to **sirolimus**. Adjust dose. Moderate Theoretical

▶ Pitolisant is predicted to decrease the exposure to **sirolimus**. Avoid. Severe Theoretical

▶ Rifampicin is predicted to decrease the concentration of **sirolimus**. Avoid. Severe Study

▶ St John's Wort is predicted to decrease the concentration of **sirolimus**. Monitor and adjust dose. Severe Theoretical

▶ Sirolimus is predicted to decrease the concentration of **tacrolimus** and **tacrolimus** increases the exposure to **sirolimus**. Severe Study

▶ Velpatasvir is predicted to increase the exposure to **sirolimus**. Severe Theoretical

Sitagliptin → see TABLE 14 p. 821 (antidiabetic drugs)

Sodium aurothiomalate

▶ ACE inhibitors are predicted to increase the risk of hypersensitivity when given with **sodium aurothiomalate**. Severe Anecdotal

▶ Sodium aurothiomalate potentially increases the risk of side-effects when given with **penicillamine** (in those who have had previous adverse reactions to gold). Avoid. Severe Study

Sodium bicarbonate

▶ Sodium bicarbonate decreases the concentration of **lithium**. Severe Anecdotal

▶ Sodium bicarbonate is predicted to decrease the efficacy of **methenamine**. Avoid. Moderate Theoretical

Sodium citrate

▶ Sodium citrate is predicted to decrease the efficacy of **methenamine**. Avoid. Moderate Theoretical

▶ Sodium citrate is predicted to increase the risk of side-effects when given with **sucralfate**. Avoid. Moderate Theoretical

Sodium clodronate → see bisphosphonates

Sodium feredetate → see iron (oral)

Sodium nitroprusside → see TABLE 8 p. 819 (hypotension)

▶ Sodium nitroprusside is predicted to increase the risk of methaemoglobinaemia when given with topical anaesthetics, local **(prilocaine)**. Use with caution or avoid. Severe Theoretical

▶ Sodium nitroprusside is predicted to increase the risk of methaemoglobinaemia when given with **dapsone**. Severe Theoretical

Sodium oxybate → see TABLE 8 p. 819 (hypotension), TABLE 11 p. 820 (CNS depressant effects)

▶ Antiepileptics **(valproate)** increase the exposure to **sodium oxybate**. Adjust sodium oxybate dose. Moderate Study

Sodium phenylbutyrate

▶ Antiepileptics **(valproate)** potentially decrease the effects of **sodium phenylbutyrate**. Moderate Anecdotal

▶ Corticosteroids potentially decrease the effects of **sodium phenylbutyrate**. Moderate Anecdotal

▶ Haloperidol potentially decreases the effects of **sodium phenylbutyrate**. Moderate Anecdotal

Sodium picosulfate → see TABLE 18 p. 822 (hyponatraemia), TABLE 17 p. 822 (reduced serum potassium)

Sodium stibogluconate

▶ Sodium stibogluconate increases the risk of cardiovascular side-effects when given with **amphotericin**. Separate administration by 14 days. Severe Study

Sofosbuvir

▶ Sofosbuvir is predicted to increase the risk of severe bradycardia or heart block when given with antiarrhythmics **(amiodarone)**. Refer to specialist literature. Severe Anecdotal

▶ Antiepileptics **(carbamazepine, fosphenytoin, oxcarbazepine, phenobarbital, phenytoin, primidone)** are predicted to decrease the exposure to **sofosbuvir**. Avoid. Severe Study

▶ H₂ receptor antagonists potentially decrease the exposure to **sofosbuvir**. Adjust dose, see sofosbuvir with ledipasvir and sofosbuvir with velpatasvir. Moderate Study

▶ HIV-protease inhibitors **(tipranavir)** are predicted to decrease the exposure to **sofosbuvir**. Avoid. Severe Theoretical

▶ Proton pump inhibitors potentially decrease the exposure to **sofosbuvir**. Adjust dose, see sofosbuvir with ledipasvir and sofosbuvir with velpatasvir. Moderate Study

▶ Rifampicin is predicted to decrease the exposure to **sofosbuvir**. Avoid. Severe Study

▶ St John's Wort is predicted to decrease the exposure to **sofosbuvir**. Avoid. Severe Study

Solifenacin → see TABLE 10 p. 820 (antimuscarinics)

▶ Antiepileptics **(carbamazepine, fosphenytoin, phenobarbital, phenytoin, primidone)** are predicted to decrease the exposure to **solifenacin**. Moderate Theoretical

▶ Antifungals, azoles **(itraconazole, ketoconazole, voriconazole)** are predicted to increase the exposure to **solifenacin**. Adjust solifenacin or tamsulosin with solifenacin dose; avoid in hepatic and renal impairment. Severe Study

▶ Cobicistat is predicted to increase the exposure to **solifenacin**. Adjust solifenacin or tamsulosin with solifenacin dose; avoid in hepatic and renal impairment. Severe Study

▶ Enzalutamide is predicted to decrease the exposure to **solifenacin**. Moderate Theoretical

▶ HIV-protease inhibitors (atazanavir, darunavir, fosamprenavir, lopinavir, ritonavir, saquinavir, tipranavir) are predicted to increase the exposure to **solifenacin**. Adjust **solifenacin** or **tamsulosin with solifenacin** dose; avoid in hepatic and renal impairment. Severe Study

▶ Idelalisib is predicted to increase the exposure to **solifenacin**. Adjust **solifenacin** or **tamsulosin with solifenacin** dose; avoid in hepatic and renal impairment. Severe Study

▶ Macrolides (clarithromycin) are predicted to increase the exposure to **solifenacin**. Adjust **solifenacin** or **tamsulosin with solifenacin** dose; avoid in hepatic and renal impairment. Severe Study

▶ Rifampicin is predicted to decrease the exposure to **solifenacin**. Moderate Theoretical

Somatropin

▶ Corticosteroids are predicted to decrease the effects of **somatropin**. Moderate Theoretical

Sorafenib → see TABLE 15 p. 821 (myelosuppression), TABLE 9 p. 820 (QT-interval prolongation)

▶ Antiepileptics (carbamazepine, fosphenytoin, phenobarbital, phenytoin, primidone) are predicted to decrease the exposure to **sorafenib**. Moderate Theoretical

▶ Sorafenib increases the anticoagulant effect of **coumarins**. Severe Anecdotal

▶ Enzalutamide is predicted to decrease the exposure to **sorafenib**. Moderate Theoretical

▶ Neomycin moderately decreases the exposure to **sorafenib**. Moderate Study

▶ Sorafenib is predicted to increase the risk of bleeding events when given with **phenindione**. Severe Theoretical

▶ Rifampicin is predicted to decrease the exposure to **sorafenib**. Moderate Theoretical

Sotalol → see beta blockers, non-selective

Spironolactone → see aldosterone antagonists

SSRIs → see TABLE 18 p. 822 (hyponatraemia), TABLE 13 p. 821 (serotonin syndrome), TABLE 9 p. 820 (QT-interval prolongation), TABLE 4 p. 818 (antiplatelet effects)

> citalopram · dapoxetine · escitalopram · fluoxetine · fluvoxamine · paroxetine · sertraline

▶ Fluvoxamine very markedly increases the exposure to **agomelatine**. Avoid. Severe Study

▶ Fluvoxamine moderately increases the exposure to **alprazolam**. Adjust dose. Moderate Study

▶ SSRIs (fluoxetine, paroxetine) are predicted to increase the exposure to **amfetamines**. Severe Theoretical → Also see TABLE 13 p. 821

▶ Fluvoxamine moderately to markedly increases the exposure to **aminophylline**. Avoid. Severe Study

▶ Fluvoxamine decreases the clearance of anaesthetics, local (**ropivacaine**). Avoid prolonged use. Moderate Study

▶ Fluvoxamine is predicted to increase the exposure to **anagrelide**. Moderate Theoretical → Also see TABLE 4 p. 818

▶ Antiarrhythmics (dronedarone) are predicted to increase the exposure to **dapoxetine**. Adjust **dapoxetine** dose. Moderate Theoretical

▶ Antiarrhythmics (dronedarone) are predicted to increase the exposure to SSRIs (**citalopram, escitalopram, fluoxetine, fluvoxamine, paroxetine, sertraline**). Severe Theoretical → Also see TABLE 9 p. 820

▶ SSRIs (fluoxetine, paroxetine) are predicted to increase the exposure to antiarrhythmics (**flecainide**). Severe Theoretical

▶ SSRIs (fluoxetine, fluvoxamine, paroxetine) are predicted to increase the exposure to antiarrhythmics (**propafenone**). Monitor and adjust dose. Moderate Study

▶ SSRIs (fluoxetine, paroxetine) are predicted to increase the exposure to anticholinesterases, centrally acting (**donepezil**). Moderate Theoretical

▶ SSRIs (fluoxetine, paroxetine) are predicted to increase the exposure to anticholinesterases, centrally acting (**galantamine**). Monitor and adjust dose. Moderate Study

▶ Antiepileptics (fosphenytoin, phenytoin) decrease the concentration of **paroxetine**. Moderate Study

▶ Sertraline potentially increases the risk of toxicity when given with antiepileptics (**fosphenytoin, phenytoin**). Monitor concentration and adjust dose. Severe Anecdotal

▶ SSRIs (fluoxetine, fluvoxamine) are predicted to increase the concentration of antiepileptics (**fosphenytoin, phenytoin**). Monitor and adjust dose. Severe Anecdotal

▶ Antifungals, azoles (fluconazole, isavuconazole, posaconazole) are predicted to increase the exposure to **dapoxetine**. Adjust **dapoxetine** dose. Moderate Theoretical

▶ Antifungals, azoles (itraconazole, ketoconazole, voriconazole) are predicted to moderately increase the exposure to **dapoxetine**. Avoid or adjust **dapoxetine** dose. Severe Study

▶ Antifungals, azoles (voriconazole) are predicted to increase the exposure to **citalopram**. Severe Theoretical → Also see TABLE 9 p. 820

▶ Antihistamines, sedating (cyproheptadine) potentially decrease the effects of **SSRIs**. Moderate Anecdotal

▶ Aprepitant is predicted to increase the exposure to **dapoxetine**. Adjust **dapoxetine** dose. Moderate Theoretical

▶ SSRIs (fluoxetine, paroxetine) are predicted to moderately increase the exposure to **aripiprazole**. Adjust **aripiprazole** dose, p. 240. Moderate Study

▶ Fluvoxamine increases the exposure to **asenapine**. Moderate Study

▶ Paroxetine moderately increases the exposure to **asenapine**. Moderate Study

▶ SSRIs (fluoxetine, paroxetine) are predicted to markedly increase the exposure to **atomoxetine**. Adjust dose. Severe Study

▶ SSRIs (fluoxetine, paroxetine) are predicted to increase the exposure to beta blockers, non-selective (**carvedilol, timolol**). Moderate Study

▶ Fluvoxamine moderately increases the concentration of beta blockers, non-selective (**propranolol**). Moderate Study

▶ SSRIs (fluoxetine, paroxetine) are predicted to increase the exposure to beta blockers, selective (**metoprolol, nebivolol**). Moderate Study

▶ Bupropion is predicted to increase the exposure to **dapoxetine**. Moderate Theoretical → Also see TABLE 13 p. 821

▶ Fluvoxamine markedly decreases the clearance of **caffeine citrate**. Monitor and adjust dose. Severe Study

▶ Calcium channel blockers (diltiazem, verapamil) are predicted to increase the exposure to **dapoxetine**. Adjust **dapoxetine** dose. Moderate Theoretical

▶ Fluvoxamine is predicted to increase the exposure to **cilostazol**. Adjust **cilostazol** dose. Moderate Theoretical → Also see TABLE 4 p. 818

▶ Cinacalcet is predicted to increase the exposure to **dapoxetine**. Moderate Theoretical

▶ Fluvoxamine is predicted to increase the exposure to **cinacalcet**. Adjust dose. Moderate Theoretical

▶ Fluvoxamine is predicted to decrease the efficacy of **clopidogrel**. Avoid. Severe Theoretical → Also see TABLE 4 p. 818

▶ Fluvoxamine increases the concentration of **clozapine**. Monitor side effects and adjust dose. Severe Study

▶ Cobicistat is predicted to moderately increase the exposure to **dapoxetine**. Avoid or adjust **dapoxetine** dose. Severe Study

▶ Crizotinib is predicted to increase the exposure to **dapoxetine**. Adjust **dapoxetine** dose. Moderate Theoretical

▶ SSRIs (fluoxetine, paroxetine) are predicted to slightly increase the exposure to **darifenacin**. Mild Study

▶ Fluvoxamine moderately increases the exposure to **diazepam**. Moderate Study

▶ Fluvoxamine is predicted to increase the exposure to dopamine receptor agonists (**ropinirole**). Adjust dose. Moderate Study

▶ Fluvoxamine markedly increases the exposure to **duloxetine**. Avoid. Severe Study → Also see TABLE 18 p. 822 → Also see TABLE 13 p. 821 → Also see TABLE 4 p. 818

▶ Fluvoxamine is predicted to increase the exposure to **erlotinib**. Monitor side effects and adjust dose. Moderate Theoretical

▶ Fluvoxamine increases the concentration of **frovatriptan**. Severe Study → Also see TABLE 13 p. 821

▶ Grapefruit juice moderately increases the exposure to **sertraline**. Avoid. Moderate Study

▶ H₂ receptor antagonists (cimetidine) slightly increase the exposure to SSRIs (**citalopram, escitalopram**). Adjust dose. Moderate Study

A1

Interactions | Appendix 1

SSRIs (continued)

▸ H$_2$ receptor antagonists **(cimetidine)** slightly increase the exposure to SSRIs **(paroxetine, sertraline)**. Moderate Study

▸ **Fluoxetine** increases the concentration of **haloperidol**. Adjust dose. Moderate Anecdotal

▸ **Fluvoxamine** increases the concentration of **haloperidol**. Adjust dose. Moderate Study

▸ HIV-protease inhibitors **(atazanavir, darunavir, fosamprenavir, lopinavir, ritonavir, saquinavir, tipranavir)** are predicted to moderately increase the exposure to **dapoxetine**. Avoid or adjust **dapoxetine** dose. Severe Study

▸ HIV-protease inhibitors **(indinavir)** are predicted to increase the exposure to **dapoxetine**. Adjust **dapoxetine** dose. Moderate Theoretical

▸ **Idelalisib** is predicted to moderately increase the exposure to **dapoxetine**. Avoid or adjust **dapoxetine** dose. Severe Study

▸ **Imatinib** is predicted to increase the exposure to **dapoxetine**. Adjust **dapoxetine** dose. Moderate Theoretical

▸ **Fluoxetine** is predicted to increase the exposure to **lomitapide**. Separate administration by 12 hours. Unknown Theoretical

▸ **Fluvoxamine** is predicted to increase the exposure to **lomitapide**. Separate administration by 12 hours. Moderate Theoretical

▸ **Fluvoxamine** is predicted to increase the exposure to **loxapine**. Avoid. Unknown Theoretical

▸ **Lumacaftor** is predicted to decrease the exposure to SSRIs **(citalopram, escitalopram, sertraline)**. Adjust dose. Moderate Theoretical

▸ Macrolides **(clarithromycin)** are predicted to moderately increase the exposure to **dapoxetine**. Avoid or adjust **dapoxetine** dose. Severe Study

▸ Macrolides **(erythromycin)** are predicted to increase the exposure to **dapoxetine**. Adjust **dapoxetine** dose. Moderate Theoretical

▸ **Fluvoxamine** very markedly increases the exposure to **melatonin**. Avoid. Severe Study

▸ **Netupitant** is predicted to increase the exposure to **dapoxetine**. Adjust **dapoxetine** dose. Moderate Theoretical

▸ **SSRIs** potentially increase the risk of prolonged neuromuscular blockade when given with neuromuscular blocking drugs, non-depolarising **(mivacurium)**. Unknown Theoretical

▸ **Nilotinib** is predicted to increase the exposure to **dapoxetine**. Adjust **dapoxetine** dose. Moderate Theoretical

▸ **Fluvoxamine** moderately increases the exposure to **olanzapine**. Adjust dose. Severe Anecdotal

▸ SSRIs **(fluoxetine, paroxetine)** are predicted to decrease the efficacy of opioids **(codeine)**. Moderate Theoretical

▸ SSRIs **(fluoxetine, paroxetine)** are predicted to decrease the efficacy of opioids **(tramadol)**. Severe Study → Also see TABLE 13 p. 821

▸ **Fluvoxamine** is predicted to increase the exposure to **pentoxifylline**. Moderate Theoretical

▸ **Paroxetine** markedly increases the exposure to phenothiazines **(perphenazine)**. Severe Study

▸ **Fluvoxamine** is predicted to moderately increase the exposure to **pirfenidone**. Avoid. Moderate Study

▸ SSRIs **(fluoxetine, paroxetine)** are predicted to moderately increase the exposure to **pitolisant**. Use with caution and adjust dose. Moderate Study

▸ **Fluvoxamine** moderately increases the exposure to **pomalidomide**. Adjust **pomalidomide** dose. Moderate Study

▸ **Paroxetine** slightly increases the exposure to **procyclidine**. Monitor and adjust **procyclidine** dose. Moderate Study

▸ Proton pump inhibitors **(esomeprazole)** are predicted to slightly to moderately increase the exposure to **citalopram**. Monitor and adjust dose. Severe Theoretical

▸ Proton pump inhibitors **(esomeprazole)** are predicted to increase the exposure to **escitalopram**. Monitor and adjust dose. Severe Theoretical

▸ **Fluvoxamine** is predicted to increase the exposure to **proton pump inhibitors**. Mild Study

▸ Proton pump inhibitors **(omeprazole)** slightly to moderately increase the exposure to SSRIs **(citalopram, escitalopram)**. Monitor and adjust dose. Severe Study

▸ **Fluvoxamine** is predicted to increase the exposure to **riluzole**. Moderate Theoretical

▸ SSRIs **(fluoxetine, paroxetine)** are predicted to increase the exposure to **risperidone**. Adjust dose. Moderate Study

▸ **Fluvoxamine** is predicted to increase the exposure to **roflumilast**. Moderate Study

▸ SSRIs **(fluoxetine, paroxetine)** are predicted to increase the exposure to SSRIs **(dapoxetine)**. Moderate Theoretical → Also see TABLE 18 p. 822 → Also see TABLE 13 p. 821 → Also see TABLE 4 p. 818

▸ **SSRIs** potentially increase the risk of prolonged neuromuscular blockade when given with **suxamethonium**. Unknown Theoretical

▸ SSRIs **(fluoxetine, paroxetine)** are predicted to decrease the efficacy of **tamoxifen**. Avoid. Severe Study

▸ **Terbinafine** is predicted to increase the exposure to **fluoxetine**. Adjust dose. Moderate Theoretical

▸ **Terbinafine** moderately increases the exposure to **paroxetine**. Moderate Study

▸ **Terbinafine** is predicted to increase the exposure to SSRIs **(citalopram, dapoxetine, escitalopram, fluvoxamine, sertraline)**. Moderate Theoretical

▸ **Fluvoxamine** moderately to markedly increases the exposure to **theophylline**. Avoid. Severe Study

▸ **Fluvoxamine** very markedly increases the exposure to **tizanidine**. Avoid. Severe Study

▸ SSRIs **(fluoxetine, paroxetine)** are predicted to increase the exposure to **tricyclic antidepressants**. Monitor for toxicity and adjust dose. Severe Study → Also see TABLE 13 p. 821 → Also see TABLE 18 p. 822

▸ **Fluvoxamine** increases the exposure to tricyclic antidepressants **(amitriptyline, imipramine)**. Adjust dose. Severe Study → Also see TABLE 18 p. 822 → Also see TABLE 13 p. 821

▸ **Fluvoxamine** markedly increases the exposure to tricyclic antidepressants **(clomipramine)**. Adjust dose. Severe Study → Also see TABLE 18 p. 822 → Also see TABLE 13 p. 821

▸ SSRIs **(fluoxetine, paroxetine)** are predicted to increase the exposure to **vortioxetine**. Monitor and adjust dose. Moderate Study → Also see TABLE 13 p. 821 → Also see TABLE 4 p. 818

▸ **Fluvoxamine** is predicted to increase the exposure to **zolmitriptan**. Adjust **zolmitriptan** dose, p. 280. Severe Theoretical → Also see TABLE 13 p. 821

St John's Wort → see TABLE 13 p. 821 (serotonin syndrome)

▸ **St John's Wort** is predicted to decrease the exposure to **afatinib**. Moderate Study

▸ **St John's Wort** is predicted to slightly decrease the exposure to aldosterone antagonists **(eplerenone)**. Avoid. Moderate Study

▸ **St John's Wort** decreases the exposure to **aliskiren**. Moderate Study

▸ **St John's Wort** moderately decreases the exposure to **alprazolam**. Moderate Study

▸ **St John's Wort** is predicted to decrease the concentration of **aminophylline**. Moderate Theoretical

▸ **St John's Wort** is predicted to decrease the exposure to antiarrhythmics **(dronedarone)**. Avoid. Severe Theoretical

▸ **St John's Wort** is predicted to decrease the exposure to antiepileptics **(brivaracetam)**. Moderate Theoretical

▸ **St John's Wort** is predicted to decrease the concentration of antiepileptics **(carbamazepine)**. Monitor and adjust dose. Moderate Theoretical

▸ **St John's Wort** is predicted to decrease the concentration of antiepileptics **(fosphenytoin, phenobarbital, phenytoin, primidone)**. Avoid. Severe Theoretical

▸ **St John's Wort** is predicted to decrease the exposure to antiepileptics **(perampanel)**. Monitor and adjust dose. Moderate Theoretical

▸ **St John's Wort** is predicted to decrease the exposure to antifungals, azoles **(isavuconazole)**. Avoid. Severe Theoretical

▸ **St John's Wort** moderately decreases the exposure to antifungals, azoles **(voriconazole)**. Avoid. Moderate Study

▸ **St John's Wort** is predicted to decrease the concentration of antimalarials **(piperaquine)**. Avoid. Moderate Theoretical

▸ **St John's Wort** is predicted to decrease the exposure to **apixaban**. Use with caution or avoid. Moderate Theoretical

▸ **St John's Wort** is predicted to decrease the exposure to **apremilast**. Avoid. Severe Theoretical

- St John's Wort is predicted to decrease the exposure to aprepitant. Avoid. Moderate Theoretical
- St John's Wort is predicted to decrease the exposure to **axitinib**. Moderate Theoretical
- St John's Wort is predicted to decrease the exposure to bedaquiline. Avoid. Severe Study
- St John's Wort is predicted to decrease the exposure to bosentan. Avoid. Moderate Theoretical
- St John's Wort is predicted to decrease the exposure to bosutinib. Avoid. Severe Theoretical
- St John's Wort is predicted to decrease the exposure to cabozantinib. Moderate Theoretical
- St John's Wort is predicted to decrease the exposure to calcium channel blockers **(amlodipine, felodipine, isradipine, lacidipine, lercanidipine, nicardipine, nifedipine, nimodipine)**. Monitor and adjust dose. Moderate Theoretical
- St John's Wort is predicted to decrease the exposure to calcium channel blockers **(diltiazem, verapamil)**. Moderate Theoretical
- St John's Wort is predicted to decrease the exposure to ceritinib. Avoid. Severe Theoretical
- St John's Wort decreases the concentration of **ciclosporin**. Avoid. Moderate Study
- St John's Wort is predicted to alter the effects of **cilostazol**. Moderate Theoretical
- St John's Wort is predicted to decrease the exposure to cobicistat. Avoid. Severe Theoretical
- St John's Wort is predicted to decrease the exposure to cobimetinib. Avoid. Severe Theoretical
- St John's Wort decreases the efficacy of **combined hormonal contraceptives**. MHRA advises avoid. For FSRH guidance, see Contraceptives, interactions p. 474. Severe Anecdotal
- St John's Wort decreases the anticoagulant effect of **coumarins**. Avoid. Severe Anecdotal
- St John's Wort is predicted to decrease the exposure to crizotinib. Avoid. Severe Theoretical
- St John's Wort is predicted to decrease the exposure to dabigatran. Avoid. Severe Study
- St John's Wort is predicted to decrease the exposure to daclatasvir. Avoid. Severe Theoretical
- St John's Wort is predicted to decrease the exposure to darifenacin. Moderate Theoretical
- St John's Wort is predicted to decrease the exposure to dasabuvir. Avoid. Severe Theoretical
- St John's Wort is predicted to decrease the exposure to dasatinib. Severe Study
- St John's Wort is predicted to decrease the efficacy of desogestrel. MHRA advises avoid. For FSRH guidance, see Contraceptives, interactions p. 474. Severe Theoretical
- St John's Wort decreases the concentration of **digoxin**. Avoid. Severe Anecdotal
- St John's Wort decreases the exposure to **dolutegravir**. Adjust dose. Severe Study
- St John's Wort is predicted to decrease the exposure to edoxaban. Moderate Study
- St John's Wort is predicted to decrease the concentration of efavirenz. Avoid. Severe Theoretical
- St John's Wort is predicted to moderately decrease the exposure to elbasvir. Avoid. Severe Study
- St John's Wort is predicted to decrease the concentration of elvitegravir. Avoid. Severe Theoretical
- St John's Wort is predicted to decrease the effects of ergotamine. Moderate Theoretical
- St John's Wort is predicted to decrease the exposure to erlotinib. Severe Theoretical
- St John's Wort is predicted to decrease the efficacy of etonogestrel. MHRA advises avoid. For FSRH guidance, see Contraceptives, interactions p. 474. Severe Theoretical
- St John's Wort is predicted to decrease the exposure to etravirine. Avoid. Severe Study
- St John's Wort is predicted to decrease the concentration of everolimus. Avoid or adjust dose. Severe Study
- St John's Wort is predicted to decrease the exposure to exemestane. Moderate Theoretical
- St John's Wort is predicted to decrease the exposure to fesoterodine. Avoid. Severe Theoretical

- St John's Wort is predicted to decrease the exposure to fingolimod. Avoid. Moderate Theoretical
- St John's Wort is predicted to decrease the exposure to fosaprepitant. Avoid. Moderate Theoretical
- St John's Wort is predicted to decrease the exposure to gefitinib. Avoid. Severe Theoretical
- St John's Wort is predicted to markedly decrease the exposure to grazoprevir. Avoid. Severe Study
- St John's Wort is predicted to decrease the concentration of guanfacine. Adjust dose. Moderate Theoretical
- St John's Wort is predicted to decrease the exposure to **HIV-protease inhibitors**. Avoid. Severe Study
- St John's Wort is predicted to decrease the efficacy of **Hormone replacement therapy**. Moderate Theoretical
- St John's Wort is predicted to decrease the exposure to ibrutinib. Avoid. Severe Theoretical
- St John's Wort is predicted to decrease the exposure to idelalisib. Avoid. Severe Theoretical
- St John's Wort is predicted to decrease the exposure to imatinib. Moderate Study
- St John's Wort slightly decreases the exposure to **irinotecan**. Avoid. Severe Study
- St John's Wort decreases the exposure to **ivabradine**. Avoid. Moderate Study
- St John's Wort is predicted to decrease the exposure to ivacaftor. Avoid. Severe Theoretical
- St John's Wort is predicted to decrease the exposure to ixazomib. Avoid. Severe Theoretical
- St John's Wort is predicted to decrease the exposure to lapatinib. Avoid. Severe Study
- St John's Wort is predicted to decrease the exposure to ledipasvir. Avoid. Severe Theoretical
- St John's Wort is predicted to decrease the efficacy of levonorgestrel. MHRA advises avoid. For FSRH guidance, see Contraceptives, interactions p. 474. Severe Theoretical
- St John's Wort is predicted to decrease the exposure to lurasidone. Monitor and adjust dose. Moderate Theoretical
- St John's Wort is predicted to decrease the exposure to macitentan. Avoid. Severe Theoretical
- St John's Wort is predicted to decrease the exposure to maraviroc. Avoid. Severe Theoretical
- St John's Wort moderately decreases the exposure to midazolam. Monitor and adjust dose. Moderate Study
- St John's Wort is predicted to decrease the exposure to naloxegol. Avoid. Moderate Theoretical
- St John's Wort is predicted to decrease the concentration of nevirapine. Avoid. Severe Theoretical
- St John's Wort is predicted to decrease the exposure to nilotinib. Avoid. Severe Theoretical
- St John's Wort is predicted to decrease the exposure to nintedanib. Moderate Study
- St John's Wort is predicted to decrease the efficacy of norethisterone. MHRA advises avoid. For FSRH guidance, see Contraceptives, interactions p. 474. Severe Anecdotal
- St John's Wort is predicted to decrease the exposure to olaparib. Avoid. Moderate Theoretical
- St John's Wort is predicted to decrease the exposure to ombitasvir. Avoid. Severe Theoretical
- St John's Wort decreases the exposure to opioids **(methadone)**. Monitor and adjust dose. Severe Study → Also see **TABLE 13** p. 821
- St John's Wort moderately decreases the exposure to opioids **(oxycodone)**. Adjust dose. Moderate Study
- St John's Wort is predicted to decrease the exposure to osimertinib. Avoid. Moderate Theoretical
- St John's Wort is predicted to decrease the exposure to palbociclib. Avoid. Severe Theoretical
- St John's Wort is predicted to decrease the exposure to panobinostat. Avoid. Moderate Theoretical
- St John's Wort is predicted to decrease the exposure to paritaprevir (with ritonavir and ombitasvir). Avoid. Severe Study
- St John's Wort is predicted to decrease the exposure to **phosphodiesterase type-5 inhibitors**. Moderate Theoretical
- St John's Wort slightly decreases the exposure to **pioglitazone**. Mild Study

St John's Wort (continued)

▸ **St John's Wort** is predicted to decrease the exposure to pitolisant. Monitor and adjust dose. Moderate Theoretical
▸ **St John's Wort** is predicted to decrease the exposure to ponatinib. Avoid. Severe Theoretical
▸ **St John's Wort** is predicted to decrease the exposure to ranolazine. Avoid. Severe Study
▸ **St John's Wort** is predicted to decrease the exposure to rilpivirine. Avoid. Severe Theoretical
▸ **St John's Wort** is predicted to decrease the exposure to ruxolitinib. Monitor and adjust dose. Moderate Theoretical
▸ **St John's Wort** is predicted to decrease the exposure to simeprevir. Avoid. Severe Study
▸ **St John's Wort** is predicted to decrease the concentration of sirolimus. Monitor and adjust dose. Severe Theoretical
▸ **St John's Wort** is predicted to decrease the exposure to sofosbuvir. Avoid. Severe Study
▸ **St John's Wort** slightly decreases the exposure to statins (atorvastatin). Mild Study
▸ **St John's Wort** moderately decreases the exposure to statins (simvastatin). Moderate Study
▸ **St John's Wort** decreases the concentration of tacrolimus. Avoid. Severe Study
▸ **St John's Wort** is predicted to decrease the exposure to taxanes (cabazitaxel). Avoid. Severe Study
▸ **St John's Wort** is predicted to decrease the concentration of temsirolimus. Avoid. Severe Theoretical
▸ **St John's Wort** potentially decreases the exposure to theophylline. Severe Anecdotal
▸ **St John's Wort** is predicted to decrease the exposure to ticagrelor. Moderate Theoretical
▸ **St John's Wort** is predicted to decrease the exposure to tolvaptan. Moderate Theoretical
▸ **St John's Wort** is predicted to decrease the exposure to topotecan. Severe Theoretical
▸ **St John's Wort** is predicted to decrease the exposure to velpatasvir. Avoid. Moderate Theoretical
▸ **St John's Wort** is predicted to decrease the exposure to vismodegib. Avoid. Moderate Theoretical

Statins → see TABLE 1 p. 818 (hepatotoxicity)

atorvastatin · fluvastatin · pravastatin · rosuvastatin · simvastatin

▸ **Atorvastatin** slightly to moderately increases the exposure to aliskiren. Moderate Study
▸ **Antacids** moderately decrease the absorption of rosuvastatin. Separate administration by 2 hours. Moderate Study
▸ **Antiarrhythmics (amiodarone)** are predicted to increase the risk of rhabdomyolysis when given with atorvastatin. Monitor and adjust dose. Moderate Theoretical
▸ **Antiarrhythmics (amiodarone)** are predicted to increase the exposure to fluvastatin. Severe Theoretical
▸ **Antiarrhythmics (amiodarone)** increase the risk of rhabdomyolysis when given with simvastatin. Adjust simvastatin dose, p. 130. Severe Study
▸ **Antiarrhythmics (dronedarone)** are predicted to increase the exposure to atorvastatin. Monitor and adjust dose. Severe Theoretical
▸ **Antiarrhythmics (dronedarone)** slightly increase the exposure to rosuvastatin. Adjust dose. Severe Study
▸ **Antiarrhythmics (dronedarone)** are predicted to increase the exposure to simvastatin. Use with caution and adjust simvastatin dose, p. 130. Severe Study
▸ **Antiepileptics (carbamazepine)** moderately decrease the exposure to simvastatin. Monitor and adjust dose. Severe Study → Also see TABLE 1 p. 818
▸ **Antiepileptics (carbamazepine, eslicarbazepine)** are predicted to decrease the exposure to atorvastatin. Monitor and adjust dose. Moderate Theoretical → Also see TABLE 1 p. 818
▸ **Antiepileptics (eslicarbazepine)** moderately decrease the exposure to simvastatin. Monitor and adjust dose. Moderate Study
▸ **Antiepileptics (fosphenytoin, phenytoin)** potentially decrease the exposure to statins (atorvastatin, simvastatin). Moderate Anecdotal
▸ **Antifungals, azoles (fluconazole, isavuconazole, posaconazole)** are predicted to increase the exposure to atorvastatin.

Monitor and adjust dose. Severe Theoretical → Also see TABLE 1 p. 818
▸ **Antifungals, azoles (fluconazole, isavuconazole, posaconazole)** are predicted to increase the exposure to simvastatin. Use with caution and adjust simvastatin dose, p. 130. Severe Study → Also see TABLE 1 p. 818
▸ **Antifungals, azoles (fluconazole, miconazole)** are predicted to increase the exposure to fluvastatin. Severe Theoretical → Also see TABLE 1 p. 818
▸ **Antifungals, azoles (itraconazole, ketoconazole, voriconazole)** are predicted to increase the exposure to atorvastatin. Avoid or adjust dose and monitor rhabdomyolysis. Severe Study → Also see TABLE 1 p. 818
▸ **Antifungals, azoles (itraconazole, ketoconazole, voriconazole)** are predicted to increase the exposure to simvastatin. Avoid. Severe Study → Also see TABLE 1 p. 818
▸ **Antifungals, azoles (miconazole)** potentially increase the exposure to atorvastatin. Severe Anecdotal
▸ **Antifungals, azoles (miconazole)** are predicted to increase the exposure to simvastatin. Avoid. Severe Theoretical
▸ **Aprepitant** is predicted to increase the exposure to atorvastatin. Monitor and adjust dose. Severe Theoretical
▸ **Aprepitant** is predicted to increase the exposure to simvastatin. Use with caution and adjust simvastatin dose, p. 130. Severe Study
▸ **Bosentan** slightly decreases the exposure to atorvastatin. Mild Study
▸ **Bosentan** moderately decreases the exposure to simvastatin. Moderate Study
▸ **Calcium channel blockers (amlodipine)** slightly increase the exposure to simvastatin. Adjust simvastatin dose, p. 130. Mild Study
▸ **Calcium channel blockers (diltiazem, verapamil)** are predicted to increase the exposure to atorvastatin. Monitor and adjust dose. Severe Theoretical
▸ **Calcium channel blockers (diltiazem, verapamil)** are predicted to increase the exposure to simvastatin. Use with caution and adjust simvastatin dose, p. 130. Severe Study
▸ **Cephalosporins (ceftobiprole)** are predicted to increase the concentration of statins. Moderate Theoretical
▸ **Ciclosporin** very markedly increases the exposure to atorvastatin. Avoid or adjust atorvastatin dose, p. 128. Severe Study
▸ **Ciclosporin** moderately increases the exposure to fluvastatin. Severe Anecdotal
▸ **Ciclosporin** markedly to very markedly increases the exposure to pravastatin. Adjust pravastatin dose, p. 129. Severe Study
▸ **Ciclosporin** markedly increases the exposure to statins (rosuvastatin, simvastatin). Avoid. Severe Study
▸ **Clopidogrel** increases the exposure to rosuvastatin. Adjust rosuvastatin dose, p. 130. Moderate Study
▸ **Cobicistat** is predicted to increase the exposure to atorvastatin. Avoid or adjust dose and monitor rhabdomyolysis. Severe Study
▸ **Cobicistat** is predicted to increase the exposure to simvastatin. Avoid. Severe Study
▸ **Colchicine** increases the risk of rhabdomyolysis when given with statins. Severe Anecdotal
▸ **Statins (fluvastatin, rosuvastatin)** increase the anticoagulant effect of coumarins. Monitor INR and adjust dose. Severe Study
▸ **Crizotinib** is predicted to increase the exposure to atorvastatin. Monitor and adjust dose. Severe Theoretical
▸ **Crizotinib** is predicted to increase the exposure to simvastatin. Use with caution and adjust simvastatin dose, p. 130. Severe Study
▸ **Danazol** is predicted to increase the risk of rhabdomyolysis when given with atorvastatin. Severe Theoretical
▸ **Danazol** increases the risk of rhabdomyolysis when given with simvastatin. Avoid. Severe Anecdotal
▸ **Statins** are predicted to increase the risk of rhabdomyolysis when given with daptomycin. Severe Theoretical
▸ **Dasabuvir** increases the exposure to rosuvastatin. Adjust rosuvastatin dose, p. 130. Moderate Study
▸ **Dasatinib** is predicted to increase the exposure to simvastatin. Moderate Theoretical

- Efavirenz slightly decreases the exposure to **atorvastatin**. Mild Study
- Efavirenz moderately decreases the exposure to **simvastatin**. Moderate Study
- Elbasvir potentially increases the exposure to **atorvastatin**. Adjust **atorvastatin** dose, p. 128. Moderate Study
- Elbasvir is predicted to increase the exposure to **fluvastatin**. Adjust **fluvastatin** dose, p. 129. Unknown Theoretical
- Elbasvir increases the exposure to **rosuvastatin**. Adjust **rosuvastatin** dose, p. 130. Moderate Study
- Elbasvir is predicted to increase the exposure to **simvastatin**. Adjust **simvastatin** dose, p. 130. Unknown Theoretical
- Eltrombopag is predicted to increase the exposure to **statins**. Monitor and adjust dose. Moderate Study
- Ezetimibe potentially increases the risk of rhabdomyolysis when given with **statins**. Severe Anecdotal
- Fibrates **(bezafibrate, ciprofibrate)** increase the risk of rhabdomyolysis when given with **pravastatin**. Avoid. Severe Study
- Fibrates **(bezafibrate, ciprofibrate)** increase the risk of rhabdomyolysis when given with **rosuvastatin**. Adjust **rosuvastatin** dose, p. 130. Severe Study
- Fibrates **(bezafibrate, ciprofibrate)** increase the risk of rhabdomyolysis when given with **simvastatin**. Adjust **simvastatin** dose, p. 130. Severe Study
- Fibrates **(ciprofibrate)** increase the risk of rhabdomyolysis when given with **atorvastatin**. Avoid or adjust dose. Severe Study
- Fibrates **(ciprofibrate)** increase the risk of rhabdomyolysis when given with **fluvastatin**. Severe Study
- Fibrates **(fenofibrate)** are predicted to increase the risk of rhabdomyolysis when given with **fluvastatin**. Adjust **fenofibrate** dose, p. 127. Severe Theoretical
- Fibrates **(fenofibrate)** are predicted to increase the risk of rhabdomyolysis when given with **pravastatin**. Avoid. Severe Theoretical
- Fibrates **(fenofibrate)** increase the risk of rhabdomyolysis when given with **rosuvastatin**. Adjust **fenofibrate** and **rosuvastatin** doses, p. 127, p. 130. Severe Anecdotal
- Fibrates **(gemfibrozil)** increase the risk of rhabdomyolysis when given with **statins**. Avoid. Severe Anecdotal
- Fibrates **(bezafibrate)** increase the risk of rhabdomyolysis when given with statins **(atorvastatin, fluvastatin)**. Severe Study
- Fibrates **(fenofibrate)** increase the risk of rhabdomyolysis when given with statins **(atorvastatin, simvastatin)**. Adjust **fenofibrate** dose, p. 127. Severe Anecdotal
- Fusidic acid increases the risk of rhabdomyolysis when given with **statins**. Avoid. Severe Anecdotal
- Grapefruit juice increases the exposure to **atorvastatin**. Mild Study
- Grapefruit juice increases the exposure to **simvastatin**. Avoid. Severe Study
- Grazoprevir increases the exposure to **atorvastatin**. Adjust **atorvastatin** dose, p. 128. Moderate Study
- Grazoprevir is predicted to increase the exposure to **fluvastatin**. Adjust **fluvastatin** dose, p. 129. Unknown Theoretical
- Grazoprevir increases the exposure to **rosuvastatin**. Adjust **rosuvastatin** dose, p. 130. Moderate Study
- Grazoprevir is predicted to increase the exposure to **simvastatin**. Adjust **simvastatin** dose, p. 130. Unknown Theoretical
- HIV-protease inhibitors **(atazanavir, darunavir, fosamprenavir, lopinavir, ritonavir, saquinavir, tipranavir)** are predicted to increase the exposure to **atorvastatin**. Avoid or adjust dose and monitor rhabdomyolysis. Severe Study
- HIV-protease inhibitors **(atazanavir, darunavir, fosamprenavir, lopinavir, ritonavir, saquinavir, tipranavir)** are predicted to increase the exposure to **simvastatin**. Avoid. Severe Study
- HIV-protease inhibitors **(indinavir)** are predicted to increase the exposure to **atorvastatin**. Monitor and adjust dose. Severe Theoretical
- HIV-protease inhibitors slightly to moderately increase the exposure to **rosuvastatin**. Avoid or adjust dose. Severe Study
- HIV-protease inhibitors **(indinavir)** are predicted to increase the exposure to **simvastatin**. Use with caution and adjust **simvastatin** dose, p. 130. Severe Study

- Idelalisib is predicted to increase the exposure to **atorvastatin**. Avoid or adjust dose and monitor rhabdomyolysis. Severe Study
- Idelalisib is predicted to increase the exposure to **simvastatin**. Avoid. Severe Study
- Imatinib is predicted to increase the exposure to **atorvastatin**. Monitor and adjust dose. Severe Theoretical
- Imatinib is predicted to increase the exposure to **simvastatin**. Use with caution and adjust **simvastatin** dose, p. 130. Severe Study
- Ledipasvir is predicted to increase the exposure to **rosuvastatin**. Avoid. Severe Theoretical
- Ledipasvir is predicted to increase the exposure to statins **(atorvastatin, simvastatin)**. Monitor and adjust dose. Moderate Theoretical
- Ledipasvir (with sofosbuvir) is predicted to increase the exposure to statins **(fluvastatin, pravastatin)**. Monitor and adjust dose. Moderate Theoretical
- Lomitapide increases the exposure to **atorvastatin**. Adjust **lomitapide** dose or separate administration by 12 hours. Mild Study → Also see **TABLE 1** p. 818
- Lomitapide increases the exposure to **simvastatin**. Monitor and adjust **simvastatin** dose, p. 130. Moderate Study → Also see **TABLE 1** p. 818
- Macrolides **(clarithromycin)** are predicted to increase the exposure to **atorvastatin**. Avoid or adjust dose and monitor rhabdomyolysis. Severe Study
- Macrolides **(clarithromycin)** moderately increase the exposure to **pravastatin**. Severe Study
- Macrolides **(clarithromycin)** are predicted to increase the exposure to **simvastatin**. Avoid. Severe Study
- Macrolides **(erythromycin)** are predicted to increase the exposure to **atorvastatin**. Monitor and adjust dose. Severe Theoretical
- Macrolides **(erythromycin)** are predicted to increase the exposure to **pravastatin**. Severe Study
- Macrolides **(erythromycin)** are predicted to increase the exposure to **simvastatin**. Use with caution and adjust **simvastatin** dose, p. 130. Severe Study
- Monoclonal antibodies **(tocilizumab)** are predicted to decrease the exposure to **atorvastatin**. Monitor and adjust dose. Moderate Theoretical
- Monoclonal antibodies **(tocilizumab)** moderately decrease the exposure to **simvastatin**. Monitor and adjust dose. Moderate Study
- Netupitant is predicted to increase the exposure to **atorvastatin**. Monitor and adjust dose. Severe Theoretical
- Netupitant is predicted to increase the exposure to **simvastatin**. Use with caution and adjust **simvastatin** dose, p. 130. Severe Study
- Nevirapine slightly decreases the exposure to **atorvastatin**. Mild Study
- Nevirapine moderately decreases the exposure to **simvastatin**. Moderate Study
- Nicotinic acid is predicted to increase the risk of rhabdomyolysis when given with **statins**. Severe Theoretical
- Nilotinib is predicted to increase the exposure to **atorvastatin**. Monitor and adjust dose. Severe Theoretical
- Nilotinib is predicted to increase the exposure to **simvastatin**. Use with caution and adjust **simvastatin** dose, p. 130. Severe Study
- Osimertinib slightly increases the exposure to **rosuvastatin**. Moderate Study
- Paritaprevir (with ritonavir and ombitasvir) is predicted to increase the exposure to **fluvastatin**. Avoid. Moderate Theoretical
- Paritaprevir (with ritonavir and ombitasvir) increases the exposure to **pravastatin**. Adjust **pravastatin** dose, p. 129. Moderate Study
- Paritaprevir (with ritonavir and ombitasvir) increases the exposure to **rosuvastatin**. Adjust **rosuvastatin** dose, p. 130. Moderate Study
- **Rosuvastatin** is predicted to increase the anticoagulant effect of **phenindione**. Monitor INR and adjust dose. Severe Theoretical

A1

Interactions | **Appendix 1**

A1

Interactions | Appendix 1

Statins (continued)
▸ Ranolazine is predicted to increase the exposure to atorvastatin. Moderate Theoretical
▸ Ranolazine slightly increases the exposure to **simvastatin**. Adjust **simvastatin** dose, p. 130. Moderate Study
▸ Regorafenib is predicted to increase the exposure to statins (atorvastatin, fluvastatin, rosuvastatin). Severe Theoretical
▸ Rifampicin markedly decreases the exposure to **atorvastatin**. **Atorvastatin** should be taken at the same time as **rifampicin**. Moderate Study
▸ Rifampicin moderately decreases the exposure to **fluvastatin**. Monitor and adjust dose. Moderate Study
▸ Rifampicin very markedly decreases the exposure to **simvastatin**. Moderate Study
▸ Sacubitril is predicted to increase the exposure to **statins**. Severe Study
▸ Simeprevir moderately increases the exposure to **atorvastatin**. Monitor and adjust dose. Moderate Study
▸ Simeprevir is predicted to increase the exposure to **pravastatin**. Monitor and adjust dose. Severe Theoretical
▸ Simeprevir moderately increases the exposure to **rosuvastatin**. Adjust **rosuvastatin** dose, p. 130. Moderate Study
▸ Simeprevir slightly increases the exposure to **simvastatin**. Monitor and adjust dose. Moderate Study
▸ St John's Wort slightly decreases the exposure to **atorvastatin**. Mild Study
▸ St John's Wort moderately decreases the exposure to **simvastatin**. Moderate Study
▸ Sulfinpyrazone is predicted to increase the exposure to **fluvastatin**. Severe Theoretical
▸ Fluvastatin slightly increases the exposure to sulfonylureas (glibenclamide). Mild Study
▸ Tedizolid is predicted to increase the exposure to **rosuvastatin**. Avoid. Moderate Theoretical
▸ Teriflunomide moderately increases the exposure to rosuvastatin. Adjust **rosuvastatin** dose, p. 130. Moderate Study
▸ Ticagrelor slightly increases the exposure to **simvastatin**. Adjust **simvastatin** dose, p. 130. Moderate Study
▸ Velpatasvir increases the exposure to **rosuvastatin**. Adjust rosuvastatin dose and monitor side effects, p. 130. Severe Study
▸ Velpatasvir is predicted to increase the exposure to statins (atorvastatin, simvastatin). Monitor side effects and adjust dose. Severe Theoretical

Stavudine → see **TABLE 12** p. 821 (peripheral neuropathy)
▸ Didanosine increases the risk of toxicity when given with **stavudine**. Avoid. Severe Study → Also see **TABLE 12** p. 821
▸ Hydroxycarbamide increases the risk of toxicity when given with **stavudine**. Avoid. Severe Study
▸ Isoniazid is predicted to increase the risk of peripheral neuropathy when given with **stavudine**. Severe Theoretical → Also see **TABLE 12** p. 821
▸ Ribavirin increases the risk of toxicity when given with **stavudine**. Avoid. Severe Study
▸ Zidovudine is predicted to decrease the efficacy of **stavudine**. Avoid. Severe Theoretical

Stiripentol → see antiepileptics
Streptokinase → see **TABLE 3** p. 818 (anticoagulant effects)
Streptomycin → see aminoglycosides
Strontium ranelate → see **TABLE 5** p. 818 (thromboembolism)
▸ Antacids decrease the absorption of **strontium ranelate**. Separate administration by 2 hours. Moderate Study
▸ Oral calcium salts decrease the absorption of **strontium ranelate**. Separate administration by 2 hours. Moderate Study
▸ Strontium ranelate is predicted to decrease the absorption of quinolones. Avoid. Moderate Theoretical
▸ Strontium ranelate is predicted to decrease the absorption of tetracyclines. Avoid. Moderate Theoretical

Sucralfate
▸ Sucralfate potentially decreases the effects of coumarins (warfarin). Separate administration by 2 hours. Moderate Anecdotal
▸ Sucralfate decreases the absorption of digoxin. Separate administration by 2 hours. Severe Anecdotal
▸ Sucralfate decreases the absorption of dolutegravir. Moderate Study

▸ Sucralfate increases the risk of blocked enteral or nasogastric tubes when given with enteral feeds. Separate administration by 1 hour. Moderate Study
▸ Sucralfate decreases the absorption of levothyroxine. Separate administration by at least 4 hours. Moderate Study
▸ Potassium citrate increases the risk of side-effects when given with **sucralfate**. Avoid. Moderate Theoretical
▸ Sucralfate decreases the exposure to quinolones. Separate administration by 2 hours. Moderate Study
▸ Sodium citrate is predicted to increase the risk of side-effects when given with **sucralfate**. Avoid. Moderate Theoretical
▸ Sucralfate decreases the absorption of sulpiride. Separate administration by 2 hours. Moderate Study
▸ Sucralfate potentially decreases the absorption of theophylline. Separate administration by at least 2 hours. Moderate Study
▸ Sucralfate is predicted to decrease the absorption of tricyclic antidepressants. Moderate Study

Sufentanil → see opioids
Sugammadex
▸ Sugammadex is predicted to decrease the exposure to oral combined hormonal contraceptives. Refer to patient information leaflet for missed pill advice. Severe Theoretical
▸ Sugammadex is predicted to decrease the exposure to desogestrel. Refer to patient information leaflet for missed pill advice. Severe Theoretical
▸ Sugammadex is predicted to decrease the efficacy of etonogestrel. Use additional contraceptive precautions. Severe Theoretical
▸ Sugammadex is predicted to decrease the exposure to levonorgestrel. Use additional contraceptive precautions. Severe Theoretical
▸ Sugammadex is predicted to decrease the exposure to medroxyprogesterone. Use additional contraceptive precautions. Severe Theoretical
▸ Sugammadex is predicted to decrease the exposure to norethisterone. Use additional contraceptive precautions. Severe Theoretical

Sulfadiazine → see sulfonamides
Sulfamethoxazole
▸ Sulfamethoxazole increases the anticoagulant effect of coumarins. Severe Study

Sulfasalazine → see **TABLE 1** p. 818 (hepatotoxicity), **TABLE 15** p. 821 (myelosuppression)
▸ Sulfasalazine decreases the concentration of digoxin. Moderate Study
▸ Sulfasalazine decreases the absorption of folates (folic acid). Moderate Study
▸ Sulfasalazine is predicted to decrease the absorption of folates (folinic acid). Moderate Theoretical
▸ Tedizolid is predicted to increase the exposure to **sulfasalazine**. Avoid. Moderate Theoretical

Sulfinpyrazone → see **TABLE 4** p. 818 (antiplatelet effects)
▸ Sulfinpyrazone increases the concentration of antiepileptics (fosphenytoin, phenytoin). Moderate Study
▸ Aspirin decreases the effects of **sulfinpyrazone**. Moderate Study → Also see **TABLE 4** p. 818
▸ Sulfinpyrazone decreases the exposure to calcium channel blockers (verapamil). Moderate Study
▸ Sulfinpyrazone decreases the concentration of ciclosporin. Severe Study
▸ Sulfinpyrazone increases the anticoagulant effect of coumarins. Avoid. Severe Study
▸ Sulfinpyrazone slightly increases the exposure to nateglinide. Mild Study
▸ Pyrazinamide is predicted to decrease the effects of sulfinpyrazone. Moderate Theoretical
▸ Sulfinpyrazone is predicted to increase the exposure to retinoids (alitretinoin). Adjust **alitretinoin** dose. Moderate Theoretical
▸ Sulfinpyrazone is predicted to increase the exposure to statins (fluvastatin). Severe Theoretical
▸ Sulfinpyrazone is predicted to increase the exposure to sulfonylureas. Use with caution and adjust dose. Moderate Study

Sulfonamides → see TABLE 15 p. 821 (myelosuppression)

co-trimoxazole · sulfadiazine

▸ **Sulfonamides** potentially increase the risk of methaemoglobinaemia when given with topical anaesthetics, local (prilocaine). Use with caution or avoid. [Severe] Anecdotal
▸ **Sulfadiazine** is predicted to increase the concentration of antiepileptics (fosphenytoin). Monitor and adjust dose. [Moderate] Study
▸ **Sulfadiazine** increases the concentration of antiepileptics (phenytoin). Monitor and adjust dose. [Moderate] Study
▸ Antimalarials (pyrimethamine) increase the risk of side-effects when given with **sulfonamides**. [Severe] Study → Also see TABLE 15 p. 821
▸ **Sulfadiazine** is predicted to increase the anticoagulant effect of coumarins. [Severe] Theoretical
▸ **Sulfonamides** are predicted to increase the risk of methaemoglobinaemia when given with dapsone. [Severe] Theoretical
▸ **Sulfonamides** are predicted to increase the exposure to methotrexate. Use with caution or avoid. [Severe] Theoretical → Also see TABLE 15 p. 821
▸ **Sulfonamides** are predicted to increase the exposure to sulfonylureas. [Moderate] Study
▸ **Sulfonamides** are predicted to increase the effects of thiopental. [Moderate] Theoretical
Sulfonylureas → see TABLE 14 p. 821 (antidiabetic drugs)

glibenclamide · gliclazide · glimepiride · glipizide · tolbutamide

▸ Antiarrhythmics (amiodarone) are predicted to increase the exposure to **sulfonylureas**. Use with caution and adjust dose. [Moderate] Study
▸ Antifungals, azoles (fluconazole, miconazole, voriconazole) are predicted to increase the exposure to **sulfonylureas**. Use with caution and adjust dose. [Moderate] Study
▸ Bosentan increases the risk of hepatotoxicity when given with glibenclamide. Avoid. [Severe] Study
▸ Cephalosporins (ceftobiprole) are predicted to increase the concentration of glibenclamide. [Moderate] Theoretical
▸ Ceritinib is predicted to increase the exposure to glimepiride. Adjust dose. [Moderate] Theoretical
▸ Chloramphenicol is predicted to increase the exposure to **sulfonylureas**. [Severe] Study
▸ Fibrates are predicted to increase the risk of hypoglycaemia when given with **sulfonylureas**. [Moderate] Theoretical
▸ Macrolides (clarithromycin) are predicted to slightly increase the exposure to **sulfonylureas**. [Moderate] Theoretical
▸ Rifampicin is predicted to decrease the exposure to **sulfonylureas**. [Moderate] Study
▸ Statins (fluvastatin) slightly increase the exposure to glibenclamide. [Mild] Study
▸ Sulfinpyrazone is predicted to increase the exposure to **sulfonylureas**. Use with caution and adjust dose. [Moderate] Study
▸ **Sulfonamides** are predicted to increase the exposure to **sulfonylureas**. [Moderate] Study
Sulindac → see NSAIDs
Sulpiride → see TABLE 8 p. 819 (hypotension), TABLE 9 p. 820 (QT-interval prolongation), TABLE 11 p. 820 (CNS depressant effects)
▸ **Sulpiride** is predicted to decrease the effects of dopamine receptor agonists. Avoid. [Moderate] Theoretical → Also see TABLE 8 p. 819 → Also see TABLE 9 p. 820
▸ **Sulpiride** is predicted to decrease the effects of levodopa. Avoid. [Severe] Theoretical → Also see TABLE 8 p. 819
▸ **Sulpiride** potentially increases the risk of neurotoxicity when given with lithium. [Severe] Anecdotal → Also see TABLE 9 p. 820
▸ Sucralfate decreases the absorption of sulpiride. Separate administration by 2 hours. [Moderate] Study
Sumatriptan → see TABLE 13 p. 821 (serotonin syndrome)
▸ **Sumatriptan** increases the risk of vasoconstriction when given with ergotamine. Ergotamine should be taken at least 24 hours before or 6 hours after sumatriptan. [Severe] Study
▸ Moclobemide moderately increases the exposure to sumatriptan. Avoid. [Moderate] Study → Also see TABLE 13 p. 821
▸ Monoamine-oxidase A and B inhibitors, irreversible are predicted to increase the exposure to **sumatriptan**. Avoid and

for 14 days after stopping the MAOI. [Severe] Theoretical → Also see TABLE 13 p. 821
Sunitinib → see TABLE 15 p. 821 (myelosuppression), TABLE 9 p. 820 (QT-interval prolongation)
▸ Antiarrhythmics (dronedarone) are predicted to increase the exposure to **sunitinib**. [Moderate] Theoretical → Also see TABLE 9 p. 820
▸ Antiepileptics (carbamazepine, fosphenytoin, phenobarbital, phenytoin, primidone) are predicted to decrease the exposure to **sunitinib**. Avoid or adjust sunitinib dose. [Moderate] Study
▸ Antifungals, azoles (fluconazole, isavuconazole, posaconazole) are predicted to increase the exposure to **sunitinib**. [Moderate] Theoretical
▸ Antifungals, azoles (itraconazole, ketoconazole, voriconazole) are predicted to slightly increase the exposure to **sunitinib**. Avoid or adjust sunitinib dose. [Moderate] Study → Also see TABLE 9 p. 820
▸ Aprepitant is predicted to increase the exposure to **sunitinib**. [Moderate] Theoretical
▸ Calcium channel blockers (diltiazem, verapamil) are predicted to increase the exposure to **sunitinib**. [Moderate] Theoretical
▸ Cobicistat is predicted to slightly increase the exposure to sunitinib. Avoid or adjust sunitinib dose. [Moderate] Study
▸ **Sunitinib** is predicted to increase the risk of bleeding events when given with coumarins. [Severe] Theoretical
▸ Crizotinib is predicted to increase the exposure to sunitinib. [Moderate] Theoretical → Also see TABLE 15 p. 821 → Also see TABLE 9 p. 820
▸ Enzalutamide is predicted to decrease the exposure to sunitinib. Avoid or adjust sunitinib dose. [Moderate] Study
▸ Grapefruit juice is predicted to increase the exposure to sunitinib. Avoid. [Moderate] Theoretical
▸ HIV-protease inhibitors (atazanavir, darunavir, fosamprenavir, lopinavir, ritonavir, saquinavir, tipranavir) are predicted to slightly increase the exposure to sunitinib. Avoid or adjust sunitinib dose. [Moderate] Study → Also see TABLE 9 p. 820
▸ HIV-protease inhibitors (indinavir) are predicted to increase the exposure to **sunitinib**. [Moderate] Theoretical
▸ Idelalisib is predicted to slightly increase the exposure to sunitinib. Avoid or adjust sunitinib dose. [Moderate] Study → Also see TABLE 15 p. 821
▸ Imatinib is predicted to increase the exposure to sunitinib. [Moderate] Theoretical → Also see TABLE 15 p. 821
▸ Macrolides (clarithromycin) are predicted to slightly increase the exposure to **sunitinib**. Avoid or adjust sunitinib dose. [Moderate] Study → Also see TABLE 9 p. 820
▸ Macrolides (erythromycin) are predicted to increase the exposure to **sunitinib**. [Moderate] Theoretical
▸ Netupitant is predicted to increase the exposure to sunitinib. [Moderate] Theoretical
▸ Nilotinib is predicted to increase the exposure to sunitinib. [Moderate] Theoretical → Also see TABLE 15 p. 821 → Also see TABLE 9 p. 820
▸ **Sunitinib** is predicted to increase the risk of bleeding events when given with phenindione. [Severe] Theoretical
▸ Rifampicin is predicted to decrease the exposure to **sunitinib**. Avoid or adjust sunitinib dose. [Moderate] Study
Suxamethonium → see TABLE 20 p. 822 (neuromuscular blocking effects)
▸ Alkylating agents (cyclophosphamide) increase the risk of prolonged neuromuscular blockade when given with suxamethonium. [Moderate] Study
▸ Aminoglycosides are predicted to increase the risk of prolonged neuromuscular blockade when given with suxamethonium. [Severe] Study → Also see TABLE 20 p. 822
▸ Antiarrhythmics (lidocaine) are predicted to increase the effects of suxamethonium. [Moderate] Study
▸ Anticholinesterases, centrally acting increase the effects of suxamethonium. [Moderate] Theoretical
▸ Antiepileptics (carbamazepine) increase the risk of prolonged neuromuscular blockade when given with suxamethonium. [Moderate] Study
▸ Antiepileptics (fosphenytoin, phenytoin) increase the effects of suxamethonium. [Moderate] Study
▸ Clindamycin increases the effects of suxamethonium. [Severe] Anecdotal

A1

Interactions | Appendix 1

Suxamethonium (continued)

▸ Colistimethate increases the effects of **suxamethonium**. Monitor and adjust dose. Moderate Study → Also see **TABLE 20** p. 822

▸ **Corticosteroids** are predicted to decrease the effects of **suxamethonium**. Severe Anecdotal

▸ **Suxamethonium** is predicted to increase the risk of cardiovascular side-effects when given with **digoxin**. Severe Anecdotal

▸ **Irinotecan** is predicted to increase the risk of prolonged neuromuscular blockade when given with **suxamethonium**. Moderate Theoretical

▸ Intravenous **magnesium** is predicted to increase the effects of **suxamethonium**. Moderate Study

▸ **Metoclopramide** increases the effects of **suxamethonium**. Moderate Study

▸ **Penicillins (piperacillin)** increase the effects of **suxamethonium**. Moderate Study

▸ **SSRIs** potentially increase the risk of prolonged neuromuscular blockade when given with **suxamethonium**. Unknown Theoretical

Sympathomimetics, inotropic

dobutamine · dopamine · dopexamine

▸ **Sympathomimetics, inotropic** are predicted to decrease the effects of **apraclonidine**. Avoid. Severe Theoretical

▸ **Beta blockers, non-selective** increase the risk of hypertension and bradycardia when given with **dobutamine**. Severe Theoretical

▸ **Beta blockers, selective** increase the risk of hypertension and bradycardia when given with **dobutamine**. Moderate Theoretical

▸ **Entacapone** is predicted to increase the risk of cardiovascular side-effects when given with sympathomimetics, inotropic **(dobutamine, dopamine)**. Moderate Theoretical

▸ **Ergometrine** potentially increases the risk of peripheral vasoconstriction when given with **dopamine**. Avoid. Severe Anecdotal

▸ **Guanethidine** is predicted to increase the effects of **dopamine**. Severe Theoretical

▸ Sympathomimetics, inotropic **(dobutamine, dopamine)** are predicted to increase the risk of elevated blood pressure when given with **linezolid**. Avoid. Severe Theoretical

▸ **Monoamine-oxidase A and B inhibitors, irreversible** are predicted to increase the risk of a hypertensive crisis when given with **sympathomimetics, inotropic**. Avoid and for 14 days after stopping the MAOI. Severe Theoretical

▸ **Monoamine-oxidase B inhibitors** are predicted to increase the risk of a hypertensive crisis when given with **sympathomimetics, inotropic**. Avoid. Severe Anecdotal

▸ **Opicapone** is predicted to increase the risk of cardiovascular side-effects when given with sympathomimetics, inotropic **(dobutamine, dopamine)**. Severe Theoretical

▸ **Tolcapone** is predicted to increase the risk of cardiovascular side-effects when given with sympathomimetics, inotropic **(dobutamine, dopamine)**. Moderate Theoretical

Sympathomimetics, vasoconstrictor

adrenaline/epinephrine · ephedrine · isomethepene · metaraminol · midodrine · noradrenaline/norepinephrine · phenylephrine · pseudoephedrine · xylometazoline

ROUTE-SPECIFIC INFORMATION Since systemic absorption can follow topical application, the possibility of interactions should be borne in mind.

▸ **Ephedrine** increases the risk of side-effects when given with **aminophylline**. Avoid in children. Moderate Study

▸ **Sympathomimetics, vasoconstrictor** are predicted to decrease the effects of **apraclonidine**. Avoid. Severe Theoretical

▸ **Atropine** increases the risk of severe hypertension when given with **phenylephrine**. Severe Study

▸ **Beta blockers, non-selective** are predicted to increase the risk of hypertension and bradycardia when given with sympathomimetics, vasoconstrictor **(adrenaline/epinephrine, noradrenaline/norepinephrine)**. Severe Study

▸ **Beta blockers, selective** are predicted to increase the risk of hypertension and bradycardia when given with sympathomimetics, vasoconstrictor **(adrenaline/epinephrine, noradrenaline/norepinephrine)**. Severe Study

▸ **Entacapone** is predicted to increase the risk of cardiovascular side-effects when given with sympathomimetics, vasoconstrictor **(adrenaline/epinephrine, noradrenaline/norepinephrine)**. Moderate Study

▸ **Ergometrine** is predicted to increase the risk of peripheral vasoconstriction when given with **noradrenaline/norepinephrine**. Severe Anecdotal

▸ **Guanethidine** increases the effects of **metaraminol**. Severe Anecdotal

▸ **Guanethidine** increases the effects of **phenylephrine**. Severe Study

▸ **Guanethidine** is predicted to increase the effects of sympathomimetics, vasoconstrictor **(adrenaline/epinephrine, noradrenaline/norepinephrine)**. Moderate Study

▸ **Pseudoephedrine** increases the risk of elevated blood pressure when given with **linezolid**. Avoid. Severe Study

▸ Sympathomimetics, vasoconstrictor **(adrenaline/epinephrine, ephedrine, isomethepene, noradrenaline/norepinephrine, phenylephrine)** are predicted to increase the risk of elevated blood pressure when given with **linezolid**. Avoid. Severe Theoretical

▸ **Mianserin** decreases the effects of **ephedrine**. Severe Anecdotal

▸ **Moclobemide** is predicted to increase the risk of a hypertensive crisis when given with sympathomimetics, vasoconstrictor **(ephedrine, isomethepene, phenylephrine, pseudoephedrine)**. Avoid. Severe Study

▸ **Monoamine-oxidase A and B inhibitors, irreversible** are predicted to increase the risk of a hypertensive crisis when given with **sympathomimetics, vasoconstrictor**. Avoid and for 14 days after stopping the MAOI. Severe Study

▸ **Monoamine-oxidase B inhibitors** are predicted to increase the risk of a hypertensive crisis when given with **sympathomimetics, vasoconstrictor**. Avoid. Severe Anecdotal

▸ **Opicapone** is predicted to increase the risk of cardiovascular side-effects when given with sympathomimetics, vasoconstrictor **(adrenaline/epinephrine, noradrenaline/norepinephrine)**. Severe Theoretical

▸ **Ephedrine** increases the risk of side-effects when given with **theophylline**. Avoid in children. Moderate Study

▸ **Tolcapone** is predicted to increase the effects of sympathomimetics, vasoconstrictor **(adrenaline/epinephrine, noradrenaline/norepinephrine)**. Moderate Theoretical

▸ **Tricyclic antidepressants** are predicted to decrease the effects of **ephedrine**. Avoid. Severe Study

▸ **Tricyclic antidepressants** increase the effects of sympathomimetics, vasoconstrictor **(adrenaline/epinephrine, noradrenaline/norepinephrine, phenylephrine)**. Avoid. Severe Study

Tacalcitol → see vitamin D substances

Tacrolimus → see **TABLE 2** p. 818 (nephrotoxicity), **TABLE 16** p. 822 (increased serum potassium)

▸ Risk of facial flushing and skin irritation with alcohol consumption in those using topical **tacrolimus** (does not apply to tacrolimus taken systemically). Pomelo might greatly increase the concentration of tacrolimus.

▸ Since systemic absorption can follow topical application, the possibility of interactions should be borne in mind.

▸ **Antiarrhythmics (amiodarone)** are predicted to increase the concentration of **tacrolimus**. Severe Anecdotal

▸ **Antiarrhythmics (dronedarone)** are predicted to increase the concentration of **tacrolimus**. Severe Study

▸ **Antiepileptics (carbamazepine, fosphenytoin, phenobarbital, phenytoin, primidone)** decrease the concentration of **tacrolimus**. Monitor and adjust dose. Severe Study

▸ **Antifungals, azoles (fluconazole, isavuconazole, posaconazole)** are predicted to increase the concentration of **tacrolimus**. Severe Study

▸ **Antifungals, azoles (itraconazole, ketoconazole, voriconazole)** are predicted to increase the concentration of **tacrolimus**. Monitor and adjust dose. Severe Study

▸ Antifungals, azoles (miconazole) are predicted to increase the concentration of **tacrolimus**. Monitor and adjust dose. Severe Theoretical

▸ Aprepitant is predicted to increase the concentration of **tacrolimus**. Severe Study

▸ Bosentan is predicted to decrease the concentration of **tacrolimus** and **tacrolimus** potentially increases the concentration of bosentan. Avoid. Severe Theoretical

▸ Calcium channel blockers (diltiazem, verapamil) are predicted to increase the concentration of **tacrolimus**. Severe Study

▸ Calcium channel blockers (nicardipine) potentially increase the concentration of **tacrolimus**. Monitor concentration and adjust dose. Severe Anecdotal

▸ Ceritinib is predicted to increase the exposure to **tacrolimus**. Avoid. Severe Theoretical

▸ Chloramphenicol increases the concentration of **tacrolimus**. Severe Study

▸ Ciclosporin increases the concentration of **tacrolimus**. Avoid. Severe Study → Also see TABLE 2 p. 818 → Also see TABLE 16 p. 822

▸ Cobicistat is predicted to increase the concentration of **tacrolimus**. Monitor and adjust dose. Severe Study

▸ Crizotinib is predicted to increase the concentration of **tacrolimus**. Severe Study

▸ Danazol potentially increases the concentration of **tacrolimus**. Severe Anecdotal

▸ Efavirenz is predicted to decrease the concentration of **tacrolimus**. Monitor and adjust dose. Moderate Theoretical

▸ Enzalutamide decreases the concentration of **tacrolimus**. Monitor and adjust dose. Severe Study

▸ Grapefruit juice increases the concentration of **tacrolimus**. Avoid. Severe Study

▸ Grazoprevir increases the exposure to **tacrolimus**. Moderate Study

▸ HIV-protease inhibitors (atazanavir, darunavir, fosamprenavir, lopinavir, ritonavir, saquinavir, tipranavir) are predicted to increase the concentration of **tacrolimus**. Monitor and adjust dose. Severe Study

▸ HIV-protease inhibitors (indinavir) are predicted to increase the concentration of **tacrolimus**. Severe Study

▸ Idelalisib is predicted to increase the concentration of **tacrolimus**. Monitor and adjust dose. Severe Study

▸ Imatinib is predicted to increase the concentration of **tacrolimus**. Severe Study

▸ Live vaccines are predicted to increase the risk of generalised infection (possibly life-threatening) when given with **tacrolimus**. Public Health England advises avoid. Severe Theoretical

▸ **Tacrolimus** is predicted to increase the exposure to lomitapide. Separate administration by 12 hours. Moderate Theoretical

▸ Lumacaftor is predicted to decrease the exposure to **tacrolimus**. Avoid. Severe Theoretical

▸ Macrolides (clarithromycin) are predicted to increase the concentration of **tacrolimus**. Monitor and adjust dose. Severe Study

▸ Macrolides (erythromycin) are predicted to increase the concentration of **tacrolimus**. Severe Study

▸ **Tacrolimus** is predicted to affect the efficacy of mifamurtide. Avoid. Severe Theoretical

▸ Netupitant is predicted to increase the concentration of **tacrolimus**. Severe Study

▸ Nevirapine is predicted to decrease the concentration of **tacrolimus**. Monitor and adjust dose. Moderate Theoretical

▸ Nilotinib is predicted to increase the concentration of **tacrolimus**. Severe Study

▸ Palbociclib is predicted to increase the exposure to **tacrolimus**. Adjust dose. Moderate Theoretical

▸ Pitolisant is predicted to decrease the exposure to **tacrolimus**. Avoid. Severe Theoretical

▸ Ranolazine increases the concentration of **tacrolimus**. Adjust dose. Severe Anecdotal

▸ Rifampicin decreases the concentration of **tacrolimus**. Monitor and adjust dose. Severe Study

▸ Sirolimus is predicted to decrease the concentration of **tacrolimus** and **tacrolimus** increases the exposure to sirolimus. Severe Study

▸ St John's Wort decreases the concentration of **tacrolimus**. Avoid. Severe Study

▸ **Tacrolimus** potentially increases the risk of serotonin syndrome when given with venlafaxine. Severe Anecdotal

Tadalafil → see phosphodiesterase type-5 inhibitors

Tamoxifen → see TABLE 5 p. 818 (thromboembolism)

▸ Bupropion is predicted to decrease the efficacy of **tamoxifen**. Avoid. Severe Study

▸ Cinacalcet is predicted to decrease the efficacy of **tamoxifen**. Avoid. Severe Study

▸ **Tamoxifen** increases the anticoagulant effect of coumarins. Severe Study

▸ Rifampicin markedly decreases the exposure to **tamoxifen**. Unknown Study

▸ SSRIs (fluoxetine, paroxetine) are predicted to decrease the efficacy of **tamoxifen**. Avoid. Severe Study

▸ Terbinafine is predicted to decrease the efficacy of **tamoxifen**. Avoid. Severe Study

Tamsulosin → see alpha blockers

Tapentadol → see opioids

Taxanes → see TABLE 15 p. 821 (myelosuppression), TABLE 12 p. 821 (peripheral neuropathy)

cabazitaxel · docetaxel · paclitaxel

▸ Antiarrhythmics (dronedarone) are predicted to increase the exposure to **cabazitaxel**. Moderate Theoretical

▸ Antiarrhythmics (dronedarone) are predicted to increase the exposure to **paclitaxel**. Severe Theoretical

▸ Antiepileptics (carbamazepine, fosphenytoin, phenobarbital, phenytoin, primidone) are predicted to decrease the exposure to **docetaxel**. Severe Theoretical → Also see TABLE 12 p. 821

▸ Antiepileptics (carbamazepine, fosphenytoin, phenobarbital, phenytoin, primidone) are predicted to decrease the exposure to **taxanes** (cabazitaxel, paclitaxel). Avoid. Severe Study → Also see TABLE 12 p. 821

▸ Antifungals, azoles (fluconazole, isavuconazole, posaconazole) are predicted to increase the exposure to **cabazitaxel**. Moderate Theoretical

▸ Antifungals, azoles (itraconazole, ketoconazole, voriconazole) are predicted to increase the exposure to **cabazitaxel**. Avoid. Severe Study

▸ Antifungals, azoles (itraconazole, ketoconazole, voriconazole) are predicted to moderately increase the exposure to **docetaxel**. Avoid or adjust dose. Severe Study

▸ Antifungals, azoles (itraconazole, ketoconazole, voriconazole) are predicted to increase the exposure to **paclitaxel**. Severe Theoretical

▸ Antifungals, azoles (miconazole) are predicted to increase the concentration of **docetaxel**. Use with caution and adjust dose. Moderate Theoretical

▸ Aprepitant is predicted to increase the exposure to **cabazitaxel**. Moderate Theoretical

▸ Bosentan is predicted to decrease the exposure to **cabazitaxel**. Avoid. Severe Study

▸ Calcium channel blockers (diltiazem, verapamil) are predicted to increase the exposure to **cabazitaxel**. Moderate Theoretical

▸ Ceritinib is predicted to increase the exposure to **paclitaxel**. Moderate Theoretical → Also see TABLE 15 p. 821

▸ Cobicistat is predicted to increase the exposure to **cabazitaxel**. Avoid. Severe Study

▸ Cobicistat is predicted to moderately increase the exposure to **docetaxel**. Avoid or adjust dose. Severe Study

▸ Cobicistat is predicted to increase the exposure to **paclitaxel**. Severe Theoretical

▸ Crizotinib is predicted to increase the exposure to **cabazitaxel**. Moderate Theoretical → Also see TABLE 15 p. 821

▸ Efavirenz is predicted to decrease the exposure to **cabazitaxel**. Avoid. Severe Study

▸ Enzalutamide is predicted to decrease the exposure to **docetaxel**. Severe Theoretical

▸ Enzalutamide is predicted to decrease the exposure to **taxanes** (cabazitaxel, paclitaxel). Avoid. Severe Study

▸ HIV-protease inhibitors (atazanavir, darunavir, fosamprenavir, lopinavir, ritonavir, saquinavir, tipranavir) are predicted to increase the exposure to **cabazitaxel**. Avoid. Severe Study

A1

Interactions | Appendix 1

Taxanes (continued)

▸ HIV-protease inhibitors (atazanavir, darunavir, fosamprenavir, lopinavir, ritonavir, saquinavir, tipranavir) are predicted to moderately increase the exposure to **docetaxel**. Avoid or adjust dose. [Severe] Study

▸ HIV-protease inhibitors (atazanavir, darunavir, fosamprenavir, lopinavir, ritonavir, saquinavir, tipranavir) are predicted to increase the exposure to **paclitaxel**. [Severe] Theoretical

▸ HIV-protease inhibitors (indinavir) are predicted to increase the exposure to **cabazitaxel**. [Moderate] Theoretical

▸ Idelalisib is predicted to increase the exposure to **cabazitaxel**. Avoid. [Severe] Study → Also see TABLE 15 p. 821

▸ Idelalisib is predicted to moderately increase the exposure to **docetaxel**. Avoid or adjust dose. [Severe] Study → Also see TABLE 15 p. 821

▸ Idelalisib is predicted to increase the exposure to **paclitaxel**. [Severe] Theoretical → Also see TABLE 15 p. 821

▸ Imatinib is predicted to increase the exposure to **cabazitaxel**. [Moderate] Theoretical → Also see TABLE 15 p. 821

▸ Lapatinib slightly increases the exposure to **paclitaxel**. [Severe] Study

▸ Live vaccines are predicted to increase the risk of generalised infection (possibly life-threatening) when given with taxanes (**docetaxel, paclitaxel**). Public Health England advises avoid. [Severe] Theoretical

▸ Lumacaftor is predicted to affect the exposure to **paclitaxel**. [Moderate] Theoretical

▸ Macrolides (clarithromycin) are predicted to increase the exposure to **cabazitaxel**. Avoid. [Severe] Study

▸ Macrolides (clarithromycin) are predicted to moderately increase the exposure to **docetaxel**. Avoid or adjust dose. [Severe] Study

▸ Macrolides (clarithromycin) are predicted to increase the exposure to **paclitaxel**. [Severe] Theoretical

▸ Macrolides (erythromycin) are predicted to increase the exposure to **cabazitaxel**. [Moderate] Theoretical

▸ Mirabegron is predicted to increase the exposure to **paclitaxel**. [Mild] Theoretical

▸ Netupitant is predicted to increase the exposure to **cabazitaxel**. [Moderate] Theoretical

▸ Nevirapine is predicted to decrease the exposure to **cabazitaxel**. Avoid. [Severe] Study

▸ Nilotinib is predicted to increase the exposure to **cabazitaxel**. [Moderate] Theoretical → Also see TABLE 15 p. 821

▸ Pitolisant is predicted to decrease the exposure to **docetaxel**. Avoid. [Severe] Theoretical

▸ Rifampicin is predicted to decrease the exposure to **docetaxel**. [Severe] Theoretical

▸ Rifampicin is predicted to decrease the exposure to taxanes (**cabazitaxel, paclitaxel**). Avoid. [Severe] Study

▸ St John's Wort is predicted to decrease the exposure to **cabazitaxel**. Avoid. [Severe] Study

▸ Velpatasvir is predicted to increase the exposure to **paclitaxel**. [Severe] Theoretical

Tazarotene → see retinoids

Tedizolid → see TABLE 13 p. 821 (serotonin syndrome)

FOOD AND LIFESTYLE Patients taking tedizolid should avoid consuming large amounts of tyramine-rich foods (such as mature cheese, salami, pickled herring, Bovril®, Oxo®, Marmite® or any similar meat or yeast extract or fermented soya bean extract, and some beers, lagers or wines).

▸ Tedizolid is predicted to increase the exposure to imatinib. Avoid. [Moderate] Theoretical

▸ Tedizolid is predicted to increase the exposure to lapatinib. Avoid. [Moderate] Theoretical

▸ Tedizolid is predicted to increase the exposure to methotrexate. Avoid. [Moderate] Theoretical

▸ Moclobemide is predicted to increase the risk of side-effects when given with **tedizolid**. [Severe] Theoretical → Also see TABLE 13 p. 821

▸ Monoamine-oxidase A and B inhibitors, irreversible are predicted to increase the risk of side-effects when given with **tedizolid**. [Severe] Theoretical → Also see TABLE 13 p. 821

▸ Monoamine-oxidase B inhibitors (**rasagiline, selegiline**) are predicted to increase the risk of side-effects when given with **tedizolid**. [Severe] Theoretical → Also see TABLE 13 p. 821

▸ Monoamine-oxidase B inhibitors (**safinamide**) are predicted to increase the risk of side-effects when given with **tedizolid**. Avoid and for 1 week after stopping **safinamide**. [Severe] Theoretical → Also see TABLE 13 p. 821

▸ **Tedizolid** is predicted to increase the exposure to statins (**rosuvastatin**). Avoid. [Moderate] Theoretical

▸ **Tedizolid** is predicted to increase the exposure to sulfasalazine. Avoid. [Moderate] Theoretical

▸ **Tedizolid** is predicted to increase the exposure to topotecan. Avoid. [Moderate] Theoretical

Tegafur

▸ **Tegafur** potentially increases the concentration of antiepileptics (**fosphenytoin, phenytoin**). Monitor concentration and adjust dose. [Severe] Anecdotal

▸ **Tegafur** increases the anticoagulant effect of coumarins. [Moderate] Theoretical

▸ Folates (**folic acid, folinic acid**) are predicted to increase the risk of **tegafur** toxicity when given with **tegafur**. [Severe] Theoretical

▸ H_2 receptor antagonists (**cimetidine**) are predicted to increase the risk of toxicity when given with **tegafur**. [Severe] Theoretical

▸ Live vaccines are predicted to increase the risk of generalised infection (possibly life-threatening) when given with **tegafur**. Public Health England advises avoid. [Severe] Theoretical

▸ Methotrexate is predicted to increase the risk of toxicity when given with **tegafur**. [Severe] Theoretical

Teicoplanin

GENERAL INFORMATION If other nephrotoxic or neurotoxic drugs are given, monitor renal and auditory function on prolonged administration.

Telavancin → see TABLE 2 p. 818 (nephrotoxicity), TABLE 19 p. 822 (ototoxicity), TABLE 9 p. 820 (QT-interval prolongation)

▸ Telavancin is predicted to increase the risk of ototoxicity when given with aminoglycosides. [Moderate] Theoretical → Also see TABLE 2 p. 818 → Also see TABLE 19 p. 822

Telbivudine

▸ Interferons (**interferon alfa**) are predicted to increase the risk of peripheral neuropathy when given with **telbivudine**. Avoid. [Severe] Theoretical

▸ Interferons (**peginterferon alfa**) increase the risk of peripheral neuropathy when given with **telbivudine**. Avoid. [Severe] Study

Telmisartan → see angiotensin-II receptor antagonists

Temazepam → see TABLE 11 p. 820 (CNS depressant effects)

Temocillin → see penicillins

Temozolomide → see alkylating agents

Temsirolimus → see TABLE 15 p. 821 (myelosuppression)

▸ Antiarrhythmics (**dronedarone**) are predicted to increase the concentration of temsirolimus. [Moderate] Theoretical

▸ Antiepileptics (**carbamazepine, fosphenytoin, phenobarbital, phenytoin, primidone**) are predicted to decrease the concentration of temsirolimus. Avoid. [Severe] Study

▸ Antifungals, azoles (**fluconazole, isavuconazole, posaconazole**) are predicted to increase the concentration of temsirolimus. [Moderate] Theoretical

▸ Antifungals, azoles (**itraconazole, ketoconazole, voriconazole**) are predicted to increase the concentration of temsirolimus. Avoid. [Severe] Theoretical

▸ Aprepitant is predicted to increase the concentration of temsirolimus. [Moderate] Theoretical

▸ Bosentan is predicted to decrease the concentration of temsirolimus. Avoid. [Severe] Theoretical

▸ Calcium channel blockers (**diltiazem, verapamil**) are predicted to increase the concentration of temsirolimus. [Moderate] Theoretical

▸ Cobicistat is predicted to increase the concentration of temsirolimus. Avoid. [Severe] Theoretical

▸ Crizotinib is predicted to increase the concentration of temsirolimus. [Moderate] Theoretical → Also see TABLE 15 p. 821

▸ Efavirenz is predicted to decrease the concentration of temsirolimus. Avoid. [Severe] Theoretical

▸ Enzalutamide is predicted to decrease the concentration of temsirolimus. Avoid. [Severe] Study

- Grapefruit juice is predicted to increase the concentration of **temsirolimus**. Use with caution or avoid. [Moderate] Theoretical
- HIV-protease inhibitors **(atazanavir, darunavir, fosamprenavir, lopinavir, ritonavir, saquinavir, tipranavir)** are predicted to increase the concentration of **temsirolimus**. Avoid. [Severe] Theoretical
- HIV-protease inhibitors **(indinavir)** are predicted to increase the concentration of **temsirolimus**. [Moderate] Theoretical
- Idelalisib is predicted to increase the concentration of **temsirolimus**. Avoid. [Severe] Theoretical → Also see **TABLE 15** p. 821
- Imatinib is predicted to increase the concentration of **temsirolimus**. [Moderate] Theoretical → Also see **TABLE 15** p. 821
- Live vaccines are predicted to increase the risk of generalised infection (possibly life-threatening) when given with **temsirolimus**. Public Health England advises avoid. [Severe] Theoretical
- Lumacaftor is predicted to decrease the exposure to **temsirolimus**. [Moderate] Theoretical
- Macrolides **(clarithromycin)** are predicted to increase the concentration of **temsirolimus**. Avoid. [Severe] Theoretical
- Macrolides **(erythromycin)** are predicted to increase the concentration of **temsirolimus**. [Moderate] Theoretical
- Netupitant is predicted to increase the concentration of **temsirolimus**. [Moderate] Theoretical
- Nevirapine is predicted to decrease the concentration of **temsirolimus**. Avoid. [Severe] Theoretical
- Nilotinib is predicted to increase the concentration of **temsirolimus**. [Moderate] Theoretical → Also see **TABLE 15** p. 821
- Pitolisant is predicted to decrease the exposure to **temsirolimus**. Avoid. [Severe] Theoretical
- Rifampicin is predicted to decrease the concentration of **temsirolimus**. Avoid. [Severe] Study
- St John's Wort is predicted to decrease the concentration of **temsirolimus**. Avoid. [Severe] Theoretical

Tenecteplase → see **TABLE 3** p. 818 (anticoagulant effects)

Tenofovir → see **TABLE 2** p. 818 (nephrotoxicity)
- **Tenofovir** increases the risk of toxicity when given with didanosine. Avoid. [Severe] Study
- Ledipasvir (with sofosbuvir) slightly increases the exposure to tenofovir. [Moderate] Study
- **Tenofovir** is predicted to increase the exposure to sacubitril. [Moderate] Theoretical
- Velpatasvir increases the exposure to tenofovir. [Moderate] Study

Tenoxicam → see NSAIDs

Terazosin → see alpha blockers

Terbinafine

> **ROUTE-SPECIFIC INFORMATION** Since systemic absorption can follow topical application, the possibility of interactions should be borne in mind.

- **Terbinafine** is predicted to increase the exposure to antiarrhythmics **(flecainide)**. [Severe] Theoretical
- **Terbinafine** is predicted to increase the exposure to antiarrhythmics **(propafenone)**. Monitor and adjust dose. [Moderate] Study
- **Terbinafine** is predicted to increase the exposure to anticholinesterases, centrally acting **(donepezil)**. [Moderate] Theoretical
- **Terbinafine** is predicted to increase the exposure to anticholinesterases, centrally acting **(galantamine)**. Monitor and adjust dose. [Moderate] Study
- **Terbinafine** is predicted to moderately increase the exposure to aripiprazole. Adjust **aripiprazole** dose, p. 240. [Moderate] Study
- **Terbinafine** is predicted to markedly increase the exposure to atomoxetine. Adjust dose. [Severe] Study
- **Terbinafine** is predicted to increase the exposure to beta blockers, non-selective **(carvedilol, timolol)**. [Moderate] Study
- **Terbinafine** is predicted to increase the exposure to beta blockers, selective **(metoprolol, nebivolol)**. [Moderate] Study
- **Terbinafine** is predicted to slightly increase the exposure to darifenacin. [Mild] Study
- **Terbinafine** is predicted to decrease the efficacy of opioids **(codeine)**. [Moderate] Theoretical
- **Terbinafine** is predicted to decrease the efficacy of opioids **(tramadol)**. [Severe] Study

- **Terbinafine** is predicted to moderately increase the exposure to pitolisant. Use with caution and adjust dose. [Moderate] Study
- Rifampicin decreases the exposure to **terbinafine**. Adjust dose. [Moderate] Study
- **Terbinafine** is predicted to increase the exposure to risperidone. Adjust dose. [Moderate] Study
- **Terbinafine** is predicted to increase the exposure to SSRIs **(citalopram, dapoxetine, escitalopram, fluvoxamine, sertraline)**. [Moderate] Theoretical
- **Terbinafine** is predicted to increase the exposure to SSRIs **(fluoxetine)**. Adjust dose. [Moderate] Theoretical
- **Terbinafine** moderately increases the exposure to SSRIs **(paroxetine)**. [Moderate] Study
- **Terbinafine** is predicted to decrease the efficacy of tamoxifen. Avoid. [Severe] Study
- **Terbinafine** is predicted to increase the exposure to tricyclic antidepressants. Monitor for toxicity and adjust dose. [Severe] Study
- **Terbinafine** is predicted to increase the exposure to vortioxetine. Monitor and adjust dose. [Moderate] Study

Terbutaline → see beta₂ agonists

Teriflunomide
- **Teriflunomide** affects the anticoagulant effect of coumarins. [Severe] Study
- Live vaccines are predicted to increase the risk of generalised infection (possibly life-threatening) when given with **teriflunomide**. Public Health England advises avoid. [Severe] Theoretical
- **Teriflunomide** increases the exposure to repaglinide. [Moderate] Study
- **Teriflunomide** moderately increases the exposure to statins **(rosuvastatin)**. Adjust **rosuvastatin** dose, p. 130. [Moderate] Study

Tetrabenazine → see **TABLE 9** p. 820 (QT-interval prolongation)
- **Tetrabenazine** is predicted to decrease the effects of levodopa. Use with caution or avoid. [Moderate] Theoretical
- **Tetrabenazine** is predicted to increase the risk of CNS toxicity when given with monoamine-oxidase A and B inhibitors, irreversible. Avoid and for 14 days after stopping the MAOI. [Severe] Theoretical

Tetracaine → see anaesthetics, local

Tetracycline → see tetracyclines

Tetracyclines → see **TABLE 1** p. 818 (hepatotoxicity)

> demeclocycline · doxycycline · lymecycline · minocycline · oxytetracycline · tetracycline · tigecycline

- ACE inhibitors **(quinapril)** (tablet) decrease the absorption of oral **tetracycline**. Avoid. [Moderate] Study
- Antacids decrease the absorption of **tetracyclines**. Separate administration by 2 to 3 hours. [Moderate] Study
- Antiepileptics **(carbamazepine, fosphenytoin, phenobarbital, phenytoin, primidone)** decrease the exposure to **doxycycline**. Monitor and adjust dose. [Moderate] Study → Also see **TABLE 1** p. 818
- **Tetracycline** decreases the concentration of antimalarials **(atovaquone)**. [Moderate] Study
- Calcium salts **(calcium carbonate)** are predicted to decrease the absorption of **tetracyclines**. Separate administration by 2 to 3 hours. [Moderate] Theoretical
- **Tetracyclines** increase the risk of bleeding events when given with coumarins. [Moderate] Anecdotal
- Dairy products decreases the exposure to tetracyclines **(demeclocycline, oxytetracycline, tetracycline)**. Avoid. [Moderate] Study
- Enzalutamide decreases the exposure to **doxycycline**. Monitor and adjust dose. [Moderate] Study
- Iron (oral) decreases the absorption of **tetracyclines**. **Tetracyclines** should be taken 2 to 3 hours after iron (oral). [Moderate] Study
- Kaolin is predicted to decrease the absorption of **tetracyclines**. [Moderate] Theoretical
- Lanthanum is predicted to decrease the absorption of **tetracyclines**. Separate administration by 2 hours. [Moderate] Theoretical
- Retinoids **(acitretin, alitretinoin, isotretinoin, tretinoin)** increase the risk of benign intracranial hypertension when given with **tetracyclines**. Avoid. [Severe] Anecdotal

Tetracyclines (continued)

‣ Rifampicin decreases the exposure to **doxycycline**. Monitor and adjust dose. Moderate Study

‣ Strontium ranelate is predicted to decrease the absorption of **tetracyclines**. Avoid. Moderate Theoretical

‣ Oral zinc is predicted to decrease the absorption of **tetracyclines**. Separate administration by 2 to 3 hours. Moderate Theoretical

Thalidomide → see TABLE 6 p. 819 (bradycardia), TABLE 15 p. 821 (myelosuppression), TABLE 12 p. 821 (peripheral neuropathy), TABLE 5 p. 818 (thromboembolism), TABLE 11 p. 820 (CNS depressant effects)

‣ Combined hormonal contraceptives are predicted to increase the risk of venous thromboembolism when given with **thalidomide**. Avoid. Severe Study

‣ Hormone replacement therapy is predicted to increase the risk of venous thromboembolism when given with **thalidomide**. Severe Theoretical

Theophylline → see TABLE 17 p. 822 (reduced serum potassium)

FOOD AND LIFESTYLE Smoking can increase theophylline clearance and increased doses of theophylline are therefore required; dose adjustments are likely to be necessary if smoking started or stopped during treatment.

‣ Aciclovir is predicted to increase the exposure to **theophylline**. Monitor **theophylline** concentration and adjust dose. Severe Theoretical

‣ **Theophylline** decreases the efficacy of antiarrhythmics (adenosine). Separate administration by 24 hours. Mild Study

‣ Antiepileptics (carbamazepine) potentially increase the clearance of **theophylline** and **theophylline** decreases the exposure to antiepileptics (carbamazepine). Adjust dose. Moderate Anecdotal

‣ Antiepileptics (fosphenytoin) are predicted to increase the clearance of **theophylline**. Adjust dose. Moderate Study

‣ Antiepileptics (phenobarbital, primidone) are predicted to increase the clearance of **theophylline**. Adjust dose. Moderate Theoretical

‣ Antiepileptics (phenytoin) are predicted to decrease the exposure to **theophylline**. Adjust dose. Moderate Study

‣ Beta blockers, non-selective are predicted to increase the risk of bronchospasm when given with **theophylline**. Avoid. Severe Theoretical

‣ Beta blockers, selective are predicted to increase the risk of bronchospasm when given with **theophylline**. Avoid. Severe Theoretical

‣ Caffeine citrate decreases the clearance of **theophylline**. Moderate Study

‣ Combined hormonal contraceptives are predicted to increase the exposure to **theophylline**. Monitor and adjust dose. Moderate Theoretical

‣ **Theophylline** increases the risk of agitation when given with doxapram. Moderate Study

‣ Enteral feeds decreases the exposure to **theophylline**. Moderate Study

‣ H₂ receptor antagonists (cimetidine) increase the concentration of **theophylline**. Adjust dose. Severe Study

‣ HIV-protease inhibitors (ritonavir) are predicted to decrease the exposure to **theophylline**. Adjust dose. Moderate Study

‣ Interferons slightly increase the exposure to **theophylline**. Adjust dose. Moderate Study

‣ Iron chelators (deferasirox) increase the exposure to **theophylline**. Avoid. Moderate Study

‣ Isoniazid is predicted to affect the clearance of **theophylline**. Severe Anecdotal

‣ **Theophylline** is predicted to decrease the concentration of lithium. Moderate Anecdotal

‣ Macrolides (azithromycin, clarithromycin) are predicted to increase the exposure to **theophylline**. Adjust dose. Moderate Anecdotal

‣ Macrolides (erythromycin) decrease the clearance of **theophylline** and **theophylline** potentially decreases the clearance of macrolides (erythromycin). Adjust dose. Severe Study

‣ Methotrexate decreases the clearance of **theophylline**. Moderate Study

‣ Monoclonal antibodies (blinatumomab) are predicted to transiently increase the exposure to **theophylline**. Monitor and adjust dose. Moderate Theoretical

‣ Pentoxifylline increases the concentration of **theophylline**. Monitor and adjust dose. Severe Study

‣ Quinolones (ciprofloxacin) are predicted to increase the exposure to **theophylline**. Monitor and adjust dose. Moderate Theoretical

‣ Quinolones (norfloxacin) are predicted to increase the exposure to **theophylline**. Adjust dose. Moderate Anecdotal

‣ Rifampicin is predicted to decrease the exposure to **theophylline**. Adjust dose. Moderate Study

‣ **Theophylline** is predicted to slightly increase the exposure to roflumilast. Avoid. Moderate Theoretical

‣ SSRIs (fluvoxamine) moderately to markedly increase the exposure to **theophylline**. Avoid. Severe Study

‣ St John's Wort potentially decreases the exposure to **theophylline**. Severe Anecdotal

‣ Sucralfate potentially decreases the absorption of **theophylline**. Separate administration by at least 2 hours. Moderate Study

‣ Sympathomimetics, vasoconstrictor (ephedrine) increase the risk of side-effects when given with **theophylline**. Avoid in children. Moderate Study

‣ Valaciclovir is predicted to increase the exposure to **theophylline**. Severe Theoretical

Thiazide diuretics → see TABLE 18 p. 822 (hyponatraemia), TABLE 8 p. 819 (hypotension), TABLE 17 p. 822 (reduced serum potassium)

bendroflumethiazide · chlortalidone · clopamide · cyclopenthiazide · hydrochlorothiazide · hydroflumethiazide · indapamide · metolazone · xipamide

‣ **Thiazide diuretics** are predicted to increase the risk of hypersensitivity reactions when given with allopurinol. Severe Theoretical

‣ Aspirin (high-dose) increases the risk of acute renal failure when given with **thiazide diuretics**. Severe Theoretical

‣ **Thiazide diuretics** increase the risk of hypercalcaemia when given with calcium salts. Severe Anecdotal

‣ **Thiazide diuretics** increase the concentration of lithium. Avoid or adjust lithium (lithium carbonate, lithium citrate) dose and monitor lithium (lithium carbonate, lithium citrate) concentration. Severe Study

‣ NSAIDs increase the risk of acute renal failure when given with **thiazide diuretics**. Severe Theoretical → Also see TABLE 18 p. 822

‣ Reboxetine is predicted to increase the risk of hypokalaemia when given with **thiazide diuretics**. Moderate Anecdotal

‣ **Thiazide diuretics** are predicted to increase the risk of hypercalcaemia when given with toremifene. Severe Theoretical

‣ **Thiazide diuretics** increase the risk of hypercalcaemia when given with vitamin D substances. Moderate Theoretical

Thiopental → see TABLE 8 p. 819 (hypotension), TABLE 11 p. 820 (CNS depressant effects)

‣ Sulfonamides are predicted to increase the effects of thiopental. Moderate Theoretical

‣ Tricyclic antidepressants increase the risk of cardiac arrhythmias and hypotension when given with **thiopental**. Moderate Study → Also see TABLE 8 p. 819

Thiotepa → see alkylating agents

Tiagabine → see antiepileptics

Tiaprofenic acid → see NSAIDs

Tibolone → see TABLE 5 p. 818 (thromboembolism)

Ticagrelor → see TABLE 4 p. 818 (antiplatelet effects)

‣ Antiarrhythmics (amiodarone) are predicted to increase the exposure to **ticagrelor**. Use with caution or avoid. Severe Study

‣ Antiepileptics (carbamazepine, fosphenytoin, phenobarbital, phenytoin, primidone) are predicted to markedly decrease the exposure to **ticagrelor**. Avoid. Severe Study

‣ Antifungals, azoles (itraconazole, ketoconazole, voriconazole) are predicted to markedly increase the exposure to **ticagrelor**. Avoid. Severe Study

‣ Bosentan is predicted to decrease the exposure to **ticagrelor**. Moderate Theoretical

‣ Ciclosporin is predicted to increase the exposure to **ticagrelor**. Use with caution or avoid. Severe Study

- Cobicistat is predicted to markedly increase the exposure to ticagrelor. Avoid. Severe Study
- Ticagrelor increases the concentration of digoxin. Moderate Study
- Efavirenz is predicted to decrease the exposure to ticagrelor. Moderate Theoretical
- Enzalutamide is predicted to markedly decrease the exposure to ticagrelor. Avoid. Severe Study
- Grapefruit juice moderately increases the exposure to ticagrelor. Moderate Study
- HIV-protease inhibitors (atazanavir, darunavir, fosamprenavir, lopinavir, ritonavir, saquinavir, tipranavir) are predicted to markedly increase the exposure to ticagrelor. Avoid. Severe Study
- Idelalisib is predicted to markedly increase the exposure to ticagrelor. Avoid. Severe Study
- Ticagrelor is predicted to increase the exposure to lomitapide. Separate administration by 12 hours. Moderate Theoretical
- Macrolides (azithromycin) are predicted to increase the exposure to ticagrelor. Use with caution or avoid. Severe Study
- Macrolides (clarithromycin) are predicted to markedly increase the exposure to ticagrelor. Avoid. Severe Study
- Nevirapine is predicted to decrease the exposure to ticagrelor. Moderate Theoretical
- Ranolazine is predicted to increase the exposure to ticagrelor. Use with caution or avoid. Severe Study
- Rifampicin is predicted to markedly decrease the exposure to ticagrelor. Avoid. Severe Study
- St John's Wort is predicted to decrease the exposure to ticagrelor. Moderate Theoretical
- Ticagrelor slightly increases the exposure to statins (simvastatin). Adjust simvastatin dose, p. 130. Moderate Study
- Vemurafenib is predicted to increase the exposure to ticagrelor. Use with caution or avoid. Severe Study

Ticarcillin → see penicillins
Tigecycline → see tetracyclines
Timolol → see beta blockers, non-selective
Tinidazole

> FOOD AND LIFESTYLE Disulfiram-like reaction is predicted to occur on the ingestion of alcohol. Ensure that alcohol is not consumed for 72 hours after stopping tinidazole.

- Tinidazole is predicted to increase the anticoagulant effect of coumarins. Monitor INR and adjust dose. Severe Theoretical

Tinzaparin → see low molecular-weight heparins
Tioguanine → see TABLE 15 p. 821 (myelosuppression)
- Live vaccines are predicted to increase the risk of generalised infection (possibly life-threatening) when given with tioguanine. Public Health England advises avoid. Severe Theoretical

Tiotropium → see TABLE 10 p. 820 (antimuscarinics)
Tipranavir → see HIV-protease inhibitors
Tirofiban → see TABLE 4 p. 818 (antiplatelet effects)
Tizanidine → see TABLE 6 p. 819 (bradycardia), TABLE 8 p. 819 (hypotension), TABLE 9 p. 820 (QT-interval prolongation), TABLE 11 p. 820 (CNS depressant effects)
- Antiepileptics (fosphenytoin, phenytoin) moderately decrease the exposure to tizanidine. Mild Study
- Combined hormonal contraceptives increases the exposure to tizanidine. Avoid. Moderate Study
- HIV-protease inhibitors (ritonavir) moderately decrease the exposure to tizanidine. Mild Study
- Iron chelators (deferasirox) are predicted to increase the exposure to tizanidine. Moderate Theoretical
- Quinolones (ciprofloxacin) increase the exposure to tizanidine. Avoid. Moderate Study
- Rifampicin moderately decreases the exposure to tizanidine. Mild Study
- SSRIs (fluvoxamine) very markedly increase the exposure to tizanidine. Avoid. Severe Study

Tobramycin → see aminoglycosides
Tocilizumab → see monoclonal antibodies
Tolbutamide → see sulfonylureas
Tolcapone
- Tolcapone increases the exposure to levodopa. Monitor and adjust dose. Moderate Study

- Tolcapone is predicted to increase the effects of monoamine-oxidase A and B inhibitors, irreversible. Avoid. Severe Theoretical
- Tolcapone is predicted to increase the risk of cardiovascular side-effects when given with sympathomimetics, inotropic (dobutamine, dopamine). Moderate Theoretical
- Tolcapone is predicted to increase the effects of sympathomimetics, vasoconstrictor (adrenaline/epinephrine, noradrenaline/norepinephrine). Moderate Theoretical

Tolfenamic acid → see NSAIDs
Tolterodine → see TABLE 9 p. 820 (QT-interval prolongation), TABLE 10 p. 820 (antimuscarinics)
- Antiarrhythmics (dronedarone) are predicted to increase the exposure to tolterodine. Mild Theoretical → Also see TABLE 9 p. 820
- Antifungals, azoles (fluconazole, isavuconazole, posaconazole) are predicted to increase the exposure to tolterodine. Mild Theoretical
- Antifungals, azoles (itraconazole, ketoconazole, voriconazole) are predicted to increase the exposure to tolterodine. Avoid. Severe Study → Also see TABLE 9 p. 820
- Aprepitant is predicted to increase the exposure to tolterodine. Mild Theoretical
- Calcium channel blockers (diltiazem, verapamil) are predicted to increase the exposure to tolterodine. Mild Theoretical
- Cobicistat is predicted to increase the exposure to tolterodine. Avoid. Severe Study
- Crizotinib is predicted to increase the exposure to tolterodine. Mild Theoretical → Also see TABLE 9 p. 820
- HIV-protease inhibitors (atazanavir, darunavir, fosamprenavir, lopinavir, ritonavir, saquinavir, tipranavir) are predicted to increase the exposure to tolterodine. Avoid. Severe Study → Also see TABLE 9 p. 820
- HIV-protease inhibitors (indinavir) are predicted to increase the exposure to tolterodine. Mild Theoretical
- Idelalisib is predicted to increase the exposure to tolterodine. Avoid. Severe Study
- Imatinib is predicted to increase the exposure to tolterodine. Mild Theoretical
- Macrolides (clarithromycin) are predicted to increase the exposure to tolterodine. Avoid. Severe Study → Also see TABLE 9 p. 820
- Macrolides (erythromycin) are predicted to increase the exposure to tolterodine. Mild Theoretical
- Netupitant is predicted to increase the exposure to tolterodine. Mild Theoretical
- Nilotinib is predicted to increase the exposure to tolterodine. Mild Theoretical → Also see TABLE 9 p. 820
- Panobinostat is predicted to increase the exposure to tolterodine. Moderate Theoretical → Also see TABLE 9 p. 820

Tolvaptan → see TABLE 16 p. 822 (increased serum potassium)

> GENERAL INFORMATION Avoid concurrent use of drugs that increase serum-sodium concentrations.

- Antiarrhythmics (dronedarone) are predicted to increase the exposure to tolvaptan. Adjust dose. Moderate Theoretical
- Antiepileptics (carbamazepine, fosphenytoin, phenobarbital, phenytoin, primidone) are predicted to decrease the exposure to tolvaptan. Avoid. Severe Study
- Antifungals, azoles (fluconazole, isavuconazole, posaconazole) are predicted to increase the exposure to tolvaptan. Adjust dose. Moderate Theoretical
- Antifungals, azoles (itraconazole, ketoconazole, voriconazole) are predicted to increase the exposure to tolvaptan. Adjust dose. Severe Study
- Aprepitant is predicted to increase the exposure to tolvaptan. Adjust dose. Moderate Theoretical
- Bosentan is predicted to decrease the exposure to tolvaptan. Moderate Theoretical
- Calcium channel blockers (diltiazem, verapamil) are predicted to increase the exposure to tolvaptan. Adjust dose. Moderate Theoretical
- Cobicistat is predicted to increase the exposure to tolvaptan. Adjust dose. Severe Study
- Crizotinib is predicted to increase the exposure to tolvaptan. Adjust dose. Moderate Theoretical
- Tolvaptan increases the concentration of digoxin. Mild Study

A1

Interactions | Appendix 1

Tolvaptan (continued)
- Efavirenz is predicted to decrease the exposure to **tolvaptan**. Moderate Theoretical
- Enzalutamide is predicted to decrease the exposure to **tolvaptan**. Avoid. Severe Study
- Grapefruit juice increases the exposure to **tolvaptan**. Avoid. Moderate Study
- HIV-protease inhibitors (atazanavir, darunavir, fosamprenavir, lopinavir, ritonavir, saquinavir, tipranavir) are predicted to increase the exposure to **tolvaptan**. Adjust dose. Severe Study
- HIV-protease inhibitors (indinavir) are predicted to increase the exposure to **tolvaptan**. Adjust dose. Moderate Theoretical
- Idelalisib is predicted to increase the exposure to **tolvaptan**. Adjust dose. Severe Study
- Imatinib is predicted to increase the exposure to **tolvaptan**. Adjust dose. Moderate Theoretical
- **Tolvaptan** is predicted to increase the exposure to lomitapide. Separate administration by 12 hours. Moderate Theoretical
- Macrolides (clarithromycin) are predicted to increase the exposure to **tolvaptan**. Adjust dose. Severe Study
- Macrolides (erythromycin) are predicted to increase the exposure to **tolvaptan**. Adjust dose. Moderate Theoretical
- Netupitant is predicted to increase the exposure to **tolvaptan**. Adjust dose. Moderate Theoretical
- Nevirapine is predicted to decrease the exposure to **tolvaptan**. Moderate Theoretical
- Nilotinib is predicted to increase the exposure to **tolvaptan**. Adjust dose. Moderate Theoretical
- Rifampicin is predicted to decrease the exposure to **tolvaptan**. Avoid. Severe Study
- St John's Wort is predicted to decrease the exposure to **tolvaptan**. Moderate Theoretical

Topiramate → see antiepileptics

Topotecan → see TABLE 15 p. 821 (myelosuppression)
- Antiarrhythmics (amiodarone, dronedarone) are predicted to increase the exposure to **topotecan**. Severe Study
- Antiepileptics (fosphenytoin, phenytoin) increase the clearance of **topotecan**. Moderate Study
- Antifungals, azoles (itraconazole, ketoconazole) are predicted to increase the exposure to **topotecan**. Severe Study
- Calcium channel blockers (verapamil) are predicted to increase the exposure to **topotecan**. Severe Study
- Ceritinib is predicted to increase the exposure to **topotecan**. Moderate Theoretical → Also see TABLE 15 p. 821
- Ciclosporin is predicted to increase the exposure to **topotecan**. Severe Study
- HIV-protease inhibitors (lopinavir, ritonavir, saquinavir) are predicted to increase the exposure to **topotecan**. Severe Study
- Lapatinib is predicted to increase the exposure to **topotecan**. Severe Study
- Live vaccines are predicted to increase the risk of generalised infection (possibly life-threatening) when given with **topotecan**. Public Health England advises avoid. Severe Theoretical
- Lumacaftor is predicted to affect the exposure to **topotecan**. Moderate Theoretical
- Macrolides are predicted to increase the exposure to **topotecan**. Severe Study
- Mirabegron is predicted to increase the exposure to **topotecan**. Mild Theoretical
- Ranolazine is predicted to increase the exposure to **topotecan**. Severe Study
- St John's Wort is predicted to decrease the exposure to **topotecan**. Severe Theoretical
- Tedizolid is predicted to increase the exposure to **topotecan**. Avoid. Moderate Theoretical
- Velpatasvir is predicted to increase the exposure to **topotecan**. Severe Study
- Vemurafenib is predicted to increase the exposure to **topotecan**. Severe Study

Torasemide → see loop diuretics

Toremifene → see TABLE 5 p. 818 (thromboembolism), TABLE 9 p. 820 (QT-interval prolongation)

- Antiepileptics (carbamazepine, fosphenytoin, phenobarbital, phenytoin, primidone) are predicted to decrease the exposure to **toremifene**. Adjust dose. Moderate Study
- Antifungals, azoles (itraconazole, ketoconazole, voriconazole) are predicted to increase the exposure to **toremifene**. Moderate Theoretical → Also see TABLE 9 p. 820
- Cobicistat is predicted to increase the exposure to **toremifene**. Moderate Theoretical
- **Toremifene** is predicted to increase the anticoagulant effect of coumarins. Severe Theoretical
- Enzalutamide is predicted to decrease the exposure to **toremifene**. Adjust dose. Moderate Study
- HIV-protease inhibitors (atazanavir, darunavir, fosamprenavir, lopinavir, ritonavir, saquinavir, tipranavir) are predicted to increase the exposure to **toremifene**. Moderate Theoretical → Also see TABLE 9 p. 820
- Idelalisib is predicted to increase the exposure to **toremifene**. Moderate Theoretical
- Macrolides (clarithromycin) are predicted to increase the exposure to **toremifene**. Moderate Theoretical → Also see TABLE 9 p. 820
- Rifampicin is predicted to decrease the exposure to **toremifene**. Adjust dose. Moderate Study
- Thiazide diuretics are predicted to increase the risk of hypercalcaemia when given with **toremifene**. Severe Theoretical

Trabectedin → see TABLE 1 p. 818 (hepatotoxicity), TABLE 15 p. 821 (myelosuppression)
- Antiepileptics (carbamazepine, fosphenytoin, phenobarbital, phenytoin, primidone) are predicted to decrease the exposure to **trabectedin**. Severe Theoretical → Also see TABLE 1 p. 818
- Antifungals, azoles (itraconazole, ketoconazole, voriconazole) are predicted to increase the exposure to **trabectedin**. Avoid or adjust dose. Severe Theoretical → Also see TABLE 1 p. 818
- Cobicistat is predicted to increase the exposure to **trabectedin**. Avoid or adjust dose. Severe Theoretical
- Enzalutamide is predicted to decrease the exposure to **trabectedin**. Avoid. Severe Theoretical
- HIV-protease inhibitors (atazanavir, darunavir, fosamprenavir, lopinavir, ritonavir, saquinavir, tipranavir) are predicted to increase the exposure to **trabectedin**. Avoid or adjust dose. Severe Theoretical
- Idelalisib is predicted to increase the exposure to **trabectedin**. Avoid or adjust dose. Severe Theoretical → Also see TABLE 15 p. 821
- Live vaccines are predicted to increase the risk of generalised infection (possibly life-threatening) when given with **trabectedin**. Public Health England advises avoid. Severe Theoretical
- Macrolides (clarithromycin) are predicted to increase the exposure to **trabectedin**. Avoid or adjust dose. Severe Theoretical
- Rifampicin is predicted to decrease the exposure to **trabectedin**. Severe Theoretical

Tramadol → see opioids

Trametinib
- Antiarrhythmics (amiodarone, dronedarone) are predicted to increase the concentration of **trametinib**. Moderate Theoretical
- Antifungals, azoles (itraconazole, ketoconazole) are predicted to increase the concentration of **trametinib**. Moderate Theoretical
- Calcium channel blockers (verapamil) are predicted to increase the concentration of **trametinib**. Moderate Theoretical
- Ciclosporin is predicted to increase the concentration of **trametinib**. Moderate Theoretical
- HIV-protease inhibitors (lopinavir, ritonavir, saquinavir) are predicted to increase the concentration of **trametinib**. Moderate Theoretical
- Lapatinib is predicted to increase the concentration of **trametinib**. Moderate Theoretical
- Macrolides are predicted to increase the concentration of **trametinib**. Moderate Theoretical
- Ranolazine is predicted to increase the concentration of **trametinib**. Moderate Theoretical
- Vemurafenib is predicted to increase the concentration of **trametinib**. Moderate Theoretical

Trandolapril → see ACE inhibitors

Tranexamic acid → see TABLE 5 p. 818 (thromboembolism)

Tranylcypromine → see monoamine-oxidase A and B inhibitors, irreversible

Trastuzumab → see monoclonal antibodies

Trastuzumab emtansine → see monoclonal antibodies

Trazodone → see TABLE 13 p. 821 (serotonin syndrome), TABLE 11 p. 820 (CNS depressant effects)

▶ Antiarrhythmics (**dronedarone**) are predicted to increase the exposure to **trazodone**. Moderate Theoretical

▶ Antiepileptics (**carbamazepine**) decrease the concentration of **trazodone**. Adjust dose. Moderate Anecdotal

▶ Antifungals, azoles (**fluconazole, isavuconazole, posaconazole**) are predicted to increase the exposure to **trazodone**. Moderate Theoretical

▶ Antifungals, azoles (**itraconazole, ketoconazole, voriconazole**) are predicted to moderately increase the exposure to **trazodone**. Avoid or adjust dose. Moderate Study

▶ Aprepitant is predicted to increase the exposure to **trazodone**. Moderate Theoretical

▶ Calcium channel blockers (**diltiazem, verapamil**) are predicted to increase the exposure to **trazodone**. Moderate Theoretical

▶ Cobicistat is predicted to moderately increase the exposure to **trazodone**. Avoid or adjust dose. Moderate Study

▶ Crizotinib is predicted to increase the exposure to **trazodone**. Moderate Theoretical

▶ HIV-protease inhibitors (**atazanavir, darunavir, fosamprenavir, lopinavir, ritonavir, saquinavir, tipranavir**) are predicted to moderately increase the exposure to **trazodone**. Avoid or adjust dose. Moderate Study

▶ HIV-protease inhibitors (**indinavir**) are predicted to increase the exposure to **trazodone**. Moderate Theoretical

▶ Idelalisib is predicted to moderately increase the exposure to **trazodone**. Avoid or adjust dose. Moderate Study

▶ Imatinib is predicted to increase the exposure to **trazodone**. Moderate Theoretical

▶ Macrolides (**clarithromycin**) are predicted to moderately increase the exposure to **trazodone**. Avoid or adjust dose. Moderate Study

▶ Macrolides (**erythromycin**) are predicted to increase the exposure to **trazodone**. Moderate Theoretical

▶ Netupitant is predicted to increase the exposure to **trazodone**. Moderate Theoretical

▶ Nilotinib is predicted to increase the exposure to **trazodone**. Moderate Theoretical

Tree pollen extract

> **GENERAL INFORMATION** Desensitising vaccines should be avoided in patients taking beta-blockers (adrenaline might be ineffective in case of a hypersensitivity reaction) or ACE inhibitors (risk of severe anaphylactoid reactions).

Treosulfan → see alkylating agents

Tretinoin → see retinoids

Triamcinolone → see corticosteroids

Triamterene → see potassium-sparing diuretics

Tricyclic antidepressants → see TABLE 18 p. 822 (hyponatraemia), TABLE 8 p. 819 (hypotension), TABLE 13 p. 821 (serotonin syndrome), TABLE 9 p. 820 (QT-interval prolongation), TABLE 10 p. 820 (antimuscarinics)

amitriptyline · clomipramine · dosulepin · doxepin · imipramine · lofepramine · nortriptyline · trimipramine

▶ Antiarrhythmics (**dronedarone**) are predicted to increase the risk of torsade de pointes when given with **tricyclic antidepressants**. Avoid. Severe Theoretical → Also see TABLE 9 p. 820

▶ Antiarrhythmics (**propafenone**) are predicted to increase the concentration of **tricyclic antidepressants**. Moderate Theoretical → Also see TABLE 10 p. 820

▶ Antiepileptics (**carbamazepine**) decrease the exposure to **tricyclic antidepressants**. Adjust dose. Moderate Study → Also see TABLE 18 p. 822

▶ Antiepileptics (**phenobarbital, primidone**) are predicted to decrease the exposure to **tricyclic antidepressants**. Moderate Study

▶ Tricyclic antidepressants (**clomipramine, imipramine**) potentially increase the risk of overheating and dehydration when given

with antiepileptics (**zonisamide**). Avoid in children. Severe Theoretical

▶ Bupropion is predicted to increase the exposure to **tricyclic antidepressants**. Monitor for toxicity and adjust dose. Severe Study → Also see TABLE 13 p. 821

▶ Cinacalcet is predicted to increase the exposure to **tricyclic antidepressants**. Monitor for toxicity and adjust dose. Severe Study

▶ Tricyclic antidepressants decrease the antihypertensive effects of **clonidine**. Monitor and adjust dose. Moderate Anecdotal → Also see TABLE 8 p. 819

▶ Cobicistat is predicted to slightly increase the exposure to **tricyclic antidepressants**. Mild Study

▶ Darifenacin is predicted to increase the exposure to **tricyclic antidepressants**. Moderate Theoretical → Also see TABLE 10 p. 820

▶ Tricyclic antidepressants are predicted to decrease the antihypertensive effects of **guanethidine**. Moderate Study → Also see TABLE 8 p. 819

▶ H₂ receptor antagonists (**cimetidine**) increase the exposure to **tricyclic antidepressants**. Moderate Study

▶ Tricyclic antidepressants are predicted to increase the effects of **histamine**. Avoid. Severe Theoretical → Also see TABLE 8 p. 819

▶ HIV-protease inhibitors (**ritonavir, tipranavir**) are predicted to increase the exposure to **tricyclic antidepressants**. Moderate Theoretical

▶ Tricyclic antidepressants potentially increase the risk of neurotoxicity when given with **lithium**. Severe Anecdotal → Also see TABLE 9 p. 820 → Also see TABLE 13 p. 821

▶ Amitriptyline decreases the effects of **metyrapone**. Avoid. Moderate Theoretical

▶ Tricyclic antidepressants are predicted to increase the effects of **moclobemide**. Avoid. Severe Theoretical → Also see TABLE 13 p. 821

▶ Tricyclic antidepressants are predicted to increase the effects of **monoamine-oxidase A and B inhibitors, irreversible**. Avoid. Severe Theoretical → Also see TABLE 8 p. 819 → Also see TABLE 13 p. 821

▶ Tricyclic antidepressants are predicted to decrease the effects of **moxonidine**. Avoid. Moderate Theoretical → Also see TABLE 8 p. 819

▶ Tricyclic antidepressants are predicted to decrease the efficacy of **pitolisant**. Mild Theoretical

▶ SSRIs (**fluoxetine, paroxetine**) are predicted to increase the exposure to **tricyclic antidepressants**. Monitor for toxicity and adjust dose. Severe Study → Also see TABLE 13 p. 821 → Also see TABLE 18 p. 822

▶ SSRIs (**fluvoxamine**) markedly increase the exposure to **clomipramine**. Adjust dose. Severe Study → Also see TABLE 18 p. 822 → Also see TABLE 13 p. 821

▶ SSRIs (**fluvoxamine**) increase the exposure to tricyclic antidepressants (**amitriptyline, imipramine**). Adjust dose. Severe Study → Also see TABLE 18 p. 822 → Also see TABLE 13 p. 821

▶ Sucralfate is predicted to decrease the absorption of **tricyclic antidepressants**. Moderate Study

▶ Tricyclic antidepressants increase the effects of sympathomimetics, vasoconstrictor (**adrenaline/epinephrine, noradrenaline/norepinephrine, phenylephrine**). Avoid. Severe Study

▶ Tricyclic antidepressants are predicted to decrease the effects of sympathomimetics, vasoconstrictor (**ephedrine**). Avoid. Severe Study

▶ Terbinafine is predicted to increase the exposure to **tricyclic antidepressants**. Monitor for toxicity and adjust dose. Severe Study

▶ Tricyclic antidepressants increase the risk of cardiac arrhythmias and hypotension when given with **thiopental**. Moderate Study → Also see TABLE 8 p. 819

Trientine

▶ Trientine potentially decreases the absorption of **iron (oral)**. Moderate Theoretical

▶ Trientine potentially decreases the absorption of **zinc**. Moderate Theoretical

Trifluoperazine → see phenothiazines

Trihexyphenidyl → see TABLE 10 p. 820 (antimuscarinics)

A1

Interactions | Appendix 1

Trimethoprim → see TABLE 18 p. 822 (hyponatraemia), TABLE 2 p. 818 (nephrotoxicity), TABLE 16 p. 822 (increased serum potassium)

▸ **Trimethoprim** increases the concentration of antiepileptics (**fosphenytoin, phenytoin**). Moderate Study

▸ **Antimalarials (pyrimethamine)** increase the risk of side-effects when given with **trimethoprim**. Severe Study

▸ **Trimethoprim** is predicted to increase the anticoagulant effect of **coumarins**. Severe Study

▸ **Dapsone** increases the exposure to **trimethoprim** and **trimethoprim** increases the exposure to **dapsone**. Severe Study

▸ **Trimethoprim** increases the concentration of **digoxin**. Moderate Study

▸ **Trimethoprim** slightly increases the exposure to **lamivudine**. Moderate Study

▸ **Trimethoprim** is predicted to increase the risk of side-effects when given with **methotrexate**. Avoid. Severe Theoretical → Also see TABLE 2 p. 818

▸ **Trimethoprim** slightly increases the exposure to **repaglinide**. Avoid or monitor blood glucose. Moderate Study

▸ **Rifampicin** decreases the exposure to **trimethoprim**. Moderate Study

▸ **Trimethoprim** is predicted to decrease the efficacy of **sapropterin**. Moderate Theoretical

Trimipramine → see tricyclic antidepressants

Tropicamide → see TABLE 10 p. 820 (antimuscarinics)

Trospium → see TABLE 10 p. 820 (antimuscarinics)

Typhoid vaccine → see live vaccines

Ulipristal

▸ **Antiarrhythmics (dronedarone)** are predicted to increase the exposure to **ulipristal**. Avoid if used for uterine fibroids. Moderate Study

▸ **Antiepileptics (carbamazepine, eslicarbazepine, fosphenytoin, oxcarbazepine, perampanel, phenobarbital, phenytoin, primidone, rufinamide, topiramate)** decrease the efficacy of **ulipristal**. For FSRH guidance, see Contraceptives, interactions p. 474. Severe Anecdotal

▸ **Antifungals, azoles (fluconazole, isavuconazole, posaconazole)** are predicted to increase the exposure to **ulipristal**. Avoid if used for uterine fibroids. Moderate Study

▸ **Antifungals, azoles (itraconazole, ketoconazole, voriconazole)** are predicted to increase the exposure to **ulipristal**. Avoid if used for uterine fibroids. Severe Study

▸ **Aprepitant** decreases the efficacy of **ulipristal**. For FSRH guidance, see Contraceptives, interactions p. 474. Severe Anecdotal

▸ **Bosentan** decreases the efficacy of **ulipristal**. For FSRH guidance, see Contraceptives, interactions p. 474. Severe Anecdotal

▸ **Calcium channel blockers (diltiazem, verapamil)** are predicted to increase the exposure to **ulipristal**. Avoid if used for uterine fibroids. Moderate Study

▸ **Cobicistat** is predicted to increase the exposure to **ulipristal**. Avoid if used for uterine fibroids. Severe Study

▸ **Ulipristal** is predicted to decrease the efficacy of **combined hormonal contraceptives**. Avoid. Severe Theoretical

▸ **Crizotinib** is predicted to increase the exposure to **ulipristal**. Avoid if used for uterine fibroids. Moderate Study

▸ **Ulipristal** is predicted to decrease the efficacy of **desogestrel**. Avoid. Severe Theoretical

▸ **Efavirenz** decreases the efficacy of **ulipristal**. For FSRH guidance, see Contraceptives, interactions p. 474. Severe Anecdotal

▸ **Enzalutamide** is predicted to markedly decrease the exposure to **ulipristal**. Avoid and for 4 weeks after stopping **ulipristal**. Severe Theoretical

▸ **Ulipristal** is predicted to decrease the efficacy of **etonogestrel**. Avoid. Severe Theoretical

▸ **Fosaprepitant** decreases the efficacy of **ulipristal**. For FSRH guidance, see Contraceptives, interactions p. 474. Severe Anecdotal

▸ **Grapefruit juice** is predicted to increase the exposure to **ulipristal**. Avoid if used for uterine fibroids. Moderate Theoretical

▸ **Griseofulvin** potentially decreases the efficacy of **ulipristal**. For FSRH guidance, see Contraceptives, interactions p. 474. Severe Anecdotal

▸ **HIV-protease inhibitors (atazanavir, darunavir, fosamprenavir, lopinavir, saquinavir, tipranavir)** are predicted to increase the exposure to **ulipristal**. Avoid if used for uterine fibroids. Severe Study

▸ **HIV-protease inhibitors (indinavir)** are predicted to increase the exposure to **ulipristal**. Avoid if used for uterine fibroids. Moderate Study

▸ **HIV-protease inhibitors (ritonavir)** decrease the efficacy of **ulipristal**. For FSRH guidance, see Contraceptives, interactions p. 474. Severe Anecdotal

▸ **Idelalisib** is predicted to increase the exposure to **ulipristal**. Avoid if used for uterine fibroids. Severe Study

▸ **Imatinib** is predicted to increase the exposure to **ulipristal**. Avoid if used for uterine fibroids. Moderate Study

▸ **Ulipristal** is predicted to decrease the efficacy of **levonorgestrel**. Avoid. Severe Theoretical

▸ **Macrolides (clarithromycin)** are predicted to increase the exposure to **ulipristal**. Avoid if used for uterine fibroids. Severe Study

▸ **Macrolides (erythromycin)** are predicted to increase the exposure to **ulipristal**. Avoid if used for uterine fibroids. Moderate Study

▸ **Modafinil** decreases the efficacy of **ulipristal**. For FSRH guidance, see Contraceptives, interactions p. 474. Severe Anecdotal

▸ **Netupitant** is predicted to increase the exposure to **ulipristal**. Avoid if used for uterine fibroids. Moderate Study

▸ **Nevirapine** decreases the efficacy of **ulipristal**. For FSRH guidance, see Contraceptives, interactions p. 474. Severe Anecdotal

▸ **Nilotinib** is predicted to increase the exposure to **ulipristal**. Avoid if used for uterine fibroids. Moderate Study

▸ **Ulipristal** is predicted to decrease the efficacy of **norethisterone**. Avoid. Severe Theoretical

▸ **Rifabutin** decreases the efficacy of **ulipristal**. For FSRH guidance, see Contraceptives, interactions p. 474. Severe Anecdotal

▸ **Rifampicin** decreases the efficacy of **ulipristal**. For FSRH guidance, see Contraceptives, interactions p. 474. Severe Anecdotal

Umeclidinium → see TABLE 10 p. 820 (antimuscarinics)

Urokinase → see TABLE 3 p. 818 (anticoagulant effects)

Ursodeoxycholic acid

▸ **Antacids** are predicted to decrease the absorption of **ursodeoxycholic acid**. Separate administration by 2 hours. Moderate Theoretical

▸ **Ursodeoxycholic acid** affects the concentration of **ciclosporin**. Use with caution and adjust dose. Severe Anecdotal

▸ **Fibrates** are predicted to decrease the efficacy of **ursodeoxycholic acid**. Avoid. Severe Theoretical

Ustekinumab → see monoclonal antibodies

Valaciclovir → see TABLE 2 p. 818 (nephrotoxicity)

▸ **Valaciclovir** is predicted to increase the exposure to **aminophylline**. Severe Anecdotal

▸ **Mycophenolate** is predicted to increase the risk of haematological toxicity when given with **valaciclovir**. Moderate Theoretical

▸ **Valaciclovir** is predicted to increase the exposure to **theophylline**. Severe Theoretical

Valganciclovir → see TABLE 15 p. 821 (myelosuppression), TABLE 2 p. 818 (nephrotoxicity)

▸ **Valganciclovir** is predicted to increase the risk of seizures when given with **carbapenems (imipenem)**. Avoid. Severe Anecdotal

▸ **Valganciclovir** is predicted to increase the exposure to **didanosine**. Moderate Study

▸ **Mycophenolate** is predicted to increase the risk of haematological toxicity when given with **valganciclovir**. Moderate Theoretical → Also see TABLE 15 p. 821

Valproate → see antiepileptics

Valsartan → see angiotensin-II receptor antagonists

Vancomycin → see TABLE 2 p. 818 (nephrotoxicity), TABLE 19 p. 822 (ototoxicity)

▸ **Vancomycin** increases the risk of nephrotoxicity when given with **aminoglycosides**. Avoid. Moderate Study → Also see TABLE 2 p. 818 → Also see TABLE 19 p. 822

Vandetanib → see TABLE 9 p. 820 (QT-interval prolongation)
▸ Antiepileptics (**carbamazepine, fosphenytoin, phenobarbital, phenytoin, primidone**) are predicted to decrease the exposure to **vandetanib**. Avoid. Moderate Study
▸ **Vandetanib** is predicted to increase the risk of bleeding events when given with **coumarins**. Severe Theoretical
▸ **Vandetanib** slightly increases the exposure to **digoxin**. Monitor ECG and adjust dose. Moderate Study
▸ **Enzalutamide** is predicted to decrease the exposure to **vandetanib**. Avoid. Moderate Study
▸ **Vandetanib** slightly increases the exposure to **metformin**. Monitor and adjust dose. Moderate Study
▸ **Vandetanib** is predicted to increase the risk of bleeding events when given with **phenindione**. Severe Theoretical
▸ **Rifampicin** is predicted to decrease the exposure to **vandetanib**. Avoid. Moderate Study
Vardenafil → see phosphodiesterase type-5 inhibitors
Varicella-zoster vaccine → see live vaccines
Vecuronium → see neuromuscular blocking drugs, non-depolarising
Vedolizumab → see monoclonal antibodies
Velpatasvir
▸ **Velpatasvir** is predicted to increase the exposure to **aliskiren**. Severe Theoretical
▸ **Antacids** are predicted to decrease the concentration of **velpatasvir**. Separate administration by 4 hours. Moderate Theoretical
▸ **Antiarrhythmics** (**amiodarone**) are predicted to increase the concentration of **velpatasvir**. Avoid or monitor. Moderate Theoretical
▸ Antiepileptics (**carbamazepine, fosphenytoin, phenobarbital, phenytoin, primidone**) are predicted to moderately decrease the exposure to **velpatasvir**. Avoid. Severe Study
▸ Antiepileptics (**oxcarbazepine**) are predicted to decrease the exposure to **velpatasvir**. Avoid. Severe Theoretical
▸ **Velpatasvir** is predicted to increase the exposure to antihistamines, non-sedating (**fexofenadine**). Severe Theoretical
▸ **Bosentan** is predicted to decrease the exposure to **velpatasvir**. Avoid. Moderate Theoretical
▸ Calcium salts (**calcium carbonate**) are predicted to decrease the concentration of **velpatasvir**. Separate administration by 4 hours. Moderate Anecdotal
▸ **Velpatasvir** is predicted to increase the exposure to **colchicine**. Severe Theoretical
▸ **Velpatasvir** is predicted to increase the exposure to **dabigatran**. Severe Theoretical
▸ **Velpatasvir** is predicted to increase the exposure to **digoxin**. Severe Study
▸ **Velpatasvir** is predicted to increase the exposure to **edoxaban**. Severe Study
▸ **Efavirenz** is predicted to decrease the exposure to **velpatasvir**. Avoid. Moderate Theoretical
▸ **Enzalutamide** is predicted to moderately decrease the exposure to **velpatasvir**. Avoid. Severe Study
▸ **Velpatasvir** is predicted to increase the exposure to **everolimus**. Severe Theoretical
▸ H₂ receptor antagonists are predicted to decrease the concentration of **velpatasvir**. Adjust dose, see sofosbuvir with velpatasvir. Moderate Study
▸ **Velpatasvir** is predicted to increase the exposure to **loperamide**. Severe Theoretical
▸ **Nevirapine** is predicted to decrease the exposure to **velpatasvir**. Avoid. Moderate Theoretical
▸ **Proton pump inhibitors** are predicted to decrease the concentration of **velpatasvir**. Adjust dose, see sofosbuvir with velpatasvir. Moderate Study
▸ **Rifampicin** is predicted to moderately decrease the exposure to **velpatasvir**. Avoid. Severe Study
▸ **Velpatasvir** is predicted to increase the exposure to **sirolimus**. Severe Theoretical
▸ **St John's Wort** is predicted to decrease the exposure to **velpatasvir**. Avoid. Moderate Theoretical
▸ **Velpatasvir** is predicted to increase the exposure to statins (**atorvastatin, simvastatin**). Monitor side effects and adjust dose. Severe Theoretical

▸ **Velpatasvir** increases the exposure to statins (**rosuvastatin**). Adjust **rosuvastatin** dose and monitor side effects, p. 130. Severe Study
▸ **Velpatasvir** is predicted to increase the exposure to taxanes (**paclitaxel**). Severe Theoretical
▸ **Velpatasvir** increases the exposure to **tenofovir**. Moderate Study
▸ **Velpatasvir** is predicted to increase the exposure to **topotecan**. Severe Theoretical
Vemurafenib → see TABLE 9 p. 820 (QT-interval prolongation)
▸ **Vemurafenib** is predicted to increase the exposure to **afatinib**. Separate administration by 12 hours. Moderate Study
▸ **Vemurafenib** is predicted to increase the exposure to **aliskiren**. Use with caution and adjust dose. Moderate Theoretical
▸ Antiepileptics (**carbamazepine, fosphenytoin, phenobarbital, phenytoin, primidone**) are predicted to decrease the exposure to **vemurafenib**. Avoid. Severe Theoretical
▸ Antifungals, azoles (**itraconazole, ketoconazole, voriconazole**) are predicted to increase the exposure to **vemurafenib**. Severe Theoretical → Also see TABLE 9 p. 820
▸ **Vemurafenib** is predicted to increase the exposure to beta blockers, non-selective (**nadolol**). Moderate Study
▸ **Cobicistat** is predicted to increase the exposure to **vemurafenib**. Severe Theoretical
▸ **Vemurafenib** is predicted to increase the exposure to **colchicine**. Avoid or adjust **colchicine** dose. Severe Theoretical
▸ **Vemurafenib** increases the exposure to **dabigatran**. Use with caution and adjust dose. Severe Theoretical
▸ **Vemurafenib** is predicted to slightly increase the exposure to **edoxaban**. Severe Theoretical
▸ **Enzalutamide** is predicted to decrease the exposure to **vemurafenib**. Avoid. Severe Theoretical
▸ **Vemurafenib** is predicted to increase the exposure to **erlotinib**. Moderate Theoretical
▸ **Vemurafenib** is predicted to increase the exposure to **fidaxomicin**. Avoid. Moderate Study
▸ HIV-protease inhibitors (**atazanavir, darunavir, fosamprenavir, lopinavir, ritonavir, saquinavir, tipranavir**) are predicted to increase the exposure to **vemurafenib**. Severe Theoretical → Also see TABLE 9 p. 820
▸ **Idelalisib** is predicted to increase the exposure to **vemurafenib**. Severe Theoretical
▸ Macrolides (**clarithromycin**) are predicted to increase the exposure to **vemurafenib**. Severe Theoretical → Also see TABLE 9 p. 820
▸ **Vemurafenib** is predicted to increase the exposure to **nintedanib**. Moderate Study
▸ **Rifampicin** is predicted to decrease the exposure to **vemurafenib**. Avoid. Severe Theoretical
▸ **Vemurafenib** is predicted to increase the exposure to **ticagrelor**. Use with caution or avoid. Severe Study
▸ **Vemurafenib** is predicted to increase the exposure to **topotecan**. Severe Study
▸ **Vemurafenib** is predicted to increase the concentration of **trametinib**. Moderate Theoretical
Venetoclax

FOOD AND LIFESTYLE Avoid Seville (bitter orange) and star fruit as they might increase the exposure to venetoclax.

▸ Antiarrhythmics (**amiodarone**) are predicted to increase the exposure to **venetoclax**. Avoid or monitor for toxicity. Severe Theoretical
▸ Antiarrhythmics (**dronedarone**) are predicted to increase the exposure to **venetoclax**. Avoid or adjust **venetoclax** dose. Severe Study
▸ Antiepileptics (**carbamazepine, fosphenytoin, phenobarbital, phenytoin, primidone**) are predicted to decrease the exposure to **venetoclax**. Avoid. Severe Study
▸ Antifungals, azoles (**fluconazole, isavuconazole, itraconazole, ketoconazole, posaconazole, voriconazole**) are predicted to increase the exposure to **venetoclax**. Avoid or adjust **venetoclax** dose. Severe Study
▸ **Aprepitant** is predicted to increase the exposure to **venetoclax**. Avoid or adjust **venetoclax** dose. Severe Study
▸ Calcium channel blockers (**diltiazem, verapamil**) are predicted to increase the exposure to **venetoclax**. Avoid or adjust **venetoclax** dose. Severe Study

Venetoclax (continued)
- Ciclosporin is predicted to increase the exposure to **venetoclax**. Avoid or monitor for toxicity. Severe Theoretical
- Cobicistat is predicted to increase the exposure to **venetoclax**. Avoid or adjust **venetoclax** dose. Severe Study
- Venetoclax slightly increases the exposure to coumarins (warfarin). Moderate Study
- Crizotinib is predicted to increase the exposure to **venetoclax**. Avoid or adjust **venetoclax** dose. Severe Study
- Enzalutamide is predicted to decrease the exposure to **venetoclax**. Avoid. Severe Study
- Grapefruit juice is predicted to increase the exposure to **venetoclax**. Avoid. Severe Theoretical
- HIV-protease inhibitors are predicted to increase the exposure to **venetoclax**. Avoid or adjust **venetoclax** dose. Severe Study
- Idelalisib is predicted to increase the exposure to **venetoclax**. Avoid or adjust **venetoclax** dose. Severe Study
- Imatinib is predicted to increase the exposure to **venetoclax**. Avoid or adjust **venetoclax** dose. Severe Study
- Lapatinib is predicted to increase the exposure to **venetoclax**. Avoid or monitor for toxicity. Severe Theoretical
- Venetoclax potentially decreases the efficacy of live vaccines. Avoid. Severe Theoretical
- Macrolides (azithromycin) are predicted to increase the exposure to **venetoclax**. Avoid or monitor for toxicity. Severe Theoretical
- Macrolides (clarithromycin, erythromycin) are predicted to increase the exposure to **venetoclax**. Avoid or adjust **venetoclax** dose. Severe Study
- Netupitant is predicted to increase the exposure to **venetoclax**. Avoid or adjust **venetoclax** dose. Severe Study
- Nilotinib is predicted to increase the exposure to **venetoclax**. Avoid or adjust **venetoclax** dose. Severe Study
- Ranolazine is predicted to increase the exposure to **venetoclax**. Avoid or monitor for toxicity. Severe Theoretical
- Rifampicin is predicted to decrease the exposure to **venetoclax**. Avoid. Severe Study

Venlafaxine → see TABLE 13 p. 821 (serotonin syndrome), TABLE 9 p. 820 (QT-interval prolongation), TABLE 11 p. 820 (CNS depressant effects), TABLE 4 p. 818 (antiplatelet effects)
- Abiraterone potentially increases the exposure to venlafaxine. Severe Theoretical
- Antifungals, azoles (itraconazole, ketoconazole, voriconazole) are predicted to increase the exposure to venlafaxine. Moderate Study → Also see TABLE 9 p. 820
- Cobicistat is predicted to increase the exposure to venlafaxine. Moderate Study
- H₂ receptor antagonists (cimetidine) slightly increase the exposure to venlafaxine. Mild Study
- Venlafaxine slightly increases the exposure to haloperidol. Severe Study → Also see TABLE 9 p. 820 → Also see TABLE 11 p. 820
- HIV-protease inhibitors (atazanavir, darunavir, fosamprenavir, lopinavir, ritonavir, saquinavir, tipranavir) are predicted to increase the exposure to venlafaxine. Moderate Study → Also see TABLE 9 p. 820
- Idelalisib is predicted to increase the exposure to venlafaxine. Moderate Study
- Macrolides (clarithromycin) are predicted to increase the exposure to venlafaxine. Moderate Study → Also see TABLE 9 p. 820
- Tacrolimus potentially increases the risk of serotonin syndrome when given with venlafaxine. Severe Anecdotal

Verapamil → see calcium channel blockers
Verteporfin

> **GENERAL INFORMATION** Caution on concurrent use with other photosensitising drugs.

Vigabatrin → see antiepileptics
Vilanterol → see beta₂ agonists
Vildagliptin → see TABLE 14 p. 821 (antidiabetic drugs)
Vinblastine → see vinca alkaloids
Vinca alkaloids → see TABLE 1 p. 818 (hepatotoxicity), TABLE 15 p. 821 (myelosuppression), TABLE 19 p. 822 (ototoxicity), TABLE 12 p. 821 (peripheral neuropathy), TABLE 5 p. 818 (thromboembolism), TABLE 9 p. 820 (QT-interval prolongation)

vinblastine · vincristine · vindesine · vinflunine · vinorelbine

- Antiarrhythmics (dronedarone) are predicted to increase the exposure to vinca alkaloids. Severe Theoretical → Also see TABLE 9 p. 820
- Antiepileptics (carbamazepine, fosphenytoin, phenobarbital, phenytoin, primidone) are predicted to decrease the exposure to vinflunine. Avoid. Severe Theoretical → Also see TABLE 12 p. 821
- Antiepileptics (carbamazepine, fosphenytoin, phenobarbital, phenytoin, primidone) are predicted to decrease the exposure to vinorelbine. Use with caution or avoid. Severe Theoretical → Also see TABLE 12 p. 821
- Antiepileptics (carbamazepine, fosphenytoin, phenobarbital, phenytoin, primidone) are predicted to decrease the exposure to vinca alkaloids (vinblastine, vincristine, vindesine). Severe Theoretical → Also see TABLE 1 p. 818 → Also see TABLE 12 p. 821
- Antifungals, azoles (fluconazole, isavuconazole, itraconazole, ketoconazole, posaconazole, voriconazole) are predicted to increase the exposure to vinca alkaloids. Severe Theoretical → Also see TABLE 1 p. 818 → Also see TABLE 9 p. 820
- Antifungals, azoles (miconazole) are predicted to increase the concentration of vinca alkaloids. Use with caution and adjust dose. Moderate Theoretical
- Aprepitant is predicted to increase the exposure to vinca alkaloids. Severe Theoretical
- Asparaginase potentially increases the risk of neurotoxicity when given with vincristine. Vincristine should be taken 3 to 24 hours before asparaginase. Severe Anecdotal → Also see TABLE 1 p. 818 → Also see TABLE 15 p. 821
- Calcium channel blockers (diltiazem, verapamil) are predicted to increase the exposure to vinca alkaloids. Severe Theoretical
- Cobicistat is predicted to increase the exposure to vinca alkaloids. Severe Theoretical
- Crisantaspase potentially increases the risk of neurotoxicity when given with vincristine. Vincristine should be taken 3 to 24 hours before crisantaspase. Severe Anecdotal → Also see TABLE 1 p. 818 → Also see TABLE 15 p. 821
- Crizotinib is predicted to increase the exposure to vinca alkaloids. Severe Theoretical → Also see TABLE 9 p. 820 → Also see TABLE 15 p. 821
- Enzalutamide is predicted to decrease the exposure to vinca alkaloids (vinblastine, vincristine, vindesine). Severe Theoretical
- Enzalutamide is predicted to decrease the exposure to vinflunine. Avoid. Severe Theoretical
- Enzalutamide is predicted to decrease the exposure to vinorelbine. Use with caution or avoid. Severe Theoretical
- HIV-protease inhibitors are predicted to increase the exposure to vinca alkaloids. Severe Theoretical → Also see TABLE 9 p. 820
- Idelalisib is predicted to increase the exposure to vinca alkaloids. Severe Theoretical → Also see TABLE 15 p. 821
- Imatinib is predicted to increase the exposure to vinca alkaloids. Severe Theoretical → Also see TABLE 15 p. 821
- Live vaccines are predicted to increase the risk of generalised infection (possibly life-threatening) when given with vinca alkaloids. Public Health England advises avoid. Severe Theoretical
- Macrolides (clarithromycin, erythromycin) are predicted to increase the exposure to vinca alkaloids. Severe Theoretical → Also see TABLE 9 p. 820
- Netupitant is predicted to increase the exposure to vinca alkaloids. Severe Theoretical → Also see TABLE 9 p. 820 → Also see TABLE 15 p. 821
- Nilotinib is predicted to increase the exposure to vinca alkaloids. Severe Theoretical
- Pegaspargase potentially increases the risk of neurotoxicity when given with vincristine. Vincristine should be taken 3 to 24 hours before pegaspargase. Severe Anecdotal → Also see TABLE 1 p. 818 → Also see TABLE 15 p. 821
- Rifampicin is predicted to decrease the exposure to vinca alkaloids (vinblastine, vincristine, vindesine). Severe Theoretical
- Rifampicin is predicted to decrease the exposure to vinflunine. Avoid. Severe Theoretical
- Rifampicin is predicted to decrease the exposure to vinorelbine. Use with caution or avoid. Severe Theoretical

Vincristine → see vinca alkaloids
Vindesine → see vinca alkaloids
Vinflunine → see vinca alkaloids

Vinorelbine → see vinca alkaloids
Vismodegib → see TABLE 15 p. 821 (myelosuppression)
► Antiepileptics (carbamazepine, fosphenytoin, phenobarbital, phenytoin, primidone) are predicted to decrease the exposure to vismodegib. Avoid. Moderate Theoretical
► Enzalutamide is predicted to decrease the exposure to vismodegib. Avoid. Moderate Theoretical
► Rifampicin is predicted to decrease the exposure to vismodegib. Avoid. Moderate Theoretical
► St John's Wort is predicted to decrease the exposure to vismodegib. Avoid. Moderate Theoretical

Vitamin A
► Retinoids (acitretin, alitretinoin, isotretinoin) are predicted to increase the risk of vitamin A toxicity when given with vitamin A. Avoid. Severe Theoretical
► Retinoids (bexarotene) are predicted to increase the risk of toxicity when given with vitamin A. Adjust dose. Moderate Theoretical
► Retinoids (tretinoin) are predicted to increase the risk of vitamin A toxicity when given with vitamin A. Avoid. Severe Study

Vitamin D substances

alfacalcidol · calcipotriol · calcitriol · colecalciferol · dihydrotachysterol · ergocalciferol · paricalcitol · tacalcitol

► Antiepileptics (carbamazepine) are predicted to decrease the effects of vitamin D substances. Moderate Study
► Antiepileptics (fosphenytoin, phenytoin) decrease the effects of vitamin D substances. Moderate Study
► Antiepileptics (phenobarbital, primidone) are predicted to decrease the effects of vitamin D substances. Moderate Theoretical
► Antifungals, azoles (clotrimazole, ketoconazole) are predicted to decrease the exposure to colecalciferol. Moderate Theoretical
► Antifungals, azoles (itraconazole, ketoconazole, voriconazole) are predicted to increase the exposure to paricalcitol. Moderate Study
► Cobicistat is predicted to increase the exposure to paricalcitol. Moderate Study
► Vitamin D substances are predicted to increase the risk of toxicity when given with digoxin. Severe Theoretical
► HIV-protease inhibitors (atazanavir, darunavir, fosamprenavir, lopinavir, ritonavir, saquinavir, tipranavir) are predicted to increase the exposure to paricalcitol. Moderate Study
► Idelalisib is predicted to increase the exposure to paricalcitol. Moderate Study
► Macrolides (clarithromycin) are predicted to increase the exposure to paricalcitol. Moderate Study
► Thiazide diuretics increase the risk of hypercalcaemia when given with vitamin D substances. Moderate Theoretical

Vitamin E substances

alpha tocopherol · alpha tocopheryl acetate

► Vitamin E substances affect the exposure to ciclosporin. Moderate Study

Volatile halogenated anaesthetics → see TABLE 8 p. 819 (hypotension), TABLE 11 p. 820 (CNS depressant effects)

desflurane · isoflurane · sevoflurane

Voriconazole → see antifungals, azoles
Vortioxetine → see TABLE 13 p. 821 (serotonin syndrome), TABLE 4 p. 818 (antiplatelet effects)
► Antiepileptics (carbamazepine, fosphenytoin, phenobarbital, phenytoin, primidone) are predicted to decrease the exposure to vortioxetine. Monitor and adjust dose. Moderate Study
► Bupropion is predicted to increase the exposure to vortioxetine. Monitor and adjust dose. Moderate Study → Also see TABLE 13 p. 821
► Cinacalcet is predicted to increase the exposure to vortioxetine. Monitor and adjust dose. Moderate Study
► Enzalutamide is predicted to decrease the exposure to vortioxetine. Monitor and adjust dose. Moderate Study
► Rifampicin is predicted to decrease the exposure to vortioxetine. Monitor and adjust dose. Moderate Study

► SSRIs (fluoxetine, paroxetine) are predicted to increase the exposure to vortioxetine. Moderate Study → Also see TABLE 13 p. 821 → Also see TABLE 4 p. 818
► Terbinafine is predicted to increase the exposure to vortioxetine. Monitor and adjust dose. Moderate Study

Warfarin → see coumarins
Wasp venom extract

GENERAL INFORMATION Desensitising vaccines should be avoided in patients taking beta-blockers (adrenaline might be ineffective in case of a hypersensitivity reaction) or ACE inhibitors (risk of severe anaphylactoid reactions).

Xipamide → see thiazide diuretics
Xylometazoline → see sympathomimetics, vasoconstrictor
Yellow fever vaccine, live → see live vaccines
Zaleplon → see TABLE 11 p. 820 (CNS depressant effects)
► Rifampicin markedly decreases the exposure to zaleplon. Moderate Study

Zidovudine → see TABLE 15 p. 821 (myelosuppression), TABLE 2 p. 818 (nephrotoxicity)
► Antiepileptics (valproate) slightly increase the exposure to zidovudine. Moderate Study
► Antimalarials (pyrimethamine) are predicted to increase the risk of side-effects when given with zidovudine. Severe Theoretical → Also see TABLE 15 p. 821
► Zidovudine increases the risk of haematological toxicity when given with aspirin (high-dose). Severe Study
► HIV-protease inhibitors (tipranavir) slightly decrease the exposure to zidovudine. Avoid. Moderate Study
► Macrolides (clarithromycin) decrease the absorption of zidovudine. Separate administration by at least 2 hours. Moderate Study
► Nevirapine is predicted to decrease the concentration of zidovudine. Refer to specialist literature. Severe Theoretical
► Zidovudine increases the risk of haematological toxicity when given with NSAIDs. Severe Study → Also see TABLE 2 p. 818
► Ribavirin increases the risk of anaemia and/or leucopenia when given with zidovudine. Avoid. Severe Study
► Zidovudine is predicted to decrease the efficacy of stavudine. Avoid. Severe Theoretical

Zinc
► Oral zinc decreases the absorption of oral bisphosphonates (alendronic acid). Zinc should be taken at least 30 minutes before alendronic acid. Moderate Study
► Oral zinc is predicted to decrease the absorption of oral bisphosphonates (ibandronic acid). Avoid zinc for at least 6 hours before or 1 hour after ibandronic acid. Moderate Theoretical
► Oral zinc decreases the absorption of oral bisphosphonates (risedronate). Separate administration by at least 2 hours. Moderate Study
► Oral zinc decreases the absorption of oral bisphosphonates (sodium clodronate). Avoid zinc for 2 hours before or 1 hour after sodium clodronate. Moderate Study
► Oral calcium salts decrease the absorption of zinc. Moderate Study
► Zinc is predicted to decrease the absorption of eltrombopag. Eltrombopag should be taken 2 hours before or 4 hours after zinc. Severe Theoretical
► Zinc is predicted to decrease the efficacy of iron (oral) and iron (oral) is predicted to decrease the efficacy of zinc. Moderate Study
► Zinc is predicted to decrease the absorption of penicillamine. Mild Theoretical
► Zinc is predicted to decrease the exposure to quinolones. Separate administration by 2 hours. Moderate Study
► Oral zinc is predicted to decrease the absorption of tetracyclines. Separate administration by 2 to 3 hours. Moderate Theoretical
► Trientine potentially decreases the absorption of zinc. Moderate Theoretical

Zoledronic acid → see bisphosphonates
Zolmitriptan → see TABLE 13 p. 821 (serotonin syndrome)
► Combined hormonal contraceptives are predicted to increase the exposure to zolmitriptan. Adjust zolmitriptan dose, p. 280. Moderate Theoretical

A1

Interactions | **Appendix 1**

Zolmitriptan (continued)

▶ H₂ receptor antagonists (**cimetidine**) slightly increase the exposure to **zolmitriptan**. Adjust **zolmitriptan** dose, p. 280. Mild Study

▶ **Moclobemide** slightly increases the exposure to **zolmitriptan**. Adjust **zolmitriptan** dose, p. 280. Moderate Study → Also see TABLE 13 p. 821

▶ Monoamine-oxidase A and B inhibitors, irreversible are predicted to increase the exposure to **zolmitriptan**. Severe Theoretical → Also see TABLE 13 p. 821

▶ Quinolones (**ciprofloxacin**) are predicted to increase the exposure to **zolmitriptan**. Adjust **zolmitriptan** dose, p. 280. Moderate Theoretical

▶ SSRIs (**fluvoxamine**) are predicted to increase the exposure to **zolmitriptan**. Adjust **zolmitriptan** dose, p. 280. Severe Theoretical → Also see TABLE 13 p. 821

Zolpidem → see TABLE 11 p. 820 (CNS depressant effects)

▶ Antiepileptics (**carbamazepine**) moderately decrease the exposure to **zolpidem**. Moderate Study

▶ **Rifampicin** moderately decreases the exposure to **zolpidem**. Moderate Study

Zonisamide → see antiepileptics

Zopiclone → see TABLE 11 p. 820 (CNS depressant effects)

▶ Antiarrhythmics (**dronedarone**) are predicted to increase the exposure to **zopiclone**. Adjust dose. Moderate Study

▶ Antiepileptics (**carbamazepine, fosphenytoin, phenobarbital, phenytoin, primidone**) are predicted to decrease the exposure to **zopiclone**. Adjust dose. Moderate Study → Also see TABLE 11 p. 820

▶ Antifungals, azoles (**fluconazole, isavuconazole, posaconazole**) are predicted to increase the exposure to **zopiclone**. Adjust dose. Moderate Study

▶ Antifungals, azoles (**itraconazole, ketoconazole, voriconazole**) are predicted to increase the exposure to **zopiclone**. Adjust dose. Moderate Theoretical

▶ **Aprepitant** is predicted to increase the exposure to **zopiclone**. Adjust dose. Moderate Study

▶ Calcium channel blockers (**diltiazem, verapamil**) are predicted to increase the exposure to **zopiclone**. Adjust dose. Moderate Study

▶ **Cobicistat** is predicted to increase the exposure to **zopiclone**. Adjust dose. Moderate Theoretical

▶ **Crizotinib** is predicted to increase the exposure to **zopiclone**. Adjust dose. Moderate Study

▶ **Enzalutamide** is predicted to decrease the exposure to **zopiclone**. Adjust dose. Moderate Study

▶ HIV-protease inhibitors (**atazanavir, darunavir, fosamprenavir, lopinavir, ritonavir, saquinavir, tipranavir**) are predicted to increase the exposure to **zopiclone**. Adjust dose. Moderate Theoretical

▶ HIV-protease inhibitors (**indinavir**) are predicted to increase the exposure to **zopiclone**. Adjust dose. Moderate Study

▶ **Idelalisib** is predicted to increase the exposure to **zopiclone**. Adjust dose. Moderate Theoretical

▶ **Imatinib** is predicted to increase the exposure to **zopiclone**. Adjust dose. Moderate Study

▶ Macrolides (**clarithromycin**) are predicted to increase the exposure to **zopiclone**. Adjust dose. Moderate Theoretical

▶ Macrolides (**erythromycin**) are predicted to increase the exposure to **zopiclone**. Adjust dose. Moderate Study

▶ **Netupitant** is predicted to increase the exposure to **zopiclone**. Adjust dose. Moderate Study

▶ **Nilotinib** is predicted to increase the exposure to **zopiclone**. Adjust dose. Moderate Study

▶ **Rifampicin** is predicted to decrease the exposure to **zopiclone**. Adjust dose. Moderate Study

Zuclopenthixol → see TABLE 8 p. 819 (hypotension), TABLE 9 p. 820 (QT-interval prolongation), TABLE 11 p. 820 (CNS depressant effects)

▶ **Zuclopenthixol** is predicted to decrease the effects of dopamine receptor agonists. Avoid. Moderate Theoretical → Also see TABLE 8 p. 819 → Also see TABLE 9 p. 820

▶ **Zuclopenthixol** is predicted to decrease the effects of histamine. Avoid. Severe Theoretical → Also see TABLE 8 p. 819

▶ **Zuclopenthixol** is predicted to decrease the effects of **levodopa**. Avoid or monitor worsening parkinsonian symptoms. Severe Theoretical → Also see TABLE 8 p. 819

▶ **Zuclopenthixol** potentially increases the risk of neurotoxicity when given with **lithium**. Severe Anecdotal → Also see TABLE 9 p. 820

A1

Appendix 2
Borderline substances

CONTENTS

In certain conditions some foods (and toilet preparations) have characteristics of drugs and the Advisory Committee on Borderline Substances (ACBS) advises as to the circumstances in which such substances may be regarded as drugs. Prescriptions issued in accordance with the Committee's advice and endorsed 'ACBS' will normally not be investigated.

Information

General Practitioners are reminded that the ACBS recommends products on the basis that they may be regarded as drugs for the management of specified conditions. Doctors should satisfy themselves that the products can safely be prescribed, that patients are adequately monitored and that, where necessary, expert hospital supervision is available.

Foods which may be prescribed on FP10, GP10 (Scotland), or WP10 (Wales)

All the food products listed in this appendix have ACBS approval. The clinical condition for which the product has been approved is included with each entry.
Note Foods included in this appendix may contain cariogenic sugars and patients should be advised to take appropriate oral hygiene measures.

Enteral feeds and supplements

For most enteral feeds and nutritional supplements, the main source of **carbohydrate** is either maltodextrin or glucose syrup; other carbohydrate sources are listed in the relevant table, below. Feeds containing residual lactose (less than 1 g lactose/100 mL formula) are described as 'clinically lactose-free' or 'lactose-free' by some manufacturers. The presence of lactose (including residual lactose) in feeds is indicated in the relevant table, below. The primary sources of **protein** or **amino acids** are included with each product entry. The **fat** or **oil** content is derived from a variety of sources such as vegetables, soya bean, corn, palm nuts, and seeds; where the fat content is derived from animal or fish sources, this information is included in the relevant table,

below. The presence of medium chain triglycerides (MCT) is also noted where the quantity exceeds 30% of the fat content.
Enteral feeds and nutritional supplements can contain varying amounts of **vitamins, minerals,** and **trace elements**—the manufacturer's product literature should be consulted for more detailed information. Feeds containing vitamin K may affect the INR in patients receiving warfarin; see **Interactions:** Appendix 1: enteral feeds.
The suitability of food products for patients requiring a vegan, kosher, halal, or other compliant diet should be confirmed with individual manufacturers.
Note Feeds containing more than 6 g/100 mL protein or 2 g/100 mL fibre should be avoided in children unless recommended by an appropriate specialist or dietician.

Nutritional values

Nutritional values of products vary with flavour and pack size—consult product literature.
Paediatric ACBS indications: Disease-related malnutrition, intractable malabsorption, growth failure, pre-operative preparation of malnourished patients, dysphagia, short-bowel syndrome, bowel fistula
Standard ACBS indications: Disease-related malnutrition, intractable malabsorption, pre-operative preparation of malnourished patients, dysphagia, proven inflammatory bowel disease, following total gastrectomy, short-bowel syndrome, bowel fistula

Other conditions for which ACBS products can be prescribed

This is a list of clinical conditions for which the ACBS has approved toilet preparations. For details of preparations see Chapter 13.
Dermatitis, eczema and pruritus
Aveeno® Bath Oil; *Aveeno*® Cream; *Aveeno*® Lotion; *E45*® Emollient Bath Oil; *E45*® Emollient Wash Cream; *E45*® Lotion
Disfiguring skin lesions (birthmarks, mutilating lesions, scars, vitiligo)

Covermark® classic foundation and finishing powder;
Dermablend® *Ultra* corrective foundation; *Dermacolor*®
Camouflage cream and fixing powder; *Keromask*® masking
cream and finishing powder; *Veil*® Cover cream and
Finishing Powder. (Cleansing Creams, Cleansing Milks,
and Cleansing Lotions are excluded).

Disinfectants (antiseptics)
May be prescribed on an FP10 only when ordered in such
quantities and with such directions as are appropriate for
the treatment of patients, but not for general hygenic
purposes.

Dry mouth (xerostomia)
For patients suffering from dry mouth as a result of having
(or having undergone) radiotherapy, or sicca syndrome.
AS Saliva Orthana®; *Biotène Oralbalance*®; *Glandosane*®;
Saliveze®

Photodermatoses (skin protection in)
Anthelios® XL SPF 50+ Melt-in cream; *Sunsense*® Ultra;
Uvistat® Lipscreen SPF 50, *Uvistat*® Suncream SPF 30 and
50

Prices quoted in Appendix 2 are basic NHS net prices; for
further information see Prices in BNFC.

Borderline substances | Appendix 2

A2

Table 1 Enteral feeds (non-disease specific)

Less than 5 g protein/100 mL

Enteral feeds: 1 kcal/mL and less than 5 g protein/100 mL

Not suitable for use in child under 1 year unless otherwise stated; not recommended for child 1–6 years

Product	Formulation	Energy	Protein	Carbohydrate	Fat	Fibre	Special Characteristics	ACBS Indications	Presentation & Flavour
Fresubin® 1500 Complete (Fresenius Kabi Ltd)	Liquid (tube feed) per 100 mL	420 kJ (100 kcal)	3.8 g cows' milk soya	13 g (sugars 0.9 g)	3.4 g	1.5 g	Gluten-free; Residual lactose; Contains fish oil	Borderline substances standard ACBS indications p. 974 except bowel fistula and pre-operative preparation of malnourished patients. Not suitable for child under 2 years	Fresubin 1500 Complete liquid: 1.5 litre = £13.52
Fresubin® Original (Fresenius Kabi Ltd)	Liquid (sip or tube feed) per 100 mL	420 kJ (100 kcal)	3.8 g cows' milk soya	13.8 g (sugars 3.5 g)	3.4 g	Nil	Gluten-free; Residual lactose; Contains fish gelatin; Feed in flexible pack contains fish oil and fish gelatin	Borderline substances standard ACBS indications p. 974	Fresubin Original drink: blackcurrant, chocolate, nut, peach, vanilla 200 ml = £2.18; Fresubin Original tube feed liquid: 1000 ml = £8.41; 500 ml = £4.25; 1500 ml = £12.61
Fresubin® Original Fibre (Fresenius Kabi Ltd)	Liquid (tube feed) per 100 mL	420 kJ (100 kcal)	3.8 g cows' milk soya	13 g (sugars 0.9 g)	3.4 g	1.5 g	Gluten-free; Residual lactose; Contains fish oil	Borderline substances standard ACBS indications p. 974 except bowel fistula and pre-operative preparation of malnourished patients. Not suitable for child under 2 years	Fresubin Original Fibre liquid: 1000 ml = £9.59; 500 ml = £4.80
Jevity® (Abbott Laboratories Ltd)	Liquid (tube feed) per 100 mL	449 kJ (107 kcal)	4 g caseinates	14.1 g (sugars 470 mg)	3.47 g	1.76 g	Gluten-free; Residual lactose	Borderline substances standard ACBS indications p. 974 except bowel fistula. Not suitable for child under 2 years	Jevity liquid: 500 ml = £5.41; 1500 ml = £15.24; 1000 ml = £10.18
Nutrison® (Nutricia Ltd)	Liquid (tube feed) per 100 mL	420 kJ (100 kcal)	4 g cows' milk	12.3 g (sugars 1 g)	3.9 g	Nil	Gluten-free; Residual lactose	Borderline substances standard ACBS indications p. 974	Nutrison liquid: 500 ml = £5.01; 1500 ml = £13.18; 1000 ml = £8.79; 500 ml = £4.51
Nutrison® Multi Fibre (Nutricia Ltd)	Liquid (tube feed) per 100 mL	420 kJ (100 kcal)	4 g cows' milk	12.3 g (sugars 1 g)	3.9 g	1.5 g	Gluten-free; Residual lactose	Borderline substances standard ACBS indications p. 974 except bowel fistula	Nutrison Multi Fibre liquid: 1000 ml = £10.18; 1500 ml = £15.25; 500 ml = £5.08; 500 ml = £5.41
Osmolite® (Abbott Laboratories Ltd)	Liquid (tube feed) per 100 mL	424 kJ (100 kcal)	4 g caseinates soy isolate	13.6 g (sugars 630 mg)	3.4 g	Nil	Gluten-free; Residual lactose	Borderline substances standard ACBS indications p. 974	Osmolite liquid: 500 ml = £5.01; 1000 ml = £8.79; 1500 ml = £13.18

SOYA PROTEIN FORMULA

Product	Formulation	Energy	Protein	Carbohydrate	Fat	Fibre	Special Characteristics	ACBS Indications	Presentation & Flavour
Fresubin® Soya Fibre (Fresenius Kabi Ltd)	Liquid (tube feed) per 100 mL	420 kJ (100 kcal)	3.8 g soya protein	13.3 g (sugars 4.1 g)	3.6 g	2 g	Gluten-free, Lactose-free, Contains fish oil	Borderline substances standard ACBS indications p. 974; also cows' milk protein intolerance, lactose intolerance	Fresubin Soya Fibre liquid: 500 ml = £4.97
Nutrison® Soya (Nutricia Ltd)	Liquid (tube feed) per 100 mL	420 kJ (100 kcal)	4 g soy isolate	12.3 g (sugars 1 g)	3.9 g	Nil	Gluten-free, Residual lactose, Milk protein-free	Borderline substances standard ACBS indications p. 974; also cows' milk protein and lactose intolerance	Nutrison Soya liquid: 500 ml = £5.40; 1000 ml = £10.82
Nutrison® Soya Multi Fibre (Nutricia Ltd)	Liquid (tube feed) per 100 mL	420 kJ (100 kcal)	4 g soy isolate	12.3 g (sugars 700 mg)	3.9 g	1.5 g	Gluten-free, Residual lactose, Milk protein-free	Borderline substances standard ACBS indications p. 974 except bowel fistula; also cows' milk protein and lactose intolerance	Nutrison Soya Multi Fibre liquid: 1.5 litre = £18.00

PEPTIDE-BASED FORMULA

Product	Formulation	Energy	Protein	Carbohydrate	Fat	Fibre	Special Characteristics	ACBS Indications	Presentation & Flavour
Nutrison Peptisorb® (Nutricia Ltd)	Liquid (tube feed) per 100 mL	425 kJ (100 kcal)	4 g whey protein hydrolysate	17.6 g (sugars 1.7 g)	1.7 g (MCT 47%)	Nil	Gluten-free, Residual lactose	Short bowel syndrome, intractable malabsorption, proven inflammatory bowel disease, bowel fistula	Nutrison Peptisorb liquid: 1000 ml = £14.20; 500 ml = £7.88; 500 ml = £7.17
Peptamen® (Nestle Health Science)	Liquid (sip or tube feed) per 100 mL	420 kJ (100 kcal)	4 g whey peptides	12.7 g (sugars 480 mg)	3.7 g (MCT 70%)	Nil	Gluten-free, Residual lactose	Short bowel syndrome, intractable malabsorption, proven inflammatory bowel disease, bowel fistula	Peptamen liquid: vanilla 800 ml = £12.14; unflavoured 500 ml = £6.82; 1000 ml = £12.80
Survimed® OPD (Fresenius Kabi Ltd)	Liquid (tube feed) per 100 mL	420 kJ (100 kcal)	4.5 g whey protein hydrolysate	14.3 g (sugars 1.1 g)	2.8 g (MCT 51%)	0.1 g	Gluten-free, Residual lactose, Contains fish oil	Borderline substances standard ACBS indications p. 974; also growth failure	Survimed OPD: HN liquid 500 ml = £6.82; liquid 500 ml = £7.09; 800 ml = £13.08; 1000 ml = £14.17

Enteral feeds: Less than 1 kcal/mL and less than 5 g protein/100 mL

AMINO ACID FORMULA (ESSENTIAL AND NON-ESSENTIAL AMINO ACIDS)
Not suitable for use in child under 1 year unless otherwise stated; not recommended for child 1-6 years

Product	Formulation	Energy	Protein	Carbohydrate	Fat	Fibre	Special Characteristics	ACBS Indications	Presentation & Flavour
Elemental 028® Extra (Nutricia Ltd)	Liquid (sip feed) per 100 mL	360 kJ (86 kcal)	2.5 g (protein equivalent)	11 g (sugars 4.7 g)	3.5 g (MCT 35%)	Nil		Short bowel syndrome, intractable malabsorption, proven inflammatory bowel disease, bowel fistula	Elemental 028 Extra liquid summer fruits: 250 ml = £3.73
	Standard dilution (20%) of powder (sip or tube feed) per 100 mL	374 kJ (89 kcal)	2.5 g (protein equivalent)	11.8 g (sugars 1.8 g)	3.5 g (MCT 35%)	Nil		Short bowel syndrome, intractable malabsorption, proven inflammatory bowel disease, bowel fistula.	Elemental 028 Extra powder: plain, orange, banana 100 gram = £7.24

Powder provides protein equivalent 12.5 g, carbohydrate 59 g, fat 17.45 g, energy 1871 kJ (443 kcal)/100 g.

A2

Borderline substances | **Appendix 2**

Borderline substances | **Appendix 2**

A2

Enteral feeds (non-disease specific): 5 g (or more) protein/100 mL

Enteral feeds: 1.5 kcal/mL and 5 g (or more) protein/100 mL

Not suitable for use in child under 1 year unless otherwise stated; not recommended for child 1-6 years

Product	Formulation	Energy	Protein	Carbohydrate	Fat	Fibre	Special Characteristics	ACBS Indications	Presentation & Flavour
Fresubin® 2250 Complete (Fresenius Kabi Ltd)	Liquid (tube feed) per 100 mL	630 kJ (150 kcal)	5.6 g cows' milk	18.8 g (sugars 1.5 g)	5.8 g	2 g	Gluten-free Residual lactose Contains fish oil and fish gelatin	Borderline substances standard ACBS indications p. 974	Fresubin 2250 Complete liquid: 1.5 litre = £15.09
Fresubin® Energy (Fresenius Kabi Ltd)	Liquid (sip feed) per 100 mL	630 kJ (150 kcal)	5.6 g cows' milk	18.8 g (sugars)	5.8 g	Nil	Gluten-free Residual lactose Contains fish gelatin Strawberry flavour may contain traces of wheat starch and egg.	Borderline substances standard ACBS indications p. 974	Fresubin Energy liquid: banana, blackcurrant, cappuccino, chocolate, lemon, strawberry, tropical fruits, vanilla 200 ml = £1.40
	Liquid (tube feed) per 100 mL	630 kJ (150 kcal)	5.6 g cows' milk	18.8 g (sugars 1.4 g)	5.8 g	Nil	Gluten-free Residual lactose Contains fish oil and fish gelatin	Borderline substances standard ACBS indications p. 974	Fresubin Energy liquid: unflavoured 500 ml = £5.20; 1000 ml = £10.21; 1500 ml = £13.69
Fresubin® Energy Fibre (Fresenius Kabi Ltd)	Liquid (sip feed) per 100 mL	630 kJ (150 kcal)	5.6 g cows' milk	18.8 g (sugars)	5.8 g	2 g	Gluten-free Residual lactose Contains fish gelatin	Borderline substances standard ACBS indications p. 974	Fresubin Energy Fibre liquid: banana, caramel, cherry, chocolate, strawberry 200 ml = £2.09
	Liquid (tube feed) per 100 mL	630 kJ (150 kcal)	5.6 g cows' milk	18.8 g (sugars 1.5 g)	5.8 g	2 g	Gluten-free Residual lactose Contains fish oil and fish gelatin	Borderline substances standard ACBS indications p. 974	Fresubin Energy Fibre liquid unflavoured: 1000 ml = £10.87; 500 ml = £5.70
Fresubin® HP Energy (Fresenius Kabi Ltd)	Liquid (tube feed) per 100 mL	630 kJ (150 kcal)	7.5 g cows' milk	17 g (sugars 1 g)	5.8 g (MCT 57%)	Nil	Gluten-free Residual lactose Contains fish oil and fish gelatin	Borderline substances standard ACBS indications p. 974; also CAPD and haemodialysis	Fresubin HP Energy liquid: 500 ml = £5.29; 1000 ml = £10.59
Jevity® 1.5 kcal (Abbott Laboratories Ltd)	Liquid (tube feed) per 100 mL	649 kJ (154 kcal)	6.38 g caseinates and soy isolate	20.1 g (sugars 1.47 g)	4.9 g	2.2 g	Gluten-free Residual lactose	Borderline substances standard ACBS indications p. 974 Not suitable for child under 2 years; not recommended for child 2-10 years	Jevity 1.5kcal liquid: 500 ml = £6.47; 1000 ml = £12.18; 1500 ml = £18.80
Nutrison® Energy (Nutricia Ltd)	Liquid (tube feed) per 100 mL	630 kJ (150 kcal)	6 g cows' milk	18.5 g (sugars 1.5 g)	5.8 g	Nil	Gluten-free Residual lactose	Borderline substances standard ACBS indications p. 974	Nutrison Energy liquid: 1500 ml = £16.41; 500 ml = £5.83; 500 ml = £5.45 (bottle); 1000 ml = £10.97
Nutrison® Energy Multi Fibre (Nutricia Ltd)	Liquid (tube feed) per 100 mL	630 kJ (150 kcal)	6 g cows' milk	18.5 g (sugars 1.5 g)	5.8 g	1.5 g	Gluten-free Residual lactose	Borderline substances standard ACBS indications p. 974	Nutrison Energy Multi Fibre liquid: 1500 ml = £18.80; 500 ml = £6.10 (bottle); 1000 ml = £12.18; 500 ml = £6.47
Osmolite® 1.5 kcal (Abbott Laboratories Ltd)	Liquid (tube feed) per 100 mL	632 kJ (150 kcal)	6.25 g cows' milk soya protein isolate	20 g (sugars 4.9 g)	5 g	Nil	Gluten-free Residual lactose	Borderline substances standard ACBS indications p. 974	Osmolite 1.5kcal tube feed liquid: 1500 ml = £16.41; 1000 ml = £10.97; 500 ml = £5.83
Resource® Energy (Nestle Health Science)	Liquid (sip feed) per 100 mL	630 kJ (150 kcal)	5.6 g cows' milk	21 g (sugars 5.2 g)	5 g	less than 0.5 g	Gluten-free Residual lactose	Borderline substances standard ACBS indications p. 974 Not suitable for use in child under 3 years	Resource Energy liquid: apricot, banana, chocolate, coffee, strawberry & raspberry, vanilla 800 ml = £7.67

Enteral feeds: Less than 1.5 kcal/mL and 5 g (or more) protein/100 mL

Not suitable for use in child under 1 year unless otherwise stated; not recommended for child 1–6 years

Product	Formulation	Energy	Protein	Carbohydrate	Fat	Fibre	Special Characteristics	ACBS Indications	Presentation & Flavour
Fresubin® 1000 Complete (Fresenius Kabi Ltd)	Liquid (tube feed) per 100 mL	420 kJ (100 kcal)	5.5 g cows' milk	12.5 g (sugars 1.1 g)	3.1 g	2 g	Gluten-free Residual lactose Contains fish oil	Borderline substances standard ACBS indications p. 974	Fresubin 1000 Complete liquid: 1 litre = £10.87
Fresubin® 1200 Complete (Fresenius Kabi Ltd)	Liquid (tube feed) per 100 mL	500 kJ (120 kcal)	6 g cows' milk	15 g (sugars 1.22 g)	4.1 g	2 g	Gluten-free Residual lactose Contains fish oil	Borderline substances standard ACBS indications p. 974	Fresubin 1200 Complete liquid: 1 litre = £13.84
Fresubin® 1800 Complete (Fresenius Kabi Ltd)	Liquid (tube feed) per 100 mL	500 kJ (120 kcal)	6 g cows' milk	15 g (sugars 1.22 g)	4.1 g	2 g	Gluten-free Residual lactose Contains fish oil	Borderline substances standard ACBS indications p. 974	Fresubin 1800 Complete liquid: 1.5 litre = £13.84
Jevity® Plus (Abbott Laboratories Ltd)	Liquid (tube feed) per 100 mL	514 kJ (122 kcal)	5.5 g caseinates soy isolates	15.1 g (sugars 890 mg)	3.93 g	2.2 g	Gluten-free Residual lactose	Borderline substances standard ACBS indications p. 974 Not suitable for child under 2 years; not recommended for child 2–10 years	Jevity Plus liquid: 500 ml = £6.48; 1000 ml = £11.80; 1500 ml = £17.63
Jevity® Plus HP (Abbott Laboratories Ltd)	Liquid (tube feed) per 100 mL	551 kJ (131 kcal)	8.13 g cows' milk soy isolates	14.2 g (sugars 950 mg)	4.33 g	1.5 g	Gluten-free Residual lactose	Borderline substances standard ACBS indications p. 974; also CAPD, haemodialysis Not suitable for child under 2 years; not recommended for child 2–10 years	Jevity Plus HP gluten free liquid: 500 ml = £6.35
Jevity® Promote (Abbott Laboratories Ltd)	Liquid (tube feed) per 100 mL	434 kJ (103 kcal)	5.55 g caseinates soy isolates	12 g (sugars 670 mg)	3.32 g	1.7 g	Gluten-free Residual lactose	Borderline substances standard ACBS indications p. 974 Not suitable for child under 2 years; not recommended for child 2–10 years	Jevity Promote liquid: 1 litre = £11.29
Nutrison® 800 Complete Multi Fibre (Nutricia Ltd)	Liquid (tube feed) per 100 mL	345 kJ (83 kcal)	5.5 g cows' milk pea protein soya protein	8.8 g (sugars 600 mg)	2.5 g	1.5 g	Gluten-free Residual lactose Contains fish oil	Borderline substances standard ACBS indications p. 974 except bowel fistula Not suitable for child under 6 years; not recommended for child 6–12 years	Nutrison 800 Complete Multi Fibre liquid: 1 litre = £10.65
Nutrison® 1000 Complete Multi Fibre (Nutricia Ltd)	Liquid (tube feed) per 100 mL	420 kJ (100 kcal)	5.5 g cows' milk	11.3 g (sugars 700 mg)	3.7 g	2 g	Gluten-free Residual lactose	Disease related malnutrition in patients with low energy and/or low fluid requirements	Nutrison 1000 Complete Multi Fibre liquid: 1 litre = £11.29
Nutrison® 1200 Complete Multi Fibre (Nutricia Ltd)	Liquid (tube feed) per 100 mL	505 kJ (120 kcal)	5.5 g cows' milk	15 g (sugars 1.2 g)	4.3 g	2 g	Gluten-free Residual lactose	Borderline substances standard ACBS indications p. 974 except bowel fistula	Nutrison 1200 Complete Multi Fibre liquid: 1000 ml = £11.95; 1500 ml = £17.94
Nutrison® MCT (Nutricia Ltd)	Liquid (tube feed) per 100 mL	420 kJ (100 kcal)	5 g cows' milk	12.6 g (sugars 1 g)	3.3 g (MCT 61%)	Nil	Gluten-free Residual lactose	Borderline substances standard ACBS indications p. 974	Nutrison MCT liquid: 1000 ml = £10.17
Nutrison® Protein Plus (Nutricia Ltd)	Liquid (tube feed) per 100 mL	525 kJ (125 kcal)	6.3 g cows' milk	14.2 g (sugars 1.1 g)	4.9 g	Nil	Gluten-free Residual lactose	Borderline substances standard ACBS indications p. 974	Nutrison Protein Plus liquid: 1 litre = £10.44

Borderline substances | **Appendix 2**

A2

Borderline substances | Appendix 2

A2

Enteral feeds: Less than 1.5 kcal/mL and 5 g (or more) protein/100 mL (product list continued)

Not suitable for use in child under 1 year unless otherwise stated; not recommended for child 1-6 years

Product	Formulation	Energy	Protein	Carbohydrate	Fat	Fibre	Special Characteristics	ACBS Indications	Presentation & Flavour
Nutrison® Protein Plus Multi Fibre (Nutricia Ltd)	Liquid (tube feed) per 100 mL	535 kJ (128 kcal)	6.3 g cow's milk	14.1 g (sugars 1.0 g)	4.9 g	1.5 g	Gluten-free, Residual lactose	Disease related malnutrition	Nutrison Protein Plus Multifibre liquid: 1 litre = £11.64
Osmolite® Plus (Abbott Laboratories Ltd)	Liquid (tube feed) per 100 mL	508 kJ (121 kcal)	5.55 g caseinates	15.8 g (sugars 730 mg)	3.93 g	Nil	Gluten-free, Residual lactose	Borderline substances standard ACBS indications p. 974. Not suitable for child under 10 years	Osmolite Plus liquid: 1500 ml = £14.80; 1000 ml = £9.89; 500 ml = £5.44
Peptamen® HN (Nestle Health Science)	Liquid (tube feed) per 100 mL	556 kJ (133 kcal)	6.6 g whey protein hydrolysates	15.6 g (sugars 1.4 g)	4.9 g (MCT 70%)	Nil	Gluten-free, Residual lactose, Hydrolysed with pork trypsin	Short bowel syndrome, intractable malabsorption, proven inflammatory bowel disease, bowel fistula. Not suitable for child under 3 years	Peptamen HN liquid: 500 ml = £7.34
Perative® (Abbott Laboratories Ltd)	Liquid (sip or tube feed) per 100 mL	552 kJ (131 kcal)	6.7 g casenate whey protein hydrolysates	17.7 g (sugars 660 mg)	3.7 g (MCT 42%)	Nil	Gluten-free, Residual lactose	Borderline substances standard ACBS indications p. 974. Not suitable for child under 5 years	Perative liquid: 1000 ml = £14.20; 500 ml = £7.69

Enteral feeds: More than 1.5 kcal/mL and 5 g (or more) protein/100 mL

Not suitable for use in child under 1 year unless otherwise stated; not recommended for child 1-6 years

Product	Formulation	Energy	Protein	Carbohydrate	Fat	Fibre	Special Characteristics	ACBS Indications	Presentation & Flavour
Ensure® TwoCal (Abbott Laboratories Ltd)	Liquid (sip or tube feed) per 100 mL	838 kJ (200 kcal)	8.4 g cows milk	21 g (sugars 4.5 g)	8.9 g	1 g	Gluten-free, Residual lactose	Borderline substances standard ACBS indications p. 974; also haemodialysis and CAPD	Ensure TwoCal liquid: banana, neutral, strawberry, vanilla 200 ml = £2.22

Enteral feeds (non-disease specific): Child under 12 years

Enteral feeds, Child: Less than 1 kcal/mL and less than 4 g protein/100 mL

Product	Formulation	Energy	Protein	Carbohydrate	Fat	Fibre	Special Characteristics	ACBS Indications	Presentation & Flavour
Nutrini® Low Energy Multi Fibre (Nutricia Ltd)	Liquid (tube feed) per 100 mL	315 kJ (75 kcal)	2.1 g whey protein and caseinate	9.3 g (sugars 600 mg)	3.3 g	800 mg	Gluten-free, Residual lactose, Contains fish oil	Borderline substances paediatric ACBS indications p. 974 except bowel fistula, in child 1-6 years, body-weight 8-20 kg	Nutrini Low Energy Multifibre liquid: 500 ml = £6.82; 200 ml = £2.69
Nutriprem® 1 (Cow & Gate Ltd)	Liquid (sip feed) per 100 mL	335 kJ (80 kcal)	2.5 g whey protein and casein	7.6 g (lactose 6.3 g)	4.4 g	800 mg	Contains soya, fish oil and egg lipid	Low birth-weight formula	Nutriprem 1: bottle 70 ml = Hospital supply only
Nutriprem® 2 (Cow & Gate Ltd)	Liquid (sip feed) per 100 mL	310 kJ (75 kcal)	2 g whey protein and casein	7.4 g (lactose 5.8 g)	4 g	600 mg	Contains soya, fish oil and egg lipid	Catch-up growth in pre-term infants (less than 35 weeks at birth) and small for gestational-age infants up to 6 months corrected age.	Nutriprem 2 liquid: 200 ml = £1.74
	Standard dilution (15.3%) of powder (sip feed) per 100 mL	315 kJ (75 kcal)	2 g whey protein and casein	7.4 g (lactose 5.9 g)	4 g (including MCT oil)	600 mg			Nutriprem 2 powder: 900 gram = £11.67

Powder provides: protein 13 g, carbohydrate 48.3 g, fat 26.7 g, fibre 5.2 g, energy 2030 kJ (485 kcal)/100 g.

Product	Formulation	Energy	Protein	Carbohydrate	Fat	Fibre	Special Characteristics	ACBS Indications	Presentation & Flavour
SMA® Gold Prem 2 (SMA Nutrition)	Standard dilution (14%) of powder (sip feed) per 100 mL	305 kJ (73 kcal)	1.9 g cows' milk	7.5 g sugars 6.4 g	3.9 g	Nil	Contains lactose	Catch-up growth in preterm and small for gestational age infants on discharge from hospital, up to 6 months corrected age.	SMA Gold Prem 2: Catch-up Formula powder 400 gram = £4.92

Powder provides: protein 14 g, carbohydrate 54 g, fat 28 g, energy 2180 kJ (524 kcal)/100 g.

Product	Formulation	Energy	Protein	Carbohydrate	Fat	Fibre	Special Characteristics	ACBS Indications	Presentation & Flavour
SMA® High Energy (SMA Nutrition)	Liquid (sip feed) per 100 mL	382 kJ (91 kcal)	2 g whey protein and casein	9.8 g lactose	4.9 g	Nil	Contains lactose	Disease related malnutrition and malabsorption, and growth failure in child from birth to 18 months	SMA High Energy milk: 250 ml = £2.46; 100 ml = £2.46

AMINO ACID FORMULA (ESSENTIAL AND NON-ESSENTIAL AMINO ACIDS)

Product	Formulation	Energy	Protein	Carbohydrate	Fat	Fibre	Special Characteristics	ACBS Indications	Presentation & Flavour
Emsogen® (Nutricia Ltd)	Standard dilution (20%) of powder (sip or tube feed) per 100 mL	368 kJ (88 kcal)	2.5 g protein equivalent (essential and non-essential amino acids)	12 g (sugars 1.6 g)	3.3 g (MCT 83%)	Nil	Lactose-free	Short-bowel syndrome, intractable malabsorption, proven inflammatory bowel disease, bowel fistula. Not suitable for child under 1 year or as sole source of nutrition in child 1-5 years	Emsogen powder unflavoured: 100 gram = £7.46

Powder provides: protein equivalent 12.5 g, carbohydrate 60 g, fat 16.4 g, energy 1839 kJ (438 kcal)/100 g.
Additional source of alpha linolenic acid needed if used as sole source of nutrition.

Enteral feeds, Child: 1 kcal/mL and less than 4 g protein/100 mL

Not suitable for use in child under 1 year unless otherwise stated

Product	Formulation	Energy	Protein	Carbohydrate	Fat	Fibre	Special Characteristics	ACBS Indications	Presentation & Flavour
Fortini® 1.0 Multi Fibre (Nutricia Ltd)	Liquid (sip feed) per 100 mL	420 kJ (100 kcal)	2.4 g cows' milk	11.8 g (sugars 4.7 g)	4.5 g	1.5 g	Gluten-free; Residual lactose	Disease-related malnutrition and growth failure in child 1-6 years, body-weight 8-20 kg	Fortini 1.0 Multi Fibre liquid: banana, chocolate, strawberry, vanilla 200 ml = £2.57
Frebini® Original (Fresenius Kabi Ltd)	Liquid (tube feed) per 100 mL	420 kJ (100 kcal)	2.5 g cows' milk	12.5 g (sugars 700 mg)	4.4 g	Nil	Gluten-free; Residual lactose; Contains fish oils and fish gelatin	Borderline substances standard ACBS indications p. 974 and growth failure in child 1-10 years, body-weight 8-30 kg	Frebini Original liquid: 500 ml = £6.27
Frebini® Original Fibre (Fresenius Kabi Ltd)	Liquid (tube feed) per 100 mL	420 kJ (100 kcal)	2.5 g cows' milk	12.5 g (sugars 700 mg)	4.4 g	0.75 g	Gluten-free; Residual lactose; Contains fish oils and fish gelatin	Borderline substances standard ACBS indications p. 974 and growth failure in child 1-10 years, body-weight 8-30 kg	Frebini Original Fibre liquid: 500 ml = £6.97
Infatrini® (Nutricia Ltd)	Liquid (sip or tube feed) per 100 mL	415 kJ (100 kcal)	2.6 g cows' milk	10.3 g (lactose 5.2 g)	5.4 g	800 mg	Gluten-free; Contains fish oil	Failure to thrive, disease-related malnutrition and malabsorption, in child from birth up to body-weight 8 kg	Infatrini liquid: 125 ml = £1.46; 500 ml = £6.28; 200 ml = £2.31
Nutrini® (Nutricia Ltd)	Liquid (tube feed) per 100 mL	420 kJ (100 kcal)	2.8 g cows' milk	12.3 g (sugars 1 g)	4.4 g	Nil	Gluten-free; Residual lactose	Borderline substances standard ACBS indications p. 974 and growth failure in child 1-6 years, body-weight 8-20 kg	Nutrini liquid: 200 ml = £2.80; 500 ml = £6.96
Nutrini® Multi Fibre (Nutricia Ltd)	Liquid (tube feed) per 100 mL	420 kJ (100 kcal)	2.8 g whey protein and caseinate	12.3 g (sugars 800 mg)	4.4 g	800 mg	Gluten-free; Residual lactose; Contains fish oil	Borderline substances standard ACBS indications p. 974 and growth failure in child 1-6 years, body-weight 8-20 kg	Nutrini Multifibre liquid: 500 ml = £7.72; 200 ml = £3.10

Borderline substances | **Appendix 2**

A2

Enteral feeds, Child: 1 kcal/mL and less than 4 g protein/100 mL (product list continued)

Not suitable for use in child under 1 year unless otherwise stated

Product	Formulation	Energy	Protein	Carbohydrate	Fat	Fibre	Special Characteristics	ACBS Indications	Presentation & Flavour
Paediasure® (Abbott Laboratories Ltd)	Liquid (sip or tube feed) per 100 mL	422 kJ (100 kcal)	2.8 g cows' milk	11.2 g (sugars 3.92 g)	4.98 g	Nil	Gluten-free; Residual lactose	Borderline substances paediatric ACBS indications p. 974 in child 1-10 years, body-weight 8-30 kg	PaediaSure liquid: vanilla 200 ml = £2.52; 500 ml = £6.96; banana, chocolate, strawberry 200 ml = £2.52 Nutritional values may vary with flavour – consult product literature
Paediasure® Fibre (Abbott Laboratories Ltd)	Liquid (sip or tube feed) per 100 mL	424 kJ (101 kcal)	2.8 g caseinates and whey protein	10.9 g (sugars 3.84 g)	4.98 g	730 mg	Gluten-free; Residual lactose	Borderline substances paediatric ACBS indications p. 974 in child 1-10 years, body-weight 8-30 kg	PaediaSure fibre liquid: banana, strawberry 200 ml = £2.67; vanilla 200 ml = £2.67; 500 ml = £7.72 Nutritional values may vary with flavour – consult product literature
Paediasure® Peptide (Abbott Laboratories Ltd)	Liquid (sip or tube feed) per 100 mL	420 kJ (100 kcal)	3 g whey protein and caseinate	13 g (sugars 2.98 g)	4 (MCT 50%) g	Nil	Gluten-free; Residual lactose	Borderline substances standard ACBS Indications p. 974 and growth failure in child 1-10 years, body-weight 8-30 kg	PaediaSure Peptide liquid: 500 ml £10.86; 200 ml £3.92
Similac® High Energy (Abbott Laboratories Ltd)	Liquid (sip or tube feed) per 100 mL	419 kJ (100 kcal)	2.6 g cows' milk and whey protein	10.1 g (sugars 5.6 g)	5.2 g	400 mg	Gluten-free; Contains lactose and soy oil	Increased energy requirements, faltering growth, and/or need for fluid restriction, in child body-weight up to 8 kg	Similac High Energy liquid: 200 ml £2.29; 60 ml = £0.69
Tentrini® (Nutricia Ltd)	Liquid (tube feed) per 100 mL	420 kJ (100 kcal)	3.3 g whey protein and caseinate	12.3 g (sugars 800 mg)	4.2 g	Nil	Gluten-free; Residual lactose; Contains fish oil	Borderline substances standard ACBS indications p. 974 and growth failure in child 7-12 years, body-weight 21-45 kg	Tentrini liquid: 500 ml = £6.13
Tentrini® Multi Fibre (Nutricia Ltd)	Liquid (tube feed) per 100 mL	420 kJ (100 kcal)	3.3 g whey protein and caseinate	12.3 g (sugars 800 mg)	4.2 g	1.1 g	Gluten-free; Residual lactose; Contains fish oil	Borderline substances standard ACBS indications p. 974 except bowel fistula, and growth failure in child 7-12 years body-weight 21-45 kg	Tentrini Multifibre liquid: 500 ml = £6.74

HYDROLYSATE FORMULA

Product	Formulation	Energy	Protein	Carbohydrate	Fat	Fibre	Special Characteristics	ACBS Indications	Presentation & Flavour
Nutrini® Peptisorb (Nutricia Ltd)	Liquid (tube feed) per 100 mL	420 kJ (100 kcal)	2.8 g whey protein hydrolysate	13.7 g (sugars 800 mg)	3.9 g (MCT 46%)	Nil	Gluten-free; Residual lactose	Borderline substances standard ACBS indications p. 974 and growth failure in child 1-6 years, body-weight 8-20 kg	Nutrini Peptisorb liquid: 500 ml = £10.86
Peptamen® Junior (Nestle Health Science)	Liquid (tube feed) per 100 mL	420 kJ (100 kcal)	3 g whey protein hydrolysate	13.2 g	4 g (MCT 60%)	Nil	Gluten-free; Residual lactose; Hydrolysed with pork trypsin	Short bowel syndrome, intractable malabsorption, proven inflammatory bowel disease, bowel fistula, in child 1-10 years	Peptamen Junior gluten free liquid: 500 ml = £6.81
	Standard dilution (22%) of powder (sip or tube feed) per 100 mL	420 kJ (100 kcal)	3 g whey protein hydrolysate	13.8 g	3.85 g (MCT 60%)	Nil	Gluten-free; Residual lactose; Hydrolysed with bacterial trypsin		Peptamen Junior powder: 400 gram = £17.86

Powder provides: protein 13.7 g, carbohydrate 62.9g, fat 17.5g, energy 1910 kJ (457 kcal)/100 g.

Enteral feeds, Child: More than 1 kcal/mL and less than 4 g protein/100 mL
Not suitable for use in child under 1 year unless otherwise stated

Product	Formulation	Energy	Protein	Carbohydrate	Fat	Fibre	Special Characteristics	ACBS Indications	Presentation & Flavour
Fortini® (Nutricia Ltd)	Liquid (sip feed) per 100 mL	630 kJ (150 kcal)	3.4 g cows' milk	18.8 g (sugars 7.4 g)	6.8 g	Nil	Gluten-free Residual lactose	Disease-related malnutrition and growth failure in child 1-6 years, body-weight 8-20 kg	Fortini liquid: strawberry, vanilla 200 ml = £3.33
Fortini® Multifibre (Nutricia Ltd)	Liquid (sip feed) per 100 mL	630 kJ (150 kcal)	3.4 g cows' milk	18.8 g (sugars 7.4 g)	6.8 g	1.5 g	Gluten-free Residual lactose	Disease-related malnutrition and growth failure in child 1-6 years, body-weight 8-20 kg	Fortini Multi Fibre liquid: banana, chocolate, strawberry, unflavoured, vanilla 200 ml = £3.50
Fortini® Smoothie Multifibre (Nutricia Ltd)	Liquid (sip feed) per 100 mL	625 kJ (150 kcal)	3.4 g cows' milk	19 g (sugars 11.5 g)	6.4 g	1.4 g	Gluten-free Residual lactose	Disease-related malnutrition and growth failure in child 1-6 years, body-weight 8-20 kg	Fortini Smoothie Multi Fibre liquid: berry fruit, summer fruit 200 ml = £3.50
Frebini® Energy (Fresenius Kabi Ltd)	Liquid (tube feed) per 100 mL	630 kJ (150 kcal)	3.75 g cows' milk	18.75 g (sugars 830 mg)	6.7 g	Nil	Gluten-free Residual lactose Contains fish oil and fish gelatin	Borderline substances standard ACBS indications p. 974 and growth failure in child 1-10 years, body-weight 8-30 kg	Frebini Energy: 500 ml = £7.86
Frebini® Energy Drink (Fresenius Kabi Ltd)	Liquid (sip feed) per 100 mL	630 kJ (150 kcal)	3.8 g cows' milk	18.7 g (sugars 4.5 g)	6.7 g	Nil	Gluten-free Residual lactose	Disease-related malnutrition and growth failure in child 1-10 years, body-weight 8-30 kg	Frebini Energy Drink: banana, strawberry 200 ml = £2.97
Frebini® Energy Fibre (Fresenius Kabi Ltd)	Liquid (tube feed) per 100 mL	630 kJ (150 kcal)	3.75 g cows' milk	18.75 g (sugars 830 mg)	6.7 g	1.13 g	Gluten-free Residual lactose Contains fish oils and fish gelatin	Borderline substances standard ACBS indications p. 974 and growth failure in child 1-10 years, body-weight 8-30 kg	Frebini Energy Fibre liquid unflavoured: 500 ml = £8.42
Frebini® Energy Fibre Drink (Fresenius Kabi Ltd)	Liquid (sip feed) per 100 mL	630 kJ (150 kcal)	3.8 g cows' milk	18.75 g (sugars 4.5 g)	6.7 g	1.1 g	Gluten-free Residual lactose	Disease-related malnutrition and growth failure in child 1-10 years, body-weight 8-30 kg	Frebini Energy Fibre liquid: chocolate, vanilla 200 ml = £3.03
Resource® Junior (Nestle Health Science)	Liquid (sip feed) per 100 mL	630 kJ (150 kcal)	3 g cows' milk	20.6 g (sugars 4.9 g)	6.2 g	Nil	Gluten-free Residual lactose	Borderline substances standard ACBS indications p. 974 in child 1-10 years. Not suitable for use in child under 1 year	Resource Junior complete sip feed: chocolate, strawberry, vanilla 200 ml = £2.14

Enteral feeds, Child: 1.5 kcal/mL and more than 4 g protein/100 mL
Not suitable for use in child under 1 year unless otherwise stated

Product	Formulation	Energy	Protein	Carbohydrate	Fat	Fibre	Special Characteristics	ACBS Indications	Presentation & Flavour
Nutrini® Energy (Nutricia Ltd)	Liquid (tube feed) per 100 mL	630 kJ (150 kcal)	4.1 g caseinate whey protein	18.5 g (sugars 1.1 g)	6.7 g	Nil	Gluten-free Residual lactose Contains fish oil	Borderline substances standard ACBS indications p. 974 and growth failure in child 1-6 years, body-weight 8-20 kg	Nutrini Energy liquid: 200 ml = £3.41; 500 ml = £8.73
Nutrini® Energy Multi Fibre (Nutricia Ltd)	Liquid (tube feed) per 100 mL	630 kJ (150 kcal)	4.1 g caseinate whey protein	18.5 g (sugars 1.1 g)	6.7 g	800 mg	Gluten-free Residual lactose Contains fish oil	Borderline substances paediatric ACBS indications p. 974 except total bowel fistula; also total gastrectomy, in child 1-6 years, body-weight 8-20 kg	Nutrini Energy Multifibre liquid: 200 ml = £3.60; 500 ml = £9.02

Borderline substances | **Appendix 2**

Borderline substances | Appendix 2

A2

Enteral feeds, Child: 1.5 kcal/mL and more than 4 g protein/100 mL (product list continued)

Not suitable for use in child under 1 year unless otherwise stated

Product	Formulation	Energy	Protein	Carbohydrate	Fat	Fibre	Special Characteristics	ACBS Indications	Presentation & Flavour
Paediasure® Plus (Abbott Laboratories Ltd)	Liquid (sip or tube feed) per 100 mL	632 kJ (151 kcal)	4.2 g caseinates whey protein	16.7 g	7.47 g	Nil	Gluten-free Residual lactose	Borderline substances paediatric ACBS indications p. 974 in child 1-10 years, body-weight 8-30 kg	PaediaSure Plus liquid: banana, strawberry, unflavoured 200 ml = £3.25; vanilla 200 ml = £3.25; 500 ml = £8.73 Sugar content varies with presentation
Paediasure® Plus Fibre (Abbott Laboratories Ltd)	Liquid (sip or tube feed) per 100 mL	635 kJ (152 kcal)	4.2 g caseinates whey protein	16.4 g (sugars 5.3 g)	7.47 g	1.1 g	Gluten-free Residual lactose	Borderline substances paediatric ACBS indications, p. 974 in child 1-10 years, body-weight 8-30 kg. Not suitable for use in child under 1 year.	PaediaSure Plus fibre liquid: banana, strawberry 200 ml = £3.50; vanilla 200 ml = £3.50; 500 ml = £9.02 Nutritional values vary with flavour - consult product literature. Sugar content varies with presentation
Peptamen® Junior Advance (Nestle Health Science)	Liquid (tube feed) per 100 mL	630 kJ (150 kcal)	4.5 g whey protein	18 g (sugars 2.1 g)	6.6 g (MCT 61%)	540 mg	Gluten-free Residual lactose Hydrolysed with pork trypsin Contains fish oil	Intractable malabsorption, short-bowel syndrome, bowel fistula, and proven inflammatory bowel disease in child 1-10 years	Peptamen Junior Advance gluten free liquid: 500 ml = £7.77
Tentrini® Energy (Nutricia Ltd)	Liquid (tube feed) per 100 mL	630 kJ (150 kcal)	4.9 g whey protein and caseinate	18.5 g (sugars 1.1 g)	6.3 g	Nil	Gluten-free Residual lactose Contains fish oil	Borderline substances standard ACBS indications p. 974 and growth failure, in child 7-12 years, body-weight 21-45 kg	Tentrini Energy liquid: 500 ml = £7.57
Tentrini® Energy Multi Fibre (Nutricia Ltd)	Liquid (tube feed) per 100 mL	630 kJ (150 kcal)	4.9 g whey protein and caseinate	18.5 g (sugars 1.1 g)	6.3 g	1.1 g	Gluten-free Residual lactose Contains fish oil	Borderline substances paediatric ACBS indications p. 974 and proven inflammatory bowel disease, in child 7-12 years, body-weight 21-45 kg	Tentrini Energy Multifibre liquid: 500 ml = £8.34

Table 2 Nutritional supplements (non-disease specific)
Less than 5 g protein/100 mL

Nutritional supplements: 1 kcal/mL and less than 5 g protein/100 mL

Not suitable for use in child under 1 year; use with caution in child 1-5 years unless otherwise stated

Product	Formulation	Energy	Protein	Carbohydrate	Fat	Fibre	Special Characteristics	ACBS Indications	Presentation & Flavour
Ensure® (Abbott Laboratories Ltd)	Liquid (sip or tube feed) per 100 mL	423 kJ (100 kcal)	4 g caseinates soy isolate	13.6 g (sugars 3.93 g)	3.36 g	Nil	Gluten-free Residual lactose	Borderline substances standard ACBS indications p. 974	Ensure liquid: vanilla, chocolate, coffee 250 ml = £2.31

Nutritional supplements: More than 1 kcal/mL and less than 5 g protein/100 mL

Not suitable for use in child under 1 year; use with caution in child 1-5 years unless otherwise stated

Product	Formulation	Energy	Protein	Carbohydrate	Fat	Fibre	Special Characteristics	ACBS Indications	Presentation & Flavour
AYMES® Shake (Aymes International Ltd)	Standard dilution of powder (57 g in 200 mL water) (sip feed) per 100 mL	530.5 kJ (126 kcal)	4.5 g cows' milk	17.5 g (sugars 8.4 g)	4.2 g	Nil	Gluten-free Contains lactose	Borderline substances standard ACBS indications p. 974. Use with caution in child 1-6 years. Not suitable for child under 1 year.	Aymes Shake Sample Pack powder: 285 gram = £4.78; Aymes Shake powder: banana, strawberry, chocolate, neutral, vanilla 399 gram = £4.27

Powder 57 g reconstituted with 200 mL whole milk provides: protein 15.8 g, carbohydrate 44.1 g, fat 16.4 g, energy 1625 kJ (388kcal)

Product	Formulation	Energy	Protein	Carbohydrate	Fat	Fibre	Special Characteristics	ACBS Indications	Presentation & Flavour
Ensure® Plus Juce (Abbott Laboratories Ltd)	Liquid (sip feed) per 100 mL	638 kJ (150 kcal)	4.8 g whey protein isolate	32.7 g (sugars 9.4 g)	Nil	Nil	Gluten-free Residual lactose Non-milk taste	Borderline substances standard ACBS indications p. 974	Ensure Plus Juce liquid: assorted 880 ml apple, fruit punch, lemon & lime, orange, peach 220 ml = £1.97
Fortijuce® (Nutricia Ltd)	Liquid (sip feed) per 100 mL	640 kJ (150 kcal)	4.0 g cows' milk	33.5 g (sugars 13.1 g)	Nil	Nil	Gluten-free Residual lactose Non-milk taste	Borderline substances standard ACBS indications p. 974 Not suitable for child under 3 years	Fortijuce Starter Pack liquid: assorted 800 ml = £8.08; Fortijuce liquid: apple, blackcurrant, forest fruits, lemon, orange, strawberry, tropical 200 ml = £2.02; Sugar content varies with flavour
Fresubin® Jucy Drink (Fresenius Kabi Ltd)	Liquid (sip feed) per 100 mL	630 kJ (150 kcal)	4 g whey protein	33.5 g (sugars 8 g)	Nil	Nil	Gluten-free Residual lactose	Borderline substances standard ACBS indications p. 974; also CAPD, haemodialysis	Fresubin Jucy drink: apple, blackcurrant, cherry, orange, pineapple 800 ml = £7.96
Paediasure® Plus Juce (Abbott Laboratories Ltd)	Liquid (sip feed) per 100 mL	638 kJ (150 kcal)	4.2 g cows' milk	33.3 g (sugars 9.4 g)	Nil	Nil	Gluten-free Residual lactose Non-milk taste	Nutritional supplement in child 1–10 years, body-weight 8–30 kg with disease-related malnutrition and, or growth failure	PaediaSure Plus Juce liquid: apple, very berry 200 ml = £3.23
Resource® Dessert Energy (Nestle Health Science)	Semi-solid per 100 g	671 kJ (160 kcal)	4.8 g cows' milk	21.2 g (sugars 9.9 g)	6.2 g	Nil	Gluten-free Contains lactose	Borderline substances standard ACBS indications p. 974; also CAPD, haemodialysis.	Resource Dessert Energy semi-solid food: caramel, chocolate, vanilla 125 gram = £1.63 Sugar content varies with flavour.
Resource® Fruit (Nestle Health Science)	Liquid (sip feed) per 100 mL	520 kJ (125 kcal)	4 g whey protein hydrolysate	27 g (sugars 9.5 g)	less than 0.2 g	less than 0.2 g	Gluten-free Residual lactose Non-milk taste	Borderline substances standard ACBS indications p. 974 Not suitable for child under 3 years.	Resource Fruit liquid: apple, orange, pear & cherry, raspberry & blackcurrant 800 ml = £7.35 Sugar and fibre content varies with flavour.

Nutritional supplements: 5 g (or more) protein/100 mL

Nutritional supplements: 1.5 kcal/mL and 5 g (or more) protein/100 mL

Not suitable for use in child under 1 year; use with caution in child 1–5 years unless otherwise stated.

Product	Formulation	Energy	Protein	Carbohydrate	Fat	Fibre	Special Characteristics	ACBS Indications	Presentation & Flavour
Altraplen® Protein (Nualtra Ltd)	Liquid (sip feed) per 100 mL	632 kJ (150 kcal)	10 g cows' milk soya protein	15 g (sugars 4.6 g)	5.6 g	Nil	Gluten-free Residual lactose	Borderline substances standard ACBS indications p. 974 Not suitable for child under 3 years; use with caution in child 3–6 years	Altraplen Protein liquid: strawberry, vanilla 800 ml = £5.96
Ensure® Plus Commence (Abbott Laboratories Ltd)	Starter pack (5–10 day's supply), contains: Ensure® Plus Commence (various flavours), 1 pack (10 × 200ml) = £11.20								
Ensure® Plus Fibre (Abbott Laboratories Ltd)	Liquid (sip or tube feed) per 100 mL	652 kJ (155 kcal)	6.25 g cows' milk soya protein isolate	20.2 g (sugars 5.5 g)	4.92 g	2.5 g	Gluten-free Residual lactose	Borderline substances standard ACBS indications p. 974; also CAPD, haemodialysis.	Ensure Plus Fibre liquid: banana, chocolate, raspberry, strawberry, vanilla 200 ml = £2.07 Nutritional values vary with flavour – consult product literature

A2

Borderline substances | **Appendix 2**

A2

Borderline substances | Appendix 2

Nutritional supplements: 1.5 kcal/mL and 5 g (or more) protein/100 mL (product list continued)

Not suitable for use in child under 1 year; use with caution in child 1-5 years unless otherwise stated.

Product	Formulation	Energy	Protein	Carbohydrate	Fat	Fibre	Special Characteristics	ACBS Indications	Presentation & Flavour
Ensure® Plus Milkshake style (Abbott Laboratories Ltd)	Liquid (sip or tube feed) per 100 mL	632 kJ (150 kcal)	6.25 g cows' milk soya protein isolate	20.2 g (sugars 6.89 g)	4.92 g	Nil	Gluten-free Residual lactose	Borderline substances standard ACBS indications p. 974; also CAPD, haemodialysis	Ensure Plus milkshake style liquid: banana, chocolate, coffee, fruits of the forest, neutral, orange, peach, raspberry, strawberry, vanilla 220 ml = £1.12 Nutritional values vary with flavour – consult product literature
Ensure® Plus Savoury (Abbott Laboratories Ltd)	Liquid (sip or tube feed) per 100 mL	632 kJ (150 kcal)	6.25 g cows' milk soy protein isolate	20.2 g (sugars 1.13 g)	4.92 g	Nil	Gluten-free Residual lactose	Borderline substances standard ACBS indications p. 974; also CAPD, haemodialysis,	Ensure Plus savoury liquid: chicken, mushroom; 220 ml = £1.40
Ensure® Plus Yoghurt style (Abbott Laboratories Ltd)	Liquid (sip feed) per 100 mL	632 kJ (150 kcal)	6.25 g cows' milk	20.2 g (sugars 11.7 g)	4.92 g	Nil	Gluten-free Residual lactose	Borderline substances standard ACBS indications p. 974; also CAPD, haemodialysis	Ensure Plus yoghurt style liquid: orchard peach, strawberry swirl 200 ml = £1.12; 220 ml = £1.12
Fortisip® Bottle (Nutricia Ltd)	Liquid (sip feed) per 100 mL	630 kJ (150 kcal)	6 g cows' milk	18.4 g	5.8 g	Nil	Gluten-free Residual lactose	Borderline substances standard ACBS indications p. 974 Not suitable for child under 3 years; use with caution in child 3-5 years.	Fortisip Bottle: banana, caramel, chocolate, neutral, orange, strawberry, tropical fruit, vanilla 200 ml = £1.40 Sugar content varies with flavour.
Fortisip® Range (Nutricia Ltd)	Starter pack contains 4 × Fortisip® Bottle, 4 × Fortijuce®, 2 × Fortisip® Yogurt Style, 1 pack (10 × 200 ml) = £20.20								
Fortisip® Yoghurt Style (Nutricia Ltd)	Liquid (sip feed) per 100 mL	630 kJ (150 kcal)	6 g cows' milk	18.7 g (sugars 10.8 g)	5.8 g	200 mg	Gluten-free Contains lactose	Borderline substances standard ACBS indications p. 974 Not suitable for child under 3 years	Fortisip Yogurt Style liquid vanilla & lemon: 200 ml = £2.06
Fresubin® Protein Energy Drink (Fresenius Kabi Ltd)	Liquid (sip feed) per 100 mL	630 kJ (150 kcal)	10 g cows' milk	12.4 g (sugars 6.4 g)	6.7 g	Nil	Gluten-free Residual lactose Contains fish gelatin	Borderline substances standard ACBS indications p. 974; also CAPD, haemodialysis.	Fresubin Protein Energy drink: cappuccino, chocolate, tropical fruits, vanilla, wild strawberry 200 ml = £2.08 Sugar content varies with flavour. Fibre content varies with flavour.
Fresubin® Thickened (Fresenius Kabi Ltd)	Liquid (sip feed) per 100 mL	630 kJ (150 kcal)	10 g cows' milk	12.2 g (sugars 7.1 g)	6.7 g	480 mg	Gluten-free Residual lactose	Dysphagia or disease-related malnutrition. Not suitable for child under 3 years; use with caution in child 3-5 years.	Fresubin Thickened Stage 1 syrup: vanilla, wild strawberry 800 ml = £9.40; Fresubin Thickened Stage 2 custard: vanilla, wild strawberry 800 ml = £9.40 Sugar content varies with consistency. Fibre content varies with consistency.
Fresubin® YOcrème (Fresenius Kabi Ltd)	Semi-solid per 100 g	630 kJ (150 kcal)	7.5 g whey protein	19.5 g (sugars 16.8 g)	4.7 g	Nil	Gluten-free Contains lactose	Dysphagia, or presence or risk of malnutrition Not suitable for child under 3 years	Fresubin YOcreme dessert: apricot-peach, biscuit, lemon, raspberry 500 gram = £8.16

Nutritional supplements: Less than 1.5 kcal/mL and 5 g (or more) protein/100 mL

Not suitable for use in child under 1 year; use with caution in child 1–5 years unless otherwise stated.

Product	Formulation	Energy	Protein	Carbohydrate	Fat	Fibre	Special Characteristics	ACBS Indications	Presentation & Flavour
Ensure® Plus Crème (Abbott Laboratories Ltd)	Semi-solid per 100 g	574 kJ (137 kcal)	5.68 g cow's milk soy protein isolates	18.4 g (sugars 12.4 g)	4.47 g	Nil	Gluten-free Residual lactose Contains soya	Borderline substances standard ACBS indications p. 974; also CAPD, haemodialysis. Not suitable for child under 3 years; use with caution in child 3–5 years.	Ensure Plus Crème: chocolate, neutral, vanilla 500 gram = £7.72 Nutritional values vary with flavour - consult product literature
Nutilis® Fruit Stage 3 (Nutricia Ltd)	Semi-Solid per 100 g	560 kJ (133 kcal)	7 g whey isolate	16.7 g (sugars 11.3 g)	4 g	2.6 g	Gluten-free Residual lactose	Borderline substances standard ACBS indications p. 974 except bowel fistula; also CAPD, haemodialysis. Not suitable for child under 3 years; use with caution in child 3–5 years.	Nutilis Fruit Stage 3: apple, strawberry 450 gram = £7.08
Oral Impact® (Nestle Health Science)	Standard dilution of powder (74 g in 250 mL water) (sip feed) per 100 mL	425 kJ (101 kcal)	5.6 g cows' milk	13.4 g (sugars 7.4 g)	2.8 g	1 g	Residual lactose Contains fish oil	Pre-operative nutritional supplement for malnourished patients or patients at risk of malnourishment Not suitable for child under 3 years; use with caution in child 3–5 years.	Oral Impact oral powder 74 g sachets: citrus, coffee, tropical 5 sachet = £16.93

Powder provides: protein 16.8 g, carbohydrate 40.2 g, fat 8.3 g, fibre 3 g, energy 1276 kJ (303 kcal)/74 g.

Nutritional supplements: More than 1.5 kcal/mL and 5 g (or more) protein/100 mL

Not suitable for use in child under 1 year; use with caution in child 1–5 years unless otherwise stated.

Product	Formulation	Energy	Protein	Carbohydrate	Fat	Fibre	Special Characteristics	ACBS Indications	Presentation & Flavour
Altraplen Compact® (Nualtra Ltd)	Liquid (sip feed) per 100 mL	1008 kJ (240 kcal)	9.6 g cows' milk soya protein	28.8 g (sugars 11.6 g)	9.6 g	Nil	Gluten-free Residual lactose	Borderline substances standard ACBS indications p. 974 Not suitable for child under 3 years; use with caution in child 3–6 years.	Altraplen Compact liquid: strawberry, vanilla 500 ml = £5.80
Complan® Shake (Nutricia Ltd)	Powder per 57 g	1057 kJ (251 kcal)	8.8 g cows' milk	35.2 g (sugars 22.7 g)	8.4 g	Trace	Gluten-free Contains lactose	Borderline substances standard ACBS indications p. 974	Complan Shake Starter Pack sachets: 5 sachet = £4.39; Complan Shake oral powder 57 g sachets: banana, chocolate, milk, strawberry, vanilla 4 sachet = £2.80

Powder 57 g reconstituted with 200 mL whole milk provides: protein 15.6 g, carbohydrate 44.5 g, fat 16.4 g, energy 1621 kJ (387 kcal).

Product	Formulation	Energy	Protein	Carbohydrate	Fat	Fibre	Special Characteristics	ACBS Indications	Presentation & Flavour
Foodlink® Complete (Nualtra Ltd)	Powder per 100 g	1826 kJ (434 kcal)	21.3 g cows' milk	56.7 g	13.5 g	Nil	Contains lactose	Borderline substances standard ACBS indications p. 974	Foodlink Complete powder: banana, chocolate, natural, strawberry 399 gram = £4.27 Nutritional values vary with flavour - consult product literature.

Recommended serving = 4 heaped dessertspoonfuls in 200 mL full cream milk provides: protein 18.9 g, carbohydrate 41.8 g, fat 15.7 g, energy 1605 kJ (383 kcal).

Product	Formulation	Energy	Protein	Carbohydrate	Fat	Fibre	Special Characteristics	ACBS Indications	Presentation & Flavour
Foodlink® Complete with Fibre (Nualtra Ltd)	Powder per 100 g	1683 kJ (400 kcal)	19.4 g cows' milk	52.7 g (sugars 27.3 g)	12.4 g	7.2 g	Contains lactose	Borderline substances standard ACBS indications p. 974	Foodlink Complete powder with fibre vanilla: 441 gram = £4.69 Nutritional values vary with flavour - consult product literature.

Recommended serving = 4 heaped dessertspoonfuls (or the contents of a 63-g sachet) in 200 mL full cream milk provides: protein 19 g, carbohydrate 42.7 g, fat 15.8 g, fibre 4.5 g, energy 1624 kJ (388 kcal).

A2

Borderline substances | **Appendix 2**

Nutritional supplements: More than 1.5 kcal/mL and 5 g (or more) protein/100 mL (product list continued)

Not suitable for use in child under 1 year; use with caution in child 1-5 years unless otherwise stated.

Product	Formulation	Energy	Protein	Carbohydrate	Fat	Fibre	Special Characteristics	ACBS Indications	Presentation & Flavour
Forticreme® Complete (Nutricia Ltd)	Semi-solid per 100 g	675 kJ (160 kcal)	9.5 g cows' milk	19.2 g (sugars 10.6 g)	5 g	0.1 g	Gluten-free Residual lactose	Borderline substances standard ACBS indications p. 974; also CAPD, haemodialysis. Not suitable for child under 3 years; use with caution in child 3-5 years.	Forticreme Complete dessert: banana, chocolate, forest fruits, vanilla 500 gram = £7.84
Fortisip® Compact (Nutricia Ltd)	Liquid (sip feed) per 100 mL	1010 kJ (240 kcal)	9.6 g cows' milk	29.7 g (sugars 15 g)	9.3 g	Nil	Residual lactose	Borderline substances standard ACBS indications p. 974 Not suitable for child under 3 years; use with caution in child 3-5 years.	Fortisip Compact liquid: apricot, banana, chocolate, forest fruit, mocha, strawberry, vanilla 500 ml = £5.80
Fortisip® Compact Fibre (Nutricia Ltd)	Liquid (sip feed) per 100 mL	1000 kJ (240 kcal)	9.4 g cows' milk	25.2 g (sugars 13.9 g)	10.4 g	3.6 g	Gluten-free Residual lactose	Borderline substances standard ACBS indications p. 974 Not suitable for child under 3 years; use with caution in child 3-5 years.	Fortisip Compact Fibre Starter Pack liquid: 500 ml = £8.36; Fortisip Compact Fibre liquid: mocha, strawberry, vanilla 500 ml = £8.36
Fortisip® Compact Protein (Nutricia Ltd)	Liquid (sip feed) per 100 mL	1010 kJ (240 kcal)	14.4 g cows' milk	24.4 g (sugars 13.3 g)	9.4 g	Nil	Gluten-free Residual lactose	Borderline substances standard ACBS indications p. 974 Not suitable for child under 3 years; use with caution in child 3-5 years.	Fortisip Compact Protein Starter Pack liquid: 750 ml = £12.00; Fortisip Compact Protein liquid: banana, mocha, strawberry, vanilla 500 ml = £8.00. Nutritional values vary with flavour - consult product literature.
Fortisip® Extra (Nutricia Ltd)	Liquid (sip feed) per 100 mL	675 kJ (160 kcal)	10 g cows' milk	18.1 g (sugars 9 g)	5.3 g	Nil	Gluten-free Contains lactose	Borderline substances standard ACBS indications p. 974 Not suitable for child under 3 years; use with caution in child 3-5 years.	Fortisip Extra liquid: strawberry, vanilla 200 ml = £2.22
Fresubin® 2 kcal Drink (Fresenius Kabi Ltd)	Liquid (sip feed) per 100 mL	840 kJ (200 kcal)	10 g cows' milk	22.5 g (sugars 5.8 g)	7.8 g	Nil	Gluten-free Residual lactose	Borderline substances standard ACBS indications p. 974; also CAPD, haemodialysis. Not suitable for use in child under 1 year; use with caution in child 1-5 years.	Fresubin 2kcal drink: apricot-peach, cappuccino, fruits of the forest, neutral, toffee, vanilla 200 ml = £2.02
Fresubin® 2 kcal Fibre Drink (Fresenius Kabi Ltd)	Liquid (sip feed) per 100 mL	840 kJ (200 kcal)	10 g cows' milk	22.5 g (sugars 5.8 g)	7.8 g	1.6 g	Gluten-free Residual lactose	Borderline substances standard ACBS indications p. 974; also CAPD, haemodialysis. Not suitable for use in child under 1 year; use with caution in child 1-5 years.	Fresubin 2kcal Fibre drink: apricot-peach, cappuccino, chocolate, lemon, neutral 200 ml = £2.02 Nutritional values vary with flavour - consult product literature.
Fresubin® Powder Extra (Fresenius Kabi Ltd)	Powder per 100 g	1764 kJ (420 kcal)	17.5 g cows' milk whey protein	63 g (sugars 24.7 g)	10.9 g	Nil	Gluten-free Contains lactose	Borderline substances standard ACBS indications p. 974 Not suitable for child under 1 year; use with caution in child 1-5 years.	Fresubin Powder Extra oral powder 62g sachets: chocolate, neutral, strawberry, vanilla 7 sachet = £5.32 Nutritional values vary with flavour - consult product literature.

Powder 62 g reconstituted with 200 ml whole milk provides: protein 17.7 g, carbohydrate 48.5 g, fat 14.8 g, energy 1658 kJ (397 kcal).

Product	Formulation	Energy	Protein	Carbohydrate	Fat	Fibre	Special Characteristics	ACBS Indications	Presentation & Flavour
Nutilis® Complete Stage 1 (Nutricia Ltd)	Liquid (pre-thickened) per 100 mL	1010 kJ (240 kcal)	9.6 g cows' milk	29.1 g (sugars 5.4 g)	9.3 g	3.2 g	Residual lactose	Borderline substances standard ACBS indications p. 974 Not suitable for child under 3 years; use with caution in child 3–5 years.	Nutilis Complete Stage 1 liquid: strawberry, vanilla 500 ml = £8.84
Nutilis® Complete Stage 2 (Nutricia Ltd)	Semi-solid per 100 g	1030 kJ (245 kcal)	9.6 g cows' milk	29.1 g (sugars 11.8 g)	9.4 g	3.2 g	Gluten-free Residual lactose	Borderline substances standard ACBS indications p. 974 Not suitable for child under 3 years; use with caution in child 3–6 years.	Nutilis Complete Stage 2 custard: chocolate, strawberry, vanilla 500 gram = £8.84 Nutritional values vary with flavour – consult product literature.
Nutricrem® (Nualtra Ltd)	Semi-solid per 100 g	756 kJ (180 kcal)	10 g cows' milk soya protein	18.8 g (sugars 9.7 g)	7.2 g	Nil	Gluten-free Residual lactose	Borderline substances standard ACBS indications p. 974 Not suitable for child under 3 years; use with caution in child 3–6 years.	Nutricrem dessert: strawberry, vanilla 500 gram = £5.76
Renilon® 7.5 (Nutricia Ltd)	Liquid (sip feed) per 100 mL	840 kJ (200 kcal)	7.5 g cows' milk	20 g (sugars 4.8 g)	10 g	Nil	Gluten-free Residual lactose	Borderline substances standard ACBS indications p. 974 Not suitable for child under 3 years; use with caution in child 3–5 years.	Renilon 7.5 liquid: apricot, caramel 500 ml = £8.80
Resource® 2.0 Fibre (Nestle Health Science)	Liquid (sip feed) per 100 mL	836 kJ (200 kcal)	9 g cows' milk	21.4 g (sugars 5.5 g)	8.7 g	2.5 g	Gluten-free Residual lactose	Borderline substances standard ACBS indications p. 974 Not suitable for child under 6 years; caution in child 6–10 years.	Resource Fibre 2.0 liquid: apricot, coffee, neutral, strawberry, summer fruit, vanilla 200 ml = £1.88

Table 3 Specialised formulas

Specialised formulas: Infant and child

Specialised formulas: Infant and child: Amino acid-based formula

Specialised formulas are suitable for infants from birth unless otherwise indicated.

Product	Formulation	Energy	Protein	Carbohydrate	Fat	Fibre	Special Characteristics	ACBS Indications	Presentation & Flavour
Alfamino® (Nestle Health Science)	Standard dilution (13.8%) of powder per 100 mL	291 kJ (69 kcal)	1.8 g protein equivalent (essential and non-essential amino acids)	7.9 g (sugars 2.2 g)	3.4 g	Nil		Severe cows' milk allergy and or multiple food allergies	SMA Alfamino powder: 400 gram = £23.00

Powder provides protein equivalent 13.3 g, carbohydrate 57 g, fat 24.6 g, energy 2105 kJ (503 kcal)/100 g.

Product	Formulation	Energy	Protein	Carbohydrate	Fat	Fibre	Special Characteristics	ACBS Indications	Presentation & Flavour
Neocate® Active (Nutricia Ltd)	Standard dilution (21%) of powder per 300 mL serving (63-g sachet made up to 300 mL with water)	1255 kJ (300 kcal)	8.3 g protein equivalent (essential and non-essential amino acids)	34 g (sugars 3.1 g)	14.5 g	Nil	Milk protein-free	Proven whole protein intolerance, short bowel syndrome, intractable malabsorption, or other gastro-intestinal disorders where an elemental diet is indicated. Nutritional supplement only. Not suitable for child under 1 year.	Neocate Active powder: blackcurrant, unflavoured 945 gram = £67.50

Powder provides: protein equivalent 13.1 g, carbohydrate 54 g, fat 23 g, energy 1992 kJ (475 kcal)/100 g.

A2

Specialised formulas: Infant and child: Amino acid-based formula (product list continued)

Specialised formulas are suitable for infants from birth unless otherwise indicated.

Product	Formulation	Energy	Protein	Carbohydrate	Fat	Fibre	Special Characteristics	ACBS Indications	Presentation & Flavour
Neocate® Advance (Nutricia Ltd)	Standard dilution (25%) of powder per 100 mL	420 kJ (100 kcal)	2.5 g protein equivalent (essential and non-essential amino acids)	14.6 g (sugars 1.3 g)	3.5 g (MCT 35%)	Nil	Milk protein-free	Proven whole protein intolerance, short bowel syndrome, intractable malabsorption, or other gastro-intestinal disorders where an elemental diet is indicated. Not suitable for child under 1 year	Neocate Advance powder: unflavoured 1000 gram = £59.40; banana & vanilla 750 gram = £46.95

Powder provides: protein equivalent 10 g, carbohydrate 58.5 g, fat 14 g, energy 1683 kJ (400 kcal)/100 g.

Product	Formulation	Energy	Protein	Carbohydrate	Fat	Fibre	Special Characteristics	ACBS Indications	Presentation & Flavour
Neocate® LCP (Nutricia Ltd)	Standard dilution (13.8%) of powder per 100 mL	279 kJ (67 kcal)	1.8 g protein equivalent (essential and non-essential amino acids)	7.2 g (sugars 650 mg)	3.4 g	Nil	Milk protein-free	Cows' milk allergy, multiple food protein intolerance, and conditions requiring an elemental diet	Neocate LCP powder: 400 gram = £28.70

Powder provides: protein equivalent 13 g, carbohydrate 52.5 g, fat 24.5 g, energy 2020 kJ (483 kcal)/100 g.

Product	Formulation	Energy	Protein	Carbohydrate	Fat	Fibre	Special Characteristics	ACBS Indications	Presentation & Flavour
Neocate® Spoon (Nutricia Ltd)	Standard dilution (38%) of powder per 97 g serving (37-g sachet diluted with 60 mL water)	733 kJ (175 kcal)	3 g protein equivalent (essential and non-essential amino acids)	24.9 g (sugars 4.6 g)	7 g	Nil	Milk protein-free	Cows' milk allergy, multiple food protein intolerance, and conditions requiring an elemental diet. Not suitable for child under 6 months.	Neocate Spoon powder: 555 gram = £39.90

Powder provides protein equivalent 8.2 g, carbohydrate 67.4 g, fat 18.8 g, energy 1981 kJ (472 kcal)/100 g.

Product	Formulation	Energy	Protein	Carbohydrate	Fat	Fibre	Special Characteristics	ACBS Indications	Presentation & Flavour
Nutramigen® Puramino (Mead Johnson Nutrition (UK) Ltd)	Standard dilution (13.6%) of powder per 100 mL	290 kJ (68 kcal)	1.89 g essential and non-essential amino acids	7.2 g	3.6 g	Nil	Gluten-free Lactose-free	For use in the management of severe protein intolerance, multiple food intolerance and other gastro-intestinal disorders where an amino acid based diet is specifically indicated for infants and young children.	Nutramigen PurAmino powder: 400 gram = £27.63

Powder provides: protein 13.9 g, carbohydrate 53 g, fat 26 g, energy 2100 kJ (500 kcal)/100 g.

Specialised formulas: Infant and child: Hydrolysate formula

Product	Formulation	Energy	Protein	Carbohydrate	Fat	Fibre	Special Characteristics	ACBS Indications	Presentation & Flavour
Althéra® (Nestle Health Science)	Standard dilution (13.2%) of powder per 100 mL	280 kJ (67 kcal)	1.7 g whey hydrolysed	7.3 g (sugars 4 g)	3.4 g	Nil	Contains lactose	Complete nutritional support from birth to 3 years or supplementary feeding from 6 months to 3 years, in cow's milk protein allergy or multiple food protein allergies	Althéra can: 450 g = £10.68

Powder provides: protein 12.5 g, carbohydrate 55.5 g, fat 26 g, energy 2119 kJ (506 kcal)/100 g.

Formula (manufacturer)	Preparation	Energy	Protein	Carbohydrate (sugars)	Fat		Special characteristics	Indications	Presentation and price
Aptamil Pepti 1 (Allergy) (Milupa Ltd)	Standard dilution (13.6%) of powder per 100 mL	280 kJ (67 kcal)	1.6 g whey hydrolysed	7.1 g (sugars 3.5 g)	3.5 g	600 mg	Contains lactose and fish oil	Established cows' milk protein intolerance, with or without secondary lactose intolerance	Aptamil Pepti 1 (Allergy) powder: 400 gram = £9.87; 800 gram = £19.73
Powder provides: protein 11.6 g, carbohydrate 52 g, fat 25.6 g, energy 2025 kJ (484 kcal)/100 g.									
Aptamil Pepti 2 (Allergy) (Milupa Ltd)	Standard dilution (14.3%) of powder per 100 mL	285 kJ (68 kcal)	1.6 g whey hydrolysed	8 g (sugars 3.6 g)	3.1 g	600 mg	Contains lactose and fish oil	Established cows' milk protein allergy or intolerance. Not suitable for child under 6 months.	Aptamil Pepti 2 (Allergy) powder: 400 gram = £9.41; 800 gram = £18.82
Powder provides: protein 11.2 g, carbohydrate 56.1 g, fat 21.8 g, energy 1985 kJ (473 kcal)/100 g.									
Cow & Gate Pepti-Junior (Cow & Gate Ltd)	Standard dilution (12.8%) of powder per 100 mL	275 kJ (66 kcal)	1.8 g whey hydrolysed	6.8 g (sugars 1.1 g)	3.5 g	Nil	Residual lactose. Contains fish oil	Disaccharide and/or whole protein intolerance, or where amino acids and peptides are indicated in conjunction with medium chain triglycerides.	Pepti-Junior powder: 450 gram = £13.36
Powder provides: protein 14 g, carbohydrate 53.4 g, fat 27.3 g, energy 2155 kJ (515 kcal)/100 g.									
Infatrini Peptisorb (Nutricia Ltd)	Liquid (sip or tube feed) per 100 mL	420 kJ (100 kcal)	2.6 g whey protein hydrolysate	10.3 g (sugars 2.7 g)	5.4 g (MCT 50%)	Nil	Gluten-free. Residual lactose. Contains fish oil	Disease-related malnutrition, intractable malabsorption, proven inflammatory bowel disease, short bowel syndrome, bowel fistula, and intolerance to whole protein feeds in child from birth to 18 months or body-weight up to 9 kg	Infatrini Peptisorb liquid: 200 mL = £3.54
Nutramigen 1 with LGG (Mead Johnson Nutrition (UK) Ltd)	Standard dilution (13.5%) of powder per 100 mL	280 kJ (68 kcal)	1.9 g casein hydrolysed	7.5 g	3.4 g	Nil	Gluten-free. Lactose-free	For the dietary management of cow's milk allergy with/or without lactose intolerance	Nutramigen 1 with LGG powder: 400 gram = £11.21
Powder provides: protein 14 g, carbohydrate 55 g, fat 25 g, energy 2100 kJ (500 kcal)/100 g.									
Nutramigen 2 with LGG (Mead Johnson Nutrition (UK) Ltd)	Standard dilution (14.6%) of powder per 100 mL	285 kJ (68 kcal)	1.7 g casein hydrolysed	8.6 g	2.9 g	Nil	Gluten-free. Lactose-free	For the dietary management of cow's milk allergy with/or without lactose intolerance. Not suitable for child under 6 months.	Nutramigen 2 with LGG powder: 400 gram = £10.99
Powder provides: protein 12 g, carbohydrate 62 g, fat 20 g, energy 2000 kJ (480 kcal)/100 g.									
Pepdite (Nutricia Ltd)	Standard dilution (15%) of powder per 100 mL	297 kJ (71 kcal)	2.1 g protein equivalent (non-milk hydrolysate)	7.8 g (sugars 700 mg)	3.5 g	Nil	Lactose-free. Contains meat (pork) and soya derivatives	Disaccharide and/or whole protein intolerance	Pepdite powder: 400 gram = £19.04
Powder provides: protein equivalent 13.8 g, carbohydrate 52 g, fat 23.2 g, energy 1977 kJ (472 kcal)/100 g.									
Pepdite 1+ (Nutricia Ltd)	Standard dilution (22.8%) of powder per 100 mL	423 kJ (100 kcal)	3.1 g protein equivalent (non-milk hydrolysate, essential amino acids)	13 g (sugars 1.2 g)	3.9 g (MCT 35%)	Nil	Lactose-free. Contains meat (pork) and soya derivatives	Disaccharide and/or whole protein intolerance, or where amino acids or peptides are indicated in conjunction with medium chain triglycerides. Not suitable for child under 1 year.	Pepdite 1+ powder: 400 gram = £19.99
Powder provides: protein equivalent 13.8 g, fat 17.3 g, energy 1844 kJ (439 kcal)/100 g.									

A2

Specialised formulas: Infant and child: Hydrolysate formula (product list continued)

Product	Formulation	Energy	Protein	Carbohydrate	Fat	Fibre	Special Characteristics	ACBS Indications	Presentation & Flavour
Pregestimil® Lipil (Mead Johnson Nutrition (UK) Ltd)	Standard dilution (13.5%) of powder per 100 mL	280 kJ (68 kcal)	1.89 g casein hydrolysed	6.9 g	3.8 g (MCT 54%)	Nil	Gluten-free Lactose-free	Disaccharide and/or whole protein intolerance, or where amino acids or peptides are indicated in conjunction with medium chain triglycerides.	Pregestimil LIPIL powder: 400 gram = £12.43

Powder provides: protein 14 g, carbohydrate 51 g, fat 28 g, energy 2100 kJ (500 kcal)/100 g.

Product	Formulation	Energy	Protein	Carbohydrate	Fat	Fibre	Special Characteristics	ACBS Indications	Presentation & Flavour
Similac® Alimentum (Abbott Laboratories Ltd)	Standard dilution (14%) of powder per 100 mL	283 kJ (67.6 kcal)	1.86 g casein hydrolysed	6.62 g (sugars 1.5 g)	3.75 g (MCT 33%)	Nil	Gluten-free Lactose-free Contains meat derivatives	Cows' milk protein allergy and other conditions where an extensively hydrolysed formula is indicated.	Similac Alimentum powder: 400 gram = £9.10

Powder provides: protein equivalent 14.4 g, carbohydrate 51.4 g, fat 29.1 g, energy 2196 kJ (525 kcal)/100 g.

Specialised formulas: Infant and child: Residual lactose formula

Product	Formulation	Energy	Protein	Carbohydrate	Fat	Fibre	Special Characteristics	ACBS Indications	Presentation & Flavour
Enfamil® O-Lac (Mead Johnson Nutrition (UK) Ltd)	Standard dilution (13%) of powder per 100 mL	280 kJ (68 kcal)	1.42 g cows' milk	7.2 g	3.7 g	Nil	Gluten-free Residual lactose	Proven lactose intolerance	Enfamil O-Lac powder: 400 gram = £5.08

Powder provides: protein 10.9 g, carbohydrate 55 g, fat 28 g, energy 2200 kJ (524 kcal)/100 g.

Product	Formulation	Energy	Protein	Carbohydrate	Fat	Fibre	Special Characteristics	ACBS Indications	Presentation & Flavour
Galactomin 17 (Nutricia Ltd)	Standard dilution (13.6%) of powder per 100 mL	295 kJ (70 kcal)	1.7 g protein equivalent (cows' milk)	7.5 g (sugars 1.4 g)	3.7 g	Nil	Residual lactose	Proven lactose intolerance in pre-school children, galactosaemia, and galactokinase deficiency.	Galactomin 17 powder: 400 gram = £17.04

Powder provides: protein equivalent 12.3 g, carbohydrate 55.3 g, fat 27.2 g, energy 2155 kJ (515 kcal)/100 g.

Product	Formulation	Energy	Protein	Carbohydrate	Fat	Fibre	Special Characteristics	ACBS Indications	Presentation & Flavour
SMA® LF (SMA Nutrition)	Standard dilution (13%) of powder per 100 mL	281 kJ (67 kcal)	1.5 g casein, whey	7.2 g (sugars 2.6 g)	3.6 g	Nil	Residual lactose	Proven lactose intolerance	SMA LF powder: 430 gram = £5.34

Powder provides: protein 12 g, carbohydrate 55.6 g, fat 28 g, energy 2185 kJ (522 kcal)/100 g.

Specialised formulas: Infant and child: MCT-enhanced formula

Product	Formulation	Energy	Protein	Carbohydrate	Fat	Fibre	Special Characteristics	ACBS Indications	Presentation & Flavour
Lipistart® (Vitaflo International Ltd)	Standard dilution (15%) of powder per 100 mL	282 kJ (68 kcal)	2.1 g protein equivalent (whey, soya)	8.3 g (sugars 700 mg)	3.1 g (MCT 81%)	Nil	Residual lactose	Dietary management of fat malabsorption, long-chain fatty acid oxidation disorders, and other disorders requiring a high MCT, low LCT formula.	Lipistart powder: 400 gram = £19.74

Powder provides: protein equivalent 13.7 g, carbohydrate 55.3 g, fat 20.6 g, energy 1883 kJ (450 kcal)/100 g.

Product	Formulation	Energy	Protein	Carbohydrate	Fat	Fibre	Special Characteristics	ACBS Indications	Presentation & Flavour
MCT Pepdite® (Nutricia Ltd)	Standard dilution (15%) of powder per 100 mL	286 kJ (68 kcal)	2 g protein equivalent (non-milk peptides, essential amino acids)	8.8 g (sugars 1.2 g)	2.7 g (MCT 75%)	Nil	Gluten-free Lactose-free Contains meat (pork) and soya derivatives	Disorders in which a high intake of MCT is beneficial	MCT Pepdite powder: 400 gram = £20.72

Powder provides: protein equivalent 13.8 g, carbohydrate 59 g, fat 18 g, energy 1903 kJ (453 kcal)/100 g.

Product	Formulation	Energy	Protein	Carbohydrate	Fat	Fibre	Special Characteristics	ACBS Indications	Presentation & Flavour
MCT Pepdite® +1 (Nutricia Ltd)	Standard dilution (20%) of powder per 100 mL	381 kJ (91 kcal)	2.8 g protein equivalent (non-milk peptides, essential amino acids)	11.8 g (sugars 1.6 g)	3.6 g (MCT 75%)	Nil	Gluten-free Lactose-free Contains meat (pork) and soya derivatives	Disorders in which a high intake of MCT is beneficial Not suitable for child under 1 year.	MCT Pepdite 1+ powder: 400 gram = £20.72

Powder provides: protein equivalent 13.8 g, carbohydrate 59 g, fat 18 g, energy 1903 kJ (453 kcal)/100 g.

Product	Formulation	Energy	Protein	Carbohydrate	Fat	Fibre	Special Characteristics	ACBS Indications	Presentation & Flavour
Monogen® (Nutricia Ltd)	Standard dilution (17.5%) of powder per 100 mL	310 kJ (74 kcal)	2.2 g protein equivalent (whey)	12 g (sugars 1.2 g)	1.9 g (MCT 80%)	Nil	Residual lactose Supplementation with essential fatty acids may be needed	Long-chain acyl-CoA dehydrogenase deficiency (LCAD), carnitine palmitoyl transferase deficiency (CPTD), primary and secondary lipoprotein lipase deficiency, chylothorax, and lymphangiectasia	Monogen powder: 400 gram = £20.59

Powder provides: protein equivalent 12.5 g, carbohydrate 68 g, fat 11 g, energy 1769 kJ (420 kcal)/100 g.

Specialised formulas: Infant and child: Soya-based formula

Product	Formulation	Energy	Protein	Carbohydrate	Fat	Fibre	Special Characteristics	ACBS Indications	Presentation & Flavour
Wysoy® (SMA Nutrition)	Standard dilution (13.2%) of powder per 100 mL	280 kJ (67 kcal)	1.8 g soya protein isolate	6.9 g (sugars 2.5 g)	3.6 g	Nil	Lactose-free	Proven lactose and associated sucrose intolerance in pre-school children, galactokinase deficiency, galactosaemia, and proven whole cows' milk sensitivity.	SMA Wysoy powder: 860 gram = £10.31

Powder provides: protein equivalent 14 g, carbohydrate 54 g, fat 27 g, energy 2155 kJ (515 kcal)/100 g.

Specialised formulas: Infant and child: Low calcium formula

Product	Formulation	Energy	Protein	Carbohydrate	Fat	Fibre	Special Characteristics	ACBS Indications	Presentation & Flavour
Locasol® (Nutricia Ltd)	Standard dilution (13.1%) of powder per 100 mL	278 kJ (66 kcal)	1.9 g cows' milk	7 g (sugars 6.9 g)	3.4 g	Nil	Contains lactose Calcium less than 7 mg/100 mL No added vitamin D	Conditions of calcium intolerance requiring restriction of calcium and vitamin D intake	Locasol powder: 400 gram = £23.69

Powder provides: protein equivalent 14.6 g, carbohydrate 53.7 g, fat 26.1 g, energy 2125 kJ (508 kcal)/100 g.

Specialised formulas: Infant and child: Fructose-based formula

Product	Formulation	Energy	Protein	Carbohydrate	Fat	Fibre	Special Characteristics	ACBS Indications	Presentation & Flavour
Galactomin 19® (Nutricia Ltd)	Standard dilution (12.9%) of powder per 100 mL	288 kJ (69 kcal)	1.9 g protein equivalent (cows' milk)	6.4 g (fructose 6.3 g)	4 g	Nil	Residual lactose, galactose and glucose	Conditions of glucose plus galactose intolerance	Galactomin 19 powder: 400 gram = £44.85

Powder provides: protein equivalent 14.6 g, carbohydrate 49.7 g, fat 30.8 g, energy 2233 kJ (534 kcal)/100 g.

Borderline substances | **Appendix 2**

A2

Specialised formulas: Infant and child: Pre-thickened infant feeds

Not to be used for a period of more than 6 months; not to be used in conjunction with any other feed thickener or antacid products.

Product	Formulation	Energy	Protein	Carbohydrate	Fat	Fibre	Special Characteristics	ACBS Indications	Presentation & Flavour
Enfamil® AR (Mead Johnson Nutrition (UK) Ltd)	Standard dilution (13.5%) of powder per 100 mL	285 kJ (68 kcal)	1.7 g cows' milk	7.6 g (lactose 4.6 g)	3.5 g	Nil	Contains lactose, pregelatinised rice starch	Significant gastro-oesophageal reflux	Enfamil AR powder: 400 gram = £3.80

Powder provides: protein 12.5 g, carbohydrate 56 g, fat 26 g, energy 2093 kJ (500 kcal)/100 g.

Product	Formulation	Energy	Protein	Carbohydrate	Fat	Fibre	Special Characteristics	ACBS Indications	Presentation & Flavour
SMA® Staydown (SMA Nutrition)	Standard dilution (12.9%) of powder per 100 mL	279 kJ (67 kcal)	1.6 g casein, whey	7 g (lactose 5 g)	3.6 g	Nil	Contains lactose, pre-cooked corn starch	Significant gastro-oesophageal reflux	SMA Staydown powder: 900 gram = £7.80

Powder provides: protein 12.4 g, carbohydrate 54.3 g, fat 28 g, energy 2166 kJ (518 kcal)/100 g.

Specialised formulas for specific clinical conditions

Product	Formulation	Energy	Protein	Carbohydrate	Fat	Fibre	Special Characteristics	ACBS Indications	Presentation & Flavour
Alicalm® (Nutricia Ltd)	Standard dilution (30%) of powder per 100 mL	567 kJ (135 kcal)	4.5 g caseinate whey	17.4 g (sugars 3.2 g)	5.3 g	Nil	Residual lactose	Crohn's disease. Not suitable for child under 1 year; use as nutritional supplement only in children 1–6 years.	Alicalm oral powder: 400 gram = £21.79

Powder provides: protein 15 g, carbohydrate 58 g, fat 17.5 g, energy 1889 kJ (450 kcal)/100 g.

Product	Formulation	Energy	Protein	Carbohydrate	Fat	Fibre	Special Characteristics	ACBS Indications	Presentation & Flavour
Forticare® (Nutricia Ltd)	Liquid (sip feed) per 100 mL	675 kJ (160 kcal)	9 g cows' milk	19.1 g (sugars 13.6 g)	5.3 g	2.1 g	Gluten-free. Residual lactose. Contains fish oil	Nutritional supplement in patients with lung cancer undergoing chemotherapy, or with pancreatic cancer. Not suitable in child under 3 years	Forticare liquid: cappuccino, orange & lemon, peach & ginger 500 ml = £9.08
Heparon® Junior (Nutricia Ltd)	Standard dilution (18%) of powder per 100 mL	363 kJ (86 kcal)	2 g cows' milk	11.6 g (sugars 2.9 g)	3.6 g	Nil	Contains lactose. Electrolytes/100 mL: Na⁺ 0.56 mmol K⁺ 1.9 mmol Ca²⁺ 2.3 mmol P⁺ 1.6 mmol	Enteral feed or nutritional supplement for children with acute or chronic liver failure	Heparon Junior powder: 400 gram = £21.95

Powder provides: protein 11.1 g, carbohydrate 64.2 g, fat 19.9 g, energy 2016 kJ (480 kcal)/100 g.

Product	Formulation	Energy	Protein	Carbohydrate	Fat	Fibre	Special Characteristics	ACBS Indications	Presentation & Flavour
KetoCal® (Nutricia Ltd)	Standard dilution (20%) of powder per 100 mL	602 kJ (146 kcal)	3.1 g cows' milk with additional amino acids	600 mg (sugars 120 mg)	14.6 g (LCT 100%)	Nil	Electrolytes/100 mL: Na⁺ 4.3 mmol K⁺ 4.1 mmol Ca²⁺ 2.15 mmol P⁺ 2.77 mmol	Enteral feed or nutritional supplement as part of ketogenic diet in management of epilepsy resistant to drug therapy, in children over 1 year, only on the advice of secondary care physician with experience of ketogenic diet.	KetoCal 4:1 powder: unflavoured, vanilla 300 gram = £30.91

Powder provides: protein 15.25 g, carbohydrate 3 g, fat 73 g, energy 3011 kJ (730 kcal)/100 g.

Product	Dilution	Energy	Protein	Carbohydrate	Fat	Fibre	Electrolytes / other	Indication	Price
KetoCal® 3:1 (Nutricia Ltd)	Standard dilution (9.5%) of powder per 100 mL	276 kJ (66 kcal)	1.5 g	680 mg (sugars 570 mg)	6.4 g	Nil	Electrolytes/100 mL: Na⁺ 1.3 mmol, K⁺ 2.4 mmol, Ca²⁺ 2 mmol, P⁺ 1.7 mmol	Enteral feed or nutritional supplement as part of ketogenic diet in management of drug resistant epilepsy or other conditions for which a ketogenic diet is indicated in children from birth to 6 years; as a nutritional supplement in children over 6 years.	KetoCal 3:1 powder: 300 gram = £29.91

Powder provides: protein 15.3 g, carbohydrate 7.2 g, fat 67.7 g, energy 2927 kJ (699 kcal)/100 g.

Product	Dilution	Energy	Protein	Carbohydrate	Fat	Fibre	Electrolytes / other	Indication	Price
KetoCal® 4:1 LQ (Nutricia Ltd)	Liquid (sip or tube feed) per 100 mL	620 kJ (150 kcal)	3.09 g casein and whey with additional amino acids	610 mg (sugars 230 mg)	14.8 g (LCT 100%)	1.12 g	Residual lactose. Electrolytes/100 mL: Na⁺ 4.9 mmol, K⁺ 4.7 mmol, Ca²⁺ 2.4 mmol, P⁺ 3.1 mmol	Enteral feed or nutritional supplement as part of ketogenic diet in management of drug resistant epilepsy or other conditions for which a ketogenic diet is indicated in children 1–10 years; as a nutritional supplement in children over 10 years.	KetoCal 4:1 LQ liquid: unflavoured, vanilla 200 ml = £4.41
Kindergen® (Nutricia Ltd)	Standard dilution (20%) of powder per 100 mL	421 kJ (101 kcal)	1.5 g whey protein	11.8 g (sugars 1.2 g)	5.3 g (LCT 93%)	Nil	Electrolytes/100 mL: Na⁺ 2 mmol, K⁺ 0.6 mmol, Ca²⁺ 2.8 mmol, P⁺ 3 mmol. Low Vitamin A	Enteral feed or nutritional supplement for children with chronic renal failure receiving peritoneal rapid overnight dialysis.	Kindergen powder: 400 gram = £29.47

Powder provides: protein 7.5 g, carbohydrate 59 g, fat 26.3 g, energy 2104 kJ (504 kcal)/100 g.

Product	Dilution	Energy	Protein	Carbohydrate	Fat	Fibre	Electrolytes / other	Indication	Price
Modulen IBD® (Nestlé Health Science)	Standard dilution (20%) of powder (sip or tube feed) per 100 mL	420 kJ (100 kcal)	3.6 g casein	11 g (sugars 3.98 g)	4.7 g	Nil	Gluten-free. Residual lactose	Crohn's disease active phase, and in remission if malnourished	Modulen IBD powder: 400 gram = £15.06

Powder provides: protein 18 g, carbohydrate 54 g, fat 23 g, energy 2070 kJ (500 kcal)/100 g.

Product	Dilution	Energy	Protein	Carbohydrate	Fat	Fibre	Electrolytes / other	Indication	Price
ProSure® (Abbott Laboratories Ltd)	Liquid (sip or tube feed) per 100 mL	536 kJ (127 kcal)	6.65 g cows' milk	18.3 g (sugars 2.95 g)	2.56 g	2.07 g	Gluten-free. Residual lactose. Contains fish oil	Nutritional supplement for patients with pancreatic cancer. Not suitable for child under 1 year; use with caution in child 1–4 years.	ProSure liquid: 220 ml = £3.34; 240 ml = £3.34
Renamil® (Stanningley Pharma Ltd)	Powder (sip or tube feed when reconstituted) per 100 g	2003 kJ (477 kcal)	4.6 g cows' milk	70.8 g	19.3 g	Nil	Contains lactose. Gluten-free. Electrolytes/100 g: Na⁺ 0.13 mmol, K⁺ 1.04 mmol, Ca²⁺ 10.22 mmol, P⁺ 1.06 mmol. Contains no vitamin A or vitamin D	Enteral feed or nutritional supplement for adults and children over 1 year with chronic renal failure.	Renamil powder: 1000 gram = £25.40

Borderline substances | **Appendix 2**

Specialised formulas for specific clinical conditions (product list continued)

Product	Formulation	Energy	Protein	Carbohydrate	Fat	Fibre	Special Characteristics	ACBS Indications	Presentation & Flavour
Renapro® (Stanningley Pharma Ltd)	Powder per 100 g	1580 kJ (372 kcal)	90 g whey protein	800 mg	1 g	Nil	Gluten-free Residual lactose Electrolytes/100 g: Na⁺ 23 mmol K⁺ 2 mmol Ca²⁺ 4.99 mmol P⁺ 4.84 mmol	Nutritional supplement for biochemically proven hypoproteinaemia and patients undergoing dialysis. Not suitable for child under 1 year.	Renapro powder: 600 gram = £69.60

Powder provides: protein 18 g, energy 316 kJ (74 kcal)/20-g sachet.

Product	Formulation	Energy	Protein	Carbohydrate	Fat	Fibre	Special Characteristics	ACBS Indications	Presentation & Flavour
Renastart® (Vitaflo International Ltd)	Standard dilution (20%) of powder per 100 mL	414 kJ (99 kcal)	1.5 g cows' milk soya	12.5 g (sugars 1.3 g)	4.8 g	Nil	Contains lactose Electrolytes/100 mL: Na⁺ 2.1 mmol K⁺ 0.6 mmol Ca²⁺ 0.6 mmol P⁺ 0.6 mmol	Dietary management of renal failure in child from birth to 10 years.	Renastart powder: 400 gram = £26.87

Powder provides: protein 7.5 g, carbohydrate 62.5 g, fat 23.8 g, energy 2071 kJ (494 kcal)/100 g.

Table 4 Feed supplements
High-energy supplements
High-energy supplements: carbohydrate

Flavoured carbohydrate supplements are not suitable for child under 1 year; liquid supplements should be diluted before use in child under 5 years.

Product	Formulation	Energy	Protein	Carbohydrate	Fat	Fibre	Special Characteristics	ACBS Indications	Presentation & Flavour
Maxijul® Super Soluble (Nutricia Ltd)	Powder per 100 g	1615 kJ (380 kcal)	Nil	95 g Glucose polymer (sugars 8.6 g)	Nil	Nil	Gluten-free Lactose-free	Disease-related malnutrition, malabsorption states, or other conditions requiring fortification with a high or readily available carbohydrate supplement.	Maxijul Super Soluble powder: 200 gram = £2.64; 25000 gram = £157.74; 528 gram = £6.56
Polycal® (Nutricia Ltd)	Powder per 100 g	1630 kJ (384 kcal)	Nil	96 g Maltodextrin (sugars 6 g)	Nil	Nil	Gluten-free Lactose-free	Disease-related malnutrition, malabsorption states, or other conditions requiring fortification with a high or readily available carbohydrate supplement.	Polycal powder: 400 gram = £4.36
	Liquid per 100 mL	1050 kJ (247 kcal)	Nil	61.9 g Maltodextrin (sugars 12.2 g)	Nil	Nil	Disease-related malnutrition, malabsorption states, or other conditions requiring fortification with a high or readily available carbohydrate supplement. Not suitable for child under 3 years.		Polycal liquid: neutral, orange 200 ml = £1.75

Product	Formulation	Energy	Protein	Carbohydrate	Fat	Fibre	Special Characteristics	ACBS Indications	Presentation & Flavour
S.O.S.® (Vitaflo International Ltd)	Powder per 100 g	1590 kJ (380 kcal)	Nil	95 g (sugars 9 g)	Nil	Nil		For use as an emergency regimen in the dietary management of inborn errors of metabolism in adults and children from birth.	S.O.S.: 15 oral powder 31g sachets 30 sachet = £11.00; S.O.S. 20 oral powder 42g sachets 30 sachet = £14.90; S.O.S. 10 oral powder 21g sachets 30 sachet = £7.45; S.O.S. 25 oral powder 52g sachets 30 sachet = £18.43

Contents of each sachet should be reconstituted with water to a total volume of 200 ml

Product	Formulation	Energy	Protein	Carbohydrate	Fat	Fibre	Special Characteristics	ACBS Indications	Presentation & Flavour
Vitajoule® (Vitaflo International Ltd)	Powder per 100 g	1590 kJ (380 kcal)	Nil	95 g Dried glucose syrup (sugars 9 g)	Nil	Nil	Gluten-free Lactose-free	Disease-related malnutrition, malabsorption states, or other conditions requiring fortification with a high or readily available carbohydrate supplement. Flavoured carbohydrate supplements are not suitable for child under 1 year; liquid supplements should be diluted before use in child under 5 years.	Vitajoule powder: 500 gram = £4.46

High-energy supplements: fat

Liquid supplements should be diluted before use in child under 5 years

Product	Formulation	Energy	Protein	Carbohydrate	Fat	Fibre	Special Characteristics	ACBS Indications	Presentation & Flavour
Calogen® (Nutricia Ltd)	Liquid (emulsion) per 100 mL	1850 kJ (450 kcal)	Nil	0.1 g	50 g (LCT 100 %)	Nil	Gluten-free Lactose-free	Disease-related malnutrition, malabsorption states, or other conditions requiring fortification with a high fat (or fat and carbohydrate) supplement. Liquid supplements should be diluted before use in child under 5 years.	Calogen emulsion: neutral, strawberry 200 ml = £4.44; 500 ml = £10.92; banana 500 ml = £10.92
Fresubin® 5 kcal Shot (Fresenius Kabi Ltd)	Liquid (emulsion) per 100 mL	2100 kJ (500 kcal)	Nil	4.0 g (sucrose)	53.8 g	400 mg	Gluten-free Lactose-free	Disease-related malnutrition, malabsorption states, or other conditions requiring fortification with a high fat (or fat and carbohydrate) supplement. Liquid supplements should be diluted before use in child under 5 years. Not suitable for child under 3 years.	Fresubin 5kcal shot drink neutral: 480 ml = £11.40
Liquigen® (Nutricia Ltd)	Liquid (emulsion) per 100 mL	1850 kJ (450 kcal)	Nil	Nil	50 g (MCT 97 %) Fractionated coconut oil	Nil	Gluten-free Lactose-free	Steatorrhoea associated with cystic fibrosis of the pancreas, intestinal lymphangiectasia, intestinal surgery, chronic liver disease, liver cirrhosis, other proven malabsorption syndromes, ketogenic diet in epilepsy, and in type 1 lipoproteinaemia Not suitable for child under 1 year	Liquigen emulsion: 250 ml = £9.39

A2

Borderline substances | **Appendix 2**

High-energy supplements: fat (product list continued)

Liquid supplements should be diluted before use in child under 5 years

Product	Formulation	Energy	Protein	Carbohydrate	Fat	Fibre	Special Characteristics	ACBS Indications	Presentation & Flavour
Medium-chain Triglyceride (MCT) Oil (Nutricia Ltd)	Liquid per 100 mL	3515 kJ (855 kcal)	Nil	Nil	MCT 100 %	Nil		Nutritional supplement for steatorrhoea associated with cystic fibrosis of the pancreas, intestinal lymphangiectasia, intestinal surgery, chronic liver disease and liver cirrhosis, other proven malabsorption syndromes, ketogenic diet in management of epilepsy, type 1 hyperlipoproteinaemia	MCT oil: 500 ml = £14.89

FAT AND CARBOHYDRATE

Product	Formulation	Energy	Protein	Carbohydrate	Fat	Fibre	Special Characteristics	ACBS Indications	Presentation & Flavour
Duocal® Super Soluble (Nutricia Ltd)	Powder per 100 g	2061 kJ (492 kcal)	Nil	72.7 g (sugars 6.5 g)	22.3 g (MCT 35 %)	Nil	Gluten-free Lactose-free	Disease-related malnutrition, malabsorption states, or other conditions requiring fortification with a high fat (or fat and carbohydrate) supplement.	Duocal Super Soluble powder: 400 gram = £18.34
Energivit® (Nutricia Ltd)	Standard dilution (15%) of powder per 100 mL	309 kJ (74 kcal)	Nil	10 g (sugars 900 mg)	3.75 g	Nil	Lactose-free With vitamins, minerals, and trace elements	For children requiring additional energy, vitamins, minerals, and trace elements following a protein-restricted diet	Energivit powder: 400 gram = £22.30

Powder provides: carbohydrate 66.7 g, fat 25 g, energy 2059 kJ (492 kcal)/100 g.

High-energy supplements: protein

Product	Formulation	Energy	Protein	Carbohydrate	Fat	Fibre	Special Characteristics	ACBS Indications	Presentation & Flavour
ProSource® Jelly (Nutrinovo Ltd)	Semi-solid per 100 mL	315 kJ (75 kcal)	16.9 g collagen protein hydrolysate whey protein isolate	Less than 1 g	Nil	Less than 1 g	Gluten-free Lactose-free Contains porcine derivatives	Hypoproteinaemia Not recommended for child under 3 years	ProSource jelly: fruit punch, orange 118 ml = £1.87
Protifar® (Nutricia Ltd)	Powder per 100 g	1580 kJ (373 kcal)	88.5 g cows' milk	less than 1.5 g	1.6 g	Nil	Gluten-free Residual lactose Electrolytes/100 mL: Na⁺ 1.3 mmol K⁺ 1.28 mmol Ca²⁺ 33.75 mmol P⁺ 22.58 mmol	Nutritional supplement for use in biochemically proven hypoproteinaemia.	Protifar powder: 225 gram = £8.86

Powder provides: protein 2.2 g per 2.5 g scoopful.

PROTEIN AND CARBOHYDRATE

Product	Formulation	Energy	Protein	Carbohydrate	Fat	Fibre	Special Characteristics	ACBS Indications	Presentation & Flavour
Dialamine® (Nutricia Ltd)	Standard dilution (20%) of powder per 100 mL	264 kJ (62 kcal)	4.3 g protein equivalent (essential and non-essential amino acids)	11.2 g (sugars 10.2 g)	Nil	Nil	Contains vitamin C	Hypoproteinaemia, chronic renal failure, wound fistula leakage with excessive protein loss, conditions requiring a controlled nitrogen intake, and haemodialysis. Not suitable for child under 6 months.	Dialamine powder: 400 gram = £74.49
	Powder provides: protein equivalent 25 g, carbohydrate 65 g, vitamin C 125 mg, energy 1530 kJ (360 kcal)/100 g.								
ProSource® Liquid (Nutrinovo Ltd)	Liquid per 30 mL	420 kJ (100 kcal)	10 g collagen protein whey protein isolate	15 g (sugars 8 g)	Nil	Nil	Gluten-free Lactose-free May contain porcine derivatives	Biochemically proven hypoproteinaemia Not recommended for child under 3 years.	ProSource liquid 30ml sachets: citrus berry, lemon, orange creme, neutral 100 sachet = £101.16
ProSource® Plus (Nutrinovo Ltd)	Liquid per 30 mL	420 kJ (100 kcal)	15 g collagen protein whey protein isolate	11 g (sugars 10 g)	Nil	Nil	Gluten-free Lactose-free May contain porcine derivatives	Hypoproteinaemia Not recommended for child under 3 years	ProSource Plus liquid 100 × 30 ml sachets: unflavoured = £143.90
Calogen® Extra (Nutricia Ltd)	Liquid per 100 mL	1650 kJ (400 kcal)	5 g cows' milk	4.5 g (sugars 3.5 g)	40.3 g	Nil	Gluten-free Residual lactose Contains vitamins and minerals	Disease-related malnutrition, malabsorption states, or other conditions requiring fortification with a high fat or carbohydrate (with protein) supplement. Not suitable for child under 3 years; use with caution in child 3–6 years. May require dilution for child 3–5 years.	Calogen Extra emulsion: neutral, strawberry 200 ml = £4.98
Calogen® Extra Shots (Nutricia Ltd)	Liquid per 100 mL	1650 kJ (400 kcal)	5 g cows' milk	4.5 g (sugars 3.5 g)	40.3 g	Nil	Gluten-free Residual lactose With vitamins and minerals	Disease-related malnutrition, malabsorption states, or other conditions requiring fortification with a high fat or carbohydrate (with protein) supplement. Not suitable for child under 3 years; use with caution in child 3–6 years. May require dilution for child 3–5 years.	Calogen Extra Shots emulsion: neutral, strawberry 240 ml = £5.75
Calshake® (Fresenius Kabi Ltd)	Powder per 87 g	1841 kJ (439 kcal)	4.1 g cows' milk	56.4 g (sugars 20 g)	22 g	Nil	Contains lactose Gluten-free	Disease-related malnutrition, malabsorption states, or other conditions requiring fortification with a high fat or carbohydrate (with protein) supplement. Not suitable for child under 1 year.	Calshake powder: chocolate 630 gram = £17.01; banana, neutral, strawberry, vanilla 609 gram = £17.01

Powder: one sachet reconstituted with 240 mL whole milk provides approx. 2 kcal/mL and protein 12 g.

A2

Borderline substances | **Appendix 2**

A2

High-energy supplements: protein (product list continued)

Product	Formulation	Energy	Protein	Carbohydrate	Fat	Fibre	Special Characteristics	ACBS Indications	Presentation & Flavour
Enshake® (Abbott Laboratories Ltd)	Powder per 100 g	1893 kJ (450 kcal)	8.4 g cows' milk, soy protein isolate	69 g (sugars 14.5 g)	15.6 g	Nil	Residual lactose Contains vitamins and minerals	Disease-related malnutrition, malabsorption states, or other conditions requiring fortification with a high fat or carbohydrate (with protein) supplement. Not suitable for child under 1 year; use with caution in child 1–6 years.	Enshake oral powder 96.5g sachets: banana, chocolate, strawberry, vanilla 6 sachet = £14.12
Powder: 96.5 g reconstituted with 240 mL whole milk provides approx. 2 kcal/mL and protein 16 g.									
MCT Procal® (Vitaflo International Ltd)	Powder per 100 g	2742 kJ (657 kcal)	12.5 g cows' milk	20.6 g (sugars 3.1 g)	63.1 g (MCT 99%)	Nil	Contains lactose	Dietary management of disorders of long-chain fatty acid oxidation, fat malabsorption, and other disorders requiring a low LCT, high MCT supplement. Not suitable for child under 1 year.	MCTprocal oral powder 16g sachets: 30 sachet = £24.21
Powder 16 g provides: protein 2 g, carbohydrate 3.3 g, fat 10.1 g, energy 439 kJ (105 kcal).									
Pro-Cal® (Vitaflo International Ltd)	Powder per 100 g	2787 kJ (667 kcal)	13.6 g cows' milk	28.2 g (sugars 16 g)	55.5 g	Nil	Contains lactose Gluten-free	Disease-related malnutrition, malabsorption states, or other conditions requiring fortification with a high fat or carbohydrate (with protein) supplement. Not suitable for child under 1 year; use with caution in child 1–5 years.	Pro-Cal powder: 510 gram = £14.95; 12500 gram = £216.41; 1500 gram = £30.45; 3000 gram = £71.88; 375 gram = £16.13
Powder 15 g provides: protein 2 g, carbohydrate 4.2 g, fat 8.3 g, energy 418 kJ (100 kcal).									
Pro-Cal® Shot (Vitaflo International Ltd)	Liquid per 100 mL	1385 kJ (334 kcal)	6.7 g cows' milk	13.4 g (sugars 13.3 g)	28.2 g	Nil	Contains lactose Gluten-free Contains soya	Disease-related malnutrition, malabsorption states, or other conditions requiring fortification with a high fat or carbohydrate (with protein) supplement. Not suitable for child under 3 years.	Pro-Cal: shot starter pack 360 ml = £7.37; shot banana, strawberry, neutral 720 ml = £14.71
Scandishake® Mix (Nutricia Ltd)	Powder per 100 g	2099 kJ (500 kcal)	4.7 g cows' milk	65 g (sugars 14.3 g)	24.7 g	Nil	Gluten-free Contains lactose	Disease-related malnutrition, malabsorption states, or other conditions requiring fortification with a high fat or carbohydrate (with protein) supplement. Not suitable for child under 3 years.	Scandishake Mix oral powder 85g sachets: banana, caramel, chocolate, strawberry, unflavoured, vanilla 6 sachet = £15.00
Powder: 85 g reconstituted with 240 mL whole milk provides: protein 11.7 g, carbohydrate 66.8 g, fat 30.4 g, energy 2457 kJ (588 kcal).									
Vitasavoury® (Vitaflo International Ltd)	Powder per 100 g	2562 kJ (619 kcal)	12 g cows' milk	22.5 g (sugars 1.4 g)	52 g	6.4 g	Contains lactose Contains soya (chicken flavour)	Disease-related malnutrition, malabsorption states, or other conditions requiring fortification with a high fat or carbohydrate (with protein) supplement. Not suitable for child under 3 years.	Vitasavoury powder: chicken, golden vegetable, leek & potato, mushroom 500 g = £19.33

Fibre, vitamin, and mineral supplements

High-fibre supplements

Product	Formulation	Energy	Protein	Carbohydrate	Fat	Fibre	Special Characteristics	ACBS Indications	Presentation & Flavour
Resource® Optifibre® (Nestle Health Science)	Powder per 100 g	323 kJ (76 kcal)	Nil	19 g guar gum, partially hydrolysed	Nil	78 g	Gluten-free Lactose-free	Borderline substances standard ACBS indications p. 974 except dysphagia Not suitable for child under 5 years	Resource Optifibre powder: 250 gram = £10.28; 80 gram = £4.18

Vitamin and Mineral supplements

Product	Formulation	Energy	Protein	Carbohydrate	Fat	Fibre	Special Characteristics	ACBS Indications	Presentation & Flavour
FrutiVits® (Vitaflo International Ltd)	Powder per 100 g	133 kJ (33 kcal)	Nil	8.3 g (sugars 400 mg)	Less than 100 mg	3.3 g		Vitamin, mineral, and trace element supplement in children 3–10 years with restrictive therapeutic diets	FruitiVits oral powder 6g sachets: 30 sachet = £65.45
Paediatric Seravit® (Nutricia Ltd)	Powder per 100 g	1275 kJ (300 kcal)	Nil	75 g (sugars 6.75 g)	Nil	Nil	Pineapple flavour not suitable for child under 6 months	Vitamin, mineral, and trace element supplement in infants and children with restrictive therapeutic diets.	Seravit Paediatric powder: unflavoured 200 gram = £18.16; pineapple 200 gram = £19.35

A2

Borderline substances | **Appendix 2**

Feed additives

Special additives for conditions of intolerance

Colief®

▸ For the relief of symptoms associated with lactose intolerance in infants, provided that lactose intolerance is confirmed by the presence of reducing substances and/or excessive acid in stools, a low concentration of the corresponding disaccharide enzyme on intestinal biopsy or by breath hydrogen test or lactose intolerance test. For dosage and administration details, consult product literature.

LIQUID, lactase 50 000 units/g

Colief 50,000units/g infant drops (Forum Health Products Ltd)
7 ml (ACBS) · NHS indicative price = £8.40

Fructose

▸ (Laevulose) For proven glucose/galactose intolerance

Glucose

▸ (Dextrose monohydrate) For use as an energy supplement in sucrose-isomaltase deficiency

VSL#3®

▸ Nutritional supplement for use under the supervision of a physician, for the maintenance of remission of ileoanal pouchitis induced by antibacterials in adults. For dosage and administration details, consult product literature.

POWDER, containing 8 strains of live, freeze-dried, lactic acid bacteria. Contains traces of soya, gluten, and lactose.

VSL#3 Probiotic Food Supplement oral powder 4.4g sachets (Ferring Pharmaceuticals Ltd)
30 sachet (ACBS) · NHS indicative price = £34.36

Feed thickeners and pre-thickened drinks

Carobel, Instant®

▸ For thickening feeds in the treatment of vomiting.
POWDER, carob seed flour.

Instant Carobel powder (Cow & Gate Ltd)
135 gram (ACBS) · NHS indicative price = £2.91

Multi-thick®

▸ For thickening of liquids and foods in dysphagia. Not suitable for children under 1 year except in cases of failure to thrive.
POWDER, modified maize starch, gluten- and lactose-free.

Multi-thick powder (Abbott Laboratories Ltd)
250 gram (ACBS) · NHS indicative price = £4.83

Nutilis® Clear

▸ For thickening of liquids or foods in dysphagia. Not suitable for children under 3 years.
POWDER, maltodextrin, xanthan gum, guar gum, gluten- and lactose-free.

Nutilis Clear powder (Nutricia Ltd)
72 gram (ACBS) · NHS indicative price = £11.04 | 175 gram (ACBS) · NHS indicative price = £8.46

Nutilis® Powder

▸ For thickening of foods in dysphagia. Not suitable for child under 3 years.
POWDER, carbohydrate 86 g, energy 1520 kJ (358 kcal)/100 g, modified maize starch, gluten- and lactose-free.

Nutilis powder (Nutricia Ltd)
240 gram (ACBS) · NHS indicative price = £6.80 | 300 gram (ACBS) · NHS indicative price = £5.11

Resource® Thickened Drink

▸ For dysphagia. Not suitable for children under 1 year.
LIQUID, carbohydrate 22 g, energy: orange 382 kJ (90 kcal); apple 376 kJ (89 kcal)/100 mL. Gluten- and lactose-free.

Resource Thickened Drink custard apple (Nestle Health Science)
114 ml (ACBS) · NHS indicative price = £0.73

Resource Thickened Drink custard orange (Nestle Health Science)
114 ml (ACBS) · NHS indicative price = £0.73

Resource Thickened Drink syrup apple (Nestle Health Science)
114 ml (ACBS) · NHS indicative price = £0.73

Resource Thickened Drink syrup orange (Nestle Health Science)
114 ml (ACBS) · NHS indicative price = £0.73

Resource® ThickenUp®

▸ For thickening of foods in dysphagia. Not suitable for children under 1 year.
POWDER, modified maize starch. Gluten- and lactose-free.

Resource ThickenUp powder (Nestle Health Science)
227 gram (ACBS) · NHS indicative price = £4.66 | 337.5 gram (ACBS) · NHS indicative price = £17.86

Resource® ThickenUp Clear

▸ For thickening of liquids or foods in dysphagia. Not suitable for children under 3 years.
POWDER, maltodextrin, xanthum gum, gluten- and lactose-free.

Resource ThickenUp Clear powder (Nestle Health Science)
28.8 gram (ACBS) · NHS indicative price = £5.28 | 125 gram (ACBS) · NHS indicative price = £8.46

SLO Drinks®

▸ Nutritional supplement for patient hydration in the dietary management of dysphagia. Not suitable for children under 3 years.
POWDER, carbohydrate content varies with flavour and chosen consistency (3 consistencies available), see product literature.

SLO Drink 1 oral powder lemon (SLO Drinks Ltd)
25 cup (ACBS) · NHS indicative price = £7.50

SLO Drink 1 oral powder orange (SLO Drinks Ltd)
25 cup (ACBS) · NHS indicative price = £7.50

SLO Drink 1 oral powder hot chocolate (SLO Drinks Ltd)
25 cup (ACBS) · NHS indicative price = £7.50

SLO Drink 2 oral powder hot chocolate (SLO Drinks Ltd)
25 cup (ACBS) · NHS indicative price = £7.50

SLO Drink 2 oral powder lemon (SLO Drinks Ltd)
25 cup (ACBS) · NHS indicative price = £7.50

SLO Drink 2 oral powder orange (SLO Drinks Ltd)
25 cup (ACBS) · NHS indicative price = £7.50

SLO Milkshakes+ ®

▸ Nutritional supplement in the dietary management of dysphagia. Not suitable for children under 3 years.
POWDER, carbohydrate content varies with flavour and chosen consistency (2 consistencies available), see product literature.

SLO Milkshake+ 1 oral powder chocolate (SLO Drinks Ltd)
7 × 50 gram (ACBS) · NHS indicative price = £5.88

SLO Milkshake+ 1 oral powder strawberry (SLO Drinks Ltd)
7 × 50 gram (ACBS) · NHS indicative price = £5.88

SLO Milkshake+ 2 oral powder chocolate (SLO Drinks Ltd)
7 × 50 gram (ACBS) · NHS indicative price = £5.88

SLO Milkshake+ 2 oral powder strawberry (SLO Drinks Ltd)
7 × 50 gram (ACBS) · NHS indicative price = £5.88

Thick and Easy®

▸ For thickening of foods in dysphagia. Not suitable for children under 1 year except in cases of failure to thrive.
POWDERModified maize starch

Thick & Easy powder (Fresenius Kabi Ltd)
225 gram (ACBS) · NHS indicative price = £5.21 | 900 gram (ACBS) · NHS indicative price = £32.00 | 4540 gram (ACBS) · NHS indicative price = £87.18

Thicken Aid®

▸ For thickening of foods in dysphagia. Not suitable for children under 1 year.
POWDER, modified maize starch, maltodextrin, gluten- and lactose-free.

Thicken Aid powder (M & A Pharmachem Ltd)
225 gram (ACBS) · NHS indicative price = £3.71 | 900 gram (ACBS) · NHS indicative price = £22.40

Thixo-D®

▸ For thickening of foods in dysphagia. Not suitable for children under 1 year except in cases of failure to thrive.
POWDER, modified maize starch, gluten-free.

Thixo-D powder (Sutherland Health Ltd)
375 gram (ACBS) · NHS indicative price = £7.65

Thixo-D Cal-Free powder (Sutherland Health Ltd)
30 gram · NHS indicative price = £3.00

Vitaquick®
▸ For thickening of foods in dysphagia. Not suitable for children under 1 year except in cases of failure to thrive.
POWDER. Modified maize starch.

Vitaquick powder (Vitaflo International Ltd)
300 gram (ACBS) · NHS indicative price = £7.27

Flavouring preparations

Flavour Mix®
POWDER

FlavourPac®
▸ For use with Vitaflo's range of unflavoured protein substitutes for metabolic diseases; not suitable for child under 3 years.
POWDER

FlavourPac oral powder 4g sachets blackcurrant (Vitaflo International Ltd)
30 sachet (ACBS) · NHS indicative price = £14.05 | 120 sachet (ACBS) · No NHS indicative price available

FlavourPac oral powder 4g sachets lemon (Vitaflo International Ltd)
30 sachet (ACBS) · NHS indicative price = £14.05 | 120 sachet (ACBS) · No NHS indicative price available

FlavourPac oral powder 4g sachets orange (Vitaflo International Ltd)
30 sachet (ACBS) · NHS indicative price = £14.05 | 120 sachet (ACBS) · No NHS indicative price available

FlavourPac oral powder 4g sachets raspberry (Vitaflo International Ltd)
30 sachet (ACBS) · NHS indicative price = £14.05 | 120 sachet (ACBS) · No NHS indicative price available

FlavourPac oral powder 4g sachets tropical (Vitaflo International Ltd)
30 sachet (ACBS) · NHS indicative price = £14.05 | 120 sachet (ACBS) · No NHS indicative price available

Foods for special diets

Gluten-free foods

ACBS indications: established gluten-sensitive enteropathies including steatorrhoea due to gluten sensitivity, coeliac disease, and dermatitis herpetiformis.

Bread

LOAVES

Barkat® Loaf
GLUTEN-FREE

Barkat gluten free brown rice bread (Gluten Free Foods Ltd)
500 gram (ACBS) · NHS indicative price = £5.73

Barkat gluten free par baked white bread sliced (Gluten Free Foods Ltd)
300 gram (ACBS) · NHS indicative price = £4.13

Barkat gluten free home fresh country loaf (Gluten Free Foods Ltd)
250 gram (ACBS) · NHS indicative price = £4.35

Barkat gluten free wheat free multigrain bread (Gluten Free Foods Ltd)
500 gram (ACBS) · NHS indicative price = £5.73

Barkat gluten free wholemeal bread sliced (Gluten Free Foods Ltd)
500 gram (ACBS) · NHS indicative price = £3.98

Barkat gluten free white rice bread (Gluten Free Foods Ltd)
500 gram (ACBS) · NHS indicative price = £5.73

Ener-G® Loaves
GLUTEN-FREE

Ener-G gluten free brown rice bread (General Dietary Ltd)
474 gram (ACBS) · NHS indicative price = £5.47

Ener-G gluten free tapioca bread (General Dietary Ltd)
480 gram (ACBS) · NHS indicative price = £5.47

Ener-G gluten free rice loaf (General Dietary Ltd)
612 gram (ACBS) · NHS indicative price = £5.47

Ener-G gluten free Seattle brown loaf (General Dietary Ltd)
454 gram (ACBS) · NHS indicative price = £6.22

Ener-G gluten free white rice bread (General Dietary Ltd)
456 gram (ACBS) · NHS indicative price = £5.47

Genius Gluten Free® Loaf
GLUTEN-FREE

Genius gluten free brown bread sliced (Genius Foods Ltd)
400 gram (ACBS) · NHS indicative price = £2.88

Genius gluten free brown bread unsliced (Genius Foods Ltd)
400 gram (ACBS) · NHS indicative price = £2.77

Genius gluten free brown sandwich bread sliced (Genius Foods Ltd)
535 gram (ACBS) · NHS indicative price = £3.73

Genius gluten free white bread sliced (Genius Foods Ltd)
400 gram (ACBS) · NHS indicative price = £2.88

Genius gluten free white bread unsliced (Genius Foods Ltd)
400 gram (ACBS) · NHS indicative price = £2.77

Genius gluten free white sandwich bread sliced (Genius Foods Ltd)
535 gram (ACBS) · NHS indicative price = £3.73

Glutafin® Loaves
GLUTEN-FREE

Glutafin gluten free fibre loaf sliced (Dr Schar UK Ltd)
300 gram (ACBS) · NHS indicative price = £2.89

Glutafin gluten free white loaf sliced (Dr Schar UK Ltd)
300 gram (ACBS) · NHS indicative price = £2.89

Glutafin® Select Loaves
GLUTEN-FREE

Glutafin gluten free Select fibre loaf sliced (Dr Schar UK Ltd)
400 gram (ACBS) · NHS indicative price = £3.43

Glutafin gluten free Select fresh brown loaf sliced (Dr Schar UK Ltd)
400 gram (ACBS) · NHS indicative price = £3.43

Glutafin gluten free Select fresh white loaf sliced (Dr Schar UK Ltd)
400 gram (ACBS) · NHS indicative price = £3.43

Glutafin gluten free Select seeded loaf sliced (Dr Schar UK Ltd)
400 gram (ACBS) · NHS indicative price = £3.72

Glutafin gluten free Select white loaf sliced (Dr Schar UK Ltd)
400 gram (ACBS) · NHS indicative price = £3.43

Juvela® Loaf
GLUTEN-FREE

Juvela gluten free fresh fibre loaf sliced (Hero UK Ltd)
400 gram (ACBS) · NHS indicative price = £3.39

Juvela gluten free fresh white loaf sliced (Hero UK Ltd)
400 gram (ACBS) · NHS indicative price = £3.69

Juvela gluten free fibre loaf sliced (Hero UK Ltd)
400 gram (ACBS) · NHS indicative price = £3.54

Juvela gluten free part baked loaf (Hero UK Ltd)
400 gram (ACBS) · NHS indicative price = £3.95

Juvela gluten free part baked fibre loaf (Hero UK Ltd)
400 gram (ACBS) · NHS indicative price = £3.80

Juvela gluten free loaf unsliced (Hero UK Ltd)
400 gram (ACBS) · NHS indicative price = £3.54

Juvela gluten free fibre loaf unsliced (Hero UK Ltd)
400 gram (ACBS) · NHS indicative price = £3.54

Lifestyle® Loaf
GLUTEN-FREE

Lifestyle gluten free brown bread sliced (Ultrapharm Ltd)
400 gram (ACBS) · NHS indicative price = £2.82

Lifestyle gluten free high fibre bread sliced (Ultrapharm Ltd)
400 gram · NHS indicative price = £2.82

Lifestyle gluten free white bread sliced (Ultrapharm Ltd)
400 gram (ACBS) · NHS indicative price = £2.82

Warburtons® Loaf
GLUTEN-FREE

Warburtons gluten free brown bread sliced (Warburtons Ltd)
400 gram (ACBS) · NHS indicative price = £3.06

Warburtons gluten free white bread sliced (Warburtons Ltd)
400 gram (ACBS) · NHS indicative price = £3.06

Wellfoods® Loaf
GLUTEN-FREE

Wellfoods gluten free loaf sliced (Wellfoods Ltd)
600 gram (ACBS) · NHS indicative price = £5.05

Wellfoods gluten free loaf unsliced (Wellfoods Ltd)
600 gram (ACBS) · NHS indicative price = £4.95

BAGUETTES, BUNS AND ROLLS

Barkat® Baguettes and rolls
GLUTEN-FREE

Barkat gluten free par baked rolls (Gluten Free Foods Ltd)
200 gram (ACBS) · NHS indicative price = £3.98

Barkat gluten free par baked baguettes (Gluten Free Foods Ltd)
200 gram (ACBS) · NHS indicative price = £3.98

Ener-G® Rolls
GLUTEN-FREE

Ener-G gluten free dinner rolls (General Dietary Ltd)
280 gram (ACBS) · NHS indicative price = £3.71

Ener-G gluten free white round rolls (General Dietary Ltd)
220 gram (ACBS) · NHS indicative price = £2.98

Ener-G gluten free white long rolls (General Dietary Ltd)
220 gram (ACBS) · NHS indicative price = £2.98

Glutafin® Baguettes and rolls
GLUTEN-FREE

Glutafin gluten free baguettes (Dr Schar UK Ltd)
350 gram (ACBS) · NHS indicative price = £3.51

Glutafin gluten free 4 white rolls (Dr Schar UK Ltd)
200 gram (ACBS) · NHS indicative price = £3.68

Glutafin gluten free part baked 4 fibre rolls (Dr Schar UK Ltd)
200 gram (ACBS) · NHS indicative price = £3.68

Glutafin® Select Rolls
GLUTEN-FREE

Glutafin gluten free part baked 4 white rolls (Dr Schar UK Ltd)
200 gram (ACBS) · NHS indicative price = £3.68

Glutafin gluten free part baked 2 long white rolls (Dr Schar UK Ltd)
150 gram (ACBS) · NHS indicative price = £2.81

Juvela® Rolls
GLUTEN-FREE

Juvela gluten free fresh fibre rolls (Hero UK Ltd)
425 gram (ACBS) · NHS indicative price = £4.42

Juvela gluten free fresh white rolls (Hero UK Ltd)
425 gram (ACBS) · NHS indicative price = £4.42

Juvela gluten free fibre bread rolls (Hero UK Ltd)
425 gram (ACBS) · NHS indicative price = £4.77

Juvela gluten free bread rolls (Hero UK Ltd)
425 gram (ACBS) · NHS indicative price = £4.77

Juvela gluten free part baked fibre bread rolls (Hero UK Ltd)
375 gram (ACBS) · NHS indicative price = £4.94

Juvela gluten free part baked white bread rolls (Hero UK Ltd)
375 gram (ACBS) · NHS indicative price = £4.94

Lifestyle® Rolls
GLUTEN-FREE

Lifestyle gluten free brown bread rolls (Ultrapharm Ltd)
400 gram (ACBS) · NHS indicative price = £2.82

Lifestyle gluten free high fibre bread rolls (Ultrapharm Ltd)
400 gram (ACBS) · NHS indicative price = £2.82

Lifestyle gluten free white bread rolls (Ultrapharm Ltd)
400 gram (ACBS) · NHS indicative price = £2.82

Proceli® Baguettes, buns and rolls
GLUTEN-FREE

Proceli gluten free part baked baguettes (Ambe Ltd)
250 gram (ACBS) · NHS indicative price = £3.24

Warburtons® Baguettes and rolls
GLUTEN-FREE

Warburtons gluten free baguettes (Warburtons Ltd)
150 gram (ACBS) · NHS indicative price = £2.86

Warburtons gluten free brown rolls (Warburtons Ltd)
220 gram (ACBS) · NHS indicative price = £2.55

Warburtons gluten free white rolls (Warburtons Ltd)
220 gram (ACBS) · NHS indicative price = £2.55

Wellfoods® Buns and rolls
GLUTEN-FREE

Wellfoods gluten free burger buns (Wellfoods Ltd)
380 gram (ACBS) · NHS indicative price = £4.03

Wellfoods gluten free rolls (Wellfoods Ltd)
360 gram (ACBS) · NHS indicative price = £3.73

Cereals

Juvela® Fibre flakes and oats
GLUTEN-FREE

Juvela gluten free fibre flakes (Hero UK Ltd)
300 gram (ACBS) · NHS indicative price = £2.78

Juvela gluten free flakes (Hero UK Ltd)
300 gram (ACBS) · NHS indicative price = £2.78

Juvela gluten free pure oats (Hero UK Ltd)
500 gram (ACBS) · NHS indicative price = £2.78

Nairns® Porridge
GLUTEN-FREE

Nairn's gluten free oat porridge (Nairn's Oatcakes Ltd)
500 gram (ACBS) · NHS indicative price = £3.05

Cookies and biscuits

Barkat® Biscuits
GLUTEN-FREE

Barkat gluten free digestive biscuits (Gluten Free Foods Ltd)
175 gram (ACBS) · NHS indicative price = £2.61

Barkat gluten free coffee biscuits (Gluten Free Foods Ltd)
200 gram (ACBS) · NHS indicative price = £3.38

Ener-G® Cookies
GLUTEN-FREE

Ener-G gluten free vanilla cookies (General Dietary Ltd)
435 gram (ACBS) · NHS indicative price = £6.23

Glutafin® Cookies and biscuits
GLUTEN-FREE

Glutafin gluten free tea biscuits (Dr Schar UK Ltd)
150 gram (ACBS) · NHS indicative price = £2.09

Glutafin gluten free digestive biscuits (Dr Schar UK Ltd)
150 gram (ACBS) · NHS indicative price = £2.13

Glutafin gluten free shortbread biscuits (Dr Schar UK Ltd)
100 gram (ACBS) · NHS indicative price = £1.73

Juvela® Biscuits
GLUTEN-FREE

Juvela gluten free digestive biscuits (Hero UK Ltd)
150 gram (ACBS) · NHS indicative price = £3.05

Juvela gluten free savoury biscuits (Hero UK Ltd)
150 gram (ACBS) · NHS indicative price = £3.82

Juvela gluten free sweet biscuits (Hero UK Ltd)
150 gram (ACBS) · NHS indicative price = £2.88

Juvela gluten free tea biscuits (Hero UK Ltd)
150 gram (ACBS) · NHS indicative price = £3.05

Crackers, crispbreads, and breadsticks

Barkat® Crackers
GLUTEN-FREE

Barkat gluten free matzo crackers (Gluten Free Foods Ltd)
200 gram (ACBS) · NHS indicative price = £3.52

Glutafin® Crackers
GLUTEN-FREE

Glutafin gluten free high fibre crackers (Dr Schar UK Ltd)
200 gram (ACBS) · NHS indicative price = £2.90

Glutafin gluten free crackers (Dr Schar UK Ltd)
200 gram (ACBS) · NHS indicative price = £3.46

Glutafin gluten free mini crackers (Dr Schar UK Ltd)
175 gram (ACBS) · NHS indicative price = £2.96

Juvela® Crispbread
GLUTEN-FREE
Juvela gluten free crispbread (Hero UK Ltd)
200 gram (ACBS) · NHS indicative price = £4.64

Warburtons® Crackers
GLUTEN-FREE
Warburtons gluten free bran crackers (Warburtons Ltd)
150 gram (ACBS) · NHS indicative price = £2.34

Flour mixes and xanthan gum
FLOUR MIXES

Barkat® Flour mix
GLUTEN-FREE
Barkat gluten free bread mix (Gluten Free Foods Ltd)
500 gram (ACBS) · NHS indicative price = £6.81
Barkat gluten free high fibre bread mix (Gluten Free Foods Ltd)
500 gram (ACBS) · NHS indicative price = £8.96
Barkat gluten free bread and cake mix (Gluten Free Foods Ltd)
500 gram (ACBS) · NHS indicative price = £8.96
Barkat gluten free all purpose flour mix (Gluten Free Foods Ltd)
500 gram (ACBS) · NHS indicative price = £4.65

Finax® Flour mix
GLUTEN-FREE
Finax gluten free coarse flour mix (Drossa Ltd)
900 gram (ACBS) · NHS indicative price = £8.85
Finax gluten free fibre bread mix (Drossa Ltd)
1000 gram (ACBS) · NHS indicative price = £10.14
Finax gluten free flour mix (Drossa Ltd)
900 gram (ACBS) · NHS indicative price = £8.85

Glutafin Select® Flour mix
GLUTEN-FREE
Glutafin gluten free Select bread mix (Dr Schar UK Ltd)
500 gram (ACBS) · NHS indicative price = £6.66
Glutafin gluten free Select fibre bread mix (Dr Schar UK Ltd)
500 gram (ACBS) · NHS indicative price = £6.66
Glutafin gluten free Select multipurpose fibre mix (Dr Schar UK Ltd)
500 gram (ACBS) · NHS indicative price = £6.66
Glutafin gluten free Select multipurpose white mix (Dr Schar UK Ltd)
500 gram (ACBS) · NHS indicative price = £6.66

Glutafin® Flour mix
GLUTEN-FREE
Glutafin gluten free multipurpose white mix (Dr Schar UK Ltd)
500 gram (ACBS) · NHS indicative price = £6.66

Heron Foods® Flour mix
GLUTEN-FREE
Heron Hi-Fibre gluten free organic bread mix (Gluten Free Foods Ltd)
500 gram (ACBS) · NHS indicative price = £8.96

Juvela® Flour mix
GLUTEN-FREE
Juvela gluten free fibre mix (Hero UK Ltd)
500 gram (ACBS) · NHS indicative price = £7.35
Juvela gluten free harvest mix (Hero UK Ltd)
500 gram (ACBS) · NHS indicative price = £7.35
Juvela gluten free mix (Hero UK Ltd)
500 gram (ACBS) · NHS indicative price = £7.35

Mrs Crimbles® Flour mixes
GLUTEN-FREE
Mrs Crimble's gluten free bread mix (Stiletto Foods (UK) Ltd)
275 gram (ACBS) · NHS indicative price = £1.09
Mrs Crimble's gluten free pastry mix (Stiletto Foods (UK) Ltd)
200 gram (ACBS) · NHS indicative price = £1.09

Orgran® Flour mix
GLUTEN-FREE
Orgran gluten free pizza & pastry mix (Naturally Good Food Ltd)
375 gram (ACBS) · NHS indicative price = £3.80
Orgran gluten free self-raising flour (Naturally Good Food Ltd)
500 gram (ACBS) · NHS indicative price = £3.10

Orgran gluten free all purpose plain flour (Naturally Good Food Ltd)
500 gram · NHS indicative price = £3.10

Proceli® Flour mix
GLUTEN-FREE
Proceli gluten free white plain flour (Ambe Ltd)
1000 gram (ACBS) · NHS indicative price = £9.95

Pure® Flour mix
GLUTEN-FREE
Innovative Solutions Pure gluten free blended flour (Innovative Solutions (UK) Ltd)
1000 gram (ACBS) · NHS indicative price = £4.35
Innovative Solutions Pure gluten free brown rice flour (Innovative Solutions (UK) Ltd)
500 gram (ACBS) · NHS indicative price = £1.63
Innovative Solutions Pure gluten free white rice flour (Innovative Solutions (UK) Ltd)
500 gram (ACBS) · NHS indicative price = £1.73
Innovative Solutions Pure gluten free potato flour (Innovative Solutions (UK) Ltd)
500 gram (ACBS) · NHS indicative price = £1.73
Innovative Solutions Pure gluten free tapioca flour (Innovative Solutions (UK) Ltd)
500gram (ACBS) · NHS indicative price = £2.33
Innovative Solutions Pure gluten free brown teff flour (Innovative Solutions (UK) Ltd)
1000 gram (ACBS) · NHS indicative price = £4.91
Innovative Solutions Pure gluten free white teff flour (Innovative Solutions (UK) Ltd)
1000 gram (ACBS) · NHS indicative price = £4.91

Tobia® Flour mix
GLUTEN-FREE
Tobia Teff gluten free brown teff flour (Tobia Teff UK Ltd)
1000 gram (ACBS) · NHS indicative price = £3.50
Tobia Teff gluten free white teff flour (Tobia Teff UK Ltd)
1000 gram (ACBS) · NHS indicative price = £3.50

Tritamyl® Flour mix
GLUTEN-FREE
Tritamyl gluten free brown bread mix (Gluten Free Foods Ltd)
1000 gram (ACBS) · NHS indicative price = £7.10
Tritamyl gluten free flour mix (Gluten Free Foods Ltd)
2000 gram (ACBS) · NHS indicative price = £14.26
Tritamyl gluten free white bread mix (Gluten Free Foods Ltd)
2000 gram (ACBS) · NHS indicative price = £14.26

Wellfoods® Flour mix
GLUTEN-FREE
Wellfoods gluten free flour alternative (Wellfoods Ltd)
1000 gram (ACBS) · NHS indicative price = £7.80

XANTHAN GUM

Ener-G® Xanthan gum
GLUTEN-FREE
Ener-G xanthan gum (General Dietary Ltd)
170 gram (ACBS) · NHS indicative price = £8.63

Pure® Xanthan gum
GLUTEN-FREE
Innovative Solutions Pure xanthan gum (Innovative Solutions (UK) Ltd)
100 gram (ACBS) · NHS indicative price = £6.85

Pasta

Barkat® Pasta
GLUTEN-FREE
Barkat gluten free pasta animal shapes (Gluten Free Foods Ltd)
500 gram (ACBS) · NHS indicative price = £5.88
Barkat gluten free pasta macaroni (Gluten Free Foods Ltd)
500 gram (ACBS) · NHS indicative price = £5.88
Barkat gluten free pasta spaghetti (Gluten Free Foods Ltd)
500 gram (ACBS) · NHS indicative price = £5.88
Barkat gluten free pasta spirals (Gluten Free Foods Ltd)
500 gram (ACBS) · NHS indicative price = £5.88

A2

Borderline substances | Appendix 2

Barkat gluten free pasta tagliatelle (Gluten Free Foods Ltd)
500 gram (ACBS) · NHS indicative price = £5.88

Barkat gluten free pasta buckwheat penne (Gluten Free Foods Ltd)
250 gram (ACBS) · NHS indicative price = £2.93

Barkat gluten free pasta buckwheat spirals (Gluten Free Foods Ltd)
250 gram (ACBS) · NHS indicative price = £2.93

BiAlimenta® Pasta
GLUTEN-FREE

BiAlimenta gluten free pasta (Drossa Ltd)
Spirals, sagnette 500 gram (ACBS) · NHS indicative price =
£6.11

Ener-G® Pasta
GLUTEN-FREE

General Dietary gluten free macaroni (General Dietary Ltd)
454 gram (ACBS) · NHS indicative price = £5.03

General Dietary gluten free spaghetti (General Dietary Ltd)
454 gram (ACBS) · NHS indicative price = £5.03

General Dietary gluten free vermicelli (General Dietary Ltd)
300 gram (ACBS) · NHS indicative price = £5.03

Glutafin® Pasta
GLUTEN-FREE

Glutafin gluten free pasta macaroni penne (Dr Schar UK Ltd)
500 gram (ACBS) · NHS indicative price = £6.73

Glutafin gluten free pasta shells (Dr Schar UK Ltd)
500 gram (ACBS) · NHS indicative price = £6.73

Glutafin gluten free pasta spirals (Dr Schar UK Ltd)
500 gram (ACBS) · NHS indicative price = £6.73

Glutafin gluten free pasta long-cut spaghetti (Dr Schar UK Ltd)
500 gram (ACBS) · NHS indicative price = £6.73

Juvela® Pasta
GLUTEN-FREE

Juvela gluten free fibre penne (Hero UK Ltd)
500 gram (ACBS) · NHS indicative price = £6.61

Juvela gluten free pasta fusilli (Hero UK Ltd)
500 gram (ACBS) · NHS indicative price = £7.21

Juvela gluten free pasta lasagne (Hero UK Ltd)
250 gram (ACBS) · NHS indicative price = £3.68

Juvela gluten free pasta macaroni (Hero UK Ltd)
500 gram (ACBS) · NHS indicative price = £7.21

Juvela gluten free pasta spaghetti (Hero UK Ltd)
500 gram (ACBS) · NHS indicative price = £7.21

Juvela gluten free pasta tagliatelle (Hero UK Ltd)
250 gram (ACBS) · NHS indicative price = £3.47

Orgran® Pasta
GLUTEN-FREE

Orgran gluten free pasta rice & corn lasagne (Naturally Good Food Ltd)
200 gram (ACBS) · NHS indicative price = £3.13

Orgran gluten free pasta rice & corn macaroni (Naturally Good Food Ltd)
250 gram (ACBS) · NHS indicative price = £2.42

Orgran gluten free pasta buckwheat spirals (Naturally Good Food Ltd)
250 gram (ACBS) · NHS indicative price = £2.42

Orgran gluten free pasta corn spirals (Naturally Good Food Ltd)
250 gram (ACBS) · NHS indicative price = £2.42

Orgran gluten free pasta brown rice spirals (Naturally Good Food Ltd)
250 gram (ACBS) · NHS indicative price = £2.42

Orgran gluten free pasta rice & corn spirals (Naturally Good Food Ltd)
250 gram (ACBS) · NHS indicative price = £2.42

Orgran gluten free pasta rice & millet spirals (Naturally Good Food Ltd)
250 gram (ACBS) · NHS indicative price = £2.42

Rizopia® Pasta
GLUTEN-FREE

Rizopia gluten free organic brown rice pasta fusilli (PGR Health Foods Ltd)
500 gram (ACBS) · NHS indicative price = £2.72

Rizopia gluten free organic brown rice pasta lasagne (PGR Health Foods Ltd)
375 gram (ACBS) · NHS indicative price = £2.72

Rizopia gluten free organic brown rice pasta penne (PGR Health Foods Ltd)
500 gram (ACBS) · NHS indicative price = £2.72

Rizopia gluten free organic brown rice pasta spaghetti (PGR Health Foods Ltd)
500 gram (ACBS) · NHS indicative price = £2.72

Pizza bases

Barkat®, Pizza crust
GLUTEN-FREE

Barkat gluten free brown rice pizza crust (Gluten Free Foods Ltd)
150 gram (ACBS) · NHS indicative price = £5.00

Barkat gluten free white rice pizza crust (Gluten Free Foods Ltd)
150 gram (ACBS) · NHS indicative price = £5.00

Glutafin® Pizza base
GLUTEN-FREE

Glutafin gluten free pizza base (Dr Schar UK Ltd)
300 gram (ACBS) · NHS indicative price = £6.56

Juvela® Pizza base
GLUTEN-FREE

Juvela gluten free pizza base (Hero UK Ltd)
360 gram (ACBS) · NHS indicative price = £8.78

Proceli® Pizza base
GLUTEN-FREE

Proceli gluten free pizza base (Ambe Ltd)
250 gram (ACBS) · NHS indicative price = £3.90

Wellfoods® Pizza base
GLUTEN-FREE

Wellfoods gluten free pizza base (Wellfoods Ltd)
600 gram (ACBS) · NHS indicative price = £9.13

Gluten- and wheat-free foods

ACBS indications: established gluten-sensitive enteropathies with coexisting established wheat sensitivity only.

Ener-G® Bread loaves, rolls and pizza bases
GLUTEN-FREE, WHEAT-FREE

Ener-G gluten free Seattle brown hamburger rolls (General Dietary Ltd)
320 gram (ACBS) · NHS indicative price = £4.08

Ener-G gluten free Seattle brown hot dog rolls (General Dietary Ltd)
320 gram (ACBS) · NHS indicative price = £4.08

Glutafin® Flour mix, fibre and crispbread
GLUTEN-FREE, WHEAT-FREE

Glutafin gluten free crispbread (Dr Schar UK Ltd)
150 gram (ACBS) · NHS indicative price = £3.25

Glutafin gluten free bread mix (Dr Schar UK Ltd)
500 gram (ACBS) · NHS indicative price = £6.66

Glutafin gluten free fibre bread mix (Dr Schar UK Ltd)
500 gram (ACBS) · NHS indicative price = £6.66

Glutafin gluten free wheat free fibre mix (Dr Schar UK Ltd)
500 gram (ACBS) · NHS indicative price = £6.66

Heron Foods® Flour mixes
GLUTEN-FREE, WHEAT-FREE

Heron gluten free organic bread mix (Gluten Free Foods Ltd)
500 gram (ACBS) · NHS indicative price = £8.96

Low-protein foods

ACBS indications: inherited metabolic disorders, renal or liver failure, requiring a low-protein diet

Bread

Ener-G® Rice bread
LOW PROTEIN

Ener-G low protein rice bread (General Dietary Ltd)
600 gram (ACBS) · NHS indicative price = £5.60

Juvela® Loaf and rolls
LOW PROTEIN

Juvela gluten free loaf sliced (Hero UK Ltd)
400 gram (ACBS) · NHS indicative price = £3.54

Juvela low protein bread rolls (Hero UK Ltd)
350 gram (ACBS) · NHS indicative price = £4.52

Juvela low protein loaf sliced (Hero UK Ltd)
400 gram (ACBS) · NHS indicative price = £3.64

Loprofin® Bread
LOW-PROTEIN

Loprofin low protein part baked bread rolls (Nutricia Ltd)
260 gram (ACBS) · NHS indicative price = £4.20

Loprofin low protein part baked loaf sliced (Nutricia Ltd)
400 gram (ACBS) · NHS indicative price = £3.98

PK Foods® Loaf
LOW PROTEIN

PK Foods low protein white bread sliced (Gluten Free Foods Ltd)
300 gram · NHS indicative price = £4.75

Cake, biscuits, and snacks

Juvela® Cookies
LOW-PROTEIN

Juvela low protein cinnamon cookies (Hero UK Ltd)
125 gram (ACBS) · NHS indicative price = £7.62

Juvela low protein chocolate chip cookies (Hero UK Ltd)
110 gram (ACBS) · NHS indicative price = £7.62

Juvela low protein orange cookies (Hero UK Ltd)
125 gram (ACBS) · NHS indicative price = £7.62

Loprofin® Wafers
LOW-PROTEIN

Loprofin low protein crackers (Nutricia Ltd)
150 gram (ACBS) · NHS indicative price = £3.67

Loprofin low protein herb crackers (Nutricia Ltd)
150 gram (ACBS) · NHS indicative price = £3.67

Loprofin low protein vanilla cream wafers (Nutricia Ltd)
100 gram (ACBS) · NHS indicative price = £2.62

PK Foods® Biscuits
LOW-PROTEIN

PK Foods Aminex low protein biscuits (Gluten Free Foods Ltd)
200 gram (ACBS) · NHS indicative price = £5.04

PK Foods Aminex low protein cookies (Gluten Free Foods Ltd)
150 gram (ACBS) · NHS indicative price = £5.04

PK Foods Aminex low protein rusks (Gluten Free Foods Ltd)
200 gram (ACBS) · NHS indicative price = £5.04

PK Foods low protein chocolate chip cookies (Gluten Free Foods Ltd)
150 gram (ACBS) · NHS indicative price = £5.04

PK Foods low protein cinnamon cookies (Gluten Free Foods Ltd)
150 gram (ACBS) · NHS indicative price = £5.04

PK Foods low protein crispbread (Gluten Free Foods Ltd)
75 gram (ACBS) · NHS indicative price = £2.42

PK Foods low protein orange cookies (Gluten Free Foods Ltd)
150 gram (ACBS) · NHS indicative price = £5.04

Promin® Cooked and flavoured pasta snax
LOW-PROTEIN

Promin low protein Snax salt & vinegar 25g sachets (Firstplay Dietary Foods Ltd)
3 sachet · No NHS indicative price available | 12 sachet (ACBS) · NHS indicative price = £10.58

Promin low protein Snax ready salted 25g sachets (Firstplay Dietary Foods Ltd)
3 sachet · No NHS indicative price available | 12 sachet (ACBS) · NHS indicative price = £10.58

Promin low protein Snax cheese & onion 25g sachets (Firstplay Dietary Foods Ltd)
3 sachet · No NHS indicative price available | 12 sachet (ACBS) · NHS indicative price = £10.58

Taranis® Cake bars
LOW-PROTEIN

Taranis low protein apricot cake (Lactalis Nutrition Sante)
240 gram (ACBS) · NHS indicative price = £6.08

Taranis low protein lemon cake (Lactalis Nutrition Sante)
240 gram (ACBS) · NHS indicative price = £6.08

Taranis low protein pear cake (Lactalis Nutrition Sante)
240 gram (ACBS) · NHS indicative price = £6.08

Vita Bite®
▸ Not recommended for any child under 1 year.
LOW PROTEIN. Bar, protein 30 mg (less than 2.5 mg phenylalanine), carbohydrate 15.35 g, fat 8.4 g, energy 572 kJ (137 kcal)/25 g.

VitaBite bar (Vitaflo International Ltd)
175 gram (ACBS) · NHS indicative price = £8.77

Vitaflo Choices® Mini crackers
LOW-PROTEIN

Vitaflo Choices mini crackers (Vitaflo International Ltd)
40 gram (ACBS) · NHS indicative price = £0.87

Cereals

Loprofin® Breakfast cereal
LOW-PROTEIN

Loprofin low protein breakfast cereal flakes apple (Nutricia Ltd)
375 gram (ACBS) · NHS indicative price = £8.09

Loprofin low protein breakfast cereal flakes chocolate (Nutricia Ltd)
375 gram (ACBS) · NHS indicative price = £8.09

Loprofin low protein breakfast cereal flakes strawberry (Nutricia Ltd)
375 gram (ACBS) · NHS indicative price = £8.09

Loprofin low protein breakfast cereal loops (Nutricia Ltd)
375 gram (ACBS) · NHS indicative price = £8.39

Promin® Hot breakfast
LOW-PROTEIN

Promin low protein hot breakfast powder sachets apple & cinnamon (Firstplay Dietary Foods Ltd)
342 gram (ACBS) · NHS indicative price = £8.09

Promin low protein hot breakfast powder sachets banana (Firstplay Dietary Foods Ltd)
342 gram (ACBS) · NHS indicative price = £8.09

Promin low protein hot breakfast powder sachets chocolate (Firstplay Dietary Foods Ltd)
342 gram (ACBS) · NHS indicative price = £8.09

Promin low protein hot breakfast powder sachets original (Firstplay Dietary Foods Ltd)
336 gram (ACBS) · NHS indicative price = £8.09

Desserts

PK Foods® Jelly
LOW-PROTEIN

PK Foods low protein jelly mix dessert cherry (Gluten Free Foods Ltd)
320 gram (ACBS) · NHS indicative price = £8.03

PK Foods low protein jelly mix dessert orange (Gluten Free Foods Ltd)
320 gram (ACBS) · NHS indicative price = £8.03

Promin® Desserts
LOW-PROTEIN

Promin low protein imitation rice pudding apple (Firstplay Dietary Foods Ltd)
276 gram (ACBS) · NHS indicative price = £6.33

Promin low protein imitation rice pudding banana (Firstplay Dietary Foods Ltd)
276 gram (ACBS) · NHS indicative price = £6.33

Promin low protein imitation rice pudding original (Firstplay Dietary Foods Ltd)
276 gram (ACBS) · NHS indicative price = £6.33

A2

Borderline substances | Appendix 2

Promin low protein imitation rice pudding strawberry (Firstplay Dietary Foods Ltd)
276 gram (ACBS) · NHS indicative price = £6.33

Flour mixes and egg substitutes

Ener-G® Egg replacer
LOW-PROTEIN

Ener-G low protein egg replacer (General Dietary Ltd)
454 gram (ACBS) · NHS indicative price = £5.17

Fate® Flour mix
LOW PROTEIN

Fate low protein all purpose mix (Fate Special Foods)
500 gram (ACBS) · NHS indicative price = £6.97

Fate low protein chocolate cake mix (Fate Special Foods)
500 gram (ACBS) · NHS indicative price = £6.97

Fate low protein plain cake mix (Fate Special Foods)
500 gram (ACBS) · NHS indicative price = £6.97

Juvela® Mix
LOW-PROTEIN

Juvela low protein mix (Hero UK Ltd)
500 gram (ACBS) · NHS indicative price = £7.79

Loprofin® Flour mixes and egg substitutes
LOW-PROTEIN

Loprofin low protein egg replacer (Nutricia Ltd)
500 gram (ACBS) · NHS indicative price = £15.72

Loprofin low protein egg white replacer (Nutricia Ltd)
100 gram (ACBS) · NHS indicative price = £10.12

Loprofin low protein cake mix chocolate (Nutricia Ltd)
500 gram (ACBS) · NHS indicative price = £9.06

Loprofin low protein mix (Nutricia Ltd)
500 gram (ACBS) · NHS indicative price = £8.43

PK Foods® Flour mix and egg substitute
LOW-PROTEIN

PK Foods low protein egg replacer (Gluten Free Foods Ltd)
200 gram (ACBS) · NHS indicative price = £4.08

PK Foods low protein flour mix (Gluten Free Foods Ltd)
750 gram (ACBS) · NHS indicative price = £10.71

Pasta

Loprofin® Pasta
LOW-PROTEIN

Loprofin low protein pasta animal shapes (Nutricia Ltd)
500 gram (ACBS) · NHS indicative price = £8.61

Loprofin low protein pasta lasagne (Nutricia Ltd)
250 gram (ACBS) · NHS indicative price = £4.35

Loprofin low protein pasta penne (Nutricia Ltd)
500 gram (ACBS) · NHS indicative price = £8.94

Loprofin low protein pasta tagliatelle (Nutricia Ltd)
250 gram (ACBS) · NHS indicative price = £4.30

Loprofin low protein pasta macaroni elbows (Nutricia Ltd)
250 gram (ACBS) · NHS indicative price = £4.30

Loprofin low protein rice (Nutricia Ltd)
500 gram (ACBS) · NHS indicative price = £8.68

Loprofin low protein pasta long cut spaghetti (Nutricia Ltd)
500 gram (ACBS) · NHS indicative price = £8.94

Promin® Pasta
LOW-PROTEIN

Promin low protein pasta alphabets (Firstplay Dietary Foods Ltd)
500 gram (ACBS) · NHS indicative price = £6.99

Promin Plus low protein pasta macaroni (Firstplay Dietary Foods Ltd)
500 gram (ACBS) · NHS indicative price = £6.99

Promin Plus low protein pasta flat noodles (Firstplay Dietary Foods Ltd)
500 gram (ACBS) · NHS indicative price = £6.99

Promin low protein pasta shells (Firstplay Dietary Foods Ltd)
500 gram (ACBS) · NHS indicative price = £6.99

Promin low protein pasta short cut spaghetti (Firstplay Dietary Foods Ltd)
500 gram (ACBS) · NHS indicative price = £6.99

Promin low protein tricolour pasta spirals (Firstplay Dietary Foods Ltd)
500 gram (ACBS) · NHS indicative price = £6.99

Promin low protein pasta spirals (Firstplay Dietary Foods Ltd)
500 gram (ACBS) · NHS indicative price = £6.99

Promin low protein imitation rice (Firstplay Dietary Foods Ltd)
500 gram (ACBS) · NHS indicative price = £6.99

Promin low protein tricolour pasta alphabets (Firstplay Dietary Foods Ltd)
500 gram (ACBS) · NHS indicative price = £6.99

Promin low protein tricolour pasta shells (Firstplay Dietary Foods Ltd)
500 gram (ACBS) · NHS indicative price = £6.99

Promin low protein lasagne sheets (Firstplay Dietary Foods Ltd)
200 gram (ACBS) · NHS indicative price = £3.03

Pizza bases

Juvela® Pizza base
LOW-PROTEIN

Juvela low protein pizza base (Hero UK Ltd)
360 gram (ACBS) · NHS indicative price = £8.61

Savoury meals and mixes

Promin® Savoury meals and mixes
LOW-PROTEIN

Promin low protein burger mix (Firstplay Dietary Foods Ltd)
248 gram (ACBS) · NHS indicative price = £12.72

Promin low protein cous cous (Firstplay Dietary Foods Ltd)
500 gram (ACBS) · NHS indicative price = £6.99

Promin low protein pasta elbows (Firstplay Dietary Foods Ltd)
500 gram · NHS indicative price = £6.99

Promin low protein pastameal (Firstplay Dietary Foods Ltd)
500 gram (ACBS) · NHS indicative price = £6.99

Promin low protein pasta macaroni (Firstplay Dietary Foods Ltd)
500 gram (ACBS) · NHS indicative price = £6.99

Promin Plus low protein pasta spirals (Firstplay Dietary Foods Ltd)
500 gram (ACBS) · NHS indicative price = £6.99

Promin low protein lamb and mint burger mix (Firstplay Dietary Foods Ltd)
248 gram (ACBS) · NHS indicative price = £12.72

Promin low protein sausage mix apple and sage (Firstplay Dietary Foods Ltd)
120 gram (ACBS) · NHS indicative price = £7.15

Promin low protein sausage mix original (Firstplay Dietary Foods Ltd)
120 gram (ACBS) · NHS indicative price = £7.15

Promin low protein sausage mix tomato and basil (Firstplay Dietary Foods Ltd)
120 gram (ACBS) · NHS indicative price = £7.15

Promin low protein pasta in cheese and broccoli sauce (Firstplay Dietary Foods Ltd)
264 gram (ACBS) · NHS indicative price = £8.31

Promin low protein pasta spirals in Moroccan sauce (Firstplay Dietary Foods Ltd)
288 gram (ACBS) · NHS indicative price = £8.31

Promin low protein pasta in tomato, pepper and herb sauce (Firstplay Dietary Foods Ltd)
288 gram (ACBS) · NHS indicative price = £8.31

Promin low protein potato pot with croutons onion (Firstplay Dietary Foods Ltd)
200 gram (ACBS) · NHS indicative price = £16.40

Promin low protein potato pot with croutons cabbage & bacon (Firstplay Dietary Foods Ltd)
200 gram (ACBS) · NHS indicative price = £16.40

Promin low protein potato pot with croutons sausage (Firstplay Dietary Foods Ltd)
200 gram (ACBS) · NHS indicative price = £16.40

Promin low protein X-Pot all day scramble (Firstplay Dietary Foods Ltd)
240 gram (ACBS) · NHS indicative price = £20.94

Promin low protein X-Pot beef & tomato (Firstplay Dietary Foods Ltd)
240 gram (ACBS) · NHS indicative price = £20.94

Promin low protein X-Pot chip shop curry (Firstplay Dietary Foods Ltd)
240 gram (ACBS) · NHS indicative price = £20.94

Promin low protein X-Pot rogan style curry (Firstplay Dietary Foods Ltd)
240 gram (ACBS) · NHS indicative price = £20.94

Spreads

Taranis® Spread
LOW-PROTEIN

Taranis low protein hazelnut spread (Lactalis Nutrition Sante)
230 gram (ACBS) · NHS indicative price = £7.87

Nutritional supplements for metabolic diseases

Glutaric aciduria (type 1)

GA1 Anamix® Infant
▸ Nutritional supplement for the dietary management of proven glutaric aciduria (type 1) in children from birth to 3 years.
POWDER, protein equivalent (essential and non-essential amino acids except lysine, and low tryptophan) 13.1 g, carbohydrate 49.5 g, fat 23 g, fibre 5.3 g, energy 1915 kJ (457 kcal)/100 g, with vitamins, minerals, and trace elements; standard dilution (15%) provides protein equivalent 2 g, carbohydrate 7.4 g, fat 3.5 g, fibre 800 mg, energy 287 kJ (69 kcal)/100 mL.

GA1 Anamix Infant powder (Nutricia Ltd)
400 gram (ACBS) · NHS indicative price = £39.45

GA Gel®
▸ Nutritional supplement for dietary management of type 1 glutaric aciduria in children 6 months–10 years.
GEL, protein equivalent (essential and non-essential amino acids except lysine, and low tryptophan) 10 g, carbohydrate 10.3 g, fat trace, energy 339 kJ (81 kcal)/24 g, with vitamins, minerals, and trace elements. To flavour unflavoured products, see FlavourPac p. 1003.

GA gel oral powder 24g sachets (Vitaflo International Ltd)
30 sachet (ACBS) · NHS indicative price = £216.48

GA1, Maxamaid®
▸ Nutritional supplement for the dietary management of type 1 glutaric aciduria.
POWDER, protein equivalent (essential and non-essential amino acids except lysine, and low tryptophan) 25 g, carbohydrate 51 g, fat less than 500 mg, energy 1311 kJ (309 kcal)/100 g, with vitamins, minerals, and trace elements.
Maxamaid products are generally intended for use in children 1–8 years.

GA1 Maxamaid powder (Nutricia Ltd)
500 gram (ACBS) · NHS indicative price = £99.61

XLYS, TRY Glutaridon®
▸ Nutritional supplement for the dietary management of type 1 glutaric aciduria in children and adults; requires additional source of vitamins, minerals, and trace elements.
POWDER, protein equivalent (essential and non-essential amino acids except lysine and tryptophan) 79 g, carbohydrate 4 g, energy 1411 kJ (332 kcal)/100 g.

XLYS TRY Glutaridon powder (Nutricia Ltd)
500 gram (ACBS) · NHS indicative price = £188.69

Glycogen storage disease

Corn flour and corn starch
▸ For glycogen storage disease

Glycosade®
▸ A nutritional supplement for use in the dietary management of glycogen storage disease and other metabolic conditions where a constant supply of glucose is essential. Not suitable for use in children under 2 years.
POWDER, protein 200 mg, carbohydrate (maize starch) 47.6 g, fat 100 mg, fibre less than 600 mg, energy 803 kJ (192 kcal)/60 g.

Glycosade oral powder 60g sachets (Vitaflo International Ltd)
30 sachet (ACBS) · NHS indicative price = £113.77

Homocystinuria or hypermethioninaemia

HCU Anamix® Infant
▸ Nutritional supplement for the dietary management of proven vitamin B6 non-responsive homocystinuria or hypermethioninaemia in children from birth to 3 years.
POWDER, protein equivalent (essential and non-essential amino acids except methionine) 13.1 g, carbohydrate 49.5 g, fat 23 g, fibre 5.3 g, energy 1915 kJ (457 kcal)/100 g, with vitamins, minerals, and trace elements; standard dilution (15%) provides protein equivalent 2 g, carbohydrate 7.4 g, fat 3.5 g, fibre 800 mg, energy 287 kJ (69 kcal)/100 mL.

HCU Anamix Infant powder (Nutricia Ltd)
400 gram (ACBS) · NHS indicative price = £39.45

HCU cooler® 15
▸ A methionine-free protein substitute for use as a nutritional supplement in children over 3 years with homocystinuria.
LIQUID, protein (essential and non-essential amino acids except methionine) 15 g, carbohydrate 7 g, fat 500 mg, energy 393 kJ (92 kcal)/130 mL, with vitamins, minerals, and trace elements.

HCU orange cooler 15 liquid (Vitaflo International Ltd)
130 ml (ACBS) · NHS indicative price = £11.42

HCU Express® 15
▸ A methionine-free protein substitute for use as a nutritional supplement in children over 8 years with homocystinuria.
POWDER, protein (essential and non-essential amino acids except methionine) 15 g, carbohydrate 3.8 g, fat 30 mg, energy 315 kJ (75.3 kcal)/25 g with vitamins, minerals, and trace elements. To flavour unflavoured products, see FlavourPac p. 1003.

HCU express 15 oral powder 25g sachets (Vitaflo International Ltd)
30 sachet (ACBS) · NHS indicative price = £336.16

HCU Express® 20
▸ A methionine-free protein substitute for use as a nutritional supplement in children over 8 years with homocystinuria.
POWDER, protein (essential and non-essential amino acids except methionine) 20 g, carbohydrate 4.7 g, fat 70 mg, energy 416 kJ (99 kcal)/34 g with vitamins, minerals, and trace elements. To flavour unflavoured products, see FlavourPac p. 1003

HCU express 20 oral powder 34g sachets (Vitaflo International Ltd)
30 sachet (ACBS) · NHS indicative price = £434.31

HCU gel®
▸ A methionine-free protein substitute for use as a nutritional supplement for the dietary management of children 1–10 years with homocystinuria.
POWDER, protein (essential and non-essential amino acids except methionine) 10 g, carbohydrate 10.3 g, fat 20 mg, energy 339 kJ (81 kcal)/24 g with vitamins, minerals, and trace elements. To flavour unflavoured products, see FlavourPac p. 1003.

HCU gel oral powder 24g sachets (Vitaflo International Ltd)
30 sachet (ACBS) · NHS indicative price = £216.42

HCU Lophlex® LQ 20
▸ Nutritional supplement for the dietary management of homocystinuria in children over 3 years.
LIQUID, protein equivalent (essential and non-essential amino acids except methionine) 20 g, carbohydrate 8.8 g, fat 440 mg, energy 509 kJ (120 kcal)/125 mL, with vitamins, minerals, and trace elements.

HCU Lophlex LQ 20 liquid (Nutricia Ltd)
125 ml (ACBS) · NHS indicative price = £16.27

HCU LV®
▸ Nutritional supplement for the dietary management of
hypermethioninaemia or vitamin B6 non-responsive
homocystinuria in children over 8 years.
POWDER, protein (essential and non-essential amino acids
except methionine) 20 g, carbohydrate 2.5 g, fat 190 mg, energy
390 kJ (92 kcal)/27.8-g sachet, with vitamins, minerals, and
trace elements.

HCU-LV oral powder 27.8g sachets tropical (Nutricia Ltd)
30 sachet (ACBS) · NHS indicative price = £500.10

HCU-LV oral powder 27.8g sachets unflavoured (Nutricia Ltd)
30 sachet (ACBS) · NHS indicative price = £500.10

XMET Homidon®
▸ Nutritional supplement for the dietary management of
hypermethioninaemia or homocystinuria in children and
adults.
POWDER, protein equivalent (essential and non-essential amino
acids, except methionine) 77 g, carbohydrate 4.5 g, fat nil,
energy 1386 kJ (326 kcal)/100 g.

XMET Homidon powder (Nutricia Ltd)
500 gram (ACBS) · NHS indicative price = £188.69

HCU Maxamaid®
▸ Nutritional supplement for the dietary management of
hypermethioninaemia or homocystinuria.
POWDER, protein equivalent (essential and non-essential amino
acids except methionine) 25 g, carbohydrate 51 g, fat less than
500 mg, energy 1311 kJ (309 kcal)/100 g, with vitamins,
minerals, and trace elements. Maxamaid products are generally
intended for use in children 1–8 years.

HCU Maxamaid powder (Nutricia Ltd)
500 gram (ACBS) · NHS indicative price = £99.61

HCU Maxamum®
▸ Nutritional supplement for the dietary management of
hypermethioninaemia or homocystinuria.
POWDER, protein equivalent (essential and non-essential amino
acids except methionine) 39 g, carbohydrate 34 g, fat less than
500 mg, energy 1260 kJ (297 kcal)/100 g, with vitamins,
minerals, and trace elements. Maxamum products are generally
intended for use in children over 8 years.

HCU Maxamum powder (Nutricia Ltd)
500 gram (ACBS) · NHS indicative price = £159.66

Hyperlysinaemia

HYPER LYS Anamix® Infant
▸ Nutritional supplement for the dietary management of proven
hyperlysinaemia in children from birth to 3 years.
POWDER, protein equivalent (essential and non-essential amino
acids except lysine) 13.1 g, carbohydrate 49.5 g, fat 23 g, fibre
5.3 g, energy 1915 kJ (457 kcal)/100 g, with vitamins, minerals,
and trace elements; standard dilution (15%) provides protein
equivalent 2 g, carbohydrate 7.4 g, fat 3.5 g, fibre 800 mg, energy
287 kJ (69 kcal)/100 mL.

HYPER LYS Anamix Infant powder (Nutricia Ltd)
400 gram (ACBS) · NHS indicative price = £39.45

HYPER LYS Maxamaid®
▸ Nutritional supplement for the dietary management of
hyperlysinaemia.
POWDER, protein equivalent (essential and non-essential amino
acids except lysine) 25 g, carbohydrate 51 g, fat less than
500 mg, energy 1311 kJ (309 kcal)/100 g with vitamins, minerals,
and trace elements. Maxamaid products are generally intended
for use in children 1-8 years.

HYPER LYS Maxamaid powder (Nutricia Ltd)
500 gram (ACBS) · NHS indicative price = £99.61

Isovaleric acidaemia

IVA Anamix® Infant
▸ Nutritional supplement for the dietary management of proven
isovaleric acidaemia or other proven disorders of leucine
metabolism in children from birth to 3 years.
POWDER, protein equivalent (essential and non-essential amino
acids except leucine) 13.1 g, carbohydrate 49.5 g, fat 23 g, fibre
5.3 g, energy 1915 kJ (457 kcal)/100 g, with vitamins, minerals,
and trace elements; standard dilution (15%) provides protein
equivalent 2 g, carbohydrate 7.4 g, fat 3.5 g, fibre 800 mg, energy
287 kJ (69 kcal)/100 mL.

IVA Anamix Infant powder (Nutricia Ltd)
400 gram (ACBS) · NHS indicative price = £39.45

IVA Maxamaid®
▸ Nutritional supplement for the dietary management of
isovaleric acidaemia.
POWDER, protein equivalent (essential and non-essential amino
acids except leucine) 25 g, carbohydrate 51 g, fat less than
500 mg, energy 1311 kJ (309 kcal)/100 g with vitamins, minerals,
and trace elements. Maxamaid products are generally intended
for use in children 1-8 years.

IVA Maxamaid powder (Nutricia Ltd)
500 gram (ACBS) · NHS indicative price = £99.61

Maple syrup urine disease

MSUD Aid III®
▸ Nutritional supplement for the dietary management of maple
syrup urine disease and related conditions in children and
adults where it is necessary to limit the intake of branched
chain amino acids.
POWDER, protein equivalent (essential and non-essential amino
acids except isoleucine, leucine, and valine) 77 g, carbohydrate
4.5 g, fat nil, energy 1386 kJ (326 kcal)/100 g.

MSUD Aid 111 powder (Nutricia Ltd)
500 gram (ACBS) · NHS indicative price = £188.69

MSUD Anamix® Infant
▸ Nutritional supplement for the dietary management of proven
maple syrup urine disease in children from birth to 3 years.
POWDER, protein equivalent (essential and non-essential amino
acids except isoleucine, leucine, and valine) 13.1 g,
carbohydrate 49.5 g, fat 23 g, fibre 5.3 g, energy 1915 kJ
(457 kcal)/100 g, with vitamins, minerals, and trace elements;
standard dilution (15%) provides protein equivalent 2 g,
carbohydrate 7.4 g, fat 3.5 g, fibre 800 mg, energy 287 kJ
(69 kcal)/100 mL.

MSUD Anamix Infant powder (Nutricia Ltd)
400 gram (ACBS) · NHS indicative price = £39.45

MSUD Anamix® Junior
▸ Nutritional supplement for the dietary management of maple
syrup urine disease in children 1–10 years.
POWDER, protein equivalent (essential and non-essential amino
acids except isoleucine, leucine, and valine) 8.4 g, carbohydrate
11 g, fat 3.9 g, energy 474 kJ (113 kcal)/29-g sachet, with
vitamins, minerals, and trace elements.

MSUD Anamix Junior oral powder 36g sachets (Nutricia Ltd)
30 sachets (ACBS) · NHS indicative price = £210.90

MSUD Anamix® Junior LQ
▸ Nutritional supplement for the dietary management of maple
syrup urine disease in children 1–10 years.
LIQUID, protein equivalent (essential and non-essential amino
acids except isoleucine, leucine, and valine) 10 g, carbohydrate
8.8 g, fat 4.8 g, fibre 310 mg, energy 497 kJ (118 kcal)/125 mL,
with vitamins, minerals, and trace elements. Lactose-free.

MSUD Anamix Junior LQ liquid (Nutricia Ltd)
125 ml (ACBS) · NHS indicative price = £9.15

MSUD cooler® 15
▸ Nutritional supplement for the dietary management of maple syrup urine disease in children over 3 years and adults.
LIQUID, protein equivalent (essential and non-essential amino acids except leucine, isoleucine, and valine) 15 g, carbohydrate 7 g, fat 500 mg, energy 393 kJ (92 kcal)/130-mL pouch, with vitamins, minerals, and trace elements.

MSUD orange cooler 15 liquid (Vitaflo International Ltd)
130 ml (ACBS) · NHS indicative price = £11.42

MSUD red cooler 15 liquid (Vitaflo International Ltd)
130 ml (ACBS) · NHS indicative price = £11.42

MSUD express® 15
▸ Nutritional supplement for the dietary management of maple syrup urine disease in children over 8 years and adults.
POWDER, protein equivalent (essential and non-essential amino acids except leucine, isoleucine, and valine) 15 g, carbohydrate 3.8 g, fat less than 100 mg, energy 315 kJ (75 kcal)/25 g, with vitamins, minerals, and trace elements. To flavour unflavoured products, see FlavourPac p. 1003.

MSUD express 15 oral powder 25g sachets (Vitaflo International Ltd)
30 sachet (ACBS) · NHS indicative price = £336.16

MSUD express® 20
▸ Nutritional supplement for the dietary management of maple syrup urine disease in children over 8 years and adults.
POWDER, protein equivalent (essential and non-essential amino acids except leucine, isoleucine, and valine) 20 g, carbohydrate 4.7 g, fat less than 100 mg, energy 416 kJ (99 kcal)/34 g, with vitamins, minerals, and trace elements. To flavour unflavoured products, see FlavourPac p. 1003.

MSUD express 20 oral powder 34g sachets (Vitaflo International Ltd)
30 sachet (ACBS) · NHS indicative price = £434.31

MSUD Gel®
▸ Nutritional supplement for the dietary management of maple syrup urine disease in children 1–10 years.
POWDER, protein equivalent (essential and non-essential amino acids except leucine, isoleucine, and valine) 10 g, carbohydrate 10.3 g, fat less than 100 mg, energy 339 kJ (81 kcal)/24 g, with vitamins, minerals, and trace elements. To flavour unflavoured products, see FlavourPac p. 1003.

MSUD gel 24g sachets (Vitaflo International Ltd)
30 sachet (ACBS) · NHS indicative price = £218.96

MSUD Lophlex® LQ 20
▸ Nutritional supplement for the dietary management of maple syrup urine disease in children over 3 years.
LIQUID, protein equivalent (essential and non-essential amino acids except isoleucine, leucine, and valine) 20 g, carbohydrate 8.8 g, fat less than 500 mg, energy 509 kJ (120 kcal)/125 mL, with vitamins, minerals, and trace elements.

MSUD Lophlex LQ 20 liquid (Nutricia Ltd)
125 ml (ACBS) · NHS indicative price = £16.27

MSUD Maxamaid®
▸ Nutritional supplement for the dietary management of maple syrup urine disease.
POWDER, protein equivalent (essential and non-essential amino acids except isoleucine, leucine, and valine) 25 g, carbohydrate 51 g, fat less than 500 mg, energy 1311 kJ (309 kcal)/100 g, with vitamins, minerals, and trace elements. Maxamaid products are generally intended for use in children 1–8 years.

MSUD Maxamaid powder (Nutricia Ltd)
500 gram (ACBS) · NHS indicative price = £99.61

MSUD Maxamum®
▸ Nutritional supplement for the dietary management of maple syrup urine disease.
POWDER, protein equivalent (essential and non-essential amino acids except isoleucine, leucine, and valine) 39 g, carbohydrate 34 g, fat less than 500 mg, energy 1260 kJ (297 kcal)/100 g, with vitamins, minerals, and trace elements. Maxamum products are generally intended for use in children over 8 years.

MSUD Maxamum powder orange (Nutricia Ltd)
500 gram (ACBS) · NHS indicative price = £159.66

MSUD Maxamum powder unflavoured (Nutricia Ltd)
500 gram (ACBS) · NHS indicative price = £159.66

Methylmalonic or propionic acidaemia

MMA/PA Anamix® Infant
▸ Nutritional supplement for the dietary management of proven methylmalonic acidaemia or propionic acidaemia in children from birth to 3 years.
POWDER, protein equivalent (essential and non-essential amino acids except methionine, threonine, and valine, and low isoleucine) 13.1 g, carbohydrate 49.5 g, fat 23 g, fibre 5.3 g, energy 1915 kJ (457 kcal)/100 g, with vitamins, minerals, and trace elements; standard dilution (15%) provides protein equivalent 2 g, carbohydrate 7.4 g, fat 3.5 g, fibre 800 mg, energy 287 kJ (69 kcal)/100 mL.

MMA / PA Anamix Infant powder (Nutricia Ltd)
400 gram (ACBS) · NHS indicative price = £39.45

MMA/PA Maxamaid®
▸ Nutritional supplement for the dietary management of methylmalonic acidaemia or propionic acidaemia.
POWDER, protein equivalent (essential and non-essential amino acids except methionine, threonine, and valine, and low isoleucine) 25 g, carbohydrate 51 g, fat less than 500 mg, energy 1311 kJ (309 kcal)/100 g, with vitamins, minerals, and trace elements. Maxamaid products are generally intended for use in children 1–8 years.

MMA/PA Maxamaid powder (Nutricia Ltd)
500 gram (ACBS) · NHS indicative price = £99.61

XMTVI Asadon®
▸ Nutritional supplement for the dietary management of methylmalonic acidaemia or propionic acidaemia in children and adults.
POWDER, protein equivalent (essential and non-essential amino acids except methionine, threonine, and valine, and low isoleucine) 77 g, carbohydrate 4.5 g, fat nil, energy 1386 kJ (326 kcal)/100 g.

XMTVI Asadon powder (Nutricia Ltd)
200 gram (ACBS) · NHS indicative price = £75.47

XMTVI Maxamum®
▸ Nutritional supplement for the dietary management of methylmalonic acidaemia or propionic acidaemia.
POWDER, protein equivalent (essential and non-essential amino acids except methionine, threonine, and valine, and low isoleucine) 39 g, carbohydrate 34 g, fat less than 500 mg, energy 1260 kJ (297 kcal)/100 g, with vitamins, minerals, and trace elements. Maxamum products are generally intended for use in children over 8 years.

MMA/PA Maxamum powder (Nutricia Ltd)
500 gram (ACBS) · NHS indicative price = £159.66

Other inborn errors of metabolism

Cystine500®
▸ Nutritional supplement for the dietary management of inborn errors of amino acid metabolism in adults and children from birth.
POWDER, cystine 500 mg, carbohydrate 3.3 g, fat nil, energy 63 kJ (15 kcal)/4 g

Cystine500 oral powder 4 g sachets (Vitaflo International Ltd)
30 sachet (ACBS) · NHS indicative price = £55.00

DocOmega®
▸ Nutritional supplement for the dietary management of inborn errors of metabolism for adults and children from birth.
POWDER, protein (cows' milk, soya) 100 mg, carbohydrate 3.2 g, fat 500 mg (of which docosahexaenoic acid 200 mg), fibre nil, energy 74 kJ (18 kcal)/4 g, with minerals

DocOmega oral powder 4g sachets (Vitaflo International Ltd)
30 sachet (ACBS) · NHS indicative price = £39.80

EAA® Supplement
▸ Nutritional supplement for the dietary management of

disorders of protein metabolism including urea cycle disorders in children over 3 years.

POWDER, protein equivalent (essential amino acids) 5 g, carbohydrate 4 g, fat nil, energy 151 kJ (36 kcal)/12.5 g, with vitamins, minerals, and trace elements.

EAA Supplement oral powder 12.5g sachets (Vitaflo International Ltd)
50 sachet (ACBS) · NHS indicative price = £207.51

Isoleucine50®
▸ Nutritional supplement for use in the dietary management of inborn errors of amino acid metabolism in adults and children from birth.
POWDER, isoleucine 50 mg, carbohydrate 3.8 g, fat nil, energy 63 kJ (15 kcal)/4 g

Isoleucine50 oral powder 4g sachets (Vitaflo International Ltd)
30 sachet (ACBS) · NHS indicative price = £55.00

KeyOmega®
▸ Nutritional supplement for the dietary management of inborn errors of metabolism.
POWDER, protein (cows' milk, soya) 170 mg, carbohydrate 2.8 g, fat 800 mg (of which arachidonic acid 200 mg, docosahexaenoic acid 100 mg), energy 80 kJ (19 kcal)/4 g.

KeyOmega oral powder 4g sachets (Vitaflo International Ltd)
30 sachet (ACBS) · NHS indicative price = £40.70

Leucine100®
▸ Nutritional supplement for the dietary management of inborn errors of amino acid metabolism in adults and children from birth.
POWDER, leucine 100 mg, carbohydrate 3.7 g, fat nil, energy 63 kJ (15 kcal)/4 g

Leucine100 oral powder sachets (Vitaflo International Ltd)
30 sachet (ACBS) · NHS indicative price = £55.00

Low protein drink
▸ Nutritional supplement for the dietary management of inborn errors of amino acid metabolism in adults and children over 1 year.
POWDER, protein (cows' milk) 4.5 g (phenylalanine 100 mg), carbohydrate 59.5 g, fat 29.9 g, fibre nil, energy 2194 kJ (528 kcal)/100 g, with vitamins, minerals, and trace elements. Contains lactose.
Termed *Milupa® lp-drink* by manufacturer.

Milupa LP drink (Nutricia Ltd)
400 gram (ACBS) · NHS indicative price = £9.36

Phenylalanine50®
▸ Nutritional supplement for use in the dietary management of inborn errors of metabolism in adults and children from birth.
POWDER, phenylalanine 50 mg, carbohydrate 3.8 g, fat nil, energy 63 kJ (15 kcal)/4 g

Phenylalanine50 oral powder sachets (Vitaflo International Ltd)
30 sachet (ACBS) · NHS indicative price = £53.40

ProZero®
▸ A protein-free nutritional supplement for the dietary management of inborn errors of metabolism in children over 6 months and adults.
LIQUID, carbohydrate 8.1 g (of which sugars 3.5 g), fat 3.8 g, energy 278 kJ (66 kcal)/100 mL. Contains lactose.

ProZero liquid (Vitaflo International Ltd)
250 ml (ACBS) · NHS indicative price = £1.46 | 1000 ml (ACBS) · NHS indicative price = £5.86

Tyrosine1000®
▸ Nutritional supplement for the dietary management of inborn errors of amino acid metabolism in adults and children from birth.
POWDER, tyrosine 1 g, carbohydrate 2.9 g, fat nil, energy 63 kJ (15 kcal)/4-g sachet.

Tyrosine1000 oral powder 4g sachets (Vitaflo International Ltd)
30 sachet (ACBS) · NHS indicative price = £5.04

Valine50®
▸ Nutritional supplement for the dietary management of inborn errors of amino acid metabolism in adults and children from birth.

POWDER, valine 50 mg, carbohydrate 3.8 g, fat nil, energy 63 kJ (15 kcal)/4 g

Valine50 oral powder 4g sachets (Vitaflo International Ltd)
30 sachet (ACBS) · NHS indicative price = £55.00

Phenylketonuria

Add-ins®
▸ Nutritional supplement for the dietary management of proven phenylketonuria in children over 4 years.
POWDER, protein equivalent (containing essential and non-essential amino acids except phenylalanine) 10 g, carbohydrate nil, fat 5.1 g, energy 359 kJ (86 kcal)/18.2-g sachet, with vitamins, minerals, and trace elements.

Add Ins oral powder 18.2g sachets (Nutricia Ltd)
60 sachet (ACBS) · NHS indicative price = £381.00

Easiphen®
▸ Nutritional supplement for the dietary management of proven phenylketonuria in children over 8 years.
LIQUID, protein equivalent (containing essential and non-essential amino acids except phenylalanine) 6.7 g, carbohydrate 5.1 g, fat 2 g, energy 275 kJ (65 kcal)/100 mL with vitamins, minerals, and trace elements.

Easiphen liquid (Nutricia Ltd)
250 ml (ACBS) · NHS indicative price = £9.79

L-Tyrosine
▸ Nutritional supplement for the dietary management of phenylketonuria in pregnant women with low plasma tyrosine concentrations.
POWDER, L-tyrosine 20 g, carbohydrate 76.8 g, fat nil, energy 1612 kJ (379 kcal)/100 g.

L-Tyrosine powder (Nutricia Ltd)
100 gram (ACBS) · NHS indicative price = £22.22

Lophlex®
▸ Nutritional supplement for the dietary management of proven phenylketonuria in children over 8 years and adults including pregnant women.
POWDER, protein equivalent (essential and non-essential amino acids except phenylalanine) 20 g, carbohydrate 2.5 g, fat 60 mg, fibre 220 mg, energy 385 kJ (91 kcal)/27.8-g sachet, with vitamins, minerals, and trace elements.

Lophlex powder 27.8g sachets berry (Nutricia Ltd)
30 sachet (ACBS) · NHS indicative price = £294.00

Lophlex powder 27.8g sachets orange (Nutricia Ltd)
30 sachet (ACBS) · NHS indicative price = £294.00

Lophlex powder 27.8g sachets unflavoured (Nutricia Ltd)
30 sachet (ACBS) · NHS indicative price = £294.00

Loprofin® PKU Drink
▸ Nutritional supplement for the dietary management of phenylketonuria in children over 1 year and adults.
LIQUID, protein (cows' milk) 400 mg (phenylalanine 10 mg), lactose 9.4 g, fat 2 g, energy 165 kJ (40 kcal)/100 mL.

Loprofin PKU drink (Nutricia Ltd)
200 ml (ACBS) · NHS indicative price = £0.76

Loprofin® Sno-Pro
▸ Nutritional supplement for the dietary management of phenylketonuria, chronic renal failure and other inborn errors of amino acid metabolism.
LIQUID, protein (cows' milk) 220 mg (phenylalanine 12.5 mg), carbohydrate 8 g, fat 3.8 g, energy 273 kJ (65 kcal)/100 mL. Contains lactose.

Loprofin SNO-PRO drink (Nutricia Ltd)
200 ml (ACBS) · NHS indicative price = £1.27

Phlexy-10® Exchange System
▸ Nutritional supplement for the dietary management of phenylketonuria.
CAPSULES, protein equivalent (essential and non-essential amino acids except phenylalanine) 416.5 mg/capsule.

Phlexy-10 500mg capsules (Nutricia Ltd)
200 capsule (ACBS) · NHS indicative price = £44.00

TABLETS, protein equivalent (essential and non-essential amino acids except phenylalanine) 833 mg tablet.

Phlexy-10 tablets (Nutricia Ltd)
75 tablet (ACBS) · NHS indicative price = £28.50

DRINK MIX, powder, protein equivalent (essential and non-essential amino acids except phenylalanine) 8.33 g, carbohydrate 8.8 g/20-g sachet.

Phlexy-10 drink mix apple & blackcurrant (Nutricia Ltd)
600 gram (ACBS) · NHS indicative price = £130.20

Phlexy-10 drink mix citrus burst (Nutricia Ltd)
600 gram (ACBS) · NHS indicative price = £130.20

Phlexy-10 drink mix tropical surprise (Nutricia Ltd)
600 gram (ACBS) · NHS indicative price = £130.20

Phlexy-Vits®
▸ For use as a vitamin and mineral component of restricted therapeutic diets in children over 11 years and adults with phenylketonuria and similar amino acid abnormalities.
POWDER, vitamins, minerals, and trace elements

Phlexy-Vits powder (Nutricia Ltd)
210 gram (ACBS) · NHS indicative price = £72.30

TABLETS, vitamins, minerals, and trace elements

Phlexy-Vits tablets (Nutricia Ltd)
180 tablet (ACBS) · NHS indicative price = £82.80

PK Aid 4®
▸ Nutritional supplement for the dietary management of phenylketonuria in children and adults.
POWDER, protein equivalent (essential and non-essential amino acids except phenylalanine) 79 g, carbohydrate 4.5 g, fat nil, energy 1420 kJ (334 kcal)/100 g.

PK Aid 4 powder (Nutricia Ltd)
500 gram (ACBS) · NHS indicative price = £145.04

PKU Anamix® First Spoon
▸ Nutritional supplement for the dietary management of proven phenylketonuria in children from 6 months to 5 years.
POWDER, protein equivalent (essential and non-essential amino acids except phenylalanine) 5 g, carbohydrate 4.8 g, fat 150 mg, fibre nil, energy 168 kJ (41 kcal)/12.5-g sachet, with vitamins, minerals, and trace elements

PKU Anamix First Spoon oral powder 12.5g sachets (Nutricia Ltd)
30 sachet (ACBS) · NHS indicative price = £93.00

PKU Anamix® Infant
▸ Nutritional supplement for the dietary management of proven phenylketonuria in children from birth to 3 years.
POWDER, protein equivalent (essential and non-essential amino acids except phenylalanine) 13.1 g, carbohydrate 49.5 g, fat 23 g, fibre 5.3 g, energy 1915 kJ (457 kcal)/100 g, with vitamins, minerals, and trace elements; standard dilution (15%) provides protein equivalent 2 g, carbohydrate 7.4 g, fat 3.5 g, fibre 800 mg, energy 287 kJ (69 kcal)/100 mL

PKU Anamix Infant powder (Nutricia Ltd)
400 gram (ACBS) · NHS indicative price = £35.86

PKU Anamix® Junior
▸ Nutritional supplement for the dietary management of phenylketonuria in children 1–10 years.
POWDER, protein equivalent (essential and non-essential amino acids except phenylalanine) 8.4 g, carbohydrate 9.9 g, fat 3.9 g, energy 455 kJ (108 kcal)/29-g sachet, with vitamins, minerals, and trace elements

PKU Anamix Junior powder chocolate (Nutricia Ltd)
1080 gram (ACBS) · NHS indicative price = £128.10

PKU Anamix Junior powder neutral (Nutricia Ltd)
1080 gram (ACBS) · NHS indicative price = £128.10

PKU Anamix® Junior LQ
▸ Nutritional supplement for the dietary supplement of phenylketonuria in children 1–10 years.
LIQUID, protein equivalent (essential and non-essential amino acids except phenylalanine) 10 g, carbohydrate 8.8 g, fat 4.8 g, fibre 310 mg, energy 497 kJ (118 kcal)/125 mL, with vitamins, minerals, and trace elements. Lactose-free.

PKU Anamix Junior LQ liquid berry (Nutricia Ltd)
125 ml (ACBS) · NHS indicative price = £5.69

PKU Anamix Junior LQ liquid orange (Nutricia Ltd)
125 ml (ACBS) · NHS indicative price = £5.69

PKU cooler10®
▸ Nutritional supplement for the dietary management of phenylketonuria in children over 3 years.
LIQUID, protein equivalent (essential and non-essential amino acids except phenylalanine) 10 g, carbohydrate 5.1 g, energy 258 kJ (62 kcal)/87-mL pouch, with vitamins, minerals, and trace elements.

PKU orange cooler 10 liquid (Vitaflo International Ltd)
87 ml (ACBS) · NHS indicative price = £4.65

PKU purple cooler 10 liquid (Vitaflo International Ltd)
87 ml (ACBS) · NHS indicative price = £4.65

PKU red cooler 10 liquid (Vitaflo International Ltd)
87 ml (ACBS) · NHS indicative price = £4.65

PKU white cooler 10 liquid (Vitaflo International Ltd)
87 ml (ACBS) · NHS indicative price = £4.65

PKU cooler15®
▸ Nutritional supplement for the dietary management of phenylketonuria in children over 3 years.
LIQUID, protein equivalent (essential and non-essential amino acids except phenylalanine) 15 g, carbohydrate 7.8 g, energy 386 kJ (92 kcal)/130-mL pouch, with vitamins, minerals, and trace elements.

PKU orange cooler 15 liquid (Vitaflo International Ltd)
130 ml (ACBS) · NHS indicative price = £6.92

PKU purple cooler 15 liquid (Vitaflo International Ltd)
130 ml (ACBS) · NHS indicative price = £6.92

PKU red cooler 15 liquid (Vitaflo International Ltd)
130 ml (ACBS) · NHS indicative price = £6.92

PKU white cooler 15 liquid (Vitaflo International Ltd)
130 ml (ACBS) · NHS indicative price = £6.92

PKU cooler20®
▸ Nutritional supplement for the dietary management of phenylketonuria in children over 3 years.
LIQUID, protein equivalent (essential and non-essential amino acids except phenylalanine) 20 g, carbohydrate 10.2 g, energy 517 kJ (124 kcal)/174-mL pouch, with vitamins, minerals, and trace elements.

PKU orange cooler 20 liquid (Vitaflo International Ltd)
174 ml (ACBS) · NHS indicative price = £9.30

PKU purple cooler 20 liquid (Vitaflo International Ltd)
174 ml (ACBS) · NHS indicative price = £9.30

PKU red cooler 20 liquid (Vitaflo International Ltd)
174 ml (ACBS) · NHS indicative price = £9.30

PKU white cooler 20 liquid (Vitaflo International Ltd)
174 ml (ACBS) · NHS indicative price = £9.30

PKU express15®
▸ Nutritional supplement for the dietary management of phenylketonuria. Not recommended for children under 3 years.
POWDER, protein equivalent (essential and non-essential amino acids except phenylalanine) 15 g, carbohydrate 2.4 g, energy 293 kJ (70 kcal)/25 g, with vitamins, minerals, and trace elements. To flavour unflavoured products, see FlavourPac p. 1003.

PKU express 15 powder lemon (Vitaflo International Ltd)
750 gram (ACBS) · NHS indicative price = £203.80

PKU express 15 powder orange (Vitaflo International Ltd)
750 gram (ACBS) · NHS indicative price = £203.80

PKU express 15 powder tropical (Vitaflo International Ltd)
750 gram (ACBS) · NHS indicative price = £203.80

PKU express 15 powder unflavoured (Vitaflo International Ltd)
750 gram (ACBS) · NHS indicative price = £203.80

PKU express20®
▸ Nutritional supplement for the dietary management of phenylketonuria. Not recommended for children under 3 years.

A2

Borderline substances | **Appendix 2**

POWDER, protein equivalent (essential and non-essential amino acids except phenylalanine) 20 g, carbohydrate 3.3 g, energy 389 kJ (93 kcal)/34 g, with vitamins, minerals, and trace elements. To flavour unflavoured products, see FlavourPac p. 1003.

PKU express 20 powder lemon (Vitaflo International Ltd)
1020 gram (ACBS) · NHS indicative price = £263.30

PKU express 20 powder orange (Vitaflo International Ltd)
1020 gram (ACBS) · NHS indicative price = £263.30

PKU express 20 powder tropical (Vitaflo International Ltd)
1020 gram (ACBS) · NHS indicative price = £263.30

PKU express 20 powder unflavoured (Vitaflo International Ltd)
1020 gram (ACBS) · NHS indicative price = £263.30

PKU gel®
▸ For use as part of the low-protein dietary management of phenylketonuria in children 1–10 years
POWDER, protein equivalent (essential and non-essential amino acids except phenylalanine) 10 g, fat less than 100 mg, energy 518 kJ (76 kcal)/24 g, with vitamins, minerals, and trace elements. To flavour unflavoured products, see FlavourPac p. 1003.

PKU gel powder orange (Vitaflo International Ltd)
720 gram (ACBS) · NHS indicative price = £140.99

PKU gel powder raspberry (Vitaflo International Ltd)
720 gram (ACBS) · NHS indicative price = £140.99

PKU gel powder unflavoured (Vitaflo International Ltd)
720 gram (ACBS) · NHS indicative price = £140.99

PKU Lophlex® LQ 10
▸ Nutritional supplement for the dietary management of phenylketonuria in children over 4 years and adults including pregnant women.
LIQUID, protein equivalent (essential and non-essential amino acids except phenylalanine) 10 g, carbohydrate 4.4 g, fibre 250 mg, energy 245 kJ (58 kcal)/62.5 mL, with vitamins, minerals, and trace elements.

PKU Lophlex LQ 10 liquid berry (Nutricia Ltd)
62.5 ml (ACBS) · NHS indicative price = £5.25

PKU Lophlex LQ 10 liquid juicy berries (Nutricia Ltd)
62.5 ml (ACBS) · NHS indicative price = £5.25

PKU Lophlex LQ 10 liquid juicy orange (Nutricia Ltd)
62.5 ml (ACBS) · NHS indicative price = £5.25

PKU Lophlex® LQ 20
▸ Nutritional supplement for the dietary management of phenylketonuria in children over 4 years and adults including pregnant women.
LIQUID, protein equivalent (essential and non-essential amino acids except phenylalanine) 20 g, carbohydrate 8.8 g, fibre 340 mg, energy 490 kJ (115 kcal)/125 mL, with vitamins, minerals, and trace elements.

PKU Lophlex LQ 20 liquid berry (Nutricia Ltd)
125 ml (ACBS) · NHS indicative price = £10.47

PKU Lophlex LQ 20 liquid juicy berries (Nutricia Ltd)
125 ml (ACBS) · NHS indicative price = £10.47

PKU Lophlex LQ 20 liquid orange (Nutricia Ltd)
125 ml (ACBS) · NHS indicative price = £10.47

PKU Lophlex® Sensation 20
▸ Nutritional supplement for the dietary management of phenylketonuria in children over 4 years and adults including pregnant women.
SEMI-SOLID, protein equivalent (containing essential and non-essential amino acids except phenylalanine) 20 g, carbohydrate 20.2 g, fibre 1 g, energy 706 kJ (166 kcal)/109 g, with vitamins, minerals, and trace elements.

PKU Lophlex Sensation 20 berries (Nutricia Ltd)
327 gram (ACBS) · NHS indicative price = £33.45

PKU Lophlex Sensation 20 orange (Nutricia Ltd)
327 gram (ACBS) · NHS indicative price = £33.45

PKU squeezie®
▸ Nutritional supplement for the dietary management of phenylketonuria in children from 6 months to 10 years.
LIQUID, protein equivalent (essential and non-essential amino acids except phenylalanine) 10 g, carbohydrate 22.5 g, fat 500 mg, energy 565 kJ (135 kcal)/85 g, with vitamins, minerals, and trace elements.

PKU squeezie liquid (Vitaflo International Ltd)
2550 gram (ACBS) · NHS indicative price = £134.78

PKU Maxamaid®
▸ Nutritional supplement for the dietary management of phenylketonuria in children 1–8 years.
POWDER, protein equivalent (essential and non-essential amino acids except phenylalanine) 25 g, carbohydrate 51 g, fat less than 500 mg, energy 1311 kJ (309 kcal)/100 g, with vitamins, minerals, and trace elements.

PKU Maxamaid powder orange (Nutricia Ltd)
500 gram (ACBS) · NHS indicative price = £58.92

PKU Maxamaid powder unflavoured (Nutricia Ltd)
500 gram (ACBS) · NHS indicative price = £58.92

PKU Maxamum®
▸ Nutritional supplement for the dietary management of phenylketonuria in children over 8 years and adults.
POWDER, protein equivalent (essential and non-essential amino acids except phenylalanine) 39 g, carbohydrate 34 g, fat less than 500 mg, energy 1260 kJ (297 kcal)/100 g, with vitamins, minerals, and trace elements.

PKU Maxamum oral powder 50g sachets orange (Nutricia Ltd)
30 sachet (ACBS) · NHS indicative price = £273.30

PKU Maxamum oral powder 50g sachets unflavoured (Nutricia Ltd)
30 sachet (ACBS) · NHS indicative price = £273.30

PKU Maxamum powder orange (Nutricia Ltd)
500 gram (ACBS) · NHS indicative price = £91.14

PKU Maxamum powder unflavoured (Nutricia Ltd)
500 gram (ACBS) · NHS indicative price = £91.14

Tyrosinaemia

Methionine-free TYR Anamix® Infant
▸ Nutritional supplement for the dietary management of proven tyrosinaemia type 1 in children from birth to 3 years.
POWDER, protein equivalent (essential and non-essential amino acids except methionine, phenylalanine, and tyrosine) 13.1 g, carbohydrate 49.5 g, fat 23 g, fibre 5.3 g, energy 1915 kJ (457 kcal)/100 g, with vitamins, minerals, and trace elements; standard dilution (15%) provides protein equivalent 2 g, carbohydrate 7.4 g, fat 3.5 g, fibre 800 mg, energy 287 kJ (69 kcal)/100 mL.

TYR Anamix Infant methionine free powder (Nutricia Ltd)
400 gram (ACBS) · NHS indicative price = £39.45

TYR Anamix® Infant
▸ Nutritional supplement for the dietary management of proven tyrosinaemia where plasma-methionine concentrations are normal in children from birth to 3 years.
POWDER, protein equivalent (essential and non-essential amino acids except phenylalanine and tyrosine) 13.1 g, carbohydrate 49.5 g, fat 23 g, fibre 5.3 g, energy 1915 kJ (457 kcal)/100 g, with vitamins, minerals, and trace elements; standard dilution (15%) provides protein equivalent 2 g, carbohydrate 7.4 g, fat 3.5 g, fibre 800 mg, energy 287 kJ (69 kcal)/100 mL.

TYR Anamix Infant methionine free powder (Nutricia Ltd)
400 gram (ACBS) · NHS indicative price = £39.45

TYR Anamix Infant powder (Nutricia Ltd)
400 gram (ACBS) · NHS indicative price = £39.45

TYR Anamix® Junior
▸ Nutritional supplement for the dietary management of proven tyrosinaemia in children 1–10 years.
POWDER, protein equivalent (essential and non-essential amino acids except phenylalanine and tyrosine) 8.4 g, carbohydrate 11 g, fat 3.9 g, energy 475 kJ (113 kcal)/29-g sachet, with vitamins, minerals, and trace elements.

TYR Anamix Junior oral powder 29g sachets (Nutricia Ltd)
30 sachet (ACBS) · NHS indicative price = £206.40

TYR Anamix® Junior LQ
▸ Nutritional supplement for the dietary management of
tyrosinaemia type 1 (when nitisinone (NTBC) is used, see
p. 585, type II, and type III, in children over 1 year.
LIQUID, protein equivalent (essential and non-essential amino
acids except phenylalanine and tyrosine) 10 g, carbohydrate
8.8 g, fat 4.8 g, fibre 310 mg, energy 500 kJ (119 kcal)/125 mL,
with vitamins, minerals and trace elements.

TYR Anamix Junior LQ liquid (Nutricia Ltd)
125 ml (ACBS) · NHS indicative price = £9.15

TYR cooler® 15
▸ Nutritional supplement for the dietary management of
tyrosinaemia in children over 3 years and adults.
LIQUID, protein equivalent (essential and non-essential amino
acids except tyrosine and phenylalanine) 15 g, carbohydrate 7 g,
fat 500 mg, energy 393 kJ (92 kcal)/130 mL, with vitamins,
minerals, and trace elements.

TYR orange cooler 15 liquid (Vitaflo International Ltd)
130 ml (ACBS) · NHS indicative price = £11.42

TYR red cooler 10 liquid (Vitaflo International Ltd)
87 ml (ACBS) · NHS indicative price = £7.32

TYR red cooler 15 liquid (Vitaflo International Ltd)
130 ml (ACBS) · NHS indicative price = £11.42

TYR red cooler 20 liquid (Vitaflo International Ltd)
174 ml (ACBS) · NHS indicative price = £15.29

TYR express15®
▸ Nutritional supplement for the dietary management of
tyrosinaemia in children over 8 years and adults.
POWDER, protein equivalent (essential and non-essential amino
acids except tyrosine and phenylalanine) 15 g, carbohydrate
3.4 g, fat less than 100 mg, energy 310 kJ (74 kcal)/25 g, with
vitamins, minerals, and trace elements. To flavour unflavoured
products, see FlavourPac p. 1003.

TYR express 15 oral powder 25g sachets (Vitaflo International Ltd)
30 sachet (ACBS) · NHS indicative price = £336.16

TYR express20®
▸ Nutritional supplement for the dietary management of
tyrosinaemia in children over 8 years.
POWDER, protein equivalent (essential and non-essential amino
acids except tyrosine and phenylalanine) 20 g, carbohydrate
4.7 g, fat less than 100 mg, energy 416 kJ (99 kcal)/34 g, with
vitamins, minerals, and trace elements. To flavour unflavoured
products, see FlavourPac p. 1003.

TYR express 20 oral powder 34g sachets (Vitaflo International Ltd)
30 sachet (ACBS) · NHS indicative price = £434.31

TYR Gel®
▸ Nutritional supplement for the dietary management of
tyrosinaemia in children 1–10 years.
GEL, protein equivalent (essential and non-essential amino
acids except tyrosine and phenylalanine) 10 g, carbohydrate
10.3 g, fat less than 100 mg, energy 339 kJ (81 kcal)/24 g, with
vitamins, minerals and trace elements. To flavour unflavoured
products, see FlavourPac p. 1003.

TYR gel oral powder 24g sachets (Vitaflo International Ltd)
30 sachet (ACBS) · NHS indicative price = £216.42

TYR Lophlex® LQ 20
▸ Nutritional supplement for the dietary management of
tyrosinaemia in children over 3 years and adults.
LIQUID, protein equivalent (essential and non-essential amino
acids except phenylalanine and tyrosine) 20 g, carbohydrate
8.8 g, fat less than 500 mg, fibre 500 mg, energy 509 kJ
(120 kcal)/125 mL, with vitamins, minerals, and trace elements.

TYR Lophlex LQ 20 liquid (Nutricia Ltd)
125 ml (ACBS) · NHS indicative price = £16.27

XPHEN TYR Maxamaid®
▸ Nutritional supplement for the dietary management of
tyrosinaemia in children 1–8 years.

POWDER, protein equivalent (essential and non-essential amino
acids except phenylalanine and tyrosine) 25 g, carbohydrate
51 g, fat less than 500 mg, energy 1311 kJ (309 kcal)/100 g, with
vitamins, minerals, and trace elements.

TYR Maxamaid powder (Nutricia Ltd)
500 gram (ACBS) · NHS indicative price = £99.61

XPHEN TYR Tyrosidon®
▸ Nutritional supplement for the management of tyrosinaemia in
children and adults where plasma-methionine concentrations
are normal.
POWDER, protein equivalent (essential and non-essential amino
acids except phenylalanine and tyrosine) 77 g, carbohydrate
4.5 g, fat nil, energy 1386 kJ (326 kcal)/100 g.

XPHEN TYR Tyrosidon Free AA Mix powder (Nutricia Ltd)
500 gram (ACBS) · NHS indicative price = £188.69

XPTM Tyrosidon®
▸ Nutritional supplement for the dietary management of
tyrosinaemia type I in children and adults where plasma-
methionine concentrations are above normal.
POWDER, protein equivalent (essential and non-essential amino
acids except methionine, phenylalanine, and tyrosine) 77 g,
carbohydrate 4.5 g, fat nil, energy 1386 kJ (326 kcal)/100 g.

XPTM Tyrosidon powder (Nutricia Ltd)
500 gram · NHS indicative price = £91.31

A2

Borderline substances **|** Appendix 2

Appendix 3
Cautionary and advisory labels for dispensed medicines

Guidance for cautionary and advisory labels

Medicinal forms within BNF publications include code numbers of the cautionary labels that pharmacists are recommended to add when dispensing. It is also expected that pharmacists will counsel patients and carers when necessary.

Counselling needs to be related to the age, experience, background, and understanding of the individual patient or carer. The pharmacist should ensure understanding of how to take or use the medicine and how to follow the correct dosage schedule. Any effects of the medicine on co-ordination, performance of skilled tasks (e.g. driving or work), any foods or medicines to be avoided, and what to do if a dose is missed should also be explained. Other matters, such as the possibility of staining of the clothes or skin, or discolouration of urine or stools by a medicine should also be mentioned.

For some medicines there is a special need for counselling, such as an unusual method or time of administration or a potential interaction with a common food or domestic remedy, and this should be mentioned where necessary.

Original packs

Most preparations are dispensed in unbroken original packs that include further advice for the patient in the form of patient information leaflets. The advice in patient information leaflets may be less appropriate when the medicine is for a child, particularly for unlicensed medicines or indications. Pharmacists should explain discrepancies to carers, if necessary. The patient information leaflet should only be withheld in exceptional circumstances because it contains other information that should be provided. Label 10 may be of value where appropriate. More general leaflets advising on the administration of preparations such as eye drops, eye ointments, inhalers, and suppositories are also available.

Scope of labels

In general no label recommendations have been made for injections on the assumption that they will be administered by a healthcare professional or a well-instructed patient. The labelling is not exhaustive and pharmacists are recommended to use their professional discretion in labelling new preparations and those for which no labels are shown.

Individual labelling advice is not given on the administration of the large variety of antacids. In the absence of instructions from the prescriber, and if on enquiry the patient has had no verbal instructions, the directions given under 'Dose' should be used on the label.

It is recognised that there may be occasions when pharmacists will use their knowledge and professional discretion and decide to omit one or more of the recommended labels for a particular patient. In this case counselling is of the utmost importance. There may also be an occasion when a prescriber does not wish additional cautionary labels to be used, in which case the prescription should be endorsed 'NCL' (no cautionary labels). The exact wording that is required instead should then be specified on the prescription.

Pharmacists label medicines with various wordings in addition to those directions specified on the prescription. Such labels include 'Shake the bottle', 'For external use only', and 'Store in a cool place', as well as 'Discard.... days after opening' and 'Do not use after....', which apply particularly to antibiotic mixtures, diluted liquid and topical preparations, and to eye-drops. Although not listed in the *BNF for Children* these labels should continue to be used when appropriate; indeed, 'For external use only' is a legal requirement on external liquid

preparations, while 'Keep out of the reach of children' is a legal requirement on all dispensed medicines. Care should be taken not to obscure other relevant information with adhesive labelling.

It is the usual practice for patients to take standard tablets with water or other liquid and for this reason no separate label has been recommended.

The label wordings recommended by the *BNF for Children* apply to medicines dispensed against a prescription. Children and carers should be aware that a dispensed medicine should never be taken by, or shared with, anyone other than for whom the prescriber intended it. Therefore, the *BNF for Children* does not include warnings against the use of a dispensed medicine by persons other than for whom it was specifically prescribed.

The label or labels for each preparation are recommended after careful consideration of the information available. However, it is recognised that in some cases this information may be either incomplete or open to a different interpretation. The *BNF for Children* will therefore be grateful to receive any constructive comments on the labelling suggested for any preparation.

Recommended label wordings

For *BNF for Children* 2011–2012, a revised set of cautionary and advisory labels were introduced. All of the existing labels were user-tested, and the revised wording selected reflects terminology that is better understood by patients.

Wordings which can be given as separate warnings are labels 1–19, 29–30, and 32. Wordings which can be incorporated in an appropriate position in the directions for dosage or administration are labels 21–28. A label has been omitted for number 20; labels 31 and 33 no longer apply to any medicines in the *BNF for Children* and have therefore been deleted.

If separate labels are used it is recommended that the wordings be used without modification. If changes are made to suit computer requirements, care should be taken to retain the sense of the original.

Welsh labels

Comprehensive Welsh translations are available for each cautionary and advisory label. These appear directly under the English label.

Labels

1 **Warning: This medicine may make you sleepy**

 Rhybudd: Gall y feddyginiaeth hon eich gwneud yn gysglyd
 To be used on *preparations for children* containing antihistamines, or other preparations given to children where the warnings of label 2 on driving or alcohol would not be appropriate.

2 **Warning: This medicine may make you sleepy. If this happens, do not drive or use tools or machines. Do not drink alcohol**

 Rhybudd: Gall y feddyginiaeth hon eich gwneud yn gysglyd. Peidiwch â gyrru, defnyddio offer llaw neu beiriannau os yw hyn yn digwydd. Peidiwch ag yfed alcohol
 To be used on *preparations for adults that can cause drowsiness*, thereby affecting coordination and the ability to drive and operate hazardous machinery; label 1 is more appropriate for children. *It is an offence to drive while under the influence of drink or drugs.*

 Some of these preparations only cause drowsiness in the

first few days of treatment and some only cause drowsiness in higher doses.

In such cases the patient should be told that the advice applies until the effects have worn off. However many of these preparations can produce a slowing of reaction time and a loss of mental concentration that can have the same effects as drowsiness.

Avoidance of alcoholic drink is recommended because the effects of CNS depressants are enhanced by alcohol. Strict prohibition however could lead to some patients not taking the medicine. Pharmacists should therefore explain the risk and encourage compliance, particularly in patients who may think they already tolerate the effects of alcohol (see also label 3). Queries from patients with epilepsy regarding fitness to drive should be referred back to the patient's doctor.

Side-effects unrelated to drowsiness that may affect a patient's ability to drive or operate machinery safely include *blurred vision, dizziness, or nausea*. In general, no label has been recommended to cover these cases, but the patient should be suitably counselled.

3 **Warning: This medicine may make you sleepy. If this happens, do not drive or use tools or machines**

Rhybudd: Gall y feddyginiaeth hon eich gwneud yn gysglyd. Peidiwch â gyrru, defnyddio offer llaw neu beiriannau os yw hyn yn digwydd

To be used on *preparations containing monoamine-oxidase inhibitors*; the warning to avoid alcohol and dealcoholised (low alcohol) drink is covered by the patient information leaflet.

Also to be used as for label 2 but where alcohol is not an issue.

4 **Warning: Do not drink alcohol**

Rhybudd: Peidiwch ag yfed alcohol

To be used on *preparations where a reaction such as flushing may occur if alcohol is taken* (e.g. metronidazole). Alcohol may also enhance the hypoglycaemia produced by some oral antidiabetic drugs but routine application of a warning label is not considered necessary.

Patients should be advised not to drink alcohol for as long as they are receiving/using a course of medication, and in some cases for a period of time after the course is finished.

5 **Do not take indigestion remedies 2 hours before or after you take this medicine**

Peidiwch â chymryd meddyginiaethau camdreuliad 2 awr cyn neu ar ôl y feddyginiaeth hon

To be used with label 25 on *preparations coated to resist gastric acid* (e.g. enteric-coated tablets). This is to avoid the possibility of premature dissolution of the coating in the presence of an alkaline pH.

Label 5 also applies to drugs such as gabapentin *where the absorption is significantly affected by antacids*. Pharmacists will be aware (from a knowledge of physiology) that the usual time during which indigestion remedies should be avoided is at least 2 hours before and after the majority of medicines have been taken; when a manufacturer advises a different time period, this can be followed, and should be explained to the patient.

6 **Do not take indigestion remedies, or medicines containing iron or zinc, 2 hours before or after you take this medicine**

Peidiwch â chymryd meddyginiaethau camdreuliad neu feddyginiaethau sy'n cynnwys haearn neu sinc, 2 awr cyn neu ar ôl y feddyginiaeth hon

To be used on *preparations containing ofloxacin and some other quinolones, doxycycline, lymecycline, minocycline, and penicillamine*. These drugs chelate calcium, iron, and zinc and are less well absorbed when taken with calcium-containing antacids or preparations containing iron or zinc. Pharmacists will be aware (from a knowledge of physiology) that these incompatible preparations should be taken at least 2 hours apart for the majority of medicines; when a

manufacturer advises a different time period, this can be followed, and should be explained to the patient.

7 **Do not take milk, indigestion remedies, or medicines containing iron or zinc, 2 hours before or after you take this medicine**

Peidiwch â chymryd llaeth, meddyginiaethau camdreuliad, neu feddyginiaeth sy'n cynnwys haearn neu sinc, 2 awr cyn neu ar ôl cymryd y feddyginiaeth hon

To be used on *preparations containing ciprofloxacin, norfloxacin, or tetracyclines that chelate calcium, iron, magnesium, and zinc*, and are thus less liable for absorption. Pharmacists will be aware (from a knowledge of physiology) that these incompatible preparations should be taken at least 2 hours apart for the majority of medicines; when a manufacturer advises a different time period, this can be followed, and should be explained to the patient. Doxycycline, lymecycline, and minocycline are less liable to form chelates and therefore only require label 6 (see above).

8 **Warning: Do not stop taking this medicine unless your doctor tells you to stop**

Rhybudd: Peidiwch â stopio cymryd y feddyginiaeth hon, oni bai fod eich meddyg yn dweud wrthych am stopio

To be used on *preparations that contain a drug which is required to be taken over long periods without the patient necessarily perceiving any benefit* (e.g. antituberculous drugs).

Also to be used on *preparations that contain a drug whose withdrawal is likely to be a particular hazard* (e.g. clonidine for hypertension). Label 10 (see below) is more appropriate for corticosteroids.

9 **Space the doses evenly throughout the day. Keep taking this medicine until the course is finished, unless you are told to stop**

Gadewch yr un faint o amser rhwng pob dôs yn ystod y dydd. Parhewch i gymryd y feddyginiaeth nes bod y cyfan wedi'i orffen, oni bai eich bod yn cael cyngor i stopio

To be used on *preparations where a course of treatment should be completed* to reduce the incidence of relapse or failure of treatment.

The preparations are antimicrobial drugs given by mouth. Very occasionally, some may have severe side-effects (e.g. diarrhoea in patients receiving clindamycin) and in such cases the patient may need to be advised of reasons for stopping treatment quickly and returning to the doctor.

10 **Warning: Read the additional information given with this medicine**

Rhybudd: Darllenwch y wybodaeth ychwanegol gyda'r feddyginiaeth hon

To be used particularly on *preparations containing anticoagulants, lithium, and oral corticosteroids*. The appropriate treatment card should be given to the patient and any necessary explanations given.

This label may also be used on other preparations to remind the patient of the instructions that have been given.

11 **Protect your skin from sunlight—even on a bright but cloudy day. Do not use sunbeds**

Diogelwch eich croen rhag golau'r haul, hyd yn oed ar ddiwrnod braf ond cymylog. Peidiwch â defnyddio gwely haul

To be used on *preparations that may cause phototoxic or photoallergic reactions* if the patient is exposed to ultraviolet radiation. Many drugs other than those listed in Appendix 3 (e.g. phenothiazines and sulfonamides) may, on rare occasions, cause reactions in susceptible patients. Exposure to high intensity ultraviolet radiation from sunray lamps and sunbeds is particularly likely to cause reactions.

12 **Do not take anything containing aspirin while taking this medicine**

Peidiwch â chymryd unrhyw beth sy'n cynnwys aspirin gyda'r feddyginiaeth hon

To be used on *preparations containing sulfinpyrazone* whose activity is reduced by aspirin.

Label 12 should not be used for anticoagulants since label 10 is more appropriate.

A3

Cautionary and advisory labels | **Appendix 3**

13 Dissolve or mix with water before taking

Gadewch i doddi mewn dŵr cyn ei gymryd

To be used on *preparations that are intended to be dissolved in water* (e.g. soluble tablets) or *mixed with water* (e.g. powders, granules) before use. In a few cases other liquids such as fruit juice or milk may be used.

14 This medicine may colour your urine. This is harmless

Gall y feddyginiaeth hon liwio eich dŵr. Nid yw hyn yn arwydd o ddrwg

To be used on *preparations that may cause the patient's urine to turn an unusual colour*. These include triamterene (blue under some lights), levodopa (dark reddish), and rifampicin (red).

15 Caution: flammable. Keep your body away from fire or flames after you have put on the medicine

Rhybudd: Fflamadwy. Ar ôl rhoi'r feddyginiaeth ymlaen, cadwch yn glir o dân neu fflamau

To be used on *preparations containing sufficient flammable solvent to render them flammable if exposed to a naked flame.*

16 Dissolve the tablet under your tongue—do not swallow. Store the tablets in this bottle with the cap tightly closed. Get a new supply 8 weeks after opening

Rhowch y dabled i doddi dan eich tafod - peidiwch â'i lyncu. Cadwch y tabledi yn y botel yma gyda'r caead wedi'i gau yn dynn. Gofynnwch am dabledi newydd 8 wythnos ar ôl ei hagor

To be used on *glyceryl trinitrate tablets* to remind the patient not to transfer the tablets to plastic or less suitable containers.

17 Do not take more than... in 24 hours

Peidiwch â chymryd mwy na... mewn 24 awr

To be used on *preparations for the treatment of acute migraine* except those containing ergotamine, for which label 18 is used. The dose form should be specified, e.g. tablets or capsules.

It may also be used on preparations for which no dose has been specified by the prescriber.

18 Do not take more than... in 24 hours. Also, do not take more than... in any one week

Peidiwch â chymryd mwy na... mewn 24 awr. Hefyd, peidiwch â chymryd mwy na... mewn wythnos

To be used on preparations containing ergotamine. The dose form should be specified, e.g. tablets or suppositories.

19 Warning: This medicine makes you sleepy. If you still feel sleepy the next day, do not drive or use tools or machines. Do not drink alcohol

Rhybudd: Bydd y feddyginiaeth hon yn eich gwneud yn gysglyd. Os ydych yn dal i deimlo'n gysglyd drannoeth, peidiwch â gyrru, defnyddio offer llaw neu beiriannau. Peidiwch ag yfed alcohol

To be used on *preparations containing hypnotics (or some other drugs with sedative effects) prescribed to be taken at night*. On the rare occasions when hypnotics are prescribed for daytime administration (e.g. nitrazepam in epilepsy), this label would clearly not be appropriate. Also to be used as an *alternative to the label 2 wording* (the choice being at the discretion of the pharmacist) *for anxiolytics prescribed to be taken at night*.

It is hoped that this wording will convey adequately the problem of residual morning sedation after taking 'sleeping tablets'.

21 Take with or just after food, or a meal

Cymerwch gyda neu ar ôl bwyd

To be used on *preparations that are liable to cause gastric irritation, or those that are better absorbed with food*.

Patients should be advised that a *small amount of food* is sufficient.

22 Take 30 to 60 minutes before food

Cymerwch 30 i 60 munud cyn bwyd

To be used on some preparations *whose absorption is thereby improved*.

Most oral antibacterials require label 23 instead (see below).

23 Take this medicine when your stomach is empty. This means an hour before food or 2 hours after food

Cymerwch y feddyginiaeth hon ar stumog wag. Mae hyn yn golygu awr cyn, neu 2 awr ar ôl bwyd

To be used on *oral antibacterials whose absorption may be reduced by the presence of food and acid in the stomach*.

24 Suck or chew this medicine

Bydd angen cnoi neu sugno'r feddyginiaeth hon

To be used on *preparations that should be sucked or chewed*. The pharmacist should use discretion as to which of these words is appropriate.

25 Swallow this medicine whole. Do not chew or crush

Llyncwch yn gyfan. Peidiwch â chnoi neu falu'n fân

To be used on *preparations that are enteric-coated or designed for modified-release*.

Also to be used on *preparations that taste very unpleasant or may damage the mouth* if not swallowed whole.

Patients should be advised (where relevant) that some modified-release preparations can be broken in half, but that the halved tablet should still be swallowed whole, and not chewed or crushed.

26 Dissolve this medicine under your tongue

Gadewch i'r feddyginiaeth hon doddi o dan y tafod

To be used on *preparations designed for sublingual use*. Patients should be advised to hold under the tongue and avoid swallowing until dissolved. The buccal mucosa between the gum and cheek is occasionally specified by the prescriber.

27 Take with a full glass of water

Cymerwch gyda llond gwydr o ddŵr

To be used on *preparations that should be well diluted* (e.g. chloral hydrate), *where a high fluid intake is required* (e.g. sulfonamides), or *where water is required to aid the action* (e.g. methylcellulose). The patient should be advised that 'a full glass' means at least 150 mL. In most cases fruit juice, tea, or coffee may be used.

28 Spread thinly on the affected skin only

Taenwch yn denau ar y croen sydd wedi'i effeithio yn unig

To be used on *external preparations* that should be applied sparingly (e.g. corticosteroids, dithranol).

29 Do not take more than 2 at any one time. Do not take more than 8 in 24 hours

Peidiwch â chymryd mwy na 2 ar unrhyw un adeg. Peidiwch â chymryd mwy nag 8 mewn 24 awr

To be used on containers of dispensed *solid dose preparations containing paracetamol for adults* when the instruction on the label indicates that the dose can be taken on an 'as required' basis. The dose form should be specified, e.g. tablets or capsules.

This label has been introduced because of the serious consequences of overdosage with paracetamol.

30 Contains paracetamol. Do not take anything else containing paracetamol while taking this medicine. Talk to a doctor at once if you take too much of this medicine, even if you feel well

Yn cynnwys paracetamol. Peidiwch â chymryd unrhyw beth arall sy'n cynnwys paracetamol tra'n cymryd y feddyginiaeth hon. Siaradwch gyda'ch meddyg ar unwaith os ydych yn cymryd gormod, hyd yn oed os ydych yn teimlo'n iawn

To be used on all containers of dispensed *preparations containing paracetamol*.

32 Contains aspirin. Do not take anything else containing aspirin while taking this medicine

Yn cynnwys aspirin. Peidiwch â chymryd unrhyw beth arall sy'n cynnwys aspirin tra'n cymryd y feddyginiaeth hon

To be used on containers of dispensed *preparations containing aspirin when the name on the label does not include the word 'aspirin'*.

Dental Practitioners' Formulary

List of Dental Preparations

The following list has been approved by the appropriate Secretaries of State, and the preparations therein may be prescribed by dental practitioners on form FP10D (GP14 in Scotland, WP10D in Wales).
Licensed **sugar-free** versions, where available, are preferred.
Licensed **alcohol-free** mouthwashes, where available, are preferred.

Aciclovir Cream, BP
Aciclovir Oral Suspension, BP, 200 mg/5 mL
Aciclovir Tablets, BP, 200 mg
Aciclovir Tablets, BP, 800 mg
Amoxicillin Capsules, BP
Amoxicillin Oral Powder, DPF
Amoxicillin Oral Suspension, BP
Artificial Saliva Gel, DPF
Artificial Saliva Oral Spray, DPF
Artificial Saliva Pastilles, DPF
Artificial Saliva Protective Spray, DPF
Artificial Saliva Substitutes as listed below (to be prescribed only for indications approved by ACBS (patients suffering from dry mouth as a result of having or, having undergone, radiotherapy or sicca syndrome):
   BioXtra ® Gel Mouthspray
   BioXtra ® Moisturising Gel
   Glandosane ®
   Saliveze ®
Artificial Saliva Substitute Spray, DPF
Aspirin Tablets, Dispersible, BP
Azithromycin Capsules, 250 mg, DPF
Azithromycin Oral Suspension, 200 mg/5 mL, DPF
Azithromycin Tablets, 250 mg, DPF
Azithromycin Tablets, 500 mg, DPF
Beclometasone Pressurised Inhalation, BP, 50 micrograms/metered inhalation, CFC-free, as:
   Clenil Modulite ®
Benzydamine Mouthwash, BP 0.15%
Benzydamine Oromucosal Spray, BP 0.15%
Betamethasone Soluble Tablets, 500 micrograms, DPF
Carbamazepine Tablets, BP
Cefalexin Capsules, BP
Cefalexin Oral Suspension, BP
Cefalexin Tablets, BP
Cefradine Capsules, BP
Cetirizine Oral Solution, BP, 5 mg/5 mL
Cetirizine Tablets, BP, 10 mg
Chlorhexidine Gluconate Gel, BP
Chlorhexidine Mouthwash, BP
Chlorhexidine Oral Spray, DPF
Chlorphenamine Oral Solution, BP
Chlorphenamine Tablets, BP
Choline Salicylate Dental Gel, BP
Clarithromycin Oral Suspension, 125 mg/5 mL, DPF
Clarithromycin Oral Suspension, 250 mg/5 mL, DPF
Clarithromycin Tablets, BP
Clindamycin Capsules, BP
Co-amoxiclav Tablets, BP, 250/125 (amoxicillin 250 mg as trihydrate, clavulanic acid 125 mg as potassium salt)
Co-amoxiclav Oral Suspension, BP, 125/31 (amoxicillin 125 mg as trihydrate, clavulanic acid 31.25 mg as potassium salt)/5 mL
Co-amoxiclav Oral Suspension, BP, 250/62 (amoxicillin 250 mg as trihydrate, clavulanic acid 62.5 mg as potassium salt)/5 mL
Diazepam Oral Solution, BP, 2 mg/5 mL

Diazepam Tablets, BP
Diclofenac Sodium Tablets, Gastro-resistant, BP
Dihydrocodeine Tablets, BP, 30 mg
Doxycycline Tablets, Dispersible, BP
Doxycycline Capsules, BP, 100 mg
Doxycycline Tablets, 20 mg, DPF
Ephedrine Nasal Drops, BP
Erythromycin Ethyl Succinate Oral Suspension, BP
Erythromycin Ethyl Succinate Tablets, BP
Erythromycin Stearate Tablets, BP
Erythromycin Tablets, Gastro-resistant, BP
Fluconazole Capsules, 50 mg, DPF
Fluconazole Oral Suspension, 50 mg/5 mL, DPF
Hydrocortisone Cream, BP, 1%
Hydrocortisone Oromucosal Tablets, BP
Hydrogen Peroxide Mouthwash, BP, 6%
Ibuprofen Oral Suspension, BP, sugar-free
Ibuprofen Tablets, BP
Lansoprazole Capsules, Gastro-resistant, BP
Lidocaine Ointment, BP, 5%
Lidocaine Spray 10%, DPF
Loratadine Syrup, 5 mg/5 mL, DPF
Loratadine Tablets, BP, 10 mg
Menthol and Eucalyptus Inhalation, BP 1980
Metronidazole Oral Suspension, BP
Metronidazole Tablets, BP
Miconazole Cream, BP
Miconazole Oromucosal Gel, BP
Miconazole and Hydrocortisone Cream, BP
Miconazole and Hydrocortisone Ointment, BP
Nystatin Oral Suspension, BP
Omeprazole Capsules, Gastro-resistant, BP
Oxytetracycline Tablets, BP
Paracetamol Oral Suspension, BP
Paracetamol Tablets, BP
Paracetamol Tablets, Soluble, BP
Phenoxymethylpenicillin Oral Solution, BP
Phenoxymethylpenicillin Tablets, BP
Promethazine Hydrochloride Tablets, BP
Promethazine Oral Solution, BP
Saliva Stimulating Tablets, DPF
Sodium Chloride Mouthwash, Compound, BP
Sodium Fluoride Mouthwash, BP
Sodium Fluoride Oral Drops, BP
Sodium Fluoride Tablets, BP
Sodium Fluoride Toothpaste 0.619%, DPF
Sodium Fluoride Toothpaste 1.1%, DPF
Sodium Fusidate Ointment, BP
Temazepam Oral Solution, BP
Temazepam Tablets, BP
Tetracycline Tablets, BP

Nurse Prescribers' Formulary

Nurse Prescribers' Formulary for Community Practitioners

List of preparations approved by the Secretary of State which may be prescribed on form FP10P (form HS21(N) in Northern Ireland, form GP10(N) in Scotland, forms WP10CN and WP10PN in Wales) by Nurses for National Health Service patients.

Community practitioners who have completed the necessary training may only prescribe items appearing in the nurse prescribers' list set out below. Community Practitioner Nurse Prescribers are recommended to prescribe generically, except where this would not be clinically appropriate or where there is no approved generic name.

Medicinal Preparations

Preparations on this list which are not included in the BP or BPC are described under Details of NPF preparations (p. 1021).

Almond Oil Ear Drops, BP
Arachis Oil Enema, NPF
Aspirin Tablets, Dispersible, 300 mg, BP (max. 96 tablets; max. pack size 32 tablets)
Bisacodyl Suppositories, BP (includes 5-mg and 10-mg strengths)
Bisacodyl Tablets, BP
Catheter Maintenance Solution, Sodium Chloride, NPF
Catheter Maintenance Solution, 'Solution G', NPF
Catheter Maintenance Solution, 'Solution R', NPF
Chlorhexidine Gluconate Alcoholic Solutions containing at least 0.05%
Chlorhexidine Gluconate Aqueous Solutions containing at least 0.05%
Choline Salicylate Dental Gel, BP
Clotrimazole Cream 1%, BP
Co-danthramer Capsules, NPF
Co-danthramer Capsules, Strong, NPF
Co-danthramer Oral Suspension, NPF
Co-danthramer Oral Suspension, Strong, NPF
Co-danthrusate Capsules, NPF
Co-danthrusate Oral Suspension, NPF
Crotamiton Cream, BP
Crotamiton Lotion, BP
Dimeticone barrier creams containing at least 10%
Dimeticone Lotion, NPF
Docusate Capsules, BP
Docusate Enema, NPF
Docusate Oral Solution, BP
Docusate Oral Solution, Paediatric, BP
Econazole Cream 1%, BP
Emollients as listed below:
  Aquadrate® 10% w/w Cream
  Arachis Oil, BP
  Balneum® Plus Cream
  Cetraben® Emollient Cream
  Dermamist®
  Diprobase® Cream
  Diprobase® Ointment
  Doublebase®
  Doublebase® Dayleve Gel
  E45® Cream
  E45® Itch Relief Cream
  Emulsifying Ointment, BP
  Eucerin® Intensive 10% w/w Urea Treatment Cream
  Eucerin® Intensive 10% w/w Urea Treatment Lotion

  Hydromol® Cream
  Hydromol® Intensive
  Hydrous Ointment, BP
  Lipobase®
  Liquid and White Soft Paraffin Ointment, NPF
  Neutrogena® Norwegian Formula Dermatological Cream
  Nutraplus® Cream
  Oilatum® Cream
  Oilatum® Junior Cream
  Paraffin, White Soft, BP
  Paraffin, Yellow Soft, BP
  Ultrabase®
  Unguentum M®
Emollient Bath and Shower Preparations as listed below:
  Aqueous Cream, BP
  Balneum® (except pack sizes that are not to be prescribed under the NHS (see Part XVIIIA of the Drug Tariff, Part XI of the Northern Ireland Drug Tariff))
  Balneum Plus® Bath Oil (except pack sizes that are not to be prescribed under the NHS (see Part XVIIIA of the Drug Tariff, Part XI of the Northern Ireland Drug Tariff))
  Cetraben® Emollient Bath Additive
  Dermalo® Bath Emollient
  Doublebase® Emollient Bath Additive
  Doublebase® Emollient Shower Gel
  Doublebase® Emollient Wash Gel
  Hydromol® Bath and Shower Emollient
  Oilatum® Emollient
  Oilatum® Gel
  Oilatum® Junior Bath Additive
  Zerolatum® Emollient Medicinal Bath Oil
Folic Acid Tablets 400 micrograms, BP
Glycerol Suppositories, BP
Ibuprofen Oral Suspension, BP (except for indications and doses that are prescription-only)
Ibuprofen Tablets, BP (except for indications and doses that are prescription-only)
Ispaghula Husk Granules, BP
Ispaghula Husk Granules, Effervescent, BP
Ispaghula Husk Oral Powder, BP
Lactulose Solution, BP
Lidocaine Ointment, BP
Lidocaine and Chlorhexidine Gel, BP
Macrogol Oral Liquid, Compound, NPF
Macrogol Oral Powder, Compound, NPF
Macrogol Oral Powder, Compound, Half-strength, NPF
Magnesium Hydroxide Mixture, BP
Magnesium Sulfate Paste, BP
Malathion aqueous lotions containing at least 0.5%
Mebendazole Oral Suspension, NPF
Mebendazole Tablets, NPF
Methylcellulose Tablets, BP
Miconazole Cream 2%, BP
Miconazole Oromucosal Gel, BP
Mouthwash Solution-tablets, NPF
Nicotine Inhalation Cartridge for Oromucosal Use, NPF
Nicotine Lozenge, NPF
Nicotine Medicated Chewing Gum, NPF
Nicotine Nasal Spray, NPF
Nicotine Oral Spray, NPF
Nicotine Sublingual Tablets, NPF
Nicotine Transdermal Patches, NPF
Nystatin Oral Suspension, BP
Olive Oil Ear Drops, BP

Paracetamol Oral Suspension, BP (includes 120 mg/5 mL and 250 mg/5 mL strengths—both of which are available as sugar-free formulations)
Paracetamol Tablets, BP (max. 96 tablets; max. pack size 32 tablets)
Paracetamol Tablets, Soluble, BP (includes 120-mg and 500-mg tablets; max. 96 tablets; max. pack size 32 tablets)
Permethrin Cream, NPF
Phosphates Enema, BP
Povidone–Iodine Solution, BP
Senna Oral Solution, NPF
Senna Tablets, BP
Senna and Ispaghula Granules, NPF
Sodium Chloride Solution, Sterile, BP
Sodium Citrate Compound Enema, NPF
Sodium Picosulfate Capsules, NPF
Sodium Picosulfate Elixir, NPF
Spermicidal contraceptives as listed below:
  Gygel® Contraceptive Jelly
Sterculia Granules, NPF
Sterculia and Frangula Granules, NPF
Titanium Ointment, BP
Water for Injections, BP
Zinc and Castor Oil Ointment, BP
Zinc Oxide and Dimeticone Spray, NPF
Zinc Oxide Impregnated Medicated Bandage, NPF
Zinc Oxide Impregnated Medicated Stocking, NPF
Zinc Paste Bandage, BP 1993
Zinc Paste and Ichthammol Bandage, BP 1993

Appliances and Reagents (including Wound Management Products)

Community Practitioner Nurse Prescribers in England, Wales and Northern Ireland can prescribe any appliance or reagent in the relevant Drug Tariff. In the Scottish Drug Tariff, Appliances and Reagents which may **not** be prescribed by Nurses are annotated **Nx**.

Appliances (including Contraceptive Devices) as listed in Part IXA of the Drug Tariff (Part III of the Northern Ireland Drug Tariff, Part 3 (Appliances) and Part 2 (Dressings) of the Scottish Drug Tariff). (Where it is not appropriate for nurse prescribers in family planning clinics to prescribe contraceptive devices using form FP10(P) (forms WP10CN and WP10PN in Wales), they may prescribe using the same system as doctors in the clinic.)

Incontinence Appliances as listed in Part IXB of the Drug Tariff (Part III of the Northern Ireland Drug Tariff, Part 5 of the Scottish Drug Tariff).

Stoma Appliances and Associated Products as listed in Part IXC of the Drug Tariff (Part III of the Northern Ireland Drug Tariff, Part 6 of the Scottish Drug Tariff).

Chemical Reagents as listed in Part IXR of the Drug Tariff (Part II of the Northern Ireland Drug Tariff, Part 9 of the Scottish Drug Tariff).

The Drug Tariffs can be accessed online at:
National Health Service Drug Tariff for England and Wales: www.ppa.org.uk/ppa/edt_intro.htm
Health and Personal Social Services for Northern Ireland Drug Tariff: www.hscbusiness.hscni.net/services/2034.htm
Scottish Drug Tariff: www.isdscotland.org/Health-topics/Prescribing-and-Medicines/Scottish-Drug-Tariff/

Details of NPF preparations

Preparations on the Nurse Prescribers' Formulary which are not included in the BP or BPC are described as follows in the Nurse Prescribers' Formulary. Although brand names have sometimes been included for identification purposes, it is recommended that non-proprietary names should be used

for prescribing medicinal preparations in the NPF except where a non-proprietary name is not available.

Arachis Oil Enema
arachis oil 100%
Catheter Maintenance Solution, Sodium Chloride
(proprietary products: *OptiFlo S; Uro-Tainer Sodium Chloride; Uriflex-S*), sodium chloride 0.9%
Catheter Maintenance Solution, 'Solution G'
(proprietary products: *OptiFlo G; Uro-Tainer Suby G; Uriflex G*), citric acid 3.23%, magnesium oxide 0.38%, sodium bicarbonate 0.7%, disodium edetate 0.01%
Catheter Maintenance Solution, 'Solution R'
(proprietary products: *OptiFlo R; Uro-Tainer Solution R; Uriflex R*), citric acid 6%, gluconolactone 0.6%, magnesium carbonate 2.8%, disodium edetate 0.01%
Chlorhexidine Gluconate Alcoholic Solutions
(proprietary products: *ChloraPrep; Hydrex Solution; Hydrex spray*), chlorhexidine gluconate in alcoholic solution
Chlorhexidine Gluconate Aqueous Solutions
(proprietary product: *Unisept*), chlorhexidine gluconate in aqueous solution
Co-danthramer Capsules [PoM]
co-danthramer 25/200 (dantron 25 mg, poloxamer '188' 200 mg)
Co-danthramer Capsules, Strong [PoM]
co-danthramer 37.5/500 (dantron 37.5 mg, poloxamer '188' 500 mg)
Co-danthramer Oral Suspension [PoM]
(proprietary product: *Codalax*), co-danthramer 25/200 in 5 mL (dantron 25 mg, poloxamer '188' 200 mg/5 mL)
Co-danthramer Oral Suspension, Strong [PoM]
(proprietary product: *Codalax Forte*), co-danthramer 75/1000 in 5 mL (dantron 75 mg, poloxamer '188' 1 g/5 mL)
Co-danthrusate Oral Suspension [PoM]
(proprietary product: *Normax*), co-danthrusate 50/60 (dantron 50 mg, docusate sodium 60 mg/5 mL)
Dimeticone Barrier Creams
(proprietary products *Conotrane Cream*, dimeticone '350' 22%; *Siopel Barrier Cream*, dimeticone '1000' 10%), dimeticone 10–22%
Dimeticone Lotion
(proprietary product: *Hedrin*), dimeticone 4%
Docusate Enema
(proprietary product: *Norgalax Micro-enema*), docusate sodium 120 mg in 10 g
Liquid and White Soft Paraffin Ointment
liquid paraffin 50%, white soft paraffin 50%
Macrogol Oral Liquid, Compound
(proprietary product: *Movicol Liquid*), macrogol '3350' (polyethylene glycol '3350') 13.125 g, sodium bicarbonate 178.5 mg, sodium chloride 350.7 mg, potassium chloride 46.6 mg/25 mL
Macrogol Oral Powder, Compound
(proprietary products: *Laxido Orange, Molaxole, Movicol*), macrogol '3350' (polyethylene glycol '3350') 13.125 g, sodium bicarbonate 178.5 mg, sodium chloride 350.7 mg, potassium chloride 46.6 mg/sachet; (amount of potassium chloride varies according to flavour of *Movicol*® as follows: plain-flavour (sugar-free) = 50.2 mg/sachet; lime and lemon flavour = 46.6 mg/sachet; chocolate flavour = 31.7 mg/sachet. 1 sachet when reconstituted with 125 mL water provides K⁺ 5.4 mmol/litre)
Macrogol Oral Powder, Compound, Half-strength
(proprietary product: *Movicol-Half*), macrogol '3350' (polyethylene glycol '3350') 6.563 g, sodium bicarbonate 89.3 g, sodium chloride 175.4 mg, potassium chloride 23.3 mg/sachet
Malathion Aqueous Lotions
(proprietary products: *Derbac-M Liquid*), malathion 0.5% in an aqueous basis
Mebendazole Oral Suspension [PoM]
(proprietary product: *Vermox*), mebendazole 100 mg/5 mL

Mebendazole Tablets PoM
(proprietary products: *Ovex, Vermox*), mebendazole 100 mg
(can be supplied for oral use in the treatment of enterobiasis
in adults and children over 2 years provided its container or
package is labelled to show a max. single dose of 100 mg and
it is supplied in a container or package containing not more
than 800 mg)

Mouthwash Solution-tablets
consist of tablets which may contain antimicrobial,
colouring and flavouring agents in a suitable soluble
effervescent basis to make a mouthwash

Nicotine Inhalation Cartridge for Oromucosal Use
(proprietary products: *NicAssist Inhalator, Nicorette
Inhalator*), nicotine 15 mg (for use with inhalation
mouthpiece; to be prescribed as either a starter pack
(6 cartridges with inhalator device and holder) or refill pack
(42 cartridges with inhalator device))

Nicotine Lozenge
nicotine (as bitartrate) 1 mg or 2 mg (proprietary product:
Nicorette Mint Lozenge, Nicotinell Mint Lozenge), or nicotine
(as resinate) 1.5 mg, 2 mg, or 4 mg (proprietary product:
NiQuitin Lozenges, NiQuitin Minis, NiQuitin Pre-quit)

Nicotine Medicated Chewing Gum
(proprietary products: *NicAssist Gum, Nicorette Gum,
Nicotinell Gum, NiQuitin Gum*), nicotine 2 mg or 4 mg

Nicotine Nasal Spray
(proprietary product: *NicAssist Nasal Spray, Nicorette Nasal
Spray*), nicotine 500 micrograms/metered spray

Nicotine Oral Spray
(proprietary product: *Nicorette Quickmist*), nicotine
1 mg/metered spray

Nicotine Sublingual Tablets
(proprietary product: *NicAssist Microtab, Nicorette Microtab*),
nicotine (as a cyclodextrin complex) 2 mg (to be prescribed
as either a starter pack (2 × 15-tablet discs with dispenser)
or refill pack (7 × 15-tablet discs))

Nicotine Transdermal Patches
releasing in each 16 hours, nicotine approx. 5 mg, 10 mg, or
15 mg (proprietary products: *Boots NicAssist Patch, Nicorette
Patch*), or releasing in each 16 hours approx. 10 mg, 15 mg, or
25 mg (proprietary products: *NicAssist Translucent Patch,
Nicorette Invisi Patch*), or releasing in each 24 hours nicotine
approx. 7 mg, 14 mg, or 21 mg (proprietary products:
Nicopatch, Nicotinell TTS, NiQuitin, NiQuitin Clear)
(prescriber should specify the brand to be dispensed)

Permethrin Cream
(proprietary product: *Lyclear Dermal Cream*), permethrin 5%

Senna Oral Solution
(proprietary product: *Senokot Syrup*), sennosides 7.5 mg/5 mL

Senna and Ispaghula Granules
(proprietary product: *Manevac Granules*), senna fruit 12.4%,
ispaghula 54.2%

Sodium Citrate Compound Enema
(proprietary products: *Micolette Micro-enema; Micralax
Micro-enema; Relaxit Micro-enema*), sodium citrate 450 mg
with glycerol, sorbitol and an anionic surfactant

Sodium Picosulfate Capsules
(proprietary products: *Dulcolax Perles*), sodium picosulfate
2.5 mg

Sodium Picosulfate Elixir
(proprietary product: *Dulcolax Liquid*), sodium picosulfate
5 mg/5 mL

Sterculia Granules
(proprietary product: *Normacol Granules*), sterculia 62%

Sterculia and Frangula Granules
(proprietary product: *Normacol Plus Granules*), sterculia 62%,
frangula (standardised) 8%

Zinc Oxide and Dimeticone Spray
(proprietary product: *Sprilon*), dimeticone 1.04%, zinc oxide
12.5% in a pressurised aerosol unit

Zinc Oxide Impregnated Medicated Bandage
(proprietary product: *Steripaste*), sterile cotton bandage
impregnated with paste containing zinc oxide 15%

Zinc Oxide Impregnated Medicated Stocking
(proprietary product: *Zipzoc*), sterile rayon stocking
impregnated with ointment containing zinc oxide 20%

Non-medical prescribing

Overview

A range of non-medical healthcare professionals can prescribe medicines for patients as either Independent or Supplementary Prescribers.

Independent prescribers are practitioners responsible and accountable for the assessment of patients with previously undiagnosed or diagnosed conditions and for decisions about the clinical management required, including prescribing. They are recommended to prescribe generically, except where this would not be clinically appropriate or where there is no approved non-proprietary name.

Supplementary prescribing is a partnership between an independent prescriber (a doctor or a dentist) and a supplementary prescriber to implement an agreed Clinical Management Plan for an individual patient with that patient's agreement.

Independent and Supplementary Prescribers are identified by an annotation next to their name in the relevant professional register.

Information and guidance on non-medical prescribing is available on the Department of Health website at www.dh.gov.uk/health/2012/04/prescribing-change.

For information on the mixing of medicines by Independent and Supplementary Prescribers, see *Mixing of medicines prior to administration in clinical practice—responding to legislative changes*, National Prescribing Centre, May 2010 (available at https://www.webarchive.org.uk/wayback/archive/2014627111725/http://www.npc.nhs.uk/improving_safety/mixing_meds/resources/mixing_of_medicines.pdf).

For information on the supply and administration of medicines to groups of patients using Patient Group Directions see Guidance on prescribing p. 1.

Nurses

Nurse Independent Prescribers (formerly known as Extended Formulary Nurse Prescribers) are able to prescribe any medicine for any medical condition.

Nurse Independent Prescribers are able to prescribe, administer, and give directions for the administration of Schedule 2, 3, 4, and 5 Controlled Drugs. This extends to diamorphine, dipipanone, or cocaine for treating organic disease or injury, but not for treating addiction.

Nurse Independent Prescribers must work within their own level of professional competence and expertise.

The Nurse Prescribers' Formulary for Community Practitioners p. 1020 provides information on prescribing.

Pharmacists

Pharmacist Independent Prescribers can prescribe any medicine for any medical condition.

They are also able to prescribe, administer, and give directions for the administration of Schedule 2, 3, 4, and 5 Controlled Drugs. This extends to diamorphine, dipipanone, or cocaine for treating organic disease or injury, but not for treating addiction.

Pharmacist Independent Prescribers must work within their own level of professional competence and expertise.

Optometrists

Optometrist Independent Prescribers can prescribe any licensed medicine for ocular conditions affecting the eye and the tissues surrounding the eye, except Controlled Drugs or medicines for parenteral administration.

Optometrist Independent Prescribers must work within their own level of professional competence and expertise.

Index of proprietary manufacturers

Alphabetical list of manufactuerers and other companies.

The following is an alphabetical list of manufacturers and other companies referenced in the BNF, with their medicines information or general contact details. For information on 'special-order' manufacturers and specialist importing companies see 'Special-order manufacturers'.

3M Health Care Ltd, Tel: (01509) 611 611

Allen & Hanburys Ltd, Tel: 0800 221 441, customercontactuk@gsk.com

A1 Pharmaceuticals Plc, Tel: (01708) 528 900, sales@a1plc.co.uk

Abbot, Tel: (01628) 773 355

Abbott Healthcare Products Ltd, Tel: (01628) 773 355, medinfo.shl@abbott.com

AbbVie Ltd, Tel: (01628) 561 090, ukmedinfo@abbvie.com

Abraxis BioScience Ltd, Tel: (020) 7081 0850, abraxismedical@idispharma.com

Acorus Therapeutics Ltd, Tel: (01244) 625 152

Actavis UK Ltd, a subsidary of Accord Healthcare Ltd, Tel: (01271) 385 267, medinfo@accord-healthcare.com

Actelion Pharmaceuticals UK Ltd, Tel: (020) 8987 3333, medinfo_uk@actelion.com

Activa Healthcare, Tel: 0845 060 6707, advice@activahealthcare.co.uk

Adienne Pharma and Biotech, Tel: 0039 (0) 335 873 8731

ADI Medical UK, Tel: (01628) 485159, info@adimedical.co.uk

Advanced Medical Solutions Group Plc, Tel: (01606) 863 500

Advancis Medical Ltd, Tel: (01623) 751 500, info@advancis.co.uk

Advantech Surgical Ltd, Tel: 0845 130 5866, customerservice@newgel.co.uk

Aegerion Pharmaceuticals Ltd, Tel: 00800 2343 7466, medinfo.emea@aegerion.com

AgaMatrix Europe Ltd, Tel: (01235) 838 639, info@wavesense.co.uk

Agepha GmbH, Tel: (020) 3239 6241, uk@agepha.com

Aguettant Ltd, Tel: (01275) 463 691, info@aguettant.co.uk

Air Products Plc, Tel: 0800 373 580

Alan Pharmaceuticals, Tel: (020) 7284 2887, info@alanpharmaceuticals.com

Alcon Laboratories (UK) Ltd, Tel: 0345 266 9363, gbmedicaldepartment@alcon.com

Alexion Pharma UK Ltd, Tel: (01932) 359 220, alexion.uk@alxn.com

Alimera Sciences Limited, Tel: 0800 019 1253, medicalinformation@alimerasciences.com

Alissa Healthcare, Tel: (01489) 80 759, enquiries@alissahealthcare.com

ALK-Abelló (UK) Ltd, Tel: (0118) 903 7940, info@uk.alk-abello.com

Alkopharma Sarl, Tel: (0041) 277 206 969, regulatory@alkopharma.com

Allergan Ltd, Tel: (01628) 494 026

Allergy Therapeutics Ltd, Tel: (01903) 844 702

Alliance Pharmaceuticals Ltd, Tel: (01249) 466 966, info@alliancepharma.co.uk

Almirall Ltd, Tel: 0800 008 7399, medinfouk@almirall.com

Altacor Ltd, Tel: (01223) 421 411, info@altacorpharma.com

Amdipharm Mercury Company Ltd, Tel: 08700 70 30 33, medicalinformation@amcolimited.com

Amgen Ltd, Tel: (01223) 420 305, gbinfoline@amgen.com

Abbot Medical Optics, Tel: 0800 376 7950

Amred Healthcare Ltd, Tel: (0330) 333 0079, info@amredhealthcare.com

Amryt Pharma, Tel: 00800 234 37466, medinfo@amrytpharma.com

Apollo Medical Technologies Ltd, Tel: (01636) 831 201, supercheck2@btinternet.com

Archimed, Tel: 0800 756 9951, enquiries@archimed.co.uk

Archimedes Pharma UK Ltd, Tel: (0118) 931 5094, medicalinformationuk@archimedespharma.com

Arctic Medical Ltd, Tel: (01303) 277 751, sales@arcticmedical.co.uk

Ardana Bioscience Ltd, Tel: (0131) 226 8550

ARIAD Pharma UK Ltd, Tel: 0800 0002 7423, eumedinfo@ariad.com

Ark Therapeutics Group Plc, Tel: (020) 7388 7722, info@arktherapeutics.com

Aspen, Tel: 0800 008 7392, aspenmedinfo@professionalinformation.co.uk

Aspen Medical Europe Ltd, Tel: (01527) 587 728, customers@aspenmedicaleurope.com

AS Pharma Ltd, Tel: 0870 066 4117, info@aspharma.co.uk

Aspire Pharma Ltd, Tel: (01730) 231 148, info@aspirepharma.co.uk

Astellas Pharma Ltd, Tel: (020) 3379 8000, medinfo.gb@astellas.com

AstraZeneca UK Ltd, Tel: 0800 783 0033, medical.informationuk@astrazeneca.com

Auden Mckenzie (Pharma Division) Ltd, Tel: (01895) 627 420

Auxilium, Tel: 0845 017 2315, auxilium@pilglobal.com

Axcan Pharma SA, Tel: (0033) 130 461 900

AYMES International Ltd, Tel: 0845 6805 496, info@aymes.com

Ayrton Saunders Ltd, Tel: (0151) 709 2074, info@ayrtons.com

BAP Medical UK Ltd, Tel: 0844 879 7689

Bard Ltd, Tel: (01293) 527 888

Basilea Pharmaceuticals Ltd, Tel: (01483) 790 023, ukmedinfo@basilea.com

Bausch & Lomb UK Ltd, Tel: (01748) 828 864, medicalinformationuk@bausch.com

Baxalta UK Limited, Tel: (01635) 798 777, medinfo.emea@baxalta.com

Baxter Healthcare Ltd, Tel: (01635) 206 345, surecall@baxter.com

Bayer Healthcare Pharmaceuticals, Tel: (01635) 563 000, medical.information@bayer.co.uk

BBI Healthcare, Tel: (01792) 229 333, info@bbihealthcare.com

B. Braun Medical Ltd, Tel: (0114) 225 9000, info.bbmuk@bbraun.com

Beacon Pharmaceuticals Ltd, Tel: (01892) 600 930, info@beaconpharma.co.uk

Beiersdorf UK Ltd, Tel: (0121) 329 8800

Besins Healthcare (UK) Ltd, Tel: (01748) 828 789, information@besins-healthcare.com

BGP Products Ltd, Tel: (01707) 853 000, medinfo.shl@mylan.com

BHR Pharmaceuticals Ltd, Tel: (024) 7637 7210, info@bhr.co.uk

Bial Pharma UK Ltd, Tel: 01753 916 010, medinfo.uk@bial.com

Biogen Idec Ltd, Tel: 0800 008 7401

Biolitec Pharma Ltd, Tel: (00353) 1463 7415

BioMarin Europe Ltd, Tel: (020) 7420 0800, biomarin-europe@bmrn.com

BioMonde, Tel: 0845 230 1810, info@biomonde.com

Biotest (UK) Ltd, Tel: (0121) 733 3393, medicinesinformation@biotestuk.com

Blackwell Supplies Ltd, Tel: (01634) 877 620

BOC Medical, Tel: 0800 111 333

Boehringer Ingelheim Ltd, Tel: (01344) 424 600, medinfo@bra.boehringer-ingelheim.com

The Boots Company PLC, Tel: (0115) 959 5165

BPC 100 Ltd, Tel: 01942 852085

Bio Products Laboratory Ltd, Tel: (020) 8957 2255, medinfo@bpl.co.uk

Brancaster Pharma Ltd, Tel: (01737) 243 407, enquiries@brancasterpharma.com

Bray Healthcare, Tel: (01367) 240 736, info@bray-healthcare.com

Bristol Laboratories Ltd, Tel: (0) 1442 200 922, info@bristol-labs.co.uk

Bristol-Myers Squibb Pharmaceuticals Ltd, Tel: (01895) 523 000, medical.information@bms.com

Britannia Pharmaceuticals, Tel: 0870 851 0207, enquiries@medinformation.co.uk

BSN Medical Ltd, Tel: 0845 122 3600

BTG International Ltd, Tel: (0207) 575 0000, medical.services@btgplc.com

Bullen Healthcare, Tel: 0800 269 327

Cambridge Medical Aesthetics Ltd, Tel: (01733) 396171, info@cambridgemedicalaesthetics.com

Cambridge Sensors Ltd, Tel: (01480) 482 920, sales-orders@cs-limited.co.uk

CareFusion UK 244 Ltd, Tel: 0800 043 7546, enquiries@chloraprep.co.uk

Casen-Fleet, Tel: (0034) 913 518 800

C D Medical Ltd, Tel: (01942) 816 184

Celgene Ltd, Tel: 0844 801 0045, medinfo.uk.ire@celgene.com

iMed Systems Ltd, Tel: (0203) 397 8020, emerade@imed-systems.com

INCA-Pharm UK, Tel: (01748) 828 812, info@inca-pharm.com

Infai UK Ltd, Tel: (01904) 435 228, info@infai.co.uk

Injex UK Ltd, Tel: 0845 126 8900, enquiries@injexuk.com

Innovative Solutions UK Ltd, Tel: (01706) 746 713, enquiries@innovative-solutions.org.uk

Insight Medical Products Ltd, Tel: (01666) 500 055, info@insightmedical.ne

InterMune, Tel: (03308) 080 960, med-info@intermune.co.uk

Internis Pharmaceuticals Ltd, Tel: 0870 851 0207, enquiries@medinformation.co.uk

Intrapharm Laboratories Ltd, Tel: (01628) 771 800, sales@intrapharmlabs.com

Ipsen Ltd, Tel: (01753) 627 777, medical.information.uk@ipsen.com

Iroko Cardio GmbH, Tel: (020) 3002 8114, info@irokocardio.com

Johnson & Johnson Ltd, Tel: (01628) 822 222, medinfo@congb.jnj.com

Janssen-Cilag Ltd, Tel: 0800 731 8450, medinfo@its.jnj.com

Jobskin Ltd, Tel: (0115) 973 4300, dw@jobskin.co.uk

Juvela (Hero UK) Ltd, Tel: (0151) 432 5300, info@juvela.co.uk

K/L Pharmaceuticals Ltd, Tel: (01294) 215 951

KCI Medical Ltd, Tel: (01865) 840 600

Kestrel Ophthalmics Ltd, Tel: (01202) 658 444, info@kestrelophthalmics.co.uk

King Pharmaceuticals Ltd, Tel: (01438) 356 924

KoRa Healthcare Ltd, Tel: 0845 303 8631, info@kora.ie

Kyowa Kirin Ltd, Tel: (01896) 664 000, medinfo@kyowakirin.com

Labopharm Europe Ltd, Tel: 0800 028 0037, medinfo@paladin-labs.com

Laboratoires CTRS, ctrsgb@pi-arm.co.uk

LaCorium Health (UK) Ltd, Tel: 0800 158 8233, ukinfo@flexitol.com

Lantor UK Ltd, Tel: (01204) 855 000, help@lantor.co.uk

LEO Laboratories Ltd, Tel: (01844) 347 333, medical-info.uk@leo-pharma.com

LifeScan, Tel: 0800 001 210

Eli Lilly & Co Ltd, Tel: (01256) 315 000, ukmedinfo@lilly.com

Lincoln Medical Ltd, Tel: (01722) 742 900, info@lincolnmedical.co.uk

Linderma Ltd, Tel: (01942) 816 184, linderma@virgin.ne

Lipomed GmbH, Tel: (0041) 6170 20200, save@lipomed.com

Livwell Ltd, Tel: 0845 120 0038, info@livwell.eu

LogixX Pharma Solutions Ltd, Tel: (01189) 011 747, medinfo@logixxpharma.com

Lornamead UK Ltd, Tel: (01276) 674000, lornamead@dhl.com

LPC Pharmaceuticals Ltd, Tel: (01582) 560 393, info@lpcpharma.com

Lucane Pharma, Tel: 0033 (0) 153 868 750, info@lucanepharma.com

Lundbeck Ltd, Tel: (01908) 649 966, ukmedicalinformation@lundbeck.com

L'Oréal Active Cosmetics UK, Tel: 0800 055 6822

M & A Pharmachem Ltd, Tel: (01942) 816 184

Manuka Medical Ltd, Tel: (01623) 600 669

Manx Healthcare, Tel: (01926) 482 511, info@manxhealthcare.com

Marlborough Pharmaceuticals, Tel: (01279) 406 759, info@marlborough-pharma.co.uk

Martindale Pharma, Tel: (01277) 266 600, medinfo@martindalepharma.co.uk

MASTA, Tel: (0113) 238 7500, medical@masta.org

McNeil Products Ltd, Tel: (01628) 822 222

Medical Diagnostics Europe Ltd, Tel: 0845 370 8077, info@mdediagnostic.co.uk

Mead Johnson Nutrition, Tel: (01895) 230 575

Meadow Laboratories Ltd, Tel: (020) 8597 1203

Meda Pharmaceuticals Ltd, Tel: (01748) 828 810, meda@professionalinformation.co.uk

Medac (UK), Tel: (01786) 458 086, info@medac-uk.co.uk

Medical Developments UK Ltd, Tel: 0870 850 1234, enquiries@ashfieldin2focus.com

Medicare Plus International Ltd, Tel: (020) 8810 8811, info@medicare-plus.com

Medicom Healthcare Ltd, Tel: (01489) 574 119, info@medicomhealthcare.com

Medihoney (Europe) Ltd, Tel: 0800 071 3912

Medisana, Tel: +49 (0) 2131/36 68 0

Medlock Medical Ltd, Tel: (0161) 621 2100

MedLogic Global Ltd, Tel: (01752) 209 955, enquiries@mlgl.co.uk

A. Menarini Farmaceutica Internazionale SRL, Tel: (01628) 856 400, menarini@medinformation.co.uk

A. Menarini Diagnostics, Tel: (0118) 944 4100

Merck Serono Ltd, Tel: (020) 8818 7200, medinfo.uk@merckserono.net

Merck Sharp & Dohme Ltd, Tel: (01992) 467 272, medicalinformationuk@merck.com

Merus Labs, Tel: 00352 (0) 2637 5878, qchs.mi@quintiles.com

Merz Pharma UK Ltd, Tel: (020) 8236 0000, info@merzpharma.co.uk

Micro Medical Ltd, Tel: (01634) 893 500

Milupa Aptamil, Tel: 0845 762 3676, careline@aptamil4hcps.co.uk

Mitsubishi Pharma, Tel: (0207) 382 9000, medinfo@mitsubishi-pharma.eu

Mölnlycke Health Care Ltd, Tel: (0161) 777 2628, info.uk@molnlycke.net

Moorfields Pharmaceuticals, Tel: (020) 7684 9090

Morningside Healthcare Ltd, Tel: (0116) 204 5950

Movianto UK, Tel: (01234) 248 500, movianto.uk@movianto.com

Mylan, Tel: (01707) 853 000, info@mylan.co.uk

Nagor Ltd, Tel: (01624) 625 556, enquiries@nagor.com

Nairn's Oatcakes Ltd, Tel: (0131) 620 7000

Napp Pharmaceuticals Ltd, Tel: (01223) 424 444

Neoceuticals Ltd, Tel: (01748) 828 865

Neolab Ltd, Tel: (01256) 704 110, info@neolab.co.uk

Neomedic Ltd, Tel: (01923) 836 379, marketing@neomedic.co.uk

Neon Diagnostics Ltd, Tel: (01376) 500 720

Nestlé Nutrition, Tel: 00800 6887 4846, nestlehealthcarenutrition@uk.nestle.com

Newport Pharmaceuticals Ltd, Tel: (00353) 1890 3011

Nicox Pharma, Tel: (01483) 549 211, ukmedicalinformation@nicox.com

Northern Ireland Blood Transfusion Service, Tel: (028) 9032 1414, inet@nibts.hscni.net

Nipro Diagnostics (UK) Ltd, Tel: 0800 08 588 08, info@homediagnostics-uk.com

Nordic Pharma UK Ltd, Tel: (0118) 929 8233, info@nordicpharma.co.uk

Norgine Pharmaceuticals Ltd, Tel: (01895) 826 600, medinfo@norgine.com

Nova Laboratories Ltd, Tel: 08707 120 655, xaluprine@aptivsolutions.com

Novartis Pharmaceuticals UK Ltd, Tel: (01276) 692 255, medinfo.uk@novartis.com

Novartis Consumer Health, Tel: (01276) 687 202, medicalaffairs.uk@novartis.com

Novartis Vaccines Ltd, Tel: 0845 745 1500, service.uk@novartis.com

Novo Nordisk Ltd, Tel: (01293) 613 555

nSPIRE Health Ltd, Tel: (01992) 526 300, info@nspirehealth.com

Nualtra Ltd, Tel: 0808 101 0926, support@nualtra.co.uk

Nutricia, Tel: (01225) 751 098, resourcecentre@nutricia.com

Nutrinovo Ltd, Tel: (01304) 829 068, info@nutrinovo.com

Nutrition Point Ltd, Tel: (07041) 544 044, info@nutritionpoint.co.uk

Nycomed UK Ltd, Tel: (01628) 646 4397, medinfo@nycomed.com

OakMed Ltd, Tel: 0800 592 786, orders@oakmed.co.uk

Octapharma Ltd, Tel: (0161) 837 3770, octapharma@octapharma.co.uk

Omega Pharma, Tel: (01748) 828 860, omega@professionalinformation.co.uk

Omron Healthcare (UK) Ltd, Tel: 0870 750 2771, info.omronhealthcare.uk@eu.omron.com

Orion Pharma (UK) Ltd, Tel: (01635) 520 300, medicalinformation@orionpharma.com

Orphan Europe (UK) Ltd, Tel: (01491) 414 333, infouk@orphan-europe.com

Otsuka Pharmaceuticals (UK) Ltd, Tel: (020) 3747 5300, ukmedinfo@otsuka.co.uk

Otsuka Novel Products GmbH, Tel: (0049) 892 0602 0500, medical@otsuka-onpg.com

Ovation Healthcare International Ltd, Tel: (00353) 1613 9707

Owen Mumford Ltd, Tel: (01993) 812 021, customerservices@owenmumford.co.uk

Oxbridge Pharma Ltd, Tel: (020) 8335 4110, enquiries@oxbridgepharma.com

Oxford Nutrition Ltd, Tel: (01626) 832 067, info@nutrinox.com

PARI Medical Ltd, Tel: (01932) 341 122, infouk@pari.de

Parkside Healthcare, Tel: (0161) 795 2792

PaxVax, Tel: 0800 088 5449, medicalinformation@paxvax.com

Peckforton Pharmaceuticals Ltd, Tel: (01270) 582 255, info@peckforton.com

Penn Pharmaceuticals Services Ltd, Tel: (01495) 711 222, penn@pennpharm.co.uk

Pfizer Ltd, Tel: (01304) 616 161, eumedinfo@pfizer.com

PGR Health Foods Ltd, Tel: (01992) 581 715, info@pgrhealthfoods.co.uk

Pfizer Ltd, Tel: (01304) 616 161, eumedinfo@pfizer.com

Pharmacosmos UK Ltd, Tel: (01844) 269 007, info@vitalineuk.co.uk

Pharma Nord (UK) Ltd, Tel: (01670) 519 989, uksales@pharmanord.co.uk

Pharmasure Ltd, Tel: (01923) 233 466, info@pharmasure.co.uk

Pharmaxis Pharmaceuticals Ltd, Tel: (01628) 902 053, med.info@pharmaxis.com.au

PharSafer Associates Ltd, Tel: 01483 212151, medinfoenquiries@pharsafer.com

Phoenix Labs, Tel: (00353) 1468 8917, medicalinformation@phoenixlabs.ie

Pinewood Healthcare, Tel: (00353) 523 6253, info@pinewood.ie

Pinnacle Biologics Inc., Tel: 1-866-248-2039, pinnaclemedinfo@optum.com

Potters Herbal Medicines, Tel: (01942) 219 960

Proceli, Tel: (01226) 713 044, admin@proceli.co.uk

Procter & Gamble (Health and Beauty Care) Ltd, Tel: (0191) 297 5000

Profile Pharma Ltd, Tel: 0800 0288 942, info.profilepharma@zambongroup.com

Protex Healthcare (UK) Ltd, Tel: 0870 011 4112, orders@protexhealthcare.co.uk

PTC Therapeutics Ltd, Tel: (0)1483 246 865, medinfo@ptcbio.com

Qdem, Tel: (01223) 426 929, medicalinformationukqdem@qdem.co.uk

Ranbaxy UK Ltd, Tel: (020) 8280 1986, medinfoeurope@ranbaxy.com

Ransom Consumer Healthcare, Tel: (01462) 437 615, info@williamransom.com

Ratiopharm UK Ltd, Tel: (023) 9231 3592, info@ratiopharm.co.uk

Reckitt Benckiser Healthcare, Tel: (01482) 326 151, info.miu@reckittbenckiser.com

Recordati Pharmaceuticals Ltd, Tel: (01491) 576 336, medinfo@recordati.co.uk

ReSource Medical UK Ltd, Tel: (01484) 531 489, info@resource-medical.co.uk

Philips Respironics (UK) Ltd, Tel: 0800 130 0840, rukmarketing@respironics.com

RF Medical Supplies Ltd, Tel: (0151) 493 1473, enquiries@rfmedicalsupplies.co.uk

Richardson Healthcare Ltd, Tel: 0800 170 1126, info@richardsonhealthcare.com

Riemser Arzneimittel AG, Tel: (0049) 383 517 6679, info@riemser.de

RIS Products Ltd, Tel: (01438) 840 135

Robinson Healthcare Ltd, Tel: (01909) 735 064, enquiry@robinsonhealthcare.com

Roche Products Ltd, Tel: 0800 328 1629, medinfo.uk@roche.com

Roche Diagnostics Ltd, Tel: (01444) 256 000

Rosemont Pharmaceuticals Ltd, Tel: 0800 919 312, rosemont.infodesk@perrigouk.com

Rowa Pharmaceuticals Ltd, Tel: (00353) 275 0077, rowa@rowa-pharma.ie

RPH Pharmaceuticals, Tel: (01483) 212 151, medinfoenquiries@pharsafer.com

Sallis Healthcare Ltd, Tel: (0115) 978 7841

Sandoz Ltd, Tel: (01276) 698 020, sandoz@professionalinformation.co.uk

Sanochemia Diagnostics UK Ltd, Tel: (0117) 906 3562

Sanofi-Aventis Ltd, Tel: 0845 372 7101, uk-medicalinformation@sanofi-aventis.com

Sanofi Pasteur MSD Ltd, Tel: (01628) 785 291

SanoMed Manufacturing BV, Tel: +32 503 93627, info@sanomed.nl

Santen UK Limited, Tel: (0345) 075 4863, medinfo@santen.co.uk

Santhera (UK) Ltd, Tel: (0)203 434 5740, santhera@pi-arm.co.uk

Schuco International Ltd, Tel: (020) 8368 1642, sales@schuco.co.uk

Schülke UK, Tel: (0114) 254 3500, mail.uk@schuelke.com

Scope Ophthamics Ltd, Tel: (01293) 897 209, info@scopeophthalmics.com

SD Biosensor, Inc., Tel: 0082 31 300 0475, sales@sdbiosensor.com

SD Healthcare, Tel: (0161) 776 7626, sales@sdhealthcare.com

Seahorse Laboratories Ltd, Tel: (020) 8257 8412, info@seahorse-labs.com

Septodont Ltd, Tel: (01622) 695 520

Servier Laboratories Ltd, Tel: (01753) 666 409, medical.information-uk@servier.com

Seven Seas Ltd, Tel: (01482) 375 234

Shermond, Tel: 0870 242 7701, sales@shermond.com

Shield TX, Tel: (01915) 118500, medinfo@shieldtx.com

Shire Pharmaceuticals Ltd, Tel: 0800 055 6614, medinfouk@shire.com

Shire Human Genetic Therapies, Tel: (01256) 894 000, hgtmedcomm@shire.com

SHS International Ltd, Tel: (0151) 228 8161

Siemens Healthcare Diagnostics Ltd, Tel: 0845 600 1966, dx-diag_sales-uk.med@siemens.com

Sigma-Tau Pharma Ltd (UK), Tel: 0800 043 1268, medical.information@sigma-tau.co.uk

SilDerm Ltd, Tel: (01260) 271 666

Sinclair IS Pharma, Tel: (01244) 625 152, enquiries@ispharma.plc.uk

Skinnies UK Ltd, Tel: (01562) 546 123, info@skinniesuk.com

SLO Drinks Ltd, Tel: 0345 222 205, info@slodrinks.com

Smith & Nephew Healthcare Ltd, Tel: (01482) 222 200, advice@smith-nephew.com

Scottish National Blood Transfusion Service, Tel: (0131) 536 5700, contact.pfc@snbts.csa.scot.nhs.uk

Sound Opinion, Tel: 0870 192 3283, enquiries@medinformation.co.uk

Speciality European Pharma Ltd, Tel: (020) 7421 7400, info@spepharma.com

SpePharm UK Ltd, Tel: 0844 800 7579, medinfo.uk@spepharm.com

Spirit Healthcare Ltd, Tel: 0800 881 5423, cs@spirit-healthcare.co.uk

SSL International plc, Tel: 0870 122 2690

Stanningley Pharma Ltd, Tel: (01159) 124 253, medinfo@stanningleypharma.co.uk

STD Pharmaceutical Products Ltd, Tel: (01432) 373 555, enquiries@stdpharm.co.uk

Steraid (Gainsborough) Ltd, Tel: (01427) 677 559

St George's Medical, Tel: (020) 7582 1015

Stiefel (a GSK company), Tel: 0800 221 441

Stiletto Foods UK Ltd, Tel: 0845 130 0869

Stragen UK Ltd, Tel: 0870 351 8744, info@stragenuk.com

Sucampo Pharma, Tel: 0800 756 3416, infoeu@sucampo.com

Su-Med International UK Ltd, Tel: (01457) 890 980, sales@sumed.co.uk

Sunovion Pharmaceuticals Europe Ltd, Tel: (020) 7821 2840, medinfo@sunovion.eu

Sutherland Health Ltd, Tel: (01635) 874 488

Swedish Orphan Biovitrum Ltd, Tel: (01638) 722 380, medical.info@sobi.com

Synergy Healthcare (UK) Ltd, Tel: (0161) 624 5641, healthcaresolutions@synergyhealthplc.com

Syner-Med (Pharmaceutical Products) Ltd, Tel: 0845 634 2100, mail@syner-med.com

Systagenix Wound Management, Tel: (01293) 842 000

Takeda UK Ltd, Tel: (01628) 537 900, medinfo@takeda.co.uk

Talley Group Ltd, Tel: (01794) 503 500

Taro Pharmaceuticals (UK) Ltd, Tel: 0870 736 9544, customerservice@taropharma.co.uk

Teofarma S.r.l., servizioclienti@teofarma.it

TEVA UK Ltd, Tel: (020) 7540 7117, medinfo@tevauk.com

The Medicines Company, Tel: 00800 8436 3326, medical.information@themedco.com

The Skin Camouflage Company Ltd, Tel: (01507) 343 091, smjcovermark@aol.com

Thea Pharmaceuticals, Tel: 0870 192 3283, thea-pharma@medinformation.co.uk

Therabel Pharma UK Ltd, Tel: 0800 066 5446, info@therabel.co.uk

The Urology Company Ltd, Tel: (020) 3077 5411, info@theurologyco.com

Thomas Blake Cosmetic Creams Ltd, Tel: (01207) 272 311, sales@veilcover.com

Thornton & Ross Ltd, Tel: (01484) 842 217

Tillomed Laboratories Ltd, Tel: (01480) 402 400, info@tillomed.co.uk

Tillotts Pharma UK Ltd, Tel: 01522 813 500, ukmedinfo@tillotts.com

TMC Pharma Services Ltd, Tel: (01252) 842 255, info@tmcpharma.com

Tobia Teff UK Ltd, Tel: (020) 7328 2045, info@tobiateff.co.uk

Torbet Laboratories Ltd, Tel: (01953) 607 856, customerservices@cambridge-healthcare.co.uk

Transdermal Ltd, Tel: (020) 8654 2251, info@transdermal.co.uk

TRB Chemedica (UK) Ltd, Tel: 0845 330 7556

Typharm Ltd, Tel: (01603) 722 480, customerservices@typharm.com

UCB Pharma Ltd, Tel: (01753) 534 655, medicalinformationuk@ucb.com

Ultrapharm Ltd, Tel: (01491) 578 016

Univar Ltd, Tel: (01908) 362 200, trientine@univareurope.com

Unomedical Ltd, Tel: (01527) 587 700

Urgo Ltd, Tel: (01509) 502 051, woundcare@uk.urgo.com

Vertex Pharmaceuticals (UK) Ltd, Tel: 0800 028 2616, eumedicalinfo@vrtx.com

Vifor Pharma UK Ltd, Tel: (01276) 853 633, medicalinfo_uk@viforpharma.com

ViiV Healthcare UK Ltd, Tel: 0800221441, customercontactuk@gsk.com

Viridian Pharma Ltd, Tel: (01633) 400 335, info@viridianpharma.co.uk

ViroPharma Ltd, Tel: (020) 7572 1222

Vitaflo International Ltd, Tel: (0151) 709 9020, vitaflo@vitaflo.co.uk

Vitalograph Ltd, Tel: (01280) 827 110, sales@vitalograph.co.uk

Wallace Cameron Ltd, Tel: (01698) 354 600, sales@wallacecameron.com

Wallace Manufacturing Chemists Ltd, Tel: (01235) 538 700, info@alinter.co.uk

Warburtons, Tel: (01204) 513 004

Warner Chilcott UK Ltd, Tel: (01932) 824 700

Welsh Blood Service, Tel: (01443) 622 000, donor.care@wales.nhs.uk

Wellfoods Ltd, Tel: (01226) 381 712, wellfoods@wellfoods.co.uk

Williams Medical Supplies Ltd, Tel: (01685) 844 739

Wockhardt UK Ltd, Tel: (01978) 661 261

Wyeth Pharmaceuticals, Tel: (01628) 604 377, eumedinfo@pfizer.com

Wynlit Laboratories, Tel: (07903) 370 130

Wyvern Medical Ltd, Tel: (01531) 631 105

Zentiva, Tel: (01483) 554 101, gb-zentivamedicalinformation@sanofi.com

Zeroderma Ltd, Tel: (01858) 525 643

Special-order manufacturers

Unlicensed medicines are available from 'special-order' manufacturers and specialist-importing companies; the MHRA maintains a register of these companies at tinyurl.com/cdslke.

Licensed **hospital manufacturing units** also manufacture 'special-order' products as unlicensed medicines, the principal NHS units are listed below. A database (*Pro-File*; www.pro-file.nhs.uk) provides information on medicines manufactured in the NHS; access is restricted to NHS pharmacy staff.

The Association of Pharmaceutical Specials Manufacturers may also be able to provide further information about commercial companies (www.apsm-uk.com).

The MHRA recommends that an unlicensed medicine should only be used when a patient has special requirements that cannot be met by use of a licensed medicine.

As well as being available direct from the hospital manufacturer(s) concerned, many NHS-manufactured Specials may be bought from the Oxford Pharmacy Store, owned and operated by Oxford Health NHS Foundation Trust.

England

London

Barts and the London NHS Trust
Mr J. A. Rickard, Head of Barts Health Pharmaceuticals
Barts Health NHS Trust
The Royal London Hospital
Pathology and Pharmacy Building
80 Newark St
Whitechapel
London
E1 2ES
(020) 3246 0394 (order/enquiry)
barts.pharmaceuticals@bartshealth.nhs.uk

Guy's and St. Thomas' NHS Foundation Trust
Mr P. Forsey, Associate Chief Pharmacist
Guy's and St. Thomas' NHS Foundation Trust
Guy's Hospital
Pharmacy Department
Great Maze Pond
London
SE1 9RT
(020) 7188 4992 (order)
(020) 7188 5003 (enquiry)
Fax: (020) 7188 5013
paul.forsey@gstt.nhs.uk

Moorfields Pharmaceuticals
Mr. T. Record, Technical Director
Moorfields Pharmaceuticals
25 Provost St
London
N1 7NH
(020) 7684 9090 (order/enquiry)
Fax: (020) 7502 2332

London North West Healthcare NHS Trust
Mr K. Wong,
London North West Healthcare NHS Trust
Northwick Park Hospital
Watford Rd
Harrow
Middlesex
HA1 3UJ
(020) 8869 2295 (order)
(020) 8869 2204/2223 (enquiry)
kwong@nhs.net

Royal Free Hampstead NHS Trust
Ms C. Trehane, Production Manager
Royal Free Hampstead NHS Trust
Pond St
London
NW3 2QG
(020) 7830 2424 (order)
(020) 7830 2282 (enquiry)
Fax: (020) 7794 1875
christine.trehane@nhs.net

St George's Healthcare NHS Trust
Mr V. Kumar, Assistant Chief Pharmacist
St George's Hospital
Technical Services
Blackshaw Rd
Tooting
London
SW17 0QT
(020) 8725 1770/1768
Fax: (020) 8725 3947
vinodh.kumar@stgeorges.nhs.uk

University College Hospital NHS Foundation Trust
Mr T. Murphy, Production Manager
University College Hospital
235 Euston Rd
London
NW1 2BU
(020) 7380 9723 (order)
(020) 7380 9472 (enquiry)
Fax: (020) 7380 9726
tony.murphy@uclh.nhs.uk

Midlands and Eastern

Barking, Havering and Redbridge University Trust
Mr N. Fisher, Senior Principal Pharmacist
Queen's Hospital
Pharmacy Department
Romford
Essex
RM7 0AG
(01708) 435 463 (order)
(01708) 435 042 (enquiry)
neil.fisher@bhrhospitals.nhs.uk

Burton Hospitals NHS Foundation Trust
Mr D. Raynor, Head of Pharmacy Manufacturing Unit
Queens Hospital
Burton Hospitals NHS Foundation Trust
Pharmacy Manufacturing Unit
Belvedere Rd
Burton-on-Trent
DE13 0RB
(01283) 511 511 ext: 5275 (order/enquiry)
Fax: (01283) 593 036
david.raynor@burtonft.nhs.uk

Colchester Hospital University NHS Foundation Trust
Mr S. Pullen, Pharmacy Production Manager
Colchester General Hospital
Main Pharmacy
Turner Rd
Colchester
Essex
CO4 5JL
(01206) 742 007 (order)
(01206) 744 208 (enquiry)
Fax: (01206) 841 249
pharmacy.stores@colchesterhospital.nhs.uk (order)
psu.enquiries@colchesterhospital.nhs.uk (enquiry)

Ipswich Hospital NHS Trust
Dr J. Harwood, Production Manager
Ipswich Hospital NHS Trust
Pharmacy Manufacturing Unit
Heath Rd
Ipswich
IP4 5PD
(01473) 703 440 (order)
(01473) 703 603 (enquiry)
Fax: (01473) 703 609
john.harwood@ipswichhospital.nhs.uk

Nottingham University Hospitals NHS Trust
Mr J. Graham, Senior Pharmacist, Production
Nottingham University Hospitals NHS Trust
Pharmacy Production Units
Queens Medical Centre Campus
Nottingham
NG7 2UH
(0115) 924 9924 ext: 66521 (enquiry/order)
Fax: (0115) 970 9780
jeff.graham@nuh.nhs.uk

University Hospital of North Staffordshire NHS Trust
Ms K. Ferguson, Chief Technician
University Hospital of North Staffordshire NHS Trust
Pharmacy Technical Services
City General Site
Stoke-on-Trent
ST4 6QG
(01782) 674 568 (order)
(01782) 674 568 (enquiry)
Fax: (01782) 674 575
caroline.ferguson@uhns.nhs.uk

North East

The Newcastle upon Tyne Hospitals NHS Foundation Trust
Mr Y. Hunter-Blair, Production Manager
Royal Victoria Infirmary
Newcastle Specials
Pharmacy Production Unit
Queen Victoria Rd
Newcastle-upon-Tyne
NE1 4LP
(0191) 282 0395 (order)
(0191) 282 0389 (enquiry)
Fax: (0191) 282 0469
yan.hunter-blair@nuth.nhs.uk

North West

Preston Pharmaceuticals

Ms A. Bolch, Deputy Chief Pharmacist (PMU)
Preston Pharmaceuticals
Royal Preston Hospital
Fulwood
Preston
PR2 9HT
(01772) 523 617 (order)
(01772) 522 593 (enquiry)
Fax: (01772) 523 645
angela.bolch@lthtr.nhs.uk

Stockport Pharmaceuticals

Mr A. Singleton, Head of Production
Stepping Hill Hospital
Stockport NHS Foundation Trust
Stockport Pharmaceuticals
Stockport
SK2 7JE
(0161) 419 5666 (order)
(0161) 419 5657 (enquiry)
Fax: (0161) 419 5426
andrew.singleton@stockport.nhs.uk

South

Portsmouth Hospitals NHS Trust

Mr R. Lucas, Product Development Manager
Portsmouth Hospitals NHS Trust
Pharmacy Manufacturing Unit
Unit D2, Railway Triangle Industrial Estate
Walton Road
Farlington
Portsmouth
PO6 1TF
(02392) 389 078 (order)
(02392) 316 312 (enquiry)
Fax: (02392) 316 316
robert.lucas@porthosp.nhs.uk

South East

East Sussex Healthcare NHS Trust

Mr P. Keen, Business Manager
Eastbourne District General Hospital
East Sussex Hospitals NHS Trust
Eastbourne Pharmaceuticals
Kings Drive
Eastbourne
BN21 2UD
(01323) 414 906 (order)
(01323) 417 400 ext: 3076 (enquiry)
Fax: (01323) 414 931
paul.keen@esht.nhs.uk

South West

Torbay Pharmaceuticals

Ms J. Bamby, Pharmacy Manufacturing
Services Manager
South Devon Healthcare NHS Foundation Trust
Torbay Pharmaceuticals
Kemmings Close, Long Rd
Paignton
TQ4 7TW
(01803) 664 707
Fax: (01803) 664 354
jane.bamby@nhs.net

Yorkshire

Calderdale and Huddersfield NHS Foundation Trust

Dr B. Grewal, Managing Director
Calderdale and Huddersfield NHS Foundation
Trust
Huddersfield Pharmacy Specials
Gate 2 - Acre Mills, School St West
Huddersfield
HD3 3ET
(01484) 355 388 (order/enquiry)
info.hps@cht.nhs.uk

Northern Ireland

Victoria Pharmaceuticals

Mr S. Cameron, Production Manager -
Pharmacy
Victoria Pharmaceuticals
Royal Hospitals
Plenum Building
Grosvenor Road
Belfast
BT12 6BA
(028) 9063 0070 (order/enquiry)
Fax: (028) 9063 5282 (order/enquiry)
samuel.cameron@belfasttrust.hscni.net

Scotland

NHS Greater Glasgow and Clyde

Ms K. Pollock, Acting Production Manager
Pharmacy Production Unit
University Place
Glasgow
G12 8TA
(0141) 451 5820 (order)
(0141) 451 5822 (enquiry)
Fax: (0141) 334 9137
pharmacyproductionunit@ggc.scot.nhs.uk

Tayside Pharmaceuticals

Mr S. Bath, Production Manager
Ninewells Hospital
Tayside Pharmaceuticals
Dundee
DD1 9SY
(01382) 632 052 (order)
(01382) 632 273 (enquiry)
Fax: (01382) 632 060
sbath@nhs.net

Wales

Cardiff and Vale University Health Board

Mr P. Spark, Principal Pharmacist (Production)
Cardiff and Vale University Health Board
20 Fieldway
Cardiff
CF14 4HY
(029) 2074 8120
Fax: (029) 2074 8130
paul.spark@wales.nhs.uk

Index

INDEX